OXFORD MEDICAL PUBLICATIONS

OXFORD TEXTBOOK
OF ONCOLOGY

OXFORD TEXTBOOK OF ONCOLOGY

VOLUME 2

Edited by

MICHAEL PECKHAM, HERBERT PINEDO,
and UMBERTO VERONESI

Oxford   New York   Tokyo
OXFORD UNIVERSITY PRESS
1995

Oxford University Press, Walton Street, Oxford OX2 6DP

Oxford   New York
Athens   Auckland   Bangkok   Bombay
Calcutta   Cape Town   Dar es Salaam   Delhi
Florence   Hong Kong   Istanbul   Karachi
Kuala Lumpur   Madras   Madrid   Melbourne
Mexico City   Nairobi   Paris   Singapore
Taipei   Tokyo   Toronto
and associated companies in
Berlin   Ibadan

Oxford is a trade mark of Oxford University Press

Published in the United States
by Oxford University Press Inc., New York

A catalogue record for this book is available from the British Library

Library of Congress Cataloging in Publication Data
(Data applied for)

ISBN 0 19 261685 4 (Two Volume Set)
ISBN 0 19 262663 9 (Vol. 1)
ISBN 0 19 262664 7 (Vol. 2)

Typeset by Dobbie Typesetting Limited, Tavistock, Devon

Printed in Great Britain by
The Bath Press, Avon

Preface

The *Oxford Textbook of Oncology* is one of the highly successful series of textbooks produced by Oxford University Press of which the best known forerunner is the *Oxford Textbook of Medicine*. This textbook of oncology is the first new, major, and comprehensive textbook on cancer to appear for more than a decade and so is an important landmark for a wide readership. It comes at a crucially important time in the evolution of cancer treatment. During the past two to three decades some forms of cancer have become curable but many common cancers still pose an intractable problem. As in the health field generally, there is a high level of interest in primary and secondary prevention. However, the most important distinguishing feature of the 1990s is the explosive and far-reaching developments in the biological and physical sciences relevant to cancer.

In selecting the authorship of the chapters in the textbook, the editors have not drawn narrowly from one country but have been concerned to provide a wide range of expertise and a broad international perspective. The coverage is not only comprehensive but 'holistic', extending from advances in molecular genetics through to societal issues such as the support systems needed by cancer patients and their families.

Particular emphasis has been given to the integration of clinical oncology and science. In addition to the sections devoted to the scientific foundations of oncology, individual chapters included in the clinical sections make reference to aetiology and biology. The clinical sections are designed not only to instruct readers but to provide practical guidance on everyday problems. In addition to common problems there is coverage of uncommon and rare tumours, less common presentations, and unusual complications of cancer and its treatment.

The expanding number of cancer journals, reviews, and books focusing on particular forms of diagnosis, on individual therapies, or on specific cancers, makes the place of the comprehensive reference source that maps the range of the oncology territory all the more important. The *Oxford Textbook of Oncology* will serve as a source of instruction and advice but also a pointer to some of the emergent areas such as the handling of genetic risk. The Textbook is designed to be relevant to a wide constituency within the general field of oncology including not only oncologists but clinicians whose day-to-day work includes the diagnosis and care of cancer patients. It will be relevant to oncologists in training as a reference source and for other clinicians in training. It will be of interest to scientists and to non-medical health professionals involved in the care of cancer patients. It will also be of value to epidemiologists and behavioural scientists.

Many have helped in this important enterprise. John Wagstaff has been an unflagging source of support and his important contribution is gratefully acknowledged. The editors are also grateful for the help provided by Jonathan Waxman and Alberto Costa. We also wish to thank Pat Price, Cyril Fisher, and Maureen Wagstaff for their editorial assistance. We owe a particular debt of gratitude to Sally Welham who has been closely involved with the Textbook since its inception and whose input, constructive advice, and hard work has greatly contributed to its success.

May 1995

Michael Peckham
Herbert Pinedo
Umberto Veronesi

Dose schedules are being continually revised and new side-effects recognized. Oxford University Press makes no representation, express or implied, that the drug dosages in this book are correct. For these reasons the reader is strongly urged to consult the drug company's printed instructions before administering any of the drugs recommended in this book.

Contents

VOLUME 2

Contributors

MATTI S. AAPRO
Director, Division of Medical Oncology, European Institute of Oncology, Milan, Italy
19.14 *Nutritional support of cancer patients*

DUNCAN ACKERY
Professor, formerly Consultant in Charge, Department of Nuclear Medicine, Southampton General Hospital, UK
4.27 *Targeted radiotherapy*

G. E. ADAMS
Professor and Director, Medical Research Council Radiobiology Unit, Chilton, Oxfordshire, UK
4.28 *Hypoxia—selective bioreductive drugs*

MÅNS AKERMAN
Associate Professor and Head, Department of Pathology and Cytology, University Hospital, Lund, Sweden
3.3 *Cytology*

MALCOLM C. ALDRIDGE
Consultant Surgeon, Queen Elizabeth II Hospital, Welwyn Garden City, Hertfordshire, UK
7.8 *Tumours of the biliary tract*

D. G. ALLEN
Visiting Specialist, Department of Gynaecological Oncology, Mercy Hospital for Women, Melbourne, Australia
9.1 *Carcinoma of the ovary*

T. D. ALLEN
Head, Department of Structural Cell Biology, Paterson Institute, Christie Hospital, Manchester, UK
12.1 *The biology of haemopoiesis*

P. L. AMLOT
Department of Haematology, Royal Free Hospital, London
19.4 *Immunological and haematological complications of cancer*

JØRGEN BACH ANDERSEN
Professor of Electrical Engineering, Aalborg University, Denmark
4.31 *Hyperthermia*

JOHN E. ANTOINE
Professor of Radiation Medicine, Loma Linda University School of Medicine, California, USA
4.25 *Intraoperative radiotherapy: an investigational approach to cancer*

J. W. ARNDT
Staff Physician, Nuclear Medicine, University Hospital Leiden, The Netherlands
3.12 *Nuclear medicine procedures*

S. J. ARNOTT
Consultant Radiotherapist, St Bartholomew's Hospital, London
7.4 *Colorectal tumours*

D. ASH
Consultant Clinical Oncologist, Cookridge Hospital, Leeds, UK
4.22 *Interstitial radiation therapy*
4.32 *Photodynamic therapy*

KENNETH D. BAGSHAWE
Emeritus Professor of Medical Oncology, Charing Cross and Westminster Medical School, London
3.11 *Circulating tumour markers*

CLIFFORD C. BAILEY
Consultant Paediatric Oncologist, St James's University Hospital Trust, Leeds, UK
15.1 *Brain tumours in children*

FRANCES BALKWILL
Principal Scientist, Imperial Cancer Research Fund, London
1.9 *Cytokines*

G. W. BARENDSEN
Professor of Radiobiology, University of Amsterdam, The Netherlands
2.3 *Cellular and molecular mechanisms in radiation carcinogenesis*

A. BARRETT
Professor of Radiation Oncology, Beatson Oncology Centre and University of Glasgow, UK
4.24 *Total body irradiation*

HARRY BARTELINK
Professor and Chairman, Radiotherapy Department, The Netherlands Cancer Institute/Antoni van Leeuwenhoek Huis, Amsterdam, The Netherlands
4.30 *Combined chemotherapy and radiotherapy*
6.13 *Management of cervical lymph nodes*

CLAIRE BARTON
Research Fellow (Honorary Senior Registrar in Medical Oncology), Royal Postgraduate Medical School, Hammersmith Hospital, London
19.10 *Effects of cancer chemotherapy on fertility*

R. H. J. BEGENT
Professor of Clinical Oncology, Royal Free Hospital School of Medicine, London
9.5 *Gestational trophoblastic tumours*

A. C. BEGG
Head, Division of Experimental Therapy, The Netherlands Cancer Institute, Amsterdam, The Netherlands
4.30 *Combined chemotherapy and radiotherapy*

FILIBERTO BELLI
Division of Surgical Oncology 'B', Istituto Nazionale Tumori, Milan, Italy
6.2 *Cutaneous melanoma*

CONTRIBUTORS

JACQUES BERNIER
Director, Cantonal Department of Radiation Oncology, Ospedale San Giovanni, Bellinzona, Switzerland
12.7.2 *Non-Hodgkin's lymphoma in adults*

MICHAEL BESSER
Professor of Medicine and Physician in Charge, Department of Endocrinology, St Bartholomew's Hospital, London
16.3 *Pituitary tumours*

HENRI BISMUTH
Professor of Surgery, Faculty of Medicine, University of South Paris, France
7.8 *Tumours of the biliary tract*

PETER BLAKE
Consultant Radiotherapist and Oncologist, Royal Marsden Hospital, London
4.23 *Intracavitary therapy*
9.6 *Carcinoma of the vagina*

STEPHEN R. BLOOM
Professor of Endocrinology, Royal Postgraduate Medical School, Hammersmith Hospital, London
16.5 *Neuroendocrine gastroenteropancreatic tumours*

WALTER F. BODMER
Director-General, Imperial Cancer Research Fund, London
1.5 *Genetics and familial cancer*

GIANNI BONADONNA
Professor of Haematology, University of Milan School of Medicine; Chairman, Department of Cancer Medicine, Istituto Nazionale Tumori, Milan, Italy
19.12 *Carcinogenic effects of cancer treatment*

THIERRY BOON
Ludwig Institute for Cancer Research, Brussels Branch, Belgium
1.7 *The cell-mediated immune response to tumours*

PIET BORST
Director of Research of The Netherlands Cancer Institute; Professor of Clinical Biochemistry, University of Amsterdam, The Netherlands
4.13 *Drug resistance*

STEPHEN G. BOWN
ICRF Professor of Laser Medicine and Surgery, University College London Medical School, UK
4.33 *Lasers in oncology*

MICHAEL J. BOYER
Staff Specialist in Medical Oncology, Royal Prince Alfred Hospital, Sydney, New South Wales, Australia
10.2 *Extragonadal germ-cell tumours*

PETER BOYLE
Director, Division of Epidemiology and Biostatistics, European Institute of Oncology, Milan, Italy
2.9 *Cancer epidemiology and prevention*

FEDERICO BOZZETTI
Associate Director, Division of Surgical Oncology 'A', Istituto Nazionale Tumori, Milan, Italy
7.7 *Liver tumours*

MICHAEL BRADA
Senior Lecturer and Consultant in Radiotherapy and Oncology, Royal Marsden Hospital and Institute of Cancer Research, Sutton, Surrey, UK
15.2 *Tumours of the brain and spinal cord in adults*
20.6 *Rehabilitation of the cancer patient*

MARC E. BUYSE
Director, International Institute for Drug Development, Brussels; Visiting Professor, Limburgs Universitair Centrum, Belgium
20.1 *Clinical trial methodology*

GRAEME M. BYDDER
Professor of Diagnostic Radiology, Royal Postgraduate Medical School, Hammersmith Hospital, London
3.8 *Magnetic resonance in oncology*

A. HILARY CALVERT
Professor of Clinical Oncology, Cancer Research Unit, University of Newcastle upon Tyne, UK
4.9 *Cisplatin and analogues: discovery, mechanism of action, and clinical pharmacology*

STEPHEN R. CANNON
Consultant Orthopaedic Surgeon, Bone Tumour Unit, Royal National Orthopaedic Hospital, Stanmore, Middlesex, UK
13.4 *Osteosarcoma*

JEAN-PAUL CANO
Marseilles, France
4.11 *Vinca alkaloids: cellular pharmacology and clinical pharmacokinetics*

PAOLO CASALI
Attending Physician, Division of Medical Oncology, Istituto Nazionale Tumori, Milan, Italy
13.5 *Malignant bone tumours other than osteosarcoma and Ewing's sarcoma*

NATALE CASCINELLI
Director, Division of Surgical Oncology 'B', Istituto Nazionale Tumori, Milan, Italy
6.2 *Cutaneous melanoma*

J. CASSIDY
Professor of Oncology, Aberdeen University, UK
4.6 *Alkylating agents and related drugs*

FRANCO CAVALLI
Professor of Medical Oncology, Ospedale San Giovanni, Bellinzona, Switzerland
12.7.2 *Non-Hodgkin's lymphoma in adults*

JEAN-CHARLES CEROTTINI
Director, Ludwig Institute for Cancer Reseach, Lausanne Branch, Switzerland
1.7 *The cell-mediated immune response to tumours*

JOCELYN CHAMBERLAIN
Director of Cancer Screening Evaluation Unit, Institute of Cancer Research, Sutton, Surrey, UK
2.8 *Evaluation of screening for cancer*

PIERRE CHAUVEL
Head of Department of Radiation Oncology, Centre Antoine-Lacassagne, Nice, France
6.9 *Tumours of the hypopharynx*

JUDITH M. CHESSELLS
Leukaemia Research Fund Professor of Paediatric Oncology, Institute of Child Health and Great Ormond Street Hospital for Children NHS Trust, London
12.2.3 *Acute leukaemia in childhood*

CLAUDIO CLEMENTE
Division of Pathology and Cytology, Istituto Nazionale Tumori, Milan, Italy
6.2 *Cutaneous melanoma*

F. J. CLETON
Professor of Medicine, University Hospital, Leiden, The Netherlands
4.1 *Chemotherapy: general aspects*

MARY M. H. CODY
Lecturer in Psychosocial Aspects of Cancer, Department of Medical Oncology, St Bartholomew's Hospital, London
20.11 *Support systems for cancer patients*

NICOLETTA COLOMBO
Deputy Director, Division of Gynaecology, European Institute of Oncology, Milan, Italy
9.1 *Carcinoma of the ovary*

R. CHARLES COOMBES
Professor, Department of Medical Oncology, Charing Cross Hospital, London
4.16 *The basis of hormonal therapy of cancer*

D. P. COOPER
Scientific Officer, Cancer Research Campaign Department of Carcinogenesis, Paterson Institute of Cancer Research, Christie Hospital, Manchester, UK
2.1 *Cell and molecular mechanisms in chemical carcinogenesis*

DAVID O. COSGROVE
Consultant in Radiology, Hammersmith Hospital, London
3.10 *Ultrasonic scanning*

ALBERTO COSTA
Surgical Oncologist and Director, European School of Oncology, Milan, Italy
2.6 *Prospects for tumour chemoprevention*

JOHN K. COWELL
Senior Scientist, ICRF Oncology Group, Institute of Child Health, London
14.1 *The molecular pathology of childhood tumours*

DEREK CROWTHER
Professor of Medical Oncology, Christie Hospital NHS Trust, Manchester, UK
12.6.2 *Hodgkin's disease in adults*

MAURIZIO D'INCALCI
Chief, Laboratory of Cancer Chemotherapy, 'Mario Negri' Institute, Milan, Italy
4.10 *Podophyllotoxins*

PAOLA DAL CIN
Centre for Human Genetics, University of Leuven, Belgium
1.4 *Chromosomes and cancer*

GEDSKE DAUGAARD
Senior Registrar, Rigshospitalet, Copenhagen, Denmark
11.4 *Other thymic tumours*

PIERO DE BESI
Department of Oncology, Padua Hospital, Italy
7.1 *Malignancies of the oesophagus*

J. C. J. M. DE HAES
Associate Professor, Department of Medical Psychology, University of Amsterdam and Department of Medical Decision Making, University of Leiden, The Netherlands
20.3 *Quality of life*

NICO DE VRIES
Otolaryngologist/Head and Neck Surgeon, Free University Hospital, Amsterdam, The Netherlands
6.7.2 *The role of surgery in the treatment of tumours of the oral cavity*

ADRIAAN W. DEKKER
Associate Professor of Haematology, University Hospital Utrecht, The Netherlands
19.9 *Complications of cytotoxic therapy*

RAFFAELE DEL BUONO
Research fellow, Histopathology Unit, Imperial Cancer Research Fund, London
1.1 *The growth of human tumours*

GABRIELLA DELLA TORRE
Division of Experimental Oncology 'A', Istituto Nazionale Tumori, Milan, Italy
6.6 *Tumours of the nasopharynx*

FRANÇOIS DEMARD
Professor of Otolaryngology—Head and Neck Surgery, Centre Antoine-Lacassagne, University of Nice, France
6.9 *Tumours of the hypopharynx*

LOUIS DENIS
Professor of Urology, Vrye Universiteit Brussel, Antwerp, Belgium
10.4 *Bladder cancer*

T. M. DEXTER
Department of Experimental Haematology, Paterson Institute, Christie Hospital, Manchester, UK
12.1 *The biology of haemopoiesis*

VOLKER DIEHL
Director, Internal Medicine, University of Cologne, Germany
12.6.1 *The cell biology of Hodgkin's disease*

LUC Y. DIRIX
Consultant, Department of Medical Oncology, University Hospital, Antwerp, Belgium
19.2 *Metabolic disturbances*

STANLEY DISCHE
Visiting Professor, University College London; Honorary Consultant, Centre for Cancer Treatment, Mount Vernon Hospital, Northwood, Middlesex, UK
4.29 *Clinical fractionation studies*

ROBERTO DOCI
Associate Director, Division of Surgical Oncology 'A', Istituto
Nazionale Tumori, Milano, Italy
7.7 *Liver tumours*

ROBERT F. DONDELINGER
Professor of Radiology, University of Liège; Head of Department
of Medical Imaging, University Hospital Sant-Tilman, Liège,
Belgium
3.9 *Interventional radiology: percutaneous tissue sampling guided by
imaging*

JOHN F. DOWSETT
VMO, Gosford and Royal North Shore Hospitals, Sydney,
Australia
7.6 *Tumours of the pancreas*

WILLIAM DUNCAN
Professor of Radiation Oncology and Head of Department of
Clinical Oncology, University of Edinburgh, Western General
Hospital, Edinburgh, UK
4.26 *Particle radiotherapy*

JERZY EINHORN
Professor Emeritus of Radiotherapy, Karolinska Institute and
Hospital, Stockholm, Sweden
20.8 *The organization of cancer services*

D. G. R. EVANS
Consultant in Medical Genetics, Christie Hospital and St Mary's
Hospital, Manchester, UK
2.7 *Practical implications of the new cancer genetics*

CAROLYN M. FAULDER
Author and Medical Journalist, Longtown, Herefordshire, UK
20.10 *Cancer and society: health education*

IAN S. FENTIMAN
Consultant Surgeon, ICRF Clinical Oncology Unit, Guy's
Hospital, London
19.5 *Serous effusions*

J. W. L. FIELDING
Consultant Surgeon, Queen Elizabeth Hospital, Birmingham,
UK
7.2 *Cancer of the stomach*

GORDON FINDLAY
Consultant Neurosurgeon, Walton Centre for Neurology and
Neurosurgery, Liverpool, UK
19.6 *Spinal metastatic disease*

MICHAEL P. N. FINDLAY
Staff Specialist in Medical Oncology, Royal Prince Alfred
Hospital, Sydney, New South Wales, Australia
18 *Cancer in the elderly*

F. FLAMANT
Department of Paediatric Oncology, Institut Gustave Roussy,
Paris, France
13.2 *Malignant mesenchymal tumours in childhood*

ALEXANDER T. FLORENCE
Professor and Dean, School of Pharmacy, University of
London
4.17 *Targeted therapy with microspheres and other carrier
systems*

CHRISTA FONATSCH
Professor of Human Genetics, and Tumour Genetics, Medical
University of Lübeck, Germany
12.6.1 *The cell biology of Hodgkin's disease*

JOHN F. FOWLER
Professor of Human Oncology and Medical Physics, University
of Wisconsin Medical School, Madison, USA
4.26 *Particle radiotherapy*

R. S. J. FRACKOWIAK
Professor of Cognitive Neurology, Wellcome Department
of Cognitive Neurology, National Hospital for Nervous Diseases,
London
3.7 *Positron emission tomography*

DAVID G. GADIAN
Professor of Biophysics, Institute of Child Health, London
3.8 *Magnetic resonance in oncology*

CHARLES S. B. GALASKO
Professor of Orthopaedic Surgery, University of Manchester,
Hope Hospital, Salford, UK
19.7 *Pathological fracture*

C. GALLAGHER
Department of Medical Oncology, Royal London Hospital,
London
9.4 *Tumours of the endometrium and adnexa*

TRIVADI S. GANESAN
Consultant Medical Oncologist and Clinical Scientist, ICRF
Department of Clinical Oncology, Churchill Hospital, Oxford
12.2.1 *Biology of leukaemia*

LEANDRO GENNARI
Professor and Head of Surgical Oncology 'A', Istituto Nazionale
Tumori, Milan, Italy
7.7 *Liver tumours*

JEAN PIERRE GERARD
Professor of Radiotherapy, CHU de Lyon, France
10.4 *Bladder cancer*

ALAIN GERBAULET
Chef de Service de Curietherapie, Institut Gustave Roussy,
Villejuif, France
6.7.3 *The role of radiotherapy in the treatment of tumours of the
oral cavity*

ELI GLATSTEIN
Professor and Chairman, Department of Radiation Oncology,
Simmons Cancer Center, University of Texas Southwestern
Medical School, Dallas, USA
4.25 *Intraoperative radiotherapy—an investigational approach to
cancer*

ULRICH GÖBEL
Professor, Department of Haematology and Oncology, Heinrich
Heine University Dusseldorf, Germany
13.3 *Ewing's sarcoma*

A. GOLDHIRSCH
Professor of Medical Oncology and Chairman, Scientific
Committee, International Breast Cancer Study Group, Bern,
Switzerland
8 *Breast cancer*

A. GOLDSTONE
Department of Clinical Haematology, University College
Hospital, London
12.3 *The chronic leukaemias*

PETER GOLDSTRAW
Consultant Thoracic Surgeon, Royal Brompton Hospital; Senior
Lecturer, National Heart and Lung Institute, London
11.1 *Tumours of the trachea and the lung*
11.5 *Surgical resection of pulmonary metastases*

MARTIN GORE
Consultant Medical Oncologist, Royal Marsden Hospital,
London and Surrey, UK
12.8 *Myeloma and other plasma cell malignancies*

ALAIN GOUYETTE
Senior Research Scientist and Deputy Scientific Director of
the Life Sciences Department, Centre National de la Recherche
Scientifique, Institut Gustave-Roussy, Villejuif, France
4.34 *Principles of pharmacokinetics*

CESARE GRANDI
Head and Neck Surgical Oncology, Istituto Nazionale Tumori,
Milan, Italy
6.6 *Tumours of the nasopharynx*

MARCO GRECO
Professor of Surgery and Vice-Director, Division of Surgical
Oncology 'B', Istituto Nazionale Tumori, Milan, Italy
5.1.1 *Achievements and obstacles to progress in cancer surgery*

ANNA GREGOR
Senior Lecturer in Clinical Oncology, University of Edinburgh,
UK
11.1 *Tumours of the trachea and the lung*

ASHLEY GROSSMAN
Professor of Neuroendocrinology, St Bartholomew's Hospital,
London
16.4 *Adrenal tumours*

BARRY GUSTERSON
Professor of Histopathology, Institute of Cancer Research,
University of London
3.2 *New techniques in pathology and their application in diagnosis
and studies of tumour biology*

JEAN-LOUIS HABRAND
Professor of Radiation Oncology, Institut Gustave Roussy,
Villejuif, France
13.2 *Malignant mesenchymal tumours in childhood*

JANE HALL
Centre for Health Economics Research and Evaluation, University
of Sydney, Australia
20.9 *Economic considerations in cancer care*

MICHAEL T. HALLISSEY
Senior Lecturer, Department of Surgery, University of Birmingham
and Honorary Consultant, Queen Elizabeth Hospital, Birmingham,
UK
7.2 *Cancer of the stomach*

G. W. HANKS
Professor of Palliative Medicine, University of Bristol, UK
20.5 *Pain and symptom control in advanced cancer*

HEINE H. HANSEN
Professor of Clinical Oncology and Physician-in-Chief, Department of Oncology, Rigshospitalet, The National University
Hospital, Copenhagen, Denmark
11.1 *Tumours of the trachea and the lung*

DONALD F. N. HARRISON
Institute of Laryngology and Otology, Royal National Throat,
Nose and Ear Hospital, London
6.5 *Carcinoma of the nasal cavity and paranasal sinuses*

MARCEL HAYAT
Professor of Medical Oncology, University of Paris XI,
France
5.2 *Staging classifications*

W. F. HENDRY
Consultant Urologist, Royal Marsden Hospital, London
10.1 *Testicular tumours*

J. MICHAEL HENK
Consultant Clinical Oncologist, Royal Marsden Hospital,
London
6.3.2 *Tumours of the orbit*
6.11 *Uncommon tumours of the head and neck region*

PAUL HERMANEK
Professor of Surgical Pathology Emeritus, University of Erlangen,
Germany
5.2 *Staging classifications*

MICHAEL HOBSLEY
David Patey Professor of Surgery, University College London,
UK
6.4 *Salivary tumours*

DIETER HOELZER
Professor of Haematology/Oncology, Department of Internal
Medicine, University of Frankfurt, Germany
12.2.2 *Acute leukaemia in adults*

D. HOLLYWOOD
Royal Postgraduate Medical School, Hammersmith Hospital,
London
1.6 *Oncogenes*

JEAN CLAUDE HORIOT
Professor of Radiotherapy, University of Dijon; Head of
Radiotherapy Department, Centre George François Leclerc,
Dijon, France
6.8 *Tumours of the oropharynx*

A. HORWICH
Professor, Academic Unit of Radiotherapy and Oncology,
The Royal Marsden NHS Trust, Sutton, Surrey, UK
10.1 *Testicular tumours*
10.6 *Tumours of the prostate*

P. J. HOSKIN
Consultant in Clinical Oncology, Mount Vernon Hospital,
Northwood, Middlesex; Senior Lecturer in Oncology, University
College London Medical School, UK
20.5 *Pain control and palliation*

ANTHONY HOWELL
Senior Lecturer in Medical Oncology, CRC Department of Medical Oncology, Christie Hospital NHS Trust, University of Manchester, UK
4.16 *The basis of hormonal therapy of cancer*

C. N. HUDSON
Professor of Obstetrics and Gynaecological Surgery, St Bartholomew's Hospital Medical School, London
9.8 *Sarcoma and melanoma of the female genital system*

JOHN HUNGERFORD
Consultant Surgeon, Moorfields Eye Hospital; Consultant Ophthalmic Surgeon, St Bartholomew's Hospital, London
6.3.1 *Melanoma of the eye and orbit*
14.3 *Retinoblastoma*

ROBERT D. HUNTER
Director of Radiotherapy, Christie Hospital and Holt Radium Institute, Manchester, UK
9.3 *Carcinoma of the cervix*

JANET E. W. HUSBAND
Consultant Radiologist, Royal Marsden Hospital, Surrey, UK
3.6 *The role of radiological imaging in the management of cancer*

CLAUDIUS IRLE
Director, Haematology-Oncology Unit, La Tour Hospital, Meyrin/Geneva, Switzerland
12.5 *Autologous bone-marrow transplantation and intensification therapies for solid tumours and lymphomas*

PETER G. ISAACSON
Professor of Histopathology, University College London Medical School, UK
12.7.1 *The pathology and biology of non-Hodgkin's lymphoma*

JEREMY R. JASS
Professor of Pathology, School of Medicine, University of Auckland, New Zealand
7.4 *Colorectal tumours*

J. JASSEM
Professor of Oncology and Radiotherapy, Medical Academy of Gdansk, Poland
4.30 *Combined chemotherapy and radiotherapy*

ANTHONY M. JELLIFFE
Emeritus Consultant in Radiotherapy and Oncology, Middlesex Hospital, London and Mount Vernon Hospital, Northwood, Middlesex, UK
6.4 *Salivary tumours*

ALISTAIR JENKINS
Consultant and Senior Lecturer in Neurosurgery, University of Newcastle upon Tyne, UK
19.6 *Spinal metastatic disease*

OLE MØLLER JENSEN
Director, Division of Cancer Epidemiology, Danish Cancer Society, Copenhagen, Denmark
2.4 *The cancer registry: organization and function*

P. W. M. JOHNSON
ICRF Cancer Medicine Research Unit, St James's University Hospital, Leeds, UK
4.14 *High-dose chemotherapy and autologous bone-marrow rescue*

COLIN H. JONES
Head of Medical Physics, Royal Marsden Hospital; Senior Lecturer in Physics, Institute of Cancer Research, London
4.23 *Intracavitary therapy*

TERRY JONES
Medical Research Council Cyclotron Unit, Hammersmith Hospital, London
3.7 *Positron emission tomography*

HERBERT F. JURGENS
Professor of Paediatric Haematology and Oncology, Westfälischen Wilhelms University, Münster, Germany
13.3 *Ewing's sarcoma*

S. B. KAYE
Professor of Medical Oncology, University of Glasgow, UK
4.12 *New and miscellaneous anticancer drugs: future developments in drug design*

S. A. KELLY
Consultant in Clinical Oncology, Freedom Fields Hospital, Plymouth, UK
1.9 *Cytokines*

DAVID J. KERR
Professor of Clinical Oncology, Queen Elizabeth Hospital, University of Birmingham, UK
4.12 *New and miscellaneous anticancer drugs: future developments in drug design*
4.34 *Principles of pharmacokinetics*

K. KIAN ANG
Professor of Radiotherapy, University of Texas M.D. Anderson Cancer Center, Houston, USA
19.8 *Complications related to radiotherapy*

JUDITH E. KINGSTON
Senior Lecturer in Paediatric Oncology, St Bartholomew's Hospital, London
14.3 *Retinoblastoma*

JEAN-CLAUDE KURDZIEL
Radiologist in Charge, Department of Diagnostic and Interventional Radiology, Centre Hospitalier de Luxembourg, Luxembourg
3.9 *Interventional radiology: percutaneous tissue sampling guided by imaging*

CARLO LA VECCHIA
Head, Laboratory of Epidemiology, Istituto 'Mario Negri' and Associate Professor of Epidemiology, University of Milan, Italy
2.9 *Cancer epidemiology and prevention*

MARIE JOSE LACOMBE
Pathologist, Institut Gustave Roussy, Villejuif, France
13.2 *Malignant mesenchymal tumours in childhood*

H. LAMBERT
Consultant Clinical Oncologist, Hammersmith Hospital, London
9.7 *Carcinoma of the vulva and its putative precursors*

TORSTEN G. LANDBERG
Professor of Oncology, University of Lund Institute for Oncology, Malmö, Sweden
5.1.2 *Radiotherapy*

J. W. H. LEER
Professor and Head of Department of Clinical Oncology, University Hospital of Leiden, The Netherlands
3.5 *Clinical approaches to precancerous states*

JEAN-LOUIS LEFEBVRE
Chief of Head and Neck Department, Centre Oscar Lambret, Lille, France
6.8 *Tumours of the oropharynx*

ALEXANDER D. LEWIS
Senior Research Fellow, CRC Department of Medical Oncology, University of Glasgow, UK
4.6 *Alkylating agents and related drugs*

G. J. LINDEMAN
Research Fellow, Walter and Eliza Hall Institute for Medical Research, Royal Melbourne Hospital, Victoria, Australia
17 *Tumours of unknown primary site*

DAVID LOWE
Reader in Histopathology, St Bartholomew's Hospital Medical College, London
9.8 *Sarcoma and melanoma of the female genital system*

VALENTINE MACAULAY
Senior Registrar in Medical Oncology, ICRF Clinical Oncology Unit, Churchill Hospital, Oxford
19.3 *Paraneoplastic syndromes*

GARY J. MACFARLANE
Deputy Director, Division of Epidemiology and Biostatistics, European Institute of Oncology, Milan, Italy
2.9 *Cancer epidemiology and prevention*

J.-P. MACH
Professor, Institute of Biochemistry, University of Lausanne; Member of the Swiss Institute for Cancer Research, Switzerland
1.8 *Monoclonal antibodies*

IAN MAGRATH
Chief, Section of Lymphoma Biology, Pediatric Branch, National Cancer Institute; Professor of Pediatrics, University of the Uniformed Services in the Health Sciences, Bethesda, Maryland, USA
12.7.3 *The non-Hodgkin's lymphomas in children*

PETER MAGUIRE
Director and Honorary Consultant Psychiatrist, Cancer Research Campaign Psychological Medicine Group, Christie Hospital, Manchester, UK
20.4 *Psychological sequelae of cancer and its treatment*

PATRICK MAISONNEUVE
Deputy Director, Division of Epidemiology and Biostatistics, European Institute of Oncology, Milan, Italy
2.9 *Cancer epidemiology and prevention*

S. T. A. MALIK
Director of Research, Thunder Bay Regional Cancer Center; Assistant Professor of Medicine, McMaster University, Ontario, Canada
1.9 *Cytokines*

M. MALONE
Consultant Histopathologist, Great Ormond Street Hospital for Children, London
12.9 *Histiocyte disorders*

JAMES S. MALPAS
Professor of Medical Oncology, Imperial Cancer Research Fund Department of Medical Oncology, St Bartholomew's Hospital, London
12.6.3 *Hodgkin's disease in childhood*

ANTHONY A. MANCUSO
Professor of Radiology, University of Florida College of Medicine, Gainesville, USA
6.8 *Tumours of the oropharynx*

HENRY J. MANKIN
Chief of the Orthopedic Service, Massachusetts General Hospital, and Edith Mashley Professor of Orthopedics, Harvard Medical School, Boston, USA
13.1 *Sarcoma of the soft tissues*

JILLIAN R. MANN
Consultant Paediatric Oncologist, The Children's Hospital, Birmingham, UK
14.5 *Germ cell tumours of childhood*

MALCOLM D. MASON
Consultant Clinical Oncologist, Vilindre Hospital, Cardiff, UK
10.1 *Testicular tumours*

PHILIP MAYLES
Physicist, Royal Marsden Hospital, Sutton, Surrey, UK
4.21 *External-beam radiation therapy, including conformational therapy*

TIM McELWAIN
Royal Marsden Hospital, Sutton, Surrey, UK
4.14 *High-dose chemotherapy and autologous bone-marrow rescue*

G. ANGUS J. McINDOE
Senior Registrar in Gynaecological Oncology, Hammersmith Hospital, London
9.7 *Carcinoma of the vulva and its putative precursors*

E. B. McNEIL
Data Manager, Department of Medical Oncology, Royal Prince Alfred Hospital, Sydney, New South Wales, Australia
18 *Cancer in the elderly*

J. GORDON McVIE
Director, Scientific Department, Cancer Research Campaign, London
4.7 *Antitumour antibiotics*
5.1.3 *Achievements of chemotherapy and obstacles to further progress*

URS F. METZGER
Professor of Surgery, Triemli Hospital, Zurich, Switzerland
7.3 *Malignancies of the small bowel*

BEN J. MIJNHEER
Head, Clinical Physics, Radiotherapy Department, The Netherlands Cancer Institute, Amsterdam, The Netherlands
4.20 *Current practice of radiotherapy: physical basis*

SAM MILLIKEN
Bone Marrow Transplant Co-ordinator, Royal Marsden Hospital, Sutton, Surrey, UK
12.4 *Bone marrow transplantation for leukaemia*

CHRISTOPHER D. MITCHELL
Consultant Paediatric Oncologist, Oxford Radcliffe Hospital, UK
14.4 *Wilms' tumour*

ROBERTO MOLINARI
Chief, Head and Neck Surgical Oncology Division, Istituto Nazionale Tumori, Milan, Italy
6.6 *Tumours of the nasopharynx*

SILVIO MONFARDINI
Chief, Division of Medical Oncology, Centro di Riferiment o Oncologico; Professor of Medical Oncology, Udine University, Aviano, Italy
12.10 *Neoplastic complications of AIDS*

P. W. MORTIMER
Consultant Skin Physician, St George's and Royal Marsden Hospitals, London
6.1 *Skin cancer other than melanoma*

CLAIRE MOYNIHAN
Royal Marsden Hospital, Sutton, Surrey, UK
20.6 *Rehabilitation of the cancer patient*

VICTORIA MURDAY
Senior Lecturer in Genetics, Department of Child Health, St George's Hospital Medical School, London
1.5 *Genetics and familial cancer*

STEPHEN NEIDLE
Professor of Biophysics; Director, CRC Biomolecular Structure Unit, Institute of Cancer Research, Sutton, Surrey, UK
4.2 *Biomolecular structure and rational drug design*

JAN P. NEIJT
Associate Professor in Internal Medicine, Utrecht University Hospital, The Netherlands
9.1 *Carcinoma of the ovary*

DAVID R. NEWELL
Senior Lecturer in Experimental Oncology, Medical School, University of Newcastle upon Tyne, UK
4.9 *Cisplatin and analogues: discovery, mechanism of action, and clinical pharmacology*

EDWARD S. NEWLANDS
Professor of Cancer Medicine, Charing Cross and Westminster Medical School, London
9.2 *Ovarian germ-cell and other rare ovarian tumours*

D. W. W. NEWLING
Professor and Chief, Department of Urology, Academic Hospital of the Free University of Amsterdam, The Netherlands
10.4 *Bladder cancer*

JACQUES NINANE
Professor in Paediatric Haematology and Oncology, Saint-Luc University Hospital, Catholic University of Louvain, Brussels, Belgium
14.2 *Neuroblastoma*

J. M. A. NORTHOVER
Consultant Surgeon, St Mark's Hospital; Honorary Director, Colorectal Cancer Unit, Imperial Cancer Research Fund, London
7.4 *Colorectal tumours*

P. J. O'CONNOR
Head, Cancer Research Campaign Department of Carcinogenesis, Paterson Institute for Cancer Research, Christie Hospital, Manchester, UK
2.1 *Cell and molecular mechanisms in chemical carcinogenesis*

P. T. D. OLIVER
Sir Maxwell Joseph Professor of Medical Oncology, Royal London Hospital, UK
10.5 *Tumours of the kidney (other than nephroblastoma)*

JULIE OLLIFF
Consultant Radiologist, Queen Elizabeth Hospital, Edgbaston, Birmingham, UK
3.6 *The role of radiological imaging in the management of cancer*

JAN OLOFSSON
Professor and Chairman, Department of Otolaryngology/Head and Neck Surgery, Haukeland University Hospital, Bergen, Norway
6.10 *Tumours of the larynx*

SUSAN M. O'REILLY
Consultant in Medical Oncology, Clatterbridge Centre for Oncology, Wirral, UK
3.4 *Flow cytometry*

JENS OVERGAARD
Professor, Danish Cancer Society, Aarhus, Denmark
4.31 *Hyperthermia*

CHRISTOPHER PAINE
Consultant Radiotherapist, Oxford Radcliffe Hospital, UK
4.22 *Interstitial radiation therapy*

JEAN PAPILLON
Professor of Radiology, University of Lyon, Centre Leon Berard, Lyon, France
7.5 *Radical radiotherapy of cancer of the rectum and anus*

FERNANDO J. PARADINAS
Senior Lecturer (Honorary Consultant), Charing Cross and Westminster Medical School, London
9.2 *Ovarian germ-cell and other rare ovarian tumours*

E. K. J. PAUWELS
Professor of Radiological Sciences (Nuclear Medicine), University Hospital Leiden, The Netherlands
3.12 *Nuclear medicine procedures*

MARTIN F. PERA
Research Scientist, Cancer Research Campaign, Department of Zoology, Oxford University
1.3 *Differentiation and cancer*

ALBERTO PERACCHIA
Professor of Surgery, School of Medicine, University of Milan, Italy
7.1 *Malignancies of the oesophagus*

GODEFRIDUS J. PETERS
Associate Professor, Department of Oncology, Free University Hospital, Amsterdam, The Netherlands
4.8 *Antimetabolites*

THIERRY O. PHILIP
Professor of Medical Oncology and Director of the Centre Leon Berard, Lyon, France
12.5 *Autologous bone-marrow transplantation and intensification therapies for solid tumours and lymphomas*

SILVANA PILOTTI
Deputy Director of Pathology, Istituto Nazionale Tumori, Milan, Italy
3.1 *Histological classification and typing of solid tumours*
6.6 *Tumours of the nasopharynx*

HERBERT M. PINEDO
Professor of Oncology, Free University Hospital and Netherlands Cancer Institute, Amsterdam, The Netherlands
4.13 *Drug resistance*

ROSS PINKERTON
Consultant Paediatric Oncologist, Royal Marsden Hospital, Sutton, Surrey, UK
4.14 *High-dose chemotherapy and autologous bone-marrow rescue*
14.6 *Liver tumours*

LUIGI PIVA
Assistant, Section of Urologic Oncology, Istituto Nazionale Tumori, Milan, Italy
10.3 *Tumours of the penis*

GIORGIO PIZZOCARO
Chief, Division of Urology, Department of Surgery, Istituto Nazionale Tumori, Milan, Italy
10.3 *Tumours of the penis*

JULIA M. POLAK
Professor of Histochemistry, Royal Postgraduate Medical School, Hammersmith Hospital, London
16.5 *Neuroendocrine gastroenteropancreatic tumours*

JACQUELINE POMP
Radiation Oncologist, Reinier de Graaf Hospital, Delft, The Netherlands
6.7.3 *The role of radiotherapy in the treatment of tumours of the oral cavity*

BRUCE A. J. PONDER
CRC Professor of Human Cancer Genetics, University of Cambridge; Honorary Consultant Physician, Addenbrooke's Hospital, Cambridge and Royal Marsden Hospital, Sutton, Surrey, UK
16.2 *Medullary carcinoma of the thyroid*

JAN PONTEN
Professor, Department of Pathology, University of Uppsala, Sweden
1.6 *Oncogenes*

ANTHONY C. POVEY
Scientific Officer, Cancer Research Campaign Department of Carcinogenesis, Paterson Institute for Cancer Research, Christie Hospital, Manchester, UK
2.3 *Cell and molecular mechanisms in chemical carcinogenesis*

RAY POWLES
Consultant Physician, Royal Marsden Hospital, Sutton, Surrey, UK
12.4 *Bone marrow transplantation for leukaemia*

CHRISTOPHER G. A. PRICE
Senior Registrar, Wessex Regional Oncology Unit, Southampton University Hospitals, UK
19.1 *Acute emergencies in oncology: general overview*

PAT PRICE
Senior Lecturer in Clinical Oncology, Royal Postgraduate Medical School, Hammersmith Hospital, London
19.1 *Acute emergencies in oncology: general overview*

JON PRITCHARD
Consultant and Honorary Senior Lecturer in Paediatric Oncology, Hospital for Sick Children and Institute of Child Health, London
12.9 *Histiocyte disorders*

J. A. RAFFERTY
Scientific Officer, Cancer Research Campaign Department of Carcinogenesis, Paterson Institute for Cancer Research, Christie Hospital, Manchester, UK
2.3 *Cell and molecular mechanisms in chemical carcinogenesis*

DEREK RAGHAVAN
Professor of Medicine and Chief of Division of Solid Tumour Oncology, Roswell Park Cancer Institute, Buffalo, New York, USA
10.2 *Extragonadal germ cell tumours*
18 *Cancer in the elderly*

ROGER RAHMANI
Director of Research, INSERM, Centre INRA d'Antibes, France
4.11 *Vinca alkaloids: cellular pharmacology and clinical pharmacokinetics*

Y. REVILLON
Professor, Hôpital des Enfants Malades, Paris, France
13.2 *Malignant mesenchymal tumours in childhood*

MICHAEL A. RICHARDS
Reader in Medical Oncology, United Medical and Dental Schools, Guy's Hospital, London
3.4 *Flow cytometry*

FRANCO RILKE
Director of Pathology and Deputy Scientific Director, Istituto Nazionale Tumori, Milan, Italy
3.1 *Histopathological classification and typing of solid tumours*

ALASTAIR W. S. RITCHIE
Consultant Urological Surgeon, Gloucestershire Royal Hospital, Gloucester, UK
10.5 *Tumours of the kidney (other than nephroblastoma)*

BORGHILD ROALD
Professor of Pathology, Ullevål University Hospital, University of Oslo, Norway
14.2 *Neuroblastoma*

FAUSTO ROILA
Vice-Director, Division of Medical Oncology, Policlinico Hospital, Perugia, Italy
19.13 *Supportive care, antiemetics, and alimentation*

MIKAEL RØRTH
Professor of Clinical Oncology, Rigshospitalet, Copenhagen, Denmark
11.4 *Other thymic tumours*

ANDREW E. ROSENBERG
Assistant Professor, Harvard Medical School; Assistant Pathologist, Massachusetts General Hospital, Boston, USA
13.1 *Sarcoma of the soft tissues*

NICOLE ROTMENSZ
Division of Epidemiology and Biostatistics, Istituto Europeo di Oncologia, Milan, Italy
20.2 *Data management*

ENRIQUE ROZENGURT
Head, Laboratory of Growth Regulation, Imperial Cancer Research Fund, London
1.2 *Polypeptide and neuropeptide growth factors: signalling pathways and role in cancer*

ALBERTO RUOL
Assistant Professor, Second Department of General Surgery, University of Padua, Italy
7.1 *Malignancies of the oesophagus*

R. C. G. RUSSELL
Consultant Surgeon, Middlesex Hospital, London
7.6 *Tumours of the pancreas*

GORDON J. S. RUSTIN
Senior Lecturer in Medical Oncology, Charing Cross Hospital, London and Consultant Physician, Mount Vernon Hospital, Northwood, Middlesex, UK
3.11 *Circulating tumour markers*

JOSE SANTINI
Professor of Oto-Rhino-Laryngology, Head and Neck Surgery, University of Nice-Sophia Antipolis, France
6.9 *Tumours of the hypopharynx*

ARMANDO SANTORO
Associate Director, Medical Oncology, Istituto Nazionale Tumori, Milan, Italy
13.5 *Bone malignant tumours other than osteosarcoma and Ewing's tumour*

RODOLFO SARACCI
Chief, Unit of Analytical Epidemiology, International Agency for Research on Cancer, Lyon, France
2.5 *Aetiological leads*

ROLF SAUER
Professor of Radiation Therapy, University of Erlangen, Germany
13.3 *Ewing's sarcoma*

MICHELE I. SAUNDERS
Reader in Oncology, University College London; Consultant, Centre for Cancer Treatment, Mount Vernon Hospital, Northwood, Middlesex, UK
4.29 *Clinical fractionation studies*

PIERRE G. M. SCALLIET
Associate Professor of Oncology, VIA, Department of Radiation Oncology, Middelheim Hospital, Antwerp, Belgium
10.4 *Bladder cancer*

M. SCHAADT
Klinik I für Innere Medizin der Universität zu Köln, Germany
12.6.1 *The cell biology of Hodgkin's disease*

MARTIN SCHLUMBERGER
Consultant Physician, Department of Nuclear Medicine, Institut Gustave Roussy, Villejuif, France
16.1 *Carcinoma of the thyroid*

FRITZ H. SCHRÖDER
Professor and Chairman, Department of Urology, Erasmus University Rotterdam, The Netherlands
10.6 *Tumours of the prostate*

GILBERTO SCHWARTSMANN
Director, South-American Office for Anticancer Drug Development, Hospital de Clinicas de Porto Alegre, Brazil
4.7 *Antitumour antibiotics*
19.9 *Complications of cytotoxic therapy*

G. R. H. SEALY
Director (retired), Mersey Regional Centre for Radiotherapy and Oncology, Clatterbridge Hospital, Merseyside, UK
6.12 *Carcinoma of the external auditory meatus and middle ear*

P. SELBY
Professor of Cancer Medicine, University of Leeds, St James's University Hospital, Leeds, UK
4.14 *High-dose chemotherapy and autologous bone-marrow rescue*
12.8 *Myeloma and other plasma cell malignancies*

YVONNE D. SENTURIA
Clinical Assistant Professor of Pediatrics, Northwestern University Medical School, Chicago, Illinois, USA
19.11 *Teratogenic effects of cancer treatment*

KAROL SIKORA
Professor of Clinical Oncology, Royal Postgraduate Medical School, Hammersmith Hospital, London
1.6 *Oncogenes*
4.18 *Monoclonal antibody targeting*

WILLIAM F. SINDELAR
Senior Investigator, Surgery Branch, National Cancer Institute, National Institutes of Health, Maryland, USA
4.25 *Intraoperative radiotherapy: an investigational approach to cancer*

CHARLES R. J. SINGER
Consultant Haematologist, Royal United Hospital, Bath, UK
12.3 *The chronic leukaemias*

MAURICE L. SLEVIN
Consultant Physician, Department of Medical Oncology, St Bartholomew's Hospital, London
20.11 *Support systems for cancer patients*

IAN E. SMITH
Consultant Cancer Physician, Royal Marsden Hospital, London
19.3 *Paraneoplastic syndromes*

O. SMITH
Department of Haematology, Royal Free Hospital, London
19.4 *Immunological and haematological complications of cancer*

GORDON B. SNOW
Professor and Chairman, Department of Otolaryngology-Head and Neck Surgery, Free University Hospital, Amsterdam, The Netherlands
6.13 *Management of cervical lymph nodes*

LESLIE H. SOBIN
Chief, Gastrointestinal Pathology, Armed Forces Institute of Pathology, Washington DC; Chairman TNM Project, International Union against Cancer
5.2 *Staging classifications*

R. SOUHAMI
Professor of Oncology, University College London Medical School, UK
13.4 *Osteosarcoma*

W. PATRICK SOUTTER
Reader in Gynaecological Oncology, Institute of Obstetrics and Gynaecology, Royal Postgraduate Medical School, Hammersmith Hospital, London
9.7 *Carcinoma of the vulva and its putative precursors*

MARGARET F. SPITTLE
Consultant Clinical Oncologist, The Middlesex Hospital, London
6.1 *Skin cancer other than melanoma*
6.5 *Carcinoma of the nasal cavity and paranasal sinuses*

DAVID SPOONER
Consultant Clinical Oncologist, The Children's and Queen Elizabeth Hospitals, Birmingham, UK
15.1 *Brain tumours in children*

G. GORDON STEEL
Professor of Radiobiology Applied to Radiotherapy, Institute of Cancer Research, Sutton, Surrey, UK
4.19 *The biological basis of radiotherapy*
4.23 *Intracavitary therapy*

ROBERT C. STEIN
Clinician Scientist, Ludwig Institute for Cancer Research and Department of Oncology, University College London Medical School, UK
4.16 *The basis of hormonal therapy of cancer*

P. M. STELL
Professor of Otorhinolaryngology, University of Liverpool, UK
6.12 *Carcinoma of the external auditory meatus and middle ear*

MICHAEL J. E. STERNBERG
Head of Laboratory of Biomolecular Modelling, Imperial Cancer Research Fund, London
4.3 *Protein modelling*

WILLIAM P. STEWARD
Senior Lecturer and Consultant in Medical Oncology, Beatson Oncology Centre, Western Infirmary, Glasgow, UK
4.15 *Clinical uses of haemopoietic growth factors*

FIONA STEWART
Radiologist, The Netherlands Cancer Institute, Amsterdam, The Netherlands
4.30 *Combined chemotherapy and radiotherapy*

HANS H. STORM
Head, Department of Cancer Registration, Division of Cancer Epidemiology, Danish Cancer Society, Copenhagen, Denmark
2.4 *The cancer registry: organization and function*

GERRIT STOTER
Professor of Medical Oncology, Rotterdam Cancer Institute, The Netherlands
10.4 *Bladder cancer*

I. J. STRATFORD
MRC Radiology Unit, Chilton, Oxfordshire, UK
4.28 *Hypoxia—selective bioreductive drugs*

MICHAEL R. STRATTON
Honorary Consultant Pathologist, Institute of Cancer Research, Sutton, Surrey, UK
3.2 *New techniques in pathology and their application in diagnosis and studies*

HERMAN D. SUIT
Andres Soriano Professor of Radiation Oncology, Harvard Medical School, Massachusetts General Hospital, Boston, USA
13.1 *Sarcoma of the soft tissues*

SIMON B. SUTCLIFFE
Professor of Radiation Oncology, University of Toronto; Vice President, Oncology Programs, Princess Margaret Hospital, Ontario Cancer Institute, Toronto, Canada
12.6.2 *Hodgkin's disease in adults*

HANS SVENSSON
Professor of Medical Radiation Physics, University Hospital, Umeå, Sweden
4.20 *Current practice of radiotherapy: physical basis*

DIANA TAIT
Consultant in Radiotherapy and Oncology, Royal Marsden Hospital, Sutton, Surrey, UK
4.21 *External beam radiation therapy including conformational therapy*

SILVIA TANA
Assistant in Radiotherapy, Istituto Nazionale Tumori, Milan, Italy
10.3 *Tumours of the penis*

IAN F. TANNOCK
Chief of Medicine, Princess Margaret Hospital and Professor of Medicine, University of Toronto, Canada
6.14 *Chemotherapy in conjunction with radiotherapy and/or surgery in head and neck cancer*

D. TARIN
Nuffield Reader in Pathology (University of Oxford), John Radcliffe Hospital, Oxford
1.10 *Cancer metastasis*

MARTIN TATTERSALL
Professor of Cancer Medicine, University of Sydney; Head, Department of Medical Oncology, Royal Prince Alfred Hospital, Sydney, Australia
17 *Tumours of unknown primary site*
20.9 *Economic considerations in cancer care*

HANS TESCH
Klinik I für Innere Medizin, Universitat Köln, Germany
12.6.1 *The cell biology of Hodgkin's disease*

D. G. T. THOMAS
Professor of Neurosurgery, Gough Cooper Department, The National Hospital for Neurology and Neurosurgery, London
15.2 *Tumours of the brain and spinal cord in adults*

R. TIFFANY
Chief Nurse and Director of Patient Services, Royal Marsden Hospital, Sutton, Surrey, UK
20.6 *Rehabilitation in the cancer patient*

M. J. TILBY
Senior Research Associate, Leukaemia Research Fund Unit, Medical School, University of Newcastle, UK
4.9 *Cisplatin and analogues: discovery, mechanism of action, and clinical pharmacology*

ADRIAN R. TIMOTHY
Consultant Clinical Oncologist, South East London Oncology Centre, St Thomas's Hospital, London
7.2 *Cancer of the stomach*

JEFFREY S. TOBIAS
Clinical Director, Meyerstein Institute of Oncology, Middlesex Hospital, London
11.6 *Uncommon intrathoracic tumours*

MAURIZIO TONATO
Professor and Director of the Division of Medical Oncology, Policlinico Hospital, Perugia, Italy
19.13 *Supportive care, antiemetics, and alimentation*

DIMITRIOS TRICHOPOULOS
Vincent L. Gregory Professor of Cancer Prevention and Professor of Epidemiology, Harvard School of Public Health, Boston, Massachusetts, USA
2.5 *Aetiological leads*

MAURICE TUBIANA
Emeritus Professor of Radiotherapy, Institut Gustave Roussy, Villejuif, France
16.1 *Carcinoma of the thyroid*

PINUCCI A. VALAGUSSA
Division of Medical Oncology, Istituto Nazionale Tumori, Milan, Italy
19.2 *Carcinogenic effects of cancer treatment*

ROELF VALKEMA
Physician, Nuclear Medicine, University Hospital Leiden, The Netherlands
3.12 *Nuclear medicine procedures*

HERMAN VAN DEN BERGHE
Director, Centre for Human Genetics, University of Leuven, Belgium
1.4 *Chromosomes and cancer*

W. VAN DEN BOGAERT
Professor of Radiation Oncology, University Hospital Leuven, Belgium
6.10 *Tumours of the larynx*

ALBERT J. VAN DER KOGEL
Professor of Experimental Radiotherapy, Institute of Radiotherapy, University of Nijmegen, The Netherlands
19.8 *Complications related to radiotherapy*

ISAÄC VAN DER WAAL
Professor of Oral Pathology, Free University/ACTA, Amsterdam, The Netherlands
6.7.1 *Epidemiology and clinicopathological aspects of premalignant and malignant lesions*

J. H. VAN DONGEN
Head of Department of Surgery, The Netherlands Cancer Institute; Professor of Surgical Oncology, University of Amsterdam, The Netherlands
3.5 *Clinical approaches to precancerous states*

CEES VAN GROENINGEN
Massachusetts General Hospital, Boston, USA
13.1 *Sarcoma of the soft tissues*

A. T. VAN OOSTEROM
Professor of Medical Oncology, Antwerp University Hospital, Belgium
19.2 *Metabolic disturbances*

RUUD E. N. VAN RIJSWIJK
Medical Oncologist, University Hospital, Maastricht, The Netherlands
19.2 *Metabolic disturbances*

JAN VERHOEF
Professor of Medical Microbiology, Eijkman-Winkler Institute for Medical Microbiology, Utrecht University, The Netherlands
19.9 *Complications of cytotoxic therapy*

JAN B. VERMORKEN
Senior Consultant, Department of Medical Oncology, Free University Hospital, Amsterdam, The Netherlands
9.1 *Carcinoma of the ovary*

UMBERTO VERONESI
Scientific Director, European Institute of Oncology, Milan, Italy
8 *Breast cancer*

LARS VINDELØV
Staff Physician, Rigshospitalet, Copenhagen, Denmark
11.1 *Tumours of the trachea and the lung*

CHRISTOF VON KALLE
Research Associate, Klinik I für Innere Medizin, Cologne University, Germany
12.6.1 *The cell biology of Hodgkin's disease*

P. A. VOÛTE
Professor of Paediatric Oncology, Emma Kinderziekenhuis, Academic Medical Centre, University of Amsterdam, The Netherlands
7.7 *Liver tumours*

DAVID A. WALKER
Senior Lecturer in Paediatric Oncology, Department of Child Health, University Hospital, Queen's Medical Centre, Nottingham, UK
14.7 *Rare tumours of childhood*

J. A. H. WASS
Professor of Clinical Endocrinology, St Bartholomew's Hospital Medical College, London
16.3 *Pituitary tumours*

GWYN T. WATKIN
Consultant Surgeon, Ysbyty Gwynedd, Bangor, North Wales, UK
6.4 *Salivary tumours*

DEIRDRE C. T. WATSON
Consultant Thoracic Surgeon, East Birmingham Hospital, UK
11.2 *Mesothelioma*

JONATHAN WAXMAN
Reader in Oncology, Royal Postgraduate Medical School, Hammersmith Hospital, London
10.6 *Tumours of the prostate*
19.10 *Effects of cancer chemotherapy on fertility*

ROBIN A. WEISS
Professor of Viral Oncology, Institute of Cancer Research, London
2.2 *Viral carcinogenesis*

TOM WEST
Medical Director (retired), St Christopher's Hospice, Sydenham, London
20.7 *Care of the dying patient*

NICHOLAS WILLCOX
Senior Research Fellow, Neuroscience Group, Institute for Molecular Medicine, Oxford
11.3 *Thymic tumours with myasthenia gravis or bone marrow dyscrasias*

NORMAN S. WILLIAMS
Professor of Surgery; Director, Academic Surgical Unit, The Royal London Hospital, London
7.4 *Colorectal tumours*

DERRY E. V. WILMAN
Drug Development Section, Institute of Cancer Research, Cancer Research Campaign Laboratory, Sutton, Surrey, UK
4.4 *Structure–activity relationships of anticancer agents*

CHARLES G. WILSON
Consultant in Clinical Oncology, Addenbrooke's Hospital, Cambridge, UK
3.7 *Positron emission tomography*

W. WINKELMANN
Professor of Orthopaedic Surgery, Westfälische-Wilhelms University, Münster, Germany
13.3 *Ewing's sarcoma*

BENJAMIN WINOGRAD
Director, Clinical Cancer Research, Europe, Bristol Myers Squibb, Pharmaceutical Research Institute, Brussels, Belgium
4.5 *New drug development*

PAUL WORKMAN
Head of Bioscience Section, Cancer Research Department, Zeneca Pharmaceuticals, Alderley Park, Macclesfield, Cheshire, UK
4.6 *Alkylating agents and related drugs*

NICHOLAS A. WRIGHT
Director, Clinical Research, Imperial Cancer Research Fund, and Professor of Histopathology, Royal Postgraduate Medical School, Hammersmith Hospital, London
1.1 *The growth of human tumours*

PETER F. M. WRIGLEY
Consultant Cancer Physician, St Bartholomew's Hospital, London
7.2 *Cancer of the stomach*

DAVID WYNICK
Clinician Scientist, Royal Postgraduate Medical School, Hammersmith Hospital, London
16.5 *Neuroendocrine gastroenteropancreatic tumours*

JOHN YARNOLD
Senior Lecturer and Honorary Consultant in Clinical Oncology, Institute of Cancer Research and Royal Marsden Hospital, Sutton, Surrey, UK
4.21 *External-beam radiation therapy, including conformational therapy*
8 *Breast cancer*

TONGZHANG ZHENG
Istituto di Biometria e Statistica Medica, University of Milan, Italy
2.9 *Cancer epidemiology and prevention*

XIAO-JIAN ZHOU
INSERM U-278, Marseilles, France
4.11 *Vinca alkaloids: cellular pharmacology and clinical pharmacokinetics*

ROBERT A. ZITTOUN
Professor and Head, Department of Haematology, Hôtel Dieu, Paris, France
20.3 *Quality of life*

MARKUS ZUBER
Staff Surgeon, Department of Surgery, University of Basel, Switzerland
7.3 *Malignancies of the small bowel*

ROBERTO ZUCALI
Director, Radiotherapy 'A', Istituto Nazionale Tumori, Milan, Italy
6.6 *Tumours of the nasopharynx*

Section 8
Breast cancer

8   Breast cancer

UMBERTO VERONESI, A. GOLDHIRSCH, AND JOHN YARNOLD

EPIDEMIOLOGY AND PREVENTION

Breast cancer is the most common cancer found in women in Europe (180 000 cases per year), the United States (130 000 cases per year), Australia, and many Latin-American countries. In European women it represents 20 per cent of all malignancies. Breast cancer is exceptional before the age of 20 years and is rare below 30 years but then the incidence rises very steadily up to the age of 50 years, after which the rate of increase slows down, although the incidence rate continues to rise. Mortality rates for breast cancer in western Europe and North America are of the order of 15–25 per 100 000 women, that is 30–40 per cent of the incidence rate, which is approximately 50–60 per 100 000 women.

The incidence of breast carcinoma is increasing in most countries at a mean rate of 1–2 per cent annually and soon nearly 1 million women will develop this disease every year throughout the world (Table 1). The annual rate of increase in incidence is more pronounced in low-risk populations than in high-risk populations, which have a tendency to level off. It is likely, therefore, that the difference in incidence between women living in Western countries and those living in the Far East will decrease with time. The highest increase in incidence rates has occurred in Canada, the United States, Sweden, Spain, and Finland (3–6 per cent annually between 1960 and 1975), while the lowest rates were observed in Norway and Denmark (1.8 per cent per year between 1965 and 1975). The mortality rates are also increasing but at a slower pace, with the lowest values in Denmark, The Netherlands, Norway, Sweden, and Switzerland (0.1–0.8 per cent increase per annum) and the highest values in Belgium, France, Germany, Italy, and Portugal (2.2–3.2 per cent increase per annum) between 1950 and 1979. Very recent reports show data in favour of a slowing down in breast cancer incidence and mortality in younger cohorts (Boyle 1988).

Geographical distribution

Breast cancer shows a wide variation in incidence and mortality in different countries (Table 2). The highest incidence rates have been observed among women living in Hawaii, British Columbia, and California. In these areas the annual incidence rate is approximately 80–90 per 100 000 women. The lowest incidence has been observed in some areas of Japan, with an incidence rate approximately 12–15 per 100 000 women. Western Europe shows rates that range from

40 to 60 cases per 100 000 women per annum, whilst Indian, African, and Chinese women show intermediate figures. Latin-American women show incidence rates either close to the European ones in some areas (Sao Paulo, Brazil) or close to the Indian ones in other areas (Puerto Rico). The incidence rates in Europe decrease from the north to the south and from west to east. Within each country, breast cancer incidence correlates well with the per capita income of the population in the various districts. In Finland, recent data (Pukkala *et al.* 1986) show that the high-risk areas for breast cancer are those in which there is a high proportion of women in the higher social classes. In Italy, the mortality rate for breast cancer in northern regions is more than twice that of the southern areas (Cislaghi *et al.* 1986).

Studies conducted on migrants (Buell 1974; Dunn 1977; Locke and King 1980) have shown the tendency of these populations to reach the incidence rates of women living in the host countries within a couple of generations, thus confirming the importance of the environment, meaning all external factors, including life-style.

Genetic factors

In the last few decades a number of studies have shown a 2–3-fold increase in the risk of breast cancer among first-degree relatives of patients with cancer of the breast (Wassink 1935; Martynova 1937; Penrose *et al.* 1948; Smithers 1948; Bucalossi *et al.* 1954; Macklin 1959; Tulinius *et al.* 1982). In particular, the Milan study (Bucalossi *et al.* 1954) showed an increased risk in relatives of patients with bilateral breast carcinoma. Anderson published studies in the early 1970s (Anderson 1972, 1976) showing that relatives of patients with breast cancer in whom the onset of the disease was in pre-menopause had a three times higher risk of breast carcinoma and that relatives of patients with bilateral carcinoma had a five times higher risk.

Table 1 Projected number of new cases of breast cancer in women in the year 2000 (modified from Parklin *et al.* 1984)

Africa	56 000
Central and South America	92 700
North America	160 600
Asia	204 400
Europe	190 500
Australia and New Zealand	8 000
ex-USSR area	46 900
Total	859 300

Table 2 Geographic variation in the annual incidence of cancer of the female breast (from Waterhouse *et al.* 1976)

	Age-standardized rate (per 100 000)	Cumulative rate[a] (%)
Japan (Osaka)	12.1	1.3
Nigeria (Ibidan)	15.5	1.7
India (Bombay)	20.1	2.2
Cuba	28.0	3.1
Finland	32.9	3.7
Norway	44.4	4.9
Sweden	52.4	5.8
New Zealand	52.5	5.8
UK (Oxford)	54.5	5.9
USA (NY)	57.2	6.2
USA (LA Whites)	79.9	8.9
Canada (Alberta)	57 4	6.2
Canada (British Columbia)	80.3	8.8
Switzerland (Geneva)	70.6	7.5

[a] Approximate cumulative lifetime risk.

A more recent study (Adami *et al.* 1981) drastically reduced the importance of the familial factor, showing a relative risk, 1.7 times higher, in mothers and sisters of breast cancer patients. When the carcinoma was bilateral and the onset of the disease occurred in pre-menopause the risk increased to 2.4 and 2.2, respectively.

It is impossible to establish how much of this increased familial risk is due to the sharing of a common life-style, including diet, among the members of the same family and how much is due to a true genetically inherited factor. Although in a disease like breast cancer, which has been defined as an environmental one, the term 'hereditary' sounds contradictory, Lynch and others have attempted to define the hereditary cases as 'the breast cancer cases with a positive family history of breast cancer and a distribution in the pedigree that is consistent with an autosomal dominant, highly penetrant, cancer susceptibility factor'. According to Lynch and Lynch (1986) the proportion of the true hereditary breast cancers is approximately 8 per cent of the total.

In recent years, familial cancer syndromes have helped to define the role of the inherited genetic defects in a number of tumours, including breast cancer. For example, an inherited mutation in the p53 tumour suppressor gene on the short arm of chromosome 17 underlies the high cancer risk, including breast cancer, in those affected by the extremely rare Li–Fraumeni syndrome (Li and Fraumeni 1969; Malkin *et al.* 1990). Of much greater practical significance is recognition that as much as 60–70 per cent of familial breast cancer predisposition in young women is linked to an unidentified locus on the long arm of chromosome 17 (Hall *et al.* 1990). Other evidence of an inherited contribution to breast cancer risk comes from examining kindreds affected by ataxia telangiectasia (Swift *et al.* 1987, 1991). These data raise the possibility that ataxia telangiectasia carriers (heterozygotes) in the general population represent a cancer-prone group with an elevated lifetime risk of breast cancer.

Reproductive history

Nulliparous women have a greater risk of breast cancer (Mustacchi 1961), whereas multiparity and a full-term pregnancy before 20 years of age protect women from the disease (MacMahon *et al.* 1970). Women who have had their ovaries removed before the age of 40 years have a reduced risk of breast cancer (Lilienfeld 1956). This shows that a relationship must exist between reproductive factors and breast carcinoma. However, it has not been clarified which specific hormones are involved in this process.

The oestrogenic hypothesis is one of the oldest and is based mainly on experimental evidence from laboratory animals. However, this hypothesis is not convincing for two reasons. First, because repeated full-term pregnancies at an early age with the consequent long-lasting increase of oestrogenic levels are associated with a decreased risk of breast cancer and, secondly, because the highest incidence of breast cancer is observed in old women when the oestrogenic level has been very low for decades.

It has been suggested that progesterone exerts a protective function and it has been proposed that the full differentiation of the mammary gland due to pregnancy allows the breasts of parous women to respond to the protective action of progesterone, whereas the breast tissue of nulliparous women is unable to respond. However, the epidemiological evidence in support of the protective hypothesis of progesterone is very weak.

Androgens have also been proposed as a possible carcinogenic factor in breast cancer. This hypothesis is mainly supported by the fact that the incidence of breast cancer is high in post-menopausal women, when androgenic levels are high, that administration of androgens for cystic disease has been shown to increase the risk of breast cancer (Veronesi and Pizzocaro 1968), and that higher levels of androgens and lower levels of progesterone have been found in pre-menopausal women with breast cancer compared to controls (Secreto *et al.* 1984). Moreover, Japanese women, who are at a lower risk of breast cancer than British women, have lower plasma androgen levels. Elevated levels of sex-hormone-binding globulin, a protein present in human serum capable of binding to both androgens and oestrogens, reduce the availability of oestrogens to the mammary epithelium (Siliteri *et al.* 1981). Sex-hormone-binding globulin would therefore play an important role in any possible type of endocrine carcinogenesis, both in the oestrogenic and in the androgenic hypothesis.

A possible association between chronic use of oral contraceptives and increased risk of breast cancer has been suggested by some studies (Paffenbarger *et al.* 1977; Kelsey *et al.* 1978), but other investigations (Ravnihar *et al.* 1979; Kelsey *et al.* 1981; Harris *et al.* 1982; Rosenberg *et al.* 1984), conducted on large populations exposed for a considerable length of time, have shown that the use of oral contraceptives is not associated with an increased risk of breast cancer. A recent case-control study on 755 women conducted in the United Kingdom showed, however, a significant trend in breast cancer risk with total duration of oral contraceptives. The same study showed that oral contraceptives containing less than 50 mg oestrogen have a lower risk associated with their use and that there may be some protective effect of progestogen-only pills.

The results of studies on the hypothetical risk of breast cancer associated with post-menopausal replacement oestrogen therapy are controversial: a number of studies reveal an increased risk of breast cancer, whereas several others failed to find any correlation (Hoover *et al.* 1976; Sartwell *et al.* 1977; Jick *et al.* 1980; Sobin and Sherif 1980; Brinton *et al.* 1981; Hulka *et al.* 1982).

Recently, Bergkvist *et al.* (1989), in a study of 23 244 post-menopausal women, showed a very limited increase in breast cancer risk with oestrogenic treatment; however, this was of some importance if the treatment was very prolonged. Nevertheless, the advantages linked to the oestrogen replacement treatment as regards protection from cardiovascular diseases and from osteoporosis seem to outweigh the limited risk of breast cancer (B. E. Henderson *et al.* 1986, 1988).

Diet

An association between a high-fat diet and breast cancer was first suggested by experimental studies on laboratory animals, which have shown that the incidence of spontaneous mammary tumours in mice is increased by the administration of a high-fat diet. This has also been proved for mammary tumours induced in rats by dimethyl-benzanthracene (DMBA) (Carroll and Hopkins 1979).

Correlation studies in female populations show that breast cancer occurs more commonly in countries with a high consumption of total and saturated fat, total calories, and animal proteins. In Japan breast cancer is increasing progressively, paralleling the mean daily increase of fat intake and the incidence rates of breast cancer of the offspring of Japanese migrants to the United States has increased with the progressive adaptation to the high-fat diet of the Americans (Dunn 1977). Among some religious groups, like the Seventh Day Adventists, who have a low-fat intake, the incidence rates of breast cancer are particularly low (Philips *et al.* 1980). Studies on these religious groups have also shown that the cohorts who entered the religious community in adult life did not show a reduction of breast

Table 3 Relationship of age at first exposure to radiation and breast cancer risk

Age at first exposure (years)	Atomic bomb series[a]	Canadian fluoroscopy series[b]
0–9	2.4	58.0
10–19	2.0	2.5
20–29	1.6	2.8
30–39	1.2	1.2
40–49	1.1	1.0
50+	1.2	0.0

[a] Ratio of observed to expected cases for those exposed to 10 rad (100 mGy) or more (Tokunaga *et al.* 1984).

[b] Ratio of death rates from breast cancer for those exposed to 100+ rad (1+ Gy) relative to the unexposed (Miller *et al.* 1989).

cancer rates, suggesting that the protective factors operate before adult life (Philips *et al.* 1980; Kinlen 1982).

The possible increased risk of breast cancer due to a high-fat diet has been explained in various ways: the increased introduction into the body, through the fat, of chemical carcinogens from the environment, an excess of adipose tissue, which in turn increases the level of circulating oestrogens, and the alteration of the intestinal microflora with increased production of potentially carcinogenic substances.

Radiation

An increased risk of breast cancer in women exposed to various doses of radiation has been shown in Japanese atomic bomb survivors (Tokunaga *et al.* 1984), in patients receiving radiotherapy for post-partum mastitis, and in patients who have had multiple fluoroscopies during treatment of pulmonary tuberculosis (Land *et al.* 1980). In these studies it has been observed that sensitivity to radiation is mainly concentrated in the first two or three decades of life. In the atomic bomb survivors the relative risk was 2.4 in women who were exposed to radiation in the first decade of life, 2.0 in women exposed during the second decade, and 1.6 in women exposed during the third decade. Women who were more than 30 years old when irradiated did not show any increase in breast cancer risk (Tokunaga *et al.* 1984). Identical results were obtained in the recent Canadian fluoroscopy study (Miller *et al.* 1989). These data are important in relation to the hypothetical risk of repeated mammograms (Table 3).

Benign breast disease

There are a few particular types of benign breast proliferations, such as diffuse papillomatosis and atypical hyperplasia, which will increase the breast cancer risk considerably. It is, however, generally accepted that the most common types of benign breast disease (fibroadenomas, cystic disease) do not represent an important risk factor. The fact that many studies have shown an increased risk of breast carcinoma among patients with cystic disease (Veronesi and Pizzocaro 1968; Donnelly *et al.* 1975; Kodlin *et al.* 1977; Page *et al.* 1978; Hutchinson *et al.* 1980) may be explained partly by other factors which are associated with cystic disease, such as pauci-parity, which in turn may increase the risk of breast cancer.

Other factors

Studies comparing the alcohol intake of women with breast cancer with that of controls showed a large number of drinkers among breast cancer patients, but this finding may be due to other dietary factors associated with alcohol intake. Case-control studies evaluating a possible increased risk due to hair dyes have produced conflicting results and no firm conclusions can be drawn at present (Nasca *et al.* 1980). In a recent paper (Al Sumidaie *et al.* 1988) reverse-transcriptase activity has been detected *in vitro* in blood monocytes from patients with breast cancer. As reverse transcriptase is strong evidence for the presence of a retrovirus, this finding is of particular interest since a retroviral causation for mammary carcinoma is known in mice.

Breast cancer prevention

In laboratory animals breast cancer can be induced by viruses, radiation, chemical carcinogens, and hormones. Moreover, genetic factors are of great importance. In humans, breast cancer may be induced by radiation but the cases due to such exposure are negligible. In humans, it is impossible to verify any hypothesis based on viral or chemical factors and many conflicting opinions about the role of hormones have been recorded. Nevertheless, breast cancer is mainly an environmental disease, as has been proved by the variability in incidence in different geographical areas and by studies on migrant populations. The identity of the specific environmental factors is unknown.

It therefore follows that all plans to reduce the incidence of breast cancer by preventive measures are theoretically weak. An empirical type of approach would be to analyse the life-style of a population with low breast cancer incidence (for instance that of Japanese women) and recommend that the high-risk populations conform their life-styles to the former. The United States' project for reducing breast cancer incidence by 25 per cent by the year 2000 is based mainly on dietary modifications. The reduction of fat consumption to 100 g/day/capita and the reduction of obesity are the main objectives of the plan (Greenwald and Sondik 1986).

A more promising preventive measure lies in the prolonged administration of anti-oestrogens (tamoxifen) or differentiating agents (retinoids), as many experimental studies have shown their ability to reduce breast cancer incidence both in chemically induced and in spontaneous mammary carcinomas in rodents.

Tamoxifen is an obvious candidate for chemoprevention studies as it decreases the incidence of contralateral breast cancer when administered for long periods (Fornander *et al.* 1989, 1991). However, the presence of some side-effects, although of mid intensity and the risk of inducing endometrial carcinoma have presented an obstacle to the implementation of long-term large randomized studies. As regards retinoids, theoretical and experimental evidence of these as chemopreventive agents has been presented in many papers (Moon *et al.* 1979, 1989; Sporn and Newton 1979; Sporn and Roberts 1991). One specific derivative of retinoid acid, hydroxyphenilretinamide, is being employed in an extensive randomized study on breast cancer patients to test its ability to reduce the incidence of contralateral breast carcinoma (Veronesi and Costa 1988; Veronesi *et al.* 1992).

NATURAL HISTORY OF BREAST CANCER

Histopathogenesis

The neoplastic transformation occurs mainly in the terminal ductal/lobular unit of the breast. According to some authors (Squartini and Sounelli 1981), the first appearance of the cancer process is *in situ*, but how long the proliferation remains intraepithelial before becoming infiltrating has never been elucidated. Certainly, in a great proportion of cases, the invasive character appears very early in the development of the cancer process. This is documented in the frequent observations by the pathologists of very tiny cancer foci (< 1 mm) with invasive features.

Due to the extensive heterogenicity of malignant cells in human breast cancer, a uniform histology has not been found within breast carcinomas and this finding is confirmed by ultrastructural studies (Tseng 1980). Biochemical markers of differentiation are irregularly distributed, as are many tumour-associated antigens and hormone receptors (Horand Hand *et al.* 1983; Natali *et al.* 1983; Oxenhandler *et al.* 1984). Flow cytometry has allowed a better study of the differences in ploidy within single breast carcinomas. One obvious sign of heterogeneity of breast carcinomas is the clinical observation of a mixed response to endocrine, chemotherapeutic, or radiological treatments. In disseminated breast carcinoma, systemic treatment induces mixed responses in 10–20 per cent of cases, some metastases disappearing completely while others remain stable or continue their progression. Sometimes the primary tumour regresses, while distant metastases may progress.

The heterogeneity of breast cancer cells may be explained by polyclonal origin. Although the monoclonal origin of cancer (that it arises from a single transformed cell) is a commonly accepted dogma (Fialkow 1979), if in a restricted area of the normal breast, under the action of a carcinogenic agent, many normal cells undergo neoplastic transformation simultaneously, the resulting carcinoma may be composed of different clonal cell subpopulations. According to another hypothesis (Nowell 1976) the cancer cells are genetically unstable and this instability is the cause of variations in phenotypic characteristics due to the generation of new cell subpopulations.

It has also been suggested that some modifications of the biological behaviour of breast carcinoma (for instance, a sudden rapid tumour growth) may be due not so much to the appearance of a new variant of cell populations but to the failure of the immune defence mechanism in the host.

Breast cancer may have a multicentric origin. In an extensive case review (Popkin and De Feo 1976) multicentric primary carcinomas, mostly non-invasive, were found in 13 per cent of the cases. In the contralateral breasts, the incidence of occult primaries is in the order of 15 per cent (Sanderson and Mackie 1979; Van Scott 1979). However, in clinical practice the finding of a double carcinoma in the same breast and of a simultaneous bilateral carcinoma is infrequent. It has also been reported that the incidence of occult carcinomas in the breasts of women over 70 years who died from other causes is 19 times greater than the incidence of clinical breast cancer (Sage and Casson 1976). Therefore, it is likely that many occult foci of carcinoma will never progress to overt disease.

Local development

Breast carcinoma spreads initially by infiltrating the surrounding breast tissue. If the tissue is homogeneous, the shape tends to be spherical, but if the tissue is of irregular density, as may happen in fibrocystic breasts, the shape is often very irregular, with extension along the planes where the tissues are softer. In a paper published by Holland *et al.* (1985), 5 mm sections of a series of 399 mastectomy specimens with invasive cancer were taken and each macrosection was radiographed. Any radiologically suspicious area was carefully examined histologically, with a mean of 20 blocks per specimen. In 37 per cent of the specimens there were no tumour

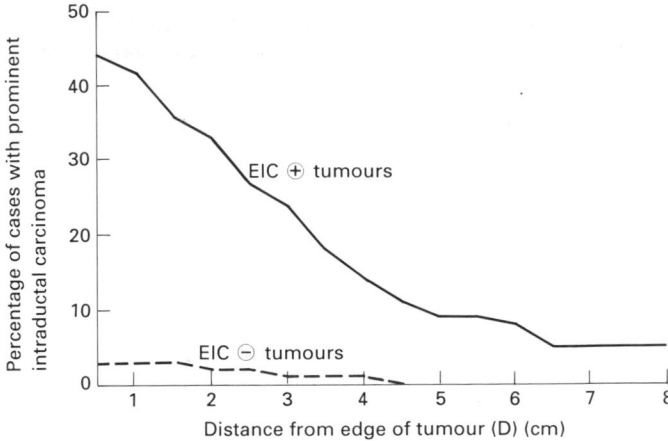

Fig. 1 Frequency of extensive intraductal carcinoma as a function of distance from the reference tumour EIC (extensive intraductal component). (Reproduced from Holland *et al.* (1990), with permission.)

foci around the primary tumour, in 20 per cent a tumour was found within 2 cm, and in 43 per cent tumour foci were found beyond 2 cm (27 per cent non-invasive, 16 per cent invasive). Invasive carcinoma were found at 3 cm in 9 per cent of the cases and in 7 per cent at 4 cm. It is possible, therefore, to predict the risk of local recurrence according to the amount of normal tissue removed around the primary carcinoma.

Local spread may also occur with intraductal extension. This extension may occasionally represent the exclusive or the major component of the proliferative process. In these cases, the mass is often impalpable, although its extension (which is generally indicated by microcalcifications at mammography) may be very large, occupying a considerable portion of the breast tissue.

In a recent paper, Holland *et al.* (1990) showed that primary carcinomas with an extensive intraductal component often have cancer beyond the edge of the primary tumour. Fourteen per cent of patients with an extensive intraductal component had intraductal carcinoma 4 cm or more away from the edge of the primary tumour, compared with only 1 per cent of patients with a primary tumour lacking an extensive intraductal component (Holland *et al.* 1990) (Fig. 1).

Very occasionally, the spread may also occur by direct permeation of lymphatic spaces, giving the clinical aspect of skin oedema and, if particularly extensive, of inflammatory carcinoma.

The amount of time from the original cell transformation to the clinical appearance has been the subject of many investigations. In their original article, Collins *et al.* (1956), assuming an exponential model for tumour growth, observed a median volume doubling time of 78 days and concluded that the time required for a malignant cell to grow to a 1 cm mass would be approximately 6–7 years. Mean doubling times of 105–215 days have been reported by other studies (Gershon-Cohen *et al.* 1963; Kusama *et al.* 1972; Fournier *et al.* 1980).

Conclusions derived from these studies are acceptable only if the growth rate is constant. If the growth rate is variable at different stages of tumour development and if the growth is better described by a gompertzian curve than by an exponential one, the results may be totally different.

Axillary node metastases

Breast carcinoma metastasizes to axillary nodes with a frequency that varies according to its size and its histological and biological

Table 4 Probability of metastases at second- and third-level lymph nodes according to the size of the primary carcinoma and to the number of involved nodes at the first level

		Involvement of second and third levels (%)
Size of	T1	28.4
primary	T2	51.3
	T3	67.9
Number of positive	1	8.0
nodes at	2	25.3
level 1	3	30.2
	>3	65.8

Table 5 Probability for patient with breast cancer to have metastases in internal mammary nodes according to age, status of axillary nodes, and maximum diameter of the tumour

	Risk of IMN metastases (%)
Less than 40 years	
>2 cm	
N+	41.2
N−	16.3
<2 cm	
N+	34.1
N−	12.6
41−60 years	
>2 cm	
N+	33.2
N−	10.9
<2 cm	
N+	26.8
N−	8.3
More than 60 years	
>2 cm	
N+	24.9
N−	8.5
<2 cm	
N+	19.7
N−	6.4

characteristics. A limited higher incidence is observed in tumours of the outer upper quadrants. The axillary lymph nodes are subdivided by most pathologists into three levels: the first includes the nodes external to the lateral margin of the minor pectoralis muscle, the second includes the nodes posterior to the minor pectoralis muscle, and the third level includes the nodes medial to that muscle. In a recent study of 1446 cases, 29 378 lymph nodes were removed, with a mean of 20.3 nodes per patient (Veronesi *et al.* 1990*b*; Kiricuta and Tausch 1992). The mean number of lymph nodes at the first level was 13.5, at the second level 4.5, and at the third level 2.3. The number of nodes was 20.7 in cases treated with Halsted mastectomy, 20.4 with modified radical mastectomy, and 20.0 with quadrantectomy and axillary dissection. In 98.7 per cent of the cases the distribution showed an orderly progression of metastatic spread from the first to the third level: the first level only was involved in 54 per cent, the first and the second levels were involved in 23 per cent, and all three levels were involved in 21 per cent of cases. An irregular distribution was observed in only 1.3 per cent of cases, with metastases skipping the first level (1.2 per cent) or the first and second levels (0.1 per cent).

The predictive value of the information obtained from the first level is excellent. When the nodes of the first level are clear, the chances that metastatic nodes are present at the second and third levels are negligible. When the first level is positive, the chances that metastases are present at the second and the third levels are high, of the order of 40 per cent. The risk of metastases at the second and third levels when the first is positive changes according to the number of nodes involved at the first level and according to the size of primary tumour (Table 4). As a general order of probabilities, one may say that in T1 cases, one-third of the patients have occult or overt axillary metastases, that in T2 cases nearly half of the patients have axillary involvement, and that in T3 cases this goes up to nearly two-thirds of the patients. The clinical diagnosis is good in the case of clinically positive nodes, with some 20 per cent of false-positivity and less good in cases of clinically negative nodes, with some 30 per cent of false-negativity.

INTERNAL MAMMARY NODE METASTASES

Dissection of the internal mammary nodes became a widely performed operation during the 1950s, with results that seemed to be encouraging (Giacomelli and Veronesi 1952; Urban and Baker 1952). However, an international randomized clinical trial, started in 1962, showed that prognosis was not improved by the radical dissection of the internal mammary chain (Veronesi and Valagussa 1981; Lacour *et al.* 1983).

Although the dissection of internal mammary nodes therefore appears uninfluential on survival, information about their metastatic involvement is of considerable importance as a prognostic factor. In 1119 cases treated by mastectomy plus internal mammary dissection, the risk of metastatic involvement of internal mammary nodes was evaluated according to various characteristics of the primary tumour (Veronesi *et al.* 1983*a*). As regards the site of the primary tumour, all quadrants had a similar frequency of internal mammary metastases, although there was a slightly higher incidence in the central quadrants (22.1 per cent) compared with internal (19.1 per cent) and external ones (18 per cent). The common belief that internal mammary node metastases are more frequent for tumours of the internal quadrants was therefore disproved. On the contrary, the size of the primary tumour accounts for a significant difference of incidence of internal mammary node metastases, as carcinomas of small size are rarely associated with internal mammary metastases. The age of the patient is another important factor: the younger the patient, the more likely the risk of internal mammary metastases. The presence or absence of axillary metastases is the dominant predicting factor: out of the 563 cases without axillary metastases, 51 (9.1 per cent) showed internal mammary involvement, while out of 556 with axillary node metastases, 162 (29.1 per cent) had internal mammary node metastases. If the three major characteristics conditioning the incidence of internal mammary node metastases (the presence of axillary metastases, the size of the primary tumour, and the age of the patient) are evaluated simultaneously, the risk of a breast cancer patient harbouring occult metastases in the internal mammary nodes can be calculated (Table 5).

Distant spread

The most common sites of distant metastases are the lungs, the bones, and the liver (Warren and Whitman 1937; Veronesi *et al.*

1957; Haagensen 1986). Metastases are rarely present at the time of first diagnosis of breast cancer and in the majority of cases they appear years after the treatment of the primary. The risk of metastases occurs mainly in the third, fourth, and fifth years after treatment. During the first year, as well as after the fifth, the patients have a lower risk of metastases. Cases with an aggressive type of disease and extensive regional metastases will obviously show an early appearance of distant metastases. In patients with less aggressive types of carcinoma, without involvement of axillary nodes, the appearance of distant metastases is delayed. In the latter cases, the likelihood of developing metastases remains present to a certain degree even after 10–20 years.

The distribution of distant metastases is regulated mainly by biological factors; whether it is also influenced by haematodynamic factors is controversial. Liver and bone metastases may be present in the absence of macroscopic lung metastases, suggesting that the malignant cells may easily go through the lung 'filter'. An analysis on post-mortem material by Veronesi et al. (1957) showed, however, that when lung metastases were present, liver metastases were also present in 64 per cent of the cases, whereas if the lungs were macroscopically free of metastases, the rate of liver metastases was lower (41 per cent). Another problem is the distribution of metastases in the bones, occurring most frequently in the spine and pelvis, whereas the long bones are relatively untouched. This distribution has suggested that bone invasion might occur mainly by way of a retrograde venous invasion through the paravertebral vein system (Batson 1940). Although this hypothesis is not convincing, no other explanation for the peculiar metastatic distribution in bones has been put forward.

As regards the timing of distant spread, no clear data are available. The fact that at the time of first diagnosis of breast cancer the great majority of patients are free from overt distant metastases, leads one to assume that the metastatic growth in distant organs starts years after the initial development of the primary carcinoma. In fact, in the hypothesis of breast cancer as a 'systemic disease', the proliferation of disseminated cells would start simultaneously or immediately after the beginning of the proliferation of the primary tumour cells. In this case, if a primary carcinoma of 1 cm is found in the breast, it is likely that metastases of the same size will be discovered in other organs. The fact that distant metastases appear later shows that their proliferation also started later, compared to the primary carcinoma.

An interesting analysis of 3000 patients treated by the Institut Gustave Roussy over a 15–30-year period has studied the relationship between pathological tumour size, the number of axillary node metastases, the histological grade, and subsequent probability of distant metastases and death (Tubiana and Koscielny 1991). This analysis supports the current model of metastases in which axillary lymph node involvement indicates a predisposition to distant metastases but not a pathway of spread to the bloodstream. The model is based on data from classic randomized trials, comparing mastectomy with and without treatment of lymphatic pathways (by surgery and/or radiotherapy), which have failed to demonstrate a survival advantage associated with treatment of the lymphatic pathways. The assumption has been that haematogenous dissemination usually occurs at about the same time as lymphatic spread. The French study shows that a high proportion of women treated by radical mastectomy with small or low-grade tumours and low numbers of axillary lymph node metastases remain disease-free for 25 years or more. Long-term survivors with positive nodes at presentation may still not be biologically cured, harbouring microscopic distant metastases that are capable of becoming clinically overt well beyond 20 years of disease-free survival. Alternatively, a proportion of patients with axillary node metastases may have truly limited disease, but untreated lymph node metastases may somehow not become a source of haematogenous spread if they are subsequently removed when they become palpably enlarged in the years following primary treatment. A third possibility is that the subset of patients cured by an axillary dissection is too small to have been detected in clinical trials.

In conclusion there are important gaps in our understanding of blood-borne spread in relation to the development of a primary breast cancer and spread to axillary lymph nodes. The uncertainty is most relevant to the management of patients with a very early stage of the disease, including those with screen-detected tumours.

PATHOLOGY OF BREAST CANCER
Non-invasive breast carcinoma

Lobular carcinoma in situ defines a proliferative lesion limited to one or more mammary lobules, composed of cells with all the characteristics of malignant cells but without invasion of the basement membrane.

The type of lesion was first described by Muir (1941) and was called acinar carcinoma. Foote and Stewart, in the same year, used the definition 'lobular carcinoma in situ' to describe a form of mammary carcinoma originating in the lobules and terminal ducts without interruption of the basement membrane. They also described some special features of the lesion like the involvement of the lobular-terminal duct complex as an anatomic unit, the multicentricity, the 'pagetoid' extension, and the central mucoid globules in the cells. Many pathologists refused to use the term 'carcinoma' for a non-invasive lesion and coined various definitions, such as 'epitheliosis', 'small cell neoplasia', and 'lobular neoplasia'.

Lobular carcinoma in situ occurs mainly in pre-menopausal women, is multicentric in 50–70 per cent of the cases, and is often bilateral. It is, in general, clinically occult and the diagnosis is occasionally made from samples removed in benign conditions. The incidence of invasive breast carcinoma in patients with lobular carcinoma in situ not treated with mastectomy was evaluated by McDivitt et al. (1967) who showed a 15 per cent risk of developing a homolateral invasive carcinoma at 10 years and a 35 per cent risk at 20 years, with figures somewhat lower for the contralateral breast. Wheeler and others (1974) showed a risk of 9.7 per cent at 10 years, with no difference between a homolateral and a contralateral invasive carcinoma. An extensive analysis of 99 cases with lobular carcinoma in situ followed up for more than two decades was published by Rosen et al. (1978). All cases had a limited resection of the breast and the frequency of invasive carcinomas was compared to the expected rates in the general population. Subsequent cancers occurred in 28 of the 99 cases, while the expected rate was 3.1, with a risk nine times higher. There was no difference in incidence of subsequent cancers between the homolateral and the contralateral breast.

Haagensen (1986) reported the results of a long-term follow-up of 287 patients with lobular carcinoma in situ not treated by mastectomy. The total number of observed invasive carcinomas was 33, whereas the expected number of breast cancers in the general population was approximately five for the same time period. The incidence of contralateral cancers appeared to be of the same order as the homolateral incidence.

'Ductal carcinoma in situ' describes a group of lesions whose common feature is the proliferation of cancer cells within the ducts, without invasion of the surrounding stromal tissue.

Information on the natural history of ductal carcinoma *in situ* is still very limited as there are no important series in which the lesion has been minimally treated and followed up. The great majority of ductal carcinomas *in situ* have been submitted to some sort of radical surgery and, although the results appear excellent (10 year survivals close to 100 per cent), the outcome of these cases, had they been treated only with limited surgery and radiotherapy, is not known. At present, many clinical trials are in progress to evaluate the possibility of conservation treatment with or without radiotherapy. Ductal carcinomas *in situ* may be simply divided into comedo and non-comedo types. The comedo type has large nuclei with mitotic figures, necrosis at the centre of the ducts, and has, in general, a greater chance of recurring than the non-comedo type, following breast conservation treatment.

Ductal carcinoma *in situ* may grow to a considerable size without becoming invasive, showing that it is a biologically different entity which should be considered separately both from lobular carcinoma *in situ* and from invasive carcinoma. It is multifocal in 30 per cent of cases, foci being present mainly in the same breast. The incidence of axillary lymph node metastasis is very low, approximately 2–3 per cent (Murad and Scarpelli 1967; Ashikari *et al.* 1971; Gallager and Martin 1971; E. R. Fisher *et al.* 1986) and is a likely expression of inadequate examination of the primary carcinoma.

Invasive breast carcinoma

Invasive ductal carcinoma is the most common type of breast cancer, accounting for 70–80 per cent of all cases and including tumours that were formerly defined as 'infiltrating carcinoma not otherwise specified'. Ductal invasive carcinoma may contain a component of intraductal carcinoma that may be so extensive as to be predominant. Multicentricity is not rare.

Invasive lobular carcinoma represents 10–20 per cent of all breast cancers and it is considered to be more frequently multicentric than ductal carcinoma. Then there are other less common types of carcinoma, such as medullary carcinoma, with its sharp tumour borders and lymphoid infiltration, mucoid carcinoma, characterized by the presence of large amounts of extracellular mucus, and papillary carcinoma, with a well-differentiated papillary structure. There are also rare types which represent little more than pathological curiosities, such as adenoid cystic carcinoma, apocrine carcinoma, and carcinoma with squamous metaplasia.

Inflammatory carcinoma (1–2 per cent of all cases) has specific histological features. The morphology is that of an invasive ductal carcinoma with extensive invasion of lymphatic vessels of the dermis.

Paget's disease of the nipple, which is also defined as 'epidermotropic intraductal carcinoma' (Veronesi *et al.* 1955), is a variant of ductal carcinoma *in situ*, with cells invading the ducts without infiltrating the basal membrane and extending into the major ducts of the nipple and the epidermis of the areola. In 90 per cent of cases an invasive carcinoma appears in the mammary gland only later in development.

Precursors of cancer

In the past, fibrocystic disease was considered a condition which carried the risk of breast cancer. Many clinical prospective or cohort studies indicated a mean increased risk of 1.5–2.0 (Stevens *et al.* 1982). A review by Love *et al.* (1982), re-evaluating 654 cases from five major studies concluded that the overall increased risk of 1.86 could be due more to the selection of patients than to the real malignant potential of the disease.

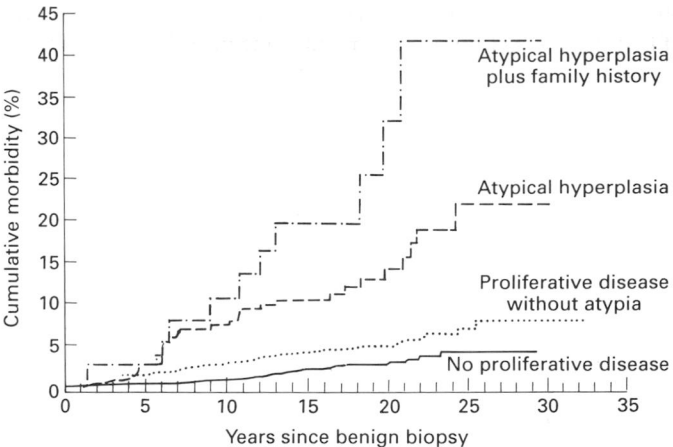

Fig. 2 Proportion of patients who have developed invasive breast cancer as a function of time since their benign breast biopsy. (Adapted from Dupont and Page 1989.)

Recently, many studies have demonstrated that the most important pathological risk for carcinoma development is the degree of epithelial proliferation and its atypical nature (Black *et al.* 1972; Page *et al.* 1978, 1985; Dupont and Page 1985). Dupont and Page, in their review on 3303 benign lesions, stated that the risk of developing cancer in benign non-proliferative cases was less than the expected incidence rates, whereas in proliferative cases it was twice the expected rates. The relative risk was, however, not very high (1.6) in proliferative disease without atypia, in cases with atypical hyperplasia the risk was higher (4.4), and it was even higher if associated with a family history of breast cancer (8.9) (Fig. 2).

Multiple intraductal papillomas also carry a high risk of breast cancer development. In surgically excised specimens subjected to three-dimensional reconstruction, an association with carcinoma was shown in 37.5 per cent of the cases. On the contrary, solitary central papillomas showed a risk of malignant transformation which was no higher than that of normal breast tissue (Ohuchi *et al.* 1984). Figure 2 shows the risk of breast cancer associated with benign lesions with and without a family history of breast cancer.

PROGNOSTIC FACTORS

Histology

Many histological types of breast carcinoma show a better prognosis than the common infiltrating carcinomas (ductal and lobular): medullary carcinomas (Richardson 1956), mucoid carcinomas (Veronesi and Gennari 1960), and papillary carcinomas (Veronesi *et al.* 1964) definitely have a better prognosis than other types. Lymphoid reactions and sinus histiocytosis have also been reported to be correlated with a better prognosis (Black and Spur 1950; Cutler *et al.* 1969). The low rate of agreement on the evaluation of sinus histocytosis (Gilchrist *et al.* 1985) and the difficulty in obtaining reproducible scores, represent a limitation to the practical application of this prognostic factor.

Histological grading shows a significant correlation with prognosis (Bloom and Field 1971; Contesso *et al.* 1989). Freedman *et al.* (1979) followed up 1759 patients with infiltrating ductal carcinoma over 10 years, showing a statistical difference in survival from 56 per cent (grade I) to 33 per cent (grade III). A recent multivariate analysis combining a number of pathological characteristics showed that the simple mitotic count is the best single predictor, followed by tumour size, lymphatic invasion, and skin invasion. Nuclear and cellular grade correlated well with survival but had no significant additional predictive value when adjusted for the mitotic count (Clayton 1991).

Peritumoral vascular invasion

The ability to invade surrounding lymphatic and blood vessels is not an uncommon characteristic of breast cancer. Peritumoral intralymphatic invasion is present in 20–40 per cent of cases, according to various pathologists (E. R. Fisher *et al.* 1975; Nime *et al.* 1977; Rosen *et al.* 1981) and represents an unfavourable prognostic factor. Blood vessel invasion is not uncommon, although it has been found in totally different percentages of cases, from 4 to 45 per cent, by various studies. As with intralymphatic invasion, tumour emboli in the blood vessels seem to be associated with a poor prognosis (Friedell *et al.* 1965). In a recent report on 506 cases of breast carcinoma with axillary negative nodes, Clemente *et al.* (1992) reported a 6.9 per cent frequency of peritumoral lymphatic invasion at routine histopathological assessment. Patients with peritumoral lymphatic invasion showed a worse prognosis than those without it, the 5 year overall survival dropping from 90 to 68 per cent.

Growth rate

The importance of the doubling time as an indicator of prognosis has been reported in many papers (Gershon-Cohen *et al.* 1963; Kusama *et al.* 1972; Fournier *et al.* 1980; Galante *et al.* 1986).

Lundgren (1983) published an extensive study on the importance of the rate of growth. In this study 139 breast cancers were diagnosed by repeated screening, but on a prior mammogram an obvious cancer had been overlooked, with a mean doubling time of 12.4 months, while 144 cases were diagnosed between screening with a mean doubling time of 2.2 months. A clear relationship between doubling time and survival was found: patients with a doubling time of less than 3 months had a 5 year survival of 56 per cent, whereas patients with a doubling time of more than 3 months were all alive at 5 years.

An interesting study was published in 1986 by Galante and co-workers on a series of 196 patients with breast cancer, who received two pre-operative mammographic examinations at an interval of 20 or more days. The cases were divided into slow-growing (doubling time more than 90 days: 81 patients), intermediate-growing (30–90 days: 84 patients), and fast growing (less than 30 days: 31 patients) and their survival was evaluated according to the number of axillary nodes involved. The data showed that the prognostic value of doubling time was applicable only in the cases with extensive node metastases. If extensive axillary involvement is a sign of the metastasizing power, the data of Galante *et al.* (1986) would suggest that the growth rate and the ability to metastasize are two independent variables. When both are present (high growth rate, extensive axillary metastases) the prognosis is bad, but when only one is present, the prognosis is much better. This conclusion, which does need confirmation, would imply that the biological factors that sustain local growth may be different from the factors responsible for metastatic implantation.

The potential proliferative activity of a cell population can be determined by the size of the fraction of S-phase cells. Therefore an important approach to prognosis is the autoradiographic evaluation of [3H] thymidine-labelled cells. The [3H] thymidine-labelling index is based on incubating fresh tumour specimens with tritiated thymidine, a radioactive pyrimidine that incorporates specifically into the DNA of the cells that are in the synthesis phase (S-phase). The subsequent use of autoradiography enables the identification of S-phase cell fractions.

Studies on the cell kinetics of breast cancer using the thymidine-labelling index have been carried out independently by different groups (Meyer *et al.* 1983; Tubiana *et al.* 1984; Silvestrini *et al.* 1985; Silvestrini 1991). The results have shown consistently that the thymidine-labelling index represents an important independent prognostic factor. This is evident mainly in patients with node-negative resectable tumours given only locoregional treatment and in locally advanced diseases (Silvestrini *et al.* 1987), whereas it is less evident in patients with positive nodes, in whom systemic therapy may have modified the natural history of the disease.

DNA flow cytometry is being used more and more to determine the proliferative rate, by the use of a DNA-specific fluorescent stain to identify S-phase cells. Flow cytometry has the advantage of speed; it can measure the DNA content of 100 000 cells in a few minutes, determining both the fraction of euploid and aneuploid cells and the fraction of cells in S-phase. Another advantage of flow cytometry is that the analysis can be performed on fixed, paraffin-embedded blocks of tumour tissue. McDivitt *et al.* (1985) found a good correlation between the S-phase fraction as determined by the thymidine-labelling index and by flow cytometry. It was also found that ploidy is an important prognostic factor, diploid tumours having a better prognosis compared to aneuploid tumours (both hypodiploid and hyperdiploid) (Coulson *et al.* 1984; Hedley *et al.* 1984). Many studies showed a correlation between hormone receptors, aneuploidy, S-phase fraction, and histology. In general, aneuploid tumours are more frequently receptor-negative, poorly differentiated, and have a high S-phase fraction (Moran *et al.* 1984; Dressler *et al.* 1986, 1987).

Size of primary

The size of the primary carcinoma is of great importance in the prognosic assessment. In a study by Koscielny *et al.* (1984), based on data from 2648 cases followed up for 10–25 years, a direct relationship between the increase of tumour size and the worsening of the prognosis was found. Adair *et al.* (1974) found a considerable difference in survival, both in patients with negative and with positive nodes, according to the size of the primary carcinoma. Russo *et al.* (1987) on a multivariate analysis of different characteristics of 646 breast carcinomas, described the size of the primary tumour as one of the most important independent prognostic variables.

As axillary involvement is also a function of the size of the primary carcinoma, it is sometimes difficult to dissociate the two variables, which have a certain independent prognostic value. For instance, Valagussa *et al.* (1978) showed that the 5 year relapse rate was 37 per cent in patients with positive nodes and small primary tumours (<2 cm) and 79 per cent in patients with positive nodes and large primary tumours (>5 cm). Cases with clinical axillary presentation without palpable or mammographically detectable primary carcinoma, have a relatively good prognosis in spite of the extensive axillary involvement and the undifferentiated character of the axillary metastases (Merson *et al.* 1992).

Regional node metastases

The prognostic significance of axillary involvement is well established. Preliminary observations reported high survival rates in node-negative patients (70–75 per cent) and low survival rates

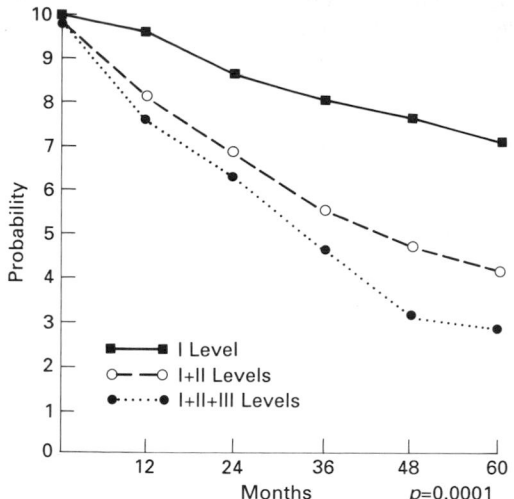

Fig. 3 Disease-free survival of breast cancer patients according to the level of axillary nodes involved. When only the first level is involved the 5 year survival is approximately 75 per cent, but when metastatic nodes are present at the third level the survival drops to 30 per cent.

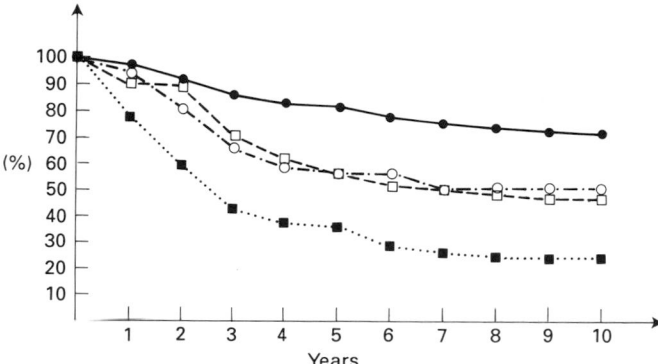

Fig. 4 Ten year disease-free survival in patients without node metastases (1), with axillary node metastases only (2), with internal mammary node metastases only (3), and with the involvement of both node groups (4) ($p = 10^{-9}$). (From Veronesi et al. 1985.)

in node-positive patients (25–30 per cent). This type of assessment appears very rough today, as the prognosis is strictly correlated to the number of metastatic nodes. (Fisher et al. 1968; Valagussa et al. 1978). If one single axillary node is involved, for example, the prognosis is very close to that of node-negative patients, but if more than 10 nodes are metastatic the prognosis becomes ominous (Salvadori et al. 1983; Cascinelli et al. 1987). The level of axillary invasion plays an important rôle, the prognosis being much worse when the third level is involved (Schottenfeld et al. 1976; Veronesi et al. 1993a; Fig. 3).

Internal mammary node involvement is an important prognostic factor (Veronesi et al. 1983a, 1985; Lacour et al. 1987). In a series of 1119 patients it was shown that the prognosis, when either the axillary nodes or the internal mammary nodes are involved separately, is similar. The prognosis is excellent when both nodal stations are free of metastases and it is very grave when both are involved (Veronesi et al. 1985; Fig. 4).

Receptor status

The oestrogen receptors in breast cancer have been utilized mainly to predict the responsiveness of breast carcinomas to endocrine therapy. Receptor assays have also been employed as prognostic factors. Tumours positive for oestrogen receptors are associated with morphological evidence of differentiation and have less aggressive biological behaviour (McCarty et al. 1980; Parl and Wagner 1980; Mohammed et al. 1986). Many studies have shown an improved prognosis in patients with tumours positive for oestrogen receptors (Wait et al. 1976; Knight et al. 1977; Osborne et al. 1981), although others have not confirmed this finding (Bloom and Degenshein 1980; Hilf et al. 1980; Pichon et al. 1980; Howat et al. 1983).

Many authors have evaluated the oestrogen-receptor status in node-negative patients with the objective of selecting those tumours destined to recur. Many studies reported higher recurrence rates and lower survival in oestrogen-receptor-negative patients (Von Maillot et al. 1982; Valagussa et al. 1984), although in one of these studies (Valagussa et al. 1984) the difference was only significant in pre-menopausal patients. However, other groups have shown no prognostic value for oestrogen receptors in node-negative patients (Butler et al. 1985; Winstanley et al. 1991).

Progesterone receptors have also been found to be associated with an improved prognosis (Clark et al. 1983; Saez et al. 1983) although, again, some studies have not found the same correlation (Allegra et al. 1979; Stewart et al. 1983).

Oncogenes and growth factors

It has been shown that oncogenes code for proteins associated with cellular growth. In breast cancer tissue some oncogenes (c-*myc*, HER-2/*neu*, int-2) were shown to be amplified in 20–35 per cent of the cases (Ali et al. 1987; Hynes et al. 1987; Kouyoumdjian et al. 1987). Theillet and others (1986) found that there was an increased Ha-*ras-1* expression in 16 out of 22 tumours tested; they also showed that 60 per cent of primary breast cancers had increased levels of ras p21 protein. In a large study published in 1987, Slamon et al. evaluated the prognostic significance of the HER-2/*neu* oncogene in patients with breast cancer. This oncogene is related to the c-*erb*-B1 proto-oncogene, which codes for the epidermal growth factor receptor and is a member of the tyrosine-kinase family. The HER-2/*neu* oncogene was found to be amplified several-fold in 30 per cent of breast tumours, the amplification being a significant predictor of lower survival.

Growth factors are considered to be of great importance in autocrine and paracrine mechanisms of breast cancer cell proliferation. Epidermal growth factor is a strong mitogen for breast cancer cells and its receptor has been found in one-third of primary breast tumours. The presence of epidermal growth factor receptor was correlated with poor differentiation and with the absence of oestrogen receptors, in support of the role of epidermal growth factor receptor as an indicator of poor prognosis in breast cancer (Rilke et al. 1991; Saccani Jotti et al. 1992).

A potentially important new prognostic factor in breast cancer is the reduced expression of a putative antimetastatic gene, called *Nm23*. So far, the data are confined to an analysis of a small group of patients, in whom a reduced level of *Nm23* gene expression is significantly correlated with positive-node status and reduced survival (Hennessy et al. 1991). If these preliminary reports are confirmed, it is likely that the cellular mechanisms whereby this altered gene affects cancer progression differ significantly from those of growth factor receptors, such as epidermal growth factor receptor and HER-2/*neu*.

In a large clinical study, Thorpe et al. (1989) showed that patients with a high concentration of the glycoprotein cathepsin D had a worse prognosis than those with lower levels, regardless of whether

Table 6 Prognostic factors reported to be of value in identifying breast cancer patients at high risk of distant recurrence

Tumour size

Lymph node status

Histological grade

Receptor status: oestrogen or progesterone level

DNA synthetic activity
  Thymidine labelling
  Flow cytometry
  Thymidine kinase
  Ki-67

Ploidy or DNA index

Receptors for growth factors or growth regulators, including oncogenes
  Epidermal growth factor receptor (c-*erb* B1)
  HER/*neu* (c-*erb* B2)
  IGF-IR
  Somatostatin receptor

Tumour suppressor genes
  p53
  Nm23

Miscellaneous
  Heat-shock protein (hsp 27)
  pS2
  Haptoglobin-related protein
  Colony formation *in vitro*
  Tumour growth factor-α
  Cathepsin D
  Urokinase-plasminogen activator
  Tissue ferritin concentration
  Laminin receptor expression
  Cyclic-AMP-binding protein
  NRCR 11

they were node negative or node positive. In a second study, however, cathepsin D was found to be a strong prognostic factor only in node-negative patients (Tandon *et al.* 1990).

The list of factors shown to be of prognostic significance is steadily growing, with selection of the more powerful and more feasible ones becoming increasingly difficult (Table 6). International agreement on this topic is needed urgently.

STAGING

The grouping of patients according to the extent of the disease is needed in clinical research to compare results and to identify the most appropriate choices of treatment. The most widely used staging system is the one adopted by both the Union Internationale Contre le Cancer (**UICC**) and the American Joint Committee (**AJC**), based on the Tumour Nodes Metastases (**TNM**) system (Hermanek and Sobin 1987). This classification, agreed by both organizations in 1987, is given in Table 7.

In the past few years the staging system, based on clinical and pathological evaluation of the extent of local, regional, and distant spread, has been considered inadequate, both because predictive biological and biomolecular parameters are becoming available and because better methods for identifying distant cellular spread have been reported. An important example in this respect is the detection of cancer cells in bone-marrow with monoclonal antibodies (Colnaghi 1988; Porro *et al.* 1988; Salvedori *et al.* 1990). Many reports have shown that occult cancer cells may be present in a

Table 7 TNM classification of breast cancer

TNM clinical classification
TX Primary tumour cannot be assessed
T0 No evidence of primary tumour
Tis Carcinoma *in situ*: intraductal carcinoma or lobular carcinoma *in situ* or Paget's disease of the nipple with no tumour
T1 Tumour 2 cm or less in greatest dimension
  T1a 0.5 cm or less in greatest dimension
  T1b More than 0.5 cm but not more than 1 cm in greatest dimension
  T1c More than 1 cm but not more than 2 cm in greatest dimension
T2 Tumour more than 2 cm but not more than 5 cm in greatest dimension
T3 Tumour more than 5 cm in greatest dimension
T4 Tumour of any size with direct extension to chest wall or skin
  T4a Extension to chest wall
  T4b Oedema (including *peau d'orange*) or ulceration of the skin of the breast or satellite skin nodules confined to the same breast
  T4c Inflammatory carcinoma

N Regional lymph nodes

NX Regional lymph nodes cannot be assessed (for example, previously removed)
N0 No regional lymph node metastasis
N1 Metastasis to movable ipsilateral axillary node(s)
N2 Metastasis to ipsilateral axillary node(s) fixed to one another or to other structures
N3 Metastasis to ipsilateral internal mammary lymph node(s)

M Distant metastasis

MX Presence of distant metastasis cannot be assessed
M0 No distant metastasis
M1 Distant metastasis (includes metastasis to supraclavicular lymph nodes)

pTNM Pathological classification
  pT Primary tumour

The pathological classification requires the examination of the primary carcinoma with no gross tumour at the margins of resection. A case can be classified pT if there is only microscopic tumour in a margin
The pT categories correspond to the T categories.

pN Regional lymph nodes

The pathological classification requires the resection and examination of at least the low axillary lymph nodes (level 1). Such a resection will ordinarily include six or more lymph nodes
pNX Regional lymph nodes cannot be assessed (not removed for study or previously removed)
pN0 No regional lymph node metastasis
pN1 Metastasis to movable ipsilateral axillary node(s)
  pN1a Only micrometastasis (none larger than 0.2 cm)
  pN1b Metastasis to lymph node(s), any larger than 0.2 cm
    pN1bi Metastasis in one to three lymph nodes, any more than 0.2 cm and all less than 2.0 cm in greatest dimension
    pN1bii Extension of tumour beyond the capsule of a lymph node metastasis less than 2.0 cm in greatest dimension
    pN1biv Metastasis to a lymph node 2.0 cm or more in greatest dimension
pN2 Metastasis to ipsilateral axillary lymph nodes that are fixed to one another or to other structures
pN3 Metastasis to ipsilateral internal mammary lymph node(s)

significant percentage (15–30 per cent) of patients with stage I and stage II breast cancer. The prognostic significance of this finding is being investigated.

DETECTION AND DIAGNOSIS

Recently there have been considerable changes in the methodologies employed for the diagnosis of breast cancer. The diagnostic process, based in the past mainly on physical examination (inspection and palpation), has been transformed into a highly sophisticated technological procedure, allowing the recognition of lesions of minimal size, which are often not palpable. The advances in methods of breast cancer diagnosis have given a considerable boost to early detection programmes. Today, a timely diagnosis of breast cancer represents one of the most important ways of reducing breast cancer mortality.

Breast cancer screening

Methodology

Screening modalities for breast cancer include clinical examination of the breast (by a doctor, by a nurse, and by the patient herself), imaging techniques (mammography, xeromammography, ultrasonography), and detection of cancer markers in the serum.

The screening test must be sensitive, specific, simple, safe, and economic. Sensitivity, defined as the power of the test to identify the disease, is measured by the proportion of true-positive examinations out of the total number of persons with the disease. The lower the percentage of false-negative tests (that is, cases with the disease not identified by the test), the higher the sensitivity. Specificity is the power of the test to detect only the disease. The lower the percentage of false-positive tests (that is, cases without the disease but considered positive or suspicious by the test), the higher the overall specificity.

Clinical examination is not a very sensitive test. The sensitivity is approximately 50 per cent, meaning that the interval cases, appearing within 1 year from a negative screen, equal the cases detected at screening. Specificity is also low, as palpation detects a large number of benign conditions which may require a biopsy to be confirmed as non-malignant.

Clinical examination is generally performed by a doctor, but well-trained nurses may well perform the examination with similar results. The examination of the breast by the woman herself (breast self-examination) is the most simple, repeatable, and economic measure of cancer screening. If one could convince women to carry out a periodic 'systemic' examination, one would expect an increased number of early cases detected by the women themselves. There is, however, a psychological barrier against breast self-examination in many women and the percentage of those who perform breast self-examination regularly varies from 15 to 40 per cent of the population, a rate too low to be effective in a screening programme. Breast self-examination may create a condition of anxiety and may produce more uncertainties than certainties. In any case, breast self-examination has never been appropriately evaluated, but it may have more potential applicability than other screening tests because it does not need auxiliary technologies (Miller *et al.* 1985).

Today, mammography fulfils the criteria for screening better than other tests. The sensitivity varies from 80 to 95 per cent and its specificity is also high. In Sweden, following a mammography programme, only 0.2 per cent of subjects with non-malignant conditions needed to be biopsied.

In the late 1970s publicity was given to the carcinogenic risk of mammography (Bailar 1976) which led to public concern resulting in its decreased acceptance by women, especially as a detection procedure. This fear appears to be unjustified because the low-dose film-screen combination now used exposes the breast to a very low dose (0.002–0.005 Gy per examination) and because the carcinogenic risk of radiation does not seem to exist for women exposed after the age of 30 years (Boyle 1988).

Ultrasonography for visualizing breast tissue has been developed recently and its performance is improving year by year. So far it has been used only in symptomatic patients to distinguish benign (especially cystic) lesions from malignant ones. The limitations of this method lie in its inability to detect tumours of less than 5 mm diameter and to identify microcalcifications, which, at mammography, are important indicators of early malignant lesions.

Screening by detection of a circulating breast cancer marker in small blood samples taken from the female population appears to be a very important objective, but, for the moment, no tests with sufficient specificity and sensitivity are available to warrant an extensive trial.

Feasibility

The feasibility of a screening programme is linked to two main factors. The first is a good logistic organization to enlist the participation of the chosen segment of the population, to perform the test, to ask for rescreening, to follow-up the women, etc. The second is a good level of acceptance by the female population, which is linked to the fear of an unpleasant truth, the fear of mutilation, and the anxiety produced by the waiting time between the test and the results. Therefore, a screening programme may be performed only in well-developed and well-organized countries. Moreover, great attention must be paid to publicizing the screening programme and to convincing women to participate in it, allaying the fears linked with the programme by appropriate communication.

Assessment of efficacy

The fact that screening will yield an increased number of early cases would suggest that it is effective and is to be recommended. However, the results of a programme of breast cancer screening must be evaluated with great objectivity as there are many pitfalls in the assessment process. There are, in fact, four major biases in evaluating mass detection procedures in general: lead time, length time, selection, and overdiagnosis (Miller 1986).

Lead time is the time at diagnosis that has been advanced by the screening test. The survival will automatically be prolonged by this interval, simply by the fact that the diagnosis is made earlier in the natural history of the disease. The resulting longer survival time must obviously not be considered an improvement. Length time bias is the selection due to the growth rate of the tumour, as rapidly growing tumours are less likely to be detected by screening tests applied at periodic intervals than slowly growing ones. The cases detected inside a screening plan might therefore have a better prognosis than the ones detected otherwise.

The selection bias reflects the self-selection in attending the screening programme, as women who are more careful about their health are more liable to participate.

The overdiagnosis bias is due to the number of borderline lesions (such as *in situ* carcinomas) detected by the screening that otherwise would never have been diagnosed.

The difficulties in assessing the efficacy of breast screening are therefore considerable, not only because of the mentioned biases but also because of the need for a very long follow-up. It is essential that a control group forms an integral part of the design and that the end-point for the assessment is the mortality rate on a population basis.

Economic aspects

The calculations of the cost—benefit evaluation vary considerably in different countries. In a calculation by Miller (1983) it was shown that the 5 year screening programme for 100 000 women, aged between 50 and 59 years, with a double-view mammography plus a biennial examination by a physician, would cost some $US 5 million: 2558 person-years of life saved, at a cost of some $US 2000 per year of life saved.

Results of screening

The detection of breast cancer at an early stage does not ensure that breast cancer mortality will be automatically reduced. In fact, screening may just detect cancers at an earlier point in time (lead time bias) and cancers which are growing more slowly and less likely to be lethal (length time bias) or in situ carcinomas that might never become clinically overt (overdiagnosis bias) and patients who participate in screening may be healthier than patients who do not (selection bias). Only accurate randomized trials will be able to assess the effect of screening on breast cancer mortality. The various trials implemented in different countries, although difficult to summarize, show that screening appears to reduce breast cancer mortality by approximately 25 per cent.

The fact that screening reduces breast cancer mortality has important implications as regards the natural history of the disease. There have been suggestions that breast cancer should be considered a systemic disease from its onset. The reduction in breast cancer mortality by screening provides apposite evidence that early diagnosis and treatment of breast cancer can avert the onset of metastasis. One unsolved issue is the effect of screening in women aged below 50 years. In all randomized studies the beneficial effects of screening are fairly consistently restricted to women aged between 50 and 69 years. Because breast cancer is less common in younger women, larger studies may be needed to demonstrate the effectiveness in women younger than 50 years. Moreover, mammographic imaging is less sensitive in younger women than in older women and the subclinical phase of the disease is estimated to be shorter. Preliminary results from a Canadian trial show an increased mortality in screened women aged between 40 and 49 years, compared to non-screened women. Although this report has been questioned, especially regarding the technical quality of the mammography used, at this time there is no evidence that screening reduces breast cancer mortality in women aged between 40 and 49 years. For women aged between 50 and 69 years, the reduction in breast cancer mortality is more consistently observed and is in the range of 30—40 per cent. The available trials assess neither the optimal periodicity of screening, nor the relative effects of mammography and physical examination in reducing breast cancer mortality. These issues are being addressed directly in a second generation of trials, including the Canadian studies.

To achieve maximal mammographic screening efficacy quality control of both the images obtained and the reading of these images must be maintained. This requires extensive training of radiology technicians, physicists, and mammographers at many steps along the process. Training and experience are also important for health professionals involved in physical examination of the breast if this is to be part of the detection process.

Breast cancer diagnosis: clinical examination

The examination starts with the patient lying supine, with her arms raised above her head. A first inspection gives an immediate evaluation of the condition of the skin and of the nipples. The entire breast must then be accurately palpated and all types of lumps, nodules, recesses, and irregularities must immediately be evaluated for their risk of being malignant. Then the patient is requested to contract the pectoralis muscles by pressing her hips firmly with her hands. This makes an additional useful examination possible.

The patient must then be examined in a sitting position. When the patient raises the arms upwards, alterations to the lower part of the breast may easily become apparent. Inspection is completed by looking at asymmetries, changes in shape, or changes in the colour or thickness of the skin.

The obvious suspicious signs are ulceration, retraction, oedema, and erythema. As regards retraction it must be observed that in post-menopausal women and in women who have recently lost weight, there may be false retractions due to fat and breast tissue atrophy, especially in the lower parts of the breast. If the patient had an axillary dissection, the breast may have areas of skin oedema, especially if she had radiotherapy on the breast. Erythema of the skin is also a grave sign and, although it may be due to an inflammatory process, a carcinomatous mastitis must always be suspected.

The nipple must be carefully examined, looking at any sign of superficial erosion or ulceration. This may be a sign of an early stage of Paget's disease, which may begin with a limited area of itching erythema around one lactiferous porus of the nipple.

The discharge or fluid from the nipple is not infrequent and is generally a benign sign. Milky, aqueous, green, or brown discharges have no pathological relevance, whereas yellow and red (serous and bloody) discharges must be given careful attention as they may be the sign of a papilloma of the ducts or, more rarely, of an intraductal carcinoma.

The axillary fossae are then carefully examined, holding the patient's arms to allow the chest wall muscles to relax. The physician must evaluate the number, the site, the size, and the consistency of the palpable nodes and mentally form a judgement on their possible involvement. The supraclavicular fossae and both sides of the neck must also be examined in the upright position in a search for any suspicious lymph node.

Mammography

Mammography is the method of choice for identification of a breast carcinoma. Its superiority over physical examination in detecting small carcinomas has been shown by the Breast Cancer Detection Demonstration Project (**BCDDP**). Not infrequently, a mammography may detect a non-palpable small carcinoma, whereas carcinomas detected by palpation and not visible by mammography, although not rare, are less frequent, with the exception of cases of cancer in young, dense, breasts. The two main direct diagnostic signs are the presence of an opacity and of microcalcifications (Figs 5—8). The malignant opacity is non-homogeneous and has irregular margins. In some cases the margins may be smooth (as in colloid carcinoma and in medullary carcinoma) and may simulate benign lesions. The microcalcifications that indicate the presence of a carcinoma are very fine, punctuated, and elongated, frequently with irregular margins. The calcifications may be associated with an opacity or may be the only sign of malignancy.

When a large number of fine calcifications are present in a limited area of the breast, the diagnosis of cancer is almost certain. Other

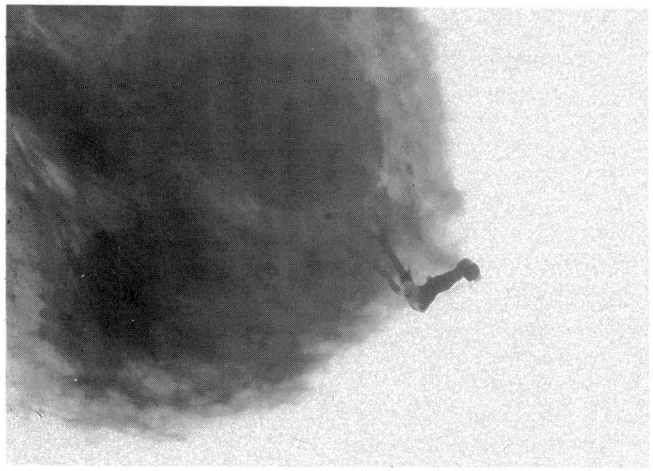

Fig. 5 Ductogalactography. An intraductal papilloma is clearly evident.

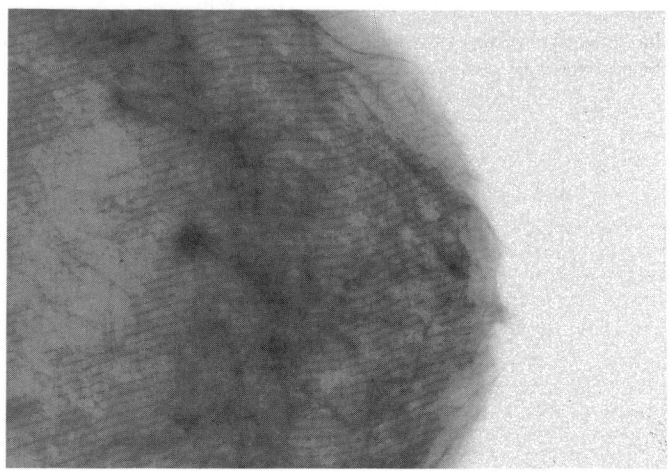

Fig. 7 Small non-palpable carcinoma, 6 mm in diameter.

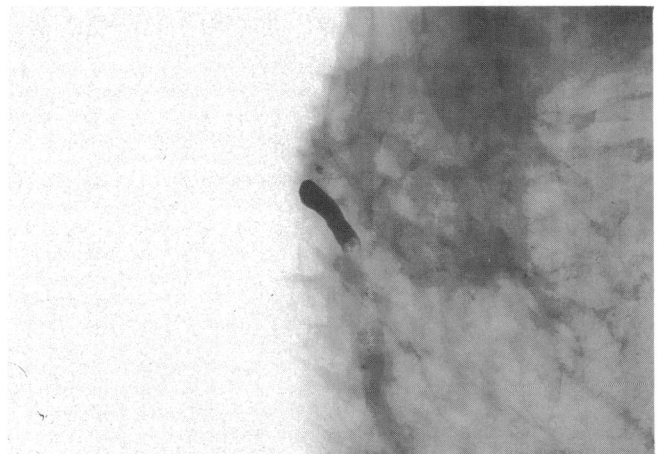

Fig. 6 Ductogalactography. The interrupted duct image as a sign of an intraductal carcinoma.

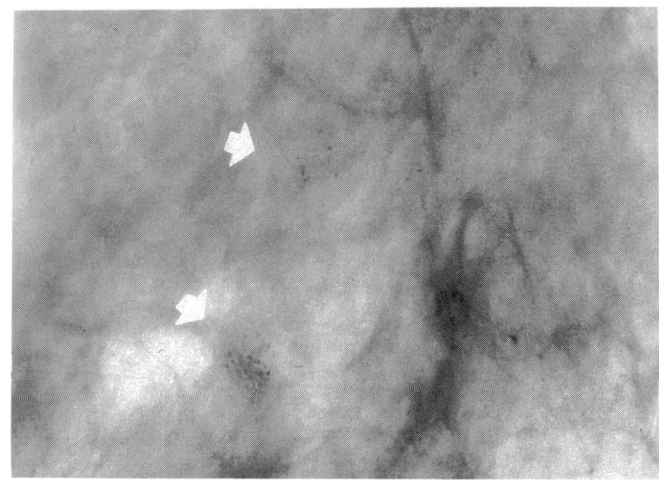

Fig. 8 Microcalcifications in a patient with intraductal carcinoma.

indirect signs of malignancy may be the hypervascularity, the structural alterations of the breast tissue, and the thickening of the skin. Sometimes plasma-cell mastitis, fat necrosis, and sclerosing adenosis may simulate a small breast carcinoma.

The radiographic size of the carcinoma is usually smaller than the clinical size and some 30 per cent of cases clinically defined as T2 are classified as T1 by mammography.

Biopsy

Fine-needle biopsy has been more and more widely utilized in the past 10 years. Large studies have shown that the risk of false-positive diagnosis is extremely low and almost non-existent in the hands of experienced cytologists.

Unfortunately false-negative cases are not infrequent, especially if the tumour to be detected is small. Therefore, a negative cytological diagnosis should not be considered if a clinical mammographic suspicion exists. Cytology cannot demonstrate that the tumour is invasive and therefore a cytological diagnosis of malignant cells could not fully justify a definitive surgical procedure. However, if there is clinical and mammographic evidence of cancer, the adjunctive evidence of malignant cells justifies definitive surgery

without an open biopsy, with the advantage of operating on an intact breast. This is particularly useful in the case of conservative surgery.

The final proof of malignancy is histology and the biopsy remains, therefore, an important step, although cytology may replace it in many cases. It may be performed by removing all the primary tumour (excisional) or a part of it (incisional). If the tumour is large, an excisional biopsy is impractical, whilst a lump of limited size is better removed by total excision.

As regards the timing, the extemporary biopsy with frozen section is performed less and less, both because fine-needle biopsy may provide the proof of malignancy and because many surgeons prefer a preliminary biopsy, which may even be performed in the doctor's office under local anaesthesia.

Localization of occult lesions

Often the only suspicious sign of a breast cancer is the presence of a number of microcalcifications at mammography. It is generally possible to localize the position of the lesion with great accuracy by inserting a needle under double-view mammographic control. The needle may leave in place either a coloured substance to be recognized by the surgeon or a spring hook wire which provides an anchored guide for the surgeon. It is then possible for the surgeon to remove only the portion of tissue that includes the lesion, which must be submitted to a specimen radiography to document the complete removal of the suspicious area. Specimen radiography must be performed while the patient is under anaesthesia, so that in the case of incomplete removal of the microcalcifications, a re-excision may be made immediately.

Other diagnostic techniques

Ultrasonography utilizes high-frequency sound waves produced by piezoelectric crystals and stimulated by electronic pulses. Although ultrasonography has the ability to differentiate between cystic and solid masses, its sensitivity to detect small carcinomas is not great. However, the technology is improving very rapidly (Dempsey 1986). Ultrasound demonstrates cysts very clearly, much better than mammography. Solid masses are also well detected by sonography, but criteria to distinguish benign from malignant lesions are not

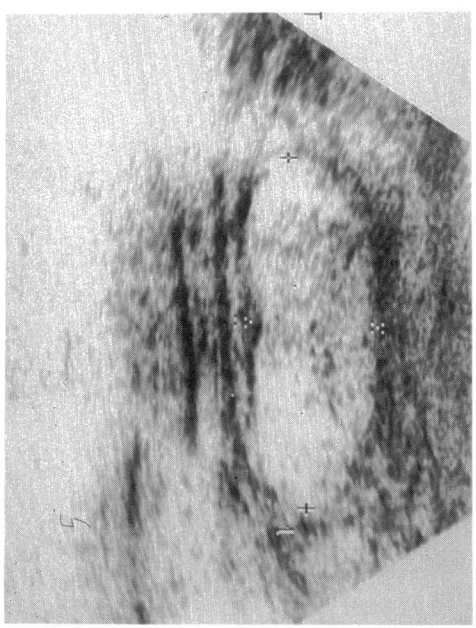

Fig. 9 Echography: fibroadenoma in a young woman.

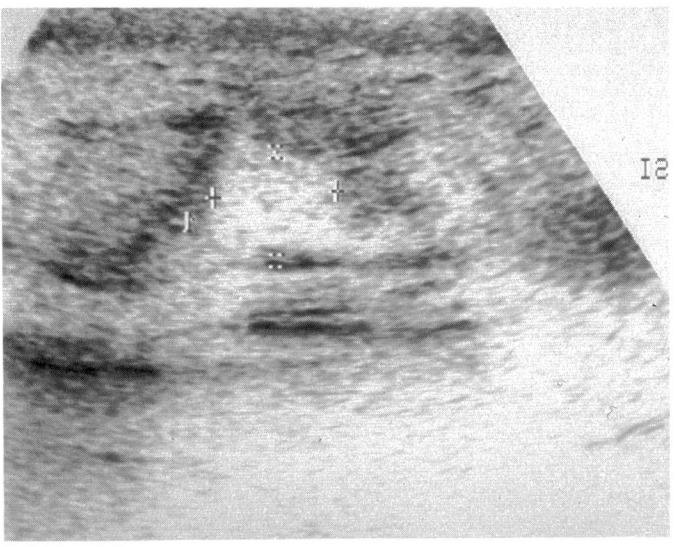

Fig. 10 Echography: a small carcinoma, 8 mm in diameter.

always sharply defined. Ultrasonic guidance can be particularly useful in obtaining aspiration material for cytology. Sonography may be particularly useful in young women, while the fatty breasts of post-menopausal women present difficulties for ultrasound (Figs 9 and 10).

Computed tomography scanning and magnetic resonance imaging are also under evaluation, but the preliminary data show that they cannot compete with mammography in accuracy, simplicity, and cost.

SURGERY OF PRIMARY BREAST CANCER

The first objective of the treatment of non-disseminated breast cancer is the locoregional control of the disease. As, at the time of diagnosis, we have no information on the possible presence of the occult cancer cells in distant organs, all the patients must, in principle, be considered as potentially curable with locoregional treatment and must benefit from a treatment that assures maximal local control of the disease. If prognostic data show that the risk that the disease is already disseminated is high, the treatment may be supplemented, but not substituted, with other measures aimed at controlling occult distant metastases.

The second objective is to obtain all possible information from surgery on the spread of the disease, both for a prognostic evaluation and for the planning of adjunctive treatments. The third objective is to minimize the extent of breast removal to obtain acceptable cosmetic and functional results. Sometimes it is difficult to fulfil all the three objectives and they have been enumerated according to a logical priority.

Surgical techniques for primary breast cancer

Halsted mastectomy

Halsted mastectomy was the type of operation most extensively applied to breast cancer patients during the first half of the century, but it has gradually been replaced by a variety of different operations. Performed by Halsted in 1882, the preliminary results were published in 1894 (Halsted 1894–1895). In the same year, Meyer (1894) reported his results with a very similar operation. This mastectomy involves an *en bloc* removal of the breast, both pectoralis muscles, and the content of all axillary fossa. Important modifications, such as the vertical type of incision, the extensive skin excision, the very thin skin flaps, and the removal of the thoraco-dorsal nerve and vessels, were introduced by Haagensen (1956).

Total mastectomy and axillary dissection

In the late 1930s, Patey in Great Britain introduced a less mutilating operation, preserving the major pectoralis muscle and its neurovascular bundle (Patey and Dyson 1948). Although, for a few decades, this operation was not considered to be appropriate by most surgeons, in the past 20 years it has gained widespread acceptability and many variations have been introduced (Scanlon and Caprini 1975; Maier *et al.* 1977; Roses *et al.* 1977; Andersson *et al.* 1979).

Extended mastectomy

The extended types of mastectomy include dissection of the regional nodes which are neglected by the Halsted mastectomy, in particular the internal mammary nodes. Early attempts were made by Handley (Handley and Thackray 1954) in London and by many other

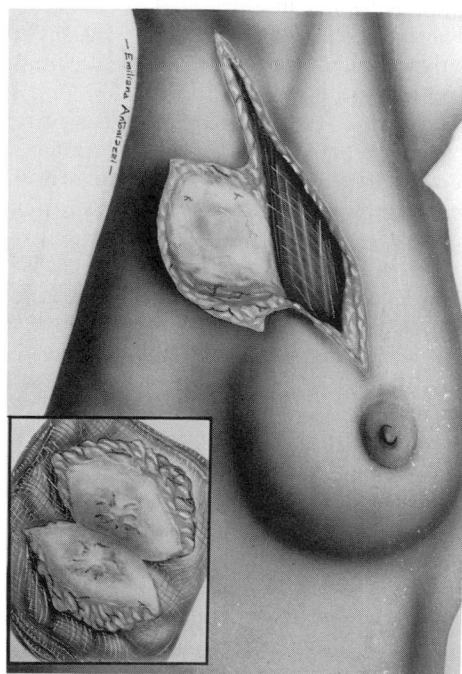

Fig. 11 Quadrantectomy with *en bloc* axillary dissection for a carcinoma of the outer upper quadrant.

European (Margottini and Bucalossi 1949; Giacomelli and Veronesi 1952; Redon and Lacour 1955) and American surgeons (Urban and Baker 1952). Superradical operations, including the dissection of internal mammary nodes, supraclavicular nodes, and, optionally, the mediastinal nodes, were devised and performed by Wangensteen (1949) in the United States and by Dahl-Iversen (1952) and Veronesi and Zingo (1967) in Europe.

Quadrantectomy

This term was coined at the beginning of the 1970s to describe an operation which involved the removal of a quadrant of the breast, including the skin and the fascia of the major pectoralis muscle (Veronesi *et al.* 1977). The aim of this operation is the radical elimination of the primary carcinoma, by its removal with a margin of 2−3 cm of normal breast tissue (Fig. 11).

Lumpectomy (or tumorectomy)

This is an operation that provides for the removal of the tumour mass with a limited portion of normal tissue (1 cm). It is generally conceived as a debulking operation to be followed by radiotherapy.

Primary chemotherapy

In the early 1970s primary chemotherapy or induction chemotherapy was introduced to treat locally advanced breast carcinomas, in combination with radiotherapy and/or surgery. The response rates appeared very high: De Lena *et al.* (1978) reported a complete or partial response of 86 per cent to four cycles of Adriamycin[R] and vincristine, Hortobagyi *et al.* (1987) found an overall response rate of 83 per cent with a combination of cyclophosphamide, Adriamycin[R], and 5-fluorouracil (CAF), and Sorace *et al.* (1985) reported a 33 per cent complete response rate with treatment with CAF plus methotrexate, leucovorin rescue + Premarin[R] and tamoxifen. Chemotherapy was able to reduce the tumour mass to allow radical surgery in cases which appeared to

be inoperable at the original examination. However, the impact of primary chemotherapy on long-term local control and survival seems to be of limited importance. The 5 year survival rate of patients treated at Joint Center for Radiation Therapy (**JCRT**) in Boston with radiation only was inferior (38 per cent) to that obtained with radiation following cyclophosphamide, methotrexate, and fluorouracil (CMF) or Adriamycin[R] (51 per cent), but the difference was not statistically significant. The median survival in the various studies varied from 30 to 65 months, not much superior to that obtained with radiotherapy alone or with radiotherapy plus surgery (Harris *et al.* 1983).

More recently, the use of chemotherapy as a primary treatment (with the bizarre name of 'neo-adjuvant') has been introduced in early breast cancer, stages I and II. The objective would be to exploit the local action of chemotherapy, in addition to the general one, which would increase the spectrum of possibilities of conservative treatments and possibly reduce the rate of local recurrences. Interesting early reports have been published by some authors (Forrest *et al.* 1986; Jacquillat *et al.* 1987) on unselected series of patients.

A recent report from the Milan Cancer Institute (Bonadonna *et al.* 1990), on 165 women who were candidates to mastectomy because of the large size of their tumour and who were treated pre-operatively with different combinations of drugs, showed a complete or partial response of the primary tumour which was so extensive as to allow conservative treatment in 88 per cent of the cases. The tumour response was unrelated to age, menopausal status, ploidy, [^{3}H]thymidine-labelling index, and type of drug combination. The response rate was greater in receptor-negative tumours.

From Halsted mastectomy to breast conservation procedures

The introduction of the so-called modified radical mastectomy, which consists of total mastectomy with dissection of axillary nodes, sparing the pectoralis muscles, was not the result of controlled studies. Only after the procedure was popular did the results of clinical trials become available. Paradoxically, the two available trials showed increased recurrence rates with the new procedure. A randomized trial, conducted by Turner *et al.* (1981) in the United Kingdom, compared 534 patients undergoing either modified radical or radical mastectomy. No difference in disease-free or overall survival was noted, but a trend of improved survival at 5 years was observed in the radical mastectomy group (85 per cent), compared to the modified radical mastectomy (78 per cent). Moreover, there was an increased incidence of local wound recurrence in those patients who had undergone modified radical mastectomy (*p* = 0.03). In the United States, Maddox *et al.* (1983) reported the results of a multicentric randomized trial comparing Halsted radical mastectomy with a modified radical mastectomy. A total of 311 patients with primary operable carcinoma of the breast were entered into the surgical and adjunctive chemotherapeutic trial between 1975 and 1978. After a median follow-up of 5 years there was no significant difference in disease-free survival or in overall survival between the two groups, although the local recurrence rate was higher in the modified mastectomy group.

The Guy's Hospital trial was the first attempt to evaluate the role of conservative treatments through a randomized control study. Three hundred and seventy stage I and II patients aged over 50 years were randomized from 1961 to 1971 in two groups. Halsted mastectomy with post-operative radiotherapy (24 Gy with orthovoltage) to axillary, supraclavicular, and internal mammary

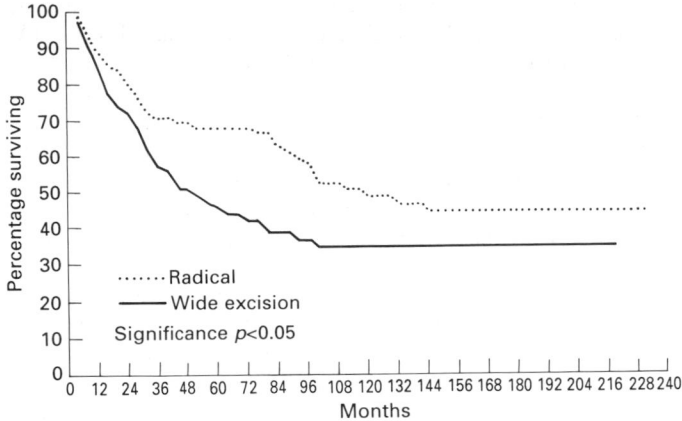

Fig. 12 Overall survival of patients treated with radical mastectomy and with wide excision and radiotherapy (38 Gy) at Guy's Hospital.

nodes was performed in 188 patients. Breast resection with radiotherapy to the breast residual tissue (35 Gy by linear accelerator) and to the regional nodes was performed in 182 patients. Until 1969, both groups received three doses of thiotepa up to a total dose of 0.7 mg/kg body weight over 4 days. In stage I patients (without palpable nodes), local excision was followed by a higher incidence of local and axillary recurrence, but the survival rates were not significantly different from those obtained in the Halsted mastectomy group. By contrast, in stage II patients (with clinically palpable nodes) the 10 year survival rate was lower in the local excision than in the mastectomy group.

A second series of 253 stage I patients was randomized between 1971 and 1975, to either wide excision or radical mastectomy. In both cases, radiotherapy was administered with a dosage similar to that used for the first series. In this second series there was a significantly higher local and distant recurrence rate after wide excision, with reduced survival. The excess of local recurrences occurred mostly in the axilla and was probably due to an insufficient dose of radiation therapy (Fig. 12). According to Hayward (1983), the increased distant recurrence rate and the diminished survival appeared to be the direct result of locoregional recurrences, suggesting that effective local control of disease is essential in the management of patients with early breast cancer.

The reduced survival after conservative treatment in the Guy's trial was considered the result of insufficiently aggressive local regional treatment (too low a dosage, no axillary dissection), so the subsequent trials had more 'radical' locoregional protocols (Table 8).

A randomized trial, known as the 'QUART' study, (QUART is an abbreviation of 'quadrantectomy, axillary dissection, radiotherapy') was designed in 1969 and implemented at the Milan Cancer Institute 4 years later (Veronesi et al. 1981). From June 1973 to May 1980, 701 evaluable patients were gathered in the trial: 349 were treated by Halsted mastectomy and 352 with the conservative procedure. Comparison of the two groups according to age, menopausal status, tumour site, dimensions of the primary cancer, and previous biopsy showed no statistically significant differences.

After 17 years from the beginning of the trial, seven patients in the Halsted group and 13 in the QUART group showed local recurrence of the primary cancer as the first sign of failure. However, only two out of the seven patients who recurred after mastectomy survived, whereas 10 out of the 13 patients who recurred after QUART are alive and well. Moreover, in the conservative group nine more cases developed a second primary cancer in the ipsilateral breast, which was treated with quadrantectomy and radiotherapy. The number of contralateral breast carcinomas was 24 in patients treated with Halsted mastectomy and 20 in those treated with QUART.

The long-term results of the trial showed similar 10 year relapse-free and overall survival rates in the two groups of patients (Veronesi et al. 1983b, 1986, 1990c). Relapse-free survival was 79 per cent in the conservative treatment and 76 per cent in the Halsted mastectomy group. Overall survival was 79 per cent in the first group and 77 per cent in the second group (Fig. 13).

At the end of 1990, 245 patients out of the 349 treated with Halsted mastectomy and 251 out of 352 patients treated with QUART were alive. The QUART technique therefore appeared acceptable, with reasonable cosmetic results and a long-term survival which was not inferior to that of mastectomy. However, these results were limited to carcinomas of less than 2 cm diameter, which account for 30–40 per cent of all breast cancers in most hospital series in Western countries. The quadrantectomy procedure, although suitable for carcinomas of limited extent, is less suitable for tumours of a larger size. In fact, the need to remove a large portion of normal tissue around the primary tumour may lead to poor cosmetic results. This is particularly true for patients with small breasts. Therefore, for larger tumours the quadrantectomy technique may be indicated only when the breast is large.

The results of a trial carried out at the Gustave Roussy Institute in Paris were published by Sarrazin et al. (1983). Patients having a breast cancer of less than 2 cm diameter (at macroscopic evaluation) with negative or positive mobile axillary nodes ($N_0–N_1$) were randomized to mastectomy or large excision plus irradiation. In both groups, low axillary dissection and histological examination of the nodes of the first level were performed. If node metastases were present, complete axillary dissection was performed. Radiotherapy to the breast was delivered with ^{60}Co teletherapy (45 Gy) plus a boost to the tumour bed of 15 Gy. Altogether, 179 patients were randomized into the two main arms; 88 to the conservative and 91 to the mastectomy group. The results after 5 years showed no difference between the groups, either in terms of locoregional recurrences or distant metastases. The overall and disease-free curves showed a slight advantage for conservatively treated patients compared to the mastectomized patients.

Table 8 Trials of first-generation studies showing no survival differences in conservative treatments compared to mutilating treatments

Reference	Number of cases	Comparison	Local recurrence	Survival
Veronesi et al. (1981)	701	Halsted v. quadrant.[a] + RT	No difference	No difference
Sarrazin et al. (1983)	179	Modif. rad. v. WE[a] and RT	No difference	No difference
B. Fisher et al. (1985a)	1843	Modif. rad. v. lumpectomy[a] ± RT	Increased in cases without RT	No difference
van Dongen (1987)	903	Modif. rad. v. wide resect.[a] + RT	No difference	No difference
Lichter et al. (1992)	237	Modif. rad. v. lumpect.[a] + RT + CT	?	No difference

[a]Axillary dissection.

Abbreviations: CT, chemotherapy; lumpect., lumpectomy; modif. rad., modified radical mastectomy; quadrant., quadrantectomy; resect., resection; RT, radiotherapy; WE, wide excision.

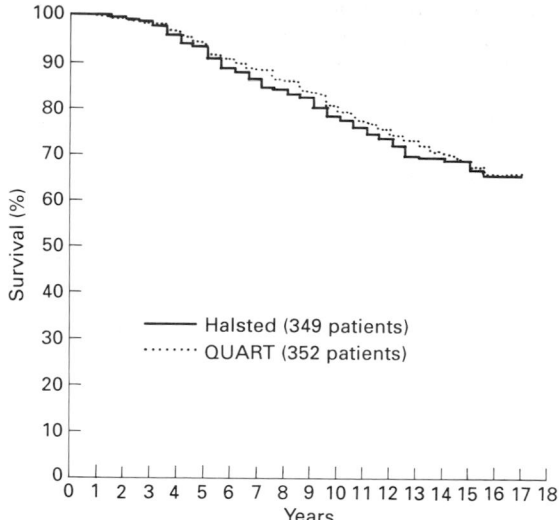

Fig. 13 Long-term overall survival in women treated with Halsted mastectomy or quadrantectomy, axillary dissection, and radiotherapy (60 Gy) at the Milan Cancer Institute.

In 1976, the National Surgical Adjuvant Breast and Bowel Project (**NSABP**) in North America started a randomized trial that compared total mastectomy with two conservative treatments (B. Fisher *et al.* 1985*a*, 1989*c*). The patients were allocated to

(1) total mastectomy with axillary dissection;

(2) mammary resection with axillary dissection;

(3) the same treatment plus radiotherapy (45 Gy) to the ipsilateral breast.

Patients with primary breast cancer up to 4 cm in diameter were considered eligible for the study. The extent of the breast resection in the two conservative groups was defined as 'wide mammary resection' or 'segmental mastectomy' or more recently 'lumpectomy'. If the specimen submitted to the pathologist showed breast cancer cells at the margins of the resected mammary tissue, a total mastectomy was performed. The results published in 1989 (B. Fisher *et al.* 1989*a*) showed no difference in survival among the three groups. However, the differences in local recurrences were striking. Some 30 per cent of patients who had been treated with partial resection without radiotherapy experienced breast recurrences; whereas 10 per cent of the patients who had a partial resection plus radiotherapy had local recurrences. True local recurrences and new primary carcinomas were computed together. Local recurrences occurred in 5 per cent of patients submitted to modified radical mastectomy.

As mentioned, one of the requirements for the conservative procedure was that the margins of the breast resection should be free from cancer cells. In fact, some 10 per cent of the cases treated with limited surgery were found to have positive margins and were immediately submitted to mastectomy. However, out of the remaining 90 per cent of cases with free margins, one-third had a local recurrence, showing that the clear margins had very limited value in predicting the risk of recurrence (B. Fisher *et al.* 1985*a*).

In 1979 at the National Cancer Institute (Bethesda) a randomized trial was started which compared total mastectomy and axillary dissection with lumpectomy plus radiotherapy and axillary dissection (Lichter *et al.* 1992). Patients were assigned either to total mastectomy plus axillary dissection or to lumpectomy followed by external radiotherapy (with a dose of 45–50 Gy to the breast, internal mammary and supraclavicular nodes, using a 4 or 6 MeV linear accelerator) and implantation radiotherapy (20–30 Gy using iridium or caesium). Patients with positive nodes, from both groups in the study, were treated with a two-drug combination chemotherapy, using doxorubicin and cyclophosphamide, for a total cumulative dose of 330 mg/m^2 of doxorubicin. Estimates at 5 years showed that 85 per cent of mastectomy-treated patients were alive compared with 89 per cent of the lumpectomy–radiation patients.

Between 1980 and 1985 the Breast Group of the European Organization for Research and Treatment of Cancer (**EORTC**) conducted a study on conservative treatment of breast cancer. Patients with stage I and II breast cancer, with a tumour diameter of less than 5 cm, were randomized to undergo a radical mastectomy (Halsted or Patey) or local excision of the tumour plus axillary dissection and radiotherapy to the breast. Beginning within 6 weeks of surgery, radiotherapy of 50 Gy in 5 weeks was administrated to the whole breast. Moreover, radiotherapy of 50 Gy to the internal mammary nodes was given to all patients in both groups, if the tumour was located medially or centrally. Within 2–6 weeks after completion of external radiotherapy, ^{192}Ir was implanted, the target volume including the whole excisional bed with a 1 cm margin. Adjuvant chemotherapy with CMF was administrated to patients with positive axillary nodes. Altogether, 903 patients were entered into the study, of whom 148 were in stage I and 755 were in stage II. The disease-free survival, evaluated by the log-rank test, was similar in both groups ($p = 0.927$). At stage I, locoregional recurrences, including supraclavicular metastases and ipsilateral second tumours, were absent in the mastectomy group and occurred at a rate of 5 per cent in the conservative group. At stage II the rates were 5 per cent in both groups (van Dongen 1987).

At the Milan Cancer Institute, between 1985 and 1987, a second randomized trial was conducted with the aim of comparing the classic QUART technique with a more reduced surgical intervention followed by aggressive radiotherapy treatment, consisting of 45 Gy delivered by an external high-energy source plus an implant of ^{192}Ir wires, which would deliver an additional 15 Gy to the tumour bed. The operation consisted of a simple 'tumorectomy', which removed the tumour mass with a limited amount of peripheral normal tissue (1 cm). Altogether, 705 cases, all with a carcinoma of less than 2.5 cm diameter at microscopic examination, were entered into the trial, 360 of whom were treated with QUART and the other 345 with TART (tumorectomy, axillary dissection, radiotherapy). In those cases found to have positive resection margins, no modifications of treatment were introduced. Preliminary results published in 1990 (Veronesi *et al.* 1990*c*) showed a similar survival in the two groups of patients, but an excess of local recurrences in the TART (24) compared to the QUART patients (13) (Fig. 14).

The possibility of withdrawing radiotherapy in the conservative methods has been explored in two different trials. The advantages of breast conservation with surgery alone, without radiotherapy, are treatment is easier and cheaper, it is easier to discover local recurrence as there is no fibrosis due to radiotherapy, and possible late effects of radiotherapy (such as pulmonary fibrosis and cardiac damage, as well as any hypothetical oncongenic risk) are avoided.

The Swedish Uppsala randomized trial on 381 patients with a small breast carcinoma (<2 cm) showed that patients treated with an extensive local resection (defined as sector resection) had a 3 year local recurrence rate of 7.6 per cent, whereas patients treated with the same surgery plus radiotherapy had a rate of 2.9 per cent,

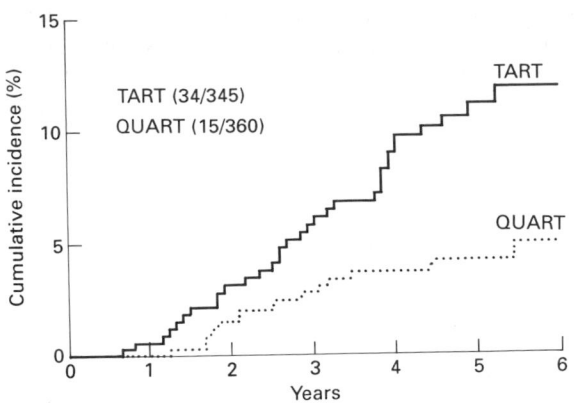

Fig. 14 Cumulative rates of local recurrences according to treatment: TART, tumorectomy, axillary dissection, and radiotherapy; QUART, quadrantectomy, axillary dissection, and radiotherapy (Milan trial II).

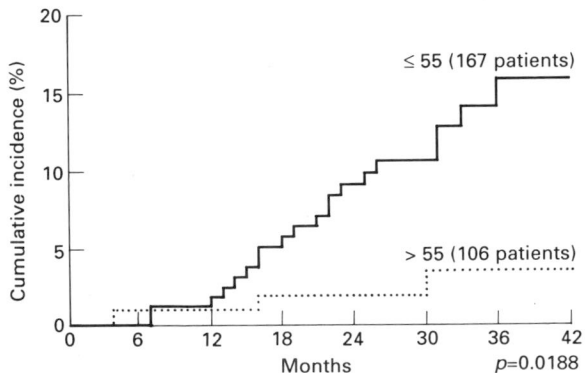

Fig. 15 Cumulative rates of local recurrences in patients treated with quadrantectomy and axillary dissection, without radiotherapy, according to age (Milan trial III).

without differences in survival (Uppsala-Orebro Breast Cancer Study Group 1990).

At the Milan Cancer Institute a similar randomized trial conducted on 567 patients showed a very low rate of local recurrence with quadrantectomy plus radiotherapy (1 per cent), whereas women treated with quadrantectomy alone suffered a much higher local recurrence rate (9 per cent). However, the trial showed that in women older than 55 years the local recurrence rate was also very low (3 per cent) in patients treated with quadrantectomy without radiotherapy (Fig.15) (Veronesi et al. 1993b).

At least three trials have recently been concluded or are in progress in the United Kingdom, comparing different conservative techniques. In the Scottish trial, which started in 1983, patients treated with breast resection plus low axillary dissection were randomized between breast radiotherapy and no further treatment.

In a trial conducted in Manchester between 1982 and 1987 stage I patients treated with breast resection (without axillary dissection) were randomized between radiotherapy to all breast tissue and limited radiotherapy by direct field. The preliminary results of the two trials were published recently, showing very clearly that traditional radiotherapy on the whole breast reduces considerably the rate of local recurrences compared either to no radiotherapy or to limited radiotherapy by direct field. Finally, in the West Midlands' trial, the patients were randomized to breast resection with or without radiotherapy (Table 9). The final objective of this research effort was the identification of the 'ideal line', when the treatment has its maximum efficacy and minimum breast ablation (Fig. 16). As an exercise, in Fig. 17 the positions of the various types of treatments (for small tumours) tested in the past century are drawn in relation to the 'ideal line'.

Treatment of axillary node metastases

The treatment of axillary nodes has been controversial. In the case of clinically positive nodes, all surgeons agree that the nodes must be removed, but the suggested type of surgical dissection is often different. In the case of clinically negative nodes, the major question is whether the dissection is necessary, as in early breast cancer the chances that the nodes are negative are very high.

That clinically positive nodes should be treated is a unanimous principle. However, although surgical dissection appears to be the most widely accepted form of treatment, for a long period of time axillary radiotherapy has been the treatment of choice, especially in the United Kingdom and northern Europe. This procedure was especially supported by McWhirter (1955) in Edinburgh, who was able to show that total mastectomy plus axillary radiotherapy may produce results similar to Halsted mastectomy. In a large randomized trial in the United Kingdom by the Cancer Research Campaign, 2268 stage I and stage II patients were randomized between mastectomy plus radiotherapy (including the axillae) and mastectomy followed by a watch policy. At 5 years there was no evidence that radiotherapy increased survival, although the rate of local recurrence was lower in the irradiated patients. The value of axillary radiotherapy was reinforced by a clinical randomized trial conducted by the National Surgical Adjuvant Breast and Bowel Project in the United States between 1971 and 1974. In this study stage II patients (with suspicious palpable nodes) were randomized between Halsted mastectomy and total mastectomy with radiotherapy. The study showed that at 10 years there was no significant difference between the two treatments in terms of locoregional or distant failures and survival.

Although axillary radiotherapy appears to be as effective as surgery in the control of the disease, it has been gradually abandoned, due to its inability to give useful information on the state of the axillary nodes. In fact, the prognostic value of the axillary node involvement is considerable and the advantage of surgical

Table 9 Trials of second-generation studies (conservative versus conservative treatments)

Reference	Comparison			Local recurrence	Survival
Milan II (Veronesi et al. 1990c)	Quadrant. + RT (ext.)	versus	Lumpect. + RT (ext. + ^{192}Ir)	Increased in lumpect.	No diff.
Uppsala (Uppsala-Orebro 1990)	Sector resection + RT	versus	Sector resection	Increased without RT	No diff.
Milan III (Veronesi et al. 1993b)	Quadrant. + RT	versus	Quadrantectomy	Increased without RT	No diff.
Scottish (Stewart et al. 1989)	Lumpect. + RT	versus	Lumpectomy	Increased without RT	No diff.
Manchester (Ribeiro et al. 1990)	Lumpect. + RT (whole breast)	versus	Lumpect. + RT (direct field)	Increased in direct field	No diff.
Milan IV (unpublished)	Lumpect. + RT (ext.)	versus	Lumpect. + RT (ext. + ^{192}Ir)	In progress	

Abbreviations: diff., difference; ext., external; lumpect., lumpectomy; quadrant., quadrantectomy; RT, radiotherapy.

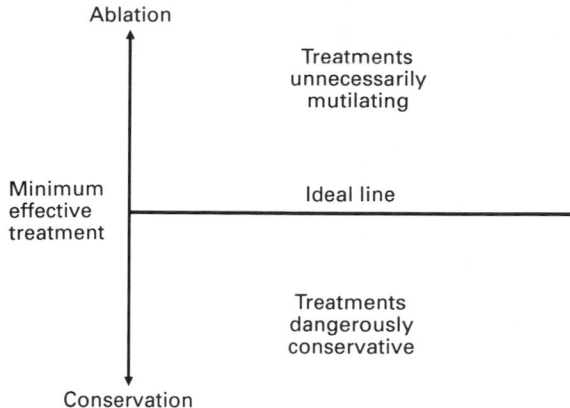

Fig. 16 The objective of trials on primary tumour management is the identification of an ideal line corresponding to the minimum effective treatment.

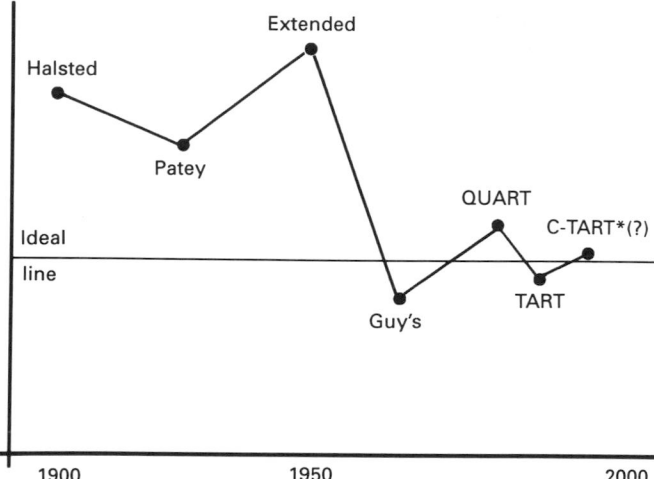

*TART after primary chemotherapy

Fig. 17 Position of the various techniques (for treatment of a small cancer) in relation to the 'ideal line'. TART = tumourectomy, axillary dissection, radiotherapy; QUART = quandrantectomy, axillary dissection, radiotherapy.

axillary dissection is to have access to this information, which is important in deciding on possible adjunctive treatments.

The 'staging' aim of axillary dissection is considered to be the main reason for the dissection in patients with clinically negative nodes. In fact, when the axillary nodes are negative at clinical examination immediate dissection does not show any superiority, in terms of survival, compared to dissection performed only at the appearance of clinical metastases (B. Fisher *et al.* 1985*b*). The 'staging' aim of the dissection has led many surgeons to reduce the extent of the dissection to removal of the first level only, as the absence or presence of metastases at the first level is highly predictive of higher axillary involvement.

The need for axillary dissection in patients with clinically negative nodes has been questioned recently (Sacks *et al.* 1992) on the following grounds:

(1) in early breast cancer the chances that the axillary nodes are not involved is of the order of 75–80 per cent;

(2) a dissection performed at the time of appearance of clinical metastases does not change the survival rate;

(3) in post-menopausal patients, positive for oestrogen receptors, in whom the indication as an adjunctive treatment is mainly limited to tamoxifen, this may be applied in all patients;

(4) in pre-menopausal patients the adjunctive therapies may be deferred at the time of clinical evidence of axillary metastases, as the timing of their application does not seem to be very important (Glucksberg *et al.* 1982);

(5) alternatively, prognostic indications to be decided for adjunctive treatments may be derived from the primary tumour (from growth rate, ploidy, oestrogen receptor status, and pathological grade peritumoral lymphatic invasion).

In consideration of a progressive reduction of surgery in the treatment of early breast cancer, these points must be carefully evaluated, as it is likely that in the near future the present policy of axillary dissection will be largely revised. The extent and the technique of axillary dissection to be employed are even more uncertain.

The 'sampling' technique advocated by many surgeons (Davies *et al.* 1980; Pigott *et al.* 1984), by which only the first level (or a portion of it) is removed, has disadvantages. In fact, if the 'sampling' shows an involvement of the first axillary level, the second and/or the third levels are likely to be involved and the problem of the treatment of these occult metastases arises (Veronesi *et al.* 1990*b*; Kiricuta and Tausch 1992). As recurrences in an operated axilla are very difficult to detect, the treatment of the occult residual disease should aim at the total destruction of the cancer cells in that site. This can be obtained either by another operation or by radiotherapy. However, surgical dissection is not easy when a portion of the axilla has already been resected and radiotherapy may create late lymphoedema of the arm. These complications may be easily avoided if the axillary dissection includes all the three levels of lymph nodes. The advantages of total dissection are:

(1) the prognostic information is excellent as the distribution by level will give the maximum information for evaluation;

(2) no additional treatment is needed;

(3) the risk of local recurrence in the axillary fossa is practically zero.

Treatment of internal mammary nodes

Internal mammary nodes as a possible site of metastases from breast cancer were neglected by surgeons until Handley, in London, inaugurated a surgical technique which included, after the classic radical mastectomy, the removal of the internal mammary nodes from the second to the fifth intercostal space, a technique which was immediately followed by a number of European surgeons. The first reports showed a rate of metastatic spread to the internal mammary nodes of approximately 20–30 per cent, indicating the importance of this nodal basin in the natural history of breast cancer. Urban and Baker (1952) developed a more extensive procedure, removing a good portion of the chest wall *en bloc*, including part of the sternum and the anterior portion of four ribs. A randomized international clinical trial was designed and implemented by five different institutions between 1962 and 1966 and the results were published in 1976 and in 1983 with clear evidence of the overall inefficacity of the extended procedure compared to the traditional Halsted mastectomy (Lacour *et al.* 1983).

Post-mastectomy reconstruction

The replacement of standard Halsted mastectomy by modified radical mastectomy has given great impetus to the practice of breast reconstruction; in fact, by preserving the pectoralis muscles, the modified mastectomy offers a basis for thorax symmetry after a breast reconstruction with appropriate techniques.

All patients operated on for breast cancer are possible candidates and breast reconstruction is possible following any kind of cancer surgery (Bohmert and Strömbeck 1986). The patient must be informed of the options of reconstruction techniques available to her and of the possible results; she must know that the reconstructed breast can never become completely normal.

As regards the timing of reconstruction, there are two choices. Primary reconstruction immediately after mastectomy for cancer is still an uncommon procedure but with the improvement of techniques it is becoming increasingly utilized, whereas the most accepted procedure is to carry out the reconstruction at least 6 months after mastectomy, when the skin cover has become soft and elastic.

Many techniques of breast reconstruction after cancer surgery are available (Bostwick 1987). The choice between different techniques depends on the prerequisites at hand following ablative surgery. Deformities may range from limited asymmetry after quadrantectomy, to an irradiated ulcer following an extended Halsted mastectomy. Also, the appearance of the oppositive breast influences the choice of a reconstructive method. For limited deformities, such as those resulting from a modified radical mastectomy, a breast reconstruction with a silicone breast implant (which may be preceded by a tissue 'expander') may be satisfactory. In other cases, with larger defects and ulceration, distant musculocutaneous flaps, either pedicled into the area or transferred by microvascular techniques, are necessary.

RADIOTHERAPY OF BREAST CANCER

Post-mastectomy radiotherapy

Radiotherapy to the chest wall and lymphatic pathways reduces the risk of locoregional relapse after mastectomy. For example, actuarial 5 year locoregional recurrence rates in 2243 women with breast cancer at clinical stages I and II, randomized to simple mastectomy plus or minus radiotherapy, were reduced from 30 to 11 per cent by radiotherapy (Cancer Research Campaign 1980). Even after radical mastectomy, post-operative radiotherapy lowers the risk of locoregional recurrence, with the absolute benefit depending on prognostic markers. In patients with positive axillary lymph nodes, the cumulative risk of locoregional recurrence 8 years after radical mastectomy was reduced from 45 to 13 per cent by post-operative radiotherapy (Wallgren et al. 1986).

The observation that post-operative radiotherapy reduces locoregional recurrence risk does not necessarily justify its routine use. Recommendations for radiotherapy after mastectomy depend on the surgical procedure and on prognostic markers of locoregional recurrence. It is reasonable to assume that reducing the lifetime risk of locoregional relapse by radiotherapy leads to a gain in life quality for those at highest risk (for example, node-positive women), but it should be remembered that radiotherapy is associated with its own risk of morbidity in terms of chest wall fibrosis, arm swelling, and reduced arm mobility. In practice, this means that radiotherapy should not be given to the axilla after radical or modified radical mastectomy. Complete axillary dissection deals effectively with the problem of axillary recurrence and post-operative axillary radiotherapy increases treatment morbidity. After radical or modified radical mastectomy, it is reasonable to confine post-operative radiotherapy to the chest wall and to patients at the highest risk of local relapse.

The current use of adjuvant systemic therapy following mastectomy does not solve the problem of locoregional recurrence and radiotherapy still has a role to play in selected groups. For example, 5 year locoregional recurrence rates were reduced from 28 to 9 per cent by post-operative radiotherapy, after mastectomy and adjuvant CMF in 1473 pre-menopausal women with node-positive early-stage disease or advanced local disease (Overgaard et al. 1990). The Danish Cooperative Group also found that post-operative radiotherapy reduced the locoregional recurrence rate from 36 to 6 per cent at 4 years in 1202 high-risk post-menopausal women treated by total mastectomy, partial axillary dissection, and adjuvant tamoxifen.

When it comes to the internal mammary chain, radiotherapy has not been shown to benefit any identifiable subgroup of women in terms of prolonged overall survival and parasternal relapse is so uncommon that prophylactic internal mammary chain irradiation is difficult to justify in terms of improving life quality. In fact, it is very likely that internal mammary chain irradiation contributes to excess mortality from ischaemic heart disease in long-term survivors. A clinically and statistically significant increase in mortality from ischaemic heart disease has been reported in long-term survivors randomized to post-mastectomy radiotherapy in clinical trials conducted since 1950 (Host et al. 1986; Haybittle et al. 1989; Jones and Ribeiro 1989). It is probably true that crude radiotherapy techniques were partly to blame in these early trials, but even with optimal field arrangements there are strong arguments for a selective use of post-mastectomy irradiation.

Advanced locoregional disease

Adjuvant systemic therapy has a proven role in reducing the odds of death in women with early breast cancer, but in patients with advanced locoregional disease (stage III) the four clinical trials carried out so far have not demonstrated an overall survival advantage for patients treated with systemic therapy. Only one out of these four trials suggests an overall survival gain for combined modalities treatment, including chemotherapy (Klefstrom et al. 1987). One factor that might limit the effect of treatment is the increased burden of clonogenic tumour cells at occult metastatic sites in these patients. Other contributory factors may include the scheduling of chemotherapy, which often follows the completion of locoregional therapy. In the absence of a clear overall survival advantage, the justification for systemic therapy rests on improving disease-free survival and life quality in a group of women having 5 year survival rates ranging from 13 to 48 per cent, depending on tumour and patient characteristics (Rubens et al. 1977; Vilcoq et al. 1984).

Responses to locoregional surgery and/or radiotherapy vary according to several tumour and patient characteristics, especially tumour size and this variability makes single-arm studies very difficult to compare. A traditional approach is to combine radiotherapy and surgery, the sequence of each modality being influenced by the operability of disease at presentation. Despite combinations of surgery and radiotherapy, locoregional failure rates occur in up to 50 per cent of women, depending on local disease stage (Harris and Hellman 1984). The type and quality of treatment delivered are likely to be important determinants of outcome, but it is very difficult to draw these conclusions from the available data. On the basis of retrospective data, it is likely that combinations of surgery and radiotherapy are superior to either modality alone for the control of locoregional disease (Bedwinek et al. 1982; Chu et al. 1984).

The impact of adjuvant systemic therapy on local control in advanced locoregional disease has been evaluated in only four trials, totalling 832 patients. In all studies, chemotherapy was commenced after the completion of local treatment by radiotherapy and/or surgery; in two trials there was a significant improvement in locoregional control arising from the addition of systemic therapy, whereas in the other two trials no such improvement in local control emerged (De Lena et al. 1981; Schaake-Koning et al. 1985; Klefstrom et al. 1987; Derman et al. 1989; Rubens et al. 1989).

In patients given induction chemotherapy as primary treatment, two trials have studied the relative effectiveness of subsequent mastectomy or radiotherapy in dealing with residual locoregional disease (De Lena et al. 1981; Perloff et al. 1988). The two trials totalled 219 patients and each reported up to 50 per cent locoregional recurrence rates regardless of whether mastectomy or radiotherapy was delivered. If locoregional disease remains unresectable after induction chemotherapy, women without overt metastases should be considered for high-dose radiotherapy. The whole breast, axilla, and supraclavicular fossa should be given the equivalent of 50 Gy in 25 daily fractions, followed by local boosts of 15–30 Gy, using shrinking-field techniques or interstitial implantation, to residual primary and axillary tumour masses. There is reasonably good evidence from retrospective studies that higher radiation doses are more effective than lower doses in controlling bulky residual disease (Arriagada et al. 1985).

In recent years, there has been increasing interest in the potential ability of primary chemotherapy and/or endocrine therapy to shrink bulky locoregional disease sufficiently to make breast conservation a testable treatment option in a substantial proportion of patients with advanced locoregional disease.

According to these protocols, systemic therapy is followed by local excision, with or without axillary dissection and radiotherapy (Forrest et al. 1986; Mansi et al. 1989; Bonadonna et al. 1990; Mauriac et al. 1991). To summarize the preliminary data, it appears a very feasible management option with a clinically significant proportion of women avoiding the need for mastectomy. Determination of the potential benefits in terms of disease-free and overall survival compared to other schedules combining surgery, radiotherapy, and systemic therapy will require large, randomized trials.

Radiotherapy in metastatic disease

Radiotherapy palliates a high proportion of patients with symptoms of bone and brain metastases. Based on patient self-assessment, up to 80 per cent of women get some relief of bone pain and 30–40 per cent get complete relief of bone pain after a conventional course of palliative treatment, viz. 30 Gy in ten daily fractions. Recent randomized clinical trials suggest that a single fraction of 8 Gy is as effective as more prolonged schedules for the short-term relief of symptoms, that is, up to 3 months post-treatment (Price et al. 1986; Hoskin et al. 1992). Where the primary aim of treatment is to restore the structural integrity of an affected bone, higher doses of fractionated radiotherapy are often employed. In patients with lytic disease in bone that threatens the pathological fracture of a weight-bearing long bone, an orthopaedic procedure prior to radiotherapy may be the way of reducing the risk of fracture.

Low-dose fractionated radiotherapy schedules similar to those used to palliate bone pain are also effective in palliating the symptoms associated with brain metastases. The probability of a

useful improvement in neurological function following treatment depends strongly on the deficit at the time of relapse. Patients with a mild deficit gain a useful response much more frequently than patients with a severe deficit. A measurable gain in neurological function is reported in at least 70 per cent of affected patients (Hendrickson 1977; Hoskin et al. 1990). Several randomized trials have evaluated the effectiveness of different radiotherapy schedules. There is no clear advantage with respect to frequency of improvement, time to progression, or survival in patients treated with high- versus low-dose schedules. Commonly used schedules include 30 Gy in ten fractions or 20 Gy in five fractions.

Radiotherapy techniques after breast-preserving surgery

The usual procedure is to irradiate the whole breast using medial and lateral glancing radiation fields delivered with the woman lying supine with one or both arms abducted out of the way of the beams to approximately a right angle. A dose of 45–50 Gy in fraction sizes of 2 Gy is recommended, with maximal sparing of the underlying lung tissue and avoidance of the heart. ^{60}Co γ-rays or 4 MeV X-rays are suitable because there is sufficient skin sparing to avoid unsightly telangiectasia. No wax build-up is needed over the excision scar. It is not known for certain whether a boost to the tumour bed is needed routinely, but prospective trials are currently under way to answer this question. Boosts are often delivered using a direct electron field 7–10 cm in diameter, but a two-plane radioactive implant is a reasonable alternative. A dose of 10–25 Gy in 2 Gy fractions is commonly prescribed, depending on the microscopic excision margins.

If there are reasons to irradiate the axilla and supraclavicular fossa, care must be taken to avoid an overlap between the anterior axillary field and the tangential breast fields, otherwise matchline fibrosis can spoil breast cosmesis. There are straightforward techniques based on half-beam blocks or asymmetric collimators which match field junctions successfully. Doses to the midplane axilla should be 45–50 Gy in 2 Gy fractions, the midplane dose to the axilla being supplemented by a smaller posterior axillary field (Yarnold and Bloom 1989).

Locoregional radiotherapy after mastectomy is delivered using exactly the same principles, except that 1 cm of wax bolus should be placed over the whole of the chest wall to ensure a maximum dose at the skin surface. All these techniques are best planned with the aid of a simulator, with subsequent portal verification on the treatment machine.

SYSTEMIC THERAPY FOR EARLY BREAST CANCER

Adjuvant systemic therapy

Many breast cancer patients who remain disease-free after local and regional treatment eventually relapse and die of or with overt metastasis. This is true regardless of whether they received an appropriate local therapy. The current hypothesis ascribes the failure to obtain freedom from disease to occult micrometastatic disease already present at the time of diagnosis and first surgery (Henderson and Canellos 1980). This hypothesis has acquired indirect support from the results of clinical trials that show no additional advantage, in terms of disease-free or overall survival, for a more radical local therapy (Veronesi et al. 1985; Fisher et al. 1989c). There is evidence that occult metastases can still be eliminated by current therapeutic means, but the overt metastatic phase of the disease is considered incurable. These observations lead to substantially different attitudes towards the treatment of patients in these two distinct clinical situations.

Long before the present hypothesis of disease spread (presence of micrometastases at diagnosis), adjuvant systemic therapy was applied in the form of hormonal ablative treatment, consisting of ovarian radiation (Cole 1970). Previous observations made of tumour regression after oophorectomy (Beatson 1896) justified the investigation of ablative therapy in patients with operable disease after the completion of local treatment.

The use of systemic adjuvant chemotherapy was based upon observations of substantial rates of response of measurable metastatic disease to cytotoxic agents. In addition, the first hypothesis concerning the value of chemotherapy as an adjuvant treatment was related to the attempt to kill those cells that detach during operation. The detached cells were considered to be responsible for the subsequent development of overt metastases. This hypothesis of perioperative migration of cells with metastatic potential has been abandoned in favour of one that argues for the presence of micrometastatic disease at the time of primary diagnosis (Berlin 1975).

Experimental observations that have helped to guide the use of adjuvant systemic therapy after surgical removal of the primary tumour were made on the basis of animal models (Martin and Fugman 1957; Martin 1960; Karrer and Humphreys 1967; Martin et al. 1970; Mayo et al. 1972). An inverse relationship was demonstrated between the number of viable tumour cells in the animal and the response to treatment with a cytotoxic agent, that is, the smaller the number of tumour cells the greater the chemotherapeutic effect. The explanation for this phenomenon was provided by experiments conducted on mouse leukaemia cells (Wilcox 1966). In this model, cell kill due to exposure to cytotoxic drugs follows first-order kinetics, that is, a given dose will kill the same percentage and not the same number of drug-sensitive cells regardless of the total burden of malignant cells. This model has been borrowed from bacterial systems and from cultures of mammalian cells. A drug may cause the destruction of 99.9 per cent of cancer cells, no matter what their numbers are within a tumour mass. Thus, in a micrometastasis of 100 cells, there is a high statistical probability that a given dose of chemotherapy will destroy all of the cancer cells. On the other hand, it is clear that if a metastasis contains 10^{10} cells (weighing approximately 10 g), then the same chemotherapy might leave 10^6 viable cells to re-grow and subsequently to kill the patient. The principle indicates that if surgery has reduced the number of cells to micrometastases consisting of no more than 100 cells, then the optimal time for chemotherapy potentially to eradicate all cells is immediately after operation. In fact, adjuvant therapy after surgery will increase the cure rate in animal models in contrast to both delayed administration of drugs and their use without surgical tumour reduction (Martin et al. 1975). In an attempt to explain the failure of adjuvant therapy to achieve a cure in most of the treated humans, despite the fact that first-order kinetics of drug action might have predicted otherwise, the following issues arise.

1. Tumours are heterogeneous as regards the cell cycle, cellular metabolism, and drug availability within a tumour mass.

2. Resistance to treatment. Among the causes for drug resistance, which may be intrinsic or acquired, are those that relate to the timing of drug administration. Based upon an experimental system, the early administration of cytotoxic drugs is hypothesized to avert the formation of resistant tumour cells (Goldie and Coldman 1979).

3. The growth of tumour cells is hypothesized to follow Gompertzian kinetics, according to which plateaux of slow or no growth are interrupted by random growth spurts (Retsky et al. 1987). The occurrence of these spurts may be favoured by treatment-free intervals and represent periods of higher susceptibility to cytotoxics. According to this latter hypothesis the best therapy for averting metastatic growth is one that follows therapy-free intervals.

Irrespective of the foregoing considerations, which describe our theoretical knowledge about why systemic therapy might or might not function, its application in operable breast cancer roughly followed an empirical pattern. All the knowledge related to the benefits of adjuvant systemic treatment is derived from randomized trials. The trials designed to define treatment benefit in terms of disease-free survival or overall survival focused upon the types of therapies that were believed likely to produce an improvement.

Three main types of treatments have been investigated during the past decades: endocrine therapies, cytotoxic therapies administered as single- or multiple-agent regimens, and combined chemoendocrine therapies (Table 10). To better understand the developments in the field of adjuvant therapy, it might be useful to list the types of treatments according to the chronological sequence of their development:

(1) adjuvant oophorectomy (either surgical- or radiation-induced);

(2) adjuvant perioperative cytotoxic therapy of short duration (given immediately after the completion of surgery of the primary tumour);

Table 10 Review of randomized trials of adjuvant therapies according to the type of treatments investigated (not all trials are published) (from Henderson (1987) modified and updated)

Trial design	Number of trials	Number of patients
Endocrine therapies		
Ovarian ablation v. nil	12	>3500
Tam v. nil	24	>15000
Tam in N− disease	18	>8000
Two tamoxifen durations	7	>2500
Other endocrine therapies v. nil	4	>600
Chemotherapies		
Perioperative CT v. nil	15	>7000
Post-operative CT v. nil (N+)	41	>17000
CT in N− disease	24	>12000
CT v. adjuvant RT	8	>2200
Multi- v. single-agent CT	15	>4000
Peri/pre-op. v. post-op. CT	7	>2600
Two multidrug regimens	23	>10000
CT +/− RT v. CT	6	>1000
Two CT durations	9	>6000
Two CT doses	2	>2000
Combined chemoendocrine therapies or chemotherapy v. endocrine therapy		
CT v. endocrine therapy	8	>3000
CT+ET v. nil	6	>1800
CT+ET v. ET	12	>4500
CT+ET v. CT	25	>10000

Abbreviations: CT, chemotherapy; ET, endocrine therapy; N−, no axillary node metastases; N+, with axillary node metastases; Peri/pre-op., Peri/pre-operative; post-op., post-operative; RT, radiotherapy; Tam., tamoxifen.

(3) adjuvant prolonged chemotherapy: mainly studied in patients with axillary node metastases (N+), definition of the role of a multidrug combination chemotherapy as opposed to that of a single agent, definition of the duration of treatment, definition of the timing of treatment, definition of 'dose intensity' of chemotherapy, and definition of the type of cytotoxics used in the combination chemotherapy regimen;

(4) adjuvant immunotherapy, usually added to chemotherapy;

(5) adjuvant endocrine therapy, mainly with prolonged administration of the anti-oestrogen tamoxifen; recently, the use of some other agents and direct comparison of chemotherapy to endocrine therapy alone;

(6) adjuvant chemoendocrine therapies, mainly the combination of multiagent chemotherapy and oophorectomy or tamoxifen;

(7) trials specifically conducted in populations of patients prospectively defined according to risk factors that might influence the outcome (that is, patients with no axillary node metastases (N−) and patients with a known oestrogen-receptor content in the primary tumour (ER+ or ER− tumours).

Definition of benefit to patients treated in clinical trials

Adjuvant systemic therapy does not provide a cure for most of the treated patients. It is estimated roughly that adjuvant therapy averts relapse in one-third of the patients, which corresponds to a reduction in death rate of approximately one-fifth to one-sixth as compared with that for patients who do not receive adjuvant therapy. This magnitude of effect is easily missed when results from individual randomized studies are analysed, even if 500–1000 patients were included in the study, because an annual death rate of approximately 5 per cent implies the capability to detect a difference of less than 1 per cent relative to the entire treated population. Cumulative figures after several years of follow-up indicate that the benefit in terms of a reduction of the risk of death is approximately 10–12 per cent (for example, the overall survival percentage at a given time increases from 40 to 52 per cent) in a population of patients with N+ disease and 2–5 per cent in a population with N− breast cancer (for example, the overall survival percentage increases at a given time from 79 to 84 per cent).

In the summing-up of the results (overview or meta-analysis) from individual trials that compared one therapy with another one can evaluate whether, in the presence of modest differences, the null hypothesis (of no treatment effect) might be rejected. The advantages of pooling the results from all available trials include the possibility of detecting small but humanly meaningful treatment effects of otherwise doubtful utility and, indirectly, of increasing the interest of physicians and communities in improving upon modest but real treatment results. Among the disadvantages of an overview is the tendency, in interpreting its results, to rely upon the magnitude of the detected treatment effects and to perform indirect comparisons between therapies which were never directly compared (in a randomized trial) (Gelber and Goldhirsch 1986a, 1991; Henderson et al. 1989a), allowing for biases. The advantage of detecting small outcome differences may be considered the strength as well as the weakness of an overview and, thus, analysis of individual trials must remain the basis for clinical and research purposes (Henderson 1991).

Some overview analyses have been conducted; the most extensive one included all available results from published and unpublished

trials in almost 30 000 patients (Early Breast Cancer Trialists' Collaborative Group 1988, 1990). This overview included randomized trials which started before 1985 and which compared tamoxifen to no adjuvant therapy or tamoxifen plus another treatment versus the other therapy alone (for example, tamoxifen plus radiation therapy versus radiation therapy alone), as well as trials that compared chemotherapy to no adjuvant therapy or chemotherapy plus another therapy versus the other therapy alone (for example, chemotherapy and tamoxifen versus tamoxifen alone). The first results showed that within the first 5 years there was a significant reduction in the odds of relapse or death obtained by the two treatments, mainly with tamoxifen for the post-menopausal and with combination chemotherapy for the pre-menopausal patients. The update of this overview also related to trials that began before 1985 (Early Breast Cancer Trialists' Collaborative Group 1992). It extended the estimated figures to the tenth year and included trials with tamoxifen (tamoxifen versus no tamoxifen; 29 892 women, 40 trials) and chemotherapy (chemotherapy versus no chemotherapy; 18 403 women, 44 trials), as well as those with ovarian ablation (ovarian ablation versus the same without ovarian ablation; 3072 women, 10 trials) and those with immunotherapy (immunotherapy versus the same without immunotherapy; 6300 women, 23 trials) (Early Breast Cancer Trialists' Collaborative Group 1992). Furthermore, the update included other trials in which the duration, timing, and type of the adjuvant therapy were studied; these were of such heterogeneity that no better conclusion was possible than that obtained by reviewing the individual trials. Subgroup analyses were attempted, to provide an estimate of treatment effects by a specific feature, such as the oestrogen-receptor content in the primary tumour, a factor which is known to predict the response to endocrine treatments.

The estimated cumulative results by treatment are described in Table 11. From the evidence of indirect comparisons, chemotherapy or oophorectomy and possibly the combination of both might represent a relevant treatment option for younger women, while tamoxifen without or with chemotherapy is the therapy that should be offered to post-menopausal patients. However, it is clear from results of some trials in N+ and especially N− breast cancer that tamoxifen can also be very useful in pre-menopausal women (Fisher et al. 1989a) and that chemotherapy yields similar results in post-menopausal and pre-menopausal patients (Fisher et al. 1989b). Further clinical research with available treatments and review of the results from individual trials, will clarify patient-care-related issues.

An example of a trial comparing surgical oophorectomy to no adjuvant treatment is the Saskatchewan trial (Bryant and Weir 1981) in which, from 1964 to 1973, 359 women (46 per cent of whom were N+) were randomly assigned to one of the two treatment options. While after 5 years of follow-up the difference between the two treatment groups was significant only in terms of disease-free survival (8 per cent difference, $p < 0.05$), after 10 years an overall survival advantage in favour of the oophorectomy group also appeared and the difference increased to 11 per cent ($p < 0.05$). The delayed appearance of a difference in outcome for oophorectomized patients seems to be a pattern common to the trial with ablative endocrine therapies (Ludwig Breast Cancer Study Group 1985; The International Breast Cancer Study Group 1990; Nissen-Meyer 1991). This feature of increasing treatment effects, especially upon mortality, emerges clearly from the overview figures (Fig. 18(a) and (b)) (Early Breast Cancer Trialists' Collaborative Group 1992). New approaches, which include ovarian suppression by means of luteinizing-hormone-releasing hormone analogues, are being studied.

Table 11 Effects of treatment for patients with oophorectomy versus no oophorectomy, prolonged adjuvant tamoxifen versus no adjuvant tamoxifen (Tam), and prolonged adjuvant multiagent chemotherapy (CT) versus no adjuvant chemotherapy; overall, by associated systemic therapy and by age; for Tam, by oestrogen receptor status (ER) (Early Breast Cancer Trialists' Collaborative Group 1992)

	Typical reduction in annual odds of recurrence or death (%±SD)					
	Recurrence			Death		
	< 50	≥ 50	Any age	< 50	≥ 50	Any age
Ovarian ablation (Ox) all < 50 yr	26±6	—[a]	—	25±7	—[a]	—
Ox v. nil	30±9	—[a]	—	28±9	—[a]	—
Ox+CT v. CT	21±9	—[a]	—	19±11	—[a]	—
Tam (all)	12±4	29±2	25±2	6±5	20±2	16±2
Tam v. nil	27±7	30±2	29±3	17±10	19±3	19±3
Tam+CT v. CT	7±4	28±3	24±3	3±5	20±4	16±3
ER poor	3±8	16±5	13±4	−5±9	16±6	11±5
ER+	19±6	36±3	32±3	13±8	23±4	21±3
ER?	12±7	26±3	22±3	8±8	17±4	15±3
poly CT (all)	36±5	23±3	28±3	24±5	13±4	17±3
CT v. nil	37±5	22±4	27±3	27±6	14±5	18±4
CT+ Tam v. Tam	26±5	28±6	24±3	−6±23	10±7	5±9

[a]Treatment effects not statistically different.

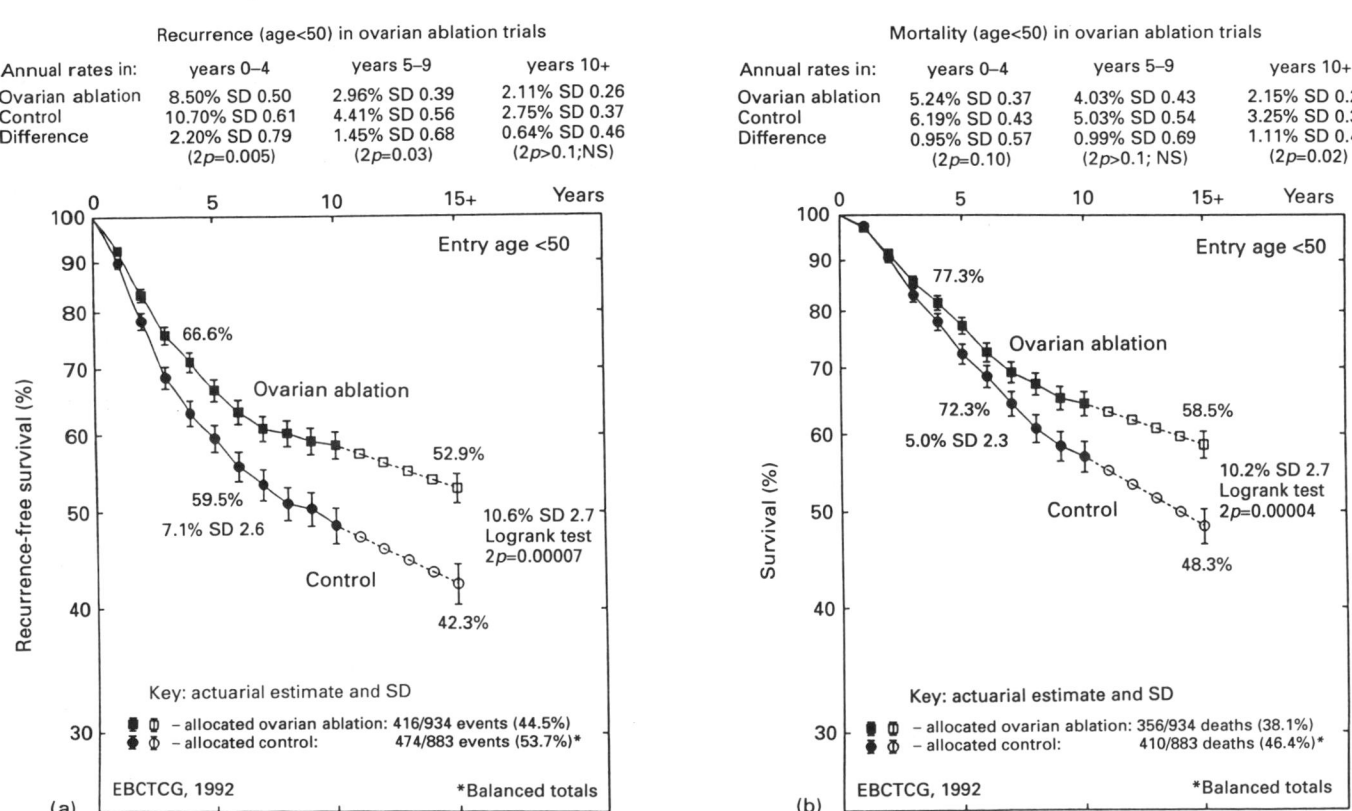

Fig. 18(a) and (b) Fifteen year outcome in ovarian ablation trials for women < 50 years of age.

An example of a trial comparing a short course of perioperative chemotherapy is Trial V of the International Breast Cancer Study Group (IBCSG: formerly the Ludwig Group) (Ludwig Breast Cancer Study Group 1988, 1989). Between 1981 and 1985, 1275 patients with N− breast cancer received either a single course of cyclophosphamide, methotrexate, and 5-fluorouracil or no adjuvant therapy. At 5 years' median follow-up the 5 year disease-free survival percentages were 74 per cent for the adjuvant therapy group and 68 per cent for the controls ($p = 0.04$). The largest magnitude of effect was shown for patients who had low or no oestrogen receptor levels in the primary tumours (ER−). The differences were seen for pre- and post-menopausal patients and the treatment may be considered effective, although additional courses of systemic adjuvant therapy increased the benefit in a cohort of 1229 patients with N+ disease within the same trial (Ludwig Breast Cancer Study Group 1988). For these patients the perioperative start of chemotherapy did not show any significant advantage. Also, using the summary data provided by the overview (4985 patients) (Early Breast Cancer Trialists' Collaborative Group 1992), the effects of perioperative therapy were of small magnitude and only marginally significant (on recurrence). Two recent trials, one of which has been published (Sertoli *et al.* 1991), in which 4-epidoxorubicin (epirubicin) was used in the perioperative regimen, showed a very early reduction in mortality for the patients treated perioperatively. Further follow-up will clarify whether a perioperative treatment with the most effective regimens has a larger impact upon outcome.

The Milan trial is an example of a study comparing prolonged chemotherapy (12 courses of CMF) to surgery alone and is considered to be one of the hypothesis-generating investigations in the field (Bonadonna and Valagussa 1989). Table 12 illustrates the highly significant difference between treatments for pre-menopausal patients, in contrast to the similar outcomes for both treatment groups in the post-menopausal populations. The lack of effect of the treatment programme in post-menopausal women has been attributed to the lower doses of cytotoxics given to the older women in the trial. This feature, of a larger treatment effect for younger women as compared to post-menopausal patients, clearly emerges from the overview data (Table 11 and Fig. 19(a) and (b)) (Early Breast Cancer Trialists' Collaborative Group 1992).

The trials of single-agent chemotherapy versus multidrug combination indicate that polychemotherapy improves outcome in terms of reduction of recurrences and prolongation of survival, especially for pre-menopausal patients. These results refer mainly to alkylating agents. Whether the same is true for anthracyclines has not been studied.

Table 12 Median disease-free survival and overall survival at 14 years for patients randomized to 1 year of CMF or no adjuvant therapy (control) in the Milan trial

Patient group	Median disease-free (months)		Median survival (months)	
	Control	CMF	Control	CMF
All	40	83	104	140
N+				
1–3 nodes	63	141	130	Not reached
4 or more	20	44	77	82
Pre-menopausal	32	141	96	Not reached
Post-menopausal	59	64	128	113

The cyclophosphamide, methotrexate, 5-fluorouracil combination (CMF) has been compared to the same combination plus either low-dose continuous or high-dose intermittent prednisone and to a drug combination which includes vincristine given weekly (cyclophosphamide, methotrexate, 5-fluorouracil, vincristine, prednisone; CMFVP) but no advantage in favour of the four- or five-drug regimens has been demonstrated. Initially the CMF regimen included the following doses (cyclophosphamide, $100\ mg/m^2$ orally, daily during days 1–14, methotrexate, $40\ mg/m^2$ intravenously, days 1 and 8, and 5-fluorouracil, $600\ mg/m^2$ intravenously, days 1 and 8; the entire cycle is repeated every 28 days). Variations included the intravenous administration of cyclophosphamide ($600\ mg/m^2$ together with methotrexate and fluorouracil, all three given on day 1 every 3 weeks or on days 1 and 8 every 4 weeks). In advanced disease the first

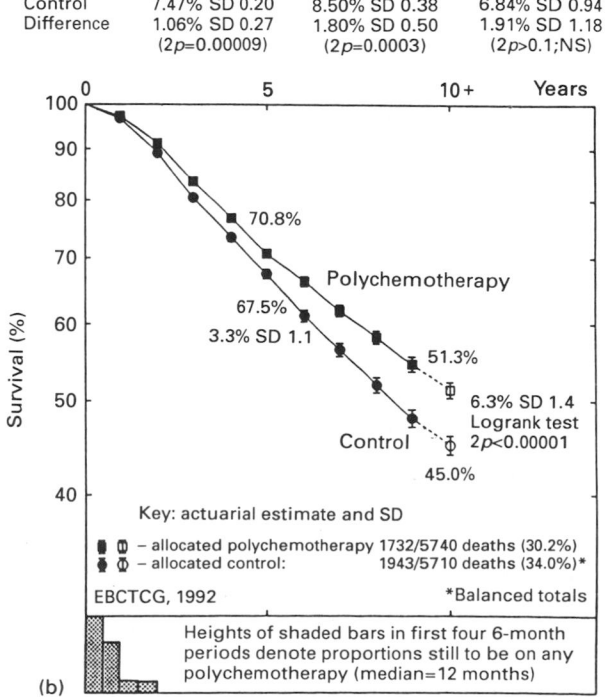

Recurrence (all ages) in polychemotherapy trials

Annual rates in:	years 0–4	years 5–9	years 10+
Polychem.	10.96% SD 0.25	6.14% SD 0.35	5.45% SD 0.84
Control	15.12% SD 0.32	7.09% SD 0.41	3.96% SD 0.85
Difference	4.16% SD 0.41 (2p<0.00001)	0.94% SD 0.54 (2p=0.08)	1.49% SD 1.19 (2p>0.1;NS)

Mortality (all ages) in polychemotherapy trials

Annual rates in:	years 0–4	years 5–9	years 10+
Polychem.	6.40% SD 0.18	6.70% SD 0.32	4.93% SD 0.71
Control	7.47% SD 0.20	8.50% SD 0.38	6.84% SD 0.94
Difference	1.06% SD 0.27 (2p=0.00009)	1.80% SD 0.50 (2p=0.0003)	1.91% SD 1.18 (2p>0.1;NS)

Fig. 19(a) and (b) Ten year outcome in polychemotherapy trials for patients of all ages.

version of CMF proved to be more effective than the all-intravenous CMF regimen given once every 3 weeks.

Comparisons of Adriamycin[R] (doxorubicin)-containing regimens with other multidrug combination therapies were based upon observations made in advanced disease. Their application was associated with higher response rates, although differences in overall survival were rare. Results are available from several studies in which an Adriamycin[R] or epirubicin combination was added in some manner to the therapy. In many of these trials the use of the anthracycline was associated with a significant improvement in the disease-free survival as compared to a CMF-type regimen. Overall survival was usually no different for the two treatments; this was because the sample size of the individual studies was too small to detect a difference which might be below 10 per cent (Carpenter *et al.* 1991). The largest of these trials was the National Surgical Adjuvant Breast and Bowel Project B-15, in which a regimen of Adriamycin[R] (60 mg/m^2 intravenously) and cyclophosphamide (600 mg/m^2 intravenously), both given on day 1 every 3 weeks for four cycles, was compared with six courses of CMF (Fisher *et al.* 1990*a*). The outcome in terms of disease-free survival and overall survival was similar for the two treatments. No sufficient data on this subject were available in the overview database, since these trials started before 1985. It is likely, however, that the next generation update will provide a definite answer to whether an anthracycline should be used initially. Some of the available data do not clarify the issue at all: one Milan trial, in patients with four or more positive axillary nodes, showed the superiority of Adriamycin[R] administered for four initial courses followed by CMF, as compared to the two types of treatment given alternately (Buzzoni *et al.* 1991). Another trial at the same institute, in women with one to three positive nodes, indicated the slight (not significant) advantage in favour of a CMF combination, compared to the same combination if followed by Adriamycin[R] (Moliterni *et al.* 1991). In view of the potential long-term cardiac toxicity of Adriamycin[R] and of the need to keep this extreme active agent in reserve for purposes of palliation in case of need, additional data are needed to assess its role as 'standard' adjuvant therapy in operable breast cancer.

It is commonly believed that the higher the dose of cytotoxic drugs, the more effective the treatment. This is based upon the increased complete response rates in trials investigating the dose–response relationship in advanced breast cancer, even though such high-dose therapies do not imply a cure. Retrospective analyses have been performed upon different data sets in an attempt to correlate the failure of response to a given treatment with the lower dose administered and the success of a therapy in patients with the higher doses given. Some of the series confirm the association between higher dose and better outcome and some do not. Several ongoing randomized trials on dose-intensity are being conducted, the largest by the Cancer and Acute Leukemia Group B, the Eastern Cooperative Oncology Group, and the National Surgical Adjuvant Breast and Bowel Project. Many other studies, the majority of which are not randomized, are being conducted with high-dose chemotherapy and the use of colony-stimulating factors (G- or GM-CSFs), usually together with autologous marrow or committed peripheral blood stem cells. These studies represent pilot series in planning randomized trials for patients with a very high risk of relapse, for whom the results of available treatments are very poor (for example, patients with ten or more positive axillary nodes).

Two trials are typical of those that addressed the question of duration of adjuvant cytotoxic therapy. The first is the Milan study of six versus 12 courses of CMF, in which 459 N+ breast cancer patients were included (Bonadonna *et al.* 1987). The 10 year results show an advantage in favour of the shorter treatment course (10 year disease-free survival percentage: 46 per cent for the 12 courses as compared to 53 per cent for the six courses). Based upon this trial, the proper duration of adjuvant cytotoxic therapy with CMF is considered to be six courses.

The second trial is related to the hypothesis that the first course of chemotherapy, if given perioperatively (immediately after surgery), might yield results in terms of outcome similar to those of the therapies of longer duration. Trial V of the International Breast Cancer Study Group (Ludwig Breast Cancer Study Group 1988) showed, in a population of 1229 N+ patients, that one course of chemotherapy is significantly inferior to the prolonged treatment of 6–7 months in terms of both disease-free survival and overall survival. The search for an 'optimal' duration, which, according to the available data, is more than one and perhaps less than six courses, is ongoing.

Studying the question of timing of adjuvant chemotherapy has entailed important practical and logistical challenges. Non-randomized pre-surgical chemotherapy has been studied under a variety of clinical conditions but has not yielded convincing evidence of benefit greater than that achieved with the established mode of therapy administered only after surgical removal of the primary and axillary nodes for histopathological staging. In a recent series, chemotherapy was given uniformly to patients with large tumours (≥ 3 cm) to reduce tumour size and, thus, improve the chances of successful breast conservation (Bonadonna and Valagussa 1989). More than 90 per cent of the patients were enabled to have a less-than-mastectomy procedure. In some trials, pre-operative chemotherapy is being compared to the post-operative administration of cytotoxic drugs. The largest study might be the National Surgical Adjuvant Breast and Bowel Project trial B-18, in which four pre-operative courses of Adriamycin[R] and cyclophosphamide are compared to the same courses administered post-operatively. Its results will be of relevance to the question of whether adjuvant therapy may improve the outcome even more if given pre-operatively.

The question of whether early administration of chemotherapy (immediately after surgery) might improve outcome, as compared to the usual delayed administration after removal of stitches and healing of the wound (4–6 weeks), has been asked in a single randomized trial (Trial V of the International Breast Cancer Study Group) (Ludwig Breast Cancer Study Group 1988). Indirect evidence from a study of the Scandinavian Group (Nissen-Meyer *et al.* 1978), using a single course of cyclophosphamide alone for 6 days, showed that in all participating hospitals where the drug had been administered immediately after surgery there was a benefit in favour of the treated patients. In the only hospital in which, due to referral patterns, the treatment started with a delay as short as 3 weeks, no advantage in terms of disease-free survival or overall survival could be observed. Trial V showed that no advantage is obtained by starting the adjuvant chemotherapy immediately after surgery compared with the usual delay provided that 6–7 months of adjuvant therapy are administered. The 6 year disease-free survival percentage, for the 815 patients with N+ breast cancer who were randomized to perioperative chemotherapy followed by prolonged 'conventionally timed' treatment, was identical (49 per cent) to that for patients who started therapy only 25–36 days after operation.

The delayed and repeated administration of cytotoxic drugs after initial courses of adjuvant systemic therapy and treatment-free intervals is the subject of recent trials (Goldhirsch and Gelber 1987; B. Fisher *et al.* 1990*a*). These trials are based on the previously mentioned hypothesis according to which cell kill is enhanced during spurts of fast tumour growth (Retsky *et al.* 1987) and on the fact that the treatment used in the adjuvant setting is still effective in subsequent metastatic disease, indicating a lack of definitive resistance to therapy of the tumour cells.

A beneficial effect of adjuvant prolonged multidrug chemotherapy in reducing relapse and mortality has been observed in pre-menopausal patients early during follow-up. Investigations aimed at correlating this effect upon outcome with the amenorrhoea observed in a large number of the pre-menopausal patients gave controversial results. While initial investigations on patients in the Milan and the National Surgical Adjuvant Breast and Bowel Project trials with CMF (78 patients) and melphalan (L-PAM), alone or with 5-fluorouracil (96 patients), showed no relationship between amenorrhoea and treatment effect, additional analyses, conducted for 1839 patients from several trials, showed some association between the cessation of menses and improved prognosis. The effects of amenorrhoea were also seen almost exclusively in the subpopulation of patients with positive oestrogen receptors. These observations have led to the speculation that adjuvant cytotoxic therapy is effective only because it causes a chemically induced oophorectomy (Goldhirsch *et al.* 1987). Evidence that adjuvant cytotoxic therapy is also effective in patients with tumours having no oestrogen receptors and that it produces effects which begin to appear early during follow-up, has been cited in support of arguments against a major role for an endocrine mechanism. An extensive analysis of a cohort of 1127 pre-menopausal patients with breast cancer, who received either no cytotoxic therapy, a single short course, or a prolonged chemotherapy (six or seven courses), has been conducted. Amenorrhoea was associated with an increased disease-free survival only in patients with prolonged cytotoxic therapy (387 N+ patients of whom 68 per cent ceased menses): the 4 year disease-free survival percentages were 68 and 61 per cent, for the groups with amenorrhoea and without amnenorrhoea, respectively ($p = 0.05$). In contrast, the comparison between prolonged chemotherapy and one single course among N+ patients (387 versus 188 N+ pre-menopausal patients included in the International Breast Cancer Study Group Trial V) (Ludwig Breast Cancer Study Group 1988) showed a much larger difference in treatment effect: 4 year disease-free survival percentages were 66 and 38 per cent, respectively ($p < 0.0001$). It might be concluded that although cytotoxic-induced amenorrhoea is associated with a better outcome, it is unlikely that this form of endocrine manipulation is the main mechanism of response to adjuvant systemic chemotherapy in pre-menopausal women.

Adjuvant systemic endocrine therapy with the anti-oestrogen, tamoxifen, was initiated in clinical trials because of the recognition of its effects on advanced disease and because of the demonstration of excellent tolerance towards this drug (Mouridsen *et al.* 1978). An example of the use of tamoxifen as an adjuvant is a trial of the Scottish group (Scottish Cancer Trials Office 1987). The drug was given as an adjuvant for at least 5 years, the results being compared with those of its use upon relapse. This study included 1312 women, of whom 242 were pre-menopausal with N− disease and 1070 were post-menopausal with both N− and N+ breast cancer. There was an advantage, in terms of disease-free survival and overall survival, at the end of the eighth year of follow-up, which was statistically significant for the entire population, for the N+ cohort and for the post-menopausal women. Table 13 describes the differences in the median disease-free and overall survival periods for the two treatment groups at 8 years' median follow-up time. This trial is important because it reports a population in which the comparison

Table 13 Median disease-free survival and overall survival at 8 years for patients randomized to 5 years' adjuvant tamoxifen (TAM) or to no adjuvant therapy and tamoxifen given only upon relapse (control) in the Scottish trial

Patient group	Median disease-free (months)		Median survival (months)	
	Control	TAM	Control	TAM
All	73	Not reached	95	Not reached
N−	Not reached	Not reached	Not reached	Not reached
N+	31	84	63	85

made is between the same treatments given either as adjuvant or as delayed therapy upon relapse (which was applied in more than 90 per cent of the patients in whom the disease reappeared). The fact that a significant overall survival difference has been demonstrated is indirect evidence that early administration of antineoplastic agents, which fail to achieve cure when applied at the advanced disease stage, may do so in the presence of a smaller tumour burden, which is assumed to be the case in the adjuvant setting. The effects of tamoxifen upon relapse-free survival and upon overall survival are confirmed by the overview update which extends this analysis at least up to the tenth year (Table 11 and Fig. 20(b)) (Early Breast Cancer Trialists' Collaborative Group 1992).

The dosage of adjuvant tamoxifen has not been studied. Doses between 20 and 40 mg a day have been given in various trials. A recent report of an excess of endometrial cancer in patients who received 40 mg a day for at least 2 years (Fornander *et al.* 1989, 1991) could not be confirmed in an analysis of the Scottish trial in which a dose of 20 mg a day was given for 5 years (Stewart and Knight 1989). Indirect comparisons within the overview show no differences between the outcome in studies in which doses of 20 mg were used as compared to those with doses of 30–40 mg/day (Early Breast Cancer Trialists' Collaborative Group 1992). Assuming equivalent antineoplastic effectiveness for these two doses of tamoxifen, the recommended dose is therefore 20 mg a day.

The question of the optimum duration of endocrine therapy with tamoxifen has not yet been clarified. Indirect evidence from non-randomized comparisons suggests that the administration of tamoxifen should continue for at least 2–5 years. This should be the basis for therapy decision-making outside of clinical investigations, at least until the results from randomized studies of 5 years versus continuous administration become available.

Data of the response to adjuvant endocrine therapy according to the oestrogen receptor content of the primary tumour are somewhat controversial. The controversy arises from data on the positive effects of tamoxifen seen in retrospective analyses of British trials for patients with ER− primaries (Nolvadex Adjuvant Trial Organisation 1985; Scottish Cancer Trials Office 1987). Data from trials III and IV of the International Breast Cancer Study Group (Goldhirsch and Gelber 1986) show that only patients who had ER+ primaries benefited from the endocrine therapy with tamoxifen and low-dose prednisone given for 1 year. Also in other trials investigating tamoxifen alone, in a population with patients whose tumours contain or lack oestrogen receptors, only the ER+ subpopulation benefited (Henderson 1991). The response to adjuvant tamoxifen for patients with ER− primaries might, however, be explained by results of recent experiments which related the drug's activity to the production of transforming growth factor β, which inhibits the growth of breast cancer cells regardless of their steroid hormone receptor content (Lippman *et al.* 1986). Transforming growth factor β is, however, produced in cells

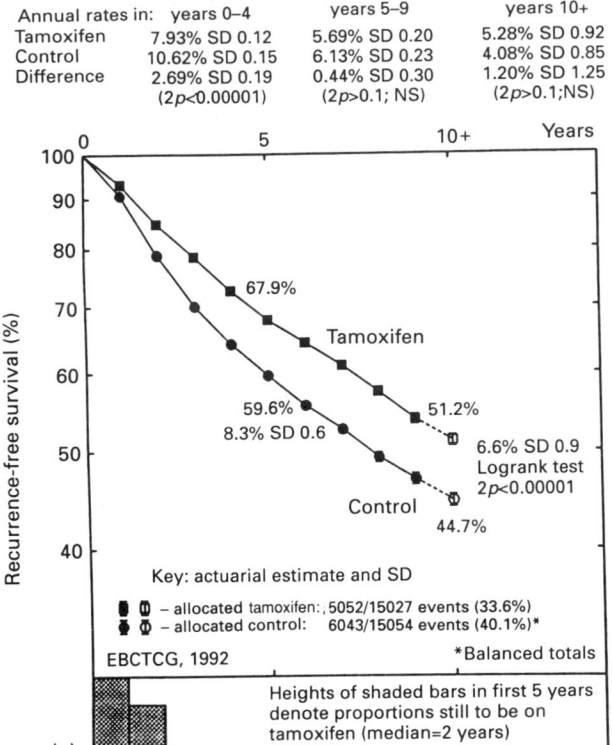

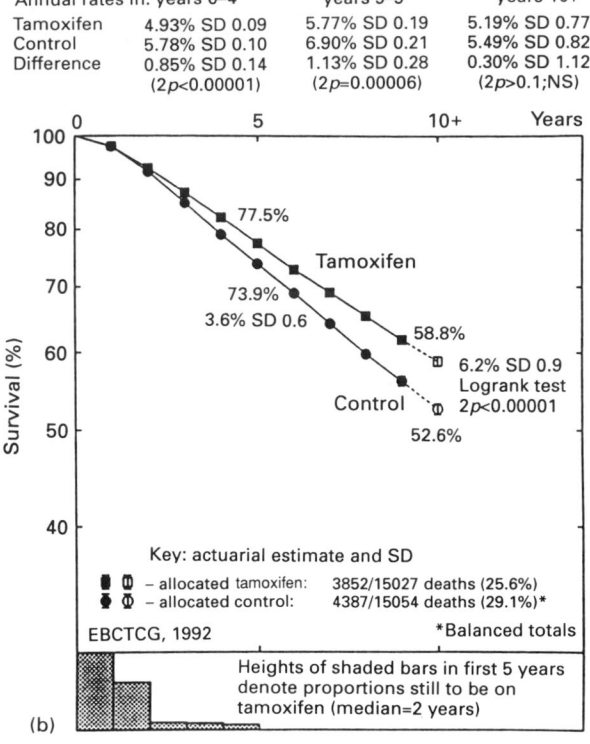

Fig. 20(a) and (b) Ten year outcome in tamoxifen trials for patients of all ages.

containing oestrogen receptors. The definition of benefit from an endocrine treatment alone to the population of patients with ER− tumour, especially those of post-menopausal age, awaits the maturation of trials specifically investigating this issue.

Combined chemoendocrine therapies have been the subject of many trials, most of which are either too small to be conclusive or which have had too brief a follow-up. The rationale for combining the two modalities was the possibility of finding synergistic or additive effects on tumour cells. The two therapies have different spectrums of toxicity which facilitate their simultaneous use. A review of chemoendocrine trials in advanced disease showed a significant advantage in terms of remission rates in 8 of the 12 studies which compared chemoendocrine to endocrine therapy alone. Only in one trial was there an overall survival advantage for the combination. In eight of the 13 published trials, the comparison of the combination versus chemotherapy alone showed an increased remission rate for the combination. There was an advantage in terms of survival in two trials. The higher response rate for the combination by itself justified its being tested in the adjuvant setting.

The overview update contains trials that started before 1985. Data on combined chemoendocrine therapies, especially in comparison to endocrine therapy alone, are therefore scarce. Table 11 describes the treatment effects observed with the combination of polychemotherapy and endocrine treatments such as oophorectomy (for pre-menopausal women) or tamoxifen (for both, pre- and post-menopausal patients). It appears that for pre-menopausal women the available data indicate a lack of response to the combination as compared to each treatment modality alone.

Factors involved in interpreting results related to this issue are illustrated by three recent trials. In the National Surgical Adjuvant Breast and Bowel Project Trial B-09, 779 patients were randomized

Table 14 Five year disease-free survival (DFS) rates and overall survival (OS) rates for patients included in the NSABP trial B-09 by menopausal and receptor status

Patient group	Five year DFS (%)			Five year OS (%)		
	PF	PFT	*p*-value	PF	PFT	*p*-value
All	47	52	0.002	67	67	0.8
Age <50	49	50	0.98	67	64	0.27
ER− PR−	41	38	0.4	56	44	0.06
ER− PR+	55	43	0.4	65	66	0.9
ER+ PR−	55	41	0.08	70	56	0.07
ER+ PR+	51	60	0.1	69	75	0.4
Age >49	44	54	0.001	67	70	0.27
ER− PR−	29	39	0.4	44	46	0.9
ER− PR+	45	48	0.9	58	59	0.7
ER+ PR−	52	48	0.6	75	67	0.3
ER+ PR+	45	56	0.002	76	74	0.9

Abbreviations: ER, oestrogen receptor; PR, progesterone receptor.

to receive either PF (melphalan and 5-fluorouracil) or the combination of the two cytotoxics with tamoxifen (PFT) (B. Fisher *et al.* 1986). The results showed a qualitative difference of response according to age and steroid hormone receptor status (Table 14): pre-menopausal women who had one of the receptors classified as negative, had a shorter disease-free and overall survival rate after receiving chemoendocrine therapy. One explanation for this derives from experiments showing a clear antagonism between tamoxifen and both melphalan and 5-fluorouracil, in which the endocrine agent inhibits the cytotoxic efficacy of the two chemotherapeutic agents (Osborne 1988). The results of the National Surgical Adjuvant

Breast and Bowel Project trial may be interpreted as related to a reduced effect of the combination, due to the antagonism between the cytotoxics and tamoxifen, being particularly evident in those who obtain the maximum of tumour cell kill with chemotherapy (that is, pre-menopausal patients), while for post-menopausal women, more responsive to tamoxifen therapy (especially if having receptor-positive tumours), the effect of the endocrine agent is sufficient to produce some benefit over chemotherapy alone. In trials with a direct comparison between the two treatments, tamoxifen and multi-agent chemotherapy, a significant advantage was described in favour of the cytotoxic regimen in the pre-menopausal cohort and for the tamoxifen therapy in the post-menopausal women (Kaufmann *et al.* 1987).

In trial III of the International Breast Cancer Study Group, the combination of chemotherapy and tamoxifen (CMF combination with low-dose continuous prednisone (7.5 mg a day) and tamoxifen: the CMFp+T regimen (administered for 12 courses)) was compared to p+T alone given for 12 months and to a surgical control group. Table 15 describes the results after 5 and 10 years, which indicate the late appearance of a significant advantage to overall survival, as compared to an early disease-free survival benefit, in favour of the patients who received the combined chemoendocrine therapy. Preliminary results of an Italian trial showed an improved control of disease, especially in post-menopausal women, by the combination as compared to both chemotherapy alone and tamoxifen alone in a patient population with N+ and ER+ disease (Boccardo *et al.* 1990). The benefit from the combination was seen in patients with a large number of positive nodes, that is, with a more aggressive presentation. Similarly, the National Surgical Adjuvant Breast and Bowel Project trial B-16 for patients aged 50 years or more, with tumours responsive to tamoxifen (according to a previous definition by the National Surgical Adjuvant Breast and Bowel Project, based on results from B-09), treated with a combination of

chemoendocrine therapy versus tamoxifen alone, showed a significant improvement of outcome for the combination (B. Fisher *et al.* 1990*b*). The toxic effects of combined chemoendocrine therapies were also studied extensively (Goldhirsch 1984; Saphner *et al.* 1991) and it is mandatory that these be taken into account in every cost–benefit evaluation for patient care purposes.

Some evidence exists that prolonging the duration of treatment with tamoxifen beyond the cessation of the initial chemoendocrine therapy might provide additional benefit, especially if disease-free survival is taken into consideration (Falkson *et al.* 1989). On the other hand, the issue of treatment of pre-menopausal patients with tamoxifen after cessation of therapy with either chemotherapy alone or with combined CMF and tamoxifen remains unsettled. Reports of increased uterine pathology in patients on tamoxifen, as well as patterns of relapse in young patients after cessation of tamoxifen treatment, require that all pre-menopausal patients who receive long-term tamoxifen be treated within the framework of clinical trials.

The combination of chemotherapy and ablative surgery was rarely studied. Trial II of the International Breast Cancer Study Group (Ludwig Breast Cancer Study Group 1985; The International Breast Cancer Study Group 1990) investigated the role of oophorectomy followed by 12 courses of chemotherapy in pre- and perimenopausal women with four or more positive axillary nodes. While the 4 year results of trial II did not differ for the two treatment groups, an analysis at 8 years' median follow-up showed some benefit in favour of the combined treatment, which appeared only after 5 years. Although not statistically significant, the difference was confined to the subpopulation with ER+ tumours. An interesting observation is that averted relapses in the oophorectomy group are exclusively in the skeleton. A second trial, conducted by the Southwestern Cooperative Oncology Group (Rivkin *et al.* 1991), compared in a N+ ER+ pre-menopausal population the combination of cyclophosphamide, methotrexate, 5-fluorouracil, vincristine, and prednisone (CMFVP) (administered continuously for 12 months) with the same combination preceded by surgical oophorectomy. Only 314 patients could be accrued in 11 years and the 5 year disease-free survival values were 61 and 67 per cent, respectively.

New approaches, including the combination of ovarian function suppression with analogues of luteinizing-hormone-releasing hormone together with adjuvant chemotherapy, are under investigation.

The use of systemic adjuvant therapy for patients with node-negative disease has been a matter of controversy in recent years, not because clinical research in this field is more difficult than in patients with positive nodes, but rather because of the way clinical data are interpreted. Patients with node-negative disease generally have a better prognosis and the absolute differences between those who receive adjuvant therapy and those who do not are likely to be small, especially during the first years after diagnosis. An attempt to identify factors which will predict a higher relapse rate and a shorter survival and thus assist in the selection of a population which might have a better chance of response, has been only partially successful. Even excluding patients with ER− primaries and with large tumours did not lead to the selection of a population which had, in the context of randomized trials, an estimated relapse rate at 5 years of less than 20 per cent. Table 16 lists some trials carried out in populations with N− breast cancer (Caffier *et al.* 1984; Senn *et al.* 1986; Bonadonna *et al.* 1987; Jakesz *et al.* 1987; Morrison *et al.* 1987; Williams *et al.* 1987; B. Fisher *et al.* 1989*a,b*; Ludwig Breast Cancer Study Group 1989; Mansour *et al.* 1989). An analysis of the data from these individual trials, in conjunction with data

Table 15 Five and 10 year disease-free survival (DFS) rates and overall survival (OS) rates for post-menopausal patients (65 years old or younger) included in trial III of the IBCSG; overall results and by oestrogen receptor status

Patient group	DFS (%)		OS (%)	
	5 year	10 year	5 year	10 year
All				
Observ.	30	18	59	35
p+T	42*	29*	63	41*
CMFp+T	58*	38*	70	49*
ER+				
Observ.	30	20	72	40
p+T	55	32	80	41
CMFp+T	60	30	74	48
ER−				
Observ.	30	21	45	33
p+T	20*	17*	37	23(*)
CMFp+T	63*	47*	63	49(*)
ER unknown				
Observ.	30	15	56	32
p+T	44(*)	31(*)	63	47
CMFp+T	57(*)	42(*)	70	50

*Pairwise comparisons of chemoendocrine therapy versus endocrine therapy alone, $p < 0.05$; (*) $p = 0.07-0.05$.
Abbreviations: CMFp+T, cyclophosphamide+methotrexate+5-fluorouracil+prednisone-+tamoxifen; ER, oestrogen receptor; Observ., observation; p+T prednisone+tamoxifen.

Table 16 Trials of adjuvant systemic therapy in node-negative breast cancer. All trials evaluate chemotherapy except NSABP Trial B-14

Trial	Therapy	No. of patients; population		Year	Disease-free survival (%) Rx	Control
OSAKO	LMF×6	122;	all	14	62	54
Midlands	LMF×8 low dose	543;	all	10	n.a.	n.a.
Mainz	CMF×12	175;	all	5	82	72
Wien	CFVbM×8 (in 3 years)	128;	all	5	86	78
Cardiff	VAC×6	52;	ER−	3	83*	71*
Milan	i.v.CMF×12	90;	ER−	7	85*	42*
NSABP B-13	M→F×13	737;	ER−	5	74*	65*
Intergroup	CMFP×6	425;	ER− or ER+ if T>3 cm	5	83*	61*
Trial V	i.v. CMF×1 (periop.)	1275;	all	5	74*	68*
NSABP B-14	Tam×5 yr	2644;	ER+	5	82*	72*

*Statistically significant difference.
n.a., not available.
Abbreviations: CMF, cyclophosphamide, methotrexate, 5-fluorouracil; CMFP, cyclophosphamide, methotrexate, 5-fluorouracil, prednisone;. CFVbM, cyclophosphamide, 5-fluorouracil, vinblastine, methotrexate; F, 5-fluorouracil; LMF, chlorambucil (Leukeran™), methotrexate, 5-fluorouracil; M, methotrexate; periop., perioperative; T, tumour; Tam, tamoxifen; VAC, vincristine, actinomycin D, cyclophosphamide.

Table 17 Effects of treatment for patients with prolonged adjuvant tamoxifen versus no adjuvant tamoxifen (Tam) and prolonged adjuvant multi-agent chemotherapy (CT) versus no adjuvant chemotherapy, by nodal status and age (Early Breast Cancer Trialists' Collaborative Group 1992)

	Typical reduction in annual odds of recurrence or death (%±SD) Recurrence <50	≥50	Any age	Death <50	≥50	Any age
Tam v. nil						
Node negative	22±8	28±4	26±4	19±12	16±5	17±5
Node positive	11±4	33±2	28±2	5±5	22±3	18±2
Poly CT v. nil						
Node negative	26±10	27±9	26±7	6±13	23±11	18±8
Node positive	41±5	23±4	30±3	30±6	11±4	18±3

labelling index (high versus low), flow cytometry analyses (aneuploid or diploid with a large S-phase component), oestrogen receptor content of the tumour (low concentrations or no detectable receptor versus high concentrations), expression of epithelial growth factor receptor (high versus low), amplification or overexpression of the c-erb-B2 oncogene (high versus low), the expression of a lysosomal enzyme, cathepsin D (high versus low), and the expression of heat shock protein (high versus low). The prognostic value of each of these factors is under investigation (McGuire 1991), as is the benefit obtainable from adjuvant systemic therapy for a N− patient population. Outside of clinical trials, the risks of acute and potentially delayed toxicities, as well as the magnitude of the benefits to be derived, must be explained to the patient before a mutual therapeutic decision is made.

Chemotherapy regimens and their toxicities

Many chemotherapy regimens were included in trials of adjuvant therapy for early breast cancer and some of them were subsequently widely used. The question of whether there are data to prove one regimen superior to the others can only partially be answered. The cyclophosphamide (100 mg/m² orally, days 1−14), methotrexate (40 mg/m² intravenously, days 1 and 8), 5-fluorouracil (600 mg/m² intravenously, days 1 and 8) combination (CMF) given every 28 days has been found to be superior to single-agent therapy, mainly melphalan (0.15 mg/kg daily for 5 consecutive days every 6 weeks) and, in one large trial, also cyclophosphamide (130 mg/m² daily for 14 days every 28 days). The acute toxicity of the CMF regimen includes gastrointestinal side-effects, nausea, vomiting, some mucositis, conjunctivitis, and diarrhoea and, in approximately 40 per cent of the patients, alopecia (which, for most of these patients, requires the use of a wig). The use of more complex regimens, including either prednisone (alone at low dose continuously or at high dose intermittently) or prednisone and vincristine (the CMFVP regimen, with cyclophosphamide and prednisone administered continuously; methotrexate, 5-fluorouracil, and vincristine weekly) did not improve the outcome in trials of direct comparison. To improve on the therapeutic index by excluding cyclophosphamide and substituting chlorambucil (LMF regimen) has been attempted, but the results of a single trial of the Swiss group are not conclusive. Late side-effects of cytotoxic drug regimens were reported almost exclusively for melphalan combinations by the National Surgical Adjuvant Breast and Bowel

available from other studies which included both node-positive and node-negative patients and which mainly investigated adjuvant tamoxifen, indicate no survival advantage. However, no difference in overall survival is to be expected due to a relatively short follow-up. The analysis of the overview data of all available trials (Early Breast Cancer Trialists' Collaborative Group 1992) shows no difference in the relative magnitude of treatment effects among N+ and N− patients (staged by axillary sampling or dissection) (Table 17). Another fact emerges from the review of trials of adjuvant therapy for N− disease. The prognoses of the no-adjuvant therapy cohorts are worse than expected. In the National Surgical Adjuvant Breast and Bowel Project trial B-14, 28 per cent of patients, all of whom had ER+ tumours, were estimated to relapse within 5 years. In the International Breast Cancer Study Group trial V, in which patients entered before histopathological determination of prognostic factors (perioperative randomization), 32 per cent of the adjuvant-untreated N− patients were estimated to relapse within 5 years.

The search for prognostic factors which might predict either a low-risk N− population or a high-risk cohort includes identification of histopathological, functional, and biological features. These include tumour size (≥ 2 cm versus smaller), site of the primary (internal quadrants of the breast versus other), nuclear and histological grade (poor and high, respectively, versus other grades),

Project. There was an 11-fold increase in acute leukaemia and a 24-fold increase in acute myelogenous leukaemia within the first 10 years of follow-up after a 2 year treatment with this drug (B. Fisher *et al.* 1985*b*). Analysis of second malignancies with CMF or LMF did not reveal differences between the treatment groups and the controls. The issue of Adriamycin^R-containing regimens has been discussed previously in this chapter. Toxic effects of anthracyclines include haematological and mucosal toxicity, nausea and vomiting, alopecia (almost universal and difficult to protect from), skin pigmentation, and, especially, cumulative cardiac toxicity.

Breast conservation and adjuvant systemic therapies

Most of the trials regarding the use of adjuvant systemic therapies were carried out in patients who had undergone mastectomy. Adjuvant therapy was therefore usually started after a delay of 4–6 weeks. The increasing proportion of patients who choose a breast-conserving procedure, which implies, in accord with our present knowledge, irradiation of the remaining breast, raises a question of priorities. Combined chemotherapy and radiation therapy has been reported by some as a feasible procedure but others observed an impaired cosmetic result (Gore *et al.* 1987). The order of the sequential use of both modalities represents a controversy. On one hand, data are available showing that radiation may be delayed until after the systemic therapy has been completed (3–6 months after surgery), since breast relapse rates for patients whose tumours were small enough for a breast-conserving therapy are below 2 per cent within this time period. On the other hand, a retrospective analysis of delaying radiation therapy beyond the completion of adjuvant systemic chemotherapy showed a detrimental effect (Recht *et al.* 1991). Ongoing trials will provide a clear answer to the questions of sequence and timing in the near future. In the meanwhile, evidence on the prognostic features of the disease should guide the sequential order of the two modalities.

Quality of life-oriented evaluation

Analysis of results from clinical trials which investigated the relevance of adjuvant therapy for the treated populations focused upon benefits in terms of disease-free survival and overall survival. A recurring theme in analysing data from individual trials is the relatively early appearance of a disease-free survival benefit for treated patients and the occasional late emergence of an overall survival advantage. Another end-point was developed which, in a comparative analysis between two or more treatments differing from each other by subjective toxicity, took into account the time spent without symptoms of recurrent disease and toxic effects of therapy (TWiST) (Gelber and Goldhirsch 1986*b*; Goldhirsch *et al.* 1989; Gelber *et al.* 1991). In this analysis, a month of TWiST was removed for any month in which subjective side-effects of therapy were recorded, even those which lasted a single day or less. Three months were removed beyond the end of adjuvant therapy to allow hair regrowth for patients with alopecia and adjustment for those with significant weight gain. The same time period was removed in case of an isolated local recurrence. The remainder of a patient's lifetime was removed from the analysis if the patient developed distant metastases or a second malignant disease other than breast cancer. The method was applied to a trial (International Breast Cancer Study Group trial III) which investigated 1 year of chemoendocrine therapy (cyclophosphamide, methotrexate, 5-fluorouracil, low-dose prednisone, and tamoxifen; CMFp+T) versus 1 year of adjuvant

Table 18 Components of Q-TWiST for the three treatments in trial III, CMFp+T, p+T, and observation (for regimens see text). Mean months of experienced toxicity (TOX), time without symptoms and toxicity (TWiST), and time with overt symptomatic relapse (REL) accumulated within 84 months of randomization, with Q-TWiST calculated for the arbitrary utility coefficient of 0.5 (u tox = u rel = 0.5) for both TOX and REL

	CMFp+T	p+T	Observation
TOX	9.6	2.0	0.0
TWiST	50.3	47.1	41.5
REL	7.1	12.9	20.9
Q-TWiST (u tox = u rel = 0.5)	58.7	54.6	51.9

endocrine therapy alone (p+T) versus no adjuvant treatment (observation). During the first years after adjuvant therapy, patients in the observation group had a much larger TWiST than did the treated patients. However, as disease-free survival benefits began to emerge and to increase for the patients who had adjuvant therapy, their TWiST increased to such an extent that after a 72 month period the mean gain was of 6 months compared to the observation patients. This advantage was statistically significant. This initial pragmatic approach, in which life with toxicity and life beyond relapse were compared to death, was then further elaborated to allow quality adjustments. A quality-adjusted TWiST method (Goldhirsch *et al.* 1989) (Q-TWiST) which better suits a quality of life-oriented approach, allowed the application of utility coefficients to every time-component spent with either toxic effects or with symptoms of disease and to describe the ranges of values for which the mean gain in terms of adjusted TWiST will indicate the significant superiority of one treatment over another. Table 18 describes the components of Q-TWiST for the three treatments in trial III. Mean months of experienced toxicity (TOX), time without symptoms and toxicity (TWiST), and time with overt symptomatic relapse (REL) accumulated within 84 months of randomization, with Q-TWiST calculated for an arbitrary utility coefficient of 0.5 for both TOX and REL, are shown. Quality of life issues were introduced in some trials of adjuvant therapy by using validated instruments to allow a better appreciation of patients' perceptions of each component of their lives after the diagnosis of breast cancer (Levine *et al.* 1988). Future research might allow the integration of patients' perceptions of toxicity, symptoms of disease, well-being, and coping for evaluating benefits from therapies (Gelber *et al.* 1989).

Treatment of elderly patients

Breast cancer in the elderly is a considerable public health problem. Approximately 45 per cent of all newly diagnosed breast cancers are estimated to occur in women above the age of 65 years. In this age-group the yearly incidence rate of breast cancer is estimated to exceed 320 per 100 000 population (Stewart and Foster 1989; Yancik *et al.* 1989). Co-morbid conditions and compromised functional status are usually the basis for the tendency to exclude the elderly from randomized clinical trials (Allen *et al.* 1986; Samet *et al.* 1986). Guidelines for treating elderly patients are usually extrapolated from the results of trials conducted in a younger population. However, a recent survey showed that in terms of survival, elderly women do as well as younger patients for locally and regionally confined disease stages, but far worse for distant metastatic disease. Data are available from three trials in which the elderly were specifically treated with an endocrine therapy (Table 19) (Mouridsen *et al.* 1986; Castiglione *et al.* 1990;

Table 19 Trials of adjuvant systemic therapy in a population of elderly women

Trial and age of population	Therapies	Number of patients reported	Year	Results (DFS %)		
				Rx	Control	Significant
ECOG 65–84 yr	Tam 20 mg ×2 yr	168	10	39	12	Yes
Danish 70–79 yr	Tam 30 mg ×1 yr	509	6	41	39	No
IBCSG Trial IV 66–80 yr	Tam 20 mg	320	10	31	20	Yes

Abbreviations: ECOG, Eastern Cooperative Oncology Group; DFS, disease-free survival; IBCSG, International Breast Cancer Study Group; p, prednisone; Tam, tamoxifen.

Cummings *et al.* 1991). These data represent the basis for the treatment recommendation in this age group.

Carcinoma of the breast in man

Breast carcinoma in man is a rare disease (Haagensen 1971); its incidence is approximately 1 per cent of that for women. It usually presents in a more advanced stage and the pectoral fascia is frequently involved, which requires a radical mastectomy for local control. Lymph node involvement has a prognostic value similar to that of female cancer, as has the presence of oestrogen receptors, which are found in approximately 85 per cent of cases (Cupta *et al.* 1980). The prognosis of male breast cancer is also similar to that in females if the nodes are found to be free of disease, but has been described to be worse in patients with nodal disease (N+). Hormonal ablative manipulations, especially orchidectomy, were reported to be associated with a 50–60 per cent response rate in advanced disease, but no reports are available about their use in the adjuvant setting. Similar response rates have been achieved by the use of tamoxifen, anti-androgens, analogues of luteinizing-hormone-releasing hormone, and (slightly lower) oestrogens. Data from a series of 24 male patients who received an adjuvant CMF combination demonstrated an increased overall survival as compared to historical controls (Bagley *et al.* 1987). The test of the role of either adjuvant tamoxifen alone or in the case of ER− disease of chemotherapy followed by tamoxifen, is reasonable.

Patterns of relapse after adjuvant systemic therapy and response to 'salvage treatment'

Patients who relapse during or soon after an adjuvant systemic therapy (with 6–12 months after its cessation) have a dire prognosis. They tend not to respond to the same systemic therapy used as an adjuvant (Valagussa *et al.* 1986). In contrast, the patients who develop metastases long after cessation of adjuvant treatment tend to have an excellent response, especially if the sites of recurrent disease are local, regional, or in soft tissue (Castiglione *et al.* 1989). The complete response rate for these patients is slightly below 50 per cent with the same therapy as given in the adjuvant setting. On the other hand, based on analysis of 818 patients with N+ disease who received adjuvant chemotherapy in International Breast Cancer Study Group trials I and II and of whom 352 patients relapsed, the 5 year survival rate for patients who had visceral metastases or metastases in multiple sites was 16 per cent. The patients with regional metastases and those with bony involvement alone had an

intermediate prognosis, with a 2 year survival rate of 41 per cent as compared to 70 per cent for those with isolated local recurrence or contralateral breast cancer (Goldhirsch *et al.* 1988).

Use of combined modality treatment in locally advanced breast cancer

Locally advanced cancer of the breast is a specific stage of the disease, with marked local or regional extension but without manifestation of distant metastases. The clinical signs which indicate a locally advanced stage are infiltration of the underlying muscles in the presence of a primary larger than 5 cm (T3b), extensive oedema of the skin over the breast, skin ulcerations, inflammatory cancer of the breast, satellite nodes on the skin, fixed axillary nodes, parasternal and supraclavicular nodes, and oedema of the arm. In the past, most of these signs predicted a survival rate at 5 years which varied from 0 to 36 per cent (Haagensen 1971). Retrospective analyses of studies using combination chemotherapy regimens as a part of the treatment strategy have suggested an improvement in outcome for the combined modality (Sheldon *et al.* 1987). Recent pilot studies showed that the use of high-dose chemotherapy, together with colony-stimulating factors and bone-marrow or peripheral committed precursors of blood cells, yields a useful regression of the tumours at that stage. The way to use combined modality together with high-dose chemotherapy and the impact of such combination upon long-term outcome, are as yet a matter of clinical research.

TREATMENT OF OVERT METASTATIC DISEASE

The fact that a patient has developed overt metastases is, with few exceptions, an indication that she will have to live with clinical manifestations of the disease and that she will eventually die of its complications. The treatment for metastatic disease must, therefore, be defined by its efficacy in providing palliation. Considering that the median survival of the population with overt metastases is approximately 2 years, but that the range of survival times extends from a few weeks to more than 35 years, the choice of treatment must take into account not only the extent of the disease and its related symptoms, but also the estimation of its duration. Furthermore, it is essential that the choice of therapy and its timing be adapted to the type of symptoms, if already present and, if not, the likelihood of such to occur. Thus, the objective of treatment should be to increase the total duration of time with no or few disease-related symptoms, using the therapy associated with the lowest cost in terms of side-effects (Goldhirsch and Gelber 1988). All treatment modalities are therefore used in the therapy of metastatic disease and an approach that includes systemic therapy, radiation therapy, or surgery must be discussed in a multidisciplinary setting.

The most frequent sites of metastatic disease have been summarized in a previous paragraph. Table 20 lists useful information for determining the therapeutic approach in metastatic breast cancer. The choice of primary treatment must also take into consideration certain biological features that define the aggressiveness of the disease. A shorter disease-free interval (from diagnosis to appearance of overt metastases), low or no steroid hormone receptor content in the tumour tissue, and multiple organ involvement are all indicators for a short survival. In addition, host-related factors, best objectively quantified by the performance status, also influence the prognosis and, therefore, the choice of first therapy

Table 20 Useful information for determining the therapeutic approach in metastatic breast cancer

Information	Remarks and consequences
Symptoms	Localized, generalized; choice of modality, for example radiation therapy for localized pain due to bone metastases
Sites of metastases (number and type)	Choice of modality and intensity of treatment, for example endocrine therapy for soft tissue metastases or chemotherapy for multiple organ involvement
Menstrual status and age	Choice of type of endocrine therapy (if indicated), for example ovarian function suppression for pre-menopausal patients
Receptor status	Choice of therapy (endocrine yes versus no)
Disease-free interval from diagnosis to first overt metastasis	Choice of therapy (for example intensive for short; 'milder' for long)
Prior therapy (chemo- or endocrine therapy) and response	Choice of therapy (endocrine versus chemotherapy), for example secondary endocrine therapy if previous response

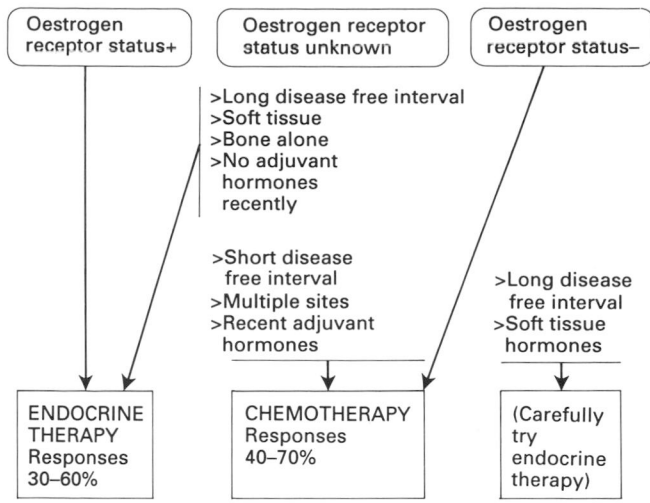

Fig. 21 An algorithm for the choice of the initial systemic therapy for metastatic disease.

upon relapse. These factors influence overall survival either because of a lower response rate to therapy or because of a shorter duration of response (Fey *et al.* 1981). Previous adjuvant therapy, especially if completed shortly before the appearance of metastases, is associated with a dire subsequent prognosis, due most frequently to resistance of the tumour cells to all available antineoplastic agents.

The subjective attitude of the patient and the physician toward systemic treatment which, in the case of chemotherapy, is associated with significant subjective side-effects, is one of the major factors influencing the choice and acceptance of a therapeutic programme. Too few studies take these factors into consideration. Personal preference, therefore, rather than data from clinical trials, guides the treatment choice when quality of life issues are concerned. The potential time lag until signs of response to treatment occur is one of the objective features which may guide the choice of therapy: endocrine manipulations require a mean of 6–12 weeks, while chemotherapy might influence disease symptoms within a shorter time. Taking into account biological and clinical features, an algorithm for choice of the initial systemic therapy of metastatic disease may be proposed (Fig. 21).

Whether the asymptomatic patient with overt metastatic disease should receive immediate systemic therapy is a controversial point, important for determination of the therapeutic approach. No trials have been conducted to answer this question, mainly because of the availability of non-toxic endocrine therapies and because therapeutic nihilism is difficult to justify. Data from two trials provide indirect evidence that the smaller the tumour burden the higher the chance of prolonging survival. The Scottish trial of adjuvant tamoxifen in operable breast cancer included 1312 evaluable patients who received the drug either as adjuvant or, in 93 per cent of the relapsing patients, upon relapse (Scottish Cancer Trials Office 1987). Thus, the trial was essentially a comparison between early and delayed tamoxifen. In this trial a significant improvement in overall survival has been observed in favour of early

tamoxifen. Since adjuvant therapy is considered effective on micrometastatic disease and since biological systems are likely to represent a quantitative continuum, it is appealing to extrapolate from this adjuvant trial that early commencement of treatment, even in overt metastatic stage, is beneficial. The trial by the Australian and New Zealand Breast Cancer Trials Group investigated two treatment options in 307 evaluable patients with metastatic disease: one was a chemotherapy given continuously until evidence of progression and the second was an interrupted treatment after three courses of chemotherapy, if a response or stable disease was observed at that time (Coates *et al.* 1987). The same therapy was reinstituted later when disease progressed (intermittent regimen). Patients on the continuous treatment had a longer survival (although of borderline statistical significance), a fact which might provide incentive for treatment before the appearance of progressing disease-related symptoms in advanced breast cancer.

Before the start of any systemic therapy it is important to evaluate by the easiest diagnostic method available (for example, radiographic assessment of sites of bone pain, assessment of single hepatic lesions by ultrasound, etc.) most tumour parameters of all sites of measurable disease. This provides a more accurate evaluation of response and will serve to avoid ineffective therapy. The use of tumour markers such as carcinoembryonic antigen or CA15-3 is valuable only within the context of the clinical situation. The increase in the blood levels of both markers reflects a progressive disease and a rise in values of more than 10 ng/ml and more than 30 μg/ml, respectively, is usually an expression of tumour growth (Hayes *et al.* 1986; Loprinzi *et al.* 1986). Assessment of response must follow in parallel with evaluation of the degree of palliation. The usefulness of assessing objective responses in advanced breast cancer is controversial (Mouridsen and Rose 1987). There is evidence that objective response and subjective palliation by chemotherapy are correlated. It was, however, shown that a substantially higher number of patients experienced relief of pain than could be defined as responders using the strict objective response criteria. Even 33 per cent of patients who had a measurably progressive disease were reported to have obtained a significant relief of pain (Brunner *et al.* 1975). While objective evaluation of the response by measurement of the tumour might be important for assessing the activity of antineoplastic drugs or drug regimens, evaluation of the impact of therapy upon the patient's quality of life requires a more subjective definition. Attempts to have the patient define her symptoms, the side-effects of the drugs, her anxiety and depression, personal relations, physical performance, sense of well-being, and efforts to cope with the disease and its symptoms have been made by various investigators using linear analogue self-assessment scales and questionnaires (Baum *et al.* 1980; Coates *et al.* 1983). An example of the use of such measurements for comparisons of systemic treatments and their impact upon patients was conducted and reported by the Australian and New Zealand Breast Cancer Group (Coates *et al.* 1987). Their trial compared a continuous regimen of chemotherapy given until progression with an intermittent one, which was interrupted in all patients with at least a stable disease obtained with the first three courses and then resumed in case of progression. The intermittent regimen was not only associated with a lower response rate and a trend for a shorter survival, but also with a surprising finding of the assessed instruments measuring aspects of quality of life. Linear analogue self-assessment scores for physical well-being, mood, pain, and appetite, as well as the physician's assessment of a quality of life index for the patient, all improved significantly during the first three treatment courses received by patients in the two treatment groups. Thereafter, patients on intermittent therapy showed a significantly worse quality of life as measured by all of the parameters mentioned above.

Endocrine therapy for overt metastatic disease

Endocrine therapy for inoperable breast cancer has been known since the end of the last century under the form of surgical oophorectomy (Beatson 1896). Novel concepts related to the increasing knowledge of endocrine-dependent growth regulatory mechanisms and the number of new endocrine agents have increased and completely changed the available hormonal treatments. Breast cancer is, in fact, responsive to a variety of endocrine agents via a poorly understood mechanism. Growth factors which have been shown to be produced by the human breast cancer cell line MCF-7 under the influence of oestrogen (transforming growth factor α) will stimulate the growth of both oestrogen receptor-rich and oestrogen receptor-poor cells.

Anti-oestrogens, such as tamoxifen, which were assumed to exert their growth-inhibiting action by competitively binding to the oestrogen receptor, appear to stimulate the formation of transforming growth factor β, which inhibits the growth of cells both with and without oestrogen hormone receptors (Dickson and Lippman 1988).

The following general features of endocrine therapies must be taken into consideration when the therapy is offered to a patient with metastatic disease.

1. Approximately one-third of an unselected patient population is likely to respond to the therapy: as mentioned, the chances of response are higher when the tumour is known to be rich in oestrogen receptors; approximately 50–60 per cent of the patients with oestrogen receptor-rich tumours respond to the endocrine therapy.

2. Patients who respond to one endocrine therapy are likely to respond to subsequent hormonal manipulations.

3. The removal of additive endocrine therapy, such as oestrogens, upon disease progression might induce a response after the withdrawal. The mechanism for this phenomenon is unknown.

4. At the start of some hormonal manipulations there can be an exacerbation of cancer-related symptoms. This manifestation might appear within hours or days and last for a month. Besides an increase in markers of tumour activity, there might be a significant increase in alkaline phosphatase levels and, in particular, the appearance of a hypercalcaemia. This phenomenon, or flare, seen with a frequency of between 3 and 9 per cent, is likely to be followed by an objective response to therapy. It has been observed after the start of therapy with oestrogens, tamoxifen, androgens, and progestins, but not after aromatase inhibitors (Henderson and Harris 1991).

Table 21 lists some available endocrine therapies, the magnitude of their effects (from a review of published results), and some of the described side-effects (Henderson 1987).

The most widely used endocrine therapy is tamoxifen. The drug is known to bind by competition to the oestradiol receptor, altering the biological effects of the receptor–hormone complex and inducing changes which result in reduced proliferation and growth (Jordan 1984). Another possible mechanism of growth inhibition of tumour cells was ascribed to the transforming growth factor β produced by tumour cells under the influence of the drug. The daily dose of tamoxifen is usually 20 mg; its half-life after a continuous administration exceeds 200 h and its blood levels remain detectable for 6–12 weeks after cessation of treatment (Fabian *et al.* 1981), an important fact for the timing of biopsies for oestrogen-receptor determination. Higher doses of tamoxifen, in excess of $60 \text{ mg/m}^2/\text{day}$, were related to the risk of impaired visual acuity and retinopathy (Kaiser-Kupfer and Lippman 1978). Data on higher doses of tamoxifen are relevant due to reports of responses in patients who were given doses of 80 mg/day after having relapsed on a lower-dose regimen. A comparison of tamoxifen and various other endocrine therapies, which attempted to find other candidates for primary endocrine therapy and especially to improve upon the response rate of the drug, yielded interesting observations, which are summarized in Table 22. In particular, the results of the two trials which compare the drug to oophorectomy indicate that, with very few exceptions, tamoxifen should be used first to predict subsequent chances of response to oophrectomy (Ingle *et al.* 1981; Buchanan *et al.* 1986). Tamoxifen is a relatively non-toxic treatment and its chronic use, mainly in the adjuvant setting, has been associated with certain rare side-effects. Thrombophlebitis has been observed in 1–3 per cent of the patients. Some protective effect upon post-menopausal-associated bone loss, due to its slight oestrogenic effect, has also been described. Long-term use of tamoxifen has been reported to be associated with an increased incidence of endometrial cancer in a large series from Sweden (Fornander *et al.* 1989, 1991). This has not been confirmed by other large studies (Stewart and Knight 1989).

Ovarian ablation is still considered by many to be the treatment of choice for most of the pre-menopausal patients. The preference for surgical ablation rather than ovarian radiation is related to the shorter time to response associated with the former. The response to oophorectomy of an unselected population of pre-menopausal women was below 20 per cent. If endocrine therapy is indicated, it is common practice today to treat pre-menopausal patients with tamoxifen and only upon progression after an initial response to consider oophorectomy. Initial oophorectomy should be considered in older pre-menopausal patients because a prolonged time in response on initial tamoxifen might also mean cessation of ovarian function and a subsequent loss of oophorectomy as an efficient endocrine treatment option.

Table 21 Available endocrine therapies, their effects in terms of response rates (RR) for unselected and selected patients, and a description of some reported side-effects. A review of published results

Endocrine therapy	Patient group (% RR)			Major toxicities
	Unselected	ER+	ER−	
Tamoxifen	32	54	9	Nausea, hot flashes, flare[a], hypercalcaemia[a], thrombocytopenia[a], thromboembolism[a]
Oophorectomy	33	62	6	Hot flashes, surgery-related complications[a]
Progestins	31	35	8	Weight gain, fluid retention, nausea[a], hot flashes[a], thrombophlebitis
Aminoglutathimide + cortisone	31	54	6	Lethargy, dizziness/ataxia, rash, Cushingoid syndrome, nausea, thrombocytopenia
LHRH analogues		42		Hot flashes, nausea, headache[a]
Pre-menopausal		45		
Post-menopausal		8		
Oestrogens	26	57	9	Nausea, hot flashes, flare[a], hypercalcaemia, water retention, cardiovascular side-effects, incontinence, vaginal bleeding
Androgens	21	43	8	Masculinization, nausea, weight gain, flare, hypercalcaemia[a]

[a]Rare side-effects.
Almost all data for endocrine manipulations relate to results in post-menopausal patients.
LHRH, luteinizing-hormone-releasing hormone.

Table 22 Randomized trials relating to the choice of endocrine therapies in advanced breast cancer

Randomized comparison	No. of trials	No. of patients	Comments
Tam v. other endocrine therapies (no progestins) (post-m.)	9	576	Oestrogens, androgens, and ablative; Tam advantageous because of lower toxicity and similar therap. effects.
Tam v. oophorectomy (Ox) (pre-m.)	2	160	No overall trend: response rate (RR) higher for Ox in one trial, duration of response longer for Tam in the other. Secondary RR to Ox after Tam=33 per cent to Tam following Ox=11 per cent
Tam low-dose v. higher dose (post-m.)	4	556	No dose–response relationship
Progestins v. other endocrine therapies	13	1424	Mainly comparison with Tam; progestins as effective as Tam In two trials high-dose MPA significantly superior to Tam
Progestins low v. high-dose	7	1018	Trend favours higher dose in three trials (two significant)
Aminoglutethimide (AG) v. other endocrine therapy	5	516	Mainly comparison with Tam; similar RR; one favours AG
Single v. combination Endocrine therapy	10	981	Some trend in favour of combination, especially Tam+prednisolone (two trials, post-m.) or Tam + Ox (one trial, pre-m.)

Abbreviations: MPA, Medroxyp.; pre-m., pre-menopausal; post-m., post-menopausal; Tam, tamoxifen; therap., therapeutic.

Progestins have a role as effective therapy in metastatic breast cancer. Their mechanism of action is attributed to either a direct effect on the cancer cell (a receptor-mediated mechanism) or an indirect effect via the pituitary-ovarian and the pituitary-adrenal axes. Initially a low response rate was observed, which might have been related to their use exclusively as secondary or tertiary treatment. Therapeutically effective doses of medroxyprogesterone acetate are considered to be 500 mg/day after an initial loading phase of 1000 mg/day. The reinstitution of a high dose upon evidence of progression after response is reported to provide additional responses. The therapeutic dose for megestrol acetate is 160 mg once daily. Higher doses have been associated with a grotesque increase in appetite and subsequent weight gain in more than 80 per cent of the patients. Other toxic effects are summarized in Table 21.

Corticosteroids are effective hormonal agents, although not considered as such; their use induces responses in approximately 25 per cent of treated patients (Stuart-Harris and Smith 1984). Their main effect of providing palliation, especially for bone pain and dyspnoea, is particularly useful for terminal care. The side-effects related to chronic administration are difficult to control and include a cushingoid appearance, diabetes mellitus, water retention, atrophic changes of the skin and its vessels, gastric and duodenal bleeding with or without ulcers, and osteoporosis.

Aminoglutathimide is given with a low-dose supplement of cortisone to avoid symptoms of adrenal suppression. It blocks steroid hydroxylation and cleavage enzymes, causing a deficient steroidogenesis with a more effective inhibition of oestrone in peripheral tissues and, thus, has a direct anti-oestrogen effect on the metastatic environment. The efficiency of the treatment in controlling disease is equal to that of tamoxifen. Its therapeutic dosage is 250 mg twice daily, with cortisone 40 mg/day. Although lower doses of aminoglutathimide without the corticosteroid supplement are effective, they seem to cause unpredictable toxic effects. The side-effects of the treatment are dose-dependent and include lethargy as well as symptoms related to steroid therapy. Thrombocytopenia, even severe and leucopenia have been described between the second and seventh week of treatment. New aromatase inhibitors, such as 4-hydroxyandrostendione, with significantly fewer toxic effects, are now under advanced evaluation.

Analogues of luteinizing-hormone-releasing hormone were recently introduced to clinical investigations and have already significant antineoplastic activity, especially in pre-menopausal but also in post-menopausal breast cancer patients. More than 420 patients were reported as evaluable after treatment with all the available compounds. These drugs are all analogues of the decapeptide that is intermittently secreted in regular pulses by the hypothalamus, causing release of luteinizing hormone and follicle-stimulating hormone. Overall response rates for pre- and post-menopausal women are described in Table 21. The responses of post-menopausal women are interesting (Harvey 1988). Peripheral oestradiol levels measured in a group of 28 post-menopausal patients treated with analogues of luteinizing-hormone-releasing hormone were significantly suppressed (Harris *et al.* 1989). The patient who had the most marked drop in oestradiol levels also had the maximal response rate. It was, therefore, suggested that the luteinizing-hormone-releasing hormone analogue might act upon tumour cells via changes in circulating oestrogen (an indirect effect, as for pre-menopausal patients) rather than via a postulated direct effect (which was hypothesized to explain the effect in post-menopausal patients). The use of this compound is associated with minimal toxic effects. For pre-menopausal patients, reversible amenorrhoea occurs within 40 days and menses resume usually within 80 days after cessation of therapy.

Oestrogens are rarely used today because of their side-effects (nausea and vomiting, water retention, and cardiovascular damage). They can still be used as fourth-line hormonal therapy in older patients who do not have cardiovascular contraindications. Diethylstilbestrol (5 mg three times daily), ethinyl oestradiol (1 mg three times daily), or Premarin[R] (2.5 mg three times daily) can be used. Dose escalation might be attempted. It is important to recognize that an estimated one-third of the patients who progress after therapy with oestrogens experience a withdrawal response.

Androgen therapy provides good palliation but is associated with side-effects which are only partially reversible: masculinization, hoarseness, hirsutism, a masculine-like boldness, acne, and seborrhoea. Fluoxymestrone acetate (30 mg/day) might, however, be a useful tertiary therapy for elderly women with congestive heart failure, because, as opposed to progestins and oestrogens, androgens do not cause water retention.

Since many of the endocrine treatments have different mechanisms of action, their concomitant or sequential use might result in an additive or even synergistic cytocidal effect. This hypothesis has been investigated in several randomized trials (Table 22). The most impressive improvements in terms of response rates were seen in trials which investigated the use of prednisolone combined with either tamoxifen or oophorectomy, compared with use of the single endocrine modality (tamoxifen or oophorectomy) (Stewart *et al.* 1982; Rubens and Knight 1985).

Chemotherapy for overt metastatic disease

Traditionally, the use of cytotoxic agents was considered for all patients whose young age or aggressive disease impressed the physician as requiring a fast and objective tumour regression. Overall response rates to chemotherapy are reported to range between 43 and 90 per cent, with some proportion being classified as complete (usually from anecdotal incidence to almost 50 per cent for the programme with intensive therapy and bone-marrow supportive measures). The median time to response is described as ranging between 7 and 14 weeks, with a maximum reported to be 16 months. The median duration of response to drug combinations ranges between 6 months and 1 year. However, some patients are described as having been in response for more than a decade. Despite these observations, there is a significant controversy concerning the prolongation of survival of patients with advanced disease who are being treated with cytotoxic drugs. In fact, a trial to answer such a question cannot be conducted because of the relevant improvement of symptoms under treatment. Some evidence does exist, however, to indicate that any improvement in overall survival might be limited to patients with aggressive tumours as opposed to those with less rapidly progressive disease (Cavalli *et al.* 1983). The most significant factor related to improvement of survival, as well as to quality of life, is the response to treatment.

Predictive factors for high response rates are

(1) a good performance status;

(2) only one or two sites of metastatic disease, especially in soft tissue;

(3) prior hormonal therapy;

(4) with some limited evidence, a fast-growing tumour as indicated by high labelling indices.

Factors which are predictive for a longer duration of response and survival are

(1) a good performance status;

(2) only one or two sites of disease, especially in soft tissue and nodular lung metastases;

(3) prior endocrine therapy or response to hormonal manipulations.

On the other hand, factors predictive for a decreased chance of response and for a shorter duration of response and survival are prior chemotherapy and/or radiation therapy, bone and visceral metastases, and low blood lymphocyte counts.

Age, menopausal status, and steroid hormone receptor status do not influence the response rate and duration of the response to chemotherapy.

The drugs most frequently used are those which were investigated in the 1950s, also because subsequent populations who were offered new drugs had already been heavily pre-treated with chemo- and radiotherapy, factors known to be associated with a poor response rate. Table 23 lists active drugs, including some new agents which have recently been added to the cytotoxic arsenal. Cyclophosphamide, doxorubicin (or Adriamycin[R]), methotrexate, and 4-fluorouracil (all used in first line regimens) are considered to be most useful.

Questions related to the choice of first chemotherapy, which have been addressed in randomized trials, are listed in Table 24. The use of combination chemotherapy yielded a higher response rate in almost all the trials comparing it to a single-agent chemotherapy. Exceptions are the use of cyclophosphamide and doxorubicin, which are considered the most active drugs for treatment of breast cancer. A survival difference in favour of the combination chemotherapy has been significant only in one trial, which compared melphalan alone versus a cyclophosphamide, methotrexate, and 5-fluorouracil combination (Canellos *et al.* 1976). The use of alternating non-cross-resistant drug combinations with available agents, such as cyclophosphamide and doxorubicin, did not appear to influence survival. Similarly, the evaluation of two trials of sequentially administered therapies with single agents, as compared with their simultaneous combination, yielded similar overall outcome figures. A careful analysis of the data revealed that the population with liver and lung metastases (that is, with a disease which generally has a worse prognosis due to a rapid evolution) had significant benefit in terms of survival, if treated with the simultaneous combination. On the other hand, the sequential use of single agents had some

Table 23 List of cytotoxic agents and data on their effectiveness in metastatic breast cancer. Years of the reported results are also given. A, active drugs which are commonly used in the treatment of the disease; B, active drugs or potentially active drugs

Agent studied	Years published	Number of patients	Remission rates (%) Overall	Pre-treated	Not pre-treated or not heavily pre-treated
A					
Chlorambucil	1959–1968	58	17	–	–
Cyclophosphamide	1961–1979	887	33	22	36
Adriamycin[R]	1974–1985	1122	32	29	43
4-Epiadriamycin	1983–1990	390	39	33	71
Mitoxantrone	1981–1989	848	21	7	27
5-Fluorouracil	1961–1981	1921	27	15	28
Melphalan	1965–1982	222	20	4	25
Methotrexate	1952–1981	547	28	17	26
Mitomycin C[R]	1976–1985	307	22	22	–
Thiotepa	1959–1968	266	29	–	25
Vinblastine	1962–1972	119	21	0	–
Vincristine	1964–1976	251	19	10	8
B					
Amonafide	1990	26	23	–	23
Bisantrene	1983–1985	306	15	15	–
Platinum	1978–1988	191	21	8	52
CBDCA (carboplatin)	1983–1990	122	15	4	26
BCNU (carmustine)	1972–1973	155	16	–	–
Etoposide	1975–1989	319	8	7	15
Elliptinium	1982–1985	228	27	22	37
Estracyt[R]	1982	97	20	–	12
Sterecyt	1980–1983	166	26	21	35
Ifosfamide	1974–1976	48	27	32	20
Floxuridine	1963–1973	152	35	–	7
Hexamethylmelamine	1969–1979	151	11	11	–
Mitolactol	1976–1984	142	17	17	–
Navelbine	1989–1990	88	48	18	70
Mustargen	1961	95	18	–	39
Pirarubicin	1988–1990	364	29	21	38
Taxol	1990–1991	25	56	–	56
Vindesine	1979–1988	218	24	22	39

advantages for disease presentations considered to be of less aggressive evolution, such as soft tissue and bone metastases (Chlebowski et al. 1989). It is, therefore, mandatory that phase III trials in advanced disease, which compare the effectiveness of two treatments or approaches, be conducted separately in groups with some prognostic uniformity because of the evidence that some qualitative interaction between treatment effects and prognosis might be real.

The available evidence for a role of some of the drugs contained in certain combinations is weak. An example is the use of vincristine. This drug has been included in treatment regimens because of an extrapolation from therapies used in Hodgkin's disease and because it is not myelosuppressive and, therefore, is easier to combine with other drugs in the regimen. Five randomized studies with either a cyclophosphamide-based combination (for example, cyclophosphamide, methotrexate, 5-fluorouracil, prednisone versus cyclophosphamide, methotrexate, 5-fluorouracil, vincristine, prednisone) (Segaloff et al. 1985) or a doxorubicin regimen (for example, doxorubicin, vincristine versus doxorubicin) (Steiner et al. 1983) showed that the addition of vincristine was not associated with an improved outcome. Its use in the treatment of metastatic breast cancer is not recommended.

The addition of prednisone to a combination chemotherapy was suggested by the superior tolerance of antineoplastic agents when administered with this drug. Despite the fact that some improvement in outcome is attributable to the addition of prednisone (Tormey et al. 1982), the issue is still open for investigation. Prednisone is currently used to improve the tolerance of combination chemotherapy.

When compared to methotrexate combinations, doxorubicin-containing regimens are associated with higher response rates, response durations, and even overall survival of subgroups with aggressive disease. The sequential use of methotrexate combinations and doxorubicin-based regimens is a common oncological procedure. Table 25 describes some widely used drug regimens. Considering the treatment with doxorubicin, data are available to suggest that its use alone or in combination with cyclophosphamide might provide the maximal benefit (O'Bryan et al. 1977; Tranum et al. 1982).

The search for new anthracyclines to replace doxorubicin and avoid part or all of its toxic effects (the most feared being cardiac toxicity), yet maintaining its degree of effectiveness, has had limited success. The comparison between 4-epidoxorubicin and doxorubicin terms of toxic effect and therapeutic efficacy involved studies in

Table 24 Randomized comparisons related to the choice of chemotherapy in advanced breast cancer: cytotoxic without (A) and with (B) endocrine therapies

Randomized comparison	Number of trials	Number of patients	Comments
A. Cytotoxic therapy comparisons			
Single agent or sequence of single agents v. the drug combination	10	1263	Favour combination for response rate, trend for duration; survival advantage only in aggressive visceral (mainly liver) disease
Single regimen v. alternating non-cross-resistant regimens	9	948	Trends favour alternating regimens for response rate and duration but not for survival
Chemotherapy v. same chemotherapy plus prednisone	2	202	Trend favours added prednisone for response rate, duration, and survival
Chemotherapy v. same chemotherapy plus vincristine	5	735	No added benefit from vincristine
Chemotherapy v. same chemotherapy plus methotrexate (CFP±M)	1	336	Higher response rate for CMFP; similar duration of response and survival
Doxorubicin combinations v. methotrexate combinations (other drugs similar)	7	1263	Favour doxorubicin for response rate, duration, and in some, survival; in studied comparisons, doxorubicin associated with significantly more toxicity
Doxorubicin combinations v. CMFVP	6	855	No significant difference
Doxorubicin–cyclophosphamide v. same plus 5-fluorouracil (F)	2	382	No added benefit with F
Mitozantrone v. doxorubicin, both either alone or in combination	12	1880+	Mitozantrone yields slightly lower remission rates; survival similar
4-Epidoxorubicin v. doxorubicin, both in combination	15	2000+	Similar outcome for the two anthracyclines
B. Cytotoxic and endocrine therapy comparisons			
Endocrine therapy (ET) v. ET plus chemotherapy	12	1177	Higher response rate for combination; no survival benefit
Chemotherapy v. chemotherapy plus ET	11	1591	Higher response rate for combination; no clear survival advantage for the combination

Abbreviations: C, cyclophosphamide; F, 5-fluorouracil; M, methotrexate; P, prednisone; V, vincristine.

Table 25 Common regimens used in the treatment of metastatic breast cancer. All drug doses are subject to changes according to current and previous myelosuppression

Regimen	Dose	Route	Schedule
CMF (P)			Repeat every 28 days
C	100 mg/m²	po	Days 1–14
M	40 mg/m²	iv	Days 1 and 8
F	600 mg/m²	iv	Days 1 and 8
(P)	40 mg/m²	po	Days 1–14
iv CMF			Repeat every 21 days
C	600 mg/m²	iv	Day 1
M	40 mg/m²	iv	Day 1
F	600 mg/m²	iv	Day 1
LMF (p)			Repeat every 28 days
L	5 mg/m²	po	Days 1–14
M	40 mg/m²	iv	Days 1 and 8
F	600 mg/m²	iv	Days 1 and 8
(p) low dose	12.5 mg	po	Days 1–14
AC			Repeat every 21–28 days
A	40 mg/m²	iv	Day 1
C	200 mg/m²	po	Day 3–6
CAF			Repeat every 3 weeks
C	400–500 mg/m²	iv	Day 1
A	40–50 mg/m²	iv	Day 1
F	400–500 mg/m²	iv	Days 1 and 8

Abbreviations: iv, intravenous; po, by mouth; C, cyclophosphamide; M, methotrexate; F, 5-fluorouracil; L, chlorambucil (Leukeran™); A, AdriamycinR, doxorubicin; p, prednisone.

more than 2000 patients, and showed some evidence of an improved therapeutic index for the analogue, especially for reduced gastrointestinal tolerance. Studies of other anthracycline analogues, such as menogaril and idarubicin, are not yet mature enough to provide data useful for routine patient care.

The use of mitozantrone as a single agent (14 mg/m² intravenously, every 3 weeks) yielded results similar to those for doxorubicin (75 mg/m² every 3 weeks), with some lesser, non-haematological toxic effects (Henderson *et al.* 1989*b*). Comparison of the two drugs (10 mg/m² mitozantrone versus 50 mg/m² doxorubicin) combined with other agents showed an advantage for the doxorubicin combination in terms of response rate. Furthermore, the high incidence of side-effects due to the chosen treatment regimens (alopecia: 49.1 per cent for the mitozantrone combination versus 85.8 per cent for the doxorubicin combination) rendered the search for a less toxic alternative to AdriamycinR unfruitful (Bennett *et al.* 1988).

The use of mitomycin C, especially with vinblastine, has not been compared in a randomized trial to other primary treatment regimens, mainly because it is almost exclusively used as a second-line therapy. The use of the drug in doses above 10–15 mg/m² intravenously every 4–6 weeks may be associated with severe myelosuppression in a pre-treated population.

Therapies with continuous infusions of cytotoxic drugs, especially doxorubicin (Legha *et al.* 1982) and 5-fluorouracil, particularly if given at a low dose (Huan *et al.* 1989), were described to be less toxic and to have significant antitumour activity even in pre-treated patients. Comparisons related to such schedule dependency are warranted to establish the role of these administration modalities. Another modality of treatment using 5-fluorouracil with leucovorin (which enhances the inhibition of fluoropyrimidines by thymidylate synthase) has been shown to be effective even in patients who were described as resistant to 5-fluorouracil combinations (Marini *et al.* 1987). The use of this combination of drugs is associated with severe toxic effects (mucositis) and its role and safety must be defined in further investigations (Loprinzi 1989).

Dose–response in metastatic breast cancer

The hypothesis that high-dose chemotherapy might induce more responses and, hence, palliate more patients and perhaps prolong survival is a subject of controversy. The methodological issues related to retrospective analyses of a dose–response relationship across trials have been discussed extensively (Henderson *et al.* 1988). A low-dose CMF combination compared with a 'standard' dose was associated in one of two randomized trials with a lower response rate and a marginally shorter survival. The same trial provided some evidence for a better palliation obtained by the full-dose combination chemotherapy, as measured by self-assessment linear analogue questionnaires administered to a cohort of the patients (Tannock *et al.* 1988). The use of very high doses of cytotoxic drugs, either in uncontrolled studies or in comparison with 'standard' doses, showed a very high remission rate for the high-dose regimens. The comparative studies (for example, with the fluorouracil, doxorubicin, cyclophosphamide (FAC) regimen) (Hortobagyi *et al.* 1987) failed, however, to show a survival advantage of the therapy with the higher dose. A review of results from single-therapy projects, with high-dose single-agent therapies and high-dose combination regimens

followed by autologous bone-marrow reinfusion, showed a large difference between the rate of complete remissions obtained with the therapies (five out of 71 (7 per cent) and 39 out of 67 (58 per cent), respectively) (Cheson *et al.* 1989), although the selection of patients to the projects was obviously the main reason for the difference. Despite their limited effect on platelets, the use of available colony-stimulating factors with or after high-dose cytotoxic drug administration might provide some additional possibilities for studying the role of high-dose therapy in breast cancer.

Combined cytotoxic and endocrine therapies are believed, at least theoretically, to act additively, if not synergistically in their antineoplastic efficacy. The assumptions that the two treatments might have separate cytocidal effects on two distinct target clones, plus the evidence that the spectrum of toxicity of the two modalities is different, were the reasons for their combination. The results for primary treatment of metastatic disease with combined chemoendocrine therapy have not shown benefit in terms of survival, despite higher response rates (Table 24B). Data show that the sequential use of endocrine therapy and chemotherapy in post-menopausal patients confers an advantage, especially in patients with slow-growing tumours (Stewart *et al.* 1982; Australian and New Zealand Breast Cancer Trials Group 1986). Only patients who were relatively young and whose metastatic disease had an aggressive presentation gained some benefit from the combination. In pre-menopausal patients, despite the existence of suggestive trends, the data do not permit definition of a subpopulation which will benefit from a primary combined approach. The general tendency is to use the modalities separately and to reserve the combined treatment for situations requiring salvage regimens. Investigations that applied the approach of 'priming' or 'recruiting' malignant cells with oestrogens, followed by combination chemotherapy, have provided

Table 26 Issues related to the therapy of specific sites of overt metastatic disease

Site (reference)	Accepted therapy	Open therapeutic questions
Local recurrence/scar alone	Surgery, if circumscribed; radiation provides control in < half of patients; high response rate with systemic therapy (62–85 per cent)	Role of radical surgery or other surgical techniques; role of adjuvant systemic therapy
Breast recurrence after breast conserving procedure	Mastectomy	Adjuvant systemic therapy
Contralateral breast	Mastectomy + axillary clearance (multicentric)	Adjuvant systemic therapy; less than mastectomy; immediate reconstruction
Bone metastases	Systemic therapy; radiation for localized pain (more effective than systemic therapy); surgery for weight-bearing and functionally important structures	Biphosphonates against bone pain and fractures; regional chemotherapy
Brain metastases	High-dose steroids and radiotherapy; surgery for uncertain or accessible single metastases	Combined systemic therapy +/− radiotherapy; high-dose chemotherapy for selected patients
Spinal cord compression	High-dose dexamethasone (given even before myelography); radiation therapy (RT); surgery on progression under RT or in irradiated areas, or if bony instability, or if questionable diagnosis	Combination systemic therapy±radiotherapy; high-dose chemotherapy
Choroidal metastases	Radiation therapy (improvement in 80–90 per cent)	Systemic therapy
Carcinomatous meningitis	Intrathecal methotrexate; thiotepa, cytosine-arabinoside; radiotherapy to symptomatic areas	
Symptomatic malignant effusions	Drainage and instillation of various compounds, including cytotoxics	Use of 'biological response modifiers' locally

some interesting observations (Benz *et al.* 1987; Lippman 1987). The approach requires randomized controlled testing.

Secondary treatments and salvage regimens

During the course of the disease most patients will require a new therapy for reattempting palliation. It is a common observation that the duration of prior treatment and the number and type of previous treatment regimens are probably the most important predictive factors for successful subsequent palliation. In patients who had no previous doxorubicin, response rates with the drug used alone are approximately 30 per cent and the median remission duration is approximately 6 months (Ingle *et al.* 1985). Mitomycin C in combination with vinblastine or other vinca alkaloids results in response rates of between 10 and 40 per cent in patients who relapsed after prior doxorubicin (Garewal *et al.* 1983). The combined chemoendocrine therapy is often applied successfully as salvage treatment, especially in patients without prior doxorubicin.

Duration of treatment with chemotherapy

While it is reasonable to continue an endocrine therapy until relapse, the optimal duration of chemotherapy is unknown. Results from trials with either a combination chemotherapy without (Smalley *et al.* 1976) or with Adriamycin^R (Coates *et al.* 1987) or a monotherapy with mitozantrone (Harris *et al.* 1990), indicate a maximal useful duration of 6 months and a possible role for some form of maintenance treatment.

Therapeutic issues related to special sites of overt metastases

The treatment of overt metastatic disease is very often influenced by a set of specific clinical problems which are entirely related to their site. Generally, data used to justify particular approaches are derived from observations and clinical experience, rather than from controlled trials. The purpose of this section has been to summarize general treatment guidelines, but also to point out some of the remaining questions that require additional investigation. The study of these special problems of breast cancer must also consider quality of life-oriented end-points, to ensure the inclusion of this concept in patient care. Table 26 describes the issues related to the therapy of specific sites of disease.

REFERENCES

Adair F, Berg J, Joubert L (1974). Long term follow-up of breast cancer patients: the thirty year report. *Cancer*, 33:1145–50.

Adami HO, *et al.* (1981). Characteristics of familial breast cancer in Sweden. Absence of relation of age and unilateral versus bilateral disease. *Cancer*, 48:1688–95.

Ali IU, Lidereau R, Theillet C, Callahan R (1987). Reduction to homozygosity of genes on chromosome 11 in human breast neoplasia. *Science*, 238:185–8.

Allegra JC, *et al.* (1979). Relationship between progesterone, androgen, and glucocorticoid receptor and response rate to endocrine therapy in metastatic breast cancer. *Cancer Research*, 39:1973–9.

Allen K, Cox E, Manton K, Cohen JH (1986). Breast cancer in the elderly: current patterns of care. *Journal of the American Geriatrics Society*, 34:637–42.

Al-Sumidaie AM, *et al.* (1988). Particles with properties of retrovirus in monocytes from patients with breast cancer. *Lancet*, i:5–8.

Anderson DE (1972). A genetic study of human breast cancer. *Journal of the National Cancer Institute*, 48:1029–34.

Anderson DE (1976). Genetic study of breast cancer – identification of high risk group. *Cancer*, 34:1090–7.

Andersson I, *et al.* (1979). Breast cancer screening with mammography. A population-based randomised trial with mammography as the only screening node. *Radiology*, 132:273–6.

Arriagada R, *et al.* (1985). Radiotherapy alone in breast cancer. I. Analysis of tumour parameters, tumour dose and local control: the experience of the Gustave-Roussy Institute and the Princess Margaret Hospital. *International Journal of Radiation Oncology — Biology — Physics*, 11:1751–7.

Ashikari R, Hajdu SI, Robbins GF (1971). Intraductal carcinoma of the breast (1960–1969). *Cancer*, 28:1182–7.

Australian and New Zealand Breast Cancer Trials Group (ANZ BCTG) (1986). A randomized trial in postmenopausal patients with advanced breast cancer comparing endocrine and cytotoxic therapy given sequentially or in combination. *Journal of Clinical Oncology*, 4:186–93.

Bagley CS, *et al.* (1987). Adjuvant chemotherapy in males with cancer on the breast. *American Journal of Clinical Oncology*, 10:55–60.

Bailar JC, III (1976). Mammography: a contrary view. *Annals International Medicine*, 84:77–84.

Batson OV (1940). The function of the vertebral venis and their role in the spread of metastasis. *Annals of Surgery*, 112:138–49.

Baum M, *et al.* (1980). A comparison of subjective responses in a trial comparing endocrine with cytotoxic treatment in advanced carcinoma of the breast. In *Breast cancer — experimental and clinical aspects* (ed. HT Mouridsen and T Palshot), pp. 223–6. Pergamon Press, Elmsford.

Beatson GT (1896). On the treatment of inoperable cases of carcinoma of the mammae — suggestions for a new method of treatment with illustrative cases. *Lancet*, ii:104–7.

Bedwinek J, *et al.* (1982). Stage III and localised stage IV breast cancer: irradiation alone vs irradiation plus surgery. *International Journal of Radiation Oncology — Biology — Physics*, 8:31–6.

Bennett JM, *et al.* (1988). A randomized multicenter trial comparing mitoxantrone, cyclophosphamide, and fluorouracil with doxorubicin, cyclophosphamide, and fluorouracil in the therapy of metastatic breast carcinoma. *Journal of Clinical Oncology*, 6:1611–20.

Benz C, Gandara D, Miller B (1987). Chemoendocrine therapy with prolonged estrogen priming in advanced breast cancer: endocrine pharmacokinetics and toxicity. *Cancer Treatment Report*, 71:283–9.

Bergkvist L, *et al.* (1989). The risk of breast cancer after estrogen and estrogen-progestin replacement. *New England Journal of Medicine*, 5:293–7.

Berlin NT (1975). Research strategy in cancer: screening, diagnosis, prognosis. *Hospital Practice*, 10:83–91.

Black MM, Spur FD (1950). Sinus histiocytosis of lymph nodes in cancer. *Surgical Gynecology and Obstetrics*, 106:163–75.

Black MM, *et al.* (1972). Association of atypical characteristics of benign breast lesions with subsequent risk of breast cancer. *Cancer*, 29:338–43.

Bloom HJG, Degenshein GA (1980). Estrogen receptors and disease-free interval: a dissenting opinion. *Breast*, 6:25–7.

Bloom HJG, Field JR (1971). Impact of tumor grade and host resistance on survival of women with breast cancer. *Cancer*, 28:1580–9.

Boccardo F, *et al.* (1990). Chemotherapy versus tamoxifen versus chemotherapy plus tamoxifen in node-positive, estrogen receptor-positive breast cancer patients: results of a multicentric Italian study. *Journal of Clinical Oncology*, 9:1310–20.

Bohmert H, Strömbeck JO (1986). Postmastectomy reconstruction. In *Surgery of the breast* (ed. JO Strombeck and FE Rosato), pp. 243–66. Thieme, Stuttgart.

Bonadonna G, Valagussa P (1989). Systemic therapy in resectable breast cancer. *Hematology/Oncology Clinics of North America*, 3, 727–42.

Bonadonna G, *et al.* (1987). Milan adjuvant trials for stage I-II breast cancer. In *Adjuvant therapy of cancer V* (ed. SE Salmon), pp. 211–22. Grune and Stratton, Orlando.

Bonadonna G, *et al.* (1990). Primary chemotherapy to avoid mastectomy in tumours with diameters of three centimetres or more. *Journal of the National Cancer Institute*, 82:1539–45.

Bostwick J (1987). Breast reconstruction after mastectomy. In *Breast diseases* (ed. JR Harris, S Hellman, IC Henderson, and DW Kinne), pp. 668–83. Lippincott, Philadelphia.

Boyle P (1988). Epidemiology of breast cancer. *Baillière's Clinical Oncology*, 2:1–57.

Brinton LA, *et al.* (1981). Menopausal estrogen and risk of breast cancer. *Cancer*, 47:2517–22.

Brunner KW, *et al.* (1975). Controlled study in the use of combined drug therapy for metastatic breast cancer. *Cancer*, 36:1208–19.

Bryant AJ, Weir JA (1981). Prophylactic oophorectomy in operable instances of carcinoma of the breast. *Surgery Gynecology and Obstetrics*, 153:660–4.

Bucalossi P, Veronesi U, Pandolfi A (1954). Il problema dell'ereditarietà neoplastica nell'uomo. Il cancro della mammella. *Tumori*, 40:365–402.

Buchanan RB, *et al.* (1986). A randomized comparison of tamoxifen with surgical oophorectomy in premenopausal patients with advanced breast cancer. *Journal of Clinical Oncology*, 4:1326–30.

Buell P (1974). Changing incidence of breast cancer in Japanese American women. *Journal of the National Cancer Institute*, 51:479–87.

Butler JA, Bretsky S, Menedez-Botet C, Kinne DW (1985). Estrogen receptor protein of breast cancer as a predictor of recurrence. *Cancer*, 55:1178–81.

Buzzoni R, *et al.* (1991). Adjuvant chemotherapy with doxorubicin plus cyclophosphamide, methotrexate, and fluorouracil in the treatment of resectable breast cancer with more than three positive axillary nodes. *Journal of Clinical Oncology*, 9:2134–40.

Caffier H, Rotte K, Haeggqwist O (1984). Adjuvant chemotherapy versus postoperative irradiation in node-negative breast cancer. In *Adjuvant therapy of cancer IV* (ed. SE Jones and SE Salmon), pp. 417–24. Grune and Stratton, Orlando.

Cancer Research Campaign Working Party (1980). CRC (King's/Cambridge) Trial for Early Breast Cancer: a detailed update at the tenth year. *Lancet*, 2:55–60.

Cannellos GP, *et al.* (1976). Combination chemotherapy for metastatic breast carcinoma. *Cancer*, 38:1882–6.

Carpenter JT, *et al.* (1991). Prospective randomized comparison of cyclophosphamide, doxorubicine (Adriamycin) and fluorouracil (CAF) vs cyclophosphamide, methotrexate and fluorouracil (CMF) for breast cancer with positive axillary nodes: a Southeastern Cancer Study Group Study. *Proceedings of the American Society of Clinical Oncology*, 10:45.

Carroll KK, Hopkins GJ (1979). Dietary polyunsaturated fat versus saturated fat in relation to mammary carcinogenesis. *Lipids*, 14:155.

Cascinelli N, *et al.* (1987). Prognosis of breast cancer with axillary node metastases after surgical treatment only. *European Journal of Cancer and Clinical Oncology*, 23:795–9.

Castiglione M, *et al.* (1989). Systemic treatment for first relapse of breast cancer after adjuvant therapy using the same treatment again. *Proceedings of the American Society of Clinical Oncology*, 8:41.

Castiglione M, Gelber RD, Goldhirsch A, for the International Breast Cancer Study Group (1990). Adjuvant systemic therapy for breast cancer in the elderly: competing causes of mortality. *Journal of Clinical Oncology*, 8:519–26.

Cavalli F, *et al.* (1983). Concurrent or sequential use of cytotoxic chemotherapy and hormone treatment in advanced breast cancer. *British Medical Journal*, i:5–8.

Cheson BD, *et al.* (1989). Autologous bone marrow transplantation. Current status and future directions. *Annals of Internal Medicine*, 110:51–65.

Chlebowski RT, *et al.* (1989). Combination versus sequential single agent chemotherapy in advanced breast cancer: associations with metastatic sites and long-term survival. *British Journal of Cancer*, 59:227–30.

Chu AM, *et al.* (1984). Non-metastatic locally advanced cancer of the breast treated with radiation. *International Journal of Radiation Oncology—Biology—Physics*, 10:2299–304.

Cislaghi C, Decarli A, La Vecchia C (1986). *Dati, Indicatori e mappe di mortalità tumorale. Italia 1975/1977*. Pitagora Editrice, Bologna.

Clark GM, *et al.* (1983). Progesterone receptors as a prognostic factor in stage II breast cancer. *New England Journal of Medicine*, 309:1343–7.

Clayton F (1991). Pathologic correlates of survival in 378 lymph node-negative infiltrating ductal breast carcinomas. *Cancer*, 68:1309–17.

Clemente C, *et al.* (1992). Peritumoral lymphatic invasion in patients with node-negative mammary duct carcinoma. *Cancer*, 69:1396–403.

Coates A, *et al.* (1983). On the receiving end—II. Linear analogue self-assessment (LASA) in evaluation of aspects of quality of life of cancer patients receiving therapy. *European Journal of Cancer and Clinical Oncology*, 19:1633–7.

Coates A, *et al.* (1987). Improving the quality of life during chemotherapy for advanced breast cancer. *New England Journal of Medicine*, 317:1490–5.

Cole MP (1970). Prophylactic compared with therapeutic x-ray artificial menopause. *Second Tenovus workshop of breast cancer*, pp. 2–11.

Collins V, Loeffler RK, Tivey H (1956). Observations on growth rates of human tumors. *American Journal of Roentgenology*, 76:988–1000.

Colnaghi MI (1988). Monoclonal antibodies in breast cancer studies. *Baillière's Clinical Oncology*, 2:85–102.

Contesso G, Saccani Jotti G, Bonadonna G (1989). Tumor grade as prognostic factor in primary breast cancer. *European Journal of Cancer and Clinical Oncology*, 25:403–9.

Coulson PB, *et al.* (1984). Prognostic indicators including DNA histogram type, receptor content, and staging related to human breast cancer patient survival. *Cancer Research*, 44:4187–96.

Cummings FJ, *et al.* (1991). Adjuvant tamoxifen versus placebo in elderly women with node-positive breast cancer: longterm follow-up and causes of death. *Proceedings of the American Society of Clinical Oncology*, 10:47.

Cupta N, Cohen JL, Rosenbaum C (1980). Estrogen receptors in male breast cancer. *Cancer*, 46:1781–4.

Cutler SJ, *et al.* (1969). Further observations on prognostic factors in cancer of the female breast. *Cancer*, 24:653–67.

Dahl-Iversen E (1952). Recherches sur les matastases microscopiques des cancers du sein dans les ganglions lymphatiques parasternaux et sousclaviculaires. *Memoires de l'Academie de Clinique*, 78:651–63.

Davies GC, Millis RR, Hayward JL (1980). Assessment of axillary lymph node status. *Annals of Surgery*, 192:148–51.

De Lena M, *et al.* (1978). Combined chemotherapy–radiotherapy approach in locally advanced (T3b–T4) breast cancer. *Cancer Chemotherapy Pharmacology*, 1:53–9.

De Lena M, *et al.* (1981). Multimodal treatment for locally advanced breast cancer. *Cancer Clinical Trials*, 4:229–36.

Dempsey PJ (1986). Breast senography: clinical applications in image interpretation. *Breast Imaging*, 99–104.

Derman DP, *et al.* (1989). Adjuvant chemotherapy (CMF) for stage III breast cancer: a randomized trial. *International Journal of Radiation Oncology—Biology—Physics*, 12:257–61.

Dickson RB, Lippman ME (1988). Control of human breast cancer by estrogen, growth factors and oncogens. In *Breast cancer: cellular and molecular biology* (ed. ME Lippman and R Dickson), pp. 119–65. Kluwer Academic Publishers, Boston.

Donnelly PK, *et al.* (1975). Benign breast lesions and subsequent breast carcinoma in Rochester, Minnesota. *Mayo Clinic Proceedings*, 50:650.

Dressler LG, Owens M, Seamer L, McGuire WL (1986). Identifying breast cancer patients for adjuvant therapy by DNA flow cytometry and steroid receptors; a 1000 patients study (Abstract 238). *Proceedings Twenty-second Annual Meeting of ASCO*, 4–6 May, Los Angeles, California.

Dressler LG, *et al.* (1987). Evaluation of a modeling system for S-phase estimation in breast cancer by flow cytometry. *Cancer Research*, 47:5294–302.

Dunn JE (1977). Breast cancer among American Japanese in the San Francisco Bay area. *National Cancer Institute Monograph*, 47:157–60.

Dupont WD, Page DL (1985). Risk factors for breast cancer in women with proliferative breast disease. *New England Journal of Medicine*, 312:146–51.

Dupont WD, Page DL (1989). Relative risk of breast cancer varies with time since diagnosis of atypical hyperplasia. *Human Pathology*, 20:723–5.

Early Breast Cancer Trialists' Collaborative Group (1988). Effects of adjuvant tamoxifen and of cytotoxic therapy on mortality in early breast cancer. An overview of 61 randomized trials among 28,896 women. *New England Journal of Medicine*, 319:1681–92.

Early Breast Cancer Trialists' Collaborative Group (1990). *Treatment of early breast cancer*, Volume 1. *Worldwide evidence 1985–1990*. Oxford University Press, Oxford.

Early Breast Cancer Trialists' Collaborative Group (1992). Systemic treatment of early breast cancer by hormonal, cytotoxic or immune therapy: 133 randomized trials involving 31000 recurrences and 24000 deaths among 75000 women. *Lancet*, 339:1–15, 71–85.

Fabian C, *et al.* (1981). Clinical pharmacology of tamoxifen in patients with breast cancer: correlation with clinical data. *Cancer*, 48:876–82.

Falkson HC, Gray R, Wolberg WH, Falkson G (1989). Adjuvant therapy of postmenopausal women with breast cancer—an ECOG phase III study. *Proceedings of the American Society of Surgical Oncology*, 8–19.

Fey MF, Brunner KW, Sonntag RW (1981). Prognostic factors in metastatic breast cancer. *Cancer Clinical Trials*, **4**:237–47.

Fialkow PJ (1979). Clonal origin of human tumors. *Annual Review of Medicine*, **30**:135–43.

Fisher B, *et al.* (1968). Surgical adjuvant chemotherapy in cancer of the breast: results of a decade of cooperative investigation. *Annals of Surgery*, **168**:337–56.

Fisher B, *et al.* (1985a). Ten year results of randomized clinical trial comparing radical mastectomy and total mastectomy with or without radiation. *New England Journal of Medicine*, **312**:674–81.

Fisher B, *et al.* (1985b). Leukemia in breast cancer patients following adjuvant chemotherapy or postoperative radiation. The NSABP experience. *Journal of Clinical Oncology*, **3**:1640–58.

Fisher B, *et al.* (1986). Adjuvant chemotherapy with and without tamoxifen: five-year results from the National Surgical Adjuvant Breast and Bowel Project Trial. *Journal of Clinical Oncology*, **4**:459–71.

Fisher B, Costantino J, Redmond C (1989a). A randomized clinical trial evaluating tamoxifen in the treatment of patients with node-negative breast cancer who have estrogen-receptor-positive tumours. *New England Journal of Medicine*, **320**:479–84.

Fisher B, *et al.* (1989b). A randomized clinical trial evaluating sequential methotrexate and fluorouracil in the treatment of patients with node-negative breast cancer who have estrogen-receptor-negative tumours. *New England Journal of Medicine*, **320**:473–8.

Fisher B, *et al.* (1989c). Eight-year results of a randomized clinical trial comparing total mastectomy and lumpectomy with or without irradiation in the treatment of breast cancer. *New England Journal of Medicine*, **320**:822–8.

Fisher B, *et al.* (1990a). Two months of doxorubicin-cyclophosphamide with and without interval reinduction therapy compared with six months of cyclophosphamide, methotrexate, and fluorouracil in positive-node breast cancer patients with tamoxifen-nonresponsive tumors: results from the National Surgical Adjuvant Breast and Bowel Project B-15. *Journal of Clinical Oncology*, **8**:1483–96.

Fisher B, *et al.* (1990b). Postoperative chemotherapy and tamoxifen compared with tamoxifen alone in the treatment of positive-node breast cancer patients aged 50 years and older with tumors responsive to tamoxifen: results from the National Surgical Adjuvant Breast and Bowel Project B-16. *Journal of Clinical Oncology*, **8**:1005–18.

Fisher ER, *et al.* (1975). The pathology of invasive breast cancer. A syllabus derived from findings of the National Surgical Adjuvant Breast Project. (Protocol No. 4). *Cancer*, **36**:1–85.

Fisher ER, *et al.* and collaborating NSABP Investigators (1986). Pathologic findings from the National Surgical Adjuvant Breast Project (Protocol 6) I. Intraductal carcinoma (DCIS) *Cancer*, **57**:197–208.

Foote FW, Stewart FW (1941). Lobular carcinoma *in situ*. A rare form of mammary cancer. *American Journal of Pathology*, **17**:491–509.

Fornander T, *et al.* (1989). Adjuvant tamoxifen in early breast cancer: occurrence of new primary cancer. *Lancet*, i:117–20.

Fornander T, *et al.* (1991). Adjuvant tamoxifen in early breast cancer: effects on intercurrent mortality. *Journal of Clinical Oncology*, **9**:1740–8.

Forrest APM, *et al.* (1986). A human tumour model. *Lancet*, ii:840–2.

Fournier DV, *et al.* (1980). Growth rate of 147 mammary carcinomas. *Cancer*, **45**:2198–207.

Freedman LS, Edwards DN, McConnell EM, Downham DY (1979). Histological grade and other prognostic factors in relation to survival of patients with breast cancer. *British Journal of Cancer*, **40**:44–5.

Friedell GH, Betts A, Sommers SC (1965). The prognostic value of blood vessel invasion and lymphocytic infiltrates in breast carcinoma. *Cancer*, **18**:164–6.

Galante E, *et al.* (1986). Growth rate of primary breast cancer and prognosis: observations on 3 to 7 year follow-up in 180 breast cancers. *British Journal of Cancer*, **54**:833–6.

Gallager HS, Martin JE (1971). An orientation to the concept of minimal breast cancer. *Cancer*, **28**:1505–7.

Garewal HS, *et al.* (1983). Treatment of advanced breast cancer with mitomycin C combined with vinblastine or vindesine. *Journal of Clinical Oncology*, **1**:772–4.

Gelber RD, Goldhirsch A (1986a). The concept of an overview of cancer clinical trials with special emphasis on early breast cancer. *Journal of Clinical Oncology*, **4**:1696–703.

Gelber RD, Goldhirsch A (1986b). A new endpoint for assessment of adjuvant therapy in postmenopausal women with operable breast cancer. *Journal of Clinical Oncology*, **4**:1772–9.

Gelber RD, Goldhirsch A (1991). Meta-analysis: the fashion of summing-up evidence. Part I. Rationale and conduct. *Annals of Oncology*, **2**:461–8.

Gelber RD, Goldhirsch A, Castiglione M, for the International Breast Cancer Study Group (1989). The duration of a life of quality should become the focus of "quality-of-life" studies. (letter). *Journal of Clinical Oncology*, **7**:542–3.

Gelber RD, Goldhirsch A, Cavalli F, for the International Breast Cancer Study Group (1991). Quality-of-life-adjusted evaluation of adjuvant therapies for operable breast cancer. *Annals of Internal Medicine*, **114**:621–8.

Gershon-Cohen J, Berger SM, Klickstein HS (1963). Roentgenography of breast cancer moderating concept of "biological predeterminism". *Cancer*, **16**:961–4.

Giacomelli V, Veronesi U (1952). Internal mammary nodes as a site for metastatic spread of breast cancer. *Tumori*, **38**:376–93.

Gilchrist NW, *et al.* (1985). Interobserver reproducibility of histopathological features in stage II breast cancer. *Breast Cancer Research and Treatment*, **5**:3–10.

Glucksberg H, *et al.* (1982). Combination chemotherapy (CMFVP) versus L-phenylalanine mustard (L-PAM) for operable breast cancer with positive axillary nodes: a Southwest Oncology Group Study. *Cancer*, **50**:423–34.

Goldhirsch A, for the Ludwig Breast Cancer Study Group (1984). Adjuvant therapy for postmenopausal women with operable breast cancer. Part I: a randomized trial of chemoendocrine versus mastectomy alone. In *Adjuvant therapy of cancer IV* (ed. SE Jones and SE Salmon), pp. 379–91. Grune and Stratton, Orlando.

Goldhirsch A, Gelber RD, for the Ludwig Breast Cancer Group (1986). Adjuvant treatment for early breast cancer: the Ludwig Breast Cancer Studies. *National Cancer Institute Monographs*, **1**:55–70.

Goldhirsch A, Gelber RD, for the Ludwig Breast Cancer Group (1987). Adjuvant therapy for breast cancer: the Ludwig Breast Cancer Trials. In *Adjuvant therapy of cancer V* (ed. SE Salmon), pp. 297–309. Grune and Stratton, Orlando.

Goldhirsch A, Gelber RD (1988). Treatment of overt metastatic breast cancer. In *Baillière's Clinical Oncology*, **3**:215–29.

Goldhirsch A, Gelber RD, Mouridsen H (1987). Adjuvant chemotherapy in premenopausal patients: a more complicated form of oophorectomy? In *European School of Oncology monographs: endocrine therapy of breast cancer II* (ed. F Cavalli), pp. 11–19. Springer Verlag, Berlin.

Goldhirsch A, Gelber RD, Castiglione M (1988). Relapse of breast cancer after adjuvant treatment in premenopausal and perimenopausal women: patterns and prognoses. *Journal of Clinical Oncology*, **6**:89–97.

Goldhirsch A, *et al.* for Ludwig Breast Cancer Study Group (1989). Costs and benefits of adjuvant therapy in breast cancer: a quality-adjusted survival analysis. *Journal of Clinical Oncology*, **7**:36–44.

Goldie JH, Coldman AJ (1979). A mathematic model for relating the drug sensitivity of tumors to spontaneous mutation rate. *Cancer Treatment Reports*, **63**:1828–33.

Gore SM, *et al.* (1987). Influence of the sequencing of the chemotherapy and radiation therapy in node-negative breast cancer patients treated by conservative surgery and radiation therapy. In *Adjuvant therapy of cancer V* (ed. SE Salmon), pp. 365–73. Grune and Stratton, Orlando.

Greenwald P, Sondik E (1986). Division of cancer prevention and control. Cancer control. Objectives for the nation 1985–2000. *National Cancer Institute Monographs*, **2**:1–105.

Haagensen CD (1956). *Diseases of the breast* (1st edn). WB Saunders, Philadelphia.

Haagensen CD (1971). Carcinoma of the male breast. In *Diseases of the breast* (2nd edn), pp. 779–92. WB Saunders, Philadelphia.

Haagensen CD (1986). *Diseases of the breast* (3rd edn), pp. 426, 864–71. WB Saunders, Philadelphia.

Hall JM, *et al.* (1990). Linkage of early-onset familial breast cancer to chromosome 17q21. *Science*, **250**:1684–9.

Halsted WS (1894–1895). The results of operations for the cure of cancer of the breast performed at the Johns Hopkins Hospital from June, 1889 to January, 1894. *Johns Hopkins Hospital Bulletin*, **4**:297.

Handley RS, Thackray AC (1954). Invasion of the internal mammary lymph nodes. *British Medical Journal*, **1**:61.

Harris AL, Carmichael J, Cantwell BMJ, Dowsett M (1989). Zoladex: endocrine and therapeutic effects in postmenopausal breast cancer. *British Journal of Cancer*, 59:97–9.

Harris AL, *et al.* (1990). Comparison of short-term continuous chemotherapy (mitozantrone) for advanced breast cancer. *Lancet*, 335:186–90.

Harris JR, Hellman S (1984). The role of radiation therapy in the management of locally advanced carcinoma of the breast. *Cancer*, 53:758–61.

Harris JR, *et al.* (1983). Management of locally advanced carcinoma of the breast by primary radiation therapy. *International Journal of Radiation Oncology — Biology — Physics*, 9:345–9.

Harris NV, *et al.* (1982). Breast cancer in relation to patterns of oral contraceptive use. *American Journal of Epidemiology*, 116:643.

Harvey HA (1988). Luteinizing hormone-releasing hormone agonists in the treatment of breast cancer. In *Endocrine therapies in breast and prostatic cancer* (ed. CK Osborne), pp. 39–49. Kluwer Academic Publishers, Boston.

Haybittle JL, *et al.* (1989). Postoperative radiotherapy and late mortality: evidence from the Cancer Research Campaign trial for early breast cancer. *British Medical Journal*, 298:1611–14.

Hayes DF, Zurawski VR Jr, Kufe DW (1986). Comparison of circulating CA 15-3 and carcinoembryonic antigen levels in patients with breast cancer. *Journal of Clinical Oncology*, 4:1542–50.

Hayward JL (1983). Prospective studies, the Guy's Hospital trials on breast conservation. In *Conservative management of breast cancer* (ed. JR Harris, S Hellman, and WJB Silen). JB Lippincott, Philadelphia.

Hedley DW, *et al.* (1984). Influence of cellular DNA content on disease free survival of stage II breast cancer patients. *Cancer Research*, 44:5395–8.

Henderson BE, Ross RK, Paganini-Hill A, Mack TM (1986). Estrogen use and cardiovascular disease. *American Journal of Obstetrics and Gynecology*, 154:1181.

Henderson BE, *et al.* (1988). Re-evaluating the role of progestogen therapy after the menopause. *Fertility and Sterility*, 49:95.

Henderson IC (1987). Adjuvant systemic therapy for early breast cancer. *Current Problems in Cancer*, 11:125–207.

Henderson IC (1991). Adjuvant systemic therapy of early breast cancer. In *Breast diseases* (2nd edn) (ed. JR Harris, S Hellman, IC Henderson, and DW Kinne), pp. 427–86. JB Lippincott, Philadelphia.

Henderson IC, Canellos GP (1980). Cancer of the breast: a past decade. *New England Journal of Medicine*, 302:17–30, 78–90.

Henderson IC, Harris JR (1991). Principles in the management of metastatic disease. In *Breast diseases* (2nd edn) (ed. JR Harris, S Hellman, IC Henderson, and DW Kinne), pp. 547–677. JB Lippincott, Philadelphia.

Henderson IC, Hayes, DF, Gelman R (1988). Dose–response in the treatment of breast cancer: a critical review. *Journal of Clinical Oncology*, 6:1501–15.

Henderson IC, Harris JR, Kinne DW, Hellman S (1989*a*). Cancer of the breast. In *Cancer. Principles and practice of oncology* (ed. VT De Vita Jr, S Hellman, and SA Rosenberg), pp. 1197–268. JB Lippincott, Philadelphia.

Henderson IC, *et al.* (1989*b*). Randomized clinical trial comparing mitoxantrone with doxorubicin in previously treated patients with metastatic breast cancer. *Journal of Clinical Oncology*, 7:560–71.

Hendrickson FR (1977). The optimum schedule for palliative radiotherapy for metastatic bone pain. *International Journal of Radiation Oncology — Biology — Physics*, 2:165–8.

Hennessy C, *et al.* (1991). Expression of the antimetastatic gene nm23 in human breast cancer: an association with good prognosis. *Journal of the National Cancer Institute*, 83:281–5.

Hermanek P, Sobin LH (ed.) (1987). *TNM classification of malignant tumours*, (4th edn). Springer, Berlin.

Hilf R, *et al.* (1980). The relative importance of estrogen receptor analysis as a prognostic factor for recurrence or response to chemotherapy in women with breast cancer. *Cancer*, 45:1993–2000.

Holland R, Veling SHJ, Mravunac M, Hendriks JHCL (1985). Histologic multifocality of Tis, T_{1-2} breast carcinomas. Implications for clinical trials of breast-conserving surgery. *Cancer*, 56:979–90.

Holland R, *et al.* (1990). The presence of an extensive intraductal component (EIC) following a limited excision correlates with prominent residual disease in the remainder of the breast. *Journal of Clinical Oncology*, 8:113–18.

Hoover R, *et al.* (1976). Menopausal estrogens and breast cancers. *New England Journal of Medicine*, 295:401–5.

Horan Hand P, *et al.* (1983). Definition of antigenic heterogeneity and modulation among human mammary carcinoma cell populations using monoclonal antibodies to tumor-associated antigens. *Cancer Research*, 43:728–35.

Hortobagyi GN, *et al.* (1987). Evaluation of high-dose versus standard FAC chemotherapy for advanced breast cancer in protected environment units: a prospective randomized study. *Journal of Clinical Oncology*, 5:354–64.

Hoskin PJ, Crow J, Ford HT (1990). The influence of extent and local management on the outcome of radiotherapy for brain metastases. *International Journal of Radiation Oncology — Biology — Physics*, 19:111–15.

Host H, Brennhovd IO, Loeb M (1986). Postoperative radiotherapy in breast cancer – long-term results from the Oslo study. *International Journal of Radiation Oncology — Biology — Physics*, 12:727–32.

Howat JMT, *et al.* (1983). The association of cytosol oestrogen and progesterone receptors with histological features of breast cancer and early recurrence of disease. *British Journal of Cancer*, 47:629–40.

Huan S, *et al.* (1989). Low-dose continuous infusion 5-fluorouracil. Evaluation in advanced breast cancer. *Cancer*, 63:419–22.

Hulka BS, *et al.* (1982). Breast cancer and estrogen replacement therapy. *American Journal of Obstetrics and Gynecology*, 143:638–44.

Hutchinson WB, *et al.* (1980). Risk of breast cancer in women with benign breast disease. *Journal of the National Cancer Institute*, 65:13–20.

Hynes MA, *et al.* (1987). Growth hormone dependence of somatomedin C/insulin-like growth factor-I and insulin-like growth factor-II messenger ribonucleic acids. *Molecular Endocrinology*, 1:233–42.

Ingle JN, *et al.* (1981). Randomized trial of bilateral oophorectomy versus tamoxifen in premenopausal women with metastatic breast cancer. *Journal of Clinical Oncology*, 4:876–82.

Ingle JN, *et al.* (1985). Randomized trial of doxorubicin alone or combined with mitolactol in women with advanced breast cancer and prior chemotherapy exposure. *American Journal of Clinical Oncology*, 8:275–82.

Jacquillat C, *et al.* (1987). Pre-operative (Neoad) chemotherapy (Chem) and radiotherapy in breast cancer (BC). *EORTC Breast Cancer Cooperative Group, 4th Working Conference*, 30 June–3 July, London, p. 4.8.

Jakesz R, *et al.* (1987). Adjuvant chemotherapy in node-negative breast cancer patients. In *Adjuvant therapy of cancer V* (ed. SE Salmon), pp. 223–31. Grune and Stratton, Orlando.

Jick H, *et al.* (1980). Replacement estrogens and breast cancer. *American Journal of Epidemiology*, 112:586.

Jones JM and Ribeiro GG (1989). Mortality patterns over 34 years of breast cancer patients in a clinical trial of postoperative radiotherapy. *Clinical Radiology*, 40:204–8.

Jordan VC (1984). Biochemical pharmacology of antiestrogen action. *Biochemical Review*, 36:245–76.

Kaiser-Kupfer MI, Lippman ME (1978). Tamoxifen retinopathy. *Cancer Treatment Report*, 62:315–20.

Karrer K, Humphreys SR (1967). Continuous and limited courses of cyclophosphamide (NSC 26271) in mice with pulmonary metastases after surgery. *Cancer Chemotherapy Report*, 51:439–49.

Kaufmann M, *et al.* (1987). Adjuvant systemic risk adapted cytotoxic +/− tamoxifen therapy in women with node-positive breast cancer. In *Adjuvant therapy of cancer V* (ed. SE Salmon), pp. 337–46. Grune and Stratton, Orlando.

Kelsey JL, *et al.* (1978). Oral contraceptives and breast disease: an epidemiological study. *American Journal of Epidemiology*, 107:236.

Kelsey JL, *et al.* (1981). Estrogenous estrogens and other factors in the epidemiology of breast cancer. *Journal of the National Cancer Institute*, 67:327–33.

Kinlen LJ (1982). Meat and fat consumption and cancer mortality: a study of strict religious orders in Britain. *Lancet*, i:946.

Kiricuta CI, Tausch J (1992). A mathematical model of axillary lymph node involvement based on 1446 complete axillary dissection in patients with breast carcinoma. *Cancer*, 69:2496–501.

Klefstrom P, *et al.* (1987). Adjuvant postoperative radiotherapy, chemotherapy and immunotherapy in stage III breast cancer. II. 5-year results and influence of Levamisole. *Cancer*, 60:936–42.

Knight WA III, Livingston RB, Gregory EJ (1977). Estrogen receptor as an independent prognostic factor for early recurrence in breast cancer. *Cancer Research*, 37:4669–71.

Kodlin D, *et al.* (1977). Chronic mastopathy and breast cancer. A follow-up study. *Cancer*, **39**:2603–7.

Koscielny S, *et al.* (1984). Breast cancer: relationship between the size of the primary tumour and the probability of metastatic dissemination. *British Journal of Cancer*, **49**:709–15.

Kouyoumdjian JC, Feuilhade F, Dupre G, Rymer JC (1987). Multiple oncogenes transcription in normal, benign and malignant human breast tissue. *Proceedings of the International Association of Breast Cancer Research*, E-04.

Kusama S, *et al.* (1972). The gross rates of growth of human mammary carcinoma. *Cancer*, **30**:594–9.

Lacour J, *et al.* (1983). Radical mastectomy versus radical mastectomy plus internal mammary dissection. Ten-year results of an international cooperative trial in breast cancer. *Cancer*, **51**:1941–3.

Lacour J, *et al.* (1987). Is it useful to remove internal mammary nodes in operable breast cancer? *European Journal of Surgical Oncology*, **13**:309–14.

Land CE, *et al.* (1980). Breast cancer risk from low-dose exposure to ionizing radiation: results of parallel analysis of three exposed populations of women. *Journal of the National Cancer Institute*, **65**:353–76.

Legha SS, *et al.* (1982). Adriamycin therapy by continuous intravenous infusion in patients with metastatic breast cancer. *Cancer*, **49**:1762–6.

Levine MN, *et al.* (1988). Quality of life in stage II breast cancer: an instrument for clinical trials. *Journal of Clinical Oncology*, **6**:1798–810.

Li FP, Fraumeni JF (1975). Soft tissue sarcomas, breast cancer, and other neoplasms: a familial syndrome? *Annals of Internal Medicine*, **83**:833–4.

Lichter AL, *et al.* (1992). Mastectomy versus breast-conserving therapy in the treatment of stage I and II carcinoma of the breast: a randomized trial at the National Cancer Institute. *Journal of Clinical Oncology*, **10**:976–83.

Lilienfeld A (1956). The relationship of cancer of the female breast to artificial menopause and marital status. *Cancer*, **9**:927–34.

Lippman M (1987). Hormone stimulation and chemotherapy for breast cancer. *Journal of Clinical Oncology*, **5**:331–2.

Lippman ME, *et al.* (1986). Autocrine and paracrine growth regulation of human breast cancer. *Breast Cancer Research and Treatment*, **7**:59–70.

Locke FB, King H (1980). Cancer mortality risk among Japanese in the United States. *Journal of the National Cancer Institute*, **64**:1149–56.

Loprinzi CL (1989). 5-Fluorouracil with leucovorin in breast cancer. *Cancer*, **63**:1045–7.

Loprinzi CL, *et al.* (1986). Prospective evaluation of carcinoembryonic antigen levels and alternating chemotherapeutic regimens in metastatic breast cancer. *Journal of Clinical Oncology*, **4**:46–56.

Love SM, Gellman RS, Silen W (1982). Fibrocystic "disease" of the breasts— a nondisease? *New England Journal of Medicine*, **307**:1010–14.

Ludwig Breast Cancer Study Group (1985). Chemotherapy with or without oophorectomy in high-risk premenopausal patients with operable breast cancer. *Journal of Clinical Oncology*, **3**:1059–67.

Ludwig Breast Cancer Study Group (1988). Combination adjuvant chemotherapy for node-positive breast cancer: inadequacy of a single perioperative cycle. *New England Journal of Medicine*, **319**:677–83.

Ludwig Breast Cancer Study Group (1989). Prolonged disease-free survival after one course of perioperative adjuvant chemotherapy for node-negative breast cancer. *New England Journal of Medicine*, **320**:491–6.

Lundgren B (1983). The growth rate of breast cancer as a dynamic indicator of prognosis. *Australasian Radiology*, **27**:178–80.

Lynch HT, Lynch JF (1986). Breast cancer genetics in an oncology clinic: 328 consecutive patients. *Cancer Genetics and Cytogenetics*, **22**:369–71.

McCarty KS, *et al.* (1980). Correlation of estrogen and progesterone receptors with histologic differentiation in mammary carcinoma. *Cancer*, **46**:2851–8.

McDivitt RW, Hutter, RVP, Foote FW, Stewart FW (1967). *In situ* lobular carcinoma of the breast. A prospective follow-up study indicating cumulative patient risks. *Journal of the American Medical Association*, **201**:82–6.

McDivitt RW, Stone KR, Craig RB, Meyer JS (1985). A comparison of human breast cancer cell kinetics measured by flow cytometric analysis. *Journal of Surgical Oncology*, **29**:35–9.

McGuire WL (1991). Breast cancer prognostic factors: evaluation guidelines. *Journal of the National Institute of Cancer*, **83**:154–5.

Macklin MT (1959). Comparison of the number of breast cancer deaths observed in relatives of breast cancer patients, and the number expected on the basis of mortality rates. *Journal of the National Cancer Institute*, **22**:927–51.

MacMahon B, *et al.* (1970). Age at first birth and cancer of the breast. A summary of an international study. *Bulletin of the World Health Organization*, **43**:209.

MacWhirter R (1955). Simple mastectomy and radiotherapy in the treatment of breast cancer. *British Journal of Radiology*, **28**:128–39.

Maddox WA, *et al.* (1983). A randomized prospective trial of radical (Halsted) mastectomy versus modified radical mastectomy in 311 breast cancer patients. *Annals of Surgery*, **198**:207–12.

Maier WP, *et al.* (1977). The technique of modified radical mastectomy. *Surgical Oncology and Obstetrics*, **145**:69–74.

Malkin D, *et al.* (1990). Germ line p53 mutations in a familial syndrome of breast cancer, sarcomas, and other neoplasms. *Science*, **250**:1233–8.

Mansi JL, *et al.* (1989). Primary medical therapy for operable breast cancer. *European Journal of Cancer and Clinical Oncology*, **25**:1623–7.

Mansour EG, *et al.* (1989). Efficacy of adjuvant chemotherapy in high-risk node-negative breast cancer. An intergroup study. *New England Journal of Medicine*, **320**:485–90.

Margottini M and Bucalossi P (1949). Le metastasi linfoghiandolari mammarie interne nel cancro della mammelia. *Oncologia*, **23**:70–83.

Marini G, *et al.* (1987). 5-Fluorouracil and high-dose folinic acid as salvage treatment of advanced breast cancer: an update. *Oncology*, **44**:336–40.

Martin DS (1960). Clinical implications of the interrelationship of tumour size and chemotherapeutic response. *Annals of Surgery*, **151**:97–100.

Martin DS, Fugman RA (1957). A role of chemotherapy as an adjunct to surgery. *Cancer Research*, **17**:1098–101.

Martin DS, Hayworth PE, Fugman RA (1970). Enhanced cures of spontaneous murine mammary tumors with surgery, combination chemotherapy, and immunotherapy. *Cancer Research*, **30**:709–16.

Martin DS, *et al.* (1975). Solid tumor animal model therapeutically predictive for human breast cancer. *Cancer Chemotherapy Report*, **59**:89–109.

Martynova RP (1937). Studies in the genetics of human neoplasms. Cancer of the breast, based on 201 family histories. *American Journal of Cancer*, **29**:530–40.

Mauriac L, *et al.* (1991). Effects of primary chemotherapy in conservative treatment of breast cancer patient with operable tumours larger than 3 cm. Results of a randomized trial in a single centre. *Annals of Oncology*, **2**:347–54.

Mayo JG, Laster WR, Andrews CM, Schable FM (1972). Success and failure in the treatment of solid tumors. III. "Cure of metastic Lewis lung carcinoma with methyl-CCNU (NSC 94551) and surgery-chemotherapy". *Cancer Chemotherapy Report*, **56**:183–95.

Merson M, *et al.* (1992). Breast carcinoma presenting as axillary metastases without evidence of a primary tumour. *Cancer*, **2**:504–8.

Meyer JS, *et al.* (1983). Prediction of early course of breast carcinoma by thymidine labeling. *Cancer*, **51**:1879–86.

Meyer W (1894). An improved method of the radical operation for carcinoma of the breast. *Medicine Records*, **46**: 746.

Miller AB (1983). Screening for breast cancer. *Breast Cancer Research and Treatment*, **3**:143–56.

Miller AB (1986). Early detection of breast cancer. In *Breast diseases* (ed. JR Harris, S Hellman, IC Henderson, and DW Kinne), pp. 122–34. Lippincott, Philadelphia.

Miller AB, Chamberlain J, Tsechkovski M (1985). Self-examination in the early detection of breast cancer. A review of the evidence, with recommendations for further research. *Journal of Chronic Diseases*, **38**:527.

Miller AB, *et al.* (1989). Mortality from breast cancer after irradiation during fluoroscopic examinations in patients being treated for tuberculosis. *New England Journal of Medicine*, **321**:1285–9.

Mohammed RH, Lakatua DJ, Haus E, Yasmineh WJ (1986). Estrogen and progesterone receptors in human breast cancer. Correlation with histologic subtype and degree of differentiation. *Cancer*, **58**:1076–81.

Moliterni A, *et al.* (1991). Cyclophosphamide, methotrexate, and fluorouracil with and without doxorubicin in the adjuvant treatment of resectable breast cancer with one to three positive axillary nodes. *Journal of Clinical Oncology*, **9**:1124–30.

Moon RC, *et al.* (1979). N-(4-Hydroxyphenyl) retinamide, a new retinoid for prevention of breast cancer. *Cancer Research*, **39**:1339–46.

Moon RC, *et al.* (1989). Suppression of rat mammary cancer development by N-(4-hydroxyphenyl)-retinamide (4-HPR) following surgical removal of first palpable tumor. *Carcinogenesis*, **10**:1645–9.

Moran RE, Black MM, Alpert L, Straus MJ (1984). Correlation of cell-cycle kinetics, hormone receptors, histopathology, and nodal status in human breast cancer. *Cancer*, **54**:1586–90.

Morrison JM, *et al.* (1987). The West Midlands Oncology Association trials on adjuvant chemotherapy for operable breast cancer. In *Adjuvant therapy of cancer V* (ed. SE Salmon), pp. 311–18. Grune and Stratton, Orlando.

Mouridsen HT and Rose C (1987). Values and limitations of current criteria for objective response in advanced breast cancer. In *European School of Oncology monographs: endocrine therapy of breast cancer II* (ed. F Cavalli), pp. 41–6. Springer Verlag, Berlin.

Mouridsen H, Palshof T, Patterson J (1978). Tamoxifen in advanced breast cancer. *Cancer Treatment Review*, **5**:131–41.

Mouridsen HT, *et al.* (1986). Adjuvant tamoxifen in post-menopausal high-risk breast cancer patients: present status of Danish Breast Cancer Cooperative Group Trials. *National Cancer Institute Monograph*, **1**:115–18.

Muir R (1941). The evolution of carcinoma of the mammary. *Journal of Pathology and Bacteriology*, **52**:155–60.

Murad TH, Scarpelli DG (1967). The ultrastructure of medullary and scirrhous mammary duct carcinoma. *American Journal of Pathology*, **50**:335–60.

Mustacchi P (1961). Ramazzini and Rigoni-Stern on parity and breast cancer. *Archives of Internal Medicine*, **108**:195.

Nasca PC, *et al.* (1980). Relationship of hair dye use, benign breast disease, and breast cancer. *Journal of the National Cancer Institute*, **64**:23–8.

Natali PG, *et al.* (1983). Heterogeneity in the expression of HLA and tumor-associated antigens by surgically removed and cultured breast carcinoma cells. *Cancer Research*, **43**:660–8.

Nime FA, *et al.* (1977). Prognostic significance of tumor emboli in intramammary lymphatics in patients with mammary carcinoma. *American Journal of Surgical Pathology*, **1**:25–30.

Nissen-Meyer R (1991). Primary breast cancer: the effect of primary ovarian radiation. *Annals of Oncology*, **2**:343–6.

Nissen-Meyer R, *et al.* (1978). Surgical adjuvant chemotherapy. *Cancer*, **41**:2088–98.

Nolvadex Adjuvant Trial Organization (1985). Controlled trial of tamoxifen as single adjuvant agent in management of early breast cancer: analysis at six years. *Lancet*, **i**:836–9.

Nowell PC (1976). The clonal evolution of tumor cell populations. *Science*, **194**:23–8.

O'Bryan RM, Baker LH, Gottlieb JE (1977). Dose–response evaluation of adriamycin in human neoplasia. *Cancer*, **39**:1940–8.

Ohuchi N, Abe R, Kasai M (1984). Possible cancerous change of intraductal papillomas of the breast. A 3-D reconstruction study of 25 cases. *Cancer*, **54**:605–11.

Osborne CK (1988). Effects of estrogens and antiestrogens on cell proliferation. Implications for treatment of breast cancer. In *Endocrine therapies in breast and prostatic cancer* (ed. CK Osborne), pp. 111–29. Kluwer Academic Publishers, Boston.

Osborne CK, *et al.* (1981). Estrogen receptor and prognosis in breast cancer. In *Breast cancer, advances in research and treatment*, Vol. 4 (ed. WL McGuire), pp. 33–49. Plenum, New York.

Overgaard M, *et al.* (1990). Evaluation of radiotherapy in high-risk breast cancer patients: report from the Danish Breast Cancer Cooperative Group (DBCG 82) trial. *International Journal of Radiation Oncology—Biology—Physics*, **19**:1121–4.

Oxenhandler RW, *et al.* (1984). Flow cytometric determination of estrogen receptors in intact cells. *Cancer Research*, **44**:2516–23.

Paffenbarger RS, *et al.* (1977). Cancer risk as related to use of oral contraceptives during fertile years. *Cancer*, **39**(Suppl.):1887–91.

Page DL, *et al.* (1978). Relationship between component parts of fibrocystic disease complex and breast cancer. *Journal of National Cancer Institute*, **61**:1055–63.

Page DL, *et al.* (1985). Atypical hyperplastic lesions of the female breast: a long-term follow-up study. *Cancer*, **55**:2698–708.

Parklin DM, Stjernsward J, Muir CC (1984). Estimates of the worldwide frequency of twelve major cancers. *Bulletin of the World Health Organization*, **62**:163.

Parl FF, Wagner RK (1980). The histopathological evaluation of human breast cancers in correlation with estrogen receptor values. *Cancer*, **46**:362–7.

Patey HD, Dyson WH (1948). The prognosis of carcinoma of the breast in relation to the type of operation performed. *British Journal of Cancer*, **2**:7.

Penrose LS, MacKenzie HJ, Karn MNA (1948). Genetical study of human mammary cancer. *Annals of Eugenics*, **14**:234–66.

Perloff M, *et al.* (1988). Combination chemotherapy with mastectomy or radiotherapy for stage III breast carcinoma: a cancer and leukaemia group B study. *Journal of Clinical Oncology*, **6**:261–9.

Philips RL, *et al.* (1980). Mortality among California Seventh-Day Adventists for selected cancer sites. *Journal of the National Cancer Institute*, **65**:1097–107.

Pichon MF, *et al.* (1980). Relationship of presence of progesterone receptors to prognosis in early breast cancer. *Cancer Research*, **40**:3357–60.

Pigott J, *et al.* (1984). Metastases to the upper levels of the axillary nodes in carcinoma of the breast and its implications for nodal sampling procedures. *Surgical Gynecology and Obstetrics*, **158**:255–9.

Popkin GL, De Feo CP Jr (1976). Basal cell epithelioma. In *Cancer of the skin: biology–diagnosis–management* (ed. R Andrade, *et al.*), pp. 821–44. WB Saunders, Philadelphia.

Porro G, *et al.* (1988). Monoclonal antibody detection of carcinoma cells in bone marrow biopsy specimens from breast cancer patients. *Cancer*, **61**:2407–11.

Price P, *et al.* (1986). Prospective randomized trial of single and multifraction radiotherapy schedules in the treatment of painful bony metastases. *Radiotherapy and Oncology*, **6**:147–55.

Pukkala E, Gustavsson N, Teppo L (1986). *Atlas of cancer incidence in Finland 1953–1982*. Cancer Society of Finland, Helsinki.

Ravnihar B, Siegel DG, Lindtner J (1979). An epidemiologic study of breast cancer and benign breast neoplasia in relation to the oral contraceptive and estrogen use. *European Journal of Cancer*, **15**:395–405.

Recht A, *et al.* (1991). Integration of conservative surgery, radiotherapy, and chemotherapy for the treatment of early-stage, node-positive breast cancer: sequencing, timing, and outcome. *Journal of Clinical Oncology*, **9**:1662–7.

Redon H and Lacour J (1955). La place du curage parasternal dans le traitement du cancer du sein. *Presse Médicine*, **63**:1173–6.

Retsky MW, *et al.* (1987). Prospective computerized simulation of breast cancer: comparison of computer predictions with nine sets of biological and clinical data. *Cancer Research*, **47**:4982–7.

Ribeiro GG, Dunn G, Swindell R, Harris M, Banerjee SS (1990). Conservation of the breast using two different radiotherapy techniques: interim report of a clinical trial. *Clinical Oncology*, **2**:27–34.

Richardson WW (1956). Medullary carcinoma of the breast. A distinctive tumour type with a relatively good prognosis following radical mastectomy. *British Journal of Cancer*, **10**:415.

Rilke F, *et al.* (1991). Prognostic significance of her-2/NEU expression in breast cancer and its relationship to other prognostic factors. *International Journal of Cancer*, **49**:44–9.

Rivkin S, *et al.* (1991). Adjuvant combination chemotherapy (CMFVP) vs oophorectomy followed by CMFVP (OCNFVP) for premenopausal women with ER+ operable breast cancer with positive axillary lymph nodes. *Proceedings of the American Society of Clinical Oncology*, **10**:47.

Rosen PP, *et al.* (1978). Lobular carcinoma *in situ* of the breast. A detailed analysis of 99 patients with average follow-up of 24 years. *American Journal of Surgical Pathology*, **2**:225–39.

Rosen PP, *et al.* (1981). Predictors of recurrence in stage I (TINOMO) breast carcinoma. *Annals of Surgery*, **193**:15–25.

Rosenberg L, *et al.* (1984). Breast cancer and oral contraceptive use. *American Journal of Epidemiology*, **119**:167.

Roses DF, Harris MN, Gumport SL (1977). Total mastectomy with axillary dissection. *American Journal of Surgery*, **134**:674–7.

Rubens RD, Knight RK (1985). The contribution of prednisone (P) to primary endocrine therapy (PET) in advanced breast cancer. *Proceedings of the American Society of Clinical Oncology*, **4**:53.

Rubens RD, *et al.* (1977). Prognosis in inoperable stage III carcinoma of the breast. *European Journal of Cancer*, **13**:805–11.

Rubens RD, *et al.* (1989). Locally advanced breast cancer: the contribution of cytotoxic and endocrine treatment to radiotherapy. An EORTC Breast Cancer Cooperative Group Trial (10792). *European Journal of Cancer and Clinical Oncology*, **25**:667–78.

Russo J, *et al.* (1987). Predictors of recurrence and survival of patients with breast cancer. *American Journal of Clinical Pathology*, **88**:123–31.

Saccani Jotti G, *et al.* (1992). Preliminary study on oncogene product immunohistochemistry (c-erbB-2, c-myc, ras p21, EGFR) in breast pathology. *International Journal of Biological Markers*, 7:35–42.

Sacks NP, Barr LC, Allan SM, Baum M (1992). The role of axillary dissection in operable breast cancer. *Breast*, 1:41–9.

Saez S, Cheix F, Asselain B. (1983). Prognostic value of estrogen and progesterone receptors in primary breast cancer. *Breast Cancer Research and Treatment*, 3:345–54.

Sage HH, Casson PR (1976). Squamous cell carcinoma of the scalp, face, and neck. In *Cancer of the skin* (ed. R Androde, *et al.*), pp. 899–915. WB Saunders, Philadelphia.

Sainsbury JRC, *et al.* (1987). Epidermal-growth-factor receptor status as predictor of early recurrence of and death from breast cancer. *Lancet*, i:1398–402.

Salvadori B, *et al.* (1983). Prognostic factors in operable breast cancer. *Tumori*, 69:477–84.

Salvadori B, *et al.* (1990). Use of monoclonal antibody MBrl to detect micro-metastases in bone marrow specimens of breast cancer patients. *European Journal of Cancer*, 26:865–7.

Samet J, *et al.* (1986). Choice of cancer therapy varies with age of patient. *Journal of the American Medical Association*, 255:3385–90.

Sanderson KV, Mackie R (1979). Tumors of the skin. In *Textbook of dermatology* (3rd edn) (ed. A Rook, DS Wilkinson, and FJS Ebling), pp. 2171–9. Blackwell Scientific, London.

Saphner T, Tormey DC, Gray R (1991). Venous and arterial thrombosis in patients who received adjuvant therapy for breast cancer. *Journal of Clinical Oncology*, 9, 286–94.

Sarrazin, D., *et al.* (1983). Conservative treatment versus mastectomy in T1 or small T2 breast cancer: a randomized trial. In *Conservative management of breast cancer* (ed. JR Harris, S Hellman, and W Silen), pp. 101–14.

Sartwell PE, Arthes FG, Tonascia JA (1977). Exogenous hormones, reproductive history, and breast cancer. *Journal of the National Cancer Institute*, 59:1589–92.

Scanlon EF, Caprini JA (1975). Modified radical mastectomy. *Cancer*, 35:710–13.

Schaake-Koning C, *et al.* (1985). Adjuvant chemo- and hormonal therapy in locally advanced breast cancer: a randomized clinical study. *International Journal of Radiation Oncology—Biology—Physics*, 11:1759–63.

Schottenfeld D, *et al.* (1976). Ten-year results of the treatment of primary operable breast carcinoma. *Cancer*, 38:1001–7.

Scottish Cancer Trials Office (1987). Adjuvant tamoxifen in the management of operable breast cancer. The Scottish trial. *Lancet*, ii:171–5.

Secreto G, *et al.* (1984). Increased androgen activity and breast cancer risk in premenopausal women. *Cancer Research*, 44:5902–5.

Segaloff A, *et al.* (1985). An evaluation of the effect of vincristine added to cyclophosphamide, 5-fluorouracil, methotrexate, and prednisone in advanced breast cancer. *Breast Cancer Research and Treatment*, 5:311–19.

Senn HJ, *et al.* (1986). Swiss adjuvant trial (OSAKO 06/74) with chlorambucil, methotrexate, and 5-fluorouracil plus BCG in node-negative breast cancer patients: nine-year results. *National Cancer Institute Monographs*, 1:129–34.

Sertoli MR, *et al.* (1991). Perioperative polichemiotherapy for primary breast cancer: a randomized study. *Proceedings of the American Society of Clinical Oncology*, 10:49.

Sheldon T, *et al.* (1987). Primary radiation therapy for locally advanced breast cancer. *Cancer*, 60:1219–25.

Siiteri PK, Hammond GL, Nisker JA (1981). Increased availability of serum estrogens in breast cancer: a new hypothesis. In *Bambury Report No. 8: hormones and cancer* (ed. Pike, *et al.*), p. 87. Cold Spring Harbor Laboratory Press, Cold Spring Harbor, NY.

Silvestrini R (1991). Feasibility and reproducibility of the (3H)-thymidine labelling index in breast cancer. *Cellular Proliferation*, 24:437–45.

Silvestrini R, Daidone MG, Gasparini G (1985). Cell kinetics as a prognostic marker in node negative breast cancer. *Cancer*, 56:1982–7.

Silvestrini R, *et al.* (1987). Cell kinetics as a prognostic marker in locally advanced breast cancer. *Cancer Treatment Reports*, 71:375–9.

Slamon DJ, *et al.* (1987). Human breast cancer: correlation of relapse and survival with amplification of the HER-2/neu oncogene. *Science*, 235:177–82.

Smalley RV, *et al.* (1976). Combination versus sequential five-drug chemotherapy in metastatic carcinoma of the breast. *Cancer Research*, 36:3911–16.

Smans M, Boyle P, Muir CS (1993). *Cancer mortality atlas of Europe*. IARC Scientific Publication No. 7, Lyon.

Smithers DW (1948). Family histories of 459 patients with cancer of the breast. *British Journal of Cancer*, 2:163–7.

Sobin LH, Sherif M (1980). Relation between male breast cancer and prostate cancer. *British Journal of Cancer*, 42:787–90.

Sorace RA, *et al.* (1985). Management of nonmetastatic locally advanced breast cancer using primary induction chemotherapy with hormonal synchronization followed by radiation therapy with or without debulking surgery. *World Journal of Surgery*, 9:775.

Sporn MB, Newton DL (1979). Chemoprevention of cancer with retinoids. *Federation Proceedings*, 38:2528–34.

Sporn MB, Roberts AB (1991). Interactions of retinoids and transforming growth factor-beta in regulation of cell differentiation and proliferation. *Minireview Molecular Endocrinology*, 5:3–7.

Squartini F, Sounelli R (1981). Structure, functional changes, and proliferative pathology of the human mammary lobule in cancerous breasts. *Journal of the National Cancer Institute*, 67:33–46.

Steiner R, *et al.* (1983). Adriamycin alone or combined with vincristine in the treatment of advanced breast cancer. *European Journal of Cancer and Clinical Oncology*, 11:1553–7.

Stevens RG, Moolgavkar SH, Lee JH (1982). Temporal trends in breast cancer. *American Journal of Epidemiology*, 115:759.

Stewart H, Foster RS (1989). Breast cancer and aging. *Seminars in Oncology*, 16:41–50.

Stewart H, Knight GM (1989). Tamoxifen and the uterus and endometrium. *Lancet*, i:375–6.

Stewart HJ, Prescott RJ, Forrest PA (1989). Conservation therapy of breast cancer. *Lancet*, 2:168–9.

Stewart JF, *et al.* (1982). Contribution of prednisolone to the primary endocrine therapy of advanced breast cancer. *European Journal of Clinical Oncology*, 18:1307–14.

Stewart JF, *et al.* (1983). Steroid receptors and prognosis in operable (stage I and II) breast cancer. *European Journal of Cancer and Clinical Oncology*, 19:1381–7.

Stuart-Harris RC, Smith IE (1984). Aminoglutethimide in the treatment of advanced breast cancer. *Cancer Treatment Reviews*, 11:189–204.

Swift M, Reitnauer PJ, Morrell D, Chase, CL (1987). Breast and other cancers in families with ataxia-telangiectasia. *New England Journal of Medicine*, 316:1289–94.

Swift M, Morrell D, Massey RB, Chase CL (1991). Incidence of cancer in 161 affected by ataxia-telangiectasia. *New England Journal of Medicine*, 325:1831–5.

Tandon A, *et al.* (1990). Cathepsin D and prognosis in breast cancer. *New England Journal of Medicine*, 322:297–302.

Tannock IF, *et al.* (1988). A randomized trial of two dose levels of cyclophosphamide, methotrexate, and fluorouracil chemotherapy for patients with breast cancer. *Journal of Clinical Oncology*, 6:1377–87.

Theillet C, *et al.* (1986). Loss of a c-H-ras-1 allele and aggressive human primary breast carcinomas. *Cancer Research*, 46:4776–81.

The International Breast Cancer Study Group (1990). Late effects of adjuvant oophorectomy and chemotherapy upon pre-menopausal breast cancer patients. *Annals of Oncology*, 1:30–5.

Thorpe SM, *et al.* (1989). Association between high concentrations of M, 52.000 cathepsin D and poor prognosis in primary human breast cancer. *Cancer Research*, 49:6008–14.

Tokunaga M, *et al.* (1984). Breast cancer among atomic bomb survivors. In *Radiation carcinogenesis: epidemiology and biological significance* (ed. JD Boice Jr and JF Fraumeni Jr), pp. 45–6. Raven Press, New York.

Tormey DC, *et al.* (1982). Comparison of induction chemotherapies for metastatic breast cancer: an Eastern Cooperative Oncology Group Trial. *Cancer*, 50:1235–44.

Tranum B, *et al.* (1982). Adriamycin combinations in advanced breast cancer. *Cancer*, 49:835–9.

Tseng MT (1980). Ultrastructure of the hormone-dependent N-nitrosomethylurea-induced mammary carcinoma of the rat. *Cancer Research*, 40:3112–15.

Tubiana M, Koscielny S (1991). Natural history of human breast cancer: recent data and clinical implications. *Breast Cancer Research and Treatment*, 18:125–40.

Tubiana M, *et al.* (1984). The long term prognostic significance of the thymidine labelling index in breast cancer. *International Journal of Cancer*, 33:441–5.

Tulinius H, *et al.* (1982). Familial breast cancer in Iceland. *International Journal of Cancer*, 29:365–71.

Turner L, Swindell R, Bell WGT (1981). Radical versus modified radical mastectomy for breast cancer. *Annals of the Royal College of Surgeons of England*, 63:239.

Uppsala-Orebro Breast Cancer Study Group (1990). Sector resection with or without postoperative radiotherapy for stage I breast cancer: a randomized trial. *Journal of the National Cancer Institute*, 82:277–82.

Urban JA, Baker HW (1952). Radical mastectomy in continuity with *en bloc* resection of the internal mammary lymph-node chain. *Cancer*, 5:992–1008.

Valagussa P, Bonadonna G, Veronesi U (1978). Patterns of relapse and survival following radical mastectomy. *Cancer*, 41:1170–8.

Valagussa P, *et al.* (1984). Are estrogen receptors alone a reliable prognostic factor in node negative breast cancer? In *Adjuvant therapy of cancer IV* (ed. SE Jones and SE Salmon), pp. 407–15. Grune and Stratton, Orlando.

Valagussa P, Tancini G, Bonadonna G (1986). Salvage treatment of patients suffering relapse after adjuvant CMF chemotherapy. *Cancer*, 58:1411–17.

van Dongen E (1987). Breast conserving therapy in operable breast cancer. *EORTC Working Conference on Breast Cancer*, 1–3 July 1987, London.

Van Scott EJ (1979). Basal cell carcinoma. In *Dermatology in general medicine* (2nd edn) (ed. TB Fitzpatrick, *et al.*), pp. 377–83. McGraw-Hill, New York.

Veronesi U, Costa A (1988). Chemoprevention of contralateral breast cancer with the synthetic retinoid fenretinide. The first international breast cancer chemoprevention workshop, New York City, November 20, 1987. *Cancer Investigation*, 6:55–7.

Veronesi U, Gennari L (1960). Il carcinoma gelatinoso della mammella. *Tumori*, 46:119–55.

Veronesi U, Pizzocaro G (1968). Breast cancer in women subsequent to cystic disease of the breast. *Surgical Gynecology and Obstetrics*, 126:529–32.

Veronesi U, Valagussa P (1981). Inefficacy of internal mammary nodes dissection in breast cancer surgery. *Cancer*, 47:170–5.

Veronesi U, Zingo L (1967). Extended mastectomy for cancer of the breast. *Cancer*, 20:677–80.

Veronesi U, Rabotti GC, Sirtori C (1955). Il carcinoma intraduttale epidermotropo della mammella (cosidetto Morbo di Paget) *Tumori*, 41:1–142.

Veronesi U, Consolandi G, Briziarelli G (1957). The metastatic spread of breast cancer. *Lavori Istituto Anatomia Patologica, Perugia*, 17:5–66.

Veronesi U, Giarrusso AM, Guarino M (1964). Il carcinoma papillifero della mammella. *Tumori*, 50:421–9.

Veronesi U, *et al.* (1977). Conservative treatment of breast cancer. *Cancer*, 39:2822–6.

Veronesi U, *et al.* (1981). Comparing radical mastectomy with quadrantectomy, axillary dissection, and radiotherapy in patients with small cancers of the breast. *New England Journal of Medicine*, 305:6–11.

Veronesi U, *et al.* (1983*a*). Risk of internal mammary lymph node metastases and its relevance on prognosis of breast cancer patients. *Annals of Surgery*, 198:681–4.

Veronesi U, *et al.* (1983*b*). Results of quadrantectomy, axillary dissection, and radiotherapy (QUART) in T1N0 patients. In *Conservative management of breast cancer* (ed. JR Harris, S Hellman, and W Silen), pp. 91–100. JB Lippincott, Philadelphia.

Veronesi U, *et al.* (1985). Prognosis of breast cancer patients after mastectomy and dissection of internal mammary nodes. *Annals of Surgery*, 202:702–7.

Veronesi U, *et al.* (1986). Comparison of Halsted mastectomy with quadrantectomy, axillary dissection, and radiotherapy in early breast cancer: long term results. *European Journal of Clinical Oncology*, 22:1085–9.

Veronesi U, *et al.* (1990*a*). Breast conservation is the treatment of choice in small breast cancer: long-term results of a randomized trial. *European Journal of Cancer*, 26:668–70.

Veronesi U, *et al.* (1990*b*). Extent of metastatic axillary involvement in 1446 cases of breast cancer. *European Journal of Surgical Oncology*, 16:127–33.

Veronesi U, *et al.* (1990*c*). Quadrantectomy versus lumpectomy for small size breast cancer. *European Journal of Cancer*, 26:671–3.

Veronesi U, *et al.* (1993*a*). Prognostic significance by level and number of involved nodes in breast cancer. *Breast*, 2:224–8.

Veronesi U, *et al.* (1993*b*). Radiotherapy after breast-preserving surgery in women with localized cancer of the breast. *New England Journal of Medicine*, 328:1587–91.

Vilcoq JR, *et al.* (1984). Prognostic significance of clinical nodal involvement in patients treated by radical radiotherapy for a locally advanced breast cancer. *American Journal of Clinical Oncology*, 7:625–8.

Von Maillot K, Horke W, Prestele H (1982). Prognostic significance of the steroid receptor content in primary breast cancer. *Archives of Gynecology*, 321:185.

Wallgren A, *et al.* (1986). Radiation therapy in operable breast cancer: results from the Stockholm trial on adjuvant radiotherapy. *International Journal of Radiation Oncology—Biology—Physics*, 12:533–7.

Walt AJ, *et al.* (1976). The surgical implications of estrophile protein estimations in carcinoma of the breast. *Surgery*, 80:506–12.

Wangensteen OH (1949). Remarks on extension of the Halsted operation for cancer of the breast. *Annals of Surgery*, 130:315.

Warren S, Whitman EM (1937). Studies on tumour metastases: the distribution of metastases in cancer of the breast. *Surgery Gynecology and Obstetrics*, 57:81.

Wassink WF (1935). Cancer et hérédité. *Genetika*, 17:103–44.

Waterhouse J, *et al.* (1976). *Cancer incidence in five continents*. IARC Scientific Publication No. 15. IARC, Lyon.

Wheeler JE, *et al.* (1974). Lobular carcinoma *in situ* of the breast. Long-term follow-up. *Cancer*, 34:554–63.

Wilcox WS (1966). The last surviving cancer cell: the chance of killing it. *Cancer Chemotherapy Report*, 50:541–2.

Williams CJ, *et al.* (1987). Adjuvant chemotherapy for T 1-2, No, Mo, estrogen receptor negative breast cancer: preliminary results of a randomized trial. In *Adjuvant therapy of cancer V* (ed. SE Salmon), pp. 233–41. Grune and Stratton, Orlando.

Winstanley J, *et al.* (1991). The long term prognostic significance of oestrogen receptor analysis in early carcinoma of the breast. *British Journal of Cancer*, 64:99–101.

Yancik R, Ries LG, Yates JW (1989). Breast cancer in aging women. A population-based study of contrasts in stage, surgery, and survival. *Cancer*, 63:976–81.

Yarnold JR, Bloom HJG (1989). Radiation after limited and radical surgery. In *UICC Series: current treatment of breast cancer* (ed. B Hoogstraten, I Burn, and HJG Bloom), pp. 181–97. Springer-Verlag, Berlin.

Section 9
Gynaecological malignancy

9.1 Carcinoma of the ovary

JAN P. NEIJT, DAVID G. ALLEN, NICOLETTA COLOMBO,
AND JAN B. VERMORKEN

INTRODUCTION

This chapter deals with epithelial ovarian carcinomas. Treatment remains problematic, mainly because most of these carcinomas are at an advanced state at the time of diagnosis and cure is seldom possible. The primary treatment of patients with early stage ovarian carcinoma is surgical, but some patients may benefit from additional treatment. Standard treatment for the advanced stages consists of cytoreductive surgery followed by platinum-based chemotherapy. Over the last 15 years there has only been a small improvement in the overall prognosis. Further improvements in survival may have to await effective screening programmes, further randomized trials to assess treatment strategies, and the use of new chemotherapeutic agents.

EPIDEMIOLOGY

The incidence of ovarian cancer is highest in the highly industrialized countries of the world, particularly Western and Northern Europe and North America. The empirical lifetime risk of developing ovarian cancer is 1:70 and the median age at diagnosis is 62 years. Women over 55 years of age have a higher incidence rate of ovarian cancer and usually have more aggressive and advanced disease (Merino and Jaffe 1993). Ovarian cancer is the fifth leading cause of death in women in the United States, with an estimated incidence of 50 cases per 100 000 women. Epithelial ovarian cancer produces 20 000 new cases and causes 12 500 deaths annually in the United States (Silverberg et al. 1990). Of the ovarian cancers, 85–90 per cent are epithelial and more than two-thirds are stage III or IV disease.

The most consistently reported risk factor is ovulation. The risk of ovarian cancer decreases with increasing parity, anovulation, and oral contraceptive use. Likewise, late menopause has been linked to an increased ovarian cancer risk. The strongest epidemological leads include anovulation, parity, and oral contraceptive use. Pregnancy has consistently been shown to protect against the development of ovarian cancer (Booth et al. 1989). Oral contraceptive use for as long as 5 years has been shown to reduce the risk of ovarian cancer by approximately half (Cramer et al. 1983b). Only contraceptives which suppress ovulation have been found to protect against ovarian cancer. Single women, women of low parity, and women with a history of prior breast cancer are at higher risk. Hyperstimulation of the ovary using clomiphene citrate or gonadotrophins resulting in raised oestrogen concentrations and multiple follicle production over many cycles may predispose infertility patients to ovarian cancer (Fishel and Jackson 1989). Infertile women who have received fertility drugs may have a risk of epithelial ovarian cancer which is three times higher than that of women with no history of infertility. At present, however, the link between ovarian cancer and fertility drugs is by no means certain (Whittemore et al. 1992). Despite several case reports, no direct or causal link has yet been established (Goldberg and Runowicz 1992). The risk of ovarian cancer is variably higher in White, affluent, and better educated societies. Hysterectomy without oophorectomy or with unilateral oophorectomy and tubal ligation have consistently been reported to reduce the risk of ovarian cancer.

From an aetiological point of view women with ovarian cancer are a heterogeneous group and include (1) women whose genetic make-up predisposes them to ovarian cancer, (2) women whose life-styles have contributed to their ovarian carcinogenesis, and (3) women who have an interaction of environmental and host factor susceptibility (Lynch et al. 1993). The familial nature of ovarian cancer is also well documented (Schildkraut and Thompson 1988). This has resulted in the establishment of familial ovarian cancer registries (Piver et al. 1984).

More variable links to ovarian cancer include socio-economic status, childhood infections such as mumps (Cramer et al. 1983a) and rubella (McGowan et al. 1979), obesity (Slattery et al. 1989), diet, and exposure to radiation and talc.

PATHOLOGY

The ovary is covered by coelomic epithelium which is of mesodermal origin. The peritoneum is of similar origin, which accounts for the similarity between ovarian and peritoneal (extra-ovarian) tumours. Approximately 85 per cent of all primary malignant ovarian tumours arise from the coelomic epithelium (Parmley and Woodruff 1974). The pathological classification of epithelial ovarian tumours is shown in Table 1. The cause of metaplasia and neoplasia of the epithelial cells of the ovary is still unknown. Ovulation appears to play a major role in the production of inclusion cysts in the ovarian cortex (Radisavljevic 1977) and may contribute to the development of epithelial neoplasms.

Histological types

Approximately 10–20 per cent of the common epithelial tumours are of borderline malignancy (or carcinomas of low malignant potential). They show papillary proliferation and multilayering of epithelial cells with nuclear abnormalities but no true stromal invasion. These tumours are neither benign nor clearly malignant. The diagnosis is based solely on histological examination and the prognosis is excellent. Most borderline tumours are either mucinous

Table 1   Classification of epithelial ovarian tumours

I	Serous tumours
II	Mucinous tumours
III	Endometrioid tumours
IV	Clear cell (mesonephroid) tumours
V	Brenner (transitional cell) tumours
VI	Mixed tumours
VII	Undifferentiated tumours
VIII	Unclassified and miscellaneous tumours

Epithelial ovarian tumours are classified as benign, borderline, or malignant.

(48 per cent) or serous (47 per cent) and only 5 per cent are of other types (Kaern *et al.* 1993). Approximately 85 per cent are FIGO stage I at presentation. These tumours can implant on peritoneum, omentum, and serosal surfaces, produce ascites, and metastasize to lymph nodes. Borderline tumours may have malignant metastases.

Serous tumours form the largest group of epithelial neoplasms and comprise approximately 50 per cent of all ovarian carcinomas. They secrete serous fluid. Approximately 10 per cent of ovarian serous tumours are of low malignant potential or borderline. The serous carcinomas tend to be large tumours, with just over half measuring more than 15 cm in diameter. Macroscopically, most of these tumours are papillary and cystic and secrete a serous fluid. Microscopically, the well-differentiated carcinomas have large vesicular nuclei with prominent nucleoli. Stromal invasion is usually obvious, but can be difficult to identify in some cases. The moderately and poorly differentiated carcinomas have more solid sheets of cells, with the least differentiated and more aggressive tumours displaying undifferentiated and large bizarre cells. Psammoma bodies are frequently associated with the serous tumours. These are small laminated calcospherites and are found in approximately one-third of these carcinomas. They are more commonly seen in the borderline and well-differentiated tumours. Serous carcinomas may arise from the pelvic peritoneum without involvement of the ovaries.

Approximately 10 per cent of primary epithelial ovarian carcinomas are mucinous. It is important to make multiple sections from many areas before a borderline mucinous tumour is diagnosed. Metastatic lesions from the gastrointestinal tract should be excluded. Bilaterality suggests a metastatic adenocarcinoma. Pseudomyxoma peritonei is a rare condition which results in accumulations of gelatinous mucus within the pelvic and abdominal cavities. It is a poorly understood condition and most patients gradually deteriorate as a result of infections and bowel obstruction.

Malignant endometrioid carcinomas are characterized by an adenomatous pattern. Macroscopically, they are more solid than the serous or mucinous carcinomas; most are 10–20 cm in diameter and contain a dark haemorrhagic fluid. Microscopically, they resemble well-differentiated adenocarcinomas of the endometrium.

Clear cell tumours are also termed mesonephric tumours, although it is now accepted that they arise from the Müllerian ducts and not the mesonephric duct system. The carcinomas have two basic histological patterns, clear cell and hobnail cell, although numerous cellular patterns are described. Approximately 10 per cent of patients with ovarian clear cell carcinomas have hypercalcaemia.

Malignant Brenner (transitional cell) tumours are rare and resemble carcinomas of the bladder and lower genital tract. Epithelial nests containing coffee-bean-shaped nuclei are seen within a proliferative stroma, with transition into carcinoma showing pleomorphic nuclei infiltrating the ovarian stroma.

Mixed epithelial tumours (mixtures of two or more cell types) are found in less than 3 per cent of epithelial carcinomas. Mixed cell types are difficult to diagnose if the tumour is poorly differentiated.

Primary ovarian carcinomas that are too poorly differentiated to be categorized are classified as undifferentiated carcinomas. The difference between a very poorly differentiated serous or endometrioid adenocarcinoma and an undifferentiated carcinoma can be subjective. Small cell carcinomas of the ovary are classified as undifferentiated tumours. They are very uncommon tumours and two-thirds are associated with hypercalcaemia. They are aggressive tumours with a poor prognosis.

Unclassified tumours generally represent mesotheliomas and unusual tumours of an uncertain nature and can be classified into four categories: fibrosarcomatous, tubopapillary, mesothelial, and mixed histological patterns.

Patterns of spread

Epithelial ovarian carcinoma spreads in three main ways: (1) direct extension, (2) exfoliation of clonogenic cells, and (3) lymphatic spread. Metastasis through the bloodstream is rare. Direct extension occurs when the carcinoma penetrates the capsule of the ovary and involves structures in the pelvis or abdomen by direct contact. Malignant cells can also escape into the peritoneal fluid and be carried throughout the abdomen, allowing the cancer to implant and grow. Diaphragmatic and omental implants are common sites of spread. Spread to the retroperitoneal lymph nodes occurs in more than 60 per cent of cases (Allen *et al.* 1992). The pelvic lymph nodes are more commonly involved than the para-aortic lymph nodes.

Flow cytometry

DNA ploidy has been shown to be a valuable prognostic indicator in patients with both early and late stage ovarian cancer. Aneuploidy predicts a significantly shorter survival time, even in patients with borderline tumours and the prognostic value of flow cytometry is likely to influence the clinical management of ovarian cancer patients in the future (Braly and Klevecz 1993). Flow cytometry may aid in determining tumour response to treatment, help the individualization of therapy, and predict which borderline tumours will progress to invasive cancers. In a recent study using image analysis to measure the DNA content and morphometric nuclear features of 21 borderline ovarian tumours, a significant association between aneuploidy and tumour recurrence was found (Drescher *et al.* 1993). This confirms the findings of earlier studies (Kaern *et al.* 1990; Padberg *et al.* 1992) In stage I–IIa ovarian cancers there is a trend towards conservative management and flow cytometric ploidy may help in the selection of those who can be observed after surgery and those who require adjuvant chemotherapy.

SCREENING

Despite advances in the evaluation and treatment of ovarian cancer, mortality has decreased minimally during the past two decades. Five year survival rates increased from 36 per cent in 1975 to 39 per cent in 1990 (Boring *et al.* 1992). However, stage I ovarian cancer is highly amenable to therapy and the outlook is excellent. Therefore, it is imperative that effective methods for the detection of early stage ovarian cancer are developed if a significant impact is to be made on survival rates. The lack of early symptoms is responsible, to a large extent, for the poor prognosis in ovarian cancer. Bimanual pelvic examination has been the most commonly used method for the detection of ovarian cancer, but it is too insensitive and cannot reliably detect early disease. The most effective screening method for ovarian cancer at present is a combination of serum CA125 levels and transvaginal sonography. In screening studies serum CA125 levels have been shown to have a reasonably high specificity but a low sensitivity. Elevated serum levels of CA125 are present in over 80 per cent of ovarian cancer patients, but elevated levels are also found in approximately 6 per cent of patients with benign disease and 1 per cent of apparently healthy women (Lynch *et al.* 1986). Transvaginal sonography has a high sensitivity but only moderate specificity. The optimal population for ovarian screening and the screening interval are at present undefined. Preliminary studies suggest that all post-menopausal women should be screened on a yearly basis. Ovarian abnormalities will be early ovarian cancers (Campbell *et al.* 1989; Bourne *et al.* 1991; Van Nagell *et al.* 1991). Multi-institutional screening trials need to be instituted (Van Nagell *et al.* 1993). The National Cancer Institute in the United States is planning a randomized study of 74 000 women to test routine medical care in women aged 60–74 years versus screening with pelvic examination, CA125, and transvaginal ultrasound (Kramer *et al.* 1993).

The link between family history and epithelial ovarian cancer is now firmly established and the mode of inheritance in site-specific ovarian cancer families appears to be autosomal dominant with transmission through either the female or male parent. At present, however, there are no genetic markers with which to screen women genetically predisposed to ovarian cancer.

PROPHYLAXIS

Oophorectomy is the only effective prophylactic measure in the prevention of ovarian cancer. A recent study of prophylactic oophorectomy in women undergoing hysterectomy at the age of 40 years or older has shown that this can prevent 5.2 per cent of ovarian cancers (Sightler *et al.* 1991). These authors recommended routine prophylactic oophorectomy in all women undergoing hysterectomy after the age of 40 years. However, this policy would not prevent the relatively rare cancers arising from the mesothelial tissue of the peritoneum, which resemble ovarian cancers. A policy of routine prophylactic oophorectomy at the time of hysterectomy remains controversial.

Prophylactic oophorectomy may be advisable in women who have at least two first-degree blood relatives diagnosed with ovarian cancer as the chance of disease developing in this situation may be as high as 50 per cent (Barber 1993). Lynch *et al.* (1986) identified three distinct hereditary syndromes in ovarian cancer families: (1) site-specific ovarian cancer, (2) breast ovarian syndrome, and (3) cancer family syndrome (Lynch syndrome II). These syndromes may account for up to 10 per cent of all ovarian cancer cases.

CLINICAL PRESENTATION

In early stage ovarian cancer there may be minimal or no symptoms, and symptoms are often non-specific even in the more advanced stages. In early stage disease the patient may complain of irregular menses if she is pre-menopausal. Other complaints may include abdominal distension, pressure, pain, bloating, constipation, nausea, anorexia, and abnormal vaginal bleeding. Pressure symptoms from a pelvic mass may include urinary frequency or constipation. Acute symptoms are unusual. The most important sign of ovarian cancer is a pelvic mass on examination, particularly one which is irregular and fixed. The ovaries in a post-menopausal woman should not be palpable. A palpable ovary in this group of women has been referred to as the 'post-menopausal palpable ovary (PMPO) syndrome' (Barber and Graber 1971) and malignancy should be excluded.

Investigations

The patient with a suspected ovarian cancer should undergo a routine investigation before any planned laparotomy is carried out. This should include haematological (complete blood count) and biochemical (renal and liver function tests) assessments, tumour markers (CA125), radiological examination (chest radiography), and blood cross-match. Initial assessment should also include a Papanicolaou smear. Tumour markers such as human chorionic gonadotrophin and α-fetoprotein should be performed in case the tumour turns out to be non-epithelial.

Other investigations are performed only if indicated. A barium enema or sigmoidoscopy/colonoscopy may be indicated to exclude a primary colonic lesion with ovarian metastasis if there are symptoms suggestive of lower gastrointestinal tract pathology. Similarly, the upper gastrointestinal tract (upper gastrointestinal series or gastroscopy) and breasts (mammography) should be investigated when relevant. An intravenous pyelogram or renal ultrasound is not routinely performed pre-operatively. Liver, bone, and brain scans are only indicated if specific symptoms suggest metastases to these sites. If ascites or a pleural effusion is present, samples should be obtained for cytological analysis prior to surgery. This information is useful for the staging classification and to confirm an intra-abdominal malignancy.

Management planning

Pre-operatively the patient should be prepared both mentally and physically for surgery. A bowel preparation should be performed. Removal of ascites and any pleural effusion may be indicted to relieve symptoms and optimize the patient's condition prior to anaesthesia. When bowel surgery is anticipated, this should be discussed with the patient and the small chance of a colostomy should also be mentioned. Positioning on the theatre table also needs to be planned. If a low rectal anastomosis is anticipated, the patient should be placed in a position with the legs slightly raised to facilitate stapling. Consideration should also be given to the placement of a central venous access line such as a Port-A-Cath or Hickman catheter which is useful for the administration of chemotherapy or total parenteral nutrition post-operatively.

STAGING CLASSIFICATION

Epithelial ovarian carcinomas are staged according to the International Federation of Gynaecology and Obstetrics (FIGO) system (FIGO 1987). This is a surgical staging system, which makes an accurate staging laparotomy of great importance as subsequent treatment of the patient is based on the stage of the disease. The FIGO system is shown in Table 2.

SURGICAL TREATMENT

Several surgical procedures in ovarian cancer patients have been described in the literature. The terminology used is not always consistent. Different types of surgery for epithelial ovarian cancers and their synonyms are shown in Table 3 and discussed below.

Staging laparotomy

A systematic technique for exploring the abdomen should be developed. At the completion of an exploratory laparotomy, the surgeon should be confident that no significant pathological lesion has been overlooked. A midline abdominal incision extending above the umbilicus is recommended to allow access to and examination of the upper abdomen. If ascites is present, this should be aspirated and submitted for cytological evaluation. If no ascites is present, then peritoneal washings should be obtained from the pelvic cul-de-sac, the paracolic gutters, and beneath the hemidiaphragms. All intra-abdominal surfaces and organs should be evaluated by inspection and palpation, including the liver and diaphragm.

Table 2 FIGO stages for primary carcinoma of the ovary

I	Growth limited to the ovaries
Ia	Growth limited to one ovary; no ascites; no tumour on the external surface; capsule intact
Ib	Growth limited to both ovaries; no ascites; no tumour on the external surfaces; capsule intact
Ic*	Tumour either stage Ia or stage Ib, but with tumour on surface of one or both ovaries or with capsule ruptured or with ascites present containing malignant cells or with positive peritoneal washings
II	Growth involving one or both ovaries with pelvic extension
IIa	Extension and/or metastases to the uterus and/or tubes
IIb	Extension to other pelvic tissues
IIc*	Tumour either stage IIa or stage IIb but with tumour on surface of one or both ovaries, or with capsule(s) ruptured or with ascites present containing malignant cells or with positive peritoneal washings
III	Tumour involving one or both ovaries with peritoneal implants outside the pelvis and/or positive retroperitoneal of inguinal nodes; superficial liver metastases equals stage III; tumour is limited to the true pelvis but with histologically proven malignant extension to small bowel or omentum
IIIa	Tumour grossly limited to the true pelvis with negative nodes but with histologically confirmed microscopic seeding of abdominal peritoneal surfaces
IIIb	Tumour involving one or both ovaries with histologically confirmed implants of abdominal peritoneal surfaces; none exceeding 2 cm in diameter; nodes are negative
IIIc	Adbominal implants greater than 2 cm in diameter and/or positive retroperitoneal or inguinal nodes
IV	Growth involving one or both ovaries with distant metastases; if pleural effusion present, there must be positive cytology to allot a case to stage IV; parenchymal livermetastasis equals stage IV

*To assess the impact prognosis of the different criteria for allotting cases to stage Ic or stage IIc it is of value to know whether the source of malignant cells was (i) peritoneal washings or (ii) ascites and whether rupture of the capsule was spontaneous or caused by the surgeon.

Suspicious areas or lesions, including adhesions, should be biopsied. If there is no evidence of disease, multiple intraperitoneal biopsies should be performed from the peritoneum of the bladder and the intestinal mesentery and diaphragms. If possible, the ovarian tumour should be removed intact. In most cases a total abdominal hysterectomy and bilateral salpingo-oophorectomy, infracolic omentectomy, and retroperitoneal lymph node sampling is then performed. The retroperitoneal spaces should be explored to evaluate the pelvic and para-aortic lymph nodes. Any enlarged nodes should be resected and submitted separately for histopathological evaluation. Up to 31 per cent of patients with apparent stage I or stage II disease are 'upstaged' after re-exploration following an inadequate initial staging procedure (Young *et al.* 1983). The importance of retroperitoneal lymphadenectomy in detecting advanced stages of disease has been documented (Allen *et al.* 1992). At the completion of a staging laparotomy, the surgeon must record the size and location of all residual tumour deposits.

Conservative surgery

Recently, it has become apparent that some early stage ovarian cancers can be treated with conservative surgery alone. In stage I, grade 1 disease, fertility can even be preserved by removing only the diseased ovary. A Dutch prospective study has shown that the disease-free survival for stage I–IIa grade 1 patients was 100 per cent after careful staging and 88 per cent without complete surgical

Table 3 Types of surgery for epithelial ovarian carcinomas

A. Primary surgery
  1. Staging laparotomy (diagnostic laparotomy)
  2. Radical cytoreductive (or debulking) surgery
  3. Conservative surgery

B. Secondary surgery
  1. Intervention (or interval) cytoreductive surgery
  2. Second-look laparotomy
  3. Secondary cytoreduction (salvage surgery)
  4. Palliative surgery

staging (Trimbos *et al.* 1991). Similar results were obtained by Monga *et al.* (1991). The Italian National Research Council recently reported no difference between optimally and suboptimally staged patients with stage I–IIa disease with regard to relapse or time to recurrence. An extensive review of stage I disease has also shown that, besides grade, only dense adhesions and large volume ascites are predictive of relapse, exluding conservative surgery in these patients (Dembo *et al.* 1990). Patients with early stage ovarian carcinoma (stage I–IIa) or borderline tumours who wish to retain their reproductive function may qualify for conservative surgery. However, these patients may be advised to undergo further surgery to remove both ovaries and the uterus once the family is complete. If this is not done, then close follow-up is mandatory.

Cytoreductive surgery

In order to minimize the tumour burden before chemotherapy or radiotherapy, cytoreductive (or debulking) surgery is performed. There are four possible benefits from cytoreductive surgery.

1. Improvement of tumour response to further therapy. Cytoreduction should improve tumour perfusion and increase the growth fraction, both of which improve response to chemotherapy or radiotherapy. Smaller tumour masses require fewer cycles of chemotherapy so that there is less chance of induced drug resistance. Clones of phenotypically resistant cells may also be removed.

2. Treatment, delay, or prevention of complications arising from tumour masses, for example bowel obstruction and ascites.

3. Enhancement of the immunological competence of the patient. The immunogenicity of ovarian cancer has been demonstrated *in vivo* and cytoreduction may help the patient to mobilize her own immune response to the cancer.

4. Psychological benefit to the patient of knowing that the tumour bulk has been removed.

The aim of cytoreductive surgery is the removal of all primary tumour and, as far as possible, the resection of the metastatic disease. If complete resection is not possible, then all individual tumour sites should be reduced to a minimal residuum. Optimal resection is achieved if tumour nodules are reduced to a diameter of 1.0 cm or less. This is associated with a significant longer survival for the patient (Griffiths 1975), which is increased further if residual lesions are less than 5 mm in diameter (Hacker *et al.* 1983; Van Lindert *et al.* 1984). Most studies of advanced ovarian cancer show that the amount of residual tumour after the first laparotomy is the most important prognostic factor and the only one on which the treating physician can have any influence. Recent studies confirm the significant survival benefits when optimal cytoreduction is achieved (Teeling *et al.* 1992; Tibben *et al.* 1992). However, Goodman *et al.* (1992) found no difference in survival between patients with stage IV disease who were optimally cytoreduced and those who were not. Bowel resections are performed in approximately 30 per cent of cytoreductive procedures (Allen *et al.* 1992), but whether this improves the survival of the patient is controversial (Potter *et al.* 1991; Miholic *et al.* 1992). Long-term survival is likely only if all macroscopic tumour can be removed without the need for aggressive surgery involving bowel or liver resections or splenectomy. The true value of primary cytoreductive surgery is difficult to assess as no randomized trials have been performed. Therefore, a fundamental question remains unanswered: is surgical resection *per se* or the complete resectability of the tumour the most important factor? This reflects the biology and aggressiveness of the tumour.

Intervention cytoreductive surgery

In those patients in whom the tumour is deemed irresectable at the initial laparotomy, maximum cytoreduction can be attempted as soon as chemotherapy response renders the tumour masses resectable. This is called intervention cytoreductive surgery and its benefits are not yet established. In a Dutch study, intervention surgery achieving a tumour residual of less than 1 cm did not result in survival benefit (Neijt *et al.* 1987). The findings suggested that if a serious attempt at cytoreduction had been made before starting chemotherapy, a second attempt by the surgeon during chemotherapy would not improve survival. Surgery may have a role only in cases in which initial debulking had not been attempted. A study from the MD Anderson Cancer Centre reported on a group of patients who were given two to four cycles of neoadjuvant chemotherapy followed by intervention debulking surgery and a further six cycles of chemotherapy. This group was compared with two matched control groups. The median survival times for the three groups were not significantly different, suggesting that patients with bulky residual disease have a uniformly poor prognosis regardless of the timing of further surgery (Jacob *et al.* 1991).

One prospective randomized study of intervention surgery has been carried out by the European Organization on Research and Treatment of Cancer (EORTC). After three cycles of cisplatin and cyclophosphamide, patients without progressive disease were randomized between intervention cycloreduction or no further surgery, followed by additional chemotherapy. The data of 278 patients have been analysed. The median progression-free and overall survival were prolonged by 5 and 6 months, respectively, in the surgical arm of the study ($p=0.01$) (Van der Burg *et al.* 1993). It must be emphasized that not all eligible patients in this study had attempted debulking at the initial laparotomy. The survival benefit noted in the group of patients operated on may thus be the result of delayed initial cycloreduction. A confirmatory study, only admitting patients with irresectable tumours at the initial laparotomy is needed.

Second-look laparotomy

Second-look laparotomy is defined as an exploratory procedure planned to assess the cancer status of a patient with no clinical evidence of disease and normal CA125 levels after a planned course of treatment. The second-look procedure includes (1) peritoneal washings for cytology, (2) inspection and palpation of the abdomen and pelvis, (3) biopsies taken from initial primary tumour sites, (4) random biopsies including the ovarian pedicles, and (5) pelvic and para-aortic lymph node sampling. In addition, if the primary surgery was incomplete, any remaining uterus, tubes, ovary, or omentum should be removed. In a research setting it is used to determine the complete pathological response to therapy. A negative second-look laparotomy may have some prognostic value, although up to 40 per cent recur within 5 years of negative findings. Persistent disease is detected in approximately 60 per cent of patients at second-look laparotomy. At present, the role of second-look laparotomy remains controversial (Luesley *et al.* 1988; Podratz and Kinney 1993). Prospective studies are required to determine the place of a second-look laparotomy with regard to consolidation therapy, salvage therapy, and overall survival times.

Secondary cytoreduction

Secondary surgery is performed on patients with clinical evidence of recurrent disease. The purpose of performing the surgery is cytoreduction before instituting salvage therapy. Although this treatment is controversial, the weight of evidence suggests that if the patient is left with only microscopic disease then survival benefit can be expected. The therapeutic value of secondary surgery depends to a large extent on the efficacy of second-line treatment. Secondary cytoreduction will become more important as better salvage regimens become available (Hoskins 1993). Other factors associated with the efficacy of secondary surgical cytoreduction are less than 55 years, a long interval from initial diagnosis to secondary cytoreduction, residual disease at initial staging laparotomy of less than 2 cm, and a complete clinical response to a cisplatin-based front-line regimen. When these factors are present, the performance of secondary cytoreductive surgery for patients who develop gross recurrent or progressive ovarian cancer following cisplatin therapy is probably justified (Segna *et al.* 1993).

Palliative surgery

Palliative surgery often involves surgery for bowel obstruction and aims to improve quality of life. Patients with recurrent epithelial ovarian cancer often develop intestinal obstruction. The life expectancy of these patients is short and decisions regarding palliative surgery must be carefully considered. Any surgery must be planned according to the patient's condition. Bowel obstruction in one area can be resected or bypassed. Multiple obstructed areas may require bypass, colostomy, or gastrostomy. Operative mortality can be high and survival is often limited.

Immediate post-operative period and morbidity

Aggressive surgery and any associated morbidity must be balanced with therapeutic benefits. In patients with advanced stage epithelial ovarian cancer, optimal cytoreduction can be achieved in approximately 80 per cent with major morbidity occurring in approximately 5–7 per cent and operative mortality in approximately 1 per cent. In experienced hands, serious morbidity can be kept to acceptably low levels (Hacker 1989). After cytoreductive surgery the immediate post-operative period can be complicated. The patient is best managed in a high dependency area where close observation can be maintained. Particular attention should be paid to fluid and electrolyte balance. A nasogastric tube is advisable for the first 24–72 h. Prophylactic antibiotics should be used, particularly if bowel surgery has been performed. Venous thrombosis and pulmonary embolism are a constant danger despite the use of prophylactic measures. Other factors to consider in the post-operative period are the need for total parental nutrition and the timing of adjuvant chemotherapy.

PROGNOSTIC FACTORS

At present one of the leading issues in the treatment of cancer is the identification of subgroups of patients with good or poor diagnosis. A better definition of these subgroups leads to the creation of less toxic treatment schedules for low-risk patients and new treatment strategies for the high-risk groups. The assessment of prognosis is valuable not only in the planning of treatment for individual patients but also for the stratification of patients in clinical trials.

The prognosis of patients is estimated on the basis of pre-treatment factors such as tumour stage, grade, and histological type, size of residual tumour after primary cytoreduction, and patient age and performance status. The surgical stage of the tumour is important. The 5 year survival is 85–100 per cent for patients in stage I, 40–50 per cent for stage II–IIIa, 20 per cent for stage IIIb, and 5–10 per cent for stages IIIc and IV. Grade 2 and 3 tumours result in poorer survivals than grade 1 tumours. The prognostic validity of the FIGO stages and of tumour grading has recently been confirmed (Partridge et al. 1993). Serous adenocarcinomas are associated with a poor prognosis and endometrioid types with a somewhat better prognosis, whilst the prognosis for mucinous and clear cell tumours is somewhere in between. The smaller the residual tumour volume after primary cytoreductive surgery the better the prognosis for the patient, with no residual or microscopic residual reflecting the best chance of survival. Older patients and patients with poor performance indices have a more unfavourable outcome (Ries 1993). For the borderline ovarian tumours important prognostic information can be obtained by measuring DNA ploidy and nuclear morphology (Drescher et al. 1993); recurrence is associated with aneuploidy and increased nuclear texture.

In the advanced stages the prognosis is directly correlated with tumour size. In a historical retrospective study, Griffiths (1975) showed that despite 'debulking', there were no long-term survivors if a mass larger than 1.5 cm in diameter was left behind. In his study of 102 patients with stage II and III ovarian carcinoma, a residual tumour mass less than 1.5 cm in diameter was an independent prognostic factor predicting survival, but this association was not present above 1.5 cm.

In later studies, sophisticated statistical analyses revealed other important factors predicting survival benefit: these were, in order of decreasing value, the performance status, the differentiation grade of the tumour, the size of the residual tumour prior to the initiation of chemotherapy, the FIGO classification of stage, and the presence or absence of ascites (Swenerton et al. 1985; Van Houwelingen et al. 1985; Redman et al. 1986; Kappen and Niejt 1993). Much work to identify prognostic factors in advanced ovarian cancer has been done by Lund and co-workers. She identified, on the basis of the results of a Cox multivariate stepwise analysis, a subset of independent significant prognostic factors in a Danish study population (Lund and Williamson 1991): residual tumour size, performance status, alkaline phosphatase, number of metastases, and histological differentiation grade and type. A major problem with studies that identify prognostic factors in a subset of patients is that these factors only apply to the group of patients used for the analyses. The factors have to be validated in other databases before they can be recommended for general use. Factors emerging from nearly all studies of this type are the performance status, the size of the residual tumour prior to chemotherapy, and the FIGO stage.

TREATMENT OF STAGES I AND IIa

The primary treatment of patients with early stage ovarian carcinoma is surgical and has been discussed earlier when considering conservative surgery. An adequate surgical procedure must be emphasized. Patients with stage Ia, Ib, or IIa grade 1 lesions can be treated with surgery alone (Young et al. 1990; Trimbos et al. 1991), whereas patients in these stages with higher grade lesions or stage Ic lesions require adjuvant therapy. The appropriate adjuvant treatment has been poorly defined and must be individualized. Chemotherapy or radiation therapy can be considered.

The role of radiation therapy (Lanciano and Randall 1991) is limited. The main problem restricting its use is the relatively high morbidity, particularly acute and chronic intestinal morbidity. Whole-abdomen radiation has been used, employing either a moving-strip technique or an open-field technique (Thomas and Dembo 1993). In a Danish study patients with FIGO stages Ib, Ic, IIa, IIb, and IIc were randomized to abdominal irradiation or pelvic irradiation plus cyclophosphamide. There was no difference between the regimens with respect to recurrence-free survival (55 per cent) and 4 year overall survival (63 per cent). Twenty-five per cent of the patients treated with pelvic irradiation plus cyclophosphamide had haemorrhagic cystitis, probably caused by radiation damage and cyclophosphamide cystitis. Eight per cent had late gastrointestinal symptoms requiring surgery. From this study of 118 patients, Sell et al. (1990) conclude that abdominal irradiation does not have a role in the treatment of early stage ovarian cancer.

The Gynecologic Oncology Group has performed a series of trials testing adjuvant treatment in carefully staged patients. One study compared patients with poorly differentiated stage I or II disease who received melphalan (less effective than cisplatin or carboplatin and cyclophosphamide) or intraperitoneal ^{32}P (Young et al. 1990). An overall disease-free survival rate of 85 per cent was observed at 5 years in both groups. In the current Gynecologic Oncology Group study patients are randomized to receive either intraperitoneal ^{32}P or 3 monthly cycles of cyclophosphamide and cisplatin (Young et al. 1993). Although the study has not been completed, it is now believed by many physicians that chemotherapy (cisplatin or carboplatin and cyclophosphamide) is preferable to radiotherapy or intraperitoneal ^{32}P for the treatment of early stage moderate and undifferentiated ovarian cancer.

TREATMENT OF STAGES IIb, III, AND IV

In this section we summarize the most important facts and try to answer the question: 'what is an optimal treatment for advanced ovarian cancer today?'. The choice of treatment is determined by the stage of the disease. In an advanced stage (FIGO stages IIb, III, and IV) chemotherapy is the treatment of choice after appropriate cytoreductive surgery has been performed. The use of radiotherapy has remained a controversial subject (Thomas and Dembo 1993). Evidence that radiation therapy is curative in advanced disease is lacking. Even in patients with small residual disease after the completion of chemotherapy, the results have been disappointing. For instance in an Italian study performed at the Istituto Nazionale per la Ricera sul Cancro, Genoa, patients with no disease or minimal residual disease at second-look laparotomy were randomized between three more courses of chemotherapy or whole-abdomen radiotherapy. At a median follow-up of 22 months, 11 out of 20 patients in the radiotherapy arm and six out of 21 in the chemotherapy arm progressed and nine and three patients, respectively died. Although the number of randomized patients was small, the trial was stopped because of the survival and progression-free survival advantage of patients treated with chemotherapy (Bruzzone et al. 1990b). Another randomized trial (117 patients) comparing single-agent carboplatin with carboplatin followed by radiotherapy showed no significant advantage for consolidation whole-abdomen radiotherapy compared with the continuation of chemotherapy, even when no macroscopic residual disease was apparent at second look (Lambert *et al.* 1993). Toxic effects during whole-abdomen radiotherapy require treatment interruption in most patients and are sometimes serious (small bowel obstruction requiring surgery). Whole-abdomen radiotherapy is not indicated in the treatment of advanced ovarian cancer because of the poor disease-free interval and the severe toxicity (Franchin *et al.* 1991).

Chemotherapy

Single drugs

Before cisplatin was introduced, the drug of choice in stages IIb, III, and IV was a single alkylating agent, usually 1-phenylalanine mustard (melphalan, alkeran) or cyclophosphamide. The response rates mentioned in the literature for these agents fluctuated from 10 to 70 per cent, with a mean response rate of 40 per cent and a median survival time of 12–14 months. In one series, the overall 5 year survival rate after treatment with melphalan is less than 10 per cent and only 16 per cent of patients who responded to chemotherapy survived (Smith and Day 1979). Several non-alkylating drugs have been found to be more or less effective in ovarian cancer. As for the alkylating agents, the response rates for most drugs vary widely because dose, prior treatment, and patient characteristics have a significant influence on outcome. As illustration, the response rates for teniposide ranged from 0 to 40 per cent in five series and from an overall response rate of less than 10 per cent to a complete response rate greater than 10 per cent in another nine studies (Muggia and Russell 1991). Etoposide (VP-16) another podophyllotoxin, administered orally in a low dose (50mg per day for 20 days, repeated every 28 days) is associated with almost no activity in platinum-refractory ovarian cancer (6 per cent partial response rate) (Markman *et al.* 1992). Hexamethylmelamine administered orally has been recognized as having single-agent activity (Foster *et al.* 1986; Schein *et al.* 1991), but in a phase 2 trial of intravenous hexamethylmelamine there were no objective responses among 15 evaluable patients (Hauge *et al.* 1992). Other drugs that may have single-agent activity are doxorubicin, epirubicin (Thigpen 1985), and probably mitomycin C (Creech *et al.* 1985).

The list of drugs judged to have no activity is much longer and includes VM-26, 5-fluorouracil and *N*-(phosphonoacetyl)-L-aspartate (PALA), vinblastine, esorubicin mitoxantrone, and mitozolomide. Data concerning ifosfamide are conflicting. Two studies have shown a negative result with ifosfamide in pre-treated ovarian cancer (Jungi *et al.* 1985; Willemse *et al.* 1990), but a Gynecologic Oncology Group study of 41 patients evaluable for response showed three (7 per cent) with a complete response and five (13 per cent) with a partial response. Response to ifosfamide was not correlated with the previous response to cisplatin-based treatment and the group concluded that further study of this drug is warranted (Sutton *et al.* 1989*a*).

Cisplatin is the most active agent for the treatment of ovarian cancer. It causes a variety of side-effects: nausea, vomiting, nephrotoxicity, electrolyte disturbances, allergic reactions, ototoxicity, neurotoxicity, and mild myelosuppression. The cisplatin dose most frequently used in previously treated and untreated patients is 50–100 mg/m^2 intravenously. It has been reported that escalation of the dose cisplatin can increase the response rate (Lambert and Berry 1985; Ozols *et al.* 1985; Wiltshaw *et al.* 1986). However, even

though hydration prevented nephrotoxicity in these studies, it did not give protection against the other side-effects such as ototoxicity and sensory neuropathy. In the higher dose ranges these disabling effects of toxicity have become dose limiting. The problems associated with the toxicity of cisplatin have encouraged research to find less toxic analogues.

Carboplatin is one such cisplatin analogue. This drug is less nephrotoxic and less emetogenic but more myelosuppressive than its parent cisplatin. Neurotoxicity, ototoxicity, and nephrotoxicity are minimal or absent. Carboplatin is excreted by the kidneys, which can lead to enhanced toxicity in patients with decreased renal function. The area under the plasma concentration versus time curve is related to the renal function. Therefore, a fixed dose, as prescribed in many trials, may lead to an overdose, unexpected toxicity, or an underdose because of variation in renal clearance between patients (Calvert *et al.* 1992). Myelosuppression, particularly thrombocytopenia, is a major side-effect and is dose limiting.

Three randomized studies of single-agent carboplatin versus cisplatin in patients with previously untreated ovarian cancer have shown that a carboplatin dose of 400 mg/m^2 monthly is equivalent to a cisplatin dose of 100 mg/m^2 monthly (Wiltshaw *et al.* 1985; Adams *et al.* 1989; Mangioni *et al.* 1989). All three of these studies concluded that carboplatin had similar antitumour activity to cisplatin but was less toxic in all respects, except for bone-marrow suppression. However, the survival results of the above studies are difficult to interpret because most patients randomized to receive carboplatin are subsequently treated with cisplatin and vice versa. The cross-over from one treatment to the other before resistant disease emerges influences the outcome in terms of progression-free and overall survival. In addition, the progression-free survival in these studies is calculated from the date of first surgery to the date of first progression, irrespective of whether progression occurred during carboplatin treatment or during subsequent cisplatin treatment. Thus, survival is also a result of the activity of both carboplatin and cisplatin.

Cisplatin-based combinations

Since the introduction of cisplatin-based combinations in the 1980s, the outcome of treatment has improved markedly. At present, up to 30 per cent of patients survive for 5 years despite advanced tumour at diagnosis. A cumulative response rate of 68 per cent was found with combinations that include cisplatin, which is clearly superior to the response rates of 47 per cent with combinations lacking this drug and of 40 per cent with alkylating agents alone (Slevin 1986). On the basis of overview analysis of randomized trials the Advanced Ovarian Cancer Trialists Group (1991) concluded that, in terms of survival, immediate platinum-based treatment was better than non-platinum regimens and that cisplatin in combination was better than single-agent cisplatin when used in the same dose.

A problem with most combination regimens is that the toxicity of the less active agents in the combination prevents the use of optimal doses of the more effective drugs such as cisplatin, carboplatin, and cyclophosphamide. So far, it has not been proved for ovarian cancer that more drugs in one combination are better than two. This was illustrated by the results of a randomized comparison of treatment with CHAP-5 (cyclophosphamide, hexamethylmelamine, doxorubicin, and cisplatin) and CP (cyclophosphamide and cisplatin) (Neijt *et al.* 1987). In this study, 191 patients were treated with either CHAP-5 or CP; remission rates were similar and progression-free, and overall survival rates were exactly the same. Overall toxicity was lower with CP and required a shorter period in hospital. Thus, the single-day regimen was preferred to CHAP-5. Data from the Mayo Clinic and a large-scale Danish study support this conclusion (Edmonson *et al.* 1985; Bertelsen *et al.* 1987). These investigators concluded from their findings that CP, HCAP (hexamethylmelamine, cyclophosphamide, doxorubicin, and cisplatin), and CAP were equally effective. The above studies also suggest that hexamethylmelamine and doxorubicin probably do not contribute to the efficacy of CP. Indeed, no clinical studies have indicated that the addition of hexamethyl-melamine to cisplatin-based combinations increases either survival or response rate (Foster *et al.* 1986).

The role of doxorubicin

An Italian study showed no statistically significant improvement of survival attributable to the addition of doxorubicin to CP (Conte *et al.* 1986). The Gynecologic Oncology Group conducted a randomized study in FIGO stage III patients, all with residual tumours of dimensions less than 1 cm, to determine whether or not there was a difference between CP (1000 mg/m^2 cyclophosphamide plus 50 mg/m^2 cisplatin) and CAP (500 mg/m^2 cyclophosphamide plus 50 mg/m^2 doxorubicin plus 50 mg/m^2 cisplatin). In 349 evaluable patients they found no significant difference in progression-free interval, frequency of negative second-look laparotomy, or survival. The authors conclude from this large study, using dose schedules with equal haematological toxicity, that the addition of doxorubicin has no significant advantage. The survival results obtained with cisplatin-based regimens with two, three, or four drugs are probably equal if equitoxic doses are delivered (Omura *et al.* 1989). However, the debate about the role of doxorubicin is fuelled by the results of meta-analysis. Although four randomized trials comparing CP with CAP failed to show a significant survival difference, in a meta-analysis pooling 1194 patients from these trials, a significant survival benefit for CAP was found. Because the dose intensity of CAP was greater then CP in three of the trials, the Ovarian Cancer Meta-Analysis Project (1991) concluded that it remains unresolved to what extent the benefit of CAP is from greater dose intensity and to what extent it is from the doxorubicin itself. New trials testing the role of doxorubicin and the analogue epirubicin are under way. According to the data available so far, the role of doxorubicin in platinum combinations remains questionable.

The role of cyclophosphamide

The role of cyclophosphamide in cisplatin combinations has also been investigated. An Italian study group compared cisplatin alone with CP and CAP. No difference in survival or disease-free survival was reported and it was concluded that the addition to cisplatin of either cyclophosphamide or doxorubicin and cyclophosphamide does not substantially increase the number of 'potentially curable' advanced ovarian cancer patients (Gruppo Interregionale Cooperativo Oncologico Ginecologia 1987). The study clearly indicates that cisplatin is the major agent in ovarian cancer, but it is not possible to draw the conclusion that cisplatin alone is preferable to com-bination CP. The cycle times (4 weeks) and dose rates of the drugs in the study were not maximal and, therefore, the possible contributions of cyclophosphamide and doxorubicin are not completely answered by these studies.

The role of carboplatin

In recent years CP has been accepted as the regimen of choice (Thigpen *et al.* 1990; Kaye *et al.* 1992), but times change and

many now prefer carboplatin to cisplatin in combination regimens (Markman *et al.* 1991; Ozols and Young 1991; Ozols 1992).

Several key studies have been performed to explore the role of carboplatin as part of combinations. A Mayo Clinic study (Edmonson *et al.* 1989) comparing cyclophosphamide plus carboplatin with CP showed better progression-free survival with CP. In this study, 103 women were randomly allocated to groups receiving monthly intravenous regimens of cyclophosphamide 1 g/m^2 plus either cisplatin 60 mg/m or carboplatin 150 mg/m^2 (a very low dose). After an interim analysis revealed superior progression-free survival for the group receiving cisplatin, the study was closed to further accrual. The authors stated that this study demonstrated the superiority of cisplatin over carboplatin when the two platinum compounds were compared at equally myelosuppressive low doses in combination with cyclophosphamide. If cisplatin is to be replaced by carboplatin, a higher dose of carboplatin will definitely be required.

Using higher doses of carboplatin (300 mg/m^2 every 4 weeks) the Southwest Oncology Group reported equal efficacy of the combinations, carboplatin plus cyclophosphamide and cisplatin (100 mg/m^2) plus cyclophosphamide. In their final report on 342 patients a clinical response rate of 61 per cent for those patients treated with the carboplatin combination and 52 per cent for those treated with the cisplatin combination was presented. Moreover, median survivals for eligible carboplatin plus cyclophosphamide and cisplatin plus cyclophosphamide patients were 20 months and 17.4 months, respectively. Pathologically complete response rates were similar in both study arms (Alberts *et al.* 1992). Unexpectedly, the analysis revealed similar percentages of granulocytopenia in both arms. This may be due to the postponement of treatment as was allowed in the protocol. Twenty to fifty per cent of the patients did not receive cisplatin from the third to the sixth course. It was not reported how many patients in the cisplatin group were subsequently treated with carboplatin.

The National Cancer Institute of Canada completed a similar study in patients with macroscopic residual disease. Of those patients who underwent repeated surgery, 34.8 per cent of cisplatin-treated and 26.2 per cent of carboplatin-treated patients achieved a histologically complete response. However, at this time in follow-up this difference did not influence survival. Overall response and survival were similar for cisplatin and carboplatin (Swenerton and Pater 1992).

Another large study using carboplatin in combination was performed by the European Organization for Research and Treatment of Cancer (EORTC) Gynaecological Group. In this study 341 patients were randomized to receive CHAP-5 or CHAC-1 (a regimen similar to CHAP-5, replacing cisplatin for 5 days with carboplatin on one day). The response rate achieved with the cisplatin regimen was 63 per cent (69 out of 110) and 48 per cent (57 out of 118) with the carboplatin combination (Ten Bokkel Huinink *et al.* 1988). It is not yet certain whether this difference will result in a survival advantage for the cisplatin regimen used in the group of patients with initially small residual disease. Long-term follow-up of this interesting subgroup of patients is not yet available (Ten Bokkel Huinink *et al.* 1992). A similar experience was reported from an Italian randomized study that investigated doxorubicin and cyclophosphamide plus either carboplatin or cisplatin (PAC). A preliminary evaluation revealed a more frequent clinical complete response rate in favour of the PAC regimen ($p < 0.05$), but the progression-free survival and survival curves were similar with a median survival time of approximately 1.5 years (Giaccone *et al.* 1989).

Opposite results have been reported by a French cooperative group. This group compared a CAP regimen (cyclophosphamide, doxorubicin, and cisplatin 75 mg/m^2) with the same schedule but replacing cisplatin with carboplatin (300 mg/m^2). The report describes the results of 144 eligible patients. The pathological and overall response rates were significantly higher for the cisplatin combination than for the carboplatin combination: 33 per cent versus 15 per cent and 73 per cent versus 47 per cent, respectively. At a median follow-up of 27 months, the median survival was significantly higher with CAP than with the carboplatin regimen: 27.9 months versus 20.6 months (Belpomme *et al.* 1992). An explanation of these results is not provided by the authors. One reason may be that, contrary to other studies, a cross-over from carboplatin to cisplatin (at relapse or earlier) was not allowed.

The question of whether carboplatin is as effective as cisplatin was also addressed by the British Advanced Ovarian Cancer Trialists Group using the tool of meta-analysis. The survival curves computed for patients treated with cisplatin or carboplatin, alone or in combination, showed a slightly better survival after 3 years for those treated with cisplatin. The authors concluded that 'at this time, platinum combinations should be accepted as optimal standard therapy' and that 'the comparison of cisplatin and carboplatin is potentially flawed by crossovers' (Williams *et al.* 1992).

When carboplatin is combined with other myelosuppressive agents, dose adjustments or delay between treatment cycles may be necessary. The advantage of cisplatin is that a dose of 75 mg/m^2 can be maintained for at least six cycles of treatment at nearly 100 per cent of the planned dose, even when combined with myelosuppressive agents. Because maximal dose intensity of cisplatin seems essential for optimal results, this may turn out to be a crucial difference between the two agents.

At present it can be concluded from the above that the position of carboplatin as part of the initial treatment has pros and cons. Data from the carboplatin studies have to be analysed with special attention to cross-over, dose delivered, postponement of treatment, and follow-up before a final decision can be made about carboplatin (Nash and Young 1991; Neijt 1991; Kaye *et al.* 1992; Williams *et al.* 1992; Kaye 1993). During an international workshop, it was accepted as a consensus statement that carboplatin-based therapy is considered to be an acceptable choice in patients with suboptimal stage III and stage IV ovarian cancer. The regimen recommended is carboplatin 300 mg/m^2 plus cyclophosphamide 600 mg/m^2 every 4 weeks (Consensus Group 1993).

Long-term results of cisplatin-based combinations

Whether the current treatment strategy of extensive primary surgery followed by cisplatin-based combinations results in long-term survival benefit remains an important question.

A retrospective analysis of cancer registry data (Illinois hospitals) for 2669 women with newly diagnosed ovarian carcinoma from 1983 to 1988 showed that use of extensive surgery and platinum-based chemotherapy improved survival for stage III patients. Forty-five per cent of 516 stage III patients underwent hysterectomy, bilateral salpingo–oophorectomy, omentectomy, sampled peritoneal washings, and node biopsy. Five year survival was 28 per cent for those in stage III after surgery and 21 per cent for those who were only clinically staged ($p=0.01$). Platinum-based combinations were given to 76 per cent of 221 patients with pathological stage III disease. Their 5 year survival was 50 per cent for the group with no residual and 20 per cent for patients not optimally debulked. Without

Table 4 Survival results of cisplatin-based chemotherapy in series with a follow-up of at least 4 years

Regimen	No. of patients	5 year survival rate	Reference
Chex-Up	62	15	Louie *et al.* (1968)
CHAP-5	92	32	Neijt *et al.* (1987)
PAC	56	23	Sutton *et al.* (1989*b*)
CAP-1	88	33	Wils (1990)
CP/CAP	266	20	Bertelsen (1990)
CP/CAP	103	26	Belinson *et al.* (1990)
CAP	46	39	Davidson *et al.* (1990)
CP	97	28	Neijt *et al.* (1991)

platinum included in the treatment, 37 per cent and 5 per cent, respectively survived. However, as the authors acknowledge, a problem with the interpretation of these data is that the patients in the groups receiving platinum were younger (Hand *et al.* 1993).

The question as to whether cisplatin treatment offers a long-term survival advantage can better be answered by randomized studies with a follow-up considerably longer than 4 years. This period is needed because patients who do not respond to treatment die within 3 years of follow-up and patients with a partial remission die within 4 years. A selection of studies covering a sufficiently long period to permit conclusions at 5 years are summarized in Table 4. Of the patients entered in these series, 8–27 per cent were disease free and 13–39 per cent were alive after 5 years of follow-up. This is unequivocally a higher rate than has been obtained with alkylating monotherapy or regimens without cisplatin.

Survival results after 5 years have now been published by several groups. The Gruppo Interregionale Cooperativo Oncologico Ginecologia, Italy, reported on the long-term results of a randomized trial comparing a combination of cisplatin, cyclophosphamide, and adriamycin with a combination of cisplatin, cyclophosphamide, and cisplatin alone. Their update on 529 cases showed estimated percentage survivals at 7 years (confidence limits) of 21.7 (14.9–28.4), 17.0 (11.0–22.9), and 12.2 (6.9–17.4), respectively (Gruppo Interregionale Cooperativo Oncologico Ginecologia 1992).

The results of two older studies by the Netherlands Joint Study Group for Ovarian Cancer have recently been updated (Neijt *et al.* 1991). These two studies were initiated in 1979 and 1981 and accrued 377 patients with advanced ovarian cancer. The first study compared a combination of hexamethylmelamine, cyclophosphamide, methotrexate, and 5-fluorouracil (Hexa-CAF) with CHAP-5 and in the second study patients were treated with either CHAP-5 or CP. At the time that both studies were reanalysed, the median follow-up of patients was 9.5 years for the first study and 7.7 years for the second. The longest follow-ups were 10.5 and 8.5 years. At 10 years 9 per cent of the patients initially treated with Hexa-CAF and 21 per cent of patients assigned to CHAP-5 were alive. Among the 10 year survivors treated with Hexa-CAF, 50 per cent had experienced progressive disease but were alive as a result of retreatment with cisplatin. The survival curves of both studies revealed that approximately 60 per cent of the patients who reach a complete remission are alive at 5 years and 40 per cent at 10 years (Table 5). These data show that relapses occur even after 5 years of follow-up and in the most favourable group of patients with an incidence of approximately 5 per cent each year. Patients with microscopic disease at second look have a less favourable outlook: 35 per cent survived 5 years. The performance status as measured

Table 5 Survival rates of all eligible patients in two subsequent studies comparing Hexa-CAF with CHAP-5 (first study) and CHAP-5 versus CP (second study)

	Survival rates		
	First study		Second study
	5 years	10 years	5 years
All eligible patients	25	15	30
Response			
Complete remission	58	39	64
Microscopic disease	61	31	35
Partial remission	7	4	12
Progression	2	0	0
FIGO stage			
III	30	20	34
IV	12	3	14
Residual tumour before chemotherapy[a]			
Microscopic	62	37	61
<1 cm	46	25	41
1–2 cm	30	17	25
2–5 cm	21	17	25
≥5 cm	13	9	18
Histological grade (Broders)			
1	48	33	50
2	24	14	26
3	16	11	27
4	28	16	39
Karnofsky index			
100	26	18	39
90	35	19	34
80	26	22	25
70	21	8	9
≤60	0	0	0

[a]Largest cross-sectional diameter.

by the Karnofsky index was among the most important pre-treatment characteristics predicting long-term survival (Neijt 1992).

Another population-based registry studied the survival of 568 Dutch patients with ovarian cancer diagnosed in the period from 1975 to 1985. Patients treated from 1981 to 1985 had a more than 10 per cent improved survival compared with those in the period 1975–1980 before cisplatin was introduced. Because 750 000 patients in Western countries are expected to die of ovarian cancer in the 1990s, the use of platinum combinations may result in long-term survival of 75 000 more patients than would have been achieved in the past decade (Balvert-Locht *et al.* 1991).

The above studies show that a number of patients with ovarian cancer may survive 10 years despite having advanced disease at the start of the treatment. Combination chemotherapy with cisplatin can enhance survival by more than 10 per cent at 5 and 10 years compared with the treatment of the pre-cisplatin era.

Current treatment

With cisplatin-based combinations the 5 and 10 year survival rates have doubled compared with the use of alkylating agents alone or combinations without cisplatin. These results have led to the acceptance of the cisplatin combinations as the standard initial treatment. Before treatment with cyclophosphamide and cisplatin is initiated, contraindications must be excluded. Serious cardiac disease or inadequate renal function (creatinine clearance lower than 70 ml/min) may be reasons not to start cisplatin-based treatment, but to use a carboplatin combination instead. A patient should have adequate white blood cell counts and follow-up must be feasible. The extent of the disease and the amount of tumour present must be documented. As many tumour variables as possible should be listed.

A dose of cisplatin 75 mg/m² and cyclophosphamide 750 mg/m² repeated every 3 weeks appears to be a reasonable standard. Cisplatin can be safely administered as a 4 h infusion in 1 litre of normal saline after prehydration with 1 litre of normal saline. Post-hydration is achieved with 2 litres of normal saline over the following 12 h. Carboplatin is probably as effective as cisplatin when the dose is calculated in relation to the renal function; comparative studies using individual dose optimization are needed. In a fixed dose caution should be exercised in accepting carboplatin-based treatment as a new standard (Nash and Young 1991; Neijt 1991; Calvert *et al.* 1992; Kaye 1993).

It is not certain how many cycles of chemotherapy should be administered to obtain an optimal effect. In the Dutch studies, the median number of courses required to reach a complete remission was six (range from two to seven courses). Thus, at least six treatment courses should be planned. For patients in clinically complete remission including a normal CA125 after six cycles, no further chemotherapy seems warranted. For patients with a partial remission, treatment can be continued; for those with stable non-resectable tumour or disease progression, salvage treatment can be considered.

The assessment of treatment and follow-up

It is advisable to evaluate all patients by physical examination and blood cell counts, serum creatinine, electrolytes, and CA125 tumour marker before each cycle of chemotherapy. Chest radiography and measurement of the tumour diameter by ultrasound should be performed after every third cycle and CT after six cycles or when indicated.

As ovarian cancer is usually limited to the peritoneal cavity, the second-look procedure appears to be a sensitive tool in detecting remaining tumour deposits. Second-look surgery is defined as an exploratory laparotomy to assess the cancer status of a patient who has completed a programme of chemotherapy and is clinically free of cancer (including normal CA125). The role of the second look is a matter of debate. The operation has never been shown to influence survival and, therefore, the procedure should be reserved for circumstances where second-line or 'salvage' therapies are undergoing clinical trials (Berek 1990; Podratz and Kinney 1993).

CA125 tumour marker

It is advisable to monitor all patients by CA125 tumour marker during the course of the disease. In patients with elevated CA125 values at the start of chemotherapy the decrease of marker levels correlates with tumour regression and as long as no rise in blood levels is seen progressive disease can virtually be excluded (Bruzzone *et al.* 1990*a*). It is important to keep in mind that CA125 levels may rise following abdominal surgery not related to ovarian cancer. A rise in CA125 will occur in approximately 80 per cent of the patients after extensive intraperitoneal abdominal surgery. The highest levels are observed in the second week after operation (range 3–336 units/ml). Thereafter the levels gradually decrease to become normal at 8 weeks after surgery (Van der Zee *et al.* 1990). The use of CA125 measurement for the follow-up of patients in remission is also useful. Progression or recurrence can be diagnosed in 73 per cent of patients by CA125 alone and in 92 per cent of patients when combining CA125, gynaecological, and general physical examination. Because CA125 levels may rise several months (median 4.5 months) before other signs of progression are clinically detectable (Van der Burg *et al.* 1990), recurrent tumour can be detected earlier in the course of the disease. Although not proven, it can be assumed that early detection of relapse will mean that the tumour is smaller and, thus, easier to control with reinduction treatment. However, it must be emphasized that it is controversial to treat a patient on the rise of CA125 alone and many wait until there is clinical evidence of relapse.

Salvage treatment

Patients with recurrent disease can be given second-line treatment or salvage treatment. In general, the effect of salvage treatment is dependent on the patient characteristics at the start. Three prognostic groups can be distinguished.

1. Patients whose tumour has never responded and who have had progressive or stable disease from the start of first-line treatment.

2. Patients who have reached a partial remission but developed tumour progression during chemotherapy.

3. Patients who have reached a complete remission and have been without treatment for a considerable time.

The results of salvage treatment are minimal or absent for the first group and modest for the second group. In these patients the disease is resistant to platinum, but for patients in the third group the tumour is theoretically still clinically sensitive to platinum and may respond a second time. The longer the time between the initial diagnosis and the institution of salvage treatment, the more chance patients have to benefit from reinduction treatment. This has been demonstrated by Markman *et al.* (1991). To ascertain the incidence of secondary responses to cisplatin-based therapy in patients previously treated with cisplatin, they undertook a retrospective review of patients at the Memorial Sloan-Kettering Cancer Center. Eighty-two patients had a cisplatin-free interval of more than 4 months between the completion of their first regimen and the start of a second cisplatin/carboplatin programme. Of the 72 assessable patients, 43 per cent responded. The overall response rates based on duration of the treatment-free interval were as follows: 5–12 months, 27 per cent; 13–24 months, 33 per cent; more than 24 months, 59 per cent. Patients without any treatment for more than 24 months from the completion of their initial therapy experienced a 77 per cent (17 out of 22) response rate. The authors concluded that secondary responses to cisplatin/carboplatin-based treatment are common in patients who have previously responded to the agents and increase in frequency with greater distance from the initial therapy (Markman *et al.* 1991). In this study the CA125 assay was not used to detect recurrent disease. Monitoring with CA125 allows detection several months (mean 3–4 months) prior to any clinical manifestation of relapse. This implies that the interval in Markman's study can be assumed to be 3–4 months shorter. Therefore, we should consider offering retreatment with a cisplatin/carboplatin-based regimen to all patients who relapse after a treatment-free period of any length. Patients with proven evidence of resistance to cisplatinum (progression during platinum-based therapy) should receive alternative treatment with one of the new drugs such as taxol.

FUTURE TREATMENT

A number of new treatments are currently being tested in clinical trials and may change the future for ovarian cancer patients. Among them are the use of dose-intensive regimens with or without growth factors and new drugs such as taxol.

Dose intensification

The effect of dose intensity (defined as mg/m^2 per time period) relative to clinical outcome in ovarian cancer has been reviewed by Levin and Hryniuk (1987). The mean relative dose intensity of cisplatin correlated significantly with clinical response and with the median survival time. Accordingly, the dose of the active drugs delivered appears to be important and the question that has to be answered by clinical studies is: will an increase above standard doses further improve the results while maintaining acceptable toxicity?

Most clinical studies addressing this question have been small and non-randomized. So far only a few randomized studies have been published (Ngan *et al.* 1989; Kaye *et al.* 1992; McGuire *et al.* 1992; Murphy *et al.* 1993). A key study addressing the question of cisplatin dose was performed by the Scottish Cancer Study Group. In this study patients received treatment with $50 \, mg/m^2$ (low dose) or $100 \, mg/m^2$ (high dose) cisplatin plus $750 \, mg/m^2$ cyclophosphamide for a maximum of six cycles. Overall median survival was 17 months in the low dose group and 28 months in the high dose group. Because of unacceptable side-effects or patient refusal, six in the low dose group and 25 in the high dose group stopped treatment. The price paid for the improvement of survival consisted of neurotoxicity, hearing loss, alopecia, vomiting, and anaemia (Kaye *et al.* 1992). In another randomized study by the Gynecologic Oncology Group increased toxicity was the only difference between the dose-intense regimen and the standard treatment (McGuire *et al.* 1992). However, in this study the total dose of cisplatin received in the two groups was kept the same at $400 \, mg/m^2$. It seems likely that both dose intensity and total dose determine treatment outcome. Moreover, in the Gynecologic Oncology Group study only patients with tumours of diameter more than 1 cm were eligible. This is a group of patients where differences between treatments are expected to be smaller compared with patients with smaller tumours at the start.

Further increase in the dose of cisplatin beyond $100 \, mg/m^2$ is not clinically relevant because of the severe toxicity. This may be completely different for the analogue carboplatin. The dose of carboplatin can be increased to $2000 \, mg/m^2$ before hepatoxicity and renal toxicity become dose limiting. Another approach to increasing the platinum dose intensity is to combine carboplatin and cisplatin. The Belgian Study Group for Ovarian Carcinoma performed a phase I–II trial of escalating doses of cisplatin ($50–100 \, mg/m^2$) plus carboplatin ($300–400 \, mg/m^2$). They concluded that the two drugs could be safely combined at reasonably high doses (cisplatin $100 \, mg/m^2$, carboplatin $300 \, mg/m^2$) over a 6 month period. The authors correctly conclude that randomized studies are needed before final conclusions can be drawn (Piccart *et al.* 1990).

Nevertheless, the above studies leave the crucial clinical question unanswered. Will an increase above the conventional dose range have an equal effect on survival whilst maintaining acceptable toxicity? If there is a benefit for survival, is it a trend towards better palliation (improved median survival and response rate without negative effect on quality of life) or an improvement in long-term survival?

Growth factors

Another development related to the dose of chemotherapy is the use of growth factors to prevent myelosuppression. The results of studies using granulocyte colony-stimulating factors and granulocyte–macrophage colony-stimulating factor have been reported and phase II studies with macrophage colony-stimulating factor and interleukin-3 have recently begun. In a Dutch study, granulocyte–macrophage colony-stimulating factor was used in a placebo-controlled trial including 15 patients with advanced ovarian cancer. Chemotherapy consisted of six cycles of carboplatin ($300 \, mg/m^2$) with granulocyte–macrophage colony-stimulating factor or placebo. Dose reduction occurred in 15 per cent of 33 cycles in the granulocyte–macrophage colony-stimulating factor group and in 32 per cent of 28 cycles in the control group. The granulocyte count at day 15 of the cycle was significantly lower in the control group than in the patients treated with granulocyte–macrophage colony-stimulating factor. It was concluded that low-dose granulocyte–macrophage colony-stimulating factor, on an out-patient basis, is feasible and diminishes chemotherapy-induced leucopenia and thrombocytopenia (De Vries et al. 1991). Rusthoven et al. (1991) explored the role of granulocyte–macrophage colony-stimulating factor in chemotherapy-naïve ovarian cancer patients. They received regimens of increasing dose levels of carboplatin (starting at $400 \, mg/m^2$) and fixed doses of cyclophosphamide ($600 \, mg/m^2$) and granulocyte–macrophage colony-stimulating factor. In the subsequent trial, the design was the same except that cyclophosphamide was omitted. Early and severe thrombocytopenia was a major problem with or without cyclophosphamide when doses of carboplatin exceeded $600 \, mg/m^2$. Carboplatin $500 \, mg/m^2$ administered every 3 weeks is the highest dose in combination with cyclophosphamide that can be given safely in the out-patient setting with granulocyte–macrophage colony-stimulating factor.

The above studies show that dose-limiting neutropenia can be overcome by using growth factors. The dose of carboplatin and other drugs can be increased until a different dose-limiting toxicity is encountered. As stated in the Newsletter of the National Cancer Institute of Canada: 'in a sense, the drug has become a new agent and should be re-explored in clinical practice' (Anonymous 1992). The question of whether the use of growth factors will result in survival advantage remains open. If it does not, it is better to prevent serious myelotoxicity by adjusting the dose instead of using growth factors. We have to await the results of studies addressing this question before any recommendations can be made about the use of growth factors in the standard treatment of ovarian cancer.

Intraperitoneal chemotherapy

Intraperitoneal chemotherapy is based on the concept that the intra-abdominal administration of drugs can produce high concentrations locally and also give adequate systemic levels. The drugs are given in large volumes of fluid instilled via a Tenckhoff catheter or Port-A-Cath device. Unfortunately, effective drug concentrations are only achieved to the depth of a few cell layers. Systemic toxicity is not avoided and local complications may be frequent. For patients with more than minimal disease (tumour diameter more than 1 cm) and for those who have not responded to systemic platinum administration, there seems to be no role for intraperitoneal treatment (Markham 1987). Agents with antineoplastic activity after intraperitoneal administration in women with ovarian cancer include cisplatin, carboplatin, mitoxantrone, taxol, α- and γ-interferon, and

interleukin-2. With these agents complete remissions have been achieved in patients with minimal disease at second-look laparotomy. However, the benefits of intraperitoneal chemotherapy for patients with small or microscopic tumours initially or following systemic chemotherapy will have to be established by randomized clinical trials (Markham et al. 1993). So far there is no place for intraperitoneal treatment outside the research setting.

New drugs

Among the many drugs tested in the last years, paclitaxel (Taxol) is the most promising. Paclitaxel is a natural product extracted from the bark of the Pacific yew (*Taxus brevifolia*). The drug inhibits the formation of the cellular microtubule network. These microtubules are an important element in the formation of the mitotic spindle. In order to assess the activity and toxicity of paclitaxel in patients with progressive refractory ovarian cancer, a non-randomized phase II trial was performed at the Johns Hopkins Hospital, Baltimore (McGuire et al. 1989). Forty patients were evaluable and 12 (30 per cent) responded to paclitaxel for periods lasting from 3 to 15 months. The dose-limiting toxicity was myelosuppression with leucocytes affected more commonly and severely than thrombocytes. Other adverse effects included myalgias, arthralgias, total alopecia, diarrhoea, nausea, vomiting, mucositis, cardiac arrhythmias, and peripheral neuropathy. A Gynecologic Oncology Group study confirmed that paclitaxel is active in cisplatin-refractory ovarian cancer (eight responses occurred in 27 patients) (Thigpen et al. 1990). These data stimulated the group to initiate a study using cisplatin ($75 \, mg/m^2$) and paclitaxel ($135 \, mg/m^2$ in 24 h) in previously untreated patients with ovarian cancer (McGuire and Rowinsky 1991).

In most studies paclitaxel was administered as a 24 h infusion. To assess its safety as a 3 h infusion, 34 European and Canadian institutions used paclitaxel in 407 patients with ovarian cancer pretreated with platinum. Patients were treated with either 135 or $175 \, mg/m^2$ of paclitaxel as a 3 or 24 h infusion. To avoid the hypersensitivity effects seen in early trials, all patients received premedication with steroid, antihistamine, and a H_2-receptor antagonist. Initial analysis revealed that neither dose nor schedule affected the frequency or severity of hypersensitivity reactions (Table 6). Only three patients had severe reactions, with respiratory distress requiring therapy. Neutropenia was more common and severe in the 24 h tests (Swenerton et al. 1993). The results suggest that a 3 h infusion is feasible and safe and it may become the standard for future study.

It is expected that paclitaxel will be generally available outside clinical trials after 1993. At first the use of the drug should be restricted to salvage therapy for patients who progress during cisplatin-based treatment. New approaches combining paclitaxel with platinum or cyclophosphamide as initial treatment require further evaluation. One randomized trial compared cisplatin plus cyclophosphamide to cisplatin plus paclitaxel and showed the paclitaxel combination to yield statistically significant improvement in clinical response rate, surgical complete response rate, and progression-free survival. At the time of presentation of these results overall survival data were too premature to draw definite conclusions (McGuire et al. 1993). The data strongly suggest that paclitaxel followed by cisplatin every 3 weeks will be at least as good as cyclophosphamide and cisplatin (Consensus Group 1993). Although a confirmatory trial is needed, it appears that the combination of cisplatin and paclitaxel is the next step forward.

Table 6 Toxicity and response data of paclitaxel in a high or low dose, short or long-term infusion in patients with recurrent ovarian cancer

	175 mg/m² (n=144)	135 mg/m² (n=154)	24 h infusion (n=163)	3 h infusion (n=135)
Toxicity				
Hypersensitivity				
Any reaction (%)	42	41	45	36
Severe reaction (%)	1.4	1.9	1.2	2.2
Any neuropathy (%)	52	33	40	45
Neutropenia grade 4	55	41	74	17
Response (%)	24	13	20	17

Modified from Swenerton *et al.* (1993).

Docetaxol (taxotee) is a semi-synthetic compound structurally related to paclitaxel. In a phase I study (with a 1 h infusion for 5 consecutive days repeated every 21 days) 39 cancer patients with advanced disease were entered. Antitumour activity was observed in six patients with ovarian cancer and in one with breast carcinoma (Pazdur *et al.* 1992). Whether this semi-synthetic drug is as active as paclitaxel in ovarian cancer has yet to be established.

2',2'-Difluorodeoxycytidine (gemcitabine) is a new deoxycytidine analogue (a new antimetabolite) with preclinical antitumour activity against various solid tumours including OVCAR-5 human ovarian carcinoma cells. A phase II trial of gemcitabine with a schedule of 30 min infusion once a week for 3 weeks followed by 1 week rest showed a meaningful number of responses in ovarian cancer (Lund *et al.* 1993). The toxicity appears to be mild, including myelosuppression, fatigue, fever, appetite loss, and skin rash.

Many other new drugs, including tetraplatin, organoplatinum, and topotecan and approaches to overcome intrinsic or acquired resistance to the conventional agents have to be explored. These advances are now being tested in clinical trials and may be expected to yield new ways of improving future treatment results.

REFERENCES

Adams M, *et al.* (1989). A comparison of the toxicity and efficacy of cisplatin and carboplatin in advanced ovarian cancer. The Swons Gynaecological Cancer Group. *Acta Oncologica*, 28(1):57–60.

Advanced Ovarian Cancer Trialists Group (1991). Chemotherapy in advanced ovarian cancer, an overview of randomised clinical trials. *British Medical Journal*, 303:884–93.

Alberts DS, *et al.* (1992). Improved therapeutic index of carboplatin plus cyclophosphamide versus cisplatin plus cyclophosphamide. Final report by the Southwest Oncology Group of a phase III randomized trial in stages III and IV ovarian cancer. *Journal of Clinical Oncology*, 10:706–17.

Allen DG, Planner RS, Grant PT (1992). Maximum effort in the management of ovarian cancer, including pelvic para-aortic lymphadenectomy. *Australian and New Zealand Journal of Obstetrics and Gynaecology*, 32(1):50–3.

Anonymous (1992). Policy on use of colony stimulating factors in studies. *NCIC-CTG Group Newsletter*, 2.

Balvert-Locht HR, Coebergh JW, Hop WC (1991). Improved prognosis of ovarian cancer in The Netherlands during the period 1975–1985, a registry-based study. *Gynecologic Oncology*, 42:3–8.

Barber HRK (1983). Prophylaxis in ovarian cancer. *Cancer*, 71:1529–33.

Barber HRK, Graber EA (1971). The PMPO syndrome (postmenopausal palpable ovary syndrome). *Obstetrics and Gynecology*, 38:921–3.

Belinson JL, Lee KR, Jarrell MA, McClure M (1990). Management of epithelial ovarian neoplasms using a platinum-based regimen, a 10-year experience. *Gynecologic Oncology*, 37:66–73.

Belpomme D, *et al.* (1992). Carboplatin versus cisplatin in association with cyclophosphamide and doxorubicin as first line therapy in stage III and IV ovarian carcinoma, results of an artac phase III trial. *Proceedings of the American Society of Clinical Oncology*, 11:227.

Berek JS (1990). Epithelial ovarian cancer. In *Practical gynecologic oncology* (ed. JS Berek and NF Hacker), pp. 327–64. Williams & Wilkins, Baltimore.

Bertelsen K (1990). Tumor reduction surgery and long-term survival in advanced ovarian cancer, a DACOVA study. *Gynecologic Oncology*, 38:203–9.

Bertelsen K, *et al.* (1987). A randomized study of cyclophosphamide and cis-platinum with or without doxorubicin in advanced ovarian carcinoma. *Gynecologic Oncology*, 28:161–9.

Booth M, Beral V, Smith P (1989). Risk factors for ovarian cancer: a case-control study. *British Journal of Cancer*, 60:592–8.

Boring C, Squires T, Tong T (1992). Cancer statistics 1992. *CA: A Cancer Journal for Clinicians*, 42:19–38.

Bourne TH, *et al.* (1991). Ultrasound screening for familial ovarian cancer. *Gynecologic Oncology*, 43:92–7.

Braly PS, Klevecz RR (1993). Flow cytometric evaluation of ovarian cancer. *Cancer*, 71(Suppl.):1621–8.

Bruzzone M, *et al.* (1990a). CA-125 monitoring in the management of ovarian cancer. *Anticancer Research*, 10:1353–9.

Bruzzone M, *et al.* (1990b). Chemotherapy versus radiotherapy in the management of ovarian cancer patients with pathological complete response or minimal residual disease at second look. *Gynecological Oncology*, 38(3):392–5.

Calvert AH, Newell DR, Gore ME (1992). Future directions with carboplatin: can therapeutic monitoring, high dose administration and hematologic support with growth factors expand the spectrum compared with cisplatin? *Seminars in Oncology*, 19:155–63.

Campbell S, *et al.* (1989). Transabdominal ultrasound screening for early ovarian cancer. *British Medical Journal*, 299:1363–7.

Consensus Group (1993). Advanced epithelial ovarian cancer: 1993 Consensus Statements. In *Ovarian cancer: where do we stand and where do we go? Annals of oncology* (ed. JP Neijt, E Wiltshaw, and B Lund), Suppl. 4. (In press.)

Conte PF, *et al.* (1986). A randomized trial comparing cisplatin plus cyclophosphamide versus cisplatin, doxorubicin and cyclophosphamide in advanced ovarian cancer. *Journal of Clinical Oncology*, 4:965–71.

Cramer DW, Welch WR, Cassells S, Scully RE (1983a). Mumps, menarche, menopause and ovarian cancer. *American Journal of Obstetrics and Gynecology*, 147:1–6.

Cramer DW, *et al.* (1983b). Determinants of ovarian cancer risk. 1. Reproductive experiences and family history. *Journal of the National Cancer Institute*, 71(4):711–16.

Creech RH, *et al.* (1985). Phase II study of low-dose mitomycin in patients with ovarian cancer previously treated with chemotherapy. *Cancer Treatment Reports*, 69:1271–3.

Davidson NG, *et al.* (1990). Long-term survival after chemotherapy with cisplatinum, adriamycin and cyclophosphamide for carcinoma of the ovary. *Clinical Oncology of the Royal College of Radiology*, 2:206–9.

Dembo AJ, *et al.* (1990). Prognostic factors in patients with stage 1 epithelial ovarian cancer. *Obstetrics and Gynecology*, 75:263–73.

De Vries EG, *et al.* (1991). A double-blind placebo-controlled study with granulocyte–macrophage colony-stimulating factor during chemotherapy for ovarian carcinoma. *Cancer Research*, 51:116–22.

Drescher CW, Flint A, Hopkins MP, Roberts JA (1993). Prognostic significance of DNA content and nuclear morphology in borderline ovarian tumors. *Gynecolic Oncology*, 48:242–6.

Edmonson JH, *et al.* (1985). Comparison of cyclophosphamide plus cisplatin versus hexamethylmelamine, cyclophosphamide, doxorubicin and cisplatin in combination as initial chemotherapy for stage III and IV ovarian carcinomas. *Cancer Treatment Reports*, 69:1243–8.

Edmonson JH, *et al.* (1989). Cyclophosphamide–cisplatin versus cyclophosphamide–carboplatin in stage III–IV ovarian carcinoma, a comparison of equally myelosuppressive regimens. *Journal of the National Cancer Institute*, 81:1500–4.

FIGO (International Federation of Gynecologists and Obstetricians) Cancer Committee (1987). Changes in FIGO staging. *Obstetrics and Gynecology*, 138.

Fishel S, Jackson P (1989). Follicular stimulation for high tech pregnancies: are we playing it safe? *British Medical Journal*, 299:309–11.

Foster BJ, et al. (1986). Role of hexamethylmelamine in the treatment of ovarian cancer: where is the needle in the haystack? *Cancer Treatment Reports*, 70:1003–14.

Franchin G, et al. (1991). Whole abdomen radiation therapy after a short chemotherapy course and second-look laparotomy in advanced ovarian cancer. *Gynecologic Oncology*, 41:206–11.

Giaccone G, et al. (1989). Cisplatin and carboplatin in combination chemotherapy for advanced ovary cancer. In: *Multimodal treatment of ovarian cancer* (ed. PF Conte et al.), pp. 219–26. Monograph Series of the EORTC 20, Raven Press, New York.

Goldberg GL, Runowicz CD (1992). Ovarian carcinoma of low malignant potential, infertility, and induction of ovulation—is there a link? *American Journal of Obstetrics and Gynecology*, 166:853–4.

Goodman HM, et al. (1992). The role of cytoreductive surgery in the management of stage IV epithelial ovarian carcinoma. *Gynecologic Oncology*, 46(3):367–71.

Griffiths CT (1975). Surgical resection of tumor bulk in the primary treatment of ovarian carcinoma. *National Cancer Institute Monographs*, 42:101.

Gruppo Interregionale Cooperativo Oncologico Ginecologia (1987). Randomised comparison of cisplatin with cyclophosphamide/cisplatin and with cyclophosphamide/doxorubicin/cisplatin in advanced ovarian cancer. *Lancet*, 2:353–9.

Gruppo Interregionale Cooperativo Oncologico Ginecologia. (1992). Long-term results of a randomized trial comparing cisplatin with cisplatin and cyclophosphamide with cisplatin, cyclophosphamide, and adriamycin in advanced ovarian cancer. *Gynecological Oncology*, 45(2):115–17.

Hacker NF (1989). Controversial aspects of cytoreductive surgery for epithelial ovarian cancer. *Bailtière's Clinical Obstetrics and Gynaecology*, 3:49–57.

Hacker NF, et al. (1983). Primary cytoreductive surgery for epithelial ovarian cancer. *Obstetrics and Gynecology*, 61:413–20.

Hand R, et al. (1993). Staging procedures, clinical management, and survival outcome for ovarian carcinoma. *Journal of the American Medical Association*, 269(9):1119–22.

Hauge MD, et al. (1992). Phase II trial of intravenous hexamethylmelamine in patients with advanced ovarian cancer. *Investigational New Drugs*, 10(4), 299–301.

Hoskins WJ (1993). Surgical staging and cytoreductive surgery of epithelial ovarian cancer. *Cancer*, 71:1534–40.

Jacob JH, et al. (1991). Neoadjuvant chemotherapy and interval debulking for advanced epithelial ovarian cancer. *Gynecologic Oncology*, 42(2):146–50.

Jungi WF, et al. (1985). Phase II trial with high-dose ifosfamide (IFO)+Mesna in advanced pretreated ovarian cancer (meeting abstract). *Proceedings of the American Society of Clinical Oncology*, 4:115.

Kaern J, et al. (1990). Cellular DNA content as a new prognostic tool in patients with borderline tumours of the ovary. *Gynecologic Oncology*, 38:452–7.

Kaern J, Trope CG, Abeler VM (1993). A retrospective study of 370 borderline tumors of the ovary treated at the Norwegian Radium Hospital from 1970 to 1982. *Cancer*, 71:1810–20.

Kappen HJ, Neijt JP (1993). Neural network analysis to predict treatment outcome. In *Ovarian cancer: where do we stand and where do we go? Annals of oncology* (ed. JP Neijt, E Wiltshaw, and B Lund), Suppl. 4. (In press.)

Kaye SB (1993). Chemotherapy for ovarian cancer. *European Journal of Cancer*, 29a:632–5.

Kaye SB, et al. (1992). Randomised study of two doses of cisplatin with cyclophosphamide in epithelial ovarian cancer. *Lancet*, 340:329–33.

Kramer BS, Gohagan J, Prorok P, Smart C (1993). A National Cancer Institute sponsored screening trial for prostatic, lung, colorectal and ovarian cancers. *Cancer*, 71:589–93.

Lambert HE, Berry BJ (1985). High dose cisplatin compared with high dose cyclophosphamide in the management of advanced epithelial ovarian cancer (FIGO stages III and IV). Report from the North Thames Cooperative Group. *British Medical Journal*, 290:889–93.

Lambert HE, Rustin GJS, Gregory WM, Nelstrop AE (1993). A randomized trial comparing single-agent carboplatin with carboplatin followed by radiotherapy for advanced ovarian cancer: a North Thames ovary group study. *Journal of Clinical Oncology*, 11(3):440–8.

Lanciano RM, Randall M (1991). Update on the role of radiotherapy in ovarian cancer. *Seminars in Oncology*, 18(3):233–47.

Levin L, Hryniuk WM (1987). Dose intensity analysis of chemotherapy regimens in ovarian carcinoma. *Journal of Clinical Oncology*, 5:756–67.

Louie KG, et al. (1968). Long-term results of a cisplatin-containing combination chemotherapy regimen for the treatment of advanced ovarian carcinoma. *Journal of Clinical Oncology*, 4:1579–85.

Luesly D, et al. (1988) Failure of second-look laparotomy to influence survival in epithelial ovarian cancer. *Lancet*, ii:599–603.

Lund B, Williamson P (1991). Prognostic factors for overall survival in patients with advanced ovarian carcinoma. *Annals of Oncology*, 2(4):281–7.

Lund B, et al. (1993). Phase II study of gemcitabine in previously platinum treated ovarian cancer patients. *Proceedings of the American Society of Clinical Oncology*, 12:262.

Lynch HT, et al. (1986). Familial ovarian carcinoma. *American Journal of Medicine*, 81:1073–6.

Lynch HT, et al. (1993). Hereditary ovarian cancer—heterogeneity in age at onset. *Cancer*, 71:573–81.

McGowan L, Parent L, Lednar W, Norris HJ (1979). The woman at risk for developing ovarian cancer. *Gynecologic Oncology*, 7:325–44.

McGuire WP, Rowinsky EK (1991). Old drugs revisited, new drugs, and experimental approaches in ovarian cancer therapy. *Seminars in Oncology*, 18:255–69.

McGuire WP, et al. (1989). Taxol, a unique antineoplastic agent with significant activity in advanced ovarian epithelial neoplasms. *Annals of Internal Medicine*, 111:273–9.

McGuire WP, et al. (1992). A phase III trial of dose intense versus standard dose cisplatin and cytoxan in advanced ovarian cancer. *Proceedings of the American Society of Clinical Oncology*, 11:226.

McGuire WP, Hoskins W, Brady M, et al. (1993). A phase III trial comparing cisplatin/cytoxan and cisplatin/taxol in advanced ovarian cancer. *Proceedings of the American Society of Clinical Oncology*, 12:255.

Mangioni C, et al. (1989). Randomized trial in advanced ovarian cancer comparing cisplatin and carboplatin. *Journal of the National Cancer Institute*, 81:1464–71.

Markman M (1987). Intraperitoneal antineoplastic agents for tumors principally confined to the peritoneal cavity. *Cancer Treatment Reviews*, 13:219–42.

Markman M, et al. (1991). Second-line platinum therapy in patients with ovarian cancer previously treated with cisplatin. *Journal of Clinical Oncology*, 9:389–93.

Markman M, et al. (1992). Phase 2 trial of chronic low-dose oral etoposide as salvage therapy of platinum-refractory ovarian cancer. *Journal of Cancer Research and Clinical Oncology*, 119(1):55–7.

Markman M, et al. (1993). Intraperitoneal chemotherapy in the management of ovarian cancer. *Cancer*, 71(Suppl. 4):1565–70.

Merino MJ, Jaffe G (1993). Age contrast in ovarian pathology. *Cancer*, 71:537–44.

Miholic J, et al. (1991). The role of intestinal resection in primary surgery of ovarian carcinoma. *Zentralblatt für Chirurgie*, 116(7),:465–70.

Monga M, et al. (1991). Surgery without adjuvant chemotherapy for early epithelial ovarian carcinoma after comprehensive surgical staging. *Gynecological Oncology*, 43:195–7.

Muggia FM, Russell CA (1991). New chemotherapies for ovarian cancer. Systemic and intraperitoneal podophyllotoxins. *Cancer*, 67(Suppl. 1):225–30.

Murphy D, et al. (1993). A randomised dose–intensity study in ovarian carcinoma comparing chemotherapy given at four week intervals for six cycles with half dose chemotherapy given for twelve cycles. *Annals of Oncology*, 4:377–83.

Nash JD, Young RC (1991). Gynecologic malignancies. In *Cancer chemotherapy and biological response modifiers*, Vol. 12 (ed. HM Pinedo, DL Longo, and BA Chabner), pp. 549–69. Elsevier, Amsterdam.

Neijt JP (1991). Ovarian cancer treatment, time for some hard thinking. *European Journal of Cancer*, 27:680–1.

Neijt JP (1992). Treatment of advanced ovarian cancer, 10 years of experience. *Annals of Oncology*, 3:17–27.

Neijt JP, et al. (1987). Randomised trial comparing two combination chemotherapy regimens (CHAP-5 vs CP) in advanced ovarian carcinoma. *Journal of Clinical Oncology*, 5:1157–68.

Neijt JP, et al. (1991). Long-term survival in ovarian cancer. Matured data from The Netherlands Joint Study Group for Ovarian Cancer. *European Journal of Cancer*, 27:1367–72.

Ngan HY, *et al.* (1989). A randomized study of high-dose versus low-dose cisplatin combined with cyclophosphamide in the treatment of advanced ovarian cancer. Hong Kong Ovarian Carcinoma Study Group. *Chemotherapy*, **35**:221–7.

Omura GA, *et al.* (1989). Randomized trial of cyclophosphamide plus cisplatin with or without doxorubicin in ovarian carcinoma. A gynaecologic oncology group study. *Journal of Clinical Oncology*, **7**:457–65.

Ovarian Cancer Meta-Analysis Project (1991). Cyclophosphamide plus cisplatin versus cyclophosphamide, doxorubicin, and cisplatin chemotherapy of ovarian carcinoma: a meta-analysis. *Journal of Clinical Oncology*, **9**(Suppl. 6): 1668–74.

Ozols RF (1992). Advances in the chemotherapy of gynecologic malignancies. *Hematological Oncology*, **10**:43–51.

Ozols RF, Young RC (1991). Chemotherapy of ovarian cancer. *Seminars in Oncology*, **18**:222–32.

Ozols RF, Ostchega Y, Myers CE, Young RC (1985). High-dose cisplatin in hypertonic saline in refractory ovarian cancer. *Journal of Clinical Oncology*, **3**:1246–50.

Padberg BC, *et al.* (1992). DNA cytophotometry and prognosis in ovarian tumors of borderline malignancy. *Cancer*, **69**:2510–14.

Parmley TH, Woodruff JD (1974). The ovarian mesothelioma. *American Journal of Obstetrics and Gynecology*, **120**:234–40.

Partridge EE, *et al.* (1993). The validity and significance of substages of advanced ovarian cancer. *Gynecological Oncology*, **48**:236–41.

Pazdur R, *et al.* (1992). Phase I trial of Taxotere: five-day schedule. *Journal of the National Cancer Institute*, **84**(23):1781–8.

Piccart MJ, *et al.* (1990). Cisplatin combined with carboplatin, a new way of intensification of platinum dose in the treatment of advanced ovarian cancer. *Journal of the National Cancer Institute*, **82**:703–7.

Piver MS, *et al.* (1984). Familial Ovarian Cancer Registry. *Obstetrics and Gynecology*, **64**:195–9.

Podratz KC, Kinney WK (1993). Second-look operation in ovarian cancer. *Cancer*, **71**(4)(Suppl.):1551–18.

Potter ME, *et al.* (1991). Primary surgical therapy of ovarian cancer: how much and when. *Gynecologic Oncology*, **40**(3), 195–200.

Radisavljevic SV (1977). The pathogenesis of ovarian inclusion cysts and cystomas. *Obstetrics and Gynecology*, **49**:424–9.

Redman JR, *et al.* (1986). Prognostic factors in advanced ovarian carcinoma. *Journal of Clinical Oncology*, **4**:515–23.

Ries LAG (1993). Ovarian cancer. Survival and treatment differences by age. *Cancer*, **71**:524–9.

Rusthoven J, *et al.* (1991). Two phase I studies of carboplatin dose escalation in chemotherapy-naive ovarian cancer patients supported with granulocyte–macrophage colony-stimulating factor. *Journal of the National Cancer Institute*, **83**:1748–53.

Schein PS, Scheffler B, McCullock W (1991). The role of hexamethylmelamine in the management of ovarian cancer. *Cancer Treatment Reviews*, **18**(Suppl. A):67–75.

Schildkraut JM, Thompson WD (1988). Familial ovarian cancer: a population-based case-control study. *American Journal of Epidemiology*, **128**:456.

Segna RA, *et al.* (1993). Secondary cytoreduction for ovarian cancer following cisplatin therapy. *Journal of Clinical Oncology*, **11**(3):434–9.

Sell A, *et al.* (1990). Randomized study of whole-abdomen irradiation versus pelvic irradiation plus cyclophosphamide in treatment of early ovarian cancer. *Gynecologic Oncology*, **37**:367.

Sightler SE, Boike GM, Estape RE, Averette HE (1991). Ovarian cancer in women with prior hysterectomy: a 14-year experience at the University of Miami. *Obstetrics and Gynecology*, **78**:681–4.

Silverberg E, Boring CS, Squires TS (1990). Cancer statistics 1990. *CA: A Cancer Journal for Clinicians*, **40**:9–26.

Slattery ML, *et al.* (1989). Nutrient intake and ovarian cancer. *American Journal of Epidemiology*, **130**:497.

Slevin ML (1986). Ovarian cancer. In: *Randomized trials in cancer: a critical review by sites* (ed. ML Slevin and MJ Staquet), pp. 385–416. Raven Press, New York.

Smith JP, Day GT (1979). Review of ovarian cancer of the University of Texas Systems Cancer Center M. D. Anderson Hospital and Tumor Institute. *American Journal of Obstetrics and Gynecology*, **135**:984–90.

Sutton GP, *et al.* (1989*a*). Phase II trial of ifosfamide and mesna in advanced ovarian carcinoma, a Gynecologic Oncology Group Study. *Journal of Clinical Oncology*, **7**(11):1672–6.

Sutton GP, *et al.* (1989*b*). Ten-year follow-up of patients receiving cisplatin, doxorubicin, and cyclophosphamide chemotherapy for advanced epithelial ovarian carcinoma. *Journal of Clinical Oncology*, **7**: 223–9.

Swenerton KD, Pater JL (1992). Carboplatin in the treatment of carcinoma of the ovary. The National Cancer Institute of Canada experience. *Seminars in Oncology*, **19**:114–19.

Swenerton KD, *et al.* (1985). Ovarian carcinoma: a multivariate analysis of prognostic factors. *Obstetrics and Gynecology*, **65**:264–70.

Swenerton K, *et al.* (1993). Taxol in relapsed ovarian cancer: high versus low dose and short versus long infusion: a European–Canadian study coordinated by the NCI Canada Clinical Trials Group. *Proceedings of the American Society of Clinical Oncology*, **12**:256.

Teeling M, Hayes Y, Fitzmaurice B, McGing P, Carney DN (1992). Carboplatin/cyclophosphamide combination chemotherapy for advanced ovarian cancer. *Seminars in Oncology*, **19** (Suppl. 2):102–6.

Ten Bokkel Huinink WW, *et al.* (1988). Carboplatin in combination therapy for ovarian cancer. *Cancer Treatment Reviews*, **15**:9–15.

Ten Bokkel Huinink WW, *et al.* (1992). Replacement of cisplatin with carboplatin in combination chemotherapy against ovarian cancer: long-term treatment results of a study of the Gynaecological Cancer Cooperative Group of the EORTC and experience at The Netherlands Cancer Institute. *Seminars in Oncology*, **19**(Suppl. 2):99–101.

Thigpen JT (1985). Single agent chemotherapy in the management of ovarian carcinoma. In *Ovarian cancer* (ed. D Alberts and E Surwit), pp. 115–46. Boston, Martinus Nijhoff.

Thigpen T, *et al.* (1990). Phase II trial of taxol as second-line therapy for ovarian carcinoma, a Gynecologic Oncology Group study. *Proceedings of the American Association of Clinical Oncology*, **9**:156 (abstract).

Thomas GM, Dembo AJ (1993). Integration radiation therapy into the management of ovarian cancer. *Cancer*, **71**(Suppl.):1710–18.

Tibben JG, Schijf CP, Beex LV (1992). Results of cyclophosphamide and cisplatin combination chemotherapy in patients with ovarian carcinoma. *European Journal of Gynaecological Oncology*, **13**(4):33–9.

Trimbos JB, *et al.* (1991). Watch and wait after careful surgical treatment and staging in well-differentiated early ovarian cancer. *Cancer*, **67**: 597–602.

Van der Burg MEL, Lammers FB, Verweij J (1990). The role of CA125 in the early diagnosis of progressive disease in ovarian cancer. *Annals of Oncology*, **1**:301–2.

Van der Burg MEL, *et al.* (1993). Intervention debulking surgery (IDS) does improve survival in advanced epithelial ovarian cancer (EOC); an EORTC Gynecological Cancer Cooperative Group (GCCG) Study. *Proceedings of the American Society of Clinical Oncology*, **12**:258.

Van der Zee AG, *et al.* (1990). The effect of abdominal surgery on the serum concentration of the tumour-associated antigen CA125. *British Journal of Obstetrics and Gynaecology*, **97**:935–8.

Van Houwelingen JC, Ten Bokkel Huinink WW, Van der Burg MEL, Neijt JP (1989). Predictability of the survival of patients with advanced ovarian cancer. *Journal of Clinical Oncology*, **7**:769–73.

Van Lindert AM, *et al.* (1984). The role of the abdominal radical tumor reduction procedure (ARTR) in the treatment of ovarian cancer. In *Surgery in gynecologic oncology* (ed. APM Heintz, CT Griffiths, and JB Trimbos), pp. 275–87. Martinus Nijhoff, The Hague.

Van Nagell JR, *et al.* (1991). Ovarian cancer screening in asymptomatic postmenopausal women by transvaginal sonography. *Cancer*, **68**(3):458–62.

Van Nagell JR, DePriest PD, Gallion HH, Pavlik EJ (1993). Ovarian cancer screening. *Cancer*, **71**(Suppl.):1523–8.

Whittemore AS, *et al.* (1992). Characteristics relating to ovarian cancer risk: collaborative analysis on 12 case control studies. II Invasive epithelial ovarian cancers in white women. *American Journal of Epidemiology*, **136**:1184–203.

Willemse PHB, *et al.* (1990). Ifosamide given as a 24-h infusion with mesna in patients with recurrent ovarian cancer, preliminary results. *Cancer Chemotherapy and Pharmacology*, **26**:51–4.

Williams CJ, Stewart L, Parmaz M, Guthrie D (1992). Meta-analysis of the role of platinum compounds in advanced ovarian carcinoma. *Seminars in Oncology*, 19:120–8.

Wils JA (1990). Long-term follow-up of patients with advanced ovarian carcinoma treated with debulking surgery and chemotherapy consisting of cisplatin, doxorubicin, and cyclophosphamide. *Oncology*, 47:115–20.

Wiltshaw E, Evans B, Harland S (1985). Phase III randomized trial cisplatin versus JM8 (carboplatin) in 112 ovarian cancer patients, stages III and IV (Meeting Abstract). *Proceedings of the American Society of Clinical Oncology*, 4:121.

Wiltshaw E, *et al.* (1986). A prospective randomized trial comparing high-dose cisplatin with low-dose cisplatin and chlorambucil in advanced ovarian carcinoma. *Journal of Clinical Oncology*, 4:722–9.

Young RC, *et al.* (1983). Staging laparotomy in early ovarian cancer. *Journal of The American Medical Association*, 250:3072–6.

Young RC, *et al.* (1990). Adjuvant therapy in stage I and II epithelial ovarian cancer. *New England Journal of Medicine*, 322:1021–7.

Young RC, Brady MF, Walton LA (1993). Localized ovarian cancer in the elderly: the Gynecologic Oncology Group experience. *Cancer*, 71(2) (Suppl.):601–5.

9.2 Ovarian germ cell and other rare ovarian tumours

EDWARD S. NEWLANDS AND FERNANDO J. PARADINAS

INTRODUCTION

Tumours of the ovary are diverse in terms of histogenesis, endocrine effects, and clinical behaviour. There is no universally accepted classification: a clinical classification is clearly unsatisfactory because the behaviour and response to therapy are better predicted by the pathological nature of the tumour; equally, there is little sense in classifying them according to the endocrine syndrome they cause because the same endocrine effects can be shared by tumours of diverse nature and behaviour. It follows that in spite of our imperfect knowledge of ovarian histogenesis, the most useful classification at present is a morphological one. In this chapter we have followed a simplified version of that proposed by Langley and Fox (1987) rather than the World Health Organization (**WHO**) classification (Serov *et al.* 1973). Our version is as follows.

1. 'Common' epithelial tumours
   serous
   mucinous
   endometrioid
   clear cell

2. 'Rare' epithelial tumours
   Brenner tumours
   small cell carcinoma

3. Mixed Müllerian (mesodermal) tumours

4. Sex cord–stromal tumours
   (a) female-directed cells
      granulosa cell tumours
      thecomas and other fibrous tumours
   (b) male-directed cells
      Sertoli–Leydig cell tumours
      pure Leydig cell tumours
      pure Sertoli cell tumours
   (c) mixed
      gynandroblastomas
   (d) uncertain histogenesis
      lipid cell tumours
      sex cord–stromal tumour with annular tubules

5. Germ cell tumours

6. Mixed germ cell/sex cord–stromal tumours (gonadoblastomas)

7. Undifferentiated and unclassified tumours

8. Metastatic tumours

The 'common' epithelial tumours are the subject of a separate chapter. The list of 'rare' tumours included here is not fully comprehensive and has been divided into four groups: germ cell tumours, sex cord–stromal tumours, rare epithelial tumours, and mixed Müllerian tumours.

GERM CELL TUMOURS

Introduction

In contrast to germ cell tumours of the testis, which are rare but nearly always malignant, germ cell tumours of the ovary are common and very frequently benign (the ovarian cystic teratoma or 'dermoid cyst'). It follows that the majority of ovarian germ cell tumours are cured by surgical excision, but there are three instances in which other forms of therapy may be necessary:

(1) when the germ cell tumour is clearly malignant;
(2) when it is composed of a mixture of immature tissues with malignant potential;
(3) when one of the components of a benign teratoma becomes malignant.

Epidemiology and aetiology

Germ cell tumours constitute approximately 25 per cent of all ovarian tumours (Fox and Langley 1976) but only 4 per cent are malignant, accounting for 1 per cent of all ovarian tumours. The incidence of malignant ovarian germ cell tumours is only approximately one-tenth of that of malignant testicular germ cell tumours, but the incidence of this cancer in both sexes may be rising (Walker *et al.* 1984). Whereas the age of presentation of benign ovarian germ cell tumours reaches a peak in the fourth and fifth decades, the mean age of patients with malignant ovarian germ cell tumours is 19 years. In women under the age of 20, 58 per cent of ovarian tumours are germ cell tumours, of which 65 per cent are malignant; under the age of 10, the proportion of malignant germ cell tumours increases to 81 per cent (Norris and Jensen 1979). It is therefore important to consider the possibility of a germ cell tumour in young patients with a pelvic mass, as modern management, which avoids radical surgery, offers an excellent chance for both long-term survival and preservation of fertility.

The cause of ovarian germ cell tumours is not known but recent evidence, including a case-controlled study (Walker *et al.* 1988), suggests that *in utero* exposure to exogenous hormones or to high oestrogen concentrations in the mother constitute risk factors of ovarian germ cell tumours in her offspring.

Pathology

Germ cell tumours derive from totipotential germ cells and can be classified according to the main line of differentiation.

1. Dysgerminoma (germinal epithelium)

2. Anaplastic germ cell tumours (primitive and extra-embryonic tissues)
   embryonal carcinoma (undifferentiated)
   polyembryoma (embryoid bodies)
   endodermal sinus or yolk sac tumour (yolk sac structures)
   hepatoid tumour (primitive liver)
   choriocarcinoma (trophoblast)

3. Teratomas (embryonic or somatic tissues)
   immature (solid) teratoma (immature tissues present)
   mature (cystic) teratoma (mature tissues only)
   monodermal teratomas (one tissue only; usually mature)

4. Mixtures of all three above

Dysgerminoma

This is the ovarian counterpart of testicular seminoma and is a solid, tan-coloured tumour, which in approximately 15 per cent of cases is bilateral. It is composed of glycogen-rich cells that resemble germinal epithelium in a stroma with abundant lymphoid cells, but in some cases lymphoid cells may be few (Fig. 1). Chorionic gonadotrophin-producing syncytial cells are rarely found. The tumour spreads mainly intraperitoneally and to regional lymph nodes, but haematogenous spread occasionally occurs.

Anaplastic germ cell tumours

Embryonal carcinoma is a highly malignant tumour composed of epithelial-like cells forming sheaths, cords, tubules, or papillae (Fig. 2(a)). The germ cell derivation of this anaplastic tumour is more obvious when it is mixed with other recognizable germ cell patterns, such as embryoid bodies (Fig. 2(b)), primitive yolk sac structures including the well-known Duval–Schiller bodies (Fig. 2(c)) and trophoblast (Fig. 2(d)). Rare tumours exclusively composed of embryoid bodies are called polyembryomas and equally rare, pure tumours of trophoblast choriocarcinomas. Those composed of yolk sac structures, yolk sac tumours or endodermal-sinus tumours, are less uncommon. Some germ cell tumours previously described as solid variants of yolk sac probably represent hepatoid differentiation (Prat *et al.* 1982*a*). Mixtures of all these patterns are more common than previously recognized, although not as frequent as in the testis. Factors common to them all are their anaplasia (they are composed of primitive cells already present before the appearance of the three embryonic layers that will form the fetus), their frequent production of oncofetal proteins

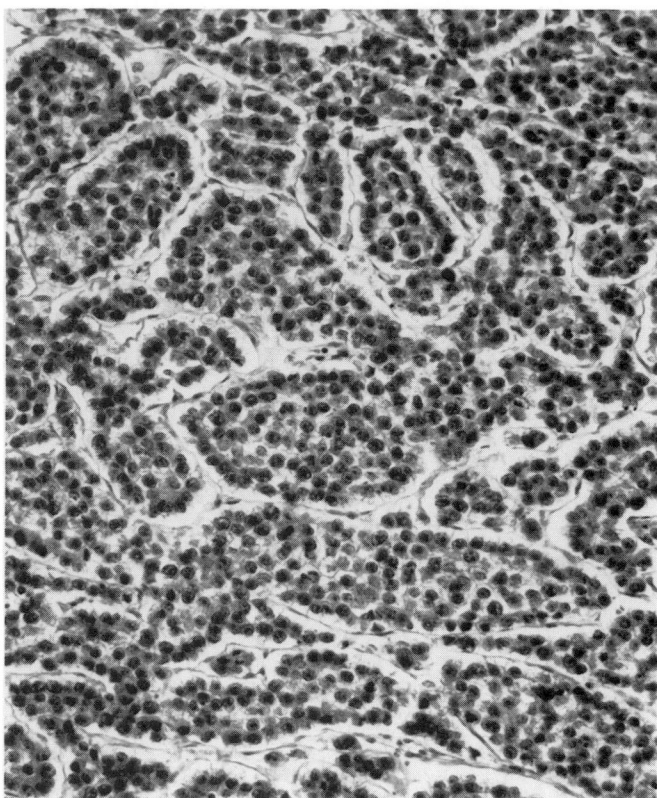

Fig. 1 Dysgerminoma. In this example the germinal cells form well-defined clusters and there is no lymphoid infiltrate.

(particularly α-fetoprotein and chorionic gonadotrophin), and their good response to chemotherapy. Because of this, we find the term anaplastic germ cell tumours useful to describe this group. Anaplastic germ cell tumours are often of large size and soft in consistency, with frequent areas of necrosis and haemorrhage. They are rarely confined to the ovary on laparotomy; ascites, peritoneal spread, and liver or lung metastases are common.

Teratomas

Solid (immature) teratomas also occur in young women and are, in spite of their name, often multicystic and composed of a mixture of immature (fetal) and mature (adult) tissues. As a result they have a variegated appearance. Histologically, they have mixtures of every possible tissue and, although all these tumours have to be regarded as potentially malignant (Talerman 1982), their prognosis worsens with an increase in the proportion of immature to mature tissues and when one of the components is frankly carcinomatous or sarcomatous. Primitive neuroepithelial tissues (Fig. 3) are most prone to disseminate throughout the peritoneal cavity. Distant metastases are rare.

Cystic teratomas are composed of mature tissues surrounding a single cyst, usually wholly or partly lined by squamous epithelium. Malignancy complicating a known or unsuspected cystic teratoma is probably no more than 0.5 per cent (Stamp and McConnell 1983) and is usually a squamous cell carcinoma but many other tumours, such as adenocarcinomas, melanomas, and sarcomas, have been reported.

Monodermal teratomas are tumours in which only one tissue type foreign to the ovary is present. Struma ovarii, composed of thyroid

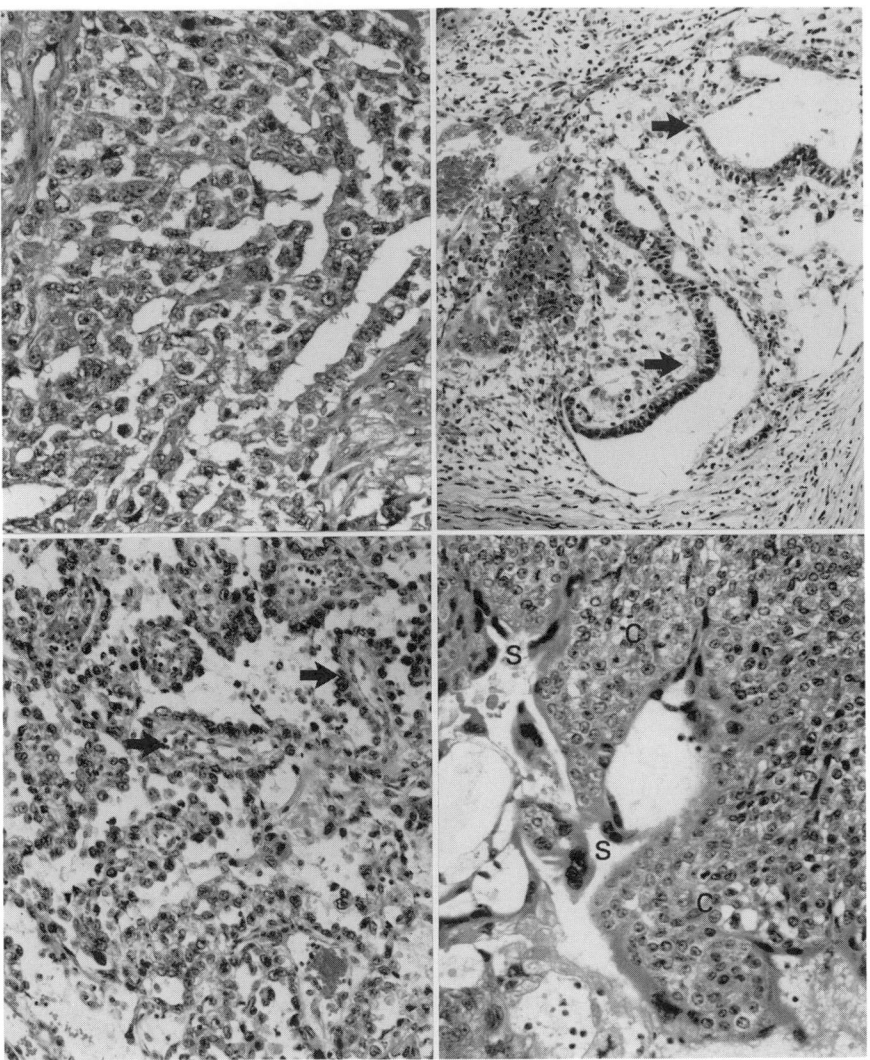

Fig. 2 Some patterns seen in anaplastic germ cell tumours. (a) Embryonal carcinoma forming cords and tubules, (b) embryoid bodies (arrow), (c) yolk sac pattern with Duval–Schiller body (arrow), (d) choriocarcinoma forming cyto- (C) and syncytiotrophoblast (S).

tissue and ovarian carcinoid are probably the best known. Most of them are benign but they can become malignant (Fox and Langley 1976).

Gonadoblastomas are uncommon tumours with a mixture of germ cells and gonadal stromal cells, usually Sertoli cells arranged in rosettes around basement membrane material (Fig. 4); they occur predominantly in XY ovarian dysgenesis with female phenotype (Adewole *et al.* 1987) and the germ cell component of the tumour eventually forms a dysgerminoma, which is often bilateral. Very rarely, mixed germ cell–stromal tumours occur in previously normal gonads, when germinal and stromal cells are usually intermingled in a haphazard way.

Biology

The evidence that human germ cell tumours are derived from germ cells comes from morphological and genetic studies. The fact that the majority of germ cell tumours occur in the gonads, where germ cells are or in the midline of the body, along which germ cells migrate to the gonadal ridges encased laterally by the foregut mesentery, speaks strongly in favour of this view. In the testis, there is also the frequent observation of *in situ* germ cell tumour (Skakkebaek 1978). Benign cystic teratomas of the ovary usually

have a 46XX chromosomal complement, but DNA and enzyme studies show that they are often homozygous for markers for which the host is heterozygous and that they do not contain genetic material foreign to the host. This is better explained if they arise from germ cells and rules out the formation of a tumour from a fertilized ovum. By further studying the homo- or heterozygosity of markers near or away from the centromere (Linder *et al.* 1975; Parrington *et al.* 1984), it has been possible to ascertain that ovarian teratomas can probably arise from germ cells before, between, and after the two meiotic divisions of the ovum. Immature and malignant germ cell tumours may have trisomies and other chromosomal abnormalities but also appear to arise from germ cells in the same fashion (Arias-Bernal and Jones 1968; Ohama *et al.* 1985).

Ovarian teratomas can arise in highly inbred strains of mice in rather similar fashion (Stevens 1983). The reasons for the predominance of benign germ cell tumours in the ovary when compared with the testis is not known, but genetic and environmental factors, as well as hormonal stimuli, are probably important.

Clinical presentation

In common with other ovarian tumours, germ cell tumours cause few symptoms until they are large enough to compress

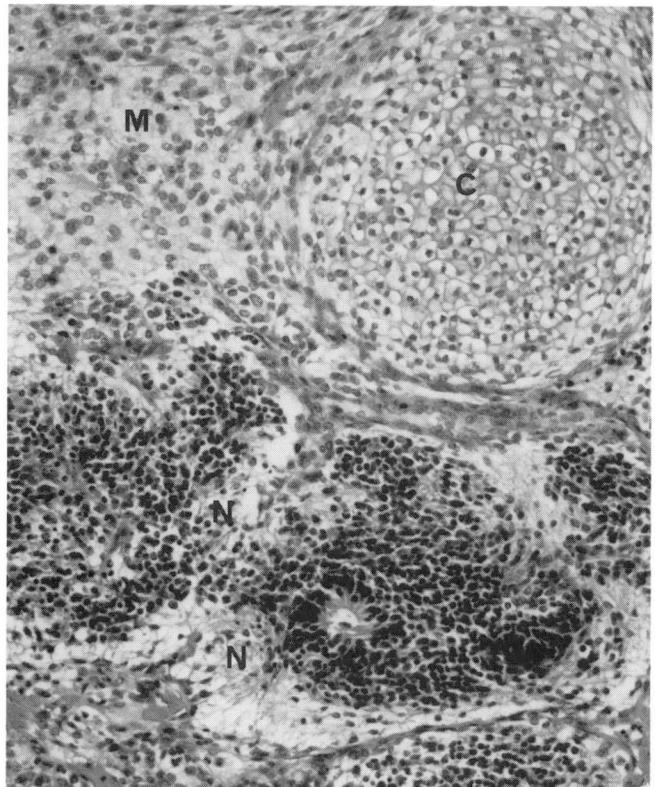

Fig. 3 Immature teratoma. The illustration includes cartilage (C), immature mesenchye (M), and immature neuroepithelial tissue (N) with an ependymal rossette.

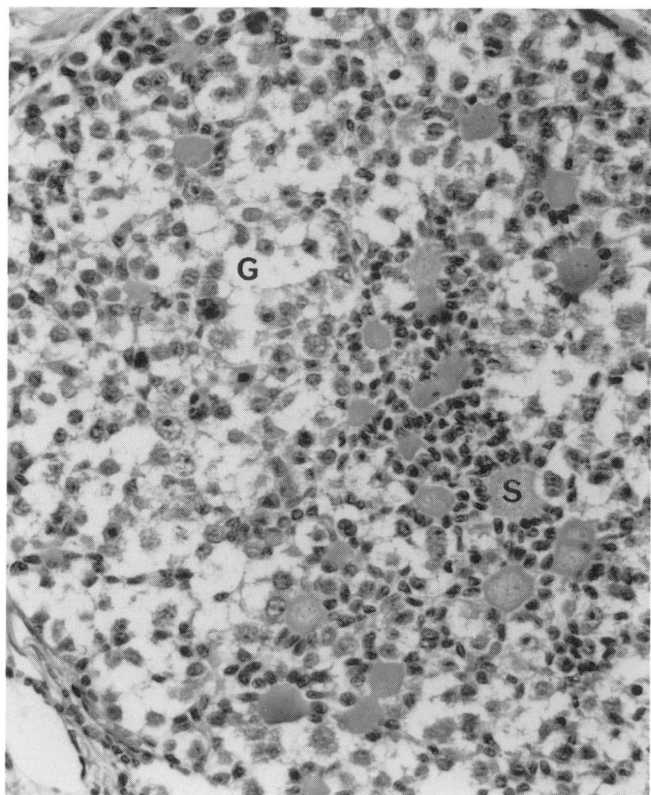

Fig. 4 Gonadoblastoma. The larger cells (G) are germinoma cells. The small cells (S) with oval nuclei surrounding hyaline material are Sertoli cells.

adjacent structures or until they disseminate. Slowly growing tumours may present with a feeling of abdominal distension or various degrees of lower abdominal pain. Tumours producing placental hormones, particularly chorionic gonadotrophin, may cause menstrual irregularities. Rapidly growing tumours can additionally present with the symptomatology of acute abdomen, often due to haemorrhage within the tumour or to haemoperitoneum.

It should be remembered that over half of malignant ovarian tumours in women under 20 are likely to be germ cell tumours and tumour markers in serum, including human chorionic gonadotrophin, α-fetoprotein, placental alkaline phosphatase, lactate dehydrogenase, and CA125 (Altaras *et al.* 1986), may be raised. Of these, chorionic gonadotrophin (produced by trophoblast) and α-fetoprotein (produced by yolk sac, embryonic liver, and primitive intestinal mucosa) remain the most useful and in an analysis of 51 patients we found that 48 (88 per cent) had raised chorionic gonadotrophin and/or α-fetoprotein (Newlands *et al.* 1988a). Placental alkaline phosphatase may be present in some germ cell tumours, particularly dysgerminomas, but it does not necessarily appear in the serum in detectable amounts. Lactate dehydrogenase is not specific for germ cell tumours but when raised, it can be useful in monitoring treatment of germ cell tumours negative for chorionic gonadotrophin and α-fetoprotein.

Management

General

Any malignant ovarian tumour in a young woman could be a germ cell tumour and if it is discovered during an emergency laparotomy and is not resectable by unilateral oophorectomy, it is important to establish the diagnosis and avoid radical surgery. A frozen section may be diagnostic, but this is not always so and in such a situation it is better to biopsy the tumour and wait for the results of histological examination and assay of serum markers before planning further surgery.

Once the diagnosis has been established, a number of additional staging investigations are indicated. These include thoracic and abdominal, computerized tomographic (**CT**) scan and ultrasonography of the liver, para-aortic region, and pelvis. In these sites, ultrasound can be more rewarding than CT scanning because young patients frequently have a limited amount of intra-abdominal fat, which makes CT definition poor. Post-operative and, if known, pre-operative serum markers should be used as a baseline. Ovarian germ cell tumours seldom metastasize to the brain but if this is suspected, a brain CT scan and assay of markers in cerebrospinal fluid can be of use (Newlands *et al.* 1988a). Germ cell tumours are staged according to the International Federation of Obstetricians and Gynaecologists (**FIGO**) classification.

If, after initial surgery and the above investigations, the tumour is shown to be stage I, we do not use chemotherapy but follow the patient closely with clinical, biochemical, and radiological investigations (Table 1). To date, none of our 13 stage-I patients with ovarian germ cell tumours has relapsed. This policy is based on our greater experience with stage-I testicular germ cell tumours: of 129 males with stage-I tumours, 25 per cent have relapsed but all have been salvaged by chemotherapy at the time of the relapse and remain in remission. In our view, the only role for adjuvant chemotherapy in patients with stage-I disease is when close follow-up is not possible.

Table 1 Follow-up of patients with germ cell tumours at Charing Cross Hospital

Stage I, from normalization of markers; stages II–IV, from end of treatment
Serum tumour markers (human chorionic gonadotrophin and α-fetoprotein)

    Year 1: weekly×10; 2-weekly×21
    Year 2: monthly
    Year 3: 2-monthly
    Years 4 and 5: 3-monthly
    Subsequent years: 6-monthly

Clinical examination with chest radiograph (or CT scan if available)

    Year 1: monthly
    Year 2: 2-monthly
    Years 3 and 4: 3-monthly
    Subsequent years: 6-monthly

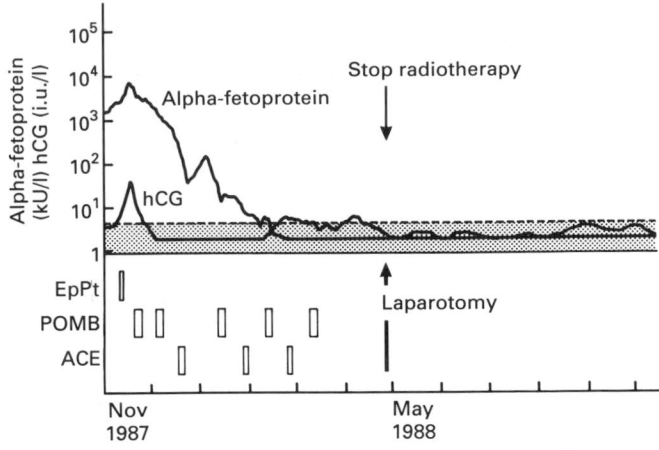

Fig. 5 Course of a patient treated for a 17 cm pelvic recurrent mixed GCT (dysgerminoma/yolk sac tumour) causing hydronephrosis. Low-dose etoposide/platinum (EpPt) was given before POMB/ACE to relieve the ureteric obstruction. After hCG and AFP fell within the normal range, a CT scan confirmed a residual mass of 5 × 5 cm. This was resected and histology showed necrotic material only.

Management of stage-II–IV, anaplastic germ cell tumours

Anaplastic germ cell tumours have been known to respond to chemotherapy for many years. During the 1970s the most widely used drug combination was vincristine, actinomycin D, and cyclophosphamide (**VAC**). The results of VAC chemotherapy have been reviewed by Slayton *et al.* (1985): 15 of 54 patients (28 per cent) who had all the apparent tumour removed surgically and 15 of 22 patients (68 per cent) known to have residual disease after surgery developed progressive disease. By current standards, it is unlikely that VAC chemotherapy is optimal but Mann *et al.* (1989) have reported a 78 per cent survival in 29 patients treated with VAC given in higher doses. This study also emphatically confirms that low-dose VAC is inadequate, giving in their pilot study an actuarial survival of only 8 per cent after 5 years.

During the 1970s, cisplatin and etoposide were introduced. Williams *et al.* (1984) reported a 54 per cent survival in 30 patients treated with cisplatin, vinblastine, and bleomycin (**PVB**). More recently, better preliminary results have been reported with cisplatin, bleomycin, and etoposide (Smales and Peckham 1987) with survival of six out of seven patients.

It should be noted that many of these studies include patients with stage-I germ cell tumours, and that the results appear better than they really are because the majority of stage-I tumours do not require chemotherapy.

Table 2 POMB/ACE chemotherapy

POMB
Day 1: Vincristine 1 mg/m² intravenously; methotrexate 300 mg/m² as a 12-h infusion
Day 2: bleomycin 15 mg as a 24-h infusion; folinic acid rescue begins 24 h after the start of methotrexate in a dose of 15 mg 12-hourly for four doses
Day 3: bleomycin 15 mg by 24-h infusion
Day 4: cisplatin 120 mg/m² as a 12-h infusion given together with hydration and a 3 g magnesium sulphate supplementation

ACE
Days 1 to 5: etoposide (VP16-213) 100 mg/m² intravenously
Days 3, 4 and 5: actinomycin D, 0.5 mg intravenously
Day 5: cyclophosphamide 500 mg/m² intravenously

OMB
Day 1: vincristine 1 mg/m² intravenously; methotrexate 300 mg/m² as a 12-h infusion
Day 2: bleomycin 15 mg as a 24 h infusion; folinic acid rescue begins 24-h after the start of methotrexate in a dose of 15 mg 12-hourly for four doses
Day 3: bleomycin 15 mg by 24-h infusion

For the last 16 years at Charing Cross Hospital (London) we have been using **POMB/ACE** (Table 2), an alternating chemotherapeutic regimen. This regimen differs from other schedules used in the treatment of ovarian germ cell tumours in that seven drugs are used in the initial management with the aim of minimizing the possibility of drug resistance. It alternates a relatively non-myelosuppressive combination (POMB) with the more myelosuppressive ACE, keeping the intervals between treatments as short as possible. Because of the alternate use of two different drug combinations, the cumulative dose of each drug has been less than when the same combination is repeated with each treatment and the possibility of complications due to cumulative toxicity, such as bleomycin pneumonitis or the induction of second tumours with cyclophosphamide are potentially less than with other regimens.

All patients received a minimum of three courses of POMB (total dose of cisplatin, 360 mg/m²). POMB has been continued until biochemical remission occurs, as shown by normalization of tumour markers (Fig. 5). Initially we continued the same combination without cisplatin (OMB), alternating with ACE for a further 12 weeks, but experience has shown that this is probably unnecessary and now we only use this second schedule for 6–8 weeks after normalization of markers.

An analysis of results in 58 patients with stage-II–IV disease and with a maximum follow-up of 12 years (1977–1989) confirms previous reports (Newlands *et al.* 1982; 1988*a,b*) that our patients do as well or better with POMB/ACE chemotherapy than those treated elsewhere with other, even more intensive, schedules (Hitchins *et al.* 1989). Our current survival rate is 83 per cent and there have been no deaths beyond the third year of entry into the study (Fig. 6). Age over 30 years is the one significantly adverse, prognostic factor. The FIGO stage at presentation and presence of liver metastases are not major prognostic factors in our series. The initial concentrations of tumour markers do not appear to influence survival to the extent they do in testicular germ cell tumours (Hitchins *et al.* 1989).

After chemotherapy, menstruation reappears within 2–6 months and fertility is preserved in most cases. A number of children have been born to mothers who have received POMB/ACE chemotherapy for ovarian germ cell tumours and no congenital abnormalities have

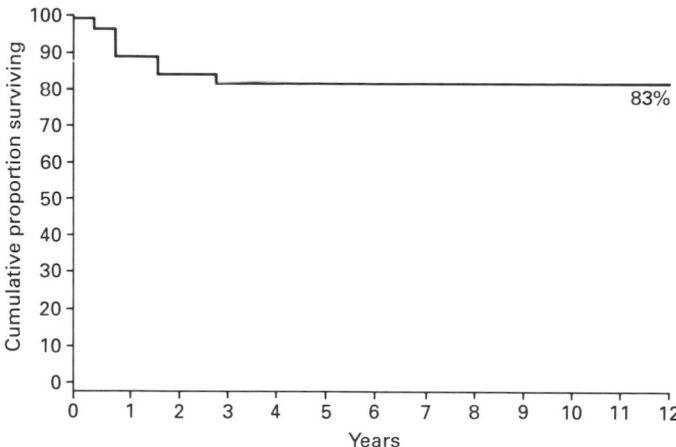

Fig. 6 Current overall survival rate for stage-II to -IV ovarian germ cell tumours at Charing Cross Hospital (58 cases) Maximum follow-up 12 years.

been reported in them (Pektasides *et al.* 1987). Fertility is also usually preserved with VAC chemotherapy (Gershenson 1988).

Specific management of dysgerminomas

As 15 per cent of dysgerminomas are bilateral the initial management of stage-I tumours should include resection of the tumour and biopsy of any suspicious lesion in the contralateral ovary. If full staging investigations are negative, our current policy is to advocate no further treatment, but we establish a meticulous follow-up system (see Table 1). So far, none of our stage-I dysgerminomas has relapsed, confirming the relatively low malignant potential of this tumour.

If a tumour relapses in the pelvis or para-aortic region, the management depends primarily on whether the patient wants to retain fertility or not. Dysgerminomas are highly radiosensitive as well as chemosensitive, but even with shielding there is considerable scatter of radiation to the uterus and contralateral ovary; if fertility is to be preserved, chemotherapy, similar to that used for other ovarian germ cell tumours, is the treatment of choice. Surgery may be necessary to remove suspicious residual masses after chemotherapy; if so, this should be done with extreme care because, like seminoma in the male, dysgerminoma shrinks with intense fibrosis after chemotherapy.

Management of immature (solid) teratomas

Stage-I tumours are treated surgically and their prognosis as a group is better than that of anaplastic germ cell tumours. When they disseminate, they seldom extend beyond the peritoneal cavity. Peritoneal seedlings may consist of mesenchymal or neuroepithelial tissue and can mature spontaneously to inactive glial implants. In addition, the malignant and immature components of these tumours often have more in common with neuroblastomas and sarcomas than with other germ cell tumours. The success of chemotherapy in anaplastic components of germ cell tumours has highlighted the fact that some of these sarcomas and neuroepithelial malignant tumours can persist as the only therapy-resistant component of a germ cell tumour (Ulbright *et al.* 1984). Experience with this problem is at present too limited to recommend a firm policy.

Management of malignancy arising in benign cystic teratomas

If this is discovered on microscopical examination of a stage-I tumour the prognosis is good and no further treatment is usually

necessary. Occasionally, a squamous cell carcinoma has pelvic or peritoneal metastases on presentation. There is little information of chemotherapy in this situation.

SEX CORD–STROMAL TUMOURS

Introduction

Tumours derived from ovarian stroma are classified according to whether they differentiate towards female-directed cells (granulosa–theca cell tumours) or to male-directed cells (Sertoli–Leydig cell tumours). Tumours with male and female sex cord differentiation are called gynandroblastomas. In the account below, lipid cell tumours have been grouped with pure Leydig cell tumours; sex cord tumours with annular tubules are studied with pure Sertoli cell tumours.

Granulosa cell stromal tumours

Introduction

Granulosa cell stromal tumours are composed of cells with various degrees of resemblance to granulosa cells. They may be pure or have a cellular fibrous stroma that may contain luteinized theca cells or Leydig cells. They are classically associated with oestrogen excess and its complications but they can be androgenic. The more common form (95 per cent) of the neoplasm is often referred to as 'adult type' because of the existence of a rarer 'juvenile type', but the adult type can be found in children and the juvenile type in adults. Even the well-differentiated forms of the tumour can behave in a malignant fashion and it is doubtful whether any granulosa cell stromal tumour can be classed as benign on morphological grounds.

Epidemiology and aetiology

These tumours have been described in all races and constitute approximately 70 per cent of all feminizing tumours of the ovary but no more than 5 per cent of all malignant ovarian tumours. Approximately 5 per cent occur in children, 40 per cent during reproductive life, and 55 per cent after the menopause (Young and Scully 1984*b*).

Nothing is known about the causation of human granulosa cell stromal tumours but parallels have been drawn between the circumstances in which human tumours arise and spontaneous or experimental animal tumours: granulosa cell tumours can be induced in mice in a variety of ways (Fox 1985) but prerequisites for tumorigenesis are an intact pituitary gland and the absence of normal ovarian tissue, particularly oocytes. The assumption is that the loss of oocytes and functioning ovarian tissue leads to a rise in pituitary gonadotrophins and this in turn leads to abnormal proliferation and eventually neoplasia of granulosa cells. A similar mechanism could explain granulosa cell stromal tumours in perimenopausal and post-menopausal women. The occurrence of such tumours in infancy and childhood is usually associated with low concentrations of gonadotrophins and resembles more closely spontaneously occurring granulosa cell tumours in inbred strains of mice or in mice with ovotestes or mosaicisms. The association of juvenile granulosa cell stromal tumours with mesenchymal dysplastic syndromes, particularly Ollier's disease (see below), points towards an underlying genetic abnormality. None of these animal models helps to explain the considerable proportion of human granulosa cell stromal tumours that occurs during reproductive life.

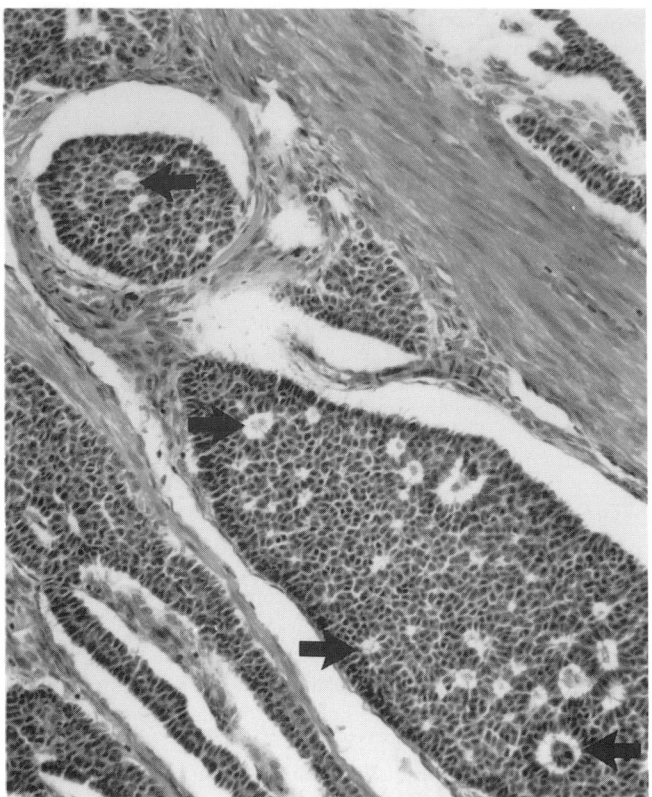

Fig. 7 Well-differentiated adult-type granulosa cell tumour composed of clusters and cords in a fibrous stroma. Note the Call–Exner bodies (arrows) formed by granulosa cells surrounding spaces which contain necrotic cell debris.

Pathology

Granulosa cell stromal tumours can be solid or cystic; solid tumours may have a yellowish hue if they contain abundant lipid. Cystic tumours are characteristically multiloculated, the cysts containing fluid or blood. In 5 per cent of cases, bilateral tumours may be found. The tumours can vary in size from those too small to be detected by gynaecological examination to huge masses over 15 kg in weight (Scully 1982).

Adult type

These neoplasms are composed of granulosa cells arranged in a variety of patterns of which the microfollicular with Call–Exner bodies (Fig. 7) is the most characteristic. Other patterns, such as macrofollicular, trabecular, insular, and diffuse, co-exist in most tumours. In approximately 2 per cent of cases, bizarre nuclei can be seen (Young and Scully 1983*b*) but this in itself does not seem to worsen prognosis. In most granulosa cell stromal tumours there are theca cells that may be luteinized. Leydig cells, with typical Reinke's crystals, can be seen in some cases, particularly those with androgen production. Sarcomatous transformation of granulosa cell stromal tumours has been described (Susil and Sumithran 1987). Adult-type tumours grow slowly and may recur many years after initial presentation. Five year survival rates are not very meaningful and data from longer follow-up suggest that granulosa cell stromal tumours have a worse prognosis than previously thought, with only 34 per cent survival after 20 years in one report (Dempster *et al.*

1987). Recurrences are usually confined to the pelvis or peritoneum, but distant metastases can occur, including to liver, lung, bone, and many other sites.

Juvenile type

These are composed of cells that are often less characteristic and more malignant looking than those of adult-type tumours (Vassal *et al.* 1988). They are either arranged in solid clusters intermixed with abundant, often luteinized, theca cells or form the lining of small follicles. The clusters are often separated by abundant oedematous stroma. In most cases the tumours occur in apparently normal children but associations with Ollier's disease, Maffuci's syndrome, Potter's syndrome, and dysmorphism have been described (see review by Velasco-Oses *et al.* (1988)). Approximately 50 per cent occur in the first decade of life, 35 per cent in the second, and the rest in adult life, including a case in a 67-year-old woman (Young *et al.* 1984*a*). Most juvenile granulosa cell stromal tumours are stage Ia on presentation (Zaloudek and Norris 1982) and prognosis is usually very good in this group. In the series of Young *et al.* (1984*a*), only four out of 91 patients with stage-I disease died of their tumours but all three patients with stage-II tumours died. Although mitoses and cellular pleomorphism may delineate the more aggressive tumours, the stage at laparotomy appears to have a greater influence on outcome. Unlike the adult type, juvenile granulosa cell stromal tumours that recur do so early and behave in an aggressive way, most deaths occurring within 3 years of diagnosis.

Biology

The majority (approximately 75 per cent) of granulosa cell stromal tumours are associated with excess oestrogen secretion by the tumour. It has been pointed out that in most cases granulosa cells lack the enzymes and organelles for complete steroid synthesis and it has been postulated that oestrogen production by them takes place by aromatization of androgenic precursors produced by theca cells (Fox 1985). The fact that oestrogens can be demonstrated immuno-cytochemically in most granulosa cell stromal tumours (Kurman *et al.* 1979) is not against this. It may also explain the predominantly androgenic secretion of some tumours. Progesterone is often present in luteinized theca cells but can also be demonstrated in granulosa cells. A report of renin production causing hypertension in a reputed granulosa cell stromal tumour (Tetu *et al.* 1988) appears exceptional.

It has been argued that only the granulosa-cell component of these tumours is neoplastic (Fox 1985) and that other cell types may derive from ovarian mesenchyme under the influence of granulosa cells. The rarity of malignant change in the fibrous or thecal component and the failure to establish tissue culture lines from thecomas or grow them in nude mice (Ishiwata *et al.* 1984), favour this view.

Clinical presentation

Granulosa cell stromal tumours in children often present before the fifth year with sexual pseudoprecocity, a term used to distinguish it from true precocity, caused by pituitary gonadotrophic stimulation of the ovary, in which oocyte maturation occurs and a pregnancy is theoretically possible. Oestrogen production by these tumours results in the development of breasts, axillary and pubic hair, and external and internal secondary sexual organs, and in accelerated skeletal growth. Irregular uterine bleeding and vaginal discharge can occur. In some patients, androgen excess and virilization can co-exist with hyperoestronism (Nakashima *et al.* 1984).

In post-menopausal women, granulosa cell stromal tumours often present with vaginal bleeding. The endometrium may show cystic hyperplasia but in some cases adenomatous (atypical) hyperplasia, frank carcinoma *in situ*, or invasive adenocarcinoma of the endometrium occur. The incidence of endometrial adenocarcinoma is difficult to establish but probably does not exceed 5 per cent (Stenwig *et al.* 1979).

During reproductive life the tumours can present with excessive uterine bleeding but amenorrhoea can precede this or be the dominant symptom, particularly in patients with tumours producing androgens. Occasionally, tenderness or fullness of the breasts is the dominant symptom. Whether the tumours secrete oestrogens or not, this may not interfere significantly with ovarian function and there are instances when the tumour has been detected during a pregnancy (Young *et al.* 1984*b*). Predominantly androgenic tumours are rare (Nakashima *et al.* 1984) and often, but not always, present with virilization. Endometrial hyperplasia and adenocarcinoma are a little less common in this group than in post-menopausal women.

In a proportion of patients, granulosa cell stromal tumours present with symptoms unrelated to their endocrine secretion, such as abdominal distension, abdominal pain, or even acute abdomen and shock resulting from rupture of a cystic tumour (Scully 1982). If the nature of the tumour is not suspected by the clinical features, radiological investigations are of little help, given the variable appearance. Reports of cytological diagnosis in ascitic fluid or needle aspirations are few (Ehya and Lang 1986) and so far appear to have had very little influence in diagnosis or management.

Management

In children with stage-Ia tumours, unilateral oophorectomy or salpingo–oophorectomy appears to be the treatment of choice. Hysterectomy and bilateral salpingo–oophorectomy have been used for more extensive disease. The value of radiotherapy or chemotherapy as co-adjuvants to surgery has not been tested. When tumours recur, combination chemotherapy has been used (Malkasian 1988) but the prognosis is poor.

In adults, but particularly in pre-menopausal and post-menopausal women, the treatment of choice is bilateral salpingo–oophorectomy and hysterectomy. In patients so treated in one study (Evans *et al.* 1980), the recurrence rate was only 6 per cent, whereas it was 25 per cent in patients in whom the ovary only was removed. In young women with either juvenile or adult-type granulosa cell stromal tumours, unilateral salpingo–oophorectomy may be justified for stage-Ia tumours if preservation of the uterus is an important consideration. If a hysterectomy is not done, endometrial curettage to exclude endometrial carcinoma is mandatory.

In stage-Ia$_{ii}$ disease, hysterectomy and bilateral salpingo–oophorectomy followed by cyclophosphamide and cisplatin have been recommended (Malkasian 1988). Oestrogen and inhibin, a protein produced by granulosa cells, have been used as tumour markers (Lappohn *et al.* 1989). The optimal treatment of recurrent tumours or those that are stage II or III on presentation is still to be determined. The results reported up to 1984 with a variety of agents have been reviewed by Malkasian (1988) and suggest that combination chemotherapy, particularly regimens including cisplatin, cyclophosphamide or doxorubicin, can achieve sustained remissions. More recent reports reinforce this view: Kaye and Davies (1986) treated two patients with cyclophosphamide, adriamycin, and cisplatin and both had partial responses and Colombo *et al.* (1986) treated 11 patients with cisplatin, vinblastin, and bleomycin and achieved six complete remissions in patients with small-volume residual disease (only one of them had a subsequent relapse 18 months later).

Thecomas and other fibrous stromal tumours

The presence of a theca cell component in granulosa cell stromal tumours has already been discussed. Pure thecomas or fibrothecomas are benign tumours more often found in perimenopausal women and which may produce oestrogens and, very rarely, androgens. They are mentioned here because, like granulosa cell stromal tumours, they are often associated with endometrial adenocarcinoma (Malkasian 1988). In young patients, resection of the tumour and diagnostic endometrial curettage is all that is needed. In perimenopausal women and those with endometrial adenocarcinoma, hysterectomy and bilateral salpingo–oophorectomy may be indicated. Sclerosing stromal tumours are very rare, benign ovarian tumours with a distinct histological appearance, which, in approximately 25 per cent of cases, may also be hormonally active (Fox 1985) and may present with menorrhagia, infertility, or endometrial cystic hyperplasia.

Ovarian fibromas are non-functioning, benign stromal tumours that can occasionally be associated with a pleural effusion of unknown pathogenesis and mimic malignancy (Meigs 1954). Cellular fibromas and fibrosarcomas have been described but are very rare (Prat and Scully 1981).

Tumours of Sertoli or Leydig cells (androblastomas)

Introduction

The WHO has recommended that the old term 'arrhenoblastoma' should no longer be used and the term 'androblastoma' or 'Sertoli–Leydig cell tumour' is to be preferred (Serov *et al.* 1973). The majority of malignant tumours of this group have a mixture of Sertoli and Leydig cells, whereas tumours of Sertoli cells only or of Leydig cells only, are seldom malignant. Lipid cell tumour is a term introduced by Scully in 1963 to describe tumours composed of polygonal cells containing abundant steroid lipid. It includes pure Leydig cell tumours and tumours of similar morphology that may produce female hormones or adrenocortical steroids.

Sertoli–Leydig cell tumours
Epidemiology and aetiology

These account for only 1 per cent of all ovarian tumours (Hughesdon 1985). The mean age of presentation is 25 years, with most tumours occurring in the third decade, but they have been reported between the ages of 2 and 75 (Young and Scully 1985). There are reports of Sertoli–Leydig cell tumours in several members of a family (Jensen *et al.* 1974). The association with endometrial carcinoma in 8 per cent of cases is probably not coincidental (Montz and Morrow 1988). The possible development of sarcomas in some of these tumours will be discussed later. Nothing is known about their causes.

Pathology

The majority of Sertoli–Leydig cell tumours are either solid or partly cystic, with no specific gross macroscopical features, but haemorrhage and necrosis are more common in poorly differentiated tumours. They vary greatly in size, with a mean diameter of 13 cm and less than 2 per cent are bilateral (Young and Scully 1985). It has been customary to classify them histologically into four groups (Serov *et al.* 1973). Their main features and incidence in the series of Young and Scully (1985), comprising 207 cases, are as follows.

1. *Well differentiated* (11 per cent) in which Sertoli cells are arranged in well-formed tubules resembling pre-pubertal gonad, separated by a variable amount of Leydig cells. They are all benign (Young and Scully 1984*c*).

2. *Intermediately differentiated* (54 per cent) in which Sertoli cells form cords and clusters resembling embryonic testicular sex cords. Again, Leydig cells are found in the interstitium (Fig. 8). Approximately 11 per cent of them behave in a malignant fashion.

3. *Poorly differentiated* (13 per cent) composed of spindle cells that resemble the stroma of the undifferentiated gonad and can be frankly sarcomatous. Clusters and cords of recognizable Sertoli and Leydig cells form a minor component. Approximately 60 per cent have behaved as malignant tumours.

4. *Tumours with heterologous elements* (22 per cent): the Sertoli–Leydig component is usually intermediately or poorly differentiated and their overall malignancy rate is 19 per cent.
   There are three major heterologous components.

   (i) Intestinal type mucinous cysts with or without carcinoid elements. Malignancy of the cyst epithelium and recurrence of the Sertoli–Leydig component are very rare (Young *et al*. 1982*b*).

   (ii) Striated muscle, cartilage, or neuroepithelial tissues, which can be immature or frankly sarcomatous. The Sertoli–Leydig component is usually poorly differentiated and approximately 80 per cent of patients die of their tumours (Prat *et al*. 1982*b*).

   (iii) Structures resembling rete testis (Young and Scully 1983*a*), which may co-exist with other heterologous elements. Approximately one-third are malignant.

These tumours spread within the abdominal cavity and metastases outside the abdomen are rare.

Biology

The cell mixtures found in this group of tumours present a challenge to embryologists and a diagnostic problem to pathologists. They probably are a manifestation of the totipotential nature of ovarian gonadal stroma. Tumours with heterologous elements could be explained as a metaplastic phenomenon rather than as teratomatous elements of germ cell derivation (Fox 1985). The majority of Sertoli–Leydig cell tumours are androgenic and there is evidence that the Leydig cells are the main site of androgen synthesis. A proportion are inert and, rarely, they can secrete oestrogens (Genton and Schmid 1981). In some cases, production of α-fetoprotein has been described (Chumas *et al*. 1984) and in a patient with a heterologous, retiform type the α-fetoprotein was traced to areas of hepatocyte differentiation (Young *et al*. 1984*c*).

Clinical presentation

This reflects the patterns of hormone production by these tumours, with varying degrees of defeminization that include amenorrhoea with atrophic changes of breasts and genitalia or frank virilization with clitoral enlargement, hirsutism, acne, voice change, and increased libido. In well-differentiated tumours the changes develop over a number of years but virilization can be rapid with more rapidly growing tumours. In the series of Roth *et al*. (1981), 39 per cent of patients were virilized and 11 per cent were hirsute. The existence of inert and oestrogenic variants has already been

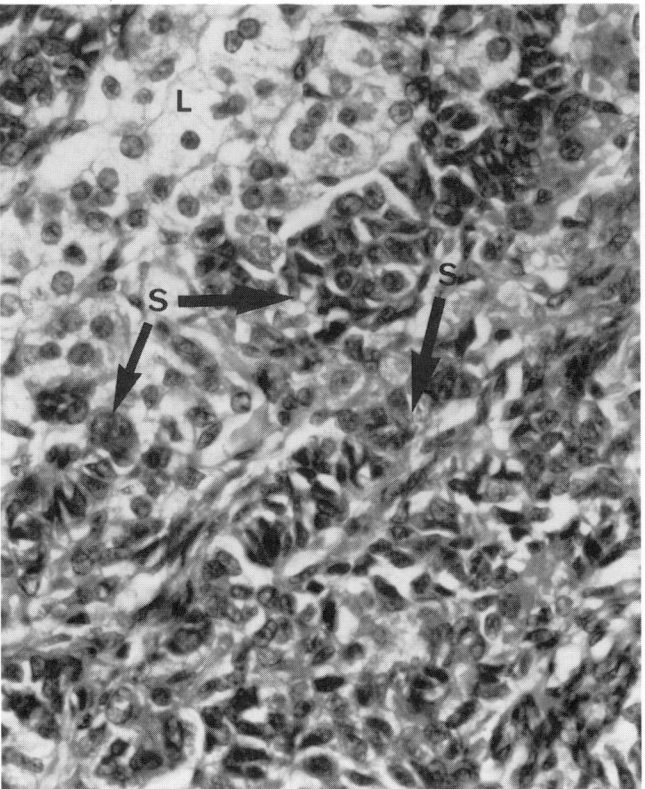

Fig. 8 Sertoli–Leydig cell tumour (androblastoma) of intermediate differentiation. Ill-defined clusters of Sertoli cells (S) are intermixed with Leydig cell (L).

mentioned. Some patients may not have symptoms related to hormone production and, in some cases, whether virilizing or not, the tumour has been discovered during pregnancy (Young *et al*. 1984*b*)

Biochemical investigations usually disclose an increase in testosterone and other steroid hormones (Munemura *et al*. 1982) and the testosterone concentration tends to be higher in the more malignant tumours (Friedman *et al*. 1985). It should be remembered that Sertoli–Leydig cell tumours are not the only tumours capable of androgen production, which can occur in granulosa cell tumours and that even epithelial and metastatic tumours of the ovary appear to have the capacity for stimulation of the ovarian stroma to produce hormones (Scully 1988). Other causes of androgen excess have been summarized by Montz and Morrow (1988) and include polycystic ovaries, Cushing's syndrome, acromegaly, pregnancy, exogenous androgens, congenital adrenal hyperplasia, and genetic abnormalities.

The implications of α-fetoprotein production by Sertoli–Leydig cell tumours in the differential diagnosis with germ cell tumours with yolk sac and hepatoid differentiation are obvious.

Management

The majority of Sertoli–Leydig cell tumours (95–97 per cent) are FIGO stage I on presentation (Roth *et al*. 1981; Young and Scully 1985) and unilateral salpingo-oophorectomy is the treatment of choice in young women or those who want to retain fertility. Because of the occasional association with endometrial adenocarcinoma, endometrial curettage is recommended. Hysterectomy and bilateral salpingo-oophorectomy is done in all other instances. The prognosis in most cases is excellent.

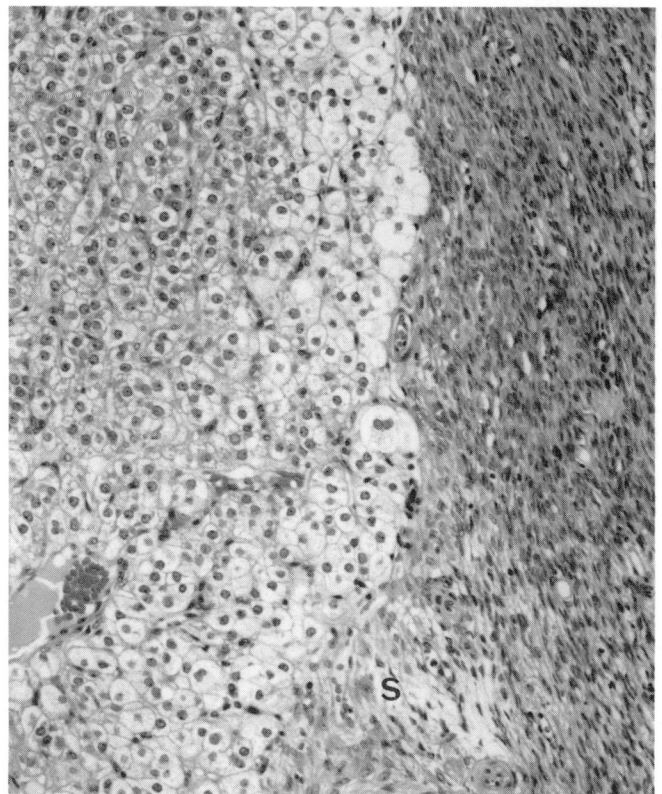

Fig. 9 Lipid cell tumour arising in ovarian stroma (S). This tumour was virilizing and composed of clear cells containing abundant lipid and resembling adrenocortical cells.

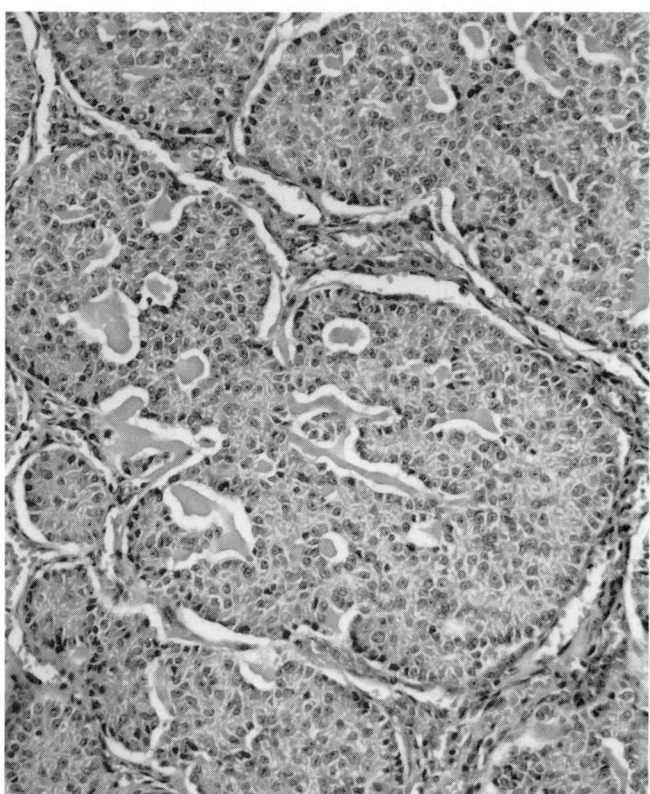

Fig. 10 Sex cord tumour with annular tubules (SCTAT). Tumours of this type in patients with Peutz–Jeghers syndrome are usually benign but a small proportion of those arising outside the syndrome can be malignant.

Approximately 20 per cent of stage-I tumours are potentially malignant histologically and some of these recur within the first year and may require further resection. The role of radiotherapy in the management of Sertoli–Leydig cell tumours is uncertain because of the limited experience with this treatment. Chemotherapy has been used in only a few cases and short-lived responses have been obtained with VAC and also with bleomycin, etoposide, and cisplatin (BEP). In a summary of results, Montz and Morrow (1988) conclude that no particular recommendation on therapy can be made on the basis of published information.

Pure Leydig cell tumours and lipid tumours

Leydig cells are usually present in small numbers in the hilum of the adult ovary and some pure Leydig cell tumours arise in the hilum (hilar tumours) but can also arise in the ovarian stroma. A proportion of these neoplasms is composed of large cells resembling luteinized theca cells or adrenocortical cells (Fig. 9). The majority, but not all, are androgenic and present with virilization but some are oestrogenic and not all can be identified as composed of Leydig cells. Because of this, the non-committal term 'lipid cell tumour' has been proposed. There is no firm evidence that some of these tumours arise in adrenal rests, but the occurrence, in some cases, of Cushing's syndrome and hyperaldosteronism is of interest. The majority of Leydig cell tumours are benign but rare malignant examples have been reported (Stewart and Woodward 1962).

Pure Sertoli cell tumours and sex cord tumour with annular tubules

Sertoli cell tumours resemble the well-differentiated Sertoli–Leydig cell tumours but without the Leydig cell component. They are all benign but one case with tubular pattern co-existing with frank carcinoma has been described (Young and Scully 1984a). Endometrioid carcinomas with a tubular pattern resembling that of Sertoli cell tumours and with or without Leydig cells can be a source of error (Roth *et al.* 1982; Young *et al.* 1982a). Some Sertoli cell tumours are associated with oestrogen production and, although virilizing examples have been described, the presence of Leydig cells has not always been excluded by careful sampling. Treatment is by surgical excision.

Sex cord tumour with annular tubules was described by Scully (1970) as a tumour associated with the Peutz–Jeghers syndrome but similar tumours can occur in women without this syndrome (Young *et al.* 1982c). The histological appearances (Fig. 10) are characteristic and resemble the annular tubules seen in cryptorchid testes and in gonadoblastomas (see Fig. 4). Morphologically and on electron microscopy (Ahn *et al.* 1986), they resemble Sertoli rather than granulosa cells, but their derivation is controversial. About half of them are associated with complications suggestive of oestrogenic secretion, such as endometrial hyperplasia, amenorrhoea, menorrhagia, or sexual pseudoprecocity. Tumours in association with Peutz–Jeghers syndrome are often small, partly calcified, bilateral, and benign. When they occur outside this syndrome they tend to be larger, unilateral, may be associated with granulosa or Sertoli–Leydig cell tumours, and some of them (probably no more than 15 per cent), are malignant (Ahn *et al.* 1986; Malkasian 1988). The role of radiotherapy and chemotherapy is yet to be established.

Gynandroblastomas

Gynandroblastoma is a term that has been used loosely in the past. It is clear that some feminizing, granulosa cell tumours contain Leydig cells and that it may be difficult to judge whether some tubular structures in tumours are composed of Sertoli cells or granulosa cells, but the term should only be used when significant proportions of both male- and female-directed cells are present. With these criteria the number of acceptable cases reported is very small (Fox 1985) and their biological behaviour and management are still to be determined.

RARE EPITHELIAL TUMOURS
Malignant Brenner tumours
Introduction

Ober (1979), wittily tells the story of how, in 1956, Fritz Brenner, who had lost contact with academic medicine 46 years before and was then practising general medicine in Johannesburg, was astonished to learn that his name was firmly attached to that of a rare ovarian tumour. Brenner's report in 1907 was not the first and his interpretation of the tumour as arising from Graafian follicles was certainly wrong, but the failure to find, in the years that followed, a satisfactory explanation for the origin of this tumour, led to use of the eponym. The majority of Brenner tumours are benign but reports of malignant examples, which began to appear in 1945 (Rybak *et al.* 1981), had reached at least 110 in 1987 (van der Weiden and Gratama). In 1971, Roth and Sternberg, coined the term 'proliferating Brenner tumour' for intermediate, potentially malignant forms.

Epidemiology and aetiology

Brenner tumours of all types constitute at most 1.7 per cent of all ovarian neoplasms and of these, no more than 5 per cent have been reported as malignant (Czernobilsky 1982). Not only are Brenner tumours rare, in addition, malignant Brenner tumours are a heterogeneous group from a pathological viewpoint, so that information available at present is likely to be modulated in the light of a more precise definition of the malignant Brenner tumour. Although Brenner tumours occur at all ages, including childhood, they are most common in perimenopausal and post-menopausal women; malignant forms have been reported between the ages of 23 and 78 years, with a mean age of 60 (Rybak *et al.* 1981). There is apparently no relationship with parity or race. Nothing is known about their aetiology.

Pathology

Benign Brenner tumours are more often solid than cystic and their size can vary from microscopical to over 20 cm in largest dimension and over 8 kg in weight. Malignant Brenner tumours are, on average, larger and a higher proportion (60 per cent) are cystic (Rybak *et al.* 1981) with polypoid projections into the cysts. Examples of bilateral, malignant Brenner tumours have been recorded (Rybak *et al.* 1981; Kennedy *et al.* 1984). It is not unusual for Brenner tumours to co-exist with other ovarian neoplasms, particularly mucinous epithelial tumours and cystic teratomas (Silverberg 1971).

Histologically they are composed of islands of transitional epithelium made up of cells with characteristic, grooved nuclei and surrounded by cellular fibrous tissue which resembles that of ovarian fibromas (Fig. 11). Mucinous and squamous metaplasia can be seen in the epithelial islands, which in some cases contain serotonin-producing, endocrine cells (Fetissof *et al.* 1983; Aguirre *et al.* 1986).

Reported cases of malignant Brenner tumours include at least three different entities: (i) transitional carcinomas in association, or in continuity, with the epithelial component of a typical, benign Brenner tumour, (ii) mucinous, serous, or squamous carcinomas in association with a benign Brenner tumour, and (iii) transitional carcinomas without any typical Brenner tumour.

It appears sensible to regard only the first of these groups as true, malignant Brenner tumours. Mucinous or other cystadeno-carcinomas of the second group could be explained as collision tumours but even if they arise by metaplasia from Brenner tumours, their biological behaviour and response to therapy could resemble those of common forms of ovarian cancer. It is also becoming increasingly clear that finding a transitional carcinoma in the ovary does not mean that it has arisen in a previous Brenner tumour and a separate category for transitional carcinoma without evidence of Brenner tumour has been suggested (Austin and Norris 1987). According to them, transitional carcinomas arising *de novo* are usually more advanced on presentation (FIGO stages II–IV) and have a worse prognosis than malignant Brenner tumours in which typical Brenner is identified in part of the mass.

Malignant Brenner tumours may be restricted to the ovary or show pelvic spread on presentation (Roth and Czernobilsky 1985). The uterus, bladder, ureters, rectum, and abdominal wall may be invaded and the tumour may spread intraperitoneally. Metastases to ileofemoral nodes, liver, bone, and lung have been reported.

Roth and Sternberg (1971) described large, unilateral, cystic Brenner tumours, which they called 'proliferating Brenner tumours', in three post-menopausal patients. The tumours were partly typical benign Brenners but the transitional epithelium lining some cysts was proliferating in a papillary fashion. There was no stromal invasion and the tumours did not recur. They pointed out that some previously reported 'malignant' cases were, in fact, of this type. More recently Roth *et al.* (1985) described two new categories: 'metaplastic' and 'Brenner tumours of low malignant potential'. The distinction of these intermediate forms from truly malignant Brenner tumour is important and based on the absence of stromal invasion (a feature often difficult to assess) but it is questionable whether subdivision of these already rare, intermediate forms into three groups serves any practical purpose.

Biology

The origin of Brenner tumours is controversial but the theories of a follicular or stromal origin are now discredited. It is indeed arguable whether their stromal component is neoplastic and the synthesis of oestrogen by some Brenner tumours and malignant Brenner tumours (Seldenrijk *et al.* 1986; Kuhnel *et al.* 1987) can also occur in other epithelial ovarian tumours and in ovarian metastases. Other less favoured theories reviewed by Czernobilsky (1982) are that they arise in mesonephric and paramesonephric rests, by metaplasia from mucinous tumours, or as the sole component of a teratoma. Electron-microscopical and immunohistochemical observations (Fetissof *et al.* 1983) now stress the similarities between Walthard-cell nests, urothelium, and the epithelial component of Brenner tumours and support the theory, already proposed by Meyer in 1932, that Brenner tumours, like other epithelial tumours of the ovary, arise by urothelial metaplasia from coelomic epithelium (Czernobilsky 1982).

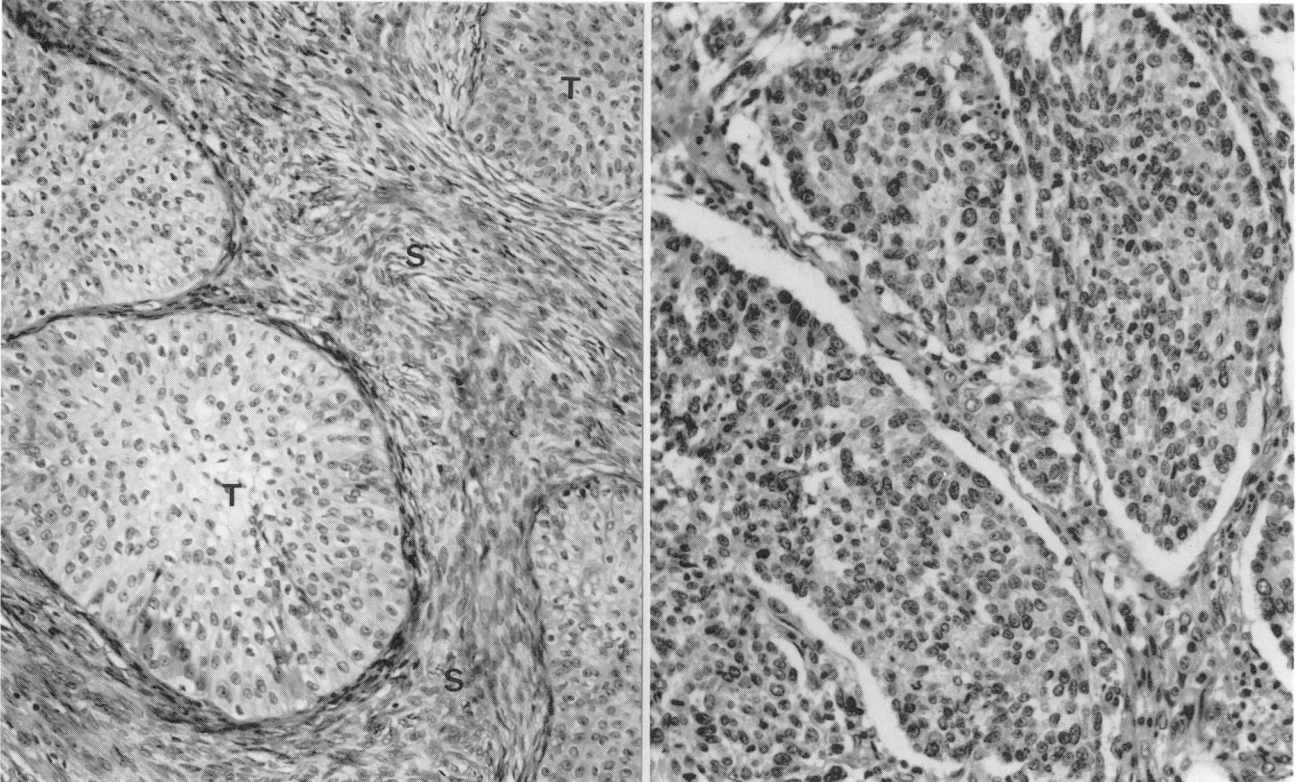

Fig. 11 (a) Benign Brenner tumour composed of islands of transitional epithelium (T) in a very cellular stroma (S) resembling that of ovarian fibromas. (b) Transitional cell carcinoma (TCC) of the ovary which was stage-III on presentation. TCC can occur with or without a pre-existing Brenner tumour.

Clinical presentation

Many benign Brenner tumours are incidental findings in ovaries removed for other reasons but a majority of patients with malignant Brenner tumours have abdominal pain or other symptoms related to the ovarian mass, such as abdominal distension, ascites, bowel or urinary symptoms, uterine prolapse, and dependent oedema. Post-menopausal bleeding or metromenorrhagia in pre-menopausal women, are reported in approximately 25 per cent of cases, which may reflect the propensity of some tumours to secrete oestrogens. Although oestrogen excess is only recorded in a few cases, endometrial hyperplasia is recorded in nearly a quarter of patients with malignant Brenner tumour and endometrial adenocarcinoma in one. Amenorrhoea is rare and only one case of Meigs' syndrome has been reported (Rybak *et al.* 1981). Other symptoms, such as anorexia and weight loss, are common to many forms of neoplasia.

On examination a pelvic mass, more often left sided, may be palpable. Radiographs, ultrasonography, or CT scan may demonstrate a solid or partly cystic tumour with focal calcification (Athey and Siegel 1987), but these features are common to many ovarian and uterine neoplasms and the diagnosis is usually histological.

Management

In the past, management has been essentially surgical and varying from unilateral salpingo-oophorectomy to hysterectomy and bilateral salpingo-oophorectomy (Rybak *et al.* 1981). The roles of radiotherapy and chemotherapy, other than palliative, in the management of a rare tumour of imprecise pathological definition are not yet established, but there are reports of apparent remissions

with irradiation and combination chemotherapy (Magrina *et al.* 1982; Haid *et al.* 1983). The majority of patients die within a year of surgery and few die of the tumour after 5 years have elapsed.

Small cell carcinoma with hypercalcaemia

Introduction

In 1982, Dickersin *et al.* reported 11 cases of a distinct form of ovarian cancer that occurred in young women and was associated with hypercalcaemia. They pointed out that three cases previously reported as granulosa cell carcinoma, gonadal stromal sarcoma, and undifferentiated sex cord tumour were, in fact, examples of this entity, which accounted for half the cases of ovarian cancer with hypercalcaemia on record. This is a very rare tumour and its nature is still controversial but it is an aggressive tumour that can be interpreted clinically and pathologically as either an anaplastic granulosa cell tumour or a germ cell tumour.

Epidemiology and aetiology

Small cell carcinoma with hypercalcaemia has been described in most races and between the ages of 10 and 55 (mean 25 years). Nothing is known about its causes.

Pathology

All reported cases have been unilateral. The tumours are predominantly solid but small cysts can be present and a 9 cm cyst is described in one case (Dickersin *et al.* 1982). They vary in size from 8 to 27 cm in largest dimension and in weight from 0.5 to

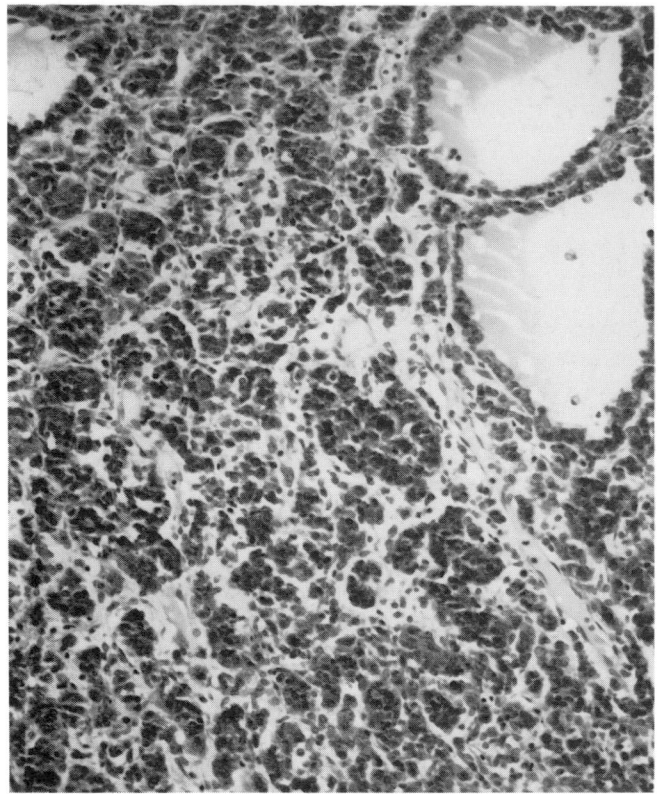

Fig. 12 Small cell carcinoma with hypercalcaemia from a 20 year old woman. Note the clusters of undifferentiated cells and the occasional cysts lined by similar cells.

2 kg. Foci of necrosis, haemorrhage, and mucoid degeneration are common.

Microscopically, small cell carcinomas are composed of hyperchromatic cells with scanty cytoplasm arranged in sheaths, cords, or islands or infiltrating singly in a cellular stroma. Sarcomatoid, spindle cell areas can be present and sometimes the tumour cells line small cavities that vaguely resemble the follicular structures seen in some granulosa cell tumours (Fig. 12). In some cases there are also larger cells with eosinophilic cytoplasm and prominent nucleoli and the name 'undifferentiated carcinoma' rather than small cell carcinoma has been suggested (Ullbright *et al.* 1987).

Small cell carcinoma behaves aggressively and peritoneal spread may be present at the time of the initial operation. The pelvic peritoneum and adjacent viscera are most often involved when the tumour recurs. Distant metastases are less common but have been reported in retroperitoneal, pelvic, and inguinal lymph nodes, liver, and lung.

Biology

Electron microscopy of these carcinomas favours an epithelial nature for this tumour, but their occurrence at an age when other epithelial ovarian neoplasms are distinctly rare and the absence of mixtures of small cell and other epithelial cancers points to an origin different from that of common, epithelial, ovarian tumours. There is no evidence to support a stromal origin. Ulbright *et al.* (1987) favour a germ cell origin but their evidence is unconvincing and, as they recognize, the tumour does not produce α-fetoprotein or chorionic gonadotrophin, nor does it respond to the

therapies for germ cell tumour. No dense core granules have been demonstrated in small cell carcinoma and, although Abeler *et al.* (1988) describe neurone-specific enolase and parathormone-like reactivity, the endocrine nature of this tumour remains to be established.

Hypercalcaemia is present in most, but not all, cases of small cell carcinoma (Patsner *et al.* 1985) and is probably due to a substance produced by the tumour, as none of the patients had bone metastases, there was no overproduction of parathormone in the cases in which this was assayed, and hypercalcaemia remits when the tumour is removed, reappearing when it recurs. Other ovarian epithelial tumours, particularly mesonephroid adenocarcinoma and serous cystadenocarcinoma, have been rarely associated with hypercalcaemia but small cell carcinomas account for half the cases reported.

Clinical presentation

The most common complaint is lower abdominal pain of short duration, other common symptoms being amenorrhoea, nausea, and abdominal swelling. An ovarian mass is usually palpable and at operation the tumour may be confined to one ovary or, more often, may have spread to the adjacent peritoneum, when ascites is usually present.

Management

In the series of Dickersin *et al.* (1982) the only patient out of 11 to survive 5 years free of disease was stage Ic on presentation and had bilateral salpingo-oophorectomy and hysterectomy followed by radiotherapy. Other patients treated similarly or with unilateral salpingo-oophorectomy, died with recurrences in periods varying from a few months to 5 years. Others have stressed the bad prognosis of this tumour (Patsner *et al.* 1985; Ulbright *et al.* 1987). Abeler *et al.* (1988) describe one patient with stage Ia who survived 14 months after radical surgery, including omentectomy and postoperative cisplatin chemotherapy. When tumours recur or are stage II or III on presentation, all authorities remark on the lack of response to the usual chemotherapy regimens for germ cell tumours, but initial responses have been reported with a seven-drug regimen (Senekjian *et al.* 1986).

MIXED MÜLLERIAN TUMOURS OF THE OVARY

Introduction

Mixed Müllerian tumours (also called mixed mesodermal tumours) are tumours with a mixture of epithelial and mesenchymal components and can occur throughout the female genital tract, but the most common sites are the uterus and (considerably less often) the ovary.

Epidemiology and aetiology

These are characteristically tumours of old age and most cases occur in the fifth to seventh decades. Approximately 200 cases in the ovary have been recorded (Marshall 1988). Nulliparity, hypertension, diabetes mellitus, and previous radiotherapy to the pelvis have been suggested as risk factors in uterine tumours (Vellacot and Shaw 1988). In the ovary, 35 per cent have occurred in nulliparas. Their aetiology is unknown.

Pathology

Macroscopically, mixed Müllerian tumours are frequently cystic, fleshy, and haemorrhagic; they have often spread to other pelvic structures and over peritoneal surfaces at the time of surgery. Microscopically, they are a combination of a carcinomatous component and a sarcomatous component (Fig. 13). The carcinomatous component can be undifferentiated or reproduce any of the patterns of endometrial or ovarian adenocarcinoma (endometrioid, serous, mucinous, squamous, and clear cell) or a mixture of them. The sarcomatous component can contain heterologous elements not normally present in the ovary (such as cartilage, bone, striated muscle, adipose tissue, or smooth muscle) or may lack these elements, when the name homologous mixed Müllerian tumour or carcinosarcoma is used. Most ovarian, mixed Müllerian tumours are heterologous (Morrow *et al.* 1984), cartilage (60 per cent) and bone (20 per cent) being the most common tissues found. Although histologically they can present differential diagnostic problems with germ cell and other ovarian tumours, their different age of presentation should be helpful in distinguishing them.

Mixed Müllerian tumours are very aggressive and metastasize widely in the peritoneal cavity, para-aortic nodes, liver and lungs.

Biology

The Müllerian ducts are formed by fusion of mesenchyme from the urogenital ridge lined by epithelium derived from the coelomic cavity. Both these structures remain in adult life as the epithelium covering the ovary and the adjacent mesenchyme and these mixed tumours are thought to be derived from them. They are sometimes grouped with endometrioid ovarian tumours.

Clinical presentation

Mixed Müllerian tumours present with symptoms similar to those of other ovarian tumours, such as increased abdominal girth, lower abdominal pain, weight loss, or anorexia. Gastrointestinal or urinary signs and symptoms may be present. Clinical examination confirms a pelvic mass, often with evidence of extension to other pelvic organs. CT scanning and ultrasonography can help to assess the extent of tumour in the pelvis and the presence of distant metastases. Staging is usually done according to the FIGO classification and more than 60 per cent are found to be stage III or IV on presentation (Marshall 1988). It has been suggested that patients with heterologous tumours tend to have more advanced disease, but evidence for this is conflicting.

Management

If the mixed Müllerian tumour is localized, the treatment of choice is hysterectomy and bilateral salpingo–oophorectomy together with omentectomy. Post-operative radiotherapy has been frequently given to the pelvis or the whole abdomen but the contribution of radiotherapy to overall results is difficult to assess (Grover *et al.* 1985).

The role of chemotherapy remains to be determined. Lele *et al.* (1980) reviewed 35 reported cases: no patient responded to single agents and the response to combinations was low. Carlson *et al.* (1983) reported the use of a combination of radiotherapy and chemotherapy with VAC in 20 patients. Although the contribution of chemotherapy in this combined approach is difficult to assess, complete tumour control was achieved in four patients. Cisplatin is clearly an active agent in mixed Müllerian tumours: Thigpen *et al.* (1986) reported five responses in a group of 28 patients (18 per cent), and Janssen *et al.* (1987) obtained responses in five out of six patients with platinum-based chemotherapy. More recently, Andersen *et al.* (1989) have reported four complete and two partial responses out of a total of six patients with a combination of cisplatin (P) together with either adriamycin (A) or cyclophosphamide (C) or with all three drugs together (PAC), however the duration of these responses lasted a maximum of 14 months. POMB/ACE chemotherapy (Table 2) has also been used in small numbers of patients; it confirms that cisplatin-based chemotherapy induces good objective responses but no long-term remissions have been obtained.

The prognosis of the majority of mixed Müllerian tumours that cannot be completely resected therefore remains poor. Perhaps the best recommendation that can be made at present is that the maximum possible amount of tumour should be resected surgically. This can be followed by cisplatin-based chemotherapy. From our current information it is probably reasonable to complete the treatment with radiotherapy to the site or sites of the initial disease, as local recurrences are common after surgery and chemotherapy.

REFERENCES

Abeler V, Kjorstad KE, Nesland JM (1988). Small cell carcinoma of the ovary. A report of six cases. *International Journal of Gynecological Pathology*, 7:315–29.
Adewole IF, Newlands ES, Lamki H, Nevin M (1987). Metastatic germ cell tumour associated with XY gonadal dysgenesis successful chemotherapy. Case report. *British Journal of Obstetrics and Gynaecology*, 94:589–91.

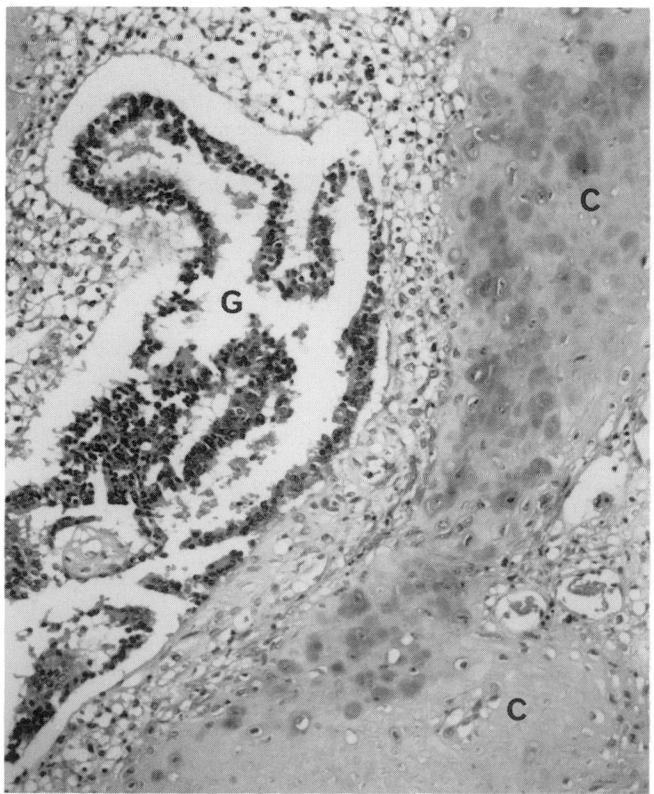

Fig. 13 Mixed Müllerian (mesodermal) tumour. Note the formation of poorly defined glands (G) and cartilage (C).

Ahn GH, Chi JG, Lee SK (1986). Ovarian sex cord tumor with annular tubules. *Cancer*, **57**:1066–73.

Aguirre P, Scully RE, Wolfe HJ, DeLellis RA (1986). Argyrophil cells in Brenner tumors: histochemical and immunohistochemical analysis. *International Journal of Gynecological Pathology*, 5:223–4.

Altaras MM, Goldberg GL, Levin W, Darge L, Bloch B, Smith JA (1986). The value of cancer antigen-125 as a tumor marker in malignant germ cell tumors of the ovary. *Gynecologic Oncology*, 25:150–9.

Andersen WA, Young DE, Peters WA, Smith EB, Bagley CM, Taylor PT (1989). Platinum-based combination chemotherapy for malignant mixed mesodermal tumors of the ovary. *Gynecologic Oncology*, 32:319–22.

Arias-Bernal L, Jones HW (1968). Chromosomes of a malignant ovarian teratoma. *American Journal of Obstetrics and Gynecology*, **100**:785–9.

Athey PA, Siegel MF (1987). Sonographic features of Brenner tumour of the ovary. *Journal of Ultrasound Medicine*, 6:367–72.

Austin RM, Norris HJ (1987). Brenner tumor and transitional carcinoma of the ovary: a comparison. *International Journal of Gynecological Pathology*, 6:29–39.

Carlson JA, Creighton E, Wharton JT, Gallager HS, Delclos L, Rutledge F (1983). Mixed mesodermal sarcoma of the ovary. *Cancer*, **52**: 1473–7.

Chumas JC, Rosenwaks Z, Mann WJ, Finkel G, Pastore J (1984). Sertoli–Leydig cell tumor of the ovary producing alpha-fetoprotein. *International Journal of Gynecological Pathology*, 3:213–19.

Colombo N, Sessa C, Landoni F, Sartori E, Pecorelli S, Mangioni C (1986). Cisplatin, vinblastine and bleomycin combination chemotherapy in metastatic granulosa cell tumor of the ovary. *Obstetrics and Gynecology*, **67**:265–8.

Czernobilsky B (1982). Brenner tumors. In *Pathology of the female genital tract* (ed. A Blaustein), pp. 547–53. Springer Verlag, New York.

Dempster J, Geirsson RT, Duncan ID (1987). Survival after granulosa and theca cell tumours. *Scottish Medical Journal*, 32:38–9.

Dickersin GR, Kline IW, Scully RE (1982). Small cell carcinoma of the ovary with hypercalcemia. A report of eleven cases. *Cancer*, 49: 188–97.

Ehya H, Lang WR (1986). Cytology of granulosa cell tumor of the ovary. *American Journal of Clinical Pathology*, 85:402–5.

Evans AT, Gaffey TA, Malkasian GD, Annegers JF (1980). Clinicopathologic review of 118 granulosa and 82 theca cell tumors. *Obstetrics and Gynecology*, **55**:231–8.

Fettissof F, Dubois MP, Arbeille-Brassart B, Lanson Y, Boivin F, Jobard P (1983). Endocrine cells in the prostate gland, urothelium and Brenner tumours. *Virchows Archives (B)*, **42**:53–64.

Fox H (1985). Sex-cord–stromal tumours of the ovary. *Journal of Pathology*, **145**:127–48.

Fox H, Langley FA (1976). *Tumours of the ovary*, pp. 173–261. Heinemann, London.

Friedman CI, Schmidt GE, Kim NM, Powell J (1985). Serum testosterone concentration in the evaluation of androgen producing tumors. *American Journal of Obstetrics and Gynecology*, **153**:44–9.

Genton CY, Schmid J (1981). Ovarian Sertoli–Leydig cell tumour with hyperoestronism. *Virchows Archives (A)*, **390**:243–8.

Gershenson DM (1988). Menstrual and reproductive function after treatment with combination chemotherapy for malignant ovarian germ cell tumors. *Journal of Clinical Oncology*, 6:270–5.

Grover V, Dhall K, Grover RK, Choudhry T (1985). Malignant mixed mesodermal tumor of the ovary. *European Journal of Obstetrics, Gynecology and Reproductive Biology*, 20:241–6.

Haid M, Victor TA, Weldon-Linne CM, Danforth DN (1983). Malignant Brenner tumor of the ovary. Electron microscopic study of a case responsive to radiation and chemotherapy. *Cancer*, 51:498–508.

Hitchins RN, Newlands ES, Smith DB, Begent RHJ, Rustin GJS, Bagshawe KD (1989). Long-term outcome in patients with germ cell tumours treated with POMB/ACE chemotherapy: comparison of commonly used classification systems of good and poor prognosis. *British Journal of Cancer*, 59: 236–42.

Hughesdon PE (1985). Rarer non-germinal ovarian malignancies. In *Ovarian cancer* (ed. CN Hudson), pp. 113–39. Oxford Medical Publications.

Ishiwata I, Ishiwata C, Soma M, Kobayashi N, Ishikawa H (1984). Establishment and characterization of an estrogen-producing human ovarian granulosa tumor cell line. *Journal of the American Cancer Institute*, 72:789–800.

Janssen RLH, van der Burgh MEL, Verweij J, Stoter G (1987). Cyclophosphamide, hexamethylmelamine, adriamycin and cisplatin combination chemotherapy in mixed mesodermal sarcoma of the female genital tract. *European Journal of Cancer*, 23:1131–3.

Jensen RD, Norris HJ, Fraumen JF (1974). Familial arrhenoblastoma and thyroid adenoma. *Cancer*, 33:218–23.

Kaye SB, Davies E (1986). Cyclophosphamide, adriamycin and cis-platinum for the treatment of advanced granulosa cell tumor, using estradiol as a tumor marker. *Gynecologic Oncology*, 24:261–4.

Kennedy M, Holck S, Bock J (1984). Bilateral malignant Brenner tumour. A light and electron microscopic study. *Acta Pathologica et Immunologica Scandinavica (A)*, 92:161–6.

Kuhnel R, Rao BR, Stolk JG, van-Kessel H, Seldenrijk CA, Willig AP (1987). Estrogen synthesizing rare malignant Brenner tumor of the ovary with the presence of progesterone and androgen receptors in the absence of estrogen receptors. *Gynecologic Oncology*, 26:263–9.

Kurman RJ, Goebelsmann U, Taylor CR (1979). Steroid localization in granulosa–theca tumors of the ovary. *Cancer*, 43:2377–84.

Langley FA, Fox H (1987). Ovarian tumours: classification, histogenesis and aetiology. In *Haines and Taylor obstetrical and gynaecological pathology* (ed. H Fox), pp. 542–55. Churchill Livingstone, Edinburgh.

Lappohn RE, Burger HG, Bouma J, Bangah M, Krans M, de Bruijn HWA (1989). Inhibin as a marker for granulosa-cell tumours. *New England Journal of Medicine*, **321**:790–3.

Lele SB, Piver MS, Barlow JJ (1980). Chemotherapy in management of mixed mesodermal tumors of the ovary. *Gynecologic Oncology*, **10**: 298–302.

Linder D, Kaiser-McCaw B, Hetch F (1975). Parthogenic origin of benign ovarian teratomas. *New England Journal of Medicine*, 292:63–6.

Magrina JF, Villamaria FJ, Masterson BJ, Lin F (1982). Malignant Brenner tumor of the ovary. A case report: negative second look laparotomy following surgery, radiation and chemotherapy. *International Journal of Gynecology and Obstetrics*, **20**:155–8.

Malkasian GD (1988). Tumors of granulosa–theca derivation. In *Textbook of uncommon cancer* (ed. CJ Williams), pp. 3–8. Wiley, Chichester.

Mann JR, Pearson D, Barrett A, Raafat F, Barnes JM, Wallendszus KR (1989). Results of the United Kingdom children's cancer study group's malignant germ cell tumor studies. *Cancer*, 63:1657–67.

Marshall RJ (1988). Mixed Müllerian tumours of the gynaecological system other than endometrial tumours. In *Textbook of uncommon cancer* (ed. CJ Williams), pp. 65–75. Wiley, Chichester.

Meigs JV (1954). Fibroma of the ovary with ascites and hydrothorax—Meigs' syndrome. *American Journal of Obstetrics and Gynecology*, 67:962–87.

Montz FJ, Morrow CP (1988). Sertoli–Leydig cell tumor, gynandroblastoma and lipid germ cell tumors of the ovary. In *Textbook of uncommon cancer* (ed. CJ Williams), pp. 15–36. Wiley, Chichester.

Morrow CP, d'Ablaing G, Brady LW, Blessing JA, Hreshchyshyn MM (1984). A clinical and pathological study of 30 cases of malignant mixed Müllerian epithelial and mesenchymal ovarian tumors: a gynecologic oncology group study. *Gynecologic Oncology*, **18**:278–92.

Munemura M, Nakamura T, Matsuura K, Maeyama M, Iwamasa T (1982). Endocrine profile of an ovarian androblastoma. *Obstetrics and Gynecology*, 59 (Suppl.):100–5.

Nakashima N, Young RH, Scully RE (1984). Androgenic granulosa cell tumors of the ovary: a clinico-pathologic analysis of 17 cases and review of the literature. *Archives of Pathology and Laboratory Medicine*, 108:786–91.

Newlands ES, Begent RHJ, Rustin GJS, Bagshawe KD (1982). Potential for cure in metastatic ovarian teratomas and dysgerminomas. *British Journal of Obstetrics and Gynaecology*, 89:555–60.

Newlands ES, Holden L, Bagshawe KD (1988a). Tumour markers and POMB/ACE chemotherapy in the management of ovarian germ cell tumours (GCTs). *International Journal of Biological Markers*, 3:185–92.

Newlands ES, Southall PJ, Paradinas FJ, Holden L (1988*b*). Management of ovarian germ cell tumours. In *Textbook of uncommon cancer* (ed. CJ Williams), pp. 37–53. Wiley, Chichester.

Norris HJ, Jensen RD (1979). Relative frequency of ovarian neoplasms in childhood and adolescence. *Cancer*, 30:713–19.

Ober WB (1979). History of the Brenner tumor of the ovary. In *Pathology annual* (ed. SC Sommers and PP Rosen), pp. 107–24. Appleton, New York.

Ohama K, Nomura K, Okamoto S, Fakuda Y, Ihara T, Fusiwara A (1985). Origin of immature teratoma of the ovary. *American Journal of Obstetrics and Gynecology*, 152:896–900.

Parrington JM, West LF, Povey S (1984). The origin of ovarian teratomas. *Journal of Medical Genetics*, 24:4–12.

Patsner B, Piver MS, Lele SB, Tsukada Y, Bielat K, Castillo NM (1985). Small cell carcinoma of the ovary: a rapidly lethal tumor occurring in the young. *Gynecologic Oncology*, 22:233–9.

Pektasides D, Rustin GJS, Newlands ES, Begent RHJ, Bagshawe KD (1987). Fertility after chemotherapy for ovarian germ cell tumours. *British Journal of Obstetrics and Gynaecology*, 94:477–9.

Prat J, Scully RE (1981). Cellular fibromas and fibrosarcomas of the ovary: a comparative clinicopathologic analysis of seventeen cases. *Cancer*, 47:2663–70.

Prat J, Bhan AK, Dickersin GR, Robboy SJ, Scully RE (1982*a*). Hepatoid yolk sac tumor of the ovary (endodermal sinus tumor with hepatoid differentiation). A light microscopic, ultrastructural and immunohistochemical study of seven cases. *Cancer*, 50:2355–68.

Prat J, Young RH, Scully RE (1982*b*). Ovarian Sertoli–Leydig cell tumors with heterologous elements. II. Cartilage and skeletal muscle: a clinicopathologic analysis of 12 cases. *Cancer*, 50:2465–75.

Roth LM, Sternberg WH (1971). Proliferating Brenner tumors. *Cancer*, 27:687–93.

Roth LM, Czernobilsky B (1985). Brenner tumors. II. Malignant. *Cancer*, 56:592–601.

Roth LM, Anderson MC, Govan ADT, Langley FA, Gowing NFC, Woodcock AS (1981). Sertoli–Leydig cell tumors: a clinicopathologic study of 34 cases. *Cancer*, 48:187–97.

Roth LM, Liban E, Czernobilsky B (1982). Ovarian endometrioid tumors mimicking Sertoli and Sertoli–Leydig cell tumors: Sertoliform variant of endometrioid carcinoma. *Cancer*, 50:1322–31.

Roth LM, Dallenbach-Hellweg G, Czernobilsky B (1985). Brenner tumors. I. Metaplastic, proliferating and of low malignant potential. *Cancer*, 56:582–91.

Rybak BJ, Ober WB, Bernacki EG (1981). Malignant Brenner tumor of the ovary. Report of three cases. *Diagnostic Gynecology and Obstetrics*, 3:61–74.

Scully RE (1970). Sex cord tumors with annular tubules: a distinctive ovarian tumor of the Peutz–Jeghers syndrome. *Cancer*, 25:1107–21.

Scully RE (1982). Sex cord-stromal tumors. In *Pathology of the female genital tract* (ed. A Blaustein), pp. 581–601. Springer Verlag, New York.

Scully RE (1988). Ovarian tumours with functioning stroma. In *Haines and Taylor obstetrical and gynaecological pathology* (ed. H Fox), pp. 724–36. Churchill Livingstone, Edinburgh.

Seldenrijk CA, *et al.* (1986). Malignant Brenner tumor: a histologic, morphometrical, immunohistochemical and ultrastructural study. *Cancer*, 58:754–60.

Senekjian EK, *et al.* (1986). Management of small cell carcinoma of the ovary (SCCO) with a multi-drug regimen: vinblastine (VB), cis-platinum (P), cytoxan (C), bleomycin (B), adriamycin (A), VP-16 and vincristine (VC) ('6 in 1'). *Proceedings of the American Society of Clinical Oncology*, 5:121.

Serov SF, Scully RE, Sobin LH (1973). *Histological typing of ovarian tumours*, International Histological Classification of Tumours No. 9, WHO, Geneva.

Silverberg SG (1971). Brenner tumor of the ovary. A clinicopathologic study of 60 tumours in 54 women. *Cancer*, 28:588–96.

Skakkebaek NE (1978). Carcinoma *in situ* of the testis: frequency and relationship to invasive germ cell tumours in infertile men. *Histopathology*, 2:157–70.

Slayton RE, Park RC, Silverberg SG, Shingleton H, Creasman WT, Blessing JA (1985). Vincristin, dactinomycin and cyclophosphamide in the treatment of malignant germ cell tumors of the ovary. A gynecologic oncology group study (a final report). *Cancer*, 56:243–8.

Smales E, Peckham MJ (1987). Chemotherapy of germ-cell ovarian tumours: first line treatment with etoposide, bleomycin and cis-platin or carboplatin. *European Journal of Cancer and Clinical Oncology*, 23:469–74.

Stamp GH, McConnell EM (1983). Malignancy arising in cystic ovarian teratomas: a report of 24 cases. *British Journal of Obstetrics and Gynaecology*, 90:671–5.

Stenwig JT, Hazekamp JT, Beecham JB (1979). Granulosa cell tumors of the ovary. A clinicopathological study of 118 cases with long-term follow-up. *Gynecologic Oncology*, 7:136–52.

Stevens LC (1983). Testicular, ovarian and embryo-derived teratomas. *Cancer Surveys*, 2:75–91.

Stewart RS, Woodward DE (1962). Malignant ovarian hilus cell tumor. *Archives of Pathology*, 73:91–9.

Susil BJ, Sumithran E (1987). Sarcomatous change in granulosa cell tumor. *Human Pathology*, 18:397–9.

Talerman A (1982). Germ cell tumors of the ovary. In *Pathology of the female genital tract* (ed. A Blaustein), pp. 602–64. Springer Verlag, New York.

Tetu B, Lebel M, Camilleri JP (1988). Renin producing ovarian tumor: a case report with immunohistochemical and electron-microscopical study. *American Journal of Surgical Pathology*, 12:634–40.

Thigpen JT, Blessing JA, Orr JW, Di Sala PJ (1986). Phase II trial of cisplatin in the treatment of patients with advanced or recurrent mixed mesodermal sarcomas of the uterus: a gynecologic group study. *Cancer Treatment Reports*, 70:271–4.

Ulbright TM, Loehrer PJ, Roth LM, Einhorn LH, Williams SD, Clark SA (1984). The development of non-germ cell malignancies within germ cell tumors: a clinicopathologic study of 11 cases. *Cancer*, 54:1824–33.

Ulbright TM, Roth LM, Stehman FB, Talerman A, Senekjian EK (1987). Poorly differentiated (small cell) carcinoma of the ovary in young women: evidence supporting a germ cell origin. *Human Pathology*, 18:175–84.

van der Weiden RM, Gratama S (1987). Proliferative and malignant Brenner tumors (BT) and their differentiation from metastatic transitional cell carcinoma of the bladder: a case report and review of the literature. *European Journal of Gynecology, Obstetrics and Reproductive Biology*, 26:251–60.

Vassal G, Flamant F, Caillaud JM, Demeocq F, Nihoul-Fekete C, Lemerle J (1988). Juvenile granulosa cell tumour of the ovary in children: a clinical study of 15 cases. *Journal of Clinical Oncology*, 6:990–5.

Velasco-Oses A, Alonso-Alvaro A, Blanco-Pozo A, Nogales FF (1988). Ollier's disease associated with ovarian juvenile granulosa cell tumor. *Cancer* 62:222–5.

Vellacot I, Shaw RW (1988). Mixed Müllerian tumours of the corpus uteri. In *Textbook of uncommon cancer* (ed. CJ Williams), pp. 55–64. Wiley, Chichester.

Walker AH, Ross RK, Pike MC, Henderson BE (1984) A possible rising incidence of malignant germ cell tumours in young women. *British Journal of Cancer*, 49:669–72.

Walker AH, Ross RK, Haile RWC, Henderson BE (1988). Hormonal factors and risk of ovarian germ cell cancer in young women. *British Journal of Cancer*, 57:418–22.

Williams S, Blessing J, Adcock C, Homesberg H (1984). Treatment of ovarian germ cell tumours with cisplatin, vinblastin and bleomycin (PVB). *Proceedings of the American Society of Clinical Oncology*, 3:175.

Young RH, Scully RE (1983*a*). Ovarian Sertoli–Leydig cell tumours with a retiform pattern: a problem in histopathologic diagnosis. *American Journal of Surgical Pathology*, 7:755–71.

Young RH, Scully RE (1983*b*). Ovarian sex-cord stromal tumors with bizarre nuclei: a clinicopathologic analysis of seventeen cases. *International Journal of Gynecological Pathology*, 1:325–35.

Young RH, Scully RE (1984*a*). Ovarian Sertoli cell tumors: a report of 10 cases. *International Journal of Gynecological Pathology*, 2:349–63.

Young RH, Scully RE (1984*b*). Ovarian sex cord–stromal tumours: recent advances and current status. *Clinics in Obstetrics and Gynecology*, 11:93–134.

Young RH, Scully RE (1984*c*). Well differentiated ovarian Sertoli–Leydig cell tumors: a clinicopathological analysis of 23 cases. *International Journal of Gynecological Pathology*, 3:277–90.

Young RH, Scully RE (1985). Ovarian Sertoli–Leydig cell tumors: a clinicopathological analysis of 207 cases. *American Journal of Surgical Pathology*, 9:543–69.

Young RH, Prat J, Scully RE (1982*a*). Ovarian endometrioid carcinomas resembling sex cord–stromal tumors: a clinicopathological analysis of 13 cases. *American Journal of Surgical Pathology*, 6:513–22.

Young RH, Prat J, Scully RE (1982*b*). Ovarian Sertoli—Leydig cell tumors with heterologous elements. I. Gastrointestinal epithelium and carcinoid: a clinicopathologic analysis of 36 cases. *Cancer*, 50:2448—56.

Young RH, Welch WR, Dickersin GR, Scully RE (1982*c*). Ovarian sex cord tumor with annular tubules: review of 74 cases including 27 with Peutz—Jeghers syndrome and four with adenoma malignum of the cervix. *Cancer*, 50:1384—402.

Young RH, Dickersin GR, Scully RE (1984*a*). Juvenile granulosa cell tumor of the ovary: a clinicopathological analysis of 125 cases. *American Journal of Surgical Pathology*, 8:575—96.

Young RH, Dudley AG, Scully RE (1984*b*). Granulosa cell, Sertoli—Leydig cell and unclassified sex cord—stromal tumors associated with pregnancy: a clinicopathological analysis of thirty-six cases. *Gynecologic Oncology*, 18:181—205.

Young RH, Perez-Atayde AR, Scully RE (1984*c*). Ovarian Sertoli—Leydig cell tumour with retiform and heterologous components. Report of a case with hepatocytic differentiation and elevated serum alpha-fetoprotein. *American Journal of Surgical Pathology*, 8:709—18.

Zaloudek C, Norris HJ (1982). Granulosa tumors of the ovary in children: a clinical and pathologic study of 32 cases. *American Journal of Surgical Pathology*, 6:503—12.

9.3   Carcinoma of the cervix

ROBERT D. HUNTER

INTRODUCTION

Carcinoma of the cervix is a very important malignant disease internationally. In part this is due to the apparently high incidence in developing countries. It also has unusual and distinctive epidemiological features and has demonstrated interesting changes of incidence and age-related incidence this century. Perhaps most importantly, because of the ease of examination of the cervix in the apparently healthy woman, the early, asymptomatic stages of the disease can be observed and monitored, giving rise to the belief that invasive carcinoma of the cervix may, through an effective cytological programme, become a preventable disease in many women.

INCIDENCE

In many countries the incidence of cervical cancer is unknown but any visitor to a hospital in Asia, Africa, or South America will be told that it is the most common malignant disease in women and is, as the infectious diseases come under control, rapidly becoming a major cause of morbidity and mortality in the Third World.

The situation in the United Kingdom, Europe, North America, and Japan is different. So-called gynaecological cancer is less important than breast and gastrointestinal malignancy. Among the gynaecological cancers, although the incidence of the different diseases varies between countries, carcinoma of the ovary is consistently a more lethal disease and endometrial cancer is more commonly curable. In the United Kingdom, invasive carcinoma of the cervix is the sixth most common malignancy in women (4 per cent of all female malignant disease) (OPCS 1993). The incidence of the disease has been approximately 15/100 000 women during the 1980s and the overall mortality of patients with invasive carcinoma of the cervix is approximately 45 per cent. In practice, just under 2000 women die of invasive carcinoma of the cervix each year in the United Kingdom.

Studies relating the incidence of carcinoma of the cervix to the decade of birth during the twentieth century suggest that incidence has varied quite considerably in the different cohorts. These studies are complicated by a failure to separate clearly endometrial from cervix cancer in early cancer registration, but they do support the thesis that it is a disease whose incidence has risen and fallen 'naturally' with peak rises in cohorts young and sexually active during the two World Wars. It has also become apparent that interesting changes are still taking place in the age incidence.

Two decades ago, in the United Kingdom, invasive carcinoma of the cervix was a disease that was uncommon before 40 and had a peak incidence in 50- and 60-year-olds. In the last decade, for reasons that will be discussed, although the overall incidence has not changed significantly, it has become increasingly common in women between 25 and 40 years of age and the old peak has been replaced by a plateau of incidence between 35 and 55 (Fig. 1). This trend is particularly tragic because these are often young married women with dependent families. In addition, being pre-menopausal, they commonly fail to notice early, significant symptoms.

ANATOMY

Cervical carcinoma is a disease that arises from the epithelium of the cervix. The cells of origin are in the basal layers of an epidermis that lines the endocervix, including the mouth of the endocervical glands, and extends over the surface of the ectocervix and merges

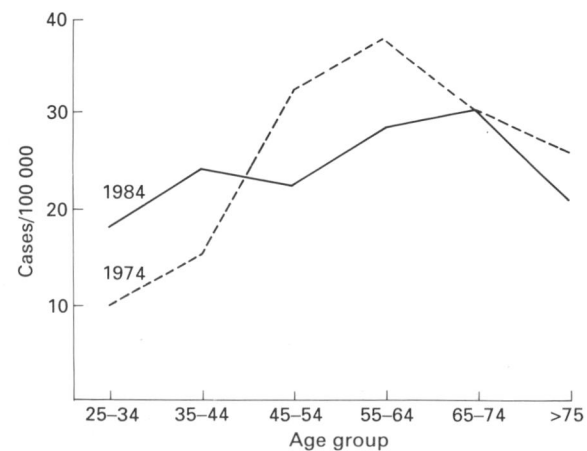

Fig. 1 United Kingdom incidence of invasive carcinoma of the cervix by age group, 1974 and 1984 (OPCS).

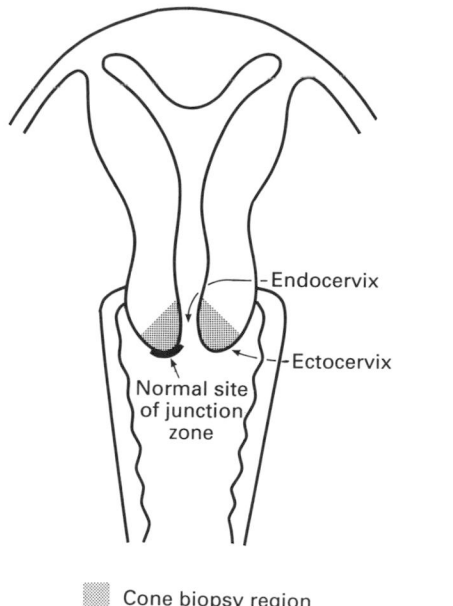

Cone biopsy region

Fig. 2 Anteroposterior diagram of anatomy of cervix.

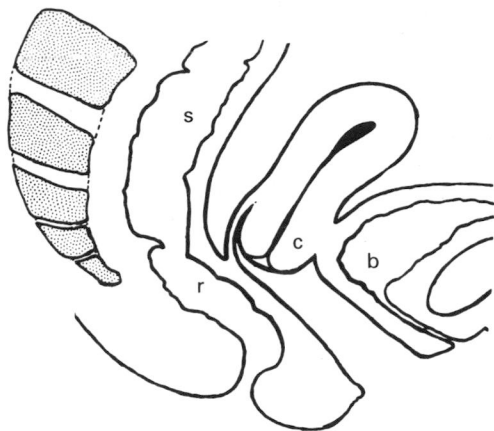

Fig. 3 Lateral diagram of female pelvis emphasizing proximity to the cervix (c), of the bladder (b), rectum (r), and sigmoid colon (s).

into the vaginal epithelium. There is general agreement that the junction between the squamous epithelium of the ectocervix and the adenomatous epithelium of the endocervix, the transformation zone, is the most common site of origin of carcinomatous change. In the young woman after the menarche this zone is in the lower endocervix or at the external os. In the older, multiparous woman it is often clearly visible on the ectocervix.

The cervix is the lower segment of the uterus. In the mature woman it is a simple structure consisting of a muscular canal controlling the entrance of the uterine cavity. The smooth muscle varies in thickness throughout life and with pregnancy. The part of the cervix visible on gynaecological examination is known as the ectocervix and is often an upper anterior vaginal wall structure. The visible entrance to the uterine canal, the external os, leads to the endocervical canal, which becomes the uterine cavity at the internal os (Fig. 2).

The epithelial lining of the cervix is cuboidal before the menarche but then undergoes metaplasia to become squamous on the ectocervix. The endocervical epithelium remains cuboidal and the meeting of the two epithelial types in the mature female at the junction zone is an important epithelial landmark. The endocervical canal has mucus-secreting glands whose epithelium is in continuity with the endocervical epithelium. These two epithelial structures and the glands can all be involved in the early changes of cervical malignancy. The vaginal epithelium in continuity with the ectocervical epithelium can also experience similar malignant change.

Important anatomical features in relation to carcinoma are that the cervix is suspended in the centre of the pelvis by the parametrium and its ligaments, which provide a line of spread for disease laterally and posterolaterally. The ureters run through the parametrium adjacent and lateral to the cervix. The posterior bladder wall becomes an anterior relation of the cervix as it distends and in older women the base of the bladder may, with shrinkage of the upper gynaecological tissues, come to lie truly anterior to the cervix. Posteriorly the pouch of Douglas may contain the sigmoid colon or small bowel (Fig. 3). The rectum lies posterior to the upper posterior vaginal wall and may, in the older woman in whom the

cervix shrinks to become a vaginal vault structure, be very close to the posterior cervix.

AETIOLOGY

Cancer of the cervix perhaps more than any other primary carcinoma has attracted the attention of epidemiologists for many years. An enormous number of studies have addressed the associations with the disease, all looking for clues to a factor or factors. The original observation in the eighteenth century was that cancer of the 'uterus' was a disease of married women, occurred in the 30–40 year age group, and increased in incidence in older women. Twentieth-century epidemiology noted the absence of carcinoma of the cervix in a large population of nuns and linked the disease more closely to sexual activity. Further studies expanded this observation to emphasize the importance of low socio–economic class, multiparity, early marriage, and multiple sexual partners. Helped by the voyeuristic interest of the press, the expression 'promiscuity' began to be associated with the disease and many patients carried that extra stigma as they fought their illness. The balance began to be redressed by studies linking the disease to other external factors like cigarette smoking and by investigators pointing out the importance of the husband's occupation. Gradually the male partner and his behaviour have emerged as potentially important factors and the idea of the 'high-risk man' who has himself had multiple partners has shifted the focus on to both partners rather than to the woman herself.

In spite of all these epidemiological studies the cause of carcinoma of the cervix is still unknown. The epidemiological evidence has helped focus attention on several possible causative factors. Early ideas involved concerns about trauma and poor hygiene. Linked to the latter was the smegma hypothesis, which highlighted the infrequency of the disease in certain Jewish communities and emphasized the importance of circumcision. This was subsequently shown to be a consequence of hygiene rather than of circumcision itself.

Although associated with sexual activity, carcinoma of the cervix is not a true, sexually transmitted disease like syphilis or gonorrhoea. There is no agreed, single, transmissible agent. There is recognition that malignant transformation is probably a multifactorial, step-wise process in which a number of factors can, but do not necessarily always, play a part. The malignant change most commonly occurs first in the transformation zone of the cervix. The squamous metaplasia that takes place on the cervix at the time of the menarche is thought to create relative 'instability' of the epithelium during which other carcinogenic influences may be able to induce changes that manifest themselves many years later. The nature of the instability at a molecular level is unknown but the susceptibility of the teenage cervix to genital infections and the association of early, unprotected intercourse with a subsequent high incidence of carcinoma of the cervix seems to support the general concept.

The important possible carcinogenic influences may be considered under the headings of genetic, chemical, infective, and immunological. To what extent any one or combination of these influences can themselves induce malignant changes without the other is unknown, but there is no reason to believe that the malignant change is a consequence of a single, common pathway in which one factor must always operate.

Genetic

There is no evidence to suggest that carcinoma of the cervix is a true, genetically inherited disease, although in practice siblings and mother/daughter combinations are regularly seen. This has often been ascribed to socio-economic factors rather than genetic, but formal genetic studies have not been undertaken. Like many other malignant diseases it seems possible that some of the other putative factors, particularly virus infection, could operate by altering DNA and releasing oncogenes from suppressor control.

Chemical

No single chemical group has been identified and linked to carcinoma of the cervix. The possibility that the sperm head of certain males contains histones that can damage the epithelial cells permanently and act as a carcinogen has been promoted by some workers without becoming internationally accepted. It would help to explain the 'high-risk male' if an associated, transmissible, infective agent could be excluded. Carcinoma of the cervix is also strongly associated with cigarette smoking. The mechanism by which cigarette smoking might chemically cause carcinoma of the cervix is unknown.

Infective

Many studies have excluded bacterial and protozoal diseases from implication in cervical carcinogenesis. Among virus groups, two have been extensively investigated. Initially the herpes simplex-2 group was considered a possible strong contender as a carcinogen. This virus group regularly produces overt infections and can induce identifiable antibody responses in patients with carcinoma of the cervix. Certainly the associations are strong but are far from being conclusive epidemiologically. The strong, biologically supportive evidence necessary to confirm opinion as to the significance of this virus group is lacking.

The virus group most strongly implicated in true carcinogenesis is human papilloma virus (**HPV**).

Human papilloma virus

This group of DNA viruses has been difficult to investigate for a number of reasons. They cannot be cultured outside the host, they are very widespread in the population, many discrete types exist, and immunological reactions are weak, even in healthy adults. Nevertheless, modern techniques in molecular biology have enabled much more investigation of their possible role in carcinogenesis.

The advent of techniques for using specific antibodies to investigate the molecular structure of the nucleus of the malignant cells has allowed different subtypes of the virus genome to be identified in patients with carcinoma of the cervix. These techniques have become widely available and allow tissue samples as small as cervical smears to be analysed for evidence of the presence of different virus types. A large amount of research has thereby been done in a short period of time; results are still inconclusive in proving causation but this virus group remains a leading contender.

The different subtypes, of which more than 60 are now known, are tissue specific for reasons that are not known. Certain types (6, 11, 16, 18, 31, and 33) show a predilection for the genital tract of both men and women. The virus causes an initial infection of the basal cell layers of the epidermis and can involve the skin of the vulva, vagina, cervix, shaft of penis, or urethra. The response of the individual to infection is variable. In some, frank, clinically recognizable, warty lesions can be present. In others the epithelium looks healthy to the naked eye. At a histological level a variable response can also be seen. Classical viral changes, koilocytes, in which large cytoplasmic vacuoles may appear due to degenerating cytoplasm in the more mature layers of the epidermis, are often identified. In others, viral particles can be identified within the cytoplasm by electron microscopy or surface viral antigens may be detected immunologically. The basal cell layers, on the other hand, may appear histologically normal but molecular biological techniques have shown that, in this form of the infection, basal cells can also harbour viral DNA within their nuclei, either in an integrated or a non-integrated, episomal form. This integrated DNA may or may not be active at any point in time.

The concept is therefore emerging that some of the subtypes of HPV, particularly types 16 and 18, can be easily transmitted to a woman and that the viral DNA becomes integrated into the DNA of the basal epithelium of the cervix without producing any overt clinical, histological, cytological, or immunological evidence of disease. The integration appears to be random and may very well be capable of inactivity or activity at different times after the initial infection. Supportive evidence suggests that this is probably an important step in carcinogenesis because of the following.

1. There are animal models in which papillomavirus can be shown to induce malignant transformation.
2. HPV is associated with benign and malignant human tumours at a number of sites.
3. HPV infections are sexually transmissible and have the same epidemiological risk factors as clinical carcinoma of the cervix.
4. The strong association of HPV types 16, 18, 31, and 33 with malignant change is difficult to ignore.

This does leave a number of unresolved questions.

1. What is the mechanism of viral malignant transformation?
2. What is the relationship between integrated and non-integrated DNA and malignant change?
3. Why do some apparently early, cytologically pre-malignant changes (cervical intraepithelial neoplasia) resolve?
4. What is the role of other agents?

In the United Kingdom, HPV type 16 is the most common type identified (approximately 60 per cent), followed by a sprinkling of the other subtypes. Only 5 per cent of malignant primary tumours of the cervix do not have any identifiable evidence of viral infection using the most sensitive, presently available, polymerase chain reaction techniques.

It is important to realize that these patients with carcinoma of the cervix are not manifesting any clinical evidence of a viral infection. Apparently healthy tissues or classical, warty lesions in the lower genital tract may contain much higher concentrations of the virus and histological evidence of viral infection but in the malignant tissue the viral DNA is integrated into the host DNA. In the genital tract the clinically recognizable lesions of papillomavirus infection are acuminate warts and flat condylomata.

Although unproven by strict criteria, strong association of the HPV group with invasive carcinoma, the fact that cell lines from the carcinoma consistently contain the papillomavirus, that pre-cancerous lesions often contain the virus, that type-16 infection induces aneuploidy and abnormal mitotic changes, that the viral DNA is transcriptionally active, and that there is an increased risk of developing the disease in virus carriers all tend to support the thesis that certain subtypes of HPV, perhaps supported by genetic and environmental factors, cause malignant transformation in the basal cells of the cervix. Present evidence suggests that the virus infection is one of the most important initiating factors.

Even if causation was proven the papillomaviruses are so widely scattered in nature and are, like the influenza group, so able to change their antigenicity, that prevention based on immunization appears an unrealistic aim. The thrust of the research activity will have a possible practical result if the investigations can be easily and consistently translated into the colposcopy clinic and the cytology and general pathology laboratory. The identification of a type-16 rather than, for example a type-6 or -11 infection in a histologically or cytologically normal or mildly abnormal tissue will allow the identification of an 'at risk' individual who can be followed more closely. At the same time the system can be relieved of the excessive screening and unnecessary treatment of patients without any evidence of those types of infection. Already such an approach holds out hope for improved cytological screening.

Another profitable area of clinical research emerging from these studies has been an appreciation of the need to screen male partners of patients with abnormal cytological results for evidence of virus infection and viral lesions. Unfortunately, the flat condylomata that harbour the virus are often only visible by colposcopy but examination and treatment of the male for benign viral lesions as well as the early diagnosis of intraepithelial neoplasia of the penile skin has become an important aspect of patient management in some centres.

Immunological

Immunological factors have been considered important in the aetiology of carcinoma of the cervix as at many other sites. A number of associated points suggest that they should not be entirely excluded.

1. Cigarette smoking, which is strongly associated with the disease, is associated with a decrease in cellular immunity.
2. Patients with renal failure who are immunosuppressed are prone to develop viral genital lesions and changes of cervical intraepithelial neoplasia.

In addition, the HPV group is notorious because it induces very poor cellular and humoral responses to its antigens and yet an intact immunological system is important in controlling latent viral infection and preventing the development of frank clinical lesions. There is also some evidence that papilloma-specific and carcinoma-specific antigens in carcinoma of the cervix are immunosuppressive. To what extent immunological factors contribute to the latency of

infections and the clinical manifestations is not understood. In spite of all this, there is also some suggestion that initial infection can assist in the development of resistance to reinfection with papillomavirus and this alone holds some long-term hope for the development of suitable vaccines that might prevent or reduce infection by a carcinoma-associated antigenic type.

SCREENING

Over the last 30 years, enormous efforts have been made to reduce the incidence of disease in North America, Scandinavia, and the United Kingdom. If the surface of the cervix is scraped or brushed, cells from the epithelial layer are removed and they can then be transferred to a slide for cytological examination. When the smear obtained is examined using a special Papanicolau (Pap) stain, then healthy squamous cells and infected and malignant cells of different types can be identified (Fig. 4).

The advantages of the examination as a test for early cancer are enormous. It can be done in a home, surgery, or hospital, by a health worker with limited but specific training. The cervix needs to be visualized using a speculum and a good light. The smear is taken

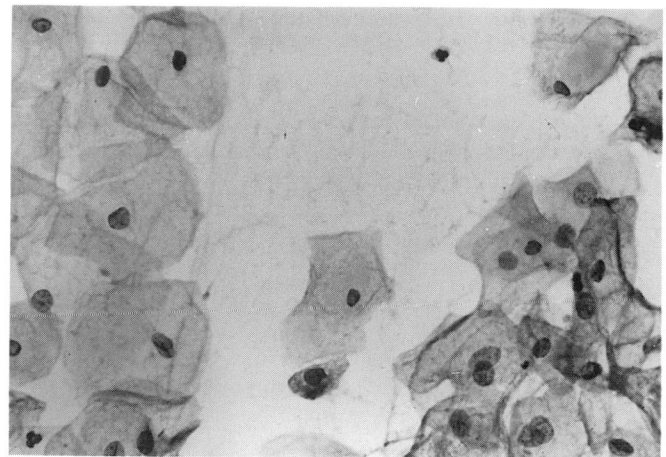

(a)

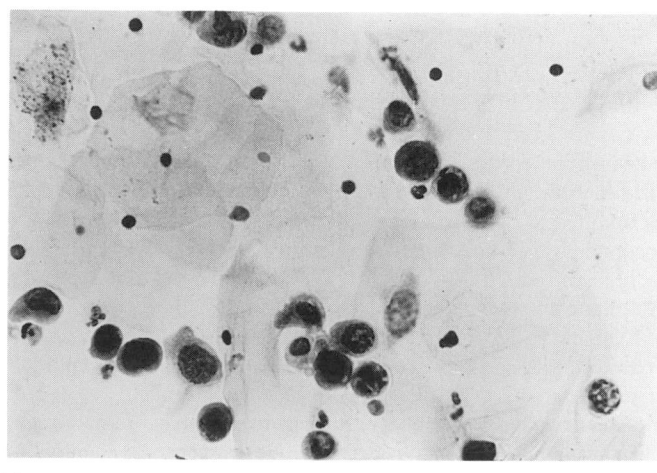

(b)

Fig. 4 (a) Good normal cervical smear: the cells are spread evenly allowing the normal architecture to be seen. (b) Cervical smear from a patient with CIN III: the majority of cells are of malignant appearance; a few normal squamous cells are visible.

from the visible ectocervix using a swab, brush, or spatula by stroking movements and the cells obtained are smeared smoothly, thinly, and evenly across a clean slide. It should be fixed, dried, and clearly marked for identification and placed in a robust container for transport to a cytology laboratory. Using special equipment, skilled workers can take a separate smear from the lower endocervical canal. From the woman's point of view the examination requires no preparation or anaesthesia, should take a few minutes, and be painless. It can be safely repeated as often as required.

The problem for the cytologist is considerable. The epithelial cells of the cervix respond to systemic hormonal changes, pregnancy, and viral and other genital infections by producing architectural abnormalities. Some of these influences may also be carcinogenic or procarcinogenic. The same cells when they become malignant can also show grades of cytological abnormality from apparently differentiated, minimally changed cells right through to frank and indisputably malignant cells. The effect is that a smear, which is only a sample of cells being shed from the cervix epithelium, may contain a variety of changes of varying significance. In addition, because of the nature of the technique, the abnormalities are mixed up together and then artificially separated on the slide. In the laboratory the smear is examined after staining by a technician trained to identify different cytological abnormalities. The report is based on a subjective impression of the cell populations on the slide. A number of regular problems arise.

1. The cervix may be difficult to see and the smear may be from the vaginal vault or not from the whole of the ectocervix (technique failure).
2. (a) The cells obtained may not be spread thinly enough on the slide (technical failure).

   (b) The presence of blood or necrotic cells may obscure the epithelial cells (technical failure).
3. The presence of inflammatory changes in the cells may mask underlying pre-malignant changes (false-negative).
4. Malignant cells may not be noted by the cytology technician (false-negative).
5. Cytological changes induced by infection or hormonal effects may be misinterpreted as being pre-malignant or malignant (false-positive).

To complicate the situation further, some changes regress, some remain static with time, and others apparently progress to more serious changes. These difficult problems have encouraged research on a more objective technique for identifying the true malignant cells from others and, therefore, improving the accuracy of the smear examination. To date, the use of biochemical and immunological techniques to allow scanning of batches of smears has not gained acceptance and only individual examination of each smear by a technician trained in cytological assessment remains an acceptable technique.

Even in the best hands the problems of technical failure and false-negative and false-positive investigations occur in 10—20 per cent of examinations. The real problem is the false-negatives because the other two results encourage further investigation. False-negatives are considerably reduced by carrying out two separate examinations within a year on the same patient and most cytological programmes encourage this approach in new entrants.

In general clinical practice these screening tests are made on a population basis. It has been found that to be successful it is necessary to investigate a high percentage (80—90 per cent) of the relevant age group. The consensus is that this is all women between the ages of 20 and 65 who have been or are sexually active. Optimum screening for the individual is two initial examinations within a year, followed by annual examinations up to the age of 65. Few health programmes achieve this frequency and 3—5 year examinations are a regular feature of the United Kingdom programmes. By screening the general population within this age group, significant cytological abnormalities are seen in 15—20/1000 examinations. When high-risk groups like female prisoners, prostitutes, and very young, sexually active women are examined the frequency of abnormalities can rise as high as 75/1000.

As a screening test for early cancer of the cervix the smear is attractive because of its simplicity, the ease of transport to a central laboratory, and the permanence of the sample. There is a need for a good technique among the initial health workers, high laboratory standards, an emphasis on quality control, and careful liaison between the laboratory and the responsible doctors about inadequate and abnormal smears if the promise is to be translated into practice.

These observations effectively allowed the previously clinically unrecognized condition of 'carcinoma in situ' or cervical intra-epithelial neoplasia to be identified. In this the malignant change is confined to the epithelium. The cervix regularly looks normal and the patient is asymptomatic.

Early investigations suggested that the peak incidence of the 'in situ' phase occurred 10—15 years before the peak incidence of invasive carcinoma. A hypothesis was developed that carcinoma of the cervix is a slowly evolving disease with a prolonged prodromal phase in which the malignant cells are confined to the epithelium and that intensive screening of healthy asymptomatic women between the ages of 35 and 45 years would allow the changes to be identified at an early and easily treatable stage and, thus, prevent the development of invasive carcinoma of the cervix.

In the last 20 years, as a result of their cytology programmes, in some parts of North America, Canada, and Scandinavia there have been very significant changes in the incidence of the disease, resulting in a reduction to levels as low as one-quarter of those seen before the start of screenings. Other countries, including the United Kingdom, have achieved much less success from their extensive programmes. In most countries, improvements have been a result of policies that initiated screening at the time of onset of sexual intercourse and allowed annual smear examinations to be made. They were helped by compliant populations interested in health care and preventative medicine. In many parts of the United Kingdom the response to screening initiatives has been much less spectacular. The United Kingdom Government has responded to patient and doctor pressure and has funded and encouraged different levels of screening, although even the most recent Department of Health advice has not endorsed the North American or Scandinavian policies in their frequency of recall. The Health Service has been unable to offer the same level of screening, the population has been less responsive, and as a result the impact has been limited. There has been a small fall in the overall incidence of the disease over the last 20 years in the United Kingdom but this is a result of two competing changes. The incidence of carcinoma of the cervix in women between 40 and 60 years has fallen in the last decade but in parallel there has been a striking increase in the incidence of the disease in women aged 20—40 years. Similar changes in the younger age groups have been seen in other countries.

There is no doubt that screening asymptomatic, sexually active women can reduce the incidence of invasive carcinoma in a population and this remains an important goal in public health, but success requires attention to detail of technique in the clinic and the laboratory, ensuring a high response to the initial call and to regular recalls.

An important consequence of the cytology programmes becoming available to young, sexually active women has been an enormous increase in the incidence of patients with cytological abnormalities which are considered to indicate that epithelial changes are taking place which may herald invasive malignant change. This was an interesting phenomenon of the 1980s whose true incidence is unknown, although in the limited systematic studies available it seems massively disproportionate to the expected incidence of invasive carcinoma. In the United Kingdom, registration is not compulsory but all gynaecology units have had to change their working practice to accommodate this group of patients. Many are treated using a variety of techniques, to be discussed later and are followed-up without the true significance of the changes and the relationship to malignant disease being fully understood.

PATHOLOGY

In many patients with carcinoma of the cervix, particularly those with early disease, there is a need for a close liaison between the cytologist/pathologist and the clinician if an accurate diagnosis is going to be made. The source of the specimen, the presence or absence of symptoms, the clinical appearance of the ectocervix, and the clinical impression of what may be wrong are all important elements in helping the pathologist to come to an opinion. Unless the whole cervix is present in the specimen the opinion can only be about the tissues sampled; the quality of the smear technique and the care taken over the biopsy can seriously influence the value of the final pathological opinion. This is particularly true in colposcopy clinics where under-assessment can lead to an invasive carcinoma of the cervix being missed. The range of pathology specimens includes cervical cytology with or without endocervical cytology, microbiopsies obtained under colposcopic control, punch biopsies, cone biopsies, and hysterectomy specimens obtained at operations of different extent.

It should be remembered that the cytological examination is of a sample of the cells lying on the surface of the ectocervix or lower endocervix. A good specimen will include cells of endo- and ectocervical origin. The effect of the technique is to mix up the abnormalities and potentially to dilute any changes with normal cells, necrotic cells, and cells responding to hormonal and even viral change. As a consequence of these limits it is accepted that 10 per cent of carefully examined smears will contain missed but significant lesions on each examination. In addition, the presence of blood and inflammatory and necrotic cells can complicate interpretation and this is a particular problem in the presence of fully developed invasive carcinoma when these elements in a smear examination can often cause confusion.

The microbiopsy is a tiny biopsy of a colposcopically abnormal looking area. A punch biopsy is based on the detection of a naked-eye abnormality on the visible cervix. A cone biopsy should remove the bulk of the ectocervix and the lower endocervical canal and a hysterectomy the whole cervix. The first three and to some extent even the fourth are samples of the whole tissue and may have missed the most important area. The cytological or histopathological opinion should, therefore, not be allowed to override clinical judgement. Whatever the real pathology it cannot be better than that revealed by the examination, but it may be worse.

Pathologically, a wide range of primary tumours has been recognized, as follows.

(1) Squamous-cell carcinoma:
    (a) large cell, keratinizing,
    (b) large cell, non-keratinizing,
    (c) small cell,
    (d) verrucous carcinoma.

(2) Adenocarcinoma:
    (a) common type,
    (b) adenoma malignum,
    (c) mucinous,
    (d) papillary,
    (e) endometrioid,
    (f) clear cell,
    (g) adenoid cystic.

(3) Adenosquamous.

(4) Stem cell carcinoma (glassy cell carcinoma).

In practice the majority of patients have squamous cell carcinomas. These are commonly divided into large cell keratinizing, large cell non-keratinizing, and small cell type. The other common varieties are common pattern adenocarcinomas or adenosquamous carcinomas of different degrees of differentiation. Traditional teaching was that 95 per cent of primary carcinomas of the cervix were squamous in origin. Improvements in pathological techniques suggest that this is not correct and more mixed pattern disease (15 per cent) and adenocarcinoma (15 per cent) are recognized both as pre-invasive and invasive disease. Not all pathologists agree about the pathological significance of the different histological types and the need to identify them. Some carcinomas contain mixtures of different patterns; this and the subjective nature of the interpretation of the histological pattern has prevented the fine details of the pathology from proving useful in day to day clinical management. Some types of carcinoma are rare and it is difficult to be dogmatic about prognosis on the basis of histology but, in general, verrucous carcinoma often follows a benign course while adenoma malignum and small cell squamous carcinoma, papillary adenocarcinoma, and stem cell, glassy carcinoma have a more sinister prognosis than the common types of squamous cell carcinoma.

In an attempt to improve the pathological contribution to the assessment of these patients, some pathologists have focused on other features visible on large punch, cone, and hysterectomy specimens, including the degrees of differentiation, cell structural changes, numbers of mitoses, the stromal response, and the vascular invasion. Attempts have been made to correlate these features individually or multifactorially with prognosis. Individually the degree of differentiation of the principal cell types and the presence of vascular invasion are, by concensus, thought to be the most important features but they are rarely used individually to determine treatment.

The best-understood disease pathologically is squamous cell carcinoma. It has been observed both at a pre-malignant and a microscopically, early malignant phase as well as in the typical, fully developed invasive carcinoma. Different possible steps in the evolution of the disease have been seen in individual patients and some have been seen to progress from one phase to another. The disease has been conceived of as an early basal cell change, typically occurring first at the squamocolumnar junction but later affecting the ectocervix and even extending on to the vaginal vault and endocervix. It gradually affects the different layers of the epidermis, breaching the basement membrane, invading the dermis and then the cervical stroma, infiltrating vascular spaces, and then behaving

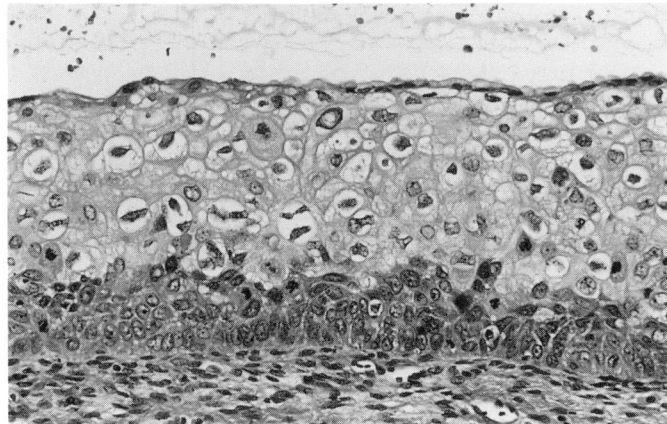

(a)

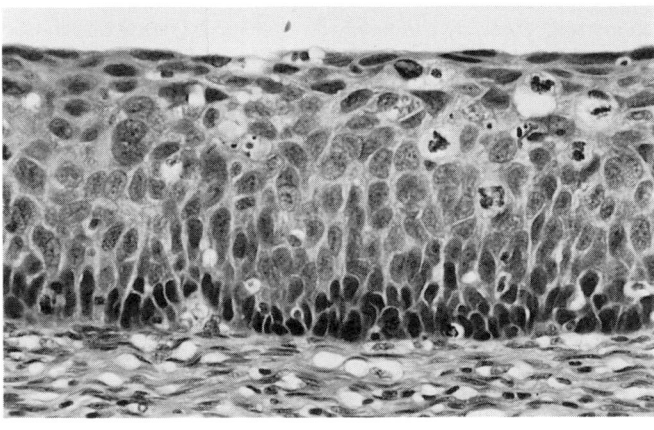

(b)

Fig. 5 Haematoxylin- and eosin-stained sections of cervical epithelium. (a) CIN I with neoplastic changes in the lower epithelium; extensive viral changes (koilocytes) are visible in the upper epithelium (original magnification × 295). (b) CIN III (original magnification × 370).

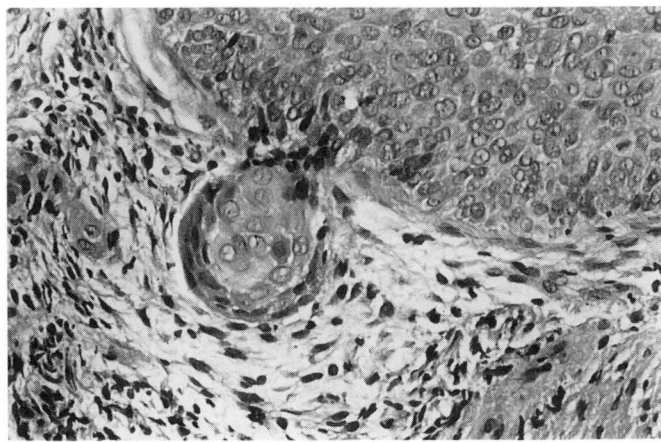

Fig. 6 Microinvasive carcinoma: early stromal invasion arising from an epithelium showing the features of CIN III (original magnification × 370) (courtesy of Dr H. Buckley).

like any other invasive carcinoma. While the disease is confined to the epithelium it is called cervical intraepithelial neoplasia (CIN). Different suffixes, I, II, and III, are ascribed to different levels of involvement of the epidermis as it gradually affects the different layers. By international agreement, changes confined to the lower third of the epithelium are known as CIN I, CIN II changes affect the lower and middle third, and CIN III the full thickness of the epidermis. The actual cellular chain certainly appears to start in the basal cell layers of the epidermis and the cells become cytologically abnormal, changing their shape and their nuclear:cytoplasmic ratio, and showing increased and abnormal mitotic activity (Fig. 5).

Provided the abnormality remains confined to the epidermis it is not classified as invasive carcinoma and is not subject to statutory notification. The process can even extend into and fill the crypts of the endocervical glands. It only becomes an invasive carcinoma if at any point it breaches the basement membrane. In the early stages these breaches may be very small and associated with a stromal abnormality and an inflammatory response (Fig. 6). Early invasion is assessed in terms of the depth of the deepest invasive element from the surface of the epithelium. Typically, this is expressed in millimetres and up to 5 mm is known as microinvasive carcinoma. Small tongues of invasion up to 5 mm probably carry

a very low risk of metastatic disease, while large confluent areas of invasion greater than 3 mm may be associated with lymph node disease. When invasion extends beyond 5 mm there is agreement that this is a true, invasive carcinoma and it can be staged as described here in the relevant section. The recognition of the steps in the evolution of squamous cell carcinoma has been followed by an understanding that adenocarcinoma of the cervix can arise in the same way. CIN of adenocarcinoma type may initially involve the endocervix and its glands but can extend to the ectocervix. The epithelial lesions do not shed cells for cytological specimens as reliably as does squamous cell carcinoma. Sometimes the intraepithelial process may be mixed in histological type and in others a 'collision' carcinomatous change may be observed in which the two adjacent intraepithelial diseases meet each other. It seems likely that the true precursor basal cells of squamous cell and adenocarcinomas are reacting to the same carcinogenic influences. The cause of the different patterns of ecto- and endocervical disease of different histological type is unknown.

While the different steps in the disease process can be viewed as a continuum and in some patients may behave that way, there are a number of problems that arise when that model is applied clinically.

1. Some of the early phases of CIN have been seen to regress to normal, either with time or in response to oestrogen therapy.

2. Not all patients progress through the stages.

3. In those who do progress the rate of evolution of the disease is very variable.

4. In some patients, different degrees of change may be present on different parts of the cervix.

5. The limits between the different phases are abitrary and not easily reproducible between different treatment centres.

PATHOLOGY OF SPREAD

The cervix lies in the centre of the pelvis surrounded by a variety of different tissues. In spite of this, invasive carcinoma of the cervix often spreads in a very sequential and predictable fashion. Initially the disease invades the underlying cervical stroma and muscle, extending through it and going on to involve the uterine cavity and the myometrium or to involve the vaginal fornices and the inner parametrium. This intitial pattern can be influenced by the site of origin of the disease and its nature. Endocervical disease most commonly involves the uterus while ectocervical disease more commonly involves the vagina.

Three general types of primary tumour are seen. A proliferative, bulky, ectocervical disease that fills the upper vagina eventually and can fall off in large pieces after clinical examination, an invasive, bulky disease that can balloon the cervix up to the point that it fills the pelvis, and an unpleasant, destructive, invasive disease that erodes the normal tissues and leads to ulcerated, excavating tumours with heavily infective, necrotic cavities. Once off the cervix the disease more commonly spreads laterally than in any other direction; it infiltrates the parametrium surrounding the ureters and extends laterally or posteriorly to infiltrate the suspensory ligaments of the cervix. Following the line of these ligaments the disease regularly reaches the pelvic side wall. Extension of the disease down the vagina is a less common, though well-described line of spread. Anteroposterior infiltration at the level of the cervix is unusual except in the presence of advanced local disease; infiltration of the posterior bladder wall and rectum therefore are not often presenting features in European patients.

The metastatic spread is predominantly lymphatic. There are small groups of lymph nodes in the inner parametrium and these drain to the internal iliac, hypogastric, and obturator groups. From these nodal areas the disease spreads to the common and external iliac groups, the para-aortic, and, typically, the nodes of the left supraclavicular fossa. Involvement of the inguinal nodes is uncommon without lower-third vaginal involvement. Occasionally an isolated vaginal or vulval mass may be present initially or appear on follow-up. Lymphatic spread can be very slow growing and the appearance of metastatic disease in a single lymph node group outside the true pelvis can occur up to 10 years after apparently successful treatment of the primary disease.

Haematogenous spread is uncommon initially and relatively less common than pelvic or para-aortic lymphadenopathy. Pulmonary metastases can be difficult to differentiate from a new primary carcinoma of the lung. Liver and bone metastases are rare and metastases to the central nervous system are very unusual, even when the patient has overt metastatic disease at other sites.

STAGING

The staging of these carcinomas is very much dominated by the relative ease of assessment of the primary tumour and the unreliability of investigations of lymph node disease. Two international systems are commonly used, the Union Internationale Contre le Cancer (**UICC**) and the International Federation of Gynaecology and Obstetrics (**FIGO**) (Table 1). In addition many centres use their 'home grown' systems, which may incorporate the radiological and pathological information not necessary to the two international systems.

Correctly to stage a patient by the UICC/FIGO approach, she should be examined under an anaesthetic, have a biopsy, a chest radiograph, and an intravenous urogram. More extensive investigations are not required but gynaecologists are encouraged to examine the bladder and/or rectum in patients with significant symptoms from either of these sites or in those whose disease appears extensive enough to involve these tissues. The systems depend heavily upon the tissues involved with the primary disease and are not concerned with the size or volume of the disease.

The classical staging systems were dominated by primary disease and contained four stages (I–IV). With the better understanding of the natural history of the disease another stage, stage 0, has been added and applied to intraepithelial disease (CIN I–III). Stage I has also been split to allow for asymptomatic, microinvasive disease to be discriminated from those patients with frank, symptomatic, invasive carcinoma of the cervix.

Improved imaging techniques and consensus about extending the investigations may eventually change the systems to make them more responsive to lymph node spread, but attempts to achieve this have to be balanced against the need for all systems to be applicable

Table 1 Carcinoma of the cervix uteri (correlation between the FIGO, UICC, and AJCC nomenclatures)

Stage 0	Carcinoma *in situ*, intraepithelial carcinoma
Stage I	The carcinoma is strictly confined to the cervix (extension to the corpus should be disregarded)
Stage Ia	Preclinical carcinomas of the cervix, that is those diagnosed only by microscopy
Stage Ia$_1$	Minimal microscopically evident stromal invasion
Stage Ia$_2$	Lesions detected microscopically that can be measured
	The upper limit of the measurement should not show a depth of invasion of more then 5 mm taken from the base of the epithelium, either surface or glandular, from which it originates
	A second dimension, the horizontal spread, must not exceed 7 mm
	Larger lesions should be staged as Ib
Stage Ib	Lesions of greater dimensions than Stage Ia$_2$ whether seen clinically or not
	Preformed space involvement should not alter the staging but should be specifically recorded so as to determine whether it should affect treatment decisions in the future
Stage II	The carcinoma extends beyond the cervix, but has not extended on to the pelvic wall
	The carcinoma involves the vagina, but not as far as the lower third
Stage IIa	No obvious parametrial involvement
Stage IIb	Obvious parametrial involvement
Stage III	The carcinoma has extended on to the pelvic wall
	On rectal examination there is no cancer-free space between the tumour and the pelvic wall
	The tumour involves the lower third of the vagina
	All cases with hydronephrosis or non-functioning kidney should be included, unless they are known to be due to another cause
Stage IIIa	No extension on to the pelvic wall, but involvement of the lower third of the vagina
Stage IIIb	Extension on to the pelvic wall or hydronephrosis or non-functioning kidney
Stage IV	The carcinoma has extended beyond the true pelvis or has clinically involved the mucosa of the bladder or rectum
Stage IVa	Spread of the growth to adjacent organs
Stage IVb	Spread to distant organs

in small centres and developing countries. This remains important because, since 1940, at regular intervals, the results of treating carcinoma of the cervix in many centres of variable size throughout the world have been published in the form of the 'FIGO Reports'. If the pattern of results over time is to be understood clearly, then the overall staging system must be simple in concept, easy to apply in practice, and consistent over decades.

SYMPTOMS

Carcinoma of the cervix can only begin to produce symptoms when the integrity of the epithelium is disturbed. Patients with the different changes of CIN I–III and microinvasion are asymptomatic. The cervix usually looks normal to the naked eye and their disease is only detectable by cervical examination with cytology or colposcopy.

The earliest symptoms are vaginal discharge and bleeding. The vaginal discharge is entirely non-specific, can be intermittent or continuous, scanty or very heavy. Sometimes due to secondary infection the discharge can be sufficiently heavy to make the patients think that it is urine. For the true post-menopausal patient the change of habit is easily recognized, though the significance may not be appreciated. Pre-menopausal and perimenopausal women often notice the changes but they or their confidants may not appreciate their significance. Bleeding may be spontaneous but, in the early stages, it is not uncommonly seen after coitus, micturition, or defecation. In addition, the patient may not be entirely certain where the blood is coming from. Some ignore scanty bleeding and go on to become anaemic through chronic blood loss or have a sudden, severe, vaginal haemorrhage that precipitates emergency admission to hospital. It is very common for patients to ascribe early symptoms to normal gynaecological dysfunction. Quite often, even if noted, this early combination of symptoms is ignored until they become persistent, severe, or associated with other new symptoms. Patients may seek a cervical cytological examination rather than a formal medical consultation on the basis of these symptoms and they and their doctors may be falsely reassured by a normal result.

The differential diagnosis of vaginal discharge and bleeding is considerable, even in the post-menopausal woman. Common reasons for vaginal discharge and irregular bleeding in the pre-menopausal woman are dysfunctional bleeding, cervical erosion, uterine fibroids, and oral and intrauterine contraceptive techniques. In the post-menopausal woman, atrophic vaginitis, endometrial hyperplasia, and endometrial carcinoma should be considered. A high incidence of suspicion and a willingness to carry out a full pelvic examination are required if the disease is not going to be missed at the stage of early symptoms.

As the disease progresses, often the next symptom to develop is pelvic discomfort or frank pain. Often this is rather poorly localized and described as dull or boring pain in the suprapubic or sacral region. It may be persistent or intermittent and may be likened to pre-menstrual discomfort. It can become a very dominant symptom and result in referral for an orthopaedic opinion if the associated gynaecological symptoms are not recognized. As the disease progresses further it moves out of the gynaecological tissues and symptoms are dictated by the line of spread. Symptoms can arise from pressure or infiltration of one of the many tissues that surround the cervix. Common symptoms are urinary frequency or change of bowel habit. Bladder invasion can produce dysuria or even haematuria. Ureteric pressure and infiltration can be remarkably asymptomatic and unilateral or bilateral obstructive uropathy causing renal failure with oligurea and uraemia are occasional presenting

features. Infiltration of the rectum or sigmoid colon is remarkably uncommon, even in the presence of advanced disease. Common problems of advanced disease therefore are urinary frequency, lateral pelvic pain, pain radiating to the thighs, unilateral oedema of the leg, and altered bowel habit. Patients with carcinoma of the cervix do not often present with symptomatic metastatic disease outside the pelvis but occasionally, even in developed countries, they present with uraemia, intestinal obstruction, or symptoms from para-aortic or pulmonary metastases. Some patients do get significant secondary pelvic infections causing parametritis, pyometritis, or salpingitis and the inflammatory feature may predominate and mask the underlying malignant disease.

SIGNS

General signs depend enormously on the stage of the disease.

In patients with pre-invasive or microinvasive disease, full examination, including speculum examination of the cervix, can be normal. Some patients with extensive intraepithelial disease may have white patches (leucoplakia) or extensive red patches (erythroplasia) on the visible cervix.

Until recently, painting the cervix and upper vagina with Lugol solution was the only way to identify abnormal epithelium (CIN), which does not take up the iodine stain owing to a lack of glycogen. This was a crude, imprecise test and has been supplanted by colposcopy. The colposcope is a stereoscopic binocular microscope that uses a green filter to accentuate the vascular patterns and colour differences between normal and abnormal epithelium. Colposcopy allows examination of the visible cervix, including the transformation zone, in many patients. Before the examination the cervix is cleaned with acetic acid, removing excess mucus and debris. The ectocervix, vaginal vault and lower endocervical canal can then be inspected, biopsied, and treated. In practice, a wide variety of normal patterns is visible on the cervix. In addition, a number of typical patterns have become recognized (Fig. 7):

(1) white epithelium (leucoplakia);

(2) mosaic structures and punctation;

(3) abnormal vascularity.

The first two suggest intraepithelial disease. Vascular changes are associated with invasive disease. Colposcopic patterns cannot be

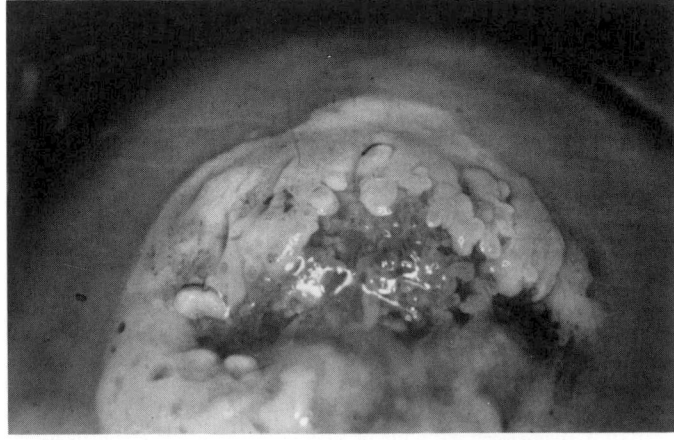

Fig. 7 White, superficially proliferative, colposcopic appearance of abnormal cervical epithelium (CIN III) on the outer ectocervix (courtesy of Mr A. Singer).

accepted as diagnostic and directed biopsies are important to substantiate the diagnosis. The ability to direct biopsy is an important advantage colposcopy has over normal cytological examination.

In practice, the majority of patients with invasive disease also look entirely well. Occasionally, signs of anaemia, particularly of the iron deficiency type, may be observed in patients with chronic or heavy bleeding or uraemia in those with locally very advanced disease. Very rarely the nodes of the left supraclavicular fossa may be significantly enlarged at the time of presentation. Pulmonary or upper abdominal abnormalities are more likely to be a consequence of intercurrent disease, particularly relating to cigarette smoking or alcohol abuse than to carcinoma of the cervix. Early, unilateral oedema of the leg is an important sign of pelvic side wall disease and very often affects the thigh rather than the ankle.

Gynaecological examination in an out-patient setting may be difficult and it should not be relied on for staging. Only when the patient's intercurrent medical condition is very poor should she not have a full examination under an anaesthetic. The vulva is usually normal. Further examination for staging, treatment assessment, and planning should involve vaginal digital examination, supplemented by speculum examination and digital examination of the central pelvic tissues *per rectum*. Particular attention should be paid initially to the size of the vagina and the site of the cervix, the size and texture and visual appearance of the cervix, and the size and mobility of the uterus. The vagina should be carefully examined for evidence of infiltration of the fornices and the walls; in particular, the level of the vaginal infiltration in relation to the upper, middle, or lower third of the vagina should be noted. Occasionally a metastatic submucosal deposit will be found on one of the lower walls, often the anterior, just inside the introitus. Early vaginal infiltration often produces a visible rather than a palpable abnormality. If the anterior vaginal wall is infiltrated in the upper half, then the disease will be close to or infiltrating the base of the bladder and close to one or both ureters and cystoscopy should be performed. The parametrium is best examined rectally. The staging system is heavily dependent on the extent of this infiltration, which should be expressed in terms of which side wall is involved and the extent and whether the disease reaches and fixes to the side wall. The presence of adnexal masses and pelvic inflammation considerably complicates this assessment. Occasionally, patients with advanced disease will also present with metastatic nodal disease in the external iliac or inguinal region or with masses involving the lateral upper pelvis. This can be difficult to distinguish initially from an enlarged bladder and/or uterus. Quite commonly the ectocervix looks macroscopically normal, even if it feels abnormal. It is mandatory that a biopsy is taken. Normally this will require a general anaesthetic. At least one specimen should be obtained from the abnormal tissue, with care that it is not from the periphery, which, particularly in carcinoma of the cervix, may give a misleading impression of the nature of the disease.

The cervix and uterus should first be examined bimanually and if possible the os should be identified and the uterus cannulated. The length of the uterine cavity and the position of the uterus in the pelvis are important pre-treatment points for radiotherapy. Regularly the ectocervix is normal but the endocervical canal feels hard and 'gritty'. The cervix should be dilated sufficiently to allow for endocervical biopsy or curettage. Subsequent curettage of the uterine body is thought by some to give information of prognostic significance relating to the uterine extension of disease but it is technically difficult and the procedure does not attract universal support. Among the problems encountered at this stage are a

pyometrium or uterine perforation. The latter may establish a false passage and complicate subsequent intrauterine brachytherapy. It may be impossible to identify the canal, owing to the proliferative or destructive nature of the tumour. Even under an anaesthetic, upper pelvic nodal masses and/or para-aortic nodes are not reliably identified. On completion of the procedure a clear description and/or diagram of the primary tumour should be prepared to aid final staging.

For many years, cystoscopy and sigmoidoscopy were advised as part of the staging investigations. Both examinations are easy to do but in early disease are so regularly normal that they are a waste of time. If, on vaginal examination, the infiltrating disease is extending anteriorly and filling the anterior fornix, then cystoscopy must be done. A number of abnormalities may be found. Commonly, the posterior wall of the bladder is pushed forward in the midline by the expanded cervix. More infrequently the base and/or posterior wall may look oedematous (bullous oedema) or, occasionally, tumour may be seen infiltrating the bladder wall. A bladder biopsy may have to be done to discriminate between oedema and infiltration. Even more infrequently the rectal examination of the central pelvic tissues may suggest that the disease is infiltrating the anterior wall at 10–15 cm from the anal verge and this will be visible on sigmoidoscopy.

INVESTIGATIONS

It is easy to write a long list of investigations that can be carried out on patients with carcinoma of the cervix but it is equally easy to overinvestigate them. There are certain investigations that all patients should have to complement the results of their examination and biopsy.

A full blood count may reveal evidence of anaemia, particularly of iron deficiency type. Renal function tests are necessary to exclude significant renal failure. In the presence of unilateral obstructive uropathy and/or bilateral early obstructive uropathy the urea is often normal. A chest radiograph will occasionally reveal early pulmonary metastases and should be done also to exclude intercurrent pulmonary disease, to assist the anaesthetist, and to provide a base line for any future situation when a radiological abnormality has been identified and needs elucidating.

It is common practice to do an intravenous urogram. Parametrial extension of disease can and regularly does block the lower ureter just before it enters the bladder (Fig. 8). This gives rise to a hydronephrosis of varying degree on the affected side and the increasing pressure in the system eventually causes obstructive uropathy and damages the function of the kidney. The whole sequence of events can be asymptomatic unless both kidneys are affected and renal failure supervenes. The recognition of ureteric obstruction is important in establishing the final stage. If significant bilateral obstructive uropathy is revealed by intravenous urography, then a transabdominal ultrasonographic examination of the abdomen should be done to identify the number and site of the kidneys, the level of the ureteric obstruction, and the thickness of the remaining cortex on each kidney.

Investigation of the patient beyond this point is not necessary to complete staging but if facilities are available and local imaging expertise is good, then further information about the disease can be obtained before starting treatment. The most widely used investigation has been lower-limb lymphangiography (Fig. 8). The weakness of this investigation from the point of view of carcinoma of the cervix is that the procedure does not fill the nodes of the true pelvis, which are the first nodal station of the disease. Nodal

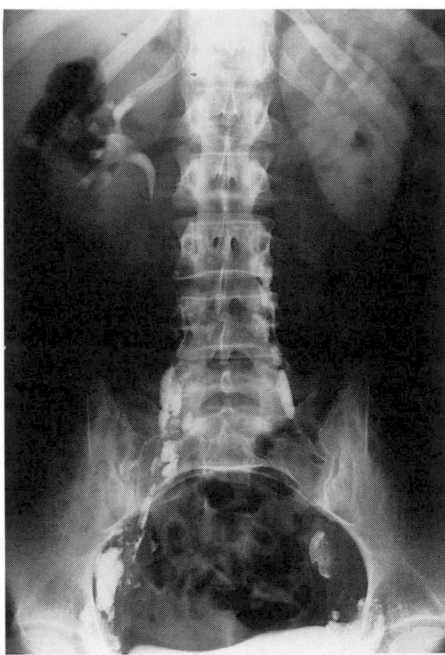

Fig. 8 Intravenous urogram in a patient with carcinoma of the cervix who has had a lower-limb lymphangiogram. A soft tissue mass in the left pelvis is displacing an abnormal group of lymph nodes that is invaded by metastatic carcinoma. There is left ureteric obstruction shown by the left nephrogram while the right pelvicalyceal system is clearly visible and normal.

involvement in the external, common iliac chains and the para-aortic region can be identified and is recognized to be associated with a poor prognosis.

Pelvic computerized tomographic scanning has been a very disappointing investigatory tool at the time of diagnosis. Even with an excellent scanning technique the extension of disease off the cervix and into the parametrium and the distinction of infiltration from pelvic inflammatory disease has proved impossible and false-positive and -negative investigations are common. A more useful aspect of this scanning is assessment of the pelvic side wall, where

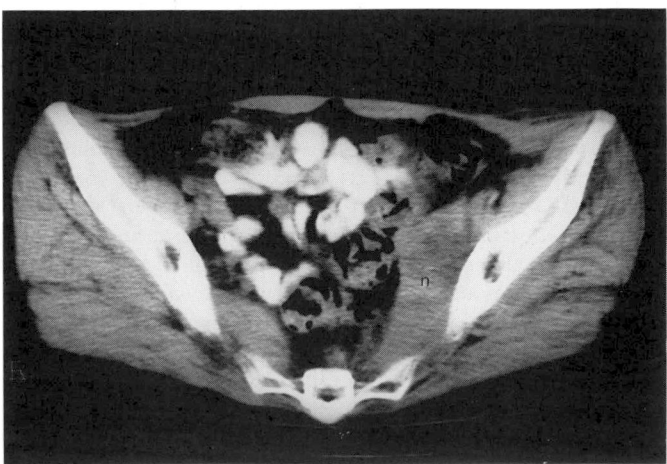

Fig. 9 Pelvic computerized tomographic scan in a patient with carcinoma of the cervix. Gastrografin is present in the small bowel. A large, left pelvic, soft tissue mass is visible, indicating an infiltrating lymph node mass.

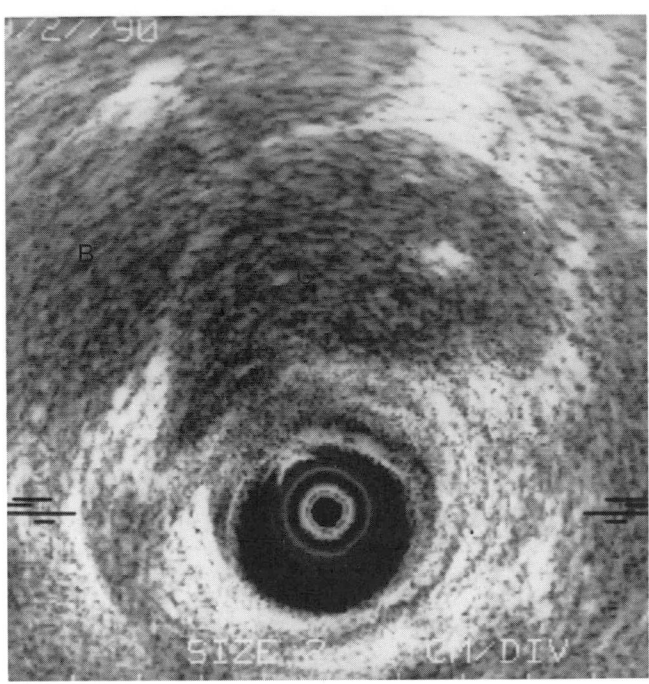

Fig. 10 Transrectal ultrasonogram in a patient with stage IIb carcinoma of the cervix. The cervix (c) shows bilateral irregularity of the margins indicating early parametrial infiltration. The bladder (b) is anterolateral to the cervix.

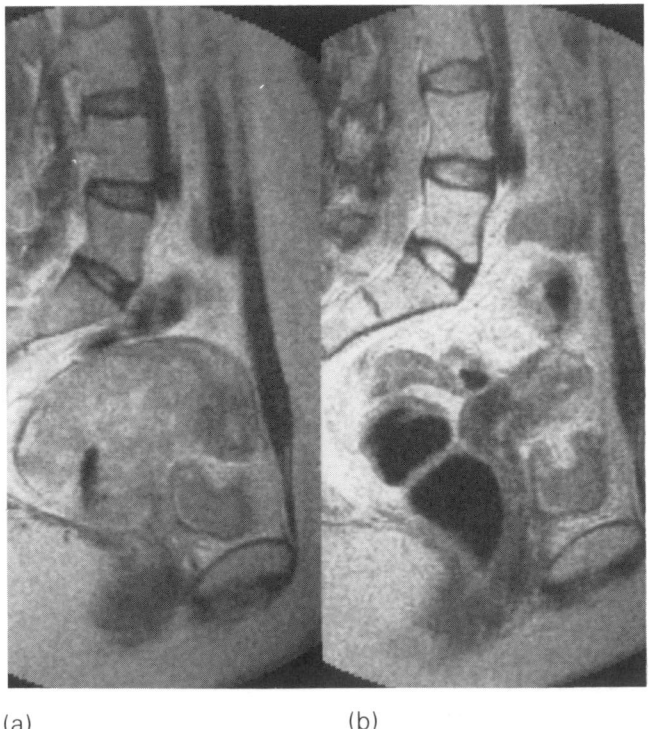

(a)   (b)

Fig. 11 Sagittal T_2-weighted (SE 1500/80) magnetic resonance scans of the pelvis in a patient with carcinoma of the cervix. (a) Pre-treatment of a large primary carcinoma involves the cervix and the middle segment of the body of the uterus. (b) Three months' post-radiotherapy. There is complete resolution of the tumour and reconstitution of the cervical stromal walls.

enlarged nodes in the obturator and internal iliac groups are quite commonly identified (Fig. 9). As nodes up to 2 cm can be inflammatory or reactive, it is difficult to use the information fully without histological confirmation of their nature and percutaneous needle aspiration biopsy of such nodes is practised in some centres.

Two other investigatory techniques have been introduced to try to improve the initial assessment of the disease. Transrectal ultrasonography carried out systematically under an anaesthetic can give an accurate, three-dimensional picture of the cervix and some idea of the parametrial and/or vaginal extension of disease (Fig. 10). The more sophisticated examination of magnetic resonance imaging can give a very clear picture of the primary tumour and pericervical infiltration, and can identify nodal enlargement in the pelvis or paraaortic region (Fig. 11(a)). As with computerized tomographic scanning, enlargement does not equal involvement and may be reactive. It is undoubtedly the investigation of the future in the assessment of new patients with carcinoma of the cervix. It is also a very useful tool for monitoring response to treatment (Fig. 11(b)).

TREATMENT: GENERAL ASPECTS

Surgery and radiotherapy, sometimes alone and sometimes in combination, are used to treat patients with cervical carcinoma of different stages. The treatment is not strictly by stage but is dependent on the patient's general condition as well as the volume and local extension of the disease. Primary radical surgery is normally directed to microinvasive carcinoma, small-volume, early stage-I and -IIa disease and very occasionally locally advanced, destructive primary tumours invading the bladder and/or rectum. Radiotherapy techniques can and sometimes are used to treat all stages of disease from microinvasive carcinoma to stage IV, although the majority of patients treated by radical radiotherapy are in stages II and III.

A range of surgical and radiotherapy techniques is available to treat these patients. Their best interests are served by a decision made after consultation between both specialties. Although the extent of the disease may be a discriminant in this decision, there are a number of points which may have emerged from the history and physical examination that should be reviewed at this time. They include the general fitness of the patient for pelvic surgery. Patients with carcinoma of the cervix are often cigarette smokers and may have some of the related chest diseases. Among them is also a number of alcoholics, particularly those who work in places where alcohol is served. Among other general medical conditions a history of colitis or Crohn's disease, pelvic inflammatory disease, previous pelvic surgery, or diabetes mellitus of significant type should be positively sought as they can be associated with abnormally severe radiation reactions. Very occasionally, carcinoma of the cervix may arise in a patient who has previously had pelvic radiotherapy for benign disease, for example menorrhagia. They may even have had treatment for a previous malignant disease involving the pelvis, for example lymphoma or carcinoma of the bladder. These will prevent further satisfactory treatment by radiotherapy.

Surgical treatment and radiotherapy are considered separately and in detail in the next sections, followed by sections on consideration of the choice of initial treatment, the management of recurrence and metastasis, and of chemotherapy.

SURGICAL TECHNIQUES

Five general levels of surgical approach are available:

(1) local destruction of abnormal epithelium by cautery, cryosurgery, or laser;

(2) cone biopsy;

(3) hysterectomy: simple;

(4) radical hysterectomy (often called Wertheim's hysterectomy);

(5) anterior, posterior, or total pelvic clearance.

Destruction of the abnormal ectocervical epithelium

This is the least damaging of any of the procedures and can be done at the time of colposcopy on an out-patient basis with local anaesthesia of the cervix. It does not normally cause cervical incompetence or prevent further pregnancy. The patients must have intraepithelial neoplasia only and the lesion must be confined to the ectocervix. Over the years in which these techniques have evolved, different types of destruction have been used, including cautery, cryosurgery, and laser. They can be equally successful in trained hands but the latter two are more commonly used, with laser preferred if available. More recently, some gynaecologists have taken to stripping the cervical epithelium using loop diathermy. This has the advantage of providing a specimen for histological examination in contrast with the earlier techniques, which really just destroy the epithelium.

Post-operatively the patient may experience discomfort, vaginal discharge, and occasionally bleeding. Healing of the damaged area can be easily observed by repeat colposcopy and should be complete in 3 months. If the procedure has been successful the epithelium will look normal and in the majority of patients will stay that way. Repeat cytological examination should be normal and the patient should remain on indefinite annual follow-up by cytology as they have an increased incidence of subsequent *in situ* and invasive cervical and vaginal carcinoma.

Cone biopsy

This became a common procedure when cytological assessment suggested CIN and before the general use of colposcopy allowed patients with non-invasive ectocervical disease to be identified easily and treated as described above. Cone biopsy is still done in patients in whom there is no ectocervical *invasive* disease but in whom there is evidence of epithelial disease extending up the cervical canal beyond the limit of colposcopic assessment. The operation involves the removal of the ectocervix and the majority of the endocervix (see Fig. 2) in a single piece of tissue that looks like a doughnut. This specimen is fixed in an orientated position and multiple sections are taken. In the majority of patients, if the wound is closed properly, so reconstructing the cervix and healing takes quickly, then there is little symptomatic problem apart from a light vaginal discharge and some central pelvic discomfort. Occasionally a secondary infection or haemorrhage complicates the post-operative course. Pregnancy is possible after this procedure provided the internal os has not been damaged.

A cone biopsy is considered a satisfactory therapeutic procedure if examination of the specimen suggests that the abnormality is confined to the epithelium and the margins of both ecto- and endocervix are clear of disease. If the operation is treated as definitive, patients should remain on indefinite, annual, cytological follow-up. Occasionally, patients treated in this way can develop new *in situ* or invasive disease on the new ectocervix or high in the endocervix; for this reason, cone biopsy is a poor therapeutic procedure in fit patients who are not interested in or are unable to have a subsequent pregnancy. Hysterectomy is to be preferred in these patients.

Hysterectomy

In carefully chosen patients with extensive intraepithelial disease who are not interested in the possibility of subsequent pregnancy or patients with microinvasive disease only (less than 5 mm infiltration), a hysterectomy can be done without any significant parametrial or nodal dissection. The size of the vaginal cuff must be determined by any intravaginal extension of disease but, in principle, the fornices need to be removed. The Fallopian tubes and ovaries are removed in the post-menopausal patient but the ovaries are left in the pre-menopausal. Post-operatively the patient remains at some risk of developing intraepithelial or invasive disease of the vagina, particularly the upper third. These women should continue to have regular vault smears.

Hysterectomy is associated with a low risk of general post-operative complications, including infections, venous thrombosis of the pelvic veins, and post-operative vault granulations and haemorrhage. It carries very little risk of long-term morbidity and is an excellent definitive procedure for a correctly staged patient. Unfortunately, because of the multifocal, field nature of carcinoma of the cervix, some patients treated in this manner are found on histological examination to have more extensive invasive disease than expected. They may need post-operative radiotherapy (see later).

Radical hysterectomy (Wertheim's hysterectomy)

This general title covers a group of operations of varying extent aiming at definitive treatment of invasive, infiltrating, and early metastatic carcinoma of the cervix. The absolute extent of the operation varies between gynaecologists and between patients, depending on philosophy, training, expertise, and the extent of the disease in the individual. The aim is excision of the primary tumour with a reasonable margin of healthy tissue (approximately 1 cm) and as '*en bloc*' as possible a resection of the principal, important, pelvic lymph node areas; the ureteric, obturator, hypogastric, and internal iliac groups. The vaginal margins may involve the removal of the upper one-third and the parametrial dissection may include the uterovesical and the uterosacral ligaments. It used to be standard practice to remove the ovaries and Fallopian tubes but in recent years, in patients who are more than 5 years pre-menopausal and in whom there is no evidence of metastatic disease, it has been common practice to leave one ovary with an intact blood supply and to mark this with a radiopaque clip. Some surgeons attempt to swing the ovary out of the true pelvis and into the hollow of the innominate bone or lower abdominal retroperitoneal tissues. If this procedure is successful then the radiotherapist may be able to avoid the ovary by careful treatment planning and post-treatment hormone replacement therapy is not required.

A number of specific problems are encountered with the regular use of this type of surgery. Post-operatively, bladder function may recover only slowly and occasionally chronic retention as a consequence of detrusor dysfunction may require further assessment and management. The central pelvic/parametrial dissection involves

clearing tissue from the lower ureters and ureteric fistulae may complicate the immediate post-operative period. Reimplantation of the ureters resolves this problem. Aggressive lymph node dissection, particularly if done transabdominally rather than retroperitoneally, can result in post-operative lymphocyst formation. Often this results in a smooth, palpable, static mass in the lateral pelvis or left iliac fossa, clearly a simple cyst on ultrasonographic examination which then resolves spontaneously. Occasionally lymphocysts can cause local pain from pressure on the pelvic side wall or become secondarily infected. In either situation, drainage relieves the immediate problem and marsupialization (deroofing the cyst and stitching the margins) may be required as a long-term solution. Other difficult complications related to the pelvic side wall include venous thrombosis or lymphatic insufficiency leading to a chronically swollen, uncomfortable leg. All these complications are reduced in incidence with practice and good surgical technique.

The careful histological examination of the radical hysterectomy specimen is assuming an increasing importance as options about adjuvant post-operative treatments and their hazards become better understood. A full report should include information about the histological type of the carcinoma, its degree of differentiation, the size and extent of the primary tumour, particularly in relation to the resection margins vaginally and parametrially, the presence or absence of vascular invasion both venous and lymphatic, the number of nodes removed, their site, the numbers invaded, and their size and type of invasion. Patients with small-volume, well-differentiated, fully resected primary tumours without evidence of vascular invasion and with no or only early lymphatic invasion are regularly cured by radical hysterectomy alone. All others may require further radiotherapy and/or chemotherapy (see below).

Anterior, posterior, or total pelvic exenteration

These operations have been developed over the last 40 years and may result in the creation of one or two stomata. They were developed for recurrent carcinoma of the cervix but can be applied to unusually advanced, primary, untreated disease confined to the soft tissues of the pelvis but invading the bladder or rectum. All three operations involve the removal of the pelvic adnexae. In the anterior procedure there is preservation of the rectosigmoid and, in the posterior, of the bladder. If the bladder is removed a small healthy segment of small or large bowel is isolated with its blood supply and the ureters are implanted into this. The new urinary stoma opens normally into the right lower anterior abdominal wall and the urine is collected in a stoma bag. If the rectosigmoid is removed a colostomy is fashioned in the left iliac fossa. If the operation is done as a primary procedure, a large layer of omentum or an artificial mesh may be drawn across the upper pelvis to prevent large and small bowel from prolapsing into the pelvis. This can be advantageous if post-operative radiotherapy proves necessary because it keeps to a minimum the amount of normal bowel that will be irradiated within the true pelvis.

The selection of patients for these extensive operations is difficult because of the need for general physical fitness for such major procedures, true resectability of the primary tumour, minimal pelvic lymph node involvement, and psychological strength to overcome the very destructive nature of the surgery. An exploratory laparotomy may be required before a final decision about resectability can be made. The preservation of either bladder or normal bowel and the reconstruction of the vagina can contribute to good long-term recovery. The most common complications are urinary tract obstruction and infection and small bowel obstruction due to post-operative adhesions.

RADIOTHERAPY

Introduction

Carcinoma of the cervix is unusual among malignant diseases being treated by radiotherapy in that radical treatment regularly employs a combination of radiotherapeutic techniques. Two very different techniques are regularly used, intracavitary brachytherapy and external-beam radiotherapy. The actual balance of the techniques in any group of patients may vary, depending on the training, experience, and philosophy of the radiotherapist, but it is most unusual in true, radical radiotherapy not to consider a combined approach. In addition to these standard approaches, there has been a recent resurgence of interest among some therapists in interstitial rather than intracavitary techniques for patients with locally advanced cancer of the cervix.

Intracavitary therapy

Introduction

Shortly after the discovery of radium it was observed empirically that the insertion of radium tubes into the vagina and uterus could induce useful regression in patients with carcinoma of the cervix. At the time, because of the inadequacy of the major surgical service and the advanced nature of the disease in the majority of patients, there was no alternative treatment available and the observation was greeted with enormous excitement internationally. Many hospitals rushed to buy radium and experiment with its use. Eventually they noticed in some of their patients major radiation damage to the central pelvic tissues as a consequence of radium treatment and they recognized the need to develop safe techniques or 'systems' for this type of therapy.

Intracavitary systems have evolved continuously from the beginning of the twentieth century. Initially, Paris and Stockholm took the lead and their approaches have been modified, refined, and developed in Manchester and Houston and continued in Paris. In the original systems, radium powder was sealed into platinum-coated tubes and mounted in metal, cork, or rubber applicators. These were inserted into the uterus and vagina and left in place, either continuously or intermittently, over a number of weeks.

By trial and error, different centres evolved their own approaches using different overall quantities of radium, different loading patterns for the uterus and vagina, and different treatment times. The result has been the development of a number of schools of intracavitary brachytherapy, each of which has been subjected to minor modifications by their users without any consensus internationally about which, if any, is the optimum approach. The most widely used approach in the United Kingdom is the Manchester system and this will be used as the basis for discussing modern treatment.

Many modifications have taken place over the years to the original system. The original applicator materials have been replaced by plastics and/or lightweight steel alloys, which are more easily fashioned and sterilized (Fig. 12). Radium has been discarded because of the problems of radiation safety caused by its high γ-ray energy, its daughter product the radioactive gas radon, and its powder form. For intracavitary brachytherapy it has been replaced by the artificial radionuclides ^{137}Cs, ^{192}Ir, and ^{60}Co. None of these is ideal. Caesium is a fission product and is freely available. Its half-life is acceptable at 30.5 years, its mean γ-energy at 660 keV

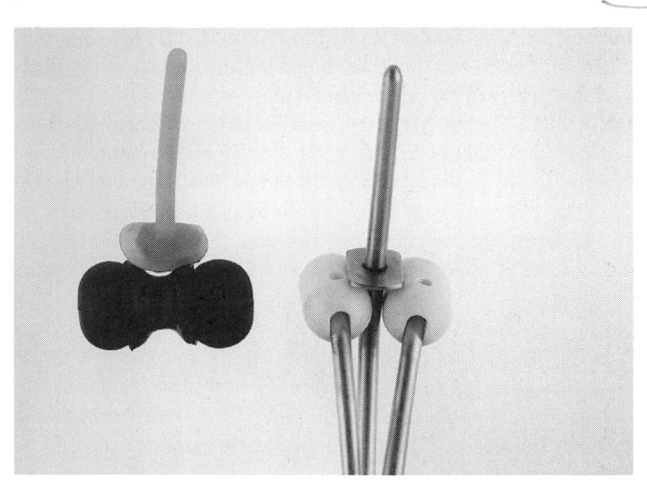

(a)

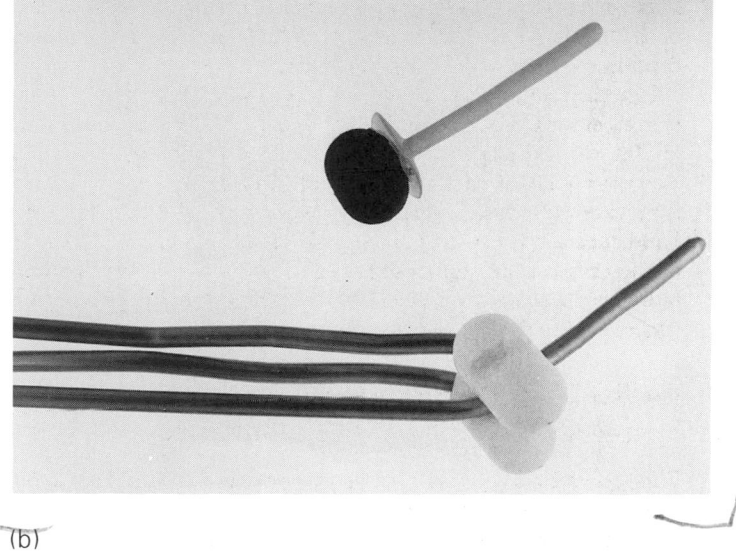

(b)

Fig. 12 (a) Anteroposterior and (b) lateral view of classical and after-loading Manchester intracavitary applicators. The preloaded radium applicators made in rubber have been replaced by lightweight metal applicators designed to allow simulation of the original system.

makes it easier to shield than radium, and it can be prepared in a solid, machinable form, but it has a low specific activity that can only be used if relatively weak sources are required. In situations where strong radiation sources are required, ^{60}Co or ^{192}Ir are preferred in spite of their short half-lives and the consequent and expensive need to replace sources more frequently.

The use of modern applicator materials and safer radionuclides has released the radiotherapist from many of the constraints of the original systems. Instead of placing radioactive sources manually in the uterus and vagina in theatre and nursing patients in open wards, empty applicators are now positioned in theatre and the patient transferred to a radiation-protected room where sources are loaded from a safe through transfer tubes into the applicators. This is normally done by remote control (remote afterloading). The use of a range of artificial radionuclides of different specific activity has allowed very much stronger sources than before to be used shortening treatments from days to hours or even minutes. To prevent any confusion associated with these changes the

International Commission on Radiation Units (ICRU) has suggested the use of the terms low, medium, and high dose rate. Low dose-rate systems are really modern equivalents of the classical radium systems in which source strengths, distribution, and treatment times are maintained. Medium dose-rate systems shorten treatment times by a factor of 4—10, while high dose-rate systems shorten the treatment times to minutes. Both medium and high dose rates are departures from the original systems and their safe usage calls for the use of dose-rate correction factors and/or increased fractionation.

In all the treatments during the active phase, γ-radiation is given off from the sources in the uterus and vagina and spreads three-dimensionally through the pelvis, giving a high dose to the tissues close to the sources and a rapidly falling dose to the different tissues as it spreads outwards. There is a very wide range of techniques in use but they all produce isodose patterns that are remarkably similar. Looked at in an anteroposterior plane the distribution is pear shaped and in the lateral plane it is more banana shaped (Fig. 13). The practical result is a unique, inhomogeneous dose distribution that has to be integrated into an external-beam treatment.

Practical intracavitary therapy

Under most circumstances the patient is placed in the lithotomy position and the cervix and vagina examined. The extent of any vaginal involvement should be noted and checked against the original examination under anaesthesia findings. If the disease is extending down the vagina it may be helpful to place a 'dead' gold seed at the lower limit to aid treatment planning. The cervix is identified and the uterus cannulated carefully. Practical problems encountered include difficulty in identifying an os, creating a false passage, and uterine perforation. It is not unusual to find the os more easily by digital examination. Sometimes the uterus may contain pus. This should be drained, cultured, and the patient rested for a few days to allow any infection to settle before introducing radiation sources. If the os cannot be identified or the endocervix is solid due to carcinoma or previous surgery, a second attempt after some external-beam therapy or in the knee—chest anaesthetic position may allow satisfactory cannulation.

The cervix is dilated sufficiently to allow the standard diameter (6 mm) intrauterine tubes to be inserted. The length of the uterus and its position in the pelvis should be noted. If the uterus is retroverted, an attempt is made to move it into a midline, anteverted position. This is not possible in the presence of advanced disease and it may encourage the therapist to abort the procedure and use further external-beam therapy to supplement the initial treatment.

Typically the uterine cavity will be 4—8 cm long. An intrauterine tube is inserted up to the length of the cavity without distending the uterus and with a flange arranged to sit on the cervix (Fig. 14). A vaginal applicator or applicators are then introduced to allow coverage of the identified vaginal disease and the combined applicators are packed with gauze or fixed by a harness or clamp into position. At this point, weak radiation sources may be introduced into the applicator and an ionization chamber inserted into the rectum and/or bladder to estimate the radiation exposure of these organs. Orthogonal anteroposterior and lateral radiographs are taken for dosimetry purposes. In an attempt to define the

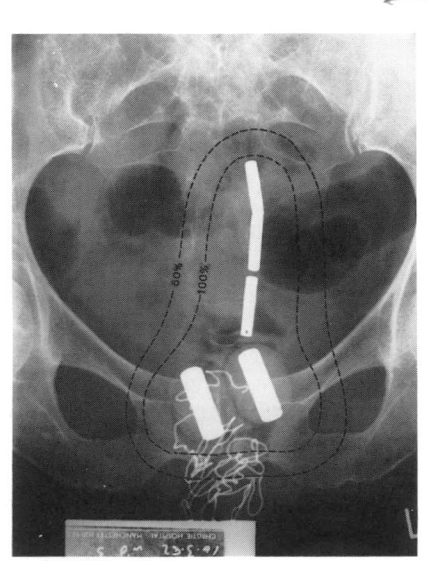

(a)

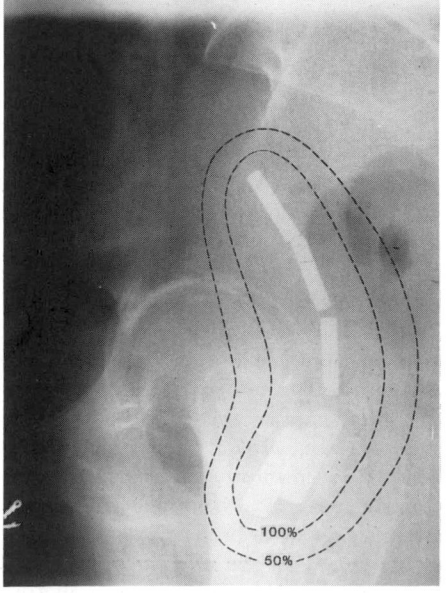

(b)

Fig. 13 (a) Anteroposterior and (b) lateral radiographs illustrating the typical distribution of dose from intracavitary applicators pre-loaded with Ra/Cs. The dotted lines illustrate all points receiving (a) 100 per cent and (b) 50 per cent of the dose rate to the dosimetry point.

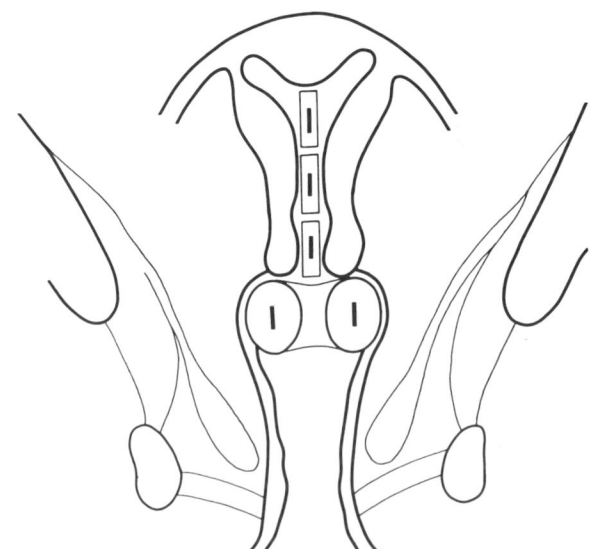

Fig. 14 Diagram illustrating the correct positioning of applicators.

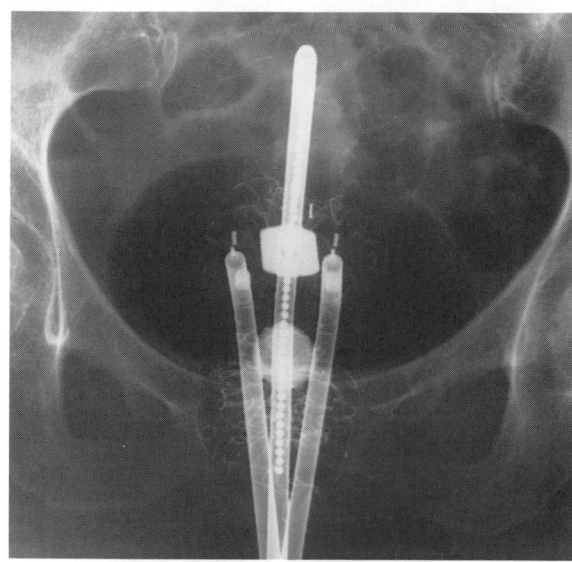

(a)

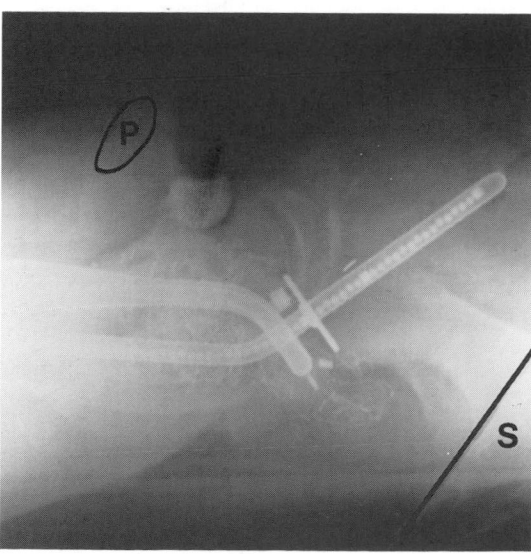

(b)

Fig. 15 (a) Anteroposterior and (b) lateral radiograph of pelvis showing cervix applicators correctly positioned with visible packing between (i) the rectum and (ii) the bladder and the sources. There is a catheter in the bladder containing 3 cc of radio-opaque contrast in the balloon. The bladder has been emptied and air introduced to allow the posterior bladder wall to be visualized.

position of normal tissues at risk from radiation injury therapists are encouraged to introduce a contrast-containing, Foley catheter balloon into the bladder; some also use rectal markers and/or air in the bladder to achieve definition of the critical walls of these organs (Fig. 15).

Dosimetry for intracavitary therapy remains in a state of evolution. The original therapists used milligrams of radium×number of hours of treatment (mg h). This was always a gross oversimplification and did not express the distribution of sources clearly. The Manchester system introduced the concept of 'point A'. This was originally conceived of as a point in a volume of steep dose gradient lateral to the cervix and was defined in ideal geometry as being 2 cm vertical to the upper surface of the vaginal

Manchester C.C.U. Treatment point A
Large ovoid, spacer, long central tube

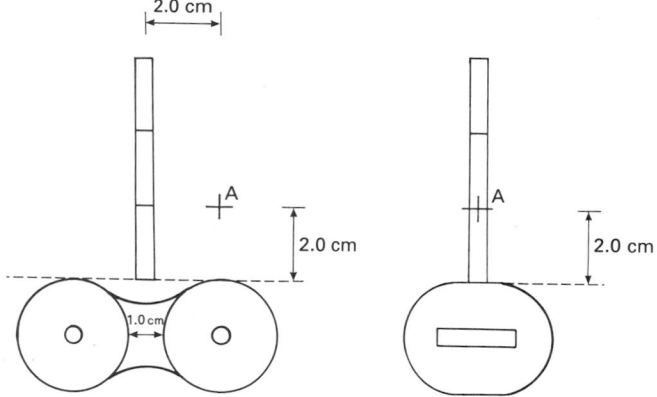

Fig. 16 The definition of point A.

applicator and 2 cm lateral to the mid-plane of the uterine applicator in the pelvis (Fig. 16). Its use was based on a series of clinical studies and involved standard dose distributions from standard radium-loading patterns. Used in this way, dosage has been shown to be closely related to cancer control and major radiation morbidity. It is, however, not freely translatable to other systems.

It is very common practice in the United Kingdom to express dosage of intracavitary therapy at point A. This must always be accompanied by a description of the radiation source-loading pattern, fractionation, overall time, and the dose rate at point A of the treatment. However, the choice of a point in a volume of rapidly changing dose rate has provoked considerable debate and criticism over many years. There is a consensus that radiation tolerance to intracavitary therapy is dependent on the tolerance of the pericervical tissues. In the absence of homogeneity of dose and with steep gradients, no practical, acceptable alternative to point A has emerged from decades of debate. Many centres internationally used point A, as well as other 'bladder', 'vaginal', or 'rectal' dosimetry points that they define themselves. North American centres following the dominant Houston School still use equivalent mg h of radium. A more radical approach emerging from the Paris school has been the concept of a 60 Gy isodose 'envelope' whose volume is defined by the maximum height, width, and depth of the 60 Gy intracavitary isodose line; this concept is under international scrutiny at the moment.

The dose distributions resulting from these intracavitary treatments are uniquely different from those in all other radiotherapy practice. The intrauterine and intravaginal sources combine to give a very high dose to the uterus and cervix, but at no point is it homogeneous and it is best represented by a series of isodose lines that can be drawn around the applicators. These demonstrate the very steep gradients of dose being delivered to the tissues and any cancer surrounding the cervix and uterus (Fig. 17). In a typical treatment the dose around the applicator is three or four times that given in any other radiotherapy treatment. Fortunately the uterus is very tolerant to these doses. As the dose falls throughout the pelvis, all the adjacent tissues are subjected to inhomogeneous exposure. In practice, the size and thickness of the cervix and uterus, the bulk of the tumour, and the position of the bladder, rectum, sigmoid, and small bowel are variable between patients, which means that standard applicators 'see' very variable amounts of these important normal tissues. Using modern systems

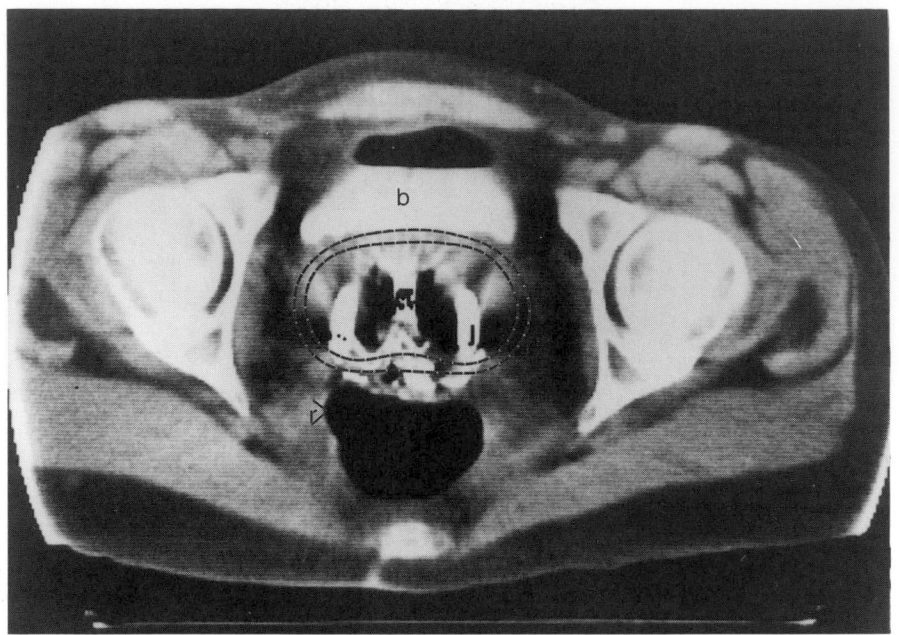

Fig. 17 Pelvic computerized tomographic scan in a patient with carcinoma of the cervix undergoing intracavitary therapy. The scan is through the level of the ovoids. The bladder (b) and rectum (r) are clearly visible. The two isodose lines shown illustrate all points receiving 100 per cent (inner) and 50 per cent (outer) of the dose to point A.

with computerized tomographic dosimetry, different dose distributions in relation to the applicators can be computed and the three-dimensional aspects of the treatment appreciated. In this way, radiotherapeutically dangerous situations that were not previously identified can be avoided.

Radiation tolerance to intracavitary therapy is expressed by the tissues of a middle zone surrounding the cervix, including the central gynaecological organs and variable amounts of bladder, terminal ureter, and large and small bowel. The combined impact of the steep dose gradients and the steep dose–response curves for control of human cancer means that, in practice, effective tumour cell 'kill' is not possible with intracavitary therapy outside a volume defined by a line approximately 4 cm lateral to the applicators.

Whatever dosimetry system is used the dose to be delivered should be qualified by a statement of the type and size of applicator, the radionuclide and its strength, the loading pattern, the fractionation, and the overall time. In addition, in modern practice the dosage should include a statement of the dose rate employed. The tolerance of normal tissue is usually expressed as a percentage of the dose delivered and typical allowances in the Manchester system are 66 per cent of the point A dose to the rectum and 80 per cent to the bladder.

With dosimetry complete the intracavitary therapy is delivered and the applicators are then carefully removed. Schedules for the management of carcinoma of the cervix may involve the use of a single or multiple (up to 12) intracavitary therapy sessions, depending on the technique being used.

The system described above is designed to treat cervical and upper vaginal disease in patients with an intact uterus that can be cannulated. Regular changes have to be introduced to cope with the patient with vaginal disease extending down the vagina, even to the introitus or the patient in whom the uterus cannot or is not available for cannulation. In the first, the lower limit of the disease

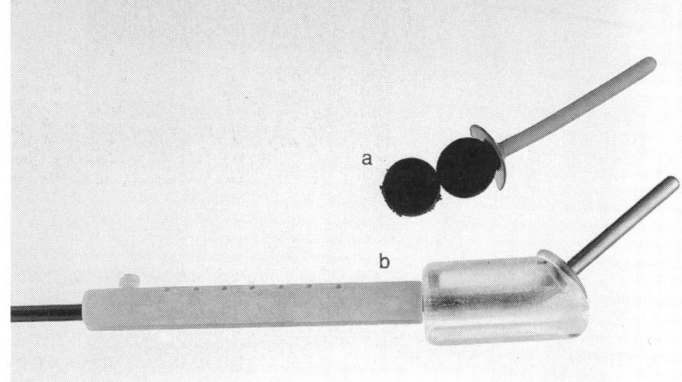

Fig. 18 Applicator arrangement in (a) classical and (b) afterloading system to allow coverage of lower vaginal extension of disease.

should have been marked at the time of the original examination. A vaginal applicator is inserted to allow coverage of that lower limit (Fig. 18). Here the vaginal component can be loaded to draw the treatment down below the disease. This approach changes the isodose pattern, flattening out and elongating the 'pear' and 'banana' distributions and reducing the dose that a standard loading and time will contribute to point A. The treatment also exposes an increased length of the urethra and the anterior rectal wall to higher doses of radiation, increasing the risk of injury to normal tissues. The effect of all these changes has to be summated and a balance between tumour dose and normal tissue dose achieved.

The second, regular, 'non-standard' treatment is that of the vaginal vault, commonly used in the post-hysterectomy patient. Here there is very little scope for significant variations in treatment because of the limited volume available for arrangement of sources. A typical approach is to use standard vaginal applicators for a single, protracted treatment. The technique is easily modified to modern

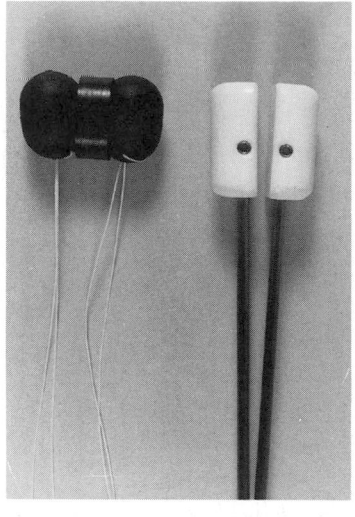

(a)

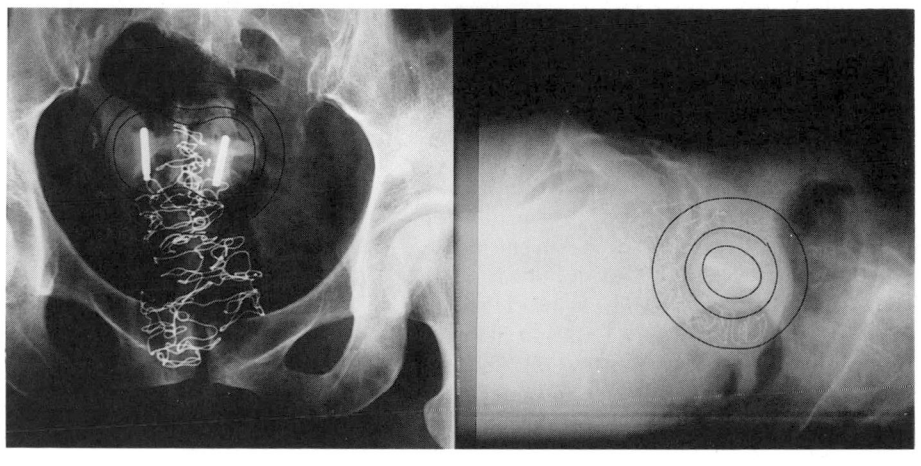

(b)

Fig. 19 (a) Anteroposterior view of classical and afterloading vaginal applicators correctly arranged; (b) dose distribution from vaginal applicators.

applicators and can be employed on an out-patient, fractionated basis using high-dose-rate equipment (Fig. 19).

Three other systems are regularly used internationally; Paris, Stockholm, and Houston. The Paris system employs weak low dose-rate sources arranged in an even, linear pattern and typically uses single, protracted, 6–8 day treatments. Standard applicators have been discarded in favour of individual, 'moulinage', vaginal applicators fashioned from vaginal impressions taken at the time of the initial examination. Dosimetry includes the concept of the volume enclosed within a 60 Gy isodose line. The Stockholm system typically employs heavier loading patterns and short (less than 24 h), multiple-fraction (2–3) treatments, and uses point A for dosimetry. The Houston (Fletcher) system employs unique applicators that incorporate shields made of tungsten within the anterior and posterior surfaces of the vaginal applicators to reduce bladder and rectal dosage. Dosimetry is based on a combination of mg h radium equivalent and bladder, rectum, and lymph node dosimetry points.

All of these systems have been adapted to modern radionuclides, applicators, and afterloading. There are enormous numbers of small differences between them but the limited size of the uterus and vagina and the radiation tolerance of the adjacent tissues severely constrain real, individual differences. As a result the functional similarities between the different treatment systems outweigh the differences. In spite of this, prospects for international rationalization are poor.

The practical result of intracavitary brachytherapy is, as outlined earlier, a unique, inhomogeneous dose distribution that has to be integrated into an external-beam treatment to produce acceptable results in terms of survival and complications.

External-beam radiotherapy

Although the unique intracavitary systems contribute importantly to the radical radiotherapy of carcinoma of the cervix, the majority of patients receive a lot of their treatment from their external-beam component. The treatment volume, dose, fractionation, and overall time varies very significantly between centres but there are a number of basic principles that guide decision making.

In modern radiotherapy all patients with carcinoma of the cervix receiving external-beam therapy are treated with megavoltage equipment. In developing countries, telecobalt techniques can be used successfully but in Europe and North America it is considered advantageous to employ megavoltage techniques on linear accelerators of 4–20 MV.

In the external-beam treatment of carcinoma of the cervix the volume to be treated initially is variable, depending on the stage and volume of the primary tumour and on any other information about possible metastatic nodal disease in the true pelvis, common iliac, or para-aortic regions. The principal problem is balancing the dose against a volume whose extent may be being dictated by increasingly insecure information. Certainly, at the end of the clinical examination under anaesthetic, there should be a clear idea of some of the components of the volume of the primary tumour and its position in the pelvis. The limits of vaginal disease identified are usefully marked by inert tissue markers. The upper limit of the fundus of the uterus normally is relatively easily identified and the whole uterus should be within the primary target volume. The upper lateral and posterolateral true pelvis is difficult to examine by any technique short of laparotomy and certainly should be included for possible primary tumour and early lymph node spread.

The lower limit of the initial target volume is normally the pelvic floor, which runs through the mid–obturator foramen or a minimum of 1 cm below the lower limit of identified vaginal disease if it extends down the vagina below this standard line. The lateral margins should clearly encompass the true pelvis. The upper limit is more difficult and variable. The practical situation is that the limit can be placed above the true pelvic brim (and uterine fundus) (Fig. 20), up to the limits of the upper sacrum, so taking in the common iliac vessels (Fig. 21) or shaped further to take in different levels of the para-aortic region. Each different upper level reduces the dose that can be delivered in any period of time without an increase in normal tissue morbidity. In routine treatment, that is when nodal status is unknown, there is no evidence of advantage in treating above the level of the upper sacrum. Patient tolerance is improved by reducing the volume of the field further in all except very thin patients by using a box technique instead of a parallel-opposed pair of fields. The lateral field dimensions depend on the primary tumour volume but the posterior fields should be a minimum of 2 cm behind the posterior fornix of the vagina and the anterior limit of the field through the posterior pubis. This type of target volume will encompass the primary tumour and the lymph node areas of the true pelvis and adjacent nodes including the common and internal iliac. It can be reduced to include only the true pelvis without identifiable detriment. Some centres attempt

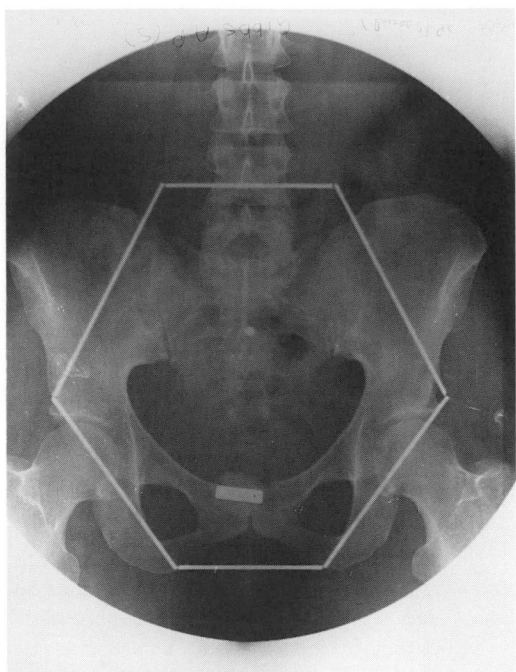

Fig. 21 Anteroposterior simulator radiograph of a large, trimmed field designed to irradiate the primary disease and the immediate draining nodes.

to reduce the initial volume further by introducing a standard or individually shaped wedge that theoretically shields the tissues to be irradiated in the intracavitary treatment. Matching the penumbra of a homogeneous beam to the inhomogeneous intracavitary dose distribution is difficult theoretically. Such a wedge can only really be used in a parallel pair set-up when external-beam therapy is given after intracavitary therapy.

Combining external-beam and intracavitary therapy

The intracavitary component of the treatment, while clinically advantageous, adds a number of special problems related to the decisions about the balance between the two types of treatment, their timing, and the difficulty of matching a potentially homogeneous treatment to an intrinsically inhomogeneous, irregular, individual treatment volume.

Balance

The balance between the external-beam and intracavitary components has evolved through empirical observation over many decades. At the end of a course of external-beam therapy the acute tolerance of the true pelvis to that style of homogeneous therapy has been reached but some limited local tolerance of the uterus, vagina, and parametrial tissues remains. This can be reached by using an intracavitary treatment in one of the standard systems. Dosage should be based on radium treatment times, modified to allow for any significant changes in dose rate, fractionation, and overall time.

Timing

Theoretically, if an attempt is to be made to match the dose distribution from intracavitary therapy to that for external-beam therapy, it would be sensible to do the intracavitary therapy first because the individual anatomy of the patient dictates some of the features of the dose distribution. In practice such an approach is

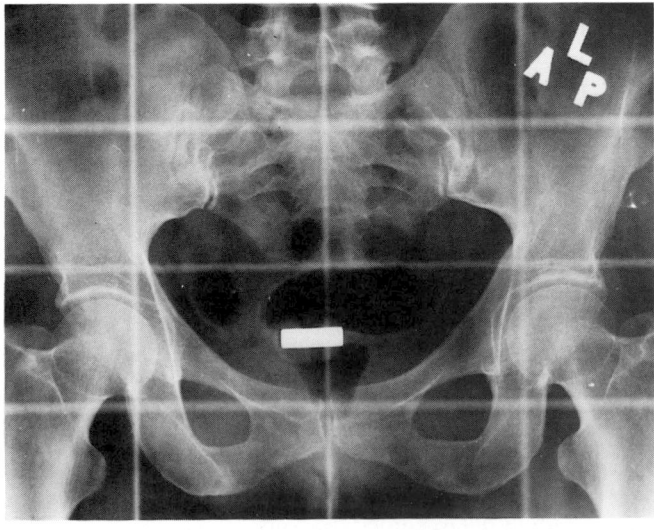

Fig. 20 Anteroposterior simulator radiograph of a small-field pelvic treatment; a vaginal ovoid has been placed against the cervix.

not usually followed because, even if the point A dosage is identical among a group of patients, the size and the position of the uterus and the size of the upper vagina added to the different 'anatomy' of the primary tumour means that a range of individual, inhomogeneous treatments occur between treatments in patients. To compound the problem, uterine cannulation and good applicator positioning are commonly inhibited by large, untreated, primary tumours. Finally, multiple treatments in the individual patient may produce different dose distributions and in low/medium dose-rate therapy the applicators may move with the pelvic floor during the time of an individual treatment. Certainly, in patients whose pelvis is not fixed the applicators tend to settle into the pelvis over the first 24 h.

As a result of the need to shrink locally advanced disease down to a mimimum volume for intracavitary therapy and to improve the anatomy from a technical point of view, the majority of centres start with external-beam therapy and add the intracavitary component towards the end or following completion of the treatment. To some extent it may depend on how many intracavitary treatments are planned. Single treatments are best given immediately or shortly after X-ray therapy; multiple, high dose-rate treatments may have to be integrated into the later part of the external-beam treatment to ensure an efficient management scheme.

Matching

It is not possible to match an irregular, inhomogeneous, three-dimensional target volume to an homogeneous external-beam therapy, even if the volume is modified by individual treatment wedges. The best that can be done is to avoid overdosage but at the expense of compounding the inhomogeneity. 'Matching' is therefore best approached in terms of the tolerance of normal tissues rather than physics and the aim is good local pelvic control with minimum morbidity.

Dose, fractionation, and time

The radiation tolerance of homogeneous pelvis/extended pelvic treatment is dictated by the tissues of the central pelvis, particularly the bladder and large and small bowel. Tolerance doses for the different types of volume described are shown in Table 2. From the point of view of the lateral pelvis/para-aortic region this is certainly acute tolerance; boost techniques in these areas have not been shown to improve cure and may increase morbidity. In addition, remembering that the majority of cancers are squamous cell carcinomas, it is immediately apparent that only small and radiosensitive nodal spread in extended pelvic fields can hope to be controlled by this type of radiation schedule.

Final dosage

A radical course of external-beam therapy does not exceed the tolerance of the gynaecological tissues and with each regimen there is some scope for intracavitary treatment. The dosage and number of fractions varies enormously, depending on factors previously described. Both the external-beam and the intracavitary dosage can be considered at one point, for example point A or at a number of chosen points; when allowances for overall treatment time, dose rate, and the number of fractions have been taken into account a balance between these treatments can be achieved, although the doses cannot truly be added together. Typical intracavitary tolerance dosages using the Manchester system are included in Table 2.

Table 2 Dose, fractionation, and time

Volume	External dose (cGy)	Fractions	Time in days	LDR Intra-cavitary fractions	Dose (cGy)
True pelvis	4500	20	28	1	200–2500
Extended pelvis	4000	20	28	1	3250–3750
Para-aortic and pelvis	3500	20	28	1	3250–3750

Variations on the standard radical radiotherapy approach

Haemorrhage

Patients who are bleeding heavily at the time of presentation can be helped considerably by an early intracavitary treatment either before or during the external-beam therapy. Bleeding normally stops within a week. It is best not to give all the available intracavitary therapy during the external-beam course if possible but reserve some for the end when optimum intracavitary conditions will exist.

Early disease

Patients with small-volume disease (stage I or even stage IIa) and of good histological type can be treated very successfully by intracavitary therapy alone. This is an excellent approach in older women when two standard insertions to radical intracavitary dosage can produce good cure rates without significant morbidity.

Destructive disease

Patients with very destructive disease are sometimes unsuitable for intracavitary therapy because the uterine canal cannot be identified and they have to be managed by external-beam therapy alone or external-beam therapy supplemented by limited intravaginal brachytherapy. They do less well and their treatment carries a danger of increased morbidity. At the end of the standard pelvic treatment, further small-volume, external-beam therapy may be focused on to the cervix and uterus and limited further treatment can be given.

Stump carcinoma

Subtotal hysterectomy is no longer an acceptable surgical treatment for benign gynaecological disease but there remains a small number of patients who developed carcinoma in a residual cervical stump following hysterectomy many years ago or patients in whom the cervix could not be removed due to technical problems. In this group there is either very little or no uterine canal and standard intracavitary therapy is not possible. External-beam therapy proceeds normally to tolerance. Sometimes a short intracanal source can be placed to complement the vaginal sources at the time of intracavitary therapy but the dose distribution is suboptimal and the risk of radiation injury as a result of the intracavitary therapy is higher.

Pregnancy

Intercurrent pregnancy is now exceptionally rare in the United Kingdom, although it remains a problem in developing countries. Early, operable carcinoma of the cervix should be dealt with by Wertheim's hysterectomy and advanced disease by radical radiotherapy. The timing of the procedures may be adjustable by a very few weeks if the pregnancy is wanted and approaching fetal viability.

Otherwise treatment should proceed normally. If the patient is treated by radical radiotherapy a spontaneous abortion will occur after a week or 10 days of external-beam treatment. Rarely it may be necessary to perform a hysterectomy if a poor cervical dilatation is anticipated or realized when radiotherapy is initiated.

Radiation reactions

All patients treated radically for carcinoma of the cervix will develop some degree of acute pelvic reaction of varying severity. The acute reaction is a consequence of radiation-induced injury of the epithelial tissues involved in the target volume. The late reaction is a consequence of arteriolar narrowing through a process of endarteritis proliferans and of mesenchymal depopulation.

Because the cervix sits in the centre of the pelvis surrounded by so many different normal genitourinary and gastrointestinal tissues, all of which may independently be included to a variable amount in the target volumes both for intracavitary and external-beam therapy, the type of reactions and their severity can be unpredictably variable, even if a standard treatment is given to a group of patients.

The most consistent, acute radiation reaction is a change of bowel habit due to the combined impact of treatment on small bowel, sigmoid, and rectum. This normally causes increased bowel movements with loose stools and some colic approximately 10–14 days after starting therapy. In most patients this appears quite quickly over approximately 24 h and can be initially quite severe but it usually settles on bulking agents containing ispaghula husk into a manageable though abnormal bowel habit. It will persist until 3–4 weeks after therapy and may then settle completely. Some patients develop a more acute severe reaction and can require admission to hospital and management as subacute intestinal obstruction. Clinically they appear to have signs of severe peritonitis but they settle quickly and well with conservative management; laparotomy should be avoided without some other evidence of intra-abdominal sepsis or perforation. In some patients the severity of the acute reaction is such that even when it settles it precludes further external-beam radiotherapy and an alternative surgical or intracavitary approach may be required.

A less consistent acute reaction is experienced by the bladder, where dysuria and/or frequency may be seen at approximately the same time as the bowel reaction. If it is radiation induced it tends to be sterile to culture. It is difficult to treat beyond the use of symptomatic measures including analgesics and antispasmodics but settles quickly unless it is complicated by infection or post-operative bladder atonia.

While these acute reactions are going on, radiation fibrin may be visible on the cervix but this is usually asymptomatic and vaginal bleeding and/or discharge are more likely to be a consequence of the primary tumour than the radiation itself. Uterine infection and parametritis can rarely be aggravated by external-beam therapy and cause increasing signs of infection needing antibiotics and/or surgical drainage. The acute radiation reactions due to intracavitary therapy are similar, although less severe and shorter lasting than those from external-beam treatment.

All acute radiation reactions are normally settled by 6–8 weeks. During these weeks the acute mucosal reaction in the vagina can cause fibrinous adhesions to form, particularly in the part exposed to intracavitary therapy (normally the upper third). If these are allowed to persist the vagina can shorten and narrow to the point where cervix examination and intercourse are impossible. It is sensible practice to encourage the patient to use a vaginal dilator every day after treatment for the first 6 weeks and two or three times weekly for 3 months; in this way, adhesions can be avoided.

Approximately 2–4 months after starting treatment, premenopausal women will develop menopausal symptoms of variable severity if their ovaries were still in the pelvis during treatment or were included in any radiotherapy field. This has become an increasing problem, since larger numbers of younger patients have developed invasive carcinoma of the cervix. A positive decision needs to be made about whether to institute hormone replacement therapy. There is no evidence that squamous carcinoma of the cervix and even adenocarcinoma of the cervix are hormone-sensitive tumours, although they can be shown to have weak oestrogen and/or progesterone receptors and a policy of active hormonal therapy should be encouraged in all women experiencing this problem under the age of 45. The problem in this group is cooperation and normal, cyclical hormone replacement therapy may not be acceptable. In the post-hysterectomy patient and in the majority of post-radiotherapy patients there is no residual viable endometrium and in these groups a policy of continuous oral oestrogen therapy or subcutaneous implant may prove the most satisfactory solution to a difficult problem.

Late tissue changes in the surrounding pelvic tissues are inevitable after radical radiotherapy but their range, severity, and time of onset are very variable.

The majority of patients settle after their acute reactions and remain well for a minimum of 6 months. From that time until the patient's death from any cause they remain at some risk from a late genitourinary or gastrointestinal complication. These are usually identified by tissue and by severity. International grading systems commonly group them into three or four categories. A useful system developed in Europe groups complications into:

- Group 1: minor symptomatic disturbance;

- Group 2: disturbance of function requiring investigation and treatment but responding usually to conservative therapy;

- Group 3: injury requiring surgical treatment or producing major long-term morbidity;

- Group 4: death from the complication.

No matter which tissue is manifesting the damage and, in most situations it is a single tissue, the radiational damage is a consequence of stromal and vascular change that produces thinning or ulceration, neovascularization, and/or fibrosis. These reactions manifest themselves as spontaneous bleeding, disordered function, ulceration, perforation, and even fistula formation. Gastrointestinal symptoms may appear from 6 months to 10 years after treatment. Genitourinary complications more commonly appear between 1 and 4 years. The earlier reactions can appear suddenly, be troublesome, and then settle spontaneously. Later reactions are more insidious, fibrotic, and rarely reversible but can stabilize with care. Common syndromes that need to be recognized and identified are:

(1) painless haematuria due to posterior bladder wall telangiectasia (usually 1–2 years after treatment);

(2) painless, fresh, rectal bleeding with or without a change of bowel habit (commonly 6–18 months after treatment);

(3) mild, chronic frequency due to reduced bladder capacity (2–4 years after treatment).

Unfortunately, some complications require surgical relief or correction. The decision has to be made on an individual basis but it is important to consider radiation-induced complications in the differential diagnosis of problems encountered after therapy as they are potentially much less lethal than recurrence and some, for example small bowel stenosis or sigmoid perforation, can be corrected completely by surgery. Unusual late complications after radiotherapy can include malabsorption syndromes, owing to small-bowel injury and second primary malignancy, particularly in the bladder or lower gastrointestinal tract. These latter tumours are particularly difficult to deal with as radiotherapy is not an option and surgically the tissues are extremely difficult to manipulate because of underlying late radiational vascular damage.

Even with very careful treatment planning and good intracavitary technique, centres treating patients with carcinoma of the cervix radically by radiotherapy see major (grades 3 and 4) complications in up to 5 per cent of cases.

Susceptibility to radiation injury

Some late radiation reactions appear to be entirely sporadic, others are a consequence of treating patients with predisposing factors. General susceptibility to severe acute and late reactions is seen in patients with well-established diabetes mellitus or generalized vasculitis. Local pelvic factors that predispose to injury are previous pelvic surgery, including minor procedures like tubal ligation, pelvic inflammatory disease, or previous severe infection. They have in common the development of adhesions between the gynaecological organs, the uterus, bowel, and bladder, which inhibits normal peristalsis and allows loops of bowel to be held close to the uterus within the target volumes during the whole of the treatment period.

THE CHOICE OF INITIAL TREATMENT

A large number of factors, including age, stage, and general medical condition, help to influence the decision about which approach should be used in the initial management of individual patients. These factors should be weighed up carefully at the time of presentation. Ideally the patient should have a single, definitive procedure that is curative on its own. Combined treatments are commonly associated with increased morbidity. The extent of the treatment both surgically and radiotherapeutically should be the minimum required to achieve cure. Radical surgery and radiotherapy are associated with an increased risk of long-term complications.

Surgical techniques have much to commend them as a radical approach to new patients presenting to the gynaecologist. The advantage to the patient is a definitive procedure carried out on one day with a post-operative healing phase and a low risk of long-term injury to normal, healthy, adjacent tissues. Thus, the majority of women with CIN can be dealt with as out-patients using nothing more than light sedation and/or a local anaesthetic. This is particularly true of ectocervical, CIN III disease. The response to treatment can be easily visualized and monitored and there is a high expectation of initial cure. This appears to be maintained in the majority of patients. The long-term natural history of this early disease of the ectocervix and the adjacent endocervix and vaginal vault is unknown but the general impression at present is that the response will be maintained in the majority of patients.

This surgical strength is continued into endocervical CIN III where cone biopsy, now often done under colposcopic control, is often definitive and simple hysterectomy is available to clear residual and intraepithelial disease. Even when microinvasion is present, simple hysterectomy with its low operative mortality and low

risk of any significant post-operative morbidity is a reliable curative approach.

The more invasive, stage-Ib disease begins to present quite a range of problems and raises some questions about the choice of initial treatment. Many of the patients are younger (30–50 years), medically fit, and may have small-volume tumours that do not significantly distort the normal anatomy. They are an ideal group for Wertheim's hysterectomy, with a greater than 90 per cent chance of cure if the pelvic lymph nodes are not involved and even a 50 per cent chance if they are. Some schools, for example Paris and Oxford, have always advocated a combined approach to this type of disease, with pre-operative intracavitary therapy given to a dose that is approximately 10–15 per cent below tolerance followed within 4–6 weeks by Wertheim's hysterectomy. This approach produces excellent results in experienced hands, with very low levels of central pelvic failure and apparently low levels of major morbidity, but it does involve the use of a significant dose of radiation, which can impair post-operative healing and will induce a menopause in pre-menopausal women. Trials comparing Wertheim's hysterectomy alone against pre-operative intracavitary therapy and Wertheim's hysterectomy have not been made, which makes a true comparison of the approaches difficult. In view of the good results from both approaches it would be a difficult trial to mount, even if there was a genuine will and would require a large number of patients.

Stage Ib, invasive carcinoma also includes patients with increasingly bulky primary tumours, distorting the normal anatomy, of both proliferating ectocervical and invasive endocervical type. These can even be large enough to fill the true pelvis without extending to the vagina and parametrium. Using modern imaging techniques and careful examination under anaesthetic they can be separated from higher stages of disease. As they become larger they become increasingly unsuitable for a primary Wertheim's hysterectomy, with or without pre-operative intracavitary therapy. A more realistic approach is a radical course of pelvic radiotherapy including external beam and intracavitary to tolerance dosage. The response to initial treatment can be watched and many patients prove to have radioresponsive disease that shrinks down during the external-beam component of the treatment. They can proceed to satisfactory intracavitary therapy. Some patients only regress partially and/or remain unsuitable for intracavitary therapy after waiting even 2–4 weeks; most experienced gynaecologists would be prepared to carry out a subfascial hysterectomy on this group. This operation is less radical than Wertheim's and is tolerated by patients who have had significant doses of radiation. The selection of patients with stage-I disease for a primary surgical or initial radical radiotherapy approach varies depending on the experience and training of the team involved and is not always easy.

Radical radiotherapy remains an acceptable approach to all degrees of stage-I disease if other factors, for example age or general condition, makes the risk of the longer anaesthetic and the surgical procedure appear too high. Radical intracavitary therapy alone can be a satisfactory technique in older patients with extensive CIN III disease, microinvasive carcinoma, and small-volume, primary invasive carcinoma of the cervix. Radiation tolerance is probably slightly reduced by cone biopsy and certainly that approach can distort the normal anatomy and delay healing. Radical external-beam and intracavitary therapy can be an effective curative treatment in more bulky carcinomas of the cervix. The use of radical radiotherapy techniques does, however, increase the chance of late radiation changes of variable degree in the pelvis.

Two other groups of patients with stage-I disease are often considered for radical pelvic X-ray therapy. The first is of patients who, after Wertheim's hysterectomy, are considered to have a poor surgical clearance (less than 1 cm margin on the primary tumour), extensive vascular invasion, high-grade disease, or poor prognostic histological type, for example adenosquamous or small cell. It also includes patients with pelvic lymph node involvement. Post-operative pelvic radiotherapy including external beam sometimes supplemented by vaginal vault treatment is often offered to this group and will help local control. Its influence on survival has never been explored in the setting of a prospective trial. The other group who will benefit from radical radiotherapy of a post-operative type is the unusual patients with recurrent central disease after radical hysterectomy. It is a problem that is difficult to detect until the recurrence is of significant volume and can occur at the vault, in the parametrium, or in the middle and lower vagina.

Stage-II disease represents a more difficult primary surgical condition. Some patients with stage-II disease have small-volume, ectocervical disease involving the vaginal fornices and can be treated by Wertheim's hysterectomy or radical radiotherapy. The majority have disease infiltrating the parametrium, usually laterally, bringing it close to the ureters and sometimes into close proximity to the bladder and rectum. The primary, successful, surgical treatment of this type of disease is difficult and runs an increasing risk of post-operative morbidity. Only the occasional gynaecological oncologist attempts this type of disease surgically and the majority of patients are treated by radical radiotherapy techniques. Patients treated by primary surgery may warrant post-operative radiotherapy if, like stage-I patients, they have poor prognostic features.

Stage-III disease is, by consensus, primarily a radiotherapeutic problem. These patients often have bulky, infected tumours that lie close to the other pelvic organs. The treatment is difficult and associated with a high risk of pelvic failure and significant morbidity. This can eventually depend on the dose and technique employed, but the majority of centres in the United Kingdom would not expect a greater than 40 per cent overall 5 year survival, with approximately 40 per cent of the patients having pelvic failure and at least 5 per cent experiencing significant complications as a result of treatment. If patients have been properly staged, then there is no real scope for surgical salvage in recurrent/residual disease, although they should be amenable to surgical correction of the post-treatment injuries. Stage-IVa disease involving normally the bladder or occasionally the rectum is fortunately rare in the United Kingdom. If the patient has a fistula at the time of presentation, then they should not be offered radiotherapy. They may be suitable for one of the pelvic exenterative techniques described above and should be investigated and even explored surgically with that in mind if they appear suitable. Few stage-IV patients prove to be operable and fewer still achieve long-term survival but the chance should not be lost. Those with stage-IV disease involving the bladder but not causing a fistula may be offered a trial of radical, pelvic, external-beam therapy supplemented, if regression is good, by post-operative intracavitary therapy. Surprisingly, these patients do not inevitably develop a vesicovaginal fistula; in practice perhaps only 20 per cent will go on to do this. Patients presenting with disease outside the pelvis are normally incurable by radical surgical and/or radiotherapeutic techniques. Occasional patients have been described with histologically proven para-aortic nodal disease who have survived after radiotherapy involving the pelvis and the para-aortic region but they remain exceptional. If there was a successful form of systemic therapy available, this would be a more suitable approach to this type of disease.

RECURRENT/METASTATIC DISEASE

Even after the best radical radiotherapy or surgery, some patients develop further problems from recurrent and/or metastatic disease.

Recurrent primary disease represents the true failure of the surgical or radiotherapy treatment. The likelihood varies with the stage of disease and ranges from less than 5 per cent in stage I to 40 per cent in stage III. The symptoms may be vaginal bleeding and discharge associated with an ulcerated vault lesion or mass symptoms from an intrapelvic, non-ulcerating recurrence. The principal questions arising are as follows.

1. How extensive is the recurrence?

2. Is it also metastatic, for example to lymph nodes, liver, or lung?

3. What was the previous treatment?

4. What is the general medical and psychological status of the patient?

5. What is the renal function and are both kidneys functioning?

It is good practice to confirm the diagnosis histologically, carry out an examination under anaesthesia and cystoscopy, a chest radiograph, and, if the patient still appears suitable for further treatment, an intravenous urogram and abdominopelvic, computerized tomographic scan. Patients initially treated radiotherapeutically and free of evidence of metastatic disease should be considered for one of the exenterative procedures listed in the surgical section. Even limited central recurrences are not usually treatable by Wertheim's hysterectomy because the extensive radiational changes in the central pelvic tissues impair healing.

Patients who were initially treated surgically may still be treatable radically by radiotherapy using a post-operative technique previously described.

A special problem of recurrence that is a consequence of the use of more extensive cytological techniques in the post-operative patient is vaginal intraepithelial neoplasia (VAIN)±microinvasion. This condition is histologically very similar to the CIN changes and is graded in the same fashion. It is a very difficult condition to manage satisfactorily after previous radical radiotherapy for carcinoma of the cervix. Normally it is identified initially on the basis of cytological examination. Diagnostic problems include the fact that patients treated for carcinoma of the cervix can shed malignant cells from the upper vagina for many months or even years after treatment. Secondly, smears are difficult to interpret in VAIN and the condition can be patchy on the vault or very extensive on one or all of the vaginal walls. Cytological examination should be repeated and colposcopy done to confirm the diagnosis and map the extent of the process. Some patients have CIN-like, dystrophic changes due to oestrogen deficiency and the application of oestrogen creams to the vagina can reverse the abnormality.

If the disease is limited in volume and not invasive, then local destructive surgical techniques, for example cryotherapy or cautery, are possible. Local laser surgery is technically difficult. Extensive and microinvasive disease are best treated by vaginectomy. If this is not possible or acceptable, then vaginal intracavitary brachytherapy may be possible but it is likely to lead to vaginal shortening and narrowing and makes further monitoring of the vaginal changes very difficult.

Patients at any stage of primary disease are susceptible to the development of metastatic disease. Commonly this is in the lymph nodes of the upper posterior pelvis or para-aortic region. The early symptom is pain, usually at first unilateral in the pelvis and radiating into the leg. Often initial investigations are uninformative and the patient may go on to develop unilateral oedema and even neurological signs in the leg, due to the development of neural damage, particularly of the sciatic nerve anterior to the sacrum or around the sciatic notch. Present experience suggests that this group of patients is incurable by standard techniques. In view of the lymphatic and/or venous obstruction they are commonly anticoagulated and fitted with support stockings. Disease is best visualized by scanning (see Fig. 8) and radiation portals can be planned to encompass the known disease. The dose and fractionation are influenced by the volume, the patient's condition, and the extent and nature of any previous therapy. Commonly there may be some overlap with the previous radiotherapy volume. Doses of 25–30 Gy in eight fractions over 10 days can achieve useful, short-term palliation in approximately half of the patients with this syndrome.

Less common metastatic problems are in the lung. Their diagnosis is complicated by the fact that many patients with carcinoma of the cervix are cigarette smokers and are susceptible to the development of primary lung cancer. On following-up a group of patients treated radically for carcinoma of the cervix a range of chest malignancy is seen, including solitary endobronchial carcinoma, solitary peripheral lung masses, multiple pulmonary metastases, or malignant effusions. Radiotherapy can be used for endobronchial obstructive disease but other types of problem must be dealt with as if one was dealing with new primary disease, for example surgically for solitary, slow-growing, peripheral metastases, drainage plus chemotherapy for effusion, and chemotherapy or symptomatic care for multiple metastases.

Relatively unusual local spread of disease is to the lower anterior vagina where metastases can appear submucosally, in the labia, or in the nodes of the external inguinal region. Local radiotherapy techniques can help to palliate these problems but they are a manifestation of metastatic disease and essentially herald a new phase in the patient's illness. Liver, bone, and cerebral metastases remain very rare in patients treated for carcinoma of the cervix; the latter two can be improved by palliative radiotherapy techniques.

CHEMOTHERAPY

Until fairly recently, patients with carcinoma of the cervix rarely received chemotherapy. The introduction of new agents, more intensive regimens, and the increasing incidence of carcinoma of the cervix in younger, generally fitter patients has prompted a reappraisal. Special problems encountered in the chemotherapeutic management of these patients include a relatively higher incidence of some degree of obstructive uropathy in many patients with recurrent/metastatic/advanced disease and the difficulty of assessing and monitoring disease response in deep-seated disease in the pelvis or abdomen in patients who have previously been subjected to radical surgical or radiotherapeutic techniques.

There is no single agent that produces better than a 30 per cent overall response and all have a very low rate of complete responses. Combination regimens of many types have been investigated. The best include cisplatin supplemented by drugs like methotrexate, iphosphamide, mitomycin C, and bleomycin. The use of nephrotoxic drugs or drugs whose excretion depends on a renal route poses some management problems and pre-chemotherapeutic management must include a careful assessment of renal function with reassessment at regular intervals throughout the course. Renal rather than marrow toxicity is the problem in many of these patients.

The optimum approach to the patient with recurrent/metastatic disease not suitable for surgery or radiotherapy is to assess for chemotherapy and then, if the patient's general condition, psyche, renal and marrow function appear suitable, to give a trial of active chemotherapy using a standard combination regimen. Initial symptomatic responses including relief of pain and leg oedema may be seen in 1 month and objective responses in 2–3 months. Only if symptomatic and objective responses are achieved by this time should the patient be offered a full 6–8 month course of combination chemotherapy. Even the best responses turn out to be palliative in time in the majority of the patients and it is unusual for even complete responses to last more than 3 years. Relapse at the initial site of tumour is the common pattern of events. Good partial and complete remission may only be evident in 20–25 per cent of patients but they are very much appreciated by the responding individuals. The response to chemotherapy following a second relapse is rare and a second intensive regimen is not often tolerable or indicated.

The relatively high initial response to chemotherapy, the poor long-term control, the poor condition of some relapsing patients, and the high incidence of relapse at the primary site in patients with advanced disease has raised the question of the use of chemotherapy earlier in the natural history of the disease. Early intervention could take place at the time of primary, radical treatment, particularly in combination with radiotherapy in locally advanced disease, post-operatively in patients with multifocal nodal involvement, either with or as an alternative to pelvic radiotherapy, or pre-operatively in patients with locally bulky but operable disease. There is no agreed advantage to any of these approaches but the first two of these options are the subject of ongoing clinical trials. Because of the relative rarity of the individual problems they do not lend themselves to local trials and multicentre international studies are really needed in this field to see whether there is a place for this type of chemotherapy in the long-term management of carcinoma of the cervix.

RESULTS

The results of treating carcinoma of the cervix are published as individual series, clinical trials, national statistics, and, regularly, since 1937, in the international FIGO report. From a purist point of view there are considerable problems in comparing results between countries and centres of variable size with different facilities for assessment and treatment. In spite of these reservations the FIGO results have value because of the enormous number of patients included (20 653 in 1988). Over the last 30 years institutions reporting regularly have noted very stable overall mean survival results (78.6 per cent stage I, 55.9 per cent stage II, 30.9 per cent stage III, 11 per cent stage IV). These means conceal enormous ranges of individual results, even in a single country like the United Kingdom (Table 3). Some of the variation is a reflection of selection and statistical variability rather than a true difference in results.

Table 3 Carcinoma of the cervix: range of 5-year survival by stage—1979–81 (FIGO)

Stage	International	United Kingdom
I	55–95	60–80
II	40–85	46–61
III	15–60	15–30
IV	0–19	5–10

The mean incidence of the disease by stage internationally is 36.4 per cent stage I, 31.9 per cent stage II, 26.6 per cent stage III, and 5.1 per cent stage IV. Early-stage patients tend to be younger (mean 48.6 years stage I vs 58.4 years stage III) and they are more commonly selected for and treated surgically. As a result, primary surgical survival figures are biased by selection on the grounds of age, tumour volume, and general fitness. The most important, general prognostic features emerging from international studies are histology and nodal status. Patients with squamous cell carcinoma overall do better than those with adenocarcinoma, for example 5 year survival, stage-IIb squamous cell carcinoma 61.7 per cent, adenocarcinoma 48.2 per cent. (FIGO 1988). In the international results the adenocarcinoma group makes up 10 per cent of the series.

Individual series and clinical trials are inevitably selected to some extent, while national figures are prone to the errors intrinsic in registration and certification. However, not all the variability is a consequence of patient selection or a reflection of clinical skill. Compounding problems include the different care with which staging has been done and the variable volume of disease within each treatment stage. Other less important factors include the age of the patient and the general fitness of the population.

General rules that help to give a clearer idea of individual prognosis within the stage survival bands are as follows.

1. Within each stage, small-volume primary disease does better than large volume.

2. Young patients (less than 40 years) with stage-I disease do statistically better than older patients with the same level of disease.

3. Degree of differentiation, except when the rarer types of carcinoma are involved (see Pathology section), does not influence prognosis.

4. Squamous cell carcinoma does better than adenocarcinoma.

5. The presence of involved lymph nodes in the pelvis, particularly in the younger patient, implies a very poor prognosis, for example patients with stage-I disease treated surgically without involved nodes have a 5 year survival of 83.1 per cent while those with positive nodes only achieve a 53.8 per cent result, even after post-operative radiotherapy.

Now that the individual surgical skills and very similar radiotherapy techniques are available in most developed countries, it is really the balance of these prognostic factors, that is age, volume, histological type, and lymph node status, that determines the outcome in the individual patient.

PALLIATIVE TREATMENT

At the time of initial presentation the majority of patients are suitable for a trial of radical surgery or radiotherapy. Occasionally an elderly or medically frail woman with relatively early disease will not be fit for full radical treatment and an abbreviated course, normally based on a single, long, intracavitary treatment, may be given. At the least this will produce haemostasis and control discharge and in some patients excellent primary control may be achieved. A more difficult problem is the unfit patient presenting with stage-III or -IV disease. In the absence of fistulae a single intracavitary treatment or a short course of external-beam treatment may be beneficial temporarily in relieving distressing symptoms, particularly vaginal

haemorrhage and discharge, but an ultimate relapse in the symptoms is likely. Patients presenting with bowel or bladder fistulae should not be irradiated. A small number may be suitable for an exenteration procedure (see the section on surgery), but more commonly the problem will arise whether to offer a palliative urinary diversion or colostomy. This is a difficult individual decision in which the wishes of the patient and an assessment of her possible prognosis play an important part. Unless she is likely to live 4–6 months after the procedure, the combined catabolic impact of the surgery and the need to learn about stoma care mean that significant palliation will not be acquired and the procedure cannot be justified.

IMPROVING RESULTS

As stage is the most important prognostic factor, major efforts to aid early diagnosis are likely to be rewarded by an improvement in regional or international results. This has been most evident in Scandinavia, Canada, and the United States where overall mortality from the disease has fallen over the last two decades, due in part to the successful cytology programmes. These programmes can never sufficiently cover the population at risk or be sufficiently frequent to eliminate carcinoma of the cervix and a reduction to below one-third of the original incidence is not expected. It has also been noticed that patients developing invasive carcinoma between cytological examinations more commonly have aggressive, poorly differentiated carcinomas or endocervical, bulky disease.

Any successful programme of management for cervix cancer should not, however, concentrate on cytology alone. Early diagnosis of symptomatic disease should be encouraged by health education and making facilities for diagnostic assessment easily available to all women. The education of medical students and doctors in the need to examine symptomatic patients, along with teaching and understanding of the relative value of speculum examination, cytology, and colposcopy, is particularly important.

Better management also follows better pre-treatment assessment and is likely to follow the extended use of ultrasonography and magnetic resonance imaging. It awaits better techniques to detect early pelvic lymph node involvement. Potentially the biggest advance in the management of early-stage disease would follow the development of techniques to separate node-positive from node-negative patients without surgical intervention. Surgically, better pre-treatment assessment techniques would reduce unnecessary, extended surgery and help to limit complications. Radiotherapeutically, the constraint is the radiation tolerance of the normal female pelvis. Attempts have been made to improve results by the use of hyperbaric oxygen, hypoxic cell sensitizers, fast-neutron therapy, hyperthermia, and mitochondrial toxins, all without any consensus that therapeutic advantage has been gained. The present approach is to attempt to improve pelvic control in advanced disease by the use of combined chemotherapy and radiotherapy, but this is not of proven value and remains the subject of clinical trials.

Finally, any society that encourages the use of hysterectomy for benign disease in late pre-menopausal women, for example the United States, will have a reduced incidence of invasive carcinoma of the cervix without any further effort. The procedure does not, of course, eliminate the need for vault examination on a regular basis to detect early intraepithelial *in situ* or early invasive disease.

SUGGESTED READING AND REFERENCES

Incidence

Gardner M, Winter P, Taylor C, Acheson E (1983). *Atlas of cancer mortality in England and Wales*. Wiley, Chichester.

Howe G (1986). *Global geocancerology*. Churchill Livingstone, Edinburgh.

Office of Population Census and Surveys (1993). *Cancer statistics*, Registrations Series MB1, No. 20. HMSO, London.

Office of Population Census and Surveys (1993). *Mortality statistics*, Series DH2, No. 18. HMSO, London.

Epidemiology

Beral V (1985). Epidemiology and aetiology of cancers of the female genital tract. In *Clinical gynaecological oncology* (ed. J Shepherd and J Monaghan). Blackwell, Oxford.

Miller AB, Rawls WE (1981). Epidemiology of gynecologic cancer: I. Cervix. In *Gynecologic oncology* (ed. M Coppleson). Churchill Livingstone, Edinburgh.

Staging

Bears OH, Henson DE, Hutter R, Kennedy B (ed.) (1992). *Manual for staging of cancer* (4th edn). Lippincott, Philadelphia.

Pathology/colposcopy

Cartier R (1977). *Practical colposcopy*. Karger, Basel.

Radiology

Eddleston B (1990). The cervix. In *Radiology in the management of cancer* (ed. RJ Johnson, BE Eddleston, and RD Hunter), pp. 295–318. Churchill Livingstone, Edinburgh.

Surgery

Monaghan J (1985). The management of advanced and recurrent cervical cancer by pelvic exenteration. In *Clinical gynaecological oncology* (ed. J Shepherd and J Monaghan), pp. 84–96. Blackwell, Oxford.

Shepherd J (1985). Cervical cancer. The surgical management of early stage disease. In *Clinical gynaecological oncology* (ed. J Shepherd and J Monaghan), pp. 63–83. Blackwell, Oxford.

Radiotherapy

Coulter C, Mason P (1990). Cervix, endometrium and uterus. In *Treatment of cancer* (2nd edn) (ed. K Sikora and K Halnan). Chapman & Hall, London.

Fletcher G (1978). Squamous cell carcinoma of the uterine cervix. In *Textbook of Radiotherapy* (3rd edn) (ed. G Fletcher). Lea & Febiger, New York.

Hunter RD (1990). Carcinoma of the cervix. In *The radiotherapy of malignant disease* (2nd edn) (ed. R Pointon and G Ribeiro). Springer-Verlag, Berlin.

International Commission on Radiation Units (1985). *Report No. (38)*. ICRU.

Chemotherapy

Hoskins W, Perez C, Young R (1989). Gynecologic tumours. In *Cancer: principles and practice* (ed. V DeVita, S Hellman, and S Roseberg). Lippincott, Philadelphia.

FIGO Reports

FIGO (1988). *Annual report on the results of treatment in gynaecological cancer*, Vol. 21. Radiumhemmet, Stockholm.

9.4 Tumours of the endometrium and adnexa

C. GALLAGHER

ENDOMETRIAL CANCER

Introduction

Carcinoma of the endometrium is the most common gynaecological cancer in the United States, accounting for 34 000 new cases and 3000 deaths per year. It is the second most common pelvic malignancy in the United Kingdom. There is evidence to suggest that the disease is increasing in incidence, with a higher proportion of cases occurring in the younger age groups. The reported incidence is inevitably influenced by increasing screening, and improved diagnosis through hysteroscopy, an increasingly aged population, a broadening of pathological criteria, and, arguably, evidence of increased oestrogen usage. Endometrial cancer is more common in the more affluent countries of the world and there has also been a true increase in developing countries worldwide.

Endometrial cancer generally presents at an early age in its evolution when it can be cured by the primary surgery. Complacency in management however is to be firmly discouraged, as survival figures are poor for the less favourable cases and it is salient that 25 per cent of all women with endometrial cancer will die within 5 years of initial diagnosis often having presented with apparently early stage disease (Burket 1990).

There is therefore a need to identify the woman at high risk of recurrence and then consistently apply accurate and appropriate surgery, followed by individualized adjuvant therapy according to prognostic criteria, in order to improve survival.

Aetiology

Age

Endometrial cancer is essentially a disease of post-menopausal women with at least 80 per cent of cases occurring after the menopause. The maximum number of cases occur in the sixth decade of life with a median age of presentation of 61 years. Less than 5 per cent of cases occur in women under the age of 40 years and there is a decrease in age-specific incidence rates after the age of 65 years.

Obesity

Increased oestrogenic stimulation of proliferation in the endometrium is thought to raise the risk of malignant transformation by diminishing the apoptotic response to DNA alterations during cell division. Overweight post-menopausal women have increased conversion of androstenedione to oestrone in their peripheral subcutaneous fat. Sex hormone binding globulin levels are decreased causing an increase in free oestrogens at a cellular level. The risk of development of endometrial cancer is proportional to the degree of obesity (Shu Xias Ou 1992). The risk has been described as being increased 3-fold if a woman is between 9.5 and 23 kg overweight and 10-fold if she is greater than 23 kg overweight.

Medical disorders

Diabetes mellitus and hypertension are risk factors associated with endometrial cancer and also occur in conjunction with obesity and increasing age. The available data suggest that the risk of endometrial cancer is increased 2.8 times in women who are diabetic. Conversely reports vary regarding the incidence of diabetes mellitus (5–45 per cent) and hypertension (25–60 per cent) in patients with endometrial cancer. Immunodeficiency disorders and immunosuppressed states have been associated with the development of endometrial cancer as has a past history of pelvic irradiation.

Abnormal hormonal status

Excessive endogenous oestrogen stimulation may occur in patients with hormone secreting tumours (for example, ovarian granulosa cell) and in such conditions as polycystic ovary disease (Kistner 1970). Exogenous oestrogen has been implicated in the aetiology of endometrial cancer in patients with Turner's syndrome, in women taking sequential oral contraception (Silverberg and Makowski 1975) and in women who have inappropriately prescribed or administered oestrogen replacement therapy (Antunes et al. 1979; Collins et al. 1980; Elwood and Boges 1980; Shapiro et al. 1980, 1985; Kaufman et al. 1984). There is evidence to suggest that the inclusion of a progestogen in 'opposed' hormone replacement regimens reduces endometrial stimulation and results in a concomitant reduction in the incidence of uterine corpus cancer in developed Western populations. The increased usage of the oestrogen receptor blocker tamoxifen in the treatment and prophylaxis of breast cancer is a cause of concern because of its agonist effect on the endometrium. Many clinicians are encountering abnormal bleeding patterns in up to 30 per cent of patients taking tamoxifen and evidence on ultrasound and curettage of hyperplasia, but whether this results in an increase in neoplastic change in the endometrium as observed in the Scottish adjuvant tamoxifen study is currently the source of much debate.

Parity

Between 21 and 34 per cent of patients with endometrial cancer are nulliparous and the risk of developing the disease diminishes with increasing number of pregnancies. A nulliparous woman is twice as likely to develop endometrial cancer as a woman who has had one child and is three times more likely to develop the disease than a woman who has had five children.

Age of menopause

The association between the delayed cessation of menstruation and the development of endometrial cancer has long been recognized. Women who experience a spontaneous menopause after the age of 52 years have a two to four times increased risk of developing endometrial cancer compound with women who cease menstruation before the age of 49 years.

Family history

Positive family histories are present in approximately 15 per cent of cases. Endometrial adenocarcinoma occurs as one component in the Lynch type II family cancer syndrome in association with non-polyposis coli colon cancer, pancreatic cancer, and ovary and breast cancer. There is an autosomal dominant pattern of inheritance with increasing penetrance over successive generations. Patients with two or more first-degree relatives with one of these cancers of young (under 45 years old) age of onset are likely to have inherited the gene and should be offered genetic counselling and appropriate screening of those at risk to allay fears which are often only too well appreciated within the family prior to medical intervention (Farhi et al. 1986).

Demography

Endometrial cancer is typically a disease with a high incidence in Western developed countries of America and northern Europe. Associations have been drawn with the typical high fat and high protein Western diet and populations from low-risk areas that adopt such a dietary modification or migrate to a country of high incidence will assume the higher incidence of the disease within one generation.

Pathology

Histology

Macroscopically, endometrial cancer may occur in a localized or a diffuse form. When localized, the neoplastic change may be confined to a solitary polyp. More usually, the gross appearance is one of a diffuse exophytic growth which may occur in conjunction with adjacent hyperplastic or atrophic endometrium. The fundus and posterior wall of the uterus is more frequently involved than the anterior wall, with extension to the cervix being found in a minority of cases.

Histologically, by far the commonest cell type is a classical adenocarcinoma, with most series quoting incidence rates between 60 and 80 per cent. Variants include adeno-acanthomas which comprise adenocarcinomatous change with co-existent benign squamous metaplasia. These account for approximately 20 per cent of endometrial tumours with a further 14 per cent being of the adenosquamous type where both the glandular and squamous elements are considered to be malignant. Both mucinous and the high-risk papillary serous variants of endometrial adenocarcinoma are described, the latter accounting for some 5 per cent of tumours. Clear cell carcinomas of the endometrium are recognized. They probably arise from Müllerian structures and are most frequently seen in the older patient. They account for no more than 1–2 per cent of endometrial cancers but are generally thought to be of a more aggressive behaviour and carry a relatively poor prognosis as a result (Webb 1987). Primary squamous cell cancer of the endometrium is a real but rare entity and is regularly associated with a pyometra.

Metastatic malignancies occur and the endometrium is a favoured site of secondary spread from primary tumours arising in the cervix, the breast, the gastrointestinal tract, and kidney. Moreover, in women with endometrioid ovarian cancer, the uterine corpus is involved in up to one-third of cases either as a function of metastatic spread or as a concomitant primary tumour.

Hormonal sensitivity

Knowledge of the cyclical effects of oestrogen and progesterone upon the uterine epithelium and the existence of benign hyperplasia and dysplasia in association with disorders of hormonal regulation lead naturally to the supposition that endometrial cancers might also be manipulated via the hormonal milieu. Hormone receptors for oestrogen and progesterone were identified as specific cytosolic binding activity (Ehrlich et al. 1981; Billiet et al. 1982) the presence of which was necessary for the action of the hormones upon the endometrium. Oestrogen acts to promote proliferation and the expression of progesterone receptors while progesterone causes differentiation and inhibits proliferation. With the availability of long-acting synthetic analogues of progesterone Kelly and Baker (1960) were able to publish their report on the clinical application with the inhibition of endometrial cancer growth by medroxyprogesterone acetate.

The effect of progesterone upon endometrial cancer is to cause the induction of several markers of differentiation, leading to cell death through apoptosis or programmed cell death, a mechanism which has been common to most hormonal responses studied to date. The efficacy of progesterone can be correlated with the expression of progesterone receptors by the tumour (Benraad et al. 1980; Creasman et al. 1980), which in turn are related to the degree of morphological differentiation (McKarty et al. 1979) and tumour type with no expression in the papillary serous variant (Carcangiu et al. 1990). However, immunohistology with antibodies to the progesterone receptor has shown that there is considerable heterogeneity of expression of the progesterone receptor between cells within each endometrial cancer as indeed there is of the oestrogen receptor. Thus while progesterone can effect a regression of the tumour which bears sufficient progesterone receptor-positive cells it may also act to provide a selective growth advantage to those cells that are progesterone independent. It seems likely that this is the underlying basis for the clinical observation that the majority of those remitting on progesterone therapy will relapse within on average 2 years from starting treatment with a progesterone insensitive tumour.

New biology
Mode of spread
Direct invasion

Approximately 50 per cent of all endometrial cancers will not have breached the basement membrane and are confined to the endometrium at the time of diagnosis, a further 26 per cent will exhibit less than one-third myometrial invasion, and 12 per cent will exhibit deep myometrial invasion (T1). The earliest spread of cancer of the corpus is by direct extension into the myometrium and progressively towards the uterine isthmus and cervix (T2). Extension beyond the uterus at the time of presentation is found in 11 per cent of cases (Reagan and Fu 1981). Adenosquamous tumours tend to be more advanced at the time of detection; in the same series only 35 per cent were limited to the endometrium at the time of diagnosis. Papillary serous tumours are also often more disseminated with a particular tendency to intraperitoneal

dissemination (T4) in the manner of the epithelial ovarian carcinomas. Routine assessment of peritoneal cytology by pelvic washings collected before removing the uterus will defect this mode of spread and the need for further adjuvant therapy.

Lymphatic spread
Lymphatic spread may involve three groups of nodes; pelvic, para-aortic, and, rarely, the inguinal lymph nodes. The incidence of nodal involvement closely correlates with the size of the central tumour, the histological grade, and the depth of myometrial invasion (Berman et al. 1980; Disaia and Creasman 1981; Bucy 1989). An understanding of the pattern of lymphatic spread in this disease is important in selecting the extent of surgical and radiotherapeutic treatment.

In the majority of instances tumour cells will pass into broad ligament lymphatics to the external iliac, internal iliac, and obturator groups of nodes at the pelvic side wall. Para-aortic node involvement may occur on a progressive and secondary basis. Tumours arising from the uterine fundus can, however, spread via lymphatic channels in the infundibulopelvic ligament and thereafter follow pathways associated with the lymphatic drainage of the ovary leading to metastatic disease in the para-aortic lymph nodes at the level of the renal vessels. Although the prevailing lymph flow is cephalad, retrograde spread is well described and disease may arise in the nodes at the aortic bifurcation by this second pathway.

Nevertheless the finding of positive aortic nodes in the absence of pelvic node disease is an uncommon event; conversely, if the pelvic nodes are involved the para-aortic nodes will be positive in approximately 60 per cent of cases (Creasman et al. 1976). It is unusual for lymphatic channels in the region of the round ligament to convey tumour to the groin nodes, but such spread patterns are occasionally encountered. Spread to the vagina, at the apex of the vaginal vault and also to the lower third of the anterior wall, is a feared complication and occurs in approximately 8 per cent of cases. This is probably a manifestation of retrograde spread in lymphatics rather than a consequence of cell spillage and implantation.

Bloodborne spread
Spread by the bloodstream tends to occur at a later stage in this disease and most commonly involves the lungs (8.3 per cent), but metastases to liver (5.9 per cent), bone (3.4 per cent), brain, and the adrenal glands are also described (Plentl and Friedman 1971).

Clinical features

Cancer of the corpus originates in the superficial layers of a thick-walled organ. Disruption of the endometrium will reveal itself at an early stage by inappropriate vaginal bleeding, which in some instances is preceded by a brownish water discharge. Because of the age distribution of this disease, the prime symptom therefore is post-menopausal bleeding. Twenty per cent of cases, however, occur in younger women and in these patients the presenting complaint is of intermenstrual bleeding or menorrhagia. However, the specificity of abnormal bleeding patterns for endometrial cancer is low. Estimates of the incidence of endometrial cancer being the underlying cause of the symptom of post-menopausal bleeding vary between 1 and 20 per cent.

Diagnosis
Traditionally, the diagnosis of endometrial cancer has been confirmed by the histological examination of the specimen obtained at dilatation and curettage. At this procedure, examination under anaesthesia will also provide the clinician with an initial assessment

of the extent of the pelvic pathology. The size of the uterus can be assessed with accuracy and evidence of adnexal pathology can be obtained. Exploration of the uterine cavity and systematic curettage will also allow an impression to be gained of the extent of the tumour burden, but gross inspection of curettings is notoriously inaccurate and the precise location and extent of tumour spread cannot be assessed with any accuracy by this technique (Janicek et al. 1994).

Some authorities advocate the use of fractional curettage in order to obtain evidence of cervical involvement by the tumour (T2), although this procedure may be very imprecise and if treatment modification is to be based on information gained from this technique it is essential that as much care as possible is taken to avoid mixing specimens obtained from the cervical canal and the uterine cavity. Prior to any manipulative procedure, therefore, the cervical canal must be carefully curetted and any specimen should be obtained prior to sounding or dilatation. In spite of this it is a rare circumstance to find convincing evidence of occult stage II disease at this pre-treatment assessment (Boronow 1990).

Hysteroscopy is advocated by some as a means of staging endometrial cancer. Both contact and standard hysteroscopy have been employed and those in support of the technique testify to its usefulness in directing biopsy and in assessing tumour characteristics (Joeslsson et al. 1971; Sugimoto 1975) such as volume and involvement of the endocervix. A persistent worry associated with hysteroscopy has always been that it could theoretically facilitate tumour spread to the peritoneal cavity via the Fallopian tubes (Romano et al. 1992). Gas hysteroscopy markedly reduces the risk of tumour dissemination and may become a useful adjuvant investigation in the pre-treatment assessment of patients with endometrial cancer.

Recently there has been increasing interest in the use of imaging techniques in the initial assessment of patients with post-menopausal bleeding (Ross 1988). Abdominal and more successfully vaginal ultrasound can detect endometrial thickening, tumour size, and grossly enlarged regional lymph nodes (Lehtovirta et al. 1987). Whether it is of value as a screening test which may be used to subselect a group of patients with post-menopausal bleeding who do not need a curettage awaits the results of current research trials. Computerized tomographic (CT) scanning and, more recently, magnetic resonance imaging (MRI) may also be employed to provide information on tumour spread. Such techniques have superseded lymphography (Galaknoffet et al. 1988) and can detect enlarged (>1 cm) lymph nodes and the extent and depth of myometrial invasion.

Further information regarding tumour spread may be obtained from a chest radiograph, which is essential, but radiological assessment of the urinary and gastrointestinal tract need not be performed on a routine basis.

Age

Evidence exists to show that older patients developing endometrial cancer have poorer survival rates. This probably reflects the detection of a disproportionately high number of tumours of poor histological differentiation and more advanced stage in women in their 60s and 70s compared with women who develop the disease in their 50s (Frick et al. 1973). The patient's age may also reflect her general health (Oster et al. 1982) and associated obesity which reduces her suitability for surgery.

Uterine size

This factor has been incorporated into a FIGO clinical substage and there is some correlation between uterine size and survival with an 84.5 per cent 5 year survival for normal sized uterus versus 66.6 per cent 5 year survival if the uterus is enlarged (>8 cm intracavity length (Jones 1975)). However, the uterus may be enlarged by pathology other than corpus cancer making size an unreliable prognostic factor. In a review of 100 cases of endometrial cancer Javert and Douglas (1956) reported that uterine enlargement was present in half, but cancer was the underlying cause of the enlargement in only eight patients.

Histological grade and cell type

Information on the histological grade of the tumour will be obtained at the initial curettage; however, this is subject to sampling error since the degree of differentiation in any malignancy is not homogenous. The tumour should be classified according to the least differentiated elements and, thus, discrepancies can arise between tumour differentiation reported at curettage and in the final hysterectomy specimen. The histopathologist's difficulties may be compounded by the inherent problems in the subjective appraisal of architectural appearance. Grade I and grade III tumours are usually easy to distinguish but grade II lesions are less easy to define using standard morphological techniques. Newer proliferative indices such as ploidy (Ambros et al. 1992), S phase fraction (Konski 1991), and labelling of nuclear proliferation antigens such as Ki67 await further assessment. Patients with a poorly differentiated or unclassifiable tumour are recognized as being at highest risk of metastasis and recurrence (Chambers et al. 1987).

Cell type is an important prognostic indicator in patients with endometrial carcinoma. Although the majority (85 per cent) are endometrioid adenocarcinomas, the less common histological variants must be recognized as these have a much poorer survival.

Serum markers

In advanced disease approximately 60 per cent of patients will have an elevated serum antigen test as detected by antibodies to CA125 and CA19.9 (Duk 1986; Neunteufel 1988; Patsner 1989). No systematic data have been published, however, for the diagnostic sensitivity and specificity of these tests especially in early stage disease when very few patients may have an elevated serum level (Rose et al. 1993). Elevation of these markers does occur in association with several other benign and malignant (ovary, pancreas, bowel, lung) diseases.

Laparotomy

At the time of the primary assessment, therefore, patients can be categorized as high risk because of obvious advanced disease, adverse histological features, or both. Other risk factors may not be defined until the time of the initial laparotomy or until the final histological assessment of the hysterectomy specimen is obtained.

While approximately 75 per cent of these tumours at the time of presentation may be designated stage I it is widely agreed that clinical staging of cancer of the corpus is inaccurate and the majority of patients dying of endometrial cancer present with apparently stage I disease. There is confusion in the earlier literature between clinical and surgicopathological staging. At the FIGO World Congress in 1988 the concept of surgical staging and an official classification was agreed (Creasman 1990).

Thorough surgical exploration and accurate clinicopathological assessment will rid us of the nosological dilemmas previously faced when clinical stage I disease was found to have occult ovarian metastases at the time of surgery, when a large uterus with apparent clinical stage IB disease at laparotomy was found to be a small tumour with a fibroid, when apparent clinical stage III disease was found to be an early endometrial cancer and a benign ovarian cyst, and, finally, surgical staging enables the critical factor of lymph node status to be taken into account (Genest 1987).

Cytological washings

On opening the peritoneal cavity, the pouch of Douglas and pelvic peritoneum can be washed with saline and the aspirate sent for cytological examination. A positive result is obtained in up to 15 per cent of endometrial cancers and has been associated with a poorer prognosis (Creasman and Rutledge 1971; Lewis 1980). Positive peritoneal cytology is more frequently associated with high-grade lesions and those tumours invading the outer third of the myometrium when a positive result may be obtained in 50 per cent of washings taken. However, there is no agreement on the significance of peritoneal cytology. Konski et al. (1988) did not find that positive cytology was an independent prognostic factor and a retrospective study of 163 patients by Kennedy et al. (1987) failed to demonstrate a significant association between positive washings and other risk factors. In the last study only two patients with early stage disease underwent treatment modification as a result of the cytology result.

Myometrial invasion

On removing the uterus the specimen should be opened carefully in a longitudinal fashion until the endometrial cavity is displayed. Macroscopic assessment enables the clinician to assess the bulk of tumour present and in most a preliminary assessment of the depth of myometrial invasion can be used to guide the search for metastatic disease. Impaired survival with increasing depth of myometrial invasion is reported by most series. Patients with superficial or less than one-third myometrial invasion have no worse a prognosis in terms of 5 year survival than patients with tumour confined to within the endometrial basement membrane; however, if there is deep myometrial involvement the survival rates fall from 80 to 60 per cent in stage I disease (Jones 1975). The proximity of tumour invasion to the serosal surface is also of prognostic significance (Lutz et al. 1978).

Adnexal spread

At the time of primary surgical assessment spread to the adnexae (T3) may be identified in 7–8 per cent of cases. Frequently this is a microscopic finding which is reported at the time of the final histological report. If it is the sole site of metastatic disease then it need not signify a worse survival, unless as most frequently occurs there are other risk factors such as poor histological differentiation, myometrial invasion, and cervical involvement.

Lymph node status

Clearly, the risk factors for lymphatic spread, that is, histological grade and myometrial invasion are interlinked. Only 12 per cent of well-differentiated lesions exhibit deep myometrial invasion compared with a 46 per cent incidence in grade III lesions. If, at the time of primary or secondary assessment, a patient is deemed to be at high risk due to any of the above risk factors then either selective lymph node sampling or more accurately pelvic lymphadenectomy may be performed to assess the degree of lymph node involvement and the indications for adjuvant radiotherapy.

Management

Screening and prevention

In purely theoretical terms endometrial cancer is a disease that should lend itself to the screening process, since there is a high likelihood of cure for early stage disease; however, no studies of large-scale screening of an asymptomatic female population have been reported. A major problem is that no single test fulfils the basic screening requirements of sensitivity, specificity, cost effectiveness, and improved survival. A variety of techniques exist which permit sampling of endometrial cells by both cytological and histological means. The standard Papanicolaou cervical smear has inadequate specificity for use as a screening test for endometrial cancer, being positive, probably, in no more than 50 per cent of cases (Jones et al. 1972; Frick et al. 1975). Cytological assessment of endometrial cells which are obtained by brushing or washing the endometrial cavity have a limited diagnostic accuracy for endometrial cancer and their ability to detect precursor lesions is even less satisfactory (Pacifico et al. 1982).

Histological analysis of specimens obtained by suction aspiration techniques provide greater accuracy and have a higher ability to identify precursor lesions and accuracy rates in excess of 96 per cent have been reported by instruments such as the Kevorikian curette and the Vabra aspirator. Cytology requires special skills in interpretation. A negative result will not necessarily exclude endometrial pathology but false-positive results are uncommon. The main limitations of these techniques, however, are the skilled operator time and cost required and the discomfort caused by the passage of the cannula through the cervical canal, particularly in post-menopausal women with a degree of atrophic change and cervical stenosis.

The incidence of hyperplasia of the endometrium in asymptomatic women is unknown but the problem is greatest in the perimenopausal age group and may occur in 30 per cent of post-menopausal women taking oestrogen without progesterone or long-term tamoxifen. Screening has been proposed for these high-risk populations and may become increasingly necessary with the prolonged use of tamoxifen in women cured of breast cancer (Ewertz et al. 1988). In practice, a form of screening in a selected population already exists if diagnostic curettage is performed on all women with abnormal bleeding patterns in their 40s and 50s. It is in this group of symptomatic women that screening techniques such as serum antigens, CA19.9 and CA125, vaginal ultrasound, hysteroscopy, or magnetic resonance imaging might be most rapidly assessed before being applied to the surveillance of the asymptomatic women at risk of endometrial hyperplasia.

The identification of atypical hyperplasia in these groups which may progress to carcinoma in up to 23 per cent of patients (Kurmen et al. 1985) would allow the better definition of the relationship of hyperplasia and dysplastic changes to the subsequent development of carcinoma and provides the information and opportunity to counsel the patient about hysterectomy and prevention of endometrial cancer (Fox and Buckley 1982; Scully 1982). Interestingly, prolonged use of depot medroxyprogesterone acetate for contraceptive purposes is associated with a lower risk of endometrial cancer offering an alternative intervention for high-risk women (WHO 1991).

FIGO stage I

Seventy-five per cent of cases of endometrial cancer present at this early stage. Many reports have served to identify the main risk factors for recurrence, that is, differentiation and depth of myometrial invasion (Marziale 1989). The major issues that influence attitudes and fire prejudices concern the use and timing of radiotherapy in relation to surgery and the degree of radicality that is required of the operative procedure. The answers to these questions based on scientific data are frequently absent because either trials of sufficient statistical power have not been done or, for instance, in well-differentiated stage 1 tumours 5 year survival rates in excess of 90 per cent are described. To detect statistically significant improvements at this level is clinically impractical. Nevertheless it is clear that survival is better when surgery is used alone than when radiotherapy is the sole treatment modality. Although endometrial cancer is radiosensitive the survival benefit of combining surgery and radiotherapy is unproven.

Radical versus non-radical surgery

Current surgical thinking dictates that endometrial cancer should be treated by extrafascial total hysterectomy with bilateral salpingo-oophorectomy. The inclusion of a cuff of upper vagina with the specimen is favoured by some in the belief that upper vaginal vault recurrence will be prevented. However, this is not borne out in practice and it is argued that for favourable tumours it is an unnecessary procedure and for more aggressive tumours it is ineffective (Price et al. 1965; Candiani 1990).

Lymphadenectomy

Poorly differentiated lesions and tumours with a one-third myometrial invasion have a high risk of lymphatic spread. Selective lymphadenectomy can provide staging information that is of prognostic importance and will modify treatment (Boronow 1990). Balanced against this is the possibility of increased morbidity from extended surgery in women who often have a poor general medical status. The technique of lymphadenectomy, whether pelvic or para-aortic is not a difficult one (Oram 1988) but is considerably hampered by obesity in many of these patients. Access is restricted, small vessel bleeding from fatty tissue is a nuisance, and landmark anatomy is obscured. The use of occlusive clips to secure both haemostasis and lymphostasis is recommended.

Pelvic lymphadenectomy

Knowledge gained from the status of the regional lymph nodes can be used to modify treatment since if following complete pelvic lymphadenectomy no evidence of metastatic nodal spread is evident, the patient can be spared unnecessary post-operative irradiation. If positive lymph nodes are found however, the situation is less clear. It is debatable whether lymphadenectomy is curative in its own right. Equally it is not clear if the addition of pelvic irradiation in these cases confers any survival benefit especially since up to 60 per cent may have para-aortic lymph node involvement.

Para-aortic lymphadenectomy

Para-aortic lymphadenectomy is indicated in high-risk cases when the patient's general medical condition permits and is the only means of accurately assessing the nodal status. These nodes lie outside conventional radiation treatment fields. The identification of para-aortic nodal disease (T3) will modify treatment, either by extending the irradiation field to include this nodal group or adding systemic hormonal and/or chemotherapy to the management plan. In the course of providing practical patient care, however, the clinical judgement of the gynaecological oncologist should acknowledge that in elderly women who are overweight and often medically unfit for radical surgery, lymphadenectomy is feasible in no more than 30–40 per cent of cases (Kneale 1979). Secondly, treatment modification based on the knowledge of nodal status has not been proven to result in improved overall survival.

In summary, selective extensive nodal sampling will identify a proportion of high-risk patients who do not require radiotherapy and a small number of women who might benefit from extended field irradiation and/or systemic chemotherapy.

Grade 1 lesions rarely invade the myometrium to any significant degree and may be regarded as minimal risk. In poorly differentiated tumours, myometrial invasion and lymphatic spread are encountered with increasing frequency. Lymphadenectomy is recommended in such instances and it is in this minority (20 per cent) of patients with endometrial cancer that tertiary referral to a gynaecological oncology centre might be considered.

Radiotherapy for stage I

Endometrial cancer is a radiocurable malignancy. Intracavitary brachytherapy is commonly used to treat patients who because of age or intercurrent disease, are considered unfit for surgery. This technique produces a corrected 10 year survival of 62 per cent for clinical stage I cases (Jones and Stout 1986).

This relative success is due to a combination of two factors. Firstly the anatomical site allows the use of intracavitary brachytherapy which can deliver a higher dose to a localized volume than is possible with external-beam therapy. Secondly endometrial cancer tends to present as a localized tumour with only 12 per cent of cases having extrauterine spread which would be outside the high-dose volume produced by sealed source therapy.

Radiotherapy cannot be recommended as the sole treatment for patients who are fit for surgery. Surgery produces a superior disease-free survival and provides prognostic information upon which the need for supplementary treatment is based. Most oncologists recommend a combination of surgery and radiotherapy for the majority of patients but there is little agreement on which technique to use, the exact time sequence of the two treatments, and the criteria used to select patients for a particular technique.

Intracavitary brachytherapy following surgery reduces the incidence of vaginal vault recurrence but confers no survival advantage compared with surgery alone.

The report incidence of vaginal recurrence following surgery which removes a vaginal cuff varies from 5 to 20 per cent. Vault brachytherapy reduces this incidence from 0 to 5 per cent (Dobbie 1965; Joslin et al. 1977). A prospective randomized study comparing surgery alone with pre-operative brachytherapy plus surgery or surgery plus post-operative brachytherapy confirmed the reduction in vault recurrence in both groups receiving brachytherapy but there was no difference in survival between the three groups (Piver et al. 1979).

However, the value of routine post-operative vault brachytherapy has been questioned (Bond 1985). An isolated vault recurrence took place in only 3.4 per cent of cases of which local control was achieved in 79 per cent with a 5 year survival of 45 per cent. Deferring brachytherapy for use in the event of relapse could ultimately provide the same level of local control as prophylactic treatment but would spare the majority of patients the inconvenience of treatment. Although this may be an extreme view, a good case can be made for deferred treatment in patients with well-differentiated tumours and no deep myometrial invasion. This policy has produced vaginal recurrence rates similar to other strategies (Meerwaldt et al. 1990).

Despite the absence of macroscopic extrauterine spread, pelvic recurrence develops in 22 per cent of patients treated by surgery alone (Nori *et al.* 1987). This is not surprising since lymph node sampling reveals involvement in 10 per cent of patients and this figure rises to 37 per cent in patients with poorly differentiated tumours. It has also been demonstrated that up to 60 per cent of patients with positive pelvic nodes will have involvement of para-aortic nodes (which will not be treated if only the pelvis is irradiated).

External-beam pelvic radiotherapy has been shown in randomized and retrospective studies to reduce the incidence of pelvic recurrence to 3–8 per cent (Onsrud *et al.* 1976; Salazar *et al.* 1978; Asalders *et al.* 1980). Retrospective studies report that the addition of external radiotherapy to surgery increases the 5 year disease-free survival from 70 to 90 per cent (Nori *et al.* 1987). Unfortunately a prospective randomized study failed to confirm this improvement (Onsrud *et al.* 1976). A subset analysis of these data, however, revealed a statistically significant improvement in survival for patients with poorly differentiated tumours and greater than 50 per cent myometrial invasion (Aalders *et al.* 1980).

A selective policy of external pelvic radiotherapy only for patients with adverse prognostic features is employed in some centres. Treating only those patients with poorly differentiated tumours or deep myometrial invasion or histological evidence of extrauterine spread produces a pelvic recurrence rate of 5–7 per cent which is similar to the rate in series which all patients are treated (Poulson and Roberts 1987).

The precise scheduling of radiotherapy and surgery is unimportant. Pre-operative and post-operative treatments are equally effective. A randomized trial of pre-operative and post-operative external pelvic radiotherapy has not been carried out. Despite the extravagant claims often made, retrospective studies show no consistent advantage for one over the other (Salazar *et al.* 1978; Nori *et al.* 1987; Poulson and Roberts 1987).

If external pelvic radiotherapy is administered, this will provide adequate protection against vaginal vault recurrence. There is no advantage in adding vault brachytherapy (Randall *et al.* 1990). To do so produces a significant increase in late morbidity with the incidence of rectal bleeding or proctitis rising from 3.8 to 18.6 per cent.

Recommended policy

If radical surgery with a Wertheim's hysterectomy including a pelvic lymphadenectomy is planned, then pre-operative or post-operative intracavitary brachytherapy is indicated to reduce the incidence of vault recurrence. External-beam therapy should not be given as this combination produces an unacceptable incidence of pelvic fibrosis and lymphoedema, that is, the surgeon must produce local control within the pelvis. If a less radical total abdominal hysterectomy and bilateral salpingo-oophorectomy is planned, then adjuvant radiotherapy will depend on the histological findings. If the patient is unfit for surgery, then she should be treated with intracavitary brachytherapy alone. Attempts to add in external-beam therapy in selected cases tend to be self-defeating as the combination is more toxic and is poorly tolerated by this group of patients.

Adjuvant hormone therapy and chemotherapy

Following the use of progesterone in advanced disease several attempts have been made to test adjuvant therapy in the post-operative setting for all patients (Lewis *et al.* 1974) or for high-risk patients. The high cure rate with surgery and radiotherapy alone, however, has meant that all the studies to date have failed

to enrol sufficient patients to achieve the power required to reject the null hypothesis (Macdonald 1988; Vergote *et al.* 1989). The results of the international collaborative study COHSA are awaited with interest. Neoadjuvant progesterone has also been employed often in uncontrolled trials between the time of diagnostic curettage and definitive hysterectomy on the supposition that it may reduce the viability and, hence, metastatic potential of the tumour at the time of surgery and coincidentally blood loss encountered during surgery. There is no compelling data to support this practice and attempts to mount trials to test it have failed over worries about the potential for down-staging the tumour and removing the conventional staging criteria upon which the decisions about adjuvant postoperative radiotherapy are made. This ignores the risks from the increased blood coagulability that has been documented following progesterone treatment and its potential effects upon perioperative morbidity and mortality.

Similar difficulties have attended the testing of adjuvant chemotherapy such as doxorubicin which has failed to show significant benefit (Morrow *et al.* 1990) although in theory progress in improving the outcome for stage I disease can only come through the addition of effective systemic treatment.

Hormone replacement therapy

Patients with well-differentiated stage I endometrial cancer showing less than one-third depth of myometrial invasion have only a 10 per cent risk of recurrence and it has been argued recently that many such patients may safely benefit from hormonal replacement therapy (Jick *et al.* 1979). Published experience would support this though follow-up is relatively short and no controlled trials have been reported (Creasman *et al.* 1986; Lee 1990). Since oestrogens may accelerate the growth of residual disease it has otherwise been generally advised that hormone replacement therapy should not be provided following treatment of endometrial cancer.

FIGO stage II

Cervical involvement by tumour in endometrial cancer is frequently undiagnosed pre-operatively. With the variable application of fractional curettage and hysteroscopy, extension to the cervix is found most commonly when the uterus is opened following its removal at surgery or upon histological examination. Treatment guidelines may be affected by the timing of this knowledge. Traditionally those patients in whom T2 disease was diagnosed pre-operatively were treated by a radical hysterectomy with pelvic lymphadenectomy. However, as previously discussed, radical surgery in these women is frequently difficult and confers no survival advantage over irradiation and simple hysterectomy. Prognosis depends as much upon the differentiation of the tumour as the actual cervical involvement (Reisinger *et al.* 1991). The pattern of recurrence in stage II disease for the majority of patients is one of distant metastases rather than recurrent pelvic disease (Larson 1987). At the present time therefore, it must be concluded that stage II corpus cancer should be treated by a combination of simple hysterectomy and bilateral salpingo-oophorectomy combined with radiotherapy to achieve local control.

Radiotherapy for stage II

Invasion of the cervix, particularly deep stromal invasion, confers an inferior probability of survival compared to stage I. This may be due to a greater propensity for spread to the pelvic nodes which is found in 23–37 per cent of cases with 5–35 per cent also having involvement of the para-aortic nodes.

No randomized trial has been carried out but retrospective studies suggest that the incidence of pelvic recurrence can be reduced by the addition of radiotherapy to surgery. The incidence of pelvic recurrence after total abdominal hysterectomy and bilateral salpingo-oophorectomy can be as high as 42 per cent (Roberts 1961). This can be reduced to 0–19 per cent by the addition of external pelvic radiotherapy plus vault brachytherapy (Bruckman et al. 1978; Larson et al. 1988). In comparison, external pelvic radiotherapy and brachytherapy without surgery produce a recurrence rate of 34 per cent (Grigsby et al. 1985).

The addition of radiotherapy to surgery in these studies produced no detectable improvement in survival. Non-randomized comparisons show 5 year disease-free survival with surgery alone varies from 61 to 85 per cent with radiotherapy alone from 42 to 65 per cent and with the combination from 60 to 85 per cent. The poorer figures for radiotherapy alone may be due to selection bias (Boothby 1989).

Recommended treatment

Two policies appear equally valid for those patients who are fit for surgery. If stage II disease is diagnosed prior to laparotomy then pre-operative intrauterine and intravaginal brachytherapy is used followed by a Wertheim's hysterectomy. Otherwise if cervical involvement is discovered post-operatively total abdominal hysterectomy and bilateral salpingo-oophorectomy should be followed by external pelvic radiotherapy with an intracavitary boost to the vault.

For patients who are unfit for surgery, the optimal treatment would be intrauterine and intravaginal brachytherapy followed by external pelvic radiotherapy with midline shielding. Judgement needs to be exercised in the selection of patients for such aggressive treatment as toxicity may be as debilitating as the morbidity of surgery in the very frail patient of poor performance status.

FIGO stage III

Fortunately, advanced stage disease at the time of presentation is relatively uncommon. Attention may be drawn to the possibility of tumour spread beyond the uterus at the time of the initial clinical appraisal but the management of patients with stage III disease will be dictated by the time at which it is identified. If the pre-operative clinical assessment provides conclusive evidence of adnexal spread, then pre-operative whole pelvic irradiation followed by total abdominal hysterectomy and bilateral salpingo-oophorectomy may improve survival. More often, adnexal spread is identified intraoperatively or post-operatively at the time of histological examination of the surgical specimen.

Radiotherapy

Most published series contain two groups of patients: those with clinical stage III disease who tend to have involvement of the cervix, parametria, and pelvic side-wall and those with pathological stage III disease who often are found to have spread limited to the ovaries or tubes. This last group of patients has an 80 per cent probability of disease-free survival at 5 years compared with 35 per cent for the former (Greven 1989).

No prospective trials have been carried out. In retrospective studies, most patients have been treated with a combination of surgery and radiotherapy or radiotherapy on its own. With the combination, the overall 5 year relapse-free survival is 50 per cent. The completeness of surgical clearance is an important predictor of outcome. With complete excision, this figure rises to 79 per cent;

with residual tumour, it falls to 23 per cent (Malkasian et al. 1977; McKillop and Pringle 1985).

The relapse-free survival for patients treated with radiotherapy alone is 32 per cent. It is inevitable that this group has a worse prognosis because it contains either those patients who were unfit for surgery or those whose tumours were inoperable.

Recommended policy

Patients fit for surgery and with technically operable tumour should be treated with total abdominal hysterectomy and bilateral salpingo-oophorectomy or a Wertheim's hysterectomy followed by external pelvic radiotherapy and vault brachytherapy. Patients unfit for surgery or technically inoperable should be treated by external pelvic radiotherapy followed by intrauterine and intravaginal brachytherapy.

Radiotherapy techniques

Intrauterine and intravaginal brachytherapy

Although other techniques have been described, the advent of mechanical afterloading equipment means that most centres now use some modification of the Manchester system. This employs either a single central line of radioactive material in the intrauterine canal plus two ovoid sources in the vaginal vault or a single central line extending from the uterine fundus to the vaginal vault.

Because of the theoretical risk of submucosal spread to the lower third of the vagina, some authors have emphasized the importance of treating the whole length of the vagina down to the introitus. Practically this seems unnecessary since recurrence in the lower third of the vagina occurs in less than 1 per cent of cases (Poulson and Roberts 1987), an incidence which seems too low to justify the increased risk of vaginal stenosis.

The vaginal vault can be treated using either two vaginal ovoids or a single line source. A total dose of 80 Gy is delivered in two insertions 1 week apart, if the traditional Manchester loadings are used.

External pelvic radiotherapy

The volume to be irradiated extends from the lower border of the obturator foramia inferiorly to the disc space between the fourth and fifth lumbar vertebrae superiorly and laterally extends to the pelvic side walls. This volume can be irradiated adequately using anterior and posterior radiation fields although some authors prefer to use a three- or four-field technique to reduce the dose received by the rectum. If this technique is employed in conjunction with high-dose brachytherapy then it is necessary to use midline shielding to avoid an excessive dose to the rectum.

The recommended dose to the whole pelvis is 40 Gy in 20 daily fractions over 4 weeks or its biological equivalent in a shorter or longer time.

Acute radiation reactions

Intracavitary brachytherapy alone produces no side-effects in most patients. A minority will experience transient bowel or bladder irritation causing diarrhoea or cystitis which settles within a few days.

External pelvic radiotherapy causes temporary side-effects in the majority of patients. Diarrhoea or cystitis will develop during the latter part of treatment and will continue for 2–3 weeks following its cessation. A transient skin reaction which often progresses to moist desquamation may develop in the vulva, perineum, and gluteal cleft, particularly if anterior and posterior fields alone are used.

Chronic radiation reactions

Vault brachytherapy produces no long-term bladder or bowel complications but 15–20 per cent of patients will develop vaginal stenosis. Intrauterine and intravaginal brachytherapy causes telangiectasia of the bladder in 2 per cent of cases. Bowel fibrosis and obstruction occurs in 0.5 per cent of cases and is more common when there has been preceding pelvic surgery.

External pelvic radiotherapy plus intracavitary brachytherapy, particularly following surgery, produces significant complications in 9–18 per cent of cases in addition to a 20 per cent incidence of vaginal stenosis. Proctocolitis has been reported in 2–18 per cent of cases, bowel obstruction in 0.5–3 per cent, and necrosis in the vaginal vault in 0.5–1 per cent. In most cases, these complications resolve with conservative management but 2–3 per cent will require surgical intervention to relieve obstruction or rectal bleeding (Greven 1991).

FIGO stage IV and recurrent disease

Surgery and radiotherapy

Stage IV disease with invasion of bladder/bowel or more distant metastases may be identified either pre-operatively or at the initial surgical assessment. Radical surgery in these cases has little place because of the high potential for distant metastatic spread.

Only the occasional patient is suitable for attempted curative radiotherapy. In the vast majority palliation is all that can be offered. External pelvic radiotherapy or intracavitary brachytherapy are appropriate to relieve vaginal bleeding or pelvic pain related to the primary or symptomatic metastases particularly in bone. Medical management with hormonal and or chemotherapy will also be required.

Tumour recurrences are more likely in the defined high-risk groups and in approximately 80 per cent of cases will occur within 2 years of primary therapy. Treatment is determined by the site of recurrence and whether it is solitary or multifocal. Isolated pelvic recurrence occurs in only 30 per cent (Burke 1990); vaginal recurrences classically occur in two sites, at the apex of the vaginal vault and in the lower third of the vagina in a retrourethral position on the anterior wall. If there is no other site of disease these can usually be treated by surgery, radiotherapy, or a combination of both. Patients frequently do well and long-term survivors are described. The place of radical or exenterative surgery is extremely limited and should only be considered if recurrent disease is confined to the centre of the pelvis with no evidence of further spread. In endometrial cancer, this is an uncommon clinical scenario.

Endocrine treatment

In the early clinical series there was a reported response rate of 30–40 per cent following progesterone treatment of endometrial cancers using either medroxyprogesterone acetate (Bonte et al. 1978) or hydroxyprogesterone caproate. Response can be correlated with differentiation and expression of progesterone receptors. Both compounds appeared to be of similar efficacy although there is only one randomized trial to support this view (Piver et al. 1980). Several studies examined dose and route of administration which seemed of particular interest because of the low bioavailability and great interpatient variation in absorption of oral progesterones. However, no clinically significant differences emerged from those somewhat flawed studies and we can conclude that 300 mg of medroxy-progesterone acetate or more recently 160 mg megestrol acetate are equivalent and optimally effective doses. Higher doses or parenteral administration although pharmacologically different have not reproducibly resulted in more responses and do increase the side-effects of fluid retention, peripheral oedema, hypertension, weight gain, hirsuitism, and gastrointestinal upset.

More recent studies have, however, reported only a 17 per cent response rate to progestagens. The difference seems to be mainly due to changes in the selection of patients; with improved early diagnosis those failing primary management by surgery and or radiotherapy are increasingly those with poor-risk disease at presentation, in particular those with poorly differentiated disease. In one series the response rate for well differentiated tumours was 40–60 per cent compared with 0–10 per cent in poorly differentiated and receptor-negative tumours (Martin et al. 1979). Those not progesterone sensitive have had a median survival of only 8 months and for the whole group the overall long-term survival is in the order of 10 per cent.

There is conflicting evidence on the use of tamoxifen in recurrent endometrial cancer following the failure of progestagens with single institution studies reporting a 30 per cent response though of short duration (Swenerton 1980; Bonte et al. 1981; Slavik et al. 1984) whilst subsequent multicentre trials found no evidence of activity (Edmonson 1986). From this it is possible to conclude only that while in a few cases tamoxifen can exert an anticancer effect, it has not proved useful in general for progesterone-resistant endometrial cancer. Continuing research has highlighted a paradoxical agonist effect of tamoxifen on endometrial cancer growth in vitro and an oestrogen-like stimulation of the expression of progesterone receptors. It has been suggested that tamoxifen combined (Carlson et al. 1984) in an alternating cyclical fashion with progesterone could even be used to take advantage of the receptor induction to increase hormonal sensitivity progesterone (Ayoub 1988). Observation of women prescribed long-term continuous adjuvant tamoxifen for early stage breast cancer has also highlighted its oestrogen-like effect on endometrial growth. Other pure anti-oestrogens and aromatase inhibitors are in the process of being evaluated in endometrial cancer and preliminary observations have suggested that gonadotrophin releasing-hormone agonists may have antitumour activity in post-menopausal women with recurrent disease.

Chemotherapy

There is a relatively limited literature on the chemotherapy of endometrial cancer but historically a variety of single agent studies have established that doxorubicin, (Thigpen et al. 1979; Trope et al. 1980; Seski et al. 1982) cisplatin, and carboplatin (Long et al. 1988) achieve the highest response rates, while hexamethylmelamine and vinblastine are less active. There is still doubt about the activity of classical alkylating agents such as cyclophosphamide (Horton et al. 1978) and 5-fluorouracil while methotrexate, mitozantrone, and etoposide appear inactive (Piver et al. 1986; Thigpen 1989). Newer agents such as the taxanes have not been tested as yet. Intra-peritoneal therapy has been investigated inconclusively for although intraperitonenal dissemination is a common form of spread for endometrial cancer, haematogenous spread is also a common reason for the failure of local therapy, hence the need for better systemic therapy. Combination chemotherapy with doxorubicin, cisplatin and cyclophosphamide, or vinblastine has enhanced the rate of response to therapy to 30 per cent but has made no impact upon survival which remains at a median of 8–10 months from the institution of chemotherapy (Seski et al. 1981; Horton et al. 1982; Trope et al. 1984; Pasmantier et al. 1985; Turbow et al. 1985; Hancock et al. 1986; Alberts 1987; Edmonson et al. 1987). Combined approaches with chemo-hormonal therapy have achieved a median survival of more than 15 months in some but not all trials (Deppe *et al.* 1981; Piver *et al.* 1991). Results from current trials examining the use of chemotherapy as adjuvant treatment for high-risk, early stage disease are awaited.

UTERINE SARCOMAS

Pathology and presentation

Uterine sarcomas comprise less than 2–5 per cent of the cancers of the corpus uteri and while much is known about their biology their rarity makes for only fragmentary knowledge of how to best treat them based on retrospective reviews spanning many years and modes of treatment.

The sarcomas of the uterus can be divided into pure sarcomas composed of homologous elements such as leiomyosarcoma and stromal sarcoma or heterologous elements such as rhabdomyosarcoma, mixed sarcomas of homologous and heterologous elements, and carcinosarcomas or mixed Müllerian sarcomas.

Uterine sarcomas usually present with vaginal bleeding, less frequently with a uterine mass or pain, and sometimes as an unexpected finding upon examination of hysterectomy specimens for supposed benign fibroadenosis. Diagnostic dilatation and curettage is accurate in only one-third of cases. The median age of incidence of leiomyosarcoma and endometrial stromal sarcoma is 45–55 years while the mixed Müllerian sarcomas tend to occur later (55–65 years). However, those tumours may occur in women in their 20s and previous irradiation to the pelvis may predispose to later uterine sarcomas in the same way it may affect other irradiated organs. No other predisposing factors have been reliably identified although the presence of oestrogen receptors especially in endometrial stroma sarcomas (Baggish 1972; Sutton *et al.* 1986) raises the possibility of a hormonal component as with endometrial carcinomas.

The conventions adopted for staging uterine sarcomas are those developed by FIGO for endometrial carcinomas with stage I involvement of corpus only, stage II corpus and cervix, stage III invasion through to serosa and involvement of other pelvic organs, and stage IV more distant spread, usually intraperitoneally or to the lungs.

Leiomyosarcoma

Leiomyosarcomas are almost twice as common as endometrial stromal and mixed Müllerian sarcomas. Leiomyosarcomas are differentiated from benign leiomyoma primarily on the cellularity, nuclear morphology, and mitotic rate. Those tumours with less than five mitoses per ten high-power fields are benign with a 99 per cent long-term survival and those with five to nine mitoses per ten high-power fields are of variable malignancy with a 30 per cent long-term survival, whereas those with more than ten mitoses per ten high-power fields are usually highly malignant with 16 per cent survival (Piver and Lurain 1981). Similar results may also be achieved by flow cytometric measurement of ploidy and S phase fraction (Malstrom *et al.* 1993; Wolfson *et al.* 1994). Overall, 20–30 per cent of those diagnosed with stage I disease are long-term survivors.

Endometrial stromal sarcomas

Differentiation between low-grade and high-grade stromal sarcomas depends upon the mitotic index plus cytological atypia, with some investigators also including the pattern of infiltration and presence of necrosis (Evans 1982). Low-grade stromal sarcomas also known as endolymphatic stromal myosis have less than ten mitoses per ten high-power fields, smaller regular cells, a pushing edge, and are more likely to be oestrogen and progesterone receptor positive (Baggish *et al.* 1972; Lantta *et al.* 1984; Piver *et al.* 1984; Katz *et al.* 1987). The median time to recurrence in low-grade stromal sarcomas is 34 months compared with 29 months for high-grade sarcomas (Berchuck *et al.* 1990) though some low-grade tumours may recur up to 12 or more years later (Norris and Taylor 1966). Some 75 per cent of patients with low-grade, compared with 0–20 per cent of high-grade endometrial stromal sarcomas will be long-term survivors. For those with stage I disease 50 per cent of those with high-grade tumours may survive 10 years (Berchuck 1990) compared with a median survival of only 43 months for patients with advanced stage III or IV high-grade tumours (de Fusco *et al.* 1989; Mansi *et al.* 1990).

Mixed Müllerian sarcomas

Mixed Müllerian sarcomas are more properly termed carcinosarcomas composed of both carcinoma and sarcoma cell types. The degree of myometrial invasion and the presence of blood and lymphatic vessel invasion correlate with the incidence of lymph node metastases. The 5 year survival for all patients with mixed Müllerian sarcoma is 20 per cent (Piver and Lurain 1981).

Müllerian adenosarcoma

Müllerian adenosarcoma (Clement and Scully 1990) is a rare variant of mixed Müllerian tumour in which there is a benign or at most atypical glandular element with a low-grade sarcomatous stroma. Also known as uterine cystosarcoma phylloides they are related to the purely benign papillary or cystadenofibroma and may be confused with benign endometrial or endocervical polyps. There may be a variety of Müllerian epithelia or sec chord elements in the tumour with the usual homologous stromal elements with less than ten mitoses per high-power field. Unlike other sarcomas distant metastasis is very uncommon (2 per cent) and typically their course is indolent with local recurrence in 26 per cent at 5 years; half of these can be salvaged by local surgical excision. The role of radiotherapy and chemotherapy has not been well defined and offers no great improvement to date.

Treatment

Total abdominal hysterectomy is the preferred surgical approach with bilateral salpingo-oophorectomy because of possible metastatic spread and the possible oestrogen dependence, especially of endometrial stromal sarcomas. It would seem logical to avoid postoperative hormone replacement therapy. Total excision of the tumour carries the greatest prognostic significance after tumour grade and metastectomy for isolated deposits may also be appropriate at presentation or recurrence as this has been associated with long-term survival.

Radiotherapy has had limited success in leiomyosarcoma either for metastatic disease or in adjuvant treatment of the pelvis after surgery (Belgrad *et al.* 1975; Salazar *et al.* 1978). Metastatic and recurrent low- or high-grade endometrial stromal sarcomas may respond to radiotherapy in 50–60 per cent of patients for a median duration of 61 months (Berchuck *et al.* 1990). For patients with endometrial stromal sarcoma, radiotherapy to the pelvis may improve local relapse rates but not survival for low- or high-grade tumours (Belgrade *et al.* 1975) although others have failed to find any benefit from radiotherapy in comparison with historical controls (de Fusco *et al.* 1989). Mixed Müllerian sarcomas may respond to radiotherapy and adjuvant treatment to the pelvis improves local control but again not overall survival (Belgrad *et al.* 1975; Sorbe 1985; Echt *et al.* 1990).

Extrapelvic spread is common in the high-grade tumours at presentation and recurrence is met commonly in the peritoneal cavity, lungs, and bone. Isolated pelvic recurrence occurs in only 20 per cent of patients (Goff *et al.* 1993). Chemotherapy has been used in small numbers of patients with uterine sarcomas with doxorubicin and cyclophosphamide with or without dacarbazine (DTIC) achieving responses in 20–50 per cent of patients and a median survival of 6–9 months (Omura *et al.* 1983). Cisplatin has shown some activity against mixed Müllerian sarcomas with responses in 20 per cent of patients. A randomized controlled trial of adjuvant chemotherapy with single agent doxorubicin (Omura *et al.* 1985) did not prove successful though the small number of cases render this and other published experience inconclusive (Covens *et al.* 1987; DeFusco *et al.* 1989).

There are several anecdotal reports correlating the expression of hormone receptors with responses in metastatic endometrial stromal sarcoma either to oophorectomy in the pre-menopausal or progesterone (O'Brien *et al.* 1970; Baggish *et al.* 1972; Lanta *et al.* 1984; Katz *et al.* 1987; Keen *et al.* 1989; Rand *et al.* 1990), however, there have been no recorded responses to tamoxifen.

For the present, early detection and complete surgical excision remain the mainstays of treatment and further progress will require the efforts of large collaborative groups to assess new treatments in these rare tumours.

FALLOPIAN TUBE CARCINOMA

Primary carcinoma of the Fallopian tube is a rare tumour occurring in approximately 0.4/100 000 women and comprises 0.5–1.0 per cent of all gynaecological malignancies. Metastatic spread, especially from adjacent pelvic organs, is the most common cause of a Fallopian tube tumour, requiring definition of a primary epithelial tumour of the Fallopian tube as being one which involves the tubal mucosa with a clear transition zone from benign to malignant. Non-epithelial and primary epithelial Fallopian tube tumours should only be diagnosed in the absence of any primary tumour of the ovary or uterus except when there is clearly different pathology (Amendola *et al.* 1983). There is an associated increase in incidence of other gynaecological and breast cancers in women with Fallopian tube carcinoma such that appropriate screening has been recommended for all patients (Peters *et al.* 1989).

The mean age of incidence is between 55 and 65 years although the disease can occur even in young women in their 20s. There is an increase incidence in association with salpingitis and infertility, especially of bilateral tumours, but no causal relationship has been established.

Pathology and presentation

The adenocarcinomas may display varying patterns of growth with solid, papillary, or alveolar tumours. The degree of differentiation is of the greater prognostic importance, but only for those lesions confined to the wall of the Fallopian tube (Hu *et al.* 1950). Other rare tumours such as leiomyosarcoma and mixed Müllerian sarcoma (Weber *et al.* 1993) may occur and lymphoma, adenosquamous carcinoma, and choriocarcinoma have been described.

Fallopian tube carcinomas tend to spread in a similar manner to other cancers in hollow organs such that local spread and prognosis can be estimated from the degree of invasion from the tubal lumen through to the serosa and abdominopelvic cavity beyond. Spread however may also occur via the tubal lumen direct

to the abdominal cavity and this is thought to explain the relatively high frequency of metastatic spread associated with even apparently localized disease (Harrison *et al.* 1989). In approximately 20 per cent of cases the carcinoma will be bilateral, occurring with equal frequency on either side. Lymphatic spread may occur via the infundibulopelvic lymphatic to para-aortic nodes or through the broad ligament to the iliac and inguinal lymph nodes as with the uterine tumours (Eddy *et al.* 1984).

Presentation

Approximately half of all patients will present with abnormal vaginal bleeding or profuse serous discharge and this together with abdominal pain and a palpable adnexal mass constitutes 'hydrops tubae profluens'. It is considered pathognomonic of tubal carcinoma although the full syndrome is rare, occurs late in the disease, and is not restricted to malignant tubal disorders. Occasionally suspicion of the diagnosis may be raised by the finding of malignant cells from cervicovaginal cytology in the presence of a normal appearance on colposcopy and normal endometrial curettage. Pre-surgical diagnosis may also be made upon the detection of an adnexal mass by vaginal ultrasound and the elevation of the serum CA125 level (Subramanyam *et al.* 1984; Tokunaga *et al.* 1990). At operation it may not be possible to distinguish tubal carcinoma macroscopically from hydrosalpinx or tubo-ovarian abscess with closure of the fimbriated end and biopsy with frozen section examination is recommended.

Staging is according to a modified ovarian FIGO type staging (Erez *et al.* 1967); approximately 40 per cent will be stage I at diagnosis, 17 per cent stage II, 30 per cent stage III, and 12 per cent stage IV. In one series (Rosen *et al.* 1993) the overall 5 year survival was 37 per cent and the two most significant prognostic factors on multivariate analysis were stage and the completeness of the surgical resection. For stage I and II completely resected disease there was a 51 per cent 5 year survival whilst for stages III and IV 5 year survival was only 14 per cent (Schiller and Silverberg 1971).

Treatment

It is recommended that the surgical management follows that of ovarian cancer with a total abdominal hysterectomy, bilateral salpingo-oophorectomy, and omentectomy with debulking of all macroscopic disease and thorough surgical staging because of the propensity for exfoliative peritoneal spread even in stage I disease (Raju *et al.* 1981; Denham and Maclennan 1984). Lymphadenectomy does not appear to add to the prognosis for tubal carcinoma since lymph node spread has not been found in stages I to IIA and when associated with more advanced stage III or IV disease, removal of the lymph nodes did not appear to improve survival (Klein *et al.* 1993).

Radiotherapy

External-beam and intracavity pelvic radiotherapy has been given as adjuvant therapy following resection of Fallopian tube carcinoma although 50 per cent of those recurring will do so in the upper abdomen and 25 per cent will develop extraperitoneal disease in addition, mostly within 2–3 years from initial diagnosis. The overall 5 year survival with radiation is reported to be between 33 and 38 per cent and compared unfavourably with historical controls not given pelvic radiotherapy who had a 6 month median survival with 15 per cent alive at 5 years. However, no randomized trials have been performed to confirm such a difference (Greene and Scully 1962; Engstrom 1967; Amendola *et al.* 1983). Abdomino-pelvic radiotherapy has been reported to result in a 3 year survival of 86 per cent for stage I, dropping, however, to 27 per cent for stage II and III in one report (McMurray *et al.* 1986) and remains of unproven benefit.

Chemotherapy

There is little more than anecdotal evidence for single agent chemotherapy in Fallopian tube carcinoma; however, it is said to be as sensitive as ovarian carcinoma to cisplatin and the combination of cisplatin, doxorubicin, and cyclophosphamide has produced a response rate of up to 75 per cent (Jacobs *et al.* 1986; Peters *et al.* 1989; Morris *et al.* 1990).

REFERENCES

Alberts DS (1987). Doxorubicin, cisplatin, vinblastine combination chemotherapy of advanced endometrial carcinoma: a southwest oncology group study. *Gynecologic Oncology*, 26:193–201.

Aalders J, Abeler V, Kolstad P, Onsrud M (1980). Postoperative external irradiation and prognostic parameters in stage I endometrial cancer. *Obstetrics*, 56:419–26.

Ambros RA, Kurman RJ (1992). Identification of patients with stage I uterine endometrioid adenocarcinoma at high risk of recurrence by DNA ploidy, myometrial invasion, and vascular invasion. *Gynecologic Oncology*, 45:235–9.

Amendola BE, *et al.* (1983). Adenocarcinoma of the fallopian tube. *Surgery, Gynecology, Obstetrics*, 158:223.

Antunes CMF, *et al.* (1979). Endometrial cancer and oestrogen use: report of a large case-controlled study. *New England Journal of Medicine*, 300:9–14.

Ayoub J (1988). Efficacy of sequential cyclical hormonal therapy in endometrial cancer and its correlation with steroid hormone receptor status. *Gynecologic Oncology*, 31:327–37.

Baggish MS, Woodruff DJ (1992). Sterine stromatosis: clinicopathologic features and hormone dependency. *Obstetrics and Gynecology*, 40:487–98.

Belgrad R, Elbadaw N, Rubin P (1975). Uterine sarcoma. *Radiology*, 114:181.

Benraad T, *et al.* (1980). Do estrogen and progestogen receptors in metastasizing endometrial cancers predict the response to gestogen therapy? *Acta Obstetrica et Gynaecologica Scandinavica*, 59:155–9.

Berchuck A, Rubin SC, Hoskins WJ, Saigo PE, Pierce VK, Lewis JL (1990). Treatment of endometrial stromal tumors. *Gynecologic Oncology*, 36:60–5.

Billiet G, *et al.* (1982). Estrogen receptors in human uterine adenocarcinoma: correlation with tissue differentiation, vaginal karyopycnotic index, and effect of progestogen on anti-estrogen treatment. *Gynecologic Oncology*, 14:33.

Bonte J, *et al.* (1981). Tamoxifen as a possible chemotherapeutic agent in endometrial adenocarcinoma. *Gynecologic Oncology*, 11:140–4.

Boothby RA (1989). Treatment of stage II endometrial carcinoma. *Gynecologic Oncology*, 33:204–8.

Boronow RC (1990). Advances in diagnosis staging and management of cervical and endometrial cancer stages I and II. *Cancer*, 65:648–59.

Bruckman JE, Goodman RK, Murthy A, Merek A (1978). Combined surgery and radiotherapy in the treatment of stage III carcinoma of the endometrium. *Cancer*, 42:1146–51.

Bucy GS (1989). Clinical stage I and II endometrial carcinoma treated with surgery and/or radiation therapy: analysis of prognostic and treatment related factors. *Gynecologic Oncology*, 33:290–5.

Burke TW (1990). Treatment failure in endometrial carcinoma. *Obstetrics and Gynecology*, 75:96–101.

Candiani GB (1990). Evaluation of different surgical approaches in the treatment of endometrial cancer at FIGO stage I. *Gynecologic Oncology*, 37:6–8.

Carcangiu MI, Chambers JT, Voynick IM, Pirro M, Schwartz PE (1990). Immunohistochemical evaluation of estrogen and progesterone receptor content in 183 patients with endometrial carcinoma. 1. Clinical and histologic correlations. *American Journal of Clinical Pathology*, 94:247–54.

Carcangiu MI, Chambers JT (1992). Uterine papillary serous carcinoma: a study on 108 cases with emphasis on the prognostic significance of associated endometrioid carcinoma, absence of invasion, and concomitant ovarian carcinoma. *Gynecologic Oncology*, 47:298–305.

Carlson JA, *et al.* (1984). Tamoxifen and endometrial carcinoma: alterations in estrogen and progesterone receptors in untreated patients and combination hormonal therapy in advanced neoplasia. *American Journal of Obstetrics and Gynecology*, 149:149.

Clement PB, Scully RE (1990). Mullerian adenosarcoma of the uterus: a clinicopathologic analysis of 100 cases with a review of the literature. *Human Pathology*, 21:363–81.

Collins J, *et al.* (1980). Oestrogen use and survival in endometrial cancer. *Lancet*, 2:961.

Covens AL, Nisker JA, Chapman WB, Allen HH (1987). Uterine sarcoma: an analysis of 74 cases. *American Journal of Obstetrics and Gynecology*, 156:370–4.

Creasman WT, McCarty KS sr, Barton TK (1980). Clinical correlates of estrogen and progesterone binding proteins in human endometrial adenocarcinoma. *Obstetrics and Gynecology*, 55:363–70.

Creasman WT (1990). New gynecologic cancer staging. *Obstetrics and Gynecology*, 75:287–8.

De Fusco PA, Gaffey TA, Malkasian GD, Long HJ, Cha SS (1989). Endometral stromal sarcoma: review of Mayo Clinic experience, 1945–1980. *Gynecologic Oncology*, 35:8–14.

Denham J, Maclennan K (1984). The management of primary carcinoma of the fallopian tube. *Cancer*, 53:166–72.

Deppe G, Jacoms AJ, Bruckner H, Cohen CJ (1981). Chemotherapy of advanced and recurrent endometrial carcinoma with cyclophosphamide doxorubicin, 5-fluorouracil, and megestrol acetate. *American Journal of Obstetrics and Gynecology*, 140:313–6.

Duk JM (1986). CA125: a useful marker in endometrial carcinoma. *American Journal of Obstetrics and Gynecology*, 155:1097–102.

Dobbie BMW, Taypov CW, Waterhouse JAG (1965). A study of carcinoma of the endometrium. *Journal of Obstetrics and Gynaecology of the British Commonwealth*, 72:659–73.

Echt G, *et al.* (1990). Treatment of uterine sarcomas. *Cancer*, 66:35–9.

Eddy GI, Copeland IJ, Gershenson DM, Atkinson EN, Wharton JT, Rutledge FN (1984). Fallopian tube carcinoma. *Obstetrics and Gynecology*, 64:546–52.

Edmonson JH (1986). Ineffectiveness of tamoxifen in advanced endometrial carcinoma after failure of progestin treatment. *Cancer Treatment Response*, 70:1019–20.

Edmonson JH, *et al.* (1987). Randomized phase 2 studies of cisplatin and a combination of cyclophosphamide doxorubicin cisplatin (CAP) in patients with progestin refractory advanced endometrial carcinoma. *Gynecologic Oncology*, 28:20–4.

Ehrlich CE, Young P, Cleary R (1981). Cytoplasmic progesterone and estradiol receptors in normal, hyperplastic, and carcinomatous endometria: therapeutic implications. *American Journal of Obstetrics and Gynecology*, 141:539–46.

Elwood JM, Boyes DA (1980). Clinical and pathological features and survival of endometrial cancer patients in relation to prior use of estrogens. *Gynecologic Oncology*, 10:173–7.

Engstrom I (1987). Primary carcinoma of the fallopian tube. *Acta Obstetrica et Gynecologica Scandinavica*, 36:289.

Erez S, Kaplan A, Wall J (1967). Clinical staging of carcinoma of the uterine tube. *Obstetrics and Gynecology*, 30:547–50.

Evans HI (1982). Endometrial stromal sarcomas and poorly differentiated endometrial sarcoma. *Cancer*, 50:2170–82.

Farhi DC, Nosanchuk J, Silverberg SG (1986). Endometrial adenocarcinoma in women under 25 years of age. *Obstetrics and Gynecology*, 68:741.

Fujimoto I, *et al.* (1993). Studies on *ras* oncogene activation in endometrial carcinoma. *Gynecologic Oncology*, 48:196–202.

Genest P (1987). Stage carcinoma of the endometrium: a review of 41 cases. *Gynecologic Oncology*, 26:77–86.

Goff BA, *et al.* (1993). Uterine leiomyosarcoma and endometrial stroma sarcoma: lymph node metastases and sites of recurrence. *Gynecologic Oncology*, 50:105–9.

Grigsby PW, Perez CA, Camel HM, Kao HS, Galakatos AE (1985). Stage II carcinoma of the endomtrium: results of therapy and prognostic factors. *International Journal of Radiation Oncology—Biology—Physics*, 11:1915–23.

Greene TH, Scully RE (1962). Tumors of the fallopian tube. *Clinical Obstetrics and Gynecology*, 5:886.

Greven KM (1991). Analysis of complications in patients with endometrial carcinoma receiving adjuvant irradiation. *International Journal of Radiation Oncology—Biology—Physics*, 21:919–23.

Greven KM (1989). Analysis of failure patterns in stage III endometrial carcinoma and therapeutic implications. *International Journal of Radiation Oncology—Biology—Physics*, 17:35–9.

Hancock KC, Freedman RS, Edwards CL (1986). Use of cisplatin, doxorubicin, and cyclophosphamide to treat advanced and recurrent adenocarcinoma of the endometrium. *Cancer Treatment Reports*, 70:789.

Harrison C, Averette H, Jarell M, Penalver M, Donato D, Sevin B-U (1989). Carcinoma of the fallopian tube: clinical management. *Gynecologic Oncology*, 32:357–9.

Hetzel DJ, Wilson TO, Keeney GL, Roche PC, Cha SS, Podratz KC (1992). Her-2/neu expression; a major prognostic factor in endometrial cancer. *Gynecologic Cancer*, 47:179–85.

Horton J, et al. (1978). Comparison of adriamycin with cyclophosphamide in patients with advanced endometrial cancer. *Cancer Treatment Reports*, 62:159–61.

Horton J, Elson P, Gordon P, Hahn R, Creech R (1982). Combination chemotherapy for advanced endometral cancer. *Cancer*, 49:2441–5.

Hu CY, Taymor ML, Hertig AT (1950). Primary carcinoma of the fallopian tube. *American Journal of Obstetrics and Gynecology*, 59:58.

Jacobs AJ, et al. (1986). Treatment of carcinoma of the fallopian tube using cisplatin, doxorubicin, and cyclophosphamide. *American Journal of Clinical Oncology*, 9:436.

Janicek M, Rosenshein NB (1994). Invasive endometrial cancer *in uteri* resected for atypical endometrial hyperplasia. *Gynecologic Oncology*, 52:373–8.

Janne O, et al. (1979). Female sex steroid receptors in normal, hyperplastic and carcinomatous endometrium: the relationship to serum steroid hormones and gonadotropins and changes during medroxyprogesterone acetate administration. *International Journal of Cancer*, 24:545.

Jick H, et al. (1979). Replacement estrogens and endometrial cancer. *New England Journal of Medicine*, 300:218.

Jones DA, Stout R (1986). Results of intracavitary radium treatment for adenocarcinoma of the body of the uterus. *Clinical Radiology*, 37:169–71.

Joslin CA, Vaishampayan GV, Mallik A (1977). The treatment of early cancer of the corpus utri. *British Journal of Radiology*, 50:38–45.

Katz I, Merino MJ, Sakamoto H, Schwartz PE (1987). Endometrial stromal sarcoma: a clinicopathologic study of 11 cases with determination of estrogen and progestin receptor levels in three tumors. *Gynecologic Oncology*, 26:87–97.

Kaufman DW, et al. (1984). Noncontraceptive estrogen sue and the risk of breast cancer. *Journal of the American Medical Association*, 252:63.

Keen CE (1989). Progestogen induced regression in low grade endometrial stromal sarcoma: case report and literature review. *British Journal of Obstetrics and Gynaecology*, 96:1435–9.

Kelly RM, Baker WH (1960). Progestational agents in the treatment of carcinoma of the endometrium. *New England Journal of Medicine*, 264:216–22.

Klein M, Rosen A, Lahousen M, Graf A, Vavra N, Beck A (1993). Radical lymphadenectomy in the primary carcinoma of the fallopian-tube. *Archives of Gynecology and Obstetrics*, 253:21–5.

Konski AA (1991). Flow cytometric DNA content analysis of paraffin block embedded endometrial carcinomas. *International Journal of Radiation Oncology—Biology—Physics*, 21:1033–9.

Korc M (1987). Divergent effects of epidermal growth factor and transforming growth factors on a human endometrial carcinoma cell line. *Cancer Research*, 47:4909–14.

Creasman WT, et al. (1986). Estrogen replacement therapy in the patient treated for endometrial cancer. *Obstetrics and Gynecology*, 67:326.

Kurman RJ, Kaminski PF, Norris HJ (1985). The behaviour of endometrial hyperplasia: a long-term study of "untreated" hyperplasia in 170 patients. *Cancer*, 56:403–12.

Lantta M, Karkkainen J, Wahlstrom T, Widholm O (1984). Estradiol and progesteone receptors in gynecologic sarcomas. *Acta Obstetrica et Gynecologica Scandinavica*, 63:505–8.

Larson DM (1987). Prognostic factors in stage II endometrial carcinoma. *Cancer*, 60:1358–61.

Larson DM, Copeland LJ, Gallagher HS, Kong JP, Wharton JT, Stringer LA (1988). Stage II endometrial cancer. *Cancer*, 61:1528–34.

Lewis GC, et al. (1974). Adjuvant progestogen therapy in the primary definitive treatment of endometial cancer. *Gynecologic Oncology*, 2:368.

Lee RB (1990). Estrogen replacement therapy following treatment for stage I endometrial carcinoma. *Gynecologic Oncology*, 36:189–91.

Long HJ, Pfeifle DM, Wieand HS, Krook JE, Edmondson JH, Buckner JC (1988). Phase 2 evaluation of carboplatin in advanced endometrial carcinoma. *Journal of the National Cancer Institute*, 80:276–8.

Macdonald RR (1988). A randomized trial of progestogens in the primary treatment of endometrial carcinoma. *British Journal of Obstetrics and Gynaecology*, 95:166–74.

Malkasian GD, McDonald TW, Pratt JH (1977). Carcinoma of endometrium—Mayo Clinic experience. *Mayo Clinic Proceedings*, 52:175–80.

Malmstrom H, Schmidt H, Persson PG, Carstensen J, Nordenskjold B, Simonsen E (1993). Flow cytometric analysis of uterine sarcoma: ploidy and s-phase rate as prognostic indicators. *Gynecologic Oncology*, 48:172–7.

Mansi JL, Ramachandra S, Wiltshaw E, Fisher C (1990). Endometrial stromal sarcomas. *Gynecologic Oncology*, 36:113–18.

Martin PM, Rolland PH, Gammere M, Serment H, Toga M (1979). Estradiol and progesterone receptors in normal and neoplastic endometriums: correlations between receptors, histopathological examinations and clinical responses under progestin therapy. *International Journal of Cancer*, 24:324–9.

Marziale P (1989). 426 cases of stage 1 endometrial carcinoma: a clinicopathological analysis. *Gynecologic Oncology*, 32:278–81.

Maudelonde T, Cathepsin D (1990). Human endometrium: induction by progesterone and potential value as a tumour marker. *Journal of Clinical Endocrinology and Metabolism*, 70:115.

McCarty KS Jr, Barton TK, Fetter BF, Creasman WT, McCarty KS Sr (1979). Correlation of estrogen and progesterone receptors with histologic differentiation in endometrial adenocarcinoma. *American Journal of Pathology*, 96:171–83.

McKillop WJ, Pringle JF (1985). Stage III endometrial cancer. *Cancer*, 56:2519–23.

McMurray E, Jacobs A, Perez C, Camel H, Cao M-S, Galakatos A (1986). Carcinoma of the fallopian tube. Management and sites of failure. *Cancer*, 58:2070–5.

Meerwaldt JH, Hoekstra CJ, Van Putten WKJ, Tjokrowardojo AJS, Koper PCM (1990). Endometrial adenocarcinoma, adjuvant chemotherapy tailed to prognostic factors. *International Journal of Radiation Oncology—Biology—Physics*, 18:229–304.

Morris M, Gershenson DM, Burke TW, Kavanagh JJ, Silva EG, Wharton T (1990). Treatment of fallopian tube carcinoma with cisplatin, doxorubicin and cyclophosphamide. *Obstetrics and Gynecology*, 6:1020–23.

Morrow CP (1990). Doxorubicin as an adjuvant following surgery and radiation therapy in patients with high-risk endometrial carcinoma, stage I and occult stage II: a gynecologic oncology group study. *Gynecologic Oncology*, 36:166–71.

Neunteufel W (1988). CA19.9, CA125, and CEA in endometrial carcinoma tissue and its relation to hormone receptor content and histological grading. *Archives of Gynecology and Obstetrics*, 244:47–52.

Nori D, Hilaris BS, Tome M, Lewis JL, Birubaum S, Fuks Z (1987). Combined surgery and radiation in endometrial carcinoma: an analysis of prognostic factors. *International Journal of Radiation Oncology—Biology—Physics*, 13:489–97.

Norris HJ, Taylor HB (1966). Mesenchymal tumors of the uterus. 1. A clinical and pathological study of 53 endometrial stromal tumors. *Cancer*, 19:755–66.

O'Brien AA, O'Brien DS, Daly PA (1970). Aggressive endometrial stromal sarcoma responding to medroxyprogesterone following failure of tamoxifen and combination chemotherapy. Case report. *British Journal of Obstetrics and Gynaecology*, 92:862–6.

O'Hanlan KA (1990). Virulence of papillary endometrial carcinoma. *Gynecologic Oncology*, 37:112–9.

Omura GA, et al. (1985). A randomized trial of adjuvant adriamycin in uterine sarcomas: a Gynecologic Oncology Group study. *Journal of Clinical Oncology*, 3:1240.

Omura GA, et al. (1983). A randomized study of adriamycin with and without dimethyltriazenomidazole carboxamide in advanced uterine sarcomas. *Cancer*, 52:626.

Onsrud M, Kolstad P, Norman T (1976). Postoperative external pelvic irradiation in carcinoma of the corpus stage I: a controlled clinical trial. *Gynaecology and Obstetrics*, 4:222–31.

Pasmantier MW, *et al.* (1985). Treatment of advanced endometrial carcinoma with doxorubicin and cisplatin: effects on both untreated and previously treated patients. *Cancer Treatment Reports*, 69:539–42.

Patsner B (1989). Use of serum CA125 levels to monitor therapy of patients with advanced or recurrent endometrial carcinoma. *European Journal of Gynaecological Oncology*, 10:322–5.

Peters III W, Andersen W, Hopkins M (1989). Results of chemotherapy in advanced carcinoma of the fallopian tube. *Cancer*, 63:836–8.

Phelps H, Chapman K (1974). Role of radiation therapy in the treatment of primary carcinoma of the uterine tube. *Obstetrics and Gynecology*, 43:669–73.

Piver MS (1986). Melphalan, 5-fluorouracil, and medroxyprogesterone acetate in metastatic endometrial carcinoma. *Obstetrics and Gynecology*, 67:261–4.

Piver MS (1991). Phase II trial of cisplatin, adriamycin, and etoposide for metastatic endometrial adenocarcinoma. *American Journal of Clinical Oncology*, 14:200–2.

Piver MS, Lurain JR (1981). Uterine sarcomas: clinical features and management. In *Gynecologic oncology: fundamental principles and clinical practice* (ed. M Coppleson), pp. 608–18. Churchill Livingstone, New York.

Piver MS, Yazigi R, Blumenson L, Tsukada Y (1979). A prospective trial comparing hysterectomy, hysterectomy plus vaginal radium and uterine radium plus hysterectomy in stage I endometrial cancer. *Obstetrics and Gynaecology*, 54:85–9.

Piver S, *et al.* (1980). Medroxyprogesterone acetate (Depo-provera) vs. hydroxyprogesterone caproate (Delalutin) in women with metastatic endometrial adenocarcinoma. *Cancer*, 45:268–72.

Piver SM, Rutledge FN, Copeland I, Webster K, Blumenson I, Suh O (1984). Uterine endolymphatic stromal myosis: a collaborative study. *Obstetrics and Gynecology*, 64:173–8.

Raju KS, Barker GH, Wiltshaw E (1981). Primary carcinoma of the Fallopian tube: report of 22 cases. *British Journal of Obstetrics and Gynaecology*, 88:1124.

Rand RJ, Lowe JW, Parker D (1990). Low-grade endometrial stromal sarcoma treated with a progestogen. *British Journal of Hospital Medicine*, 43:154–6.

Reisinger SA (1991). Survival and failure analysis in stage 2 endometrial cancer using the revised 1988 FIGO staging system. *International Journal of Radiation Oncology—Biology—Physics*, 21:1027–32.

Risinger JI (1993). Genetic instability of microsatellites in endometrial carcinoma. *Cancer Research*, 53:5100–3.

Roberts DWT (1961). Carcinoma of the body of the uterus at Chelsea Hospital for Women. *Journal of Obstetrics and Gynaecology*, 68:132–8.

Romano S, Shimoni M, Yuralee D, Shalev E (1992). Retrograde seeding of endometrial carcinoma during hysteroscopy. *Gynecologic Oncology*, 44:116–18.

Randell ME, Wilder J, Grevan K, Raben M (1990). Role of intracavitary cuff boost after adjuvant external irradiation in early endometrial carcinoma. *International Journal of Radiation Oncology—Biology—Physics*, 19:49–54.

Rosenberg P (1993). A new aggressive treatment approach to high-grade endometrial cancer of possible benefit to patients with stage I uterine papillary cancer. *Gynecologic Oncology*, 48:32–7.

Rosen A, Klein M, Lahousen M, Graf AH, Rainer A, Vavra N (1993). For the Austrian cooperative study group for Fallopian tube carcinoma. Primary carcinoma of the Fallopian tube—a retrospective analysis of 115 patients. *British Journal of Cancer*, 68:605–9.

Rose PG, Reale ML, Beurskens ML, Hunter RE (1993). Preoperative CA-125 levels predict poor prognostic pathologic features in early stage, FIGO grade 1 and 2 endometrial adenocarcinoma. *International Journal of Gynecological Cancer*, 3:259–62.

Salazar OM, *et al.* (1978). Uterine sarcomas. Analysis of failures with special emphasis on the use of adjuvant radiation therapy. *Cancer*, 42:1161.

Scambia G (1993). Expression of ras p21 oncoprotein in normal and neoplastic human endometrium. *Gynecologic Oncology*, 50:339–46.

Schiller HM, Silverberg STG (1971). Staging and prognosis in primary carcinoma of the Fallopian tube. *Cancer*, 28:389–95.

Seski JC, Edwards CL, Gershenson DM, Copeland LJ (1981). Doxorubicin and cyclophosphamide chemotherapy for disseminated endometrial cancer. *Obstetrics and Gynecology*, 58:88–91.

Seski J, *et al.* (1982). Cisplatin chemotherapy for disseminated endomerial cancer. *Obstetrics and Gynecology*, 59:225–8.

Shapiro S, *et al.* (1980). Recent and past use of conjugated estrogens in relation to adenocarcinoma of the endometrium. *New England Journal of Medicine*, 303:485.

Shapiro S, *et al.* (1985). Risk of localized and widespread endometrial cancer in relation to recent and discontinued use of conjugated estrogens. *New England Journal of Medicine*, 313:969.

Shu Xiao Ou (1992). Relation of obesity and body fat distribution to endometrial cancer in Shanghai, China. *Cancer Research*, 52:3865–70.

Silverberg SG, Makowski EL (1975). Endometrial carcinoma in young women taking oral contraceptive agents. *Obstetrics and Gynecology*, 46:503.

Slavik M, Petty WM, Blessing JA, Creasman WT, Homesley HD (1984). Phase 2 clinical study of tamoxifen in advanced endometrial adenocarcinoma: a Gynecologic Oncology Group study. *Cancer Treatment Reports*, 68:809–11.

Sorbe B (1985). Radiotherapy and/or chemotherapy as adjuvant treatment of uterine sarcomas. *Gynecologic Oncology*, 20:271–89.

Subramanyam B, Raghavendra B, Whalen C, Yee J (1984). Ultrasonic features of fallopian tube carcinoma. *Journal of Ultrasound Medicine*, 3:391–3.

Sutton GP, Stehman FB, Michael H, Young PCM, Ehrlich CE (1986). Estrogen and progesterone receptors in uterine sarcomas. *Obstetrics and Gynecology*, 68:709–14.

Swenerton K (1980). Treatment of advanced endometrial adenocarcinoma with tamoxifen. *Cancer Treatment Reports*, 64:805.

Thigpen T, Buchsbaum A, Mangan C, Blessing JA (1974). Phase 2 trial of adriamycin in the treatment of advanced recurrent endometrial carcinoma. *Cancer Treatment Reports*, 63:21–7.

Thigpen T (1989). Systemic therapy with single agents for advanced or recurrent endometrial carcinoma. In *Endometrial cancer* (ed. EA Surwit and DS Alberts), pp. 93–106. Kluwer Academic Publishers, Boston.

Tokunaga T, Miyazaki K, Matsuyama S, Okamura H (1990). Serial measurement of CA 125 in patients with primary carcinoma of the fallopian tube. *Gynecologic Oncology*, 36:335–7.

Trope C, *et al.* (1980). A phase 2 study of cisplatinum for recurrent corpus cancer. *European Journal of Cancer*, 16:1025–6.

Trope C, *et al.* (1984). Treatment of recurrent endometrial adenocarcinoma with a combination of doxorubicin and cisplatin. *American Journal of Obstetrics and Gynecology*, 149:379–81.

Turbow MM, Ballon SC, Sikic BI, Koretz MM (1985). Cisplatin, doxorubicin and cyclophosphamide chemotherapy for advanced endometrial carcinoma. *Cancer Treatment Reports*, 69:465–7.

Vergote I (1989). A randomized trial of adjuvant progestagen in early endometrial cancer. *Cancer*, 64:1011–6.

Weber AM, Hewett WF, Gajewski WH, Curry SI (1993). Malignant mixed Müllerian tumors of the fallopian tube. *Gynecologic Oncology*, 50:239–43.

Webb GA (1987). Clear cell carcinoma of the endometrium. *American Journal of Obstetrics and Gynecology*, 156:1486–91.

WHO Collaborative. Depot-medroxyprogesterone acetate (DMPA), and risk of endometrial cancer. *International Journal of Cancer*, 49:186–90.

Young PCM, Cleary RE (1974). Characterization and properties of progesterone binding components in human endometrium. *Journal of Clinical Endocrinology and Metabolism*, 89:425.

9.5   Gestational trophoblastic tumours

R. H. J. BEGENT

INTRODUCTION

One of the first tissues to differentiate in the fetus, trophoblast, at first grows rapidly, with invasion of the endometrium and uterine vasculature. In the second and third trimesters of a normal pregnancy this aggressive behaviour is moderated. Its gestational nature gives trophoblast a unique relationship with the host and the immunological basis of this is only partly understood.

Gestational trophoblastic tumours belong to a group of trophoblastic diseases not all of which are malignant. They include hydatidiform mole, which comprises complete and partial hydatidiform mole, invasive mole, gestational choriocarcinoma, and placental-site trophoblastic tumour. Choriocarcinoma arising in germ cell tumours and common epithelial carcinomas is excluded because it is not gestational in origin.

This classification, defined by a World Health Organization (**WHO**) Scientific Group (WHO 1983) acknowledges the existing WHO 'Histological Classification of Tumours' (Poulsen 1975) but modifies it because of the subsequent discovery (Vassilakos *et al.* 1977) that complete and partial hydatiform mole are separate entities of different aetiology.

COMPLETE HYDATIDIFORM MOLE
Origin

Complete hydatidiform mole originates from fertilization of an ovum from which the maternal genetic material is lost or inactivated

(Fig. 1). A single sperm bearing a 23X set of chromosomes produces the fertilization and then duplicates to 46XX in approximately 90 per cent of cases (Vassilakos *et al.* 1977; Kajii and Ohama 1977; Lawler *et al.* 1979, 1982*a*; Davis *et al.* 1984; Lawler and Fisher 1986). Occasionally, fertilization takes place with two spermatozoa, resulting in the XY configuration (Ohama *et al.* 1981). The 46XX constitution can probably also originate in this way. A 46YY conceptus would be theoretically possible by this mechanism but is not described and is presumably non-viable. The most frequent variants are shown in Fig. 1(a) and (b). Whilst the nuclear genetic material is paternal, the mitochondrial DNA is of maternal origin (Edwards *et al.* 1984). The conceptus in complete hydatiform mole is thus entirely paternally derived and a total allograft in the mother. Twin pregnancies with a complete hydatiform mole and normal fetus have been reported (Fisher *et al.* 1982; Berrebi *et al.* 1988). The Berrebi paper reviewed this literature and found birth of a viable fetus in 27 per cent, fetal death *in utero* in 46 per cent, and birth of a non-viable fetus in 23 per cent.

Historical note

Hydatidiform mole was recognized as a cause of abortion by Hippocrates and his pupil, Diocles. Its origin from the chorion was recognized in Paris in the nineteenth century (Ober 1987). The macroscopic structure of multiple hydropic vesicles probably led the attendants of Margeret Countess of Henneberg in 1276 to

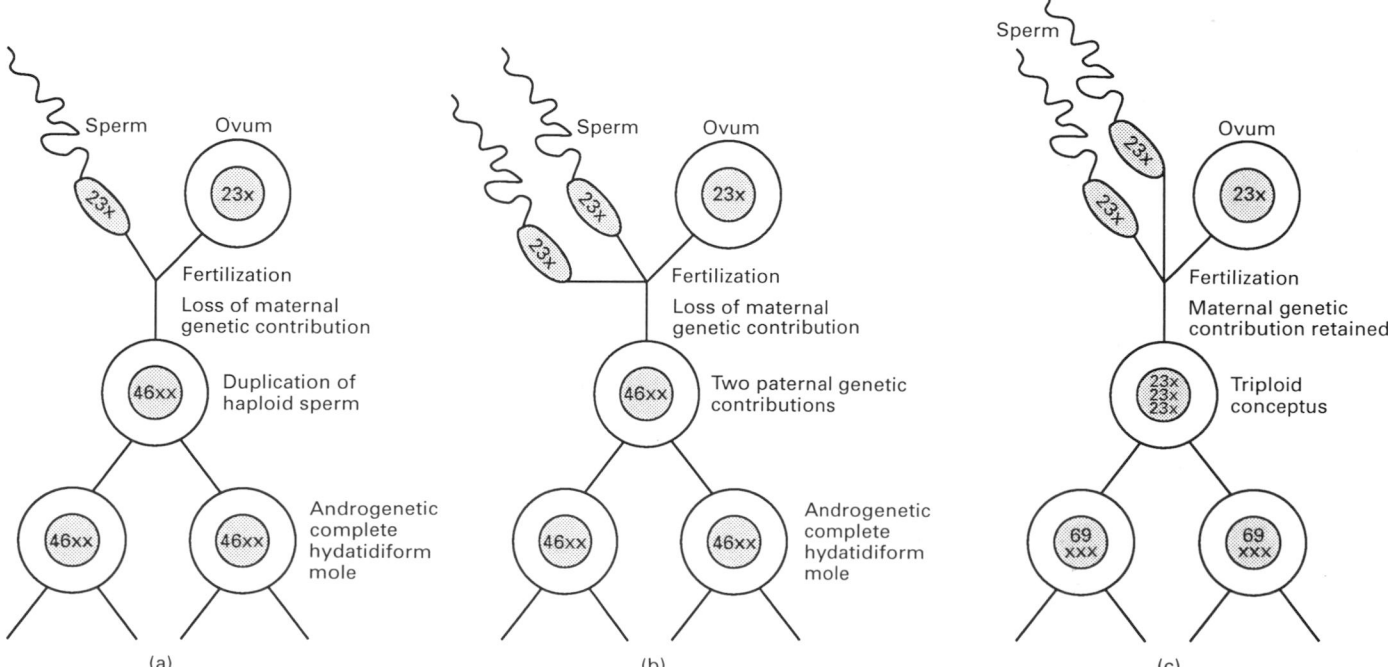

Fig. 1   The genetic origin of (a) complete hydatidiform mole originating from fertilization by a single sperm, (b) complete hydatidiform mole originating from dispermy (this form can also be XY), and (c) partial hydatidiform mole, which is triploid. (Reproduced from Begent (1990), with permission.)

believe that each vesicle was a separate conception and to christen half John and half Mary.

Morphology

The universal, hydropically dilated, trophoblastic villi connected by narrow bridges bear hyperplastic syncitio- and cytotrophoblast on their surface, with varying degrees of exuberance. The villi initially contain oedematous mesenchyme. Cisterns form within the mesenchyme, which involutes with increasing gestational age. Any blood vessels in the mesenchyme also tend to die out leaving the fluid-filled cistern as the feature causing hydropic villous dilatation. There being no fetus, nucleated fetal erythrocytes are not seen in any vessels present.

PARTIAL HYDATIDIFORM MOLE
Origin

Cytogenetic and biochemical studies show that partial moles are triploid, differing from complete hydatidiform mole by retaining a maternal genetic contribution. They most often arise by diandry, with two paternal and one maternal set of chromosomes (Jacobs et al. 1982; Lawler et al. 1982b; Lawler and Fisher 1987) (Fig. 1(c)). Triploidy occurs in 1–3 per cent of all recognized conceptions and in approximately 20 per cent of spontaneous abortions with abnormal karyotype. Not all of these become partial hydatidiform mole. Exceptionally, partial mole can be tetraploid, with three paternal contributions (Sheppard et al. 1982). Flow cytometry can now be used to determine whether trophoblastic disease is triploid or diploid. This offers a practical solution to the problem of discriminating complete and partial mole because it can be done on formalin-fixed, paraffin-embedded tissue (Fisher et al. 1987; Lage et al. 1988).

Morphology

Discrimination from complete hydatidiform mole by morphology is not always straightforward. There is evidence of a fetus as part of the same conception, in which the placenta contains some normal and some abnormal villi. These villi are swollen, showing trophoblastic hyperplasia and cistern formation. In older examples (more than 18–20 weeks), a maze-like outline is sometimes seen in the cisterns. If the fetus is alive the vessels in the villi contain nucleated, fetal red blood cells. There is a characteristic scalloping of the outline of the villi and stromal trophoblastic inclusions are common. The affected villi are mixed in the form of a mosaic, with normal trophoblastic villi within the placenta. The trophoblastic hyperplasia is often less marked than in complete hydatidiform mole and is usually confined to the syncytiotrophoblast. The fetus usually dies at 8–9 weeks of menstrual age. This is followed by fibrosis of the villous mesenchyme in unaffected and affected villi.

It is not certain whether partial hydatidiform mole can give rise to choriocarcinoma. However, after evacuation the concentration of human chorionic gonadotrophin has failed to fall to normal in some patients (Berkowitz et al. 1985; Watson et al. 1987), indicating persistent growth of trophoblast, which could be explained by the development of choriocarcinoma or invasive mole. However, metastatic choriocarcinoma was not reported and there is doubt whether this ever occurs.

INVASIVE MOLE

Invasive mole occurs when complete or partial hydatidiform mole invades deep into the myometrium. This extension is well beyond the usual decidual site of implantation and has been likened to placenta accreta or percreta in the non-molar placenta (Szulman 1987). Invasive mole is distinguished from choriocarcinoma by the presence of chorionic villae. However, the diagnosis is often obscure because uterine curettage cannot gain access to the tumour deep in the myometrium. Similarly, it is not possible to determine whether a pulmonary metastasis after hydatidiform mole is choriocarcinoma or hydatidiform mole without resecting it. This is hardly ever justified.

The principal risk is of uterine perforation or severe uterine bleeding. Invasive mole may metastasize to the lungs, cervix, vulva, and vagina. It may regress spontaneously and, although it can occasionally progress to choriocarcinoma, it does not usually exhibit the progression of true malignancy. There is some evidence that heterozygosity is more common in moles subsequently requiring chemotherapy because of invasive mole or choriocarcinoma (Davis et al. 1984; Sheppard et al. 1985; Lawler and Fisher 1986).

CHORIOCARCINOMA
Origin

Choriocarcinoma may originate from hydatidiform mole, being of paternal genetic origin or from a normal conception. It is still uncertain whether it can follow partial hydatidiform mole.

Morphology

Choriocarcinoma is a malignant tumour made up of, principally, villous trophoblast. It has the essential features of the rapidly dividing and invasive trophoblast of the implanting blastocyst but maintains these features instead of differentiating to a more stable form as occurs in the progress of a normal pregnancy. Chorionic villi are absent. The characteristic morphology is of pleomorphic cytotrophoblast surrounded by some syncytium with extensive areas of haemorrhage and necrosis. The syncitiotrophoblast is largely responsible for production of human chorionic gonadotrophin and other hormones of pregnancy. Because of the similarity to early trophoblast in normal pregnancy, caution is needed in making the diagnosis on scanty uterine curettings when an early pregnancy is possible. Viable choriocarcinoma cells may comprise only a rim on a mass of necrotic and haemorrhagic tissue. The tumour has no stroma or vasculature of its own and relies on vessels of the tissue which it invades. Choriocarcinoma may follow normal pregnancy, non-molar abortion, ectopic pregnancy, or hydatidiform mole. It is not practical to make the diagnosis on uterine curettings after hydatidiform mole because it is necessary to obtain more comprehensive material in order practically to exclude the presence of chorionic villi. For this reason, doubt often exists at the time the patient comes to treatment whether she has invasive mole or choriocarcinoma. Gestational choriocarcinoma must also be distinguished from choriocarcinoma arising in an ovarian germ cell tumour or from trophoblastic differentiation in a common epithelial carcinoma. Gestational choriocarcinoma metastasizes widely, particularly to the lungs, pelvic organs, and brain.

PLACENTAL-SITE TROPHOBLASTIC TUMOUR

Placental-site trophoblastic tumours (PSTT) may follow term delivery, non-molar abortion, or complete hydatidiform mole. They are slow growing and may present many years after the causative gestation.

Morphology

These are slow-growing, malignant tumours of placental-site (intermediate) trophoblast. In the normal placenta, placental-site trophoblast is separate from villous trophoblast and infiltrates the deciduum, myometrium, and spiral arteries of the placental site (Kurman *et al.* 1976). The cells are mostly mononuclear, though multinucleate forms occur. Their appearance in the normal placenta and PSTT has been reviewed by Mazur and Kurman (1987). Discrimination between PSTT and the non-malignant, exaggerated placental-site reaction and placental nodule may present considerable difficulties. Young *et al.* (1988) and Lathrop *et al.* (1988) attempted to define the morphology of the two conditions but difficulties still arise. There is little human chorionic gonadotrophin in the cells of PSTT but abundant human placental lactogen is present. This can be valuable in diagnosis and in discriminating from carcinomas or sarcomas by immunohistochemistry.

HYDROPIC DEGENERATION

This is characterized by dilatation, with increased fluid content or liquefaction, of placental villi. It has also previously been known as molar degeneration and hydropic change. The trophoblastic proliferation and other characteristic features of complete or partial hydatidiform mole are absent and there is no increased risk of neoplastic sequelae compared with a normal pregnancy. It is mentioned here in order to exclude it from the definition of trophoblastic disease.

INCIDENCE OF TROPHOBLASTIC DISEASE

Complete hydatidiform mole

The incidence of hydatidiform mole has been reviewed by a WHO Scientific Group (WHO 1983) and Bracken *et al.* (1984). Epidemiological studies have not, in general, taken into account the fact that complete or partial hydatidiform mole have a different pathological basis. The situation is further complicated by variation in the classification of hydropic degeneration, a harmless condition (see above), which is sometimes included in studies of hydatidiform mole. There is probably a tendency for hospital-based studies to exaggerate the incidence of hydatidiform mole, particularly in the developing countries where the hospital population will reflect a selected group of patients with a greater incidence of complications of pregnancy. Reports are also difficult to compare because some relate the incidence of hydatidiform mole to the number of pregnancies, others to normal deliveries, and still others to the number of live births.

Overall incidence

The incidence from hospital-based studies varies between 0.7 and 10 cases of hydatidiform mole per 1000 pregnancies. The highest values have been from South-East Asia and Western Africa, where the effect of the selection of hospital is likely to be high. Population-based studies do not reflect the same differences, with the exception of Japan where higher incidences have been reported than in other parts of the world. There are not enough studies to establish with certainty that incidence does vary substantially in different parts of the world; the incidence in the order of 1/1000 pregnancies appears representative.

Information on temporal trends of hydatidiform mole is more conflicting and again tends to suffer from the problems of hospital-based studies. No clear trend emerges.

Ethnic origin

Large differences in the incidence of hydatidiform mole do seem to be present in various ethnic groups. In the United States, for 1970–1977, hydatidiform mole was only half as frequent in Black women as in others (Hayashi 1982); in Singapore, from 1963 to 1965, Eurasian women had a rate of hydatidiform mole twice as high as that of Chinese, Indian, or Malaysian (Teoh *et al.* 1971). A higher incidence was also seen in Jewish women over 45 years old who lived in Israel and came from Europe than in those of the same age who were born in Africa, Asia, or Israel (Matalon and Modan 1972). A study by Jacobs *et al.* (1982) showed that Filipinos seem to maintain the high risk of hydatidiform mole that prevails in their own country, whereas Japanese and other East Asians seem to lose the high incidence of their own countries when they live in Hawaii. This suggests that cultural factors affect the immigrants when they move to a new environment.

Age

In the United Kingdom the lowest incidence appears to be between 25 and 29 years of age, with a 6-fold increase in relative risk in pregnancies in girls under 15 years. There is also an increased risk above the age of 40 years, with a relative risk of 3-fold between 40 and 45 years, 26-fold between 45 and 49, and more than 400-fold over 50 years of age (Bagshawe *et al.* 1986). The effect of paternal age is difficult to separate from that of maternal age and conflicting studies of the independent effect of paternal age have been reported (Yen and McMahon 1968; La Vecchia *et al.* 1984). No clear effect from gravidity seems to apply, but women who have had a previous hydatidiform mole have a substantially increased risk of having another. For instance, in the United Kingdom the incidence rises from 1 in 1000 pregnancies for the first mole to 1 in 74 in women who have already had one mole (Bagshawe *et al.* 1986).

Incidence of partial mole

Partial mole was found to be less frequent than complete hydatidiform mole (24 per cent of the total) in a series in which cases were selected because of suspicion of hydatidiform mole (Lawler and Fisher 1986). Similarly, Berkowitz and Goldstein (1981) found 3 per cent of partial hydatidiform moles in their series. However, in patients presenting as spontaneous abortion the frequency of partial hydatidiform mole was 69 per cent relative to complete hydatidiform mole (Jacobs *et al.* 1982).

Incidence and epidemiology of choriocarcinoma

This is influenced by the incidence of hydatidiform mole and approximately 3 per cent of patients with hydatidiform mole finally develop choriocarcinoma. Problems with definition arise in this group where histological diagnosis is not always available and discrimination between invasive mole and choriocarcinoma is not possible. Hydatidiform mole is probably the most common antecedent to choriocarcinoma, comprising 29–83 per cent in studies from various parts of the world, abortion or ectopic pregnancy being the next most common (11–42 per cent), followed by live births (5–34 per cent) (WHO 1983). The incidence following term delivery without hydatidiform mole is of the order of 1 in 50 000. No very clear trends emerge for greater frequency in particular parts of the world (Bracken *et al.* 1984) but more extensive, population-based studies are needed.

Genetic factors

Cytogenetic studies show 4.6 per cent of balanced translocations in women with complete hydatidiform mole compared with 0.6 per cent of normal populations. The ABO blood groups of women with hydatidiform mole and their spouses do not appear to differ from normal populations. However, choriocarcinoma after term delivery is approximately twice as common when patient and partner have different A and O blood groups as when they are the same (for a review, see WHO (1983)).

Incidence of placental-site trophoblastic tumours

Although only approximately 50 cases have been reported, PSTT is thought to constitute approximately 1 per cent of trophoblastic tumours.

CLINICAL FEATURES

Hydatidiform mole

Hydatidiform mole, including the complete and the partial, presents in the first trimester, most commonly with vaginal bleeding that may be fresh or altered, light or heavy enough to require transfusion, and frequently associated with anaemia. The uterus may be enlarged or small for gestational age. Hyperemesis and toxaemia (Newman and Eddy 1988) occur with greater frequency than in normal pregnancy. Passage of vesicles is not infrequent and occasionally the entire mole is evacuated spontaneously. Theca lutein cysts are frequently found when the concentrations of human chorionic gonadotrophin are high. Pulmonary, vaginal, and cervical metastases may occur but do not necessarily imply development of invasive mole or choriocarcinoma, as they may resolve after evacuation of the mole. Hyperthyroidism (Fradken *et al.* 1989) and pulmonary emboli of trophoblast occur occasionally. The clinical features of hydatidiform mole have been reviewed by Goldstein *et al.* (1981). Pregnancy terminated for medical or social reasons may be a mole and escape detection when no histological examination is done (Kiel 1986).

Partial mole

Vaginal bleeding is the most frequent presentation, the diagnosis usually being made on histological examination of curettings from a presumed missed or incomplete abortion. Presentation is often made relatively late in pregnancy, at a mean of 23 weeks' gestation in the series of Watson *et al.* (1987). The uterus is small or of appropriate size for gestational age and the human chorionic gonadotrophin is under 100 000 iu/l at diagnosis in over 90 per cent of patients. Ultrasonography commonly does not show a fetal heart (Berkowitz *et al.* 1985).

In the series of Berkowitz *et al.* (1985) and Watson *et al.* (1987), 10 and 14 per cent were considered to have persistent trophoblastic disease in the uterus and were treated with chemotherapy. The experience at Charing Cross Hospital is that the serum human

chorionic gonadotrophin returns to normal concentrations without treatment in almost all these patients and that chemotherapy is rarely required. It is uncertain whether metastases ever occur. Doubt exists because the series reported were diagnosed by morphology, which is not reliable at discriminating between complete and partial hydatidiform mole. Series in which the diagnosis of partial mole is confirmed by the presence of triploidy or tetraploidy will be more reliable in determining the clinical behaviour.

Invasive mole

This is usually diagnosed in the weeks following evacuation of hydatidiform mole because invasion of the myometrium produces heavy bleeding, lower abdominal pain, or intraperitoneal haemorrhage. These life-threatening presentations of invasive mole should not be awaited before treatment is started because they can be predicted in most cases by monitoring human chorionic gonadotrophin in urine or serum. Occasionally the bladder or rectum is infiltrated, producing haematuria or rectal bleeding. Enlarging pulmonary, vulval, or vaginal metastases may occur.

Choriocarcinoma

Choriocarcinoma is 1500 times more common after a molar pregnancy than after a term delivery. In the former case it should be suspected if the concentration of human chorionic gonadotrophin is not normal 6 months after evacuation. It may occur sooner than this after a mole but then is often difficult to distinguish from invasive mole without doing a hysterectomy to determine the diagnosis histologically. Hysterectomy is only rarely justified or necessary at this stage, so there remain many cases in which it is never known whether the patient had invasive mole or choriocarcinoma, even after treatment. Choriocarcinoma and placental-site tumour are the only possible gestational trophoblastic tumours originating from a term delivery or a non-molar abortion.

Presentation

The majority of patients with choriocarcinoma present within a year of an apparently normal pregnancy or non-molar abortion. The presentation may be delayed for several years, however; in the Charing Cross Hospital series the longest interval was 17 years. Vaginal bleeding or blood-stained discharge, sometimes with abdominal pain and mass, are most common. Extrauterine masses and ovarian involvement are frequent. In approximately one-third of cases, however, the presenting features are not gynaecological but originate from distant metastases (McGrath *et al.* 1971). Pulmonary, cerebral, and hepatic deposits are most frequent (Table 1) (Begent and Bagshawe 1982). Pulmonary deposits (see Fig. 5) may cause dyspnoea, or haemoptysis, and when widespread can be associated with pneumonia. Choriocarcinoma can grow within the pulmonary artery and cause pulmonary hypertension (Bagshawe and Begent 1981). Cerebral metastases may present with focal neurological signs, convulsions, and evidence of raised intracranial pressure or of haemorrhage intracerebrally or into the subarachnoid space (Athanassiou *et al.* 1983). These features are not specific for choriocarcinoma and it may be many years since the causative pregnancy. It is important, therefore, to remember to measure the concentration of human chorionic gonadotrophin (see below) when cerebral metastases occur in women who have had a pregnancy. Metastases in viscera such as the liver, kidney, spleen, or bowel may also present with haemorrhage intraperitoneally or into the lumen of the bowel. Skin metastases are usually purple and most

Table 1 Sites of metastases outside the pelvis detected at presentation in 72 patients with high-risk gestational choriocarcinoma

Site	No. of patients
Lungs	57
Brain	11
Liver	9
Breast	1
Spleen	1
Cauda equina	1
Not detected	8

frequently occur late in the course of the disease. Lymph node and bone metastases are so rare that their presence should lead to review of the evidence for the diagnosis.

Occasionally, thyrotoxicosis is present in patients with very high concentrations of human chorionic gonadotrophin because of cross-reaction between the α-subunit of the gonadotrophin and thyroid-stimulating hormone (Fradken *et al.* 1989).

Production of human chorionic gonadotrophin by a common epithelial malignancy such as a bronchial or gastrointestinal carcinoma may be difficult to discriminate from gestational choriocarcinoma, especially if it presents with lung, brain, or intra-abdominal metastases.

Choriocarcinoma in the fetus

This is a rare accompaniment to choriocarcinoma in the mother, 13 cases being recorded. Flam *et al.* (1989), reviewing the literature and reporting a case, noted presentation usually in the first 6 months of the child's life and some cases in which choriocarcinoma was not found in the mother. Diagnosis was usually made in the child before the mother and all of the children died. Hepatomegaly was common in the children and tumour was found in the liver in some cases. This may cause sudden death from intraperitoneal haemorrhage. It is probably wise to measure the human chorionic gonadotrophin in babies whose mothers have choriocarcinoma following term delivery and to search for evidence of choriocarcinoma in mothers of children with the diagnosis.

Placental-site trophoblastic tumour

PSTT has a slow growth rate and may present years after term delivery, non-molar abortion, or complete hydatidiform mole. Only approximately 50 cases have been reported. PSTT usually presents with vaginal bleeding or amenorrhoea (Finkler *et al.* 1988). Cases following hydatidiform mole may come to light because of resistance to cytotoxic chemotherapy (Heyderman *et al.* 1989). Nephrotic syndrome or haematuria may occur and appear to be related to glomerular deposition of fibrin (Eckstein *et al.* 1982; Young *et al.* 1985). Disseminated intravascular coagulation has been reported in relation to this syndrome. Nagelberg and Rosen (1985) reported virilization with raised testosterone levels, which appeared to be an ovarian response to gonadotrophin drive from the tumour.

PSTT is usually confined to the uterus and was originally thought to be benign, being then called trophoblastic pseudotumour. However, later experience shows that PSTT may metastasize and is usually resistant to cytotoxic chemotherapy (Scully and Young 1981; Eckstein *et al.* 1982; Finkler *et al.* 1988). Metastases can occur in the vagina, extrauterine pelvic tissues, retroperitoneum, lymph nodes, lungs, and brain (Eckstein *et al.* 1985; Hopkins *et al.* 1985; Samlowski *et al.* 1985).

INVESTIGATION

Human chorionic gonadotrophin

This hormone is only one of a range produced by normal and neoplastic trophoblast. It is a polypeptide composed of two subunits with a combined molecular weight of 37 000. It is excreted in the urine with a half-life of approximately 24–36 h and has so far proved the most sensitive and specific marker for trophoblastic tumours when compared with other placental proteins (PP) such as PP5 and β_1-SP1. Pregnancy tests employing haemagglutination inhibition or complement fixation methods have a lower limit of sensitivity of approximately 2000 iu/l whereas the best radioimmunoassays are sensitive to 1 iu/l in serum and 20 iu/l in urine (Kardana and Bagshawe 1976). Immunoenzymatic, immunochemiluminescent, and fluoroimmunoassays also have the potential to match or improve on this sensitivity. It is important to be aware that simple pregnancy tests can also give false-negative results when values for human chorionic gonadotrophin are very high.

When it is wished to exclude a trophoblastic tumour, one of the more sensitive assays must be used. Assays for human chorionic gonadotrophin do not discriminate between trophoblastic tumours and normal pregnancy, although very high values outside the range for twin pregnancy may lead to suspicion of a trophoblastic tumour. The concentrations of the chorionic gonadotrophin are frequently within the pregnancy range. Considering that pregnancy is much the more common cause of a raised chorionic gonadotrophin, this possibility must always be considered before embarking on investigation or treatment of a suspected trophoblastic tumour. Germ cell tumours containing trophoblastic elements can produce concentrations of chorionic gonadotrophin as high as with gestational trophoblastic tumours (for a review, see Bagshawe and Begent (1983)). Approximately 15 per cent of common epithelial malignancies produce measurable amounts of human chorionic gonadotrophin (Vaitukaitis 1979) and, exceptionally, levels can exceed 20 000 iu/l.

In gestational trophoblastic disease, the amount of chorionic gonadotrophin gives an indication of the volume of tumour. It has been estimated from tissue culture experiments that a serum chorionic gonadotrophin of the order of 5 iu/l corresponds to $10^4–10^5$ viable tumour cells, making these assays orders of magnitude more sensitive than the most sensitive imaging methods. Total tumour volume can be estimated from measurements of the gonadotrophin and used to determine prognosis (Bagshawe 1976). Serial measurements allow progress of the disease or response to therapy to be monitored (Fig. 2). Development of drug resistance can be detected at an early stage. Estimates may be made of the time for which chemotherapy should be continued after chorionic gonadotrophin is undetectable in serum in order theoretically to eradicate all tumour cells. In these respects it is the best tumour marker known and is of wider interest as a model for the way in which tumour markers may eventually be used in other diseases.

Ultrasonography

Ultrasonography has transformed the investigation of the uterus and pelvic organs in trophoblastic tumours. It has largely displaced arteriography, which was used previously to show the distinctive circulation of hydatidiform mole and choriocarcinoma. Ultrasonography is used to discriminate between normal pregnancy and hydatidiform mole, not solely by the pattern of echogenicity (Fig. 3), which is not entirely specific, but by the presence of this pattern when there is a history consistent with hydatidiform mole or normal

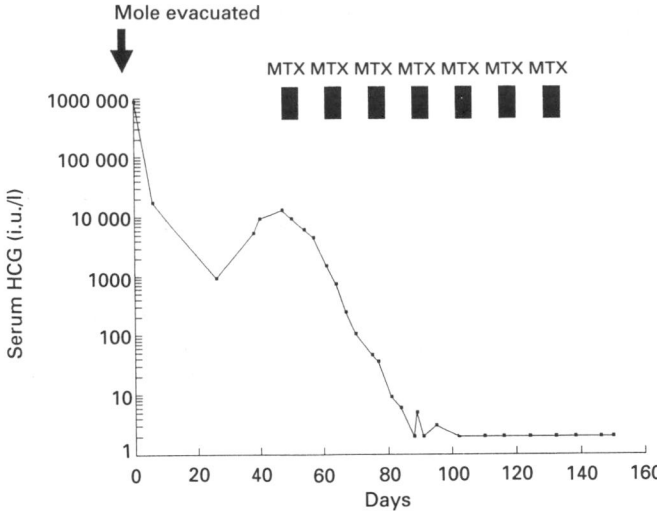

Fig. 2 Chart showing a fall in human chorionic gonadotrophin (HCG) concentrations after evacuation of a hydatidiform mole. The serum HCG later increased, indicating post-molar trophoblastic disease. The patient fell into the low-risk group and was successfully treated with methotrexate (MT) and folinic acid (see Table 6).

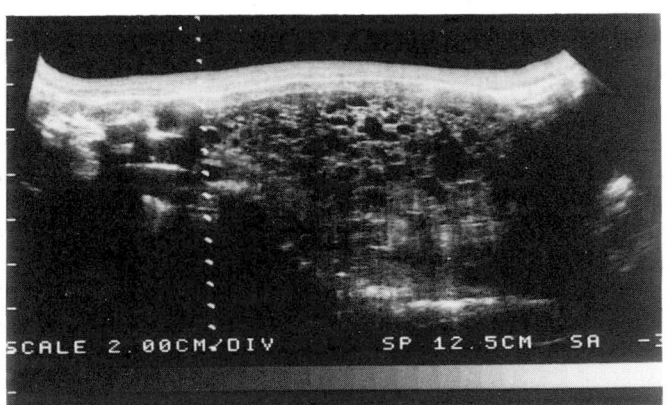

Fig. 3 Ultrasonographic appearances of complete hydatidiform mole. The vesicular nature of the mole can be seen. There is no evidence of a fetus. (Illustration kindly provided by Dr J. E. Boultbee.)

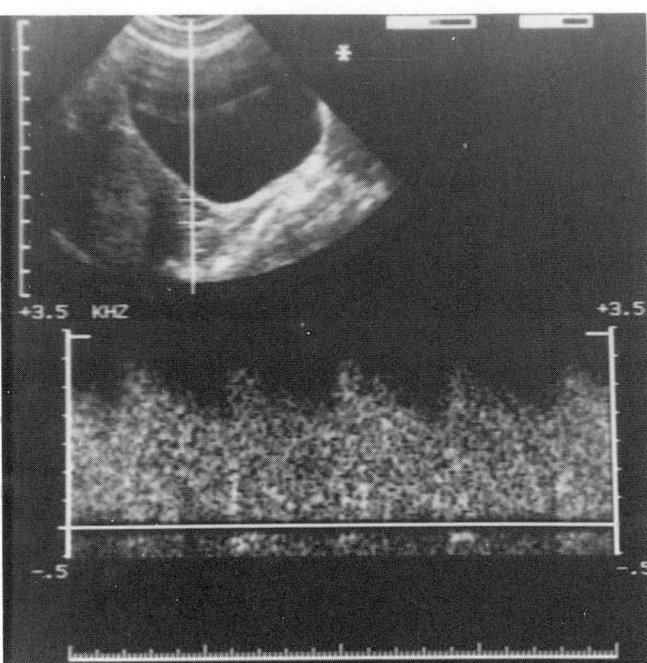

Fig. 4 Ultrasonographic appearances in choriocarcinoma in the uterus (arrowed in the upper section). Doppler ultrasonogram of the myometrium (lower section) gives a waveform typical of the vascular flow which may develop in response to trophoblastic disease. (Illustration kindly provided by Dr J. E. Boultbee.)

pregnancy and when the chorionic gonadotrophin is raised. Romero *et al.* (1985) found that the absence of a fetal heart movement in the presence of a serum chorionic gonadotrophin over 82 350 iu/l predicted hydatidiform mole in 88 per cent of cases, whereas ultrasonography alone only led to a definitive diagnosis on the first examination in 41 per cent.

An example of the appearances of choriocarcinoma is given in Fig. 4. An indication of uterine volume can be obtained that is more accurate than estimations obtained by palpation and is useful as a prognostic indicator. It is helpful in showing extension of the tumour through the uterine wall and separate extrauterine masses. Doppler ultrasonography can be used to study blood flow characteristics in the uterine artery, where abnormalities are found with gestational trophoblastic tumours. These are attributed to the large vascular channels forming in the myometrium, which change the waveform of the uterine artery and may be expressed as an altered pulsatility index (Long *et al.* 1989, 1992). Doppler signals are also produced in the myometrium by invasive mole and choriocarcinoma, which

can help to discriminate these from other uterine conditions (Long *et al.* 1987). However, the abnormal vasculature producing these findings may persist after eradication of the trophoblastic tumour as shown by a persistently normal serum chorionic gonadotrophin.

Theca lutein cysts of the ovary and other ovarian masses are well seen by ultrasonography. Hepatic and renal deposits can be identified and shown to have an abnormal Doppler signal. Ultrasonography is convenient to use for monitoring the progress of the disease (Requard and Mettler 1980), although it does not match the sensitivity of measurements of chorionic gonadotrophin and should not be used as a substitute. When uterine or ovarian masses are present at the start of treatment it is worth repeating the ultrasonogram at the end of treatment to ensure that the changes were not due to some other pathology.

Arteriography

Arteriography has a very limited place since the introduction of Doppler ultrasonography. It shows the great vascularity of trophoblastic tumours and the arteriovenous malformations that exist within them. This vascular pattern sometimes persists after eradication of the mole and can cause severe haemorrhage. Arteriography is useful in determining the extent and vascular supply of deposits of choriocarcinoma in the liver if resection is planned for drug-resistant disease.

Plain radiography of the chest

This demonstrates the diverse patterns of metastases of gestational trophoblastic tumours. The most common appearance (Fig. 5) is of multiple, discrete, rounded lesions but large solitary lesions or a miliary pattern can occur (Bagshawe and Begent 1981). Pleural effusions are rare but dilatation of the pulmonary arteries occurs in patients with pulmonary hypertension.

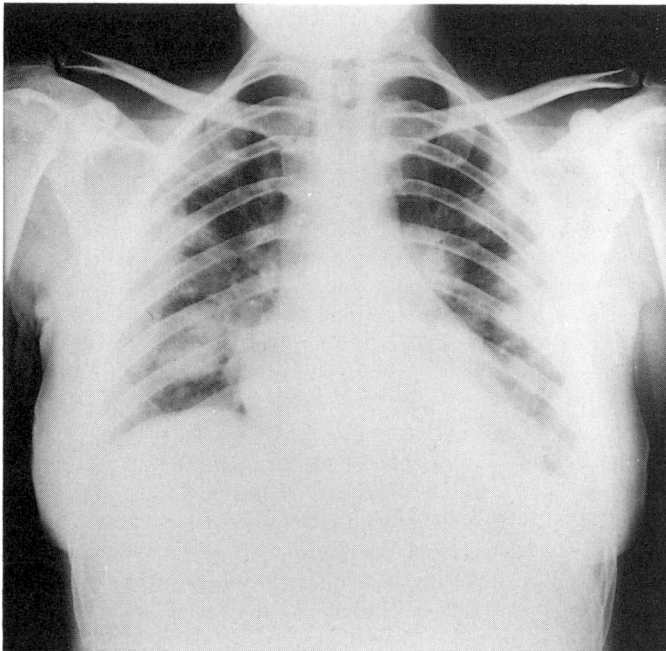

Fig. 5 Chest radiograph showing multiple lung metastases of choriocarcinoma.

Computerized tomography

Computerized tomography is more sensitive than plain radiography, being able to detect metastases of 3–4 mm in the lungs (Fig. 6). It is not necessary to make this investigation routinely but it is invaluable in determining the extent of disease if resection of drug-resistant deposits of choriocarcinoma is being considered. It is also valuable along with ultrasonography in assessing intra-abdominal disease, particularly in the liver and pelvis. In the brain,

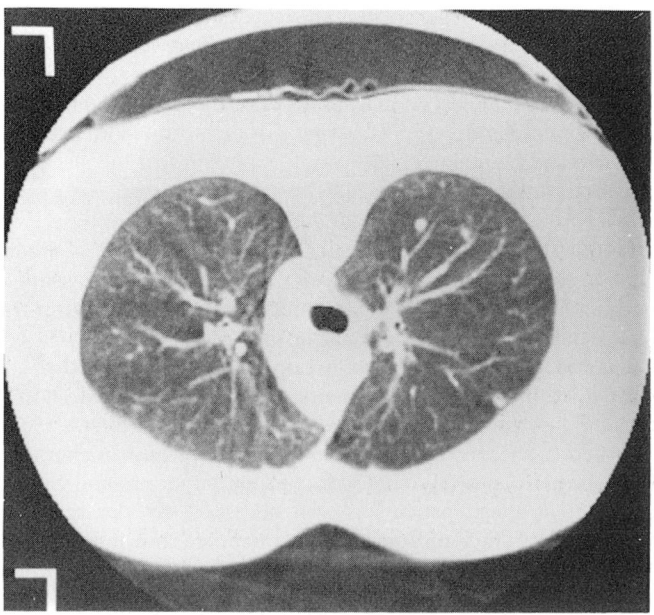

Fig. 6 Computerized tomogram showing small lung metastases (arrowed).

computerized tomography is better than isotope scanning (Athanassiou *et al.* 1983) and is now the standard method for imaging cerebral metastases.

Magnetic resonance imaging

This type of imaging (Steiner and Radda 1983) can also be used to give images of choriocarcinoma in the pelvis and liver. It is not yet clear whether it will be superior to computerized tomography in these areas but it does have advantages in the brain, where better images of the posterior fossa are obtained. In imaging of choriocarcinoma in the cerebral hemispheres it is able to locate deposits close to the bone of the skull that have been undetectable by computerized tomography. These have been resected, eradicating drug-resistant disease.

Antibody imaging

In this method, radiolabelled antibody directed against human chorionic gonadotrophin (**anti-HCG**) is given intravenously. Anti-HCG is retained in chorionic gonadotrophin producing tumours but is cleared more rapidly from the circulation and normal tissues. Tumour deposits can then be located by gamma-camera imaging, appearing as areas of concentration of radioactivity (Begent *et al.* 1980, 1987; Goldenberg *et al.* 1980; Begent 1989). In practice, much of the radiolabelled antibody persists in the circulation and normal tissues. In order to image small tumours it is necessary either to simulate this background with a different radiolabelled medium and perform computer subtraction or to remove non-tumour antibody from the circulation with a second antibody directed against the first (Begent *et al.* 1982; Begent 1989). Deposits of choriocarcinoma can be localized in this way and the method is unique in that it depends on a specific biochemical feature of the tumour, implying viability in the tumour deposit thus localized. Tumour deposits that could not be localized by computerized tomography or ultrasonography have been found in this way and drug-resistant tumours resected (Table 2). The technique has proved most valuable in locating disease in the uterus and lung. However, the yield of positive images is low when the serum chorionic gonadotrophin is below 100 iu/l (Begent 1989). This is not surprising when it is considered that as few as 10^6–10^7 tumour cells can produce this concentration of the hormone.

Deposits of placental-site trophoblastic tumour that could not be located by other means have been detected by imaging with antibody to human chorionic gonadotrophin (Heyderman *et al.* 1989). False-negatives and false-positives do occur, however and the investigation would be regarded as complementary to computerized tomography and ultrasonography.

Table 2 Surgery guided by immunoscintigraphy in gestational choriocarcinoma

	Tumour site			
	Lung	Uterus	Brain	Total
Tumour located and resected	7	2	2	11
Relapse after resection or incomplete resection	2	1	1	4
Disease free when last seen	6	2	1	9

MANAGEMENT

Evacuation of hydatidiform mole

As soon as the diagnosis is strongly suspected on the basis of clinical features and ultrasonography, any significant blood loss should be replaced and the uterus evacuated by suction. This has the advantage that even a large hydatidiform mole can be evacuated with little blood loss (Brandes *et al.* 1966; Schlaerth *et al.* 1988).

Risks of sequelae

The risk of sequelae requiring chemotherapy is relatively small with suction evacuation (Stone and Bagshawe 1979). Medical induction involving repeated contraction of the uterus induced by oxytocin or prostaglandin increases the risk of requiring chemotherapy by 2- to 3-fold compared with suction evacuation. The risk is also greater by a similar amount when hysterectomy or hysterotomy are done (Curry *et al.* 1975; Stone and Bagshawe 1979). This is thought to be because tumour is more likely to be disseminated by uterine contraction or manipulation. If bleeding is severe after uterine evacuation, use of ergometrine on one occasion can sometimes not be avoided. This seems to be acceptable on the grounds that a single uterine contraction produced by this agent is less likely to produce embolization of trophoblast to distant sites than repeated contractions induced by the other agents. If bleeding persists after two curettages, chemotherapy is very likely to be needed for invasive mole or choriocarcinoma and further curettages are unlikely to be beneficial. Hysterectomy can be dangerous in patients with invasive mole before chemotherapy because of the intense vascularity of the tissue, which may be invading outside the uterus. Uncontrollable bleeding has occurred during such operations and if there is some definite reason for hysterectomy it is better to delay the operation until the tumour mass has been greatly reduced or eliminated by chemotherapy.

Management after uterine evacuation

The majority of patients require no more treatment after uterine evacuation but in good circumstances some 8 per cent develop invasive mole or choriocarcinoma (Bagshawe *et al.* 1986). These must be identified and treatment started at any early stage. Factors increasing the chance of requiring treatment should be avoided where possible. These are listed in Table 3. More data are needed about the importance of oral contraceptives but until these are available we advise patients not to take oral contraceptives until the chorionic gonadotrophin has been normal for 3 months.

Uterine size greater than gestational age and bilateral cystic ovarian enlargement have been found to increase the risk of complications requiring chemotherapy (Curry *et al.* 1975; Zongfu

Table 3 Factors increasing the risk of sequelae of hydatidiform mole requiring chemotherapy

Factor	Reference
Uterine size >gestational age	Curry *et al.* (1975)
Bilateral cystic ovarian enlargement	Zongfu *et al.* (1979)
	Berkowitz and Goldstein (1981)
Pre-evacuation serum HCG[a] >100 000 iu/l	Berkowitz and Goldstein (1981)
Oral contraceptives given before HCG falls to undetectable levels	Stone *et al.* (1976)

[a]HCG, human chorionic gonadotrophin.

et al. 1979). Pre-evacuation concentrations of chorionic gonadotrophin greater than 100 000 iu/l also predict a greater than mean risk of sequelae requiring therapy. Pathological classifications intended to predict prognosis have been successful in some reports but not in the majority.

Prophylactic chemotherapy

As approximately 8 per cent of patients have invasive mole or choriocarcinoma after complete hydatidiform mole (Bagshawe *et al.* 1986), it has been proposed that it would be better if all patients received cytotoxic chemotherapy as soon as the uterus has been evacuated. Given that over 90 per cent of the patients probably do not require any treatment, it is essential that the chemotherapy is not toxic. Methotrexate has proved unsatisfactory for this purpose because of significant toxicity to the liver and other sites (Goldstein 1971). A study in Singapore found a higher mortality in patients receiving methotrexate prophylaxis than a control group (Ratnam *et al.* 1968). This is probably because the dosages used are insufficient to eradicate those tumours with malignant potential and yet can induce drug resistance, making later therapy more difficult. However, a non-randomized Italian study found no deaths among 104 patients treated with methotrexate for 7 weeks and a lower incidence of those subsequently requiring chemotherapy than in untreated patients (Fasoli *et al.* 1982). Actinomycin D probably provides a more satisfactory agent. In one study it reduced the proportions subsequently requiring chemotherapy (Goldstein *et al.* 1981). Xia *et al.* (1988) and Kashimura *et al.* (1986) have defined groups of patients more likely to require chemotherapy than others after evacuation of hydatidiform mole and given prophylactic chemotherapy only to them. However, mortality is lower in the series of Bagshawe *et al.* (1986), in which prophylactic chemotherapy was not given, and prophylactic chemotherapy is not recommended.

Follow-up of human chorionic gonadotrophin

The preferred management after evacuation of hydatidiform mole is to follow up the urine and serum concentrations of chorionic gonadotrophin and only give chemotherapy if there is evidence of invasive mole or choriocarcinoma. Such a scheme has existed in the United Kingdom since 1972 under the auspices of the Royal College of Obstetricians and Gynaecologists. Patients are registered by their gynaecologist at one of three centres where chorionic gonadotrophin is assayed (Charing Cross Hospital in London, Sheffield and Dundee). Urine samples are then sent by post every 2 weeks until the hormone's concentrations are normal. In a study of 4205 patients, these fell to undetectable levels within 56 days of uterine evacuation in 42 per cent of patients, none of whom required chemotherapy (Bagshawe *et al.* 1986). Follow-up is continued for 6 months in these patients and for 2 years after the concentrations have been normal in the remainder.

A number of indications for treatment have evolved that are designed to pick out those patients who have developed chorio-carcinoma or are at risk of dangerous sequelae of invasive mole. They depend heavily on the results of assays for human chorionic gonadotrophin but other clinical factors are important and clinical follow-up of these patients is also necessary by the referring gynaecologist. The indications for treatment are shown in Table 4. A very high chorionic gonadotrophin concentration, in the order of 20 000 iu/l, 4 weeks after evacuation of a mole or rising values in this range at an earlier stage, indicate the patient is at risk of severe haemorrhage or uterine perforation with intraperitoneal bleeding. These complications can be life-threatening and the ability

Table 4 Indications for chemotherapy of gestational trophoblastic tumours

Rising HCG[a] after evacuation
Very high HCG after evacuation (for example, 20 000 iu/l after 4 weeks)
HCG not falling 4 months after evacuation
Raised HCG 6 months after evacuation even if still falling slowly
Pulmonary, vulval, or vaginal metastases unless HCG falling
Metastases at any other site
Heavy vaginal bleeding or evidence of gastrointestinal or intraperitoneal bleeding
Histological evidence of choriocarcinoma
Raised HCG with a clinical picture strongly suggestive of choriocarcinoma if the patient is too ill for a suitable biopsy

[a]HCG, human chorionic gonadotrophin.

to predict them to some extent with assays of the gonadotrophin usually enables treatment to be started before complications develop. Chemotherapy is, in general, the best way of dealing with heavy bleeding. Repeated dilatation and curretage has not been shown to be beneficial provided that the uterus was thoroughly evacuated on the first occasion.

Metastases in the lungs, vulva, or vagina are not necessarily indications for treatment provided that the concentrations of chorionic gonadotrophin are falling. However, chemotherapy should be started if metastases are present and those concentrations are not dropping. Metastases at other sites are an indication of the development of choriocarcinoma and chemotherapy is required. Although choriocarcinoma cannot be diagnosed on uterine curettings, as described, histological evidence of choriocarcinoma from other specimens is an indication for chemotherapy because it is known that this tumour will not die out spontaneously. The development of choriocarcinoma can also be predicted if concentrations of the gonadotrophin are rising 4 months after evacuation of a mole or if the hormone is detectable at all 6 months after evacuation. Mortality from the sequelae of hydatidiform mole was 0.1 per cent in patients followed-up according to this scheme.

Patients requiring chemotherapy

All trophoblastic tumours requiring chemotherapy are dealt with as a group that is divided according to various prognostic factors. Although complete hydatidiform mole, partial hydatidiform mole, and choriocarcinoma following normal conception are of different cytogenetic origins, they respond to the same cytotoxic drugs. The tendency to drug resistance between these pathological groups is probably no greater than that within groups. Empirically derived prognostic factors appear to predict this satisfactorily when applied to the assembled group. PSTT is an exception, showing a substantial degree of drug resistance in all cases.

Staging

Anatomical staging systems such as that of the International Federation of Gynaecology and Obstetrics (**FIGO**) would be relevant if surgical treatment was appropriate after the diagnostic evacuation. As surgery is virtually never indicated at this time, these systems play no part in treatment planning.

Prognostic factors

Patients are divided into risk groups that express the prospects for eradication of the tumour by cytotoxic drugs. It was noted in the 1960s that the proportion of patients achieving long-term complete remission was lower if the concentrations of chorionic gonadotrophin were markedly raised and if there was a long interval after the

Table 5 Scoring system based on prognostic factors

Prognostic factors	Score[b]			
	0	1	2	4
Age (years)	<39	>39		
Antecedent pregnancy	HM[c]	Abortion	Term	
Interval[a]	4	4–6	7–12	>12
HCG (i.u.)/l	10^3	10^3–10^4	10^4–10^5	>10^5
ABO groups (female×male)		O×A	B	
		A×O	AB	
Largest tumour, including uterine tumour		3–5 cm	>5 cm	
Site of metastases		Spleen	GI tract	Brain
		Kidney	Liver	
No. of metastases identified		1–4	4–8	>8
Prior chemotherapy			Single drug	2 or more drugs

[a]Interval time (months) between end of antecedent pregnancy and start of chemotherapy.
[b]The total score for a patient is obtained by adding the individual scores for each prognostic factor. Total score: <4, low-risk; 5–7, middle risk; >8, high risk.
[c]HM, hydatidiform mole.

antecedent pregnancy. It subsequently became clear that there are several factors influencing prognosis in this context and a scoring system incorporating them and giving due weight to each was described by Bagshawe (1976). A system applicable to patients with metastases was also described by Hammond et al. (1973). Since that time, attempts have been made to simplify the system in the light of further experience of chemotherapy. Azab et al. (1988) have used multivariate analysis to try and improve on the univariate methods of others but their patients were already treated differently according to previously identified risk factors. This makes their system less satisfactory than that adopted by the WHO (1983) (Table 5). Patients are divided on the basis of these scores into three risk groups.

The whole topic of chemotherapy and risk groups is assigned to the next, separate section.

CHEMOTHERAPY

The immediate threat to life

Examination of the criteria for treatment and prognostic factors identifies a group of patients with life-threatening complications of a trophoblastic tumour, as follows.

Haemorrhage

Heavy vaginal or intraperitoneal bleeding is the most frequent, immediate threat to life. It is usually possible to control uterine bleeding with chemotherapy. It may, however, be necessary to transfuse many units of blood whilst waiting for the chemotherapy to be effective. Control is usually achieved within a few days. It is important to be ready to do a hysterectomy if bleeding cannot be controlled but fortunately this is usually avoided.

Intraperitoneal bleeding may come from invasive mole or choriocarcinoma that has invaded through the myometrium, from tubal choriocarcinoma or from metastases of choriocarcinoma in the liver or kidneys. Patients sometimes present in this way, the diagnosis being made at laparotomy. As with vaginal bleeding it is usually possible to control intraperitoneal haemorrhage with chemotherapy and blood transfusion. These patients are sometimes considered too unwell for intensive chemotherapy on presentation, particularly if there is hepatic or renal impairment. Actinomycin D has a reputation for producing early cessation of bleeding and can be used as a single agent for the first course in the most seriously ill patients. Usually, however, it is possible to use the chemotherapy regimen dictated by the risk group in which the patient is classified. Particular attention must be paid here to hepatic and renal function. Seriously ill patients, especially if they have lost a lot of blood, are prone to significant renal impairment. The excretion of drugs such as methotrexate by the kidney will be delayed and this can easily produce fatal toxicity. Similarly, hepatic impairment delays metabolism of methotrexate and vincristine, with heightening of toxicity. It is essential, therefore, that the metabolism of the drugs to be used is well understood, and that reversible conditions such as prerenal uraemia are detected and treated at the earliest possible stage.

Respiratory failure

Pulmonary metastases producing significant respiratory impairment at the start of treatment should also be handled with caution. When the disease is diffuse it is often accompanied by fever, with or without purulent sputum. In many of these cases the patients have superadded infection in the lungs and if there is any doubt about this, antibiotic therapy should be given after taking cultures of blood and sputum. Respiratory function often deteriorates after beginning cytotoxic chemotherapy and it is thought that this is because of oedema and inflammation around tumour deposits that are becoming necrotic. Serial measurements of arterial blood gases provide the best means of monitoring such patients. Dyspnoea can often be relieved by giving oxygen but if this is not sufficient, artificial ventilation has to be considered but is rarely successful. It is thought that vigorous combination chemotherapy at the outset of treatment often precipitates a more severe initial deterioration than if treatment is started in a less aggressive fashion. This is very difficult to submit to a randomized study but it does appear that nearly all patients will respond at first to a simple therapy with one or two drugs. After the initial crisis is over, intensive therapy can be instituted.

Cerebral oedema and intracranial haemorrhage

Central nervous metastases also present special problems during the first few weeks of treatment. This topic will be dealt with separately below.

Tumour eradication by chemotherapy

It is necessary to develop a strategy that gives the best chance of tumour eradication in the shortest time with the minimum of toxicity. Placing the patient in an appropriate risk group is the basis of this approach. However, the duration of treatment will need to be different for each patient and some will develop drug resistance and then require to change to other therapy. Twice weekly measurements of the serum chorionic gonadotrophin provides a basis for making these decisions in any individual. The rate of fall of this hormone is monitored and when it becomes normal an estimate is made of the duration for which chemotherapy should be continued in order to reduce the tumour mass theoretically to zero cells. This is done on the assumption that a value for the gonadotrophin at the limit of detectability of the most sensitive assays corresponds to $10^4–10^5$ tumour cells. For the average patient in the low-risk group who has responded reasonably rapidly to therapy, approximately 8 weeks further treatment is required (see Fig. 2). With a slow fall, patients in the high-risk group may require treatment for as much as 12 or 16 weeks after the concentrations of the hormone become normal. If drug resistance develops during treatment, then this can be seen by a failure of

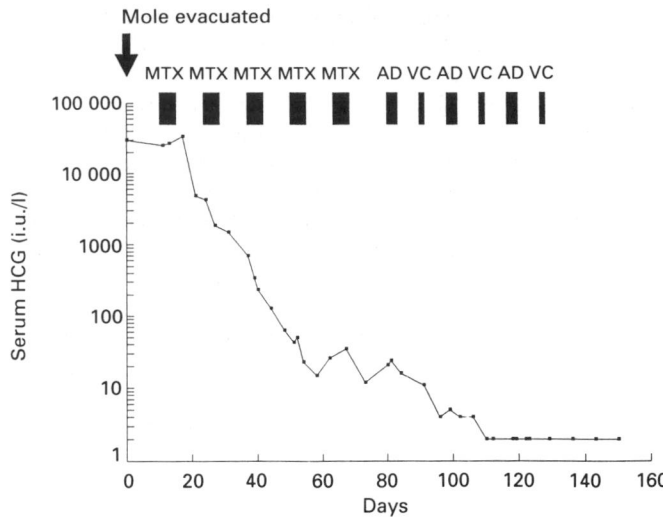

Fig. 7 Chart showing an initial fall in human chorionic gonadotrophin (HCG) concentrations response to methotrexate and folinic acid (MTX) (see Table 6) in a patient in the low-risk group. However, there was evidence of drug resistance with HCG concentrations failing to fall to normal. The tumour was eradicated after a change in therapy to actinomycin D (AD) alternating with vincristine (VC) and cyclophosphamide (see Table 7).

the gonadotrophin to fall. Normally, it should fall by approximately half a log with each course of chemotherapy; rates of fall below this are suggestive of a degree of drug resistance. Very slow rates of fall or a sustained rise are an indication to change chemotherapy (Fig. 7). In this context it is important that patients are treated where results of the gonadotrophin assays can be obtained rapidly, otherwise significant delays tend to occur between development of resistance and an appropriate change of treatment.

In order to be sure that the patient is responding in the initial weeks of therapy and to minimize risks associated with haemorrhage or respiratory deterioration that may occur after the start of treatment, patients are kept in hospital for the first 3–5 weeks of their treatment. Later they are admitted only as necessary for the administration of chemotherapy. In parts of the world where it is difficult for patients to come back repeatedly to hospital they may receive the entire course of therapy as an in-patient.

Low-risk therapy

The regimen used for this group for the last 17 years at Charing Cross Hospital and widely followed in other centres is shown in Table 6. It is simple to administer and in the later stages can sometimes be given by the district nurse in the patient's own home. Toxicity is either absent or modest. There is no alopecia but oral ulceration may occur in patients with fluid intake below 2–3 l/day and in some others presumably due to individual variations in the

Table 6 Regimen for low-risk patients

MX/FA

Methotrexate	50 mg (or 1 mg/kg with maximum 70 mg) by i.m. injection repeated every 48 h×4
Calcium folinate	6 mg, 30 h after each injection of methotrexate by i.m. injection

Courses repeated after a 1 week interval without treatment, i.e. days 1, 15, 29, etc.

rate of methotrexate metabolism. If this is a problem then folinic acid can be given earlier than 30 h after giving methotrexate but not usually less than 24 h after methotrexate. Some patients experience pleuritic chest pains and vaginal or, rarely, perianal ulceration. Allergic reactions occur in a small proportion of patients. Methotrexate induces photosensitivity and patients are advised to avoid sunbathing. Myelosuppression is infrequent but it is essential to measure haemoglobin, white cell, and platelet counts before each course of chemotherapy. Renal and hepatic function should be measured at least every week during treatment. An example of a patient successfully treated in this way was shown in Fig. 2.

In approximately three-quarters of 'low-risk' patients the tumour will be eradicated by this treatment alone, 20 per cent need to change to the medium-risk regimen because of drug resistance, and approximately 5 per cent do so because of intolerance to methotrexate (Bagshawe et al. 1989).

Medium risk

This regimen is shown in Table 7, the alternating courses comprising etoposide and actinomycin D, being the second and third most important agents after methotrexate. This strategy of including several effective agents reduces the chances of development of drug resistance. Etoposide is an important, recent addition to the drugs with high response rates in trophoblastic tumours (Newlands and Bagshawe 1982; Newlands et al. 1986; Hitchins et al. 1988). As well as being used for patients falling into the medium-risk group from the outset, the 'medium-risk' regimen is also used for those showing evidence of drug resistance on the low-risk regimen. In those patients, if it is clear that concentrations of chorionic gonadotrophin are rising during methotrexate therapy, then the methotrexate-containing component is omitted. The medium-risk regimen produces alopecia and is occasionally associated with myelosuppression. Oral ulceration with etoposide is rare but actinomycin D sometimes produces this and nausea or vomiting. Some 86 per cent of patients had complete response with no modification of the regimen and the remainder did so with some modification; 4 per cent of patients relapsed but all achieved sustained complete remission with EMA/CO therapy (see High-risk disease, below). No deaths occurred in 76 patients treated in this way (Newlands et al. 1986).

High-risk disease

These patients require intensive combination chemotherapy because deaths from drug resistance are still a significant problem. The aim is to give chemotherapy with the highest practical dosages as rapidly and consistently as possible. The CHAMOCA regimen (Bagshawe and Begent 1981) was developed for this purpose, containing the best drugs available in the early and mid 1970s. It has now been superceded by EMA/CO (Newlands et al. 1986), as explained in Table 8. An example of the response achieved with this therapy is shown in Fig. 8. Complete remission has been achieved in 67 per cent of patients receiving this regimen whereas only approximately half of patients treated with CHAMOCA achieved a sustained complete remission (Bagshawe and Begent 1981). Relapse after treatment occurred in 3 per cent who had no prior chemotherapy and in 19 per cent who had. Sustained complete remission was eventually achieved in 93 per cent of patients who had no prior chemotherapy and 74 per cent who had prior chemotherapy (Newlands et al. 1986). Similar results have also been reported with EMA/CO by Bolis et al. (1988). Most patients are able to have this therapy with only one night in hospital every 2 weeks. With a weekly regimen it is sometimes necessary to maintain treatment despite a low white cell and platelet count. Chemotherapy is continued unless the total white cell count falls below $1.5 \times 10^9/l$ or platelets below $60 \times 10^9/l$ or unless mucosal ulceration develops. The combination of neutropenia and mucosal ulceration seems to be particularly associated with development of febrile episodes, presumably because there is already a portal for entry of bacteria into the circulation through the ulcerated mucosa. Other therapy regimens used have been reviewed by Rustin and Bagshawe (1984).

Chemotherapy of PSTT

PSTT is best treated by hysterectomy if still localized to the uterus. The prognosis is very poor if metastases have developed but one

Table 7 Regimens for medium-risk patients

EHMMAC

Regimen 1	Etoposide (VP16–213)
	Day 1–5: etoposide 100 mg/m^2 in 200 ml saline by i.v. infusion over 30 min daily
Regimen 2	HU,MX/FA,MP
	Day 1: hydroxyurea, 0.5 g repeated after 12 h (2 doses) orally
	Day 2–8: methotrexate 50 mg i.m. (or 1 mg/kg (max. 70 mg)) repeated every 48 h×4; calcium folinate (folinic acid), 6 mg i.m. 30 h after each dose of methotrexate; mercaptopurine, 75 mg orally on alternate days×4 (on calcium folinate days only)
Regimen 3	Actinomycin D
	Day 1–5: actinomycin D 0.5 mg i.v. daily
Regimen 4	VC,CY
	Day 1 and 3: vincristine, 1 mg/m^2 i.v.
	Day 1 and 3: cyclophosphamide, 400 mg/m^2 i.v.

The sequence of regimens in EHMMAC is 1,2,3,4,1,2, etc.
Alternatively, regimen 4 may be held in reserve, to be used if one of the other regimens proves ineffective or toxic. The preferred sequence then is 1,2,3,2,1,2,3, etc.
The interval between the end of one course and the start of the next should not be less than 7 days or more than 10 days, but some extension is sometimes necessary.

Table 8 Regimen for high-risk patients

EMA/CO
(This regimen consists of two courses. Course 1 is given on days 1 and 2. Course 2 is given on day 8. Course 1 may require overnight admission, course 2 does not)

Course 1	(EMA)	
Day 1	Etoposide	100 mg/m^2, by i.v. infusion in 200 ml 0.9% saline over 30 min
	Actinomycin D	0.5 mg, i.v. stat
	Methotrexate	300 mg/m^2, in 1 l 0.9% saline by i.v. infusion over 12 h
Day 2	Etoposide	100 mg/m^2, by i.v. infusion in 200 ml 0.9% saline over 30 min
	Actinomycin D	0.5 mg, i.v. stat
	Calcium folinate (folinic acid)	15 mg, i.m. or orally every 12 h for four doses beginning 24 h after starting methotrexate
Course 2	(CO)	
Day 8	Vincristine	1.0 mg/m^2, i.v. stat
	Cyclophosphamide	600 mg/m^2, i.v. in saline

These courses can usually be given on days 1 and 2,8,15, and 16,22, etc. and the intervals should not be extended without cause.

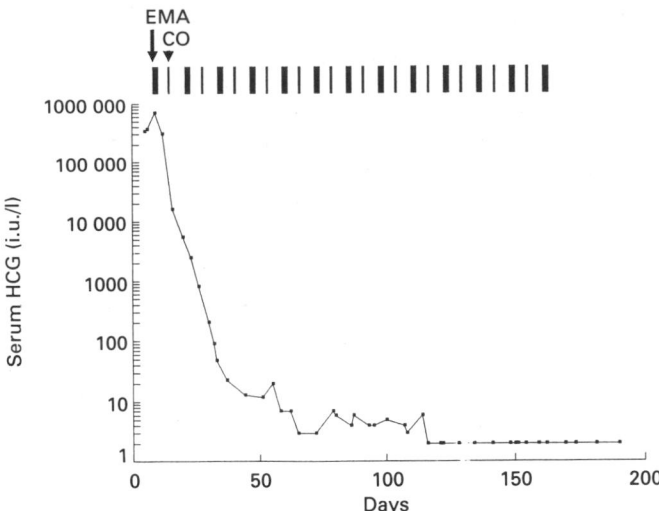

Fig. 8 Chart showing EMA/CO therapy with the response in human chorionic gonadotrophin (HCG) concentrations in a patient in the high-risk group.

patient in the Charing Cross Hospital series is in sustained complete remission after treatment of pulmonary metastases with EMA/CO. The majority, while responding initially to this regimen, subsequently have progressive, drug-resistant disease.

Drug-resistant disease

The development of drug resistance in any of the three risk groups is shown by failure of the chorionic gonadotrophin to fall at a satisfactory rate or by its sustained rise. This is an indication to change to a regimen of the next highest group. Occasionally patients in a low-risk group will require high-risk therapy, having failed to respond to the medium-risk regimen. This is very unusual, however, if etoposide is used in the medium-risk group. Patients in the high-risk group have only one remaining major drug, that is cisplatin (Newlands and Bagshawe 1979; Begent and Bagshawe 1983). Those who fail on the EMA/CO regimen receive cisplatin in combination with vincristine and methotrexate. If cisplatin fails, there are few promising options for therapy.

Surgery for drug-resistant disease

When chemotherapy fails to eradicate the tumour, surgical resection of truly localized disease can sometimes lead to sustained complete response (Begent and Bagshawe 1982). This depends, of course, on the residual tumour being localized and it being technically possible to resect it. Sensitive and specific imaging methods become of great importance in this context. First, the major sites of the tumour must be defined and, secondly, the imaging methods must be sufficiently sensitive, within reason, to exclude metastases at other sites.

Hammond *et al.* (1980) have advocated surgery at the start of treatment for high-risk patients. In our experience this is sometimes dangerous, owing to the profuse vasculature around an infiltrating choriocarcinoma and also because some patients are left unnecessarily infertile.

Computerized tomographic scanning is important in this context, being able to detect lesions of a few millimetres in the lungs and being a sensitive indicator of brain metastases. Outside the pelvis, these are the two sites most likely to contain metastases that can

be resected. The uterus is the most common site in which drug-resistant disease can be resected by hysterectomy (Begent and Bagshawe 1982). Computerized tomography or ultrasonography may show the uterus to be enlarged. If both investigations are negative and no other sites of disease can be found, a hysterectomy should be done. It is unusual for it to be possible to resect disease at sites other than the pelvis, lung, and brain but exceptions do exist in other intra-abdominal sites, particularly the bowel. Antibody imaging has particular attraction in this context because it shows the site at which chorionic gonadotrophin is being produced. Choriocarcinoma frequently leaves mass lesions visible by conventional radiography after tumour has been eradicated from the site concerned. Histological examination of these lesions shows them to contain only necrotic disease. Here antibody imaging could discriminate between viable and necrotic deposits of tumour, giving important information for selection for surgery. Study of antibody imaging using radiolabelled antibody directed against human chorionic gonadotrophin in this context at Charing Cross Hospital has shown that it is sometimes possible to locate tumour when computerized tomographic scanning or ultrasonograms are negative (Begent *et al.* 1980, 1987; Begent 1989). An example is shown in Fig. 9. A positive result is evidence of gonadotrophin production in the site. Unfortunately, some false-negative and false-positive results do occur. This investigation should be seen as complementary to the other imaging methods and if both are positive in one site then the probability of there being viable tumour present in that location is very high. The results of use of antibody imaging in this context are shown in Table 2. It has been the experience at Charing Cross Hospital that multiple metastases may appear within a few weeks of such surgery, suggesting that there has been a spread of tumour at the time of the operation. For this reason it is our practice to give methotrexate, 50 mg intravenously, at the time of operation.

Central nervous metastases

The central nervous system is the second most common site of metastases in the high-risk group (Begent and Bagshawe 1982). In the study of patients treated at Charing Cross Hospital over a period of 23 years (Athanassiou *et al.* 1983), nearly all those with brain

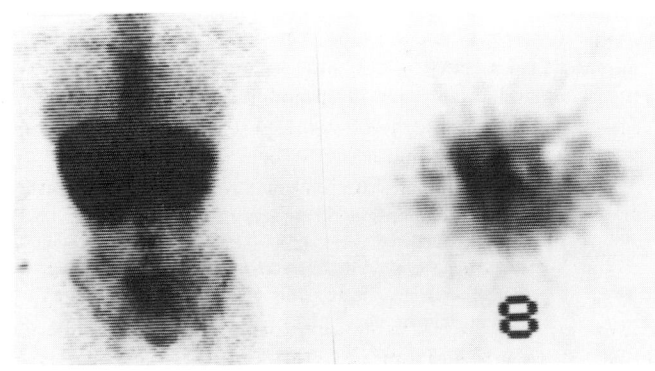

(a)   (b)

Fig. 9 Antibody imaging in a patient with drug resistance. (a) Anterior gamma-camera image showing localization of ^{111}In-labelled antibody to human chorionic gonadotrophin (HCG) in the uterus. (b) Single-photon emission tomography confirms the position of the tumour in the uterine area. Computerized tomography and ultrasonography failed to show the tumour but sustained complete remission was achieved by hysterectomy, which confirmed the presence of tumour. (Reproduced with permission, from Heyderman *et al.* 1989.)

metastases also had lung deposits. Also, if lung metastases developed during chemotherapy the chance of their eradication was very small, whereas if they were diagnosed at the start of treatment prospects of cure were good. For these reasons, prophylactic intrathecal methotrexate is now given to all patients at risk of cerebral metastases, namely those with pulmonary metastases in any risk group and those in the high-risk group regardless of whether lung metastases are detected. Since this policy has been in use, development of brain metastases without evidence of drug resistance elsewhere has been much less frequent (Athanassiou et al. 1983). In order to increase the chance of detection of central nervous metastases, the concentrations of chorionic gonadotrophin are measured in the cerebrospinal fluid at the start of treatment. A concentration of greater than 1/60 the serum value suggests the presence of central nervous metastases. The poor penetration of most cytotoxic drugs into the central nervous system means that conventional chemotherapy is not effective against brain metastases. In the regimen for prophylaxis in the central nervous system, 12.5 mg of methotrexate are given intrathecally with each course of chemotherapy until the chorionic gonadotrophin concentration becomes normal. In the case of the EMA/CO regimen, this is given with the CO part of each course.

Established central nervous metastases

Patients with metastases to the central nervous system on presentation sometimes already have serious neurological signs. This accounts for the fact that approximately one-quarter of these patients die within 2 weeks of starting treatment (Athanassiou et al. 1983). Some patients present with extremely severe neurological damage, whilst others develop this soon after starting treatment, often as a result of haemorrhage into the area or tumour. Early resection of solitary deposits in patients presenting with serious neurological signs can sometimes be life saving (Ishizuka 1983; Song and Wu 1988; Rustin et al. 1989). Earlier consideration of a diagnosis of choriocarcinoma could probably also improve this situation.

Dexamethasone is given at the start of treatment to reduce oedema. The EMA/CO regimen is modified with the dose of methotrexate in EMA being increased to $1 g/m^2$ as a 24 h intravenous infusion on day 1. Folinic acid, 30 mg, is given intravenously at 8-hourly intervals for 3 days, starting 32 hours after the beginning of the methotrexate infusion. If there is no evidence of raised intracranial pressure, intrathecal methotrexate, 12.5 mg, is given with each course of CO and followed, after 24 h by a single dose of folinic acid, 15 mg, orally or intravenously. Patients surviving the first 3 weeks of treatment have a good prognosis, the chance of tumour eradication then being 89 per cent (Athanassiou et al. 1983; Rustin et al. 1989). This therapy is continued until the end of treatment.

Cerebral metastases developing during chemotherapy

Prospects of tumour eradication for this group are poor because the development of cerebral tumour during chemotherapy implies that it is already drug resistant. The patients who have been cured in these circumstances in our series have had the tumour deposit resected as soon as it was diagnosed (Athanassiou et al. 1983; Rustin et al. 1989). Whilst computerized tomography is usually sufficient for location of brain deposits, magnetic resonance imaging has located deposits of choriocarcinoma in the cerebral hemispheres close to the skull that were not detected by computerized tomography and which have been successfully removed. A raised cerebrospinal fluid : serum ratio of chorionic gonadorophin often gives a guide to the presence of a central nervous deposit.

Radiation therapy

Radiation therapy has some activity against cerebral deposits of choriocarcinoma but has not been shown to eradicate tumour without chemotherapy in addition. Regimens that include radiation (Weed et al. 1982; Ishizuka 1983) with cytotoxic chemotherapy have been less successful than those depending on chemotherapy alone (Athanassiou et al. 1983; Rustin et al. 1989).

Survival

One hundred per cent of patients in the low-risk group can be expected to be completely cured (Bagshawe et al. 1986). In the medium-risk group, an analysis in 1981 showed 98 per cent long-term survival and there have been no fatalities since etoposide has been introduced into the regimen (Newlands et al. 1986). In the high-risk group, survival has progressively improved since the introduction of methotrexate in the 1950s, when 30–50 per cent survival could be expected. This figure has risen progressively and with the EMA/CO regimen it is currently 93 per cent for patients who have not had prior chemotherapy and 74 per cent for those who have (Newlands et al. 1986). This figure is only achieved, however, by the use of the additional drugs such as cisplatin and appropriate use of surgery in those showing evidence of drug resistance. Relapse after apparently successful intitial therapy does not necessarily imply a fatal outcome, even in the high-risk group. Complete responses can often be achieved by chemotherapy with or without surgery.

Many of the deaths are among patients who present to a specialized unit with disease so advanced that they are close to death and there is no time for chemotherapy to be effective. The number of such patients can be diminished by a greater awareness of the possibility of the diagnosis of choriocarcinoma and by measurement of human chorionic gonadotrophin. The other major problem is drug-resistant disease months or years after the initial treatment. Patients still die for this reason and it is probable that new drugs are necessary before the problem can be completely overcome.

Follow-up and sequelae of the therapy

Because of the potential of choriocarcinoma to recur after a period of several years it is necessary to continue follow-up of human chorionic gonadotrophin. It is our policy to do this for the rest of the patient's life. Serum or urine samples can be mailed into the central laboratory.

Patients are advised against subsequent pregnancy for a year after completion of chemotherapy in order to avoid confusion between relapse and pregnancy and the possible adverse effects on the ovum induced by chemotherapy. When a patient becomes pregnant it is important to confirm by ultrasonography and other appropriate means that the pregnancy is normal. Follow-up is then discontinued until the end of the pregnancy, being resumed in the normal way 3 weeks after delivery. Patients who have not received chemotherapy should have the chorionic gonadotrophin measured 3 weeks and 3 months after the end of any further pregnancy because of the increased risk of a second hydatidiform mole.

Effects on fertility

The study of patients receiving chemotherapy for gestational trophoblastic tumours has shown that with the regimens described here, 68 per cent of patients wishing to have a further pregnancy have succeeded in having at least one live birth. The patients all receive methotrexate and it seems that, given in the way described here, this drug and etoposide have little effect on subsequent fertility (Rustin *et al.* 1984; Adewole *et al.* 1987). Song *et al.* (1988) have reported similar findings from China. Neither study showed an increased incidence of fetal abnormalities.

The incidence of second malignancies in the Charing Cross series is also of the order that would be expected in the normal population, there having been only one case of breast cancer and one of acute myeloid leukaemia (Rustin *et al.* 1983). In that series the expected figure would be 3.5 cases.

Contraceptive advice

Studies in the United Kingdom have found that patients given oral contraceptives before the chorionic gonadotrophin falls to normal after evacuation of hydatidiform mole have an increased incidence of sequelae requiring chemotherapy (Stone *et al.* 1976). For this reason patients are advised to avoid oral contraceptives until that hormone has been normal for 3 months if they have had a hydatidiform mole not requiring chemotherapy or for 6 months after completion of chemotherapy. The mechanisms by which oestrogens and progestogens may influence trophoblastic tumours are unclear.

CONCLUSIONS

Until the first successes of chemotherapy in the 1950s, trophoblastic tumours could only be treated by hysterectomy. Those with locally invasive or metastatic tumour died and the remainder lost their fertility. The finding of drugs that cured some patients gave new impetus to the study of the pathology, natural history, and diagnostic and monitoring methods in trophoblastic tumours. The result is an understanding of the extraordinary cytogenetic basis of gestational trophoblastic diseases, an appreciation of the risks of different clinical situations, a knowledge of prognostic factors, and systems for monitoring and imaging based on a tumour marker. These have played a crucial role in conjunction with developments in chemotherapy and surgery in giving a 95 per cent chance of tumour eradication in those treated and in letting us understand when chemotherapy is not needed. This model is worthy of study by those seeking to improve treatment of other types of cancer.

The 33 years since cytotoxic chemotherapy came into use for treatment of gestational trophoblastic tumours have seen great advances in our understanding of these diseases. Approximately 90 per cent of patients with hydatidiform mole do not need chemotherapy and can be followed-up by their gynaecologist in conjunction with a central laboratory that monitors human chorionic gonadotrophin in samples sent by post. Long-term, disease-free survival is now expected for the great majority of patients requiring chemotherapy but this is only achieved with careful attention to detail by experienced staff. Even though treatment may mean spending time away from their homes and families, there can be little doubt that the chances of long-term survival are greater if the small proportion of patients who need chemotherapy are managed in special centres.

REFERENCES

Adewole IF, Rustin GJS, Newlands ES, Dent J, Bagshawe KD (1987). Fertility in patients with gestational trophoblastic tumours treated with etoposide. *European Journal of Cancer and Clinical Oncology*, **22**:1479.

Athanassiou A, Begent RHJ, Newlands ES, Parker D, Rustin GJS, Bagshawe KD (1983). Central nervous system metastases of choriocarcinoma: 23 years' experience at Charing Cross Hospital. *Cancer*, **52**:1728–35.

Azab MB, *et al.* (1988). Prognostic factors in gestational trophoblastic tumours. A multivariate analysis. *Cancer*, **62**:585–92.

Bagshawe KD (1976) Risk and prognostic factors in trophoblastic neoplasia. *Cancer*, **38**:1373–85.

Bagshawe KD, Begent RHJ (1981). Trophoblastic tumours: clinical features and management. In *Gynaecologic oncology*, Vol. 2 (ed. M Coppleson), pp. 757–72. Churchill Livingstone, Edinburgh.

Bagshawe KD, Begent RHJ (1983). Staging markers and prognostic factors in germ cell tumours. In *Clinics in oncology 2, Germ cell tumours* (ed. KD Bagshawe, ES Newlands, and RH Begent), pp. 159–81.

Bagshawe KD, Dent J, Webb J (1986). Hydatidiform mole in the United Kingdom 1973–1983. *Lancet*, **ii**:673.

Bagshawe KD, Dent J, Newlands ES, Begent RHJ, Rustin GJS (1989). The role of low-dose methotrexate and folinic acid in gestational trophoblastic tumours (GTT). *British Journal of Obstetrics and Gynaecology*, **96**:795–802.

Begent RHJ (1989). Immunoscintigraphy with radiolabelled antibody directed against HCG. In *Monoclonal antibodies in immunoscintigraphy* (ed. J-F Chatal). CRC Press, Boca Raton, FA.

Begent RHJ (1990). Trophoblastic disease. In *Clinical gynaecological oncology*, (2nd edn) (ed. J Shepherd and J Monaghan), pp. 299–332. Blackwell, Oxford.

Begent RHJ, Bagshawe KD (1982). The management of high risk choriocarcinoma. *Seminars in Oncology*, **9**:198–203.

Begent RHJ, Bagshawe KD (1983). Treatment of advanced trophoblastic disease. In *Gynecologic oncology* (ed. CT Griffiths and AF Fuller), pp. 155–86. Martinus Nijhoff, Boston.

Begent RHJ, *et al.* (1980). Radioimmunolocalization of tumours by external scintigraphy after administration of ^{131}I antibody to human chorionic gonadotrophin. *Journal of the Royal Society of Medicine*, **73**:624–30.

Begent RHJ, *et al.* (1982) Liposomally entrapped antibody improves imaging with radiolabelled (first) antitumour antibody. *Lancet*, **ii**:739–42.

Begent RHJ, Bagshawe KD, Green AJ, Searle F (1987). The clinical value of imaging with antibody to human chorionic gonadotrophin in the detection of residual choriocarcinoma. *British Journal of Cancer*, **55**:657–60.

Berkowitz RS, Goldstein DP (1981). Pathogenesis of gestational trophoblastic neoplasms. In *Pathobiology annual* (ed. HL Ioachim), pp. 391–411. Raven Press, New York.

Berkowitz RS, Goldstein DP, Bernstein MR (1985). Natural history of partial molar pregnancy. *Obstetrics and Gynecology*, **66**:677–81.

Berrebi A, *et al.* (1988). A new case of hydatidiform mole occurring on one of the ova of a twin pregnancy. *Revue Français de Gynecologie et d'Obstetrique*, **83**:439–41.

Bolis C, *et al.* (1988). EMA/CO regimen in high-risk gestational trophoblastic tumor (GTT). *Gynecologic Oncology*, **31**:439–44.

Bracken MB, Brinton LA, Hayashi K (1984). Epidemiology of hydatidiform mole and choriocarcinoma. *Epidemiologic Review*, **6**:52–74.

Brandes JM, Grunstein S, Peretz A (1966). Suction evacuation of the uterine cavity in hydatidiform mole. *Obstetrics and Gynecology*, **28**:689–91.

Curry SL, Hammond CB, Tyrey L, Creasman WT, Parker RT (1975). Hydatidiform mole; diagnosis, management and long term follow up of 347 patients. *Obstetrics and Gynecology*, **45**:1–8.

Davis JR, Surwit EA, Garay JP, Fortier KJ (1984). Sex assignment in gestational trophoblastic neoplasia. *American Journal of Obstetrics and Gynecology*, **148**:722–5.

Eckstein RP, Paradinas FJ, Bagshawe KD (1982). Placental site trophoblastic tumour: a study of four cases requiring hysterectomy, including one fatal case. *Histopathology*, **6**:211–26.

Eckstein RP, Russell P, Friedlander ML, Tattersall MH, Bradfield A (1985). Metastasizing placental site trophoblastic tumor: a case study. *Human Pathology*, **16**:632–6.

Edwards YH, *et al.* (1984). Complete hydatidiform moles combine maternal mitochondria with a paternal nuclear genome. *Annals of Human Genetics*, **48**:119–27.

Fasoli M, Ratti E, Franceschi S, La Vecchia C, Pecorelli S, Mangioni C (1982). Management of gestational trophoblastic disease: results of a cooperative study. *Obstetrics and Gynecology*, **60**:205–9.

Finkler NJ, Berkowitz RS, Driscoll SG, Goldstein DP, Bernstein MR (1988). Clinical experience with placental site trophoblastic tumors at the New England Trophoblastic Disease Center. *Obstetrics and Gynecology*, **71**:854–7.

Fisher RA, Sheppard DM, Lawler SD (1982). Twin pregnancy with complete hydatidiform mole (46,XX) and fetus (46,XY): genetic origin proved by analysis of chromosome polymorphism. *British Medical Journal*, 1:1218–20.

Fisher RA, Lawler SD, Ormerod MG, Imrie PR, Povey S (1987). Flow cytometry used to distinguish between complete and partial hydatidiform moles. *Placenta*, 8:249–56.

Flam F, Lundstrom V, Silfversward C (1989) Choriocarcinoma in mother and child. *British Journal of Obstetrics and Gynaecology*, 96:241–4.

Fradken JE, Eastman RC, Lesniak MA, Roth J (1989). Specificity spillover at the hormone receptor—exploring its role in human disease. *New England Journal of Medicine*, 320:640–5.

Goldenberg DM, Kim EE, DeLand FM, Van Nagell JR, Javadapour N (1980). Clinical radioimmunodetection of cancer with radiolabelled antibodies to human chorionic gonadotrophin. *Science*, 208:1284–6.

Goldstein DP (1971). Prophylactic chemotherapy with molar pregnancy. *Obstetrics and Gynecology*, 38:817–22.

Goldstein DP, Berkowitz RS, Bernstein MR (1981). Management of molar pregnancy. *Journal of Reproductive Medicine*, 26:208–12.

Hammond CB, Borchert LG, Tyrey L, Creasman WT, Parker RT (1973). Treatment of metastatic trophoblastic disease: good and poor prognosis. *American Journal of Obstetrics and Gynecology*, 115:451–7.

Hammond CB, Weed JC, Currie JL (1980). The role of operation in the current therapy of gestational trophoblastic disease. *American Journal of Obstetrics and Gynecology*, 136:844–58.

Hayashi H (1982) Hydatidiform mole in the United States (1970–1977): a statistical and theoretical analysis. *American Journal of Epidemiology*, 115:67–77.

Heyderman RS, Begent RHJ, Buckley RG, Searle F, Southall P, Bagshawe KD (1989). Antibody imaging to locate a placental site trophoblastic tumour following a complete hydatidiform mole. *Journal of the Royal Society of Medicine*, 82:299–300.

Hitchins RN, Holden L, Newlands ES, Begent RHJ, Rustin GJS, Bagshawe KD (1988). Single agent etoposide in gestational trophoblastic tumours. Experience at Charing Cross Hospital 1978–1987. *European Journal of Cancer and Clinical Oncology*, 24:1041–6.

Hopkins M, Nunez C, Murphy JR, Wentz WB (1985). Malignant placental site trophoblastic tumor. *Obstetrics and Gynecology*, 66 (Suppl.):95–100S.

Ishizuka T (1983). Intracranial metastases of choriocarcinoma: a clinicopathologic study. *Cancer*, 52:1896–903.

Jacobs PA, Hunt PA, Matsuuro JS, Wilson CC (1982). Complete and partial hydatidiform mole in Hawaii: cytogenetics, morphology and epidemiology. *British Journal of Obstetrics and Gynaecology*, 89:258–66.

Kajii T, Ohama K (1977). Androgenetic origin of hydatidiform mole. *Nature*, 268:633–4.

Kardana A, Bagshawe KD (1976). A rapid, sensitive and specific radioimmunoassay of human chorionic gonadotrophin. *Journal of Immunology Methods*, 9:297–305.

Kashimura Y, et al. (1986). Prophylactic chemotherapy of hydatidiform mole. *Cancer*, 58:624–9.

Kiel FW (1986). The medical value of examining tissue from therapeutic abortions: an analysis of 13,477 cases. *British Journal of Obstetrics and Gynaecology*, 93:594–6.

Kurman RJ, Scully RE, Norris HJ (1976). Trophoblastic pseudotumour of the uterus. *Cancer*, 38:1214–26.

Lage JM, Driscoll SG, Yavner DL, Olivier AP, Mark SD, Weinberg DS (1988). Hydatidiform moles. Application of flow cytometry in diagnosis. *American Journal of Clinical Pathology*, 89:596–600.

Lathrop JC, Lauchlan S, Nayak R, Ambler M (1988). Clinical characteristics of placental site trophoblastic tumor (PSTT). *Gynecologic Oncology*, 31:32–42.

La Vecchia C, et al. (1984). Age of parents and risk of gestational trophoblastic disease. *Journal of the National Cancer Institute*, 73:639–42.

Lawler SD, Fisher RA (1986). Genetic aspects of gestational trophoblastic tumors. In *Trophoblastic diseases* (ed. K Ichinoe), pp. 23–33. Igaku-Shoin Tokyo, New York.

Lawler SD, Fisher RA (1987). Genetic studies in hydatidiform mole with clinical correlations. *Placenta*, 8:77–88.

Lawler SD, Pickthall VG, Fisher RA, Povey S, Wyn Evans M, Szulman AE (1979). Genetic studies of complete and partial hydatidiform mole. (Letter) *Lancet*, ii:580.

Lawler SD, Fisher RA, Pickthall VG, Povey S, Wyn Evans M (1982a). Genetic studies on hydatidiform moles. I. The origin of partial moles. *Cancer Genetics and Cytogenetics*, 4:309–20.

Lawler SD, Povey S, Fisher RA, Pickthall VG (1982b). Genetic studies on hydatidiform moles. II. The origin of complete moles. *Annals of Human Genetics*, 46:209–22.

Long MG, Boultbee JE, Begent RHJ, Bagshawe KD (1987). Doppler ultrasound of the uterine artery and uterus in invasive mole and choriocarcinoma. Proceedings of the British Medical Ultrasound Society. *British Journal of Radiology*, 60:621.

Long MG, Boultbee JE, Hanson ME, Begent RHJ (1989). Doppler time velocity waveform studies of the uterine artery and uterus. *British Journal of Obstetrics and Gynaecology*, 96:588–93.

Long MG, Boultbee JE, Langley R, Newlands ES, Begent RHJ, Bagshawe KD (1992). Doppler assessment of the uterine circulation and the clinical behaviour of gestational trophoblastic tumours requiring chemotherapy. *British Journal of Cancer*, 66:882–7.

McGrath IT, Golding PR, Bagshawe KD (1971). Medical presentations of choriocarcinoma. *British Medical Journal*, 2:633–7.

Matalon M, Modan B (1972). Epidemiologic aspects of hydatidiform mole in Israel. *American Journal of Obstetrics and Gynecology*, 112:107–12.

Mazur MT, Kurman RJ (1987). Choriocarcinoma and placental site trophoblastic tumour. In *Gestational trophoblastic disease* (ed. AE Szulman and HJ Buchsbaum). Springer Verlag, New York.

Nagelberg SB, Rosen SW (1985). Clinical and laboratory investigation of a virilized woman with placental-site trophoblastic tumor. *Obstetrics and Gynecology*, 65:527–34.

Newlands ES, Bagshawe KD (1979). Activity of high dose platinum (NCI 119875) in combination with vincristine and methotrexate in drug resistant choriocarcinoma. A report of 17 cases. *British Journal of Cancer*, 40:943–5.

Newlands ES, Bagshawe KD (1982). Role of VP16–213 (etoposide; NSC 141540) in gestational choriocarcinoma. *Cancer Chemotherapy and Pharmacology*, 7:211–14.

Newlands ES, Bagshawe KD, Begent RHJ, Rustin GJS, Holden L, Dent J (1986). Developments in chemotherapy for medium- and high-risk patients with gestational trophoblastic tumours (1979–1984). *British Journal of Obstetrics and Gynaecology*, 93:63–9.

Newman RB, Eddy GL (1988). Association of eclampsia and hydatidiform mole: case report and review of the literature. *Obstetrics and Gynecology Survey*, 43:185–90.

Ober WB (1987). Choriocarcinoma: historical notes. In *Gestational trophoblastic tumours* (ed. AE Szulman and HJ Buchsbaum), p. 1. Springer Verlag, New York.

Ohama K, et al. (1981). Dispermic origin of XY hydatidiform mole. *Nature*, 292:551–2.

Poulsen HE (1975). *Histological typing of female genital tract tumours*, International Histological Classification of Tumours, No. 13, pp. 70–3. WHO, Geneva.

Ratnam SS, Teoh ES, Dawood MY (1968). Methotrexate for prophylaxis of choriocarcinoma. *American Journal of Obstetrics and Gynecology*, 111:1021–7.

Requard CK, Mettler FA (1980). The use of ultrasound in the evaluation of trophoblastic disease and its response to therapy. *Radiology*, 135:419–22.

Romero R, Horgan JG, Kohorn EI, Kadar N, Taylor JJ, Hobbins JC (1985). New criteria for the diagnosis of gestational trophoblastic disease. *Obstetrics and Gynecology*, 66:553–8.

Rustin GJS, Bagshawe KD (1984). Gestational trophoblastic tumours. In *Critical review in oncology*. CRC Press, Boca Raton, FA.

Rustin GJS, Rustin F, Dent J, Booth M, Salt J, Bagshawe KD (1983). No increase in second tumors after chemotherapy for gestational trophoblastic tumors. *New England Journal of Medicine*, 308:473–6.

Rustin GJS, Booth M, Dent J, Salt S, Rustin F, Bagshawe KD (1984). Pregnancy after cytotoxic chemotherapy for gestational trophoblastic tumours. *British Medical Journal*, 288:103–6.

Rustin GJS, Newlands ES, Begent RHJ, Dent J, Bagshawe KD (1989). Weekly alternating chemotherapy (EMA/CO) for treatment of central nervous systems of choriocarcinoma. *Journal of Clinical Oncology*, 7:900–3.

Samlowski WE, Abbott TM, Kepas DE, Eyre HJ (1985). Placental-site trophoblastic tumor (trophoblastic pseudotumor): case report demonstrating failure of chemotherapy, surgery, and radiotherapy to control metastatic disease. *Gynecologic Oncology*, 21:111–17.

Schlaerth JB, Morrow CB, Montz EJ, d'Ablaing G (1988). Initial management of hydatidiform mole. *American Journal of Obstetrics and Gynecology*, **158**:1299–306.

Scully RE, Young RH (1981). Trophoblastic pseudotumour: a reappraisal. *American Journal of Surgical Pathology*, **5**:75–6.

Sheppard DM, Fisher RA, Lawler SD, Povey S (1982). Tetraploid conceptus with three paternal contributions. *Human Genetics*, **62**:371–4.

Sheppard DM, Fisher RA, Lawler SD (1985). Karyotypic analysis and chromosome polymorphisms in four choriocarcinoma cell lines. *Cancer Genetics and Cytogenetics*, **16**:251–8.

Song HZ, Wu BZ (1988). Treatment of brain metastases in choriocarcinoma and invasive mole. In *Studies in trophoblastic diseases in China* (ed. HZ Song and PC Wu), pp. 231–7. Pergamon, Oxford.

Song HZ, Wu PC, Wang YE, Yang XY, Dong SY (1988). Pregnancy outcomes after successful chemotherapy for choriocarcinoma and invasive mole: long term follow-up. *American Journal of Obstetrics and Gynecology*, **158**:538–45.

Steiner RE, Radda G (ed.) (1983). Nuclear magnetic resonance and its clinical applications. *British Medical Bulletin*, **40**(2).

Stone M, Bagshawe KD (1979). An analysis of the influence of maternal age, gestational age, contraceptive method, and the mode of primary treatment of patients with hydatidiform moles on the incidence of subsequent chemotherapy. *British Journal of Obstetrics and Gynaecology*, **86**:782–92.

Stone M, Dent J, Kardana A, Bagshawe KD (1976). Relationship of oral contraception to development of trophoblastic tumour after evacuation of a hydatidiform mole. *British Journal of Obstetrics and Gynaecology*, **83**:913–16.

Szulman AE (1987). Complete hydatidiform mole: clinicopathologic features. In *Gestational trophoblastic disease* (ed. AE Szulman and HJ Buchsbaum). Springer Verlag, New York.

Teoh ES, Dawood MY, Ratnam SS (1971). Epidemiology of hydatidiform mole in Singapore. *American Journal of Obstetrics and Gynecology*, **110**:415–20.

Vaitukaitis JL (1979). Human chorionic gonadotrophin—a hormone secreted for many reasons. *New England Journal of Medicine*, **301**:324–6.

Vassilakos P, Riotton G, Kajii T (1977). Hydatidiform mole: two entities. A morphologic and cytogenetic study with some clinical considerations. *American Journal of Obstetrics and Gynecology*, **127**:167–70.

Watson EJ, Hernandez E, Miyazawa K (1987). Partial hydatidiform moles: a review. *Obstetrics and Gynecology Surveys*, **42**:540–4.

Weed JC, Kent TW, Hammond CB (1982). Choriocarcinoma metastatic to the brain: therapy and prognosis. *Seminars in Oncology*, **9**:208–12.

World Health Organization (1983). *Gestational trophoblastic diseases*, Technical Report Series 692. WHO, Geneva.

Xia ZF, Song HZ, Tang MY (1988). Risk of malignancy and prognosis using a provisional scoring system in hydatidiform mole. In *Studies in trophoblastic diseases in China* (ed. HZ Song and PC Wu), pp. 175–85. Pergamon, Oxford.

Yen S, MacMahon B (1968). Epidemiological features of trophoblastic disease. *American Journal of Obstetrics and Gynecology*, **101**:126–32.

Young RH, Scully RE, McCluskey RT (1985). A distinctive glomerular lesion complicating placental site trophoblastic tumor: report of two cases. *Human Pathology*, **16**:35–42.

Young RH, Kurman RJ, Scully RE (1988). Proliferations and tumors of intermediate trophoblast of the placental site. *Seminars in Diagnostic Pathology*, **5**:223–37.

Zongfu X, Hongzhao S, Minyi T (1979). Risk of malignancy and prognosis using a provisional scoring system in hydatidiform mole. *China Medical Journal*, **93**:605–12.

9.6   Carcinoma of the vagina

PETER BLAKE

INTRODUCTION

Primary neoplasms of the vagina are rare and comprise only 1–2 per cent of all gynaecological malignancies, the incidence being less than 1/100 000 women or approximately 200 cases per annum in England and Wales. Malignant disease of the vagina is most commonly secondary to direct spread from neoplasms of the cervix and vulva, but can also be involved by tumours of the body of the uterus, bladder, rectum, or sigmoid colon. Occasionally, lymphatic spread from the cervix and body of the uterus may give rise to discrete vaginal metastases and, similarly, blood-borne metastasis to the vagina may occur from distant neoplasms, such as carcinoma of the breast. In addition to carcinoma, other primary neoplasms of the vagina are the rare sarcoma botryoides in young girls, melanoma, sarcoma, and lymphoma.

Invasive squamous carcinoma of the vagina is often preceded by vaginal intraepithelial neoplasia (commonly abbreviated to VAIN), just as invasive carcinoma of the cervix is preceded by cervical intraepithelial neoplasia (commonly abbreviated to CIN). However, the aetiological causes of vaginal carcinoma are not as clearly defined as for cervical carcinoma, although age, low socio-economic class, and a history of trauma or chronic irritation are implicated. A very small number of women presenting in their second or third decade

with adenocarcinoma of the vagina may give a history of their mothers having been exposed to diethylstilboestrol during pregnancy.

More than 90 per cent of vaginal carcinomas are squamous and most occur in elderly women, in whom they are often asymptomatic until in an advanced stage. It is this late presentation that gives vaginal carcinoma the reputation of carrying a very poor prognosis. Local control of advanced disease is difficult and death is commonly due to haemorrhage, uraemia from ureteric obstruction, or infection secondary to the vesicovaginal or rectovaginal fistula.

Treatment aims to effect local control, either by surgery in early disease (stage I) or by radiotherapy, both external beam and brachytherapy, in more advanced stages. Preservation of bladder and bowel function is achieved whenever possible but diversion of the urinary or gastrointestinal tract may be necessary, both as part of a planned surgical approach to primary treatment or for palliation of refractory or recurrent disease. In young women with small primary tumours, vaginal function can sometimes be retained.

Problems in reducing the morbidity and mortality of vaginal carcinoma are related to inadequate knowledge of the risk factors, which prevents an at-risk population from being identified and screened for intraepithelial or early invasive disease and delays by both patients and general practitioners in referral for investigation of apparently minor vaginal symptoms. Early-stage disease can be cured whilst advanced disease may not only be difficult to cure but may also be difficult to palliate effectively.

EPIDEMIOLOGY

The epidemiology of squamous carcinoma of the vagina is not the same as that of adenocarcinoma of the vagina. Whilst the mean age of presentation with the squamous carcinoma is approximately 60 years (Al-Kurdi and Monaghan 1981), in the 5 per cent of women presenting with the adenocarcinoma the incidence is biphasic, with a small subgroup developing this disease at around the age of 20 years and the majority at approximately the same age as for squamous carcinoma.

Squamous carcinoma of the vagina is seen most commonly in women in their sixth and seventh decades and from low socio-economic groups. Although the incidence in Black women has been reported to be higher than that in White, a case-controlled study has failed to show this to be a factor separate from socio-economic status (Brinton et al. 1990). This same study has shown similarities between the epidemiology of both intraepithelial and invasive disease of the vagina and that of the cervix with regard to socio-economic status, a history of vaginal irritation, and previously abnormal cervical cytology. However, the study was not able to show sexual history or smoking to be important for vaginal disease, whilst these are recognized epidemiological factors in cervical neoplasia. Interestingly, whilst the frequency of bathing appeared not to reflect on the incidence of vaginal carcinoma, an increased frequency of washing the genital area or of using a vaginal douche was associated with increased neoplasia. An association has been seen between previous hysterectomy and the subsequent development of vaginal neoplasia, even when the hysterectomy was for a non-malignant condition (Bell et al. 1984).

AETIOLOGY

Squamous carcinoma

The cervix and the vagina, in common with the vulva, show a range of malignant changes in the squamous epithelium from mild through moderate to severe dysplasia or carcinoma in situ (Table 1). This intraepithelial neoplasia precedes the development of invasive carcinoma.

The aetiology of vaginal carcinoma is unknown but the similarity between the epidemiology of vaginal and cervical neoplasia would suggest that both areas are at risk from the same carcinogenic agents. In support of this, a patient with cervical cancer may develop vaginal cancer some time after initial treatment, suggesting that the carcinogenic agent that caused neoplasia in the cervix continued to affect the vagina (Rose et al. 1987).

It is difficult to discern why hysterectomy, even for apparently benign uterine conditions, should be associated with an increased incidence of intraepithelial and invasive vaginal neoplasia. However, the reported increased incidence of vaginal neoplasia after total hysterectomy may be accounted for by controlling for the presence of malignancy in the removed cervix (Stuart et al. 1987). The

Table 1 Intraepithelial neoplasia of the lower genital tract

	Cervix	Vagina	Vulva	Cytological description
Grade	1	1	1	Mild dysplasia
	2	2	2	Moderate dysplasia
	3	3	3	Severe dysplasia/carcinoma in situ

incidence of intraepithelial vaginal neoplasia after hysterectomy may not only be raised in women with previous evidence of cervical malignancy because of inadequate primary treatment and residual cervical intraepithelial neoplasia at the margins of excision, but also because of a 'field change' throughout the epithelium of the lower genital tract, suggesting a common aetiological agent.

However, there is a difference in the importance of sexual history in vaginal and cervical neoplasia, with smoking, the age of first intercourse, and the number of sexual partners being prominent factors in the epidemiology of cervical but not vaginal cancer. This may indicate a different aetiology or may simply be a product of the small numbers of women with vaginal carcinoma available for study (Brinton et al. 1990).

An association with human papilloma virus (**HPV**) has been sought and, in common with cervical neoplasia, HPV types 16 and 18 have been found in vaginal carcinoma tissue (Campion 1987). However, as techniques for the detection of HPV DNA within cells have improved, the frequency with which this virus can be found in normal women with no evidence of either vaginal or cervical neoplasia has increased, throwing doubt on its role as an important aetiological agent. Herpes simplex virus type 2 is also now found so ubiquitously in the female population that it would seem unlikely that it is associated with the aetiology of vaginal carcinoma. It may be that several factors are needed to cause neoplasia in the vagina, viral infection being only one of them.

Classically, vaginal carcinoma is associated with procidentia, which causes the vaginal mucosa to be constantly traumatized and long-term use of ring pessaries, which produce local irritation, both physical and chemical. However, it is actually uncommon to find either of these factors in the history of most patients seen nowadays, although many complain of long-term vaginal irritation (Al-Kurdi and Monaghan 1981). The association with increased washing of the genital area and especially the use of vaginal douches (Brinton et al. 1990), would appear to confirm that continued trauma to the vagina plays a part in the development of some cases of intraepithelial neoplasia and of invasive disease. Very rarely, vaginal carcinoma arises after pelvic radiotherapy (Pride et al. 1979).

Adenocarcinoma of the vagina

The young subgroup of women developing adenocarcinoma is more evident in North America than in the United Kingdom. These are the children of women given diethylstilboestrol during pregnancy. Particularly in North America, this treatment began to be used in 1940 with the intention of reducing complications of pregnancy such as abortion, toxaemia, prematurity, and perinatal mortality. In 1970 the first report of a possible association between maternal exposure to diethylstilboestrol during pregnancy and a raised incidence of clear cell adenocarcinoma of the vagina in the female offspring appeared (Herbst and Scully 1970). Subsequent reports indicated that exposure before the eighteenth week of pregnancy carried the greatest risk; this is the time at which epithelialization of the vagina takes place. The problems seen in these offspring include an increased incidence of developmental abnormalities, dysplasia, and both pre-invasive and invasive neoplasia of the vagina. Developmental abnormalities include vaginal adenosis (the abnormal presence of glandular tissue in the squamous epithelium), whilst neoplasia is seen as an increase in adenocarcinoma of the vagina and both intraepithelial and invasive squamous neoplasia of the vagina and cervix. The risk to exposed daughters of developing vaginal and cervical clear cell adenocarcinoma is 0.14–1.4/1000, which, although low, is between 100 and 1000 times more than the natural

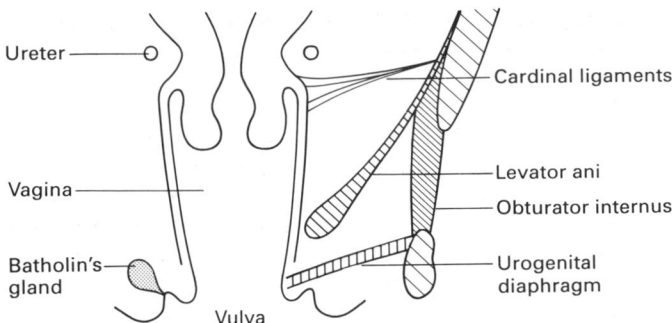

Fig. 1 Coronal section of the vagina and vulva showing the relationship of the vagina to the muscles of the pelvic floor and Bartholin's gland

incidence (Melnick *et al.* 1987). An association with diethylstilboestrol has not been identified in the women developing adenocarcinoma of the vagina late in life.

ANATOMY

Embryologically, the upper two-thirds of the vagina develops separately from the lower third, the upper part growing down from the Müllerian ducts and the lower third developing upwards from the cloaca. The upper two-thirds therefore share their blood supply and lymphatic drainage with the cervix whilst the lower third shares its blood and lymphatic system with that of the vulva. The vagina is lined throughout by stratified squamous epithelium.

Superiorly, the cervix protrudes into the vaginal vault and, inferiorly, the vagina meets the vulva at the vestibule (Fig. 1). Anteriorly, the vagina is related to the bladder and urethra posteriorly, where it is covered by peritoneum, to loops of bowel in the pouch of Douglas. Below the peritoneal cavity it is in close proximity to the rectum and anus. Laterally, the ureters pass near to the vaginal vault.

Lymphatic drainage

The lymphatic drainage of the upper two-thirds of the vagina is the same as that of the cervix, draining to the internal and external iliac and obturator nodes and to the common iliac and lower para-aortic nodes. The drainage of the lower third is the same as the vulva, draining to the inguinal and femoral nodes. However, there are many variations on this drainage pattern (Al-Kurdi and Monaghan, 1981).

PATHOLOGY

Before making a diagnosis of primary vaginal cancer, the following criteria must be met: the primary site of growth must be in the vagina, the uterine cervix and vulva must not be involved, and there must be no clinical evidence that the vaginal tumour is metastatic from a primary elsewhere.

Like the cervix, the vagina is affected by pre-malignant lesions, although, after hysterectomy, some may be previously unrecognized extensions of cervical abnormalities. Coincident with the rise in prevalence of cervical intraepithelial neoplasia is an increase in the frequency of recognition of vaginal intraepithelial neoplasia.

Vaginal intraepithelial neoplasia

This, like cervical intraepithelial neoplasia, must be considered to have malignant potential and requires treatment, although neither the proportion of patients with lower grades of vaginal intraepithelial neoplasia who would proceed to develop invasive disease nor the rate of this progression is known. Vaginal intraepithelial neoplasia usually occurs in the upper third of the vagina and the diagnosis is made on exfoliative cytological examination or biopsy at colposcopy. Many of these women have undergone hysterectomy and most of the lesions occur in the suture line or arise in the angles of the vault where it is difficult to take a biopsy and determine whether or not there is underlying invasive disease (Soutter 1988).

Carcinoma of the vagina

More than 90 per cent of primary invasive tumours are squamous carcinomas, whilst adenocarcinoma accounts for only 4–5 per cent. Malignant melanomas and sarcomas comprise the remainder. The posterior wall of the upper third of the vagina is the site of invasive disease in 50 per cent, whilst 25–30 per cent arise on the anterior wall in the lower third. It is difficult to postulate why the distribution of the disease should favour these two sites.

CLINICAL FEATURES

By exfoliative cytological means, vaginal carcinoma can be detected at an early stage, but this method is seldom used in the asymptomatic, elderly women who usually develop this disease and, although some cases are found incidentally, most present because of symptoms.

Symptoms and signs

The most common symptom is vaginal bleeding, which, in the greater majority of patients, will be post-menopausal. Approximately 15 per cent of patients complain of an offensive discharge and 8 per cent of pain, suggesting that advanced disease is already present.

Clinical assessment should include inspection of the vagina using a speculum, and both vaginal and rectal digital examination to determine the size and mobility of the tumour.

Spread of disease

Vaginal cancer spreads by local invasion to the rest of the vagina and to the vulva, paravaginal tissues, and parametria. Haematogenous spread is unusual and occurs late in the disease.

Lymphatic spread is dependent upon the site of tumour, to pelvic or groin nodes or both. Pelvic and para-aortic node involvement is reported as uncommon (6 per cent) in stage I disease but occurs in one-quarter (26 per cent) of patients with stage II disease in whom the nodes are assessed surgically (Davis *et al.* 1991). Tumours in the lower third of the vagina are associated with inguinal node involvement in up to 38 per cent, whilst these nodes are very seldom involved from tumours of the middle and upper thirds (Al-Kurdi and Monaghan 1981; Perez *et al.* 1988).

INVESTIGATIONS

Colposcopy will identify tumour and co-existing intraepithelial neoplasia but, as with other gynaecological tumours, a careful examination under anaesthesia is essential. This should include a careful inspection of the vulva, vagina, and cervix, biopsy of the tumour and any abnormal areas elsewhere in the vagina or on the cervix, curetting of the uterine cavity and endocervical canal, and cystoscopy and sigmoidoscopy to assess involvement of the bladder and rectum. The size and mobility of the tumour should be assessed

Table 2 Modified FIGO staging of vaginal carcinoma

Stage 0	Pre-invasive carcinoma
Stage I	Tumour limited to vaginal wall
Stage II	Tumour involving subvaginal tissues
	Not extending to pelvic side wall
Stage III	Tumour extending to pelvic side wall
Stage IVa	Tumour involving the mucosa of the bladder or rectum or
	extending beyond the true pelvis
IVb	Blood-borne spread to distant organs.

and, in particular, any submucosal spread or deep invasion or fixation should be noted. These findings will provide the basis for tumour staging.

A chest radiograph and renal ultrasonographic scan or intravenous urogram are the only radiological investigations needed routinely, but computerized tomographic scanning or lymphography can help identify nodal involvement in advanced disease. Transrectal ultrasonographic scanning and magnetic resonance imaging can help to define the size and extent of the primary tumour.

CLINICAL STAGING

The International Federation of Gynaecology and Obstetrics (**FIGO**) staging system is shown in Table 2. However, vaginal cancer is often described differently by clinicians with a particular interest in the disease (Perez and Camel 1982). This particularly is the case for early-stage disease where FIGO stage I applies to all sizes of invasive tumours confined to the vagina.

Stage distribution varies widely in reported series but approximately one-third of patients present with stage I tumours, one-third with stage II tumours, and the remaining third with stage III and IV disease.

TREATMENT

Vaginal intraepithelial neoplasia

This can be treated by several methods including excision, laser vaporization, and the cytotoxic agent 5-fluorouracil, which is applied topically as a cream. However, the majority of patients will have had a previous hysterectomy and the last method is only suitable if the area of intraepithelial neoplasia is clearly demarcated and does not involve the suture line. If the suture line is involved or if there is any suggestion of underlying invasive disease, then partial or total vaginectomy may be required (Ireland and Monaghan 1988). Occasionally, local intracavitary radiotherapy is used for persistent lesions in the vault (Woodman et al. 1988).

In young, sexually active women, vaginal reconstruction is possible but major sexual problems may still arise, as can further malignant change within the reconstructed vagina.

Invasive disease

In early-stage disease the aim of treatment is to eradicate local tumour and remove or sterilize involved lymph nodes. In late-stage disease a decision must be made as to whether curative therapy is a realistic aim for the patient, especially if they are very elderly or whether palliative treatment would be more appropriate.

Treatment options include surgery and radiotherapy, both external beam and brachytherapy, either alone or combined. As yet, chemotherapy has little place in the management of carcinoma of the vagina as there is limited experience. However, the drugs most likely to be effective are those with the highest response rates in

cervical cancer, namely cisplatin and ifosfamide, both of which are too toxic for most of these elderly patients.

Surgery

Stage I carcinoma of the vagina can be treated by surgery, entailing a radical hysterectomy, vaginectomy, and pelvic lymphadenectomy. This procedure is usually more suitable for lesions in the upper and middle thirds of the vagina rather than the lower third. However, patients are often too old to allow this approach, in which case radiotherapy should be used.

Stage II and III disease is not suitable for surgery, although stage II disease may be operated on in the belief that the tumour is less advanced than proves to be the case histologically. These patients should be referred for post-operative radiotherapy if the margins of excision are not clear.

Occasionally, stage IV tumours invading the bladder or rectum, but without involvement of the pelvic side walls may be suitable for pelvic exenteration with the diversion of the urinary or gastrointestinal tract or both (Al-Kurdi and Monaghan 1981). Equally, if a tumour recurrent after radiotherapy remains sufficiently localized, exenteration may be considered in younger patients.

Radiotherapy

The usual treatment for invasive carcinoma of the vagina is radiation therapy, which is particularly effective in the early stages. Radiotherapy can be given by megavoltage external beam, interstitial implant, or vaginal mould or, for small local lesions, by a transvaginal 'cone' using orthovoltage X-rays (100–250 keV). Because of the rarity of the tumour few protocols have accrued enough patients to define ideal treatment schedules for each stage of disease.

Small, accessible, stage I tumours in the middle and lower thirds of the vagina may be suitable for an interstitial implant. This uses either 'live' sources, usually caesium needles or hollow needles after-loaded, either manually or mechanically, with iridium wire. The use of 'live' sources is declining, for reasons of staff protection and mechanical afterloading systems are widely used. These introduce the possibility of using radioactive sources of higher activity than was possible when sources had to be manually inserted. Higher-activity sources allow shorter treatment times and, therefore, less discomfort for the patient and less time for displacement of the needles, a serious consideration for elderly patients in whom prolonged bed-rest carries a high morbidity. However, the dose of radiation that is tolerated by the normal tissues is less when using high-activity sources than when using those of standard activity. There is still uncertainty about the 'dose-rate' effect, even for carcinoma of the cervix, which has been treated by high dose-rate brachytherapy for more than 20 years (Fu and Phillips 1990) and recommendations for the treatment of vaginal cancer by high dose-rate brachytherapy are, therefore, lacking. Using standard activity iridium wire it would be usual to deliver 60–70 Gy to the target volume, which should include a margin around the tumour of at least 0.5 cm, over 6–7 days. The geometry of this implant may be improved by the use of a plastic template to hold rigidly the steel tubes that carry the iridium wires (Fig. 2) (Branson et al. 1985), as otherwise the needles tend to splay cranially whilst crowding together caudally when the legs are lowered from the lithotomy position used during the insertion.

Tumours of the upper third of the vagina may be treated in the same way as cervical carcinoma by a combination of external-beam and intracavitary therapy, the latter with an intrauterine tube and vaginal applicators. The dose would be that used for the radical radiotherapy of stage IIa cervical cancer.

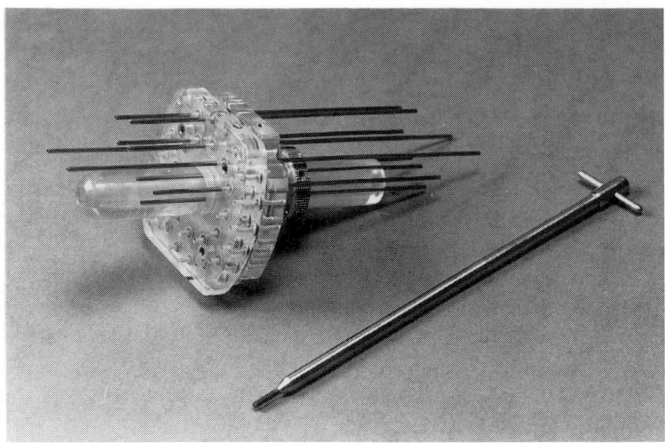

Fig. 2 The Perspex perineal template for holding parallel, after-loading tubes for use with ^{192}Ir wire. The template is stitched to the perineum with the central obturator in the vagina. The afterloading tubes are introduced with the aid of a trochar and held in place by rubber 'O' rings compressed by screwing the two Perspex plates together using a large Allen key.

Larger, stage I and II tumours and stage III disease require both external-beam therapy to the pelvis, 40–50 Gy in 20–28 fractions and a boost to residual tumour by an implant, to give a total dose of 65–75 Gy to the tumour. The external-beam treatment should be by megavoltage radiotherapy, using either a cobalt machine or a linear accelerator, and should encompass the entire vagina and pelvic nodes if the tumour is stage II or III, although many radiotherapists would also cover these nodes when treating a bulky, stage I tumour. In addition, the treatment volume should include the inguinal nodes if the tumour is in the lower third of the vagina.

The implant may be by intracavitary applicators rather than an interstitial technique if, after external-beam treatment, the tumour has completely regressed. The dose prescribed would be such as to take the rectal mucosa to its tolerance dose, which, with the external-beam component, is 60–65 Gy.

Equally, if the tumour is still very bulky at the time of brachytherapy or if there is proven disease on the pelvic side wall, then a parametrial boost after the brachytherapy should be considered. The total dose to the pelvic side wall from the initial external treatment, the brachytherapy, and the parametrial boost should be in the region of 60 Gy.

Stage IV disease may be treated by external-beam therapy alone or may be more suitable for radical exenterative surgery with or without pre-operative radiotherapy. Most of these patients will be suitable for palliative therapy only.

Palliative treatment is usually best delivered by a parallel, opposed pair of external-beam fields to cover the primary tumour and any symptomatic local metastases. A short course of 20–30 Gy in 5–10 fractions over 1 or 2 weeks will, in most cases, produce good haemostasis and pain relief. Very occasionally, disease recurrent after external-beam therapy can be treated by an intracavitary insertion to palliate local symptoms.

Complications of radiotherapy

Vaginal stenosis can occur in up to 30 per cent of patients and is more likely when advanced tumours are treated. This is a problem for sexually active patients but may be reduced by the regular use of vaginal douches during treatment and dilators afterwards. Mucosal ulceration is an uncommon but distressing complication

Table 3 Results of treatment of carcinoma of the vagina

Stage	Percentage of total	5 year survival (%)
I	30	53.0
II	31	43.0
III	26	28.0
IV	12	12.5

Modified from FIGO (1988).

that usually resolves with conservative therapy, especially the use of antibiotics active against Gram-negative bacteria. Late damage to the rectum and bladder may occur, especially when a combination of external-beam and interstitial radiotherapy is needed and is related to the relatively large volumes that have to be treated and the proximity of these to the rectum and bladder (Perez *et al.* 1988; Kucera and Vavra 1991).

RESULTS

There is a wide range of results because reported series are small. The results collected from many centres and reported by FIGO are shown in Table 3. Individually reported series quote higher survival rates than FIGO for stage I disease in particular, 82 per cent at 5 years (Davis *et al.* 1991), 81 per cent at 5 years (Kucera and Vavra 1991), and 75 per cent at 10 years (Perez *et al.* 1988). These series are all of patients treated by radiotherapy. Surgical series would appear to be able to produce similar results in stage I disease, as with 84 per cent 5 year survival (Ball and Berman 1982). However, there has not been a randomized trial comparing primary surgery with radiotherapy for early-stage disease and most series contain an element of patient selection.

The results for more advanced disease show less variation from the FIGO data, with particularly low survival rates for patients with stage III and IV disease.

Whilst stage is the most powerful prognostic factor, the tumour grade of squamous carcinomas may also be important, with, in one series, almost twice as many patients surviving 5 years with well-differentiated tumours (62.5 per cent) as with poorly differentiated tumours (34.9 per cent) (Kucera and Vavra 1991). However, the histological type of carcinoma, squamous, adeno-, or adenosquamous, appears not to be important (Davis *et al.* 1991). The presence of involved lymph nodes, whether pelvic or inguinal, carries a poor prognosis.

CONCLUSIONS

The majority of vaginal neoplasms are metastases from tumours in others parts of the gynaecological tract and primary vaginal carcinoma is rare. The majority of patients present when elderly with squamous carcinomas, although there has been a very small incidence of adenocarcinoma in young women associated with exposure to diethylstilboestrol whilst *in utero*.

The aetiology of squamous carcinoma of the vagina is uncertain but the association with chronic irritation of the mucosa is well recognized. Viruses may play a part in carcinogenesis at this site as they may at the cervix. Tumours are often advanced when diagnosed because of the occult nature of the disease and inappropriate primary therapy for supposed vaginal infection.

Early-stage disease may be treated by surgery alone or in combination with interstitial or intracavitary brachytherapy. More advanced disease requires external-beam radiotherapy and brachytherapy when possible. Treatment may be tolerated poorly and chemotherapy is relatively untried for this disease because of the advanced age of most patients.

Except for early-stage disease the results of treatment are poor. The outlook for this disease will only improve if tumours are found at an earlier stage either by screening or by increasing doctors' awareness of the disease to avoid unnecessary delay in diagnosis.

REFERENCES

Al-Kurdi M, Monaghan JM (1981). Thirty-two years experience in management of primary tumours of the vagina. *British Journal of Obstetrics and Gynaecology*, 88:1145–50.

Ball HG, Berman ML (1982). Management of primary vaginal carcinoma. *Gynecologic Oncology*, 14:154–63.

Bell J, Sevin B, Averette H, Nadjii M (1984). Vaginal cancer after hysterectomy for benign disease: value of cytologic screening. *Obstetrics and Gynaecology*, 54:699–701.

Branson AN, Dunn P, Kam K, Lambert HE (1985). A device for interstitial therapy for low pelvic tumours—the Hammersmith perineal hedgehog. *British Journal of Radiology*, 58:537–9.

Brinton LA, et al. (1990). Case-control study of *in situ* and invasive carcinoma of the vagina. *Gynecologic Oncology*, 38:49–54.

Campion MJ (1987). Clinical manifestations and natural history of genital human papillomavirus infection. *Obstetric and Gynecologic Clinics of North America*, 14:363–87.

Davis KP, Stanhope CR, Garton GR, Atkinson ES, O'Brien PC (1991). Invasive vaginal carcinoma: analysis of early-stage disease. *Gynecologic Oncology*, 42:131–6.

Fu, KK, Phillips TL (1990). High dose-rate versus low dose-rate intracavitary brachytherapy for carcinoma of the cervix. *International Journal of Radiation Oncology—Biology—Physics*, 19:791–6.

Herbst AL, Scully RE (1970). Adenocarcinoma of the vagina in adolescence: a report of seven cases including six clear-cell carcinomas (so-called mesonephromas). *Cancer*, 25:745–7.

Ireland D, Monaghan JM (1988). The management of the patient with abnormal vaginal cytology following hysterectomy. *British Journal of Obstetrics and Gynaecology*, 95:973.

Kucera H, Vavra N (1991). Radiation management of primary carcinoma of the vagina: clinical and histopathological variables associated with survival. *Gynecologic Oncology*, 40:12–16.

Melnick S, Cole P, Anderson D, Herbst A (1987). Rates and risks of diethylstilboestrol-related clear-cell adenocarcinoma of the vagina and cervix. *New England Journal of Medicine*, 316:514–16.

Perez CA, Camel HM (1982). Long-term follow-up radiation therapy of carcinoma of the vagina. *Cancer*, 49:1308–15.

Perez CA, et al. (1988). Definitive irradiation in carcinoma of the vagina: long-term evaluation of results. *International Journal of Radiation Oncology—Biology—Physics*, 15:1288–90.

Pride GL, Shultz AE, Chuprevich TW, Bucher DA (1979). Primary invasive squamous carcinoma of the vagina. *Obstetrics and Gynaecology*, 53:218–25.

Rose PG, Heterick EE, Boutselis JG, Moeshburger M, Sachs L (1987). Multiple primary gynaecologic neoplasms. *American Journal of Obstetrics and Gynaecology*, 157:261–7.

Soutter WP (1988). The treatment of vaginal intra-epithelial neoplasia after hysterectomy. *British Journal of Obstetrics and Gynaecology*, 95:961.

Stuart GC, Allen HH, Anderson RJ (1987). Squamous cell carcinoma of the vagina following hysterectomy. *American Journal of Obstetrics and Gynecology*, 139:311.

Woodman CB, Mould JS, Jordan JA (1988). Radiotherapy in the management of vaginal intra-epithelial neoplasia after hysterectomy. *British Journal of Obstetrics and Gynaecology*, 95:976.

9.7 Carcinoma of the vulva and its putative precursors

W. PATRICK SOUTTER, H. LAMBERT, AND G. ANGUS J. McINDOE

INTRODUCTION

Invasive vulval cancer is an uncommon and unpleasant disease, but is potentially curable even in elderly unfit women if it is referred early and managed correctly from the outset. If mismanaged, the patient with vulval cancer is condemned to a miserable degrading death. The surgical treatment appears deceptively simple, but few gynaecologists and their nursing colleagues acquire sufficient experience of this disease to offer the highest quality of care for these women. All too often, an initial attempt at surgery is made and the patient is referred for specialist care only after recurrent disease is evident.

There are approximately 750 new cases of carcinoma of the vulva each year in England and Wales and the annual incidence is approximately 3.1 in 100 000, making it approximately five times less common than cervical cancer (Office of Population Censuses and Surveys 1985). The majority of these women are elderly; only 7.5 per cent are less than 55 years of age and 78 per cent are over 65 years (Office of Population Censuses and Surveys 1985). With increased life expectancy this cancer will be seen more frequently.

AETIOLOGY

Little is known of the aetiology of vulval cancer. There is some evidence of viral factors. Antigens induced by herpes simplex virus type 2 and DNA from type 16/18 human papillomavirus have been detected in vulval intraepithelial neoplasia and invasive lesions (Brinton et al. 1990). Vulval cancer is associated with a history of genital warts, but the significance of this association remains uncertain. The majority of genital condylomata contain human papillomavirus 6/11, which is not now considered to have any oncogenic potential and very few contain HPV 16, the type found in invasive lesions (Bergeron et al. 1987). Cigarette smoking is more common in women with vulval intraepithelial neoplasia and the mean age of smokers with this condition (39 years) is significantly less than that of their non-smoking counterparts (51 years) (Ferenczy 1992). A study of renal allograft patients showed a 31-fold increase in the incidence of cancer of the vulva (Disney 1989), suggesting that immunosuppression may play an important part in the aetiology of this disease.

ANATOMY

The vulva includes the mons pubis, the labia majora and minora, the clitoris, the vestibule of the vagina, the bulb of the vestibule, and the greater vestibular glands (Bartholin's glands).

The mons pubis is a pad of fat anterior to the pubic symphysis and covered by hair-bearing skin. The labia majora extend posteriorly from the mons on either side of the pudendal cleft into which the urethra and vagina open. They merge with one another and the perineal skin anterior to the anus. They consist largely of areolar tissue and fat. On their lateral aspects the skin is pigmented and covered with crisp hairs. On the medial side the skin is smooth and has many sebaceous glands. The labia minora are small folds of skin that lie between the labia majora and divide anteriorly to envelop the clitoris. The medial surfaces contain many sebaceous glands. The clitoris is an erectile structure analogous to the male penis. Partly hidden by the anterior folds of the labia minora, it consists of a body of two corpora cavernosa lying side by side and connected to the pubic and ischial rami and a glans of sensitive spongy erectile tissue. The vestibule is that area between the labia minora into which the urethra and vagina open. The bulbs of the vestibule are elongated masses of erectile tissue lying on either side of the vaginal opening. The greater vestibular glands lie posterior to the bulbs of the vestibule and are connected to the surface by short ducts.

VULVAL LESIONS BELIEVED TO HAVE MALIGNANT POTENTIAL

Vulval dystrophies

There is great controversy and little hard evidence on the malignant potential of chronic vulval dystrophies. It is hardly surprising that squamous cell hyperplasia is often seen beside invasive lesions, given that this is the skin's response to chronic irritation and scratching. In this situation the rubbing is probably induced by the cancer.

Lichen sclerosus is the commonest condition found in elderly women complaining of vulval itch, but may also be seen in children and less commonly in younger women. The cause is not known, but the condition is associated with autoimmune disorders. Although it most commonly affects the vulva and perianal skin, lesions do appear elsewhere. The lesion is white and the skin looks thin, with a crinkled surface. The contours of the vulva slowly disappear and labial adhesions form. If the patient has been rubbing the area the skin will become thickened (lichenified). The diagnosis can usually be made clinically, but a biopsy should be performed whenever possible. Even in a typical case, the histology is sometimes not characteristic.

There is much uncertainty about the risk to patients with lichen sclerosus of developing vulval cancer. Vulval intraepithelial neoplasia and lichen sclerosus can co-exist in the same patient and many patients with invasive carcinoma also have lichen sclerosus in the surrounding skin. Approximately 4 per cent of women with lichen sclerosus develop invasive cancer (Meyrick-Thomas et al. 1988). In one study, progression to invasive cancer occurred in 13 out of 92 patients with chronic vulval dystrophy followed for up to 19 years (Elliott 1992).

Vulval intraepithelial neoplasia

Vulval intraepithelial neoplasia are seen more commonly than was the case 10–20 years ago. It is not certain whether this represents a real increase or is simply the result of greater awareness of the problem.

Histology

Squamous vulval intraepithelial neoplasia and, more rarely, adenocarcinoma *in situ* (Paget's disease) occur on the vulva. The histological features and terminology of vulval intraepithelial neoplasia are analogous to those of CIN (cervical intraepithelial neoplasia) and VAIN (vaginal intraepithelial neoplasia). In the same way, the histological appearance of Paget's disease is similar to the lesion seen in the breast. In a third of cases of Paget's disease, there is an adenocarcinoma in underlying apocrine glands and these carry a particularly poor prognosis (Creasman et al. 1975).

Natural history

Forty per cent of women with vulval intraepithelial neoplasia are less than 41 years of age (Buscema et al. 1980a). Although histologically very similar to CIN and often occurring in association with it, vulval intraepithelial neoplasia are said not to have such a high malignant potential (Buscema et al. 1980b; Kaufman and Gordon 1986a). However, this opinion is based largely on studies of women who have been treated by excision biopsy or vulvectomy. This may not be true of untreated or inadequately treated patients; five such women were reported to have progressed to invasive cancer in 2–8 years (Jones and McLean 1986).

Presentation and diagnosis

Intraepithelial disease of the vulva often presents as pruritus vulvae, but 20–45 per cent of cases are asymptomatic and are frequently found after treatment of pre-invasive or invasive disease at other sites in the lower genital tract, particularly the cervix (Jones and McLean 1986; Kaufman and Gordon 1986b).

These lesions are often raised above the surrounding skin and have a rough surface. The colour is variable: white because of hyperkeratinization, red because of thinness of the epithelium, or dark brown because of increased melanin deposition in the epithelial cells. However, the full extent of the abnormality is often not apparent until 5 per cent acetic acid is applied. After 2 min, the lesion turns white and mosaic or punctation may be visible. While these changes can be seen with the naked eye in a good light, it is much easier to use a hand lens or a colposcope. Some gynaecologists also use toluidine blue as a nuclear stain, but areas of ulceration give false-positive results and hyperkeratinization gives false-negatives.

Adequate biopsies must be taken from abnormal areas to rule out invasive disease. This can usually be done under local anaesthesia in the out-patient clinic using a disposable 4 mm Stiefel biopsy punch or a Keyes punch.

Treatment

The treatment of vulval intraepithelial neoplasia is difficult. Uncertainty about the malignant potential, the multifocal nature of the disorder, and the discomfort and mutilation resulting from therapy suggest that recommendations should be cautious and conservative to avoid making the treatment worse than the disease. The youth of many of these patients is a further important consideration. None the less, the documented progression of untreated cases to invasive cancer underlines the potential importance of these lesions (Jones and McLean 1986). If the patient has presented with symptoms, therapy is required. Asymptomatic patients, particularly under the age of 50 years, are probably best observed closely with biopsies repeated if there are any suspicious changes.

If the lesion is small, an excision biopsy may be both diagnostic and therapeutic. If the disease is multifocal or covers a wide area, a skin graft may improve the cosmetic result of a skinning vulvectomy (Caglar *et al.* 1986). However, the donor site is often very painful and in many patients a satisfactory result can be obtained without grafting.

An alternative approach is to vaporize the abnormal epithelium with a carbon dioxide laser. Given the very irregular surface of the vulva, it is extremely difficult to achieve a uniform depth of destruction. Moreover, the depth of treatment required for vulval intraepithelial neoplasia is still unclear (Dorsey 1986). In some cases hair follicles may be involved for several millimetres below the surface (Mene and Buckley 1985). Even with carefully controlled depth of treatment, re-epithelialization of large areas treated with a laser will take several weeks. The other main disadvantage is the absence of histopathological assessment.

Results of treatment

Assessment of the results of treatment should include a consideration of the length of follow-up. Surgical excision is associated with recurrence rates of 13–43 per cent (Jones and McLean 1986; Shafi *et al.* 1989). Short-term results from patients treated by laser were very promising (Leuchter *et al.* 1984), but longer follow-up showed a recurrence rate similar to that of surgery (Shafi *et al.* 1989). Close observation and rebiopsy are essential to detect invasive disease among those who relapse. Early invasion was detected in three out of 21 patients (14 per cent) with persisting signs of disease (Shafi *et al.* 1989). Repeated treatments are commonly required.

Conclusions

Vulval intraepithelial neoplasia are becoming more common, particularly in young women. The treatment must be carefully tailored to the individual to avoid mutilating therapy whenever possible. In view of the uncertainty about the malignant potential of these lesions there is a place for careful observations, particularly for young women without severe symptoms. However, it must not be forgotten that some of these patients will develop vulval cancer if untreated and so the importance of close follow-up must be emphasized to the patient and her general practitioner.

Paget's disease

Paget's disease is an uncommon condition, similar to that found in the breast. Pruritus is the presenting complaint. The lesion is indistinguishable clinically from squamous intraepithelial neoplasia and the diagnosis must be made by biopsy.

Associated malignancies

In approximately one-third of patients there is an adenocarcinoma in the apocrine glands (Boehm and Morris 1971; Creasman *et al.* 1975). This has a poor prognosis if the groin lymph nodes are involved and none survive for 5 years (Boehm and Morris 1971). Excluding underlying adnexal carcinomas, concomitant genital malignancies are found in 15–25 per cent of women with Paget's disease of the vulva (Degefu *et al.* 1986). These are most commonly vulval or cervical, but transitional cell carcinoma of the bladder (or kidney) and ovarian, endometrial, vaginal, and urethral carcinomas have all been reported (Degefu *et al.* 1986).

Treatment

The treatment of Paget's disease is very wide local excision, usually involving total vulvectomy, because of the propensity of this condition to involve apparently normal skin (Creasman *et al.* 1975). The specimen must be examined histologically with great care to exclude an apocrine adenocarcinoma.

INVASIVE DISEASE OF THE VULVA

Pathology

Most invasive cancers (85 per cent) are squamous. Approximately 5 per cent are melanomas and the remainder are made up of carcinomas of Bartholin's gland, other adenocarcinomas, basal cell carcinomas, and the very rare verrucous carcinomas, rhabdomyosarcomas, and leiomyosarcomas.

In a third of cases of Paget's disease there is an adenocarcinoma in underlying apocrine glands and these carry a particularly poor prognosis (Boehm and Morris 1971; Creasman *et al.* 1975).

Natural history

Invasive disease involves the labia majora in approximately two-thirds of cases and the clitoris, labia minora, or posterior fourchette and perineum in the remainder (Cavanagh *et al.* 1985). The tumour usually spreads slowly, infiltrating local tissue before metastasizing to the groin nodes.

The lymph drains from the vulva to the inguinal and femoral glands in the groin and then to the external iliac glands in the pelvis. It is thought that lymphatic drainage from the vulva passes first to the superficial inguinal nodes before subsequently going to the femoral nodes deep to the cribriform fascia (Way 1948; Parry-Jones 1960; Borgno *et al.* 1990). Drainage to both groins occurs from the midline structures, the perineum and the clitoris, but some contralateral spread may take place from other parts of the vulva (Iversen and Aas 1983). Direct spread to the pelvic nodes along the internal pudendal vessels occurs only very rarely and no direct pathway from the clitoris to pelvic nodes has been demonstrated consistently (Iversen and Aas 1983).

Spread to the contralateral groin occurs in 25–30 per cent of those cases with positive groin nodes and so bilateral groin node dissection is required in all such cases (Monaghan 1985; Homesley *et al.* 1991) (Table 1). If the groin nodes are positive, 17–34 per cent of women will have positive pelvic nodes (Homesley *et al.* 1986; Shimm *et al.* 1986; Hopkins *et al.* 1991). Pelvic nodes are very seldom involved if the groin nodes are negative (Shimm *et al.* 1986; Hopkins *et al.* 1991). Haematogenous spread to bone, lung, or other distant sites occurs in apppproximately 5 per cent of cases (Podratz *et al.* 1982).

Death is a long and unpleasant process and is often due to sepsis and inanation or haemorrhage. Uraemia from bilateral ureteric obstruction may supervene first. Such is the abject misery of this

Table 1 Inguinal node metastases in women with carcinoma of the vulva

Nodal status	Midline lesion		Unilateral lesion		Total
Negative	184		201		385
Ipsilateral			62	(21.6%)	
Contralateral			8	(2.8%)	
Unilateral	71	(23.5%)	70	(24.4%)	141
Bilateral	46	(15.3%)	16	(5.6%)	62
Total positive	117	(38.9%)	86	(30.0%)	203
Total	301	(100.0%)	287	(100.0%)	588

Modified from Homesley *et al.* (1991).

Table 2 The FIGO staging of vulval cancer

Stage I	Confined to vulva and/or perineum, maximum diameter 2 cm or less
Stage II	Confined to vulva and/or perineum, maximum diameter more than 2 cm
Stage III	Extends beyond the vulva (vagina, lower urethra, or anus) or unilateral regional lymph node metastasis
Stage IVa	Involves the mucosa of rectum or bladder, upper urethra, or pelvic bone and/or bilateral regional lymph node metastases
Stage IVb	Any distant metastasis including pelvic lymph node

demise that all patients with resectable vulval lesions should be offered surgery regardless of their age and general condition.

Clinical staging

The current FIGO classification is shown in Table 2. Despite its apparent limitations, it does give a reasonable guide to the prognosis. Formerly, the main drawback was a reliance on clinical palpation of the groin nodes, which is notoriously inaccurate (Monaghan 1985). Now that the surgical findings are incorporated in the staging evaluation, the prognostic value is greatly improved.

Diagnosis and assessment

Most patients with invasive disease (71 per cent) complain of irritation or pruritus and 57 per cent note a vulval mass or ulcer (Monaghan 1985). Medical advice is not usually sought until the mass appears. Bleeding (28 per cent) and discharge (23 per cent) are less common presentations (Monaghan 1985). One of the major problems in invasive vulval cancer is the delay between the first appearance of symptoms and referral for gynaecological opinion. This is only partly due to the patient's reluctance to attend. In many cases the doctor fails to recognize the gravity of the lesion and prescribes topical therapy, sometimes without examining the woman. Delays of over 12 months occurred in 33 per cent of a large series collected in Florida (Cavanagh et al. 1985).

Because of the multicentric nature of female lower genital tract cancer (Hammond and Monaghan 1983), the investigation of a patient with vulval cancer should include inspection of the cervix and cervical cytology. The groin nodes must be palpated carefully and any suspicious nodes sampled by fine-needle aspiration. Chest radiography is always required, but an intravenous pyelogram or lymphangiography may sometimes be helpful. Thorough examination under anaesthesia and a generous full-thickness biopsy are the most important investigations. The examination should note the size and distribution of the primary lesion, particularly the involvement of the urethra or anus and secondary lesions in the vulval or perineal skin must be sought. The groin should be re-examined under general anaesthesia, as previously undetected nodes may be palpated at that time.

Treatment

Surgery

Surgery is the mainstay of treatment. The introduction of radical vulvectomy reduced the mortality from 80 to 40 per cent (Taussig 1940; Way 1960). However, these techniques removed large areas of normal skin from the groins and primary wound closure was rarely achieved. Modifications of this *en bloc* excision were devised to allow primary closure and to reduce the considerable morbidity (Monaghan 1986; Cavanagh et al. 1990). Although these variations

reduced the rate of wound breakdown without any apparent loss of efficacy, the morbidity remained high and impaired psychosexual function was common (Andersen and Hacker 1983).

Separate groin incisions

In pursuit of an effective treatment with lower morbidity, the *en bloc* dissection of the groin nodes in continuity with the vulva was replaced by an operation using three separate incisions. This technique was originally suggested by Taussig (1940) and depended on the principle that lymphatic metastases developed initially by embolization. Therefore, in the early stages of spread there would be no residual tumour in the lymphatic channels between the tumour and the local lymph nodes in the groin. Many studies have since attested to the reduced morbidity of this method without loss of efficacy (Byron et al. 1962; Ballon and Lamb 1975; Hacker et al. 1981; Cavanagh et al. 1990; Helm et al. 1992; Grimshaw et al. 1993). Recurrent tumour in the bridge of skin between the groin and the vulva has been reported occasionally (Hacker et al. 1981; Schulz and Penalver 1989; Sutton et al. 1991; Grimshaw et al. 1993). This is most likely to occur when the lymph nodes are extensively involved and such women are better treated with an *en bloc* technique.

Ipsilateral lymphadenectomy

Spread to the contralateral groin from a lesion placed on one side of the vulva without the ipsilateral nodes being involved is very unusual (Homesley et al. 1991; Grimshaw et al. 1993) (Table 1). This has led to the suggestion that, in the absence of clinical suspicion of groin node involvement, ipsilateral lymphadenectomy is sufficient to detect lymph node disease.

Superficial inguinal lymphadenectomy

A further modification of groin node lymphadenectomy, applicable to women without clinical evidence of nodal disease, is limitation of the dissection to the superficial nodes lying anterior to the cribriform fascia (DiSaia et al. 1979). The rationale for this suggested change is the belief that lymphatic drainage from the vulva passes first to the superficial inguinal nodes before subsequently going to the femoral nodes deep to the cribriform fascia (Way 1948; Parry-Jones 1960; Borgno et al. 1990). The superficial nodes are sent for frozen section. Deep femoral lymphadenectomy is performed only if the pathologist identifies lymphatic metastases. This places a great responsibility upon the pathologist who will have to identify and examine rapidly a mean of 18 nodes from each groin (Helm et al. 1992). Inevitably, mistakes will occur with tragic consequences (Berman et al. 1989). It is unlikely that post-operative radiotherapy will prove an adequate substitute for complete surgical clearance of the groin in this situation (see below).

Superficial lymphadenectomy reduces still further the risk of troublesome lymphoedema and wound breakdown (DiSaia et al. 1979; Helm et al. 1992). However, because few women survive after recurrence in the groin, it is essential to ensure that this modified lymphadenectomy is as effective as standard inguinofemoral lymphadenectomy (Podratz et al. 1982; Lingard et al. 1992; Tilmans et al. 1992; Piura et al. 1993). Most of the experience with this technique has been obtained in women with a low risk of nodal disease, but several authors have commented upon an apparent increase in nodal recurrences (Table 3).

Hacker et al. (1984a) noted that three out of 26 patients who had a modified lymphadenectomy (one) or no lymphadenectomy (two) developed a groin recurrence. All three died, as did one other woman treated with radical local excision, giving a mortality rate

Table 3 Groin recurrence in women who had undergone unilateral or bilateral superficial inguinal lymphadenectomy (none had clinically suspicious groin nodes)

Reference	Depth of lesion (mm)	Diameter of lesion (cm)	Other criteria	Vulval surgery	Number evaluable	Groin recurrence	DOD with groin disease
DiSaia *et al.* (1979)	≤5	≤1	Non-clitoral, nodes negative	WLE	16	0	0
Hacker *et al.* (1984*a*)	≤5	≤2	No suspicious nodes	WLE	3	1	1
Berman *et al.* (1989)	36/37 assessable <5	≤2	No suspicious or positive nodes	WLE	50	1	1
Burke *et al.* (1990)	>1	0.5–6.5	No suspicious nodes	WLE	32	1	0
Sutton *et al.* (1991)	1–5	≤2	No suspicious nodes	MRV	36	1	1
Kelly *et al.* (1992)	<1	≤2	No suspicious nodes	Various	11	1	0
Stehman *et al.* (1992*a*)	≤5	≤2	No suspicious or positive nodes	WLE	121	9	5
Helm *et al.* (1992)			All stages	Various	32	3	1
					301	17 (5.7%)	9 (3.0%)

DOD, died of disease; WLE, wide local excision; MRV, modified radical vulvectomy.

of 15.4 per cent for the conservative treatment of superficially invasive tumours. No groin recurrence was seen in 58 patients who were treated with inguinofemoral lymphadenectomy because of more advanced disease and only one of these women died (mortality rate 1.7 per cent). Hacker *et al.* commented that 'patients with greater than 1 mm of stromal invasion require at least ipsilateral inguinal–femoral lymphadenectomy'.

Berman *et al.* (1989) reported one nodal recurrence, who died, in 50 superficially invasive stage I vulval cancers. The M. D. Anderson group described the results of radical wide excision and selective inguinal node dissection in 32 women with tumours invading more than 1 mm into the stroma (Burke *et al.* 1990). They excluded all patients with invasion less than 1 mm because most of them 'had no clinically identifiable tumour and were undergoing resection for suspected carcinoma *in situ*'. Only two patients were found to have groin node disease and the dissection was extended to include the deep femoral glands. Both received post-operative radiotherapy to the groins and whole pelvis and were alive with no evidence of disease at 32 and 56 months. Helm *et al.* (1992) described a similar experience in their matched retrospective comparison of traditional radical vulvectomy with a triple-incision technique incorporating superficial lymphadenectomy in most cases. The outcome in the 32 women in each group was similar, but they expressed concern that the four women with positive nodes in the conservative group seemed to have done rather badly.

At Indiana University, modified radical hemivulvectomy and superficial inguinal lymphadenectomy was performed on 36 women with lesions of diameter 2 cm or less invading less than 5 mm into the stroma and without clinically suspicious nodes (Sutton *et al.* 1991). In one case tumour recurred in the groin and the vulva less than 3 months after surgery and this woman died a few months later despite further surgery and radiotherapy. These authors expressed concern at a possible increase in recurrent disease.

The M. D. Anderson Centre reported their experience with 24 cases of minimally invasive carcinoma, defined as lesions invading less than 1 mm (Kelly *et al.* 1992). Most of these were women without a clinical tumour who were thought to have only vulval intraepithelial neoplasia III. However, four patients (17 per cent) developed recurrent vulval intraepithelial neoplasia and four more (17 per cent) developed an invasive recurrence! One of the invasive recurrences was in the groin of a woman whose superficial node dissection had been negative. She was treated with surgery and radiotherapy and was disease free at 27 months. Two other cases of groin node recurrence in women with lesions invading less than 1 mm have been reported, one following wide local excision only (Atamdede and Hoogerland 1989) and one after a superficial

lymphadenectomy (van der Velden *et al.* 1992). The present authors have themselves seen a third woman with a tiny minimally invading lesion on the vulva who presented with groin node disease. Two of these women died of their disease and the third almost certainly did so, as she had multiple groin and pelvic nodes involved, but no follow-up was reported.

The only prospective study of conservative surgery has been performed by the Gynecological Oncology Group (Stehman *et al.* 1992*a*). In this study the role of ipsilateral inguinal lymphadenectomy and modified radical hemivulvectomy was examined in 121 women with primary carcinoma of the vulva 2 cm or less in maximum diameter, 5 mm or less in thickness, without vascular space invasion, and with no suspicious groin nodes. Patients found to have positive lymph nodes at primary surgery were withdrawn. Although this was a highly selected low-risk group of patients, invasive disease recurred in 19 women (15.6 per cent). There were nine (7.3 per cent) groin and ten (8.3 per cent) vulval recurrences. Six of the groin recurrences occurred on the same side as the lymphadenectomy. At the time of the report, five of the nine women with recurrence in the groin had died, as had two of the ten vulval recurrences. These results were compared with a historical group of 96 similar patients who had been treated with radical vulvectomy and bilateral inguinofemoral lymphadenectomy. Six (6.3 per cent) of these developed a vulval recurrence and one (1.0 per cent) developed a pelvic recurrence, but none recurred in the groin. The recurrence-free survival was significantly better in the controls ($p=0.0028$). After 5 years the disease-free survival in the control and study groups was approximately 91 and 81 per cent, respectively. Surprisingly, there was no significant difference in the survival, corrected for death from intercurrent disease. After 5 years the corrected survival in the control and study groups was approximately 92 and 83 per cent, respectively. Given that only 50 per cent of the study group as opposed to 88 per cent of the control group had died or had been followed for 3 years, more prolonged follow-up may reveal a survival difference. Indeed, the survival in the control group is surprisingly low given that two recent series of radical vulvectomy and inguinofemoral lymphadenectomy in unselected women with FIGO (1988) stage I disease reported 5 year corrected survivals of 96.7 and 98 per cent (Homesley *et al.* 1991; Grimshaw *et al.* 1993). The authors themselves expressed concern at the high rate of recurrent disease and noted the groin recurrences in particular. They speculated very reasonably that this may be due to undetected disease in the femoral nodes.

This combined experience of superficial lymphadenectomy is not very reassuring. Even when applied to a low-risk population, it seems

Table 4 Groin recurrences in women who did not undergo any form of groin node surgery (all were believed to have no clinically suspicious lesions in the groin and, in many, groin node surgery was omitted because the patient had associated medical problems)

Reference	Depth of lesion (mm)	Diameter of lesion (cm)	Number evaluable	Groin recurrence	DOD with groin disease
Magrina et al. (1979)	≤5	≤2	35	4	3
Hacker et al. (1984a)	>1	≤2	23	2	2
Bryson et al. (1991)	NK	≤2	27	6	NK
Sutton et al. (1991)	≤1	≤2	10	0	0
Kelly et al. (1992)	≤1	≤2	13	0	0
Lingard et al. (1992)	NK	NK	20	7	7
			128	19	

DOD, died of disease; NK, not known.

to be associated with an unexpectedly high risk of recurrent disease in the groin, which is ultimately fatal in most cases.

Deep femoral lymphadenectomy with preservation of the cribriform fascia

A study in Turin has suggested that the deep femoral nodes can be excised without removing the fascia lata or the cribriform fascia (Micheletti et al. 1990). An earlier study of 50 female cadavers confirmed that these nodes lie medial to the femoral vein and can be seen through the fossa ovalis (Borgno et al. 1990). The altered technique suggested by this anatomical information was used in 42 women with vulval cancer. A mean of nine nodes were removed from each groin, a number similar to cadaver studies. The 5 year survival rates of 91.4 and 86.7 per cent in 14 and 18 women with stage I and stage II disease, respectively, are comparable with those reported in the literature. However, the wound complication rate remained high owing to retention of the 'butterfly' incision in the first 25 patients. This technique may allow the radical removal of superficial and deep groin lymph nodes with less morbidity and is worthy of investigation.

'Microinvasive' disease

The definition of 'microinvasion' of the vulva has proved extremely problematical. The purpose is to identify a group of women with invasive carcinoma who could safely be treated without inguinofemoral lymphadenectomy. The potential for disaster if lymphadenectomy is wrongly omitted is all too clear (Table 4). Although it was initially suggested that up to 5 mm invasion into the stroma might be acceptable (Rutledge et al. 1970; Wharton et al. 1974), subsequent reports have suggested lower limits. Some have suggested 2 mm (Friedrich and Wilkinson 1982), but most others preferred 1 mm (Iversen et al. 1981; van der Velden et al. 1992). Further reports emphasize the importance of lymphatic or vascular invasion and the degree of differentiation (Parker et al. 1975) or confluence (Hoffman et al. 1983). However, all these have been retrospective studies and most of the subjects were women in whom invasive disease was not suspected initially but found in a specimen removed in the treatment of vulval intraepithelial disease.

The Gynaecological Oncology Group undertook a prospective study of women with vulval cancer treated with radical vulvectomy and groin node dissection between November 1977 and February 1984. Superficial vulval cancer was identified in 272 of 558 women (Sedlis et al. 1987). These authors chose tumour thickness rather than depth of stromal invasion, which they found impracticable in their material. They found positive nodes even in women with tumours less than 1 mm thick (Table 5). They concluded that the risk of nodal disease was best assessed by a combination of factors. A later study of the whole group of 558 patients concurred that

Table 5 Tumour thickness and positive groin nodes

Tumour thickness (mm)	Positive nodes	Total
<1	1 (3.1%)	32
2	5 (8.9%)	56
3	11 (18.6%)	59
4	21 (30.9%)	68
5	19 (33.3%)	57

Modified from Sedlis et al. (1987).

several factors were independent predictors of positive groin nodes (Homesley et al. 1992). They did not attempt to define a group free of risk. Finally, it is important to remember that prognostic factors worked out on one population must be tested against a second population of patients to confirm their general applicability. This has never been done in this disease.

Modified radical vulvectomy

The major cause of psychosexual morbidity and damage to body image comes from the vulvectomy, particularly the removal of the clitoris and mons pubis. This has led some surgeons to devise more limited operations on the primary tumour when this has been small and unifocal (DiSaia et al. 1971; Hacker et al. 1984a). In all these, the objective has been to obtain a margin of 2–3 cm of apparently healthy tissue all round the lesion. This is often impossible with lesions adjacent to the urethra or anus, but every effort must be made to maximize the margins even if this means sacrificing the lower 1–2 cm of urethra or parts of the anus. The latter will sometimes make a colostomy necessary. Pre-operative radiotherapy may allow less radical surgery by shrinking the tumour. The risk of local recurrence is related to the size of the tumour-free margin (Heaps et al. 1990). These authors recommended aiming for a tumour-free margin of only 1 cm, but the lesion may extend far further than is obvious to naked-eye inspection and so obtaining a wider zone of healthy tissue would be prudent. Not only are wide lateral margins required, but the dissection must be taken down to the deep fascia in exactly the same way as a traditional radical vulvectomy. These 'wide local excisions', 'hemivulvectomies', or 'modified radical vulvectomies' are very radical operations indeed but, in suitable cases, do permit preservation of the clitoris and part of the vulva. The effect on psychosexual function has not been studied in depth, but it does seem likely that these procedures are less damaging (DiSaia et al. 1979).

The reported vulval recurrences following radical local excision are shown in Table 6. The recurrence rate of 6.3 per cent is a little disappointing for what are generally small low-risk tumours. However, very few of these women subsequently died of their disease because vulval recurrences are fairly readily treated (Tilmans

Table 6 Vulval recurrences and deaths following conservative vulval surgery

Reference	Depth of lesion (mm)	Diameter of lesion (cm)	Other criteria	Vulval surgery	Groin surgery	Number evaluable	Vulval recurrence	DOD with vulval disease
DiSaia et al. (1979)	≤5	≤1	Non-clitoral, nodes negative	WLE	SIL	16	0	0
Hacker et al. (1984a)	9/10<1	≤2	No suspicious nodes	WLE	None	11	1	1
Hacker et al. (1984a)	≤5	≤2	No suspicious nodes	WLE	SIL	3	0	0
Hacker et al. (1984a)	≤5	≤2	No suspicious nodes	WLE/MRV	IFL	14	0	0
Burrell et al. (1988)	>1	0.7–4.5	Included suspicious nodes	MRV	IFL	28	0	0
Berman et al. (1989)	36/37 assessable <5	≤2	No suspicious or positive nodes	WLE	SIL	50	4	0
Burke et al. (1990)	>1	0.5–6.5	No suspicious nodes	WLE	SIL	32	2	0
Hoffman et al. (1991)	>1	up to 6	Included suspicious nodes	MRV	Various	45	1	0
Sutton et al. (1991)	≤1	≤2	No suspicious nodes	WLE	None	10	0	0
Sutton et al. (1991)	1–5	≤2	No suspicious nodes	MRV	SIL	36	3	0
Kelly et al. (1992)	>1	≤2	No suspicious nodes	WLE	Various	18	3	0
Stehman et al. (1992a)	≤5	≤2	No suspicious or positive nodes	WLE	SIL	121	10	2
						384	24 (6.3%)	3 (0.8%)

DOD, died of disease; WLE, wide local excision; MRV, modified radical vulvectomy; SIL, superficial inguinal lymphadenectomy; IFL, inguinofemoral lymphadenectomy.

et al. 1992; Piura et al. 1993). A retrospective comparison of radical vulvectomy with modified radical vulvectomy found no difference in recurrence rates or cancer deaths in a small study with 45 patients in each group (Hoffman et al. 1991). However, there were differences between the groups, not least in the length of follow-up which was much shorter in the modified vulvectomy patients. More importantly it was impossible to say why the women had been assigned to a particular form of treatment. There must be a substantial risk of an undetected bias in any study of this sort.

A similar, but much larger, study was undertaken at the M. D. Anderson Centre (Rutledge et al. 1991). This consisted of an analysis of the records of 365 women with carcinoma of the vulva treated between 1944 and 1990. A Cox proportional hazards model was used to identify factors which predicted recurrence and death. This technique allows the effect of all known variables to be evaluated individually and together. An analysis of the 176 stage I and stage II lesions treated with curative intent showed no difference in the disease-free survival or the survival corrected for death from intercurrent disease between women treated with radical vulvectomy and those who underwent radical local excision. While this is reassuring, it should be noted that only 27 women were treated with radical local excision and few of the patients had been followed for more than 2 years (Mitchell, personal communication).

Complications

The complication rate depends on the surgical method but all share common problems. The most common complication is wound breakdown and infection. With the triple-incision technique this is seldom more than a minor problem. Conservative therapy with liquid honey packs is all that is required for the occasional dehiscence. Osteitis pubis is a rare but very serious complication which requires intensive and prolonged antibiotic therapy. Thromboembolic disease is always a greatly feared complication of surgery for malignant disease, but the combination of pre-operative epidural analgesia to ensure good venous return with subcutaneous heparin begun 12–24 h before the operation seems to reduce this risk. Secondary haemorrhage occurs from time to time. Chronic leg oedema may be expected in 14–21 per cent of women (Hacker et al. 1981; Grimshaw et al. 1993). Numbness and paraesthesia over the anterior thigh is common owing to the division of small cutaneous branches of the femoral nerve. Loss of body image and impaired sexual function undoubtedly occur, but the

responses of patients to surgery are extremely variable and probably depend on the woman's age, upbringing, and attitudes to life.

Conclusions

The emphasis of current research in the surgical treatment of vulval carcinoma is in reducing morbidity, particularly for young women in whom the disease appears to be becoming more common. However, there is little solid evidence on which to base a decision as to the best practice. While most agree that an en bloc dissection of the inguinofemoral nodes and the vulva through a modified incision remains the optimum treatment for women with clinically suspicious nodes, there is no general agreement as to the best management for early invasive disease.

Groin node dissection

Given the nature of the evidence available, the lack of consistent results and the very high mortality associated with groin recurrences, it seems that the safest course is to perform a groin node dissection in all cases with more than 1 mm stromal invasion and to remove both superficial and deep nodes (Hacker et al. 1984a; Monaghan 1985). A possible exception might be women with vulval intraepithelial neoplasia III being treated by excision in whom a small, superficial focus of invasion is found. These might not require lymphadenectomy. Individual women with selected stage I and stage II lesions may prefer unilateral superficial lymphadenectomy, but very careful pathological and clinical assessment would be necessary to advise on the degree of risk. Separate incisions in the groin are recommended in cases without clinically suspicious nodes, but en bloc excision with the vulva is required in other cases. The technique of deep femoral lymphadenectomy which preserves the cribriform fascia is worth investigation.

Vulval dissection

Because recurrent disease on the vulva does not carry such a high risk of mortality and because vulval surgery has the greatest impact upon a woman's body image and sexuality, there is more to be gained and less to lose from a conservative approach. Although the evidence supporting radical local excision is far from conclusive, it would seem to offer a reasonable approach provided that the principles of wide lateral and deep margins are observed. The benefits will be far less in anterior and clitoral lesions. Large or multicentric lesions may still require radical vulvectomy to achieve adequate local control. Such tumours may well benefit from pre-operative irradiation (see below).

Radiotherapy

Although the main therapy for carcinoma of the vulva is surgery, radiotherapy alone or given concurrently with chemotherapy is playing an expanding role in the management of this malignancy. Occasionally it is given with radical intent (Backstrom *et al.* 1972; Thomas *et al.* 1989; Hoffman *et al.* 1990), but it is mainly used pre- and post-operatively. It is also of value in the management of recurrent and metastatic disease.

Radiotherapy to the vulva

For many years radiotherapy to the vulva was avoided because severe late morbidity was common with the machines available and the techniques used. Modified techniques now permit radiation to the vulva without undue morbidity (Thomas *et al.* 1989), but this mode of therapy is being accepted only slowly.

Severe acute reactions in the vulval epithelium and severe late radiation reactions, such as vulvar fibrosis, atrophy, or even necrosis, have made radiotherapy to this organ difficult. These are avoidable by limiting each daily treatment fraction to 1.6–1.7 Gy and by limiting the total dose (Thomas *et al.* 1991). Thomas *et al.* (1991) recommend a maximum of 55 Gy for pre-operative radiotherapy to the vulva in order not to interfere with healing and a maximum total dose of 65 Gy in combination with 5-fluorouracil for radical treatment. The total dose for post-operative radiotherapy is 45–50 Gy if there is no macroscopic residual disease.

In Toronto, the size of the area to be irradiated and the radiation technique used depend on the size of the lesion. Perineal portals, localized to the site of disease, are used for smaller lesions and the application of opposed anterior and posterior fields is restricted to those cases that require the whole vulva to be included in the radiation field.

At Hammersmith Hospital we have adopted a similar policy with regard to radiation fields but a different approach to fractionation of radiotherapy. Instead of a daily fractionation scheme, radiotherapy is given in two fractions per day at least 6 h apart. This approach enables a large percentage of the total dose to be given over a short period of time and avoids delays in treatment due to acute local reactions. Pre-operative treatment consists of 1.5 Gy per fraction given to a total dose of 45 Gy in 30 fractions, 5 days per week for 3 weeks. Surgery can be carried out 2–3 weeks later when healing is usually complete. Women who are unsuitable for surgery receive 45 Gy to the vulva in 3 weeks, followed by a 2 week break before continuing with the same fractionation regimen to a total dose of 65 Gy. While photons are used for opposed radiation fields to the whole of the vulva, smaller vulval lesions are treated with electrons on direct perineal fields because of their limited depth of penetration, thus reducing the radiation effect on organs close to the vulva. This regime is well tolerated and the reduced treatment time allows the prescribed dose to be given without interruption. This contrasts with the experience of Thomas *et al.* (1989) where, with daily fractionation, 16 out of 27 patients had treatment suspended for 10–34 days.

Interstitial radiotherapy has a place in the non-surgical management of cancer of the vulva as an alternative to electrons, particularly if the lower vagina is involved. It is carried out by the insertion of needles afterloaded with ^{192}Ir. A plastic template, such as the Hammersmith Hedgehog (Fig. 1), ensures an even distribution. The procedure is carried out under general anaesthesia. For small lesions, when interstitial therapy is used alone, the total dose should be no higher than 65 Gy given over 6–7 days to prevent serious morbidity. Sometimes external and interstitial radiotherapy

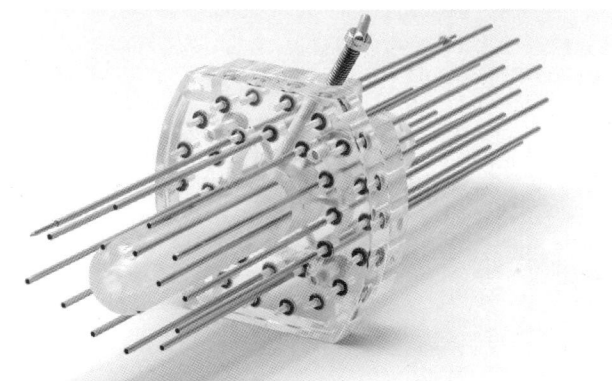

Fig. 1 The Hammersmith Hedgehog: a template for the interstitial treatment of carcinoma of the vagina. (Reproduced with permission from Shaw *et al.* 1992.)

are used sequentially, with the interstitial treatment being given 2 weeks after the end of external-beam therapy. The total dose remains 65 Gy. The importance of the size of the total dose was shown in a report of interstitial radiotherapy combined in most cases with external radiation in which six out of ten patients developed radionecrosis when doses of 70–90 Gy were given (Hoffman *et al.* 1990).

Primary radical radiotherapy

Radiotherapy is considered as primary radical treatment only for patients who are unfit for surgery. With modern anaesthesia and present surgical techniques, such cases are very few.

Pre-operative radiotherapy to the vulva

Surgery for some women may have to be very extensive and may give a poor cosmetic result and poor function. Patients with large tumours which extend very close to or involve the urethra, vagina, or anus may benefit from pre-operative radiotherapy alone or with chemotherapy to facilitate subsequent surgery and reduce its morbidity. Pre-operative radiotherapy can be given without serious complications and substantially reduces the size of the lesions (Acosta *et al.* 1978; Hacker *et al.* 1984*b*; Boronow *et al.* 1987; Rotmensch *et al.* 1990).

Post-operative radiotherapy to the vulva

Heaps *et al.* (1990) concluded that a surgical disease-free margin of less than 8 mm was associated with a 50 per cent chance of recurrence. If further surgery is not possible, post-operative radiotherapy to the vulva should be considered. The radiotherapy field may not always need to cover the whole vulva but can be confined to the site of disease in early lateral lesions (Thomas *et al.* 1991).

Groin node disease

Some 20 per cent of women with positive groin nodes will have metastatic disease in the pelvic lymph nodes. Radiotherapy to the groin and pelvic nodes is effective in the management of women with positive groin nodes if given after a complete inguinofemoral lymphadenectomy (Homesley *et al.* 1986) and is now offered to all women with more than microscopic disease of one groin node. In this randomized study all subjects underwent a radical vulvectomy and inguinofemoral groin node dissection and those with positive groin nodes were randomized to pelvic lymphadenectomy or radiotherapy. The radiotherapy was started within 6 weeks of surgery and encompassed bilateral groin, obturator, and external and internal iliac nodes even if only unilateral groin node metastases were detected. A total dose of 45–50 Gy in 1.8–2.0 Gy fractions was administered to the midplane of the pelvis in opposed anterior and posterior fields using a midline block to protect the vulva. The dose was measured halfway between the superior border of the obturator foramen and the L5–S1 junction. In addition, 45–50 Gy, measured 2–3 cm from the anterior surface, was given to the centre of the inguinal and femoral nodes. Using this technique, both the time to recurrence and the survival were improved compared to pelvic lymphadenectomy, particularly when more than one node was involved. Although both groins and the whole pelvis were treated in this study, ipsilateral radiotherapy to the groin and hemipelvis may well be sufficient when bilateral inguinofemoral lymphadenectomy has shown only unilateral groin node disease. When the vulva is also being irradiated, a similar technique is used but the midline block to exclude the vulva is omitted.

Pre-operative radiotherapy to the groins and pelvis is of value in women with clinically detectable disease in the nodes (Boronow et al. 1987). Only one of seven had residual disease at surgery following radiotherapy, compared with seven out of nine to whom radiotherapy was not given. Some authors have even suggested radiotherapy as an alternative to inguinofemoral lymphadenectomy (Perez et al. 1993). However, this opinion was based upon a retrospective review of a highly selected group of 37 women treated over a period of 22 years. In contrast, the Gynecological Oncology Group terminated prematurely a prospective randomized controlled trial comparing radiotherapy with inguinofemoral lymphadenectomy in a group of women with clinically non-involved nodes because of the higher recurrence rate ($p=0.033$) and mortality ($p=0.035$) in the radiation group (Stehman et al. 1992b). The 20 per cent of cases who were found to have positive nodes at surgery received post-operative radiotherapy to the groin and pelvis. Five (18.5 per cent) groin relapses occurred in the radiation-only group compared with none in the groin dissection regimen. While radiation is a useful supplement to inguinofemoral lymphadenectomy, it is not an effective substitute.

Concurrent chemoradiotherapy

Concurrent radiotherapy and chemotherapy have been used for vulval carcinoma in a small number of cases (Thomas et al. 1989). In this study of 33 patients, the combination was given pre-operatively in nine cases, after surgery in nine cases, and for recurrent disease in 15 cases. 5-Fluorouracil was given, with or without mitomycin C, as a continuous intravenous infusion for 4–5 days at 1 g/m^2 every 24 h. One or two courses were given every 4 weeks. When it was included in the regimen, mitomycin C was given at a dose of 6 mg/m^2 as an intravenous bolus which was repeated 4 weeks later in some patients. This regimen was based on the study of squamous carcinoma of the anus which resulted in disease control in over 90 per cent of patients (Cummings et al. 1984). Seven of the nine patients who received chemoradiotherapy prior to surgery were alive at the time of writing, three having achieved a complete response with chemoradiotherapy alone. None of the nine patients who received this regime post-operatively relapsed within the radiation field and eight out of 15 women treated for recurrence in the vulva or inguinal nodes had a complete response. A similar regime using 5-fluorouracil and mitomycin C with radiotherapy caused one treatment-related death in 12 patients with advanced or recurrrent disease (Whitaker et al. 1990).

Concurrent cisplatin, 5-fluorouracil, and radiation therapy to the pelvic and groin nodes were given as primary treatment to 12

patients with stage III and stage IV disease (Berek et al. 1991). Complete responses were seen in six of the eight stage III patients and in two of the four stage IV patients. Only one patient showed no response and four patients required salvage surgery. With a median follow-up of 37 months, ten patients were alive and disease free. No serious morbidity was reported with this combined approach. It seems that some advanced vulval carcinomas may be cured by chemoradiotherapy, thus reserving salvage surgery for those with an incomplete response. However, randomized studies comparing chemoradiotherapy with radiotherapy alone are required.

Recurrent disease

While most women with recurrence in the groin die of their disease despite treatment, surgical excision of a vulval recurrence can be effective, particularly if the recurrence is delayed for more than 2 years (Shimm et al. 1986; Grimshaw et al. 1993). However, in the majority of patients only palliative treatment is possible and this is usually external or interstitial radiotherapy. Chemotherapy may be given with the radiotherapy or alone. As well as regimens using 5-fluorouracil, other cytotoxic combinations have been assessed. The European Organization for the Research and Treatment of Cancer (EORTC) used a continuous low-dose regimen designed for elderly women consisting of bleomycin, methotrexate, and CCNU (lomustine) given as a 6 week cycle repeated three times depending on response and toxicity (Durrant et al. 1990). Although 60 per cent of 28 women with inoperable or recurrent tumours showed a response, toxicity was unacceptably high, particularly stomatitis and infection secondary to myelosuppression. Single-agent chemotherapy using bleomycin or cisplatin can give a few partial responses but is usually ineffective (Deppe et al. 1979; Thigpen et al. 1986).

Conclusion

Surgery remains the mainstay of treatment, but radiotherapy has a proven role in the treatment of groin node disease after inguinofemoral lymphadenectomy. It can also prevent local recurrence in the vulva when there is an insufficient tumour-free margin. Radiotherapy, with or without chemotherapy, is an effective treatment for some cases of cancer of the vulva and can be given without excessive acute morbidity and with minimal late sequelae. It will not replace surgery for early stage disease, even in the very elderly, but it will be used increasingly for the pre-operative treatment of advanced disease. Chemotherapy may add to the efficacy of radiotherapy when used concurrently, but this has not yet been demonstrated by randomized studies. Chemotherapy for recurrent disease is usually too toxic for the elderly women who develop this tumour.

Results of treatment

Corrected survival rates from two recent publications (Homesley et al. 1991; Grimshaw et al. 1993) are shown in Table 7. These

Table 7 Survival by FIGO (1988) stage

FIGO stage	Corrected 5 year survival (%)	
	Grimshaw et al. (1993)	Homesley et al. (1991)
I	97	98
II	85	85
III	46	74
IV	50	31

1391

use the 1988 FIGO staging which includes the surgical findings, so that stages I and II do not have groin lymph node involvement. However, stages III and IV are more heterogeneous. The overall 5 year corrected survival in the British study was 74.6 per cent (Grimshaw *et al.* 1993).

UNCOMMON TUMOURS OF THE VULVA

Melanoma

Approximately 5 per cent of melanomas in women occur on the vulva. It is the second most common carcinoma of the vulva (Morrow and DiSaia 1976; Monaghan and Hammond 1984). Melanin production is variable and the lesions range from black to completely amelanotic. The most usual presenting complaint is of a lump or an enlarging mole. Pruritus and bleeding are less common.

The prognosis is strongly related to the depth of invasion (Clark *et al.* 1969; Breslow 1970; Podratz *et al.* 1983). Because of the absence of a well-defined papillary dermis in much of the vulval skin, levels of invasion, as defined by Clark *et al.* (1969), are unsuitable for use on vulval skin (Chung *et al.* 1975) and measurement of the thickness of the lesion, as suggested by Breslow (1970), may be more reproducible. No patient from the Sloan-Kettering series died with a lesion with less than 1 mm penetration, but thereafter the outlook was bleak (Chung *et al.* 1975).

Local invasion occurs in an outward direction as well as downward and so excision margins must be very wide, with 3–5 cm being suggested for all but the most superficial lesions (White and Polk 1986). Approximately one-third of patients have inguinal lymph node metastases at presentation and 2.6 per cent have distant spread (Morrow and DiSaia 1976). When the nodes are negative the 5 year survival rate is approximately 56 per cent, falling to 14 per cent when the nodes are positive (Morrow and DiSaia 1976). Involvement of the urethra or vagina or the presence of satellite lesions all worsen the prognosis.

It is probable that the minimum therapy should be wide local excision (this usually requires a radical vulvectomy) without lymphadenectomy unless there is clinical evidence of groin disease (White and Polk 1986; Davidson *et al.* 1987). If the groin nodes are removed, the operation should be performed *en bloc* rather than through separate incisions because of the melanoma's propensity to spread unseen by lateral intradermal infiltration (Karlen *et al.* 1975). Radiation therapy is ineffective (White and Polk 1986) and adjuvant chemotherapy and immunotherapy have no proven value. Chemotherapy has not proved effective in the treatment of recurrent disease (Seeger *et al.* 1986).

Verrucous carcinoma

This slowly growing neoplasm is seen rarely on the vulva (Gallousis 1972; Isaacs 1976). Both macroscopically and histologically it resembles condyloma accuminata and the diagnosis can be difficult. Generous biopsies are required to provide sufficient material for the pathologist. The treatment is surgery, usually a radical vulvectomy but very occasionally wide local excision. The place of lymphadenectomy is debatable as lymph node metastases are uncommon. Radiotherapy is ineffective and might cause anaplastic transformation (Kraus and Perezi-Mesa 1966).

Basal cell carcinoma

This tumour is rarely found on the vulva. Wide local excision gives excellent results.

Bartholin's gland carcinoma

This tumour, which is usually an adenocarcinoma, may be squamous transitional-cell type or even mixed squamous and adenocarcinoma (Cavanagh *et al.* 1985). It has often spread widely to pelvic and groin nodes before the diagnosis is made. It must be distinguished from adenoid cystic carcinoma which is similar to the tumour found in salivary glands and which seldom gives rise to metastatic disease (Webb *et al.* 1984; Cavanagh *et al.* 1985). The treatment is surgery but, because of its deep origin, part of the vagina, the levatores ani, and the ischiorectal fat must be removed.

Sarcoma

This is a particularly rare tumour. Leiomyosarcomata may be difficult to distinguish from their benign counterparts histologically, but the presence of more than ten mitoses per high-power field serves to differentiate the two. These tumours tend to grow slowly and metastasize late. In contrast, rhabdomyosarcomata are rapidly growing aggressive tumours. A radical vulvectomy and groin node dissection is the usual treatment, but local recurrence is common and haematogenous spread is unaffected by this treatment (DiSaia *et al.* 1971; Cavanagh *et al.* 1985).

CONCLUSIONS

The main problems with carcinoma of the vulva are delay in presentation and diagnosis and inadequate initial therapy. Surgery remains the cornerstone of treatment but, in carefully selected cases, this can be made less extensive than in the past. Even when radical surgery is necessary, new techniques have reduced the morbidity enormously. Radiotherapy has an important role to play, particularly in the treatment of patients with metastatic groin node disease.

REFERENCES

Acosta A, Given FT, Frazier AB, Cordoba RB, Luminari A (1978). Preoperative radiation therapy in the management of squamous cell carcinoma of the vulva: preliminary report. *American Journal of Obstetrics and Gynecology*, **132**:198–206.

Andersen BL, Hacker NF (1983). Psychosexual adjustment after vulvar surgery. *Obstetrics and Gynecology*, **62**:457–62.

Atamdede F, Hoogerland D (1989). Regional lymph node recurrence following local excision for microinvasive vulvar carcinoma. *Gynecologic Oncology*, **34**:125–8.

Backstrom A, Edsmyr F, Wickland H (1972). Radiotherapy of carcinoma of the vulva. *Acta Obstetrica Gynecologica Scandinavica*, **51**:109–15.

Ballon SC, Lamb EJ (1975). Separate incisions in the treatment of carcinoma of the vulva. *Surgery, Gynecology and Obstetrics*, **140**:81–4.

Berek JS, *et al.* (1991). Concurrent cisplatin and 5-fluorouracil chemotherapy and radiation therapy for advanced-stage squamous carcinoma of the vulva. *Gynecologic Oncology*, **42**:197–201.

Bergeron C, Ferenczy A, Shah K, Naghashfar Z (1987). Multicentric human papillomavirus infections of the female genital tract: correlation of viral types with abnormal mitotic figures colposcopic presentation and location. *Obstetrics and Gynecology*, **69**:736–42.

Berman ML, Soper TJ, Creasman WT, Olt GT, DiSaia PJ (1989). Conservative surgical management of superficially invasive stage I vulvar carcinoma. *Gynecologic Oncology*, **35**:352–7.

Boehm F, Morris JM (1971). Paget's disease and apocrine gland carcinoma of the vulva. *Obstetrics and Gynecology*, **38**:185–92.

Borgno G, *et al.* (1990). Topographic distribution of groin lymph nodes. *Journal of Reproductive Medicine*, **35**:1127–9.

Boronow RC, *et al.* (1987). Combined therapy as an alternative to exenteration for locally advanced vulvovaginal cancer. *American Journal Clinical Oncology*, **10**:171–81.

Breslow A (1970). Thickness cross-sectional areas and depth of invasion in the prognosis of cutaneous melanoma. *Annals of Surgery*, 172:902–8.

Brinton LA, Nasca PC, Mallin K, Baptiste MS, Willbanks GD, Richart RM (1990). Case control study of cancer of the vulva. *Obstetrics and Gynaecology*, 75:859–66.

Bryson SC, Dembo AJ, Colgan TJ, Thomas GM, DeBoer G, Lickrish GM (1991). Invasive squamous cell carcinoma of the vulva: defining low and high risk groups for recurrence. *International Journal of Gynecological Cancer*, 1:25–31.

Burke TW, Striner CA, Gershenson DM, Edwards CL, Morris M, Wharton JT (1990). Radical wide excision and selective inguinal node dissection for squamous cell carcinoma of the vulva. *Gynecologic Oncology*, 38:328–32.

Burrell MO, Franklin EW, Campion MJ, Crozier MA, Stacy PW (1988). The modified radical vulvectomy with groin dissection: an eight year experience. *American Journal of Obstetrics and Gynecology*, 159:715–22.

Buscema J, Woodruff JD, Parmley TH, Genadry R (1980a). Carcinoma *in situ* of the vulva. *Obstetrics and Gynecology*, 55:225–30.

Buscema J, Stern J, Woodruff JD (1980b). The significance of the histologic alterations adjacent to invasive vulvar carcinoma. *American Journal of Obstetrics and Gynecology*, 137:902–8.

Byron RL, Lamb EJ, Yonemoto RH, Kase S (1962). Radical inguinal node dissection in the treatment of cancer. *Surgery, Gynecology and Obstetrics*, 114:401–8.

Caglar H, Delgado G, Hreshchyshyn MM (1986). Partial and total skinning vulvectomy in treatment of carcinoma *in situ* of the vulva. *Obstetrics and Gynecology*, 68:504–7.

Cavanagh D, Ruffolo EH, Marsden DE (1985). Cancer of the vulva. In *Gynecologic cancer—a clinicopathological approach* (ed. D Cavanagh, EH Ruffolo, and DE Marsden), pp. 1–40. Appleton–Century–Crofts, Norwalk.

Cavanagh D, Fiorica JV, Hoffman MS, Roberts WS, Bryson P, LaPolla JP, Barton DPJ (1990). Invasive carcinoma of the vulva—changing trends in surgical management. *American Journal of Obstetrics and Gynecology*, 163:1007–15.

Chung AF, Woodruff JM, Lewis JL (1975). Malignant melanoma of the vulva—a report of 44 cases. *Obstetrics and Gynecology*, 45:638–46.

Clark WH, From L, Bernadino EA, Mihm MC (1969). The histogenesis and biologic behaviour of primary human malignant melanomas of the skin. *Cancer Research*, 29:705–26.

Creasman WT, Gallacher HS, Rutledge F (1975). Paget's disease of the vulva. *Gynecological Oncology*, 3:133–48.

Cummings B, *et al.* (1984). Results and toxicity of the treatment of anal carcinoma by radiation therapy or radiation and chemotherapy. *Cancer*, 54:2062–8.

Davidson T, Kissin M, Westbury G (1987). Vulvo-vaginal melanoma—should radical surgery be abandoned? *British Journal of Obstetrics and Gynaecology*, 94:473–6.

Degefu S, O'Quinn AG, Dhurandhar HN (1986). Paget's disease of the vulva and urogenital malignancies: a case report and review of the literature. *Gynecological Oncology*, 25:347–54.

Deppe G, Cohen CJ, Bruckner HW (1979). Chemotherapy of squamous cell carcinoma of the vulva: a review. *Gynecologic Oncology*, 7:345–8.

DiSaia PJ, Rutledge F, Smith JP (1971). Sarcoma of the vulva. *Obstetrics and Gynecology*, 38:180–4.

DiSaia PJ, Creasman WT, Rich WM (1979). An alternative approach to early cancer of the vulva. *American Journal of Obstetrics and Gynecology*, 133:825–32.

Disney APS (1989). *Twelfth report of the Australia and New Zealand combined dialysis and transplant registry (ANZDATA)*. Australian Kidney Foundation, Sydney.

Dorsey JH (1986). Skin appendage involvement and vulval intraepithelial neoplasia. In *Gynaecological laser surgery* (ed. F Sharp and JA Jordan), pp. 193–5. Perinatology Press, New York.

Durrant KR, *et al.* (1990). Bleomycin, methotrexate, and CCNU in advanced inoperable squamous cell carcinoma of the vulva: a phase II study of the EORTC Gynaecological Cancer Cooperative Group (GCCG). *Gynecologic Oncology*, 37:359–62.

Elliott PM (1992). Early invasive carcinoma of the vulva: definition, clinical features and management. In *Gynecologic oncology* (2nd edn) (ed. M Coppleson), pp. 465–77. Churchill Livingstone, Edinburgh.

Ferenczy A (1992). Intraepithelial neoplasia of the vulva. In *Gynecologic oncology* (2nd edn) (ed. M Coppleson), pp. 443–63. Churchill Livingstone, Edinburgh.

Friedrich EG, Wilkinson EJ (1982). The vulva. In *Pathology of the female genital tract* (2nd edn) (ed. A Blaustein), pp. 13–58. Springer-Verlag, New York.

Gallousis S (1972). Verrucous carcinoma—report of three vulvar cases and review of the literature. *Obstetrics and Gynecology*, 40:502–7.

Grimshaw RN, Murdoch JB, Monaghan JM (1993). Radical vulvectomy and bilateral inguinal–femoral lymphadenectomy through separate incisions—experience with 100 cases. *International Journal of Gynecological Cancer*, 3:18–23.

Hacker NF, Leuchter RS, Berek JS, Castaldo TW, Lagasse LD (1981). Radical vulvectomy and bilateral inguinal lymphadenectomy through separate groin incisions. *Obstetrics and Gynecology*, 58:574–9.

Hacker NF, Berek JS, Lagasse LD, Neiberg RK, Leuchter RS (1984a). Individualisation of treatment for stage I squamous cell vulvar carcinoma. *Obstetrics and Gynecology*, 63:155–62.

Hacker NF, Berek JS, Juillard GJF, Lagasse LD (1984b). Preoperative radiation therapy for locally advanced vulvar cancer. *Cancer*, 54:2056–61.

Hammond IG, Monaghan JM (1983). Multicentric carcinoma of the female genital tract. *British Journal of Obstetrics and Gynaecology*, 90:557–61.

Heaps JM, Fu YS, Montz FJ, Hacker NF, Berek JS (1990). Surgical–pathological variables predictive of local recurrence in squamous cell carcinoma of the vulva. *Gynecologic Oncology*, 38:309–14.

Helm CW, Hatch K, Austin JM, Partridge EE, Soong S-J, Elder JE, Shingleton HM (1992). A matched comparison of single and triple incision techniques for the surgical treatment of carcinoma of the vulva. *Gynecologic Oncology*, 46:150–6.

Hoffman JS, Kumar NB, Morley GW (1983). Microinvasive squamous carcinoma of the vulva: search for a definition. *Obstetrics and Gynecology*, 61:615–18.

Hoffman M, *et al.* (1990). Interstitial radiotherapy for the treatment of advanced or recurrent vulvar and distal vaginal malignancy. *American Journal of Obstetrics and Gynecology*, 162:1278–82.

Hoffman MS, Roberts WS, Finan MA, Fiorica JV, Bryson SCP, Ruffolo EH, Cavanagh D (1991). A comparative study of radical vulvectomy and modified radical vulvectomy for the treatment of invasive squamous cell carcinoma of the vulva. *Gynecologic Oncology*, 45:192–7.

Homesley HD, Bundy BN, Sedlis A, Adcock L (1986). Radiation therapy versus pelvic node resection for carcinoma of the vulva with positive groin nodes. *Obstetrics and Gynecology*, 68:733–40.

Homesley HD, Bundy BN, Sedlis A, Yordan E, Berek JS, Jahshan A, Mortel R (1991). Assessment of current International Federation of Gynecology and Obstetrics staging of vulvar carcinoma relative to prognostic factors for survival (a Gynecological Oncology Group Study). *American Journal of Obstetrics and Gynecology*, 164:997–1004.

Homesley HD, Bundy BN, Sedlis A, Yordan E, Berek JS, Jahshan A, Mortel R (1992). Prognostic factors of groin node metastasis in squamous cell carcinoma of the vulva (a Gynecologic Oncology Group Study), *Gynecologic Oncology*, 49:279–83.

Hopkins MP, Reid GC, Vettrano I, Morley GW (1991). Squamous cell carcinoma of the vulva: prognostic factors influencing survival. *Gynecologic Oncology*, 43:113–17.

Isaacs JH (1976). Verrucous carcinoma of the female genital tract. *Gynecologic Oncology*, 4:259–69.

Iversen T, Aas M (1983). Lymph drainage from the vulva. *Gynecologic Oncology*, 16:179–89.

Iversen T, Abeler V, Aalders J (1981). Individualized treatment of stage I carcinoma of the vulva. *Obstetrics and Gynecology*, 57:85–9.

Jones RW, McLean MR (1986). Carcinoma *in situ* of the vulva: a review of 31 treated and five untreated cases. *Obstetrics and Gynecology*, 68:499–503.

Karlen JR, Piver MS, Barlow JJ (1975). Melanoma of the vulva. *Obstetrics and Gynecology*, 45:181–5.

Kaufman R, Gordon A (1986a). Squamous cell carcinoma *in situ* of the vulva. Part II. *British Journal of Sexual Medicine*, 13:55–8.

Kaufman R, Gordon A (1986b). Squamous cell carcinoma *in situ* of the vulva. Part I. *British Journal of Sexual Medicine*, 13:24–7.

Kelly JL III, Burke TW, Tornos C, Morris M, Gershenson DM, Silva EG, Wharton JT (1992). Minimally invasive vulvar carcinoma: an indication for conservative surgical therapy. *Gynecologic Oncology*, 44:240–4.

Kraus FT, Perezi-Mesa C (1966). Verrucous carcinoma—clinical and pathological study of 105 cases involving oral cavity larynx and genitalia. *Cancer*, **19**:26–38.

Leuchter RS, Townsend DE, Hacker NF, Pretorius RG, Lagasse LD, Wade ME (1984). Treatment of vulvar carcinoma *in situ* with the CO_2 laser. *Gynecologic Oncology*, **19**:314–22.

Lingard D, Free K, Wright RG, Battistutta D (1992). Invasive squamous cell carcinoma of the vulva: behaviour and results in the light of changing management regimens. *Australian and New Zealand Journal of Obstetrics and Gynaecology*, **32**:137–45.

Magrina JF, Webb MJ, Gaffey TA, Symmonds RE (1979). Stage I squamous cell cancer of the vulva. *American Journal of Obstetrics and Gynecology*, **134**:453–9.

Micheletti L, *et al.* (1990). *Journal of Reproductive Medicine*, **35**:1130–3.

Mene A, Buckley CH (1985). Involvement of the vulval skin appendages by intraepithelial neoplasia. *British Journal of Obstetrics and Gynaecology*, **92**:634–8.

Meyrick TRH, Ridley CM, McGibbon DH, Black MM (1988). Lichen sclerosus and autoimmunity—a study of 350 women. *British Journal of Dermatology*, **118**:41–6.

Monaghan JM (1985). Management of vulvar carcinoma. In *Clinical gynaecological oncology* (ed. JH Shepherd and JM Monaghan), pp. 133–53. Blackwell, London.

Monaghan JM (1986). Radical surgery for carcinoma of the vulva. In *Bonney's gynaecological surgery* (9th edn) (ed. JM Monaghan), pp. 121–8. Baillière Tindall, Eastbourne.

Monaghan JM, Hammond IG (1984). Pelvic node dissection in the treatment of vulvar carcinoma—is it necessary? *British Journal of Obstetrics and Gynaecology*, **91**:270–4.

Morrow CP, DiSaia PJ (1976). Malignant melanoma of the female genitalia: a clinical analysis. *Obstetrical and Gynecologic Survey*, **31**:233–71.

Office of Population Censuses and Surveys (1985). *Cancer statistics—registrations*, pp. 27, 39. HMSO, London.

Parker RT, Duncan I, Rampone J, Creasman W (1975). Operative management of early invasive epidermoid carcinoma of the vulva. *American Journal of Obstetrics and Gynecology*, **123**:349–55.

Parry-Jones E (1960). Lymphatics of the vulva. *Journal of Obstetrics and Gynaecology of the British Commonwealth*, **67**:919–28.

Perez CA, Grigsby PW, Galakatos A, Swanson R, Camel HM, Kao M-S, Lockett MA (1993). Radiation therapy in management of carcinoma of the vulva with emphasis on conservative therapy. *Cancer*, **71**:3707–16.

Piura B, Masotina A, Murdoch J, Lopes A, Morgan P, Monaghan J (1993). Recurrent squamous cell carcinoma of the vulva: a study of 73 cases. *Gynecologic Oncology*, **48**:189–95.

Podratz KC, Symmonds RE, Taylor WF (1982). Carcinoma of the vulva: analysis of treatment failures. *American Journal of Obstetrics and Gynecology*, **143**:340–51.

Podratz KC, Gaffey TA, Symmonds RE, Johansen KL, O'Brien PC (1983). Melanoma of the vulva: an update. *Gynecological Oncology*, **16**:153–68.

Rotmensch J, *et al.* (1990). Preoperative radiotherapy followed by radical vulvectomy with inguinal lymphadenectomy for advanced vulvar carcinomas. *Gynecologic Oncology*, **36**:181–4.

Rutledge FN, Smith JP, Franklin EW (1970). Carcinoma of the vulva. *American Journal of Obstetrics and Gynecology*, **106**:1117–30.

Rutledge FN, Mitchell MF, Munsell MF, Atkinson EN, Bass B, McGuffee V, Silva E (1991). Prognostic indicators for invasive carcinoma of the vulva. *Gynecologic Oncology*, **42**:239–44.

Schulz MJ, Penalver M (1989). Recurrent vulvar carcinoma in the intervening tissue bridge in early invasive stage disease treated by radical vulvectomy and bilateral groin node dissection through separate incisions. *Gynecologic Oncology*, **35**:383–6.

Sedlis A, *et al.* (1987). Positive groin nodes in superficial squamous cell vulvar cancer. *American Journal of Obstetrics and Gynecology*, **156**:1159–64.

Seeger J, Richman SP, Allegra JC (1986). Systemic therapy of malignant melanoma. *Medical Clinics of North America*, **70**:89–94.

Shafi MI, Luesley DM, Byrne P, Samra JS, Redman CW, Jordan JA, Rollason TP (1989). Vulval intraepithelial neoplasia—management and outcome. *British Journal of Obstetrics and Gynaecology*, **96**:1339–44.

Shaw R, Soutter P, Stanton S (1992). *Gynaecology*. Churchill Livingstone, London.

Shimm DS, Fuller AF, Orlow EL, Dosoretz DE, Aristizabal SA (1986). Prognostic variables in the treatment of squamous cell carcinoma of the vulva. *Gynecologic Oncology*, **24**:343–58.

Stehman FB, Bundy BN, Dvoretsky PM, Creasman WT (1992a). Early stage I carcinoma of the vulva treated with ipsilateral superficial inguinal lymphadenectomy and modified radical hemivulvectomy: a prospective study of the Gynecologic Oncology Group. *Obstetrics and Gynecology*, **79**:490–7.

Stehman FB, *et al.* (1992b). *International Journal of Radiation Oncology—Biology—Physics*, **24**:389–96.

Sutton GP, Miser MR, Stehman FB, Look KY, Ehrlich CE (1991). Trends in the operative management of invasive squamous carcinoma of the vulva at Indiana University, 1974 to 1988. *American Journal of Obstetrics and Gynecology*, **164**:1472–81.

Taussig FJ (1940). Cancer of the vulva—an analysis of 155 cases (1911–1940). *American Journal of Obstetrics and Gynecology*, **40**:764–79.

Thigpen JT, Blessing JA, Homesley HD, Lewis GC (1986). Phase II trials of cisplatin and piperazinedione in advanced or recurrent squamous cell carcinoma of the vulva: a Gynecologic Oncology Group Study. *Gynecologic Oncology*, **23**:358–63.

Thomas G, *et al.* (1989). Concurrent radiation and chemotherapy in vulvar carcinoma. *Gynecologic Oncology*, **34**:263–7.

Thomas G, *et al.* (1991). Changing concepts in the management of vulvar cancer. *Gynecologic Oncology*, **42**:9–21.

Tilmans AS, Sutton GP, Look KY, Stehman FB, Ehrlich CE, Hornback NB (1992). Recurrent squamous carcinoma of the vulva. *American Journal of Obstetrics and Gynecology*, **167**:1383–9.

van der Velden J, Kooyman CD, van Lindert ACM, Heintz APM (1992). A stage Ia vulvar carcinoma with an inguinal lymph node recurrence after local excision. A case report and literature review. *International Journal of Gynecological Cancer*, **2**:157–9.

Way S (1948). The anatomy of the lymphatic drainage of the vulva and its influence on the radical operation for carcinoma. *Annals of the Royal College of Surgeons of England*, **3**:187–209.

Way S (1960). Carcinoma of the vulva. *American Journal of Obstetrics and Gynecology*, **79**:692–8.

Webb JB, Lott M, O'Sullivan JC, Azzopardi JG (1984). Combined adenoid cystic and squamous carcinoma of Bartholin's gland. *British Journal of Obstetrics and Gynaecology*, **91**:291–5.

Wharton JT, Gallagher S, Rutledge FN (1974). Microinvasive carcinoma of the vulva. *American Journal of Obstetrics and Gynecology*, **118**:159–62.

Whitaker SJ, *et al.* (1990). A pilot study of chemo-radiotherapy in advanced carcinoma of the vulva. *British Journal of Obstetrics and Gynaecology*, **97**:436–42.

White MJ, Polk HC (1986). Therapy of primary cutaneous melanoma. *Medical Clinics of North America*, **70**:71–87.

9.8 Sarcoma and melanoma of the female genital system

DAVID LOWE AND C. N. HUDSON

INTRODUCTION

It is unlikely that many clinicians will encounter large numbers of sarcomas and other rare tumours of the female genital system, but one or two cases a year might be expected to present in an active oncology or gynaecological oncology practice. Even so, any one clinician's experience is likely to be very limited. It is very difficult to establish the biological behaviour of these rare tumours in adults, though sarcomas account for over 80 per cent of all malignant tumours of the female genital system that arise in childhood (La Vecchia *et al.* 1984).

Patients with a rare malignancy of the female genital system such as sarcoma should ideally be managed in a tertiary referral centre where the necessary surgical and pathological expertise can be accumulated. In practice there are several reasons why this may not easily be achieved. For anatomical and other reasons the female genital system presents problems with clinical and surgical access, so that the diagnosis of a sarcoma of the upper genital system may be established only after another condition has been wrongly diagnosed. Sarcomas of the vulva or vagina are more accessible but are covered by squamous epithelium and so can be difficult to diagnose clinically. An exception to this is malignant melanoma, but even with these tumours an atypical appearance can result in the true diagnosis being overlooked.

Table 1   Sarcomas of the female genital system

Pure sarcomas
  Homologous sarcomas of the female genital system
    Pure:
      Leiomyosarcoma
      Fibrosarcoma and variants
      Vascular tumours
    Mixed

  Heterologous sarcomas of the female genital system
    Pure
      Rhabdomyosarcoma
      Osteosarcoma
      Chondrosarcoma
    Mixed

  Mixed homologous and heterologous sarcomas

  Other
    Synovial sarcoma-like tumour
    Alveolar soft part sarcoma
    Lymphoma
    Epithelioid sarcoma
    Kaposi's sarcoma
      (Aggressive angiomyxoma)

Sarcomas with epithelial elements
  Adenosarcoma
  Malignant mixed Müllerian tumour

Sarcomas of the female genital system are classified according to their histological features and in particular by the cell type or types present. Sarcomas of a single tissue type include tumours of cells normally present in the female genital system, such as smooth muscle, stromal cells, and cells of vessels, nerves, and fibrous tissue, tumours of cells not normally found at that site, for example of striated muscle, bone, and cartilage, and tumours that occur in almost any part of the body, such as lymphoma (Table 1). Sarcomas of more than one cell type include adenosarcoma and malignant mixed Müllerian tumours.

Sarcomas that occur in the female genital system often have counterparts in other tissues of the body and the histological features are in most cases very similar. Extrapolation of the behaviour of these to the female genital system may not always be valid, but in most cases will provide some clue to the likely clinical features, histological characteristics, and eventual behaviour of these rare tumours.

CLINICAL PRESENTATION AND DIAGNOSIS

There are rarely any specific features of the presentation of these unusual tumours. The clinical manifestations of any form of ovarian malignancy, even the more common types, are protean: pain and abdominal swelling are the most prominent. Bleeding *per vaginam* is rare. Even at operation, specimens taken for frozen section are seldom suitable for precise diagnosis. Tumours of the uterine corpus vary in presentation according to their relation with the endometrium. If the endometrium is involved, either by a primary tumour or invasion by a smooth muscle malignancy, bleeding is likely.

With myometrial lesions the clinical distinction between leiomyoma and leiomyosarcoma is not easily made. Benign tumours are not commonly painful and the symptom of pain suggests that there has been either a complication of a benign lesion or that a malignant tumour is present. More likely than the last is the possibility that two pathological processes account for the pain, such as a leiomyoma associated with endometriosis or pelvic inflammatory disease. Expensive and complicated imaging techniques such as computerized tomography or magnetic resonance imaging are not usually used before operation when there is a firm clinical diagnosis of fibroids. Ultrasonographic scans, on the other hand, are commonly used, chiefly to investigate the possibility of adnexal pathology that comes into the differential diagnosis of a pelvic mass.

A positive finding will necessitate revision of the surgical plan. Leiomyomas have different echogenicity from normal uterine muscle but the picture can be very variable because of degeneration that occurs in these tumours and a firm diagnosis of malignancy on ultrasonographic scanning may not be possible. However, one clinical situation is suggestive of malignancy: leiomyomas regress after the menopause and if a woman presents post-menopausally with symptoms and physical signs of a fibroid uterus, the possibility of malignancy must be seriously entertained.

On the vulva or vagina, a pigmented lesion may be a malignant melanoma and this must be considered in the differential diagnosis of pigmented skin tumours, the most common of which are basal cell papilloma and basal cell carcinoma. Melanoma is more commonly polypoid or nodular than elsewhere on the skin and bleeding is more commonly seen in melanoma than in squamous cell or basal cell carcinoma of the vulva or vagina. Melanoma can occasionally be plum coloured or red and an important differential diagnosis in these cases is metastatic tumour, which is usually adenocarcinoma and rarely choriocarcinoma.

IMMUNOHISTOCHEMISTRY

Immunohistochemical stains are useful in the differential diagnosis of sarcoma of the female genital system: antibodies to desmin, laminin, and myoglobin stain some sarcomas in a specific or helpful manner and stains for epithelial markers are negative. Undifferentiated and very poorly differentiated carcinomas can have spindle cell areas and resemble sarcoma, but their epithelial nature can be confirmed by staining with antikeratin antibodies (Kahn *et al.* 1984). The diagnosis is more reliable if a panel of antikeratin antibodies is used rather than just one and care must be taken in the choice of antibody: smooth muscle tumours can contain cytokeratins and stain positively with the antibody CAM 5.2 (Norton *et al.* 1987).

Most of the cells in leiomyosarcoma, rhabdomyosarcoma, and endometrial stromal sarcoma are positive for desmin, the muscle type of intermediate filament protein (Om and Ghose 1987; Sahin and Benda 1988). Rhabdomyosarcomas also stain with the antiskeletal muscle antibody found in patients with myasthenia gravis, which appears to be a more sensitive and specific detector for these tumours than the standard antimyoglobin and antidesmin antibodies (Om and Ghose 1987). Staining for vimentin is not helpful: it can be present in carcinoma and lymphoma as well as solid sarcoma of the female genital system and even then is expressed patchily (Bonazzi del Poggetto *et al.* 1983).

Malignant mixed mesodermal tumours of the uterus and ovary express several different types of intermediate filament protein (Sahin and Benda 1988). Most of the stromal cells stain positively for desmin and vimentin and, occasionally, myoglobin; the epithelial elements express cytokeratin (Bonazzi del Poggetto *et al.* 1983) and this is also seen occasionally in stromal cells. α_1-Antitrypsin and α_1-antichymotrypsin, markers of fibrohistiocytic differentiation, may be present in areas resembling the so-called malignant fibrous histiocytoma of skin and elsewhere (Marshall and Braye 1985; Auerbach *et al.* 1988). Glial fibrillary acidic protein, found in normal astrocytes, is also present in the stromal cells of malignant mixed Müllerian tumours (Liao and Choi 1986).

S100 protein, which is present in normal glial cells, Schwann cells, melanocytes, and Langerhans cells, is found in melanoma of the female genital system (Kahn *et al.* 1983), in some of the cells of phaeochromocytoma (Kahn *et al.* 1983), and in some cases of malignant mixed Müllerian tumour (Auerbach *et al.* 1988; Sahin and Benda 1988). The differential diagnosis of these three tumours seldom overlaps and immunostaining for S100 can therefore be diagnostically helpful.

LEIOMYOSARCOMA

Leiomyosarcoma is the most common sarcoma of the female genital system, accounting for over 80 per cent of malignant connective tissue neoplasms in that site. The prevalence overall is approximately $0.67/10^5$ women over the age of 20 years (Vardi and Tovell 1980). The condition is slightly more common in Blacks than Whites, which may reflect the fact that leiomyoma is also more common, but there is no definite racial predisposition and the incidence is unrelated to gravidity or parity. Leiomyosarcoma is most common in the corpus of the uterus but in the female genital system has been described also in the cervix, vagina, vulva, broad ligament, Fallopian tube, and ovary (Peters *et al.* 1985; Prat and Fox 1987).

The incidence of leiomyosarcoma in the uterus is far lower than the incidence of leiomyoma (fibroid) and leiomyosarcoma is rarely important in the differential diagnosis of these tumours. In practice, many gynaecologists advise surgical removal of uterine smooth muscle tumours that are larger than a certain size, usually that equivalent to a 14 week pregnancy, because the pressure effects and complications of fibroids are more common. Some cases of leiomyosarcoma are therefore discovered by chance. The incidence in such cases shows a gradient with age from 0.2 per cent at the age of 36 to 1.7 per cent at the age of 62 years (Liebsohn *et al.* 1990).

Oestrogen receptors have been found in normal myometrium and leiomyomas (Kornyei *et al.* 1986) and medical methods of shrinking fibroids with gonadotrophin partial agonist therapy have been tried. Some of the diagnoses in these studies were not confirmed by biopsy. It was inevitable that misdiagnosis of a leiomyosarcoma should occur (Liebsohn *et al.* 1990) and, although shrinkage of the leiomyosarcoma was observed, viable sarcoma was demonstrable in the uterus when it was eventually excised.

The macroscopical features of leiomyosarcomas when small may resemble those of leiomyomas. Larger tumours may be intramural, submucosal, or subserosal; they are soft and pink with poorly circumscribed borders. Haemorrhage and necrosis are common. The gross appearances may give an indication of the extent of their spread but contribute nothing to the diagnosis, which rests purely on the histological features.

Microscopically, leiomyosarcomas have a range of cellular appearances from uniform, fusiform cells with a relatively normal density of distribution and occasional mitoses to densely crowded, pleomorphic cells with hyperchromatic nuclei that have numerous mitoses, areas of necrosis and haemorrhage, and obvious vascular invasion. Invasion of the surrounding myometrium can be difficult to delineate, especially with well-differentiated tumours and lack of local invasion does not mean that the tumour will not metastasize.

The mitotic count per 10 high-power microscope fields is the cornerstone of the diagnosis of smooth muscle tumours of the female genital system. This numerical approach is appealing but the problems involved should be appreciated. Most reported series assess the mitotic count in 10 high-power fields of the tumour but the area of a high-power field is not always stated and, moreover, may not correspond with the area defined by the microscope used for diagnosis. The thickness of the section has a great bearing on the number of mitoses that are likely to be available for counting. Distinguishing a mitotic figure from a pyknotic or karyorrhectic nucleus can be difficult. When the tumour has very numerous mitoses these problems are less important, but in clinicopathological practice, confident prediction of the behaviour of a smooth muscle tumour can be very difficult.

A smooth muscle tumour that has 10 or more mitoses per 10 high-power fields of tumour is considered to be leiomyosarcoma, irrespective of the degree of atypia of the tumour cells. In fact, tumours with a high mitotic count are almost always obviously malignant, with pleomorphic, multinucleate, and hyperchromatic cells.

Subtypes

Leiomyosarcoma may have the typical histological features described above or may be myxoid, epithelioid, or haemangiopericytoma-like (Kurman and Norris 1976; Gray *et al.* 1986). When a smooth muscle tumour has epithelioid elements, malignancy is defined by a smaller number of mitoses per 10 high-power fields than for typical leiomyosarcoma: the presence of two or more mitoses per 10 high-power fields in a tumour with epithelioid cells is highly suggestive of the potential to metastasize.

As leiomyosarcoma is the most common sarcoma of the female genital system there is more experience in treating these tumours than many of the other sarcomas. Post-operative radiotherapy has been widely used and may be efficacious in some cases to reduce the rate of local relapse (Salazar and Dunne 1980). Chemotherapeutic regimens have been devised and can have a useful place in palliation in cases that have relapsed. Whether to give adjuvant, post-operative chemotherapy after notionally complete surgery or to give chemotherapy for documented but unevaluable residual disease, remain controversial (Marchetti and Piver 1988), as for all soft tissue sarcomas.

The most efficacious drug is probably doxorubicin (Kolstad 1983). Repeat surgery can also be useful in certain cases; together with radiotherapy and chemotherapy, surgery for accessible tumour recurrence may prolong life. As discussed above, hormonal treatment may theoretically be an option, but tamoxifen has been used without notable success and leiomyosarcoma has not been shown to be usefully sensitive to hormonal manipulation.

STROMAL SARCOMAS OF THE VAGINA, CERVIX, AND ENDOMETRIUM

Endometrial stromal sarcoma has been recognized as a discrete entity only relatively recently and so data on its incidence and prevalence are difficult to obtain from reported cases. The term stromatosis has been used for a benign tumour by some and for a malignant tumour by others (Hart and Yoonessi 1977; Thatcher and Woodruff 1982). A classification of abnormalities of growth of endometrial stroma has now become established and three categories are recognized: benign stromal nodule, low-grade stromal sarcoma, and high-grade stromal sarcoma. Stromal sarcoma of the cervix (Jaffe *et al.* 1985; Young *et al.* 1988) and of the vagina (Goyert *et al.* 1987) has been described by analogy and has similar histological features to endometrial stromal sarcoma. The tumour can be associated with endometriosis (Berkowitz *et al.* 1978).

Both low and high grades of endometrial stromal sarcoma infiltrate the adjacent endometrial stroma and the underlying myometrium; the low-grade tumour can be distinguished from an endometrial stromal nodule by this infiltration. Stromal sarcomas have three principal growth patterns: they can grow as clearly defined, rounded, polypoid tumours that indent the endometrial cavity and compress the adjacent myometrium, they can diffusely infiltrate the myometrium without forming a discrete tumour mass, so that they resemble involvement of the corpus by adenomyosis, or they can be poorly defined tumours that extend as cords of soft pink or brown tissue into the adjacent tissues. This last growth pattern is the most common for both low- and high-grade tumours.

A high-grade stromal sarcoma rarely forms a well-defined tumour. They tend to be larger and more friable than low-grade tumours and expand the endometrial cavity in the manner of malignant mixed Müllerian tumours of the uterus (see below).

Histologically, endometrial stromal sarcoma resembles the stroma of proliferative phase endometrium. High-grade tumours usually have the morphological features of endometrial stroma sufficient to permit diagnosis without difficulty and the degree of cellular pleomorphism and number of mitoses makes differentiation from normal endometrium and low-grade stromal sarcoma reasonably simple.

Low-grade stromal sarcomas are composed of uniform cells with little nuclear or cytoplasmic atypia. Because of the great similarity with normal endometrium it may be impossible to diagnose a low-grade stromal sarcoma with certainty on curettage fragments. The myometrium is characteristically invaded and may be widely infiltrated by sarcoma cells, either by direct invasion or by involvement of thin-walled, vascular channels in the myometrium. This produces the cords of tissue that give the tumour its characteristic macroscopical appearance. Infarction is not commonly seen and is present only in small areas. There may rarely be decidualization of the tumour cells as a response to endogenous or administered progesterone. Most low-grade endometrial sarcomas have mitotic counts of fewer than three mitoses per 10 high-power fields, though as many as nine may be present if there is no significant pleomorphism or necrosis (Norris and Taylor 1966; Kempson and Bari 1970; Hart and Yoonessi 1977; Fekete and Vellios 1984). Recurrent lesions often develop after many years and can be treated surgically (Hart and Yoonessi 1977).

Surgery followed by an indefinite course of progestogen therapy appears to be the treatment of choice. Radiotherapy may be indicated when there is residual pelvic disease. Chemotherapy has been found to be unrewarding (Piver *et al.* 1984).

High-grade stromal sarcoma histologically shows considerably more pleomorphism than the low-grade variety and the mitotic count per 10 high-power fields is more than 10 and usually more than 20. Myometrial penetration is more aggressive and destructive than with the low-grade sarcoma and necrosis is common.

Some authorities accept areas of epithelial differentiation in the category of stromal sarcoma; this occurs more commonly in the low-grade variety and consists of structures resembling endometrial glands, collections of clear, polygonal cells, or solid cords of epithelial cells. Epithelial cell areas have been reported in approximately 25 per cent of cases. Strictly these areas should be sparse and obviously only a very minor component of the tumour: if there is more than this, a diagnosis of malignant mixed Müllerian tumour or adenosarcoma should be made.

MIXED MESODERMAL TUMOURS

Mixed mesodermal tumour is a term that encompasses neoplasms of the female genital system that have both epithelial and mesenchymal elements and are derived, if only presumptively, from cells that differentiate from primitive mesoderm and not from germ cells.

Examples of mixed mesodermal tumours include adenofibroma, adenosarcoma, carcinofibroma, and mixed Müllerian tumour (carcinosarcoma). In the first two the epithelial element is benign, paired with benign and malignant mesenchymal cells, respectively, in carcinofibroma, a very rare tumour, there is malignant epithelial proliferation with apparently benign and fully differentiated fibrous tissue as a significant part of the neoplasm, and in mixed Müllerian tumours, the epithelial and mesenchymal elements are both malignant. The last is also called malignant mixed Müllerian tumour to indicate this. Adenofibroma and carcinofibroma are discussed elsewhere.

Adenosarcoma

Adenosarcoma occurs in the uterine corpus (Dekel *et al.* 1988; Clement 1989) and cervix (Hirschfield *et al.* 1986) and has been reported in the pelvic peritoneum in relation to the broad ligament (Kerner *et al.* 1989). High levels of circulating oestrogen have been implicated in the development of these tumours (Press and Scully 1985) but most cases arise without. Adenosarcoma of the corpus has been described in association with adenomyosis (Oda *et al.* 1984).

The tumour almost always forms a polypoid mass that protrudes into the endometrial cavity and into the endocervical canal. Adenosarcoma can grow very large and develop cystic spaces containing clear or blood-stained mucus. The epithelial element is usually endometrioid, but the tumour may be covered by endocervical-type or stratified squamous epithelium, especially when the cervix is the site of origin. The connective tissue element can resemble low- or high-grade endometrial stromal sarcoma or fibrosarcoma, and occasionally the sarcoma overgrows the glandular element (Clement 1989). Areas of chondrosarcoma, rhabdomyosarcoma, and liposarcoma may also occasionally be found and trophoblastic differentiation has been reported (Barua and Richmond 1988). Fibrosarcoma is the most common mesodermal element. Four or more mitoses per 10 high-power fields of stroma are needed for a confident diagnosis, but the mitotic rate can be variable and extensive sampling of these tumours is essential.

The prognosis of adenosarcoma is relatively good, with patients surviving apparently disease free for more than 5 years (Hajnal Papp and Szilagyi 1988; Clement 1989), but tumours in which there has been overgrowth of the sarcomatous element have a worse prognosis, with frequent local recurrences and widespread metastases (Clement 1989).

Malignant mixed Müllerian tumours

Malignant mixed Müllerian tumours have been reported at many sites in the female genital system, including the ovary (Barua and Richmond 1988; Motoyama *et al.* 1987), Fallopian tube (Buchino and Buchino 1987; Muntz *et al.* 1989), uterine corpus (Vlahoussis *et al.* 1983; Ben Baruch *et al.* 1984; Izumi *et al.* 1985; Macasaet *et al.* 1985; Marshall and Braye 1985; Press and Scully 1985; Kahanpaa *et al.* 1986; Liao and Choi 1986; Hajnal Papp and Szilagyi 1988), cervix (Tokunaga *et al.* 1985; Sugimura *et al.* 1986), and vagina (Peters *et al.* 1985). The prevalence of malignant mixed Müllerian tumour is approximately 3 per cent of malignant tumours of the female genital system. Most tumours occur in postmenopausal women and children are very rarely affected (La Vecchia *et al.* 1984; Amr *et al.* 1986). Pelvic irradiation, especially with intracavitary sources that have been used to induce a 'radiation menopause', has been implicated as an aetiological agent (Hoffman *et al.* 1985), although curiously the same has not been found with radiotherapy for cervical carcinoma. There is also an association with obesity and high levels of circulating oestrogen (Press and Scully 1985). Malignant transformation of the ectopic endometrium in pelvic endometriosis can result in malignant mixed Müllerian tumour (Mostoufizadeh and Scully 1980).

As with adenosarcoma, malignant mixed Müllerian tumour can be diagnosed on endometrial curettage but the definitive diagnosis with characterization of all of the cell types in the tumour can be made only on a hysterectomy specimen. The tumour has been called carcinosarcoma because of the combination of malignant epithelial and mesenchymal elements and this is in fact a better term for a malignant mixed tumour with heterologous elements (see below) that are not Müllerian.

The epithelium may resemble that in a serous, mucinous, endometrioid, or clear cell carcinoma of the ovary or squamous cell carcinoma of the cervix. In both the corpus and cervix, endometrioid carcinoma is the most common, but the prevalence of squamous cell carcinoma is higher in malignant mixed Müllerian tumour of the cervix.

In the uterine corpus the mesenchymal component may be homologous or heterologous. Homologous mixed malignant tumour is the most common and fibrosarcoma or endometrial stromal sarcoma are the most frequent mesodermal cell types. Leiomyosarcoma can occur rarely and areas of malignant smooth muscle cells can be mixed with the first two homologous tumour cell types. Heterologous sarcomatous components include rhabdomyosarcoma, osteosarcoma, and liposarcoma.

The differential diagnosis of malignant mixed Müllerian tumour includes carcinoma with spindle cell differentiation, pure sarcoma such as leiomyosarcoma or endometrial stromal sarcoma with enveloped non-neoplastic epithelium that becomes hyperplastic or atypical, and possibly immature teratoma of ovary with primitive epithelial and mesodermal components. Immunohistochemical markers for epithelial cells, smooth muscle, and myoglobin may be necessary to resolve the diagnosis.

The most important prognostic factors for malignant mixed Müllerian tumour of the uterus are the extent of tumour spread and the presence of vascular invasion in the myometrium (Macasaet *et al.* 1985). Interestingly, in one study (Hajnal Papp and Szilagyi 1988) no difference in prognosis was found between patients who had tumours with only homologous elements and those with tumours with heterologous tissues, a finding at variance with other workers. As with leiomyosarcoma, hormonal therapy with antioestrogens and progestogens has been tried but with little success. The most consistent indicator of a poor prognosis is extragenital spread. Lymph nodes are involved in one-third of the cases in which they are examined. Cure depends on the possibility of complete surgical removal of the tumour and, therefore, on the clinical stage (Kahanpaa *et al.* 1986). Cytological examination of peritoneal washings can reveal the presence of malignant cells, even when the tumour is apparently limited to the uterus (Geszler *et al.* 1986).

Radiotherapy has not been found to affect the long-term prognosis significantly, though this may have a role in containing the expansion of local and metastatic disease, particularly of pelvic recurrence after surgery. There have been several reports of the use of chemotherapy for malignant mixed Müllerian tumour. Successful management with vincristine, actinomycin D, and cyclophosphamide has been reported (Carlson and Day 1985). Doxorubicin was favoured at one time but response rates were low (Morrow *et al.* 1986). A combination of cisplatin with other chemotherapeutic agents is the current treatment of choice.

RHABDOMYOSARCOMA

Embryonal rhabdomyosarcoma and its variant botryoid rhabdomyosarcoma are rare tumours of the vulva, vagina, and cervix. It is a tumour of children, adolescents, and young adults (La Vecchia *et al.* 1984; Brand *et al.* 1987); in the vagina most occur in girls under 5 years old, the first 2 years of life being the most common time for the tumour to appear (Hays *et al.* 1988). The most frequent site of origin is the anterior wall of the vagina. In the cervix and corpus the onset is later, peaking at 14–18 years (Brand *et al.* 1987). Embryonal rhabdomyosarcoma may be associated with chromosomal abnormalities (such as trisomy 8) and cystic nephroblastoma (Nakamura *et al.* 1985). Alveolar rhabdomyosarcoma may be found as a pelvic tumour in girls and is associated with 2;13 translocation which is not random (Rowe *et al.* 1987; Engel *et al.* 1988).

Embryonal rhabdomyosarcoma commonly presents as a shiny polyp protruding from the introitus or vaginal bleeding or both. The naked-eye appearances can resemble the benign mucoid polyp of the adult cervix. Any such lesion in a prepubertal girl should be regarded with suspicion. Under an epithelial surface, such as in the vagina or vulva, it may form smooth, fleshy, polypoid masses resembling a bunch of grapes, hence the term botryoid rhabdomyosarcoma.

Microscopically the tumour can have a range of appearances. There is usually a myxoid stroma around groups of small, darkly-staining, spindle and stellate cells and in a small proportion of these tumours plumper, strap-shaped or rounded, eosinophilic cells with open nuclei and prominent nucleoli give evidence of rhabdomyoblastic differentiation. Cross-striations are not usually visible and are not required for the diagnosis. Tumour cells crowding around blood vessels and below the overlying epithelium may form a 'cambium layer' (named by analogy with the growth of a tree). Focal haemorrhage is common. The tumour has the potential to metastasize but in most cases death results from local pelvic extension.

Alveolar rhabdomyosarcoma has a more open arrangement of tumour cells, with alveolar patterns and solid areas. These tumours are very rare and are usually considered to be more aggressive than the embryonal variant (Rowe *et al.* 1987; Dodd *et al.* 1989). Metastatic alveolar rhabdomyosarcoma to the ovary has been described (Young and Scully 1989) and an extensive search for disease elsewhere must be made before the ovary is accepted as the primary site of one of these tumours.

The differential diagnosis of vulval and vaginal tumours includes fibroepithelial polyp, which resembles botryoid rhabdomyosarcoma macroscopically and can have atypical spindle and stellate cells in its stroma (Ostor *et al.* 1988). The clustering of tumour cells and the cambium layer of rhabdomyosarcoma are not a feature. In infancy the possibility of yolk sac tumour has also to be considered clinically (Copeland *et al.* 1985), although the histological features of this and the serum and tissue expression of tumour markers are usually quite different.

Rhabdomyosarcoma can be treated with surgery, chemotherapy, and radiotherapy. In view of the young age of many of the patients, the long-term sequelae and morbidity from treatment have considerable importance. Radical surgery, which may necessitate some form of pelvic exenteration, can result in cure in children with localized disease. In various sites, radical radiotherapy has produced similar survival figures of approximately 70 per cent at 5 years, which has obvious implications for the long-term preservation of pelvic function. In the early 1970s, combination chemotherapy with the **VAC** (vincristine, actinomycin D, and cyclophosphamide) regimen was introduced and some 20 years experience of this is now available. Multimodal therapy can now be applied, with individual tailoring (Kingston *et al.* 1983) and exenteration can be avoided in many cases (Dewhurst 1985).

Conventional management nowadays includes radical excision only where this is easily achievable and this is followed sequentially by radiotherapy and adjuvant VAC chemotherapy. Otherwise, a 'sandwich' approach is used: the initial treatment is pulsed chemotherapy, followed by surgery and radiotherapy or both, and then a further course of pulsed chemotherapy. The extent of disease is the most important prognostic factor and there is a 5 year survival of over 85 per cent when the disease is confined to the organ of origin. Embryonal rhabdomyosarcoma has a somewhat more favourable prognosis than the other types, but age at diagnosis does not appear to be an important prognostic factor (Ragab *et al.* 1986). Relapse at the primary site is more likely than tumour appearance elsewhere and radiotherapy can have an important prophylactic role in this context (Plowman 1988).

Recently, interest has focused on the preservation of as much normal pelvic function as possible. Although female reproductive function can be retained after combination chemotherapy that includes cyclophosphamide (Ward *et al.* 1982), this alkylating agent is known to have an adverse effect on the ovary (Warne and Fairley 1973) and on spermatogenesis and combination chemotherapy for Hodgkin's disease has resulted in ovarian failure (Chapman *et al.* 1978); it is suspected that mustine and procarbazine are the most potent factors in this. At all events, the International Rhabdomyosarcoma Study has suggested that in early disease the combination of vincristine and actinomycin D is as effective and possibly less damaging to oocytes (Hays *et al.* 1988).

An additional measure has been the reintroduction of modified brachytherapy using a vaginal applicator. When combined with oophoropexy, ovarian function can be preserved and the need for external-beam teletherapy is obviated (Plowman *et al.* 1989). These important developments emphasize the need for tertiary referral of such cases to special centres so that optimum individual management can be devised.

To some extent, similar considerations apply to the less common occurrence of these tumours in adolescents and young adults. There are conflicting reports on prognosis (Daya and Scully 1988; Hays *et al.* 1988).

AGGRESSIVE ANGIOMYXOMA OF THE VULVA

This gelatinous soft tissue tumour of young women characteristically presents as a vulval mass and may be mistaken clinically for a Bartholin's cyst (Begin *et al.* 1985). Histologically the tumour appears bland, with large amounts of myxoid stroma in which spindle and stellate cells and blood vessels with prominent endothelial lining cells are scattered. There is a high incidence of local recurrence but metastases do not occur.

KAPOSI'S SARCOMA

Kaposi's sarcoma has been reported in the vagina (Lee *et al.* 1988) and cervix (Audouin *et al.* 1988; Lopes *et al.* 1988). The histological features of the disease are the same as those of Kaposi's sarcoma elsewhere. ^{201}Tl scintigraphy can be used to detect deposits of the sarcoma in the female genital system and nodal sites (Lee *et al.* 1988). Organ transplantation and the immunosuppression associated with it appear to be an aetiological factor: there are reports of two patients who developed Kaposi's sarcoma of the cervix after cardiac transplantation (Audouin *et al.* 1988; Lopes *et al.* 1988). One of these patients also had atypical condylomas in association with the sarcoma (Audouin *et al.* 1988).

HAEMANGIOPERICYTOMA

These rare tumours of the female genital system have gross features similar to those of leiomyosarcoma. They may be overdiagnosed clinically when a vascular malignant tumour is encountered (Buscema *et al.* 1985). The histological features are the same for this lesion elsewhere. Because of the rarity of the lesion and difficulty in diagnosis, there are no useful guidelines for therapy other than extirpative surgery.

MALIGNANT FIBROUS HISTIOCYTOMA AND RELATED TUMOURS

Malignant fibrous histiocytoma is a tumour classically of the skin and soft tissues of the extremities that very rarely affects the vulva (Santala *et al.* 1987). The histological features are the same as when this tumour occurs elsewhere. The differential diagnosis includes nodular fasciitis of the vulva and dermatofibrosarcoma protuberans (Bock *et al.* 1985).

ALVEOLAR SOFT PART SARCOMA

Alveolar soft part sarcoma is a rare tumour that characteristically arises in the subcutis in the upper and lower limbs of young adults. It tends to grow slowly and remains confined to the site of origin, though metastasis to regional lymph nodes, the liver, and lungs has been described (Flint *et al.* 1985). Recurrence after limited surgery is common, both in extragenital and the much rarer genital sites (Shen *et al.* 1982; Chapman *et al.* 1984). In the female genital system, alveolar soft part sarcoma has been reported in the labium minus (Shen *et al.* 1982), the vagina (Kasai *et al.* 1980; Chapman *et al.* 1984; O'Toole *et al.* 1985; Zaleski *et al.* 1986), the cervix (Flint *et al.* 1985; Gray *et al.* 1986; Kopolovic *et al.* 1987; Foschini *et al.* 1989), and uterine corpus (Gray *et al.* 1986).

The histological appearances of these tumours does not depend on their site of origin and is the same in female genital organs as in the extremities. The tumour is composed of relatively uniform, oval or polyhedral cells with clear cytoplasmic borders. These contain crystalloid structures composed of glycoprotein that is periodic acid–Schiff positive after diastase digestion but negative with alcian blue stains; the precise chemical nature is unknown. Mitoses are not usually a feature. The tumour cells are arranged in an alveolar arrangement around apparently empty spaces. There may also be papillary structures with fibrous cores.

The differential diagnosis includes primary adenocarcinoma of the vagina, metastatic renal cell carcinoma, metastatic clear cell carcinoma of ovary, and alveolar rhabdomyosarcoma. Alveolar soft part sarcoma should be distinguished from the aggressive ('malignant') variant of granular cell tumour. Infiltrative granular cell tumours of the vagina may be composed of polygonal cells resembling those of alveolar soft part sarcoma but they are not arranged in the alveolar or papillary growth patterns that are characteristic of that tumour.

There are few established guidelines for the surgical treatment of alveolar soft part sarcoma because of the paucity of reports. The 5 year survival is approximately 80 per cent (Shen *et al.* 1982), death almost always being due to metastatic rather than local disease. On the other hand, local recurrence can be a major management problem; radical reoperation may be necessary for local recurrence after radiotherapy and chemotherapy (Chapman *et al.* 1984). Recurrences can appear after many years and prolonged follow-up is therefore essential.

EPITHELIOID SARCOMA

This very rare tumour, which like alveolar soft part sarcoma predominantly affects the extremities of young adults, has been described in the vulva (Ulbright *et al.* 1983) at the posterior aspect of the labium majus, where it can closely resemble a cyst of Bartholin's gland or duct. It is therefore important clinically to be aware of the condition for the differential diagnosis of swellings in that area.

The tumour develops in the subcutis and may extend well beyond the area in which it is palpable clinically. Wide excision is therefore essential, and re-excision should be considered if an epithelioid sarcoma is found on biopsy or excision of what was thought to be a Bartholin's cyst. The small number of genital cases reported have had a worse prognosis than extragenital lesions, with a higher proportion of metastases. Benefit from radiotherapy or chemotherapy has been found, but this is seldom curative.

SYNOVIAL SARCOMA-LIKE TUMOUR

This is also known as synovial-like sarcoma, but this name is gramatically poor. Synovial sarcoma-like tumours have been reported in the vagina (Okagaki *et al.* 1976). As with alveolar soft part sarcoma, these tumours histologically and behaviourally resemble synovial sarcoma at other sites in the body. There is the typical biphasic cell pattern, with epithelioid cells in islands and tubules and sheets of closely packed spindle cells. The electron microscopic features of the tumour cells are very similar to those of synovial sarcoma and suggest that the tumour is of mesothelial origin.

MELANOMA

At the beginning of this century, malignant melanoma was known as melanotic sarcoma and involvement of the external genitalia and anal region by primary tumour is described in the St Bartholomew's Hospital pathology museum catalogue of 1929.

Melanoma of 'non-specialized' skin (rather than that of the vulva) is rare and accounts for approximately 2–7 per cent of melanomas in women and 4–11 per cent of all malignant vulval tumours (Bradgate *et al.* 1990). In a series of over 3000 cases reported in 1981, there were 48 melanomas that arose in the female genital tract, a proportion that corresponds with the relative surface area of the vulva compared with the total surface area of the body (Ariel 1981). Development of melanoma is related to exposure to sunlight; this aetiological factor is unlikely to be important for melanoma in female genital tissues.

Though it is rare, vulval melanoma is the second most common malignant tumour at that site (Silvers and Halperin 1978; Bradgate *et al.* 1990). The vulvovaginal junction at the introitus is considered to be a high-risk site in terms of development of melanoma (Glaser *et al.* 1989) and, indeed, melanoma of the vagina usually occurs in the lower aspect (Reid *et al.* 1989), although the upper third can also be affected (Cappello *et al.* 1989). Melanoma can be associated with pigmentation elsewhere in the vagina and this can make delineation of the tumour at surgery very difficult; conversely, amelanotic melanoma has been reported and would cause diagnostic difficulties (Scambia *et al.* 1989). Melanoma of the cervix is even rarer, with only sporadic case reports and a small series in the literature. The predominant types of melanoma in the lower female genital system are superficial spreading melanoma and nodular melanoma (Brand *et al.* 1989; Ronan *et al.* 1990) and the stage of the disease is typically advanced, with development of metastatic disease and local recurrences.

When melanoma arises on the vulva, predictors of survival have been found to include the patient's age, the clinical stage of the tumour (which is related to the depth of spread into the dermis or submucosa), the cell type and mitotic rate, and the presence of ulceration (Bradgate *et al.* 1990). In this series, no relation was found between survival and the type of surgery performed. Systemic recurrence is more common in melanoma of the anorectum, vulva, and vagina than in melanoma of the mucosal surfaces of the head and neck (McKinnon *et al.* 1989) and the survival rate at 5 years is approximately 35 per cent (Das Gupta and d'Urso 1964).

In a series of 15 patients with vaginal melanoma, tumour thickness significantly affected the disease-free interval and tumour size influenced survival, whereas age, stage, and site of the tumour did not (Reid *et al.* 1989). Patients treated by surgical resection, irradiation, or both had no difference in survival times, though a good result was found in one patient who was treated with high-dosage irradiation. Whether the surgery was radical or conservative did not influence survival.

Traditionally, routine radical surgery of the vulva has been applied to melanoma and the results have been disappointing (Monaghan 1987). The validity of this approach has been questioned and it is more logical to use the principles of surgical therapy that are currently applied elsewhere in the body. Wide local excision is the key to the primary management of the primary lesion. The fact that radical vulvectomy does not achieve this in some cases may be due to a 'compartmentalized' approach to the vulva, overlooking its proximity to the vestibule (including the urethra) and the vagina. These are often shaved off well within the accepted excision margin (see below) (Townsend 1988). By contrast, wide excision of the contralateral skin of the vulva will add little and cause further mutilation.

Wide local excision of a unilateral lesion on the vulva will require hemivulvectomy with a 5 cm clear margin, which should include resection of the terminal urethra and the equivalent distance up the ipsilateral vaginal wall. The urethral stump just distal to the pubo-urethral (triangular) ligaments can be anastomosed to the advanced upper vaginal stump. The hemivulvectomy incision can often be closed by rotational flaps, which reduces the subsequent complications of surgical treatment of a disease with a poor prognosis and at the same time conforms to currently accepted, optimal surgical principles. Lymphadenectomy can be done synchronously or serially as indicated by the particular case (Poderantz *et al.* 1983).

LYMPHOMA

Patients with lymphoma of the female genital system usually present with an abdominal mass, bleeding *per vaginam* or a mass below the mucosa of the vagina or cervix with no apparent ulceration or epithelial abnormality (Chorlton *et al.* 1974*b*). The most common primary manifestation is in the ovary, where it is bilateral in approximately 55 per cent of cases (Osborne and Robboy 1983). The presence of ascites is very rarely reported. In most cases these tumours are Burkitt's lymphoma, but may be misdiagnosed histologically at first as granulosa cell tumour, dysgerminoma, or undifferentiated carcinoma.

Unusual tumours feature disproportionately in accounts of second malignancies arising in patients who have been treated with chemotherapy for lymphoma and the female genital system may be involved by these (Lowe and Hudson 1988). Lymphoma of the cervix and vagina is approximately half as common as in the ovary (Chorlton *et al.* 1974*a*). They are diffuse and usually composed of large neoplastic cells (Harris and Scully 1984). Because of the differences in classification of lymphomas used by workers over the last 20 years, comparison of their data is difficult; most lymphomas of the female genital system appeared to be of high-grade type, although sclerosis, a feature associated with a good prognosis, is often prominent in lymphoma of the cervix and vagina. Patients may have quite limited disease with, for example tumour in only the cervix and one lymph node or in the cervix and ovary. Lymph node involvement is not common, in contrast to secondary

lymphoma of the female genitalia (Miketic *et al.* 1988). Biopsy is the most reliable method of diagnosis, but positive results can be obtained with cytological investigation. Computerized tomography gives images similar to those of other primary neoplasms in these sites, but the extent of the disease can be assessed to aid treatment planning (Miketic *et al.* 1988).

The 5 year survival overall for tumours of the lower female genital system is approximately 75 per cent (Miketic *et al.* 1988); the survival of patients with lymph node or ovarian involvement is considerably less, with 20 per cent survival after 5 years. Local surgery with or without radiotherapy to the affected sites is a worthwhile practice and recurrence is low (Miketic *et al.* 1988). Disease localized to the ovary will commonly be diagnosed only after surgical excision. The presence of extensive pelvic and intra-abdominal lymphadenopathy should always suggest the possibility of lymphoma.

PHAEOCHROMOCYTOMA

The behaviour of these very rare tumours of the female genital system is similar to that at other sites in the body, and the means of investigation with computerized tomography and *meta*-iodobenzylguanidine scanning is also the same. The treatment will depend on the site involved but is essentially surgical.

REFERENCES

Amr SS, Tavassoli FA, Hassan AA, Isa AA, Madanat FF (1986). Mixed mesodermal tumor of the uterus in a 4 year old girl. *International Journal of Gynecological Pathology*, 5:371–8.

Ariel IM (1981). Malignant melanoma of the female genital system: a report of patients and review of the literature. *Journal of Surgical Oncology*, 16:371–83.

Audouin AF, Lopes P, Lenne Y (1988). Sarcome de Kaposi du col uterin associé à un condylome atypique chez une femme transplantée cardiaque (lors du post-partum). *Archives d'Anatomie et de Cytologie Pathologiques*, 36:226–8.

Auerbach HE, LiVolsi VA, Merino MJ (1988). Malignant mixed Müllerian tumors of the uterus: an immunohistochemical study. *International Journal of Gynecological Pathology*, 7:123–30.

Barua R, Richmond D (1988). Trophoblastic differentiation in a malignant mixed mesodermal tumor of the ovary. *Human Pathology*, 19:1235–6.

Begin LR, Clement PB, Kirk ME, Jothy S, McCaughey WT, Ferenczy ATI (1985). Aggressive angiomyxoma of pelvic soft parts: a clinicopathologic study of nine cases. *Human Pathology*, 16:621–8.

Ben Baruch G, Amir G, Menczer J, Bubis JH (1984). Uterine sarcomas in Israeli patients: a clinicopathological study. *Israel Journal of Medical Sciences*, 20:211–15.

Berkowitz RS, Ehrmann RL, Knapp RC (1978). Endometrial stromal sarcoma arising from vaginal endometriosis. *Obstetrics and Gynecology*, 51:34–37S.

Bock JE, Andreasson B, Thorn A, Holck S (1985). Dermatofibrosarcoma protuberans of the vulva. *Gynecologic Oncology*, 20:129–35.

Bonazzi del Poggetto C, Virtanen I, Lehto VP, Wahlstrom T, Saksela E (1983). Expression of intermediate filaments in ovarian and uterine tumors. *International Journal of Pathology*, 1:359–66.

Bradgate MG, Rollason TP, McConkey CC, Powell J (1990). Malignant melanoma of the vulva: a clinicopathological study of 50 women. *British Journal of Obstetrics and Gynaecology*, 97:124–33.

Brand E, Berek JS, Nieberg RK, Hacker NF (1987). Rhabdomyosarcoma of the uterine cervix. Sarcoma botryoides. *Cancer*, 60:1552–60.

Brand E, Fu YS, Lagasse LD, Berek JS (1989). Vulvovaginal melanoma: report of seven cases and literature review. *Gynecologic Oncology*, 33:54–60.

Buchino JJ, Buchino JJ (1987). Malignant mixed Müllerian tumor of the Fallopian tube. *Archives of Pathology and Laboratory Medicine*, 111:386–7.

Buscema J, Rosenheim NB, Taqi F, Woodruff JD (1985). Vaginal haemangiopericytoma. *Obstetrics and Gynecology*, 66:82–5.

Cappello F, Pomari R, Corradi G (1989). Melanoma relapse of the upper third of the vagina treated with BCG and β-interferon. *Clinical and Experimental Obstetrics and Gynecology*, 16:88–92.

Carlson JA, Day TG (1985). Five year survival following combination radiotherapy for recurrent mixed mesodermal sarcoma of the ovary. *Gynecology and Oncology*, 22:129–32.

Chapman GW, Benda J, Williams T (1984). Alveolar soft part sarcoma of the vagina. *Gynecologic Oncology*, 18:125–9.

Chapman R, Sutcliffe S, Malpas JS (1978). Cytotoxic drug induced ovarian failure in women with Hodgkin's disease. *Journal of the Royal Society of Medicine*, 71:96–8.

Chorlton I, Norris HJ, King FM (1974a). Malignant reticuloendothelial disease involving the ovary as a primary manifestation: a series of 19 lymphomas and 1 granulocytic sarcoma. *Cancer*, 34, 397–407.

Chorlton I, Karnei RF, King FM, Norris HJ (1974b). Primary malignant reticuloendothelial disease involving the vagina, cervix, and corpus uteri. *Obstetrics and Gynecology*, 44:735–48.

Clement PB (1989). Müllerian adenosarcomas of the uterus with sarcomatous overgrowth. A clinicopathological analysis of 10 cases. *American Journal of Surgical Pathology*, 13:28–38.

Copeland LJ, et al. (1985). Endodermal sinus tumor of the vagina and cervix. *Cancer*, 55:2558–65.

Das Gupta T, d'Urso J (1964). Melanoma of the female genitalia. *Surgery, Gynecology and Obstetrics*, 119:1074–8.

Daya DA, Scully RE (1988). Sarcoma botryoides of the uterine cervix in young women: a clinicopathological study of 13 cases. *Gynecologic Oncology*, 29:290–304.

Dekel A, Dicker D, Kugler D, Ben David M, Gal R, Goldman JA (1988). Müllerian adenosarcoma of the uterus: report of a rare case and review of the literature. *Gynecologic Oncology*, 30:291–7.

Dewhurst J (1985). Malignant disease of the genital organs in childhood. In *Clinical gynaecological oncology* (ed. JH Shepherd and JM Monaghan), pp. 270–85. Blackwell, Oxford.

Dodd S, Malone M, McCulloch W (1989). Rhabdomyosarcoma in children: a histological and immunohistochemical study of 59 cases. *Journal of Pathology*, 158:13–18.

Engel R, Ritterbach J, Schwabe D, Lampert F (1988). Chromosome translocation (2;13)(q37;q14) in a disseminated alveolar rhabdomyosarcoma. *European Journal of Pediatrics*, 148:69–71.

Fekete PS, Vellios F (1984). The clinical and histologic spectrum of endometrial stromal neoplasms: a report of 41 cases. *International Journal of Gynecological Pathology*, 3:198–212.

Flint A, Gikas PW, Roberts JA (1985). Alveolar soft part sarcoma of the uterine cervix. *Gynecologic Oncology*, 22:263–7.

Foschini MP, Eusebi V, Tison V (1989). Alveolar soft part sarcoma of the cervix uteri: a case report. *Pathology Research Practice*, 184:354–8.

Gallop DG, Cordray DR (1979). Leiomyosarcoma of the uterus: case report and a review. *Obstetrical and Gynecological Survey*, 34:300–14.

Geszler G, Szpak CA, Harris RE, Creasman WT, Barter JF, Johnston WW (1986). Prognostic value of peritoneal washings in patients with malignant mixed Müllerian tumors of the uterus. *American Journal of Obstetrics and Gynecology*, 155:83–9.

Glaser D, Huth F, Schwedhelm A, Mast H (1989). Metastasierendes malignes Melanom der Vagina. *Geburtshilfe und Frauenheilkunde*, 49:1014–16.

Goyert G, Budev H, Wright C, Jones A, Deppe G (1987). Vaginal Müllerian stromal sarcoma: a case report. *Journal of Reproductive Medicine*, 32:129–30.

Gray GF, Glick AD, Kurtin PJ, Jones HW, III (1986). Alveolar soft part sarcoma of the uterus. *Human Pathology*, 17:297–300.

Hajnal Papp R, Szilagyi I (1988). Malignant Müllerian tumours of the uterus. *Archives of Gynecology and Obstetrics*, 241:209–19.

Harris NL, Scully RE (1984). Malignant lymphoma and granulocytic sarcoma of the uterus and vagina. A clinicopathologic analysis of 27 cases. *Cancer*, 53:2530–45.

Hart WR, Yoonessi M (1977). Endometrial stromatosis of the uterus. *Obstetrics and Gynecology*, 49:393–403.

Hays DM, et al. (1988). Clinical staging and treatment results in rhabdomyosarcoma of the female genital tract among children and adolescents. *Cancer*, 61:1893–903.

Hirschfield L, Kahn LB, Chen S, Winkler B, Rosenberg S (1986). Müllerian adenosarcoma with ovarian sex cord like differentiation. A light and electron microscopic study. *Cancer*, 57:1197–200.

Hoffman M, Roberts WS, Cavanagh D (1985). Second pelvic malignancies following radiation therapy for cervical cancer. *Obstetrical and Gynecological Survey*, 40:611–17.

Izumi S, Hasegawa T, Tsutsui F, Kurihara S (1985). Carcinosarcoma of the uterus. Cytologic and ultrastructural features. *Acta Cytologica*, 29:602–6.

Jaffe R, Altaras M, Bernheim J, Ben Aderet N (1985). Endocervical stromal sarcoma: a case report. *Gynecologic Oncology*, 22:105–8.

Kahanpaa KV, Wahlstrom T, Grohn P, Heinonen E, Nieminen U, Widholm O (1986). Sarcomas of the uterus: a clinicopathologic study of 119 patients. *Obstetrics and Gynecology*, 67:417–24.

Kahn HJ, Marks A, Thom H, Baumal R (1983). Role of antibody to S100 protein in diagnostic pathology. *American Journal of Clinical Pathology*, 79:341–7.

Kahn HJ, Huang SN, Hanna WM, Baumal R, Phillips MJ (1984). Immunohistochemical localization of epidermal and Mallory body cytokeratin in undifferentiated epithelial tumors. Comparison with ultrastructural features. *American Journal of Clinical Pathology*, 81:184–91.

Kasai K, Yoshida Y, Okumura M (1980). Alveolar soft part sarcoma in the vagina. Clinical features and morphology. *Gynecologic Oncology*, 9:277–36.

Kempson RL, Bari W (1970). Uterine sarcoma. Classification, diagnosis and prognosis. *Human Pathology*, 1:331–49.

Kerner H, Lichtig C, Beck D (1989). Extrauterine Müllerian adenosarcoma of the peritoneal mesothelium: a clinicopathologic and electron microscopic study. *Obstetrics and Gynecology*, 73:510–31.

Kingston JE, McElwain TJ, Malpas JS (1983). Childhood rhabdomyosarcoma. *British Journal of Cancer*, 48:195–207.

Kolstad P (1983). Adjuvant chemotherapy in sarcoma of the uterus. In *Recent clinical developments in gynecologic oncology* (ed. C Morrow), pp. 125–9. Raven Press, New York.

Kopolovic J, Weiss DB, Dolberg L, Brezinsky A, Ne'eman Z, Anteby SO (1987). Alveolar soft part sarcoma of the female genital tract. Case report with ultrastructural findings. *Archives of Gynecology*, 240:125–9.

Kornyei J, Csermely T, Szekely JA, Vertes M (1986). Two types of nuclear oestradiol binding sites in human myometrium and leiomyoma during the menstrual cycle. *Experimental and Clinical Endocrinology*, 87:256–64.

Kurman RJ, Norris HJ (1976). Mesenchymal tumors of the uterus. VI. Epithelioid smooth muscle tumors including leiomyoblastoma and clear cell leiomyoma: a clinical and pathologic analysis of 26 cases. *Cancer*, 37:1853–65.

La Vecchia C, Draper GJ, Franceschi S (1984). Childhood nonovarian female genital tract cancers in Britain, 1962–1978. Descriptive epidemiology and long term survival. *Cancer*, 54:188–92.

Lee VW, Rosen MP, Baum A, Cohen SE, Cooley TP, Liebman HA (1988). AIDS-related Kaposi sarcoma: findings on thallium-201 scintigraphy. *American Journal of Roentgenology*, 151:1233–5.

Liao SY, Choi BH (1986). Expression of glial fibrillary acidic protein by neoplastic cells of Müllerian origin. *Virchows Archives B*, 52:185–93.

Liebsohn S, d'Ablaing G, Mishell DR, Schlaerth JB (1990). Leiomyosarcoma in a series of hysterectomies performed for presumed uterine leiomyomas. *American Journal of Obstetrics and Gynecology*, 162:968–76.

Lopes P, Petit T, Audoin AF, Lenne Y (1988). Sarcoma de Kaposi du col uterin chez une transplantée cardiaque. *Presse Medicale*, 17:1539.

Lowe DG, Hudson CN (1988). Rare tumours of the cervix. In *Textbook of uncommon cancer* (ed. CJ Williams, JG Krikorian, MR Green, and D Rhagavan), pp. 167–82. Wiley, Chichester.

McKinnon JG, Kokal WA, Neifeld JP, Kay S (1989). Natural history and treatment of mucosal melanoma. *Journal of Surgical Oncology*, 41:222–5.

Macasaet MA, et al. (1985). Prognostic factors in malignant mesodermal (Müllerian) mixed tumors of the uterus. *Gynecologic Oncology*, 20:32–42.

Marchetti DL, Piver MS (1988). Management of gynaecological sarcomas. In *Texbook of uncommon cancer* (ed. CJ Williams, JG Krikorian, MR Green, and D Rhagavan), pp. 151–66. Wiley, Chichester.

Marshall RJ, Braye SG (1985). α_1 Antitrypsin, α_1 antichymotrypsin, actin, and myosin in uterine sarcomas. *International Journal of Gynecological Pathology*, 4:346–54.

Miketic LM, Carroll R, Harris NL, Linggood RM (1988). Computed tomography in the evaluation of lymphoma of the uterine cervix. *Journal of Computed Tomography*, 12:154–8.

Monaghan JM (1987). Vulvar carcinoma: the case for individualisation of treatment. *Baillières Clinical Obstetrics and Gynecology*, 1:263–76.

Morrow CP, *et al.* (1986). Adriamycin chemotherapy for malignant mixed mesodermal tumor of the ovary. *American Journal of Clinical Oncology*, 9:24–6.

Mostoufizadeh M, Scully RE (1980). Malignant tumors arising in endometriosis. *Clinical Obstetrics and Gynecology*, 23:51–63.

Motoyama T, Watanabe H, Yamamoto T, Sekiguchi M (1987). Production of alpha-fetoprotein by human germ cell tumors *in vivo* and *in vitro*. *Acta Pathologica Japan*, 37:1263–77.

Muntz HG, Rutgers JL, Tarraza HM, Fuller AF Jr (1989). Carcinosarcomas and mixed Müllerian tumors of the Fallopian tube. *Gynecologic Oncology*, 34:109–15.

Nakamura Y, Nakashima H, Fukuda S, Hashimoto T, Maruyama M (1985). Bilateral cystic nephroblastomas and multiple malformations with trisomy 8 mosaicism. *Human Pathology*, 16:754–6.

Norris HJ, Taylor HB (1966). Mesenchymal tumors of the uterus. I. A clinical and pathological study of 53 endometrial stromal tumors. *Cancer*, 19:755–66.

Norton AJ, Thomas JA, Isaacson PG (1987). Cytokeratin-specific monoclonal antibodies are reactive with tumours of smooth muscle derivation. An immunohistochemical and biochemical study using antibodies to intermediate filament cytoskeletal proteins. *Histopathology*, 11:487–99.

Oda Y, Nakanishi I, Tateiwa T (1984). Intramural Müllerian adenosarcoma of the uterus with adenomyosis. *Archives of Pathology and Laboratory Medicine*, 108:798–803.

Okagaki T, Ishida T, Hilgers RD (1976). A malignant tumor of the vagina resembling synovial sarcoma. *Cancer*, 37:2306–20.

Om A, Ghose T (1987). Use of antiskeletal muscle antibody from myasthenic patients in the diagnosis of childhood rhabdomyosarcomas. *American Journal of Surgical Pathology*, 11:272–6.

Osborne BM, Robboy SJ (1983). Lymphoma or leukemia presenting as ovarian tumors: an analysis of 42 cases. *Cancer*, 52:1933–43.

Ostor AG, Fortune DW, Riley CB (1988). Fibroepithelial polyps with atypical stromal cells (pseudosarcoma botryoides) of vulva and vagina. A report of 13 cases. *International Journal of Gynecological Pathology*, 7:351–60.

O'Toole RV, Tuttle SE, Lucas JG, Sharma HM (1985). Alveolar soft part sarcoma of the vagina: an immunohistochemical and electron microscopic study. *Journal of Gynecological Pathology*, 4:258–65.

Peters WA, III, Kumar NB, Andersen WA, Morley GW (1985). Primary sarcoma of the adult vagina: a clinicopathologic study. *Obstetrics and Gynecology*, 65:699–704.

Piver MS, *et al.* (1984). Uterine endolymphatic stromal myosis. *Obstetrics and Gynecology*, 64:173–8.

Plowman PN (1988). Radiotherapy of pediatric genitourinary tumours. In *Pediatric tumors of the genitourinary tract*, pp. 263–81. Liss, New York.

Plowman PN, Dougherty D, Hadnett AN (1989). Paediatric brachytherapy. *British Journal of Radiology*, 62:218–22.

Poderantz KC, *et al.* (1983). Melanoma of the vulva: an update. *Gynecologic Oncology*, 16:153–9.

Prat J, Fox H (1987). Mesenchymal tumours of the ovary. In *Haynes and Taylor obstetrical and gynaecological pathology* (ed. H Fox), pp. 701–2. Churchill Livingstone, Edinburgh.

Press MF, Scully RE (1985). Endometrial 'sarcomas' complicating ovarian thecoma, polycystic ovarian disease and estrogen therapy. *Gynecologic Oncology*, 21:135–54.

Ragab AH, Heyn R, Tefft M, Hays DN, Newton WA Jr, Beltangady M (1986). Infants younger than 1 year of age with rhabdomyosarcoma. *Cancer*, 58:2606–10.

Reid GC, Schmidt RW, Roberts JA, Hopkins MP, Barrett RJ, Morley GW (1989). Primary melanoma of the vagina: a clinicopathologic analysis. *Obstetrics and Gynecology*, 74:190–9.

Ronan SG, Eng AM, Briele HA, Walker MJ, Das Gupta TK (1990). Malignant melanoma of the female genitalia. *Journal of the American Academy of Dermatology*, 22:428–35.

Rowe D, Gerrard M, Gibbons B, Malpas JS (1987). Two further cases of t(2;13) in alveolar rhabdomyosarcoma indicating a review of the published chromosome breakpoints. *British Journal of Cancer*, 56:379–80.

Sahin A, Benda JA (1988). An immunohistochemical study of primary ovarian sarcoma. An evaluation of nine tumors. *International Journal of Gynecological Pathology*, 7:268–79.

Salazar OM, Dunne ME (1980). The role of radiotherapy in the management of uterine sarcomas. *International Journal of Radiation Oncology–Biology–Physics*, 6:899–902.

Santala M, Suonio S, Syrjanen K, Uronen MT, Saarikoski S (1987). Malignant fibrous histiocytoma of the vulva. *Gynecologic Oncology*, 27:121–6.

Scambia G, *et al.* (1989). A primary amelanotic melanoma of the vagina diagnosed by immunocytochemistry. *International Journal of Gynecology and Obstetrics*, 29:159–64.

Shen JT, D'Ablaing G, Morrow T (1982). Aveolar soft part sarcoma of the vulva. Report of first case and review of literature. *Gynecologic Oncology*, 13:120–8.

Silvers DH, Halperin AJ (1978). Cutaneous and vulvar melanoma—an update. *Clinics in Obstetrics and Gynecology*, 21:1117–18.

Sugimura H, Mohri N, Urano Y, Yamamoto E, Kawana T, Hagino Y (1986). A case report of mixed mesodermal tumor of the uterine cervix (mixed heterologous and homologous sarcoma of the uterine cervix). *Japan Journal of Clinical Oncology*, 16:391–6.

Thatcher SS, Woodruff JD (1982). Uterine stromatosis: a report of 33 cases. *Obstetrics and Gynecology*, 59:428–34.

Tokunaga T, Matsuyama S, Kuwahara S, Himeno R, Terao K (1985). Mixed mesodermal tumor of the uterine cervix: a trial search for intermediate forms between carcinoma and sarcoma. *Asia and Oceania Journal of Obstetrics and Gynaecology*, 11:429–35.

Townsend DE (1988). Malignant melanoma. Paget's disease and sarcoma of the vulva. In *Textbook of uncommon cancer* (ed. CJ Williams, JG Krikorian, MR Green, and D Rhagavan), pp. 211–22. Wiley, Chichester.

Ulbright TM, Brokaw SA, Stehman FB, Roth LM (1983). Epithelioid sarcoma of the vulva. Evidence suggesting a more aggressive behavior than extra-genital epithelioid sarcoma. *Cancer*, 52:1462–9.

Vardi JR, Tovel HM (1980). Leiomyosarcoma of the uterus: clinicopathologic study. *Obstetrics and Gynecology*, 56:428–34.

Vlahoussis AP, Katsoulis ME, Dwitsas SJ, Papadimitriou GC (1983). Sarcoma of the uterus: a ten year experience. *International Surgery*, 68:263–6.

Ward BG, Harvey VJ, Shepherd JH (1982). Pregnancy after treatment of endodermal sinus tumour. *British Journal of Obstetrics and Gynaecology*, 89:769–70.

Warne GI, Fairley KF (1973). Cyclophosphamide induced ovarian failure. *New England Journal of Medicine*, 289:1159–62.

Young N, Damien M, Schwartz PE, Carter D, Mittal KR (1988). Carcinosarcoma of the uterine cervix initially interpreted as high grade sarcoma. *Human Pathology*, 19:605–8.

Young RH, Scully RE (1989). Alveolar rhabdomyosarcoma metastatic to the ovary. A report of two cases and a discussion of the differential diagnosis of small cell malignant tumors of the ovary. *Cancer*, 64:899–904.

Zaleski S, Setum C, Benda J (1986). Cytologic presentation of alveolar soft part sarcoma of the vagina. A case report. *Acta Cytologica*, 30, 665–70.

Section 10
Urological cancer

10.1　Testicular tumours

A. HORWICH, MALCOLM D. MASON, AND W. F. HENDRY

INTRODUCTION

In the 1970s and 1980s, the conceptual framework within which we consider the management of testicular tumours was altered by the impact of combination cytotoxic chemotherapy. This change has been most dramatic for metastatic non-seminoma, where the great majority of patients are now cured. The chemosensitivity of this tumour type has contributed to the investigation of general principles of medical oncology with regard to dose response, the role of maintenance therapy, duration of chemotherapy, the investigation of alternating schedules, and also the investigation of dose intensity. As the majority of non-seminomas express one of the relatively specific tumour markers, α-fetoprotein or human chorionic gonadotrophin, they have also provided the model for how a serum marker should be used in the assessment of malignant disease and in monitoring response and relapse. Important remaining questions relate to the improvement of treatment required for adverse presentations, the role of surgery after chemotherapy, and the mitigation of acute and late toxicity.

The success of chemotherapy in metastatic non-seminoma has led to a re-evaluation of the management of patients presenting with disease apparently confined to the testis. A policy that has been extensively explored, especially within the United Kingdom, is that of surveillance post-orchidectomy, with chemotherapy deferred for relapse; more recently, adjuvant chemotherapy post-orchidectomy has been investigated. The results of these programmes need to be compared with the more traditional approaches of lymph node dissection or retroperitoneal node radiotherapy. However, it is unlikely that any of these policies will demonstrate a clear survival advantage; thus the basis of comparison will be acceptability, side-effects, and quality of life.

The management of seminoma is similarly successful. Radiotherapy is extremely effective in the management of more localized stages, which represent the majority of presentations of seminoma. For the 10–20 per cent of patients who present with advanced disease, the cure rate using platinum-based combination chemotherapy is extremely high. Again, there is some controversy over the role of chemotherapy in earlier stages of the disease but the high success rate of radiotherapy makes this question less compelling.

The success of treatment of germ cell tumours is particularly important because the incidence of these diseases is rising rapidly in Western societies, especially in the young adult age group. They have been described as 'the model of a curable tumour' and this is not only for the analysis of the principles of treatment efficacy but also because they permit the evaluation of the long-term impact of the diagnosis and treatment of malignant disease. For this reason they continue to be a focus of academic research in oncology.

EPIDEMIOLOGY AND AETIOLOGY

The causes of germ cell tumours are unknown. The incidence of testicular tumours has been rising steadily over the past few decades in several populations (Waterhouse 1985; Osterlind 1986) and the mortality has diminished with the advent of effective treatment. Testicular tumours are more common in developed countries, with the highest incidences being reported in Denmark, Israel, the United States, and the United Kingdom. It is interesting that within developed countries the incidence is highest in the higher socio-economic groups and, furthermore, data from migrant populations, though scarce, point towards an environmental component to the causation of testicular tumours. Though the incidence rate in the United Kingdom is only 1 : 100 000 men per year, the mean lifetime risk of developing a testicular tumour is approximately 1 in 500; while uncommon, testicular cancer is hardly a rare disease.

The age-specific incidence of testicular tumours is striking. There is a small peak of incidence in infancy, predominantly due to yolk sac tumours, after which testicular cancer is extremely uncommon until puberty. Thereafter the incidence rates of both seminoma and malignant teratoma rise sharply to a peak between 20 and 30 years for malignant teratoma and 30–40 years for seminoma (Fig. 1), while the peak age for combined tumours is in between these two (Pugh 1976). These data suggest that causative factors operate early in life, either in the pre-natal period or during early childhood. The onset of testicular tumours after puberty raises the possibility that the production of pituitary hormones or testosterone might also contribute to their development, but this remains hypothetical and the sharp fall in the incidence rates of testicular tumours at older ages contrasts with most other hormone-dependent malignancies.

The association between testicular maldescent and testicular cancer has been known for over 40 years. The risk of testicular cancer in men with maldescent was thought to be 40 times higher than in the general population, though more recent estimates of the relative risk are only 5–10 times higher (Giwercman et al. 1987; Strader et al. 1988). Interestingly, in cases where the maldescent is unilateral, the increased risk is not confined to the maldescended testicle, suggesting that maldescent per se is not a cause of testicular cancer but rather that both maldescent and testicular cancer have common aetiological factors. Consistent with the latter view is the observation that the surgical correction of maldescent does not abolish the risk of testicular cancer (Senturia 1987).

Germ cell tumours are associated with other abnormalities of testicular development including gonadal dysgenesis, androgen insensitivity, and various intersex states; they are also associated with testicular atrophy and infertility.

In mice susceptible to malignant teratomas there is a strong genetic component to the aetiology of their spontaneously arising testicular tumours and this has raised the question of whether such a genetic predisposition exists in man. The relative rarity of documented families with more than one member affected by testicular tumours suggests that a genetic component is less important in man than in mice, but it has recently been demonstrated that first-degree relatives of patients with testicular germ cell tumours are at increased risk of developing the disease themselves (Forman et al. 1992). Linkage analysis coupled with cytogenetic advances in germ cell tumours described later may assist

Supported by grants from the Cancer Research Campaign and the Bob Champion Cancer Trust.

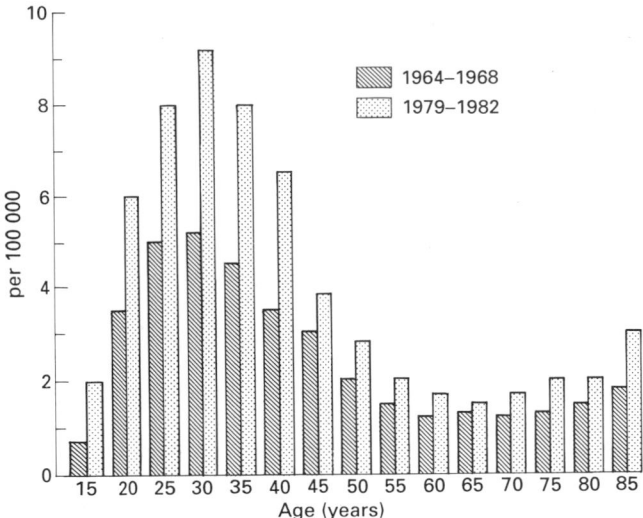

Fig. 1 Age-specific incidence of testicular cancer in England and Wales showing the increase in 1979–1982 compared to 1964–1968.

in the identification of the gene or genes responsible for an inherited predisposition.

It has been suggested that exposure to maternal oestrogens *in utero* might be related to the risk of testicular cancer later in life (Depue 1984). Such a hypothesis would fit the observed differences in incidence geographically and between social classes, as higher-fat diets in mothers in developed countries and higher social classes might be expected to be associated with higher levels of circulating oestrogen. Interestingly, it has been observed that exposure to exogenous oestrogen *in utero* causes maldescent of the testes in newborn mice. However, the widespread use of diethyl stilboestrol in pregnant women in Denmark in the 1960s has not resulted in an epidemic of testicular cancer in their male offspring, in contrast to the appearance of clear cell adenocarcinoma of the vagina in their female offspring. Other possible aetiological factors for testicular cancer include torsion, mumps orchitis, injury, and occupational exposure to wood dust, degreasing agents, chromate- and zinc-based dyes, and dimethylformamide. The consensus is that as yet the evidence implicating these various factors is limited, though mumps orchitis in particular has been suspected in the past (for a review, see Depue 1984).

There is now good evidence that testicular carcinoma *in situ* is the precursor of both seminoma and malignant teratoma, though the nature of the event responsible for the final step transforming this lesion to invasive cancer is unknown. It would be expected that the factors described above in relation to invasive testicular cancer would also be associated with testicular carcinoma *in situ* and indeed this is the case. From studies of testicular biopsies in the United Kingdom and in Denmark it has been shown that carcinoma *in situ* is found in infertile men and in association with testicular maldescent, atrophy, and in maldevelopmental states including gonadal dysgenesis and androgen insensitivity. Patients who develop one testicular tumour are also at higher risk of developing a contralateral testicular tumour at any time up to 20 years after the development of the first. The 5 per cent incidence of contralateral testicular tumours seen in patients with stage I seminoma (Hamilton *et al.* 1986) seems to correspond well with the 5 per cent incidence of contralateral carcinoma *in situ* found on routine biopsy of the contralateral testis in patients with testicular tumours and approximately 50 per cent

Table 1 WHO classification of testicular tumours

I: Germ cell tumours
    A. Tumours of one histological type
        1. Seminoma
        2. Spermatocytic seminoma
        3. Embryonal carcinoma
        4. Yolk sac tumour (embryonal carcinoma, infantile type; endodermal sinus tumour)
        5. Polyembryoma
        6. Choriocarcinoma
        7. Teratomas
            (a) Mature
            (b) Immature
            (c) With malignant transformation

    B. Tumours of more than one histological type
        1. Embryonal carcinoma and teratoma (teratocarcinoma)
        2. Choriocarcinoma and any other types (specify type)
        3. Other combinations (specify)

II: Sex cord/stromal tumours
    Tumours containing both germ cell and sex cord/stromal elements
    Miscellaneous tumours
    Lymphoid and haematopoietic tumours
    Secondary tumours
    Tumours of collecting ducts, rete, epididymis, spermatic cord, capsule, supporting structures, and appendices

Reproduced from Mostofi and Sobin (1977), with permission.

of those patients with documented carcinoma *in situ* progress to subsequent contralateral tumours within 5 years (Berthelsen *et al.* 1982).

PATHOLOGY

Testicular germ cell tumours characteristically contain a variable mixture of cell types. This complexity has led to different classification systems, comparisons between which can be confusing. It should be recognized at the outset that the two most commonly used classifications were developed with different aims. The World Health Organization (WHO) classification aimed to describe in detail the cell types present in a particular tumour (Table 1), while the British Testicular Tumour Panel (**BTTP**) classification was developed from a need to classify testicular tumours according to their clinical behaviour in the era before platinum-containing chemotherapy was available (Table 2). It is not surprising, therefore, that cell biologists favour the WHO classification, while the BTTP classification has remained in common clinical usage in the United Kingdom.

Non-seminomatous germ cell tumours

Malignant teratomas are caricatures of normal mammalian embryogenesis, in which somatic differentiation gives rise to tissues that will form the fetus and subsequently the animal itself and extraembryonic differentiation gives rise to supporting tissues, such as trophoblast and yolk sac, that do not form the animal itself.

Embryonal carcinoma has been widely viewed as the malignant stem cell of non-seminomatous germ cell tumours and its phenotype in terms of cell structural antigens has been well characterized. Embryonal carcinoma cells within a tumour are heterogeneous in their capacity for differentiation, varying from nullipotent cells that are apparently incapable of differentiating to multipotent cells that differentiate into a variety of somatic and extraembryonic cell types.

Table 2 British Testicular Tumour Panel classification of testicular tumours

Germ cell tumours
   Seminoma
      Classical
      Spermatocytic

   Non-seminomatous germ cell tumours
      Teratoma, differentiated (TD)
      Malignant teratoma, intermediate (MTI)
      Malignant teratoma, undifferentiated (MTU)
      Malignant teratoma, trophoblastic (MTT)

      Combined seminoma/non-seminoma

      Yolk sac carcinoma

Non-germ cell tumours
   Sertoli cell tumour

   Leydig cell tumour

   Malignant lymphoma

   Others
      Paratesticular rhabdomyosarcoma
      Carcinoma of the rete testis

Reproduced from Pugh (1976), with permission.

Table 3 Histology of germ cell tumours (Royal Marsden Hospital 1980–1989)

Teratoma, differentiated (TD)	17	(2%)
Malignant teratoma, intermediate (MTI)	181	(21%)
Malignant teratoma, undifferentiated (MTU)	170	(19%)
Malignant teratoma, trophoblastic (MTT)	34	(4%)
Combined teratoma and seminoma	127	(14%)
Seminoma	346	(40%)
Total	876	

Histologically, tumours composed of pure embryonal carcinoma can adopt a variety of morphologies: solid, papillary, acinar, or tubular. Embryonal carcinoma cells are not the only malignant stem cells found in non-seminomatous germ cell tumours, as malignant yolk sac and choriocarcinoma stem cells have also been isolated from testicular tumours. It is not clear whether these extraembryonic malignant stem cells are always derived from embryonal carcinoma cells or whether they also arise *de novo* from carcinoma *in situ*.

Choriocarcinoma can be understood as an attempt to mimic normal trophoblastic differentiation in which dividing cytotrophoblast cells differentiate into non-dividing syncytiotrophoblast cells that secrete human chorionic gonadotrophin. In choriocarcinoma it is the cytotrophoblast stem cell that is malignant and dividing, whereas the syncytiotrophoblast is post-mitotic, though as in normal trophoblast, chorionic gonadotrophin is mainly a product of syncytiotrophoblast. Syncytiotrophoblast giant cells are also seen not infrequently in seminomas, where their origin is obscure and are probably responsible for the phenomenon of chorionic gonadotrophin-producing seminoma. The malignant cytotrophoblast cell is not seen in these circumstances and this distinguishes such seminomas from combined seminoma/malignant teratoma (trophoblastic).

The human yolk sac is poorly developed in comparison to that in rodent embryos and, interestingly, the morphological patterns seen in yolk sac carcinoma are highly reminiscent of rodent primitive endoderm. Thus, yolk sac carcinoma can be present in a number of forms, including a 'solid' form and the form referred to as endodermal sinus tumour, characterized by a lacy network of cells and by characteristic 'Schiller–Duval bodies', which consist of glomeruloid structures with a fibrovascular stalk lined by flattened 'hobnail' cells. As in the mammalian embryo, the secretion of α-fetoprotein is a characteristic of cells of the yolk sac lineage, though areas of primitive gut-like and liver-like epithelium can also express α-fetoprotein. The finding of a raised α-fetoprotein in a patient with what is histologically a pure seminoma must be taken as evidence of occult non-seminomatous elements and treated as such; to describe such a tumour as an α-fetoprotein-producing seminoma

is probably inaccurate in cellular terms and possibly dangerous in clinical terms. This is discussed further below.

When the BTTP classification was evolved it was clear that pure testicular choriocarcinoma behaved as a distinct clinical entity, with widespread, often rapidly growing metastatic disease involving such diverse sites as skin and brain in addition to the more usual sites such as lung and lymph nodes. It was therefore classified separately as malignant teratoma, trophoblastic (**MTT**), had a particularly poor prognosis, and indeed still does when associated with its characteristic advanced presentation (Stoter *et al.* 1987). Metastatic non-seminomatous germ cell tumours in general had a poor prognosis in the era before effective chemotherapy, but it was clear from the studies of the BTTP and others that when there was evidence of somatic differentiation as a component (that is, teratocarcinoma in the WHO classification), the prognosis was better than when there was none. Therefore, teratocarcinoma was classified as **MTI** (malignant teratoma, intermediate). All other non-seminomatous germ cell tumours were classified as malignant teratoma, undifferentiated (**MTU**), a term not strictly true because yolk sac carcinoma, included in this group, represents a malignant stem cell with a distinct type of differentiation with respect to embryonal carcinoma cells. Teratoma, differentiated (**TD**) often follows an indolent course and metastatic disease is uncommon. Table 3 shows the histological subtypes in 526 patients with testicular non-seminoma who presented to the Royal Marsden Hospital, London, between 1980 and 1989.

Features that relate to the probability of occult metastatic disease in a patient who appears to be clinical stage I (disease confined to testis on computerized tomographic (**CT**) scanning and marker negative) include the presence within the primary tumour of vascular or lymphatic invasion (Hoskin *et al.* 1986; Freedman *et al.* 1987). It has also been suggested that the presence of yolk sac elements within the primary tumour reduces the risk of metastatic relapse in the stage I patients managed by surveillance. However, this may be an artefact of late registration, as these tumours are associated with the presence in the serum of α-fetoprotein with a long half-life of 5–7 days, which is cleared after orchidectomy. Relapse is rare when the primary tumour does not contain undifferentiated (that is, embryonal carcinoma) cells.

Germ cell tumours are often composed of both seminomatous and non-seminomatous elements, accounting for some 20 per cent of cases in Pugh's original BTTP series. These combined tumours have a peak age of occurrence in between that of seminoma and non-seminomatous germ cell tumour. They resemble non-seminomas in their clinical behaviour and response to treatment.

Seminoma

Macroscopically, classical seminomas appear as a pale, creamy, homogeneous tumour, often with well-developed fibrous septa. Microscopically, too, they are uniform, composed of small round cells with dark-staining nuclei. Classical seminoma may be associated with a lymphocytic infiltration, which has been shown to be mainly with cells of a helper/suppressor phenotype. The presence of a lymphocytic infiltrate is not clearly relevant to prognosis. Seminoma characteristically has an indolent clinical course and metastases only occur in 20–30 per cent of patients.

The most frequent sites of metastases are the first-station nodes, which are in the para-aortic area unless there has previously been inguinal or scrotal surgery, when the pelvic or inguinofemoral nodes may be involved (Mason *et al.* 1991). Occasionally, seminoma may metastasize to bizarre sites such as pancreas and prostate.

Of 876 patients with testicular primary germ cell tumours presenting to the Royal Marsden Hospital between 1980 and 1988, 350 (40 per cent) were pure seminomas (Horwich 1991). Five of these were spermatocytic seminomas, a subtype not associated with carcinoma *in situ* and which occurs predominantly in elderly men. Metastasis from spermatocytic seminoma is very rare (Talerman 1980).

TUMOUR MARKERS

Germ cell tumours are associated with relatively specific and sensitive tumour markers and approximately 75 per cent of non-seminomas express α–fetoprotein, human chorionic gonadotrophin, or both. α-Fetoprotein is associated with evidence of yolk sac differentiation, whereas the gonadotrophin is associated with trophoblastic elements.

A high proportion of seminomas stain with antibodies to placental-like alkaline phosphatase, which has also been shown to stain the abnormal cells in testicular carcinoma *in situ* (Jacobsen and Norgaard-Padersen 1984). This enzyme and lactate dehydrogenase have also been investigated as serum markers.

α-Fetoprotein is an embryonic protein produced by the yolk sac and then by fetal liver. It is related to albumin and is the major serum protein in the fetus. Its production in the primary tumour may be identified by immunohistochemical techniques and it is usually associated with the yolk sac pattern of differentiation (Mostofi 1984). α-Fetoprotein is not produced by classical seminoma. It is conventionally assayed in the serum by a double-antibody radioimmunoassay (Waldman and McIntire 1974). Now enzyme-linked immunosorbent assays are commercially available. Elevated serum α-fetoprotein is found in 45–65 per cent of non-seminomatous germ cell tumours (Bosl *et al.* 1983; Norgaard-Padersen *et al.* 1984; Horwich *et al.* 1987). It is also produced by hepatocellular carcinoma and rarely by other tumours of the upper gastrointestinal tract. Occasionally, moderately raised serum concentrations are found in liver damage from various causes; this can be particularly confusing if patients with germ cell tumours are treated with hepatoxic drugs, in which case a persistent, abnormal serum concentration may be mistakenly interpreted as an indicator of tumour persistence (Coppac *et al.* 1983). Human chorionic gonadotrophin is a moderately small polypeptide consisting of both an α- and a β-subunit. The α–chain is closely related to a number of other hormones such as luteinizing hormones, but the β–chain is specific and the molecule is conventionally assayed with antibodies to the β-chain specifically (Vaitukaitis *et al.* 1972; Javadpour 1986). An elevated serum chorionic gonadotrophin is found in 30–60 per cent of patients with germ cell tumours (Bosle *et al.* 1983; Norgaard-Padersen *et al.* 1984; Horwich *et al.* 1987) and in approximately 10 per cent of seminomas. The serum concentration in metastatic seminoma is rarely more than 200–300 iu/l and higher levels raise suspicion of a non-seminomatous component in the tumour. In seminoma, an elevated chorionic gonadotrophin is associated with relatively bulky disease and as a tumour marker it is not more sensitive than conventional radiology.

Markers and prognosis

The amount of serum markers at presentation is linked to the volume of metastatic disease (Horwich *et al.* 1987). The serum marker concentration has been shown to have independent prognostic significance in patients treated with chemotherapy (Medical Research Council (**MRC**) Working Party 1985) (see below). The second MRC analysis of 793 patients treated between 1982 and 1986 revealed that the 204 patients with either an α-fetoprotein concentration of more than 1000 u/l or a chorionic gonadotrophin of more than 10 000 u/l had a 3 year survival of 67 per cent compared to 91 per cent in the remaining 589 patients ($p < 0.001$).

Lactate dehydrogenase has also provided useful prognostic information, though it is not used so extensively to monitor testicular germ cell tumours because its concentration can be influenced by so many other medical conditions. Serum concentrations of lactate dehydrogenase are elevated in 20–75 per cent of patients with testicular tumour (Javadpour 1986).

Placental alkaline phosphatase was first identified as a tumour marker in a patient with lung cancer (the Reagan isoenzyme). Its serum concentrations have been found to be elevated especially in patients with seminoma (Lange *et al.* 1982; Epenetos *et al.* 1985; Horwich *et al.* 1985); however, false-positive assays are found in patients who smoke. Preliminary investigation has not suggested that it will prove a sensitive measure of small-volume metastatic seminoma and its clinical role is as yet uncertain.

Tumour markers can also give prognostic information following treatment. As serum concentrations of α-fetoprotein and human chorionic gonadotrophin appear to reflect tumour extent, they can be used to measure treatment response and sequential measurements can define response kinetics. In patients who truly have stage I disease the serum markers should decline in concentration after orchidectomy at a rate determined by the physiological half-life; that is, 5 days for α-fetoprotein and 36 h for chorionic gonadotrophin. Slower rates usually apply to the production of the metastatic marker. In patients treated with chemotherapy for the metastatic germ cell tumour, as expected, a lack of fall or a relatively slow fall in tumour markers indicate a poor response and are harbingers of early disease progression. A problem in evaluation of early response is the patient whose drug-resistant disease comprises only a small component at the time of treatment and, thus, does not influence the initial pattern of marker fall at that time. Rates of regression for tumour markers do not identify most patients destined to relapse after chemotherapy, though occasionally a slow initial fall in marker is of adverse prognostic significance (Horwich and Peckham 1984). This appears to be even more important with the VAB (see below) chemotherapy regimens (Toner *et al.* 1990), possibly because of the long cycle interval and is used to select patients for a change to more intensive chemotherapy (Motzer *et al.* 1991). A further complication in the evaluation of initial marker regression is the phenomenon termed the 'marker surge' (Bagshaw 1973; Vogelzang *et al.* 1982; Horwich and Peckham 1986). This temporary rise in marker, usually for only the first 5–10 days after the start of chemotherapy, is more common with human chorionic gonadotrophin than with α-fetoprotein. Dramatic rises up to four times the original concentration have been seen and though the prognostic significance of this event is unclear it can cause difficulty in the interpretation of post-treatment marker concentrations. The phenomenon was thought originally to be due to tumour cell lysis; however, tissue culture experiments have suggested that it may be caused by differentiation of tumour stem cells (Browne and Bagshawe 1982).

The serum concentration of marker represents the balance between production and degradation. With the assumption that a constant proportion of a tumour will produce a particular marker in a consistent way, it can be taken that changes in the rate of tumour marker production per day reflect changes in tumour volume and, thus, can provide an estimate of tumour growth. Price *et al.* (1990*a,b*) have investigated the prognostic significance of rates of tumour marker production at presentation and have suggested that rapidly growing tumours have a poor prognosis.

THE BIOLOGY OF GERM CELL TUMOURS

To date it has not been possible to establish cell lines or xenografts that are unequivocally representative of seminoma and many laboratory studies are therefore restricted to non-seminomatous germ cell tumours. Much of our understanding of these has resulted from early studies of mouse teratocarcinoma, which led to the identification of many cell lines and of strains of mice with a high incidence of spontaneous teratomas. Whether the genes associated with such inherited mouse tumours have homologues in man remains to be determined, but meanwhile the nature of the mutation at the so-called *ter* gene locus in susceptible mice would be of great interest (Noguchi and Noguchi 1985).

Early studies confirmed that embryonal carcinoma cells were the malignant stem cells of mouse teratocarcinoma and also that some embryonal carcinoma cells were pluripotent because they differentiated into a variety of somatic tissues when transplanted *in vivo* (Kleinsmith and Pierce 1964). Furthermore, such cells could be reimplanted into early mouse embryos and could participate in development, resulting in apparently normal chimeric mice whose adult tissues were partly composed of embryonal carcinoma-derived cells in tissues of mesodermal, ectodermal, and endodermal origin and even included testicular germinal epithelium (Martin 1980). Further confirmation of the close relation between murine embryonal carcinoma cells and cells of the early pre-implantation embryo came from the culture *in vitro* of pluripotential cells from the inner cell mass of normal mouse embryos, so-called embryonic stem cells. There are a number of similarities between embryonal stem and carcinoma cells and, interestingly, transplantation of embryonic stem cells into extrauterine sites resulted in the development of a teratocarcinoma (Martin 1981). It seems likely that human embryonal carcinoma cells are also closely related to early embryonic cells, though they may be more similar to early extraembryonic endoderm cells than cells of the inner cell mass (Pera *et al.* 1987).

Differentiation of embryonal carcinoma cells occurs *in vitro* as well as *in vivo*. However, the pathway of differentiation depends both on the agent used to trigger it and the target cell type. Retinoic acid is a potent inducer of differentiation in mouse teratocarcinoma cell lines, the most notable being the F9 cell line, which differentiates into primitive endoderm on treatment with retinoic acid (Strickland and Sawey 1980). Such *in vitro* differentiation is also seen in human embryonal carcinoma cells such as TERA-2, but exposure to retinoic acid in these cells results in differentiation into neurone-like cells. By contrast, exposure of TERA-2 cells to hexamethylbisacetamide induces them to differentiate into primitive mesenchymal cells (Andrews 1988). Spontaneous differentiation can also occur *in vitro*

in the absence of any exogenous agent. The embryonal carcinoma cell line GCT 27 maintains its phenotype under normal growth conditions, but a clonal derivative of this cell line, GCT 27X, differentiates spontaneously in the appropriate culture conditions into cells representative of all three germ layers (Pera *et al.* 1989). The precise factors that trigger somatic differentiation in embryonal carcinoma cells and which determine the cell lineage pathway that differentiation will follow are unknown. Retinoic acid presumably exerts its effects through its nuclear receptors, but some embryonal carcinoma cells are unresponsive to retinoic acid despite expressing receptors.

Early cytogenetic studies indicated a major difference between testicular and ovarian germ cell tumours in that testicular tumours arose from cells that were pre-meiotic whereas benign ovarian teratomas arose from cells that had completed the first though not the second meiotic division (Linder 1983). More recent cytogenetic studies have identified a common chromosomal abnormality in testicular non-seminomatous germ cell tumours, the isochromosome of the short arm of chromosome 12 (Atkin and Baker 1983). This appears to be the most common cytogenetic abnormality that is regularly seen in non-seminomatous germ cell tumours and raises the hope that rather than being an epiphenomenon, it might be somehow related to the genesis of these tumours. It has also been suggested that the number of copies of i(12p) in a germ cell tumour relates to prognosis (Bosl *et al.* 1989*a*). Subsequently the evidence for this has weakened. Cytogenetics have also shown that an early event in the genesis of a germ cell tumour is the acquisition of aneuploidy; mean chromosome numbers are highest in carcinoma *in situ* and lowest in non-seminomatous germ cell tumours and in between these two in seminoma (Oosterhuis *et al.* 1990).

Many cell lines are now available from non-seminomatous germ cell tumours; their abundance and the relative ease with which they can be established, give grounds for some degree of confidence in extrapolating from cell-line data to the situation *in vivo*. Our understanding of the cell-lineage relations in lymphoid malignancies was greatly facilitated by the use of monoclonal antibodies and other probes to cellular antigens and a similar approach is proving useful in the study of germ cell tumours. Such studies have clearly identified embryonal carcinoma cells as one distinct type of malignant stem cell in non-seminomatous germ cell tumours, but they are not the only one. Yolk sac carcinoma may be derived from two distinctive types of malignant stem cell, distinguished by their morphology, growth characteristics, and cytostructural antigens (Pera *et al.* 1987, 1988). The first, giving rise in nude mice to yolk sac tumours resembling rodent visceral endoderm, produces copious amounts of α-fetoprotein. The second, giving rise to yolk sac carcinomas resembling rodent partial endoderm (endodermal sinus tumour), has characteristics suggestive of a particularly aggressive phenotype and, interestingly, produces only modest amounts of α-fetoprotein (Pera *et al.* 1987). As expected from the clinical syndrome of trophoblastic teratoma, a further distinct malignant stem cell has been identified which gives rise to choriocarcinoma, and which, as described above, is equivalent to what is recognizable in histological sections as malignant cytotrophoblast (Yamazaki *et al.* 1987).

Figure 2 shows one possible model for the cell-lineage relations in germ cell tumours. However, there are alternative views: one was based on the isolation of cell lines and xenografts that were thought to represent seminoma, but which produced α-fetoprotein and this led to the suggestion that seminoma and yolk sac carcinoma were related to each other and represented extremes of the same histological continuum. However, a cell line derived from these 'α-fetoprotein-producing seminomas' has now been shown to have the *in vitro* characteristics of the yolk sac carcinoma resembling visceral endoderm (Pera *et al.* 1987) and some pathologists felt that all of the tumours in the original series were yolk sac carcinomas and not seminomas (Mostofi 1984). Another view of cell-lineage relations states that all non-seminomatous germ cell tumours pass through a seminoma stage in their development and that seminoma represents an intermediate stage between carcinoma *in situ* and the non-seminomatous tumour (Oliver 1990; Oosterhuis *et al.* 1990). This is based, first, on the chromosome numbers in carcinoma *in situ*, seminoma, and non-seminomatous germ cell tumour and, second, on the observation that the peak age for combined tumours is between that of seminoma and non-seminomatous germ cell tumour and such data certainly fit this hypothesis. However, the hypothesis explains less easily why seminomas very rarely occur in teenagers in contrast to their proposed derivative, non-seminomatous germ cell tumour, why a high proportion of the non-seminomas have no seminomatous components though they do have carcinoma *in situ* components, why patients relapsing after surveillance for stage I seminoma almost invariably relapse as seminomas and not as non-seminomatous germ cell tumours (Thomas *et al.* 1989; Duchesne *et al.* 1990; see below), and why the peak age of seminomas is as much as 10 years later than that of non-seminomatous germ cell tumours. What can be said with more certainty is that seminoma closely resembles its precursor, carcinoma *in situ* and that both seminoma and carcinoma *in situ* resemble embryonic germ cells. Studies using *in situ* hybridization have suggested that differences between teratoma and seminoma can be detected even at the *in situ* stage, suggesting that the theory that all teratomas evolve from seminomas is not universally correct, though it is still possible that such a pathway can occur sometimes (Looijenga *et al.* 1993). We must await further *in vitro* characterization of seminoma before speculating too much on its exact relation to non-seminomatous germ cell tumour.

Studies of oncogenes in germ cell tumours have led to confusing results. Given that the cKi-*ras*$_2$ gene is located on chromosome 12p it was hoped that this oncogene might be implicated in the genesis of germ cell tumours, but evidence for this view has been difficult to obtain (Dimitrovsky *et al.* 1990). Nevertheless, this abnormality provides a focus for the identification of specific candidate tumour suppressor genes (Murty *et al.* 1992). Studies of c-*myc* expression in human tumour biopsies showed much expression in seminoma and in areas of somatic and yolk sac differentiation in non-seminomas, but less in embryonal carcinoma cells (Sikora *et al.* 1987). More inconsistent results have been found in murine teratocarcinomas and in human embryonal carcinoma cells *in vitro*, in which no such pattern emerged (Schofield *et al.* 1987; Finkelstein and Weinberg 1988). More promising, perhaps, will be studies on the expression of genes such as *Hst-1* (Dimitrovsky *et al.* 1990; Sugimura *et al.* 1990; Strohmeyer *et al.* 1991). There is some controversy over the frequency of p53 mutations in germ cell tumours (Peng *et al.* 1993; Ye *et al.* 1993). Similarly, data on growth factors are confusing because although human embryonal carcinoma cells produce a number of growth factors (platelet-derived growth-factor-α, tumour growth factor-β, basic fibroblast growth factor, and insulin-like growth factor II (**IGF-II**)), it has not been shown as yet that any of these have biological effects on either stem cells or on their differentiated derivatives. TERA-2 human embryonal carcinoma cells have high-affinity receptors for IGF-II and produce IGF-II transcripts and yet the effect of IGF-II on these cells in culture is not mitogenic, but merely survival enhancing (Biddle *et al.* 1988). In the mouse it is felt that growth factors produced by embryonal carcinoma cells may regulate the growth of their

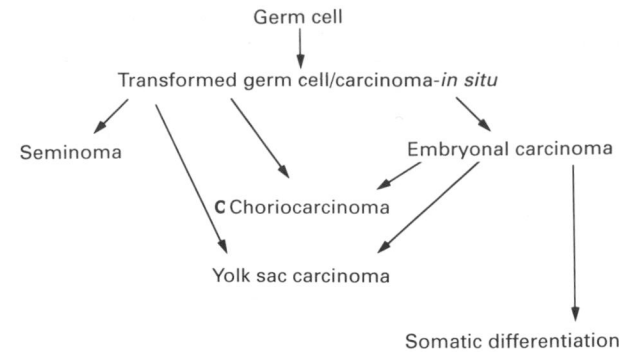

Fig. 2 Possible cell-lineage relations in germ cell tumours.

differentiated derivatives, though the embryonal carcinoma cells themselves are growth factor-independent for growth (Pera *et al.* 1990).

Laboratory studies have so far not explained the most striking clinical observation about germ cell tumours, namely their exquisite drug sensitivity. It seems that the amount of platinum bound to treated embryonal carcinoma cells is similar to the amount bound to more resistant cells. The basis of etoposide sensitivity is also unknown. Conversely, the biological basis of treatment failure is also obscure. The cell biological studies described above would indicate that the presence of aggressive cell types such as choriocarcinoma and endodermal sinus tumour stem cells might be reflected in the clinical outcome and there is some evidence that rapidly proliferating tumours might carry a worse prognosis (Sledge *et al.* 1988). Acquired drug resistance, though widely postulated clinically, is difficult to demonstrate *in vitro*; platinum-resistant, embryonal carcinoma cell lines have been reported, but in general they are difficult to generate, requiring periods of up to 1 year of continuous exposure to platinum (Roth *et al.* 1989; Walker *et al.* 1990).

PRESENTATION, CLINICAL FEATURES, DIAGNOSIS, AND DIFFERENTIAL DIAGNOSIS OF THE PRIMARY TUMOUR

There is increasing evidence that the excellent results now being reported from specialist cancer centres depend upon the initial choice of treatment regimen being correct for the stage of the disease in the individual patient. Once a mistake in management has occurred that allows metastases to become bulky the chance of cure is reduced. It is therefore essential that the surgeon who first meets the patient, who first gains his confidence, is aware of the developments that have occurred in this field, which make it a rarity for a young man to die of a testicular tumour today, provided he is treated correctly from the outset. A recent observational study based on 440 men with non-seminoma showed that the risk of dying was more than doubled if the patient was not managed in a specialist testicular tumour unit (Harding *et al.* 1993). Cure is also dependent upon vigilant follow-up so that relapse can be detected early and any residual disease left after completion of chemotherapy can be dealt with. In 1947, Gordon-Taylor and Wyndham concluded that 'in the matter of testicular malignancy, all is simplicity in surgery'. As we shall see, successful modern management is dependent upon

Table 4 Delay in diagnosis of testicular teratoma and prognostic factors at presentation (Royal Marsden Hospital 1980–1986)

Prognostic factor	Delay (days)			
	0–49	50–99	100 or more	All
Stage				
I	45 (54%)	42 (55%)	39 (41%)	126 (49%)
II	17 (20%)	15 (19%)	27 (28%)	56 (23%)
III and IV	22 (26%)	20 (26%)	30 (31%)	72 (28%)
Total	84 (100%)	77 (100%)	96 (100%)	257 (100%)
Markers				
Low[a]	25 (60%)	22 (61%)	32 (5%)	79 (58%)
High	17 (40%)	14 (39%)	26 (45%)	57 (42%)
Total	42 (100%)	36 (100%)	58 (100%)	136 (100%)
Tumour volume				
Stage I marker-negative	42 (50%)	41 (53%)	38 (40%)	121 (47%)
Small[b]	29 (35%)	23 (30%)	26 (27%)	38 (30%)
Large[b]	7 (8%)	8 (10%)	16 (17%)	31 (12%)
Very large[b]	6 (7%)	5 (6%)	16 (17%)	27 (11%)
Total	84 (100%)	77 (100%)	96 (100%)	257 (100%)

Reproduced from Chilvers *et al.* (1989), with permission.
[a]α-Fetoprotein <500 iu/l and human chorionic gonadotrophin <1000 iu/l.
[b]MRC classification (MRC 1985).

effective collaboration between the oncologist and surgeon and the tasks now presented to the latter may be anything but simple.

The importance of early diagnosis

The most important variables affecting the outcome of treatment for testicular tumours are tumour volume and the concentrations of serum marker at presentation and these correlate directly with delay from the first symptom to the start of treatment. For example, Bosl *et al.* (1981) showed that the median patient-plus-physician delay for stage I tumours was 75 days, for stage II, 101 days, and for stage III, 134 days, a highly significant correlation. Sadly, many patients wait a long time before seeking medical advice. Thompson *et al.* (1961) reported that 83 per cent of 178 patients delayed for over 1 month, 59 per cent for over 3 months, and 37 per cent for more than 6 months. Unfortunately the delay does not stop there. Even when these patients went to their doctors, 36 per cent of 155 patients with testicular tumours were misdiagnosed: 19 as epididymo-orchitis, 16 as post-traumatic, and 11 as hydrocele. Similarly, Stephen (1962) reported that the initial diagnosis was wrong in 56 out of 100 cases, even in the well-supervised ranks of the British Army. In a study from Stockholm, Erman (1980) found a similar delay in presentation and reported that the correct diagnosis was established at the first consultation in only 43 per cent of 526 cases seen between 1940 and 1979; no reduction of the doctor's delay was discernible during this period. Despite editorials in both the *British Medical Journal* (Editorial 1980a) and *The Lancet* (Editorial 1980b) and the preparation of films demonstrating self-examination of the testes, we still see men with advanced disease and huge testicular lumps brought to the clinic by their wives, protesting that they feel nothing wrong. The need for more public education is self-evident.

In an MRC study (MRC Working Party 1985), the 3 year survival rate for men with a history of less than 3 months was 81 per cent compared with 61 per cent when the history was more than 3 months

($p=0.02$). This difference was due to the association of more advanced disease with delay in diagnosis. Thus, when the history was less than 6 months, 54 per cent of patients had small-volume metastases and 65 per cent low serum markers, compared with 39 and 51 per cent, respectively, for patients with a history of more than 6 months. In 257 Royal Marsden Hospital patients with testicular teratoma, the median delay between the initial symptom and diagnosis was 2.5 months (mean 3.9 months). As shown in Table 4, of those presenting within 100 days of onset of symptoms, 54 per cent had stage I tumours compared with 41 per cent who delayed longer ($p=0.05$) (Chilvers *et al.* 1989). Of men delaying 100 days or more, 13 per cent had very large-volume metastatic disease with high marker concentrations compared to only 3 per cent of those with less delay. Some have found that a delay in diagnosis reduced the probability of survival (Oliver 1985; Thornhill *et al.* 1987). However, the Royal Marsden Hospital analysis showed an inverse relationship between delay and survival (Chilvers *et al.* 1989), possibly because very rapidly progressing tumours lead to a short time to presentation.

In the Danish testicular carcinoma study there was a significant increase between 1979 and 1980 in the proportion of seminoma patients with stage I disease at presentation; 70 and 78 per cent, respectively. Furthermore, there was a degree between 1976 and 1980 in the mean maximum diameter of primary tumours at diagnosis from 5.7 to 4.8 cm for seminoma and 5.1 to 4.0 cm for teratoma. Finally, the size of primary tumour could be correlated with the probability of metastases. Thus, 71 per cent of men with primary tumours smaller than 2.5 cm had stage I disease compared with 52 per cent with a tumour larger than 2.5 cm (Krag Jacobsen *et al.* 1984).

These changes are likely to be due to an increase in public awareness of testicular cancer in Denmark and suggest that prompt diagnosis can result in a significant increase in early-stage presentations with corresponding improvements in prognosis.

The importance of early diagnosis relates to the adverse prognostic influence of bulky metastatic disease and high serum concentrations of α-fetoprotein and/or human chorionic gonadotrophin, as well as to the possibility of avoiding chemotherapy if tumour is confined to the testis. In the MRC study, 91 per cent of patients with small-volume metastases and low serum markers were alive at 3 years compared with 47 per cent of those with very bulky disease and high markers. Fortunately, the latter group accounts for only 15 per cent of patients with metastases. The study also shows that between 1976 and 1982, treatment results improved significantly and with further progress in chemotherapy differences between the various prognostic subgroups are likely to become less marked. However, in order to achieve cure in patients with bulky metastases and high markers, more intensive chemotherapy is required than is the case for patients with a small tumour burden.

The avoidance of chemotherapy in stage I disease and of unnecessarily toxic chemotherapy in patients with metastatic disease is particularly desirable in patients with decades of life ahead of them in whom treatment-related morbidity, including recovery of fertility and the fathering of normal children, is of great importance.

Clinical diagnosis

There are several reasons why the diagnosis of testicular tumours is so treacherous. Although they usually present as a painless enlargement, the most common error is to mistake a tumour for epididymitis because the swollen testis is tender. In fact, Stephen (1962) noted that 13 out of 92 cases with a swollen testicle

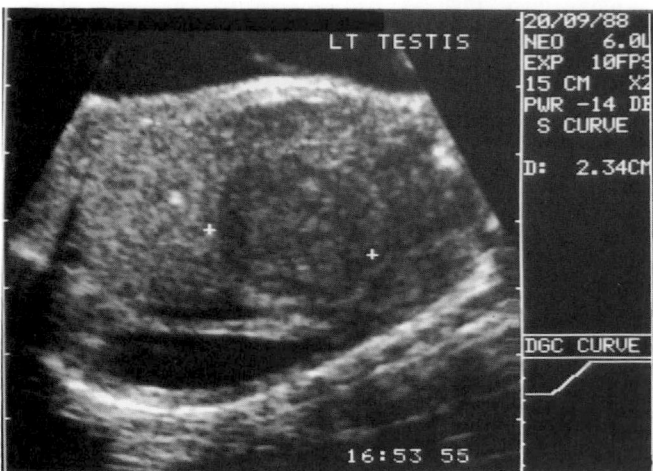

Fig. 3 Testicular ultrasonogram showing hypoechoic area characteristic of a germ cell tumour.

complained of pain from the outset. Many of these testes were found to show evidence of haemorrhage on pathological examination and it seems likely that a small bleed into or adjacent to the tumour not only causes pain and sudden swelling, but its subsequent reabsorption may also account for later subsidence of the swelling, which may coincide with antibiotic therapy, thus reinforcing the wrong diagnosis of infection. Sandeman (1979) analysed the symptomatology and early management of 502 tumours in Australia and also noted that pain was commonly a presenting feature, which led to the condition being treated as inflammatory for too long. Once again, delay was associated with higher-stage disease and poorer results.

A history of trauma, recent or remote, is recorded in 17–21 per cent of cases (Thompson *et al.* 1961; Stephen 1962) and this 'red-herring' should not be allowed to distract attention from the true underlying condition. Previous surgery to the testis or inguinal canal may make the findings more difficult to interpret and may alter the pattern of lymphatic spread (Mason *et al.* 1991). Orchidopexy, for example, may deflect metastases to the inguinal or iliac lymph nodes; sometimes the resulting lymphoedema may lead to a swollen leg as the presenting feature.

The patient who has had a testicular tumour before represents a particular problem: he has only one testicle and he is usually acutely aware of any changes that may occur in it. Twenty-one (2.75 per cent) out of 760 men with testicular tumours attending the Royal Marsden Hospital between 1952 and 1976 developed tumour in the contralateral testis, in two instances synchronously and in the remainder at intervals from 4 months to 15 years (Sokal *et al.* 1980). Carcinoma *in situ* has been demonstrated in 24 (5.6 per cent) out of 425 such patients submitted to biopsy of the contralateral testis, seven of whom subsequently developed invasive tumours (Von der Maase *et al.* 1985). Of 1219 patients seen at the Royal Marsden Hospital between 1962 and 1984, 38 (3.1 per cent) developed second tumours and eight died. Seventeen out of 26 assessable patients (65 per cent) exhibited at least one of the known aetiological risk factors for carcinoma *in situ* (infertility, atrophic testis, or a history of cryptorchidism) (Fordham *et al.* 1990). We now offer testicular biopsy to all patients with one or more of these risk factors.

Careful clinical examination of the testis still remains the best method of detecting a tumour. It is worth starting the physical examination of the testes with the patient standing: a testis with a tumour usually lies lower than normal, whereas inflammatory lesions or torsion tend to raise the testis. Once the patient is lying down, the entire outline of the body of the testis can be defined between the thumb, index, and middle fingers, gently sliding the organ from one examining hand to the other to assess its consistency and localize any induration. A tumour is identifiable first because it is a firm or hard swelling in the body of the testis, secondly because it enlarges the testicle, which may feel relatively heavy, and, thirdly, because it causes the testicle to lose its normal sensation on gently squeezing it.

Abnormal firmness in the body of the testis is the most reliable finding; however, difficulty may arise when the tumour lies in the groove between the testis and epididymis. In cases of doubt, scrotal ultrasonography (Fig. 3) (Tiptaft *et al.* 1982; Vick *et al.* 1982) or tumour marker assay may help to elucidate the situation. However, the false-negative rate is 5–12 per cent (Lightner *et al.* 1989) and so in all cases where doubt persists, the testicle should be explored without delay. The diagnosis might also be made by needle aspirate or fine-needle biopsy of a metastasis.

The differential diagnosis includes epididymitis, torsion, tuberculosis, gumma, and granulomatous orchitis. No harm will come from exploring these conditions and there is much to support the view that all non-transilluminable testicular swellings should be explored unless the swelling is strictly confined to the epididymis or there are pus cells in the urine to confirm the diagnosis of epididymitis.

Occasionally, patients present with metastatic germ cell malignancy in whom no primary tumour can be palpated in either testis. Study of 18 such patients at the Royal Marsden Hospital indicated that many had advanced disease, presenting with abdominal pain and systemic symptoms (Powell *et al.* 1983). Eight patients had a history of testicular atrophy. The diagnosis was established by biopsy of enlarged abdominal or cervical lymph nodes or lung biopsy or by the finding of high concentrations of serum markers. In three out of four patients in whom the testicle was examined histologically following a history of atrophy or pain, there was evidence of a microscopic primary tumour. It is known that in other cases the primary tumour can disappear, leaving only a scar (Azzopardi *et al.* 1961).

Metastasis

The most common sites of metastases are the retroperitoneal nodes (MRC Working Party 1985). These may cause backache unrelieved by postural changes. Renal obstruction may lead to loin pain and urinary symptoms. Rarely, high para-aortic nodes may lead to gastric outflow obstructions.

Though lung metastases are common in non-seminomatous germ cell tumours, they are virtually always asymptomatic except in the advanced trophoblastic teratoma syndrome where multiple small-volume metastases lead to dyspnoea, respiratory failure, haemoptysis, and occasionally pneumothorax. In particular, if the primary tumour is small, there are widespread other metastases in retroperitoneal nodes and possibly also in the liver and brain. There may be gynaecomastia and the serum chorionic gonadotrophin is very grossly elevated. This presentation of metastatic trophoblastic teratoma constitutes an oncological emergency and may be fatal within days. Brain metastasis is an exceptionally rare presentation except in the context of trophoblastic tumours.

INVESTIGATION OF THE PATIENT WITH A TESTICULAR GERM CELL TUMOUR

Germ cell tumours of the testis have a relatively consistent pattern of spread. It is exquisitely rare for testicular seminoma to bypass the first-station nodes in the para-aortic regions unless there has been previous inguinoscrotal surgery, which disturbs the usually lymphatic pathways (Mason *et al.* 1991). Non-seminomas metastasize most commonly to retroperitoneal lymph nodes in the para-aortic or retrocrural regions, but in some cases metastasis occurs to the lung field alone or even more rarely to the supradiaphragmatic node or liver. Metastatic disease at other sites such as bone, skin, or brain is very rare except in the context of widespread dissemination.

Pattern of lymph node metastasis

Tumours of the right testis metastasize to the interaorticocaval nodes, the pre-caval nodes, and the right para-aortic region. Left-sided tumours spread to the left para-aortic nodes and pre-aortic nodes, typically just beneath the left renal vessel. Right-sided tumours involve contralateral para-aortic nodes in approximately 20 per cent of patients (Ray *et al.* 1974; Dixon *et al.* 1986), but left-sided tumours rarely cross over to the right para-aortic region. Spread may also occur to the 'eschelon' node characteristically adjacent to the right renal hilum (Rouviere 1938).

Staging investigation

The most important staging investigations for testicular germ cell tumours are physical examination, chest radiography, lymphography (but this not usually part of British staging practice), CT scanning of thorax and abdomen, and assay of serum tumour markers, especially α-fetoprotein and human chorionic gonadotrophin, as discussed previously. In early-stage non-seminoma these can be supplemented by retroperitoneal lymph node dissection. In some patients there may be indications for contralateral testicular ultrasonography and biopsy. Abdominal and especially liver ultrasound may be helpful in distinguishing equivocal lesions seen on CT scan. The place of magnetic resonance imaging and radioimmunoscintigraphy has not been established.

Physical examination

This should be directed especially towards abnormalities of contralateral testis, inguinofemoral node region, para-aortic region, and the supraclavicular fossae and axillae. Presence of gynaecomastia should be noted.

Lymphography

The usual technique (where this technique is used in staging) is bipedal lymphography, which identifies lymph nodes in the external iliac, common iliac, and para-aortic chains. Metastases usually appear as a filling defect when small, but when larger the usual appearance of lymph nodes can be distorted such that only a thin crescentic rim of node is visible. The procedure is technically difficult and uncomfortable for the patient. Lymph node opacification rarely extends above the level of the first lumbar vertebra and the eschelon node is not identified. Lymphography has the advantage of demonstrating the internal architecture of normal sized nodes and has been reported to reveal metastasis in one in seven patients whose abdominal CT scans were normal (Lien *et al.* 1983).

Computerized tomography of the abdomen

Lymph node metastasis is diagnosed by node enlargement. Though this might be expected to increase the false-negative rate compared with lymphography, in practice reported rates are similar (Thomas *et al.* 1981; Lien *et al.* 1983; Tesoro-Tess *et al.* 1986). Sensitivity and specificity depend upon the criteria for defining the lymph node size to be abnormal. At the conventional level of 15 mm diameter the sensitivity (proportion of true positives) was similar to when the criterion was 5 mm (68 versus 71 per cent) whereas the specificity was 98 per cent for 15 mm compared to 67 per cent for 5 mm (Lien *et al.* 1986). In practice, nodes 1 cm in diameter in an appropriate position for metastatic disease are regarded as suspicious and should either be biopsied, aspirated, or followed closely unless there is other evidence of metastatic disease.

The abdominal scan also can reveal evidence of renal outflow obstruction and metastatic disease in the liver. The investigation is well tolerated and reveals both the eschelon nodes and the upper retroperitoneal and retrocrural nodes. For staging and prognostic purposes it provides a better definition of lymph node size than does lymphography.

Abdominal ultrasonography

Evaluation of the retroperitoneum is limited by bowel gas and adipose tissue in approximately 20 per cent of patients. It is equal to CT scanning in identifying bulky retroperitoneal disease (Poskitt *et al.* 1985). In experienced hands, ultrasound examination of the liver is as sensitive as CT scanning (Husband *et al.* 1980) and has an important role in elucidating equivocal abnormalities seen on that scan.

Retroperitoneal lymph node dissection

This is a highly sensitive though rigorous method of detecting involvement of retroperitoneal lymph nodes. It is widely employed in the United States and some European countries though not in the United Kingdom. The traditional approach of bilateral dissection removes nodes from around the inferior vena cava, the aorta, and around the ipsilateral iliac vessels (Whitmore 1982). In some centres, lymph nodes above the renal vessels are also dissected (Skinner 1978). It has predominantly been used in patients with non-seminomatous tumours, though an early series of patients with clinical stage I seminoma has been reported (Maier *et al.* 1968). Of patients with testicular non-seminoma with normal abdominal CT scans, 20–30 per cent have retroperitoneal lymph node metastases (Pizzocaro *et al.* 1986; Donohue *et al.* 1988; Fossa 1988; Klepp *et al.* 1989; Donohue *et al.* 1993). The risk of metastasis can be predicted by the presence of lymphatic/vascular invasion in the primary tumour (Fossa 1988; Klepp *et al.* 1989). Relapse in the abdomen following this procedure is rare and especially so when nodes were not involved. The extent of the node involvement is predictive for relapse at other sites and can be used as a basis for considering adjuvant chemotherapy.

The disadvantages of retroperitoneal lymph node dissection are the acute side-effects of major abdominal surgery and, in addition, the high incidence of loss of ejaculation, which is almost invariable after the bilateral dissection (Donohue and Rowland 1981). This is due to dissection of autonomic nerves and nerve-sparing techniques have now been developed for more limited dissection (Donohue *et al.* 1988; Jewett *et al.* 1988). Technical aspects of this development are described by Donohue and Thornhill (1991). Published results on 73 patients having the nerve-sparing dissection at Indiana University Medical Centre (Donohue *et al.* 1988) have indicated that 59 patients were pathological stage I, the remaining 14 having involved retroperitoneal nodes. Four of these subsequently relapsed and required chemotherapy. As none of the 59 patients with pathological stage I disease relapsed, it would appear that the modified technique did not miss any involved nodes. Seventy-two patients retained normal ejaculatory function. There are many complications of this retroperitoneal dissection and its use in staging is becoming controversial (Sujka *et al.* 1991; Horwich 1993).

Staging of the thorax

Advanced thoracic disease is most easily detected by chest radiographs; however, a significant proportion of patients with abnormal chest radiographs have either mediastinal or lung involvement on CT scan of the thorax (Husband and Grimer 1985). Lien *et al.* (1988) studied 47 patients with lung metastases from testicular tumours and found that in 20 these were detected by CT scan but not by chest radiograph. Problems of differential diagnosis of small nodules may occur with granulomas and areas of inflammation; in the hilar region, major blood vessels create diagnostic difficulty that can often be resolved by intravenous contrast.

Strategy of investigation

Seminoma

After the physical examination, patients should have assessment of abdominal nodes by CT scan, assessment of the thorax with chest radiograph and thoracic CT scan, and assay of serum tumour markers. The case for thoracic CT scanning is stronger in patients with evidence of retroperitoneal node involvement. Patients with raised serum α-fetoprotein should be staged and managed as combined testicular tumours, that is as non-seminomatous tumours.

Non-seminoma

Standard current staging would include a CT scan of the thorax and abdomen and assay of serum markers α-fetoprotein and human chorionic gonadotrophin. In some centres, assay of lactate dehydrogenase would be used as a basis for prognosis.

Further assessments depend upon the management strategy. In early-stage disease this may be with surveillance alone or with retroperitoneal lymph node dissection. More advanced stages are managed initially with chemotherapy and subsequently re-evaluated for possible surgical excision of residual masses as discussed below.

Investigation of equivocal liver abnormalities can be extended by the use of liver ultrasonography. CT scanning or magnetic resonance imaging of the brain are indicated in patients with neurological symptoms or in those with high risk of brain metastasis by virtue of presentations with a high serum chorionic gonadotrophin ($>20\,000$ u/l) or multiple (more than 20) lung metastases.

Investigation of the contralateral testis

As approximately 5 per cent of patients treated successfully for a testicular germ cell tumour subsequently develop a contralateral testicular germ cell tumour, it would be desirable to identify these

Table 5 Royal Marsden Hospital (RMH) staging classification

RMH stage		Definition
I	M	Rising postorchidectomy markers only
II		Abdominal lymphadenopathy
	A	<2 cm
	B	2–5 cm
	C	>5 cm
III		Supradiaphragmatic lymphadenopathy
	0	No abdominal disease
	ABC	Abdominal node size as in stage II
IV		Extralymphatic metastases
	L_1	$\leqslant 3$ lung metastases
	L_2	>3 lung metastases, all <2 cm diameter
	L_3	>3 lung metastases, 1 or more >2 cm
	H^+	Liver involvement

patients prospectively. In a series of routine contralateral testicular biopsies in 500 patients the presence of testicular carcinoma *in situ* was found to predict those at risk of developing contralateral tumours accurately (Berthelsen *et al.* 1982). The risk of carcinoma *in situ* was significantly higher in patients with a history of testicular maldescent or with an atrophic contralateral testis and it is recommended that these patients have a testicular biopsy. It appears that a 3 mm biopsy is sufficient. Patients with carcinoma *in situ* have a risk of developing overt neoplasia of approximately 50 per cent over the subsequent 5 years. This can be managed either by close surveillance, by orchidectomy, or by low-dose testicular irradiation. There is a risk of developing antisperm antibodies as a result of biopsy.

Occult presentation

Approximately 10 per cent of patients with germ cell tumours present without an overt testicular abnormality. They present with the effects of metastatic disease, the diagnosis being established by biopsy of the metastasis. General staging investigations should be carried out as for testicular primaries, although the poor prognosis of patients with mediastinal masses makes their investigation and treatment urgent. Additionally, it may be relevant to investigate the possibility of an occult testicular primary by testicular ultrasonography, possibly supplemented by biopsy if an abnormality in one testis is suspected. A high incidence of carcinoma *in situ* of the testis has been found in patients with extragonadal presentations in the retroperitoneal area (Von der Maase 1991).

New investigative techniques

Magnetic resonance imaging

As with CT imaging, magnetic resonance can demonstrate node involvement where there is enlargement and has the advantage of imaging in multiple planes. It is also easy to distinguish blood vessels without the need for intravenous contrast. It has not yet proved more successful at characterizing benign rather than malignant node enlargements.

Radioimmunoscintigraphy

The production of specific tumour markers from germ cell tumours offers the potential for sensitive imaging using radioimmunoscintigraphy (Javadpour *et al.* 1981; Begent 1986). Interpretation of

Table 6 The Indiana University staging system

Minimal disease
1. Elevated human chorionic gonadotrophin and/or α-fetoprotein only
2. Cervical nodes (±non-palpable retroperitoneal nodes)
3. Unresectable, but non-palpable, retroperitoneal disease
4. Minimal pulmonary metastases; less than five per lung field and the largest <2 cm (±non-palpable abdominal disease)

Moderate disease
5. Palpable (≥10 cm) abdominal mass as only disease
6. Moderate pulmonary metastases; five to ten pulmonary metastases per lung field and the largest <3 cm or a mediastinal mass <50% of the intrathoracic diameter or a solitary pulmonary metastasis >2 cm (±non-palpable abdominal disease)

Advanced disease
7. Advanced pulmonary metastases; mediastinal mass >50% of the intrathoracic diameter or greater than 10 pulmonary metastases, largest >3 cm (±non-palpable abdominal disease)
8. Palpable abdominal mass plus pulmonary metastases
   8.1: minimal pulmonary
   8.2: moderate pulmonary
   8.3: advanced pulmonary
9. Hepatic, osseous, or CNS metastases

Table 7 Modification of Samuels' staging criteria for advanced disease

IIIA	Disease confined to supraclavicular nodes
IIIB$_1$	Either one or more biomarker elevated or gynaecomastia, unilateral or biolateral; both may be present together; no demonstrable mass
IIIB$_2$	Minimal pulmonary disease: up to five nodules in each lung field and the largest diameter of any single lesion no greater than 2.0 cm (total tumour volume does not exceed 40 cm^3)
IIIB$_3$	Advanced pulmonary disease: presence of any mediastinal or hilar mass, neoplastic pleural effusion, or intrapulmonary mass greater than 40 cm^3
IIIB$_4$	Advanced abdominal disease, defined as abdominal mass greater than 10 cm$^+$
IIIB$_5$	Visceral disease (excluding lung), most often liver but also gastrointestinal tract and brain

the scans has been difficult and the technique is evolving in a research setting. It is particularly relevant to the patient unresponsive to chemotherapy who has rising serum markers without any radiological indication of the site of persisting malignant disease.

STAGING CLASSIFICATIONS

The staging classifications in most widespread use are the Royal Marsden Hospital classification (Table 5), the Indiana University classification (Table 6), and the Samuels (MD Anderson) classification (Table 7). All three systems are successful in dividing patients into good and poor prognostic groups; however, it is important to realize that other factors are as important as stage in defining prognosis and also that there is no consensus on criteria dividing the good- from the poor-prognosis patient; indeed, this may depend upon the era of treatment and on the details of treatment employed. It will also depend upon the end-point, which may be complete remission, relapse-free survival, or survival.

In early-stage disease the Royal Marsden system is based on radiological evaluation following orchidectomy, that is predominantly on CT scan. In American centres the stage definitions are influenced by retroperitoneal node dissection and are not usually equivalent.

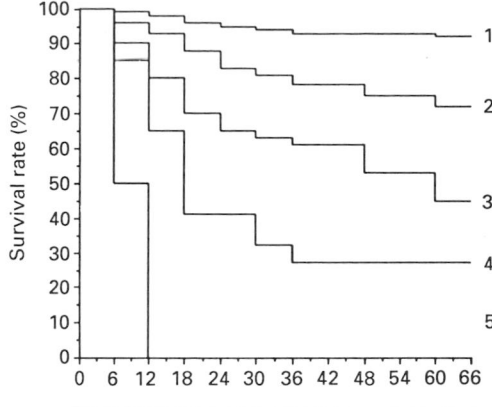

1. None of the 'poor prognosis' A,B,C, or D above features (n =531).
2. Any of the features (n =169).
3. Any two of the features (n =67).
4. Any three of the features (n =26).
5. All four features (n =2).

Fig. 4 MRC second prognostic-factor analysis of survival after chemotherapy for metastatic non-seminoma: 1, no adverse factors (n = 531); 2, any one factor (n = 169); 3, any two factors (n = 67); 4, any three factors (n = 26); 5, all four factors (n = 2). The independent adverse factors were (a) the presence of 20 or more lung metastases, (b) high concentration of serum markers defined either as human chorionic gonadotrophin >10^4 iu/l or α-fetoprotein >10^3 iu/l, (c) the presence of a mediastinal mass >5 cm in diameter, or (d) the presence of liver, bone, or brain involvement.

Clinical stage I patients have microscopic node metastases in 20–30 per cent of cases, whereas patients with stage I following node dissection represent a subset of good prognosis among the clinical stage 1 patients.

Prognosis in advanced disease

A range of factors influences the prognosis of patients treated with chemotherapy for advanced metastatic germ cell tumours including histological features, extent or volume of metastatic disease, initial serum concentrations of α-fetoprotein, human chorionic gonadotrophin, and lactate dehydrogenase, age, involvement of certain organs, site of primary, and time from diagnosis to treatment. There has been some difficulty in reaching international agreement on the definition of prognostic subgroups using all these criteria, partly because different analyses have emphasized different criteria, but also because of variability in the method of their assessment. For example, tumour markers have been analysed in both iu/l and in μg/ml. Assays for lactate dehydrogenase are very variable from different laboratories. The bulk of the disease may depend upon whether assessment has been by radiograph or by CT scan. Levels of markers may be in discrete categories or continuous, as may the number of metastatic sites or number of lung nodules. Finally, the prognosis of patients treated with chemotherapy has improved during the last 15 years (MRC Working Party 1985).

Ten different multivariate analyses of prognostic factors in advanced non-seminomatous germ cell tumours have been reviewed by Bajorin (1991) with the conclusion that the most significant factors include serum concentrations of α-fetoprotein and human chorionic gonadotrophin and extent of metastatic disease. This conclusion is supported by a recent analysis by the MRC Testicular

Table 8   Medical Research Council (MRC) Prognostic Factors Analysis based on Royal Marsden staging system

MRC categories	Stages	Treatment period[a] 1976–1982 No. of patients	3 year survival (%)	Treatment period[b] 1982–1986 No. of patients	3 year survival (%)
Small volume	IM	18	83	78	95
	II III AB	106	87	253	92
	IV L_1 L_2 AB	70	75	200	90
Large volume	IIC IIIC	104	85	82	82
	IV L_1 L_2 C	43	77	37	89
Very large volume	IV L_3 H$^+$	117	54	145	60

[a]MRC (1985).
[b]Mead et al. (1992).

Tumour Working Party of 795 patients treated with chemotherapy between 1982 and 1986, during which time the prognosis did not change with time of treatment. The 3 year survival was influenced by a range of factors; however, on multiple-factor regression analysis the significant adverse features were the presence of 20 or more lung metastases, high serum markers (defined either as chorionic gonadotrophin $> 10^4$ iu/l or α-fetoprotein $> 10^3$ iu/l), the presence of a mediastinal mass of more than 5 cm in diameter, or the presence of liver, bone, or brain involvement (Fig. 4). The presence of any one of these factors indicated a 3 year survival of 67 per cent compared with 94 per cent if no factor was present (Mead et al. 1992). This investigation examined the Royal Marsden Hospital classification and the prognoses of various substages are shown in Table 8.

Criteria for entering patients in trials for poor-prognosis metastatic teratoma

A comparison of the criteria used by the European Organization for Research on Treatment of Cancer (**EORTC**), Indiana University, the National Cancer Institute, and the Memorial Sloan-Kettering Cancer Centre was made in 118 patients treated on MSKCC protocols by Bajorin et al. (1988). Patients had previously been prospectively allocated to good- and poor-risk groups using the MSKCC system (Bosl et al. 1983). (This system is based on serum concentrations of lactate dehydrogenase and human chorionic gonadotrophin, and the total number of metastatic sites; it identifies, as poor prognosis, the patient with a less than 50 per cent probability of achieving complete remission.) Allocation of patients into either good- or poor-risk categories by all four sets of criteria was concordant in only 66 patients (56 per cent); the major differences occurred among patients allocated to the poor-risk subgroup, with the proportion of these same patients allocated to poor risk ranging from 31 to 72 per cent. For example, the EORTC allocated 61 per cent of all patients to the poor-risk category and succeeded in predicting response and non-responders in only 60 per cent of patients. The consequent differences in patient selection in poor-risk studies emphasize the need to evaluate these studies by prospective, randomized trial.

MANAGEMENT

Carcinoma in situ of the testis

At present the diagnosis of carcinoma in situ is based on biopsy of the testis, though it has been suggested that it may also be detected in seminal fluid, either by fluorescent-activated sorting of any aneuploid cells (Giwercman et al. 1988a) or by use of a monoclonal antibody (Giwercman et al. 1988b); these methods are not as reliable as biopsy.

Carcinoma in situ is found in less than 1 per cent of subfertile men (Nuesch-Bachmann and Hedinger 1977; Pryor et al. 1983; Schütte 1988), approximately 2–8 per cent of patients with corrected testicular maldescent (Krabbe et al. 1979; Ford et al. 1985; Pedersen et al. 1987; Giwercman et al. 1989), and approximately 5 per cent of contralateral testes in men who have had an orchidectomy for testicular cancer (Von der Maase et al. 1987; Kleinschmidt et al. 1989). It is very common in patients with gonadal dysgenesis and common in those with androgen-insensitivity syndrome.

In patients with germ cell tumours of the testis and carcinoma in situ of the contralateral testis, the risk of developing a contralateral cancer is approximately 50 per cent within 5 years (Von der Maase et al. 1986). In these patients the risk of carcinoma in situ of the testis was particularly high (23 per cent) in those with testicular atrophy or a history of maldescent.

The management of carcinoma in situ of the testis may be by orchidectomy, by close surveillance with orchidectomy should an evasive tumour develop, or by low-dose testicular irradiation. The appropriate management depends upon the patient's age and personal wishes and also on whether the condition is unilateral or bilateral and on whether the patient is available for close follow-up.

Orchidectomy offers a rapid, simple, and safe treatment of carcinoma in situ; however, if as in the case of contralateral germ cell tumour there is only one remaining testis, then this will lead to abrogation of both fertility and physiological hormone production.

Surveillance has the advantage of allowing normal sperm production should this be present. The option of definitive treatment remains should the patient either develop an evasive tumour in the testis or should he in the meantime complete his family. There is a risk that the patient may develop an invasive germ cell tumour and metastatic disease even though on surveillance.

Localized low-dose radiation has been explored in the treatment of carcinoma in situ of the testis, mainly by Von der Maase et al. (1986, 1987). Their technique employs 14–20 MeV electrons to the scrotum, which is placed in a cup of lead. This is treated to a total dose of 20 Gy in ten fractions of 2 Gy, giving five fractions per week. Post-irradiation biopsy revealed eradication of carcinoma in situ changes in eight out of eight reported cases. On relatively short follow-up there was no impact on testosterone production, libido, or other sexual functions. So far, 20 patients have been treated, with no impact on testicular hormone production after short follow-up (Von der Maase 1991). Further support for the long-term efficacy of radiation in treating carcinoma in situ of the testis comes from the experience of the Christie Hospital in Manchester, where the standard radiation field for early testicular tumours encompassed the contralateral testis (Read 1987). None of more than 1000 patients treated in this way developed a contralateral testicular cancer. The disadvantage of low-dose testicular irradiation is that the treatment induces sterility; however, most of the patients with testicular cancer and contralateral carcinoma in situ have very impaired fertility anyway.

Chemotherapy is probably not effective in eradicating carcinoma in situ of the testis permanently, which has been reported to reappear 2 years after cessation of cisplatin-based, intensive chemotherapy (Von der Maase et al. 1988).

Table 9 Histology of masses resected post chemotherapy

Reference or source	No. of patients	Histology of residual mass		
		Fibrosis/ necrosis	TD	MTU
Bracken et al. (1983)	60	25 (42)	14 (23)	17 (28)
Donohue and Rowland (1984)	123	34 (28)	46 (37)	43 (35)
Staehler et al. (1989)	65	23 (35)	25 (39)	17 (26)
Herr et al. (1991)	122	57 (47)	45 (39)	17 (14)
Kulkarni et al. (1991)	67	18 (27)	20 (43)	20 (30)
Royal Marsden Hospital (1976–1990)	231	52 (22)	131 (57)	48 (21)

TD, teratoma differentiated; MTU, malignant teratoma undifferentiated.

Surgery of primary tumour

Investigations that should precede orchidectomy

Three-quarters of non-seminomatous germ cell tumours produce either α-fetoprotein or β-human chorionic gonadotrophin. This information is invaluable for follow-up purposes, as the concentration of one or other of these markers may rise later, indicating recurrence long before metastases are visible on radiographs or scanning; of course, this is the time that chemotherapy is most effective. It follows that blood should be taken for estimation of these two markers before the testicle is explored. There is really no need to delay for other investigations apart from a chest radiograph.

The technique of orchidectomy

In planning the surgical approach to the testicle, the surgeon must bear two factors in mind. The first concerns the pathways of spread of these tumours and the second is related to the patient's future fertility. The tunica albuginea will contain the tumour locally until it is far advanced, even though distant spread may occur via the lymphatics or bloodstream. Once this fibrous sheath is punctured, however, the local defences are breached and a scrotal recurrence may arise (Dean 1925; Blandy et al. 1970). If the orchidectomy is done through the inguinal region, however, and the testis is removed by gently withdrawing it through the neck of the scrotum, local recurrence is exceptionally rare. When radiotherapy was employed and the scrotal sac was irradiated, the risk of sterility was high, whereas fertility could be preserved in patients receiving lymph node irradiation after an inguinal incision. Thus, Smithers et al. (1973) report 52 children fathered by 34 men after pelvic and para-aortic irradiation with protection to the contralateral testis.

Ideally, the surgical approach should be through a standard or skin-crease inguinal incision. If inspection and palpation confirm the presence of a firm area in the body of the testis, often associated with dilated overlying veins, the cord is divided between clamps and the testis is removed. Biopsy is only necessary with a solitary testicle. Under these circumstances, the testicle should be mobilized through an inguinal incision after applying a soft clamp to the cord. It is then bisected and a biopsy taken from any firm areas to obtain histological confirmation of the diagnosis before removing the testis.

If there is a hydrocele it should not be tapped: it too should be explored, with a view to examining the testis, if it occurs for no apparent reason in a young man; an operation for cure of the hydrocele can be done if the testis is normal. The temptation to needle the scrotum or to do transcrotal biopsy should be resisted, as the tunica albuginea will contain the primary tumour provided it is not surgically breached. It is reasonable to explore the testes through a scrotal incision in the first instance, to inspect them and establish the diagnosis; if a tumour is present, a second incision can easily be made in the groin to remove the testis and cord. Provided that the tunica albuginea has not been opened, there is no increased risk of scrotal dissemination.

Once the testicle has been removed the patient can be referred for further treatment as soon as the pathology report is available. Further local surgery is not necessary after inguinal orchidectomy, but difficulties may arise if a scrotal orchidectomy has been done. Not uncommonly a firm nodule is left in the scrotum adjacent to the cut end of the cord and there may be considerable concern as to whether this is haematoma or residual tumour. It is our policy in these cases to excise the stump of cord through an inguinal incision, which is extended as a 'tennis racket' incision around the scrotum to excise the original scar and the underlying nodule completely as a partial or hemiscrotectomy. Markland et al. (1973) found residual tumour in six out of 19 patients with non-seminomatous tumours treated by hemiscrotectomy after primary scrotal biopsy or orchidectomy. Boileau and Steers (1984) found no adverse effect on prognosis after prompt adequate local managment in such cases. Kennedy et al. (1986) reported on 36 patients with clinical stage I tumours followed at the Royal Marsden Hospital who had had scrotal interference before or at the time of removal of the primary tumour and who had no further treatment. None developed local recurrence during an observation period of 37 months, although scrotal recurrence has been seen in such a case since completion of the study. Clearly, scrotal interference with tumours is best avoided, although the consequences may not be so horrendous as previously imagined.

Surgical excision of residual masses

We have always avoided routine para-aortic lymphadenectomy in early-stage malignant teratoma, preferring surveillance in stage I and chemotherapy in stage II disease (Peckham and Hendry 1985). On the other hand, 73 (23.8 per cent) out of 307 patients who completed chemotherapy for advanced disease between 1976 and 1983 had residual masses in the para-aortic region or in the chest or in both sites. The resected tissue contained residual malignancy in 16 (22 per cent) out of 73 cases (Tait et al. 1984). Further analysis (Hendry et al. 1993) has confirmed that active cancer was present in 48 (21 per cent) out of 231 patients followed-up to the end of 1990. These findings are similar to those reported from other centres (Table 9). After follow-up for 0–13 years (median 4 years), 93 per cent of 52 cases with necrosis and fibrosis and 88 per cent of 131 with differentiated teratoma are alive at 5 years, compared to only 41 per cent of 48 patients with active disease in the residual masses (Fig. 5). However, amongst the patients with active malignancy in para-aortic lymph nodes, 53 per cent survived for at least 5 years after complete excision, with or without follow-up chemotherapy, whereas all six patients who had incomplete excision died (Fig. 6). The results are clearly better in the 182 patients treated electively after initial chemotherapy (5 year survival, 86 per cent) than in the 49 patients whose surgery was a component of salvage treatment after relapse (5 year survival, 50 per cent; $p < 0.005$) (Hendry et al. 1993). We believe that all residual metastatic masses should be removed after completion of chemotherapy, first to define whether or not there is residual active malignancy in the lump and, secondly, because complete surgical removal and follow-up chemotherapy appears to offer the best chance of cure for the 20 per cent of patients who do have active residual tumour. This view is shared by Herr et al. (1991).

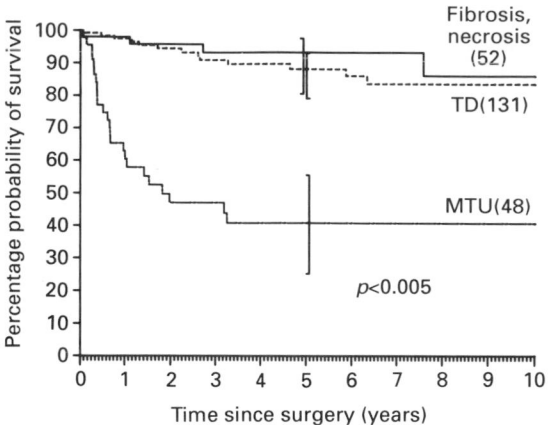

Fig. 5 Survival after post-chemotherapy lymphadenectomy showing impact of histological features of resected mass.

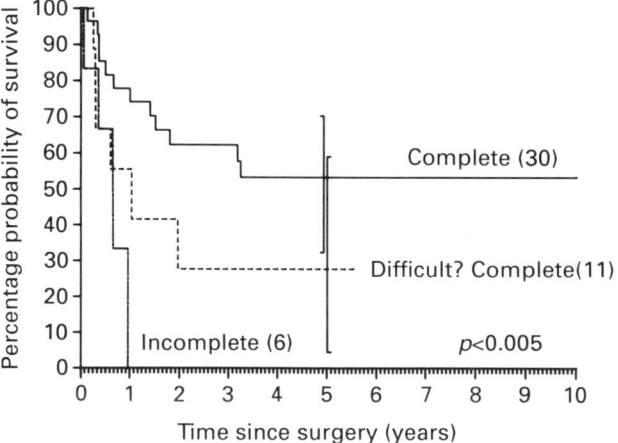

Fig. 6 Survival after post-chemotherapy lymphadenectomy showing impact of completeness of excision in patients whose resected masses contained undifferentiated tumour.

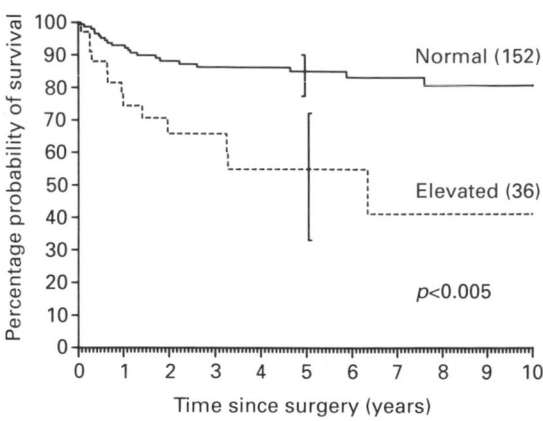

Fig. 7 Survival after post-chemotherapy lymphadenectomy showing impact of serum marker status at time of surgery.

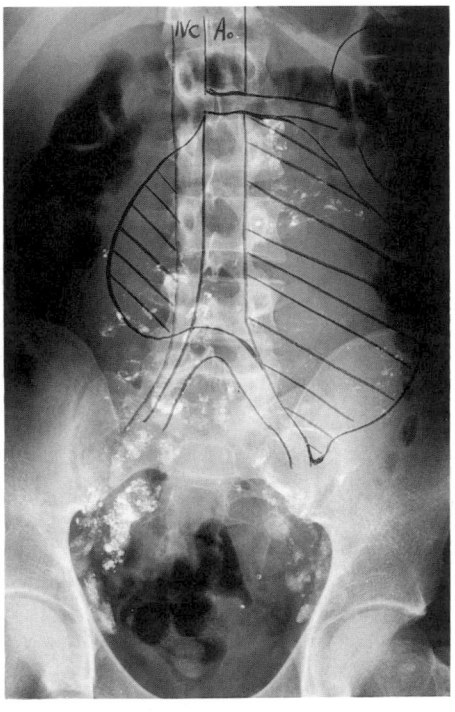

Fig. 8 'Topogram' representing site of tumour mass to be resected; this is derived from axial CT slices.

In practice, implementation of a policy of removal of all residual masses after chemotherapy has raised a number of questions: which patients require surgery, how much chemotherapy should be given, is there a place for radiotherapy, when should the surgery be done in relation to completion of chemotherapy and to sequential studies of serum markers, how complete must the surgery be, and what complications may arise? Analysis of the 231 patients treated at the Royal Marsden Hospital has provided some answers to these questions.

Four cycles of chemotherapy produce complete remission in 70–75 per cent of patients with advanced-stage disease (Donahue and Rowland 1984; Tait *et al.* 1984). To operate before completion of four cycles would require a considerable number of unnecessary operations on masses that would ultimately have resolved spontaneously. The addition of further cycles of chemotherapy beyond four, provided that the serum markers have returned to normal, seems pointless and the addition of radiotherapy in a small, uncontrolled series of observations did not produce significant reduction in the proportion of cases with residual active malignancy (Hendry *et al.* 1981). Our practice, therefore, is to remove residual masses 4–6 weeks after completion of four cycles of chemotherapy, provided that the serum markers have returned to normal. If the surgery is done while the serum markers are still elevated there is every likelihood that the excised mass will contain

active tumour; however, concentrations of serum markers were normal within 1 month of surgery in almost half of our patients who had residual malignancy (21 out of 43 in whom this information was available). Thus, normalization of serum markers is no guarantee that a residual mass is tumour free. Overall, 85 per cent of 152 patients whose marker concentrations were normal at surgery were alive at 5 years, compared to only 55 per cent of 36 whose serum markers were up within 1 month of surgery (Fig. 7).

Excision of these residual masses requires careful pre-operative localization by CT scanning, so that the optimum surgical approach can be planned. This information is most conveniently presented in the form of a 'topogram' (Fig. 8), relating the site of the residual mass to the surrounding vital structures. The residual masses were confined to the para-aortic area in 211 patients and 20 had additional masses removed from lung or mediastinum. During the same time period, residual masses confined to the chest were removed in 80

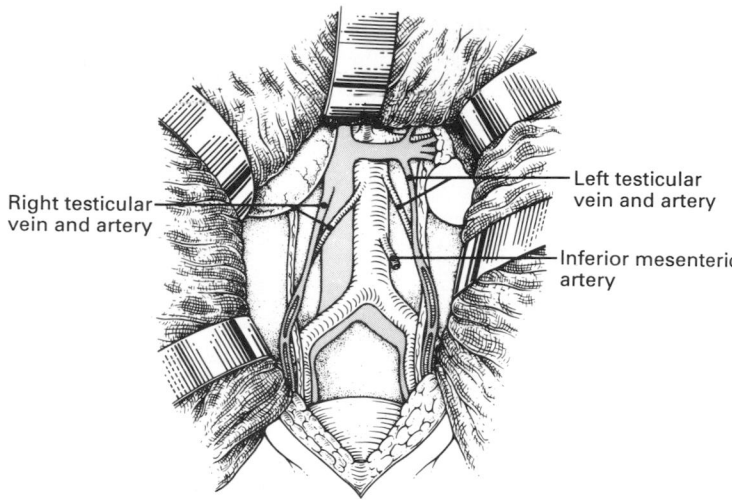

Fig. 9 Surgical field following paramedian incision.

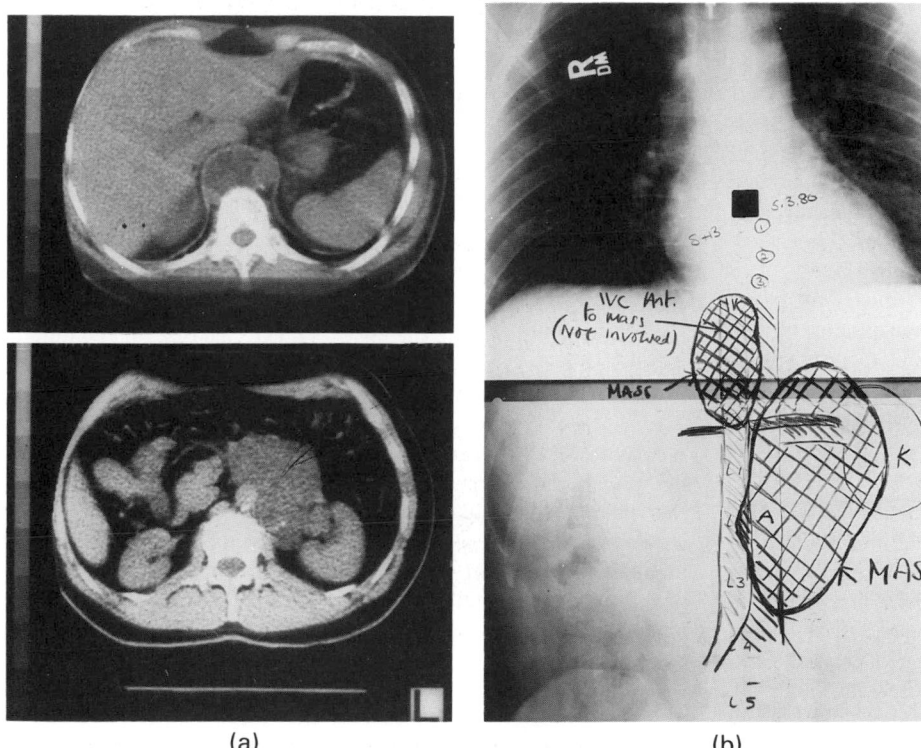

(a) (b)

Fig. 10 Retrocrural and para-aortic lymphadenopathy requiring a modified surgical approach (see text): (a) CT axial slices; (b) 'topogram' (see Fig. 7).

cases (Goldstraw 1991). The relation of the mass to the renal vessels is of paramount importance: irrespective of the size of the mass, a long midline incision provides excellent access below this level (Fig. 9). In our series a midline incision was used in 195 out of 231 cases. However, if retrocrural or mediastinal nodes are involved (Fig. 10), a thoracoabdominal incision is required, but the improved exposure is at the expense of poorer access to tumour lower down on the far side of the great vessels. Our present practice is to make a separate, staged approach to widespread disease rather than trying to do too much through one incision, which may provide suboptimal access to difficult areas of tumour. Two recent patients have undergone no less than four separate procedures before achieving macroscopic tumour clearance. The significance of leaving a little

differentiated teratoma behind is not clear, although there is evidence that this tissue is probably unstable (Logothetis *et al.* 1982; Loehrer *et al.* 1983) and our present belief is that every effort should be made to remove it to avoid the so-called growing teratoma syndrome (Jeffery *et al.* 1991).

The technical aspects of removal of these masses has been described by Hendry (1991) and the potential hazards are well documented (Donohue and Rowland 1981; Skinner *et al.* 1982). The problems encountered relate first to the size of the mass and, secondly to involvement of adjacent structures. Some correlation can be demonstrated between the size of the mass and the likelihood of cure (Fig. 11), although this is obviously less important than its histological composition. In 18 per cent of cases, adjacent structures

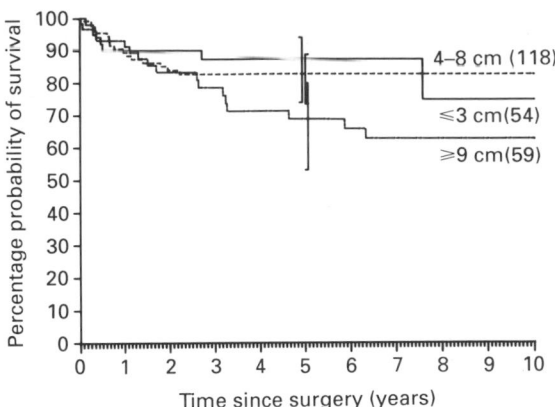

Fig. 11 Survival after post-chemotherapy lymphadenectomy showing the impact of the diameter of resected mass.

were involved: 29 kidneys had to be removed, most of which were poorly functioning, in seven cases the vena cava was invaded (no complications followed sleeve resection), the aorta or common iliac artery was involved in ten cases and arterial grafts had to be inserted, and the renal artery was damaged in one case in whom the contralateral kidney was hydronephrotic (this patient died 1 year later after regular dialysis and a failed kidney transplant). Two patients died post-operatively: one of respiratory failure after thoracoabdominal surgery and one of secondary haemorrhage 10 days after operation. Our immediate operative mortality of 0.9 per cent may be compared with 2 per cent recorded by Donohue and Rowland (1984) and 4 per cent (2/52) for similar cases described by Skinner *et al.* (1982) and by Kulkarni *et al.* (1991).

Forty (29 per cent) out of 138 patients who underwent para-aortic lymphadenectomy reported loss of ejaculation after operation. Analysis of these patients showed that this complication was most likely to occur when the residual para-aortic mass was very large or when it extended on both sides of the great vessels (Jones *et al.* 1993). These figures may be used as a basis for advising these patients on the likelihood of this complication, a medicolegal requirement that should always precede this type of surgery. Loss of ejaculation is probably caused by division of the sympathetic nerves on both sides of the great vessels or removal of the hypogastric plexus, which lies just below the bifurcation of the aorta (Leiter and Brendler 1967). Despite optimistic reports of return of ejaculation after the use of drugs such as ephedrine (Lynch and Maxted 1983) or imipramine (Nijman *et al.* 1982), we have had little success in treating this complication, which probably should be regarded as permanent. However, electroejaculation (Bennett *et al.* 1987) on insertion of a sperm reservoir (Brindley *et al.* 1986) may produce viable spermatozoa for artificial insemination.

SEMINOMA

Radiotherapy

Radiotherapy for stage I seminoma of the testis

Important features of seminoma are its exquisite radiosensitivity and the rarity with which the illness progresses beyond the retroperitoneal lymph nodes. These features have led to the traditional treatment of stage I testicular seminoma by orchidectomy followed by adjuvant nodal irradiation to a field encompassing para-aortic and ipsilateral pelvic nodes (Boden and Gibb 1951; Thomas *et al.* 1982; Hamilton *et al.* 1986; Zagars 1991).

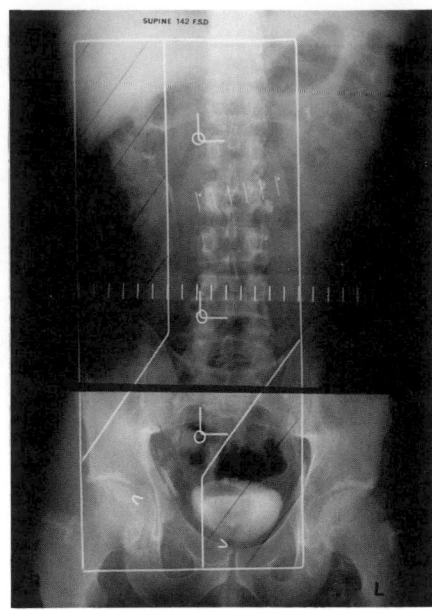

Fig. 12 Radiotherapy field for stage I seminoma.

Radiation field

The standard radiation volume is illustrated in Fig. 12 and extends from the lower border of the tenth dorsal vertebra superiorly encompassing the para-aortic region to include the widest lumbar transverse process and the ipsilateral renal hilum; in the pelvis the field is shaped to include the ipsilateral external iliac and common iliac lymph nodes and extends inferiorly to the level of the obturator foramen. There has been some controversy over whether the entire inguinal orchidectomy scar should be included, but as scar recurrence does not arise, it appears unnecessary to treat this area definitively though most of the scar would anyway be included in the field. The field is modified in patients with previous inguinoscrotal surgery because of the risk of metastasis to the inguinofemoral region. Additionally, it has been recommended that patients having scrotal surgery for their testicular tumour should have either hemiscrotectomy or hemiscrotal irradiation; the disadvantage of the latter is the scattered radiation to the contralateral testis. Data on surveillance of patients with this form of scrotal violation would suggest that local recurrence is very uncommon (Kennedy *et al.* 1985). A further indication for local treatment to the scrotum is the rare case of locally advanced tumour extending to the scrotal skin.

The Royal Marsden Hospital planning technique incorporates an intravenous urogram to delineate the position of the kidneys. Patients are treated by single parallel opposed anterior and posterior fields at 100 cm focus skin distance (FSD) and lying supine. The fields are shaped by blocks. Treatment is carried out on 6–8 MeV linear accelerators.

Dose

Despite a variety of techniques and doses, local failure within the field or field margin is exceptionally rare. In a compilation of series including 1765 patients, only two were reported to have failed in the irradiated volume (Zagars 1991); in one patient the total dose

Table 10 Radiotherapy alone in seminoma of testis (results Royal Marsden Hospital 1962–1983)

Stage	Era	No. of patients	% recurrence	% disease-specific survival	Reference
I	1962–1983	232	2	100	Hamilton *et al.* (1986)
II	1970–1984	A 28	11	95	Gregory and Peckham (1986)
		B 11	18	75	
		C 14	28		
III & IV	1963–1975	15	67	33	Peckham (1981)

was 15 Gy (Lester *et al.* 1986) and in the other it was 21 Gy in 22 fractions over 35 days (Dosoretz *et al.* 1981). The most common prescriptions lie between 25 Gy in 15 fractions and 30 Gy in 15–20 fractions over 3–4 weeks.

Results

As indicated previously, after careful staging and treatment with adjuvant radiotherapy, recurrence from stage I seminoma is uncommon (Table 10). A number of recent series have been reviewed by Zagars (1991). In five series of 1059 patients the recurrence rate was 3.6 per cent and the cause-specific mortality 1 per cent. Recurrences are equally distributed within supradiaphragmatic nodes and lung fields; relapse at other sites is rare. The great majority of recurrences can be salvaged, especially in recent years after the development of effective chemotherapy (see below).

Recurrences are too few for detailed prognostic analysis; however, it does seem clear that the histological subtype of seminoma, the local extent of the primary, and the production of human chorionic gonadotrophin by *in situ* trophoblastic cells are not of critical importance (Zagars and Babaian 1987).

Side-effects

Acute side-effects are uncommon and consist predominantly of a mild feeling of nausea lasting for 1–2 h and beginning soon after each fraction of treatment. In approximately 20 per cent of patients this may be more severe and associated with retching. Late gastrointestinal complications are also uncommon; however, an association between radiation and the development of peptic ulceration has been proposed (Hamilton *et al.* 1987; Coia and Hanks 1988; Fossa *et al.* 1989).

The impact of adjuvant radiotherapy on subsequent fertility depends upon the extent of the radiation field and the consequent scattered dose to the contralateral testis. With the standard technique the contralateral testis should receive less than 100 cGy and though temporary suppression of spermatogenesis may occur, in most patients this would have recovered within 2 years of treatment. Because of the theoretical risk of genetic damage, patients are counselled to avoid conception for 2 years after treatment. Finally, there is controversy over the carcinogenic potential of radiation and this is discussed more fully in the rationale for surveillance.

Surveillance for stage I seminoma

The conventional management of stage I seminoma by adjuvant radiotherapy is simple, effective, and established. The background to surveillance in this context includes the possibility of reducing treatment toxicity, the desirability of documenting the number of patients with clinical stage I seminoma who have subclinical metastases at presentation, and the availability of highly successful treatments for relapse with overt metastatic disease. Some of the

side-effects of adjuvant radiotherapy have been discussed above; the most worrisome is the risk that radiotherapy might lead to second malignancy. Hay *et al.* (1984) analysed second-cancer risk in 547 patients treated with radiotherapy for testicular tumours between 1950 and 1969. In five Scottish radiotherapy centres, two cases of leukaemia were observed (not significant); within the high-dose radiation volume 19 tumours were observed (expected 9.81; $p < 0.05$). The excess risk was confined to solid tumours of the genital, urinary, and gastrointestinal tracts and the peak time of these was 15–19 years after irradiation.

The South-West Thames Cancer Registry Study of 2013 patients registered between 1961 and 1980 found a relative risk of second malignancy of 0.7 (observed 27, expected 36). Two cases of leukaemia were observed (expected 0.8).

In a collaborative study among 11 population cancer registries, Kaldor *et al.* (1987) reported on 17 730 patients with testicular tumours registered between 1945 and 1984. Apart from tumours of the second testis there was an increased incidence of rectal cancer, connective tissue tumours, malignant melanomas, non-Hodgkin's lymphomas, and acute leukaemia. It must be emphasized that these patients were not treated with radiation alone. The evidence of second-tumour induction is suggestive and is supported by long-term follow-up of patients treated with radiotherapy for Hodgkin's disease. There would appear to be little excess risk within the first 10–15 years after treatment and also it seems clear that the excess risk after this time is small.

Surveillance policy

The policy is influenced by the absence of a sensitive serum tumour marker and by the relative slow natural history of the tumour. The Royal Marsden policy involves out-patient visits with tumour marker assays and chest radiograph every 2 months for the first year, every 3 months for the second year, every 4 months for the third year, every 6 months for the fourth year, and then annually. Abdominal CT scan or ultrasound is done every 6 months for the first 2 years and then annually until 5 years. The Princess Margaret Hospital policy involves more frequent abdominal CT scans (Thomas *et al.* 1989). In the early period of the surveillance investigation, patients were staged and monitored by lymphography; however, this was very rarely useful and has now been abandoned at the Royal Marsden Hospital.

To evaluate surveillance of stage I seminoma at the Royal Marsden Hospital, a cohort of 113 sequential patients with this tumour has been analysed (Duchesne *et al.* 1990). The median follow-up was 33 months (range 60–64 months). The probability of recurrence by 3 years was 14.9 per cent (95 per cent confidence intervals, 7.1 per cent). This is very similar to the results from a national Danish study (H. Von der Maase, personal communication), which was based on 274 patients, 43 of whom had relapsed. A low risk of recurrence was found in the Princess Margaret Hospital series (Thomas *et al.* 1989). Of 81 patients followed for 3–43 months (median 19 months) only three had relapsed, at 3, 5, and 18 months after orchidectomy. The predominant site of relapse was the para-aortic nodes and there is a suggestion that delayed treatment of these nodes may lead to a higher incidence of supradiaphragmatic metastasis. In the Royal Marsden series, 11 para-aortic node recurrences were treated with retroperitoneal irradiation in a two-phase treatment to a total dose of 35 Gy in 20 fractions over 4 weeks. Four of these patients relapsed in supradiaphragmatic lymph nodes and all have been successfully salvaged. In a recent update of the Princess Margaret Hospital study (G. M. Thomas, personal communication), six out of seven recurrences were in the retroperitoneal region and one in both retroperitoneum and mediastinum. In the Danish study, 41 out of 43 recurrences were confined to para-aortic nodes; all are currently in remission.

Recent reports have suggested that factors predicting recurrence may include vascular invasion (Horwich et al. 1992a), larger size of the primary tumour (Von der Maase et al. 1993), and older age (Warde et al. 1993). These three series comprise 512 patients and were in agreement that the actuarial 4–5 year risk of relapse was 80–82 per cent.

Conclusions

Though surveillance may avoid side-effects of radiation it should be appreciated that these side-effects are extremely uncommon and that surveillance may be time-consuming, prolonged, and stressful for both patient and physician. It is difficult to monitor the retroperitoneal nodes and a delay in treatment may lead to increased tumour stage. As the alternative management with adjuvant radiotherapy appears so effective, surveillance and other approaches should be regarded as research investigations rather than alternatives in management.

Radiotherapy for metastatic seminoma

As seminoma is highly responsive to radiotherapy and to platinum-based combination chemotherapy, there is some controversy in stage II disease over the optimal initial treatment. Furthermore, in patients with bulky seminomatous metastases treated with combination chemotherapy, a residual opacity is frequently detected on CT scan and radiotherapy may be considered for the adjuvant treatment of these masses.

Stage II seminoma

This encompasses a wide range of disease bulk and there is some evidence that recurrence after radiotherapy is related to the size of the abdominal mass (Gregory and Peckham 1986). Unfortunately an accurate delineation of retroperitoneal node size was difficult before the era of CT scanning. However, in the Royal Marsden series the relapse rate after radiotherapy was 28 per cent in patients with masses of more than 5 cm in diameter. In many centres this size criterion has been used to define the indication for initial chemotherapy, a further problem being the difficulty in irradiating large retroperitoneal masses without radiation damage to the kidneys. Other centres using careful CT-based planning techniques have reported successful irradiation of larger retroperitoneal masses of seminoma (Green et al. 1983).

The success of radiotherapy in various size categories of metastatic seminoma has been reviewed by Thomas (1991), who found in a cumulative series that, in 106 patients with stage II disease of less than 5 cm in diameter, the relapse rate was 8 per cent and

that the rate was similar in 48 patients with masses between 5 and 10 cm in diameter. The relapse rate rose to 35 per cent in 49 patients with abdominal masses of more than 10 cm in diameter.

The initial sites of relapse are commonly the supradiaphragmatic lymph nodes and the issue as to whether these patients should receive prophylactic mediastinal irradiation is controversial. Reports have not shown a survival benefit for this policy (Ball et al. 1982; Thomas et al. 1982; Herman et al. 1983; Evensen et al. 1985). Many centres are reluctant to extend the radiation field to the supradiaphragmatic region for fear of compromising bone-marrow reserve should chemotherapy be required. Furthermore, there is concern that more widespread radiation might predispose to second malignancies.

Chemotherapy for advanced seminoma

It is generally accepted that stage III and stage IV seminoma are treated with initial chemotherapy, but as previously discussed there is some controversy as to the optimum management for stage II disease. Most centres employ radiotherapy for small-volume abdominal lymphadenopathy up to 5 cm in diameter and use initial chemotherapy for abdominal masses of more than 10 cm in diameter. Some centres employ radiotherapy for masses between 5 and 10 cm in diameter (Thomas 1991). This requires careful, computer-based planning and a shrinking-field technique to avoid renal damage. The Royal Marsden policy is to use initial chemotherapy for stage IIc, stage III, and stage IV seminoma.

Development of chemotherapy for seminoma

Before the era of cisplatin, seminomas were widely treated with alkylating agents (Golbey 1970; Calman et al. 1979). Complete remissions were seen; however, they were predominantly of short duration. More recently, similar responses have been reported with ifosfamide (Schmoll 1989).

The combination chemotherapy of seminoma has derived from that employed for non-seminomatous testicular tumours. The combination of vinblastine and bleomycin was unsuccessful in seminoma; however, with bleomycin, cyclophosphamide, vincristine, methotrexate and 5-fluorouracil (Bleo-COMF), ten complete remissions were reported in 18 patients, five of these remissions being prolonged (Samuels et al. 1976, 1983).

The current era of chemotherapy for advanced seminoma

Cisplatin-based combination chemotherapy for testicular cancer was developed by Einhorn and Donohue (1977). An early report indicated that the combination of cisplatin, vinblastine, and bleomycin was strikingly effective in advanced seminoma (Einhorn and Williams 1980). A range of reports has indicated that 75–95 per cent of patients with cisplatin-based combination chemotherapy remained free from any evidence of disease progression (Friedman et al. 1985; Peckham et al. 1985; Stanton et al. 1985; Pizzocaro et al. 1986; Fossa et al. 1987; Clemm et al. 1989). Results of a number of series are illustrated in Table 11. It can be seen that the results from a multicentre review were inferior, with only 66 per cent survival in 60 treated patients (Loehrer et al. 1987). This is likely to be a consequence of less-selective patient entry. Results in Table 11 are presented more in terms of progression-free survival than in terms of remission rates. A particular problem with judging remission in advanced bulky seminoma is the probability that there will be a residual mass at the site of the previous bulky disease

Table 11 Chemotherapy for advanced seminoma

Reference	Drug(s)	No. of patients	Continuous disease-free survival (%)	Survival (%)
Peckham et al. (1985)	PVB or BEP	39	90	92
Stanton et al. (1985)	VAB-6 EP	30	80	80
Friedman et al. (1985)	PVB or EP	20	65	70
Fossa et al. (1987)	PVB or BEP	55	78	78
Loehrer et al. (1987)	PVB+A or BEP	62	60	63
Logothetis et al. (1987)	Cy+P	42	92	92
Horwich et al. (1989b)	Ca	33	79	91
Oliver (1988)	P	27	77	85
Clemm et al. (1989)	VIP	24	83	87
Mencel et al. (1994)	VAB-6, EP or ECa	142	85	88

The drug abbreviations are explained in the text.

(Peckham et al. 1985; Horwich et al. 1989b; Fossa 1991). It has been claimed that residual masses of more than 3.5 cm in diameter are more likely to contain residual seminoma (Motzer et al. 1988). Other reports have not confirmed that recurrences are more common from residual masses than from complete remission (Horwich et al. 1989b; Schultz et al. 1989).

Such is the activity of platinum drugs in this disease that it has been suggested that single-agent therapy may be as effective as combination chemotherapy. The impetus for this direction of chemotherapy research came from the MD Anderson Hospital, where Samuels and colleagues reported long-term experience of the combination of cisplatin and cyclophosphamide in advanced disease (Samuels and Logothetis 1983; Logothetis et al. 1986). These reports included eight patients treated with cisplatin alone by a weekly infusion of 100 mg/m^2; all eight were treated successfully. This experience was confirmed by Oliver et al. (1990), who reported 22 patients followed for a median of 4 years in whom the continuous disease-free survival was 82 per cent.

More recently, single-agent carboplatin has been evaluated at the Royal Marsden Hospital. Patients were treated once every 3 or 4 weeks at a dose of 400 mg/m^2, with dose modifications for patients with abnormal renal function (Horwich et al. 1989b). After treatment with single-agent carboplatin, 82 per cent of 33 patients with a minimum of 12 months' follow-up remain continuously disease free. With single-agent therapies, relapses appeared more common in those who had previously been treated with radiotherapy and then relapsed before treatment with chemotherapy. Salvage of the patients who relapsed on carboplatin was particularly effective, with five out of the six relapsing patients achieving long-term remission with intensive bleomycin, vincristine, and cisplatin (Horwich et al. 1989a). The actuarial survival of the group was 94 per cent at 2 years. A multicentre study from Germany has subsequently confirmed the activity of single-agent carboplatin (Schmoll et al. 1991). A current randomized MRC trial is prospectively comparing single-agent carboplatin with the combination of etoposide and cisplatin in patients with advanced seminoma. In the meantime cisplatin-based combination chemotherapy should be regarded as standard.

Adjuvant radiotherapy following chemotherapy

The role of adjuvant radiotherapy to sites of original bulk disease has not been established. It is a logical treatment to consider as

10–20 per cent of patients relapse after chemotherapy and the predominant pattern of initial relapse is in the same or an adjacent nodal group as was previously involved with bulk disease. Also, the extreme radiosensitivity of seminoma allows adjuvant treatment to be carried out with relatively little morbidity. Paradoxically, it is easier to argue for adjuvant radiotherapy to follow chemotherapy in stage II seminoma than in more advanced stages, as adjuvant radiotherapy for stage III disease involves extensive irradiation of the bone-marrow. In some centres, adjuvant radiotherapy after chemotherapy is used routinely (Fossa et al. 1987), but there is as yet no evidence that this approach improves survival. There is no doubt that single-agent carboplatin is a treatment of particularly low toxicity and one study has suggested that adjuvant radiotherapy will reduce the recurrence rate in this context (Horwich et al. 1992b). A full discussion of the toxicity of chemotherapy of germ cell tumours is included in the section on chemotherapy of non-seminomatous tumours.

Non-seminomatous testicular tumours

Management of stage I non-seminoma

Treatment options for stage I non-seminoma include:

(1) surveillance, with chemotherapy reserved for patients who relapse;

(2) retroperitoneal lymph node dissection followed by surveillance;

(3) retroperitoneal lymph node dissection with adjuvant chemotherapy for node-positive patients;

(4) immediate adjuvant radiotherapy to retroperitoneal lymph nodes;

(5) immediate adjuvant chemotherapy.

Until 10 years ago the standard approach in the United Kingdom was to employ adjuvant radiotherapy (Peckham 1971), whereas in the United States and in a number of European countries, treatment was with retroperitoneal lymph node dissection as discussed above. In the last decade these approaches have been challenged by the policy of surveillance. This is a particularly unusual approach in oncology, allowing as it does the tumour to progress to overt relapse and it is only feasible because of the efficacy of chemotherapy in small-volume, metastatic, non-seminomatous tumours.

The surveillance protocol

Surveillance was first investigated at the Royal Marsden Hospital (Peckham 1981). It is important that it be followed as an active protocol rather than be regarded as a policy of clinical neglect. It is necessary to diagnose recurrence as sensitively as possible in order to ensure the efficacy of salvage chemotherapy. The policy is based on regular monitoring by physical examination, radiological investigation, and tumour marker assay, especially of α-fetoprotein and human chorionic gonadotrophin. A current surveillance policy is illustrated in Fig. 13. It can be seen that patients are assessed each month in the first year after orchidectomy and every 2 months in the second year. When surveillance was first investigated, CT scanning was more frequent; it now appears unnecessary to repeat the CT scan of thorax and abdomen more often than every 3 months in the first year after orchidectomy, with a further scan at the end of the second and third years.

TESTICULAR TUMOURS
Teratoma stage I surveillance

Month:	0	1	2	3	4	5	6	7	8	9	10	11	12
OPD		+		+		+		+		+		+	
Markers		+	+	+	+	+	+	+	+	+	+	+	+
CXR		+	+	+	+	+	+	+	+	+	+	+	+
CT chest and abdomen				+			+			+			+

Year 2   OPD q 3/12 (if originally marker negative, CT abdomen @ 24/12)

Year 3   OPD q 4/12

Year 4   OPD q 6/12

Then annually

Teratoma post-chemotherapy F/U

Year 1   q 2/12

Year 2   q 3/12

Year 3   q 6/12

Then annually

Fig. 13 Surveillance protocol for stage I teratoma.

The earlier reports from the Royal Marsden Hospital indicated that the policy was practical and safe (Peckham *et al.* (1982). Twenty-six per cent of patients relapsed, but in the first 199 patients managed by surveillance, only one patient was not successfully cured with chemotherapy. The early pattern of relapse is demonstrated in Fig. 14 (Horwich and Peckham 1988). An analysis of presentation factors revealed that patients with stage I non-seminoma who had lymphatic or vascular invasion within the primary tumour were at higher risk of recurrence (Hoskin *et al.* 1986). This form of analysis raised the possibility that some patients with a particularly high risk of recurrence might better be treated by immediate adjuvant chemotherapy.

The MRC Testicular Tumour Working Party undertook a coordinated investigation of surveillance in two trials. The first was a retrospective analysis of data accumulated from six centres in the United Kingdom and incorporated the early series from the Royal Marsden Hospital (Peckham *et al.* 1982) and from the Christie Hospital in Manchester (Read 1987). Two hundred and fifty-nine patients registered between 1979 and 1983 were analysed (Freedman *et al.* 1987); the median follow-up of this group is now 54 months and 90 per cent of the cases have been followed for more than 2 years. Seventy patients (27 per cent) relapsed, predominantly in the first year after orchidectomy. After 18 months the risk of relapse decreased to 4 per cent per year. The relapse-free rate at 4 years was 68 per cent (95 per cent confidence intervals, 60–75 per cent). Despite the early era of this investigation and the number of centres involved, the great majority of recurrences were detected with small-volume disease; only three recurrences were with nodal disease of more than 5 cm in diameter and only two were with what the MRC classifies as very large-volume disease, one with multiple, large, lung metastases and one with liver and brain metastases. Detailed multivariate analysis of presentation and histological variables identified four factors independently predictive of relapse: (i) lymphatic invasion, (ii) vascular invasion, (iii) undifferentiated

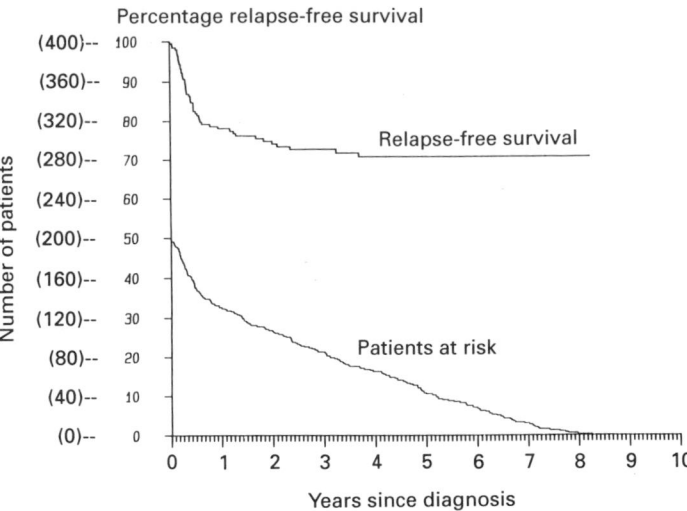

Fig. 14 Relapse-free survival after surveillance of 199 patients with clinical stage I teratoma (Royal Marsden Hospital 1979–1988).

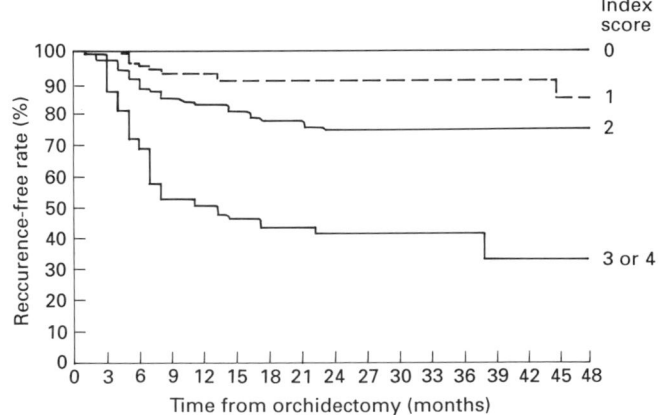

Fig. 15 Relapse-free survival relative to the number of histological risk factors in clinical stage I teratoma managed by surveillance (after Freedman *et al.* 1987).

cells, (iv) absence of yolk sac elements. Figure 15 shows the relapse-free survival curve based on the number of these factors present in the individual tumour. The small group of patients with none of these risk factors was composed of patients with teratoma differentiated together with a small group of patients with malignant teratoma entirely composed of yolk sac elements. None relapsed. For patients with either three or four risk factors the relapse-free rate at 2 years was only 42 per cent. This high-risk group comprised 21.2 per cent of the patients and a recent MRC study has investigated two courses of adjuvant combination chemotherapy for these patients and has shown a very low recurrence rate (Cullen *et al.* 1992).

After this retrospective surveillance study, the MRC initiated a prospective study involving 16 United Kingdom centres and one Norwegian centre in order to independently validate the prognostic index. This study was made between 1984 and 1987 and included 373 patients followed for a median of 37 months. The 2 year, relapse-free rate was 75 per cent (95 per cent confidence interval, 71–79 per cent). Of the 100 patients who have relapsed, two have died and two are alive with active disease. Three patients died of

Table 12 Chemotherapy regimens for testicular tumours

BEP

Cisplatin	20 mg/m²/day	Days 1–5
Etoposide	120 mg/m²/day	Days 1–3
Bleomycin	30 mg	Days 2, 8, 15

(In USA, etoposide given at 100 mg/m²/day, days 1–5)
Repeat every 21 days for four courses

VAB-6

Vinblastine	4 mg/m²	Day 1
Cyclophosphamide	600 mg/m²	Day 1
Acintomycin D	1 mg/m²	Day 1
Bleomycin	30 u	Day 1
Bleomycin	20 u/m²	Days 1–3 by continuous infusion
Cisplatin	120 mg/m²	Day 4

Repeat every 4 weeks for 3 months
No bleomycin on third cycle

unrelated intercurrent causes and the overall 4 year survival rate was 98 per cent. The previously defined prognostic index was evaluated, the high-risk group (three or four risk factors) showing a 3 year relapse-free survival rate of 50 per cent.

The conclusion from these studies was that surveillance for clinical stage I non-seminoma appeared to be a practicable and safe method of management, offering a survival probability equivalent to other treatments. A Danish National trial randomized stage I patients between surveillance and adjuvant radiotherapy (Roth 1987). The radiation was given to para-aortic and ipsilateral pelvic nodes to a dose of 40 Gy in 20 fractions over 4 weeks. This dose prevented abdominal relapse and, thus, dramatically reduced the overall relapse rate. However, there was no survival difference.

The problem with surveillance is that some patients find the persisting threat of relapse stressful (Moynihan 1987). Also, the policy requires regular and reliable follow-up with appropriate facilities for CT scanning and tumour marker assay. Just over one-quarter of patients are treated with combination chemotherapy; however, fewer than 10 per cent require lymphadenectomy (for residual masses post-chemotherapy) and, thus, long-term sexual problems are rare.

Immediate adjuvant chemotherapy

This approach can be considered in stage I non-seminoma following orchidectomy in most patients with a particularly high risk of relapse. The MRC studies of surveillance described above would suggest that patients with three or four of the unknown independent risk factors for recurrence would have, overall, at least a 50 per cent chance of recurrence and it is therefore appropriate to offer adjuvant treatment to this group. An MRC study has investigated the use of two cycles of chemotherapy in this early setting, based upon the report from the Testicular Cancer Intergroup study (Williams *et al.* 1987*b*), in which patients found to have involvement of abdominal nodes following retroperitoneal dissection were randomized between two courses of chemotherapy (mainly cisplatin, vinblastine and bleomycin) or to no further treatment. In this trial of 195 patients, the recurrence rate in the 'no further treatment' group was 49 per cent. In the adjuvant chemotherapy arm there were six recurrences, but five of these were before any chemotherapy had been given. It thus appears that two cycles of chemotherapy are sufficient to sterilize subclinical extents of metastatic non-seminoma

and this has been supported by early results in clinical stage I patients (Cullen *et al.* 1992).

Metastatic non-seminoma

The chemotherapy of non-seminomatous germ cell tumours represents one of the most exciting and successful stories in modern oncology. Before 1975 the cure rate of bulky abdominal or more advanced metastatic disease was under 10 per cent and this has risen to between 80 and 90 per cent on current management. Historically the major advances in the development of combination chemotherapy were the combinations based on vinblastine and bleomycin developed by Samuels *et al.* (1976) and subsequently the incorporation of high doses of cisplatin into the platinum, vinblastine, and bleomycin (**PVB**) schedule by Einhorn and Donohue (1977). Nichols and Roth (1991) have reviewed the historical development of this field, including the modifications of the PVB regimen evaluated by the Indiana University Group and the sequence of **VAB** (vincristine, actinomycin D, and bleomycin) regimens investigated at the Memorial Sloan-Kettering Hospital. Currently the most widely used combinations and bleomycin, etoposide, and cisplatin (**BEP**) (Peckham *et al.* 1983; Williams *et al.* 1987*b*) and the VAB-6 regimen (Vugrin *et al.* 1983; Bosl *et al.* 1986). These schedules are illustrated in Table 12.

It is now more than a decade since the introduction of the PVB regimen and sufficient long-term results of chemotherapy have been reported to indicate the likelihood that long-term remission can be equated with cure (Peckham *et al.* 1988; Roth *et al.* 1988; Hitchins *et al.* 1989).

From these and other reports it is clear that a large proportion of patients with small-volume, metastatic, non-seminomatous germ cell tumours are cured with chemotherapy. It is important to recognize this group and to minimize treatment side-effects. In patients with small volume stage II disease there is controversy over whether to treat with primary chemotherapy or with node dissection (Horwich *et al.* 1994*b*). Patients with more advanced presentations have gained from advances in chemotherapy techniques (Williams *et al.* 1987*b*; Peckham *et al.* 1988) and from a better understanding of the role of post-chemotherapy surgery for residual masses (Donohue *et al.* 1982; MRC Working Party 1985; Hendry *et al.* 1987). However, as some 10–20 per cent of patients with metastatic non-seminomatous tumour still die of their malignant disease, a current challenge is to increase the efficacy of chemotherapy. It is logical to divide patients with metastatic non-seminoma into good and poor prognostic groups for 'risk-related' chemotherapy (Horwich 1989). The exact definition of these groups varies in different centres and depends upon the treatment being employed. For example, centres exploring high-dose chemotherapy and bone-marrow transplantation for an adverse subgroup would tend to have a very rigorous definition of adverse subgroup, considering this approach only for patients whose prognosis on conventional treatment would be very poor. For those centres where the adverse subgroup is treated by less toxic schedules the definition of adverse is more broad, as the approach is relevant to those whose prognosis is moderate as well as those whose prognosis is very poor. For example, the MRC Testicular Tumour Working Party has based its designation of prognostic groups on a prognostic-factor analysis of 795 patients treated with chemotherapy between 1982 and 1986. Multivariate analysis of survival revealed that the significant adverse features at presentation are the presence of 20 or more lung metastases, high serum markers (defined either as human chorionic gonadotrophin $> 10^4$ iu/l or α-fetoprotein $> 10^3$/iu/l), the presence of a mediastinal mass of more than 5 cm in diameter, or the presence of liver, bone, or brain involvement. The presence of any one of those features implied a 3 year survival of 68 per cent, whereas if none was present 3 year survival was 94 per cent (Mead *et al.* 1992).

With better understanding of tumour biology these simple assessments of tumour bulk can be supplemented by measurements of tumour proliferation (Sledge *et al.* 1988; Price *et al.* 1990*a*) or by characterization of extent of chromosome abnormality (Bosl *et al.* 1989*b*) or oncogene expression (Watson *et al.* 1986).

Chemotherapy for the poor-prognosis subgroup

The era of modern chemotherapy for metastatic non-seminoma was heralded by the reports of Einhorn and his colleagues on the efficacy of the cisplatin, vinblastine, and bleomycin combination (PVB) (Einhorn and Donohue 1977; Einhorn and Williams 1980). Four courses of chemotherapy were employed on a 3 week cycle time. Prospective, randomized studies did not demonstrate any benefit from additional adriamycin (Einhorn and Williams 1980) or from maintenance vinblastine (Einhorn *et al.* 1981). There is, however, good evidence that the substitution of etoposide for vinblastine (Peckham *et al.* 1983) is more effective than PVB in advanced disease. Pizzocaro *et al.* (1985) reported excellent results of BEP chemotherapy in 40 patients with advance bulky disease and Williams *et al.* (1987*a*) reported a prospective, randomized comparison of PVB and BEP, in which patients with advanced disease on the Indiana University staging system had a 2 year survival probability after BEP of 76 per cent versus 48 per cent with PVB ($p < 0.05$).

The second approach to improving chemotherapy has been the investigation of dose escalation. It has been shown that doses less than the standard 100 mg/m^2 of cisplatin every 3 weeks are disadvantageous (Samson *et al.* 1984). As the renal toxicity of high-dose cisplatin can be mitigated by hypertonic saline hydration (Ozols *et al.* 1984), this drug has been tested at double the usual dose, i.e. 200 mg/m^2 per course. Severe toxicity has been demonstrated (Daugaard and Rorth 1986; Ozols *et al.* 1988). There have been two prospective, randomized trials of double-dose cisplatin. The first from the National Cancer Institute (Ozols *et al.* 1988) assessed high-dose cisplatin combined with etoposide, vinblastine, and bleomycin (**PVeBV**) and the regimen was compared with PVB in the poor-risk patients. Only 52 patients were randomized and the median follow-up at time of reporting was 4 years. The complete remission rate was 88 per cent with PVeBV versus 67 per cent with PVB and also relapse was less common; however, the intensive treatment was also very toxic, 91 per cent of patients had nadir total white counts of less than 1×10^9/l and 88 per cent had neutropenic sepsis. Furthermore, ototoxicity was severe, with 12 patients requiring hearing aids; also there was severe peripheral neuropathy. The interpretation of the high-dose component of treatment was compromised, as this arm also contained etoposide; this has been previously shown to improve results in advanced disease (Williams *et al.* 1987*a*). The second prospective trial of high-dose cisplatin reported by Nichols *et al.* (1991*b*) was rigorously designed and the two arms of the trial differed only in respect of the dose of cisplatin, namely 100 mg/m^2 per course versus 200 mg/m^2 per course. The trial was carried out in patients classified as advanced on the Indiana University system (Nichols *et al.* 1991*a*). One hundred and fifty-nine patients entered the randomized trial and were evaluable and the median follow-up of these patients was 24 months. Sixty-eight per cent of patients on the high-dose platinum arm became free

of disease, compared to 73 per cent of those on conventional dose. With the high-dose therapy, 74 per cent were alive and 63 per cent continuously free of disease, whereas on conventional dose 74 per cent were alive and 61 per cent continuously disease free. The essential conclusion was that doubling the dose of cisplatin did not contribute to improving the therapeutic efficacy of the BEP regimen.

Dose escalation has been investigated further in the context of autologous bone-marrow-transplant support (Ahlgren *et al.* 1988; Mulder *et al.* 1988; Nichols *et al.* 1989; Broun *et al.* 1992). The most extensive investigation was by the Indianapolis and Vanderbilt University groups and involves the dose-escalation and phase-2 study of combined high-dose carboplatin and high-dose etoposide. The dose-escalation study defined the appropriate doses for phase-2 evaluation in patients with relapsed germ cell tumours as etoposide 1200 mg/m^2 and carboplatin 1500 mg/m^2, each dose divided into three injections on days -7, -5, and -3 with marrow infusion on day 0 (Nichols *et al.* 1989). There is provision for repeating this treatment in patients who responded. Thirty-three patients were treated altogether; 20 at the phase-2 dose were given 31 courses of treatment. Myelosuppression was severe at all doses with a median time to granulocyte counts of more than 0.5×10^9/l of 24 days after the marrow infusion and a median time to a platelet count of more than 50×10^9/l of 26 days. All patients had granulocytopenic fevers with each course and seven died of treatment, five from granulocytopenic infection and two from thrombocytopenic haemorrhage. Other toxic effects included hypomagnesaemia, pancreatitis, stomatitis, nausea, vomiting, and alopecia, there was no clinically significant hearing loss, and decline of renal function was uncommon and usually associated with a pre-terminal syndrome. Eight out of 32 evaluable patients achieved a complete remission, six a partial remission, with four patients remaining in continuous complete remission at the time of reporting, three of them being disease free for more than 1 year. As all patients in this study had failed or were refractory to a cisplatin-based conventional regimen and have been deemed incurable with standard chemotherapy, the efficacy of high-dose treatments was felt to be encouraging and the study continues (Broun *et al.* 1992). The approach is also being explored by other groups (Barnett *et al.* 1991; Siegert *et al.* 1991).

A different approach to treatment intensification has been the reduction of the interval between cycles of chemotherapy, as delay appears to be an adverse prognostic factor (Peckham *et al.* 1985; Crawford *et al.* 1989). Wettlaufer (1984) demonstrated tolerance of a 7-day cycle of a PVB (platinum, vincristine, and bleomycin) regimen and this experience has been extended in high-risk patients (Daniels *et al.* 1987; Murray *et al.* 1987; Horwich *et al.* 1989*a*). The Royal Marsden Study employed four cycles of PVB at 7 day intervals followed by three cycles of conventional BEP; the initial analysis revealed that 82 per cent of the 29 treated patients remained free from progressive disease after a median follow-up of 2 years (Horwich *et al.* 1989*a*). To date, 61 patients have been treated with intensive induction chemotherapy for adverse presentations of metastatic non-seminoma at the Royal Marsden. Nineteen of the 57 evaluable patients (32 per cent) had complete remission with chemotherapy alone and a further 20 (34 per cent) following resection of residual masses. There have been only two recurrences in the 39 patients entering complete remission. Currently, 71 per cent of patients are alive and disease free (Dearnaley 1991). The major toxicity was myelosuppression and two patients died from sepsis during the first month of chemotherapy; another two patients died of bleomycin lung toxicity.

A further approach to improving efficacy has been the use of alternating regimens (Logothetis *et al.* 1985; Newlands *et al.* 1986).

Table 13 CEB chemotherapy regimen (see text) in good-prognosis non-seminomatous germ cell tumour (Royal Marsden Hospital, 1984–1988)

	n	%
Patients	76	
Follow-up (months)		
Range	6–54	
Median	24	
Complete remission	72	95
Relapse after chemotherapy	1	
Toxic deaths	1	
Cause-specific survival		98.5

POMB/ACE involving cisplatin, vincristine, methotrexate, bleomycin, actinomycin D, cyclophosphamide, and etoposide was developed in the Charing Cross Hospital in 1977 and was reported to be effective in adverse subgroups of patients. This has been investigated independently by Cullen *et al.* (1988), who also found it to be effective in adverse subgroups. Hitchins *et al.* (1989) reported on 237 consecutive patients treated with POMB/ACE. In this study the first 31 patients were treated less intensively and were excluded; 193 of the remaining 206 patients were assessable. A number of prognostic classifications were compared and the best discriminator of survival was the group with either a serum α-fetoprotein of more than 5000 ku/l or a serum human chorionic gonadotrophin of more than 50 000 iu/l. In patients with lower markers there was a 95 per cent 5 year survival compared to 78 per cent in those with high markers.

Logothetis *et al.* (1985) also report excellent results with an alternating regimen of CISCA (adriamycin, cyclophosphamide, and cisplatin) and VB-4 (vinblastine and bleomycin), with complete remission in 44 out of 48 patients. Myelosuppressive complications were common, with infections after 45 per cent of chemotherapy courses. On the other hand, the Memorial Sloan-Kettering Cancer Centre study of alternating EP/VAB-6 (Bosl *et al.* 1987) did not suggest any benefit from alternation and the EORTC randomized trial showed alternating BEP and PVB to be no better than BEP (Stoter *et al.* 1986). Nevertheless, these approaches are promising and merit prospective evaluation using the more intensive alternating regimens. The VIP (etoposide, ifosfamide, and cisplatin) regimen is equivalent in efficacy to BEP (Stoter *et al.* 1993) and the alternating BOP–VIP-B approach (Lewis *et al.* 1991) has been investigated in a MRC/EORTC trial to be analysed at the end of 1994. The C-BOP–BEP regimen has performed well in adverse patients in a pilot study (Horwich *et al.* 1993) and will be tested in an EORTC multicentre pilot in 1994 and 1995.

Chemotherapy of good-prognosis patients

The major life-threatening complications of the drug regimens employed for germ cell tumours include myelosuppression and bleomycin-induced penumonitis. Some long-term side-effects may have their full impact years after completion of treatment and these include the renal damage and ototoxicity due to cisplatin (Daugaard *et al.* 1988; Hamilton *et al.* 1989) and Raynaud's phenomenon due to bleomycin (Roth *et al.* 1988). Amongst the attempts to reduce the toxicity of chemotherapy are reduction of drug dose, reductions in the number of drugs in the schedule, and the use of less toxic drugs or drug analogues. There has also been a careful study of maintenance chemotherapy and the total number of induction courses required.

An early, prospective, randomized trial from Indiana University addressed the question of vinblastine dosage in the PVB schedule and found that the lower dose of 0.3 mg/kg/course was equivalent to 0.4 mg/kg (Einhorn and Williams 1980). This has been confirmed in a large EORTC trial (Stoter and Denis 1985). On the other hand, dose reduction of cisplatin (Samson *et al.* 1984) and of etoposide (Brada *et al.* 1987) may compromise treatment efficacy. Total drug dosage can also be reduced by avoiding maintenance chemotherapy (Einhorn *et al.* 1981) or by reducing the total number of induction courses. Thus, there was no difference in the prospective randomized comparison of three versus four courses of BEP chemotherapy (Einhorn *et al.* 1989).

The life-threatening lung toxicity of bleomycin has led to a number of studies exploring the deletion of this drug. An early pilot study from the Royal Marsden Hospital suggested that dose compromise of bleomycin would impair treatment efficacy (Brada *et al.* 1987); however, reports of three trials have now shown a significant reduction in the number of patients free from disease on follow-up (Levi *et al.* 1986; Stoter 1987; Bosl *et al.* 1988). Further follow-up from these trials is required before the need for bleomycin can be evaluated fully though it is clearly needed if only three cycles of chemotherapy are employed (Loehrer *et al.* 1991).

Much of the toxicity of cisplatin can be avoided by the use of the analogue carboplatin (Calvert *et al.* 1985), which does not cause significant renal toxicity, neurotoxicity, or ototoxicity. The drug is more myelosuppressive than cisplatin and optimal dosage is based on assessment of renal function (Calvert *et al.* 1985). A pilot study at the Royal Marsden Hospital has investigated the combination of carboplatin, etoposide, and bleomycin (**CEB**) in good-prognosis patients (Table 13). Its activity appears comparable with cisplatin in combination and these regimens formed the basis of two prospective randomized trials: BEP against CEB which was undertaken jointly by the MRC and EORTC and CE versus PE, coordinated by the Memorial Sloan-Kettering Cancer Centre and the Southwestern Oncology Group (Bajorin *et al.* 1991). Both have found the carboplatin-based regimen to be inferior in activity (Bajorin *et al.* 1993; Horwich *et al.* 1994a).

The studies of the reduction of treatment toxicity are particularly important in view of the good prognosis and young age of patients with non-seminomatous tumours. However, it is important to ensure there is no associated compromise of antitumour effect, as even in good-prognosis subgroups the risk of the patients dying from progressive malignant disease is higher than the risk of dying from treatment toxicity.

Brain metastases

The treatment of brain metastases presents a particular problem because of the possibility of drug access being limited by the blood–brain barrier. They are rare at presentation and were detected in only 17 out of 746 patients (2 per cent) in the MRC prognostic factor analysis of patients with metastatic non-seminoma (Mead *et al.* 1992). They occur at presentation almost exclusively in the context of metastatic trophoblastic teratoma presenting with multiple lung metastases and a high serum chorionic gonadotrophin (Lester *et al.* 1984; Rustin *et al.* 1986; Andreyev *et al.* 1993). Relapse in brain metastases is occasionally an isolated event but more commonly is part of disease dissemination.

Presentation with central nervous involvement is an indicator of poor prognosis. In the MRC analysis the 3 year survival of 17 patients with such involvement was 38 per cent compared with 86 per cent in 729 patients without involvement.

(a)

(b)

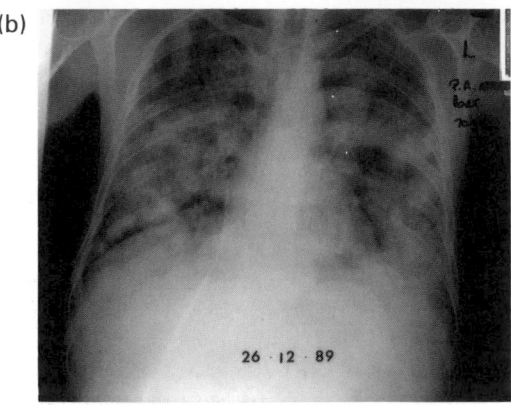

Fig. 16 (a) and (b) Tumour flare after chemotherapy.

Treatment of brain metastases

Lester *et al.* (1984) reported a treatment based on standard PVB followed by whole-brain radiotherapy, usually to a dose of 50 Gy in 25 fractions. Patients with isolated relapse in the central nervous system and maintained systemic remission had surgical excision of metastatic disease when feasible. Survival at the time of analysis was reported in four out of five patients who presented initially with brain metastases and three out of five developing an isolated relapse after systemic remission. There are no survivors amongst 12 patients with associated systemic relapse after chemotherapy. Logothetis *et al.* (1982), also using chemotherapy and radiotherapy, reported the better prognosis of patients with single brain lesions, with four out of six surviving compared to no survivors in patients with multiple lesions.

Raghavan *et al.* (1987) reported on four patients managed by an approach including surgery, radiotherapy, and cisplatin-based chemotherapy; there were two long-term survivors. Rustin *et al.* (1986) reported on 12 patients presenting with brain metastases and it is particularly interesting that these patients were treated with chemotherapy alone with excellent results. The chemotherapy consisted basically of the POMB/ACE regimen (Newlands *et al.* 1983), modified by changing the intravenous methotrexate to a dose of 1 g/m², given as a 24 h infusion followed 32 h after the start of methotrexate with folinic acid and also modified by the incorporation of intrathecal methotrexate with each course of ACE. Nine of the 12 patients were alive at the time of analysis 12–63 months after diagnosis.

The Charing Cross experience would suggest that adjuvant cranial irradiation following POMB/ACE chemotherapy is unnecessary for patients presenting with brain metastases. For patients who relapse

after previous chemotherapy, this level of chemosensitivity should not be assumed and it remains appropriate to consider excision and radiotherapy if the relapse appears restricted to one or two brain deposits.

Tumour flare

Occasionally there is a transient exacerbation of symptoms and signs from metastatic non-seminoma which immediately follows the start of chemotherapy and this is of critical importance when the extent of metastatic disease threatens all in failure. In practice this is very uncommon and mainly of concern in the patient with multiple lung metastases to the extent that dyspnoea is caused before the start of chemotherapy. In this situation, rapid deterioration can occur within a few days of starting chemotherapy (Fig. 16). These patients should only be treated where facilities are available for resuscitation and respiratory support by artificial ventilation.

Chemotherapy side-effects

As with other drug combinations the toxicity of chemotherapy for germ cell tumour represents a summation of the side-effects of whichever individual drugs are employed. The particular features of chemotherapy for germ cell tumour are the relatively high doses of cisplatin and bleomycin that are frequently employed. At the same time the excellent prognosis of patients treated with these drugs heightens issues of long-term toxicity. Second cancers were discussed in general but elsewhere there is particular concern over leukaemia after etoposide (Nichols *et al.* 1993).

Cisplatin

Though cisplatin is only of moderate bone-marrow toxicity it nevertheless represents, in the doses used for germ cell tumours, one of the most toxic cytotoxic agents in use. The major subjective toxicity is severe nausea and vomiting, though this can be considerably ameliorated by recent anti-emetic developments such as high-dose metoclopramide (Gralla *et al.* 1981), combinations of dexamethasone and metoclopramide (Kris 1989), or 5-hydroxy-tryptamine type 3 (Einhorn 1990) antagonists. The addition of lorazepam is said to reduce the problem of anticipatory nausea and vomiting and dexamethasone of delayed nausea.

Neurotoxicity of cisplatin causes peripheral numbness, especially severe in the soles of the feet and is associated with loss of vibration sense (Mollman 1990). Ototoxicity may be manifested by tinnitus or high-tone hearing loss, though it is rarely symptomatic at conventional dosage. Neurotoxicity is particularly severe if cisplatin is administered at double dose (200 mg/m²) per course (Ozols *et al.* 1988). The renal toxicity of cisplatin is reduced considerably by forced hydration and diuresis (Hayes *et al.* 1977). At standard doses of 100 mg/m² per course ×4 courses, patients lose a mean of 25 per cent of their glomerular filtration and it appears that this lesion does not recover after completion of chemotherapy (Hansen *et al.* 1988; Hamilton *et al.* 1989).

The toxicity of cisplatin has led to the development of an analogue carboplatin, which at standard dosage does not appear to cause neurotoxicity, renal toxicity, or severe gastrointestinal toxicity (Calvert *et al.* 1985; Horwich *et al.* 1989b, 1991; Mason *et al.* 1991). It is, however, more bone-marrow suppressive than cisplatin.

Bleomycin

This antibiotic has an unusual pattern of toxicity rarely affecting bone-marrow but causing skin rashes and pigmentation, pneumonitis,

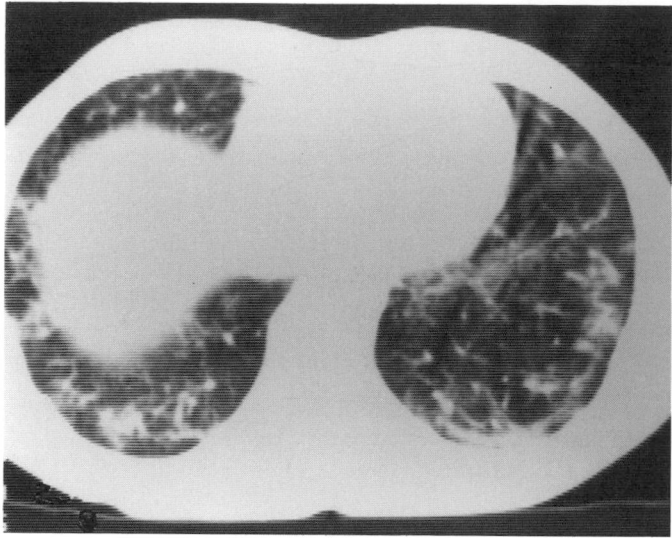

Fig. 17 CT scan illustrating bleomycin-induced lung toxicity.

and pulmonary fibrosis and as a late effect of treatment a vascular sensitivity syndrome similar to Raynaud's phenomenon. With bleomycin given at 30 u/week for 12 weeks approximately 15–20 per cent of the patients experience dyspnoea and 1 per cent develop an irreversible pulmonary fibrosis, which is usually fatal (Peckham *et al.* 1987; Williams *et al.* 1987*b*). It has been suggested that toxicity is less with an infusion than a bolus administration (Van Barneveld *et al.* 1985), though direct comparisons have not been made at equivalent doses. In practice, careful monitoring of lung function is important in patients having high doses of bleomycin. It should also be noted that the frequent consequence of bleomycin therapy is the induction of small, pleural-based, inflammatory nodules that may possibly be mistaken for metastases (Fig. 17).

Cutaneous toxic effects of bleomycin are varied and most patients experience some hyperpigmentation especially at sites of trauma or inflammation. Thickening of subcutaneous tissues, especially in the fingers, is common.

Raynaud's phenomenon occurs after treatment in 15–20 per cent of patients having bolus doses of bleomycin on the standard PVB or BEP schedule (30 u/week×12). Subclinical Raynaud's phenomenon is more common (Hansen and Olsen 1989).

Infections

Though neutropenic sepsis is a risk with most regimens used for the germ cell tumours, opportunistic fungal or protozoal infections are rare. This may relate to the relatively short treatment period. A particular syndrome of infected differentiated teratoma cyst has been reported (Fig. 18). These require drainage and appropriate antibiotics.

Fertility

Fertility is often grossly impaired in patients presenting with testicular tumours; normal sperm counts (more than 10 million spermatozoa per ml) were observed in only 22 per cent of 54 patients with seminomas and 29 per cent of 154 patients with teratomas or mixed tumours, presenting to the Royal Marsden Hospital between 1976 and 1983 (Hendry *et al.* 1983). Similar observations have been made by Bracken and Smith (1980), Jewett *et al.* (1983), and Berthelsen and Skakkebaek (1983). Interestingly, very low sperm counts were sometimes observed in men who had previously fathered children, suggesting that depression of spermatogenesis was an acquired phenomenon accompanying the development of the tumour.

The sperm count recovered to normal in 24 per cent of 80 patients, up to 3 years after chemotherapy: surprisingly, such recovery was seen in 35 per cent of 23 men with initially poor sperm counts, but in only 26 per cent of 19 with good initial counts (Hendry *et al.* 1983). This observation led to the hypothesis that reversible temporary depression of spermatogenesis may protect the sperm precursor cells from the toxic effects of chemotherapy and this possibility is now under detailed investigation.

Altogether 34 pregnancies have been produced by men who had testicular tumours and who received chemotherapy, mostly 2 or more years after completion of treatment. Cryopreservation of semen in liquid nitrogen has been done in some patients with

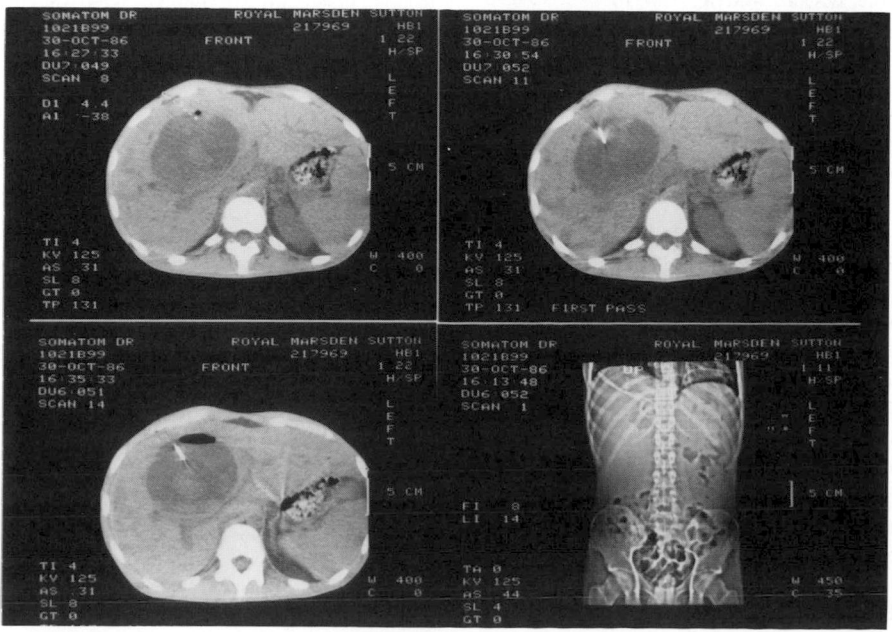

Fig. 18 CT scans of an infected teratoma cyst and the diagnostic aspiration.

testicular tumours before treatment, but in our practice so far only three pregnancies have been produced after thawing and insemination. We continue to offer this service to young men with advanced testicular tumours, however, especially if they have bulky para-aortic masses that may require excision.

Standard PVB, BEP, or CEB schedules rarely cause permanent sterility (Fossa *et al.* 1987; Horwich *et al.* 1991). The risk of impaired spermatogenesis is higher in regimens using alkylating agents.

Rare testicular tumours

These include non-Hodgkin's lymphoma of the testis, gonadal stromal tumours, and adenocarcinoma of the rete testis (Hamilton and Horwich 1988). Paratesticular rhabdomyosarcoma frequently presents with a testicular mass. It usually presents early and radical inguinal orchidectomy is feasible. The pattern of disease and management are similar to embryonal rhabdomyosarcomas presenting at other sites.

Non-Hodgkin's lymphoma

This usually presents in patients over the age of 50 years and may be bilateral (Duncan *et al.* 1980). It may be difficult to distinguish primary testicular lymphoma from metastatic involvement; however, in the British Testicular Tumour Registry 15 out of 124 patients treated by orchidectomy alone survived disease free for 5 years, implying that this was truly the primary site (Gowing 1976).

Most of these tumours are high grade and the prognosis appears poorer than for presentations at other extranodal sites (Gowing 1976; Jackson and Montessori 1980; Read 1981); survival of patients who present with stage IV disease is poor (Duncan *et al.* 1980; Tepperman *et al.* 1982). In the past, stage I or II disease was usually managed by orchidectomy followed by retroperitoneal irradiation. Survival in stage I was of the order of 50 per cent, but stage II patients had a poor prognosis (Hamilton *et al.* 1988).

The current view is that these tumours require extensive staging of retroperitoneal nodes, mediastinal nodes, liver, bone-marrow, and cerebrospinal fluid. Patients with early-stage disease who are fit for aggressive combinations of chemotherapy should be managed with a regimen appropriate for high-grade lymphoma and in this context the role of adjuvant radiotherapy has not been established.

Gonadal stromal tumours

This category includes Sertoli and Leydig cell tumours. The majority are benign but approximately 10 per cent metastasize (Javadpour 1988); they produce testosterone or human chorionic gonadotrophin. Oestrogen levels may be high as a result of peripheral aromatization of testosterone. Leydig cell tumours represented 1.6 per cent of those in the British Testicular Tumour Panel Series (Symington and Cameron 1976). Pathological indicators of malignancy include large size, lack of encapsulation, presence of satellite nodules, areas of necrosis, a high mitotic index, and vascular or lymphatic invasion. The pattern of spread is to regional (para-aortic) lymph nodes, liver, lung, and bone (Kim *et al.* 1985). Metastatic disease seems resistant to both radiotherapy (Feldman *et al.* 1982) and chemotherapy (Grem *et al.* 1986).

Sertoli cell tumours occasionally present in infancy. Again, the pattern of spread appears initially to be retroperitoneal nodes and long-term survivors have been reported following resection of metastatic nodal disease (Weitzner *et al.* 1979). Sensitivity to radiotherapy or chemotherapy is unknown. The majority of patients with metastatic disease have died within 18 months (Symington and Cameron 1976).

Adenocarcinoma of the rete testis

This tumour is excessively rare, Sarma and Weillbaecher (1985) reporting the twenty-first case and indicating that long-term survival post-orchidectomy was possible. There is no information on the treatment of metastatic disease and a reasonable approach is therefore to base the management on surgery. Primary tumours should be managed with radical inguinal orchidectomy with hemiscrotectomy if the disease is locally advanced. If there is no clinical or radiological evidence of metastases then retroperitoneal node dissection should be considered.

REFERENCES

Ahlgren P, Langleben A, Fauser A, Shustik C (1988). Autologous bone marrow transplantation (ABMT) as primary therapy for poor prognosis germ cell cancer. *Proceedings of the American Society of Clinical Oncology*, 7:133.

Andrews PW (1988). Human teratocarcinomas. *Biochimica et Biophysica Acta*, 948:17–36.

Andreyev HJN, Dearnaley DP, Horwich A (1993). Testicular non-seminoma with high serum human chorionic gonadotrophin: the trophoblastic teratoma syndrome. *Diagnostic Oncology*, 3:67–71.

Atkin NB, Baker MC (1983). i (12): specific chromosomal marker in seminoma and malignant teratoma of the testis? *Cancer Genetics and Cytogenetics*, 10:199–204.

Azzopardi JG, Mostofi FK, Theiss EA (1961). Lesions of testes observed in certain patients with widespread choriocarcinoma and related tumors. *American Journal of Pathology*, 38:207–25.

Bagshawe KD (1973). Recent observations related to the chemotherapy and immunology of gestational choriocarcinoma. *Advances in Cancer Research*, 18:231–63.

Bajorin DF (1991). Prognostic classification in metastatic non-seminoma. In *Testicular cancer—clinical investigation and management* (ed. A Horwich), pp. 125–45. Chapman & Hall, London.

Bajorin D, Katz A, Chan E, Geller N, Vogelzang N, Bosl GJ (1988). Comparison of criteria for assigning germ cell tumour patients to 'good risk' studies and 'poor risk' studies. *Journal of Clinical Oncology*, 6:786–92.

Bajorin DF, Sarosdy MF, Bosl GJ, Weisen S, Heller G (1991). A randomized trial of etoposide+carboplatin (EC) vs etoposide+cisplatin (EP) in patients (PTS) with metastatic germ cell tumors (GCT). *Proceedings of the American Society of Clinical Oncology*, 10:168.

Bajorin DF, *et al.* (1993). Randomized trial of etoposide and cisplatin versus etoposide and carboplatin in patients with good-risk germ cell tumours: a multiinstitutional study. *Journal of Clinical Oncology*, 11(4):598–606.

Ball D, Barrett A, Peckham MJ (1982). The management of metastatic seminoma testis. *Cancer*, 50:2289–94.

Barnett MJ, *et al.* (1991). Intensive therapy and autologous bone marrow transplantation (BMT) for patients with poor prognosis nonseminomatous germ cell tumors. *Proceedings of the American Society of Clinical Oncology*, 10:165.

Begent RHJ (1986). Radioimmunolocalisation of germ cell tumours. In *Germ cell tumours II* (ed. WG Jones, M Ward, and CK Anderson). Pergamon, Oxford.

Bennett CJ, Seager SWT, McGuire EJ (1987). Electroejaculation for recovery of semen after retroperitoneal lymph node dissection: case report. *Journal of Urology*, 137:513–15.

Berthelsen JG, Skakkebaek NE (1983). Gonadal function in men with testis cancer. *Fertility and Sterility*, 39:68–75.

Berthelsen JG, Skakkebaek NE, Von der Maase H, Sorensen BL (1982). Screening for carcinoma *in situ* of the contralateral testis in patients with germinal testicular cancer. *British Medical Journal*, 285:1683–6.

Biddle C, *et al.* (1988). Insulin-like growth factors and the multiplication of tera-2, a human teratoma-derived cell line. *Journal of Cell Science*, 90:475–84.

Blandy JP, Hope-Stone HF, Dayan AD (1970). *Tumours of the testicle*. Heinemann, London.

Boden G, Gibb R (1951). Radiotherapy and testicular neoplasms. *Lancet*, ii:1195–7.

Boileau MA, Steers WD (1984). Testis tumors: the clinical significance of the tumor-contaminated scrotum. *Journal of Urology*, 132:51–4.

Bosl GJ, et al. (1981). Impact of delay in diagnosis on clinical stage of testicular cancer. *Lancet*, ii:970–2.

Bosl GJ, et al. (1983). Serum tumour markers in patients with metastatic germ cell tumours of the testis: a ten year experience. *American Journal of Medicine*, 75:29–35.

Bosl GJ, et al. (1986). VAB-6: an effective chemotherapy regimen for patients with germ-cell tumors. *American Journal of Clinical Oncology*, 4:1493–9.

Bosl GJ, et al. (1987). Alternating cycles of etoposide plus cisplatin and VAB-6 in the treatment of poor-risk patients with germ cell tumors. *Journal of Clinical Oncology*, 5:436–40.

Bosl GJ, et al. (1988). A randomized trial of etoposide+cisplatin versus VAB-6 (vinblastine+bleomycin+cisplatin+cyclophosphamide+dactinomycin) in patients with good prognosis germ cell tumor. *Journal of Clinical Oncology*, 6:1231–8.

Bosl GJ, et al. (1989a) Isochromosome of chromosome 12: clinically useful marker for male germ cell tumours. *Journal of the National Cancer Institute*, 81:1874–8.

Bosl GJ, Dmitrovsky E, Reuter V, Samaniego F, Murty VVVS, Chaganti RSK (1989b). A specific karyotypic abnormality in germ cell tumors (GCT). *Proceedings of the American Society of Clinical Oncology*, 8:131.

Bracken RB, Smith KD (1980). Is semen cryopreservation helpful in testicular cancer? *Journal of Urology*, 15:581–3.

Bracken RB, Johnson DE, Frazier OH, Logothetis CJ, Trindade A, Samuels ML (1983). The role of surgery following chemotherapy in stage III germ cell neoplasms. *Journal of Urology*, 129:39–43.

Brada M, Horwich A, Peckham MJ (1987). Treatment of favourable prognosis nonseminomatous testicular germ cell tumours with etoposide, cisplatin and reduced dose of bleomycin. *Cancer Treatment Reports*, 7:655–6.

Brindley GS, Scott GI, Hendry WF (1986). Vas cannulation with implanted sperm reservoirs for obstructive azoospermia or ejaculatory failure. *British Journal of Urology*, 58:721–3.

Broun ER, et al. (1991). Long term follow-up of salvage chemotherapy in relapsed and refractory germ cell tumors using high dose carboplatin and etoposide with autologous bone marrow rescue (ABMR). *Proceedings of the American Society of Clinical Oncology*, 10:167.

Broun ER, Nichols CR, Kneebone P, Williams SD, Loehrer PJ, Einhorn LH, Tricot GJ (1992). Long-term outcome of patients with relapsed and refractory germ cell tumors treated with high-dose chemotherapy and autologous bone marrow rescue. *Annals of International Medicine*, 117(2):124–8.

Browne P, Bagshawe KD (1982). Enhancement of human chorionic gonadotrophin production by antimetabolites. *British Journal of Cancer*, 46:22–9.

Calman FMB, Peckham MJ, Hendry WF (1979). The pattern of spread and treatment of metastases in testicular seminoma. *British Journal of Urology*, 51:154–60.

Calvert AH, Harland SJ, Newell D, Siddik ZH, Harrap KR (1985). Phase I studies with carboplatin at The Royal Marsden Hospital. *Cancer Treatment Reviews*, 12 (Suppl. A):51–7.

Chilvers CED, Saunders M, Bliss JM, Nicholls J, Horwich A (1989). Influence of delay in diagnosis on prognosis in testicular teratoma. *British Journal of Cancer*, 59:126–8.

Clemm C, Schmidkunz P, Mair W, Hartenstein R, Wilmanns W (1989). Combination chemotherapy in bulky seminoma with cisplatin/ifosfamide and vinblastine or etoposide. *Proceedings of the European Conference on Clinical Oncology*, 5:P-0813.

Coia LR, Hanks GE (1988). Complications from large field intermediate dose in infradiaphragmatic radiation: an analysis of the patterns of care outcome studies for Hodgkin's disease and seminoma. *International Journal of Radiation Oncology—Biology—Physics*, 15:29–35.

Coppac S, Newlands ES, Dent J, Mitchell H, Goka G, Bagshawe KD (1983). Problems of interpretation of serum concentrations of alpha-fetoprotein (AFP) in patients receiving cytotoxic chemotherapy for malignant germ cell tumours. *British Journal of Cancer*, 48:335–40.

Crawford SM, Newlands ES, Begent RHJ, Rustin GJ, Bagshawe KD (1989). The effect of intensity of administered treatment on the outcome of germ cell tumours treated with POMB/ACE chemotherapy. *British Journal of Cancer*, 59:243–6.

Cullen MH, Harper PG, Woodroffe CM, Kirkbridge P, Clarke J (1988). Chemotherapy of poor risk germ cell tumours: an independent evaluation of POMB/ACE regime. *British Journal of Urology*, 62:454–60.

Cullen MH, Stenning S, Fossa SD, Horwich A, Kaye SB, MRC Testicular Tumour Working Party (1992). Short course adjuvant chemotherapy in high risk stage I non-seminoma germ cell tumours of the testis (NSGCTT): preliminary report of an MRC study. *British Journal of Cancer*, 65 (Suppl. XVI):8.

Daniels JR, Russell C, Skinner DG (1987). Malignant germinal neoplasms: intensive weekly chemotherapy with cisplatin, vincristine, bleomycin and etoposide. *Proceedings of the American Society of Clinical Oncology*, 6:104.

Daugaard G, Rorth M (1986). High-dose cisplatin and VP-16 with bleomycin, in the management of advanced metastatic germ cell tumors. *European Journal of Cancer and Clinical Oncology*, 22:477–85.

Daugaard G, Rossing N, Roth M (1988). Effects of cisplatin on different measures of glomerular function in the human kidney with special emphasis on high dose. *Cancer Chemotherapy and Pharmacology*, 21:163–7.

Dean AL (1925). The treatment of teratoid tumors of the testis with radium and the X-ray. *Journal of Urology*, 13:149–65.

Dearnaley DP (1991). Intensive induction treatment for poor risk patients. In *Testicular cancer—clinical investigation and management* (ed. A Horwich), pp. 396–417. Chapman & Hall, London.

Depue RH (1984). Maternal and gestational factors affecting the risk of cryptorchidism and inguinal hernia. *International Journal of Epidemiology*, 13:311–18.

Dixon AK, Ellis M, Sikora K (1986). Computed tomography of testicular tumours: distribution of abdominal lymphadenopathy. *Clinical Radiology*, 37:519–23.

Dmitrovsky E, Bosl GJ, Chaganti RSK (1990). Clinical and genetic features of human germ cell cancer. *Cancer Surveys*, 9:369–86.

Donohue JP, Rowland RG (1981). Complications of retroperitoneal lymph node dissection. *Journal of Urology*, 125:338–40.

Donohue JP, Rowland RG (1984). The role of surgery in advanced testicular cancer. *Cancer*, 54:2716–21.

Donohue JP, Thornhill JA (1991). Retroperitoneal lymphadenectomy in staging and treatment of the development of nerve-sparing techniques. In *Testicular cancer—clinical investigation and management* (ed. A Horwich), pp. 304–20. Chapman & Hall, London.

Donohue JP, Zachary JM, Maynard BR (1982). Distribution of nodal metastases in nonseminomatous testis cancer. *British Journal of Urology*, 128:315–20.

Donohue JP, Foster RS, Geier G, Rowland RG, Bihrle R (1988). Preservation of ejaculation following nerve sparing retroperitoneal lymphadenectomy (RPLND). *Journal of Urology*, 139:176.

Donohue JP, Thornhill JA, Foster RS, Rowland RG, Bihrle R (1993). Primary retroperitoneal lymph node dissection in clinical stage A non-seminomatous germ cell testis cancer. Review of the Indiana University experience 165-1989. *British Journal of Urology*, 71(3):326–35.

Dosoretz DE, et al. (1981). Megavoltage irradiation for pure testicular seminoma: results and patterns of failure. *Cancer*, 48:2184–90.

Duchesne GM, Horwich A, Dearnaley D (1990). Orchidectomy alone for stage I seminoma of the testis. *Cancer*, 65:1115–18.

Duncan PR, Checa F, Gowing NFC, McElwain TJ, Peckham MJ (1980). Extranodal non-Hodgkin's lymphoma presenting in the testicle: a clinical and pathologic study of 24 cases. *Cancer*, 45:1578–4.

Editorial (1980a). Earlier diagnosis of testicular tumours. *British Medical Journal*, 1:961.

Editorial (1980b). Early testicular cancer. *Lancet*, ii:1175.

Einhorn LH (1990). Ondansetron: a new antiemetic for patients receiving cisplatin chemotherapy. *Journal of Clinical Oncology*, 8:731–5.

Einhorn LH, Donohue J (1977). *Cis*-diammine-dichloroplatinum, vinblastine, and bleomycin combination chemotherapy in disseminated testicular cancer. *Annals of Internal Medicine*, 87:293–8.

Einhorn LH, Williams SD (1980). Chemotherapy of disseminated testicular cancer: a random prospective study. *Cancer*, 46:1339–44.

Einhorn LH, Williams SD (1980). Chemotherapy of disseminated seminoma. *Cancer Clinical Trials*, **3**:307.

Einhorn LH, Williams SD, Troner M (1981). The role of maintenance therapy in disseminated testicular cancer: a Southeastern Cancer Study Group evaluation. *New England Journal of Medicine*, **305**:727–31.

Einhorn LH, Williams SO, Loehrer P, Birch R, Greco A (1988). A comparison of four courses of cisplatin, VP16 and bleomycin (PVP16B) in favorable prognosis disseminated germ cell tumors: a Southeastern Cancer Study Group (SECSG) protocol. *Proceedings of the American Society of Clinical Oncology*, **7**:120.

Einhorn LH, Williams SD, Loehrer PJ, Birch R, Drasga R, Omura G, Greco FA (1989). Evaluation of optimal duration of chemotherapy in favorable-prognosis disseminated germ cell tumors: a Southeastern Cancer Study Group Protocol. *Journal of Clinical Oncology*, **23**:219–22.

Epenetos AA, *et al.* (1985). Indium-111 labelled monoclonal antibody to placental alkaline phosphatase in the detection of neoplasms of testis, ovary and cervix. *Lancet*, **ii**:350–3.

Erman P (1980). Delay in the diagnosis of testicular cancer. *Lakaratidningen*, **77**:4275–7.

Evensen JF, Fossa SD, Kjellevold K, Lien HH (1985). Testicular seminoma: analysis of treatment and failure for stage II disease. *Radiotherapy and Oncology*, **4**:55–61.

Feldman PS, Kovacs K, Horvath E, Adelson GL (1982). Malignant Leydig cell tumor: clinical, histologic and electron microscopic features. *Cancer*, **49**:714–21.

Finkelstein R, Weinberg RA (1988). Differential regulation of N-*myc* and C-*myc* expression in Fa teratomcarcinoma cells. *Oncogene Research*, **3**:287–92.

Ford TF, Parkinson MC, Pryor JP (1985). The undescended testis in adult life. *British Journal of Urology*, **57**:181–4.

Fordham MVP, Mason MD, Blackmore C, Hendry WF, Horwich A (1990). Management of the contralateral testis in patients with testicular germ cell cancer. *British Journal of Urology*, **65**:290–3.

Forman D, *et al.* (1992). Familial testicular cancer: a report of the UK family register, estimation of risk and an HLA Class 1 sib-pair analysis. *British Journal of Cancer*, **65**:255–62.

Fossa S (1988). Testicular cancer in young Norwegians. *Journal of Surgical Oncology*, **39**:43–63.

Fossa SD (1991). Response evaluation in seminoma. In *Testicular cancer—clinical investigation and management* (ed. A Horwich), pp. 252–68. Chapman & Hall, London.

Fossa S, Borge L, Aass N, Johannessen NB, Stenwia AE, Kaalhus O (1987). The treatment of advanced metastatic seminoma: experience in 55 cases. *Journal of Clinical Oncology*, **5**:1071–7.

Fossa SD, Aass N, Kaalhus O (1989). Radiotherapy for testicular seminoma stage I: treatment results and long-term post-irradiation morbidity in 365 patients. *International Journal of Radiation Oncology—Biology—Physics*, **16**:383–8.

Freedman LS, *et al.* (1987). Histopathology in the prediction of relapse of patients with stage I testicular teratoma treated by orchidectomy alone. *Lancet*, **ii**:294–8.

Friedman EL, Garnick MB, Stomper PC, Mauch PM, Harrington DP, Ritchie JP (1985). Therapeutic guidelines and results in advanced seminoma. *Journal of Clinical Oncology*, **3**:1325–32.

Giwercman A, Berthelsen JG, Muller J, Von der Maase H, Skakkebaek NE (1987). Screening for carcinoma-*in-situ* of the testis. *International Journal of Andrology*, **10**:173–80.

Giwercman A, Clausen OPF, Skakkebaek NE (1988*a*). Carcinoma *in situ* of the testis: aneuploid cells in semen. *British Medical Journal*, **296**:1762–4.

Giwercman A, Marks A, Skakkebaek NE (1988*b*). Carcinoma-*in-situ* germ-cells exfoliated from seminiferous epithelium into seminal fluid. *Lancet*, **i**:530.

Giwercman A, Bruun E, Frimodt-Moller C, Skakkebaek NE (1989). Prevalence of carcinoma *in situ* and other histopathological abnormalities in testes of men with a history of cryptorchidism. *Journal of Urology*, **142**:998–1002.

Golbey RB (1970). The place of chemotherapy in the treatment of testicular tumors. *Journal of the American Medical Association*, **213**:101–3.

Goldstraw P (1991). Thoracotomy post-chemotherapy in non-seminoma patients. In *Testicular cancer—clinical investigation and management* (ed. A Horwich), pp. 475–86. Chapman & Hall, London.

Gowing NFC (1976). Malignant lymphoma of the testis. In *Pathology of the testis* (ed. RCB Pugh), pp. 334–55. Blackwell Scientific, London.

Gralla RJ, *et al.* (1981). Antiemetic efficacy of high-dose metoclopramide: randomized trials with placebo and prochlorperazine in patients with chemotherapy induced nausea and vomiting. *New England Journal of Medicine*, **305**:905–9.

Green N, *et al.* (1983). Radiation therapy in bulky seminoma. *Journal of Urology*, **21**:467–9.

Gregory C, Peckham MJ (1986). Results of radiotherapy for stage II testicular seminoma. *Radiotherapy and Oncology*, **6**:285–92.

Grem JL, Robins I, Wilson KS, Gilchrist K, Trump DL (1986). Metastatic Leydig cell tumor of the testis. *Cancer*, **58**:2116–19.

Hamilton CH, Horwich A (1988). Rare tumours of the testis and paratesticular tissues. In *Uncommon cancer* (ed. CJ Williams, JGG Krikorian, MR Green, and D Raghavan), pp. 225–48. Wiley, London.

Hamilton CR, Horwich A, Easton D, Peckham MJ (1986). Radiotherapy for stage I seminoma testis: results of treatment and complications. *Radiotherapy and Oncology*, **6**:115–20.

Hamilton CR, Horwich A, Bliss JM, Peckham MJ (1987). Gastrointestinal morbidity of adjuvant radiotherapy in stage I malignant teratoma of the testis. *Radiotherapy and Oncology*, **10**:85–90.

Hamilton CR, Bliss JM, Horwich A (1989). The late effects of cisplatinum on renal function. *European Journal of Cancer and Clinical Oncology*, **25**:185–9.

Hansen SW, Olsen N (1989). Raynaud's phenomenon in patients treated with cisplatin, vinblastin and bleomycin for germ cell cancer: measurement of vasoconstrictor response to cold. *Journal of Clinical Oncology*, **7**:940–3.

Hansen SW, Groth S, Daugaard G, Rossing N, Rorth M (1988). Long-term effects on renal function and blood pressure of treatment with cisplatin, vinblastine and bleomycin in patients with germ cell cancer. *Journal of Clinical Oncology*, **16**:1728–31.

Harding MJ, Paul J, Gillis CR, Kaye SB (1993). Management of malignant teratoma: does referral to a specialist unit matter? *Lancet*, **341**:999–1002.

Hay JH, Duncan W, Kerr GR (1984). Subsequent malignancies in patients irradiated for testicular tumours. *British Journal of Radiology*, **57**:597–602.

Hayes DM, Cvitkovic E, Golbey RB, Scheiner E, Helson L, Krakoff IH (1977). High dose *cis*-platinum diammine dichloride: amelioration of renal toxicity by mannitol diuresis. *Cancer*, **39**:1372–81.

Hendry WF (1991). Abdominal surgery post-chemotherapy: metastatic teratoma. In *Testicular cancer—clinical investigation and management* (ed. A Horwich), pp. 449–74. Chapman & Hall, London.

Hendry WF, Goldstraw P, Husband JE, Barrett A (1981). Elective delayed excision of bulky para-aortic lymph node metastases in advanced non-seminoma germ cell tumours of testis. *British Journal of Urology*, **53**:648–53.

Hendry WF, Stedronska J, Jones CR, Blackmore AA, Barrett A, Peckham MJ (1983). Semen analysis in testicular cancer and Hodgkin's disease: pre- and post-treatment findings and implications for cryopreservation. *British Journal of Urology*, **55**:769–73.

Hendry WF, Goldstraw P, Peckham MJ (1987). The role of surgery in the combined management of metasatases from testicular teratomas of testis. *British Journal of Urology*, **59**:358.

Hendry WF, A'Hern RP, Hetherington JW, Peckham MJ, Dearnaley DP, Horwich A (1993). Para-aortic lympadenectomy after chemotherapy for metastatic non-seminomatous germ cell tumours: prognostic value and therapeutic benefit. *British Journal of Urology*, **71**(2):208–13.

Herman JG, Sturgeon J, Thomas GM (1983). Mediastinal prophylactic irradiation in seminoma. *Proceedings of the American Society of Clinical Oncology*, **2**:133.

Herr HW, Toner GC, Geller NL, Bosl GT (1991). Patient selection for retroperitoneal lymph node dissection after chemotherapy for nonseminomatous germ cell tumours. *European Urology*, **19**:1–5.

Hitchins RN, Newlands ES, Smith DB, Begent RHJ, Rustin GIS, Bagshawe KD (1989). Long-term outcome in patients with germ cell tumours treated with POMB/ACE chemotherapy: comparison of commonly used classification systems of good and poor prognosis. *British Journal of Cancer*, **59**:236–42.

Horwich A (1989). Germ cell tumour chemotherapy. *British Journal of Cancer*, **59**:156–9.

Horwich A (1991). Surveillance for stage I seminoma of the testis. In *Testicular cancer—clinical investigation and management* (ed. A Horwich), pp. 197–210. Chapman & Hall Medical, London.

Horwich A (1993). Comments and critique—current issues in the management of clinical stage I testicular teratoma. *European Journal of Cancer*, 29A(7):933–4.

Horwich A, Peckham MJ (1984). Serum tumour marker regression rate following chemotherapy for malignant teratoma. *European Journal of Cancer and Clinical Oncology*, 20:1463–70.

Horwich A, Peckham MJ (1986). Transient tumour marker elevation following chemotherapy for germ cell tumours of the testis. *Cancer Treatment Reports*, 70:1329–31.

Horwich A, Peckham MJ (1988). Surveillance after orchidectomy for clinical stage I germ cell A tumours of the testis. In *Progress and controversies in oncological urology II*. Liss, New York.

Horwich A, Tucker DF, Peckham MJ (1985). Placental alkaline phosphatase as a tumour marker in seminoma using the H17E2 monoclonal antibody assay. *British Journal of Cancer*, 51:625–9.

Horwich A, Easton D, Husband J, Nicholas D, Peckham MJ (1987). Prognosis following chemotherapy for metastatic malignant teratoma. *British Journal of Urology*, 59:578–83.

Horwich A, *et al.* (1989*a*). Intensive induction chemotherapy for poor risk non-seminomatous germ cell tumours. *European Journal of Cancer and Clinical Oncology*, 25:177–84.

Horwich A, Dearnaley DP, Duchesne GM, Williams M, Brada M, Peckham MJ (1989*b*). Simple non-toxic treatment of advanced metastatic seminoma with carboplatin. *Journal of Clinical Oncology*, 7:1150–6.

Horwich A, *et al.* (1990). Prognostic factors for survival in advanced non seminomatous germ cell tumours (NSGCT): a study by the Medical Research Council (MRC) Testicular Tumour Subgroup. *Proceedings of the American Society of Clinical Oncology*, 9:132.

Horwich A, Dearnaley DP, Nicholls J, Jay G, Mason M, Harland S (1991). Effectiveness of carboplatin, etoposide, bleomycin (CEB) combination chemotherapy in good prognosis metastatic testicular nonseminomatous germ cell tumours. *Journal of Clinical Oncology*, 9:62–9.

Horwich A, Alsanjari N, A'Hern R, Nicholls J, Dearnaley DP, Fisher C (1992*a*). Surveillance following orchidectomy for stage I testicular seminoma. *British Journal of Cancer*, 65:775–8.

Horwich A, Dearnaley DP, A'Hern R, Mason M, Thomas G, Jay G, Nicholls J (1992*b*). The activity of single-agent carboplatin in advanced seminoma. *European Journal of Cancer*, 28A(8/9):1307–10.

Horwich A, Wilson C, Cornes P, Gildersleve J, Dearnaley DP (1993). Increasing the dose intensity of chemotherapy in poor-prognosis metastatic non-seminoma. *European Urology*, 23:219–22.

Horwich A, Norman A, Fisher C, Hendry WF, Nicholls J, Dearnaley DP (1994*a*). Primary chemotherapy for stage II nonseminomatous germcelltumors of the testis. *Journal of Urology*, 151:72–8.

Horwich A, Sleifer D, Fossa S, Stenning S, Cooker P, Sylvester R, Vermeijlen K on behalf of the UK Medical Research Council Testicular Tumour Working Party and EORTC Genito-Urinary Group (1994*b*). A trial of carboplatin-based combination chemotherapy in good prognosis metastatic testicular non seminoma. *Proceedings of the American Society of Clinical Oncology*, 13:231.

Hoskin P, Dilly S, Easton D, Horwich A, Hendry WF, Peckham MJ (1986). Prognostic factors in stage I non seminomatous germ cell testicular tumours managed by orchidectomy and surveillance: implications for adjuvant chemotherapy. *Journal of Clinical Oncology*, 4:1031–6.

Husband JE, Grimer DP (1985). Staging testicular tumours: the role of CT scanning. *Journal of the Royal Society of Medicine*, 58:429–36.

Husband JE, Peckham MJ, MacDonald JS (1980). The role of abdominal computed tomography in the management of testicular tumours. *Journal of Computer Assisted Tomography*, 4:1–16.

Jackson SM, Montessori GA (1980). Malignant lymphoma of the testis: review of 17 cases in British Columbia with survival related to pathological subclassification. *Journal of Urology*, 123:881–3.

Jacobsen GK, Norgaard-Padersen B (1984). Placental alkaline phosphatase in testicular germ cell tumours and carcinoma *in situ* of the testis: an immunohistochemical study. *Acta Pathologica, Microbiologica et Immunologica Scandinavica*, 92(A):323–9.

Javadpour N (1986). Serum and cellular markers in testicular cancer. In *Principles and management of testicular cancer* (ed. N Javadpour), pp. 155–65. Thieme, New York.

Javadpour N (1988). Gonadal stromal tumours of the testis. In *Testicular cancer* (ed. N Javadpour), pp. 383–6. Thieme, New York.

Javadpour N, Kim EE, Deland FH, Salyer JR, Shah U, Goldenberg DM (1981). The role of radioimmunodetection in the management of testicular cancer. *Journal of the American Medical Association*, 246:45–9.

Jeffery GM, Theaker JM, Lee AHS, Blaquiere RM, Smart CJ, Mead GM (1991). The growing teratoma syndrome. *British Journal of Urology*, 67:195–202.

Jewett MAS, Thachil JV, Harris JF (1983). Exocrine function of testis with germinal testicular tumour. *British Medical Journal*, 286:1849–50.

Jewett MAS, Kong YS, Goldberg SD, Sturgeon JF (1988). Retroperitoneal lymphadenectomy for testis tumor with nerve sparing for ejaculation. *Journal of Urology*, 139:1220–4.

Jones DR, Norman AR, Horwich A, Hendry WF (1993). Ejaculatory dysfunction after retroperitoneal lymphadenectomy. *European Urology*, 23:169–71.

Kaldor JM, Day NE, Band P (1987). Second malignancies following testicular cancer, ovarian cancer and Hodgkin's disease: an international collaborative study among cancer registries. *International Journal of Cancer*, 39:571–85.

Kennedy CL, Husband JE, Bellamy EA (1985). The accuracy of CT scanning prior to para-aortic lymphadenectomy in patients with bulky metastases from testicular teratoma. *British Journal of Urology*, 57:755–8.

Kennedy CL, Hendry WF, Peckham MJ (1986). The significance of scrotal interference in stage I testicular cancer managed by orchiectomy and surveillance. *British Journal of Urology*, 58:705–8.

Kim I, Young RH, Scully RE (1985). Leydig cell tumours of the testis. *American Journal of Surgical Pathology*, 19:177–92.

Kleinschmidt K, Kemper J, Holstein AF (1989). Carcinoma *in situ* of the testis in the presence of contralateral germ cell tumor. *European Urology*, 16:74–7.

Kleinsmith LJ, Pierce GB (1964). Multipotentiality of embryonal carcinoma cells. *Cancer Research*, 24:1544–51.

Klepp O, *et al.* (1989). Predicting metastases in clinical stage I testicular teratoma: multivariate analysis of a large multicentric study (SWENOTECA). *Fifth European Conference on Clinical Oncology*, London. GCC Ltd, Macclesfield, Cheshire.

Krabbe S, *et al.* (1979). High incidence of undetected neoplasia in maldescended testes. *Lancet*, i:999–1000.

Krag Jacobsen G, *et al.* (1984). Testicular germ-cell tumours in Denmark 1976–1980 pathology of 1058 consecutive cases. *Acta Radiologica*, 23:239–47.

Kris MG (1989). Double-blind, randomized trial comparing placebo, dexamethasone alone, and metoclopramide plus dexamethasone in patients receiving cisplatin. *Journal of Clinical Oncology*, 7:108–11.

Kulkarni RP, *et al.* (1991). Cytoreductive surgery in disseminated nonseminomatous germ cell tumours. *British Journal of Surgery*, 78:226–9.

Lange PH, Millan JL, Stigbrand T, Vessella L, Ruoslahti E, Fishman WH (1982). Placental alkaline phosphatase as a tumour marker for seminoma. *Cancer Research*, 42:3244–7.

Leiter E, Brendler H (1967). Loss of ejaculation following bilateral retroperitoneal lymphadenectomy. *Journal of Urology*, 98:375–8.

Lester SG, Morphis JGI, Hornback NB, Williams SD, Einhorn LH (1984). Brain metastases and testicular tumors: need for aggressive therapy. *Journal of Clinical Oncology*, 2:1397–403.

Lester SG, Morphis JG, Hornback NB (1986). Testicular seminoma: analysis of treatment results and failures. *International Journal of Radiation Oncology—Biology—Physics*, 12:353–8.

Levi J, *et al.* (1986). Deletion of bleomycin from therapy for good prognosis advanced testicular cancer: a prospective randomized study. *Proceedings of the American Society of Clinical Oncology*, 5:97.

Lewis CR, *et al.* (1991). BOP/VIP—a new platinum-intensive chemotherapy regimen for poor prognosis germ cell tumours. *Annals of Oncology*, 2(3):203–11.

Lien HH, Fossa SD, Ous S (1983). Lymphography in retroperitoneal metastases in non-seminoma testicular tumor patients with a normal CT scan. *Acta Radiologica*, 24:319–22.

Lien HH, Stenwig AE, Ous S (1986). Influence of different criteria for abnormal lymph node size on reliability of computed tomography in patients with nonseminomatous testicular tumor. *Acta Radiologica*, 27:199–203.

Lien HH, Lindskold L, Fossa SD, Aass N (1988). Computed tomography and conventional radiography in intrathoracic metastases from non-seminomatous testicular tumor. *Acta Radiologica*, 29:547–9.

Lightner DJ, Grund F, Lange PH (1989). Noninvasive scrotal imaging techniques. In *Difficult diagnosis in urology* (ed. DL McCullough), pp. 249–48. Churchill Livingstone, New York.

Linder D (1983). The origin of teratomas. In *The human teratomas; experimental and clinical biology* (ed. I Damganov, BB Knowles, and D Solter), pp. 67–80. Humana, Clifton, NJ.

Loehrer PJ, Williams SD, Clark SA (1983). Teratoma following chemotherapy for non-seminomatous germ-cell tumor: a clinicopathologic correlation. *Proceedings of the American Society of Clinical Oncology*, 2:139.

Loehrer PJ, Birch R, Williams SD, Greco A, Einhorn LH (1987). Chemotherapy of metastatic seminoma: the Southeastern Cancer Study Group experience. *Journal of Clinical Oncology*, 5:1212–20.

Loehrer PJ, Elson P, Johnson DH, Williams SD, Trump DL, Einhorn LH (1991). A randomised trial of cisplatin plus etoposide with or without bleomycin in favorable prognosis disseminated germ cell tumours: ECOG study. *Proceedings of the American Society of Clinical Oncology*, 10:169.

Logothetis CJ, Samuels ML, Trindale A, Johnson DE (1982). The growing teratoma syndrome. *Cancer*, 50:1629–35.

Logothetis CJ, Samuels ML, Selig DE, Swanson D, Johnson DE, Von Eschenbach AC (1985). Improved survival with cyclic chemotherapy for non-seminomatous germ cell tumors of the testis. *Journal of Clinical Oncology*, 3:326–35.

Logothetis CJ, et al. (1986). Cyclic chemotherapy with cyclophosphamide, doxorubicin and cisplatin plus vinblastine and bleomycin in advanced germinal tumors: results with 100 patients. *American Journal of Medicine*, 81:219–28.

Logothetis CJ, Samuels ML, Ogden SL, Dexeus FH, Chong C (1987). Cyclophosphamide and sequential cisplatin for advanced seminoma: long-term follow-up in 52 patients. *Journal of Urology*, 138:789–94.

Looijenga LH, Gillis AJ, Van Putten WL, Oosterhuis JW (1993). *In situ* numeric analysis of centromeric regions of chromosomes 1, 12 and 15 of seminomas, nonseminomatous germ cell tumours, and carcinoma in situ of human testis. *Laboratory Investigation*, 68(2):211–19.

Lynch JH, Maxted WC (1983). Use of ephedrine in post-lymphadenectomy ejaculatory failure: a case report. *Journal of Urology*, 129:379.

Maier JG, Sulak MH, Mittemeyer BT (1968). Seminoma of the testis: analysis of treatment success and failure. *American Journal of Roentgenology*, 102:596–602.

Markland C, Kebia K, Fraley EE (1973). Inadequate orchiectomy for patients with testicular tumours. *Journal of the American Medical Association*, 224:1025–6.

Martin GR (1980). Teratocarcinomas and mammalian embryogenesis. *Science*, 209:768–76.

Martin GR (1981) Isolation of a pluripotent cell line from early mouse embryos cultured in medium conditioned by teratocarcinoma stem cells. *Proceedings of the National Academy of Sciences USA*, 78:7634–8.

Mason MD, Featherstone J, Olliff JAH (1991). Inguinal iliac lymph node involvement in germ cell tumours of the testis: implications of radiological investigation and for therapy. *Clinical Oncology*, 3:147–50.

Mason MD, Nicholls J, Horwich A (1991). The effect of carboplatin on renal function in patients with metastatic germ cell tumours. *British Journal of Cancer*, 63:630–3.

Mencel PJ, Motzer RJ, Mazumdar M, Vlamis V, Bajorin DF, Bosl GJ (1994). Advanced seminoma: treatment results, survival, and prognostic factors in 142 patients. *Journal of Clinical Oncology*, 12(1):120–6.

Mollman JE (1990). Cisplatin neurotoxicity. *New England Journal of Medicine*, 322:126–7.

Mostofi FK (1984). Tumor markers and pathology of testicular tumors. *Progress in Clinical and Biological Research*, 153:69–87.

Mostofi FK, Sobin LH (1977). *International histological classification of tumours of testes*. WHO, Geneva.

Motzer RJ, et al. (1988). Advanced seminoma: the role of chemotherapy and adjunctive surgery. *Annals of Internal Medicine*, 108:513–18.

Motzer RJ, et al. (1991). High-dose (HD) carboplatin (C)+etoposide (E) with autologous bone marrow rescue (AUBMAR) in poor risk nonseminomatous germ cell tumor (NSGCT) patients (PTS) with slow serum tumor marker decline induction with cyclophosphamide, bleomycin, actinomcyin D, vinblastine cisplatin (VAB-6). *Proceedings of the American Society for Clinical Oncology*, 10:164.

Moynihan CM (1987). Testicular cancer: the psychosocial problems of patients and their relatives. *Cancer Surveys*, 6:477–510.

MRC Working Party on Testicular Tumours (1985). Prognostic factors in advanced non-seminomatous germ-cell testicular tumours: results of a multicentre study. *Lancet*, i:8–12.

Mulder POM, et al. (1988). Chemotherapy with maximally tolerable doses of VP 16-213 and cyclophosphamide followed by autologous bone marrow transplantation for the treatment of relapsed or refractory germ cell tumors. *European Journal of Cancer and Clinical Oncology*, 24:675–9.

Murray N, Coppin C, Swenerton K (1987). Weekly high intensity cisplatin etoposide (HIPE) for far advanced germ cell cancers (GCC). *Proceedings of the American Society of Clinical Oncology*, 6:101.

Murty VV, et al. (1992). Allelic deletions in the long arm of chromosome 12 identify sites of candidate tumor suppressor genes in male germ cell tumors. *Proceedings of the National Academy of Sciences USA*, 89(22):11006–10.

Newlands ES, Begent RHJ, Rustin GJS, Parker D, Bagshawe KD (1983). Further advances in the management of malignant teratomas of the testis and other sites. *Lancet*, i:948–51.

Newlands ES, Bagshawe KD, Rustin GJ, Crawford SM, Holden L (1986). Current optimum management of anaplastic germ cell tumours of the testis and other sites. *British Journal of Urology*, 58:307–14.

Nichols CR, Roth BJ (1991). Management of metastatic non-seminoma: development of effective chemotherapy. In *Testicular cancer—clinical investigation and management* (ed. A Horwich), pp. 321–50. Chapman & Hall, London.

Nichols CR, et al. (1989). Dose-intensive chemotherapy in refractory germ cell cancer—a phase I/II trial of high-dose carboplatin and etoposide with autologous bone marrow transplantation. *Journal of Clinical Oncology*, 7: 932–9.

Nichols CR, et al. (1991a). Randomized study of cisplatin dose intensity in poor-risk germ cell tumors: a Southeastern Cancer Study Group and Southwest Oncology Group protocol. *Journal of Clinical Oncology*, 9:1163–72.

Nichols CR, et al. (1991b). Randomized study of cisplatin dose intensity in poor-risk germ cell tumors: a Southeastern Cancer Study Group and Southwest Oncology Group Protocol. *Journal of Clinical Oncology*, 9(7):1163–72.

Nichols CR, Breeden ES, Loehrer PJ, Williams SD, Einhorn LH (1993). Secondary leukemia associated with a conventional dose of etoposide: review of serial germ cell tumor protocols. *Journal of the National Cancer Institute*, 85(1):36–40.

Nijman JM, Jager S, Boer PW, Kremer J, Oldhoff J, Koops HS (1982). The treatment of ejaculation disorders after retroperitoneal lymph node dissection. *Cancer*, 50:2967–71.

Noguchi T, Noguchi M (1985). A recessive mutation (*ter*) causing germ cell deficiency and a high incidence of congenital testicular teratoma. *Journal of the National Cancer Institute*, 75:385–9.

Norgaard-Padersen B, et al. (1984). Tumour markers in testicular germ cell tumours: five year experience from the DATECA study 1976–1980. *Acta Radiologica Oncologica*, 23:287–94.

Nuesch-Bachmann IH, Hedinger C (1977). Atypische Spermatogonien als Prakanzerose. *Schweizerische Medizinische Wochenschrift*, 107:795–801.

Oliver RTD (1985). Factors contributing to delay in diagnosis of testicular tumours. *British Medical Journal*, 290:356.

Oliver RTD (1988). The clinical potential of interleukin-2. *British Journal of Cancer*, 58:405–9.

Oliver RTD (1990). Atrophy, hormones, genes and viruses in aetiology of germ cell tumours. *Cancer Surveys*, 9:263–86.

Oliver RTD, Lore S, Ong J (1990). Fixed and potentially reversible risk factors for treatment response in patients with metastatic malignant teratoma. *Journal of Clinical Oncology*, 9:598.

Oosterhuis JW, Castedo SMMJ, De Jong B (1990). Cytogenetics, ploidy and differentiation of human testicular, ovarian and extragonadal germ cell tumours. *Cancer Surveys*, 9:321–32.

Osterlind A (1986). Diverging trends in incidence and mortality of testicular cancer in Denmark. *British Journal of Cancer*, 53:501–5.

Ozols RF, et al. (1984). Randomized trial of PV BV [high dose (HD) *cis*-platinum (P), vinblastine (Ve), bleomycin (B), VP.16 (V)] versus PVeB in poor prognosis non-seminomatous testicular cancer (NSTC). *Proceedings of the American Society of Clinical Oncology*, 3:155.

Ozols RF, Linehan WM, Jacob J, Ostchega Y, Young RC (1988). A randomized trial of standard chemotherapy v a high-dose chemotherapy regimen in the treatment of poor prognosis nonseminomatous germ-cell tumors. *Journal of Oncology*, 6:1031–40.

Peckham MJ (1971). Investigations and staging: general aspects and staging classification. In *The management of testicular tumours* (ed. MJ Peckham), pp. 89–101. Arnold, London.

Peckham MJ (1981) Investigation and staging: general aspects and staging classifications; non-seminomas: current treatment results and future prospects. In *The management of testicular tumours* (ed. MJ Peckham), pp. 89–101; 218–239. Arnold, London.

Peckham MJ, Hendry WF (1985). Clinical stage II non-seminomatous germ cell testicular tumours: results of management by primary chemotherapy. *British Journal of Urology*, 57:763–8.

Peckham MJ, Barrett A, Husband JE, Hendry WF (1982). Orchidectomy alone in testicular stage I non-seminomatous germ-cell tumours. *Lancet*, ii:678–80.

Peckham MJ, *et al.* (1983). The treatment of metastatic germ-cell testicular tumours with bleomycin, etoposide and *cis*-platinum (BEP). *British Journal of Cancer*, 47:613–19.

Peckham MJ, Horwich A, Hendry WF (1985). Advanced seminoma: treatment with *cis*-platinum-based combination chemotherapy or carboplatin (JM8). *British Journal of Cancer*, 52:7–13.

Peckham MJ, Hamilton CR, Horwich A, Hendry WF (1987). Surveillance after orchidectomy for stage I seminoma of the testis. *British Journal of Urology*, 59:343–7.

Peckham MJ, Horwich A, Easton DF, Hendry WF (1988). The management of advanced testicular teratoma. *British Journal of Urology*, 62:63–8.

Pedersen KV, Boiesen P, Zetterlund CG (1987). Experience of screening for carcinoma-*in-situ* of the testis among young men with surgically corrected maldescended testes. *International Journal of Andrology*, 10:181–5.

Peng HQ, *et al.* (1993). Mutations of the p53 gene do not occur in testis cancer. *Cancer Research*, 53(15):3574–8.

Pera MF, Blasco-Lafita MJ, Mills J (1987). Cultured stem cells from human testicular teratomas: the nature of embryonal carcinoma, and its comparison with two types of yolk sac carcinoma. *International Journal of Cancer*, 40:334–43.

Pera MF, Blasco-Lafita MJ, Cooper S, Mason M, Mills J, Monaghan P (1988). Analysis of cell differentiation lineage in human teratomas using new monoclonal antibodies to cytostructural antigens of embryonal carcinoma cells. *Differentiation*, 39:139–49.

Pera MF, Cooper S, Mills J, Parnington JM (1989). Isolation and characterisation of multipotent clone of human embryonal carcinoma cells. *Differentiation*, 42:10–23.

Pera MF, Roach S, Ellis CJ (1990). Comparative biology of mouse and human embryonal carcinomas. *Cancer Surveys*, 9:243–62.

Pizzocaro G, Piva L, Salvioni R, Zanoni F, Milani A (1985). Cisplatin, etoposide, bleomycin first-line therapy and early resection of residual tumor in far-advanced germinal testis cancer. *Cancer*, 56:2411–15.

Pizzocaro G, Salvioni R, Piva L, Zanoni F, Milani A, Faustini M (1986). Cisplatin combination chemotherapy in advanced seminoma. *Cancer*, 58:1625–9.

Poskitt KJ, Cooperberg PL, Sullivan LD (1985). Sonography and CT in staging nonseminomatous testicular tumors. *American Journal of Roentgenology*, 144:939–44.

Powell S, Hendry WF, Peckham MJ (1983). Occult germ-cell testicular tumours. *British Journal of Urology*, 55:440–4.

Price P, Hogan SJ, Bliss JM, Horwich A (1990a). The growth rate of metastatic non-seminomatous germ cell testicular tumours measured by marker production doubling time. II. Prognostic significance in patients treated by chemotherapy. *European Journal of Cancer*, 26:453–6.

Price P, Hogan SJ, Bliss JM, Horwich A (1990b). The growth rate of metastatic non-seminomatous germ cell testicular tumours measured by marker production doubling time. II. Prognostic significance in patients treated by chemotherapy. *European Journal of Cancer*, 26:453–7.

Pryor JP, *et al.* (1983). Carcinoma *in situ* in testicular biopsies from men presenting with infertility. *British Journal of Urology*, 55:780–4.

Pugh RCB (1976). Testicular tumours. In *Pathology of the testis* (ed. RCB Pugh), pp. 139–59. Blackwell Scientific, Oxford.

Raghavan D, Mackintosh JF, Fox RM, Rogers J, Duval P, Besser M (1987). Improved survival after brain metastases in non-seminomatous germ cell

tumours with combined modality treatment. *British Journal of Urology*, 60:364–7.

Ray B, Steven I, Hajdu SI, Whitemore WF, Jr (1974). Distribution of retroperitoneal lymph node metastases in testicular germinal tumors. *Cancer*, 33:340–8.

Read G (1981). Lymphomas of the testis—results of treatment 1960–1977. *Clinical Radiology*, 32:687–92.

Read G (1987). Carcinoma *in situ* of the contralateral testis. *British Medical Journal*, 294:121.

Rorth M (1987). Orchiectomy alone versus orchiectomy plus radiotherapy in stage I nonseminomatous testicular cancer: a randomized study by the Danish Testicular Carcinoma Study Group. *International Journal of Andrology*, 10:255–62.

Roth BJ, Greist A, Kublilis PS (1988). Cisplatin-based combination chemotherapy for disseminated germ cell tumors: long term follow-up. *Journal of Clinical Oncology*, 6:1239–47.

Roth BJ, Sledge GWJ, Heerema NA, Schultz S (1989). Establishment and initial characterisation of a human testicular cancer cell line with acquired resistance to *cis*-diamminedichloroplatinum. *Proceedings of the American Association for Cancer Research*, 30:2094.

Rouviere H (ed.) (1938). *Anatomy of the human lymphatic system*, pp. 216–26. Edward Brothers, Ann Arbor, MI.

Rustin GJS, Newlands ES, Bagshawe KD, Begent RHJ, Crawford SM (1986). Successful management of metastatic and primary germ cell tumours in the brain. *Cancer*, 57:2108–13.

Samson MK, *et al.* (1984). Dose–response and dose–survival advantage for high versus low-dose cisplatin combined with vinblastine and bleomycin in disseminated testicular cancer: a Southwest Oncology Group study. *Cancer*, 53:1029–35.

Samuels ML, Logothetis CJ (1983). Follow-up study of sequential weekly pulse *cis*-platinum for advanced seminoma. *Proceedings of the American Society of Clinical Oncology*, 2:137.

Samuels ML, Lanzotti VJ, Holoye PY, Boyle LE, Smith TL, Johnson DE (1976). Combination chemotherapy in germinal cell tumor. *Cancer Treatment Reviews*, 3:185–204.

Sandeman TF (1979). Symptoms and early management of germinal tumours of the testis. *Medical Journal of Australia*, 2:281–4.

Sarma DP, Weillbaecher TG (1985). Adenocarcinoma of the rete testis. *Journal of Surgical Oncology*, 30:67–71.

Schmoll HJ (1989). Ifosamide in testicular cancer. *Seminars in Oncology*, 16:82–95.

Schmoll H-J, *et al.* (1991). Single agent carboplatinum (CBDCA) for advanced seminoma: a phase II study. *Proceedings of the American Society of Clinical Oncology*, 10:181.

Schofield PN, Engstom W, Lee AJ, Biddle C, Graham CF (1987). Expression of c-*myc* during differentiation of the human teratocarcinoma cell line tera-2. *Journal of Cell Science*, 88:57–64.

Schultz SM, Einhorn LH, Conces DJJ, Williams SD, Loehrer PJ (1989). Management of postchemotherapy residual mass in patients with advanced seminoma: Indiana University experience. *Journal of Clinical Oncology*, 7:1497–503.

Schütte B (1988). Early testicular cancer in severe oligozoospermia. In *Carl Schirren Symposium: advances in andrology* (ed. AF Holstein, F Leidenberger, KH Hölzer, and G Bettendorf). Diesbach Verlag, Berlin.

Senturia YD (1987). The epidemiology of testicular cancer. *British Journal of Urology*, 60:285–91.

Siegert W, *et al.* (1991). High dose carboplatin (C), etoposide (E) and ifosfamide (I) with autologous stem cell rescue (ASCR) for relapsed and refractory non-seminomatous germ cell tumors (NSGCT). *Proceedings of the American Society of Clinical Oncology*, 10:163.

Sikora K, Evans G, Watson J (1987). Oncogenes and germ cell tumours. *International Journal of Andrology*, 10:57–67.

Skinner DG (1978). Management of nonseminomatous tumors. In *Genitourinary cancer* (ed. DG Skinner and JG de Kernion), pp. 470–93. Saunders, Philadelphia, PA.

Skinner DG, Melamud A, Lieskovsky G (1982). Complications of thoraco-abdominal retroperitoneal lymph node dissection. *Journal of Urology*, 127:1107–10.

Sledge GW, Eble JN, Roth BJ, Wuhrman BP, Fineberg N, Einhorn LH (1988). Relation of proliferative activity to survival in patients with advanced germ cell cancer. *Cancer Research*, 48:3864–8.

Smithers DW, Wallace DM, Austin DE (1973). Fertility after unilateral orchidectomy and radiotherapy for patients with malignant tumours of the testis. *British Medical Journal*, 4:77–9.

Sokal M, Peckham MJ, Hendry WF (1980). Bilateral germ cell tumours of the testis. *British Journal of Urology*, 52:158–62.

Staehler G, Weisel M, Clemm C, Gokel JM, Marchner M (1989). Significance of salvage lymphadenectomy in the therapeutic concept of advanced nonseminomatous germ cell tumours. *Urology International*, 44:84–6.

Stanton GF, *et al.* (1985). VAB-6 as initial treatment of patients with advanced seminoma. *Journal of Clinical Oncology*, 3:336–9.

Stephen RA (1962). The clinical presentation of testicular tumours. *British Journal of Urology*, 34:448–50.

Stoter G (1987). Preliminary results of BEP (bleomycin, etoposide, cisplatin) versus EP in low volume metastatic (LVM) testicular non-seminomas: an EORTC study. *Proceedings of the American Society of Clinical Oncology*, 6:110.

Stoter G, Denis L (1985). The chemotherapy of disseminated testicular nonseminomatous germ cell tumors and the clinical research of the EORTC Genitourinary Group. *Acta Urologica Belgica*, 53:428–35.

Stoter G, *et al.* (1986). Preliminary results of BEP (bleomycin, etoposide, cisplatin) versus an alternating regimen of BEP and PVB (cisplatin, vinblastine, bleomycin) in high volume metastatic (HVM) testicular non-seminomas. *Proceedings of the American Society of Clinical Oncology*, 5:106.

Stoter G, *et al.* (1987). Multivariate analysis of prognostic factors in patients with disseminated nonseminomatous testicular cancer: results from a European Organization for Research on Treatment of Cancer multiinstitutional phase III study. *Cancer Research*, 47:2714–18.

Stoter G, Sleijifer DTh, Schormagel JH, Ten Bokkel-Huinink WW, Vermeijlen K, Sylvester R on behalf of the EORTC Genito-Urinary Group (1993). BEP versus VIP in intermediate risk patients with disseminated non-seminomatous testicular cancer (NSTC). *Proceedings of the American Society of Clinical Oncology*, 12:232.

Strader CH, Weiss NS, Daling JR, Karagas MR, McKnight B (1988). Cryptorchism, orchiopexy, and the risk of testicular cancer. *American Journal of Epidemiology*, 127:1013–18.

Strickland S, Sawey MJ (1980). Studies on the effect of retinoids on the differentiation of teratocarcinoma stem cells *in vitro* and *in vivo*. *Developmental Biology*, 78:76–85.

Strohmeyer T, Peter S, Hartmann M, Munemitsu S, Ackermann R, Ullrich A, Slamon DJ (1991) Expression of the HST-1 and C-KIT protoonocogenes in human testicular germ cell tumors. *Cancer Research*, 51(7):1811–16.

Sugimura T, Yoshida T, Sakamoto H, Katoh O, Mattori Y, and Terada M (1990). Molecular biology of the *list 1* gene. In *Proto-oncogenes in cell development* (ed. GJM Bock), pp. 89–105. Wiley, London.

Sujka SK, Huben RP (1991). Clinical stage I nonseminomatous germ cell tumors of testis. Observation vs retroperitoneal lymph node dissection. *Urology*, 38(1):29–31.

Symington T, Cameron KM (1976). Testicular diseases. In *Pathology of the testis* (ed. RCB Pugh), pp. 259–303. Blackwell Scientific Publications, London.

Tait D, Peckham MJ, Hendry W, Goldstraw P (1984). Post-chemotherapy surgery in advanced non-seminoma germ cell tumours: the significance of histology with particular reference to differentiated (mature) teratoma. *British Journal of Cancer*, 50:601–9.

Talerman A (1980). Spermatocytic seminoma: clinicopathological study of 22 cases. *Cancer*, 45:2169–76.

Tepperman BS, Gospodarowicz MK, Bush RS, Brown TC (1982). Non-Hodgkin's lymphoma of the testis. *Radiology*, 142:203–8.

Tesoro-Tess JD, Pizzocaro G, Zanoni F, Musumeci R (1986). Lymphangiography and computerized tomography in testicular carcinoma: how accurate in early state disease? *Journal of Urology*, 133:967–70.

Thomas G (1991). Management of metastatic seminoma: role of radiotherapy. In *Testicular cancer—clinical investigation and management* (ed. A Horwich), pp. 211–31. Chapman & Hall, London.

Thomas GM, *et al.* (1982). Seminoma of the testis: results of treatment and patterns of failure after radiation therapy. *International Journal of Radiation Oncology—Biology—Physics*, 8:165–74.

Thomas GM, *et al.* (1989). A study of post-orchidectomy surveillance in stage I testicular seminoma. *Journal of Urology*, 142:313–16.

Thomas JL, Bernardino ME, Bracken RB (1981). Staging of testicular carcinoma: comparison of CT and lymphangiography. *American Journal of Roentgenology*, 137:991–6.

Thompson IM, Wear J, Almond C, Schewe EJ, Sala J (1961). An analytical survey of one hundred and seventy-eight testicular tumours. *Journal of Urology*, 85:173–9.

Thornhill JA, Fennelley JJ, Kelly DG, Walsh A, Fitzpatrick JM (1987). Patients delay in the presentation of testis cancer in Ireland. *British Journal of Urology*, 59:447.

Tiptaft RC, Nicholls BM, Hately W, Blandy JP (1982). The diagnosis of testicular swelling using water-path ultrasound. *British Journal of Urology*, 54:759–64.

Toner GC, Geller NL, Tan C, Nisselbaum J, Bosl GJ (1990). Serum tumor marker half-life during chemotherapy allows early prediction of complete response and survival in non-seminomatous germ cell tumors. *Cancer Research*, 50:5904–10.

Vaitukaitis JL, Braunstein GD, Ross GT (1972). A radioimmunoassay which specifically measures human chorionic gonadotrophin in the presence of human luteinizing hormone. *American Journal of Obstetrics and Gynecology*, 113:751–8.

Van Barneveld PWC, *et al.* (1985). Changes in pulmonary function during and after bleomycin treatment in patients with testicular carcinoma. *Cancer Chemotherapy and Pharmacology*, 14:168–71.

Vick CW, Bird KI, Rosenfield AT, Richter J, Taylor KJ (1982). Ultrasound of the scrotal contents. *Urologic Radiology*, 4:147–53.

Vogelzang NJ, Lange PH, Goldman A, Vessela RH, Fraley EE, Kennedy BJ (1982). Acute changes of alpha-fetoprotein and human chorionic gonadotrophin during induction chemotherapy of germ cell tumours. *Cancer Research*, 42:4855–61.

Von der Maase H (1991). Diagnosis and management of carcinoma *in situ* of the testis. In *Testicular cancer—clinical investigation and management* (ed. A Horwich), pp. 532–51. Chapman & Hall, London.

Von der Maase H, *et al.* (1985). Carcinoma-*in-situ* of testis eradicated by chemotherapy. *Lancet*, ii:98.

Von der Maase H, *et al.* (1986). Carcinoma *in situ* of contralateral testis in patients with testicular germ cell cancer: study of 27 cases in 500 patients. *British Medical Journal*, 293:1398–401.

Von der Maase H, Giwercman A, Muller J, Skakkebaek NE (1987). Management of carcinoma-*in-situ* of the testis. *International Journal of Andrology*, 10:209–20.

Von der Maase H, Meinecke B, Skakkebaek NE (1988). Residual carcinoma-*in-situ* of contralateral testis after chemotherapy. *Lancet*, i:477–8.

Von der Maase H, *et al.* (1993). Surveillance following orchiedectomy for stage I seminoma of the testis. *European Journal of Cancer*, 29A(14):1931–4.

Vugrin D, Whitmore WF, Golbey RB (1983). VAB-6 combination chemotherapy without maintenance in the treatment of disseminated cancer of the testis. *Cancer*, 51:211–15.

Waldman T, McIntire KR (1974). The use of a radioimmunoassay for alpha-fetoprotein in the diagnosis of malignancy. *Cancer*, 34:1510–15.

Walker MC, Povey S, Parringto JM, Riddle PN, Knuechel R, Masters JRW (1990). Development and characterization of cisplatin-resistant human testicular and bladder tumour cell lines. *European Journal of Cancer*, 26:742–7.

Warde PR, *et al.* (1993). Results of a policy of surveillance in stage I testicular seminoma. *International Journal of Radiation Oncology—Biology—Physics*, 27(1):11–15.

Waterhouse JAH (1985) Epidemiology of testicular tumours. *Journal of Social Medicine*, 78 (Suppl. 6):3–7.

Watson JV, Stewart J, Evan GI, Ritson A, Sikora K (1986). The clinical significance of flow cytometric c-*myc* oncoprotein quantitation in testicular cancer. *British Journal of Cancer*, 53:331–7.

Weitzner S, Addridge JE, Lamar Weems W (1979). Sertoli cell tumour of the testis. *Journal of Urology*, 13:87–9.

Wettlaufer JN (1984). The management of advanced seminoma. *Seminars in Urology*, 2:257–63.

Whitmore WFJ (1982). Surgical treatment of clinical stage I non-seminomatous germ cell tumors of the testis. *Cancer Treatment Reports*, 66:5–10.

Williams SD, Birch R, Einhorn LH (1987a). Disseminated germ cell tumors: chemotherapy with cisplatin plus bleomycin plus either vinblastine or etoposide: a trial of the Southeastern Cancer Study Group. *New England Journal of Medicine*, **316**:1435–40.

Williams SD, *et al.* (1987*b*). Immediate adjuvant chemotherapy versus observation with treatment at relapse in pathological stage II testicular cancer. *New England Journal of Medicine*, **317**:1433–8.

Yamazaki H, Kotera S, Ishikawa H, Machida T (1987). Characterisation of a human chorionic gonadotrophin-producing testicular choriocarcinoma cell line. *Journal of Urology*, **137**:548–51.

Ye DW, Zheng J, Qian SX, Ma Y, Zheng X, Li D, Gu S (1993). p53 gene mutations in Chinese human testicular seminoma. *Journal of Urology*, **150**(3):884–6.

Zagars GK (1991). Management of stage I seminoma: radiotherapy. In *Testicular cancer—clinical investigation and management* (ed. A Horwich), pp. 146–96. Chapman & Hall, London.

Zagars GK, Babaian RJ (1987). Stage I testicular seminoma: rationale for post-orchiectomy radiation therapy. *International Journal of Radiation Oncology—Biology—Physics*, **13**:155–2.

10.2 Extragonadal germ cell tumours

MICHAEL J. BOYER AND DEREK RAGHAVAN

INTRODUCTION

Extragonadal germ cell tumours are rare neoplasms with histological features analogous to those of gonadal germ cell tumours but arising in sites other than the gonads, most commonly the mediastinum, retroperitoneum, sacrococcygeal region, and the pineal.

The histogenesis and management of extragonadal germ cell tumours have been the subject of much controversy for many years. Initial debate centred on whether or not this group of tumours existed at all; some workers suggested that they represented metastases from primary gonadal neoplasms. Many early case reports no longer stand up to critical scrutiny. Prym (1927) first suggested that a fibrous nodule in the testicle of a patient with disseminated choriocarcinoma represented spontaneous regression of a primary tumour. Since that time, 'burnt out' primary lesions of the testis have been documented in patients with apparent extragonadal primary tumours (Friedman and Moore 1946; Rather *et al.* 1954; Azzopardi *et al.* 1961; Azzopardi and Hoffbrand 1965; Meares and Briggs 1972).

More recently, however, it has become apparent that true extragonadal germ cell tumours do exist. Numerous cases have been reported in which the testes of patients with suspected extragonadal tumours have been carefully examined and found to contain neither tumour nor scarring (Utz and Buscemi 1971; Johnson *et al.* 1973; Cox 1975; Luna and Valenzuela-Tamariz 1976; Raghavan and Barrett 1980). These reports of patients with germ cell tumours and histologically normal testicles confirm that the extragonadal types exist independently of their gonadal counterparts. With the demonstration that these tumours are a discrete entity, the focus of interest has shifted. The questions of importance now relate to the optimal management of patients with these rare neoplasms.

HISTOGENESIS

A number of hypotheses have been proposed to account for the occurrence of extragonadal germ cell tumours, although their precise histogenesis remains unclear. It is generally accepted that they arise from primordial germ cells that have been misplaced during ontogeny for unknown reasons. Thus, tumours of different sites originate from germ cells that, during their passage from the yolk sac endoderm, have migrated to the mediastinum or pineal or sacrococcygeal regions rather than to the gonadal ridge. The demonstration of the pathway of germ cell migration (Witschi 1948) has lent support to this theory, which was first proposed by Askanazy (1907). The propensity of these tumours to arise in midline structures is explained by the passage of primordial germ cells in the midline.

An alternative hypothesis proposes that extragonadal germ cell tumours result from the local displacement of germ cell layers during embryogenesis (Schlumberger 1946). Neoplasia develops in rests of totipotential cells left during the blastular or morular stages. For example, mediastinal germ cell tumours would arise, according to this hypothesis, from the third branchial pouch, which is the anlage of the thymus. Other discredited hypotheses include the suppressed twin theory and the concept of fetus *in fetu*, as reviewed elsewhere (Gonzalez-Crussi 1982).

One clinical feature that is not explicable on the basis of either of these hypotheses of histogenesis is the striking male predominance of malignant germ cell tumours. This contrasts with benign extragonadal germ cell tumours, which occur with similar frequency in both sexes. Although explanations for this observation have been offered, including a greater propensity for differentiation in the female related to the endocrine environment (Luna 1976), none is convincing. This difference in frequency is also apparent at gonadal sites, with malignant testicular germ cell tumours occurring much more frequently than their ovarian counterpart; possible reasons for this have been reviewed by Erickson and Gondos (1976).

PATHOLOGY

The histology of the extragonadal germ cell tumours is identical to that of the gonadal. In fact, the intimate admixture of classical elements of seminomatous and non-seminomatous germ cell tumours at extragonadal sites lends support to the view that these tumours have a common origin (Raghavan and Neville 1982). When biopsy specimens of the extragonadal tumours are examined histologically, it is very difficult to distinguish them from their gonadal counterparts without the aid of surrounding tissues. The detailed histopathology of germ cell tumours is beyond the scope of this review and is dealt with elsewhere.

The differentiation between seminomatous and non-seminomatous extragonadal germ cell tumours is one of the most important aspects of the histopathological assessment of these tumours. This distinction carries with it greater therapeutic and prognostic

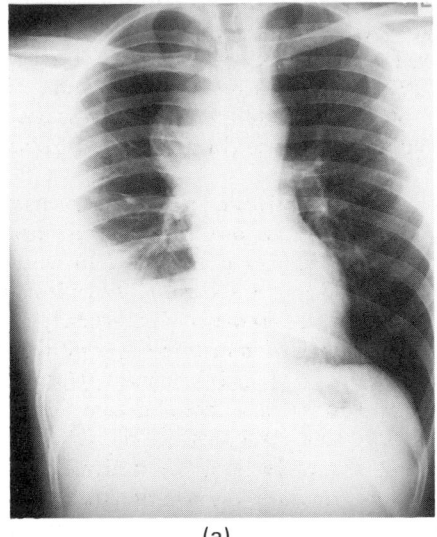
(a)

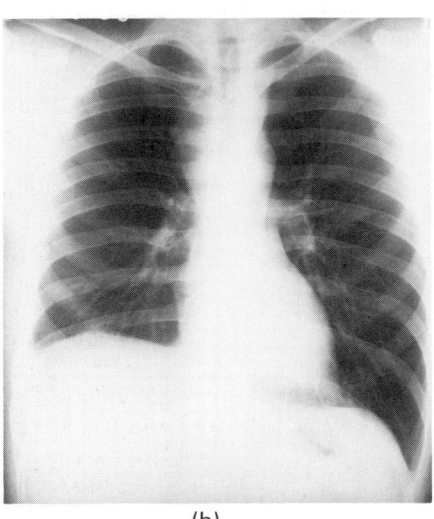
(b)

Fig. 1 (a) and (b) Mediastinal germ cell tumour before and after treatment with chemotherapy.

significance than the site of extragonadal presentation of the tumour.

The most common sites of the extragonadal tumours are mediastinum, retroperitoneum, sacrococcygeal region, and pineal. Histological diagnosis may be difficult; in particular, differentiation of mediastinal germ cell tumours from thymoma may pose problems (Lattes 1962). There are numerous case reports of these tumours arising in other locations, although many of these do not stand up to critical scrutiny with respect to the absence of testicular involvement. Reported sites are prostate (Benson *et al.* 1978), bladder (Hyman and Leiter 1943), liver (Misugi and Reiner 1965; Hart 1975), oesophagus (Kikuchi *et al.* 1988), and stomach (Holt *et al.* 1965).

CLINICAL FEATURES

Mediastinum

Primary mediastinal germ cell tumours are rare, accounting for only 2–6 per cent of mediastinal tumours and 5–13 per cent of malignant mediastinal tumours (Joseph *et al.* 1966; Wychulis *et al.* 1971; Conkle and Adkins 1972; Cox 1975). These tumours have been reported with equal frequency in males and females, although there is an excess of malignancy in males (Cox 1975; Martini *et al.* 1974; Polansky *et al.* 1979). Usually they occur in the second to fourth decades of life (Martini *et al.* 1974; Luna and Valenzuela-Tamariz 1976), but they have also been reported in childhood, accounting for 10–20 per cent of mediastinal tumours (Canty and Siemens 1978).

The symptoms and signs produced by mediastinal germ cell tumours relate to their anatomical location adjacent to vital intrathoracic structures (Fig. 1), with direct local extension being a more common cause of symptoms than metastatic disease (Vogelzang *et al.* 1982). The most common presenting feature is chest pain, although up to 25 per cent are detected by routine chest radiographs (Leading Article 1969; Martini *et al.* 1974; Cox 1975) (Table 1). Other common clinical features include dyspnoea, cough (with or without haemoptysis), constitutional upset with fevers, and weight loss. In patients with mediastinal choriocarcinoma, gynaecomastia occurs commonly (Leading Article 1969). Obstruction of the superior vena cava is noted in 10–25 per cent of patients (Polansky *et al.* 1979; Vogelzang *et al.* 1982). Typically, by the time of presentation there is advanced local disease (Jain *et al.* 1984).

The pattern of metastasis is outlined in Table 2. There is a difference in the sites of metastases detected in autopsy series from clinical series, reflecting the propensity of germ cell tumours to metastasize widely when uncontrolled and the lack of symptoms associated with certain sites of presentation. From autopsy series, the common sites of metastasis include lung, liver, lymph nodes, and bone (Oberman and Libcke 1964; Cox 1975; Luna and Valenzuela-Tamariz 1976; Recondo and Libshitz 1978; Aliotta *et al.* 1988). By contrast, clinical series report only the lung, lymph nodes, and pleura as frequent metastatic sites (Martini *et al.* 1974; Walden *et al.* 1977; Burt and Javadpour 1981) and in one series, no patient had metastatic disease (Vogelzang *et al.* 1982).

Retroperitoneum

The second most common site of origin of extragonadal germ cell tumours is the retroperitoneum (MacKay and Sellers 1966). Approximately 10 per cent of primary retroperitoneal tumours are reported to be teratomas and 6.8–10 per cent of these are malignant (Palumbo *et al.* 1949; Arnheim 1951). However, these reports preceded the introduction of modern pathological techniques and non-invasive staging investigations and may be inaccurate. Seminomas, non-seminomas, and mature teratomas all occur in the retroperitoneum (Palumbo *et al.* 1949; Abell *et al.* 1965; Engel *et al.* 1968; Pantoja *et al.* 1976).

Table 1 Presentation of mediastinal germ cell tumours (seminoma and non-seminoma)

Presentation	%
Chest pain	40
Cough	24
Routine chest radiograph	21
Dyspnoea	10
Constitutional	9
Superior vena caval obstruction	5
Haemoptysis	3
Gynaecomastia	3

Data from Oberman and Libcke (1964), Patcher and Lattes (1964), Martini *et al.* (1974), Cox (1975), Bush *et al.* (1981), Hurt *et al.* (1982), and Kay *et al.* (1987).

Table 2 Sites of metastasis of mediastinal non-seminomatous germ cell tumours

Site	Combined autopsy series (%)	Combined clinical series (%)
Lung	75.0	67.0
Liver	62.5	13.8
Lymph nodes	60.0	31.0
Bone	27.5	2.7
Kidney	15.0	5.5
Central nervous system	12.5	8.3
Spleen	7.5	
Adrenal	5.0	
Muscle	2.5	
Heart	2.5	
Pleura[a]	2.5	38.8
Pericardium[a]		27.7

[a]Possibly direct extension.

Data from Schlumberger (1946), Oberman and Libcke (1964), Martini et al. (1974), Luna et al. (1976), Walden et al. (1977), Recondo (1978), Burt and Javadpour (1981), and Kay et al. (1987).

Retroperitoneal non-seminomatous germ cell tumours occur predominantly in teenage children, with the most common lesion being a mature teratoma and only 10 per cent demonstrating malignant features. These tumours are slightly more common in females (Palumbo et al. 1949; Engel et al. 1968). Seminomas at this site, by contrast, are more common in an older age group, with the mean age in reported series ranging from 42 to 48 years (Abell et al. 1965; Medini et al. 1979; Feun et al. 1980; Jain et al. 1984).

The most common presenting features are abdominal pain (80 per cent) or a palpable mass (40–75 per cent). In addition, abdominal distension (15–20 per cent), back pain (10 per cent), weight loss (10 per cent), nausea and vomiting (5–10 per cent), and constipation (5 per cent) may occur. Rarely, urinary tract symptoms and vascular obstruction may be present. Occasional patients present with an asymptomatic mass detected on routine physical examination.

The major diagnostic difficulty with retroperitoneal germ cell tumours is the exclusion of a testicular primary. Reports of patients with apparent primary retroperitoneal germ cell tumours who are later shown to have a testicular focus of tumour emphasize the need for careful physical examination, supplemented by the use of high-resolution ultrasonography, before a firm diagnosis is made (Kirschling et al. 1983; Bohle et al. 1986; Saltzman et al. 1986). Because of the usual pattern of spread of testicular germ cell tumours, this distinction is a greater problem in the case of retroperitoneal germ cell tumours, particularly if lateralized, as it raises the issue of the management of the testicular primary lesion. That issue is of less importance in mediastinal germ cell tumours, as isolated anterior mediastinal metastasis from testicular cancer is a most unusual occurrence (Peckham 1981). For example, Bohle et al. (1986) reported occult testicular primary tumours, noted by ultrasonography or biopsy, in 10 of 12 men with retroperitoneal germ cell tumours and in none (of four) with mediastinal germ cell tumours; however, of importance, five of these 10 men had a clinically abnormal testicle.

Sacrococcygeal region

Germ cell tumours of the sacrococcygeal and presacral regions are rare. They occur predominantly in infants, with an incidence of approximately 1 in 40 000 births (Ross 1948; Dillard et al. 1970;

Izant and Filston 1975). There is a marked female preponderance (4 : 1), although as at other sites, malignancy is more common in males (Gross et al. 1951; Donellan and Swenson 1968; Altman et al. 1974; Schey et al. 1977). In adults the tumour is rare, with a reported incidence of 1 in 87 000 hospital admissions and malignancy is an unusual occurrence (Marcuse 1959; Miles and Stewart 1974).

Germ cell tumours arising in this site are unusual in that they frequently are benign. The precise incidence of malignancy is difficult to define because of varying criteria used to make this diagnosis. While Donellan and Swenson (1968) have relied on the demonstration of invasion for the diagnosis of malignancy, others have only required the presence of immature or primitive tissue in order to classify a tumour as 'potentially malignant' (Conklin and Abell 1967). Overall, the reported incidence of malignancy ranges from 9 to 40 per cent (Donellan and Swenson 1968; Whalen et al. 1985; Dewan et al. 1987). The frequency of malignancy is age related and these tumours are much less common under the age of 2 months and in adults (Donellan and Swenson 1968; Altman et al. 1974; Miles and Stewart 1974).

The clinical picture in these patients is dominated by the presence of a large pelvic mass, often detected pre-natally or at birth. Sacrococcygeal teratomas, especially those which are benign, may be asymptomatic. If the tumour is large, progressive obstructive symptoms may occur, owing to rectal compression or involvement of the bladder neck (Donellan and Swenson 1968; Whalen et al. 1985). The young age group in which these tumours frequently occur may account, to a large extent, for the lack of reported symptoms. Occasionally, lower-limb weakness or pain may occur as a result of peripheral nerve encroachment or when there is an intraspinal component (Gwinn et al. 1955), which may be found in both benign and malignant tumours. Local complications of these tumours may include haemorrhage, necrosis, and infection.

The tumour may have variable intra- and extrapelvic components. In an attempt to classify these tumours, the American Academy of Pediatrics has divided them, based on the degree of intrapelvic tumour (Altman et al. 1974). Type I tumours are those with predominantly sacrococcygeal tumour and only a minimal presacral component, whereas type IV have no external component. Types II and III have increasing volumes of intrapelvic disease. Type I and II tumours were the most common in a review of 405 patients, accounting for 46 and 35 per cent of cases (Altman et al. 1974).

Clinical associations have been reported with sacrococcygeal teratomas, including a family history of twins (Gross et al. 1951; Izant and Filston 1975; Schey et al. 1977) and coccygeal or sacral agenesis (Kenefick 1973). Six families have been reported with a syndrome of type IV teratoma, anal stenosis, and an autosomal dominant pattern of inheritance. In these families, the sex incidence was almost equal (Ashcraft and Holder 1965; Hunt et al. 1977).

Intracranial germ cell tumours

In Western countries, primary germ cell tumours of the pineal and suprasellar regions are rare, accounting for 0.4–3.4 per cent of all primary intracranial neoplasms (Jellinger 1973). By contrast, in Japan and Taiwan, comparable rates of 2.1–9.4 per cent exist (Koide et al. 1980). The reason for this difference and the aetiology of these tumours is unknown. Intracranial germ cell neoplasms occur most commonly in the first two decades of life (Jenkin et al. 1978; Jennings et al. 1985; Edwards et al. 1988), although a case has been reported in a 69-year-old (Jennings et al. 1985). Whilst pineal germinomas are twice as common in males (Jenkin et al. 1978; Wara (a)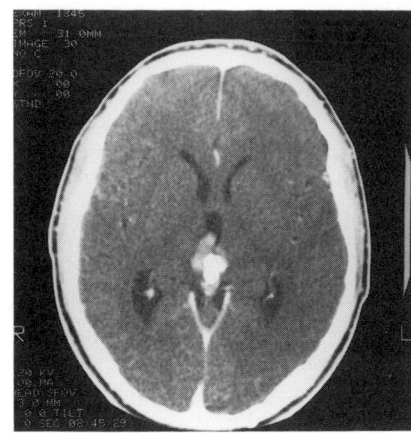

(b)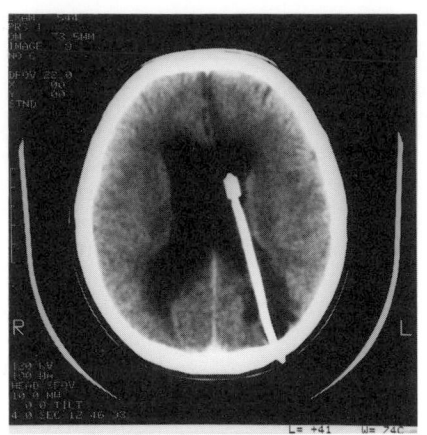

Fig. 2 (a) and (b) CT scans of pineal tumours.

et al. 1979; Jennings *et al.* 1985), no such sex difference exists for suprasellar germ cell tumours (Simson *et al.* 1968; Jenkin *et al.* 1978; Sung *et al.* 1978).

Both seminomatous and non-seminomatous germ cell tumours may originate intracranially (Russell 1944; Friedman 1947; Dayan *et al.* 1966; Borit 1969; Beeley *et al.* 1973; Ho and Rassekh 1979). The most common sites are the pineal and suprasellar regions, which together account for 95 per cent of cases (Jennings *et al.* 1985). Other sites include the third ventricle, basal ganglia/thalamus, and other ventricular regions (Jennings *et al.* 1985). Germinomas (seminomas) are the most common tumours at both pineal and suprasellar sites, but when they do occur, non-seminomatous germ cell tumours are more frequently pineal in location (Jennings *et al.* 1985).

Typically, there is a prolonged symptomatic period (which may be longer than 2 years) before the diagnosis is made (Jennings *et al.* 1985). Symptoms and signs are related to the nearby anatomical structures and, thus, differ for suprasellar and pineal tumours. Pineal tumours, with their location close to the midbrain and aquaduct, frequently present with headache (80–100 per cent), and nausea and vomiting (50–100 per cent), indicative of raised intracranial pressure (Fig. 2). Signs on physical examination include papilloedema (50–65 per cent) and features of Parinaud's syndrome (paralysis of conjugate upward deviation of the eyes) (20–60 per cent). In contrast, suprasellar tumours, located in the region of the optic chiasm, pituitary and hypothalamus, commonly present with symptoms of visual disturbance (20–100 per cent), polyuria and polydipsia (40–80 per cent), and lethargy and somnolence (40–50 per cent). Signs of hypopituitarism (20–70 per cent) are often present, as are those of visual field loss (35–60 per cent) (Simson *et al.* 1968; Sung *et al.* 1978; Abay *et al.* 1981; Amendola *et al.* 1984; Jennings *et al.* 1985; Sakai *et al.* 1988; Legido *et al.* 1989).

The most common site of metastatic disease is the spinal subarachnoid space, although systemic metastases have been reported in patients with and without ventriculosystemic shunts (Giuffre and Di Lorenzo 1975; Jennings *et al.* 1985). Spinal metastasis occurs in 15 per cent of cases (range, 5–57 per cent) (Wara *et al.* 1977; Jenkin *et al.* 1978; Sung *et al.* 1978; Chapman and Linggood 1980). It has been suggested that this is more common after biopsy of the primary tumour (Wara *et al.* 1977; Jenkin *et al.* 1978; Sung *et al.* 1978; Leibel and Sheline 1987).

INVESTIGATION

In general the investigation of patients with extragonadal germ cell tumours is similar to that of patients with the gonadal counterparts.

The major goal of assessment is to delineate the histological type and extent of the tumour.

In addition, however, exclusion of a testicular origin for the neoplasm is mandatory, especially in retroperitoneal germ cell tumour. Careful clinical examination of the testicles can be supplemented by high-resolution ultrasonography, as the discovery of a testicular primary site will affect subsequent therapy. The testis represents a 'sanctuary' site and tumour within it may remain viable after aggressive multiagent chemotherapy (Greist *et al.* 1984). By contrast, if both clinical examination and ultrasonograms of the testicles are normal, there is no routine indication for orchidectomy.

The applications of the serum tumour markers, β-human chorionic gonadotrophin and α-fetoprotein, are identical in the management of gonadal and extragonadal germ cell tumours and this is described in detail elsewhere. Of importance, however, has been the recognition that pure seminoma does not produce α-fetoprotein and elevated amounts imply the presence of non-seminomatous elements (Raghavan *et al.* 1982). This is of therapeutic significance (see below), as the results of radiotherapy for non-seminomatous extragonadal germ cell tumours are generally poor and these patients are best managed with combination chemotherapy.

A further application of tumour markers is their measurement in the cerebrospinal fluid. If chorionic gonadotrophin is not being produced in the central nervous system, its concentration in the cerebrospinal fluid should be less than 2.5 per cent of that in serum (Kaye *et al.* 1979). Simultaneous measurement of serum and cerebrospinal fluid concentrations may help to determine whether disease is present outside the central nervous system in cases of primary intracranial non-seminomatous germ cell tumour. In other extragonadal germ cell tumours, raised concentrations may be an indicator of central nervous metastasis. This is of particular value in patients with mediastinal or retroperitoneal choriocarcinoma. In this context, we routinely screen for central nervous involvement with computerized tomography (**CT**) followed by lumbar puncture.

Difficulties exist in the interpretation of marker concentrations in cerebrospinal fluid in two settings: after placement of a ventriculosystemic shunt, serum concentrations of human chorionic gonadotrophin may be falsely elevated in patients with disease limited to the central nervous system; measurement of α-fetoprotein in the cerebrospinal fluid is unreliable (Kaye *et al.* 1979), and thus of limited use.

TREATMENT

Accounts of the management of extragonadal germ cell tumours are complicated by the variety of nomenclature used and the failure,

Table 3 Results of radiotherapy (with or without surgery) for extragonadal seminoma (based on initial treatment; some patients received chemotherapy at relapse)

Author	Year	No. of patients	Site	Alive		Dead
				No disease	Disease	
Abell et al.	1965	10	R	6 (6–288 months)		4 (5–12 months)
El-Domeiri et al.	1968	9	M	4 (90–216 months)	1	4 (12–96 months)
Schantz et al.	1972	17	M	16 (4–240 months)		1 (operative)
Martini et al.	1974	10	M	3 (144–288 months)	2	5 (9–150 months)
Cox	1975	6	M	4 (26–216 months)		2 (4–28 months)
Recondo et al.	1978	5	M	2 (96–108 months)	2	1 (96 months)
Medini et al.	1979	8	M, R	4 (60–204 months)		4 (2–192 months)
Polansky et al.	1979	4	M	3 (6–18 months)		1 (8 months)
Raghavan et al.	1980	6[a]	M	2 (58–132 months)	1	2 (35–43 months)
Bush et al.	1981	13	M	54 % (actuarial)		31% (actuarial)
Economou et al.	1982	11	M	9 (36–180 months)		2 (3, 9 months)
Hurt et al.	1982	16	M	9 (14–336 months)		7 (6–130 months)
Jain et al.	1984	10	M, R	6 (55–104 months)[b]		4 (13–36 months)

M, mediastinum; R, retroperitoneum.
[a]One patient too early to assess.
[b]One patient lost to follow-up at 55 months.

in earlier series, to distinguish between seminomatous and non-seminomatous tumours. Due to the rarity of the condition, most reported series include patients treated over a long time-span, with a variety of different surgical or radiotherapeutic techniques or chemotherapeutic regimens.

Mediastinal germ cell tumours

Benign teratomas

Left untreated, benign teratomas of the mediastinum may cause a variety of complications; compression of adjacent structures such as the great vessels, malignant degeneration, and infection or haemorrhage may all occur. Furthermore, the diagnosis in such cases is often established by percutaneous needle biopsy. Although this is a useful technique, malignancy may be overlooked as a result of sampling error; even with surgical biopsy the same problem may occur. Consequently, all mediastinal germ cell tumours should be resected if possible, even if apparently benign. Careful histological examination is then required to exclude malignancy in any part of the tumour. For truly benign teratomas, surgical resection alone is adequate treatment. If histological evidence of malignancy is detected, however, management should be along the lines described below.

Seminoma

Traditionally, the management of mediastinal seminoma was based upon locoregional therapy, with radiotherapy either being used alone or after surgery (Bagshaw et al. 1969; Medini et al. 1979; Polansky et al. 1979; Raghavan and Barrett 1980; Bush et al. 1981; Hurt et al. 1982). A dose of 35–40 Gy, in fractions of 1.5–2 Gy, was recommended as the treatment of choice (Bagshaw et al. 1969; Medini et al. 1979; Economou et al. 1982). The results of treatment varied, but in an analysis of 106 patients reported in the literature, the 5 year survival rate was 58 per cent (Nickels and Franssila 1972; Schantz et al. 1972; Besznyak et al. 1973; Martini et al. 1974; Sterchi and Cordell 1975).

The results of surgery and radiotherapy for extragonadal seminoma are presented in Table 3. Most deaths occurred as a result of metastases, with treatment proving effective in controlling locoregional disease. Although chemotherapy was used in some patients in these series, it was given late in the course of the illness, and with relatively ineffective drugs such as thiotepa, melphalan, nitrogen mustard, chlorambucil, and cyclophosphamide (Martini et al. 1974; Raghavan and Barrett 1980). However, many of these reports preceded the introduction of modern imaging techniques such as CT scanning, and some of the treatment failures may have represented the inappropriate treatment of patients with metastatic disease by using only local therapy.

With the introduction of cisplatin in the 1970s, there was a change in the approach to the treatment of mediastinal seminoma. The recognition that seminoma, whether of gonadal or extragonadal origin, is exquisitely chemosensitive has led to the proposition that high-dose (100–120 mg/m^2 per cycle) cisplatin-based combination chemotherapy should be the mainstay of treatment in mediastinal seminoma (Jain et al. 1984; Logothetis et al. 1985; Motzer et al. 1988). This is followed, where appropriate, by radiotherapy or, less frequently, surgery for residual tumour masses. On using this combined approach, complete remission and long-term survival has been achieved in more than 80 per cent of patients. Furthermore, in a series of patients with advanced seminoma (44 with testicular primary, 17 with extragonadal primary), there was no significant difference in survival following cisplatin-based chemotherapy between the two groups (Motzer et al. 1988). Table 4 summarizes the published experience of cisplatin-based chemotherapy in patients with mediastinal seminoma.

Our approach to the management of such patients is to treat them with radiotherapy to the mediastinum if a thorough evaluation fails to reveal evidence of metastatic spread and the maximum horizontal diameter of the tumour is less than 50 per cent of the width of the thorax. Radiotherapy is delivered with a 'shrinking field' technique, where the fields are modified as the tumour mass regresses; the exposure of normal lung to radiation is thus decreased. If metastases are present at diagnosis or if the tumour occupies more than half of the thoracic diameter, combination chemotherapy is used routinely, followed by radiotherapy to residual masses.

High response rates have now been demonstrated in men with metastatic testicular seminoma treated with carboplatinum-based chemotherapy (Peckham et al. 1985). Although we have not used carboplatinum in extragonadal seminoma, it is likely to have similar

Table 4 Results of chemotherapy (with or without post-chemotherapy surgery) for mediastinal germ cell tumours

Author	Year	No. of patients	Chemotherapy	Alive — No disease	Disease	Dead
Mediastinal seminoma						
Feun et al.[a]	1980	2	VBP			2 (? follow-up)
Jain et al.	1984	5	VAB-6	5 (19–23 months)		0
		2	CP	2 (29, 46 months)		0
Logothetis et al.	1985	1	CISCA$_{II}$	1 } Duration		0
		3	CP	3 }		0
Motzer et al.[b]	1988	17	VAB-6 or EP	?	?	2 (<2 years)
Mediastinal non-seminoma						
Feun et al.[a]	1980	7	VBP	PR 3 (mean 4 months), no response 4		
Vogelzang et al.	1982	7	PVB	3 (12–30 months)		4 (3–9 months)
		5	No cDDP	1 (56 months)		4 (2–12 months)
Hainsworth et al.[c]	1982	31	PVB	19 (5–52 months)	2	10 (2–9 months)
Kuzur[d]	1982	10	Various	1 (60 months)	1	8 (9–23 months)
Garnick et al.	1983	8	PVB	1 (24 months)	1	6 (3–15 months)
Parker et al.	1983	8	POMB/ACE	5 (13–136 months)		3 (1–15 months)
Logothetis et al.	1985	4	No cDDP			4 }
		6	CISCA$_{II}$	1 } ? time		5 } ? time
		5	CISCA$_{II}$/VB$_{IV}$	3 }		2 }
Israel et al.[e]	1985	12	VAB-3	1 (8 months)		11
		6	VAB-5			6
		11	VAB-6	4 (median 36 months)		7
Kay et al.[f]	1987	12	PVB/BEP	5 (48–84 months)	2	3 (3–6 months)
Mcleod et al.[e]	1988	7	VAB/VV	3 (24–57 months)		4 (5–25 months)
		2	Other	1 (23 months)	1	

Abbreviations: PR, partial response; VBP, vinblastine, bleomycin, cisplatin (also PVB); VAB 3–6, see VAB/VV; no cDDP, non-cisplatin-containing chemotherapy; CISCA$_{II}$, cyclophosphamide, adriamycin and cisplatin; CP, cyclophosphamide and cisplatin; EP, etoposide and cisplatin; POMB/ACE, see text; VAB/VV, cyclophosphamide, vinblastine, actinomycin D, bleomycin, cisplatin, etoposide, vincristine; VB$_{IV}$, continuous-infusion vinblastine and bleomycin; BEP, bleomycin+EP.
[a] Some patients had prior radiotherapy; cisplatin dose, 75 mg/m^2 per cycle.
[b] Ten cases retroperitoneal and seven cases mediastinal seminoma.
[c] Retroperitoneal non-seminomatous germ cell tumours included; endodermal sinus tumours excluded; includes six patients with seminoma; six patients had prior radiotherapy and seven also received adriamycin.
[d] All endodermal sinus tumours.
[e] Includes cases of retroperitoneal non-seminomatous germ cell tumours.
[f] Two patients lost to follow-up.

efficacy to cisplatin-based regimens. The decreased oto- and nephrotoxicity compared to cisplatinum may facilitate the use of carboplatinum in combination with radiotherapy in the future, although further experience with this drug is required.

Non-seminoma

In general, the results of the treatment of non-seminomatous mediastinal germ cell tumours have been disappointing compared with those for seminomas. Interpretation of the literature is once again hampered by the small numbers of patients reported in each series and the variety of treatment regimens used. In addition, some groups have excluded endodermal sinus tumours and included seminomas in their results, making comparisons difficult (Hainsworth et al. 1982). However, since the introduction of cisplatin, regimens have become more standardized and the results of series employing cisplatin-based therapy are summarized in Table 4.

A variety of regimens such as cisplatin, vinblastine, bleomycin (**PVB**), vincristine, actinomycin D, bleomycin and cisplatin (**VAB-6**), vincristine, methotrexate, bleomycin, cisplatin/actinomycin D, cyclophosphamide, etoposide (**POMB/ACE**), and cyclophosphamide, adriamycin, cisplatin with continuous-infusion vinblastine and bleomycin (**CISCA$_{II}$/VB$_{IV}$**) has been used (Hainsworth et al. 1982;

Newlands et al. 1983; Logothetis et al. 1985; Bosl et al. 1986); although differing in some details, they are similar in that they employ cisplatin in a dose of 100–120 mg/m^2 per cycle. There are no data available that directly compare any of these treatment programmes. More recently, the use of a regimen containing cisplatin, 200 mg/m^2 per cycle, for the treatment of poor-prognosis testicular cancer, including extragonadal germ cell tumours, has been reported (Ozols et al. 1988). Overall, there was a statistically significant improvement in survival when compared to standard PVB, but data relating to the subgroup of patients with extragonadal tumours were not provided.

The role of post-chemotherapy surgery in extragonadal germ cell tumours is also unclear. However, using testicular cancer as a model, most groups have advocated its use (Parker et al. 1983; Kay et al. 1987). In the case of mediastinal germ cell tumours, however, the location of the primary tumour may make adequate resection impossible.

Durable complete remissions are achieved in only 20–40 per cent of patients (Vogelzang et al. 1982; Garnick et al. 1983; Israel et al. 1985; Logothetis et al. 1985). Although numbers are small, patients treated with recent more intensive regimens (VAB-6, CISCA$_{II}$/VB$_{IV}$, POMB/ACE) may have a higher rate of complete remission (Newlands et al. 1983; Israel et al. 1985; Logothetis et al.

Table 5 Results of chemotherapy (with or without post-chemotherapy surgery) for retroperitoneal germ cell tumours

Author	Year	No. of patients	Chemotherapy	Alive — No disease	Disease	Dead
Retroperitoneal seminoma						
Feun et al.[a]	1980	2	VBP			2
Jain et al.	1984	1	PVB			1 (16 months)
		3	VAB-6	3 (21–38 months)		
Logothetis et al.	1985	1	No cDDP			1 ⎫
		1	CISCA$_{II}$	1		⎬ ? duration
		13	CP	11	1	1 ⎭
Retroperitoneal non-seminoma						
Feun et al.[a]	1980	4	VBP	1 CR, 2 PR and 1 no response		
Garnick et al.	1983	5	PVB	3 (26–58 months)	0	2 (15, 44 months)
Logothetis et al.	1985	6	No cDDP	2 ⎫		4
		3	VB$_{III}$+P	2 ⎪ ? time		1 ⎫ ? time
		3	CISCA$_{II}$	1 ⎪		2 ⎭
		3	CISCA$_{II}$/VB$_{IV}$	3 ⎭		
Tondini and Garnick[b]	1989	13	PVB/PEB(A)	7 (14–48 months)	?	?

Abbreviations: CR, complete response; PR, partial response; no cDDP, non-cisplatin-containing chemotherapy; CP, cyclophosphamide and cisplatin; CISCA$_{II}$, cyclophosphamide, adriamycin and cisplatin; PVB/PEB(A), alternating PVB and PEB (see Table 4 for these and other abbreviations) with or without adriamycin; VB$_{IV}$, continuous-infusion vinblastine and bleomycin.
[a] Some patients had prior radiotherapy; cisplatin dose, 75 mg/m^2 per cycle.
[b] Includes two patients with seminoma, and two with mediastinal extragonadal germ cell tumours.

Table 6 Results of therapy of malignant sacrococcygeal germ cell tumours

Author	Year	No. of patients	Number receiving: Surgery	Radiotherapy	Chemotherapy	Alive — NED	Disease	Dead
Applebaum et al.	1979	6	6	4	6	4 (17–96 months)	1 (66 months)	1 (14 months)
Brodeur et al.	1981	12		9	11	2 (86/122 months)	0	10 (2–28 months)
Noseworthy et al.	1981	21	19	14[a]	14[a]	0	0	21 (7 days–19 months)
Raney et al.	1981	12	8	10	12	2 (72–96 months)	0	10 (6 days–36 months)
Whalen et al.	1985	19	19	13	14	1 (25 years)	0	18
Dewan et al.	1987	19	18	7	14	6 (7–120 months)	1 (6 months)	12 (0–81 months)
Total		89				15 (17%)	2 (2%)	72 (81%)

[a] Fourteen patients received radiotherapy ± chemotherapy.
NED, no evidence of disease.

1985) and these approaches will require further validation in structured studies. Another possible option may be afforded by the recent demonstration of tumour responses in association with high-dose therapy and autologous bone-marrow transplantation.

Retroperitoneal germ cell tumours

The approach to management of retroperitoneal germ cell tumour is dependent on both the histological type and size of the tumour. For the same reasons as described above for mediastinal teratomas, benign retroperitoneal teratomas should be resected. The need for further therapy after resection is, once again, determined by the histological findings.

It has been suggested that seminomas of the retroperitoneal space without evidence of metastatic disease should be treated with radiotherapy, if less than 5 cm in largest extent. Doses of 18–40 Gy have been used (Abell et al. 1965; Medini et al. 1979) with excellent outcomes. However, because of the lack of symptoms associated with masses in the retroperitoneum, seminomas at this site are more frequently large. In testicular seminoma with retroperitoneal lymph-node metastases, the results of radiotherapy alone in patients with masses greater than 5 cm in diameter are poor (Lederman et al. 1989). Furthermore, if relapse occurs after radiotherapy, delivery of subsequent chemotherapy may be compromised (Loehrer et al. 1987). Based on this, the initial treatment in patients with large retroperitoneal seminoma should be chemotherapy. The regimens used are similar to those for mediastinal seminoma. Table 5 outlines the results of treatment, which, similar to mediastinal seminomas, results in a large proportion of long-term survivors. It is our practice to irradiate residual masses after chemotherapy.

We believe that non-seminomatous germ cell tumours of the retroperitoneum should be treated initially with combination chemotherapy, using one of the dose-intensive regimens as described for the mediastinal type. Residual masses should be resected surgically; further chemotherapy may be necessary in those with viable tumour at resection. Although reported results (Table 5), particularly from older series, are poor, improved survival may occur after treatment with more intensive regimens (Garnick et al. 1983; Logothetis et al. 1985). Despite this, late relapses may occur in the retroperitoneum or even in the testes (Boyer et al. 1990).

Sacrococcygeal tumours

The mainstay of management of sacrococcygeal tumours in children has been immediate radical surgical resection. Excision of the coccyx

Table 7 Results of radiotherapy for intracranial germ cell tumours

Author	Year	Type	Continuous NED/treated	Survival[a] (%)	Follow-up
Wara *et al.*	1977	Germinoma	5/6	83.0	10 months–21 years
		P & S, no biopsy	11/13	76.0	2–20 years
Jenkin *et al.*	1978	P, germinoma	8/10	100.0	
		S, germinoma	2/6		2 months–10 years
		<25 years, no biopsy	12/15	81.0	
		>225 years, no biopsy	5/16	37.0	
Sung *et al.*	1978	All P & S tumours	44/72	78.0	5–23 years
Salazar *et al.*	1979	P+ectopic	13/22	54.0	1–16 years
Wara *et al.*	1979	All P & S tumours	69/118	65.0	2–15 years
		P & S, germinoma	?	72.0	?
Abay *et al.*	1981	P, no biopsy	14/27	48.0	2–30 years
Amendola *et al.*	1984	P, germinoma	5/15	40.0	6–288 months
		P, no biopsy	12/12	83.0	144–360 months
Rich *et al.*	1985	P & S, germinoma	3/4	75.0	6–64 months
		P & S, non-germinoma	4/7	57.0	7–32 months
		No biopsy	12/14	93.0	4–127 months
Edwards *et al.*	1988	P, germinoma	9/11	91.0	1–12 years
		P, non-germinoma	2/8[b]	37.5	1–5 years
Sakai *et al.*	1988	IC, germinoma	20/24	83.0	1–11.5 years
		IC, non-germinoma	2/7	71.0	
Legido *et al.*	1989	S, germinoma	9/10	100.0	2–9.3 years

P, pineal; S, suprasellar; G, germinoma; IC, intracranial.
[a] Percentage alive at time of report, varying follow-up.
[b] Some patients received adjuvant chemotherapy.

should be included as part of the operative procedure because relapse is common if this is not done (Donellan and Swenson 1968; Whalen *et al.* 1985; Dewan *et al.* 1987). This should be carried out irrespective of the age of the patient (even in the neonate), as delay increases the probability of malignant transformation. The results of this approach in benign tumours are excellent, with almost all patients being cured (Conklin and Abell 1967; Donellan and Swenson 1968; Izant and Filston 1975; Schey *et al.* 1977; Whalen *et al.* 1985). Even in a series where 12 out of 40 patients had excision delayed for up to 24 months the outcome was excellent, with 33 being long-term survivors (Dewan *et al.* 1987). Most sacrococcygeal tumours are resectable via a sacral approach, although in those with a large intrapelvic component, a combined abdominoperineal operation may be necessary (Donellan and Swenson 1968).

Occasionally there is local recurrence that requires further surgery (Altman *et al.* 1974); in a small number of cases the recurrence may be malignant (Dewan *et al.* 1987). The major risks of radical surgery are incomplete removal of the coccyx (with a high rate of subsequent recurrence), hypotensive shock due to inadequate fluid replacement in the neonate, and unrecognized dural injury in tumours with intraspinal components (Gross *et al.* 1951; Donellan and Swenson 1968).

In adults, where the risk of malignancy is lower, the need for surgical resection is less pressing, although most will require resection for the relief of symptoms. As in children, the prognosis after complete resection of a benign sacrococcygeal teratoma is excellent.

In contrast to benign sacrococcygeal teratomas, the results of treatment of malignant germ cell tumours of this site are unsatisfactory (Table 6). Surgery, as single therapy, is inadequate: the primary tumours are often incapable of resection (Dewan *et al.* 1987; Mahour 1988) and distant metastases are often present, sometimes at diagnosis (Altman *et al.* 1974; Brodeur *et al.* 1981; Dewan *et al.* 1987). Although combined approaches employing surgery together with chemotherapy and/or radiotherapy have been used, the outcome has been disappointing. Even with modern multiagent chemotherapy, only 5–31 per cent of patients achieve lasting remissions (Brodeur *et al.* 1981; Whalen *et al.* 1985; Dewan *et al.* 1987). However, in a preliminary report, better results have been documented, with four out of six patients remaining disease free for periods of 17 months to 8 years after more aggressive multimodality therapy (Appelbaum *et al.* 1979).

Intracranial germ cell tumours

The 'standard' approach to the management of incracranial germ cell tumours has been a shunting procedure to relieve hydrocephalus, followed by radiotherapy (Simson *et al.* 1968; Jenkin *et al.* 1978; Sung *et al.* 1978; Abay *et al.* 1981). A histological diagnosis has only occasionally been achieved because of the location of the tumour and this has contributed substantially to the controversy over treatment outcomes. The specific therapeutic role of surgery has been thought to be limited in view of substantial morbidity and mortality (Schmidek 1977).

The techniques of irradiation vary, with different groups recommending various field sizes and doses. Most commonly a dose to the tumour volume of 50 Gy in 25 fractions has been used (Jenkin *et al.* 1978; Sung *et al.* 1978; Rich *et al.* 1985), although doses as low as 35 Gy (Jenkin *et al.* 1978) and as high as 72 Gy (Edwards *et al.* 1988) have been reported. Furthermore, little agreement exists as to the need for adjuvant craniospinal irradiation (Jenkin *et al.* 1978; Edwards *et al.* 1988; Legido *et al.* 1989). Its proponents emphasize a rate of metastasis via cerebrospinal fluid of 37 per cent (particularly in suprasellar germinomas) and use this as justification for the extended radiation field (Legido *et al.* 1989). Opponents of this approach point out that in the absence of biopsy, metastasis by cerebrospinal fluid is rare and that craniospinal irradiation is associated with increased toxicity (Wara *et al.* 1977; Salazar *et al.* 1979; Leibel and Sheline 1987).

Overall the results of this approach to management have been good, with 60–90 per cent 5 year survival (Table 7) (Wara *et al.* 1977; Jenkin *et al.* 1978; Sung *et al.* 1978; Wara *et al.* 1979; Rich *et al.* 1985; Legido *et al.* 1989). It has long been recognized, however, that patients with pineal or suprasellar, non-seminomatous germ cell tumours have a worse prognosis; variations in the proportions of these patients in reported series could, in fact, account for some of the differences in reported treatment outcomes.

The approach to the management of intracranial germ cell tumours has begun to change in recent years (Edwards *et al.* 1988) with improvements in surgical techniques, an understanding of the implications of tumour markers, the recognition of the long-term toxicity of cranial irradiation in children, and the establishment of curative, cisplatin-based chemotherapy for testicular germ cell neoplasms. Increasingly, an attempt is being made in these patients to identify the histological subtype of tumour, in an effort to tailor therapy more appropriately.

The disappointing results obtained with radiotherapy for intracranial non-seminomatous germ cell tumours, in contrast to the successful management of cerebral metastases from testicular non-seminomas (Rustin *et al.* 1986; Raghavan *et al.* 1987), have prompted the evaluation of systemic chemotherapy as first-line treatment (Rustin *et al.* 1986; Allen *et al.* 1987). We do not know of any large published series of intracranial germ cell tumours treated by chemotherapy alone. However, Kobayashi *et al.* (1989) have reported the successful treatment of recurrent intracranial non-seminomatous germ cell tumours with cisplatin and etoposide. Three out of four patients achieved a complete response and all are alive without further recurrence during follow-up of 9–22 months. A series of 17 patients with α-fetoprotein-secreting, intracranial germ-cell tumours had previously been reported from the same institution (Kida *et al.* 1986). Four out of 10 patients treated with cisplatin-based chemotherapy achieved complete remission, with two remaining disease-free beyond 2 years. Before the introduction of cisplatin, all such patients had died (Kida *et al.* 1986).

In the presence of markedly elevated amounts of tumour markers in cerebrospinal fluid, indicative of a non-germinoma, chemotherapy has a central role in management. Thus, patients who have detectable α-fetoprotein in their blood and/or cerebrospinal fluid proceed to either chemotherapy or surgery, depending on the clinical circumstances (Edwards *et al.* 1988). Patients with high amounts of human chorionic gonadotrophin are at risk of having non-seminomatous germ cell tumours, although the syncytiotrophoblastic giant cells sometimes found in pure testicular seminoma are able to secrete the gonadotrophin (Heyderman and Neville 1976); where biopsy is not feasible, it is probably safer to employ chemotherapy, with or without radiotherapy, on the presumption that this may be the case.

Radiotherapy remains the treatment of choice for patients with tumours not producing markers, or those with a histological diagnosis of germinoma. It also has a role after chemotherapy in patients with persistently elevated tumour markers, although the outlook for this group of patients is poor. Whether radiotherapy should be used electively as part of a combined approach with multidrug chemotherapy has not yet been resolved.

PROGNOSIS

Notwithstanding the difficulties of interpreting the literature, at all extragonadal sites, stage for stage, the prognosis for patients with seminomatous tumours is better than for those with non-seminomas.

Extragonadal seminomas, with their marked radio- and chemosensitivity, have a similar prognosis to their gonadal counterparts, with a large proportion of patients being long-term survivors.

The situation for non-seminomas of extragonadal origin is quite different. As is apparent from the results of treatment summarized above and in Tables 4 and 5, the prognosis of patients with non-seminomatous extragonadal germ cell tumours is poor. Initially, it was thought that this may be due to inherent resistance to therapy of these tumours (Feun *et al.* 1980). More recently, however, it has been proposed from the use of multivariate analysis that extragonadal primary site may not be an adverse prognostic factor *per se* (Bosl *et al.* 1983; Medical Research Council 1985; Birch *et al.* 1986; Levi *et al.* 1988). Rather, the poor outcome of patients with extragonadal tumours may relate in part to the bulk of disease at the time of presentation, which is often greater than in patients with gonadal primary sites. This issue remains unresolved.

THE 'ATYPICAL TERATOMA SYNDROME' ('UNRECOGNIZED EXTRAGONADAL GERM CELL CANCER SYNDROME')

A syndrome in young men with metastatic, undifferentiated carcinoma, sometimes responsive to the chemotherapy regimens developed for germ cell tumours, was first reported by Fox *et al.* (1979) and later confirmed by others (Richardson *et al.* 1981; Greco *et al.* 1986). In these and subsequent reports it was suggested that these tumours represented cases of unrecognized extragonadal germ cell tumours. Histological review of the five cases of Fox *et al.* (1979) reportedly confirmed this view. By contrast, review of the light- and electron-microscopic features of the series from Vanderbilt University revealed only one case out of 113 to be a definite germ cell tumour (Hainsworth *et al.* 1987). A further five cases were felt to represent possible germ cell tumours, but only one of these had a complete response to chemotherapy.

Logothetis *et al.* (1985) have studied such cases, but have failed to confirm the diagnosis of extragonadal germ cell tumour in the majority. While the original cases reported by Fox *et al.* (1979) may have represented true extragonadal tumours, it has become clear from these detailed histological reviews that only a minority of young men with undifferentiated metastatic malignancy truly have an extragonadal germ cell tumour. The remainder have poorly differentiated carcinoma, which fortuitously may respond to cisplatin-based chemotherapy and the syndrome should no longer be considered within the spectrum of extragonadal germ cell tumours. A detailed discussion of the management of this group of patients is beyond the scope of this review. However, we believe that considerable caution should be exercised in extrapolating the end-results of therapy of testicular germ cell tumours, via a tenuous similarity to extragonadal germ cell tumours, to the care of these patients.

SUMMARY

Extragonadal germ cell tumours constitute a group of malignancies that occur either in childhood or in the prime of life. By analogy to gonadal germ cell tumours, they are potentially curable in a large proportion of cases. Yet despite major advances in both the understanding and treatment of metastatic testicular germ cell tumour, major challenges remain in the care of patients with extragonadal tumours. A clearer understanding of the differences between gonadal and extragonadal germ cell tumours and their response to management is crucial. Of particular interest is the prognostic similarity of extragonadal seminoma to metastatic testicular carcinoma, in contrast to extragonadal non-seminomatous germ cell tumours. For non-seminomatous extragonadal germ cell tumours the major therapeutic challenge is to improve the long-term survival rate, while in seminomatous extragonadal germ cell tumours, reduction of the toxicity of therapy with maintenance of an excellent outcome, remains the goal. Ultimately, the greatest chance for success in the care of these uncommon tumours will be achieved by collaborative intergroup studies that address these issues.

REFERENCES

Abay EO, et al. (1981). Pineal tumors in children and adolescents: treatment by CSF shunting and radiotherapy. *Journal of Neurosurgery*, **55**:889–95.

Abell MR, Fayos JV, Lampe I (1965). Retroperitoneal germinomas (seminomas) without evidence of testicular involvement. *Cancer*, **18**:273–90.

Aliotta PJ, Castillo J, Englander LS, Nseyo UO, Huben RP (1988). Primary mediastinal germ cell tumors: histologic patterns of treatment failure at autopsy. *Cancer*, **62**:982–4.

Allen JC, Kim JH, Packer RJ (1987). Neoadjuvant chemotherapy for newly diagnosed germ-cell tumors of the central nervous system. *Journal of Neurosurgery*, **67**:65–70.

Altman RP, Randolph JG, Lilly JR (1974). Sacrococcygeal teratoma: American Academy of Pediatrics section survey—1973. *Journal of Pediatric Surgery*, **9**:389–98.

Amendola BE, McClatchey K, Amendola M (1984). Pineal region tumors: analysis of treatment results. *International Journal of Radiation Oncology—Biology—Physics*, **10**:991–7.

Applebaum H, Exelby PR, Wollner N (1979). Malignant presacral teratoma in children. *Journal of Pediatric Surgery*, **14**:352–5.

Arnheim EE (1951). Retroperitoneal teratomas in infancy and childhood. *Pediatrics*, **8**:309–27.

Ashcraft KW, Holder TM (1965). *Annals of Surgery*, **162**:1091.

Askanazy M (1907). Die Teratome nach ihrem bau, ihrem Verlauf, ihrer Genese und in Vergleich zum experimentellen Teratoid. *Verhandlungen der Deutschen Gesellschaft für Pathologie*, **1**:39–82.

Azzopardi JG, Hoffbrand AV (1965). Retrogression in testicular seminoma with viable metastases. *Journal of Clinical Pathology*, **18**:135–41.

Azzopardi JG, Mostofi FK, Thiess EA (1961). Lesions of testes observed in certain patients with widespread choriocarcinoma and related tumours. *American Journal of Pathology*, **38**:207–19.

Bagshaw MA, McLaughlin WT, Earle JD (1969). Definitive radiotherapy of primary mediastinal seminoma. *American Journal of Roentgenology*, **105**:86–94.

Beeley JM, Daly JJ, Timperley WR, Warner J (1973). Ectopic pinealoma: an unusual clinical presentation and a histochemical comparison with a seminoma of the testis. *Journal of Neurology, Neurosurgery and Psychiatry*, **36**:864–73.

Benson RC, Segura JW, Carney JA (1978). Primary yolk sac (endodermal sinus) tumor of the prostate. *Cancer*, **41**:1395–8.

Besznyak I, Sebesteny M, Kuchar F (1973). Primary mediastinal seminoma: a case report and review of the literature. *Journal of Thoracic and Cardiovascular Surgery*, **65**:930.

Birch R, et al. (1986). Prognostic factors for favourable outcome in disseminated germ cell tumors. *Journal of Clinical Oncology*, **4**:400–7.

Bohle A, Studer UE, Sonntag RW, Scheidegger JR (1986). Primary or secondary extragonadal germ cell tumors? *Journal of Urology*, **135**:939–43.

Borit A (1969). Embryonal carcinoma of the pineal region. *Journal of Pathology*, **97**:165–9.

Bosl GJ, et al. (1983). Multivariate analysis of prognostic variables in patients with metastatic testicular cancer. *Cancer Research*, **43**:3403–7.

Bosl GJ, et al. (1986). VAB-6: an effective chemotherapy regimen for patients with germ-cell tumors. *Journal of Clinical Oncology*, **4**:1493–9.

Boyer M, et al. (1990). Lack of late toxicity in patients treated with cisplatin-containing combination chemotherapy for metastatic testicular cancer. *Journal of Clinical Oncology*, **8**:1–6.

Brodeur GM, Howarth CB, Pratt CB, Caces J, Hustu HO (1981). Malignant germ cell tumors in 57 children and adolescents. *Cancer*, **48**:1890–8.

Burt ME, Javadpour N (1981). Germ-cell tumors in patients with apparently normal testes. *Cancer*, **47**:911–1015.

Bush SE, Martinez A, Bagshaw MA (1981). Primary mediastinal seminoma. *Cancer*, **48**:1877–82.

Canty TG, Siemens R (1978) Malignant mediastinal teratoma in a 15-year-old girl. *Cancer*, **41**:1623–6.

Chapman PH, Linggood RM (1980). The management of pineal area tumor: a recent reappraisal. *Cancer*, **46**:1253–7.

Conkle DM, Adkins RB (1972). Primary malignant tumors of the mediastinum. *American Thoracic Surgery*, **14**:553–67.

Conklin J, Abell MR (1967). Germ cell neoplasms of sacrococcygeal region. *Cancer*, **20**:2105–17.

Cox JD (1975). Primary malignant germinal tumors of the mediaastinum; a study of 24 cases. *Cancer*, **36**:1162–8.

Dayan AD, Marshall AHE, Miller AA, Pick FJ, Rankin NE (1966). Atypical teratomas of the pineal and hypothalamus. *Journal of Pathology and Bacteriology*, **92**:1–28.

Dewan PA, Davidson PM, Campbell PE, Tiedemann K, Jones PG (1987). Sacrococcygeal teratoma: has chemotherapy improved survival? *Journal of Pediatric Surgery*, **22**:274–7.

Dillard BM, Mayer JH, McAlister WH, McGarvin M, Strominger DB (1970). Sacrococcygeal teratoma in children. *Journal of Pediatric Surgery*, **5**:53.

Donnellan WA, Swenson O (1968). Benign and malignant sacrococcygeal teratoma. *Surgery*, **64**:834–46.

Economou JS, Trump DL, Holmes EC, Eggleston JE (1982). Management of primary germ cell tumours of the mediastinum. *Journal of Thoracic and Cardiovascular Surgery*, **83**:643–9.

Edwards MSB, Hudgins RJ, Wilson CB, Levin VA, Wara WM (1988). Pineal region tumors in children. *Journal of Neurosurgery*, **68**:689–97.

El-Domeiri AA, Hutter RVP, Pool JL, Foote FW (1968). Primary seminoma of the anterior mediastinum. *Annals of Thoracic Surgery*, **6**:513–21.

Engel RM, Elkins RC, Fletcher BD (1968). Retroperitoneal teratoma. *Cancer*, **22**:1068–73.

Erickson RP, Gondos B (1976). Alternative explanations of the differing behaviour of ovarian and testicular teratomas. *Lancet*, **1**:407–10.

Feun LG, Samson MK, Stephens RL (1980). Vinblastine (VLB), bleomycin (BLEO), cis-diamminedichloroplatinum (DDP) in disseminated extragonadal germ cell tumors: a Southwest Oncology Group study. *Cancer*, **45**:2543–9.

Fox RM, Woods RL, Tattersall MHN, McGovern VJ (1979). Undifferentiated carcinoma in young men: the atypical teratoma syndrome. *Lancet*, **i**:1316–18.

Friedman NB (1947). *Cancer Research*, **7**:363.

Friedman NB, Moore RA (1946). Tumors of the testis: a report of 921 cases. *Military Surgery*, **99**:573–93.

Garnick MB, Canellos G, Ritchie JP (1983). Treatment and surgical staging of testicular and primary extragonadal germ cell cancer. *Journal of the American Medical Association*, **250**:1733–41.

Giuffre R, Di Lorenzo N (1975). Evolution of a primary intrasellar germinomatous teratoma into a choriocarcinoma. *Journal of Neurosurgery*, **42**:602–4.

Gonzalez-Crussi F (1982). *Extragonadal teratomas*, pp. 9–25; 33–35. Armed Forces Institute of Pathology, Washington DC.

Greco FA, Vaughn WK, Hainsworth JD (1986). Advanced poorly differentiated carcinoma of unknown primary site: recognition of a treatable syndrome. *Annals of Internal Medicine*, **104**:547–53.

Greist A, Einhorn LH, Williams SD, Donohue JP, Rowland RG (1984). Pathologic findings at orchiectomy following chemotherapy for disseminated testicular cancer. *Journal of Clinical Oncology*, **2**:1025–7.

Gross RE, Clatworthy HW, Meeker IA (1951). Sacrococcygeal teratomas in infants and children: a report of 40 cases. *Surgery, Gynecology and Obstetrics*, **92**:341–54.

Gwinn JL, Dockerty MB, Kennedy RLJ (1955). Presacral teratomas in infancy and childhood. *Pediatrics*, **36**:239–49.

Hainsworth JD, Einhorn LH, Williams SD, Stewart M, Greco FA (1982). Advanced extragonadal germ cell tumours. Successful treatment with combination chemotherapy. *Annals of Internal Medicine*, **97**:7–11.

Hainsworth JD, Wright EP, Gray GF, Greco FA (1987). Poorly differentiated carcinoma of unknown primary site: correlation of light microscopic findings with response to cisplatin-based combination chemotherapy. *Journal of Clinical Oncology*, **5**:1275–80.

Hart WR (1975). Primary endodermal sinus (yolk sac) tumour of the liver: first reported case. *Cancer*, **35**:1453–8.

Heyderman E, Neville AM (1976). Syncytiotrophoblast in malignant testicular tumours. *Lancet*, ii:103.

Ho KL, Rassekh ZS (1979). Endodermal sinus tumor of the pineal region: case report and review of literature. *Cancer*, **44**:1081–6.

Holt LP, Melcher DH, Colquhoun J (1965). Extragonadal choriocarcinoma in the male. *Postgraduate Medical Journal*, **41**:134–41.

Hunt PT, Davidson KC, Ashcraft KW, Holder TM (1977). Radiography of hereditary presacral teratoma. *Radiology*, **122**:187–91.

Hurt RD, Bruckman JE, Farrow GM, Bernatz PE, Hahn RG, Earle JD (1982). Primary anterior mediastinal seminoma. *Cancer*, **49**:1658–63.

Hyman A, Leiter HE (1943). Extratesticular chorioepithelioma in male probably primary in urinary bladder. *Journal of the Mount Sinai Hospital*, **10**:212–16.

Israel A, Bosl GJ, Golbey RB, Whitmore W, Martini N (1985). The results of chemotherapy for extragonadal germ-cell tumors in the cisplatin era: the Memorial Sloan-Kettering Cancer Center experience (1975 to 1982). *Journal of Clinical Oncology*, **3**:1073–8.

Izant RJ, Filston HC (1975). Sacrococcygeal teratomas: analysis of forty-three cases. *American Journal of Surgery*, **130**:617–21.

Jain KK, Bosl GJ, Bains MS, Whitmore WF, Golbey RB (1984). The treatment of extragonadal seminoma. *Journal of Clinical Oncology*, **2**:820–7.

Jellinger K (1973). Primary intracranial germ cell tumours. *Acta Neuropathologica*, **25**:291–306.

Jenkin RD, Simpson WJK, Keen CW (1978). Pineal and suprasellar germinomas: results of radiation treatment. *Journal of Neurosurgery*, **48**:99–107.

Jennings MT, Gelman R, Hochberg F (1985). Intracranial germ-cell tumors: natural history and pathogenesis. *Journal of Neurosurgery*, **63**:155–67.

Johnson DE, Laneri JP, Mountain CF, Luna M (1973). Extragonadal germ cell tumors. *Surgery*, **73**:85–90.

Joseph WL, Murray JF, Mulder DG (1966). Mediastinal tumors—problems in diagnosis and treatment. *Diseases of the Chest*, **50**:150–60.

Kay PH, Wells FC, Goldstraw P (1987). A multidisciplinary approach to primary nonseminomatous germ cell tumours of the mediastinum. *Annals of Thoracic Surgery*, **44**:578–82.

Kaye SB, Bagshawe KD, McElwain TJ, Peckham MJ (1979). Brain metastases in malignant teratoma: a review of four years' experience and an assessment of the role of tumour markers. *British Journal of Cancer*, **39**:217–23.

Kenefick JS (1973). Hereditary sacral agenesis associated with presacral tumours. *British Journal of Surgery*, **60**:271–4.

Kida Y, Kobayshi T, Yoshida J, Kato K, Kageyama N (1986). Chemotherapy with cisplatin for AFP-secreting germ-cell tumors of the central nervous system. *Journal of Neurosurgery*, **65**:470–5.

Kikuchi Y, Tsuneta Y, Kawai T, Aizawa M (1988). Choriocarcinoma of the esophagus producing chorionic gonadotrophin. *Acta Pathologica Japan*, **38**:489–99.

Kirschling RJ, Kvols LK, Charboneau JW, Grantham JG, Zincke H (1983). High-resolution ultrasonographic and pathologic abnormalities of germ cell tumors in patients with clinically normal testes. *Mayo Clinic Proceedings*, **58**:648–53.

Kobayashi T, Yoshida J, Ishiyama J, Noda S, Kito A, Kida Y (1989). Combination chemotherapy with cisplatin and etoposide for malignant intracranial germ cell tumors: an experimental and clinical study. *Journal of Neurosurgery*, **70**:676–81.

Koide O, Watanabe Y, Sato K (1980). A pathologic survey of intracranial germinoma and pinealoma in Japan. *Cancer*, **45**:2119–30.

Kuzur ME, Cobleigh MA, Greco FA, Einhorn LH, Oldham RK (1982). Endodermal sinus tumor of the mediastinum. *Cancer*, **50**:766–74.

Lattes R (1962). Thymoma and other tumours of the thymus. *Cancer*, **15**:1224–60.

Leading Article (1969). Primary mediastinal choriocarcinoma. *British Medical Journal*, ii:135–6.

Lederman GS, *et al.* (1989). Radiation therapy of seminoma: 17 year experience at the Joint Center for Radiation Therapy. *Radiotherapy and Oncology*, **14**:203–8.

Legido A, *et al.* (1989). Suprasellar germinomas in childhood: a reappraisal. *Cancer*, **63**:340–4.

Leibel SA, Sheline GE (1987). Radiation therapy for brain tumours. *Journal of Neurosurgery*, **66**:1–22.

Levi JA, *et al.* (1988). A prospective study of cisplatin-based combination chemotherapy in advanced germ cell malignancy: role of maintenance and long-term follow-up. *Journal of Clinical Oncology*, **6**:1154–60.

Loehrer PJ, Birch R, Williams SD, Greco FA, Einhorn LH (1987). Chemotherapy of metastatic seminoma: the Southeastern Cancer Study Group experience. *Journal of Clinical Oncology*, **5**:1212–20.

Logothetis CJ, *et al.* (1985). Chemotherapy of extragonadal germ cell tumours. *Journal of Clinical Oncology*, **3**:316–25.

Luna MA (1976). Extragonadal germ cell tumors. In *Testicular tumors* (ed. DE Johnson), pp. 261–91. Medical Examination, New York.

Luna MA, Valenzuela-Tamariz J (1976). Germ-cell tumors of the mediastinum, postmortem findings. *American Journal of Clinical Pathology*, **65**:450–4.

MacKay EN, Sellers AH (1966). A statistical review of malignant testicular tumours based on the experience of the Ontario Foundation clinics, 1938–1961. *Canadian Medical Association Journal*, **94**:889–99.

McLeod DG, Taylor HG, Skoog SJ, Knight RD, Dawson NA, Waxman JA (1988). Extragonadal germ cell tumors: clinicopathologic findings and treatment experience in 12 patients. *Cancer*, **61**:1187–91.

Mahour GH (1988). Sacrococcygeal teratomas. *CA—A Cancer Journal for Clinicians*, **38**:362–7.

Marcuse PM (1959). Malignant presacral teratoma in an adult. *Cancer*, **12**:889–93.

Martini N, Golbey RB, Hajdu SI, Whitmore WF, Beattie EJ (1974). Primary mediastinal germ cell tumors. *Cancer*, **33**:763–9.

Meares EM, Briggs EM (1972). Occult seminoma of the testis masquerading as a primary extragonadal germinal neoplasm. *Cancer*, **30**:300–6.

Medical Research Council Working Party on Testicular Tumours (1985). Prognostic factors in advanced non-seminomatous germ-cell testicular tumours: results of a multicenter study. *Lancet*, i:8–11.

Medini E, Levitt SH, Jones TK, Rao Y (1979). The management of extratesticular seminoma without gonadal involvement. *Cancer*, **44**:2032–8.

Miles RM, Stewart GS (1974). Sacrococcygeal teratomas in adults. *Annals of Surgery*, **179**:676–83.

Misugi K, Reiner CB (1965). A malignant true teratoma of liver in childhood. *Archives of Pathology*, **80**:409–12.

Motzer RJ, *et al.* (1988). Advanced seminoma: the role of chemotherapy and adjunctive surgery. *Annals of Internal Medicine*, **108**:513–18.

Newlands ES, Begent RHJ, Rustin GJS, Parker D, Bagshawe KD (1983). Further advances in the management of malignant teratomas of the testis and other sites. *Lancet*, i:948–51.

Nickels J, Franssila K (1972). Primary seminoma of the anterior mediastinum. *Acta Pathologica et Microbiologica Scandinavica*, **80**:260.

Noseworthy J, Lack EE, Kozakewich HPW, Vawter GF, Welch KJ (1981). Sacrococcygeal germ cell tumors in childhood: an updated experience with 118 patients. *Journal of Pediatric Surgery*, **16**:358–64.

Oberman HA, Libcke JH (1964). Malignant germinal neoplasms of the mediastinum. *Cancer*, **17**:498–507.

Ozols RF, Ihde DC, Linehamn WM, Jacob J, Ostchega Y, Young RC (1988). A randomized trial of standard chemotherapy v a high dose chemotherapy regimen in the treatment of poor prognosis nonseminomatous germ-cell tumors. *Journal of Clinical Oncology*, **6**:1031–40.

Pachter MR, Lattes R (1964). 'Germinal' tumors of the mediastinum: a clinicopathologic study of adult teratomas, teratocarcinomas, choriocarcinomas and seminomas. *Diseases of the Chest*, **45**:301–10.

Palumbo LT, Cross KR, Smith AN, Baronas AA (1949). Primary teratomas of the lateral retroperitoneal spaces. *Surgery*, **26**:149–59.

Pantoja E, Llobet R, Gonzalez-Flores B (1976). Retroperitoneal teratoma: historical review. *Journal of Urology*, **115**:520–3.

Parker D, *et al.* (1983). Effective treatment for malignant mediastinal teratoma. *Thorax*, **38**:897–902.

Peckham, M. J. (1981). Investigation and staging: general aspects and staging classification. In *The management of testicular tumours* (ed. MJ Peckham), pp. 89–101. Arnold, London.

Peckham MJ, Horwich A, Hendry WF (1985). Advanced seminoma: treatment with cis-platinum-based combination chemotherapy of carboplatin (JM8). *British Journal of Cancer*, **52**:7–13.

Polansky SM, Barwick KW, Ravin CE (1979). Primary mediastinal seminoma. *American Journal of Roentgenology*, **132**:17–21.

Prym P (1927). Spontanheilung eines bosartigen wahrscheinlich chorionepitheliomatosen Gewachs im Hoden. *Virchows Archiv für Pathologische Anatomie und Physiologie*, **265**:239–58.

Raghavan D, Barrett A (1980). Mediastinal seminomas. *Cancer*, **46**:1187–91.

Raghavan D, Neville AM (1982). The biology of testicular tumours. In *Scientific foundations of urology* (2nd edn) (ed. D Innes Williams and GD Chisholm), pp. 785–96. Heinemann Medical, London.

Raghavan D, Mackintosh JF, Fox RM, Rogers J, Duval P, Besser M (1987). Improved survival after brain metastases in non-seminomatous germ-cell tumours with combined modality treatment. *British Journal of Urology*, **60**:364–7.

Raney BR, *et al.* (1981). Treatment strategies for infants with malignant sacrococcygeal teratoma. *Journal of Pediatric Surgery*, **16** (Suppl. 1):573–7.

Rather LJ, Gardiner WR, Frerichs JB (1954). Regression and maturation of primary testicular tumors with progressive growth of metastases; report of 6 new cases and review of the literature. *Stanford Medical Bulletin*, **12**:12–25.

Recondo J, Libshitz HI (1978). Mediastinal extragonadal germ cell tumors. *Urology*, **11**:369–75.

Rich TA, Cassady JR, Strand RD, Winston KR (1985). Radiation therapy for pineal and suprasellar germ cell tumors. *Cancer*, **55**:932–40.

Richardson RL, *et al.* (1981). The unrecognized extragonadal germ cell cancer syndrome. *Annals of Internal Medicine*, **94**:181–6.

Ross ST (1948). Sacral and presacral tumors. *American Journal of Surgery*, **76**:687.

Russell DS (1944). The pinealoma: its relationship to teratoma. *Journal of Pathology and Bacteriology*, **56**:145–50.

Rustin GJS, Newlands ES, Bagshawe KD, Begent RHJ, Crawford SM (1986). Successful management of metastatic and primary germ cell tumours in the brain. *Cancer*, **57**:2108–13.

Sakai N, Yamada H, Andoh T, Hirata T, Shimizu K, Shinoda J (1988). Primary intracranial germ cell tumors: a retrospective analysis with special reference to long-term results of treatment and the behaviour of rare types of tumors. *Acta Oncologica*, **27**:43–50.

Salazar OM, Castro-Vita H, Bakos RS, Feldstein ML, Keller B, Rubin P (1979). Radiation therapy for tumours of the pineal region. *International Journal of Radiation Oncology—Biology—Physics*, **5**:491–9.

Saltzman B, Pitts WR, Vaughan ED (1986). Extragonadal retroperitoneal germ cell tumors without apparent testicular involvement: a search for the source. *Urology*, **27**:504–7.

Schantz A, Sewall W, Castleman B (1972). Mediastinal germinoma: a study of 21 cases with an excellent prognosis. *Cancer*, **30**:1189–94.

Schey WL, Shkolnik A, White H (1977). Clinical and radiographic considerations of sacrococcygeal teratomas: an analysis of 26 new cases and review of the literature. *Radiology*, **125**:189–95.

Schlumberger HG (1946). Teratoma of the anterior mediastinum in the group of military age: a study of sixteen cases and a review of theories of genesis. *Archives of Pathology*, **41**:398–444.

Schmidek HH (1977). Surgical management of pineal region tumors. In *Pineal tumors* (ed. HH Schmidek). Masson, New York.

Simson LR, Lampe I, Abell MR (1968). Suprasellar germinomas. *Cancer*, **22**:533–44.

Sterchi M, Cordell AR (1975). Seminoma of the anterior mediastinum. *Annals of Thoracic Surgery*, **19**:371–7.

Sung DI, Harisiadis L, Chang CH (1978). Midline pineal tumors and suprasellar germinomas: highly curable by irradiation. *Radiology*, **128**:745–51.

Tondini C, Garnick MB (1989). Chemotherapy for extragonadal and poor-prognosis germ cell cancers: the Dana-Farber Cancer Institute approach. In *Systemic therapy for genitourinary cancers* (ed. DE Johnson, CJ Logothetis, and AC Von Eschenbach), pp. 370–9. Year Book Medical Publishers, Chicago.

Utz DC, Buscemi MK (1971). Extragonadal testicular tumors. *Journal of Urology*, **105**:271–4.

Vogelzang NJ, Raghavan D, Anderson RW, Rosai J, Levitt SH, Kennedy BJ (1982). Mediastinal nonseminomatous germ cell tumors: the role of combined modality therapy. *Annals of Thoracic Surgery*, **33**:333–9.

Walden PAM, Woods RL, Fox B, Bagshawe KD (1977). Primary mediastinal trophoblastic teratomas. *Thorax*, **32**:752–8.

Wara WM, Fellows CF, Sheline GE, Wilson CB, Townsend JJ (1977). Radiation therapy for pineal tumours and suprasellar germinomas. *Radiology*, **124**:221–3.

Wara WM, *et al.* (1979). Tumors of the pineal and suprasellar region: Children's Cancer Study Group Treatment results 1960–1975. *Cancer*, **43**:698–701.

Whalen TV, Mahour GH, Landing BH, Woolley MM (1985). Sacrococcygeal teratomas in infants and children. *American Journal of Surgery*, **150**:373–5.

Witschi E (1948). Migration of the germ cells of human embryos from the yolk sac to the primitive gonadal folds. *Contributions to Embryology* (Publication of the Carnegie Institution), **209**:67–80.

Wychulis AR, Payne WS, Clagett OT, Woolner LB (1971). Surgical treatment of mediastinal tumors; a 40 year experience. *Journal of Thoracic and Cardiovascular Surgery*, **62**:379–92.

10.3 Tumours of the penis

GIORGIO PIZZOCARO, LUIGI PIVA, AND SILVIA TANA

MAJOR FEATURES

Squamous cell carcinoma is the most common tumour of the penis. It is a rare disease in Western countries and it is often associated with phimosis, poor hygiene, or human papilloma virus infection. It could be prevented or diagnosed early in most cases, but, for cultural and educational reasons, it is often diagnosed late. Nodal metastases are relatively common, but distant dissemination is very rare.

Radical surgery (some type of amputation) gives the best control of the primary tumour, but it is a mutilating procedure. Laser surgery for limited superficial lesions and sophisticated radiotherapy for relatively small (less than 4 cm) infiltrating tumours have been successfully employed, alone or in combination with chemotherapy. Therefore, the use of radical surgery can be restricted to relapses or to cases which are unsuitable for conservative treatment.

Survival mainly depends on nodal metastases, but the management of the regional lymph nodes is controversial. Radical inguinal (and pelvic) lymphadenectomy can cure approximately 40–50 per cent of patients with positive nodes, but nearly half of the patients with clinically enlarged nodes actually have no metastases. Invalidating leg (and genital) oedema is a frequent complication of (bilateral) inguinal lymphadenectomy. The point is to restrict the operation to patients with positive nodes. Expectant policy can be dangerous, as many of these patients are not reliable for a careful follow-up. Therefore, the results of delayed lymphadenectomy are usually poor. Fine-needle aspiration biopsy and imaging may be of help in diagnosing nodal metastases. Modified surgical procedures have been advocated in order to obtain a pathological staging of the inguinal nodes which avoids invalidating sequelae, but results seem to be controversial. T category and tumour grade seem to be of help in identifying patients at a very high risk of harbouring nodal metastases.

Squamous cell carcinoma of the penis is responsive to chemotherapy to some extent. Limited experiences suggest that adjuvant chemotherapy can improve the long-term survival of patients with radically resected positive nodes and primary (neoadjuvant) chemotherapy can make resectable approximately 50 per cent of cases with fixed inguinal metastases. However, no chemotherapeutic regimen alone seems to be curative for metastatic disease.

EPIDEMIOLOGY AND AETIOLOGY

Carcinoma of the penis accounts for less than 1 per cent of all malignant tumours in the male in Western countries. The tumour is found occasionally in young men and the highest incidence occurs in the seventh decade. The disease has been reported in all races, but it is more common in Asia, Africa, and South America. Other epithelial and connective tumours are extremely rare.

Social and cultural habits seem to be more important than racial factors in cancer of the penis. Phymosis and poor hygiene are commonly associated with this tumour. Circumcision performed in infancy gives almost 100 per cent protection against the disease, while circumcision performed later in life is less protective.

There is an increasing body of evidence that cancer of the penis can be associated with human papilloma virus infection (Barrasso *et al.* 1987). In the majority of the cases DNA of human papilloma virus type 16 was found (Iwasawa *et al.* 1993). Penile cancer associated with human papilloma virus seems to occur at a younger age. Men exposed to psoralens and ultraviolet radiation for psoriasis are also at risk of developing penile cancer (Stern *et al.* 1990).

PATHOLOGY

The pathology of penile cancer has been reviewed by Lucia and Miller (1992). Neoplasms of the penis arise most frequently from the covering epithelium of the preputial sac; rarely they originate in the skin of the shaft or in the connective tissues that comprise the bulk of the organ.

Benign lesions of the penile epithelium

Condyloma acuminata are soft papillomatous growths of viral origin. Buschke–Loewenstein tumour or giant condyloma, differs from benign condyloma in its propensity to destroy adjacent tissues by compression. An actual invasion is not documented. Although locally aggressive, it does not metastasize. Sometimes it is difficult to differentiate from verrucous carcinoma.

Leucoplakia appears as scaly patches or plaques on the glans penis and may involve the urethral meatus. It is usually associated with chronic irritation and may precede or co-exist with carcinoma. Therefore, surgical or laser excision with histological examination is indicated and a careful follow-up is important.

Balanitis xerotica obliterans is a localized variant of lichen sclerosus and atrophicus that is usually limited to the glans and prepuce. It presents with white atrophic plaques that may result in phymosis or meatal stenosis.

Carcinoma *in situ*

Carcinoma *in situ* of the penis appears more commonly as erythroplasia of Queyrat in the preputial sac or, rarely, as Bowen's disease of the skin of the shaft.

Erythroplasia of Queyrat presents as a red velvety plaque on the glans or the prepuce. It can be solitary or multiple. Erosion and ulceration usually signify the development of invasive carcinoma, which occurs in as many as one-third of patients.

Bowen's disease is a common carcinoma *in situ* of the skin which resembles a plaque with crusting and ulceration. Development of squamous cell carcinoma is relatively rare, but simultaneous systemic malignancies can occur in 25 per cent of patients. When occurring in the penis, only the skin of the shaft is involved.

Squamous cell carcinoma

The site of origin is nearly always the glans or the inner surface of the prepuce. It develops as a small ulcer, nodule, or verruca and rapidly invades underlying tissues. Histologically, squamous cell carcinoma of the penis is usually well to moderately differentiated. Verrucous carcinoma is a variant of squamous cell carcinoma. It is extremely well differentiated and has a pronounced papillary and verrucous pattern. It actually invades underlying tissues along a broad front. Penile verrucous carcinoma demonstrates characteristic and uniform morphological features and does not contain the human papilloma virus types typically associated with condyloma, giant condyloma, or carcinoma.

Other epithelial tumours

Basal cell carcinoma of the penis is rare and usually involves the skin of the shaft. Metastatic carcinoma of the penis usually originates from the bladder, the prostate, and the kidney and involves the corpora. Malignant melanoma of the penis is also quite rare (Stillwell *et al.* 1988). It may originate from both the preputial sac and the skin of the shaft. Prognosis is usually severe.

Soft tissue sarcomas

Soft tissue sarcomas of the penis represent less than 5 per cent of all penile malignancies.

Most angiosarcomas of the corpora cavernosa tend to be relatively well differentiated, to have an indolent behaviour, and to respond to surgical management. However, high grade tumours do exist and they metastasize to distant sites. Haemangioendotelioma may represent low-grade angiosarcoma.

Kaposi's sarcoma of the penis usually presents as multiple small blue–red nodules or patches within the skin of the shaft or glans penis. As many as 3 per cent of AIDS patients initially present with penile Kaposi's sarcoma. The non-epidemic form has an indolent behaviour.

Leiomyosarcoma of the penis may present as a slowly growing subcutaneous nodule or as a less common deep mass which arises from the smooth muscle of corpora cavernosa and tends to metastasize early. Most penile rhabdomyosarcomas occur in children and are of the embryonal type. They form asymptomatic masses on the shaft near the root of the penis and are responsive to chemotherapy.

Fibrosarcoma of the penis can be superficial or deep and usually presents as a slow-growing firm non-tender mass on the dorsum of the shaft or on the glans. Deep fibrosarcoma can metastasize.

Primary lymphomas of the penis are extremely rare. They are usually of the non-Hodgkin type and they respond very well to local low-dose irradiation (Stewart et al. 1985). They must be managed as extranodal lymphomas.

NATURAL HISTORY

Despite the vascularity of the penis, the spread of penile carcinoma via the blood vessels is rare. Carcinoma of the penis metastasizes via the lymphatic system. Metastases usually occur to regional lymph nodes by lymphatic embolization, rarely as a process of lymphatic permeation. However, this process may occur, as concomitant metastases are usually present in the rare event of relapse on the penile stump following partial amputation (Zanoni et al. 1989). The regional lymph nodes for carcinoma of the penis are the superficial, the deep inguinal, and the pelvic nodes, particularly those located in the obturator fossa. Approximately 20 per cent of patients with metastases in more than one inguinal node also have pelvic nodal involvement (Horenblas et al. 1993). Pelvic metastases in the absence of inguinal involvement are exceptionally rare (Riveros and Gorostiaga 1962). Metastases to the common iliac and para-aortic nodes are very rare and are considered to be distant metastases.

Although half of patients present with enlarged inguinal nodes at diagnosis, less than 30 per cent actually have nodal metastases. Regional metastases will develop during the follow-up in another 10–15 per cent of category N0 cases. Thus, approximately 40–50 per cent of patients with penile cancer will develop nodal metastases during the course of the disease (Ekstrom and Edsmyr 1958; Zanoni et al. 1989). Corpus cavernosum invasion and tumour grade have been related to the occurrence of nodal metastases (Solsona et al. 1992).

The penile urethra is only exceptionally invaded by the tumour. We have seen only one instance of urethral involvement in 120 consecutive cases (Zanoni et al. 1989). In very advanced disease a perineal dissemination en cuirasse may occur. To our knowledge tumour invasion into the prostate has never been reported.

Death from cancer of the penis is usually a consequence of local complications such as infection and haemorrhage of the ulcerated tumour or of ulcerated nodal metastases. Cachexia from distant dissemination is extremely rare.

CLINICAL FEATURES AND DIAGNOSIS

The first symptom of cancer of the penis is usually the appearance of an exophytic growth or an ulcerated nodule or a flat ulcer which does not heal but enlarges progressively. In phymotic patients, the first symptoms are swelling and discharge from the prepuce. Rarely, the first sign is the appearance of an enlarged inguinal node. Repeated episodes of belanoposthitis followed by acquired phimosis may precede the occurrence of cancer of the penis.

Although the penis can easily be inspected and palpated, too often the diagnosis of cancer in this organ is late. Major causes of late diagnosis are preceding episodes of balanoposthitis, poor self-care, and misdiagnosis. At present diagnosis in over 50 per cent of cases is made at least 6 months after the onset of the first symptom.

Carcinoma in situ must be differentiated from other superficial epithelial lesions. Early ulcerated tumours must be differentiated from venereal ulcer and primary syphiloma. Early exophytic tumours must be differentiated from condylomata and giant condyloma. A tumour in a phimotic patient must be differentiated from acute or chronic balanoposthitis.

The only way to make a diagnosis is to take a biopsy. In phimotic patients, the prepuce must be divided longitudinally on the dorsal side in order to expose the lesion and take the biopsy. The procedure can be performed under local anaesthesia on an out-patient basis.

INVESTIGATIONS

The minimal requirements for the diagnosis and staging of cancer of the penis are biopsy and clinical examination (UICC 1978). Ascertainment of infiltration of the corpora cavernosa by clinical examination is usually difficult. Cavernosography has been found to be useful in evaluating infiltrating tumours (Ragavaiah 1978), but it is an invasive procedure. Ultrasound examination can give a clear insight into the anatomical relations of the tumour with other penile structures (Yamashita and Ogawa 1989). This easy, accessible, and cheap examination may be very helpful in deciding whether penis conservation is feasible (Horenblas 1993, pp. 71–83). Magnetic resonance imaging (MRI) also shows great promise (Vapnek et al. 1992).

Involvement of inguinal nodes may be assessed by direct palpation, but palpable nodes are found to be cancerous in only approximately 50 per cent of cases and clinically normal nodes contain unsuspected metastases in approximately 15 per cent of cases (Persky and de Kernion 1986). Fine-needle aspiration cytology may add very useful information in the presence of palpable inguinal nodes. In the event of enlarged nodes and negative cytology, the patients should be re-examined 3–4 weeks after treatment of the primary tumour in order to allow inflammatory reactions to subside.

Bipedal lymphangiography, CT of the abdomen and pelvis, or fine-needle aspiration cytology were found to be unable to detect regional lymph node invasion that had escaped clinical examination (Horenblas et al. 1991). We do not use penile lymphangiography (Kuisk 1971) or sentinel node biopsy (Cabanas 1977, 1992) because the first procedure is difficult to perform and inguinal metastases have been reported following negative sentinel node biopsy (Perinetti et al. 1980; McDougal et al. 1986). Bipedal lymphangiography or CT scan of the abdomen and pelvis may be of some help in detecting pelvic node invasion and in the determination of the extent of the disease in patients with unequivocal evidence of inguinal metastases (Horenblas et al. 1991).

STAGING CLASSIFICATION

Several staging classifications have been proposed for cancer of the penis. Those most frequently used are Jackson's classification (Jackson 1966) and the TNM system (UICC 1978, 1987).

Jackson's classification (Jackson 1966) is as follows.

- Stage I: tumour limited to the glans and/or prepuce.
- Stage II: tumour invading the shaft.
- Stage III: tumour with operable metastatic nodes.
- Stage IV: tumour invading adjacent structures or with unoperable nodes or distant metastases.

The TNM classification (UICC 1987) prescribes the following procedures for the assessment of T, N, and M categories in penile carcinoma.

- T categories: physical examination and endoscopy.
- N categories: physical examination and imaging.
- M categories: physical examination and imaging.

Table 1 UICC TNM classifications of penile cancer

Category	1978 edition	1987 edition
T0	No evidence of primary tumour	Unchanged
Tis	Carcinoma *in situ*	Unchanged
Ta	Carcinoma *in situ*	Unchanged
T1	Strictly exophytic (<2 cm)	Invasion of subepithelial tissue
T2	2–5 cm or minimal invasion	Invasion of corpora
T3	>5 cm or deep invasion	Invasion of urethra or prostate
T4	Invasion of adjacent structures	Unchanged
N0	No evidence of regional node involvement	Unchanged
N1	Involved moveable unilateral nodes	Metastases in a single superficial inguinal node
N2	Involved moveable bilateral nodes	Multiple or bilateral superficial nodes
N3	Fixed inguinal nodes	Metastases to deep inguinal or pelvic nodes
M0	No evidence of distant metastases	Unchanged
M1	Evidence of distant metastases	Unchanged
Regional nodes	Inguinal	Inguinal and pelvic

Both TNM classifications are shown in Table 1. The major criticisms of the 1978 TNM classification of penile cancer were that there was no difference between a large (more than 5 cm) exophytic tumour and a deep (corpora cavernosa) invasion and only the inguinal nodes were reported as regional. The 1987 edition introduced the Ta category for non-invasive verrucous carcinoma and clearly divided limited invasion of subepithelial tissue (T1 category) from invasion of the corpora (T2). However, it introduced invasion of urethra or prostate (T3 category), which are respectively very rare or almost impossible and required endoscopy to assess the T category. Furthermore, the 1987 edition correctly considers the superficial, the deep inguinal, and the pelvic nodes as regional, but the N category for fixed inguinal metastases has disappeared. Consequently, all three classifications of cancer of the penis are difficult to apply (Maiche and Pyrhoenen 1990). However, the 1987 UICC TNM classification will be considered in this chapter.

MANAGEMENT

In the management of cancer of the penis we shall discuss the treatment of the primary tumour, the management of nodal metastases, and palliation separately. The quality of life issue will be considered in each section.

Primary tumour

The treatment of the primary tumour is extremely controversial, particularly as far as small tumours (less than 4 cm) in category T1 (UICC 1987) are concerned.

Surgery (Pizzocaro 1989)

The standard surgical treatment of category T1 cancer of the penis is partial amputation carried out as a guillotine resection 2 cm from the proximal margin of the tumour. The urethra is left 1.5 cm longer, in order to perform a comfortable everted tip urethrostomy (Klein 1991).

In patients with documented invasion of the corpora (T2 category), a total penectomy is advised. The operation is concluded with a perineal urethrostomy (Klein 1991). The urethra is sectioned at the base of the penis in order to leave at least 5 cm of the bulb and to have enough length to perform a comfortable everted nipple urethrostomy following elliptical excision of 1 cm of skin in the perineum. Total amputation is also indicated in the occasional patient with tumour infiltration into the urethra (category T3).

Emasculation is only exceptionally performed. It is mandatory only in category T4 tumours. As the inguinal nodes are always involved in this category, emasculation is routinely performed *en bloc* with bilateral inguinal lymphadenectomy. The pelvic nodes may be removed extraperitoneally through a separate suprapubic incision (Whitmore and Vagaiwala 1984).

Circumcision is sufficient treatment for carcinoma *in situ* and small category T1 N0 cancers entirely limited to the foreskin (Bissada 1992). Circumcision should also be performed before referring patients to radiotherapy for cancer of the glans.

Laser surgery is routinely performed nowadays for superficial pre-malignant and malignant lesions of the squamous epithelium of the penis (Bandieramonte *et al.* 1992; Malek 1992). We prefer a CO_2 laser to a Nd:YAG laser because it is possible to perform an almost bloodless surgical resection with minimal tissue coagulation with the former, with the further advantages of resection under microscopic control (magnification 6–12×) and subsequent histological examination. CO_2 laser resection is usually performed under local anaesthetic 5 mm from the lateral margins of the lesion and to a depth of 2.5 mm (Bandieramonte *et al.* 1987). Even the total surface of the glans penis and the prepuce can be excised with the CO_2 laser with good secondary healing and satisfactory cosmetic and functional results (Bandieramonte *et al.* 1988). Neither patients with carcinoma *in situ* nor those with histological verification of infiltration into the subepithelial connective tissue and clear resection deep margins need be submitted to any further therapy. Patients with uncleared margins are treated with post-operative external-beam irradiation (Bandieramonte *et al.* 1992). However, relatively large category T1 N0 exophytic tumours can be submitted to CO_2 laser surgery following total or partial remission to primary (neoadjuvant) chemotherapy in order to resect the base of the tumour and to verify the histological response (Bandieramonte *et al.* 1993). However, absolute indications for laser surgery are superficial pre-malignant lesions and carcinoma *in situ* of the penis. Circumcision is also recommended in these cases.

Radiotherapy

Radiotherapy is the most traditional form of conservative therapy for cancer of the penis. Category T1 N0 tumours with the largest diameter (less than 4 cm) are usually selected and circumcision is always recommended as the first step in order to achieve complete exposure of the tumour and to decrease the risk of some side-effects (Gerbaulet and Lambin 1992).

Various techniques are now available because of major improvements in equipment and radiation sources. Both external radiation and brachytherapy are widely used. Brachytherapy is preferred in France and the United Kingdom (Pierquin *et al.* 1971; Hope-Stone 1975; El-Demiry *et al.* 1984; Mazeron *et al.* 1984); external radiation therapy is the treatment of choice in Scandinavia and North America (Sagerman *et al.* 1984; Edsmyr *et al.* 1985).

Brachytherapy can be performed with either an external isotope mould technique or interstitial radiotherapy. Circumcision is mandatory before brachytherapy and ^{192}Ir is now preferred to radium sources. The mould radioactive technique (contact brachytherapy) is preferred in the United Kingdom (Hope-Stone 1975; El-Demiry et al. 1984). An inner Perspex cylinder is worn over the penis and an outer cylinder, loaded with ^{192}Ir wires and designed to be fitted over the penis, is kept beside the patient in a lead box. In the privacy of his room the patient is taught to place the outer cylinder over the inner cylinder and to make a note of the time that it is held in place. The timing of the applications and the length of the iridium wire is calculated to give 60 Gy to the tumour, but only 50 Gy to the urethra. The applicator is removed by the patient when he wishes to urinate and in practice is worn for 12 h a day for 1 week. Of course, this technique demands good cooperation by the patient. With this limitation, the technique is painless, easy to apply, and safe for both the patient and the nursing staff.

The interstitial technique is commonly used by French radiotherapists (Pierquin et al. 1971; Mazeron et al. 1984; Delannes et al. 1992). Implants of ^{192}Ir wires are performed under general or spinal anaesthesia. The radioactive lines are maintained parallel by perforated Plexiglas plates and the number, length, and spacing of the sources are determined as a function of the diameter and infiltration of the tumour. An original plastic box device has also been described (Gerbaulet et al. 1992). Usually, four or six wires of length 40 mm are disposed in two parallel planes 15 mm apart. A dose ranging from 50 to 70 Gy (median dose 60 Gy) is usually given at a low dose rate (reference isodose, 0.5–1.0 Gy/h).

External radiation therapy can be performed with both a conventional low-energy X-ray device and high-energy photons. The orthovoltage ranged widely from 60 to 250 kV_p, with quite different fractionation regimes (7–20 fractions over 2–6 weeks), and a total dose of 4.000–8.000 R has usually been administered through opposed lateral fields (Edsmyr et al. 1985) or, less frequently, by a single direct field (Haile and Delclos 1980). In more recent series (Sagerman et al. 1984; Kausal and Sharma 1987) patients have mainly been treated with megavoltage beams from cobalt or caesium units or 6 MV linear accelerators. High-energy photon doses ranging from 45 to 60 Gy have been administered in 15–30 fractions over a period of 3–8 weeks, always through two opposed lateral fields including the whole penis. In general, the patients wear an individualized wax mould (Haile and Delclos 1980; Kausal and Sharma 1987) to ensure a uniform dose distribution. Some authors (Sagerman et al. 1984) have described original devices, usually water-filled plastic containers, designed to allow the penis to be held up or suspended during irradiation.

Complications following radiotherapy for penile cancer are very common (Jones et al. 1989). Acute reactions include mucosistis, oedema of the prepuce, and local infections. Previous circumcision, careful daily toilet, and antibiotics minimize these side-effects (Kausal and Sharma 1987). Minor late complications such as telangiectasia, dyscromia, and superficial necrosis are noted in more than 40 per cent of cases (Gerbaulet et al. 1992). The most frequent late complication is urethral meatal stenosis, which occurs in up to 30 per cent of cases following either brachytherapy or external radiation therapy (Edsmyr et al. 1985; Kausal and Sharma 1987; Delannes et al. 1992). Post-radiation meatal stenosis usually recovers by means of repeated instrumental dilatations, but sometimes requires surgical repair (Mazeron et al. 1984). Deep fibrosis is dose and volume dependent and is almost exclusively reported in patients treated for tumours which are larger than 4 cm or which have

Table 2 Weekly vincristine–bleomycin–methotrexate combination chemotherapy

Drug	Dosage (mg)	Administration
Vincristine	1	IV, day 1
Bleomycin	15	IM, 6 and 24 h after vincristine[a]
Methotrexate	30	Orally in divided doses, day 3

IV, intravenous; IM, intramuscular.
[a]In patients with chronic lung disease, bleomycin is omitted on day 2 and methotrexate is anticipated on the same day.

invaded the corpora cavernosa (Gerbaulet et al. 1992). Circumcision is necessary to prevent annular sclerosis of the foreskin (Edsmyr et al. 1985). The most serious radiation complication is necrosis, which very often occurs after a biopsy has been taken in the irradiated area. This complication is also dose and volume dependent and is particularly prevalent in patients treated for larger tumours (Delannes et al. 1992). It is more frequent in patients treated with brachytherapy (15 per cent) than in those treated with external radiation therapy (8 per cent). These necroses are poorly inclined to heal with medical care and amputation is necessary in up to 50 per cent of cases.

Combined treatment modalities

Squamous cell carcinoma of the penis is responsive to chemotherapy to some extent. The most active agents are bleomycin, methotrexate, and cisplatin (Ahmed et al. 1984). These agents have been employed in combination with radiotherapy or laser surgery to improve the results in the conservative management of (selected) tumours in category T1 N0 (UICC 1987).

Edsmyr et al. (1985) suggested single-agent bleomycin in combination with external irradiation for the control of the primary tumour. Bleomycin 15 mg was given intramuscularly 2 h before irradiation on each of 5 days during the first, third, and fifth weeks of radiotherapy. A total tumour dose of 58 Gy was given, which is approximately 10–15 per cent less than the usual full course. The whole penis was irradiated from two opposed lateral fields with a conventional X-ray device.

At our institute, relatively large exophytic T1 N0 tumours are being treated with weekly courses of neoadjuvant low-dose vincristine+bleomycin+methotrexate combination chemotherapy (Table 2). The therapy is delivered at home with the cooperation of the family doctor. Patients are checked every 4 weeks for both toxicity and response. Patients are admitted to the day clinic for CO_2 laser surgery after 8–12 weeks of therapy. If residual cancer is found in the deep margin, patients are treated with external-beam irradiation (50 Gy in 5 weeks). No further treatment is given to patients with clear margins (Bandieramonte et al. 1993).

Regional lymph nodes

The management of regional lymph nodes in squamous cell carcinoma of the penis is controversial (Abi-Aad and deKernion 1992). The price to pay for a successful block dissection is high: delayed healing is common and distressing lymphoedema of the lower limbs and external genitalia is a frequent late and permanent complication (McDougal et al. 1986; Fraley et al. 1989; Ornellas et al. 1991; Horenblas et al. 1993). However, there is no evidence that radiotherapy is a satisfactory treatment for the inguinal nodes; the cure rate in patients with metastasis is extremely low and prophylactic irradiation does not prevent the risk of subsequent metastases (Jones *et al.* 1989). Surgical healing following unsuccessful radiotherapy is even more difficult (Gursel *et al.* 1978; Gerbaulet *et al.* 1992). At present, surgery remains the main therapy for nodal metastases in cancer of the penis. Recent work suggests that adjuvant and neoadjuvant chemotherapy may be able to improve the results of radical surgery (Pizzocaro and Piva 1988).

Indications to lymphadenectomy

As only 30–50 per cent of all patients with cancer of the penis will develop nodal metastases during the disease and the price to pay for a radical dissection is high, routine prophylactic lymphadenectomy cannot be recommended except for the very few patients with category T3–T4 tumours (UICC 1987). However, the results of secondary lymphadenectomy in patients who develop nodal metastases during follow-up are usually poor (Johnson and Lo 1984; Fraley *et al.* 1989; Zanoni *et al.* 1989; Horenblas *et al.* 1993). The aim is to select patients at a very high risk of harbouring nodal metastases for nodal dissection. This risk increases significantly with the G grade (Blandy 1989; Fraley *et al.* 1989; Horenblas *et al.* 1993) and invasion of the corpora cavernosa (Crawford and Dawkins 1988). Solsona *et al.* (1992) recently reported nodal metastases in 80 per cent of 25 G2–3-T2 tumours, in 41 per cent of 17 G1 T2 tumours, and in 4 per cent of 24 G1T1 cases. These data, if confirmed by further studies, could allow a selection of patients with N0 tumours to submit to primary lymphadenectomy or to (close) observation.

Catalona (1988) proposed a modified groin dissection with preservation of the saphenous vein as prophylactic lymphadenectomy in patients with N0 tumours. However, all patients suffered mild to moderate lower-extremity oedema and four out of six patients required long-term support stockings. Furthermore, the dissection was revealed to be insufficient in patients with positive nodes. The aim remains the selection of high-risk patients for radical surgery.

En bloc surgery is indicated only in the rare T4 tumours, while contemporary penile amputation and lymphadenectomy are mandatory only when there is obvious evidence of nodal involvement. In all other cases the regional nodes can be re-evaluated a few weeks after the treatment of the primary tumour and a decision taken on the basis of the G,T categories, the clinical evolution of doubtful adenopathies following adequate antimicrobial therapy, and eventually the report of fine-needle aspiration cytology. We do not advise sentinel node biopsy (Cabanas 1987) because of frequent false-negative reports (Perinetti *et al.* 1980; McDougal *et al.* 1986).

Extension and technical considerations

The aim is to identify patients who need a bilateral groin dissection and a pelvic lymphadenectomy. As reported previously, the regional nodes of cancer of the penis are the superficial and deep inguinal nodes, the obturator nodes, and the external iliac nodes (UICC 1987). However, contralateral and pelvic metastases do not usually occur in patients with negative nodes (Srivinas *et al.* 1987), although they are relatively frequent in patients with positive nodes (Riveros and Gorostiaga 1962; Livne and Pontes 1986) and their frequency increases with increasing metastatic spread (Srivinas *et al.* 1987; Horenblas *et al.* 1993). Bilateral and pelvic lymphadenectomy are indicated in patients with documented metastatic disease. From a practical point of view, in the event of a very high-risk patient the most suspect site should be operated on first, while in the presence of obvious metastases a bilateral inguinopelvic lymphadenectomy should be planned.

Whitmore's technique (Whitmore and Vagaiwala 1984), with two parainguinal incisions for the inguinal nodes and a separate suprapubic extraperitoneal approach for the pelvic nodes, is recommended for contemporary bilateral lymphadenectomy. We prefer a longitudinal incision lateral to the femoral vessels for unilateral lymphadenectomy. It can easily be extended upwards and, by dividing the inguinal ligament and abdominal muscles close to the superior iliac spine, the pelvic nodes can easily be reached on retracting the peritoneal sac medially (Pizzocaro 1989). Furthermore, as the major risk of inguinal lymphadenectomy is extensive skin necrosis with exposure of the femoral artery, it has been recommended that the femoral vessels are covered with the sartorius muscle (Blandy 1989).

Combined treatment modalities

Pre- and post-operative radiotherapy

As has been stated before, prophylactic bilateral groin irradiation (50 Gy using mixed gamma rays and electron beams) is no longer recommended (Gerbaulet and Lambin 1992) and pre-operative irradiation leads to delayed healing, cutaneous sclerosis, and lymphoedema (Gursel *et al.* 1978). In contrast, some authors (Gerbaulet and Lambin 1992) advise post-operative irradiation for patients with extensive extracapsular spread or multiple nodal metastases. The inguinal and iliac regions should be treated with a dose of 45–50 Gy in fractions of 2 Gy with cobalt or high-energy photons. Special skin care must be instituted to prevent moist epidermitis and serious discomfort to the patient. Nowadays, post-operative irradiation tends to be replaced by adjuvant chemotherapy.

Adjuvant and neoadjuvant chemotherapy

Starting in 1979, we introduced adjuvant vincristine+bleomycin+methotrexate chemotherapy (Table 2) for radically resected inguinal metastases from penile cancer (Pizzocaro and Piva 1988, 1991). The chemotherapy is administered at home with the cooperation of the family doctor. Patients are checked for toxicity in the out-patient department every 4 weeks. A total of 12 cycles are administered at weekly intervals. The therapy is extremely well tolerated and in the rare event of moderate myelotoxicity or mucositis it is delayed for a week. In the event of documented lung toxicity, bleomycin is withdrawn.

A little more experience on primary therapy is available in the literature. We have been using vincristine+bleomycin+methotrexate as neoadjuvant therapy in patients with fixed inguinal nodes since 1979 (Pizzocaro and Piva 1988, 1992). Fisher *et al.* (1990) introduced neoadjuvant therapy with cisplatin and 5-fluorouracil

Table 3 Cisplatin–5-fluorouracil combination chemotherapy

Drug	Dosage (mg/m^2)	Administration
Cisplatin	100	IV day 1 with high-volume hydration, mannitol-induced diuresis, and intensive anti-emetics
5-Fluorouracil	1000 (daily)	IV continuous infusion for 96–120 h

IV, intravenous.
Repeat every 3–4 weeks for at least two courses. Give two more courses after maximal response has been achieved. Withhold cisplatin if the serum creatinine level is greater than 2 mg/100 ml. Reduce 5-fluorouracil infusion for stomatis and/or granulocytopenia.

Table 4 Methotrexate–bleomycin–cisplatin combination

Drug	Dosage (mg/m^2)	Administration
Methotrexate	200	IV on days 1,15, and 22 with leucovorin rescue 25 mg orally every 6 h starting on the following day for 3 days
Bleomycin	10	IV continuous infusion on days 1–5
Cisplatin	20	IV 1 h infusion with hydration, mannitol-induced diuresis, and anti-emetics on days 1–5

IV, intravenous.

Repeat every 4 weeks, provided that haematological recovery has occurred, for five courses. Deliver methotrexate on days 15 or 22 if there is stable serum creatinine, no mucositis, granulocytes over 1000/mm^3 and platelets >75 000/mm^3. Reduce cisplatin to 50 per cent for creatinine clearance between 40 and 50 ml/min. Withdraw bleomycin for lung toxicity.

(Table 3) for Jackson stage III disease and other authors (Hussein et al. 1990; Shammas et al. 1992) have used the same combination in patients with fixed inguinal nodes with or without distant metastases (Jackson stage IV). The treatment requires high-volume hydration for single-dose cisplatin and 5 days continuous intravenous infusion of 5-fluorouracil. It must be administered on an in-patient basis and requires good renal function and careful monitoring. The treatment is poorly tolerated by the elderly and mild to severe mucositis has been universally reported. Impaired renal function, neutropenic infections, and neurological toxicity are relatively rare.

Dexeus et al. (1991) used a combination of methotrexate, bleomycin, and cisplatin (Table 4) in 14 patients with inoperable inguinal nodal involvement or distant metastases. Also, this rather complicated regimen must be delivered on an in-patient basis for the first 5 days and patients must be evaluated and followed very carefully. Bleomycin and cisplatin have been administered intra-arterially in a few patients. Toxicity was significant: mucositis and myelotoxicity were nearly universal, with two episodes of neutropenic infections. Renal or pulmonary toxicities occurred in one-third of cases.

Palliation for disseminated and advanced disease

Combination chemotherapy (Pizzocaro and Piva 1988; Hussein et al. 1990; Dexeus et al. 1991; Shammas et al. 1992) seems to be more effective than single-agent chemotherapy in advanced squamous cell carcinoma of the penis (Eisenberg 1992), even though an occasional complete remission has been reported with single-agent high-dose methotrexate (Garnick et al. 1979). Combination chemotherapy is the treatment of choice for the rare instances of distant dissemination. As responses are usually of short duration, we advise an in-patient regimen followed by vincristine+bleomycin+methotrexate administered at home.

More commonly, advanced squamous cell carcinoma of the penis remains a locoregional problem with fixed (ulcerated) nodes, multiple nodular recurrences, and en cuirasse dissemination. In these cases, external radiation therapy may be of help for palliation of unresectable patients following systemic chemotherapy. Furthermore, cisplatin has shown a very important synergistic effect with radiotherapy (O'Hara et al. 1986).

FOLLOW-UP AND RESULTS

Control of the primary tumour

A very careful follow-up for recurrences of the primary tumour is very important in patients undergoing conservative treatment as local relapses occur in 20–50 per cent of patients treated with radiotherapy (Gerbaulet and Lambin 1992), 5–15 per cent of those treated by laser (Malek 1992; Bandieramonte et al. 1993), and approximately 30 per cent of those undergoing circumcision alone (Zanoni et al. 1989). While local recurrences following conservative surgery can occur within 2 or 3 years, local relapse following radiotherapy may also occur after 5 years (Gerbaulet and Lambin 1992). Most of these relapses are not concomitant with nodal metastases and they can be cured with surgery. Therefore, it is obvious that patients treated conservatively need a very careful and a very long follow-up. Finally, we have recently seen new occurrences of penile cancer related to human papilloma virus in a few patients more than 10 years after radiotherapy or post-chemotherapy conservative surgery.

In contrast, local recurrences following penile amputation are extremely rare. We observed none following total amputation in 43 patients treated between 1950 and 1987 and four out of 67 (6 per cent) following partial amputation during the same period of time (Zanoni et al. 1989). Nodal metastases were concomitant in all four cases and all relapses occurred within 3 years. Only one of these four patients could be salvaged with radical surgery. Nodal metastases alone occur after a disease-free interval which never exceeds 3 years (Zanoni et al. 1989; Horenblas et al. 1993). They develop in 10–15 per cent of N0 cases and they progress rapidly. Therefore, the necessity for a very careful follow-up of category N0 patients during the first 3 years is obvious; poor follow-up is probably the main reason for the poor results of secondary lymphadenectomy in penile cancer (McDougal et al. 1986).

Long-term survival

Survival of patients with cancer of the penis has been mainly related to nodal involvement. Srivinas et al. (1987) reported 85 per cent disease-free survival following lymphadenectomy in 34 patients with negative nodes compared with 32 per cent in 69 patients with positive histology who had not been lost at follow-up for at least 5 years. Also, the extent of nodal involvement was important; patients with unilateral inguinal nodal metastases, no extranodal tumour extension nor iliac nodal involvement had a median 5 year survival rate of 56 per cent. In particular, five out of six patients with only one positive node survived disease free for over 5 years.

The management of regional lymph nodes according to tumour stage also seems to be important. None of the 19 Jackson stage I patients in the series reported by McDougal et al. (1986) had a lymph node dissection and none died of cancer. Of the nine patients with clinical stage II disease who had a groin dissection as part of the initial treatment (positive nodes in six), only one died of cancer, while nine out of 14 stage II patients who initially had no lymphadenectomy died of the disease. Furthermore, the 5 year survival in 15 stage III patients submitted to lymphadenectomy was 67 per cent compared with zero in eight unresected or irradiated patients. Similarly, Fraley et al. (1989) reported no cancer-related death in 15 Jackson stage I patients treated with or without ileoinguinal lymphadenectomy, while in clinical stage II the 5 year disease-free survival was 100 per cent in the nine patients with negative nodes, 75 per cent in the eight patients with positive nodes, and only 15 per cent in the 20 cases not initially treated with lymphadenectomy. Not only patients with (extensive) positive nodes but also clinical Jackson stage II patients seem to have a poor survival if they do not undergo primary lymphadenectomy.

Recently, both tumour grade and extension of the primary tumour have been found to be significantly related to nodal metastases (Solsona *et al.* 1992; Horenblas *et al.* 1993) and the extent of nodal involvement, assessed both clinically and pathologically, seems to be significantly correlated with survival (Horenblas *et al.* 1993). Furthermore, Horenblas (1993, pp. 145–60) has statistically analysed several prognostic factors for survival in a series of 118 squamous cell carcinomas of the penis treated between 1956 and 1989. Age group and type of treatment of the primary tumour were not statistically significant, in contrast with all the other factors. The 5 year (disease-specific) survival figures for T1, T2, and T3 tumours (UICC 1978) were 94, 59, and 52 per cent, respectively. A statistically significant survival difference was seen between patients with and without clinically suspected nodes. The 5 year survival figures according to the clinical N categories (UICC 1978) were 93, 57, 50, and 17 per cent for N0, N1, N2, and N3, respectively. Grade 3 tumours showed a statistically significant difference in 5 year survival compared with grade 1 tumours (47 and 79 per cent, respectively). No significant difference was shown between grade 3 and grade 2 tumours (5 year survival of 68 per cent). Cox's proportional hazard analysis showed that only N category and grade were highly statistically significant independent prognostic factors of survival.

The introduction of combination chemotherapy in a multidisciplinary approach to the management of nodal metastases from squamous cell carcinoma of the penis seems to be able to improve the prognosis in these patients (Pizzocaro and Piva 1988). During the period 1979–1988 we treated 18 patients consecutively with 12-weekly courses of home-administered adjuvant vincristine–bleomycin–methotrexate (Table 2) following radical ileoinguinal lymphadenectomy for histologically documented nodal metastases (Pizzocaro and Piva 1991). The majority of cases (14 or 78 per cent) had extranodal spread and six had pelvic node involvement. After a follow-up of 3–12 years, only two patients (11 per cent) had relapsed. Both had extranodal spread and pelvic metastases. During the same period of time we treated 11 patients consecutively with neoadjuvant chemotherapy for fixed inguinal metastases (Pizzocaro and Piva 1992). The size of the metastases ranged from 6 to 11 cm and they were bilateral in eight cases. Nine patients were treated with vincristine+bleomycin+methotrexate and five of them had a partial remission. The four patients who were unresponsive to vincristine+bleomycin+methotrexate and another two with chronic bronchitis were treated with cisplatin+5-fluorouracil (Table 3). Four of them achieved a partial remission. The nine responsive patients underwent surgery, which was radical in eight of them. All resected patients had residual cancer, with six also affected in the pelvic nodes. Four patients are alive disease free after 24+, 60+, 72+, and 120+ months, respectively. Fisher *et al.* (1990) treated five patients with cytologically documented Jackson stage II penile cancer with two courses of neoadjuvant cisplatin+5-fluorouracil. One unresponsive patient progressed and died of the disease. The four responders were submitted to radical lymphadenectomy and no viable tumour was found in two of them. All four patients are alive disease free after a follow-up of 6–40 months. Hussein *et al.* (1990) and Shammas *et al.* (1992) treated a total of 13 patients with Jackson stage IV disease with the same combination chemotherapy. Seven patients (54 per cent) achieved a partial remission. Three of them were able to undergo radical surgery: one relapsed after 18 months

and two are alive disease free at 32+ and 57+ months, respectively. The median duration of survival for all patients was 15 months. Dexeus *et al.* (1991) reported two clinically complete responses and eight partial responses out of 14 men with inoperable or metastatic squamous cell carcinoma of the genital tract treated with a mean of five courses of methotrexate+bleomycin+cisplatin (Table 4). The median response duration was 5.9 months, and the median duration of survival for all patients was 10 months (range from 4 to 24+ months). One patient with complete remission relapsed with distant metastases after 4 months and three partial responders were submitted to surgery. However, in all three cases it was impossible to remove all of the remaining disease.

It can be concluded that combination chemotherapy in metastatic squamous cell carcinoma of the penis is promising, but results in patients with unresectable disease are of short duration.

REFERENCES

Abi-Aad AS, deKernion JB (1992). Controversies in the ileoinguinal lymphadenectomy for cancer of the penis. *Urologic Clinics of North America*, **19**:319–24.

Ahmed T, Sklaroff R, Jagoda A (1984). Sequential trials of methotrexate, cisplatin and bleomycin for penile cancer. *Journal of Urology*, **132**:465–8.

Bandieramonte G, Lepera P, Marchesini R, Andreola S, Pizzocaro G (1987). Laser microsurgery for superficial lesions of the penis. *Journal of Urology*, **138**:315–19.

Bandieramonte G, Santoro O, Baracchi P, Piva L, Pizzocaro G, De Palo G (1988). Total resection of glans penis surface by CO_2 laser microsurgery. *Acta Oncologica*, **27**:575–8.

Bandieramonte G, *et al.* (1992). Excisional laser surgery for *in situ* and initially invasive neoplasia of the penis. In *Urology 1992* (ed. L Giuliani and P Puppo), pp. 649–62. Monduzzi, Bologna.

Bandieramonte G, Lepera P, Moglia D, Faustini M, Pizzocaro G (1993). Neoadjuvant chemotherapy and conservative surgery for exophytic T1 N0 carcinoma of the penis. *Abstracts of the 4th International Congress on Anticancer Chemotherapy, Paris 1993*, p. 102, Abstract 178.

Barrasso R, De Brux J, Croissant O, Orth G (1987). High prevalence of papilloma virus associated penile intraepithelial neoplasia in sexual partners of woman with cervical intraepithelial neoplasia. *New England Journal of Medicine*, **317**:916–23.

Bissada NK (1992). Conservative extirpative treatment of cancer of the penis. *Urologic Clinics of North America*, **19**:283–90.

Blandy JP (1989). Carcinoma of the penis. In *Surgical oncology* (ed. U Veronesi), pp. 746–55. Springer Verlag, Berlin.

Cabanas RM (1977). An approach for the treatment of penile carcinoma. *Cancer*, **39**:456–60.

Cabanas RM (1992). Anatomy and biopsy of sentinel lymphnodes. *Urologic Clinics of North America*, **19**:267–76.

Catalona WJ (1988). Modified inguinal lymphadenectomy for carcinoma of the penis with preservation of saphenous vein: technique and preliminary results. *Journal of Urology*, **140**:306–10.

Crawford ED, Dawkins CA (1988). Cancer of the penis. In *Diagnosis and management of genitourinary cancer* (ed. DG Skinner and G Lieskovsky), pp. 549–63. WB Saunders, Philadelphia, PA.

Delannes M, *et al.* (1992). Iridium-192 interstitial therapy for squamous cell carcinoma of the penis. *International Journal of Radiation Oncology—Biology—Physics*, **24**:479–83.

Dexeus FH, *et al.* (1991). Combination chemotherapy with methotrexate, bleomycin and cisplatin for advanced squamous cell carcinoma of the male genital tract. *Journal of Urology*, **146**:1284–7.

Edsmyr F, Anderson L, Espositi PL (1985). Combined bleomycin and radiotherapy in carcinoma of the penis. *Cancer*, **56**:1257–63.

Eisenberg MA (1992). Chemotherapy for carcinoma of the penis and urethra. *Urologic Clinics of North America*, **19**:333–8.

Ekstrom R, Edsmyr F (1958). Cancer of the penis: a clinical study of 229 cases. *Acta Chirurgica Scandinavica*, **115**:24–5.

El-Demiry MIN, *et al.* (1984). Reappraisal of the role of radiotherapy and surgery in the management of carcinoma of the penis. *British Journal of Urology*, 56:724–8.

Fisher HAG, Barada JH, Horton J, von Roemeling R (1990). Neoadjuvant therapy with cisplatin and 5-fluorouracil for stage III squamous cell carcinoma of the penis. *Journal of Urology*, 143:352A, Abstract 653.

Fraley EE, Zhang G, Manuvel C, Niehans GA (1989). The role of ileo-inguinal lymphadenectomy and significance of histological differentiation in treatment of carcinoma of the penis. *Journal of Urology*, 142:1478–82.

Garnick M, Skain AT, Steele GD (1979). Metastatic squamous cell carcinoma of the penis: complete response after high dose MTX chemotherapy. *Journal of Urology*, 122:265–6.

Gerbaulet A, Lambin P (1992). Radiotherapy of cancer of the penis. Indications, advantages, pitfalls. *Urologic Clinics of North America*, 19:325–32.

Gerbaulet A, *et al.* (1992). La curiethérapie du cancer de la verge. A propos d'un nouveau GAG (gland applicateur de Gerbaulet). *Bulletin du Cancer/Radiotherapie*, 79(1):95–100.

Gursel ED, *et al.* (1978). Penile cancer: clinicopathological study of 64 cases. *Urology*, 1:569–78.

Haile K, Delclos L (1980). The place of radiation therapy in the treatment of carcinoma of the distal and of the penis. *Cancer*, 45:1980–4.

Hope-Stone HF (1975). Carcinoma of the penis. External radiation mould technique. *Proceedings of the Royal Society of Medicine*, 68:777–9.

Horenblas S (1993). The management of penile squamous cell carcinoma. A retrospective and prospective study. Thesis, Universiteit van Amsterdam, BV Export drukkerij, Zoetermeer.

Horenblas S, *et al.* (1991). Squamous cell carcinoma of the penis: accuracy of tumor nodes and metastasis classification system, and role of lymphangiography, computed tomography scan and fine needle aspiration cytology. *Journal of Urology*, 146:1279–83.

Horenblas S, *et al.* (1993). Squamous cell carcinoma of the penis—III. Treatment of regional lymph nodes. *Journal of Urology*, 149:492–7.

Hussein AM, Benedetto P, Sridhar KS (1990). Chemotherapy with cisplatin and 5-fluorouracil for penile and urethral squamous cell carcinoma. *Cancer*, 65:433–8.

Iwasawa A, Kumamoto Y, Fujinaga K (1993). Detection of human papilloma virus deoxyribonucleic acid in penile carcinoma by polymerase chain reaction and *in situ* hybridization. *Journal of Urology*, 149:59–63.

Jackson SM (1966). Treatment of carcinoma of the penis. *British Journal of Surgery*, 53:33–5.

Johnson DE, Lo RK (1984). Management of regional lymph nodes in penile carcinoma: five-year results following therapeutic groin dissection. *Urology*, 24:308–11.

Jones WG, Fossa SD, Harmers H, van den Bogaert W (1989). Penis cancer: a review by the Joint Committee of the European Organization for Research and Treatment of Cancer (EORTC), Genito-urinary and Radiotherapy Groups. *Journal of Surgical Oncology*, 40:227–31.

Kausal V, Sharma SC (1987). Carcinoma of the penis. *Acta Oncologica*, 26:413–17.

Klein EA (1991). Partial and total penectomy for cancer. *Urologic Clinics of North America*, 18:161–9.

Kuisk H (1971). Penile lymphography. In *Technique of lymphography*, pp. 135–40. HG Warren, St Louis, MO.

Livne PM, Pontes JE (1986). Tumors of penis, scrotum and spermatic cord. In *Urologic oncology* (ed. SD Graham Jr), pp. 369–82. Raven Press, New York.

Lucia MF, Miller GJ (1992). Histopathology of malignant lesions of the penis. *Urologic Clinics of North America*, 19:227–46.

McDougal WS, Kirchner FK, Edwards RH, Killion LT (1986). Treatment of carcinoma of the penis: the case for primary lymphadenectomy. *Journal of Urology*, 136:38–41.

Maiche AG, Pyrhoenen S (1990). Clinical staging of cancer of the penis: by size? by location? or by depth of infiltration? *European Urology*, 18:16–22.

Malek RS (1992). Laser treatment of premalignant and malignant squamous cell lesions of the penis. *Lasers in Surgery and Medicine*, 12:246–53.

Mazeron JJ, *et al.* (1984). Interstitial radiation therapy for carcinoma of the penis using iridium-192 wires. The Henry Mondor experience (1970–1979). *International Journal of Radiation Oncology—Biology—Physics*, 10:1891–5.

O'Hara JA, Doule EB, Richmond RC (1986). Enhancement of radiation induced cell kill by platinum complexes in V 79 cells. *International Journal of Radiation Oncology—Biology—Physics*, 12:1419–22.

Ornellas AA, Correa Seixas AL, De Morales JR (1991). Analysis of 200 lymphadenectomies in patients with penile carcinoma. *Journal of Urology*, 146:330–2.

Perinetti E, Crane DB, Catalone WT (1980). Unreliability of sentinel lymph node biopsy for staging penile carcinoma. *Journal of Urology*, 124:734–5.

Persky L, De Kernion J (1986). Carcinoma of the penis. *CA—A Cancer Journal for Clinicians*, 36(5):258–73.

Pierquin B, Chassagne D, Cex JD (1971). Toward consistent local control of certain malignant tumours. *Radiology*, 99:661–7.

Pizzocaro G (1989). I tumori dell'apparato genitale maschile. In *Trattato di Chirurgia Oncologica* (ed. U Veronesi), pp. 571–618. UTET, Torino.

Pizzocaro G, Piva L (1988). Adjuvant and neoadjuvant vincristine, bleomycin and methotrexate for inguinal metastases from squamous cell carcinoma of the penis. *Acta Oncologica*, 27:823–4.

Pizzocaro G, Piva L (1991). Adjuvant home vincristine, bleomycin, methotrexate (VBM) in resected nodal metastases from squamous cell carcinoma of the penis. *Journal of Urology*, 145:367A, Abstract 619.

Pizzocaro G, Piva L (1992). Primary chemotherapy and surgery for fixed inguinal metastases from squamous cell carcinoma of the penis. *Journal of Urology*, 147:369A, Abstract 627.

Ragavaiah NV (1978). Corpus cavernosogram in the evaluation of carcinoma of the penis. *Journal of Urology*, 120:423.

Riveros M, Gorostiaga R (1962). Cancer of the penis. *Archives of Surgery*, 85:377–82.

Sagerman RH, *et al.* (1984). External-beam irradiation of carcinoma of the penis. *Radiology*, 152:183–5.

Shammas FV, Ons S, Fossa SD (1992). Cisplatin and 5-fluorouracil in advanced cancer of the penis. *Journal of Urology*, 147:630–2.

Solsona E, *et al.* (1992). Corpus cavernosum invasion and tumor grade in the prediction of lymph node metastases. *European Urology*, 22:115–18.

Srivinas V, Morse MJ, Herr HW, Sogani PC, Whitmore WF (1987). Penile cancer relation of extent of nodal metastases to survival. *Journal of Urology*, 137:880–2.

Stern RS, Members of the Photochemotherapy Follow-up Study (1990). Genital tumors among men with psoriasis exposed to ultraviolet radiation. *New England Journal of Medicine*, 332:1093–7.

Stewart AL, Grieve RJ, Banarjee SS (1985). Primary lymphoma of the penis. *European Journal of Surgical Oncology*, 11:179–81.

Stillwell TJ, Zinke H, Gaffey TA, Woods JE (1988). Malignant melanoma of the penis. *Journal of Urology*, 140:72–5.

UICC (Union Internationale Contre le Cancer) (1978). *TNM classification of malignant tumours* (3rd edn) (ed. H Harmer), pp. 126–8. SA Buren, Geneva.

UICC (Union Internationale Contre le Cancer) (1987). *TNM classification of malignant tumours* (4th edn) (ed. P Hermaneck and H Sobi), pp. 130–2. Springer-Verlag, Berlin.

Vapnek JM, Hricak H, Caroll PR (1992). Recent advance in imaging studies for staging of penile and urethral carcinoma. *Urologic Clinics of North America*, 19:257–66.

Whitmore WF, Vagaiwala MR (1984). A technique of ileoinguinal lymph node dissection for carcinoma of the penis. *Surgery, Gynaecology and Obstetrics*, 159:573–8.

Yamashita T, Ogawa A (1989). Ultrasound in penile cancer. *Urologic Radiology*, 11:174–7.

Zanoni F, *et al.* (1989). Chirurgia radicale nel carcinoma spinocellulare del pene. In *I Tumori Genito-Urinari* (ed. U Veronesi, G Pizzocaro, and E Pisani), pp. 233–8. CEA, Milan.

10.4   Bladder cancer

D. W. W. NEWLING, LOUIS DENIS, JEAN PIERRE GERARD,
PIERRE G. M. SCALLIET, AND GERRIT STOTER

INTRODUCTION

In Europe, bladder cancer is the fourth most common cancer in males and the fifth most common cause of cancer death. Worldwide, the vast majority of bladder cancer is of the transitional cell type, but in certain Middle Eastern and tropical countries, where bilharzia infestation is endemic, it is mainly of the squamous cell type. The incidence of bladder cancer worldwide continues to increase by 5–10 per cent every 5 years and this rise may well be related to the increase in tobacco abuse, particularly in Third World countries.

AETIOLOGY AND EPIDEMIOLOGY

Although transitional cells line the urinary tract from the calyces to the proximal third of the urethra, transitional cell carcinoma is far more common in the bladder than in other parts of the urinary tract. Logically, the cause or aetiological agent for bladder cancer must reside in the urine. Bladder cancer is almost three times as common in men as in women and the highest incidence is in the sixth decade. Although it is tempting to suggest that the increased incidence is simply related to the increasing mean age of the population in Western countries, it is far more likely to be related to the increasing incidence of tobacco abuse worldwide. A hospital-based controlled study has shown that the risk of bladder cancer for a man smoking more than 20 cigarettes per day is 2.5 times greater than the risk for a non-smoker. In both sexes the risk increases with duration of smoking (Augustine *et al.* 1988).

The second group of patients with a well-known aetiology for their bladder cancer comprises those who have been exposed to industrial carcinogens. Workers in the rubber, petrochemical, oil, paint, dyeing, and metal-refining industries have an increased incidence of bladder cancer and in many cases the exact aetiological agent has been identified (British Association of Urological Surgeons 1988).

Because of the long latent period in the development of bladder cancer, with some tumours occurring more than 30 years after exposure to a known carcinogen, there must be many risk factors and carcinogenic agents which have eluded identification. This long latent period also suggests a two-step developmental process in bladder cancer: the first step probably causes a mutation of the DNA and the second step promotes the growth of the altered cells. It is likely that in many instances the carcinogen and the promoting agent are the same.

A number of drugs have been identified as aetiological agents in bladder cancer. Phenacetin, which was in general use as an antipyretic analgesic 20 years ago, appears unique in that it causes almost as many tumours in the upper as in the lower urinary tract. Cytotoxic and antimetabolic agents used in the treatment of cancer are themselves carcinogenic, as are many of their metabolites. Probably the best known of these is cyclophosphamide, which gives rise to a cystitis-like condition which is known to be pre-carcinogenic.

Although aetiological agents have been identified in a number of patients with bladder cancer, many more remain who neither smoke nor have been exposed to industrial or other identifiable carcinogenic substances. The search for compounds with a similar chemical formulation to known carcinogens in the urine of normal people has led to the identification of a number of carcinogenic metabolites of tryptophan (Brown *et al.* 1960). Some patients with a slightly abnormal tryptophan metabolism have been shown to produce significantly high concentrations of kynurenine, acetyl-kynurenine, and xanthurenic acid, which are all identifiable carcinogens, in their urine (Bryan *et al.* 1964).

Alterations of the levels of these metabolites by administration of pyridoxine in one randomized study (Byar and Blackard 1977) resulted in a diminished incidence of recurrent tumour in patients treated for superficial bladder cancer. Although these findings were not confirmed in a subsequent study (Newling *et al.* 1983), there must be a strong possibility that carcinogens which give rise to a large number of bladder cancers in patients not exposed to known industrial or other carcinogenic agents may exist within the metabolic pathway of tryptophan and similar substances.

ONCOGENES AND GROWTH FACTORS

The role of growth factors and oncogenes in the development of bladder cancer has been investigated. Epidermal growth factor has been identified as a promoter of urothelial cancer. It is excreted in increased amounts in the bladder urine early in the development of tumour. Epidermal growth factor may function as an early tumour marker which could be used for screening the disease and monitoring the treatment results of both superficial and invasive tumours (Momose *et al.* 1991; Kawamata *et al.* 1992; Messing 1992).

Acidic and basic fibroblast growth factors have also been identified as regulatory peptides inolved in the biology of transitional cell cancer. Acidic fibroblast growth factor has been demonstrated in epithelial cells and basic fibroblast growth factor on basal membranes and stromal vessels (Ravery *et al.* 1992). In a rat model, acidic fibroblast growth factor appears to have a dual function: at high cell density it is a potent mitogen, but at low density it converts bladder cancer cells into motile fibroblast-like cells. These different modes of action appear to be related to the level of cAMP (Boyer and Thiery 1993). Whether these findings reflect the situation in the human is unknown.

Human bladder cancer has been shown to secrete increased amounts of vascular permeability factor, which enhances the nutritional status of the tumour (Nguyen *et al.* 1993; Roberts and Hasan 1993).

Numerous genetic alterations have been associated with the development and evolution of bladder cancer. Non-random aberrations of chromosomes 1, 5, 7, 9, 11, and 17 have been reported (Borland *et al.* 1992). These genetic alterations include the epidermal growth factor receptor, *erbB*-2, *int*-2, *hst*, H-*ras*, and the suppressor genes Rb-1 and p53 (Jones *et al.* 1992; Sridansky and Messing 1992; Tennant *et al.* 1993). Overexpression of H-*ras*

Table 1 Proposed guidelines for histopathological evaluation of biopsy specimens of bladder cancer

Biopsy: each specimen submitted should be described separately (gross and microscopic), evaluated, and diagnosed separately

A. Gross description
 1. Number of pieces and greatest dimension of each
 2. Configuration; papillary or not
 3. Tissue embedded: all
   If not, specify the number of pieces in relationship to the whole, e.g. 5/10

B. Microscopic description
 1. Epithelial surfaces
   Intact
   Denuded: partially or completely
   Ulcerated
 2. Amount of bladder wall present
   (a) Fronds only
   (b) Lamina propria present
   (c) Muscularis propria present
 3. Patterns of growth (WHO)
   (a) Not determinable
   (b) Papillary
   (c) Infiltrating
   (d) Non-papillary, non-infiltrating (flat)
   (e) Papillary and infiltrating
   (f) Papillary and flat
   (g) Infiltrating and flat
   (h) Papillary, infiltrating, and flat
 4. Histology (WHO)
   (a) Transitional cell papilloma
   (b) Transitional cell papilloma (inverted)
   (c) Squamous cell papilloma
   (d) Adenoma (specify type)
   (e) Transitional cell carcinoma
   (f) Transitional cell carcinoma and
     (1) Squamous elements
     (2) Glandular elements (columnar)
     (3) Tubular elements (cuboidal)
     (4) Squamous and glandular elements
     (5) Squamous and tubular elements
     (6) Undifferentiated elements
   (g) Squamous carcinoma
   (h) Adenocarcinoma
   (i) Undifferentiated carcinoma
   (j) Spindle
   (k) Others (specify)
 5. Grade (based primarily on nuclear appearance)
   (a) Slight anaplasia (grade 1)
   (b) Moderate anaplasia (grade 2)
   (c) Marked anaplasia (grade 3)

 6. Inflammatory cell infiltration
   (a) Present
   (b) Absent
   (c) Peripheral to the tumour
   (d) Intermingled with the tumour
   (e) Type
     (1) Lymphocytes
     (2) Plasma cells
     (3) Eosinophils
     (4) Monocytes
     (5) Atypical fibroblasts
     (6) Granuloma
 7. Extent of invasion
   (a) No invasion: papillary or flat lesion
   (b) Subepithelial connective tissue (lamina propria)
   (c) Superficial muscle
   (d) Deep muscle
   (e) Perivesical adipose tissue
   (f) Adjacent organs or structures, if present
     (1) Prostate
     (2) Cervix
     (3) Vagina
     (4) Pelvis
     (5) Others
 8. Location of spread
   (a) Lymphatics
   (b) Vascular
   (c) Subjacent
   (d) Lateral
 9. Mode of spread
   (a) Broad front (pushing)
   (b) Tentacular
   (c) Mixed: (a) and (b)
   (d) Undetermined
 10. Status of mucosa
   (a) Normal
   (b) Brunn's nests
   (c) Papillary cystitis
   (d) Cystitis cystica
   (e) Hyperplasia, atypia, atypical hyperplasia, dysplasia
   (f) Carcinoma *in situ* II
   (g) Carcinoma *in situ* III
   (h) Cystitis glandularis
   (i) Squamous metaplasia
   (j) Tubular metaplasia
   (k) Others

upregulates the expression of epidermal growth factor receptor (Theodorescu *et al.* 1991). More recently, it has been suggested that deletions at chromosome 9q are associated with superficial bladder tumours (Ta-1) and deletions at 3q, 5q, and 17p are associated with invasive tumours (T2-4). The conclusion must be that more attention should be focused on the elucidation of genetic markers in order to predict the course of the disease and the response to treatment (Dalbagni *et al.* 1993).

HISTOPATHOLOGY

Transitional cell carcinoma is a heterogeneous disease with a wide variation in prognosis according to individual tumour cell characteristics, even in tumours of comparable stage and grade. Most

clinical studies fail to take these variables into account, which makes central pathology monitoring an essential part of clinical research studies.

Specific pathological guidelines for the evaluation of specimens of bladder cancer have been developed in a succession of Consensus Conferences on Bladder Cancer organized by the European Organization for Research and Treatment of Cancer (EORTC GU Group). The agreed minimum criterion for the diagnosis of transitional cell carcinoma was a neoplastic formation more than seven cell layers thick showing anaplasia characterized by increased cellularity, nuclear crowding, disturbances of cellular polarity, failure of differentiation, irregularity in size, and variation in shape and chromatin distribution of the nuclei. It was further agreed that there should be four grades of differentiation (Hermanck and Sobin 1987):

grade 1, well differentiated; grade 2, moderately differentiated; grade 3, poorly differentiated; grade 4, undifferentiated.

The ten guidelines for a histopathological description of a biopsy specimen (Table 1) illustrate the complexity of the problem. The possibility that the common histological subtypes under 4(f) probably arise from a common progenitor cell should be noted. However, it is believed that focal areas of squamous or glandular differentiation should still be classified and treated as transitional cell carcinoma. Interest in the mucosa adjacent to the tumour and in the normal mucosa of the bladder has been generated by the longitudinal studies of the National Bladder Cancer Collaborative Group A program (NBCCG) (National Bladder Cancer Collaborative Group A 1977) which suggested that unsuspected carcinoma *in situ* is frequently present in the bladder mucosa of patients with papillary tumours, particularly those of a high grade.

These observations led to a definite conclusion that transitional cell epithelium transforms into neoplastic epithelium by two main pathways. Approximately two-thirds of all bladder cancers are papillary in configuration and develop from normal or hyperplastic epithelium without nuclear abnormalities. Sometimes diagnosis is based only on the number of cell layers. These tumours exhibit low-grade cytological atypia and, of course, are not detected in cytological examinations of the urine. They are labelled as papillary carcinomata and were formerly called papillomata. Not all papillary tumours are so innocent and some present with cell anaplasia with the inclusion of nuclear abnormalities among other morphological features. These tumours form a poor prognosis subgroup of superficial bladder tumours.

The flat carcinoma *in situ* is superficial as a tumour but quite distinct in its biological behaviour (Friedell 1976).

Confusion still apparently exists over the terms atypia, hyperplasia, atypical hyperplasia, and dysplasia. The majority of pathologists would now accept that the first three terms, atypia, hyperplasia, and atypical hyperplasia, should be reserved for benign disorders. Dysplasia implies alterations in the nucleus which are commonly seen in association with frank carcinoma *in situ*. Therefore, it is not only a definite pre-malignant condition but is also predictive of a tumour with many features carrying a poor prognosis.

A third of bladder cancers at presentation have already invaded into the subepithelial connective tissue. Even the initial invasion of the subepithelial connective tissue (basement, membrane) is a poor prognostic factor and defines a specific subset of patients. These tumours invariably progress to higher stages of disease and, in the majority of cases, metastasize within a year of deep muscle invasion. A large number of these tumours, once diagnosed, should be treated as systemic disease (Prout and Kopp 1984). A particularly poor prognosis is associated with poorly differentiated (grade 3) or undifferentiated (grade 4) tumours. Cytological examination of collected urine specimens plays a key role in the diagnosis of these tumours and in experienced hands malignant cells are found in the urine in 100 per cent of cases of carcinoma *in situ* and in 80–90 per cent of all tumours (Koss *et al.* 1985). It should be emphasized that both cytological and histological examinations must be performed for adequate quality control and all cytological diagnoses of bladder cancer must be confirmed by biopsy prior to definitive therapy. Bladder washings or washings of the upper urinary tract can yield abundant cellular material to give information to confirm a suspected diagnosis. Bladder irrigation specimens are required for flow cytology analysis. Once again, it must be emphasized that bladder washings, like voided urine cytology, cannot identify low-grade papillary tumours. The correlation of visual, histological, and

Table 2 Correlation of cytology, cystoscopy, and histology

Cytology	Cystoscopy	Histology	Decision
Positive	Negative	—	Repeat cytology
			Upper-tract imaging
			Random biopsies
Negative	Papillary tumour	Low grade	Treat as low grade
		High grade	Random biopsies
	Sessile tumour	Low grade	Upper-tract imaging
			Random biopsies
		High grade	Repeat cytology

cytological findings is presented in Table 2. The false-positive cytology reports are usually caused by other instrumentation (brushing), poor cell preservation, prior radiotherapy, or urinary tract lithiasis. In conclusion it can be stated again that accurate sampling of urine cytology and subsequent biopsy/definitive specimen is a prerequisite for proper diagnosis and treatment.

STAGING

Spread of bladder cancer occurs by direct infiltration of the bladder wall, where invasion of the subepithelial connective tissue is the first marker of invasive potential and invasion of the bladder muscle is the start of a lethal cascade. Lymphatic spread occurs to the regional nodes and then to the para-aortic, mediastinal, and supraclavicular nodes. Metastasis by vascular dissemination most commonly affects lungs, bone, and liver. As recognized by the histopathological examination, although bladder cancer is a very heterogeneous tumour, a gross relationship exists between prognosis and the extent of the tumour and its metastasis. The TNM system proposed by the Union Internationale Contre le Cancer (UICC), where T stands for tumour, N for nodes, and M for metastasis, is now univerally accepted as a global staging system. A 1987 revision of the TNM classification of malignant tumours was intended to simplify the classification by utilizing principles applicable to all sites. The classification aims to help the clinician in the planning of the treatment and to give some indication of prognosis and should assist in the evaluation of results and facilitate the communication between treatment centres.

The addition of numbers to the TNM indicates the extent of the disease by rating T0–4, N0–3, M0, and M1. The M1 category can be further specified as nodal (M1 Lym), osseous (M1 Oss), etc. Two classifications are described for each site. The clinical or pre-treatment classification designated TNM is based on physical examination, imaging, endoscopy, biopsy, surgical exploration, and other relevant examinations and is a classification of the tumour before definitive treatment. The pathological classification is designated pTNM. It is based on subsequent evidence acquired from surgery and from the pathological specimens obtained after cystectomy. The pathological assessment entails the resection of the primary tumour or wide and deep biopsy to evaluate the highest pT category. Assessment of the nodes entails removal of the nodes sufficient to evaluate the highest N category. The assessment of pM1 entails microscope examination of a metastasis. The TNM categories can be used in clincial stages to select and evaluate therapy. Lack of proof should classify a tumour in the classification or the stage group in the lower category (for example, T1 instead of T2 or T3 instead of T2).

Table 3 TNM categories in bladder cancer (ICD.0188)

T Primary tumour
  TX   Primary tumour cannot be assessed
  T0   No evidence of primary tumour
  Tis Carcinoma *in situ*: 'flat tumour'
  Ta   Non-invasive papillary carcinoma
  T1   Tumour invades subepithelial connective tissue
  T2   Tumour invades muscle (inner half)
  T3   Tumour invades deep muscle or perivesical fat
  T3a Tumour invades deep muscle (outer half)
  T3b Tumour invades perivesical fat
  T4   Tumour invades any of the following: prostate, uterus, vagina, pelvic wall, abdominal wall

N Regional lymph nodes
  NX Regional lymph nodes cannot be assessed
  N0 No regional node metastasis
  N1 Metastasis in a single lymph node 2 cm or less in greatest dimension
  N2 Metastasis in a single lymph node more than 2 cm but not more than 5 cm in greatest dimension, or multiple nodes, none more than 5 cm in greatest dimension
  N3 Metastasis in a lymph node more than 5 cm in greatest dimension

M Distant metastasis
  MX Presence of distant metastasis cannot be assessed
  M0 No distant metastasis
  M1 Distant metastasis

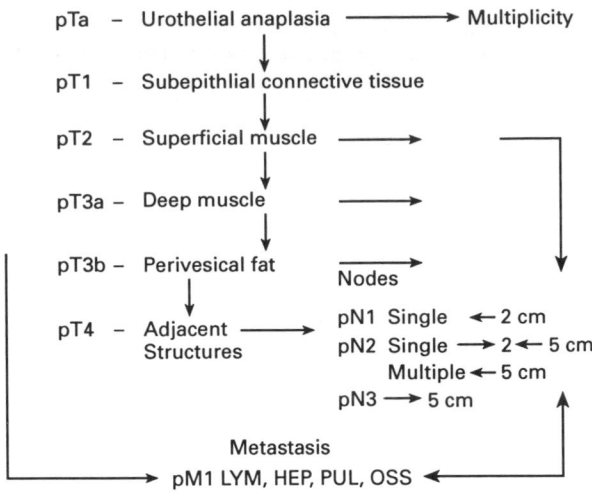

Fig. 1 Pathological (p) classification of bladder cancer. pTis may be concomitant with all T. Regional lymph node invasion pN1–3 and pM1 LYM (extraregional lymph nodes), HEP (lung), PUL (lung), and OSS (bone) should be evaluated as lethal disease.

There has been considerable criticism of the new classification by international and national urological groups. The EORTC urological group specifically suggested retaining the presence or absence of a palpable mass in extravesical cancer after transurethral resection and a division of the T4 category where the stage grouping was rejected as grossly inaccurate (Schröder *et al.* 1988). The TNM categories (fourth edition) are presented in Table 3 with pathological classification in Fig. 1. The suffix (m) can be added to any T category to indicate multiple tumours or the presence of associated carcinoma *in situ*.

The following changes to the current classification have now been recommended.

1. T3b tumour invades perivesical fat (i) microscopically or (ii) macroscopically (mass).

2. T4a tumour invades any of the following: prostate, uterus, vagina.

3. T4b tumour invades the pelvic wall and/or the abdominal wall.

The agreed stage grouping is shown in Table 4.

It is agreed that a substantial percentage of invasive tumours are understaged as primary tumours and the correct nodal staging is reliably obained only by surgical lymphadenectomy. Fine-needle aspiration under CT scan control or through laparoscopy may obviate the need for surgery. Chest radiography, liver ultrasound, and bone scan are used to identify clinical distant metastases. However, it must be recognized that a number of other factors, such as DNA ploidy, the absence of ABH blood group isoantigens, and the proportion of S-phase nuclei or chromosomal markers, predict the biological activity of the tumour. Further clinical research in carefully controlled studies will add to the categorization and staging of tumours.

NATURAL HISTORY

Tumour grade and stage are two determinants of the natural history of the disease. The two tumour types of transitional cell carcinoma show distinctly different development.

Low-grade papillary tumours have a low potential for invasion. They often recur, depending on multiplicity and size, but remain non-invasive. Only 10 per cent of patients with recurrent superficial bladder cancer showed invasion in a 10 year follow-up (Bouffioux *et al.* 1992). Histological evidence of disease is seldom found in random mucosal biopsies and their follow-up and treatment have been simplifed in the last decade after general recognition of the 'benign' course of this disease (Schröder and Richards 1983).

Superficial papillary tumours usually appear in the lower part of the bladder and are multiple in approximately 50 per cent of cases. Sixty to eighty per cent of these experience recurrent disease after destruction of the papillary lesions at initial diagnosis. Synchronous tumours of the upper tract are discovered in 5 per cent of the patients and of the prostate and urethra in another 5 per cent. These tumours progress from hyperplastic areas to papillary lesions, possibly over a long period of time. A number eventually invade the superficial connective tissue (T1 disease) and are characterized by a different prognosis and survival. The presence of a high-grade (grade 3) tumour or its subsequent development changes the picture completely since approximately one-third of

Table 4 Proposed stage grouping for the UICC TNM staging for bladder cancer (ICD.0188)

Stage 0	Ta	N0	M0
Stage 'is'	Tis	N0	M0
Stage I	T1	N0	M0
Stage II	T2	N0	M0
	T3a	N0	M0
Stage III	T3b	N0	M0
	T4a	N0	M0
Stage IV	T4b	N0	M0
	Any T	N1–3	M0
	Any T	Any N	M1

Table 5 Multivariate analysis of EORTC studies 30782 and 30790 for prognostic factors: tumour progression in Ta and T1 tumours according to risk group

Group	No. of patients	Progression	Percentage
1	281	20	7.1
2	218	38	17.4
3	36	15	41.6
Total	535	73	13.6

$p=30.000$ (log rank overall); $p>0.000$ (log rank trend).

Table 6 Measurable lesions in metastatic bladder cancer

Site[a]	Method
Lymph nodes	Caliper+CT
Subcutaneous masses	Caliper+CT
Pulmonary metastases	Radiography+CT
Hilar/mediastinal masses	CT+tomography
Liver metastases	CT+MRI+US
Retroperitoneal nodes	CT
Abdominal/pelvic masses	CT

MRI, magnetic resonance imaging; US, ultrasonography.
[a]Always >25 mm

these patients progress to invasive disease in a few years (Kurth 1984).

Although considered as superficial disease, carcinoma *in situ* (Tis) of the bladder is a different pathological entity. It is classified as primary Tis, where it occurs in isolation, secondary Tis, where it occurs after treatment of a papillary tumour, or concomitant Tis, where it occurs simultaneously with a papillary lesion. The term Tis should be reserved for a flat lesion of the urothelium with enough cellular anaplasia to be recognized as carcinoma grade 2 at least and usually grade 3–4. In concomitant Tis, which is recognized as a poor prognostic factor, treatment will be dictated by the associated gross cancer (Smith *et al.* 1983). Treatment of carcinoma *in situ* usually depends on the extent and location of lesions. Aggressive intravesical treatment is preferred since half the tumours progress to invasive disease. The *in situ* cancers are considered to be the precursors of invasive bladder cancers (Melamed *et al.* 1964).

Approximately one-third of all cancer invades muscle at initial diagnosis and is usually of the solid variety or mixed papillary and solid. They are usually biologically active and invade and metastasize readily. It is accepted that 30 per cent of patients with transitional cell carcinoma and deep muscle invasion (T3a) have regional lymph node metastasis and the great majority of these develop metastases within the first year of diagnosis irrespective of local therapy (Prout *et al.* 1979). Few patients survive for 5 years if left untreated and half of treated patients are dead after 5 years.

PROGNOSTIC FACTORS

Many studies have shown that tumour grade and stage have a predictive value for recurrence and survival (Lutzeyer *et al.* 1982). A prognostic factor analysis of two EORTC studies examining different intravesical therapies in the prophylaxis of recurrence of superficial bladder cancer (Sylvester 1985) revealed a correlation between recurrence rate and time to invasion. The multivariate analysis showed that three main factors determined prognosis: the prior recurrence rate, the grade, and the number and location of tumours. The most important factor is the presence or absence of recurrence at first cystoscopy at 3 months. Based on these figures three risk groups can be identified. The percentage of patients who experienced tumour progression to at least T2 is given in Table 5 (Sylvester 1985). The combination of grade 3, T1, or Tis and recurrent disease at 3 months was associated with muscle invasion in 82 per cent of patients after a median interval of 8.4 months (Richards 1986). These observations highlight the importance of the proper evaluation of these factors in treatment decisions and clinical follow-up. Linked to prognostic factors are the response criteria which in turn define the end-points. The end-points in superficial bladder cancer are destruction of the primary

visible tumour(s), prophylaxis against recurrence, which is a common feature in multiple tumours, and, as mentioned, progression of or death from the disease.

The prime parameter of tumour destruction is visible absence of tumour, no mass under bimanual examination, negative biopsies of the tissue left after complete resection, and negative urine cytology in the follow-up. The reverse, which is a recurrence, is usually established by control cystoscopy and urine cytology. The success of treatment can be expressed in several ways as percentage of patients with recurrence, disease-free interval, and recurrence rate per year. This is an abstract number which is the preferred form of analysis from a statistical point of view since it takes into consideration all recurrences during a defined follow-up period. A recurrence rate of 0.2 means one recurrence every 5 years.

The use of a marker lesion intentionally left after resection in therapeutic trials allows the effect of ablative chemotherapy to be examined. This method was first introduced by the NBCCGA and accepted by the EORTC for evaluation of new agents in phase II protocols. Complete and partial response as well as treatment failure are the critical standards. The concept faced resistance from some ethical committees, but the chances of progression during the observation period in a 'worst case scenario' has been shown to be less than 2 per cent (R. R. Hall, personal communication). These patients are all in clinical studies and under stricter surveillance than in routine treatment. The response criteria for the treatment of Tis are of course based on the destruction of all visible lesions, negative cytology, and negative random biopsies.

The important prognostic indicators, independent of treatment, are tumour stage and grade, as well as certain radiological and biochemical findings such as upper tract dilatation and the absence of ABH antigens on the tumour cells. The extent of disease as assessed by the TNM system should be the strongest pre-treatment prognostic parameter and, thus, is a minimal requirement in the report of clinical stage. Unfortunately, a correct assessment utilizing newer imaging techniques such as transvesical ultrasonography and CT probably leaves a significant percentage of error in the staging which should be incorporated in clinical decisions. One important aspect of the assessment of the prognosis of the tumour is the relationship between pT stage and regional lymph node invasion (Smith and Whitmore 1981a). Indeed, distant metastases are subsequently found in most patients with regional lymph node metastases. Again, grade plays an important role in determining the rate of metastatic spread, together with tumour configuration, the completeness or otherwise of the transurethral resection, ureteral obstruction, and the size of the tumour mass.

The performance status and haemoglobin characterize the host and their resistance to the biological aggression. Tumour response to treatment is usually a strong prognostic parameter in most

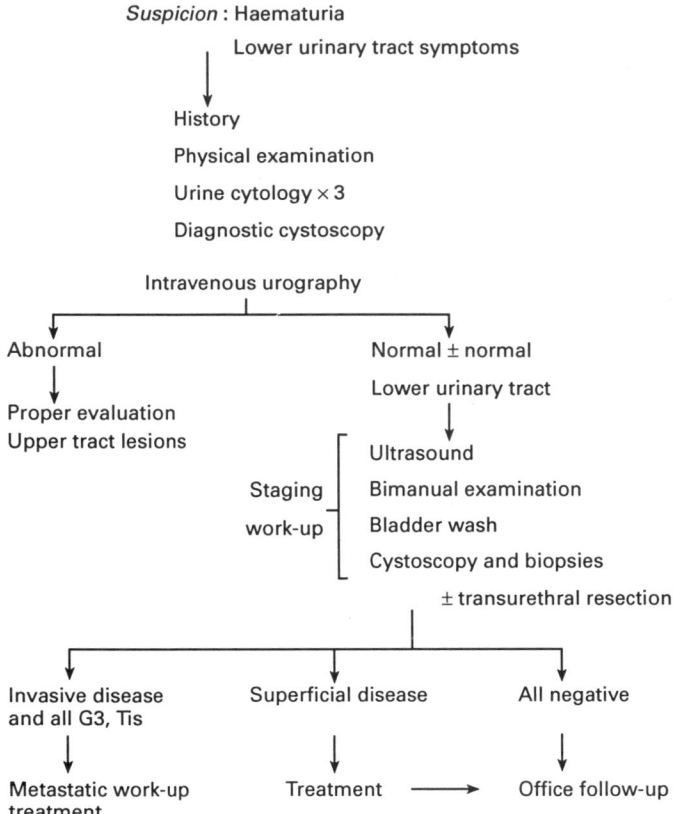

Suspicion : Haematuria
        Lower urinary tract symptoms

History
Physical examination
Urine cytology × 3
Diagnostic cystoscopy

Intravenous urography

Abnormal   Normal ± normal
                         Lower urinary tract

Proper evaluation
Upper tract lesions

Staging   Ultrasound
             Bimanual examination
work-up   Bladder wash
             Cystoscopy and biopsies

± transurethral resection

Invasive disease   Superficial disease   All negative
and all G3, Tis

Metastatic work-up   Treatment ⟶ Office follow-up
treatment

Fig. 2 Algorithm of diagnostic work-up of bladder cancer.

reported studies (Slack and Prout 1980). A number of prognostic factors have been evaluated in research studies.

Tumours that elaborate ABH antigens are usually associated with a better prognosis, while the presence of the Thomsen–Friedenreich (T) antigen is associated with a poor prognosis. Assessment of chromosomal complement or DNA content has been widely studied, particularly in flow cytometry procedures. The development of bladder cancer seems to be associated with aneuploidy (Raghavan *et al.* 1990). The enhanced expression (or specific mutation) of certain oncogenes may lead to better indicators of prognosis based on genotypic rather than phenotypic features. Placental protein production has been reported as a feature of increasing dedifferentiation of transitional cell carcinoma related to nodal and distant metastases (Mead 1990).

Response is easier to assess in patients with metastatic disease than in patients with the primary tumour as sole indicator lesion. Bidimensionally measurable lesions may include cutaneous or peripheral nodal masses, pulmonary metastases defined by chest radiography, abdominal masses measured by CT, and liver metastases measured by CT. The measurable lesions are presented in Table 6. The criteria for response and the definition of treatment toxicity are those recommended by the World Health Organization (WHO 1979). The methods used to measure response in the primary tumour include cytoscopy, cytology, CT, ultrasound, and multiple deep biopsies at the site of previously resected lesions. The last of these should be the most reliable. The final pathological report can only be obtained from complete resections of the bladder wall by total or partial cystectomy. Standardization in our clinical routine and research studies will create the medium for comparability of results.

PRESENTATION AND DIAGNOSIS OF BLADDER CANCER

Haematuria, either macroscopic or microscopic, must lead to suspicion of urothelial cancer until proved negative. A radiological imaging study is one of the first examinations. If no gross abnormalities are detected, it is still prudent to request cytology of the urine in a patient over the age of 50 years because this examination is capable of detecting cells shredded by small grade 2 or grade 3 tumours and cystoscopy is mandatory. Screening for bladder cancer is not cost effective and only high-risk groups of patients with a previous diagnosis of urothelial tumours or workers exposed to carcinogens over a number of years are recommended to undergo regular urine cytology examinations. The utilization of transabdominal ultrasound and the flexible cytoscope may facilitate compliance in long-term follow-up.

A structured diagnostic work-up such as that presented in Fig. 2 (Niijima *et al.* 1986) is advisable and cytohistological diagnosis must be followed by sufficient investigation to ascertain the proper stage and grade of the newly diagnosed tumour, to determine its other prognostic factors, and to evaluate the host before embarking upon final decisive treatment in bladder cancer. Symptoms other than painless haematuria are usually late symptoms in bladder cancer, although frequency and dysuria without obstructing hypertrophy of the prostate can be a first clear signal of a primary symptomatic carcinoma *in situ*.

Once a visual image or a suspicious mass or cell type in the urine is noted, a staging cytoscopy is planned which is scheduled under anesthaesia. This assessment starts with a bimanual examination of the empty bladder to evaluate the size and mobility of the palpable tumours. Physical examination of the genital tract in females and the prostate in males should be performed at the same time. This examination is repeated after the endoscopic procedure if a mass is felt. This is also an appropriate time, if cytology was forgotten in the out-patient clinic, to collect at least one sample before treatment. The cystoscopy evalutes the capacity of the bladder, the mucosa, and possible field changes such as hyperaemic patches, oedema, cystitis cystica, ulcerative lesions, and of course all obvious exophytic tumours. The location of the visible tumours should be carefully recorded on a diagram available in the operating room. It is easiest to mark the location relative to fixed structures such as the trigone and the bladder neck. The size and the growth pattern of the tumours are important. The next step involves cold cup biopsies of all suspicious areas of bladder mucosa, followed by biopsies of normal mucosa next to the tumour and distant from the tumour of healthy mucosa. A biopsy of the prostatic urethra and of the prostate may be indicated for sessile tumours located near the bladder neck. Only then can complete tumour destruction be considered. In dealing with small papillary tumours a cup biopsy can be taken and the rest of the tumour(s) destroyed by coagulation or laser. It is recommended that at least one tumour is removed with its base containing underlying muscle to give a representative sample of possible invasion to the pathologist. Errors of omission or commission abound here and this is the critcal phase in the procedure since T classification will be based on these samples. The complete resection is followed by a deep biopsy of the muscle to exclude deep invasion of tumour. It is customary to make wide excisions in broad-based sessile tumours to include submucosal outgrowth of the tumour. In some instances one papillary lesion, usually on the trigone, can be left in place as a tumour marker for subsequent treatment with intravesical chemo- or immunotherapy. Even clearly invasive lesions can be left untouched except for a deep

Complete this form and indicate cystoscopical findings on the scheme. Keep one copy for yourself and send the two other copies to your local pathologist with the specimen(s)

Protocol number:................... Responsible urologist..

Institution:...

Patient's name:... Birthdate:...

Clinical T category:...

Date of specimen ☐☐☐☐☐ (day, month, year)

Material: ☐ TUR
         ☐ Smear preparation(s)
         ☐ Lymph node(s)
         ☐ Other, specify:.............................

INDICATE ON THE SCHEME:

TUMOUR(S) WITH ☐T
BIOPSY(IES) OF SUSPECTED AREAS WITH ☐S
RANDOM BIOPSIES WITH ☐R
SELECTED BIOPSIES WITH ☐B

TICK THE NAME OF THE REFEREE PATHOLOGIST FOR THIS STUDY:

☐ Dr. J. BULTINCK
AZ Middalheim
Dep. of Pathology
Lindendreef 1
B 2020 Antwerpen (Belgium)

☐ Dr. F. J. ten KATE
Erasmus University
Dep. of Pathology
Dr. Molewaterplein 40
NL 3015 GD Rotterdam (Nederland)

☐ Dr. J. R. READ
Dep. of Histopathology
Castle Hill Hospital
Cottingham North Humberside
E HU 16 SJQ (England)

☐ Dr. P. J. SPAANDER
Dep. of Pathology
Rode Kruls Ziekanhuis
Sportleen 600
NL 2566 MJ Den Haag (Nederland)

LEGEND

A: TRIGONE
B: RIGHT URETERAL ORIFICE
C: LEFT URETERAL ORIFICE
D: RIGHT WALL
E: LEFT WALL
F: ANTERIOR WALL
G: POSTERIOR WALL
H: DOME
I: NECK
J: PROSTATIC URETHRA
K: PROSTATIC SUBSTANCE

Name and address of local pathologist:...
....

Please send a copy of your histological report to the referee pathologist of this protocol together with three unstained slides from EACH block and if possible an (unstained) smear preparation. Keep one form for yourself and send the other form to the referee pathologist.

For each case there will be a refund for the local pathologist. Please indicate to whom the check must be made payable:

....

DATE:.................................SIGNATURE:...

Fig. 3 EORTIC Genito-urinary Tract Cooperative Group standard bladder cancer pathology form (September 1986).

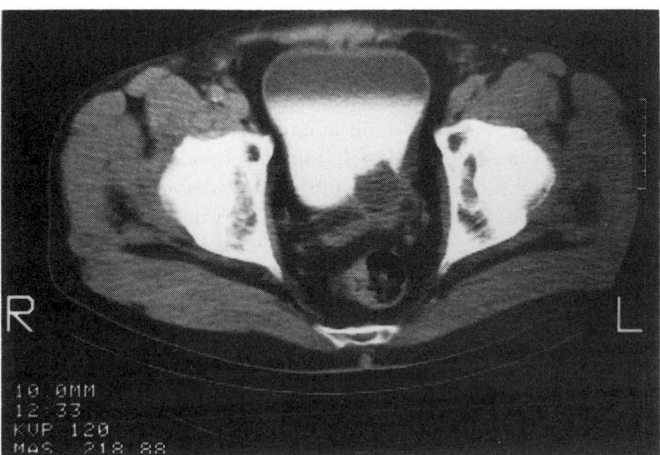

Fig. 4 Image of mass invading bladder base after chemotherapy. Surgical specimen was negative, underlining the need for histological diagnosis.

biopsy procedure if a primary tumour marker is required for neoadjuvant systemic chemotherapy. All this information is recorded on a bladder endoscopy programme sheet which forms an integral part of the patient's hospital record. An example utilized by the EORTC GU Group is shown in Fig. 3. All tumours with invasion of the muscle require a search for metastases which includes an abdominal CT scan, a chest radiograph, liver ultrasonography, a bone scan, and laboratory examinations. An example of a typical CT scan of a grossly invasive tumour is presented in Fig. 4. A CT has become an integral part of this section of the work-up and is sometimes followed by fine-needle aspiration or pelvioscopy of the regional lymph nodes. It is obvious that the CT images are not representative of tumour extent and should be followed by biopsy procedures. Even the new upgraded magnetic resonance imaging (MRI) lacks the precision necessary for accurate staging.

Early consultation with a medical or radiation oncologist, with a mutual review of pathology and other diagnostic information, is essential for good strategical treatment planning.

Table 7 Chemoresection studies in superficial bladder cancer

Drug	CR (%)	PR (%)	LT	ST
Thiotepa	50	70	++	+
Adriamycin	66	78	++	−
Mitomycin C	47	81	+	−
BCG	65	81	+++	+
4-Epirubicin	50	70	+	−
Mitoxantrone	55	72	+++	−

CR, complete remission; PR, partial remission; LT, local toxicity (mainly chemocystitis); ST, systemic toxicity.

Table 8 Place of intravesical chemo-immunotherapy in the treatment of superficial bladder cancer

Ta, grades 1–2	Single; no indication
Ta, grades 1–2	Multiple; short courses to reduce recurrent disease
T1, grades 1–2	Single; no indication
T1, grades 1–2	Multiple; indication; toxicity acceptable; prevents progression–recurrence
Tis	Indication; toxicity acceptable; prevents progression; saves bladder
T1, grade 3	Indication; in case of failure more aggressive treatment (interstitial radiation, systemic chemotherapy, cystectomy)

TREATMENT

Superficial bladder cancer

The term 'superficial' includes by definition not only non-invasive tumours (Ta) and tumours invading the subepithelial tissue (T1), but also high-grade urothelial lesions (Tis). The term 'superficial' has relevance with regard to the choice of treatment, but these three classes of tumour will appear in different stages of the next TNM classification because of their differing prognosis. The long-term survival difference between Ta and T1 disease is at least 30 per cent, which makes it imperative to separate these patients in clinical trials. This fact was ignored in the early prospective studies, which makes comparisons for survival or even recurrence of disease of questionable value. Ta tumours are found in up to 40 per cent of patients at initial diagnosis, but only a few develop progressive disease and the recurrence rate is dictated by the rate of previous recurrence and the grade and size of the tumour as already stated. A number of randomized trials reported by the EORTC GU Group and several other authors have established the fact that single low-grade Ta tumours seldom recur and deserve no additional treatment after destruction (England *et al.* 1981; Denis *et al.* 1987). The primary treatment usually comprises transurethral resection or coagulation. The neodymium:YAG laser has been advocated as a viable alternative although prospective data to back this claim are lacking. A more aggressive method used principally for the treatment of Tis is photodynamic therapy after intravenous injection of the photosensitizing dye haematoporphyrin derivative. Irradiation of tumour tissue containing this dye with laser radiation at a wavelength of 630 mm creates general tumour tissue destruction. Some groups still feel that a single low-grade Ta tumour could be treated by a single cytostatic instillation after complete resection, hoping to gain additional advantage for patients in terms of less recurrences over a long-term follow-up. The EORTC GU Group recently closed a randomized trial that recruited over 400 patients who received a single instillation of 80 mg of 4-epirubicin intravesically within 24 h of resection. The preliminary results show an advantage for additional therapy in terms of a lower recurrence rate compared with the control group. Indeed, it might be expected that the problem of recurrent tumours in superficial bladder cancer, whether they are new tumours emanating from the mucosa altered by carcinogens or recurrent tumours emanating from the implanted cells at the time of the first resection, could be diminished by the application of intravesical chemotherapy.

It has been demonstrated that intravesical chemotherapy can be used for chemoresection or chemoprophylaxis in ablating and preventing the recurrence of superficial tumours. A number of active agents are currently used but mitomycin C and 4-epirubicin have emerged as the most popular drugs in the field (Denis *et al.* 1989).

All of these drugs and the immunomodulator BCG are effective in obtaining complete remissions in approximately half the patients with marker lesions. Chemoresection is only indicated in Tis or in phase II studies aiming to measure the efficacy of the drug in destroying the tumour. A scheme of their activity and toxicity is presented in Table 7. Another series of trials organized by the EORTC GU Group initially demonstrated that intravesical instillation was superior to placebo in diminishing the recurrence rate of tumours and a definite regime of early versus delayed or mid-term versus long-term maintenance therapy showed no difference in an interim analysis (Newling 1990). However, a final analysis of these studies has shown that early administration with 6 months' maintenance therapy is as good as delayed therapy with 12 months' maintenance using mitomycin C or adriamycin in preventing recurrence of Ta and T1 tumours (K. H. Kurth and C. H. Bouffioux, personal communication). Intravesical BCG has also been used for many years in both therapeutic and prophylactic treatment (Lamm *et al.* 1980; Herr *et al.* 1987). It seems to change the natural history of the disease, but questions remain concerning the optimal strain and the viability, dose, and duration of treatment. The production of interleukin 2 by BCG instillation, as demonstrated in the urine of the treated patients, has been postulated to correlate with treatment efficacy. Instillations with α-interferon have been successfully used with minimal toxicity in patients with tumours exhibiting poor prognostic features (Torti and Lum 1987).

The use of immunomodulators has been very successful in Tis disease where repeated courses with BCG after initial failure increased the success rate of eradication overall to 89 per cent (Sarosdy and Lamm 1989). Again, failures after BCG administration may respond to interferon instillation treatment (Glashan 1990), which suggests the need for further proper randomized trials in this condition. Immunomodulation by BCG is effective and is more efficient than thiotepa and adriamycin in reducing recurrences in Ta and T1 tumours as well as in bringing about complete remission in Tis patients. The principal problems of BCG therapy are the side-effects which are local and systemic. The local side-effect is chemocystitis, which occurs in over 90 per cent of the treated patients and the systemic side-effects include fever, malaise, and nausea. Severe side-effects are seen in 5 per cent of the patients, but only a few fatal complications have been reported (Witjes and Debruyne 1991). Although BCG seems to be the drug of choice in the United States and Canada for prophylaxis against recurrence in Ta and T1 tumours as well as in the treatment of Tis, randomized EORTC studies comparing BCG and mitomycin remain inconclusive as far as a prevention of recurrence of these tumours is concerned (Debruyux *et al.* 1988). It may be prudent to use the known chemotherapy drug to reduce recurrence in Ta and T1 and

Table 9 Initial management of T3 transitional cell carcinoma by specialty

Treatment preference	Percentage responders	Urologists		Medical oncologists (%)	Radiation oncologists (%)
		UK (%)	USA (%)		
Cystectomy	32	11	60	29	4
Radiotherapy + cystectomy	22	15	8	18	39
Radiotherapy alone	14	44	0	0	31
Chemotherapy + cystectomy	12	4	20	25	8
Other combinations	20	26	12	29	19

to treat an initial Tis and to switch to BCG or interferon in the latter case if a response is not obtained in 6 weeks. There still remains a worry over precisely what the optimal treatment for all T1 lesions is. A third of these tumours do not recur, another third recur, and a third, or possibly more, go into progression in a defined time, particularly if the tumour is of high grade.

Some authors have suggested treating grade 3 T1 tumours by radical cystectomy, and their policy is supported by the fact that out of 17 patients with T1G3 tumours, 14 (82 per cent) developed muscle invasion after BCG treatment in the first year. Again, this emphasizes the fact that a recurrence at the first control cystoscopy at 3 months is a poor prognostic factor which necessitates more aggressive treatment than watchful waiting (Herr 1991).

A few studies using systemic chemotherapy such as methotrexate have proved unsuccessful (Scher 1989). However, intravesical radium or iridium implantation gave superior long-term results compared with transurethral resection only (Van der Werf-Messing *et al.* 1984). A randomized control of these treatment options would be appropriate.

In conclusion, we can state that intravesical chemo-immunotherapy has clinical efficacy and a potential to delay progression of disease. Only one-third of the patients should receive this treatment and they should have adequate and intensive follow-up studies to prevent the development of invasive disease. A summary is presented in Table 8. Clinical research in superficial bladder cancer is not complete since we still need to be able to identify those tumours that look harmless but carry biological invasive potential and to investigate the action of the different intravesical treatments.

The final warning is that these patients stay in the high risk category for recurrent disease, which makes an extended follow-up imperative. Cytoscopy, cytology, and ultrasound of the bladder are the three follow-up parameters of disease which, if repeated every 3 months in the first 2 years and then every 6 months for a lifetime, should normally prevent the insidious recurrence of invasive tumours. Repeat intravenous urography every 3–5 years in the case of haematuria or suspicious cytology seems indicated.

Invasive bladder cancer

The optimal treatment of invasive bladder cancer is not definitely known. Single-modality treatments, that is, surgery, chemotherapy, or radiotherapy alone, all give less than satisfactory responses. Therefore it is likely that the best approach will be multimodality combination therapy, which will be considered later in this section. First, each of the three principal therapeutic options will be discussed separately.

Surgery

Jewitt and Strong (1946) performed the pioneering work which established the relationship between muscle invasion and potential curability of bladder cancer following an autopsy study of 107 patients. They found that 80 per cent of tumours confined to the muscularis were potentially curable, while 80 per cent where the tumour infiltrated the perivesical fat were thought to be incurable by locoregional treatments (Jewett and Strong 1946). The subsequent demonstration of a link between depth of invasion and histological grade of the tumour, linking tumour mass to dedifferentiation, was reflected in the dependence of 5 year survival rates on the stage of invasion (Marshall 1952).

It is obvious that muscle infiltration is the first step towards systemic disease and is indicated by positive regional nodes or microscopic metastases at the time of diagnosis. The heterogeneity seen in superficial bladder cancer occurs in invasive disease. In the past a certain lack of perception of the natural history of bladder cancer has led to confusion over treatment strategies. On the one hand many T1 and T4b tumours were subjected to very aggressive therapy, usually inappropriately, while on the other hand many tumours with identifiable poor prognostic factors and invasive features were treated too conservatively. This confusion was well illustrated by the answers to a questionnaire on the management of invasive disease given by urologists, medical oncologists, and radiation oncologists (Moor *et al.* 1988). The answers are summarized in Table 9.

These results provide an indirect confirmation of the clinician's perception of the heterogeneity of the tumour, since some patients do survive, even after stage progression where the ultimate survival is clearly dependent on the prognostic factors and not necessarily the treatment. The prognostic factors which are universally accepted are extent and bulk of disease in all categories of disease, tumour morphology and grade, the anticipated completeness of surgery, concomitant carcinoma *in situ*, vascular space involvement, and finally performance status and haemoglobin at diagnosis. The type of invasion is of importance as papillary tumours tend to invade on a broad front and not nearly as deeply as the solid nodular tumours which tend to invade in a tentacular fashion.

Most of the early literature reports were retrospective which, as in other situations, commonly confirms the pre-set hypothesis defined by the investigator. This led to rôle models of therapy which were only questioned with the introduction of proper randomized trials. Very few surgical trials were randomized, but the prospective data collected by the NBCCG raised the question of the biological activity of invasive tumours treated by pre-operative radiotherapy (Slack and Prout 1980). This study showed a 3:1 preponderance of solid versus papillary invasive tumours and a deeper invasion for vascular positive tumours which did not regress under radiotherapy.

Table 10 Surgery for primary tumour

Partial cystectomy
 Resection of part of the bladder wall with inclusion of perivesical fat and
  peritoneum

Simple cystectomy
 Removal of the bladder with or without the perivesical fat and/or
  peritoneum

Total cystectomy
 Prostate and seminal vesicles are included in the specimen; complete
  resection of female urethra and resection of the uterus, ovaries, and
  part of the vagina

Radical cystectomy
 Similar to total cystectomy, but the plane of dissection is the pelvic wall;
  no residual fat or tissue is left in the perivesical space

Table 11 Lymph node staging

Radical node dissection
 Dissection from the aortic bifurcation down to Cloquet's node in an *en
  block* dissection with the inclusion of the nodes around the common
  and external iliac vessels down to the obturator fossa

Selective node dissection
 Dissection of the lymph nodes in the broad 'triangle' formed by the
  external and internal iliac vessels down to the obturator fossa

Sampling node dissection
 Dissection or biopsy of suspicious regional nodes

Table 12 Urinary diversion

External diversion
 (1) Cutaneous ureterostomy
 (2) Ileal conduit (Bricker)
   Colon conduit
 (3) Continent pouch (Kock)
   Variations: Mainz, Indiana, Florida, VIP

Internal diversion
 (1) Ureterosigmoidostomy (Coffey)
 (2) Bladder substitutes (Couvelaire)
   Variations: Camey, Studer, S bladder, Mainz

The conclusion is that all studies should be stratified for these data to allow comparison. It is now well known, as outlined earlier in this chapter, that the surgical treatment of an invasive tumour should be preceded by a complete diagnostic and staging work-up of the patient before definitive therapy is contemplated.

Technical aspects

There are several options of surgery for invasive bladder cancer where the balance rests between radical treatment of the tumour and conservative treatment for the patient (Table 10). The different stages of surgery involve lymph node dissection, which is an obligatory first step before attempting ablative surgery, surgical removal of the primary tumour, and finally urinary diversion or replacement by a substitute bladder. Approaches to the first and the third stages are summarized in Tables 11 and 12.

The technique of radical cystectomy advocated by Marshall and Whitmore at the Memorial Sloan-Kettering Institute in the 1960s started with careful dissection of the lymphatics down from the bifurcation of the aorta, through the space of Marciel, and down to the nodes of Cloquet. This surgery was carried out following the pelvic wall and not the pelvic organs. It became clearer in the next three decades that this extensive and meticulous node dissection did not improve survival and that the only confirmed benefit for the patient came from careful dissection of the nodes close to the bladder. There is agreement that the presence of macroscopic positive nodes signals disseminated disease, but Skinner (1982) demonstrated a possible 30 per cent survival after 5 years for patients with microscopic foci in their nodes.

Apart from nodal dissection, most surgeons perform adequate cystectomies where radicalism is dictated by the stage of disease and the desire in low-stage disease to spare the neurovascular bundles for preservation of potency. The technique of radical cystectomy is routine in urological hands (Skinner *et al.* 1990). The mortality and morbidity of ablative sugery are minimal with the improvement of anaesthesia and systemic support of the patient before, during, and after surgery.

Urinary diversion has been radically changed by the introduction of a variety of procedures aimed at the creation of a continent reservoir with an abdominal stoma or substituting the bladder by intestinal emptying through the normal intact urethral mechanism. The older procedure included implantation of the ureters in the sigmoid colon as prescribed by Coffey (1925) and improved with

antireflux implantation by Goodwin (1980). A more recent internal derivation was initiated by Couvelaire (1951) and perfected by Camey and Leduc (1979). These techniques were derived from early European experiments on bladder substitution (Lemoine 1912). Salvage of the membranous urethra is necessary for this type of orthotopic bladder replacement. Tumours in the prostate or urethra or carcinoma in the urethral margins on frozen section exclude this type of surgery.

The learning curve for these procedures takes its toll, but a perioperative mortality of 1 per cent is possible in experienced hands. The morbidity can be considerably reduced by patient selection, with pre- and post-operative treatment extending for many months. A bladder substitute reconstructed from 40 cm of ileum, opened along its antimesenteric border and folded twice to create a low pressure cup, has been advocated by the Bern group (Studer *et al.* 1989). Their system, which is based on the physiological principles of bowel pressure, worked well, in the first series of patients with a 6 year follow-up. However, detailed post-operative surveillance, care, and advice must be continued for at least the first 9 months. A number of variations utilizing the ileum, ileocaecal conduits and the colon, with modifications, have been reported (Van Velthoven 1991).

When bladder replacement or the construction of a continent reservoir is impossible, most surgeons employ the ileal conduit devised by Bricker (1950). This supravesical derivation utilizes a short segment of ileum to bring the urine from the implanted ureters to the skin. It replaced the nephrostomies and ureterostomies of earlier days and rapidly became popular. Variations in the technique of conduit diversion have utilized sigmoid or transverse colon segments. Long-term problems with the urinary stoma led to the concept of the continent stoma, where intussusceptions or the coecal valve of Baubin were initially utilized as continence mechanisms. The various methods used to obtain continence rely on sphincteric compression, peristaltic activity, equilibrated pressure, and valvular action (Hinman 1990). All these possibilities have resulted in a number of different pouches, such as the Mainz pouch, the Florida pouch, the Indiana pouch, and the vesical interna Paduensis (VIP) pouch. This large number of procedures highlights the lack of a best procedure accepted by all. The continent ileostomy utilized by Kock (1969) was the original form of the procedure.

The Mainz pouch seems to have become the most popular form of continent diversion, but it is obvious that the cosmetic effect and reflux prevention results in a number of complications inherent in more complex surgery. Long-term results of continent diversions are required before they can be compared with the known long-term complications of the Bricker ileal conduit. These complications will include metabolic disorders and histological differentiation in the bowel mucosa. Again, the final choice of surgery will depend upon prognosis, the patient's preference and performance status, and the experience of the surgeon in bladder substitution procedures.

In selected cases of invasive disease the surgeon may opt for a segmental resection which, however, is limited to specific indications. The classic indications are patients with low-grade unifocal disease away from the bladder neck and negative randomized biopsies of the bladder mucosa or unifocal tumours in the dome of the bladder. Segmental resections may also be indicated in patients with unifocal high-grade tumours in complete remission after systemic pre-operative chemotherapy (Denis 1987).

Finally, as a last resort, salvage cystectomy may be performed after repeated failures of transurethral resection and radiotherapy. The operative morbidity is usually more pronounced, but some patients may be cured.

Survival after surgery

Most T1 tumours and some T2 tumours are treated by transurethral resection only. The category of these tumours is established on the resected material which leaves room for understaging. This is a major problem of therapeutic decision since resection is unlikely to cure deeply invasive disease.

An estimate for cure of T1 and T2 tumours treated by transurethral resection alone ranges from 20 to 40 per cent (Wolff et al. 1987). This estimate leaves 60–80 per cent of recurrent tumours which need more radical therapy. The overall 5 year survival rate hovers around 70 per cent for T1 tumours and 50 per cent for T2 tumours. However, these results may be greatly improved by combination with effective systemic chemotherapy and leave this form of bladder-saving surgery a place in the therapeutic options for invasive disease. It is not surprising that some centres prefer the aggressive approach of radical cystectomy for these patients, obtaining 80 per cent survival for pT1 tumours and 76 per cent survival for pT2 tumours, including in one report 11 patients who had positive nodes (Malkowicz et al. 1990). Although the presence of Tis was confirmed in a large number of these latter cases, and required cystectomy, it is still felt that patients with T2 tumours whose disease was downstaged by chemotherapy and were followed conservatively had a 5 year survival rate of 70 per cent (Herr 1987). At present it can only be concluded that aggressive therapy for superficial disease should be reserved for T2 and high-risk T1 with high-grade lesions at the most and longer follow-up periods are necessary to establish a valid therapeutic option.

Partial cystectomy has the same limitations as TUR but it does provide a pathological stage. The procedure is acceptable for solitary tumours of limited size, but is contraindicated for multifocal tumours, inability to obtain adequate margins, the presence of Tis, and inability to maintain a reasonable functional bladder volume.

Table 13 Five year survival after cystectomy for T2–T3 disease

Reference	Five year survival (%)		
	pT2	pT3a	pT3b
Pagano et al. (1991)	63	50	15
Montie et al. (1984)[a]	50	63	29
Skinner and Lieskowsky (1984)	64	44	

[a]Some lost to follow-up.

Wound implantation has been reported and pre-operative radiation in high-grade disease has been recommended. The overall 5 year survival rate has been reported to reach 50 per cent in selected cases. The 5 year survival results of cystectomy are presented in Table 13 for the different stages. Treatment comparisons are difficult since many of these patients have been pre-treated by transurethral resection and other forms of treatment which deal with clinical rather than pathological stages.

Operative mortality has decreased significantly over the last decades and the problems associated with removal of the bladder have been eased by the newer approaches of nerve-sparing surgery for potency and orthotopic bladder replacement, but the quality of life due to a functional bladder is lost (Prout et al. 1979). Failure of surgery because of existing undetected metastatic disease occurs in 25 per cent of the patients in the first year. In summary, half the patients with invasive disease will die, primarily of metastatic disease, in the 3 years following diagnosis. The apparently excellent results obtained are mainly due to patient selection and the reporting of results by clinical stage. This gloomy picture is confirmed by the enormous interest in adjuvant and particularly neoadjuvant chemotherapy in M0 invasive bladder cancer.

Radiotherapy

Introduction

The patient presenting with a transitional cell bladder cancer is usually elderly. This important fact has often resulted in a recruitment selection between younger patients, who are frequently treated by radical surgery and older patients, in poorer general condition, who are more often referred to the radiation oncologist. Data from retrospective series of radical radiotherapy must then be examined in the context of this particular pattern of patient selection. Indeed, the radiotherapeutic series were potentially biased by the preferential inclusion of patients with a shorter life expectancy, whereas the surgical series benefited from a surgical rather than clinical staging and the ability to undergo a planned cystectomy. However, some radiological series have also included salvage cystectomy, which improved the long-term survival statistics.

Thus, a simple comparison of the results of surgery and radiotherapy is not straightforward and this must be remembered when analysing the available literature data on the treatment of bladder cancer.

Experience with external radiotherapy alone

A number of series (Miller and Johnson 1973; Rousseau et al. 1974; Goffinet et al. 1975; Morrison 1975; Blandy et al. 1980; Radwin 1980; Bloom et al. 1982; Shipley et al. 1985; Yu 1985) have shown that long-term local control and cure can be achieved in 60–80 per cent of TaT1/A, 27–58 per cent of T2/B1, and 20–38 per cent

Table 14 Results of bladder-sparing treatment of clinical stage Ta and T1 bladder cancer

Institution	No. of patients	Treatment	Five year local control (%)	Five year survival (%)
Tokyo (Matsumoto et al. 1981)	66	RT + IORT	91	96
Rotterdam (Van der Werf-Messing 1978)	196	RT + Ra-226	88	81
Amsterdam (Batterman and Tierce 1986)	34	RT + Ra-226	83	72
Creteil (Mazeron et al. 1985)	31	RT + Ir-192	77	74
Rotterdam (Van der Werf-Messing 1978)	143	TURB alone	20	75
NBCG (Cutler et al. 1982)	259	TURB + CTG intravesical	39	—

RT, radiotherapy; IORT, intraoperative electron irradiation; TURB, transurethral resection of bladder tumour.

of T3/B2.C with doses in the range of 60–70 Gy (Raghavan et al. 1990). The best results were reported in series including salvage cystectomy. In T4 tumours or in the presence of ureterohydronephrosis (reflecting the bulky nature of the tumour), complete sterilization is uncommon.

There is a clear dose–effect relationship, as demonstrated for instance by the downstaging of the operative specimen after pre-operative radiotherapy (Sagerman et al. 1968; Prout et al. 1973; Prout 1976; Miller 1980). In the study by Batata et al. (1981), downstaging was observed in 27 per cent of 86 patients after doses of 20 Gy in 1 week and in 40 per cent of 119 patients after doses of 40 Gy in 4 weeks. Pre-operative tumour sterilization reaches 50 per cent after 60 Gy. This supports the use of high-dose radiotherapy (60–70 Gy) in the treatment of bladder cancer with curative intent. Indeed, local control and patient survival have both been related to the total dose delivered to the primary tumour (Morrison 1975; Parsons et al. 1980) and also to the more precise delivery of radiation through CT scan-assisted planning.

Two randomized trials comparing pre-operative irradiation and cystectomy versus radical irradiation in advanced bladder cancer produced conflicting results. The smaller trial reported radiotherapy as being significantly inferior (Miller 1977), whereas the larger failed to demonstrate a difference in long-term survival between the two arms (Wallace and Bloom 1976; Bloom et al. 1982). It is important to remember that these studies were carried out before CT scanning and computer dosimetry were in common use. A more recent Danish study (Sell and Jacobsen 1990), performed with more accurate therapy, concluded there was an equivalence between pre-operative irradiation followed by cystectomy and radical radiotherapy.

Recent experience indicates that the success of radiotherapy may be favourably influenced by certain prognostic factors such as the absence of ureteral obstruction (Greiner et al. 1977; Van der Werf-Messing 1979; Shipley et al. 1985), the achievement of a complete transureteral resection before irradiation (Miller and Johnson 1973; Shipley et al. 1985), the presence of a papillary rather than a sessile tumour (Goffinet et al. 1975; Van der Werf-Messing 1979; Van der Werf-Messing et al. 1983; Shipley et al. 1985), and the clinical stage (Goffinet et al. 1975; Van der Werf-Messing et al. 1983; Yu et al. 1985). A good response after the first 40 Gy in radical radiotherapy is also well correlated with long-term local control and prolonged survival (Blandy et al. 1980; Shipley et al. 1985).

Some biological tumoral factors have also been reported as predictors of tumour response to radiotherapy. Beta human chononic gonadotrophin staining on a pathological specimen and/or the presence of squamous metaplasia predicted a bad response to irradiation: 26 out of 28 patients with both features failed to respond to treatment, whereas 40 out of 45 who had neither feature responded to treatment (Jenkins et al. 1989). Hypertetraploidy, as assessed by DNA flow cytometry, also correlated with a higher response rate to irradiation in 140 patients (Vindelov et al. 1989). Confirmation that these prognostic factors will also predict a better survival requires longer follow-up. Definitive irradiation with curative intent by an external beam involves treating the true pelvis with a four-field technique to include the external iliac, obturator, and hypogastric lymph nodes at a dose of 46 Gy in 5 weeks (1.8–2 Gy per fraction, five fractions per week) followed by a boost to the bladder tumour at a dose of 66 Gy in 7 weeks (same fractionation parameters). The external boost can be replaced by an intraoperative boost with electrons or iridium (see later). The need for extensive staging by a trained urologist before planning the treatment is obvious, making collaboration between the radiation oncologist and the urologist the cornerstone of good radiotherapy. The irradiation usually begins 3–4 weeks after the debulking transurethral resection.

A three- or four-field technique can be used for the pelvis irradiation. The size of the anterior field is in the range of 14 cm×14 cm (the posterior field is the same if the tumour is centrally located in the pelvis). These dimensions are only provisional, since the extact field sizes are defined directly from the patient's anatomy and the tumour parameters. The upper limit is L5–S1 and the lower limit is the prostate in the male patient (excluding the anal canal) and the distal part of the urethra in the female patient. Lateral borders 1–2 cm from the pelvic rim. The lateral fields need a very careful simulation with an opacified bladder. Their height should match the height of the anterior field and their width should be approximately 10–11 cm. The anterior part of the rectum in the male and the uterus in the female are included in the field. The lateral fields must be wedged in the three-field technique. According to the different diameters of the patient, the first 46 Gy will be given with a loading of 30–36 Gy by the anteroposterior fields and 10–16 Gy by the lateral fields. The boost field must be directed toward the tumoral bed only, sparing as much normal bladder as possible. Two fields, three fields with lateral wedges, or four-field box techniques in thick patients (the arc rotation technique is an alternative) may be chosen according to the tumour location. Accurate simulation, CT-assisted dosimetry, and megavoltage irradiation are mandatory (>10 MV with

Table 15 Intraoperative results for clinical stage T2 bladder cancer

Institution	No. of patients	Treatment	Five year local control (%)	Five year survival (%)
Rotterdam (Van der Werf-Messing 1978)	328	RT + Ra-226	77	58
Amsterdam (Batterman and Tierce 1986)	85	RT + Ra-226	74	55
Creteil (Mazeron et al. 1985)	24	RT + Ir-192[a]	92	58
Tokyo (Matsumoto et al. 1981)	28	IORT + RT	82	62
French Co-op. (Rozan et al. 1989)	205	RT + Ir-192[a]	—	66.8

RT, radiotherapy; IORT, intraoperative electron irradiation.
[a]Partial resection.

photons). Portal films will confirm the correct set-up of the patient.

It should be remembered that, although the bladder has a good tolerance to radiation, a diseased bladder may be more liable to side-effects, either acute (frequent micturition) or late (haematuria, contracted bladder). Therefore, care must be taken to protect non-tumoral areas of the bladder during the boost to 66 Gy. The rectosigmoid, small bowel, pelvic bones, and femoral heads are also critical organs which must not be injured by radiotherapy. The dose to the anterior rectal wall should not exceed 60 Gy, while the anus and proximal femorae should be limited to less than 45 Gy. However, those dose limits are only guidelines and must be adapted according to each individual clinical situation. The planned schedule of 2 Gy per fraction, five fractions per week, must be accurately followed, in particular without gaps in the treatment which could lengthen the total irradiation time. Indeed, tumours repopulate during radiotherapy and 6–7 weeks of irradiation represents a delicate trade-off between tumour sterilization and normal tissue sparing. Any gap in the treatment will break the equilibrium in favour of tumour repopulation. For example, in the radiotherapy series of Symonds et al. (1990), a 2–3 week split in the treatment significantly decreased the 5 year survival from 35 to 22 per cent.

Pure squamous cell carcinoma and adenocarcinoma of the bladder, which are quite infrequent, are slightly less radiosensitive than transitional cell carcinoma.

Intraoperative radiotherapy

Radiotherapy has definitely proved its value in one type of treatment of transitional cell carcinoma of the bladder: the conservative treatment of small superficial or infiltrative tumours with interstitial brachytherapy or intraoperative external radiotherapy. Again, close collaboration between the surgeon and the radiation oncologist is extremely important. Results are summarized in Tables 14 and 15.

Brachytherapy

Brachytherapy was introduced by Darget in 1920 (Darget 1951) and popularized by Van der Werf-Messing in Rotterdam (Van der Werf-Messing 1979; Van der Werf-Messing et al. 1983; Van der Werf-Messing and Van Putten 1989), who treated more than 1000 patients by radium and later by caesium needle implants, through an opened bladder. Five year survival was 58 per cent in T2 and 23 per cent in T3 tumours.

A similar technique, but with flexible miniaturized sources (iridium wires), has become associated with tumorectomy or partial

cystectomy (Gérard et al. 1985; Mazeron et al. 1985; Straus et al. 1988). [192]Ir wires have the advantage of a low energy gamma–ray emission which allows less traumatic implants and source removal at the patient's bed, without the need for narcosis. More important is the possibility of the use of afterloading techniques (manual or automatic), thus totally protecting the surgical and the nursing staff against stray irradiation and allowing for accurate predetermined dosimetry. With such an approach, it is possible to treat conservatively some T2 and T3 tumours with good bladder preservation giving 5 year survival rates between 50 and 70 per cent. In the French series (Rozan et al. 1989), 5 year survival in 205 patients was 66.8 per cent (T1, 70.4 per cent; T2, 62.9 per cent; T3, 46.8 per cent). The procedure must always be preceded by a short course of external irradiation, as demonstrated by Van der Werf-Messing and Van Putten (1989) and must be restricted to highly selected patients with solitary tumours (after careful random biopsies in the bladder) not exceeding 5 cm in diameter (T2 or T3). Tumours located on the mobile part of the bladder, particularly on the dome, are ideal candidates for partial cystectomy and iridium implants.

Pre-operative irradiation is given through two parallel opposed fields of high-energy photons, following the recommendations for radical radiotherapy. The classical Rotterdam dose is 3×3.5 Gy at mid-thickness on 3 consecutive days. Surgery follows the day after the last session (partial cystectomy in the mobile part of the bladder and tumorectomy in the fixed part) and two (sometimes three) plastic tubes are inserted pre-operatively, parallel to the incision, with a 1–2 cm spacing (depending on the volume to be treated). A week after surgery, the patient is transferred to the brachytherapy department for ^{192}Ir loading. Wires of length 4–8 cm with an activity of 4–8 μGy/cm are inserted in the plastic tubes under fluoroscopy. A dose of 40–60 Gy is delivered on the 85 per cent isodose (Paris system) in 2–5 days.

For large tumours, the contribution of the external dose can be increased to 46 Gy in 23 sessions in order to downstage the tumour before boosting with a local implant, in which case the boost dose is reduced to 20 Gy (Van der Werf-Messing and Van Putten 1989). Carcinoma developing in a bilharzian bladder is usually quite radioresistant.

Intraoperative electron irradiation

The first report of this elegant technique came from Japan (Matsumoto et al. 1981). After careful clinical staging, a single dose boost was delivered directly on the tumour by open cystotomy, followed by an external pelvic irradiation of 30–40 Gy in 15–20

Table 16 Three week treatment cycle with cisplatin and methotrexate (EORTC)

Cisplatin	70 mg/m² IV daily
Methotrexate	40 mg/m² IV on days 8 and 15

IV, intravenous.
Source: Stoter *et al.* (1987).

Table 17 Three week treatment cycle with cisplatin, methotrexate, and vinblastine (NCOG)

Methotrexate	30 mg/m² IV on days 1 and 8
Vinblastine	4 mg/m² IV on days 1 and 8
Cisplatin	100 mg/m² IV on day 2

NCOG, Northern California Oncology Group; IV, intravenous.
Source: Harker *et al.* (1985).

Table 18 Four week treatment cycle with cisplatin, methotrexate, vinblastine, and adriamycin (MSKCC)

Methotrexate	30 mg/m² on days 1, 15, and 22
Vinblastine	3 mg/m² on days 2, 15, and 22
Adriamycin	30 mg/m² on day 2
Cisplatin	70 mg/m² on day 2

MSKCC, Memorial Sloan-Kettering Cancer Centre.
Source: Sternberg *et al.* (1988).

fractions. In 57 patients followed for more than 5 years, the disease-free survival was 81 per cent (stages Ta, T1, and T2 grouped), a substantially better long-term result than obtained with the classical transurethral resection plus intravesical chemotherapy management. More important, this local control was obtained with a very low complication rate; only one out of the 57 patients developed a contracted bladder. A short pilot study has also been performed in Boston (Shipley *et al.* 1987*b*).

The technique requires an easy access to the linear accelerator bunker from the operating theatre. A cystostopy is performed under anaesthetic; the patient is then transferred, still anaesthetized, to the irradiation room and positioned under the accelerator collimator. The intraoperative electron irradiation dose is 25–30 Gy in a single delivery by electron beams directed through sterile cylinders of internal diameter 4, 5, or 6 cm. These cylinders are positioned in the bladder, through the cystotomy incision, directly on the tumoural bed. They must be angled lateroinferiorly so that the anus, rectum, and prostate or lower vagina are not in the path of the exit beam. The choice of electron energy is critical and requires good assessment of the tumour invasion depth.

It is obvious that both brachytherapy and intraoperative electron irradiation need the collaboration of very skilled radiotherapists and surgeons. An amateur approach is always dangerous, but can be catastrophic in this special case.

Fast neutron therapy

Fast neutron beams have been tested in transitional cell carcinoma of the bladder. The large Edinburgh randomized trial failed to demonstrate any advantage of d(15)+Be neutrons over photons in invasive bladder cancer in terms of long-term survival. The local control rates were similar in the two arms, but neutrons showed a higher complication rate (Duncan *et al.* 1985). However, the physical and geometrical performances of the neutron beam were far from optimal and these data cannot be extrapolated to modern high-energy, isocentric neutron facilities. At present neither the EORTC Radiotherapy Group, nor the Medical Research Council or the Radiation Therapy and Oncology Group, regard bladder cancer as suitable for new trials of this therapy.

Hyperfractionation

A greater radiation effectiveness against tumour, at a lower cost in normal tissue toxicity, has been predicted with multifractionated radiotherapy; that is, more than one fraction per day (Thames *et al.* 1983). This approach has been tested with some success in other indications, triggering a phase II study in invasive transitional cell carcinoma of the bladder at the Royal Marsden Hospital in Sutton (A. Horwich, personal communication). A high complete response rate has been achieved, but long-term survival is still unknown.

The key word in any form of radiotherapy, either alone or in combination with other treatment modalities, is 'bladder preservation' and most of the current trials investigate not only more effective schedules but also better prognostic factors to identify those patients who can be treated safely without radical surgery. It is worth noting that all these new approaches require a close collaboration between medical, radiological, and surgical oncologists.

Palliative radiotherapy

Owing to the high incidence of distant metastases in the evolution of invasive bladder cancer, a number of patients are referred to the radiation oncologist for palliative irradiation. The indications are generally aspecific, for instance pain from bone metastases, vascular compression from pelvic nodes, or bladder haemorrhage in locally advanced tumours. The success rate is good, with a preference for concentrated irradiation schedules (a small number of large fractions) in order to interfere as little as possible with the patient's life. The risk of late sequelae from such concentrated regimens must be appreciated in the context of the remaining life expectancy of the patient, the critical organs involved, and previous or concomitant treatments.

Chemotherapy

The majority of urothelial tract tumours are transitional cell cancers. The most active single agents against this type of tumour are cisplatin and methotrexate: overall response rates vary from 30 to 40 per cent and the median duration of response is approximately 6 months. Adriamycin and vinblastine are active to a lesser degree, with overall response rates of 15–20 per cent for a median response duration of 3 months. There is suggestive evidence that cisplatin combination chemotherapy including methotrexate with or without adriamycin and vinblastine is superior to single-agent treatment, with overall response rates varying from 40 to 70 per cent, including 15–35 per cent complete responses. The treatment schemes most widely used are presented in Tables 16–18.

It appears that complete responses are translated into prolonged survival, exceeding a median of 1 year (Harker *et al.* 1985; Stoter *et al.* 1987; Sternberg *et al.* 1988) (Table 19). Patients with partial response and stable disease do not benefit in terms of survival, but palliation of symptoms and improvement of performance status can be achieved.

Although combination chemotherapy based on cisplatin and methotrexate is generally considered to be superior to either drug alone, this has not been clearly proved in randomized controlled studies. To date, one randomized study of cisplatin alone versus

Table 19 Treatment results with regimens from Tables 16, 17, and 18

Investigator	No. of patients	Response Complete	Partial	Median survival of complete responders (months)	Toxic death rate (%)
EORTC	43	10 (23%)	10 (23%)	18	2
NCOG	50	14 (28%)	14 (28%)	11	4
MSKCC	123	43 (35%)	41 (33%)	48	3

Table 20 Comparison of MVAC with CISCA

	MVAC	CISCA
Number of patients	54	48
Complete response	19 (35%)	12 (25%)
Partial response	16 (30%)	10 (21%)

Data from MD Anderson Hospital.

Table 21 Three week treatment cycle for cisplatin and methotrexate with citrovorum factor

Methotrexate	200 mg/m^2 IV over 24 h, day 1
Citrovorum factor	9 mg/m^2 IV four times daily, days 2 and 3
Cisplatin	100 mg/m^2 IV 6 h after methotrexate, day 2

IV, intravenous.
Data from the Medical Research Council.

Table 22 Four week treatment cycle for escalated MVAC with granulocyte–macrophage colony-stimulating factor

Methotrexate	30 mg/m^2 IV on days 1, 15 and 22
Vinblastine	4 mg/m^2 IV on days 2, 15 and 22
Adriamycin	60 mg/m^2 IV on day 2
Cisplatin	100 mg/m^2 IV on day 2

IV, intravenous.
Data from MD Anderson Hospital.

cisplatin and methotrexate did not show a difference in treatment results (Hillcoat et al. 1989). However, data from a randomized comparison of cisplatin, cyclophosphamide, and adriamycin (CISCA) versus cisplatin, methotrexate, vinblastine, and adriamycin (MVAC) indicated a superior complete response rate to MVAC (Logothetis et al. 1988, 1989a, 1990a) (Table 20). A recent study has randomly investigated cisplatin as a single agent at a dose of 70 mg/m^2 every 4 weeks compared with MVAC (Loehrer et al. 1992). MVAC yielded a response rate of 39 per cent and cisplatin alone induced an overall response of 12 per cent. Disease-free and overall survival were superior with the MVAC combination. This study can be criticized for the use of suboptimal cisplatin therapy in the single-agent arm.

Transitional cell tumours of the bladder, the ureter, and the renal pelvis are more sensitive to chemotherapy than are those of the urethra. Adenocarcinoma and squamous cell cancer of the urothelium are usually unresponsive to chemotherapy.

The major side-effects of combination chemotherapy regimens used at present are nausea, vomiting, bone-marrow depression, and mucositis. This toxicity profile will prohibit adequate treatment of patients with a poor performance status, reduced bone-marrow reserve, and impaired renal function. Since hyperhydration and forced diuresis are a prerequisite for cisplatin chemotherapy, patients with compromised cardiac function should not receive this treatment. Provided that these precautions are observed, cisplatin and methotrexate combination chemotherapy can be recommended as standard treatment. Other measures to alleviate or prevent severe side-effects include the administration of citrovorum factor (leucovorin) and the use of haematological growth factors.

Citrovorum factor compensates for the methotrexate-induced inhibition of folate reductase and should be given 24 h after the administration of methotrexate to allow for the adequate antitumour efficacy of this cytotoxic agent. The Medical Research Council has reported the results of such a regime (Table 21) and found identical treatment results to those observed in other studies, but significantly less bone-marrow toxicity and mucositis (Carmichael et al. 1985).

Haematological growth factors such as granulocyte and granulocyte–macrophage colony stimulating factor have recently been introduced in the clinic. A study from the Memorial Sloan-Kettering Cancer Center with the use of MVAC and granulocyte colony-stimulating factor has shown that myelotoxicity and mucosal toxicity are reduced and that full protocol treatment can be given

adequately (Gabrilove et al. 1988). This opens the possibility of dose escalation and cycle-time reduction in order to increase the antitumour efficacy of chemotherapy. Preliminary data from the MD Anderson Hospital with MVAC, including escalated doses of adriamycin and vinblastine (Table 22) with granulocyte–macrophage colony-stimulating factor given to chemotherapy refractory patients, seem to confirm this concept (Logothetis et al. 1989b, 1990b).

Non-metastatic invasive bladder cancer

The development of active chemotherapy in metastatic disease has led to investigations of the use of chemotherapy before radical local treatments; that is, radiotherapy and/or cystectomy. The rationale for this so-called neoadjuvant chemotherapy is to increase the local control rate and to eradicate systemic micrometastases. Complete local control, that is, complete killing of the primary tumour, would allow the avoidance of mutilating cystectomy, whereas the destruction of micrometastases would lead to prolonged survival and even cure.

The combination of single-agent cisplatin and full-dose radiotherapy in T2–T4 tumours has been studied by the National Bladder Cancer Project. A complete response rate as high as 70 per cent was observed, evaluated by repeated cystoscopy and biopsy. The local control rate at 3 years was 80 per cent in T2 and 50 per cent in T3–T4 tumours. However, the overall 3 year survival in T3–T4 tumours was only 35 per cent, indicating that cisplatin alone is not effective in the eradication of micrometastases outside the radiation field (Shipley et al. 1987a) (Table 23). This is also apparent from a similar type of study with cisplatin and adriamycin with

Table 23 Cisplatin and radiotherapy in clinical stage T2–T4

No. of patients	Stage	Survival 2 years (%)	3 years (%)	4 years (%)	Median (months)
70	All	52	43	35	30
22	T2	75	64	64	>48
48	T3+T4	42	35	24	18

radiotherapy, where 80 per cent of the patients with T2–T4 tumours achieved a complete response, but a third of them developed progression within 18 months (Jakse and Frommhold 1988). In addition, a randomized study from Australia and the United Kingdom did not show a significant difference in survival between patients treated with either full-dose radiotherapy or with cisplatin and radiotherapy (Raghavan et al. 1989). These outcomes demonstrate that invasive bladder cancer should be regarded as a systemic disease. This emphasizes the need to preserve the bladder and apply more effective systemic treatment, probably in combination with local radiotherapy (Prout et al. 1990). Chemotherapy before cystectomy is under intensive investigation. Most reports confirm the findings reported from the Memorial Sloan-Kettering Cancer Center, with approximately 30 per cent pathological complete responses. Responding patients appear to have significantly better survival rates than non-responders (Splinter et al. 1989).

It is not yet clear which prognostic factors are the most important variables for the prediction of complete response, but stage and diameter of the tumour play an important role (Fung et al. 1991). At present the administration of neoadjuvant chemotherapy should be regarded as investigational and should be performed in randomized controlled studies.

Bilharzial bladder cancer

In countries where bilharziasis is endemic (for example, Egypt) a high incidence of bladder cancer is caused by this infectious disease. The histology of these tumours is predominantly squamous cell cancer. Bilharzial bladder cancer has a low tendency for distant spread. In contrast with transitional cell cancer, this tumour type is not sensitive to cisplatin and methotrexate, but hexamethylmelamine and 4-epi-adriamycin exert antitumour activity (Gad-el-Mawla et al. 1978).

Future prospects

Combination chemotherapy with regimens containing cisplatin and methotrexate is probably more effective than single-agent and other combination chemotherapy. However, this contention has not been convincingly proved by properly conducted randomized trials. The side-effects can be ameliorated with modern anti-emetics, citrovorum factor, and haematological growth factors. Since no new effective agents against urothelial cancer are available at present, improvement of results should be attempted with dose escalation and cycle-time reduction of chemotherapy under the protection of haematological growth factors.

Neoadjuvant chemotherapy for muscle-invasive bladder cancer is aimed at local tumour control as well as eradication of distant micrometastases. There is suggestive evidence that the combination of radiotherapy and chemotherapy is the most effective way of achieving this and avoiding cystectomy. However, randomized prospective studies are needed to demonstrate whether survival can be prolonged and which proportion of patients maintain a complete response in the bladder during their remaining lifetime.

Combination therapies

Surgery and radiotherapy

Patterns of failure after radical cystectomy include local recurrences and tumoral cell scar implants at the time of surgery and these form the rationale for the different radiosurgical combination therapies proposed in the literature. Metastatic evolution is also frequent, but its prevention is beyond the possibilities of radiotherapy. It has generally been agreed that pre-operative irradiation is the logical combination, although no direct comparative data between pre- and post-operative radiotherapy are available.

The randomized trial performed by Miller (1977) in Houston, which included 67 patients, showed a better survival in patients treated with cystectomy and pre-operative irradiation (50 Gy in 5 weeks) than in patients treated with irradiation alone (46 per cent versus 22 per cent after 5 years).

The London trial (Wallace and Bloom 1976; Bloom et al. 1982) included 189 patients between 1966 and 1975 and compared pre-operative irradiation (40 Gy in 4 weeks) followed by radical cystectomy with irradiation alone (60 Gy in 6 weeks) eventually followed by salvage cystectomy in case of local failure. This trial demonstrated a small advantage for the radiosurgical combination, which was almost significant in males less than 60 years old. However, in patients aged 70 years or more radical radiotherapy gave similar results to the radiosurgical combination and was able to preserve a normal bladder in 40 per cent of cases. Salvage cystectomy was feasible after 60 Gy with an acceptable morbidity (post-operative mortality 3.7 per cent in 54 patients). Similar results with salvage cystectomy have been reported by others (Crawford and Skinner 1980; Smith and Whitmore 1981b). The general philosophy of these two trials is that surgery is preferable for patients who are under 70 years or in very good general condition and irradiation alone should be offered to old and frail patients.

During the past decade many institutions have claimed that pre-operative irradiation improved the results compared with surgery alone (De Weerd and Colbt 1973; Reid et al. 1976; Whitmore et al. 1977; Skinner et al. 1982; Van der Werf-Messing 1982). Different schedules were used, with 50–45 Gy in 4–5 weeks being the most popular. Accelerated schedules also gave satisfactory results (20 Gy in five fractions in 1 week or 16 Gy in four fractions in 1 week). The historical series reported by Van der Werf-Messing (1982) clearly demonstrated the value of pre-operative irradiation to prevent scar implant in the case of partial cystectomy. With no irradiation, a rate of local relapse of 9 per cent was seen; 10.5 Gy in three fractions of 3.5 Gy given post-operatively reduced that rate to 3 per cent and the same dose immediately before surgery totally prevented scar implant and possibly some distant metastatic seeding.

Two randomized trials addressed the question of the value of pre-operative irradiation (Prout et al. 1973; Slack et al. 1977; Crawford et al. 1987). Neither of them were able to demonstrate a clear advantage of pre-operative irradiation in terms of survival. Indeed, local control and long-term survival are not directly correlated, since most patients eventually die from metastatic disease. In the trial reported by Prout (1976), including 488 patients, 45 Gy pre-operatively led to fewer local recurrences (37 per cent) than cystectomy alone (48 per cent) and survival was also slightly improved (36 per cent versus 28 per cent at 5 years). Nevertheless, different methodological biases make it impossible to draw definitive conclusions from this trial.

Few data are available on the value of post-operative irradiation. Such treatment is logical when a high risk of local relapse is suspected after surgery. Doses of 45–55 Gy in 5–6 weeks seem to be able to control subclinical disease (Mohiuddin et al. 1985; Spera et al. 1988). In view of these data, pre-operative irradiation may be advised if the planned treatment is cystectomy, although it remains difficult to choose between the different schedules (the logical choice would be the shortest and the simplest).

Table 24 Rationale for pre-operative chemotherapy

1. Dissatisfaction with treatment results in T3–T4 tumours
2. Early treatment of unrecognized micrometastasis
3. Availability of effective drug combination CMV
4. Long-term results in responders
5. Possibility of leaving primary tumour as measurable marker
6. Definitive treatment is delayed but not hampered
7. Downstaging to T0 N0 offers chance of bladder preservation

CMV, cisplatin + methotrexate + vinblastine.

Surgery and chemotherapy

The promising results obtained by combination chemotherapy in metastatic disease led to the concept of adjuvant chemotherapy after surgery. Earlier trials provided no advantage and toxicity proved a serious obstacle in the randomization and evaluation of the patients after surgery (Prout and Kopp 1984).

More encouraging results have been reported with the post-surgical administration of cyclophosphamide, adriamycin, and cisplatin (CAP) in patients with high risk of recurrent disease. Preliminary data suggested advances which, however, were unable to pass the test of a critical analysis (Tannock 1991). These studies showed that the concept is feasible but that randomized trials are needed to define the optimal scheduling. This state of affairs led quite naturally to the concept of pre-operative chemotherapy or neoadjuvant chemotherapy. This was based on the presumption that as soon as 20 per cent of patients with metastatic disease regressed to complete remission, it was ethical to attempt adjuvant chemotherapy in phase II studies (Bertino 1982).

A prospective phase II study employing both cisplatin and methotrexate as pre-operative chemotherapy reported clinical complete response rates in up to 30 per cent of patients with measurable lesions. The rationale for the concept is presented in Table 24. A 5 year follow-up of 25 patients who completed the first trial revealed a complete response in ten (40 per cent) and partial response in four (16 per cent). Twelve out of 14 patients survived with a minimum follow-up of 60 months with no evidence of disease. One patient died from a brain metastasis after 22 months and one (PR T1) died from cancer after 63 months. All non-responders died within a mean of 28 months (D'Hont *et al.* 1990).

It is possible that there is no causal relationship between response and survival, but response stands out as a powerful prognostic indicator with an influence on further treatment. At least 40 different phase II trials have been reported on the results of more than 1000 patients. They all seem to confirm the possibility of downstaging, particularly in transitional cell carcinoma after a minimum of two effective courses of chemotherapy. The response rate seems more pronounced for smaller tumours with no effect on any Tis present. In a recent update of 147 patients from eight different centres, a major pathological response of 41.5 per cent was established where 75 per cent of these patients survived for 5 years in contrast with 20 per cent of the non-responders. The immediate conclusion is that bladder sparing might be achieved in responders, while non-responders require alternative treatment (Splinter *et al.* 1990).

Chemotherapy before cystectomy is under intensive investigation. Most reports confirm the findings reported from the Memorial Sloan-Kettering Cancer Center with approximately 30 per cent pathological complete responses. Responding patients appear to have significantly better survival rates than non-responders (Splinter *et al.* 1989). It is not yet clear which prognostic factors are the most important variables for the prediction of complete response, but stage and diameter of the tumour play an important role. At present the administration of neoadjuvant chemotherapy should be regarded as investigational.

A randomized trial has been launched by a number of international groups from Europe (EORTC, Medical Research Council, Norway, Spain, and Finland), Australia, and Canada. The preferred regimen is cisplatin, methotrexate, and vinblastine (CMV) for three cycles, followed by definitive surgery or radiotherapy. The first objective of the trial is to randomize 400 patients to look for the survival advantage of pre-operative chemotherapy, for the morbidity of the definitive treatment and the prognostic significance to T0 downstaging (Hall 1991).

Radiotherapy and chemotherapy

Approximately half the patients treated by any individual therapy alone will relapse, either locally or with metastases, within 3 years. Many patients who have apparently been cured of their primary tumour relapse with metastatic disease. In order to try and improve overall survival while at the same time sparing mutilating surgery, various combinations of radiotherapy and chemotherapy have been investigated. In a comparison of the results of radical cystectomy, radical radiotherapy, and combined treatment, the survival rate appears to be broadly similar (Raghavan 1988). In this context, it appears that it would be difficult to set up an ideal randomized trial to resolve the important issue of any differences.

Concomitant radiochemotherapy has proved to be able to induce high complete response rates in invasive bladder cancer (Yagoda *et al.* 1976; Shipley *et al.* 1984, 1988; Jakse *et al.* 1985; Raghavan *et al.* 1985; Sauer *et al.* 1988). Indeed, the development of new chemotherapy regimens, usually with a cisplatin combination, has stimulated many trials with induction chemotherapy. The rationale is to combine the efficiency of cisplatin-containing regimens in increasing local response and to benefit from the systemic effect of chemotherapy against micrometastasis.

Favourable and encouraging results have been reported with protracted external irradiation and cisplatin-based regimens (Jakse *et al.* 1985; Raghavan *et al.* 1985; Sauer *et al.* 1988; Shipley *et al.* 1988; Wajsman *et al.* 1989). The MGH phase II trial (Shipley *et al.* 1988) is one of the best examples of this philosophy. Fifty-three patients, staged cT2–T4, were treated by two induction courses of CMV (cisplatin 70 mg/m^2, methotrexate 30 mg/m^2, and vinblastine 3 mg/m^2), followed by 40 Gy on the pelvis in 4 weeks with two concomitant cycles of cisplatin (same dosage). A thorough evaluation of response with cystoscopy plus biopsies and urine cytology was performed at the end of this schedule. Complete responders were further irradiated to 66 Gy (boost technique) with a third course of cisplatin. Incomplete responders benefited from an immediate salvage cystectomy. Response to chemoradiotherapy was thus used as a selecting factor for bladder-preserving treatment. Out of the 53 patients, 42 completed the protocol. Thirty-four received the complete chemoradiotherapy combination therapy and eight were operated on because of incomplete response. After 26 months median follow-up (range 15–42 months), 82 per cent of patients were alive in the chemoradiotherapy arm versus 38 per cent in the salvage cystectomy arm. Metastases developed in 21 per cent of the former (Kaufman *et al.* 1989; Shipley 1990). Because of the high local response rate, even in advanced tumours, a randomized protocol has been activated to test this association further. Indeed, whether high local response rates will be translated into higher survival rates is still unclear and these regimens must be considered investigational at present.

With respect to the precise timing of cisplatin (and other drugs) and irradiation, the definition of an optimal association remains an area of research (Pearson and Steel 1984). So far, concomitant cisplatin-containing chemotherapy seems to be the most efficient association (Raghavan *et al.* 1990). Adriamycin should be omitted when irradiation is scheduled because of additional toxicity (Richards *et al.* 1986).

Radiotherapy, surgery, and chemotherapy

It might be thought that this is the final and most logical solution to utilizing the best of all therapeutic options.

As early as 1983, Herr showed that 70 mg/m^2 cisplatin given once with 20 Gy in five fractions in 1 week of external irradiation followed by cystectomy within 2 days was able to improve the therapeutic index of radiotherapy with no tumour in the surgical specimen in 21 per cent of patients (Herr *et al.* 1983). However, the majority of trials which have employed all three modalities of treatment, while showing minimal improvement in the therapeutic effect on the tumours because of overwhelming toxicity, have not been found to be a practical alternative. Perhaps with the diminution of the toxicity of chemotherapy by the use of growth factors plus leucovorin rescue and the increased accuracy of radiotherapy, triple combination therapy will again become a viable alternative.

Prospects for combination therapy

Combination chemotherapy with cisplatin and methotrexate as basic ingredients in the regimens is certainly more effective than single-agent chemotherapy, but has not yet been proved to prolong survival when combined with other modalities of treatment. With the discovery of modern anti-emetics, haematological growth factors, and the use of citrovorum factor, the toxicity of powerful chemotherapy regimens can be considerably reduced and thus their use in combination regimens becomes a more viable prospect. The combination of these effective chemotherapeutic regimens with radiotherapy for single tumours appears to be the optimal treatment where possible. In multiple tumours the combination of chemotherapy (with or without radiotherapy) and cystectomy seems to be the most promising approach. The results of the EORTC trial already mentioned (Hall 1991) are eagerly awaited, as this will prove once and for all whether modern combination chemotherapy prolongs survival in patients regardless of the definitive local therapy chosen.

Since no new effective agents against urothelial cancer are available at present, improvement of results should be attempted with dose escalation and cycle-time reduction of chemotherapy under the protection of haematological growth factors. Neoadjuvant chemotherapy for muscle-invasive bladder cancer is aimed at local tumour control as well as eradication of distant micrometastases. There is suggestive evidence that the combination of radiotherapy and chemotherapy is the most effective way of achieving this and avoiding cystectomy. However, randomized prospective studies are needed to demonstrate whether survival can be prolonged and which proportion of patients maintain a complete response in the bladder during their remaining lifetime.

CONCLUSIONS

Significant changes in the treatment of bladder cancer have come from an increased knowledge of prognostic factors in the superficial disease and the introduction of immunomodulation therapy. The development of effective systemic combination chemotherapy combined with new methods of urinary diversion have improved the outlook for patients with more advanced disease. These new avenues of treatment have been matched by new technology in imaging as well as in the development of tumour markers.

Survival is clearly the most important end-point. Those patients with biologically more favourable tumours may be amenable to less aggressive, ablative surgery and bladder preservation. However, patients whose tumours have poor prognosis features may deserve more aggressive surgery with the formation, if possible, of a continent urine reservoir. The many questions surrounding the treatment of bladder cancer will only be solved by the performance of prospective randomized trials. It seems that the heterogeneity of bladder cancer will mean that multimodality therapy is going to be necessary for all advanced tumours, although precisely which combination is the best is unclear at the present time.

REFERENCES

Augustine A, Hebert JR, Kabat GC, Wynder EL (1988). Bladder cancer in relation to cigarette smoking. *Cancer Research*, 37:4405–8.

Batata MA, *et al.* (1981). Factors of prognostic and therapeutic significance in patients with bladder cancer. *International Journal of Radiation Oncology—Biology—Physics*, 7:575–9.

Batterman JJ, Tierie AH (1986). Results for implantation of T1 and T2 bladder tumors. *Radiotherapy and Oncology*, 5:85–90.

Bertino JR (1982). Adjuvant chemotherapy and cancer cure. *International Journal of Radiation Oncology—Biology—Physics*, 8:109–13.

Blandy JP, *et al.* (1980). T3 bladder cancer—the case for salvage cystectomy. *British Journal of Urology*, 52:506–10.

Bloom HJ, Hendry WF, Wallace DM, Skeet RG (1982). Treatment of T3 bladder cancer: controlled trial of preoperative radiotherapy and radical cystectomy versus radical radiotherapy, second report and review. *British Journal of Urology*, 54:136–51.

Borland RN, Brendier CB, Isaacs WB (1992). Molecular biology of bladder cancer. *Hematology and Oncology Clinics of North America*, 6(1):31–9.

Bouffioux CH, *et al.* (1992). *Journal of Urology*, 148:297–301.

Boyer B, Thiery JP (1993). Cyclic AMP distinguishes between two functions of acidic FGF in a rat bladder carcinoma cell line. *Journal of Cell Biology*, 120(3):767–76.

Bricker EM (1950). Bladder substitution after pelvic evisceration. *Surgical Clinics of North America*, 30:1511.

British Association of Urological Surgeons Subcommittee on Industrial Bladder Cancer (1988). Occupational bladder cancer: a guide for clinicians. *British Journal of Urology*, 61:183–91.

Brown RR, Price JM, Salter EJ, Wear JB (1960). The metabolism of tryptophan in patients with bladder cancer. *Acta Unio Internationalis Contra Cancrum*, 16:299–303.

Bryan GT, Brown RR, Price JM (1964). Mouse: bladder carcinogenicity of certain tryptophan metabolites and other aromatic nitrogen compounds suspended in cholesterol. *Cancer Research*, 24:596–602.

Byar D, Blackard C (1977). Comparisons of placebo, pyridoxine and topical thiotepa in preventing recurrence of stage 1 bladder cancer. *Urology*, 10:556–60.

Camey M, Leduc A (1979). L'entéro-cystoplastie après cystoprostatectomie totale pour cancer de vessie. *Annales d'Urologie*, 13:114.

Carmichael J, Cornbleet MA, MacDougall RH, Allan SG, Dunwan W, Chisholm GD, Smyth JF (1985). Cisplatin and methotrexate in the treatment of transitional cell carcinoma of the urinary tract. *British Journal of Urology*, 57:299–302.

Coffey RC (1925). A technique for simultaneous implantation of the right and left ureters into the pelvic colon which does not obstruct the ureters or disturb kidney function. *Northwest Medicine*, 24:211.

Couvelaire R (1951). Le réservoir iléal de substitution après la cystectomie totale chez l'homme. *Journal d'Urologie (Paris)*, 57:408.

Crawford ED, Skinner DG (1980). Salvage cystectomy for irradiation failure. *Journal of Urology*, **123**:32.

Crawford ED, Das S, Smith JA (1987). Preoperative radiation therapy in the treatment of bladder cancer. *Urological Clinics of North America*, **14**:781–7.

Cutler SJ, Heney NM, Friedell GH (1982). Longitudinal study of patients with bladder cancer: factors associated with disease recurrence and progression. In *Bladder cancer*, AUA Monograph Vol. 3 (ed. WW Bonney and GR Prout), pp. 35–48. Williams and Wilkins, Baltimore, MD.

Dalbagni G, Presti J, Reuter V, Fair WR, Cordon-Cardo C (1993). Genetic alterations in bladder cancer. *Lancet*, **342**:469–71.

Darget R (1951). *Tumeurs malignes de la vessie. Traitement par le radium-thérapie à vesse ouverte*. Masson, Paris.

Debruyux FMJ, et al. (1988). BCG rival vs MMCC intravesical therapy in patients with superficial bladder cancer. *Urology*, **31** (Suppl.):20–5.

Denis LJ (1987). Deeply invasive transitional cell cancer of the bladder. In *Current therapy in genito-urinary surgery* (ed M Resnick), pp. 63–9. Decker, Toronto.

Denis L, et al. (1987). Current status of intravesical chemotherapy trials in the EORTC Urological Group. An overview. *Cancer Chemotherapy and Pharmacology*, **20**:67–71.

Denis L, Stoter G, Gerard JP (1989). Cancers of the urinary bladder, ureters and urethra. In *Oxford textbook of oncology* (ed. M Peckham, H Pinedo, and U Veronesi), pp. 705–19. Oxford University Press.

De Weerd JR, Colbt MY Jr (1973). Bladder carcinoma treated by irradiation surgery. Interval report. *Journal of Urology*, **109**:409.

D'Hont C, Keuppens F, Denis L (1990). Preoperative chemotherapy in deeply invasive M0 bladder cancer: the case for a marker lesion. *Poster, 9th Congress of the European Association of Urology*, Amsterdam 13–16 June 1990.

Duncan W, et al. (1985). A report of a randomized trial of d(15)+Be neutrons compared with mega-voltage X-ray therapy of bladder cancer. *International Journal of Radiation Oncology—Biology—Physics*, **11**:2043–9.

England HR, Paris AMI, Blandy JP (1981). The correlation of T1 bladder tumour history with prognosis and follow-up requirement. *British Journal of Urology*, **53**:593–602.

Friedell G (1976). Cancer, carcinoma *in situ* and 'early lesions' of the uterine and urinary bladder: introduction and definition. *Cancer Research*, **36**:2482–4.

Fung CY, et al. (1991). Prognostic factors in invasive bladder carcinoma in a prospective trial of preoperative adjuvant chemotherapy and radiotherapy. *Journal of Clinical Oncology*, **9**:1533–42.

Gabrilove JL, et al. (1988). Effect of granulocyte colony-stimulating factor on neutropenia and associated morbidity due to chemotherapy for transitional cell carcinoma of the urothelium. *New England Journal of Medicine*, **318**:1414–22.

Gad-el-Mawla NM, Muggia FM, El-Morsi B, Sherif M, Mansour MA, Khafagy M, El-Sabai IT (1978). Chemotherapeutic management of carcinoma of the bilharzial bladder: a phase II trial with hexamethylmelamine and VM-26. *Cancer Treatment Reports*, **62**:993–6.

Gad-el-Mawla NM, Mansour MA, Eissa S, Ali NN, Habboubi N, Nagrath J (1988). Epirubicin in bilharzial bladder cancer: a phase II and neoadjuvant trials. *Proceedings of the American Society of Clinical Oncology*, **7**:123.

Gérard JP, et al. (1985). La curiethérapie á l'iridium dans le traitement conservateur des cancers infiltrants de vessie. *Journal d'Urologie (Paris)*, **91**:139–44.

Glashan RW (1990). A randomized controlled study of intravesical alfa-2b-interferon in carcinoma *in situ* of the bladder. *Journal of Urology*, **144**:658–61.

Goffinet DR, et al. (1975). Bladder cancer: results of radiation therapy in 384 patients. *Radiology*, **117**:149–53.

Goodwin WE (1980). Ureterosigmoidostomy. *Bulletin of the New York Academy of Medicine*, **56**:734.

Greiner R, et al. (1977). The prognostic significance of ureteral obstruction in carcinoma of the bladder. *International Journal of Radiation Oncology—Biology—Physics*, **2**:1095–1100.

Hall RR (1991). *EORTC 30894: a phase III study of primary chemotherapy in T2(G3), T3 and T4a; N0 or NX; M0 transitional cell carcinoma of the bladder*. EORTC, Brussels.

Harker WG, et al. (1985). Cisplatin, methotrexate, and vinblastine (CMV): an effective chemotherapy regimen for metastatic transitional cell carcinoma of the urinary tract. A Northern California Oncology Group study. *Journal of Clinical Oncololgy*, **3**:1463.

Hermanek P, Sobin LH (1987). *TNM classification of malignant tumours* (4th edn). Springer-Verlag, London.

Herr HW (1987). Conservative management of muscle-infiltrating bladder cancer: prospective experience. *Journal of Urology*, **138**:1162.

Herr HW (1991). Progression of stage T1 bladder tumors after intravesical chemotherapy for superficial bladder tumours. *Journal of Urology*, **145**:40–4.

Herr HW, Yagoda A, Batata M, Sogani PC, Whitmore WF (1983). Planned preoperative cisplatin and radiation therapy for locally advanced bladder cancer. *Cancer*, **52**:2205–8.

Herr HW, Laudone VP, Whitmore FW Jr (1987). An overview of intravesical chemotherapy for superficial bladder tumours. *Journal of Urology*, **138**:1363–8.

Hillcoat BL, et al. (1989). A randomised trial of cisplatin versus cisplatin plus methotrexate in advanced cancer of the urothelial tract. *Journal of Clinical Oncology*, **7**:706–9.

Hinman F Jr (1990). Functional classification of conduits for continent diversion. *Journal of Urology*, **144**:27–30.

Jakse G, Frommhold H (1988). Treatment of locally advanced bladder cancer by hyperfractionated radiotherapy and chemotherapy. In *Management of advanced cancer of prostate and bladder* (ed. PH Smith and M Pavone-Macaluso), pp. 431–6. Liss, New York.

Jakse G, et al. (1985). Combined radiation and chemotherapy for locally advanced transitional cell carcinoma of the urinary bladder. *Cancer*, **55**:1659–64.

Jenkins BJ, Martin JE, Baithun SI, Doran H, Blandy JP (1989). The prediction of response to radiotherapy in invasive bladder cancer (abstract). *Proceedings of the 5th European Conference on Clinical Oncology (ECCO)*. Pergamon Press, London.

Jewett HJ, Strong GH (1946). Infiltrating carcinoma of bladder: relation of depth of penetration of bladder wall to incidence of local extension and metastases. *Journal of Urology*, **55**:366–72.

Jones RF, Debiec-Rychter M, Wang CY (1992). Chemical carcinogenesis of the urinary bladder—a status report (editorial). *Journal of Cancer Research and Clinical Oncology*, **118**(6):411–19.

Kaufman DS, et al. (1989). Upfront MCV chemotherapy + cisplatin and radiotherapy: its efficacy in successful preservation in 50 patients with invasive cancer (abstract). *Proceedings of the American Society of Clinical Oncology*, 500.

Kawamata H, Azuma M, Kameyama S, Nan L, Oyasu R (1992). Effect of epidermal growth factor/transforming growth factor alpha and transforming growth factor beta 1 on growth *in vitro* of rat urinary bladder carcinoma cells. *Cell Growth Differentiation*, **3**(11):819–25.

Kock NG (1969). Intraabdominal 'reservoir' in patients with permanent ileostomy. *Archives of Surgery*, **99**:223.

Koss LG, Deitch D, Ramanathan R, Sherman A (1985). Diagnostic value of cytology of voided urine. *Acta Cytologica*, **29**:810–16.

Kurth KH (1984). Superficial TCC bladder cancer: the impact of tumor differentiation of recurrence, progression and survival. In *Bladder cancer. A. Pathology, diagnosis and surgery* (ed. R Küss, S Khoury, L Denis, GP Murphy, and JP Karr), pp. 307–18. Liss, New York.

Kurth KH, Singe T, Ay R, Sylvester R, Ten Kate F, DePaul M and the EORTC GU Group (1989). Adjuvant chemotherapy of supplements of TCL—final analysis of a randomized trial. *Journal of Urology*, **147**:333.

Lamm DL, Thor DE, Harris SC, Reyna JA, Stogdill VD, Radwin HM (1980). BCG immunotherapy with superficial bladder cancer. *Journal of Urology*, **124**:38.

Lemoine G (1912). Création d'une vessie nouvelle par un procédé personnel après cystectomie totale pour cancer. *Journal d'Urologie Médicale et Chirurgicale*, **4**:367.

Loehrer PGJ, et al. (1992). A randomized comparison of cisplatin alone or in combination with methotrexate, vinblastine, and doxorubicin in patients with metastatic urothelial carcinoma: a cooperative group study. *Journal of Clinical Oncology*, **10**:1066–73.

Logothetis CJ, Choug C, Dexeus F, Sella A, Finn L (1988). Preliminary results of a prospective randomized trial comparing CISCA to MVAC chemotherapy for patients with advanced transitional cell carcinomas of the urothelium. *Proceedings of the American Society of Clinical Oncology*, **7**:134.

Logothetis CJ, Dexeus FH, Chong C, Sella A, Ayala AG, Ro JY, Pilat S (1989a). Cisplatin, cyclophosphamide and doxorubicin chemotherapy for unresectable urothelial tumors: the M. D. Anderson experience. *Journal of Urology*, **141**:33–7.

Logothetis CJ, Dexeus F, Sella A, Amato R, Finn J, Gutterman J (1989*b*). Escalated MVAC with recombinant human granulocyte–macrophage stimulating factor for patients with advanced and chemotherapy refractory urothelial tumors. *Proceedings of the American Society of Clinical Oncology*, 8:132.

Logothetis CJ, Dexeus FH, Finn L, Sella A, Amato RJ, Ayala AG, Kilbourn RG (1990*a*). A prospective randomized trial comparing MVAC and CISCA chemotherapy for patients with metastatic urothelial tumors. *Journal of Clinical Oncology*, 8:1050–5.

Logothetis CJ, Dexeus FH, Sella A, Amato RJ, Kilbourn RG, Finn L, Gutterman JU. (1990*b*). Escalated therapy for refractory urothelial tumors: methotrexate–vinblastine–doxorubicin–cisplatin plus unglycosylated recombinant human granulocyte–macrophage-colony-stimulating factor. *Journal of the National Cancer Institute*, 82:667–72.

Lutzeyer W, Rubben H, Dahm J (1982). Prognostic parameters in superficial bladder cancer: an analysis of 315 cases. *Journal of Urology*, 127:250–2.

Malkowicz SB, Nichols P, Lieskovsky G, Boyd SD, Huffman J, Skinner DG (1990). The role of radical cystectomy in the management of high grade superficial bladder cancer (Pa, P1, Pis and P2). *Journal of Urology*, 144:641–5.

Marshall VF (1952). Relation of preoperative estimate to pathological demonstration of extent of vesical neoplasms. *Journal of Urology*, 68:714–23.

Matsumoto L, *et al.* (1981). Clinical evaluation of intra-operative radiotherapy for carcinoma of the urinary bladder. *Cancer*, 47:509–13.

Mazeron JJ, *et al.* (1985). Treatment of bladder tumors by iridium 192 implantation. The Creteil technique. *Radiotherapy and Oncology*, 4:111–19.

Mead GM (1990). Bladder cancer. *Current Science*, 2:514–19.

Melamed MR, Voutsa NG, Grabstald H (1964). Natural history and clinical behavior of *in situ* carcinoma of the human urinary bladder. *Cancer*, 17:1535–45.

Messing EM (1992). Growth factors and bladder cancer: clinical implications of the interactions between growth factors and their urothelial receptors. *Seminars in Surgical Oncology*, 8(5):285–92.

Miller LS (1977). Bladder cancer: superiority of pre-operative irradiation therapy and cystectomy in clinical stages B2 and C. *Cancer*, 39:973–80.

Miller LS (1980). T3 bladder cancer. The case for higher radiation dosage. *Cancer*, 45:1875–8.

Miller LS, Johnson DE (1973). Megavoltage radiation for bladder carcinoma: alone, postoperative, or preoperative. *Proceedings of the 7th National Cancer Conference*, pp. 771–82. JB Lippincott, Philadelphia, PA.

Mohiuddin M, *et al.* (1985). Combined preoperative and postoperative irradiation for bladder cancer, results of RTOG/Jefferson study. *Cancer*, 55:963–6.

Momose H, Kakinuma H, Shariff SY, Mitchell GB, Rademaker A, Oyasu R (1991). Tumor-promoting effect of urinary epidermal growth factor in rat urinary bladder carcinogenesis. *Cancer Research*, 15(20):5487–90.

Montie JE, Straffon RA, Stewart BH (1984). Radical cystectomy without radiation therapy for carcinoma of the bladder. *Journal of Urology*, 131:477–82.

Moore MJ, O'Sullivan B, Tannock IF (1988). How expert physicians would wish to be treated if they had genitourinary cancer. *Journal of Clinical Oncology*, 6:1736–45.

Morrison R (1975). The results of treatment of cancer of the bladder: a clinical contribution of radiobiology. *Clinical Radiology*, 76:67–78.

National Bladder Cancer Collaborative Group A (1977). Cytology and histopathology of bladder cancer cases in a prospective longitudinal study. *Cancer Research*, 37:2911–15.

Newling D (1990). Intravesical therapy in the management of superficial transitional cell carcinoma of the bladder: the experience of the EORTC GU Group. *British Journal of Cancer*, 61:497–9.

Newling D, *et al.* (1983). Tryptophan metabolites in superficial bladder cancer: the background to and preliminary report on EORTC trial 30781. *Controlled Clinical Trials in Urological Oncology*, 13:296.

Nguyen M, Watanabe H, Budson AE, Richie JP, Folkman J (1993). Elevated levels of the angiogenic peptide basic fibroblast growth factor in urine of bladder cancer patients. *Journal of the National Cancer Institute*, 85(3):241–2.

Nijima T, *et al.* (1986). Diagnostic work-up. In *Developments in bladder cancer* (ed. L Denis, T Niijima, GR Prout, and FH Schröder), pp. 211–22. Liss, New York.

Pagano F, Bassi P, Galetti TP, Meneghini A, Milani C, Artibani W, Garbeglio A (1991). Results of contemporary radical cystectomy for invasive bladder cancer: a clinico-pathological study with an emphasis on the inadequacy of the tumor, nodes and metastases classification. *Journal of Urology*, 145:45–50.

Parsons JT, Thar TL, Bova FJ, Million RR (1980). An evaluation of split-course irradiation for pelvic malignancies. *International Journal of Radiation Oncology—Biology—Physics*, 6:175–81.

Pearson AE, Steel GG (1984). Chemotherapy in combination with pelvic irradiation: a time-dependence study in mice. *Radiotherapy and Oncology*, 2:49–55.

Prout GR Jr (1976). The surgical management of bladder cancer. *Urologic Clinics of North America*, 3:149–75.

Prout GR Jr, Kopp J (1984). Evaluation and management of patients with primary bladder carcinoma: protocols of the National Bladder Cancer Collaborative Group A. In *Controlled clinical trials in urologic oncology* (ed. L Denis, GP Murphy, GR Prout, and F Schröder), pp. 221–40. Raven Press, New York.

Prout GR Jr, *et al.* (1973). Preoperative irradiation and cystectomy for bladder carcinoma. IV. Results in a selected population. *Proceedings of the 7th National Cancer Conference, Philadelphia*. JB Lippincott, Philadelphia, PA.

Prout GR Jr, Griffin PP, Shipley WU (1979). Bladder carcinoma as a systemic disease. *Cancer*, 43:2532–9.

Prout GR Jr, *et al.* (1990). Preliminary results in invasive bladder cancer with transurethral resection, neoadjuvant chemotherapy and combined pelvic irradiation plus cisplatin chemotherapy. *Journal of Urology*, 144:1128–45.

Radwin HM (1980). Radiotherapy and bladder cancer: a critical review. *Journal of Urology*, 124:43–6.

Raghavan D (1988). *The management of bladder cancer*, pp. 317–22. Arnold, London.

Raghavan D, *et al.* (1985). Initial intravenous *cis*-platinum therapy: improved management for invasive high risk bladder cancer. *Journal of Urology*, 133:399–402.

Raghavan D, *et al.* (1989). First randomised trials of pre-emptive (neoadjuvant) intravenous cisplatin for invasive transitional cell carcinoma of the bladder. *Proceedings of the American Society of Clinical Oncology*, 8:133.

Raghavan D, Shipley WU, Garnick MB, Russell PJ, Richie JP (1990). Biology and management of bladder cancer. *New England Journal of Medicine*, 322(16):1129–38.

Ravery V, Jouanneau J, Gil Diez S, Abbou CC, Caruelle JP, Barritault D, Chopin DK (1992). Immunohistochemical detection of acidic fibroblast growth factor in bladder transitional cell carcinoma. *Urological Research*, 20(3):211–14.

Reid EC, *et al.* (1976). Pre-operative irradiation and cystectomy in 135 cases of bladder carcinoma. *Urology*, 85:247.

Richards B, *et al.* (1986). Prognostic factors in infiltrating bladder cancer. In *Developments in bladder cancer* (ed. L Denis, T Niijima, GR Prout Jr, and FH Schröder), pp. 271–86. Liss, New York.

Roberts WG, Hasan T (1993). Tumor-secreted vascular permeability factor/vascular endothelial growth factor influences photosensitizer uptake. *Cancer Research*, 53(1):153–7.

Rousseau J, *et al.* (1974). La radiothérapie transcutanée des cancers de la vessie. *Journal de Radiologie et d'Electrologie*, 55:834–40.

Rozan R, *et al.* (1989). Curietherapie interstitielle des cancers de la vessie par iridium 192: etude multicentrique portant sur 279 cas (abstract). *Proceedings of the 17th International Congress of Radiology (ICR 89)*, Paris.

Sagerman RH, *et al.* (1968). Preoperative irradiation in carcinoma of the bladder. *American Journal of Roentgenology*, 102:577–80.

Sarosdy MF, Lamm DL (1989). Long-term results of intra-vesical bacillus Calmette–Guérin therapy for superficial bladder cancer. *Journal of Urology*, 142:719–22.

Sauer R, *et al.* (1988). Preliminary results of treatment of invasive bladder carcinoma with radiotherapy and cisplatin. *International Journal of Radiation Oncology—Biology—Physics*, 15:871–5.

Scher HI (1989). Should single agents be standard therapy for urothelial tumors. *Journal of Clinical Oncology*, 10:694–7.

Scher HI, *et al.* (1988). Neoadjuvant M-VAC (methotrexate, vinblastine, doxorubicin and cisplatin) effect on the primary bladder lesion. *Journal of Urology*, 139:470–4.

Schröder FH, Richards B (1983). *Superficial bladder tumours*. Liss, New York.

Schröder FH, *et al.* (1988). TNM classification of genitourinary tumours 1987—position of the EORTC Genitourinary Group. *British Journal of Urology*, 62:502–10.

Sell A, Jacobsen A (1990). Preoperative irradiation and cystectomy versus radical irradiation in advanced bladder cancer (abstract). *Proceedings of the 9th Annual Meeting of the European Society for Therapeutic Radiology and Oncology (ESTRO)*, Montecattini.

Shipley WU (1990). Data presented at *ESO Seminar on Advanced Bladder Cancer*, Venice, 17 April 1990.

Shipley WU, *et al.* (1984). Cisplatin and full-dose irradiation for patients with invasive bladder carcinoma: a preliminary report of tolerance and local response. *Journal of Urology*, 132:899–903.

Shipley WU, *et al.* (1985). Full-dose irradiation for patients with invasive bladder carcinoma: clinical and pathological correlates of improved survival. *Journal of Urology*, 134:679–83.

Shipley WU, Prout GR, Einstein AB, Coombs LJ, Wajsman Z, Soloway MS, Englander L (1987*a*). Treatment of invasive bladder cancer by cisplatin and radiation in patients unsuited for surgery. *Journal of the American Medical Association*, 258:931–5.

Shipley WU, *et al.* (1987*b*). Intraoperative therapy in patients with bladder cancer. *Cancer*, 60:1485–8.

Shipley WU, *et al.* (1988). Combined chemotherapy and radiation therapy in the treatment of patients with muscle invasive bladder carcinoma following transurethral surgery: an update of bladder sparing effort. *International Journal of Radiation Oncology—Biology—Physics*, 15:132.

Sidransky D, Messing E (1992). Molecular genetics and biochemical mechanisms in bladder cancer. Oncogenes, tumor suppressor genes, and growth factors. *Urological Clinics of North America*, 19(4):629–39.

Skinner DG (1982). Management of invasive bladder cancer. A meticulous pelvic node dissection can make a difference. *Journal of Urology*, 128:34–6.

Skinner DG, Lieskovsky G (1984). Temporary cystectomy with pelvic node dissection compared to preoperative radiation therapy plus cystectomy in management of invasive bladder cancer. *Journal of Urology*, 131:1069–72.

Skinner DG, *et al.* (1982). High dose, short course preoperative radiation therapy and immediate single stage radical cystectomy with pelvic node dissection in the management of bladder cancer. *Journal of Urology*, 27:671–4.

Skinner EC, Lieskovsky G, Skinner DG (1990). The technique of radical cystectomy. *AUA Update Series Lesson 7*, 9:50–5.

Slack NH, Prout GR Jr (1980). The heterogeneity of invasive bladder carcinoma and different responses to treatment. *Journal of Urology*, 123:644–52.

Slack NH, *et al.* (1977). Five-year follow up results of collaborative studies of therapies for carcinoma of the bladder. *Journal of Surgical Oncology*, 9:3963.

Smith G, Elton RA, Beynon LL, Newson JE, Chisholm GD, Hargreaves TB (1983). Prognostic significance of biopsy results of normal-looking mucosa in cases of superficial bladder cancer. *British Journal of Urology*, 55:665–9.

Smith JA Jr, Whitmore WF Jr (1981*a*). Regional lymph node metastasis from bladder cancer. *Journal of Urology*, 126:591–3.

Smith JA Jr, Whitmore WF Jr (1981*b*). Salvage cystectomy for bladder cancer after failure of definitive irradiation. *Journal of Urology*, 125:643.

Spera JA, *et al.* (1988). A comparison of preoperative radiotherapy regimens for bladder cancer. *Cancer*, 61:255–62.

Splinter TAW, *et al.* (1989). EORTC GU Group study 30851. A phase II study of upfront chemotherapy in patients with invasive bladder cancer. *Proceedings of the American Society of Clinical Oncology*, 8:139.

Splinter TAW, *et al.* (1990). The prognostic value of the pT-category after combination chemotherapy for patients with invasive bladder cancer who underwent cystectomy. In *Neoadjuvant chemotherapy in invasive bladder cancer* (ed. TAW Splinter and HI Scher), pp. 219–24. Wiley-Liss, New York.

Sternberg CN, *et al.* (1988). M-VAC (methotrexate, vinblastine, doxorubicin and cisplatin) for advanced transitional cell carcinoma of the urothelium. *Journal of Urology*, 139:461–9.

Stoter G, *et al.* (1987). Combination chemotherapy with cisplatin and methotrexate in advanced transitional cell cancer of the bladder. *Journal of Urology*, 137:663.

Straus KL, *et al.* (1988). Treatment of bladder cancer with interstitial iridium 192 implantation and external beam irradiation. *International Journal of Radiation Oncology—Biology—Physics*, 14:265–71.

Studer UE, Ackerman D, Casanova GA, Zingg EJ (1989). Three years experience with an ileal low pressure bladder substitute. *British Journal of Urology*, 63:43–52.

Sylvester R (1985). The analysis of results in prophylactic superficial bladder cancer studies. In *Superficial bladder tumors* (ed. FH Schroder and B Richards), pp. 3–11. Liss, New York.

Tannock IF (1991). The current status of adjuvant chemotherapy for bladder cancer. *Seminars in Urology*.

Tennant RW, Rao GN, Russfield A, Seilkop S, Braun AG (1993). Chemical effects in transgenic mice bearing oncogenes expressed in mammary tissue. *Carcinogenesis*, 14(1):29–35.

Thames HD, Peters LJ, Withers HR (1983). Accelerated fractionation versus hyperfractionation: rationales for several treatments per day. *International Journal of Radiation Oncology—Biology—Physics*, 9:127.

Theodorescu D, Cornil I, Sheehan C, Man MS, Kerbel RS (1991). Ha-*ras* induction of the invasive phenotype results in up-regulation of epidermal growth factor receptors and altered responsiveness to epidermal growth factor in human papillary transitional cell carcinoma cells. *Cancer Research*, 51(16):4486–91.

Torti FM, Lum BL (1987). Superficial bladder cancer. Risk of recurrence and potential role for interferon. *Cancer*, 59:613–19.

Van der Werf-Messing BVD (1975). Carcinoma of the bladder T3 NX M0 treated by preoperative irradiation followed by cystectomy. *Cancer*, 36(Suppl.): 712–22.

Van der Werf-Messing B (1978). Cancer of the urinary bladder treated by interstitial radium implant. *International Journal of Radiation Oncology—Biology—Physics*, 4:373.

Van der Werf-Messing B (1979). Preoperative irradiation followed by cystectomy to treat carcinoma of the urinary bladder category T3NX, 0–4 M. *International Journal of Radiation Oncology—Biology—Physics*, 5:394–401.

Van der Werf-Messing B (1982). Carcinoma of the urinary bladder T3 NX M0 treated by preoperative radiation followed by simple cystectomy. *International Journal of Radiation Oncology—Biology—Physics*, 8:1849–55.

Van der Werf-Messing B, Van Putten W (1989). Carcinoma of the urinary bladder category T2 T3 treated by 40 Gy external irradiation followed by cesium 137 implant at reduced dose. *International Journal of Radiation Oncology—Biology—Physics*, 16:369–71.

Van der Werf-Messing B, *et al.* (1983). Carcinoma of the urinary bladder category T3 NX M0 treated by the combination of radium implant and external irradiation. *International Journal of Radiation Oncology—Biology—Physics*, 9:177–80.

Van der Werf-Messing BHP, Menon RS, Hop WCJ (1984). Intestitial radiotherapy of carcinoma of the bladder at the Rotterdam Radiotherapy Institute (RRTI). In *Bladder cancer, part B: radiation, local and systemic chemotherapy and new treatment modalities* (ed. R Küss, S. Khoury, LJ Denis, GP Murphy, and JP Karr), pp. 71–85. Liss, New York.

Van Velthoven R (1991). Le remplacement vésical et la dérivation urinaire continente après cystectomie. *Acta Urologica Belgica*, 59:1–349.

Vindelov I, Christensen IJ, Engelholm SA, Guldhammer B (1989). Prognosis and DNA content determined by flow-cytometry in 251 patients with bladder cancer (abstract). *Proceedings of the 5th European Conference on Clinical Oncology (ECCO 5)*, London.

Wajsman Z, *et al.* (1989). Bladder sparing treatment for muscle invasive transitional cell carcinoma: systemic chemotherapy followed by radiation therapy with adjunctive cisplatin (abstract). *Proceedings of the American Society of Clinical Oncology* p. 513.

Wallace DM, Bloom HJG (1976). The management of deeply infiltrative (T3) bladder carcinoma: controlled trial of radical radiotherapy versus preoperative radiotherapy and radical cystectomy (first report). *British Journal of Urology*, 48:587–94.

WHO (1979). *Handbook for reporting results of cancer treatment*. World Health Organization, Geneva.

Whitmore WF, *et al.* (1977). A comparative study of two preoperative radiation regimens with cystectomy for bladder cancer. *Cancer*, 40:1077.

Witjes JA, Debruyne FMJ (1991). Optimal management of superficial bladder cancer. *European Journal of Cancer*, 27(3):330–3.

Wolff H, Iversen HG, Rosenhilde P, Schröder T (1987). Transurethral surgery in the treatment of invasive bladder cancer (T1 and T2). *Scandinavian Journal of Urology and Nephrology (Suppl.)*, 104:127–33.

Yagoda A, *et al.* (1976). Cisplatin in advanced bladder cancer. *Cancer Treatment Reports*, 60:917–18.

Yu WS, Sagerman RH, Chung CT, Dalad PS, King GA (1985). Bladder carcinoma: experience with radical and preoperative radiotherapy in 421 patients. *Cancer*, 56:1293–9.

10.5 Tumours of the kidney (other than nephroblastoma)

ALASTAIR W. S. RITCHIE AND P. T. D. OLIVER

INTRODUCTION

Mass lesions in the kidney are common. The majority are cystic and benign. Tumours of the renal parenchyma account for approximately 85 per cent of all malignant renal lesions. Overall, renal tumours account for only 2–3 per cent of all adult cancers. Renal carcinoma has reported age-standardized incidence rates of 3.6–5.6 per 100 000 males and 1.7–3.4 per 100 000 females in the United Kingdom. The range of incidence rates illustrates regional variation in the United Kingdom. There are also marked international variations in incidence, which are high in northern Europe and North America and low in Africa, Asia, and South America (Waterhouse et al. 1976). There is some evidence of increasing incidence in males (Kantor et al. 1973; Ritchie et al. 1984) and that the incidence is increasing faster than most malignancies other than carcinoma of the lung, leukaemia, and brain tumours in the United Kingdom (Alderson 1982). The disease affects males more often than females (approximately 2 : 1) and can occur at any age, although it is most common in the sixth and seventh decades.

The results of surgical management are good if the tumour is confined to the kidney. There is no consistently effective systemic treatment for metastatic renal carcinoma.

CLASSIFICATION OF RENAL TUMOURS

As in other anatomical sites, tumours of the kidney can be primary or secondary and benign or malignant. The commoner tumours are benign cystic lesions of the parenchyma, malignant tumours of the renal parenchyma (renal carcinoma), tumours of the renal urothelium, and Wilms' tumour (nephroblastoma). A variety of sarcomas account for approximately 1 per cent of renal tumours (Table 1).

PATHOLOGY

Benign tumours

Unequivocally benign lesions such as lipomas, angiomyolipomas and fibromas are rare and are usually grouped with small, clear cell tumours classified as benign adenomas. In a surgical pathology-based tumour registry, only 38 from a series of 3270 were benign, indicating that benign tumours are an uncommon clinical problem. Post-mortem studies have shown a much higher incidence, with 'adenomatous' lesions being found in approximately 25 per cent of males over the age of 50 years (Reese and Winstanley 1958).

Adenoma

Historically, the term adenoma has been bestowed on well-differentiated renal cortical glandular tumours of less than 3 cm maximum diameter. Bell (1950) reported a direct relationship between size and the frequency of distant metastases. However, he did note metastases in 3 out of 65 (4.6 per cent) tumours of diameter less than 3 cm. Further justification for the distinction of benign from malignant, was the greater frequency with which the adenomas were reported in autopsy series, compared to carcinomas. The shared cell of origin, the absence of histological differentiating features, the shared male predominance and age range, and the occurrence of metastases from small lesions, have led some pathologists to express the view that adenomas are simply small carcinomas (Bennington 1973; Petersen 1986). Conversely, Mostofi and Davis (1986) have stated that they believe in the existence of adenomas but use both clinical aspects of the lesions' behaviour and histology to distinguish between the two. However, for the clinician there is no reliable method to identify which lesions have metastatic potential. Size alone is not a good criterion, since widespread metastases have been reported from a collected series of ten tumours less than 3 cm in diameter (Petersen 1986) and the histology of nine renal neoplasms first visible when less than 3 cm in diameter showed that only one lesion was 'benign' (oncocytoma). The remainder were all classified as carcinomas and two produced metastases (Curry et al. 1986).

Angiomyolipoma

Angiomyolipoma is an uncommon benign tumour of the kidney, also referred to as hamartoma. The tumour consists of smooth muscle, thick-walled blood vessels, and mature adipose tissue. The lesion may be associated with tuberous sclerosis or may occur in a sporadic form. Lesions associated with tuberous sclerosis are commonly multiple and may be bilateral. The sporadic form of tumour is usually single. Many small lesions are asymptomatic and the true incidence of the tumour is therefore unknown. The tumour is more common in females than males and may produce massive haemorrhage or rupture spontaneously, necessitating urgent nephrectomy.

Renal carcinoma may rarely co-exist with angiomyolipoma; Huang et al. (1988) found nine such cases in the English literature.

Prolonged observation with repeated ultrasound and computed tomography has shown that the lesions do not normally progress. In a minority of cases the tumour may grow and produce pain and haemorrhage. Local extension, venous involvement, and even lymph node involvement have been reported but the lesion is not known to produce metastases (reviewed by Blute et al. 1988).

Malignant parenchymal tumours

Oncocytoma

Oncocytomas have a characteristic appearance, being usually well circumscribed with a uniform tan colour and, in some cases, a central scar, with radiations into the surrounding tumour. The lesions may be multicentric and bilateral. The term adenoma has also been

Table 1 Classification of renal tumours (based on Studer and deKernion 1986)

	Benign	Malignant
Parenchymal tumours		
Epithelium	Adenoma	Carcinoma
	Oncocytoma	
Mesenchymal	Fibroma	Fibrosarcoma
and	Haemangioma	Haemangiosarcoma
capsular		Haemangioendothelioma
	Juxtaglomerular cell tumour (angioreninoma)	Haemangiopericytoma
	Lymphangioma	Lymphangiosarcoma
	Leiomyoma	Leiomyosarcoma
	Rhabdomyoma	Rhabdomyosarcoma
	Lipoma	Liposarcoma
	Chondroma	Osteogenic sarcoma
	Angiomyolipoma (hamartoma)	
Neurogenic	Neurofibroma	Neuroblastoma
Developmental	Mesoblastic nephroma	Nephroblastoma (Wilms' tumour)
		Embryonic carcinoma
Miscellaneous	Dermoid	Deposits of haemato-logical tumours
	Adrenal rests	
	Endometriosis	
	Carcinoid	
	Granulomas	Metastases
	Phaeochromocytoma	
	Cysts	
Collecting system tumours		
Epithelial	Papilloma	Transitional cell carcinoma
	Leukoplakia	Squamous carcinoma
	Glandular metaplasia	Adenocarcinoma
Mesenchymal	Fibroma	Fibrosarcoma
	Haemangioma	Haemangiosarcoma
	Leiomyoma	Leiomyosarcoma

applied to tumours containing cells with oncocytic features, devoid of mitoses, and with no evidence of local extension, metastases, or haemorrhage and necrosis (Klein and Valensi 1976). The 'adenomas' with oncocytic elements have been renamed oncocytomas (Lieber *et al.* 1981). Renal oncocytomas comprise approximately 4 per cent of all parenchymal tumours previously grouped together as renal carcinoma. Oncocytes are altered epithelial cells that have an abundant homogeneous eosinophylic cytoplasm and usually a small, round nucleus. The cells contain abundant mitochondria with a paucity of other cytoplasmic organelles. Oncocytes have been described in other tissues and apparently increase with advancing age. The origin of renal oncocytes is controversial (Klein and Valensi 1976; Eble and Hull 1984). Oncocytomas are incidental findings in approximately 70 per cent of cases and have a low but not absent potential for local penetration and metastases. Many renal carcinomas have oncocytic features in certain areas but may have aggressive clinical behaviour. Thus, the term oncocytoma has to be reserved for a tumour composed solely of oncocytes.

The deoxyribonucleic acid content of renal tumours has a certain prognostic value (see below). The DNA content of oncocytomas however, is heterogeneous. Rainwater *et al.* (1986) found that 39 per cent of 51 typical specimens of oncocytoma had a marked increase in the DNA tetraploid peak and 11 per cent showed a distinct DNA aneuploid peak. Among 21 grade 2 oncocytomas, 43 per cent showed a marked increase in the tetraploid peak and 24 per cent showed a distinct aneuploid peak. The majority of cases

with an abnormal flow pattern had easily identifiable cells, containing large abnormal nuclei on light microscopy. No instances of tumour progression or death were noted in the patients having tumours with normal ploidy or aneuploidy. Three tumours showed evidence of progression from the group with tetraploid flow patterns. These findings are surprising in view of the clinical behaviour of these lesions and would appear to preclude the use of flow cytometry on fine-needle aspirates for pre-operative distinction of oncocytoma from carcinoma.

Juxtaglomerular tumour

The rare juxtaglomerular tumour is associated with the clinical syndrome of hypertension and hypokalaemia. This tumour is thought to arise from the renin-secreting juxtaglomerular cells. The tumours are usually small (3–5 cm in diameter) situated in the cortex and appear to be well circumscribed. Neither local recurrence nor metastases have been described with this tumour.

Renal carcinoma

The commonest malignant tumour of the kidney is the renal carcinoma, which is also referred to as renal cell carcinoma, renal adenocarcinoma, and hypernephroma. The latter name derives from the erroneous concept that such tumours arose from the suprarenal gland. The term hypernephroma, although in common usage, is therefore misleading and should be deleted from the medical vocabulary.

The gross appearance of renal carcinoma is variable but the typical appearance is of a yellow tumour with areas of haemorrhage and necrosis. The necrosis may be extensive, leading to a lesion with a dirty brown semi-liquid centre, the only viable tumour being at the periphery of the lesion. The tumour may produce a pseudocapsule, caused by compression of surrounding healthy kidney by mechanical expansion. Areas of tumour infiltration may be obvious and evidence of penetration of the capsule and Gerota's fascia should be sought. Intrarenal veins may show invasion and extension of tumour which may extend into the main renal vein(s) and vena cava. Spread via lymphatics to hilar, para-aortic, mediastinal, and iliac nodes is erratic (see below). Haematogenous spread may occur from any size of primary tumour and the lungs are the commonest site of metastases.

Renal carcinoma has a number of cell types but any one tumour is rarely homogeneous. As noted above, the tumour was originally confused with adrenal tumours due to the common clear cell pattern. Papillary, granular, alveolar, spindle cell, and mixed types also exist. Nuclear pleomorphism and mitotic activity are usually prominent.

There is no clear relationship between the predominate cell type and prognosis, although the presence of spindle cells in conjunction with poor grade has been reported to imply a poor outcome.

Transitional cell tumours of the collecting system

Tumours arising from the transitional epithelium of the collecting system account for up to 10 per cent of all renal tumours. Over 90 per cent are transitional cell carcinomas, with true benign transitional tumours (papilloma) being very rare. Squamous cell carcinomas account for 7–9 per cent of renal urothelial tumours and are associated with chronic inflammation usually caused by calculi. It was only with the revised classification of disease sponsored by WHO in 1967 that ICD 189 was subdivided into 189.0

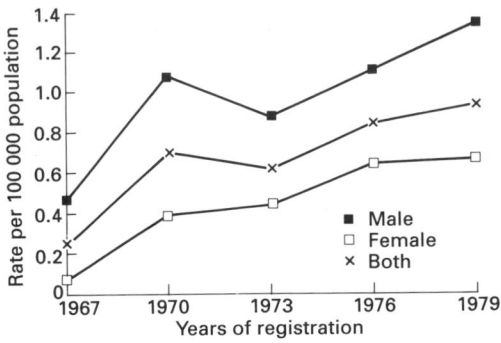

Fig. 1 Age-standardized incidence rates for tumours of the renal pelvis and ureter 1967–1979.

(parenchymal tumours) and 189.1,2 (tumours of the pelvis and ureter). Accurate data on the relative incidence of such tumours has therefore only been available for a short time. Available data suggest that the number of registered cases of upper-tract urothelial tumours is increasing in both sexes (Fig. 1 shows age-standardized incidence rates based on Scottish Cancer Registration data 1967–1979), but it is not clear whether this represents a genuine increase in incidence or reflects better diagnostic methods. For example, the recent availability of good quality urine cytology may have stimulated a more thorough search for upper-tract tumours in patients with negative cystoscopy and positive urine cytology.

Urothelial tumours of the kidney occur most commonly in the sixth and seventh decades and the data shown in Fig. 1 indicate that they occur more commonly in males (M : F = 2.1 : 1).

The tumours show international variation in incidence and are classically associated with residence in the Balkan countries and excessive analgesic ingestion (especially phenacetin). The latter two associations are also related to a higher incidence of bilateral tumours. Other aetiological factors are similar to those of bladder urothelial cancer (Wallace 1988). Upper-tract tumours may occur in association with bladder tumours and vice versa. The implication of this observation is that the patient who has had a urothelial tumour requires follow-up and supervision of the entire urinary tract or at least those parts left behind by the surgeon.

Renal metastases

Metastases to the kidney are usually clinically silent (Table 2). Although it is not possible to differentiate a renal carcinoma from a metastasis to the kidney on clinical and imaging data, the factors favouring the diagnosis of renal metastases are small, multifocal, avascular renal masses in association with widespread metastases elsewhere in the body. Renal metastases do not tend to enhance with contrast on computerized tomography studies and do not usually involve the renal venous system (Pagani 1983). When both kidneys are involved, the commonest primary is a lymphoma, whereas if one kidney is involved the commonest primary is the lung (Klinger 1951). Other primary sources are the breast and uterus.

Prognostic factors

Renal carcinoma has an unusual natural history. Prediction of the outcome for individual patients must therefore be guarded. Many attempts at prediction have been based on pathological analysis of the tumour specimen. The tumour size, stage, predominant cell

Table 2 Characteristics of patients with renal metastases

No. of patients	No symptoms (%)	Normal urinalysis	Normal renal function	Reference
27	23(85)	9(33)	25(93)	Choyke et al. (1987)
116	115/142ᵃ(81)	43(37)	96(83)	Klinger (1951)
10	8(80)	NS	NS	Bhatt et al. (1983)

ᵃ115/142 patients with metastases to the urinary tract: the proportion of 116 with renal metastases was not specified.
NS, not stated.

type, grade, mitotic rate, and DNA ploidy have all been reported as influential.

Grading of malignant tumours

There have been a number of attempts at grading renal carcinoma (Hand and Broders 1932; Riches et al. 1951; Arner et al. 1965; Skinner et al. 1971). These have included analysis of both histological and cytological features and, in the authors' hands, have a significant correlation to the outcome. The grading systems are, however, subjective and are not easily reproduced by another pathologist. In addition, such systems face the difficult problem of heterogeneity of cell type, architectural pattern, and cytological features within any one tumour.

DNA content

Dissatisfaction with the reproducibility of grading has led to a search for more objective indicators of prognosis. The prognostic significance of the DNA content of renal tumour cells has been reported in recent studies (Otto et al. 1984; Ljunberg et al. 1986a,b; Rainwater et al. 1987; deKernion et al. 1989). Analysis of DNA ploidy can be performed on fresh, fresh frozen, or paraffin-embedded tissues using flow cytometry. Use of paraffin-embedded tissue has the obvious advantage of allowing analysis of tumour material from patients whose outcome has been determined (Hedley et al. 1983). Better prognosis, in terms of tumour recurrence and survival, has been noted for patients with diploid or near diploid DNA content when compared to patients with an aneuploid pattern.

The question of whether DNA flow cytometry adds prognostic information independent of other predictors of outcome has been addressed in a multivariate analysis of 103 cases (Grignon et al. 1989). Statistically significant prognostic variables were Robson stage, DNA ploidy, mitotic rate, worst nuclear grade, predominant nuclear grade, and sex. Tumour size, cell type, and architectural pattern were also assessed but did not prove to be significant. Cox proportional hazards regression analysis revealed that Robson stage, ploidy, and mitotic rate were independent, significant predictors of outcome.

The implications of such findings are that DNA content may be useful in a prospective fashion in helping to select patients for adjunctive nephrectomy and in stratifying patients entering clinical trials. Pathological information should be used in conjunction with relevant clinical data such as the presence or absence of metastases and performance status.

AETIOLOGY, EPIDEMIOLOGY, AND PREVENTION

Little is known of the cause of renal carcinoma, although there are some animal models demonstrating causation by viruses (Granoff

1972), radiation (Rosen and Cole 1962), and carcinogens (reviewed by Murphy *et al.* 1966). In addition, there are high-incidence strains of mice (Claude 1958) and rats, the latter showing dominant inheritance (Eker and Mossige 1961). This mode of inheritance has also been well documented in the rhesus monkey (Ratcliffe 1940). Furthermore, there are at least 114 familial cases reported in man (Reddy 1981), suggesting that some human tumours may have a genetic factor in their aetiology. Such cases are, however, a minority of most tumours presenting clinically. In a series of 102 patients treated by one of us (RTDO) over the past decade, there were only two familial cases.

There have been few formal genetic studies of these families, although associations have been shown with blood group A, chromosome 3 deletions (Cohen *et al.* 1979; Zbar *et al.* 1987), colour blindness (Griffin *et al.* 1967), and HLA (Tiwari and Terasaki 1985). In view of these observations, there is now a need for more intensive genetic studies, including study of tumour chromosome abnormalities.

Over the past century, the issue of viruses in human cancer has been very contentious. However, the 1980s saw increasing recognition of, for example, the promoting role of Epstein–Barr virus in Burkitt's lymphoma and, more recently, papilloma virus in carcinoma of the cervix. Little work has been reported on the subject of viral involvement in the aetiology of human renal carcinoma, despite the observation that there is a clear-cut association between a herpes-type virus and renal tumours in the toad, *Rana pipiens* (Marlow and Mizell 1972). The virus is a well-documented member of the herpes group and although nearly all toads carry the infection, only 10 per cent of animals develop tumours (Skinner and Mizell 1978). The virus is spread mostly through the germ-line but can also spread horizontally. The observation that only when infected frogs are stressed by being cooled to 4–9 °C, can free virus be found is of particular interest, in view of the difficulty of demonstrating any virus in human renal tumours. At summer temperatures, the virus may be demonstrated by DNA hydridization but free virus is undetectable. The finding that the virus in this animal tumour was a DNA herpes virus led to a search in human renal tumours for evidence of herpes virus proteins. Although herpes simplex proteins were found in the only study reported to date (Cocchiara *et al.* 1980), these observations have not been repeated or related to pathological subtypes of clinical behaviour. The ubiquity of this virus makes it difficult to interpret these observations without DNA hybridization studies: even then, if the history of herpes genitalis involvement in carcinoma of the cervix is anything to go by, it will be difficult to prove that the virus is involved (Kessler 1984). Only if vaccination against herpes simplex in early life led to a reduction in the incidence of the tumour could the issue of virus involvement be resolved. A testing ground for such theories may be the current programme of vaccination against hepatitis B and the subsequent incidence of hepatoma in East Africa.

Evidence for involvement of carcinogens in human renal carcinoma is even more indirect. However, in animal models there is no shortage of proven active agents, including heavy metals such as cadmium and lead and carcinogens such as nitrosamines, aflatoxins, alkylating agents, and even chloroform if given in low doses for prolonged periods (reviewed by Pavone-Macaluso *et al.* 1982; Sufrin 1982). None of these classes of compound has ever been tested prospectively in chronic low-dose exposure, human studies with a 5 year follow-up or more. Their role as initiators or co-factors acting with an as yet undefined virus, remains speculative.

Clues to the aetiology may be gained from intensive study of younger patients who may display increased sensitivity to the putative causative agent. Three out of ten patients treated by one of us (RTDO) had been exposed to excessive amounts of agricultural pesticides. One had greatly elevated blood levels of DDT following accidental overexposure due to a crop-spraying accident and came from an agricultural area in which the local community physician had identified a cluster of patients with renal carcinoma.

CLINICAL PRESENTATION

Renal carcinoma has a diverse presentation, which can be classified on the basis of mechanical and systemic effects of the tumour or its secretions (see Table 3). Being deep-seated in the retroperitoneum, tumours may reach the size of a football before producing any symptoms. The majority of patients present with haematuria and the renal mass is detected by subsequent investigation. Loin pain, from expansion of the tumour, clot colic, or the presence of a mass are other common mechanical features. Tumour extension into the renal vein and vena cava may produce an acute varicocele and later induce features of vena caval obstruction. In the absence of

Table 3 Clinical presentation of renal carcinoma

Mechanical effects
  Local
    Haematuria
    Loin pain
    Palpable mass
    Varicocele
    Caval obstruction
    Non-functioning kidney
  Metastatic
    Pain
    Pathological fracture
    Focal neurological signs
    Pulmonary mass

Systemic effects
  Non-specific
    Weight loss
    Fever
    Anorexia
    Anaemia
    Raised erythrocyte sedimentation rate
    Hepatic dysfunction
    Hypercalcaemia
    Thrombocytosis
    Thrombocytopenia
    Disorders of coagulation
    Plasma protein abnormalities (for example, alpha-2 globulin)
    Amyloid
    Nephrotic syndrome
    Neuromyopathy
    Polymyositis and dermatomyositis
    x light-chain nephropathy

Paraneoplastic syndromes
  Hypersecretion of substances with effects such as the following
    Renin
    Erythropoietin
    Parathormone
    Prostaglandins
    Enteroglucagon
    Gonadotrophin
    Prolactin
    ACTH

specific symptoms resulting from mechanical effects, patients may present to virtually any department with non-specific symptoms such as fatigue, malaise, anorexia, and weight loss. These non-specific symptoms occur in patients with and without metastases. Approximately 25 per cent of patients present with metastases which may cause neurological symptoms and signs, pathological fractures, and localized pain. Metastases from renal carcinoma may also occur in odd sites, such as the iris, the vagina, the subungual skin, and the soft palate. The symptoms of such lesions will be correspondingly variable.

Males are affected approximately twice as often as females and the disease usually presents in the sixth and seventh decades. However, renal carcinoma can occur at any age (Dehner et al. 1970). In childhood the disease has to be distinguished from Wilms' tumour but is a distinct entity. There is no sex difference in incidence in children and the common presenting feature is an abdominal mass.

Von Hippel–Lindau syndrome, one of the phakomatoses, places patients at increased risk of renal tumour formation and screening with computerized tomography may be justifiable in this select group of patients (Levine et al. 1983). Tumours present at a younger age than normal in up to 45 per cent of patients and have a tendency to be multifocal. These patients also have a high incidence of renal cysts, phaeocromocytoma, and papillary cystadenomas of the epididymis (Horton et al. 1976). Autosomal dominant inheritance of this syndrome means that family members should also be screened for occult tumours.

Paraneoplastic syndromes

Paraneoplastic syndromes are thought to result from release of 'hormone-like' substances from the tumour (Chisholm 1980; Sufrin et al. 1989). The most frequent of these syndromes is hypercalcaemia resulting from the secretion of parathyroid hormone-related peptide, isolated and originally sequenced from a human renal cell carcinoma and mapped to the short arm of chromosome 12 (Burtis et al. 1987). Although 10 per cent of patients at presentation have elevated calcium levels (Friocourt et al. 1982), the incidence in terminal metastatic patients may be as high as 34 per cent (Oliver 1989, unpublished).

Two other relatively rare effects of tumour products are polycythemia due to erythropoietin production by the tumour and hypertension due to renin production by the tumour. Although the full-blown clinical picture is rare, results using radioimmunoassays for erythropoietin and renin found elevated levels in 63 and 37 per cent of patients, respectively, without overt clinical effects (Sufrin et al. 1977), suggesting that the tumour might be producing an inert precursor, as is often seen in the tumour products, such as ACTH, secreted by patients with oat cell carcinoma of the lung.

Stauffer's syndrome (hepatic dysfunction syndrome)

The association of reversible hepatic dysfunction with non-metastatic renal carcinoma was first reported by Stauffer (1961). The syndrome encompasses the following features: hepatospleno-megaly, increased serum alkaline phosphatase, hypoalbuminaemia, hypoprothrombinaemia, prolonged prothrombin time, and hyper-gammaglobulinaemia. Various of these features are present in the absence of demonstrable metastases. Liver biopsy may show a variety of non-specific histological features, including Kupffer cell proliferation, focal lymphocytic infiltration, and focal necrosis.

The renal tumour is usually of the clear cell type (Utz et al. 1970).

Other rare syndromes resulting from systemic effects of renal carcinoma are listed in Table 3. The importance of these fascinating syndromes is that their presence does not necessarily imply metastatic spread and should not be taken as a contraindication to nephrectomy.

Renal carcinoma as an incidental finding

Most clinical series of patients with renal carcinoma contain a proportion which were discovered by chance, usually during investigation for some unrelated pathology. The proportion depends on the source of data. Careful post-mortem studies on hospital in-patients have shown that a significant number of cases are not diagnosed during life (Hajdu and Thomas 1967; Hellsten et al. 1981a,b). A series of 16 294 autopsies performed in Malmo, Sweden, revealed 350 cases of renal carcinoma, 235 of which were unrecognized during life (Hellsten et al. 1981a,b). This series included patients with metastatic disease. From the literature, it would appear that the proportion of tumours discovered incidentally is increasing. Riches et al. (1951) reported that 4 per cent of 1746 tumours were an incidental discovery, Skinner et al. (1971) detailed 7 per cent of 309 carefully studied patients. Ueda and Mihara (1987) found that two out of 16 (13 per cent) patients presenting between 1976 and 1980 had their tumour found by chance, compared with 13 out of 37 (35 per cent) between 1981 and 1985. In a small series, Konnak and Grossman (1986) described seven out of 56 (13 per cent) tumours discovered incidentally during the period 1961–1973, compared with 22 out of 46 (48 per cent) during the 4 years from 1980.

An increasing proportion of the submerged part of the 'iceberg' of renal tumour incidence is thus coming to light and most likely reflects the increasing use of sophisticated imaging techniques such as computer assisted tomography, ultrasound, and magnetic resonance imaging.

DIAGNOSIS AND INVESTIGATIONS

Cystic or solid?

Renal cystic masses are common and malignant tumours relatively uncommon. The majority of renal mass lesions do not therefore require treatment but must be accurately diagnosed. This imposes a heavy responsibility on those involved with generating and reporting the investigative images. There are now well-established criteria for distinguishing suspicious from non-suspicious renal masses and these must be applied methodically if malignancy is not to be overlooked.

The commonest mass lesions are cysts and a classification of renal cysts proposed by Bosniak (1986) is depicted in Table 4.

The first suspicion of a renal mass may be aroused by clinical examination, plain radiography, intravenous urogram, ultrasound, or computerized tomography. Ultrasound and/or computerized tomography will usually resolve the nature of the lesion. If not, then radionuclide imaging, angiography, magnetic resonance imaging, or fine-needle aspiration cytology may be required to define the diagnosis. In the occasional patient the best of imaging techniques fail to give a clear answer. The options are to repeat the investigations after a set period of 3–4 months or to undertake surgical exploration. If the patient is fit, the latter approach is

Table 4 Classification and management of renal cystic masses (modified from Bosniak 1986)

Category	Description	Management
I	Simple benign cyst (sharply marginated, smooth thin walls, homogeneous water density content (0–20 HU[a]), no enhancement with contrast	None
II	Minimally complicated benign cyst (septated, minimal calcification, infected cysts, high-density cyst)	None
III	Complicated cyst	Further evaluation
IV	Malignant lesions with cystic components (irregular margins, solid or vascular elements)	Excision

[a]Hounsfield units.

recommended as surprisingly large tumours may be present in spite of dubious imaging. In addition to diagnostic information, imaging reveals evidence of tumour stage, the reliability of which is discussed below.

Pseudotumours

Felson and Moskowitz (1969) described 'a real or simulated renal mass, roentgenologically resembling neoplasm, but histologically consisting of normal renal parenchyma'. Such lesions are referred to as renal pseudotumours and are usually first detected by intravenous urogram. The differentiation from more sinister lesions is not always possible on the intravenous urogram appearances but radionuclide imaging will usually resolve the issue, with absence of any 'cold' areas in the region of the mass, after administration of the isotope (Pollack *et al.* 1974). Ultrasound, computed tomography with and without contrast and, rarely, angiography may also be necessary to distinguish lobation, regenerate nodules, and columns of Bertin from pathological lesions. Renal sinus fat and compression of the collecting system by overlying blood vessels are other sources of pseudotumours (Feldman *et al.* 1978).

A normal intravenous urogram does not exclude the diagnosis of renal carcinoma; 5–10 per cent of tumours may be missed by this imaging technique (Glen *et al.* 1989). Three of nine small neoplasms, less than 3 cm in diameter when first imaged, were not visible on the intravenous urogram, even in retrospect, and a further three were overlooked (Curry *et al.* 1986). Ultrasound can be used to evaluate patients with persistent haematuria after intravenous urogram and cystoscopic examination have failed to show a lesion.

Angiomyolipoma

These lesions are usually asymptomatic and may be discovered incidentally during imaging for other pathology. The characteristic features on imaging are hyperechogenicity on ultrasound and fat attenuation on computerized tomography. Complex features on imaging raises the possibility of the rare combination of angiomyolipoma and renal carcinoma and should suggest further investigation and exploration.

Transitional cell carcinoma

The diagnosis of collecting system lesions depends heavily on good quality intravenous urography in a suitably prepared patient. This investigation should be done in all patients with haematuria and periodically in those being followed after a previous diagnosis of urothelial cancer at other sites. The presence of a filling defect, distortion of the calyces, and the finding of a poorly or non-functioning kidney all raise the possibility of urothelial tumour. Filling defects may require better definition with retrograde ureteropyelography, which is best done with a combination of

screening under image intensification and single-shot radiographs. Oblique views, use of dilute contrast, and post-drainage images may be helpful in the identification of small lesions.

Urine cytology by an experienced cytologist is most helpful when unequivocally positive, but may be negative in the presence of well-differentiated tumours. The combination of a typical filling defect on intravenous urogram and positive voided urine cytology can establish the diagnosis. If the voided urine cytology is negative or equivocal, then urine samples can be obtained from the upper tract at the time of retrograde studies. The acquisition of the sample can be assisted by lavage of the renal pelvis with saline or by brushing the lesion. This is best performed before injection of contrast as this may distort the cytological appearances, producing a false-positive result. False-positive cytology may also result from coincidental inflammatory lesions of the urinary tract, such as calculi and infection. Sarnacki *et al.* (1971) have reported a 6 per cent false-positive rate and a false-negative rate of up to 38 per cent in a study of 2400 urine specimens from 1400 patients. The diagnosis of urothelial malignancy cannot therefore be made by cytological studies in isolation.

Diagnostic ureteroscopy can be performed if the foregoing studies fail to establish a diagnosis. Ureteroscopy using rigid instruments is more likely to produce valuable additional information for ureteric lesions than caliceal lesions, as the view above the pelvi-ureteric junction (PUJ) is limited. Flexible ureteroscopes are not widely available but may give a better view of the pelvis and calices.

In the presence of ureteric obstruction, antegrade pyelography, using percutaneous needle puncture, may occasionally be necessary. This technique should be used with caution, however, as there is a small but definite risk of tumour implantation after puncture of the collecting system. This caveat should be extended to the risk of perforation of the ureter at the time of ureteroscopy.

Ultrasound is less useful for urothelial lesions than in the diagnosis of parenchymal renal tumours, but may be performed in the evaluation of a non-functioning kidney. Similarly, computerized tomography is less sensitive in the diagnosis of small collecting-system tumours and is not usually necessary in making the diagnosis. Tumours of the collecting system may invade the renal parenchyma and vice versa. When it is not clear from the intravenous urogram whether a lesion arises from the parenchyma or the collecting system, then computerized tomography with and without contrast may be of considerable value (Gatewood *et al.* 1982). The distinction of parenchymal from urothelial tumours is of practical importance as the necessity for complete removal of the ureter depends upon the nature of the tumour.

Pre-operative biopsy or fine aspiration cytology is not usually necessary or desirable on account of the risks of malignant cellular extravasation. The procedures recommended by the UICC for assessment are physical examination, imaging, and endoscopy.

Table 5 Robson staging system

Stage 1
  Confined to kidney
Stage 2
  Perirenal fat involvement but confined to Gerota's fascia
Stage 3
  A Gross renal vein or inferior vena cava involvement
  B Lymphatic involvement
  C Vascular and lymphatic involvement
Stage 4
  A Adjacent organs other than adrenal involved
  B Distant metasases

STAGING

Pre-operative staging

Imaging for staging purposes has included nephrotomography, arteriography, digital subtraction angiography, inferior vena cavography, ultrasound, lymphangiography, conventional and dynamic computerized tomography, radionuclide imaging, and magnetic resonance imaging. A number of studies have reported comparisons of information derived from each method (Frohmuller *et al.* 1987; London *et al.* 1989). Ideally, the least expensive, least invasive method should be employed to obtain the necessary information about size, site(s), local extension, nodal masses, liver metastases, and venous extension. In current practice, ultrasound and computerized tomography will provide adequate information in 90 per cent of patients. Angiography has been largely displaced by the less invasive methods, but retains an important place if parenchymal preserving surgery is considered or if embolization techniques are to be used. Magnetic resonance imaging has the advantage of displaying the renal vessels without the need for contrast injection, but has the disadvantages of long imaging times and motion artefact (Karstaedt *et al.* 1986).

From the surgeon's viewpoint, the essential pre-operative staging includes information on the presence or absence of renal vein and caval tumour extension and the status of the opposite kidney. The upper level of any caval extension must be imaging to allow planning of the surgical approach. Ultrasound is the simplest investigation and has been shown to demonstrate adequately the inferior vena cava from the renal veins to the diaphragm in 36 per cent of patients (Webb *et al.* 1987). In the same study, 12 out of 28 ultrasound examinations failed to show the whole of the cava and in six the cava was completely obscured by bowel gas or obesity. No case of caval extension was missed. If ultrasound is technically incomplete or doubt remains, then computerized tomography or inferior vena cavography is required. If the cava is obstructed, then the upper limit of the tumour extension can be visualized with echocardiography or superior vena cavography. Different surgeons will have differing opinions on what is resectable and what inoperable. The presence of a huge nodal mass around the renal vessels may make complete resection difficult if not impossible and such patients will have a poor prognosis with or without surgery (see below).

Post-operative staging

Flocks and Kadesky (1958) proposed one of the first staging systems for renal carcinoma, based on an analysis of 353 patients followed for 5 years or more. This system was subsequently modified by

Table 6 TNM classification of renal carcinoma

T Primary tumour
  TX Primary tumour cannot be assessed
  T0 No evidence of primary tumour
  T1 Tumour 2.5 cm or less in greatest dimension, limited to the kidney
  T2 Tumour >2.5 cm in greatest dimension, limited to the kidney
  T3 Tumour extends into the major veins or invades the adrenal gland or perinephric tissues but not beyond Gerota's fascia
      T3a Tumour invades the adrenal gland or perinephric tissues but not beyond Gerota's fascia
      T3b Tumour grossly extends into renal vein(s) or vena cava
  T4 Tumour invades beyond Gerota's fascia

N Regional lymph nodes (The regional lymph nodes are the hilar, abdominal para-aortic, and paracaval nodes. Laterality does not affect the N categories.)
  NX Regional lymph nodes cannot be assessed
  N0 No regional lymph nodes
  N1 Metastasis in a single lymph node 2 cm or less in greatest dimension
  N2 Metastasis in a single lymph node >2 cm but not >5 cm in greatest dimension or multiple lymph nodes, none >5 cm in greatest dimension
  N3 Metastases in a lymph node >5 cm in greatest dimension

M Distant metastasis
  MX Presence of distant metastasis can not be assessed
  M0 No distant metastasis
  M1 Distant metastasis
The categories M1 and pM1 can be further specified according to the site of the metastasis

Stage grouping

Stage	T	N	M
Stage I	T1	N0	M0
Stage II	T2	N0	M0
Stage III	T1	N1	M0
	T2	N1	M0
	T3a	N0, N1	M0
	T3b	N0, N1	M0
Stage IV	T4	Any N	M0
	Any T	N2, N3	M0
	Any T	Any N	M1

Robson *et al.* (1969) and is depicted in Table 5. The appreciation that venous extension and lymph node metastases have differing effects on the outcome (see below) led to subdivision of stage 3 into 3A, B, and C.

The TNM system is shown in Table 6. The fourth edition of the TNM classification of malignant tumours (Hermanek and Sobin 1987) applies to renal carcinoma only. The recommended procedures for the assessment of the T, N, and M categories are physical examination and imaging, without specification. The pathological classification (pTNM) categories correspond to the clinical classification (T, N, M).

Staging of transitional cell carcinoma

Pre-operative staging should include a chest radiograph. Bone scintiscan and abdominal computerized tomography may be added if the symptoms or imaging studies raise the possibility of local invasion and if cytology suggests a high-grade lesion. The TNM clinical and pathological classifications are similar to those used in bladder cancer and are shown in Table 7. Assessment of function in the opposite kidney is necessary before planning definitive management.

Table 7 TNM classification for renal pelvis and ureter

T   Primary tumour
  TX   Primary tumour cannot be assessed
  T0   No evidence of primary tumour
  Tis   Carcinoma *in situ*
  Ta   Papillary non-invasive carcinoma
  T1   Tumour invades subepithelial connective tissue
  T2   Tumour invades muscularis
  T3   Tumour invades beyond muscularis into peri-ureteric or peri-pelvic fat or renal parenchyma
  T4   Tumour invades adjacent organs or through the kidney into the peri-nephric fat

N   Regional lymph nodes
  NX   Regional lymph nodes cannot be assessed
  N0   No regional lymph nodes
  N1   Metastasis in a single lymph node 2 cm or less in greatest dimension
  N2   Metastasis in a single lymph node >2 cm but not >5 cm in greatest dimension, or multiple lymph nodes, none >5 cm in greatest dimension
  N3   Metastases in a lymph node >5 cm in greatest dimension

M   Distant metastasis
  MX   Presence or distant metastasis can not be assessed
  M0   No distant metastasis
  M1   Distant metastasis
The categories M1 and pM1 can be further specified according to the site of the metastasis

Stage grouping

Stage	T	N	M
Stage 0	Tis	N0	M0
	Ta	N0	M0
Stage I	T1	N0	M0
Stage II	T2	N0	M0
Stage III	T3	N0	M0
Stage IV	T4	N0	M0
	Any T	N1, N2, N3	M0
	Any T	Any N	M1

SURGICAL MANAGEMENT

Management of benign tumours

Much will depend on the confidence to be placed in the imaging results. Conservative management of, for example angiomyolipoma, has been recommended provided the lesion is asymptomatic and there are no complex features to suggest carcinoma. However, the patient should be followed to ensure that the tumour is not silently enlarging or producing symptoms or loss of renal function. In reality many mass lesions are not accurately diagnosed pre-operatively and the surgeon must proceed on the assumption of malignancy. Conservative resection by parenchymal sparing surgery can be recommended for von Hippel–Lindau syndrome and angiomyolipoma. Renal arterial embolization has also been advocated for the management of angiomyolipoma (Oesterling *et al.* (1986).

Management of malignant parenchymal tumours

Surgical excision is recommended for all solid and suspicious renal neoplasms unless the patient is unfit for surgery or there is good evidence of a benign nature of the mass.

Radical nephrectomy

The principles of surgery for renal tumours are to gain early access to the vessels and ligate them before manipulation and dissection of the tumour and to remove the tumour, kidney, and adrenal with a margin of healthy tissue. The anatomical plane between Gerota's fascia and the surrounding structures provides a convenient method of achieving this aim in the majority of cases. Local extension of tumour into the mesentery, colon, pancreas, duodenum, and diaphragm may involve a more extensive dissection. In the absence of metastases or involved lymph nodes, such extended local resection is justified by improved survival and local control. Whether an anterior transperitoneal, thoracoabdominal, or loin approach is used is dependent on the preference of the surgeon, the build of the patient, and the site and size of the tumour. Large, upper-pole tumours may be best approached with a thoracoabdominal incision.

For small, polar tumours, the extent of the surgical procedure is currently debated and it is not clear whether the standard radical nephrectomy is necessary in every case. The issue of conservative surgery is discussed under the heading Bilateral tumours. In the absence of a controlled comparison of the alternatives, radical nephrectomy seems likely to remain the standard treatment if the opposite kidney is normal.

Lymphadenectomy in renal carcinoma

There is continuing debate about the role of lymphadenectomy as part of the primary treatment for renal carcinoma. The procedure is recommended in order to obtain pathological information which may be of prognostic value and, by some, as a therapeutic procedure with the hope of completely excising disease confined to the surgical specimen. The reported incidence of lymph node metastases depends on the source of the data. A review of surgical reports has shown that regional node metastases are present in 5–10 per cent of tumours confined by the renal capsule, approximately 30 per cent of tumours extending beyond the capsule, and 50 per cent of those with distant metastases (Pizzocaro *et al.* 1983). Post-mortem studies have shown a variable distribution of involved nodes. Hulten *et al.* (1969) reported that most involved lymph nodes were in the renal hilum or near the origin of the renal vessels from the aorta and vena cava. However, involved nodes were also found on the contralateral side of the great vessels or in the supraclavicular area. The ipsilateral iliac nodes were the sole site of lymphatic metastases in one case. Hellsten *et al.* (1983) reported lymphatic spread in 37 out of 235 (16 per cent) of clinically unrecognized cases found at post-mortem. Nodal metastases were usually multiple and multifocal, being almost as common in the mediastinum as in the retroperitoneum. Concomitant metastases were common in subjects with positive nodes. One possible explanation for this irregular pattern of lymphatic spread may be the pronounced neovascularity that occurs in many renal tumours. It appears that lymphatics, developing with the new blood vessels, can disseminate tumour to any part of the retroperitoneum and posterior mediastinum. This unpredictable pattern of lymphatic spread complicates the composition of surgical strategies for lymphadenectomy, although some authors continue to claim therapeutic benefit from extensive lymphadenectomy (Pizzocaro *et al.* 1983). It is noteworthy that patients in the series by Robson *et al.* (1969), who had the best-reported survival after radical nephrectomy plus clearance of the ipsilateral abdominal nodes, had pre-operative mediastinoscopy and biopsy of suspicious nodes. Patients with positive mediastinal nodes were then excluded from analysis. Without such selection, any benefit from lymphadenectomy

Table 8 Relationship of anatomical extent of tumour to survival (based on data from Skinner *et al.* 1971)

Anatomical extent of tumour	Survival (%)	
	5 year	10 year
Confined by renal capsule	65	56
Renal vein alone	66	49
Renal vein+perinephric fat	50	33
Renal vein+regional nodes	0	0
Perinephric fat alone	47	20
Regional nodes alone	33	17
Direct extension to nearby structures	0	0

must be small and has to be balanced against the extra time, morbidity, and mortality involved with the larger dissection. No controlled data have been reported on this subject, although a multicentre study is currently in progress. The majority of British urological surgeons do not undertake extensive lymphadenectomy (Ritchie and Chisholm 1983).

Since the majority of patients having involved nodes will have these around the hilum and vascular pedicle, biopsy of such nodes will help in identifying those patients at risk of relapse or progression after nephrectomy.

Management of tumour extension to the vena cava

Tumour extension to the vena cava is a distinctive feature of renal carcinoma, it occurs in up to 10 per cent of patients, and requires careful pre-operative assessment. Imaging must always take account of the possible presence of renal vein and caval extension (see the section entitled Pre-operative staging). It is possible to fragment a tumour and induce pulmonary tumour embolism by manipulation of the veins in ignorance of the existence of tumour extension.

The presence of tumour in the vena cava used to be considered as implying a poor prognosis and many such patients were deemed inoperable. Studies by Skinner *et al.* (1972), Cherrie *et al.* (1982), and Libertino *et al.* (1987) have shown that venous extension alone, does not impart a poor prognosis, if it is completely removed. Positive lymph nodes in association with the venous extension are linked to diminished survival (Table 8).

Successful surgery involves accurate assessment of the upper level of the caval extension. Extension to the first few centimetres of the suprarenal cava can be managed by exclusion of the tumour using a vascular clamp. Larger subhepatic extension involves dissection to control the opposite renal vein and clamping the cava above or below the liver. Extension above the level of the hepatic veins usually necessitates a combined cardiac and urological approach, usually with cardiopulmonary bypass, to avoid the risks of a large loss of blood and fragmentation of the tumour thrombus. Direct invasion of the wall or complete obstruction may require resection of the cava. This does not usually produce post-operative problems if the caval obstruction has been chronic. Such procedures are usually performed for right-sided tumours and the left renal veins must be ligated close to the cava to allow for venous drainage from the left kidney via the adrenal/azygous systems. In the case of left-sided tumours, ligation of the right renal vein is much more likely to produce renal failure and anastomosis to the portal vein may be necessary.

Adjuvant treatment of localized disease

Radiotherapy has been used in the perioperative period as an adjunct to surgery. Early, uncontrolled studies suggested that pre-operative

adjuvant radiotherapy improved survival, but a randomized study performed by van der Werf-Messing (1973) showed no difference in survival at 5 years if 30 Gy or no therapy was given before surgery. Similar results are available for post-operative radiotherapy, with uncontrolled reports suggesting improved survival but a controlled study by Finney (1973), comparing surgery alone with surgery and post-operative radiotherapy, showing that the survival of those treated with post-operative radiotherapy was worse. Although still a controversial topic there seems little objective evidence to support the use of radiotherapy in the management of local disease. Use of adjuvant hormonal therapy in M0 disease is discussed in the section on management of metastatic disease. Adjuvant biological therapy with interferon is currently under trial.

Bilateral tumours and tumour in a solitary kidney

Bilateral renal carcinoma occurs with a frequency as high as 3 per cent. Wickham (1975) reported on 25 patients with bilateral tumours. In 16 patients where no attempt was made to remove the tumours, all were dead within 5 months. In seven patients the tumours were treated aggressively by total nephrectomy on one side and partial nephrectomy on the other; five of these patients remained alive at 23 months' mean follow-up. Two patients had died after a mean follow-up of 12 months.

Some authors have suggested that bilateral synchronous disease has a better prognosis than asynchronous disease (Jacobs *et al.* 1980; Zincke and Swanson 1982). Zincke and Swanson (1982) reported a 5 year survival of 77.8 per cent for synchronous tumours compared with 37.5 per cent survival for asynchronous disease. They did, however, note a tendency for the synchronous tumours to be of lower grade and stage. Smith *et al.* (1984) have disputed this difference in survival and state that survival seems to be related more to the stage of the tumour and the adequacy of tumour resection that the fate of the opposite kidney.

In operable patients with bilateral tumours, the usual approach is to perform a radical nephrectomy on the side with the more advanced lesion and conservative surgery on the other side. The options for conservative resection include, enucleation, partial nephrectomy *in situ*, extracorporeal partial nephrectomy (bench surgery) with autotransplantation, or complete nephrectomy with post-operative dialysis. Tumour enucleation has been reported to produce a 90 per cent 3 year survival in 33 patients with bilateral disease or tumour in a solitary kidney (Novick *et al.* 1986). This group of patients was carefully selected from 1286 undergoing treatment for renal tumours over the same time period and comprised only low-grade lesions. Five of the patients had von Hippel–Lindau syndrome. After a mean follow-up of 45 months, there were two local recurrences. In contrast to the latter authors' enthusiastic support for enucleation, is the reported experience of three local recurrences after enucleation (Smith *et al.* 1984) and the demonstration by Marshall *et al.* (1986) that there was residual tumour in six out of 15 kidneys after *ex vivo* enucleation of the tumour. The size of the tumours in this latter study varied from 5 to 12 cm and all grade 1 tumours had negative tumour beds, whereas all grade 3 tumours were associated with residual disease. In another study, careful microscopic examination revealed that neoplastic cells invaded the pseudocapsule in 23 out of 25 tumours ranging in size between 1.2 and 12 cm. Even in a well-differentiated lesion with a diameter of only 1.2 cm, it was possible to demonstrate breakthrough of the pseudocapsule and spreading into the adjacent normal renal tissue (Rosenthal *et al.* 1984). These latter studies indicate that resection of a margin of normal kidney is necessary to avoid leaving malignant cells in the bed and, thus, partial nephrectomy may be a better procedure. For small, well-differentiated lesions, enucleation gives short-term survival, close to that of radical nephrectomy (Zincke *et al.* 1985) and it is suggested that partial nephrectomy should improve on this experience and be worthy of further careful evaluation in patients with suitably placed, small, well-differentiated, asymptomatic lesions, and a normal contralateral kidney. Topley *et al.* (1984) have reported 5 year cancer survival of 70 per cent after partial nephrectomy, but there was a 13 per cent incidence of local recurrence in the renal remnant. If possible, the partial nephrectomy should be performed *in situ* as the complication rate (17 per cent) is increased to 43 per cent if bench surgery is required (Marberger *et al.* 1981).

Highly selective arterial embolization and instillation of radioactive seeds or microspheres containing mitomycin have also been undertaken in situations where it is imperative to preserve renal tissue, but no long-term results have been reported.

Overall, the data suggest that the natural course of bilateral tumours and tumour in a single kidney, is to progress with early death of the patient and that aggressive intervention can be performed safely with a significant improvement in survival. If parenchymal sparing surgery is not possible, bilateral nephrectomy followed by dialysis can be considered. Most programmes accepting such patients will insist on a period of approximately 2 years before transplantation will be considered. Such patients raise numerous clinical and ethical problems and the quality of life should be a major factor in formulating the management plan.

Management of urothelial tumours

Definitive management is by surgical removal of the kidney, ureter, and a cuff of bladder mucosa around the ureter. Subtotal removal of the upper urinary tract on the side of the lesion is associated with a significant risk (up to 84 per cent) of recurrent malignancy in the ureteric stump (Droller 1986).

Traditionally the nephroureterectomy has been performed by a retroperitoneal approach through two incisions. The kidney and upper ureter are mobilized through a standard loin approach to the kidney. Maintaining continuity of the ureter, the kidney is placed in a pouch in the retroperitoneum and the superior incision closed. Using a separate incision, the distal ureter is then dissected from within and outside the bladder to allow *en bloc* removal.

A modification of the two-incision approach has been suggested by Abercrombie (1972). This modified nephroureterectomy involves transurethral resection of the intramural ureter using a resectoscope. The resection is carried through the full thickness of the bladder until the ureter is seen lying free in the perivesical fat. The bladder is drained with a catheter and the patient turned for a standard loin approach to the kidney. A ligature is placed around the ureter early in the dissection. After mobilization of the kidney, the ureter can be removed from above by careful finger dissection. This approach has the obvious advantage of avoiding the lower incision and ensures complete removal of the ureter. The defect in the bladder wall heals readily with catheter drainage for 8 days. Concern expressed about a higher incidence of local tumour recurrence at the site of the distal resection (Hetherington *et al.* 1986) has not been confirmed (Abercrombie *et al.* 1988). Both the modified approach and conventional nephroureterectomy are associated with a 30 per cent probability of subsequent bladder tumours. However, the modified approach should be confined to renal tumours; ureteric tumours are not considered suitable.

Endoscopic management

Patients with bilateral tumours or compromised renal function in the opposite kidney may not be suitable for definitive management by nephroureterectomy. In such patients, local management may be effected by segmental resection or endoscopic techniques, either using the ureteroscope or by percutaneous access to the collecting system. Percutaneous approaches have the advantage of a better view and the ability to insert larger instruments for resection or coagulation of the tumour. The disadvantage of this approach, however, is the difficulty of assessment of the depth of tumour penetration and the need to irradiate the percutaneous tract to prevent tumour implantation. Long-term follow-up of patients treated by endoscopic surgery is not available and, as yet, these techniques can not be recommended for patients with a normal contralateral kidney and ureter.

Chemotherapy and biological therapy

Where surgical resection is not possible, chemotherapy may be used by both systemic and topical application. Infusion of drugs with proven efficacy against urothelial lesions of the bladder (for example, mitomycin and bacille Calmette–Guérin) can be performed via a nephrostomy tube in patients with multifocal non-invasive urothelial renal tumours and responses have been reported. Systemic therapy for patients with invasive transitional cell carcinoma of the upper tract, metastases, or those unsuitable for surgery has not been thoroughly investigated as a separate entity. There have been cases of upper-tract tumours included in most series of transitional cell carcinoma treated with combination chemotherapy (Sternberg *et al.* 1988). There has been little evidence that the response rate is any different from that seen for bladder cancer metastases. In the series reported by Oliver *et al.* (1985) two of the best responses were in patients with metastases from upper-tract tumours, one with 18 months' complete remission of supraclavicular lymph nodes after single-agent methotrexate and one with 9 months' near complete remission of massive liver metastases.

Evidence for the value of biological therapy is less clear-cut, although there was one anecdotal report of a patient with multifocal superficial transitional cell carcinoma who achieved durable complete remission beyond 3 years of renal pelvic ureteric and bladder tumours after 3 months' treatment with α-interferon (Oliver *et al.* 1986a; Oliver 1989).

RESULTS OF SURGERY

Renal carcinoma

Survival after nephrectomy for renal carcinoma is related to the anatomical extent of the disease and the pathological prognostic factors discussed above. The presence or absence of metastases is the most important determinant of survival. Patients with no evidence of metastases have a 90 per cent 2 year survival, compared with 20 per cent for those with metastases (Selli *et al.* 1983).

For patients without distant metastases, survival is also related to the local anatomical extent of the disease, with involved lymph nodes having a significant adverse effect on survival (Table 8). Five year survival rates of up to 93 per cent have been reported for tumours confined by the renal capsule (Selli *et al.* 1983). For all other stages, there is a significant decline in survival, suggesting the presence of undetected metastatic disease at the time of nephrectomy. Patients at particular risk of recurrent or metastatic

Table 9 Extent of disease compared with symptomatic status in 3232 renal tumours

	Localized	Direct extension	Regional nodes	Distant metastases	Unknown
Asymptomatic (*n*=489)	77.5[a]	10.4	1.4	9.4	1.2
Symptoms unknown (*n*=295)	28.8	10.2	1.7	17.6	41.3
Symptomatic (*n*=2448)	43.9	21.9	4.7	28.0	1.5

[a]Figures are percentages.

disease are those with obvious tumour extension to nearby structures, those with positive regional lymph nodes, and those with evidence of tumour penetration into the perinephric fat. Such patients are therefore candidates for adjuvant therapy after nephrectomy.

Tumours discovered incidentally have a better prognosis (Thompson and Peek 1988) but this is most likely a reflection of the fact that they are of lower stage than those producing symptoms. Additional data have been obtained from the Cancer Surveillance Program, University of Southern California. This programme obtains information from hospital pathology reports for Los Angeles County, a population of approximately 7.5 million. Benign and malignant renal parenchymal tumours were separately identified using ICD9 codes and analysed according to presenting symptoms, sex, and extent of disease at presentation. Cases of Wilms' tumour were excluded from the analysis. Of 3232 histologically confirmed cases of renal carcinoma, 77.5 per cent of those without symptoms had disease confined to the kidney and only 9.4 per cent had distant metastases. By comparison, only 43.9 per cent of those with symptoms had localized disease and 28 per cent had metastases at presentation (*p*=0.001) (Table 9).

Transitional cell carcinoma

Evaluation of the results of nephroureterectomy for transitional cell tumours of the kidney is complicated by the variety of staging systems reported in the literature. Furthermore, factors which may influence the outcome, such as tumour grade, ploidy (Oldbring *et al.* 1989), and the association with urothelial tumours or carcinoma *in situ* at other sites, are not reported consistently. Within these limitations, it appears that the prognosis for patients having low-grade tumours with no evidence for muscle invasion is excellent (5 year survival approximately 90 per cent). Penetration of tumour into the peripelvic or perirenal area, in association with high tumour grade, carries a poor prognosis (5 year survival 5–10 per cent) (Mufti *et al.* 1989).

MANAGEMENT OF METASTATIC RENAL CARCINOMA

Natural history of metastases

There are few well-documented instances where large cohorts of unselected patients with malignant tumours have been followed without intervention to establish the natural history of the disease. For breast cancer (Bloom 1960) and bladder cancer (Marshal *et al.* 1956) reasonable reliable data exist and allow a confident assertion that, in addition to its palliative value, surgery does improve

survival. For renal carcinoma, Riches (1964) reported on a series of 443 untreated patients selected on the basis of being either 'inoperable' or unfit for surgery. The crude survival rate was 4.4 per cent at 3 years and 1.7 per cent at 5 years. Without more details of the precise staging, it is difficult to extrapolate this survival to current surgical results, but the data strongly suggest a significant survival advantage for surgical management. In addition, the unpleasant local symptoms and high incidence of extrarenal manifestation of this tumour, even in the absence of metastases, provide adequate justification for surgical intervention.

For patients who present with metastases or develop them after surgical removal, the evidence for value of therapeutic intervention is considerably more controversial, despite the wide range of therapy reported to have benefit, such as surgery, hormone therapy, chemotherapy, and various immunological treatments. The reason for this is the lack of data from large-scale studies of untreated patients. It has long been known that patients with metastatic renal carcinoma can, even untreated, have prolonged periods of 'stable' disease and some even demonstrate spontaneous regression of measurable metastases. This has been well documented since the observations of Everson and Cole (1966) that renal carcinoma had one of the highest incidences of spontaneous regression, although there is disagreement in the literature as to the precise frequency with which it occurs. Bloom (1972), in a review of 200 personal cases of renal carcinoma, reported two unexplained regressions (1 per cent) but, on review of the literature, estimated that the frequency was 0.3 per cent. Montie *et al.* (1977), reviewing the results of nephrectomy in patients with established metastases, reported four regressions out of 474 patients (0.8 per cent). Van der Werf-Messing and van Gilse (1971), investigating a series of 33 patients with established measurable metastases with frequent follow-up examination, reported a 24 per cent incidence of regression or non-progression of pulmonary metastases.

Many of these differences can be explained by the selection of cases, particularly the extent of the metastases and whether the primary tumour had been removed. In the review by Freed *et al.* (1977), 38 out of 51 of the documented regressions occurred after nephrectomy performed in the presence of metastases; 45 of the 51 patients who showed regression had lung metastases only, but three had metastases in bone and three in soft tissues, which completely regressed.

Tumour ploidy

A further characteristic of patients with longer survival is a diploid or near diploid DNA content of the tumour cells. In addition to use in patients with localized disease a statistically significant difference in survival has been noted after 15 months of follow-up in patients with metastases and diploid or near diploid tumours, when compared with aneuploid tumours (see the section entitled Prognostic factors). Although this study was performed using a variety of fresh, autopsy, aspiration biopsy, and paraffin-embedded material, a more recent study using fresh frozen samples of 32 primary renal tumours from patients who had metastases at the time of presentation has confirmed that ploidy accurately predicted those patients with a longer survival (Mukamel *et al.* 1988). Given its predictive value, the authors have suggested that measurement of tumour ploidy should be routinely used for future stratification of patients in clinical trials and a selection of those patients who are suitable for aggressive surgical therapy, such as excision of limited metastases. Golimbu *et al.* (1986) have related survival after aggressive treatment of metastases to a prognostic index, which may well reflect the ploidy of the tumour. Ten out of 21 patients had a primary tumour with a low prognostic index. Metastases developed in these patients a mean of 45.5 months after nephrectomy and they survived a mean of 69 months after excision of the initial metastasis. By comparison, 11 patients had a high prognostic index and developed their metastases on average 13.5 months after nephrectomy and they survived, on average, only 20 months.

Surgery for metastatic disease

Adjunctive nephrectomy in the face of established metastases at the time of diagnosis

If the patient has large-volume distant metastases or obvious bulky lymph node involvement so that metastatic disease volume exceeds that of the primary tumour, removal of the primary is usually not justifiable. For patients with operable primaries where primary tumour volume exceeds the volume of metastases, particular if small-volume lung disease, the situation is less clear-cut. Although there is no overall demonstrable survival benefit (Johnson et al. 1975), there is some suggestion that removal of the primary may increase the chance of 'spontaneous' regression of metastases, possibly by altering the immunological balance possibly by reducing tumour antigen load. There have been no series addressing this issue prospectively with regular chest radiographs, although in a retrospective literature review, Montie et al. (1986) reported a 0.8 per cent incidence of regression of metastases in patients undergoing nephrectomy, although in their own personal series of patients the incidence was 2 per cent. Although nephrectomy in a patient with metastatic disease has a measurable mortality and variable morbidity, a survey of British urologists showed that 89 per cent did not consider the presence of metastases an absolute contraindication to nephrectomy (Ritchie and Chisholm 1983). Patients with symptoms related to the primary and patients with knowledge of the existence of the primary, may benefit symptomatically and psychologically from surgery. Middleton (1967) has suggested that nephrectomy is only effective if the metastases involve only one organ (with the exception of the brain). Onishi et al. (1989) found that four out of 80 (5 per cent) patients having nephrectomy in the presence of metastases, survived for more than 3 years, whereas 51 out of 80 (64 per cent) died within 1 year. Patients with survival over 3 years had better performance status at presentation and a slower doubling time of pulmonary metastases. Retrospective analyses of data from clinical trials of immunotherapy, have shown some survival advantage in those in whom the primary was completely removed, especially those with small pulmonary metastases and nephrectomy may therefore be justified in the context of a clinical trial or where there are local symptoms.

Renal arterial embolization

Renal arterial embolization of the primary tumour is an alternative to nephrectomy in the presence of metastases, as symptoms from the primary tumour can be alleviated. However, this technique is not entirely without risk as it causes frequent side-effects including pain, ileus, and fever. Occasionally infection leading to abscess formation and inadvertent embolization of other structures can lead to death. When pre-operative embolization was combined with delayed radical nephrectomy and post-operative medroxyprogesterone acetate in 50 patients, there was regression of metastases in 24 per cent (Wallace et al. 1981), although in a subsequent cohort of 50 patients the response rate was 6 per cent (Swanson et al. 1983).

Excision of solitary metastases at time of diagnosis

Although surgical excision of solitary metastases has produced long-term disease-free survival, it is difficult to be sure how much of the beneficial response claimed for such treatment may relate to tumour biology rather than the surgical procedure, particularly in those patients presenting with metastases late after nephrectomy.

The first report of this approach was 1939 when Barney and Churchill reported excision of a primary renal tumour and a solitary pulmonary metastasis. The patient survived for 23 years before dying of ischaemic heart disease. This report stimulated an analysis of patients with apparent solitary metastases and a search for those suitable for aggressive treatment. Solitary metastases have been reported to occur in 1.6–3.2 per cent of patients at diagnosis (Middleton 1967; Tolia and Whitmore 1975). All of these series were reported from referral centres and may therefore be an overestimate of the true incidence.

Several authors have drawn attention to the difference in survival of those presenting with metastasis, only 4 out of 18 survived longer than 24 months, compared with 18 out of 26 in whom the metastasis developed after nephrectomy (O'Dea et al. 1978).

Radiotherapy for metastatic disease

Most studies of surgical treatment of patients with solitary metastases have been in symptomatic patients and it is far from clear how much the occasional long survivor is a reflection of the natural history of the disease or the effects of intervention.

Radiotherapy in contrast, although also used for patients with localized problems, has mainly been used to treat painful local recurrences in the renal bed or for metastases, so comparison with the results of surgery are not possible. Although a response does occur, it has been poorly documented in terms of frequency and duration. However, there are several reports of the abscopal effects of radiation (Freed et al. 1977).

Cytotoxic chemotherapy

Among agents considered to be effective in the treatment of renal cell carcinoma, vinblastine and lomustine (CCNU®) are the most active. However, the order of response is low, at less than 10 per cent (deKernion 1983). In order to improve upon the results obtained, these agents have been applied in unconventional schedules and in combination. Lomustine at a dosage of 120 mg/m^2 was given on day 1 and vinblastine at a dosage of 0.1 mg/kg on days 1 and 8 of a 6 week treatment cycle. No responses were seen in 15 patients (Sommer et al. 1985). Vinblastine was given as an infusion at a dosage of 1.5 mg/m^2 daily for 5 days, 3-weekly to 14 patients, one of whom responded (Tannock and Evans 1985). Methotrexate given in combination with vinblastine and bleomycin with or without tamoxifen resulted in ten partial responses of median duration (57 weeks) in 34 treated patients (Bell et al. 1984). Vinblastine at a dosage of 5 mg/m^2 on day 1, lomustine at 60 mg/m^2 on day 2, and hydroxyurea at 400 mg/m^2 twice daily on days 3 and 14 of a 4 week treatment cycle, together with medroxyprogesterone acetate, 1 g intramuscularly, weekly led to three partial responses in 26 patients (Brubaker et al. 1983).

Other newer agents have been applied to the treatment of renal cell carcinoma with almost as little effect as more established therapies. Mitozantrone is an anthracycline with less cardiotoxicity than Adriamycin®, which does not result in significant nausea nor alopecia. Fifty-eight patients with advanced renal cell carcinoma were treated with this agent at a dosage of 5 mg/m² weekly; no responses were seen (Garns *et al.* 1986). 4-Demethoxydaunorubicin, an Adriamycin® derivitive without significant cardiac toxicity was given at a dosage of 12.5 mg/m² 3-weekly to 19 patients, none of whom responded (Scher *et al.* 1985). Streptozocin was given to 18 evaluable patients at a dosage of 500 mg/m² for 5 days every month and one partial response was reported (Licht and Garnick 1987).

The response rate to chemotherapy is low, and provides an impetus and justification for the investigation of new therapies for renal cell cancer.

Hormone therapy and chemotherapy for metastases

The 7 per cent frequency of unexplained response makes it difficult to accept many previous reports suggesting that renal tumours are sensitive to progestogens or chemotherapy. Despite this, a survey of British urologists established that Provera® (medroxyprogesterone acetate) is the mainstay of treatment of patients with metastases in the United Kingdom (Ritchie and Chisholm 1983). This arose because of the observation that oestrogens induced renal cancer in hamsters and that progesterone would protect them from this effect. Using a tumour cell line developed from one of these tumours, which grew best in males, Bloom *et al.* (1963*b*) demonstrated that orchidectomy induced temporary regressions, which were overcome by oestradiol or testosterone. Because progesterone suppressed the original induction of this tumour in hamsters (Bloom *et al.* 1963*a*), this group then went on to use medroxyprogesterone acetate in patients and originally reported that 27 per cent responded for 2–35 (median 9) months (Bloom 1972, 1973).

With the discovery of progesterone receptors in renal tumours as well as in normal kidney, there developed a scientific rationale for this approach and a randomized trial using Provera® as adjuvant treatment after nephrectomy was undertaken (Pizzocaro *et al.* 1986). In the event the treatment arm actually did worse than the control: moreover, although those patients whose tumours had the highest level of receptor did better, so did receptor-positive patients in the control group. As the level of receptor was higher in the rim of normal kidney than in the tumour, the favourable prognosis seen in receptor-positive tumours presumably reflected the degree of differentiation of the tumour. This suggestion is supported by the most recent report of high-dose medroxyprogesterone (500 mg daily intramuscularly for 6 weeks) where a response was only seen in diploid tumours (Ljungberg *et al.* 1989).

Despite this observation and the fact that with time the response to medroxyprogesterone in patients with metastases fell from 17 to 5 per cent (Hrushesky and Murphy 1977), this progestogen is still used quite extensively. In part this is due to its effect on the appetite and general well-being of patients, which has always been more pronounced than its action on measurable tumour. There are two aspects of this work that need emphasis. First, unlike patients who undergo unexplained 'spontaneous' regression, more than 50 per cent of the responses in Bloom's original series (Bloom 1972, 1973) were in sites outside the lung. The second observation comes from the animal studies. To date there are three species, mouse (Murphy 1982), hamster (Bloom *et al.* 1963*a,b*), and rat (Jasmin and Riopelle 1970), in which hormones have been demonstrated to affect the growth rate of renal adenocarcinomas. Castration consistently works in all three models and exogenous oestrogen or testosterone induces growth of the tumours in both mouse (Murphy 1982) and hamster (Bloom *et al.* 1963*b*).

Table 10 Recent chemotherapy studies for metastatic renal carcinoma

	No. of cases	No. of responses
Cimetidine/coumarin (Marshall *et al.* 1987)	42	3+11 (33%)
Circadian modified 5-fluoropyrimidine (Hrushesky *et al.* 1989)	61	6+12 (30%)

Although there are human renal cell lines which grow in nude mice, none has so far been examined systemically for hormone sensitivity, although one *in vitro* study showed no response to medroxyprogesterone of a tumour from a patient who clinically responded (Cummings *et al.* 1977). Clearly, without more data surgical castration of patients with renal carcinoma would be excessive. However, there is now a wide range of medical hormone treatments available for prostatic cancer (Oliver 1985). Given the conflicting evidence from experimental animal models of renal carcinoma hormone therapy, further exploration of hormone therapy in human renal carcinoma in the nude mouse model should be an early priority for the future.

Although most phase 1 or 2 studies of new chemotherapeutic agents include patients with renal carcinoma, the frequency of response in the chemotherapy studies is no different from the observed spontaneous regression rate (Malpas 1982). So far none of the studies has been controlled, to exclude the possibility that treatment may actually accelerate tumour growth. There have been two recent reports using relatively simple non-toxic treatments (Table 10). The first (Marshall *et al.* 1987) used cimetidine and coumarin on the basis that this treatment would be shown to interfere with tumour angiogenesis and the second (Hrushesky *et al.* 1989) used fluoropyrimidine given by a 'time-modified infusion' (sinusoidal with peak centred around 18.00 h) to take advantage of observations on the circadian rhythm of rats suggesting that the therapeutic ratio could be increased.

Although these initial reports were encouraging, studies using increased numbers with a longer follow-up are required as preliminary results from the initial follow-up studies have not been as encouraging.

Biological therapy for renal carcinoma

Introduction

The concept that host factors can influence resistance to cancer has been in existence for a long time (Oliver *et al.* 1983; Oliver 1989). Renal carcinoma, because of the high incidence of spontaneous remission, has figured prominently in this history. It is of interest that with the more prolonged follow-up of transplant patients on immunosuppressive therapy, an increased incidence of renal cancer has been reported (Penn 1987).

Immunology of tumour rejection

So far there has been little evidence for abnormal cellular immunity against autologous tumour in patients with renal cell cancer. The most convincing data come from work by Vanky *et al.* (1986) who demonstrated (Table 11) that assays of autologous renal cancer/lymphocyte proliferation were more frequently positive than assays of autologous tumour cell lysis. It has long been known from studies of tumour cell suspensions that some kidney tumours had as much as 25 per cent of mononuclear cells consisting of infiltrating

Table 11 Assay of antitumour cellular immunity in patients with renal cancer (Vanky *et al.* 1986)

		No. of cases	Positive assay (%)
Antitumour lymphocyte	Renal cancer	18	72
proliferation	Other tumours	342	42
Antitumour lymphocyte	Renal cancer	57	32
cytotoxicity	Other tumours	139	38

Table 12 Biological treatment of renal cancer and response of measurable metastases

	No. of cases	No. of responses (CR+PR)	Alive at 2 years (%)
BCG vaccine			
Minton *et al.* (1976)	9	1+0	NA
Montie *et al.* (1982)	4	0+0	NA
Eidinger and Morales (1978)	8	1+2	NA
Oliver *et al.* (1988)	19	2+1	
Autologous tumour vaccine			
Tykka *et al.* (1978)	16	6+2	4
Control patients	12	0+1	22
Sahasrabudhe *et al.* (1986)	20	1+4	NA
Neidhart *et al.* (1980)	30	2+2	NA
Prager *et al.* (1980)	11	2+0	NA
Scharfe *et al.* (1989)	114	6+4	NA
Interferon			
(Natural leucocyte)	141	6+20 (18%)	NA
(Natural lymphoblastoid)	398	4+57 (15%)	NA
(Recombinant)	573	10+73 (14%)	NA
Interferon[a]	31	0+3 (10%)	NA
Interferon[a]	121	1+10 (9%)	NA
Interleukin-2[b]			
Low dose	77	0+8 (10%)	NA
High dose alone	109	7+15 (20%)	NA
High dose+LAK	131	10+18 (21%)	NA

[a] Data from Horoszewitz and Murphy (1989).
[b] Data from Bradley *et al.* (1989).
Abbreviations: CR+PR, complete response+partial response; LAK, lymphokine-activated killer cells; NA, not available.

T-lymphocytes, some of which produced autorosettes with T-cells *in vitro* (Oliver *et al.* 1983). Recent experience using interleukin-2 to clone out tumour-infiltrating lymphocytes has provided important insights into understanding the variability of immune defects that may contribute to the escape of tumour cells from immune surveillance. In contrast to melanoma, where approximately 50 per cent of studies on tumour-infiltrating lymphocytes yielded cytotoxic CD8$^+$ cells, showing a degree of selectivity for the specific autologous tumour (Topalian *et al.* 1987, 1988), no renal carcinoma tumour-infiltrating lymphocytes have shown any evidence for cytotoxicity restricted to autologous tumours (Belldegrun *et al.* 1988). This is of interest, in light of Vanky's observation that peripheral blood lymphocytes from patients with renal carcinoma demonstrate more frequent positivity in cell proliferation assays with the autologous tumour than in autologous tumour cell cytotoxicity assays. Recently interleukin-4, known to be important in helper cell regulation of cytotoxic cell specificity (Spitz *et al.* 1988), in part due to its ability to upregulate selectively class II HLA antigens or target cells, has also been shown to augment the cytotoxic activity of tumour-infiltrating lymphocytes grown from renal tumours when combined *in vitro* with interleukin-2. Such tumour-infiltrating lymphocytes also had more restricted cytotoxicity against the specific autologous tumour cells (Belldegrun *et al.* 1989). This suggests that a qualitative difference in class II expression in renal cancers compared to melanoma may be responsible for the lack of specificity of renal cancer tumour-infiltrating lymphocytes generated by interleukin-2 alone.

Active immunotherapy

Over the past 20 years, autologous tumour cell vaccine, BCG, interferon, and interleukin-2 have all been used to a greater or lesser extent in active immunotherapy (Table 12). Only for interleukin-2 and α-interferon is there a sufficiently large and consistent database from more than one centre to be confident of the true response rate in patients with measurable metastases. Most of the other studies have had relatively small numbers of cases, making it difficult to judge whether there was any difference in response rates. None of these studies had randomized, untreated controls, except the vaccine study of Tykka *et al.* (1978) and as the control patients in this case did not receive purified protein derivative (PPD) (which was the adjuvant used), it is not possible to say whether the improvement was a specific immunological response rather than a placebo response to the increased care and attention associated with receiving treatment. The response rates in all these studies are greater than the 7 per cent seen in patients observed without treatment. However, selection using exclusion criteria such as performance status and normal calcium, which have been entry criteria for some of these studies, makes it difficult to be absolutely sure of the response rates, as pointed out by Maladazys and deKernion (1986). Given this uncertainty, in the future it may be necessary to do a double-blind

cross-over study, with patients receiving immediate versus delayed treatment on progression, to exclude completely a placebo effect of treatment.

Passive (adoptive) immunotherapy

Passive specific therapy of cancer may be defined as any treatment involving immune sera or cells with specific activity against the patient's tumour. Most experience in passive immune therapy of infectious disease would suggest that such treatment is of limited value unless associated with a treatment aimed also at boosting specific immune memory involving T-cells. This observation and the lack of serologically well-defined tumour antigens in man has meant that more work has been done with adoptive cellular therapy rather than adoptive sero-therapy. Animal studies support the same view, though the number of experiments that have been performed in animal models to confirm the widely held concept that memory for immune resistance to malignant tumours is mediated by lymphocytes is relatively small. However, there are more lasting responses to adoptive cellular therapy than to adoptive serological therapy. In man there have been few direct comparisons (Rosenberg and Terry 1977). Most passive therapy has used lymphokine-activated killer cells, usually in combination with active therapy with systemic interleukin-2 because the original animal studies of Rosenberg demonstrated strong evidence of the benefit of combination therapy (Rosenberg *et al.* 1986). In man, as demonstrated in Table 12, the cumulative results in patients with renal carcinoma provide no evidence for benefit from lymphokine-activated killer cells, as compared with that achieved with interleukin-2 alone.

Table 13 The impact of schedule and dose on the response of metastatic renal cell carcinoma to α-interferon (modified from Horoszewitz and Murphy 1989)

Frequency of treatment	<3 mu/m²		3–10 mu/m²		>10 mu/m²	
	No. of cases	CR+PR (%)	No. of cases	CR+PR (%)	No. of cases	CR+PR (%)
>5/week	153	4+14	203	2+16	494	2+13
<5/week	51	2+8	54	0+13	147	0+13
<5/week+ vinblastine q 3 week	NA	–	NA	–	207	3+22

Abbreviations: CR+PR, complete response+partial response; NA, not available.

However, in the only randomized trial there was a small but statistically higher incidence of complete remission (Rosenberg *et al.* 1988). Given the logistic problems in preparing lymphokine-activated killer cells and the relative expense, this difference is insufficient to justify the routine use of these cells in therapy, particularly as there is no evidence that these cells home to tumour sites. Furthermore, biopsy studies of regressing lesions show that regression is associated with increased T-lymphocyte infiltration and augmented expression of tumour cell class II antigens (Cohen *et al.* 1986), suggesting that T-cells rather than lymphokine-activated killer cells are the ultimate mediators of rejection.

The lack of major gain from non-specific adoptive therapy led to studies aimed at developing specific cellular therapy, following the discovery that tumour-infiltrating lymphocytes showed greater specific anti-autologous tumour killing *in vitro*.

The initial clinical studies in melanoma with these specific tumour-infiltrating lymphocytes combined with interleukin-2 showed a 50 per cent response (Topalian *et al.* 1988), but there were very few complete remissions and the partial responses that occurred were relatively short-lived. Although similar responses have been reported from preliminary studies of tumour-infiltrating lymphocyte therapy for renal cancer (Kradin *et al.* 1989), the logistic problems and cost of tumour-infiltrating lymphocyte production exceed those of the production of lymphokine-activated killer cells and make it highly unlikely that such therapy will be widely used, although studies of tumour-infiltrating lymphocyte function are clearly very important in understanding the mechanism of action of cytokines.

Future developments in biological therapy

While a 15 per cent response to α-interferon treatment (Horoszewitz and Murphy 1989) and a 20 per cent response to treatment with interleukin-2 (Bradley *et al.* 1989) are better than any responses achieved consistently with any treatment previously used to treat this condition, these are certainly not major advances when compared to the 50 per cent 3 year survival for cardiac transplantation and in today's economic climate these treatments cannot easily be justified on a service basis. Recently there have been several laboratory-based studies demonstrating synergy between cytokines, most notably α-interferon and interleukin-2, but also interleukin-2 and tumour necrosis factor, interleukin-2 and interleukin-4, and γ-interferon and tumour necrosis factor. For the future, evaluation of combination cytokine therapy will be the major priority, although these studies will take time given the number of cytokines and the need to study dosage schedules in combination; the limited results to date suggest that the optimum dose in combination may not be the same as in single-agent treatment. Recent results suggest that, contrary to current practice, a low dose for prolonged periods produced more frequent and better responses (see Table 13). However, despite these difficulties, the preliminary results from combination studies are already looking encouraging, particularly in terms of the percentage of complete remissions, although it will be some time before the final results are available.

For the future, given the large number of possible combinations needing to be tested, it would seem important to define separate strategies for phase 2 and 3 testing. Thus, in view of the overall general low level of response, it would be reasonable to define a good-risk population using, for example DNA ploidy and clinical features such as metastatic site, extent of disease, and time to relapse. Poorer risk patients could be entered into phase 1 or 2 studies of experimental combinations.

CONCLUSION

Renal carcinoma, though relatively rare, has long been a tumour that provides interest to surgeon, physician, and biologist, alike. To the biologist, the myriad of extrarenal effects of tumour products continue to offer insights into the cellular function of normal renal cells as well as the nature of the malignant process, particularly in the area of oncogenes and their products. The lack of real insight into its cause, despite excellent animal models, is another area for future research, given our increasing understanding of the role of viruses in malignancy and the single report of herpes simplex protein in renal tumours.

To the surgeon, unresolved issues, such as the need for lymph node dissection and nephrectomy in the presence of metastases, will continue to raise controversy, but the real challenge is to develop a cost-effective way to diagnose this deep-seated tumour early. To the physician, the mounting evidence that this tumour responds to immunotherapy will focus attention on the newer immune modulators and the need for appropriate trial methodology to find ways of assessing the multiple options for using them in combination.

REFERENCES

Abercrombie GF (1972). Nephro-ureterectomy. *Proceedings of the Royal Society of Medicine*, **65**:1021–2.

Abercrombie GF, Eardley I, Payne SR, Walmsley BH, Vinnicombe J (1988). Modified nephro-ureterectomy. Long term follow-up with particular reference to subsequent bladder tumours. *British Journal of Urology*, **61**:198–200.

Alderson M (1982). The extent of the problem. In *Prevention of cancer* (ed. M Alderson), pp. 3–19. Edward Arnold, London.

Arner O, Blanck C, van Schreeb T (1965). Renal adenocarcinoma. Morphology, grading of malignancy, prognosis. A study of 197 cases. *Acta Chirugica Scandinavia*, **346** (Suppl.).

Barney JD, Churchill EJ (1939). Adenocarcinoma of the kidney with metastasis to the lung: cured by nephrectomy and lobectomy. *Journal of Urology*, **42**:269–76.

Bell DR, Aroney RS, Fisher RJ, Levi JA (1984). High dose methotrexate with leucovorin rescue vinblastine and bleomycin with or without tamoxifen in metastatic renal cell carcinoma. *Cancer Treatment Reports*, **68**:587–90.

Bell ET (1950). *Renal disease* (2nd edn). Lea and Febiger, Philadelphia.

Belldegrun A, Muul LM, Rosenberg SA (1988). Interleukin-2 expanded tumour infiltrating lymphocytes in human renal cell. Cancer: isolation, characterization and antitumour activity. *Cancer Research*, 48:206.

Bhatt GH, Bernadino ME, Graham SD (1983). CT diagnosis of renal metastases. *Journal of Computer Assisted Tomography*, 7:1032–4.

Bloom HJG (1964). The natural history of untreated breast cancer. *Annals of the New York Academy of Science*, 114:747–54.

Bloom HJG (1972). Renal cancer. In *Endocrine therapy in malignant disease*, pp. 339–67. W. B. Saunders, Philadelphia.

Bloom HJG (1973). Hormone-induced and spontaneous regression of metastatic renal cancer. *Cancer*, 32:1066–71.

Bloom HJG, Dukes CE, Mitchley BCV (1963a). Hormone-dependent tumours of the kidney. I The oestrogen-induced renal tumour of the Syrian hamster. Hormone treatment possible relationship to carcinoma of the kidney in man. *British Journal of Cancer*, 17:611–45.

Bloom HJG, Baker WH, Dukes CE, Mitchley BCV (1963b). Hormone-dependent tumours of the kidney. II Effect of endocrine ablation procedures on the transplanted oestrogen-induced renal tumour of the Syrian hamster. *British Journal of Cancer*, 17:646–56.

Blute ML, Malek RS, Segura JW (1988). Angiomyolipoma: clinical metamorphosis and concepts for management. *Journal of Urology*, 139:20–4.

Bosniak MA (1986). The current radiological approach to renal cysts. *Radiology*, 158:1–10.

Bradley M (1989). Cetus interleukin-2 studies in renal cell cancer. *Proceedings of the American Society of Clinical Oncology*, 8:C-519.

Brubaker LH, Troner MB, Birch R (1983). Advanced adenocarcinoma of the kidney: therapy with lomustine, vinblastine, hydroxyurea, and medroxyprogesterone acetate and regression analysis of factors relating to survival. *Cancer Treatment Reports*, 67(7/8):741–2.

Burtis W, et al. (1987). Identification of a novel 1700 Dalton parathyroid hormone-like adenylate cyclase-stimulating protein from a tumor associated with humoral hypercalcaemia of malignancy. *Journal of Biological Chemistry*, 262:7151–6.

Cherrie RJ, et al. (1982). Prognostic implications of vena caval extension of renal cell carcinoma. *Journal of Urology*, 128:910–12.

Chisholm GD (1980). Clinical and biochemical markers in renal carcinoma. In *Renal adenocarcinoma* (ed. G Sufrin and SA Beckley), UICC Report No. 10, pp. 182–98. WHO, Geneva.

Choyke PL, White EM, Zeman RK, Jaffe MH, Clark LR (1986). Renal metastases: clinicopathologic and radiologic correlation. *Radiology*, 162:359–63.

Claude A (1958). Adenocarcinoma renal endemique chez une souche de souris. *Revue Francaise d'Etudes Cliniques et Biologiques*, 3:261–2.

Cocchiara R, Tarro G, Flaminio G, Di Gioia M, Smeraglia R, Geraci D (1980). Purification of herpes simplex virus tumor associated antigen from human kidney carcinoma. *Cancer*, 46:1594–601.

Cohen AJ, et al. (1979). Hereditary renal cell carcinoma associated with a chromosome translocation. *New England Journal of Medicine*, 301:592–5.

Cohen PJ, Lotze MT, Roberts JR, Rosenberg SA, Jaffe ES (1987). Immunopathology of sequential tumour biopsies in patients on IL-2. *American Journal of Pathology*, 129:208–16.

Cummings KB, Wheelis RG, Nelson FW (1977). Role of hormones in growth kinetics of renal cell carcinoma *in vitro*. *Journal of Urology*, 117:269–71.

Curry NS, Schabel SI, Betsill WL (1986). Small renal neoplasms: diagnostic imaging, pathologic features and clinical course. *Radiology*, 158:113–17.

Dehner LP, Leestma JE, Price EB (1970). Renal cell carcinoma in children: a clinicopathological study of 15 cases and review of the literature. *Journal of Pediatrics*, 76:358–68.

deKernion JB (1982). Immunobiology of renal carcinoma. In *Scientific basis of urology* (2nd edn) (ed. GD Chisholm and D Innes Williams), pp. 690–9. William Heinemann, London.

deKernion JB (1983). Treatment of advanced renal cell carcinoma—traditional methods and innovative approaches. *Journal of Urology*, 130:2–7.

deKernion JB, Mukarnel E, Ritchie AWS, Blyth B, Hannah J, Bohman R (1989). The prognostic significance of the DNA content of renal carcinoma. *Cancer*, 64:1669–73.

Droller MJ (1986). Transitional cell cancer: upper tracts and bladder. In *Campbell's urology* (5th edn) (ed. PC Walsh, RF Gittes, AD Perlmutter, and TA Stamey), pp. 1343–4. WB Saunders, Philadelphia.

Eble JN, Hull MT (1984). Morphological features of renal oncocytoma: a light and electron microscopic study. *Human Pathology*, 15:1054–61.

Eidinger D, Morales A (1978). BCG immunotherapy of metastatic adenocarcinoma of the kidney. Workshop on Genitourinary Cancer Immunology, Iowa (ed. WW Bonney). *National Cancer Institute Monograph*, 49:339–41.

Eker R, Mossige J (1961). A dominant gene for renal adenoma in the rat. *Nature*, 189:858–9.

Everson TC, Cole WH (1966). *Spontaneous regression of cancer*, pp. 11–87. WB Saunders, Philadelphia.

Feldman AE, Pollack HM, Perri AJ, Karafin L, Kendall AR (1978). Renal pseudotumors: an anatomic-radiologic classification. *Journal of Urology*, 120:133–9.

Felson B, Moskowitz M (1969). Renal pseudotumors: the regenerated nodule and other lumps, bumps and dromedary humps. *American Journal of Roentgenology*, 107:720–9.

Finney R (1973). The value of radiotherapy in the treatment of hypernephroma—a clinical trial. *British Journal of Urology*, 45:258–69.

Flocks RH, Kadesky MC (1958). Malignant neoplasms of the kidney: an analysis of 353 patients followed five years or more. *Journal of Urology*, 79:196–201.

Freed SZ, Halperin JP, Gordon M (1977). Idiopathic regression of metastases from renal cell carcinoma. *Journal of Urology*, 118:538–42.

Friocourt L, Jouquan J, Khoury S, Richard R, Chomette G, Godea R (1982). Fever in adult renal cancer. In *Renal tumour: Proceedings of the First International Symposium on Kidney Tumours*, pp. 283–91. Alan R. Liss, New York.

Frohmuller HGW, Grups JW, Heller V (1987). Comparative value of ultrasonography, computerized tomography, angiography and excretory urography in the staging of renal cell carcinoma. *Journal of Urology*, 138:482–4.

Garns RA, Nelson O, Birch R (1986). Phase II evaluation of mitoxantrone in advanced renal cell carcinoma: a Southeastern Cancer Study Group trial. *Cancer Treatment Reports*, 70(7):921–2.

Gatewood OMB, Goldman SM, Marshall FF, Siegelman SS (1982). Computerized tomography in the diagnosis of transitional cell carcinoma of the kidney. *Journal of Urology*, 127:876–87.

Glen DA, Gilbert FJ, Bayliss AP (1989). Renal carcinomas missed by urography. *British Journal of Urology*, 63:457–9.

Golimbu M (1986). Aggressive treatment of metastatic renal cancer. *Journal of Urology*, 136:805–7.

Granoff A (1972). Herpes virus and the frog renal adenocarcinoma. *Federation Proceedings*, 31:1612–16.

Griffin JP, Hughes GV, Peeling WB (1967). A survey of the familial incidence of adenocarcinoma of the kidney. *British Journal of Urology*, 39:63–9.

Grigon DJ, et al. (1989). Renal cell carcinoma: a clinicopathologic and DNA flow cytometric analysis of 103 cases. *Cancer*, 64:2133–40.

Hajdu SI, Thomas AG (1967). Renal cell carcinoma at autopsy. *Journal of Urology*, 97:978–82.

Hand JR, Broders AC (1932). Carcinoma of the kidney: the degree of malignancy in relation to factors bearing on prognosis. *Journal of Urology*, 28:199–216.

Hedley DW, Friedlander ML, Taylor IW, Rugg CA, Musgrove EA (1983). Method for analysis of cellular DNA content of paraffin-embedded material using flow cytometry. *Journal of Histochemistry and Cytochemistry*, 31:1333–5.

Hellsten S, Berge T, Wehlin L (1981a). Unrecognized renal cell carcinoma. Clinical and diagnostic aspects. *Scandinavian Journal of Urology and Nephrology*, 8:269–72.

Hellsten S, Berge T, Wehlin L (1981b). Unrecognized renal cell carcinoma. Clinical and pathological aspects. *Scandinavian Journal of Urology and Nephrology*, 8:273–8.

Hellsten S, Berge T, Linell F (1983). Clinically unrecognized renal carcinoma: aspects of tumour morphology, lymphatic and haematogenous metastatic spread. *British Journal of Urology*, 55:166–70.

Hermanek P, Sobin LH (ed.) (1987). *TNM classification of malignant tumours* (4th edn), pp. 136–8. Springer Verlag, Berlin.

Hetherington JW, Ewing R, Philp NH (1986). Modified nephroureterectomy: a risk of tumour implantation. *British Journal of Urology*, 58:368–70.

Horoszewitz JS, Murphy GP (1989). An assessment of the current use of human interferons in therapy of urological cancers. *Journal of Urology*, **142**:1173–8.

Horton WA, Womg V, Elridge R (1976). Von Hippel–Lindau disease: clinical and pathological manifestations in nine families with 50 affected members. *Archives of Internal Medicine*, **136**:769–77.

Hrushesky WJM, Murphy GP (1977). Current status of the therapy of advanced renal carcinoma. *Journal of Surgical Oncology*, **9**:277–88.

Hrushesky WJM, Lanning R, Roemeling R, Fraley E, Wesen C, Grage T (1989). Circadian modified FUDR infusion controls progressive metastatic renal cell cancer (RCC). *Proceedings of the American Society of Clinical Oncology*, **8**.

Huang J, Ho DM, Wang J, Chou Y, Chen M, Chang S (1988). Coincidental angiomyolipoma and renal carcinoma—report of 1 case and review of the literature. *Journal of Urology*, **140**:1516–18.

Hulten L, *et al.* (1969). Occurrence and localization of lymph node metastases in renal carcinoma. *Scandinavian Journal of Urology and Nephrology*, **3**:129–33.

Jacobs SC, Berg SI, Lawson RK (1980). Synchronous bilateral renal cell carcinoma: total surgical excision. *Cancer*, **46**:2341–5.

Jasmin, Riopelle JL (1970). Nephroblastomas induced in ovariectomised rats by dimethyl-benzanthracene. *Cancer Research*, **30**:321–6.

Johnson DE, Kaesler KE, Samuels ML (1975). Is nephrectomy justified in patients with metastatic renal carcinoma? *Journal of Urology*, **114**:27–9.

Kantor ALF, Meigs JW, Heston JF, Flannery JT (1976). Epidemiology of renal cell carcinoma in Connecticut, 1935–1973. *Journal of the National Cancer Institute*, **57**:495–500.

Karstaedt N, McCullough DL, Wolfman NT, Dyer RB (1986). Magnetic resonance imaging of the renal mass. *Journal of Urology*, **136**:566–70.

Kessler II (1984). Natural history and epidemiology of cervical cancer with special reference to the role of herpes genitalis. In *Cancer of the uterine cervix* (ed. DCH McBrien and TF Salter), pp. 31–54. Academic Press, London.

Klein MJ, Valensi QJ (1976). Proximal tubular adenomas of kidney with so-called oncocytic features; a clinico-pathologic study of 13 cases of a rarely reported neoplasm. *Cancer*, **38**:906–14.

Klinger ME (1951). Secondary tumours of the genitourinary tract. *Journal of Urology*, **65**:144–53.

Konnack JW, Grossman HB (1986). Renal cell carcinoma as an incidental finding. *Journal of Urology*, **134**:1094–6.

Kradin RL, *et al.* (1989). Tumour infiltrating lymphocytes and interleukin-2 in the treatment of advanced cancer. *Lancet*, **1**:577–80.

Levine E, Weigel JW, Collins DL (1983). Diagnosis and management of asymptomatic renal cell carcinomas in von Hippel–Lindau syndrome. *Urology*, **21**:146–50.

Libertino JA, Zinman L, Watkins E (1987). Long-term results of resection of renal cell cancer with extension into inferior vena cava. *Journal of Urology*, **137**:21–4.

Licht JD, Garnick MB (1987). Phase II trial of streptozocin in the treatment of advanced renal cell carcinoma. *Cancer Treatment Reports*, **71**(1):97–8.

Lieber MM, Tomera KM, Farrow GM (1981). Renal oncocytoma. *Journal of Urology*, **125**:481–5.

Ljungberg B, Tomic R, Roos G (1989). Deoxyribonucleic acid content and medroxyprogesterone acetate treatment in metastatic renal cell carcinoma. *Journal of Urology*, **141**:1308–10.

London NJM, *et al.* (1989). A prospective study of the value of conventional CT, dynamic CT, ultrasonography and arteriography for staging renal carcinoma. *British Journal of Urology*, **64**:209–17.

Maladazys JD, deKernion JB (1986). Prognostic factors in metastatic renal carcinoma. *Journal of Urology*, **136**:376–9.

Malpas JS (1982). Cytotoxic therapy for renal tumours. In *Scientific basis of urology* (2nd edn) (ed. GD Chisholm and D Innes Williams), pp. 680–3. William Heinemann, London.

Marberger M, *et al.* (1981). Conservative surgery of renal carcinoma: the EIRSS experience. *British Journal of Urology*, **53**:528–32.

Marlow PB, Mizell J (1972). Incidence of Lucke renal adenocarcinoma in *Rana pipiens* as determined by histological examination. *Journal of the National Cancer Institute*, **48**:823–9.

Marshall VF, Holden J, Ma KT (1956). Survival of patients with bladder carcinoma treated by simple segmental resection. *Cancer*, **9**:568–70.

Marshall EM, *et al.* (1987). Treatment of metastatic renal cell carcinoma with coumarin (1,2-benzopyrone) and cimetidine: a pilot study. *Journal of Clinical Oncology*, **5**:862–6.

Marshall FF, Taxy JB, Fishman EK, Chang R (1986). The feasibility of surgical enucleation for renal cell carcinoma. *Journal of Urology*, **135**:231–4.

Middleton R (1967). Surgery for metastatic renal cell carcinoma. *Journal of Urology*, **97**:973–7.

Minton JP, Pennlins K, Nowrocki JF (1976). Immunotherapy of kidney cancer. *Proceedings of the American Society of Clinical Oncology and ADCR*, **17**:301.

Montie JE, Stewart BHm, Straffon RA, Banowsky LHW, Hewitt CB, Montague DK (1977). The role of adjunctive nephrectomy in patients with metastatic renal cell carcinoma. *Journal of Urology*, **117**:272–5.

Montie JE, Bukowski RM, James RE, Straffon RA, Stewart BH (1982). A critical review of immunotherapy of disseminated renal adenocarcinoma. *Journal of Surgical Oncology*, **21**(1):5–8.

Mostofi FK, Davis C (1986). Tumours and tumor-like lesions of the kidney. *Current Problems in Cancer*, **10**:53–114.

Mufti GR, *et al.* (1989). Transitional cell carcinoma of the renal pelvis and ureter. *British Journal of Urology*, **63**:135–40.

Murphy GP (1982). Murine renal cell carcinoma: a suitable human model. In *Renal tumours: Proceedings of the First International Symposium on Kidney Tumours*, pp. 175–206. Alan R. Liss, New York.

Murphy GP, Mirand EA, Johnson GS, Schmidt JD, Scott WW (1966). Renal tumours induced by a single dose of dimethylnitrosamine: morphologic, functional, enzymatic and hormonal characterization. *Investigative Urology*, **4**:39–56.

Neidhart JA, Samuel MD, Murphy G, Hennick LA, Wise HA (1980). Active specific immunotherapy of stage IV renal carcinoma with aggregated tumour antigen adjuvant. *American Cancer Society*, **46**:1128–34.

Novick AC, Zincke H, Neves RJ, Topley HM (1986). Surgical enucleation for renal cell carcinoma. *Journal of Urology*, **135**:235–8.

O'Dea MJ, *et al.* (1978). The treatment of renal cell carcinoma with solitary metastases. *Journal of Urology*, **120**:540–2.

Oesterling JE, Fishman EK, Goldman SM, Marshall FF (1986). The management of renal angiomyolipoma. *Journal of Urology*, **135**:1121–4.

Oldbring J, Hellsten S, Lindholm K, Mikulowski P, Tribukait B (1989). Flow DNA analysis in the characterization of carcinoma of the renal pelvis and ureter. *Cancer*, **64**:2141–5.

Oliver RTD (1985). Dilemmas in the management of prostatic carcinoma. *Lancet*, **2**:1219–20.

Oliver RTD (1988). A phase 2 study of surveillance in patients with metastatic renal cell carcinoma and assessment of response of such patients to therapy on progression. *Molecular Biotherapy*, **1**:14–20.

Oliver RTD (1989*a*). Medical management of bladder cancer with an emphasis on the role of immune modulators and chemotherapy. In *Urological and genital cancer* (ed. RTD Oliver), pp. 115–26. Blackwell Scientific, Oxford.

Oliver RTD (1989*b*). Medical management of renal cell carcinoma. In *Urological and genital cancer* (ed. RTD Oliver), pp. 180–191. Blackwell Scientific, Oxford.

Oliver RTD (1989*c*). Tumour cell vaccines: has their time arrived? *Lancet*, **2**:955–2.

Oliver RTD, Stuart-Harris R, Wrigley PFM (1983). Spontaneous regression of metastatic renal cell carcinoma and its significance in assessing the response of such patients to chemotherapy. In *Cancer of the prostate and kidney* (ed. M Pavone-Macaluso and PH Smith), pp. 625–99. Plenum Publishing, London.

Oliver RTD, Waxman JH, Kwok H, Fowler CG, Mathewman P, Blandy JP (1986*a*). Alpha lymphoblastoid interferon for non-invasive bladder cancer. *British Journal of Cancer*, **53**:432.

Oliver RTD, Kwok HK, Highman WJ, Waxman J (1986*b*). Methotrexate, cisplatin and carboplatin as single agents and in combination for metastatic bladder cancer. *British Journal of Urology*, **58**:31–5.

Onishi T, *et al.* (1989). Nephrectomy in renal carcinoma with distant metastasis. *British Journal of Urology*, **63**:600–4.

Pagani JJ (1983). Solid renal mass in the cancer patient: second primary renal cell carcinoma versus renal metastasis. *Journal of Computer Assisted Tomography*, **7**:444–8.

Pavone-Macaluso M, Ingargiola GB, Lamartina M (1982). Aetiology of kidney tumours. In *Cancer of the prostate and kidney* (ed. M Pavone-Macaluso and PH Smith), pp. 475–88. Plenum Publishing, London.

Penn I (1982). Malignancies following the use of cyclosporin A in man. *Cancer Surveys*, **1**:621–4.

Petersen RO (1986). *Urologic pathology*, p. 86. JB Lippincott, Philadelphia.

Pizzocaro G, Piva L, Salvioni R (1983). Lymph node dissection in radical nephrectomy for renal cell carcinoma. is it necessary? *European Urology*, 9:10–12.

Pizzocaro G, *et al.* (1986). Adjuvant medroxyprogesterone acetate and steroid hormone receptors in category MD renal cell carcinoma. An interim report of a prospective randomised study. *Journal of Urology*, 135:18–21.

Pollack HM, Edell S, Morales JO (1974). Radionuclide imaging in renal pseudotumors. *Radiology*, 111:639–44.

Prager MD, Peters PC, Baechtel FS, Brown G (1980). Specific immunotherapy of metastatic human renal cell carcinoma: preliminary results. *Proceedings of the American Association Cancer Research*, 21:213.

Rainwater LM, Farrow GM, Lieber MM (1986). Flow cytometry of renal oncocytoma: common occurrence of deoxyribonucleic acid ploidy and aneuploidy. *Journal of Urology*, 135:1167–71.

Ratcliffe HL (1940). Familial occurrence of renal carcinoma in rhesus monkey (*Macaca mulatta*). *American Journal of Pathology*, 16:619–24.

Reddy ER (1981). Bilateral renal cell carcinoma, unusual occurrence in three members of one family. *British Journal of Radiology*, 54:8–11.

Reese AJM, Winstanley DP (1958). The small tumour-like lesions of the kidney. *British Journal of Cancer*, 12:507–16.

Riches E (1964). The natural history of renal tumours. In *Tumours of the kidney and ureter*, pp. 124–34. E. and S. Livingston, Edinburgh.

Riches EW, Griffiths IH, Thackray AC (1951). New growths of the kidney and ureter. *British Journal of Urology*, 23:297–356.

Ritchie AWS, Chisholm GD (1983). Management of renal carcinoma—a questionnaire survey. *British Journal of Urology*, 5:591–4.

Ritchie AWS, Kemp IW, Chisholm GD (1984). Is the incidence of renal carcinoma increasing? *British Journal of Urology*, 56:571–3.

Robson CJ, Churchill BM, Anderson W (1969). The results of radical nephrectomy for renal cell carcinoma. *Journal of Urology*, 101:297–301.

Rosen VJ Jr, Cole LJ (1962). Accelerated induction of kidney neoplasms in mice after X-irradiation (690 rad) and unilateral nephrectomy. *Journal of the National Cancer Institute*, 28:1031–41.

Rosenberg SA (1986). Adoptive immunotherapy of cancer using lymphokine activated cells and recombinant interleukin-2. In *Important advances in oncology* (ed. VT DeVita Jr, S Hellman, and SA Rosenberg), pp. 55–91. JB Lippincott, Philadelphia.

Rosenberg SA, Terry W (1977). Passive immunotherapy of cancer in animals and man. *Advances in Cancer Research*, 25:323–88.

Rosenberg SA, *et al.* (1987). A progress report on treatment of 157 patients with advanced cancer using lymphokine-activated killer cells and interleukin-2 or high-dose interleukin-2 alone. *New England Journal of Medicine*, 316:889–97.

Rosenberg SA, *et al.* (1989). Combination therapy with interleukin-2 and alpha-interferon for the treatment of patients with advanced cancer. *Journal of Clinical Oncology*, 7:1863–74.

Rosenthal CL, Kraft R, Zingg EJ (1984). Organ-preserving surgery in renal cell carcinoma: tumour enucleation versus partial kidney resection. *European Urology*, 10:222–8.

Sahasrabudhe DM, *et al.* (1986). Specific immunotherapy with suppressor function inhibition for metastatic renal cell carcinoma. *Journal of Biological Response Modifiers*, 5:581–94.

Sarnacki CT, McCormack LJ, Kiser WS, Hazard JB, McLaughlin TC, Belovich DM (1971). Urinary cytology and the clinical diagnosis of urinary tract malignancy: a clinicopathologic study of 1,400 patients. *Journal of Urology*, 106:761–4.

Scharfe T, Miller S, Riedmiller H, Jacobi GH, Hohenfellner R (1989). Immunotherapy of metastasizing renal cell carcinoma. *Urology International*, 44:1–4.

Scher HI, Yagoda A, Ahmed T, Budman D, Sordillo P, Watson RC (1985). Phase-II trial of 4-demethoxydaunorubicin (DMDR) for advanced hypernephroma. *Cancer Chemotherapy and Pharmacology*, 14:79–80.

Selli C, *et al.* (1983). Stratification of risk factors in renal cell carcinoma. *Cancer*, 52:899–903.

Skinner DG, Colvin RB, Vermillion CD, Pfister RC, Leadbetter WF (1971). Diagnosis and management of renal cell carcinoma. A clinical and pathological study of 309 cases. *Cancer*, 28:1165–77.

Skinner DG, Pfister FG, Colvin R (1972). Extension of renal cell carcinoma into the vena cava: the rationale for aggressive surgical management. *Journal of Urology*, 107:711–16.

Skinner MS, Mizell M (1978). The effect of different temperatures on herpes virus induction and replication in Lucke explants. *Laboratory Investigation*, 26:671–5.

Smith RB, deKernion JB, Ehrlich RM, Skinner DG, Kaufmann JJ (1984). Bilateral renal cell carcinoma and renal cell carcinoma in the solitary kidney. *Journal of Urology*, 132:450–4.

Sommer HH, Fossa SD, Lien HH (1985). Combination chemotherapy of advanced renal cell cancer with CCNU and vinblastine. *Cancer Chemotherapy and Pharmacology*, 14:277–8.

Spitz H, Yssel H, Paliard X, Kastelein R, Figdor C, De Vries JE (1988). IL-4 inhibits IL-2 mediated induction of human lymphokine activated killer cells, but not the generation of antigen-specific cytotoxic T lymphocytes in mixed leukocyte cultures. *Journal of Immunology*, 141:29–36.

Stauffer MH (1961). Nephrogenic hepatosplenomegaly. *Gastroenterology*, 40:694.

Sternberg CN, *et al.* (1988). M-VAC (methotrexate, vinblastine, adriamycin and cisplatin) for advanced transitional cell carcinoma of the urothelium. *Journal of Urology*, 139:461–9.

Studer UE, deKernion JB (1986). Mesenchymal and capsular tumours of the kidney. In *Tumours of the kidney* (ed. JB deKernion and M Pavone-Macaluso), *International Perspectives in Urology* Vol. 13, pp. 297–305.

Sufrin G (1982). Experimental models of renal parenchymal neoplasms. In *Scientific basis of urology* (2nd edn) (ed. GD Chisholm and DI Williams), pp. 67–77. Heinemann, London.

Sufrin G, Mirand EA, Moore RH, Chu TM, Murphy GP (1977). Hormones in renal cancer. *Journal of Urology*, 117:433–8.

Sufrin G, Chasan S, Golio A, Murphy G (1989). Paraneoplastic and serologic syndromes of renal adenocarcinoma. *Seminars in Urology*, 7:158–71.

Swanson DA, Johnson DE, von Eschenbach AC, Chuang VP, Wallance S (1983). Angioinfarction plus nephrectomy for metastatic renal cell carcinoma—an update. *Journal of Urology*, 130:449–52.

Tannock IF, Evans WK (1985). Failure of 5-day vinblastine infusion the treatment of patients with renal cell carcinoma. *Cancer Treatment Reports*, 69(2):227–8.

Thompson IM, Peek M (1988). Improvement in survival of patients with renal cell carcinoma—the role of the serendipitously detected tumour. *Journal of Urology*, 140:487–90.

Tiwari JL, Terasaki PI (1985). Renal cell carcinoma. In *HLA and disease associations*, pp. 292–3. Springer Verlag, New York.

Tolia BM, Whitmore WF (1975). Solitary metastases from renal carcinoma. *Journal of Urology*, 114:836–8.

Topalian SL, Muul IM, Solomon D, Rosenberg SA (1987). Expansion and human tumour infiltrating lymphocytes for use in immunotherapy trials. *Journal of Immunological Methods*, 102:127–41.

Topalian SL, *et al.* (1988). Immunotherapy of patients with advanced cancer using tumour infiltrating lymphocytes and recombinant interleukin-2; a pilot study. *Journal of Clinical Oncology*, 6:839–53.

Topley M, Novick AC, Montie JE (1984). Long-term results following partial nephrectomy for localized renal adenocarcinoma. *Journal of Urology*, 131:1050–2.

Tykka H, Oravisto KH, Lehtonen T, Sarna S, Tallberg T (1978). Active specific immunotherapy of advanced renal cell carcinoma. *European Journal of Urology*, 4:250–8.

Ueda T, Mihara Y (1987). Incidental detection of renal carcinoma during radiological imaging. *British Journal of Urology*, 59:513–15.

Utz DC, Warren MM, Gregg JA, Ludgwig J, Kelalis PP (1970). Reversible hepatic dysfunction associated with hypernephroma. *Mayo Clinic Proceedings*, 45:161–9.

van der Werf-Messing B (1973). Carcinoma of the kidney. *Cancer*, 32:1056–61.

van der Werf-Messing B, van Gilse HA (1971). Hormonal treatment of metastases of renal carcinoma. *British Journal of Cancer*, 25:563–7.

Vanky F, *et al.* (1986). Lysis of autologous tumour cells by blood lymphocytes tested at the time of surgery. Correlation with the postsurgical clinical course. *Cancer Immunology and Immunotherapy*, 21:69–766.

Wallace S, *et al.* (1981). Embolisation of renal carcinoma. *Radiology*, 138:563–7.

Waterhouse J, Muir C, Cornea P, Powell J (ed.) (1976). *Cancer incidence in five continents*, Vol. II. IARC Scientific Publication No. 15, Lyon.

Webb JAW, Murray A, Bary PR, Hendry WF (1987). The accuracy and limitations of ultrasound in the assessment of venous extension in renal carcinoma. *British Journal of Urology*, **60**:14–17.

Wickham JEA (1975). Conservative renal surgery for adenocarcinoma. The place of bench surgery. *British Journal of Urology*, **47**:25–36.

Zbar B, Brauch H, Talmadge C, Linehan M (1987). Loss of alleles at loci on the short arm of chromosome 3 in renal cell carcinoma. *Nature*, **327**:721–4.

Zincke H, Swanson SK (1982). Bilateral renal cell carcinoma; influence of synchronous and asynchronous occurrence on patient survival. *Journal of Urology*, **128**:913–15.

Zincke H, Engen DE, Henning KM, McDonald MW (1985). Treatment of renal cell carcinoma by *in situ* partial nephrectomy and extracorporeal operation with autotransplantation. *Mayo Clinic Proceedings*, **60**:651–62.

10.6   Tumours of the prostate

A. HORWICH, JONATHAN WAXMAN, AND FRITZ H. SCHRÖDER

INTRODUCTION

In the West carcinoma of the prostate is the second most common malignancy in men over 55 years of age and from the age of 70 years it becomes the most frequent. The incidence and stage distribution is affected by the practice of screening; there is a real difference in incidence between the West and Japan or other eastern countries. It is predominantly a disease of the elderly and only approximately 15 per cent of cases occur under the age of 65 years.

A particular challenge to the oncologist is the variable natural history of prostatic cancer and optimal management of early stages requires a precise judgement of prognosis as well as a thorough appreciation of the management roles of surgery, radiotherapy, and ormonal ablation (Dearnaley *et al.* 1993). In advanced and metastatic disease the gratifyingly frequent remission caused by hormonal therapies is tempered by the inevitability of relapse and the grim prospect of subsequent chronically painful metastatic bone disease.

Unfortunately, more than half of all prostate cancers and in some areas of the world more than 80 per cent present in an advanced stage. Although screening measures lead to a higher rate of diagnosis when the disease is locally confined, it remains uncertain whether early detection and early treatment will lead to an overall decrease in mortality.

The diagnosis of prostate cancer is based on rectal examination and biopsy. Transrectal sonography, assay of serum markers such as prostatic acid phosphatase and prostate-specific antigen, isotope bone scans, and pelvic lymph node dissection are important tools in diagnosis and staging. The most important prognostic factors for localized disease are the T (tumour) stage, the estimated tumour volume, the degree of differentiation, ploidy, and the N (node) stage. Serum prostatic-specific antigen (PSA) concentration is increasingly proving valuable. For metastatic disease the important factors include performance status, extent of metastases, alkaline phosphatase concentration, and presence of a T4 tumour.

The management of disease confined to the prostate is controversial and options including surveillance, radiotherapy, or radical prostatectomy are widely employed as initial therapy. There are no valid prospective randomized studies and historical comparison of extensive data, even though specified by stage and grade, has left the issue of initial management inconclusive (Whitmore 1994). Trials in prostate cancer are made difficult by its slow natural history and by the predominant incidence in the elderly, such that the necessary long-term follow-up is confounded

by the incidence of death from other causes. Presentation variables appear to influence survival to a far greater extent than choice of initial treatment. Therefore, quality of life considerations are important in determining therapy and recent technical advances in both radiotherapy and surgery have reduced the risks of toxicity.

Patients who present with metastatic disease are eligible for endocrine management. The disease is exquisitely sensitive to hormonal therapies and 80 per cent of treated patients have a subjective and 50 per cent an objective response. However, endocrine treatment is palliative. If the natural lifespan of the patients is long enough, all tumours progress. The median time to progression is 12 months and median survival after the start of endocrine therapy for metastatic disease is 30 months. The optimal timing of endocrine treatment is still a subject of controversy. While there is no doubt that hormonal treatments are effective at alleviating disease symptoms, including pain and urinary obstruction, it remains unclear whether earlier therapy of the asymptomatic patient leads to longer survival. Therefore, in view of the side-effects of endocrine management, it may be desirable to delay such treatment until symptoms occur.

A recent controversy has been the question of whether 'total' androgen blockade, which aims to eliminate adrenal as well as testicular sources of androgenic steroids, is superior as initial endocrine therapy to medical or surgical castration alone. Published trials relating to this question will be discussed, but at present they give conflicting results. A major unresolved problem concerns those patients who relapse after endocrine management, since cytotoxic chemotherapy only achieves transient partial remissions in 10–30 per cent of patients.

Developments in our understanding of basic mechanisms controlling prostatic cancer have provided new insights into this disease. The recent discovery of the importance of oncogene expression and of new hormonal receptors, which suggests a direct effect of some of the new agents used in the treatment of the disease, has meant that we are nearer to discovering the scientific basis for response and relapse. It is hoped that these advances will soon achieve clinical significance.

EPIDEMIOLOGY

Geographical and racial factors and age

Age is the single most important risk factor for the development of prostatic cancer. There is an almost exponential increase in the age-related incidence and mortality from prostatic cancer, reaching its zenith at 85 years. Between 65 and 70 years the incidence of prostatic cancer is 358 cases per 100 000 population and for men aged 80–85 years it is 1035. The mortality rates are 76 and 410, respectively (Waterhouse *et al.* 1982).

Prostatic cancer has an extraordinarily varied geographical incidence and age-standardized mortality rates vary from 0.1 per 100 000 in Thailand to 30 per 100 000 in some parts of the West Indies. The overall incidence also varies markedly from 0.8 per 100 000 in China to 100 per 100 000 in Blacks living in North America (Waterhouse *et al.* 1982). Superficially, it would seem to be extremely difficult to separate out environmental factors from racial factors to explain this difference in worldwide incidence. However, it seems clear from studies of migrant populations that environmental factors are more significant than racial origin. At the end of the last century there was a large wave of migration of Japanese peoples to North America and Hawaii. The incidence of carcinoma of the prostate in Japan is at least ten times less than that of the White populations in North America. The incidence of prostatic cancer increased in succeeding generations of Japanese in North America and Hawaii such that in the first generation of migrants it was 5 : 1 and in the second generation 1.4 : 1 compared with North Americans of Caucasian origin (Buell and Dunn 1965). Similarly, comparison of Americans of African origin, who have the highest incidence of prostatic cancer in the world, with similar populations in Africa shows an incidence increased by up to a factor of 20 in Black Americans (Zaridze and Boyle 1987) (Table 1). Overt prostatic cancer presenting with symptoms has to be differentiated from carcinoma of the prostate that is not clinically manifest and is found incidentally at post-mortem where the patient has died from another cause. Microscopic prostatic cancers are very common and these 'tumours' do not vary with age or geographic location in the population studied. Their clinical significance is unknown and their relationship to overt cancer is unclear. Small foci are present in approximately 10–20 per cent of normal men aged over 45 years (Breslow *et al.* 1977).

Prostate cancer and environmental factors

There is clear-cut evidence that our own behaviour causes the diseases that we develop and this is particularly true with regard to prostatic cancer. The overall incidence of prostatic cancer in vegetarians compared with omnivores is significantly less, with a 25–50 per cent reduction in the chance of developing this malignancy. In a prospective study of 120 000 men in Japan specific

protective effects were observed in those men who had diets high in green and yellow vegetables, suggesting that vitamin A may be a factor implicated in the protection of some men from the development of prostatic cancer (Hirayama 1979).

Libido and bachelor status has been implicated in the development of prostatic cancer, but the studies demonstrating associations are of small numbers of patients and poorly case controlled (Steele *et al.* 1971). It is difficult to be convinced that there is any association between libido and the development of prostatic cancer because libido is so difficult to quantitate retrospectively.

Radiation exposure has been implicated in the development of prostatic cancer and in an analysis of deaths amongst 39 546 employees of the United Kingdom Atomic Energy Authority the only malignancy clearly related to radiation exposure was prostatic cancer for which the standardized mortality ratio was 115. This increased incidence was particularly evident in young men (Beral *et al.* 1985).

Recently, case reports have appeared implicating anabolic steroids with the early development of prostatic cancer in young weight-lifters. It is extremely difficult to know whether this association is real because the cases reported are few and the disease is increasing in incidence within the populations of the first and second worlds.

Prostatic cancer hormones and age

There are obvious changes in the levels of hormones with increasing age of the population studied. Plasma testosterone and free testosterone decrease with age, whilst testosterone binding capacity increases. Follicle-stimulating hormone and luteinizing hormone both increase, as do serum 17β oestradiol levels (Baker *et al.* 1976). However, virtually all cancers increase with age; this increased incidence is not ascribed to a hormonal cause so whether these changes relate to the development of prostatic cancer is not clear.

BIOLOGICAL RESEARCH

There is a surprising lack of scientific research into the origins of prostate cancer. It is the second most common malignancy of men over 55 years and should stimulate the same level of interest in its molecular origin as is the case for breast carcinoma. Indeed, its sensitivity to hormonal therapies is such that clues to the biochemical basis for response in hormone-dependent malignancies might be easier to detect in this condition than in any other cancer.

Steroid receptors

Recently the genes encoding steroid hormone receptors have been cloned. The genes for the receptors for dihydrotestosterone, 17β oestradiol, progesterone, thyroid-stimulating hormone, retinoic acid, and vitamin A have considerable sequence homology and are considered part of a single supergene family. This supergene family has sequence homology with the oncogene for the avian erythro-blastosis virus v-*erb* A (O'Malley 1990). Hormone receptor assays are technically difficult in prostatic cancer and this relates to the problems in separating stroma from tumour, a high concentration of endogenous steroids which lead to receptor saturation, and the presence of two non-specific binding proteins, albumin and sex-hormone-binding globulin. The active tissue metabolite of testosterone is dihydrotestosterone. There seems to be conflicting evidence for the presence of receptors for dihydrotestosterone in benign hypertrophy. In one series of 23 patients dihydrotestosterone binding was absent (Nijis and Hawkins 1976), in contrast to the finding of receptor positivity in 14 out of 17 patients in another study

Table 1 Age-specific incidence of prostatic cancer 1972–1973

Age	Japan	San Francisco White population	San Francisco Black population
40–44	0.5	1.5	2.3
45–49	0.9	5.4	10.8
50–54	1.0	14.3	62.1
55–59	3.2	64.8	174.2
60–64	8.3	153.1	290
65–69	27.5	286.4	418.5
70–74	51.1	484.9	1007
75–79	65.4	721.5	1009.7
80–84	80.3	909.3	1486.2
>85	110.5	938.4	865.2

Adapted from Waterhouse *et al.* (1982).

(Geller *et al.* 1975). In prostatic cancer the situation is more clear-cut and dihydrotestosterone receptor positivity corresponds to hormonal responsiveness. Receptor concentration correlates with response and in 23 patients in whom dihydrotestosterone binding was greater than 110 fmol/mg the mean response time was 17 months and mean survival was 24 months. In patients with binding less than 110 fmol/mg of DNA, the mean response time was 7 months and mean survival was 17 months (Trachtenberg and Walsh 1982). Oestrogen and progestogen receptor positivity does not correlate with response to treatment. In a series of 22 patients with prostate cancer, only six were found to contain 17β oestradiol receptors (Martelli *et al.* 1980) and in a further series tumours in 14 out of 26 patients contained oestrogen receptors and 13 out of 15 contained progesterone receptors (Concolino *et al.* 1982).

Gonadotrophin-releasing hormone receptors

Gonadotrophin-releasing hormone agonists are effective therapies of prostatic cancer. There has been recent interest in the possibility that the response to treatment may relate to a direct effect of these agonists at the level of the tumour itself. Two human prostatic cancer cell lines have been examined for the presence of the receptor for this peptide. High-affinity binding was found in membrane preparations from the LNCaP line. This is a human hormone-sensitive prostatic carcinoma line which is derived from a lymph node. In contrast, low-affinity binding was found in the DU145 cell line which is derived from brain metastases from a patient with hormone-unresponsive prostatic cancer (Qayum *et al.* 1990). This contrast between hormone-dependent and hormone-independent cell lines is of interest, particularly in relation to the observation that both cell lines produced a peptide with gonadotrophin-releasing hormone-like radio-immunoactivity in amounts directly related to the number of cells in culture. Although this peptide has not yet been sequenced, it has a very close homology to the native hormone in terms of its high performance liquid chromatography (HPLC) characteristics both before and after digest with various peptide-degenerative enzymes (Qayum *et al.* 1990). This result fits in well with the autocrine hypothesis of cell regulation in which cancers are believed to produce factors that are stimulatory for their own growth and have specific receptors for these growth factors on their cell surface. It may well be that gonadotrophin-releasing hormone agonists interfere with this autocrine network, down-regulating cell surface receptors in hormone-dependent lines and that the difference between hormone dependence and independence is in the characteristics of this receptor.

Oncogenes and prostate cancer

Oncogene expressions have been examined in four prostatic cancer cell lines. 'Large amounts' of c-*myc* and H-*ras* mRNA were present in all the cell lines and c-*fos* mRNA was present in the hormone-dependent line alone. Withdrawal of androgens from the growth medium led to a dramatic reduction in c-*fos* and H-*ras* mRNA with no change in c-*myc* mRNA concentrations. Therefore, androgens may act directly to regulate the expression of these oncogenes which are essential for growth (Rijinders *et al.* 1985). Viola *et al.* (1986) have investigated the expression of the p21 product by the *ras* oncogene using the RAP-5 antibody. P21 positivity was found in 23 out of 29 prostatic carcinoma specimens and the extent of positivity correlated with differentiation. In this study there was no positive staining in all 19 cases of benign hypertrophy. The expression of c-*myc* was examined in seven patients with carcinoma of the prostate and 11

with benign hypertrophy. The level of c-*myc* expression, as assessed by hybridization studies with a ^{32}P-labelled c-*myc* probe, was significantly higher in the carcinoma group (Fleming *et al.* 1986). In a recent publication only one out of 24 prostatic cancer tumours had *ras* oncogene mutations (Carter *et al.* 1990).

Tumour suppressor genes

The expression of the retinoblastoma (RB) tumour suppressor gene and its product has been examined in prostatic cancer cell lines. Aberrant expression of the RB gene was found in one of three lines and normal levels of expression were achieved by transfection of the normal gene. This resulted in a decrease in the ability of the transfected cells to form tumours in nude mice (Bookstein *et al.* 1990). Mutations of the tumour suppressor, gene *p53*, were examined in patients with benign hypertrophy or prostatic cancer and were found to be infrequent (Uchida *et al.* 1993). This is in contrast to the high frequency of aberrant *p53* expression in most human tumours.

Growth factors

Epidermal growth factor is secreted throughout the urinary tract. Its receptor is present in many human tumours where it correlates with response. Epidermal growth factor receptor mRNA expression has been found to be significantly higher in prostatic cancer than in benign hypertrophy (Morris and Green Dodd 1990). The transforming growth factors are a unique class of regulatory peptides which may in different circumstances act to inhibit or stimulate tumour growth. There are two main classes of transforming growth factors (TGFs) and these are termed alpha and beta. There are at least five beta transforming growth factors. In carcinoma of the breast, TGF-β has been shown to inhibit the growth of tumour cell lines and antibodies to this peptide have been used to abolish its inhibitory effect on this growth (Knabbe *et al.* 1987). It has been suggested that the response to endocrine therapies in breast cancer is related to the secretion of inhibitory growth factors by stromal elements with local autocrine loops operating between fibroblasts and epithelial cells. This may explain the discrepancies between the finding of hormone responsiveness in oestrogen receptor negative patients and the lack of hormone response in a significant proportion of patients with hormone receptor negative tumours. In prostatic cancer the DU145 cell line has been shown to secrete TGF-α as well as epidermal growth factor (MacDonald *et al.* 1990). The exact relevance of this finding is not known, but it suggests future avenues of exploration in this cancer.

PATHOLOGY

Adenocarcinoma of the prostate

Site of origin

Adenocarcinoma of the prostate arises from the epithelial lining of the true prostatic gland and small tumours are usually found near the outer margins of the gland, particularly in the posterolateral portion (Moore 1935; Rich 1935; Edwards *et al.* 1953; Franks 1954). The tumour is frequently multicentric (Moore 1935; Edwards *et al.* 1953; Blennerhassett and Vickery 1966) and in step-section examination of total prostatectomy specimens this was found in 85 per cent of cases (Byar and Mostofi 1972).

Pathology

The World Health Organization (WHO) classification of prostatic tumour histology (Mostofi *et al.* 1980) categorizes small acinar, large acinar, cribriform, solid/trabecular, and other tumours; that is, endometrioid carcinoma, mucinous carcinoma, and adenoid cystic carcinoma.

In small acinar adenocarcinoma, the small acinae are usually spread irregularly through the stroma of the prostate, although in some cases the acinae are closely packed with stroma obliterated. The acinae may be adjacent to smooth muscle bundles without intervening collagen and immunohistological study of type IV collagen and laminin suggest a lack of basement membrane between the acinae and the stroma (Barsky *et al.* 1983). Invasion of lymph and vascular channels is less common in well-differentiated than in poorly differentiated adenocarcinoma. Invasion of perineural space occurs early (Moore 1935; Kahler 1939) but may not be of prognostic importance (Byar and Mostofi 1972). The acinae are lined by columnar or cuboidal epithelial cells with a clear or vaculated cystoplasm which may be basophilic or eosinophilic. The nuclei form a single row next to the basement membrane. In well-differentiated tumours the nuclei are uniform with prominent nucleoli and it has been suggested that nucleolar size does have prognostic significance; patients with larger nucleolar surface area measured by scanning electron microscope are more likely to develop metastases (Tannenbaum *et al.* 1982).

Cell divisions are rare in well-differentiated prostatic cancer although they are seen more commonly in moderate and poorly differentiated tumours.

Large acinar adenocarcinoma is less common. The glands are approximately the same size as normal prostatic acinae and may be associated with microcystic changes and the epithelial cysts often show secretory activity. Cribriform adenocarcinoma refers to a growth pattern associated with round or ovoid lumina which may contain sialomucin (Franks *et al.* 1964).

In the solid trabecular form of adenocarcinoma tumour cells are arranged in nests, sheets, or cords and the differential diagnosis is with a transitional cell carcinoma of the prostate except that the malignant cells show some irregular prostatic acid phosphatase and prostate-specific antigen immunostaining.

In undifferentiated or poorly differentiated adenocarcinoma, the growth pattern is irregular with cells in cords, sheets, or large solid aggregates. There is no attempt at gland formation. There may be patchy prostatic acid phosphatase or prostate-specific antigen immunostaining.

Grading of carcinoma of the prostate

Grading is based on glandular differentiation and cellular anaplasia. Thus, if acinar structures are formed resembling the glands of the normal prostate, the tumour is considered well differentiated and low grade. If no gland formation is seen, the carcinoma is termed poorly differentiated or high grade. Anaplasia is represented by variations in size, shape, and the chromatin content of the nuclei. A number of grading systems are in use for carcinoma of the prostate. The Gleason system (Gleason and Veterans Administration Cooperative Urological Research Group 1977) is based on glandular differentiation, whereas other systems (Utz and Farrow 1969; Mostofi 1975, 1976; Gaeta *et al.* 1980; Gaeta 1981; Bocking *et al.* 1982) are based on both differentiation and the degree of anaplasia.

The Mostofi system

The Mostofi system has three grades.

Grade 1. Well-differentiated glands with slight nuclear anaplasia.

Grade 2. Gland formation with moderate nuclear anaplasia.

Grade 3. Gland formation with severe nuclear anaplasia or alternatively undifferentiated tumour.

This system has been found to predict prognosis well, with the prognosis being determined predominantly by the least differentiated element in the tumour (Schröder *et al.* 1985).

The Gleason system

The Gleason system was devised for the Veterans Administration Cooperative Urological Research Group (VACURG) (Gleason *et al.* 1974).

Grade 1. Well-differentiated carcinoma with uniform gland pattern.

Grade 2. Well-differentiated carcinoma with glands varying in size and shape.

Grade 3. Moderately differentiated carcinoma with either (a) irregular acinae often widely separated or (b) well-defined papillary/cribriform structures. This is the commonest pattern seen in carcinoma of the prostate.

Grade 4. Poorly differentiated carcinoma with fused glands widely infiltrating the prostatic stroma. Neoplastic cells may grow in cords or sheets and the cytoplasm is clear.

Grade 5. Very poorly differentiated carcinoma with no or minimal gland formation. Tumour cell masses may have central necrosis.

Approximately 50 per cent of tumours exhibit more than one pattern. The commonest pattern is called the primary and the less common pattern is called the secondary. The two patterns can be recorded separately or, alternatively, they can be summed to produce an average pattern called the pattern score which correlates well with mortality (Gleason and Veterans Administration Cooperative Urological Research Group 1977).

The Gaeta system

The Gaeta system is used by the National Prostatic Cancer Project and is based on both differentiation and nuclear anaplasia on a four-point scale (Gaeta *et al.* 1980; Gaeta 1981).

Grade 1. Well-defined acinae with uniform normal-sized neoplastic cells.

Grade 2. Irregular infiltration of stroma by acinae structures with slightly pleomorphic tumour cells containing discernible nucleoli.

Grade 3. Small irregular poorly formed acinae or cribriform pattern with pleiomorphic neoplastic cells. The nuclei are often vacuolated with large nucleoli.

Grade 4. Round masses of tumour with absent glandular differentiation. There may be considerable mitotic activity, usually with more than three divisions per high power field.

Comparison of grading systems

Murphy and Whitmore (1979) compared four major systems: the Mostofi system, the Gleason system, the Gaeta system, and the Mayo Clinic system. The consensus viewpoint was to recommend the Gleason system, possibly incorporating cytological information. This was also the conclusion reached in a comparison of the Gleason system and a modified Gaeta system (Gaeta *et al.* 1986).

Heterogeneity of prostatic cancer histology

The difficulty in grading tumours on the basis of a single-needle biopsy is that a variety of histological patterns are seen in a single carcinoma (Byar and Mostofi 1972). When the grading score from a needle biopsy was compared with that from the radical prostatectomy specimen, it was found that the needle biopsy grade was too low in 33 per cent of patients and too high in 8 per cent when a three-point grading scale was used (Catalona *et al.* 1982). Similar results are reported for Gleason grade comparison (Lange and Narayan 1983; Garnett *et al.* 1984; Mills and Fowler 1986). Grading errors were less likely with larger biopsy specimens.

Local extension

From the site of origin in the subcapsular region, the tumour spreads both centrally towards the urethra and peripherally to the prostatic capsule (Byar and Mostofi 1972). Extension to the capsule does not influence prognosis; however, penetration predisposes to metastasis and influences survival (McNeal 1969; Byar and Mostofi 1972). The tumour also extends locally into the bladder neck, the trigone, the seminal vesicles, and occasionally the rectum. An autopsy study showed bladder invasion in 50 per cent of cases and seminal vesicle invasion in 58 per cent (Mintz and Smith 1934). Invasion of the rectum is deterred by Denonvilliers' fascia. Occasionally, there is difficulty in differential diagnosis from a primary rectal tumour in which case immunohistological staining for prostatic acid phosphatase or prostate-specific antigen is helpful.

Other prostatic tumours

Transitional cell carcinoma

This pattern is usually secondary to a primary in the urinary bladder or the prostatic urethra (Goebbels *et al.* 1985; Mahadevia *et al.* 1986) and primary transitional carcinoma of the prostate is very rare (Ortega *et al.* 1953; Kopelson *et al.* 1978). Patients are usually in the sixth decade and present with obstructive symptoms and haematuria. The prognosis is poor with invasive tumours (Schellhammer *et al.* 1977).

Squamous cell carcinoma

Squamous cell carcinoma represents less than 1 per cent of prostatic carcinomas (Mott 1979) and is associated with both transitional carcinoma and treated prostatic adenocarcinoma. There is a variant exhibiting pseudosarcomatous change which is called spindle cell carcinoma (Battifora 1976). Clinically, the tumour presents with prostatism. There is no elevation of serum prostatic acid phosphatase and bone metastases are osteolytic (Mott 1979).

Adenosquamous carcinoma

Adenosquamous carcinoma is extremely rare and appears to derive from adenocarcinoma of the prostate. The reported cases had prior radiotherapy and two of the three had prior oestrogen therapy (Moyana 1987).

Adenocarcinoma of ductal origin

Pure ductal carcinoma represents approximately 1 per cent of prostatic carcinomas, although a further 5 per cent of tumours have a pattern of ductal carcinoma together with acinar carcinoma. The tumour cells may grow in a papillary or cribriform pattern and there may be central necrosis in cribriform tumours. Ductal carcinoma with both papillary and glandular patterns has been called 'endometrial carcinoma' (Melicow and Pachter 1967) and shows complex glandular formations lined by a multilayered epithelium. It often co-exists with acinar carcinoma (Epstein and Woodruff 1986). The proposal that this tumour arose from the Müllerian epithelium led to the idea that orchidectomy or oestrogen therapy were contraindicated; however, not only have responses to orchidectomy been reported (Young and Lagios 1973) but it is also clear that the tumour stains for both prostatic acid phosphatase and prostate-specific antigen (Pillarisetti *et al.* 1983).

Mucinous carcinoma of the prostate

This is a form of adenocarcinoma in which part of the tumour contains extensive mucin (Epstein and Liebermann 1985). The tumour cell stains for both prostatic acid phosphatase and prostate-specific antigen. The disease behaves aggressively and is said to respond poorly to endocrine treatment.

Carcinoid and small cell carcinoma of the prostate

It is uncertain whether these subtypes are distinct. In some, there are argentaffin or argyrophil granules and electron microscopy reveals dense core granules (Wasserstein and Goldman 1981). In two cases of carcinoid tumour the neoplastic cells stained for prostatic acid phosphatase and prostate-specific antigen (Azumi *et al.* 1984; Ghali and Garcia 1984) and in one of these cells also contained ACTH (Ghali and Garcia 1984).

Prostate-specific antigen and prostatic acid phosphatase may be negative in small cell carcinoma of the prostate, although this also appears to be an APUD tumour with ACTH production (Schron *et al.* 1984; Tetu *et al.* 1987). This tumour may respond to chemotherapy in a fashion similar to its lung counterpart (Hindson *et al.* 1985).

Sarcomas of the prostate

Sarcomas represent approximately 0.1 per cent of prostatic malignancy and are predominantly either rhabdomyosarcoma or leiomyosarcoma, with the former occurring in young patients (Smith and Dehner 1972; Hays *et al.* 1982). Leiomyosarcoma occasionally occurs in children but the main incidence peak is between 40 and 70 years of age (Christofferson 1973).

Leukaemia and lymphoma of the prostate

Chronic lymphocytic leukaemia cells may infiltrate the prostate more commonly than the incidence of overt symptoms would suggest (Cachia *et al.* 1987). Prostatic involvement with acute leukaemia is rare and local resection may cause haemorrhage (Frame *et al.* 1987).

Non-Hodgkin's lymphoma of the prostate is also uncommon. Most are of intermediate grade and occur in the elderly (Bostwick and Mann 1985).

Secondary tumours of the prostate

Secondary tumours constitute approximately 1 per cent of prostatic cancers, with the most common primaries being malignant melanoma and bronchial carcinoma (Johnson *et al.* 1974).

Staging classifications

As described below the staging of prostatic cancer is based upon rectal examination, laboratory tests, plain radiographs, and radio-isotope bone scans. Pathological staging may follow prostatectomy

Table 2 Staging of carcinoma of the prostate

UICC 1978/1982		AUS stage		UICC 1987		
T0	Occult carcinoma	A	Occult carcinoma	T1		Incidental
		A1	One lobe		T1a	Three foci or less
		A2	Multifocal or diffuse		T1b	More than three foci
T1	Intracapsular tumour					
		B	Confined to prostate	T2		Clinically or grossly, limited to gland
		B1	One lobe		T2a	$\leqslant 1.5$ cm
		B2	Diffuse		T2b	> 1.5 cm/ $>$ one lobe
T2	Tumour (?) but does not breach capsule					
T3	Extraprostatic extension	C	Extracapsular extension	T3		Invades prostatic apex/beyond capsule/bladder neck/seminal vesical/not fixed
T4	Fixed invading adjacent organs			T4		Fixed or invades other adjacent structures
N 1	Single regional node involved	D1	Pelvic node metastasis	N1		Single $\leqslant 2$ cm
2	Multiregional nodes			N2		Single > 2 cm $\leqslant 5$ cm, multiple $\leqslant 5$ cm
3	Fixed node mass			N3		> 5 cm
4	Juxta-regional nodes					
M 1	Distant metastasis	D2	Distant metastasis	M1		Distant metastasis

Source: Wallace *et al.* (1975) and Whitmore (1984).

and/or node sampling or dissection. Table 2 shows the International Union Against Cancer (UICC) system (Wallace *et al.* 1975; UICC 1978, 1987) and also the American urologic system based on that described by Whitmore (1984). The extension of prostate cancer at the time of diagnosis is variable and depends on many parameters. Stages T1a and T1b (UICC 1978) are focal or more extensive tumours found on histological examination of specimens removed for apparently benign obstructive prostatic disease. Rectal examination is normal in these cases. In the United States this disease is commonly classified as stages A1 and A2. Obviously, the incidence depends on the indication for surgery for benign prostatic hyperplasia, the distribution of age at the time of surgery, the pathological techniques applied, and a number of other variables. Categories T2a and T2b, which correspond exactly to stages B1 and B2 in the American system, characterize tumours that are identifiable on rectal examination, appear to be confined to the prostate, and have a diameter of less than or more than 1.5 cm, respectively. Stage T3, which also includes confined disease involving the apex of the prostate, corresponds to the American stage C and stands for disease which has penetrated through the capsule of the prostate. Metastatic disease is differentiated as N+ and M1 disease depending on the presence of tumour deposits in lymph nodes or at a distance. This corresponds to stages D1 and D2 in the American system.

Since prostatic cancer in stages A, B, and C is usually asymptomatic, the incidence of the corresponding diagnoses depends on factors that are mainly related to the patterns of medical practice in given geographical areas. Table 3 gives an indication of the incidence of stages A, B, and C in the United States in 1974 and 1979. In many European countries and certainly in less developed countries, prostate cancer is more frequently diagnosed in the more advanced stages.

Examination of surgical specimens suggests that clinical staging is far from perfect and there is a significant risk of understaging extracapsular extension, seminal vesicle involvement, and pelvic node metastasis (Byar and Mostofi 1972; Spellman 1977; Walsh 1988).

A modification of the TNM classification has recently been proposed (UICC 1987). This has not been fully accepted by urological oncologists (Hall *et al.* 1988; Schröder *et al.* 1988) because it does not contain specified minimum investigations for ascribing

Table 3 Clinical stages of prostate cancer in 20 166 cases diagnosed in 1974–1975 (long-term study) and 14 079 cases diagnosed in 1979–1980 in the United States (short-term study)

Study	Stage (%)				
	A	B	C	D	Unknown
1974	20.8	30.7	17.7	21.5	9.2
1979	25.9	28.9	14.9	25.9	4.3

Source: Mettlin *et al.* (1982).

stage. Other criticisms include concern that confusion may derive from the classification of occult carcinoma as T1 and the inclusion of invasion of the prostatic apex within T3.

NATURAL HISTORY

The natural history of prostate cancer by stage

The classical article on this subject was written by Whitmore (1973). Since that time much more knowledge has been obtained and a clearer picture can be drawn of prognosis without treatment. In dealing with natural history by disease extension, it must be realized that each of these steps is associated with morphological changes which again probably reflect genetic events of unknown nature. In comparing prostatic tissue obtained in the same patient population with a mean interval of 2.4 years, Cumming *et al.* (1990) clearly showed that there is dedifferentiation of prostatic cancer with time.

Categories T1a and T1b

Tumours that are not palpable on rectal examination are usually found at the time of transurethral or open prostatectomy for benign prostatic hyperplasia. Categories T1a and T1b roughly correspond to the American stages A1 and A2. Their incidence depends on the completeness of the surgical removal of the benign prostatic hyperplasia specimen, on age, and on the pathological review of the specimen. This tumour is commonly called 'incidental carcinoma' and is found in 8–12 per cent of patients undergoing prostatic surgery. Jewett (1975) first drew attention to the different prognosis of focal and extensive incidental carcinoma. This lesion

Table 4 Progression rates (PD), median time to progression, and prostate cancer death rates in patients with untreated incidental prostate cancer (TNM 1987)

Reference	N	Stage	PD (percentage)	Median time to PD (months)	Cancer deaths per total deaths
Blackard et al. (1971)	45		13 (28.8)	62	2
Cantrell et al. (1981)	48	A1	1 (2.0)	>48	0
	34	A2	11 (32.0)	>48	5/23
Epstein et al. (1986)	50	A1	8 (16.0)	>96	6/26
Blute et al. (1986)	15	A2	4 (26.6)	134	1/8
(age <60 years)	8	A2	2 (25.0)	134	1/8
Lowe and Liström (1988a)	143	A1	(50)[a]	162	3
	55	A2	(50)[a]	54	12/38
Johansson et al. (1989)	72	T1a[b]	7 (10)		3/22
	34	T1b[b]	11 (32)	78	5/10

Categories T1a and T1b are comparable with A1 and A2.
[a]Figures are related to median time to progression.
[b]Eight patients with G2 and G3 tumours were excluded.

has been studied by a number of groups in longitudinal studies of otherwise untreated patients. The results of such studies are summarized in Table 4. In most instances, the definition of Cantrell (1981), using the amount of slide surface positive for cancer, has been applied to differentiate between T1a and T1b disease. In addition to the data reported in Table 2, Johansson (1989) used a univariate analysis to calculate the relative risks of dying of prostate cancer which amounted to 1.0 for T1a and 3.7 for T1b. Most authors report higher progression rates for the T1b lesions. However, owing to competing causes of death in the age group involved, patients with T1a and T1b disease rarely die from prostatic cancer. Lowe and Liström (1988a) found median times to progression of 162 months for A1 lesions and 54 months for A2 lesions. Five year progression rates for A2 lesions are reported to be in the range 25–30 per cent.

These data can be seriously distorted by inaccurate rectal examination. Transrectal ultrasonography and tumour markers such as prostate specific antigen may be helpful in excluding more extensive disease. A number of the authors cited, in addition to Adolfsson et al. (1990) and George (1988), have reported progression rates separately for local and systemic disease. It seems that local progression occurs more frequently than progression to metastatic disease. Since local progression can be detected by rectal examination and since the risk of progression is low, most clinicians will follow patients with T1a disease clinically without active treatment. As pointed out by Epstein et al. (1986) and Blute et al. (1986), very young patients may deserve a different approach because the period of time that they are at risk may be considerably longer. Most clinicians agree that, with rates of progression in the range of 25 per cent within 5 years, some kind of treatment is warranted.

Categories T2a, T2b (B1, B2, B3)

The definition of this T category, which usually occurs without the presence of obvious metastatic disease, corresponds exactly to the American stages B1 and B2. If lymph node dissection is carried out in patients with this disease, regional lymph node metastases are found with an incidence of 10–25 per cent. T2a and T2b tumours are usually confined to the prostate and are considered potentially curable. Radical prostatectomy and radiotherapy are competing forms of treatment. No conclusive randomized trials exist. Treatment results reveal significant differences according to T subcategories and the grade of differentiation (G category). As Whitmore (1988a) elegantly elaborated, there is little doubt that many of these lesions are curable. However, it remains doubtful whether, in view of our knowledge of the natural history, potentially curative treatment is always necessary.

Table 5 shows some of the available data for groups of patients who have been followed after diagnosis of T2a or T2b prostatic cancer without any form of treatment until progression occurred. The series of Warner and Whitmore (1990) was established by a retrospective review of a large number of records from the Memorial Sloan-Kettering Cancer Center. In each of these patients the wait and see approach was adopted for some specific reason. In this particular series local progression occurred in 48 out of 75 patients (64 per cent) and progression to distant metastases occurred in 25 out of 75 (33 per cent) with a mean follow-up of almost 10 years. The 20 patients reported by Byar et al. (1981) represent the control arm of an incomplete randomized study of the Veterans Administration Cooperative Urological Research Group (VACURG). These patients were identified by biopsy or TUR and metastases were excluded by means of acid phosphatase determinations and bone radiographs.

Table 5 Progression rates (PD), duration of follow-up, and prostate cancer death rates in patients with locally confined prostate cancer

Author		N	Stage	PD (percentage)	Follow-up (mean months)	Cancer deaths per total deaths
Warner and Whitmore (1990)		29	B1	19 (66)	124	—
		37	B2	29 (78)	120	—
		9	B3	4 (44)	96	—
	Total	75		52 (69)	114	
Byar et al. (1981)		20	T2	7 (35)	91	1/6
		13	T1	3 (23)	78	1/3
Johansson et al. (1989)		104	T2	44 (42)	(36–120)	7/32

TNM category T2a, T2b (1987) corresponds to B1 and B2.

The patients of Johansson *et al.* (1989) were collected prospectively and were carefully staged according to the 1982 TNM system. Unfortunately, during a 2 year period, grade 3 patients were excluded from the study because it was felt that these patients should be actively treated. Extrapolation from these data reveals a median time to progression of 7–8 years and progression rates of 30–35 per cent at 5 years and 56–70 per cent at 10 years. In all reported series local progression rates are more frequent than distant metastases. Death rates from prostate cancer are low. Local progression can be prevented in most cases by surgery, radiotherapy, and endocrine treatment at the price of side-effects to be referred to later in this chapter. It is evident from the data shown that if an advantage in survival is ever to be demonstrated in a prospective randomized study, this advantage can only be small if the relatively small proportion of patients dying of prostate cancer is considered. Competing causes of death overrule in this age group; prostate cancer seems to be a slowly progressing disease. The literature is controversial about the impact of age on prostate cancer. However, the predominant opinion is that there is no correlation of younger age or older age with more or less aggressive prostate cancer. On this background it seems sensible to consider more aggressive and active treatment in locally confined prostate cancer occurring in younger age groups with a higher natural life expectancy.

Progression rates over 5 and 10 year periods are high and worrying. It is difficult to judge the impact of uncertainty and the amount of suffering resulting from the experience of progressive disease. Undoubtedly, if any of the treatment modalities were to achieve a degree of tolerability and lack of side-effects which would positively balance this amount of suffering, there could be a role for palliative surgery, radiotherapy, or any other form of potentially curative management of this disease.

Category T3 M0

T3 tumours extend through the capsule of the prostate or are localized in the apex. They are just at the limit of potential curability or have passed this stage. It is probably because of more sensitive techniques of detecting metastases that the incidence of this class of tumours has decreased in recent years. It is known that lymph node metastases occur in approximately 50 per cent of these patients. If this is the case, prognosis is determined by the N category rather than by the T category. T3 tumours without lymph node metastases have a prognosis which is clearly poorer compared with the smaller intraprostatic lesions. As Bosch *et al.* (1987) pointed out, cure rates by means of surgery cannot be expected to be above 30 per cent. Very little is known about the natural history of category T3 disease. If lymph node metastases are present, these are of overruling prognostic significance. Progression rates of lymph node negative disease have never been determined. In VACURG study II a median time to progression of 48 months was found in the placebo group. However, in this study no attempt was made to rule out or confirm the presence of lymph node metastases. Available data from the literature are summarized in Table 6. Median survival in this group

Table 6 Progression rates and median time to progression in patients with locally extensive non-metastatic prostate cancer

Reference	N	Stage	Mean time to PD (months)	No. with PD (%)
Byar and Corle (1988)	262	III	84[a]	50
Byar (1977)	75	III	48[a]	50

[a] Extrapolated from time to progression curves.

Table 7 Incidence of pelvic node metastasis documented in 452 patients with staging lymphadenectomy

Clinical stage	WD	Total MD	Grade (%) PD	(%)
A1	0	0	0	0
A2	0	26	43	24
B1	4	14	33	12
B2	18	27	43	28
C	50	41	93	58
Total	10	24	54	23

WD, well differentiated=Gleason grades 2–4; MD, moderately differentiated=Gleason grades 5–7; PD, poorly differentiated=Gleason grades 8–10.
Source: Smith *et al.* (1983).

of patients was found in prospective studies to be approximately 4 years.

There is no doubt that if effective treatment were available, this disease should be attacked aggressively, particularly in younger males. However, most patients seem to fail attempts at treatment and progress to metastatic disease with time. A complete review of this issue was recently given by Schröder *et al.* (1989).

N+ and M+ disease

Lymph node metastases are frequently identified at the time of surgical staging lymphadenectomy (Table 7). These patients were often asymptomatic and therefore treatment was deferred. Table 8 summarizes such data. There is a remarkable uniformity of median times to progression which are in the range of 11–24 months. It does not seem to matter whether delayed endocrine treatment, radiotherapy, or radical prostatectomy is applied. Regional lymph node metastases lead to a pattern of progression that is independent of regional treatment efforts. It has been shown by van Aubel *et al.* (1985) and Bosch *et al.* (1987) that with early endocrine treatment the median time to progression can be prolonged to 5 years. Despite some reports of long-term survival of patients with minimal lymph node involvement, the general consensus is that cure of this disease is impossible or extremely unlikely.

The natural history of M1 disease (that is, patients with distant metastases beyond the regional lymph nodes), is unknown. Placebo groups from early VACURG studies are not very useful because up to 44 per cent of these patients had been treated endocrinologically and still remained in the originally assigned treatment group. Furthermore, metastases were only identified by radiography, which leads to a sample which is not comparable with M1 patients identified by more recent standards. Following endocrine treatment, median times to progression of M1 patients are in the range of 1–1.5 years and median survival is 2–3 years. After the stage of

Table 8 Progression rates (PD) in patients with regional nodal metastases under delayed endocrine treatment

Reference	N	Time to PD (months)	Treatment (besides node dissection)
Kramer *et al.* (1981)	11	18.3	Radical prostatectomy
	20	15.8	Radiotherapy
	13	22.5	Delayed treatment
Paulson *et al.* (1982)	36	23.9	Radical prostatectomy
	41	12.2	Radiotherapy
Bagshaw (1980)	32	11–18.3	Radiotherapy
deVere White (1983)	25	11.6	Delayed endocrine

hormone independence of metastatic lesions has been reached, independent of the type of treatment that may be applied, the mean life expectancy is in the range of 1 year.

PRESENTATION AND DIAGNOSIS

Prostate cancer is a slowly developing malignancy in most patients. On the basis of longitudinal observations of prostate-specific antigen values reported by Stamey et al. (1989) for locally confined disease and ultrasound studies of similar groups of patients (F. H. Schröder, unpublished observations), volume doubling times of 2 years are estimated. Because of this slow development, at least during the early stage of the disease and because of the fact that only large tumours lead to urethral obstructive symptoms, early diagnosis is often made incidentally and rarely as a result of symptoms. Even metastatic disease is often not associated with symptoms. This leads to a delay of diagnosis in a very large proportion of patients, as indicated in Table 3 by the large number of patients diagnosed with metastatic disease.

Symptoms and physical examination

Symptoms of locally confined non-metastatic prostate cancer are rare because most tumours develop in the periphery of the prostate gland and do not lead to early obstructive symptoms. Such symptoms if they occur, are identical to those seen in patients with prostatic hyperplasia and consist of a slow stream and hesitancy, frequency, and urgency of micturition. Patients with locally confined prostate cancer sometimes present with perineal discomfort. This symptom clearly overlaps with the symptomatology of prostatitis which is an important differential diagnosis of this disease. Perineal discomfort, if due to prostate cancer, disappears with treatment but tends to recur with recurrence. Some patients will present with acute or chronic urinary retention as their initial symptom. This symptomatology will usually occur in patients with rapidly progressing tumours and is associated with a poor prognosis.

Regional and subregional lymph nodes are the most frequent sites of metastatic spread. Again, lymph node metastases are usually asymptomatic. However, physical examination may reveal an inguinal or suprapubic mass or very rarely a palpable fixed abdominal mass. Bone is the second most frequent site of metastases. Usually the pelvic bones and the axial skeleton are involved initially. Bone metastases may result in bone pain but this is not always the case. Metastases to the lumbar spine and the true pelvis may present with neurological symptoms which can be clearly related to lumbar or sacral roots. Paraplegia may result from compression of the spinal cord. Pain related to bone metastases is the most frequent symptom of prostate cancer. Obviously, degenerative changes of the spinal column and herniation of intervertebral discs leading to sciatic pain are important in the differential diagnosis. Unfortunately, tumour-related anorexia, anaemia, and decrease of performance status are frequently the first symptoms of prostate cancer. The prognosis of patients presenting in this fashion is usually poor.

On physical examination the only specific findings are on rectal examination. Prostatic carcinoma leads to changes in the consistency of the prostatic tissue and in the more advanced stages to deformations of the symmetry and architecture of the gland. A normal prostate has a transverse diameter of approximately 2.5 cm and a craniocaudal diameter of approximately 2 cm. In the age groups involved, benign prostatic hyperplasia is often present. The presentation of prostate cancer on rectal examination can vary from very small differences in tissue consistency through nodular changes to diffuse enlargement and hardening of the whole prostate. T categories are assigned by means of rectal examination as previously described.

Rectal examination can be carried out in several positions of which three have distinct advantages and disadvantages. Probably the best penetration and greatest depth of examination can be achieved with the patient standing upright and his elbows leaning on an examining table. The disadvantage of this position is that the pelvic musculature is tense, firm areas are accentuated, and even the normal prostate will always feel rather firm. The knee–elbow position offers relaxation and good depths of penetration but is less acceptable to patients. The lithotomy position, with the patient on his back and his legs pulled up, represents a compromise. Important differential diagnostic findings of rectal examination are benign prostatic hyperplasia, which may be irregular and nodular but not usually firm, prostatitis, prostatic calculi, and, rarely, tuberculosis. Granulomatous prostatitis is the most difficult differential diagnosis particularly since pathologists sometimes fail to differentiate this entity from poorly differentiated prostatic cancer. Forty to fifty per cent of all lesions that are believed to be suspicious on rectal examination are confirmed as prostatic adenocarcinomas by biopsy.

Rectal examination can accurately differentiate between extensive local disease infiltrating neighbouring organs (T4 and lower categories). Reliable differentiation between potentially curative disease and patients who are eventually shown to have gross penetration through the fibrous capsule of the prostate or invasion of the seminal vesicles is not possible by means of rectal examination. Data reported by Bosch et al. (1987) are in agreement with findings of others and show that in diagnosing T2 disease understaging occurs in approximately 50 per cent of cases. In diagnosing T3 disease overstaging may occur in up to 20 per cent of cases.

Transrectal ultrasonography and prostate specific antigen in the diagnosis of prostate cancer and screening

It has been claimed that these two diagnostic tools play a role in diagnosis and even in early diagnosis and screening studies of prostate cancer. The two techniques are also considered to be important in the staging and follow-up of prostate cancer patients. Comments here will be limited to their possible role in diagnosis.

Transrectal ultrasonography

Frentzel-Beyme (1985) and Lee et al. (1985) were the first authors to point out that most prostate cancers seem to present as hypoechogenic areas on transrectal ultrasound scanning of the prostate. This is at variance with earlier observations. Rifkin et al. (1989) believe that hypoechogenic lesions in general correlate well with the presence of better differentiated cancers. In their study of 51 cancers evaluated by ultrasound guided biopsy, they identified six isoechoic cancerous areas and ten which showed a mixed pattern. They are of the opinion that isoechoic cancers and those with hyperechoic areas more often have poor cellular differentiation and a larger stromal fraction. Lee et al. (1985) studied 784 men who were worried about the possible presence of prostate cancer by means of rectal examination and ultrasound. Seventy-seven cases were biopsied, 64 because of suspicion on transrectal ultrasonography and 23 because of suspicion by DRE. Twenty-two cancers were detected; the detection rate with transrectal ultrasonography was 2.6 versus 1.3 per cent with direct rectal examination. Carter et al. (1989) studied the contralateral lobe of 59 patients with proven carcinoma of the prostate in one lobe. Unexpected tumour on histological examination was found in 25 patients. A hypoechogenic area was mistaken for cancer not shown in histology in 11 cases, resulting in a false-positive rate of 32 per cent. Transrectal ultrasound detected 13 out of 25 unsuspected cancers. The sensitivity was 52 per cent and the specificity was 68 per cent. The authors concluded that transrectal ultrasonography may not be an adequate technique to detect clinically unsuspected prostate cancer, particularly because of the high false-positive rate.

A higher incidence of prostate cancer diagnosed with ultrasound guided biopsy of hypoechogenic or otherwise suspicious lesions on ultrasonography has also been reported by other authors. With new technology, particularly with the use of fine-needle aspiration and fine-needle core biopsy, more specimens are usually taken. It is not clear at present whether these changes in biopsy technique will have an effect on the higher detection rate seen with ultrasound-based diagnostic procedures. The fear is that with more extensive biopsies of prostates that are normal to direct rectal examination, lesions may be diagnosed which normally would not be found and that may not require any form of treatment. The role of ultrasonography in the diagnosis of prostate cancer needs to be more clearly defined.

Magnetic resonance imaging

Magnetic resonance imaging (MRI) is another novel interesting technique whose diagnostic contribution to prostate cancer needs to be further defined. Schiebler et al. (1989) have correlated radical prostatectomy specimens to MRI findings in 14 cases of previously diagnosed carcinoma of the prostate. They found that all carcinomas had a low signal intensity that led to suspicion of malignancy in all 14 cases. MRI is an expensive diagnostic tool. Its role in diagnosis and staging requires further assessment.

Prostate-specific antigen (PSA)

After having been in use for almost half a century, acid phosphatase as a marker for prostate cancer (Pontes et al. 1981) has been replaced by prostate-specific antigen (PSA) for most clinical situations. The sensitivity of PSA in identifying the presence of prostate cancer is approximately 20 per cent higher than that of the immunologically determined prostatic acid phosphatase, as shown by Hetherington et al. (1988), van Dieijen-Visser et al. (1988), and Oosterom et al. (1989). Serum PSA is not specific for prostate cancer; benign prostatic hyperplasia also leads to elevation of the substance in the serum. PSA is higher in patients with large volumes of benign prostatic hyperplasia; however, the volume correlation is poor. Stamey et al. (1989) have described a strong correlation with the volume of prostate cancer tissue in patients who have undergone radical prostatectomy. Therefore, several authors have recommended increasing the normal value to 10 ng/ml which is 2.5 times the recommended normal value. This leads to an increase in the specificity of the test and a decrease in the number of false-positive diagnoses. Cooner et al. (1988) applied PSA as a single screening procedure and found, for cut-off points of 4.0 and 10.0 ng/ml, sensitivities and specificities of 75.0 and 79.7 per cent, respectively, compared with 35.7 and 95.9 per cent for the higher normal value. Several authors have determined PSA in benign prostatic hyperplasia patients; values were above 10 ng/ml in 10–20 per cent of cases. In a preclinical screening study Powell et al. (1989) used PSA as a single parameter in patients with obstructive urinary symptoms. Of 36 patients with a PSA above 10 ng/l, 17 were proved to have carcinoma of the prostate and nine of these had

distant metastases. In this study the specificity of PSA for detecting prostate cancer was 90 per cent and the sensitivity was 98.5 per cent.

Cooner et al. (1990) used direct rectal examination, PSA, and transrectal ultrasonography together in a population of 1807 patients from a urology out-patient clinic. Patients were selected by urological complaint or by their desire to be screened. Rectal examination was carried out after the decision for inclusion in the study had been taken. A total of 267 carcinomas were identified (14.7 per cent); 203 diagnoses resulted from suspicion on rectal examinations. PSA and transrectal ultrasonography added a further 64. The combination of the three tests had the highest efficiency; PSA (above 10 ng/ml) and transrectal ultrasonography contributed equally. The distribution of stages is indicated in the original paper.

The role of PSA in the diagnosis of prostate cancer needs to be investigated further. When combined with an abnormal rectal examination or an abnormal ultrasound study, an elevation of PSA above normal or above 10 ng/ml certainly warrants a biopsy evaluation of the prostate. If PSA were used alone and there is no good reason to do so because a rectal examination is usually readily available, an undesirably high number of patients would have to undergo prostatic biopsy which would result in the diagnosis of benign prostatic hyperplasia. An elevated PSA in the absence of benign prostatic hyperplasia and of a palpable abnormality should be sufficient reason for prostatic biopsy.

Biopsy is usually carried out with a biopsy needle which can be used transrectally or transperineally and which provides a histological specimen. The use of fine-needle aspiration, which is applied transrectally, necessitates the availability of a well-trained cytologist and of a person who is skilful and trained in taking such biopsies. Under optimal conditions the results of the two techniques may be identical. Both biopsy techniques allowing grading which is reliable in identifying poorly differentiated tumours in only approximately 50 per cent of cases. Thus, undergrading is very common. Transrectal biopsies in particular may be associated with infectious complications. These complications and patient discomfort limit the indications for this procedure to extremely suspicious cases. If a biopsy is negative in the presence of strongly suspicious findings on rectal examination, it should be repeated. With very few exceptions a positive biopsy of the primary tumour remains a requirement for instituting treatment for prostatic cancer.

Screening for prostatic cancer

The availability of a blood test for prostatic cancer has major implications for the screening of normal populations. Assays have recently been developed for prostate-specific antigen which is a glycoprotein of molecular weight 34 kDa. PSA levels are elevated in the serum of patients with carcinoma of the prostate. Levels are within the normal range in normal men, but are elevated in 30 per cent of patients with benign prostatic hypertrophy. Thus, even if there were any survival advantage to early detection, which is arguable, this antigen cannot be used as a disease marker. PSA cannot be used to distinguish reliably between patients with or without metastatic spread. Although PSA levels are much more likely to be elevated in patients with metastatic cancer, being increased in approximately 95 per cent of patients, it is also elevated in 66 per cent of patients with localized cancer (Ferro et al. 1987). In this same study 95 per cent of patients with localized prostatic cancer had normal prostatic acid phosphatase levels. PSA levels do not reflect histological grade, prostatic acid phosphatase level, or alkaline phosphatase level (Emtage et al. 1987); however, cancers detected by PSA screening have a relatively low incidence of pelvic node involvement (Petros and Catalona 1992). In view of these findings, it is unlikely that levels of this antigen will be clinically useful in screening for prostate cancer, though accuracy may be improved by adjusting the PSA value for prostate volume (Benson *et al.* 1992).

Populations have been screened in an attempt to detect what some consider to be potentially curable prostatic cancer with the hope of altering the natural course of this malignancy. In a randomly selected population of 1494 normal men aged between 50 and 69 years, 13 early cancers were detected (Johansson *et al.* 1989). Ten of this group chose to be treated by radical prostatectomy and one chose radical radiotherapy. One patient was treated with endocrine therapies for advanced disease and another was untreated. The value of this screening technique, with an estimated cost of nearly 24 ECUs for each normal man and of 2500 ECUs for each case treated, is not clear, particularly as there is no evidence that the treatment of localized prostatic cancer bears any relationship to overall survival (Chodak 1993; Schröder 1993). A recent survey in the USA revealed dramatic increases in the detection rate of early prostate cancer during the 1980s, paralleled by increases in prostatectomy rates; however, there was no apparent correlation between the incidence and mortality rates for particular areas and the conclusion was that there was no evidence that screening and prostatectomy are effective in reducing mortality (Lu-Yao and Greenberg 1994).

ASSESSMENT AND INVESTIGATION

In the majority of patients a careful clinical history and examination will define disease extent. The presence of bone pain and weight loss implies metastatic cancer and a rectal examination will determine local disease extent. Plain radiographs of the chest and pelvis will show the presence of the characteristic sclerotic and lytic deposits that occur with prostatic cancer. Radio–isotope bone scanning using ^{99}Tc should proceed where the radiographs show no evidence of metastatic disease. Where solitary bone secondaries are present, it is important to distinguish between metastatic cancer and Paget's disease. Paget's disease tends to affect the whole of a bone, occupying, for example all of the ileum, whereas prostatic cancer metastases generally involve part of a bone. In prostatic cancer, where there is extensive involvement of bone, a characteristic scan known as a 'superscan' is described. All the tracer is taken up by bone so that the kidneys are not defined as they would be in a 'normal' bone scan. These scans are said to be absolutely characteristic of prostatic cancer and very unusual in any other condition.

The diagnosis of nodal metastasis in the pelvis or para-aortic areas is difficult without biopsy. The usual techniques of bipedal lymphography and CT scanning have high false-positive (10–30 per cent) and false-negative (20–40 per cent) rates unless grossly abnormal.

The staging of prostatic cancer is assisted by measurement of serum levels of prostatic acid phosphatase. Prostatic acid phosphatase is a sialoglycoprotein. It is a dimer of molecular weight 100 kDa which is in high concentration in prostatic tissue and present in many normal tissues. Its elevation in prostatic cancer was first noted in 1938. It is also present in many other tissues, but at levels 100 times lower than that in the prostate. Its first-phase serum half-life is approximately 1 h and its second-phase half-life is 11 days. The enzyme is not stable and delays in handling the specimen or freezing without acidification will result in falsely low values. Acid

phosphatase levels can be measured by enzymatic techniques or by radio–immunoassay (Heller 1987). Recently, immunoperoxidase techniques for staining histological specimens have become available, allowing precise histological diagnosis in cases with atypical presentations where there is difficulty in defining the primary site of the metastatic tumour.

Serum acid phosphatase levels have been used to define the extent of disease elevated levels correlate with the presence of metastatic cancer. However, normal serum levels do not invariably indicate disease confined to the prostate and values may be normal in metastatic prostatic cancer. Overall, approximately 15 per cent of patients with clinically localized prostatic cancer have elevated prostatic acid phosphatase levels (Robey *et al.* 1985). This may reflect the limitations of conventional staging techniques. If clinical staging is more extensive, it is found that those patients with clinically localized disease who have elevated prostatic acid phosphatase levels do not have localized cancer. Thus, in 20 patients proceeding to radical prostatectomy, none with prostatic disease alone had elevated serum prostatic acid phosphatase levels whereas elevated levels indicated extraprostatic disease (Pontes *et al.* 1981). Normal prostatic acid phosphatase levels are not necessarily indicative of disease confined to the prostate and approximately 20 per cent of patients with metastatic cancer will have normal acid phosphatase at presentation (El-Shirbiny *et al.* 1984).

Investigation of the patient is incomplete without measurement of PSA concentration. As well as contributing to staging information (Pantelides *et al.* 1992; Oesterling *et al.* 1993) PSA levels provide important prognostic information, especially for localized presentations (Ritter *et al.* 1992; Pisansky *et al.* 1993). The monitoring of serum PSA after local therapy may be even more specific and it should be noted that the expected rate of PSA decline after successful therapy is with a half-life of 2–3 days after prostatectomy and approximately 43 days after radiotherapy (Meek *et al.* 1990; Stein *et al.* 1992).

ROLE AND RESULTS OF SURGERY

In the management of any disease, particularly malignant disease, a risk–benefit analysis has to be made for the patient who is to be treated. The risk of the disease in question has to be balanced against the potential benefit and the side-effects of the treatment. Treatment should only be instituted if this risk–benefit analysis is clearly positive for the patient.

Because of the relatively low risk of dying from locally confined prostate cancer, which has been outlined above, straightforward decision-making in the various stages has been difficult in the past. It is evident from the low death rates that any improvement in overall survival can only be marginal. However, some patients, whether untreated or treated, will experience early progression and death from this disease. As with other malignant tumours, somewhere in the course of events there has to be a situation where even such aggressive tumours must be curable provided that they are completely removed. Unfortunately, at this time very few parameters are available to predict the course of individual tumours. Although tumour mass, grade of differentiation, and DNA ploidy may be such parameters, the reliability of their pre-treatment evaluation leaves much to be desired. In this situation the individual physician is confronted with the necessity of deciding treatment for patients with an incomplete knowledge of the risk of the given tumour to progress and to kill. Obviously, in any clinical situation in which overtreatment of a large proportion of patients is likely

Table 9 Selected results of radical prostatectomy and radiotherapy in locally confined prostate cancer

Treatment stage	N	Overall survival (%)		
		5 years	10 years	15 years
Surgery[a]				
B	132	76	61	39
C	213	64	36	20
Radiotherapy[b]				
T1	125	75	58	46
T2	119	75	50	36
T3	242	61	42	30

[a]Schröder and Belt (1975): some patients received adjuvant endocrine treatment; no node dissections were performed.
[b]Bagshaw (1984).

it is of paramount importance that the treatment itself has minimal side-effects. Considerable improvement has been achieved concerning the surgical technique of radical prostatectomy. The side-effects of impotence and incontinence have decreased considerably and have become manageable if they occur. A smaller and more purposeful lymph node dissection has fewer side-effects. However, the decision on how to treat locally confined prostate cancer remains difficult and variable recommendations are made to patients by different urologists in different parts of the world.

End-point analysis in locally confined disease

Obviously, prolongation of overall survival should be the goal of management of any life-threatening disease. However, in situations where considerable suffering may result from the disease itself on the one hand and where competing unrelated causes of death generally determine the remaining lifespan on the other hand, treatment policies must also be directed towards improvement of parameters other than overall survival.

Tables 9 and 10 show the dilemma. Historical comparison of even very large series of patients treated by radiotherapy, radical prostatectomy, or even a delayed treatment policy remain inconclusive despite a maximum effort of clinical staging. No large differences emerge that would make the pendulum swing in one or the other direction on the basis of overall survival figures. In a series of 191 patients treated by the late Dr Elmer Belt of Los Angeles and which had been followed for more than 15 years, 191 patients were found to be dead at a given time. The analysis of causes of death is shown in Table 10. Approximately two-thirds of these patients were believed to have locally extensive stage C

Table 10 Causes of death in 191 patients treated by radical prostatectomy for locally confined prostatic carcinoma

Causes of death	No. of patients	Percentage
Cardiovascular	87	45.6
Prostate cancer	46	24.2
Other malignancy	21	10.9
Pulmonary	5	2.6
Post-operative	4	2.1
Other known causes	15	7.8
Renal	3	1.6
Unknown	10	5.2
Total	191	100.0

disease and one-third appeared to be confined to the prostate. Despite total perineal prostatectomy, 24.2 per cent of the patients died of prostate cancer. However, most patients died of cardiovascular causes. Since cardiovascular disease, other malignancies, pulmonary disease, renal disease, and other known non-malignant causes together amounted to most causes of death, it would be very difficult to detect the influence of a 10–20 per cent improvement in prostate cancer mortality on overall mortality.

Cancer-specific survival and morbidity

Recently, Chodak et al. (1994) analysed reports on 828 patients with prostate cancer managed by surveillance. The median age was 69 years and median follow-up was 78 months. The 10 year actuarial disease-free survival was 87 per cent for those with grade 1 or grade 2 tumours, but only 34 per cent for those with grade 3 tumours and the 10 year mortality was 13 and 66 per cent, respectively. The incidence of metastatic disease by 10 years was 19 per cent in grade 1 tumours, 42 per cent in grade 2, and 74 per cent in grade 3. In the situation just described it is necessary to reconsider the position of the patient. Certainly, everybody wants to escape an untimely death due to cancer. Statistically the risk may be low. However, the situation is entirely different for the unfortunate individual patient who suffers from the more aggressive type of prostate cancer. In this case it is important to consider the quality of the patient's life with and without treatment for his disease. What are the sequelae of untreated disease and what is the chance of serious suffering? Warner and Whitmore (1990) described 66 and 87 per cent progression of B1 and B2 lesions, respectively, during a 10 year period. Two-thirds of these patients suffered local progression and one-third suffered progression to systemic disease. Local progression can be managed by transurethral resection with or without palliative radiotherapy. Also, endocrine control of the progression of the primary tumour is possible. However, this treatment is associated with repeated admission to hospital, considerable potential side-effects, and an amount of suffering that is difficult to appreciate. Systemic progression will put the patient into a different category. He will be confronted with a significantly shortened lifespan of 2.5–3.5 years and all the suffering that is associated with the distant spread of prostate cancer. In addition, an unknown amount of psychological suffering comes with the knowledge of the presence of cancer and the associated uncertainties. There is little doubt that, in addition to the cure of a number of patients, much of this suffering, particularly the local problems, can be avoided by radical prostatectomy. This view is also shared by Whitmore (1988b).

Therefore, in patients with locally confined prostate cancer it seems advisable to consider not just overall survival as an end-point. An improvement in cancer mortality and the inconvenience resulting from the tumour that is left behind should be balanced against the effectiveness of radical prostatectomy and radiotherapy in preventing the suffering associated with local and distant progression.

Selection of patients

Patients with prostate cancer in categories T1a, T1b, T2a, and T2b are, with certain limitations, eligible for potentially curative management. In patients with T3 disease, radiotherapy is usually applied whereas radical surgery is rarely attempted. Bosch et al. (1987) have reported on a series of 48 T3 patients in whom surgical cure was the goal. After exclusion of those patients who had positive lymph nodes and other prognostic factors that were thought to preclude the chance of cure, a projected cure rate of 29 per cent was estimated. Obviously, T3 patients are at the limits of curability or are already incurable by local regional management.

Category T1, T2 (A1, A2)

Progression rates in A1 and A2 disease as reported by Johansson *et al.* (1989) amount to 10 and 32 per cent, respectively. Cancer deaths at 5 years are estimated to occur in 4 and 15 per cent of cases, respectively. These data are in good agreement with those of Epstein *et al.* (1986, 1988*b*) who showed for A1 and A2, respectively, 5 and 10 year progression rates of 2 and 16 per cent as opposed to 39 and 68 per cent. In the A1 disease group at 10 years 12 per cent cancer deaths were projected. Provided that tumour foci are well differentiated, observation is indicated, at least in the older patient. It is important to consider life expectancy in this particular group. The exceptional very young patient who presents with this disease may be a candidate for treatment because he may outlive the 15 year risk of an even higher progression rate, as pointed out by Blute *et al.* (1986). Results of treatment by radical prostatectomy in A1 and A2 disease have been reported by Paulson *et al.* (1988). This group carefully analysed the pathological findings of the surgical specimens and found that of 11 patients with specimen-confined disease no treatment failure occurred. Of 41 patients with organ-confined disease four (9.7 per cent) failed despite radical prostatectomy at periods of up to 11.9 years. Twenty-four patients had positive margins and six of those failed within 8 years. If anything, this study shows that the group of A1 and A2 patients is heterogeneous and contains high-risk patients which again seem to be difficult to identify.

In this situation the question is often considered as to whether a second transurethral resection prostate would help to identify residual tumour. The issue was recently reviewed by Epstein *et al.* (1988*a*). In an analysis of 21 radical prostatectomy specimens of clinical A1 disease, the authors show that no tumour was found in three cases, 13 had minimal residual tumour, and five had a substantial amount of tumour. After radical prostatectomy all patients were continent and 93 per cent were potent. They believe that although some patients would have been upstaged by a repeat transurethral resection, others would have remained at stage A1 despite a more extensive tumour mass due to the peripheral location of the residual tumour which might not be accessible to transurethral resection. If tumour is present in the second transurethral resection specimen, this will not indicate complete removal or tumour still remaining. A negative retransurethral resection specimen will not mean that there is no tumour left. If observation is chosen as the mode of treatment in A1 disease, it is necessary to remember that, while local recurrence is more frequent, distant progression may occur primarily in approximately one-third of patients. Rectal examination and PSA determinations should detect both events when combined with bone scans at the time of a rising PSA.

There is some uncertainty about the best management of T1b (A2) disease. Lymph node dissection combined with radical prostatectomy as well as radiotherapy may be indicated. The proper identification of A2 disease strongly depends on a previous careful rectal examination. Prostate cancer missed or misinterpreted on rectal examination will lead to the inclusion of far more advanced cases in this category.

Stage T2a, T2b (B1, B2)

Radical prostatectomy was first introduced into clinical medicine by Young in 1905. Jewett (1970, 1984) has pointed out that the palpable nodule of prostate cancer which is limited to the prostate gland is the classical and most appropriate indication for radical prostatectomy. Belt and Schröder (1972) revealed survival rates of 78, 55, 31, and 20 per cent in 185 patients and histologically confined prostate cancer at 5, 10, 15, and 20 years. These data turned out to be identical with the expected age-corrected survival period and at that time represented strong evidence for the effectiveness of radical surgery. These data need to be contrasted with estimated rates of progression at 5, 10, and 15 years of 54, 66, and 100 per cent and with the associated cancer death rates at 5, 10, and 15 years of 0, 17, and 50 per cent in Whitmore's (1988*b*) patients with stage B1 disease. Although some of Belt and Schröder's (1972) patients were treated with adjuvant endocrine techniques, the long-term follow-up reporting of overall survival and the lack of node dissection make this series useful for comparison.

The only prospective randomized study ever attempted in locally confined palpable prostate cancer was that of VACURG reported by Byar *et al.* (1981). Unfortunately, this trial was never completed and has therefore remained inconclusive. Twenty patients received placebo and 30 received placebo plus radical prostatectomy in a randomized fashion. Seven of the placebo group and six of the radical prostatectomy group progressed within a 7.7 year period. Five year survival was 48 per cent in the placebo and 67 per cent in the radical surgery group. No significant differences were found. Another randomized study in this disease compared radical prostatectomy with radiotherapy. A significant difference in favour of the radical prostatectomy group occurred after 30 months (Paulson *et al.* 1982) and the study was discontinued for ethical reasons. This study was later criticized for various reasons as described fully below in the section on radiotherapy.

Category T3 (C)

As mentioned before, the natural history of this disease is not well known. Five year progression rates are estimated to be in the range of 40–50 per cent. Obviously, if effective treatment were available this is a group of patients that should be treated aggressively. A recent review by Schröder *et al.* (1989) reveals that only a small subgroup of patients within this category can be expected to be cured. The best palliation in stage C disease is not known. Again, complications of surgical treatment and radiotherapy will have to be matched against the natural course of the disease.

Grade and ploidy

de Voogt *et al.* (1989) have shown conclusively in 436 patients with advanced prostatic cancer recruited to the European Organization for Research on Treatment of Cancer (EORTC) Genitourinary Group protocols that grade of differentiation has a significant influence on cancer-related mortality. However, in a multivariate analysis, performance status, M category, elevation of alkaline phosphatase, and the presence of a T4 category had a stronger prognostic impact. It has been shown by several authors that grade of differentiation is a very important, maybe the most important, routinely evaluated prognostic factor in localized prostate cancer. This is shown in virtually every reported series. T category and grade of differentiation can be combined to become an even more powerful predictor of prognosis. This is shown in Table 11 which correlates death from prostatic carcinoma to T, PT, and G categories in a series of 342 patients treated by radical prostatectomy. It can be seen that in patients with truly focal and well-differentiated tumours the risk of dying of prostate cancer in this series was zero. At the other end of the spectrum, 30–45 per cent of patients with G3 tumours, virtually independent of tumour extension, died despite

Table 11 Identification of risk groups by correlating T and P categories with the grade of differentiation (nuclear pleomorphism) with disease-related mortality

T, P category	G1			G2			G3		
	No. of patients	Deaths	No. with cancer (%)	No. of patients	Deaths	No. with cancer (%)	No. of patients	Deaths	No. with cancer (%)
T0	10	0	0	23	6	26.1	5	2	40.0
P1	6	0	0	4	0	0	0	0	0
T1–2	33	3	9.1	125	18	14.4	31	10	32.3
P2	28	2	7.1	72	7	9.7	14	2	14.3
T3	15	1	6.7	73	21	28.8	27	12	44.4
P3	22	1	4.6	146	38	26.0	51	22	43.1

radical prostatectomy. In considering the uncertainties of the natural history and the related risk of locally confined prostatic cancer, at first glance this type of information seems to be extremely useful for patient selection. Unfortunately, however, the pre-operative determination of the grade of differentiation is extremely inaccurate. If a G3 tumour is diagnosed, this will certainly indicate a poor prognosis. However, as shown by Ackermann and Müller (1981) and Kastendieck (1980), the finding of a well-differentiated tumour in a biopsy specimen is associated with the presence of moderately or poorly differentiated adenocarcinoma in the radical prostatectomy specimen in 50–65 per cent of cases. Narayan et al. (1989) compared the diagnostic accuracy of core biopsies and fine-needle aspiration biopsies in 121 patients. The findings were related to the pathological specimens obtained at radical prostatectomy or transurethral resection of the prostate. Although fine-needle aspiration was superior in identifying prostate cancer, it did not show superiority in identifying the correct grade of differentiation. Although the volume of prostatic cancer present in histological specimens after radical prostatectomy provides excellent correlation with the incidence of nodal and distant metastases, this parameter is not easily available for pre-operative evaluation as was shown by Partin et al. (1989).

Twenty to fifty per cent of patients with locally confined prostate cancer have non-diploid tumours. Several centres in the United States, including the Mayo Clinic, have carefully elaborated the prognostic impact of ploidy as reported by Nativ et al. (1989). The preliminary data show that ploidy is a very powerful prognostic factor in locally confined prostate cancer. However, almost no data exist on pre-operative evaluation and the role of ploidy in decision-making in these patients needs to be determined in the future. One possible solution of the dilemma of management of locally confined prostate cancer would be the availability of a set of prognostic factors which have a high sensitivity and specificity and which can be evaluated with great accuracy in the pre-operative situation. Unfortunately, most available factors are not ready for daily use in patient selection.

Patient-related factors

Obviously, in selecting patients for radical prostatectomy, age, biological age, associated chronic illnesses, and the general condition of the patient have to play an important role. To give an extreme example, it certainly does not make sense to carry out a radical prostatectomy in a 75 year old patient with stage T1 disease in whom the 10 year progression rate may be in the range of 20 per cent. The chance of this patient suffering and even dying of cancer is too small to warrant radical surgery. It is the authors' experience that in patients who are intellectually capable of understanding the most important factors of decision-making, patient involvement is a very useful, motivating, and important factor in selection. Patients should be confronted with the risk of the tumour, the complications of surgery, the chance of eradication of the tumour by radical prostatectomy and radiotherapy, and the potential complications of both forms of treatment. The decision-making process is very complicated because so many factors are involved. All prognostic and patient-related factors should be compiled prior to the decisive conversation and should be discussed whenever possible with the patient and, if desired, with family members.

N+ (D1) disease

As shown in the previous section and indicated in Table 8, the prognosis of patients with lymph node involvement is not determined by the primary tumour but by distant spread. Time to progression is in the range of 10–20 months and is not influenced by any treatment modality except endocrine therapy. In this situation radical prostatectomy does not seem to be indicated, except if there is good reason to expect a significant palliative effect of radical surgery. This concept was recently confirmed by a careful study of 511 patients reported by Gervasi et al. (1989).

There is still controversy about this subject, since Zincke et al. (1987) have reported a significantly better survival in patients undergoing node dissection, radical prostatectomy, and early endocrine treatment as opposed to node dissection and early endocrine treatment alone. Recently, the differences in overall survival have been explained by differences in ploidy distribution (Zincke 1988). Bosch and Schröder (1990), in an analysis of the data of Zincke (1988), also conclude that the difference seen is due to patient selection and to a different distribution of prognostic factors in the two treatment groups. In agreement with other findings reported in the literature, there is no doubt that early endocrine treatment prolongs time to progression. However, an advantage in survival for this combination has not been shown.

Lymphadenectomy and radical prostatectomy

The purpose of this chapter is not to give a detailed description of surgical techniques. A recent update of the technical aspects has been given by Walsh et al. (1986). Whitmore (1984) made an important contribution by showing in 130 patients that a modified and very limited lymph node dissection gives a representative lymph node sampling. There is general agreement that lymph node dissection does not contribute to the cure of patients, except in a few exceptions. It is recommended that lymph node dissection is carried out in the area between the inguinal ligament, the obturator vessels, the internal iliac artery, and the external iliac vein. With this limited dissection morbidity has markedly decreased.

Important modifications to the technique of radical prostatectomy have been made and reported by Walsh and his associates. These modifications have led to a significant decrease in morbidity resulting from radical prostatectomy and to widespread general acceptability of this operation. These modifications include the following. Reiner and Walsh (1979) described a surgical approach to the anatomy of Santorini's plexus which helps to avoid blood loss and allows proper anatomical dissection of the neurovascular bundles which were described by Walsh and Donker (1982). Walsh (1988) has subsequently shown that preservation of potency is possible in 74 per cent of 482 patients treated in this way. Even with retention of one neurovascular bundle, preservation of potency is reported to be possible in 69 per cent of cases. Different ways of handling the bladder neck and the apex of the prostate have resulted in higher continence rates. Incontinence occurs in 2–4 per cent of cases and can be effectively treated with indwelling sphincter prosthesis if this complaint persists for prolonged periods of time.

Results of radical prostatectomy

The data available in the literature on the results of radical prostatectomy have recently been given in *National Cancer Institute Monograph 7* which is dedicated to a consensus development conference on the management of clinically localized prostate cancer. In the resulting consensus statement radiotherapy and radical prostatectomy are both characterized as being active and suitable ways of managing this disease. As mentioned above, conclusive randomized studies of radical prostatectomy, delayed treatment policy, and radiotherapy are unfortunately not available. Phase II results are strongly dependent on prognostic factors such as T category, G category, age of the patients, accompanying disease, etc. Most authors find that 5, 10, and 15 year survivals for patients with stage A and B1 disease are identical or superior to the life expectancy calculated for the group of patients involved. Figure 1 can be considered representative for these results except that lymph node dissection was not employed (Belt and Schröder 1972). Positive lymph nodes can be expected in the group of patients thought to be eligible for radical surgery in approximately 25–30 per cent of

cases. If these patients are excluded from radical surgery, this will result in a considerable improvement of survival. However, local extension and grade of malignancy remain important prognostic factors, leading to significant differences in overall and corrected survival (Gibbons 1993). A review of available data including series with and without lymphadenectomy has been given by Walsh and Lepor (1987). In our opinion it does not make any sense to attempt historical comparison. As pointed out earlier, in view of the natural history, whatever differences in time to progression, disease-specific survival, and overall survival are found, these differences will be small. For this reason it seems more important to consider early and late complications of radical prostatectomy.

Palliative surgical treatment of prostate cancer, particularly obstructive symptoms, plays an important role in daily clinical practice. Transurethral resection in non-metastatic prostate cancer is controversial. Hanks *et al.* (1983) and McGowan (1988) have suggested that transurethral resection of the prostate is associated with a higher incidence of distant metastases. However, this view is disputed and rejected by a report by Meacham *et al.* (1989).

Transurethral resection of the prostate may be necessary for urinary obstruction. The complication rate of this procedure is clearly higher as far as secondary bleeding and incontinence is concerned, as in similar cases of prostatic hyperplasia. This is probably due to the more difficult visual orientation with regard to the usual landmarks and to the lack of re-epitheliazation of cancerous areas after transurethral resection. To avoid repeated transurethral resections in locally progressive disease, palliative radiotherapy may be useful.

Early and late complications of lymph node dissection and radical prostatectomy

A summary of complications seen at the Department of Urology, Erasmus University, Rotterdam, is given in Tables 12 and 13 for radical prostatectomy and lymph node dissection. A large number of reports are available in the literature.

As far as impotence is concerned, the excellent results of Walsh are not always achieved by every surgeon. Catalona and Bigg (1990) described preservation of potency in 71 out of 112 patients (63 per cent). Preservation of potency correlated with patient age and was higher in patients with organ-confined tumours. Walsh *et al.* (1986) showed that, with the unilateral preservation of the

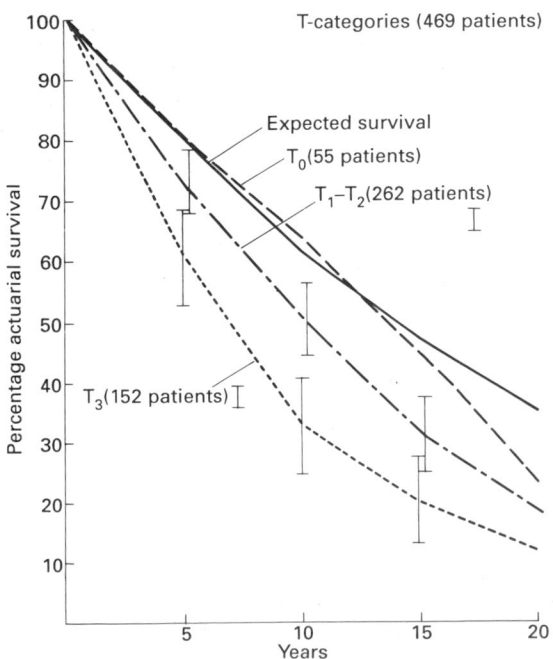

Fig. 1 Actuarial overall survival of 469 patients treated by radical prostatectomy without node dissection. T stage is by 1982 TNM classification.

Table 12 Course and complications encountered in 33 patients after lymphadenectomy alone

Follow-up 4.1 years (1.0–9.8)
Ten (30%) suffered early post-operative complications (prolonged drainage, lymphocele, thrombosis, embolism (2×), no deaths (<6 weeks)
Eleven (33%) later required treatment of prostatic obstruction
Fourteen (42%) progressed, eight (24%) died of prostate cancer

Table 13 Course and complications of 109 patients after node dissection and radical prostatectomy

Follow-up 3.8 years (1.0–12.0)
Twenty (18%) required dilatations of the bladder neck
Five (5%) still wear pads (>2)
Four (4%) required an artificial sphincter for incontinence
Forty-one per cent lost potency in spite of attempts to preserve the neurovascular bundles
Sixty-three (60%) suffered some kind of early post-operative or intraoperative complications with no long-term sequelae

neurovascular bundle, 69 per cent of potency in previously potent men can be obtained. Pontes *et al.* (1986) described an overall erectile potency in 54 per cent of 45 patients. In the authors' own experience 59 per cent of preservation of potency was seen.

In treatment utilizing advanced techniques incontinence has been reported in 2–5 per cent of cases (Walsh 1988; Catalona and Bigg 1990).

Both these major long-term complications of radical prostatectomy can be managed effectively. Impotence can be treated by repeated papaverine injections which have been shown by Dennis and McDougal (1988) to be effective in 12 out of 14 patients. At the Mayo Clinic the AMS 800 artificial urinary sphincter was implanted in 117 patients with incontinence after radical prostatectomy. The results indicated a 90 per cent continence and satisfaction rate. A recent report on early post-operative morbidity has been given by Donohue *et al.* (1990). This review is comprehensive and representative. Early post-operative complications include wound infection and associated problems, lymphoceles, urinary tract infection, epididymitis, urethral anastomotic stricture, pulmonary embolus, and, very rarely, weakness of the adductor muscles due to injury of the obturator nerve. Frohmüller and Grups (1985) reported on complications in 175 patients. The complication of stricture of the anastomosis was found to occur in 11.5 per cent of 156 patients (Surya *et al.* 1990). This early post-operative complication is usually transient and disappears after several dilatations of the involved area.

Total perineal prostatectomy is rarely practised because of the disadvantage of having to perform lymph node dissections in a separate position and possibly at a different time. Also, preservation of potency with this procedure is not as readily possible, although some promising results have been reported by Weldon and Tavel (1988) who preserved potency in five out of nine patients. The complications of total perineal prostatectomy are different and will not be reported in this context.

Adjuvant treatment

Adjuvant treatment may be applied as initial endocrine therapy with the purpose of shrinking the prostate to facilitate surgery and to improve resectability of more extensive tumours. Adjuvant treatment is also used in situations where positive margins indicate incomplete resection of the primary tumour and in cases of local recurrence after radical prostatectomy.

Initial endocrine treatment

This approach was developed by Monfette *et al.* (1989) who treated 50 patients who were eligible for radical prostatectomy with immediate total androgen blockade. The authors describe a significant decrease of prostatic volume, as expected and a facilitation of surgery and speculate about an advantage in survival. The issue was recently reviewed by Bosch and Schröder (1990). While surgery may be facilitated, those patients who remain potent after radical prostatectomy will have to suffer from a 7 months' delay in return of potency because of the immediate endocrine treatment. In those patients whose tumour is not resectable, a survival advantage could not be demonstrated in the series of Belt and Schröder (1972), where a comparison between adjuvant endocrine treatment and no adjuvant treatment is possible. An advantage in survival which was encountered at 5 years disappeared after 10 and 15 years.

Adjuvant treatment after incomplete resection

The management of this situation has remained controversial despite a large volume of literature dealing with this problem. It has been shown that even in the presence of positive margins only 20–30 per cent of such patients will ever experience local recurrence. However, several authors (Gibbons *et al.* 1986; Lange *et al.* 1988; Anscher and Prosnitz 1989; Carter *et al.* 1989) who compared results from patients who were treated immediately with those who were treated after local recurrence was clinically evident have shown an advantage for early adjuvant radiotherapy in this situation. Walsh (1987) reviewed the issue and came to the contrary conclusion. Complications of radiotherapy in the post-surgical situation are not negligible. Those 70–75 per cent who will never suffer local recurrence will have to bear these complications for no good reason. It is a disturbing fact that local recurrence is frequently associated with distant progression which will necessitate endocrine treatment anyway. The news to the patient that resection was incomplete has a severe psychological impact. Obviously, there is much to be said against delaying treatment in the situation of positive margins.

An analysis of local relapse after prostatectomy was performed in 273 patients of whom 46 developed local recurrence (Anscher and Prosnitz 1991). The independent risk factors were poorly differentiated histology, positive margins, and elevated acid phosphatase (PSA was not analysed). It was suggested that these could provide indications for adjuvant radiotherapy. Alternatively it has been argued that monitoring serum PSA after prostatectomy allows selection of patients for radiotherapy on the basis of rising PSA with no evidence of metastatic disease. In seven of the 11 patients reported by Schild *et al.* (1992) this led to a fall in PSA to normal levels.

Once local recurrence is manifest and demonstrated by means of cytology or histology, radiotherapy and/or endocrine therapy are clearly indicated.

Adjuvant treatment in D1 disease

It has been shown by van Aubel *et al.* (1985) and more recently by Kramolowsky (1988), together with the data from the Mayo Clinic reported by Zincke (1988), that adjuvant endocrine treatment in this situation leads to a significant prolongation of time to progression. With delayed endocrine treatment progression will occur within 10–22 months of lymph node dissection. With immediate endocrine treatment the median time to progression ranges from 60 to 100 months. It is uncertain at present whether early or delayed endocrine treatment may be associated with an advantage in disease-related overall survival. However, the patient has a choice. Many may opt for a longer initial symptom-free interval at the price of impotence. If potency is of a great importance, delayed endocrine treatment is advisable.

ROLE AND RESULTS OF RADIOTHERAPY
History

The first radiotherapy for prostatic malignancy was undertaken in the early years of this century (Von Paschkis and Tittinger 1910; Pasteau 1911) by implantation of radium needles through a perineal fistula. Later developments employed applicators *per urethrum* or *per rectum* (Young and Fronz 1917; Deming 1922). A combination of brachytherapy with external-beam irradiation was employed by Caulk (1937). Significant advances followed the development of higher-energy external-beam equipment which appeared able to control the primary tumour (del Regato 1967; Bennett 1968; Ray *et al.* 1973; Bagshaw *et al.* 1993).

Anatomy

The prostate gland is shaped like an inverted pyramid and surrounds the urethra distal to the bladder neck, posterior to the pubic bone, and anterior to the rectum from which it is separated by Denonvilliers' fascia. The seminal vesicles enter the prostate gland posterosuperiorly.

The great majority of carcinomas arise in the peripheral part of the gland and the tumour is frequently multinodular (Jewett 1980). Invasion of prostatic capsule occurs early and extension in to the seminal vesicle is common. The incidence of pelvic lymph node involvement is associated with both primary stage and grade of the tumour (Table 7). Local nodes include those in periprostatic, obturator, internal iliac, external iliac, hypogastric, and pre-sacral groups.

Although the prostate appears to tolerate radiation well, histologically there is fibrosis and loss of glandular structure and calcification may occur (Leach *et al.* 1982). The relatively slow cycle time of many prostatic tumours (Trott and Kummermehr 1985) may account for the frequency of biopsy evidence of persisting carcinoma after radiotherapy, particularly since the incidence of positive biopsy seems to decrease with time (Cox and Kline 1983). In assessing the significance of post-irradiation biopsy, it is important not to base results only on prostates which feel abnormal in which the incidence of persistent cancer is much higher than in the total population irradiated (Freiha and Bagshaw 1984). Nevertheless, if post-irradiation biopsy is performed more than 6 months after radiation therapy, the result does convey prognostic information. Scardino and Wheeler (1988) found that the rate of local recurrence was 19 per cent in patients with negative biopsy and 60 per cent in those with a positive biopsy.

Indications for radiotherapy

The rationale for local treatment is discussed above in the section on the role of surgery. Radical radiotherapy is regarded as an alternative to surgery in the radical treatment of T1 and T2 N0M0 tumours and is used at radical doses for local control of more advanced primaries. Radiotherapy also has an important palliative role, particularly for painful bone metastases refractory to hormone therapy when low-dose single-fraction treatments are able to reduce pain in more than three-quarters of patients (Price *et al.* 1986). Pelvic radiotherapy is employed for obstructive lymphadenopathy or haematuria.

Radiation therapy techniques

External-beam radiation therapy

Planning

Traditionally, planning has involved localization of the bladder neck using intravesical contrast on orthogonal anterioposterior and lateral radiographs. The incorporation of rulers allows a correction for magnification and translation of the patient's axial body outline with the position of the target volume located accurately within it. Barium in the rectum outlines the relationship of this organ to the prostate on a lateral film.

Alternatively the prostate can be localized using CT imaging (Fig. 2). It is important that this is performed in the treatment position and that a marker is placed on the skin tattoo, so that this

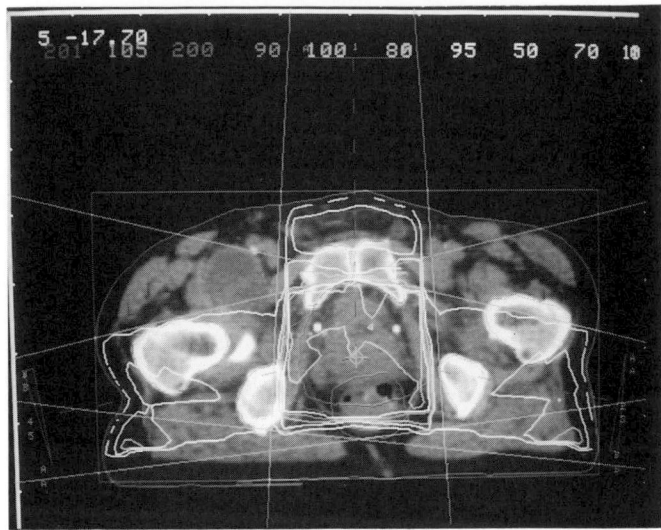

Fig. 2 Radiation isodose distribution calculated and displayed on the central axial CT slice for radical radiotherapy for an early prostatic carcinoma.

can be located on the CT image and used to relate the image to the patient. Cuts of 1 cm through the prostate suffice except for the accurate definition of the upper and lower borders. Oral and rectal contrast help the delineation of bowel within the pelvis and usually planning and treatment are carried out with bladder full in order to move both the dome of the bladder and as much bowel as possible away from the high-dose area.

Conventional planning has been compared with CT localization (Kuruvilla *et al.* 1989) which was believed to show advantages in demonstrating local tumour extension. CT scanning is most accurate in defining the lateral and anterior extents of the tumour in a central slice. The prostatic apex can be difficult to discern on an axial slice and it has been proposed that this can be marked by placement of a gold seed in the urogenital diaphragm (Murphy and Porter 1988). As shown in Figs 3 and 4 the ability of MRI techniques to image in coronal and sagittal planes may give them a useful role in planning carcinoma of the prostate because of their precise delineation of the vertical extent of the tumour.

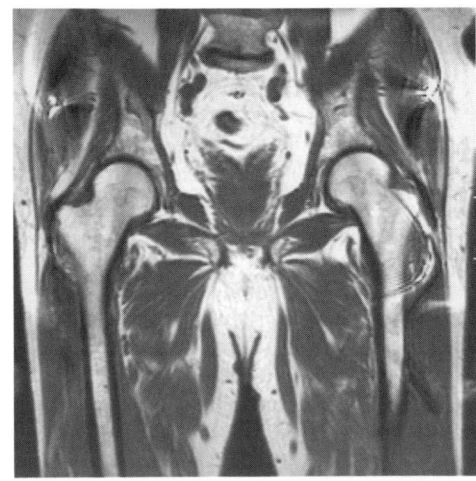

Fig. 3 Coronal magnetic resonance image through prostate and seminal vesicles.

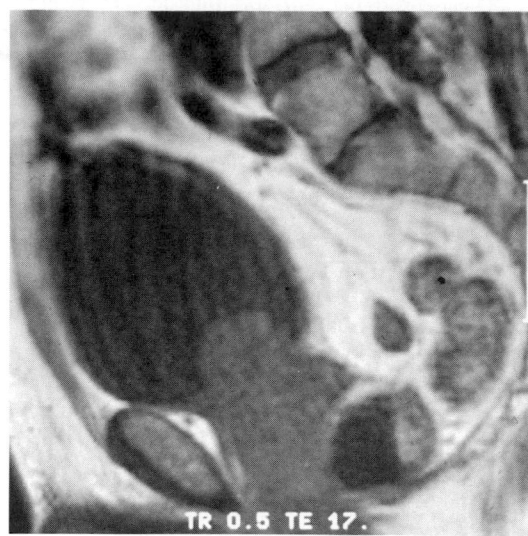

Fig. 4 Sagittal magnetic resonance image through T4 prostate carcinoma invading the bladder.

Table 14 Radiation dose and local recurrence

| Dose (Gy) | In-field failure rates (%) | |
	Stage B (n=724)	Stage C (n=624)
<60	24	25
60–64	13	28
65–69	13	23
70+	14	17

Source: Hanks *et al.* (1988).

outcome similar to that of patients without evidence of lymphatic involvement, suggesting a beneficial effect of pelvic irradiation in patients with nodal involvement (Pilepich 1988).

Radiation dose

There is evidence that the dose required for local control is related to the volume of primary tumour treated (Hanks 1985; Hanks *et al.* 1985), as shown in Table 14. The recurrence rates vary from greater than 20 per cent for doses below 55 Gy to less than 10 per cent for doses above 65 Gy (Perez 1983; Aristizabal *et al.* 1984). Doses of 60–64 Gy led to 87 per cent local-recurrence-free survival in 17 patients with T2 tumours and a 75 per cent local-recurrence-free survival in 29 patients with T3 tumours (Hanks *et al.* 1985). For T1 tumours there is no evidence that doses over 60 Gy improve local control (Hanks *et al.* 1988). The issue of dose is important since there is evidence in prostate cancer that local control influences the rate of metastasis (Fuks *et al.* 1991).

Field arrangements

A range of techniques have been used to irradiate the prostate, including multiple fixed-field techniques, rotational therapy, and brachytherapy which is discussed further below. A quality assurance study of external-beam therapy compared 20 radiotherapy centres in The Netherlands (Wittkamper *et al.* 1987). For reference ^{60}Co or megavoltage X-ray beams, the mean difference between measured and stated dose values was only 0.5 per cent with a standard deviation of 1.9 per cent. When the local planning system was used to simulate the treatment of prostate cancer on an anthropomorphic phantom, differences between the measured and stated doses at the isocentre were on average 1.5 per cent with a standard deviation of 1.5 per cent. Differences between stated and measured doses at several points in the target volume averaged 0.4 per cent with a standard deviation of 5.2 per cent. The most marked differences were found in the rectum with a mean of 4 per cent and a larger standard deviation of 18 per cent.

A simple three-field plan which can be used throughout the treatment course is shown in Fig. 5. Radiobiological considerations would suggest that all three fields are treated at each fraction. There is evidence of increased complications from utilization of a simple parallel opposed anterior and posterior field arrangement (Leibel *et al.* 1984; Forman *et al.* 1985) and there is also evidence for increased complications with larger radiation fields (Dewit *et al.* 1983; Mameghan *et al.* 1990). Analysis of the RTOG prospective study of the extent of radiation fields in stage A2 and B carcinoma of the prostate suggested that parallel opposed anterior and posterior portal treatment of pelvic lymphatics was associated with an increased incidence of bowel complications and in more advanced tumours the RTOG study found an increased incidence of bowel

It is unclear that treating the patient in a prone position more effectively separates the prostate from the rectum and the convention at the Royal Marsden Hospital is to apply treatment with the patient supine (Dobbs and Barrett 1985). Planning and treatment are carried out with a full bladder to displace the dome of the bladder and the small intestine from the treatment volume. Alignment is to skin tattoos placed in the midline over the pubic symphysis and laterally over each iliac crest. Beam alignment is checked using an anterior laser beam for the midline and two lateral lasers to align the lateral skin tattoos in order to prevent rotation.

Target volume

Conventional external-beam treatment has been to either the whole pelvis with a boost dose to the prostate or the prostate and the immediately surrounding tissues alone. There is no strong evidence to support treatment of pelvic lymph nodes despite retrospective studies suggesting advantage for this (McGowan 1981; Polysongsang *et al.* 1986). This was not supported by the Patterns of Care Study (Leibel *et al.* 1984). Also, between 1978 and 1983 the Radiation Therapy Oncology Group (RTOG) conducted a prospective randomized study in patients with stage A2 and stage B carcinoma of the prostate. Patients received 65 Gy to the prostate in 1.8–2 Gy fractions over a period of 6.5 weeks or pelvic node irradiation of 45 Gy with a boost of 20 Gy to the prostate. After a median follow-up of 7 years 445 patients were evaluated (Asbell *et al.* 1988). There was no statistically significant benefit of pelvic node irradiation in terms of local control, rate of development of distant metastases, or survival. Concurrently the RTOG conducted a second prospective randomized trial in patients with stage C tumour or with evidence of pelvic node involvement, comparing pelvic irradiation with pelvic plus para-aortic radiotherapy, again treating the prostate with 65 Gy and lymph nodes with 40–45 Gy (Pilepich *et al.* 1986). Analysis of 523 patients was performed with a median follow-up of 4 years and no statistically significant difference between the treatment arms was demonstrated for either relapse or survival. Although these studies would not suggest any benefit from enlarging the radiation target volume beyond the prostate and periprostatic tissues, it was noted that patients with extracapsular extension of the primary tumour and evidence of pelvic lymph node involvement had an

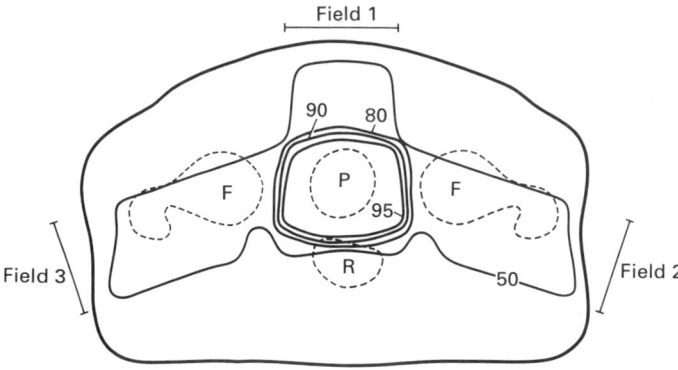

Fig. 5 Three-field plan with shaped blocks providing a small conformal radiation volume.

injuries if the prostatic boost was given by lateral fields alone or by a perineal field (Pilepich *et al.* 1987*a*).

Brachytherapy

Interstitial implantation techniques for the brachytherapy of carcinoma of the prostate also have a long history (Young and Fronz 1917). The potential advantages of brachytherapy are the reduction in treated volume with the radiobiological advantages of continuous low-dose rate irradiation and shortened overall treatment time (Horwich 1989). Various techniques have been employed including combination of radioactive gold (^{198}Au) with external-beam therapy (Carlton *et al.* 1976), interstitial ^{125}I (Hilaris *et al.* 1977), and implantation of ^{192}Ir (Court and Chassagne 1977). These techniques for implantation of the prostate have often been combined with either external-beam irradiation or pelvic lymph node dissection.

As with all interstitial treatments, the geometry of the implant is critically important and the technique is most appropriate for small, well-defined, and regularly shaped tumours.

There has been extensive recent experience with low-energy ^{125}I seeds. The half-life of ^{125}I is 60 days and the usual recommended dose to the periphery of the prostate is 180 Gy delivered over 1 year. In contrast, gold seeds are of high activity with a half-life of only 2.7 days and, thus, confer a hazard on staff. A dose of 35 Gy has been employed combined with 45 Gy by fractionated external-beam treatments (Carlton *et al.* 1976; Rosenberg *et al.* 1985). In the past, isotopes were usually implanted at the time of lymphadenectomy. An alternative approach is the transperineal insertion of hollow needles to allow afterloading of isotopes to improve safety (Carlton *et al.* 1976; Khan *et al.* 1983; Rosenberg *et al.* 1985).

Leibel *et al.* (1994) reviewed 1078 patients with stage B or C prostate cancer treated by pelvic node dissection and interstitial ^{125}I. 345 patients had nodal involvement. Overall, the 15 year disease-free survival probability was 27 per cent; however, this figure rose to 70 per cent in those achieving local control.

Radiation toxicity

Transient acute side-effects of irradiation relate to the extent of the irradiation field and include rectal discomfort and diarrhoea secondary to proctitis, dysuria, frequency of micturition due to cystitis, and occasionally skin reactions, particularly in the natal cleft and perineum.

The incidence of acute gastrointestinal side-effects is related to technique. Thus, van der Werf-Messing (1978) reported that only

five out of 84 patients (6 per cent) had mild side-effects and none had severe side-effects and this high tolerance may relate to the use of a split course technique and therefore a long overall treatment time. However, McGowan (1977) treated a relatively large field with a dose of 60 Gy in 6 weeks using telecobalt apparatus and reported mild bowel symptoms in 40 out of 107 patients (37 per cent). Acute genitourinary symptoms occur in approximately 40 per cent of patients (Ray *et al.* 1973; McGowan 1977) but are severe in only 3 per cent.

The incidence of late effects of radiotherapy is often underestimated by reporting complications as a proportion of patients treated, rather than actuarially as a proportion of patients who are alive at the late time period and could thus experience the complications. Late gastrointestinal side-effects include a persistent rectal discharge, tenesmus, bloody diarrhoea, and rectal stricture. Severe injuries are usually treated by performing a colostomy and in a series of patients treated with external-beam radiotherapy the larger series report colostomies in 0.2–0.3 per cent of patients (Pistenma *et al.* 1976; Pilepich *et al.* 1987*a*). However, a number of smaller series report the incidence to be 5–6 per cent (del Regato 1979; Hussey 1979). The development of severe bowel injury is more common when the dose to the posterior rectal wall is 65–76 Gy and the length of the treated rectum is at least 10 cm (Dewit *et al.* 1983).

The major late severe genitourinary side-effects are urethral stricture, urinary incontinence, bladder ulceration, chronic cystitis, and, rarely, penile and scrotal oedema. These may be more common when tumour invades the urethra (Harisiadis *et al.* 1978) or in patients who have had prostatectomy (Perez *et al.* 1977*a*; Taylor *et al.* 1979). Genitourinary complications appear to be influenced by the local extent of the tumour and by previous surgical manipulations. A dose of over 70 Gy to the prostatic area may increase the risk of late urethral stricture and penile scrotal oedema (del Regato 1979; Taylor *et al.* 1979) and the dose to the anterior bladder wall correlates with other types of genitourinary complications, particularly if it is more than 65 Gy (Dewit *et al.* 1983).

The third type of late complication of radiation is erectile impotence. The reported incidence of this is broad in different series of patients treated by external-beam radiotherapy. Since impotence is also a consequence of local spread of prostatic cancer the reported incidence may relate to the accuracy of pre-treatment history, the local control of the tumour, and the method of obtaining post-treatment history from the patient (Zinreich *et al.* 1990).

It has been claimed that complications of treatment are much rarer as a consequence of interstitial brachytherapy than of external-beam radiation (Hilaris *et al.* 1977; Morton and Peschel 1988). However, these patients have usually had a pelvic lymphadenectomy which may compound interpretation of post-treatment problems. The radiation side-effects of ^{125}I implantation may be delayed because of the slow treatment time. Approximately one-quarter of patients experience delayed cystitis; however, bowel complications are rare (Abadir *et al.* 1984). Major intestinal complications occurred in 3–5 per cent of patients (Fowler *et al.* 1979; Schellhammer *et al.* 1985). An earlier report indicated that potency was preserved in more than 90 per cent of patients who were potent before therapy (Herr 1980); however, Schellhammer *et al.* (1985) reported problems with potency in approximately one-quarter of patients.

Results of radiotherapy

T0 tumours

As discussed above, a proportion of patients with T0 or stage A carcinoma of the prostate have a significant risk of progression and are identifiable by histological and staging criteria (Epstein *et al.* 1986; Goodman *et al.* 1988; Lowe and Listrom 1988*b*). Radical radiotherapy to a dose of 60 Gy over 6 weeks leads to a very high rate of local control of the order of 94–100 per cent (Perez 1983; Aristizabal *et al.* 1984; Hanks *et al.* 1985) and these translate to approximately 80 per cent of patients surviving 5 years free of disease. A case-control study suggests that these results are significantly better than equivalent patients managed expectantly (Lowe and Listrom 1988*b*).

For 60 patients treated in 1973 and 1974 and followed as part of the Patterns of Care Survey, 5 and 10 year survivals were identical with those expected from an age- and sex-matched population without cancer, namely 85 per cent at 5 years and 61 per cent at 10 years (Hanks *et al.* 1987).

T1/T2 tumours (stage B)

In the Patterns of Care Survey survival of 312 stage B patients was 73 per cent at 5 years and 46 per cent at 10 years. At 5 and 10 years 86 and 74 per cent, respectively, remained free of local recurrence (Hanks *et al.* 1987). Perez (1983) reported a local control rate in 93 patients of 90 per cent and Aristizabal *et al.* (1984) confirmed this, reporting 95 per cent local control in 101 patients (both figures analysed at 5 years). Long-term results from Zagars *et al.* (1988) support these figures, with 10 years' disease-free survival of 86 per cent in 114 patients. One of the largest single-institute experiences has been reported by Bagshaw *et al.* (1985). In the B1 subcategory of a discrete nodular lesion approximately 1 cm in diameter limited to one lateral lobe, the actuarial 15 year survival in 40 patients was 62 per cent compared with the 51 per cent estimated survival after surgery reported by Walsh and Jewett (1980). They found little difference between B1 and B2 disease, although this distinction is clearly important for surgical management of carcinoma of the prostate since so many B2 tumours are found on histological examination to have extracapsular extension and a worse prognosis (Elder *et al.* 1982). Both Stanford Hospital and MD Anderson Hospital report survival in stage A and B patients treated with radiotherapy to be equivalent to that of men in the general population (Bagshaw *et al.* 1985; Zagars *et al.* 1988).

A prospective trial of prostatectomy versus radical radiotherapy in stages A2 and B carcinoma of the prostate was performed by the Uro-Oncology Research Group in patients staged by bone scan and pelvic lymphadenectomy (Paulson *et al.* 1982). The end-point analysed was time to progression at any site and, although the report suggested significantly worse results for radiotherapy, it has been strongly criticized on the following and other grounds (Hanks 1988).

1. The randomization was unequal.

2. Analysis was by treatment given rather than treatment assigned. Only 52 out of 59 patients received their assigned radiotherapy and 38 out of 47 their assigned surgery.

3. Patients with tumour at the surgical resection margins were deemed non-evaluable.

4. Fifty-six per cent of patients were lost to follow-up or died of intercurrent disease within 4–7 years of entry.

5. The radiation therapy members of the committee had no input to the data analysis or review report.

6. No patients had a local recurrence recorded.

7. Patients treated with radiation therapy had too high a rate of development of distant metastases if their primary tumours were really stage A or B (Pilepich *et al.* 1987*b*).

The issue of optimum management of early stage carcinoma of the prostate remains unresolved. It is probable that both local control and survival are equivalent with surgery or radiotherapy and the treatment decision will depend on local resources and expertise and on the different patterns of toxicity.

The RTOG analysed 484 patients with stage A2 or stage B carcinoma of the prostate treated between 1978 and 1983. There was a steady local recurrence rate of approximately 2 per cent per year and this rate was relatively constant during the first 10 years of follow-up (Asbell *et al.* 1988). The rate of developing metastatic disease was also fairly constant over 10 years at approximately 3 per cent per year and the 5 year survival was approximately 65 per cent. In this study staging could be by either lymphangiography (328 patients) or staging lymphadenectomy (117 patients) and any patients with evidence of pelvic node involvement were excluded. The group staged by lymphadenectomy had a better prognosis demonstrated by better disease-free survival and overall survival despite no difference in local control (Asbell *et al.* 1988); presumably this was due to understaging of pelvic nodes by lymphangiograms.

T3 tumours (stage C)

The Patterns of Care Study showed that, following extended field radiotherapy of stage C carcinoma of the prostate, 74 per cent of patients remained free from local recurrence at 5 years and 69 per cent at 10 years (Hanks *et al.* 1987). Single-institute reports support these figures, with 70–90 per cent local control at 5 years (Neglia *et al.* 1977; Aristizabal *et al.* 1984; Forman *et al.* 1985), 81 per cent at 10 years, and 75 per cent at 15 years (Zagars *et al.* 1987). The systemic relapse rate is high: approximately 50 per cent within 5 years (Perez 1983; Rounsaville *et al.* 1987). Overall survival is 58–62 per cent at 5 years and 36–38 per cent at 10 years (Bagshaw *et al.* 1985; Hanks *et al.* 1987). The high and continuous metastatic recurrence rate leads to the hypothesis that the great majority of these patients have subclinical dissemination at the time of presentation and, thus, the main function of radiotherapy at this stage is to achieve long-term local control.

Results of brachytherapy

These techniques achieve high control rates in pathologically staged patients with stage A2 and B disease (Hilaris *et al.* 1978; Scardino and Carlton 1983; Schellhammer *et al.* 1985; Whitmore *et al.* 1985) with little apparent difference between the use of ^{125}I and ^{198}Au seeds plus external beam. For patients in these stages of disease treated by node dissection and ^{125}I implantation the 5 year survival is over 80 per cent, falling to 55–60 per cent for more advanced lesions. Local control averages 85 per cent and, as shown in Table 15, 60–90 per cent of early stage patients are disease free at 5 years (Grossman *et al.* 1982; Schellhammer *et al.* 1985). Brachytherapy with ^{125}I may not be as effective in larger tumours (Giles and Brady 1986; Morton and Peschel 1988).

Prognostic factors for radiotherapy

The major factors indicating prognosis after radical radiotherapy are the primary stage (Table 16), the nodal status, and histological differentiation of the tumour (Bagshaw *et al.* 1985; Preston *et al.*

Table 15 Interstitial implantation with [125]I

Series	Stage[a]	No. of patients	Disease free at 5 years (%)
Grossman et al. (1982)	CS A and B	52	60
	C	38	24
Whitmore (1984)	CS A and B	463	70
	C	124	29
Giles and Brady (1986)	PS A and B	78	85
Schellhammer et al. (1985)	PS A and B	49	82
	C	15	66

[a]CS, clinical stage; PS, pathological stage.

Table 16 Local control of carcinoma of the prostate following external-beam radiotherapy

Stage	Patients	Local control (%) At 5 years	At 10 years
A	60	97	97
B	312	85	71
C	296	72	65

Source: Hanks et al. (1987).

1986; Hanks et al. 1987; Pilepich et al. 1987c). Although serum prostatic acid phosphatase levels are correlated with more advanced disease, a more accurate serum marker of extracapsular extension is serum PSA (Ercole et al. 1987). The serum level of PSA both before and after radiotherapy gives important prognostic information (Landmann and Hunig 1989; Stamey et al. 1989). If PSA is going to fall to normal levels after radiotherapy it usually does so within 6 months and patients with persistently raised levels at 1 year have a high incidence of metastatic disease detected by isotope bone scan (Landmann and Hunig 1989; Stamey et al. 1989). An analysis of PSA regression after radiotherapy suggests that it occurs slowly with an apparent half-life of 43 days (Meek et al. 1990). A multivariate model of prognostic variables based on radical radiotherapy of 1078 patients has been derived at the Princess Margaret Hospital, Toronto (W. Duncan and M. Gospodarowicz, personal communication) and is illustrated in Table 17.

A current controversy is whether prior transurethral resection confers an adverse prognosis (Hanks et al. 1983; Pilepich et al. 1987c; McGowan 1988) or whether the need for this treatment merely indicates a more advanced primary (Meacham et al. 1989). In the Pattern of Care Study the effect was confined to T3 and T4 patients with moderately or poorly differentiated histology (Hanks et al. 1983). Of 87 patients with prior transurethral resection, 60 per cent were metastasis free at 5 years compared with 85 per cent if no transurethral resection had been performed. However, a

Table 18 Biopsy of the prostate more than 1 year after radiotherapy

Series	Negative biopsy	Recurrence (%)	Positive biopsy	Recurrence (%)
Sewell et al. (1975)	6	17	10	80
Kurth et al. (1977)	9	0	14	14
Nachtsheim et al. (1978)	14	0	15	53
Kiesling et al. (1980)	29	14	39	28
Freiha and Bagshaw (1984)	25	24	39	72
Total	79	14	117	39

multivariate analysis which included as prognostic variable the degree of symptomatic obstruction to micturition found no significance in the method of initial biopsy (Meacham et al. 1989). The resolution of this issue requires a prospective randomized trial.

Response assessment by prostatic biopsy after radiotherapy

Although persistent positive biopsies are reported after radiotherapy for prostatic carcinoma, the proportion decreases with time after irradiation and this has been interpreted to indicate that persisting malignant cells may represent a dormant pool rendered reproductively sterile (Cox and Stoffel 1977). The incidence of positive biopsies is related to the initial stage and also to whether the biopsy was performed routinely or because of clinical suspicion of local recurrence, with the latter identifying a particularly adverse subgroup. However, as shown in Table 18, if the biopsy is performed more than 1 year after treatment, the persistence of malignant cells confers a high risk of recurrence compared with a negative biopsy.

Radiotherapy post-prostatectomy

Thirty-five to fifty per cent of patients having radical prostatectomy demonstrate capsular penetration by carcinoma and 22–45 per cent of these will suffer local recurrence (Belt and Schröder 1972; Meyers and Fleming 1983). Adjuvant radiotherapy has been considered for these pathological stage C patients and also for patients found to have seminal vesicle involvement in whom there is a high risk of nodal disease. With adjuvant irradiation doses of 60 Gy in 30–35 fractions over 6–7 weeks, local control is achieved in more than 90 per cent of patients (Belt and Schröder 1972; Meyers and Fleming 1983; Pilepich et al. 1984; Ray et al. 1984; Gibbons et al. 1986). The treatment of overt local recurrence requires higher doses and is less successful (Ray et al. 1984; Forman et al. 1986; Gibbons et al. 1986).

The combination of hormone and radiation therapy

Limited in vitro studies do not suggest that hormones radiosensitize prostatic carcinoma cell lines (Wollin et al. 1989) and there is no

Table 17 Prognosis after radical radiotherapy for carcinoma of the prostate

Group	Definition	No. of patients	5 year survival (%)	10 year survival (%)	Median survival (years)
1	Age <60 years and T1 or T2 and WD or MD	79	91	83	14.1
2	T1/2 <60 years PD or T1/2/3 <69 years WD & MD	474	77	49	9.7
3	T3 PD <60 years or T4 WD or MD	389	61	23	6.7
4	or T1, 2, 3 ≥70 years T4 PD	53	34	5	2.7

PD, poorly differentiated histology; MD, moderately differentiated histology; WD, well-differentiated histology.
Data from Princess Margaret Hospital, Toronto, 1971–1985 (W. Duncan and M. Gospodarowicz, personal communication).

clinical evidence that concurrent therapy with hormones and radiation improve either local control or survival (Neglia *et al.* 1977; Perez *et al.* 1977*b*, 1980). The trial performed by Neglia *et al.* (1977) was predominantly in T3 patients and 154 were randomized to radiation alone or to radiation plus oestrogens. After a mean follow up 4.5 years from entry into the study, there was no difference in the rate of development of distant metastases. For stages B and C1 there was no difference in local control or survival, but for stage C2 local control and survival were inferior for combined treatment. This may have been due to longer prior history of prostate cancer in this group.

A Medical Research Council (MRC) trial comparing orchidectomy, orchidectomy plus radiotherapy, and radiotherapy alone in T2–T4 tumours showed no difference in local control or survival, but predictably there is a delay in the appearance of metastatic disease in patients with initial hormone manipulation (Fellows *et al.* 1992).

A distinct approach to combining hormone and radiation treatments is hormonal cytoreduction prior to radiation therapy, with the aim of downstaging the primary tumour to improve local control, reducing the target volume and, hence, the side-effects of radiotherapy, and providing early treatment of any subclinical metastatic disease. Green *et al.* (1984) studied oestrogen therapy prior to radiation in 25 patients with bulky primary disease and found that a higher complete response rate was obtained than would have occurred with radiotherapy alone. The RTOG has completed pilot studies of initial oestrogen therapy and confirm a response rate before radiotherapy of 95 per cent (Pilepich *et al.* 1989). A current prospective trial in stages B2, C, and D1 is examining hormonal cytoreduction with a luteinizing-hormone-releasing hormone (LHRH) analogue for 12 weeks prior to radical radiotherapy. At the Royal Marsden Hospital a pilot study of hormonal ablation prior to radical radiotherapy has been performed (Shearer *et al.* 1992). Regression of the primary tumour was measured by monthly transrectal ultrasonography. A mean reduction of 61 per cent in prostate volume was documented (Fig. 6), and the validity of a consequent reduction in radiation field size will be investigated.

Experimental radiation techniques

Conformal radiotherapy

Modern imaging techniques and the new generation of linear accelerators allow three-dimensional planning and conformal

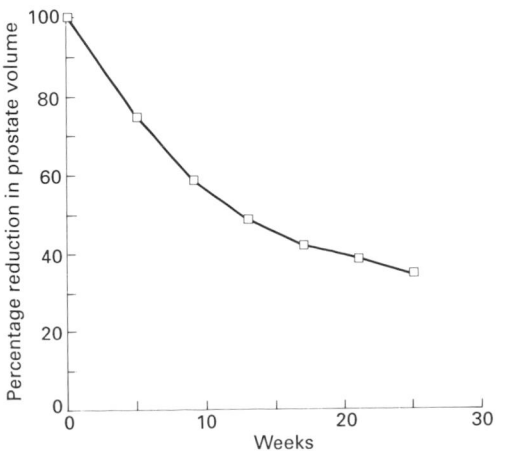

Fig. 6 The effect of hormonal cytoreduction on mean prostatic volume in 21 patients with prostate cancer assessed by monthly rectal ultrasonography (D. P. Dearnaley, personal communication).

radiotherapy. This reduces by up to 50 per cent the amount of normal tissue included within the target volume (Tait *et al.* 1988), which should allow either a reduction in radiation side-effects (Dewit *et al.* 1983; Mameghan *et al.* 1990) or dose escalation at currently acceptable levels of toxicity. A prospective randomized trial of conformal versus standard radiotherapy is being pursued at the Royal Marsden Hospital to determine the extent of toxicity reduction and this is based at present on customized blocking. This technique has been applied to shaping of the boost-field for carcinoma of the prostate by ten Haken *et al.* (1989), who also found that the volume of bladder and rectal tissue in the 95 per cent isodose volume was halved.

There is already evidence that the volume of normal tissue in pelvic radiotherapy is a determinant of toxicity (Soffen *et al.* 1992; Benk *et al.* 1993; Tait *et al.* 1993). A number of centres have embarked on dose escalation studies in prostate cancer (Sandler *et al.* 1992; Leibel *et al.* 1994) and it seems clear already that doses in excess of 75 Gy in daily 1.8 Gy fractions are tolerated with conformal techniques.

Altered fractionation

Primary carcinoma of the prostate is usually a relatively slowly proliferating tumour (Trott and Kummermehr 1985) and there is no conclusive evidence of reduction of local control using protracted or split-course techniques (Lai *et al.* 1990) or of improved control using multiple fractions per day (Vanuytsel *et al.* 1986). Indeed, in the latter study the relatively short interfraction time of 4 h may have led to an increase in late toxicity.

The RTOG performed a pilot study of hyperfractionation between 1983 and 1986, applying a 1.2 Gy fraction twice per day to total doses of 60.0, 64.8, and 69.6 Gy (Cox *et al.* 1988). The level of activity and toxicity was believed to justify a prospective trial at 69.6 Gy, at which dose level the cumulative probability of grade 3 or 4 late toxicity was 11 per cent.

There has also been a study of hypofractionated therapy based on six fractions given over a 3 week period (Collins *et al.* 1991) and a trial involving neutron beam therapy (Russell *et al.* 1994).

Palliative radiotherapy

The commonest symptom in hormone-failed metastatic carcinoma of the prostate is bone pain, particularly in the spine and pelvis. Local radiotherapy is indicated unless pain relief is obtained with mild and well-tolerated analgesics and radiotherapy is most effective for single sites of pain (Benson *et al.* 1982). This retrospective review noted complete pain relief in 42 per cent of 62 patients and partial relief in 35 per cent. Conventionally, pain has been treated to 20 Gy in five fractions or to 30 Gy in ten fractions; however, the Royal Marsden Hospital prospective randomized trial of 30 Gy in ten fractions versus 8 Gy in one fraction did not detect any difference in efficacy (Price *et al.* 1986).

Multiple painful sites are treated with wide-field (that is, hemibody), irradiation to a dose of 6 Gy for the upper half and 8 Gy to the lower half. If sequential hemibody radiotherapy is planned, it is important to leave 6–8 weeks between treatments to allow recovery of marrow suppression. Complete pain relief is less common when multiple sites are treated, but some benefit occurs in approximately 70–80 per cent of patients (Keen 1980; Rowland *et al.* 1981; Hoskin *et al.* 1989). Toxicity includes marrow suppression, particularly prolonged thrombocytopenia and pneumonitis. Acute gastrointestinal problems can be largely circumvented by hydration and steroids.

An alternative approach to whole-skeletal irradiation is the use of systemic radiochemicals. Most experience has been with ^{32}P

(Smart 1965); its concentration in new bone can be increased by prior parathormone or testosterone (Corwin *et al.* 1970; Morales *et al.* 1970). More recently, ^{89}Sr has been investigated. This element is handled like calcium and thus concentrates selectively in osteoblastic deposits. The therapy dose is 1.5–3.0 MBq/kg and improvement in bone pain has been reported in 77 per cent of patients although only 10 per cent become pain free (Robinson 1986; Dearnaley *et al.* 1992). A trial in the United Kingdom coordinated by Amersham International has prospectively compared external-beam radiotherapy with systemic ^{89}Sr. There was little difference in pain relief but patients treated with ^{89}Sr developed fewer new painful bone sites (Bolger *et al.* 1993). This was in agreement with the trial of ^{89}Sr reported by Porter *et al.* (1993). A side-effect of both radiochemical treatments is bone-marrow depression, which is particularly severe in those with peripheral blood evidence of marrow infiltration, but otherwise systemic ^{89}Sr is very well tolerated.

Bisphosphonates have a potential role in inhibiting bone resorption and, thus, reducing the incidence of symptoms from bone metastases (Morton and Howell 1988). Sodium etidronate inhibits both mineralization and resorption but has been disappointing in relieving bone pain. A double-blind randomized trial showed no difference from placebo (Smith 1989).

Clodronate and pamidronate (APD) mainly prevent resorption. A prospective study in patients with bone metastases from breast cancer has shown a reduction in new episodes of bone pain in patients on maintenance APD (van Holten-Verzantvoort *et al.* 1987), and bisphosphonates are now being evaluated extensively in prostate cancer.

Other problems treated for palliation include spinal cord compression (Kuban *et al.* 1986), although it remains unclear whether decompressive laminectomy is more effective than radiotherapy (Bruckman and Bloomer 1978). Ureteric obstruction can be relieved in approximately 70 per cent of patients (Carlton *et al.* 1972; Kraus *et al.* 1972) but high doses of more than 50 Gy were used. Similar doses have been effective in treating leg oedema; however, it may well be possible to relieve symptoms with lower doses. Radiotherapy is particularly useful in the control of haematuria (Carlton *et al.* 1972; Kraus *et al.* 1972).

THE ROLE AND RESULTS OF HORMONAL TREATMENT AND OF CHEMOTHERAPY

The treatment of metastatic prostatic cancer remains controversial. The main controversies relate to the timing of therapy and the treatment modality itself. The reasons for this are that all treatments for metastatic cancer have some disadvantage to the patients and early treatment has not been clearly shown to prolong life. Within the last decade the investigation of patients with prostatic cancer and the assessment of quality of life have been stimulated by the development of new treatments for this disease. These treatments have led to a reassessment of the meaning of response and its precise delineation. The more accurate staging and follow-up assessment by standard criteria have shown that, although approximately 80 per cent of patients have a subjective response to treatment, only 50 per cent have an objective response for a median duration of 1 year. The median duration of survival is 2.5 years for patients with metastatic cancer and 4.5 years for those with locally advanced disease.

It is commonly believed that the first treatments for prostatic cancer date from the 1940s following the pioneering work of

Huggins and Hodges (1941) who treated patients by orchidectomy and oestrogen therapy. These treatments, given in the context of disease for which there was no previous cure, were miraculous in effect, with patients rising Lazarus-like from their deathbeds. In fact, orchidectomy was first performed for prostatic diseases at the turn of century (White 1893). In 1950 Nesbitt and Baum published a retrospective analysis of 1818 patients and described a survival advantage to treatment. The results of this analysis were not disputed until the VACURG investigations of prostatic cancer were published. These series of studies led to a refutation of the findings of Nesbitt and Baum (1956) whose conclusions are now believed to be invalid because the study was retrospective, was not randomized, and made a comparison with a historic case-control group. In the first VACURG study 266 patients with locally advanced disease and 223 patients with metastatic prostatic cancer were randomized to orchidectomy, whilst 262 patients with locally advanced disease and 223 patients with metastatic disease received placebo. The long-term survival of the two groups was identical: 20 per cent of patients with metastatic cancer and 50 per cent of patients with locally advanced disease survived for 5 years (VACURG 1967).

Later analysis of this first VACURG study cast doubt upon the conclusion. The reason for this was that all patients randomized to placebo treatment eventually received some form of therapy outside the trial from their local clinicians. The main conclusion of this study was that there is an equivalence of survival for early compared with delayed treatment.

The second VACURG publication described the effects of oestrogen therapy in the treatment of prostatic cancer. In this trial 265 patients with locally advanced disease and 211 patients with metastatic prostatic cancer received 5 mg of diethylstilboestrol daily. Their survival was compared with 262 patients with locally advanced disease and 223 patients with metastatic disease who received placebo. Although the overall survival from prostatic cancer was similar in both groups there was an excess of death from cardio-vascular causes in patients treated with diethylstilboestrol. One hundred and twelve patients with locally advanced disease and 76 patients with metastatic cancer died from cardiovascular causes compared with 88 patients with locally advanced disease and 55 with metastatic disease who were treated with placebo (Blackard *et al.* 1973). This dose of diethylstilboestrol is slightly higher than that in current use, which is 1 mg three times a day. However, even this dosage has significant effects on antithrombin III levels and plasma volume such that, although not clearly documented, it would be expected that treatment would cause a similar increase in cardio-vascular morbidity and mortality (Varenhorst *et al.* 1981).

The Coronary Drug Project Research Group (1970) investigated the effects of oestrogen treatment upon cardiovascular morbidity in patients with histories of myocardial infarction. The reason for this study was that the group were investigating the reduced incidence of cardiac disease in women compared with men. They observed cardiac morbidities of between 38 and 66 per cent in the oestrogen-treated patients compared with 11 per cent in controls. There are other side-effects from oestrogen therapy, including gastrointestinal symptoms in 30 per cent of patients and breast swelling in virtually all patients, such that in the view of these authors oestrogen therapy is absolutely contraindicated in the treatment of prostatic cancer.

There has been considerable pressure to develop new medical treatments for prostatic cancer because of the side-effects of oestrogen treatment and the unacceptability of orchidectomy. These are reviewed below in the order of their historical development.

Cyproterone acetate and progestogen therapies

Cyproterone acetate was introduced into the treatment of prostatic cancer in the mid-1960s. It is a complex compound and has many endocrine effects: it is progestogenic, decreasing luteinizing hormone and follicle-stimulating hormone levels, it inhibits testicular and adrenal hydroxylase activity, decreasing testosterone synthesis, it competes with testosterone for its cytoplasmic receptor, it displaces the androgen steroid receptor complex from the cell nucleus, and, finally, it has inherent androgenicity itself. Its long-term use may be associated with hypoadrenalism and, paradoxically, it may also produce Cushing's syndrome (Neumann and Jacobi 1982).

Early studies of cyproterone acetate assessed response by criteria not included nowadays in either the National Prostatic Cancer Project Group or the British Prostate Group evaluation systems. In one study of 95 patients treated with cyproterone acetate and 96 patients treated with oestradiol undecylate, equivalent subjective response rates occurred with both treatments and serial cytological assessment of the prostate showed a regression to a more differentiated histological pattern in 18 per cent of both patient groups (Tunn *et al.* 1983).

The EORTC have compared the treatment of 75 patients with cyproterone acetate 250 mg daily and 71 with medroxyprogesterone acetate 500 mg intramuscularly for 8 weeks and then 200 mg orally daily thereafter, with 64 patients treated with 3 mg of diethylstilboestrol daily. Patients either had locally advanced disease or metastatic prostate cancer. In those patients with metastatic disease two out of 38 patients (5 per cent) treated with cyproterone acetate had a complete response and three (8 per cent) had a partial response. None out of 35 patients treated with medroxyprogesterone acetate had a complete response and one (3 per cent) had a partial response. One out of 28 patients (4 per cent) treated with diethylstilboestrol had a complete response and four (14 per cent) had a partial response. Local responses were evaluated, and nine out of 68 evaluable patients (15 per cent) treated with cyproterone acetate had a complete response and 15 (25 per cent) had a partial response compared with one complete response (2 per cent) and 14 partial responses (24 per cent) in 58 patients treated with medroxyprogesterone acetate. Of 57 evaluable patients treated with diethylstilboestrol, nine (16 per cent) had a complete response and 22 (39 per cent) had a partial response. In terms of local response cyproterone acetate and diethylstilboestrol were equivalent and better than medroxyprogesterone acetate. In terms of metastatic disease there was no significant difference between the treatment arms in terms of initial response rate. However, when patients were compared for progression rates, the time to first progression was significantly shorter with medroxyprogesterone acetate compared with diethylstilboestrol or cyproterone acetate which had similar progression rates. Overall survival between the different treatment arms was comparable (Pavone-Macaluso *et al.* 1986).

In a second report of this study cardiovascular toxicity was described but the numbers of patients treated were slightly different from those in the original report: 4 per cent of 82 patients treated with cyproterone acetate had myocardial infarcts, 2 per cent had fluid retention, and 2 per cent had thromboembolic lesions, but 90 per cent had no toxicity whatsoever; 6 per cent of 73 patients treated with medroxyprogesterone acetate had fluid retention and 6 per cent had thromboembolism, but 82 per cent had no toxicity; 11 per cent of the diethylstilboestrol-treated patients had fluid retention, 1 per cent had myocardial infarction, 5 per cent had hypertension, and 8 per cent had thromboembolism, but 66 per cent

of 140 patients had no toxicity. The risk of cardiovascular complications was highest during the first 6 months of treatment (de Voogt *et al.* 1986). This study documented the relative lack of toxicity of cyproterone acetate and taken in conjunction with the equivalence of effect with diethylstilboestrol reinforces the fact that diethylstilboestrol should never be used in the first-line treatment of prostate cancer.

Flutamide

Flutamide is a 'pure' anti-androgen that exerts its effects by competitive inhibition of androgen uptake and nuclear binding in target tissues. Its lack of pituitary effects leads to increased levels of luteinizing hormone and follicle-stimulating hormone with progressive rises in serum testosterone concentrations. Initial reports of the activity of flutamide appeared in the mid-1970s (Sogani *et al.* 1975) and an update of the initial trials at the Memorial Sloan Kettering Hospital showed a response in 63 out of 72 patients who were previously untreated with endocrine therapies (Sogani *et al.* 1984). Until recently flutamide was not in use in the treatment of prostate cancer for two reasons. The first was that responses to therapy were believed to be of shorter duration than other agents, although the evidence for this is not convincing. Second, a high incidence of nausea and depression was reported in the British reports of the activity of flutamide (MacFarlan and Tolley 1985).

Gonadotrophin-releasing hormone analogues

The synthesis and release of luteinizing and follicle-stimulating hormones by the pituitary is dependent upon the pulsatile output of gonadotrophin-releasing hormone from the hypothalamus. This hypothalamic hormone is a decapeptide and structural modifications lead to compounds with altered properties to the parent molecule. Substitutions at residues 6 and 10 produce a group of peptides which are termed 'agonists' which result in the supraphysiological release of hormone and follicle-stimulating hormone if given as a single dosage. The antagonist analogues of gonadotrophin-releasing hormone have substitutions mainly at amino acid residues 2 and 3 and a single injection causes a decrease in the pituitary gonadotrophins. The repeated administration of agonist analogues has a paradoxical effect due to down-regulation of the pituitary gonadotroph and after initial supraphysiological increase in the gonadotrophins there is a decrease and concomitant fall in gonadal steroids (Waxman 1987).

There is a need for an effective medical therapy without side-effects for prostate cancer and because of this there has been interest in the development of the gonadotrophin-releasing hormone analogues as treatment for this disease. Initial reports of the activity of gonadotrophin-releasing hormone analogues in prostatic cancer appeared in the early 1980s (Labrie *et al.* 1980; Tolis *et al.* 1982; Allen *et al.* 1983; Waxman *et al.* 1983). The first randomized study to be reported contrasted the responses of 101 patients with metastatic prostatic cancer treated with 3 mg of diethylstilboestrol daily with 98 patients treated with 1 mg of D-Leu[6]-LHRH ethylamide daily. Responses were judged according to the National Prostatic Cancer Project criteria and were equivalent in both arms of the study. One per cent of the leuprolide group and 2 per cent of the diethylstilboestrol group had a complete response and 37 per cent of the leuprolide group and 44 per cent of the oestrogen-treated group showed a partial response to treatment (Leuprolide Study Group 1984). The long-term follow-up of these patients showed an exact equivalent of response duration and survival. The median duration of survival was 146 weeks in the leuprolide group and 136 weeks in the diethylstilboestrol-treated patients. There was a marked difference in the side-effects reported. Cardiovascular toxicity was seen in 33 of the diethylstilboestrol-treated patients and ten of the leuprolide-treated patients. Twenty diethylstilboestrol-treated patients had gastrointestinal toxicity compared with ten in the leuprolide group. Thirteen per cent of the diethylstilboestrol group discontinued treatment because of side-effects compared with 3 per cent of the leuprolide group (Garnick 1986). In a small study gonadotrophin-releasing hormone agonist therapy with decapeptile was compared with orchidectomy, again with a similar response rate. Forty-one per cent of patients treated by orchidectomy responded compared with 50 per cent of those treated with decapeptile. In this paper the survival analysis is slightly unconventional and reported as being equivalent, but gives the median survival in patients failing treatment as 16 months in those treated with decapeptile and 13 months in those treated by orchidectomy (Parmar et al. 1987).

A major controversy in prostatic cancer that has sparked innumerable debates and still remains unresolved is the concept of 'total androgen ablation'. The hypothesis behind this concept is that in a disease that is androgen dependent it is important to eliminate all sources of androgen from the prostate. Gonadotrophin-releasing hormone agonists limit testicular gonadal steroid production but do not affect the adrenal glands. The adrenal glands make a contribution of 5 per cent to circulating androgen levels, but owing to concentrating mechanisms in the prostate there are relatively higher proportions of androgens of adrenal than of testicular origin in the 'castrate'. The main protagonist of this theory used evidence from normal animal models to support the hypothesis showing a synergy of effect of gonadotrophin-releasing hormone agonists and antiandrogens in decreasing prostate and seminal vesicle weight (Povet and Labrie 1985). This was countered by studies of transplanted tumours in which no synergy of effect was demonstrable (Redding and Shally 1985). A number of reports claiming an advantage for combination therapy have appeared, but these were generally uncontrolled (Labrie et al. 1987, 1988). Such was the controversy generated that a large randomized trial was initiated at the National Cancer Institute to investigate this. Three hundred patients with metastatic prostatic cancer were randomized to receive leuprolide and placebo, whilst 303 patients received leuprolide and flutamide. Progression-free survival was prolonged at 16.5 months compared with 13.9 months in the combination therapy group and the median duration of survival was longer at 35.6 months compared with 28.3 months in the combination group (Crawford et al. 1989). This meticulously documented study provided supporting evidence for a hypothesis which still causes some unease amongst clinicians, particularly because of continuing investigations of this concept that seem to disprove it. In general, most of these studies are not yet complete and are reported in abstract format. The EORTC has recently published its study comparing goserelin acetate and flutamide with orchiectomy in 327 patients with metastatic cancer. Response assessment was unconventional; however, combination therapy led to significantly improved time to progression and overall survival. Overall response rates were identical (Denis et al. 1993). Taken together with the NCI study and observations with regard to tumour flare, one can only conclude that Labrie's hypothesis is vindicated and that combination endocrine treatment is the therapy of first choice for prostatic cancer.

Gonadotrophin-releasing hormone agonists were initially given as daily injections or as nasal insufflations five or six times daily.

This is obviously suboptimal and pharmacological developments have led to the introduction of depot preparations of agonist that can be given monthly (Williams et al. 1984), two monthly (Waxman et al. 1989a), or three monthly (Waxman et al. 1989b). Currently, there is litigation over the depot material used and this has meant that the longer-acting depot preparations have not become generally available. This is obviously to the detriment of the patients and it is hoped that the issue will soon be resolved.

One problem with gonadotrophin-releasing hormone agonists is the development of tumour flare. This is the initial exacerbation of the symptoms and signs of disease and has a strict temporal relationship with the start of treatment, usually occurring within the first week of treatment (Waxman et al. 1985). The incidence of this syndrome is variably reported at between 3 and 40 per cent of patients. A randomized study comparing different dosages of cyproterone acetate with flutamide has shown that cyproterone acetate at a dosage of 100 mg three times a day given for 1 week prior to and for the first month of gonadotrophin-releasing hormone agonist treatment prevents the development of tumour flare (Waxman et al. 1988).

There has been considerable interest in the mechanism of effect of these compounds in prostatic cancer and it has been recently shown that there may be a direct effect at the level of the tumour. High-affinity binding of gonadotrophin-releasing hormone agonist has been demonstrated in a hormone-sensitive prostate cancer cell line. This binding was absent in insensitive lines and present in human tumours. In the absence of androgens, gonadotrophin-releasing hormone agonist directly stimulated the short-term growth of hormone-sensitive lines but had no stimulatory effect on hormone-insensitive lines. It is of interest that both lines secreted gonadotrophin-releasing-hormone-like peptides, suggesting that there is some role for this peptide as an autocrine stimulatory factor in this disease (Qayum et al. 1990).

Hormonal treatment of recurrent refractory prostate cancer

The median survival of patients from symptomatic relapse of metastatic disease after hormone therapy is 6 months. Unfortunately there is absolutely no evidence that any second-line endocrine therapy will prolong survival. However, useful palliation of symptoms may occur in up to one-third of patients treated and so these manoeuvres are worthwhile if they have limited toxicity (Stone et al. 1980).

Surgical manoeuvres

It used to be common clinical practice to proceed to orchidectomy after the failure of oestrogen therapy. There is no evidence to support its continued use, although up to 10 per cent of patients may have a minimal subjective response to therapy (Biorn et al. 1979). Adrenalectomy was introduced as a second-line therapy for carcinoma of the prostate by Huggins and Hodges (1941) and was reported to produce a subjective improvement in between 50 and 70 per cent of patients (Bhanalaph et al. 1974). This is a major procedure and, because less invasive methods of pain relief are available to clinicians, adrenalectomy is not part of current clinical practice in the management of patients with recurrent prostatic cancer. Similarly, hypophysectomy is not part of clinical practice. However, transphenoidal hypophysectomy in experienced hands has very limited morbidity and an extraordinarily high and inexplicable response rate with up to 75 per cent of patients having significant pain relief post-operatively (Silverberg 1977). Objective responses to hypophysectomy are more difficult to quantify because many of the studies were performed without applying the stringent response criteria used today. In one review of hypophysectomy 18 objective responses were seen in 50 patients treated in nine series of clinical studies. Responses were not found to relate to previous responses to endocrine therapy (Brendler 1973).

Aminoglutethimide and cortisone acetate

Aminoglutethimide has been used as second-line therapy for patients with carcinoma of the prostate. The original reason for employing this agent was its potential role as a substitute for surgical adrenalectomy. Aminoglutethimide was introduced into the treatment of epilepsy in 1959, but was found to cause hypoadrenalism in a significant number of patients and so was withdrawn from use. Because of this side-effect it was later employed to treat breast cancer and prostatic cancer. However, paradoxically the effect of aminoglutehamide on the adrenal glands is transient due to hepatic enzyme induction and its real activity is at the level of the peripheral aromatase system where it inhibits the conversion of androstendione to oestradiol and oestrone sulphate. In men there is very little peripheral aromatase activity, in contrast with the situation in women and it is postulated that the 'real' effect of aminoglutethimide is due to the steroids given as replacement therapy. Approximately 20 per cent of patients overall have a subjective response to aminoglutethimide and steroids (Stanford et al. 1976; Ponder et al. 1984). Recently, there have been reports that this level of activity can be obtained using low-dose steroids alone (Plowman et al. 1987).

Other endocrine agents

In a disease that responds to androgen withdrawal it seems strange that anti-oestrogens should be effective, but seven responses to tamoxifen were seen in 31 patients with advanced disease who had relapsed following orchidectomy or oestrogen therapy and two responses were seen in another group of 41 patients. Responses tend to be short, ranging up to approximately 5 months (Glick et al. 1979; Spremulli et al. 1982). There are no case-controlled trials. Thirty-seven evaluable patients treated with megestrol acetate (160 mg daily) were assessed for response. Only one partial response was seen. All patients had been previously treated with hormonal therapy (Crombie et al. 1987). Suramin, a growth factor inhibitor, has been used to treat prostatic cancer in relapse. Subjective responses and improvements in PSA levels have been reported with the use of this agent which is very toxic (Myers et al. 1992). It should be noted that hydrocortisone is given to patients treated with suramin, to limit allergic and other side-effects. As steroids are effective agents in this condition it may be that the responses reported are due to these compounds rather than suramin.

Chemotherapy for prostatic cancer

Almost invariably chemotherapy is given to patients with prostatic cancer as a last resort. These are patients with poor performance status and minimal marrow reserve. In this context it is not surprising that chemotherapy has a poor reputation when used to treat prostatic cancer. However, this poor reputation is not entirely justified and if, for example, a comparison is made with other treatment modalities given at the time of relapse, similar responses

Table 19 Chemotherapy for prostatic cancer

Agent	No. evaluated	CR + PR (percentage)	95% confidence limits (%)
Adriamycin	214	31 (14)	10–19
Cisplatin	209	26 (12)	8–17
Cyclophosphamide	151	7 (5)	1–8
Estramustine	561	109 (19)	16–23
Methotrexate	82	6 (10)	2–13
5-Fluorouracil	124	11 (9)	4–14
Vinblastine	39	8 (21)	8–33
Vindesine	27	5 (19)	4–33
Mitomycin C	48	10 (21)	9–32
Mitoguazone	25	6 (24)	7–41
Etoposide	19	2 (12)	0–24
Gallium nitrate	13	1 (7)	0–22

CR, complete response; PR, partial response.
After Scher and Sternberg (1985).

and identical lack of survival advantages is seen. These response rates are succinctly summarized in Table 19.

In almost all the studies reported, comparison of treatment and control groups shows no survival advantage. The median duration of survival is approximately 6 months from the initiation of treatment. Of the newer agents used to treat prostatic cancer, mitozantrone seems to have promise. Approximately 10–20 per cent of patients respond and the responses show little toxicity (Osborne et al. 1983). It should be noted that combination chemotherapy offers no advantage to patients with prostatic cancer and has the additional problems of increased toxicity.

Androgen priming has been investigated with the idea of enhancing the effect of cytotoxic agents by stimulating the division of androgen-responsive cells. One study has shown a slightly increased initial response rate to androgen priming compared with control. However, responses included those patients with disease stabilization and no difference in response duration was found between the two patient groups (Manni et al. 1986). Androgen priming has considerable morbidity with significant increases in bone pain and reports of spinal cord compression with treatment (Prout and Brewer 1967). In the view of the present authors, treatment with androgens is contraindicated.

REFERENCES

Abadir R, Ross Y Jr, Weinstein SH (1984). Carcinoma of the prostate treated by pelvic and node dissection, iodine-125 seed implant and external irradiation: a study of rectal complications. *Clinical Radiology*, 35:359–61.

Ackermann R, Müller HA (1981). Der Wert der perinealen Stanzbiopsie zur Beurtelung des histologischen Differenzierungsgrades des Prostata-Carcinoms. *Verhandl. Deutsch Ges. Urol.*, 32:79–81.

Adolfsson J, et al. (1990). The natural course of low grade, non-metastatic prostatic carcinoma. *British Journal of Urology*, 65:611–14.

Allen JM, O'Shea JP, Mashiter K (1983). Advanced carcinoma of the prostate: treatment with a gonadotrophin releasing hormone agonist. *British Medical Journal*, 286:1607–9.

Anscher MS, Prosnitz LR (1989). Radiotherapy vs. hormonal therapy for the management of locally recurrent prostate cancer following radical prostatectomy. *International Journal of Radiation Oncology — Biology — Physics*, 17(5):953–8.

Anscher MS, Prosnitz LR (1991). Multivariate analysis of factors predicting local relapse after radical prostatectomy — possible indications for postoperative radiotherapy. *International Radiation Oncology — Biology — Physics*, 21.941–7.

Aristizabal SA, Steinbronn D, Hensinkveld RS (1984). External beam radiotherapy in cancer of the prostate. *Radiotherapy and Oncology*, 1:309–15.

Asbell SO, et al. (1988). Elective pelvic irradiation in stage A2, B carcinoma of the prostate: analysis of RTOG 77-06. *International Journal of Radiation Oncology — Biology — Physics*, 15:1307–16.

Azumi N, Shibuya H, Ishikura M (1984). Primary prostatic carcinoid tumor with intracytoplasmic prostatic acid phosphatase and prostate-specific antigen. *American Journal of Surgical Pathology*, 8:545–50.

Bagshaw MA (1980). External radiation therapy of carcinoma of the prostate. *Cancer*, 45:1912–21.

Bagshaw MA (1984). Radiotherapy of prostatic cancer: Stanford University experience. In *Progress in clinical and biological research: progress and controversies in oncological urology* I, Vol. 153 (ed. K Kurth, F Debruyne, F Schröder, T Splinter, and T Wagener), pp. 493–512. Alan R Liss, New York.

Bagshaw MA, Ray GR, Cox RS (1985). Radiotherapy of prostatic carcinoma: long- or short-term efficacy. *Urology*, 25:17–23.

Bagshaw MA, Kaplan ID, Cox RC (1993). Prostate cancer. Radiation therapy for localised disease. *Cancer*, 71 (Suppl. 3):939–52.

Baker HW, Burger HG, De Kretser DM (1976). Changes in the pituitary–testicular system with age. *Clinical Endocrinology*, 5:349–72.

Barsky SH, Siegal, GP, Jannotta F, Liotta LA (1983). Loss of basement membrane components by invasive tumors but not by their benign counterparts. *Laboratory Investigation*, 49:140–7.

Battifora H (1976). Spindle cell carcinoma. Ultrastructural evidence of squamous origin and collagen production by the tumor cells. *Cancer*, 37:2275.

Belt E, Schröder FH (1972). Total perineal prostatectomy for carcinoma of the prostate. *Journal of Urology*, 107:91–6.

Benk AV, et al. (1993). Late rectal bleeding following combined x-ray and proton high dose irradiation for patients with stage T3–T4 prostate carcinoma. *International Journal of Radiation Oncology — Biology — Physics*, 26(3):551–7.

Bennett JE (1968). Treatment of carcinoma of the prostate by cobalt beam therapy. *Radiology*, 90:532–5.

Benson RC Jr, Hasan SM, Jones AG, Schlise S (1982). External beam radiotherapy for palliation of pain from metastatic carcinoma of the prostate. *Journal of Urology*, 127:69–71.

Benson MC, Whang IS, Olsson CA, McMahon DJ, Cooner WH (1992). The use of prostate specific antigen density to enhance the predictive value of intermediate levels of serum prostate specific antigen. *Journal of Urology*, 147:817–21.

Beral V, Inskip H, Fraser P (1985). Mortality of employees of the United Kingdom Atomic Energy Authority. *British Medical Journal*, 291:440–7.

Bhanalaph T, Varkarakis MJ, Murphy GP (1974). Current status of bilateral adrenalectomy on advanced prostatic carcinoma. *Annals of Surgery*, 179:17–23.

Biorn GL, Gray CP, Strauss E (1979). Orchiectomy after presumed oestrogen failure in treatment of carcinoma of the prostate. *Western Journal of Medicine*, 130:363–4.

Blackard CE, Mellinger GT, Gleason DF (1971). Treatment of stage 1 carcinoma of the prostate: a preliminary report. *Journal of Urology*, 106:729–33.

Blackard CE, Byar DP, Jordan WP Jr (1973). Orchiectomy for advanced prostatic carcinoma: a re-evaluation. *Urology*, 1(6):553–60.

Blennerhassett JB, Vickery AL (1966). Carcinoma of the prostate gland. An anatomical study of tumor location. *Cancer*, 19:980–4.

Blute ML, Zincke H, Farrow GM (1986). Long-term follow-up of young patients with stage A adenocarcinoma of the prostate. *Journal of Urology*, 136:840–3.

Bocking A, Kiehn J, Heinzel-Wach M (1982). Combined histologic grading of prostatic carcinoma. *Cancer*, 50:288.

Bolger JJ, et al. (1993). Strontium-89 (Metastron) versus external beam radiotherapy in patients with painful bone metastases secondary to prostatic cancer: preliminary report of a trial. UK Metastron Investigators Group. *Seminars in Oncology*, 20 (3 Suppl. 2):32–3.

Bookstein R, Shew JY, Chen PL, Scully P, Lee WH (1990). Suppression of tumorigenicity of human prostate carcinoma cells by replacing a mutated RB gene. *Science*, 247(4943):712–15.

Bosch R, Schröder FH (1990). Radical prostatectomy and adjuvant endocrine treatment: a review. In *EORTC Genitourinary Group Monograph 8. Treatment of prostatic cancer, facts and controversies* (ed. FH Schröder), pp. 239–47. Wiley-Liss, New York.

Bosch RJLH, Kurth KH, Schröder FH (1987). Surgical treatment of locally advanced (T3) prostatic carcinoma — early results. *Journal of Urology*, 138:816–22.

Bostwick DG, Mann RB (1985). Malignant lymphomas involving the prostate: a study of 13 cases. *Cancer*, 56:2932.

Brendler H (1973). Adrenalectomy and hypophysectomy for prostatic cancer. *Urology*, 2:99–102.

Breslow N, Chan CW, Dhom G (1977). Latent carcinoma of prostate at autopsy in seven areas. *International Journal of Cancer*, 20:680–88.

Bruckman JE, Bloomer WD (1978). Management of spinal cord compression. *Seminars in Oncology*, 5:135–40.

Buell P, Dunn JE (1965). Cancer mortality against Japanese Issei and Nisei of California. *Cancer*, 18:656–65.

Byar DP, Corle DK (1988). Hormone therapy for prostate cancer: results of the Veterans Administration Cooperative. Urological Research Group Studies. *NCI Monograph*, 7:165–70.

Byar DP, Mostofi FK (1972). Carcinoma of the prostate: prognostic evaluation of certain pathologic features in 208 radical prostatectomies. *Cancer*, 30:5–13.

Byar DP, Corle DK, Veterans Administration Cooperative Urological Research Group (1981). VACURG randomized trial of radical prostatectomy for stages I and II prostate cancer. *Urology*, 17(4):7–11.

Byar DP (1977). VACURG studies on prostatic cancer and its treatment. In *Urologic pathology: the prostate* (ed. M Tannenbaum), pp. 241–67. Lea & Febiger, Philadelphia.

Cachia PG, McIntyre MA, Stockdill G (1987). Prostatic infiltration in chronic lymphatic leukaemia. *Journal of Clinical Pathology*, 40:342.

Cantrell BB, et al. (1981). Pathological factors that influence prognosis in stage A prostatic cancer: the influence of extent versus grade. *Journal of Urology*, 125:516–20.

Carlton CE Jr, Dawoud F, Hudgins P (1972). Irradiation treatment of carcinoma of the prostate: a preliminary report based on 8 years of experience. *Journal of Urology*, 108:924–7.

Carlton CE Jr, Hudgins PT, Guerriero WG, Scott R (1976). Radiotherapy in the management of stage C carcinoma of the prostate: 452 patients over 11 years. *Journal of Urology*, 116:206–10.

Carter BS, Epstein JI, Isaacs WB (1990). *ras* gene mutations in human prostate cancer. *Cancer Research*, 50:6830–2.

Carter HB, et al. (1989). Evaluation of transrectal ultrasound in the early detection of prostate cancer. *Journal of Urology*, 142:1008–10.

Catalona WJ, Biggs SW (1990). Nerve-sparing radical prostatectomy: evaluation of results after 250 patients. *Journal of Urology*, 143:538–43.

Catalona WJ, Stein AJ, Fair WR (1982). Grading errors in prostatic needle biopsies: relation to the accuracy of tumor grade in predicting pelvic lymph node metastases. *Journal of Urology*, 127:919–22.

Caulk JR (1937). Carcinoma of the prostate. *Journal of Urology*, 37:832–9.

Chodak GW (1993). Questioning the value of screening for prostrate cancer in asymptomatic men. *Urology*, 42:116–18.

Chodak GW, et al. (1994). Results of conservative management of clinically localised prostate cancer. *New England Journal of Medicine*, 330(4):242–8.

Christofferson J (1973). Leiomyosarcoma of the prostate. *Acta Chirurgica Scandinavica (Supplement)*, 433:75.

Collins CD, Lloyd Davies RW, Swan AV (1991). Radical external beam radiotherapy for localised carcinoma of the prostate using a hypofractionation technique. *Clinical Oncology*, 3(3):127–32.

Concolino G, Marocchi A, Margitta G (1982). Steroid receptors and hormone responsiveness of human prostatic carcinoma. *Prostate*, 3(5):475–82.

Cooner WH, et al. (1988). Clinical application of transrectal ultrasonography and prostate specific antigen in the search for prostate cancer. *Journal of Urology*, 139:758–61.

Cooner WH, et al. (1990). Prostate cancer detection in a clinical urological practice by ultrasonography, digital rectal examination and prostate specific antigen. *Journal of Urology*, 143:1146–54.

Coronary Drug Project Research Group (1970). The Coronary Drug Project. Initial findings leading to modifications of its research protocol. *Journal of the American Medical Association*, 214:1030–313.

Corwin SH, Malament M, Small M, Strauss HD (1970). Experiences with P-32 in advanced carcinoma of the prostate. *Journal of Urology*, 104:745.

Court B, Chassagne D (1977). Interstitial radiation therapy of cancer of the prostate using iridium 192 wires. *Cancer Treatment Reports*, 61:329–30.

Cox JD, Kline RW (1983). Do prostate biopsies 12 months or more after external irradiation for adenocarcinoma, stage III, predict long-term survival? *International Journal of Radiation Oncology — Biology — Physics*, 9:299–303.

Cox JD, Stoffel TJ (1977). The significance of needle biopsy after irradiation for stage C adenocarcinoma of the prostate. *Cancer*, 40:156–60.

Cox JD, *et al.* (1988). Tolerance of pelvic normal tissues to hyperfractionated radiation therapy: results of protocol 83-08 of the radiation therapy oncology group. *International Journal of Radiation Oncology — Biology — Physics*, 15:1331–6.

Crawford ED, Eisenberger MA, McLeod GD (1989). A controlled trial of leuprolide with and without flutamide in prostatic carcinoma. *New England Journal of Medicine*, 321:419–24.

Crombie C, Raghavan D, Page J (1987). Phase II study of megestrol acetate for metastatic carcinoma of the prostate. *British Journal of Urology*, 59:443–6.

Cumming JA, *et al.* (1990). De-differentiation with time in prostate cancer and the influence on the course of the disease. *British Journal of Urology*, 65:271–4.

de Voogt HJ, *et al.* (1986). Cardiovascular side effects of diethylstilbestrol, cyproterone acetate, medroxyprogesterone acetate and estramustine phosphate used for the treatment of advanced prostatic cancer: results from European Organization for Research of Treatment of Cancer Trials 30761 and 30762. *Journal of Urology*, 135:303–7.

de Voogt HJ, *et al.* (1989). Multivariate analysis of prognostic factors in patients with advanced prostatic cancer: results from two European organizations for research on treatment of cancer trials. *Journal of Urology*, 141(4):883–8.

Dearnaley DP, Bayly RJ, A'Hern RP, Gadd J, Zivanovic MM, Lewington VJ (1992). Palliation of bone metastases in prostate cancer, hemibody irradiation or strontium-89? *Clinical Oncology*, 42(2):101–7.

Dearnaley DP, *et al.* (1993). Prostate cancer (Grand Round). *Lancet*, 342:901–5.

del Regato JA (1967). Radiotherapy in the conservative treatment of operable and locally inoperable carcinoma of the prostate. *Radiology*, 88:761–6.

del Regato JA (1979). Long term curative results of radiotherapy of patients with inoperable carcinoma of the prostate. *Radiology*, 131:291–7.

Deming CL (1922). Results of 100 cases of cancer of the prostate and seminal vesicles treated with radium. *Surgery, Gynecology and Obstetrics*, 34:99–118.

Denis LJ, Carneiro de Moura JL, Bono A, Sylvester R, Whelan P, Newling D, Depauw M (1993). Goserelin acetate and flutadmide versus bilateral orchiectomy a phase III EORTC trial (30853). EORTC GU Group and EORTC Data Center. *Urology*, 41(2):119–29.

Dennis RL, McDougal WS (1988). Pharmacological treatment of erectile dysfunction after radical prostatectomy. *Journal of Urology*, 139:775–6.

deVere White R (1983). Radiation and chemotherapy for stage D1 prostate cancer. *Seminars in Urology*, 1:261–4.

Dewit L, Ang KK, van der Schueren E (1983). Acute side effects and late complications after radiotherapy of localized carcinoma of the prostate. *Cancer Treatment Reviews*, 10:79–89.

Dobbs J, Barrett A (1985). *Prostate*. Edward Arnold, London.

Donohue RE, *et al.* (1990). Intraoperative and early complications of staging pelvic lymph node dissection in prostatic adenocarcinoma. *Urology*, 35:223–7.

Edwards CN, Steinthorsson E, Nicholson D (1953). An autopsy study of latent prostatic cancer. *Cancer*, 6:531–54.

Elder JS, Jewett HJ, and Walsh PC (1982). Radical perineal prostatectomy for clinical stage B2 carcinoma of the prostate. *Journal of Urology*, 127:704–6.

El-Shirbiny A, Bhargava A, Beckley S (1984). Comparison of immunologic and enzymatic assay of prostatic acid phosphatase for follow-up and assessment of clinical status of stage D prostate cancer. *Journal of Surgical Oncology*, 26:256.

Emtage LA, Lewis PW, Blackledge GRP (1987). The role of prostate specific antigen in the baseline assessment of patients undergoing hormone therapy for advanced prostate cancer. *British Journal of Urology*, 60:572–7.

Epstein JI, Liebermann PH (1985). Mucinous adenocarcinoma of the prostate gland. *American Journal of Surgical Pathology*, 9:299–308.

Epstein JI, Woodruff JM (1986). Adenocarcinoma of the prostate with endometroid features. A light microscopic and immunohistochemical study of ten cases. *Cancer*, 57:111.

Epstein JI, Paull G, Eggleston JC, Walsh PC (1986). Prognosis of untreated stage A1 prostatic carcinoma: a study of 94 cases with extended follow-up. *Journal of Urology*, 136:837–9.

Epstein JI, Oesterling JE, Walsh PC (1988a). Tumor volume versus percentage of specimen involved by tumor correlated with progression in stage A prostatic cancer. *Journal of Urology*, 139:980–4.

Epstein JI, Oesterling JE, Walsh PC (1988b). The volume and anatomical location of residual tumor in radical prostatectomy specimens removed for stage A1 prostate cancer. *Journal of Urology*, 139:975–9.

Ercole CJ, *et al.* (1987). Prostatic specific antigen and prostatic acid phosphatase in the monitoring and staging of patients with prostatic cancer. *Journal of Urology*, 138:1181.

Fellows GJ, *et al.* (1992). Treatment of advanced localised prostatic cancer by orchiectomy, radiotherapy, or combined treatment — a Medical Research Council Study. *British Journal of Urology*, 70(3):304–9.

Ferro MA, Barnes I, Roberts JBM (1987). Tumour markers in prostatic carcinoma. A comparison of prostate-specific antigen with acid phosphatase. *British Journal of Urology*, 60:69–73.

Fleming WH, Hamel A, MacDonalt R (1986). Expression of the c-*myc* proto-oncogene in human prostatic carcinoma and benign prostatic hyperplasia. *Cancer Research*, 46:1538.

Forman JD, *et al.* (1985). Improving the therapeutic ratio of external beam irradiation for carcinoma of the prostate. *International Journal of Radiation Oncology — Biology — Physics*, 11:2073–80.

Forman JD, *et al.* (1986). Definitive radiotherapy following prostatectomy: results and complications. *International Journal of Radiation Oncology — Biology — Physics*, 12:185–9.

Fowler JE Jr, Barzell WW, Hilaris BS, Whitmore WF (1979). Complications of ^{125}I implantation and pelvic lymphadenectomy in the treatment of prostatic cancer. *Journal of Urology*, 121:447–51.

Frame R, *et al.* (1987). Granulocytic sarcoma of the prostate. *Cancer*, 59:142.

Franks LM (1954). Latent carcinoma of the prostate. *Journal of Pathology and Bacteriology*, 68:603.

Franks LM, O'Shea JD, Thompson AER (1964). Mucin in the prostate: a histochemical study in normal glands, latent, clinical, and colloid cancers. *Cancer*, 17:983–91.

Freiha FS, Bagshaw MA (1984). Carcinoma of the prostate: results of post-irradiation biopsy. *Prostate*, 5:19–25.

Frentzel-Beyme B (1985). Die transrektale Prostatasonographie. *Fortschritte der Röntgenstrasse*, 142(3):298–303.

Frohmüller H, Grups J (1985). Complications of radical prostatectomy. *Urology*, 24(3):142–7.

Fuks Z, *et al.* (1991). The effect of local control on metastatic dissemination in carcinoma of the prostate: long-term results in patients treated with 125I implantation. *International Journal of Radiation Oncology — Biology — Physics*, 21:537–47.

Gaeta JF (1981). Glandular profiles and cellular patterns in prostatic cancer grading. *Urology*, 17 (Suppl.):33.

Gaeta JF, Asirwatham JE, Miller G, Murphy GP (1980). Histologic grading of primary prostatic cancer: a new approach to an old problem. *Journal of Urology*, 123:689.

Gaeta JF, Englander LC, Murphy GP (1986). Comparative evaluation of national prostatic cancer treatment group and Gleason systems for pathologic grading of primary prostatic cancer. *Urology*, 27:306.

Garnett JE, Oyasu R, Grayhack JT (1984). The accuracy of diagnostic biopsy specimens in predicting tumor grades by Gleason's classification of radical prostatectomy specimens. *Journal of Urology*, 131:690–3.

Garnick M (1986). Leuprolide versus diethylstilboestrol for previously untreated stage D2 prostate cancer. *Urology*, 27:21–6.

Geller J, Cantor T, Albert J (1975). Evidence of a specific dihydro-testosterone-binding cytosol receptor in the human prostate. *Journal of Clinical Endocrinology and Metabolism*, 41:854–62.

George NJR (1988). Natural history of localised prostatic cancer managed by conservative therapy alone. *Lancet*, i:494–7.

Gervasi LA, Mata J, Easley JD (1989). Prognostic significance of lymph nodal metastases in prostate cancer. *Journal of Urology*, 142:332–6.

Ghali VS, Garcia RL (1984). Prostatic adenocarcinoma with carcinoidal features producing adrenocorticotropic syndrome: immunohistochemical study and review of the literature. *Cancer*, 54:1043.

Gibbons RP (1993). Localised prostate carcinoma — surgical management. *Cancer*, 72(10):2865–72.

Gibbons RP, et al. (1986). Adjuvant radiotherapy following radical prostatectomy: results and complications. Journal of Urology, 135:65–8.

Giles GM, Brady LW (1986). ^{125}Iodine implantation after lymph-adenectomy in early carcinoma of the prostate. International Journal of Radiation Oncology—Biology—Physics, 12:2117–25.

Gleason DF, Veterans Administration Cooperative Urological Research Group (1977). Histologic grading and clinical staging of prostatic carcinoma. In Urologic pathology: the prostate (ed. M Tannenbaum), p. 171. Lea & Febiger, Philadelphia.

Gleason DF, Mellinger GT, Veterans Administration Cooperative (1974). Prediction of prognosis for prostatic adenocarcinoma by combined histological grading and clinical staging. Journal of Urology, 111:58.

Glick J, et al. (1979). Tamoxifen in metastatic prostate and renal cancer. Proceedings of the American Society of Clinical Oncology, 84:311.

Goebbels R, Amberger L, Wenert N (1985). Urothelial carcinoma of the prostate. Applied Pathology, 3:242.

Goodman CM, Busuttil A, Chisholm GD (1988). Age, and size and grade of tumour predict prognosis in incidentally diagnosed carcinoma of the prostate. British Journal of Urology, 62:576–80.

Green N, et al. (1984). Improved control of bulky prostate cancer with sequential estrogen and radiation therapy. International Journal of Radiation Oncology—Biology—Physics, 10(7):971–6.

Grossman HB, Batata M, Hilaris B, Whitmore WF Jr (1982). ^{125}I implantation for carcinoma of the prostate. Urology, 20:591–8.

Hall RR, et al. (1988). Urology and the TNM classification. Lancet, ii:1145–6.

Hanks GE (1985). Optimizing the radiation treatment and outcome of prostate cancer. International Journal of Radiation Oncology—Biology—Physics, 11:1235–54.

Hanks GE (1988). More on the Uro-Oncology Research Group report of radical surgery vs radiotherapy for adenocarcinoma of the prostate. International Journal of Radiation Oncology—Biology—Physics, 14:1053–7.

Hanks GE, Leibel S, Kramer S (1983). The dissemination of cancer by transurethral resection of locally advanced prostate cancer. Journal of Urology, 129:309–11.

Hanks GE, Leibel SA, Krall JM (1985). Patterns of care studies: dose—response of observations for local control of adenocarcinoma of the prostate. International Journal of Radiation Oncology—Biology—Physics, 11:153–7.

Hanks GE, et al. (1987). A ten year follow-up of 682 patients treated for prostate cancer with radiation therapy in the United States. International Journal of Radiation Oncology—Biology—Physics, 13:499–505.

Hanks GE, Martz KL, Diamond JJ (1988). The effect of dose on local control of prostate cancer. International Journal of Radiation Oncology—Biology—Physics, 15:1299–1305.

Harisiadis L, et al. (1978). Carcinoma of the prostate: treatment with external radiotherapy. Cancer, 41:2131–42.

Hays DM, et al. (1982). Bladder and prostatic tumours in the intergroup rhabdomyosarcoma study (IRS-1). Results of therapy. Cancer, 50:1472.

Heller JE (1987). Prostatic acid phosphatase: its current clinical status. Journal of Urology, 137:1091–103.

Herr HW (1980). Iodine-125 implantation in the management of localized prostatic carcinoma. Urologic Clinics of North America, 7:606–12.

Hetherington JW, Siddall JK, Cooper EH (1988). Contribution of bone scintigraphy, prostatic acid phosphatase and prostate-specific antigen to the monitoring of prostatic cancer. European Urology, 14:1–5.

Hilaris BS, Whitmore WF Jr, Batata MA, Barzell W (1977). Behavior patterns of prostatic adenocarcinoma following ^{125}I implant and pelvic node dissection. International Journal of Radiation Oncology—Biology—Physics, 2:631–7.

Hilaris BS, Whitmore WF, Batata MA (1978). Iodine-125 implantation of the prostate: dose response consideration. Frontiers of Radiation Therapy and Oncology, 12:82–90.

Hindson DA, Knight LL, Ocker JM (1985). Small cell carcinoma of the prostate: transient complete remission with chemotherapy. Urology, 26:182.

Hirayama T (1979). Epidemiology of prostate cancer with special reference to the role of diet. National Cancer Institute Monographs, 53:149–55.

Horwich A (1989). Clinical aspects of radiation dose rate. In The biological basis of radiotherapy (ed. GG Steel and A Horwich), pp. 237–47. Elsevier, Amsterdam.

Hoskin PJ, Ford HT, Harmer CL (1989). Hemibody irradiation (HBI) for metastatic bone pain in two histologically distinct groups of patients. Journal of Clinical Oncology, 1:67–9.

Huggins C, Hodges CV (1941). The effect of castration, of estrogen and of androgen injection on serum phosphatases in metastatic carcinoma of the prostate. Cancer Research, 1:292.

Hussey D (1979). Experience with limited field irradiation for adenocarcinoma of the prostate. In Cancer of the genito-urinary tract (ed. DEJ Samuels and ML Samuels), pp. 217–28. Raven Press, New York.

Jewett HJ (1970). The case of radical perineal prostatectomy. Journal of Urology, 103:195–9.

Jewett HJ (1975). The present status of radical prostatectomy for stage A and B prostatic cancer. Urologic Clinics of North America, 2:105–24.

Jewett HJ (1980). Radical perineal prostatectomy for palpable, clinically localized, non-obstructive cancer. Journal of Urology, 124:492–4.

Jewett HJ (1984). Prostatic cancer: a personal view of the problem. Journal of Urology, 131:845–9.

Johansson JE, et al. (1989). Natural history of localised prostatic cancer. Lancet, i:799–803.

Johnson DE, Chalbaud R, Ayala AG (1974). Secondary tumors of the prostate. Journal of Urology, 112:507.

Kahler JE (1939). Carcinoma of the prostate gland: a pathologic study. Journal of Urology, 41:557.

Kastendieck H (1980). Morphologie des prostatacarcinoms in Stanzbiopsien und totalen Prostatektomien. Pathologe, 2:31–43.

Keen CW (1980). Half body radiotherapy in the management of metastatic carcinoma of the prostate. Journal of Urology, 123:713.

Khan K, Crawford ED, Johnson EL (1983). Transperineal percutaneous iridium-192 implant of the prostate. International Journal of Radiation Oncology—Biology—Physics, 9:1391–5.

Kiesling VJ, McAninch JW, Goebel JL, Agee RE (1980). External beam radiotherapy for adenocarcinoma of the prostate: a clinical follow-up. Journal of Urology, 124:851–4.

Knabbe C, Lippman ME, Wakefield L (1987). Evidence that transforming growth factor-B is a hormonally regulated negative growth factor in human breast cancer cells. Cell, 48:417–28.

Kopelson G, et al. (1978). Periurethral duct carcinoma. Clinical features and treatment results. Cancer, 42:2894.

Kovi J (1985). Microscopic differential diagnosis of small acinar adenocarcinoma. Pathology Annual, 20(1):157.

Kramer SA, et al. (1981). Prognosis of patients with stage D1 prostatic adenocarcinoma. Journal of Urology, 125:817–19.

Kramolowsky EV (1988). The value of testosterone deprivation in stage D1 carcinoma of the prostate. Journal of Urology, 139:1242–4.

Kraus PA, Lytton B, Weiss RM, Prosnitz LR (1972). Radiation therapy for local palliative treatment of prostatic cancer. Journal of Urology, 108:612–14.

Kuban DA, et al. (1986). Characteristics of spinal cord compression in adenocarcinoma of prostate. Urology, 28:364.

Kurth KH, Altwein JE, Skoluda D (1977). Follow-up of irradiated prostatic carcinoma by aspiration biopsy. Journal of Urology, 117:615–17.

Kuruvilla AM, et al. (1989). Radiotherapy planning for simulation of prostate cancer: computerized tomographic scanning vs conventional radiographic localization. Medical Dosimetry, 14(4):277–84.

Labrie F, Belanger A, Cusan L (1980). Antifertility effects of LHRH agonists in the male. Journal of Andrology, 1:209–28.

Labrie F, Dupont A, Giguere M (1987). Combination therapy with flutamide and castration (orchiectomy or LHRH agonist): the minimal endocrine therapy in both untreated and previously treated patients. Journal of Steroid Biochemistry, 27:525–32.

Labrie F, Dupont A, Cusan L (1988). Combination therapy with flutamide and castration (LHRH agonist or orchiectomy) in previously untreated patients with clinical stage D 2 prostate cancer: today's therapy of choice. Journal of Steroid Biochemistry, 29:385–96.

Lai PP, Perez CA, Shapiro SJ, Lockett MA (1990). Carcinoma of the prostate stage B and C: lack of influence of duration of radiotherapy on tumor control and treatment morbidity. International Journal of Radiation Oncology—Biology—Physics, 19:561–8.

Landmann C, Hunig R (1989). Prostatic specific antigen as an indicator of response to radiotherapy in prostate cancer. *International Journal of Radiation Oncology — Biology — Physics*, 17:1073–6.

Lange PH, Narayan P (1983). Understaging and undergrading of prostate cancer. Argument for postoperative radiation as adjuvant therapy. *Urology*, 21:113.

Lange PH, Reddy PK, Medini E (1988). Radiation therapy as adjuvant treatment after radical prostatectomy. *National Cancer Institute Monographs*, 335(7):141–9.

Leach GE, Cooper JF, Kagan AR (1982) Radiotherapy for prostatic carcinoma: post irradiation prostatic biopsy and recurrent patterns with longterm followup. *Journal of Urology*, 128:505–9.

Lee F, Gray JM, McLeary RD (1985). Transrectal ultrasound in the diagnosis of prostate cancer: location, echogenicity, histopathology and staging. *Prostate*, 7:117–29.

Leibel SA, Hanks GE, Kramer S (1984). Patterns of care outcome studies: results of the national practice in adenocarcinoma of the prostate. *International Journal of Radiation Oncology — Biology — Physics*, 10:401–9.

Leibel SA, et al. (1994). Three-dimensional conformal radiation therapy in locally advanced carcinoma of the prostate: preliminary results of a phase I dose-escalation study. *International Journal of Radiation Oncology — Biology — Physics*, 28(1):55–65.

Leuprolide Study Group (1984). Leuprolide versus diethylstilboestrol for metastatic prostatic cancer. *New England Journal of Medicine*, 331:1271–86.

Lowe BA, Liström MB (1988a). Incidental carcinoma of the prostate: an analysis of the predictors of progression. *Journal of Urology*, 140:1330–44.

Lowe BA, Liström MB (1988b). Management of stage A prostate cancer with a high probability of progression. *Journal of Urology*, 140:1345–7.

Lu-Yao GL, Greenberg ER (1994). Changes in prostate cancer incidence and treatment in USA. *Lancet*, 343:251–4.

MacDonald A, Chisholm GD, Habib FK (1990). Production and response of a human prostatic cancer line to transforming growth factor-like molecules. *British Journal of Cancer*, 62:579–84.

MacFarlan JR, Tolley DA (1985). Flutamide therapy for advanced prostatic cancer: a phase II study. *British Journal of Urology*, 57:172–4.

McGowan DG (1977). Radiation therapy in the management of localized carcinoma of the prostate. *Cancer*, 39:98–103.

McGowan DG (1981). The value of extended field radiation therapy in carcinoma of the prostate. *International Journal of Radiation Oncology — Biology — Physics*, 7:1333.

McGowan DG (1988). The effect of transurethral resection on prognosis in carcinoma of the prostate: real or imaginary? *International Journal of Radiation Oncology — Biology — Physics*, 15:1057–64.

McNeal JE (1969). Origin and development of carcinoma of the prostate. *Cancer*, 23:24–34.

Mahadevia PS, Koss LG, Tar IJ (1986). Prostatic involvement in bladder cancer: Prostate mapping in 20 cystoprostatectomy specimens. *Cancer*, 58:2096.

Mameghan H, et al. (1990). Bowel complications after radiotherapy for carcinoma of the prostate: the volume effect. *International Journal of Radiation Oncology — Biology — Physics*, 18(2):315–20.

Manni A, Santen RJ, Boucher AE (1986). Androgen priming and response to chemotherapy in advanced prostatic cancer. *Journal of Urology*, 136:1242–6.

Martelli A, Soli M, Bercovich E (1980). Correlation between clinical response to anti-androgenic therapy and occurrence of receptors in human prostatic cancer. *Urology*, 16:245–9.

Meacham RB, et al. (1989). The risk of distant metastases after transurethral resection of the prostate versus needle biopsy in patients with localized prostate cancer. *Journal of Urology*, 142(2):320–5.

Meek AG, Park TL, Oberman E, Wielopolski L (1990). A prospective study of prostate specific antigen levels in patients receiving radiotherapy for localized carcinoma of the prostate. *International Journal of Radiation Oncology — Biology — Physics*, 19:733–41.

Melicow MM, Pachter MR (1967). Endometrial carcinoma of prostatic utricle (uterus masculinus). *Cancer*, 20:1715–22.

Mettlin C, Natarajan M, Murphy GP (1982). Recent patterns of care of prostate cancer patients in the United States: results from the survey of the American College of Surgeons Commission on Cancer. *International Advances in Surgical Oncology*, 5:277–321.

Meyers RP, Fleming TR (1983). Course of localized adenocarcinoma of the prostate treated by radical prostatectomy. *Prostate*, 4:461–72.

Mills SE, Fowler JE Jr (1986). Gleason histologic grading of prostatic carcinoma. Correlations between biopsy and prostatectomy specimens. *Cancer*, 57:346.

Mintz ER, Smith GG (1934). Autopsy findings in 100 cases of prostatic cancer. *New England Journal of Medicine*, 211:479.

Moore RA (1935). The morphology of small prostatic carcinoma. *Journal of Urology*, 33:224.

Morales A, Connolly JG, Burr RC, Bruce AW (1970). The use of radioactive phosphorous to treat bone pain in metastatic carcinoma of the prostate. *Canadian Medical Association Journal*, 103:372.

Morris GL, Green Dodd J (1990). Epidermal growth factor receptor mRNA levels in human prostatic tumors and cell lines. *Journal of Urology*, 143:1272–4.

Morton AR, Howell A (1988). Bisphosphonates and bone metastases. *British Journal of Cancer*, 58:556–7.

Morton JD, Peschel RE (1988). Iodine-125 implants versus external beam therapy for stages A2, B, and C prostate cancer. *International Journal of Radiation Oncology — Biology — Physics*, 14:1153–7.

Mostofi FK (1975). Grading of prostatic carcinoma. *Cancer Chemotherapy Reports*, 59:111–17.

Mostofi FK (1976). Problems of grading carcinoma of the prostate. *Seminars in Oncology*, 3:161–9.

Mostofi FK, Sesterhenn I, Sobin LH (1980). Histological typing of prostate tumors. In *International histological classification of tumors*, p. 22. World Health Organization, Geneva.

Mott LJM (1979). Squamous cell carcinoma of the prostate: report of two cases and review of the literature. *Journal of Urology*, 121:833.

Moyana TN (1987). Adenosquamous carcinoma of the prostate. *American Journal of Surgical Pathology*, 11:403–7.

Murphy DJ Jr, Porter AT (1988). Prostate localization for the treatment planning of prostate cancer: a comparison of two techniques. *Medical Dosimetry*, 13(1):11–12.

Murphy GP, Whitmore WF Jr (1979). A report of the workshops on the current status of histologic grading of prostate cancer. *Cancer*, 44:1490.

Myers C, et al. (1992). Suramin: a novel growth factor antagonist with activity in hormone-refractory metastatic prostate cancer. *Journal of Clinical Oncology*, 10(6):881–9.

Nachtsheim DA Jr, McAninch JW, Stutzman RE, Goebel JL (1978). Latent residual tumor following external radiotherapy for prostate adenocarcinoma. *Journal of Urology*, 120:312–14.

Narayan P, Jojodia P, Stein R, Tanagho EA (1989). A comparison of fine needle aspiration and core biopsy in diagnosis and preoperative grading of prostate cancer. *Journal of Urology*, 141:560–3.

Nativ O, Winkler HZ, Raz Y (1989). Stage C prostatic adenocarcinoma: flow cytometric nuclear DNA ploidy analysis. *Mayo Clinic Proceedings*, 64(8):911–19.

Neglia WJ, Hussey DH, Johnson DE (1977). Megavoltage radiation therapy for carcinoma of the prostate. *International Journal of Radiation Oncology — Biology — Physics*, 2:873–82.

Nesbit RM, Baum WC (1950). Endocrine control of prostatic carcinoma. *Journal of the American Medical Association*, 143:1317–20.

Neumann F, Jacobi GH (1982). Antiandrogens in tumour therapy. *Journal of Clinical Oncology*, 1:41–64.

Nijis M, Hawkins EF (1976). Binding of 6 alpha dihydrotestosterone in human prostatic cancer: examination by agar gel electrophoresis. *Journal of Endocrinology*, 69:18–19.

Oesterling JE, Jacobsen SJ, Chute CG, Guess HA, Girman CJ, Panser LA, Lieber MM (1993). Serum prostate-specific antigen in an community-based population of healthy men: establishment of age-specific reference ranges. *Journal of the American Medical Association*, 270(7):860–4.

O'Malley B (1990). The steroid receptor superfamily: more excitement predicted for the future. *Molecular Endocrinology*, 4(3):363–9.

Oosterom R, Bogdanowicz J, Schroder FH (1989). Evaluation of prostate specific antigen in untreated prostatic carcinoma. *European Urology Annals of Surgery*, 16:253–7.

Ortega LG, Whitmore WF Jr, Murphy AI (1953). *In situ* carcinoma of the prostate with intra-epithelial extension into the urethra and bladder: Paget's disease of the urethra and bladder. *Cancer*, 6:898–923.

Osborne CK, Drelichman A, von Hoff D (1983). Mitoxantrone: modest activity in a phase II trial in advanced prostate cancer. *Cancer Treatment Reports*, 67:1133–5.

Pantelides ML, Bowman SP, George NJ (1992). Levels of prostate specific antigen that predict skeletal spread in prostate cancer. *British Journal of Urology*, 70(3):299–303.

Parmar H, Edwards L, Phillips RH (1987). Orchidectomy versus long-acting D-Trp-6-LHRH in advanced prostatic cancer. *British Journal of Urology*, 59:248–54.

Partin AW, Epstein JI, Cho KR (1989). Morphometric measurement of tumor volume and per cent of gland involvement as preditors of pathological stage in clinical stage B prostate cancer. *Journal of Urology*, 141:341–5.

Pasteau O (1911). Traitement du cancer de la prostate par le radium. *Revues de Maladies de la Nutrition*, 363.

Paulson DF, Lin G, Hinshaw W, Stephani S (1982). Radical surgery versus radiotherapy for adenocarcinoma of the prostate. *Journal of Urology*, 128:502–4.

Paulson DF, Robertson JF, Daubert LM, Walther PJ (1988). Radical prostatectomy in stage A prostatic adenocarcinoma. *Journal of Urology*, 140:535–9.

Pavone-Macaluso M, de Voogt HJ, Viggiano G (1986). Comparison of diethylstilboestrol, cyproterone acetate and medroxyprogesterone acetate in the treatment of advanced prostatic cancer: final analysis of a randomized phase III trial of the European Organization for Research on Treatment of Cancer Urological Group. *Journal of Urology*, 136:624–31.

Perez CA (1983). Carcinoma of the prostate: a vexing biological and clinical enigma. *International Journal of Radiation Oncology—Biology—Physics*, 9:1427–38.

Perez CA, Bauer W, Garza R, Royce RK (1977a). Complications and regression of primary tumor site with radiotherapy in prostate cancer. *Journal of Urology*, 108:921–47.

Perez CA, Bauer W, Garza R, Royce RK (1977b). Radiation therapy in the definitive treatment of localized carcinoma of the prostate. *Cancer*, 40:1425–33.

Perez CA, Walz BJ, Zivnuska FR (1980). Irradiation of carcinoma of the prostate localized to the pelvis: analysis of tumor response and prognosis. *International Journal of Radiation Oncology—Biology—Physics*, 6:555–63.

Petros JA, Catalona WJ (1992). Lower incidence of unsuspected lymph node metastases in 521 consecutive patients with clinically localised prostate cancer. *Journal of Urology*, 147:1574–5.

Pilepich MV (1988). Radiation therapy oncology group studies in carcinoma of the prostate. *National Cancer Institute Monographs*, 7:61–5.

Pilepich MV, Walz BJ, Baglan RJ (1984). Postoperative irradiation in carcinoma of the prostate. *International Journal of Radiation Oncology—Biology—Physics*, 10:1869–73.

Pilepich MV, et al. (1986). Extended field (periaortic) irradiation in carcinoma of the prostate analysis of RTOG 75-06. *International Journal of Radiation Oncology—Biology—Physics*, 12(3):345–51.

Pilepich MV, et al. (1987a). Correlation of radiotherapeutic parameters and treatment related morbidity—analysis of RTOG study 77-06. *International Journal of Radiation Oncology—Biology—Physics*, 13:1007–12.

Pilepich MV, et al. (1987b). Radical prostatectomy or radiotherapy in carcinoma of prostate, the dilemma continues. *Urology*, 30(1):18–21.

Pilepich MV, et al. (1987c). Prognostic factors in carcinoma of the prostate-analysis of RTOG study 7506. *International Journal of Radiation Oncology—Biology—Physics*, 13(3):339–49.

Pilepich MV, et al. (1989). Hormonal cytoreduction in locally advanced carcinoma of the prostate treated with definitive radiotherapy: preliminary results of RTOG 83-07. *International Journal of Radiation Oncology—Biology—Physics*, 16(3):813–17.

Pillarisetti SG, Esplinoza CG, Richman AV (1983). Prostatic adenocarcinoma with focal 'endometrial' features. Histopathologic and immunocytochemical findings. *Laboratory Investigations*, 48:68A.

Pisanksy TM, Cha SS, Earle JD, Durr ED, Kozelsky TF, Wieand HS, Oesterling JE (1993). Prostate-specific antigen as a pretherapy prognostic factor in patients treated with radiation therapy for clinically localised prostate cancer. *Clinical Journal of Urology*, 11:2158–66.

Pistenma DA, Ray GR, Bagshaw MA (1976). The role of megavoltage radiation therapy in the treatment of prostatic cancer. *Seminars in Oncology*, 3:115–22.

Plowman PN, Perry LA, Chard T (1987). Androgen suppression by hydrocortisone without aminoglutethimide in orchiectomised men with prostatic cancer. *British Journal of Cancer*, 50:757–63.

Polysongsang S, et al. (1986). Comparison of whole pelvis versus small field radiation therapy for carcinoma of the prostate. *Journal of Urology*, 27:10–16.

Ponder BAJ, Shearer RJ, Pocock RD (1984). Response to aminoglutethimide and cortisone acetate in advanced prostatic cancer. *British Journal of Cancer*, 50:757–63.

Pontes JE, Choe BK, Rose NR (1981). Clinical evaluation of immunological methods for detection of serum prostatic acid phosphatase. *Journal of Urology*, 126:363–5.

Pontes JE, Huben R, Wolf R (1986). Sexual function after radical prostatectomy. *Prostate*, 8:123–6.

Porter AT, McEwan AJ (1993). Strontium-89 as an adjuvant to external beam radiation improves pain relief and delays disease progression in advanced prostate cancer: results of a randomised controlled trial. *Seminars in Oncology*, 20 (3 Suppl. 2):38–43.

Powell CS, Field AM, Rosser K (1989). Prostate specific antigen—a screening test for prostatic cancer? *British Journal of Urology*, 64:504–6.

Poyet P, Labrie F (1985). Comparison of the antiandrogenic/androgenic activities of flutamide, cyproterone acetate and megestrol acetate. *Molecular and Cellular Endocrinology*, 42:283–8.

Preston CI, Duncan W, Kerr GR (1986). Radical treatment of prostatic carcinoma by megavoltage X-ray therapy. *Clinical Radiology*, 37:473–7.

Price P, et al. (1986). Prospective randomised trial of single and multi-fraction schedules in the treatment of painful bone metastases. *Radiotherapy and Oncology*, 6:247–55.

Prout GR, Brewer WR (1967). Response of men with advanced prostatic carcinoma to exogenous administration of testosterone. *Cancer* 20:1871–8.

Qayum A, et al. (1990). The effects of gonadotrophin releasing hormone analogues in prostate cancer are mediated through specific tumour receptors. *British Journal of Cancer*, 62(1):96–9.

Ray GR, Cassady R, Bagshaw MA (1973). Definitive radiation therapy of carcinoma of the prostate—a report on 15 years of experience. *Radiology*, 106:407–18.

Ray GR, Bagshaw MA, Freiha F (1984). External beam radiation salvage for residual or recurrent local tumor following radical prostatectomy. *Journal of Urology*, 132:926–30.

Redding T, Shally A (1985). Investigation of the combination of the agonist D-TRP⁶-LHRH and the antiandrogen flutamide in the treatment of the Dunning prostate cancer model. *Prostate*, 6:218–32.

Reiner WG, Walsh PC (1979). An anatomical approach to the surgical management of the dorsal vein and Santorini's plexus during radical retropubic surgery. *Journal of Urology*, 121(2):198–200.

Reynoso G, Murphy GP (1972). Adrenalectomy and hypophysectomy in advanced prostatic cancer. *Cancer*, 29:941.

Rich AR (1935). On the frequency of occult carcinoma of the prostate. *Journal of Urology*, 33:215.

Rifkin MD, McGlynn ET, Choi H (1989). Echogenicity of prostate cancer correlated with histologic grade and stromal fibrosis: endorectal US studies. *Radiology*, 170(2):549–52.

Rijinders AW, et al. (1985). Expression of cellular oncogenes in human prostatic carcinoma cell lines. *Biochemical and Biophysical Research Communications*, 132:548–54.

Ritter MA, Messing EM, Shanahan TG, Potts S, Chappell RJ, Kinsella TJ (1992). Prostate-specific antigen as a predictor of radiotherapy response and patterns of failure in localised prostate cancer. *Journal of Clinical Oncology*, 10(8):1205–7.

Robey EL, Schellhammer PF, Wright GL Jr (1985). Cancer serum index and prostatic acid phosphatase for detection of progressive prostatic cancer. *Journal of Urology*, 134:787–90.

Robinson RG (1986). Radionuclides for the alleviation of bone pain in advanced malignancy. *Clinics in Oncology*, 5(1):39–49.

Rosenberg SA, et al. (1985). Radical prostatectomy with adjuvant radioactive gold for prostatic cancer: a preliminary report. *Journal of Urology*, 133:225–7.

Rounsaville MC, et al. (1987). Prostatic carcinoma: limited field irradiation. *International Journal of Radiation Oncology—Biology—Physics*, 13:1013–20.

Rowland CG, Bullimore JA, Smith P, Roberts JBM (1981). Half body irradiation in the treatment of metastatic prostatic carcinoma. *British Journal of Urology*, **53**:628–9.

Russell KJ, *et al.* (1994). Photon versus fast neutron external beam radiotherapy in the treatment of locally advanced prostate cancer: results of a randomised prospective trial. *International Journal of Radiation Oncology—Biology—Physics*, **28**(1):47–54.

Sandler HM, Perez-Tamayo C, Ten Haken RK, Lichter AS (1992). Dose escalation for stage C(T3) prostate cancer: minimal rectal toxicity observed using conformal therapy. *Radiotherapy and Oncology*, **23**:53–4.

Scardino P, Carlton C Jr (1983). Combined interstitial and external radiation for prostatic cancer. In *Principles and management of urologic cancer* (ed. N Javadpour), pp. 392–408. Williams & Wilkins, Baltimore.

Scardino PT, Wheeler TM (1988). Local control of prostate cancer with radiotherapy: frequency and prognostic significance of positive results of postirradiation prostate biopsy. *National Cancer Institute Monographs*, **7**:95–103.

Schellhammer PF, Bean MA, Whitemore WF Jr (1977). Prostatic involvement by transitional cell carcinoma. Pathogenesis, patterns and prognosis. *Journal of Urology*, **118**:399.

Schellhammer P, El-Mahdi AE, Ladaga LE (1985). ^{125}Iodine implantation for carcinoma of the prostate: 5 year survival free of disease and incidence of local failure. *Journal of Urology*, **134**:1140–5.

Scher HI, Sternberg CN (1985). Chemotherapy of urologic malignancies. *Seminars in Urology*, **3**:239.

Schiebler ML, *et al.* (1989). Prostatic carcinoma and benign prostatic hyperplasia: correlation of high-resolution MR and histopathologic findings. *Radiology*, **172**(1):131–7.

Schild SE, Buskirk SJ, Robinow JS, Tomera KM, Ferrigni RG, Frick LM (1992). The results of radiotherapy for isolated elevation of serum PSA levels following radical prostatectomy. *International Journal of Radiation Oncology—Biology—Physics*, **23**(1):141–5.

Schröder FH (1993). Prostate cancer: to screen or not to screen? *British Medical Journal*, **306**:407–8.

Schröder FH, Belt E (1975). Carcinoma of the prostate: a study of 213 patients with stage C tumors treated by total perineal prostatectomy. *Journal of Urology*, **114**:257–60.

Schröder FH, Blom JHM, Hop WCJ, Mostofi FK (1985). Grading of prostatic cancer. II. An analysis of the prognostic significance of the presence of multiple architectural patterns. *Prostate*, **6**:403.

Schröder FH, *et al.* (1988). TNM classification of genitourinary tumours 1987—position of the EORTC genitourinary group. *British Journal of Urology*, **62**:502–10.

Schröder FH, Blom JHM, Bosch JLHR (1989). Considerations on surgical management of locally advanced prostatic carcinom. In *Prostatic disorders* (ed. DF Paulson), pp. 330–1. Lea & Febiger, Philadelphia.

Schron DS, Gipson T, Mendelsohn G (1984). The histogenesis of small cell carcinoma of the prostate: an immunohistochemical study. *Cancer*, **53**:2478.

Sewell RA, Braren V, Wilson SK, Rhamy RK (1975). Extended biopsy follow-up after full-course radiation for resectable prostatic carcinoma. *Journal of Urology*, **113**:371–3.

Shearer RJ, Davies JH, Gelister JSK, Dearnaley DP (1992). Hormonal cytoreduction and radiotherapy for carcinoma of the prostate. *British Journal of Urology*, **69**(5):521–4.

Silverberg GD (1977). Hypophysectomy in the treatment of disseminated prostate carcinomas. *Cancer*, **39**:1727–37.

Smart JG (1965). The use of ^{32}P in the treatment of severe pain from bone metastases of carcinoma of the prostate. *British Journal of Urology*, **37**:139–47.

Smith BH, Dehner LP (1972). Sarcoma of the prostate gland. *American Journal of Clinical Pathology*, **58**:43.

Smith JA (1989). Palliation of painful bone metastases from prostate cancer using sodium etidronate: results of a randomized, prospective, double-blind, placebo-controlled study. *Journal of Urology*, **141**:85–7.

Smith JA Jr, Seaman JP, Gleidman JB, Middleton RG (1983). Pelvic lymph node metastases from prostatic cancer. Influence of tumor grade and stage in 452 consecutive patients. *Journal of Urology*, **130**:290–2.

Soffen FM, Hanks GE, Hunt MA (1992). Epstein BE conformal static field radiation therapy treatment of early prostate cancer versus non-conformal techniques. A reduction in acute morbidity. *International Journal of Radiation Oncology—Biology—Physics*, **24**:485–8.

Sogani PC, Ray B, Whitmore WF (1975). Advanced prostatic carcinoma. *Urology*, **6**:164–6.

Sogani PC, Vagaiwala MR, Whitmore WF Jr (1984). Experience with flutamide in patients with advanced prostatic cancer without prior endocrine therapy. *Cancer*, **54**(4):744–50.

Spellman MC (1977). An evaluation of lymphography in localized carcinoma of the prostate. *Radiology*, **125**:637.

Spremulli E, DeSimone P, Durant J (1982). A phase II study of novadex tamoxifen citrate in the treatment of advanced prostatic adenocarcinoma. *American Journal of Clinical Oncology*, **5**:149–53.

Stamey TA, Kabalin JN, Ferrari M (1989). Prostate specific antigen in the diagnosis and treatment of adenocarcinoma of the prostate. III. Radiation treated patients. *Journal of Urology*, **141**:1084–90.

Stanford EJ, Drago JR, Rohner TJ (1976). Aminoglutethimide medical adrenalectomy for advanced prostatic carcinoma. *Journal of Urology*, **115**:170–4.

Steele R, Lees RE, Kraus AS, Rao S (1971). Sexual factors in the epidemiology of cancer of the prostate. *Journal of Chronic Diseases*, **24**:29–37.

Stein A, deKernion JB, Smith RB, Dorey F, Patel H (1992). Prostate specific antigen levels after radical prostatectomy in patients with organ confined and locally extensive prostate cancer. *Journal of Urology*, **147**(3 part 2):942–6.

Stone AR, Hargreave TB, Chisholm GD (1980). The diagnosis of oestrogen escape and the role of secondary orchiectomy in prostatic cancer. *British Journal of Urology*, **52**:535–8.

Surya BV, Provet J, Johanson KE, Brown J (1990). Anastomic strictures following radical prostatectomy: risk factors and management. *Journal of Urology*, **143**:755–8.

Tait D, *et al.* (1988). Benefits expected from simple conformal RT in the treatment of pelvic tumours. *Radiotherapy and Oncology*, **13**:23–30.

Tait DM, Nahum AE, Rigby L, Chow M, Mayles WPM, Dearnaley DP, Horwich A (1993). Conformal therapy of the pelvis: assessment of acute toxicity. *Radiotherapy and Oncology*, **29**(2):117–26.

Tannenbaum M, Tannenbaum S, DeSanctis PN (1982). Prognostic significance of nucleolar surface area in prostatic cancer. *Urology*, **19**:546.

Taylor WJ, Richardson RG, Hafermann MD (1979). Radiation therapy for localized prostatic cancer. *Cancer*, **43**:1123–7.

ten Haken RK, *et al.* (1989). Boost treatment of the prostate using shaped, fixed fields. *International Journal of Radiation Oncology—Biology—Physics*, **16**:193–200.

Tetu B, *et al.* (1987). Small cell carcinoma of the prostate part 1. A clinicopathologic study of 20 cases. *Cancer*, **59**:1803.

Tolis G, Ackman D, Stellos A (1982). Growth inhibition in patients with prostatic cancer treated with luteinizing hormone releasing hormone agonists. *Proceedings of the National Academy of Sciences USA*, **79**:1658–62.

Trachtenberg J, Walsh PC (1982). Correlation of prostatic nuclear androgen receptor content with duration of response and survival following hormonal therapy in advanced prostatic cancer. *Journal of Urology*, **127**:466–71.

Trott KR, Kummermehr J (1985). What is known about tumour proliferation rates to choose between accelerated fractionation or hyperfractionation? *Radiotherapy and Oncology*, **3**:1–9.

Tunn UW, Graff J, Senge TH (1983). Treatment of inoperable prostatic cancer with cyproterone acetate. In *Androgens and anti-androgens* (ed. FH Schroder), pp. 149–59. Schering, The Netherlands.

Uchida T, Wada C, Shitara T, Egawa S, Koshiba K (1993). Infrequent involvement of p53 gene mutations in the tumourigenesis of Japanese prostate cancer. *British Journal of Cancer*, **68**(4):751–5.

UICC (1978). *TNM classification of malignant tumours.* Springer-Verlag, Geneva.

UICC (1987). *TNM classification of malignant tumours.* Springer-Verlag, Geneva.

Utz DC, Farrow GM (1969). Pathologic differentiation and prognosis of prostatic carcinoma. *Journal of the American Medical Association*, **209**:1701.

van Aubel OGJM, Hoekstra WJ, Schroder FH (1985). Early orchicctomy for patients with stage D1 prostatic carcinoma. *Journal of Urology*, **134**:292–4.

van der Werf-Messing B (1978). Prostatic cancer treated at the Rotterdams Institute. *Strahlentherapie*, **154**:537–41.

van Dieijen-Visser MP, van Delaere KPJ, Gijzen AHJ, Brombacher PJ (1988). A comparative study on the diagnostic value of prostatic acid phosphatase (PAP) and prostatic specific antigen (PSA) in patients with carcinoma of the prostate gland. *Clinica Chemica Acta*, 174:131–40.

van Holten-Verzantvoort ATH, Bijvoet OLM, Hermans J (1987). Reduced morbidity from skeletal metastases in breast cancer patients during long-term bisphosphonate (APD) treatment. *Lancet*, ii:983–5.

Vanuytsel L, *et al.* (1986). Radiotherapy in multiple fractions per day for prostatic carcinoma: late complications. *International Journal of Radiation Oncology—Biology—Physics*, 12(9):1589–95.

Varenhorst E, Wallentin L, Risberg B (1981). The effects of orchidectomy, oestrogens and cyproterone acetate on the antithrombin-III concentration in carcinoma of the prostate. *Urological Research*, 9:25–8.

Veterans Administration Cooperative Urological Research Group (1967). Treatment and survival of patients with cancer of the prostate. *Surgery, Gynecology and Obstetrics*, 124:1011–17.

Viola MV, *et al.* (1986). Expression of *ras* oncogene p21 in prostatic cancer. *New England Journal of Medicine*, 314(3):133–7.

von Paschkis R, Tittinger W (1910). Radiumbehandlung eines prostatasarkoms. *Wiener Klinische Wochenschrift*, 48:1715–16.

Wallace DM, Chisholm GD, Hendry WF (1975). TNM Classification for urological tumours (UICC) 1974. *British Journal of Urology*, 47:1–12.

Walsh PC (1987). Editorial: adjuvant radiotherapy after radical prostatectomy: is it indicated? *Journal of Urology*, 138:1427–8.

Walsh PC (1988). Radical retropubic prostatectomy with reduced morbidity: an anatomical approach. *National Cancer Institute Monographs*, 7:133–7.

Walsh PC, Donker PJ (1982). Impotence following radical prostatectomy: insight into etiology and prevention. *Journal of Urology*, 128:492–9.

Walsh PC, Jewett HJ (1980). Radical surgery for prostatic cancer. *Cancer*, 45:1906–11.

Walsh PC, Lepor H (1987). The role of radical prostatectomy in the management of prostatic cancer. *Cancer*, 60:526–37.

Walsh PC, Gittes RF, Perlmutter AD, Stamey TA (1986). *Campbell's urology.* WB Saunders, Philadelphia.

Warner W, Whitmore WF Jr (1990). *Expected management of localized prostatic cancer. Abstract and oral communication.* Canadian Urological Association, Vancouver.

Wasserstein PW, Goldman RL (1981). Diffuse carcinoid of prostate. *Urology*, 18:407.

Waterhouse JA, Muir CA, Shanmugaratnam K (1982). *Cancer incidence in five continents.* IARC Scientific Publications, Lyon.

Waxman J (1987). Gonadotrophin hormone releasing analogues open new doors in cancer treatment. *British Medical Journal*, 295:1084–5.

Waxman JH, Wass JA, Hendry WF (1983). Treatment with gonadotrophin releasing hormone analogue in advanced prostatic cancer. *British Medical Journal*, 286:1309–12.

Waxman HH, Man A, Hendry WF (1985). Importance of early tumour exacerbation in patients treated with long acting analogues of gonadotrophin releasing hormone for advanced prostatic cancer. *British Medical Journal*, 291:1387–8.

Waxman J, Williams G, Sandow J (1988). The clinical and endocrine assessment of three different antiandrogen regimens combined with a very long-acting gonadotrophin-releasing hormone analogue. *American Journal of Clinical Oncology*, 11(2):152–5.

Waxman HH, Sandow J, Abel P (1989a). Two-monthly depot gonadotrophin releasing hormone agonist (buserelin) for treatment of prostatic cancer. *Acta Endocrinologica (Copenhagen)*, 120:315–18.

Waxman J, Sandow J, Thomas H (1989b). A pharmacological evaluation of a new 3-month depot preparation of buserelin for prostatic cancer. *Cancer Chemotherapy and Pharmacology*, 25:219–20.

Weldon VE, Tavel FR (1988). Potency-sparing radical perineal prostatectomy: anatomy, surgical technique and initial results. *Journal of Urology*, 140:559–62.

White JW (1893). The present position of the surgery of the hypertrophied prostate. *Annals of Surgery*, 18:152–88.

Whitmore WF Jr (1973). The natural history of prostatic cancer. *Cancer*, 32:1104–12.

Whitmore WF Jr (1984). Natural history and staging of prostate cancer. *Urologic Clinics of North America*, 11:205–20.

Whitmore WF Jr (1988a). Overview: historical and contemporary. *National Cancer Institute Monographs*, 7:7–11.

Whitmore WF Jr (1988b). Panel discussion: management of stage B1 and B2 disease. In *Multidisciplinary analysis of controversies in the management of prostate cancer* (ed. DS Coffey, MI Resnick, FA Door, and JP Karr), pp. 143–4. Plenum Press, New York.

Whitmore WF (1994). Localised prostatic cancer: management and detection issues. *Lancet*, 343:1263–7.

Whitmore WF Jr, *et al.* (1985). Interstitial radiation: short-term palliation or curative therapy? *Urology*, 25 (Suppl.):24–9.

Williams G, *et al.* (1984). Biodegradable polymer luteinising hormone releasing hormone agonist for prostatic cancer: use of a new peptide delivery system. *British Medical Journal*, 289:1580–1.

Wittkamper FW, Mijnheer BJ, van Kleffens HJ (1987). Dose intercomparison at the radiotherapy centres in The Netherlands. 1. Photon beams under reference conditions and for prostatic cancer treatment. *Radiotherapy and Oncology*, 9(1):33–44.

Wollin M, *et al.* (1989). Radiosensitivity of human prostate cancer and malignant melanoma cell lines. *Radiotherapy and Oncology*, 15:285–93.

Young BW, Lagios MD (1973). Endometrial (papillary) carcinoma of the prostatic utricle: response to orchiectomy. A case report. *Cancer*, 32:1293–1300.

Young HH, Fronz W (1917). Some new methods in the treatment of carcinoma of the lower genitourinary tract with radium. *Journal of Urology*, 1:505–36.

Zagars GK, von Eschenbach AC, Johnson DE, Oswald MJ (1987). Stage C adenocarcinoma of the prostate: an analysis of 551 patients treated with external beam radiation. *Cancer*, 60:1489–99.

Zagars GK, von Eschenbach AC, Johnson DE, Oswald JM (1988). The role of radiation therapy in stages A2 and B adenocarcinoma of the prostate. *International Journal of Radiation Oncology—Biology—Physics*, 14:701–9.

Zaridze DG, Boyle P (1987). Cancer of the prostate: epidemiology and aetiology. *British Journal of Urology*, 59(6):493–502.

Zincke H (1988). Bilateral pelvic lymphadenectomy and radical retropubic prostatectomy for stage C or D1 adenocarcinoma of the prostate: possible beneficial effect of adjuvant treatment. *National Cancer Institute Monographs*, 7:109–15.

Zincke H, Utz DC, Thule PM, Taylor WF (1987). Treatment options for patients with stage D1 (T0-3 N1-2 M0) adenocarcinoma of prostate. *Urology*, 30:207–315.

Zinreich ES, *et al.* (1990). Pre- and post-treatment evaluation of sexual function in patients with adenocarcinoma of the prostate. *International Journal of Radiation Oncology—Biology—Physics*, 19:729–32.

Section 11
Thoracic tumours

11.1   Tumours of the trachea and the lung

HEINE H. HANSEN, PETER GOLDSTRAW, ANNA GREGOR, AND
LARS VINDELØV

INTRODUCTION

Primary lung tumours are now a global health problem. Almost unheard of before this century, their incidence has risen dramatically during the last five to six decades, reflecting the popularity of cigarette smoking and effects of urbanization and pollution. Lung cancer is now the most frequent cancer among men in most European countries and it is increasing rapidly in women. More than 800 000 people die annually from lung cancer worldwide and its incidence is rising, especially in the so-called developing countries (Stanley and Stjernswärd 1989).

In spite of the fact that many of the aetiological factors in lung cancer have been known for years, it is only within the last few years that preventive and antismoking programmes have been initiated and only in some countries. With the long lag between exposure and the clinical development of the tumour, lung cancer will continue to be frequently seen long into the next century. In spite of increased insight into the biology of the disease and some therapeutic advances in the last two decades, it will also remain a major therapeutic challenge for many years to come.

EPIDEMIOLOGY

It has been estimated that in 1990 approximately 270 000 cases of respiratory-tract malignancies were diagnosed in Europe. Among these, tracheal cancer constitutes approximately 0.2 per cent and it is thus a rare disease. Life-long probability of developing lung cancer varies from 4 to 12 per cent for European men, depending on the country of residence. The corresponding probabilities for women are 0.5 to 3 per cent (Muir *et al.* 1987; Parkin *et al.* 1988; Jensen *et al.* 1990).

On average, one out of 10–15 European men and one out of 80–90 European women develops lung cancer before the age of 75, if they do not die before this age of other causes. As the incidence of lung cancer is still increasing in most countries, the lifetime risk for young European men and women is probably closer to the upper range of these estimates. In the absence of major changes in risk factors, we may expect 300 000 cases per year of lung cancer in Europe by the year 2000 (Hansen 1991).

The mortality trends for men and women for some of the European countries are given in Figs 1 and 2, respectively (Hansen 1991). In the United Kingdom the rates increased until the early 1970s; they then reached a plateau, followed by a gradual decline. In contrast, the rates, although much lower, in Southern Europe are rapidly increasing. The countries in Central Europe already had relatively high rates in the 1950s, with a steady increase in the following years. Belgium and The Netherlands have shown a greater increase than the other countries and in recent years have had higher rates than England (Hansen 1991).

In women, mortality rates for lung cancer are increasing everywhere. The highest rates are found in the United Kingdom, Ireland, and Denmark. In Central and Southern Europe the incidence is still low, in the range of 2–5 per 100 000 per year. As smoking is increasing steadily in these countries among the younger female population, a dramatic increase in lung cancer is to be expected in Southern Europe within the next two to three decades (Hansen 1991).

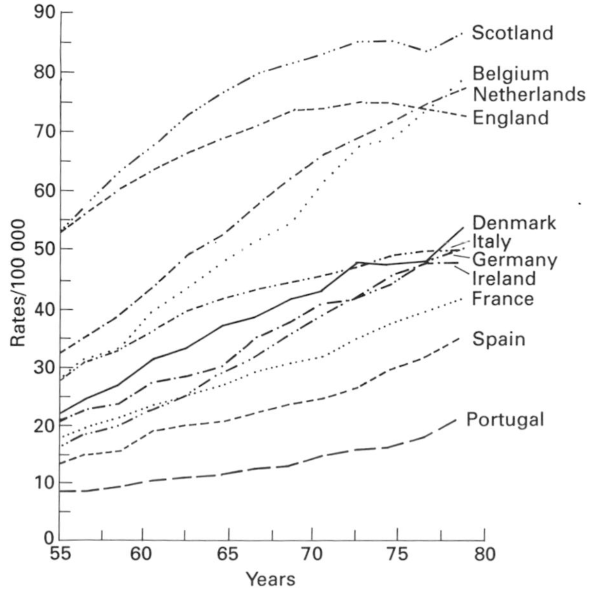

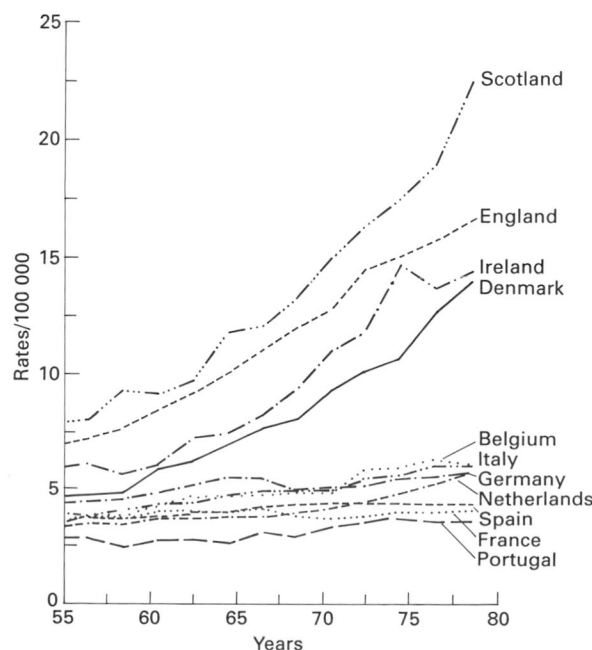

Fig. 1 Age-adjusted lung cancer mortality rates in 11 European countries (males).

Fig. 2 Age-adjusted lung cancer mortality rates in 11 European countries (females).

AETIOLOGY

It has long since been established that tobacco and particularly cigarette smoking is the major cause of lung cancer (Loeb *et al.* 1984). In most countries of the world the elimination of tobacco would result in a reduction in lung cancer risk to 10–15 per cent of the present incidence; that is, the abolition of lung cancer as a major health problem. Since the early studies in the 1950s which showed that lung cancer patients smoked more than healthy controls, the association has been fully corroborated in cohort studies, that is, by prolonged follow-up of populations with different smoking habits, in order to compare lung cancer incidence or mortality rates. One of the most important studies is the 20 year prospective observation of more than 30 000 male British doctors whose smoking habits were repeatedly established by questionnaire between 1951 and 1972 (Doll and Peto 1976). Mortality rates for lung cancer are up to 25 times higher in smokers than in non-smokers, increasing with the number of cigarettes per day (Fig. 3).

The lung cancer risk depends more strongly on the duration of smoking than on the daily dose of cigarettes. For example, a 3-fold increase in the daily number of cigarettes may produce only approximately a 3-fold increase in risk, while 45 years of smoking against 15 might produce a 100-fold effect (Lubin *et al.* 1984). In terms of lifelong risk, therefore, smoking 30 cigarettes a day for 15 years is far less dangerous than smoking 10 cigarettes a day for 45 years. Even among people who have been smoking for many years, those who have not yet developed lung cancer can, by giving up smoking, significantly reduce their subsequent risk of tobacco-induced cancer (Fig. 4).

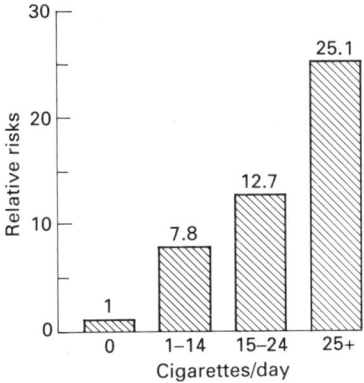

Fig. 3 Relative risks of lung cancer versus daily consumption of cigarettes.

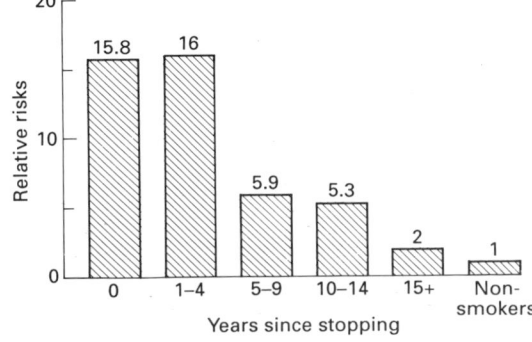

Fig. 4 Relative risks of lung cancer versus years since stopping smoking.

When a person stops smoking, the excess risk of developing lung cancer appears to remain approximately constant for many years, instead of increasing, as would have been the case if smoking was continued. For reasons that are not yet established, cigarette smoking has a greater effect on lung cancer risk than do cigar and pipe smoking.

Specific preventive activities have lately been established, for example in the United States among physicians trying to influence heavy smokers and with some success (Lubin *et al.* 1984; Kottke *et al.* 1988; Cohen *et al.* 1989; Cummings *et al.* 1989). The programmes include education and counselling in order to prevent the onset of the smoking habit (Cullen 1989).

Passive smoking (that is, breathing other people's smoke) must be presumed to carry some risk, as ambient smoke contains the same chemicals as those inhaled by smokers. It is generally accepted that a safe threshold is very unlikely to exist for carcinogenic chemicals. The risk is mostly too small to be detectable on national mortality statistics. A small but measurable effect on the lung cancer risk can be found in non-smokers living together with smokers. A number of studies have shown rather consistently that a non-smoking spouse of a smoker has a 20–50 per cent higher risk than a non-exposed subject. Overall, approximately one-fourth of all lung cancer cases in non-smokers, that is approximately 2 per cent of all lung cancer cases, might be due to passive smoking (Akiba *et al.* 1986; Dalager *et al.* 1986).

Lung cancer in non-smokers is rare; less than 10 per cent of patients with respiratory malignancy in large series never smoked.

A number of chemicals to which people may be exposed in the occupational environment increase the risk of lung cancer, sometimes dramatically (Table 1) (Merletti *et al.* 1984; Pastorini *et al.* 1984). In a few cases the occupational exposure interacts synergistically with tobacco smoking, in such a way that the combined exposure is associated with a lung cancer risk far exceeding that expected from the separate exposure to each of the agents (Pastorini *et al.* 1984). The lung cancer risk for insulation workers, for instance, who are heavily exposed to a variety of asbestos fibres, is five times the risk for unexposed persons, whatever their smoking habits, while the risk for smokers is 10 times that for non-smokers, whether they are exposed to asbestos or not. As a consequence, the lung cancer incidence among smokers exposed to asbestos is 50 times higher than that among unexposed non-smokers. From a practical, preventive point of view, this means that most of the excess risk can be abolished by eliminating or decreasing either exposure. A similar multiplicative interaction has been described for tobacco and ionizing radiation and for tobacco and arsenic compounds. Furthermore, poorly defined factors, such as urban air pollution or non-specific occupational exposures to dust, gases, or fumes may be potentially relevant to cancer aetiology, but whether they do increase the risk and to what extent is not known.

A fairly large number of studies have consistently shown that the incidence of lung cancer can be reduced by approximately

Table 1 Occupational risk factors for lung cancer

Arsenic compounds
Asbestos
Alkylating agents (mechlorethamine hydrochloride and bis-chloromethylether)
Chromium compounds
Mustard gas (sulphur mustard)
Nickel compounds
Ionizing radiation (γ-rays and radon)
Soots, tars, and some mineral oils

30 per cent when the proportion of foods rich in β-carotene in the diet is increased. It is not clear whether β-carotene is responsible for this protection or whether long-term dietary changes would be sufficient to yield any protection (Menkes *et al.* 1986; Pisani *et al.* 1986; Miller and Risch 1989).

HISTOPATHOLOGY

Cancer of the lung is caused by neoplastic transformation of the normal bronchial lining epithelium. Most of the cells in the lung are clearly of endodermal origin, but in the adult lung as in the fetal lung tissue, endocrine cells (Kulchitsky cells) of more uncertain origin can be demonstrated. The properties of these cells in terms of hormone production qualify them as members of the *amine precursor uptake and decarboxylation* (APUD) cell system as defined by Pearse (1969). Their origin has been thought to be ectodermal, for instance from the neural crest, but ultrastructural studies have cast doubt on this (Mackay *et al.* 1989).

It is most likely that bronchogenic carcinoma originates as a single malignant clone, but rapid cell proliferation and mutations result in the creation of heterogeneous tumours with many subpopulations (Gazdar and Linnoila 1988). This heterogeneity is reflected by the presence of a variety of histological patterns and types, indicating differentiation in more than one direction, even in the same patient.

The vast majority of bronchial tumours (over 95 per cent) are readily classified into four major cell types: squamous cell carcinoma (WHO I), adenocarcinoma (WHO III), large cell carcinoma (WHO IV), and small cell carcinoma (WHO II) (World Health Organization (**WHO**) 1981) Table 2. The remaining 5 per cent of malignant lung tumours include mesothelioma, carcinoids, and muco-epidermoid carcinoma. The same histological types are found in the trachea, with squamous cell carcinoma being the most dominant followed by adenoid cystic carcinoma (cylindroma). The latter tumour occurs in patients younger than the typical patient with squamous cell carcinoma and is equally common among men and women.

Among the various cell types, small cell carcinoma and possibly also carcinoids of the lung arise from the Kulchitsky cells and accordingly possess a number of endocrine features.

For practical therapeutic reasons, WHO I, III, and IV are commonly referred to as 'non-small' cell lung cancer in contrast to small cell lung cancer, which during the last decades has emerged as a separate entity among the other histological varieties of lung cancer, with specific biological and clinical characteristics. The relative frequency of each type varies considerably among different series and different countries and at different times. Table 3 gives the incidence from some countries and great variations are noted (Watkin 1989). The variations might not only be based on geographic differences, for example related to different aetiological factors, but it might also reflect variations in histopathological classification, including criteria used for classification. In many European countries and in North America there appears to have been an increase during the last decade in the frequency of adenocarcinoma, especially among women (Wu *et al.* 1985; McDuffie *et al.* 1987; Watkin 1989).

The diagnosis of lung cancer is usually based on histopathological biopsy material obtained at bronchoscopy, mediastinoscopy, lung biopsy, or the like. The larger the biopsy, the better the possibility of a correct diagnosis, including histopathological classification. In some cases it may be difficult to obtain material for histopathological evaluation and the diagnosis of lung cancer is then based on cytological evaluation. The cytological method is less precise for classification purposes, especially for poorly differentiated tumours. Overall, cytotyping accuracy compared with histological classification is above 75 per cent, exceeding 90 per cent for highly differentiated tumours (Liang 1989).

The most commonly used histopathological classification is the World Health Classification, first published in 1967 and revised in 1981 (Table 2) (WHO 1981). The classification is based on light-microscopic criteria using 'standard' staining procedures. The four major cell types are demonstrated in Figs 5–8. Results of electron microscopy and immunohistochemistry are not included as diagnostic criteria in the WHO classification, but they may in some cases clarify the diagnosis.

The histopathological classification constitutes a strong, independent prognostic factor, with the best prognosis obtained for squamous cell carcinoma. The impact of the subtyping remains uncertain, but studies have now shed further light on this issue. For instance, two studies have indicated that the response rate and the median survival for patients with small cell lung cancer combined with large cell is significantly lower than in patients with small cell carcinoma of the other subtypes (Radice *et al.* 1982; Hirsch *et al.*

Table 2   WHO classification of malignant lung tumours

Squamous cell carcinoma
  Variant
  1. Spindle cell carcinoma

Small cell carcinoma
  1. Oat cell carcinoma
  2. Intermediate-cell type
  3. Combined small cell carcinoma

Adenocarcinoma
  1. Acinar adenocarcinoma
  2. Papillary adenocarcinoma
  3. Bronchiolo-alveolar carcinoma
  4. Solid carcinoma with mucus formation

Large cell carcinoma
  1. Solid carcinoma without mucin
  2. Giant cell carcinoma
  3. Clear cell carcinoma

Carcinoids

Mesothelioma
  1. Epithelial
  2. Fibrous (spindle cell)
  3. Biphasic

Table 3   Incidence of major histological cell types of lung cancer in various countries

Population	Period	No. of cases	WHO grouping (%)			
			I	II	III	IV
Iceland	1931–64	136	17	34	23	17
Finland	1968–71	175	54	30	9	1
Singapore	1968–72	522	37	26	20	14
Switzerland	1974–76	223	56	19	13	12
Western Europe	1976–80	7804	51	18	12	9
Eastern USA	1974–81	8897	30	17	29	7
Hong Kong	1973–82	1055	37	22	22	16
Scotland	1981–84	2117	48	24	13	10

Modified from Watkin (1989).

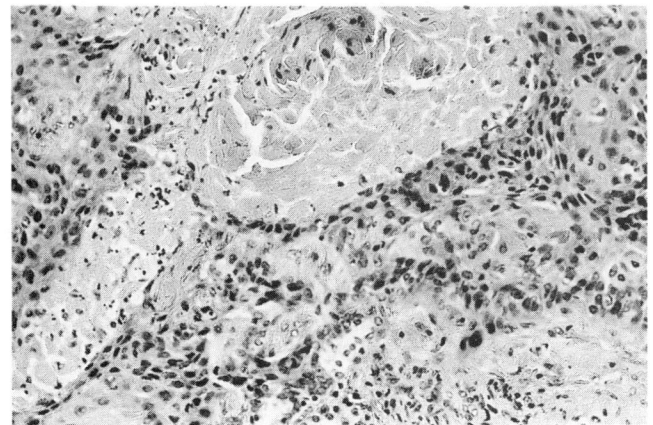

Fig. 5 Squamous cell carcinoma; WHO I.

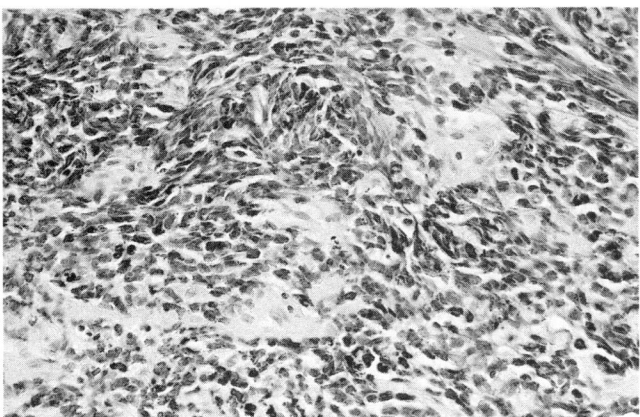

Fig. 6 Small cell carcinoma; WHO II.

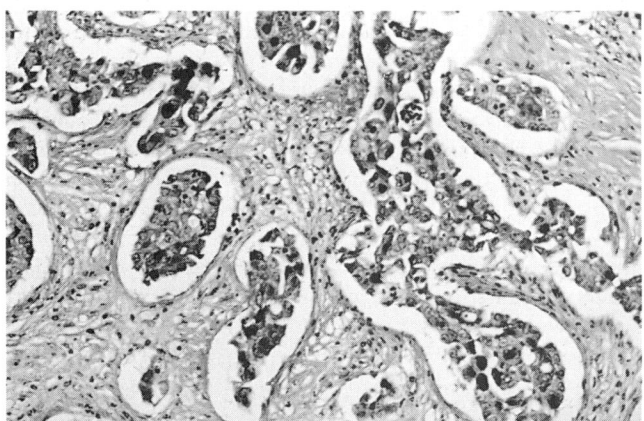

Fig. 7 Adenocarcinoma; WHO III.

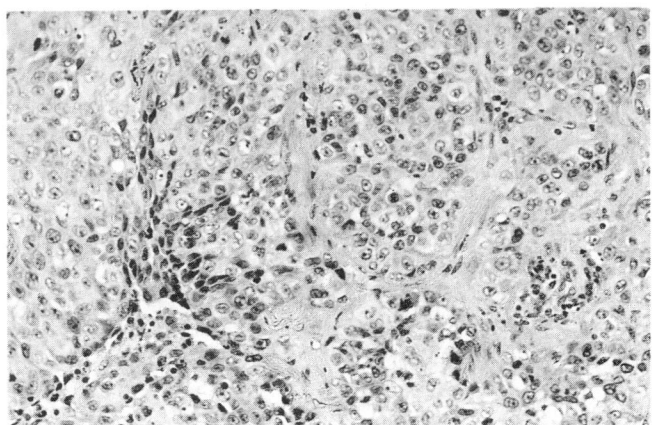

Fig. 8 Large cell carcinoma; WHO IV.

Table 4 Histopathological classification of small cell lung cancer

World Health Organization (1981)	International Association for the Study of Lung Cancer (Hirsch *et al.* (1988))
Oat cell carcinoma	Small cell
Intermediate cell type	Small cell with large cell elements
Combined oat cell carcinoma	Combined small cell+adenocarcinoma+ squamous carcinoma

1983). In accordance with these observations the pathology committee of the International Association for the Study of Lung Cancer (IASLC) has proposed a new classification of small cell carcinoma (Table 4) (Hirsch *et al.* 1988). A more recent study reviewing 550 patients with extensive small cell lung cancer has disputed these results (Aisner *et al.* 1990).

Among the adenocarcinomas, the bronchiolo-alveolar carcinoma appears to have a better prognosis than the other subtypes (Sørensen *et al.* 1988). For both squamous cell carcinoma and adenocarcinoma the outcome for the well-differentiated tumours is better than for the poorly differentiated.

BIOLOGY

Experimental models of lung cancer

Our present knowledge of the biology of lung cancer is to a large extent derived from studies made in model systems, that is, *in vitro* cell lines and tumours xenografted to athymic nude mice. Small cell lung cancer, with its high sensitivity to antineoplastic treatment and interesting neuroendocrine properties, has been studied much more intensively than non-small cell lung cancer.

Several publications have now described in detail methods for the establishment of cell lines of small cell lung cancer (Carney *et al.* 1985; Carney and Leij 1988). Using a chemically defined medium (HITES), with or without serum supplementation, cell lines have been reproducibly established from 75 per cent of all tumour-containing biopsy specimens. More than 100 cell lines, from a variety of organ sites, have been established and characterized; in general they retain the properties of small cell lung cancer (Gazdar 1989). This includes the morphology, the presence of cytoplasmic dense-core granules, and secretion of the enzymes L-dopa decarboxylase, neurone-specific enolase, the BB isozyme of creatine kinase, and secretion of peptide hormones. It has been suggested that the cell lines can be classified into two major categories, classic and variant. The classic cell lines, which account for approximately 70 per cent of all lines, grow as tightly packed, floating aggregates, have a relatively long doubling time (72 h), a low plating efficiency in agarose (1–5 per cent), are relatively radiosensitive, and have the above-mentioned properties of small cell carcinoma. The variant cell lines grow as looser aggregates, have a shorter doubling time (32 h), a higher plating efficiency (10–15 per cent), are relatively radioresistant, and lack L-dopa decarboxylase. Furthermore, the variant cell lines do not produce the hormone gastrin-releasing peptide, which is found in classic cell lines. Amplification of the c-*myc* oncogene is a characteristic of variant cell lines. Not all cell lines fall into these two categories. Some lines grow as monolayer cultures. Many of the lines reported are very slow growing and have extremely low plating efficiencies.

Although the non-small cell lung cancers account for approximately 70 per cent of all lung cancers, fewer cell lines have been established from these tumours. Adenocarcinomas can be grown in fully defined media. This is not the case for squamous cell carcinomas and the success rate is low. The cell lines generally exhibit adherent growth with plating efficiencies of 0.5–40 per cent. Expression of neuroendocrine properties such as L-dopa decarboxylase and neurone-specific enolase is low or absent. The cells are generally resistant to radiation and most chemotherapeutic agents.

The athymic nude mouse will accept xenografts of small and non-small cell cancers. It therefore offers a possibility for study of human tumours in an '*in vivo*' system. Great skill and patience are required to work with this model, as the mice are frail and may succumb to infections during experiments (Gazdar 1989). As in the *in vitro* system, the tumours generally retain their properties. The nude mouse model is an important link between studies of therapy *in vitro* and in patients, as it offers an opportunity to compare tumour reduction and toxicity.

Cytogenetics, oncogenes, and tumour-suppressor genes

The fundamental change(s) that transform a normal cell into a malignant cell is now recognized as genetic damage. With the discovery of oncogenes and tumour-suppressor genes a final common pathway to neoplastic growth seems to be in sight. It is currently believed that lung cancer cells, through the action of carcinogens, have accumulated a series of genetic changes that activate proto-oncogenes while inactivating a second class of genes, referred to as tumour-suppressor genes (Minna 1989; Slebos and Rodenhuis 1989). Changes in both types of genes appear necessary for malignant transformation. The dominantly acting proto-oncogenes, which are present in all normal cells, control metabolic pathways that involve peptide growth factors and their receptors, as well as post-receptor signalling mechanisms. The genetic damage can affect the function of the proto-oncogene so that it is expressed at wrong times or places or in deleterious quantities or it may change the function of the protein encoded by the oncogene. The damage may be chromosomal translocations, gene amplifications, or point mutations. In small cell lung cancer the cell cycle-related family of *myc* oncogenes has been studied most extensively. One study found one of the *myc* genes amplified and/or expressed in approximately 60 per cent of the cell lines; c-*myc* amplification was associated with the variant subtype of small cell cancer with more aggressive growth behaviour. In a retrospective review of all patients who had a cell line established during their clinical course, amplification of either c-*myc* or N-*myc* was associated with a significantly shorter survival than of patients whose specimens lacked these changes. L-*myc* was first discovered in small cell lung cancers, but like c-*myc* can be expressed in non-small cell cancers as well. A comparison in small cell cancer of fresh specimens from treated and untreated patients with cell lines showed abnormalities in *myc* family oncogenes more frequently in cell lines. In addition, fresh specimens obtained at relapse showed more abnormality than specimens obtained before treatment. These results suggest that the changes are not important early events, but may contribute to

the more aggressive behaviour of the tumours often observed at relapse. Other oncogenes activated in small cell lung cancer include c-*raf*1 and c-*jun* and in non-small cell cancer the *ras* oncogene family and *erb* B. Mutational activation of K-*ras* seems to be specific for adenocarcinomas from patients with a history of heavy smoking. The *erb* B oncogene, which encodes for epidermal growth-factor receptor, is often highly expressed in epidermoid carcinomas (Carney 1989).

Genetic changes in small cell lung cancer have been demonstrated by flow cytometry and karyotype analysis. Flow cytometric DNA analysis has shown aneuploidy in up to 85 per cent of all tumour specimens (Vindeløv *et al.* 1980; Salvati *et al.* 1989). The ploidy is not scattered at random but grouped into near-diploid, near-triploid, and near-tetraploid values. In 20 per cent of the patients, different subpopulations can be found. Considering the detection limit of the analysis, this is a conservative estimate and the true degree of heterogeneity is likely to be much higher. Karyotype analysis of small cell lung cancer has demonstrated numerical abnormalities involving chromosomes 1, 3, 9, 13, 14, and 15, in addition to chromosomal rearrangements and deletions, hetero-geneously staining regions, and double minutes suggestive of gene amplification (Birrer and Minna 1988). The presence of the latter abnormalities may in some instances be related to gene amplification and drug resistance; in other cases they appear to be associated with amplification and increased expression of specific oncogenes. A consistent cytogenetic abnormality, a deletion of part of the short arm of chromosome 3, 3p (14–23) was originally described as being specific for small cell lung cancer. More recent studies using restriction fragment length polymorphism probes have revealed this deletion in almost all small cell and most non-small cell specimens (Carney 1989). The data suggest that this deletion is an important early event in the pathogenesis of lung cancer. It is speculated that the deletion uncovers an inactivating mutation in the remaining copy of a recessive tumour-suppressor gene. A similar mechanism is known for Wilms' tumour and for retinoblastoma. Interestingly, an abnormality in both structure and expression of the human retinoblastoma gene located on chromosome 13 has been detected in small cell but not in non-small cell lung cancer (Carney 1989). Much work remains to clarify the relations between chromosomal abnormalities, expression of oncogenes, deletion of tumour-suppressor genes, and the malignant phenotype of lung cancer.

Heterogeneity

Morphological heterogeneity of lung cancer has been recognized by pathologists for decades and is now taken into account in the WHO subtyping of small cell lung cancer. The realization that genetic instability and heterogeneity are essential properties of most malignant tumours and that problems of successfully treating malignant tumours are essentially caused by this heterogeneity, is more recent. According to the theory of clonal evolution, as formulated by Nowell, malignant tumours are monoclonal in origin, that is, they arise from a single cell (Nowell 1976). This original tumour cell has two basic characteristics: it has a growth advantage over the normal cells and therefore overgrows these and it is genetically unstable, so that new variants are produced as the tumour population expands. One implication of this is that tumours may be heterogeneous and contain different, although related, subpopulations of cells. Because of the random nature of the evolution, a further implication is that each individual tumour is unique. There is also evidence of heterogeneity of small cell lung cancers in regard to chromosome constitution, DNA content, growth characteristics, antigenic properties, enzyme and peptide hormone production, and sensitivity to radiation and chemotherapy. The last-mentioned type of heterogeneity is of particular interest, as treatment failure in initially responsive tumours such as small cell lung cancers is readily explained by the selection and overgrowth of resistant subpopulations. The fact that chemotherapy may result in perhaps 99.9 per cent tumour reduction in sensitive subpopulations at each treatment cycle, while resistant subpopulations grow unaffected, indicates that rapid changes in tumour constitution can take place during treatment. The theory of Coldman and Goldie (1985) is of interest here. Their mathematical model describes the probability of resistant variant cells being present in a tumour cell population as a function of the mutation rate toward resistance and tumour burden. Not surprisingly, this probability increases with an increasing mutation rate. The interesting prediction of the theory is that the likelihood of there being at least one resistant tumour cell present will go from low to high over a very short interval of the tumour's growth. The finding that patients with limited disease have a better response to treatment and a better prognosis than those with extensive disease is in agreement with the theory. The predictions of the theory and the occasional very rapid progression of small cell lung cancers (see below) indicate that diagnostic and staging procedures should be done with as little delay as possible and efficacious systemic treatment started immediately after diagnosis. The importance of these theoretical considerations has been emphasized by the results of assessing new drugs by single-drug treatment of previously untreated patients with small cell carcinoma. Patients treated with inactive drugs did very poorly in spite of a policy of switching quickly to conventional combination therapy. Non-small cell lung cancer seems to be as heterogeneous as small cell but is less well described and of less clinical importance because of the primary resistance of this group of tumours to the currently available antineoplastic drugs.

Cell kinetics

Cell kinetic data from patients with lung cancer are limited to doubling times for the clinical range of growth, estimates of the S-phase size by labelling index or flow cytometric DNA analysis, and the study of a few patients with the percentage labelled-mitosis technique. Circumstantial evidence on the growth of small cell cancers has been derived from cell lines in culture and tumours grown as xenografts in nude mice. The emerging picture is characterized by great variability. Doubling times *in vitro* and in nude mice, which may give an indication of growth at the subclinical level of tumour sizes, range from 2 to 35 days. The mean doubling time in nude mice was 10 days in one study. Doubling times in patients range from 17 to 264 days, with a mean of 55 days. In comparison, the mean doubling times for large cell, squamous, and adenocarcinoma are 92, 100, and 183 days, respectively (Vindeløv *et al.* 1985). Small cell lung cancer is thus the most rapidly growing, as previously thought. This fact does not exclude the possibility that it is rapidly proliferating. High S phases, 14−43 per cent in one study with flow cytometric DNA analysis and a high spontaneous cell loss found in nude mice, support this notion. It is possible that the high responsiveness to chemotherapy of small cell cancer is partly based on rapid proliferation, which in general is correlated to drug sensitivity. DNA flow cytometric studies have now also revealed that patients with diploid tumours have a superior survival to those with aneuploid tumours (Cibas *et al.* 1989; Isobe *et al.* 1990; Sahin *et al.* 1990).

Enzymes and peptide hormones

Neoplastic cells may produce and release several substances that correspond with those of their normal counterparts. In some cases the substances have not been found in normal cells of that organ, leading to the term 'ectopic production'. In addition, substances similar but not identical to the genuine hormone may be released. When substances are characteristic of fetal development, they are referred to as oncofetal antigens. A great number of substances are consistently produced by small cell lung cancers and less often by non-small cell, but there is considerable overlap of properties, suggesting a common origin for all lung cancer. The substances are of interest as possible markers of tumour burden, for diagnostic purposes, for their role as autocrine or paracrine growth stimulators, and as the cause of endocrine syndromes.

Serum specimens from patients with small cell lung cancer show elevated concentrations of calcitonin, adrenocorticotropic hormone (**ACTH**), antidiuretic hormone, carcinoembryonic antigen, neurophysin, oxytocin, β-endorphin, neurone-specific enolase (the neuronal form of the glycolytic enzyme enolase), and the BB isoenzyme of creatine kinase in 25−75 per cent of cases (Hansen and Pedersen 1986). The amount of these markers is related to the stage of the disease in groups of patients and elevated pre-treatment concentrations decrease with tumour regression. However, the marker concentrations are not valid in defining the tumour load and the presence of disease in the individual patient and it has not yet been documented that the markers can be used for clinical decisions on antineoplastic therapy (Hansen and Hansen 1987).

A development is the finding that measurement of cerebro-spinal fluid and plasma concentrations of antidiuretic hormone, calcitonin, creatine kinase-BB, gastrin-releasing peptide, and neurone-specific enolase may contribute to the diagnosis of central nervous metastases, including meningeal carcinomatosis (Hansen and Pedersen 1986). Neurone-specific enolase has also been applied in the diagnosis of malignant pleural effusion in patients with small cell lung cancer (Shimokata *et al.* 1989).

Growth factors are defined as polypeptides that stimulate cell proliferation or differentiation by binding to high-affinity, cell membrane receptors. The phenomenon that a cell produces and secretes growth factors that interact with specific membrane receptors on the surface of the cell and thereby induces proliferation has been termed 'autocrine growth stimulation' (Mulshine *et al.* 1989). Four autocrine growth factors, gastrin-releasing peptide, insulin–like growth factor-I, transferrin, and epidermal growth factor, have been described in lung cancer. Gastrin-releasing peptide, which stimulates the normal bronchial epithelial cells, may function as an autocrine growth factor contributing to the transformed growth properties of small cell carcinoma. Antibodies to the peptide and peptide antagonists have been reported to block the growth of small cell carcinoma cell lines and to be cytotoxic against small cell cancers grown in nude mice. A clinical phase I−II trial to determine if a monoclonal antibody against gastrin-releasing peptide can inhibit proliferation of small cell lung carcinoma is ongoing (Mulshine *et al.* 1990). Transferrin stimulates the growth of small cell cancer and the growth of cell lines from that tumour can be inhibited to approximately 50 per cent by an antitransferrin receptor monoclonal antibody. Both small and non-small cell lines express insulin–like growth factor-I receptor. Monoclonals against that receptor have a weak growth-inhibitory effect. Epidermal growth-factor (**EGF**) receptor is frequently expressed by squamous cell carcinoma and a clinical trial using a radioconjugate of an anti-EGF receptor antibody is ongoing.

The endocrine syndromes are described elsewhere in this chapter.

Monoclonal antibodies

Monoclonal antibodies have potential application in diagnosis, staging and treatment of lung cancer (Souhami *et al.* 1988; Stahel 1989). The focus has been on monoclonals against cell-surface membrane antigens, generated against whole cells or membrane extracts of cell lines or tumour tissue. The antibodies have then been selected by phenotypic criteria based on differential binding between tumours of various lineages or between tumours and normal cells. The biological or functional significance of the antigens identified in this way remains largely unknown. Most of the antibodies have been found to identify antigens present on a wide range of epithelial tumours or normal epithelial cells. A smaller number of antibodies appear to identify antigens of a certain lineage relationship. This includes antigens that have preferential reactivity with non-small cell but not small cell lung cancers and antigens selectively expressed in adenocarcinoma but not in squamous cell carcinoma. An antigen that allows positive discrimination between mesothelioma and adenocarcinoma has been reported.

Most normal human tissues express the class 1 histocompatibility antigens, HLA-A, -B, and -C and β_2-microglobulin. In contrast, cell lines from small cell carcinoma either do not express these antigens or do so weakly. Thus, antibodies to these antigens can be used to distinguish between small cell and non-small cell tumours. A number of cells with neuroendocrine properties share an antigen recognized by monoclonal antibodies HNK-1 and NKH-1, which also recognize natural killer cells. These antigens are often expressed in small cell but not non-small cell lung cancers and may be used to distinguish between the two (Souhami *et al.* 1988).

On using the monoclonal SMI, cells of small cell lung cancer could be detected in 19 out of 30 bone-marrow specimens pathologically considered to be free of tumour. There is thus a potential use of monoclonal antibodies in staging this cancer (Stahel *et al.* 1985).

Several monoclonals that are cytotoxic to small cell lung cancer *in vitro* have been described. Attempts at purging tumour-contaminated bone-marrow *ex vivo* before autologous bone-marrow transplantation have been made with some success.

As mentioned above, monoclonal antibodies against autocrine growth factors are being investigated for therapeutic use.

In vitro phase II trials

Sensitivity testing of individual tumours before the start of chemotherapy would be ideal, if possible. Attempts at this using the clonogenic assay have not been successful for the following reasons: (a) biopsies of viable tumour tissue must be available; (b) only a fraction of the tumours will grow in primary culture; (c) the test takes 2–3 weeks. Even more serious are the theoretical limitations caused by tumour heterogeneity. Only the most dominant subpopulation will be tested and as chemotherapy in most cases must be started before the results of the test are ready, the composition of the tumour may already have changed significantly.

An approach that seems more promising is phase II testing *in vitro*, using a panel of established cell lines to screen new drugs for activity (Roed and Vindeløv 1989). It is assumed that new drugs with activity against small cell lung cancer and without cross-resistance to the best drugs used against it today could improve the treatment results. The aim is to select drugs that in combination would be able to eradicate the whole panel of cell lines. Preferentially, drugs with different types of toxicity should be combined to minimize the need for dose reduction. Some reports have shown that *in vitro* phase II testing of drugs for activity is possible. In addition to information on relative sensitivity, cross-resistance, and collateral sensitivity, the data contain information about cell-cycle specificity and consequently about the most rational way of drug administration. Clinical trials will eventually determine the value of this approach.

CLINICAL PRESENTATIONS AND SYMPTOMS

The majority of patients with lung cancer are symptomatic at the time of diagnosis (Table 5) (Hawson *et al.* 1990). Less than 10–15 per cent of lung cancers will be detected in the asymptomatic state, usually by chest radiographs taken for other purposes (routine pre-operative films, insurance examinations, etc.). Asymptomatic lung cancers are associated with a much higher rate of resectability and a much better 5 year survival rate than are symptomatic cancers.

Symptoms that may be related to the local effects of the cancer include cough, haemoptysis, dyspnoea, and chest pain. Development of a cough or change in the character of a pre-existing cough is the most common symptom. Haemoptysis may be secondary to ulceration of the primary tumour and is usually not severe. Occasionally, brisk haemoptysis is present, owing to erosion of a blood vessel. Massive haemoptysis may occur as a terminal event, related to erosion of a major vessel such as the aorta or pulmonary artery. Haemoptysis is less frequent among patients with small cell carcinoma than with other types because of its tendency to submucosal growth.

The causes of dyspnoea are varied and include pleural effusion, diaphragmatic paralysis due to phrenic nerve involvement, obstructive pneumonitis, and lymphangitic metastasis. Frequently, patients with lung cancer have co-existent chronic obstructive pulmonary disease that contributes to their dyspnoea.

Chest pain may be present as a consequence of invasion of the pleura or chest wall. Less frequently encountered symptoms related to the local effects of lung cancer include hoarseness, superior vena cava syndrome, stridor, dysphagia, and shoulder pain. Pronounced stridor suggests a localization of tumour in either the trachea or main bronchus. Hoarseness may be the initial symptom and is caused by vocal cord paralysis. The left recurrent laryngeal nerve

Table 5 Presenting signs and symptoms for 1024 patients with lung cancer

Tumour-related symptoms	Percentage of patients	
	NSCLC	SCLC
Cough	45	49
Dyspnoea	37	53
Haemoptysis	33	30
Chest pain	27	48
Anorexia	22	37
Fatigue	22	37
Weight loss (>10% body weight)	16	21
Wheeze	10	23
Bone pain	10	13
Hoarseness	7	21
Dysphagia	3	9
Asymptomatic	15	5

NSCLC, non-small cell lung cancer; SCLC, small cell lung cancer.
Modified from Hawson *et al.* (1990).

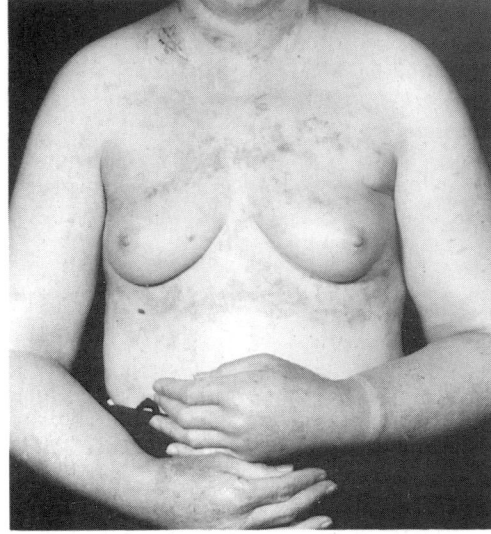

(a)

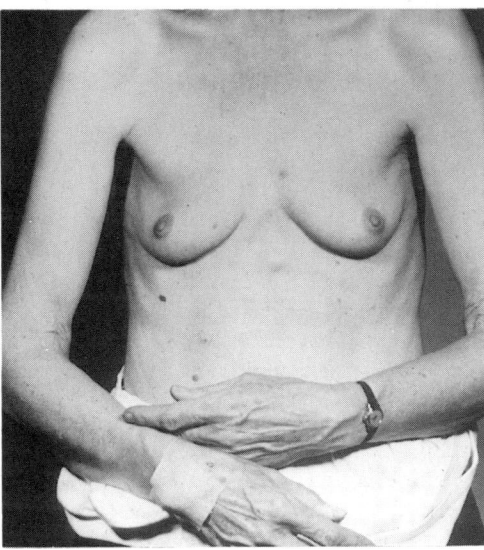

(b)

Fig. 9 Patient with superior vena cava syndrome. (a) Before and (b) after treatment.

passes through the mediastinum and loops around the aortic arch. It is susceptible to compression from mediastinal nodal metastasis or from direct invasion by the primary tumour.

The syndrome of obstruction of the superior vena cava consists of oedema of the face and upper extremities, along with dilated superficial veins in the neck, arms, and thorax (Fig. 9). It may be caused either by direct invasion of the superior vena cava or by compression from mediastinal metastases. Superior vena cava syndrome is most frequently observed in small cell lung cancer.

Stridor may be caused by narrowing of the trachea or a mainstem bronchus by intraluminal tumour or by extraluminal compression. Dysphagia is usually a late symptom, but it can be present initially. It is secondary to compression of the oesophagus by mediastinal lymphadenopathy or to direct invasion of the oesophagus by the primary lung cancer. The so-called Pancoast syndrome (or superior sulcus syndrome) is related to cancer in the apex of the lung that may also be associated with involvement of

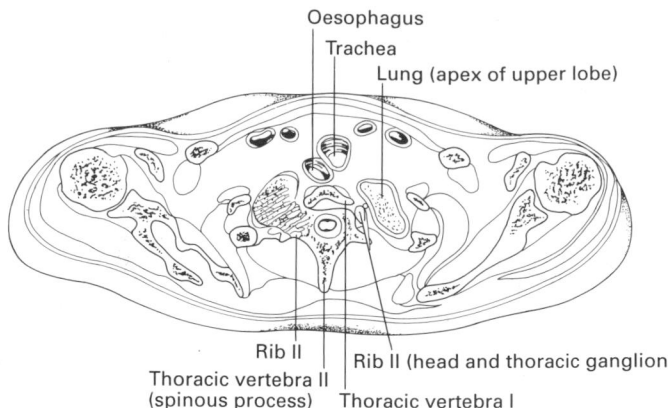

Fig. 10 Illustration of a superior sulcus tumour (Pancoast syndrome).

the first and second ribs, vertebral column, spinal cord, and brachial plexus (Fig. 10). The tumour is frequently overlooked during its early stages. Patients may complain of pain in the shoulder, scapula, or interscapular area. There may also be pain in the arm, neck, and axilla. Horner's syndrome (ptosis, miosis, enophthalmus) may be present in patients with a Pancoast tumour and is due to involvement of the cervical sympathetic nerves. Pancoast tumours are often associated with the squamous and adenocarcinomatous cell types.

Lung cancer frequently presents with evidence of extrathoracic metastases. Lymph node enlargement in the supraclavicular and cervical regions may be the initial finding. Pain due to bony metastasis is another common presenting symptom. The bones most frequently involved are the spine, pelvis, femur, ribs, and skull, although any bone may be affected. Hepatomegaly is a relatively uncommon presenting complaint, but when it is a presenting symptom the patient usually has small cell lung cancer.

Evidence of metastases to the central nervous system is the initial manifestation in 10–15 per cent of lung cancer. Cerebral and cerebellar metastases are frequently observed in small cell lung cancer. Symptoms may include headache, personality changes, seizures, mono- or hemiparesis, ataxia due to cerebellar metastasis or, occasionally, cranial nerve paralysis due to metastasis to the brainstem or base of the skull.

The systemic effects of lung cancer include non-specific constitutional symptoms of anorexia, weakness, and weight loss. Weight loss is a poor prognostic sign and often associated with distant metastases.

Paraneoplastic syndromes are more specific entities. They are caused by remote, non-metastatic effects of the tumour and may be present in 10–20 per cent of all cases of lung cancer. The more well-established paraneoplastic syndromes are listed in Table 6, correlated if possible to histological cell type.

Haematological abnormalities are generally not dramatic. The anaemia of chronic disease and thrombocytosis are the most common. Thrombocytopenia usually heralds the presence of bone-marrow metastasis, most frequently observed in small cell lung carcinoma.

Cardiovascular syndromes include arterial thrombosis, non-bacterial thrombotic (marantic) endocarditis and recurrent venous migratory thrombophlebitis (Trousseau's syndrome).

Cutaneous manifestations include acanthosis nigricans and dermatomyositis, while musculoskeletal syndromes may include digital clubbing, hypertrophic pulmonary osteoarthropathy, and polymyositis. Hypertrophic pulmonary osteoarthropathy is due to periostitis with periosteal new-bone formation. It usually involves the distal ends of the tibia and fibula or radius and ulna. Patients

Table 6 Paraneoplastic syndromes associated with bronchogenic carcinoma

Haematological
   Haemolytic anaemia
   Red cell aplasia
   Polycythaemia
   Thrombocytosis[a]
   Eosinophilia
   Leucoerythroblastic reaction[b] including thrombocytopenia

Endocrine
   Cushing's syndrome[a]
   Inappropriate ADH secretion[b]
   Hypercalcaemia[c,d]
   Carcinoid syndrome[b]
   Gynaecomastia[a]
   Hyperglycaemia
   Hypoglycaemia
   Galactorrhea
   Growth hormone excess[a]
   Secretion of thyroid-stimulating hormone[b]
   Calcitonin secretion[c]

Others
   Nephrotic syndrome[b]
   Hyperuricaemia
   Amyloidosis

Neuromuscular
   Polymyositis[b]
   Myasthenic syndrome[b]
   Sensory–motor neuropathy
   Encephalopathy[b]
   Myelopathy
   Psychosis
   Dementia

Musculoskeletal and cutaneous
   Hypertrophic osteoarthropathy[d]
   Clubbing[d]
   Dermatomyositis[b]
   Acanthosis nigricans
   Pruritus
   Urticaria
   Erythema multiforme
   Hyperpigmentation

Cardiovascular
   Superficial thrombophlebitis
   Arterial thrombosis
   Marantic endocarditis

[a]Most frequently observed with large cell carcinoma.
[b]Most frequently observed with small cell carcinoma.
[c]Most frequently observed with squamous cell carcinoma.
[d]Most frequently observed with adenocarcinoma.

complain of pain and tenderness over the affected areas and will frequently believe that they have arthritis. Radiographs demonstrate periosteal new-bone formation (Fig. 11). The osteoarthropathy is usually accompanied by digital clubbing, but clubbing in lung cancer may occur in its absence. Polymyositis may present as slowly progressive weakness in the proximal muscles or as muscular pain.

Neurological paraneoplastic syndromes are quite varied. The myasthenic syndrome of Eaton and Lambert is now a well-recognized entity, but it can be confused with myasthenia gravis. Electromyography differentiates between the two entities. The myasthenic syndrome is usually associated with the small cell type of lung cancer. In some cases the syndrome will improve significantly or even resolve after treatment of the cancer. Peripheral sensorimotor

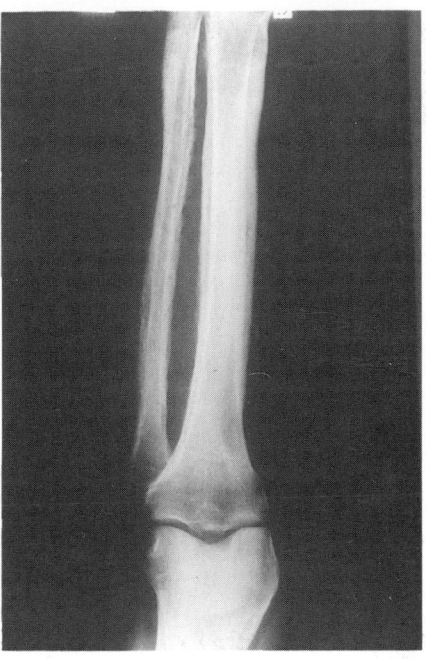

Fig. 11 Digital clubbing and periosteal new bone formation.

neuropathies may be evident 2–3 years before the initial diagnosis of cancer. Ataxia due to cerebellar degeneration or decreased cognitive function due to cerebral atrophy may be presenting symptoms.

Endocrine syndromes are demonstrable in 5–10 per cent of patients with lung cancer at the time of initial diagnosis (Hansen and Pedersen 1986). These syndromes are also most commonly associated with small cell cancer. So-called 'ectopic' production of ACTH may produce Cushing's syndrome. Because small cell cancers tend to grow very rapidly, patients may not have enough time to develop the typical Cushingoid appearance, but may present with hypertension, fluid retention, and hyperglycaemia.

Occasionally, patients with lung cancer present with mental confusion and in such instances one must consider the possibility of metastasis to the central nervous system as well as electrolyte imbalance. Hyponatraemia and hypercalcaemia are other well-recognized endocrine manifestations of lung cancer. The syndrome of inappropriate antidiuretic hormone secretion (inappropriate antidiuresis) results in hyponatraemia and is most strongly associated with small cell lung cancer.

The manifestations of hypercalcaemia include anorexia, constipation, polyuria, and stupor. Hypercalcaemia may be caused by bony metastases or by ectopic secretion of a parathyroid-like hormone, an osteolytic substance, or prostaglandin. Unlike the other syndrome of ectopic hormone secretion, the secretion of parathyroid-like hormone is usually associated with the squamous and adenomatous histological types of lung cancer (Bender and Hansen 1974).

Less frequently encountered entities associated with ectopic hormone secretion are the carcinoid syndrome, gynaecomastia, and hypoglycaemia.

DIAGNOSTIC EVALUATION
Primary tumour and locoregional spread

A careful history and physical examination are important when evaluating a patient suspected of having lung cancer. Visual examination may disclose evidence of superior vena caval obstruction, Cushing's syndrome, or cutaneous signs of malignancy.

Palpation may lead to discovery of lymphadenopathy, subcutaneous nodules or masses, or organomegaly related to metastases. While examination of the thorax is frequently normal, the absence of breath sounds or the presence of a localized wheeze may be manifestations of an obstructing endobronchial tumour. Absent breath sounds and dullness to percussion of the lower hemithorax may indicate the presence of pleural effusion.

A chest radiograph and a sputum cytological test are often the next procedures to follow clinical examination. To be detectable by chest radiograph, most tumours need to be at least 1 cm in greatest diameter. The chest radiograph is best at detecting peripherally located cancers, while sputum cytological examination is best for centrally located cancers, especially squamous cancers involving major airways.

The diagnostic accuracy of cytology is heavily dependent on the expertise of the cytopathologist. Generally, sputum is positive in less than 20 per cent of patients with peripheral lung cancers, that is, those cancers that are more than 2–3 cm from the hilum on chest radiograph and are not visible endoscopically. Centrally located cancers may yield a positive sputum in over 50 per cent of cases, but the yield is directly related to cell type. Squamous cell carcinoma is the most likely cell type to yield a positive finding cytologically. Occasionally, small cell carcinomas and adenocarcinomas will be positive.

In most patients, the initial abnormal test is the chest radiograph. The location of the abnormality suggests the histological cell type. Centrally located or hilar lesions are more likely to be small cell or squamous cell carcinomas (Fig. 12). In contrast, large cell carcinomas and adenocarcinomas are likely to be present as peripheral lesions (Fig. 13). The chest radiograph may also suggest the anatomical extent of the cancer. Mediastinal metastases, chest wall involvement, rib metastasis, pleural effusion, tracheal compression, and atelectasis are frequently detectable by standard chest radiographs. Lateral chest radiographs may reveal small central tumours hidden in the mediastinum on the anteroposterior view, while lateral decubitus views of the chest may detect free pleural effusion not obvious on standard views.

Chest tomography may be useful, especially in the evaluation of the solitary pulmonary nodule. Tomography will help localize the lesion as well as determine the presence of calcification, cavitation, or an air bronchogram.

Computerized tomography (**CT**) of the thorax has greatly aided the physician's clinical evaluation of patients with suspected lung cancer (Grant *et al.* 1988; Glazer 1989). CT scanning improves localization of tumours and is better than standard chest radiographs for detecting multiple intrapulmonary lesions and mediastinal lymphadenopathy. While the criteria for mediastinal lymph node involvement may vary depending on the resolution of the CT scanner employed and the size of lymph node considered abnormal, that is more than 1, 1.5, or 2 cm, there is no disagreement about the value of CT in determining diagnostic and therapeutic approaches. Moreover, the ability of CT to define more accurately multiple nodules and chest wall or mediastinal invasion aids greatly in patient evaluation. Extension of the chest CT examination to include the liver and adrenal glands has become standard in many medical centres. This enhances detection of occult metastases, thus eliminating non-curative thoracotomies.

Bronchoscopy with the flexible fibre-optic scope is the primary means of diagnosis of most cases of tracheal/bronchogenic carcinoma. The flexible scope has greatly expanded the visualized endobronchial distance to include third- and fourth-order bronchi and, thus, has expanded the number of patients with lung cancer

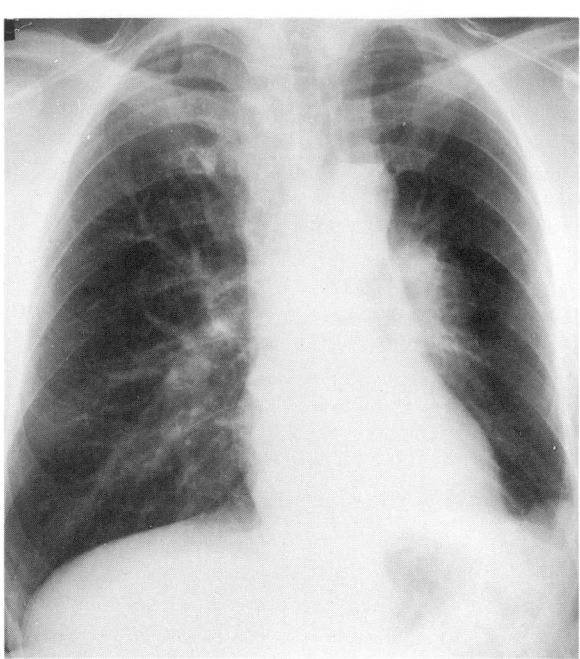

Fig. 12 Radiograph of typical small cell carcinoma.

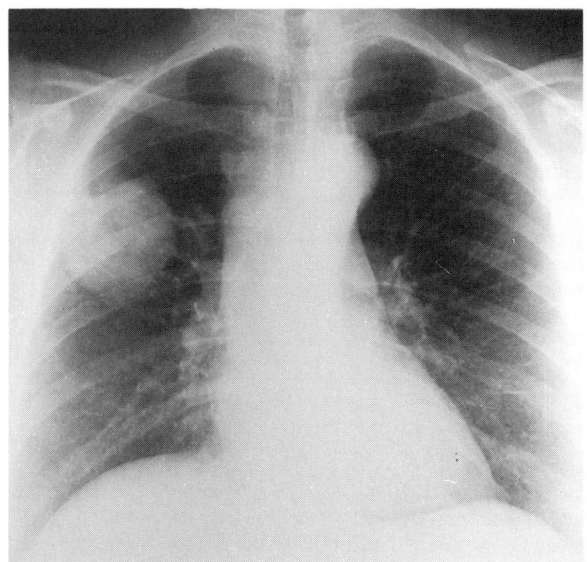

Fig. 13 Radiograph of typical bronchogenic adenocarcinoma.

in whom the diagnosis can more easily be obtained. If bronchogenic carcinomas are endoscopically visualized, then the rate of positive diagnosis from bronchial brushings and biopsy is generally 70–90 per cent. If lung lesions are not visible endoscopically, then the rate of successful diagnosis with brushing and biopsies under fluoroscopic guidance is dependent on the diameter of the lesion. In most series, lesions less than 2 cm have a less than 25 per cent diagnostic rate. If the lesion is 2 cm or greater, then a positive histological or cytological diagnosis can be obtained in 50–70 per cent of these patients. Specialized needles have now been developed to obtain transbronchial cytological samples through the fibre-optic bronchoscope from intrapulmonary lesions as well as from mediastinal lymph nodes (Brynitz *et al.* 1985; Blainey *et al.* 1988). The demonstration of malignant cells in transcarinal or transtracheal aspirate confirms mediastinal metastasis.

In patients who have undergone a non-diagnostic bronchoscopy, consideration can be given to transthoracic needle aspiration for obtaining a cytologic diagnosis. This method is not indicated for all patients with negative bronchoscopic findings, but may be appropriate in some cases (Poe and Tobin 1980; Veake *et al.* 1988). In patients with a lung lesion less than 2 cm in diameter, transthoracic needle aspiration should be the diagnostic procedure of choice if a tissue diagnosis is indicated. The yield of tissue diagnosis in lesions of 1–2 cm is approximately 60–80 per cent and greatly exceeds the diagnostic rate with flexible bronchoscopy. The principal limiting factor of transthoracic aspiration is the visibility of the lesion under fluoroscopy, although lesions that are not visible with fluoroscopy may be accessible with CT guidance. Complications are rare in skilful operative hands, but may include pneumothorax.

Pleural effusion frequently accompanies bronchogenic carcinoma and is usually secondary to pleural metastases or due to lymphatic obstruction from mediastinal metastases. In evaluation of patients with pleural effusion, thoracocentesis is the procedure of choice. In large series of patients with malignant pleural effusion proven by subsequent testing and follow-up, the pleural fluid cytology is positive in 55–60 per cent of cases. If the initial pleural fluid cytology is negative, a repeat is indicated. The rate of positivity is still approximately 50 per cent with repeat thoracocentesis. Pleural biopsy can add to the diagnostic yield when evaluating possibly malignant effusions. In several series the pleural biopsy has been positive for malignancy in 40–50 per cent of cases. When the biopsy is combined with cytological evaluation, the diagnostic yield has been reported to be between 60 and 90 per cent of all cases with malignant effusions. Pleuroscopy or thoracoscopy is a technique used increasingly and is a means of directly visualizing the pleural space. This technique of direct visualization and biopsy has yielded superior results to those of blind or random pleural biopsy.

Distant metastases

Systemic manifestations of lung cancer are present in more than 50 per cent of cases at the outset; the clinical course of lung cancer after apparent curative resection shows that such a figure is an underestimate of the actual degree of dissemination.

The application of the various diagnostic procedures differs according to the patient's clinical presentation, the histological type of lung cancer, the yield of the procedure relative to its morbidity, and, finally, but often most important, to the availability of the various techniques, the skills of the investigator, and the therapeutic implications attached to the results of staging.

The scheme of diagnostic procedures should not be too rigid, but the diagnostic work-up for the different types of lung cancer can be generalized to a certain extent depending on preferred site of metastases according to histological type. Preferred sites of distant metastases in relation to histological type before treatment and at autopsy are depicted in Tables 7 and 8, respectively (Hansen 1982). The limitations of the diagnostic procedures are strikingly shown in the investigation by Matthews *et al.* (1973), who carried out a careful autopsy investigation of patients dying within 1 month of curative resection. Sixty-three per cent of patients with small cell carcinoma were shown to have distant metastases. The corresponding numbers for squamous, adeno- and large cell carcinoma were 17, 40, and 14 per cent. As these patients represent a special group selected for resection, it is certainly indicative of a high degree of dissemination in lung cancer, especially in small cell lung cancer at presentation.

Table 7 Preferred sites of distant metastases at autopsy in relation to histological features (percentages)

Cell type	Liver[a]	Adrenal[a]	Bone[a]	Brain[b]	Other
Squamous cell	30.5	27.4	24.4	13.7	
Small cell	61.9	39.2	37.5	30.5	56.6 (abdominal lymph nodes)
Adenocarcinoma	44.8	42.9	39.9	25.4	
Large cell	39.6	36.4	28.9	29.4	36.0 (abdominal lymph nodes)

[a]Data accumulated from the literature.
[b]Data from 247 consecutive patients of the NCI-VA Medical Oncology Service, Washington, DC, including all clinical and autopsy incidence.

Table 8 Site of distant metastases in relation to histological features before treatment

Cell type	No. with distant metastases	Percentage with metastases to:					
		Liver	Bone[a]	Brain	Thorax[b]	Lymph nodes[c]	Skin
Squamous cell	25	8.0	16	20	36	24	8.0
Small cell	25	40.0	72	8	20	8	8.0
Adenocarcinoma	24	12.5	46	21	29	20	12.5
Large cell	31	6.0	26	13	38	35	13.0
Total	105[d]	16	40	15	30	22	10

[a]Excludes direct extension.
[b]Refers to contralateral lung and mediastinum and pericardium.
[c]Refers to non-regional peripheral lymph nodes.
[d]Data from 105 consecutive patients of the NCI-VA Medical Oncology Service, Washington, DC.

As shown in Table 7, liver, bone, and brain metastases are the most frequent signs of dissemination. The measures to identify these metastases will be evaluated below.

Detection of liver metastases

Evaluation of biochemical variables, such as transaminases, bilirubin, alkaline phosphatase, and coagulation factors, is routinely used in the follow-up of patients with lung cancer in order to detect liver metastases. The specificity of these measurements is, however, very low, in that, for example cirrhosis or fatty degeneration of the liver and several other diseases, can give positive tests. Furthermore, the number of false-negative results is also rather high. In the presence of verified liver metastases in small cell carcinoma, it was found that alkaline phosphatase was increased in 70 per cent and transaminase in 56 per cent of patients. The more non-specific lactate dehydrogenase was elevated in 79 per cent of the cases (Hansen 1982).

Other non-invasive diagnostic procedures include imaging techniques such as radionuclide scanning, CT scan, and ultrasonography (Hansen *et al.* 1987; Jensen *et al.* 1992). The latter two are superior to radionuclide imaging and the last is rarely done any more. For detection of liver metastases, ultrasonography with biopsy was shown to be superior to CT scan in a comparative study of patients with small cell carcinoma (Hansen *et al.* 1987). On the other hand, CT scanning reveals more frequently abnormalities located in the adrenals, pancreatic region, and retroperitoneal lymph nodes than does ultrasonography (Jensen *et al.* 1992).

Detection of bone and bone-marrow metastases

The skeletal system consists, in principle, of two organs, namely the bone-marrow and the osseous tissue. These two organs are obviously intimately connected, but in terms of seeding of metastases there seem to be distinct differences between them. Clinically, metastases to the osseous tissue are characterized by pain, while metastases to the bone-marrow primarily affect the haemopoietic tissue, which clinically may lead to thrombopenia or anaemia, but seldom pain. Of the lung cancer types, small cell carcinoma has a higher propensity for bone-marrow involvement than the others, especially squamous cell carcinoma. This type, on the other hand, when disseminated, fairly often involves the osseous tissue.

Evaluation of bone-marrow is therefore usually a part of the diagnostic work-up for patients with small cell carcinoma, in which group the number of positive biopsies is usually from 15–25 per cent depending on patient selection. The number of positive tests increases by approximately 10 per cent when using bilateral aspiration and biopsy from the iliac crest as compared to ipsilateral aspiration.

The osseous part of the bones can be evaluated by scans and radiographs. Radiography is far too insensitive to be used for screening or surveying. It is, however, desirable in cases of bony symptoms (pain) or in order to confirm tumour involvement in areas positive on bone scans. In a differential diagnosis between benign and malignant causes of abnormalities in bone scans, radiography is obviously needed. Usually metastases to the bones from primary lung cancer are manifested by the presence of osteolytic lesions. In small cell carcinoma, osteoblastic changes can be observed quite frequently in patients with documented bone-marrow metastases responding to treatment.

Routine use of bone scintigrams in asymptomatic patients adds little information to the diagnostic work-up in patients with lung cancer.

Detection of central nervous metastases

Among the lung cancers, small cell cancer most frequently has brain metastases, including an especially high incidence of metastases in the cerebellar and pituitary region. Central nervous system metastases also occur in significant numbers in the other types. In order to detect such metastases the following techniques are at hand: a thorough clinical neurological examination, lumbar puncture with investigation of the cerebrospinal fluid, CT scan, myelography, and, recently, also magnetic resonance imaging. Isotope brain scanning has gradually been replaced by CT scan; by using contrast medium in the vascular system during the CT scan of the brain, a high sensitivity and specificity can be obtained.

Leptomeningeal involvement can be confirmed by investigation of the crebrospinal fluid. This should include cytological evaluation for tumour cells and protein content.

As mentioned earlier, staging procedures may vary from institution to institution and no standard recommendations have been made, with the exception of small cell carcinoma, for which Table 9 gives the recommendations as outlined at an international workshop (Stahel *et al.* 1989).

PROGNOSTIC FACTORS AND STAGING

Prognostic factors

Multivariate analysis of large populations of patients shows that performance status; stage of disease according to WHO classification, and histological cell types are the most important influences to be taken into account. Women tend to do better than men and the under 60s better than the over 60s. Pre-treatment weight loss of more than 3 kg indicates a substantially worse prognosis. Routine biochemical values such as serum lactate dehydrogenase, albumin, or alkaline phosphatase enable identification of prognostic subgroups.

Table 9 Staging procedures in small cell carcinoma

Procedure	Clinical practice Local treatment modality under consideration		Clinical trial
	No	Yes	
General procedures			
Patient history	+	+	+
Physical examination	+	+	+
Blood counts	+	+	+
Serum biochemistry	+	+	+
Cytological or histological documentation of small cell lung cancer	+	+	+
Procedures for local disease			
Chest radiograph	+	+	+
Chest CT scan	−	−	+[a]
Fibre-optic bronchoscopy	−	−	+[b]
Mediastinoscopy	−	−	+[c]
Cytology of effusion	−	−	+
Cytology of supraclavicular node	−	−	+[d]
Procedures for distant disease			
Bone			
Scan	−	+[e]	+
Radiographs	−	+[f]	+[f]
Liver and retroperitoneal organs			
Ultrasound or abdominal CT	−	+[e]	+
Fine-needle aspiration/biopsy	−	+[e]	+[d]
Bone-marrow: aspirate and biopsy	−	+[e]	+
Brain: CT	−	+[e]	+

[a]Especially for trials of limited disease.
[b]If use of bronchoscopy is anticipated at restaging, surgery for limited disease is considered or diagnosis cannot be obtained otherwise.
[c]Only if needed by surgeon for pre-operative work-up.
[d]If the findings are doubtful and the establishment of a positive finding affects the treatment.
[e]If one of tests is positive further evaluation can be discontinued.
[f]Only in areas of increased uptake on bone scan.

The application of modern molecular biological methods such as for K-*ras* oncogene (Rodenhuis *et al.* 1987) and H/Le^y/Le^b antigen (Miayke *et al.* 1992) has also now been shown to be of prognostic value in patients with non-small cell lung cancer.

All the above-mentioned features may prove helpful for stratification of patients in large trials, although they cannot replace a detailed anatomical staging as the main influence on the choice of treatment. The clinician will find them helpful for decision making in the individual patient, for example when deciding between toxic therapy, which is indicated for patients in whom long-term tumour control is a realistic goal and less toxic, palliative therapy for elderly patients with advanced disease.

TNM staging

Various staging systems have been designed, mainly to assess the suitability and results of surgery. The TNM system is the most commonly used: it describes by T subsets the localization and the size of the primary tumour (T), including possible local invasion, while N is used to describe the degree of nodal involvement and M to inform about the presence of distant metastases (Table 10).

Information about the anatomy of the primary site, local lymph node involvement, and metastatic sites is important for optimal staging and for lung cancer these factors vary considerably from one histological type to another.

Table 10 TNM clinical classification

N: regional lymph nodes
NX   Regional lymph nodes cannot be assessed
N0   No regional lymph node metastasis
N1   Metastasis in ipsilateral peribronchial and/or ipsilateral hilar lymph nodes, including direct extension
N2   Metastasis in ipsilateral mediastinal and/or subcarinal lymph node(s)
N3   Metastasis in contralateral mediastinal, contralateral hilar, ipsilateral or contralateral scalene or supraclavicular lymph node(s)

M: distant metastasis
MX   Presence of distant metastasis cannot be assessed
M0   No distant metastasis
M1   Distant metastasis
The category M may be further specified according to the following notation

Pulmonary	PUL	Bone-marrow	MAR
Osseous	OSS	Pleura	PLE
Hepatic	HEP	Peritoneum	PER
Brain	BRA	Skin	SKI
Lymph nodes	LYM	Other	OTH

Staging can be subdivided into five categories:

(1)   clinical diagnostic staging (cTNM);

(2)   surgical evaluation (sTNM);

(3)   surgical resection: pathological staging (pTNM);

(4)   retreatment staging (rTNM);

(5)   autopsy staging (aTNM).

The rules for the above classification have been worked out jointly by the Union Internationale Contre le Cancer and the American Joint Committee for Cancer Staging and End Results Reporting (American Joint Committee 1979; Mountain 1986; Miayke *et al.* 1992).

Clinical staging (cTNM) permits the incorporation of information from all investigations before treatment. If treatment entails thoracotomy, then further staging information is obtainable to permit a surgical/evaluation classification (sTNM). If resection is undertaken, then a detailed histological assessment is available and post-surgical pathological staging (pTNM) is possible, taking into account additional histopathological information. If further treatment becomes necessary a re-evaluation staging (rTNM) may include additional investigations. Should death occur and autopsy be performed, a final staging (aTNM) may be done. The staging categories should not be altered in the light of subsequent information.

Table 11 Stage grouping of lung tumours

	Stage grouping		
Occult carcinoma	TX	N0	M0
Stage 0	Tis	N0	M0
Stage I	T1	N0	M0
	T2	N0	M0
Stage II	T1	N1	M0
	T2	N1	M0
Stage IIIA	T1	N2	M0
	T2	N2	M0
	T3	N0, N1, N2	M0
Stage IIIB	AnyT	N3	M0
	T4	Any N	M0
Stage IV	Any T	Any N	M1

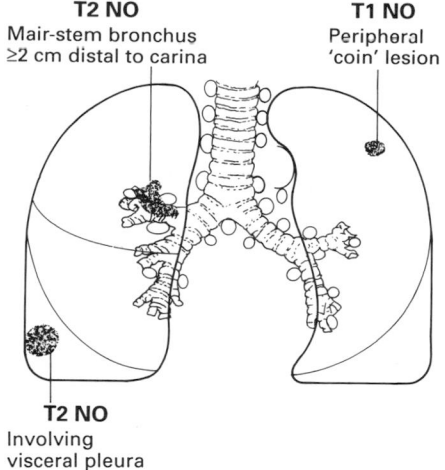

Fig. 14 Examples of TNM stage grouping: stage I and II (modified from Mountain 1986).

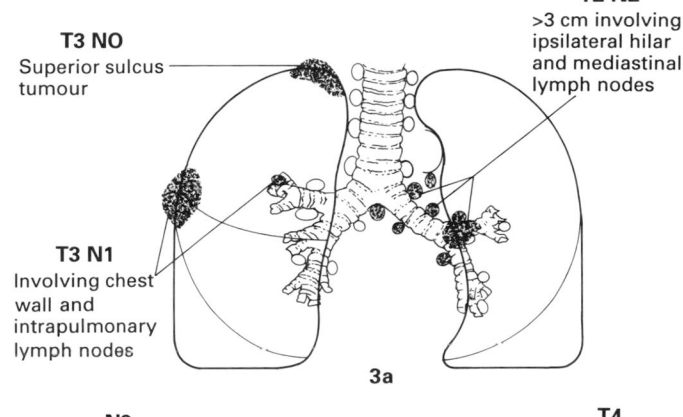

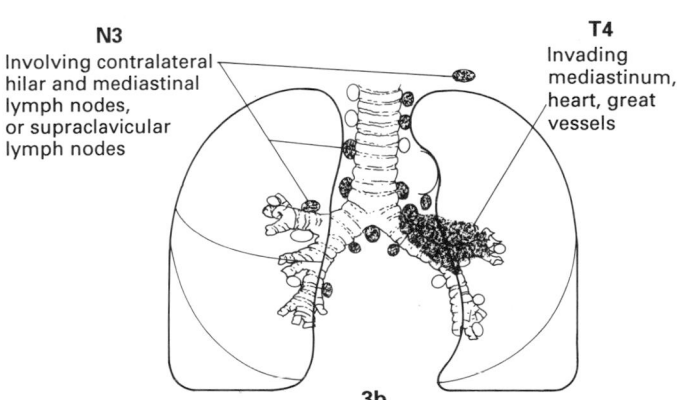

Fig. 15 Example of TNM stage grouping: stage IIIa and IIIb.

With the TNM classification as background it is possible to stage patients with lung cancer into various groups (Table 11) which include (a) occult-stage carcinoma; (b) stage 0; (c) stage I; (d) stage II; (e) stage III a and b; (f) stage IV. Further subdivision can take place in some of the groups.

The definitions of the stages are as follows (Table 11), (Figs 14 and 15).

Occult stage: TX, N0, M0. An occult carcinoma with broncho-pulmonary secretions containing malignant cells but without other evidence of tumour, metastasis to the regional lymph nodes, or distant metastasis.

Stage 0: Tis, N0, M0. Carcinoma *in situ*.

Stage I: T1, N0, M0, T2, N0, M0. A tumour that can be classified T1 without any metastases or a tumour that can be classified T2 without any metastases to nodes or distant organs (Note: TX, N1, M0 is also theoretically possible, but such a clinical diagnosis would be difficult if not impossible to make. If such a diagnosis is made, it would be included in stage I.)

Stage II: T1, N1, M0 and T2, N1, M0. A tumour classified as either T1 or T2 with metastases to the lymph nodes in the peribronchial or ipsilateral hilar region only.

Stage IIIa: T1, N2, M0; T2, N2, M0; T3, N0, N1, N2, M0 with any N or M; N2 with any T or M; M1 with any T or N. Any tumour with ipsilateral mediastinal lymph nodes only or T3 tumour without contralateral mediastinal, scalene, supraclavicular or distant metastases.

Stage IIIb: Any T, N3 M0, T4, any N1 M0. Any tumour with contralateral, mediastinal scalene or supraclavicular lymph nodes or any T4 tumour without spread beyond the thorax.

Stage IV: Any tumour with distant metastases.

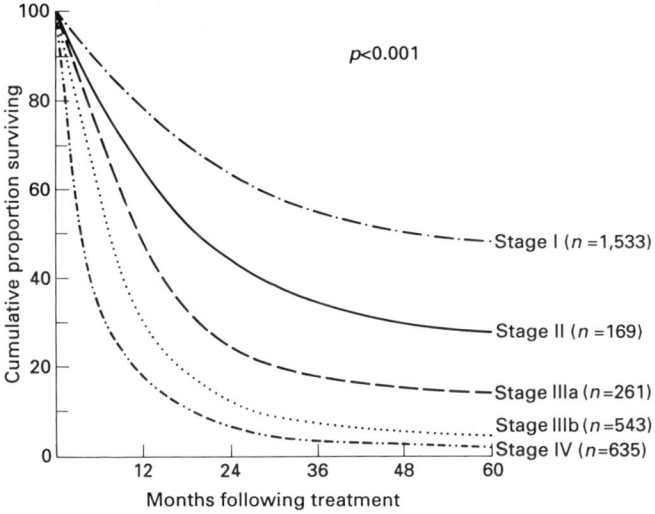

Fig. 16 Survival of 'non-small cell' lung cancer according to clinical diagnostic stage.

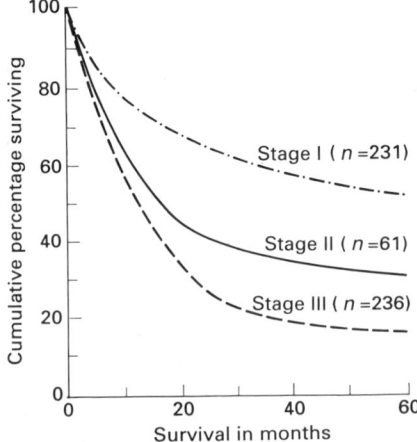

Fig. 17 Survival of patients with squamous cell carcinoma of lung by clinical diagnostic stage.

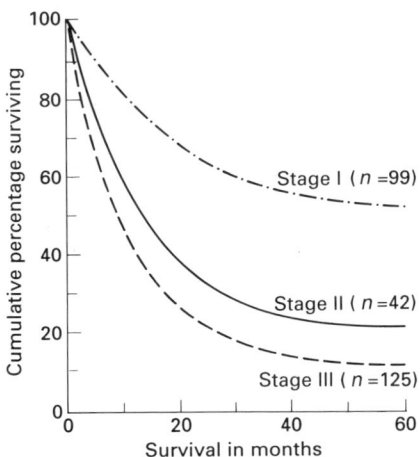

Fig. 18 Survival of patients with adenocarcinoma and undifferentiated large cell carcinoma of lung by clinical diagnostic stage.

Stage grouping is significant for all cell types listed under histopathology above except undifferentiated small cell carcinoma, in which there is a poor correlation between TNM stage and survival rates. The anatomical extent of small cell cancers may, however, be recorded by the TNM system for future reference.

The correlation between the stage and survival is quite evident when one analyses the overall survival both by data for clinical stage and for the various cell types such as squamous cell carcinoma, adenocarcinoma, and large cell carcinoma, as shown in Figs 16–18.

Veterans' Administration Lung Cancer Study Group staging

For unresectable patients, a more simplified staging system is generally used, with division of patients between localized (limited disease, LD) or extensive disease (ED). This staging system was first used by the Veterans Administration Lung Cancer Group (**VALG**) in the United States and it remains the most widely used for staging patients who are not candidates for surgery. Limited disease is defined as tumour confined to one hemithorax, with or without local extension, including mediastinal and supraclavicular lymph nodes, while extensive disease is defined as demonstrable tumour beyond these limits. The extensive disease classification is thus equivalent to stage IV of the international system. The VALG staging system was originally proposed because of its suitability for radiotherapy, which was the main type of non-surgical therapy at the time when the system was introduced.

TREATMENT

The treatment of lung cancer should be considered in accordance with the histopathological type and the stage of disease.

For practical reasons, the treatment will be presented for the following two categories of patients: group 1, patients with squamous cell, large cell carcinoma, and adenocarcinoma ('non-small cell' lung cancer) and group 2, small cell lung cancer.

Treatment of squamous cell, adeno-, and large cell carcinoma

Surgery

The primary curative treatment for these cell types is surgery. The success of surgical treatment is highly dependent on the appropriate selection of patients. The selection criteria relate the anatomical extent of disease to the biological nature of the tumour and the patient's physiological status (Markos *et al.* 1989; Salvatierra *et al.* 1990). Candidates for definitive resection include only patients with stage I and stage II disease and a small group of patients with stage IIIa, where the disease is confined to the ipsilateral hemithorax and in whom complete resection is considered technically feasible.

Evaluation of the pulmonary function is mandatory before surgical resection is undertaken in order to ensure that the patient has sufficient lung function after resection (Gass and Olsen 1986; Drings 1989). An adequate evaluation should thus indicate the patients who are at high risk for simple thoracotomy, but also estimate the maximum tolerated extent of pulmonary resection possible and predict the post-resection ventilatory capacity.

Of the tests used to evaluate the function of the airways, the flow–volume relationship, the forced expiratory volume in 1 s (**FEV**) and the forced vital capacity (**FVC**) are considered the most reliable (Stahel *et al.* 1989). The function of the alveolar capillary surface can be evaluated by measuring the carbon monoxide diffusion capacity and the blood gases, while the ventilation/perfusion of the given area of the lung can be evaluated by the use of radio-active isotopes. If the P_{CO_2} is elevated at rest, chest surgery cannot be recommended, while a decrease in P_{O_2} is not inconsistent with surgery and P_{O_2} often increases when tumour-related shunting is removed surgically.

If the FVC is equal to 2.5 litres or more, the patient has essentially normal lung function and can tolerate a pneumonectomy. If the FVC is below 2.5 litres, a ventilation and perfusion scan should be made in order to ensure a normal ventilation/perfusion relationship in the non-affected lung and to maintain the blood gases within a normal range. If the calculated FEV_1 after operation is less than 1.0 litre the patient is considered to have severe ventilatory impairment and a surgical resection of a large amount of lung tissue cannot be considered.

The extent of the resection should be carefully planned pre-operatively on the basis of the foregoing evaluation, even though final selection of the operative procedures must take place at the time of exploration. A procedure that encompasses all existent neoplastic tissue and provides the maximum conservation of lung tissue, is usually the one of choice. It is well established that surgical mortality is increased with the more radical procedures, however, potential for cure should not be compromised by strictly accommodating a conservative policy.

The choice of surgical procedure is usually indicated by the site of tumour involvement as determined by intraoperative evaluation. The following general guidelines hold true in most situations.

1. A *wedge* or *segmental resection* will be selected for patients with small peripheral tumours (less than 2 cm in greatest diameter), with no evidence of extension or metastases (T1, N0, M0, stage I disease). In some of these patients, the pre-operative diagnosis of cancer may be doubtful. A conservative resection for this extent of disease is particularly applicable in a patient whose pulmonary status is severely compromised.

2. A *lobectomy* is usually the choice for a patient with a centrally located tumour mass, completely contained within the lobe. The lobar bronchus may be involved, but there must be an adequate tumour-free margin for resection. There may be lymph node extension or metastases that are limited to intrapulmonary or immediate hilar lymphatic drainage that can be totally encompassed by an *en bloc* dissection. These tumours are usually classified as stage I or II disease.

3. *Pneumonectomy* is the procedure of choice for all physiologically able patients having more extensive disease than described above. This will include tumours extending to the orifice of the lobar bronchus (see Sleeve resection below) and tumours originating within or extending to the main stem bronchus. Furthermore, when the primary tumour involves more than one lobe, pneumonectomy is generally undertaken. Extended pneumonectomy is recommended in the presence of mediastinal lymph node involvement, stage III N2 disease (a) if the involvement is limited to the node of the ispilateral tracheobronchial angle or subcarinal space; (b) the histopathological evaluation of the nodes at mediastinoscopy and thoracotomy shows that the capsules of the nodes are intact with no perinodal disease; (c) the histopathological classification is squamous cell carcinoma.

4. *Radical pneumonectomy*, defined as resection with intrapericardial ligation of vessels, is applicable in selected patients where the disease extends proximal to the major vessels, but in whom technical resection remains possible.

5. *Bronchoplastic or sleeve resection* (Naruke 1989).

The results of surgery for non-small cell cancer are given according to stage and histopathology in Figs 19 and 20. Survival rates are highly dependent on tumour extent, particularly lymph node involvement (Williams *et al.* 1981; Naruke *et al.* 1988; Ginsberg 1989). It is noteworthy that the best results can be obtained for squamous cell carcinoma, in particular when one is comparing stages II and III of this histological type with adenocarcinoma and undifferentiated large cell carcinoma.

Adjuvant therapy to surgery

The results of surgical treatment of lung cancer have essentially been unchanged during the past two decades, for which reason great interest has been focused on the use of adjuvant therapy, such as radiotherapy, chemotherapy, and immunotherapy given either pre- or post-operatively (Evans 1989; Holmes 1989). Numerous prospective randomized trials have been performed, even combining three or four forms of therapy, but the results have generally been very disappointing.

More encouraging results have now been published by the Lung Cancer Study Group in North America. One randomized study involved 130 patients with stage II and III adenocarcinoma and large cell undifferentiated carcinoma (Holmes and Gail 1986). Patients were randomized to receive either chemotherapy (CAP, cyclophosphamide, 400 mg/m²; doxorubicin, 40 mg/m²; cis-platinum 40 mg/m²) monthly for 6 months after surgery while patients in the immunotherapy group received an intrapleural injection of 10^7 Tice BCG organisms via a chest tube, or thoraco-centesis. Median time to recurrence was approximately 7 months longer in the chemotherapy group, which is statistically significant ($p=0.018$; log rank).

A detrimental effect of BCG cannot be excluded in the study and, accordingly, results from future studies are needed to elucidate further the potential value of chemotherapy in this group of patients. At present, routine use of adjuvant chemotherapy cannot be advocated.

The same group of investigators has also evaluated post-operative chemotherapy and radiotherapy in resected, non-small cell lung cancer with microscopical residual disease or extensive lymph node involvement at the time of surgery (Lung Cancer Study Group 1988). Thoracic radiation was given on a split-dose schedule with 20 Gy in five fractions over 5 days, with each of the two

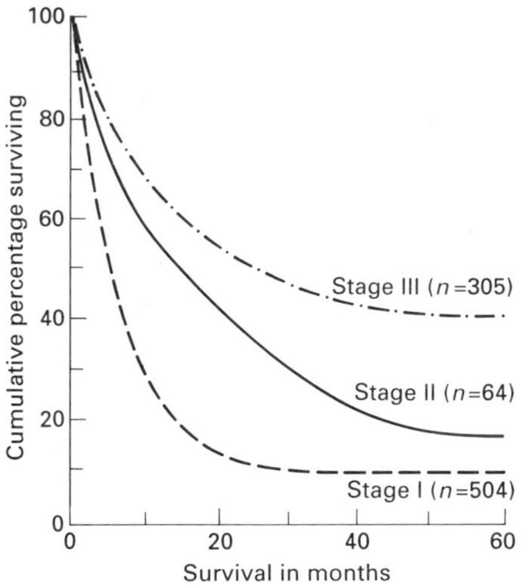

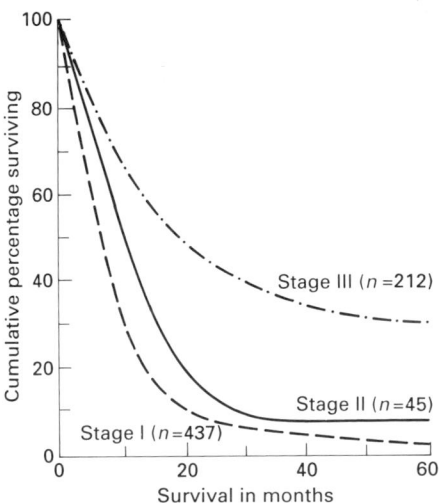

Fig. 19 Survival of patients with resected squamous cell carcinoma of lung by post-surgical treatment stage of disease.

Fig. 20 Survival of patients with resected adenocarcinoma and undifferentiated large cell carcinoma of lung by post-surgical treatment stage of disease.

courses separated by 3 weeks. Chemotherapy (cyclophosphamide, 400 mg/m²; doxorubicin, 40 mg/m²; cisplatinum, 60 mg/m²) was given every 4 weeks for six cycles. The mean time since randomization was 3.7 years and mean follow-up was 1.5 years; 164 patients were included in the study. The 18 month disease-free survival was 40 per cent for those undergoing combined therapy and 25 per cent for those receiving radiotherapy. The chemotherapy group experienced significantly fewer recurrences. Analysis also indicated that chemotherapy had a greater effect on non-squamous cell than on squamous cell tumours. In addition, chemotherapy was more beneficial for patients who had mediastinal disease (N2) than those with N1 disease. The combined therapy thus significantly prolongs disease-free survival compared with radiotherapy alone, but not overall survival.

For pre-operative chemotherapy a number of studies have shown that disease localized to the thorax responds better than systemic disseminated disease. The pathological complete response rates have been as high as 30 per cent in some of the studies (Strauss et al. 1992). Pre-operative chemotherapy has in some patients converted

technically unresectable tumours to resectable ones, but it is still unclear if it prolongs life.

Radiotherapy when combined with surgery has also now been subjected to prospective trials (Lung Cancer Study Group 1986). While radiotherapy definitely reduces the local recurrence rate, none of the studies shows any improvement in survival.

Radiotherapy

The vast majority of patients with lung cancer have tumours too advanced for surgery. For these, radiotherapy is the most frequently used treatment.

Radiotherapy can be very useful in controlling troublesome symptoms caused by local tumour effects or metastases. The palliative value of radiotherapy is undisputed. What is much less clear is the role of curative radiotherapy. This is partly due to methodological problems with the available information on patient staging and other prognostic factors, difficulties with assessment of response and local control, and often suboptimal radiotherapy.

The most important problem is the unsuitability of the majority of patients for any attempt at curative local therapy. They are generally old, ill, and have advanced tumours at presentation. This has led to understandable pessimism amongst referring clinicians and radiotherapists. The few patients who may benefit from radical radiotherapy may easily get lost among the vast majority for whom only symptom control is realistic. That there is a small population for whom radical radiotherapy can be useful has been confirmed by a number of small studies reporting survival rates comparable to surgery in highly selected groups of patients (Burt et al. 1989; Newaisky and Kerr 1989; Zhang et al. 1989).

The aim of curative radiotherapy is to deliver a tumoricidal dose to the primary tumour and to locoregional areas of spread. The treatment volume should therefore include the radiographically visible tumour, hilar, and mediastinal lymph node areas, with a margin allowing for the microscopic extension of tumour. A compromise often has to be reached between the necessary dose, large volume, the patient's tolerance, and the radiation tolerance of normal intrathoracic structures. In practice, this means irradiating the smallest possible volume of normal lung tissue and not exceeding the tolerance of the spinal cord.

Treatment planning

With the patient in the treatment position and by using either X-ray films with appropriate magnification or a treatment simulator, the proximal and distal extent and the width of treatment volume are determined. An outline of the chest is taken through the centre of the volume to be irradiated. On this cross-section is drawn the position of the high-dose target volume, the critical organs to be avoided when positioning the beams, and the outline of surrounding normal lung. This plan is then available for dose calculation. Various field arrangements are used, depending on the shape and position of the high-dose volume relative to the spinal cord. An example of a radical treatment plan is shown in Fig. 21.

This method can be greatly simplified and improved by using a CT scanner to demonstrate accurately the cross-sectional anatomy. It is linked to the planning computer and allows direct superimposition of dosimetry and accurate dose calculations.

Megavoltage treatment apparatus is used, a 4–10 MeV energy linear accelerator or ⁶⁰Co being the most frequently used machines. This energy gives a relatively low entrance skin dose, adequate penetration to deeper tissues, and excellent collimation of the beam, thus permitting very little scatter to adjacent normal tissues.

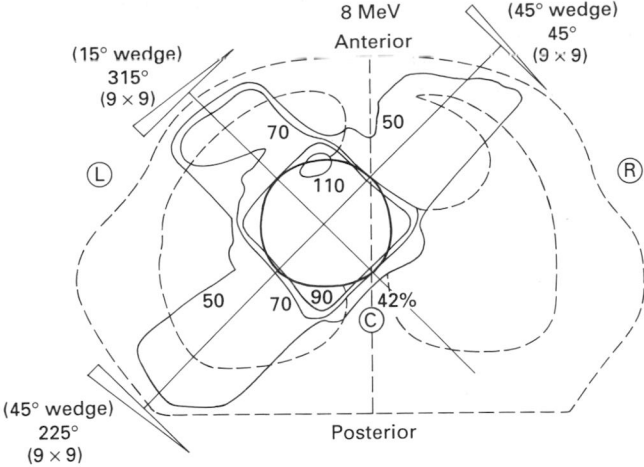

Fig. 21 Three-field plan. (All fields are wedged. Anterior and posterior oblique fields are opposed and placed to avoid irradiation of the spinal cord.)

Dose inhomogeneity can be avoided by the use of wedge filters as compensators and the dose calculations corrected for greater transmissions through normal aerated lung. The dose to sensitive normal structures (spinal cord, pericardium) can be limited by careful placement of treatment beams.

When a satisfactory dose distribution has been checked to see if it remains within radiation tolerance, radiotherapy is prescribed. Prescription specifies radiation dose, number of fractions, and overall time and gives clear indications as to the position of the individual beams in relation to the reference points marked on the patient. Port films obtained on the treatment machine may be used to verify final beam positions.

Various doses and fractionation schedules are used in the treatment of lung cancer. Despite an extensive literature and some firmly held opinions, optimal conditions have not been universally established. Commonly used fractionation schedules with their comparative total-dose fractions (**TDF**) are given in Table 12 (Perez 1985).

Studies from the Radiation Therapy Oncology Group (Bleehen 1991) report detailed information concerning the use of various fractionation regimens. Patients were randomized to receive either 40 Gy as a split course over 4 weeks or 40, 50, and 60 Gy as continuous fractionation (five fractions per week). Complete radiological regression was rare: 8 per cent in the split-course group; 20–24 per cent for the continuous regimens. The lowest incidence

Table 12 Fractionation schedules commonly used in treatment of bronchial carcinoma

Dose (cGy)	No. of fractions	Time (weeks)	NSD
4000	20	4	1351
5000	25	5	1562
6000	30	6	1758
3200	8	4	1347
3000	10	2	1291
2000	5	1	1139 (5/7)
			1097 (7/7)
4500	20	4	1528 (28/7)
			1532 (26/7)
4000	10	4[a]	1608 } split course
5000	24	9[b]	1490 }

[a]2-, [b]4-weeks' rest period. NSD, normal standard dose.

of intrathoracic failures was seen in patients treated with 60 Gy (33 per cent) with a dose–response curve for the lower TDF fractionations. Applying 40 Gy in 4 weeks, 49 per cent of patients relapsed locally. The split-course and the high-dose, continuous regimens were associated with a higher incidence of radiation-related complications. The same group of investigators has also shown that once-a-week radiotherapy (5 Gy) for 12 weeks yields results that appear no different from those achieved with conventional radiotherapy (60 Gy using 2 Gy fractions daily for 6 weeks) in locally non-metastatic lung cancer (Perez *et al.* 1980).

Radical radiotherapy

When considering the indications for radical radiotherapy, the small proportion of possible candidates can be divided into following groups.

1. Operable patients in whom there is a medical contraindication to thoracotomy or who refuse surgery. It should be emphasized that an attempt to give curative irradiation will compromise the patient's pulmonary reserve, but severe respiratory embarrassment is rare (fewer than 10 per cent of cases).

2. Findings by Burt *et al.* (1989) and Zhang *et al.* (1989) now suggest that results comparable to those of surgery can be achieved.

3. Stage II lung cancer found unresectable at thoracotomy.

4. Patients at high risk of local relapse following incomplete resections (stump, chest wall involvement).

Palliative radiotherapy

For the majority of patients with non-small cell lung cancer, the extent of disease makes the prospect of cure by any available treatment method unrealistic. Patients with extrathoracic disease at presentation have a life expectancy of 3–4 months. In most cases, the presence of advanced local disease or metastases will give rise to distressing symptoms. The use of palliative radiotherapy may greatly improve the quality of remaining life.

Palliative treatment must be given with the aim of minimum morbidity and inconvenience to the patient. Successful palliation of symptoms is almost always caused by tumour regression and it is therefore necessary to use techniques and doses that reliably produce a tumour response. The general philosophy of palliative irradiation is aimed at growth restraint, rather than at tumour 'sterilizations'. It uses relatively large fields and short, simple, fractionation schedules. Resolution of treated symptoms for the duration of the patient's life is the aim.

Numerous doses and fractionation schedules are in use, for example 30 Gy in 10 fractions over 2 weeks, 20 Gy in five fractions over 1 week, and a single fraction of 7.5–10 Gy. A number of studies have shown little difference between the effectiveness of various schedules, which appear to be dictated more by local traditions than based on scientific assessment (Perez 1985). A large, randomized trial by the British Medical Research Council Lung Group showed no significant difference in survival or palliative effect between 17 Gy in two fractions of 8.5 Gy 1 week apart or 10 Gy in a single fraction; the first schedule caused substantially more dysphagia (Bleehen 1991).

Palliative radiotherapy of intrathoracic disease
Haemoptysis and cough, perhaps the most common distressing symptoms, are easily controlled by radiotherapy. Up to 75 per cent of patients will experience a significant degree of relief. Dyspnoea caused by bronchial obstruction can be improved in approximately half of patients, depending on the site and duration of the block.

In cases where mediastinal lymph node enlargement causes compression of the oesophagus, the dysphagia can be relieved in 80 per cent of the patients.

The syndrome of a superior vena caval obstruction can also be relieved by radiotherapy. More than half of the patients will experience complete relief. In our experience, there is no reason to combine radiotherapy with the use of steroids or chemotherapy.

Local pain due to chest wall or rib involvement can be partially relieved in the majority of patients, while pain due to brachial plexus involvement in apical lesions is much less responsive to radiation.

Hoarseness due to compression of the recurrent laryngeal nerve is not responsive to radiotherapy.

Palliative radiotherapy of extrathoracic disease

Radiotherapy is often widely used in treating metastatic lesions secondary to lung cancer, for example in the brain, spinal cord, and bones.

Irradiation of the central nervous system is usually given as whole-brain irradiation with a dose of 30 Gy in 10 fractions over 2 weeks or 20 Gy in five fractions, which achieves a good, short-lasting (median 2–3 months) palliation in 50 per cent of all cases. The application of corticosteroids (for example, dexamethasone, 12 mg daily) will further give symptomatic benefit by reducing the intracranial pressure and oedema surrounding the intracerebral deposit.

Compression of the spinal cord is observed in 8–10 per cent of all patients with lung cancer. If it occurs, surgical decompression, followed by radiotherapy, remains the treatment of choice for obtaining rapid relief. Radiotherapy alone is used in patients with slowly evolving or stable compression syndromes or where the general condition of the patient precludes the possibility of surgical intervention. Its effectiveness depends on pre-treatment neurofunctional status, but is usually poor, often lasting only 1–3 months. Once paraplegia occurs, significant recovery is unlikely and prevention of neurological catastrophy should be the aim. A dose of 30 Gy in 10 daily fractions is most frequently used.

The effectiveness of radiotherapy in pain relief in patients with bone metastases secondary to lung cancer is well known. Approximately 35–50 per cent of the patients can be rendered pain-free and the remainder experience a considerable improvement. In non-weight-bearing areas where the risk of subsequent pathological fracture is minimal, single fractions of radiotherapy may be sufficient, for example 8 Gy; otherwise the simple course of low-dose irradiation, for example 20 Gy in five fractions, is sufficient.

Radiotherapy side-effects

Among the most commonly observed acute side-effects are radiation oesophagitis, which is dose and schedule dependent. It has a predictable course and dysphagia can be relieved by modifying the diet and by the use of topical anaesthetics and lubricants.

The frequency with which symptomatic oesophagitis develops is dose related. The normal oesophagus can tolerate doses up to 60 Gy. At doses in excess of 55 Gy, 40–50 per cent of all patients develop this complication. Concomitant use of chemotherapy can potentiate this complication, leading to stricture.

More serious side-effects include pneumonitis and pulmonary fibrosis. Between 5 and 15 per cent of patients receiving high-dose chest radiotherapy become breathless and develop an accompanying non-productive cough 2–6 months afterwards. A chest radiograph will frequently demonstrate soft, irregular shadowing in the irradiated zone. The syndrome is usually self-limiting and symptomatic relief may be obtained by giving systemic steroids.

The frequency and severity of pulmonary fibrosis are related to the radiation dose and to the volume of the lung encompassed in the high-dose area. Assessment of the physiological changes demonstrates severe abnormalities, which are the consequence of post-radiation fibrosis, tumour, and pre-existing lung disease. Loss of lung volume is the common radiological abnormality (Choi et al. 1990).

Other complications, which are rarely seen, include radiation myelitis, radiation myelopathy, and radiation-induced pericarditis. The latter two complications are seen in less than 5 per cent of all cases and should be completely avoidable.

Adjuvant therapy to radiotherapy

Over the years, numerous trials have exploited the effect of combined radio- and chemotherapy in patients with non-small cell, non-resectable, locoregional disease, but usually with negative results. Four publications have now presented additional and more positive data than before. Three of the studies revealed a significant survival advantage for chemotherapy+radiotherapy versus radiotherapy alone, with the chemotherapy consisting of either cisplatin given weekly (30 mg/m^2) concurrent with irradiation, a combination of vindesine, cyclophosphamide, cisplatin, and lomustine given both before and after irradiation, or a combination of cisplatin and vinblastine (Arriagada et al. 1991; Le Chevalier et al. 1992; Schaake et al. 1992; Dillman et al. 1993). The fourth study applied also a four-drug combination (methotrexate, doxorubicin, cyclophosphamide, and lomustine), but was not able to show a difference in survival data (Morton et al. 1991). The studies are summarized in Table 13.

Chemotherapy in 'non-small cell' lung cancer

Chemotherapy has as yet no established role in the routine treatment of non-small cell lung cancer. Single agents produce a response rate in the region of 10–20 per cent and combinations of cytostatic drugs will result in a larger percentage of responders. Most of these are partial and short-lasting, of 3–5 months' duration (Ruckdeschel 1988). However, response to chemotherapy does not equate simply with prolongation of survival (Sorensen et al. 1989). At present, no specific recommendations can therefore be made for any single agent or combination of chemotherapeutic agents for the treatment of non-small cell lung cancer. More recent studies with combination chemotherapeutic regimens have reportedly found objective remissions with more than a 50 per cent reduction of tumours in 20–40 per cent of previously untreated patients. Complete remissions are rare (Ruckdeschel 1988).

The literature now contains seven studies where chemotherapy is compared with an untreated, closely matched, control population receiving supportive therapy alone without chemotherapy (Table 14). In a couple of the studies a marginal difference was shown in favour of the chemotherapy group versus the non-treated group, while the majority of the studies were unable to show a similar advantage (Cellerino et al. 1990).

At the present time, chemotherapy in patients with non-small cell lung cancer should therefore be considered as an experimental treatment. In patients with poor prognostic features, such as low-performance status, extensive disease, massive weight loss, and previous radiotherapy, the likelihood of tumour regression is very low. Accordingly, treatment with cytostatic agents should only be instituted in highly selected, unresectable patients who have been informed completely about the limitations of the treatment. It is preferable that the patient be included in a controlled clinical trial.

Table 13 Radiotherapy and chemotherapy: recent randomized trials

Treatment		No. of patients	Median survival (months)	% survival (years)				Reference (see notes)
Radiotherapy	Chemotherapy			1	2	3	5	
65 Gy/26 fractions+45 days	VDS, CTX, CCNU, DDP before and after irradiation	176	12	41	14	4		(1)
	0	177	10	51	21	12		(2)
55 Gy (3 Gy×10 in five fractions a week followed by 3 weeks' rest and then 2 Gy×10 in five fractions a week	Cisplatin, 30 mg/m² weekly concurrently	110		44	19	13		(3)
	6 mg/m² daily concurrently	107		54	26	16		(3)
	0	114		46	13	2	0	(3)
50 Gy in 5 weeks with 10 Gy boost in five fractions	CCNU, CTX, MTX, DOX		10	46	21		5	(4)
	0		10	45	16		7	(4)
60 Gy	Cis-platinum+vinblastine	78	13.8	55	26	23		(5)
	0	77	9.7	40	13	11		(5)

Abbreviations: CCNU, N-(2-chloroethyl)-N'-cyclohexyl-N-nitrosourea (lomustine); CTX, cyclophosphamide; DDP, *cis*-diamminedichloroplatinum (cisplatin); DOX, doxorubicin; MTX, methotrexate; VDS, vindesine.
References: (1) Arriagada *et al.* (1991); (2) Le Chevalier *et al.* (1992); (3) Schaake-Koning *et al.* (1992); (4) Morton *et al.* (1991); (5) Dillmann *et al.* (1993).

Table 14 Non-small cell lung cancer: overview of randomized trials comparing best supportive care vs chemotherapy

Treatment	No. of evaluable patients	Response rate	Median survival (weeks)	Reference (see notes)
MACC	20	20	30	(1)
BSC	17	0	9	
Supportive care vs	50	0	17	
VDS/CDDP vs	91	25	32	(2)
CTX/DX/CDDP	92	15	17	
CTX/Epi Dx/CDDP alternating VP16/CCNU/MTX vs	44	21	36	(3)
Supportive care	45	0	21	
CDDP/VDS vs	97	28	27	(4)
Supportive care	91	0	21	
VLB/CDDP	31	22	20	(5)
BSC	32	0	14	
VDS/CDDP	23	23	27	(6)
BSC	20	0	10	
VLB/CDDP	44		19	(7)
BSC	43		19	

Abbreviations: MACC, methotrexate/adriamycin/cyclophosphamide/CCNU; BSC, best supportive care; VDS, vindesine; Epi Dx, 4-epi-doxorubicin; VLB, vinblastine; CDDP, cisplatin; VP16, etoposide; DX, doxorubicin; CCNU, lomustine; CTX, cyclophosphamide; MTX, methotrexate.
References: (1) Cornier *et al.* (1982); (2) Rapp *et al.* (1988); (3) Cellerino *et al.* (1991); (4) Woods *et al.* (1990); (5) Ganz *et al.* (1989); (6) Quoix *et al.* (1991); (7) Kaassa *et al.* (1991).

Small cell lung cancer

Chemotherapy

The realization that small cell lung cancer is a systemic disease has logically led to the use of systemic treatment as the main therapy. Less than 5 per cent of accurately staged patients will be candidates for a primary surgical resection.

Systemic treatment consisted, at first, of single-agent therapy. At least two randomized trials have shown that single-agent therapy with alkylating agents is superior to no treatment on the basis of both median survival time and estimation of quality of life (Bunn *et al.* 1989; Hansen and Kristjansen 1991). Activity has been found for many single agents, and the most effective agents at present are listed in Table 15. Responses are defined as a greater than 50 per cent reduction in tumour size. During the 1970s the median survival was prolonged by four to five times and cure was obtained in 5–10 per cent of all patients. Major additional improvement has not been observed in the 1980s, but a vast amount of studies have consolidated the early results.

Among the most commonly used combinations are (Aisner and Wiernik 1980; Catane *et al.* 1981; Wolf *et al.* 1987):

(1) etoposide and cisplatin;

(2) vincristine, etoposide, and cyclophosphamide;

(3) cyclophospamide, doxorubicin, and vincristine.

Examples of these regimens are given in Table 16. During the last few years etoposide has been used increasingly, as randomized studies have shown that its substitution for other drugs in existing combinations is often associated with small survival gains, especially in extensive disease. When administering etoposide the dose scheduling is highly important, with some work showing the efficacy of etoposide given orally over a more prolonged period (Slevin *et al.* 1989). Whether that schedule of administration is superior to standard methods is at present uncertain and can only be answered by a randomized study with the drugs given in equitoxic doses.

Table 15 Active agents in small cell lung cancer

Alkylating agents
  Cyclophosphamide
  Iphosphamide
  Nitrogen mustard
  Hexamethylmelamine
  Lomustine

Vinca alkaloids
  Vincristine
  Vindesine

Podophyllotoxin derivatives
  Etoposide (VP-16)
  Teniposide (VM-26)

Platinum analogues
  Cisplatinum
  Carboplatin (JM-8)

Miscellaneous
  Doxorubicin
  Methotrexate

Table 16 Commonly used regimens of combination chemotherapy for small cell lung cancer

(1) Etoposide	115 mg/m² i.v. days 3–5 q. 3 weeks
Cisplatin	60–80 mg/m² i.v. q. 3 weeks, day 1
(2) Etoposide	50 mg/m² i.v. daily×5 q. 3 weeks
Doxorubicin	45 mg/m² i.v. q. 3 weeks
Cyclophosphamide	1000 mg/m² i.v. q. 3 weeks
(3) Cyclophosphamide	1000 mg/m² i.v. q. 3 weeks
Doxorubicin	50 mg/m² i.v. q 3 weeks
Vincristine	2 mg i.v. q. 3 weeks

References: (1) Wolf *et al.* (1987); (2) Aisner and Wiernik (1980); (3) Catane *et al.* (1981).

Treatment regimens will result in a response rate in excess of 80 per cent for small cell lung cancer. Complete response is produced in 30–40 per cent of patients with limited disease and in more than 15–20 per cent of patients with extensive disease (Bunn *et al.* 1989; Hansen and Kristjansen 1991). Chemotherapy is also effective as single-modality treatment in patients presenting with involvement of the central nervous system (Kristensen *et al.* 1992). Provided that an adequate staging procedure has been used, the median survival for patients with limited disease should be in excess of 12 months, while median survival of patients with extensive disease should be 8 or more months. Long-term survival is reached in 10–15 per cent of patients with limited disease and in 3–5 per cent of patients with extensive disease although these results depend on selection criteria. In large national studies, which are more representative of the study population as a whole than cooperative group studies, the results are less encouraging. For example, studies from England and Italy show 5 year survival of only 4 and 2–3 per cent, respectively (Bunn *et al.* 1989; Souhami *et al.* 1990; Hansen and Kristjansen 1991; Rosti *et al.* 1991).

The duration of treatment needed to produce optimal results is uncertain; most trials are for periods of 6 months, with a tendency during the last few years to shorten therapy (Spiro and Souhami 1990). Approximately one-third of all patients will eventually relapse, but survival of more than 5 years after diagnosis offers some hope of cure.

New approaches to chemotherapy

A variety of options to improve treatment results is under investigation. These include:

(1) alternating 'non-cross-resistant' chemotherapy (Elliott *et al.* 1984; Østerlind 1989);

(2) scheduling of drug administration based on cell cycle analysis (Hirsch *et al.* 1981);

(3) incorporation of new agents with high activity in the combination chemotherapy regimens (Green 1989);

(4) intensive high-dose chemotherapy with or without autologous bone-marrow transplantation and with or without granulocyte–macrophage colony-stimulating factor (Klastersky and Sculier 1989);

(5) anticoagulants in combination with chemotherapy (Chahinian *et al.* 1989);

(6) biological modifiers such as interferon and growth factors (Carney *et al.* 1989).

These methods are at present subject to investigation and cannot be recommended in the routine management of patients with small cell lung cancer. The initial trials focusing on option (4) are disappointing. The methods are considered in more detail next.

Alternating non-cross-resistant chemotherapy
This has in some trials demonstrated modest superiority to continuous therapy. A review by Elliot *et al.* (1984) concluded that (i) treatment schedules applying cyclic, alternating, non-cross-resistant drug combinations in small cell lung cancer yield tumour responses comparable to those obtained with continuous regimens with a similar level of toxicity; (ii) controlled trials have failed to demonstrate major advantages in terms of improved survival; details of trial design, especially the scheduling, may, however, be of critical importance; (iii) further controlled studies are warranted; careful attention to the trial design with elimination of confounding variables such as radiotherapy, re-evaluation of disease-free status, and prolonged follow-up of large numbers of patients will be necessary; (iv) increased recognition of tumour cell heterogeneity as a major reason for treatment failure together with *in vitro* determination of drug sensitivity in cross-resistance may lead to a more rational future application of alternating chemotherapy.

Scheduling of drugs based on cell kinetic observations
This has been the subject of a single clinical trial, which demonstrated the superiority of etoposide scheduling based on data from flow cytometric DNA analyses (Hirsch *et al.* 1987).

New drugs
An extensive and critical update on the present status of new drugs in the treatment of small cell lung cancer has been given by Joss *et al.* (1986) and Johnson (1989) and a further update is given in Table 17 (Aisner and Wiernik 1980; Catane *et al.* 1981; Wolf *et al.* 1987). The most active of the new drugs include carboplatin (JM-8) and VM-26 (teniposide). The latter compound was shown by the Copenhagen Lung Cancer Study Group to be highly active, with a response rate of 90 per cent in untreated patients with small cell cancer. A subsequent randomized study revealed equal activity of etoposide and teniposide when given as a single agent in equitoxic doses in elderly patients with small cell carcinoma (Bork *et al.* 1991). The marked difference in response rates observed by the same group of investigators for the same compound (for example, VM-26) in

Table 17 New agents in chemotherapy of small cell carcinoma

Active agents	Inactive agents	Investigational agents
ACNU	Amonafide	Carbonyloxycamptothecin (CPT-II)
Carboplatin	Ara-C	Flutamide (antiandrogens)
Epirubicin	Idarubicin	Menogaril
Ifosphamide	Mitoxantrone	Merbarone
Teniposide (VM-26)	TGU	Navelbine
Vindesine	(Insufficient data)	Piritrexim/trimetrexate
	Lonidamine	10-EDAM

untreated (90 per cent) and previously treated (18 per cent) patients reveals that there are major methodological problems in the design and execution of clinical phase II trials with new agents in pre-treated patients with small cell lung cancer, as discussed by Cullen (1989).

Anticoagulants

The role of anticoagulants has been the subject of a small, prospective, randomized evaluation by the Veterans Administration Lung Cancer Study Group (Chahinian et al. 1989). Fifty patients were randomized to receive chemotherapy and radiotherapy with or without warfarin. Median survival was 24 weeks for control patients and 50 weeks for the warfarin group. The warfarin-treated group also demonstrated a significant increase in time before progression, suggesting an influence of warfarin on the metastatic potential of the tumour. The use of warfarin in combination chemotherapy regimens is now under large-scale evaluation by several cooperative groups in the United States. Preliminary results from a large Cancer and Acute Leukaemia Group B (CALGB) study on this topic, comprising 328 patients with extensive small cell lung cancer, show advantage in objective response rates for the warfarin-treated group, while overall survival also seems in favour of the warfarin group, but without reaching the conventional levels of significance. Because of the increased risk of serious haemorrhage, the use of warfarin should still remain experimental.

Biological-response modifiers

The clinical evaluation of these in small cell lung cancer is still in an early phase and the experience is very modest. Phase I studies with growth factors have been initiated based on in vitro data and xenografts using panels of established and well-characterized small cell carcinoma cell lines (Mulshine et al. 1989).

The therapeutic activity of interferon in small cell lung cancer has yet to be established but preliminary data suggest a potential role for it in the maintenance phase (Mattson et al. 1992).

Clinical trials with colony-stimulating factors have also been initiated, evaluating their effect on the haematological toxicity of the chemotherapy (Crawford et al. 1991; Green et al. 1991). At present it has been shown in a randomized trial that granulocyte colony-stimulating factor (G-CSF) can lessen the severity of neutropenic episodes; treatment delays can be eliminated, reduction of cytotoxic drug doses can be avoided in some patients, and the number and duration of hospital admissions for infectious complications may be reduced. Improvements in survival have not yet been observed.

Treatment of relapse

When a patient relapses from primary therapy, second-line treatment should be considered (Andersen et al. 1990). The results with combination chemotherapy are generally disappointing, which is a major problem, as most patients will relapse within a period

of 10–12 months. The first recognizable clinical relapse may be either locally or in metastatic sites and subsequent treatment depends on this localization. A multifocal relapse will usually lead to a change of chemotherapy to include other active agents not used in the primary treatment. The response rates are 20–25 per cent, with a median duration of 3–4 months. If the patient with relapse has not received chemotherapy containing etoposide+cisplatin, the response rate might increase to 50 per cent (Andersen et al. 1990). Local relapse can be usefully palliated by irradiation in 30–40 per cent of patients, but again with disappointing results for survival.

Radiotherapy

Among the different types of lung cancer, the small cell variant is by far the most radiosensitive and radiotherapy was, until the early 1970s, the main mode of therapy for this disease entity. The recognition that small cell lung cancer is disseminated early and widely and the advent of chemotherapy, have changed the role of radiotherapy considerably. It has now been shown in several randomized studies that it is systemic treatment that determines the outcome of therapy, at least in terms of median survival.

Today, radiotherapy is used in two important areas in the treatment of small cell lung cancer. Locoregional irradiation (40–50 Gy given as a 3- to 4-week course) has been found to increase local control (that is, decrease the number of local relapses) but no major beneficial effect on median survival has been found. Some studies have now indicated a small but definite benefit of 5–15 per cent in disease-free survival at 2 years, when locoregional irradiation was applied together with combination chemotherapy compared with chemotherapy alone in patients with limited disease (Perry et al. 1987). Similar data have been obtained from a meta-analysis (Pignon et al. 1992). It is also apparent that a dose–response relationship exists up to 45–50 Gy with conventional 2-Gy daily fractions and that there is an increased acute and late toxicity when chest irradiation is added to chemotherapy (Perry et al. 1987; Payne et al. 1989). The exact timing of the irradiation as related to the chemotherapy is uncertain at present, but the trend is in favour of early irradiation given concurrently or alternating with the cytostatic agents (Murray et al. 1993).

Elective cranial irradiation

The other area of clinical importance is cerebral irradiation (Pedersen et al. 1988, 1989). The preferred time is at complete remission after 3–6 months of treatment. Whether prophylactic cranial irradiation influences overall length of survival has never been shown, but an impact on the frequency of brain relapses is evident. The lack of survival data is not surprising, as none of the studies published so far had enough patients to allow detection of any such difference. Other major methodological flaws and interpretive problems account for the general lack of information (Pedersen et al. 1988). On the basis of available literature, a general delay in time until occurrence of brain relapse is apparent after prophylactic cranial irradiation. Accordingly, the reduction in central nervous relapse in patients so treated has to be weighed against the increasing evidence of severe neurological toxicity in long-term survivors. Prospective multinational trials focusing on these problems are currently being conducted.

Modifications to existing radiotherapy techniques and the introduction of new methods are under investigation, including the use of radiosensitizers, superfractionation, and whole-body irradiation, but so far there has been no indication of improved results with any of these approaches.

Surgery

The few patients presenting at TNM stage I and II with small peripleural tumours can be considered candidates for curative surgery (Ginsburg and Karrer 1989). With the knowledge of early and widespread dissemination in the vast majority of patients, most of the major centres give post-operative systemic therapy, even though no signs of residual tumour can be found. The role of secondary surgery, that is, surgery after systemic treatment in patients with regional disease when restaging indicates that the residual tumour is resectable, is now the subject of several studies. The small number of patients who have been treated in this way in a controlled trial precludes any conclusion as to the role of secondary surgery in the management of patients with small cell cancer.

Carcinoma of the trachea

The primary treatment is surgery if technically possible, usually with resection and end-to-end reconstruction of the trachea or implantation. Median survival times have been reported to be 2–5 years, with an occasional patient being cured.

For radiotherapy the doses and schedule are similar to the treatment of primary bronchogenic carcinoma. Response rates vary in the range of 50–60 per cent, including complete response.

More recently, endotracheal brachytherapy has been applied. Other local treatment methods to relieve symptoms are cryotherapy, electrocautery, Nd-yAg and CO_2 laser photoresection, or laser photodynamic therapy with sensitizers.

Experience with chemotherapy is very limited, but where histological examination reveals a small cell carcinoma, its use should be explored (Pairolero 1989).

TREATMENT COMPLICATIONS

As stated earlier, intensive treatment is necessary to obtain good results, especially with regard to complete remissions and long-term disease-free survival. It is therefore to be expected that toxicity will be seen and will inevitably lead to significant clinical problems including therapy-related deaths (Feld 1989; Feld et al. 1989). These clinical problems are, of course, not specific to lung cancer and all attempts to minimize these are a part of the practice of clinical oncology.

Bone-marrow depression is often encountered, leading to anaemia, thrombocytopenia, and/or granulocytopenia. The duration of granulocytopenia is often relatively short and documented infections are encountered in only 5–10 per cent of treated patients.

Oesophagitis occurs in many patients treated with mediastinal irradiation. In the management of patients with small cell anaplastic carcinoma, this is especially important when radiotherapy is given together with anthracyclines such as doxorubicin. In such cases, it has been reported that more than half of patients develop moderate to severe oesophagitis.

Pneumonitis and pulmonary fibrosis are generally caused by radiotherapy but can be intensified by concomitant chemotherapy. Radiation pneumonitis seems to be irreversible when total doses exceed 30 Gy and careful planning of the target volume is very important.

Late toxicity

Although unfortunately not relevant for the majority of patients, long-term toxicity should be kept in mind in the follow-up of patients with small cell lung cancer.

Secondly, smoking-related primary tumours, including 'non-small cell' lung cancer, should be looked for and histologically confirmed, as they are particularly curable by surgery. Based on available data the frequency of acute leukaemia is probably increased in patients with small cell lung cancer, related to the use of alkylating agents (Pedersen-Bjergaard et al. 1985).

CONCLUSIONS

Within the last two decades, basic research has contributed vastly to our knowledge of lung cancer. Although the clinical impact of this development at present is indeed very modest, as measured by survival data, it is to be hoped that this will result in a change within the next decade.

Although surgery and irradiation contribute significantly to disease control locally and result in cures and extension of survival, overall progress in the treatment of this highly malignant neoplasm will ultimately depend on the development of more effective and selective systemic treatment. Emphasis should thus be given to the establishment of valid screening systems for preclinical testing of new cytostatic agents and/or biological modifiers, including a proper set-up for clinical testing of such therapies.

At the same time it is important to pursue treatment strategies that also focus on the palliative effect of therapy, including quality-of-life studies. With the increase in the elderly population and the economic restrictions on the health care system in general, these issues should also be the subject for future studies in lung cancer.

Last, but not least, more than 85 per cent of all cases of lung cancer can be prevented; we as physicians should play a greater part in providing the public (and the politicians) with the necessary information. Recent information from the United States and some European countries clearly demonstrates the importance of such initiatives.

REFERENCES

Aisner J, Wiernik PH (1980). Chemotherapy versus chemoimmunotherapy for small-cell undifferentiated carcinoma of the lung. Cancer, 46:2543–9.

Aisner SC, Finkelstein DM, Ettinger DS, Abeloff MD, Ruckdeschel JC, Eggleston JC (1990). The clinical significance of variant-morphology small-cell carcinoma of the lung. Journal of Clinical Oncology, 8:402–8.

Akiba S, Kato H, Blot WJ (1986). Passive smoking and lung cancer among Japanese women. Cancer Research, 46:4804–7.

American Joint Committee of Cancer (1979). Task force on staging of lung cancer. AJCC, Chicago.

Andersen M, Kristjansen PG, Hansen HH (1990). Second line chemotherapy in small cell lung cancer. Cancer Treatment Reviews, 17:427–36.

Arriagada R, et al. (1991). Astro Plenary. Effect of chemotherapy on locally advanced non-small cell carcinoma: a randomized study of 353 patients. International Journal of Radiation Oncology — Biology — Physics, 20:1183–90.

Bender RA, Hansen HH (1974). Hypercalcemia in bronchogenic carcinoma. A prospective study of 200 patients. Annals of Internal Medicine, 80:205–8.

Birrer MJ, Minna JD (1988). Molecular genetics of lung cancer. Seminars in Oncology, 15:225–35.

Blainey AD, Cuvering M, Green M (1988). Transbronchial aspiration of subcarinal lymph nodes. British Journal of Diseases of the Chest, 82:149–54.

Bleehen NM (British Medical Research Council Lung Cancer Working Party) (1991). Prospective randomised trial of palliative radiotherapy (RT) given in two fractions (F2) or one fraction (F1) for patients with inoperable non-small-cell lung cancer (NSCLC) and poor performance status. (Abstract.) Lung Cancer, 7:89.

Bork E, et al. (1991). Teniposide and etoposide in previously untreated small-cell lung cancer: a randomized study. Journal of Clinical Oncology, 9:1627–31.

Brynitz S, et al. (1985). Transcarinal mediastinal needle biopsy compared with mediastinoscopy. Journal of Thoracic and Cardiovascular Surgery, 90:21–4.

Bunn PA, *et al.* (1989). Chemotherapy in small cell lung cancer. *Lung Cancer*, 5:127–34.

Burt PA, Hancook BM, Stout R (1989). Radical radiotherapy for carcinoma of the bronchus: an equal alternative to radical surgery? *Clinical Oncology*, 1:86–91.

Carney DN (1989). Oncogenes and genetic abnormalities in lung cancer. *Chest*, 96 (Suppl.):25–27S.

Carney DN, Leij LD (1988). Lung cancer biology. *Seminars in Oncology*, 15:199–214.

Carney DN, *et al.* (1985). Establishment and identification of small cell lung cancer cell lines having classic and variant features. *Cancer Research*, 45:2914–30.

Carney DN, *et al.* (1989). Biological response modifiers in the management of SCLC. *Lung Cancer*, 5:143–5.

Catane R, *et al.* (1981). Small cell lung cancer: analysis of treatment factors contributing to prolonged survival. *Cancer*, 48:1936–43.

Cellerino R, Tummarillo D, Piga A (1990). Chemotherapy or not in advanced non-small cell lung cancer. *Lung Cancer*, 6:99–110.

Cellerino R, *et al.* (1991). Non small cell lung cancer (NSCLC). A prospective randomized trial of alternating chemotherapy versus best supportive area in advanced non-small cell lung cancer. *Journal of Clinical Oncology*, 9:1453–61.

Chahinian AP, *et al.* (1989). A randomized trial of anticoagulation with warfarin and of alternating chemotherapy in extensive small-cell lung cancer by the Cancer and Leukemia Group. *British Journal of Clinical Oncology*, 7:993–1002.

Choi NC, Kanarek D, Grillo HC (1990). Effect of postoperative radiotherapy on changes in pulmonary function in patients with stage II and IIIA lung carcinoma. *International Journal of Radiation Oncology—Biology—Physics*, 18:95–9.

Cibas ES, Melamed MR, Zaman MB, Kimmel M (1989). The effect of tumor size and tumor cell DNA content on the survival of patients with stage I adenocarcinoma of the lung. *Cancer*, 63:1552–6.

Cohen SJ, Stookey GK, Katz BP, Drook CA, Smith DM (1989). Encouraging primary care physicians to help smokers quit: a randomized, controlled trial. *Annals of Internal Medicine*, 110:648–52.

Coldman AJ, Goldie JH (1985). Role of mathematical modelling in protocol formulation in cancer chemotherapy. *Cancer Treatment Research*, 69:1041–5.

Cornier Y, *et al.* (1982). Benefits of polychemotherapy in advanced small bronchogenic carcinoma. *Cancer*, 50:845–9.

Crawford J, *et al.* (1991). Reduction by granulocyte colony-stimulating factor of fever and neutropenia induced by chemotherapy in patients with small-cell lung cancer. *New England Journal of Medicine*, 325:164–70.

Cullen JW (1989). The impact of prophylactic methods in the control of lung cancer in the U.S.A. In *Basic and clinical concepts of lung cancer* (ed. HH Hansen), pp. 15–33. Kluwer, Dordrecht.

Cullen M (1989). The design of phase II trials. *Lung Cancer*, 5:214–20.

Cummings SRE, *et al.* (1989). Training physicians in counseling about smoking cessation. A randomized trial of the 'Quit for Life' program. *Annals of Internal Medicine*, 110:640–7.

Dalager NA, *et al.* (1986). The relation of passive smoking to lung cancer. *Cancer Research*, 46:4808–11.

Doll R, Peto R (1976). Mortality in relation to smoking: 20 years' observations on male British doctors. *British Medical Journal*, 2:1525–36.

Drings R (1989). Preoperative assessment of lung cancer. *Chest*, 96 (Suppl.):42–45.

Elliott JA, Østerlind K, Hansen HH (1984). Cyclic alternating 'non-cross resistant' chemotherapy in the management of small cell anaplastic carcinoma of the lung. *Cancer Treatment Reviews*, 11:103–13.

Evans WK (1989). Adjuvant therapy for non-small cell lung cancer. *Chest*, 96 (Suppl.):87–91S.

Feld R (1989). Late complications associated with the treatment of small cell lung cancer. In *Lung cancer IV* (ed. HH Hansen), pp. 301–25. Kluwer, Boston.

Feld R, *et al.* (1989). Toxicity and supportive care in small cell lung cancer. *Lung Cancer*, 5:146–51.

Friedman PJ (1988). Lung cancer: update on staging classifications. *American Journal of Roentgenology*, 150:261–4.

Ganz PA, *et al.* (1989). Supportive care versus supportive care and combination chemotherapy in metastatic non-small cell lung cancer. Does chemotherapy make a difference? *Cancer*, 63:1271–8.

Gass DG, Olsen GN (1986). Preoperative pulmonary function testing to predict postoperative morbidity and mortality. *Chest*, 89:127–35.

Gazdar AF (1989). Advances in the biology of lung cancer. *Chest*, 96 (Suppl.):39–41S.

Gazdar AF, Linnoila RI (1988). The pathology of lung cancer—changing concepts and newer diagnostic techniques. *Seminars in Oncology*, 15:215–25.

Ginsberg RJ (1989). Limited resection in the treatment of stage I non-small cell lung cancer; an overview. *Chest*, 96 (Suppl.):50–1S.

Ginsberg RJ, Karrer KK (1989). Surgery in small cell lung cancer. *Lung Cancer*, 5:139.

Glazer GM (1989). Radiologic staging of lung cancer using CT and MRI. *Chest*, 96 (Suppl.):44–47S.

Grant D, Edwards D, Goldstraw P (1988). Computed tomography of the brain, chest, and abdomen in the preoperative assessment of non-small cell lung cancer. *Thorax*, 43:883–6.

Green JA, Trillet VN, Manegold C for the European G-CSF Lung Cancer Study Group (1991). r-metHuG-CSF (G-CSF) with CDE chemotherapy (CT) in small cell lung cancer (SCLC): interim results from a randomized, placebo controlled trial. *Proceedings ASCO*, 10:243.

Green M (1989). Phase III chemotherapy trials in small cell lung cancer. *Lung Cancer*, 5:177–85.

Hansen HH (1982). Diagnosis in metastatic sites. In *Lung cancer: clinical diagnosis and treatment* (2nd edn) (ed. MJ Straus), pp. 185–200. Grune & Stratton, New York.

Hansen HH (ed.) (1991). *Textbook for general practitioners: lung cancer*, EEC monograph. Springer-Verlag, Berlin.

Hansen HH, Hansen M (1987). Tumor markers in small cell lung cancer. *European Journal of Clinical Oncology*, 23:1585–7.

Hansen HH, Kristjansen PEG (1991). Chemotherapy of small cell lung cancer. *European Journal of Cancer*, 27:342–9.

Hansen M, Pedersen AG (1986). Tumor markers in patients with lung cancer. *Chest*, 89 (Suppl.):219–24S.

Hansen SW, *et al.* (1987). Detection of liver metastases in ultrasonography with fine needle aspiration. *Journal of Clinical Oncology*, 5:255–9.

Hawson G, Firouz-Abadi A, Ford CA, Johnson NG, Zimmerman (1990). Primary lung cancer: characterisation and survival of 1024 patients treated in a single institution. *Australian Journal of Medicine*, 152:230–7.

Hirsch FR, Østerlind K, Hansen HH (1983). The prognostic significance of histopathologic subtyping of small cell carcinoma of the lung according to the World Health Organization classification. *Cancer*, 52:2144–60.

Hirsch FR, *et al.* (1987). The superiority of combination chemotherapy including etoposide based on *in vivo* cell cycle analysis in the treatment of extensive small cell lung cancer. *Journal of Clinical Oncology*, 5:585–91.

Hirsch FR, *et al.* (1988). Histopathologic classification of small cell lung cancer—changing concepts and terminology. *Cancer*, 62:973–7.

Holmes CE (1989). Surgical adjuvant therapy of non-small cell lung cancer. *Chest*, 89:295–300.

Holmes EC, Gail M (1986). Lung Cancer Study Group: surgical adjuvant therapy for Stage II and III adenocarcinoma and large cell undifferentiated carcinoma. *Journal of Clinical Oncology*, 4:710–15.

Isobe H, *et al.* (1990). Prognostic and therapeutic significance of the flow cytometric nuclear DNA content in non-small cell lung cancer. *Cancer*, 65:1391–5.

Jensen LI, Hirsch FR, Peters K, Jensen F, Thomsen C (1992). Diagnosis of abdominal metastases in small cell carcinoma of the lung: a prospective study of computer tomography and ultrasonography. *Lung Cancer*, 8:37–46.

Johnson DH (1989). New drugs in the management of SCLC. *Lung Cancer*, 5:221–31.

Joss RA, Cavalli F, Goldbrush A, Brunner KW (1986). New drugs in small cell lung cancer. *Cancer Treatment Reviews*, 13:157–76.

Kaasa S, Lund E, Thorud E, Hatlevoll R, Höst H (1991). Symptomatic treatment versus combination chemotherapy for patients with extensive non-small cell lung cancer. *Cancer*, 67:2443–7.

Klastersky JA, Sculier J-P (1989). Intensive chemotherapy of SCLC. *Lung Cancer*, 5:196–206.

Klastersky J, Feld R, Kleisbauer JP, Rocmans P (1989). Treatment of N2 non-small cell lung cancer (NSCLC). *Chest*, 96 (Suppl.):83–5S.

Kottke TE, Battista RN, DeFriese GH, Brekke ML (1988). Attributes of successful smoking cessation interventions in medical practice. A meta-analysis of 39 controlled trials. *Journal of the American Medical Association*, **259**:2883–9.

Kristensen C, Kristjansen PEG, Hansen HH (1992). Systemic chemotherapy of brain metastases from small cell lung cancer (SCLC). *Journal of Clinical Oncology*. (In press.)

Le Chevalier T, *et al.* (1992). Significant effect of adjuvant chemotherapy on survival in locally advanced non-small-cell lung carcinoma. *Journal of the National Cancer Institute*, **84**:58.

Liang XM (1989). Accuracy of cytologic diagnosis and cytotyping of sputum in primary lung cancer: analysis of 161 cases. *Journal of Surgical Oncology*, **40**:107–11.

Loeb LA, Ernster VL, Warner KE, Abbots J, Laslo J (1984). Smoking and lung cancer: an overview. *Cancer Research*, **44**:5940–8.

Lubin JH, *et al.* (1984). Modifying risk of developing lung cancer by changing habits of cigarette smoking. *British Medical Journal*, **288**:1953–6.

Lung Cancer Study Group (1986). Effects of postoperative mediastinal radiation on completely resected stage II and stage III epidermoid cancer of the lung. *New England Journal of Medicine*, **315**:1377–81.

Lung Cancer Study Group (1988). The benefit of adjuvant treatments for resected local advanced non-small-cell lung cancer. *Journal of Clinical Oncology*, **6**:9–17.

McDuffie HH, Klaassen DJ, Dosman JA (1987). Female–male differences in patients with primary lung cancer. *Cancer*, **59**:1825–30.

Mackay B, Ordonez NG, Dugan CC (1989). Ultrastructural and morphometric studies of lung carcinomas. *Ultrastructural Pathology*, **13**:561–71.

Markos J, *et al.* (1989). Prospective assessment as a predictor of mortality and morbidity after lung cancer. *American Review of Respiratory Diseases*, **139**:902–10.

Matthews MJ, Kanhouwa S, Picken J, Robinette D (1973). Frequency of residual and metastatic tumor in patients undergoing curative surgical resection for lung cancer. *Cancer Chemotherapy Reports*, **4**:63–7.

Mattson K, Niivanew A, Pyrhönen S, Holsti LR, Holsti P, Kumpulanen E, Cantell K (1992). Natural alpha-interferon as maintenance therapy for small cell lung cancer. *European Journal of Cancer*, **28**:1387–91.

Menkes MS, Comstock GW, Vuilleumier JP, Helsing KJ, Rider AA, Brookmeyer R (1986). Serum beta-carotene, vitamins A and E, selenium, and the risk of lung cancer. *New England Journal of Medicine*, **315**:1250–5.

Merletti F, Heseltine E, Saracci R, Simonato L, Vainio H, Wilbourn J (1984). Target organs for carcinogenicity of chemicals and industrial exposures in humans: a review of results in the IARC Monographs on the Evaluation of the Carcinogenic Risk of Chemicals to Humans. *Cancer Research*, **44**:2244–50.

Miayke M, Taki T, Hitomi S, Hakomori S-I (1992). Correlation of expression of H/Le^y/Le^b antigens with survival in patients with carcinoma of the lung. *New England Journal of Medicine*, **327**:14–18.

Miller AB, Risch HA (1989). Diet and lung cancer. *Chest*, **96** (Suppl.):8–9.

Minna JD (1989). Genetic events in the pathogenesis of lung cancer. *Chest*, **96** (Suppl.):17–23S.

Morton RF, *et al.* (1991). Thoracic radiation therapy alone compared with combined chemoradiotherapy for locally unresectable non-small cell lung cancer. *Annals of Internal Medicine*, **115**:681–6.

Mountain CF (1986). A new international staging system for lung cancer. *Chest*, **4**:2255–335.

Muir CS, Waterhouse J, Mack T, Powell J, Whelan S (1987). *Cancer incidence in five continents*, Vol. V, IARC Scientific Publications No. 88. IARC, Lyon.

Mulshine JL, Natale RB, Avis I, Cuttita F (1989). Autocrine growth factors as therapeutic targets in lung cancer. *Chest*, **96** (Suppl.):31–4S.

Mulshine J, *et al.* (1990). Phase I study of an antigastrin releasing peptide (GRP) monoclonal antibody in patients with lung cancer. *Proceedings ASCO*, **9**:230.

Murray N, *et al.* for the National Cancer Institute of Canada Clinical Trials Group (1993). Importance of timing for thoracic irradiation in the combined modality treatment of limited-stage small-cell lung cancer. *Journal of Clinical Oncology*, **11**:336–44.

Naruke T (1989). Bronchoplastic and bronchovascular procedures of the tracheobronchial tree in the management of primary lung cancer. *Chest*, **96** (Suppl.):53–6S.

Naruke T, Goya T, Tsuchiya R, Suemasu K (1988). The importance of surgery to non-small cell carcinoma of lung with mediastinal lymph node metastasis. *Annals of Thoracic Surgery*, **46**:603–10.

Newaishy GA, Kerr GR (1989). Radical radiotherapy for bronchogenic carcinoma: five year survival rates. *Clinical Oncology*, **1**:80–6.

Nowell PC (1976). The clonal evolution of tumor cell populations. *Science*, **194**:23–8.

Østerlind K (1989). Alternating versus sequential chemotherapy in SCLC. *Lung Cancer*, **5**:173–7.

Pairolero PC (1989). Benign and malignant neoplasms of the trachea. In *Thoracic oncology* (ed. A Roth, JC Ruchdeschel, and TH Weisenburger), pp. 513–19. Saunders, Philadelphia.

Parkin DM, Läärä E, Muir CS (1988). Estimates of the worldwide frequency of sixteen major cancers in 1980. *International Journal of Cancer*, **41**:184–97.

Pastorino U, Berrino F, Gervasio A, Pesenti V, Riboli E, Crosignani P (1984). Proportion of lung cancers due to occupational exposure. *International Journal of Cancer*, **33**:231–7.

Payne D, *et al.* (1989). The role of thoracic radiation therapy in small cell carcinoma of the lung. *Lung Cancer*, **5**:135–8.

Pearse AGE (1969). The cytochemistry and ultrastructure of polypeptide producing cells of the APUD-series and the embryologic physiologic and pathologic implications of the concept. *Journal of Histochemistry and Cytochemistry*, **17**:303–13.

Pedersen AG, Kristjansen PEG, Hansen HH (1988). Prophylactic cranial irradiation in small cell lung cancer: a critical review. *Cancer Treatment Reports*, **15**:85–103.

Pedersen AG, *et al.* (1989). Management of CNS metastases in small cell lung cancer. *Lung Cancer*, **5**:140–2.

Pedersen-Bjergaard J, *et al.* (1985). Acute non-lymphocytic leukemia, preleukemia and solid tumors following intensive chemotherapy of small cell carcinoma in the lung. *Blood*, **66**:1393–7.

Perez CA (1985). Non-small cell carcinoma of the lung: dose–time parameters. *Cancer Treatment Symposium*, **2**:131–42.

Perez CA, *et al.* (1980). A prospective randomized study of various irradiation doses and fractionation schedules in the treatment of inoperable non-oat cell carcinoma of the lung. *Cancer*, **45**:2744–53.

Perry MC, *et al.* (1987). Chemotherapy with or without radiation therapy in limited small-cell carcinoma of the lung. *New England Journal of Medicine*, **316**:912.

Pignon J-P, *et al.* (1992). A meta-analysis of thoracic radiotherapy for small-cell lung cancer. *New England Journal of Medicine*, **327**:1618–24.

Pisani P, Berrino F, Macaluso M, Pastorino U, Crosignani P, Baldasseroni A (1986). Carrots, green vegetables and lung cancer: a case control study. *International Journal of Epidemiology*, **15**:463–8.

Poe RH, Tobin RE (1980). Sensitivity and specificity of needle biopsy in lung malignancy. *American Review of Respiratory Disease*, **122**:725–9.

Quoix E, *et al.* (1991). La chimiothérapie comportant du cisplatine estelle utile dans le cancer bronchique on microcellulaire au stade IV? Résultats d'une étude randomisée. *Bulletin Cancer*, **78**:341–6.

Radice PA, *et al.* (1982). The clinical behavior of 'mixed' small cell/large cell bronchogenic carcinoma compared to 'pure' small cell subtypes. *Cancer*, **50**:2894–2.

Rapp E, *et al.* (1988). Chemotherapy can prolong survival in patients with advanced non-small cell lung cancer—report of a Canadian multicenter randomized trial. *Journal of Clinical Oncology*, **6**:633.

Rodenhuis S, *et al.* (1987). Mutational activation of the K-*ras* oncogene: a possible pathogenetic factor in adenocarcinoma of the lung. *New England Journal of Medicine*, **317**:929–35.

Roed H, Vindeløv LL (1989). Can human small-cell lung cancer cell lines be applied for optimizing chemotherapy. In *Basic and clinical concepts of lung cancer* (ed. HH Hansen), pp. 151–72. Kluwer, Dordrecht.

Rosti G, *et al.* (1991). Long survivors in small cell lung cancer (SCLC): Italian report on 3245 cases. *Proceedings ASCO*, **10**:268.

Ruckdeschel JC (1988). Chemotherapy of disseminated non-small cell lung cancer. In *Lung cancer: a comprehensive treatise* (ed. JD Bitran, HM Golomb, AG Little, and RR Weischelbaum), pp. 233–41. Grune & Stratton, New York.

Sahin AA, *et al.* (1990). Flow cytometric analysis of the DNA content of non-small cell lung cancer. *Cancer*, **65**:530–7.

Salazar OM, *et al.* (1986). A prospective randomized trial comparing once-a-week VS daily radiation therapy for locally-advanced, non-metastatic lung cancer: a preliminary report. *International Journal of Radiation Oncology—Biology—Physics*, **12**:779–87.

Salvati F, Teodori L, Gagliardi L, Signora M, Aquilini M, Storniello G (1989). DNA flow cytometric studies of 66 human lung tumors analyzed before treatment. *Chest*, **96**:1092–8.

Salvatierra A, Baamonde C, Llama JM, Cruz F, Lopez-Pujol J (1990). Extrathoracic staging of bronchogenic carcinoma. *Chest*, **97**:1052–8.

Schaake-Koning C, *et al.* (1992). Effects of concomitant cisplatin and radiotherapy on inoperable non-small-cell lung cancer. *New England Journal of Medicine*, **326**:524–30.

Shimokata K, Niwa Y, Yamamoto M, Sasou H, Morishita M (1989). Pleural fluid neuron-specific enolase. A useful diagnostic marker for small cell lung cancer pleurisy. *Chest*, **95**:602–3.

Slebos RJ, Rodenhuis S (1989). The molecular genetics of human lung cancer. *European Respiratory Journal*, **2**:461–9.

Slevin *et al.* (1989). A randomized trial to evaluate the effect of schedule on the activity of etoposide in small-cell lung cancer. *Journal of Clinical Oncology*, **7**:1333–40.

Sørensen JB, Hirsch FR, Olsen J (1988). Prognostic implication of histologic subtyping of pulmonary adenocarcinoma according to the classification of World Health Organization. An analysis of 259 consecutive patients with advanced disease. *Cancer*, **62**:361–7.

Sørensen JB, Badsberg JH, Hansen HH (1989). Response to cytostatic treatment in inoperable adenocarcinoma of the lung: critical implications. *British Journal of Cancer*, **60**:389–93.

Souhami RL, Law K (1990). Longevity in small cell lung cancer: a report to the Lung Cancer Subcommittee of the United Kingdom. Coordinating Committees for Cancer Research. *British Journal of Cancer*, **61**:584–9.

Souhami RL, Beverley PCL, Bobrow L (ed.) (1988). Proceedings of the First International Workshop on the Small Cell Lung Cancer Antigens. *Lung Cancer*, **4**:1–116.

Spiro SG, Souhami RL (1990). Duration of chemotherapy in small cell lung cancer. *Thorax*, **1**:1–2.

Stahel RA (1989). Monoclonal antibodies in lung cancer. *Chest*, **96** (Suppl.):27–9S.

Stahel RA, *et al.* (1985). Detection of bone marrow metastases in small cell lung cancer by monoclonal antibody. *Journal of Clinical Oncology*, **3**:455–61.

Stahel R, *et al.* (1989). Staging and prognostic factors in small cell lung cancer. *Lung Cancer*, **5**:119–26.

Stanley K, Stjernswärd J (1989). Lung cancer in developed and developing countries. In *Basic and clinical concepts of lung cancer* (ed. HH Hansen), pp. 1–14. Kluwer, Dordrecht.

Strauss GM, Langer MP, Elias AD, Skarin AT, Sugarbaker DJ (1992). Multimodality treatment of stage IIIA non-small-cell lung carcinoma: a critical review of the literature and strategies for future research. *Journal of Clinical Oncology*, **10**:829–38.

Veake D, *et al.* (1988). Prospective evaluation of fine needle aspiration in the diagnosis of lung cancer. *Thorax*, **43**:540–4.

Vindeløv LL, *et al.* (1980). Clonal heterogeneity of small-cell anaplastic carcinoma of the lung demonstrated by flow cytometric DNA analysis. *Cancer Research*, **40**:4295–300.

Vindeløv L, Hansen HH, Spang-Thomsen M (1985). Growth characteristics and heterogeneity of small cell carcinoma of the lung: recent results. *Cancer Research*, **97**:47–54.

Watkin SW (1989). Temporal demographic and epidemiologic variation in histologic subtypes of lung cancer: a literature review. *Lung Cancer*, **5**:69–81.

Williams DE, *et al.* (1981). Survival of patients surgically treated for stage I lung cancer. *Journal of Thoracic and Cardiovascular Surgery*, **82**:70–6.

Wolf M, *et al.* (1987). Cisplatin/etoposide versus iphosphamide/etoposide combination chemotherapy in small cell lung cancer: a general randomized trial. *Journal of Clinical Oncology*, **5**:1880–6.

Woods RL, Williams CJ, Levi J, Page J (1990). A randomized trial of cisplatin/vindesine versus supportive care only in advanced non-small cell lung cancer. *British Journal of Cancer*, **61**:608–11.

World Health Organization (1981). *Histological typing of lung tumors* (2nd edn), *International histological classification of tumors, 1*. WHO, Geneva.

Wu AH, Henderson BE, Pike MC, Yu MC (1985). Smoking and other risk factors for lung cancer in women. *Journal of the National Cancer Institute*, **74**:747–51.

Zhang HX, *et al.* (1989). Curative radiotherapy of early operable non-small cell lung cancer (RTO 00544). *Radiotherapy and Oncology*, **14**:89–95.

11.2 Mesothelioma

DEIRDRE C. T. WATSON

Mesotheliomata are rare tumours which arise from serosal surfaces and are therefore seen in the pleura, pericardium, peritoneum, testis, ovary, and atrioventricular node. Diffuse malignant pleural mesothelioma is the most common form, occurring more than three times as frequently as peritoneal mesothelioma, but deaths from all types of mesothelioma occur in only 12.5 people per million.

It is one of the more difficult malignancies to diagnose and, once diagnosed, to treat successfully. The difficulty in diagnosis is partly because unusual diagnoses do not always occur to the physician, and partly because its histological features are so variable.

EPIDEMIOLOGY AND AETIOLOGY

The occurrence of mesotheliomata in people who have previously been exposed to asbestos was first described in 1960 in the asbestos mining areas of South Africa. Since then an epidemic of mesothelioma has been noted in workers using asbestos in North America, western Europe, and Australia. Those at highest risk are employed in the asbestos industry itself, shipyard workers, industrial workers involved with insulation and boiler work, and people employed in the demolition and building industries. The use of asbestos as insulation in railway carriages, for gas masks during the Second World War, and in motor vehicle brake parts has also been associated with a higher incidence of mesothelioma than expected in the workers involved in these industries.

Crocidolite, also known as Cape blue asbestos, is the principal tumorigenic form of asbestos but amosite, which is also produced in South Africa, has also been incriminated in a few cases. Chrysotile has a different crystalline structure from other asbestos and has not been shown to be a causative factor in mesothelioma.

The tumorigenicity of the asbestos fibres has been shown to be related to their physical shape and size. The fibres of crocidolite are straight, up to 30 μm in length with a diameter of less than 0.2 μm; in animal experiments using asbestos and other fibres only those that conform to this structure have been shown to be tumorigenic. A non-asbestos fibre known as erionite found in central Turkey has similar dimensions and mesothelioma is relatively common in the natives of that area.

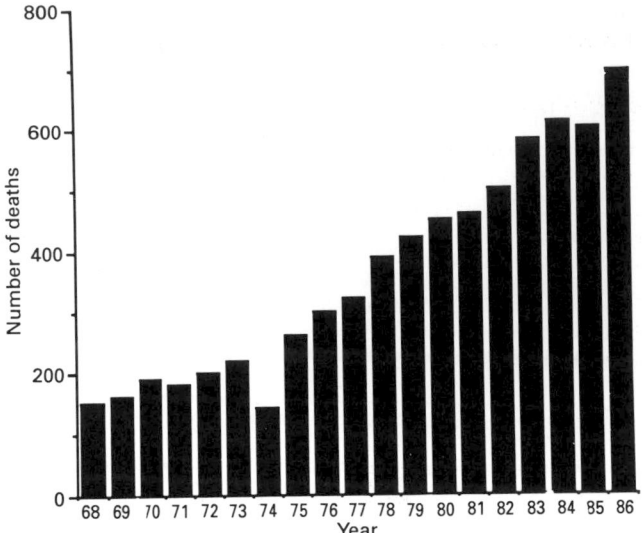

Fig. 1 The number of deaths from mesothelioma in England and Wales 1968–86 (from *Hansard*).

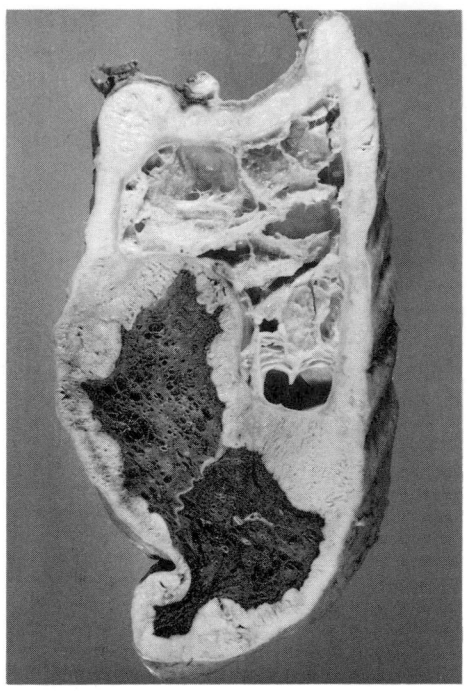

Fig. 2 An autopsy specimen showing extensive pleural mesothelioma with chest wall impression and a loculated basal effusion. Note the involved diaphragm inferiorly.

In spite of the close association between asbestos exposure and the development of mesothelioma, usually at least 20 years elapse after exposure before the development of the tumour. There are approximately 30 per cent of mesothelioma patients in whom no evidence of asbestos can be found.

The incidence of mesothelioma in the United Kingdom is approximately 12.5 cases per million (1986) with the majority in males, presumably because of their industrial exposure. The incidence is higher (39.5 per million) in shipyard areas (Hulks *et al.* 1989). The incidence of the disease has shown a steady rise over the past 20 years (Fig. 1) and this has been mirrored in the United States. It has been estimated there that the peak incidence will occur between 1990 and 1994 and that a gradual decline will then take place as the effects of more rigorous controls to prevent industrial asbestos exposure are seen (Walker *et al.* 1983).

Exposure to asbestos is also associated with other pleural and lung disease, in particular carcinoma of the lung. In asbestos-exposed smokers the risk of lung carcinoma is between 50 and 100 times higher than in smokers without asbestos exposure, but this additive carcinogenic effect has not been demonstrated for mesothelioma (Berry *et al.* 1985).

PATHOLOGY
Gross pathology
Pleural

There are two types of mesothelioma: the localized, which may be benign or malignant and frequently arises from the visceral pleura as a pendunculated mass and the diffuse. The latter is always malignant and starts as nodules on the parietal and visceral pleura. These eventually coalesce and envelop the underlying lung. The tumour is usually imprinted by the overlying chest wall unless the latter has been invaded. Similarly the underlying lung is usually only invaded superficially until the very late stages of the disease. Direct invasion of the diaphragm and mediastinum is common and may extend into the peritoneum and contralateral hemithorax. The tumour varies in consistency from gritty to gelatinous and is usually greyish in colour. There may be associated hyaline pleural plaques but there is no evidence that these, which are common in

asbestos-exposed individuals, are pre-malignant. There is frequently a pleural effusion which, when associated with the diffuse malignant disease, is often loculated and haemorrhagic.

Pericardial

The pericardium is most frequently involved by direct extension from adjacent pleural mesothelioma but a few tumours arise *de novo* on the parietal pericardium.

Microscopic pathology
Benign mesothelioma

These are rare tumours and there has been considerable histological variation amongst the tumours that have been reported. Three types have been described: cellular varieties with spindle-shaped cells, collagenous, and hyaline types (Burrig and Kastendick 1984), but in another series (Okike *et al.* 1978) all the tumours showed a whorled cut surface with spindle-shaped cells of variable density. The tumour is usually covered by a layer of mesothelial cells.

Malignant mesothelioma

There are three main types of malignant pleural mesothelioma: epithelial, sarcomatous, and mixed. Approximately two-thirds of diffuse tumours are epithelial (Suzuke 1980) but in the rarer localized malignant tumours the sarcomatous type predominates (Okike *et al.* 1978).

The epithelial tumours may form well-differentiated tumours, exhibiting a tubular–papillary pattern with cystic spaces lined by cuboidal or flattened cells with uniform vesicular nuclei, to poorly differentiated ones made up of sheets of cells which may be arranged in rests or cords (Adams and Unni 1984). The well-differentiated forms mimic carcinoma (Burns *et al.* 1985). The sarcomatous or fibrous type of mesothelioma contains spindle-shaped cells amongst

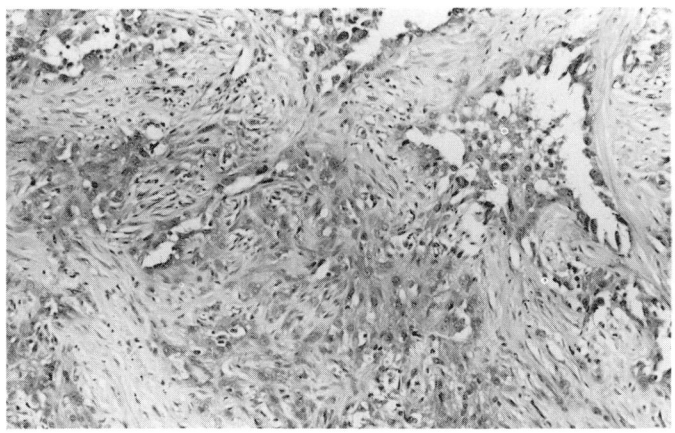

Fig. 3 A mixed tumour, showing an epithelial area with cystic spaces and tubular–papillary pattern (broad arrow) and a sarcomatous area (narrow arrow).

hyaline material which may be very difficult to distinguish from a secondary sarcoma.

PRESENTATION

Pleural malignant mesothelioma

The majority of patients presenting with malignant pleural mesothelioma have rather non-specific complaints of gradually worsening symptoms. The symptoms usually relate to progressive pleural disease with or without effusion and are thus of a vague ache involving one side of the chest which eventually progresses to pain. The discomfort or pain is not pleuritic in nature, is diffuse, and may radiate to the abdomen, shoulder, or back. Since the symptoms are vague, the patients may have had them some time before seeking medical advice and, because of the pain referral, pleural disease is not always suspected initially.

Progression of the pleural mesothelioma or development of an effusion results in shortness of breath and a non-productive cough and these are the most common presenting symptoms after pain.

Rarely the presenting symptoms arise as a result of the invasion of mediastinal structures (Brenner *et al.* 1982). Dysphagia, hoarseness (secondary to recurrent laryngeal nerve palsy), superior vena caval obstruction, and Horner's syndrome are such examples and paraplegia from invasion of the spinal canal has been seen (Cooper 1974).

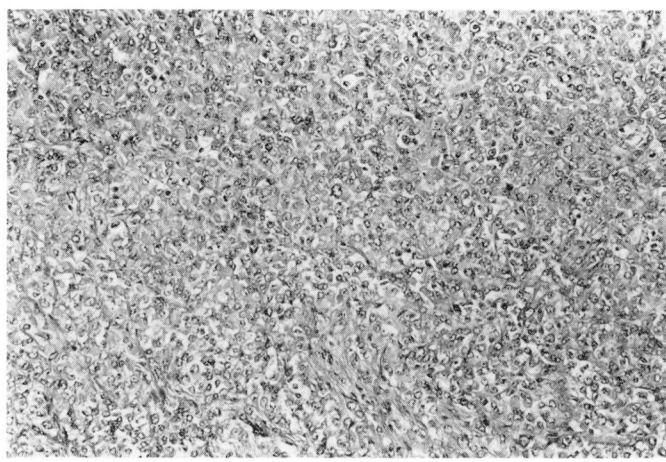

Fig. 4 A poorly differentiated mesothelioma.

Distant metastatic disease is always late in malignant mesothelioma and is rarely responsible for the presenting symptoms.

Pericardial

Primary malignant mesothelioma of the pericardium usually presents with the features of constrictive pericarditis or tamponade, but there may be a febrile element. This is seen most often in children and the diagnosis is often difficult because of the more common pericardial involvement by metastatic tumours. In adults the pericardium is most frequently invaded directly by a pleural or even peritoneal mesothelioma rather than being the original site of the disease.

Benign mesothelioma

Usually found in adults, these rare tumours are often pedunculated and 80 per cent of them arise from the visceral pleura.

The majority are detected as asymptomatic lesions on a chest radiograph, but as they grow they compress the lung, an effusion develops, and the patient may then present with dyspnoea.

Clubbing and hypertrophic pulmonary osteoarthropathy occur with large tumours and a few patients present because of inappropriate hormone secretion leading to hypoglycaemia (Nelson *et al.* 1975) or hyponatraemia (Perks *et al.* 1979).

INVESTIGATIONS AND DIAGNOSIS

Computerized tomography (CT) will provide far more detail of the parietal and pleural involvement than conventional chest radiography (Fig. 5). It may show involvement of the underlying lung and will demonstrate the presence of discrete nodules or masses (Fig. 6). If these are parenchymal, the diagnosis is more likely to be that of metastatic carcinoma or an underlying pulmonary carcinoma. The CT scan will also demonstrate the presence of fluid and will show extension of the disease process to the pericardium and contralateral hemithorax. Involvement of the peritoneum is difficult to detect in its early stages except by CT scanning.

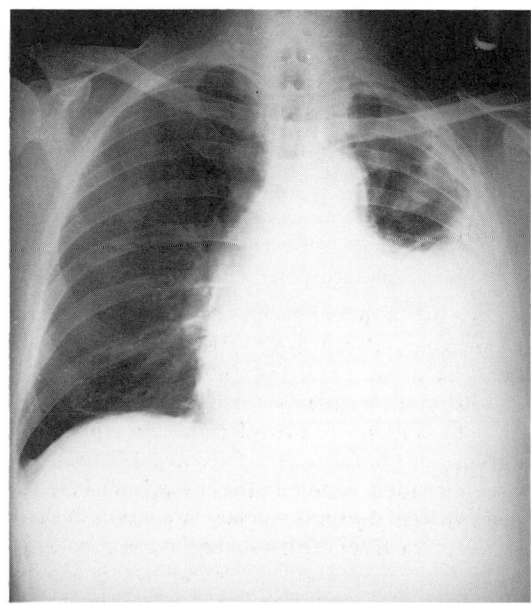

Fig. 5 Chest radiograph, showing left pleural nodules and effusion.

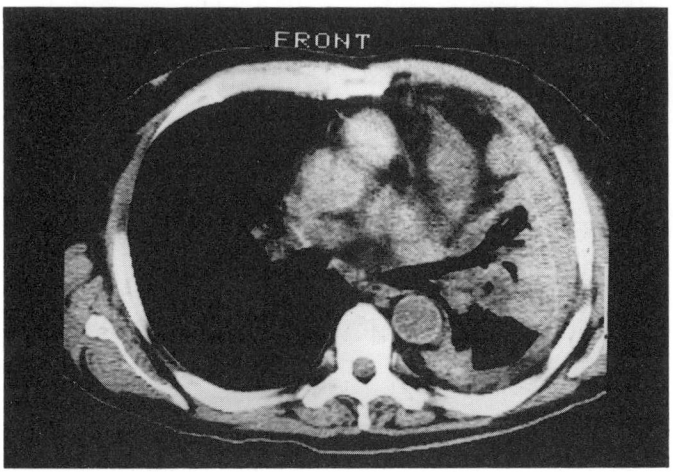

Fig. 6 A CT scan showing parietal pleural nodules and generalized thickening.

CT evidence of extensive pleural tumour is suggestive of malignant mesothelioma, but there are no specific signs and histological confirmation is necessary.

In patients presenting with a pleural effusion, cytological examination of the effusion, which is usually an exudate and is blood-stained in 50 per cent of cases, may provide the diagnosis. A pleural biopsy taken at the time of aspiration may also give the diagnosis, but histological uncertainty is a characteristic of this disease. Thoracoscopy or open pleural biopsy may be necessary to provide sufficient material for the histopathologist to make a diagnosis. In many patients with a combination of diffuse pleural thickening, with or without effusion, pain, and general debility, in the absence of primary disease elsewhere, invasive efforts to obtain histological proof are deferred to the time of autopsy. The main differential diagnosis is that of secondary malignant involvement of the pleura from tumours of the lung, breast, or ovary and is far more common than mesothelioma.

The site and timing of biopsy are bones of contention in some circles because of the well-publicized propensity for malignant mesothelioma to spread along needle tracks or incisions. Cutaneous deposits are not uncommon in patients who have had no invasive procedure and their appearance in those who have them may simply be coincidental, so the possible risk is not a reason to omit making a histological diagnosis.

STAGING

Butchart *et al.* (1976) suggested a staging for malignant mesothelioma (Table 1). Modifications incorporated by Chahanian (1982) resulted in a proposed TNM classification. CT scanning is essential for proper staging.

Table 1 Clinicopathological staging of diffuse malignant mesothelioma

Stage	
I	Tumour confined to ipsilateral pleura, lung, and pericardium
II	Tumour invading chest wall or involving mediastinal structures, for example oesophagus, heart, and opposite pleura
	Lymph node involvement within the chest
III	Tumour penetrating diaphragm to involve peritoneum directly
	Lymph node involvement outside the chest
IV	Distant blood-borne metastases

Stage I disease is that limited to the parietal and visceral pleura, with or without effusion. Invasion of the diaphragm or endothoracic fascia or involvement of hilar nodes is stage II disease and more extensive chest wall invasion or mediastinal involvement, either direct or nodal, becomes stage III. Direct extension beyond the hemithorax or metastatic disease is designated stage IV.

As in all types of malignant disease, accurate staging is essential to allow comparisons to be made between different treatments, but need only be undertaken if treatment is to be offered or if the patient is part of a study. Thus, palliative radiotherapy is useful in relieving the symptoms of superior vena caval obstruction, dysphagia, and dyspnoea due to major airway compression in approximately 66 per cent of patients so treated.

MANAGEMENT

Localized benign mesothelioma

These present as discrete but sometimes large masses in one hemithorax and should be excised surgically. No additional therapy is required since recurrence is extremely rare.

Pericardial mesothelioma

Primary pericardial mesothelioma is extremely rare and never amenable to curative resection. Parietal pericardiectomy may be indicated to relieve constriction or tamponade (Sytman and MacAlpin 1971).

Diffuse malignant pleural mesothelioma

The progression of this disease is inexorable and, except for the very rare early or localized case, treatment is palliative rather than curative.

Surgery

A variety of surgical procedures have been tried, with variable success and some have achieved long-term cures. Even in patients with apparently early disease extensive surgical excision has failed to control the disease completely. The two main surgical options, apart from simple biopsy, are parietal pleurectomy and extrapleural pneumonectomy with excision of the diaphragm and pericardium *en bloc*.

The latter is an extensive procedure and carries an operative mortality rate of approximately 12 per cent in the best hands. In all published series the patients undergoing pleuropneumonectomy have a lengthy post-operative course with its associated morbidity and, because of the variable behaviour of these tumours, the exact benefit in terms of increased survival is difficult to estimate. However, Worn (1974) did compare 248 patients who had either pleurectomy or extrapleural pneumonectomy with 128 patients managed conservatively. Of the surgical group, 9 per cent were alive at 5 years, compared with none alive at 18 months in the conservative group. There was no significant difference in survival between the two types of surgical treatment. Pleurectomy is successful in the palliation of dyspnoea due to effusion and pain, but the latter returns with continuing tumour growth (DeLaria *et al.* 1978; McCormack *et al.* 1982). Similar palliation is achieved in the extrapleural pneumonectomy group, although the post-operative mortality and the higher incidence of serious post-operative complications such as bronchopleural fistula mean that its use is restricted to curative attempts in early disease or as part of treatment protocols in controlled clinical trials.

Radiotherapy

Since malignant pleural mesothelioma is usually a diffuse disease, the use of radiotherapy has been limited until recently because it was impossible to avoid high-dose irradiation of the underlying lung. With more modern computer-assisted planning and computer-controlled dynamic techniques it is possible to deliver a uniform dose to the pleural tumour while sparing the underlying tissue. Conventional doses to the apex and diaphragm can be delivered using parallel opposing field, but to date palliation of symptoms is only temporary and survival patterns are unchanged.

Chemotherapy

The use of chemotherapeutic agents in diffuse malignant mesothelioma has been limited because of disappointing results *in vivo* and *in vitro*. All published studies have been inadequate because of the small numbers of patients admitted (due to the rarity of the disease), inadequate staging, and errors in diagnosis. The drugs with the most activity are doxorubicin, cyclophosphamide, mitomycin, and cisplatin.

In many studies using single agents as well as combination or cross-over therapy, there has been a large proportion of patients with no demonstrable response. The patients who do show a measurable response have had improved survival (Samson *et al.* 1985).

Systemic chemotherapy should not be used in the routine treatment of patients with mesothelioma until randomized studies have demonstrated their usefulness.

Intrapleural bleomycin has been shown to have some effect on the control of symptoms of pleural effusion but does not otherwise alter the course of the disease (Law *et al.* 1984).

Combined modality treatments

Surgery and radiotherapy

External-beam radiotherapy or implantation techniques have been used to treat residual disease after surgical debulking. In the best series from the Memorial Hospital in New York (Karakousis *et al.* 1980) the median survival of 41 patients treated after pleurectomy was 21 months, with 65 per cent of patients alive at 1 year and 40 per cent at 2 years.

Radiotherapy and chemotherapy

No randomized studies of any size have been reported, but the Eastern Co-operative Oncology Group has a study in progress comparing radiotherapy alone with radiotherapy followed by doxorubicin 60 mg/m^2 every 3 weeks to a maximum dose of 420 mg/m^2.

Surgery, radiotherapy, and chemotherapy

After pleurectomy, external radiation, and systemic chemotherapy, Martini *et al.* (1975) achieved a 1 year survival rate of 79 per cent and Wanebo *et al.* (1976) improved a mean survival of 14 months for epithelioid tumours treated by pneumonectomy and radiotherapy to 30 months by adding systemic chemotherapy. The equivalent figures for sarcomatous tumours were 16 and 20 months, respectively. The results from all forms and combinations of treatment are disappointing, although pleurectomy provides useful palliation of pleural effusion and, in the early case, may be followed by combined radio- and chemotherapy to improve the quality and length of life. However, for the majority of patients with diffuse malignant mesothelioma who are diagnosed late in the course of the disease, the mainstay of management is the support of the patient and his or her family. The course of the disease is inexorable, with inanition and pain being the main problems. These are best treated by the combined efforts of the terminal-care team experienced in providing pain relief and psychological support.

REFERENCES

Adams VI, Unni K (1984). Diffuse malignant mesothelioma of pleura: diagnostic criteria based on an autopsy study. *American Journal of Clinical Pathology*, **82**:15.

Ashcroft T, Barnsley WC, Butchart EG, Holden MP (1976). Pleuropneumonectomy in the management of diffuse malignant mesothelioma of the pleura. Experience with 29 patients. *Thorax*, **31**:15.

Baker L, Borden E, Samson M, Wanebo H, Wasser L (1985). Randomised comparison of cyclophosphamide DTIC and adriamycin (CIA) versus cyclophosphamide and adriamycin (CA) in patients with advanced malignant mesothelioma. A sarcoma intergroup study (meeting abstract C-448). *Proceedings of the American Society of Clinical Oncology*, **4**:128.

Beattie EJ, Hilaris B, Martini N, Melamed MR, Wanebo HJ (1976). Pleural mesothelioma. *Cancer*, **38**:2481.

Berry G, Newhouse ML, Antonis P (1985). Combined effect of asbestos and smoking on mortality from lung cancer and mesothelioma in factory workers. *British Journal of Industrial Medicine*, **42**:12.

Brenner J, Golbey RB, Magill GP, Sordillo PP (1982). Malignant mesothelioma of the pleura: review of 123 patients. *Cancer*, **49**:2431.

Burman SO, Cantave I, Chertow BS, Kiani R, Nelson R, Shah J (1975). Hypoglycemic coma associated with benign pleural mesothelioma. *Journal of Thoracic and Cardiovascular Surgery*, **69**:306.

Burns TR, *et al.* (1985). Ultrastructural diagnosis of epithelial malignant mesothelioma. *Cancer*, **56**:2036.

Burrig KF, Kastendick H (1984). Ultrastructural observations on the histogenesis of localized fibrous tumours of the pleura (benign mesothelioma). *Virchows Archive—Pathological Anatomy*, **403**:413.

Butchart EG, *et al.* (1976). Pleuropneumonectomy in the management of diffuse malignant mesothelioma of the pleura: experience with 29 patients. *Thorax*, **31**:15.

Chahanian AP (1982). Malignant mesothelioma. In *Clinical interpretation and practice of cancer chemotherapy* (ed. EM Greenspan). Raven Press, New York.

Cooper D (1974). Malignant mesothelioma invading the spinal canal. *Postgraduate Medical Journal*, **50**:718.

DeLaria GA, Faber P, Jensik R, Kittle CF (1978). Surgical management of malignant mesothelioma. *Annals of Thoracic Surgery*, **26**:375.

Dreyer NA, Friedlander ER, Loughlin JE, Rothman KJ, Walker AM (1983). Projections of asbestos related disease. 1980–2009. *Journal of Occupational Medicine*, **25**:409.

Hilaris BS, McCormack PM, Martini N, Negasaki F (1982). Surgical treatment of pleural mesothelioma. *Journal of Thoracic and Cardiovascular Surgery*, **84**:834.

Hulks G, Thomas JStJ, Waclawski E (1989). Malignant pleural mesothelioma in Western Glasgow 1980–6. *Thorax*, **44**:496.

Karakousis P, Seddiq M, Moore R (1980). Malignant mesothelioma and chemotherapy. *Journal of Surgical Oncology*, **15**:181.

Law MR, Hodson ME, Turner-Warwick M (1984). Malignant mesothelioma of the pleura: clinical aspects and symptomatic treatment. *European Journal of Respiratory Diseases*, **65**:1628.

McCormack PM, *et al.* (1982). Surgical treatment of pleural mesothelioma. *Journal of Thoracic and Cardiovascular Surgery*, **84**:834.

Martini N, Bains MS, Beattie EJ (1975). Indications for pleurectomy in malignant effusion. *Cancer*, **35**:734.

Nelson R, *et al.* (1975). Hypoglycemic coma associated with benign pleural mesothelioma. *Journal of Thoracic and Cardiovascular Surgery*, **69**:306.

Okike N, Bernatz PE, Woolner LB (1978). Localized mesothelioma of the pleura. *Journal of Thoracic and Cardiovascular Surgery*, **75**:363.

Perks WH, Stanhope R, Green M (1979). Hyponatremia and mesothelioma. *British Journal of Diseases of the Chest*, **78**:89.

Samson M, *et al.* (1985). Randomized comparison of cyclophosphamide, DTIC, and adriamycin (CIA) vs. cyclophosphamide and adriamycin (CA) in patients with advanced malignant mesothelioma: a sarcoma intergroup study (meeting abstract C-498). *Proceedings of the American Society of Clinical Oncology*, **4**:128.

Suzuke Y (1980). Pathology of human malignant mesothelioma. *Seminars in Oncology*, **8**:268.

Sytman A, MacAlpin R (1971). Primary pericardial mesothelioma: report of two cases and review of the literature. *American Heart Journal*, **81**:760.

Walker AM, *et al.* (1983). Projections of asbestos related disease 1980–2009. *Journal of Occupational Medicine*, **25**:409.

Wanebo JH (1976). Pleural mesothelioma. *Cancer*, **38**:2481.

Worn H (1974). Möglichkeiten und Ergebnisse der chirurgischen Behandlung des malignen Pleuramesothelioms. *Thorax Chirugie*, **22**:391.

11.3 Thymic tumours with myasthenia gravis or bone-marrow dyscrasias

NICHOLAS WILLCOX

Myasthenia gravis is an important diagnosis to consider for practical reasons in patients with mediastinal tumours and its effective treatment has immediate practical importance. Its association with thymoma also poses a fascinating theoretical challenge to the immunologist. Thymoma is rare overall, but occurs in approximately 10 per cent of all myasthenics in the United Kingdom and United States of America and is the only neoplasm that is consistently associated with myasthenia gravis. It is normally slow growing and of low-grade malignancy, although its clinical behaviour is not always predictable. Blood spread is very rare, while pleural metastases occur in approximately 5 per cent of cases and the myasthenia is usually the principal problem in day-to-day management. The association with myasthenia gravis is particularly interesting as the normal thymus is the primary site of T lymphocyte generation and it is intriguing to speculate on how epithelial tumours there might lead to this classic autoantibody-mediated disease or indeed to other autoimmune complications, especially selective bone-marrow aplasias. Finally, there is a wealth of specific monoclonal antibodies to various thymic epithelial and lymphoid cell subsets that are potentially valuable both in histological diagnosis and in imaging or targeted immunotherapy.

PATIENT SUBGROUPS, AETIOLOGY, AND AUTOANTIBODIES IN MYASTHENIA GRAVIS

In the United Kingdom, thymoma patients constitute one of the four main subgroups of myasthenia gravis cases (Table 1). However, in Japan and Taiwan, predominantly ocular muscle weakness ('ocular myasthenia gravis') starting at a very early age (< 10 years) generates a fifth non-thymomatous subset that largely replaces the European post-pubertal peak (Compston *et al.* 1980; Chiu *et al.* 1987) and may imply differences in provoking factors in these countries. In Caucasians with a thymoma, symptoms of myasthenia gravis may begin at any age from 15 to 80 years, perhaps with some female bias after the age of 50 years (Verley and Hollman 1985), but with no obvious genetic association (Table 1; Rosai and Levine 1976). There is also no striking increase in antibodies to common viruses (Klavinskis *et al.* 1985). However, in the Far East, where thymoma apparently occurs in a higher proportion of cases, there are hints that Epstein–Barr virus is implicated in its aetiology (McGuire *et al.* 1988; but see also Wu and Kuo 1993). Japanese myasthenics with thymoma show the same immunoglobulin heavy-chain gene

Table 1 Subgroups of myasthenia gravis patients

		Thymoma absent		
	Thymoma present	Early onset[a]	Late onset	Ocular myasthenia gravis
Patients (percentage in Caucasians)	10–15	50	15	10–15
Age at onset (years)	20–70	2–40	40–70	10–70
Predominant HLA association (percentage; Caucasians)[b]	None (*n*=45)	HLA-A1 (66) -B8 (78) -DR3 (68)	HLA-A3 (37) -B7 (42) -DR2 (37)	None (*n*=40)
Predominant Gm association[d] (Japanese)	1 : 2 : 21	1 : 2 : 21	nd	Insufficient cases
Anti-AChR titre (percentage of patients positive)	High (100)	High (100)	Moderate (90)	Low (60)
Antistriated muscle antibody (percentage of patients positive)[c]	92	21	50	23

[a]This subgroup typically shows 'hyperplasia' in the thymic medulla.
[b]Newsom-Davis, J., Lang, C., and Willcox, N., unpublished.
[c]From Compston *et al.* (1980).
[d]From Nakao *et al.* (1980); Gm, IgG heavy-chain allotypes.
nd, not done.

association as in those without (Table 1). Apart from that, little is known of the aetiology of thymoma: the genesis of the associated autoimmunity is discussed later.

The autoantibodies responsible for the clinical weakness

Myasthenics with a thymoma almost always have generalized muscle weakness very similar to that in the two other major patient subsets (see below), thus the combination of purely extraocular muscle involvement with low autoantibody levels (Table 1) is very rarely associated with a thymoma. Myasthenia gravis is characterized by IgG autoantibodies to the acetylcholine receptor in the postsynaptic muscle membrane. They are usually readily detectable in the serum by a highly sensitive radioimmunoassay and are very heterogeneous (Willcox and Vincent 1988). They lead to a reduced number of functional acetylcholine receptors which is sufficient to account for the patient's weakness and they do so via three main mechanisms. Activation of complement results in endplate damage and, ultimately, in simplification of the normally convoluted synaptic folds. Antibodies that can cross-link adjacent acetylcholine receptor molecules may accelerate the normal very slow degradation of the acetylcholine receptors and certain antibodies in some cases may cause a pharmacological block of transmitter binding or actions (Willcox and Vincent 1988). In addition, almost all cases of myasthenia gravis with a thymoma have autoantibodies to striational muscle antigens (Table 1; Aarli et al. 1981, 1990) that are probably coincidental, but may rarely produce a myopathic picture. Possible contributions of the thymoma to the generation of these autoantibodies are discussed later.

THE ORIGIN OF THE THYMOMA CELLS

The normal thymus

The thymus develops as a pair of buds from the third and fourth pharyngeal pouches, which migrate caudally to the upper anterior mediastinum (reviewed by von Gaudecker 1986; Lampert and Ritter 1988). It is thus an epithelial organ and, during fetal life, it is colonized in waves by stem cells, initially from the liver but then from the bone-marrow (second trimester into adulthood). Substantial numbers of liver- or bone-marrow-derived macrophages and interdigitating reticular 'dendritic' cells appear very early, but they are greatly outnumbered by immature T lymphocytes, that is, cortical thymocytes, which are generated initially near the outermost (subcapsular) epithelium from immigrant 'pre-T' stem cells (reviewed by Janossy et al. 1989). At about this stage the several gene segments encoding the T-cell antigen-recognizing receptors are rearranged and these clonally unique products are expressed in the cytoplasm and then on the surface. Soon these thymocytes become enmeshed in the quite distinct deeper network of cortical epithelium, which expresses HLA class I and II antigens and apparently selectively expands those clones that can subsequently recognize foreign antigens in the context of self-class I or -class II (reviewed by Sprent et al. 1988). As the nascent T-cells then emerge into the medulla, potentially autoaggressive clones are apparently deleted, probably on contact with the dendritic cells, though the cortical or even the medullary epithelium (which is similar to the subcapsular) may also be involved (Sprent et al. 1988). Finally, the surviving mature T-cells are released into the periphery, while the great majority that die during these 'positive and negative

selection' steps are destroyed by macrophages resident in both cortex and medulla.

Thymoma pathology

The associated tumour in myasthenia gravis is nearly always an epithelial thymoma. Interestingly, this typically retains the capacity to generate T lymphocytes, sometimes in such great numbers as to obscure its epithelial nature and justifying its 'lymphoepithelial' label (Willcox et al. 1987; Willcox 1989).

The gross features of thymomata are very variable (see preceding chapter); in colour, they range from fawn to grey or pink and, in consistency, from hard, fibrotic, and even calcified through tough and rubbery to soft and cerebelloid. They are usually encapsulated and may be lobulated and/or partly cystic (Rosai and Levine 1976). They may contain haemorrhagic or necrotic areas, and range from approximately 2000 cm^3 (Rosai and Levine 1976) to microscopic size (Pescarmona et al. 1992).

There are numerous histological classifications of thymomata (Rosai and Levine 1976, see below), but, in most cases of myasthenia gravis, the overall appearances are of disorganized cortex, with disrupted islands of epithelial network (see below) in an ocean of densely packed thymocytes. These mainly have the characteristic markers of typical cortical thymocytes (Fig. 1; reviewed by Willcox et al. 1987). Furthermore, in cell suspension, they are clearly not monoclonal as judged by the heterogeneous rearrangements of their T-cell receptor DNA segments (Katzin et al. 1988). In the numerous perivascular spaces and in areas resembling normal medulla, lymphocytes are usually more loosely packed and express the markers of mature T-cells (CD3$^+$, CD1$^-$). These could be generated in the thymoma or could be blood-borne immigrants.

The neoplastic cell type

The epithelial cells (by both nuclear morphological and immuno-histological criteria) simultaneously express some or all of the features of the normally distinct cortical and subcapsular epithelia (Figs 1 and 2), often in unusual combinations seen rarely, if at all, in the normal thymus (Willcox et al. 1987). Moreover, these combinations may be very variable within a single tumour as well as between patients. These findings are consistent with the widely held view that the neoplasm does indeed arise from epithelial cells rather than from the extremely abundant, but phenotypically normal lymphocytes. They further suggest to us that these diverse epithelial cells are derived from a single tumour stem cell type with combined subcapsular/cortical features (Willcox et al. 1987) that might correspond to a rare common ancestor of all thymic epithelium (Lampert and Ritter 1988; see also Fukai et al. 1992). Even when thymomata comprise almost pure spindle cells, the phenotype is similar (Willcox et al. 1987).

Immunohistological appearances are very similar in pleural deposits (Willcox et al. 1987; Kirchner and Müller-Hermelink 1989) and so was routine histopathology in a tibial metastasis in one case (Batata et al. 1974). Our interpretation is that the metastatic deposits are primarily epithelial and are colonized by blood-borne pre-lymphoid stem cells from which typical cortical lymphocytes are subsequently generated. In one case, our ability to identify these and the epithelial cells with specific monoclonal antibodies established that the tumour indeed derived from the original thymoma rather than from a new lymphoma as at first suspected (Willcox et al. 1987).

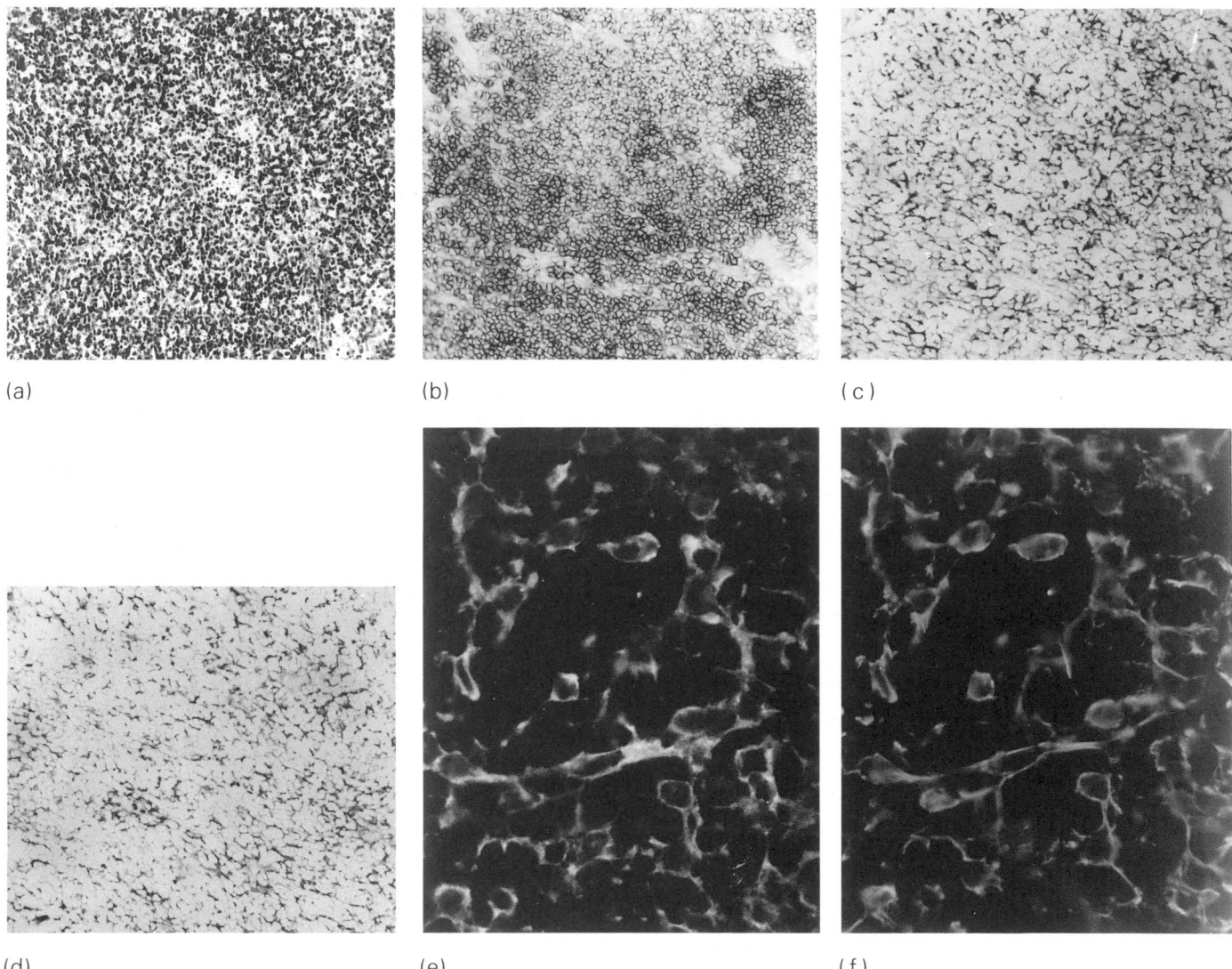

(a)   (b)   (c)

(d)   (e)   (f)

Fig. 1 Sections of a myasthenia gravis thymoma (a) stained with haematoxylin and eosin and (b–d) stained by immunoperoxidase, using monoclonal antibodies. Small CD1$^+$ thymocytes are very numerous (b), while most of the epithelium labels with antibodies to cortical (c, MR6) and subcapsular epithelium (d, Leu-7). In another myasthenia gravis thymoma, most epithelial cells label simultaneously with antibodies to cortical (e, MR6) and medullary/subcapsular epithelium (f, MR19) (by immunofluorescence). (Reproduced from Willcox et al. (1987), with permission.)

Classification and prognosis

Table 2 summarizes the main conclusions from an important clinicopathological study of 200 thymoma cases by Verley and Hollman (1985). As others have found, the commonest histological type showing bone-marrow aplasias was the spindle cell tumour (type 1), whereas for myasthenia gravis it was either the lymphocyte-rich (type 2) or the predominantly epithelial thymoma (type 3, with variable lymphocyte numbers). A somewhat different view of the lymphocyte-rich tumours was taken by Kirchner and Müller-Hermelink (1989), who particularly focused on the relative proportions of cortical- and medullary-type areas in them. They recognized a spectrum ranging from almost purely cortical (approximately 20 per cent of cases) to medullary subtypes (5 per cent), with many intermediates (40 per cent) and often considerable heterogeneity within a single tumour. They also distinguished 'well-differentiated thymic carcinoma' (25 per cent) as a separate entity;

it probably corresponds to type 3 of Verley and Hollman, whose undifferentiated type 4 (5 per cent) is essentially the only one to show marked nuclear atypia. The types most associated with myasthenia gravis are further discussed below.

Most histopathologists agree that it is very difficult to predict the invasiveness and prognosis of a thymoma from its histological appearances (for example, Rosai and Levine 1976), although, in their retrospective study, Kirchner and Müller-Hermelink (1989) found that almost all the tumours that subsequently spread locally or recurred were of the thymic carcinoma or more cortical types. While Verley and Hollman (1985) also found that their type 4 had a uniformly bad outlook (none of the 11 cases studied had survived for 4 years), in most other cases the overriding influence on prognosis was the tumour invasiveness assessed macroscopically at operation (see also Lewis et al. 1987). Ten year survival was approximately 40 per cent where the thymoma had grown through its capsule, compared with approximately 80 per cent where it had

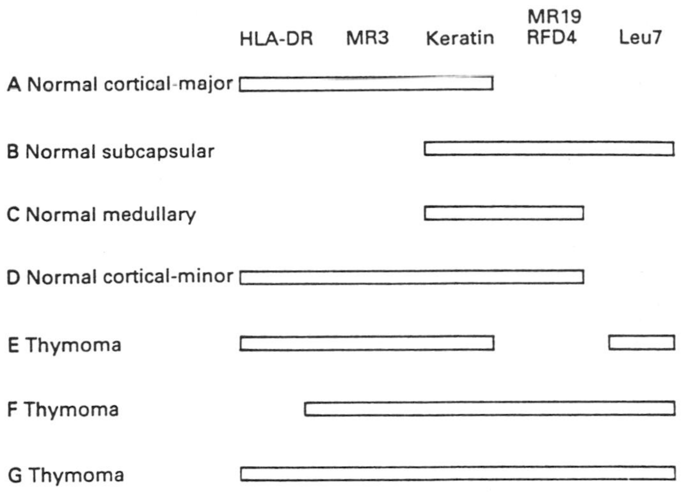

```
                          MR19
     HLA-DR   MR3  Keratin RFD4  Leu7
A Normal cortical-major
B Normal subcapsular
C Normal medullary
D Normal cortical-minor
E Thymoma
F Thymoma
G Thymoma
```

Fig. 2 Epithelial phenotypes in normal human thymus and thymoma. Leu-7 labelling is variable in the normal thymus and both Leu-7 and HLA-DR labelling may be weak or absent in some thymomata. (Reproduced from Willcox (1987), with permission.)

not and the histological classification into types 1–3 had little further influence. Many other groups have reached a similar conclusion. As Daugaard and Rørth state, all thymomata should be considered potentially invasive and malignant (Chapter 11.4).

Effects of corticosteroids

The interpatient variability in histology cannot usually be explained. However, it emerged that pre-treatment with corticosteroids drastically depletes the thymoma of lymphocytes in most cases, as they are apparently even more steroid sensitive than in the normal or the hyperplastic myasthenia gravis thymus (Willcox et al. 1987, 1989; Willcox 1989). The remaining epithelium is greatly enriched and usually appears healthy, with the same characteristics as in untreated cases, although the extensive lymphocyte necrosis, cystic degeneration, and/or fibrosis sometimes makes immunolabelling unsatisfactory. The tumours may temporarily shrink in size after this therapy, often only to recrudesce later as a result of continued epithelial growth (Shellito et al. 1987; Willcox 1989; Kirkove et al. 1990; see also preceding chapter).

Comparison with tumours from non-myasthenics

Thymomata from non-myasthenia gravis cases may show identical features to the above (Kirchner et al. 1988), even when the donor shows no detectable serum anti-acetylcholine receptor antibodies (Willcox et al. 1987). However, in the retrospective survey of Kirchner and Müller-Hermelink (1989), the incidence of myasthenia gravis was lower when the thymoma was more purely medullary, with fewer thymocytes, than in the more cortical tumours. Finally, both in the latter authors' 'well-differentiated thymic carcinoma', with fewer thymocytes and in the Verley and Hollman type 3, the incidence of myasthenia gravis was similarly high (Table 2). We suspect that, in some cases at least, this may be a sign of prior corticosteroid therapy for myasthenia gravis and consequent lymphocyte deletion, in otherwise typically cortical tumours (see Kirchner et al. 1992). Other explanations for the occurrence of myasthenia gravis in some but not all thymoma cases are discussed below.

Other pathology

The adjacent uninvolved thymus often shows a hyperplastic picture identical to that in young-onset myasthenia gravis, with no obvious echoes of the abnormalities in the thymoma (Willcox et al. 1987). This combination of lymph node-type T-cell areas and germinal centres in the medulla is rarely seen if the donor is non-myasthenic (Rosai and Levine 1976; Kirchner and Müller-Hermelink 1989); it could be an effect of an attack on thymic myoid cells provoked by the autoantibodies or autoreactive T-cells in the myasthenics (see Schluep et al. 1988 for further discussion). Finally, in skeletal muscle there may be focal lymphocytic infiltration or 'lymphorrhages' in myasthenia gravis cases with thymoma, not especially related to the endplates, but possibly provoked by the antistriated muscle antibodies. The endplates themselves show simplification of the junctional folds and loss of acetylcholine receptors in the muscle membrane, just as in any myasthenia gravis case (Santa et al. 1972).

THE GENESIS OF THE AUTOIMMUNE COMPLICATIONS OF THYMOMA
Myasthenia gravis

It is particularly intriguing that so many thymoma patients present with autoimmune syndromes. As these often lead to early presentation, whereas an uncomplicated thymoma may easily remain undetected for years (Rosai and Levine 1976; Willcox et al. 1987), it is difficult to assess their real frequency precisely, but it may well exceed 50 per cent (Souadjian et al. 1974). Interestingly, however, their repertoire is limited, myasthenia gravis being much the commonest, occurring in approximately 30–40 per cent of cases. Selective bone-marrow aplasias and hypogammaglobulinaemia are less common and polymyositis, systemic lupus erythematosus, and pemphigus vulgaris are rarer still (Souadjian et al. 1974; see also preceding chapter). However, they are important both practically and theoretically (see below).

Table 2 Classification of thymomata (after Holmes-Sellors et al. 1967; Verley and Hollman 1985)

| Histological type | Frequency (%) | Lymphocyte content | Incidence (%)[a] of | | Tendency to recur and spread |
			MG	RBC aplasia	
Type 1 Oval or spindle cell	30	+ − ++	28	7	Low
Type 2 Lymphocyte rich	30	+++	58	–	Low
Type 3 Epithelial rich, differentiated	33	+ − ++	75	1.5	Moderate (c. 20%)
Type 4 Epithelial rich, undifferentiated	7	+	29	–	High

[a]As Verley and Hollman point out, their series may have had a modest bias in favour of MG cases, reflected in an overall incidence of 105/200 cases.
MG, myasthenia gravis; RBC, red blood cells.

Two main kinds of explanation have been suggested for the association between myasthenia gravis and thymoma and they may be applicable to these other disorders too. First, T-cells are clearly being generated in great excess and in a highly disorganized and abnormal environment. Quite possibly the positive and/or negative selection processes mentioned above might be perverted or defective, so that some of the cells exported have not been properly rendered self-tolerant (Chilosi *et al.* 1986) and could initiate autoantibody responses after encountering self-antigens in the periphery. Cyclosporin A treatment of rats depletes the tolerizing medullary 'dendritic' cells and can result in an autologous 'graft-versus-host' syndrome (Glazier *et al.* 1983), so this is not just a theoretical possibility. However, the disorders described in thymoma patients are quite different and their narrow spectrum argues against such generalized 'status autotoxicus'.

The alternative is that some components of the thymoma actually sensitize the developing T-cells against self-antigens. For example, the antistriated muscle and related antibodies found in almost all thymomatous myasthenia gravis cases cross-react with antigens in the tumour (Gilhus *et al.* 1984). So do monoclonal antibodies to one cytoplasmic epitope of the acetylcholine receptor α-chain; moreover, these usually label many more epithelial cells in tumours from donors with myasthenia gravis than without (Kirchner *et al.* 1988; Geuder *et al.* 1992). The striking coincidence of two different muscle antigens present in thymoma, both of them targets of autoantibodies, makes this hypothesis particularly attractive. It also fits well with our preliminary evidence that thymoma cell suspensions include many T-cells reactive to the acetylcholine receptor and rather few specific for extraneous (recall) antigens (Sommer *et al.* 1990). If it is correct, a delay between the emigration of the sensitized T-cells and the induction of peripheral B-cells to produce pathological levels of anti-acetylcholine receptor antibodies might also explain how myasthenia gravis sometimes begins only months or even years after removal of a thymoma (Namba *et al.* 1978).

Thymoma with pure red cell aplasia

Approximately 5 per cent of thymoma patients develop pure red cell aplasia and a thymoma, which is usually spindle celled, is found in approximately half of all patients with this disorder (reviewed by Ammus and Yunis 1987). Pure red cell aplasia is characterized by severe anaemia (usually normochromic, normocytic) with very few reticulocytes, a cellular bone-marrow that is grossly deficient in nucleated erythroid precursors and with no evidence of extramedullary haematopoiesis. It may rarely coincide with myasthenia gravis (and/or even hypogammaglobulinaemia). If so, its onset is usually several years after the myasthenia gravis has been well controlled (reviewed by Bailey *et al.* 1988).

Some pure red cell aplasia cases with thymoma have a variety of antibodies to erythroid precursors (Ammus and Yunis 1987). Others have excessive CD8+ T-cells in the bone-marrow, blood, and probably the thymoma itself, which can inhibit erythroid colony formation in culture (Mangan *et al.* 1986) perhaps by releasing inhibitory cytokines or by some other 'suppressive' or cytotoxic action. In some cases, there is a gross deficiency of erythroid progenitor cells in the bone-marrow; in others, their frequencies become relatively normal once they are liberated from the inhibitory effects *in vitro*.

The pathogenetic mechanisms suggested above for myasthenia gravis could also be relevant here. The idea of a simple failure of self-tolerance induction in the T-cells generated and exported by the thymoma fits with the late onset of pure red cell aplasia in the course of tumour growth; these relatively immature T-cells might take a long time to affect the bone-marrow. If, alternatively, something in the thymoma actively sensitizes developing T-cells against erythroid precursor cells, it would be very interesting to look for antigens shared by these and thymoma cells.

While the anaemia remits in up to 30 per cent of cases after removal of the thymoma, most patients require immunosuppression with corticosteroids and even cyclophosphamide for effective control of this condition (Ammus and Yunis 1987).

CLINICAL PRESENTATION OF MYASTHENIA GRAVIS CASES WITH THYMOMA

The smaller tumour size in myasthenics, and their slightly lower age at diagnosis (Rosai and Levine 1976; Verley and Hollman 1985), suggest that these thymoma patients present earlier than those without autoimmune complications (Willcox *et al.* 1987). Typically, they show fatiguable weakness of the cranial nerve-innervated, trunk and even limb muscles, with diminished tone and normal or brisk tendon reflexes. Their myasthenia gravis is thus indistinguishable clinically from that of other patients with generalized symptoms but without any tumour, though a more myopathic picture is rarely seen (Rowland *et al.* 1973). However, tests for serum anti-acetylcholine receptor and antistriated muscle antibodies are both almost always positive (Aarli *et al.* 1981; Newsom-Davis *et al.* 1987). Since the latter are much less common in the other subgroups of patients with myasthenia gravis (Table 1), their presence should serve as a warning to check at regular (yearly) intervals for a thymoma in any patient with generalized myasthenia gravis. However, we have observed initially undetectable thymomata to appear very rarely during the follow-up of approximately 50 cases over 5–10 years. One should bear in mind that antistriated muscle antibodies may escape detection if rat, rather than human muscle is used as the target antigen in the assay (Aarli *et al.* 1981) and their absence does not therefore prove the absence of a thymoma. Signs of anaemia or recurrent infection should obviously also be pursued appropriately. Otherwise, these syndromes may lead to unexpected post-operative complications (including hypersensitivity to muscle relaxants).

The diagnosis of myasthenia gravis is established by the presence of serum anti-acetylcholine receptor antibody and can be confirmed by electromyography. Edrophonium testing is usually required only in the extremely rare cases without detectable anti-acetylcholine receptor antibodies. The absence of antistriated muscle antibodies makes the diagnosis of thymoma less likely, especially in young patients. A large thymoma can be seen on routine chest radiography but the detection of smaller tumours requires anterior mediastinal tomography or, preferably, CT scanning.

MANAGEMENT
Management of the thymoma

The tumour should, if possible, be resected through a trans-sternal approach. In most cases, recurrence and metastases do not occur; prognosis and surgical and adjunctive management are discussed in detail elsewhere.

Management of the myasthenia

Weakness in mild cases is treated initially with anticholinesterase preparations only (e.g. pyridostigmine), but in most severe cases immunosuppressive drug treatment is also required, with alternate-day prednisolone and/or azathioprine. In patients with very severe weakness, particularly when it affects respiratory or bulbar muscles, plasma exchange may be needed.

Removal of the tumour is undertaken as soon as the patient is fit for surgery, although exceptions are sometimes made in the very old. Most clinical studies show, paradoxically, that tumour excision does not ameliorate the myasthenia and the clinician should therefore be prepared for a subsequent increase in myasthenic symptoms or indeed for their appearance *de novo* (Namba *et al.* 1978).

In the majority of cases, the outcome is very satisfactory with full repression of myasthenic symptoms, often at lower doses of immunosuppressive drugs than those required initially to gain control. It is, however, exceptional to be able to withdraw the drugs completely without a recurrence of weakness. Nevertheless, according to recent surveys (for example, Verley and Hollman 1985), the myasthenia gravis scarcely affects the prognosis of a thymoma patient, whereas, in a few cases, recurrent or metastatic tumour may shorten life. Follow-up radiography is needed every 1–2 years in those whose tumours seem likely to be invasive and all patients should also be monitored for signs of anaemia or immunodeficiency.

FUTURE PROSPECTS

If these tumours were commoner or more aggressive, there would be a strong case for using some of the very specific monoclonal antibodies available for imaging and drug targeting (see Al Jabaari *et al.* 1989).

REFERENCES

Aarli JA, Lefvert A-K, Tonder O (1981). Thymoma-specific antibodies in sera from patients with myasthenia gravis demonstrated by indirect haemagglutination. *Journal of Neuroimmunology*, 1:421–7.

Aarli JA, Stefansson K, Marton LSG, Wollmann RL (1990). Patients with myasthenia gravis and thymoma have in their sera IgG autoantibodies against titin. *Clinical and Experimental Immunology*, 82:284–8.

Al Jabaari B, Ladyman HM, Larché M, Sivolapenko GB, Epenetos AA, Ritter MA (1989). Elevated expression of the interleukin 4 receptor in carcinoma: a target for immunotherapy? *British Journal of Cancer*, 59:910–14.

Ammus SS, Yunis AA (1987). Acquired pure red cell aplasia. *American Journal of Hematology*, 24:311–26.

Bailey RO, Dunn HG, Rubin AM, Ritaccio AL (1988). Myasthenia gravis with thymoma and pure red blood cell aplasia. *American Journal of Clinical Pathology*, 89:687–93.

Batata MA, Martini N, Huvos AG, Aguilar RI, Beattie EJ (1974). Thymomas: clinicopathologic features, therapy, and prognosis. *Cancer*, 34:389–96.

Chilosi M, *et al.* (1986). Myasthenia gravis: immunohistological heterogeneity in microenvironmental organization of hyperplastic and neoplastic thymuses suggesting different mechanisms of tolerance breakdown. *Journal of Neuroimmunology*, 11:191–204.

Chiu H-C, Vincent A, Newsom-Davis J, Hsieh K-H, Hung T (1987). Myasthenia gravis: population differences in disease expression and acetylcholine receptor antibody titres between Chinese and Caucasians. *Neurology*, 37:1854–7.

Compston DAS, Vincent A, Newsom-Davis J, Batchelor JR (1980). Clinical, pathological, HLA antigen and immunological evidence for disease heterogeneity in myasthenia gravis. *Brain*, 103:579–601.

Fukai I, *et al.* (1992). An immunohistologic study of the epithelial components of 81 cases of thymoma. *Cancer*, 69:2463–8.

Geuder KI, Marx A, Witzemann V, Schalke B, Kirchner T, Müller-Hermelink HK (1992). Genomic organization and lack of transcription of the nicotinic acetylcholine receptor subunit genes in myasthenia gravis-associated thymoma. *Laboratory Investigation*, 66:452.

Gilhus NE, Aarli JA, Christensson B, Matre R (1984). Rabbit antiserum to a citric acid extract of human skeletal muscle staining thymomas from myasthenia gravis patients. *Journal of Neuroimmunology*, 7:55–64.

Glazier A, Tutschka PJ, Farmer ER, Santos GW (1983). Graft-versus-host disease in cyclosporin A-treated rats after syngeneic and autologous bone marrow reconstitution. *Journal of Experimental Medicine*, 158:1–8.

Holmes-Sellors T, Thackray AC, Thomson AD (1967). Tumours of the thymus; a review of 88 operation cases. *Thorax*, 22:193–220.

Janossy G, Campana D, Akbar A (1989). Kinetics of T lymphocyte development. *Current Topics in Pathology*, 79:59–99.

Katzin WE, Fishleder AJ, Linden MD, Tubbs RR (1988). Immunoglobulin and T cell receptor genes in thymomas: genotypic evidence supporting the non-neoplastic nature of the lymphocytic component. *Human Pathology*, 19:323–8.

Kirchner T, Müller-Hermelink HK (1989). New approaches to the diagnosis of thymic epithelial tumours. *Progress in Surgical Pathology*, X:107–89.

Kirchner T, Tzartos S, Hoppe F, Schalke B, Wekerle H, Müller-Hermelink HK (1988). Pathogenesis of myasthenia gravis: acetylcholine receptor-related antigenic determinants in tumor-free thymuses and thymic epithelial tumors. *American Journal of Pathology*, 130:268–80.

Kirchner T, Schalk B, Buchwald J, Ritter M, Marx A, Müller-Hermelink HK (1992). Well-differentiated thymic carcinoma. *American Journal of Surgical Pathology*, 16:1153–69.

Kirkove C, Berghmans J, Noel H, Van de Merckt J (1992). Dramatic response of recurrent invasive thymoma to high doses of corticosteroids. *Clinical Oncology*, 4:64–6.

Klavinskis LS, Willcox N, Oxford J, Newsom-Davis J (1985). Anti-virus antibodies in myasthenia gravis. *Neurology*, 35:1381–4.

Lampert I, Ritter MA (1988). The origin of the diverse epithelial cells of the thymus: is there a common stem cell? *Thymus Update*, 1:2–25.

Lewis JE, Wick MR, Scheithauer BW, Bernatz PE, Taylor WF (1987). Thymoma: a clinicopathologic review. *Cancer*, 60:2727–43.

McGuire LJ, Huang DP, Teoh R, Arnold M, Wong K, Lee JCK (1988). Epstein–Barr virus genome in thymoma and thymic lymphoid hyperplasia. *American Journal of Pathology*, 131:385–90.

Mangan KF, Volkin R, Winkelstein A (1986). Autoreactive erythroid progenitor—T suppressor cells in the pure red cell aplasia associated with thymoma and panhypogammaglobulinemia. *American Journal of Hematology*, 23:167–73.

Nakao Y, *et al.* (1980). Gm allotypes in myasthenia gravis *Lancet*, i:677–80.

Namba T, Brunner NG, Grob D (1978). Myasthenia gravis in patients with thymoma, with particular reference to onset after thymectomy. *Medicine*, 57:411–33.

Newsom-Davis J (1982). Autoimmune diseases of neuromuscular transmission. *Clinics in Immunology and Allergy*, 2:405–24.

Newsom-Davis J, *et al.* (1987). Immunological heterogeneity and cellular mechanisms in myasthenia gravis. *Annals of the New York Academy of Science*, 505:12–26.

Pescarmona E, Rosati S, Pisacane A, Rendina EA, Venuta F, Baroni CD (1992). Microscopic thymoma: histological evidence of multifocal cortical and medullary origin. *Histopathology*, 20:263–6.

Rosai J, Levine GD (1976). Tumors of the Thymus. In *Atlas of tumor pathology*. US Armed Forces, Institute of Pathology, 2nd series, Fascicle 13.

Rowland LP, Lisak RP, Schotland DL, DeJesus PV, Berg P (1973). Myasthenic myopathy and thymoma. *Neurology*, 23:282–8.

Santa S, Engel AG, Lambert EH (1972). Histometric study of neuromuscular junction ultrastructure 1. Myasthenia gravis. *Neurology*, 22:71–82.

Schluep M, Willcox N, Ritter MA, Newsom-Davis J, Larche M, Brown AN (1988). Myasthenia gravis thymus: clinical, histological and culture correlations. *Journal of Autoimmunity*, 1:445–67.

Shellito J, Khandekar JD, McKeever WP, Vick NA (1987). Invasive thymoma responsive to oral corticosteroids. *Cancer Treatment Reports*, 62:1397–400.

Sommer N, Willcox N, Harcourt GC, Newsom-Davis J (1990). Myasthenic thymus and thymoma are selectively enriched in acetylcholine receptive-reactive T cells. *Annals of Neurology*, 28:312–19.

Souadjian JV, Enriquez P, Silverstein MN, Pepin J-M (1974). The spectrum of diseases associated with thymoma. *Archives of Internal Medicine*, 134:374–9.

Sprent J, Lo D, Gao E-R, Ron Y (1988). T cell selection in the thymus. *Immunological Reviews*, 101:173–90.

Verley JM, Hollman KH (1985). Thymoma: a comparative study of clinical stages, histologic features and survival in 200 cases. *Cancer*, **55**:1074–86.

Von Gaudecker B (1986). The development of the human thymus microenvironment. *Current Topics in Pathology*, **75**:1–41.

Willcox N, Vincent A (1988). Myasthenia gravis as an example of an organ-specific autoimmune disease. In *B lymphocytes in human disease* (ed. G Bird and JE Calvert), pp. 469–506. Oxford University Press.

Willcox N (1989). The thymus in myasthenia gravis patients, and the *in vivo* effects of corticosteroids on its cellularity, histology and functions. *Thymus Update*, **2**:105–24.

Willcox N, Schluep M, Ritter MA, Schuurman HJ, Newsom-Davis J, Christensson B (1987). Myasthenic and nonmyasthenic thymoma: an expansion of a minor cortical epithelial subset? *American Journal of Pathology*, **127**:447–60.

Willcox N, *et al.* (1989). Variable coticosteroid sensitivity of thymic cortex and medullary peripheral-type lymphoid tissue in myasthenia gravis patients: structural and functional effects. *Quarterly Journal of Medicine*, **73**:1071–87.

Wu T-C, Kuo TT (1993). Study of Epstein–Barr virus early RNA 1 (EBER 1) expression by in situ hybridization in thymic epithelial tumors of Chinese patients in Taiwan. *Human Pathology*, **24**:235–8.

11.4　Other thymic tumours

GEDSKE DAUGAARD AND MIKAEL RØRTH

Thymoma refers to tumours of epithelial and lymphocytic origin in the thymus. The thymus gland develops as a pair of solid buds arising predominantly from the third branchial pouch at approximately the sixth week of embryonic life. It migrates caudally during intrauterine development to lie in the upper part of the anterior mediastinum.

Thymomas comprise approximately 20 per cent of all mediastinal tumours and cysts and they are the most common anterior mediastinal tumour (Silverman and Sabiston 1977). Hodgkin's and non-Hodgkin's lymphomas, germ cell tumours, malignant lymphomas, primary carcinomas, and carcinoid tumours may involve the thymus gland and must be differentiated from true thymomas.

Thymomas may occur at any age but are rare before the age of 20 years. Only 20 well-documented cases of thymoma involving children have been reported in the literature (Kaplinsky *et al.* 1992). They occur with equal frequency in both sexes. Peak incidence occurs between 40 and 60 years of age. A rate of 0.4 new cases per year per 100 000 people has been observed by the Cancer Registry of Isére (Exbrayat *et al.* 1989).

PATHOLOGY

Thymomas are slow-growing tumours. Extrathoracic metastases occur rarely. Thymomas express their malignant potential by invading surrounding tissues and by developing local recurrences and implants in the chest. The malignant potential of the tumour is best evaluated by the surgeon rather than the pathologist (Fechner 1969). Invasion as determined by the surgeon, however, must be supplemented by histologic search by the pathologist for evidence of capsular invasion or the presence of microscopic foci within mediastinal fat. This is particularly true for stage II thymoma, which might otherwise be understaged and which has a propensity for recurrence (Wilkins *et al.* 1991).

Macroscopically, these neoplasms are usually solid, occasionally cystic, lobulated, well-circumscribed, white-grey, soft masses located in the anterior compartment. Generally they measure 5–10 cm in greatest diameter.

Microscopic examination reveals epithelial reticular cells arranged in nests of solid cords surrounded by a varying number of lymphocytes. Most thymomas are surrounded by a thick fibrous capsule that is continuous with broad fibrous tissue septa, separating the tumour into nodules of various sizes and shapes (Rosai and Levine 1976; Bergh *et al.* 1978). Three principal histological groups have been described (Lattes and Jones 1957; Bernatz *et al.* 1961).

1. The epithelial type in which up to 80 per cent of the cells are epithelially derived (subgroups of this class are sometimes referred to as spindle cell, oval cell, or epidermoid).

2. The lymphocytic type in which up to 80 per cent of cells are lymphocytically derived.

3. The mixed or lymphoepithelial, type in which neither cell type predominates.

Lewis *et al.* (1987) defined the lymphocytic type as consisting of more than 66 per cent lymphocytes and less than 33 per cent epithelial cells and vice versa for the predominantly epithelial type. These cellular characteristics do not, however, appear to influence prognosis, which is governed more by gross appearance, whether or not the tumour has an intact capsule (Silverman and Sabiston 1977). It is generally accepted that the epithelial cells of thymomas are the neoplastic components of these tumours and lymphocytes present in the thymomas are considered non-neoplastic (Rosai and Levine 1976; Baroni *et al.* 1980, 1983). The morphological features of the epithelial cells have been taken into consideration in the newer classification proposed by Marino and Müller-Hermelink (1985). This classification consists of the following groups

1. Cortical thymomas mainly composed of medium-sized to large epithelial cells with round-oval nuclei, finely dispersed chromatin, evident nucleoli, and ill-defined cytoplasm; lymphocytes are usually numerous and sometimes have a blastic appearance.

2. Medullary thymoma consisting of small to medium-sized epithelial cells with irregular and sometimes spindle-shaped nuclei, usually without nucleoli.

3. Mixed thymoma in which both the epithelial cortical and medullary cell types are present, intermingled with a variable amount of usually small lymphocytes.

In a study by Pescarmona *et al.* (1990) the classification by Marino and Müller-Hermelink (1985) was applied and a statistically significant relationship between histologic results and age, surgical stage, and prognosis was demonstrated. Medullary thymoma had the best prognosis (100 per cent 5 year survival), cortical thymoma had the worst prognosis (52 per cent 5 year survival), and mixed thymoma showed an intermediate prognosis (85 per cent 5 year survival). Others have failed to confirm the usefulness of this classification (Kornstein *et al.* 1988; Wick 1990).

Thymomas possess the characteristic ultrastructural features of thymic epithelial cells, including long cellular processes surrounding lymphocytes, prominent well-formed desmosomes, and variable numbers of tonofilament bundles within the cytoplasm. The epithelial cells may closely resemble cortical thymocytes or medullary thymocytes or may have intermediate characteristics (Hammond and Flinner 1991).

Thymic epithelial cells can be distinguished from non-epithelial cells such as histiocytes by means of antibodies to keratin and epithelial membrane antigen (Battifora *et al.* 1980; Lewis *et al.* 1987; Hammond and Flinner 1991). Another family of antigens, the desmoplakins, has been advocated recently in differentiating epithelial from non-epithelial malignancies (Moll *et al.* 1986). Their use in mediastinal tumours is highly attractive because desmosomes form an important basis for the diagnosis of thymoma. Cortical epithelial cells of thymus and malignancies derived from them may express markers of cortical thymic epithelial cells. They express MHC class II antigen, p19 (core antigen of human immuno-deficiency virus) and Leu7 (myelin associated glycoprotein), a marker of natural killer cells that cross-reacts with neuroendocrine neoplasms (Marino and Müller-Hermelink 1985). By contrast, medullary epithelial cells express little if any HLA-DR or Leu7 but do express p19 and neurofilament protein epitopes, features that are shared by mixed thymomas and medullary type thymomas.

Thymomas, particularly those associated with myasthenia gravis, are likely to express increased amounts of nicotinic acetylcholine receptor protein, a unique epitope not to be found in other types of epithelial malignancies (Kirchner and Müller-Hermelink 1989). Lymphocytes in thymomas also may possess distinctive phenotypes. Cortical lymphocytes are immature and consistently express CD1 and TdT. Thymocytes that reside in the medulla are usually more mature, do not express CD1, and show CD3 expression, as do lymphocytes of peripheral blood (Kirchner and Müller-Hermelink 1989). These characteristics often persist in thymomas: cortical thymomas and the malignancies derived from them are likely to contain lymphocytes that express CD1 and TdT, features that are not shared by any other type of epithelial neoplasm (Kirchner and Müller-Hermelink 1989).

In order to find a marker of aggressiveness in thymoma, 21 cases (nine non-invasive, eight invasive, and four metastatic thymomas) were examined for expression of the *ras* oncogene product p21 by immunohistochemistry and immunoblot analysis (Mukai *et al.* 1990). It was demonstrated that neoplastic thymoma cells generally contained more p21 than normal thymic epithelial cells. The increased amount of p21 in thymomas suggested that this protein may have a role in the oncogenesis or progression of thymoma and may be a possible marker of aggressive behaviour.

In a study of 39 cases of thymoma, including benign thymoma, invasive thymoma, and thymic carcinoma, Asamura *et al.* (1988) found that 92 per cent of thymic carcinomas were aneuploid, in contrast to invasive and non-invasive thymomas. Only one invasive thymoma and none of the benign thymomas were aneuploid. Because DNA ploidy analysis cannot separate invasive

from benign tumours, it is not helpful in predicting malignant behaviour.

A 'benign' thymoma has been defined as a tumour that is well encapsulated and does not invade adjacent mediastinal structures. Fifty to 65 per cent of thymomas fit this definition. The distinction between 'benign' and 'malignant' thymomas is artificial and should be discarded. All thymomas are potentially invasive and therefore they should be considered malignant.

PRESENTATION AND CLINICAL FEATURES

Approximately two-thirds of patients with thymomas are symptomatic when the lesion is discovered. Some complain of chest pain, cough, dyspnoea and frequently recurrent respiratory infections, dysphagia, hoarseness, stridor, and haemoptysis. Vena caval obstruction from the local invasive and compressive effects of the tumours is also observed. The majority, however, present with symptoms related to one of the many associated syndromes, the most common of which is myasthenia gravis (Lewis *et al.* 1987). Myasthenia is reported in 10–50 per cent of patients having thymomas. Conversely, the reported incidence of thymoma in patients having myasthenia gravis ranges from 8 to 23 per cent (Oldham 1971; Rubush *et al.* 1973; Ohmi and Ohuchi 1990).

Pure red cell aplasia occurs in approximately 5 per cent of cases of thymoma. One-third to one-half of all patients with red cell aplasia will have a thymoma (Zeok *et al.* 1979). An associated decrease in the number of platelets or leucocytes is found in 30 per cent of patients with red cell aplasia. Ninety-six per cent of the patients who develop this syndrome are older than 40 years. Red cell precursors are absent in the bone-marrow, whereas platelet and leucocytic elements are normal. Thymectomy results in remission of this disease in 25–30 per cent of the patients (Zeok *et al.* 1979).

Hypogammaglobulinaemia is present in 5–10 per cent of patients with thymoma (Souadjian *et al.* 1974). Patients with hypogammaglobulinaemia have a 10 per cent incidence of thymoma. More than one-third of these patients also have red cell hypoplasia. Combined humoral and cellular immunodeficiencies are present. Practically all patients are older than 40 years of age. Thymectomy has not proven to be beneficial in this condition.

Nearly 70 per cent of patients with thymomas and other diseases will have disorders related to immunological phenomena. Approximately 5 per cent will have an endocrine disorder and 15 per cent will have a severe infection or another seemingly unrelated condition such as megaloesophagus (Table 1). Whether an increase in non-thymic malignancies is associated with thymoma has not been clarified (Souadjian *et al.* 1968; Vessey and Doll 1972). The presence of secondary tumours in approximately 10 per cent of patients with thymomas has been suggested.

Thymomas are located largely or completely in the anterior mediastinum. Approximately 15 per cent occupy both the anterior and superior mediastinum and 6 per cent are primarily in the superior mediastinum. No more than 5–10 per cent of thymomas occur in other locations, such as the neck and middle or posterior mediastinum.

Radiographically, these tumours present as round, smooth, or lobulated densities, usually occurring near the junction of the heart and the great vessels. Approximately 20 per cent demonstrate calcification by standard radiography or tomography. CT scans allow more precise definition of the extent of involvement and the nature of a tumour mass suspected as being a thymoma (Zerhouni *et al.*

Table 1 Syndromes and diseases associated with thymomas

Autoimmune or immune phenomena	Endocrine disorders
Myasthenia gravis	Cushing's syndrome
Cytopenias (pure red cell aplasia)	Hyperthyroidism
Hypogammaglobulinaemia	Addison's disease
Polymyositis	Panhypopituitarism
Systemic lupus erythematosus	
Rheumatoid arthritis	Severe infections and miscellaneous
Thyroiditis	diseases
Sjögren's syndrome	Myocarditis
Chronic ulcerative colitis	Megaloesophagus
Pernicious anaemia	Chronic macrocutaneous candidiasis
Raynaud's disease	
Regional enteritis	
Rheumatic endocarditis	
Sarcoidosis	
Dermatomyositis	
Scleroderma	
Takayasu's syndrome	

1982). The information from a CT scan is useful in directing surgical intervention, planning radiotherapy treatment, evaluating treatment response, and monitoring for recurrence of disease (Zerhouni et al. 1982). MR imaging may also turn up to be an excellent technique for identifying and defining the extent of thymic tumours (Molina et al. 1990).

Thoracotomy plays an important role, not only as a diagnostic procedure but as a major mode of therapy. Because of the propensity of thymomas to recur or develop local metastases when the integrity of the capsule is violated, biopsy of these tumours is best avoided. The tumour should be removed *in toto* whenever possible. At the time of operation, local invasion or distant metastases is observed in 30–70 per cent of cases (Table 2).

The differential diagnosis of thymoma ranges from small cell malignant lymphomas (predominantly lymphocytic tumours) to large cell lymphoma or carcinoma (predominantly epithelial tumours). However, neoplasms with obviously malignant cytological characteristics should be excluded from consideration as true thymomas.

STAGING

The following staging system has been suggested by Bergh et al. (1978).

Stage I: Intact capsule or growth within the capsule.
Stage II: Pericapsular growth into the mediastinal fat tissue.
Stage III: Invasive growth into the surrounding organs, intrathoracic metastases, or both.

In a series by Bergh et al. (1978), 40 per cent were stage I thymomas, 19 per cent stage II, and 41 per cent stage III.

A slightly different classification has been suggested by Masaoka et al. (1981).

Stage I: Macroscopically completely encapsulated and microscopically no capsular invasion.
Stage II: 1. Macroscopic invasion into surrounding fatty tissue or mediastinal pleura; or
2. microscopic invasion into capsule.
Stage III: Macroscopic invasion into neighbouring organ (pericardium, great vessels, or lung).
Stage IVa: Pleural or pericardial dissemination.
Stage IVb: Lymphogenous or haematogenous metastases.

The classification suggested by Masaoka et al. (1981) is commonly used with slight modifications (Varley and Hollmann 1985; Curran et al. 1988).

Table 2 Results of treatment

References:	1		2		3		4		5		6[a]		7		8	Total	
No. of patients	96		56		200		165		283		103		141		77	1121	
Histological type																	
Lymphoepithelial	47	(49)					107	(65)	122	(43)			77	(55)		353	(40)
Lymphocytic	16	(17)			59	(30)	20	(12)	72	(25)			36	(26)		203	(23)
Epithelial	24	(25)			141	(70)	36	(22)	87	(31)			26	(18)		314	(35)
Unknown	9	(9)					2	(1)	2	(1)			2	(1)		15	(2)
Invasiveness																	
No	37	(39)			133	(67)	106	(64)			43	(42)	45	(32)		364	(46)
Yes	59	(61)	56	(100)	67	(33)	59	(36)			60	(58)	96	(68)	77	418	(53)
Surgery																	
Non-invasive																	
Radical	37	(100)					106	(100)	228[b]		43	(100)	45	(100)			
Invasive																	
Radical	31	(60)	6	(11)			34	(58)			26	(45)	68	(71)	33		
Subtotal	13	(25)	22	(39)			16	(27)	47	(17)	14	(25)	16	(17)	36		
Biopsy	8	(15)	28	(50)			9	(15)			17	(30)	12	(12)	8		
Five-year survival																	
Non-invasive	89%				85%		85%		75%				100%[c]				
Invasive			46%		50%		67%		50%				82%[c]				
Ten-year survival																	
Non-invasive	75%				80%		71%		63%				100%[c]				
Invasive					35%		53%		30%				75%[c]		58%		

[a]Whether the tumours are invasive or non-invasive is not mentioned.
[b]Extent of surgery unknown in three cases.
[c]Patients dying from other causes than tumour recurrence are not included.
Number in brackets are percentages.
References: 1, Masaoka et al. (1981); 2, Arriagada et al. (1984); 3, Verley and Hollmann (1985); 4, Maggi et al. (1986); 5, Lewis et al. (1987); 6, Curran et al. (1988); 7, Nakahara et al. (1988); 8, Urgesi et al. (1990).

Metastases to regional nodes or distant organs are uncommon. The organs reported to be involved have been the liver, bone, colon, kidney, brain, and spleen (Gravanis 1968). The most common metastases occur in the pleura or pericardium.

TREATMENT

The most effective therapy of a thymoma is its complete removal (Sawyers and Foster 1968; Salyers and Eggleston 1976; Cohen *et al.* 1984; Nakahara *et al.* 1988). Median sternotomy is the preferred incision for thymectomy, since it provides excellent exposure of the heart, great vessels, and pleural cavities. A left or right thoracotomy is used in some cases and sometimes in combination with a median sternotomy. The surgeon is usually in the best position to determine whether a thymoma has infiltrated the surrounding tissue. Adherence to pleura and pericardium is not uncommon and occasionally it is difficult to differentiate between actual invasion and the mere adherence of a benign neoplasm. Recent advantages in vascular and thoracic surgery have made possible a more radical surgical procedure for invasive thymoma. The superior vena cava can now be removed and reconstructed and pneumonectomy and pleurapneumonectomy can be performed when needed.

Some data are available concerning the prognosis after surgery alone. Legg and Brady (1965) observed no deaths due to thymoma in a group of 37 patients with non-invasive tumours treated by total excision of the tumour (observation time 0–10 years) and neither did Salyer and Eggleston (1976) in a survey of 25 patients or Batata *et al.* (1974) in a group of 16 patients (observation time 5–17 years). In another series of 14 patients, three out of five patients with complete excision of their non-invasive thymomas were alive after 7–12 years (Sawyers and Foster 1968), whereas 89 per cent of patients with incomplete resection died. Curran *et al.* (1988) observed a relapse rate of 38 per cent within the mediastinum in invasive thymoma treated with radical surgery alone, while Batata *et al.* (1974) observed a relapse rate of 100 per cent within 5 years.

In the past, the presence of myasthenia gravis represented a greater threat to the immediate success of the operation than that imposed by the presence of a thymic tumour (Braitman *et al.* 1971; Masaoka *et al.* 1981; Maggi *et al.* 1986; Curran *et al.* 1988). Complications related to surgery have been observed in 4–71 per cent of the patients (Braitman *et al.* 1971; Appelquist *et al.* 1982; Cohen *et al.* 1984; Maggi *et al.* 1986) and in some studies the reported mortality rate has been between 8 and 12 per cent (Bergh *et al.* 1978; Appelquist *et al.* 1982).

Reoperation is a valid accessory to an unsuccessful initial operation. Also response of initially inoperable thymoma to chemotherapy or radiotherapy or both favours successful reoperation (Kirschner 1990).

Although surgical extirpation remains the mainstay of therapy for invasive thymoma, adjunctive irradiation and chemotherapy have been widely advocated. Radiotherapy is recommended in doses of 40–60 Gy given in 20–30 fractions (Marks *et al.* 1978; Arriagada *et al.* 1984; Uematsu and Kondo 1986). Treatment has often been delivered via a linear accelerator or ^{60}Co unit, using an opposing anterior–posterior technique until spinal cord tolerance has been approached. When the prescribed dose exceeded 40 Gy, the additional therapy has been delivered using angled fields, sparing the spinal cord (Curran *et al.* 1988). In order to prevent recurrence, it has been recommended that the fields include the bilateral supraclavicular fossae and whole mediastinum down to the diaphragmatic crura (Uematu and Kondo 1986). However, whole-mediastinal irradiation may be insufficient for invasive thymomas, since recurrence often develops at the pleural surface and sometimes in the lung remote from the primary lesion. In a few cases of pleural metastases, the entire hemithorax and lung has been irradiated with success (14–21 Gy) (Ariaratnam *et al.* 1979; Uematsu and Kondo 1986).

The optimal radiation dose is at present unknown. Better local control could not be demonstrated within a dose range of 40–59 Gy (Arriagada *et al.* 1984). Only a small number of patients received 60 Gy.

The results of treatment from some of the larger series published in recent years are shown in Table 3. In these studies nearly all patients with invasive thymoma have been treated with radiotherapy, except for the study by Maggi *et al.* (1986). Radical surgery has been possible in all cases of non-invasive thymoma (Table 3). Prophylactic radiotherapy for stage I tumours was used in the study by Masaoka *et al.* (1981). The 5 and 10 year survival rates were not improved by this treatment. Local relapse occurred in up to 12 per cent of patients with non-invasive thymomas (Fechner 1969; Verley and Hollmann 1985; Maggi *et al.* 1986; Lewis *et al.* 1987; Curran *et al.* 1988).

Approximately 50–60 per cent of patients with invasive thymoma can be treated radically with surgery and radiotherapy. When radical operation alone was considered, no difference between the prognosis for invasive or non-invasive thymoma was apparent (Maggi *et al.* 1986; Nakahara *et al.* 1988). Cohen *et al.* (1984) were unable to demonstrate any significant difference in survival between patients who received post-operative irradiation and those who did not, when complete resection of the tumour was obtained. However, the most common finding was that patients with invasive thymomas benefited from post-operative radiotherapy (Table 3). The intrathoracic relapse rate following total resection alone was 24 per cent compared with 8 per cent after total resection and radiotherapy.

In patients who had incomplete excision of the thymoma, Cohen *et al.* (1984), Arriagada *et al.* (1984), and Curran *et al.* (1988) observed no difference between patients having partial excision (of most of their tumour) and those having only a biopsy, provided they received post-operative radiotherapy. These data imply that there is no value in so-called 'debulking procedures' and that this could be due to the effectiveness of radiation therapy in the local control of thymoma. On the other hand, Maggi *et al.* (1986) found that the type of surgery had a clear impact on survival: 80 per cent of patients with radically resected invasive thymoma survived at 5 years and 73 per cent at 10 years, as compared to 59 per cent at 5 years and 44 per cent at 10 years for those with subtotally resected tumours and 42 per cent at 5 years and 21 per cent at 8 years for patients when only a biopsy was performed. Comparable data were

Table 3 Thoracic failure following total resection±radiotherapy (RT) for invasive thymoma (stages II to IV)

Series	Total resection without RT	Total resection with RT
Batata *et al.* (1974)	6/6	–
Marks *et al.* (1978)	–	0/3
Masaoka *et al.* (1981)	3/21	3/47
Chahinian *et al.* (1981)	3/3	–
Arriagada *et al.* (1984)	–	1/6
Cohen *et al.* (1984)	3/5	3/6
Monden *et al.* (1985)	4/26	4/75
Maggi *et al.* (1986)	1/34	0/2
Curran *et al.* (1988)	8/21	0/5
Total	28/116	11/144

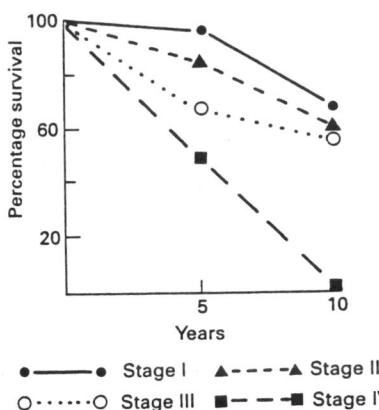

Fig. 1 Survival according to stage (data from Masaoka *et al.* 1981; Curran *et al.* 1988).

obtained by Nakahara *et al.* (1988) who reported that six out of 113 (5.3 per cent) patients undergoing complete resection died of tumour, seven out of 16 patients (43.8 per cent) undergoing subtotal resection, and 10 out of 12 patients (83.3 per cent) undergoing biopsy only, despite radiotherapy.

Local recurrence has been observed in 20–30 per cent of patients with invasive thymomas treated with radiotherapy (Arriagada *et al.* 1984; Monden *et al.* 1985; Verley and Hollmann 1985). The rate of recurrence/persistence in the study by Monden *et al.* (1985) according to stage was 3 per cent with stage I disease, 13 per cent with stage II disease, 27 per cent with stage III disease, and 54 per cent with stage IV. Recurrence of non-invasive thymomas has been observed at a median of 3.8–8 years and for invasive thymomas at a median of 3 years (Verley and Hollmann 1985; Curran *et al.* 1988). Survival according to stage and overall survival for patients with thymoma are shown in Figs 1 and 2.

The available data on systemic treatment of invasive thymoma are limited (Daugaard 1989). Cisplatin has documented efficacy, with a response in seven out of nine patients (three complete remissions). A response rate of 60 per cent has been demonstrated for ifosfamide. Experience with other single agents is limited. Nitrogen mustard, maytansine, chlorambucil, and doxorubicin have been tested without convincing effect.

Corticosteroid treatments have resulted in tumour regression in 10 out of 11 reported cases (Daugaard 1989). Two patients have achieved complete remission. In general, the thymoma recurs immediately after cessation of corticoid therapy. The mechanism

of action of corticosteroids in the treatment of invasive thymoma remains speculative. Corticosteroids have been demonstrated to have both an oncolytic (Gurcay *et al.* 1971; Postner *et al.* 1977) and a direct thymolytic effect (Claman 1972). In addition, glucocorticoid receptors have been found in radiation-induced mouse thymomas (Leinen *et al.* 1974). Although such receptors have not been found in human thymomas, it is conceivable that the thymolytic effect of corticosteroids is related to the presence of such receptors.

Combination chemotherapy has been used in the treatment of invasive thymoma, with a variety of different treatment programmes (Daugaard 1989). Studies involving more than four patients are referred to in Table 4. For regimens containing platinum, treatment results of 96 patients were reported. Twenty-eight patients (29 per cent) obtained complete remission and 44 patients (46 per cent) partial remission. The median duration of the responses was 11 months (range 2–96 months).

Most of the regimens without cisplatin included cyclophosphamide, vincristine, doxorubicin, and prednisone. Treatment results for 54 patients were reported. Twenty patients (37 per cent) obtained complete remission and 15 patients (28 per cent) partial remission. The median duration of the responses was 15 months (range 2–117+ months).

Most of the patients presented in Table 4 had relapsed after previous treatment with radiotherapy. The results obtained with chemotherapy either as first- or second-line treatment are sufficiently encouraging to explore this treatment modality for invasive thymomas. In a small study by Macchiarini *et al.* (1991), seven patients were treated with neoadjuvant chemotherapy (cisplatin, epirubicin, and etoposide) followed by surgery and post-operative radiation therapy (4600–6000 Gy). Two year disease-free survival was 80 per cent.

It appears that the best single agents for the systemic treatment of invasive thymomas are prednisone and cisplatin. Other cytotoxic agents have been used largely in combination with these drugs. Because of the unknown or limited efficacy of the other drugs as single agents, it is difficult to assess their additional value in combination with prednisone and cisplatin.

Autologous bone-marrow transplantation after treatment with carmustine–etoposide–cytosine arabinoside and melphalan has been used in at least two patients with thymomas (Gaspard *et al.* 1988). This treatment resulted in a continuous complete response in one patient.

It can be concluded that radical surgery is by far the most important factor in the treatment of thymoma. The presence of invasion has been cited by many authors as the single most important factor in predicting recurrence. Total resection alone is adequate therapy for stage I thymomas and there is no rationale for the use of adjuvant radiotherapy in this group of patients. Complete surgical excision appears to offer a better chance of long-term survival than partial resection plus irradiation. Radiotherapy seems to decrease the rate of local recurrence in invasive carcinoma of the thymus.

At present it is unknown whether radiation therapy or chemotherapy is the most effective post-operative treatment for invasive thymoma. In order to elucidate this problem further, randomized studies between these treatment modalities should be performed and the chemotherapy regimen should probably include both cisplatin and prednisone.

The histological type of a thymoma appears to bear no relationship to prognosis. Late recurrence of thymoma is common (Fechner 1969; Cohen *et al.* 1984). Therefore, lifetime surveillance and follow-up of patients who have previously been treated for invasive thymoma is essential.

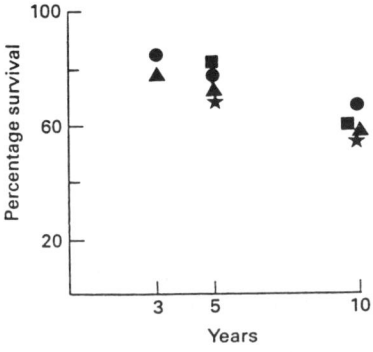

Fig. 2 Overall survival (data from: ▲, Masaoka *et al.* 1981; ■, Appelquist *et al.* 1982; ●, Maggi *et al.* 1986; and ★, Lewis *et al.* 1987).

Table 4 The effect of combination chemotherapy on invasive thymomas

Regimen	No. of patients	No. of complete remissions	Response frequency (%)	Reference
Cisplatin-containing regimens				
CDDP–CTX–DX–VCR	37	16	91	Fornasiero *et al.* (1991)
CDDP–VP–16	4	0	25	Giaccone *et al.* (1985)
CDDP–DX–Bleo–P	6	0	50	Chahinian *et al.* (1981); Göldel *et al.* (1989)
CDDP–CTX–DX	21	4	67	Campbell *et al.* (1981); Loehrer *et al.* (1990)
PVB	4	2	100	Dy *et al.* (1988)
Non-cisplatin containing regimens				
CTX–VCR–CCNU–P	9	4	56	Daugaard *et al.* (1983)
CTX–DX–VCR	12	5	92	Loehrer *et al.* (1985); Kosmidis *et al.* (1988)
CHOP	10	3	30	Hu and Levine (1986); Uematsu and Kondo (1986); Göldel *et al.* (1989)
COPP	10	2	70	Evans *et al.* (1980); Göldel *et al.* (1989)
CHOP–Bleo	4	3	75	Göldel *et al.* (1989)

Abbreviations: Bleo, bleomycin; CCNU, lomustine; CDDP, cisplatin; CHOP, cyclophosphamide–doxorubicin–vincristine–prednisone; COPP, cyclophosphamide–vincristine–procarbazine–prednisone; CTX, cyclophosphamide; DX, doxorubicin; P, prednisone; PVB, cisplatin–vinblastine–bleomycin; VCR, vincristine; VP-16, etoposide.

Taking the infrequency of this tumour type into account, the many problems concerning the treatment of thymoma can obviously only be solved in multicentre studies.

REFERENCES

Appelquist P, Kostiainen S, Franssila K, Mattila S, Gröhn P (1982). Treatment and prognosis of thymoma: a review of 25 cases. *Journal of Surgical Oncology*, **20**:265–8.

Ariaratnam LS, Kalnicki S, Mincer F, Botstein C (1979). The management of thymoma with radiation therapy. *International Journal of Radiation Oncology—Biology—Physics*, **5**:77–80.

Arriagada R, *et al.* (1984). Invasive carcinoma of the thymus. A multicenter retrospective review of 56 cases. *European Journal of Cancer and Clinical Oncology*, **20**:69–74.

Asamura H, Nakajima T, Mukai K, Noguchi M, Shimosato Y (1988). Degree of malignancy of thymic epithelial tumors in terms of nuclear DNA content and nuclear area. *American Journal of Pathology*, **133**:615–22.

Baroni CD, Rigato P, Ruco LP, Uccini S, Mineo TC (1980). A lymphocytes response in normal, hyperplastic and neoplastic thymuses. Morphologic and functional correlations. *Cancer*, **46**:2055–62.

Baroni CD, Valtieri M, Stoppacciaro A, Ruco LP, Uccini S, Ricci C (1983). The human thymus in aging: the histologic involution is paralleled by increased mitogen response and by enrichment of OKT3+ lymphocytes. *Immunology*, **50**:519–28.

Batata MA, Martini N, Huvos AG, Aquilar RI, Beattie EJ (1974). Thymomas: clinicopathologic features, therapy and prognosis. *Cancer*, **34**:389–96.

Battifora H, Sun TT, Bahn RM, Rao S (1980). The use of antikeratin antiserum as a diagnostic tool: thymoma versus lymphoma. *Human Pathology*, **11**:635–41.

Bergh NP, Gatzinsky P, Larsson S, Lundin P, Ridell B (1978). Tumors of the thymus and thymic region: I. Clinicopathological studies on thymomas. *Annals of Thoracic Surgery*, **25**:91–8.

Bernatz PE, Harrison EG, Clagett OT (1961). Thymoma: a clinicopathologic study. *Journal of Thoracic Surgery*, **42**:424–44.

Braitman H, Herrmann C, Mulder DG (1971). Surgery for thymic tumors. *Archives of Surgery*, **103**:14–16.

Campbell MG, Pollard R, Al-Saraf M (1981). A complete response in metastatic thymoma to *cis*-platinum, doxorubicin and cyclophosphamide: a case report. *Cancer*, **48**:1315–17.

Chahinian AP, Bhardway S, Meyer RJ, Jaffrey IS, Kirschner PA, Holland JF (1981). Treatment of invasive or metastatic thymoma: report of eleven cases. *Cancer*, **47**:1752–61.

Claman HN (1972). Corticosteroids and lymphoid cells. *New England Journal of Medicine*, **287**:388–97.

Cohen DJ, *et al.* (1984). Management of patients with malignant thymoma. *Journal of Thoracic and Cardiovascular Surgery*, **87**:301–7.

Curran WJ, Kornstein MJ, Brooks JJ, Turrisi AT (1988). Invasive thymoma: the role of mediastinal irradiation following complete or incomplete surgical resection. *Journal of Clinical Oncology*, **6**:1722–7.

Daugaard G (1989). The effect of chemotherapy in the treatment of malignant thymoma. In *Thymic tumors* (ed. R Sarrazin, C Vrousos, and F Vincent), pp. 112–19. Karger, Basel.

Daugaard G, Hansen HH, Rørth M (1983). Combination chemotherapy for malignant thymoma. *Annals of Internal Medicine*, **99**:189–90.

Dy C, *et al.* (1988). Undifferentiated epithelial-rich invasive malignant thymoma: complete response to cisplatin, vinblastine and bleomycin therapy. *Journal of Clinical Oncology*, **6**:536–42.

Evans WK, Thompson DM, Simpson WJ, Feld R, Philips MJ (1980). Combination chemotherapy in invasive thymoma, role of COPP. *Cancer*, **46**:1523–7.

Exbrayat C, Colonnat M, Ménégoz F (1989). Descriptive epidemiology of thymoma. In *Thymic tumors* (ed. R Sarrazin, C Vrousos, and F Vincent), pp. 14–19. Karger, Basel.

Fechner RE (1969). Recurrence of non-invasive thymomas. Report of four cases and review of the literature. *Cancer*, **23**:1423–7.

Fornasiero A, *et al.* (1991). Chemotherapy for invasive thymoma. *Cancer*, **68**:30–3.

Gaspard MH, *et al.* (1988). Intensive chemotherapy with high doses of BCNU, etoposide, cytosine arabinoside, and melphalan (BEAM) followed by autologous bonemarrow transplantation: toxicity and antitumour activity in 26 patients with poor-risk malignancies. *Cancer Chemotherapy and Pharmacology*, **22**:256–62.

Giaccone G, Musella R, Bertello O, Donadio M, Calciati A (1985). Cisplatin-containing chemotherapy in the treatment of invasive thymoma: report of 5 cases. *Cancer Treatment Reports*, **69**:695–7.

Göldel N, Böning L, Fredrik A, Hölzel D, Hartenstein R, and Wilmanns W (1989). Chemotherapy of invasive thymoma. A retrospective study of 22 cases. *Cancer*, **63**:1493–500.

Gravanis MB (1968). Metastasizing thymoma. *American Journal of Clinical Pathology*, **49**:690–6.

Gurcay O, Wilson C, Barker M, Eliason J (1971). Corticosteroid effect on transplantable rat glioma. *Archives of Neurology*, **24**:266–9.

Hammond EH, Flinner RL (1991). The diagnosis of thymoma: a review. *Ultrastructural Pathology*, **15**:419–38.

Hu E, Levine J (1986). Chemotherapy of malignant thymoma. *Cancer*, **57**:1101–4.

Kaplinsky C, *et al.* (1992). Childhood malignant thymoma: clinical, therapeutic, and immunohistochemical considerations. *Pediatric Hematology and Oncology*, **9**:261–8.

Kirchner T, Müller-Hermelink H (1989). New approaches to the diagnosis of thymic epithelial tumors. *Progress in Surgical Pathology*, **10**:167–89.

Kirschner PA (1990). Reoperation for thymoma: report of 23 cases. *Annals of Thoracic Surgery*, **49**:550–5.

Kornstein MJ, *et al.* (1988). Cortical versus medullary thymomas: a useful morphologic distinction? *Human Pathology*, **19**:1335–9.

Kosmidis PA, Iliopoulos E, Pentea S (1988). Combination chemotherapy with cyclophosphamide, adriamycin and vincristine in malignant thymoma and myasthenia gravis. *Cancer*, **61**:1736–40.

Lattes R, Jones S (1957). The pathological and clinical features in eighty cases of thymoma. *Bulletin of the New York Academy of Medicine*, **33**:145–7.

Legg MA, Brady WJ (1965). Pathology and clinical behaviour of thymomas. A survey of 51 cases. *Cancer*, **18**:1131–44.

Leinen JG, Wittliff JL, Kostyn JA, Brown RC (1974). Glucocorticoid-binding components in an irradiation-induced thymoma of the C57BL/6J mouse. *Cancer Research*, **34**:2779–83.

Lewis JE, Wick MR, Scheithauer BW, Bernatz PE, Taylor WF (1987). Thymoma, a clinicopathologic review. *Cancer*, **60**:2727–43.

Loehrer PJ, *et al.* (1985). Remission of invasive thymoma due to chemotherapy. Two patients treated with cyclophosphamide, doxorubicin and vincristine. *Chest*, **87**:377–80.

Loehrer PJ, Perez CA, Roth LM, Greco FA, Livingston RB, Einhorn LH (1990). Chemotherapy for advanced thymoma. *Annals of Internal Medicine*, **113**:520–4.

Macchiarini P, *et al.* (1991). Neoadjuvant chemotherapy, surgery, and postoperative radiation therapy for invasive thymoma. *Cancer*, **68**:706–13.

Maggi G, *et al.* (1986). Thymomas. A review of 169 cases, with particular reference to results of surgical treatment. *Cancer*, **58**:765–76.

Marino M, Müller-Hermelink HK (1985). Thymoma and thymic carcinoma: relation of thymoma epithelial cells to the cortical and medullary differentiation of thymus. *Virchows Archives Pathological Anatomy*, **407**:119–49.

Marks RD, Wallace KM, Pettit HS (1978). Radiation therapy control of nine patients with malignant thymoma. *Cancer*, **41**:117–19.

Masaoka A, Monden Y, Nakahara K, Tanioka T (1981). Follow-up study of thymomas with special reference to their clinical stages. *Cancer*, **48**:2485–92.

Molina PL, Siegel MJ, Glazar HS (1990). Thymic masses on MR imaging. *American Journal of Radiology*, **155**:495–500.

Moll R, Cowin P, Kapprell HP, Franke WW (1986). Desmosomal proteins: new markers for identification and classification of tumors. *Laboratory Investigation*, **54**:4–25.

Monden Y, *et al.* (1985). Recurrence of thymoma: clinicopathologic features, therapy and prognosis. *Annals of Thoracic Surgery*, **39**:165–9.

Mukai K, Sato Y, Hirohashi S, Shimosato Y (1990). Expression of ras p21 protein by thymoma. *Virchows Archive B Cell Pathology*, **59**:11–16.

Nakahara K, *et al.* (1988). Thymoma: results with complete resection and adjuvant postoperative irradiation in 141 consecutive patients. *Journal of Thoracic and Cardiovascular Surgery*, **95**:1041–7.

Ohmi M, Ohuchi M (1990). Recurrent thymoma in patients with myasthenia gravis. *Annals of Thoracic Surgery*, **50**:243–7.

Oldham HN, Jr (1971). Mediastinal tumors and cysts. *Annals of Thoracic Surgery*, **11**:246–75.

Pescarmona E, Rendina EA, Venuta F, Ricci C, Ruco LP, Baroni CD (1990). The prognostic implication of thymoma histologic typing. A study of 80 consecutive cases. *American Journal of Clinical Pathology*, **93**:190–5.

Posner JB, Howieson J, Cvitkovic E (1977). "Disappearing" spinal cord compression: oncolytic effect of glucocorticoids (and other chemotherapeutic agents) on epidural metastases. *Annals of Neurology*, **2**:409–13.

Rosai J, Levine GD (1976). Tumors of the thymus. In *Atlas of tumor pathology* (2nd series), Fascicle 13. Armed Forces Institute of Pathology, Washington DC.

Rubush JL, Gardner IR, Boyd WC, Ehrenhoft JL (1973). Mediastinal tumors. *Journal of Thoracic and Cardiovascular Surgery*, **65**:216–22.

Salyer WR, Eggleston JC (1976). Thymoma, a clinical and pathological study of 65 cases. *Cancer*, **37**:229–49.

Sawyers JL, Foster JH (1968). Surgical treatment of thymomas. *Archives of Surgery*, **96**:814–17.

Silverman NA, Sabiston DC (1977). Primary tumors and cysts of the mediastinum. *Current Problems in Cancer*, **2**, 3–16.

Souadjian JV, Silverstein MN, Titus JL (1968). Thymoma and cancer. *Cancer*, **22**:1221–5.

Souadjian JV, Enriquez P, Silverstein MN, Pépin JM (1974). The spectrum of diseases associated with thymoma. *Annals of Internal Medicine*, **134**:374–9.

Uematsu M, Kondo M (1986). A proposal for treatment of invasive thymoma. *Cancer*, **58**:1979–84.

Urgesi A, Monetti U, Rossi G, Ricardi U, Casardio C (1990). Role of radiation therapy in locally advanced thymoma. *Radiotherapy and Oncology*, **19**:273–80.

Verley JM, Hollmann KH (1985). Thymoma, a comparative study of clinical stages, histologic features and survival in 200 cases. *Cancer*, **55**:1074–86.

Vessey MP, Doll R (1972). Thymectomy and cancer—a follow up study. *British Journal of Cancer*, **26**:53–8.

Wick MR (1990). Assessing the prognosis of thymomas. *Annals of Thoracic Surgery*, **50**:521–2.

Wilkins EW, Hermes CG, Scannell JG, Moncure AC, Mathisen DJ (1991). Role of staging in prognosis and management of thymoma. *Annals of Thoracic Surgery*, **51**:888–92.

Zeok JV, Todd EP, Dillon M, DeSimone P, Utley JR (1979). The role of thymectomy in red cell aplasia. *Annals of Thoracic Surgery*, **28**:257–60.

Zerhouni EA, Scott WW, Baker RR, Wharam MD, Siegelman SS (1982). Invasive thymomas: diagnosis and evaluation of computed tomography. *Journal of Computer Assisted Tomography*, **6**:92–100.

11.5 Surgical resection of pulmonary metastases

PETER GOLDSTRAW

For patients receiving treatment for the vast majority of malignant neoplasms the development of pulmonary metastases signals the end of any hope of cure. Few disseminated tumours are chemocurable. Although there are anecdotal reports of long-term survival in these circumstances (Casciato *et al.* 1983), the great majority of patients will survive for less than 2 years (Joseph *et al.* 1971). The realization that surgical resection of pulmonary metastases may, in carefully selected cases, extend the survival of some of these patients, has led to a rapid rise in referrals for such surgery. Inevitably such selection will favour patients with fewer metastases, those with better performance status, and those whose tumours have longer doubling times, factors known to improve survival. The results of pulmonary metastasectomy are now comparable to those achieved by the surgical treatment of many primary tumours and randomized, prospective trials with a control arm would be impractical and unethical. This unsatisfactory fact has to be recognized, but only the most cynical would disregard the impressive results obtained with this surgical contribution to the cure of disseminated malignancy.

In this chapter the term 'pulmonary metastasectomy' is reserved for the planned excision, by one or more operations, of all pulmonary metastases with curative intent. We would not use this term in other circumstances; where the excision of a solitary pulmonary nodule

Table 1 Surgery for pulmonary metastases

	N	Operation	Years	(%) Carcinoma	(%) Sarcoma	Mortality	5 year survival
McCormack and Martini (1979)	448	663	17	55	45	1%	Carcinoma 25% Sarcoma 30%
Takita (1981)	234	286	27	75	25	2.4%	Median 21 month
Wright and Brandt (1982)	142	153	22	70	30	0.7%	Carcinoma 24% Sarcoma 29%
Wilkins (1982)	200	239	47	NA	NA	0.8%	10 year 22%
Mountain and McMurtney (1984)	556	772	20+	55	32	1.5%	Carcinoma 39% Sarcoma 38%
Total	1580	2113					

reveals the presence of a previously occult primary, where in a patient with a previously treated primary tumour a pulmonary nodule is found to be benign or a new pulmonary primary, or where the excision of a pulmonary metastasis is undertaken only as a biopsy to confirm the metastatic nature of the lesion(s). Although the excision of other thoracic metastases, such as chest wall deposits, might on occasions be justified by the relief of symptoms, we have not as yet undertaken the excision of pulmonary metastases for palliation.

The first successful pulmonary resection for known metastatic disease was undertaken by Barney and Churchill in 1939. Following this report, single-case reports (Mair and Taylor 1947; Effler and Blades 1948) were followed by series in which solitary (Alexander and Haight 1947; Wilkins *et al.* 1961; Holmes Sellors 1970; Rees and Cleland 1971) and multiple (Seilor *et al.* 1950; Thomford *et al.* 1965) metastases had been successfully excised. In the past two decades five large series from North America have reported the long-term results of pulmonary metastasectomy, with over 2000 operations in over 1500 patients (Table 1). These cases were, however, collected over a long period, up to 47 years and during this period, selection, investigative techniques, and other treatments must have changed considerably.

SELECTION

The selection of patients for pulmonary metastasectomy must be rigorous if perioperative mortality and morbidity are to be kept low and the chance of cure offered is to be reasonable. Inevitably this will dash the hopes of many patients hoping for cure, but in the past we have mistakenly undertaken surgery in circumstances we now know to be futile. To be suitable for such surgery each case must satisfy all of the following criteria.

1. The primary tumour must have been reliably controlled. In the vast majority of cases this will have entailed surgical excision. Local recurrence should be excluded by the most sensitive means available. Careful clinical examination may suffice, but increasingly, especially with deep-seated primaries, it is necessary to undertake computerized tomography (CT) of the primary site. If there is doubt as to local control, the situation should be clarified by a period of observation or surgical exploration and biopsy. In most such circumstances the thoracic surgeon must look for guidance from the colleague who treated the primary.

2. Extrathoracic metastases must be excluded by the most sensitive and appropriate tests. These tests will vary depending on the organ of origin and the cell type, but whole-body CT scanning, isotope bone scanning, and ultrasound facilities must be freely available. If any extrathoracic disease is found, its control must be assured before undertaking pulmonary metastasectomy. This usually entails surgical excision. The sequence of such operations

will be decided in discussion with the other surgeon(s), but in general the more difficult and less certain resection should be performed first. There is little point in undertaking the easier procedure, only to find that complete excision of the other deposits then proves impossible. If the pre-operative search for extrathoracic metastases is inconclusive, the suspicious area should be biopsied. In some circumstances it may be preferable to undertake a period of observation followed by re-evaluation.

3. The extent of the intrathoracic disease must be documented using the most sensitive tests available. While others have relied on conventional tomography, we have found CT to be more accurate. We now insist on contiguous or overlapping CT cuts of both lung fields, from the very apex to the bottom of the costodiaphragmatic recesses. The surgeon then makes his own assessment of the number, size, and disposition of the metastatic deposits and compares this with the radiologist's report. The surgeon must judge that the total excision of all pulmonary metastases is possible, by one or more operations.

4. The patient must be sufficiently robust to tolerate the proposed resection(s). If sequential operations are thought necessary, psychological resilience is also necessary. The patient's lung function must be adequate for the proposed pulmonary resection. Although the extent of resection can only be finally determined at thoracotomy, it is usually possible, with experience, to make a reasonably accurate prediction. Simultaneous bilateral resections will contuse both lungs, and better lung function is necessary if such an approach is being considered. Simple spirometric tests prove adequate to assess lung function. As a rough guide, a pre-operative forced expired volume in 1 s (FEV_1) of 1 litre will allow the safe excision of several unilateral deposits by local excision. If more extensive resection is thought necessary or if bilateral deposits are to be tackled, then proportionally better lung function must be demanded.

Our selection has not been influenced by disease-free interval, tumour doubling time, cell type, or by the number of deposits. Inevitably, however, referring physicians will have been more reticent to refer patients with short disease-free intervals, with tumours having more rapid doubling times, and those with more numerous deposits. There have been occasions when we have felt that the removal of multiple, large, and centrally placed deposits was not feasible. We are aware that others have found long-term survival to be adversely affected by tumour doubling time (Joseph *et al.* 1971; Huth *et al.* 1980; Takita *et al.* 1981) and disease-free interval (Takita *et al.* 1981), but this has not been substantiated by other studies (McCormack and Martini 1979; Wright *et al.* 1982; Mountain *et al.* 1984). Takita *et al.* (1981) found an association between survival and the number of deposits resected, but somewhat paradoxically patients with nine or more deposits fared better than those with four to eight deposits. We and others (McCormack and Martini 1979) have not found the number of deposits to influence survival.

DELAYED METASTASECTOMY

It might be argued that once pulmonary metastases are discovered there should be a period of observation before metastasectomy, to allow other, presently occult, metastases to develop, thus saving futile surgery or allowing more effective tumour clearance. There is some evidence that this is not the case (Mountain *et al.* 1984) but others have found such a delay useful in pre-operative selection (Morton 1983). There is also the concern that, during this delay, metastases may metastasize. This has been shown to occur in the experimental situation (Hoover and Ketcham 1975) and we had one patient in whom events suggested that this can also occur in the clinical setting. This patient underwent a liver transplant for cholangiocarcinoma. Pulmonary deposits became evident later and were excised. Further pulmonary metastases occurred as part of more generalized relapse, with deposits in the brain and skeleton. At 2 years after transplantation, liver metastases were detected in the transplant.

Delay might still prove useful if the initial evaluation leaves one in doubt as to the wisdom of metastasectomy. One may not be convinced that the primary is controlled or there may be suggestions of extrathoracic metastases which cannot be more rapidly resolved by biopsy. In such circumstances we find it of value to repeat the evaluation after 3 or 4 months.

CHOICE OF APPROACH

Once the patient has been accepted for surgery and the extent of intrathoracic disease has been assessed, one can plan surgery so as to excise all the metastases with as few operations as thought safe. In some circumstances it may be possible to cooperate with other surgeons to excise intrathoracic and extrathoracic metastases at a combined operation. Where the pulmonary metastases are thought to be unilateral, we and most other thoracic surgeons would choose a lateral thoracotomy incision. Other surgeons, however, might undertake a median sternotomy incision to inspect the contralateral lung. Johnston (1983) used this approach in 18 patients with apparently unilateral pulmonary metastases from sarcoma and found unsuspected contralateral deposits in 11 patients. One could criticize these results as conventional tomography was used to assess the extent of pulmonary disease. As far as we can judge by the incidence of pulmonary relapse, these results were not superior to those we have obtained with a unilateral approach. Clearly, despite the original operation dealing with unsuspected contralateral deposits, tumour clearance was no more effective, a further example that increasing the scale of surgery cannot compensate for inaccurate evaluation. We have reviewed retrospectively the fate of 60 patients who presented with pulmonary metastases, judged to be unilateral on CT scanning, who underwent lateral thoracotomy. Twenty-one of these patients subsequently relapsed. Ipsilateral pulmonary deposits occurred in seven patients, bilateral pulmonary deposits developed in four patients, relapse was systemic in three patients, and relapse was limited to the opposite lung in only seven patients. Of these, relapse in three patients occurred within 12 months and might have been prevented if the initial surgery had been bilateral. We do not believe that a 5 per cent reduction in relapse rate justifies the routine use of median sternotomy. The handling of the opposite lung greatly increases the physiological upset, as evidenced by the high incidence of prolonged ventilation in the series of Johnston (1983) and complicates further CT evaluation and subsequent surgery.

In 23 per cent of our patients, the initial assessment for metastasectomy showed bilateral pulmonary deposits. These were dealt with at sternotomy in the majority of cases. We would still be selective in the use of sternotomy, preferring staged lateral thoracotomies, if:

(1) the number of deposits in each lung was sufficient to result in extensive bilateral post-operative contusion;

(2) large deposits lay posteriorly in the basal segments, which are less accessible at sternotomy (Fig. 1);

(3) large deposits lay close to hilar structures, such that the improved exposure at lateral thoracotomy might make more conservative resection possible or at least make segmentectomy or lobectomy safer (Fig. 2);

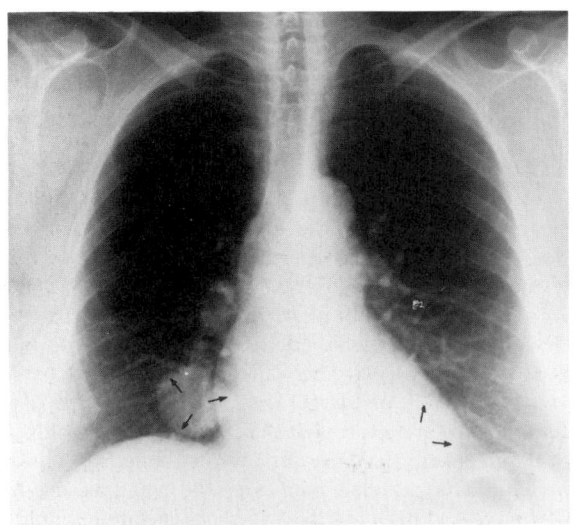

(a)

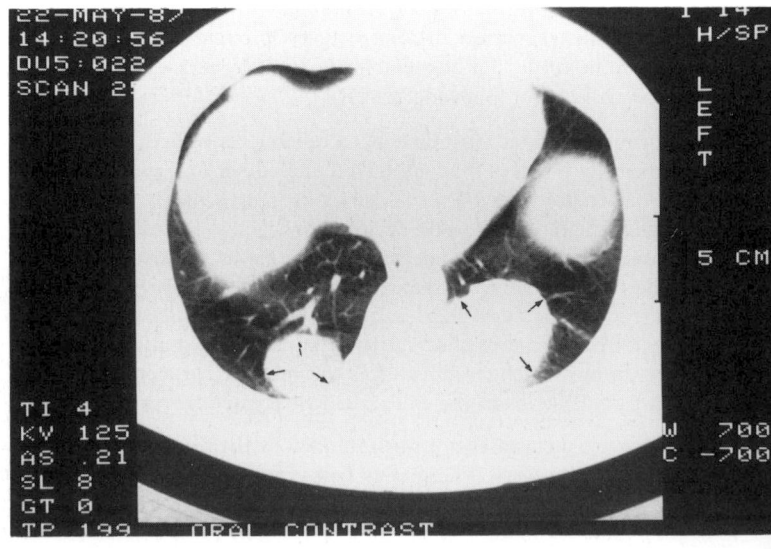

(b)

Fig. 1 (a) Radiograph and (b) CT scan showing large deposits of metastases lying posteriorly in the basal segments.

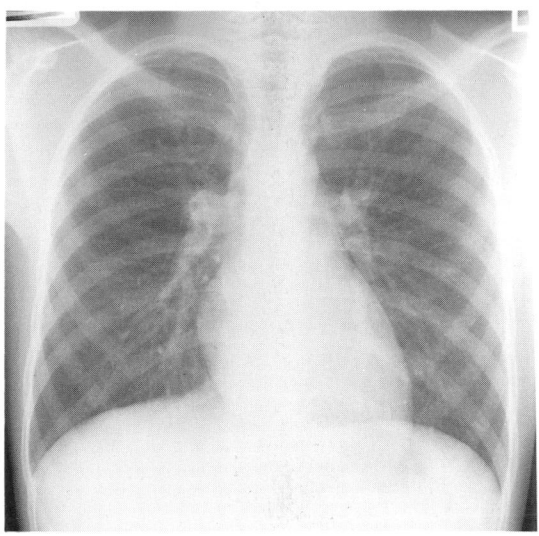

(a)

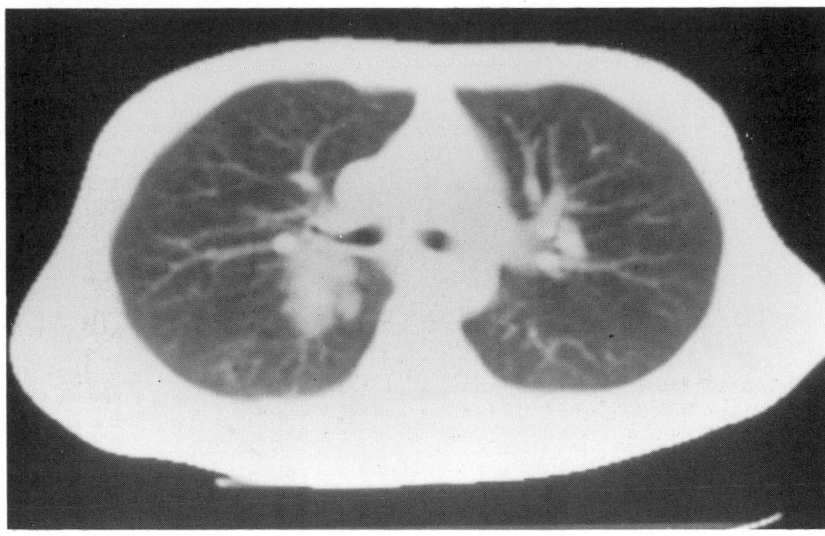

(b)

Fig. 2 (a) Radiograph and (b) CT scan showing large deposits of metastases lying close to hilar structures.

(4) the consistency of the deposits is similar to lung tissue, as can occur with synovial sarcoma and the lateral thoracotomy approach results in less contusion to obscure the deposit at surgery;

(5) there are other extrapulmonary deposits to be excised.

SURGICAL TECHNIQUE

The surgical resection is essentially conservative there is no advantage in removing more lung tissue than is necessary to excise the tumour deposit with a thin rim of surrounding normal tissue.

Preliminary bronchoscopy is performed to exclude the rare occurrence of an intrabronchial metastasis and the less uncommon occurrence of intrabronchial extension. An endobronchial, double-lumen tube is inserted by the anaesthetist to allow collapse of the lung during surgery. During bilateral resections, first one lung can be collapsed and then the other. After the appropriate incision, the lung is palpated by the surgeon and then the assistant, first while it is aerated and then when collapsed. All deposits located are tagged with stay sutures. Although in this the surgeons are guided by the CT scan, all other areas are carefully inspected, including the whole of the lung, the pleura, the mediastinum, and the hilum. Special care is taken in those areas where the CT scan is less reliable, at the apex of the lung and the fringes of the basal segments. Once this evaluation has been made, the number and disposition of deposits is compared with the pre-operative prediction. Each deposit is then excised. In 75 per cent of cases this can be accomplished by wedge excision(s), removing the deposit(s) and a thin rim of surrounding lung tissue. We excise such deposits using diathermy resection, but larger vessels and bronchi will be sutured. The resulting lung defect is then sutured using monofilament material. The use of stapling devices is popular, but does not allow one to curve the line of excision around spherical deposits and the metal staples will make subsequent CT scans difficult to interpret. In the other 25 per cent of our cases, the proximity of the deposit to hilar structures has necessitated that some deposits be resected by more formal excision; segmentectomy, lobectomy, bilobectomy, or a combination of these procedures. Whereas this is more likely with large, centrally positioned deposits, it is occasionally necessary with small deposits, close to hilar structures. The pre-operative CT scan

is most helpful in warning the surgeon that this is a possibility, allowing the patient to be forewarned and the surgical approach to be tailored accordingly. On occasions we have undertaken pneumonectomy, but this operation has given poor results and we would now use it only in the most unusual circumstances.

THE ACCURACY OF CT SCANNING

Clearly, thoracic CT scanning is of great importance in the selection of patients for this type of surgery and in the choice of incision used. We have analysed retrospectively the accuracy of the CT prediction for 121 lungs where we have a correlation with the number of deposits found at operation and confirmed histologically. The results are analysed according to cell type in Table 2 and are remarkably consistent, with an accuracy of 62–70 per cent, rising to 77–79 per cent for solitary deposits. CT scanning underestimated the number of deposits in 25 per cent of cases and overestimated the number in 5–13 per cent of cases. It was rare for these errors to be greater than one or two deposits, such as to undermine the rationale of surgery.

Table 2 Accuracy of CT scanning

	Number of comparisons	Overall accuracy	Under-estimate by CT	Over-estimate by CT	Accuracy for solitary metastases
Carcinoma	40	70%	25%	5%	79%
Sarcoma	28	64%	25%	11%	77%
Teratoma	53	62%	26%	13%	78%

PERSONAL EXPERIENCE

Between 1980 and 1987 we have undertaken pulmonary metastasectomy at 156 operations in 118 patients. There were 80 male and 38 female patients, aged from 5 to 74 years, with a mean age of 38.8 years. The primary tumour was a sarcoma in 43 patients, a teratoma in 42 patients, a carcinoma in 29 cases, and a melanoma in four cases. In 91 patients the metastases were unilateral and approached by a lateral thoracotomy incision, extended into the abdomen in nine patients who had disease above and below the diaphragm. In the 27 patients with bilateral disease, 16 underwent a single operation to

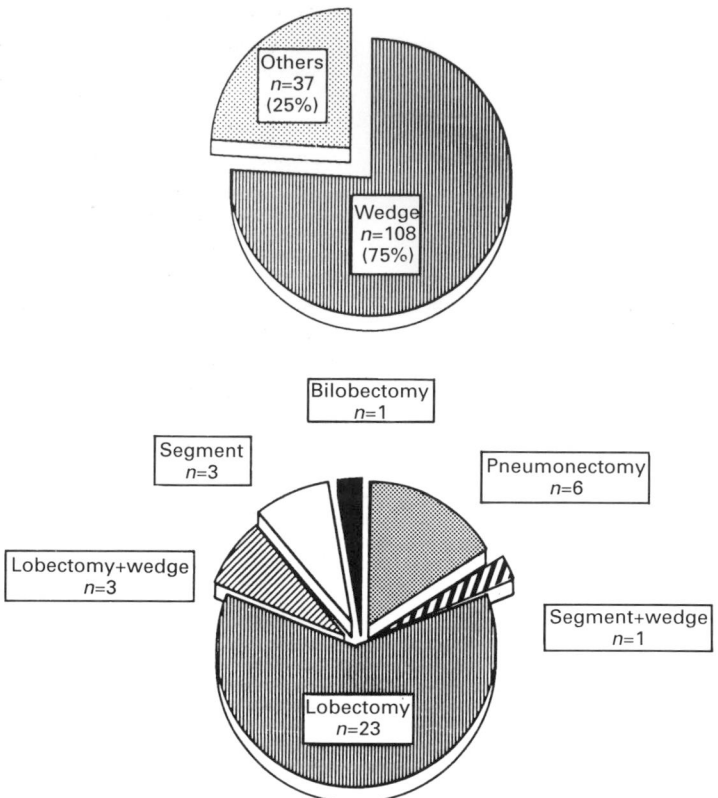

Fig. 3 Pulmonary resections.

excise deposits from both lungs. In 11 patients sequential, staged, lateral thoracotomies were thought to be more prudent. The resections performed are shown in Fig. 3. With subsequent relapse, 23 patients underwent repeat evaluation and further surgery and four patients have undergone a third pulmonary metastasectomy. Since this analysis two patients have had a fourth procedure on the lungs. Two patients died following surgery, an in-hospital mortality of 1.6 per cent per patient and 1.2 per cent per operation. One patient died following lobectomy, due to infection by multiple resistant *Staphylococcus aureus* and one patient died with right heart failure following an ill-advised pneumonectomy. Other morbidity has been low and infection, which was a problem early in our experience, is now controlled by prophylactic antibiotics. We have had three nodules recur after wedge excision, two required lobectomy and the third was treated by more extensive local excision. The local recurrence rate with this conservative approach is therefore 2.7 per cent per operation, 0.8 per cent per wedge excision.

The number of deposits excised at each operation ranged from 1 to 19, with a mean of 3.4 per operation. The maximum number of pulmonary deposits excised at one operation was 19 when bilateral procedures were performed and 13 from one lung. The maximum number of deposits excised with repeated surgery was 26.

SURVIVAL

The results of surgery reported in five other studies are shown in Table 1. The defects of these reports have already been discussed but they remain as important and valid studies. In these studies, survival following pulmonary metastasectomy for carcinoma and sarcoma at 5 years is 24–39 per cent and 20–38 per cent respectively, with a 10-year survival of 22 per cent.

Follow-up in our series (Venn *et al.* 1989) has been 92.4 per cent, with only 11 patients lost to follow-up. The actuarial 5 year survival

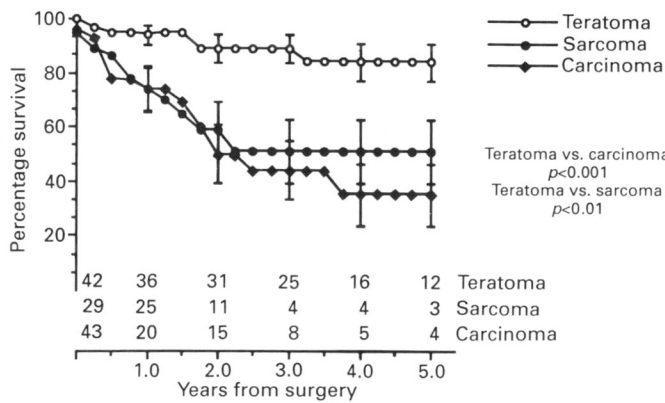

Fig. 4 Actuarial survival.

for our patients, including perioperative deaths, is shown in Fig. 4, with figures for teratoma, sarcoma, and carcinoma of 84 ($\pm$7), 51 ($\pm$12), and 35 per cent ($\pm$12 per cent), respectively. We felt it important to separate out the teratoma patients as their prognosis has been vastly improved with effective chemotherapy and we did not want them to artificially elevate the results obtained for the other cell types. The results in the melanoma group are poor, with only one patient surviving beyond 1 year, to die 16 months after surgery. Others have found the results of treatment for melanoma to be disappointing (Takita *et al.* 1981; Mountain *et al.* 1984). Our relapse-free survival is shown in Fig. 5. Survival did not correlate with the number of deposits, nor was survival worse when multiple rather than solitary deposits were resected (Fig. 6). It is our unsubstantiated belief that the success of this surgery is related to the accuracy of the preoperative evaluation and that success falls as the number of unexpected

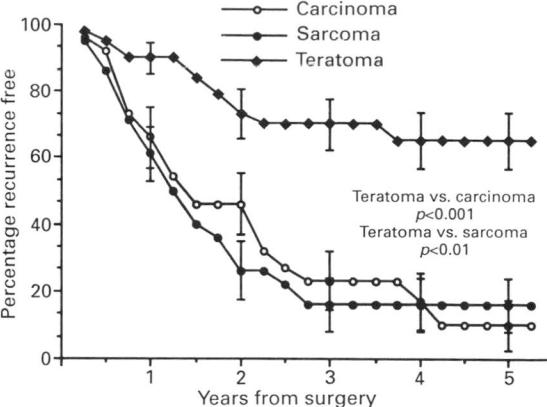

Fig. 5 Recurrence-free survival.

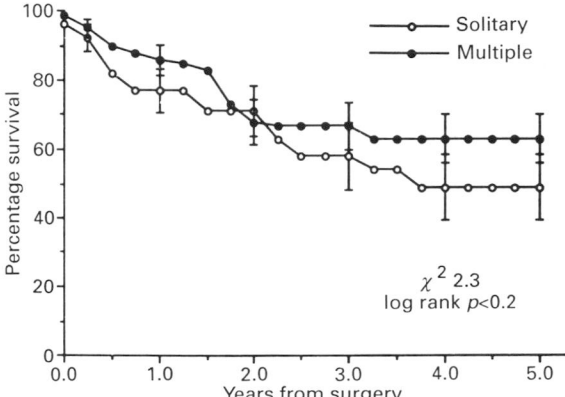

Fig. 6 Solitary versus multiple occurrence.

deposits found at surgery rises. These deposits are too small to be seen on CT scan but palpable to the surgeon and one suspects that in this situation there is a high risk of other deposits which are impalpable to the surgeon.

ADJUVANT THERAPY

The rôle of adjuvant therapy in pulmonary metastasectomy is not clear. Prior treatment of pulmonary metastases by radiotherapy produces considerable surrounding scarring and relapse within this area is most difficult to detect. Usually any such radiotherapy makes conservative resection by wedge excision impossible. For those tumours where effective chemotherapy exists, the oncologist may well wish to assess the response with one or two courses of treatment prior to surgery. Mountain *et al.* (1984) and Huth *et al.* (1980) have found survival to be improved when adjuvant chemotherapy is given in conjunction with metastasectomy. We have had no fixed policy in this respect, but all our cases have been treated in cooperation with oncologists and any adjuvant therapy has been at their discretion. Certainly in the teratoma patients, surgery has only been considered when disease control has been achieved with chemotherapy. In this unusually chemoresponsive tumour, 78 per cent of patients (Tait *et al.* 1984) will have no viable malignancy in the resected deposits, but we believe that surgery is necessary to identify those who have residual malignancy despite normal tumour markers and who need additional chemotherapy, that surgery prevents relapse from unstable differentiated deposits, and that surgery aids tumour control even when malignancy is confirmed (Hendry *et al.* 1987).

Pulmonary metastasectomy is a safe and effective technique, offering reasonable prospects of cure in a carefully selected subset of patients with disseminated malignancy. Pre-operative evaluation must be rigorous. Experience has taught us not to be too ambitious in our surgery and on occasions a sequence of operations will prove necessary. Melanoma patients fare badly and we must be especially cautious in accepting these patients for surgery. Patients with tumours having a rapid doubling time do less well, as they do with all forms of treatment, but we do not take any arbitrary doubling time as a contraindication if the patient is otherwise suitable. Conservative resection is possible in the majority of cases, but more extensive resection is necessary in a quarter of patients. Pneumonectomy is only justified in the most unusual situations. Adjuvant chemotherapy is probably of value if effective regimes exist for the cell type. The timing and duration of chemotherapy should be left to the discretion of the oncologist.

ACKNOWLEDGEMENT

The author wishes to acknowledge the help of the Cancer Research Campaign in funding the collection of his data.

REFERENCES

Alexander J, Haight C (1947). Pulmonary resection for solitary metastatic sarcomas and carcinomas. *Surgery, Gynaecology and Obstetrics*, **85**:129–46.

Barney JE, Churchill EJ (1939). Adenocarcinoma of the kidney with metastasis to the lung. *Journal of Urology*, **42**:269–76.

Casciato DA, Nagurka C, Tabbarah HJ (1983). Prolonged survival with unresected pulmonary metastases. *Annals of Thoracic Surgery*, **36**:202–8.

Effler DB, Blades B (1948). *Journal of Thoracic Surgery*, **17**:27.

Hendry WF, Goldstraw P, Peckham MJ (1987). The role of surgery in the combined management of metastases from teratomas of testis. *British Journal of Urology*, **59**:358.

Holmes Sellors T (1970). The treatment of isolated pulmonary metastases. *British Medical Journal*, 1:253–6.

Hoover HC, Ketcham AS (1975). Metastasis of metastases. *American Journal of Surgery*, **30**:405–11.

Huth JF, Holmes EC, Vernon SE, Callery CD, Ramming KP, Morton DL (1980). Pulmonary resection for metastatic sarcoma. *American Journal of Surgery*, **140**:9–16.

Johnston MIR (1983). Median sternotomy for resection of pulmonary metastases. *Journal of Thoracic and Cardiovascular Surgery*, **85**:516–22.

Joseph WL, Morton DL, Adkins PC (1971). Prognostic significance of tumour doubling time in evaluating operability in pulmonary metastatic disease. *Journal of Thoracic and Cardiovascular Surgery*, **61**:23–32.

McCormack PM, Martini N (1979). The changing role of surgery for pulmonary metastases. *Annals of Thoracic Surgery*, **28**:139–45.

Maier HC, Taylor HC (1947). Metastatic choriocarcinoma of the lung treated by lobectomy. *American Journal of Obstetrics and Gynecology*, **53**:674–7.

Morton DL (1983). In the discussion of Johnston, M. I. R. (1983). Median sternotomy for resection of pulmonary metastases. *Journal of Thoracic and Cardiovascular Surgery*, **85**:516–22.

Mountain CF, McCurtney MJ, Hermes KE (1984). Surgery for pulmonary metastases: a 20 year experience. *Annals of Thoracic Surgery*, **38**:323–30.

Rees GM, Cleland WP (1971). The surgical treatment of pulmonary metastases from testicular tumours. *British Medical Journal*, 2:467–70.

Seilor HH, Claggett OT, MacDonald JR (1950). The surgery of pulmonary metastases. *Journal of Thoracic Surgery*, **19**:655–75.

Tait D, Peckham MJ, Hendry W, Goldstraw P (1984). Post-chemotherapy surgery in advanced non-seminomatous germ-cell testicular tumours: the significance of histology with particular reference to differentiated (mature) teratoma. *British Journal of Cancer*, **50**:601–9.

Takita H, Edgerton F, Karakousis Z, Douglass HO, Vincent RJ, Beckley S (1981). Surgical management of metastases to the lung. *Surgery, Gynecology and Obstetrics*, **152**:191–4.

Thomford NR, Woolner LB, Claggett OT (1965). The surgical treatment of metastatic tumours of the lungs. *Journal of Thoracic and Cardiovascular Surgery*, **49**:357–70.

Venn GE, Sarin S, Goldstraw P (1989). Survival following pulmonary metastasectomy. *European Journal of Cardiothoracic Surgery*, **3**:105–10.

Wilkins EW, Burke JF, Head JM (1961). The surgical management of metastatic neoplasms in the lung. *Journal of Thoracic and Cardiovascular Surgery*, **42**:298–303.

Wright JO, Brandt B, Ehrenhaft JL (1982). Results of pulmonary resection for metastatic lesions. *Journal of Thoracic and Cardiovascular Surgery*, **83**:94–9.

11.6   Uncommon intrathoracic tumours

JEFFREY S. TOBIAS

INTRODUCTION

The uncommon intrathoracic tumours are a widely heterogeneous group of malignancies, arising from the chest wall, mediastinum, and from the lung itself. Occasionally, the tumour is so large or unusually situated that it is difficult to be certain as to the precise primary origin. This chapter will consider separately the unusual tumours of lung, mediastinum, and chest wall using the anatomical classification outlined in Table 1.

UNCOMMON TUMOURS OF THE LUNG

This group of tumours represents a spectrum of disorders from benign to highly malignant. Of the malignant group, both Hodgkin's disease and non-Hodgkin's lymphomas are occasionally encountered, but very rarely as parenchymal tumours without obvious mediastinal involvement as well. In patients with advanced lymphoma, both pleural effusion and scattered pulmonary lymphomatous nodules may be present. Their clinical behaviour is described elsewhere.

Of the less malignant neoplasms, the bronchial gland tumours ('bronchial adenomas') form an important group, comprising up to 1 per cent of all primary bronchial tumours (Burcharth and Axelsson 1972). They are derived from the epithelial and glandular structures of the bronchi and include bronchial carcinoids which are easily the commonest type of bronchial adenoma, as well as adenoid cystic carcinomas, mucoepidermoid tumours, and other mixed types.

Bronchial carcinoids

These constitute 90 per cent of the bronchial adenoma group, tend to be centrally located in main, lobar, or segmental bronchi (85 per cent of all cases), and share the common characteristics of all carcinoid tumours; that is, the presence of fluorogenic amines and/or the ability to take up amine precursors, together with the presence of specific neurosecretory granules and aminodecarboxylases within the cells (Hirsch 1988). It is currently believed that these endocrine cells originate from the neural crest, although other explanations are possible. The central carcinoid group develops as polypoid exophytic lesions projecting into the lumen of the bronchus, with a characteristic histological appearance of trabecular or ribbon–like patterns of cells containing abundant clear or granular cytoplasm. The peripheral group has a more variable histological appearance, with a more disordered cellular pattern and frequent inclusion of spindle cell elements. A further group of atypical bronchial carcinoids has a more puzzling appearance with increased cellularity and nuclear pleomorphism,

Table 1   Classification of uncommon lung tumours

Tumours of blood and reticuloendothelial system
  Hodgkin's lymphoma
  Non-Hodgkin's lymphoma
  Leukaemias
  Plasmacytoma
  Histiocytic tumours
  Lymphoproliferative conditions

Tumours of epithelium
  Carcinoid
  Cylindroma
  Mucoepidermoid tumour
  Melanoma
  Papilloma
  Clear cell tumour
  Adenoma
  Sclerosing pneumocytoma

Tumours of vascular tissue
  Haemangiopericytoma
  Intravascular bronchioloalveolar tumour
  Angiosarcoma
  Lymphangioleiomyoma
  Tuberous sclerosis
  Arteriovenous malformations
  Lymphangiectasis

Tumours of muscle and connective tissue
  Leiomyoma (sarcoma)
  Rhabdomyosarcoma
  Fibroma (sarcoma)
  Lipoma (sarcoma)
  Chondroma (sarcoma)
  Myxoma

Tumours of neural tissue
  Neurofibroma
  Neurilemmoma
  Neurosarcoma
  Chemodectoma

Tumours of mixed cell origin
  Teratoma
  Hamartoma
  Carcinosarcoma
  Blastoma

Reproduced from Crofton and Douglas (1981), with permission.

often accompanied by a greater than expected degree of mitotic activity. Lymphatic involvement is unusual though demonstrable in up to 20 per cent of cases (McCaughan *et al.* 1985), but haematogenous spread is very unusual, occurring in less than 5 per cent of patients with primary bronchial carcinoid.

Clinically the group of central carcinoids is more likely than the others to result in specific symptoms, often present for many years in view of the relatively benign nature of the lesion and the low level of metastatic spread. In approximately 50 per cent of cases, there is a history of recurrent infection, haemoptysis, or wheezing (Hurt and Bates 1984), though pain, cough, and dyspnoea may also occur and only 20 per cent are entirely asymptomatic. Carcinoid syndrome is rarely associated with these tumours (Ricci *et al.* 1973) and is almost invariably associated with distant metastases.

Careful anatomical staging is of particular importance since adequate surgical resection carries an excellent prognosis. Most patients have tumours which are visible at rigid bronchoscopy; the majority of these prove resectable. Although notorious for risk of haemorrhage, most bronchial carcinoids can be biopsied safely in order to establish the diagnosis before resection is attempted (Hurt and Bates 1984).

Peripherally located carcinoids are more difficult to diagnose and indeed to distinguish from carcinoma of the bronchus, particularly small-cell lung cancer. Occasionally, resection of a peripheral small cell lung cancer unexpectedly confirms that the tumour is indeed a carcinoid; perhaps more commonly, the correct diagnosis comes to light after the failure of chemotherapy to provide tumour shrinkage in what was assumed to be a peripheral small-cell lung cancer. Computerized tomography (CT) and formal lung function testing should generally be undertaken before surgical resection of both the central and peripheral group of tumours, although the demonstration of mediastinal lymphadenopathy should not necessarily preclude an attempt at resection since a long-term cure is still sometimes possible.

Thoracotomy and resection is essential for cure and endobronchial procedures should be avoided. Lobectomy is generally required, with routine mediastinal lymph node dissection both for staging and also resection of involved node groups. Although the long-term prognosis is excellent, with 5 year survival rates of over 92 per cent (Hurt and Bates 1984; McCaughan *et al.* 1985), the likelihood of long survival clearly relates to the type of tumour. In the British series, chiefly of patients with central tumours, the high survival rate was well maintained at 10 years, although in the series from New York the 10 year survival rate had fallen to 77 per cent, presumably a reflection of the greater degree of lymphatic involvement, peripheral primary sites, larger tumour size, and atypical carcinoids.

Bronchial adenoid cystic carcinoma ('cylindroma')

This is much less common and frequently arises from the trachea, especially the upper third. As with adenoid cystic carcinomas at other sites, these tumours are characterized by cellular growth in lengthy cylinders, with small, darkly staining tumour cells sometimes clustered around a lumen and often with perineural infiltration, which is thought to account for the pain they cause in a large proportion of patients. Because of their proximal location, they frequently produce symptoms of upper airway obstruction including stridor, hoarseness, or late-onset asthma. Unlike bronchial carcinoids, they are often locally invasive, sometimes with a surprisingly distant degree of perineural or other planar spread. Naturally this will often make adequate resection much more difficult, particularly where tracheal resection is required. None the less, surgical resection offers the best means of local control and should never be excluded without good reason. However, as with adenoid cystic carcinomas elsewhere, it is now clear that the long-established view that radiotherapy is ineffective should be abandoned (Price *et al.* 1979). Post-operative radiotherapy should be strongly considered when tumour resection is inadequate or where there is obvious perineural or local lymphatic invasion. For the occasional case where resection is contraindicated, radiotherapy offers a reasonable alternative without the risk of surgical morbidity, although admittedly with a less certain probability of adequate local control. Although chemotherapy has only rarely been used for these tumours, there are one or two encouraging reports (Stuart-Harris and McCaughan 1988).

Mucoepidermoid tumours

These are very rare, arising from the bronchial epithelium most frequently in proximal bronchi. Low-grade tumours have a very low metastatic potential, whereas high-grade mucoepidermoid tumours may spread to regional lymph nodes or more distant sites. Wherever possible, complete surgical resection should be carried out, although radiotherapy is worth considering for irresectable cases.

Myoblastomas (granular cell tumours)

Other tumours in the 'occasionally malignant' category are much less common. Myoblastomas are very rare, chiefly occurring in large bronchi as polypoid single growths but occasionally occurring as multiple tumours. The tumour is more common in females and in dark-skinned races, has a very low malignant potential, and presents only occasionally as a lung or tracheobronchial tumour. At this site, it may be difficult to distinguish from secondary carcinoma from thyroid, pancreatic, or hepatic primary sites (Brooks 1988), although special stains may prove conclusive. Malignant granular cell tumours can only be diagnosed in the presence of metastatic disease; by contrast, the benign granular cell tumour is generally cured by surgical excision, with a local recurrence rate of well under 10 per cent.

Pulmonary neurofibromas

Pulmonary neurofibromas or other intrapulmonary neurogenic tumours are excessively rare, although they do seem to occur in some patients with generalized neurofibromatosis or von Recklinghausen's disease. Indeed, both these and also the schwannoma group may sometimes undergo malignant change and for this reason are generally resected wherever possible.

Primary lung sarcomas

These are extremely unusual and often difficult to distinguish from pulmonary deposits of sarcoma from other primary sites. They occur from early infancy to adult life but are most frequently encountered in middle-aged or elderly patients. Most of them arise from the bronchial walls, but some apparently occur as parenchymal tumours, often remaining asymptomatic until a large size has been reached or chest wall extension has occurred. There is no known relationship to cigarette smoking and the clinical course is generally slower than in patients with bronchogenic carcinomas. Although, of course, much rarer than carcinomas, a cluster of chest radiographic features has been described which may suggest a sarcomatous lesion, including large size and peripheral location, clear margins to the tumour, and lack of central cavitation (Nascimento and Unni 1982). The commoner pathological subtypes include leiomyosarcoma, fibrosarcoma, chondrosarcoma, and carcinosarcoma. It is generally possible to make a firm diagnosis with the appropriate special staining techniques (Wick and Manivel 1988). Both leiomyosarcoma and fibrosarcoma generally occur as an endobronchial or intrapulmonary mass, with typical histological appearances. Electron microscopy may be helpful for distinction from other intrathoracic sarcomas. Other types of primary thoracic sarcoma, such as haemangiopericytoma, malignant fibrous histiocytoma of the lung, angiosarcoma, and rhabdomyosarcoma, are even less common. However, the epithelioid haemangioendothelioma, initially described as a primary chondrosarcoma of the lung, may be more common and is now recognized as an endothelial low-grade malignancy, also found with an identical histological appearance in other sites, such as liver and soft tissues. Sometimes referred to as an intravascular broncho-alveolar tumour, most of these, when presenting as lung primaries, are peripheral and multifocal but, occasionally, endobronchial tumours have also been recognized. In some respects, these tumours closely resemble angiosarcoma, particularly in their electron microscopic and immunocytochemical features. Finally in the sarcoma group, the rapid increase in cases of Kaposi's sarcoma related to infection by the human immunodeficiency virus has led to the recognition of primary Kaposi's sarcoma of the lung (Nash and Fligiel 1984). In addition, as pointed out by Wick and Manivel (1988), several cases of 'inflammatory pseudo-tumour' of the lung have now been reported, which histologically seem to resemble fibrous histiocytoma most closely.

True primary lung sarcomas tend to be aggressive and rapidly malignant, although local progression is more common than distant metastasis. Some types of sarcoma, particularly malignant fibrous histiocytoma and angiosarcoma, appear more aggressive than the epithelioid haemangioendothelioma or endobronchial fibrosarcoma. Wherever possible, adequate surgical resection should be undertaken, even if this requires pneumonectomy. Non-surgical methods of treatment have, for the most part, been unhelpful, although adjuvant chemotherapy is often employed, using appropriate soft tissue sarcoma regimens.

Primary melanoma of the lung

This is exceptionally uncommon and particularly difficult to document in view of the extreme frequency of the lung as a site of secondary spread in melanoma arising elsewhere. None the less, approximately 20 cases have now been described (Herbert 1988), most of which were accepted by this author as genuine cases. Most of the tumours were polypoid, intraluminal, or had infiltrated the bronchial wall and were generally described as pleomorphic or polygonal or spindle-celled tumours. Interestingly, 60 per cent of 12 patients with surgically resected primary lung melanoma were alive and well after 5 years of follow-up, a very much better prognosis than would be expected if these had indeed been lung metastases from another primary site.

UNCOMMON MEDIASTINAL TUMOURS

An understanding of mediastinal anatomy is important in the consideration of all mediastinal tumours and the simplest approach is to divide the mediastinum into three portions, the anterosuperior, middle, and posterior sections. The anterosuperior compartment is bounded inferiorly by the diaphragm, anteriorly by the sternum, and posteriorly by the vertebral column down to the fourth thoracic vertebra and then by the anterior pericardium. It contains the upper trachea and oesophagus, the aortic arch, and the thymus and may also include a retrosternal portion of normal thyroid gland, with parathyroid structures and embryonic cell rests. The middle compartment is bounded anteriorly by the anterior pericardium and posteriorly by the oesophagus and extends downwards to the diaphragm. It contains the heart, ascending aorta, main bronchi,

Table 2 Types and major location of mediastinal tumours

Anterosuperior
  Thymoma
  Teratoma
  Thyroid and parathyroid tumours
  Sarcoma (haemangiosarcoma, haemangiopericytoma)
  Mesothelioma
  Lipomas

Middle
  Malignant lymphoma
  Tumours of the heart
  Secondary lymph node involvement
  Pericardial tumours

Posterior
  Neurofibroma, neurilemmoma, schwannoma
  Neuroblastoma
  Neurofibrosarcoma
  Phaeochromocytoma
  Chordoma
  Paraganglioma

Reproduced from Souhami and Tobias (1986), with permission.

hila and carina, and the subcarinal and other closely related tracheo-bronchial lymph nodes. The posterior mediastinum lies between the vertebral column and posterior pericardium, containing the oesophagus, the descending thoracic aorta, and the sympathetic nerve chains. The pattern of tumours arising in the mediastinum reflects these anatomical divisions (Souhami and Tobias 1986). Table 2 outlines the commoner types of mediastinal tumour.

Thymic tumours and mesothelioma have been dealt with earlier in this section. Thymomas are the most common tumours of the anterior mediastinum (Harper and Addis 1988) but other non-thymic anterior mediastinal malignant tumours include three important groups: the germ cell tumours, malignant lymphomas, and paragangliomas. In addition, in the more superior aspect of the anterosuperior compartment of the mediastinum, thyroid and parathyroid tumours (and hyperplasias) both occur.

In a large series of anterior mediastinal tumours reported by Mullen and Richardson (1986), thymic tumours accounted for just under half (47 per cent), lymphomas 23 per cent, endocrine tumours 16 per cent, and germ cell tumours 15 per cent of cases. In children and young adults, lymphomas and germ cell tumours were particularly important.

Anterosuperior mediastinum

In view of the central nature of this tumour location, the majority of patients present with specific chest symptoms, chiefly pain, dyspnoea, and cough due to compression of local structures. Dysphagia, superior vena caval obstruction, cardiac arrhythmia, and Horner's syndrome are also common. Tumours of the most superior part of the mediastinum sometimes cause respiratory distress and stridor due to direct tracheal pressure or invasion. From the point of view of aetiology, pathology, and clinical behaviour, the thyroid and parathyroid tumours are similar to the same tumours at their more common primary sites in the neck. With regard to management, surgical and radiotherapeutic approaches will naturally be modified. Surgical resection of retrosternal intrathoracic thyroid or parathyroid tumours is generally a more hazardous procedure than when the tumour is confined to the neck; in other respects the indications for surgery are identical. Adequate removal of anaplastic tumours is likely to prove even more difficult in the case of retrosternal primaries, generally leading to a greater reliance on definitive or post-operative radiotherapy.

Thymic tumours, including the important lymphomatous and germ cell groups, are dealt with elsewhere, though it is worth pointing out that some of these disorders, for example Hodgkin's disease of the thymus, most frequently exhibit widespread anterior mediastinal involvement beyond the thymus itself. Similarly, mediastinal germ cell tumours are frequently extrathymic and, indeed, germ cell malignancies constitute 2–3 per cent of all mediastinal tumours.

Although paragangliomas sometimes develop in the anterior mediastinum, deriving from the parasympathetic aortopulmonary bodies, they are described together with the other neurogenic tumours of the posterior mediastinum, the more characteristic primary location (see below).

Of the non-thymic tumours of the true anterior mediastinum, the most important groups are the extragonadal (mediastinal) germ cell tumours and the mediastinal lymphomas.

Mediastinal germ cell tumours

Primary germ cell tumours of the mediastinum are now increasingly recognized and constitute between 1 and 5 per cent of all germ cell malignancies, together accounting for approximately 3 per cent of mediastinal tumours. They often arise within the thymus and thymic tissue is frequently intermixed, giving a histologically varied appearance with respect to the more common gonadal sites (Addis 1988). Presumably they develop as a result of malignant change within cell 'rests' left during the early stages of embryogenesis as a result of incomplete migration of germ cell elements. Important associations are with Klinefelter's syndrome (Sogge et al. 1979; McNeil et al. 1981) and acute leukaemia (Nichols et al. 1985). All types of germ cell tumour are seen, including pure seminomas, mixed tumours, and both mature and immature non-seminomatous germ cell tumours.

Pure seminomas constitute approximately half of all mediastinal germ cell tumours, occurring almost invariably in males, at a mean age of 30 years (Hurt et al. 1982). The non-seminomatous germ cell tumours occur in a younger age group, as with gonadal primary non-seminomatous germ cell tumours and all the common histological types are represented (see Chapter 3.1 for a discussion of histological features). Benign mediastinal teratoma ('dermoid cyst') also occurs chiefly in adult life and, unlike the malignant group, is equally frequent in women. This is a very unusual mediastinal tumour of bizarre histology, with skin, hair follicles, cartilage, smooth muscle, and other organs often well represented.

As with primary gonadal germ cell tumours, tumour markers are often prominent although, even in marker-negative cases, immuno-histochemical techniques may demonstrate small foci of yolk sac or choriocarcinomatous elements which stain readily with antibodies to α-fetoprotein or β-human chorionic gonadotropin. With pure seminoma, staining for placental alkaline phosphatase is often clearly visible.

In view of the extreme chemosensitivity of malignant germ cell tumours, both seminoma and non-seminomatous germ cell tumours, the principles of management of mediastinal germ cell tumours are similar to those of the primary gonadal group of tumours. Chemotherapy is clearly the mainstay of treatment, using cisplatin- or carboplatin-based regimens similar to those developed for malignant gonadal germ cell tumours (Hainsworth et al. 1982). However, unlike the primary gonadal group, surgical resection of a mediastinal germ cell tumour is much more hazardous and chemotherapy is essentially required for every case. A policy of surveillance, which has become commonplace in stage 1 gonadal

patients post-orchidectomy, is clearly inappropriate in the mediastinal group. Although chemoresponsive, the proportion of complete responders to chemotherapy is somewhat lower than with primary germ cell tumours, possibly because of residual masses of mature teratoma or fibrous-stromal residue. In the Hainsworth series, for instance, the complete remission rate was 15 out of 32 patients (47 per cent) and an additional six patients (19 per cent) were rendered disease free with surgical resection. Although these results were felt to be worse than those for testicular tumours, they are broadly similar to the results in metastatic testicular tumours of similar bulk (Einhorn et al. 1985). It is also worth remembering that radiotherapy may play a useful rôle, particularly, of course, in mediastinal pure seminoma, although chemotherapy should always be offered in the first instance for bulky tumours. For monitoring the progress and response to treatment, serial tumour marker estimations and CT scanning are invaluable. Chemotherapy combinations are further discussed in detail elsewhere and the detailed choice of agents should clearly follow current guidelines for gonadal primary tumours, with particular emphasis on regimens appropriate to bulky tumours. In patients with small-volume pure seminoma who are unwilling or unable to tolerate chemotherapy, mediastinal irradiation is a satisfactory alternative, with a high response and cure rate using the relatively modest dosage of 40 Gy in 20 daily fractions in 4 weeks as a midline dose.

With radiologically visible residual disease after chemotherapy, surgery should always be considered, particularly in the case of non-seminomatous germ cell tumours (Kay et al. 1987) because, as with testicular teratoma, mature teratoma is frequently encountered without evidence of residual undifferentiated disease. Although most of such patients are cured, there are certainly documented instances in which a late relapse has occurred. Operations of this type may be hazardous in view of the previous exposure of most patients to bleomycin, with its associated pulmonary toxicity and reduced pulmonary compliance and reserve.

Malignant lymphoma of the thymus and anterior mediastinum

Hodgkin's disease

In approximately 10 per cent of all patients with Hodgkin's disease, the mediastinum is the only site of involvement (Fig. 1). Approximately half of these cases are confined to the thymus alone (Addis 1988), the remainder involving the mediastinum more widely. Mediastinal involvement, to the exclusion of other sites, seems more common in females and is frequently asymptomatic, the disease manifesting either because of lymphoma-related symptoms or recognized as a chance finding on a chest radiograph. Large lymphoma centres occasionally encounter patients who have been referred from the dermatology clinic with an initial clinical presentation of pruritus, in whom mediastinal Hodgkin's disease is diagnosed without any other evidence of superficial or distant lymphadenopathy. Staging investigations are mandatory, as with any patient with newly diagnosed Hodgkin's disease, but are generally negative. Laparotomy is nowadays rarely advised, although there are certainly cases where it might be justified, for instance in the case of a large but asymptomatic mediastinal tumour occurring in a young patient with anxieties about fertility, chemotherapy might be avoidable provided there is no evidence of infradiaphragmatic involvement.

Microscopically, mediastinal Hodgkin's disease is almost always of the nodular sclerosis variety, often with prominent lacunar cells and rather scanty Reed–Sternberg cellular infiltration, together with an admixture of residual thymic epithelium.

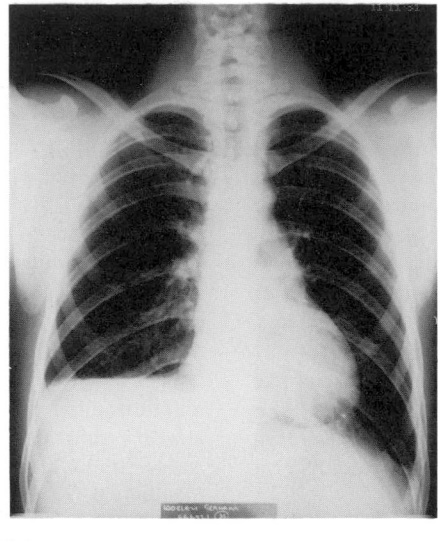

(a)   (b)

Fig. 1 (a) Presenting chest radiograph of a male patient with nodular sclerosing Hodgkin's disease. This 24 year old asymptomatic patient was diagnosed in 1979 and treated by radiotherapy. (b) Chest radiograph 2 years later; the patient remains alive and well.

Clinical management follows standard guidelines as for Hodgkin's disease at other sites with local radiotherapy generally advised for small-bulk mediastinal involvement (less than one-third of the transverse diameter of the thorax) and chemotherapy as the initial treatment for more bulky disease (Mauch *et al.* 1978; Johnson *et al.* 1983).

Non-Hodgkin's lymphoma

Mediastinal or hilar lymphadenopathy occurs in approximately 20 per cent of patients overall, but is much less commonly present at diagnosis. Mediastinal non-Hodgkin's lymphoma is commoner in children and adolescents and approximately 70 per cent of cases are of T-cell origin, the others being of pre-B-cell type (Addis 1988). Many of these predominantly lymphoblastic cases are associated with a substantial thymic mass, the so-called Sternberg sarcoma (Smith *et al.* 1973). This highly malignant tumour frequently involves bone-marrow and may present as a rapidly progressive acute leukaemia. It is much more common in males. Finally, a more recently recognized form of mediastinal non-Hodgkin's lymphoma is the large cell mediastinal lymphoma with sclerosis, thought to be a B-cell neoplasm of true thymic origin (Addis and Isaacson 1986) and chiefly affecting patients in middle age, predominantly female. Unlike the T-cell lymphoblastic lymphoma, extrathoracic spread is generally to viscera such as kidney, liver, or thyroid, rather than to bone-marrow or other lymph node groups. The tumour may cause superior vena caval obstruction and can be extremely bulky at presentation. Characteristically, the histological picture is one of large tumour cells with features of high-grade lymphoma, a high mitotic rate, folded or lobulated nuclei, and with stromal fibrosis and areas of non-neoplastic T lymphocytes.

As with non-Hodgkin's lymphoma at other sites, management is non-surgical. Combination chemotherapy is invariably required, particularly for high-grade lesions, though treatment failure is common, particularly with the aggressive T-cell lymphoblastic lymphoma of adolescents, for whom treatment should probably be instituted as for acute lymphoblastic leukaemia from the outset. Local irradiation is generally employed for residual disease and there are documented cases in which an incomplete chemotherapy response has been 'converted' into a long-lasting complete remission with the addition of mediastinal irradiation.

Miscellaneous tumours of the anterior mediastinum

This group includes benign tumours such as thymolipoma (rare, benign, well under 10 per cent of all thymic tumours), thymic sarcoma (extremely rare; see Addis 1988), and histiocytosis X. This last entity is extremely unusual as a thymic tumour, but may occur in the absence of lesions elsewhere.

Mediastinal sarcomas of non-thymic origin are a little more common and occur in both the anterior and posterior mediastinal compartments. Liposarcoma is the commonest primary cell type; leiomyosarcoma and angiosarcoma are also occasionally encountered, although they may be difficult to distinguish from the primary pulmonary sarcomas described above. Primary liposarcoma of the mediastinum is perhaps the best understood of these diseases, a tumour affecting both sexes at a mean of 45 years and presenting chiefly with respiratory distress, chest pain, cough, and weight loss. In the childhood age group, mediastinal rhabdomyosarcoma is also well recognized though extremely unusual. Combinations of surgery, chemotherapy, and radiotherapy should probably be employed in all cases, although the prognosis remains very poor (Crist *et al.* 1982).

Castleman's disease (angiofollicular lymph node hyperplasia)

This curious and essentially non-malignant condition was first reported by Castleman and colleagues (Castleman *et al.* 1954; Keller *et al.* 1972), who described patients with a relatively benign hyperplastic mediastinal lymph node enlargement, initially thought to resemble thymoma. The condition generally presents as a large asymptomatic mediastinal mass and true thymic involvement is now thought to be rare (Addis 1988). Other sites include retroperitoneum and superficial node groups and, more recently, a systemic syndrome has been recognized in association with this lesion, which includes fever, anaemia, and hyperglobulinaemia. Two main types of Castleman's disease have been described, a hyaline vascular type, the commonest variety, generally with a single, rounded mass of nodes with small follicular centres and prominent vessels surrounded by sheaths of hyalinized collagen. The second type, the plasma cell variant, has large numbers of mature plasma cells between the follicles and the lymphoid sinuses are usually effaced although

Table 3 Mediastinal lymph node enlargement simulating lymphoma from causes other than Castleman's disease

Follicular histology
  Reactive hyperplasia
  Rheumatoid arthritis and related arthritides
  Angiofollicular hyperplasia
  Toxoplasmosis

Diffuse histology
  Phenytoin sensitivity
  Dermatopathic lymphadenopathy
  Angioimmunoblastic lymphadenopathy with dysproteinaemia
  Metastatic carcinoma

Other histologies
  Sinus histiocytosis with massive lymph node enlargement
  Infectious mononucleosis
  Cat scratch fever
  Metastatic carcinoma (especially melanoma)

Reproduced from Souhami and Tobias (1986), with permission.

follicular centres may be present. It is this latter type which is particularly associated with the systemic symptoms. Other associated conditions include nephrotic syndrome, myasthenia gravis, and unexplained peripheral neuropathy.

The disease can occur at any age and in both sexes. Most of the lymph node enlargement is central (hilar–mediastinal) although intrapulmonary lesions are sometimes seen. The clinical pattern of evolution is often very indolent, with static lesions for many years which may appear to be cured by surgical excision. The response to radiotherapy and chemotherapy is poor, although steroids may be helpful in minimizing the symptoms.

Other non-malignant causes of mediastinal lymph node enlargement simulating lymphoma are shown in Table 3. It is sometimes necessary to undertake mediastinal biopsy in order to exclude a possible lymphoma and reactive hyperplasia, in particular, may cause real diagnostic difficulty, although the monoclonal nature of a true lymphoma is usually apparent with immunohistochemical staining. It is particularly important to distinguish reactive hyperplasia from non-Hodgkin's lymphoma in patients with persistent lymphadenopathy related to human immunodeficiency virus infection. Totally benign conditions, such as phenytoin hypersensitivity, may also cause difficulties, since the typical histological picture in this condition may closely resemble Hodgkin's disease. In a separate condition, *angioimmunoblastic lymphadenopathy*, there is evidence that some cases may develop into a diffuse T-cell non-Hodgkin's lymphoma. Notwithstanding this worrying eventuality, it is still generally felt unwise to treat these patients in the early phase of the disease, since even intensive chemotherapy will not produce a durable regression or any alteration in its outcome. As with Castleman's disease, a response to steroids is sometimes symptomatically helpful.

Posterior mediastinum

A large majority of these tumours, whether benign, borderline, or unequivocally malignant, derive from nervous tissue and approximately 75 per cent of posterior mediastinal tumours are benign. In general, they are either of nerve-sheath origin (schwannomas, often termed neurilemmomas) or neurofibromas. In addition, tumours of the autonomic nervous system also occur, although less commonly, at least in adults. The most frequent types of autonomic nerve tumour are neuroblastoma, ganglioneuroblastoma, ganglioneuroma, and paraganglioma. The tumours may be single or multiple and are undoubtedly more common in patients with neurofibromatosis.

Nerve sheath tumours

These arise from the intercostal or vagus nerves and can present histological difficulties since the distinction between posterior mediastinal node tumours is frequently indistinct. Most are benign schwannomas or neurofibromas, both of which frequently occur as fusiform swellings although the neurofibroma has no true capsule, which is often a feature of the schwannoma, having a uniform appearance visible on the cut surface.

Malignant nerve sheath tumours are far less common and generally occur in patients with neurofibromatosis. The malignant equivalents of the two benign tumours described above are the malignant schwannoma and neurofibrosarcoma, usually showing obvious areas of malignant cellular morphology. Immunocytochemical staining has improved diagnostic accuracy and, in particular, S-100 protein is a useful marker for Schwann cells. It is unclear whether or not the malignant tumours can arise from benign neurofibromas, but there are certainly patients with neurofibromatosis in whom this seems likely, particularly where a large plexiform neurofibroma is present.

Tumours of the autonomic nervous system

These include neuroblastoma, a common childhood tumour fully described in Chapter 14.2 and the most malignant of this group, as well as more benign lesions such as ganglioneuroma and paraganglioma. Benign ganglioneuromas are most frequently encountered in adolescence, with a histological appearance very similar to that of a normal ganglion but generally occurring as a fairly large encapsulated tumour. Although generally of low malignant potential, foci of neuroblastoma have been reported as present within these tumours (Addis 1988). In ganglioneuroblastoma, the histology typically shows a far greater degree of cellular maturation than in the true neuroblastoma and in a large review of 80 cases (Adams and Hochholzer 1981) the authors described specific subtypes with differing patterns of behaviour.

Paragangliomas (chemodectoma, Fig. 2) also occur most typically in the posterior mediastinum, where they arise from the sympathetic chain. These curious tumours, which also occur at other sites in the body, arise from paraganglia associated with the arteries and nerves of the branchial arches (Harper and Addis 1988). They also occur in the anterior mediastinum and are often attached in this site to the pericardium and other local structures. Unlike the equivalent adrenal tumour, it is unusual for a mediastinal paraganglioma to be functioning, but those arising in the costovertebral sulcus, although less common, are more likely to be functional. From both the histological and the endocrine points of view, these tumours are similar to adrenal phaeochromocytoma and may produce symptoms due to adrenalin and noradrenalin release. Macroscopically, these are typically pink, vascular, and sometimes haemorrhagic lesions, with large chief cells of typical appearance. They are highly active with neurosecretory granules visible on electron microscopy and generally showing antibody staining to neurone-specific enolase and S-100 protein positivity. As with many thymic tumours, the presence of histological features typical of malignancy bears a rather uncertain relationship to clinical behaviour. Important metastatic sites include bone, bone-marrow, and lung.

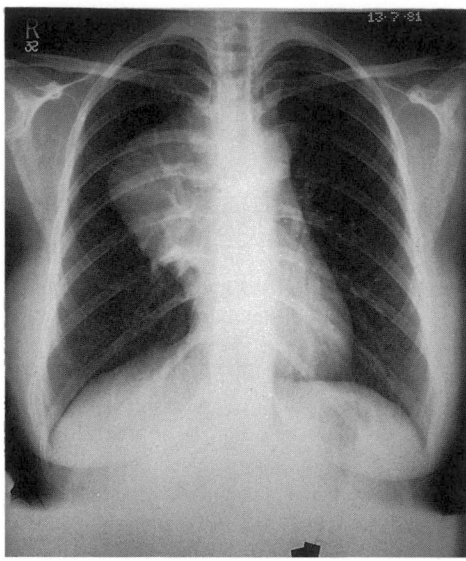

Fig. 2 Chest radiograph showing a large well-defined posterior mediastinal mass, diagnosed as chemodectoma at thoracotomy.

For all posterior mediastinal tumours, adequate localization with CT scanning is essential, with particular reference to surgical resectability since this clearly remains the treatment of choice. Adequate surgical resection is necessary not only for local control but also to allow careful examination of the complete specimen, often the only means of determining that no malignant foci are present within what at first sight appears to be a benign tumour. Tumours adherent to pericardium, chest wall, or paravertebral and vertebral structures may represent a major surgical challenge and may even require extensive thoraco-abdominal resection techniques with appropriate reconstruction of the chest wall, diaphragm, and other structures. It is exceedingly unusual for a tumour to be so large as to be unresectable, particularly bearing in mind the young age and uncertain prognosis of many of these tumours, particularly if resected only incompletely. For tumours which cannot be fully removed, the rôle of post-operative radiotherapy remains uncertain, although as with thymomas and other anterior mediastinal tumours, it seems likely that post-operative radiotherapy may in some cases be helpful (Mantell 1976). A few case reports have appeared suggesting that some of the more malignant tumours may respond to chemotherapy (Cairnduff and Smith 1986). Monoclonal antibody techniques have also been used for localization and therapy (*Lancet* 1984).

UNCOMMON TUMOURS OF THE CHEST WALL

Malignant mesothelioma, the commonest malignant chest wall tumour, is dealt with in Chapter 11.2. All of the other primary chest wall tumours are uncommon and for the most part tend to be soft tissue or primary bone sarcomas more frequently encountered at other sites. All of the major tissue types may be represented since the chest wall is a composite structure, its tissues including bone and cartilage (rib), fibrous tissue and fascial layers, nervous tissue (chiefly intercostal nerves and their branches), and muscular and vascular structures and it is bounded medially by parietal pleura and superficially by skin and its appendages. Primary adult soft tissue sarcomas of the chest wall are extremely uncommon and may indeed be difficult to differentiate from each other and, occasionally, from

benign chest wall lesions (Eng *et al.* 1990). In this primary surgical series, the commonest tumours were chondrosarcomas and plasmacytomas and treatment by radical surgical excision resulted in 5 and 10 year survival rates of 43 and 27 per cent, respectively.

In adults, secondary involvement, generally by local extension of a more deeply placed tumour, is very much more common. Carcinoma of the bronchus, particularly adenocarcinomas arising at peripheral sites, may develop essentially as pleural-based tumours with a clinical behaviour very similar to mesothelioma and, in particular, with a pattern of spread involving the pleural cavity and chest wall, often with an adjacent malignant pleural effusion. The histological distinction from mesothelioma is generally clear-cut, although in a proportion of cases even an experienced lung pathologist may be unable to give an unequivocal final opinion, though pleural biopsy is generally adequate. The cytological appearance of effusion fluid from these two tumours is usually distinct. Other intrathoracic metastatic tumours may present with pleural deposits with or without a malignant effusion. These are most commonly adenocarcinomas of breast, ovary, pancreas, bowel, and other typical primary sites, although the primary tumour may remain undetected until death. Both Hodgkin's disease and non-Hodgkin's lymphomas can involve either the pleura or chest wall, nodules of lymphoma occurring most frequently subpleurally rather than as a true chest wall tumour, being encountered most frequently in patients with advanced disease (Kaplan 1981; Press *et al.* 1985).

Of the soft tissue sarcomas occurring on or just beneath the chest wall, the malignant nerve sheath tumours form an important group, particularly since many patients with von Recklinghausen's disease have multiple lesions situated on the trunk, any of which can exhibit malignant change (Fig. 3). Other soft tissue sarcomas occasionally occur as primary chest wall tumours. In particular, the dermato-fibrosarcoma protruberans is a low-grade sarcoma which is encountered quite frequently on the chest wall and is characterized

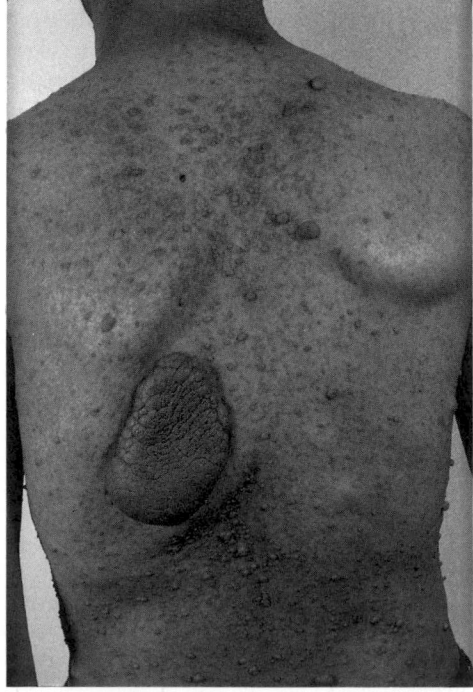

Fig. 3 Neurofibrosarcoma of the chest wall in a patient with von Recklinghausen's disease; this proved fatal after unsuccessful surgery.

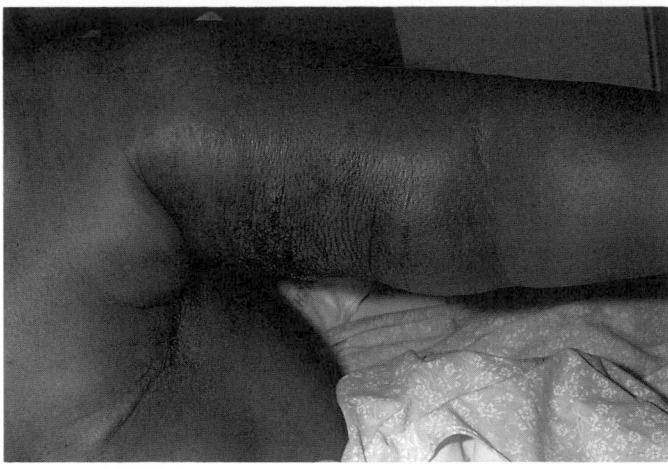

Fig. 4 Lymphangiosarcoma of the chest wall and upper arm in a patient with chronic lymphoedema, recurrent cellulitis, and a previous history of chest wall irradiation for breast cancer.

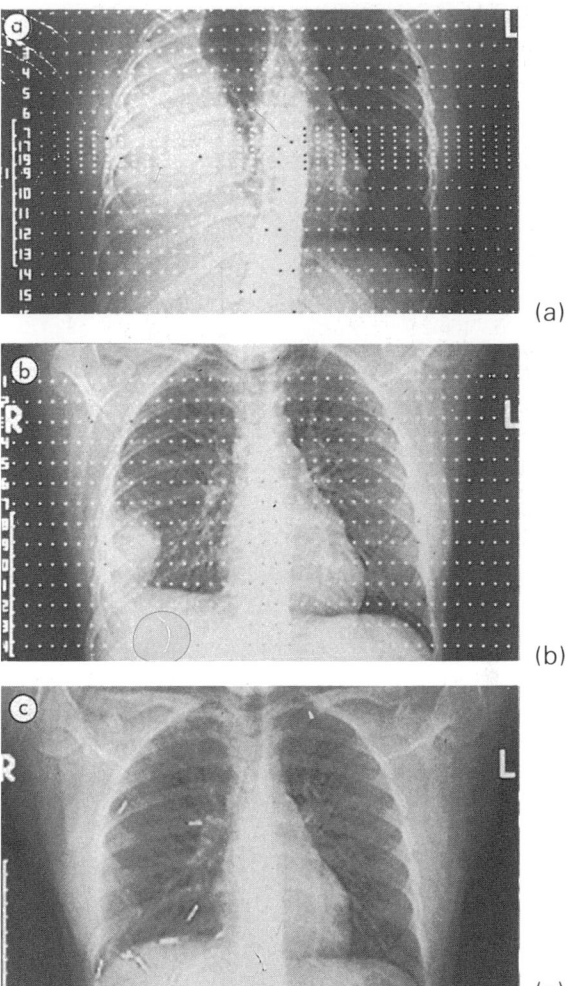

Fig. 5 Askin's tumour (a) at diagnosis, (b) after 3 months of treatment with combination chemotherapy, and (c) after surgery for residual bulk disease. (By courtesy of Professor R. L. Souhami.)

by a locally extensive subcutaneous infiltration of a sarcoma with a rather uniform spindle cell (sometimes storiform) pattern and with a marked tendency to local recurrence after excision. The metastatic potential is relatively low. In cases of desmoid tumour, arising from deep fascia and muscular connective tissue, the upper chest wall is again a relatively common site. The tumours appear as hard, fixed masses invading and replacing muscle (Addis 1988). Histologically, this is another spindle cell tumour within a collagenous stroma, generally without cartilagenous or bone formation. Malignant fibrous histiocytoma and fibrosarcomas also occur in this site. Despite the frequency of benign lipoma of the trunk, the malignant counterpart is rare. Angiosarcoma is also extremely uncommon, but the well-known haemangioendotheliosarcoma of Stewart and Treves, a classic post-irradiation sarcoma following mastectomy and post-operative radiotherapy for breast cancer, only occurs at this site (Fig. 4). Most patients have a lengthy period of lymphoedema of the arm, preceding the onset of the malignant tumour by some years.

In childhood, three important chest wall tumours have been described. Askin's tumour (Barson *et al.* 1978; Askin *et al.* 1979) occurs as a primary chest wall tumour of adolescence (Fig. 5), with a higher frequency in girls (75 per cent of all cases), specific radiological features (Burge *et al.* 1990), and a tendency to local recurrence without widespread dissemination, unlike the other typical small-cell malignant childhood tumours, such as Ewing's sarcoma, rhabdomyosarcoma, malignant lymphoma, and neuroblastoma. Askin's original description suggested a neuroepithelial derivation and, more recently, immunohistochemical stains have supported this view since these cells are positive to S-100 protein and neurone-specific enolase (Gonzalez-Crussi *et al.* 1984). As noted in the original description by Askin, massive involvement of the lung, pleura, or soft tissues of the chest wall resulted in a dismal outcome in nearly all patients, despite aggressive treatment and a rather low potential for widespread dissemination, although bone, lung, and other secondary sites are sometimes affected. In a recent series of 31 patients with primary chest wall tumours (13 with Askin's tumour), treated by intensive combination modality treatment, patients with localized disease at presentation appeared to enjoy improved disease-free and overall survival (Young *et al.* 1989). Combinations of intensive chemotherapy and high-dose localized irradiation are now routinely employed for this condition, although patients presenting with metastatic disease still clearly represent a major challenge. For patients both with localized and with extensive disease, the achievement of a complete clinical remission following treatment was strongly predictive of eventual outcome.

Ewing's sarcoma of bone occasionally arises from a rib and extraosseous Ewing's sarcomas, generally affecting a slightly older age group than the classical bone primaries, occur not uncommonly as primary chest wall or paravertebral tumours. These are discussed more fully in Chapter 13.3. Approximately 6 per cent of all cases of Ewing's tumour occur as primary rib lesions (Thomas *et al.* 1983). The third important chest wall tumour of childhood, rhabdomyosarcoma, occasionally occurs as a primary chest wall lesion.

Other bone and cartilagenous sarcomas quite frequently occur on the chest wall, notably benign and malignant cartilagenous tumours, osteosarcoma, and primary bone lesions of 'borderline' malignancy, such as the aneurysmal bone cyst, osteoclastoma or giant cell tumour, and osteoid osteoma. Approximately one in five chondrosarcomas occur on the trunk, sometimes appearing to arise from a pre-existing benign chondroma. Less than 5 per cent of osteosarcomas occur as a primary chest wall malignancy. Occasionally, these bone and cartilagenous tumours occur as radiation-induced neoplasms, following post-operative chest wall

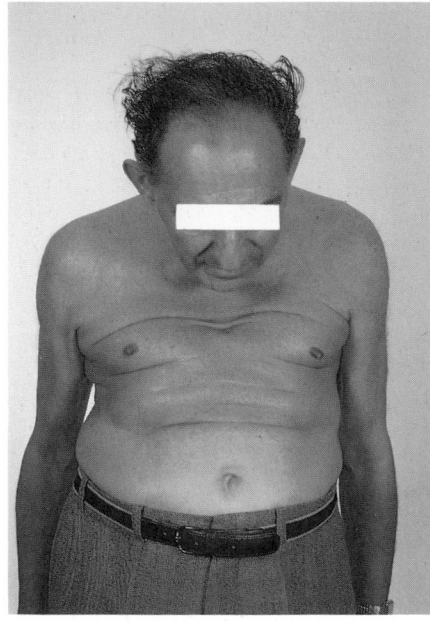
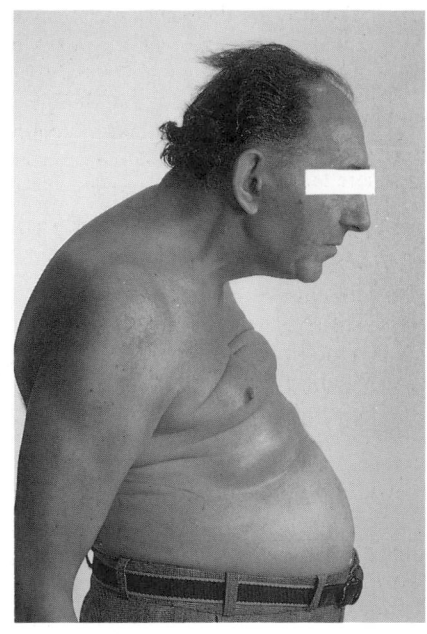

(a)   (b)

Fig. 6 Anterior and lateral views of a patient with sternal fracture from multiple myeloma.

irradiation for breast cancer and typically with a lag period of 10–20 years. Another important bone lesion of the chest wall is the solitary plasmacytoma, although sternal and rib deposits of multiple myeloma are more common (Fig. 6).

Treatment of chest wall tumours

With few exceptions, treatment should be by radical surgical removal wherever possible. A prior biopsy is essential since secondary deposits and radiosensitive tumours, such as non-Hodgkin's lymphoma or plasmacytoma, are clearly best treated by radiotherapy. However, the largest single category of primary malignant chest wall tumours is chondrosarcoma, generally regarded as a tumour with little, if any, response to non-surgical treatment. Tumours of the sternum itself are almost invariably malignant (Treasure 1988).

Normal surgical principles are obviously essential, particularly when planning a wide excision. CT scanning of the chest is mandatory both to define the anatomy pre-operatively and also to exclude pulmonary secondary deposits. When planning surgical resection, local recurrence is the problem that has to be anticipated most frequently. A full-thickness panel of chest wall is generally removed and primary closure may be effected without prosthestic material in most cases, although closure of large chest wall defects may be impossible without it; myocutaneous flaps may also be necessary.

In a few cases, primary treatment by local irradiation may be preferable (Tobias 1988). First, a number of these tumours are at least partly radiosensitive, for example squamous cell carcinoma arising at the apex of the lung and involving the chest wall with rib and brachial plexus involvement (Pancoast tumour). Secondly, surgical resection may be difficult or impossible, particularly with extensive tumours. Even where surgery has been performed, there may still be evidence of residual disease. This may not be clinically evident and it is important to confirm that the resection margins of the excised specimen have been carefully inspected histologically and are free of disease. Thirdly, chest wall tumours may produce severe symptoms, particularly pain, a characteristic feature of the Pancoast syndrome. In these cases, radiotherapy may be particularly valuable for symptomatic relief.

There are no specific contraindications to radiotherapy for chest wall and pleural tumours, although the following guidelines should always be considered.

1. Is the tumour surgically resectable? If so, then surgery should be the treatment of choice in most clinical situations. However, if the tumour is known to be highly radiosensitive, for example non-Hodgkin's lymphoma, surgical resection is unnecessary. Tumours such as Ewing's sarcoma and Askin's tumour are clearly radiosensitive. Ewing's sarcoma is usually treated by multimodality approaches using chemotherapy, radiotherapy, and, quite frequently, radical surgery. Other specific tumours should be treated along normal guidelines, for example the rare osteosarcoma of the chest wall is best treated by pre-operative chemotherapy with wide local removal and radiotherapy should be avoided unless surgical resection is incomplete.

2. Has the tumour been completely surgically resected? In most cases, where complete surgical excision has been achieved, there is no role for routine post-operative radiotherapy. Opinions are divided as to whether post-operative radiotherapy should routinely be given following surgery for a melanoma of the chest wall. In general, if there has been wide excision of the primary site, radiotherapy is probably best avoided, although post-operative treatment of the surrounding area is sometimes given, particularly if the primary melanoma was large, in an attempt to avoid local recurrence or satellite skin deposits. For soft tissue sarcomas arising on the chest wall, wide local excision is probably best followed by local irradiation of the tumour bed. Although there are no firm data to support this approach, the analogy is with compartmental resection of soft tissue sarcoma of the extremity, which has now largely replaced amputation.

3. Most patients are fit for radiotherapy even where there is evidence of distant disease. However, in patients with widespread metastases the role of radiotherapy is clearly limited to palliation. If the primary tumour is painful, local irradiation is particularly valuable, especially if surgical resection is incomplete. Where pleural effusion is the only evidence of disease, palliative treatment should

again be considered since neither surgery nor radical irradiation are likely to be curative.

4. Is the tumour likely to be radiosensitive? The question is an important one. Some tumours (for example, Ewing's tumour, seminoma, and lymphoma) are highly responsive to radiotherapy and therefore a low or modest dose may be sufficient to ensure local control, although there is increasing evidence that, in the case of Ewing's tumour, an absolute minimum of 50 Gy in 25 fractions in 5 weeks should be given and preferably a still higher dose, to avoid the problem of late local recurrence. On the other hand, tumours such as melanoma and soft tissue sarcoma are much less sensitive and higher doses will be necessary, with the risk of damage to local normal tissues. Tumour bulk is of great importance; the smaller the tumour the more likely is control by radiotherapy.

5. Are there alternatives to radiotherapy? Patients with chemosensitive tumours such as non-Hodgkin's lymphoma, Askin's tumour, neuroblastoma, embryonal rhabdomyosarcoma, and Ewing's tumour should be considered for chemotherapy in the first instance, particularly where the tumour is bulky and radiotherapy alone is unlikely to be curative. However, in most of these situations, local treatment with radiotherapy should be offered as well, in order to maximize the chance of local control.

6. What are the disadvantages of radiotherapy? Radiotherapy-induced side-effects vary sharply with the dose administered. At low dosage, it is unusual to encounter side-effects at all, particularly if the treatment is fractionated carefully over several days or weeks. At higher doses or if the treatment is given more briskly over a shorter period, skin reactions of varying intensity will occur, ranging from mild erythema to mild and then moist desquamation, sometimes with permanent pigmentation. Later skin changes include subcutaneous fibrosis, loss of elasticity, and telangiectasia. All of these changes are common where a superficial chest wall tumour has been treated with deliberate intent to raise the skin surface itself to a high dose. Rib fractures will also occur in a proportion of the patients treated for chest wall or pleural disease and supervoltage equipment should obviously be preferred in tumours at this site. Brachial plexus radiation damage is also important as a radiation side-effect following treatment of apical chest wall or pleural tumours and the risk is at least as high as the well-recognized complication of radiation brachial plexopathy occurring following treatment for carcinoma of the breast (Stoll and Andrews 1966). Radiotherapy of apical or axillary tumours may also lead to local lymphatic obstruction and lymphoedema, particularly where axillary lymph node dissection has taken place, for example as part of the surgical treatment of a melanoma of the chest wall. In children, local growth failure should be anticipated if wide-field irradiation has been necessary and there may be loss of height, together with scoliosis if part of the spine has been included in the radiation beam. For more laterally placed tumours, reduction in rib growth may result in a local and permanent loss of pulmonary volume and distortion of the chest wall. In girls, such treatment may also lead in later life to failure of breast development on the affected side.

The radiation technique is generally by means of a two-field wedged-pair arrangement using supervoltage equipment. It is important to minimize the dose to the underlying lung, without compromising the dose to the chest wall itself. Treatment by a direct field is unsatisfactory because of inevitable damage to the lung, though a single electron beam may be suitable. More sophisticated techniques, such as the use of mixed photon and electron-beam therapy have also been recommended, though the deepest part of the pleura may be inaccessible even with these techniques and will require surgical resection or implantation of radioactive sources, such as ^{125}I (Habrand et al. 1988).

Radiation dosage should follow guidelines applicable to the tumour under treatment (see, for example, specific chapters on Ewing's sarcoma, non-Hodgkin's lymphoma, soft tissue sarcomas, and osteosarcoma). Likewise, chemotherapy schedules will follow specific guidelines. The uncommon Askin's tumour, generally confined entirely to the chest wall, is generally treated using similar schedules to those employed for Ewing's sarcoma and other malignant small, round cell tumours.

CONCLUSION

Uncommon intrathoracic tumours represent a diverse group of cancers which often pose exceptional problems both in diagnosis and management. The histopathologist may have difficulty in identification since a number of these tumours are very unusual indeed, although accurate diagnosis is critical for proper management. For the clinician, a full understanding of the relative rôles of surgical resection, radiotherapy, and chemotherapeutic management is essential. As techniques of both diagnosis and management continue to advance, it becomes increasingly important to maintain a close liaison between the many members of the clinicopathological team.

REFERENCES

Adams SA, Hochholzer L (1981). Ganglioneuroblastoma of the posterior mediastinum. A clinico-pathologic review of eighty cases. Cancer, 47:373–81.

Addis B (1988). Pathology of mediastinal tumors. In Lung tumors (ed. B Hoogstraten, BJ Addis, HH Hansen, N Martini, and SG Spiro), pp. 169–204. Springer-Verlag, Berlin.

Addis BJ, Isaacson PG (1986). Large cell lymphoma of the mediastinum: a B-cell tumour of probable thymic origin. Histopathology, 10:379–90.

Askin FB, Rosai J, Sibley RK, Dehner LP, McAlister WG (1979). Malignant small cell tumor of the thoracopulmonary region in childhood. Cancer, 43:2438–51.

Barson AJ, Ahmed A, Gibson AAM, MacDonald AM (1978). Chest wall sarcoma of childhood with a good prognosis. Archives of Disease in Childhood, 53:882–9.

Brooks JJ (1988). Malignant schwannomas with divergent differentiation including 'triton tumor'. In Textbook of uncommon cancer (ed. CJ Williams, JG Krikorian, MR Green, and D Raghavan), pp. 669–81. John Wiley & Sons, Chichester.

Burcharth F, Axelsson C (1972). Bronchial adenomas. Thorax, 27:442–9.

Burge HJ, Novotny DB, Schiebler ML, Delaney MD, McCartney WH (1990). MRI of Askin's tumour. Chest, 97:125–54.

Cairnduff F, Smith IE (1986). Carboplatin chemotherapy for malignant paraganglioma. Lancet, ii:982.

Castleman B, Iversen L, Menendez VP (1954). Localised mediastinal lymph node hyperplasia resembling thymoma. Cancer, 9:822–30.

Crist WM, Raney RB, Newton W, Lawrence W, Tefft M, Foulkes MA (1982). Intrathoracic soft tissue sarcomas in children. Cancer, 50:598–604.

Crofton Sir J, Douglas A (1981). Respiratory diseases (3rd edn). Blackwell Scientific, Oxford.

Einhorn LH, Donohue JP, Peckham MJ, Williams SD, Loehrer PJ (1985). Cancer of the testes. In Cancer—principles and practice of oncology (2nd edn) (ed. VT DeVita Jr, S Hellman, and SA Rosenberg), pp. 979–1012. JB Lippincott, Philadelphia.

Eng J, Sabanathan S, Pradhan GN, Mearns AJ (1990). Primary bony chest wall tumours. Journal of the Royal College of Surgeons of Edinburgh, 35:44–7.

Gonzalez-Crussi F, Wolfson SL, Misingi K, Nakajima T (1984). Peripheral neuroectodermal tumors of the chest wall in childhood. Cancer, 54:2519–27.

Habrand JL, Nasr E, Couanet D, Teissier E (1988). Pleural irradiation in thoracic malignancies. International Journal of Radiation Oncology—Biology—Physics, 15:1050.

Hainsworth J, Einhorn LH, Williams SD, Stewart M, Greco A (1982). Advanced extra-gonadal germ cell tumors: successful treatment with combination chemotherapy. *Annals of Internal Medicine*, **97**:7–11.

Harper PG, Addis B (1988). Unusual tumours of the mediastinum. In *Textbook of uncommon cancer* (ed. CJ Williams, JG Krikorian, MR Green, and D Raghavan), pp. 411–46. John Wiley & Sons, Chichester.

Herbert A (1988). Primary malignant melanoma of the lung. In *Textbook of uncommon cancer* (ed. CJ Williams, JG Krikorian, MR Green, and D Raghavan), pp. 383–97. John Wiley & Sons, Chichester.

Hirsch FR (1988). Histopathology, ultrastructure and cytology. In *Lung tumors* (ed. B Hoogstraten, BJ Addis, HH Hansen, N Martini, and SG Spiro), pp. 37–56. Springer-Verlag, Berlin.

Hurt R, Bates M (1984). Carcinoid tumours of the bronchus: a 33 year experience. *Thorax*, **39**:617–23.

Hurt RD, Bruckman JE, Farrow GM, Benatz PE, Hahn RG, Earle JD (1982). Primary anterior mediastinal seminoma. *Cancer*, **49**:1658–63.

Johnson DW, Hoppe RT, Cox RS, Rosenberg SA, Kaplan HS (1983). Hodgkin's disease limited to intra-thoracic sites. *Cancer*, **52**:8–13.

Kaplan H (1981). *Hodgkin's disease*. Harvard University Press, Cambridge, MA.

Kay PH, Wells FC, Goldstraw P (1987). A multidisciplinary approach to primary nonseminomatous germ cell tumors of the mediastinum. *Annals of Thoracic Surgery*, **44**:578–82.

Keller AR, Hochholzer L, Castleman B (1972). Hyaline-vascular and plasma-cell types of giant lymph node hyperplasia of the mediastinum and other locations. *Cancer*, **29**:670–83.

Lancet (1984). Iodobenzylguanidine for location and treatment of phaeochromocytoma ii:905–7.

McCaughan BC, Martini N, Bains MS (1985). Bronchial carcinoids. *Journal of Thoracic and Cardiovascular Surgery*, **89**:8–17.

McNeil MM, Leong AS-Y, Sage RE (1981). Primary mediastinal embryonal carcinoma in association with Klinefelter's syndrome. *Cancer*, **47**:343–5.

Mantell BS (1976). Tumours of the chest and mediastinum. In *Radiotherapy in modern clinical practice* (ed. HF Hope-Stone) Crosby, Lockwood and Staples, London.

Mauch P, Goodman R, Hellman S (1978). The significance of mediastinal involvement in early stage Hodgkin's disease. *Cancer*, **42**:1039–45.

Mullen B, Richardson JD (1986). Primary anterior mediastinal tumours in children and adults. *Annals of Thoracic Surgery*, **42**:338–45.

Nascimento AG, Unni KK (1982). Sarcomas of the lung. *Mayo Clinic Proceedings*, **57**:355–9.

Nash G, Fligiel S (1984). Kaposi's sarcoma presenting as pulmonary disease in the acquired immunodeficiency syndrome: diagnosis by lung biopsy. *Human Pathology*, **15**:999–1001.

Nichols CR, Hoffman R, Einhorn LH, Williams SD, Wheeler LA, Garnick MB (1985). Hematologic malignancies associated with primary mediastinal germ-cell tumours. *Annals of Internal Medicine*, **102**:603–9.

Press GA, Glazer HS, Wasserman TH, Aronberg DJ, Lee JKT, Sagel SS (1985). Thoracic wall involvement by Hodgkin's disease and non-Hodgkin's lymphoma: CT evaluation. *Radiology*, **157**:195–8.

Price JC, Percarpio B, Murphy PW, Henderson RL (1979). Recurrent adenoid cystic carcinoma of the trachea: intraluminal radiotherapy. *Otolaryngology—Head and Neck Surgery*, **87**:614–23.

Ricci C, Patrassi N, Massa R, Mineo C, Benedetti-Valentini F Jr (1973). Carcinoid syndrome in bronchial adenoma. *American Journal of Surgery*, **126**:671–7.

Smith JL, Clein GP, Barker CR, Collins RD (1973). Characterisation of mediastinal malignant lymphoid neoplasm (Sternberg sarcoma) as thymic in origin. *Lancet*, i:74–7.

Sogge MR, McDonald SD, Cofard PB (1979). The malignant potential of the dysgenetic germ cell in Klinefelter's syndrome. *American Journal of Medicine*, **66**:515–18.

Souhami RL, Tobias JS (1986). *Cancer and its management*. Blackwell Scientific, Oxford.

Stoll BA, Andrews JT (1966). Radiation-induced peripheral neuropathy. *British Medical Journal*, **1**:834–7.

Stuart-Harris R, McCaughan BC (1988). Bronchial gland tumours ('bronchial adenomas'). In *Textbook of uncommon cancer* (ed. CJ Williams, JG Krikorian, MR Green, and D Raghavan), pp. 399–410. John Wiley & Sons, Chichester.

Thomas PRM, *et al.* (1983). Primary Ewing's sarcoma of the ribs: a report from the Intergroup Ewing's sarcoma study. *Cancer*, **51**:1021–7.

Tobias JS (1988). Radiotherapy of mediastinal and chest wall tumors. In *Lung tumors* (ed. B Hoogstraten, BJ Addis, HH Hansen, N Martini, and SG Spiro), pp. 247–60. Springer-Verlag, Berlin.

Treasure T (1988). Chest wall tumors. In *Lung tumors* (ed. B Hoogstraten, BJ Addis, HH Hansen, N Martini, and SG Spiro), pp. 233–6. Springer-Verlag, Berlin.

Wick MR, Manivel JC (1988). Primary sarcomas of the lung. In *Textbook of uncommon cancer* (ed. CJ Williams, JG Krikorian, MR Green, and D Raghavan), pp. 335–81. John Wiley & Sons, Chichester.

Young MM, *et al.* (1989). Treatment of sarcomas of the chest wall using intensive combined modality therapy. *International Journal of Radiation Oncology—Biology—Physics*, **16**:49–57.

Section 12
Lymphoid and myeloid neoplasia, histiocytosis, and AIDS-related malignancy

12.1　The biology of haemopoiesis

T. D. ALLEN AND T. M. DEXTER

INTRODUCTION

The continued supply of mature differentiated elements into the bloodstream is one of the most crucial requirements for the maintenance of good health. The numbers and rate at which blood cells are produced are staggering, equivalent to the entire body weight of the individual every 2 years. Despite the relative longevity of red blood cells (a half-life of some 60–120 days in the circulation), they are replaced at a rate of approximately 2 million per second. White cells, some of which have an ephemeral existence of a few hours, are replaced at a lower rate (500 000 per second). Thus, in the half minute taken to read this paragraph so far, 60 million red and 15 million white cells will have been freshly added to the peripheral circulation. Translated into the DNA replication (at approximately 2 m per cell) required for this cellular production, enough DNA to stretch three and a half times around the globe would have been produced. It is against these enormous and continual rates of production that the biology of haemopoiesis must be set.

STEM CELLS

The source of all haemopoietic populations is a single cell type termed a pluripotential stem cell, which has the ability to differentiate and develop into at least nine cell lineages: erythrocytes, and platelets, eosinophils, neutrophils, basophils, monocytes, osteoclasts, T and B lymphocytes. With the exception of osteoclasts, all these different mature cell types are found in the circulation. Another feature that distinguishes stem cells from other haemopoietic cells is their ability to self-renew (otherwise the 'stock' would be quickly depleted) and, thus, maintain the stem cell 'pool'. The division potential of stem cells does not appear to be a limiting factor in terms of the longevity of haemopoietic production, as stem cells can be transferred successfully through several generations of experimental animals. The first stage in the differentiation of a stem cell is its 'commitment' to produce cells that are more limited in their developmental options. These cells undergo further differentiation to produce tri, bi, and unipotent progenitor cells. These proliferate further to produce mature blood cells, competent in the various differentiated functions, into the bloodstream. Just how stem cells 'choose' (or are chosen) to stay stem cells or become differentiated along the various blood cell lineages is still far from being completely understood, but many of the influences and mechanisms involved in these processes, such as haemopoietic growth factors, have come to light over the last few years. The cellular hierarchy, together with the influences of particular growth factors, is illustrated in Fig. 1. What is also apparent from this diagram is that different sites are associated with different lines of production, for instance T-lymphocyte maturation in the thymus and B-lymphocyte maturation in lymphoid organs. Both these examples exhibit a fundamental characteristic of blood formation, namely the association with fixed tissue cells, as an essential aspect of haemopoiesis. As many experimental protocols in basic haemopoietic research involve isolated blood cell populations cultured in liquid or semi-solid culture conditions, it is worth restating that haemopoiesis

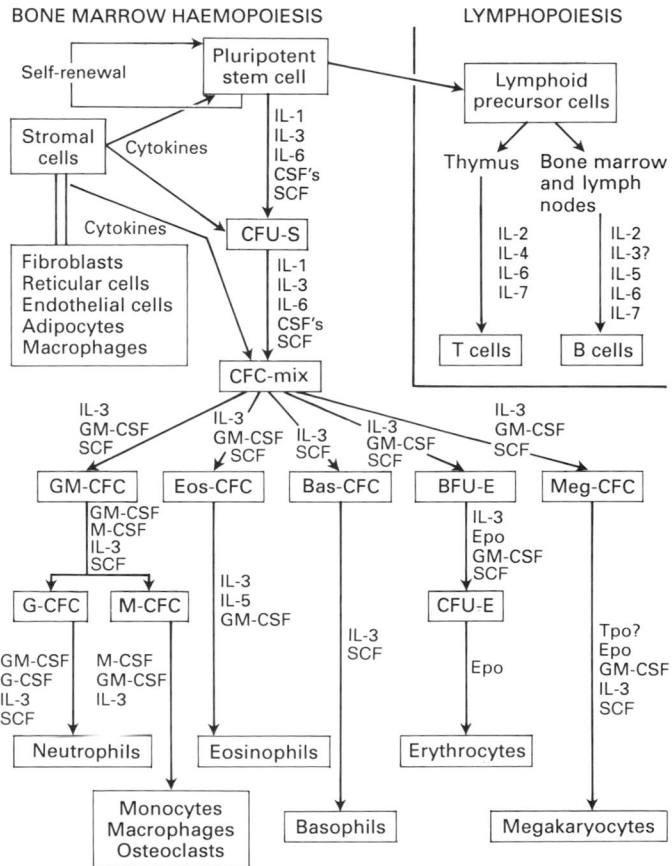

Fig. 1　Hierarchical structure of haemopoiesis and the influence of growth factors: CFU-S, spleen colony-forming cells (a murine assay for multipotent cells); CFC-Mix, colony-forming cell-mixed (*in vitro* multipotential clonogenic cell); GM-CFC, granulocyte macrophage colony-forming cell (a tripotent progenitor cell able to produce neutrophils, monocytes, and osteoclasts); Eos-CFC, eosinophil colony-forming cell; Bas-CFC, basophil colony-forming cell; BFU-E, burst-forming unit-erythroid (a primitive erythroid progenitor cell that develops into erythroid colony-forming units termed CFU-E that proliferate further to produce mature erythrocytes); Meg CFC, megakaryocyte colony-forming cell (proliferates to produce mature megakaryocytes and platelets); IL, interleukin; CSF, colony-stimulating factor; G, granulocyte; M, macrophage; Epo, erythropoietin; Tpo, thrombopoietin; SCF, stem cell factor. For reviews of these growth factors and their biological and clinical significance, the reader is referred to Ciba Foundation (1990), Dexter *et al.* (1990*b*), and Whetton and Dexter (1989).

in vivo (and *in vitro* in certain circumstances) cannot take place without the involvement of associated fixed tissue 'stromal' cells. These associations appear to be necessary at all stages of development, starting with haemopoiesis in the embryonic yolk sac, then the fetal liver, and, finally, the adult bone-marrow. These associations will be considered in more detail below. Perhaps the clearest example of haemopoietic cell–stromal cell association *in vivo* is demonstrated in the spleen colony assay, where lethally irradiated mice have their blood systems reconstituted by an injection of haemopoietic cells, which 'home' to the spleen and produce colonies containing multiple myeloid cell lineages. The phenomenon of site-specific blood cell production was initially described by Trentin (1970), based on the observation that erythropoiesis was favoured in mouse spleen whereas myelopoiesis occurred mainly in the marrow. From this work, the idea of the haemopoietic inductive microenvironment emerged to complement the view that commitment to a particular line in haemopoietic development was stochastic (due to chance). Further modifications of the microenvironmental influence over haemopoietic development have been suggested in the form of stem cell 'niches' (Schofield 1978). Within these 'niches' the local environment inhibits or restrains differentiation, thus maintaining stem cells in an undifferentiated state, whereas those cells which leave the stem cell niche become committed to other lines of development as a result of encountering differentiating influences in other locations.

STEM CELLS, COMMITTED PRECURSORS, AND MATURING CELLS

As the basic raw material of haemopoiesis, stem cells have been intensively studied for many years. This has not been without difficulty, as stem cells comprise perhaps less than 0.1 per cent of the total haemopoietic cells (Dexter 1987) and have no specific morphological features allowing direct recognition. Furthermore, when cell populations are separated by fluorescence-activated cell sorting and enriched for stem cells, they display morphological features which resemble small lymphocytes, a population of cells which comprises in excess of 20 per cent of the bone-marrow cells from which the stem cells were enriched. Stated simply, only one haemopoietic cell in 1000 may be a stem cell, but 200 of those 1000 cells look very much alike. Consequently the presence of stem cells is usually inferred from functional assays, which involve growth of isolated populations either *in vitro*, where colony-forming cells can be scored by their overall growth and colony formation or in the spleens of lethally irradiated mice, where a single cell (colony-forming unit) develops into a visible colony on the surface of the spleen that can be scored between 8 and 14 days after injection of the test population. Despite the fact that the spleen colony assay is restricted to a single species (the mouse) and measures a heterogeneous population of cells (some of them multipotential and others more developmentally restricted), much of our knowledge of the basic biology of stem cells in haematology has been produced by this technique.

Committed precursor cells are derived from stem cells which have not 'self-renewed' (that is, divided and retained their stem cell characteristics) but, as a result of the intrinsic and/or extrinsic influences (for example, growth factors), have become developmentally restricted and finally committed to a single line of development. This population forms approximately 3 per cent of the total marrow haemopoietic cell population and, as in the case of their stem cell precursors, cannot be morphologically characterized and are consequently assessed by their growth in colony assays *in vitro*. Growth factors which are specific for individual lines of development will promote colony growth *in vitro* and biotechnology-derived recombinant growth factors have also been shown to produce stimulation of specific haemopoietic lineages *in vivo*. However, the exact pathways and mechanisms by which growth factors act in physiological steady-state haemopoiesis are not well characterized.

Committed precursor cells will divide a few times and subsequently become morphologically recognizable as early stages of particular haemopoietic lineages, namely lymphocytes, erythroid cells, granulocytes, macrophages, and megakaryocytes (which produce platelets). These complete the recognizable subpopulations of maturing cells which, as a whole, comprise 95 per cent of all bone-marrow cells. Maturing cells then undergo the amplifying divisions necessary to produce sufficient numbers of mature post-mitotic products that enter the bloodstream. In some cases the final stages of differentiation are fairly dramatic, for instance the cytoplasmic fragmentation of the megakaryocyte to form platelets or nuclear expulsion in the case of red cells.

DISTRIBUTION OF STEM CELLS IN THE MARROW

Weiss (1970) characterized bone-marrow as having the unique capacity to 'trap' circulating stem cells. Within the bone-marrow itself, the distribution of primitive cells is heterogeneous. Colony-forming units are found in much greater concentration (two and a half times more frequently) at the inner surface of the bone shaft than in the central axis of the marrow (Lord *et al.* 1975). Furthermore, investigations have shown that the majority of colony-forming unit proliferation takes place close to the bone surface. However, these bone-associated colony-forming units have less facility to self-renew than the colony-forming units found in the centre. This variation in stem cell 'quality' and behaviour is most probably accounted for by the associated fixed stromal cell populations in these areas, which make up the local microenvironmental stem cell niches (Lord and Testa 1988).

THE MECHANISMS OF HAEMOPOIESIS

In moving away from the still largely theoretical concepts of stem cells and their modulation by a mixture of both short-range (microenvironmental) and long-range (hormonal, growth factor) influences, we can consider the recognizable constituents of the haemopoietic process and draw potential parallels from the cellular interactions where the cell types involved are readily identifiable, in contrast with those earlier in the hierarchy. Cells in sites of haemopoietic activity can be broadly divided into haemopoietic and non-haemopoietic. Non-haemopoietic cells, which form an integral part of the tissue framework for blood cell production, are termed stromal cells. From their initial perception as providing a structural framework for haemopoietic development only, it has become generally accepted that the stromal cells are crucial to the processes of haemopoiesis and intimately involved at a cell-to-cell level throughout all stages of blood cell development. Much of the evidence that has led to this view has come from an experimental system of bone-marrow grown in tissue culture conditions. This system of long-term bone-marrow culture (Dexter *et al.* 1984) has shown that not only are stromal cell populations required to support continued stem cell and differentiated cell production, but that these processes are not maintained unless direct interaction can occur between the haemopoietic and stromal cells. Clearly, the stromal cells which grow in tissue culture conditions are derived from the original marrow innoculum and are responsible for the establishment of the supportive environment. In the present state of knowledge, the types of stromal cell and roles they play *in vitro* and *in vivo* are less than completely characterized, but consideration of their associations with developing haemopoietic cells are beginning to elucidate their possible roles.

MARROW STROMAL CELLS *IN VIVO* AND *IN VITRO* AND THEIR ROLES IN HAEMOPOIESIS

Sections through haemopoietically active bone-marrow display many non-haemopoietic cell types. Vascular elements and neural structures form two clearly defined populations and the neural tissue can be subdivided into myelinated and unmyelinated nerve fibres and Schwann cells. Neural involvement in haemopoiesis has long been an intriguing possibility, and a neuroreticular complex has recently been described (Yamazaki and Allen 1992). The vasculature comprises nutrient arteries and veins and sinuses into which the products of haemopoiesis are transported. The remaining category of fixed non-haemopoietic bone-marrow population can be termed stromal cells and are classified according to their sites and functions (if known). The generally accepted 'standard' stromal cell of bone-marrow has been termed the reticular cell, not to be confused with reticulum cells (an early term for stem cells) or elements of the reticuloendothelial system. Having also made a clear separation between haemopoietic and non-haemopoietic cell types, there is also a qualification to be made in the case of fixed tissue macrophages within the bone-marrow, which are of haemopoietic origin but play crucial roles in the stromal support of haemopoiesis.

STROMAL–VASCULATURE INTERACTIONS IN HAEMOPOIESIS

Marrow vasculature can be separated into nutrient vessels and capillaries which run throughout the entire marrow, in contrast with the radially oriented individual venous sinuses which open into a single central venous sinus. It is between the radial sinuses where haemopoiesis takes place and as mature blood cells are produced they are 'fed' into the bloodstream across sinus walls by a process called extravasation. In some areas these venous sinus walls have three layers, formed from sinus lining endothelium and a basal lamina between the endothelium and a population termed adventitial reticular cells. Adventitial reticular cells (Weiss 1970) form a proportion of the overall reticular cell population of stromal cells which permeate the entire bone marrow and secrete the silver staining 'reticulin' fibres. The term 'adventitial' denotes their position against the venous sinus wall. *In vivo* studies of these cells show that they may well have an influence on the passage of cells into the bloodstream, as they appear to alter the amount of their coverage of the sinus walls and consequently influence the ease of access into the bloodstream for freshly matured red and white cells. This coverage is estimated to be approximately 65 per cent in mice in the steady state, but the adventitial reticular cells can be induced to round up and thus reduce their coverage dramatically as a result of blood loss or administration of bacterial endotoxin (Chamberlain *et al.* 1975). With the adventitial cell coverage reduced, increased cell migration into the bloodstream is facilitated. This mechanism may be partially responsible for the rapid mobilization of mature myeloid cells into the bloodstream of patients treated with colony-stimulating factors (Crowther *et al.* 1990).

RETICULAR CELLS AND MARROW FAT

Reticular cells form the major population of bone-marrow stromal cells, including those in contact with the sinus endothelia (adventitial reticular cells). They are not themselves capable of developing into haemopoietic cells, although it has been suggested that both stromal and haemopoietic cells may be descendants of a common precursor. Reticular cells show no mitotic activity in adult marrow, unless damage occurs. They also possess the ability for extensive lipogenesis and are thus the precursor population themselves for the adipocyte (fat cell) populations of 'fatty marrow'. The long bones of larger mammals, including humans, are not involved in haemopoietic activity and are filled with fat cells. In smaller mammals such as the mouse, all medullary space is taken up with haemopoietic marrow so that fatty marrow only tends to occur when haemopoiesis is depressed. In humans where there appears to be ample 'volume' for haemopoiesis in ribs and pelvic bone-marrow, loss of marrow production in aplastic anaemia results in the replacement of haemopoietic cells with fat cells. Fat cells in marrow are different from adipocytes in other sites of the body, leading to the suggestion that they may serve a different function from other stores of potential energy as they do not undergo lipolysis in response to acute starvation. Marrow fat cells themselves may comprise either stable yellow marrow cells or more labile 'white' fat cells which can undergo lipolysis to become reticular cells during periods of intense haemopoiesis. Fat cells will also develop when bone-marrow is grown in tissue culture, where they appear to arise from a fibroblast cell type in both human and mouse cultures. In mouse cultures the fibroblast precursor also appears to give rise to a 'blanket cell' which is thought of as the *in vitro* equivalent of the reticular cell in marrow *in vivo* (Allen and Dexter 1984). A further similarity of *in vivo* fat cell behaviour is shown by *in vitro* fat cells in mouse long-term bone-marrow cultures, where lipolysis occurs as a result of the addition of serum from anaemic mice (which also stimulates erythropoiesis). *In vivo*, chronic hypertransfusion of red cells in mice can also lead to the development of adipocytes in areas where the erythropoiesis

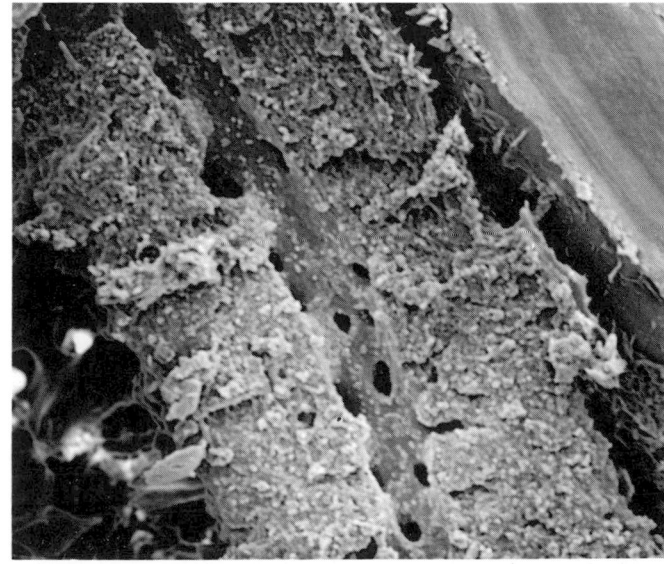

Fig. 2 Scanning electron micrograph of mouse femur, split longitudinally, revealing radial sinuses opening into a central venous sinus amongst the packed haemopoietic tissue.

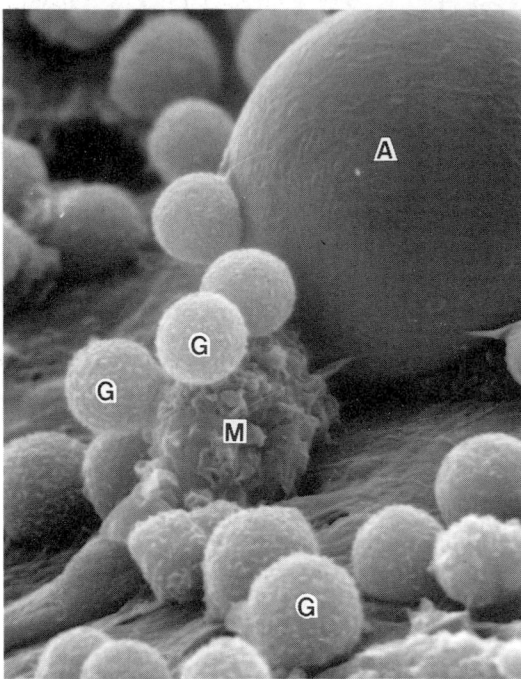

Fig. 3 Scanning electron micrograph of long-term bone-marrow culture showing a large adipocyte (A), maturing granulocytes (G), and a macrophage (M).

has been suppressed. However, the relationship that might exist between fat cell populations and haemopoietic activity is not cause and effect; that is, increase in fat cells inhibits proliferation of progenitor cells. Perhaps the simplest concept for marrow fat cells is a 'space-filling' role and, thus, they proliferate as a secondary response to marrow aplasia rather than being the reason for it. This suggestion may also account for the massive growth of adipocytes in mouse marrow long-term cultures, where they have much greater growing space in comparison with the tightly packed haemopoietic populations of mouse femur *in vivo* where adipocytes are not seen (Figs 2 and 3).

STROMAL–HAEMOPOIETIC INTERACTIONS IN HAEMOPOIESIS

The close affinity of developing blood cells with the specific elements of the fixed (stromal) populations of bone-marrow is well established, originally as a result of observations in marrow *in vivo* but more recently and rather more extensively as a result of observations of associations in long-term marrow cultures (Fig. 3) (Bentley 1981). It should be stressed that all associations observed to date *in vivo* have also been observed *in vitro* and that as the long-term cultures retain virtually all aspects of haemopoiesis *in vivo*, it is a very reasonable postulate to assume that the increased experimental access to cell interactions facilitated by long-term bone-marrow cultures (Allen 1981) are a true indication of phenomena which also occur *in vivo*. Long-term bone-marrow cultures also allow a further investigation of the mechanisms of interaction in those associations already characterized *in vivo*.

THE BIOLOGY OF ERYTHROPOIESIS

The existence of a substance in the circulation which modulates red cell production was first postulated by Carnot in 1906 and subsequently verified some 30 years later. This substance, erythropoietin, is the most investigated of all haemopoietic factors, having originally been available as an experimental tool from the urine of patients with aplastic anaemia and more recently from recombinant technology in amounts which have already shown promising results in clinical trials. Despite the wealth of information gathered over this period, the actual cellular mechanisms of the role of erythropoietin in red cell differentiation (or for that matter the whole family of haemopoietic growth factors) have still to be elucidated.

Erythropoiesis in bone-marrow can be recognized from the appearance of the morphologically characterized precursors of red cells, the proerythrocytes. The proerythrocytes develop into mature red cells via a series of maturing stages over 3 days, involving four or five divisions with increasing differentiation of the daughter cells, culminating in the expulsion of the nucleus and the formation of the mature erythrocyte which is now little more than a bag of haemoglobin when liberated into the circulation (Fig. 4). Approximately 60–120 days later, at the end of the red cell lifespan, it will be phagocytosed by macrophages in the bone-marrow or other haemopoietic organs. The sequence of maturing red cells is proerythroblasts, basophilic erythroblasts I and II, polychromatophilic erythroblasts I and II, reticulocytes (the last nucleated stage), and erythroblasts. 'Basophilic' and 'polychromatophilic' refer to light microscope staining characteristics at the various stages. Throughout the final red cell maturation sequence, there is a continuing reduction in cell size, accompanied by increasing amounts of heterochromatin in the nucleus and a gradual reduction in the cytoplasmic organelles including a reduction in mitochondria. The final period of differentiation is also characterized by increasing amounts of cytoplasmic ferritin. The mechanism by which the reticulocyte nucleus is 'expelled' is not dissimilar to a mitotic division, in that two 'daughter' cells are produced. However, one of these products of division is a nucleus covered with a minimal surface coat of cytoplasm and cell membrane, whereas the other product is the newly formed erythrocyte. Thus, the description 'nuclear expulsion' is not absolutely correct, as it may indicate the exocytic mechanism of a 'naked' nucleus from within the cell, but clearly a cell cannot eject a naked nucleus without undergoing lysis (Fig. 4).

Erythropoietic development has long been characterized *in vivo* by the association between the developing erythroblasts and a central macrophage. This combination is termed an erythroblastic islet and can be observed readily in freshly prepared bone-marrow smears. It can also be maintained for a short time in culture and more recently erythroblastic islets have been formed *de novo* in long-term bone-marrow cultures when erythropoiesis is stimulated *in vitro* (Allen and Dexter 1982). Time-lapse observations of the behaviour of the central macrophage and erythrocytes within these associations have confirmed some of the original reports from fixed or short-term cultured preparations. The erythroblastic islet is formed by the association of a proerythroblast with an erythroblastic islet macrophage. Whether there is a subpopulation of macrophages specifically differentiated for this purpose is unknown. Subsequently all erythroid maturation from the proerythroblast takes place in intimate association with the macrophage, occurring as a synchronous

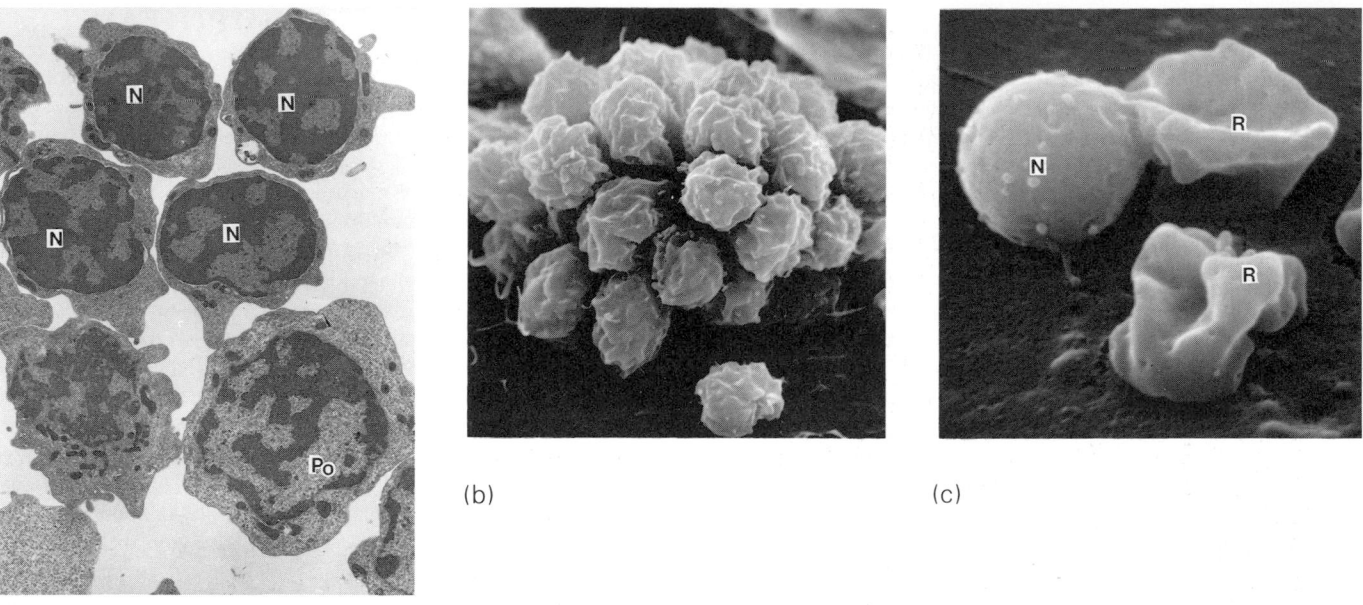

Fig. 4 (a) Transmission electron micrograph of a section through a region of maturing red cells, showing a polychromatophilic erythroblast (Po) and four normoblasts (the last nucleated stage of the erythroid series). (b) Scanning electron micrograph of an erythroblastic islet at a late stage of red cell maturation. The islet macrophage is obscured by the packed developing red cells over its surface. (c) Scanning electron micrograph of the later stages of red cell maturation. Enucleation is occurring, separating the normoblast into a nuclear remnant (N) and freshly formed reticulocyte (R) with another newly formed reticulocyte in the foreground.

cohort of division and maturation which results in 16 or 32 mature erythrocytes. The significance of this association is still unclear, but there are several interesting possibilities. Macrophages have been shown to produce erythropoietin, so that a direct transfer from the cell of production (the macrophage) to the target cells (developing erythroblasts) is possible. The central islet macrophage could also play a part in maintaining the observed synchrony of maturation. An advantage in efficiency of synchronous erythroid maturation could well accrue from the fact that erythroid development occurs some distance from the venous sinuses (the point of entry into the circulation) and the erythroblastic islet macrophages migrate towards the sinus wall as their erythroid cohorts mature. Upon reaching the sinus wall, the entire mature erythroid cohort will be ready for introduction into the circulation at once, minimizing the time spent at the venous sinus wall and also allowing other mature blood cells to enter the circulation without delay. Reference to the rates of red cell production at the beginning of this chapter will remind the reader of the need for efficient delivery of the final products of haemopoiesis. A third interaction between the islet macrophage and the differentiating red cells has been observed in living cells in long-term bone-marrow cultures by time-lapse video. At the conclusion of nuclear expulsion, which occurs on the surface of the islet macrophage, contrasting behaviour is observed between the freshly formed reticulocyte, which undergoes a very involved and active series of shape changes (termed polylobulations (Bessis *et al.* 1983)) and the nuclear remnant, which is largely inert and is subsequently phagocytosed by the islet macrophage within minutes of nuclear expulsions taking place. This process leads to two further as yet unanswered questions: Why do red cells lose their nuclei? What happens to the nucleus itself? The usual response to the first question is that as the cell nucleus is a relatively bulky and rigid structure, the nucleus-free erythrocyte is much more flexible with respect to negotiating the finest capillary networks in the tissue and

is thus highly efficient in the distribution of oxygen. Against this view, however, we should consider avian red cells, which retain their nuclei and the fact that bird flight muscle is generally recognized as the most efficient vertebrate musculature and therefore must be considered as efficiently oxygenated. With respect to the phago-cytosis of expelled nuclei, there can be little doubt that this forms part of a recycling system for fresh DNA synthesis. Red cell production is not unique as a tissue in which conservation of DNA is practised, as the squames that are shed from the surface of the epidermis have had their nuclear content removed prior to final differentiation and loss.

THE BIOLOGY OF MYELOID DEVELOPMENT

Production of granulocytes, monocytes, and megakaryocytes occurs as a result of stem cell commitment to produce (functionally) recognizable lineage-restricted progenitor cells. These progenitor cells are acted upon by a series of interleukins and colony-stimulating factors that, *in vitro*, drive proliferation and development, resulting in the production of the various mature cell lineages (Fig. 1). The nature, characteristics, target cells, and clinical uses for these growth factors comprise an extensive literature that is reviewed elsewhere (Allen and Dexter 1990; Dexter *et al.* 1990*c*). What is often forgotten, however, is that these growth factors are *essential* for maintaining the viability of the stem cell and progenitor cell populations *in vitro*; in their absence the cells die through a mechanism involving apoptosis (Williams *et al.* 1990). This could well represent one of the natural mechanisms for maintaining homeostasis *in vivo*, ensuring an equilibrium between the availability of growth factors and the size of the maturing cell compartments.

Granulocytes show a series of differentiating alterations from their first recognizable precursor, the myeloblast, through promyelocyte,

myelocyte, metamyelocyte, and mature granulocyte. These morphological changes involve an alteration in nuclear morphology from spherical to multilobed and the accumulation of a specific granule population in the cytoplasm. It is these granules that separate the granulocyte population into neutrophils, eosinophils, and basophils. This process takes approximately 14 days in the marrow, but the mature neutrophil has a half-life of only approximately 8 h in the circulation.

Macrophage maturation can also be separated into morphologically distinct stages, namely monoblast, promonocyte, monocyte, and macrophage, with an 'immature' macrophage stage still capable of mitosis before final differentiation to a mature macrophage. In contrast with granulocytes and erythrocytes, however, maturation only progresses to the monocyte stage within the marrow and this is also the only stage normally encountered in the circulation. The monocyte—macrophage maturation takes place after the monocyte leaves the circulation and enters various tissues, which have a resident fixed-tissue mature macrophage population (sometimes termed histiocytes). While overall maturation involves an increase in cell size and in numbers of organelles such as mitochondria and lysosomes, some of the final characteristics are specific for the tissue in which the macrophage has matured. Thus, specific differences exist between lung macrophages (alveolar macrophages), skin macrophages (Langerhans' cells), and liver macrophages (Kupffer cells) according to the functions required of the macrophages in particular tissue locations. By the same token, mature macrophages within the bone-marrow appear to be involved in the processes of haemopoiesis, and thus represent the fixed-tissue macrophages of marrow itself. In this way, a cell of haemopoietic origin joins the stromal population and subsequently influences haemopoiesis itself.

Cellular interactions in granulopoiesis involve both stromal macrophages and reticular cells. The association between developing granulocytes and reticular cells has been reported regularly in marrow *in vivo*, but is more accessible to direct observation in long-term bone-marrow cultures, where it represents the best characterized example of cell behaviour in microenvironmental activity described to date (Allen and Dexter 1990). Briefly, during the formation of the stromal adherent layers in marrow cultures, the reticular cells give rise to a population of flattened epithelial cells which have been termed 'blanket cells'. As the blanket cells develop, they appear to attract adjacent macrophages which remain in association throughout the culture. By the third week of culture, granulocyte precursors can also be observed (by time-lapse video) migrating beneath the blanket cells to make intimate membrane association with the fixed macrophages in these 'cobblestone' regions. 'Cobblestone regions', characterized as regions of granulocyte proliferation and maturation, develop in these areas and time-lapse observations of living cultures show that active membrane-to-membrane association occurs between the developing granulocytes and fixed macrophages 2–3 h prior to division of the developing granulocytes. At these sites, concentrations of several hundred granulocytes can be produced within 3–5 days. After such a burst of proliferation has occurred, the mature granulocytes will migrate away from these regions and other foci will develop. If this activity is indicative of marrow granulopoiesis or site-specific haemopoiesis in general, then all the individual haemopoietic microenvironments may not participate continuously in blood cell production, with only a small proportion involved at any one time. Such an arrangement would lead to a vast 'reserve capacity' which could be switched into production at times of haemopoietic stress, such as blood loss or major infection.

BIOLOGY OF LYMPHOPOIESIS

The precursors of lymphocytes are stem cell products which become committed to lymphoid differentiation. T lymphocytes are so termed because of their maturation period spent in the thymus. B lymphocytes were initially identified in the bursa of Fabricius in birds and subsequently in the bone-marrow of mammals. Lymphocytes in general do not show the same well-marked series of morphologically characterized differentiation as myeloid and erythroid cells, but B lymphocytes are the precursors for plasma cells, a cell type strikingly characterized by its specialization of endoplasmic reticulum for antibody production. From the original morphological classification of all lymphocytes as small, medium, or large, B and T lymphocytes are now characterized more functionally, with the T lymphocytes giving rise to various populations of helper, suppressor, and cytotoxic cells. In the absence of clear morphological differences, a wide range of specific monoclonal antibodies to cell surface antigens are used to characterize cell types amongst the lymphoid populations.

As with the myeloid cell populations, lymphoid differentiation occurs in close association with stromal cells. Lymphoid microenvironments occur at other sites in addition to bone-marrow and thymus, namely the spleen and lymph nodes. Both these sites possess cells termed reticular or fibroblastic reticular as their primary stromal population, forming the overall framework of the organs and providing an overall 'scaffolding' for lymphopoiesis. Specific antibodies for these cell types have shown their exact distribution in lymphoid tissue, although their association and mechanisms of interaction with the lymphoid cells themselves is still obscure. Within the spleen, however, T and B lymphocytes each have their own domains, with B cells localized in follicles in the peripheral part of the white pulp and also in the marginal zone which separates the white pulp from the red pulp. T-cells in spleen occupy the periarteriolar lymphoid sheath. In lymph nodes B-cells are found in the follicles of the outer cortex and T-cells are found in the paracortical area. Other non-lymphoid stromal cells which have been described in both spleen and lymph nodes, such as interdigitating cells, follicular cells, and the ubiquitous macrophage, may help the lymphocytes to 'home' to their specific sites, but by unknown mechanisms (Van Vleit *et al*. 1984). In long-term bone-marrow cultures the culture conditions can be modified so that B lymphopoiesis is stimulated. In these cultures, similar associations to those described between the blanket cells, macrophages, and developing granulocytes have been reported for lymphocytes (Kincade 1988). Whether modification of the cultures to encourage lymphoid production also involves conversion of the stromal population to support lymphopoiesis is not known, but the idea of specific microenvironmental sites for individual blood cell development would suggest that this should be the case. Long-term bone-marrow cultures converted to lymphopoiesis show very similar cobblestone areas of lymphoid production to those observed in granulopoiesis. In these sites the groups of developing B lymphocytes are found in tightly packed association with stromal cells, but not apparently requiring the involvement of macrophages. Furthermore, the developing lymphocytes appeared to crawl under the spread stromal cells in the same way as the developing granulocytes, but to the point that they seemed to become completely encapsulated (Dorshkind 1986) by the cytoplasm of the stromal cells, in a very similar way to the descriptions of T lymphocytes within thymic 'nurse' cells. It seems unlikely that the long-term bone-marrow cultures conditions provide a complete microenvironment for lymphocyte maturation, with the majority of lymphocytes arrested at or before a relatively immature B-cell stage.

THE ROLE OF GROWTH FACTORS, STROMAL CELLS, AND EXTRACELLULAR MATRIX MOLECULES IN HAEMOPOIESIS: A UNIFYING CONCEPT

From the discussion so far, it is clear that specific cell associations occur between stromal cells and developing haemopoietic cells. What is the nature of these interactions and how do they regulate haemopoietic cell development? From *in vitro* studies, it is known that the survival, proliferation, and development of isolated haemopoietic stem cells and their progeny, immobilized in a soft-gel matrix, require the continual presence of either colony-stimulating factors or interleukin; in the absence of these factors, the cells die. In long-term bone-marrow cultures, in contrast, haemopoiesis can be maintained for several months in the *absence* of added growth factors, suggesting that the stromal cells themselves are supplying the various factors necessary for haemopoiesis. In these cultures, however, direct cell-to-cell contact is required between the stromal cells and the haemopoietic cells in order for stem cell self-renewal, differentiation, and development to occur; when this contact is prevented, the haemopoietic cells die. This suggests that the factors necessary for haemopoiesis are in some way localized to the membrane of the stromal cells and can exert their influence only via direct cell association. A clue to the mechanism underlying this phenomenon was provided by the observation that molecules of the extracellular matrix can sequester growth factors (Gordon *et al.* 1987). Subsequently, it was shown that this ability resided in the cell-membrane-associated heparan sulphate proteoglycan on the resident marrow stromal cells (Roberts *et al.* 1988). Therefore, it seems likely that the marrow stromal cells themselves are producing a range of cytokines which are exported to the cell membrane and become sequestered by the extracellular matrix molecules (Dexter *et al.* 1990a; De Wynter *et al.* 1993). These are then 'presented' to the haemopoietic cells in a biologically active form. In other words, when considering stromal cell-mediated haemopoiesis, several regulatory components need to be considered: first, the known heterogeneity of the stromal cells, which may well differ in their ability to produce and/or sequester different growth factors; second, the cell adhesion molecules, present on both stromal cells and haemopoietic cells, that allow *specific* cell association to be made (Gordon 1988; Kincade *et al.* 1989; Clarke *et al.* 1992); third, the nature and distribution of cell matrix molecules that may well serve to localize growth factors to discrete sites. In this way, it is possible to envisage the bone-marrow (and also the sites promoting T- or B-cell development) as consisting of a series of anatomically discrete environments where particular developmental options occur at the expense of others, such as environments promoting preferential stem cell self-renewal and other environments facilitating preferential development of stem cells into erythrocytes or neutrophils and so on. The problem now, of course, is to define these environments at the molecular level.

REFERENCES

Allen TD (1981). Haemopoietic microenvironments *in vitro*: ultrastructural aspects. In *Microenvironments in haemopoietic and lymphoid differentiation* (ed. R Porter and J Whelan), pp. 38–67. Ciba Foundation Symposium 84. Pitman Medical, London.

Allen TD, Dexter TM (1982). Ultrastructural aspects of erythropoietic differentiation in long-term bone marrow culture. *Differentiation*, **21**:86–94.

Allen TD, Dexter TM (1984). The essential cells of the haemopoietic microenvironment. *Experimental Hematology*, **12**:517–21.

Allen TD, Dexter TM (1990). Marrow biology and stem cells. In *Colony-stimulating factors: molecular and cellular biology* (ed. TM Dexter, JM Garland, and GG Testa), pp. 1–38. Dekker, New York.

Bentley SA (1981). A close range cell: cell interaction required for stem cell maintenance in continuous bone marrow culture. *Experimental Hematology*, **9**:303–12.

Bessis M, Lessin LS, Beutler E (1983). Morphology of the erythron. In *Hematology* (3rd edn) (ed. WJ Williams, E Beutler, AJ Erselv, and MA Lichtman), pp. 257–79. McGraw-Hill, New York.

Chamberlain JK, Leblond PF, Weed RI (1975). Reduction of adventitial cell cover: an early direct effect of erythropoietin on bone marrow ultrastructure. *Blood Cells*, **1**:655–74.

Ciba Foundation (1990). *Molecular control of haemopoiesis*, Ciba Foundation Symposium 148. Wiley, Chichester.

Clarke BR, Gallagher JT, Dexter TM (1992) Cell adhesion in the stromal regulation of haemopoiesis. In *Clinical haematology*, Vol. 5, No. 3, *Growth factors in haemopoiesis* (ed. BI Lord and TM Dexter). Baillière Tindall, London.

Crowther D, *et al.* (1990). Growth factor assisted chemotherapy, the Manchester experience. In *Molecular control of haemopoiesis*, pp. 201–14. Ciba Foundation Symposium 148. Wiley, Chichester.

De Wynter E, Allen TD, Coutinho L, Flavell D, Flavell SU, Dexter TM (1993). Localisation of granulocyte marophage colony stimulating factor in human long-term bone marrow cultures. Biological and immunocytochemical characterisation. *Journal of Cell Science*, **106**:761–9.

Dexter TM (1987). Stem cells in normal growth and disease. *British Medical Journal*, **295**:1192–4.

Dexter TM, Spooncer E, Simmons PJ, Allen TD (1984). Long-term marrow culture: an overview of techniques and experience. In *Long term bone marrow culture* (ed. DG Wright and JS Greenberger) pp. 57–97. Kroc Foundation Series 18. Alan R. Liss, New York.

Dexter TM, *et al.* (1990a). Stromal cells in haemopoiesis. In *Molecular control of haemopoiesis*, pp. 76–95. Ciba Foundation Symposium 148. Wiley, Chichester.

Dexter TM, Garland JM, Testa NG (1990b). *Colony stimulating factors: molecular and cellular biology*. Dekker, New York.

Dexter TM, Heyworth CM, Spooncer E, Ponting ILO (1990c). The role of growth factors in self renewal and differentiation of haemopoietic stem cells. *Philosophical Transactions of the Royal Society of London, Series B*, **327**:85–98.

Dorshkind K (1986). *In vitro* differentiation of B lymphocytes from primitive haemopoietic precursors present in long term bone marrow cultures. *Journal of Immunology*, **136**:422–31.

Gordon MY (1988). Adhesive properties of haemopoietic stem cells. *British Journal of Haematology*, **68**:149–51.

Gordon MY, Riley GP, Watt SM, Greaves MF (1987). Compartmentalization of a haemopoietic growth factor (GM-CSF) by glycosaminoglycans in the bone marrow microenvironment. *Nature, London*, **326**:403–5.

Kincade PW (1988). Experimental models for understanding B lymphocyte formation. *Advances in Immunology*, **41**:181–267.

Kincade PW (1988). Experiment models for understanding B lymphocyte formation. *Advances in Immunology*, **41**:181–267.

Kincade PW, Lee G, Pietrangeli CE, Hayashi S, Gimble JM (1989) Cells and molecules that regulate B lymphopoiesis in bone marrow. *Annual Reviews in Immunology*, **7**:111–43.

Lord BI, Testa NG (1988). The hemopoietic system: structure and regulation. *Hematology*, **8**:1–26.

Lord BI, Testa NG, Hendry JH (1975). The relative spatial distribution of CFU-S and CFU-C in the normal mouse femur. *Blood*, **46**:65–72.

Roberts R, Gallagher J, Spooncer E, Allen TD, Bloomfield F, Dexter TM (1988). Heparan sulphate bound growth factor: a mechanism for stromal cell mediated haemopoiesis. *Nature, London*, **332**:376–8.

Schofield R (1978). The relationship between the spleen colony-forming cell and the haemopoietic stem cell. A hypothesis. *Blood Cells*, **4**, 7–25.

Trentin JJ (1970). Influence of hemopoietic organ strom (hemopoietic microenvironment) on stem cell differentiation. In *Regulation of hematopoiesis* Vol. 1 (ed. AS Gordon), pp. 161–86. Meredith, New York.

Weiss L (1970). The histology of the bone marrow. In *Regulation of hematopoiesis*, Vol. 1 (ed. AS Gordon), pp. 79–92. Appleton-Century-Crofts, New York.

Whetton AD, Dexter TM (1989). Myeloid haemopoietic growth factors. *Biochimica Biophysica Acta*, **989**(2):111–32.

Williams GT, Smith CA, Spooncer E, Dexter TM, Taylor D (1990).

Haemopoietic colony-stimulating factors promote survival by suppressing apoptosis. *Nature, London*, **343**:76–9.

Yamazaki K, Allen TD (1992). Ultrastructural morphometric study of efferent nerve terminals on murine bone marrow stromal cells and the recognition of a novel anatomical unit: the "neuroreticular complex". *American Journal of Anatomy*, **187**:261–76.

12.2.1 Biology of leukaemia

TRIVADI S. GANESAN

Leukaemia was first recognized as an entity by Virchow and Bennet independently in 1845 (Virchow 1845; Bennet 1985). The definition of leukaemia by Virchow in 1849 still remains valid today:

This is what we know about leukaemia: during normal blood cell production, the blood cells differentiate into specific types. In a pathological situation, the differentiation into specific cells is blocked. This disturbance of normal differentiation—so called *leukaemia*—is a disease *sui generis*. We know the sequelae of this disease, but we do not know its origin.

An important additional characteristic is that it is a neoplastic proliferation.

Since the original description 150 years ago, considerable effort has been made to classify and characterize leukaemic cells. However, leukaemia is a generic term given to a number of diseases, clinically and morphologically different from one another. Correspondingly the aetiology and biology are unique to each subtype. The 'how' and 'when' of leukaemogenesis will be closely inter-related as the understanding of leukaemia improves. The many factors associated with leukaemogenesis suggest that the disease arises in individuals in whom multiple events and conditions are concatenated in a precise spatial and temporal relationship, leading sooner or later to an overt clinical leukaemic state (Henderson 1982). This is best exemplified by the current hypothesis for an aetiology and development of childhood acute lymphoblastic leukaemia (Greaves 1988, 1993; Greaves and Alexander 1993).

CLONAL DEVELOPMENT AND STEM CELL ORIGIN

The origin of the leukaemic cell, an important issue, has been approached in different ways. According to the current view, the leukaemic process is assumed to begin in a single haemopoietic cell of any lineage, varying in maturity from the multipotential primitive stem cell to the more differentiated cell. This critical defect is intrinsic to the cell and inheritable by its progeny. The clonal nature of the leukaemic process has been proved indirectly by analysis of leukaemic cells for glucose-6-phosphate dehydrogenase (G_6PD) isoenzymes, cytogenetics and restriction fragment length polymorphisms. At present, only X-linked markers are definitive markers for the extent of a leukaemic clone (Busque and Gilliland 1993). Lineage-specific markers like immunophenotype are helpful in identifying the clone, but they can be misleading as to its extent because of the necessity of interpreting such studies appropriately for differentiation and clonal evolution.

The ability to distinguish isoenzyme variants of G_6PD by electrophoresis was the basis for the application of this technique in tracing the origin of the leukaemic cell. In comparison with other markers, G_6PD polymorphisms have the advantage of being independent of lineage, post-embryonic differentiation, and clonal evolution. Technically, only a few cells, even enucleated, are required to detect activity of the enzyme. The clonal nature of leukaemia was first established in chronic myeloid leukaemia by G_6PD enzyme analysis. The leukaemic cells expressed only one type of enzyme, whereas non-malignant tissues expressed an equal mixture of the two normal isoenzymes (Fialkow *et al.* 1977). Thus in chronic myeloid leukaemia, at the stage of disease when it is studied, it is clonal. The observation that the same single-enzyme phenotype was found in all lineages of haemopoietic cells in chronic myeloid leukaemia indicated that the leukaemic process originated in a multipotential primitive stem cell (Fialkow *et al.* 1981; Greaves 1982). This was corroborated by the presence of the Philadelphia chromosome (Ph), consistent cytogenetic abnormality observed in chronic myeloid leukaemia, in lineages of cells other than granulocytes. In acute myeloid leukaemia, however, G_6PD enzyme analysis reveals the existence of two subtypes. In elderly patients the leukaemia originates in multipotential stem cells, whereas in younger patients it arises in a more restricted progenitor cell of the granulocytic lineage (Fialkow *et al.* 1987). The clonal nature of lymphoid leukaemias was similarly established by using G_6PD isoenzyme analysis, immunoglobulin expression with cell surface markers, and, more recently, by immunoglobulin and T-cell receptor gene rearrangement. In leukaemias where a complete drug-induced remission was possible the existence of both clonal and non-clonal normal haemopoietic cell progenitors was identified (Coulombel *et al.* 1983; Fialkow *et al.* 1987; Busque and Gilliland 1993). These studies of leukaemic cells have resulted in three major conclusions: (a) haematological malignancies are clonal when diagnosed clinically, i.e. they either arise from one cell or are the result of overgrowth of progeny from one cell and are not the result of transformation or stimulation of many haemopoietic progenitors; (b) the maturity of the primary cell involved in the transformation varies from disease to disease; (c) leukaemias develop by a multistep process.

KINETICS OF LEUKAEMIA

Normal cell production by the bone marrow is characterized by an orderly process of controlled cell proliferation in which cells mature progressively as they divide. This process of differentiation is irreversible, ultimately producing mature cells which are released

Table 1 Abnormalities of cellular proliferation in leukaemia

Stem cells	Normal	Abnormal
Maturation	Synchronous with proliferation	Asynchronous does not terminate in division
Feedback	Controls production	Absent or ineffective
Steady state	Yes	No
Release	Orderly	Random
End product	Mature cells	Immature cells

into the blood. For each cell type, maturation and release into and disappearance from the blood is in a steady state. Contrary to earlier views, leukaemia is not a wild disorder of cellular proliferation. It is now widely accepted that leukaemic cells divide normally or more slowly than normal haemopoietic precursors and also take longer to synthesize DNA (Andreeff 1986; Vincent 1989). The kinetic behaviour of leukaemic cells in human disease can best be represented as an intermediate between maximum exponential growth and the steady state characteristic of normal haemopoiesis (Table 1). Leukaemic cells gradually accumulate in most patients and compete with normal haematopoietic cellular proliferation. The fraction of leukaemic cells with stem cell capability must vary greatly among different populations, and it is this variability that partly accounts for the differences in the rate of progression of the disease. Other factors influencing the rate of progression are the growth fraction, or proportion of actively dividing cells, and the fact that many leukaemic populations have a substantial spontaneous death rate. The kinetic status of the target cell may be important in determining the extent to which the change due to the leukaemogenic agent is expressed. For instance, in one hypothesis (sleeper to feeder/stem cell) the damage to a stem cell in G_0 produced leukaemia only if that cell subsequently entered the cell cycle (Killmann 1968). Alternatively, the primary leukaemogenic event may alter the responsiveness of a G_0 stem cell to normal control mechanisms, increasing its cycling rate and decreasing the time in G_0 (Lajtha 1981). Shortening the duration of G_0 may carry the risk of accumulating additional errors, as it is during this phase that the cell undertakes 'genetic housekeeping'. In some leukaemic populations, such as those in the chronic leukaemias and myelodysplastic syndromes, the majority of cells may mature to the extent of losing their ability to divide. In such instances their behaviour may closely resemble that of normal haemopoietic cells, and the leukaemic population may expand very slowly. The failure of normal haemopoiesis as leukaemic cell mass increases is not completely understood. Current evidence suggests that leukaemic cells inhibit the proliferation of normal colony-forming unit cells in coculture experiments owing to the development of a soluble inhibitor called the leukaemia inhibitory factor. The identity of this factor is uncertain, but it has been claimed to be isoferritin, prostaglandins, and various other factors (Broxmeyer and Williams 1988; Vincent 1989). Another important characteristic of the leukaemic state is that leukaemic cells are relatively unresponsive to normal regulatory mechanisms which maintain the size of the haemopoietic compartments within normal limits, as in chronic myeloid leukaemia (Eaves et al. 1986). The degree of escape from normal control varies widely, partly explaining the relative behaviour of the leukaemic process in individual patients. The effectiveness of chemotherapy in acute leukaemias is essentially due to the relatively faster proliferative rate of normal progenitor cells when leukaemic cells are suppressed or destroyed.

The recent discovery of genes critical to the control of the cell cycle promises to reveal more about their function in leukaemic states where cellular kinetics are altered (Hartwell and Weinert 1989; Laskey et al. 1989; Murray and Kirschner 1989; Pardee 1989).

IMMUNOLOGY OF LEUKAEMIC CELLS

Immunological study of leukaemic cells was originally undertaken to identify leukaemia-specific antigens. Despite intensive efforts over the last 20 years, most of the antigens originally thought to be leukaemia specific have turned out to be normal gene products: differentiation-linked antigens expressed on cells in extremely small numbers in normal blood and bone marrow. However, the study of these cell-surface antigens in leukaemia has been useful in the clinical management of individual patients, as in acute lymphoblastic leukaemia (Chan et al. 1985). Fundamentally, their discovery has enormously improved the understanding of normal haemopoietic cell differentiation. The explosion of research over the last 15 years started with the demonstration of surface membrane immunoglobulin and restriction of the light chain expression in chronic lymphatic leukaemia. Extension of such analysis into acute lymphoblastic leukaemia revealed the marked phenotypic heterogeneity from patient to patient and also within a single patient. The major conclusions drawn from the analysis of childhood and adult lymphoid leukaemias are as follows.

1. Acute lymphoblastic leukaemia arises in the B- or T-cell progenitor compartments during the phase of clonal diversification and receptor gene rearrangement. In contrast, the chronic lymphocytic leukaemias, adult T-cell leukaemias, derive from subsets of mature immunocompetent B or T lymphocytes. The malignant cell population is monoclonal and is frozen at a particular stage of differentiation for that lineage, which is of variable stringency (Sallan et al. 1980; Korsmeyer et al. 1983; Chan et al. 1985; Greaves 1985).

2. The hypothesis of lineage fidelity proposes that leukaemic blast cells arise from clonal expansion of a transformed haemopoietic progenitor cell with exclusively myeloid or lymphoid characteristics. Essentially this model holds good for the majority of acute leukaemias, except for a significant subset where blasts express both lymphoid and myeloid features (mixed lineage leukaemia). In addition to patients with acute leukaemia, who demonstrate lineage infidelity, there is a second group who undergo a lineage switch, providing a further example of lineage heterogeneity. Such a lineage switch usually occurs at relapse of leukaemia after intensive chemotherapy and during the blast crisis of chronic myeloid leukaemia (Greaves et al. 1986; Stass and Mirro 1986).

The above conclusions had major implications for acute lymphoblastic leukaemia. They underlined the hypothesis that in the leukaemic state proliferation is uncoupled from differentiation with the result that a normally rare and transient progenitor cell phenotype is stabilized. By analogy such a concept has been extended to other leukaemias.

Similarly, surface marker analysis of blast cells from acute myeloid leukaemia have demonstrated the existence of lineage-restricted antigens which have their counterparts on normal haemopoietic progenitor cells. However, a panel of markers is necessary to establish the myeloid or lymphoid origin of the leukaemia (Griffin et al. 1982; Messner and Griffin 1986).

Thus the immunological view of the cell has reinforced the maturation arrest hypothesis, though not necessarily improving the understanding of how such an event occurs.

Immunological studies of leukaemia, however, have been useful clinically in improving the precision of diagnosis and in raising the possibility of a more defined antibody based therapy (Pui *et al.* 1993).

COLONY-STIMULATING FACTORS

The colony-stimulating factors described in detail earlier are important regulators of normal haemopoiesis. Naturally their role is under increasing scrutiny in understanding leukaemogenesis. The *in vitro* growth of leukaemic blast cells in semisolid media or in liquid suspension is critically dependent on a supply of exogenous colony-stimulating factors. Thus a simple autocrine model of increased secretion of an appropriate colony-stimulating factor by the leukaemic blast cell acting on its own receptor on the cell membrane has not been held valid (Metcalf 1988). Despite this proviso, there is now clear evidence in acute myeloid leukaemia of constitutive expression of the GM-CSF and G-CSF genes and secretion of their respective factors by blast cells in a proportion of cases (Young *et al.* 1987). The role played by colony-stimulating factor in the initiation and maintenance of leukaemia is still far from clear, but undoubtedly will be investigated in detail. The following experimental evidence suggests possible roles for colony-stimulating factor in the induction of leukaemias.

1. Cells that synthesize abnormal numbers or types of receptors, with or without growth factor binding, are able to elicit the metabolic cascade that normally occurs following binding of a growth factor to its receptor. This is observed in HTLV-1, transformed T lymphocytes which express high levels of IL-2 receptor (Kronke *et al.* 1985).

2. Intracellular activation of the receptor by its growth factor in blast cells, without excessive secretion or display of receptors. Such a mechanism has been postulated when FDC-P$_1$ cells transfected by a retrovirus containing the GM-CSF gene are rendered leukaemogenic in mice (Lang *et al.* 1985; Pierce *et al.* 1985).

3. Leukaemic cells may produce intermediate messengers in the metabolic cascade initiated following growth factor—receptor binding, thus delivering a proliferative signal bypassing normal receptor—ligand interactions (Cook *et al.* 1985).

4. The translocations or deletions involving chromosome 17 or 5 respectively, affecting the colony-stimulating factor gene cluster, may result in a low but quite crucial level of autonomous production of colony-stimulating factor by blast cells.

Thus the colony-stimulating factors may play a critical role in the biology of leukaemias. Myeloid leukaemic cells remain dependent on the colony-stimulating factors for proliferative stimulation in the majority of instances, and are essential cofactors in the development of leukaemia. However, the exact inter-relationship between the primary genetic change altering the balance between proliferation and differentiation versus self-renewal and the requirement for colony-stimulating factors is still to be determined.

SIGNIFICANCE OF KARYOTYPE ABNORMALITIES

It has long been recognized, since the original observation by Boveri (1914), that chromosomal abnormalities are important in the genesis of cancer. The first specific cytogenetic abnormality to be detected

Table 2 Karyotypic abnormalities in leukaemia

Type	Gains	Losses	Rearrangement
Chronic myeloid leukaemia			
CP			t(9;22)(q34;q11)
B/C	+8,+Ph	Rare; −7	t(9;22),i(17q)
Acute myeloid leukaemia			
M2	+8	−7; −5	t(8;21)(q22;q22)
M3	—	—	t(15;17)(q22;q12−21)
M4 (eosinophilia)	+8, +22	−7	inv(16)(p13q22);t(16;16), del(16q)
M5	—	—	t(9;11)(p22;q23), t(11q), del(11q)
M2/M4 (basophilia)	—	—	t(6;9)(p23;q34)
M4 (platelets)	—	—	t(3;3)(q21;q26),inv(3)
Chronic lymphoblastic leukaemia			
B-cell	+12	—	14q+(q32)
T-cell	—	—	t(8;14)(q24;q11), inv(14)(q11;q32)
Acute lymphoblastic leukaemia			
B lymphoid/ myeloid			t(4;11)(q21;q23)
Precursor B	+21, +6	Rare	t(9;22),del(6q)(q15−q21), near haploid
Pre-B	—	—	t(1;19)(q23;p13)
B-cell	—	—	t(8;14)(q24;q32), t(2;8)(p13;q24) t(8;22)(q24;q11)
Early T-cell precursor			t(9p),del(9p)(p21−22)
T-cell			inv(14)(q11;q32), t(7;7)(p15;q11) t(8;14)(q24;q11) t(7;9)(q36;q34) t(10;14)(q24;q11) t(11;14)(p13;q11) t(7;14)(q35−36;q11)

was the Philadelphia chromosome in chronic myeloid leukaemia (Nowell and Hungerford 1960; Rowley 1973). Since then a number of consistent cytogenetic abnormalities have been associated with specific types of leukaemias (Table 2) (Sandberg 1986). The primary karyotypic change may be a translocation, deletion, or gain of a whole or part of a chromosome, and other structural rearrangements. This diversity of abnormalities implies an equal diversity of mechanisms of genetic changes that can be associated with malignant cell transformation. Thus a gain of all or part of a chromosome implies amplification of a gene or genes; deletion suggests loss of genes. However, consistent translocations imply a more complex process as two chromosomes are involved in the rearrangement. It is now apparent that consistent translocations pinpoint chromosome segments that contain genes critically involved in malignant cell transformation. The primary karyotypic changes play a crucial part in leukaemogenesis and underline the clonal nature of leukaemias. Secondary karyotypic changes in the leukaemic cells are observed with evolution of the leukaemic process and often herald a more aggressive state as in chronic myeloid leukaemia. The question of how and when consistent chromosomal abnormalities occur has not been satisfactorily resolved. They probably occur continuously and randomly. In a given cell some are lethal while others may be neutral, and selection acts to eliminate the majority of chromosomal abnormalities. Some changes in the appropriate cell type may provide the cell with a proliferative advantage over normal cells, or these may occur preferentially allowing them to be observed. The stage at which chromosomal abnormalities occur in the development of leukaemia is unclear because of the lack of independent markers for the malignant cell. In chronic myeloid leukaemia and acute myeloid leukaemia, based on G_6PD data, the hypothesis is that there is proliferation of a chromosomally normal clone that has some selective advantage compared with all other myeloid cells. The relevant chromosomal change occurs in this initiated clone which leads to overt leukaemia (Fialkow and Singer 1985). It is the analysis of translocations, and particularly the study of breakpoints on chromosome segments, using modern biological techniques that has revealed new insights into leukaemogenesis.

The identification of consistent reciprocal translocations in the leukaemic cell has been enormously useful in further genetic analysis and isolation of genes. This area of research has rapidly increased over the last few years, with several individual participating genes in translocations being identified. The molecular analysis of the Philadelphia chromosome in chronic myeloid leukaemia is an excellent example (see later). Similarly, the analysis of the t(11;14) translocation observed in B-cell chronic lymphoblastic leukaemia has revealed the existence of new genes which may be determinant in initiating or maintaining the leukaemic process. An interesting translocation involves the 11q23 region as a constant partner in association with other chromosomes. Another interesting abnormality seen in leukaemias secondary to a myelodysplastic state is the 5q-syndrome. The genes for the colony-stimulating factors M-CSF, GM-CSF, and IL-3 are located on the arm which is deleted in these leukaemias (Bunn 1986; Le Beau et al. 1986a). Thus chromosomal abnormalities increasingly are the starting point for the genetic analysis of the primary defect in the leukaemic cell.

HUMAN RETROVIRUSES AND LEUKAEMOGENESIS

Retroviruses have long been implicated in the pathogenesis of feline leukaemia, bovine leukaemia and avian leukaemia (Jarret and Onions 1984). The discovery of reverse transcriptase, and T-cell growth factor (IL-2) set the scene for the discovery of human retroviruses. The two human retroviruses HTLV-I and HTLV-II are now implicated in the pathogenesis of adult T-cell leukaemia/lymphoma diseases (Shaw et al. 1984). This aggressive form of leukaemia is observed in the United States, Japan, the Caribbean Islands, and Caribbean immigrants in the United Kingdom (Blattner et al. 1983a). The proof that the virus is closely associated with the development of leukaemia and lymphoma comes from several lines of evidence. First, HTLV-I transforms T lymphocytes in vitro and the provirus is integrated into the genome in leukaemic cells obtained from patients. The site of integration is uniform in each patient, though it may vary from patient to patient. In addition, the provirus is integrated only in the genome of leukaemic cells, and the monoclonality has been confirmed by both phenotype and T-cell receptor gene rearrangements. The transformation of T_H lymphocytes by HTLV-I in vitro has been elegantly substantiated by coculture experiments with umbilical cord lymphocytes (Blattner et al. 1983b). The transformed T cells have been shown to express constitutively an increased amount of IL-2 receptors, though levels of IL-2 are not increased. Further serological evidence of antibodies to HTLV-I are detected in over 90 per cent of patients with a diagnosis of adult T-cell leukaemia (Gallo et al. 1983; Yoshida et al. 1984). The strong epidemiological evidence from Japan, where it is endemic, supports a causative role for HTLV-I in adult T-cell leukaemia.

The current view based on serology and epidemiological data is that infection by HTLV-I occurs at an early age, when the virus (and disease) is endemic, with immortalization of T_4 cells. The virus is probably transmitted horizontally and requires intimate contact or through blood transfusions. Further, the virus is transmitted from males to females but not the converse. Constitutive expression of the IL-2 receptor and IL-2 secretion in T_4 lymphocytes sets the stage for the first step in the development of leukaemia. It appears that the transformation results from an increased number of permanently stimulated IL-2 receptors, possibly because of deregulation of the IL-2 receptor gene (Kronke et al. 1985). Secondary genetic events including other cofactors are probably necessary for the full development of the disease in view of the long incubation period. Studies of immigrant populations provide evidence for a latency period of over 30 years for leukaemia to develop (Greaves et al. 1984). Consistent cytogenetic abnormalities involving trisomy 7, 14q- and 6q have been reported, although the relationship to the disease is unclear. Further research in this area will improve the understanding of events leading from infection with HTLV-I to frank acute leukaemia (Kueffler and Bunn 1986). None of the other leukaemias has been shown to have a causal relationship to human or other retroviruses.

ONCOGENES

The foundation for the genetic basis of cancer and leukaemias was laid by the discovery of oncogenes. Proto-oncogenes, the cellular progenitors of retroviral transforming genes (oncogenes), have been highly conserved throughout vertebrate evolution. It is presumed that the normal role of the products encoded by these genes is to regulate the processes involved in cell proliferation, differentiation, and death. When incorporated within the retroviral genome, such transduced sequences acquire the ability to induce neoplastic transformation as viral oncogenes, an observation that initially linked these genes to the neoplastic process (Bishop 1983; Varmus 1984). It is quite evident now that proto-oncogenes may be frequent targets for genetic alterations that lead normal cells along the pathway to malignancy under natural conditions. This conversion of proto-oncogenes into 'oncogenes' can be caused by DNA rearrangements due to chromosomal translocations, gene amplifications, point mutations, deletions, and other mechanisms affecting their normal regulation and expression. Another important mechanism is the loss or inactivation of a class of genes termed tumour suppressor genes. These, though less commonly identified as a pathogenetic mechanism in leukaemia, play an important role in progression of leukaemia. The genes identified with leukaemias are listed in Table 3. The involvement of such oncogenes and tumour suppressor genes in human leukaemia, their possible association with specific phenotypes, and the genetic changes responsible for their alteration are areas of intense research (Rowley 1983).

Activation of oncogenes by chromosomal translocations

The association between specific chromosomal translocations and oncogenes was derived from initial mapping of retroviral oncogenes to human chromosomes. It was found that proto-oncogenes were often located at or near the breakpoint of several translocations. The prime example of such a translocation altering (structurally and functionally) a proto-oncogene in human leukaemia involves the c-ABL gene and the Ph translocation associated with chronic myeloid leukaemia. In this reciprocal translocation involving chromosomes 9

Table 3 Genetic changes in leukaemia

Type of gene	Function	Molecular alteration	Common chromosomal abnormality	Approximate percentage of leukaemias with genetic alteration
ras	Signal transduction	*N-ras* mutations	None	AML, 15–50% ALL, 14% Blast crisis of CML, <5%
Tyrosine kinases	Membrane signal transduction	Fusion of c-*abl* to *bcr*	t(9;22)(q34;q11)	CML, >95%
Transcriptional control element	Gene transcription	Fusion of *myc* to immunoglobulin genes	t(8;14)(q24;q32)	Burkitt's lymphoma, 100% Pre-B-cell ALL, T-ALL, <10%
		Fusion of *E2A* to *PBX* or *HLF*	t(1;19)(q23;p13) t(17;19)(q22;p13)	Pre-B-cell ALL, <10%
		Fusion of *SCL (tal-1)* to TCR or *SIL* genes	t(1;14)(p32;q11)	T-ALL, 15–25%
		Fusion of *tal-2* to TCR genes	t(7;9)(q35;p13)	T-ALL, <10%
		Fusion of *lyl-1* to TCR genes	t(7;19)(q35;p13)	T-ALL, <5%
		Fusion of *Ttg-1, Ttg-2* to TCR genes	t(11;14)(p15;q11) t(11;14)(p13;q11)	T-ALL, <10%
Homeodomain	Differentiation and gene transcription	Fusion of *HOX-11* to TCR genes	t(10;14)(q24;q11)	T-ALL, 7%
		HRX translocation	t(11q23)	Multilineage leukaemia?
Receptor	Differentiation	Fusion of α-retinoic acid-receptor gene to *PML*	t(15;17)(q21;q21)	PML, 100%
bcl	Apoptosis, other functions?	Fusion of *bcl-2* immunoglobulin genes	t(14;18)(q32;q21)	>75% CLL, 5%
	Cell-cycle control	Fusion of *bcl-1* immunoglobulin genes	t(11;14)(q13;q32)	CLL, 2–5%
	Inhibition of gene transcription	Fusion of *bcl-3* to immunoglobulin genes	t(14;19)(q32;q13)	CLL, <10%
Anti-oncogenes	Tumour suppression, transcription, cell-cycle control, apoptosis	Mutation, loss, or rearrangement of p53	del 17	Blast crisis of CML >20% AML, 3–7% Pre-B-cell ALL, 2% T-ALL, <2% CLL, 15%
		Disruption of *RB1*	13q	Ph¹-positive ALL, >30% AML, <3%; AMML, 25% Pre-B-cell ALL, T-ALL, 20%
Other	Function unknown	Fusion of *DEKICAN, SETICAN*	t(6;9)(p23;q34)	AML, MDS, <2%
		Fusion of *MLL*	t(11q23)	AML?, ALL?
		Rearrangement of *TAN-1*	t(7;9)(q34;q34.3)	T-ALL?
		Fusion of *AML1*	t(8;21)	AML?
	Regulation of growth	Fusion of interleukin-3	t(5;14)(q31;q32)	Pre-B-cell ALL?

AML, acute myeloid leukaemia (acute non-lymphocytic leukaemia); ALL, acute lymphoblastic leukaemia; CML, chronic myelocytoblastic leukaemia; TCR, T-cell-receptor; CLL, chronic lymphocytic leukaemia; AMML, acute myelomonocytic leukaemia (stage M4 or M5) syndromes.

and 22, the c-ABL gene normally located at the segment of the break on chromosome 9 is translocated to the breakpoint cluster region (bcr) on the long arm of chromosome 22. The breakpoints on chromosome 9 are variable in individual patients, while on 22 they occur in a defined region 'bcr'. This is part of a larger gene called BCR with unknown function. This gene, along with the translocated c-ABL, forms a hybrid BCR-ABL gene which transcribes an abberrant 8 Kb transcript observed in leukaemic cells. This transcript encodes for an abnormal protein of 210 kDa with constitutively activated tyrosine kinase function. This fusion protein has both *in vivo* and *in vitro* phosphorylation activity predominantly on tyrosine residues, similar to that associated with the viral gag-v-abl fusion proteins. The BCR-ABL protein p210 differs from the normal unaltered c-ABL product p145 which is not detectably phosphorylated *in vivo* or *in vitro*. Thus the translocation results in the alteration of the structure and function of the c-ABL protein which at present is the only known biochemical difference between

normal and leukaemic cells in chronic myeloid leukaemia. In acute lymphoblastic leukaemia, the same translocation results in the production of a different protein P190 in leukaemic cells from some patients, whilst others express P210. So far no critical changes have been observed in the levels of expression of these proteins during the transition from the chronic to the acute phase of chronic myeloid leukaemia (Groffen and Heisterkamp 1987; Kurzrock *et al.* 1988). It has now been shown that the pathway of signal transduction by these abnormal proteins in leukaemic cells mimics the normal (Pendergast *et al.* 1993).

The biological effects of the BCR-ABL gene products have been tested in several systems. The BCR-ABL gene was able to induce clonal pre-B cell proliferation, conferring transforming potential to some clones after continued *in vitro* propagation. In addition, the BCR-ABL gene has also been shown to render factor-dependent cell lines independent of factor requirements. It has recently been demonstrated that reconstitution of mouse bone marrow cells carrying the virus encoding the BCR-ABL gene leads to the development of a leukaemic state similar to chronic myeloid leukaemia (Daley *et al.* 1990), whilst another construct carrying the P190 variant gives rise to acute leukaemia in transgenic mice (Heisterkamp *et al.* 1990). Ultimately, the function of these genes and their role in intracellular physiology would determine their contribution to leukaemogenesis (Pendergast and Witte 1987; Ramakrishman and Rosenberg 1989).

The other consistent translocation wherein an oncogene is activated by a translocation is the t(8:14) translocation in Burkitt's lymphomas. Here c-MYC from chromosome 8 is translocated to 14 and lies in a head-to-head configuration with the heavy chain locus of the immunoglobulin gene. The c-*myc* gene is constitutively activated as a result. The contribution of this to the development of leukaemia is linked with the role of the Epstein–Barr virus, and the geographical locale of Burkitt's lymphoma (Klein 1983; Croce and Nowell 1985). Similar translocations have been shown to involve the T-cell receptor genes in some T-cell leukaemias (Rabbits *et al.* 1988; Boehm and Rabbits 1989). The aberrant expression of oncogenes resulting from the fusion to immunoglobulin or T-cell receptor genes is common in T-cell and B-cell leukaemias.

Analysis of similar translocations associated with specific leukaemias has been revealing. The t(11;14) translocation observed in B-cell chronic lymphocytic leukaemia, involves the bcl-1 locus on chromosome 11 and the immunoglobulin heavy chain locus on chromosome 14 (Tsujimoto *et al.* 1984). The specific translocation of acute promelocytic leukaemia t(15:17), has been shown to result in a fusion protein between α-retinoic acid receptor gene and a gene called PML (Kakisuka *et al.* 1991). A more general translocation found in leukaemias, lymphomas, and secondary leukaemias (exposure to etoposide) involve the region 11q23 in partnership with other chromosomes. The gene involved, HRX, is a novel gene with homology to the trilthorax gene in fruitfly implicated in development (Trachuk *et al.* 1992).

The identification of genes involved in a translocation, has been made easier with advances in genetic techniques over the last 5 years.

Activation of oncogenes by point mutations

The *ras* gene family comprising N-*ras*, K-*ras*, and H-*ras* has been investigated in detail because of its involvement in human leukaemias (Barbacid 1986). Point mutations of this gene involving single base changes confer malignant potential to these genes in *in vitro* systems. In leukaemias, particularly in acute myeloid leukaemia, mutations of the N-*ras* gene have been noted to occur in pre-leukaemia as well as in frank leukaemia, and to disappear on restoration of normal haemopoiesis after intensive chemotherapy. The normal function of *ras* is to provide an important conduit for flow of information from the surface of the cell to nucleus. Mutations at these codons alter the normal biological function and are thought to affect their role in normal signal transduction.

Mutations in the p53 gene, have now been detected in leukaemias. The p53 gene is involved in maintaining the integrity of the genome and also in apoptosis. Mutations in this gene in leukaemia, though less common in frequency than in solid tumours, may contribute to progression of leukaemia rather than initiation. Another important gene *Rb*, implicated in retinoblastoma, is altered in 10 to 30 per cent of all types of acute leukaemia, especially AML (M4,M5). The phosphoprotein encoded by the *Rb* gene is important in the development of the haemopoeitic system (Cline 1994).

Deletions

Deletion of the long arm of chromosome 5 is frequently observed in therapy-related myelodysplastic syndrome and acute myeloid leukaemias. The interstitial deletions from 5q13–5q33 involve a critical region of 5q23–5q31 involved in all leukaemias. The genes for GM-CSF, IL-3, M-CSF, IL-4, IL-5, and the receptor for M-CSF have been mapped to these regions. At least one allele is lost in these abnormalities, and at the present time it is not known whether this is critical to the development of myeloid leukaemias (Le Beau *et al.* 1986*a*,*b*). Loss of 7q is another chromosomal abnormality identified in therapy related leukaemias, where the gene is yet to be identified.

The evidence that certain proto-oncogenes code for either growth factor or its receptor (c-FMS codes for M-CSF receptor) implies that the normal metabolic pathways by which cell proliferation and differentiation is controlled can be subverted. This has been experimentally proven in *in vitro* systems where oncogenes transform appropriate cell lineages, blocking further differentiation or at the same time rendering factor-dependent cell lines independent of factor requirements. Thus a critical way in which oncogenes may act is to subvert normal growth regulatory pathways.

The impact of a variety of disciplines in understanding the biology of leukaemia has been described. It is evident from a number of *in vitro* and *in vivo* experiments that multiple stages can be identified in the evolution of leukaemia. According to the current view, the critical initial event in leukaemogenesis is the transformation of a single cell, either a multipotential stem cell or a progenitor for a particular lineage. The initial mutation in a cellular gene may affect the probability of stem cell renewal at the expense of further differentiation. This mutation could be the result of an environmental carcinogen, a virus, radiation, or chromosomal instability. Expansion of this clone proceeds with gradual accumulation of immature cells dependent on colony-stimulating factors or other cytokines for growth. Further genomic instability with evolution of subclones occurs, marked by new karyotypic abnormalities with growth advantage over the original clone. The increase in the probability of self-renewal over differentiation results in accumulation of blasts and frank leukaemia. It is possible that the acquisition of the ability to produce colony-stimulating factors would provide such a growth advantage. This can be by a number of different mechanisms, eventually leading to an autonomous evolution to acute leukaemia. This model, currently widely accepted, explains the role of many of the cofactors necessary in initiating and maintaining the leukaemic state.

The initial causative agents which alter the genetic structure of the haemopoietic cell are yet to be identified in the common acute and chronic leukaemias. In the majority of instances it is unlikely that radiation or chemicals play a significant role. Radiation can cause leukaemia, as has been shown by studies of the survivors of the atomic bomb explosion in Nagasaki and Hiroshima (Heysell *et al.* 1960). The dose of irradiation and the age of the individual determine the type of leukaemia. Similarly, patients who have received irradiation for ankylosing spondylitis and carcinoma of the cervix have an increased relative risk of developing leukaemia (Court-Brown and Abbatt 1965; Boice *et al.* 1987). The leukaemia clusters around nuclear waste installations have not been conclusively proven to be due to irradiation (Beral 1990). Chemicals like benzene and, more recently, chemotherapy with alkylating agents in Hodgkin's disease and ovarian cancer confer an increased risk of development of leukaemia (Vigliani and Saita 1964; Kaldor *et al.*

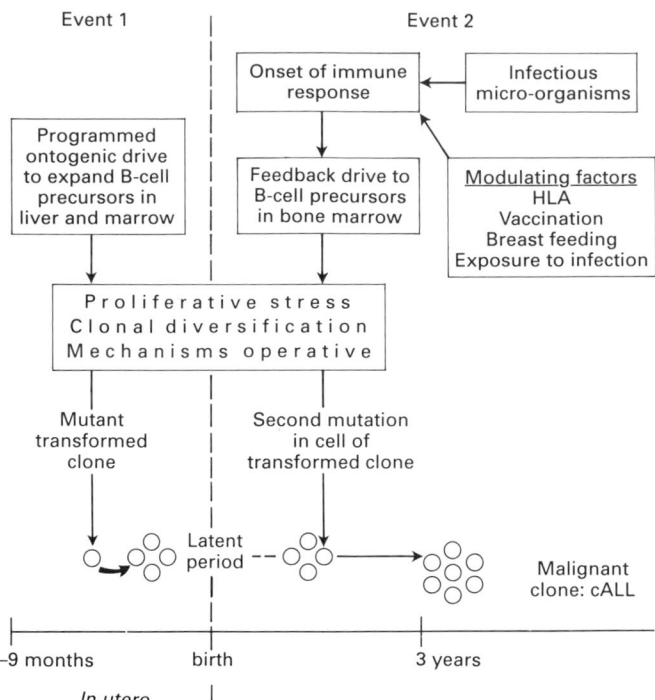

Fig. 1 Hypothetical model for the aetiology of childhood common (B cell precursor) acute lymphoblastic leukaemia. (Reproduced from Greaves 1988, with permission.)

1990*a*,*b*). Retroviruses, especially HTLV-I and HTLV-II, are the only agents causally related to human leukaemia so far.

It is in this context that the development of a unified hypothesis for the cause and development of leukaemia is inherently difficult. The model proposed by Greaves (1988, 1993; Greaves and Alexander 1993) for the aetiology and development of acute lymphoblastic leukaemias, though not entirely proven, illustrates the complexity and the synthesis of a number of related events before leukaemia is established (Fig. 1). Childhood acute lymphoblastic leukaemia originates in B- or T-lymphocyte precursors. These cells are important in the development of the immune system and such a process starts *in utero*. Sufficient biology of the normal development of B and T cells and the mechanism for generating antibody diversity and antigen recognition is now known. The combination of a high proliferation rate, together with developmentally regulated intrinsic and receptor gene rearrangement, promotes the occurrence of spontaneous mutations in such cells. The factors which promote the normal development of the immune system are exogenous and include feeding practices, infections, vaccinations in infancy and childhood, and, more indirectly, the socio-economic status of the family and genetic factors (HLA). The direct stress of developmental proliferation of B-cell precursors *in utero* and the later addition of exogenous factors in infancy increase the risk (or 'promote') spontaneous mutations. Essentially, the hypothesis proposes that spontaneous mutation (one or two events), as distinct from that due to exogenous leukaemogenic (i.e. mutagenic) agents, may explain the development of acute lymphoblastic leukaemia. The natural immune response thus increases the risk for the development of leukaemia by indirectly upregulating the number of target B cells at risk. Thus, if the small number of patients for whom clear inherited genetic defects or other factors operate are excluded, such a model would explain the aetiology and development of acute lymphoblastic leukaemia in the majority of instances. Another

mathematical model based on estimated mutation rates in man, particularly the lymphoid system, suggests the loss of two pairs of regulatory genes for the development of leukaemia (Morris 1989).

The biology of leukaemia is definitely better understood than it was 15 years ago, but the major causes remain elusive. However, the various methods adopted to examine the leukaemic cell, be they cytogenetics, morphology, immunology, or, more recently, molecular biology, have demonstrated subsets of disease amenable to current chemotherapy. The aim of studying leukaemia should necessarily be that, in the final analysis, outcome in patients is improved with cure for the majority. The exciting recent discoveries in understanding leukaemogenesis increasingly point that way.

REFERENCES

Andreef MA (1986). Cell kinetics of leukaemia. *Seminars in Hematology*, **23**:300–14.

Barbacid M. (1986). Human oncogenes. In *Important advances in oncology* (ed. PD Vincent, T De Vita, S Hellman, and SA Rosenberg), pp. 2–22. Lippincott, Philadelphia.

Bennett JH (1985). Case of hypertrophy of the spleen and liver, in which death took place from suppuration of the blood. *Edinburgh Medical and Surgical Journal*, **64**:413.

Beral V (1990). Leukaemia and nuclear installations. *British Medical Journal*, **300**:411–12.

Bishop JM (1983). Cellular oncogenes and retroviruses. *Annual Reviews of Biochemistry*, **52**:301–54.

Blattner WA, Blayney DW, Gwroff M, *et al.* (1983*a*). Epidemiology of the human T-cell leukaemia-lymphoma virus. *Journal of Infectious Diseases*, **147**(3): 404–16.

Blattner WA, Takatsuki K, Gallo RC (1983*b*). Human T-cell leukaemia-lymphoma virus and adult T-cell leukaemia. *Journal of the American Medical Association*, **250**:1074–80.

Boehm T, Rabbits TH (1989). A chromosomal basis for lymphoid malignancy in man. *European Journal of Biochemistry*, **185**:1–17.

Boice JD Jr, Blettner M, Kleinerman RA, *et al.* (1987). Radiation dose and leukaemia risk in patients treated for cancer of the cervix. *Journal of the National Cancer Institute*, **79**:1295–1311.

Boveri T (1912). Beitrag zum Studum des Chromatins in den Epithelzellen der Carcinoma. *Beiträge zur Pathologie*, **14**:249.

Broxmeyer HE, Williams DE (1988). The production of myeloid blood cells and their regulation during health and disease. *CRC Critical Reviews in Oncology and Hematology*, **8**:173–226.

Bunn HF (1986). 5q- and disordered haemopoiesis. *Clinics in Haematology*, **15**:1023–35.

Chan LC, Pegram SM, Greaves MF (1985). Contribution of immunophenotype to the classification and diagnosis of acute lymphoblastic leukaemia. *Lancet*, i:475–9.

Cline MJ (1994). The molecular basis of leukaemia. *New England Journal of Medicine*, **330**:328–36.

Cook WD, Metcalf D, Nicola NA, Burgess AW, Walker F (1985). Malignant transformation of a growth factor dependent myeloid cell line by Abelson virus without evidence of an autocrine mechanism. *Cell*, **41**:677–83.

Coulombel L, Eaves C, Kalousek DK, Gupta CM, Eaves AC. (1983). Long term bone marrow culture reveals chromosomally normal haemopoietic progenitor cells in patients with Philadelphia chromosome-positive chronic myelogenous leukaemia. *New England Journal of Medicine*, **308**:1493–8.

Court-Brown WM, Abbat JD (1965). Mortality from cancer and other causes after radiotherapy for ankylosing spondylitis. *British Medical Journal*, **2**:1327–9.

Croce CM, Nowell PC (1985). Molecular basis of human B cell neoplasia. *Blood*, **65**:1–7.

Daley GQ, van Etten RA, Baltimore D (1990). Induction of chronic myelogenous leukaemia in mice by the P210 bcr/abl gene of the Philadelphia chromosome. *Science*, **247**:824–9.

Eaves AC, Cashman JD, Gabowry LA, Kalowsek DK, Eaves CJ (1986). Unregulated proliferation of primitive chronic myeloid leukaemia progenitors in the presence of normal marrow adherent cells. *Proceedings of the National Academy of Sciences of the USA*, **83**:5306–10.

Fialkow PJ, Singer JW (1985). Tracing developing and cell lineages in human haemopoietic neoplasia. In *Leukaemia. Dahlem Konferenzen* (ed. H Weissman), p. 203. Springer-Verlag, Berlin.

Fialkow PJ, Jacobson RJ, Pappayannopoulou T (1977). Chronic myelocytic leukaemia: clonal origin in a stem cell common to the granulocyte, erythrocyte platelet, and monocyte/macrophage. *American Journal of Medicine*, 63:125–30.

Fialkow PJ, Martin PJ, Najfeld V, *et al.* (1981). Evidence for a multistep pathogenesis of chronic myelogenous leukaemia. *Blood*, 58:158–63.

Fialkow PJ, Singer RW, Raskind WH, *et al.* (1987). Clonal development, stem cell differentiation and clinical remissions in acute non-lymphocytic leukaemia. *New England Journal of Medicine*, 317:468–73.

Gallo RC, Kalyananaman VS, Sarangadharan MG, *et al.* (1983). Association of the human type C retrovirus with a subset of adult T-cell cancers. *Cancer Research*, 43:3892–9.

Greaves MF (1982). Target cell, differentiation and clonal evolution in chronic granulocytic leukaemia—a model for understanding the biology of malignancy. In *Chronic granulocytic leukaemia* (ed. MT Shaw), pp. 15–47. Praeger, London.

Greaves MF (1985). Phenotypic heterogeneity and the origins of lymphoid malignancy in man. Biological and clinical implications. In *Leukaemia. Dahlem Konferenzen* (ed. IL Weissman), pp. 95–110. Springer-Verlag, Berlin.

Greaves MF (1988). Speculations on the cause of childhood acute lymphoblastic leukaemia. *Leukaemia*, 2:120–5.

Greaves MF (1993). A natural history for pediatric acute leukaemia. *Blood*, 82:1043–51.

Greaves MF, Alexander FE (1993). An infectious etiology for common acute lymphoblastic leukaemia in childhood. *Leukaemia*, 7:349.

Greaves MF, Verbi W, Tilley R, *et al.* (1984). Human T-cell leukaemia virus (HTLV) in the United Kingdom. *International Journal of Cancer*, 33:795–806.

Greaves MF, Chan LC, Furley AJW, Watt SM, Molgaard HV (1986). Lineage promiscuity in haemopoietic differentiation and leukaemia. *Blood*, 67:1–11.

Griffin JD, Ritz J, Madler LM, Schlossman SF (1982). Expression of myeloid differentiation antigens on normal and malignant myeloid cells. *Journal of Clinical Investigation*, 68:932–41.

Groffen J, Heisterkamp N (1987). The BCR/ABL gene. *Baillière's Clinical Haematology*, 1:983–99.

Hartwell LH, Weinert TA (1989). Checkpoints: controls that ensure the order of cell cycle events. *Science*, 240:629–33.

Heisterkamp N, Jenster G, Hoeve J, Zovich D, Pattengale PK, Groffen J (1990). Acute leukaemia in BCR/ABL transgenic mice. *Nature, London*, 344:251–3.

Henderson ES (1982). Etiology of leukaemia: a persisting puzzle. In *Leukaemia* (4th edn) (ed. FW Gunz and ES Henderson), pp. 287–8. Grune and Stratton, New York.

Heysell R, Brill B, Woodbury LA (1960). Leukaemia in Hiroshima atomic bomb survivors. *Blood*, 15:313–31.

Jarrett O, Onions DE (1984). Retroviruses in leukaemia of animals and man. In *Haematology*, Vol 1, *Leukaemias* (ed. JM Goldman and HD Preisler), pp. 1–34. Butterworth, Boston.

Kakisuka A, Miller Jr, WH, Umesonak, *et al.* (1991). Chromosomal translocation t(15-17) in human acute promyelocytic leukaemia fuses RAR alpha with a novel putative transcription factor, PML. *Cell*, 66:663–74.

Kaldor JM, Day NE, Petersson F, *et al.* (1990*a*). Leukaemia following chemotherapy for ovarian cancer. *New England Journal of Medicine*, 322:1–6.

Kaldor JM, Day NE, Clarke A, *et al.* (1990*b*) Leukaemia following Hodgkin's disease. *New England Journal of Medicine*, 322:7–14.

Killmann SA (1968). Acute leukaemia: development, remission/relapse pattern, relationship between normal and leukaemic haemopoiesis, and the sleeper to feeder/stem cell hypothesis. *Seminars in Hematology*, 1:103.

Klein G (1983). Specific chromosomal translocations and the genesis of B-cell derived tumours in mice and men. *Cell*, 32:311–15.

Korsmeyer SJ, Arnold A, Bakshi A, *et al.* (1983). Immunoglobulin gene rearrangement and cell surface antigen expression in acute lymphocytic leukemias of T cell and B cell precursor origins. *Journal of Clinical Investigation*, 71:301–3.

Kronke M, Leonard WJ, Depper JM, Greene WC (1985). Deregulation of interleukin-2 gene expression in HTLV-1 induced acute leukaemia. *Science*, 228:1215–17.

Kueffler PR, Bunn PA (1986). Adult T-cell leukaemia/lymphoma. *Clinics in Hematology*, 15:695–726.

Kurzrock R, Gutterman JU, Talpaz M (1988). The molecular genetics of Philadelphia chromosome positive leukaemias. *New England Journal of Medicine*, 319.990–8.

Lajtha LG (1981). Which are the leukaemic cells? *Blood Cells*, 7:45.

Lang R, Metcalf N, Gough N, Dunn AR, Gonda TJ (1985). Expression of a haemopoietic growth factor cDNA in a factor-dependent cell line results in autonomous growth and tumorigenicity. *Cell*, 43:531–42.

Laskey RA, Fairman MP, Blow JJ (1989). S phase of the cell cycle. *Science*, 240:609–14.

Le Beau MM, Aebain KS, Larson RA, *et al.* (1986*a*). Clinical and cytogenetic correlations in 63 patients with therapy-related myelodysplastic syndromes and acute non-lymphocytic leukemias—further evidence for characteristic abnormalities of chromosome 5 and 7. *Journal of Clinical Oncology*, 4:325–45.

Le Beau MM, Westbrook CM, Diaz MO, *et al.* (1986*b*). Evidence for the involvement of GM-CSF, and FMS in the deletion (5q) in myeloid disorders. *Science*, 231:984–7.

Messner HA, Griffin JD (1986). Biology of acute myeloid leukaemia. *Clinics in Hematology*, 15:641–67.

Metcalf D (1988). *The molecular control of blood cells*, pp. 124–47. Harvard University Press, Cambridge, MA.

Morris JA (1989). A mutational theory of leukaemogenesis. *Journal of Clinical Pathology*, 42:337–40.

Murray AW, Kirschner MW (1989). Dominoes and clocks: the union of the cell cycle. *Science*, 240:614–21.

Nowell PC, Hungerford DA (1960). A minute chromosome in human chronic granulocytic leukaemia. *Science*, 132:1497.

Pardee AB (1989). G_1 events and regulation of cell proliferation. *Science*, 240:603–8.

Pendergast AM, Witte ON (1987). Role of the ABL oncogene tyrosine kinase activity in human leukaemias. *Baillière's Clinical Haematology*, 1, 1001–20.

Pendergast AM, Quilliam LA, Cripe LD, *et al.* (1993). Bcr-abl induced oncogenesis is mediated by direct interaction with the SH-2 domain of the GRB-2 adapter protein. *Cell*, 75:175–85.

Pierce JH, Defiore PP, Aaronson SA, *et al.* (1985) Neoplastic transformation of mast cells by Abelson virus: abrogation of IL3 dependence by a non-autocrine mechanism. *Cell*, 41:685–93.

Pui CH, Behm FG, Crist WM (1993). Clinical and biological relevance of immunological marker studies in childhood acute lymphoblastic leukaemia. *Blood*, 82:343–62.

Rabbits TH, Boehm T, Mengle-Gaw L. (1988). Chromosomal abnormalities in lymphoid tumours: mechanism and role in tumour pathogenesis. *Trends in Genetics*, 4:300–4.

Ramakrishman L, Rosenberg N (1989). 'abl' genes. *Biochemica et Biophysica Acta*, 989:209–24.

Rowley JD (1973). A new consistent chromosomal abnormality in chronic myelogenous leukaemia identified by quinacrine fluorescence and Giemsa staining. *Nature, London*, 243:290–91.

Rowley JD (1983). Human oncogene locations and chromosome aberrations. *Nature, London*, 301:290.

Sallan SE, Ritz J, Pesando J, *et al.* (1980). Cell surface antigens: prognostic implications in childhood acute lymphoblastic leukaemia. *Blood*, 55:395–402.

Sandberg AA (1986). The chromosomes in human leukemia. *Seminars in Hematology*, 23:201–17.

Shaw GM, Broden S, Essex M, Gallo RC (1984). Human T-cell leukaemia virus: its discovery and role in leukaemogenesis and immuno-suppression. *Blood*, 64(2):482–90.

Stass SA, Mirro J (1986). Lineage heterogeneity in acute leukaemia: acute mixed lineage leukaemia and lineage switch. *Clinics in Haematology*, 15:811–27.

Tkachuk DC, Kohler S, Cleary ML (1992). Involvement of a homolog of *Drosophila trithorax* by 11q23 chromosomal translocations in acute leukaemias. *Cell*, 71:691–700.

Tsujimoto Y, Yunis J, Onarato Showe L, *et al.* (1984). Molecular cloning of the chromosomal breakpoint of B-cell lymphomas and leukaemia with the (11;14) chromosome translocation. *Science*, 224:1403–6.

Varmus HE (1984). The molecular genetics of cellular oncogenes. *Annual Review of Genetics*, 18:553–612.

Vigliani EC, Saita G (1964). Benzene and leukaemia. *New England Journal of Medicine*, 271:872.

Vincent PC (1989). Kinetics of leukaemia and control of cell division and replication. In *Leukaemia*, 5th edn. (ed. ES Henderson and TA Lister), pp. 55–104. Grune and Stratton, New York.

Virchow R (1845). Weisses Blut. *Froriep's Notizen*, **36**:151.

Yoshida M, Saiki M, Yamaguchi K, Takatsuki K (1984). Monoclonal integration of human T-cell leukaemia provirus in all primary tumours of adult T-cell leukaemia suggests causative role of human T-cell leukaemia virus in the disease. *Proceedings of the National Academy of Sciences, USA*, **81**:2534–7.

Young D, Wagner K, Griffin J (1987). Constitutive expression of the granulocytic-macrophage colony stimulating factor in acute myeloblastic leukaemia. *Journal of Clinical Investigation*, **79**:100–6.

12.2.2 Acute leukaemias in adults

DIETER HOELZER

STATUS AND PROSPECTS

In adults, approximately 80 per cent of acute leukaemias are acute myeloblastic (AML) and 20 per cent are acute lymphoblastic (ALL). The acute leukaemias are a heterogeneous group of disorders in which the malignant clone arises from progenitors in the bone-marrow or lymphatic system, resulting in an increase of immature, non-functioning leukaemic cells. Infiltration of bone-marrow leads to anaemia, granulocytopenia, and thrombocytopenia, with the clinical manifestations of fatigue, weakness, infection, and haemorrhages. These symptoms are more often the reason a patient first seeks medical advice than are other organomegalies, such as lymph node enlargement or hepatosplenomegaly caused by leukaemic infiltration.

The diagnosis of acute leukaemia is basically made morphologically from smears of peripheral blood or bone-marrow. The classification includes cytochemistry, immunological markers, cytogenetic analysis, and molecular genetic methods. For AML the major diagnostic criteria are still morphology and cytochemistry, revealing a large heterogeneity as expressed in the morphological FAB classification (see below) types M1–M7, whereas for the acute lymphoblastic leukaemias immunological phenotyping to discriminate between those of the B- or T-cell lineage is more relevant.

Treatment results

Considerable progress has been made in the treatment of acute leukaemias. In 1955, with supportive treatments only, the survival of patients with this disease was less than 2 months (Tivey 1955). By using treatment stategies that have been developed for childhood ALL, rates of complete remission of 70–80 per cent can now be achieved in adult ALL and disease-free survival at 5 or more years is 20–40 per cent. In acute myeloblastic leukaemia treated with intensive induction therapy, complete remissions of 60–70 per cent can be obtained and 20–30 per cent of patients are disease free at 3 or 5 years. After successful induction therapy a consolidation therapy has proved to be necessary in both ALL and AML. Maintenance therapy seems of no benefit in AML. In ALL trials this approach has been adopted from experience in childhood ALL and its value in adult ALL is still not established.

Prognostic factors

Factors predictive of disease-free survival have been identified in adult ALL; they are mainly the time to achieve complete remission, age, initial white blood count, immunological subtype, and karyotype. On using these prognostic factors, patients with adult ALL can, similarly to children with ALL, be identified as being standard risk, with a projected disease-free survival of 50 per cent or more at 5 years or high risk, with a disease-free survival of 25 per cent. In AML, prognostic factors for disease-free survival are less well defined; they may include specific morphological features according to FAB subtype or chromosome abnormalities, an antecedent disease such as myelodysplastic syndrome, or a previous toxic exposure leading to secondary AML. Whereas in ALL the stratification of patients into high- and low-risk groups and risk-adapted therapy are possible, this is not yet routine in AML.

Bone-marrow transplantation

This is now an accepted effective procedure in the treatment of adult leukaemias but when it is most profitable for the patient, in first or in second remission, remains to be evaluated. The definition of risk groups may give more precise guidelines, such as allogeneic marrow transplantation in ALL for high-risk ALL patients in first remission and for standard-risk patients in second complete remission, whereas in AML, owing to the lack of well-defined risk groups, allogeneic transplantation in first remission is generally considered. Whether autologous marrow transplantation, a successful new approach, is more advantageous in first or second remission in either disease is still undecided.

Future aspects

Future strategies that may improve the outcome for patients with adult acute leukaemia may be the use of haemopoietic growth factors to shorten regeneration after chemotherapy or bone-marrow transplantation, the use of differentiation inducers such as *trans*-retinoic acid in acute promyelocytic leukaemia, giving complete remission rates of 80–90 per cent, or adoptive immunotherapy with interleukin-2 as a maintenance therapy to suppress or eradicate minimal residual disease. Peripheral blood stem cell transplantation and unrelated BMT now also offer new chances for the patient.

Incidence and age

The mean annual incidence rate of acute leukaemias is 4–7 persons/100 000.

Acute lymphoblastic leukaemia

ALL is the most frequent neoplastic disease in children, with an early peak at the age of 3–4 years. Only approximately one-quarter of the patients with ALL are aged 15 years or more but the incidence seems to increase over the age of 50 years (McKinney *et al.* 1989). The median age in most treatment reports for adult ALL ranges from 25 to 37 years. Immunological subtypes in adult ALL are age correlated, T-ALL being more frequent in younger adults, 15–35 years of age. Although male predominance is general for ALL it is particularly marked for T-ALL.

Acute myeloblastic leukaemia

AML is infrequent in children and 80 per cent of patients are adults above 15 years of age. The incidence increases after the age of 15 and the peak incidence is above the age of 55–65 years; although two-thirds of patients with AML are more than 50 years old, the median age in most treatment trials is below that age. There is also a slight male predominance in AML.

Aetiology

The aetiology of acute leukaemia is unknown. There are, however, intrinsic and extrinsic factors that influence the incidence of leukaemia. Inheritance of certain diseases and exposure to ionizing radiation or to chemicals are associated with an increased risk of developing leukaemia.

Congenital disorders

Patients with some rare congenital chromosomal abnormalities have an increased risk for development of acute leukaemia. A 20-fold increased incidence of leukaemia is reported for patients with Down's syndrome, who develop ALL in childhood or AML at a later stage. There is also a higher risk of acute leukaemias in rare familial diseases such as Klinefelter's syndrome, Fanconi's anaemia, Bloom's syndrome, ataxia telangiectasia, and neurofibromatosis. A genetic predisposition may exist, as the identical twin of a leukaemic child has a 5-fold greater risk of developing acute leukaemia than a child in the general population (Falletta *et al.* 1973). Simultaneous development of ALL in identical twins (Chaganti *et al.* 1979) may indicate that an intrauterine event affected both twins (Keith and Brown 1971). There are many anecdotal reports of an increased incidence of leukaemia within families. However, such evidence is only circumstantial because common environmental factors may also be responsible.

Infectious agents

Although there is no direct evidence that a virus causes human acute leukaemia, the nature of the adult T-cell leukaemia/lymphoma suggests that a virus might probably be involved.

That the human T-cell leukaemia virus I is associated with adult T-cell leukaemia/lymphoma is mainly based on sero-epidemiological evidence suggesting person-to-person spread of the virus in areas of endemic disease in Japan, the Caribbean, and elsewhere. The mode of transmission is controversial.

No definite association of leukaemia with chronic infection, influenza, or other viral infections has been observed up to now. There is, however, a highly speculative hypothesis that in the aetiology of common ALL in young children, infections may play a role as promoter of a second event in disease development whereas the first is a spontaneous mutation *in utero* (Greaves 1988).

Ionizing radiation

Exposure to ionizing radiation in appreciable doses leads to an increased risk of developing leukaemia, mainly AML but at a lower frequency also ALL (Heath 1982). This is evident from survivors of atomic bombs in Japan or of nuclear reactor accidents and from patients receiving radiotherapy or diagnostic radiation. The incidence of leukaemia in survivors of the Hiroshima atomic bomb (> 1 Gy exposure) indicated an increased risk of more than 20-fold. The peak incidence of leukaemia occurred at 6–7 years after exposure. Of major interest is the minimal radiation dose that may have a leukaemogenic effect. From the survivors of atomic bombs in Japan it was calculated that when less than 0.05 Gy was received the incidence of leukaemia was still 3–4 per cent higher than in an unexposed population. The establishment of a 'threshold' dose, however, is not possible. Although thyroid cancers have increased, there has so far been no rise in the incidence of ALL following the Chernobyl nuclear power station accident. The increased incidence of leukaemia in children living near nuclear power stations could not be directly related to radioactive emission (Haesman *et al.* 1984) and has since been shown to be related to the preconceptual radiation exposure of fathers working at the nuclear plant (Gardner *et al.* 1990). However, no increased incidence of leukaemia was found in children of Japanese men who survived the atomic bomb explosions, so some additional factor(s), such as dosage rate or duration of exposure, must be involved.

Chemical agents

Agents associated with an increased risk of leukaemia might be either those to which people are continuously exposed, such as benzene used in industry or those used as therapeutic agents (Rosner and Grünwald 1980; Kyle 1982), such as chloramphenicol or, most particularly, alkylating agents. Most of these chemical agents cause bone-marrow hypoplasia, which in some cases is followed by the development of an acute leukaemia. Such secondary AMLs often have specific chromosome abnormalities involving chromosomes 5 and 7. Alkylating agents used alone or in combination with radiotherapy have increased the frequency of such secondary malignancies, for example in Hodgkin's disease where the cumulative risk after treatment ranges from 2 to 7 per cent at 10 years. Secondary AML also occurs after exposure to cyclophosphamide and to epipodophyllotoxins used in the treatment of ALL (Kantarjian *et al.* 1993). Also in patients with non-neoplastic diseases the majority with rheumatoid arthritis, renal transplants, nephrotic syndrome, and others have an increased risk of developing acute leukaemia following immunosuppressive chemotherapy. The mean interval from the cytotoxic therapy to the development of acute leukaemia in these patients is 5 years.

DIAGNOSIS AND CLASSIFICATION

The diagnosis of acute leukaemia is made by examination of the peripheral blood and bone-marrow. A considerable number of other investigations are also needed for the further identification of the patient's disease in preparation for therapy; these include cytochemical stains, immunological markers, enzyme markers, and cytogenetic analysis with, if possible, molecular markers. The major aim of classification is to distinguish between AML and ALL because of the different treatments. Morphology and cytochemical stains are still the main methods for categorizing AMLs into their morphological subtypes, whereas immunological markers are the major criteria for subdividing ALL into disease of B- or T-cell lineage.

Morphology

The morphological diagnosis of acute leukaemia is made from smears of bone-marrow and peripheral blood stained with Romanowsky dyes, usually May–Grünwald and Giemsa stains. Leukaemic cells are classified according to size, nuclear chromatin, nuclear shape, nucleoli, amount and basophilia of cytoplasm, and cytoplasmic vacuolization.

The morphology of the leukaemic blast cells differs widely and therefore, in 1976, the French–American–British (**FAB**) committee classified AML and ALL into subgroups on the basis of cytomorphology (Bennett *et al.* 1976), using the degree of maturation of the leukaemic blast cells compared to their normal counterparts.

Morphology of AML

The FAB classification originally distinguished six subtypes (M1–M6) for AML, later extended and revised to include M7 (Bennett *et al.* 1985*a*) and some subvariants (Bennett *et al.* 1985*b*). FAB subtypes for AML are subdivided depending on the predominant differentiation pathway and the degree of maturation. For the M1, M2, and M3 subtypes, granulocytic differentiation is predominant, for M4 the differentiation pathway is mixed granulocytic/monocytic, for M5 predominantly monocytic, for M6 eosinophilic, and for M7 the megakaryocytic lineage is predominant.

1. M1 (acute myeloblastic leukaemia without maturation) is very poorly differentiated and characterized by a predominance of immature myeloblasts with less than 10 per cent promyelocytes/myelocytes or monocytes. Auer rods may be present and these confirm the diagnosis. Otherwise cytochemical staining may be needed to demonstrate myeloid differentiation of subtype M1, which accounts for approximately 20 per cent of cases.

2. M2 (acute myeloblastic leukaemia with maturation) is characterized by myeloblasts but in addition more differentiated cells (> 10 per cent promyelocytes/myelocytes). Auer rods may be present; most cells are peroxidase positive. Monocytic cells are less than 20 per cent. This is the most common subvariant with a frequency of 30 per cent of all AML cases.

3. M3 (acute promyelocytic leukaemia) is morphologically well characterized, with a predominance of promyelocytes (> 30 per cent) showing marked granulation. The cells are large, the cytoplasm contains azurophilic granules and often Auer bodies. An M3 variant (M3v), in which the cytoplasm contains more granules, can be detected by electron microscopy. The M3 subtype accounts for 10 per cent of all adult cases of AML.

4. M4 (acute myelomonocytic leukaemia) shows a mixture of abnormal monocytoid cells (< 20 per cent) and of myeloblasts/promyelocytes (> 20 per cent). Corresponding to monocytic/myeloid differentiation the cytochemical stain non-specific esterase is positive as well as peroxidase, Sudan black, and chloracetate-esterase. Auer rods may be present. In the variant M4$_{EO}$, eosinophilia is present in up to 30 per cent of the cells. The frequency of this subtype is 20 per cent.

5. M5 (acute monocytic leukaemia) is a poorly differentiated subtype with predominantly monocytoid cells (> 80 per cent) characterized by large blast cells with a more greyish cytoplasm (M5a). In a more mature form (M5b), more than 20 per cent of cases have well-recognizable monocytes. The immature form

can often only be identified by cytochemical stains or immunological markers. The poorly differentiated monoblastic M5a and the differentiated promonocytic/monocytic M5b account for 15 per cent of AMLs.

6. M6 (acute erythroleukaemia) is a rare form (frequency 5 per cent) characterized by bizarre erythroblasts (> 50 per cent) and abnormal, multinucleated erythroblasts. In addition there is a population of myeloblasts, sometimes with Auer rods. There are often nucleated red cells in the peripheral blood. Bone-marrow erythroblasts have strong positivity for periodic acid–Schiff (**PAS**) stain.

7. M7 (acute megakaryoblastic leukaemia) (< 5 per cent) is a variant that mostly cannot be recognized by morphology. The mega-karyocytic precursor cells are identified by the platelet peroxidase reaction on electron micrography or with platelet-specific antibodies (J15, AN51, C17). Bone-marrow aspiration may be difficult because there is often increased bone-marrow reticulin.

Morphology of ALL

In ALLs three subgroups are distinguished morphologically by the FAB classification (see Table 1, Chapter 12.2.3).

1. L1 (small, monomorphic type) consists mainly of small blasts with occasional large blasts. The nuclear outline is regular, the nucleoli inconspicuous or small, the cytoplasm scanty.

2. L2 (large, heterogeneous type) is more heterogeneous. The blasts are large, the nucleoli often large, and the cytoplasm more abundant than in L1.

3. L3 (Burkitt cell type) is characterized by larger cells of homogenous size; the nucleus is round to oval with a loose nuclear chromatin. The nucleoli are prominent and the deeply basophilic cytoplasm is moderately abundant.

The incidence of the three subgroups differs widely between adult and childhood ALL: L1 is less frequent (27 per cent) in adults than in children (84 per cent), L2 is more frequent in adults (68 vs 15 per cent) and L3 is only observed in 5 and 1 per cent, respectively.

Cytochemistry

The cytochemical stains used to discriminate between AML and ALL are Sudan black, myeloperoxidase, and esterase (chloracetate and non-specific). These reactions are positive in AML and negative in ALL. Negativity is mostly defined as 3 per cent or less of leukaemic blast cells being positive. Cytochemical stains to confirm ALL are PAS and acid phosphatase. PAS will show coarse granules or block positivity in at least some cells of most patients with adult ALL of the L1 or L2 type. Approximately 60–70 per cent of L1 or L2 cases are PAS positive (Löffler *et al.* 1987). The acid phosphatase reaction is positive in 20–30 per cent of all ALL, being more specific for T-ALL. Approximately 70 per cent of patients with T-ALL will show strong and localized paranuclear staining with acid phosphatase. PAS or acid phosphatase reactivity is, however, not restricted to ALL and because it can be observed occasionally in cases of AML (M5) the additional reactions for peroxidase and acetate esterase have to be negative to confirm ALL.

Immunological markers

Heterologous antisera have been used as immunological markers, but now a series of monoclonal antibodies has been generated, which

Table 1 Immunological subtypes of ALL

B-cell lineage	
Pre-pre-B-ALL	+HLA-DR, TdT, *CD19*
	±CD24
Common-ALL	+HLA-DR, TdT, *CD10*, *CD19*, CD24
	±CD20
Pre-B-ALL	+HLA-DR, TdT, *cyIgM*, CD19, CD24, CD10, CD20
B-ALL	+HLA-DR, *CD19*, *CD20*, CD24, *SIg*
	±CD10, TdT
T-cell lineage	
Pre-T-ALL	+TdT, *CD7*, *cyCD3*
	±CD5, CD10, HLA-DR, CD34
T-ALL	+TdT, *CD7*, *cyCD2*, *CD2*, CD5
	±CD1, CD3, CD4, CD8, CD10

Abbreviations as in text. The most important markers are in italics

identifies antigens expressed on the surface of normal or leukaemic cells (Thiel *et al.* 1980; Greaves 1981; Sobol *et al.* 1985; Foon and Todd 1986). The main aim of immunological classification is the identification of ALL subtypes according to the presence of B-cell or T-cell markers, but also the identification of precursor acute leukaemia, megakaryoblastic AML, or biphenotypic or hybrid acute leukaemia. Methods to identify markers are immunofluorescence, immunoperoxidase, alkaline phophatase–antialkaline phosphatase; a typical panel of monoclonal antibodies includes those for (Hoffbrand and Pettit 1988)

1. precursor (stem cell) associated, CD34, TdT, HLA-DR;

2. myeloid, CD11, CD13, CD14, CD33;

3. monocytic, CD11, CD14;

4. erythroid, antiglycophorin;

5. megakaryocytic, J15, AN51, CD17;

6. B-cell associated, CD10, CD19, CD20, CD22, SmIg;

7. T-cell associated, CD2, CD5, CD7, cyCD3.

Immunological subtypes of ALL

The immunological subtypes of ALL are listed in Table 1.

B-cell lineage

More than 70 per cent of adult ALLs are of B-cell origin and the most frequent immunological subtype, common ALL, is characterized by the presence of the common-ALL antigen, a glycoprotein (gp100/CD10). Common-ALL blast cells do not carry markers of relatively mature B-cells such as cytoplasmic immunoglobulins (**cyIg**) or surface membrane immunoglobulins (**SmIg**). Pre-B-ALL (also termed early B-ALL) is characterized by the expression of cyIg, being negative in common ALL but otherwise identical with all other cell markers and only very rarely may the common-ALL antigen be absent in this subtype. Mature B-ALL comprises approximately 3 per cent of adult ALL patients. The blast cells express surface antigens of mature B-cells including the SmIg. Common-ALL antigen may also be present and also occasionally cyIg. Pre-pre-B-ALL, also termed early B-precursor ALL, is a leukaemia that was formerly termed non-T, non-B-ALL, or null ALL because neither T- nor B-cell features could be demonstrated. This subtype is HLA-DR, terminal deoxynucleotidyl transferase (**TdT**), and CD19 positive and forms approximately 11 per cent of adult ALL.

T-cell lineage

Nearly a quarter of adult ALL belongs to the T-cell lineage. All cases express the T-cell antigen (gp40, CD7). They may, according to their stage of T-cell differentiation, express other T-cell antigens, for example the E-rosette receptor (CD2) and/or the cortical thymocyte antigen T6 (CD1). A minority of T-ALL blast cells may also express common-ALL antigen together with other T-cell antigens. According to these markers it is possible to distinguish a pre-T-ALL (also termed early T-precursor ALL) and a more mature T-ALL.

Mixed or hybrid leukaemias

These are leukaemias in which blast cells express lymphoid as well as myeloid antigens; they were also called biphenotypic or bilineal leukaemias. Biphenotypic leukaemias are defined as those in which markers of lymphoid and myeloid lineages are co-expressed on the same leukaemic cells. Bilineal leukaemias are those with two populations of blast cells with either lymphoid or myeloid antigens. The detection of leukaemic cells that express both lymphoid and myeloid antigens is increasing, as might be expected with the more detailed marker analysis now available, reaching a reported 33 per cent in adult ALL (Sobol *et al.* 1987) but probably a more realistic level is 18 per cent (Drexler *et al.* 1991).

Gene rearrangements

The diagnosis of ALLs of B-cell origin can be confirmed by the demonstration of clonal rearrangement of their immunoglobulin genes. In most cases of T-ALL one or more of the T-cell receptor genes is rearranged. The distinction between T-cell and B-cell lineage is occasionally difficult. Thus, immunoglobulin gene rearrangements occur in 10 per cent of T-ALL cases and in a few cases with B-cell lineage ALL the blast cells have a T-cell receptor gene rearrangement. Acute leukaemias that remain unattributable to either the B-cell or T-cell lineage constituted only 1.4 per cent in a series of 500 cases of acute leukaemia (Janossy *et al.* 1989).

Biochemical markers

The enzyme most studied is TdT; earlier adenosine deaminase and the intermediate isoenyzme of hexosaminidase were also used. Elevated TdT levels are found in most patients with adult ALL, except in mature B-ALL. A positive TdT reaction is also found in approximately 10 per cent of AML cells, however, they show only moderate values compared to ALL.

Cytogenetics

Cytogenetic analysis should be made in all cases of acute leukaemia, as the demonstration of a specific karyotype may be required to confirm the diagnosis and also because chromosome abnormalities are the most independent prognostic variables for disease-free survival (Bloomfield *et al.* 1986; Sandberg 1987).

For cytogenetic analysis, bone-marrow must be examined directly as well as after 1 or 2 day culture (Second MIC Cooperative Study Group 1988). Evaluation should preferentially be with a high-resolution banding technique. A sufficient number of 20–30 metaphases must be karyotyped. In patients with AML, banding techniques now available identify an abnormal karyotype in 70–80 per cent. Of these, 60 per cent have specific cytogenetic abnormalities. In ALL, banding techniques detect chromosomal abnormalities in two-thirds of newly diagnosed patients; 20 per cent show only normal metaphases and 10 per cent cannot be analysed for a variety of technical reasons. By giving careful attention to the collection of the bone-marrow, to rapid transport, and with well-trained staff the identification of clonal abnormalities is possible in more than 90 per cent of patients with ALL (Williams *et al.* 1985).

Specific chromosomal abnormalities in AML

1. t(8;21)(q22;q22). This karyotype occurs almost exclusively in the M2 subtype and makes up 40 per cent of chromosome abnormalities seen in M2.

2. t(15;17)(q22;q12). The karyotype t(15;17) and its association with hypergranular promyelocytic leukaemia (M3) has proved to be the most specific anomaly. It has never been observed in any of the other acute leukaemias and is of particular interest because only patients with this translocation respond to the differentiation agent all-*trans* retinoic acid.

3. t/del(11)(q23). This is a heterogeneous group comprising a variety of translocations and deletions, such as t(9;11), t(11;19), t(10;11), and t(11;17), always with involvement of 11q23. This chromosome abnormality characterizes AML cases with a predominant monocytic component and approximately 50 per cent of the M5a type.

4. inv/del(16). Abnormalities of chromosome 16, which comprise inversions, deletions, and rarely translocations, are uniquely associated with abnormal eosinophils. Most patients with these abnormalities have the morphological subtype M4$_{EO}$.

5. Other cytogenetic abnormalities not clearly associated with FAB subtypes include trisomy 8 (+8). This is the most common cytogenetic anomaly in AML. Monosomy 7 (−7) and deletion of q (7q−) is the second most common anomaly in AML. Both −7 and 7q− are observed with a high incidence in patients who have received cytotoxic treatment or were exposed to toxic agents. In patients with this anomaly a careful exposure history must be taken. The deletion of 5q (5q−) has a total incidence of approximately 8 per cent in AML. As the sole anomaly the aberration is also observed after exposure to toxic agents.

6. t(9;22)(34;q11). The occurrence of the Philadelphia (Ph^1) chromosome is a rare event in AML and when present is predominantly seen in M1.

Further chromosome abnormalities are listed in detail in Table 2, Chapter 12.2.1.

Specific chromosomal abnormalities in ALL

The main cytogenetic abnormalities in ALL cases can be divided into patients with clonal abnormalities, patients with one of the structural aberrations t(4;11), t(9;22), t(8;14), 14q+, and 6q−, or when none of the structural aberrations was present, according to the modal chromosomal number (<46, 46 with structural abnormalities, 47–50, >50).

Approximately 5 per cent of children and 25 per cent of adults with ALL are Ph^1 positive. The Ph^1 chromosome is a result of the t(9;22)(q34;q11) translocation. This translocation leads to a break within the break-point cluster region gene (*BCR*) on chromosome 22 and transfer of the *ABL* proto-oncogene from chromosome 9 to a position adjacent to the truncated *BCR* gene, forming a chimeric *BCR–ABL* gene. In one-third of the *BCR–ABL*-positive patients

a 210 kDa *BCR–ABL* protein is expressed as in chronic myelocytic leukaemia; in two-thirds the translocation results in expression of a 190 kDa *BCR–ABL* protein. It remains unsolved whether Ph^1-positive ALL with the 210 kDa *BCR–ABL* protein is related to a lymphoid acute phase of chronic myeloid leukaemia or whether it is a distinct disorder.

DIAGNOSTIC INVESTIGATIONS
Peripheral blood

The diagnosis of acute leukaemia is made by examination of the peripheral blood and bone-marrow. Peripheral blood counts and a differential count from a May–Grünwald- and Giemsa-stained bloodsmear are essential at the time of presentation. The demonstration of clear granules or Auer rods enables the diagnosis of AML to be made and if there are characteristic large granules, even of the subtype M3. The white blood-cell count is reduced or normal in approximately 40 per cent of patients with either AML or ALL (Table 2). Thus, in the automatic cell counting frequently used, the diagnosis may be overlooked. One-third of the patients have a moderately increased initial white count, between 10×10^9 and 50×10^9/l. The higher values (above 50×10^9) are somewhat more frequent in ALL than in AML. Leukaemic blast cells in the peripheral blood are largely responsible for the rise in the white-cell count but it is noteworthy that in 8 per cent of patients with ALL no circulating leukaemic blast cells are observed. This is also true for some patients with AML.

Peripheral blood examination characteristically shows anaemia, thrombocytopenia, and/or neutropenia, whereby the extent is only

Table 2 Laboratory values at diagnosis of acute leukaemia

	ALL (%) ($n=1273^a$)	AML (%) ($n=1271^b$)
Initial white-cell count ($\times10^9$/l)		
<10	41	44
10–50	31	33
>50	28	23
Platelets ($\times10^9$/l)		
<20	22	18
21–40	22	26
41–100	29	34
<100	27	22
Haemoglobin (g/dl)		
<7		20
<8	28	
7–9		33
>8	72	
>9		47
Leukaemic blasts in peripheral blood		
0%	8	5
<25%	30	41
25–75%	34	37
>75%	36	22
Leukaemic blasts in bone-marrow		
>50%	96	
>75%		30

^{a}Data from three consecutive German multicentre adult (15–65 years) ALL trials.
^{b}Pooled data from four adult AML trials: British MRC trials (Report of the MRC's Working Party on Leukaemia in Adults 1974), Cancer and Leukemia Group B (Carey *et al.* 1975), Memorial Sloan-Kettering Cancer Center (Passe *et al.* 1982), and Fourth International Workshop on Chromosomes in Leukemia (1984).

partly correlated with the total white count. The reduction in the concentration of haemoglobin is mild to moderate, but nearly one-third of the patients have a haemoglobin below 7 or 8 g/dl (Table 2).

A platelet count below the critical number of $20 \times 10^9/l$ is seen in one-fifth of patients with AML and ALL (Table 2). The higher frequency of haemorrhages seen in AML might be due to platelet functional abnormalities or additional impairment of the coagulation system, as myeloblasts, promyelocytes, or monoblasts have more plasminogen activator and fibrinolytic activity than lymphoblasts. The proportion of patients with a granulocyte count below $0.5 \times 10^9/l$, usually associated with high risk of infection, was only one-fifth in an adult ALL series and is somewhat higher in AML.

Bone-marrow examination

Direct smears from the bone-marrow are essential to confirm the diagnosis of acute leukaemia and to distinguish between AML and ALL. Bone-marrow aspiration provides further material for diagnostic assessment, including morphology, cytochemical stains, immunological markers, cytogenetic analysis, and molecular analysis.

In ALL the bone-marrow is usually heavily packed with leukaemic blast cells. Nearly all patients with adult ALL have a bone-marrow infiltration with leukaemic blast cells of above 50 per cent and the majority show an infiltration of above 90 per cent. In AML only 30 per cent of patients have infiltration with more than 75 per cent blast cells.

The normal haemopoietic elements are greatly reduced or absent. In ALL they have, in contrast to AML, an essentially normal morphology. A biopsy of the bone-marrow will further demonstrate marked hypercellularity with replacement of fat spaces and normal elements by infiltration with leukaemic cells. A slight or even massive increase in marrow reticulin is common in AML but is seen in only a small proportion of patients with ALL. Whereas formerly it was controversial whether every patient with acute leukaemia should have a biopsy in addition to the bone-marrow smear, now, mainly due to easier and less painful techniques (for example, with the Jamshidi needle), a biopsy is obligatory. It is undoubtedly needed in cases with 'dry tap', which may be due to heavily packed leukaemic cells, increased reticulin fibres, or inadequate techniques. In an ALL series, aspiration was not possible in 15 per cent of patients.

Lumbar puncture

Examination of the cerebrospinal fluid is an essential diagnostic procedure in acute leukaemia to exclude or confirm initial involvement of the central nervous system, which is sometimes clinically asymptomatic. It is optional for ALL, where the incidence of initial disease in the central nervous system is approximately 6 per cent. It is not a routine diagnostic measure in AML but should be done in patients with AML when clinically indicated and is recommended in special, cytogenetically defined subtypes with a high risk for leukaemia of the central nervous system, for example in patients with AML with monocytic features.

There are different opinions as to when the first lumbar puncture should be done. One procedure is to delay the examination until remission is achieved in order to avoid seeding of the central nervous system by circulating leukaemic blast cells from the peripheral blood and not to deliver intrathecal therapy at the time of first lumbar puncture in case a second diagnostic test is required. On the other hand, early recognition of central nervous disease will lead to immediate and specific therapy, which is required for such patients. Also some patients' involvement of the central nervous system can

only be substantiated by microscopic examination of the cerebrospinal fluid. Thus, other clinicians prefer to make the lumbar puncture earlier, if possible before treatment starts. This procedure is restricted to patients with an adequate platelet count ($> 20 \times 10^9/l$), an absence of manifest clinical haemorrhages, and without a high white blood-cell count. For safety reasons such patients should receive intrathecal methotrexate at the first lumbar puncture. Clearly this procedure necessitates an atraumatic lumbar puncture.

Laboratory investigations

These may reveal metabolic abnormalities, which require correction before cytostatic treatment is started. The serum lactate dehydrogenase is markedly elevated in most patients with ALL. Fasting or random estimations of blood glucose should be made, especially if L-asparaginase is to be included in the treatment protocol. A full haemostatic profile should be acquired to detect disseminated intravascular coagulation or patients with an incidental clotting abnormality related to pre-existing liver disease or liver infiltration. Besides cultures from any clinically infected site, surveillance cultures from the nose, throat, axillae, groin, vagina, perianal area, and of sputum and urine are taken to detect clinically occult infection and to provide useful information about the microbiological background if septicaemia or severe infection subsequently develop. A sample of serum should be stored that can be used to provide baseline antibody titres in the assessment of infection during the induction phase. In patients with a past medical history of heart disease and in elderly patients in whom treatment with an anthracycline is anticipated, an echocardiograph with myocardial function, including the ejection fraction, should be recorded.

Initial complications and supportive therapy

The management of adult patients undergoing induction for acute leukaemia requires intensive treatment of initial complications and supportive care to prevent and manage the infective, haemorrhagic, metabolic, and psychological problems that may arise. The treatment of initial complications and prophylaxis for expected complications must be started immediately. In only a few cases is the leukaemic process so far advanced that immediate cytostatic treatment of the leukaemia is necessary. Sufficient fluid intake to guarantee urine production of at least 100 ml/h throughout induction therapy reduces the danger of uric acid formation. This may require parenteral fluids when the patient's oral intake is inadequate because of nausea or difficulty in swallowing. If the venous system does not offer easy access, a catheter for long-term vascular access is advantageous when anticipating a long induction and is useful when part of the therapy is given on an out-patient basis.

The most frequent metabolic abnormality is hyperuricaemia, which further increases during therapy and exacerbates cell destruction. Patients should receive allopurinol to reduce the formation of uric acid and avoid the danger of urate nephropathy. It should be given at a dose of 100 mg every 8 h and may be increased to 600 mg/day if high leucocyte counts or organomegaly persist. Allopurinol has to be discontinued when 6-mercaptopurine is given or the dosage of the latter must be reduced. Allopurinol can cause skin rashes but rarely causes severe allergic reactions.

In patients presenting with renal impairment an attempt must be made to re-establish renal function before chemotherapy is commenced. The renal failure often observed in patients with Burkitt's lymphoma or B-ALL with abdominal tumour masses can be resolved by a gentle pre-treatment with cyclophosphamide combined with prednisolone alone. The acute tumour lysis syndrome is most frequently seen in patients with B-ALL or T-ALL but may also occur in AML cases with high white-cell counts. Massive and rapid tumour lysis leads to hyperkalaemia, hyperphosphataemia, hyperuricaemia, and hypocalcaemia, which must be frequently checked and corrected.

Infection and prophylactic measures

Approximately one-third of patients with adult acute leukaemia present with infections, which are a major problem of management. Fever or infection present at the time of admission are mainly caused by severe granulocytopenia, especially if the granulocyte count is less than $5\times10^9/l$, but may also be due to immunological deficiency or mucosal lesions.

Combination chemotherapy causes additional haematological toxicity and at least 50 per cent of adults undergoing induction treatment will experience severe or life-threatening infections. In patients with severe infections, broad-spectrum antibiotics should be given empirically and immediately, even before the results of cultures are available. Much attention has been paid to prophylactic measures against infection. They include oral hygiene using antiseptic soaps and mouthwashes and disinfection of the anogenital region. Other precautions include reverse protective isolation and air filtration, if available, which can reduce the risk, in particular, of *Aspergillus* infections. Simple precautions that can always be taken are no live plants in the room, no humidifiers, no intramuscular or subcutaneous injections if avoidable, no uncooked vegetables, no unpeeled fruits, and no visitors having any kind of infection. Prophylactic medication includes agents against bacterial and fungal infection. Gastrointestinal decontamination with non-absorbable antibiotics seems of reasonable benefit. For patients with no fever or infection but having granulocytes below $0.5\times10^9/l$, prophylactic treatment with broad spectrum antibiotics such as co-trimoxazole and nystatin or polymixin B, should be commenced. Viral prophylaxis, for example against herpes simplex virus for selected patients, is currently under trial in some centres. For prophylaxis of fungal infections oral polyenes and the new triazoles, particularly fluconazole for prevention of *Candida* infections, seem effective. Also aerosol application of amphotericin B is under investigation.

Haemorrhage

Bleeding is the other life-threatening problem in the management of patients with acute leukaemia. The thrombocytopenia present in one-third of them at diagnosis will worsen after chemotherapy. Bleeding is usually due to this, but hyperleucocytosis and plasma clotting deficiency may exacerbate it. Platelet transfusions should be given for bleeding and to prevent bleeding when counts are below $20\times10^9/l$, especially during febrile periods that interfere with platelet function. Most often, four to eight platelet packs are given daily until bleeding stops and HLA-matched platelets from plateletpheresis are given to patients who become refractory to random-donor platelets.

L-Asparaginase treatment leads to a decrease in fibrinogen, which should be substituted if its concentration falls below approximately 100 mg/dl. In those few patients with an initially decreased concentration of fibrinogen, L-asparaginase can be begun if the fibrinogen is substituted and the concentrations closely followed. In some patients with adult ALL, the concentration of antithrombin III decreases induction therapy, thereby increasing the risk of thromboembolism; in these cases antithrombin III should be substituted.

Disseminated intravascular coagulation (DIC)

The majority of patients with M3 leukaemia and some with other types of AML develop consumption coagulopathy and are at high risk of life-threatening haemorrhage. It is assumed that the release of procoagulants from the azurophilic granules causes the DIC, which is characterized in the laboratory by a prolonged prothrombin and partial prothrombin time and a reduction in platelet count and in plasma fibrinogen, depending on the stage of DIC. As laboratory evidence of this complication is often obtained before actual bleeding, all patients with AML should, at first diagnosis and for the first 3 days after the beginning of induction chemotherapy, have a complete evaluation of coagulation. Clinically, DIC may lead to bleeding and to renal and respiratory failure, most probably due to microthrombi in the kidney and lung.

The role of heparin in the treatment of DIC remains controversial, particularly as prophylaxis. The main aim is a rapid reduction of the leukaemic cell mass. The occurrence and management of DIC in patients with promyelocytic leukaemia has changed recently. With all-*trans*-retinoic acid not only can this type of leukaemia be successfully treated but DIC also prevented.

CLINICAL FEATURES

The leading clinical symptoms in acute leukaemia are infections, haemorrhages, and weakness as a result of bone-marrow infiltration. Careful examination will detect that more than half of the patients also have symptoms due to organ enlargement by infiltration of leukaemic cells.

In Table 3 the initial symptoms and clinical features for a large number of adult patients with ALL or AML are listed. In AML, weakness is a leading symptom; fever and haemorrhages as initial symptoms are slightly more frequently seen in AML than in ALL.

Infections at presentation are mostly bacterial; viral or fungal infections are more frequent under chemotherapy after long granulocytopenic periods and treatment with antibiotics. Bacterial infections include ulceration of the mucosa of the mouth, tongue, and throat; infections of the skin, perianal, or perineal regions are

Table 3 Initial symptoms and clinical findings of patients with acute leukaemia (sex ratio and percentages)

	ALL ($n=1273$[a])	AML ($n=1271$[b])
Sex (male : female)	1.6 : 1	1.3 : 1
Age (years)		
<20	24	15
20–60	65	54
>60	11	31
Presenting symptoms		
Weakness		81
Fever	36	43
Bleeding	33	44
Lymphadenopathy	55	17
Splenomegaly	49	24
Hepatomegaly	45	20
Findings		
Mediastinal involvement	15	
CNS involvement	6	
Gingival hypertrophy		13
Skin infiltration		6
Other organ infiltration	10	

[a,b]Sources as in Table 2.

less frequent. Rectal examination could lead to a fissure spreading infection and should therefore be avoided. The infected lesions are also often atypical; owing to the lack of granulocytes there is no pus formation.

Haemorrhagic lesions are also slightly more often seen in AML than in ALL. They usually present as petechiae, but bruising, nose bleeds, and, in post-pubertal females, menorrhagia may also be presenting features. Sometimes haemorrhage after a dental extraction leads to the diagnosis. Haemorrhages are more frequent in patients with severe anaemia. An ecchymosis should suggest the possibility of DIC.

In AML, lymphadenopathy, splenomegaly, and hepatomegaly are less frequent than in ALL. Hypertrophy of the gums due to infiltration with leukaemic cells is a feature of the monocytic forms of AML (M4, M5). For these leukaemias, skin infiltrations, often in the form of widespread pinkish plaques, is also characteristic.

In ALL, lymphadenopathy is seen in the majority of patients and mediastinal tumour or involvement of the central nervous system are more frequent than in AML. Clinical symptoms as well as age and sex distribution are, however, different for the major immunological subtypes, common ALL, T-ALL, and B-ALL.

Clinical characteristics in adult ALL in relation to subtype

Patients with T-ALL are characterized by significantly younger age, male predominance, higher white blood-cell count, and lymphadenopathy. Mediastinal enlargement is also typical for T-ALL and seen in 48 per cent of patients. In some cases it is associated with pleural or even cardiac effusions. A mediastinal mass with pleural effusions may cause dyspnoea and obstruction. Mediastinal tumours are not exclusive to T-ALL but are also seen in a few patients with common ALL or B-ALL. Also the incidence of central nervous disease is higher in T-ALL (approximately 15 per cent).

B-ALL is similar in clinical appearance to Burkitt's non-Hodgkin's lymphoma and is partly discovered by initial surgery of large abdominal masses. In this subtype there is a high male predominance. A high white blood-cell count and splenomegaly are less frequent than in other subtypes. Abdominal lymph nodes, with renal involvement, are typical for B-ALL. The incidence of central nervous involvement B-ALL differs greatly between studies, varying from 9 to 48 per cent. Such involvement may present as nausea, vomiting, headaches, visual disturbances, and features of cranial nerve palsies.

Other manifestations of ALL, such as testicular or bone infiltration, often observed in childhood ALL, are rare in adults. In a large series only 0.3 per cent had testicular and 1.2 per cent bone infiltration.

TREATMENT OF ACUTE LEUKAEMIA
Principles and remission criteria

The initial therapeutic objective is to destroy leukaemic cells and to achieve a complete haematological remission. Complete remission is a state in which there is no clinical or laboratory manifestation of leukaemia.

Complete remission is defined as normal marrow cellularity with 5 per cent or less leukaemic blast cells and a normal representation of erythroid, myeloid, and megakaryocytic elements, that is, erythroid activity of at least 15 per cent and granulocytic elements of at least 25 per cent. In ALL the distinction between lymphocytes and lymphoblasts is occasionally difficult, so complete remission

is here defined as 5 per cent lymphoblasts or less and a combination of lymphoid cells of less than 40 per cent. Complete remission also includes normalization of the peripheral blood count, with no blast cells, a granulocyte count of at least $1.5 \times 10^9/l$, a platelet count of at least $100 \times 10^9/l$, and a haemoglobin concentration of more than 10 g/dl.

In ALL, a cytospin of cerebrospinal fluid also has to be free of blast cells. Complete remission also requires the disappearance of organomegalies but it should be noted that the persistence of splenomegaly in ALL is not always due to leukaemic infiltration.

Clonality of remission

When complete remission is achieved it is assumed that the leukaemic cell clone is eliminated. There is, however, increasing evidence that mature granulocytes in patients with AML and complete remission are not only derived from the normal stem cell clone but also from the leukaemic. This has been proved by glucose 6-phosphate dehydrogenase analysis (Fearon et al. 1986) and more recently by the restriction fragment length polymorphism. Patients with AML in complete remission with persistence of clonal leukaemic haemopoiesis have a higher rate of relapse but long-term remissions are possible.

Evaluation of therapeutic response

Intensive combination treatment in AML as well as in ALL leads to marrow aplasia with a concomitant pancytopenia before restoration of normal haemopoiesis takes place. In general, but depending on the duration and intensity of the first induction cycle, bone-marrow should be assessed at 2 (or 3) weeks after the beginning of therapy and 2–4 weeks in ALL. The therapeutic procedure when blast cells are still present is uniformly to continue with a second induction cycle, independent of whether there is still marrow aplasia or the beginning of regeneration. Some current treatment strategies prefer an early second induction cycle with the intention of shortening the total regeneration time.

Post-remission therapy

There is evidence that patients with acute leukaemia in complete remission still have a significant leukaemic cell burden (that is, 10^8–10^9 cells) and consequently these patients may expect to relapse very soon afterwards. Therefore, the general opinion is that when complete remission has been achieved the therapy has to be continued to maintain it. Continuation or post-remission therapy consists of intensification, consolidation, and maintenance therapy. Consolidation and intensification refer either to the use of multiple new agents or high-dose therapy less often to the readministration of the induction regimen. Maintenance is usually a less intensive therapy (Bloomfield 1985). In most studies that involve repeated consolidation cycles over the entire treatment period it is difficult to analyse critically the effect of the different treatment phases on outcome.

TREATMENT OF AML

Progress in the treatment of AML has been achieved by the intensification and combination of effective chemotherapeutic agents but is also the result of improved supportive care, such as antimicrobial therapy, platelet transfusions, and specialized nursing care.

A variety of chemotherapeutic regimens has been proposed for AML. Since its availability in the mid-1960s, most induction

Table 4 Results of induction chemotherapy for *de novo* AML in adults

Group	Number of patients	Induction therapy	Patients of all ages (%)		Patients >60 years (%)			DFS/CCR >3 years (%)
			CR	ED	CR	ED	MRD	
CALGB 1981 (Rai *et al.* 1981)	211	DA 3+7	55	26	42	35	12	22
CALGB 1982 (Yates *et al.* 1982)	653	DA 3+7	55	32	38	52		
SAKK 1984 (Sauter *et al.* 1984)	162	DA 3+7	72					
SECSG 1984 (Vogler *et al.* 1984)	508	DA 3+7	66				9	10
ECOG 1984 (Cassileth *et al.* 1984)	285	DA 3+7	65	17	58	27	8	
EORTC 5 1986 (Hayat *et al.* 1986)	295	ADM, V, A	64	15	47			
BMRC 1986 (Rees *et al.* 1986)	1044	DAT	66	17	48	32	15	19
CALGB 1987 (Preisler *et al.* 1987)	668	DA 3+7	53	21	41	37	12	22
		DA 3+10	57	26				
		DAT	57	26				
ECOG 1990 (Cassileth *et al.* 1990*a*)	439	DAT 3+5	67		54		9	22–33
AMLCG 1990 (Büchner *et al.* 1991)	1311	DAT DAT+DAT DAT+HAM	64	18	50	28		
EORTC 6 1990 (Jehn *et al.* 1990)	515	DAV 1+5	67	14	53	27	13	23
SHG 1990 (Kurrle *et al.* 1990)	132	DAE	67	11			20	39
ALSG 1990 (Bishop *et al.* 1990)	264	DA	56	13			12	15
		DAE	59	17			18	36

CR, complete remission; ED, early death; MRD, median remission duration (months); DFS/CCR, probability of disease free survival or continuous CR.
Drug abbreviations: DA, daunorubicin+cytosine arabinoside; DAT, DA+thioguanine; ADM, adriamycin; V, vincristine; A, asparaginase; HAM, high dose cytosine arabinoside+mitoxantrone; DAE, DA+etoposide.
Study groups: CALGB, Cancer and Leukemia Group B; SAKK, Schweizerische Arbeitsgruppe für Klinische und epidemiologische Krebsforschung; SECSG, Southeastern Cancer Study Group; ECOG, Eastern Cooperative Oncology Group; European Organisation for Research and Treatment of Cancer; BMRC, British Medical Research Council; AMLCG, AML Cooperative Group; SHG, Süddeutsche Hämoblastose Gruppe; ALSG, Australian Leukemia Study Group.

regimens for adult AML have included cytosine arabinoside. Later this was combined with 6-thioguanine and in the early 1970s the anthracycline daunorubicin was added. Most experience in AML is with the two-drug combination, **DA**, of daunorubicin and cytosine arabinoside and with the three-drug combination of these two and 6-thioguanine, **DAT** but the role of 6-thioguanine remains unclear. The most widely used chemotherapy combination, DA, typically comprises cytosine arabinoside, 100 mg/m^2 per day by continuous infusion for 7 days and daunorubicin, 45 mg/m^2 per day given on days 1, 2, and 3 and is generally designated by the abbreviation DA 7 and 3.

Induction therapy

There are now cumulative data for more than 5000 adult patients with AML treated mostly in prospective trials with a variety of cytostatic drug combinations. A complete remission rate of somewhat above 60 per cent can be realistically achieved (Table 4). The rate of complete remission is correlated with the patient's age. For the younger patients below 60 years the rate is above 70 per cent and for the older above 60 years only 46 per cent. Comparing the DA or DAT regimens, there is neither a difference in the overall rate of complete remission, 62 vs 65 per cent, nor in the rate for the different age groups: 71 vs 71 per cent for patients under 60 years and 45 vs 49 per cent for those over 60 years of age.

The results of the DA and DAT combinations now form a standard for treatment of adult AML against which other chemotherapeutic combinations including new drugs have to be compared.

Anthracyclines form a substantial part of the induction therapy. Daunorubicin is preferred to doxorubicin because of a significantly greater appearance of necrotizing colitis in patients given doxorubicin, particularly in those older than 60 years. Other anthracyclines and

also non-anthracycline intercalators are now under investigation (Table 5). For AML, idarubicin–cytosine arabinoside appears to have a superior efficacy to daunorubicin–cytosine arabinoside regimens. Amasacrine and mitoxantrone seem to have similar activity to daunorubicin. These drugs have as yet not undergone final analysis (Stone and Mayer 1993*a*). Etoposide is now used in combination with daunorubicin and cytosine arabinoside where it acts synergistically with the former. In such studies etoposide has not increased the remission rate but a significant prolongation of remission duration has been reported (Bishop *et al.* 1990).

Post-remission therapy

Patients with AML in complete remission still have a significant leukaemic cell burden and will consequently relapse very soon. In

Table 5 Selected single agents in chemotherapy of AML

	Number of studies	Number of patients	Complete remission (%)
HD-AraC[a]			
Refractory/relapsed	10	276	31
De novo	3	112	49
Mitoxantrone			
Refractory/relapsed	13	258	24
Amsacrine			
Refractory/relapsed	5	116	21
Etoposide			
Refractory/relapsed	7	74	38
Idarubicin			
Refractory/relapsed	3	95	20

[a]HD-AraC, high-dose cytosine arabinoside.

a few studies in which no post-induction therapy was given to such patients after complete remission, the median duration of remission was considerably shorter (4–8 months) than in those who received post-induction therapy (10–15 months).

There is no best approach to improve long-term survival in AML, however, there is some agreement that an intensive therapy producing bone-marrow hypoplasia or even aplasia is superior to a less myeloablative maintenance therapy. In most studies, therefore, post-induction therapy is followed by one or two courses of consolidation without maintenance therapy. The question of how many cycles of consolidation are necessary was addressed in the Medical Research Council (Great Britain) AML VIII trial in which patients were randomized to receive either two or six cycles of consolidation before maintenance. No difference, in particular in the use of more consolidation cycles, has been established (Rees et al. 1986).

High-dose cytosine arabinoside
Rationale

From the several consolidation and intensification treatments, high-dose cytosine arabinoside seems to be the most promising in AML. This treatment consists of doses up to $3\,g/m^2$, which is 15- to 30-fold higher than the conventional doses of $100–200\,mg/m^2$. With high doses the resistance to intracellular uptake of arabinoside can be overcome, because it may probably enter cells by passive transfer. The leukaemic cell is able to phosphorylate this drug and retain its triphosphate form as **Ara-CTP**; higher Ara-CTP concentrations are achieved with higher doses of cytosine arabinoside. A correlation between Ara-CTP retention and duration of remission has been demonstrated.

Schedules

The standard regimen for high-dose cytosine arabinoside introduced by Herzig et al. (1983) is $3\,g/m^2\times12$ mostly for a total of 12 doses given as a 3 or 2 h infusion every 12 h. The number of doses is usually decreased when the high dose is used in combination with other agents such as daunorubicin, mitoxantrone, asparaginase, or amsacrine. Several variations with lower doses down to $1\,g/m^2$ or shorter courses have been studied.

Results

The results of single-agent therapy in relapsed or refractory AML (see Table 5) indicate that high-dose cytosine arabinoside had the highest antileukaemic activity. When it was used alone in 112 patients with de novo AML, the rate of complete remission was 49 per cent and when used in combination in 329 patients a rate of 74 per cent could be reached. The median duration of remission in de novo AML using high-dose arabinoside alone or in combination has increased from 12 to 30 months and the 2 year survival is above 40 per cent. These promising results reflect patient selection, especially patients of younger age. However, high-dose cytosine arabinoside in reduced dosages of $0.5–1\,g/m^2$, alone or in combination, is also applicable and effective in older patients (over 50 years), particularly if it is considered that with haemopoietic growth factors the duration of severe neutropenia may be shortened and thereby the risk of infection can be decreased.

Toxicity

Most cytostatic drugs used in the treatment of AML can cause side-effects. Nearly all patients suffer neutropenia, hair loss, and other effects, but some side-effects are more specific, for example with anthracyclines or high-dose cytosine arabinoside. Anthracyclines can cause cardiotoxicity. High-dose cytosine arabinoside causes significant toxicity. Severe conjunctivitis occurs in approximately 50 per cent of patients, which may be prevented or reduced by using eye-drops usually every 6 h and continuing for 24 h after the end of the high-dose therapy. Cerebellar dysfunction, sometimes beginning with nystagmus, is especially observed in older patients on higher cumulative total doses and may be reduced by decreasing single dose levels or the total dose. Other side-effects are occasionally respiratory distress syndromes, somnolence, liver damage, diarrhoea, or skin rash. As the major toxicities appear to be correlated with dose and as pharmacokinetic and intracellular studies have now indicated that $2\,g/m^2$ or even $1\,g/m^2$ may be of equal efficacy in some trials, a reduced dosage is now used.

Treatment of resistant disease and relapse
Resistant disease

Despite intensification of induction therapy a proportion of patients will not enter remission. Most predictive for not achieving a complete remission are certain chromosome abnormalities (Bloomfield et al. 1986). If, after two cycles of induction chemotherapy, leukaemic blast cells persist, patients are considered to have resistant disease. Continuation with the same induction regimen is not very successful and, therefore, either escalation of dose, for example high-dose cytosine arabinoside or a combination of new drugs is considered, but the remission duration for these patients is still very poor. Therefore, allogeneic bone-marrow transplantation has been applied successfully in some younger patients with resistant disease (Forman and Blume 1990).

Relapse

The majority of patients with AML in remission will experience relapse. The aim is to obtain a second complete remission and approximately 50 per cent of younger patients with AML will achieve it. Median survival is, however, only 6 months and long-term survival less than 5 per cent. Because chemotherapy is evidently unable to sustain second or further remissions, allogeneic or autologous marrow transplantation is the option for younger patients.

The reported results for single agents, but also combined treatments, in relapsed or refractory AML differ widely because several factors influence the response. Results for second-remission therapy are better in younger patients and in those with a first remission of longer than 6 months and are also dependent on the intensity of first-line remission induction therapy and on pre-therapeutic variables such as FAB subtype, white blood-cell count, and karyotype. Therefore, it is difficult to derive comparative data for refractory and relapsed AML.

Special treatment problems
Hyperleucocytosis

Patients with hyperleucocytosis ($>100\times10^9/l$) at diagnosis are at high risk for early death. Hyperleucocytosis affects mainly two organs, the brain and the lungs. Cerebral leucostasis leads to leucocyte aggregation, thrombi, tissue infiltration, and vascular rupture with cerebral haemorrhage. Clinically this results in headaches, visual disturbances, lethargy, or coma. Pulmonary leucostasis can lead to severe dyspnoea.

Reduction of the leucocyte count is urgently needed in patients with hyperleucocytosis. Several treatments have been used: leucapheresis is successful and recommended; treatment with hydroxyurea, but also with single therapy with cytosine arabinoside (100 mg/m^2 as 24 h continuous infusion) can successfully reduce the leucocyte count, usually corresponding with a dramatic clinical improvement in respiratory and cerebral function. As hyperleucocytosis can, rarely, cause a hyperviscosity syndrome, red cell transfusions to correct anaemia should be postponed until the leucocyte count is reduced.

Central nervous system disease

The incidence of central nervous involvement at presentation is low in adults with AML. Patients with myelomonocytic (M4) or monocytic AML have a higher incidence. The generally low CNS relapse rate in AML does not justify prophylactic CNS treatment as in ALL, except in a few childhood AML studies. In adult AML, using prophylactic CNS therapy has been considered for those patients who show specific chromosome abnormalities that predict for higher risk of central nervous system relapse.

Therapy of elderly patients with AML

Duration of remission and survival for patients with AML are strictly correlated with age (Stone and Mayer 1993b). The rate of complete remission in adults above 60 years of age is 40–50 per cent, mainly due to a higher rate of death during induction therapy, which in the DA and DAT trials could reach more than 30 per cent (see Table 4). This early death and a higher rate of relapse, most probably due to a lesser amount of total therapy received, accounts for the poor overall survival of elderly patients. There is, however, no evidence that such patients receiving the full induction and consolidation therapy fare less well with regard to duration of remission. Therefore, the attitude towards treatment of elderly patients is changing. Whereas low-dose cytosine arabinoside (usually 10 mg/m^2 subcutaneously every 12 h for 14–28 days) was often used, giving a complete remission rate of only approximately 15–25 per cent and an insignificant proportion of survivors, now the approach is to give short intensive therapy, thereby reducing the duration of aplasia and the associated risk of life-threatening infections and bleedings. A necessary condition for such treatment is good supportive care, including improved blood products and antimicrobial support as well as trained and specialized nursing care. An advance is promised with the use of the haemopoietic growth factors granulocyte–macrophage or granulocyte colony-stimulating factor, which in pilot studies have significantly reduced the duration of neutropenia in elderly patients (see also Haemopoietic growth factors below). Supportive therapy only or therapy at very moderate dosage should be restricted to elderly patients in poor physical condition and those who refuse to undergo intensive therapy.

Hypoplastic leukaemia

In a small proportion (less than 5 per cent of patients with AML) the marrow biopsy reveals a hypocellular bone-marrow, a so-called aleukaemic leukaemia. Often such patients are men over 50 years of age. The marrow is characterized by a low leukaemic blast cell content. Treatment results are contradictory.

Secondary AML

Aetiology

Secondary AMLs may develop after exposure to ionizing radiation or to cytotoxic agents, including cytostatic therapy (Pui et al. 1989,

1991). It is estimated that up to 20 per cent of AMLs are now secondary and present a significant problem. They have become more frequently observed after chemotherapy, owing to the increase in the cure fraction and prolonged survival, the use of more intensive regimens, and the widespread adjuvant therapy and chemotherapy in benign diseases. Nearly half of the patients have a preceding myelodysplastic phase, characterized by cytopenia and specific morphological abnormalities in the bone-marrow and blood.

In more than 50 per cent of secondary leukaemias and myelodysplastic syndromes with a history of exposure to toxic agents, abnormalities of chromosome 5 and/or 7 are observed; monosomy 7 (−7), deletions of 7q (7q−) and 5q (5q−). As the growth factor gene for granulocyte–macrophage–colony stimulating factor has been mapped to 5q23–5q31, it has been suggested that the loss of the growth regulatory gene from the long arms of chromosomes 5 or 7 may play a physiological role in the disease.

Treatment

Secondary leukaemias are characterized by resistant disease and long-lasting cytopenias due to delayed and impaired marrow regeneration, leading to a high induction death rate. When low- or moderate-dose chemotherapy schedules were applied, complete remissions and survival rates were low. For younger patients with secondary AML there is a tendency to apply intensive chemotherapy as for de novo AML (Preisler et al. 1983; Kantarjian et al. 1993). By using an anthracycline and cytosine arabinoside or high-dose arabinoside, complete remission rates of over 60 per cent were achieved; however, the rate of relapse is still very high. Although the number of patients is still limited, allogeneic bone-marrow transplantation appears the most promising therapeutic approach in patients with secondary AML.

Whether treatment for secondary AML or myelodysplastic syndromes (refractory anaemia with excess of blasts (**RAEB**), RAEB-T) should be different from that for de novo AML is questionable. Experience from the Houston group (Keating et al. 1990) as well as from the Cancer and Leukaemia Group B (**CALGB**) (Bloomfield et al. 1990) shows that with equal treatment patients having the same cytogenetic abnormality do equally well (for example, with t(8;21)) or poorly, independent of whether they have myelodysplasia or de novo AML.

Differentiation therapy in AML

Acute leukaemias are characterized by an accumulation of immature blast cells with impaired maturation and differentiation. However, leukaemic cells from patients with AML can, to some extent, mature under appropriate in vitro conditions. Therefore attempts have been made to overcome this differentiation block and to induce maturation in vivo as a therapeutic principle, especially in a situation with low leukaemic cell burden and slow progression (for example, in myelodysplastic syndromes). Attempts with agents such as vitamin D analogues and low-dose cytosine arabinoside have failed to show substantial progress with regard to induction of differentiation of AML cells.

Clinically, the differentiation approach is promising for patients with acute promyelocytic leukaemia (APL) using all-trans-β-retinoic acid (ATRA). This concept is of value only in this disease characterized cytogenetically by the translocation t(15;17)(q21;q11–22) involving the α-retinoic acid receptor on chromosome 17 and the PML gene on chromosome 15. Chinese (Huang et al. 1988), French (Castaigne et al. 1990), and American (Warrell et al. 1991) studies have shown convincingly that with ATRA in 80–90 per cent of relapsed or refractory patients with APL complete remission could be obtained. Serial blood and bone-marrow smears revealed the maturation of the leukaemic cell clone without marrow hypoplasia. In a European cooperative trial with ATRA followed by intensive chemotherapy for *de novo* APL the complete remission rate was 96 per cent and disease-free survival promising (Fenaux *et al.* 1993). Since, unfortunately, ATRA alone cannot maintain remission in APL patients due to the emergence of resistance (Delva *et al.* 1993), its best combination schedule is being explored in prospective trials.

TREATMENT OF ALL

The approach to therapy of adult ALL has evolved along similar lines to that successfully employed in childhood ALL. An induction therapy is followed by a post-remission, usually consisting of consolidation and maintenance treatment. In addition, there is a prophylactic treatment of the central nervous system during induction and maintenance.

Induction of remission

A number of drugs, including vincristine, prednisone, daunorubicin, L-asparaginase, and adriamycin, were shown during the 1960s and early 1970s to have activity against adult ALL, giving complete remission rates of 25–50 per cent when used as single agents (Hoelzer 1984). The combination of vincristine and prednisone improved the response rate to 70–90 per cent in childhood ALL and to 40–60 per cent in adult ALL. When an anthracycline (Gottlieb *et al.* 1984) and L-aparaginase are added to the two-drug combination, a complete remission rate of approximately 80 per cent can be achieved in adults. To what extent L-aparaginase increases the response rate remains unclear but it may improve the quality of remission and thereby its length in adults, as has been proven in children (Sallan *et al.* 1983). The addition of other cytostatic agents such as cyclophosphamide, cytarabine, 6-mercaptopurine, or methotrexate to vincristine and prednisone in induction does not increase the rate of complete remission substantially but may affect the quality. With different induction

Table 6 Overall results of chemotherapy for *de novo* ALL in adults

Group	Year	Patients (n)	Median age (years)	Induction	Consolidation	Maintenance	CR rate (%)	MRD (months)	DFS/CCR (%)	(years)
SWOG	1989	168	28	V, P, Ad, C	M, AC, TG A, V, P, C	V, P, Ad, MP, M actD, C, BCNU	68	23	30	7
Hussein *et al.*										
GIMEMA 0183	1989	358	31	V, P, A, D	V, IdM, IdAC, P VM, AC	V, P, M, MP (A, Ac, VM, IdAC)	79	15	25	5
Mandelli *et al.*										
MDACC	1990	105	30	V, Ad Dx, C	M, A, Ad, HdAC, V, P	IdM, D, MP, P C, BCNU, VP	84	22	34	5
Kantarjian *et al.*										
MSKCC	1990	199	25	V, P, (D, A Ad, C)	AC, TG, A, V, P, M, C, BCNU	actD, BCNU V, P, Ad, M, MP, C	82	28	33	18
Clarkson *et al.*										
GATLA	1991	145	29	V, P, D, A C, AC, MP	Ad, V, Dx, A, AC, C, MP	MP, M, V, P	78	28	34	6
Lluesma-Gonalons *et al.*										
JALSG	1991	117	38	V, P, Ad, A, C	VP, Mi +other	MP, M, A +other	81		30	4
Tomonaga *et al.*										
Swedish ALL	1991	113	38	V, P, A, D, C	V, D, VP, AC, P	MP, M, V, P, (Ac, C, Ad)	77			
Smedmyr *et al.*										
FGTALL	1991	467		V, P, Ac/R, C	Ad, AC, A	MP, M, V, C, P, Ad, Ac	76		39	4
Fière *et al.*										
CALGB 8011	1991	277	33	V, P, A, D	(AC, D), M, MP	V, P, MP, M	64	21	29	9
Ellison *et al.*										
CALGB 8513	1992	164	32	V, P, Mi/D HdM	V, P, D/Mi, HdM AC, MP, A	none	64	11	18	3
Cuttner *et al.*										
GMALL 01	1992	368	25	V, P, A, D, C AC, M, MP	V, Dx, Ad AC, C, TG	MP, M	74	24	35	10
Hoelzer *et al.*										
GMALL 02	1992	562	28	V, P, A, D, C AC, M, MP	V, Dx, Ad AC, C, TG VM, AC	MP, M	75	27	40	7
Hoelzer *et al.*										
EORTC	1992	106	27	V, P, Ad, (HdAC)	A, HdC, (M, TG, AC)	V, P, M, Ad, BCNU, C, MP, M	74	32	40	8
Stryckmans *et al.*										
L+B+V	1992	212	27	V, P, Ad, A, (HdC/HdAC)	V, P, Ad, A, (HdC/HdAC)	MP, M, C	71	23	32	10
Bassan *et al.*										
		3361	29[a]				74[a]	23[a]	33[a]	

[a]Weighted mean; CR, complete remission; CCR, continuous complete remission; DFS, disease-free survival; MRD, median remission duration ( ), with or without; X/Y, either X or Y.
Drug abbreviations: V, vincristine; P, prednisone; A, asparaginase; D, daunorubicin; Ad, adriamycin; C, cyclophosphamide; AC, cytosine arabinoside; MP, mercaptopurine; M, methotrexate; BCNU, carmustine; TG, thioguanine; Dx, dexamethasone; HdM, high-dose M; IdM, intermediate-dose M; HdAC, high-dose AC; IdAC, intermediate-dose AC; VM, teniposide; VP, etoposide; Mi, mitoxantrone; actD, actinomycin D.
Study groups: SWOG, Southwest Oncology Group; GIMEMA, Gruppo Italiano Malattie Ematologiche Maligne Adupo; MDACC, M D Anderson Cancer Center; MSKCC, Memorial Sloan-Kettering Cancer Center; GATLA, Argentine Group for Treatment of Acute Leukemia; JALSG, Japan Adult Leukemia Study Group; Swedish ALL, Swedish ALL Group; FGTALL, French Group for Treatment of Adult Acute Lymphoblastic Leukemia; CALGB, Cancer and Leukemia Group B; GMALL, German multicentre trials in adult ALL; EORTC, European Organisation for Research and Treatment of Cancer; L+B+V, London (St Bartholomew's Hospital)+Bergamo (Ospedale Riuniti)+Vicenza (Ospedale San Bartolo).

regimens, usually using at least a four-drug combination with vincristine, prednisone, and daunorubicin as a basis, rates of complete remission from 65 to 85 per cent can be achieved. Despite varying post-remission approaches, long-term disease-free survival is 30–35 per cent with a wide range from 25 to 40 per cent (Table 6).

High-dose treatment in the induction therapy of adult ALL

In some, more recent series of adult ALL, intermediate or high doses of cytostatic drugs have been used to increase the rate of complete remissions and their duration. These strategies include moderate-to high-dose methotrexate ($0.6–1.5$ g/m^2), resulting in a complete remission rate of 75 per cent (Esterhay et al. 1982), intermediate-dose prednisone (350 mg/m^2), with a complete remission rate of 80 per cent (Omura and Raney 1985), high-dose rubidazone (450 mg/m^2), resulting in a rate of 73 per cent (Fière et al. 1987), or high-dose cytosine arabinoside ($1–3$ g/m^2), giving a rate of 68–100 per cent (Stryckmans et al. 1987; Willemze et al. 1988; Cassileth et al. 1990). These high-dose treatments failed to improve substantially the complete remission rate. Their impact on duration of remission is difficult to judge because other cytostatic drugs were used in addition.

Failure to respond to induction therapy

Some 20–30 per cent of patients with adult ALL do not achieve a complete remission, in contrast to the less than 5 per cent of children with ALL. The main reason is not resistant disease but mortality during induction, which is age-dependent, increasing from less than 2 per cent in children to 25 per cent or more in adults over 60 years of age. The major cause of death is infection, whereby fungal infections increase with the duration of neutropenia and use of antibiotics. For patients who are still refractory to induction therapy after an adequate time, different regimens including high-dose cytostatics or new agents should be considered. Allogeneic bone-marrow transplantation, even when done in patients not in remission, seems the most promising approach (Blume et al. 1990).

Post-remission therapy

In adult ALL there are considerable data from uncontrolled trials suggesting an advantage of consolidation and/or intensification for duration of remission. Also, in one randomized trial where some patients received an early intensive consolidation (Stryckmans et al. 1987), their median duration of remission was superior to those without but not their disease-free survival at 5 years and in another randomized trial (Fière et al. 1987), patients with consolidation therapy had a clearly superior outcome to those without. This is supported by two other large non-randomized ALL series with either intensive consolidation and maintenance therapy (Gaynor et al. 1988) or with intensive re-induction therapy (Hoelzer et al. 1984), where a disease-free survival of 35–40 per cent could be achieved (Fig. 1). Thus, there is evidence that early consolidation or intensification can prolong disease-free survival in adult ALL but neither the most suitable drugs nor the optimal duration of consolidation or intensification are known.

Maintenance therapy

Maintenance therapy usually consists of 6-mercaptopurine and methotrexate, a strategy transferred from childhood ALL. In most series of adult ALL it is combined with other drugs on a cyclic basis.

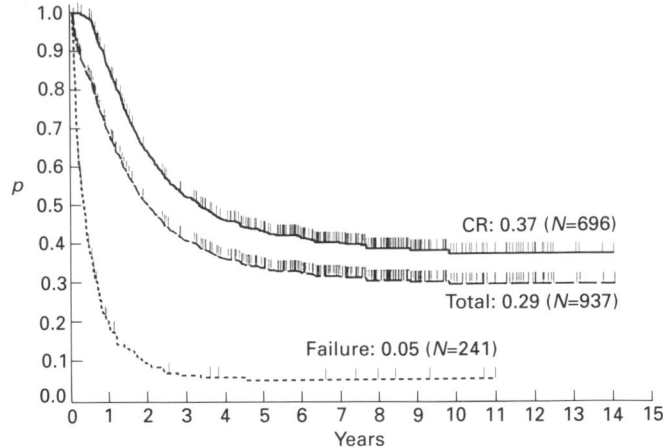

Fig. 1 Overall survival, survival after complete remission (CR), and for patients with failure in two German multicentre therapy trials (01/81 and 02/84) for adult ALL.

It is still unsolved in adult ALL whether such maintenance is of benefit after adequate induction and consolidation therapy and for how long it should be continued. In addition, the advantage of having different maintenance approaches for the varying biological subtypes in ALL is under consideration. For mature B-ALL it seems that after successful repeated cycles of intensive chemotherapy, maintenance therapy adds no benefit. Similarly, in adult T-ALL after intensive induction and consolidation the benefit of a maintenance period is questionable and is at present under study in prospective trials. Thus, the established role of maintenance therapy in its present form seems valuable only for the common ALL (Ph[1]-negative). The duration of maintenance therapy is between 1.5 and 2.5 years, but the optimal procedure remains to be established in prospective trials.

Leukaemia of the central nervous system

Prophylactic therapy

Without some form of prophylactic therapy for the central nervous system, 27–50 per cent of adults with ALL will develop overt leukaemia of that system (Table 7). In the only randomized prospective trial of prophylaxis in adult ALL (Omura et al. 1980) a higher incidence of central nervous relapse was seen in patients not receiving this therapy, although no advantage for duration of remission and survival was observed (Table 7). However, two arguments favour the continued use of this type of prophylactic therapy in adult ALL. Firstly, with improved survival rates, late-occurring relapses in the central nervous system are of increasing importance. Secondly, the prophylactic therapy also has its justification in the fact that leukaemia of the central nervous system is more easily prevented than treated and that once it has developed it has a high rate of relapse.

Routine prophylaxis for the central nervous system usually takes the form of cranial irradiation (24 Gy in 12 fractions over a period of 2–3 weeks) and, in addition, intrathecal methotrexate, 10 mg/m^2 (usual maximum dose, 15 mg) twice weekly, by lumbar puncture. A variety of different approaches to this prophylactic therapy has been reported, including the use of intrathecal methotrexate alone (without irradiation), given via an implanted Ommaya reservoir (Clarkson et al. 1985) or in combination with intrathecal cytosine arabinoside and/or hydrocortisone or dexamethasone. The question of whether intrathecal therapy should

Table 7 Central nervous system (CNS) relapse (isolated and combined) rate in relation to CNS prophylaxis in adult ALL

	Number of studies	Number of patients	CNS prophylaxis	CNS relapses[a] (%)
Without CNS prophylaxis	2	107	None	31 (27–50)
With cranial irradiation and intrathecal therapy	5	1227	24 Gy+IT-MTX (±IT-AraC/P)	14 (11–16)
Without cranial irradiation but with intrathecal therapy	3	675	IT-MTX, OM-MTX	12 (7–14)
Without specific CNS prophylaxis but with high-dose systemic therapy	4	270	HD-AraC, HD-MTX	15 (6–19)

[a]Isolated CNS and combined CNS and bone-marrow relapses; weighted mean (range) in percentages.
AraC/P, cytosine arabinoside/prednisone; HD, high dose; IT, intrathecal; MTX, methotrexate; OM, Ommaya reservoir.

be given alone or combined with prophylactic irradiation has not been formally or prospectively assessed in adult ALL.

In some adult ALL series, prophylaxis with intrathecal therapy or irradiation was substituted by systemic high-dose therapy such as high-dose intravenous methotrexate (Esterhay *et al.* (1982) or high-dose systemic cytosine arabinoside (Barnett *et al.* 1987; Cassileth *et al.* 1990*b*). These attempts were equivalent to conventional prophylactic therapy for the central nervous system, including CNS irradiation. In a retrospective analysis where patients with adult ALL received intensive chemotherapy but without specific central nervous prophylaxis, the rate of relapse in that system was 21 per cent at 1 year, ranging from 4 to 54 per cent according to differing risk groups (Kantarjian *et al.* 1988), which could lead to a risk-adapted prophylaxis for the central nervous system.

Therapy of established disease

Approximately 5–10 per cent of patients with adult ALL present with manifestations of leukaemia in the central nervous system (Morra *et al.* 1986). Treatment of overt leukaemia in that system is usually undertaken with either intrathecal methotrexate alone, intraventricular methotrexate in combination with cytosine arabinoside or hydrocortisone, or with cranial irradiation. Intrathecal methotrexate is continued over 2 or 3 weeks until two consecutive examinations of cerebrospinal fluid show no evidence of leukaemic infiltration. Continued maintenance intrathecal chemotherapy at less frequent intervals may be beneficial in prolonging the duration of remission in the central nervous system. When patients with adult ALL with leukaemia of the central nervous system at diagnosis are treated adequately they have no inferior outcome with regard to disease-free survival or relapse rate in that system (Hoelzer and Gale 1987).

Toxicity of central nervous therapy

Cranial irradiation of adult patients rarely produces a 'somnolence syndrome' similar to that in children, which is due to a transient radiation encephalopathy and is self-limiting. Cranio-spinal irradiation may produce profound and prolonged bone-marrow suppression, which may severely limit continued systemic therapy. Intrathecal chemotherapy, in particular the implantation of an Ommaya reservoir, may be complicated by infection and haemorrhage. Intrathecal methotrexate frequently causes meningeal irritation and chemical arachnoiditis, as may intrathecal cytosine arabinoside. The severity of the symptoms is variable; they include backache, headache, vomiting, fever, and leg pain. Steroids (either oral dexamethasone or intrathecal hydrocortisone) will largely prevent these symptoms. Care should be taken to use preservative-free methotrexate in Elliot's B solution or lactated Ringer's, as the use of other preparations may be responsible for some cases of

arachnoiditis. In contrast to childhood ALL, prophylaxis of the central nervous system, including cranial irradiation, is associated with only minimal subclinical neuropsychological toxicity without severe late effects (Tucker *et al.* 1989).

Relapse time and sites

More than half the adult patients with ALL will relapse despite treatment. The overall relapse rate is highest within the first 2 years and continues thereafter with a lower probability. Patterns of relapse seem to depend on immunophenotype. For common ALL, 'last' relapses are seen at 5–6 years, for T-ALL at 3–4 years, and for B-ALL within 1 year, however, the relapse pattern with regard to immunophenotype has only been analysed in few adult ALL series.

Approximately 80 per cent of all relapses occur in the bone-marrow and the remainder in extramedullary sites, predominantly the central nervous system. Other extramedullary relapses, such as in lymph nodes, skin, or other organ sites, comprise less than 3–5 per cent in adult ALL series. Relapses in the mediastinum are rare, even in those patients with initial mediastinal involvement. That testicular relapse in adult ALL is less than 1 per cent could be an underestimate because it might not be as carefully and closely controlled as in male children. Patients with isolated extramedullary relapse are at high risk for subsequent haematological relapse and require local treatment followed by systemic re-induction therapy.

Therapy of relapsed and resistant leukaemia

Patients who fail to achieve complete remission and those who subsequently relapse have been treated with a wide variety of different protocols. With combination therapy, 50–60 per cent of patients will achieve a second complete remission, although the duration of this is short, usually less than 6 months and the long-term disease-free survival less than 5 per cent. The combination of the teniposide VM-26 and cytosine arabinoside, being probably synergistic, is very effective in relapsed and resistant childhood ALL. Similar combinations of an epipodophyllotoxin and the arabinoside have been used in the treatment of *de novo* adult ALL (Jacobs *et al.* 1990) and have improved the outcome for elderly patients with ALL when used as mild consolidation therapy (Hoelzer *et al.* 1987). The combination of moderate- to high-dose methotrexate with asparaginase is based on pharmacological studies demonstrating therapeutic synergism and modulation of methotrexate toxicity. Folinic acid is effective in reducing the haematological and gastrointestinal toxicity of high-dose methotrexate and is used together with it. Response rates of 33–75 per cent have been reported using these drug combinations in resistant ALL (Amadori *et al.* 1980). High dose cytarabine alone is probably less effective in advanced ALL than in AML, with a CR rate of 37 per cent in refractory or relapsed ALL. When high-dose cytosine arabinoside is combined with asparaginase (Capizzi et al. 1984) or with amsacrine, mitoxantrone, adriamycin, or other agents, complete remission rates of 50–60 per cent can be achieved (Hoelzer 1991). As, however, such remissions are very short, it seems advisable for eligible patients to have an allogeneic or autologous bone-marrow transplantation.

Special treatment problems: hyperleucocytosis

In patients with a large leukaemic cell burden (that is, a high white blood-cell count and/or massive organomegaly), cell reduction with a cautious 'pre-induction' therapy is recommended. Patients with a high white count ($>100\times10^9$/l), where hyperviscosity due to leucostasis with cerebral impairment may rarely occur, were successfully managed with leucopheresis (Lichtmann and Rowe 1982). Such technical facilities may not be available everywhere and these patients can also be managed with a gentle chemotherapy consisting of vincristine and prednisone (for example, vincristine, 0.75 mg/m^2 on day 1 and prednisone, 30 mg/m^2, days 1–7) in nearly all cases without complications. For patients with mature B-ALL and high tumour burden an initial therapy with cyclophosphamide and prednisone is recommended (for example, cyclophosphamide, 200 mg/m^2 and prednisone, 60 mg/m^2, each on days 1–5). Thus, leucopheresis in adult ALL might not be necessary except on very rare occasions, such as for leukaemia in an expectant mother.

Prognostic factors in ALL

With the improvement of the rate of complete remission in adult ALL to 80 per cent, prognostic factors for the achievement of complete remission have lost their power, except for the lower rates for older patients. There is, however, still a variety of factors affecting the duration of remission and survival. In adult ALL series with intensive but different treatment regimens, similar prognostic factors emerge (Table 8); these include time to achieve complete remission, age, initial white blood-cell count, immunological subtype, and cytogenetic abnormalities (Clarkson et al. 1985; Hoelzer and Gale 1987).

Immunophenotype

As in childhood ALL, in most adult ALL series, patients with common ALL had the best prognosis, with a complete remission rate of 78 per cent and a probability of being in continuous remission of 34 per cent (Table 9). For adult T-ALL the prognosis has changed substantially within the last decade. In earlier studies, the rate of complete remission was 72 per cent and disease-free survival less

Table 8 Major adverse prognostic factors for remission duration in adult ALL

- Complete remission not achieved within 4 or 5 weeks
- White blood-cell count $>10–25/35–100\times10^9$/l[a]
- Age $>20–>25/35–>60$ years[a]
- Immunological subtypes:
  B-ALL (?)
  Mixed AL or hybrid ALL (?)
- Chromosomal abnormalities:
  Ph+ALL [t(9;22)] or BCR-ABL+ALL
  t(4;11)
  t(8;14)

[a]Continuous variables.

Table 9 Immunological subtype and outcome in adult ALL

Subtype	Number of trials	Number of patients	CR rate[a] (%)	CCR[a] (%)
c-ALL	10	702	78	34
T-ALL:				
−AraC/C	5	47	72	<10
+AraC/C	5	253	85	46
B-ALL:				
'ALL'-therapy	9	62	44	<10
'NHL'-therapy	5	62	79	53

[a]Weighted means.
CR, complete remission; CCR, continuous complete remission.
AraC/C, cytosine arabinoside/cyclophosphamide; NHL, non-Hodgkin's lymphoma.

than 10 per cent. In more recent studies, complete remission rates exceed 80 per cent and disease-free survival may approach 40 per cent or more. It is suggestive but not conclusive that the use of cytarabine and/or cyclophosphamide early in induction or consolidation therapy is responsible for this improvement. For adult B-ALL the rate of complete remission was only 44 per cent and disease-free survival less than 10 per cent. This poor prognosis may change when short, very intensive protocols (Müller-Weihrich et al. 1984; Patte et al. 1986) are used, which have achieved complete remission rates of 60–100 per cent and disease-free survival of 50 or more per cent in children. When such protocols are applied to adults with B-ALL, complete remission rates are 79 per cent and disease-free survival 53 per cent (Pees et al. 1985; Fenaux et al. 1989; Schaison et al. 1989; Kath et al. 1990). Few clinical studies or follow-ups are known for adult patients with mixed or hybrid acute leukaemia. Patients with this form of leukaemia had an inferior prognosis (Sobol et al. 1987). However, in more recent paediatric trials, hybrid leukaemia seems to carry no disadvantage (Pui et al. 1990).

Age

In most adult ALL series, increasing age is associated with shorter duration of remission and survival. However, as for the rate of complete remission, it is difficult to define an age limit. Unequivocally, in patients above 50 or 60 years the survival is very poor.

White blood-cell count

A high white cell count at presentation has adversely influenced the remission rate in only a few studies but, in contrast, it had an adverse impact on duration of remission in the majority. The limits are set continuously from a white count of $10–100\times10^9$/l. In recent studies the critical level was $25–35\times10^9$, similar to that in childhood ALL.

Time to response

Longer time to achieve complete remission is prognostic for a shorter duration of remission in both childhood and adult ALL. In two adult series (Clarkson et al. 1985; Hoelzer et al. 1988), patients achieving complete remission within 4 or 5 weeks had a significantly better long-term outcome than those requiring additional therapy to reach complete remission. In studies with overall complete remission rates of 70–80 per cent, the proportion of patients who need more than 4 weeks' treatment is approximately 10 per cent and it is obvious that these patients have a poorer quality of remission.

Cytogenetics

Specific chromosome abnormalities have an adverse influence on outcome in adult ALL independent of age, immunophenotype, and initial leucocyte count (Bloomfield *et al.* 1986, 1989; Heim and Mitelman 1987; Sandberg 1987). Whereas for adults with a normal karyotype and for those with chromosomal abnormalities the complete remission rates are similar, the latter group are associated with a significantly inferior survival. Of particular interest are patients with the translocations t(9;22), t(4,11), or those with a *BCR-ABL* rearrangement (Maurer *et al.* 1991) who carry a very poor prognosis with a survival rate of 0–15 per cent at 5 years after chemotherapy. Ph[1]-positive ALL or *BCR-ABL* positive ALL is observed in half of adult patients with common ALL or pre-B-ALL but not in T-ALL except in rare cases. These 25–30 per cent of all patients with adult ALL will have a very poor outcome. This is evidently the major reason for the inferior outcome of adult compared to childhood ALL where the proportion with Ph[1]-positive ALL is 3–5 per cent.

Other features

There is a tendency toward higher remission rates for female patients in most adult ALL series. Median duration of remission is not different between the sexes but when long-term outcomes are compared the survival rate is lower in males. This trend is similar to that seen in children, where the poorer outcome for male children may be partly accounted for by testicular relapses. Reports on the incidence of testicular relapse in adults with ALL are scarce; in three studies with intensive therapy it was 1 per cent or less. Thus, the inferior outcome for adult male patients with ALL remains unexplained.

Other factors reported to have an adverse influence in adult ALL include leukaemia of the central nervous system, mediastinal involvement, the number of immature cells in the peripheral blood, low platelet count at diagnosis, high serum lactate dehydrogenase, elevated serum glutamic-oxalacetic transaminase, and weight loss. Most of these variables except elevated serum lactate dehydrogenase have been evaluated in single studies only and require confirmation.

Stratification into risk groups

These prognostic factors for duration of remission can now, as in childhood ALL, identify low-risk and high-risk patients in adult ALL (Fig. 2). For low-risk patients, defined in recent studies as having younger age, complete remission within 4 or 5 weeks, low initial white blood-cell count, common ALL or T-ALL, the probability of disease-free survival at 10 years may approach 50 per cent or more (Clarkson *et al.* 1985; Hoelzer *et al.* 1988) whereas for high-risk patients characterized by older age, delayed achievement of complete remission, high initial white blood-cell count, B-ALL or null ALL, Ph[1]-positive ALL or *BCR-ABL* rearrangement, the survival is only 25 per cent or less. Such a stratification may give indications for bone-marrow transplantation in first or in second remission. In addition, it demonstrates that not all patients with adult ALL are poor risk.

Prognostic factors in AML

Although a large number of variables for entrance and course in patients with AML have been tested for prognostic significance (Gale and Foon 1986), they do not predict for outcome as in adult ALL and have not led to stratification of AML patients into risk groups for different therapeutic approaches. Age is closely correlated

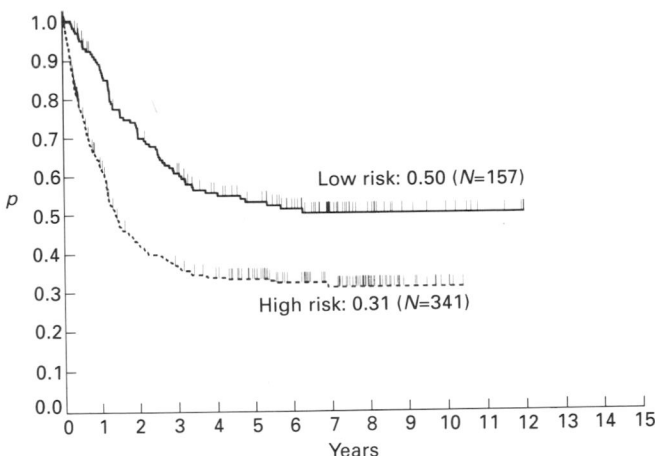

Fig. 2 Survival of patients in complete remission (CR) at standard risk or high risk in two German multicentre therapy trials (01/81 and 02/84) for adult ALL.

with the achievement of complete remission. Other prognostic factors are the FAB subtype (M3, favourable) and in some but not all studies, white blood-cell count, peripheral promyelocytes or blast cells, leukaemic cell mass, the presence or absence of Auer rods, and *in vitro* colony/cluster growth. Combined-factor analysis by multivariate analysis has been introduced, but the predictive value of such mathematical models is as yet unproven.

Recent investigations show that some variables might provide a reliable prediction of outcome. One is an antecedent myelodysplastic syndrome before overt AML or a secondary AML following exposure to toxic agents. The most important predictive factor in AML is the karyotype which is strictly correlated with the achievement of complete remission and with survival. AML patients with the chromosome aberrations t(8;21), inv(16), or t(15;17) have a favourable prognosis, whereas abnormalities of chromosomes 5 or 7, trisomy 8, abnormalities of 11q;23, or complex karyotypes are unfavourable. Therefore, in future trials stratification of AML patients according to chromosome abnormalities might be used and the treatment approaches adjusted to these risk groups.

BONE-MARROW TRANSPLANTATION

The most intensive form of post-remission treatment is high-dose chemoradiotherapy followed by allogeneic or autologous bone-marrow transplantation.

Allogeneic marrow transplantation

The antileukaemic effect of bone-marrow transplantation is achieved by an ablative therapy consisting of total-body irradiation and high-dose chemotherapy. In addition, there is evidence for an antileukaemic effect by the graft versus host disease or graft versus leukaemia effect (Horowitz *et al.* 1990). Allogeneic marrow transplantation is only applicable to a small proportion of patients, that is, those with an HLA-identical donor, usually a sibling (compatibility in 25–30 per cent) and below an age limit of 50–55 years because of the higher incidence of complications in older patients. Morbidity and death result from transplant-related problems, particularly infections including interstitial pneumonitis and graft versus host disease.

Autologous marrow transplantation

For patients without a suitable HLA-matched donor an autologous marrow transplant is a new and promising approach. Bone-marrow cells are harvested in remission, with or without purging, then cryopreserved and, after the patient has been conditioned as for allogeneic transplantation, are re-infused. The potential risk is that leukaemic cells may also be retransfused. Therefore, several methods for marrow purging to eliminate residual leukaemic cells are currently under investigation (Gorin *et al.* 1990), for example chemopurging, mainly with maphosphamide and 4-hydroxycyclophosphamide, by immunological methods with antibodies or immunotoxins, or by physical methods such as the use of magnetic beads. The absence of an antileukaemic effect from lack of graft versus host disease might be disadvantageous for autologous transplants.

Bone-marrow transplantation in AML

Allogeneic

Survival in adult patients with AML after allogeneic marrow transplantation in first complete remission ranges from 40 per cent to over 65 per cent (Table 10). This is clearly superior to the 20–30 per cent overall survival in such patients after chemotherapy alone. However, when only the younger patients on intensive chemotherapy, that is, those comparable with patients eligible for marrow transplants, are considered the results are not significantly different. Therefore, the role of allogeneic marrow transplantation in adults with AML in first remission has to be investigated further in prospective trials. As up to 30 per cent of patients who relapse after chemotherapy can be salvaged with chemotherapy, the alternative approach is to use the transplant in second remission of AML, particularly as patients at the start of relapse have also been successfully transplanted without preceding chemotherapy for the relapse.

Autologous

In patients with AML after autologous bone-marrow transplantation in first complete remission, the survival rate at 3 years is very promising (25–41 per cent) (Table 10). So far, no clear advantage of using purged vs unpurged marrow has been established.

Survival rates after autologous marrow transplants in second complete remission are 28–30 per cent and this is clearly

Table 10 Chemotherapy vs allogeneic or autologous bone-marrow transplantation (BMT)

	Disease-free survival at 3 years	
	First CR (%)	Second CR (%)
ALL		
Chemotherapy	35	5
Low risk	50	
High risk	25	
BMT		
Allogeneic	21–61	15–45
Autologous	21–65	10–40
AML		
Chemotherapy	20–30	<5
BMT		
Allogeneic	40–66	15–50
Autologous	25–41	28–30

superior to those obtained with chemotherapy. Autologous marrow transplantation in second complete remission should be recommended for every AML patient without an allogeneic donor.

Several ongoing trials compare chemotherapy with allogeneic or autologous marrow transplantation in first complete remission; others allocate all AML patients in complete remission to either allogeneic or autologous transplants but most trials suffer from refusals or exclusions, rendering this comparison difficult.

Bone-marrow transplantation in ALL

Allogeneic

Survival for adult patients with ALL transplanted in first remission ranges from 39 to 61 per cent and in second remission from 26 to 45 per cent (Table 10) (Thomas *et al.* 1983). From these results it is obvious that all such patients with second or later remission should have an allogeneic transplant if an HLA-matched donor is available. The strategy for patients in first remission is more controversial (Gale and Champlin 1984; Mayer 1988). Survival after bone-marrow transplantation seems superior to that obtained with chemotherapy alone; if, however, results are adjusted for age, other risk factors, and time to transplant, the results for chemotherapy and marrow transplantation are very similar (Horowitz *et al.* 1989). It therefore seems advisable that in studies where low-risk patients can be defined, having a survival of more than 50 per cent after chemotherapy, bone-marrow transplantation should be reserved for second remission. For high-risk, adult patients with ALL, characterized by a high initial white-cell count, late achievement of complete remission, immunological subtype B-ALL, Ph'-positive or *BCR-ABL*-positive ALL, marrow transplantation in first remission is superior to chemotherapy.

For patients without a HLA-identical donor, transplantation of unrelated but closely HLA-matched bone-marrow provides a possible treatment. National programmes have been developed to facilitate the identification of suitable donors and increasing numbers of patients are treated in this way with long-term results which do not differ substantially from results of matched sibling transplants.

Autologous

After autologous marrow transplantation in first-remission ALL, survival at 3 years ranges from 21–65 per cent (Table 10), being somewhat lower than the results obtained with allogeneic transplantation and similar to those with intensive chemotherapy. The survival after autologous transplantation in second remission is perhaps less than that achieved for allogeneic but clearly superior to results with chemotherapy alone. Thus, an advantage of autologous bone-marrow transplantation in adult ALL in first remission compared to chemotherapy is as yet unproven. It is recommended for patients with adult ALL in second remission.

An alternative to autologous BMT is the collection of haematological stem cells from the peripheral blood of the patient, with or without mobilization by growth factors and later transplantation. The haemopoietic reconstitution achieved is promising and this method may have the advantage of lower contamination with leukaemic cells.

HAEMOPOIETIC GROWTH FACTORS IN ACUTE LEUKAEMIA

The recombinant human haemopoietic growth factors, particularly G-CSF (granulocyte colony-stimulating factor) and GM-CSF (granulocyte–macrophage colony-stimulating factor) have been shown to increase the neutrophil count and to accelerate neutrophil recovery after chemotherapy, thereby reducing to some extent the duration of neutropenia, the risk of infection, the need for antibiotics, and the days in hospital.

The value of GM-CSF and G-CSF in the treatment approach for acute leukaemia is currently being intensively studied (Seipelt et al. 1990) with the aims of:

(1) shortening the time of severe neutropenia during intensive therapy, thereby reducing the infectious complications;

(2) synchronizing leukaemic blast cells for more effective treatment with cell cycle-specific chemotherapy;

(3) alteration of cellular uptake and intracellular metabolism of cytotoxic drugs;

(4) possible induction of maturation of myeloblastic leukaemic cells;

(5) enhancement of marrow recovery after chemotherapy, allowing adherence to the dose and schedule of treatment regimens;

(6) protection of normal haemopoietic stem cells from cell-cycle specific drugs by negative regulatory factors.

G-CSF in acute leukaemias

G-CSF has been applied mainly after chemotherapy to improve restoration of normal haemopoiesis. Trials of G-CSF in patients with relapsed or refractory acute leukaemias showed significantly faster recovery of neutrophil counts in the group treated with G-CSF. In a randomized trial (Ohno et al. 1990) G-CSF could significantly reduce the duration of febrile neutropenia from 6.5 days in the control group to 4 days in the G-CSF treated group. Complete remission rates were 50 and 36 per cent in the G-CSF and placebo treated groups, respectively. Since the two groups did not differ concerning the regrowth of leukaemic blast cells, the application of G-CSG after completion of chemotherapy seemed to be safe.

The effectiveness of G-CSF during standard induction for ALL, often delayed by neutropenia, has been demonstrated (Scherrer et al. 1993). Also in a randomized study (Ottmann et al. 1993) G-CSF administered concomitantly with chemotherapy and radiotherapy (CNS) resulted in a significant shortening of neutropenia, fewer febrile episodes, and closer adherence to the treatment schedule.

GM-CSF in acute leukaemias

Clinical experience with the combination of haemopoietic growth factors and cytosine arabinoside in the treatment of AML aimed at overcoming quiescence is presently limited to GM-CSF. In vivo administration of GM-CSF in de novo AML patients prior to chemotherapy resulted in leukaemic cell recruitment from the resting phase of the cell cycle into active division in all patients tested. The complete remission rate after one cycle of treatment was 83 per cent. There was no difference in leukaemic cell growth in this study.

In other trials in which GM-CSF was used following cytotoxic treatment a significant shortening of the neutropenia phase with a reduction of infectious episodes could be demonstrated (Büchner et al. 1991; Heil et al. 1993). In the study by Büchner and co-workers (1991) the chemotherapy-induced nadir in the white blood-cell count was followed by reversible regrowth of blast cells in three

AML patients. The early death rate was 14 per cent in the GM-CSF treated group versus 39 per cent in historical controls. After 2.5 years of follow-up the complete remission rate is 78 per cent with remission duration showing a trend in favour of the GM-CSF group (Büchner et al. 1993). Further trials are necessary to investigate the schedule of growth factor administration needed to achieve maximal enhancement of the sensitivity of leukaemic blast cells to cytosine arabinoside.

FUTURE ASPECTS OF THERAPY

There are several experimental and clinical approaches that might improve the outcome for adult patients with acute leukaemia. New chemotherapeutic agents of significance are not available; however, high-dose cytosine arabinoside alone or in combination seems promising for AML. In ALL, chemotherapy might be more tailored according to risk groups defined by immunophenotype or karyotype instead of using a uniform protocol for all patients. Detection of minimal residual disease with molecular methods may be used to determine the efficacy of therapy or to monitor the duration of maintenance therapy. Detection of minimal residual disease may also be used to measure the efficacy of marrow purging for autologous transplantation. For chemotherapy and bone-marrow transplantation, predictive factors for the outcome have to be more precisely defined to establish the optimal sequence of each. The role of autologous bone-marrow transplantation in adult AML and ALL in first remission needs to be determined. Immunotherapy, not successful in the last decade, may have a new future if immunotoxins conjugated to leukaemia-related monoclonal antibodies can be applied. The effect of lymphokines such as interleukin-2 in maintenance therapy of AML are at present being explored. Haemopoietic growth factors, such as GM-CSF or G-CSF, will shorten the period of granulocytopenia (interleukin-3 probably that of thrombocytopenia) after myelosuppressive chemotherapy and may allow further intensification of treatment. All these approaches need critical evaluation but may, one hopes, increase the cure rate in adult leukaemic patients.

REFERENCES

Amadori S, et al. (1980). Combination chemotherapy for acute lymphocytic leukemia in adults: results of a retrospective study in 82 patients. American Journal of Haematology, 8:175–83.

Bassan R, et al. (1992). Treatment of adult acute lymphoblastic leukaemia (ALL) over a 16 year period. Leukemia, 6(Suppl. 2):186–90.

Barnett MJ, et al. (1987). A phase I study of high-dose cytosine arabinoside in the treatment of acute leukaemia in adults. Cancer Chemotherapy and Pharmacology, 19:169–71.

Bennett JM, et al. (1976). Proposals for the classification of the acute leukaemias. British Journal of Haematology, 33:451–8.

Bennett JM, et al. (1985a). Proposed revised criteria for the classification of acute myeloid leukemia. A report of the French–American–British Group. Annals of Internal Medicine, 103:620–5.

Bennett JM, et al. (1985b). Criteria for the diagnosis of acute leukemia of megakaryocyte lineage (M7). A report of the French–American–British Group. Annals of Internal Medicine, 103:460–2.

Bishop JF, et al. (1990). Etoposide in acute nonlymphocytic leukemia. Blood, 75:27–32.

Bloomfield CD (1985). Postremission therapy in acute myeloid leukemia. Journal of Clinical Oncology, 3:1570–2.

Bloomfield CD, et al. (1986). Chromosomal abnormalities identifying high-risk and low-risk patients with acute lymphoblastic leukemia. Blood, 67:415–20.

Bloomfield CD, et al. (1989). Six-year follow-up of the clinical significance of karyotype in acute lymphoblastic leukemia. Cancer Genetics and Cytogenetics, 40:171.

Bloomfield CD, Rohatiner AZS, Hoelzer D (1990). Acute leukemia: recent advances in management. In *Hematology 1990* (ed. JM Rappeport, JR McArthur, and DI Feinstein), pp. 15–20. American Society of Hematology, Seattle.

Blume KG, *et al.* (1990). Bone marrow transplantation for acute lymphoblastic leukemia. In *Acute lymphoblastic leukemia* (ed. RP Gale and D Hoelzer), p. 279–93. Liss, New York.

Büchner T, Hiddemann W (1990). Treatment strategies in acute myeloid leukemia (AML). A. First-line chemotherapy. *Blut*, **60**:61–7.

Büchner T, *et al.* (1991). Recombinant human granulocyte–macrophage colony-stimulating factor after chemotherapy in patients with acute myeloid leukemia at higher age or after relapse. *Blood*, **78**:1190–7.

Büchner T, *et al.* (1993). GM-CSF in acute leukemia. *Annals of Hematology*, **66**:A116.

Cappizzi RL, *et al.* (1984). Treatment of poor risk acute leukemia with sequential high-dose ARA-C and asparaginase. *Blood*, **63**:694–700.

Carey RW, *et al.* (1975). Comparative study of cytosine arabinoside therapy alone and combined with thioguanine, mercaptopurine, or daunorubicin in acute myelocytic leukemia. *Cancer*, **36**:1560–6.

Cassileth PA, *et al.* (1984). A randomized study of the efficacy of consolidation therapy in adult acute nonlymphocytic leukemia. *Blood*, **63**:843–7.

Cassileth PA, *et al.* (1990*a*). Comparison of postremission therapies in adult acute myeloid leukemia: preliminary analysis of an ECOG study. *Haematology and Blood Transfusion*, **33**:267–70.

Cassileth PA, *et al.* (1990*b*). High-dose cytarabine therapy in adult acute lymphocytic leukemia. In *Acute lymphoblastic leukemia* (ed. RP Gale and D Hoelzer), p. 197–203. Liss, New York.

Castaigne S, *et al.* (1990). All *trans* retinoic acid as a differentiating therapy for acute promyelocytic leukemias. I. Clinical results. *Blood*, **76**:1704–9.

Chaganti RSK, *et al.* (1979). Cytogenetic evidence of the intrauterine origin of acute leukemia in monozygotic twins. *New England Journal of Medicine*, **330**:1032–4.

Clarkson B, *et al.* (1985). Acute lymphoblastic leukemia in adults. *Seminars in Oncology* **12**:160–79.

Clarkson B, *et al.* (1990). Importance of long-term follow-up in evaluating treatment regimens for adults with acute lymphoblastic leukemia. *Haematology and Blood Transfusion*, **33**:397–408.

Cuttner J, *et al.* (1991). Phase III trial of brief intensive treatment of adult acute lymphocytic leukemia comparing daunorubicin and mitoxantrone: a CALGB study. *Leukemia*, **5**:425–31.

Delva L, *et al.* (1993) Resistance to all-*trans* retinoic acid (ATRA) therapy in relapsing acute promyelocytic leukemia: study of *in vitro* ATRA sensitivity and cellular retinoic acid binding protein levels in leukemic cells. *Blood*, **82**:2175–81.

Drexler HG, Thiel E, Ludwig WD (1991). Review of the incidence and clinical relevance of myeloid antigen-positive acute lymphoblastic leukemia. *Leukemia*, **5**:637–45.

Ellison RR, *et al.* (1991). The effects of postinduction intensification treatment with cytarabine and daunorubicin in adult acute lymphocytic leukemia: a prospective randomized clinical trial by Cancer and Leukemia Group B. *Journal of Clinical Oncology*, **9**:2002–15.

Esterhay RJ, *et al.* (1982). Moderate dose methotrexate, vincristine, asparaginase, and dexamethasone for treatment of adult acute lymphocytic leukemia. *Blood*, **59**:334–5.

Falletta JM, Starling KA, Fernbach DJ (1973). Leukemia in twins. *Pediatrics*, **52**:846–9.

Fearon ER, *et al.* (1986). Differentiation of leukemia cells to polymorphonuclear leukocytes in patients with acute nonlymphoblastic leukemia. *New England Journal of Medicine*, **315**:15–24.

Fenaux P, *et al.* (1989). Burkitt cell acute leukaemia (L3 ALL) in adults: a report of 18 cases. *British Journal of Haematology*, **71**:371–6.

Fenaux P, *et al.* (1993). Effect of all *trans*retinoic acid in newly diagnosed acute promyelocytic leukemia. Results of a multicenter randomized trial. *Blood*, **82**:3241–9.

Fière D, *et al.* (1987). Treatment of 218 adult acute lymphoblastic leukemias. *Seminars in Oncology*, **14** (Suppl. 1):64–6.

Fière D, *et al.* (1991). Adult acute lymphoblastic leukemia (ALL). First interim analysis of the evolution of 467 patients (French Multicentric Trial LALA 87). *Haematologica*, **76** (Suppl. 4):108.

Foon KA, Todd FR (1986). Immunologic classification of leukemia and lymphoma. *Blood*, **68**:1.

Forman SJ, Blume KG (1990). Allogeneic bone marrow transplantation (BMT) as therapy for primary induction failure for patients with acute leukemia. *Proceedings of the American Society of Clinical Oncology*, **9**:204.

Fourth International Workshop on Chromosomes in Leukemia 1982 (1984). *Cancer Genetics and Cytogenetics*, **11**:251–360.

Gale RP, Champlin RE (1984). How does bone marrow transplantation cure leukemia. *Lancet*, **ii**:28–30.

Gale RP, Foon KA (1986). Acute myeloid leukaemia: recent advances in therapy. *Clinics in Haematology*, **15**:781–810.

Gardner MJ, *et al.* (1990). Results of case-control study of leukaemia and lymphoma among young people near Sellafield nuclear plant in West Cumbria. *British Medical Journal*, **1**:423–9.

Gaynor J, *et al.* (1988). A cause-specific hazard rate analysis of prognostic factors among 199 adults with acute lymphoblastic leukemia: the Memorial Hospital experience since 1969. *Journal of Clinical Oncology*, **6**:1014–30.

Gorin NC, Aegerter P, Auvert B (1990). Autologous bone marrow transplantation for acute leukemia in remission: an analysis on 1322 cases. *Haematology and Blood Transfusion*, **33**:660–6.

Gottlieb AJ, *et al.* (1984). Efficacy of daunorubicin in the therapy of adult acute lymphocyte leukemia: a prospective randomized trial by Cancer and Leukemia Group B. *Blood*, **64**:267–74.

Greaves MF (1981). Analysis of the clinical and biological significance of lymphoid phenotypes in acute leukemia. *Cancer Research*, **41**:4752–66.

Greaves MF (1988). Speculations on the cause of childhood acute lymphoblastic leukemia. *Leukemia*, **2**:120–5.

Haesman MA, *et al.* (1984). Incidence of leukaemia in young persons in West of Scotland. *Lancet*, **i**:1188–9.

Hayat M, *et al.* (1986). A randomized comparison of maintenance treatment with androgens, immunotherapy and chemotherapy in adult acute myelogenous leukemia. A Leukemia-Lymphoma Group Trial of the EORTC. *Cancer*, **58**:617–23.

Heath CW (1982). Leukemogenesis and low-dose exposure to radiation and chemical agents. In *Advances in comparative leukemia research* (ed. DS Yohn and JR Blakeslee), p. 23. North-Holland/Elsevier, Amsterdam.

Heil G, *et al.* (1993). GM-CSF in a double-blind randomized placebo controlled trial in therapy of adult patients with *de novo* acute myeloid leukemia (AML). *Annals of Hematology*, **66**:A117.

Heim S, Mitelman F (1987). *Cancer cytogenetics*. Liss, New York.

Herzig RH, *et al.* (1983). High-dose cytosine arabinoside therapy for refractory leukemia. *Blood*, **62**:361–9.

Hoelzer D (1984). Current status of ALL/AUL therapy in adults. *Recent Results in Cancer Research*, **93**:182–203.

Hoelzer D (1991). High-dose chemotherapy in adult acute lymphoblastic leukemia. *Seminars in Hematology*, **28** (Suppl. 4):84–9.

Hoelzer D, Gale RP (1987). Acute lymphoblastic leukemia in adults: recent progress, future directions. *Seminars in Hematology*, **24**:27–39.

Hoelzer D, *et al.* (1984). Intensified therapy in acute lymphoblastic and acute undifferentiated leukemia in adults. *Blood*, **64**:38–47.

Hoelzer D, *et al.* (1987). Teniposide (VM-26) and cytosine arabinoside as consolidation therapy in adult high-risk patients with acute lymphoblastic leukemia. *Seminars in Oncology*, **14** (Suppl. 1):92–7.

Hoelzer D, *et al.* (1988). Prognostic factors in a multicenter study for treatment of acute lymphoblastic leukemia in adults. *Blood*, **71**:123–31.

Hoelzer D (1991). High dose chemotherapy in adult acute lymphoblastic leukemia. *Seminars in Hematology*, **28** (Suppl. 4):84–9.

Hoelzer D, *et al.* (1992). The German multicentre trials for treatment of acute lymphoblastic leukemia in adults. *Leukemia*, **6** (Suppl. 2):175–7.

Hoffbrand AV, Pettit JE (1988). *Sandoz atlas of clinical haematology*. Gower Medical, London.

Horowitz MM, *et al.* (1991). Chemotherapy compared with bone marrow transplantation for adults with acute lymphoblastic leukemia in first remission. *Annals of Internal Medicine*, **115**:13–18.

Huang ME, *et al.* (1988). Use of all-*trans* retinoic acid in the treatment of acute promyelocytic leukemia. *Blood*, **72**:567–72.

Hussein KK, *et al.* (1989). Treatment of acute lymphoblastic leukemia in adults with intensive induction, consolidation, and maintenance chemotherapy. *Blood*, **73**:57–63.

Jacobs P, Wood L, Novitzky N (1990). Treatment of adult acute lymphoblastic leukemia. *Haematology and Blood Transfusion*, 33:428–31.

Janossy G, Coustan-Smith E, Campana D (1989). The reliability of cytoplasmic CD3 and CD33 antigen expression in the immunodiagnosis of acute leukemia: a study of 500 cases. *Leukemia*, 3:170–81.

Jehn U, *et al.* (1990). A randomized comparison of intensive maintenance treatment for adult acute myelogenous leukemia using either cyclic alternating drugs or repeated courses of the induction-type chemotherapy: AML-6 trial of the EORTC Leukemia Cooperative Group. *Haematology and Blood Transfusion*, 33:277–84.

Kantarjian HM, *et al.* (1988). Identification of risk groups for development of central nervous system leukemia in adults with acute lymphoblastic leukemia. *Blood*, 72:1784–9.

Kantarjian HM, *et al.* (1990). Results of the vincristine, doxorubicin, and dexamethasone regimen in adults with standard- and high-risk acute lymphocytic leukemia. *Journal of Clinical Oncology*, 8:994–1044.

Kantarjian HM, *et al.* (1992). Granulocyte-colony stimulating factor (G-CSF) supportive care following intensive chemotherapy consolidation in acute lymphocytic leukemia (ALL) in first remission. *Blood*, 80 (Suppl. 1):112a.

Kantarjian HM, *et al.* (1993). Treatment of therapy related leukemia and myelodysplastic syndrome. *Hematology/Oncology Clinics of North America*, 7:81–107.

Kath R, *et al.* (1990). Chemotherapy of non-endemic Burkitt's lymphoma. *Journal of Cancer Research and Clinical Oncology*, 116 (Suppl.):608.

Keating MS, *et al.* (1990). Karyotype of leukemia cells consistently predicts for response to therapy and survival following salvage therapy in acute myeloblastic leukemia. *Haematology and Blood Transfusion*, 33:593–603.

Keith L, Brown E (1971). Epidemiological study of leukemia in twins (1928–1969). *Acta Genetica et Medica Gemmellologiae*, 20:9–22.

Kurrle E, *et al.* (1990). Consolidation therapy with high-dose cytosine arabinoside: experiences of a prospective study in acute myeloid leukemia. *Haematology and Blood Transfusion*, 33:254–60.

Kyle RA (1982). Second malignancies associated with chemotherapeutic agents. *Seminars in Oncology*, 9:131–42.

Lichtman MA, Rowe JM (1982). Hyperleukocytic leukemias: rheological, clinical, and therapeutic considerations. *Blood*, 60:279–83.

Lluesma-Gonalons M, *et al.* (1991). Improved results of an intensified therapy in adult acute lymphocytic leukemia. *Annals of Oncology*, 2:33–9.

Löffler H, *et al.* (1987). Morphological and cytochemical classification of adult acute leukemias in two multicenter studies in the Federal Republic of Germany. *Haematology and Blood Transfusion*, 30:21–7.

McKinney PA, *et al.* (1989). The Leukaemia Research Fund data collection study: descriptive epidemiology of acute lymphoblastic leukaemia. *Leukemia*, 3:880–5.

Mandelli F, *et al.* (1989). GIMEMA ALL 0183: a multicentric study on adult acute lymphoblastic leukaemia in Italy. *British Journal of Haematology*, 71:377–86.

Maurer J, *et al.* (1991). Detection of chimeric *BCR-ABL* genes in acute lymphoblastic leukemia by polymerase chain reaction. *Lancet*, 337:1055–8.

Mayer RJ (1988). Allogeneic transplantation versus intensive chemotherapy in first-remission acute leukemia: is there a 'best' choice? *Journal of Clinical Oncology*, 6:1532–6.

Morra E, *et al.* (1986). Systemic high-dose ara-C for the treatment of meningeal leukemia in adult acute lymphoblastic leukemia and non-Hodgkin's lymphoma. *Journal of Clinical Oncology*, 4:1207–11.

Müller-Weihrich S, *et al.* (1984). Kindliche B-Zell-Lymphome und -Leukämien. Verbesserung der Prognose durch eine für B-Neoplasien konzipierte Therapie der BFM-Studiengruppe. *Onkologie*, 7:205–8.

Ohno R, *et al.* (1990). Effect of granulocyte colony-stimulating factor after intensive induction therapy in relapsed or refractory acute leukemia. *New England Journal of Medicine*, 323:871–7.

Omura GA, Raney M (1985). Long-term survival in adult acute lymphoblastic leukemia: follow-up of a Southeastern Cancer Study Group trial. *Journal of Clinical Oncology*, 3:1053–8.

Omura GA, *et al.* (1980). Combination chemotherapy of adult acute lymphoblastic leukemia with randomised central nervous system prophylaxis. *Blood*, 55:199–204.

Ottmann OG, *et al.* (1993). Concomitant R-metHuG-CSF (Filgrastim) and intensive chemoradiotherapy as induction treatment in adult ALL: a randomized multicenter phase III trial. *Blood*, 82 (Suppl. 1):193a.

Passe S, *et al.* (1982). Acute nonlymphoblastic leukemia: prognostic factors in adults with long-term follow-up. *Cancer*, 50:1462–71.

Patte C, *et al.* (1986). Improved survival rate in children with stage III and IV B cell non-Hodgkin's lymphoma and leukemia using multi-agent chemotherapy: results of a study of 114 children from the French Pediatric Oncology Society. *Journal of Clinical Oncology*, 8:1219–29.

Pees HW, Riehm HJ, Schwamborn J (1985). Effective treatment of lymphomas of Burkitt's type and B-ALL in adults. *Blut*, 50:213–18.

Preisler HD, *et al.* (1983). Therapy of secondary acute nonlymphocytic leukemia with cytarabine. *New England Journal of Medicine*, 308:21–3.

Preisler H, *et al.* (1987). Comparison of three remission induction regimens and two postinduction strategies for the treatment of acute nonlymphocytic leukemia: a Cancer and Leukemia Group B Study. *Blood*, 69:1441–9.

Pui C-H, *et al.* (1989). Secondary acute myeloid leukemia in children treated for acute lymphoid leukemia. *New England Journal of Medicine*, 321:136–42.

Pui C-H, *et al.* (1990). Myeloid-associated antigen 15 expression lacks prognostic value in childhood acute lymphoblastic leukemia treated with intensive multiagent chemotherapy. *Blood*, 75:198–202.

Pui C-H, *et al.* (1991). Acute myeloid leukemia in children treated with epipodophyllotoxins for acute lymphoblastic leukemia. *New England Journal of Medicine*, 325:1682–7.

Rai KR, *et al.* (1981). Treatment of acute myelocytic leukemia: a study by Cancer and Leukemia Group B. *Blood*, 58:1203–12.

Rees JKH, *et al.* (1986). Principal results of the Medical Research Council's 8th acute myeloid leukemia trial. *Lancet*, ii:1236–41.

Report of the Medical Research Council's Working Party on Leukaemia in Adults. (1974). *British Journal of Haematology*, 27:373–89.

Rosner F, Grünwald HW (1980). Cytotoxic drugs and leukaemogenesis. *Clinics in Haematology*, 9:663–81.

Sallan SE, *et al.* (1983). Influence of intensive asparaginase in the treatment of childhood non-T-cell acute lymphoblastic leukemia. *Cancer Research*, 53:5601–7.

Sandberg AA (1987). Prognostic significance of chromosome changes in acute leukemia. *Haematology and Blood Transfusion*, 30:15–20.

Sauter C, *et al.* (1984). Acute myelogenous leukaemia: maintenance chemotherapy after early consolidation treatment does prolong survival. *Lancet*, i:379–82.

Schaison G, *et al.* (1989). Short and aggressive treatment for B. acute lymphoblastic leukemia (B.ALL). Good results of protocol LMB 86. *Blood*, 74 (Suppl.):369a.

Scherrer R, *et al.* (1993). Granulocyte colony-stimulating factor (G-CSF) as an adjunct to induction chemotherapy of adult acute lymphoblastic leukemia (ALL). *Annals of Hematology*, 66:283–9.

Second MIC Cooperative Study Group (1988). Morphologic, immunologic and cytogenetic (MIC) working classification of the acute myeloid leukaemias. *British Journal of Haematology*, 68:487–94.

Seipelt G, Ganser A, Hoelzer D (1990). Hemopoietic growth factors in the treatment of acute leukemias and myelodysplastic syndromes. *Recent Results in Cancer Research*, 121:141–54.

Smedmyr B, *et al.* (1991). Treatment of adult acute lymphoblastic and undifferentiated (ALL/AUL) leukemia, according to a national protocol, in Sweden. *Haematologica*, 76 (Suppl. 4):107.

Sobol RE, *et al.* (1985). Adult acute lymphoblastic leukemia phenotypes defined by monoclonal antibodies. *Blood*, 65:730–5.

Sobol RE, *et al.* (1987). Clinical importance of myeloid antigen expression in adult acute lymphoblastic leukemia. *New England Journal of Medicine*, 316:1111–17.

Stone RM, Mayer RJ (1993a). Treatment of the newly diagnosed adult with *de novo* acute myeloid leukemia. *Hematology/Oncology Clinics of North America*, 7:47–64.

Stone RM, Mayer RJ (1993b). The approach to the elderly patient with acute myeloid leukemia. *Hematology/Oncology Clinics of North America*, 7:65–79.

Stryckmans P, *et al.* (1987). Cytosine arabinoside for induction, salvage, and consolidation therapy of adult acute lymphoblastic leukemia. *Seminars in Oncology*, 14 (Suppl. 1):67–72.

Stryckmans P, *et al.* (1992). Therapy of adult ALL: overview of 2 successive EORTC studies: (ALL-2 & ALL-3). *Leukemia*, **6** (Suppl. 2):199–203.

Thiel E, *et al.* (1980). Multimarker classification of acute lymphoblastic leukemia: evidence for further T subgroups and evaluation of their clinical significance. *Blood*, **56**:759–72.

Thomas ED, *et al.* (1983). Marrow transplantation for patients with acute lymphoblastic leukemia: a long-term follow-up. *Blood*, **62**:1139–41.

Tivey H (1955). The natural history of untreated acute leukaemia. *Annals of the New York Academy of Sciences*, **60**:322–58.

Tomonaga M, *et al.* (1991). Individualized induction therapy followed by intensive consolidation and maintenance including asparaginase in adult ALL: JALSG-ALL87 study. *Haematologica*, **76** (Suppl. 4):68.

Tucker J, *et al.* (1989). Minimal neuropsychological sequelae following prophylactic treatment of the central nervous system in adult leukaemia and lymphoma. *British Journal of Cancer*, **60**:775–80.

Vogler WR, *et al.* (1984). A randomized comparison of postremission therapy in acute myelogenous leukemia: a Southeastern Cancer Study Group Trial. *Blood*, **63**:1039–45.

Warrell RP, *et al.* (1991). Differentiation therapy of acute promyelocytic leukemia with tretinoin (all-*trans*-retinoic acid). *New England Journal of Medicine*, **324**:1385–93.

Willemze R, Peters WG, Colly LP (1988). Short-term intensive treatment (V.A.A.P.) of adult acute lymphoblastic leukemia and lymphoblastic lymphoma. *European Journal of Hematology*, **41**:489–95.

Williams DL, *et al.* (1985). Presence of clonal chromosome abnormalities in virtually all cases of acute lymphoblastic leukemia. *New England Journal of Medicine*, **313**:640–1.

Yates J, *et al.* (1982). Cytosine arabinoside with daunorubicin or adriamycin for therapy of acute myelocytic leukemia: a CALGB study. *Blood*, **60**:454–62.

12.2.3 Acute leukaemia in childhood

JUDITH M. CHESSELLS

ACHIEVEMENTS AND CHALLENGES

The dramatic improvement in outlook for children with acute leukaemia represents one of the major triumphs of paediatric oncology. Twenty-five years ago acute leukaemia was almost uniformly fatal; today two-thirds of children with acute lymphoblastic leukaemia and an increasing proportion of those with acute myeloid leukaemia experience long-term survival and many of these are cured. These advances have hitherto been obtained by means of prospective randomized trials and careful studies involving large numbers of clinicians. In the United Kingdom and many countries in Western Europe 80–90 per cent of children with leukaemia are treated on such collaborative protocols.

This improved outlook has been paralleled by improved classification systems which facilitate a common language, although, sadly, there has been no real agreement about staging as yet. The immunological classification of acute lymphoblastic leukaemia has facilitated a rational approach to management of lymphoproliferative disease in childhood. This has already led to the development of more appropriate therapy, as, for example in the recognition of the special therapeutic challenge of the 1–2 per cent of leukaemias with B-cell acute lymphoblastic leukaemia features, which are unresponsive to conventional treatment for acute lymphoblastic leukaemia but are curable with a short-term high dose chemotherapy programme, as used in non-Hodgkin's lymphoma of childhood.

Morphological and immunological classifications have been complemented in turn by the use of cytogenetics and molecular biology. These techniques have helped to identify patients at high risk of treatment failure, but at a more fundamental level they should improve our understanding of leukaemogenesis and normal haemopoiesis.

Many tasks remain. As more children are cured and survival improves for many others it becomes increasingly difficult to mount trials of therapy which have a real chance of detecting a difference between various regimens. International collaboration will be necessary for such trials. Long-term follow-up is needed to determine whether new treatments cure more patients or merely postpone relapse.

The introduction of innovative regimens or the abolition of traditional planks of treatment such as 'maintenance therapy' in acute lymphoblastic leukaemia, is naturally restrained by the fact that results are already good and the knowledge that, if such treatment fails, the chance of cure after relapse is small. Radical new approaches to treatment are thus likely to find most acceptance in the high-risk patients in the first instance.

The study of long-term survivors to monitor late effects, ascertain fertility, and determine the risk of second neoplasms will form an increasingly important task. The results of such studies have already given fresh impetus to refining treatment and particularly to the avoidance of radiotherapy. However, it must be said that the late effects of many of the more intensive chemotherapeutic regimens have as yet been insufficiently monitored.

An important challenge for the next decade is to apply advances in basic research to improve patient management. Monoclonal antibodies now have an established role in diagnosis and some place in therapy, particularly in the context of bone-marrow transplantation; their wider role in treatment remains to be determined. Advances in molecular biology will facilitate the improved detection of minimal residual disease and further research will determine whether this is feasible and useful in clinical practice. The place of growth factors in reducing myelotoxicity and of immunomodulators in treatment awaits clarification. Improved understanding of pharmacology and of the mechanisms of drug resistance has yet to be translated effectively into clinical practice. Many tasks thus remain to ensure that the work of the past is consolidated and that advances in treatment are incorporated to ensure the cure of most children at least cost.

EPIDEMIOLOGY

Incidence: age and sex

Leukaemia is the most common type of childhood malignancy, accounting for almost one-third of cases under the age of 15. The annual incidence is 30–40 cases per 10^6 children (Stiller 1985). Approximately 80 per cent of cases are of acute lymphoblastic leukaemia, approximately 18 per cent are acute myeloid leukaemia, and the remainder comprise a variety of rare chronic myeloproliferative disorders. The older literature on childhood leukaemia contains numerous references to acute undifferentiated or stem cell leukaemia, a term which has been rendered obsolete by modern methods of classification and should now be reserved for the tiny minority of cases which defy classification by cytology, cytochemistry, and immunology. Most of the cases described in this way were probably acute lymphoblastic leukaemia.

Acute lymphoblastic leukaemia, with a sex ratio of 1.28, shows a peak incidence in childhood between the ages of 3 and 5 years. With the advent of immunological classification, it has become apparent that this peak is entirely due to cases of early B-cell acute lymphoblastic leukaemia (common acute lymphoblastic leukaemia). It is reported not to occur in some developing countries, although it has been argued that this deficit may be, at least in part, due to a failure of diagnosis in an environment where anaemia and death from infection are common in the young child. Immunological classification has also shown the relatively higher incidence of T-cell acute lymphoblastic leukaemia in the older child and the prevalence of males in this subtype, accounting at least in part for the more frequent occurrence of leukaemia in males. In contrast the sex ratio in acute myeloid leukaemia is 1.1 and the incidence, after peaking at 1 year, is low thereafter in childhood although it increases after the age of 12 years (Stiller 1985).

Genetic and familial predisposition

The risk of leukaemia occurring in siblings has been estimated at two to four times that of the general population and the risk of occurrence in monozygotic twins is very high in the first year of life and is estimated as approximately one in five for the first 10 years (Neglia and Robison 1988). Apart from specific families in whom there is a history of leukaemia (often acute myeloid leukaemia), there also appears to be an association of leukaemia in families of children with brain tumours (Farwell and Flannery 1984). Children with Down's syndrome have a 10–15-fold increased risk of development of leukaemia, with a relative preponderance of cases of the common type of acute lymphoblastic leukaemia and the megakaryoblastic subtype of acute myeloid leukaemia (Levitt et al. 1990). There is a well-described transient myeloproliferative disorder of infancy which occurs in infants with Down's syndrome and which is associated with megakaryoblastic proliferation. The precise frequency of this disorder is not known, and it is now clear that some of the so-called transient cases may develop acute myeloid leukaemia later (Eguchi et al. 1989).

Other rare congenital disorders with an increased risk of acute leukaemia include Fanconi's anaemia (acute myeloid leukaemia), Schwachman's syndrome (acute myeloid leukaemia, acute lymphoblastic leukaemia), Kleinfelter's syndrome, Bloom's syndrome, and ataxia–telangiectasia (acute lymphoblastic leukaemia) (Neglia and Robison 1988).

Geographical variations

Studies in the United States have shown that acute lymphoblastic leukaemia is 20–30 per cent more common in the White population than in the Black population. There appears to be a lower incidence of acute lymphoblastic leukaemia in Africa and the Middle East than in Europe, the United States, and the Far East. Studies of acute lymphoblastic leukaemia among Arabs in the Gaza Strip have shown an apparent evolution of the pattern of childhood lymphoproliferative malignancy, progressing with increasing prosperity from a dominance of B-cell lymphomas to common acute lymphoblastic leukaemia (Ramot and Magrath 1982). It remains unclear how much these variations represent true environmental or genetic influences or, as has been argued by some, are due to failure of diagnosis of common acute lymphoblastic leukaemia. Childhood acute myeloid leukaemia is so rare that evidence of true geographical variation is scarce. However, there does seem to be a relative increase of acute myeloid leukaemia in some populations, such as Black American children and in certain geographical areas (for example, Africa) acute myeloid leukaemia in association with chloromas is frequently seen (Fleming 1985).

Environmental factors

Studies of pre-natal factors in children with acute lymphoid leukaemia have identified advanced maternal age, previous fetal loss, and high birth weight as possibly associated with an increased incidence of leukaemia. More clearly defined is the risk of exposure to ionizing radiation in pregnancy, with an increased risk of childhood leukaemia of 1.5–2 times that of the general population (Neglia and Robison 1988).

Post-natal exposure to irradiation, as in the aftermath of the Japanese nuclear explosions, increased the risk of acute lymphoblastic leukaemia and acute myeloid leukaemia and the vogue for therapeutic thymic irradiation and treatment of spondylitis with radiotherapy both increased the incidence of leukaemia. The evidence from studies of leukaemia near nuclear power plants and weapons establishments remains controversial. There does seem to be a true increase in the incidence of childhood leukaemia, but it has been argued that this may not be due to radiation per se but to other characteristics in the population at risk or their environment, for example a relative isolation from exposure to common viruses influencing immunological response to infections.

The latest suggestion, based on studies near Sellafield in Cumbria, is that exposure of fathers to radiation may have caused germ cell mutagenesis which acts as one step in the development of leukaemia (Gardner et al. 1990). These studies are not supported by the findings after Hiroshima and Nagasaki, but the type and duration of exposure would not have been similar. There is little information about the role of chemicals and toxins, although a recent report from the United States links the development of acute myeloid leukaemia in childhood with maternal abuse of marijuana (Neglia and Robison 1988).

The well-studied role of viruses in the development of animal leukaemias has naturally led to extensive searches for an association between virus infection and human leukaemia. The involvement of the Epstein–Barr virus in the genesis of Burkitt's lymphoma and the HTLV group of viruses in adult T-cell acute lymphoblastic leukaemia remain the only proven associations at present. It is tempting to speculate that pre-natal or post-natal viral infections may play a role in the development of childhood acute lymphoblastic leukaemia, a disease that has its peak incidence at a time of maximum immunological proliferation. Greaves has produced the hypothesis that acute lymphoblastic leukaemia in this age group may be the result of random mutation in a lymphoid precursor, a prospect which does not lead to hope of prevention (Greaves 1988). Further large-scale international studies are clearly needed to clarify these environmental issues.

PATHOLOGY AND BIOLOGY

Morphology and cytochemistry

The morphological and cytochemical characteristics of acute leukaemia, as seen in well-stained films of blood and bone-marrow, have been clearly described by the French-American-British (FAB) subgroup and are summarized in Tables 1 and 2. The FAB classification is based on morphology, although there are characteristic associations between certain morphological subtypes of leukaemia and the immunological and cytogenetic findings. The distinction between acute lymphoblastic leukaemia and acute myeloid leukaemia is usually readily apparent but problems may arise in paediatric practice between L2 acute lymphoblastic leukaemia, in which the blast cells appear larger and more undifferentiated and acute myeloid leukaemia of undifferentiated (M1) or monocytic (M5) subtype. These problems should be easily resolved by the routine use of Sudan black or myeloperoxidase stains, which are positive in most myeloid leukaemias and the fluoride-inhibited non-specific esterase, which is positive in most leukaemias with a monocytic component. The periodic acid–Schiff reagent stain, although frequently showing block positivity in childhood acute lymphoblastic leukaemia, is not always positive. Occasional diagnostic problems may arise with erythroleukaemia (M6), when the blasts may not show typical morphology and may exhibit block periodic acid–Schiff reagent positivity and with the more recently recognized megakaryoblastic leukaemia (M7), but these should be overcome with the application of appropriate monoclonal antibodies.

Table 1 FAB classification of acute lymphoblastic leukaemia

Features	L1	L2	L3
Cell size	Small	Large, heterogeneous	Large
Nucleoli	None or one small	One or more prominent	Prominent
Nuclear chromatin	Homogenous	Variable	Homogenous
Cytoplasm	Scanty	Often moderate	Abundant and basophilic
Nuclear shape	Regular	Irregular	Regular
Cytoplasmic vacuolation	Variable	Variable	Prominent

Reproduced from Bennett *et al.* (1981), with permission.

The significance of the morphological classification of acute lymphoblastic leukaemia remains controversial. Clearly the 1–2 per cent of cases with L3 Burkitt-type cells forms a distinct immunological, cytological, and chromosomal subgroup and it is important to identify them in order to effect appropriate treatment (see below). However, the distinction between the smaller lymphocyte-like L1 blasts and the large more pleomorphic L2 blasts is rather subjective, although rendered more precise by a scoring system (Bennett *et al.* 1981). The distinction, as seen in Table 1, bears no relationship to immunological type of acute lymphoblastic leukaemia but it persists because of evidence that the morphological subtype of acute lymphoblastic leukaemia is of independent prognostic significance although this may be less than previously supposed (Lilleyman *et al.* 1992). The biological basis for the worse prognosis of L2 acute lymphoblastic leukaemia is not clear, but probably these leukaemias have a larger proportion of cells in DNA synthesis (Scarffe *et al.* 1980) and may thus represent more aggressive disease. The morphological subtyping of acute myeloid leukaemia into myeloid or monocytic subtypes is usually straightforward (Table 2), but examination of both blood and bone-marrow is essential (Bennett *et al.* 1985a). The distinction between acute myeloid leukaemia and certain types of myelodysplasia, notably refractory anaemia with excess of blasts, is somewhat arbitrary (Bennett *et al.* 1982). It is important to identify acute myeloid leukaemia subtypes because of the early haemorrhagic and thrombotic complications seen in hypergranular promyelocytic leukaemia (M3) and the tendency for early central nervous system infiltration and other extramedullary infiltration in monocytic leukaemias (M4, M5).

Preparations of cerebrospinal fluid or of leukaemic effusions may often show a predominance of the relevant blast cell and present no diagnostic problems. However, it may prove difficult to distinguish leukaemic cells in the cerebrospinal fluid from reactive mononuclear cells, particularly in patients receiving intrathecal chemotherapy; the diagnosis may be confirmed by immunophenotyping.

Histology

Trephine biopsy of the bone-marrow plays little part in the routine management of childhood leukaemia, but it is essential to obtain biopsy material if aspiration proves impossible. In such cases trephine biopsy generally shows extensive fibrosis but the specific

Table 2 FAB classification of acute myeloid leukaemia

Type	Description	Dominant cell type	Associated features	Cytochemistry
M1	Undifferentiated AML	Myeloblast	Scanty differentiation, no Auer rods	SB+(>3% cells) NSE−
M2	AML with differentiation	Myeloblasts and promyelocytes	Differentiation, Auer rods	SB+ NSE−
M3	Promyelocytic leukaemia	Promyelocytes	Granulation prominent, Auer rods faggot like; variant has folded nuclei	SB+ NSE−
M4	Myelomonocytic leukaemia	Promyelocytes and myelocytes >20 per cent monocytic component	Both myeloid- and monocytoid-derived cells	SB+ NSE+
M5	Monoblastic leukaemia	Monoblasts	Promonocytes, monocytes	SB− NSE+
M6	Erythroleukaemia	>50 per cent erythroblasts	>30 per cent non-erythroid cells are blasts	SB± NSE− PAS±
M7	Megakaryoblastic leukaemia	Undifferentiated blasts	Blast cells may have cytoplasmic blebs, myelofibrosis	SB− NSE+

AML, acute myeloid leukaemia; SB, Sudan black, NSE, non-specific esterase.
From Bennett *et al.* (1985a,b), with permission.

nature of the infiltrate is usually apparent. This fibrosis is of no clinical or prognostic significance and tends to decrease with response to therapy. Extensive myelofibrosis is a feature of megakaryoblastic leukaemia (Bennett *et al.* 1985*b*) and also tends to improve with achievement of remission. In some protocols the response to treatment has been assessed by routine biopsy, but this is not recommended for standard practice. It is not customary or necessary to biopsy other organs at diagnosis in acute lymphoblastic leukaemia, although sometimes lymph node biopsy will have been performed in a child who presents with lymphadenopathy and a normal blood film. In such cases the node biopsy will be identical to appearances of lymphoblastic non-Hodgkin's lymphoma or, in the 1–2 per cent of cases with B-cell acute lymphoblastic leukaemia, of undifferentiated non-Hodgkin's lymphoma. Leukaemic infiltration of the testicle shows a uniform pattern which is interstitial in origin.

The pattern of leukaemic infiltration of the central nervous system determines the clinical features of central nervous system leukaemia and was well described in the early literature (Price and Johnson 1973). Focal intracerebral lesions are rare, although less so in acute myeloid leukaemia. The usual pattern is of infiltration of the arachnoid mater starting from the walls of the superficial veins and progressing to destruction of the arachnoid trabeculae and contamination of the cerebrospinal fluid. This is followed by denser infiltration of the deep arachnoid with interference with local perfusion, obstruction to cerebrospinal fluid flow, and raised intracranial pressure. Infiltration of the cerebrospinal fluid probably starts at the time of presentation when large numbers of leukaemic cells are present and conventional systemic therapy does not penetrate the central nervous system. The cells may proliferate slowly and in the absence of any central nervous system-directed therapy overt leukaemia may not become apparent for months or years. Children with acute lymphoblastic leukaemia with a high initial leucocyte count are at highest risk of central nervous system relapse (West *et al.* 1972), but there is no group of children with acute lymphoblastic leukaemia who are not at risk of this complication.

Immunology

The acute lymphoblastic leukaemias of childhood can be classified immunologically into abnormal proliferation of early B- or T-lymphoid cells (Foon and Todd 1986). The gradual recognition of this fact, which has paralleled the development of immunological techniques, has led to certain inconsistencies in nomenclature. The first immunological classification recognized the 10–15 per cent of cases of T-cell acute lymphoblastic leukaemia by their ability to form rosettes with sheep red cells, a property that is paralleled by the presence of the CD2 antigen. A tiny minority (1–2 per cent) of cases were recognized by the presence of surface membrane immunoglobulin as B-cell acute lymphoblastic leukaemia. The remainder, comprising the majority of cases, were classed as non-T, non-B acute lymphoblastic leukaemia, with a large majority, recognized by the presence of heterospecific antisera, as common acute lymphoblastic leukaemia. With the advent of monoclonal antibodies and techniques of molecular biology, it is now clear that the majority of these cases represent early B-cell acute lymphoblastic leukaemia.

Table 3 shows the main immunological subtypes of acute lymphoblastic leukaemia with the designation that will be given to them in this chapter. The recognition of these immunological subtypes has led to improved understanding of the biology of lymphoproliferative disease in childhood and emphasized the close relationship of childhood acute lymphoblastic leukaemia and non-Hodgkin's lymphoma. These subtypes are also of clinical significance, in that children with T-cell acute lymphoblastic leukaemia frequently present with a high leucocyte count, relatively high haemoglobin, and a relatively high incidence of mediastinal masses and have a relatively poor prognosis, although this is not independent of leucocyte count (Chessells *et al.* 1977). The 20–30 per cent of children with common acute leukaemia and cytoplasmic immunoglobulin (that is, with pre-B acute lymphoblastic leukaemia), have no distinct clinical features but have an apparently worse prognosis (Crist *et al.* 1989) which may, however, be overcome by more effective therapy (Raimondi *et al.* 1990).

The availability of monoclonal antibodies has helped to clarify diagnostic problems, in acute leukaemia (Chan *et al.* 1985). The immunological typing of cells in cerebrospinal fluid and other effusions may help in distinguishing between normal reactive and malignant cells. Of course, it must be emphasized that none of these antibodies is leukaemia specific and that viral infections, particularly in the young child, may cause a lymphocytosis or lymphocytic infiltration with a predominance of early B-cells.

In the myeloid leukaemias the use of monoclonal antibodies may identify cells of predominantly myeloid or monocytic lineage, but perhaps they are most useful in identifying the more unusual subtypes of acute myeloid leukaemia, for example glycophorin in M6 acute myeloid leukaemia and glycoprotein IIb/IIIa and factor VIII-related antigen in M7 acute myeloid leukaemia. There are many reports of acute leukaemia in which the leukaemic cells co-express markers normally believed to be restricted to a single lineage. It has been argued that such examples of apparent lineage infidelity reflect the existence of a transient phase of 'promiscuity' of gene expression which occurs in normal cells and remains as a relic in the leukaemic cell population (Greaves *et al.* 1986). The term hybrid acute leukaemia has been proposed for such cases (Gale and Bassat 1987) and it has been suggested that a distinction should be made between cases in which cells demonstrate both lymphoid and myeloid features and those in which there appear to be two distinct populations of cells. A relatively large number of well-described cases of hybrid acute leukaemia have been reported in

Table 3 Immunological classification of all main childhood subtypes

Immunological type	HLA DR	CD19 (B4)	CD10 (CALLA)	CD7 (WT1)	Cytoplasmic μ	Surface membrane Ig	TdT
Early B-cell acute lymphoblastic leukaemia							
Null	+	+	−	−	−	−	±
Common	+	+	+	−	−	−	+
(Pre-B)	+	+	+	−	+	−	+
B-cell acute lymphoblastic leukaemia	+	+	−	−	−	+	−
T-cell acute lymphoblastic leukaemia	±	−	±	+	−	−	+

CALLA, common acute lymphoblastic leukaemia antigen; TdT, terminal deoxynucleotidyl transferase.

association with the 4;11 translocation, either in infancy or in young adults; these tend to have a very poor prognosis (Arthur *et al.* 1982).

However, with the routine use of panels of monoclonal antibodies in phenotyping leukaemias there are increasing reports that a significant proportion of acute leukaemias exhibit some characteristics of mixed lineage or at least express unexpected antigen positivity. In one recent series of adult acute lymphoblastic leukaemia, 35 per cent of cases were reported to have expressed myeloid antigen positivity and this was associated with a worse prognosis (Sobol *et al.* 1987). A recent report from St Jude's Children's Hospital showed that in 372 cases of childhood acute lymphoblastic leukaemia 61 cases expressed at least one and 16 cases at least two myeloid antigens, usually CD11b and CD13. In contrast with the adult experience there was no relationship between myeloid antigen expression and prognosis (Pui *et al.* 1990*a*).

There are also reports of lymphoid antigen expression in acute myeloid leukaemia, in particular the CD2 and CD7 T-cell lineage markers; it has been reported that such cases may not respond to chemotherapy with a protocol designed for acute myeloid leukaemia but achieve remission with treatment as for acute lymphoblastic leukaemia (Cross *et al.* 1988). These observations about the response to treatment of mixed leukaemias require confirmation from larger studies. There is no evidence at present that the finding of both myeloid and lymphoid antigens should influence management and the choice of initial treatment.

Cytogenetics

Cytogenetic analysis of leukaemic blast cells is helpful in classification and assessment of prognosis and, at a more fundamental level, in focusing attention on specific areas of the genome where analysis may improve understanding of leukaemogenesis. Cytogenetic analysis is technically more difficult in acute lymphoblastic leukaemia than in acute myeloid leukaemia and failure to obtain an analysable result is not uncommon except in laboratories dedicated to this work. Before the advent of satisfactory banding techniques chromosomes in acute lymphoblastic leukaemia were classified by their modal number and it has been consistently shown that patients with high hyperdiploidy (>50 chromosomes) have a good prognosis; this finding is common in low count common acute lymphoblastic leukaemia (Secker Walker *et al.* 1989). There is evidence that ploidy of lymphoblasts is a strong predictor of treatment response and DNA index is relatively simple way of measuring this (Trueworthy *et al.* 1992). The outlook for hypodiploid and near-haploid acute lymphoblastic leukaemia is poor (Pui *et al.* 1990*b*). A large number, perhaps one-third, of patients in the early literature are described as having blast cells which are normal cytogenetically, but with improved techniques this proportion is decreasing and many of these cases are really pseudodiploid. At the same time it has become apparent that a number of non-random translocations and other changes which are of clinical and theoretical relevance occur in acute lymphoblastic leukaemia. A list of some of these changes is shown in Table 4, which also includes some of the commoner changes described in acute myeloid leukaemia. Some of these translocations are or have been associated with a poor prognosis and it has even been claimed that the presence of any translocation in acute lymphoblastic leukaemia is of adverse prognostic significance (Williams *et al.* 1986). However, this claim remains unconfirmed and seems unlikely, although it must also be recognized that improved therapy may influence the prognostic significance of cytogenetic abnormalities (Fletcher *et al.* 1989).

Table 4 More common non-random cytogenetic findings in acute leukaemia

Abnormality	Associated features	Significance
t(9;22)(q24;q23)	ALL or AML	Poor prognosis
t(4;11)(q21;q23) t(11;19)(q23;p13)	Null ALL often in infancy	Poor prognosis
t(1;19)(q23;p13)	Pre-B ALL	Prognosis uncertain
t(11;14)(p13;q13)	T-ALL	Uncertain
t(8;14)(q24;q32) t(8;22)(q24;q11) t(2;8)(p12;q24)	B-ALL	Previously poor prognosis; improved with modern therapy
12p12 break-point	Common ALL	Frequent finding
6q-	Common ALL	Frequent
t(8;21)(q22;q22)	M1/M2 AML	Chloromas
t(15;17)(q22;q12)	M3 AML	Early DIC and haemorrhage
Trisomy 8	AML	
Monosomy 7	AML	Poor response to induction
t(9;11) (p22;q23)	M5 AML	
inv(16) (p13;q22)	M4 eosinophilia	Good prognosis

ALL, acute lymphoblastic leukaemia; AML, acute myeloid leukaemia; B-ALL, B-cell lymphoblastic leukaemia; T-ALL, T-cell acute lymphoblastic leukaemia; DIC, disseminated intravascular coagulation.
Derived from Woods *et al.* (1985), Bloomfield *et al.* (1986), Raimondi *et al.* (1986), Williams *et al.* (1986), Secker Walker *et al.* (1989), and Kalwinsky *et al.* (1990).

Cytogenetic analysis in acute myeloid leukaemia has shown a number of translocations, usually associated with various morphological subtypes (Woods *et al.* 1985; Kalwinsky *et al.* 1990). Some of these may be associated with a poor response to treatment, but there is no firm evidence yet to decide treatment strategy on the basis of initial cytogenetic findings. As molecular analysis of cytogenetic abnormalities proceeds apace it seems highly likely that routine cytogenetic analysis in acute leukaemia will be replaced by use of a limited number of probes to identify clinically important cytogenetic abnormalities.

Molecular biology

The two main areas of interest in the molecular biology of childhood leukaemia have involved investigation of the rearrangements of the immunoglobulin and T-cell receptor genes in classification of acute lymphoblastic leukaemia and investigation of the regions of the genome associated with particular translocations. There have been a number of reports of other diverse abnormalities of oncogene mutation, amplification, and transcription in acute leukaemia. However, the significance of these is uncertain and they will not be considered here.

Chromosomal DNA in normal lymphoid cells contains non-contiguous germ-line loci for the immunoglobulin and T-cell receptor genes. These undergo a similar and complex series of changes in response to an immune stimulus involving rearrangement of so-called variable diversity and joining segments, resulting in the formation of a structurally distinct continuous VDJ region; thus the DNA in lymphocytes which have undergone rearrangement is no longer the same as that in unrearranged cells. Analysis of lymphocyte DNA by Southern blotting will not detect these myriad rearrangements in a population of normal lymphoid cells but the residual germ-line band of the cells which have not rearranged. In contrast, in cells which have undergone leukaemic transformation a consistent pattern of rearrangement, detected by Southern blotting, can be detected because acute lymphoblastic leukaemia is a clonal disease. The frequency of immunoglobulin (Ig) and T-cell receptor gene rearrangements has been studied with a variety of probes and restriction enzymes. The majority of cases of childhood acute lymphoblastic leukaemia of B-cell lineage show rearrangement of Ig heavy-chain genes, but only half show rearrangement of light-chain and T-cell receptor genes. In early B-cell acute lymphoblastic leukaemia of infancy a smaller proportion of cases show IgL rearrangements. Thus it is increasingly possible to combine molecular and immunological classification of acute lymphoblastic leukaemia, although the practical relevance of this approach is as yet unclear.

A further application of these techniques is in investigation of bone-marrow samples in apparent remission for the presence of minimal residual disease. Morphological examination of remission bone-marrows is extremely insensitive: the limit of detection of abnormal cells is at best 1–5 per cent, although with appropriate probes Southern blotting may increase this sensitivity to 0.5–1 per cent (Katz *et al.* 1989).

The sensitivity of molecular detection is enhanced dramatically by use of the polymerase chain reaction. The sensitivity of molecular detection is enhanced dramatically by use of the polymerase chain reaction. Preliminary reports show that, unsurprisingly, residual disease is detectable at the end of induction therapy in children in apparent remission (Wasserman *et al.* 1992). However, the absence of detectable residual disease at the end of chemotherapy may not ensure freedom from later relapse (Ito *et al.* 1993). Clearly large prospective studies are needed to discern the clinical value of these techniques.

The investigation of specific translocations is providing possible insights into leukaemogenesis. The most notable example is the Ph[1] chromosome, where the c-*abl* gene is translocated from chromosome 9 to chromosome 22 disrupting the *bcr* gene on that chromosome. The resulting fusion of the two genes codes for the production of a protein activating as a tyrosine-specific protein kinase. In Ph[1]-positive acute lymphoblastic leukaemia the break-point on chromosome 22 occurs at a different site and fusion products and proteins of lower molecular weight are produced (Kurzrock *et al.* 1988).

Similarly, in the translocation 8;14 seen in B-cell leukaemia the c-*myc* proto-oncogene which is encoded on chromosome 8q24 is fused near the Ig heavy chain gene at 14q32 (Davis *et al.* 1984). The c-*myc* proto-oncogene acts in the nucleus and may be involved in the regulation of transition of cells from resting to proliferative state. It has been suggested that deregulation of c-*myc* expression may contribute to malignant transformation. More recent analysis of specific translocations has identified other genetic abnormalities, most notably rearrangement of the MLL gene in a variety of leukaemias with 11q23 involvement (Thirman *et al.* 1993) and the retinoic acid receptor-alpha gene in the t15;17 (Warrell *et al.* 1993).

PRESENTATION AND DIAGNOSIS

Clinical features

The clinical features of acute leukaemia arise from the effects of marrow failure and the accumulation of malignant cells. The symptoms may precede the diagnosis by weeks or months. Certain clinical features may be suggestive of a particular type of leukaemia, but there are no specific clinical features predictive of a diagnosis of either acute myeloid leukaemia or acute lymphoblastic leukaemia. The symptoms are usually non-specific and include lethargy, pallor,

easy or spontaneous bruising, fever, or an infection. Breathlessness is usually due to anaemia, but it may be indicative of respiratory obstruction or a pleural effusion. Headache or giddiness in an older child may also be suggestive of anaemia, but occasionally of leucostasis or overt central nervous system infiltration. Bone pain and/or limping are extremely common symptoms. Rarely, polydipsia and polyuria may be symptomatic of hypercalcaemia.

Clinical examination may show no abnormal features other than pallor, petechiae, and bruises. Large lumpy bruises are suggestive of disseminated intravascular coagulation, a feature of hypergranular promyelocytic leukaemia but also seen in other forms of acute myeloid leukaemia. Slight to moderate enlargement of lymph nodes is common and the liver and or spleen may be enlarged, sometimes markedly so. Bilateral renal enlargement may mimic hepatospleno-megaly; in such cases there may be hypertension. Bony tenderness is common and, if symptoms have been long-standing, there may be muscle wasting. Joint effusions may be seen in some children in association with bone pain. Pleural effusions are most frequently found in children with T-cell acute lymphoblastic leukaemia but also, like pericardial effusions, may occur in acute myeloid leukaemia with a monocytic component. Skin infiltration, typical of this variant in infancy, is also a feature of the rare case of pre-B-cell acute lymphoblastic leukaemia in the young infant.

Examination of the mouth may show ulceration, bleeding, candida, gingivitis, or gum hypertrophy. Infiltration of the central nervous system may be suggested by the presence of papilloedema, which must be distinguished from retinal infiltration, cranial nerve palsies, or occasionally spinal cord compression. Leukaemic iritis is associated with photophobia, irregular pupils, and the presence of cells in the anterior chamber. Both retinal deposits and iritis are rare at presentation, although well-recognized sites of relapse (Ninane *et al.* 1980).

Similarly painless swelling of one or both testicles, a frequent sign of relapse in acute lymphoblastic leukaemia, may occur as a presenting feature in perhaps 1–2 per cent of boys.

Diagnosis

The diagnosis of acute leukaemia is confirmed by examination of the blood film and bone-marrow. It is absolutely essential to obtain adequate samples of blood and marrow before starting specific treatment. While urgent measures to ensure supportive care, such as treatment of infection, are always indicated, there is usually no reason to start antileukaemic therapy until results of investigations have been obtained and no harm is done by awaiting these results.

The distribution of haematological findings in a national trial of treatment of acute lymphoblastic leukaemia (Medical Research Council UKALL X) is shown in Table 5. Since the trial included over 90 per cent of cases in the United Kingdom, the findings are probably representative. The majority of children with acute

Table 5 Haematological findings in acute lymphoblastic leukaemia at presentation

WBC (×10⁹/l)	< 20	20–	50–	100+
	62%	16%	9%	13%
Hb (g/dl)	< 7	10–	10+	
	54%	33%	13%	
Platelets (×10⁹/l)	< 50	50–	100	150+
	53%	21%	11%	15%

From 1300 children aged 0–15 years.
Data from Medical Research Council UKALL X with permission.

Table 6 Age and FAB class in acute myeloid leukaemia

Age	M1	M2	M3	M4	M5	M6	M7	Unclassified	Total
<6 months	0	0	0	1	3	2	2	0	8
6 months–1 year	2	1	0	3	6	2	1	0	15
1–2 years	1	5	2	4	11	2	1	0	26
2–10 years	7	25	4	20	11	7	0	1	75
7–10 years	6	13	4	9	5	2	0	2	41
Totals	16	44	10	37	36	15	4	3	165
	(10%)	(27%)	(6%)	(22%)	(22%)	(9%)	(2%)	(2%)	

Data from Hospital for Sick Children, Great Ormond Street, 1972–1987.

lymphoblastic leukaemia are anaemic and thrombocytopenic, but the platelet count is normal in 15 per cent of patients. There is virtually always an absolute neutropenia in acute lymphoblastic leukaemia, but the white cell count is frequently raised with the majority of the cells being lymphoblasts and lymphocytes. The findings in acute myeloid leukaemia are more diverse, depending on the subtype, with abnormal myeloid precursors, neutrophils, and monocytes in addition to blast cells. The frequency of acute myeloid leukaemia subtypes in childhood is shown in Table 6.

Bone-marrow aspiration is mandatory in all cases and whenever adequate marrow cannot be obtained by aspiration a trephine biopsy should be performed. The distinction between acute lymphoblastic leukaemia and acute myeloid leukaemia is usually apparent, but should always be supplemented by cytochemistry, especially Sudan black and non-specific esterase and immunological and cytogenetic analysis should be performed whenever possible.

Differential diagnosis

Infections in childhood

Infectious mononucleosis and other viral infections in childhood may bear a superficial resemblance to acute lymphoblastic leukaemia, particularly if there is associated anaemia and thrombocytopenia. However, the blood film in such infections usually shows pleomorphic mononuclear cells and the diagnosis is confirmed by appropriate virological investigations. The bone-marrow in young children contains a high proportion of lymphoid cells, which, particularly in viral infections, may be CD10 and Tdt positive. The enlarged lymph nodes in such children will show reactive change on biopsy, whereas in acute lymphoblastic leukaemia lymph node biopsy will show appearances of a lymphoblastic lymphoma.

Serious sepsis in the young child may be associated with pancytopenia and a predominance of early myeloid cells in the bone-marrow, thus particularly mimicking acute myeloid leukaemia. More unusual infections such as kala-azar, associated with fever and splenomegaly, may also pose diagnostic problems.

In summary, a variety of haematological abnormalities can occur in the young child with infection. If there is the slightest concern about infection as a possible primary diagnosis, a period of observation and supportive care is essential.

Juvenile rheumatoid arthritis

Bone and joint pain are common in acute leukaemia and may be suggestive of Still's disease. In such cases there may be a moderate anaemia, but the platelet and leucocyte count are normal. Bone and joint radiography, when performed in children with an arthritic type of presentation, often show the characteristic changes suggestive

of leukaemia: periosteal reaction, metaphyseal bands, and single or multiple lytic lesions. Occasionally a child is treated with steroids after an erroneous diagnosis of juvenile arthritis; the resultant remission is subsequently followed by leukaemic relapse. Children inappropriately treated in this way probably have a poor prognosis and it is imperative that the differential diagnosis of leukaemia is considered in every child with bone pains.

Aplastic anaemia and pure red cell aplasia

Children with acute leukaemia may present with pancytopenia and no blast cells in the blood or with a normochronic normocytic anaemia. The distinction should be resolved by bone-marrow aspiration or trephine biopsy. The hypocellularity of the trephine in marrow aplasia should be readily distinguished from the cellular infiltrate, with or without associated fibrosis, seen in acute leukaemia. The residual lymphocytes seen in aplastic anaemia may have the immunological features of early lymphoid cells, CD10 positive and Tdt positive. The bone-marrow in pure red cell aplasia (Diamond Blackfan anaemia), particularly in the young child, contains many lymphoid cells which may suggest acute lymphoblastic leukaemia to the unwary.

There are a number of reports in the literature of children with aplastic anaemia responding to steroid therapy and then developing acute lymphoblastic leukaemia, but these cases almost certainly represent steroid-induced remissions. Children may also present with pancytopenia (a hypoplastic marrow), undergo spontaneous remission, and subsequently develop acute lymphoblastic leukaemia, which is nearly always of the common subtype; this aplastic prodrome does not have a worse prognosis (Breatnach *et al.* 1981).

Megaloblastic anaemia

Megaloblastic anaemia is rare in childhood and in the young infant is as often due to metabolic defects such as transcobalamin II deficiency as to lack of folic acid or B12. Severe megaloblastic change in the bone-marrow in a child with pancytopenia may be confused with acute myeloid leukaemia, but the diagnosis can be confirmed by appropriate investigations such as the DU suppression test.

Other lymphoproliferative disorders

Non-Hodgkin's lymphomas of childhood are a group of disorders of early B- and T-cells which are histologically, cytologically, and immunologically indistinguishable from acute lymphoblastic leukaemia. The distinction between non-Hodgkin's lymphoma and acute lymphoblastic leukaemia in childhood is thus somewhat arbitrary, usually based on the presence of more than 25 per cent blasts in the bone-marrow or of blasts in the blood. Some protocols make this distinction with additional emphasis on the presence or absence of bulk disease and the American Children's Cancer Study Group defines a group of children with so-called leukaemia–lymphoma syndrome (Miller *et al.* 1983) who usually have features of T-cell acute lymphoblastic leukaemia.

Despite some evidence that patients with T-cell non-Hodgkin's lymphoma may have blast cells of a more mature phenotype than those with T-cell acute lymphoblastic leukaemia, there is no real evidence that these are distinct entities. In practice the difference between non-Hodgkin's lymphoma and acute lymphoblastic leukaemia is not as important as the choice of an appropriate treatment strategy (see below) and in this context the most important distinction is between those children with massive abdominal tumours with or without marrow infiltration together with those with B-cell acute lymphoblastic leukaemia and the great majority of others with either early B-cell acute lymphoblastic leukaemia or T-cell acute lymphoblastic leukaemia.

Other myeloproliferative disorders

Chronic myeloproliferative disorders in children are rare. The most common are adult Ph[1]-positive chronic myeloid leukaemia, which resembles the disease seen in adults, juvenile chronic myeloid leukaemia, and the syndrome of monosomy 7. Juvenile chronic myeloid leukaemia may usually be suspected on clinical grounds by the presence of a facial rash, suppurative lymph nodes, prominent bleeding, and high fetal haemoglobin. The blood and bone-marrow appearances are usually those of chronic myelomonocytic leukaemia, but in some cases the picture may be predominantly one resembling M6 erythroleukaemia. It is important to recognize this distinction because juvenile chronic myeloid leukaemia responds very poorly to chemotherapy and the treatment of choice is allogeneic bone-marrow transplantation.

The myelodysplastic syndromes have not been as well characterized in children as in adults (Bennett *et al.* 1982), but all the recognized variants have been described. If there is doubt about the rate of progression to acute myeloid leukaemia, then observation and supportive care are appropriate.

Disseminated tumours

Bone-marrow infiltration with disseminated tumours of childhood may mimic the appearance of an unusual leukaemia. Over half of children with neuroblastoma have disseminated disease at presentation and the findings of bone and joint pain, lytic lesions on radiography, and marrow infiltration resemble those of acute leukaemia. However, the blood film usually shows a leucoerythroblastic anaemia, the marrow infiltration shows characteristic clumping, and the diagnosis may be confirmed by the finding of raised urinary catecholamines and identification of the primary tumour, frequently a calcified suprarenal mass. Bone-marrow infiltration may also be seen in soft tissue sarcomas, Ewing's tumour, and occasionally retinoblastoma.

Occasionally a child may present with bone pain, skeletal lesions, and marrow infiltration with tumour cells and no obvious primary tumour. Examination of the tumour cells may show positivity with desmin or some other antibody suggestive of a connective tissue origin. It is important to distinguish some cases from those of leukaemia since they may respond to appropriate therapy and will not remit on protocols devised for acute leukaemia.

INVESTIGATIONS AND MANAGEMENT STRATEGY

Once the diagnosis of acute leukaemia has been confirmed by examination of the blood and bone-marrow, appropriate investigations should be performed to determine whether there is any overt infiltration of the central nervous system or any derangement of hepatic or renal function and to establish baseline investigations to facilitate management of possible future infections.

Radiology

Chest radiography, both posteroanterior and lateral, should be performed in all cases to determine whether there is thymic enlargement, mediastinal widening due to lymph node enlargement, or pleural effusion. Enlargement of the thymus or a pleural effusion are suggestive of T-cell acute lymphoblastic leukaemia and in some reports are of adverse prognostic significance. A pleural effusion may occasionally occur in acute myeloid leukaemia; in monocytic leukaemias this is a leukaemic effusion, but in M3 acute myeloid leukaemia it may be a haemorrhagic effusion associated with pulmonary infarction.

Ultrasound of the abdomen is useful in the child with acute leukaemia to assess renal size and occasionally to distinguish renal infiltration from enlargement of the liver and spleen. Children with extensive renal involvement may be at increased risk of metabolic complications after treatment is started. There is no real need for any other routine radiological investigation in children with acute leukaemia. Skeletal radiography and/or bone scan may have been prompted by the finding of bone pain or tenderness, but abnormal findings, while common, do not affect management, choice of therapy, or prognosis in the vast majority of patients. Radiography of the wrist for bone age may provide a useful baseline for subsequent long-term follow-up of growth.

CT of the brain has been used to monitor the neurotoxicity of central nervous system directed therapy, but is of little or no value in the diagnosis of central nervous system infiltration. The place of magnetic resonance imaging (MRI) in this context is not clearly established.

Cerebrospinal fluid

Lumbar puncture is essential to determine whether there is overt infiltration of the central nervous system, which is present in 1–2 per cent of cases at presentation. Since this dictates subsequent management, it is essential that a clear sample of cerebrospinal fluid is obtained. A cell count is performed and then a cytocentrifuged sample of cerebrospinal fluid is examined to determine whether leukaemic blasts are present. Involvement of the cerebrospinal fluid is usually defined by the finding of more than 5 cells/mm^3 which must be recognizable blast cells; this definition is of necessity somewhat arbitrary.

Biochemistry

Blood should be taken for tests of serum urea, creatinine, electrolytes, liver function, and serum proteins including calcium, phosphate, and plasma urate. The most common finding in the presence of a large tumour mass is of a raised plasma uric acid, but urea and creatinine may be raised in children with renal infiltration. Hypercalcaemia is rare, but may occur in children with acute lymphoblastic leukaemia, usually of the common acute lymphoblastic leukaemia subtype; not all have obvious bony lesions.

Microbiology

Appropriate cultures of blood, urine, and any lesions are necessary if the patient is febrile, but it is also important to take a history of previous childhood infections and note previous immunizations. Serum should be taken for investigation of immunity to varicella-zoster, measles, and cytomegalovirus and for storage to act as a baseline in the event of future infections.

Management strategy

The child with acute leukaemia is usually anaemic, thrombocytopenic, and febrile and may be acutely ill at presentation. Approximately 1–2 per cent of children with acute lymphoblastic leukaemia and at least 5 per cent with acute myeloid leukaemia die in the first few weeks of treatment without achieving a remission. The first aim of management is to prevent such deaths by treating any presumed infection and bleeding, correcting profound anaemia if present, identifying and preventing metabolic derangements, and obtaining material for diagnosis. Once the patient's condition has been stabilized, a more leisurely appraisal for the choice of protocol for remission induction and post-remission therapy can ensue. The management of these early problems is considered here and details of specific treatment are given later.

Biochemical problems

Electrolyte disturbances

Patients most at risk of electrolyte disturbances are those with a large leukaemic cell mass, enlarged kidneys, or both and particularly those with T-cell and B-cell acute lymphoblastic leukaemia. Children with M4 and M5 acute myeloid leukaemia may, in addition, have tubular leak of electrolytes due to renal damage by lysosymes.

The rapid lysis of leukaemic cells in response to cytotoxic chemotherapy may cause hyperkalaemia, hyperphosphataemia, and hypocalcaemia. Electrolytes should be monitored and any abnormality corrected before starting any cytotoxic chemotherapy and potential hyperkalaemia should be monitored by ECG in vulnerable patients since lysis of cells may cause spurious values. Regular monitoring during the period of lysis is essential and if abnormalities cannot be corrected dialysis may be indicated. Continuing abnormalities during the induction period are usually exacerbated by the inevitable use of antibiotics and amphotericin.

Some believe that these complications are minimized by the gradual introduction of chemotherapy, for example steroids preceding cytotoxics for 24 h in high-risk patients, but there is little evidence for or against this approach.

Urate nephropathy

The serum uric acid may be raised before treatment, particularly in children with a large cell mass. The lysis of tumour cells at the start of chemotherapy liberates purines which are converted to hypoxanthine, xanthine, and uric acid by the action of xanthine oxidase. Deposition of uric acid in the renal parenchyma may then cause renal failure which can be prevented in the majority of cases by ensuring adequate hydration of, for example 3 l/m² per day, and by administration of the xanthine oxidase inhibitor allopurinol at a dose of 300–600 mg/m² for 24 h before starting chemotherapy. Despite these measures, haemodialysis may be needed in some patients if renal function deteriorates.

Abnormalities of haemostasis

Bleeding in a child with acute leukaemia is usually due to thrombocytopenia and should be prevented by administration of platelet concentrates at an initial dose of 4–5 units/m². During induction and intensive treatment, as for acute myeloid leukaemia it is desirable to keep the count above 30×10⁹/l; bleeding is more likely to occur in the presence of infection.

A proportion of early deaths in acute leukaemia, particularly acute myeloid leukaemia, may be due to bleeding, particularly in association with disseminated intravascular coagulation, which may occur in any type of leukaemia, most often in association with a high leucocyte count, but is most dramatic in patients with M3 acute myeloid leukaemia. The liberation of thromboplastins from the abnormal myeloid cells induces intravascular coagulation which may cause fatal bleeding before the onset of treatment but is exacerbated once treatment starts and may sometimes cause thrombosis or pulmonary embolus. It is therefore essential to recognize this variant of acute myeloid leukaemia and to perform initial screening tests of haemostasis in all patients. The mainstay of management is liberal use of platelet concentrates, which may need to be given twice daily, and correction of coagulation abnormalities with fresh frozen plasma. Treatment with ALL *trans* retinoic acid (Warrell *et al.* 1993) frequently produces improvement in the coagulopathy.

Leucostasis and hyperviscosity

Patients with a high initial leucocyte count, greater than 100×10⁹/l and particularly greater than 200×10⁹/l, are at increased risk of early death from cerebrovascular leucostasis and haemorrhage. Such children, if older, will complain of lethargy, headache, giddiness, and disturbed vision and in extreme cases may be comatose. Even if these children are anaemic, simple transfusion of packed cells may exacerbate symptoms by increasing blood viscosity and should be avoided. This is one of the few circumstances where urgent cytoreduction is indicated and should proceed with adequate platelet support to prevent bleeding. A variety of measures have been advocated in these circumstances, including leucopheresis and low-dose irradiation, but in most cases a safe reduction in count can be achieved by adequate hydration, maintaining haemostasis and reduction of the count with steroids in acute lymphoblastic leukaemia and cytotoxics or hydroxyurea in acute myeloid leukaemia. If it is essential to raise the haemoglobin level to prevent heart failure, a modest rise in haemoglobin level can be achieved by partial exchange transfusion. This conservative approach to management is usually more satisfactory than an inexperienced attempt to leucophorese a sick child.

Other emergencies at presentation

Occasionally children with T-cell acute lymphoblastic leukaemia may present with respiratory embarrassment due to a pleural effusion or mediastinal obstruction. Such patients improve rapidly with steroid therapy, which should be accompanied by adequate hydration and allopurinol.

Spinal cord compression is a rare emergency at presentation, requiring prompt treatment with systemic cytotoxics if the compression is extradural and concurrent intrathecal therapy if associated with blast cells in the cerebrospinal fluid. However, this presentation is more common in non-Hodgkin's lymphoma of the B-cell type.

Early infective complications

Most children with acute leukaemia are either pyrexial on admission or become so within 2 weeks of starting treatment. There may be few or no signs of local infection in the absence of neutrophils and fever or malaise may be the only symptoms of a septicaemia which, if untreated, may lead to death within hours. The child who is febrile and neutropenic ($<0.5 \times 10^9$/l) requires urgent examination, cultures of blood and any suspicious focus of infection, and broad spectrum intravenous antibiotic therapy pending the results of microbiological investigations; this therapy must provide adequate cover against Gram-negative organisms and a suitable combination would comprise a combination of an aminoglycoside and either a cephalosporin or ureidopenicillin. The increasing use of intravenous catheters has been followed by an increase in Gram-positive infections and some authors recommend the use of vancomycin in early empirical therapy. However, the combination suggested has some Gram-positive cover and these Gram-positive catheter-associated infections do not have the rapid course associated with Gram-negative septicaemia.

Children undergoing induction therapy for acute myeloid leukaemia have prolonged and profound neutropenia and are at risk of systemic fungal infection with *Aspergillus* and *Candida* species. The neutropenic child with fever who is unresponsive to antibiotics should, like adults, be considered at high risk of fungal infection and in the absence of any obvious cause for fever be treated empirically with intravenous amphotericin.

RISK GROUPS AND PROGNOSIS

Unfortunately, despite various international efforts, there is no real uniformity in reporting the results of therapeutic trials in childhood leukaemia and no general agreement about the definition of an average or poor risk patient. Children with acute leukaemia who are cured are, in general, those in whom the first remission is achieved and maintained for 6–8 years of follow-up. Thus, the most useful measure of potential cure is that of event-free survival, which represents all children achieving and remaining in first remission.

Acute lymphoblastic leukaemia

Over 90 per cent of children with acute lymphoblastic leukaemia achieve remission and for over 20 years there have been attempts to identify prognostic factors, that is, those clinical and laboratory findings at presentation which influence the chance of long-term remission. Some of these are indicated in Table 7. The factors have varied in ease of comparison from age at presentation and highest pre-treatment leucocyte count to the presence or absence of a

Table 7 Some adverse prognostic factors in acute lymphoblastic leukaemia

Clinical features	Age <1 and >10 years*
	Organomegaly
	Mediastinal mass on radiography
	Negro race
	Male sex*
	CNS disease at presentation
Laboratory features	High initial leucocyte count*
	High Hb level
	Low immunoglobulin
	L2-ALL
	T-ALL
	Pre-B-ALL*
	Certain translocations
Speed of response	Residual blasts on day 14*

See references in text.
CNS, central nervous system; ALL, acute lymphoblastic leukaemia; B-ALL, B-cell acute lymphoblastic leukaemia; T-ALL, T-cell acute lymphoblastic leukaemia.
*Prognostic features which in most series are retained on multivariate analysis.

translocation in the leukaemic cells. Of course, none of these factors take account of treatment, which is one of the most important determinants of prognosis and the fact that prognostic factors may vary according to treatment protocol. Thus, as modern treatment has cured more children with acute lymphoblastic leukaemia, it has become apparent that girls have benefited more than boys (Medical Research Council 1978a; Sather *et al.* 1981). The recognition of B-cell acute lymphoblastic leukaemia as a separate subtype of leukaemia, which is similar immunologically and cytogenetically to B-cell non-Hodgkin's lymphoma, has led to the development of new protocols for B-cell acute lymphoblastic leukaemia, with cure of what was previously a uniformly fatal disease (Hann *et al.* 1990).

Clinical and laboratory features

As shown in Table 7, age is an important prognostic factor in acute lymphoblastic leukaemia, with infants under 1 year and children over 10 years having a particularly poor prognosis (Sather 1986). Infants tend to have a distinct type of acute lymphoblastic leukaemia characterized by organomegaly, high leucocyte counts, and early B-cell phenotype associated with cytogenetic translocations involving chromosome 11 in the region of q23 (Katz *et al.* 1990). Biological differences in acute lymphoblastic leukaemia are not as apparent in older children and adolescents, who, however, also respond less well to treatment (Santana *et al.* 1990).

There is a direct relationship between the extent of disease at presentation and the chances of long-term remission and this is most readily measured in the height of the initial leucocyte count but is seen in other measures of bulk disease such as organomegaly. Thus, it has been suggested that reports of all protocols for acute lymphoblastic leukaemia should review infants under 1 year separately and give the results of treatment in two main groups of patients: children between 2 and 10 years of age with an initial leucocyte count of $<50 \times 10^9$/l and the remainder (Mastrangelo *et al.* 1986).

Response to treatment

Response is most readily assessed by looking at the proportion of blast cells remaining in the marrow at 14 days or in some reports at 7 days from the start of treatment. Slow response to treatment is predictive for both early and late relapse of acute lymphoblastic leukaemia (Miller *et al.* 1989).

Immunology and cytology

The importance of recognizing B-cell acute lymphoblastic leukaemia has been mentioned and it is clear that, overall, children with T-cell acute lymphoblastic leukaemia have a worse prognosis than those with common acute lymphoblastic leukaemia. However, multivariate analysis, which is essential in determining whether prognostic factors are truly independent, shows in most reports that the influence of T-cell acute lymphoblastic leukaemia on prognosis is largely related to leucocyte count. There have been numerous reports that patients with larger and more anaplastic L2 blast cells have a worse prognosis than those with L1 acute lymphoblastic leukaemia and this may relate to the fact that L2 blasts have a greater proportion of cells in DNA synthesis.

Cytogenetics

It is apparent that modal chromosome number influences prognosis and that patients with a high number of hyperdiploid cells have a good prognosis most readily identified by measurement of ploidy. A number of non-random translocations have been identified in acute lymphoblastic leukaemia (see above), but it is probably premature to claim, as the St Jude's group has done, that all translocations carry an adverse prognosis.

Staging systems for acute lymphoblastic leukaemia thus remain unsatisfactory, with various national groups stratifying patients for treatment according to a variety of systems which vary in complexity from the algorithm of the American Children's Cancer Study Group, allocating patients to one of five protocols (Miller *et al.* 1980) through the German risk score (Riehm *et al.* 1987) to the Medical Research Council which still relies on leucocyte count.

Acute myeloid leukaemia

Hitherto, the poor prognosis for acute myeloid leukaemia has really precluded the identification of risk groups. There is some evidence (Creutzig *et al.* 1987*b*; Grier *et al.* 1987) that patients with high leucocyte counts and with monocytic leukaemia have a worse prognosis, but these indications await confirmation in larger series.

MANAGEMENT OF ACUTE LEUKAEMIA

The overwhelming majority of children with acute leukaemia who are cured are those who have achieved and remained in a first remission. Some children may be cured after relapse, but the morbidity of retreatment is considerable and the risk of recurrence after a relapse persists for many years (Chessells *et al.* 1987*a*).

Therefore it is absolutely imperative that an appropriate management plan is made by the physician first involved in treatment. It is strongly recommended that all children with acute leukaemia are managed in collaboration with a paediatric oncology centre or at least in clinical trials or standard protocols. The benefits of this approach have been shown again recently in an independent analysis in the United Kingdom (Stiller and Draper 1989). There is overwhelming evidence that children treated in this way do better than those managed by the casual therapist.

With the obsession with risk groups, particularly in acute lymphoblastic leukaemia, there is an increasing tendency to stratify patients at diagnosis and treat them on standard or high-risk protocols. This approach is used in almost all clinical trials. The discussion below will not focus on risk groups but will review the role of various phases of treatment in the management plan.

Remission induction

The initial chemotherapeutic approach in the child with acute leukaemia, whatever the subsequent management involves one of three treatment approaches: for acute lymphoblastic leukaemia, for acute myeloid leukaemia, and for the 1–2 per cent of cases with acute lymphoblastic leukaemia and L3 SmIg+ B-cell acute lymphoblastic leukaemia, usually associated with the characteristic translocations.

The combination of oral prednisolone and weekly intravenous vincristine induces remission in over 90 per cent of children with acute lymphoblastic leukaemia and with the addition of L-asparaginase the remission rate rises to over 95 per cent (Ortega *et al.* 1977). There is evidence that the use of a third drug in induction improves the chances of long-term remission so that all children with acute lymphoblastic leukaemia should receive, as a minimum, these three drugs in induction. A variety of other combinations, such as methotrexate (Clavell *et al.* 1986), etoposide, and cytarabine (Rivera *et al.* 1985) or an anthracycline (van der Does-van den Berg 1989), have been added early in treatment, particularly in high-risk patients. The benefits of any of these drugs are not clear and they are not recommended outside the context of a clinical trial. However, it is advisable to start central nervous system-directed therapy during induction and this is most conveniently achieved with intrathecal methotrexate.

The main problems encountered during this type of induction treatment are those of bone-marrow suppression, but the blood count will start to recover after 2–3 weeks of treatment. Thrombotic episodes have been described during induction with L-asparaginase (Priest *et al.* 1980), but are rare and are not usually followed by long-term neurological deficit. Most children achieve remission with a cellular marrow by 4 weeks; failure to remit is most often seen in children with high initial leucocyte counts and Ph[1]-positive acute lymphoblastic leukaemia and is a very poor prognostic sign. More intensive induction therapy may prolong myelosuppression and increase the risk of sepsis, but with proper supportive care the death rate during induction should not exceed 1 per cent.

Children with B-cell acute lymphoblastic leukaemia do not usually achieve remission with standard acute lymphoblastic leukaemia therapy or, if they do, will rapidly relapse. Treatment should comprise a protocol with cyclophosphamide, anthracyclines, cytarabine, and methotrexate as used for non-Hodgkin's lymphoma of childhood; with this type of short-term intensive treatment, including central nervous system-directed therapy, most children achieve remission and many may be cured (Hann *et al.* 1990).

The most effective combination of drugs for remission induction in acute myeloid leukaemia is an anthracycline plus cytarabine, with the latter given by 12 hourly push or continuous intravenous infusion for 7–10 days; daunorubicin is less toxic and as effective as adriamycin in this context (Buckley *et al.* 1989*b*). There is uncertainty about the benefit of adding a third drug such as etoposide or thioguanine. The present Medical Research Council acute myeloid leukaemia trial for both children and adults involves a randomized comparison of either thioguanine or etoposide with a combination of daunorubicin for 3 days and cytarabine for 10 days. This type of regimen produces severe myelosuppression for up to 5 or 6 weeks and inevitably causes weight loss and gastrointestinal toxicity. If possible, a Hickman catheter should be inserted before the start of specific therapy to facilitate blood product support, intravenous antibiotics, and parenteral nutrition. With proper supportive care, remission should be achieved after one to two courses in at least 85 per cent of children. It is particularly important to evaluate the reason for induction failure in acute myeloid leukaemia and the criteria defined by Preisler (1978) distinguishing between early death from haemorrhage or leucostasis, failure of blast cell regression or early regrowth of blasts, and death from prolonged marrow hypoplasia are useful in this respect.

Definition of remission

The conventional definition of remission in both acute lymphoblastic leukaemia and acute myeloid leukaemia is the achievement of a normal blood count (neutrophils, $> 1.0 \times 10^9$/l; platelets, $> 100 \times 10^9$/l), no evidence of extramedullary disease, and less than 5 per cent blasts in a cellular marrow. In practice, it can be difficult to distinguish between normal blast cells and leukaemic blasts and the limitations of conventional light microscopy are obvious. There have been efforts to improve the detection of minimal residual disease by immunological analysis with double labelling of cells, for example with CD10 and CD19 or by Southern blotting to detect rearrangements of the Ig or T-cell receptor genes. These methods are more sensitive than light microscopy, while the use of the polymerase chain reaction has the potential ability to increase

ACUTE LEUKAEMIA IN CHILDHOOD

sensitivity many-fold. However, it remains to be determined whether systematic attempts to detect minimal residual disease will prove feasible and useful in clinical practice.

In acute myeloid leukaemia there is conflicting evidence as to whether remission involves re-emergence of normal bone-marrow cells or maturation of the leukaemic clone (Fialkow *et al.* 1987), but most evidence favours the former.

Post-remission therapy

Acute lymphoblastic leukaemia

Intensification

There is increasing evidence that following intensive induction some form of post-remission intensification improves event-free survival, at least in children with high-risk acute lymphoblastic leukaemia. The first strong proponents of the benefits of this phase of treatment were the West German BFM group whose original protocol incorporated a four-drug induction and a 4 week period of intensification (Riehm *et al.* 1980). The group introduced a period of intensification for high-risk patients in a subsequent unrandomized study and found that survival had improved in the patients in comparison with historical controls (Riehm *et al.* 1987). These results were in marked contrast with most previous randomized trials, which had failed to show a benefit for post-remission intensification; when reviewed in retrospect the majority of these early schedules were not very intensive, involving, for example a course of parenteral mercaptopurine and methotrexate or modest doses of cyclophosphamide and cytarabine (Chessells 1986).

Many of the strongest claims for the benefits of intensive treatment and the best results have, as is commonly the case, been derived from non-randomized single-arm studies such as that recently reported by Clavell *et al.* (1986). However, recent attempts by the BFM group to modify treatment by randomizing low-risk patients to omit intensification resulted in a worse outcome (Henze *et al.* 1990). A prospective randomized trial by the American Children's Cancer Study Group has shown that for children with high-risk acute lymphoblastic leukaemia (the most important determinant being an initial WBC of $>50\times10^9/l$) treatment with a modified BFM protocol with early and late intensification and simple continuing (maintenance) therapy or with a complicated multiple rotating drug schedule is statistically superior to standard three-drug induction and continuing treatment. Other randomized trials in the United States and the United Kingdom (Medical Research Council UKALL X) are addressing this question and show a significant benefit for one or more periods of intensification (Chessells *et al.* 1992; Tubergen *et al.* 1993).

Thus, on balance, there is evidence that, outside the context of a clinical trial, a period of post-remission intensification is of benefit, at least in the high-risk child. Further randomized trials are needed to clarify the optimum timing, dose intensity, and need for repeated courses of such intensification.

Maintenance therapy

The concept of so-called maintenance therapy (long-term low-dose continuing therapy on an out-patient basis) is perhaps unique to acute lymphoblastic leukaemia. Most early protocols for acute lymphoblastic leukaemia, even those comprising combination chemotherapy which involved treatment for up to 15 months, were associated with an extremely high relapse rate once treatment was stopped (Chessells 1986). Thus, it became customary to treat children with acute lymphoblastic leukaemia on completion of induction and intensification with low-dose continuing treatment for 2–3 years. Clearly, an infinite number of protocols can be and have been devised for continuing treatment and it may be that the optimum type of treatment depends on the biological characteristics of the leukaemia and the initial treatment. For example, B-cell acute lymphoblastic leukaemia is curable after short-term intensive protocols and patients do not receive maintenance therapy after bone-marrow transplantation in first remission. The role of bone-marrow transplant in children with acute lymphoblastic leukaemia is ill defined at present and the indications for bone-marrow transplantation in first remission are discussed below. However, for the vast majority of children with acute lymphoblastic leukaemia a period of continuing (maintenance) therapy appears essential. There is no evidence that any regimen is superior to a combination of daily 6-mercaptopurine and weekly methotrexate given to the limits of tolerance as determined by the absolute neutrophil count and pulsed by additional vincristine and prednisolone every 4–6 weeks. Numerous attempts to improve on this approach by giving the same drugs as intermittent therapy (Medical Research Council 1986*a*), addition of other drugs such as cytarabine and cyclophosphamide (Aur *et al.* 1978), or substitution of more complicated regimens, most notably perhaps the Memorial Sloane Kettering LSA2L2 with a multiple-drug rotating regimen based originally on cell-kinetic principles (Miller *et al.* 1980), have proven superior, particularly for standard-risk patients. Routine bone-marrow examination during treatment is of no benefit and is not recommended unless in the context of a formal study (Rogers *et al.* 1984).

There remain many unresolved issues about continuing therapy. It seems intuitively likely that, for maximum efficacy, drugs should be given in the maximum tolerated dose and in one early randomized trial full dose treatment was superior to half dose (Pinkel *et al.* 1971). Patients who have been treated to the limits of tolerance, as suggested by neutropenia during treatment, seem to have a better prognosis than others (Dolan *et al.* 1989). Little attention has been given to the issue of compliance, either of the patient or the physician (Peeters *et al.* 1988). There is significant variation in absorption of both methotrexate and mercaptopurine.

Methotrexate levels show wide variability in children receiving a single oral dose under standard conditions (Pearson *et al.* 1987), although a randomized trial comparing oral and intramuscular methotrexate in continuing treatment achieved more reproducible methotrexate levels with intramuscular methotrexate, but this was not reflected in an improvement in event-free survival (Chessells *et al.* 1987*b*). Plasma levels of 6-thioguanine in patients on oral 6-mercaptopurine, while correlating with the degree of neutropenia, show less correlation with drug dose, thus reflecting variations in metabolism, due at least in part to genetic variations in metabolism (Lennard and Lilleyman 1989).

Duration of treatment

There have been a number of randomized trials addressing the issue of the optimum duration of treatment and these have usually involved patients treated with this conventional continuing regimen. These trials frequently have a significant number of non-compliers because of the problems involved in late randomizations with strong parental or physician prejudice. Usually these trials show a marginal benefit for longer treatment, particularly in boys, although in many cases relapse appears to be deferred rather than abolished and in some the lower relapse rate with continued therapy has been outweighed by deaths on treatment. Thus, the American Children's

Cancer Study Group has compared 3 and 5 years of treatment (Nesbit *et al.* 1983) and shown no significant benefit for 5 years. Medical Research Council UKALL trials have shown that 18 months of treatment is probably inferior to 3 years of treatment and that 2 and 3 years are equivalent (Medical Research Council 1982). At present children in Medical Research Council trials all receive treatment for 2 years. The BFM group recently tried to reduce treatment to 18 months and found, in a small randomized trial, that the results were inferior to 2 years (Riehm *et al.* 1990).

A significant impetus to stopping treatment is, of course, the risk of serious non-bacterial infection (see below) and in the child who is not on a standard protocol it would seem reasonable to stop at 2 years. It may be that future attempts to define the state of continued remission will be more refined, but at present a bone-marrow and lumbar puncture should be performed before treatment is stopped. Testicular biopsy is not recommended because of the high false-negative rate, but regular examination of the testicles is essential in boys who have stopped treatment and any suspicious swelling should be biopsied forthwith.

The risk of relapse after ceasing continuing chemotherapy has been maximal in the first 12–18 months off treatment and has decreased thereafter, occurring very rarely in patients more than 6–8 years from diagnosis (Chessells *et al.* 1987*a*). Occasional relapses have been reported up to 12 years off treatment (Nygaard *et al.* 1989), but it remains uncertain whether such events represent a late relapse or a second leukaemia. However, there is some anxiety that modern more intensive schedules may just defer relapse in some patients; this issue should soon be resolved. There is no doubt that boys have a higher relapse rate off treatment than girls; this is due in part to testicular relapse, but boys also have a higher marrow relapse rate (Medical Research Council 1978*a*). It has been postulated that this may be due to marrow infiltration via occult testicular relapse, but there is no clear evidence to support this hypothesis and prophylactic testicular irradiation does not reduce the marrow relapse rate (Eden *et al.* 1990).

Acute myeloid leukaemia

Certain types of patient with acute myeloid leukaemia are at increased risk of failure to achieve remission. These include patients with pre-existing myelodysplasia, some with cytogenetic abnormalities such as monosomy 7, some in whom chemotherapy failure is common, and some with hyperleucocytosis and with M3 acute myeloid leukaemia who are at risk of early death. However, there is insufficient evidence about prognosis and treatment response following induction to recommend an individualized approach for any subgroup of patients with acute myeloid leukaemia except those with M3 acute myeloid leukaemia in whom treatment with ALL *trans* retinoic acid may improve coagulopathy and achieve remission without specific cytotoxic therapy. Children with a monocytic component should receive some central nervous system treatment; this may be given effectively with intrathecal chemotherapy. Childhood acute myeloid leukaemia is such a rare disease that whenever possible patients should be treated on clinical trials so that treatment and understanding of the disease improves.

The choice of post-remission therapy in childhood acute myeloid leukaemia is complicated by the fact that the results of both chemotherapy and allogeneic bone-marrow transplantation with a histocompatible sibling donor appear superior to those obtained in adults and that the results of chemotherapy appear to be steadily improving. The most impressive results have been reported in non-randomized single-arm studies of short-term intensive chemotherapy for approximately 15 months (Weinstein *et al.* 1983) or prolonged

induction and intensification with simpler continuing treatment (Creutzig *et al.* 1987*a*). However, there is little evidence that low-dose continuing therapy after intensive induction and consolidation is of any benefit in acute myeloid leukaemia. The results of allogeneic marrow transplantation in childhood acute myeloid leukaemia are also encouraging, with up to 64 per cent of children remaining alive and in remission after bone-marrow transplantation (Sanders *et al.* 1985). Treatment failures in children with acute myeloid leukaemia receiving chemotherapy are mainly due to relapse whereas in bone-marrow transplantation failure is due more to graft versus host disease, interstitial pneumonia, or other infections. Moreover, the balance is complicated by consideration of the late effects of bone-marrow transplantation.

Most children treated by bone-marrow transplantation have hitherto received fractionated or unfractionated total body irradiation as part of their conditioning and the resultant late effects are significant (see below). It is possible that preparative regimens involving chemotherapy alone, such as the combination of busulphan and cyclophosphamide used by the Baltimore group (Geller *et al.* 1989) will produce less disturbance, at least of growth, but these have not yet been fully evaluated. A prospective trial in adult myeloid leukaemia showed that busulphan and cyclophosphamide were inferior to total body irradiation and cyclophosphamide in preparation for bone-marrow transplantation but as yet there have been no paediatric comparisons (Blaise *et al.* 1992). However, so far there have been few if any systematic attempts to evaluate long-term morbidity in children treated with the very intensive regimens now used in acute myeloid leukaemia.

Despite the absence of any firm evidence of benefit, it seems appropriate that following remission induction all patients should receive one or two courses of further intensive chemotherapy with a similar protocol to that used for induction or alternative drugs in equal intensity. The choice between allogeneic marrow transplantation and chemotherapy has hitherto been rendered easy in two-thirds of children by the absence of a histocompatible sibling donor. Series comparing bone-marrow transplant and chemotherapy have tended to show that bone-marrow transplant is superior, although not necessarily statistically so (Buckley *et al.* 1989*a*).

However, the situation is becoming more complicated because of the increasing availability of matched unrelated donors and by increasing interest in autologous bone-marrow transplantation. There have been a number of reports of unrandomized studies in adults in which autologous marrow, either purged or unpurged, is given to assist marrow recovery after high-dose chemotherapy and/or total body irradiation (Burnett *et al.* 1984; Korbling *et al.* 1989). Review of the results so far suggests that autologous bone-marrow transplantation is more effective when given after several courses of chemotherapy; thus, it might be argued, given to a selected group of patients who are already at decreased risk of relapse. The benefit of autologous bone-marrow transplantation can clearly only be assessed by prospective randomized trials and such trials in children are already in progress in the United States and the United Kingdom (Stevens *et al.* 1992; Woods *et al.* 1993).

Thus, at present, the optimum treatment choice for children with acute myeloid leukaemia remains uncertain. The situation is complicated by the fact that there is relatively little information on which to base selection of children for bone-marrow transplantation. In practice, the choice of treatment after remission induction lies between further intensive chemotherapy and, in those with a histocompatible sibling donor, bone-marrow transplantation. At present the author recommends bone-marrow transplantation in first remission for those with a donor, although if results of chemotherapy improve this might arguably be performed at the first sign of relapse, an approach which has been shown to achieve some success (Appelbaum *et al.* 1983).

Bone-marrow transplantation in first remission

As discussed above, at the time of writing there is a strong argument to advocate bone-marrow transplantation in first remission for children with acute myeloid leukaemia and particularly those few children with generally recognized worse features such as monosomy 7. Recently published results from the American Children's Cancer Study Group tend to support this approach (Buckley *et al.* 1989*a*).

The situation is more difficult with respect to acute lymphoblastic leukaemia. There is a small group of patients with unquestionable poor prognosis (for example, Ph-positive acute lymphoblastic leukaemia and t4;11) in whom bone-marrow transplantation is clearly justified. Some have advocated selection on the basis of initial leucocyte count, perhaps with additional criteria such as initial treatment response on day 7 or day 14 marrow, but bone-marrow transplantation in acute lymphoblastic leukaemia requires careful clinical studies. Patients in the previous national trial in the United Kingdom (Medical Research Council UKALL X) with an initial leucocyte count in excess of 100×10^9/l all received similar induction and intensification and those with a histocompatible sibling donor could receive bone-marrow transplantation in first remission; the others proceeded to receive standard treatment with additional late intensification. The advantage of a lower relapse rate after transplantation was offset by treatment-related mortality and the benefit of transplantation did not achieve statistical significance (Chessells *et al.* 1992).

It is important that the option of bone-marrow transplantation in both acute myeloid leukaemia and acute lymphoblastic leukaemia should be evaluated in a standard way in comparison with other best options. The vast majority of reports from transplant centres report results from the time of bone-marrow transplantation, thus introducing significant bias. In both present United Kingdom trials an attempt is made to give standard initial treatment and to standardize the time of transplant, thus enabling a direct comparison with alternative treatments.

Most reports of bone-marrow transplantation have utilized cyclophosphamide and total body irradiation, but this treatment is not appropriate for young children and alternative approaches might include busulphan and cyclophosphamide with additional central nervous system-directed treatment for young children with acute lymphoblastic leukaemia.

Central nervous system-directed treatment

Treatment to prevent overt leukaemic infiltration of the central nervous system, sometimes inaccurately called central nervous system prophylaxis, is an essential component in the management of childhood acute lymphoblastic leukaemia. Long-term follow-up of early trials of central nervous system-directed treatment has confirmed the advantage in terms of survival and cure of treating all children with acute lymphoblastic leukaemia rather than those who develop overt disease (Ortega *et al.* 1987). Although the risk of central nervous system relapse is related to the height of the leucocyte count at presentation and relapse is more likely in children with a low platelet count (West *et al.* 1972), it is not possible to define a group of children who are at no risk of central nervous

system relapse and this complication may occur late off treatment in apparent low-risk children who have received no central nervous system-directed therapy.

The incidence of central nervous system relapse as a first event in acute myeloid leukaemia appears lower than in acute lymphoblastic leukaemia, although this could, at least in part, be a reflection of the lower mean length of survival. In the author's experience central nervous system infiltration at diagnosis or central nervous system relapse is virtually confined to children whose leukaemia has a monocytic component (Chessells *et al.* 1986*b*), although occasional patients with other types of acute myeloid leukaemia may present with focal intracranial lesions.

A variety of methods have been used to prevent or treat central nervous system relapse. These include intrathecal chemotherapy, high-dose intravenous therapy, radiotherapy, and any combination of these modalities. When central nervous system treatment was first introduced there were a number of trials using whole neuraxis irradiation (Aur *et al.* 1973; Medical Research Council 1978*a*). This approach, although valuable in patients with central nervous system disease at presentation and after central nervous system relapse, is myelotoxic and immunosuppressive and has been abandoned in routine use. The most widely used treatment in acute lymphoblastic leukaemia has comprised a course of cranial irradiation in a dose of 24 Gy given in 15 fractions over 3 weeks combined with up to six intrathecal methotrexate injections in a dose based on estimated cerebrospinal fluid volume (Bleyer *et al.* 1983). Reduction in the dose of radiotherapy to 18 Gy, particularly in patients with a low leucocyte count, does not compromise event-free survival (Nesbit *et al.* 1981).

However, it has become apparent that, particularly in the young child, the late effects of cranial irradiation in terms of learning problems, growth disturbance, and early puberty are considerable and have not been significantly decreased by reduction of the radiotherapy dose to 18 Gy. These considerations have led to a reappraisal of central nervous system-directed treatment in acute lymphoblastic leukaemia and increasing emphasis on tailoring such treatment to the age and risk group of the patient.

Short-term intrathecal methotrexate therapy alone is inadequate to prevent central nervous system relapse, but a course of initial injections combined with regular intrathecal methotrexate provides adequate treatment for low-risk children (Littman *et al.* 1987). Intrathecal methotrexate provides adequate treatment for low- and average-risk children as defined by initial leucocyte count (Littman *et al.* 1987; Tubergen *et al.* 1993*b*). In children with higher leucocyte counts the relative merits of intrathecal chemotherapy alone, high-dose intravenous methotrexate, and cranial irradiation with intrathecal methotrexate remain unclear. Many trials in this field have been unsatisfactory because various other aspects of treatment have varied. Many have also shown a 'swings and roundabouts' effect, for example that of Freeman *et al.* (1983) where moderate-dose intravenous methotrexate and intrathecal methotrexate resulted in a higher central nervous system relapse rate and lower testicular and marrow relapse rate than cranial irradiation. Many questions about intrathecal therapy remain unanswered; there has been no comparison of intrathecal methotrexate alone with triple intrathecal chemotherapy. The intravenous doses of methotrexate have varied from 33 g/m^2 to 500 mg/m^2 (Balis and Poplak 1989). Thus, there is a continuing need for randomized trials to determine the optimum central nervous treatment in acute lymphoblastic leukaemia and these should be accompanied by neuropsychological evaluation and assessment of growth. At present, intrathecal methotrexate alone probably provides adequate treatment for the child with standard risk acute lymphoblastic leukaemia (WBC $<50\times10^9/l$), while the child with a higher leucocyte count should either receive cranial irradiation or additional high-dose intravenous methotrexate. Radiotherapy should be avoided in children under 2 years because of the high risk of intellectual impairment. Children with acute myeloid leukaemia should receive intrathecal chemotherapy, but there is no evidence to support the benefit of cranial irradiation in the absence of central nervous system disease.

Management after stopping treatment

Once treatment has been electively stopped, regular follow-up is essential to detect possible relapse, to monitor growth and development, and to alleviate possible late effects of treatment. It is usual practice to perform monthly blood counts and clinical examination for 18–24 months and thereafter at decreasing frequency. Routine bone-marrow tests are not indicated. The most important clinical assessment is a regular examination of the testicles.

All children should have regular measurement of height, weight, and growth velocity, and pubertal progression should be systematically staged. Reimmunizations should be given after 6–12 months off treatment.

Management of relapse

Despite improvements in management, relapse still occurs in a large number of patients. The chance of cure is then dramatically reduced and the morbidity of treatment is significantly increased.

Bone-marrow relapse

The symptoms of bone-marrow relapse resemble those at presentation and relapse may be suspected because of these or indicated on a routine blood film. The diagnosis should usually be confirmed by bone-marrow examination. Reinduction may be achieved with a similar schedule to that used initially in the majority of cases of acute lymphoblastic leukaemia and some with acute myeloid leukaemia, but the main problem is that of achieving a sustained remission. The duration of second remission is proportional to the duration of first remission and very few children relapsing within 1 year of diagnosis will become long-term survivors.

A large number of treatment protocols have been devised for children relapsing on treatment or soon after stopping treatment. These tend to be more intensive and good results have been claimed, for example in one series in children relapsing after 18 months from diagnosis (Rivera et al. 1986). Such schedules will no doubt multiply with increased availability of marrow-stimulating factors. However, very-long-term follow-up is needed to determine whether such patients will be truly cured and they remain at continuing relapse for many years (Chessells et al. 1987a).

Allogeneic marrow transplantation from a sibling donor offers the best chance of survival after marrow relapse, although even with this form of treatment the chances of success are limited by the instability of second remissions and the high relapse rate in most series after transplantation (Chessells et al. 1986a). Despite the results from transplant centres claiming survival after bone-marrow transplantation of up to 60 per cent (Brochstein et al. 1987), these factors significantly reduce the impact of bone-marrow transplantation on the problem of relapsed acute lymphoblastic leukaemia. Autologous bone-marrow transplantation has been used in relapsed acute lymphoblastic leukaemia with some claims of success (Kersey et al. 1987; Sallan et al. 1989), but this form of treatment urgently needs evaluation by randomized trial. The increased availability of

matched unrelated donors is likely to lead to more transplants, but one additional problem will be the delay inherent in finding a donor.

Central nervous system relapse

The symptoms of central nervous system relapse include headache, vomiting, signs of raised intracranial pressure, and increase in appetite and weight; convulsions and focal central nervous system signs other than cranial nerve palsies are rare. CT scans are usually unhelpful in diagnosis and there is little experience yet with magnetic resonance imaging. The diagnosis is usually confirmed by the finding of blast cells in the cerebrospinal fluid, although these may be absent in patients with the hypothalamic syndrome. It may occasionally be difficult to distinguish leukaemic blasts from reactive lymphocytes, but the distinction is helped by monoclonal antibodies. A bone-marrow test is essential to exclude concurrent relapse.

Symptomatic improvement is rapidly obtained in the majority of patients with weekly intrathecal methotrexate, but further more intensive treatment is needed to prevent recurrent central nervous system disease and bone-marrow relapse, a common subsequent event. The management must thus include reinduction and further intensification of systemic chemotherapy and radiotherapy. The most established method of treating isolated central nervous system relapse is by radiation of the whole neuraxis with 24 Gy to the cranium and 10–20 Gy to the spinal cord. An alternative approach is total body irradiation and either allogeneic or autologous marrow transplantation. The relative merits of these treatments are unknown, but the conventional approach is most likely to be effective in children with late relapses; those relapsing early are frequently high-risk patients and achieve a short second remission (Ortega et al. 1987).

Testicular relapse

The testis is a common site of relapse and is involved in up to 13 per cent of boys off treatment and a small number during treatment (Medical Research Council 1978b). Relapse presents as a painless swelling of one or both testicles. The diagnosis should be confirmed by biopsy, which will frequently show bilateral infiltration. Provided that the relapse has occurred off treatment and the bone-marrow is in remission, testicular leukaemia should be treated conventionally with systemic induction and intensification, central nervous system treatment, and local irradiation of approximately 24 Gy to both testicles. By using this approach and a further 2 years of continuing treatment, long remissions can be obtained in many patients (Tiedeman et al. 1982). In contrast, relapse during treatment has a poor prognosis and we have arbitrarily recommended bone-marrow transplantation in such patients.

Other sites

Other extramedullary sites of relapse include the eye, the ovary, and skin; any of these may occur in acute lymphoblastic leukaemia or acute myeloid leukaemia. These may occur as isolated sites or in combination with marrow or central nervous system. The approach to treatment must include further chemotherapy, usually with local irradiation and further intrathecal chemotherapy. In most instances, however, the prognosis is poor, particularly with relapse occurring during treatment and high-dose chemotherapy, radiotherapy, and marrow transplantation would be reasonable treatment in such patients.

Palliative care

In clinical practice, once the decision has been made to abandon attempts at cure the most distressing symptom faced by children with relapsed leukaemia is pain and every effort should be made to control this. Sometimes it is appropriate to attempt partial regression of disease with out-patient chemotherapy because this may alleviate pain, but there should be no hesitation in prescribing regular analgesics and we have found oral slow-release morphine sulphate of great use in this respect. Local irradiation may produce dramatic relief in focal bone pain. With adequate support we have found that the majority of children can, if they and their parents wish, receive all such palliative and terminal care at home (Goldman *et al.* 1990).

RESULTS OF TREATMENT

The aim of treating children with acute leukaemia is not palliation but cure. With a few exceptions to be discussed below, most children cured are those who achieve and remain in their first remission. This section will focus on remission rate, event-free survival, and the medical cost of cure. Since remission rates are high in both types of leukaemia and second-line therapy is in general unsuccessful, the most important measure of outcome is event-free survival. Thus, induction failures, deaths in remission, and relapses represent failures and event-free survival after X years should approximate to cure.

How many years should elapse before a child is deemed cured? There is surprisingly little hard information on this issue. Results of most clinical trials, even well-conducted phase 3 trials, tend to be published too early and long-term follow-up may not be reported. The results of such trials must inevitably have a degree of selection bias and, thus, not represent the true outcome for all children with leukaemia. The most accurate estimates are provided by national cancer registries, if these are complete and exist and by organizations such as the Childhood Cancer Research Group.

Acute lymphoblastic leukaemia

The remission rate in acute lymphoblastic leukaemia exceeds 95 per cent with failures being due to haemorrhage or metabolic problems, infection, and occasional drug resistance. Up to 5 per cent of children die in remission from the immunosuppressive effects of treatment. These tragic and usually preventable deaths are generally due to non-bacterial infection such as measles, chickenpox, and *Pneumocystis carinii* pneumonitis (Ninane and Chessells 1981).

Children with adverse prognostic features are at high risk of relapse for the first 12–18 months, but thereafter their relapse rate approximates to that of other patients and in B-cell acute lymphoblastic leukaemia is virtually zero. The 'cure rate' in acute lymphoblastic leukaemia in the United Kingdom has risen from 30–40 per cent in patients diagnosed 15–20 years ago to 50–60 per cent in the era of Medical Research Council UKALL VIII (1979–1984) (Medical Research Council 1986*b*). More recent results show further improvement (Fig. 1). These results, which were independently confirmed by the Children's Cancer Study Group, were inferior to those obtained in the United States during the earlier period but are now equivalent (Stiller and Bunch 1990). They accord reasonably well with the estimates of 60–70 per cent from the Children's Cancer Study Group (Poplack and Reaman 1988) and the West German BFM group (Riehm *et al.* 1990).

The outcome after relapse remains very poor. Estimates of 30–40 per cent survival after allogeneic transplant in second remission or even higher estimates from selected centres are given from the time of transplant; our own results are similar but, of course, apply to a minority of the total population. The author's original experience

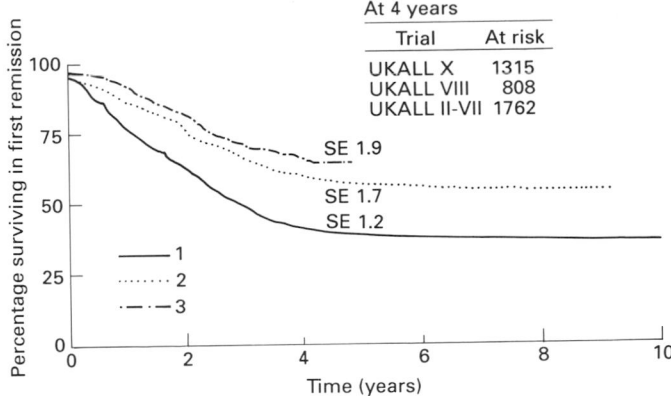

Fig. 1 Results of Medical Research Council UKALL Trials in Childhood Lymphoblastic Leukaemia. Event-free survival in three consecutive series. The bottom line refers to UKALL II–VII inclusive. The next line refers to UKALL VIII and the top line refers to UKALL X. Figures refer to numbers at risk at 4 years and the standard error at that time.

that 80 per cent of children with marrow relapse during therapy are dead within 1 year has sadly not altered with the passage of time and, moreover, while children with late relapses may have much longer survival, they remain at continued risk for many years.

Long-term follow-up of children after central nervous system or testicular relapse after stopping treatment is more encouraging, although our original experience of 85 per cent survival after late isolated testicular relapse may not be applicable for children who have received modern more intensive protocols.

Acute myeloid leukaemia

At least 85 per cent of children with acute myeloid leukaemia should achieve remission with intensive chemotherapy and good supportive care. Failures are due to early death from haemorrhage and leucostasis, infection, and, more frequently than in acute lymphoblastic leukaemia, resistance to chemotherapy. As has been pointed out, the real truth about the curability of acute myeloid leukaemia is obscured in many articles by distorted referral patterns and failure to register early deaths (Toronto Leukaemia Study Group 1986). Our own attempts to assess results in the era 1972–1982 showed a remission rate of 66 per cent and a cure rate of 12 per cent (Chessells *et al.* 1986). United Kingdom national statistics show that survival in acute myeloid leukaemia has improved from 8 per cent at 4–5 years during 1974–1976 to 25 per cent for children diagnosed between 1983 and 1985 (Stiller and Bunch 1990). Our own more recent results are shown in Fig. 2.

Recent reported results using more intensive chemotherapy show event-free survival of the order of 30–40 per cent for patients receiving chemotherapy (Buckley *et al.* 1989*a*). There is some evidence that the cure rate is higher in patients receiving allogeneic marrow transplantation. For the minority of children who have a sibling donor and survive to undergo marrow transplantation, the chance of survival from the time of transplant is of the order of 60–70 per cent (Sanders *et al.* 1985).

The chance of achieving a second remission in children with acute myeloid leukaemia depends on the time of relapse, but if this occurs early remission is not readily achieved and is of brief duration. There have been encouraging reports of results of bone-marrow transplantation in early relapse and this should be pursued if a donor

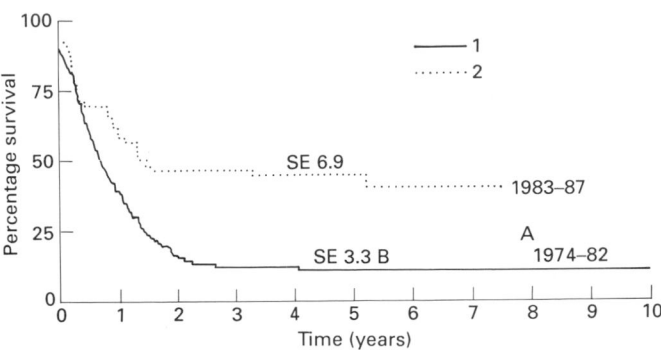

Fig. 2 Event-free survival in children with acute myeloid leukaemia, Hospital for Sick Children, Great Ormond Street, London. Series A, 1974–1982; series B, 1983–1987.

is available. The present United Kingdom trial for acute myeloid leukaemia is exploring autologous bone-marrow transplantation in patients who achieve a second remission.

MORBIDITY OF TREATMENT

Early morbidity

The early morbidity of treatment is greatest during induction and intensification therapy or marrow transplantation. Over 85 per cent of children with acute lymphoblastic leukaemia and all children with acute myeloid leukaemia develop fever during induction and require appropriate investigations and intravenous antibiotics: children with sustained fever and neutropenia are at risk of systemic fungal infection. The management of infections in the neutropenic patient, gut toxicity, and nutrition are described elsewhere. It remains to be seen in the next few years what impact the increasingly available cytokines will have on the management of patients undergoing intensive chemotherapy.

The unusual aspect of treatment morbidity in childhood acute lymphoblastic leukaemia lies in the period of continuing (maintenance) treatment. There is no evidence that children on such treatment are more susceptible to the usual viral respiratory infections and normal social intercourse and school attendance should be encouraged. However, the immunosuppressive effects of this treatment render children vulnerable to certain infections, of which some, such as varicella–zoster and herpes simplex, are now treatable with acyclovir but others, such as measles, remain a significant cause of death in countries such as the United Kingdom without compulsory immunization (Ninane and Chessells 1981). Cytomegalovirus does not carry the same risks as in the transplant recipient, although chronic lung disease, hepatosplenomegaly, intolerance of chemotherapy, and retinitis may rarely occur. Chronic infection with parvovirus is a recently recognized cause of chronic anaemia in children with acute lymphoblastic leukaemia (Kurtzman *et al.* 1988).

The most worrying complication seen during treatment is interstitial pneumonia, most often due to *Pneumocystis carinii*, but also caused by measles, *Mycoplasma pneumoniae*, cytomegalovirus, and, very rarely in this context, fungal infection. An aggressive approach to diagnosis and treatment is indicated since this complication represents the commonest cause of death in remission.

The psychosocial morbidity ensuing from admission to hospital, intensive treatment, absence from school, and frequent hospital visits is significant for most children and their families. Every effort should be made to mitigate this by ensuring the availability of psychological and social work support; these members are an essential part of the team.

Late effects of treatment

Our own survey of all children attending the department who had completed treatment for acute lymphoblastic leukaemia and been followed up for at least 6 years from diagnosis showed that two-thirds were problem free (Wheeler *et al.* 1988). The most important late effects of treatment in this group of children who had received chemotherapy of moderate intensity and cranial irradiation were neuropsychological problems and disorders of growth. Children who have been treated with cranial irradiation may have an IQ within the normal range, but may show specific difficulties with learning concentration and mathematics; the problems are greatest in those receiving cranial irradiation at a young age (Jannoun 1983). There is some correlation between these findings and the presence of abnormalities on CT scans (Brouwers *et al.* 1985). A recent analysis of our own patients has confirmed the relationship between CT scan findings and IQ deficit, shown the vulnerability of younger children to both, and shown that intramuscular methotrexate is more damaging than oral methotrexate (Chessells *et al.* 1990). These learning problems have not been reduced by reduction in radiotherapy from 24 to 18 Gy. They are, of course, exacerbated by a second course of irradiation, whether as conventional treatment or total body irradiation.

Similarly, children who have received one course of cranial irradiation may have impaired growth; many have suboptimal growth hormone secretion but relatively few require treatment. Early onset of puberty may occur in up to 13 per cent of girls and, if unnoticed and combined with the absence of a pubertal growth spurt, may result in significant reduction of final height (Leiper *et al.* 1987). A second course of radiotherapy has significant effects on growth. A much greater proportion of children will require growth hormone treatment after further irradiation.

Spinal irradiation will cause shortening and, like total body irradiation, may cause clinical or biochemical hypothyroidism. Children who have received total body irradiation will, of course, have all these complications with the additional failure of pubertal progression and sterility (Sanders *et al.* 1986). This catalogue of abnormalities emphasizes the need for non-radiotherapeutic central nervous system treatment strategies, although it must be admitted that there is a paucity of follow-up information on children treated using other approaches.

Most clinics now have a number of patients who have completed successful pregnancy and there is at present no evidence that infants born to ex-patients are more at risk of cancer or congenital abnormalities.

Clearly, most of this long-term follow-up information is derived from patients who have received relatively modest chemotherapy. As treatment becomes progressively more intensive, close monitoring of late effects is essential; of particular concern perhaps is the increasingly wide use of anthracyclines and their unknown potential for late cardiac toxicity.

The incidence of second neoplasms is as yet unknown, but among those recorded are acute myeloid leukaemia, lymphoma, and brain tumours (Meadows *et al.* 1985). It is not clear whether the latter are associated with the use of cranial irradiation (Ron *et al.* 1988) or have a genetic basis. The pattern of second neoplasms may, of course, be altered by changing chemotherapy schedules as in the reports of secondary acute myeloid leukaemia after treatment with epipidophylotoxins (Pui *et al.* 1989).

These results serve to emphasize the need for continued long-term surveillance of children who have been treated for acute leukaemia and for development of protocols which avoid radiotherapy whenever possible. A sensitive and positive attitude to counselling the young adult survivor would seem both appropriate and justified in the light of present knowledge and such an attitude appears to be taken by many employers and insurance companies. There are no grounds to advise against pregnancy and childbirth in the majority of patients whose fertility is unimpaired. It is encouraging to think that by the year 2000 one in 1000 children will be a long-term cancer survivor and a significant number of these will be adults who have been treated for childhood leukaemia.

REFERENCES

Applebaum FR, et al. (1983). Allogeneic marrow transplantation for acute nonlymphoblastic leukaemia after first relapse. Blood, 61:949–53.

Arthur DC, Bloomfield CD, Lindquist LL, Nesbit ME Jr (1982). Translocation 4;11 in acute lymphoblastic leukemia: clinical characteristics and prognostic significance. Blood, 59:96–9.

Aur RJA, Hustu HO, Verzosa MS, Wood A, Simone JV (1973). Comparison of two methods of preventing central nervous system leukaemia. Blood, 42:349–57.

Aur RJA, et al. (1978). Childhood acute lymphoblastic leukemia—study VIII. Cancer, 42:2123–34.

Balis FM, Poplack DC (1989). Central nervous system pharmacology of antileukemic drugs. American Journal of Pediatric Hematology and Oncology, 11:74–86.

Bennett JM, et al. (1981). The morphological classification of acute lymphoblastic leukaemia: concordance among observers and clinical correlations. British Journal of Haematology, 47:553–61.

Bennett JM, et al. (1982). Proposals for the classification of the myelodysplastic syndromes. British Journal of Haematology, 51:189–99.

Bennett JM, et al. (1985a). Proposed revised criteria for the classification of acute myeloid leukemia. Annals of Internal Medicine, 103:626–9.

Bennett JM, et al. (1985b). Criteria for the diagnosis of acute leukemia of megakaryocyte lineage (M7). Annals of Internal Medicine, 103:460–2.

Blaise D, et al. (1992). Allogeneic bone marrow transplantation for acute myeloid leukemia in first remission: a randomized trial of a busulfan–cytoxan versus cytoxan–total body irradiation as preparative regimen: a report from the Groupe d'Etudes de la Greffe de Moelle Osseuse. Blood, 79:2578–82.

Bleyer WA, et al. (1983). Reduction in central nervous system leukaemia with a pharmacokinetically derived intrathecal methotrexate dosage regimen. Journal of Clinical Oncology, 1:317–25.

Bloomfield CD, et al. (1986). Chromosomal abnormalities identify high-risk and low-risk patients with acute lymphoblastic leukemia. Blood, 67:415–20.

Breatnach F, Chessells JM, Greaves MF (1981). The aplastic presentation of childhood leukaemia: a feature of common-acute lymphoblastic leukaemia. British Journal of Haematology, 49:387–93.

Brochstein JA, et al. (1987). Allogeneic bone marrow transplantation after hyperfractionated total-body irradiation and cyclophosphamide in children with acute leukemia. New England Journal of Medicine, 317:1618–24.

Brouwers P, Riccardi R, Fedio P, Poplack DG (1985). Long-term neuropsychologic sequelae of childhood leukemia: correlation with CT brain scan abnormalities. Journal of Pediatrics, 106:723–8.

Buckley JD, et al. (1989a). Improvement in outcome for children with acute nonlymphocytic leukemia. Cancer, 63:1457–65.

Buckely JD, et al. (1989b). Remission induction in children with acute non-lymphocytic leukaemia using cytosine arabinoside and doxorubicin or daunorubicin: a report from the Children's Cancer Study Group. Medical and Pediatric Oncology, 17:382–90.

Burnett AK, et al. (1984). Transplantation of unpurged autologous bone-marrow in acute myeloid leukaemia in first remission. Lancet, ii:1068–70.

Chan LC, Pegram SM, Greaves MF (1985). Contribution of immunophenotype to the classification and differential diagnosis of acute leukaemia. Lancet, i:475–9.

Chessells JM (1986). Acute leukaemia in children. Clinics in Haematology, 15:727–53.

Chessells JM, Hardisty RM, Rapson NT, Greaves MF (1977). Acute lymphoblastic leukaemia in children: classification and prognosis. Lancet, ii:1307–9.

Chessells JM, et al. (1986a). Bone-marrow transplantation has a limited role in prolonging second marrow remission in childhood lymphoblastic leukaemia. Lancet, i:1239–41.

Chessells JM, O'Callaghan U, Hardisty RM (1986b). Acute myeloid leukaemia in childhood: clinical features and prognosis. British Journal of Haematology, 63:555–64.

Chessells JM, Hardisty RM, Richards S (1987a). Long survival in childhood lymphoblastic leukaemia. British Journal of Cancer, 55:315–19.

Chessells JM, Leiper AD, Tiedemann K, Hardisty RM, Richards S (1987b). Oral methotrexate is as effective as intramuscular in maintenance therapy of acute lymphoblastic leukaemia. Archives of Disease in Childhood, 62:172–6.

Chessells JM, Cox TCS, Kendall B, Cavanagh NPC, Jannoun L, Richards S (1990). Neurotoxicity in lymphoblastic leukaemia: comparison of oral and intramuscular methotrexate and two doses of radiation. Archives of Disease in Childhood, 65:416–22.

Chessells JM, Bailey C, Wheeler K, Richards SM (1992a). Bone marrow transplantation for high-risk childhood lymphoblastic leukaemia in first remission: experience in MRC UKALL X. Lancet, 340:565–8.

Chessells JM, Bailey CC, Richards SM (1992b). MRC UKALL X. The UK protocol for childhood ALL: 1985–1990. Leukaemia, 6 (Suppl. 2):157–61.

Clavell LA, et al. (1986). Four-agent induction and intensive asparaginase therapy for treatment of childhood acute lymphoblastic leukemia. New England Journal of Medicine, 315:657–63.

Creutzig U, Ritter J, Budde M, Jurgens H, Riehm H., Schellong G (1987a). Treatment results in childhood acute myeloid leukaemia, with special reference to the German studies BFM-78 and BFM-83. Haematology and Blood Transfusion, 31:30–4.

Creutzig U, Ritter J, Riehm H, Budde M, Schellong G (1987b). The childhood acute myeloid leukaemia studies BFM-78 and -83: treatment results and risk factor analysis. Haematology and Blood Transfusion, 30:71–5.

Crist W, et al. (1989). Prognostic importance of the pre-B-cell immunophenotype and other presenting features in B-lineage childhood acute lymphoblastic leukaemia: a Pediatric Oncology Group study. Blood, 74:1252–9.

Cross AH, et al. (1988). Acute myeloid leukaemia with T-lymphoid features: a distinct biologic and clinical entity. Blood, 72:579–87.

Davis M, Malcolm S, Rabbitts TH (1984). Chromosomal translocation can occur on either side of the c-myc oncogene in Burkitt lymphoma cells. Nature, 308:286–8.

Dolan G, Lilleyman JS, Richards SM (1989). Prognostic importance of myelosuppression during maintenance treatment of lymphoblastic leukaemia. Archives of Disease in Childhood, 64:1231–4.

Eden OB, Lilleyman JS, Richards S (1990). Testicular irradiation in childhood lymphoblastic leukaemia. British Journal of Haematology, 75:496–8.

Eguchi M, et al. (1989). Ultrastructural and ultracytochemical differences between transient myeloproliferative disorder and megakaryoblastic leukaemia in Down's syndrome. British Journal of Haematology, 73:315–22.

Farwell J, Flannery JT (1984). Cancer in relatives of children with central nervous system neoplasms. New England Journal of Medicine, 311:749–53.

Fialkow PJ, et al. (1987). Clonal development, stem-cell differentiation, and clinical remissions in acute nonlymphocytic leukaemia. New England Journal of Medicine, 317:468–73.

Fleming AF (1985). The epidemiology of lymphomas and leukaemias in Africa—an overview. Leukemia Research, 9:735–40.

Fletcher JA, et al. (1989). Prognostic implications of cytogenetic studies in an intensively treated group of children with acute lymphoblastic leukemia. Blood, 74:2130–5.

Foon KA, Todd RF (1986). Immunologic classification of leukaemia and lymphoma. Blood, 68:1–31.

Freeman AI, et al. (1983). Comparison of intermediate-dose methotrexate with cranial irradiation for the post-induction treatment of acute lymphocytic leukemia in children. New England Journal of Medicine, 3038:477–84.

Gale RP, Bassatt B (1987). Hybrid acute leukaemia. British Journal of Haematology, 65:261–4.

Gardner MJ, Snee MP, Hall AJ, Powell CA, Downes S, Terrell JD (1990). Results of case–control study of leukaemia and lymphoma among young people near Sellafield nuclear plant in West Cumbria. *British Medical Journal*, **300**:423–9.

Gaynon PS, *et al.* (1993). Improved therapy for children with acute lymphoblastic leukemia and unfavourable presenting features: a follow-up report on the Childrens Cancer Group study CCG-106. *Journal of Clinical Oncology*, **11**:2234–42.

Geller RB, *et al.* (1989). Allogeneic bone marrow transplantation after high-dose busulfan and cyclophosphamide in patients with acute nonlymphocytic leukemia. *Blood*, **73**:2209–18.

Goldman A, Beardsmore S, Hunt J (1990). Palliative care for children with cancer—home, hospital or hospice? *Archives of Disease in Childhood*, **65**:641–3.

Greaves MF (1988). Speculations on the cause of childhood acute lymphoblastic leukaemia. *Leukemia*, **2**:120–5.

Greaves MF, Chan LC, Furley AJW, Watt SM, Molgaard HV (1986). Lineage promiscuity in hemopoietic differentiation and leukemia. *Blood*, **67**:1–11.

Grier HE, *et al.* (1987). Prognostic factors in childhood acute myelogenous leukemia. *Journal of Clinical Oncology*, **5**:1026–32.

Hann IM, Eden OB, Barnes J, Pinkerton CR (1990). 'Macho' chemotherapy for stage IV B-cell lymphoma and B-cell acute lymphoblastic leukaemia of childhood. *British Journal of Haematology*, **76**:359–65.

Henze G, Fengler R, Reiter A, Ritter J, Riehm H (1990). Impact of early intensive reinduction therapy on event-free survival in children with low-risk acute lymphoblastic leukaemia. *Haematology and Blood Transfusion*, **33**:483–8.

Ito Y, *et al.* (1993). Molecular residual disease status at the end of chemotherapy fails to predict subsequent relapse in children with B-lineage acute lymphoblastic leukemia. *Journal of Clinical Oncology*, **11**:546–53.

Jannoun L (1983). Are cognitive and educational development affected by age at which prophylactic therapy is given in acute lymphoblastic leukaemia? *Archives of Disease in Childhood*, **58**:953–8.

Kalwinsky DK, *et al.* (1990). Prognostic importance of cytogenetic subgroups in de novo pediatric acute nonlymphocytic leukemia. *Journal of Clinical Oncology*, **8**:75–83.

Katz F, Ball L, Gibbons B, Chessells JM (1989). The use of DNA probes to monitor minimal residual disease in childhood acute lymphoblastic leukaemia. *British Journal of Haematology*, **73**:173–80.

Katz F, Ball S, Gibbons B. (1990). Acute lymphoblastic leukaemia in infancy: clinical and biological features. *Leukemia and Lymphoma*, **2**:259–69.

Kersey JH, *et al.* (1987). Comparison of autologous and allogeneic bone marrow transplantation for treatment of high-risk refractory acute lymphoblastic leukemia. *New England Journal of Medicine*, **317**:461–6.

Korbling M, *et al.* (1989) Disease-free survival after autologous bone marrow transplantation in patients with acute myelogenous leukemia. *Blood*, **74**:1898–1904.

Kurtzman GJ, Cohen B, Meyers P, Amunullah A, Young NS (1988). Persistent B19 parvovirus infection as a cause of severe chronic anaemia in children with acute lymphocytic leukaemia. *Lancet*, **ii**:1159–62.

Kurzrock R, Gutterman JU, Talpaz M (1988). The molecular genetics of Philadelphia chromosome-positive leukemias. *New England Journal of Medicine*, **319**:990–8.

Leiper AD, Stanhope R, Kitching P, Chessells JM (1987). Precocious and premature puberty associated with the treatment of acute lymphoblastic leukaemia. *Archives of Disease in Childhood*, **62**:1107–12.

Lennard L, Lilleyman JS (1989). Variable mercaptopurine metabolism and treatment outcome in childhood lymphoblastic leukaemia. *Journal of Clinical Oncology*, **7**:1816–23.

Levitt GA, Stiller CA, Chessells JM (1990). Prognosis of Down's syndrome with acute leukaemia. *Archives of Disease in Childhood*, **65**:212–16.

Lilleyman JS, *et al.* (1992). Cytomorphology of childhood lymphoblastic leukaemia: a prospective study of 2000 patients. *British Journal of Haematology*, **81**:52–7.

Littman P, *et al.* (1987). Central nervous system (CNS) prophylaxis in children with low risk acute lymphoblastic leukaemia (ALL). *International Journal of Radiation Oncology—Biology—Physics*, **13**:1443–9.

Mastrangelo R, Poplack DG, Bleyer WA, Riccardi R, Sather H, D'Angio G (1986). Report and recommendations of the Rome Workshop concerning poor-prognosis acute lymphoblastic leukemia in children: biologic bases for staging, stratification, and treatment. *Medical and Pediatric Oncology*, **14**:191–4.

Meadows AT, *et al.* (1985). Second malignant neoplasms in children: an update from the Late Effects Study Group. *Journal of Clinical Oncology*, **3**:532–8.

Medical Research Council (1978a). Effects of varying radiation schedule, cyclophosphamide treatment, and duration of treatment in acute lymphoblastic leukaemia. *British Medical Journal*, **2**:787–91.

Medical Research Council (1978b). Testicular disease in acute lymphoblastic leukaemia in childhood. *British Medical Journal*, **1**:334–8.

Medical Research Council (1982). Duration of chemotherapy in childhood acute lymphoblastic leukaemia. *Medical and Pediatric Oncology*, **10**:511–20.

Medical Research Council (1986a). Medical Research Council Leukaemia Trial—UKALL V: an attempt to reduce the immunosuppressive effects of therapy in childhood acute lymphoblastic leukemia. *Journal of Clinical Oncology*, **4**:1758–64.

Medical Research Council (1986b). Improvement in treatment for children with acute lymphoblastic leukaemia. *Lancet*, **i**:408–11.

Miller DR, *et al.* (1980). Use of prognostic factors in improving the design and efficiency of clinical trials in childhood leukemia: Children's Cancer Study Group report. *Cancer Treatment Reports*, **64**:381–92.

Miller DR, Leikin S, Albo V, Sather H, Karon M, Hammond DG (1983). Prognostic factors and therapy in acute lymphoblastic leukemia of childhood: CCG-141. *Cancer*, **51**:1041–9.

Miller DR, *et al.* (1989). Early response to induction therapy as a predictor of disease-free survival and late recurrence of childhood acute lymphoblastic leukemia: a report from the Children's Cancer Study Group. *Journal of Clinical Oncology*, **7**:1807–15.

Neglia JP, Robison LL (1988). Epidemiology of the childhood acute leukemias. *Pediatric Clinics of North America*, **35**:675–92.

Nesbit ME Jr, *et al.* (1981). Presymptomatic central nervous system therapy in previously untreated childhood acute lymphoblastic leukaemia: comparison of 1800 RAD and 2400 RAD. *Lancet*, **i**:461–5.

Nesbit ME Jr, Sather HN, Robison LL, Ortega JA, Hammond DG, Children's Cancer Study Group (1983). Randomized study of 3 years versus 5 years of chemotherapy in childhood acute lymphoblastic leukaemia. *Journal of Clinical Oncology*, **1**:308–16.

Ninane J, Chessells JM (1981). Serious infections during continuing treatment of acute lymphoblastic leukaemia. *Archives of Disease in Childhood*, **56**:841–4.

Ninane J, Taylor D, Day S. (1980). The eye as a sanctuary in acute lymphoblastic leukaemia. *Lancet*, **1**:452–3.

Nygaard R, *et al.* (1989). Late relapses after treatment for acute lymphoblastic leukemia in childhood: a population-based study from the Nordic countries. *Medical and Pediatric Oncology*, **17**:45–7.

Ortega JA, *et al.* (1977). L-Asparaginase, vincristine and prednisone for induction of first remission in acute lymphocytic leukemia. *Cancer Research*, **37**:535–40.

Ortega JA, Nesbit ME, Sather HN, Robison LL, D'Angio GJ, Hammond DG (1987). Long-term evaluation of a CNS prophylaxis trial—treatment comparisons and outcome after CNS relapse in childhood acute lymphoblastic leukaemia: a report from the Children's Cancer Study Group. *Journal of Clinical Oncology*, **5**:1646–54.

Pearson ADJ, Mills S, Amineddine HA, Long DR, Craft AW, Chessells JM (1987). Pharmacokinetics of oral and intramuscular methotrexate in children with acute lymphoblastic leukaemia. *Cancer Chemotherapy and Pharmacology*, **20**:243–7.

Peeters M, Koren G, Jakubovicz D, Zipursky A (1988). Physician compliance and relapse rates of acute lymphoblastic leukemia in children. *Clinical Pharmacology and Therapeutics*, **43**:228–32.

Pinkel D, *et al.* (1971). Drug dosage and remission duration in childhood lymphocytic leukemia. *Cancer*, **27**:247–56.

Poplack DG, Reaman GH (1988). Acute lymphoblastic leukemia in childhood. *Pediatric Clinics of North America*, **35**:903–32.

Preisler HD (1978). Failure of remission induction in acute myelocytic leukemia. *Medical and Pediatric Oncology*, **4**:275–6.

Price RA, Johnson WW (1973). The central nervous system in childhood leukaemia 1. The Arachnoid. *Cancer*, **31**:520–33.

Priest JR, *et al.* (1980). Thrombotic and hemorrhagic strokes complicating L-asparaginase therapy for childhood acute lymphoblastic leukemia. *Cancer*, **46**:1548–54.

Pui CH, *et al.* (1989). Secondary acute myeloid leukemia in children treated for acute lymphoid leukemia. *New England Journal of Medicine*, 321:136–42.

Pui CH, *et al.* (1990*a*). Myeloid-associated antigen expression lacks prognostic value in childhood acute lymphoblastic leukemia treated with intensive multiagent chemotherapy. *Blood*, 75:198–202.

Pui CH, *et al.* (1990*b*). Clinical presentation, karyotypic characterization, and treatment outcome of childhood acute lymphoblastic leukemia with a near-haploid of hypodiploid <45 line. *Blood*, 75:1170–7.

Raimondi SC, Williams DL, Callihan T, Peiper S, Rivera GK, Murphy SB (1986). Nonrandom involvement of the 12p12 breakpoint in chromosome abnormalities of childhood acute lymphoblastic leukemia. *Blood*, 68:69–75.

Raimondi SC, *et al.* (1990). Cytogenetics of pre-B-cell acute lymphoblastic leukemia with emphasis on prognostic implications of the t(1;19). *Journal of Clinical Oncology*, 8:1380–8.

Ramot B, Magrath I (1982). Hypothesis: the environment is a major determinant of the immunological subtype of lymphoma and acute lymphoblastic leukaemia in children. *British Journal of Haematology*, 50:183–9.

Riehm H, Langermann HJ, Gadner H, Odenwald E, Henze G (1980). The Berlin childhood acute lymphoblastic leukemia therapy study, 1970–1976. *American Journal of Pediatric Hematology and Oncology*, 2:299–306.

Riehm H, Feickert HJ, Schrappe M, Henze G, Schellong G (1987). Therapy results in five ALL-BFM studies since 1970: implications of risk factors for prognosis. *Haematology and Blood Transfusion*, 30:139–46.

Riehm H, *et al.* (1990). Results and significance of six randomized trials in four consecutive ALL-BFM studies. *Haematology and Blood Transfusion*, 33:439–50.

Rivera GK, Evans WE, Kalwinsky DK (1985). Unexpectedly severe toxicity from intensive early treatment of childhood lymphoblastic leukemia. *Journal of Clinical Oncology*, 3:201–6.

Rivera G, *et al.* (1986). Intensive retreatment of childhood acute lymphoblastic leukemia in first bone marrow relapse. *New England Journal of Medicine*, 315:273–8.

Rogers PCJ, *et al.* (1984). Yield of unpredicted bone-marrow relapse diagnosed by routine marrow aspiration in children with acute lymphoblastic leukaemia. *Lancet*, i:1320–2.

Ron E, *et al.* (1988). Tumors of the brain and nervous system after radiotherapy in childhood. *New England Journal of Medicine*, 319:1033–9.

Sallan SE, *et al.* (1989). Autologous bone marrow transplantation for acute lymphoblastic leukemia. *Journal of Clinical Oncology*, 7:1594–1601.

Sanders JE, Thomas ED, Buckner CD (1985). Marrow transplantation for children in first remission of acute nonlymphoblastic leukemia: an update. *Blood*, 66:460–2.

Sanders JE, *et al.* (1986). Growth and development following marrow transplantation for leukemia. *Blood*, 68:1129–35.

Santana VM, *et al.* (1990). Presenting features and treatment outcome of adolescents with acute lymphoblastic leukemia. *Leukemia*, 4:87–90.

Sather HN (1986). Age at diagnosis in childhood acute lymphoblastic leukemia. *Medical and Pediatric Oncology*, 14:166–72.

Sather H, Miller D, Nesbit M, Heyn R, Hammond DG (1981). Differences in prognosis for boys and girls with acute lymphoblastic leukaemia. *Lancet*, i:741–3.

Scarffe JH, *et al.* (1980). Relationship between the pretreatment proliferative activity of marrow blast cells and prognosis of acute lymphoblastic leukaemia of childhood. *British Journal of Cancer*, 41:764–71.

Secker Walker LM, Chessells JM, Stewart EL, Swansbury GJ, Richards S, Lawler SD (1989). Chromosomes and other prognostic factors in acute lymphoblastic leukaemia: a long-term follow-up. *British Journal of Haematology*, 72:336–42.

Sobol RE, *et al.* (1987). Clinical importance of myeloid antigen expression in adult acute lymphoblastic leukemia. *New England Journal of Medicine*, 316:1111–17.

Stevens RF, Hann IM, Wheatley K, Gray R (1992). Intensive chemotherapy with or without additional bone marrow transplantation in paediatric AML: progress report on the MRC AML 10 trial. *Leukaemia*, 6 (Suppl. 2):55–8.

Stiller CA (1985). Descriptive epidemiology of childhood leukaemia and lymphoma in Great Britain. *Leukemia Research*, 9:671–4.

Stiller CA, Bunch KJ (1990). Trends in childhood cancer survival in Britain 1971–1985. *British Journal of Cancer*, 62:806–15.

Stiller CA, Draper GJ (1989). Treatment centre size, entry to trials, and survival in acute lymphoblastic leukaemia. *Archives of Disease in Childhood*, 64:657–61.

Thirman MJ, *et al.* (1993). Rearrangement of the MLL gene in acute lymphoblastic and acute myeloid leukemias with 11q23 chromosomal translocations. *New England Journal of Medicine*, 329:909–14.

Tiedemann K, Chessells JM, Sandland RM (1982). Isolated testicular relapse in boys with acute lymphoblastic leukaemia: treatment and outcome. *British Medical Journal*, 285:1614–16.

Toronto Leukemia Study Group (1986). Results of chemotherapy for unselected patients with acute myeloblastic leukaemia: effect of exclusions on interpretation of results. *Lancet*, i:786–8.

Trueworthy R, *et al.* (1992). Ploidy of lymphoblasts is the strongest predictor of treatment outcome in B-progenitor cell acute lymphoblastic leukemia of childhood: a Pediatric Oncology Group study. *Journal of Clinical Oncology*, 10:606–13.

Tubergen DG, *et al.* (1993*a*). Improved outcome with delayed intensification for children with acute lymphoblastic leukemia and intermediate presenting features: a Childrens Cancer Group Phase III trial. *Journal of Clinical Oncology*, 11:527–37.

Tubergen DG, *et al.* (1993*b*). Prevention of CNS disease in intermediate-risk acute lymphoblastic leukemia: comparison of cranial radiation and intrathecal methotrexate and the importance of systemic therapy: a Childrens Cancer Group report. *Journal of Clinical Oncology*, 11:520–6.

van der Does-van den Berg A, *et al.* (1989). Effectiveness of rubidomycin in induction therapy with vincristine, prednisone, and L-asparaginase for standard risk childhood acute lymphocytic leukemia: results of a Dutch phase III study (ALL V). *American Journal of Pediatric Hematology and Oncology*, 11:125–33.

Warrell RP, De The H, Wang Z-Y, Degos L (1993). Acute promyelocytic leukemia. *New England Journal of Medicine*, 329:177–88.

Wasserman R, *et al.* (1992). Residual disease at the end of induction therapy as a predictor of relapse during therapy in childhood B-lineage acute lymphoblastic leukemia. *Journal of Clinical Oncology*, 10:1879–88.

Weinstein HJ, Mayer RJ, Rosenthal DS, Coral FS, Camitta BM, Gelber RD (1983). Chemotherapy for acute myelogenous leukemia in children and adults: VAPA update. *Blood*, 62:315–19.

West RJ, Graham-Pole J, Hardisty RM, Pike MC (1972). Factors in pathogenesis of central-nervous-system leukaemia. *British Medical Journal*, 3:311–14.

Wheeler K, Leiper AD, Jannoun L, Chessells JM (1988). Medical cost of curing childhood acute lymphoblastic leukaemia. *British Medical Journal*, 296:162–6.

Williams DL, *et al.* (1986). Chromosomal translocations play a unique role in influencing prognosis in childhood acute lymphoblastic leukaemia. *Blood*, 68:205–12.

Woods WG, *et al.* (1985). Correlation of chromosome abnormalities with patient characteristics, histologic subtype, and induction success in children with acute nonlymphocytic leukemia. *Journal of Clinical Oncology*, 3:3–11.

Woods WG, *et al.* (1993). Intensively timed induction therapy followed by autologous or allogeneic bone marrow transplantation for children with acute myeloid leukemia or myelodysplastic syndrome: a Childrens Cancer Group pilot study. *Journal of Clinical Oncology*, 11:1448–57.

12.3 The chronic leukaemias

CHARLES R. J. SINGER AND A. H. GOLDSTONE

INTRODUCTION

The term 'chronic' was applied to these leukaemias in the era prior to the development of chemotherapeutic agents as a result of the longer survival observed in patients with these conditions when compared with the survival of patients with the 'acute' leukaemias. They share the feature that the cells of the neoplastic clone retain a capacity to differentiate, which results in the accumulation of cells with a mature appearance in the peripheral blood and bone-marrow. In almost no other respect are these diseases similar: in chronic myeloid leukaemia 'marrow-like' granulocyte precursors accumulate and in chronic lymphatic leukaemia apparently mature lymphoid cells accumulate. In recent years laboratory advances have resulted in the further subclassification of diseases originally designated on morphological grounds simply as chronic myeloid leukaemia or chronic lymphatic leukaemia. In addition, significant advances have been made in the understanding of the molecular basis of these diseases. Although curative therapy is possibly still restricted to patients with chronic myeloid leukaemia who have a compatible sibling and are thus eligible for bone-marrow transplant, a number of promising new therapeutic options have recently emerged for the treatment of these conditions.

CHRONIC MYELOID LEUKAEMIA

Epidemiology

Chronic myeloid leukaemia has an annual incidence of 1 per 100 000 of the normal population and represents approximately 25 per cent of all cases of leukaemia in adults (Young *et al.* 1981). There appears to be no geographical variation in this incidence. The peak incidence is in the fifth decade and there is a slight male excess. There is an increased incidence in survivors of the Japanese atomic bomb explosions and an association with therapeutic exposure to radiation (Gunz 1983). However, there appears to be no link with exposure to toxic chemicals or any clear viral aetiology, though there are animal models which have implicated the latter (Tanaka and Craig 1970). A small number of families with a high incidence of the disease have been reported. Nevertheless, it is extremely uncommon for an aetiological factor to be identified in a patient with chronic myeloid leukaemia.

It has been proposed, though not yet generally accepted, that the term chronic myeloid leukaemia, traditionally used as a synonym with the terms chronic myelogenous leukaemia, chronic myelocytic leukaemia, and chronic granulocytic leukaemia, should be used as a generic term to include both classical and atypical forms of chronic leukaemia involving the myeloid lineage. The term chronic granulocytic leukaemia should be reserved for patients with the classical disease in the vast majority of whom the Philadelphia chromosome is detected and who make up 90 per cent of all cases of chronic myeloid leukaemia. The conditions which may be included in the chronic myeloid leukaemias are listed in Table 1.

Table 1 The chronic myeloid leukaemias

Chronic granulocytic leukaemia (Ph+, bcr+)
Chronic granulocytic leukaemia (Ph−, bcr+)
Juvenile chronic myeloid leukaemia
Chronic neutrophilic leukaemia
Eosinophilic leukaemia
Chronic myelomonocytic leukaemia
Atypical chronic myeloid leukaemia

Ph, Philadelphia chromosome; bcr, break-point cluster region.

Table 2 The myeloproliferative disorders

Chronic myeloid leukaemia
Polycythaemia rubra vera
Myelofibrosis
Essential thrombocythaemia

Chronic myeloid leukaemia has long been recognized to be related to polycythaemia rubra vera and idiopathic myelofibrosis and these conditions have been classified as the myeloproliferative disorders (Table 2). Chronic granulocytic leukaemia is most frequently associated with polycythaemia, thrombocytosis, and myelofibrosis, but all the conditions listed in Table 1 are clearly disorders of myeloproliferation.

CHRONIC GRANULOCYTIC LEUKAEMIA

Cytogenetic and molecular pathogenesis

The report by Nowell and Hungerford (1960) that myeloid cells from a patient with chronic granulocytic leukaemia showed deletion of the long arms of one of the G group chromosomes was the first association between neoplasia and a chromosomal abnormality in man. The abnormal chromosome, subsequently designated 22, became known as the Philadelphia (Ph, formerly Ph^1) chromosome. Rowley (1973) demonstrated that cells with a Ph chromosome had elongation of the long arms of a chromosome 9 and it was subsequently recognized that the Ph chromosome was the result of a reciprocal translocation of genetic material between one of the 9 chromosome pair and one of the 22 chromosome pair (Fig. 1). The break-points on chromosomes 9 and 22 were consistently found to be at positions 34 and 11 on the respective long arms and this translocation is described by the notation t(9;22)(q34;q11).

The Ph chromosome is found in 90–95 per cent of patients with the clinical features of chronic granulocytic leukaemia and is usually detected in all metaphases examined at diagnosis. A small proportion of patients have complex translocations involving up to three chromosomes in addition to 9 and 22. An even smaller proportion were believed to have variant translocations involving chromosome 22 and a chromosome other than chromosome 9, but recent molecular studies have shown that the Ph translocation invariably

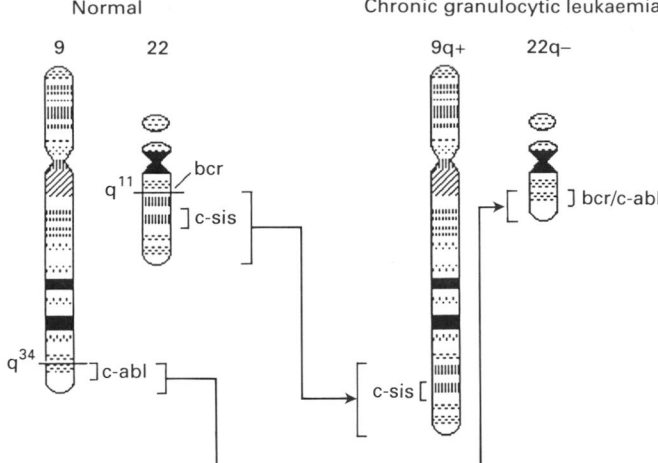

Normal   Chronic granulocytic leukaemia

Fig. 1 The cytogenetic features of the (9;22) translocation showing the Ph chromosome and the juxtaposition of fragments containing the c-*abl* and *bcr* genes.

involves chromosome 9 (Hagemeijer 1987). The Ph chromosome was also found to occur in approximately 20 per cent of adults and 2 per cent of children with acute lymphoblastic leukaemia and in 2 per cent of patients with acute myeloblastic leukaemia (Hagemeijer 1987). For almost three decades this chromosomal abnormality has provided a useful marker for the diagnosis of chronic granulocytic leukaemia, but more recently it has become clear that the exchange of genetic material between chromosomes 9 and 22 involves the translocation of two proto-oncogenes which may have an important role in its pathogenesis. This subject has been reviewed in detail by Kurzrock *et al.* (1988) and Cannistra (1990).

The breaks on the long arm of chromosome 22 which result in the Ph chromosome of chronic granulocytic leukaemia were found to be restricted to a short 5.8 kb segment which has been labelled the 'break-point cluster region' or bcr (Groffen *et al.* 1984). This is part of a gene of at least 90 kb which has become known as the *bcr* gene (Fig. 2). The translation product of the normal *bcr* gene is a 160 kDa protein (p160) which has protein kinase activity. The t(9;22) reciprocal translocation results in the movement of the c-*abl* proto-oncogene from chromosome 9 to the bcr on chromosome 22. The c-*abl* proto-oncogene is the human homologue of the Abelson B-cell murine leukaemia virus oncogene (v-*abl*) which confers upon this virus the ability to cause neoplastic transformation in

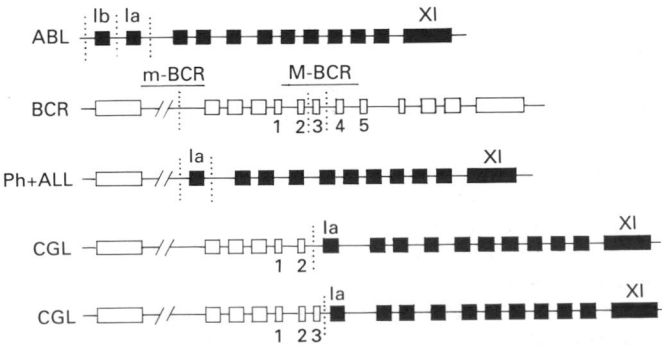

Fig. 2 Schematic representation of the normal c-*abl* and *bcr* genes and the hybrid fusion products which can result from the (9;22) translocation in chronic granulocytic leukaemia and in Ph+ acute lymphatic leukaemia. (From Gale and Goldman 1988.)

haemopoietic cells. The c-*abl* proto-oncogene spans at least 230 kb, contains at least 11 exons (Fig. 2), and has two alternative first exons (Ia and Ib), either of which can be transcribed with exons II to XI. Thus, there are two alternative mRNA transcripts of 6 or 7 kb depending on the first exon transcribed, although only one c-abl protein translation product has been identified in normal cells (see below). The c-*abl* proto-oncogene is situated close to the break-point on chromosome 9 and is thus brought into close proximity to the *bcr* gene on chromosome 22 by the t(9;22) translocation.

In common with a large number of other proto-oncogenes first identified through viral oncogenes, c-*abl* is a normal component of the human genome. It is a highly conserved structure in the genome of all vertebrates and is therefore likely to be important in the ontogeny of these species. Like many proto-oncogenes which have been characterized, it produces a protein which may have an important role in the control of normal cell proliferation (Pierce *et al.* 1986). In common with several retroviral oncogenes, the normal translation product of the human c-*abl* gene is a tyrosine protein kinase with a molecular weight of 145 kDa (p145). Protein kinases catalyse the phosphorylation of proteins on amino acid residues of the substrate protein. Tyrosine phosphorylation is an uncommon cellular event and such proteins may function as second messengers within the cytoplasm of activated cells. The receptors for several growth factors have been shown to have intracellular domains with tyrosine kinase activity (Hunter and Cooper 1985) and a cascade of biochemical events may follow an increase in tyrosine kinase activity thereby transducing the growth factor signal from the surface receptor to the cell nucleus (Kurzrock *et al.* 1988). Abnormal expression of such a protein may lead to increased cellular proliferation. Retrovirus transformation of cells frequently results in higher levels of tyrosine kinase activity than can be detected in the untransformed normal cell (Hunter *et al.* 1984).

The reciprocal t(9;22) translocation also results in the transfer of the c-*sis* proto-oncogene from chromosome 22 to chromosome 9. The c-*sis* proto-oncogene is not situated near the break-point on chromosome 22 and there is no evidence of altered protein structure or expression in chronic granulocytic leukaemia cells. c-*sis* is the human homologue of the Simian sarcoma virus oncogene (v-*sis*) and encodes sequences on the β-chain of platelet–derived growth factor which results in fibroblast stimulation. It is possible that a subtle alteration in the expression of this gene may produce the myelofibrosis which occurs in some patients with chronic granulocytic leukaemia, but this has not yet been demonstrated.

Although the Ph chromosome abnormalities seen in chronic granulocytic leukaemia, acute lymphoblastic leukaemia, and acute myeloid leukaemia appear identical by the conventional cytogenetic techniques, molecular studies have revealed that the c-*abl* proto-oncogene may be translocated to different sites on the long arm of chromosome 22 in these different conditions (Rodenhuis *et al.* 1985; Kurzrock *et al.* 1987*b*). The precise site of breakage within the bcr on chromosome 22 in chronic granulocytic leukaemia is unique to each patient, but generally occurs between exons 2 and 3 or exons 3 and 4 (Fig. 2) (Kurzrock *et al.* 1988) in a region which has been designated the major break-point cluster region (M-bcr). The t(9;22)(q34;q11) balanced translocation of chronic granulocytic leukaemia results in the juxtaposition of c-*abl* to the *bcr* gene on the Ph chromosome. The proximal *bcr* gene sequences are juxtaposed to c-*abl* sequences in a head-to-tail fashion forming a *bcr*–*abl* hybrid gene (Fig. 2) which is expressed in the leukaemic cells (Shtivelman *et al.* 1985).

The chromosome 9 breakage may occur within a region extending over more than 200 kb and the transposed fragment may include exons Ia and Ib of c-*abl* in addition to exons II–XI which are always included (Fig. 2) (Kurzrock *et al.* 1988). This hybrid gene produces an abnormal 8.5 kb mRNA, omitting c-*abl* exons Ia and Ib even if they have been included in the translocation. This occurs as a result of the ability of the splice acceptor site of c-*abl* exon II to accept multiple exon donor sites and ignore nearby exons in favour of those further away (Kurzrock *et al.* 1988). The mRNA transcript consists of the proximal *bcr* exons, extending to exon 2 or 3, fused to c-*abl* exons II–XI (Fig. 2) and the translocation product has a molecular weight of 210 kDa (p210) and is a tyrosine kinase with markedly enhanced activity compared with its normal counterpart (p145) (Konopka *et al.* 1984). Two different RNA messages are produced depending on the site of the M-bcr break-point: (b3a2 or b2a2) though some patients with 5' break-points (that is, including *bcr* exon 2) produce the b3a2 message (reviewed in Kantarjian *et al.* 1993).

The p210 hybrid gene product is expressed in virtually all patients with chronic granulocytic leukaemia but in no other forms of leukaemia. If it is capable of causing uncontrolled proliferation of the cells in which it is expressed, the t(9;22) translocation and its p210 product clearly play a major role in the pathogenesis of chronic granulocytic leukaemia. *In vitro* transformation of murine haemopoietic cells by the p210 *bcr*–*abl* oncogene product of the Ph chromosome has been reported in an experimental system (Daley *et al.* 1990) and experimental data suggest that the abnormal p210 tyrosine kinase may induce secondary activation of growth factors such as interleukin 3 (IL-3) and granulocyte colony-stimulating factor which could then induce the development and progression of chronic granulocytic leukaemia (Kurzrock *et al.* 1988; Goldman *et al.* 1990). It has been suggested that patients with break-points placed downstream of 3' in the M-bcr may be more likely to progress to the accelerated phase after a short chronic phase (Schaefer-Rego *et al.* 1987), although this has not been a universal finding (Dreazen *et al.* 1988; Mills and Birnie 1991).

Ph-negative chronic granulocytic leukaemia

The Ph chromosome is not detected in approximately 5 per cent of patients who are believed to have the diagnosis of chronic granulocytic leukaemia on clinical and haematological grounds. The majority of these patients are found to have a normal karyotype, with various other abnormalities, commonly trisomy 8, detected in approximately one-third of patients. Recent molecular studies have clarified the pathological basis on which these patients can be reclassified.

Some of these patients have clinical and haematological features and a subsequent clinical course identical to that of patients with Ph-positive chronic granulocytic leukaemia. These patients have also been shown to have expression of the hybrid p210 protein and other molecular features pathognomonic for Ph-positive chronic granulocytic leukaemia (Bartram *et al.* 1985; Wiedemann *et al.* 1988). It appears that in these patients, interstitial insertion of the c-*abl* gene next to the *bcr* gene has occurred on chromosome 22 without the reciprocal translocation of genomic material to chromosome 9 and formation of the characteristic Ph chromosome (Morris *et al.* 1986; Kantarjian *et al.* 1987). Nevertheless, the presence of the hybrid protein and the identical clinical features, course, and response to therapy in Ph-positive patients with chronic granulocytic leukaemia and the subgroup of *bcr*–*abl*-positive Ph-negative patients indicates that these patients have the same disease.

A further group of Ph-negative chronic myeloid leukaemia patients have distinct clinical features on closer examination. Early analyses suggested that the whole group labelled Ph-negative

chronic myeloid leukaemia had short survival, poor response to chemotherapy, thrombocytopenia, and absence of basophilia, but these features appear to be characteristic only of patients who are found to be negative for the p210 hybrid protein (Kantarjian *et al.* 1987; Wiedemann *et al.* 1988). In contrast, these features are often associated with chromosomal abnormalities other than t(9;22) and many of these patients can be reclassified as suffering from myelodysplastic syndromes (see below).

A small proportion of patients with otherwise typical chronic granulocytic leukaemia have been found to be negative for both the Ph chromosome and the bcr rearrangement after extensive molecular analysis (Kurzrock *et al.* 1988). The identification of an aberrant *bcr* mRNA in a single patient (Bartram 1985) without c-*abl* juxtaposition raises the possibility that alternative molecular events may have precipitated leukaemogenesis in these patients.

Ph-positive acute lymphoblastic leukaemia

Standard cytogenetic technology shows blast cells in a proportion of patients with otherwise typical acute lymphoblastic leukaemia contain a Ph chromosome with an identical t(9;22) translocation. This occurs in approximately 20 per cent of adults and 2 per cent of children with acute lymphoblastic leukaemia and patients with this feature have a poorer prognosis than those in whom no Ph chromosome is detected. The majority of these patients have no features to suggest that they have had antecedent chronic granulocytic leukaemia and, unlike patients with chronic granulocytic leukaemia blast crisis, the Ph chromosome disappears in most of those who achieve complete remission. A small proportion of patients who achieve complete remission develop chronic granulocytic leukaemia chronic phase with persistent Ph chromosome expression. The clinical and haematological differentiation of *de novo* Ph-positive acute leukaemia from chronic granulocytic leukaemia in blast crisis is often difficult. The latter diagnosis is strongly favoured by the presence of basophilia or marked splenomegaly.

Recent molecular studies have conclusively demonstrated that approximately 50 per cent of adults and 10 per cent of children with Ph-positive acute lymphoblastic leukaemia (Kurzrock *et al.* 1988) have a chromosome break-point within the M-bcr region and probably represent transformed chronic granulocytic leukaemia, but the others do not have the bcr rearrangement and have a break-point in the DNA upstream of 5' (Fig. 2) (Rodenhuis *et al.* 1985; Kurzrock *et al.* 1987*a*). This break-point is in the large first intron of the *bcr* gene and has been labelled the minor break-point cluster region or m-bcr (Fig. 2). These patients have expression of a different hybrid gene involving only the first exon of the *bcr* gene (Fig. 2); that is, only a portion of the genetic material from the *bcr* gene contributing to the p210 hybrid protein of chronic granulocytic leukaemia. This produces a 7.0 kb mRNA and a p190 protein distinct from both the p145 protein product of the c-*abl* gene in normal cells and the p210 *bcr*–*abl* hybrid product of classical chronic granulocytic leukaemia. The p190 protein is also a highly active tyrosine kinase (Clark *et al.* 1987).

It is possible that the site to which the c-*abl* gene is translocated on chromosome 22 may determine the malignant phenotype expressed by the abnormal clone, though a similar hybrid protein to that of acute lymphoblastic leukaemia has been described in a case of acute myeloid leukaemia (Kurzrock *et al.* 1987*b*). In view of the consistent molecular rearrangements it also seems possible that the translocation itself is the transforming event from which the malignant clone emerges in these conditions. However, the occurrence of similar clinical phenotypes in the absence of these molecular rearrangements suggests that other pathogenetic mechanisms must exist. A similar spectrum of leukaemia is seen in animals inoculated with cells bearing either of the *bcr–abl* fusion genes. However, animals inoculated with cells producing the p190 protein develop a more aggressive disease with a shorter latent period than those inoculated with cells with the p210 product (Kelliher *et al.* 1991). This may suggest that the type of *bcr–abl* fusion product does not dictate the phenotype of disease produced but does influence the potency of the oncogenic signal.

Pathophysiology of chronic granulocytic leukaemia

The development of chronic granulocytic leukaemia is believed to be a multistep process where the leukaemic stem cell in which the initial neoplastic event occurs is pluripotent. This acquires a proliferative advantage over the normal stem cells whose proliferation appears to be suppressed. In the chronic phase there is an increase of 3–30-fold in the peripheral granulocyte count and an increase of 10–100-fold in the total granulocyte mass with increased numbers of progenitor cells in the blood and bone-marrow (Spiers *et al.* 1977). This is due in part to a mean half-life for chronic granulocytic leukaemia granulocytes that is five to ten times longer than that for normal granulocytes. There is evidence in the chronic phase of at least partial responsiveness to regulatory control mechanisms, demonstrated by cyclical oscillations in the leucocyte and platelet counts (Spiers *et al.* 1977). However, there is some *in vitro* evidence that chronic granulocytic leukaemia cells are relatively insensitive to feedback inhibition through decreased chronic granulocytic leukaemia granulocyte production of lactoferrin which inhibits normal myelopoiesis, decreased sensitivity of chronic granulocytic leukaemia monocytes to regulation by lactoferrin, and decreased sensitivity of chronic granulocytic leukaemia progenitor cells to prostaglandin E and acidic isoferritins which are other putative regulators of normal myelopoiesis (Broxmeyer *et al.* 1977; Pelus *et al.* 1980). These observations may explain the apparent proliferative advantage of the chronic granulocytic leukaemia clone over normal haemopoiesis.

Suppression of non-leukaemic haemopoiesis is suggested by the presence of only Ph-positive metaphases at the time of diagnosis in almost all patients and the observation that presumably normal Ph-negative metaphases can be detected later in patients treated with intensive chemotherapy. The pluripotential nature of the chronic granulocytic leukaemia stem cell is suggested not only by the clonal involvement of the granulocyte lineage, including eosinophils and basophils, but also by demonstration of involvement of monocytes, megakaryocytes, erythroid cells, B lymphocytes, and some T lymphocytes by cytogenetic, glucose-6-phosphate dehydrogenase enzymatic and molecular studies (Barr and Fialkow 1973; Fialkow *et al.* 1977; Golde *et al.* 1977; Denegri *et al.* 1978; Koeffler *et al.* 1980; Martin *et al.* 1980). Marrow fibroblasts are Ph negative and therefore are probably not involved in the neoplastic clone. Thus, the increase in bone-marrow reticulin and collagen fibrosis which develops in a proportion of patients with chronic granulocytic leukaemia appears to be a secondary phenomenon.

It is not yet clearly established that the t(9;22) is the initiating event in chronic granulocytic leukaemia and the Ph-negative metaphases which may be reinduced in the marrow of patients are not necessarily normal. It is clear that the Ph-positive clone is chromosomally unstable and a number of other characteristic non-random chromosomal abnormalities occur during the course of chronic granulocytic leukaemia. Rarely, the clinical and haematological features of chronic granulocytic leukaemia have persisted after treatment while the Ph abnormality has disappeared. However, there is clear evidence from *in vitro* studies that the Ph-negative cells which may be found in chronic granulocytic leukaemia are non-clonal (Singer *et al.* 1980) and molecular studies have confirmed the absence of the p210 protein (Yoffe *et al.* 1987). This suggests that there is a suppressed residual normal stem cell pool, at least in the early stages of the condition.

Clinical features

Chronic granulocytic leukaemia is a biphasic or triphasic disease. Most patients present in a stable 'chronic phase', but this inexorably progresses to 'blast transformation' after a median period of 44 months either directly or following a period of 'accelerated phase'. Blast transformation is generally fatal in 3–6 months. The median survival of patients with chronic granulocytic leukaemia is now in the region of 60–65 months with 75–85 per cent of patients alive at 3 years (Kantarjian *et al.* 1993).

Symptoms

The commonest presenting symptoms are those of anaemia or discomfort due to splenomegaly. Less commonly a patient will complain of weight loss, sweating, bone pain, bruising, bleeding, or neurological symptoms due to leucostasis. Many patients are now diagnosed as a result of routine blood testing and patients with a very high leukaemia cell load are less common.

Physical findings

Splenomegaly is present in 90 per cent of patients and is occasionally massive. A few patients also have hepatomegaly at diagnosis, but lymphadenopathy due to chronic granulocytic leukaemia is uncommon. Low-grade fever, ecchymoses, and sternal tenderness may be present. Signs related to leucostasis (focal neurological signs, papilloedema, retinal haemorrhages) are occasionally seen in patients with marked elevation of the leucocyte count.

Natural history and prognostic factors

Chronic phase

The elevated leucocyte count of chronic phase chronic granulocytic leukaemia is generally easily controlled by therapy. The median duration of chronic phase from diagnosis to transformation is 44 months, though the range is wide and prolonged survival for periods as long as 20 years has been reported in a small number of patients. Accurate prediction of the prognosis of an individual patient is extremely difficult, although numerous attempts have been made to devise prognostic classifications.

There has been little unanimity on prognostic criteria between different study groups and only spleen size has been uniformly accepted as an indicator of poor prognosis. Multivariate analysis of data derived from six retrospective studies has identified age, spleen size, platelet count, and percentage of circulating blasts as highly significant prognostic features for patients with chronic granulocytic leukaemia (Sokal *et al.* 1984). These parameters were used to derive a 'hazard ratio formula' which has been shown to have prognostic value in a large Italian prospective study (Italian Cooperative Study Group 1988). Sex and haemoglobin become significant and age loses significance when only patients eligible for bone-marrow transplantation (younger than 46 years) are considered (Sokal *et al.* 1985). The results of the Italian

Table 3 Poor risk features at diagnosis of chronic granulocytic leukaemia

Marked splenomegaly (>15 cm)
Hepatomegaly (>6 cm)
High leucocyte count (>100×10⁹/l)
Thrombocytopenia (<150×10⁹/l)
Thrombocytosis (>500×10⁹/l)
High proportion of blasts or promyelocytes in the peripheral blood

prospective study were less conclusive with the formula derived for this younger group.

An earlier study identified the features listed in Table 3 as likely to be associated with early transformation (Tura *et al.* 1981). In addition, a patient who requires regular chemotherapy to maintain near-normal leucocyte counts can be expected to transform earlier than a patient in whom control is easily achieved.

The prognostic significance of chromosomal mosaicism, that is, the presence of residual normal metaphases in addition to Ph-positive metaphases either at diagnosis or as a result of therapy, is unclear. Although a small number of patients with mosaicism have had prolonged survival (Singer *et al.* 1984; Nowell *et al.* 1988), studies of deliberate induction of marrow hypoplasia to produce mosaicism on regeneration have not conclusively been associated with either delay in blast transformation or improved survival (Cunningham *et al.* 1979; Sharp *et al.* 1979). Interferon therapy may also permit Ph-negative clones to re-emerge in a proportion of patients (Talpaz *et al.* 1986) and early data suggest that this treatment may prolong survival (Kantarjian *et al.* 1993) although this remains controversial.

Accelerated phase

An accelerated phase lasting weeks or months may precede frank blast transformation. It is often difficult to recognize the onset of the accelerated phase and the diagnosis is often made retrospectively. This phase is associated with increasing resistance to therapy, more rapid cellular proliferation, and maturation arrest in the neoplastic clone. Features which may indicate the onset of accelerated phase in a patient with chronic phase chronic granulocytic leukaemia are listed in Table 4. Accelerated phase should always be suspected in a patient with chronic phase chronic granulocytic leukaemia who presents with vague symptoms (for example, fever, weight loss, or bone pain).

Blast transformation

Blast transformation may occur suddenly in a patient who was apparently in a stable chronic phase or may be recognized by a gradual increase in the number of blast cells in the blood and bone-marrow. Blast transformation can be defined by the presence of

Table 4 Features suggesting the onset of accelerated phase in chronic granulocytic leukaemia

Leucocyte count resistant to control with busulphan or hydroxyurea
Very rapid leucocyte doubling time (<5 days)
More than 5 per cent blasts in blood
More than 20 per cent blasts plus promyelocytes in marrow
More than 20 per cent basophils plus eosinophils in blood
Anaemia or thrombocytopenia despite adequate chemotherapy
Thrombocytosis above 100×10¹⁰/l· (in the absence of splenectomy)
Further chromosomal abnormalities in addition to the Ph chromosome
Persistent or increasing splenomegaly
Development of marrow failure associated with myelofibrosis
Unexplained fever

more than 30 per cent blasts plus promyelocytes in the blood or marrow. Patients are often unwell and may complain of fever, night sweats, weight loss, bone pain, and splenic pain. In addition, they may have symptoms of anaemia, infection, bleeding, or bruising. Occasionally a patient will present with generalized lymphadenopathy, neurological symptoms, and signs suggesting central nervous system involvement or symptoms of hyperviscosity due to leucostasis. Survival of 2–6 months is usual, with survival of over 1 year uncommon.

Laboratory features

At the time of diagnosis, the leucocyte count is generally between 100×10⁹/l and 300×10⁹/l, but may range from 20×10⁹ to 1000×10⁹/l. All stages of myeloid maturation are found in the peripheral blood, but there are characteristic peaks of myelocytes and mature neutrophils (Fig. 3). By definition blasts and promyelocytes constitute less than 10 per cent of peripheral blood cells in chronic phase. Basophils and occasionally eosinophils are prominent. There is almost invariably a relative reduction in the numbers of monocytes. The absolute numbers of lymphocytes are normal. The leucocyte alkaline phosphatase score is characteristically reduced and will swiftly differentiate chronic granulocytic leukaemia from a leukaemoid reaction due to sepsis. The leucocyte alkaline phosphatase score can be expected to increase in haematological remission induced by chemotherapy, during infection, and with progression to accelerated phase disease.

The haemoglobin is often reduced, particularly in association with leucocyte counts over 150×10⁹/l or large spleens. In contrast, the platelet count is usually moderately increased. Biochemical investigations generally reveal elevated serum lactate dehydrogenase, uric acid, vitamin B_{12}, and vitamin B_{12} binding capacity (transcobalamin I). The changes in B_{12} and B_{12} binding capacity reflect the increased production of transcobalamin I by the expanded granulocyte pool.

The bone-marrow is hypercellular with loss of fat spaces and expansion of cellular bone-marrow throughout the long bones. The marrow aspirate shows an increased myeloid to erythroid ratio with increased numbers of all myeloid progenitor cells. Megakaryocytes are also usually increased and may show left shift. Various degrees of basophilia and eosinophilia occur in the bone-marrow. Lipid-laden reticuloendothelial cells resembling those present in storage

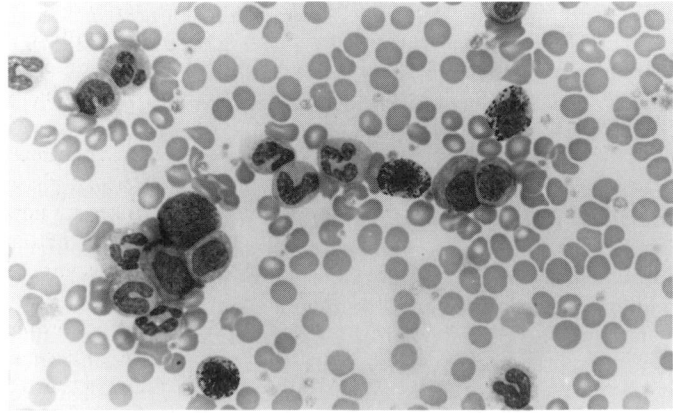

Fig. 3 Peripheral blood in chronic granulocytic leukaemia showing promyelocytes, myelocytes, and mature granulocytes. Basophils are prominent and there is thrombocythaemia with giant platelets.

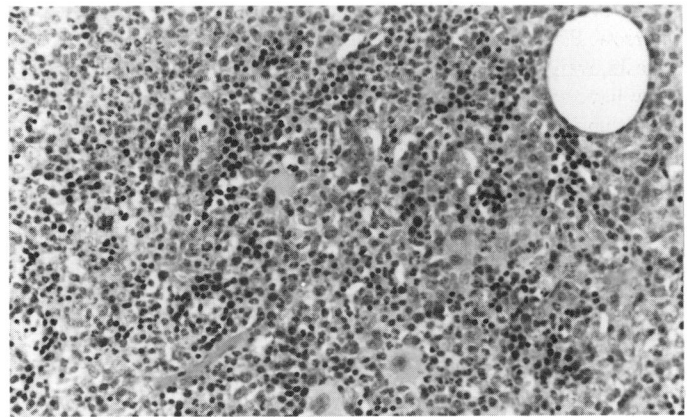

Fig. 4 Bone-marrow trephine biopsy (haematoxylin and eosin stain) in chronic granulocytic leukaemia with complete elimination of fat spaces due to gross trilineage hypercellularity. Granulopoiesis and megakaryocytes are particularly prominent. A blood vessel is also seen.

disorders (pseudo-Gaucher cells) are occasionally seen in the bone-marrow aspirate or trephine biopsy; they may reflect an increase in cell death within the hyperplastic bone-marrow.

A bone-marrow trephine biopsy will demonstrate marrow hypercellularity, increased myelopoiesis and megakaryocytopoiesis, and loss of fat spaces (Fig. 4). It frequently also shows increased reticulin staining. Occasionally extensive fibrosis is seen at diagnosis and this will eventually develop in 30–40 per cent of patients during the course of the disease.

Cytogenetic analysis confirms the presence of the Ph chromosome in 90–95 per cent of patients with a clinical and haematological diagnosis of chronic granulocytic leukaemia. The classical t(9;22)(9q34;q11) translocation is found in 95 per cent of patients who are Ph positive.

Progression to blast transformation is associated with an increase in the percentage of bone-marrow blasts and promyelocytes to over 30 per cent. The accelerated phase may be associated with a smaller increase in the proportion of blasts and promyelocytes or increased proportions of basophils or eosinophils. The blast cells have the morphological, cytochemical, and surface phenotypic features of myeloblasts in over 60 per cent of patients, features of pre-B cells equivalent to common acute lymphoblastic leukaemia in up to 30 per cent, and features of both myeloid and lymphoid cells in 10 per cent. Under 10 per cent of cases develop megakaryoblastic or erythroid blast crisis. A few cases of blast transformation with cells bearing T-lymphoid markers have been reported. In some cases all immunocytochemical stains are negative and these blasts probably represent more primitive undifferentiated cells.

Clonal evolution in the form of additional chromosomal abnormalities is seen in up to 80 per cent of patients in accelerated phase or blast transformation. Characteristic non-random changes are now recognized, the most frequent of which are duplication of the Ph chromosome, trisomy 8, trisomy 19, and isochromosome 17 (Hagemeijer 1987). It seems likely that the development of these abnormalities is related to the change in the character of chronic granulocytic leukaemia which accompanies them. The molecular events involved in clonal evolution are currently under intensive study; possible mechanisms include excessive expression of c-*myc* with trisomy 8, *bcr–abl* with the double Ph chromosome, and granulocyte colony-stimulating factor or P53 with isochromosome 17 (reviewed by Kurzrock *et al.* 1988). Other groups have attempted

to correlate the exact molecular site of the break within the 5.8 kb *bcr* on chromosome 22 and the clinical course, in particular the duration of chronic phase, but the results to date are inconclusive (Mills *et al.* 1991). Deletion of *bcr–abl* sequences has been documented in cells from a patient who entered blast crisis, which indicates that the p210 hybrid protein may not be necessary to sustain the leukaemic state once chronic granulocytic leukaemia has progressed beyond the chronic phase. It is clear that the Ph-positive clone is chromosomally unstable and secondary genetic abnormalities may be required for the development of blast transformation.

In some patients, marrow fibrosis may progressively increase and finally result in blood and marrow appearances indistinguishable from primary myelofibrosis except for the presence of the Ph chromosome. Some 10–20 per cent of patients die of bone-marrow failure due to increasing fibrosis without entering 'blast crisis'.

Treatment

Treatment in chronic phase

Although there has been an increase in survival duration compared with historical reports of untreated patients, there is no undisputed evidence that any treatment apart from bone-marrow transplantation has any impact on long-term survival of patients with chronic granulocytic leukaemia. Control of the elevated leucocyte count through chemotherapy does not delay the onset of blast transformation and conventional treatment should be used to treat or prevent the onset of symptoms rather than simply render the leucocyte count normal. However, some recent studies suggest that patients who obtain a minor cytogenetic response with α-interferon may have prolongation of both chronic phase and overall survival (Kantarjian *et al.* 1993) but this remains controversial (Ozer *et al.* 1993).

Prior to the development of the chemotherapeutic agents, irradiation of the spleen was the mainstay of treatment. It provided symptomatic relief and improved clinical and haematological abnormalities but did not substantially alter survival. Since the first report of the value of busulphan (Galton 1953), conventional treatment of chronic granulocytic leukaemia has been single-agent therapy with either busulphan or hydroxyurca which was developed in 1960.

Single-agent chemotherapy

Busulphan is a sulphonic acid alkylating agent and is a clearly superior treatment to radiotherapy (Medical Research Council 1968). This drug may be administered as a regular daily oral dose, usually beginning at 6 or 8 mg which is reduced as the leucocyte count falls. It should be discontinued when the leucocyte count falls below $50 \times 10^9/l$ as its therapeutic effect continues for some 2–3 weeks and prolonged aplasia may result. This is thought to be due to action on the early progenitor compartment which explains the slow but prolonged disease control obtained with this agent. Patients receiving busulphan should be closely monitored as some are highly sensitive to this drug. An alternative approach is the use of pulsed higher doses of busulphan; that is, 50–100 mg at monthly intervals. When normal or near normal leucocyte counts are attained, patients may be maintained on low doses of busulphan (0.5–2.0 mg/day) or the drug may be discontinued until the leucocyte count rises again. The side-effects of prolonged treatment with busulphan are skin pigmentation, infertility, and interstitial fibrosis of the lung.

Hydroxyurea is an alternative therapy for chronic phase chronic granulocytic leukaemia and its use has become more widespread in recent years. It is a ribonucleotide reductase inhibitor of DNA synthesis and acts on the late progenitor compartment. The initial daily dosage is 1.5–2.0 g orally and its effect is more rapid than that of busulphan. Thus, it can reduce a markedly elevated leucocyte count more swiftly. However, the effect of busulphan is more prolonged and hydroxyurea must be continued indefinitely at a dose of 0.5–1.0 g/day to control the leucocyte count. An alternative approach is to commence at a dose of 10 g daily, halving the dose with each halving of the leucocyte count and discontinuing therapy at a leucocyte count of 10×10^9–15×10^9/l. The side-effects of hydroxyurea are nausea, vomiting, and headache.

Until recently there has been no convincing evidence of superiority for either agent (Rushing et al. 1982) and the more severe side-effects of busulphan were balanced by the need to take continuous therapy when hydroxyurea is used. However, a German multicentre randomized comparison of busulphan and hydroxyurea treatment in 441 patients (Hehlman et al. 1993) has demonstrated a significant survival advantage for hydroxyurea-treated patients in all risk groups (58.2 months versus 45.4 months, $p=0.008$). Busulphan may be best reserved for use as second-line therapy for patients with disease resistant to hydroxyurea. In addition, previous treatment with busulphan has been identified as an adverse risk factor in patients undergoing a subsequent bone-marrow transplant (Goldman et al. 1993). In view of the more frequent use of allogeneic bone-marrow transplantation, the lower toxicity of hydroxyurea, particularly to the lungs, makes it a better initial choice for patients for whom transplantation may be considered later. Haematological response to either of these agents is associated with persistence of the Ph chromosome in all metaphases in the vast majority of patients. Only infrequently are normal metaphases found after busulphan therapy. The median survival of patients treated with single-agent chemotherapy is 3–4.5 years in most series and most patients die as a result of blast transformation (Rushing et al. 1982). The risk of transformation and death in patients who receive conventional treatment is approximately 10 per cent in each of the first 2 years after diagnosis and 20–25 per cent per year thereafter (Sokal et al. 1985).

Other chemotherapeutic agents have been used. Single-agent 6–mercaptopurine, chlorambucil, melphalan, or dibromomannitol offer no advantage over busulphan and several have given shorter median survivals. The addition of 6-mercaptopurine or 6–thioguanine to busulphan increases the speed at which a normal leucocyte count is achieved and reduces the amount of busulphan administered, but may result in increased hepatotoxicity.

Intensive combination chemotherapy

Intensive combination chemotherapy has been used in chronic phase chronic granulocytic leukaemia in an attempt to reinduce the presence of Ph-negative haemopoiesis and in the hope of eradicating the Ph-positive clone. Reductions in Ph-positive metaphases to 20–50 per cent was achieved in approximately one-third of patients by a number of groups using cycles of combination chemotherapy similar to those used in the treatment of the acute leukaemias (Cunningham et al. 1979; Sharpe et al. 1979). Sadly, this was usually transient and the intensive therapy used in these studies appeared neither to delay blast transformation nor to prolong survival significantly.

A longer median survival for patients with intermediate and high risk features (58 months and 33 months, respectively) has been claimed for the combination of vincristine, cytosine arabinoside, prednisolone, and rubidazone with suppression of Ph-positive metaphases to less than 35 per cent in over 50 per cent of patients

(Kantarjian et al. 1985). Cyclical courses of intensive chemotherapy at 6–12 month intervals have been suggested to improve these results further. However, there is a significant morbidity and mortality associated with intensive therapy and the benefits of this therapeutic approach have yet to receive universal recognition.

More recently it has been demonstrated that pure Ph-negative haemopoietic stem cells can be harvested by leucopheresis from the peripheral blood of at least a proportion of patients with chronic phase chronic granulocytic leukaemia who have received myeloablative chemotherapy (Sessarego et al. 1992). This offers the prospect of Ph-negative stem cell autografts for some patients who cannot receive an allograft due to the absence of a compatible donor. A number of studies of this approach are now in progress.

Leucopheresis

Leucopheresis has been used to induce a rapid reduction in the circulating leucocyte count, but without the addition of chemotherapy the effect is transient. This treatment offers symptomatic benefit but there is no evidence for prolongation of the chronic phase. This technique has been used in the past to obtain marrow progenitors during chronic phase for cryopreservation for subsequent autologous bone-marrow rescue after intensive therapy of blast crisis (see below). The demonstration that Ph-negative stem cells can be obtained after myeloablative therapy has rekindled interest in autologous peripheral blood stem cell collection to provide a source of haemopoietic rescue after high-dose therapy.

Splenic irradiation or splenectomy

The use of splenic irradiation was not found to have a significant impact upon survival and there was no survival advantage for splenectomized patients in randomized trials of chemotherapy with or without splenectomy (Medical Research Council 1983; Italian Cooperative Study Group 1988).

Interferon therapy

The mode of action of the interferons is unknown. Interferons suppress the in vitro growth and differentiation of myeloid progenitor cells.from patients with chronic granulocytic leukaemia (Oladipupo-Williams et al. 1981). α-Interferon appears preferentially to inhibit the late progenitor compartment which may be the major phase of chronic granulocytic leukaemia clonal expansion (Galvani and Cawley 1989). α-Interferon binding to cell surface receptors has been found to induce a marked increase in the cellular content of 2',5'-oligoadenylate synthetase, though this did not occur when the patients became resistant (Rosenblum et al. 1986). Reduction of c-abl oncogene expression has been reported after therapy with α-interferon (Brodsky et al. 1987) and this correlates with suppression of oncogene expression in other cell lines by interferons.

Recently there has been considerable interest in the use of α-interferon therapy in chronic phase chronic granulocytic leukaemia and the topic is discussed in detail by Talpaz et al. (1988) and Kantarjian et al. (1993). Initial studies used a partially pure natural α-interferon prepared by the Finnish Red Cross from donated blood and 51 newly diagnosed patients received this preparation as a daily intramuscular injection. Complete haematological response (normal blood and marrow, impalpable spleen) occurred in 36 patients and 20 patients also showed a reduction in the proportion of Ph-positive metaphases, eight patients to less than 35 per cent and some for prolonged periods. Subsequent studies have generally used recombinant α-interferon at a dose of 5 mu/m² /day.

Studies of α-interferon therapy in chronic granulocytic leukaemia have been reviewed by Kantarjian et al. (1993). Therapy with α-interferon achieves a complete haematological response (normalization of blood count and bone-marrow appearances) in 37–84 per cent of patients, with some cytogenetic response in 49–63 per cent, and a major cytogenetic response in 30–40 per cent (defined as suppression of the proportion of Ph-positive metaphases in the marrow to <35 per cent). A cytogenetic response generally takes some 9–12 months of continuous interferon therapy to emerge and up to 15 per cent of patients may develop a complete cytogenetic response with no detectable Ph-positive metaphases in the bone-marrow (Talpaz et al. 1991). Differences in the responses obtained by different study groups may relate to the stage of disease of the patients treated, pre-treatment characteristics, or the dose schedule of α-interferon used. A clear dose–response relationship has been demonstrated (Alimena et al. 1988). Durable cytogenetic responses have been obtained in 30 per cent of patients and the longest durations are seen in those patients who achieve a complete cytogenetic response. Although molecular studies have been reported suggesting that the abnormal clone has been completely eliminated after α-interferon therapy (Oguma et al. 1992), it is more usual for patients with complete cytogenetic remission to have evidence of persistent, albeit minimal, disease when analysed for the bcr–abl using the polymerase chain reaction (PCR) (Lee et al. 1992; Mahon et al. 1992). Patients with early chronic phase (<1 year from diagnosis) appear to achieve better response rates to α-interferon. Median survivals of 60–65 months and durable cytogenetic responses in 25 per cent of these patients have been reported and Kantarjian et al. (1993) have suggested that α-interferon may be superior to conventional single-agent chemotherapy. However, benefit may only be obtained in those patients who achieve a reduction in Ph-positive metaphases of over 50 per cent after 12 months and it is perhaps this group who should continue long-term α-interferon.

The observation that mosaicism has been most marked in patients treated early correlates with the results of long-term liquid in vitro cultures, where there is a higher yield of Ph-negative clones from bone-marrow taken in early chronic phase compared with that taken later and suggests that there may be gradual depletion and eventual loss of the suppressed Ph-negative normal stem cell pool with time (Coulombel et al. 1983). Response to α-interferon therapy, Ph-suppression, and 3 year survival have been better among low-risk patients than among patients in the intermediate and high-risk groups (Talpaz et al. 1987). It is too early to state conclusively whether this new approach has any impact on either the onset of blast crisis or survival, though an association between cytogenetic response and survival has been reported by several groups (reviewed by Kantarjian et al. 1993) but not all (Ozer et al. 1993).

The side-effects of therapy with α-interferon are influenza-like symptoms, lethargy, poor memory, and myalgia. The influenza-like febrile reaction is only marked during the initial days of therapy in most patients and is usually suppressed by paracetamol. Serious late side-effects of anorexia and weight loss, neurotoxicity and parkinsonian syndromes, and immune thrombocytopenia occur in under 10 per cent of patients. The majority of patients easily adapt to self-administration of interferon by subcutaneous injection, but it remains less convenient than oral hydroxyurea. Dose reductions are required in up to 40 per cent of patients particularly those aged over 60 years. If the ongoing studies confirm prolongation of survival, then these disadvantages will be acceptable.

A combined modality approach exploiting the different modes of action and therapeutic effects of chemotherapy and interferon has been examined in a small number of patients. The combination of low-dose cytosine arabinoside and α-interferon has been reported to produce better responses than α-interferon alone (Kantarjian et al. 1992) but combination with other agents has not been shown to be advantageous. More recently the sequential use of intensive cytoreduction by chemotherapy followed by α-interferon has been explored. The additional prospect of harvesting Ph-negative stem cells from the peripheral blood after intensive therapy may offer patients without compatible donors the opportunity of a subsequent 'transplant'. The results of these studies are awaited with much interest.

Investigational therapies

The plant alkaloid homoharringtonine has significant activity in chronic granulocytic leukaemia, producing haematological responses in 95 per cent of patients with early and 68 per cent of patients with late chronic phase disease and cytogenetic responses in 62 and 31 per cent, respectively (O'Brien et al. 1993). The mechanism of action of this agent is unknown.

A small number of patients have been treated with the recombinant γ-interferon which has similar in vitro properties to α-interferon. γ-Interferon is a structurally distinct molecule which binds to a separate cell surface receptor. The response rate has been lower than that obtained with α-interferon, though some patients resistant to α-interferon have achieved complete haematological responses. The converse has also been reported. Studies using both interferons in combination have shown no added benefit.

Bone-marrow transplantation

The aims of allogeneic bone-marrow transplantation are

(1) eradication of the leukaemic clone with myelo-ablative doses of chemotherapy and radiotherapy (which also provides the immunosuppression necessary for engraftment);

(2) restoration of normal haemopoiesis with normal donor bone-marrow;

(3) exploitation of the graft versus leukaemia effect of the normal donor marrow system.

Most patients have received cyclophosphamide (two doses of 60 mg/kg with total body irradiation (usually 10 Gy) or busulphan (16 mg/kg over 4 days) as cytoreduction. Because of the potential toxicity of the procedure, many centres restrict this treatment to patients under the age of 45 years. Nevertheless, matched sibling allografts for chronic granulocytic leukaemia have been used successfully in patients between the ages of 50 and 60 years (McGlave 1992) and the Seattle group recommend an upper age limit of 60 years on the basis of excellent results up to this age (Clift et al. 1993). The major risk of bone-marrow transplantation is the development of fatal graft versus host disease. Graft versus host disease prophylaxis has improved in recent years by the use of a combination of cyclosporin A and methotrexate or by T-cell depletion of the graft. However, graft versus host disease is a double-edged sword and, provided that it is not fatal, produces a graft versus leukaemia effect which provides a major component of the curative value of bone-marrow transplantation.

It is clear that allogeneic bone-marrow transplantation in the chronic phase provides the best chance of prolonged survival for younger patients with chronic granulocytic leukaemia. The actuarial probability of 3 year survival is 49–56 per cent for recipients in the chronic phase, falling to 15–28 per cent for recipients in the accelerated phase, and to 14–16 per cent for recipients with blast transformation (Goldman et al. 1986; Thomas et al. 1986). Relapse after bone-marrow transplantation is more common in patients grafted in the accelerated phase (50 per cent) or in blast crisis (60 per cent) than in chronic phase recipients (7–20 per cent). Bone-marrow transplantation beyond the chronic phase is also associated with a higher procedure-related mortality, which can rise to 20 per cent for chronic phase patients. However, it is clear that some patients who received bone-marrow transplantation beyond chronic phase 5–10 years ago have probably been cured and bone-marrow transplantation remains the best treatment option for the patient in this position who has a compatible donor (Thomas and Clift 1989).

There is now universal agreement that bone-marrow transplantation is best carried out in the chronic phase but the optimum timing within this phase has not been established until recently. Clearly, procedure-related mortality of up to 20 per cent has prevented bone-marrow transplantation from being undertaken quickly in young patients who could remain well in the chronic phase for several years. Studies in Seattle (Thomas et al. 1986) have suggested that the interval from diagnosis to transplantation in the chronic phase also has an effect on outcome: 70 per cent of patients transplanted in the first year after diagnosis will be long-term survivors. This would justify early transplantation in all patients aged under 45 years who have a compatible donor (Thomas and Clift 1989). Only recently has an International Bone Marrow Transplant Registry analysis of 450 patients transplanted in chronic phase between 1985 and 1990 confirmed this observation that leukaemia-free survival is better in patients transplanted within 1 year of diagnosis (Goldman et al. 1993). This review also identified previous treatment with busulphan rather than hydroxyurea as a poor risk factor for leukaemia-free survival after transplantation. It is possible that prolonged busulphan therapy contributes to the poorer outcome in patients transplanted later in chronic phase (Clift et al. 1993). The Seattle group have reported a 90 per cent probability of survival at 1 year and 81 per cent probability of survival at 5 years for patients transplanted in chronic phase within 1 year of diagnosis. This analysis suggests that delay over 2 years is associated with an adverse impact on survival and the improved results of patients transplanted between 1 and 2 years from diagnosis compared to earlier analyses may reflect the more widespread use of hydroxyurea as first line therapy (Clift et al. 1993). Meanwhile some groups have used mathematical models to assess relative risk and prognostic formulae to identify the patients for whom early transplantation should be recommended. Wagner et al. (1992) evaluated the outcome after transplantation in chronic phase against recognized risk factors at diagnosis and concluded that all patients with compatible sibling donors should be transplanted early after diagnosis.

The precise timing of bone-marrow transplantation for a patient in chronic phase chronic granulocytic leukaemia with a compatible donor remains a difficult decision as the time to transformation cannot be predicted with certainty. However, every patient who has a normal identical twin should be considered for early bone-marrow transplantation, regardless of age or stage of the disease, as the procedural risks are less, and younger patients with a compatible sibling donor should receive a transplant within 1–2 years of diagnosis.

Reduction in the incidence of severe graft versus host disease has been achieved by the use of monoclonal antibodies to deplete T lymphocytes from the donor bone-marrow. Unfortunately, the benefits have been outweighed by an increased incidence of graft rejection and a marked increase in the incidence of recurrent chronic granulocytic leukaemia following bone-marrow transplantation. The International Registry review found that the 3 year probability of relapse for 318 recipients of non-T-cell depleted marrow was 9 per cent compared with 48 per cent for 87 recipients of T-cell-depleted marrow (Goldman et al. 1988). This is presumably due to a reduction in a T-lymphocyte-mediated graft versus leukaemia effect. The same analysis identified the occurrence of chronic graft versus host disease as being associated with a 3-fold reduction in the risk of recurrence. A similar 3-fold increase is found in the incidence of recurrent disease after syngeneic bone-marrow transplantation from an identical twin which has a lower procedure-related morbidity and mortality in the absence of graft versus host disease. However, this has not been reported by all groups (Thomas et al. 1986).

Residual leukaemic cells are commonly detectable by polymerase chain reaction (PCR) for several months after transplantation in patients who are in complete cytogenetic remission but in many cases the marrow subsequently becomes negative (Cross et al. 1993a). Detection of PCR-positive cells over 1 year after transplantation is associated with a higher risk of relapse. A semi-quantitative PCR assay has been developed to assist in monitoring patients after transplantation and may permit the identification of patients in whom further therapeutic intervention may be necessary before the onset of overt relapse (Cross et al. 1993b). It is not yet clear whether α-interferon therapy could be beneficial for such patients with minimal residual disease after a bone-marrow transplant.

A number of alternative approaches are being explored for young patients with chronic granulocytic leukaemia who do not have a compatible sibling donor. A sibling donor mismatched at a single HLA locus appears to offer as good a prospect of success as a fully compatible donor (Beatty et al. 1985). Increasing degrees of mismatch in family donor grafts are associated with an increasing incidence of graft rejection. This can be reduced by increased dosage of radiotherapy in the pre-transplant conditioning regimen, but is accompanied by an increase in the incidence of severe graft versus host disease and higher morbidity and mortality. Although the results of transplantation using family donors mismatched at two or more loci have been relatively poor to date, this may be the only transplant option (and, hence, the only prospect of cure) for a young patient with uncommon HLA haplotypes. This remains an experimental approach at present.

Another alternative is a matched unrelated donor transplant obtained through one of the many volunteer donor panels. At the time of writing over 250 000 volunteers are registered with European panels (70 000 are fully HLA A, B, and DR typed) and there is collaboration on a worldwide basis between panels to improve the prospects of obtaining compatible donors. However, two problems impede this approach. First, the degree of polymorphism at the human HLA locus is so great that it may prove difficult to obtain a well-matched donor for more than 60 per cent of patients. It appears that, irrespective of the panel size, patients who do not have common haplotypes will probably obtain donors who are, at best, mismatched by modern tissue-typing techniques. The second problem implicit in the panel system is the delay necessary in identifying the most suitable donor and organizing the transplant procedure. This delay has normally been in excess of 6 months. Clearly, a number of patients can be expected to progress to acclerated phase or blast transformation during this period.

Transplantation from an unrelated donor is associated with a higher incidence of graft rejection (16 per cent) than for a matched sibling graft, where it can be expected to occur in up to 10 per cent of cases. There is also a higher incidence of grade III and IV acute graft versus host disease (54 per cent) and extensive chronic graft versus host disease which occurs in 52 per cent is also increased (McGlave et al. 1993). The incidence and severity of graft versus host disease correlates with the degree of match between donor and recipient and is reduced by T-cell depletion (McGlave 1992). Results of this approach have improved in good-risk patients in the chronic phase in particular and there appears to be a low recurrence rate (11 per cent at 2 years) and improved disease-free survival (45 per cent at 2 years for early chronic phase transplants). At the present time a transplant from a well-matched unrelated donor may offer a better prospect of success than a graft from a family member mismatched at two or more loci. More studies are required in this area to establish the role of unrelated and mismatched bone-marrow transplantation in the management of patients with chronic granulocytic leukaemia. Optimal donor–recipient matching criteria have yet to be determined for these kinds of transplant but preliminary analysis suggests that when serological screening is used alone, better outcomes are obtained in recipients of 'matched' unrelated donor bone-marrow (McGlave 1992).

Relapse after bone-marrow transplantation

Relapse after transplantation in accelerated phase or blast transformation generally takes the form of florid haematological relapse with return of the disease features present prior to bone-marrow transplantation. After bone-marrow transplantation in the chronic phase, relapse may occur with return to florid chronic phase, but occasionally a purely cytogenetic relapse occurs in which a low proportion of Ph-positive marrow metaphases are found which remain a minority population without progression to haematological relapse (Thomas et al. 1986). Univariate analysis of European Bone Marrow Transplant Group (EBMT) data shows a 6 year probability of survival of 52 per cent following cytogenetic relapse and 30 per cent following a haematological relapse. Treatment of patients with cytogenetic relapse with α-interferon significantly delays the onset of haematological relapse (Arcese et al. 1993) with cytogenetic response in 25 per cent. Survival is directly related to the interval between transplantation and subsequent relapse. Relapse in cells of the donor sex after brother–sister bone-marrow transplantation has also been documented. This may be explained by the persistence of a transmissible oncogenic factor or exposure to a causative environmental factor. A number of patients have had successful second transplants (Thomas and Clift 1989) and the EBMT review projected a survival of 28 per cent 4 years after a second allograft.

Autologous transplantation in chronic phase

Although autologous transplantation was initially studied as a treatment for patients in blast transformation and was found to be of only short-term benefit (Haines et al. 1984), it was recognized that this technique could be used, as in acute leukaemia, to obtain the curative potential of high-dose therapy in patients ineligible for an allograft as a result of age or donor unavailability. Only a relatively small number of patients have received an autograft in chronic phase with the aim of delaying transformation. However, this approach has become a focus of interest as a result of an increasing general interest in the use of peripheral blood haemopoietic progenitors (PBSC) to provide support to high-dose therapy and the demonstration that Ph-negative progenitors can be obtained in patients with chronic granulocytic leukaemia in chronic phase and blast transformation following treatment with intensive

myeloablative therapy (Sessarego et al. 1992). Only a proportion of patients with blast transformation had Ph-negative stem cells harvested (8/26) but in two of these patients the cells were also PCR negative and a higher proportion of chronic phase patients may yield stem cells suitable for autologous transplantation (2/3 both PCR negative). Durable clinical and cytogenetic remissions have been obtained following high-dose chemoradiotherapy and reinfusion of these 'normal' autologous stem cells (Carella et al. 1992).

An alternative approach to obtaining normal autologous haemopoietic stem cells for transplantation has followed the observation that long-term liquid (Dexter) cultures of bone-marrow may favour the growth of Ph-negative progenitors (Coulombel et al. 1983). A number of autografts have been performed using marrow 'purged' in this way to produce only Ph-negative cells after 10 days in liquid culture (Barnett et al. 1992). Thirty-three out of 88 patients screened (38 per cent) were found to have suitable marrow and 20 underwent an autograft with subsequent graft failure in five (20 per cent), complete cytogenetic remission in 12 out of 14 evaluable patients (86 per cent) but recurrence of Ph-positive haemopoiesis in eight of those after a median follow-up period of 15 months.

Comparison of the survival of 21 patients treated with unmanipulated autologous PBSC with 636 matched controls demonstrated a significantly longer survival 5 years after the autograft (56 versus 28 per cent) and suggests that autologous transplantation in chronic phase may be of value (Hoyle et al. 1994). A number of studies are now in progress with the aim of evaluating the role of high-dose therapy supported by an autograft as intensification therapy following initial treatment with chemotherapy and α-interferon. Interest in this approach is motivated by the recognition that transplantation remains the only curative therapy despite the cytogenetic responses to α-interferon but only a minority of patients have suitable donors. Moreover the tantalizing prospect that the unique bcr–abl rearrangement may be exploited using antisense oligonucleotides and conjugated toxins offers the possibility of specfic in vitro therapy to 'purge' the autograft.

Treatment in accelerated phase

Patients in whom the leucocyte count has previously been readily controlled by busulphan but who have now entered an accelerated phase may respond, albeit usually temporarily, to hydroxyurea and vice versa. Hydroxyurea may be useful in higher or more frequent doses than were required during chronic phase. Splenectomy has been advocated at this time to reduce the dose of chemotherapy required, to facilitate treatment in patients with thrombocytopenia and for patients with progressive myelofibrosis. However, this operation has no proven value.

Initially many physicians regarded the accelerated phase as the most acceptable stage at which to carry out allogeneic bone-marrow transplantation, that is, the risks of the transplant procedure had become acceptable in the face of clear evidence that the chronic phase had ended and that blast crisis could be expected in the near future. Unfortunately, the results of allogeneic bone-marrow transplantation at this stage are less good than can be achieved prior to acceleration of the disease (see above) and it is now generally accepted that bone-marrow transplantation should be performed before this stage is reached.

Treatment in blast transformation

The treatment of myeloid blast transformation has been disappointing. The prognosis is worst for those patients with a myeloid or undifferentiated blast cell type and in those who have developed thrombocytopenia or cytogenetic clonal evolution (Kantarjian *et al.* 1987). The results of treatment with conventional first-line regimens for acute myeloblastic leukaemia have been poor. The overall complete response rate ranges from 10 to 30 per cent with a median survival of 2–6 months (reviewed by Talpaz *et al.* 1988). Perhaps the most encouraging recent results have been obtained using the combination of mitozantrone and high-dose cytosine arabinoside. Although initial responses are frequently obtained, the remission is universally brief and the incidence of prolonged pancytopenia and infective complications is high. The term 'second chronic phase' is a misnomer as stability is not a feature of this stage. The use of autologous stem cells to permit the administration of more intensive regimens is discussed below. Allogeneic transplantation during 'second chronic phase', though yielding better results than during frank blast transformation, is also disappointing (see above).

It is generally believed that the prognosis following lymphoid blast transformation is better than that following myeloid transformation. The number of patients who achieve remission following lymphoid blast transformation after therapy with vincristine- and prednisolone-containing regimens designed for acute lymphoblastic leukaemia is higher (40–70 per cent) and median survival can be longer (6–12 months) (Walters *et al.* 1987). However, this may reflect the lower toxicity of these treatment regimens rather than an intrinsic biological difference in the underlying disease. Patients in whom remission is induced should then receive maintenance therapy as for *de novo* adult acute lymphoblastic leukaemia and a case can also be made for craniospinal prophylaxis.

Attempts to promote differentiation of the blast cells of transformed chronic granulocytic leukaemia have been made and Koller and Miller (1986) reported six remissions in nine patients treated with mithramycin and hydroxyurea with no intervening period of pancytopenia. This combination requires further evaluation. α-Interferon appears to have limited therapeutic value beyond the chronic phase but may play an adjuvant role with chemotherapy or bone-marrow transplantation.

Autologous transplantation in blast transformation

The use of high-dose therapy for blast transformation followed by the infusion of autologous chronic phase bone-marrow or peripheral blood stem cells did not produce durable responses (Haines *et al.* 1984) and this therapeutic approach has virtually ceased. The major problem with autologous bone-marrow transplantation at this stage is rapid recurrence of the blastic phase. There is now more interest in the use of high-dose therapy and autologous bone-marrow transplantation during chronic phase as a means of delaying blast transformation. Some patients autografted with Ph-positive cells have regenerated Ph-negative haemopoiesis, at least transiently. This approach has been further stimulated by the reports that long-term liquid culture of chronic phase bone-marrow may re-establish Ph-negative haemopoiesis (Coulombel *et al.* 1983) and that cytosine arabinoside may exert selective toxicity on the chronic granulocytic leukaemia clone and permit purging of the autologous bone-marrow. At the present time the value of such an approach remains unproven.

Therapeutic strategy in chronic granulocytic leukaemia

All patients under 55 years should be screened for sibling donors to permit bone-marrow transplantation to be carried out in early chronic phase once the proliferative process is controlled. Older patients with an identical twin could also be considered as candidates for transplantation if both donor and recipient are otherwise fit. Hydroxyurea should be used if pre-transplant therapy is necessary. Patients in chronic phase who do not have a sibling donor or well-matched unrelated donor should be treated with α-interferon. Consideration should be given to peripheral blood stem cell collection prior to α-interferon therapy and participation in a randomized study of autologous bone-marrow transplantation in chronic phase. Patients with any cytogenetic response to α-interferon at 6 months and less than 50 per cent Ph-positive metaphases at 12 months should probably continue this treatment until progression occurs. Those who do not achieve an adequate response to α-interferon should be considered for investigational treatments such as autologous bone-marrow transplantation or unrelated donor or mismatched bone-marrow transplantation. Patients who present at later stages of the disease should receive intensive therapy including a matched sibling or unrelated donor bone-marrow transplant if they are candidates by virtue of age and donor availability.

ATYPICAL CHRONIC MYELOID LEUKAEMIA

Up to 10 per cent of patients with clinical and haematological features suggestive of chronic granulocytic leukaemia have no detectable Ph chromosome. In some patients minor differences exist from the typical features of chronic granulocytic leukaemia, for example prominent monocytes, dysplastic granulocytes, low platelets, or the absence of basophilia or eosinophilia. The survival of this group of patients is poorer than that of patients with Ph-positive chronic granulocytic leukaemia. Other patients have a clinical phenotype indistinguishable from that of patients with Ph-positive chronic granulocytic leukaemia. On cytogenetic analysis, some of these patients have apparently normal karyotypes while others have a variety of other abnormalities.

Molecular analysis has permitted the division of these patients into two distinct groups (Wiedemann *et al.* 1988). Some patients, though lacking the Ph chromosome, express the same mRNA and p210 translation product as in classical chronic granulocytic leukaemia, and these findings correlate with clinical features similar to those of classical chronic granulocytic leukaemia. These patients clearly have the same translocation on a molecular level with formation

Table 5 Haematological features of chronic granulocytic leukaemia, atypical chronic myeloid leukaemia, and chronic myelomonocytic leukaemia

Chronic granulocytic leukaemia
  'Peaks' in differential count of neutrophils and of myelocytes+metamyelocytes
  Monocytes usually <3 per cent of leucocyte count
  Dyshaemopoiesis absent or minimal
  Basophilia

Atypical chronic myeloid leukaemia
  Promyelocytes, myelocytes, and metamyelocytes >15 per cent of leucocyte count
  Monocytes >3 per cent of leucocyte count (unless all other features present)
  Dysgranulopoiesis (myelocytes, metamyelocytes, neutrophils) prominent
  Absolute basophil counts not increased

Chronic myelomonocytic leukaemia
  Promyelocytes, myelocytes, and metamyelocytes <15 per cent of leucocyte count (typically <5 per cent)
  Monocytes >10^9/l (almost always >10 per cent of leucocyte count)
  Dysgranulopoiesis common but not obligatory

of the hybrid *bcr–abl* gene typical of chronic granulocytic leukaemia but without the gross translocation of the additional genetic material which results in the easily identifiable Ph chromosome. These patients have the same clinical course and response to treatment as patients with Ph-positive chronic granulocytic leukaemia. The other patients with Ph-negative p210-negative disease have no consistent molecular abnormality, respond poorly to therapy, and have a poorer prognosis. Many have been reclassified as chronic myelomonocytic leukaemia and others as atypical chronic myeloid leukaemia (Wiedemann *et al.* 1988). Atypical chronic myeloid leukaemia has features intermediate between those of classical chronic granulocytic leukaemia and chronic myelomonocytic leukaemia, with prominent dysplastic features in the granulocytic series. Individual cases may be difficult to classify. The haematological criteria used by the Medical Research Council study group are shown in Table 5.

CHRONIC MYELOGENOUS LEUKAEMIAS OF CHILDHOOD

Adult-type chronic granulocytic leukaemia

Adult-type chronic granulocytic leukaemia is a rare disorder in childhood and accounts for 3–5 per cent of all cases of childhood leukaemia. It is extremely rare in infancy and 80 per cent of cases occur after the age of 4 years (Altman 1988). The clinical and laboratory features, natural history, and therapy of this condition in childhood are identical to those described for adults with Ph-positive chronic granulocytic leukaemia. Children with chronic granulocytic leukaemia are more likely to be anaemic at presentation, with a higher leucocyte count (median 250×10^9/l), and are more likely to have symptoms of leucostasis. The differential diagnosis includes leukaemoid reaction (infective focus, minimal or absent splenomegaly, high leucocyte alkaline phosphatase score, and Ph negative), juvenile chronic myeloid leukaemia (less marked leucocytosis and splenomegaly, greater skin and lymphoid involvement, monocytosis, and Ph negative), and other myeloproliferative states (less marked granulocytosis and Ph negative).

Juvenile chronic myeloid leukaemia

Juvenile chronic myeloid leukaemia is an uncommon condition with an acute course which occurs in infancy and early childhood. Most patients are diagnosed before their second birthday and 95 per cent of patients are aged under 4 years. Juvenile chronic myeloid leukaemia must be distinguished from classical chronic granulocytic leukaemia which occurs rarely in this age group. However, this is not generally difficult as the clinical, haematological, and cytogenetic features are distinct.

A child with juvenile chronic myeloid leukaemia is generally unwell with fever, weight loss, night sweats, and sepsis. An eczematous rash unresponsive to steroid therapy is frequently present on the face or trunk and may precede the diagnosis of juvenile chronic myeloid leukaemia by 1 year. Biopsy reveals a leukaemic infiltrate in the dermis. This condition may also be associated with xanthomata or *café au lait* spots. Respiratory symptoms with an interstitial pattern on the chest radiograph occur commonly due to a peribronchial and intra-alveolar leukaemic infiltrate. Haemorrhagic complications due to thrombocytopenia are common at presentation. Splenomegaly is a constant feature and is frequently marked. Hepatomegaly and generalized lymphadenopathy are less common. The course of the disease is generally rapid with a median survival of untreated or undertreated patients of 10 months (Freedman *et al.* 1988).

The blood film shows leucocytosis with blasts and left-shifted granulocytes; monocytes may be prominent and the platelet count is often reduced. The leucocytosis is usually less pronounced (median 49.5, range 11.5–960) than that of chronic granulocytic leukaemia (median 250, range 8–800) and the characteristic myelocyte peak, basophilia, and eosinophilia of chronic granulocytic leukaemia are absent. The leucocyte alkaline phosphatase score is often unhelpful in differentiating this condition from classical chronic granulocytic leukaemia as it may be low though it is characteristically normal or increased.

The erythrocytes show many features characteristic of fetal erythropoiesis: a high level of fetal haemoglobin, a fetal glycine to alanine ratio in the gamma chain of haemoglobin F, a fetal glycolytic enzyme pattern, and a low expression of the I antigen on the erythrocyte cell membrane. Immunoglobulin levels are frequently markedly elevated and there is a high incidence of antibodies to nuclear antigen and to immunoglobin G (IgG).

The bone-marrow shows myeloid and erythroid hyperplasia with prominent immature monocytes and scanty megakaryocytes. The predominant cell in the blood and bone-marrow is a primitive monocyte precursor, although there is evidence of a clonal panmyelopathy involving all lineages except lymphocytes (Estrov *et al.* 1986a). The karyotype is generally normal, though 18 per cent of published cases have been reported to show various abnormalities (Freedman *et al.* 1988). No case of juvenile chronic myeloid leukaemia with a Ph chromosome has been reported.

This condition has an extremely poor prognosis and responds poorly to chemotherapy (Laver *et al.* 1987). Oral 6-mercaptopurine alone or in combination with subcutaneous cytosine arabinoside appears to be marginally more effective than busulphan or hydroxyurea in providing symptomatic relief, but simple supportive therapy is often as effective (Altman 1988). The median survival is less than 9 months and most patients succumb to infection. A small proportion of patients develop an erythroleukaemic terminal phase with erythroblastosis and marrow megaloblastic hyperplasia. Recently more intensive protocols designed for the treatment of acute myeloblastic leukaemia have been used and remissions lasting over 12 months were obtained in a proportion of patients (Chan *et al.* 1987). However, this approach does not seem likely to alter the ultimate outcome. Patients with a suitable donor should be treated with high-dose chemoradiotherapy and bone-marrow transplantation which offers the only prospect of prolonged disease-free survival (Sanders *et al.* 1988).

Familial chronic myeloid leukaemia

Differentiation of this syndrome from juvenile chronic myeloid leukaemia is difficult. It has been reported in three pairs of infant siblings (Altman 1988). The course is unpredictable, with one early death from progressive leukaemia and one prolonged asymptomatic survivor in each pair reported to date.

EOSINOPHILIC LEUKAEMIA

Eosinophilic leukaemia is an uncommon and poorly defined condition associated with marked eosinophilia, malaise, sweats, weight loss, skin rashes, and cardiac abnormalities. Splenomegaly is frequently, though not invariably, present. The blood film shows atypical, degranulated, and primitive eosinophils and blasts. Cytogenetic analysis has revealed a number of abnormalities, including the Ph chromosome in some patients. It is clear that some patients with this diagnosis have a condition which is a variant of chronic granulocytic leukaemia and molecular analyses should assist in fully characterizing the syndrome.

The differential diagnosis is the hypereosinophilic syndrome which is a self-perpetuating eosinophilic proliferation with a progressive course and organ involvement in which immature eosinophils are not seen and cytogenetic analysis is normal (Rickles and Miller 1972). However, it has been suggested that eosinophilic leukaemia, the hypereosinophilic syndrome, Loeffler's endocarditis parietalis fibroplastica, and eosinophilic collagen disease represent a continuum of disease differing only in the target organs predominantly affected. There is considerable support for the concept that the hypereosinophilic syndrome is also a haematological neoplasm (da Silva *et al.* 1988). However, the following criteria have been suggested as diagnostic of eosinophilic leukaemia rather than hypereosinophilic syndrome in a paediatric setting:

(1) pronounced and persistent eosinophilia, associated with immature forms, in either the peripheral blood or bone-marrow;

(2) more than 5 per cent blasts in the bone-marrow;

(3) tissue infiltration by immature cells of predominantly eosinophilic type;

(4) an acute natural history measured in months, accompanied by anaemia, thrombocytopenia, increased susceptibility to infection, and/or haemorrhage.

The clinical course is variable, but a long period of stability followed by blast transformation as in chronic granulocytic leukaemia is not uncommon. Cytotoxic drugs such as hydroxyurea are indicated for the treatment or prevention of symptoms.

CHRONIC NEUTROPHILIC LEUKAEMIA

This very rare condition may be diagnosed in a patient who maintains a raised neutrophil count in the absence of a precipitating cause (You and Weisbrot 1979). The important differential diagnosis is a leukaemoid reaction due to underlying infection or tumour. Immature granulocytes are not seen in the peripheral blood and there is no increase in basophils or eosinophils. Modest splenomegaly is usually present. Most patients also have hepatomegaly. The leucocyte alkaline phosphatase score is normal or increased and the marrow cytogenetic studies are normal. A case with such a diagnosis, in whom blast transformation occurred, has been reported. In the absence of symptoms, no treatment is indicated. It remains to be seen whether molecular studies will confirm this as a separate entity.

CHRONIC MYELOMONOCYTIC LEUKAEMIA

This condition is included in the French-American-British (FAB) classification of myelodysplastic syndromes (Bennet *et al.* 1982). This group of conditions share the common feature of low-grade clonal neoplastic proliferation of haemopoietic stem cells with progression to cytopenia or transformation to florid acute leukaemia. The defining feature of chronic myelomonocytic leukaemia is the presence of an absolute monocytosis ($>1\times10^9/l$).

Patients are generally elderly and present with symptoms of anaemia and weight loss. There may be moderate splenomegaly and lymphadenopathy and a few patients have skin infiltration. Some

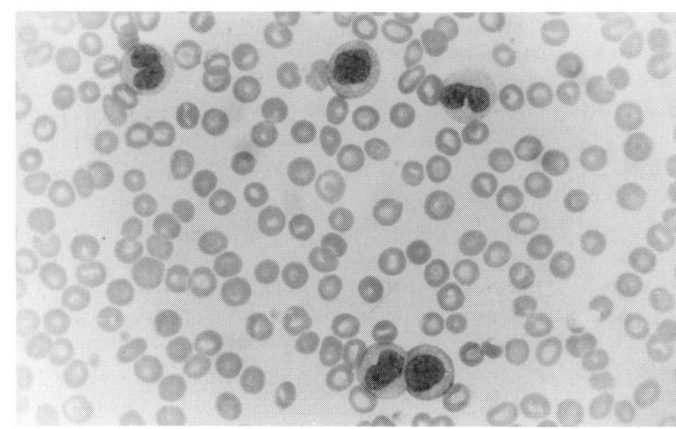

Fig. 5 Peripheral blood in chronic myelomonocytic leukaemia showing prominent abnormal monocytes. The neutrophils are hypogranular and have bilobed nuclei (the pseudo-Pelger–Huet anomaly) which are features of dysgranulocytopoiesis.

patients have gum hypertrophy or serous effusions. The blood film shows an increase in the number of mature monocytes, while the granulocytes are often also increased and frequently show dysplastic features (for example, hypogranularity or bilobulated pseudo-Pelger forms), but blasts are less than 5 per cent (Fig. 5). There are usually giant platelets and megakaryocyte fragments. The serum lysozyme is elevated and there may be associated hypokalaemia, due to increased renal potassium loss consequent upon tubular damage caused by the lysozyme.

The bone-marrow is hypercellular due to an infiltrate of mature monocytes, promonocytes, and monoblasts and, in addition, dysplastic features can be seen in all the haemopoietic lineages, that is, dyserythropoiesis, ringed sideroblasts, multisegmented neutrophils, and micromegakaryocytes. The bone-marrow frequently contains less than 5 per cent blasts but these may reach 20 per cent of cells as in refractory anaemia with excess blasts. Cytogenetic analysis reveals no Ph chromosome though other abnormalitites are found in approximately 30 per cent of patients, most notably monosomy 7, trisomy 8, and structural rearrangements of the short arm of chromosome 12 (Heim and Mitelman 1986). It is of interest that 5q−, the single most common aberration in the other myelodysplastic syndromes, is uncommon in chronic myelomonocytic leukaemia.

The course of the disease is not dissimilar from that of classical chronic granulocytic leukaemia. There is often a prolonged stable period where the features of bone-marrow failure gradually supervene and blood product support may be required on a regular basis. The reported median survival varies from 8.5 months to over 60 months (Kerkhofs *et al.* 1987), which may reflect either differences in diagnostic criteria or wide variation in the clinical course of the disease. There have been a number of attempts to identify prognostic factors (Mufti *et al.* 1985; Kerkhofs *et al.* 1987; Ribera *et al.* 1987). Increased blasts in the bone-marrow, anaemia, thrombocytopenia, high peripheral monocyte count, and splenomegaly appear to predict a poor prognosis. A simple scoring system allocating one point for haemoglobin $< 10\,g/dl$, neutrophils $<2.5\times10^9/l$ or $>16\times10^9/l$, platelets $<100\times10^9/l$, or marrow blasts >5 per cent was suggested by Worsley *et al.* (1988) to identify patients who would have an indolent course and long survival without treatment (low monocyte count and score below 2).

Some patients with a very high monocyte count or marked splenomegaly may benefit from chemotherapy with hydroxyurea or low–dose cytosine arabinoside. Etoposide at a dose of 50 mg orally on alternate days is said to be a useful agent in this condition. There has been much interest in agents which have been shown capable of inducing differentiation *in vitro* (generally on the highly inducible HL-60 cell line). Low-dose cytosine (3–10 mg/m² 12 hourly for 21 days) has been used in myelodysplastic syndromes on this basis, but no randomized study demonstrating improved survival has yet been reported. Similarly, there is no conclusive evidence to support the use of other so-called 'differentiating agents' (13-*cis*-retinoic acid and 1,25-dihydroxycholecalciferol) either singly or in combination. The same is true of the biological response modifier α-interferon, while early studies with the growth factor GM-CSF suggest that this agent may stimulate blast proliferation. The use of more intensive treatment regimens has not been found to improve the outlook of patients with myelodysplastic syndromes (Armitage *et al.* 1981), but younger patients with poor prognostic features and a compatible donor may be best treated with bone-marrow transplantation (Appelbaum *et al.* 1987).

Transformation to florid acute leukaemia may eventually supervene with increasing proportions of monoblasts. Acute myeloid leukaemia occurs in 15–40 per cent of cases and is associated with younger age at diagnosis, splenomegaly, thrombocytopenia, and excess of bone-marrow blasts. This stage is generally refractory to chemotherapy. The use of treatment regimens designed for *de novo* acute myeloid leukaemia is often associated with prolonged pancytopenia and infective complications and has not been shown to prolong survival.

THE MYELOPROLIFERATIVE DISORDERS

Polycythaemia rubra vera

Polycythaemia rubra vera is an uncommon clonal haematological neoplasm characterized by excessive proliferation of erythroid, myeloid, and megakaryocytic elements in the bone-marrow. This results in increased peripheral counts of all three formed elements of the blood. Frequent presenting features are fatigue, weight loss, plethora, epistaxis, headache, and pruritis. Up to 25 per cent of patients are found to have a chromosomal abnormality. There is associated splenomegaly and untreated patients have a short life expectancy of 18–36 months with a high incidence of haemorrhage, thrombosis, and gangrene. Other complications include splenic infarction, hypersplenism, gout, renal calculi, and peptic ulceration.

The Polycythaemia Vera Study Group have developed diagnostic criteria (Table 6) to exclude reliably patients with relative polycythaemia and secondary polycythaemia (Berk *et al.* 1986). A combination of heavy smoking and excessive alcohol consumption leads to the most likely cause of a false-positive diagnosis due to smoker's polycythaemia and alcoholic liver disease with splenomegaly, elevated serum B₁₂ levels, leucocytosis, and occasionally elevated leucocyte alkaline phosphatase score. The criteria were developed

Table 6 Polycythaemia Vera Study Group parameters for the diagnosis of polycythaemia rubra vera

A1 Red cell mass >36 ml/kg for males, >32 ml/kg for females
A2 Normal arterial O₂ saturation >92 per cent
A3 Splenomegaly
B1 Thrombocytosis >400×10⁹/l
B2 Leucocytosis >12×10⁹/l
B3 Leucocyte alkaline phosphatase >100 (no fever or infection)
   Serum B₁₂ >900 pg/ml or unbound B₁₂ binding capacity >2200 pg/ml

to minimize false-positives and it is common for patients with early polycythaemia rubra vera to fail to meet them. The diagnosis of polycythaemia rubra vera is acceptable if all three parameters in category A are present or if A1, A2, and any two category B parameters are present.

The disease can be regarded as having three phases (Silverstein 1976). Diagnosis is most frequently made during the 'proliferative phase' when therapeutic intervention is necessary to reduce elevated peripheral blood counts and prevent complications. Some patients progress to a 'stable phase' during which near normal counts are maintained without specific therapy. This may result from progressive myelofibrosis constraining the excessive proliferation and decreasing the proliferative capacity of the residual marrow. The 'spent phase' occurs as a result of extensive myelofibrosis and is characterized by progressive hepatosplenomegaly pancytopenia and transfusion dependence.

The Polycythaemia Vera Study Group have carried out a large randomized controlled study in 431 patients with active polycythaemia rubra vera comparing the efficacy of phlebotomy alone with radioactive phosphorus or chlorambucil combined with phlebotomy for a haematocrit above 45 per cent. The minimum follow-up is now over 11 years. Median survival was poorest for the chlorambucil-treated group at 8.9 years, whilst that of the ³²P-treated group at 11.8 years was not significantly different from the 13.9 years attained by the phlebotomy-only group. The principal reason for the differences was found to be the incidence of fatal events late in the study. The most frequent causes of death were thrombosis (31 per cent of reported deaths), acute leukaemia (19 per cent), other neoplasms (15 per cent), haemorrhage (5 per cent), and myelofibrosis (5 per cent). In the initial 5–7 years of follow-up the group treated with phlebotomy alone had a significantly higher incidence of fatal thrombosis (cerebrovascular accidents account for one-third overall) with increased phlebotomy rate, advanced age, and a history of prior thrombosis as additional risk factors. The association between chlorambucil treatment for polycythaemia rubra vera and the development of acute leukaemia in 13.5 per cent of patients was reported in 1981 and the association with non-Hodgkin's lymphoma in 3 per cent of patients was recognized subsequently. It is now recognized that a comparable incidence of acute leukaemia (10 per cent) occurs later among patients treated with ³²P and that the incidence of both groups who received myelosuppressive therapy markedly exceeds the incidence in the group treated with phlebotomy alone (2 per cent). When compared with an age- and sex-matched population, the rate of all malignancies in the chlorambucil group is 3–3.5 times that of a control population and that in the ³²P group is 2–2.5 times the control values, whilst the group treated with phlebotomy alone is comparable with that expected. This is principally due to haematological neoplasia, gastrointestinal cancer, and skin cancer. Another ongoing study is evaluating treatment with hydroxyurea, which appears to produce adequate control in 80–90 per cent of patients and at a median follow-up of 5 years did not appear to be associated with an increased incidence of malignant disease (Kaplan *et al.* 1986). Further follow-up of this group is clearly important.

The current therapeutic recommendations of the Polycythaemia Vera Study Group are as follows:

(1) ³²P and phlebotomy for patients over 70 years due to thrombosis risk;

(2) phlebotomy alone for patients under 50 years, unless thrombosis risk factors are present when hydroxyurea should be added;

(3) phlebotomy alone in the 'young' 50–70 year old without risk factors, otherwise add hydroxyurea;

(4) other indications for myelosuppression are excessive splenic enlargement with local symptoms, bone tenderness, intractable pruritus, or poor veins.

The Polycythaemia Vera Study Group studies have not associated thrombocytosis with thrombotic complications and it is not seen as an indication for myelosuppression. Additional treatments which may be helpful for intractable pruritus are H_1 and H_2 histamine blockers, alone or in combination. However, many patients find this symptom unrelieved by any medication. Allopurinol is frequently necessary to prevent gout. The use of aspirin or dipyridamole has not been associated with a reduction in thrombotic complications but is clearly associated with an increased incidence of serious gastrointestinal haemorrhage.

Essential thrombocythaemia

Essential thrombocythaemia is a clonal myeloproliferative disorder characterized by excessive megakaryocyte proliferation and increased platelet count in the absence of an increased red cell mass, marrow fibrosis, or leucocytosis. An increased platelet count is commonly present in all the myeloproliferative disorders and may also occur as a reactive phenomenon in response to blood loss, inflammation, or neoplasia. Although essential thrombocythaemia is now recognized as a discrete entity within the myeloproliferative disorders, establishing the diagnosis unequivocally may be difficult in practice. The Polycythaemia Vera Study Group have produced strict diagnostic criteria for essential thrombocythaemia to exclude polycythaemia rubra vera, chronic granulocytic leukaemia, idiopathic myelofibrosis, and reactive causes (Table 7) (Murphy et al. 1986). Careful exclusion of the causes of reactive thrombocytosis (chronic inflammation, infection, hyposplenism, iron deficiency, and malignancy) is an important first step in establishing the diagnosis.

The median age at diagnosis is 61 years with a range from 21 to 84 years and the condition is often diagnosed incidentally on routine testing. Neurological symptoms are frequent and the condition is often recognized during investigation of transient ischaemic attacks or paraesthesiae. Microvascular thrombosis is the cause of the characteristic syndrome of erythromelalgia (red, burning palms and soles). Multiple placental infarctions are the cause of recurrent abortions and fetal growth retardation in young women with essential thrombocythaemia. Thrombotic complications of large vessels are less frequent. Haemorrhage occurs in approximately one-third of patients due to altered haemostasis as a consequence of the increased numbers of abnormally functioning circulating platelets. Pruritus is markedly less common than in polycythaemia rubra vera (14 per cent versus 43 per cent) as is splenomegaly (38 per cent versus 70 per cent) which, when present, was only 2–4 cm

Table 7 Polycythaemia Vera Study Group diagnostic criteria for essential thrombocythaemia

1 Platelet count $>600\times10^9/l$
2 Haemoglobin 13 g/dl or normal red cell mass
3 Stainable iron in marrow or failure of iron trial
4 No Ph chromosome
5 Collagen fibrosis of the bone-marrow
  A Absent
  B Less than one-third biopsy area without splenomegaly or leucoerythroblastic blood film
6 No known cause of reactive thrombocytosis

below the costal margin. Hepatosplenomegaly occurs in less than 10 per cent of patients.

The platelet count is typically 1000×10^9–$1500\times10^9/l$, and in a few cases rises as high as $3000\times10^9/l$. The ESR is usually low in contrast to reactive thrombocytosis. Platelet morphology is often abnormal with many giant forms and platelet aggregates. Platelet aggregation is abnormal with complete loss of both primary and secondary response to epinephrine (due to absence of membrane α-adrenergic receptors) in almost all patients. Electron microscopy examination of platelets in essential thrombocythaemia has shown abnormal dense bodies and α-granules which may explain increased plasma levels of β-thromboglobulin. Mild anaemia is occasionally present and is often due to gastrointestinal blood loss. However, the Polycythaemia Vera Study Group have stressed the considerable overlap between essential thrombocythaemia and polycythaemia rubra vera in the haematocrit range 40–60 per cent and the importance of the red cell mass to distinguish these two conditions (Murphy et al. 1986). The leucocyte count is frequently also elevated at approximately $12\times10^9/l$, but on occasion may reach $40\times10^9/l$. An increased proportion of basophils of 3 per cent or more has not been found in patients meeting all the Polycythaemia Vera Study Group criteria and is associated with an atypical presentation of Ph-positive chronic granulocytic leukaemia. Marrow cellularity is normal or increased due to trilineage hyperplasia but increased megakaryocytes may be found in both primary and reactive thrombocytosis. There is often evidence of fibrosis and there are no marrow features which distinguish essential thrombocythaemia from polycythaemia rubra vera. Cytogenetic studies have shown few abnormalities.

Survival is of the order of 65 per cent at 10 years and 50 per cent at 15 years. Acute leukaemia may supervene, but it is not yet clear to what extent this is due to natural progression or is related to treatment.

Choice of therapy is difficult because of the necessity for prevention of both haemorrhage and thrombosis in a patient who may be asymptomatic for many years. A platelet count in excess of $1000\times10^9/l$ should be reduced as there is a significant risk of thrombotic complication although neither the absolute platelet count nor any other parameter of haemostasis reliably predicts thrombotic or haemorrhagic complications. However, in one large study older age, prior thrombosis, and duration of thrombocytosis were major risk factors for future thrombotic complications (Cortelazzo et al. 1990). The incidence of serious thrombotic complications in younger patients (<45 years) was 33 per cent in a review of 123 reported patients (McIntyre et al. 1991). The Polycythaemia Vera Study Group have compared melphalan and ^{32}P (up to 5 mCi 3 monthly as required) therapy for patients with platelet counts in excess of $1000\times10^9/l$ (Murphy et al. 1986). Melphalan produced a superior complete response rate (normalization of the platelet count) at 3 and 6 months. More than one-third of patients treated with ^{32}P had no response or a poor response at 6 months. A further study evaluated hydroxyurea at an initial dose of 30 mg/kg/day, reducing to 15 mg/kg/day after 1 week and thereafter dosing according to platelet and leucocyte counts. Control was achieved in most patients in 2–6 weeks with a complete or good partial response in 91 per cent of patients at 6 months. Responsiveness appears to be long-term and dose related. Quickly reversible leucopenia and chronic macrocytosis are the only frequent side-effects. More prolonged follow-up will be necessary to establish whether there is an increased incidence of malignancy in these patients. None of these studies has compared myelosuppressive therapy with an untreated control group because many of the vague symptoms of essential thrombocythaemia may be attributed to thrombocytosis. Nevertheless, hydroxyurea is now widely regarded as the treatment of choice and continuous treatment with this agent provides effective long-term control without severe marrow toxicity or serious side-effects. Busulphan and ^{32}P are no longer regarded as first-line alternatives even in older patients because of their leukaemogenic potential.

An alternative therapeutic approach has been the use of α-interferon which has been shown to lower the platelet count significantly and to control the count satisfactorily with a thrice weekly dose of 3 mu or less (Giles *et al.* 1988). Response rates of between 77 and 100 per cent have been reported (Lazzarino *et al.* 1990) and a greater than 50 per cent reduction in the platelet count can be obtained within 4 weeks. Maintenance treatment with α-interferon is usually required after initial cytoreduction and discontinuation leads to recurrence of thrombocytosis and related symptoms. Influenza-like side-effects are occasionally severe enough to necessitate cessation of therapy. Interferon may have the advantage for younger patients of not increasing the risk of future neoplasia, but has the inconvenience of parenteral dosage. Anagrelide is another agent which has been shown to control thrombocytosis associated with the myeloproliferative disorders. It is a quinazolin compound which inhibits platelet aggregation but also lowers the platelet count. However, there is no evidence of a decrease in the marrow megakaryocyte mass, myelofibrosis, or splenomegaly. One of its modes of action is to shorten platelet survival, possibly through an increase in the activity of splenic macrophages. The Anagrelide Study Group (1992) has reported that over 90 per cent of patients with myeloproliferative thrombocytosis who received 0.5–1.0 mg four times daily orally had their platelet counts reduced by at least 50 per cent or to less than $600\times10^9/l$ despite most being refractory to other agents. Side-effects included nausea, headaches, palpitations, 'forceful pulse', fluid retention and severe diarrhoea and necessitated discontinuation of therapy in 16 per cent. Despite the potent antiplatelet effect of anagrelide, significant haemorrhagic complications have not been described. This agent appears extremely promising and has the advantage of not being mutagenic.

The use of aspirin in essential thrombocythaemia is controversial as it can precipitate severe haemorrhage. It should not be used indiscriminately in essential thrombocythaemia even in patients with extremely high platelet counts. On the other hand, patients with recurrent thrombotic complications such as erythromelalgia, digital ischaemia, cerebrovascular ischaemia, or recurrent abortions will benefit from aspirin in conjunction with reduction in the platelet count to normal levels. It should probably not be used in asymptomatic patients with a history of both thrombosis and haemorrhage and must be actively avoided in patients with active haemorrhage. The decision to prescribe aspirin for essential thrombocytosis must be made on an individual patient basis with consideration of the present and past clinical situations.

Idiopathic myelofibrosis

Idiopathic myelofibrosis is a relatively uncommon myeloproliferative disorder with a variable clinical course characterized by splenomegaly, a leucoerythroblastic blood film, polychromatic and tear-drop-shaped red cells, and bone-marrow fibrosis. Bone-marrow fibrosis is seen as a secondary phenomenon in a number of conditions including the acute leukaemias, Hodgkin's disease, myeloma, carcinoma, renal osteodystrophy, hyperparathyroidism, hypothyroidism, systemic lupus erythematosus, and the grey platelet syndrome. Variable

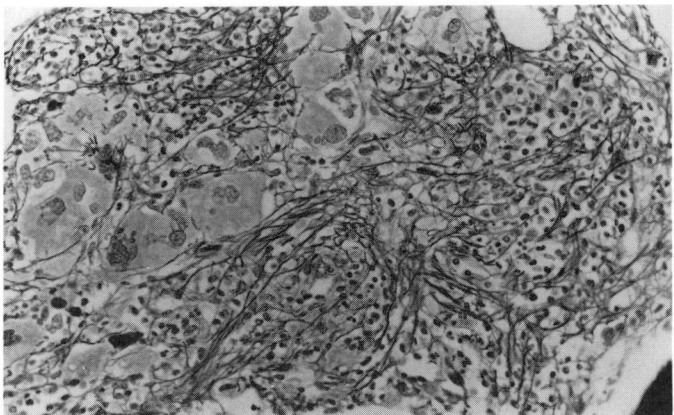

Fig. 6 Reticulin-stained bone-marrow trephine biopsy in idiopathic myelofibrosis showing early fibrosis and prominent clumps of megakaryocytes.

degrees of fibrosis are seen in all the myeloproliferative syndromes (chronic granulocytic leukaemia, polycythaemia rubra vera, and transitional myeloproliferative syndromes) but idiopathic myelofibrosis is a well-characterized syndrome in which bone-marrow fibrosis is the dominant feature (Fig. 6). However, it has been established that here too the fibrosis is secondary to a neoplastic clonal expansion of haemopoietic stem cells (Jacobson *et al.* 1978; Sato *et al.* 1986).

Patients commonly present beyond the age of 50 years, with symptoms of anaemia, abdominal discomfort due to splenomegaly, or bleeding. Other common symptoms include bone pain, night sweats, weight loss or gout due to hypermetabolism, thrombosis, and abdominal expansion due to ascites. Hepatomegaly is found in 60 per cent. Up to 30 per cent of patients are asymptomatic at the time of diagnosis. Osteosclerosis is seen in approximately 50 per cent of patients radiologically. Anaemia is almost invariable and neutropenia or thrombocytosis may also be present in 25–50 per cent of patients diagnosed early. The leucocyte alkaline phosphatase is usually high and increased numbers of basophils may be present. Attempts to obtain a bone-marrow aspirate usually result in a 'dry tap'.

The appearance of bone-marrow on trephine biopsy has been divided into three categories (Manoharan 1988):

(1) haemopoietic hypercellularity with trilineage hyperplasia and minimal fibrosis;

(2) haemopoietic normocellularity and obvious fibrosis, sometimes with osteosclerosis;

(3) haemopoietic hypocellularity with islands or clumps of mega-karyocytes, marked fibrosis, and osteosclerosis.

These categories may represent early, intermediate, and late idiopathic myelofibrosis with progressively decreasing haemopoietic cellularity and increasing fibrosis. A number of cytogenetic abnormalities have been described (Miller *et al.* 1985).

Survival of a patient with idiopathic myelofibrosis following diagnosis is extremely variable and may range from under 1 year to over 30 years. Progressive weight loss is almost invariable and anaemia becomes more severe as the disease progresses. Increasing proportions of blasts are frequently seen in the peripheral blood in the later stages of the disease. Cutaneous nodules due to extramedullary haemopoiesis in the skin develop in some patients (Mizoguchi *et al.* 1990). The commonest causes of death are infection, bleeding, and thrombosis. Up to 25 per cent of patients die as a result of transformation to acute leukaemia. A short-lived group with a median survival of approximately 2 years and a long-lived group with a median survival of approximately 10 years can be identified (Manoharan 1988). Features associated with a good prognosis are younger age (fifth and sixth decades), absence of purpura, absence of fever, night sweats, and weight loss, haemoglobin above 10 g/dl, normal or increased platelet count, and bone-marrow hypercellularity with minimal fibrosis.

There is no effective therapy for this condition. Asymptomatic patients with stable disease may simply be observed with transfusion support and folate supplements when required. Anabolic steroids (Danazol 200 mg tid orally) have been used to improve erythropoiesis and may be effective in up to 50 per cent of patients (Besa *et al.* 1982). Splenic irradiation is often useful treatment for splenic pain and tenderness. Radiotherapy may also be very useful treatment for extramedullary fibrohaemopoietic tumours. Splenectomy is often advocated when there is evidence of hypersplenism, haemolytic anaemia and a frequent transfusion requirement, severe thrombocytopenia, painful splenic infarction, or portal hypertension (Weinstein 1991). Thrombocytosis is a contraindication to splenectomy. Good responses have been reported when splenectomy is performed soon after diagnosis. However, massive symptomatic hepatomegaly may follow early splenectomy and the associated mortality of the procedure remains high.

Chemotherapy has been utilized in symptomatic patients or those with a progressive decrease in haemoglobin. The combination of chlorambucil and prednisolone or single-agent busulphan, thioguanine, or hydroxyurea (Manoharan 1988) has been reported to keep patients well with resolution of constitutional symptoms, reduced or static hepatosplenomegaly, and reversal of bone-marrow and splenic fibrosis. Following busulphan or thioguanine therapy, prolonged stable unmaintained remissions have occurred. Proof of the efficacy of this approach requires a randomized controlled trial, but chemotherapy can be expected to reduce leucocytosis or thrombocytosis, ameliorate weight loss and sweating, and may have a modest effect on splenomegaly.

A small number of patients have been treated with α-interferon with minimal evidence of efficacy (Hasselbach 1988). The clinical use of 1,25-dihydroxyvitamin D_3 has not been as effective as the initial *in vitro* studies promised. A small number of patients have been successfully treated with bone-marrow transplantation (Dokal *et al.* 1989) and this should be considered in young patients.

Table 8   Chronic B-lymphoproliferative disorders

1 B-chronic lymphocytic leukaemia
2 B-prolymphocytic leukaemia
3 Hairy cell leukaemia
4 Splenic lymphoma with villous lymphocytes
5 Follicular lymphoma

Table 9   Chronic T-lymphoproliferative disorders

1 T-chronic lymphocytic leukaemia
2 T-prolymphocytic leukaemia
3 T-hairy cell disease
4 Sézary syndrome
5 Adult T-cell leukaemia/lymphoma

CHRONIC LYMPHATIC LEUKAEMIA

Chronic lymphoproliferative disease can be conveniently divided into those derived from the B-lymphocyte lineage (Table 8), which are more common and those derived from the T-lymphocyte lineage (Table 9). The chronic lymphatic leukaemias have traditionally been classifed on a morphological basis and the morphological subtype generally correlates with the clinical course. Further classification has been possible through immunological studies of surface antigen expression in these disorders which have also yielded information on lymphocyte ontogeny.

B-CELL CHRONIC LYMPHOCYTIC LEUKAEMIA
Epidemiology

Chronic lymphocytic leukaemia, alias chronic lymphatic leukaemia, may account for 25–30 per cent of all leukaemias in the West, but for no clear reason the incidence is much lower in the Far East. Chronic lymphatic leukaemia is by far the most common of the so-called lymphoproliferative disorders with an annual incidence of 3 per 100 000. It affects twice as many males as females, with a peak incidence between 60 and 80 years. Approximately 70 per cent of patients are over 60 years of age at the time of diagnosis and only approximately 6 per cent are less than 50 years. There is a tendency for older patients to present with less advanced disease. In over 95 per cent of patients surface marker studies show that the chronic lymphatic leukaemia originates from a clone of B lymphocytes (B-cell chronic lymphatic leukaemia) and in under 5 per cent, surface marker and functional studies show a T lymphocyte origin (T-cell chronic lymphatic leukaemia).

Genetic factors may be responsible for some of the ethnic and racial variations of the disease. There have been many reports of familial aggregation. Affected members generally have a leukaemia cell type concordant with that of the proband. There is a 2–7-fold excess of leukaemia in first-degree relatives of chronic lymphatic leukaemia cases compared with controls. Studies have attempted to correlate HLA frequencies in chronic lymphatic leukaemia, but few associations have been identified except for a significant increase in HLA B18 and a possible excess of DR5. However, these associations are weak and there is no really strong link between any particular HLA type and the occurrence of chronic lymphocytic leukaemia.

Although there have been reports during the last 30 years of an increased risk of lymphoproliferative malignancy of various kinds, with a variety of chronic infections and inflammatory, connective tissue, autoimmune, or allergic disorders, a population-based control study found no association between chronic lymphatic leukaemia and a history of subacute or chronic infections, connective tissue disorders, or autoimmune disorders. Many of the investigations of early years have not been adequate epidemiological studies but primarily clinical reports which may have focused on highly selected cases with lymphoproliferative malignancies. As yet there is no accepted epidemiological study which points to chronic antigenic stimulation as a causal factor in chronic lymphocytic leukaemia.

There have been many clinical reports linking chronic lymphatic leukaemia with several occupations and occupation-related exposures. These include farming, in which correlation studies have noted a chronic lymphatic leukaemia mortality excess amongst White male farmers residing in high soya bean producing counties in Iowa.

Interestingly, farmers also seem to be at high risk for related B-cell neoplasms and non-Hodgkin's lymphoma. There has also been an association between farm herbicide use and non-Hodgkin's lymphoma in Kansas. An increased incidence of chronic lymphatic leukaemia has been found in rubber manufacturing workers in whom exposure to solvents, including benzene and xylene, may be relevant. Very strong associations have also been found for exposure to carbon tetrachloride and five cases of chronic lymphatic leukaemia were diagnosed in members of one family all of whom worked in a dry-cleaning business. However, the evidence linking chronic lymphatic leukaemia with exposure to environmental toxins is weak when compared with the substantial body of literature demonstrating a strong association between acute myeloid leukaemia and benzene exposure. Chronic lymphatic leukaemia is the only leukaemia type which has not been linked with occupational exposure to radiation or other environmental sources of high- or low-level radiation.

There is no evidence of a viral aetiology in chronic lymphatic leukaemia. However, the leukaemic cells from some patients with T-cell chronic lymphatic leukaemia have been shown to have clonal integration of HTLV-1, a retrovirus more usually associated with adult T-cell leukaemia/lymphoma (see below) (Gallo *et al.* 1983). More recently, antibodies to HTLV-1 were reported in six out of 17 patients in Jamaica with B-cell chronic lymphatic leukaemia, but there was no integration of provirus in these cases suggesting that HTLV-1 was not the aetiological agent. The possible role of DNA viruses such as the Epstein–Barr virus and cytomegalovirus in the development of chronic lymphatic leukaemia is unknown, but direct involvement of the Epstein–Barr virus seems unlikely.

Laboratory features

Haematology

The diagnosis of chronic lymphatic leukaemia should be considered in anyone whose lymphocyte count consistently exceeds $4.5 \times 10^9/l$. The National Cancer Institute Working Group (Cheson *et al.* 1988) and International Workshop on Chronic Lymphatic Leukaemia (1989) have suggested $5 \times 10^9/l$ and $10 \times 10^9/l$, respectively, as the threshold lymphocyte count for a diagnosis of chronic lymphocytic leukaemia. Usually there is a persistent lymphocytosis of at least $10 \times 10^9/l$ and a lymphocytic infiltration of the bone-marrow of at least 30 per cent. The lymphocyte count may exceed $400 \times 10^9/l$. In over 90 per cent of cases these small lymphocytes can be shown to be a monoclonal B-cell population by the demonstration of antibody light chain restriction. The leukaemic cells are small, have little cytoplasm, and a characteristic pattern of clumped nuclear chromatin and indistinct nucleoli. The presence of smear cells on the MGG-stained blood film is often of diagnostic value (Fig. 7) and the proportion of smear cells correlates with the lymphocyte count. Although most of the lymphocytes appear homogeneous, most patients have a small proportion of larger more immature or prolymphocytic forms. Isoenzyme studies in females heterozygous for glucose-6-phosphate dehydrogenase (G_6PD) demonstrate that the neoplastic clone is restricted to B lymphocytes with no involvement of red cells or T lymphocytes.

As the disease advances, patients develop anaemia and thrombocytopenia and these are important prognostic features at diagnosis (see below). Approximately 50 per cent of patients have mild anaemia at presentation. In advanced disease, there is bone-marrow failure with complete replacement of the marrow space by lymphocytes. However, it is also important to exclude iron or folate deficiency, hypersplenism, or an autoimmune component in the aetiology of the anaemia or thrombocytopenia.

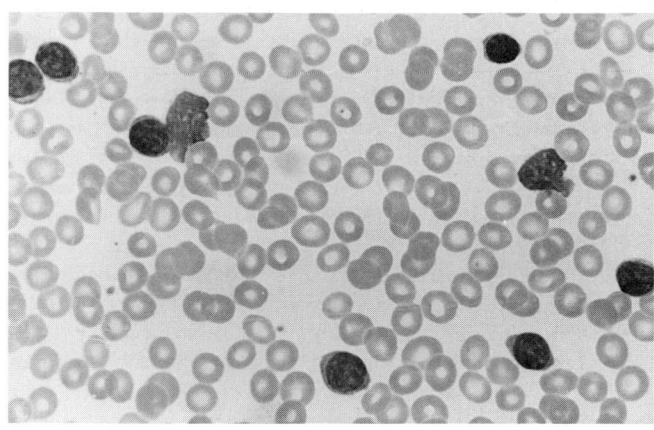

Fig. 7 Peripheral blood in chronic lymphatic leukaemia showing lymphocytes of mature appearance. Several 'smear cells' characteristic of this condition are seen.

Bone-marrow examination is rarely required to make the diagnosis of B-cell chronic lymphatic leukaemia. The bone-marrow of patients with intermediate or advanced B-cell chronic lymphatic leukaemia shows a characteristic near total replacement of haemopoietic cells with lymphocytes, many of which appear larger and more immature than those in the blood film. The bone-marrow trephine biopsy may show four different patterns which roughly correlate with disease stage: a nodular pattern is least common and is associated with early or intermediate disease, an interstitial infiltration of lymphocytes into normal haemopoietic tissue with preservation of normal architecture or a mixture of nodular and interstitial infiltration is found in two-thirds of patients, most of whom have intermediate disease and a proportion of whom require chemotherapy to maintain adequate haemopoiesis, and diffuse infiltration with a 'packed marrow' is found in one-quarter of patients and the majority require prompt therapeutic intervention. Similar infiltration of the bone-marrow with small lymphocytes in the absence of peripheral blood lymphocytosis suggests the diagnosis of well-differentiated (small lymphocytic) non-Hodgkin's lymphoma.

Cytogenetics and molecular biology

The indolent nature of chronic lymphocytic leukaemia and its low mitotic rate have delayed successful cytogenetic studies of this disease until comparatively recently. The employment of a number of B lymphocyte mitogens such as pokeweed mitogen, lipopolysaccharide, Epstein–Barr virus, tetradecanoyl phorbol acetate (**TPA**), and cytochalasin B has demonstrated the erroneous nature of the long-standing belief that there were no chromosome abnormalities in this disorder. Clonal chromosome abnormalities are found in approximately 50 per cent of patients (reviewed in Juliusson and Gahrton 1993). The most common abnormality is trisomy 12 which occurs in approximately one-third of those with an abnormal karyotype and as an isolated finding in half of those. Structural abnormalities of chromosome 12 occur most commonly at p11, q13, and q22 and several result in partial trisomy. The oncogenes which have been identified on chromosome 12 have not yet been shown to be activated in chronic lymphocytic leukaemia.

Structural abnormalities of the long arm of chromosome 13 occur in approximately 20 per cent of patients with abnormal karyotypes but the break-point is not consistent. The majority of these abnormalities involve deletion of band 13q14 which is the site of the retinoblastoma suppressor gene (RB1). The significance of this is not clear as the other allele usually has a normal RB1 gene (Liu *et al.* 1992) and the gene product is expressed normally. A region telomeric to this gene has been shown to be homozygously disrupted in cells from patients with chronic lymphocytic leukaemia (Brown *et al.* 1993) and may be the site of a tumour suppressor gene. The long arm of chromosome 14 carries the genes for the immunoglobulin heavy chain at band q32. Structural abnormalities of chromosome 14 occur in 15 per cent of patients with karyotypic abnormalities and q32 is the most commonly involved site. Most chromosome 14 abnormalities involve translocation of additional chromosomal material from a variety of sources. The most frequent source of material at 14q32 is 11q13 which juxtaposes the *bcl*-1 gene and the gene for the immunoglobulin heavy chain (Tsujimoto *et al.* 1985). This translocation may be more characteristic of prolymphocytic leukaemia and certain lymphomas. Abnormalities of the long arm of chromosome 11 are found in 14 per cent of cases of chronic lymphatic leukaemia with karyotypic abnormalities. Chromosome 6 is the next most frequently involved chromosome with deletions of the long arm or translocations involving either arm. Complex abnormalities are found in 10–15 per cent of patients.

No clear pathogenetic relationship has been established to date for the chromosomal abnormalities described. Karyotypic evolution during the course of the disease is uncommon in sequential analytical studies of patients with chronic lymphocytic leukaemia (Oscier *et al.* 1991). However, the observation that trisomy 12 has not been acquired on sequential analysis but may be commonly found in early stage patients has been interpreted as evidence that this abnormality may not be a secondary change (Juliusson and Gahrton 1993). Nevertheless, its absence in the majority of patients studied indicates that the pathogenesis of chronic lymphocytic leukaemia is initiated by another mechanism.

Activation of dominantly acting oncogenes such as *bcl*-1 and *bcl*-2 associated with other indolent lymphoproliferative disorders does not appear to be associated with the pathogenesis of chronic lymphocytic leukaemia. Inactivation of the p53 tumour suppressor gene is detected in approximately 10 per cent of patients and the frequency of p53 mutations appears to increase with Richter's transformation.

Karyotypic abnormalities are less frequent in patients with early stage disease (Binet stage A) while complex abnormalities are more common in advanced disease (Binet stage C). In addition, there is a strong correlation between karyotype and prognosis. Any clonal chromosome abnormality is associated with a poorer prognosis compared to a normal karyotype (Han *et al.* 1984). Single abnormalities are associated with a longer survival than multiple abnormalities and a high proportion of abnormal metaphases in the sample is a strong indicator of a poor prognosis (Juliusson *et al.* 1990). Despite the strong prognostic association of chromosomal abnormalities, cytogenetic studies have not yet found a routine place in the investigation of patients with chronic lymphocytic leukaemia.

Immunology

The immunology of the neoplastic cell in B-cell chronic lymphocytic leukaemia has been studied extensively over a considerable number of years. Chronic lymphatic leukaemia lymphocytes were initially thought to be the neoplastic counterparts of a subgroup of normal peripheral blood lymphocytes, a view largely based on the morphological appearance of the tumour cells. The surface antigens (Table 10) which occur on the majority of B-cell chronic lymphatic leukaemia cells have been studied in detail and comprise the following (Freedman and Nadler 1987; Dighiero 1993):

Table 10 Immunophenotype of B-cell lymphoproliferative disorders

	CLL	PLL	SLVL	HCL	FL
Surface Ig	±	++	++	++	++
HLA-DR	++	++	+	+	+
CD5	+	±	±	−	−
CD10	−	±	±	−	+
CD11c	±	−	+	+	−
CD19	++	++	++	++	++
CD23	+	±	±	−	±
CD24	+	+	+	±	+
CD25	±	−	−	+	−
FMC7	±	+	+	+	+
Mouse rosettes	++	±	±	+	+

CLL, chronic lymphocytic leukaemia; PLL, prolymphocytic leukaemia; SLVL, splenic lymphoma with villous lymphocytes; HCL, hairy cell leukaemia; FL, follicular lymphoma.

(1) antigens expressed on all B-cells (pan-B antigens);

(2) antigens expressed on resting B-cells only;

(3) B-cell 'activation antigens';

(4) antigens appearing on terminally differentiated B-cells;

(5) antigens expressed on limited stages of B-cell ontogeny;

(6) antigens expressed on minor subpopulations of B-cells only.

The cells in B-cell chronic lymphatic leukaemia commonly express the pan-B-cell antigen Ia and the antigens identified by the CD19, CD20, and CD24 monoclonal antibodies. Cell surface immunoglobulin (sIg) expression is typical and this observation established the B-cell lineage of B-cell chronic lymphatic leukaemia several years ago. The clonality of B-cell chronic lymphatic leukaemia was demonstrated by cellular synthesis of immunoglobins with a single V_H region, a single V_L region, and a single light chain type. Almost all sIg-positive B-cell chronic lymphatic leukaemia cells express surface IgM or co-express IgM and IgD. Surface immunoglobulin expression on B-cell chronic lymphatic leukaemia cells is of very low intensity, much less than that seen on normal resting B-cells found in blood or lymphoid tissues. The total cellular IgM content of B-cell chronic lymphatic leukaemia cells may be equivalent to most normal cells, as B-cell chronic lymphatic leukaemia cells have a high cytoplasmic IgM whereas normal B-cells have lower cytoplasmic IgM and higher surface IgM expression. Weak expression of surface IgM alone suggests that B-cell chronic lymphatic leukaemia cells correspond to an early B-cell, but the additional presence of surface IgD on a significant number of chronic lymphatic leukaemia cells suggests a slightly later stage of B lymphocyte differentiation. In B-cell chronic lymphatic leukaemia, clonal differentiation appears to be arrested between cytoplasmic immunoglobulin-positive pre-B-cells and sIgM-, sIgD-positive mature B-cells.

The receptor for the C3d component of complement (CD21 antigen) which is expressed on normal resting B-cells is also expressed on the majority of B-cell chronic lymphatic leukaemia cells. However, B-cell chronic lymphatic leukaemia cells do not express C3b receptors (CD35 antigen), whilst normal peripheral blood B-cells express both C3d and C3b receptors. The absence of C3b receptors on most B-cell chronic lymphatic leukaemia cells also suggests that normal peripheral blood B-cells are not the normal cellular counterpart of B-cell chronic lymphatic leukaemia cells.

The lineage-restricted antigen recognized by the monoclonal antibody FMC-7 is not present on most B-cell chronic lymphatic leukaemia cells (approximately 20 per cent of cases are positive), whereas all cells from B-cell prolymphocytic leukaemia and hairy cell leukaemias are positive. B-cell activation antigens expressed on B-cell chronic lymphatic leukaemia cells are CD23, CD25, B5, and blast 1, whereas BB-1 and the CD71 antigen (the transferrin receptor) are infrequently expressed. Expression of several activation antigens suggests that the cells of B-cell chronic lymphatic leukaemia may be the neoplastic counterpart of a small subpopulation of activated normal B-cells though retaining the morphological features of small resting B-cells (Freedman and Nadler 1987). B-cell chronic lymphatic leukaemia cells uniformly lack the antigen expressed on terminally differentiated B-cells (CD38) proving that the B-cell chronic lymphatic leukaemia cell does not correspond to a terminally differentiated secretory B-cell. The CD10 antigen demonstrated on some other B-cell tumours such as acute lymphoblastic leukaemia, nodular poorly differentiated lymphocytic lymphoma, and Burkitt's lymphoma has not been demonstrated on B-cell chronic lymphatic leukaemia cells.

A number of antigens expressed on minor subpopulations of normal B-cells are expressed on the majority of B-cell chronic lymphatic leukaemia cells and are useful in making the diagnosis of B-cell chronic lymphatic leukaemia more specific. They include a receptor for mouse red blood cells which produces spontaneous rosettes between murine erythrocytes and 95 per cent of B-cell chronic lymphatic leukaemia cells. This useful marker is restricted within the B-cell malignancies to B-cell chronic lymphatic leukaemia and some cases of hairy cell leukaemia, but has been largely superseded as a diagnostic tool since the development of monoclonal antibodies. A heteroantibody prepared against T lymphocytes which recognizes the CD5 antigen cross-reacts with the cells of B-cell chronic lymphatic leukaemia. This antigen is strongly expressed on mature T lymphocytes and B-cell chronic lymphatic leukaemia cells but is less well expressed on thymocytes. The CD5 antigen is not expressed on circulating B lymphocytes from normal individuals though a normal counterpart of the CD5+ B lymphocyte has been identified at the edge of the germinal centres of lymph nodes (Caligaris-Cappio et al. 1985) and in fetal lymph node and spleen (Bofil et al. 1985). B-cells expressing CD5 have been observed in the peripheral blood of patients following allogeneic bone-marrow transplantation and in patients with rheumatoid arthritis. These cells are therefore also putative candidates for the normal cellular counterparts of B-cell chronic lymphatic leukaemia cells.

In summary, the majority of cells from patients with B-cell chronic lymphatic leukaemia can be assigned a common antigenic phenotype including the expression of the pan-B-cell antigens HLA-DR, CD19, CD20, and CD24, the resting B-cell antigens CD21 and surface Ig (sIgM and sIgD), the B-cell activation antigen B5, and the T lymphocyte-associated CD5 antigen. In addition, B-cell chronic lymphatic leukaemia cells regularly express the mouse red blood cell receptor. However, there is clearly some heterogeneity between different clonal populations in patients with B-cell chronic lymphatic leukaemia and there is no uniform point of maturation arrest. Indeed, in an individual patient there can be mild fluctuation in the degree of differentiation of the dominant clone over time. No clear correlation has yet been established between the cellular phenotype and prognosis.

The use of these surface markers to immunophenotype the cells of a patient with lymphocytosis helps to differentiate B-cell chronic lymphatic leukaemia from a variety of other disorders which may resemble it (Table 10), including B-prolymphocytic leukaemia in which more than 55 per cent of the cells are prolymphocytes, hairy cell leukaemia (both T- and B-cell types), splenic lymphoma with villous lymphocytes, follicular centrocytic lymphoma with blood spill, and diffuse centrocytic lymphoma with blood spill (Melo et al. 1988). A number of T-cell lymphoproliferative disorders which are much less common must also be excluded: T-cell chronic lymphatic leukaemia, otherwise known as large granular lymphocyte leukaemia, T-prolymphocytic leukaemia, the adult T-cell leukaemia/lymphoma syndrome, Sézary syndrome, and HTLV-1 negative T-cell non-Hodgkin's lymphoma.

Clinical features

The clinical course of chronic lymphatic leukaemia is extremely variable. During the evolution of the disease there is a gradual increase in the total body mass of lymphocytes leading to infiltration of blood, bone-marrow, lymph nodes, spleen, and liver until in the final stages the bone-marrow reserve is so compromised that bone-marrow failure occurs. The clinical symptoms and signs are determined by the mass of leukaemic B-cells and by associated disturbances of immunity. The rate and extent of lymphocyte accumulation varies widely between patients. A patient with early chronic lymphatic leukaemia is generally asymptomatic, but as the lymphocyte mass expands gross lymphadenopathy and organomegaly become evident, the symptoms of pancytopenia develop, and the patient eventually succumbs to infection, bleeding, or organ failure unless other causes supervene.

In 25 per cent of patients, the disease is initially diagnosed by chance when a routine blood count is performed. Sometimes a patient presents as a result of the symptoms of anaemia or the finding of painless lymphadenopathy. The severity of the symptoms and signs generally parallels the lymphocyte count. Other systemic symptoms are rare at the onset. However, severe infection may be the first clinical manifestation of the disease as a result of compromised immunity. Lymph node enlargement is usually symmetrical and involves cervical, axillary, and inguinal regions. Two-thirds of patients with B-cell chronic lymphatic leukaemia have splenomegaly, which is usually less pronounced than in chronic granulocytic leukaemia or idiopathic myelofibrosis. Hepatomegaly is much less common at presentation though it is a not infrequent finding in patients with advanced disease.

Complications

The most common complication of B-cell chronic lymphatic leukaemia is infection, with chest infection being particularly common. The increased incidence of infection in these patients is believed to be due to defective immunity, the mechanism of which is complex and incompletely understood. The T lymphocytes, although not involved in the neoplastic clone, display numerous intrinsic functional defects. Hypogammaglobulinaemia is present in over 50 per cent of patients at diagnosis and this appears to be due to defective B lymphocyte function rather than to defective T-cell 'helper' function. The incidence of infection in patients with B-cell chronic lymphatic leukaemia can be reduced by monthly intravenous administration of normal immunoglobulin. In 5 per cent of patients hypogammaglobulinaemia may be associated with a monoclonal M-band, usually IgM, on protein electrophoresis. More sensitive techniques, such as immunofixation, identify a higher proportion of patients (up to 60 per cent) with monoclonal gammopathies. In a small proportion of these patients the para-protein may cause cryoglobulinaemia or a hyperviscosity syndrome similar to Waldenström's macroglobulinaemia.

Autoimmune haemolytic anaemia occurs not infrequently in patients with B-cell chronic lymphatic leukaemia and may occasionally be severe. Up to 20 per cent of patients with B-cell chronic lymphatic leukaemia are positive on the Coombs direct antiglobulin test because of a warm IgG antibody, but only a small proportion of these develop severe haemolysis. Autoimmune haemolytic anaemia may occasionally precede the diagnosis of B-cell chronic lymphatic leukaemia and there is no direct relationship between the severity of the haemolysis and the severity of the leukaemia. Prednisolone and chemotherapy are usually effective, but splenectomy is required to control the process in some patients. Autoimmune thrombocytopenia may also occur, sometimes in combination with autoimmune haemolysis (Evans' syndrome). Thrombocytopenia in B-cell chronic lymphatic leukaemia is more commonly due to marrow infiltration or sequestration by the enlarged spleen.

Bulky lymphadenopathy may cause local pressure effects on vital structures such as trachea, bronchus, or major vessels. Retroperitoneal or pelvic lymphadenopathy may cause ureteric obstruction, venous thrombosis, or lymphoedema. Cholestatic jaundice may result from lymphadenopathy at the porta hepatis or from hepatic infiltration. The result of infiltration of the skin ranges from isolated macules to generalized exfoliation, whilst infiltration of the small intestine may result in ulceration, bleeding, diarrhoea, or malabsorption. Central nervous system involvement is uncommon and usually restricted to patients with very advanced disease; it may cause headache, cranial nerve palsy, spinal cord compression, obtundation, or coma.

A second malignancy occurs relatively commonly in patients with B-cell chronic lymphatic leukaemia and is found in up to 20 per cent of patients at autopsy. Carcinomas arising in the skin or large bowel occur most frequently, but there is also an increased incidence of myeloma. Poor immune surveillance is thought to be the reason for the increased incidence of second malignancy which was noted prior to the introduction of cytotoxic chemotherapy. In contrast with chronic granulocytic leukaemia, transformation to acute leukaemia is uncommon. Most of these patients develop acute myeloid leukaemia and have been previously treated with alkylating agents and radiotherapy. The incidence of acute leukaemia in patients with B-cell chronic lymphatic leukaemia is under 2 per cent and it is not clear whether there is a true disease association or whether the development of acute leukaemia is secondary to treatment. A small number of patients with chronic lymphatic leukaemia develop prolymphocytoid transformation which is associated with increased numbers of prolymphocytes in the blood, more splenomegaly, and lymphadenopathy (Melo et al. 1986a). A proportion of patients have increased numbers of prolymphocytes at diagnosis (11–54 per cent) and clinical findings intermediate between classical B-chronic lymphocytic leukaemia and prolymphocytic leukaemia (Melo et al. 1986b). The diagnostic label chronic lymphatic leukaemia–prolymphocytic leukaemia has been applied to such patients (Litz and Brunning 1993).

Richter's syndrome is the development of a high-grade lymphoma in a patient with chronic lymphatic leukaemia. This is generally a diffuse large cell (immunoblastic) lymphoma and may occur in up to 10 per cent of patients. It is believed to develop through clonal evolution of malignant subclones in immature foci in nodal sites. The cells of Richter's syndrome bear monotypic sIg which is clonally distinct from the patient's B-cell chronic lymphatic leukaemia cells but are not found in the peripheral blood. Richter's syndrome should be suspected when a patient with B-cell chronic lymphatic leukaemia develops unexplained fever, weight loss, or rapidly progressive lymphadenopathy or hepatosplenomegaly. Extranodal infiltration eventually develops, most notably of the bone-marrow, bone, and

Table 11 Clinical staging systems for chronic lymphocytic leukaemia

Rai et al. (1975) and Rai (1987)

Level of risk	Stage	Clinical features	Median survival (years)
Low	0	Lymphocytosis alone	>15
Intermediate	I	Lymphocytosis+ lymphadenopathy	9
	II	Lymphocytosis, spleen, and/or liver enlargement	5
High	III	Lymphocytosis+anaemia (Hb <11 g/dl)	2
	IV	Lymphocytosis+ platelet count <100×10^9/l	2

Binet et al. (1981)

Stage	Lymphoid involvement[a]	Haemoglobin (g/dl)	Platelets (×10^9/l)
A	0, 1, or 2 areas		
B	3, 4, or 5 areas	>10	>100
C		<10 and/or	<100

[a]Lymphoid areas include cervical, axillary, or inguinal nodes, spleen, or liver.

gastrointestinal tract, but lymph node biopsy is often necessary to confirm the diagnosis in the early stages. The median interval from the diagnosis of B-cell chronic lymphatic leukaemia to the development of Richter's syndrome is 24 months and many patients have early B-cell chronic lymphatic leukaemia and have received no prior treatment. Median survival is only 4 months despite chemotherapy. Extensive lymphoma and heavy previous chemotherapy for B-cell chronic lymphatic leukaemia are very poor prognostic features. The results of therapy are poorer than those obtained in patients with de novo diffuse immunoblastic lymphoma.

Prognostic criteria and clinical staging

In 1975 Rai and his co-workers (Rai et al. 1975) proposed a five-stage system for chronic lymphatic leukaemia subsequently simplified into three major prognostic groups (Rai 1987). Patients with lymphocytosis alone (stage 0) and those with associated lymphadenopathy (stage I) had a median survival of greater than 10 years and greater than 8 years, respectively. However, those with more advanced disease who had splenomegaly (stage II), anaemia (stage III), or thrombocytopenia (stage IV) had a progressively shorter median survival of under 7 years, 2–5 years, and under 2 years, respectively. Anaemia or thrombocytopenia with an autoimmune basis are excluded from the classification as they do not have such a profound effect on prognosis.

The initial classification by Rai and co-workers was modified in 1981 by Binet et al. (1981) who proposed a new simpler system in which the patients were divided into three stages: A, B, and C. Patients with anaemia (less than 10 g/dl) or thrombocytopenia (less than 100×10^9/l) were designated stage C and they had the worst prognosis with a median survival under 3 years. Survival in the other 80 per cent depends on the number of lymph node sites involved. Patients with two or less sites involved were designated stage A, with a median survival of over 7 years and those with three or more sites were designated stage B (median survival 5 years or less).

An International Workshop on Chronic Lymphatic Leukaemia (1989) has proposed an integrated classification subclassifying the Binet system according to the corresponding Rai stage which has been found to be of value in several large studies (reviewed by Montserrat and Rozman 1993a) but has not been widely adopted.

A number of other parameters have emerged as reliable indicators of prognosis (reviewed by Montserrat and Rozman 1993a). The absolute lymphocyte count in the peripheral blood is a strong independent predictor of survival with a cut-off level of $40-50 \times 10^9/l$ dividing patients into low- and high-risk groups. The peripheral blood lymphocyte doubling time (**LDT**) calculated by extrapolation from the lymphocyte counts obtained over a few months untreated follow-up, is another independent prognostic variable and a useful parameter of the pace of the disease in an individual patient. Patients with a low doubling time (LDT <12 months) have an aggressive course and a short survival. The LDT appears to correlate with the cellular expression of myelomonocytic and activation antigens and a proliferating cell nuclear antigen. An increased proportion of large and immature lymphocytes (>5–10 per cent prolymphocytes) is an independent poor prognostic factor. The extent of bone-marrow involvement on the trephine biopsy usually correlates with the clinical stage but is another strong independent prognostic factor (Rozman *et al.* 1984). Patients with diffuse infiltration have a median survival of under 2–4 years compared with survival over 8–10 years for those with non-diffuse patterns. A diffuse pattern may correlate with the expression of myelomonocytic antigens. The presence of a chromosomal abnormality including a single chromosome defect, most commonly trisomy 12, is associated with a poor prognosis. The prognosis for younger patients (<50 years) has been controversial and has been the subject of several recent large studies reviewed by Montserrat and Rozman (1993a). These studies suggest that contrary to earlier reports suggesting a poorer prognosis in younger patients, the relative median survival of young and old patients is not significantly different.

Treatment

Complete remission, as understood in many other haemopoietic malignancies, is a very rare event in B-cell chronic lymphatic leukaemia. Therapy for B-cell chronic lymphatic leukaemia is generally given with palliative rather than curative intent and the advanced age of many patients and the perceived indolent nature of the condition have discouraged a more intensive approach. Indeed, treatment is not always necessary in B-cell chronic lymphatic leukaemia and once the diagnosis is established it is then necessary to decide whether to initiate therapy at once or to withhold treatment until problems develop. The management of patients with chronic lymphocytic leukaemia is an art in which there are a wide variety of therapeutic options available to the physician, each of which must only be introduced in circumstances where they may prolong the survival of the patient or alleviate immediate symptoms. Since there is a significant possibility that overaggressive treatment may further compromise haemopoiesis or immunological competence, there is no role for it in the early phases of the disease. The wise physician should consider therapeutic options very carefully in the treatment of this disease.

There is no evidence that therapeutic intervention in patients with either lymphocytosis or lymphadenopathy prolongs survival. If possible, patients with stage A or B disease should simply be kept under review without therapy. However, when lymph node enlargement causes symptoms, local or systemic therapy is often helpful. Systemic therapy is necessary in patients with more advanced disease or those who have developed cytopenia or symptomatic organomegaly, systemic symptoms (night sweats, fever, weight loss, or lethargy), autoimmune haemolysis, or thrombocytopenia or those who have diffuse infiltration on trephine biopsy or a low lymphocyte doubling time irrespective of clinical stage.

Corticosteroids

Single-agent prednisolone in moderately high dosage (60–100 mg daily) will produce a reduction in lymphocytic infiltration after a transient rise in peripheral blood lymphocytosis and results in improvements in cytopenia and symptomatic improvement in nearly all patients with B-cell chronic lymphatic leukaemia. This approach has major merit in patients with significant haemopoietic impairment prior to therapy in whom cytotoxic chemotherapy and exacerbation of cytopenia would carry additional risk. Following a short period of single-agent prednisolone therapy, haemopoiesis may regenerate sufficiently to permit treatment with alkylating agents. However, prolonged prednisolone therapy will aggravate the immuno-deficiency of B-cell chronic lymphatic leukaemia and may induce or aggravate hypertension, diabetes, tuberculosis, and osteoporosis in this elderly population. Single-agent prednisolone is a short-term measure for patients unable to tolerate or are resistant to alkylating agents.

Alkylating agents

Chlorambucil has become the conventional first-line chemotherapy for B-cell chronic lymphatic leukaemia. It has the advantages of good absorption following oral administration, absence of gastro-intestinal upset or alopecia, and preferential toxicity for lymphoid rather than myeloid cells. However, it does have cumulative toxicity on normal haemopoiesis which may aggravate cytopenia and in time the B-cell chronic lymphatic leukaemia clone frequently develops resistance. Cyclophosphamide offers no advantage over chlorambucil.

Chemotherapy should only be initiated in B-cell chronic lymphatic leukaemia when the benefits outweigh the risks. In French cooperative trials, 612 patients with stage A chronic lymphatic leukaemia were randomized between chlorambucil and no therapy (French Cooperative Group 1986). A slight survival advantage was observed in the untreated group. Chlorambucil therapy is indicated in patients with

(1) persistent constitutional symptoms (night sweats, fevers, or weight loss);

(2) rapidly progressive or painful lymphadenopathy or splenomegaly;

(3) cytopenia due to diffuse marrow infiltration;

(4) autoimmune haemolysis or thrombocytopenia.

Chlorambucil may be administered continuously at low dosage (0.1–0.2 mg/kg/day) in 7–14 day courses or at higher dosage up up to 2.5 mg/kg over 1–4 days each month. Intermittent higher dose therapy may be associated with lower haematological toxicity. It produces a reduction in lymphocytosis, shrinkage of lymphadenopathy, and improvement in constitutional symptoms in over 50 per cent of patients, irrespective of the regimen used. Chlorambucil should be discontinued when a normal lymphocyte count is achieved. Although prompt resurgence of the lymphocytosis is not infrequent, the symptoms for which treatment was initiated may not recur for some time and further therapy can be delayed. No survival advantage has been reported for continuous maintenance therapy and haematological toxicity is an inevitable result of such an approach. Higher doses of chlorambucil (15 mg/day until maximum response or unacceptable toxicity) may be associated with better responses and survival than cyclophosphamide, adriamycin, vincristine, and prednisolone (**CHOP**) chemotherapy (Jaksic *et al.* 1990). There is no evidence that the addition of prednisolone to chlorambucil improves either response or survival.

Combination chemotherapy

The UK Medical Research Council trial found no difference between single-agent chlorambucil and a combination of cyclophosphamide, vincristine, and prednisolone (COP) in treating advanced progressive chronic lymphatic leukaemia. In Spanish Cooperative trials it was found that COP is equivalent to chlorambucil and prednisolone together in patients with stage C disease. In patients with stage B disease, the French group (French Cooperative Group 1986, 1989) showed that treatment with COP was not superior to chlorambucil alone and that stage C patients treated with CHOP had a significantly higher response rate and better survival (51 versus 18 per cent at 5 years) than those treated with COP. However, this has by no means been universally found and remains controversial (reviewed by Binet *et al.* 1993). Combination therapy can induce complete remission in a small proportion of patients but relapse is common shortly after therapy is discontinued. Therapy with COP or CHOP is often attempted in patients who have developed resistance to chlorambucil, but any benefit is usually small and transient and the associated marrow toxicity is often marked.

Radiotherapy

Radiation is a frequently used and usually effective local treatment for lymph nodes compromising vital organ function. Without additional chemotherapy, lymphadenopathy is likely to recur after irradiation. Irradiation of the spleen is effective therapy for painful splenomegaly and provides systemic benefit as a result of lymphocyte trafficking. However, splenectomy is a superior treatment for massive splenomegaly if the patient is fit enough for surgery. Splenic irradiation may also be transiently effective in patients with autoimmune haemolysis or thrombocytopenia who are unfit for splenectomy and in whom chemotherapy has failed. In the late 1960s interest was revived in the use of whole-body irradiation in patients with advanced disease. Good responses have been reported in previously untreated patients, but severe haematological toxicity is a frequent problem in patients treated in this way once they have become refractory to chemotherapy. Randomized studies will determine whether this approach is superior to chemotherapy.

Purine analogues

There has been a great deal of recent interest in the therapeutic role of analogues of purine nucleosides that are either resistant to deamination by or inhibitory to the enzyme adenosine deaminase. These agents are highly lymphocytotoxic and offer the prospect of improved responses to treatment and thereby possibly also improved survival. Fludarabine, 2-chloro-deoxyadenosine (**2-CdA**) and 2' deoxycoformycin (**DCF**) are structurally similar compounds and all interfere with the purine degradation pathway through the accumulation of the triphosphorylated derivatives of fludarabine or 2-CdA or ATP as a result of DCF which may trigger apoptosis (Keating 1990; Beutler 1992; Plunkett and Gandhi 1993).

Fludarabine, an adenosine analogue, is the most widely studied of these agents in chronic lymphocytic leukaemia and early studies have demonstrated its value in this disease. This drug has produced complete responses in 15 per cent of previously treated patients with chronic lymphocytic leukaemia and an overall response rate of 56 per cent and complete responses in 37 per cent of untreated patients with an 80 per cent overall response (Keating *et al.* 1991). The median time to relapse is 21 months. Clinical stage is predictive for response to treatment and there is a significant correlation between survival and response to treatment. Febrile episodes and infection due to myelosuppression and profound CD4 lymphocyte depletion (a feature of all purine analogues) are the major side-effects and occur in up to 22 per cent of treatment episodes. Infective problems are increased by the addition of prednisolone which does not improve the response rate. Fludarabine has produced the highest remission rates ever reported for a single agent in chronic lymphocytic leukaemia. Whilst the durability of response and the effect on long-term survival is not yet clear (complete remissions appear to last over 2 years), this drug represents a major development in the treatment of this disease. It is administered by intravenous infusion at a dose of 25 mg/m^2/day for 5 consecutive days every 4 weeks for four to six cycles. An oral preparation is under development.

2-CdA is an effective agent in hairy cell leukaemia and has an overall response rate of 48 per cent in patients with refractory chronic lymphocytic leukaemia who received 0.1 mg/kg/day by continuous intravenous infusion for 7 days at 4 week intervals until maximum response or toxicity. Complete remissions were achieved in 4 per cent (Piro *et al.* 1988). Juliusson *et al.* (1992) have reported a small number of patients with disease refractory to fludarabine but responsive to 2-CdA and postulated a lack of cross-resistance between these drugs. DCF is a potent inhibitor of adenosine deaminase and has been established as an effective therapy in hairy cell leukaemia. A dose of 4 mg/m^2 intravenously every 1–2 weeks has produced partial responses in some 25 per cent of patients with chronic lymphocytic leukaemia most of whom had previously received treatment. Serious infections due to myelosuppression occur in up to one-third of patients (reviewed in Montserrat and Rozman 1993*b*).

Allogeneic bone-marrow transplantation

A relatively small number of patients with chronic lymphocytic leukaemia have been treated with allogeneic bone-marrow transplantation. This is due both to the advanced age of most patients with this condition and the relatively indolent nature of the disease as a result of which the risks associated with bone-marrow transplantation appear unacceptable. Nevertheless, most patients with chronic lymphocytic leukaemia succumb to the disease itself and this is particularly true of younger patients aged under 60 years. The median age of patients treated with bone-marrow transplantation is 40 years and most patients have received HLA-compatible sibling grafts after high-dose cyclophosphamide and total-body irradiation as treatment for advanced refractory disease. Remission was obtained in approximately 75 per cent and was more commonly achieved in patients with stable or responsive disease before the transplant. Median leukaemia-free survival of up to 7 years and survival of 30 per cent at 7 years post-transplant have been reported (reviewed by Gale and Montserrat 1993).

Approximately 40 per cent of patients have significant acute graft versus host disease (grades II–IV). These results are promising and as with other conditions may be improved if transplantation is used earlier in the course of the disease at a time when there is minimal residual leukaemia after effective initial therapy such as fludarabine. However, at the present time transplantation should probably be reserved for young patients with adverse risk factors who have failed conventional treatments. Randomized controlled studies will be necessary to establish the value of allogeneic transplantation in other situations.

Autologous bone-marrow transplantation

Although autologous bone-marrow transplantation can be safely used as treatment for older patients than are eligible for allografts, this approach has been restricted by the difficulty in achieving an acceptable degree of minimal disease in the bone-marrow to permit bone-marrow harvest in patients with aggressive enough disease to justify the risks. Autologous bone-marrow which had been purged with a cocktail of monoclonal antibodies to B-cell antigens has been reinfused after high-dose cyclophosphamide and total-body irradiation to 19 patients with a good remission to conventional treatment. A high complete remission rate (17/19) and low toxicity was reported and molecular studies suggested that this treatment may be curative (Rabinowe *et al.* 1993). Nevertheless, longer follow-up and randomized controlled studies will be necessary to establish a role for autologous transplantation.

Other therapies

Regular intravenous infusion of normal human immunoglobulin (400 mg/kg 3 weekly for 1 year) has been shown to reduce the incidence of minor bacterial infections. However, the number of severe infections does not seem to be reduced and this treatment has no impact on survival. This treatment is not widely used because of the high cost of this product but it may be of value for selected patients with profound hypoglobulinaemia and recurrent infection.

Novel approaches to treatment of chronic lymphocytic leukaemia include the use of monoclonal antibodies, α-interferon, and cytokines. The effect of monoclonal antibodies alone or conjugated to toxins, cytotoxic drugs, or radio-isotopes is usually partial and transient. Interferon has only modest activity in patients with early disease (Rozman *et al.* 1988) but cannot produce clinically useful responses as a single agent. It may prove to be of value as maintenance therapy following initial response to treatment but proof of this will require randomized controlled studies. Interleukin-2 (IL-2) has some activity *in vitro* but no major therapeutic value. Recombinant haemopoietic growth factors may permit more intensive chemotherapy but the value of this approach remains unproven.

Criteria for assessment of response to treatment

In an attempt to standardize the response criteria used by study groups in chronic lymphocytic leukaemia, the International Workshop in Chronic Lymphocytic Leukaemia (1989) and National Cancer Institute Working Group (Cheson *et al.* 1988) have defined complete remission, partial remission, stable disease, and progressive disease as detailed in Table 12. The use of more sophisticated immunological and molecular techniques are necessary to establish truly a compete remission. These would include flow cytometric analysis of CD5+ CD19+ cells for $\varkappa/\lambda$ clonal excess or analysis for clonal genetic markers by PCR. However, if adopted the criteria would improve the comparability of the therapeutic trials conducted in this disease.

Treatment strategy in chronic lymphocytic leukaemia

Patients with stage A or B disease should not be treated unless there is evidence of diffuse infiltration on the trephine biopsy, a rapid

Table 12 Response criteria for chronic lymphocytic leukaemia

Response	IW CLL criteria	NCI criteria
Complete remission	No evidence of disease	Absence of lymphadenopathy, hepatomegaly, splenomegaly, or constitutional symptoms. Normal blood count. Normal bone-marrow biopsy; marrow lymphocytes < 30 per cent
Partial remission	Change from stage C to stage A or B or stage B to stage A	Fifty per cent reduction in blood lymphocytes and lymphadenopathy and/or splenomegaly or hepatomegaly. Neutrophils >1.5×10⁹/l, Hb >11.0 g/dl and platelets >10×10⁹/l or 50 per cent improvement over baseline
Stable disease	No change in stage	No complete remission, partial remission, or progressive disease
Progressive disease	Change from stage A to B or C or from stage B to C	One of the following: >50 per cent increase in size of ≥2 nodes or new nodes; ≥50 per cent increase in spleen or liver; >50 per cent increase in lymphocyte count; transformation to more aggressive histology, Richter, or prolymphocytic leukaemia

rate of increase in lymphocyte numbers with a lymphocyte doubling time under 12 months, autoimmune cytopenias, or systemic symptoms. All stage C patients should receive immediate therapy. At the time of writing, intermittent oral chlorambucil remains first choice treatment, preceded in patients with severe cytopenias by 1–2 weeks of prednisolone with or without a single dose of intravenous vincristine. Combination regimens such as COP or CHOP are best reserved for second-line therapy. Fludarabine is currently available as second-line therapy on a named-patient basis but will clearly have a role as initial therapy in the near future.

T-CELL CHRONIC LYMPHOCYTIC LEUKAEMIA–LARGE GRANULAR LYMPHOCYTE LEUKAEMIA

It has become apparent that T-cell chronic lymphocytic leukaemia is not a distinct disorder but that all post-thymic T-cell lymphoproliferative disorders can be categorized as large granular lymphocyte leukaemia, prolymphocytic leukaemia, Sézary syndrome, or HTLV-I-related adult T-cell leukaemia (Litz and Brunning 1993). These conditions can often be differentiated by morphology and clinical features but immunophenotyping, cytogenetic analysis, and serological studies for HTLV-I are the definitive investigations in establishing the diagnosis of these disorders (Table 13).

Large granular lymphocyte leukaemia accounts for approximately 2 per cent of all cases of chronic lymphatic leukaemia and, unlike B-cell chronic lymphatic leukaemia, is found in patients of all ages (Foa *et al.* 1988). Patients generally have few specific symptoms but may present with fatigue or recurrent bacterial infection. Splenomegaly is found in 80 per cent of cases. Lymphadenopathy is very rare. Skin lesions are present in 25 per cent of cases and there is an association with seropositive rheumatoid arthritis in approximately 20 per cent of cases. The peripheral blood leucocyte count is generally only modestly elevated to between 10×10^9 and 20×10^9/l owing to large granular lymphocytes. Neutropenia is usually present and may be marked although anaemia or thrombocytopenia only occurs in 30 per cent of patients. Polyclonal hypergammaglobulinaemia, positive rheumatoid factor, and antinuclear antibodies occur in over 50 per cent of patients. Unlike B-cell chronic lymphatic leukaemia, the marrow may not be heavily infiltrated. The marrow usually contains 30–50 per cent lymphocytes and in a small proportion of cases may be near normal. Marrow and lymph node infiltration eventually develop, but this condition is only slowly progressive and its neoplastic nature has been disputed in the past. It is important to differentiate this disorder from a reactive lymphocytosis particularly in young adults and a prolonged period of observation may be required. All patients should be screened serologically for evidence of Epstein–Barr virus infection (Litz and Brunning 1993). Mild lymphocytosis and neutropenia, often associated with rheumatoid arthritis, which may persist for over 10 years may be a pre-leukaemic variant of large granular lymphocyte leukaemia. Therapy is not indicated until complications arise.

The morphology of the lymphoid cells in large granular lymphocyte leukaemia is characteristically that of mature lymphocytes with abundant cytoplasm and numerous azurophilic granules in the cytoplasm. The granules correspond to distinct structures known as parallel tubular arrays, the function of which remains unclear. Cytochemistry typically produces strong acid phosphatase staining localized to the granules and the PTA; β-glucuronidase and β-glucosaminidase are also positive. The cells display a mature post-thymic immunological phenotype which is terminal deoxyribonucleotide transferase (TdT) negative and E rosette positive. In most cases the cells express the Fc-binding receptor for IgG (T gamma cells). The majority are also CD3 positive, CD4 negative, CD1 negative, CD8 positive, and CD2 positive. The HNK-1 antigen is variably expressed. The CD7 and CD5 monoclonal antibodies, which are usually positive in normal T cells, are negative or weakly expressed in many cases of large granular lymphocyte leukaemia. Studies of T-lymphocyte function often show *in vitro* killing activity whilst natural killer function is usually absent. A few cases display a different phenotype with negative CD3, CD4, and CD8 antigen, but are positive for E rosettes, CD2 antigen, and NK markers. Often these cases have a high natural killer activity and show no helper or suppressor activity. These appear to be cases of natural killer cell-type large granular lymphocyte leukaemia and do not usually have severe neutropenia or rheumatoid arthritis.

The monoclonality of large granular lymphocyte leukaemia and, hence, its neoplastic nature has been established by studies at DNA level. The granular cells show unique clonal rearrangement of the β and the γ chain genes for the T-cell antigen receptor. Isoenzyme studies of females heterozygous for G_6PD demonstrate that the neoplastic proliferation is restricted to T lymphocytes. Chromosome abnormalities are found in large granular lymphocyte leukaemia but, unlike T-cell prolymphocytic leukaemia, no consistent abnormality characteristic of the disease has yet been described.

The chronic T-cell disorders are sometimes not easy to distinguish from one another and immunophenotyping is often helpful. The surface phenotypes of these T-lymphoproliferative disorders are summarized in Table 13. T-cell prolymphocytic leukaemia has lymphocytes with basophilic cytoplasm, a single prominent nucleolus, and no azurophilic granules. Typically, there is a high white cell

Table 13 Immunophenotype of T-cell chronic lymphoproliferative disorders

	LGLL	TPLL	ATLL	SS
TdT	–	–	–	–
CD3	++	++	++	++
CD4	–	++	++	++
CD5	–	+	+	+
CD7	–/+	+++	–	–
CD8	++	–	–	–
CD25	–	–/+	++	–/+
Other		ANAE+ inv(14)(q11 32)	HTLV-1+	

LGL, large granular lymphocyte leukaemia; TPLL, T-cell prolymphocytic leukaemia; ATLL, adult T-cell leukaemia; SS, Sézary syndrome; TdT, terminal deoxynucleotidyl transferase; ANAE, alpha-naphthol acetate esterase.

count, marked splenomegaly, and an aggressive clinical picture. T-cell prolymphocytic leukaemia cells usually express the CD4 and CD7 antigens, unlike T-cell chronic lymphatic leukaemia which is CD4 negative and shows negative or weak expression of CD7.

Sézary's syndrome is often also confused with these two disorders, but skin lesions are typically prominent in this condition and the pathological cells in the blood and skin are usually CD4 positive with demonstrable helper function *in vitro*. Classical cerebriform cells are often seen in blood films. The cells of Sézary's syndrome are CD7 negative as in large granular lymphocyte leukaemia. In adult T-cell leukaemia/lymphoma there is an association with the retrovirus HTLV-1 and the patients have lymphadenopathy, hypercalcaemia, and a polylobated nucleus with notable pleomorphism in cell size and nuclear shape. Occasional blasts are seen in the blood and the cells are CD4 positive, CD7 negative, and CD25 positive but display *in vitro* suppressor function.

HAIRY CELL LEUKAEMIA

Hairy cell leukaemia which has also been known under the name leukaemia reticuloendotheliosis is an extremely well-characterized chronic lymphoproliferative disorder associated with splenomegaly, pancytopenia, recurrent infections, and typical 'hairy cells' in the blood and bone-marrow. Although first described by Bouroncle *et al.* (1958), it is only in recent years that significant advances have occurred in the understanding of this condition and its treatment.

The morphological features of hairy cells are distinctive and easily seen in a well-stained peripheral blood film (Fig. 8), although the characteristic appearance of the electron microscopic preparations (Fig. 9) generated the descriptive title of 'hairy cell'. In addition to the fine cytoplasmic projections, another characteristic feature seen on electron microscopy are cytoplasmic inclusions known as ribosome–lamella complexes. There is a lacy chromatin pattern in the nucleus and the cytoplasm is abundant, pale, and may contain small vacuoles. The most prominent cellular feature is the presence of numerous fine short filaments or villae around the whole circumference of the cell. A variable proportion of these cells contain tartrate-resistant acid phosphatase isoenzyme 5 (TRAP). This cytochemical feature was initially thought to be diagnostic for hairy cell leukaemia, but it has also been described more recently in B-cell prolymphocytic leukaemia and some chronic T-cell disorders. The origin of the hairy cell has been vigorously debated for some years and evidence has been provided to support B-lymphocyte, monocyte, or hybrid lymphocyte–monocyte lineage. The normal counterpart of the hairy cell is as yet unknown.

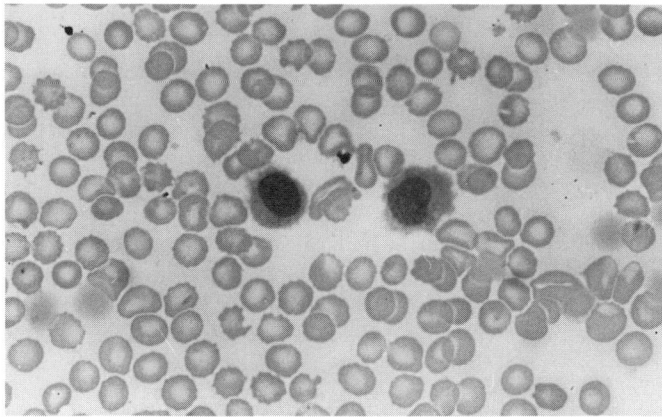

Fig. 8 Peripheral blood in hairy cell leukaemia showing two typical hairy cells. These cells have a round nucleus and shaggy pale cytoplasm with ragged cytoplasmic processes resembling pseudopods.

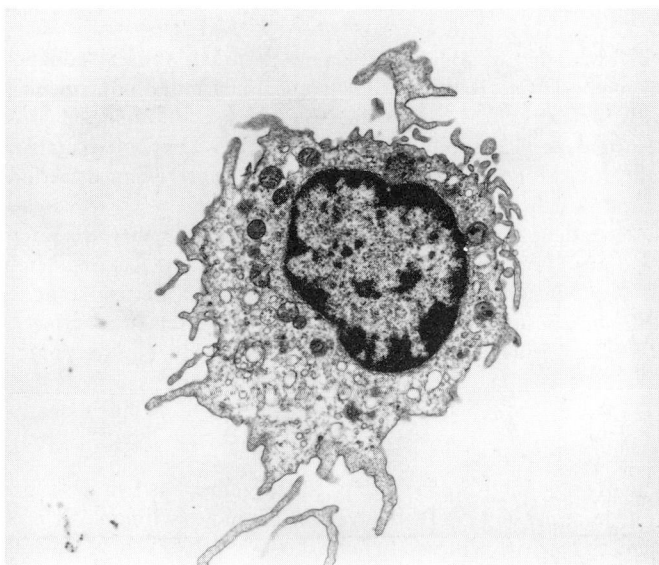

Fig. 9 Transmission photoelectron micrograph of a hairy cell from the blood of a patient with hairy cell leukaemia. This cell has the characteristic features of delicate cytoplasmic projections and chromatin clumping on the nuclear membrane. (Kindly donated by Mrs J. Price, Department of Cellular Pathology, Royal United Hospital, Bath.)

The nature of the hairy cell

The evidence for the cell of origin of the hairy cell comes from cell surface markers, cell membrane characteristics, and intracellular characteristics (reviewed in Jansen 1987). Monoclonal antibody studies of cell surface markers provide strong evidence in favour of a B-cell origin in the overwhelming majority of patients. Hairy cells are recognized by antibodies against HLA DR determinants, the CD20 antigen, the CD19 antigen, the CD22 antigen, and the Y29/55 antigen, which are found at most stages of B-cell differentiation. These cells also react with antibodies that are limited to certain particular stages of B-cell development, with almost 50 per cent of cases being positive to the antibody CD24. The HC2 monoclonal antibody raised against hairy cells reacts with normal activated B lymphocytes and monocytes. Another antigen expressed

on activated B lymphocytes (also by activated T lymphocytes and monocytes) is the CD25 antigen (TAC) which is the interleukin-2 (IL-2) receptor. Most hairy cells express an antigen recognized by the antibody FMC7 which identifies a rather mature stage of B-cell differentiation. They may also express the plasma-cell-associated antigen PCA1, another feature which suggests that the hairy cell corresponds to a late stage of B-cell ontogeny.

Although all these observations suggest that the hairy cell has a B-cell origin, hairy cells also react with the antibodies CD11b and Leu-M5 (CD11c), which are associated with the monocyte and granulocyte lineages. These results suggested some relationships with the monocyte line, but a large panel of other antibodies to monocytes and macrophages have been uniformly negative with hairy cells. The CD11b antigen may be expressed during a brief stage of B-cell ontogeny and this may coincide with the appearance of the antigen FMC7 and the developmental stage equivalent to the hairy cell. The glycolipid pattern of the membrane structure of hairy cells provides additional evidence that hairy cells are lymphoid cells, probably related to chronic lymphocytic leukaemia. A number of studies of the intracellular characteristics of hairy cells have revealed that these cells can synthesize and secrete immunoglobulin *in vivo* and *in vitro*. The hairy cells have rearranged heavy and light chains and contain the corresponding mRNA for heavy and light chain immunoglobulin production (Korsmeyer *et al.* 1983).

In conclusion, there is now very strong evidence that hairy cell leukaemia is a B-lymphoid neoplasm, although the hairy cells possess certain features such as ultrastructural peroxidase activity, procoagulant activity, and phagocytosis of small particles which are not typical of normal B cells. The most important immunological markers of hairy cells are the monoclonal antibodies CD5, FMC7, CD11c, CD25, HC2, and PCA-1 (Table 13). These antibodies not only assist in the diagnosis of hairy cell leukaemia but suggest that the hairy cell is the neoplastic equivalent of an activated B lymphocyte.

Clinical and haematological features

Hairy cell leukaemia may represent approximately 2 per cent of all leukaemias (reviewed in Golomb *et al.* 1978; Cawley *et al.* 1980b). It occurs predominantly in males, with a sex ratio of 4 : 1 and usually occurs in patients over the age of 45 years. No clear aetiology has been defined. There has been an occasional case report of familial occurrence, but this is rare. Patients present with non-specific symptoms such as weakness, weight loss, infection, and dyspnoea. They may occasionally present as a result of an abnormal blood count or the finding of unsuspected splenomegaly. On examination, the most prominent abnormal feature is splenomegaly, which occurs in approximately 80 per cent of patients and is massively enlarged by more than 10 cm beyond the left costal margin in 20–30 per cent. Lymphadenopathy is rare, being found in less than 5 per cent of patients and serves to distinguish this disorder clinically from many other lymphoproliferative disorders. If significant lymphadenopathy is seen, then the diagnosis of hairy cell leukaemia must be made with caution. Hepatomegaly is also uncommon.

The haematology at diagnosis typically shows pancytopenia and marked reduction in haemoglobin to less than 8.5 g/dl in approximately 35 per cent of patients. The white cell count is less than $4.0 \times 10^9/l$ in 50–60 per cent of cases and a leucocytosis greater than $10 \times 10^9/l$ is found in only 15–20 per cent of cases. There is neutropenia of less than $0.5 \times 10^9/l$ in approximately one-third of patients. Profound monocytopenia is usual and the presence of a normal monocyte count may coincide with the presence of other atypical features which make the diagnosis of hairy cell leukaemia questionable. More than 80 per cent of patients have a platelet count of less than $150\times10^9/l$ and severe thrombocytopenia of less than $50\times10^9/l$ is found in 20–30 per cent. The diagnosis is made from the typical appearance of hairy cells in the blood (Fig. 8) and from the TRAP cytochemistry. Confirmation comes from histological examination of involved tissue and bone-marrow biopsy is the most accessible. Bone-marrow aspiration is unsuccessful in approximately half the patients. The bone-marrow biopsy shows an infiltrate with mononuclear cells intermingled with normal haemopoietic elements. The abnormal cells are clearly separated from one another by finely reticulated zones of abundant cytoplasm which impart a 'halo' appearance. There is an increase in bone-marrow reticulin fibres. Other findings include a high leucocyte alkaline phosphatase score, hypergammaglobulinaemia, and elevated hepatic transaminases. The spleen is always involved in hairy cell leukaemia usually with diffuse infiltration of the red pulp by hairy cells in contrast to other lymphoproliferative disorders that primarily involve the white pulp.

There are a significant number of clinical complications, with infection being the major cause of morbidity and death. Pyogenic infections are most common, but unusual pathogens are also encountered in hairy cell leukaemia. These include atypical mycobacteria, toxoplasmosis, and histoplasmosis, suggesting a defect in cell-mediated immunity. Haemorrhagic complications occur because of thrombocytopenia and also because of a qualitative platelet defect which is considered to be a granule storage pool disorder. Osteolytic lesions are a well-known but rare complication of hairy cell disease with lesions of the femoral neck most typical. These generally manifest themselves through hip pain and occasionally through spontaneous fracture. Radiotherapy is the treatment of choice for these lesions. There have been an increasing number of recent reports associating a hairy cell leukaemia with autoimmune vasculitic polyarthritis.

The overall median survival for a patient with hairy cell disease has been reported as between 2 and 5 years. Patients with a high haemoglobin and neutrophil count have a median survival of more than 6 years, whilst patients in whom either the haemoglobin or the neutrophil count is low have a median survival of approximately 5 years. Patients with both low haemoglobin and low neutrophils have a median survival of approximately 16 months.

Variants of hairy cell leukaemia

Variants of hairy cell leukaemia occur (type 2 hairy cell leukaemia) (Cawley *et al.* 1980*a*). This represents a minority of patients who usually have a high white cell count (50×10^9–$80\times10^9/l$) and marked splenomegaly. The cells have a prominent nucleolus, lack the HC2 and CD25 antigens, and express IgG or no immunoglobulin on the membrane. The hairy cells in many of these patients do not exhibit cytochemical positivity to the TRAP stain and monocytopenia may be absent. The variant form of hairy cell leukaemia has a tendency to affect older patients and females and it may respond less well to α-interferon and deoxycoformycin (Sainati *et al.* 1990; Catovsky 1993).

A T-cell variant has also been described in a small number of patients. This is morphologically and clinically indistinguishable from B-cell hairy cell leukaemia, but the hairy cells unequivocally express T-cell markers. The human retrovirus HTLV-II has been isolated from T-cell lines isolated from two patients with the T-cell variant. Cells from a proportion of these patients may co-express B-cell and T-cell antigens.

Treatment

There are now several therapeutic options available for the treatment of hairy cell leukaemia and sound clinical judgement is required to determine which way to proceed in an individual patient (reviewed by Golomb 1987; Golomb and Ratain 1987; Platanias and Golomb 1993). In approximately 10 per cent of patients, more often the elderly patients with an impalpable spleen, it may be best not to initiate any treatment at all since those patients tend to have a very indolent course. These are the patients who do not suffer any serious infections, have a stable granulocyte count greater than $1.5\times10^9/l$, and have no transfusion requirement and no bleeding tendency since their platelets are greater than $100\times10^9/l$. Treatment should be initiated in patients with anaemia (Hb <10 g/dl), neutropenia ($<1\times10^9/l$), thrombocytopenia ($<100\times10^9/l$), symptomatic splenomegaly, recurrent infection, extra-lymphatic disease, autoimmune complications, or presentation in a florid leukaemic phase (Platanias and Ratain 1992). Most patients will require treatment eventually.

Splenectomy

This was the treatment of choice prior to the introduction of α-interferon. Response to splenectomy does not correlate with splenic size but with the degree of bone-marrow involvement. Patients with under 85 per cent bone-marrow cellularity respond well to splenectomy for prolonged periods and this may still be considered the treatment of choice for these patients as they may not require any further treatment for up to 10 years (Platanias and Golomb 1993). Approximately 50 per cent of patients will obtain a good partial response with normalization of blood counts after splenectomy and a further 40 per cent will obtain a minor response and may require systemic therapy.

Interferon

The use of α-interferon in hairy cell leukaemia was first described by Quesada *et al.* (1984). In a variety of studies with α-interferon blood counts have returned to normal in over 70 per cent of patients, although hairy cells are only eradicated from the bone-marrow of under 20 per cent. Interferon, although highly effective, is rarely if ever curative, but treatment with interferon results in excellent palliation of the cytopenia and its associated complications. Complete remission occurs in under 5 per cent of patients treated with α-interferon and many patients considered to have achieved a clinical complete remission will have residual splenic disease if this is sought (Pangalis *et al.* 1991).

The dose of α-interferon used in hairy cell leukaemia has generally ranged from 2 mu/m² three times weekly to 3 mu/day until maximum response has been achieved. It is administered by subcutaneous injection. Lower doses (0.2 mu/m²) have been evaluated and toxicity is less but the response rate is clearly inferior. There appears to be no significant difference between the two different recombinant forms of α-interferon, α-2a, and α-2b, either in terms of efficacy or toxicity. Haematological normalization occurs in 80 per cent of patients within 6 months of commencing therapy but several months of treatment may be required to obtain an adequate response. Treatment should be continued for at least 12 months and blood counts can be expected to remain normal for 12–15 months after stopping α-interferon. Prolongation of therapy decreases the relapse rate during treatment but does not prolong the duration of response after the treatment is discontinued. Patients who have relapsed after α-interferon is stopped will usually respond again. Relapse usually develops with a gradual onset of cytopenia.

Toxic effects of α-interferon include an influenza-like syndrome, fatigue, dry mouth, and reversible myelosuppression with less common occurrence of skin rash or gastrointestinal upset. Occasional reversible central nervous system toxicity, peripheral neuropathy, and mental disturbances occur. Mild toxic effects may respond to dose reduction or decreased frequency of administration but a proportion of patients are unable to tolerate this therapy.

The mechanism of action of α-interferon in hairy cell leukaemia is unknown but both a direct antiproliferative effect on hairy cells and an indirect effect through activation of the immune system have been postulated. The cells of patients who respond to α-interferon have been shown to express receptors for α-interferon and refractoriness to α-interferon has been associated with a lack of expression of these receptors in a small number of patients. Numerous effects on hairy cells *in vitro* have been described for α-interferon but the mechanism through which the marked therapeutic effect is achieved has yet to be elucidated (reviewed by Platanias and Golomb 1993).

Purine analogues

2-Deoxycoformycin (pentostatin)

This purine analogue is a potent inhibitor of adenosine deaminase. Inhibition of adenosine deaminase results in single-stranded DNA breaks, depletion of NAD levels, and inhibition of intracellular methylation and intracellular ATP levels. Although this agent has been shown to be effective in a number of lymphoproliferative disorders hairy cells appear to be much more sensitive to DCF at low drug levels which permits the use of non-toxic dose schedules.

Spiers *et al.* (1984) first reported the effect of DCF in hairy cell leukaemia and subsequent trials have demonstrated a complete response rate of 50–80 per cent with more rapid improvement in blood counts than had been seen with α-interferon (reviewed by Platanias and Golomb 1993). The regimen now widely used is 4 mg/m² every 2 weeks to maximum response followed by two further consolidation courses and most patients receive six to ten courses of treatment. Toxic effects at this dosage are acceptable in contrast to earlier schedules where profound immunosuppression and concomitant serious infection were common. Nausea, vomiting, rashes, neutropenia, fever, and reversible renal impairment may occur. The most notable toxic effect remains an increased number of serious infectious complications which may be related to a profound reduction in the number of circulating CD4 lymphocytes. DCF should not be used in patients with active infection.

2-Chlorodeoxyadenosine

The mechanism of action of this adenosine deaminase-resistant purine analogue is unknown but the efficacy of this agent in hairy cell leukaemia as well as chronic lymphocytic leukaemia, low-grade non-Hodgkin's lymphoma, and cutaneous T-cell lymphoma has been clearly demonstrated. An 80 per cent complete response rate and 20 per cent partial response rate have been obtained following a single 7 day course of 2-CdA at a dose of 0.1 mg/kg/day with minimal toxicity. Prolonged remissions up to 4 years have been obtained (Saven and Piro 1992). It seems probable that some patients have been cured by this extremely active drug but longer follow-up in larger groups of patients will be necessary to establish 2-CdA as the treatment of choice in hairy cell leukaemia.

SPLENIC LYMPHOMA WITH VILLOUS LYMPHOCYTES

Splenic lymphoma with villous lymphocytes is another recently described B-cell lymphoproliferative disorder which is often confused with hairy cell leukaemia but is even rarer (Melo *et al.* 1987). The patients are usually some 20 years older than those with hairy cell leukaemia (mean age 72 years). They have an enlarged spleen, which is often massive and they rarely have lymphadenopathy. The peripheral leucocytosis is a constant feature, with the highest lymphocyte count being 35×10^9/l and two-thirds of the patients have a monoclonal band. Lymphocytes in the blood have long and short villae rather suggestive of hairy cell leukaemia but have less cytoplasm and are not usually TRAP positive. Unlike hairy cell leukaemia, there is no monocytopenia, but plasmacytoid cells may be present. The marrow appearance is distinct from that seen in hairy cell leukaemia and, unlike in hairy cell leukaemia, it is nearly always possible to aspirate bone-marrow fragments. Spleen histology shows the main difference from hairy cell leukaemia with primarily white pulp involvement with evidence of lymphoplasmacytic differentiation. The villous lymphocytes show strong staining with sIg but few mouse red cell rosettes and express the HLA-DR antigen and the B-cell antigens CD19, CD20, CD22, and CD24 as well as FMC7. These cells are negative for CD5, CD23, and CD25 (Table 13).

The disorder has a benign clinical course and many patients may not need any treatment. Chlorambucil may be useful in some but the role of α-interferon or deoxycoformycin in this disorder is unknown.

B-CELL PROLYMPHOCYTIC LEUKAEMIA

The clinical and haematological features of B-cell prolymphocytic leukaemia are quite different from those of T-cell prolymphocytic leukaemia which accounts for approximately 20 per cent of all cases of prolymphocytic leukaemia (Melo *et al.* 1986). Both these diseases are relatively uncommon as prolymphocytic leukaemia accounts for only 2 per cent of all cases of chronic lymphoid leukaemia. The median age at diagnosis is 67 years and there is a male:female ratio of 2:1. Its distinctive features are massive enlargement of the spleen without significant lymph node enlargement accompanied by a rising leucocyte count, which is usually over 100×10^9/l at presentation and may well progress to between 500×10^9 and 1000×10^9/l. Prolymphocytes comprise 55 per cent or more of the lymphocytes. While B-cell chronic lymphatic leukaemia often progresses very slowly and remains indolent for long periods, B-cell prolymphocytic leukaemia is a relentlessly progressive disease in which patients almost always present with symptoms of bone-marrow failure. Most patients are anaemic and thrombocytopenic at diagnosis.

The blood film shows the presence of a homogeneous population of large lymphocytes with a large centrally placed nucleolus conspicuous because of perinucleolar chromatin (Fig. 10). These cells usually have far more abundant cytoplasm than do typical B-cell chronic lymphatic leukaemia cells and the nucleus is often slightly larger also. The immunophenotype of B-cell prolymphocytic leukaemia is very different from that of chronic lymphatic leukaemia. B-cell prolymphocytic leukaemia cells strongly express surface Ig and do not form a significant number or rosettes with mouse erythrocytes. In approximately one-third of cases there is a high proportion of CD5-positive cells but strong reactivity with FMC7

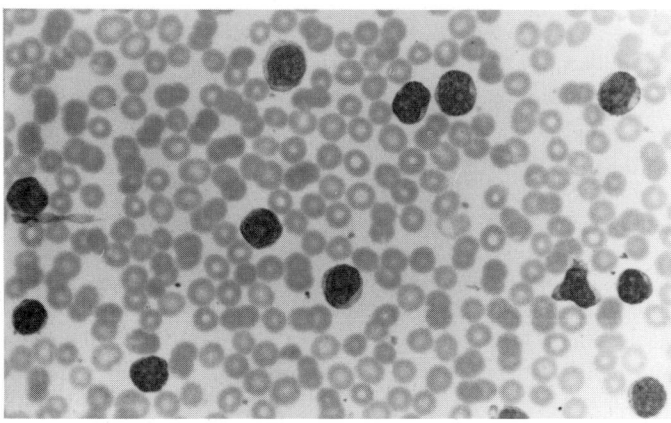

Fig. 10 Peripheral blood in B-cell prolymphocytic leukaemia showing large cells with abundant cytoplasm and immature nuclei containing a single prominent nucleolus.

and CD22 is almost invariably present. Prolymphocytes also express the pan-B-cell markers CD19, CD20, and CD24. B-cell prolymphocytic leukaemia can be distinguished from hairy cell disease by failure to react to CD25 (Table 10). The bone-marrow infiltration is diffuse, as in advanced chronic lymphatic leukaemia and spleen histology shows extensive red and white pulp involvement with large proliferative nodules. In both hairy cell leukaemia and its variants the red cell pulp is predominantly involved.

The treatment of B-cell prolymphocytic leukaemia is unsatisfactory. The chemotherapy regimens used in chronic lymphatic leukaemia, either singly or in combination, are of little value in B-cell prolymphocytic leukaemia. Splenectomy may often be helpful as this may remove the major proliferative focus. Up to 50 per cent of patients respond to splenic irradiation (100 cGy weekly for 10 weeks) and combinations including adriamycin (CHOP) may help a third of the patients. Deoxycoformycin has been reported to be of value in some patients.

T-CELL PROLYMPHOCYTIC LEUKAEMIA

It became apparent during the 1970s that almost a quarter of the prolymphocytic leukaemias expressed T-cell markers (Volk *et al.* 1983). These patients present with symptoms of short duration and most of them have splenomegaly with hepatomegaly in 50 per cent. Unlike hairy cell leukaemia or splenic lymphoma with villous lymphocytes, generalized lymphadenopathy is present in 50 per cent of patients with T-cell prolymphocytic leukaemia. Skin lesions are found in 25 per cent of cases and serous effusions in approximately 20 per cent. These patients also have a very high white cell count with a median count of $200 \times 10^9/l$. Approximately 50 per cent of patients are anaemic and thrombocytopenic (Matutes *et al.* 1991). The serum calcium is normal and HTLV-1 serology is negative (Table 13).

Membrane markers are very useful in confirming the diagnosis: 75 per cent of cases are CD4+, CD8−, whilst a small group (15−20 per cent) co-express CD4 and CD8. Whilst there are other T-cell malignancies expressing CD4, T-cell prolymphocytic leukaemia is almost unique in also expressing CD7 and membrane CD3. The T-cell prolymphocytic leukaemia cell cytochemistry is usually strongly α-naphthyl acetate esterase (ANAE) positive. Biopsy of the skin will show dense cellular infiltrates not involving the epidermis which differentiates T-cell prolymphocytic leukaemia from the infiltration seen in the Sézary syndrome. Cytogenetic studies have revealed abnormalities of chromosome 14 in 76 per cent of patients with T-cell prolymphocytic leukaemia involving break-points of 14q11 and 14q32 usually in the form of a partially inverted long arm (inv(14)(q11 32)). It is of interest that the genes for the T-lymphocyte a and d receptors are located at 14q11. Approximately 50 per cent of cases also have trisomy 8 in addition (Matutes *et al.* 1991).

Therapy of this disorder is difficult and, as in B-cell prolymphocytic leukaemia, the disease is relentlessly progressive, with the majority of the patients surviving less than a year or so. The mean survival is only 6 months. Aggressive combination chemotherapy with regimens such as CHOP may benefit some patients and most recently significant responses have been seen with deoxycoformycin. These responses have only been observed in those patients whose cells are CD4 and CD8 positive.

ADULT T-CELL LEUKAEMIA–LYMPHOMA

The association of adult T-cell leukaemia–lymphoma with the human T-cell leukaemia virus HTLV-1, first described by Takatsuki *et al.* (1977), makes this a very important disorder. C-type particles were initially grown from an adult T-cell leukaemia–lymphoma cell line and this observation established the association between this disease with HTLV-1. Subsequent elucidation of the aetiology and epidemiology has been extremely rapid though the development of effective therapy has not kept pace. An aetiological association between the retrovirus HTLV-1 and adult T-cell leukaemia–lymphoma has been established by the occurrence of a high incidence of this condition in areas of Japan with a high prevalence of HTLV-1 infection, the observation that HTLV-1 infection of human CD4 T-lymphocytes results in immortalization of those cells, the demonstration of HTLV-1 provirus in the neoplastic cells of adult T-cell leukaemia–lymphoma, and the observation that all patients with this condition have antibodies against HTLV-1 (Yamaguchi and Takatsuki 1993). The unique *tax* gene of the HTLV-1 virus induces in T-cell lines expression of the gene for the IL-2 receptor and this may be a factor in the uncontrolled proliferation of the cells of adult T-cell leukaemia–lymphoma. The site of integration of the proviral DNA in the host genome varies between individuals though it is monoclonal in the individual patient with adult T-cell leukaemia–lymphoma. Integrated provirus is not found in carriers of HTLV-1 without adult T-cell leukaemia–lymphoma. A number of chromosomal abnormalities have been reported but no consistent pattern has emerged.

A high incidence of HTLV-1 infection has been found in the Kyushu district of south-western Japan and in the Caribbean islands and countries bordering the Caribbean Sea. Many of the patients with adult T-cell leukaemia–lymphoma reported in non-endemic areas have originally come from the Caribbean. In endemic areas of Japan, antibodies to HTLV-1 are found in up to 37 per cent of healthy adults over 40 years. In these districts the incidence rate of adult T-cell leukaemia–lymphoma is estimated as 2 per 1000 seropositive males and 0.5 per 1000 seropositive females with a cumulative risk of 2.5 per cent at 70 years (Kondo *et al.* 1989). Transmission of HTLV-1 appears to be restricted to vertical transmission from mother to infant, predominantly through breast milk and horizontal transmission through sexual intercourse in an overwhelmingly male to female direction and by transfusion of seropositive blood. A small number of patients have been described with negative serology for HTLV-1 and a CD4-positive T-cell neoplasm with a similar clinical course to adult T-cell leukaemia–lymphoma. A diagnostic label of 'adult T-cell leukaemia–lymphoma not associated with HTLV-1' has been applied to these patients and there is no geographical clustering.

Clinical and haematological features

Adult T-cell leukaemia–lymphoma occurs in adults with a male:female ratio of 1.4:1 and an age range from 20 to 90 years and a mean age at diagnosis of 58 years. Lymphadenopathy occurs in 60 per cent of patients with hepatomegaly in 26 per cent, splenomegaly in 22 per cent, and skin lesions in 39 per cent. Hypercalcaemia is present in 32 per cent whilst other features include abdominal pain, diarrhoea, pleural effusions, ascites, and respiratory symptoms.

A markedly elevated leucocyte count is usual and it may reach $500 \times 10^9/l$. The cells of adult T-cell leukaemia–lymphoma characteristically resemble Sézary cells and have lobulated or indented nuclei and may be designated flower cells (Fig. 11). Cytoplasmic vacuoles are seen in approximately one-third of cases but azurophilic granules are not present. The phenotype of these cells is usually CD3+, CD4+, CD7−, CD8− CD25+, and HLA-DR+ (Table 13) though variable expression of T-cell antigens other than CD4 has been reported. Occasionally a mixed CD4+/CD8+ phenotype or rarely CD4−/CD8+ is found. Patients with adult T-cell leukaemia–lymphoma are seropositive for HTLV-1.

The prognosis of adult T-cell leukaemia–lymphoma is extremely poor and ranges from less than 2 weeks to 1 year. Death is usually due to infection, notably *Pneumocystis carinii* pneumonia, cryptococcus meningitis, and disseminated herpes zoster, DIC, or hypercalcaemia.

Four clinical subtypes are described with acute, chronic, smouldering, or lymphomatous features (Yamaguchi and Takatsuki 1993). There appears to be no correlation between cell morphology, immunophenotype, and clinical behaviour. The acute form is most common and occurs in approximately two-thirds of cases. Poor prognostic features are elevated LDH, hypercalcaemia which occurs in two-thirds, hyperbilirubinaemia, and high leucocyte count. The smouldering and chronic forms may be restricted to skin and pulmonary lesions and an elevated leucocyte count but often progress to the acute form after a variable period. Lymphomatous adult T-cell leukaemia–lymphoma occurs in approximately one-quarter of cases and is characterized by prominent lymphadenopathy and no lymphocytosis in the blood or bone-marrow. Pulmonary symptoms are frequently a result of leukaemic infiltration and this occurs in approximately 50 per cent. Hypercalcaemia will also develop in 50 per cent of patients at some point during the course of their disease. This has been shown to be due to overproduction of parathyroid hormone-related protein (**PTHrP**) by the neoplastic cells of adult T-cell leukaemia–lymphoma as a result of transactivation of the gene for PTHrP by p40tax, the transcriptional transactivator of HTLV-1 (Watanabe *et al.* 1990).

Treatment

Patients with acute or lymphomatous adult T-cell leukaemia–lymphoma have generally been treated with combination chemotherapy regimens such as CHOP, VEPA, or COMLA, but patients with hypercalcaemia, an elevated LDH, and high leucocyte count have a median survival of under 6 months despite therapy. Some short-lived remissions are obtained but infective complications frequently follow therapy in this condition. Hypercalcaemia can only be controlled if the underlying disease responds to chemotherapy. A response rate of almost 33 per cent has been reported with single-agent deoxycoformycin in the treatment of relapsed or refractory adult T-cell leukaemia–lymphoma and a study of a combination regimen including this agent is in progress. The durability of these responses has not been established. Intensive chemotherapy is often associated with life-threatening infection in patients with the smouldering and chronic forms of adult T-cell leukaemia–lymphoma. As these patients have a more indolent course and can remain static for several years an alternative approach would be more appropriate.

SÉZARY SYNDROME

Another chronic malignancy of mature T-lymphocytes which sometimes involves the blood is the Sézary syndrome. Patients with this condition present with an exfoliative erythroderma and lymphomatous infiltration of the epidermis and dermis (mycosis fungoides). In the early stages of the disease the abnormal cells are confined to the skin and skin biopsy shows infiltration of the epidermis with typical epidermotropism and Pautrier's micro-abscesses. The bone-marrow and blood become involved later with more advanced disease. Haemoglobin and platelet counts are usually normal and the leucocyte count is usually $<20 \times 10^9/l$. Lymphadenopathy occurs in 50 per cent and hepatomegaly in approximately 30 per cent. The typical Sézary cell is the key for diagnosis of the condition and when seen in the blood has a highly convoluted nucleus with deep and narrow indentations (Fig. 12). The pathological cells in the blood and in the skin are almost always CD3+, CD4+, CD8−, CD25−, and HLA-DR− (Table 13) and some show helper function *in vitro*.

Patients with the Sézary syndrome have received many different forms of treatment including chemotherapy, local irradiation, and photoactivation in combination with ultraviolet light.

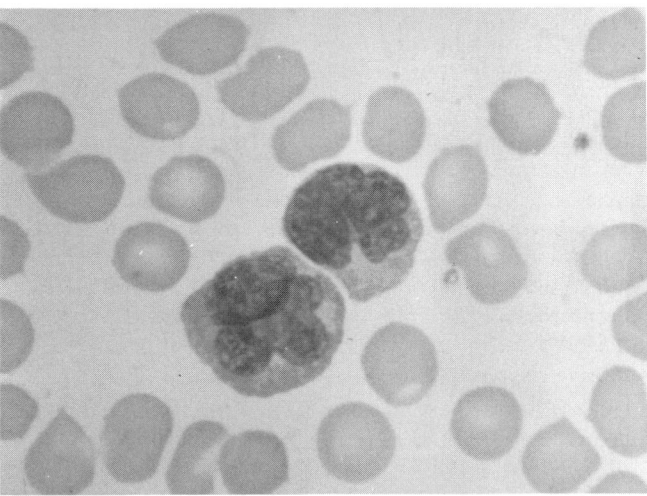

Fig. 11 Lymphoid cells in the peripheral blood of a patient with adult T-cell leukaemia–lymphoma showing the marked nuclear irregularity characteristic of this condition. (Kindly donated by Professor D. Catovsky, Department of Haematology, Royal Marsden Hospital, London.)

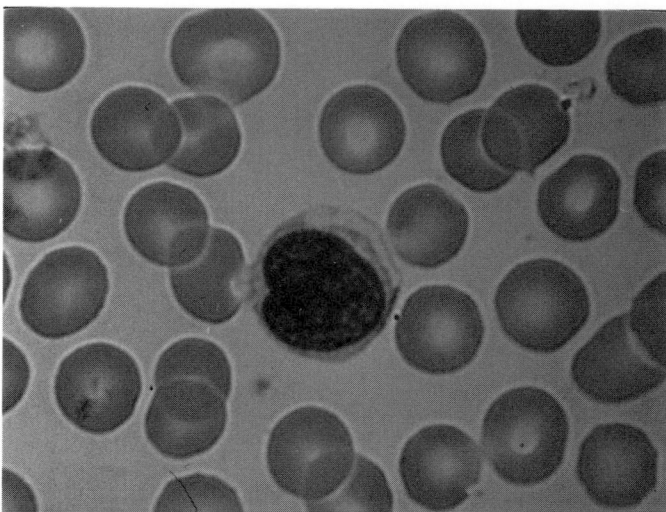

Fig. 12 A large lymphoid cell in the peripheral blood of a patient with the Sézary syndrome. The characteristic cerebriform nucleus of the Sézary cell is well shown in this example. (Kindly donated by Professor D. Catovsky, Department of Haematology, Royal Marsden Hospital, London.)

Deoxycoformycin has been reported to show some activity in this condition as in many other T-cell malignancies (Ho *et al.* 1988), although it is not certain yet whether it can improve the long-term prognosis of patients with this disease.

REFERENCES

Alimena G, *et al.* (1988). Interferon α2B as therapy for Ph-positive chronic myelogenous leukaemia. A study of 82 patients treated with intermittent or daily administration. *Blood*, **72**:642–7.

Altman J (1988). Chronic leukaemias of childhood. *Pediatric Clinics of North America*, **35**:765–76.

Anagrelide Study Group (1992). Anagrelide, a therapy for thrombocythemic states: experience in 577 patients. *American Journal of Medicine*, **92**:69–76.

Appelbaum FR, *et al.* (1987). Treatment of preleukaemic syndromes with marrow transplantation. *Blood*, **69**:92–6.

Arcese W, *et al.* (1993). Outcome of patients who relapse after allogeneic bone marrow transplantation for chronic myeloid leukaemia. *Blood*, **82**:3211–19.

Armitage JO, *et al.* (1981). Effect of chemotherapy for the dysmyelopoietic syndrome. *Cancer Treatment Reports*, **65**:601–5.

Barnett MJ, *et al.* (1992). Autografting in chronic myeloid leukaemia with cultured marrow. *Leukaemia*, **6** (Suppl. 4):118–19.

Barr RD, Fialkow PJ (1973). Clonal origin of chronic myelocytic leukaemia. *New England Journal of Medicine*, **289**:307–12.

Bartram CR (1985). bcr rearrangement without juxtaposition of c-abl in chronic myelocytic leukaemia. *Journal of Experimental Medicine*, **162**:2175–9.

Bartram CR, *et al.* (1985). c-abl and bcr are rearranged in a Ph¹-negative CML patient. *EMBO Journal*, **4**:683–6.

Beatty PG, *et al.* (1985). Marrow transplantation from related donors other than HLA-identical siblings. *New England Journal of Medicine*, **313**:765–71.

Bennett JM, *et al.* (1982). Proposals for the classification of the myelodysplastic syndromes. *British Journal of Haematology*, **51**:189–99.

Berk PD, *et al.* (1986). Therapeutic recommendations in polycythaemia vera based on the Polycythaemia Vera Study Group protocols. *Seminars in Hematology*, **23**:132–43.

Besa EC, Nowell PC, Geller NL, Gardner FH (1982). Analysis of the androgen response of 23 patients with agnogenic myeloid metaplasia: the value of chromosomal studies in predicting response and survival. *Cancer*, **49**:308–13.

Beutler E (1992). Cladribine (2-chlorodeoxyadenosine). *Lancet*, **340**:952–6.

Binet JL, *et al.* (1981). Chronic lymphocytic leukaemia: proposals for a revised prognostic staging system. *British Journal of Haematology*, **48**:365–7.

Binet JL and the French Co-operative Group on Chronic Lymphocytic Leukaemia (1993). Treatment of chronic lymphocytic leukaemia. *Bailliere's Clinical Haematology*, **6**:867–78.

Bofil M, *et al.* (1985). Human B cell development. Subpopulations in the human fetus. *Journal of Immunology*, **134**:1531–6.

Bouroncle BA, Wiseman BK, Doak CA (1958). Leukaemic reticuloendotheliosis. *Blood*, **13**:609–29.

Brodsky I, Hubbell HR, Strayer DR, Gillespie DH (1987). Implications of retroviral and oncogene activity in chronic myelogenous leukaemia. *Cancer Genetics and Cytogenetics*, **26**:15–23.

Brown AG, *et al.* (1993). Evidence for a new tumour suppressor locus (DBM) in human B-cell neoplasia telomeric to the retinoblastoma gene. *Nature Genetics*, **3**:67–72.

Broxmeyer HE, Mendelsohn N, Moore MAS (1977). Abnormal granulocytic feedback regulation of colony forming and colony stimulating activity-producing cells from patients with chronic myelogenous leukaemia. *Leukaemia Research*, **1**:3–10.

Caligaris-Cappio E, Gobbi M, Bofill M, Janossy G (1985). Unfrequent normal B-lymphocytes express features of B-chronic lymphocytic leukaemia. *Journal of Experimental Medicine*, **155**:623–7.

Cannistra S (1990). Chronic myelogenous leukaemia as a model for genetic basis for cancer. *Hematology and Oncology Clinics of North America*, **4**:337–53.

Carella AM, *et al.* (1992). Intensive conventional chemotherapy can lead to a precocious overshoot of cytogenetically normal blood stem cells in chronic myeloid leukaemia and acute lymphoblastic leukaemia. *Leukaemia*, **6** (Suppl. 4):120–3.

Catovsky D (1993). Diagnosis and treatment of CLL variants. In *Chronic lymphocytic leukaemia. Scientific advances and therapeutic developments* (ed. BD Cheson), pp. 369–97. Marcel Dekker, New York.

Cawley JC, Burns GF, Hayhoe FGJ (1980a). A chronic lymphoproliferative disorder with distinctive features: a distinct variant of hairy cell leukaemia. *Leukaemia Research*, **4**:547.

Cawley JC, Burns GF, Hayhoe FGJ (1980b). *Hairy cell leukaemia*. Springer-Verlag, New York.

Chan HSL, Estrov Z, Weitzman SS, Freedman SH (1987). The value of intensive combination chemotherapy for juvenile chronic myelogenous leukaemia. *Journal of Clinical Oncology*, **5**:1960.

Cheson BD, *et al.* (1988). Guidelines for clinical protocols for chronic lymphocytic leukaemia (CLL). Recommendations of the NCI-sponsored working group. *American Journal of Hematology*, **29**:152–63.

Clark SS, McLaughlin J, Crist WM, Champlin R, Witte ON (1987). Unique forms of the abl tyrosine kinase distinguish Ph¹-positive CML from Ph¹-positive ALL. *Science*, **235**:85–8.

Clift RA, Applebaum FR, Thomas ED (1993). Treatment of chronic myeloid leukaemia by bone marrow transplantation. *Blood*, **82**:1954–6.

Cortellazo S, Viero P, Finazzi G, D'Emilio A, Rodeghiero F, Barbui T (1990). Incidence and risk factors of thrombotic complications in a historical cohort of 100 patients with essential thrombocythaemia. *Journal of Clinical Oncology*, **8**:556–61.

Coulombel L, Kalousek DK, Eaves CJ, Gupta CM, Eaves AC (1983). Long term marrow culture reveals chromosomally normal haemopoietic progenitor cells in patients with Philadelphia chromosome-positive chronic myelogenous leukaemia. *New England Journal of Medicine*, **308**:1493–8.

Cross NCP, *et al.* (1993a). Minimal residual disease after allogeneic bone marrow transplantation for chronic myeloid leukaemia in first chronic phase: correlations with acute graft-versus-host disease and relapse. *British Journal of Haematology*, **84**:67–74.

Cross NCP, Lin F, Chase A, Bungey J, Hughes TP, Goldman JM (1993b). Competitive polymerase chain reaction to estimate the number of BCR–ABL transcripts in chronic myeloid leukaemia patients after bone marrow transplantation. *Blood*, **82**:1929–36.

Cunningham I, *et al.* (1979). Results of treatment of Ph¹ positive chronic myelogenous leukaemia with an intensive treatment regimen (L-5 protocol). *Blood*, **53**:375–93.

Daley GQ, Van Etten RA, Baltimore D (1990). Induction of chronic myelogenous leukaemia by the p210 *bcr/abl* gene of the Philadelphia chromosome. *Science*, **247**:824.

da Silva MAP, Heerema N, Schwenk GR Jr, Hoffman R (1988). Evidence for the clonal nature of hypereosinophilic syndrome. *Cancer Genetics and Cytogenetics*, 32:109–15.

Denegri JF, *et al.* (1978). *In vitro* growth of basophils containing the Philadelphia chromosome in the acute phase of chronic myelogenous leukaemia. *British Journal of Haematology*, 40:351–5.

Dighiero G (1993). Biology of the neoplastic lymphocyte in B-CLL. *Bailliere's Clinical Haematology*, 6:807–20.

Dokal I, Jones L, Deenamonde M, Lewis SM, Goldman JM (1989). Allogeneic bone marrow transplantation for primary myelofibrosis. *British Journal of Haematology*, 71:158–9.

Dreazen O, Berman M, Gale RG (1988). Molecular abnormalities of bcr and c-abl in chronic myelogenous leukaemia associated with a long chronic phase. *Blood*, 71:797–9.

Estrov Z, Grunberger T, Chan HSL, Freedman MH (1986). Juvenile chronic myelogenous leukaemia: characteristics of the disease using cultures. *Blood*, 67:1382.

Fialkow PJ, Jacobson RJ, Papayannopolou T (1977). Chronic myelocytic leukaemia. Clonal origin in a stem cell common to the granulocyte, erythrocyte, platelet and monocyte/macrophage. *American Journal of Medicine*, 63:125–30.

Foa R, Matutes E, Brito-Babapulle V, *et al.* (1988). T-cell chronic lymphocytic leukaemia. A proliferation of large granular lymphocytes. Immunological, clinical, ultrastructural and molecular studies. In *Chronic lymphocytic leukaemia* (ed. A Polliack and D Catovsky). Harwood, Chur.

Freedman AS, Nadler LM (1987). B cell development in chronic lymphocytic leukaemia. *Seminars in Hematology*, 24:230–9.

Freedman MH, Estrov Z, Chan HSL (1988). Juvenile chronic myelogenous leukaemia. *American Journal of Pediatric Hematology and Oncology*, 10:261–7.

French Co-operative Group in Chronic Lymphocytic Leukaemia (1986). Effect of CHOP regimen in advanced untreated chronic lymphocytic leukaemia. *Lancet*, i:1346–9.

French Co-operative Group on Chronic Lymphocytic Leukaemia (1989). Long-term results of the CHOP regimen in stage C chronic lymphocytic leukaemia. *British Journal of Haematology*, 73:334–40.

Gale RP, Goldman JM (1988). Rapid progress in chronic myelogenous leukaemia. *Leukaemia*, 2:321–4.

Gale RP, Montserrat E (1993). Intensive therapy of chronic lymphocytic leukaemia. *Bailliere's Clinical Haematology*, 6:879–85.

Gallo RC, *et al.* (1983). Association of the human type C retrovirus with a subset of adult T-cell cancers. *Cancer Research*, 43:3892–9.

Galton DAG (1953). Myeleran in chronic leukaemia. *Lancet*, i:208–13.

Galvani DW, Cawley JC (1989). Mechanism of action of α interferon in chronic granulocytic leukaemia: evidence for preferential inhibition of late progenitors. *British Journal of Haematology*, 73:475–9.

Giles FJ, *et al.* (1988). Alpha-interferon therapy for essential thrombocythaemia. *Lancet*, ii:71–3.

Golde DW, *et al.* (1977). The Philadelphia chromosome in human macrophages. *Blood*, 46:367–71.

Goldman JM, *et al.* (1986). Bone marrow transplantation for patients with chronic myeloid leukaemia. *New England Journal of Medicine*, 314:202–8.

Goldman JM, *et al.* (1988). Bone marrow transplantation for chronic myelogenous leukaemia in chronic phase. *Annals of Internal Medicine*, 108:806–14.

Goldman JM, Grosveld G, Baltimore D, Gale RP (1990). Chronic myelogenous leukaemia—the unfolding saga. *Leukaemia*, 4:163–9.

Goldman JM, *et al.* (1993). Choice of pretransplant treatment and timing of transplants for chronic myelogenous leukaemia in chronic phase. *Blood*, 82:2235–8.

Golomb HM (1987). The treatment of hairy cell leukaemia. *Blood*, 69:979–83.

Golomb HM, Ratain MJ (1987). Recent advances in the treatment of hairy cell leukaemia. *New England Journal of Medicine*, 316:870–1.

Golomb HM, Catvosky D, Golde DW (1978). Hairy cell leukaemia. A clinical review based on 71 cases. *Annals of Internal Medicine*, 89:677.

Groffen J, *et al.* (1984). Philadelphia chromosomal breakpoints are clustered within a limited region, bcr, on chromosome 22. *Cell*, 36:93–9.

Gunz FW (1983). Ionising radiation and human leukaemia. In *Leukaemia* (4th edn) (ed. W Gunz and ES Henderson), pp. 359–74. Grune and Stratton, New York.

Hagemeijer A (1987). Chromosomal abnormalities in CML. *Clinical Haematology*, 1:963–81.

Haines ME, *et al.* (1984). Chemotherapy and autografting for patients with chronic granulocytic leukaemia in transformation: probable prolongation of life in some patients. *British Journal of Haematology*, 58:711–12.

Han T, *et al.* (1984). The prognostic importance of cytogenetic abnormalities in patients with chronic lymphocytic leukaemia. *New England Journal of Medicine*, 310:288–92.

Hasselbach H (1988). Interferon in myelofibrosis. *Lancet*, i:355.

Hehlman R, *et al.* (1993). Randomised comparison of busulphan and hydroxyurea in chronic myelogenous leukaemia: prolongation of survival by hydroxyurea. *Blood*, 82:398–407.

Heim A, Mitelman F (1986). Chromosome abnormalities in the myelodysplastic syndromes. *Clinics in Haematology*, 15:1003–22.

Ho AD, *et al.* (1988). Clinical response to deoxycoformycin in chronic lymphoid neoplasms and biochemical changes in circulating malignant cells *in vivo*. *Blood*, 72:1884–90.

Hoyle C, Gray R, Goldman JM (1994). Autografting for patients with CML in chronic phase: an update. *British Journal of Haematology*, 86:76–81.

Hunter T, Cooper JA (1985). Protein-tyrosine kinase. *Annual Reviews in Biochemistry*, 54:897–930.

Hunter T, Gould K, Cooper JA (1984). Tyrosine protein kinases, viral transformation and the control of cell proliferation. *Biochemical Society Transactions*, 12:757–9.

International Workshop on Chronic Lymphocytic Leukaemia (1989). Recommendations for diagnosis, staging and response criteria. *Annals of Internal Medicine*, 110:236–8.

Italian Cooperative Study Group on Chronic Myeloid Leukaemia (1988). Prospective confirmation of a prognostic classification for Ph+ chronic myeloid leukaemia. *British Journal of Haematology*, 69:463–6.

Jacobson RS, Salo A, Fialkow PS (1978). Agnogenic myeloid metaplasia: a clonal proliferation of hemopoietic stem cells with secondary myelofibrosis. *Blood*, 51:189–94.

Jacksic B, Brugiatelli M, for the IGCI (Vienna) Chronic Lymphocytic Leukaemia Study Group (1990). High dose chlorambucil for the treatment of advanced B-chronic lymphocytic leukaemia. Results of two multicentric randomised trials. *Blood*, 76 (Suppl.):284 (abstract).

Jansen J (1987). Hairy cell leukaemia. *Critical Reviews in Oncology and Haematology*, 7:183–217.

Juliusson G, Gahrton G (1993). Cytogenetics in CLL and related disorders. *Bailliere's Clinical Haematology*, 6:821–48.

Juliusson G, *et al.* (1990). Prognostic subgroups in B-cell chronic lymphocytic leukaemia defined by specific chromosomal abnormalities. *New England Journal of Medicine*, 323:720–4.

Juliusson G, Elmhorn-Rosenborg A, Lillemark J (1992). Response to 2-chlorodeoxyadenosine in patients with B-cell chronic lymphocytic leukaemia resistant to fludarabine. *New England Journal of Medicine*, 327:1056–61.

Kantarjian HM, *et al.* (1985). Intensive chemotherapy (ROAP 10) and splenectomy in patients with Philadelphia positive chronic myelogenous leukaemia. *Journal of Clinical Oncology*, 3:192–200.

Kantarjian HM, *et al.* (1987). Chronic myelogenous leukaemia in blast crisis. Analysis of 242 patients. *American Journal of Medicine*, 83:445–54.

Kantarjian HM, *et al.* (1992). Treatment of advanced stages of Ph-positive chronic myelogenous leukaemia with interferon and low dose cytarabine. *Journal of Clinical Oncology*, 10:772–8.

Kantarjian HM, Deisseroth A, Kurzrock R, Estrov Z, Talpaz M (1993). Chronic myelogenous leukaemia: a concise update. *Blood*, 82:691–703.

Kaplan ME, Mack K, Goldberg JD, Donovan PB, Berk PD, Wasserman LR (1986). Long-term management of polycythaemia vera with hydroxyurea: a progress report. *Seminars in Hematology*, 23:161–71.

Keating MJ (1990). Fludarabine phosphate in the treatment of chronic lymphocytic leukaemia. *Seminars in Oncology*, 17 (Suppl. 8):49–62.

Keating MJ, Kantarjian H, O'Brien S, Robertson L, Huh Y (1991). New agents and strategies in chronic lymphocytic leukaemia. *Leukaemia and Lymphoma*, Suppl.:139–47.

Kelliher M, Knott A, McLaughlin J, Witte ON, Rosenberg N (1991). Differences in oncogenic potency but not target cell specificity distinguish the two forms of the BCR/ABL oncogene. *Molecular and Cellular Biology*, 11:4710–16.

Koeffler HP, et al. (1980). Chronic myelocytic leukaemia: eosinophils involved in the malignant clone. Blood, 55:1063–8.

Koller CA, Miller DM (1986). Preliminary observations in the therapy of myeloid blast phase of chronic granulocytic leukaemia with plicamycin and hydroxyurea. New England Journal of Medicine, 315:1433–8.

Kondo T, et al. (1989). Age and sex specific cumulative rate and risk of ATLL for HTLV-I carriers. International Journal of Cancer, 43:1061–4.

Konopka JB, Watanabe SM, Witte ON (1984). An alteration of the human c-abl protein in K562 leukaemia cells unmasks associated tyrosine kinase activity. Cell, 37:1035–42.

Korsmeyer SJ, Greene WC, Waldmann TA (1983). Rearrangement and expression of immunoglobulin genes and expression of Tac antigen in hairy cell leukaemia. Proceedings of the National Academy of Sciences USA, 80:4522.

Kurzrock R, et al. (1987a). Molecular analysis of chromosome 22 breakpoints in adult Philadelphia positive acute lymphoblastic leukaemia. British Journal of Haematology, 67:55–9.

Kurzrock R, Shtalrid M, Talpaz M, Kloetzer WS, Gutterman JU (1987b). Expression of c-abl in Philadelphia-positive acute myelogenous leukaemia. Blood, 70:1584–8.

Kurzrock R, Gutterman JU, Talpaz M (1988). The molecular genetics of Philadelphia chromosome positive leukaemias. New England Journal of Medicine, 319:990–8.

Laver J, Kushner BH, Steinherz PG (1987). Juvenile chronic myeloid leukaemia: therapeutic insights. Leukaemia, 1:730–3.

Lazzarino M, et al. (1990). Therapy of essential thrombocythaemia with alpha-interferon. European Journal of Haematology, 45 (Suppl. 52):15–20.

Lee MS, et al. (1992). Detection of minimal residual disease by polymerase chain reaction in Ph-positive chronic myelogenous leukaemia following interferon therapy. Blood, 79:1920–3.

Litz CE, Brunning RD (1993). Chronic lymphoproliferative disorders: classification and diagnosis. Bailliere's Clinical Haematology, 6:767–83.

Liu Y, et al. (1992). Retinoblastoma gene deletions in B-cell chronic lymphocytic leukaemia. Genes, Chromosomes and Cancer, 4:250–6.

McGlave PB (1992). Therapy of chronic myelogenous leukaemia with related or unrelated donor BMT. Leukaemia, 6 (Suppl. 4):115–17.

McGlave PB, et al. (1993). Unrelated donor marrow transplantation therapy for chronic myelogenous leukaemia: initial experience of the national donor program. Blood, 81:543–50.

McIntyre K, Hoagland HC, Silverstein MN, Petitt RM (1991). Essential thrombocythaemia in adults. Mayo Clinic Proceedings, 66:149–53.

Mahon F-X, et al. (1992). Polymerase chain reaction detection of residual disease in chronic myeloid leukaemia patients in complete cytogenetic remission under interferon with or without chemotherapy. Leukaemia, 6:1232–4.

Manoharan A (1988). Myelofibrosis: prognostic factors and treatment. British Journal of Haematology, 69:295–8.

Martin PJ, et al. (1980). Involvement of the B-lymphoid system in chronic myelogenous leukaemia. Nature, London, 287:49–50.

Matutes E, et al. (1991). Clinical and laboratory features of 78 cases of T-prolymphocytic leukaemia. Blood, 78:3269–74.

Medical Research Council Working Party for Therapeutic Trials in Leukaemia (1968). Chronic granulocytic leukaemia: comparison of radiotherapy and busulphan therapy. British Medical Journal, 1:201–8.

Medical Research Council Working Party for Therapeutic Trials in Leukaemia (1983). Randomised trial of splenectomy in Ph^1 positive chronic granulocytic leukaemia, including an analysis of prognostic factors. British Journal of Haematology, 54:415–20.

Melo JV, Catvosky D, Galton DAG (1986a). The relationship between chronic lymphocytic leukaemia and prolymphocytic leukaemia I: clinical and laboratory features of 300 patients and characterisation of an intermediate group. British Journal of Haematology, 63:377–87.

Melo JV, Catovsky D, Galton DAG (1986b). The relationship between chronic lymphocytic leukaemia and prolymphocytic leukaemia II: patterns of evolution of 'prolymphocytoid' transformation. British Journal of Haematology, 64:77–86.

Melo JV, Hegde U, Parreira A, Thompson I, Lambert IA, Catovsky D (1987). Splenic B-cell lymphoma with circulating villous lymphocytes: differential diagnosis of B-cell leukaemia with a large spleen. Journal of Clinical Pathology, 40:642–51.

Melo JV, Robinson DSF, Catovsky D (1988). The differential diagnosis between chronic lymphatic leukaemia and other B-cell lymphoproliferative disorders. In Chronic lymphocytic leukaemia (ed. A Polliack and D Catovsky). Harwood, Chur.

Miller JB, Testa JR, Lindgren V, Rowley JD (1985). The pattern and clinical significance of karyotypic abnormalities in patients with idiopathic and postpolycythaemic myelofibrosis. Cancer, 55:582–91.

Mills KI, Benn P, Birnie GD (1991). Does the breakpoint within the major breakpoint cluster region (M-bcr) influence the duration of the chronic phase in chronic myeloid leukaemia? An analytic comparison of current literature. Blood, 78:1155–61.

Mizoguchi M, Kawa Y, Minami T, Nakayama H, Mizoguchi H (1990). Cutaneous extramedullary haematopoiesis in myelofibrosis. Journal of the American Academy of Dermatology, 22:351–5.

Montserrat E, Rozman C (1993a). Chronic lymphocytic leukaemia: prognostic factors and natural history. Bailliere's Clinical Haematology, 6:849–66.

Montserrat E, Rozman C (1993b). Chronic lymphocytic leukaemia: treatment. Blood Reviews, 7:164–75.

Morris CM, Reeve AE, Fitzgerald PH, Hollings PE, Beard ME, Heaton DC (1986). Genomic diversity correlates with clinical variation in Ph1-negative chronic myeloid leukaemia. Nature, London, 320:281–3.

Mufti GJ, Stevens JR, Oscier DB, Hamblin TJ, Machin D (1985). Myelodysplastic syndromes: a scoring system with prognostic significance. British Journal of Haematology, 59:425–33.

Murphy S, Ilano H, Rosenthal D, Laszlo J (1986). Essential thrombocythaemia: an interim report for the Polycythaemia Vera Study Group. Seminars in Hematology, 23:177–82.

Nowell PC, Hungerford DA (1960). A minute chromsome in human chronic granulocytic leukaemia. Science, 132:1497.

Nowell PC, Jackson L, Weiss A, Kurzrock R (1988). Historical communication: Philadelphia positive chronic myelogenous leukaemia followed for 27 years. Cancer Genetics and Cytogenetics, 34:57–61.

O'Brien S, et al. (1993). Homoharringtonine induces apoptosis in chronic myelogenous leukaemia cells. Blood, 82 (Suppl. 1), 555 (abstract).

Oguma N, et al. (1992). Molecular elimination of minimal residual Ph^1 clone in chronic myelogenous leukaemia. Lancet, 339:557.

Oladipupo-Williams CK, et al. (1981). Inhibitory effects of human leucocyte and fibroblast interferons on normal and CML granulocyte progenitor cells. Oncology, 38:356–60.

Oscier DG, Fitchett M, Herbert T, Lambert R (1991). Karyotypic evolution in B-cell chronic lymphocytic leukaemia. Genes, Chromosomes and Cancer, 3:16–20.

Ozer H, et al. (1993). Prolonged subcutaneous administration of recombinant α-2b interferon in patients with previously untreated Ph-positive chronic myelogenous leukaemia: effect on remission duration and survival. Blood, 82:2975–84.

Pangalis GA, et al. (1991). Hairy cell leukaemia: splenectomy after alpha-2b interferon. Blood, 78:1385.

Pelus LM, et al. (1980). Abnormal responsiveness of granulocyte-macrophage committed colony-forming cells from patients with chronic myeloid leukaemia to inhibition by prostaglandin E. Cancer Research, 40:2512–19.

Pierce JH, Eva A, Aaronson SA (1986). Interactions of oncogenes with haemopoietic cells. Clinics in Haematology, 15:573–96.

Piro LD, Carrera CJ, Beutler E, Carson DA (1988). Chlorodeoxyadenosine: an effective new agent for the treatment of chronic lymphocytic leukaemia. Blood, 72:1069–73.

Platanias LC, Golomb HM (1993). Hairy cell leukaemia. Bailliere's Clinical Haematology, 6:887–98.

Platanias LC, Ratain MJ (1992). Hairy cell leukaemia. In Current therapy in haematology–oncology (ed. P Carbone and M Brain), pp. 73–9. BC Decker, Philadelphia.

Plunkett W, Gandhi V (1993). Cellular metabolism of nucleoside analogues in CLL: implications for drug development. In Chronic lymphocytic leukaemia: scientific advances and clinical developments (ed. BD Cheson), pp. 197–219. Marcel Decker, New York.

Quesada JR, et al. (1984). Alpha interferon for induction of remission in hairy cell leukaemia. New England Journal of Medicine, 310:15.

Rabinow SN, Grossbard ML, Nadler LM (1993). Innovative treatment strategies for chronic lymphocytic leukaemia: monoclonal antibodies, immunoconjugates and bone marrow transplantation. In *Chronic lymphocytic leukaemia: scientific advances and clinical developments* (ed. BD Cheson), pp. 337–67. Marcel Dekker, New York.

Rai KR (1987). A critical analysis of staging in CLL. In *Chronic lymphocytic leukaemia: recent progress and future directions* (ed. RP Gale and KR Rai), pp. 253–64. Alan R. Liss, New York.

Rai KR, *et al.* (1975). Clinical staging of chronic lymphocytic leukaemia. *Blood*, 46:219–34.

Ribera JM, Cervantes F, Rozman C (1987). A multivariate analysis of prognostic factors in chronic myelomonocytic leukaemia. *British Journal of Haematology*, 65:307–11.

Rickles FR, Miller DR (1972). Eosinophilic leukaemoid reaction: report of a case, its relationship to eosinophilic leukaemia and review of the literature. *Journal of Pediatrics*, 80:418–28.

Rodenhuis S, Smets LA, Slater RM, Behrendt H, Verman AJ (1985). Distinguishing the Philadelphia chromosome of acute lymphoblastic leukaemia from its counterpart in chronic myelogenous leukaemia. *New England Journal of Medicine*, 313:51–2.

Rosenblum MG, Maxwell BL, Talpaz M, Kelleher PJ, McCredie KB, Gutterman JU (1986). *In vivo* sensitivity and resistance of chronic myeloid leukaemia cells to α-interferon: correlation with receptor binding and induction of 2',5'-oligoadenylate synthetase. *Cancer Research*, 46:4848–52.

Rowley JD (1973). A new consistent chromosomal abnormality in chronic myelogenous leukaemia identified by quinacrine fluorescence and Giemsa staining. *Nature, London*, 243:290–91.

Rozman C, *et al.* (1984). Bone marrow pattern—the best single prognostic parameter in chronic lymphocytic leukaemia: a multivariate analysis of 329 cases. *Blood*, 64:642–8.

Rozman C, *et al.* (1988). Recombinant alpha-interferon in the treatment of B chronic lymphocytic leukaemia in early stages. *Blood*, 71:1295–8.

Rushing D, Goldman A, Gibbs G, Howe R, Kennedy BJ (1982). Hydroxyurea versus busulphan in the treatment of chronic myelogenous leukaemia. *American Journal of Clinical Oncology*, 5:307–13.

Sainati L, *et al.* (1990). A variant form of hairy cell leukaemia resistant to α-interferon: clinical and phenotypic characteristics of 17 patients. *Blood*, 76:157–62.

Sanders JE, *et al.* (1988). Allogeneic marrow transplantation for children with juvenile chronic myelogenous leukaemia. *Blood*, 71:1144–6.

Saven A, Piro LD (1992). Treatment of hairy cell leukaemia. *Blood*, 79:1111–20.

Schaefer-Rego K, *et al.* (1987). Chronic myeloid leukaemia patients in blast crisis have breakpoints localised to a specific region in the bcr. *Blood*, 70:448–55.

Sharp JC, *et al.* (1979). Karyotypic conversion in Ph' positive chronic myeloid leukaemia with combination chemotherapy. *Lancet*, i:1370–2.

Shtivelman E, Lifshitz B, Gale RP, Canaani E (1985). Fused transcripts of abl and bcr genes in chronic myelogenous leukaemia. *Nature, London*, 315:550–4.

Silverstein MN (1976). The evolution into and the treatment of late stage polycythaemia vera. *Seminars in Hematology*, 13:79–84.

Singer CRJ, Douglas AS, McDonald GA (1984). Twenty-five year survival of chronic granulocytic leukaemia with spontaneous karyotype conversion. *British Journal of Haematology*, 57:309–13.

Singer JW, *et al.* (1980). Restoration of nonclonal hematopoiesis in chronic myelogenous leukaemia (CML) following a chemotherapy induced loss of the Ph' chromosome. *Blood*, 56:356–60.

Sokal JE, *et al.* (1984). Prognostic discrimination in 'good risk' chronic granulocytic leukaemia. *Blood*, 63:789–99.

Sokal JE, *et al.* (1985). Prognostic discrimination amongst younger patients with chronic granulocytic leukaemia: relevance to bone marrow transplantation. *Blood*, 66:1352–7.

Spiers ASD, Bain BJ, Turner JE (1977). The peripheral blood in chronic granulocytic leukaemia: study of 50 untreated Philadelphia positive cases. *Scandinavian Journal of Haematology*, 18:25–38.

Spiers ASD, Parekh SJ, Bishop MB (1984). Hairy cell leukaemia: induction of complete remission with pentostatin (2'-deoxycoformycin). *Journal of Clinical Oncology*, 2:1336–42.

Takatsuki K, *et al.* (1977). Adult T-cell leukaemia in Japan. In *Topics in haematology* (ed. S Seno, F Takaku, S Imino), pp. 73–7. Excerpta Medica, Amsterdam.

Talpaz M, Kantarjian HM, McCredie K, Trujillo JM, Keating MJ, Gutterman J (1986). Hematologic remission and cytogenetic improvement induced by recombinant human interferon alpha A in chronic myelogenous leukemia. *New England Journal of Medicine*, 314:1065–9.

Talpaz M, Kantarjian HM, McCredie K, Keating MJ, Trujillo JM, Gutterman J (1987). Clinical investigation of human alpha interferon in chronic myelogenous leukaemia. *Blood*, 69:1280–8.

Talpaz M, Kantarjian HM, Kurzrock R, Gutterman J (1988). Therapy of chronic myeloid leukaemia: chemotherapy and interferons. *Seminars in Hematology*, 25:62–75.

Talpaz M, Kantarjian HM, Kurzrock R, Trujillo JM, Gutterman JU (1991). Interferon-α produces sustained cytogenetic responses in chronic myelogenous leukaemia. *Annals of Internal Medicine*, 114:532–8.

Tanaka T, Craig AW (1970). Cell-free transmission of murine myeloid leukaemia. *European Journal of Cancer*, 6:329–33.

Thomas ED, Clift RA (1989). Indications for marrow transplantation in chronic myelogenous leukaemia. *Blood*, 73:861–4.

Thomas ED, *et al.* (1986). Marrow transplantation for the treatment of chronic myelogenous leukaemia. *Annals of Internal Medicine*, 104:155–63.

Tsujimoto Y, Jaffe E, Cossman J, Gorham J, Nowell PC, Croce CM (1985). Clustering of breakpoint on chromosome 11 in human B cell neoplasm with the t(11,14) chromosome translocation. *Nature, London*, 315:340.

Tura S, *et al.* (1981). Staging of chronic myeloid leukaemia. *British Journal of Haematology*, 47:105–19.

Volk JR, *et al.* (1983). T-cell prolymphocytic leukaemia: clinical and immunological characterisation. *Cancer*, 52:2049–54.

Wagner JE, *et al.* (1992). Bone marrow transplantation of chronic myelogenous leukaemia in chronic phase: evaluation of risks and benefits. *Journal of Clinical Oncology*, 10:779–89.

Walters RS, *et al.* (1987). Therapy of lymphoid and undifferentiated chronic myelogenous leukaemia in blast crisis with continuous vincristine and adriamycin infusions plus high dose decadron. *Cancer*, 60:1708–12.

Watanabe T, *et al.* (1990). Constitutive expression of parathyroid hormone-related protein (PTHrP) gene in HTLV-I carriers and adult T-cell leukaemia patients which can be transactivated by HTLV-I tax gene. *Journal of Experimental Medicine*, 172:759–65.

Weinstein IM (1991). Idiopathic myelofibrosis: historical review, diagnosis and management. *Blood Reviews*, 5:98–104.

Wiedemann LM, *et al.* (1988). The correlation of breakpoint cluster region rearrangement and p210 phl/abl expression with morphological analysis of Ph-negative chronic myeloid leukaemia and other myeloproliferative diseases. *Blood*, 71:349–55.

Worsley A, *et al.* (1988). Prognostic features of chronic myelomonocytic leukaemia: a modified Bournemouth score gives the best prediction of survival. *British Journal of Haematology*, 68:17–21.

Yamaguchi K, Takatsuki K (1993). Adult T-cell leukaemia–lymphoma. *Bailliere's Clinical Haematology*, 6:899–915.

You W, Weisbrot W (1979). Chronic neutrophilic leukaemia: report of two cases and review of the literature. *American Journal of Clinical Pathology*, 72:233–42.

Young JL, Percy CL, Asire AJ (1981). Cancer incidence and mortality in the United States, 1973–1977. In *Surveillance, epidemiology and end results program*, National Cancer Institute Monograph No. 57, p. 1082. National Cancer Institute, Washington, DC.

12.4 Bone-marrow transplantation for leukaemia

SAM MILLIKEN AND RAY POWLES

GENERAL BACKGROUND

Bone-marrow can be aspirated from the pelvic bones of a donor using a wide-based needle. If infused intravenously into a recipient, it will colonize the marrow space and, under the right circumstances, a donation of as little as 2 per cent of marrow will repopulate the recipient fully in 3–6 weeks. The donor can be an identical twin (syngeneic), a donor other than a twin (allogeneic), or the patient him/herself (autologous). For allogeneic bone-marrow transplantation some degree of tissue antigen matching is crucial and the human leucocyte antigen (HLA) system is the key to this end. The bone-marrow and immune system often recognizes organs in the host as foreign, producing an attack by the graft against the host. This graft-versus-host disease can be modified by using immunosuppressive agents and within 1 year successfully grafted patients are invariably off all treatment. The most suitable allogeneic donors are fully matched siblings.

The most attractive direction for bone-marrow transplantation for the treatment of leukaemia is autografting. It can be given to all patients, the age range can be extended, and it may even be applicable to chronic granulocytic leukaemia (rendered partially Ph-negative by interferon). Growth factors may be used to reduce the length of time of bone-marrow failure, so that the length of time in hospital may be dramatically reduced. Ultimately, the use of growth factors may render bone-marrow transplantation itself redundant.

HISTORY

The therapeutic use of bone-marrow has occupied the efforts of clinicians for nearly a century, although marrow transplantation has only been possible within the past three decades. The history of bone-marrow transplantation has been extensively reviewed by Santos (1983). Brown-Séquard and d'Arsonaval are recorded to have administered marrow orally to patients with anaemia as early as 1891 (Quine 1986). The first use of viable bone-marrow has been attributed to Schretzenmayr in 1937 and Rasjok in 1939 who first injected marrow into the intramedullary space of patients with leukaemia (Santos 1983). The first successful bone-marrow transplant may have occurred in 1940, when Morrison and Samwick infused marrow from a sibling donor to a patient with aplastic anaemia who later recovered. In 1957 Thomas et al. demonstrated that a large volume of marrow could be infused safely and were able to achieve a transient engraftment in man. However, Mathe et al. (1959) were responsible for the first report of a series of patients undergoing marrow transplantation. They gave allogeneic marrow (marrow from a donor other than an identical twin) to four out of six victims of radiation overexposure and demonstrated short-term red cell engraftment in all four.

Mathe et al. (1963) were also the first to report long-term survival in a patient with leukaemia following bone-marrow transplantation. The patient died of viral encephalitis, but free of leukaemia, 20 months after the procedure. This group was also the first to characterize the clinical and pathological features of acute graft-versus-host disease (see below) as well as the susceptibility of these patients to life-threatening infections particularly due to viral and fungal pathogens (Mathe 1968; Mathe et al. 1974). In 1970 Thomas and colleagues in Seattle commenced allogeneic bone-marrow transplantation using HLA-matched sibling donors for end-stage patients with acute leukaemia and the clinical era of bone-marrow transplantation was established. For ethical reasons, these early studies were initially on end-stage patients with little hope of long-term survival. Transplant-related problems or recurrent leukaemia occurred in most patients and mortality was high. In 1977 this group published the results of the first 100 patients treated for acute leukaemia, with 13 long-term survivors (Thomas et al. 1977). By the middle of the decade, bone-marrow transplantation for patients in remission had commenced and markedly improved survival rates were noted.

THE HUMAN HISTOCOMPATIBILITY SYSTEM

In the 1960s, the success of syngeneic (identical-twin) bone-marrow transplantation for patients with aplastic anaemia (Robins and Noyes 1961) could not be duplicated for patients with active leukaemia (Thomas et al. 1959, 1961, 1975), with relapse of leukaemia despite temporary engraftment being a universal finding. It was not until the human leucocyte antigen (HLA) system was delineated that bone-marrow transplantation became a viable therapy for acute leukaemia. The description of the first HLA antigen was published in 1958 by Dausset. Subsequently a number of workers in what was a major international collaborative effort were able by 1968 to establish a reliable system of nomenclature and testing that included the HLA-A and HLA-B loci on chromosome 6, as well as the mixed lymphocyte culture (Santos 1983). By 1980 the HLA-C and HLA-D loci were also serologically defined (Dupont 1980). By the early 1970s it was possible to select logically a 'suitable' donor for allogeneic bone-marrow transplantation.

These four HLA loci have been found to be linked closely on the short arm of chromosome 6 and, within the immediate family, could be used to identify the chromosome haplotype. Each individual possesses two haplotypes inherited individually from each parent. Consequently, as long as a patient possesses siblings, he or she has a one in four chance of having an HLA-identical donor. The demonstration of these antigens and the realization of their rôle in the immune recognition of 'self' and 'non-self' removed a major stumbling block to the successful progress of bone-marrow transplantation. Currently, over 100 alleles for class I (HLA A, B, and C) and class II (HLA-DR and DP) antigens have been described (Table 1). New class I genes HLA-E, p5.4 and p6.0 and a number of new minor histocompatibility antigens (minor H antigens) have been described (Kaminski 1989). Their rôle in transplantation is currently under scrutiny. Because graft-versus-host disease usually occurs in the majority of patients receiving HLA 'matched' sibling marrow (see below) it is clear that genes on chromosome(s) other than chromosome 6 are involved in immunological function.

Table 1 Complete listing of recognized HLA specificities

A	B	C	D	DR	DQ	DP
A1	B5	Cw1	Dw1	DR1	DQ1	DPw1
A2	B7	Cw2	Dw2	DR103	DQ2	DPw2
A203	B703	Cw3	Dw3	DR2	DQ3	DPw3
A210	B8	Cw4	Dw4	DR3	DQ4	DPw4
A3	B12	Cw5	Dw5	DR4	DQ5(1)	DPw5
A9	B13	Cw6	Dw6	DR5	DQ6(1)	DPw6
A10	B14	Cw7	Dw7	DR6	DQ7(3)	
A11	B15	Cw8	Dw8	DR7	DQ8(3)	
A19	B16	Cw9(w3)	Dw9	DR8	DQ9(3)	
A23(9)	B17	Cw10(w3)	Dw10	DR9		
A24	B18		Dw11(w7)	DR10		
A403	B21		Dw12	DR11(5)		
A25(10)	B22		Dw13	DR12(5)		
A26(10)	B27		Dw14	DR13(6)		
A28	B35		Dw15	DR14(6)		
A29(19)	B37		Dw16	DR1403		
A30(19)	B38(16)		Dw17(w7)	DR1404		
A31(19)	B39(16)		Dw18(w6)	DR15(2)		
A32(19)	B3901		Dw19(w6)	DR16(2)		
A33(19)	B3902		Dw20	DR17(3)		
A34(10)	B40		Dw21	DR18(3)		
A36	B4005		Dw22			
A43	B41		Dw23	DR51		
A66(10)	B42					
A68(28)	B44(12)		Dw24	DR52		
A69(28)	B45(12)		Dw25			
A74(19)	B46		Dw26	DR53		
	B47					
	B48					
	B49(21)					
	B50(21)					
	B51(5)					
	B5102					
	B5103					
	B52(5)					
	B53					
	B54(22)					
	B55(22)					
	B56(22)					
	B57(17)					
	B58(17)					
	B59					
	B60(40)					
	B61(40)					
	B62(15)					
	B63(15)					
	B64(14)					
	B65(14)					
	B67					
	B70					
	B71(70)					
	B72(70)					
	B73					
	B75(15)					
	B76(15)					
	B77(15)					
	B7801					
	Bw4					
	B46					

CONSIDERATIONS PRIOR TO BONE-MARROW TRANSPLANTATION

Preparation of the patient recipient

Patient age is the major limiting factor to successful outcome in bone-marrow transplantation (Gale and Champlin 1986).

Transplantation mortality increases dramatically with increasing patient age, mainly because of a concurrent increase in the risk of transplant-related problems, particularly severe graft-versus-host disease. Long-term survival in acute myeloid leukaemia following allogeneic bone-marrow transplantation is 40 per cent for patients aged 30–50 years, compared to 75 per cent for patients less than 20 years of age (Gale and Champlin 1986). Most units do not accept patients over 50 years of age because of unacceptable mortality and morbidity in these patients.

The intensity of therapies involved in bone-marrow transplantation dictates that the patient must be as 'fit' as possible before the procedure. It is important to ascertain that the patient has normal or 'acceptable' cardiac, respiratory, hepatic, and renal function, and no evidence of infection prior to bone-marrow transplantation. Conditioning regimens may need to be altered to avoid specific toxicities, for example no total-body irradiation in patients who have already received local radiotherapy. As well as a thorough physical, the routine work-up before bone-marrow transplantation should include a chest radiograph, electrocardiogram, full blood count and serum biochemistry, and microbial cultures and serology. Satisfactory dental hygiene should be ensured and reinforced. A bone-marrow examination should be performed prior to bone-marrow transplantation to ensure that the patients' leukaemia has not relapsed or progressed. Ascertaining psychological well-being is as important as physical fitness. Patients should be carefully counselled and informed as to the nature of bone-marrow transplantation, its potential for success, and the risks of complications, before a decision is made to proceed with transplantation.

All bone-marrow transplantation patients will require blood product support, intravenous fluids, and antibiotics and many may require parenteral nutrition. Consequently, most units provide their patients with long-term central venous catheters, such as the Hickman or Broviac catheter (Andover et al. 1982). It is routine practice to insert these catheters electively under aseptic conditions 1 or 2 weeks prior to bone-marrow transplantation to ensure adequate healing. They are inserted through a skin tunnel on the chest wall into the subclavian vein and right atrium.

Patient preparation for autologous bone-marrow transplantation (the patient's own marrow) is almost identical to that for allogeneic bone-marrow transplantation. However, autologous bone-marrow transplantation may be offered to older patients as marrow rejection and graft-versus-host disease, do not occur, abrogating the need for prolonged immunosuppressive therapy and making the procedure much safer. Many units now accept fit patients in their sixties into their autologous bone-marrow transplantation programme. It is probably important that autologous marrow is disease-free prior to bone-marrow transplantation to ensure patients are not reseeded with leukaemia, although the possibility that tiny amounts of reseeded leukaemia may be eliminated by the patients has been a recent hypothesis. Unfortunately, the ability to detect minimal malignant disease in bone-marrow is poor and results of marrow 'purging' remain controversial.

Preparation of the donor

Adequate assessment of the bone-marrow donor before bone-marrow transplantation is essential to ensure his or her safety during a procedure that is not without risk. The need to harvest a significant volume of marrow via multiple bone aspirates requires general or spinal anaesthesia with its attendant risks. A detailed history and thorough physical examination are necessary to minimize this risk and a chest radiograph, full blood count, and serum chemistry should be done. When the bone-marrow is aspirated, it is diluted by the aspiration of up to 1 U of blood and so blood volume replacement is often necessary during or following harvest. The risk of blood transfusion to the donor may be abrogated by taking autologous blood 1–2 weeks prior to the procedure. Supplemental oral iron and folic acid therapy should be given to ensure prompt marrow and peripheral blood recovery following venesection and harvest. Because only approximately 2 per cent of the donor bone-marrow is removed, the donor is capable of replacing this loss within hours and there is no detectable loss of bone-marrow function.

Any potential risk to the patient recipient must be identified in the donor. The donor should be screened for evidence of past or current hepatitis B or C, cytomegalovirus, or human immunodeficiency virus. A positive serology for these infections may make the donor unsuitable or specific precautions necessary in the recipient. ABO blood group differences between donor and recipient do not prevent bone-marrow transplantation but the marrow harvest may require the removal of incompatible red cells or exchange transfusion of the recipient to remove antibodies and so prevent haemolytic reations. Where a choice of donor is available, identical sex and cytomegalovirus status with the recipient are beneficial.

It is essential to explain the procedure fully to the donor and to reassure him or her as to its safety and limited discomfort. It is also important to assess the reliability and commitment of the donor, as he or she may be needed to give further marrow or blood product support to the recipient.

BONE-MARROW COLLECTION

Between 500 and 1500 ml of blood and marrow are collected, with a nucleated cell count of between 1×10^8 and 3×10^8/kg of recipient weight. Multiple aspirates from the anterior and posterior iliac crests are usually adequate. Sternal aspiration may also be necessary. Infants and small children may be safely and easily used as donors because the cortex of their bones is thin and they are rich in marrow stem cells. However, special consideration must be given to their blood volume replacement. Intravenous heparin (3000–5000 iu) is usually given immediately before commencing collection. The procedure has a very low morbidity, usually consisting of transient pain and bleeding from the aspiration sites (Filshie et al. 1984). Stem cells may also be collected from a donor by leucopheresis (Juttner et al. 1985). However, as this requires multiple collections over 1 or 2 weeks and the best collections are obtained after a period of myelosuppression, this technique has been limited to autologous bone-marrow transplantation.

Harvested marrow is given to the recipient via intravenous infusion. After passing through the lungs implantation and growth occurs in the medullary cavities of bone, probably because the local microenvironment produces specific growth factors. In allogeneic bone-marrow transplantation the marrow may be given unmanipulated. However, red cell or plasma depletion may be necessary if ABO incompatibility is present. Also mature T lymphocyte depletion may also be undertaken to abrogate graft-versus-host disease. With autologous collections, various manipulative techniques may be employed in an effort to remove any residual malignant cells. Autologous bone-marrow may be cryopreserved in the presence of dimethyl sulphoxide and stored at −19°C in liquid nitrogen until the patient is ready for bone-marrow transplantation. In this situation the marrow should be red cell depleted to avoid haemolysis.

THE BONE-MARROW TRANSPLANTATION PROCEDURE
Conditioning

Leukaemic patients are generally immunologically competent and therefore able to reject donor marrow. Consequently, they require immunosuppression to prevent rejection, as well as antileukaemia therapy to reduce the risk of relapse. In practice, both of these requirements can be achieved using high doses of chemotherapy and/or total-body radiotherapy and is termed conditioning. Immunosuppressive agents such as cyclosporin, methotrexate, and corticosteroids are used after bone-marrow transplantation, mainly to ameliorate graft-versus-host disease but they will also help engraftment. The most commonly employed conditioning agent is cyclophosphamide, which was used initially as an immunosuppressive agent in bone-marrow transplantation for aplastic anaemia, in doses of 120–200 mg/kg of body weight (Storb et al. 1980). Although cyclophosphamide is a powerful suppressive agent, it is inadequate alone as an antileukaemic agent. However, the combination of cyclophosphamide with total-body irradiation, first described by the Seattle group (Thomas et al. 1977), is an effective regimen in bone-marrow transplantation for leukaemia and is still widely employed today. A total-body irradiation dose of approximately 10 Gy is necessary to achieve adequate immunosuppression and may be given as a single dose or as multiple fractions. Other commonly employed conditioning regimens are the combination of high-dose melphalan and total-body irradiation (Helenglass et al. 1987) and cyclophosphamide with busulphan without total-body irradiation (Santos et al. 1983). A vast number of regimens have been investigated in both allogeneic and autologous bone-marrow transplantation, with little attempt to compare their efficacy. It is beyond the scope of this work to discuss them all in detail.

Toxic effects of total-body irradiation

If total-body irradiation is given as a single fraction over approximately 3–4 h, then nausea and vomiting would inevitably occur. These problems can be controlled adequately with anti-emetics and steroids. The day following total-body irradiation, the patient no longer feels sick, but swelling and tenderness in the parotid glands occur and the skin becomes erythematous. During the next 1–2 weeks pain and soreness in the mouth and oesophagus occur and the irradiation produces some diarrhoea. The patient becomes severely neutropenic and requires antibiotics 5–6 days after total-body irradiation and platelet transfusions are required 2–3 days later. The other effects of total-body irradiation are discussed below.

Engraftment

Engraftment is signalled by an increase in granulocytes and platelets in the blood and the appearance of reticulocytes. Median times to granulocyte counts over 1×10^9/l are between 25 and 30 days, with normal counts seen by 40–50 days. Platelet counts usually follow by 7–14 days and the patient no longer requires red cell transfusions after 3 months. The reappearance of monocytes and tissue macrophages is also prompt and, as with the rest of the haematopoietic recovery, this is generally stable and entirely of donor origin (that is, the cells are chimeric). All cells derived from monocytes, such as osteoclasts, are also of donor origin. Although lymphocytes are of donor origin, functional immune impairments will persist while the patient receives immunosuppression to prevent graft-versus-host disease (Lum 1987). The majority of patients have profoundly impaired immunity for up to 6 months after bone-marrow transplantation; this may be prolonged indefinitely in some individuals in the presence of chronic graft-versus-host disease.

CONSIDERATIONS FOLLOWING BONE-MARROW TRANSPLANTATION

Graft-versus-host disease

As many as 70 per cent of patients undergoing allogeneic bone-marrow transplantation may develop a donor immunological reaction against the host (graft-versus-host disease) and 10–20 per cent of patients may die as a direct consequence of its severe manifestations. It is subclassified into acute and chronic forms on the basis of clinical features and onset of presentation. Although a major cause of morbidity and mortality in bone-marrow transplantation, evidence now strongly supports an antileukaemic effect for graft-versus-host disease (Weiden *et al.* 1981; Goldman *et al.* 1988; Pollard *et al.* 1988). Recipients of HLA-identical marrow who develop acute or chronic graft-versus-host disease have reduced relapse rates compared to similar patients who do not develop graft-versus-host disease. Therefore the diagnosis, treatment, and possible prevention of graft-versus-host disease has important implications to the final outcome of the patient and careful consideration must be given to overall benefits and dangers when treatment programmes are planned. One study attempting to utilize a graft-versus-leukaemia effect has been unsuccessful as increased mortality from graft-versus-host disease has abrogated any improvement due to reduced relapse rate (Sullivan *et al.* 1989). Animal studies suggest that a graft-versus-leukaemia effect may be achievable without significant graft-versus-host disease (Truitt *et al.* 1987) via manipulation of donor T lymphocyte subpopulations and/or the addition of lymphokines (Greenberg *et al.* 1981). These approaches are currently under investigation in man.

Acute graft-versus-host disease

Acute graft-versus-host disease usually occurs between 7 and 100 days after bone-marrow transplantation but is usually evident by 20 days. It is triggered by engrafted T lymphocytes which then create a local reaction against specific host tissues. The skin, gastrointestinal tract, and liver are the main organs involved (Table 2). Skin rash is usually the first manifestation with a faint, erythematous, maculopapular eruption on the extremities, which may progress to involve the entire body; it often involves the palms of the hands and soles of the feet. When severe it resembles burns, with blistering, ulceration, and exfoliation. When a rash develops, early skin biopsy is safe and helpful by excluding other diagnoses such as drug toxicity, herpes infections, or epidermal necrolysis and may give prognostic information as to the likely severity of graft-versus-host disease. Involvement of the gastrointestinal tract is characterized by diarrhoea, perhaps up to 10 l/day and usually having a 'mincemeat' appearance; that is, containing blood, mucus, and tissue. If the condition progresses, the diarrhoea becomes associated with abdominal pain, usually of a cramping or colic type, leading to ileus. There is some severe albumin loss with ascites and ultimately perforation and death. Hepatic involvement usually

Table 2 Grading of acute graft-versus-host disease

Skin
- Grade +1: a maculopapular eruption involving less than 25 per cent of the body surface
- Grade +2: a maculopapular eruption involving 25–50 per cent of the body surface
- Grade +3: generalized erythroderma
- Grade +4: generalized erythroderma with bullous formation and often with desquamation

Liver
- Grade +1: moderate increase of SGOT (150–750 IU) and bilirubin (2.0–2.9 mg/dl)
- Grade +2: bilirubin rise (3.0–5.9 mg/dl) with or without an increase in SGOT
- Grade +3: bilirubin rise (6.0–14.9 mg/dl) with or without an increase in SGOT
- Grade +4: bilirubin rise to >15 mg/dl with or without an increase in SGOT

Gut
- Grade +1: >30 ml/kg or >500 ml of stool/day or +biopsy for graft-versus-host disease
- Grade +2: >60 ml/kg or >1000 ml of stool/day
- Grade +3: >90 ml/kg or 1500 ml stool/day
- Grade +4: >90 ml/kg with abdominal pain or >2000 ml of stool/day

(Modified from Glucksberg *et al.* 1974)

Overall staging of acute graft-versus-host disease

Degree of organ involvement	Grade
Grade 1–2 skin rash with no liver or gut involvement and no clinical impairment	I (mild)
Grade 1–3 skin rash with grade 1 gut and/or liver involvement and mild clinical impairment or grade 3 skin only	II (moderate)
Grade 2–3 gut and/or liver involvement with or without grade 1–3 skin rash and marked clinical impairment	III (severe)
Grade 2–4 gut and/or liver involvement with or without grade 1–4 skin rash and extreme clinical impairment or grade 4 skin rash, and extreme clinical impairment or grade 4 skin with desquamation with or without gut or liver involvement and extreme clinical impairment	IV (life-threatening)

manifests later and is initially characterized by asymptomatic rises in serum bilirubin and alkaline phosphatase, due to a disappearance of bile canaliculi. Hepatocellular damage does not usually occur and the patients do not develop liver failure. Liver graft-versus-host disease may occur as an isolated problem with the serum bilirubin level rising to 1200–1400 μg/l, causing progressive coma, convulsions, and death. At autopsy the brain appears bright yellow due to the presence of bilirubin, which has crossed the blood–brain barrier. Graft-versus-host disease may be graded both clinically and histologically (Glucksberg *et al.* 1974) with prognostic significance (Table 2). Mortality rates for patients with moderate or severe graft-versus-host disease (grade II or greater) have been reported in excess of 50 per cent, compared to less than 10 per cent for patients with mild graft-versus-host disease. Risk factors for acute graft-versus-host disease include older patient age, female donor with male recipient, withholding immunoprophylaxis and co-trimoxazole prophylaxis, low performance status before bone-marrow transplantation, and a large number of transfusions after bone-marrow transplantation (Gale *et al.* 1989).

Management of acute graft-versus-host disease

The major emphasis in managing graft-versus-host disease has been prophylaxis using two entirely different strategies: the first has been the use of immunosuppressive agents given to the patient after bone-marrow transplantation to moderate immune function and the second has been the removal of mature T lymphocytes (and sometimes other cells) from the bone-marrow before it is given to the patient. Neither option is designed to immunosuppress the patient permanently because, ideally, the patient should ultimately become fully immunocompetent and off all treatment. The rationale is that as primitive lymphocytic stem cells ultimately repopulate the patient with a mature immunological system, immunological tolerance is induced, probably mediated by the generation of a suppressor T-cell population.

Methotrexate was the first useful prophylactic agent given to man, its use being based upon empirical experiments in dogs (Storb et al. 1970). It was injected weekly for 100 days after bone-marrow transplantation but its use was limited by suppression of graft function and mucositis. Cyclosporin has been shown to attenuate the course of graft-versus-host disease (Powles et al. 1978, 1980a). The main effect of cyclosporin appears not to be a reduction in the incidence of graft-versus-host disease, but in its severity (Bortin 1987; Deeg et al. 1987). It has not been shown clearly to be superior to methotrexate, but initially was thought to be less toxic (McGlave et al. 1985). However, it might impair renal function, although this is usually reversible with reduced dosage or cessation of the drug. It might also cause hepatic impairment, fluid retention, hypertension, convulsions (particularly in children), and hirsutism. Occasionally intractable nausea and anorexia with weight loss occurs. It is usually given for 4–6 months after bone-marrow transplantation and toxicity is reversible with discontinuation of the drug. Serum levels may be monitored to assess adequate absorption as well as to avoid toxic effects. Some patients develop graft-versus-host disease when the drug is stopped: it then needs to be re-administered. Recently the combination of cyclosporin and methotrexate has been demonstrated to be superior to either drug alone, with a survival advantage for the combined therapy in a prospective study (Storb et al. 1987). However, there is concern that this combination may exacerbate methotrexate-induced mucositis (Prentice and Brenner 1988). Similarly, the combination of methotrexate with corticosteroids has been demonstrated to be particularly effective in reducing graft-versus-host disease (Filipovich et al. 1985). Recent uncontrolled data suggest that the combination regimens (Clift et al. 1987; Gale et al. 1987) may affect the graft-versus-leukaemia phenomenon adversely and therefore increase the rates of leukaemic relapses.

Lymphocyte depletion of donor marrow virtually abrogates acute graft-versus-host disease. Various techniques of mature T-cell depletion have been employed effectively including E rosetting with sheep red cells (Reisner et al. 1981), monoclonal antibodies (Filipovich et al. 1982; Prentice et al. 1982; Hale et al. 1983), physical separation (Treleaven and Kemshead 1985), and immunotoxins (Filipovich et al. 1984). Unfortunately these cases have been associated with high rates of graft failure as well as leukaemic relapse. As both of these occurrences are invariably fatal, survival rates for such transplants have generally been inferior to non-T-cell-depleted bone-marrow transplantation (Apperley et al. 1986; Mitsuyasu et al. 1986; Pollard et al. 1986). However, the ability to abrogate severe acute graft-versus-host and its attendant morbidity and toxicity remains attractive if these problems can be overcome. Many workers are currently investigating this approach by trying to improve the anti-leukaemic effect of conditioning regimens and identifying the particular cell subsets responsible for engraftment, graft-versus-host disease and the graft-versus-leukaemia effect.

The management of established acute graft-versus-host disease remains difficult. More than 50 per cent of patients with severe disease will not survive (Gale and Champlin 1986). Treatment has been attempted with corticosteroids, cyclosporin, azathioprine, anti-lymphocyte globulin, specific anti-T-cell antibodies, and thalidomide, with only variable success (Vogelsang et al. 1988; Storb 1989). These results are clearly disappointing, indicating that new approaches to preventing graft-versus-host disease are required.

Chronic graft-versus-host disease

Chronic graft-versus-host disease occurs at least 100 days after allogeneic bone-marrow transplantation. Under variable circumstances it occurs in 15–40 per cent of patients (Sullivan et al. 1981, 1987). Clinical manifestations range from mild to extreme and include skin involvement, mucositis, keratoconjunctivitis, pulmonary insufficiency, chronic liver disease, and wasting. A scleroderma-like syndrome may occur, with oesophageal stricture and small and large intestinal involvement, causing malabsorption. Skin disease occurs in up to 75 per cent of cases, ranging from one or more localized pigmented or depigmented nodules through to a generalized erythematous rash that may progress to hyper-pigmentation, skin sclerosis, atrophy, and eventual contractures. Solar radiation may exacerbate skin changes and sun exposure should be avoided. Dry eyes and mucous membranes are common. Erosion of cartilage can occur, causing gross disfiguration of the face. Hepatic changes usually present a cholestatic picture, with characteristic biopsy changes resembling primary biliary cirrhosis. Both humoral and cellular immunity are persistently suppressed and up to 25 per cent of affected patients may die as a result of infection, usually due to encapsulated organisms. Grading of chronic graft-versus-host disease is based upon the extent of involvement of the various organ systems (Table 3).

Management of chronic graft-versus-host disease

Untreated moderate to severe chronic graft-versus-host disease usually has a relentless and often fatal outcome. The most effective treatment appears to be azathioprine in combination with prednisone and cyclosporin may also confer an additional benefit (Sullivan et al. 1988). Therapy may be required for 1–2 years

Table 3 Grading of chronic graft-versus-host disease

Limited chronic graft-versus-host disease
  Either or both of
    Localized skin involvement
    Hepatic dysfunction

Extensive chronic graft-versus-host disease
  Either of
    1. Generalized skin involvement
    2. Localized skin involvement and/or hepatic dysfunction, plus one or more of
        Liver histology showing chronic aggressive hepatitis, bridging necrosis, or cirrhosis or
        Involvement of eye: Schirmer's test with <5 mm wetting or
        Involvement of minor salivary glands or oral mucosa demonstrated on labial biopsy specimen or
        Involvement of any other target organ (for example, oesophageal abnormalities, polymyositis)

and over 80 per cent of patients should benefit. However, 20 per cent of patients will continue to have disabling and disfiguring disease. Recent anecdotal reports of the use of thalidomide in the treatment of this condition are of interest (Vogelsang *et al.* 1989) and this agent is now undergoing prospective evaluation.

Because prolonged immunodeficiency occurs with chronic graft-versus-host disease, antibiotic prophylaxis against *Pneumocystis carinii* and bacterial infection is generally recommended. Artificial tears and saliva may be necessary to relieve atrophic, dry mucous membranes.

Failure of engraftment

If T-cell depletion is not undertaken, then graft failure or rejection is rare following HLA-matched sibling bone-marrow transplants (Thomas *et al.* 1975). Poor graft function is seen occasionally and may be related to infection, drug toxicity, and possibly relapse (Bolger *et al.* 1986). If the failure of engraftment is not due to relapse, then it usually responds well to a second marrow infusion without the need for further conditioning. Graft rejection and failure to take are more common in HLA-mismatched and T-cell-depleted bone-marrow transplants. In HLA-mismatched bone-marrow transplants, graft failure occurs in 5–25 per cent of transplants, the risk increasing with the degree of mismatch (Storb 1989). In T-cell-depleted bone-marrow transplants the risk of rejection may be as high as 65 per cent (Martin *et al.* 1985). In these settings, graft rejection has an exceptionally high mortality because regrafted marrow is promptly destroyed immunologically. Strategies to reduce this problem in mismatched bone-marrow transplantation include the addition of intensified conditioning regimens and adding specific immunotherapies to the conditioning regimen, such as adding antithymoctye globulin or monoclonal antibodies directed against immune cells (such as anti-Ia bodies) (Prentice 1988).

Infection

Conditioning for bone-marrow transplantation results in severe neutropenia for 2–4 weeks and immunosuppression for many months. Immunosuppression in allogeneic transplantation is more intense where graft-versus-host disease prophylaxis is employed and prolonged graft-versus-host disease is associated with continued immunosuppression. As a consequence, bone-marrow transplant patients are at significant risk of infection from a broad spectrum of micro-organisms including viruses, bacteria, protozoa, and fungi.

Although treating the patient in a microbiologically protected environment has not been shown to improve overall survival, it reduces the risk of acquisition and colonization by patients of exogenous micro-organisms and may decrease the number of infective episodes (Jameson *et al.* 1971; Bodey *et al.* 1979). The use of high-efficiency particulate air filtration reduces the risk of aspergillosis. All transplant units utilize microbiological protection to some extent. Strict attention to patient hygiene, with the use of bactericidal skin washes and antiseptic and antifungal mouth care, is employed. Many units attempt gastrointestinal tract sterilization with absorbable antibiotics (such as Septrin®) and non-absorbable (polyenes for example, amphotericin and nystatin) antibiotics and in this situation a sterile diet should be provided. Prophylactic anti-microbial therapy has proven useful in bone-marrow transplantation (Watson and Jameson 1979) and it is likely that a number of new agents will be of most benefit in a prophylactic rôle. Prophylactic intravenous immunoglobulin may also prevent infection (Petersen *et al.* 1987; Graham-Pole *et al.* 1988) and confirmatory studies are awaited. Conveniently, the course after bone-marrow transplantation may be divided into three periods, characterized by different expectations of infective problems (Meyers and Thomas 1981).

During the first 30 days the initial neutropenic period is characterized by bacterial and, latterly, fungal, infections. As such infections may be life-threatening in a matter of hours, any suspicion of sepsis during this period must be treated aggressively with broad-spectrum antibiotics. The design of the appropriate antibiotics protocols will depend upon the design of the unit, the type of hospital it is in, and, to a considerable extent, on the type of bacteria commonly seen in the unit. However, regimens should include cover for skin staphylococci commonly associated with intravenous catheters, Gram-positive organisms arising in the respiratory tract and Gram-negative organisms arising from the gastrointestinal tract. Cultures from infected patients are commonly negative, particularly from patients already receiving antibiotics, and several changes of antibiotics may be necessary. Deep fungal infection may develop with little in the way of clinical signs and any patient with persistent unexplained fever or signs of infection beyond 7–10 days should receive intravenous amphotericin B (Milliken and Powles 1990). *Candida* sp. and *Aspergillus* sp. are the most common infective fungi. New, safer, parenterally absorbable antifungal agents such as itraconazole and fluconazole are currently undergoing assessment in clinical trials as prophylactic agents against fungal infection. Isolation in high-efficiency particulate air-filtered rooms remains the only reliable means of limiting injection by *Aspergillus*, which is a ubiquitous micro-organism. Infection by the herpes simplex virus commonly occurs in this initial period and is easily controlled with acyclovir therapy (Saral *et al.* 1981).

The second and third months after bone-marrow transplantation mark the second period, where viral and protozoal infections are more common. A major lung problem can occur with the characteristic picture of interstitial pneumonitis, that is dyspnoea, hypoxia, and small stiff lungs without necessarily having a cough, sputum, or added chest sounds. There is a characteristic 'white out' on the chest radiograph. It is the greatest infective risk following bone-marrow transplantation and usually occurs at this time. It occurs in 20–40 per cent of recipients of allogeneic bone-marrow transplants in different programmes and may be fatal in over 80 per cent of cases (Winston 1983). Cytomegalovirus is the commonest associated microbiological agent, accounting for as many as 70–80 per cent of cases. It is more common in patients who are seropositive for cytomegalovirus prior to bone-marrow transplantation (Meyers *et al.* 1986). It is much less common in autologous transplantation, presumably due to the absence of graft-versus-host disease (and its treatment) in these patients. Other causes are parainfluenza, mycoplasma, adenoviruses (Ljungman *et al.* 1989), and *Pneumocystis carinii*, but no causative agent may be identified in as many as 30 per cent of cases. The use of prophylactic low-dose co-trimoxasole has successfully prevented *Pneumocystis carinii* pneumonitis, which previously accounted for as many as 10 per cent of cases (Watson and Jameson 1979). Several factors increase the risk of interstitial pneumonitis. They are the presence of graft-versus-host disease, older patient age (over 40 years), poor patient performance status prior to bone-marrow transplantation, and methotrexate immunoprophylaxis (Gale and Champlin 1986). The use of cytomegalovirus-negative blood products in seronegative patients reduces the risk of cytomegalovirus infection but only 10 per cent of patients (or their donors) fulfil these criteria. Leucocyte depletion of blood products and prophylaxis with cytomegalovirus immunoglobulin may reduce the risk of infection but current results remain inconclusive (Meyers 1988). To date no effective therapy for established cytomegalovirus infection has been established. Results of the effect of cytomegalovirus immunoglobulin are controversial. Foscarnet (Akesson-Johansson *et al.* 1986) or dihydroxypropoxymethyl guanine (ganciclovir) may be of benefit if given early (Ettinger *et al.* 1989) but not in established cases. Currently these agents are undergoing investigation as prophylactic agents. The combination of either foscarnet or ganciclovir with cytomegalovirus immunoglobulin appears to be beneficial (Meyers 1988). High-dose acyclovir given prophylactically may reduce the incidence of cytomegalovirus pneumonitis (Meyers 1988) and currently prospective trials are investigating this finding. However, the lungs of allogeneic transplant recipients are damaged by total-body irradiation, particularly during the first 6 months after bone-marrow transplantation and it seems likely that infective agents, even when promptly treated, cause further damage that leads to progressive intractable idiopathic interstitial pneumonitis. Assisted ventilation does not help these patients. Herpes zoster virus infection is commonly seen (40 per cent of patients); it is only very rarely fatal when encephalitis or myocarditis occurs, but it does cause significant morbidity. If treated early with acyclovir, the response is dramatic (Selby *et al.* 1979) and that may be a prophylactic role for this agent (Perren *et al.* 1988). Beyond 3 months infections tend to be uncommon unless chronic graft-versus-host disease occurs. Late herpes virus, bacterial, and fungal infections may occur and are more common if graft-versus-host disease persists. Prophylactic broad-spectrum antibiotics have been recommended for patients with chronic graft-versus-host disease (McGlave *et al.* 1985). For up to 2 years after allogeneic bone-marrow transplantation, pneumococcal infections can occur, mimicking a post-splenectomy syndrome. Prophylactic penicillin should be given during this period.

Impaired nutrition

Poor nutrition is likely following the common acute toxicities of nausea, vomiting, and stomatitis associated with conditioning regimens and immunosuppression. Complications such as infections and graft-versus-host disease exacerbate the problem. Stomatitis requires aggressive pain control to enable patients to remain compliant with oral medication, mouth care, and food intake, so as to limit patient debility which increases their risk and their ability to cope with other complications. If simple measures such as diet supplementation and careful review of medications are insufficient to improve a patient's nutritional state or the patient loses 10 per cent of body weight, then parenteral feeding is required.

Blood product support

Without the advances in blood collection and the separation and storage of blood products in the past 40 years bone-marrow transplantation would have been virtually impossible. Generally, packed red cells are given to maintain patient haemoglobin above 10 g/dl. As long as the platelet count remains supported above $20 \times 10^9/l$ haemorrhage is unlikely unless drugs or complications affecting platelet function are introduced. Prophylactic white-cell transfusions are of no benefit in preventing infection. In established bacterial infection their rôle remains controversial. All blood products should be irradiated to prevent transfused T-lymphocytes inducing graft-versus-host disease which may be fatal (Mulder 1989). Fresh frozen plasma may be necessary for any acquired coagulation defects. Hypoalbuminaemia is common and plasma protein solutions may be required if levels of serum albumin fall below 30 g/l. Accurate fluid balance with maintenance of serum albumin protects against pulmonary oedema.

Rarer complications

Hepatic veno-occlusive disease

Veno-occlusive disease of the liver may be seen in as many as 28 per cent of patients and may have a morbidity of 30 per cent. First described in patients who received total-body irradiation (Berk *et al.* 1979), it is more common in patients who have underlying liver damage (McDonald *et al.* 1986) and may be exacerbated by immunosuppression, in particular by the use of cyclosporin. It has also been associated with the cyclophosphamide–busulphan conditioning regimen (Atkinson *et al.* 1987). The major pathological finding is thrombosis of small hepatic venules, leading to hepatic congestion and enlargement. Ascites and peripheral oedema are common. Characteristically, tests of liver function are only mildly elevated initially, gradually progressing to marked increases of bilirubin in particular. Heparin anticoagulation may be of benefit in the management of this condition.

Haemorrhagic cystitis

This is a well-recognized complication of high-dose cyclophosphamide (Thomas *et al.* 1975); metabolites of this drug directly damage the bladder mucosa when excreted in the urine. It may be prevented largely by the use of copious hydration fluids, urinary alkinalization, and mesna during and after administration (Scheef *et al.* 1979). The conditioning agent, busulphan, has also been implicated in promoting the occurrence of this complication (Atkinson *et al.* 1987).

Haemolytic uraemic syndrome

Over 20 severe cases of the haemolytic uraemic syndrome have now been reported associated with bone-marrow transplantation, although the incidence of milder forms of the syndrome is very much more common (Chappell *et al.* 1988). Characteristically there is evidence of intravascular haemolysis, with fragmented red cells and usually a raised bilirubin. There is initially a sharp rise in blood urea and, subsequently, oliguric renal failure. The pathological lesion is associated with the vascular endothelium. The haemolytic uraemic syndrome may occur with both allogeneic and autologous transplantation, but appears to be much less common and have a less aggressive course in autologous bone-marrow transplantation. This may be because the syndrome arises from a multiplicity of renal microvascular insults, more commonly occurring with allogeneic bone-marrow transplantation. Aetiological factors in the development of the haemolytic uraemic syndrome include the use of cyclosporin, cytomegalovirus infection, acute graft-versus-host disease, bacterial sepsis, cyclophosphamide, and total-body irradiation. Mortality is high, particularly if severe renal failure is a clinical feature. Management of the syndrome is centred around removal, when possible, of the aetiological factor. Aspirin and other antiplatelet agents appear of limited value (Byrnes and Moatic 1986). Anticoagulation with heparin and plasma exchange may be beneficial. Hypertension must be treated aggressively and progressive renal impairment, if it occurs, requires haemodialysis or haemofiltration. Peritoneal dialysis is difficult in bone-marrow transplant patients because of thrombocytopenia and leucopenia.

LATE EFFECTS OF BONE-MARROW TRANSPLANTATION

Recovery of immune function and tolerance

Following bone-marrow transplantation, the absolute lymphocyte count usually returns to normal levels by 6 months. However, it may take years for qualitative defects of both cellular and humoral immune function to return to normal (Witherspoon *et al.* 1981). Numerous factors may be responsible for immunodeficiency (Witherspoon *et al.* 1982). In allogeneic transplantation both graft-versus-host disease and the immunosuppressive drugs used to prevent it are important factors. It was hoped initially that T-cell depletion of transplants would not be associated with the same degree of immune dysfunction, as therapy for graft-versus-host disease would not be necessary. Although there are differences in the patterns of dysfunction in both forms of transplantation, immune recovery times are similar. Other factors, such as the conditioning regimens, infections, and the fact that only 2 per cent of the marrow and immune system is available to reconstitute the host, are also important. This is illustrated by the impaired immune function also seen in patients after syngeneic and autologous transplantation (Baumgartner *et al.* 1988).

Active immunization following bone-marrow transplantation is generally unsuccessful in the first year or longer if chronic graft-versus-host disease is present. It is generally considered advisable not to give live vaccines to bone-marrow transplant patients for at least 2 years post-transplant. Ultimately the immunological memory following allogeneic bone-marrow transplantation will be due to the adoptive transfer of antibody-secreting B-cells to the recipient. Immunity to tetanus toxoid and measles, for example, will be from the donor and it has been demonstrated that specific immunization of the marrow as little as 1 week prior to transplant allows antibody transfer to the recipient (Saxon *et al.* 1986). This ability could allow transfer of immunity to cytomegalovirus if an appropriate vaccine were available.

A fascinating occurrence in bone-marrow transplantation, generally not seen in solid-organ transplantation, is the development of immune tolerance. Usually by 6 months post-transplant all immunosuppressive therapy may be discontinued with little likelihood of the development of graft-versus-host disease. The mechanism for this is not well understood but is probably multifunctional, with a suppressor T lymphocyte population central to the effect.

Second malignancy

It has been realized for some time that second malignancy may follow chemotherapy and/or radiotherapy for lymphomas and other cancers (Tucker *et al.* 1988) and the commonest second malignancy is leukaemia. However, in bone-marrow transplantation, the transplanted marrow is given after drug therapy and total-body irradiation and so, theoretically, secondary leukaemia should not occur. Although leukaemia developing in donor marrow was first noted in the early 1970s (Fialkow *et al.* 1971) only a handful of cases have been reported. In a recent review of 2246 patients who underwent bone-marrow transplantation (Witherspoon *et al.* 1989) 35 patients developed secondary cancers. These were most commonly non-Hodgkin's lymphomas (16 patients) with glioblastoma, melanoma, and squamous cell carcinoma comprising almost all remaining cases. For the group overall, the age-adjusted increase in risk of secondary malignancy was nearly 7-fold. It is interesting to note that the cases of acute leukaemia and lymphoma tended to occur early after bone-marrow transplantation, while solid tumours tended to occur some years post-transplant, paralleling observations made in the victims of atomic bomb explosions. The occurrence of acute graft-versus-host disease treated with anti-thymocyte globulin or an anti-CD3 monoclonal antibody and the use of total-body irradiation, predicted for second malignancy,

while T-cell depletion and HLA-mismatched bone-marrow transplantation also predicted for lymphoma. This may reflect a greater degree of immunosuppression in patients who develop second cancers. For patients with acute leukaemia it needs be remembered that their induction chemotherapy would also increase their risk of second malignancy. This risk may be as high as 20-fold (Hawkins *et al.* 1987). As these factors will only affect a small number of patients adversely, they should not dissuade the clinician from considering bone-marrow transplantation as a curative therapy.

Ocular cataracts

Ocular cataracts may occur in up to 80 per cent of patients who receive total-body irradiation as a single fraction and it appears to be a speeding up of the natural ageing process. If total-body irradiation is fractionated, the incidence falls below 20 per cent (Deeg *et al.* 1984). The occurrence of ocular cataracts is uncommon within a year of bone-marrow transplantation. The use of high doses of prednisolone to treat graft-versus-host disease may exacerbate the occurrence of cataracts. Fortunately, modern surgical techniques are excellent in restoring satisfactory vision.

Endocrine dysfunction and sterility

Bone-marrow transplantation and, in particular, total-body irradiation may be associated with abnormal pituitary, thyroid, and adrenocortical function, with impaired growth and sexual development in children (Urban *et al.* 1988). Careful follow-up and monitoring is important to identify these problems. Growth hormone should be used to correct short stature. After total-body irradiation almost all women will lose ovarian function and develop an artificial menopause. Hormonal replacement therapy with oestrogens, progestogens, and sometimes additional androgens is crucial to avoid osteoporosis and restore libido and counselling is also required to avoid psychosexual problems. Sterility after bone-marrow transplantation is almost universal if total-body irradiation is part of the conditioning regimen. However, surveillance of patients is still necessary as unexpected pregnancies have occurred (Sanders *et al.* 1988). Succesful pregnancy has occurred (Milliken *et al.* 1990) after bone-marrow transplantation in the absence of total-body irradiation and the increasing numbers of transplants being undertaken without total-body irradiation make it likely that this will not remain a rare occurrence. For male patients, sperm samples may be cryopreserved prior to bone-marrow transplantation, but spermatogenesis can reoccur in some males several years after total-body irradiation.

Psychological function after bone-marrow transplantation

A number of functional and psychological problems following bone-marrow transplantation have been reported, including sexual problems, failure to return to work, emotional distress, low self-esteem, less than optimal life satisfaction, and mood disturbance (Andrykowski *et al.* 1989). Younger age at transplant is related to better outcome, with patients less than 30 years old reporting better functional quality of life and less mood disturbance than older patients. These impairments do not appear to improve with time. Despite these problems it is uncommon for patients to indicate that they would not make the same choice again to undergo bone marrow transplantation. Currently a number of centres are examining whether any forms of prophylactic psychological intervention may be of benefit to patients undergoing bone-marrow transplantation to improve their quality of life.

CLINICAL RESULTS OF BONE-MARROW TRANSPLANTATION

Allogeneic bone-marrow transplantation for acute myeloblastic leukaemia

In first remission

Controversy continues as to the optimal timing of bone-marrow transplantation for acute myeloblastic leukaemia. Improvements in conventional chemotherapy regimens as well as conditioning for bone-marrow transplantation are likely to aggravate rather than resolve the controversy. For acute myeloblastic leukaemia in first remission, several non-randomized studies have shown a highly significant reduction in relapse rate following HLA-matched sibling bone-marrow transplantation compared to chemotherapy alone (Powles *et al.* 1980*b*; Santos *et al.* 1983; Appelbaum *et al.* 1984; Champlin *et al.* 1985). However, in all instances there was a relatively high death rate in the bone-marrow transplant patients due to the transplant itself and these studies failed to demonstrate significantly improved leukaemia-free survival with bone-marrow transplantation because of the limited numbers in each study. In general, the cure rate for patients with acute myeloblastic leukaemia in remission undergoing bone-marrow transplantation is 55 per cent for patients under the age of 55 years (75 per cent for patients below 16 years of age).

Data from the International Bone Marrow Transplantation Registry (IBMTR) for 879 patients receiving HLA-matched sibling allografts indicate a 5 year disease-free survival probability of 48 per cent (Gale *et al.* 1989). For the same group of patients the 5 year actuarial relapse rate was 21 per cent. Similar results have been described by the Seattle group (Clift *et al.* 1987). For 231 patients there was an event-free (leukaemia-free) survival beyond 6 years of 43 per cent, with a probability of relapse of 25 per cent. Significantly improved survival was seen in young patients; however, the decrease in survival with increasing age was slight above 20 years. These data contain multiple different conditioning regimens and, to date, subset analysis has not demonstrated any clearly superior regimen in terms of survival probability. One single-centre study has addressed the issue of conditioning in a randomized fashion (Helenglass *et al.* 1988). The effect of a combination of cyclophosphamide ($3.6 \, \text{g/m}^2$) with single-fraction total-body irradiation was compared to that of melphalan ($100 \, \text{mg/m}^2$) plus single-fraction total-body irradiation. The latter regimen was superior in terms of reduced relapse rate but was more toxic, resulting in an improved probability of survival that escaped statistical significance ($p=0.1$).

Recently, almost as high disease-free survival figures have been claimed for the use of chemotherapy alone with 22–51 per cent of patients alive at 3–6 years for adults (Yates *et al.* 1982; Rees *et al.* 1986; Wolff *et al.* 1987) and 41–50 per cent for children (Creutzig *et al.* 1985; Weinstein *et al.* 1987). Almost all failures after chemotherapy were due to disease relapse and in this respect bone-marrow transplantation is obviously superior, so the elimination of non-relapse complications from bone-marrow transplantation would end the controversy. A prospective randomized study comparing the two approaches in first remission acute myeloblastic leukaemia is far beyond the scope of any single institution. It seems unlikely that the necessary international collaborative effort needed would be possible and by the time the results of such a trial were available the interpretation would be invalidated by further improvements in both treatment options.

In second or greater remission

For acute myeloblastic leukaemia beyond first remission the results of chemotherapy regimens have been disappointing, with less than 5 per cent of patients likely to achieve cure (Weinstein *et al.* 1983). Results of allogeneic bone-marrow transplantation have been shown clearly to be superior for these patients. Data from the IBMTR on 229 patients in second or subsequent remission indicate a disease-free probability of survival at 5 years of 26 per cent, with a relapse rate of 48 per cent (Gale *et al.* 1989). Data from the Seattle group (Clift *et al.* 1987) are similar, with a survival probability of 28 per cent and a relapse rate of 37 per cent in 49 patients receiving bone-marrow transplants in second remission. However, these results must be qualified by bearing in mind that only approximately 50 per cent of patients in first relapse respond sufficiently well to intensive reinductive cytotoxic chemotherapy to pass into a full second haematological remission.

In relapse

The Seattle experience in first relapse of acute myeloblastic leukaemia would indicate this to be optimal timing for bone-marrow transplantation rather than after a second remission has been achieved (Clift *et al.* 1987). The probabilities of leukaemia-free survival of 54 patients with untreated relapse and 29 patients in relapse resistant to chemotherapy were 30 and 21 per cent, respectively, with relapse rates of 36 and 56 per cent, respectively. These results are comparable to the results for second remission patients, 28 per cent and 37 per cent, respectively. These data suggest that patients should undergo bone-marrow transplantation early in first relapse rather than after an attempt to achieve a second remission, particularly as some patients could be expected to die undergoing remission chemotherapy. But these data must be interpreted with great caution. The referral pattern of patients to Seattle is often from great distances and the possibility that these 'early' untreated relapse patients are highly selected cannot be ignored. Almost certainly many of them have slowly proliferating disease and they have been able to preserve normal bone-marrow function and remain well. They may only represent 10 per cent of the first relapse population at large. The IBMTR data on 321 relapse patients (Gale *et al.* 1989) reveal a probability of disease-free survival at 5 years of 15 per cent, with a 67 per cent relapse risk, compared to 26 and 48 per cent for 229 patients in second or subsequent remission, these differences achieving statistical significance.

Acute lymphoblastic leukaemia

In first and second remission

In adults the outlook for treatment of acute lymphoblastic leukaemia following chemotherapy alone is generally considered poor. In the 1980s two studies published results with chemotherapy alone which were more encouraging and with demonstrated disease-free survivals beyond 4 years of 39 per cent (Hoelzer *et al.* 1984) and 57 per cent at 5 years (Clarkson *et al.* 1985). In both of these studies younger patients did significantly better, with disease-free survivals greater than 50 per cent. Unfortunately, these results are yet to be confirmed by other centres and in most studies cure rates of higher than 30 per cent are rare. In children the prospects for cure with chemotherapy are excellent; more than 60 per cent may expect cure. Some subgroups of child patients have been identified as having a worse prognosis. Poor prognostic features are less than 2 years or greater than 15 years old, white cell count at presentation greater than 50×10^9/l, central nervous system involvement, B-cell or T-cell phenotype, and specific chromosome abnormalities such as t(4;11), t(8;14), and t(9;22) (Weinstein *et al.* 1987). Barrett *et al.* (1988) have reported results from the IBMTR of allogeneic matched-sibling bone-marrow transplants in first remission for children of high risk and demonstrated a leukaemia-free survival of 56 per cent. IBMTR analysis (Gale *et al.* 1989) of 369 patients of all ages undergoing bone-marrow transplantation in first remission demonstrated a probability of 5 year leukaemia-free survival of 43 per cent, with a relapse rate of 30 per cent, whereas the probability of similar survival for 592 patients in second or subsequent remission was only 26 per cent, with a relapse rate of 54 per cent. All patients were adults or children of poor risk and there was a clear benefit for bone-marrow transplantation in first rather than second remission (Herzig *et al.* 1987), with probabilities of leukaemia-free survivals of 45 and 22 per cent, respectively. The Seattle group (Doney *et al.* 1987) have reported a 28 per cent probability of leukaemia-free survival at 5 years, with a relapse risk of 41 per cent in 46 patients in first remission. Results are superior when bone-marrow transplantation is carried out in remission (Thomas *et al.* 1983; Prentice and Grob 1986).

Bone-marrow transplantation is probably the treatment of choice in children with acute lymphoblastic leukaemia transplanted beyond first remission (Bacigalupo *et al.* 1985; Storb 1985). However, children who relapse from the first remission when not on maintenance chemotherapy still have a good survival probability with chemotherapy alone (Butturini *et al.* 1987*b*). Brochstein *et al.* (1987) from the Memorial Sloan Kettering Cancer Centre have presented impressive results in children transplanted in second remission and beyond. Leukaemia-free survivals at 5 years were 64, 42, and 23 per cent for second, third, and fourth remission patients, respectively.

Leukaemia-free survival is poor in adults who relapse from first remission with cure being less than 5 per cent (Hoelzer and Gale 1987). Results for bone-marrow transplantation in these patients are clearly superior, with an expected 22–36 per cent leukaemia-free survival in adults transplanted in second remission (Herzig *et al.* 1987).

Chronic granulocytic leukaemia

At present allogeneic bone-marrow transplantation is the only curative therapy for chronic granulocytic leukaemia. The optimal time for transplantation is in the chronic phase of the disease. Leukaemia-free survivals at 5 years are 41, 17, and 14 per cent for patients in the chronic phase, accelerated phase, and blast transformation, respectively. Relapse rates for these same groups are 27, 49 and 49 per cent, respectively (Gale *et al.* 1989). The probability of remaining in remission was lower for patients receiving T-cell-depleted marrows, irrespective of the grade of acute or chronic graft-versus-host disease. Data from the Seattle group indicate disease-free survivals of 49–56 per cent in the chronic phase, 15–28 per cent in the accelerated phase, and 15 per cent in blast crisis, with actuarial relapse rates of 12–20 per cent, 40–56 per cent, and 50–75 per cent, respectively (Storb 1989). The majority of patients transplanted in blast crisis die of complications related to the bone-marrow transplant (Doney *et al.* 1981). The optimal time for bone-marrow transplantation in the chronic phase

is not entirely clear. Data from the Seattle group (Thomas *et al.* 1986) indicate an inverse relationship between duration of the disease before bone-marrow transplantation and survival. However, data from the IBMTR in over 600 chronic-phase patients showed no such relationship (Gale *et al.* 1989).

Given the poorer results of bone-marrow transplantation for the accelerated phase and blast crisis, together with the toxic risk of bone-marrow transplantation, a number of investigators have attempted to predict the likelihood of transformation from the chronic phase. Factors at diagnosis that may determine a short chronic phase are being male, having a large spleen size, a high platelet count, a high percentage of circulating blast cells (Sokal *et al.* 1985), and a greater amount of chemotherapy to control chronic-phase disease in the first year of diagnosis (Wareham *et al.* 1982). Complex mathematical models have been developed to determine the risk of transformation and the risk of bone-marrow transplantation (Segel *et al.* 1986); however, these are unlikely to replace subjective patient preference.

BONE-MARROW TRANSPLANTATION USING UNRELATED DONORS

The success of HLA-matched sibling bone-marrow transplantation led to the investigation of strategies of bone-marrow transplantation for the majority of patients who do not possess a suitable sibling donor. One such strategy has been the use of autologous bone-marrow transplantation (see below) and early results appear promising. However, certain diseases are not amenable to this approach as true marrow remission is almost never achievable as in chronic granulocytic leukaemia and the myelodysplastic syndromes. A number of donor registries are now in existence around the world. It has been estimated that a donor pool of 100 000 would have a 43 per cent chance of providing a fully HLA-matched donor (Bradley *et al.* 1987). The degree of HLA match for successful unrelated donor transplantation is not fully known but mismatches of greater than one HLA antigen would appear to be associated with an unacceptable degree of fatal graft-versus-host disease and infection (Gingrich *et al.* 1988). Consequently, there are major logistic problems in handling a panel of 100 000 donors with the inevitable long delay in finding a suitable donor and therefore the resulting high cost.

In a retrospective study of 51 matched, unrelated-donor bone-marrow transplants compared to 51 matched sibling transplants for chronic granulocytic leukaemia, acute leukaemia, and severe aplastic anaemia, the actuarial patient survivals at 1 year were 32 per cent for the matched, unrelated-donor and 63 per cent for the sibling-matched bone-marrow transplants (Kaminski 1989). Graft failure was increased in the matched, unrelated-donor transplants (25 versus 16 per cent) but not graft-versus-host disease. Currently an international prospective study is underway to evaluate the place of matched, unrelated-donor transplants, particularly for chronic granulocytic leukaemia.

BONE-MARROW TRANSPLANTATION USING MISMATCHED DONORS

The prospects of using any member of the immediate family of the patient is attractive because it opens up the possibility of bone-marrow transplantation to almost all patients, and removes logistic and ethical problems. Unfortunately the results of mismatched transplants using family donors have been disappointing, with a cure rate of only 30 per cent for first remission acute myeloblastic leukaemia (Powles *et al.* 1980*b*). Transplant-related complications increase with the degree of mismatch. Within a family, genetically the commonest mismatch configuration for chromosome 6 would be a one-haplotype-identical donor (both parents, half the sibs, all the progeny). In another series of 28 patients, using very intensive conditioning and T-cell depletion, receiving one-haplotype-matched grafts, 39 per cent were alive at 7 months (Ash *et al.* 1987), although others have been less successful (Prentice and Brenner 1988). Within the mismatched haplotype of these patients the number of loci that match the donor may be important (Kaminski 1989). The risk of graft-versus-host disease increases with the degree of mismatch, being 60, 70, and 85 per cent for one, two, and three locus mismatches, respectively. Survival for one locus mismatch is equivalent to that for HLA-identical transplants, the increased risk of graft-versus-host disease being balanced by a reduced relapse risk. However, the occurrence of one and two matched loci in a mismatched haplotype is relatively uncommon within families and severely limits the widespread application of mismatched bone-marrow transplantation. Consequently attention has been directed more at the application of autologous BMT.

AUTOLOGOUS BONE-MARROW TRANSPLANTATION

Autologous bone-marrow transplantation has a long and dismal history in the treatment of cancer and has until recently been doomed to failure because of an inability of ridding the patient of the cancer before giving back his or her own marrow. The principle was that the patient could be given what would otherwise be a lethal dose of treatment but could be rescued from fatal bone-marrow failure using stored marrow. For solid tumours even these doses of treatment fail. However, autologous bone-marrow transplantation for leukaemia is currently being reinvestigated by a large number of centres worldwide. The disappointing results of HLA-mismatch transplants and the inability of unrelated donor panels to provide adequate donors for patients led many investigators to re-examine this strategy, particularly because now, through allogeneic bone-marrow transplantation, we have developed much more effective methods of treating the patient before the marrow is returned.

Theoretically, intensive antileukaemic therapy with autologous marrow rescue should benefit leukaemia patients if a linear response relationship exists for the cure of this disease. The procedure should be safer than allogeneic bone-marrow transplantation as no graft-versus-host disease would be expected and it can therefore be offered to older patients. In simple terms, 2 per cent of the patient's marrow is harvested once he or she has achieved remission, then this is utilized as a haematological 'rescue' after marrow ablation with chemotherapy and/or radiotherapy. Disadvantages of the technique are the absence of a graft-versus-leukaemia effect and the risk of reseeding occult leukaemic cells with the remission marrow. Concerns over the ability of 'manipulated' bone-marrow to reconstitute normal haematopoiesis have not been realized (Prentice and Brenner 1988). As little as 5×10^7 nucleated cells/kg are sufficient to restore haematopoiesis (Spitzer *et al.* 1980), although there may be a delay of several weeks before full re-constitution occurs.

Many investigators have developed techniques to 'purge' autologous bone-marrow of residual leukaemia. Techniques have included the use of pharmacological agents such as the cyclophosphamide derivatives 4-hydroxyperoxycyclophosphamide

(Santos and Colvin 1986) and mafosfamide (Asta-Z) (Douay *et al.* 1984), immunological purging with monoclonal antibodies such as the Campath antibodies (Hale *et al.* 1983), and the use of long-term marrow culture (Chang *et al.* 1989). Currently, immunological methods are limited to lymphoblastic leukaemia as no appropriate specific myeloid leukaemia antigen has been identified in acute myeloblastic leukaemia and non-specific manipulations may jeopardize stem cell survival. An alternative approach has been the use of peripheral blood stem cells leucapheresed from the patient during the recovery phase following chemotherapy. This may allow an adequate stem cell harvest with a reduced risk of leukaemic contamination without the need for manipulation and avoiding the risk of stem cell loss. In acute myeloblastic leukaemia, marrow (presumably with acute myeloblastic leukaemia cells present in very small numbers) can be given back without purging, presumably because when this 2 per cent of marrow proliferates 50-fold over the 3 weeks following transplantation there is such a proliferative advantage to normal marrow that the leukaemic cells die out. It is difficult to postulate another reason why 40 per cent of patients with acute myeloblastic leukaemia are cured if autografted during first remission, whereas without autologous bone-marrow transplantation only 15 per cent are cured.

Current results of autologous bone-marrow transplantation must be assessed in the light of relatively short follow-up times, small numbers of patients in individual studies, and the diversity of treatment strategies employed. At best, the results of autologous bone-marrow transplantation do not exceed those of syngeneic transplantation for acute myeloblastic leukaemia and acute lymphoblastic leukaemia, with long-term survival rates of 40 per cent and risk of relapse of 50 per cent.

Up to 45 per cent survival in first remission patients at 2 years following autologous bone-marrow transplantation have been reported (Linch and Burnett 1986; Yeager *et al.* 1986). Increased relapse rates are in part balanced by the reduced mortality of the procedure compared to allogeneic transplantation. Linch and Burnett (1986) described a 43 per cent 2 year survival following autologous bone-marrow transplantation for patients in second remission acute myeloblastic leukaemia, a group not expected to do well. The relapse risk was 46 per cent. Kersey *et al.* (1987) compared results of autologous and allogeneic bone-marrow transplantation for patients with high-risk acute lymphoblastic leukaemia in remission. At 4 years, leukaemia-free survival was 20 and 27 per cent, respectively. The relapse risk was 79 per cent for the autologous group, 37 per cent for allografted patients who developed graft-versus-host disease, and 75 per cent for allografted patients with no graft-versus-host disease.

A report from the European Cooperative Group for bone-marrow Transplantation (Gorin *et al.* 1989) analysed registry data on 1322 autologous transplants for acute leukaemia. Of 448 patients with acute non-lymphocytic leukaemia considered to be at 'standard risk' first remission, the actuarial disease-free survival at 7 years was 36 per cent. In 'high-risk' first remission patients, it was 33 per cent at 3 years. These results appear equivalent to recent reports for chemotherapy alone. In second remission patients, actuarial survivals were 30 per cent at 4 years and 28 per cent at 7 months, respectively, for standard high-risk groups, somewhat better than could be expected for chemotherapy alone. There also appeared to be a survival advantage in patients receiving mafosfamide-purged marrow for standard-risk acute non-lymphocytic leukaemia in first remission. In 125 'purged' patients the leukaemia-free survival was 60 per cent at 5 years, compared to 39 per cent in 303 'non-purged' patients. Those results await confirmation in a prospective study. For acute lymphoblastic leukaemia, actuarial leukaemia-free survivals were 42, 41, 31, and 23 per cent for first remission standard risk, first remission high risk, second remission standard risk, and second remission high risk, respectively. Patients undergoing autologous bone-marrow transplantation in relapse appear to do uniformly poorly, with little chance of prolonged leukaemia-free survival (Herve 1984).

The exact role for autologous bone-marrow transplantation remains to be determined. Preliminary results indicate that it is likely to benefit patients in remission. However, only a large, prospectively randomized trial will determine its role for first remission patients.

PERIPHERAL BLOOD STEM CELL TRANSPLANTATION

Pluripotent haematopoietic progenitor cells circulate in the peripheral blood during recovery from myelosuppressive chemotherapy and after treatment with growth factors such as granulocyte and granulocyte–macrophage colony-stimulating factor. These cells can be harvested using a cell separator and are capable of reconstituting haematopoiesis after myeloablative therapy (Sheridan et al. 1992). The period of pancytopenia following peripheral blood stem cell transplantation is significantly shorter than that after autologous bone-marrow transplantation resulting in decreased transfusion and antibiotic requirements and shorter hospitalization. While the use of peripheral blood stem cells is increasing dramatically, the issue of tumour cell contamination of the harvested material and the need for post-transplant therapy have not been adequately addressed.

FUTURE DEVELOPMENTS

For the immediate future, we are committed to allogeneic bone-marrow transplantation for the treatment of acute myeloblastic leukaemia, chronic granulocytic leukaemia, and bad-risk acute lymphoblastic leukaemia patients who have a matched sibling donor, because there are no other forms of treatment that can give comparable success. This, however, only represents a small proportion (15 per cent) of the patients with those diseases and, clearly, a wider application of bone-marrow transplantation is required. Matched, unrelated-donor panels are seen at present to have major logistic problems and only a very small proportion of initiated searches end up with a cured patient. More refined tissue typing for other antigens (on chromosome 6 and other chromosomes) will also only serve to limit the number of transplants further. Better conditioning regimens and better control of graft-versus-host disease is inevitable, although the latter may produce increased relapse rates because of the abolition of the graft-versus-leukaemia effect.

REFERENCES

Akesson-Johansson A, Lerestedt J-O, Ringdon O, Lonnqvist B, Wahren B (1986). Sensitivity of cytomegalovirus to intravenous foscarnet treatment. *Bone Marrow Transplantation*, 1:215–20.

Andover MA, et al. (1982). The double lumen Hickman catheter. *American Journal of Nursing*, 82:272–3.

Andrykowski MA, Henslee PJ, Barnett RL (1989). Longitudinal assessment of psychological functioning of adult survivors of allogeneic bone marrow transplantation. *Bone Marrow Transplantation*, 4:505–9.

Appelbaum FR, et al. (1984). Bone marrow transplantation or chemotherapy after remission induction for adults with acute nonlymphoblastic leukaemia. A prospective comparison. *Annals of Internal Medicine*, 101:581–8.

Apperley JF, et al. (1986). Bone marrow transplantation for patients with chronic myeloid leukaemia: T-cell depletion with Campath-1 reduces the incidence of graft-versus-host disease but may increase the risk of leukaemic relapse. *Bone Marrow Transplantation*, 1:53–66.

Ash RC, et al. (1987). Successful allogeneic marrow transplantation utilizing HLA-closely matched unrelated donors. *Blood*, 70 (Suppl. 1):289a.

Atkinson K, Biggs J, Noble G, Ashby M, Concannon A, Dodds A, (1987). Preparative regimens for bone marrow transplantation containing busulphan are associated with haemorrhagic cystitis and hepatic veno-occlusive disease but a short duration of leucopaenia and little oropharyngeal mucositis. *Bone Marrow Transplantation*, 2:385–94.

Bacigalupo A, Frassoni F, Van Lint MT (1985). Bone marrow transplantation for chronic granulocytic leukaemia. *Cancer*, 58:2307–11.

Barrett AJ, et al. (1988). Marrow transplantation for acute lymphoblastic leukaemia: factors affecting relapse and survival. *Blood*, 74:862–71.

Baumgartner C, et al. (1988). Humoral immune function in paediatric patients treated with autologous bone marrow transplantation for B cell non-Hodgkin's lymphoma. The influence of *ex-vivo* marrow decontamination with anti-Y 29/55 monoclonal antibody and complement. *Blood*, 71:1211–17.

Berk PD, Popper H, Krueger GR, Decter J, Herzig G, Graw RGJ (1979). Veno-occlusive disease of the liver after allogeneic bone marrow transplantation: possible association with graft-versus-host disease. *Annals of Internal Medicine*, 90:158–64.

Bodey GP, et al. (1979). Treatment of acute leukaemia in protected environment units. *Cancer*, 44:431–6.

Bolger GB, et al. (1986). Second marrow infusion for poor graft function after allogeneic transplantation. *Bone Marrow Transplantation*, 1:21–30.

Bortin MM (1987). In *Progress in bone marrow transplantation* (ed. RP Gale and R Champlin), pp. 243–64. Alan R. Liss: New York.

Bradley BA, et al. (1987). How many HLA typed unrelated donors for bone marrow transplantation are needed to provide an effective service? *Bone Marrow Transplantation*, 2 (Suppl. 1):79.

Brochstein JA, et al. (1987). Allogeneic bone marrow transplantation after hyperfractionated total-body irradiation and cyclophosphamide in children with acute leukaemia. *New England Journal of Medicine*, 817:1618–24.

Butturini A, Bortin MM, Gale RP (1987a). Graft-versus-leukaemia following bone marrow transplantation. *Bone Marrow Transplantation*, 2:233–42.

Butturini A, Rivera GK, Bortin MM, Gale RP (1987b). Which treatment for childhood acute lymphoblastic leukaemia in second remission? *Lancet*, i:429–32.

Byrnes JJ, Moatic JL (1986). Thrombotic thrombocytopaenic purpura and the haemolytic uraemic syndrome: evolving concepts of pathogenesis and therapy. *Clinics in Haematology*, 15:413–42.

Champlin RE, et al. (1985). Treatment of acute myelogenous leukaemia. A prospective controlled trial of bone marrow transplantation versus consolidation chemotherapy. *Annals of Internal Medicine*, 102:285–91.

Chang J, et al. (1989). The use of bone marrow cells grown in long-term culture for autologous bone marrow transplantation in acute myeloid leukaemia: an update. *Bone Marrow Transplantation*, 4:5–9.

Chappell ME, Keeling DM, Prentice HG, Sweny P (1988). Haemolytic uraemic syndrome after bone marrow transplantation: an adverse effect of total body irradiation? *Bone Marrow Transplantation*, 3:339–47.

Clarkson B, et al. (1985). Acute lymphoblastic leukaemia in adults. *Seminars in Oncology*, 12(2):160–79.

Clift RA, et al. (1987). The treatment of acute non-lymphoblastic leukaemia by allogeneic marrow transplantation. *Bone Marrow Transplantation*, 2:243–58.

Creutzig U, et al. (1985). Improved treatment results in childhood acute myelogenous leukaemia: a report of the German cooperative study AML-BFM-78. *Blood*, 65:298–304.

Dausset J (1958). Iso-leuco-anticorps. *Acta Haematologica (Basel)*, 20:156–66.

Deeg HJ, Storb R, Thomas ED (1984). Bone marrow transplantation: a review of delayed complication. *British Journal of Haematology*, 57:185–208.

Deeg HJ, et al. (1987). In *Progress in bone marrow transplantation* (ed. RP Gale and R Champlin), pp. 265–76. Alan R. Liss, New York.

Dicke KA, Van Bekkum DW (1978). *Experimental Haematology*, 20:126.

Doney K, et al. (1981). Allogeneic bone marrow transplantation for chronic granulocytic leukaemia. *Experimental Haematology*, 9:966–71.

Doney K, et al. (1987). Marrow transplantation for patients with acute lymphoblastic leukaemia in first marrow remission. *Bone Marrow Transplantation*, 2:355–63.

Douay L, Gorin NC, Laporte J-P, Lopez M, Najman A, Duhamel G (1984). ASTA Z 7557 (INN Mafosfamide) for the *in vitro* treatment of human leukaemic bone marrows. *Investigational New Drugs*, 2:187–90.

Dupont B (1980). HLA factors and bone marrow grafting. In *Cancer: achievements, challenges and prospects for the 1980's* (ed. JH Burchenal and HF Oettgen), pp. 683–93. Grune and Sratton, New York.

Ettinger, NA, *et al.* (1989). Cytomegalovirus pneumonia: the use of ganciclovir in marrow transplant recipients. *Journal of Antimicrobial Chemotherapy*, 24:53–62.

Fialkow PJ, Thomas ED, Bryant JI, Nieman PE (1971). Leukaemic transformation of engrafted human marrow cells *in vivo*. *Lancet*, i:251–5.

Filipovich AH, *et al.* (1982). Pretreatment of donor bone marrow with monoclonal antibody OKT3 for prevention of acute-graft-versus-host disease in allogeneic histocompatible bone marrow transplantation. *Lancet*, 1:1266–9.

Filipovich AH, *et al.* (1984). *Ex-vivo* treatment of donor bone marrow with anti-T-cell immunotoxins for prevention of graft-versus-host disease. *Lancet*, i:469–72.

Filipovich AH, *et al.* (1985). Allogeneic bone marrow transplantation with related donors other than HLA MLC-matched siblings, and the use of anti-thymocyte globulin, prednisone and methotrexate for prophylaxis of graft-versus-host-disease.*Transplantation*, 39:282–5.

Filshie J, Pollock AN, Hughes RG, Omar YA (1984). The anaesthetic management of bone marrow harvest for transplantation. *Anaesthesia*, 39:480–4.

Gale RP, Champlin R (1986). Bone marrow transplantation in acute leukaemia. *Clinics in Haematology*, 15(3):851–72.

Gale RP, Horowitz MM, Bortin MM (1987). Bone marrow transplants in acute myelogenous leukaemia. *Blood*, 70(5):293a.

Gale RP, Horowitz MM, Bortin MM (1985). IBMTR analysis of bone marrow transplants in acute leukaemia. Advisory Committee of the International Bone Marrow Transplant Registry (IBMTR). *Bone Marrow Transplant*, 4 (Suppl. 3):83–4.

Gingrich RD, *et al.* (1988). Allogeneic marrow grafting with partially matched unrelated donors. *Blood*, 71:1375–81.

Glucksberg H, *et al.* (1974). Clinical manifestations of graft-versus-host disease in human recipients of marrow from HLA-matched sibling donors. *Transplantation*, 18(4):295–304.

Goldman JM, *et al.* (1988). Bone marrow transplantation for chronic myelogenous leukaemia in chronic phase. Increased risk for relapse associated with T-cell depletion. *Annals of Internal Medicine*, 108:806–14.

Gorin NC, Aegerter P, Auvert B (1989). Autologous bone marrow transplantation (ABMT) for acute leukaemia in remission: an analysis of 1322 cases. *Bone Marrow Transplantation*, 4 (Suppl. 2):3–5.

Graham-Pole J, *et al.* (1988). Intravenous immunoglobulin may lessen all forms of infection in patients receiving allogeneic bone marrow transplantation for acute lymphoblastic leukaemia: a paediatric oncology group study. *Bone Marrow Transplantation*, 3:559–66.

Greenberg PD, Cheever MA, Fefer A (1981). Eradication of disseminated murine leukaemia by chemoimmunotherapy by cyclophosphamide and adoptively transferred immune syngeneic Lyt 1+ 2− T lymphocytes. *Journal of Experimental Medicine*, 154:953–63.

Hale G, *et al.* (1983). Removal of T cells from bone marrow for transplantation: a monoclonal anti-lymphocyte antibody that fixes human complement. *Blood*, 62:873–82.

Hawkins MM, Draper GJ, Kingston JE (1987). Incidence of secondary primary tumours among childhood cancer survivors. *British Journal of Cancer*, 56:339–47.

Helenglass G, *et al.* (1987). Bone marrow transplantation—The Royal Marsden experience. *Haematological Oncology*, 5:245–54.

Helenglass G, *et al.* (1988). Melphalan and total body irradiation (TBI) versus cyclophosphamide and TBI as conditioning for allogeneic matched sibling bone marrow transplants for acute myeloblastic leukaemia in first remission. *Bone Marrow Transplantation*, 3:21–9.

Herve P, The French Study Group on Autologous Bone Marrow Transplantation in Acute Leukaemia (1974). In *Autologous bone marrow transplantation in acute leukaemia: a French review of 120 patients* (ed. KA Dicke, G Spitzer, and AR Zander), p. 23. The University of Texas and MD Anderson Hospital and Tumour Institute, Houston.

Herve P (1984). Current status of autologous bone marrow grafting in man. *Pathologie Biologie Paris*, 32:5–8.

Herzig RH, *et al.* (1987). Bone marrow transplantation in high-risk acute lymphoblastic leukaemia in first and second remission. *Lancet*, i:786–8.

Hoelzer D, Gale RP (1987). Acute lymphoblastic leukaemia in adults: recent progress, future directions. *Seminars in Haematology*, 24:27–39.

Hoelzer D, *et al.* (1984). Intensified therapy in acute lymphoblastic and acute undifferentiated leukaemia in adults. *Blood*, 64:38–47.

Jameson B, *et al.* (1971). Five year analysis of protective isolation. *Lancet*, i, 1034.

Juttner CA, To LB, Haylock DN, Branford A, Kimber RJ (1985). Circulating autologous stem cells collected in very early remission from acute non-lymphoblastic leukaemia produce prompt but incomplete haematopoietic reconstitution after high dose melphalan or supralethal chemoradiotherapy. *British Journal of Haematology*, 61:739–45.

Kaminski ER (1989). How important is histocompatibility in bone marrow transplantation? *Bone Marrow Transplantation*, 4:439–44.

Kersey J, *et al.* (1987). Comparison of autologous and allogeneic bone marrow transplantation for treatment of high risk refractory acute lymphoblastic leukaemia. *New England Journal of Medicine*, 317:461–7.

Linch DC, Burnett AK (1986). Clinical studies of ABMT in acute myeloid leukaemia. *Clinics in Haematology*, 15:167–86.

Ljungman P, Gleaves CA, Meyers JD (1989). Respiratory virus infection in immunocompromised patients. *Bone Marrow Transplantation*, 4:35–40.

Lum LG (1987). A review: the kinetics of immune reconstitution after human marrow transplantation. *Blood*, 69:369–80.

McDonald GB, Shulman HM, Sullivan KM, Spencer GD (1986). Intestinal and hepatic complications of human bone marrow transplantation. Part I and II. *Gastroenterology*, 90:460–77, 770–84.

McGlave PB, Ramsay N, Kersey J (1985). Allogeneic and autologous bone marrow transplantation. In *Recent advances in haematology* (ed. AV Hoffbrand), pp. 171–97. Churchill Livingstone, Edinburgh.

Martin PJ, *et al.* (1985). Effects of *in vitro* depletion of T cells in HLA identical allogeneic marrow grafts. *Blood*, 66:664–72.

Mathe G (1968). Bone marrow transplantation. In *Human transplantation* (ed. FI Rappaport and J Dausset), pp. 384–403. Grune and Stratton, New York.

Mathe G, *et al.* (1959). Transfusions of grafts of homologous bone marrow in humans accidentally irradiated to high doses. *Revue Française des Etudos Cliniques Biologiques*, 4:226–38.

Mathe G, *et al.* (1963). Haematopoietic chimera in man after allogeneic (homologous) bone marrow transplantation. *British Medical Journal*, ii:1633–5.

Mathe G, *et al.* (1974). Bone marrow transplantation for aplasias and leukaemias. In *Clinical immunobiology* (ed. FH Bach and RA Good), pp. 33–62. Academic Press, New York.

Meyers JD (1988). Prevention and treatment of cytomegalovirus infection after bone marrow transplantation. *Bone Marrow Transplantation*, 3:95–104.

Meyers JD, Thomas ED (1981). Infections complicating bone marrow transplantation. In *Clinical approach to infection in the compromised host* (ed. RH Rubin and LS Young), pp 507–52. Plenum, London.

Meyers JD, Flournoy N, Thomas ED (1986). Risk factors for cytomegalovirus infection after human marrow transplantation. *Journal of Infectious Diseases*, 153:478–88.

Milliken ST, Powles RL (1990). Antifungal prophylaxis in bone marrow transplantation. *Reviews of Infectious Diseases*, 12 (Suppl. 3):5374–9.

Milliken ST, *et al.* (1990). Successful pregnancy following bone marrow transplantation for leukaemia. *Bone Marrow Transplantation*, 5:135–7.

Mitsuyasu RT, *et al.* (1986). Treatment of donor bone marrow with monoclonal anti-T-cell antibody and complement for the prevention of graft-versus-host disease. A prospective, randomized, double-blind trial. *Annals of Internal Medicine*, 105:20–6.

Morrison M, Samwick AA (1940). Intramedullary (sternal) transfusion of human bone marrow. *Journal of the American Medical Association*, 111:1708–11.

Mulder NH, Elema JD, Postmus PE (1989). Transfusion associated graft-versus-host disease in autologous bone marrow transplantation. *Lancet*, 1:735–6.

Perren TJ, Powles RL, Easton D, Stolle K, Selby PJ (1988). Prevention of herpes zoster in patients by long-term oral acyclovir after allogeneic bone marrow transplantation. *American Journal of Medicine*, 85:99–101.

Petersen FB, *et al.* (1987). The effect of prophylactic intravenous immune globulin on the incidence of septicaemia in marrow transplant recipients. *Bone Marrow Transplantation*, 2:141–8.

Pollard CM, *et al.* (1986). Leukaemic relapse following Campath 1 treated bone marrow transplantation for leukaemia. *Lancet*, 2:1343–4, 1404.

Powles RL, *et al.* (1978). Cyclosporin A for the treatment of graft-versus-host-disease in man. *Lancet*, ii:1327–31.

Powles RL, *et al.* (1980*a*). Cyclosporin A to prevent graft-versus-host disease in man after allogeneic bone marrow transplantation. *Lancet*, i:327–9.

Powles RL, *et al.* (1980*b*). The place of bone marrow transplantation in acute myelogenous leukaemia. *Lancet*, i:1047–50.

Prentice HG, Brenner MK (1988). In *Recent advances in bone marrow transplantation in the treatment of leukaemia* (ed. AV Hoffbrand), pp. 153–77. Churchill Livingstone, Edinburgh.

Prentice HG, Grob JP (1986). Acute lymphoblastic leukaemia in adults. *Clinics in Haematology*, 15(3):755–88.

Prentice HG, *et al.* (1982). Use of anti-T-cell monoclonal antibody OKT3 to prevent acute graft-versus-host-disease in allogeneic bone-marrow transplantation for acute leukaemia. *Lancet*, i:700–4.

Quine WE (1986). The remedial application of bone marrow. *Journal of the American Medical Association*, 26:1012–13.

Rees JKH, Gray RG, Swirsky D, Hayhoc FGJ (1986). Principal results of the Medical Research Council's 8th acute myeloid leukaemia trial. *Lancet*, ii:1236–41.

Reisner Y, *et al.* (1981). Transplantation for acute leukaemia with HLA-A and B non identical parental marrow cells fractionated with soybean agglutinin and sheep red blood cells. *Lancet*, 2:327–31.

Robins MN, Noyes WD (1961). Aplastic anaemia treated with bone marrow transfusion from an identical twin. *New England Journal of Medicine*, 265:974–9.

Sanders JE, *et al.* (1988). Ovarian function following marrow transplantation for aplastic anaemia or leukaemia. *Journal of Clinical Oncology*, 6:813–17.

Santos GW (1983). History of bone marrow transplantation. *Clinics in Haematology*, 12:611–39.

Santos G, Colvin OM (1986). Pharmaceutical purging of bone marrow with reference to autografting. *Clinics in Haematology*, 15:67–83.

Santos GW, *et al.* (1983). Marrow transplantation for acute nonlymphoblastic leukaemia after treatment with busulphan and cyclosporin. *New England Journal of Medicine*, 309:1347–53.

Saral R, Burns WH, Laskin OL, Santos GW, Liefman, PJ (1981). Acyclovir prophylaxis of herpes simplex virus infections. *New England Journal of Medicine*, 305:63–7.

Saxon A, Mitsuyasu R, Stevens R, Champlin RE, Kimata H, Gale RP (1986). Designed transfer of specific immune responses with bone marrow transplantation. *Journal of Clinical Investigation*, 78:959–67.

Scheef W, *et al.* (1979). Controlled clinical studies with an antidote against the urotoxicity of oxazaphosphorines: preliminary results. *Cancer Treatment Reports*, 63:501–5.

Segel GB, Simon W, Lichtman MA (1986). Variables influencing the timing of marrow transplantation in patients with chronic myelogenous leukaemia. *Blood*, 68:1055–64.

Selby PJ, *et al.* (1979). Parenteral acyclovir therapy for herpes virus infection in man. *Lancet*, ii:1267–70.

Sheridan WP, *et al.* (1992). Effect of peripheral-blood progenitor cells mobilised by Filgrastin (G-CSF) on platelet recovery after high-dose chemotherapy. *Lancet*, 339:640–4.

Sokal JE, *et al.* (1985). Prognostic discrimination among younger patients with chronic granulocytic leukaemia: relevance to bone marrow transplantation. *Blood*, 66:1352–7.

Spitzer G, *et al.* (1980). The myeloid progenitor cell—its value in predicting haematopoietic recovery after autologous bone marrow transplantation. *Blood*, 55:317–23.

Storb R (1985). Marrow grafting for leukaemia. *Experimental Haematology*, 13 (Suppl. 17):6–8.

Storb R (1989). Bone marrow transplantation. In *Cancer principles and practice of oncology* (ed. VT Devita, S Hellman, and SA Rosenberg), pp. 2474–89. JB Lippincott, Philadelphia.

Storb R, Epstein RB, Graham TC, Thomas ED (1970). Methotrexate regimens for control of graft-versus-host disease in dogs with allogeneic marrow grafts. *Transplantation*, 9:240–6.

Storb R, *et al.* (1980). Marrow transplantation in thirty 'untransfused' patients with severe aplastic anaemia. *Annals of Internal Medicine*, 92:30–6.

Storb R, *et al.* (1987). Marrow transplantation for leukaemia and aplastic anaemia. Two controlled trials of a combination of methotrexate and cyclosporine versus cyclosporine alone or methotrexate alone for prophylaxis of acute graft-versus-host disease. *Transplantation Proceedings*, 19:2608–13.

Sullivan KM, *et al.* (1987). Chronic graft-versus-host disease in man. In *Progress in bone marrow transplantation* (ed. RP Gale and R Champlin), pp. 473–87. Alan R Liss, New York.

Sullivan KM, *et al.* (1988). Alternating-day cyclosporine and prednisilone for treatment of high risk chronic graft-versus-host disease. *Blood*, 72:555–61.

Sullivan KM, *et al.* (1989). Graft-versus-host disease as adoptive immunotherapy in patients with advanced hematologic neoplasms. *New England Journal of Medicine*, 320:828–34.

Thomas ED, Lochte HL, Lu WC, Ferrebee JW (1957). Intravenous infusion of bone marrow in patients receiving radiation and chemotherapy. *New England Journal of Medicine*, 257:491–6.

Thomas ED, *et al.* (1959). Supralethal whole body irradiation and isologous marrow transplantation in man. *Journal of Clinical Investigation*, 38:1709–16.

Thomas ED, *et al.* (1961). Irradiation and marrow infusion in leukaemia. *Archives of Internal Medicine*, 107:829–45.

Thomas ED, *et al.* (1975). Bone marrow transplantation. *New England Journal of Medicine*, 292:832–43, 895–902.

Thomas ED, *et al.* (1977). One hundred patients with acute leukaemia treated by chemotherapy, total body irradiation and allogeneic bone marrow transplantation. *Blood*, 49:511–33.

Thomas ED, *et al.* (1983). Marrow transplantation for patients with acute lymphoblastic leukaemia: a long term follow up. *Blood*, 62:1139–41.

Thomas ED, *et al.* (1986). Marrow transplantation for the treatment of chronic myelogenous leukaemia. *Annals of Internal Medicine*, 104:155–63.

Treleaven JG, Kemshead JT (1985). Removal of tumour cells from bone marrow: an evaluation of the available techniques. *Hematology and Oncology*, 3:65–75.

Truitt RL, LeFever AV, Shih CC-Y (1987). Graft-versus-leukaemia reactions: experimental models and clinical trials. In *Progress in bone marrow transplantation* (ed RP Gale and R Champlin), pp. 219–32. Alan R Liss, New York.

Tucker MA, Coleman CN, Cox RS, Varghese A, Rosenberg SA (1988). Risk of second cancers after treatment for Hodgkin's disease. *New England Journal of Medicine*, 318:76–81.

Urban C, *et al.* (1988). Endocrine function after bone marrow transplantation without the use of preparative total body irradiation. *Bone Marrow Transplantation*, 3:291–6.

Vogelsang GB, Hess AD, Santos GW (1988). Thalidomide for treatment of graft-versus-host disease. *Bone Marrow Transplantation*, 3:393–8

Vogelsang GB, Hess AD, Friedman KJ, Santos GW (1989). Therapy of chronic graft-v-host disease in a rat model. *Blood*, 74:507–11.

Wareham NJ, Johnson SA, Goldman JA (1982). Relationship of the duration of the chronic phase in chronic granulocytic leukaemia to the need for treatment during the first year after diagnosis. *Cancer Chemotherapy and Pharmacology*, 8:205–10.

Watson JG, Jameson B (1979). Antibiotic prophylaxis for patients in protective isolation. *Lancet*, i:1183.

Weiden PL, *et al.* (1981). Anti-leukaemia effect of graft-versus-host disease. *New England Journal of Medicine*, 25:1529–33.

Weinstein HJ, *et al.* (1983). Chemotherapy for acute myelogenous leukaemia in children and adults VAPA update. *Blood*, 62:315–19.

Weinstein H, *et al.* (1987). *Haematology and Blood Transfusion*, 30:88–92.

Winston DW (1983). Prevention and treatment of cytomegalovirus infection in bone marrow transplant recipients. In *Recent advances in bone marrow transplantation* (ed. RP Gale), pp. 425–44. Alan R. Liss, New York.

Witherspoon RP, *et al.* (1981). Recovery of antibody production in human allogeneic marrow graft recipients: influence of time post transplantation, the presence or absence of chronic graft-versus-host disease and anti-thymocyte globulin treatment. *Blood*, **58**:360–8.

Witherspoon RP, Lum LG, Storb R, Thomas ED (1982). *In vitro* regulation of immune globulin synthesis after human marrow transplantation. II Deficient T and non-T lymphocyte function within 3–4 months of allogeneic, syngeneic or autologous marrow grafting for haematologic malignancy. *Blood*, **59**:844–50.

Witherspoon RP, *et al.* (1989). Secondary cancers after bone marrow transplantation for leukemia or aplastic anemia. *New England Journal of Medicine*, **321**:784–9.

Wolff SN, *et al.* (1987). High dose cytosine arabinoside and daunorubicin as consolidation therapy for acute nonlymphocytic leukaemia in first remission: an update. *Seminars in Oncology*, **14**:12–17.

Wright SE, *et al.* (1976). Experience with second marrow transplants. *Experimental Haematology*, **4**:221–6.

Yates J, *et al.* (1982). Cytosine arabinoside with daunorubicin or adriamycin for therapy of acute myelocytic leukaemia: a CALGB study. *Blood*, **60**:454–62.

12.5 Autologous bone-marrow transplantation and intensification therapies for solid tumours and lymphomas

CLAUDIUS IRLE AND THIERRY O. PHILIP

INTRODUCTION

Survival and the hope of cure after chemotherapy are related to the attainment of complete responses (Philip and Pinkerton 1989*a*). According to one theory, tumours consist of cells that vary in their resistance to drugs (Goldie and Coldman 1985*a,b*). Thus, dosage as well as the amount of drug delivered over a given time (the dose intensity) are significant factors in determining the outcome of chemotherapy (Skipper *et al.* 1964; Frei and Canellos 1980; Thomas 1982; De Vita *et al.* 1989; Philip and Pinkerton 1989*a*). Most drugs at present used for treatment of human cancer show a linear relation between their ability to kill tumour cells (the response rate) and the dose intensity (Skipper *et al.* 1964). The importance of dose in achieving complete responses has been shown in a variety of human malignancies (Gorin and Duhamel 1987; Frei *et al.* 1988; Hagenbeek *et al.* 1988; Hryniuk 1988; Armitage 1989; Armitage and Gale 1989; Chabner and Fojo 1989; Cheson *et al.* 1989; Dalton *et al.* 1989; Frei *et al.* 1989; Hall *et al.* 1989; Ivy *et al.* 1989; Philip and Pinkerton 1989*a,b*; Philip *et al.* 1989*b*; Shea *et al.* 1989; Antman *et al.* 1990; Canon *et al.* 1990; Elias *et al.* 1990; Goldstein *et al.* 1990; Yaniv *et al.* 1990). This appears to be the case for alkylating agents such as cyclophosphamide, as well as for vincristine, etoposide, 5-fluorouracil, methotrexate, and platinum compounds (Hryniuk 1988; Philip and Pinkerton 1989*a*; Philip *et al.* 1989*c*). It must be cautioned that these observations are from limited studies and involve tumours known to have relatively steep dose–response curves to cytotoxic drugs (Hryniuk 1988). Most treatments are delivered over a short time. This factor, described as the intensity of a given treatment, can be influential. The mean dose intensity of some combinations has been calculated and shown to correlate with outcome in a variety of malignancies (Hryniuk 1988), such as acute leukaemias, high-grade non-Hodgkin's lymphoma, Hodgkin's lymphoma, multiple myeloma, embryonic carcinomas, osteosarcoma, Ewing's sarcoma, embryonic rhabdomyosarcoma, neuroblastoma, and aggressive breast cancers (Philip *et al.* 1989*a*). When first-line treatments have failed, the use of increased dose intensities has been frequently explored (Philip and Pinkerton

1989*a*). However, the use of potentially curative, high-dose chemotherapy and radiotherapy results in dose-limiting, haematological toxicity. Therefore, the reinfusion of bone marrow has been used to circumvent the unacceptably high treatment-related mortality due to prolonged marrow aplasia brought about by these treatments (Thomas 1982).

The infused bone marrow should be free of all clonogenic tumour cells. For this reason, marrow grafts were in general taken from a healthy, HLA-compatible donor. The clinical application of such allogeneic, HLA-compatible transplants is, however, restricted to patients for whom a compatible donor can be identified; less than 20 per cent of all patients. Studies in animals showed that pluripotent bone-marrow stem cells could be frozen in a viable state in the presence of the cryoprotective agent dimethylsulphoxide and retain the ability to reconstitute haemopoiesis after thawing and reinfusion. This has led to the application of autotransplantation in man (Gorin and Duhamel 1987). Bone-marrow is harvested from the patient, cryopreserved in liquid nitrogen, and reinfused later. The chief appeal of autologous bone-marrow transplantation is the universal availability of the tissue and the elimination of prolonged immunosuppression together with the risk of graft-versus-host disease and bone-marrow rejection that complicates allogeneic transplantation (Philip and Pinkerton 1989*a*). A major concern is the risk of reinfusing tumour cells contaminating the bone-marrow and the loss of the graft-versus-tumour effect that is associated with allogeneic transplantation (Favrot and Philip 1989). The clinical experience with allogeneic bone-marrow transplantation in solid tumours is limited. No evidence for an antitumour effect could be shown in other than acute non-lymphocytic leukaemias and perhaps chronic myelogenous leukaemias (Thomas 1982). From the clinical experience of over 20 000 autologous bone-marrow transplantations now available it is not yet clear whether small numbers of malignant cells that may contaminate bone-marrow can engraft and are capable of self-renewal (Favrot and Philip 1989). Indeed, only isolated case reports describe relapses due to reinfused tumour cells contaminating the marrow (Favrot and Philip 1989). None the less, efforts to remove tumour cells from marrow before reinfusion are being actively pursued. Numerous researchers have investigated a variety of purging techniques, applying monoclonal antibodies together with complement, toxin-conjugated antibodies, antibodies cross-linked to particle substrates with diverse physical properties, or *in vitro* incubations with cytotoxic drugs. The feasibility of these techniques has been demonstrated. Their toxicity is generally acceptable, as manipulated bone-marrow results in satisfactory, although somewhat delayed, haemopoietic reconstitution. However, there is as yet no convincing evidence in support of tumour cell purging from autologous bone-marrow (Favrot and Philip 1989). Despite the increasing effectiveness of antimicrobal agents, infectious complications are still common causes of death among patients undergoing marrow ablation (Bouffet 1986; Bouffet *et al.* 1988). The increasing availability of mass-produced recombinant forms of several haemopoietic regulatory factors provides hope for more effective stimulation of the formation of granulocytes and monocytes, thereby decreasing the risks of life-threatening infections in compromised patients (Daniel and Dexter 1989). Apart from direct, drug-related toxicity in various organs, the prolonged hospital stay of patients undergoing massive chemotherapy with autologous marrow rescue is also related to thrombocytopenia and severe haemorrhage remains a serious consideration (Bouffet 1986), which is a limiting factor in the wider application of massive chemotherapy. Neither of the growth factors studied so far appears to shorten dependence on platelet transfusion.

We now review in further detail some practical aspects and the present experience in tumours for which high-dose chemotherapy followed by autologous bone-marrow rescue are used.

STEM CELL COLLECTION AND STORAGE

Bone-marrow, which is the richest source of haemopoietic stem cells, is usually harvested from the anterior and posterior iliac crests by multiple needle aspirations and suspended in heparin or a mixture of citrate/phosphate/dextrose and heparin. In some instances, sternal bone marrow may also be obtained, although this is rarely necessary (Beaujean 1985; Lopez *et al.* 1985). The procedure is done in an operating theatre under either general or spinal anaesthesia. Approximately 3×10^8 nucleated cells/kg body weight of the recipient are obtained, typically representing 15 ml of marrow blood/kg body weight. Thus, in an adult, 800–1000 ml of marrow are aspirated. If a purging procedure is contemplated, many transplant teams will try to obtain a greater volume. This procedure carries a low risk for the donor, usually limited to post-operative fever in approximately 15 per cent and rarely bleeding and local infection.

For autologous bone-marrow transplantation, the cryopreservation techniques require the preparation of cell suspensions depleted of red cells. To this end, mononuclear cell suspensions are obtained by density flotation over a Ficoll–Hypaque gradient, or by a sedimentation step of buffy coat over hydroxyethyl–starch. Specifically designed elutriation equipment allows the automatic preparation of suspensions of purified mononuclear cells, resulting in a slightly better yield and improving asepsis (Hervé *et al.* 1979; Wells *et al.* 1979; Schaeffer 1980; Gilmore *et al.* 1983; Beaujean *et al.* 1984; Beaujean 1985).

The restitution of red blood cells to the patient is necessary in order to compensate for the immediate loss of volume during marrow harvesting. For patients undergoing allografting, the reinfusion of stored, autologous blood obtained from them earlier, usually several weeks before the transplant is harvested, may be considered in order to avoid exposing a healthy donor to blood-borne viral infections. Similarly, restitution of red blood cells to patients undergoing marrow harvesting for autologous bone-marrow transplantation can be done. This is accomplished by reinfusing processed bone-marrow red cells (prepared, for example by a cell separator) taken from the marrow before its cryopreservation (Beaujean 1985).

Factors influencing the quality and quantity of stem cells recovered by marrow aspiration are the intensity of and the distance from preceding chemotherapy, the marrow cellularity, extent of myelofibrosis, and the presence of hepatitis antigen. The time-lapse between harvesting and reinfusion influences marrow recovery and this is an important factor for unrelated donor transplants and for autologous transplants using non-cryopreserved marrow. Similarly, the time-lapse between high-dose chemotherapy and marrow infusion is a critical, although still insufficiently explored, factor bearing on marrow recovery and engraftment. This issue has become increasingly important as more and more multiagent conditioning regimens are being used (Gerota *et al.* 1982; Lopez *et al.* 1985).

Stem cells can also be obtained from the peripheral blood (Armitage *et al.* 1989). This approach is based on the notion that the likelihood of contamination with malignant cells is reduced in comparison to bone marrow. The known rebound of circulating stem cells after chemotherapy allows one to increase the yield of harvested stem cells by using a cell separator and is an additional reduction of the risk of contamination with malignant cells. Peripheral stem cell collection may be used for haematological rescue after high-dose chemoradiotherapy. Until recently, this approach was very cumbersome and required numerous applications of cytopheresis and cryopreservation, owing to the small quantity of circulating stem cells. The stem cell rebound that follows chemotherapy can now be dramatically accentuated with haemopoietic growth factors that increase several-fold the number of circulating stem cells. This approach may simplify the laborious task of repetitive harvesting and cryopreservation of stem cells. The greater availability of marrow growth factors will result in increased application of this approach in the future (Daniel and Dexter 1989; Migliaccio *et al.* 1990).

Engraftment of peripheral stem cells is usually rapid, but seems to be associated with tenuous long-term recovery when compared to bone-marrow grafts. These observations have led to the concept that the reinfusion of cryopreserved bone-marrow and peripheral blood mononuclear cells obtained after chemotherapy, together with *in vivo* treatment with haemopoietic growth factors, may represent the best supportive approach after massive chemotherapy. This is now being explored in several institutions.

After the harvesting of bone-marrow and the elutriation of the nucleated cell fraction of peripheral blood, samples are further purified to isolate mononuclear cells. The mononuclear cell suspensions obtained either from the bone-marrow or from the elutriation of peripheral blood are carefully frozen at a controlled rate, using dimethylsulphoxide as a cryoprotective agent; these can then be stored for a long time in liquid nitrogen (Beaujean 1985). The rate of freezing certainly appears to be a critical factor for the optimal recovery of stem cells (Hervé *et al.* 1979). This can be appreciated *in vitro* when using cultures of granulocyte colony-forming units (CFU-C); experiments show an inverse linear relation between recovery of CFU-C and rate of freezing (Schaeffer 1980). Initially, the freezing rate must not exceed 1°C/min until the plateau of diffusion heat is reached. Rebound warming is avoided by adjusting the rate of refrigeration, as controlled by the rate of liquid nitrogen injection into the freezing chamber during the release of fusion heat. Thereafter, when marrow is frozen at a rate of less than 5°C, the CFU-C recovery is generally better than 90 per cent, while it decreases to less than 20 per cent when the rate is faster than 10°C/min. To ensure adequate freezing it is essential to monitor the temperature and to adjust the addition of liquid nitrogen continuously.

When necessary, the frozen cells are thawed rapidly and reinfused intravenously (Beaujean 1985; Lopez *et al.* 1985). This can be done safely only when the contamination of the marrow by red cells is very low, as the freezing that allows the preservation of marrow stem cells results in haemolysis of the companion red cells (Hervé *et al.* 1979). The load of circulating haemoglobin may, in some instances, result in acute renal failure secondary to haemoglobinuria. The reinfusion of dimethylsulphoxide used at 10 per cent final concentration does not result in significant tissue damage (Lopez *et al.* 1985).

PURGING OF TUMOUR CELLS FROM BONE-MARROW

Methods aimed at the depletion of tumour cells potentially contaminating the bone-marrow have been devised in order to minimize the risk of their reinfusion. Physical, chemical, and immunological techniques are used.

1. *Physical separation.* Techniques such as Percoll or bovine serum albumin gradients were the first methods described and, more recently, techniques such as counterflow centrifugation have been recorded (De Witte *et al.* 1986). The selection of haemopoietic precursors for reinfusion is based on their density and these methods can be used as a preliminary step in purging. Sheep red blood rosetting or soybean lectin separation have more restricted applications in T-cell depletion (Reisner *et al.* 1983), although soybean lectin separation allows only poor elimination of neuroblastoma cells or T and B acute lymphoblastic leukaemia cells (Reisner 1983).

2. *Chemical methods.* Chemotherapeutic agents may destroy malignant cells with at least a partial preservation of normal haemopoietic progenitors (Korbling *et al.* 1987). Although this last point is still very unclear (Kluin-Nelemans *et al.* 1984), active derivatives of cyclophosphamide, either 4-hydroperoxycyclophosphamide or mafosfamide (ASTA Z 7557), are now extensively used in clinical trials for autografting in acute lymphoblastic or acute myeloid leukaemia, as well as for non-Hodgkin's lymphoma or neuroblastoma (Hervé *et al.* 1984; Hartmann *et al.* 1985; Kaizer *et al.* 1985; Gorin *et al.* 1986; Yeager *et al.* 1986). Other chemotherapeutic agents, such as etoposide, which have been tested experimentally, have not yet been used systematically in clinical trials (Chang *et al.* 1985). Some non-chemotherapeutic agents are of potential interest, among them merocyanine 540, a DNA dye with lytic activity after photoactivation (Sieber *et al.* 1984) and 6-hydroxydopamine (Reynolds *et al.* 1982).

3. *Immunological methods.* Unwanted cells are specifically targeted by monoclonal antibodies directed against cell surface antigens. These cells are then eliminated by various mechanisms (Favrot and Philip 1989), as follows.

(a) Complement-dependent lysis: monoclonal antibodies (IgM or IgG2$_a$ isotypes) lyse targeted cells in the presence of rabbit complement (Bast *et al.* 1985; Lebien *et al.* 1985; Favrot *et al.* 1986; Janossy *et al.* 1987). Some of these monoclonals, such as rat antibodies CAMPATH-1 or AL$_2$ and mouse RFAL$_3$, RFB$_7$,

BA$_1$, BA$_2$, BA$_3$, and BG$_6$, are claimed to be lytic in the presence of human complement (Stepan *et al.* 1984; Waldman *et al.* 1984; Saarinenu *et al.* 1985; Janossy *et al.* 1987).

(b) Immunomagnetic depletion: magnetic particles (either macroparticles or colloids) covered with antimouse immunoglobulins bind malignant cells through a linkage between the antimouse immunoglobulins and the monoclonal antibodies. The magnetic particles, coated with cells, are removed by a magnetic field (Poynton *et al.* 1983; Treleaven *et al.* 1984; Reynolds *et al.* 1986; Combaret *et al.* 1987; Favrot *et al.* 1987). A few other methods come from the same principle, for example malignant cells can be absorbed in a column via monoclonals attached to a solid phase through avidin–biotin linkages (Berenson *et al.* 1986*a*,*b*; Favrot and Philip 1989).

(c) Immunotoxins: monoclonal antibodies are conjugated to various plant toxins; ricin, from the castor bean *Ricinus communis*, is the one most commonly used in clinical trials (Filipovich *et al.* 1984). This consists of two chains: the toxic A-chain acts inside the cell by inhibiting protein synthesis on the 60 S subunit of ribosomes; the B-chain permits entry into the cell because it binds to galactose and *N*-galactosamine residues on the cell surface, like a monovalent lectin. The lytic activity of the ricin A-chain is persistent (1 or 2 days) and is influenced by the presence or absence of the B-chain, the affinity of the monoclonal, and the temperature and pH of incubation (Muirhead *et al.* 1983; Myers *et al.* 1984; Stong *et al.* 1984; Casellas *et al.* 1985). In spite of these disadvantages, immunotoxins are probably the most efficient agents. Other toxins coupled to monoclonals or activators with potential clinical interest have been more recently described (Ramakrishnan and Houston 1984; Uckun *et al.* 1985; Bjorn *et al.* 1986; Coombes *et al.* 1985; Favrot and Philip 1989).

Until recently, in most clinical trials, there was no proof that the bone-marrow was infiltrated by tumour and, thus, needed to be purged and also no method of demonstrating total freedom from tumour. Partial answers will be obtained in clinical models only if rigorously controlled purging procedures are used and if the presence or absence of residual malignant cells in the bone-marrow is assayed with very sensitive methods before and after purging. Such a rigorous analysis of the clinical value of purging methods is fundamental both to the future prospects of this approach and to a meaningful assessment of the role of high-dose chemotherapy and autologous marrow transplantation in the management of malignant proliferations.

Selective *in vitro* maintenance of normal haemopoietic progenitors (Chang *et al.* 1986) or the positive selection or such progenitors with relevant monoclonal antibodies (Berenson *et al.* 1986) could be an alternative to the reinjection of the whole mononuclear cell fraction of the marrow after purging.

Some experimental therapeutic approaches, such as *in vitro* immunostimulation of the patient's effector cells, involve *ex vivo* manipulation of either peripheral or bone-marrow mononuclear cells (Rosenberg *et al.* 1985), thus, the autografting techniques developed in the last decade appear to be a preliminary but essential step that may permit the introduction of new immunological approaches to therapy (Favrot and Philip 1989).

PHASE-I/II STUDIES OF VERY HIGH-DOSE CHEMOTHERAPY

As shown in Table 1, a linear dose–effect relation has been demonstrated without bone-marrow support for methotrexate (40

Table 1 Phase I/II escalation dose studies with or without autologous bone-marrow transplantation (ABMT) in solid tumours and lymphomas

| Drug | Maximum tolerated dose | | | |
	Usual dose (mg/m^2)	Without ABMT (mg/m^2)	With ABMT (mg/m^2)	Dose effect
Cyclophosphamide	500	8000	8000	×15
Etoposide (VP16)	300	2100	3000	×10
BCNU	200	600	1250	×6
Melphalan	40	100	200	×5
Cisplatin	100	250	250	(>2.5)
Carboplatin	400	1000	2000	×5
Mitomycin	10	40	90	×9
Thiotepa	30	240	1100	×38
AZQ (aziridinyl-benzoquinone)	20		150	×7
Methotrexate	500	20 000		×40
Cytosine arabinoside	500	20 000		×40

times the usual dose) (Djerassi 1975), cytosine arabinoside (40 times the usual dose) (Duff 1985), and cisplatin (Hayes *et al*. 1977). The real significance (in terms of a dose effect) of doubling the dose is not always clear because of the binding of the metabolites to serum protein (Hayes *et al*. 1977). With bone-marrow support, a clear dose effect was reported for cyclophosphamide, etoposide, mitomycin C, melphalan, aziridinylbenzoquinone (**AZQ**), 1,3-bis(2-chloroethyl)-1-nitrosourea (**BCNU**), and amsacrine as extensively reviewed by Appelbaum and Buckner (1986). It has to be noted that for cyclophosphamide, etoposide and mitomycin C, autologous marrow reinfusion has little to contribute, at least when the single drug is used, whereas with agents such as melphalan, AZQ, and BCNU, autologous bone-marrow transplantation limits the period of marrow suppression. The phase II studies of multiagent regimens have been reviewed by Appelbaum and Buckner (1986) and Pinkerton *et al*. (1986).

Conditioning regimens such as **BACT** (BCNU, aracytosine, cyclophosphamide, thioguanine), **BEAM** (BCNU, etoposide, aracytosine, melphalan), and CBV (cyclophosphamide, BCNU, etoposide (VP16)) are very extensively used with autologous bone-marrow transplantation to reduce the duration of aplasia (Pinkerton *et al*. 1986). One of the major achievements in these patients with lymphomas was to show that even in progressive disease, clear responses could be observed with these protocols, using the dose–effect relation. As with the animal experiments, this dose-related response was usually insufficient to produce cure in advanced disease, whereas in relapsed patients with less aggressive disease, response and cure may be observed (Gehan 1984; Pinkerton *et al*. 1986). In heavily pre-treated patients, studies from Boston have shown rapid and complete responses, resembling those of lymphomas, in solid tumours (Eder *et al*. 1986; Antman *et al*. 1987). These studies, considered together with the animal and human lymphoma models, suggest that cure may be possible if high-dose therapy is applied earlier in the course of evolution of solid tumours.

ROLE OF TOTAL-BODY IRRADIATION

The feasibility of total-body irradiation was first demonstrated when it was used for marrow ablation in conditioning regimens for leukaemia. Many conventional treatment regimens that use local irradiation take advantage of the radiosensitivity of most solid tumours and lymphomas and it is a logical step, therefore, to study the efficacy of this method as a systemic therapy. Early studies with either hemicorporeal irradiation or low-dose, hyperfractionated,

total-body irradiation evaluated its effectiveness in high-risk patients (D'Angio and Evans 1983). The necessity of total-body irradiation in massive therapy regimens for solid tumours remains an area of debate. There is an understandable reluctance to use such therapy in young children because of the considerable early and as yet ill-defined long-term toxicity. Similarly, the advantages of fractionated total-body irradiation remain controversial: although pulmonary toxicity is reduced (Pino *et al*. 1982), the relative cytotoxic effect in tumours with shouldered response curves remains to be clarified. Alternative strategies to total-body irradiation are further intensification of multiple chemotherapy and the use of double autografts (Goldstone *et al*. 1984; Hartmann *et al*. 1985). Although the long-term consequences of high-dose alkylating agents should also be taken into account (Hartmann *et al*. 1984), these treatment regimens are being used in cases where the likelihood of cure with conventional treatment is minimal and choice is thus limited. Such considerations are, however, of considerable importance if the indications for massive therapy are broadened to include its use as a consolidation treatment in first complete remissions.

DEFINITION OF PATIENTS' STATUS AT AUTOLOGOUS BONE-MARROW TRANSPLANTATION

Previous therapy is mostly not clearly reported in the world literature; however, this is obviously a major problem when comparing the results of different series. Confusion is also frequent between first and subsequent complete remissions and between first partial remission and primarily refractory patients and also subsequent partial remission (patients with sensitive relapses). The relevant information should be clearly stated if possible in future reports in this area.

VERY HIGH-DOSE THERAPY IN LYMPHOMAS

A retrospective study of data from the French Autogreffe study group and investigators in London was made in July 1983 (Philip *et al*. 1985*a*,*b*; Rebattu *et al*. 1985) and a review of the world literature was given by Appelbaum *et al*. (1985) and by Singer and Goldstone (1986). From these data, as shown, for example in Fig. 1, several conclusions can be drawn. Patients with true resistant relapses (that is, those whose disease is still progressing at the time of the autologous bone-marrow transplantation) will usually not be cured by massive therapy. Responses were observed in 73 per cent of the cases in Lyon, but as shown in Fig. 1, only one out of 16

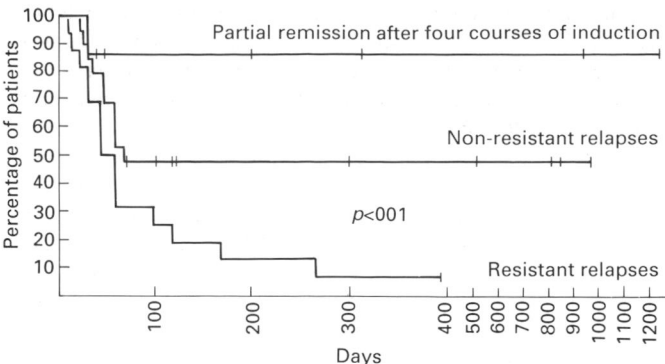

Fig. 1 Disease-free survival for 42 patients with non-Hodgkin's lymphoma (reproduced from Philip *et al.* (1984) with permission).

patients is still alive 4 years after the transplant (that is, 6 per cent). In patients with non-resistant relapses (that is, all other patients, excluding those with stable disease and those with a minor response on a rescue protocol), long-term survival appeared to be achieved in approximately one-half. Our initial data, for example concerned 15 of 19 patients in the group with non-resistant relapses who had relapsed on therapy (that is, clearly a group with a very bad prognosis). These data showed that there is no difference in outcome between patients who achieved partial or complete remission before autologous transplantation if complete remission is obtained after it. We concluded that patients in relapse have to be separated into two groups: those with resistant relapses (patients with progressive or stable disease or a minor response on salvage chemotherapy) and those with non-resistant or sensitive relapses (patients achieving a partial or complete response within the first two courses of salvage chemotherapy). Two major criticisms have been levelled at this retrospective study: the inclusion of both adults (two-thirds) and children (one-third) and the analysis of the mixture of histological types as a single group. Our series included a high proportion of childhood non-Hodgkin's lymphoma of the Burkitt's type (of 42 cases, 12 were Burkitt's lymphoma, 15 intermediate, and 15 high-grade non-Burkitt's lymphoma).

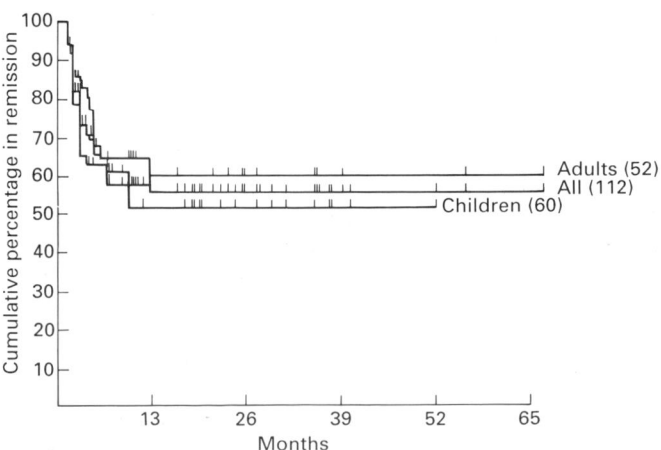

Fig. 2 Disease-free survival of children and adults, both with non-Hodgkin's lymphoma, who underwent autologous bone-marrow transplantation in European Bone Marrow Transplantation group trials (data compiled January 1984). (Reproduced from Goldstone *et al.* 1984 with permission.)

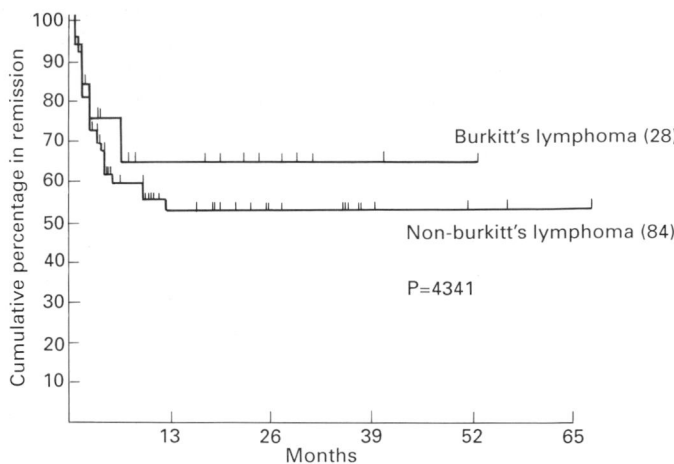

Fig. 3 Autologous bone-marrow transplantation in non-Hodgkin's lymphoma (data from EBMT, January 1984).

As shown in Figs 2 and 3, a European study by Goldstone (1985) later concluded that no statistical difference could be found either between adults and children (Fig. 2) or between Burkitt's and non-Burkitt's lymphoma (Fig. 3). The concept of resistant and sensitive relapse has been subsequently confirmed in a review of 42 cases of Burkitt's lymphoma in France (Philip *et al.* 1985*b*), a review of 42 cases of adult diffuse lymphoma from France and England (Philip *et al.* 1985*a,b*), and a review of 39 cases of non-Hodgkin's lymphoma from Houston and Omaha (Armitage *et al.* 1985).

In 1986, data from bone-marrow transplant centres in Europe and America were pooled to determine the outcome of autologous transplants in adult patients with relapsed diffuse, intermediate, or high-grade non-Hodgkin's lymphoma (excluding Burkitt's lymphoma) and to identify the prognostic significance of response to therapy preceding the bone-marrow transplantation (Philip *et al.* 1987*a*). The patients were treated with either high-dose chemotherapy alone (61 patients) or high-dose chemotherapy plus total-body irradiation (39 patients). The median age was 35 years and the median Karnofsky performance score was 80 per cent. Of these patients, 34 had progressive disease that was primarily refractory to chemotherapy (that is, they never achieved complete remission),

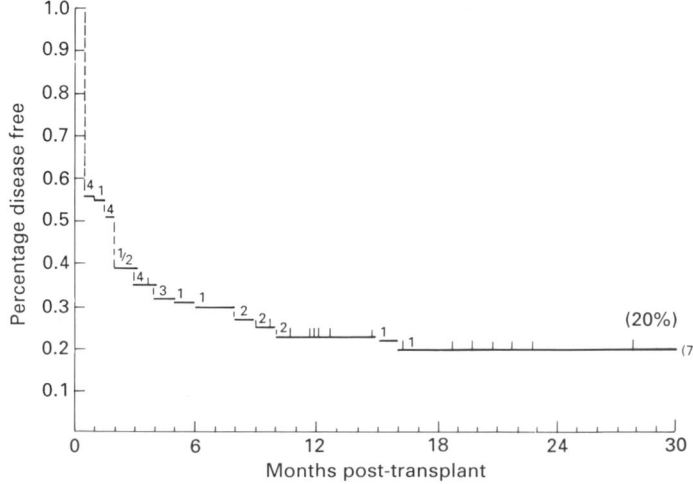

Fig. 4 Actuarial 2 year disease-free survival for 100 patients.

while 66 achieved complete remission with primary chemotherapy but later relapsed. After receiving further chemotherapy (salvage) at traditional doses, 22 patients had no response or disease progression (that is, resistant relapse), and 44 responded partially or completely (that is, sensitive relapse).

The actuarial 2 year disease-free survival rate for the entire group was 20 per cent, with the last death at 31 months and a median observation time of 33 months (Fig. 4). Disease-free survival was significantly related to previous response to chemotherapy. The 2 year disease-free survival rate was 0 per cent in the no complete remission group, 14 per cent in the resistant relapse group, and 38 per cent in the sensitive relapse group (Fig. 5). In patients who had achieved complete remission with initial chemotherapy, the disease-free survival rate after autologous bone-marrow transplantation was superior to that in those never achieving it (Fig. 6). Patients with sensitive relapse had a better disease-free survival rate than those with resistant relapse; outcome was not affected by treatment regimen and histological grade. Whether relapse occurred on or off therapy was not of significance to survival either, but the probability of responding to salvage therapy was significantly higher

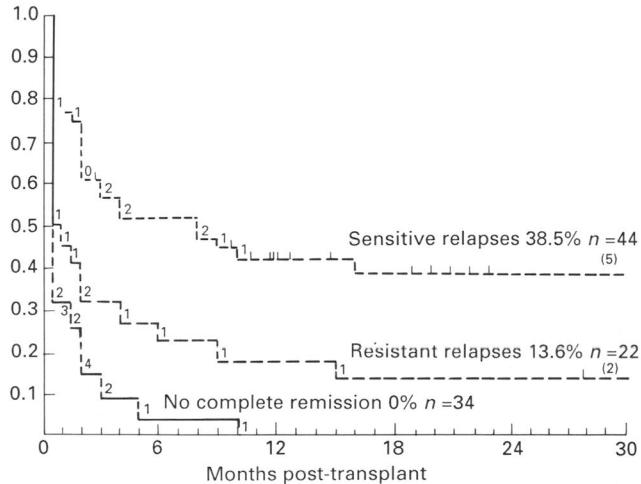

Fig. 5 Actuarial 2 year disease-free survival according to response to salvage chemotherapy.

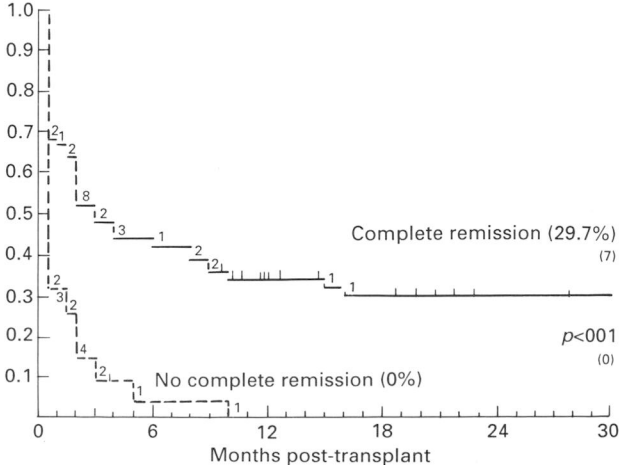

Fig. 6 Outcome after autologous bone-marrow transplantation in relation to whether patients had reached complete remission with initial therapy.

for those patients who relapsed off therapy. In conclusion, it appears that prior response to chemotherapy is an important prognostic variable in patients with intermediate or high-grade non-Hodgkin's lymphoma undergoing autologous bone-marrow transplantation (Philip *et al.* 1987a).

There remains the question of whether cures can be obtained with conventional salvage regimens without autologous bone-marrow transplantation, as there are reports of occasional long-term survivors after relapses treated with **MIME** (methyl gag, ifosfamide, methotrexate, etoposide) or **DHAP** (dexamethasone, aracytosine, platinum) (Cabanillas *et al.* 1982, 1984a,b, 1985). A randomized study is now in progress to compare conventional and high-dose treatments (Philip *et al.* 1988a). Several conclusions can, however, be drawn from the literature. The response rate after high-dose therapy and autologous bone-marrow transplantation (72 per cent achieving complete or partial remission) in the group of patients who have never reached complete remission and whose disease is progressing on conventional salvage therapy is a clear argument in favour of the dose–effect relation in non-Hodgkin's lymphoma and of investigating autologous transplantation procedures (Philip *et al.* 1987a). The significantly better survival rate achieved when patients are still responding to conventional rescue before autologous transplantation suggests that conventional rescue and high-dose therapy with such transplantation are complementary procedures. Their combination in a group of relapsed patients who previously reached complete remission may be synergistic and it led to the achievement of a survival rate of at least 40 per cent (Philip *et al.* 1988b). The difference between MIME or DHAP and autologous bone-marrow transplantation, with an overall expected survival rate in relapsing patients of approximately 5 per cent vs 20–40 per cent, cannot, however, be used definitively in support of transplantation because of selection bias (patients with better performance status, no marrow or central nervous involvement, and minimal disease being selected for bone-marrow transplantation). As an example, the response rate of 44 of 66 patients (66 per cent) in our recent data for adults indicates a large selection bias, considering that the maximum expected response rate with MIME would be in the range of 40–50 per cent in such a group (Philip *et al.* 1987a).

Several questions are still unclear and cannot be answered on the basis of the world literature review (Singer and Goldstone 1986). These concern the rôle of total-body irradiation and of involved-field radiotherapy before or after autologous transplantation, the indications for purging, and whether allogeneic marrow should be used if available (despite no difference being found in the Seattle studies (Appelbaum *et al.* 1985). In our study of autologous bone-marrow transplantation in adult lymphoma (Philip *et al.* 1987a), 39 patients received a regimen containing total-body irradiation, whereas the other 61 did not. The two groups are comparable in their number of primarily refractory cases, histological types, and bulk disease. The actuarial survival rate at 2 years is 20 per cent in both groups. In the group with primarily refractory disease (no complete remissions) and resistant relapses, response rates are identical with and without total-body irradiation (68 vs 72 per cent). Also, 75 per cent of the relapses were isolated and occurred primarily at the initial site involved before the salvage therapy, indicating that local control is a major factor. Involved-field radiotherapy (15–20 Gy) has been advocated by Phillips (1983) and Phillips *et al.* (1984), following a non-randomized comparative study favouring this strategy.

In all the published series on autologous bone-marrow transplantation, patients with marrow involvement were excluded and marrow relapses were not a major problem after the transplant. It is impossible to distinguish between relapse due to failure to eradicate the tumour and that due to reinfused tumour cells. However, experience with allogeneic marrow transplantation suggests that failure of the preparative regimen is at present responsible for the majority of relapses (Appelbaum *et al.* 1985; Singer and Goldstone 1986). Encouraging results have been reported with marrow purging in adult patients with B-cell non-Hodgkin's lymphoma and we would advocate that this issue be evaluated in a comparative study (Philip *et al.* 1988*a*). (If regimens not containing total-body irradiation are used, it is possible that spontaneous marrow recovery could occur and intensification therapy without autologous bone-marrow transplantation is thus also a possible alternative.)

The current status of autologous bone-marrow transplantation as used in the treatment of childhood lymphomas has been extensively reviewed (Pinkerton *et al.* 1986; Philip *et al.* 1988*b*) and the general conclusions are comparable to those for adults, as pointed out in an early report by our group (Philip *et al.* 1985*a*).

The indications for very high-dose therapy in Burkitt's lymphoma are, in our opinion, restricted to 20 per cent of patients and should be divided into two groups.

1. *Massive therapy and autologous bone-marrow transplantation are currently the best treatment for Burkitt's lymphoma in partial remission after initial induction therapy or in relapse when patients are still responding to rescue protocols.* The only question that remains unclear is whether the high efficacy of second-line rescue protocols will still be observed when relapses follow more aggressive initial therapy (Philip *et al.* 1988*a*).

2. *Massive therapy and autologous bone-marrow transplantation is still an experimental treatment for Burkitt's lymphoma with initial involvement of the central nervous system*, a group for which results remain disappointing with conventional regimens. Preliminary results, however, are quite promising.

Massive therapeutic regimens such as BACT or BEAM are clearly not able to cure patients with progressive disease. For this group of patients, new phase II studies are urgently needed and should be carried out through a multicentre cooperative trial. These studies could be based on conventional chemotherapy regimens tested without autologous bone-marrow transplantation to determine whether a dose–effect relation can improve the results. New massive therapeutic combinations, including high-dose *cis*-dichloraminoplatinum, melphalan, ifosfamide, BCNU, aracytosine, and high-dose methotrexate, should be explored. Combinations of various alkylating agents, as proposed by the Baltimore group, may also be a useful avenue to explore (Santos *et al.* 1985). The role of total-body irradiation remains unclear in Burkitt's lymphoma, despite results reported in other lymphomas (Philip *et al.* 1986). However, it is clear that such phase II studies will be the basis of any future progress in Burkitt's lymphoma with either conventional or massive regimens.

The role of very high-dose therapy in lymphoblastic lymphoma in children and young adults is less clear than in Burkitt's lymphoma. However, results with cyclophosphamide and total-body irradiation in relapsed patients appear to be superior to those with regimens not containing total-body irradiation (Singer and Goldstone 1986). This kind of therapy is most clearly indicated in the groups of patients who relapse with tumours still sensitive to rescue protocols. However, patients with initial disease in the central nervous system and leukaemic presentations with a very high number of circulating blast cells are also good candidates for these programmes.

The role of very high-dose therapy in Hodgkin's lymphoma was extensively reviewed by Canellos (1985) and Phillips and Reece (1986) and it appears that in approximately one-half of all patients with advanced Hodgkin's lymphoma resistant to conventional chemotherapy, remission can be achieved with existing intensive therapy regimens and autologous bone-marrow transplantation. It also appears that regimens including total-body irradiation are not better than those not containing it. The best results reported are with the cyclophosphamide/BCNU/etoposide programmes initially described by Spitzer and colleagues from the MD Anderson Hospital (Spitzer *et al.* 1980; Carella *et al.* 1984). These results are similar to those in early studies in non-Hodgkin's lymphomas and this area is probably one of the most promising for the future.

VERY-HIGH-DOSE THERAPY IN CHILDHOOD SOLID TUMOURS

We will mainly summarize the current status of the very-high-dose therapeutic programmes in rhabdomyosarcoma, Ewing's sarcoma, and neuroblastoma and describe the preliminary results in other tumours.

Rhabdomyosarcoma

Non-metastatic rhabdomyosarcoma when treated with ifosfamide/vincristine/adriamycin or vincristine/actinomycin/cyclophosphamide regimens achieves cure rates of at least 50 per cent. For metastatic disease (usually lung or bone), or with the unfavourable alveolar histological type, long-term survival is approximately 20 per cent with several new protocols including platinum derivatives, etoposide, or high-dose ifosfamide combinations.

In relapsing or resistant forms, high-dose melphalan and autologous bone-marrow transplantation had given good responses in phase II studies. On adding total-body irradiation the Lyon team reported six out of nine disease-free survivals in children with metastatic disease at 20 months. For patients in complete remission, pilot studies show 3 year survivals of approximately 40 per cent, which is better than with standard chemotherapy (Garaventa *et al.* 1989; Philip and Pinkerton 1989*a*; Yaniv *et al.* 1990).

The last report from the European Bone Marrow Transplantation Group Solid Tumours' Registry encompasses 95 patients (64 in consolidation and 31 in relapse), 21 double grafted. There are 46 rhabdomyosarcomas and 44 other soft tissue sarcomas. The overall survival is 30 per cent at 30 months. As usual, sensitive relapses do better than resistant relapses (20 vs 0 per cent). Patients in complete remission had an overall survival of 34 per cent at 40 months (Philip *et al.* 1989).

Very interesting results for rhabdomyosarcoma came from the National Cancer Institute (USA) programme with VACA (VAC plus adriamycin) plus total-body irradiation. At 12 months' follow-up the survival of some selected cases (initial stage IV, relapses, resistant relapse 93 per cent) was 45 per cent (Philip and Pinkerton 1989*a*; Yaniv *et al.* 1990).

Conclusion

The present-day overall survival at 3 years of patients treated with high-dose chemotherapy and autologous bone-marrow transplantation in rhabdomyosarcoma is better than published reports for stage IV with conventional chemotherapy. The indications for total-body irradiation are controversial because what is missing is local radiotherapy in the site(s) of metastatic disease and yet the bone-marrow, if searched by immunological methods, would reveal tumour cells. Several randomized studies of autologous bone-marrow transplantation are in progress for this small population of patients.

Neuroblastoma

This is the second most common solid tumour of childhood and the outlook in patients with limited disease (25 per cent of the cases) is good. However, with more advanced or metastatic disease, complex and demanding combinations of surgery, chemotherapy, and radiotherapy are required. Even with these, the elusive goal of cure remains a frustratingly distant objective in many patients.

The outcome with surgical treatment alone is good in the rare stage-1 patient and also in stage 2 where there is no associated lymph node involvement. Chemotherapy and/or radiation therapy is highly effective in remaining stage-2 patients, with long-term survival in excess of 75 per cent. With more advanced, initially unresectable disease (stage 3) the outcome appears to depend at least to some extent upon the completeness of eventual surgical resection after primary chemotherapy (Le Tourneau et al. 1985). The wide variation in long-term survival for this stage (40–70 per cent) thus reflects both the activity of the chemotherapy and surgical expertise. In stage-4 patients, age remains an important prognostic factor and for patients under 1 year, even with metastatic disease, cure rates may exceed 50 per cent. Between 1 and 2 years the prognosis is intermediate but for patients over 2 years of age at diagnosis there is almost universal agreement that the likelihood of long-term survival with standard chemotherapy is approximately 10 per cent. The initial response to chemotherapy is often encouraging and with most modern regimens up to 80–90 per cent will achieve at least a partial response, with clearing or improvement of metastatic disease. Unfortunately, even with surgery and radiotherapy this is rarely converted to a complete response and there is usually disease progression within the following year.

Apart from clinical staging, a number of other measures that may provide prognostic information have been introduced. Elevated serum neurone-specific enolase, raised ferritin, and high copy number of the N-myc oncogene in tumour tissue all correlate with an adverse prognosis. The Shimada classification, based upon details of stromal elements, cell differentiation, mitotic index, and age, has been shown to identify accurately poor-prognosis subgroups within clinical stages. Scintigraphy with meta-iodobenzylgunidine (**MIBG**) (Moyes et al. 1989) or magnetic resonance imaging (Couanet and Geoffray 1988) has thrown the classic staging systems for neuroblastoma somewhat into disarray. The International Staging System Working Party is currently engaged in keeping up with these changes and has produced an interim working system (Brodeur et al. 1988). Such measures are of help in making treatment decisions for the lower stages (such as stages 2 and 3) where more aggressive approaches may be warranted, but in stage-4 disease the outlook is so poor that there is little scope at the moment for a reduction in treatment intensity. Such subclassification does, however, permit better characterization of the small group of survivors. The improvement of therapy in stage 4 remains the major goal of the treatment of neuroblastoma (Graham-Pole 1989; Michon et al. 1989; Pinkerton 1990; Vossen 1990).

Until recently, most chemotherapy regimens were variations of standard sarcoma combinations with adriamycin, cyclophosphamide, and vincristine. The addition of cisplatin and the epidophyllotoxins VP16 (etoposide) and VM26 (teniposide) has had a significant impact on the initial response rate but durable remissions remain difficult to achieve (Shaffort et al. 1984). To date the most effective drugs in the treatment of neuroblastoma are cyclophosphamide, cisplatin, adriamycin, etoposide, teniposide, vincristine, peptichemio, and melphalan (Carli et al. 1982). Investigators at St Jude, Memphis, Tennessee have clearly shown that combinations are more effective than single drugs and also that the sequence of drug administration plays a major part in the response rate (that is, cisplatin followed by teniposide is superior to the reverse order). Despite clear evidence of efficacy in phase II studies as a single agent the role of adriamycin in drug combination remains controversial (Ninane et al. 1981; Philip and Pinkerton 1989b).

The dose–response relation was clearly demonstrated by a trial conducted at Villejuif, Paris, with a 2–3-fold increase in the dose of cyclophosphamide and adriamycin improving response rates from 40 to 90 per cent. Similarly, clear responses with a high dose of cisplatin (200 mg/m^2) are reported in patients progressing on conventional doses of cisplatin (100 mg/m^2) (Philip et al. 1987b). The sequential administration of non-cross-resistant drugs, based on the Goldie–Coldman hypothesis (for example, cyclophosphamide, adriamycin, vincristine, alternating with cisplatin and etoposide) has not been shown to be superior to a standard combination (Bernard et al. 1987). Drug combinations incorporating a number of agents, often in a randomized manner (dacarbazine, peptichemio, low-dose melphalan at induction), have failed to show any survival advantages (Dini et al. 1989a).

Because of the limited availability of matched, related donors in this group of very young patients, experience with autologous marrow is greater than with allogeneic marrow. Moreover, unlike leukaemia, neuroblastoma only secondarily involves the bone marrow, which may be cleared of overt tumour by effective chemotherapy before marrow harvest. Various purging techniques have been developed which, in vitro, are capable of removing residual tumour cells from marrow (Pinkerton et al. 1986). The need for such purging in practice remains a contentious issue as the clonogenic potential of reinfused neuroblastoma cells is difficult to demonstrate (Favrot and Philip 1989). The main limiting effect in the use of the megatherapeutic procedure remains its ability to ablate completely the malignant cell population.

The potential value of total-body irradiation is suggested by the finding of 20 per cent progression-free survival at 2 years in a group of highly selected patients with recurrent disease when it was used in the conditioning regimen. No progression-free survivors were reported when a regimen without this irradiation was used (Philip and Pinkerton 1989b; Philip et al. 1989). With or without total-body irradiation, with single or two sequential graft procedures, 40–45 per cent progression-free survivors at 2 years were reported in patients grafted either in complete remission or in partial remission (Hartmann et al. 1987; Philip et al. 1987b). No advantage was shown at 2 years in this group for the regimen containing total-body irradiation. The mortality rate is similar for each conditioning regimen. It is clear that in all studies no plateau has yet been reached in the survival curves at or beyond 2 years. Survival of approximately 20 per cent at 5 years and 15 per cent at 6–7 years is expected. However, O. Hartmann (unpublished) had shown 40 per cent survival at 5 years with no late relapse in a small subgroup of patients (complete remission for bone, bone-marrow, and catecholamines before surgery). This was also shown retrospectively in the Léon-Bérard/Marseille/Curie/Est de France (**LMCE**) group and the Italian group (unpublished data).

Interest in the concept of a double-graft procedure in neuroblastoma has been kindled by the timing of early relapse after bone-marrow transplantation (that is, between 3 and 12 months post-graft for the majority of the cases). Among selected patients in partial remission after induction therapy who received a double graft without total-body irradiation there were no reported survivors at 2 years. This differs from the Lyon/Marseille/Curie pilot study in which a double graft and total-body irradiation were used instead of a single graft with survivors reported up to 5 years (Hartmann *et al.* 1987; Philip *et al.* 1989).

The European Neuroblastoma Study Group has made a prospective, randomized study of high-dose melphalan in stage-3 and -4 patients who achieved at least partial remission after a standardized, platinum-containing induction regimen. There was a significant advantage at 2 years for the melphalan group, both in terms of median survival and disease progression-free duration. This provides a rational basis for the inclusion of this agent at high dose in future protocols (Pritchard *et al.* 1986). Total-body irradiation is still included in many pre-transplant regimens because of *in vitro* radiosensitivity data and early clinical experience. However, because of concern about the contribution of this irradiation to both short- and long-term morbidity, its inclusion requires prospective evaluation. It is possible that the substitution of other drugs at high dose might provide a better therapeutic index. Late effects such as second malignancies are beginning to be described and avoidance, if possible, of this problem must be a consideration in the design of new regimens. However, for the present the first concern is to achieve prolonged, good-quality remission in patients with neuroblastoma.

Results

More than 400 autologous bone-marrow transplants have been done in Europe, more than 200 in the United States, and approximately 200 in other countries (Graham-Pole *et al.* 1989; Philip *et al.* 1989).

Of the 439 grafts in the 1990 European Bone Marrow Transplantation (**EBMT**) Group review, 385 were as consolidation of first-line therapy (complete remission and very good partial remission, 212; partial remission, 173) and 50 after relapse or progression (including 35 at salvage therapy). In 80 per cent of patients the marrow was purged using immunomagnetic beads (40 per cent) or mafosfamide (40 per cent).

Clear conclusions can be drawn from this large European review.

1. Resistant relapses are not worthwhile to treat with such therapy. None of the children is alive and progression free at 2 years.

2. Forty per cent of the grafted patients are alive without progression 2 years after bone-marrow transplantation. Conditioning regimens with or without total-body irradiation give equivalent results, as do one or two autologous bone-marrow transplantations and purged or unpurged techniques. Partial response did as well as complete remission or very good partial remission and quality of surgical excision and age did not contribute either. Patients with negative MIBG bone scans at transplantation did better than all the other patients together.

3. Patients alive without progression at 2 years are not cured and no more than 20 per cent are still alive at 5 years. Patients with no bone-marrow involvement at diagnosis (stage IVS; over 1 year of age) did better, with a survival of 50 per cent at 5 years.

4. Patients with sensitive relapse could be alive without progression in 30 per cent of cases after 2 years; additional studies in this group are warranted.

Toxicity

The death rate from toxicity was 18 per cent for 'relapses' and 11 per cent for 'consolidation'. No difference was found in toxic effects between one and two grafts but total-body irradiation was more toxic (16 vs 8 per cent; $p < 0.05$).

Other studies

In the United States, during the period 1984–1989, the Pediatric Oncology Group had enrolled 74 patients with disseminated neuroblastoma from 1 to 15 years of age (median 4 years). Seven additional patients had allogeneic bone-marrow transplantation. The myeloablative treatment consisted of LPam (Melphalan), total-body irradiation, and immunomagnetic purging. Of the 81 patients grafted, 37 (46 per cent) relapsed at 1–21 months (median 6 months), while 12 (15 per cent) died of treatment-related toxicity. Thirty-two (31.8 per cent) of the children are in continuous complete remission with a short median follow-up of 14 months (range 6–47 months) (August and Auble 1989). The Children's Hospital of Philadelphia presented concordant results in 28 patients, aged from 2 to 30 years; 35 per cent are in continuous complete remission at 9–90 months (Reynolds *et al.* 1989). The Child Cancer Study Group entered 31 patients (stages II–IV) with poor prognosis in a limited pilot study. The regimen included cisplatin, etoposide, doxorubicin, and LPam plus total-body irradiation. At 23 months the overall survival probability is near 50 per cent (Philip *et al.* 1990).

The International Bone Marrow Transplant Registry has shown similar results with allogeneic bone-marrow transplantation compared to autologous bone-marrow transplantation at 17 months of follow-up (Graham-Pole *et al.* 1989).

A review of 62 patients by the LMCE group with a medium follow-up up of 59 months after autologous bone-marrow transplantation shows that continuous complete remission is 40 per cent at 2 years, 25 per cent at 5 years, and 13 per cent at 7 years. For a subgroup of 18 children with complete regression of metastasis the disease-free survival is 37 per cent at 4 years, with no relapses up to 5 years after autologous bone-marrow transplantation. Thus, a small group of patients with stage IV neuroblastoma can be cured with this type of therapy (Philip *et al.* 1987*b,c*).

Discussion

Fundamental conclusions are as follows: the most effective first-line therapy includes a large number of non-cross-resistant drugs, prognosis improves if patients are intensified and grafted early, autologous and allogeneic bone-marrow transplantations give similar results, purging appears not to be critical, total-body irradiation does not produce any advantages, and double grafting does not improve survival rates (Pinkerton 1990; Yaniv *et al.* 1990).

The optimal timing for the graft is still unclear. Controversy still surrounds all these matters and the arguments and research of concerned medical specialists should be followed attentively in the medical literature.

Ewing's sarcoma

Peripheral, non-bulky Ewing's sarcoma has a generally very good prognosis. For other axial and large-volume tumours, chemotherapy is usually only temporarily effective. Metastatic disease at diagnosis presents poor survival at 2 years (15 per cent) and no survival at 4 years with conventional chemotherapy, with the exception of the Memphis protocol (Dini *et al.* 1989*b*). European teams had shown a general pattern of response to high-dose chemotherapy plus autologous bone-marrow transplantation similar to the outcome in patients with lymphoma after massive chemotherapy: 80 per cent of continuous complete remissions at 12 months for patients in complete remission, a good response for sensitive relapse, and a very bad one for resistant relapse (Philip and Pinkerton 1989a).

The experience of the National Cancer Institute with autologous bone-marrow transplantation is probably one of the largest: with the VACA plus total-body irradiation regimen, 26 of 56 selected patients with very bad prognosis were in continuous remission at 2 years (Kinsella et al. 1983).

In 1990 the EBMT Solid Tumours Registry reported results from 90 patients (50 per cent of children). There were 52 consolidations and 38 relapses (26 sensitive relapse and 18 resistant relapse). Total-body irradiation was applied to 40 per cent of the patients. With a median follow-up from grafting of 3 months, overall survival is 30 per cent; resistant relapse had no survivors at 2 years whereas 46 per cent of patients consolidated from 185 complete remissions are alive at 30 months (Philip et al. 1989b; Hartmann et al. 1990).

The group from the Institute Gustave-Roussy reported on results of a phase II trial with 32 children treated with high-dose chemotherapy and marrow rescue from 1982 to 1987. In 14 patients with measurable targets, 61 per cent had a good response. The better protocols included HDBUS (busulphan high dose) plus other alkylating agents. Four out of 18 patients in consolidation obtained prolonged survivals (one is alive at 6 years) (Pinkerton et al. 1989).

Conclusion

Considering the results of semi-continuous conventional chemotherapy (St Jude protocol), which is still the first choice for these patients, the place of high-dose chemotherapy plus autologous bone-marrow transplantation is still unclear. The present situation is very dynamic and perhaps some good opportunities from phase II studies aimed at patients in first relapse will allow prospective studies to be set up (Philip and Pinkerton 1989a; Yaniv et al. 1990).

Other tumours

The multidisciplinary approach to treatment of Wilms' tumour is very successful; 80 per cent of children attain long-term survival. Present objectives are towards reducing the side-effects of treatment.

Nearly 20 per cent of Wilms' tumours are not curable by conventional methods. This population comprises patients with unfavourable histological types, metastatic disease, or resistance to first-line therapy.

In the experience of the Royal Marsden group, HDL-Pam resulted in six out of six complete remissions and two long-term survivors. HDC-DDP plus etoposide and whole-lung or local radiotherapy produced three out of seven complete remissions in patients treated by the Italian group. The EBMT Solid Tumours Registry studied 19 patients from 1982 to 1988. There were 15 relapses (14 salvage therapy) and four consolidations (three complete remissions; one partial remission). Overall the survival is 40 per cent at 31 months. Most regimens consisted of melphalan plus VCR or etoposide (Garaventa et al. 1989; Philip and Pinkerton 1989a; Yaniv et al. 1990).

Other solid tumours have been said to respond to high-dose chemotherapy plus autologous bone-marrow transplantation. In general, the same principles of early intensification or consolidation and of selection of chemosensitive relapses apply.

VERY-HIGH-DOSE THERAPY FOR SOLID TUMOURS IN ADULTS

A number of phase-II studies of high-dose, single-agent therapy with autologous bone-marrow transplantation have been made or are in progress in adult patients with solid tumours. From the extensive review by Appelbaum and Buckner (1986), some facts are clear. BCNU at doses of approximately $800-1500 \text{ mg/m}^2$ produces a good response rate in melanoma (45 per cent response; 16 per cent complete remissions), lung cancer (46 per cent response; no complete remissions), brain cancer (44 per cent response; 7 per cent complete remissions), and sarcoma (75 per cent response; no complete remissions). Melphalan at doses of $140-200 \text{ mg/m}^2$ has also been reported to produce a good response rate in melanoma (74 per cent response; 31 per cent complete remissions), neuroblastoma (70 per cent response; 50 per cent complete remissions), Ewing's sarcoma (80 per cent response; 20 per cent complete remissions), germ cell tumour (67 per cent response; 17 per cent complete remissions), ovarian carcinoma (56 per cent response; 14 per cent complete remissions), breast cancer (67 per cent response; mostly complete remissions), and colon carcinoma (56 per cent response; 14 per cent complete remissions). Etoposide at doses of $1500-2000 \text{ mg/m}^2$ also showed good response rates in germ cell cancer (83 per cent response; 16 per cent complete responses), small-cell lung cancer (85 per cent response; 31 per cent complete remissions), and brain cancer (50 per cent response; no complete remissions).

Studies of high-dose combinations have been reviewed by Antman et al. (1987a) but are still in their early days and are a direct continuation of the phase I dose-escalation studies. These schedules mainly use combinations of alkylating agents (Eder et al. 1986), as first proposed for leukaemia by the Baltimore group (Santos et al. 1985). The STAMP 1 and 2 programmes (solid tumour autologous marrow programme) from Boston are very encouraging because rapid complete remission was observed; this result is similar to the early experience in lymphomas with very-high-dose therapy in resistant patients. These protocols, the first to achieve such rapid complete remissions in advanced solid tumours, are very promising in spite of the short duration of the response (Eder et al. 1986; Antman et al. 1987a). Although most of these regimens have no proven clinical benefit in end-stage disease, the high response rate may provide important leads for the development of new combinations to be used in a setting of minimal residual disease (Antman et al. 1987b).

Small cell lung cancer

A study from the Ludwig Institute of Brussels is of particular note because after standard induction treatment, patients with small cell lung cancer were randomized to a further course of chemotherapy at conventional dosage versus late intensification with autologous marrow support (Humblet et al. 1987). In the transplantation arm, the rate of complete remission increased from 39 per cent before randomization to 79 per cent. Median relapse-free survival after randomization was 68 vs 55 weeks in favour of consolidation. The conclusion is that very-high-dose therapy results in a significant increase in the rate of complete remission and a significant increase in the relapse-free survival, but with no major improvement in the overall survival. In another study by Farha et al. (1983) at the MD Anderson Hospital in Texas, untreated patients initially received high-dose therapy followed by marrow rescue. They then received prophylactic cranial irradiation and four courses of the same drugs at standard dosage, followed by radiotherapy to the primary tumour. All patients responded (54 per cent completely), with a median time to treatment failure and a median survival of 41 and 56 weeks, respectively.

At University College Hospital, London, 25 newly diagnosed patients were given high-dose cyclophosphamide and radiotherapy to the primary site (Souhami *et al.* 1983). Of these patients, 56 per cent attained complete remission, with a median duration of 43 weeks and a median survival of 69 weeks. These results are comparable to those of a standard regimen for small-cell lung cancer but were obtained with a single treatment.

At the MD Anderson Hospital, 32 patients with untreated, limited, small-cell lung cancer have been studied. The patients received three cycles of induction therapy, followed by two courses of intensification with autologous bone-marrow transplantation (Spitzer *et al.* 1986). Of the 13 patients who were in complete remission at the time of transplant, five remain disease free at 4 or more years, whereas only one of nine partial responders before transplant remains disease free. Contrasts between reports are found in the relapse pattern. In Humblet's patients, relapse was mainly at the primary site, while relapses were mainly systemic in Spitzer's patients. This difference may stem from the absence of thoracic irradiation in Humblet's study.

Melanoma

The relatively promising results in small-cell lung cancer contrast with those for the chemotherapy-resistant tumour, melanoma. A significant rate of complete remission for high-dose melphalan is first seen at doses of 180 mg/m^2. There appears to be a dose–response relation in the study by Lazarus *et al.* (1985) of doses of 180 and 225 mg/m^2; however, in a larger study, patients treated with 260 mg/m^2 melphalan achieved only an 8 per cent rate of complete remission, with a 43 per cent response rate overall (Cornbleet *et al.* 1983). Melphalan or BCNU at standard doses produce responses in 10–20 per cent of patients. When these drugs are given at high doses with autologous bone-marrow transplantation, response rates of 40–65 per cent occur and there is a significant proportion of complete remissions. High-dose chemotherapy without marrow transplantation in melanoma has also been reported by the Baltimore group (Tchekmedyian *et al.* 1986).

Breast cancer

Advanced breast cancer is at present incurable and palliative hormonal or chemotherapeutic treatments are generally given, depending on the receptor status and the relation to menopause. In oestrogen or progesterone receptor-rich tumours, hormonal manipulations are the treatment of first choice, while in the receptor-negative tumours, systemic combination chemotherapy is most widely used. There is no consensus as to the best combination regimen, although anthracycline-containing combinations appear more effective. However, complete responses were only rarely obtained with these treatments, and all patients died of progressive disease (Peters *et al.* 1988).

Considerable interest has now arisen in the use of high-dose chemotherapy for metastatic stage-3 and -4 breast cancer presenting poor prognostic factors, as this is a common and generally chemosensitive tumour that appears not to be curable at conventional dosages (Antman *et al.* 1987*b*; Frei *et al.* 1988; Spinolo *et al.* 1989). However, alkylating agents display a steep response curve *in vivo* and *in vitro* and dose escalation using single alkylating agents, as well as combinations, has been undertaken. Dose intensification treatments have been investigated either at relapse or as a consolidation treatment after induction chemotherapy, similar to the approach that has resulted in cures for lymphoma (Spitzer *et al.* 1980; Antman and Gale 1988; Peters *et al.* 1988). Drug evaluation studies have shown that thiotepa and cyclophosphamide

are the most active agents. Combination regimens and particularly those including combinations of alkylating agents resulted in higher response rates than single-drug regimens and particularly in a higher proportion of complete remissions (over 70 per cent complete remissions in previously untreated patients) (Antman and Gale 1988). The role of non-alkylating agents such as platinum, etoposide, and anthracycline in combination with alkylating agents remains to be defined (McGuire *et al.* 1988). In several studies, total-body irradiation was included but its contribution remains undetermined (Armitage and Bierman 1989). As bone-marrow infiltration by tumour is a serious concern in breast cancer, efforts to remove potentially contaminating cells from the marrow have been undertaken, using gradient fractionation and allowing the removal of 1–2 logs of tumour cells (Kies *et al.* 1988). However, the need for this procedure is controversial as multimetastatic cancer was not observed in a review of over 300 procedures. In all these studies, complete responses were unfortunately of short duration, as overall median time to treatment failure was generally disappointingly short (less than 10 months). Relapses were predominantly at the sites of primary bulk disease or within previous irradiation fields. However, there appears to be a small subset of patients that can derive long-term benefit from this approach, as several groups have reported prolonged survival of some patients. Thus and by analogy with the results obtained in lymphoma autologous bone-marrow transplantation may be curative for a subset of women with stage-4 breast cancer. Future clinical trials are necessary to define the treatment timing, drug combination and dosage and circumscribe the subset that benefits the most from this approach (Antman and Gale 1988; Hortobagyi 1988).

Germ cell tumours

The prognosis of metastatic non-seminomatous germ cell tumours has been considerably improved by the advent of combined treatments, with multidrug chemotherapy of cisplatin, bleomycin, and either etoposide or vinblastin followed by surgery for metastases. However, after relapse, conventional rescue treatments are often of little efficacy, and the prognosis of patients that fail to reach complete remission is dismal (Schots *et al.* 1988; Armitage *et al.* 1989; Carella *et al.* 1989). In this group, investigations are directed to more aggressive treatments involving marrow rescue because marrow involvement is rare. As these recurrent tumours frequently retain some drug sensitivity, intensive chemotherapy with marrow rescue has been explored by a number of groups. Several agents, such as carboplatinum, ifosfamide, cyclophosphamide, and etoposide, are known to induce a steep dose response, which allows remissions in patients who were already treated and refractory to conventional doses of these drugs. However, their combined use is limited by marrow toxicity. This can be circumvented by rescue marrow reinfusion. To date, the experience with high-dose chemotherapy for relapsed non-seminomatous germ cell tumours is still limited. As previously found for lymphomas, only sensitive relapses benefit from intensification treatments, although most patients (60 per cent) will reach a complete remission. Even in the presence of poor prognostic factors such as large tumour mass, raised β-human chorionic gonadotrophin, and increased number of metastatic sites, results are encouraging, as more than 50 per cent are still alive after 1.5 years in a recent French study.

Ovarian cancers

Similar to the experience with testicular cancer, bone marrow metastasis is rare in ovarian cancer. The discovery of residual disease at a second look after optimal multidrug chemotherapy bears a poor prognosis. In this situation, high-dose chemotherapy with marrow rescue has been evaluated in a limited number of series, using a variety of regimens based on alkylating agents (BCNU, melphalan, nitrosourea) without major improvement in survival. Studies exploring novel conditioning regimens are in progress and preliminary results appear promising.

Brain tumours

Virtually all of the larger series of autologous bone-marrow transplantations for brain tumours have included high-dose BCNU. Hilderbrand *et al.* (1980) from Brussels reported on the first group of seven patients treated with lomustine (CCNU) but observed no responses by computed tomography of the brain. Of 20 patients treated with 1050 mg/m² BCNU and 60 Gy whole-brain radiotherapy, 85 per cent were still alive between 1 and 28 months later (Takvorian *et al.* 1983). When, in another study, a dose of 1200 mg/m² BCNU was used, two of 27 patients who previously failed to respond were disease free at over 3.5 years, but six of 12 patients treated adjuvantly were disease free between 7 and 59 months later (Phillips *et al.* 1985, 1986). Perren *et al.* (1987) also reported very promising results in high-grade gliomas, using high-dose BCNU before radiotherapy and very early after surgery. They found that 11 of 67 patients with grade IV gliomas were alive and disease free 26–84 months after diagnosis. In Biron's report on 100 patients, the results were similar. These studies are at least a promising start; however, toxicity was substantial, with the development of BCNU-associated pulmonary fibrosis and hepatic necrosis (Phillips *et al.* 1985, 1986). The role of high-dose BCNU and whole-brain radiotherapy has not been assessed and we can conclude that treatment duration is short, quality of life good but median survival not dramatically improved.

FUTURE PROSPECTS FOR VERY HIGH-DOSE THERAPY IN LYMPHOMAS AND SOLID TUMOURS

Studies of experimental tumour systems *in vitro* and *in vivo* have demonstrated clearly that the ability to kill tumour cells is directly related to the dose of radio- or chemotherapeutic agents (Frei and Canellos 1980). Goldie and Coldman (1979, 1985a,b) and Norton (Norton and Simon 1977; Norton 1985), have also shown, with others (Pinkerton *et al.* 1986), that minimal residual disease provides the best opportunity for the dose–effect relations to be explored. Results obtained in human models of very high-dose therapy, with or without autologous bone-marrow transplantation, for leukaemia are consistent with these theoretical assumptions (Pinkerton *et al.* 1986). Because of the success of marrow transplantation in the treatment of leukaemia, there has been increased interest in its possible application in non-Hodgkin's lymphoma; here, too, descriptions of definite success can be found in the literature. Lymphoma is on the borderline between leukaemia and solid tumours and this model is thus encouraging for oncologists.

However, several questions still remain with regard to solid tumours. In the majority of phase-II studies, impressive response rates are observed in progressive disease resistant to conventional drug doses, thus, there is clinical confirmation of a dose–effect relation in the solid tumours. However, the majority of these responses are incomplete, whereas for leukaemia and lymphoma they are usually complete, even in resistant disease. It appears that the best combinations of drugs for solid tumours have yet to be found. In this context, the report from Boston of rapid achievement of complete remission in breast cancer with the STAMP programme may provide a significant lead (Antman *et al.* 1987b). Because of the contamination of autologous marrow by malignant cells, the question of whether these regimens can be explored without autologous bone-marrow transplantation is open (Pinkerton *et al.* 1986). If total-body irradiation is not included in a conditioning regimen, this question is a realistic one because there is clear evidence that many protocols of this kind are not completely ablative (Pinkerton *et al.* 1986).

These open questions still leave room for the use of very high-dose therapy in future therapy of solid tumours, but the place and role of autologous bone-marrow transplantation, which is merely a means of lessening severe marrow toxicity, will be dependent upon the answers.

REFERENCES

Antman K, Gale RP (1988). Advanced breast cancer: high-dose chemotherapy and bone marrow autotransplants. *Annals of Internal Medicine*, 108:570–4.

Antman K, Eder JP, Frei E (1987a). High dose chemotherapy with bone marrow support for solid tumors. In *Important advances in oncology* (ed. V de Vita, S Hellman, and S Rosenberg), pp. 221–36. JB Lippincott, New York.

Antman K, *et al.* (1987b). A high dose combination alkylating agent preparative regimen with autologous bone marrow support: the DCFI/BIN experience. *Cancer Treatment Report*, 71:19–25.

Antman K, *et al.* (1990). High-dose thiotepa alone and in combination regimens with bone marrow support. *Seminars in Oncology*, 1:33–8.

Appelbaum FR, Buckner CD (1986). Overview of the clinical relevance of autologous bone marrow transplantation. *Clinical Haemotology*, 1:1–10.

Appelbaum FR, *et al.* (1985). Marrow transplantation as treatment for patients with recurrent malignant lymphoma. *International Journal of Cell Cloning*, 4:216–20.

Armitage JO (1989). Bone marrow transplantation in the treatment of patients with lymphoma. *Blood*, 73:1749–58.

Armitage JO, Bierman PT (1989). Is there an optimum conditioning regimen for patients with lymphoma undergoing autologous bone marrow transplantations? In *ABMT: Proceedings of the Fourth International Symposium* (ed. KA Dicke, G Spitzer, S Jagannath, and MJ Evinger-Hodges), pp. 299–303. University of Texas M. D. Anderson Hospital and Tumor Institute, Houston.

Armitage JO, Gale RP (1989). Bone marrow autotransplantation. *American Journal of Medicine*, 86:203–6.

Armitage JO, *et al.* (1985). Which patients with lymphoma can be salvaged with high-dose reduction and autologous marrow rescue? In *Autologous bone marrow transplantation: Proceedings of the First International Symposium* (ed. KA Dicke, G Spitzer, and AR Zander), pp. 57–60. University of Texas M. D. Anderson Hospital and Tumor Institute, Houston.

Armitage JO, *et al.* (1989). Bone marrow transplantation in the treatment of Hodgkin's lymphoma: problems, remaining challenges, and future prospects. *Recent Results in Cancer Research*, 117:246–53.

Athanasou NA, *et al.* (1990). Origin of marrow stromal cells and haemopoietic chimaerism following bone marrow transplantation determined by *in situ* hybridisation. *British Journal of Cancer*, 61:385–9.

August CS, Auble B (1989). Autologous bone marrow transplantation for advanced neuroblastoma at the Children's Hospital of Philadelphia: an update. In *ABMT: Proceedings of the Fourth International Symposium* (ed. KA Dicke, G Spitzer, S Jagannath, and MJ Evinger-Hodges), pp. 567–73. University of Texas M. D. Anderson Hospital and Tumour Institute, Houston.

Bast RC, *et al.* (1985). Elimination of malignant clonogenic cells from human bone marrow using multiple monoclonal antibodies and complement. *Cancer Research*, 45:499–502.

Beaujean F (1985). Freezing methods. *Blood Transfusion and Immunohaematology*, 5:391–6.

Beaujean F, Hartmann O, Le Forestier C, Bayet S, Duedari N, Parmentier C (1984). Successful infusion of 40 cryopreserved autologous bone marrow. *In vitro* studies of the freezing procedure. *Biomedicine*, **38**:348–51.

Berenson RJ, Andrews RG, Bensinger WI, Kalamasz D, Knitter G, Bernstein ID (1986*a*). *In vivo* reconstitution of hematopoiesis in baboons using 1.8 positive marrow cells isolated by avidin–biotin immunoadsorption. *Blood*, **68**:287–90.

Berenson RJ, Bensinger WI, Kalamasz D, Martin P (1986*b*). Elimination of Daudi lymphoblasts from human bone marrow using avidin–biotin immunoadsorption. *Blood*, **67**:509–11.

Bernard JL, *et al.* (1987). Sequential cisplatin/VM26 and vincristine/ cyclophosphamide/doxorubicin in metastatic neuroblastoma: an effective alternating non-cross resistant regimen? *Journal of Oncology*, **5**:1952–9.

Bjorn MJ, Groetsema G, Scalapino L (1986). Antibody–pseudomonas exotoxin A conjugates cytotoxic to human breast cancer cells *in vitro*. *Cancer Research*, **46**:3262–8.

Bouffet E (1986). Complications de la chimiothérapie lourde avec greffe de moelle. Etude de 103 observations consécutives au Centre Léon Bérard. Thèse. Lyon.

Bouffet E, Biron P, Frappaz D, Philip T (1988). Toxic deaths after autologous bone marrow transplantations: rate and etiology. In *Proceedings of the Third International Conference on Autologous Bone Marrow Transplantation* (ed. KA Dicke, G Spitzer, S Jagannath, and MJ Evinger-Hodges), pp. 633–8. University of Texas M. D. Anderson Hospital and Tumor Institute, Houston.

Brodeur GM, *et al.* (1988). International criteria for diagnosis, staging, and response to treatment in patients with neuroblastoma. *Journal of Clinical Oncology*, **6**:1874–81.

Brodsky I, Bulova S, Crilley P (1989). The role of busulfan/cyclophosphamide regimens in allogeneic and autologous bone marrow transplantation. *Cancer Investigation*, **7**:509–13.

Cabanillas F, Hagemeister FB, Bodey GP, Freireich EJ (1982). IMVP-16: an effective regimen for patients with lymphoma who have relapsed after initial combination chemotherapy. *Blood*, **60**:693–9.

Cabanillas F, Hagemeister FB, Bodey GP (1984*a*). M. D. Anderson experience with VP16 for therapy of refractory or recurrent lymphoma. In *Etoposide (VP-16); current status and new developments* (ed. BF Issel, FM Muggia, and SK Carter), pp. 313–20. Academic, New York.

Cabanillas F, *et al.* (1984*b*). MIME combination chemotherapy or refractory or recurrent lymphomas. *Proceedings of the American Society of Clinical Oncology*, **3**:250–6.

Cabanillas F, *et al.* (1985). Results of ifosfamide–etoposide combinations for patients with recurrent or refractory aggressive lymphoma. In *Malignant lymphomas and Hodgkin's disease: experimental and therapeutic advances* (ed. F Cavalli), pp. 485–90. Nijhoff, Boston.

Canellos P (1985). Bone marrow transplantation as salvage therapy in advanced Hodgkin disease: allogenic or autologous? *Journal of Clinical Oncology*, **11**:1451–6.

Canon JL, Humblet Y, Symann M (1990). Resistance to cisplatin: how to deal with the problem? *European Journal of Cancer*, **26**:1–3.

Carella AM, *et al.* (1984). High dose chemotherapy and non-frozen ABMT in resistant or relapsed malignant lymphomas. *Cancer*, **54**:2836–40.

Carella AM, *et al.* (1989). Optimal timing of autologous bone marrow transplantation for patients with Hodgkin's lymphoma. In *ABMT: Proceedings of the Fourth International Symposium* (ed. KA Dicke, G Spitzer, S Jagannath, and MJ Evinger-Hodges), pp. 261–7. University of Texas M. D. Anderson Hospital and Tumour Institute, Houston.

Carli M, Green AA, Hayes FA, Rivera G, Pratt CB (1982). Therapeutic efficacy of single drugs for childhood neuroblastoma: a review. In *Proceedings of the XIIIth SIOP meeting, Marseille* (ed. C Raybaud), pp. 141–50. Excerpta Medica, Amsterdam.

Casellas P, *et al.* (1985). Optimal elimination of leukemic T cells from human bone marrow with T101-ricin A chain immunotoxin. *Blood*, **65**:289–91.

Chabner BA, Fojo A (1989). Multidrug resistance: P-glycoprotein and its allies— the elusive foes. *Journal of the National Cancer Institute*, **81**:910–13.

Chang J, *et al.* (1986). Reconstitution of haemopoietic system with autologous marrow taken during relapse of acute myeloblastic leukaemia and grown in long-term culture. *Lancet*, **i**:294–5.

Chang TT, *et al.* (1985). Synergistic effect of 4-hydroperoxycyclophosphamide and etoposide on a human promyelocytic leukemia cell line (HL-60) demonstrated by computer analysis. *Cancer*, **45**:2434–7.

Cheson BD, Lacerna L, Leyland-Jones B, Sarosy G, Wittes RE (1989). Autologous bone marrow transplantation. *Annals of Internal Medicine*, **110**:51–65.

Combaret V, Favrot MC, Kremens B, Laurent JC, Philip I, Philip T (1987). Elimination of Burkitt cells from excess bone marrow with an immunomagnetic purging procedure. Selection of monoclonal antibodies is a critical step. In *Proceedings of the Third International Symposium on Autologous Bone Marrow Transplantation* (ed. K Dicke, G Spitzer, and S Jagannath), pp. 443–8. University of Texas M. D. Anderson Hospital and Tumor Institute, Houston.

Coombes RC, *et al.* (1986). *In vitro* and *in vivo* effects of a monoclonal antibody–toxin conjugate for use in autologous bone marrow transplantation for patients with breast cancer. *Cancer Research*, **46**:4217–20.

Cornbleet MA, McElwain TJ, Kumar PJ (1983). Treatment of advanced malignant melanoma with high dose melphalan and autologous bone marrow transplantation. *British Journal of Cancer*, **48**:329–33.

Couanet D, Geoffray A (1988). Etude en imagerie par résonance magnétique (IRM) des métastases ostéomédullaires des neuroblastomes. *Bulletin du Cancer*, **75**:91–6.

D'Angio GH, Evans AE (1983). Cyclic low dose total body irradiation for metastatic neuroblastoma. *International Journal of Radiation Oncology— Biology—Physics*, **9**:1961–4.

Dalton WS, *et al.* (1989). Drug-resistance in multiple myeloma and non-Hodgkin's lymphoma: detection of *p*-glycoprotein and potential circumvention by addition of verapamil to chemotherapy. *Journal of Clinical Oncology*, **7**:415–24.

Daniel CP, Dexter TM (1989). The role of growth factors in haemopoietic development: clinical and biological implications. *Cancer and Metastasis Reviews*, **8**:253–62.

De Vita V, Hellman S, Rosenberg SA (ed.) (1989). *Principles and practice of oncology* (3rd edn), p. 20. Lippincott, Philadelphia.

De Witte T, *et al.* (1986). Depletion of donor lymphocytes by counterflow centrifugation successfully prevents acute graft-versus-host disease in matched allogeneic marrow transplantation. *Blood*, **67**:1302–6.

Dini G, *et al.* (1989*a*). Bone marrow transplantation for neuroblastoma: a review of 513 cases. In *Bone marrow transplantation in children and adults* (ed. C Bernasconi and GR Burgion), p. 23. Pavia.

Dini G, Hartmann O, Pinkerton R, Dallorso S, Philip T (1989*b*). Autologous bone marrow transplantation in Ewing's sarcoma: an analysis of phase II studies from the European Bone Marrow Transplantation Group. In *ABMT: Proceedings of the Fourth International Symposium* (ed. KA Dicke, G Spitzer, S Jagannath, and MJ Evinger-Hodges), pp. 593–9. University of Texas M. D. Anderson Hospital and Tumor Institute, Houston.

Djerassi I (1975). High dose methotrexate and citrovorum factor rescue. Background and rationale. *Cancer Chemotherapy Report*, **6**:3–6.

Duff Y (1985). How much is too much high dose cytosine arabinoside? *Journal of Clinical Oncology*, **5**:601–3.

Eder JP, *et al.* (1986). High dose combination alkylating agent chemotherapy with autologous bone marrow support for metastatic breast cancer. *Journal of Clinical Oncology*, **4**:1592–4.

Elias AD, Eder JP, Shea T, Begg CB, Frei E III, Antman KH (1990). High-dose ifosfamide with mesna uroprotection: a phase I study. *Journal of Clinical Oncology*, **8**:170–8.

Farha P, Spitzer G, Valdivieso M (1983). High dose chemotherapy and autologous bone marrow transplantation for the treatment of small cell lung carcinoma. *Cancer*, **52**:1351–6.

Favrot MC, Philip T (1989). Bone marrow purging. In *New directions in cancer treatment* (ed. I Magrath), pp. 343–75. Springer-Verlag, Berlin.

Favrot MC, *et al.* (1986). Bone marrow purging procedure in Burkitt lymphoma with monoclonal antibodies and complement. Quantification by a liquid cell culture monitoring system. *British Journal of Cancer*, **64**:161–4.

Favrot MC, Philip I, Combaret V, Maritaz O, Philip T (1987). Experimental evaluation of an immunomagnetic bone marrow purging procedure using the Burkitt lymphoma model. *Bone Marrow Transplantation*, **21**:56–9.

Filipovich AH, Vallera DA, Youle RJ, Quinones RR, Neville DM, Kersey JH (1984). *Ex-vivo* treatment of donor bone marrow with anti-T cell immunotoxins for prevention of graft-versus-host disease. *Lancet*, i:469–72.

Frei E III (1985). Curative cancer chemotherapy. *Cancer Research*, 45:6523–37.

Frei E III, Canellos GP (1980). Dose: a critical factor in cancer chemotherapy. *American Journal of Medicine*, 69:585–94.

Frei E III, Teicher BA, Holden SA, Cathcart KNS, Wang Y (1988). Preclinical studies and clinical correlation of the effect of alkylating dose. *Cancer Research*, 48:4717–23.

Frei E III, Antman K, Teicher B, Eder P, Schnipper L (1989). Bone marrow autotransplantation for solid tumors—prospects. *Journal of Clinical Oncology*, 7:515–26.

Garaventa A, Bernard JL, Badell I, Hartmann O, Lanino E, Philip T (1989). High-dose chemotherapy with autologous bone marrow transplantation in Wilms' tumor: a survey of the European Bone Marrow Transplantation Group. In *ABMT: Proceedings of the Fourth International Symposium* (ed. KA Dicke, G Spitzer, S Jagannath, and MJ Evinger-Hodges), pp. 601–7. University of Texas M. D. Anderson Hospital and Tumor Institute, Houston.

Gehan E (1984). Dose–response relationship in clinical oncology. *Cancer*, 54:1204–7.

Gerota J, Bonnak H, Bunthor H, Douay L, Reviron J, and Pillier C (1982). Concentration of bone marrow stem cells using the Haemonetics system. *Cryobiology*, 19:675–8.

Gilmore MJ, Prentice HG, Corringham RE, Blacklock HA, Hoffbrand AV (1983). A technique for the concentration of nucleated bone marrow cells for *in vitro* manipulation or cryopreservation using the IBM 2991 Blood Cell Processor. *Vox Sanguis*, 45:294–301.

Goldie JH, Coldman AJ (1979). A mathematical model for relating the drug sensitivity of tumors to their spontaneous mutation rate. *Cancer Treatment Reports*, 63:1727–9.

Goldie JH, Coldman AJ (1985a). A model for tumor response to chemotherapy: an integration of the stem cell and somatic mutation hypotheses. *Cancer Investigation*, 3:553–64.

Goldie JH, Coldman AJ (1985b). Genetic instability in the development of drug resistance. *Seminars in Oncology*, 13:222–30.

Goldstein LJ, *et al.* (1990). Expression of the multidrug resistance, *MDR1*, gene in neuroblastomas. *Journal of Clinical Oncology*, 8:128–36.

Goldstone AH (1985). Autologous bone marrow transplantation for non Hodgkin's lymphoma. In *Autologous bone marrow transplantation: Proceedings of the First International Symposium* (ed. KA Dicke, G Spitzer, and AR Zander), pp. 67–72. University of Texas M. D. Anderson Hospital and Tumor Institute, Houston.

Goldstone AH, Souhami RL, Lynch DC (1984). Intensive chemotherapy and autologous bone marrow transplantation for relapsed lymphoma. *Experimental Hematology*, 12:137–9.

Gorin NC, Duhamel G (1987). *L'autogreffe de moelle osseuse*, p. 41. Masson, Paris.

Gorin NC, *et al.* (1986). Autologous bone marrow transplantation using marrow incubated with Asta Z 7557 in adult acute leukemia. *Blood*, 67:1367–70.

Graham-Pole J (1989). The role of marrow autografting in neuroblastoma. *Bone Marrow Transplantation*, 4:3–7.

Graham-Pole J, *et al.* (1989). Myeloablative treatment for children with metastatic neuroblastoma supported by bone marrow infusions: progress and problems. In *ABMT: Proceedings of the Fourth International Symposium* (ed. KA Dicke, G Spitzer, S Jagannath, and MJ Evinger-Hodges), pp. 559–66. University of Texas M. D. Anderson Hospital and Tumor Institute, Houston.

Hagenbeek A, Martens ACM, and Schultz FW (1988). How to prevent a leukemia relapse after bone marrow transplantation in acute leukemia: preclinical and clinical model studies. In *Experimental haematology today* (ed. SJ Baum, KA Dicke, E Iotzova, and DH Pluznik), pp. 147–51. Springer-Verlag, Berlin.

Hall A, Cattan AR, Proctor SJ (1989). Mechanisms of drug resistance in acute leukaemia. *Leukaemia Research*, 13:351–6.

Hartmann O, Oberlin O, Lemerle J (1984). Acute leukemia in two patients treated with high dose melphalan and autologous bone marrow transplantation for malignant solid tumours. *Journal of Clinical Oncology*, 2:1424–8.

Hartmann O, Kalifa C, Beaujean F, Bayle C, Benhamou E, Lemerle J (1985). Treatment of advanced neuroblastoma with two consecutive high-dose chemotherapy regimens and ABMT. In *Advances in neuroblastoma research* (ed. AE Evans, O D'Angio, and RC Seeger), pp. 565–8. Liss, New York.

Hartmann O, *et al.* (1987). Repeated high-dose chemotherapy followed by purged autologous bone marrow transplantation as consolidation therapy in metastatic neuroblastoma. *Journal of Clinical Oncology*, 5:1205–11.

Hartmann O, *et al.* (1990). Place de la chimiothérapie à hautes doses suivie d'autogreffe médullaire dans le traitement des sarcomes d'Ewing métastatiques de l'enfant. *Bulletin du Cancer*, 77:181–7.

Hayes DM, Cvitkovic E, Golbey R, Schneider E, Helson L, Krakoff R (1977). High dose *cis*-platinum diaminedichloride. *Cancer*, 39:1372–9.

Hervé P, Tamayo E, Coffe C, Lenus R, Peters A (1979). Cryopreservation of human bone marrow with a view to autologous bone marrow transplantation. In *Bone marrow transplantation in Europe* (ed. JL Touraine), p. 36. Excerpta Medica (80), Amsterdam.

Hervé P, *et al.* (1984). Autologous bone marrow transplantation for acute leukemia using transplant chemopurified with metabolite of oxazaphosphorines (ASTA Z 7557, INN mafosfamide): first clinical results. *New Drugs*, 2:245–50.

Hildebrand J, Badjou R, Collard-Ronge E (1980). Treatment of brain gliomas with high dose of CCNU and autologous bone marrow transplantation. *Biomedicine*, 32:71–4.

Hortobagyi GN (1988). The role of high-dose chemotherapy with autologous bone marrow transplantation in the treatment of breast cancer. *Bone Marrow Transplant*, 3:526–30.

Hryniuk WM (1988). The importance of dose intensity in the outcome of chemotherapy. In *Important advances in oncology* (ed. VT de Vita, S Hellman, and SA Rosenbert), p. 121–41. Lippincott, Philadelphia.

Humblet Y, *et al.* (1987). Transplantation in selected small cell carcinoma of the lung: a randomized study. *Journal of Clinical Oncology*, 12:1921–30.

Ivy SP, Ozols RF, Cowan KH (1989). Drug resistance in cancer. In *New directions in cancer treatment* (ed. I Magrath), pp. 191–215. Springer-Verlag, Berlin.

Janossy G, *et al.* (1987). Applications of monoclonal antibodies in bone marrow transplantation (BMT). In *Leucocyte typing III* (ed. A Mc Mickael), pp. 942–8. Oxford University Press, Oxford.

Kaizer H, *et al.* (1985). Autologous bone marrow transplantation in acute leukemia: a phase I study of *in vitro* treatment of marrow with 4-hydroperoxy-cyclophosphamide to purge tumor cells. *Blood*, 65:1504–7.

Kics MS, Gordon LI, Rosen ST, Kucuk O, Vriesendorp HM (1988). Autologous bone marrow transplantation in breast cancer: separation of clonogenic tumor cell colonies by gradient fractionation. *Experimental Hematology*, 16:190–4.

Kinsella TJ, Glaubicher D, Diesseroth A, Mukuch R, Waller B, Pizzo P, Glatstein E (1983). Intensive combined modality therapy including low-dose TBI in high-risk Ewing's sarcoma patients. *International Journal of Radiation Oncology—Biology—Physics*, 9:1955–60.

Kluin-Nelemans HC, Martens ACM, Lowenberg B, Hagenbeek A (1984). No preferential sensitivity of clonogenic AMG cells to Asta Z 7557. *Leukaemia Research*, 8:723–5.

Korbling M, Hess AD, Tutshka PJ, Kaiser H, Colvin MO, Santos GW (1987). 4-Hydroperoxycyclophosphamide: a model for eliminating residual human tumour cells and T-lymphocytes from the bone marrow graft. *British Journal of Haematology*, 52:89–90.

Lazarus H, Herzig R, Wolff S (1985). Treatment of metastatic malignant melanoma with intensive melphalan and autologous bone marrow transplantation. *Cancer Treatment Report*, 69:473–6.

Lebien TW, Stepan DE, Bartholomew RM, Stong RC, Anderson JM (1985). Utilization of a colony assay to assess the variables influencing elimination of leukemic cells from human bone marrow with monoclonal antibodies and complement. *Blood*, 65:945–9.

Le Tourneau JN, Bernard JL, Hendren WH, Carcassonne M (1985). Evaluation of the role of surgery in 130 patients with neuroblastoma. *Journal of Pediatric Surgery*, 3:244–7.

Lopez M, Andreu G, Beaujean F, Ehrsam A, Gerota J, Herve P (1985). Human bone marrow processing in view of further *in vitro* treatment and cryopreservation. *Blood Transfusion and Immunohaematology*, 5:411–25.

McGuire WL, Herzig RH, Lemaistre CF, Peters WP (1988). Autologous bone marrow transplantation in breast cancer: a panel discussion. *Breast Cancer Research and Treatment*, 11:7–17.

Michon J, *et al.* (1989). NB 87—a new protocol using an alternating non-cross-resistant induction regimen and two different modalities of massive consolidation chemotherapy in treatment of metastatic neuroblastoma in children. In *ABMT: Proceedings of the Fourth International Symposium* (ed. KA Dicke, G Spitzer, S Jagannath, and MJ Evinger-Hodges), pp. 529–41. University of Texas M. D. Anderson Hospital and Tumor Institute, Houston.

Migliaccio AR, Migliaccia G, Johnson G, Adamson JW, Torok-Storb B (1990). Comparative analysis of hematopoietic growth factors released by stromal cells from normal donors or transplanted patients. *Blood*, 75:305–12.

Moyes J, McCready VR, Fullbrook A (1989). Neuroblastoma: mIBG in its diagnosis and management. In *Neuroblastoma*, p. 26. Springer-Verlag, London.

Muirhead M, Martin PJ, Torok-Storb B, Uhr JW, Vitetta ES (1983). Use of an antibody-ricin A-chain conjugate to delete neoplastic B cells from human bone marrow. *Blood*, 62:327–30.

Myers CD, *et al.* (1984). An immunotoxin with therapeutic potential in T cell leukemia: WT1-ricin A. *Blood*, 63:1178–81.

Ninane J, Pritchard J, Malpas JS (1981). Chemotherapy of advanced neuroblastoma: does adriamycin contribute? *Archives of Diseases of Childhood*, 56:544–8.

Norton L (1985). Implications of kinetic heterogeneity in clinical oncology. *Seminars in Oncology*, 12:232–6.

Norton L, Simon R (1977). Tumor size, sensitivity to therapy and design of treatment schedules. *Cancer Treatment Report*, 61:1307–9.

Perren TJ, Mbidde E, Selby P, Workman P, Whitton A, McElwan TJ (1987). High dose BCNU with ABMT and full dose radiotherapy for grade IV astrocytoma. In *Proceedings of the EBMT Meeting* (ed. Hinterberger), p. 49. Interlaken.

Peters WP, *et al.* (1988). High-dose combinant alkylating agents with bone marrow support as initial treatment for metastatic breast cancer. *Journal of Clinical Oncology*, 6:1368–76.

Philip T, Pinkerton R (1989a). Very high dose therapy in lymphomas and solid tumors. In *New directions in cancer treatment* (ed. I Magrath), pp. 119–42. Springer-Verlag, Berlin.

Philip T, Pinkerton R (1989b). Neuroblastoma. In *New directions in cancer treatment* (ed. I. Magrath), pp. 605–8. Springer-Verlag, Berlin.

Philip T, *et al.* (1984). Role of massive chemotherapy and ABMT in NHL. *Lancet*, ii:391.

Philip T, *et al.* (1985a). Purging autologous bone marrow transplantation in 25 cases of advanced neuroblastoma. *Lancet*, ii:576–7.

Philip T, *et al.* (1985b). Massive chemotherapy with ABMT in 50 cases of bad prognosis non Hodgkin's lymphoma. *British Journal of Haematology*, 60:599–601.

Philip T, *et al.* (1985c). Massive chemotherapy with autologous bone marrow transplantation in Burkitt's lymphoma (a review of 50 patients treated in France). *Blood Transfusion and Immunohaematology*, 5:521–7.

Philip T, *et al.* (1986). The role of massive therapy with autologous bone marrow transplantation in Burkitt's lymphoma. *Clinical Haematology*, 1:205–7.

Philip T, *et al.* (1987a). High dose therapy and ABMT in 100 adults with intermediate or high grade non Hodgkin's lymphoma. *New England Journal of Medicine*, 316:1493–7.

Philip T, *et al.* (1987b). High-dose chemotherapy with bone marrow transplantation as consolidation treatment in neuroblastoma: an unselected group of stage IV patients over 1 year of age. *Journal of Clinical Oncology*, 5:266–71.

Philip T, *et al.* (1987c). A phase II study of high dose *cis*-platinum and VP16 in neuroblastoma. *Journal of Clinical Oncology*, 5:941–50.

Philip T, *et al.* (1988a). Background for an international randomized study on relapsed diffuse intermediate and high grade lymphoma in adults. In *Proceedings of the Third International Symposium on Autologous Bone Marrow Transplantation* (ed. K Dicke, G Spitzer, and S Jagannath), pp. 313–33. University of Texas M. D. Anderson Hospital and Tumor Institute, Houston.

Philip T, *et al.* (1988b). Autologous bone marrow transplantation in Burkitt's lymphoma (50 cases in the Lyon protocol). In *Proceedings of the Third International Symposium on Autologous Bone Marrow Transplantation* (ed. K Dicke, G Spitzer, and S Jagannath), pp. 249–61. University of Texas M. D. Anderson Hospital and Tumor Institute, Houston.

Philip T, Chauvin F, Abdelbost Z (1989a). Report of the EBMT working party on autologous BMT (Badgastein).

Philip T, *et al.* (1989b). A pilot study of double ABMT in advanced neuroblastoma (32 patients). In *ABMT: Proceedings of the Fourth International Symposium* (ed. KA Dicke, G Spitzer, S Jagannath, and MJ Evinger-Hodges), pp. 799–805. University of Texas M. D. Anderson Hospital and Tumor Institute, Houston.

Philip T, Bouffet E, Biron P, Brunat-Mentigny M (1989c). Facteur dose/facteur temps en chimiothérapie. *Bulletin Cancer*, 76:979–94.

Philip T, *et al.* (1991). Improved survival at two and five years in the LMCE1 unselected group of 72 children with stage IV neuroblastoma over one year of age at diagnosis: is cure possible in a small subgroup. *Journal of Clinical Oncology*, 9:1037–44.

Phillips GL (1983). Current clinical trial with intensive therapy and autologous bone marrow transplantation for lymphomas and solid tumors. In *Recent advances in bone marrow transplantation*, UCLA symposia (new series) (ed. RP Gale), p. 43. Liss, New York.

Phillips GL, Reece DE (1986). Clinical studies of autologous bone marrow transplantation in Hodgkin's disease. *Clinical Haematology*, 15:151–8.

Phillips GL, *et al.* (1984). Treatment of resistant malignant lymphoma with cyclophosphamide total body irradiation and transplantation of cryopreserved autologous marrow. *New England Journal of Medicine*, 31:1557–61.

Phillips GL, Fay J, Herzig G (1985). Autologous bone marrow transplantation in malignant glioma. *International Journal of Cell Cloning*, 3:257–60.

Phillips GL, *et al.* (1986). Intensive 1,3 bis-(2 chloroethyl)1-nitrosourea (BCNU) monochemotherapy and autologous marrow transplantation for malignant glioma. *Journal of Clinical Oncology*, 4:639–43.

Pinkerton CR (1990). Where next with therapy in advanced neuroblastoma? *British Journal of Cancer*, 61:351–3.

Pinkerton CR, Philip T, Bouffet E, Lashfort L, Kemshead J (1986). Autologous bone marrow transplantation in paediatric solid tumours. *Clinical Haematology*, 15:187–90.

Pinkerton CR, Philip T, Hartmann O, Zucker JM, Valteau D, Brugieres L (1989). High-dose chemo-radiotherapy with autologous bone marrow rescue in pediatric soft tissue sarcomas. In *ABMT: Proceedings of the Fourth International Symposium* (ed. KA Dicke, G Spitzer, S Jagannath, and MJ Evinger-Hodges), pp. 617–20. University of Texas M. D. Anderson Hospital and Tumor Institute, Houston.

Pino Y, Torres JL, Bross DS (1982). Risk factors in interstitial pneumonitis following allogeneic bone marrow transplantation. *International Journal of Radiation Oncology—Biology—Physics*, 8:1301–4.

Poynton CH, Dicke KA, Culbert S, Frankel LS, Jagannath S, Reading CL (1983). Immunomagnetic removal of CALLA positive cells from human bone marrow. *Lancet*, i:524–5.

Pritchard J, Germond S, Jones D, De Kraker J, Love S (1986). Is high dose melphalan of value in treatment of advanced neuroblastoma? Preliminary results of a randomized trial by the European Neuroblastoma Study Group. *Proceedings of ASCO*, 5:205–6.

Ramakrishnan S, Houston LL (1984). Inhibition of human acute lymphoblastic leukemia cells by immunotoxins: potentiation by chloroquine. *Science*, 223:58–9.

Rebattu P, *et al.* (1985). Indications et résultats de l'autogreffe de moelle dans les lymphomes malin non Hodgkiniens (étude de 92 cas). *Nouvelle Revue Francaise d'Hématologie*, 27:252–60.

Reisner Y (1983). Differential agglutination by soybean agglutinin of human leukemia and neuroblastoma cell lines: potential application to autologous bone marrow transplantation. *Proceedings of the National Academy of Sciences USA*, 80:6657–9.

Reisner Y, *et al.* (1983). Transplantation for severe combined immunodeficiency with HLA-A,B,D,DR, incompatible parental marrow cells fractionated by soybean agglutinin and sheep red blood cells. *Blood*, 61:341–4.

Reynolds CP, Reynolds DA, Frenkel EP, Graham Smith R (1982). Selective toxicity of 6-hydroxydopamine and ascorbate for human neuroblastoma *in vitro*: a model for clearing marrow prior to autologous transplant. *Cancer Research*, 42:1331–6.

Reynolds PC, Seeger RC, Vo DD, Black AT, Wells J, Ugelstad J (1986). Model system for removing neuroblastoma cells from bone marrow using monoclonal antibodies and magnetic immunobeads. *Cancer Research*, 46:5882–4.

Reynolds CP, *et al.* (1989). Treatment of poor prognosis neuroblastoma with intensive therapy and autologous bone marrow transplantation. In *ABMT: Proceedings of the Fourth International Symposium* (ed. KA Dicke, G Spitzer, S Jagannath, and MJ Evinger-Hodges), pp. 575–83. University of Texas M. D. Anderson Hospital and Tumor Institute, Houston.

Rosenberg SA, *et al.* (1985). Observations on the systemic administration of autologous lymphokin-activated killer cells and recombinant interleukin-2 to patients with metastatic cancer. *New England Journal of Medicine*, 313:1485–8.

Saarinenu M, Coccia PF, Gerson SL, Pelley R, Cheung NKV (1985). Eradication of neuroblastoma cells *in vitro* by monoclonal antibody and human complement: method for purging autologous bone marrow. *Cancer Research*, 45:5969–70.

Santos GW, Tutschka PJ, Brookmeyer R (1985). Marrow transplantation for acute non lymphocytic leukemia after treatment with busulfan and cyclophosphamide. *New England Journal of Medicine*, 309:1347–9.

Schaeffer YW (1980). Bone marrow stem cells. In *Low temperature preservation in medicine and biology* (ed. MJ Ashwood-Smith and J Smith), pp. 139–41. University Park Press, Baltimore.

Schots R, Biron P, Bailly C, Mornex F, Philip T (1988). Treatment strategies for advanced aggressive non-Hodgkin's disease. In *Proceedings of the Third International Conference on Bone Marrow Transplantation* (ed. KA Dicke, G Spitzer, S Jagannath, and MJ Evinger-Hodges), pp. 297–305. University of Texas M. D. Anderson Hospital and Tumor Institute, Houston.

Shaffort EA, Roger DW, Pritchard J (1984). Advanced neuroblastoma: improved response-rate using a multiagent regimen (OPEC) including sequential *cis* platinum and VM26. *Journal of Clinical Oncology*, 2:742–4.

Shea TC, *et al.* (1989). A phase I clinical and pharmacokinetic study of carboplatin and autologous bone marrow support. *Journal of Clinical Oncology*, 5:651–61.

Sieber F, Spivak JL, Sutcliffe AM (1984). Selective killing of leukemic cells by merocyanine 540-mediated photosensitization. *Proceedings of the National Academy of Sciences USA*, 81:7584–6.

Singer CR, Goldstone AH (1986). Non Hodgkin's lymphomas. *Clinical Haematology*, 15:105–6.

Skipper HE, Schabel FM Jr, Wilcor WS (1964). Experimental evaluation of potential anticancer agents XII. On the criteria and kinetics associated with 'curability' of experimental leukemia. *Cancer Chemotherapy Report*, 35:1–111.

Souhami RL, Harper PG, Linch D (1983). High dose cyclophosphamide with autologous marrow support for treatment of small cell carcinoma of the bronchus. *Cancer Chemotherapy and Pharmacology*, 10:205–17.

Spinolo JA, *et al.* (1989). High dose combination chemotherapy with cyclophosphamide, carmustine, etoposide and autologous bone marrow transplantation in 60 patients with relapsed Hodgkin disease. The M. D. Anderson experience. *Recent Results in Cancer Research*, 117:233–7.

Spitzer G, *et al.* (1980). High dose combination chemotherapy with autologous bone marrow transplantation in adult solid tumors. *Cancer*, 45:3075–7.

Spitzer G, Dicke K, Zander AR, Farha P, Valdivieso M (1986). High dose intensification therapy with autologous bone marrow support for limited small cell bronchogenic carcinoma. *Journal of Clinical Oncology*, 4:4–7.

Stepan DE, Bartholomew RM, Lebien TW (1984). *In vitro* cytodestruction of human leukemic cells using murine monoclonal antibodies and human complement. *Blood*, 63:1120–4.

Stong RC, Youle RJ, Vallera DA (1984). Elimination of clonogenic T-leukemic cells from human bone marrow using anti-M_r 65,000 protein immunotoxins. *Cancer Research*, 44:3000–6.

Takvorian T, Parker LM, Hockberg FH (1983). Autologous bone marrow transplantation: host effects of high dose BCNU. *Journal of Clinical Oncology*, 1:610–14.

Tchekmyedian JS, Tait N, Van Echo D, Aisner J (1986). High dose chemotherapy without bone marrow transplantation in melanoma. *Journal of Clinical Oncology*, 4:1811–13.

Thomas ED (1982). The role of marrow transplantation in the eradication of malignant disease. *Cancer*, 49:1963–9.

Treleaven JG, *et al.* (1984). Removal of neuroblastoma cells from bone marrow with monoclonal antibodies conjugated to magnetic microspheres. *Lancet*, ii:70–3.

Uckun FM, Ramakrishnan S, Houston LL (1985). Increased efficiency in selective elimination of leukemia cells by a combination of stable derivative of cyclophosphamide and a human B-cell-specific immunotoxin containing pokeweed antiviral protein. *Cancer Research*, 45:69–72.

Vossen JM (1990). Autologous bone marrow rescue as part of a curative approach for pediatric solid tumors: the case of neuroblastoma. *Pediatric Hematology and Oncology*, 7:iii–vii.

Waldman H, *et al.* (1984). Elimination of graft-versus-host disease by *in vitro* depletion of alloreactive lymphocytes with a monoclonal rat anti-human lymphocyte antibody (CAMPATH-1). *Lancet*, ii:483–6.

Wells JR, Sullivan A, Lcine MJ (1979). A technique for the separation and cryopreservation of myeloid stem cells from human bone marrow. *Cryobiology*, 16:201–6.

Yaniv I, *et al.* (1990). Autologous bone marrow transplantation in pediatric solid tumors. *Pediatric Hematology and Oncology*, 7:35–46.

Yeager AM, *et al.* (1986). Autologous bone marrow transplantation in patient with acute non-lymphocytic leukemia, using *ex vivo* marrow treatment with 4-hydroperoxycyclophosphamide. *New England Journal of Medicine*, 315:141–7.

12.6.1 The cell biology of Hodgkin's disease

VOLKER DIEHL, CHRISTOF VON KALLE, CHRISTA FONATSCH, HANS TESCH, AND M. SCHAADT

INTRODUCTION

Although there have been significant advances in the treatment of Hodgkin's disease, basic research has provided no major insight into the origin and nature of this malignancy. The reasons for this lie in the unique biological features of the disease, whose clinical entity represents a polymorphic disorder and where the identity of tumour cells is masked by a preponderance of non-malignant, reactive cells. Because of this we have not been able to identify whether the Hodgkin cell is infectious, reactive, or malignant in nature.

Therapeutic strategies in Hodgkin's disease are very successful but toxic, with severe side-effects and ultimately not life-saving for a third of the patients affected. It is important therefore that more should become known about the cellular pathogenesis of Hodgkin's disease, the repercussions of which would be more effective treatment.

In vitro cell lines

Within the 1980s, the successful application of new techniques has shed light on some of the pertinent questions. As a research tool, cell culture has provided virtually unlimited amounts of tumour cell equivalents. Nine tumour cell lines are likely to be Hodgkin-derived (reviewed in Schaadt *et al.* 1989), after histological confirmation

Table 1 Derivation and important characteristics of all Hodgkin's-disease-derived cell lines

Line	Clinical stage	Source	Phenotype (markers[a])	Genotype (rearrangements)	Reference
L428	IV	PE[b]	B (CD19)	B (Ig$_{H,L}$, TCR-β[e])	Schaadt et al. (1980)
L540	IV	BM	T (CD2,4)	T (TCR)	Diehl et al. (1982)
L591	IV	PE	B (CD19,20)	B (Ig)	Diehl et al. (1982)
Co	IV	LN	T (CD3,5,7)	T (TCR-β, -γ)	Jones et al. (1985)
DEV	II	PE	B (CD19,20)	B (Ig$_{H,L}$)	Poppema et al. (1985)
HD-LM2	IV	PE	T (CD2)	T (TCR)	Drexler et al. (1988)
KM-H2	IV[c]	PE	B (CD19,21)	B (Ig$_H$)	Kamesaki et al. (1986)
Ho	II	LN	T (CD3,4,7)	T (TCR-β, -γ)	Jones et al. (1985)
Zo	II	PF	B (B-IB-Ab[d])	B (Ig$_{H,L}$)	Poppema et al. (1989)

[a]Important for differentiation.
[b]PE, pleural effusion; BM, bone-marrow; LN, lymph node; PF, pericardial fluid.
[c]Histology: mixed cellularity, all others nodular sclerosing.
[d]B-immunoblastic-NHL-antibody.
[e]TCR, T-cell receptor.

by two independent pathologists and having fulfilled criteria of monoclonality and aneuploidy (Diehl et al. 1982). The establishment of a cell line (Table 1) is favoured by the presence of advanced clinical disease, nodular sclerosing subtype, and the clinical setting of an effusion.

Findings obtained by examination of cell lines in vitro do not necessarily represent biological events in vivo. This is because the establishment of the cell lines is difficult and growth in culture selects cells that have growth characteristics different from their counterparts in vivo. It is possible that the lymph node affected by Hodgkin's disease provides a congenial microenvironment for the growth of Hodgkin and Reed–Sternberg cells and this is difficult to reproduce in a culture system in vitro, so that only atypical cells survive. Although the cells retain their basic phenotypic characteristics (Athan et al. 1989), Hodgkin's disease-derived cell lines frequently undergo additional chromosomal abnormalities in culture (Diehl et al. 1985).

HODGKIN AND REED–STERNBERG CELLS: CHARACTERISTICS IN VITRO AND IN VIVO

If our 100-year quest for the cell of origin of Hodgkin's disease has taught us anything, it is the importance of maintaining an open mind, preferably with a cheerful capacity for changing it according to fashion. Every cell has had its day. As prospective candidates, all cells are equal. As we shall see, some are more equal than others. (Taylor 1983) (Table 2).

Phenotype

Morphology

The diagnosis and correct classification of any lymphoma requires surgical biopsy and morphological examination (DeVita et al. 1985). Although morphological characteristics alone do not define the cell of origin in Hodgkin's disease, some of the histological characteristics are helpful to keep in mind when evaluating other findings.

In general, Hodgkin's disease frequently involves supradiaphragmatic lymph nodes and the spleen. Initial spread is limited to contiguous lymphatic organs. In later stages, blood-borne spread to other organs is possible.

In Hodgkin's disease, tumours represent a majority of non-malignant lymphocytes, histiocytes, plasma cells, eosinophils, and others that prevail over a minority of characteristic Hodgkin and Reed–Sternberg tumour cells. The typical appearance of 'large

Table 2 Historical overview of the theory formation concerning the proposed cell of origin in Hodgkin's disease

Suggestion	Group[a]
Lymphoid origin	
Lymphoblast	Mallory (1914)
Lymphoid subpopulation, activated	
T-cell	Order (1972), Biniaminow, (1974)
B-cell	Leech (1973), Garvin (1974), Boecker (1975), Poppema et al. (1989)
Lymphoid cell (T- or B-)	Stein (1982?, 1984, 1985)
Immature lymphoid precursor	Falk (1987), Kamesaki (1989), Athan (1989), Herbst (1989)
Myelomonocytic origin	
Monocytoid cell	McJunkin (1928)
Myeloblast, myeloid precursor cell,	Lewis (1941), Stein (1982),
Myelomonocytic precursor cell	Diehl (1982)
Other origin	
Sinus endothelial cell	Reed (1902)
Megakaryocyte	Medlar (1931)
Histiocyte	Bessis (1948), Rappaport (1966), Mori (1969), Kaplan (1977), Kadin (1978)
Follicular dendritic cell	Curran (1978)
Dendritic ('Steinmann') cell,	
Antigen-presenting cell	Fischer (1983, 1985)
Interdigitating cell	Hansmann (1981), Kadin (1982), Hsu (1985)
Pluripotent precursor cell	Falk (1983)

[a]Not listed references.

inclusion-like nucleoli, thick nuclear membrane with perinucleolar halos, and abundant eosinophilic to amphoteric cytoplasm' (Lukes et al. 1966) is not pathognomonic and has also been found in several reactive lymphoid and malignant diseases, including infectious mononucleosis, non-Hodgkin's lymphoma, carcinomas, and sarcomas (Lukes et al. 1969; Strum and Rappaport 1971).

Although the distribution pattern and ratio of reactive cells and fibrosis are equally important for the diagnosis of Hodgkin's disease, Hodgkin's lymphoma is rarely diagnosed in the absence of mononuclear Hodgkin's disease cells or their polynucleated Reed–Sternberg counterpart.

The potential cell of origin of Hodgkin's disease has to fulfil three criteria, which include the induction of reactive cell proliferation, collagen/fibrillar reticulum synthesis, and relative specificity for lymphatic organs.

Immunophenotype of Hodgkin cells

Since 1980 several markers have been identified as being regularly expressed on Hodgkin and Reed–Sternberg cells, two of which were at first thought to be specific for the disease (Schwab *et al.* 1982; Stein *et al.* 1982) (Table 3). Hodgkin and Reed–Sternberg cells stain positively for the granulocyte-staining X-hapten (CD15) and the lectin peanut agglutinin (Hsu and Jaffe 1984), the interleukin-2 receptor (CD25), the Hodgkin's disease-associated activation antigen Ki-1 (CD30), the B-cell-associated antigen detected by the LN-2 antibody, and the transferrin receptor (OKT9, CD71). Major histocompatibility complex (**MHC**) class IIa (HLA-DR) antigens are constantly expressed *in vivo* and *in vitro* (Burrichter *et al.* 1985).

All of these antigens were initially defined on unrelated cells except for the CD30 antibodies that were produced by immunizing with the Hodgkin's-disease-derived cell line L428 (Stein *et al.* 1982). Except for Hodgkin and Reed–Sternberg cells, the CD30 antigen is only expressed on activated or transformed (human T-lymphotrophic virus-1; Epstein–Barr virus) T and B lymphocytes (Stein *et al.* 1985), activated (Pfreundschuh *et al.* 1988) and differentiated macrophages (Andreesen *et al.* 1989), and a distinct subentity of

large-cell, non-Hodgkin's lymphoma, the so-called 'Ki-1-Lymphoma' (O'Connor *et al.* 1987). This reaction pattern makes CD30 antibodies a valuable diagnostic tool.

The CD30 antigen is now known to exist as a 120 kDa, membrane-bound, phosphorylated glycoprotein with a non-phosphorylated, 84 kDa, intracellular apoprotein and a 90 kDa degradation residue released into the supernatant (Hansen *et al.* 1989). Additionally, an independently synthesized 57 kDa intracellular molecule has the same antigenicity. Interestingly, this second intracellular molecule is also observed in myeloma, Burkitt's lymphoma, and HL60 leukaemia cell lines (Hansen *et al.* 1989).

CD30 so far has always been associated with activated cells. Hodgkin and Reed–Sternberg cells seem to comply with that rule, as the nuclear proliferation antigen Ki67 correlates well with CD30 positivity in those cells *in situ* (Gerdes *et al.* 1987). Other functional data are not yet available.

There are, however, other data justifying interest in the antigen. Soluble CD30 (sCD30) antigen with a molecular weight of 90 kDa as well as soluble interleukin-2 receptor (**sII-2R**) can be detected in the serum of a certain percentage of patients with untreated Hodgkin's disease (Gause *et al.* 1991). In childhood Hodgkin's disease, sII-2R has been assigned prognostic validity (Pui *et al.* 1989). The clinical significance of elevated concentrations of sCD30 and sII-2R is currently being tested.

Table 3 Immunophenotype of *in vivo* and *in vitro* Hodgkin cells

Association	Cluster of differentiation	Function/derivation	Typical occurrence	Reactivity *in vivo*	Reactivity *in vitro*
T phenotype					
	CD2	LFA3-R.	T-Ly[a]	NS++[b]	L540, L591, HDLM2
	CD3	TCR-ass.-Ag	T-Ly	NS+, MC+	Co, Ho
	CD4	T-helper	T-Ly Mo	NS+, MC+	N540, Ho
	CD5	Pan-T	T- B-Ly CLL	NS+	Co
	CD7	T-diff, Pan-T	T-Ly Mo		Co, Ho
B phenotype					
	CD9	B-Pre	Mo Gran		KMH2
	CD19	Pan-B, B4	B-Ly		L428, L591, DEV, KMH2
	CD20	Pan-B, B1	B-Ly FDC	LP+++, Others (+)	L591, DEV
	CD21	C3d-R	B-Ly DRC		KMH2
	CD22	Pan-B	B-Ly		L591
	CD75	LN1	B- T-Ly Gran	LP+++, Others (+)	
	CD74	LN2	B-Ly Mo	All+++	
		L26	Ig+B-Ly	LP+++, Others (+)	KMH2
Immunoglobulins		Anti-IgA$_H$	B-Ly		L591, DEV
		Anti-λ	B-Ly		L591
Others					
Activation markers	CD30	HD der. Ag[c]	Act Ly Mo	All+++	All
	CD25	Il-2R	Act Ly Mo	All+++	All except Co, Ho
	CD71	(OKT9)Trans-ferrin-R.	Pro	All+++	All
	CD24	Pre-B	B-Ly Gran Mo		L428
	CD15	X-Hapten	Gran (Pre)	All+++	All except Ho
	CD45	LCA[d]	Leu	NS(+), MC++, LP++	All
MHC (Class II)		HLA-DR	B- T-Ly Mo	All+++	All except DEV
EBV		EBNA	B-Ly Burkitt	[+][e]	L591
ICAM1	CD54	Adhesion molecule	T-Ly B-CLL	All+++	?
LFA3	CD58	CD2-Ligand	Leu Ery	All+++	L428
Lectin		PNA	B-Ly, Mo	All+++	Co, Ho, L428, L591
Esterase		ANAE		All++	All except DEV

[a]Act, activated; Ly, lymphocytes; Mo, monocytes/macrophages; Gran, granulocytes; Pre, precursor; Pro, proliferating cells; FDC, follicular dendritic cells; DRC, dendritic reticular cells; Leu, leucocyte; ep Lh, epidermal Langerhans cell.

[b](+) <10%; + <30%; ++ <60%; +++ >60% positive cells; NS, nodular sclerosing; MC, mixed cellularity; LP, lymphocyte predominant.

[c]AG, antigen; R, receptor.

[d]Leucocyte common antigen.

[e]As detected by *in situ* hybridization.

Attempts are being made to develop CD30 antibody conjugates for the diagnosis and therapy of Hodgkin's disease (Engert *et al.* 1990). An immunoscintigraphy pilot study using radioiodine-labelled HRS-1 antibody has been completed with promising results (Carde *et al.* 1989).

Data have been more conflicting concerning T- and B-cell markers. Whereas all of the cell lines do stain positively for at least one T-cell (CD2–5, 7) or B-cell (CD19, 20, 21) antibody cluster, until recently only 11 (T) and 15 per cent (B) of Hodgkin and Reed–Sternberg cells in biopsy specimens were considered positive for the related antigens (Drexler *et al.* 1988). Further optimization of antibodies and techniques in the last 2 years has more than doubled the fraction of primary Hodgkin's cells binding lymphocyte-associated antibodies. Depending on antibodies and methods, more than 60 per cent of Hodgkin tumour cells bind either T- (40 per cent) or B-cell (20 per cent) markers (Falini *et al.* 1987; Casey *et al.* 1988; Oka *et al.* 1988; Agnarsson and Kadin 1989; Herbst *et al.* 1989; Stein *et al.* 1989). Differences between histological subtypes have been reported (Table 3). Nodular sclerosing Hodgkin's disease, the most frequent subtype and mixed cellularity cells often have a T-cell-associated immunophenotype. Lymphocyte-predominant Hodgkin's disease has a definite B-cell phenotype with constant expression of B-cell antigens (CD20, LN1, 2, L26) and J-chain (Stein *et al.* 1986; Coles *et al.* 1988; Agnarsson and Kadin 1989). These findings, together with the distinct morphology and the clinical course, distinguish lymphocyte predominance from the other subentities of Hodgkin's disease (Poppema *et al.* 1985; Wright 1989).

The relevance of some markers has not yet been evaluated in detail. In 50 per cent of mixed cellularity and lymphocyte-predominant subtypes, CD45, the common leukocyte antigen (**CLA**) can be detected (Agnarsson and Kadin 1989). CD24, M2, and colony-forming unit–granulocyte/macrophage (**CFU–G(EM)M**)-associated antigens occur on L428 (Athan *et al.* 1989).

Other markers

Rosetting of T-cells with Hodgkin cells occurs both *in vivo* (Stuart *et al.* 1977) and *in vitro* (Diehl *et al.* 1982). On L428 cells, both LFA3 and ICAM1 antigens are expressed (own data, unpublished). The presence of these ligands for T-cell structures (CD2 and CD11/18 might explain the adhesion mechanism responsible for T-cell rosettes (Sanders *et al.* 1988).

Hodgkin cells are known to stimulate mixed lymphocyte reactions both *in vivo* (Engelmann *et al.* 1980) and *in vitro* (Fischer *et al.* 1983). They are positive for non-specific esterase (Diehl *et al.* 1982). Phagocytotic properties as well as polyclonal Ig chains in primary Hodgkin's disease may be considered artefacts (Stein 1988).

Genotype

Cytogenetics

Cytogenetic analysis of primary Hodgkin and Reed–Sternberg cells is hampered by the low number of obtainable mitoses and their poor chromosome banding qualities (Fonatsch *et al.* 1990). A significant number of dividing cells with a normal karyotype most probably represent reactive lymphoid cells (Rowley 1982). Depending on the histological subtype, between 75 (nodular sclerosing) and 42 per cent (lymphocyte predominant) of cases studied yielded evaluable metaphases. Short-term cultures of 12 involved lymph nodes exhibited an uncommonly high number (75 per cent) of non-clonal

karyotype abnormalities (Dennis *et al.* 1989). In the 40 cases so far reported in complete karyotype banding studies, the percentage of abnormal karyotypes varied considerably by 22–83 per cent between studies (Thangavelu and Le Beau 1989). Although numerical and structural cytogenetic abnormalities were reported in a portion of cases (Kaplan 1980; Rowley 1982; Cabanillas *et al.* 1988; Thangavelu and Le Beau 1989), a specific chromosomal marker of Hodgkin's disease, like the Philadelphia chromosome in chronic myeloid leukaemia, has not yet been defined.

As visualized by simultaneous morphology, immunophenotype, and karyotype, abnormalities were confined to the Hodgkin and Reed–Sternberg cell in a study of two cases (Teerenhovi *et al.* 1988). Chromosome abnormalities of relapsed or treated patients' karyotypes did not differ from examinations at the time of diagnosis (Schouten *et al.* 1989; Thangavelu and Le Beau 1989). Among Hodgkin's disease-associated chromosomal abnormalities, aneuploidy (100 per cent) with hyperdiploidy (70 per cent) is the most frequent (Anastasi *et al.* 1987). Chromosomes 5, 2, 1, 12, and 21 are often triplicated. In a few cases a loss of chromosomes is reported, for example chromosomes 22, 10, 13, 17, and 21. Rearrangements, especially translocations or deletions, were found in two-thirds of cases, often involving 1p, 1q, 2q, 6q, 8q, 11q, 11p, 14q, and Xq (Thangavelu and Le Beau 1989). However, with the number of evaluable studies still low, the non-random involvement pattern has to be defined and correlated with clinical features in more detail. Break-points 11q23, 14q32, 6q, 8q24, and 11q13 have frequently been associated with B- and T-cell lymphomas (Cabanillas *et al.* 1988).

Non-random karyotype abnormalities have also been found in Hodgkin's disease-derived cell lines (Table 4). In four of the seven chromosome marker regions cellular oncogenes have been localized. In cell lines L428 and L540, chromosome abnormalities comprise the chromosome segments involved in Ig (L428; 14q32) and T-cell receptor (**TCR**) (L540; 7q11–36) gene rearrangements. In L540; 14q11, which bears the locus of TCR-α and -δ and which contains the TCR-β locus, is involved in chromosomal translocations.

Table 4 Localization of non-random chromosome abnormalities detected in all available banding studies on primary tumour material, Hodgkin's-disease-derived cell lines, and lymphoblastoid cell lines from patients with Hodgkin's disease

Primary Hodgkin tumour tissue	Hodgkin-derived cell lines	Hodgkin-derived LCLs[a]	Interesting genes localized in the region
1p21–22	1p22		N-*ras*, *B-lym-1*, L-*myc*
1q			
2q	2q33	2p23/25	
		3q27/29	
5p15			
6q11–21,24			c-*myb*
	7q11–36	7q22–36	*met*, TCR-β, T3, δ-, ε- chain
8q22–24		8q24	c-*myc*
		9q34	
11p13			
11q13			*bcl*-1
11q23	11q21–23		c-*ets*-1
14q32	14q32		Ig$_H$
	15p12		*rRNA3*
		16q22/24	
18p			
	21q21–22		c-*ets*-2
Xq			

[a]Lymphoblastoid cell line, EBV-transformed B-lymphocytic cell line.

In situ hybridization on L540 has revealed a previously unidentified translocation of the *met* oncogene and TCR-β from the long arm of chromosome 7 on to the short arm of chromosome 21 (marker chromosome XIp) (Fonatsch *et al.* 1990). In this line, TCR-α is translocated to another marker chromosome. Active nucleolus organizer regions and active ribosomal RNA genes are detectable in the centromere region of both marker chromosomes IX and XI (Fonatsch *et al.* 1990). The involvement of nucleolus organizer regions bearing chromosomes in marker formation has also been reported in Hodgkin's disease-derived cell lines L428, Cole, and KM-H2, as well as in primary Hodgkin's disease (Hossfeld and Schmidt 1978; Jones *et al.* 1985; Fonatsch *et al.* 1986; Kamesaki *et al.* 1986). As in other malignant cell lines (Holden *et al.* 1986; Takahashi *et al.* 1986), nucleolus organization genes might be responsible for the aberrant transcription of normally silent genes such as proto-oncogenes in Hodgkin's disease-derived cell lines (Fonatsch *et al.* 1990).

Peripheral blood lymphocytes from patients with Hodgkin's disease show a much greater number of abnormal metaphases when incubated with cytostatic drugs than do normal controls. Furthermore, some of these break-points have so far been seen in leukaemic cells (Fonatsch *et al.* 1990). From a knowledge of familial clustering and the tendency to develop secondary neoplasias in Hodgkin's disease, one might speculate about genetic instability as an aetiological factor in Hodgkin's disease and this hypothesis requires future investigation.

Gene rearrangements

Current phenotypic methods do not lead to the exact location of the Hodgkin cell within the haemopoietic differentiation system. Assuming that the tumour cell retains properties of its non-malignant progenitor, genetic differentiation markers may be helpful in placing the Hodgkin's cell ontogeny (Athan *et al.* 1989; Stein *et al.* 1989).

During differentiation of T and B lymphocytes, recombinations of Ig or TCR genes precede the formation of functional Ig or TCR molecules; that is, antigen-specific T- and B-cell antigen receptors (Leder *et al.* 1982; Hedrick *et al.* 1984). These recombinations join V (variable), D (diversity), and J (joining) gene segments. The resulting VDJ rearrangements together with C (constant) gene segments encode for IG_H (heavy chain) or Ig_L (light chain) $\varkappa$ or λ. Similar rearrangements occur in the TCR genes during differentiation of T-cells (Lefranc and Rabbitts 1985). These

rearrangements are specific for each B- and T-cell. By Southern blot, cells of a single clone can be detected when they represent as little as 1–2 per cent of the total cell population (Cleary *et al.* 1984; Minden and Mak 1986). The specific order of rearrangements (Ig_H before Ig_L $\varkappa$, then λ; TCR-γ, δ before TCR-β, then -α) allows definition of the differentiation stage of such a cell clone more precisely.

In the nine available Hodgkin's-disease-derived cell lines the results of differentiation studies of T or B lymphocytes are heterogeneous (Tables 1 and 5). Five of the lines show Ig and four have TCR rearrangements (Falk *et al.* 1987; Drexler *et al.* 1989). Some of these lines also express Ig or TCR mRNA.

In primary biopsy tissue, again, the percentage of malignant cells within the tumour sample is close to the detection threshold, thus limiting the reliability of clonality studies in primary tumour materials. However, in 4 per cent of cases, Ig and in 11 per cent, TCR rearrangements were detected (Table 5).

As B- as well as T-cell rearrangements occur in tested cell lines and fresh tumour material, we cannot finally determine whether the cell of origin in Hodgkin's disease is a B or T lymphocyte. Furthermore, clonal Ig or TCR rearrangements are neither specific for malignancy nor for derivation of a specific lineage. Clonal Ig rearrangements can be found in benign tissue under certain conditions, for example lymphoproliferative or lymphoepithelial lesions (Cleary *et al.* 1984; Pelicci *et al.* 1986; Fishleder *et al.* 1987). In non-lymphocytic leukaemias, Ig and TCR rearrangements have also been reported (Rovigatti *et al.* 1984; Cheng *et al.* 1986). It has not been finally determined if the rearrangements detected in primary tissue studies relate to Hodgkin and Reed–Sternberg cells (Knowles *et al.* 1986) so that we do not know if these observations pertain to normal or malignant cells.

With these important reservations, the data available from *in vitro* and *in vivo* experiments favour a lymphoid origin for the Hodgkin and Reed–Sternberg cells (Schaadt *et al.* 1988; Drexler *et al.* 1989; Stein *et al.* 1989). Although Ig or TCR gene rearrangements have also been detected in cell lines of myeloid origin (Hsu and Hsu 1989), the observation that the Hodgkin cell lines have either Ig or TCR gene rearrangements (Table 1), which are often transcribed, points to an immature lymphoid origin for these cells (Drexler *et al.* 1989; Tesch *et al.* 1990a).

Table 5 Rearrangements of the immunoglobulin supergene family in Hodgkin (HD) cells

Rearrangement	Primary HD cells DNA	HD cell lines DNA	HD cell lines RNA
TCR or Ig	+[a]	All	L428, L540,L591,Co,Ho,HDLM2
TCR	+	Co,HDLM2,Ho,L540	
α		HDLM2,L540	HDLM2,L540,L428
β	+	Co,HDLM2[+],Ho,L540,L428	Co,Ho
γ	(+)	Co,HDLM2+[b],Ho,L540	
δ	Frequently deleted		
Ig	+	DEV,KM-H2,L428,L591,Zo	L428
Ig_H[c]	+	L428,L591,DEV[+],KMH2[d],Zo	L428
Ig_L[e]	(+)	DEV,L591,Zo	L591
$Ig_L\varkappa$	(+)	DEV,L428,L591	L591
$Ig_L\lambda$		L428,L591	L591
EBV discovered	15%	L591	

[a] (+) <10%; + <30%; ++ <60%; +++ >60% positive cells.
[b] Both alleles rearranged.
[c] Heavy chain gene.
[d] Second allele deleted.
[e] Light chain gene.

Oncogenes and oncogene products

Proto-oncogenes are cellular genes potentially involved in tumorigenesis. Upon activation, they may affect malignant transformation by either point mutation (Weinberg 1984), gene amplification (Schwab et al. 1984), translocation (Leder et al. 1983), nearby insertion of a viral promoter (Hayward et al. 1981), or inactivation of a suppressor gene (Klein 1987). Each of these events can lead either to the deregulation of expression or to the formation of a structurally altered product resulting in an activated oncogene. Proto-oncogenes closely associated with certain malignancies include translocated c-myc in Burkitt's lymphoma, c-abl in Philadelphia-positive chronic myeloid and acute lymphocytic leukaemia, and bcl2 in follicular lymphoma (Klein 1983; Collins et al. 1984; Cleary et al. 1986; Fainstain et al. 1987).

The analysis of proto-oncogenes in Hodgkin's-disease-derived cell lines has revealed a heterogeneous pattern of expression. Some of the proto-oncogenes (c-myc, c-myb, c-raf, and N-ras) appeared in all of the four tested cell lines (Jücker et al. 1991). However, these proto-oncogenes are often also detected in leukaemia cell lines or non-malignant haemopoietic cells. Other genes could only be detected in some of the Hodgkin's-derived cell lines. Transcripts of c-met, a proto-oncogene originally described in an osteosarcoma cell line (Dean et al. 1985), are expressed in Hodgkin's-disease-derived cell lines L428 and L540. The gene is translocated into the vicinity of a transcriptionally active locus on marker chromosome XI in L540 but not in L428 (see the above subsection for details; Fonatsch et al. 1990). Evidence for a rearrangement or an amplification involving c-met in these lines could not be detected. Remarkably, this proto-oncogene is not transcribed in any of the leukaemic or normal controls, except for the Burkitt's lymphoma cell line Raji. It has hitherto not been analysed if c-met has transforming capability in haemopoietic cells.

Aberrant transcripts of the proto-oncogene c-fes occur in the L428 and Cole cell lines. A deletion or rearrangement of the gene was not detectable (Jücker et al. 1991). Whether these aberrant transcripts encode a transforming protein is not clear yet.

L540 and L428 express high levels of transcripts specific for the proto-oncogene c-fms as well as the resulting protein, the colony-stimulating factor (CSF)-1 receptor. It may be involved in autocrine stimulation of these cell lines (see above; Paietta et al. 1989).

The reason for the non-homogeneous pattern of expression of proto-oncogenes in Hodgkin's-disease-derived cell lines is not clear. It might represent different differentiation stages of the cells or in certain cases deregulated and probably activated proto-oncogenes (Jücker et al. 1991; Paietta et al. 1989).

Oncogene expression in primary Hodgkin's cells has to date only been studied to a limited extent: ras protein was detected in Reed–Sternberg cells and activated N-ras oncogenes (Sklar and Kitchingman 1985) have been observed in two Hodgkin's cases by transfection experiments. It cannot be defined whether these mutations occurred in the Hodgkin and Reed–Sternberg cells. Point mutations in codons 12, 13, and 61, which can activate ras proto-oncogenes, were not identified in any of 25 primary tissue samples (Steenvorden et al. 1988). High levels of c-myc protein (Mitani et al. 1988) appeared in the nuclei of Reed–Sternberg cells as well as in surrounding lymphocytes and histiocytes.

The influence of oncogenes on the tumourigenesis of Hodgkin's disease has to be clarified.

EBV infection

Epstein–Barr virus infection has long been suspected to exist in Hodgkin's disease. In addition to the clinical incidence of elevated anti-EBV antibody titres (Diehl and Johansson 1974) and detection of EBV in the Hodgkin's-disease-derived cell line L591 (Diehl et al. 1982), monoclonal or oligoclonal proliferation of EBV is present in part of the biopsy specimen in Hodgkin's disease (Weiss et al. 1987; Staal et al. 1989). By in situ hybridization, viral DNA was detected in 19 per cent of Hodgkin and Reed–Sternberg cells (Weiss et al. 1989). This incidence may be higher in acquired immune deficiency disease-associated Hodgkin's disease, where four out of seven cases displayed EBV DNA in the tumour cells (Uccini et al. 1989). Although EBV is known for its transforming capacity in B-cells (Diehl et al. 1968), its functional relevance in the pathogenesis of Hodgkin's disease remains to be elucidated.

EBV-transformed lymphocytes may be an interesting model for cellular transformation in Hodgkin's disease (Herbst et al. 1989). As already mentioned, the divergence between activated mature phenotype and pre B-cell genotype is a feature frequently described in Hodgkin's disease (Falk et al. 1987). Analogous to that, some lymphoblastoid cell lines present incomplete or no Ig rearrangements (Katamine et al. 1984; Gregory et al. 1987) while expressing activation markers (CD25, CD30, Ki-24).

Cytokine production

The humoral interaction of immunocompetent cells via cytokines is a fascinating focus of interest. Judging from the intense local and systemic reactions a Hodgkin's tumour inflicts on its organism, the tumour cells may interfere directly or via accessory cells with the immune system through mediators. Some aspects of the typical biology of Hodgkin's disease suggest the involvement of particular cytokines (Table 6).

Well in line with these theoretical considerations concerning the pathophysiology of Hodgkin's disease, several biological activities, mediators, and receptors have been proved to be produced by Hodgkin's-derived cell lines (Table 6). Cell lines do have several conceptual advantages when studying humoral mediators. Due to the inherent purity of the cell population, any measurable phenomena have to stem from the tumour cell clone. Unlike tissue in vivo, cells can be extensively manipulated in vitro. Reactions to any form of intervention can be observed over time as well as by the use of methods that are not compatible with the life of an organism.

Table 6 Cytokines that could be involved in Hodgkin's disease as derived from cell line research

Biological features in Hodgkin's disease	Possible mediators	Molecular weight (kDa)	In vitro evidence
Lymphoproliferation*, fever, night sweats, immunodeficiency	IL-1*	30–32	Immunostaining[a], bioassay[b]
	IL-2*	15.5	IL-2R (CD25), ZO growth
	IL-6*	26	Northern blot
	TNF-α	17	Immunostaining, bioassay
	TNF-β	20	Bioassay[c]
Leucocyte/eosinophil infiltration, myeloproliferation	GM-CSF	18–22	Protein sequencing
	G-CSF	19	Bioassay[d]
	M-CSF	70–90	Northern blot, M-CSF-R[e] Autocrine function
Fibrosis	TGF-β	16.5?	Northern blot[f]

[a]Hsu (1985).
[b]IL-1-dependent cell line.
[c]Cytotoxicity assay.
[d]Human and murine stem cell assay.
[e]Product of c-fms proto-oncogene.
[f]HD-derived TGP-β active at physiological pH.

Diverse biological activities have been discovered in the supernatant of Hodgkin's-disease-derived cell lines. These include inhibition of T-cell rosettes and co-stimulation of T-cells, fibroblast growth inductions, EBV-positive B-cell blast proliferation, and leucocyte migration inhibition (Schaadt *et al.* 1988; Schell-Frederick *et al.* 1988). Whether these effects can be ascribed to any of the known cytokines is currently being investigated.

Strong evidence for the involvement of interleukins and tumour necrosis factor, the interleukin-2-receptor α-chain (CD25) antigen present on both most primary tumours and cell lines, is provided by the observation that the Hodgkin's-disease-derived cell line L540 expresses functional, high-affinity, interleukin-2 receptors consisting of both β- and α-chains (Tesch *et al.* 1990a). Any further relation to growth or activation of cells has not yet been established. The concentration of the soluble CD25 molecule is elevated in the sera of patients with Hodgkin's disease (see immunocytology section for details).

Fibrosis is a characteristic feature of nodular sclerosing Hodgkin's disease and of relevance to this, the cell line L428 produces a high molecular-weight transforming growth factor-β (TGF-β). In contrast to previously described TGF-β receptor-binding cytokines, it is active at physiological pH (Newcom *et al.* 1988).

Several growth factors are released by the cell lines, including both GM-CSF and G-CSF (Byrne *et al.* 1986). Autocrine pathways involving a CSF-1 stimulation circle have been demonstrated in L540 and L428 cells using a CSF-1 assay system and mRNA probes for CSF-1 and the CSF-1 receptor (Paietta *et al.* 1989). The CSF-1 receptor itself is the product of the proto-oncogene c-*fms*.

Until now, the existence of mediators for interleukin-1 in primary Hodgkin's material has only been demonstrated by cell surface or cytoplasmic immunostaining (Hsu and Zhao 1986). In the future, *in situ* detection techniques for mRNA and proteins will help to verify the outcome of the cell line *in vivo*. At present, because cytokine production can be induced by a variety of activation mechanisms (Weir 1986), their production is no criterion of lineage specificity. Nevertheless, there is little doubt that cytokine interactions determine the pathophysiology of Hodgkin's disease.

CONCLUSIONS

The origin of Hodgkin's disease is still a mystery more than 150 years after the original description (Hodgkin 1832). In the 1980s, however, results were obtained that provide insights on this puzzle (Diehl 1989). The assumption that Hodgkin and Reed–Sternberg cells are the neoplastic cells in Hodgkin's disease is, due to the lack of other candidates, widely accepted (Diehl *et al.* 1982, 1985). The availability of cultured cells from patients with Hodgkin's disease has led to a deeper understanding of the geno- and phenotypical characteristics of the Hodgkin tumour cell. The identity of *in vivo* and *in vitro* cultured counterparts and the presence of monoclonal EBV DNA in Hodgkin and Reed–Sternberg cells have demonstrated that those are of clonal origin (Diehl *et al.* 1982; Stein *et al.* 1989). The generation of antibodies against epitopes of these cells *in vitro* (L428, L540) has expanded our knowledge of the heterogeneity of Hodgkin's disease. Remarkably, the findings from primary material at no point openly contradict those from cell line data and it is likely that these cell lines indeed stem from the tumour cell in Hodgkin's disease (Diehl *et al.* 1982, 1985; Schaadt *et al.* 1985).

Bearing in mind that the available data are not complete, a working hypothesis on the descent of the Hodgkin's cell can be contrived. In brief, the morphologically distinct Hodgkin and Reed–Sternberg cell has an immunophenotype characteristic of activated, immature T- or B-cells (Falk *et al.* 1987; Herbst *et al.* 1989; Tesch *et al.* 1990b). In Hodgkin's disease, rearrangements and expressions of the immunoglobulin supergene family are frequently incomplete or irregular (Herbst *et al.* 1989; Tesch *et al.* 1990b). The heterogeneity of the clinical and histological appearance of Hodgkin's disease and the multitude of different and somewhat controversial cellular markers might be explained by Hodgkin's disease being a group of pathophysiologically associated but not identical entities. The origin might be the same target cell transformed at different stages of maturation or, alternatively, several biologically related diseases each with a different aetiopathogenesis.

The present data may well be explained by the Hodgkin's lymphoma cell being derived from an immature lymphoid stage of differentiation that is transformed before or during the rearrangement of the B- or T-cell receptor gene (Falk *et al.* 1987; Herbst *et al.* 1989; Kamesaki *et al.* 1989). The transformation could then superimpose maturation characteristics on to the cells. A similarly dissociated geno- and phenotypic pattern of differentiation occurs in EBV-transformed fetal lymphocytes (Gregory *et al.* 1987). Myelomonocytic features could evolve in analogy to mechanisms demonstrated in other haematological models (Davidson *et al.* 1988; Klinken *et al.* 1988), where conversion of B-cells into myelomonocytoid cells by oncogenes or after treatment with lipopolysaccharide was seen. As described above, cytogenetic changes, evidence for proto-oncogene involvement, and EBV infection and/or activation have been described in Hodgkin's disease. The cell populations arising from transforming processes may stimulate their own growth by means of cytokine production. Such cytokine–receptor interactions with the immune system are likely to produce the typical morphological and clinical manifestations of Hodgkin's disease.

REFERENCES

Agnarsson BA, Kadin ME (1989). The immunophenotype of Reed–Sternberg cells. A study of 50 cases of Hodgkin's disease using fixed frozen tissues. *Cancer*, 63:2083–7.

Anastasi J, Bauer KD, Variakojis D (1987). DNA aneuploidy in Hodgkin's disease. A multiparameter flow-cytometric analysis with cytologic correlation. *American Journal of Pathology*, 128:573–82.

Andreesen R, Brugger W, Löhr GW, Bross KJ (1989). A Hodgkin cell associated antigen (Ki-1, CD30) is expressed on normal human macrophages and malignant histiocytes. *American Journal of Pathology*, 134(1):187–92.

Athan E, Paietta P, Papenhausen PR, Augenlicht L, Wiernik PH, Gallagher RE (1989). Stability of multiple antigen receptor gene rearrangements and immunophenotype in Hodgkin's disease derived cell line L428 and variant subline L428KSA. *Leukemia*, 3:505–10.

Burrichter H, Schaadt M, Heit W, Seidel K, Diehl V (1985). Hodgkin cell factors. In *Mediators in oncology*, Serono Symposia Meetings. Raven, New York.

Byrne PV, Heit WF, March CJ (1986). Human granulocyte-macrophage colony stimulating factor purified from a Hodgkin's tumor cell line. *Biochemica et Biophysica Acta*, 874(3):266–73.

Cabanillas F, *et al.* (1988). Cytogenetic features of Hodgkin's disease suggest possible origin from a lymphocyte. *Blood*, 71:1615–17.

Carde P, *et al.* (1989). Radiolabeled monoclonal antibodies against Reed–Sternberg cells for *in vivo* imaging of Hodgkin's disease by immuno-scintigraphy. *Recent Results in Cancer Research*, 117:101–11.

Casey TT, Fairfield SJ, Cousar JB, Collins RD (1988). Immunophenotypes of Reed–Sternberg cells in plastic sections: a study of nine cases of nodular sclerosing Hodgkin's disease. *Laboratory Investigation*, 58:16a.

Cheng GY, Minden MD, Toyonaga B, Mak TW, McCulloch EA (1986). T cell receptor and immunoglobulin rearrangements in acute myeloblastic leukemia. *Journal of Experimental Medicine*, 163:414–24.

Cleary ML, Chao J, Warnke R, Sklar J (1984). Immunoglobulin gene rearrangement as a diagnostic criterion of B cell lymphoma. *Proceedings of the National Academy of Sciences USA*, 81:593–7.

Cleary ML, Smith SD, Sklar J (1986). Cloning and structural analysis of cDNAs for *bcl-2* and a hybrid *bcl-2*/immunoglobulin transcript resulting from the t(14;18) translocation. *Cell*, 47:19–28.

Coles FB, Cartun RW, Pastuszak WT (1988). Hodgkin's disease, lymphoctye-predominant type: immunoreactivity with B-cell antibodies. *Modern Pathology*, 1:274–8.

Collins SJ, Kubonishi I, Miyoshi I, Groudine MT (1984). Altered transcription of the *c-abl* oncogene in K-562 and other chronic myelogenous leukemia cells. *Science*, 225:72–4.

Davidson WF, Pierce JH, Rudikoff F, Morse HC III (1988). Relationships between B cell and myeloid differentiation. Studies with a B lymphocyte progenitor line, HAFTL-1. *Journal of Experimental Medicine*, 168:389–407.

Dean M, *et al.* (1985). The human *met* oncogene is related to the tyrosine kinase oncogenes. *Nature*, 318:385–8.

Dennis TR, Stock AD, Winberg CD, Sheibani K, Rappaport H (1989). Cytogenetic studies of Hodgkin's disease: analysis of involved lymph nodes from 12 patients. *Cancer Genetics and Cytogenetics*, 37:201–8.

DeVita V, Jaffe E, Hellman S (1985). Hodgkin's disease and the non-hodgkin's lymphoma. In *Cancer: principles and practice of oncology*, (2nd edn) (ed. V DeVita, S Hellman, and S Rosenberg). J. B. Lippincott, Philadelphia.

Diehl V (1985). Hodgkin's disease: the remaining challenge. *European Surgical Research*, 17:388–98.

Diehl, V. (1989). Preface. In *Recent results in cancer research*, 117.

Diehl V, Johansson B (1974). Epstein–Barr-virus (EBV) in lymphoid cells from patients with Hodgkin's disease. In *Recent results in cancer research*, 46: 59–61.

Diehl V, Henle G, Henle W, Kohn G (1968). Demonstration of a herpes group virus (EBV) in cultures of peripheral leukocytes from patients with infectious mononucleosis. *Journal of Virology*, 2:663–9.

Diehl V, Henle W, Henle G, Kohn G (1969). Effect of a herpes group virus (EBV) on growth of peripheral leukocyte cultures. *In Vitro*, 4:92–9.

Diehl V, *et al.* (1982). Characteristics of Hodgkin's disease derived cell lines. *Cancer Treatment Reports*, 66:615–32.

Drexler HG, *et al.* (1988). Genotypes and immunophenotypes of Hodgkin's disease derived cell lines. *Leukemia*, 2:371–6.

Drexler HG, Jones DB, Diehl V, Minowada J (1989). Is the Hodgkin cell a T- or a B-lymphocyte? Recent evidence from geno- and immunophenotypic analysis and *in vitro* cell lines. *Hematological Oncology*, 7:95–113.

Engelmann EG, Benike CJ, Hoppe RT (1980). Autologous mixed lymphocyte reaction in patients with Hodgkin's disease. *Journal of Clinical Investigation*, 66:149–58.

Engert A, *et al.* (1990). Evaluation of ricin A chain-containing immunotoxins directed against the CD30 antigen as potential reagents for the treatment of Hodgkin's disease. *Cancer Research*, 50(1):84–8.

Fainstain E, *et al.* (1987). A new fused transcript in Philadelphia chromosome positive acute lymphoblastic leukemia. *Nature*, 330:386–8.

Falini B, Stein H, Pileri S (1987). Expression of lymphoid-associated antigens on Hodgkin's and Reed–Sternberg cells of Hodgkin's disease; an immunocytochemical study on lymph node cytospins using monoclonal antibodies. *Histopathology*, 11:1229–42.

Falk MH, *et al.* (1987). Phenotype versus immunoglobulin and T cell receptor genotype of Hodgkin-derived cell lines: activation of immature lymphoid cells in Hodgkin's disease. *International Journal of Cancer*, 40:262–9.

Fischer RI, Bostick-Bruton F, Sander DN, Scala G, Diehl V (1983). Neoplastic cells from Hodgkin's disease are potent stimulators of human primary mixed lymphocyte cultures. *Journal of Immunology*, 130:2666–70.

Fishleder A, Tubbs RO, Hesse B, Levine H (1987). Uniform detection of immunoglobulin gene rearrangement in benign lymphoepithelial lesions. *New England Journal of Medicine*, 316:1118–21.

Fonatsch C, Diehl V, Schaadt M, Burrichter H, Kirchner HH (1986). Cytogenetic investigation in Hodgkin's disease: I. Involvement of specific chromosomes in marker formation. *Cancer Genetics and Cytogenetics*, 20: 39–52.

Fonatsch C, Gradl G, Kolbus U, Rieder H, Tesch H (1990). Chromosomal *in situ* hybridization of a Hodgkin's disease derived cell line (L540) using

DNA probes for TCR alpha, TCR beta, *met* and rRNA. *Human Genetics*, 84(5):427–34.

Gause A, *et al.* (1991). Clinical significance of soluble CD30 antigen in the sera of patients with untreated Hodgkins disease. *Blood*, 77:1983–8.

Gerdes J, van Baarlen J, Pileri S, Schwarting R, van Unnik JAM, Stein H (1987). Tumor growth fraction in Hodgkin's disease. *American Journal of Pathology*, 129:390–3.

Gregory CD, *et al.* (1987). Epstein–Barr virus-transformed human precursor B cell lines: altered growth phenotype of lines with germline or rearranged but nonexpressed heavy chain genes. *European Journal of Immunology*, 17:1199–207.

Hansen H, Lemke H, Bredfeldt G, Konnecke I, Havsteen B (1989). The Hodgkin-associated Ki-1 antigen exists in an intracellular and a membrane-bound form. *Biol Chem Hoppe Seyler*, 370, 409–16.

Hayward WS, Neel BG, Astrin SM (1981). Activation of a cellular *onc* gene by promoter insertion in ALV-induced lymphoid leukosis. *Nature*, 290:475–80.

Hedrick SM, Cohen DI, Nielson E, Davis MM (1984). Isolation of cDNA clones encoding T cell specific membrane associated proteins. *Nature*, 308:149–53.

Herbst H, *et al.* (1989). Immunoglobulin and T cell receptor gene rearrangements in Hodgkin's disease and Ki-1 positive large cell lymphoma: dissociation between phenotype and genotype. *Leukemia Research*, 13:103–16.

Hodgkin T (1832). On some morbid appearances of the absorbent glands and spleen. *Medico-Chirurgical Transactions*, 17:68–114.

Holden JJA, Reimer DL, Roder JC, White BN (1986). Rearrangements of chromosomal regions containing ribosomal RNA genes and centromeric heterochromatin in the human melanoma cell line MeWo. *Cancer Genetics and Cytogenetics*, 21:221–37.

Hossfeld DK, Schmidt CG (1978). Chromosome findings in effusions from patients with Hodgkin's disease. *International Journal of Cancer*, 21:147–56.

Hsu S, Hsu P (1989). Aberrant expression of T and B cell markers in myelocyte/monocyte/histiocyte derived lymphoma and leukemia cells. *American Journal of Pathology*, 134:203–12.

Hsu SM, Jaffe ES (1984). Leu M1 and peanut agglutinin stain the neoplastic cells of Hodgkin's disease. *American Journal of Clinical Pathology*, 82:29–32.

Hsu SM, Zhao X (1986). Expression of interleukin-1 in H-RS cells and neoplastic cells from true histiocytic lymphomas. *American Journal of Pathology*, 186:331–6.

Jones DB, *et al.* (1985). Phenotype analysis of an established cell line derived from a patient with Hodgkin's disease. *Hematologic Oncology*, 3:133–45.

Jücker M, Schaadt M, Diehl V, Poppema S, Jones D, Tesch H (1991). Heterogeneous expression of proto-oncogenes in cell lines derived from patients with Hodgkin's disease. *Blood*, 77(11):2413–18.

Kamesaki H, *et al.* (1986). Cytochemical immunologic, chromosomal and molecular genetic analysis of a novel cell line derived from Hodgkin's disease. *Blood*, 68:285–92.

Kamesaki H, Fukuhara S, Uchino H, Nosaka T (1989). A new hypothesis on the cellular origin of Reed–Sternberg and Hodgkin cells based on the immunological and molecular genetic analysis of the KM-H2 line. *Recent Results in Cancer Research*, 117:83–90.

Kaplan HS (1980). *Hodgkin's disease*. Harvard University Press.

Katamine S, *et al.* (1984). Epstein–Barr virus transforms precursor B cells even before immunoglobulin gene rearrangements. *Nature*, 309:369–72.

Klein G (1983) Specific chromosomal translocations and the genesis of B cell derived tumors in mice and men. *Cell*, 32:311–15.

Klein G (1987). The approaching era of the tumor suppressor genes. *Science*, 238:1539–45.

Klinken SP, Alexander WS, Adams JM (1988). Hemopoietic lineage switch: v-*raf* oncogene converts N-*myc* transgenic B cells into macrophages. *Cell*, 53:857–67.

Knowles DM, *et al.* (1986). Immunoglobulin and T cell receptor β-chain gene rearrangement analysis of Hodgkin's disease: implications for lineage determination and differential diagnosis. *Proceedings of the National Academy of Sciences USA*, 83:7942–6.

Leder P, *et al.* (1983). Translocations among antibody genes in human cancer. *Science*, 222:766–71.

Lefranc MP, Rabbitts TH (1985). Two tandemly organized human genes encoding the T-cell gamma constant region sequences show multiple rearrangements in different T cell types. *Nature*, 316:464–6.

Lukes RJ, Craver LF, Hall TC, Rappaport H, Ruben P (1966). Report of the nomenclature committee. *Cancer Research*, 26:1311.

Lukes RJ, Tindlc BH, Parker JW (1969). Reed–Sternberg-like cells in infectious mononucleosis. *Lancet*, ii:1000–4.

Minden MD, Mak TW (1986). The structure of the T cell antigen receptor genes in normal and malignant T cells. *Blood*, 68:327–36.

Mitani S, Sugawara I, Shiku H, Mori S (1988). Expression of the c-*myc* oncogene product and *ras* family oncogene products in various human malignant lymphomas defined by immunohistochemical techniques. *Cancer*, 62:2085–93.

Newcom S, Kadin M Ansari A, Diehl V (1988). L428 nodular sclerosing Hodgkin's cell secretes a unique transforming growth factor beta active at physiologic pH. *Journal of Clinical Investigations*, 82:1915–21.

O'Connor NTJ, *et al.* (1987). Genotypic analysis of large lymphomas which express the Ki-1 antigen. *Histopathology*, 11:733–40.

Oka K, Mori N, Kojima M (1988). Anti-Leu-3a antibody reactivity with Reed–Sternberg cells of Hodgkin's disease. *Archives of Pathology and Laboratory Medicine*, 112:139–42.

Paietta E, Racevskis J, Stanley ER, Wiernik PH (1989). Hodgkin's disease cells: origin from a bipotential lymphoid/macrophage progenitor cell? *Proceedings of the American Association for Cancer Research*, 30:430.

Pelicci PG, Knowles DM, Dalla-Farvera R (1986). Lymphoid tumors displaying rearrangements of both immunoglobulin and T cell receptor genes. *Journal of Experimental Medicine*, 162:1015–24.

Pfreundschuh M, *et al.* (1988). Hodgkin and Reed–Sternberg cell associated monoclonal antibodies HRS-1 and HRS-2 react with activated cells of lymphoid and monocytoid origin. *Anticancer Research*, 8:217–24.

Poppema S, De Jong B, Atmosoerodjo J, Idenburg V, Visser L, De Ley L (1985). Morphologic, immunologic, enzymehistochemical and chromosomal analysis of a cell line derived from Hodgkin's disease. Evidence for a B-cell origin of Sternberg–Reed cells. *Cancer*, 55:683–90.

Poppema S, Visser L, de Jong B, Brinker M, Atmosoerodja J, Timens W (1989). *Recent Results in Cancer Research*, 117:67–74.

Pui C-H, *et al.* (1989). High serum interleukin-2 levels correlate with a poor prognosis in children with Hodgkin's disease. *Leukemia*, 3:481–4.

Rovigatti U, Mirro J, Kitchingman J (1984). Heavy chain immunoglobulin gene rearrangements in acute nonlymphocytic leukemia. *Blood*, 63:1023–7.

Rowley JD (1982). Chromosomes in Hodgkin's disease. *Cancer Treatment Reports*, 66:639.

Sanders ME, Makgoba MW, Sussman EH, Luce GA, Cossman J, Shaw S (1988). Molecular pathways of adhesion in spontaneous rosetting of T lymphocytes to the Hodgkin's cell line L428. *Cancer Research*, 48:37–40.

Schaadt M, Diehl V, Stein H, Fonatsch C, Kirchner HH (1980). Two neoplastic cell lines with unique features derived from Hodgkin's disease. *International Journal of Cancer*, 26:723–31.

Schaadt M, Burrichter H, Stein H, Pfreundschuh M, Fonatsch C, Diehl V (1985). The cell of origin in Hodgkin's disease: conclusions from *in vivo* and *in vitro* studies. *International Review of Experimental Pathology*, 27:185.

Schaadt M, von Kalle C, Tesch H, Burrichter H, Diehl V (1988). Immunlogic, functional and molecular genetic properties of Hodgkin's disease derived cell lines. *Cancer Reviews*, 10:108–22.

Schaadt M, *et al.* (1989). Biology of Hodgkin cell lines. *Recent Results in Cancer Research*, 117:53–61.

Schell-Frederick E, *et al.* (1988). Inhibition of human neutrophil migration by supernatants from Hodgkin's disease derived cell lines. *European Journal of Clinical Investigation*, 18:290–6.

Schouten H, Sanger W, Duggan M, Weisenburger D, MacLennan KA, Armitage JO (1989). Chromosomal abnormalities in Hodgkin's disease. *Blood*, 73:2149–54.

Schwab U, *et al.* (1982). Production of a monoclonal antibody specific for Hodgkin and Sternberg–Reed cells on Hodgkin's lymphoma and a subset of normal lymphoid cells. *Nature*, 299:65–7.

Schwab M, Ellison J, Busch M, Rosenau W, Varmus HE, Bishop JM (1984). Enhanced expression of the human gene N-*myc* consequent to amplification of DNA may contribute to malignant progression of neuroblastoma. *Proceedings of the National Academy of Sciences USA*, 81:4940–4.

Sklar MD, Kitchingman GR (1985). Isolation of activated *ras* transforming genes from two patients with Hodgkin's disease. *International Journal of Radiation Oncology — Biology — Physics*, 11:49–55.

Staal SP, Ambinder R, Beschorner WE, Hayward GS, Mann R (1989). A survey of Epstein–Barr virus DNA in lymphoid tissue: frequent detection in Hodgkin's disease. *American Journal of Clinical Pathology*, 91:1–5.

Steenvorden ACM, *et al.* (1985). *Ras* mutations in Hodgkin's disease. *Leukemia*, 2:325.

Stein H (1988). Comments on Hodgkin's disease: the Reed–Sternberg cell by P. Bucsky. *Blut*, 57:143–6.

Stein H, *et al.* (1982). Identification of Hodgkin and Reed–Sternberg cells as a unique cell type derived from a newly detected small-cell population. *International Journal of Cancer*, 30:445–9.

Stein H, *et al.* (1985). The expression of the Hodgkin's disease associated antigen Ki-1 in reactive and neoplastic lymphoid tissue. Evidence that Reed–Sternberg cells and histiocytic malignancies are derived from activated lymphoid cells. *Blood*, 66:848–58.

Stein H, *et al.* (1986). Reed–Sternberg cells and Hodgkin cells in lymphocyte predominant Hodgkin's disease of nodular subtype contain J chain. *American Journal of Clinical Pathology*, 86:292–7.

Stein H, Schwarting R, Dallenbach F, Dienemann D (1989). Immunology of Hodgkin and Reed–Sternberg cells. *Recent Results in Cancer Research*, 117:14–26.

Strum SB, Rappaport H (1971). Interrelations of the histologic types of Hodgkin's disease. *Archives of Pathology*, 91:127–39.

Stuart AE, Jones DB, Wright DH (1977). Reed–Sternberg cell/lymphocyte interaction. *Lancet*, ii:768–9.

Takahashi R (1986). Secondary activation of c-*abl* may be related to translocation to the nuclear organizer region in an *in vitro* cultured rat leukemia cell line (K3D). *Proceedings of the National Academy of Sciences USA*, 83:1079–83.

Taylor CR (1983). Upon the enigma of Hodgkin's disease and the Reed–Sternberg cell. In *Controversies in the management of lymphomas* (ed. JM Bennet), p. 91. Nijhoff, Boston.

Teerenhovi L, Lindholm C, Pakkala A, Franssila K, Stein H, Knuutila S (1988). Unique display of a pathologic karyotype in Hodgkin's disease by Reed–Sternberg cells. *Cancer Genetics and Cytogenetics*, 34:305–11.

Tesch H, May P, Krueger GRF, Fischer R, Diehl V (1990*a*). Analysis of immunoglobulin, T cell receptor and *bcr* rearrangements in human malignant lymphoma and Hodgkin's disease. *Oncology*, 47:215–23.

Tesch H, Hermann T, Abts H, Diamantstein T, Diehl V (1990*b*). Expression of high affinity II-2 receptors on a Hodgkin's derived cell line. *Leukemia Research*, 14:953–60.

Thangavelu M, Le Beau MM (1989). Chromosomal abnormalities in Hodgkin's disease. *Hematology/Oncology Clinics of North America*, 3:221–36.

Uccini S, *et al.* (1989). High frequency of Epstein–Barr virus genome in HIV-positive patients with Hodgkin's disease. *Lancet*, 1:1458.

Weinberg RA (1984). *ras* oncogenes and the molecular mechanisms of carcinogenesis. *Blood*, 64:1143–5.

12.6.2   Hodgkin's disease in adults

DEREK CROWTHER, SIMON B. SUTCLIFFE, AND GIANNI BONADONNA

HISTORY

Thomas Hodgkin (1798–1866) came from a staunch Quaker family maintaining the standards of this sect in their household and daily activities. The history has been told by Michael Rose in his book *Curator of the dead* (1981). Hodgkin worked at Guy's Hospital in London as Lecturer in Morbid Anatomy and Curator of the Museum. In 1832 he published his paper 'On some morbid appearances of the absorbent glands and spleen'. In it, Hodgkin described six cases which he had encountered at Guy's. In 1926 the pathological material from these six patients was re-examined using the criteria for the microscopic distinction and diagnosis of Hodgkin's disease identified by Greenfield, Sutton, and Turner which appeared in the *Transactions of the Pathological Society* in 1878. In their cases these microscopists had identified certain bizarre cells which seemed characteristic of Hodgkin's disease and without which the condition could not be diagnosed. These cellular hallmarks of Hodgkin's disease are now most commonly known as Reed–Sternberg cells after Dorothy Reed (Mrs Mendenhall) of Baltimore, Maryland, who described them in 1902 and Carl Sternberg of Vienna, who described them in 1898. Hodgkin's disease was found in three of Thomas Hodgkin's six cases, tuberculosis in one, syphilis in one, and non-Hodgkin's lymphoma in one.

In 1837 Thomas Hodgkin was the outstanding candidate for the post of Assistant Physician at Guy's Hospital in succession to Dr Thomas Addison who had been promoted to the post of Physician. Hodgkin had spent 10 years as Curator of the Dead and had published a great deal including a two-volume work on the *The morbid anatomy of serous and mucous membranes*, considered to be the first attempt to treat morbid anatomy as a separate discipline in the English medical curriculum. In 1829 he described retroversion of the aortic valves, although credit for the discovery is generally attributed to Corrigan whose description was published approximately 20 years later. He was established amongst the most eminent figures in the medical profession and many of his colleagues concurred with this view. Richard Bright, a physician of eminence of Guy's Hospital, had selected Hodgkin to care for his patients in his absence. He became a Fellow of the Royal College of Physicians in 1836 and a year later was invited by the Home Secretary to serve on the Senate of the new University of London.

On Wednesday 6 September 1837 it was not Thomas Hodgkin but a lesser man, Benjamin Babington, who was called by the General Court of the hospital to receive the congratulations of the Governor. The decision had nothing to do with medicine, since Hodgkin's growing eminence was well recognized, but much to do with another passion in his life and a clash with a powerful man. Nineteen years before, Hodgkin had pledged himself to the service and protection of aboriginal tribal people throughout the world against their ruthless exploitation by the growing flood of European traders. He had written a pamphlet entitled *Essay on the protection of civilisation*, dealing particularly with the evil influence of European settlers on the North American Indian and was one of the founders of The Aboriginal Protection Society. The wealthy Treasurer of Guy's, Benjamin Harrison, exercised an autocratic rule over the hospital and presided at the appointment of the Assistant Physician made by the General Court. Unfortunately, he was also the Deputy Governor of the Hudson's Bay Company about which Hodgkin, acting in his other capacity, had sent him a report describing the terrible consequences to the Indians of monopoly trading and the inhuman treatment they received at the hands of the trappers and officials of his Company. Thomas Hodgkin did not get the job and the next day he resigned all his appointments at Guy's Hospital.

Most of the last 30 years of his life were devoted to social work. He saw the injustice of dark-skinned races bearing the brunt of contact with a superior civilization which took their land, slew their game, and destroyed their freedom. Dogging the steps of the missionary came the trader bringing gifts of rum and syphilis. Hodgkin saw these things and felt the injustice. His efforts in those last years of his life were not wasted. He died in Jaffa in his 68th year.

EPIDEMIOLOGY

Hodgkin's disease is an uncommon disorder accounting for only approximately 1 per cent of cancers registered in developed countries in each year. The incidence is approximately one-half to one-third of that for non-Hodgkin's lymphoma. The annual incidence ranges from 3 per 100 000 in Europe and the United States to less than 1 per 100 000 in Japan.

Hodgkin's disease shows an unusual variation in incidence with age. There is a striking bimodality in incidence with peaks in young adulthood and in older adulthood (MacMahon 1966; Grufferman and Delzell 1984). The cumulative incidence shows two log-linear intervals rising steeply until the 20–24 age interval and gradually after that (Fig. 1(a)). This pattern is quite different from those of non-Hodgkin's lymphoma and the leukaemias. The pattern also varies with the histological subtype and a bimodal pattern is less evident for the lymphocyte-depleted histology (Fig. 1(b)). In young adults the nodular-sclerosing subtype predominates, but in older persons the mixed cellularity form is as frequent as the nodular-sclerosing form (Keller *et al.* 1968). These epidemiological features have led to the suggestion that the disease might have a different aetiology in the young and older age groups. There have been reports of a seasonal variation in incidence, with a greater number of diagnoses being made in the winter months. However, it is likely that patients would be evaluated more frequently for upper respiratory tract infections in winter rendering the diagnosis more common during these periods.

There is evidence of familial aggregation of Hodgkin's disease. Siblings of young adult cases are at increased risk, whereas siblings of older adult cases have no increase in risk. There is a 3-fold risk for first-degree relatives and a 7-fold increase for siblings of young adult cases (Razis *et al.* 1959; Grufferman *et al.* 1977). Among sibling pairs with Hodgkin's disease there is a marked excess of sex-concordant pairs with a 9-fold relative risk compared with 5-fold for unlike-sex siblings. This pattern is hard to explain on a simple genetic basis and some component of the increased risk is likely to be due to shared environmental exposures. Families with

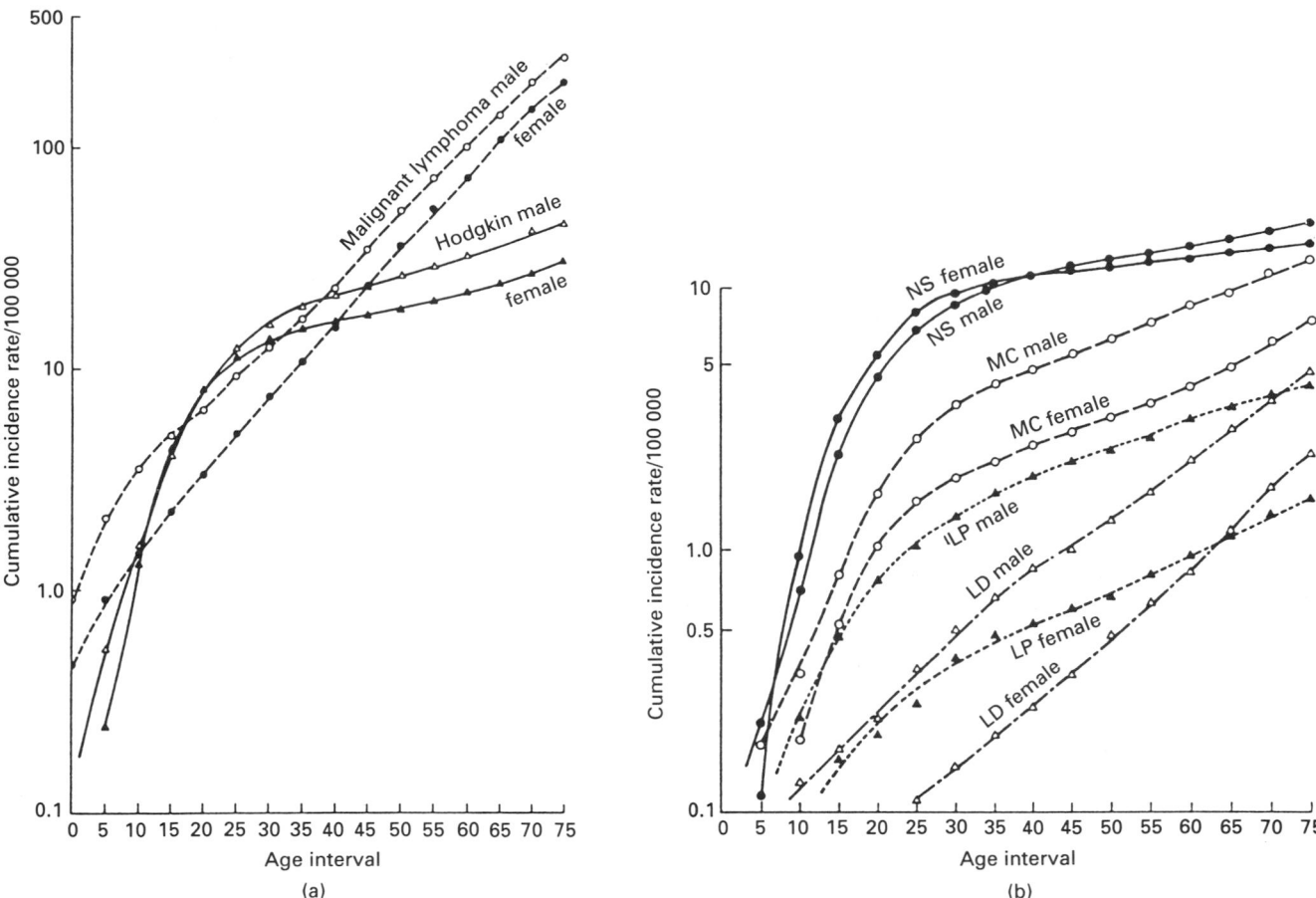

Fig. 1 (a) Lifetime cumulative incidence rates taken from the Surveillance Epidemiology and End Results (SEER) programme of the National Cancer Institute, United States (1973–1981). Malignant lymphoma shows a log-linear increase, whereas for Hodgkin's disease the cumulative incidence rates show a steep linear climb until age 20–24 years and then a much more gradual increase. Decreased rates for females are apparent after 20–24 years. (b) Cumulative incidence rate of Hodgkin's disease by histological subtype. There is a log-linear relationship with age for the lymphocyte-depleted (LD) subtype, whereas other histological types (nodular sclerosis (NS), mixed cellularity (MC), lymphocyte predominant (LP)) show a bimodal relationship with age. (Reproduced with permission from Watanabe *et al.* (1986).)

more than one case of Hodgkin's disease may share a human leucocyte antigen (HLA) haplotype between affected members (Robertson *et al.* 1987). However, it is known that the major histocompatibility complex can influence the manifestation of disease following retroviral infection and these genetic data do not rule out an environmental component.

An increased frequency of HLA 4c (an antigen subsequently split into the HLA B locus antigens B5, B15, B18, and B35) was noted in patients with Hodgkin's disease more than 20 years ago and since then other studies have recorded small increases in the frequency of HLA antigens which, collectively, are significant (Tiwari and Terasaki 1985). The most convincing evidence for the role of HLA in susceptibility to Hodgkin's disease comes from data which, when combined, indicate a highly significant excess of HLA identity in pairs of affected siblings (Hors *et al.* 1980). The exact location of this susceptibility within the HLA region is not yet known. Studies have also attempted to correlate HLA with pathological type, extent of disease, and response to therapy. The haplotypes AI and B8 seem to predominate in long-term survivors.

At all ages there is a higher incidence in males than in females. This is particularly marked for the middle aged and there is a decrease in the incidence of females with mixed cellularity and lymphocyte-predominant subtypes after 20–24 years. It has been suggested that childbearing might have a protective effect. These

features suggest that hormonal factors have a role in the aetiology of Hodgkin's disease. A large sex difference in the incidence of Hodgkin's disease occurs in childhood. Males account for the overwhelming majority (85 per cent) of childhood cases (MacMahon 1966). This could be related to the known male susceptibility to infection in the early years of life.

There is an unusual geographical pattern in the occurrence of Hodgkin's disease with marked international variation. The interesting feature is that the variation from country to country is different for the three major groups—childhood, young adult, and older adult. In less developed countries childhood incidence of Hodgkin's disease is greater than young adult incidence, whereas the converse is true for technically advanced Western countries (Fig. 2). There are racial differences in the incidence of Hodgkin's disease. Black populations in the United States have a lower incidence but a worse survival rate for the disease than White Americans. Orientals also have a lower incidence of the disease. There is some evidence that populations migrating from low-risk to high-risk areas have an increased risk of developing Hodgkin's disease. The mortality from Hodgkin's disease for Japanese living in the United States is much greater than for Japanese living in Japan (a low-risk area), suggesting the possible role of environmental factors (Mason and Fraumeni 1974).

A further interesting characteristic of Hodgkin's disease patients is that they appear to be of high socio-economic status and to have

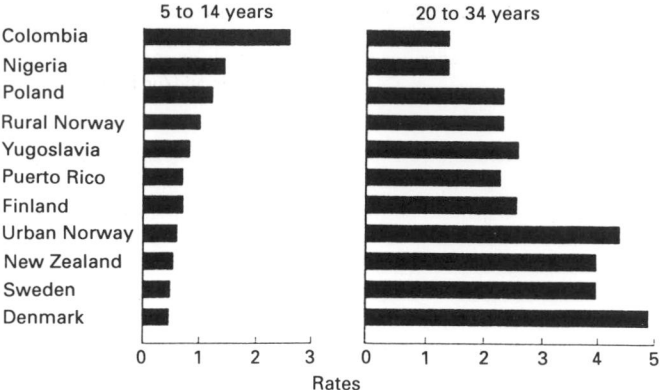

Fig. 2 Mean annual incidence rates of Hodgkin's disease per 100 000 population for children (5–14 years) and young adults (20–34 years). Calculated for males in selected countries. (Reproduced with permission from Correa and O'Connor (1971).)

high intelligence quotients. In a study of Second World War military personnel, Hodgkin's disease patients had significantly higher scores on the Army General Classification Test when compared with the army population mean test (LeShan et al. 1959). Cases were found to be better educated and were more likely to have been of higher pre-service occupational class than a comparable group of army men without the disease (Cohen et al. 1964). In the United Kingdom, mortality was highest in social class I and lowest in social class V (as defined by the Registrar General) (MacMahon 1966). It seems that the increased risk associated with high socio-economic status is confined to the young adult disease, but the relationship between risk and socio-economic status has diminished with time.

The descriptive epidemiology of Hodgkin's disease suggests an infectious disease process underlying its aetiology in young adulthood and childhood. In 1971 there was a report of 31 cases of Hodgkin's disease in a group of friends and relatives from the 1954 graduating class of a high school in Albany, New York State (Vianna et al. 1971). This aggregate of cases was defined on the basis of shared exposures. Other studies have attempted to evaluate clustering of Hodgkin's disease in time and place. Unfortunately, such studies are difficult to interpret because the various reports have been inconsistent and several apparently positive studies contained methodological flaws. For these reasons the studies cannot be used to provide evidence of an infectious aetiology. It is probable that there is no direct person to person spread of Hodgkin's disease. This is suggested by several negative studies of linkages between cases, time–space clustering, and aggregation of exposures at schools. Studies have shown that neither physicians nor nurses, groups with a greater likelihood of encountering Hodgkin's disease patients than the general public, have an increased risk.

Persons with a history of infectious mononucleosis have an increased risk of Hodgkin's disease and the proportion of patients with Hodgkin's disease who have high titres of antibody against viral capsid antigen of Epstein–Barr (**EBV**) virus is significantly greater than expected. In addition, a study of sera taken several years before diagnosis showed elevated levels of Epstein–Barr virus antibody during a period before the onset of recognizable disease (Mueller et al. 1989). The joint presence of elevated levels of IgG and IgA antibodies against capsid antigen and of early antigen D and Epstein–Barr nuclear antigen suggests an enhanced level of viral activity for an extended period before the onset of overt disease, raising the possibility that Epstein–Barr virus infection might trigger the development of Hodgkin's disease. An alternative explanation

for the association is that both prolonged Epstein–Barr virus infection and Hodgkin's disease occur with increased frequency in individuals with abnormalities of their immune response. The recent finding of Epstein–Barr virus genome within the Reed–Sternberg cells of some patients with Hodgkin's disease provides further evidence of an association between Epstein–Barr virus infection and Hodgkin's disease and, since the viral receptor is identical with the receptor for the complement component C3d found on most mature B lymphocytes, the findings are consistent with a B-cell origin for Hodgkin's disease (Weiss et al. 1989). However, not all patients have evidence of infection by Epstein–Barr virus. In this study only 19 per cent of Hodgkin's tissue contained the Epstein–Barr virus genome and several derived cell lines have been negative for the Epstein–Barr virus nuclear antigen (Drexler et al. 1987). Approximately 20–25 per cent of cases are positive using Southern blot analysis although, using the polymerase chain reaction, Epstein–Barr virus DNA can be detected in almost 90 per cent of involved tissue. However, positive results can be obtained from 'normal lymph nodes since the majority of adults are latently infected with EBV'.

There is a significant association between age and Epstein–Barr virus positivity (Jarrett et al. 1991; Armstrong et al. 1993). In the older age group (>50 years) over 70 per cent of cases were Epstein–Barr virus positive and paediatric cases showed a similar incidence. However, in the group 15–34 years only 15 per cent were positive. There is also an association with histological subtype; mixed cellularity is positive in 70 per cent, nodular-sclerosing in 40 per cent, but in lymphocyte-predominant disease of B-cell origin only 14 per cent were positive. When Hodgkin's disease tissue is involved all the tumour cells in that sample contain the virus. Several studies have assessed clonality and in the majority of cases the infected cells have been found to be monoclonal with respect to Epstein–Barr virus integration. In a proportion of Hodgkin's disease cases Reed–Sternberg cells are a clonal expansion of a single Epstein–Barr virus-infected cell. However, there is no evidence of Epstein–Barr virus in the malignant cells of some patients.

The Epstein–Barr virus genome has the capacity to encode over 80 proteins. In the latent state only a restricted group of genes are expressed. B-cells which have been immortalized by Epstein–Barr virus in vitro are known to express nine proteins. There are six nuclear proteins, the EBNAs, and three latent membrane proteins (LMP-1, 2A, and B); in addition, two RNAs, EBER-1 and 2 are transcribed. There are three different patterns of latent gene expression.

1. Hodgkin's disease and nasopharyngeal carcinoma: +EBNA-1, −EBNA-2 and +LMP-1.
2. Immortalized B-cells and lymphomas in the immunosuppressed: +EBNA-1, +EBNA-2 and +LMP-1.
3. Burkitt's lymphoma: +EBNA-1, −EBNA-2 and −LMP-1.

A predisposition to develop Hodgkin's disease could be induced by Epstein–Barr virus immortalizing a Reed–Sternberg cell precursor, mostly likely an immature lymphoid cell, conferring a growth advantage to that cell. Alternatively Epstein–Barr virus could infect a cell clone already containing genetic alternations and induce an activated phenotype possibly in cooperation with other genes such as c-myc, IL-6, IL-9 and p53 (for a review see Herbst et al. 1993).

Tonsillectomy has been reported as a possible risk factor for the development of Hodgkin's disease, but several studies show inconsistencies and the observed associations may be related, at least in part, to socio-economic factors.

Certain studies have suggested that occupational exposures in wood-related industries are associated with an increased risk of Hodgkin's disease, but other studies have failed to confirm these findings. In Scandinavia an association between Hodgkin's disease and exposures to organic solvents, phenoxy acids, and chlorophenols has been reported; however, the effect is small and confirmation is required before any causal relationship can be suggested.

HISTOPATHOLOGY

The appearance of a lymph node involved with Hodgkin's disease is unusual for a malignant neoplasm since the tumour mass usually contains only a small proportion of identifiable 'malignant' cells. The neoplastic cells take the form of mononuclear Hodgkin cells and the characteristic multinucleate Reed–Sternberg cells. These cells are large with an eosinophilic cytoplasm and contain one or more nuclei with a large eosinophilic nucleolus, pale staining chromatin, and a well-defined darkly staining nuclear membrane. The Reed–Sternberg cells classically have two mirror-image nuclei with prominent nuclear lobation, but often three or four may be present (occasionally more). These cells are characteristic and should be identified in order to substantiate the diagnosis of Hodgkin's disease. The diagnosis cannot be made with any confidence in their absence. Similar cells may be seen occasionally in other conditions such as infectious mononucleosis and non-Hodgkin's lymphoma. It is necessary to identify these cells in the appropriate histological setting. The associated non-neoplastic cells consist of variable numbers of lymphocytes, histiocytes, plasma cells, and eosinophils, considered to be a reactive element in the tumour. The polymorphic cellular infiltrate, which is a characteristic feature of lymph nodes involved by Hodgkin's disease, may be the result of cytokines secreted by Reed–Sternberg and Hodgkin cells. Variations in lymphokines secreted by these cells could account for the wide variety of histologic patterns seen in Hodgkin's disease.

An enigma in this unique form of cancer is the paucity of 'malignant' cells found in affected tissue (less than 1 or 2 per cent of the total cell population are Reed–Sternberg cells and their variants). This imbalance in comparison with the large number of normal inflammatory cells has raised questions over whether the process is neoplastic or inflammatory and, if neoplastic, whether the inflammatory reaction is a prelude to the development of the disease or a reaction to neoantigens expressed on the malignant cells.

The Rye Classification

The histological classification in current use is based on that of Lukes and Butler (1966) which was modified at the Rye Conference of 1966 and has since been known as the Rye Classification (Lukes et al. 1966) (Table 1). The histological features of the different subtypes are shown in Fig. 3.

Lymphocyte predominant

In this histological subtype the predominating cells are lymphocytes, histiocytes, or both. Eosinophils and plasma cells are uncommon and there is no necrosis or fibrosis. The pattern may be nodular or diffuse; in the original Lukes classification nodular and diffuse variants were defined separately, but they have been combined in the Rye Classification. The atypical cells in this variant are usually scarce and differ morphologically from classical Reed–Sternberg and Hodgkin cells. They are often referred to as L- and H- cells, and are characterized by lobed vesicular ('popcorn') nuclei with multiple small basophilic nuclei. Classical Reed–Sternberg cells are

Table 1 The Rye Classification for Hodgkin's disease

Lymphocyte predominance	(Including nodular and diffuse variants of lymphocytic and/or histiocytic proliferation)
Mixed cellularity	
Nodular sclerosis	(Including variant where sclerosis is sparse: cellular phase)
Lymphocyte depletion	(Including diffuse fibrosis and reticular categories)

usually very difficult to find. Recent evidence has suggested that there are not only morphological but also phenotypical differences between nodular lymphocyte-predominant Hodgkin's disease and the mixed cellularity and nodular-sclerosing forms of the disease. These differences are found in both the atypical cells and the associated population of small lymphocytes with a predominance of B-cells in lymphocyte-predominant forms and T-cells in mixed cellularity and nodular-sclerosing forms (Abdulaziz et al. 1983).

Nodular lymphocyte-predominant Hodgkin's disease has histological, ultrastructural, and phenotypic affinities with progressive transformation of germinal centres suggesting a B-cell origin for the tumour cells (Poppema et al. 1979). Immunostaining has demonstrated that the L- and H-cells of nodular lymphocyte-predominant Hodgkin's disease are usually positive for leucocyte common antigen, B-cell markers, and epithelial membrane antigen, but negative for CD15 and CD30 (Ki-1 antigen), whereas the reverse is true for the classical Reed–Sternberg, Hodgkin, and lacunar cells of the mixed cellularity and nodular-sclerosing varieties (Pinkus and Said 1985; Chittal et al. 1988; Hall et al. 1988; Stein et al. 1988). There is also some evidence to suggest that there are phenotypic differences between the nodular and diffuse variants of lymphocyte-predominant Hodgkin's disease. In the diffuse variant the atypical cells are not infrequently CD15 and CD30 positive.

One study has reported a difference in the clinical course between the nodular and diffuse variants with a chronic relapsing course for the nodular disease suggesting similarities to follicular B-cell non-Hodgkin's lymphoma (Regula et al. 1988), but others have shown the variants to be clinically similar in terms of disease distribution, relapse pattern, and overall survival (Borg-Grech et al. 1989). Patients with both the nodular and diffuse variants tend to present with stage I and II disease with a peripheral nodal distribution and an excellent prognosis.

Nodular sclerosis

This subtype is characterized by bands of dense collagen dividing nodules of neoplastic and reactive cells. The amount of fibrosis is variable, however and a variant nodular sclerosis 'cellular phase' has been described where fibrotic bands are absent or limited to one part of the specimen. Lacunar cells are an important and characteristic feature of nodular-sclerosing Hodgkin's disease. These are variants of Reed–Sternberg cells with abundant cytoplasm which often undergoes artificial shrinkage during fixation, giving the appearance of a cell within a lacuna. The nuclei differ from classical Reed–Sternberg cells in having a delicate chromatin pattern and small nucleoli. Classical Reed–Sternberg cells are less frequent in number and may be sparse. This subtype is the commonest histological type of Hodgkin's disease, particularly in the young adult. Young patients with substantial mediastinal disease are frequently of the nodular-sclerosing subtype and this association is more common among young female patients.

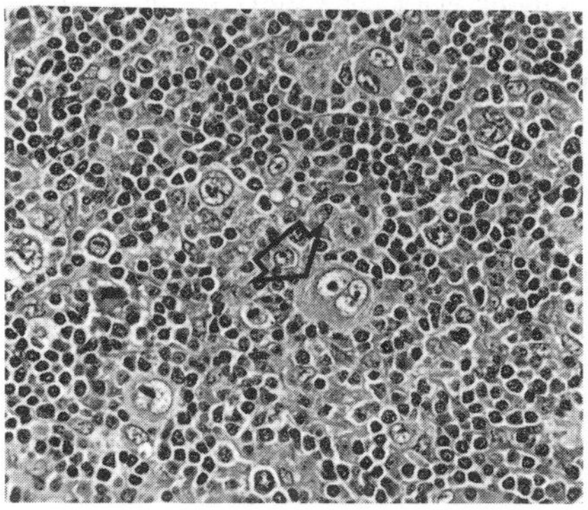

(a)

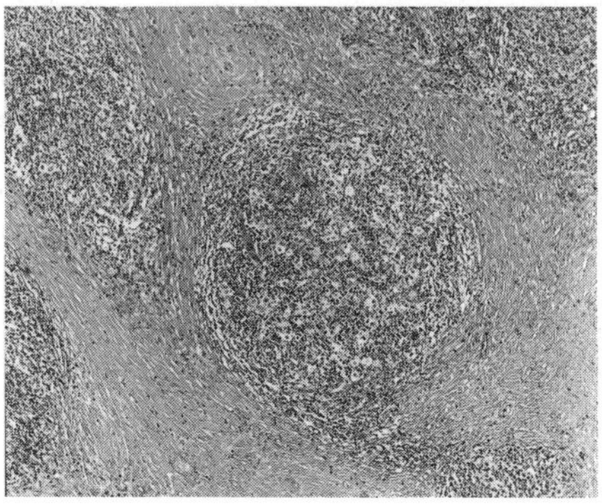

(b)

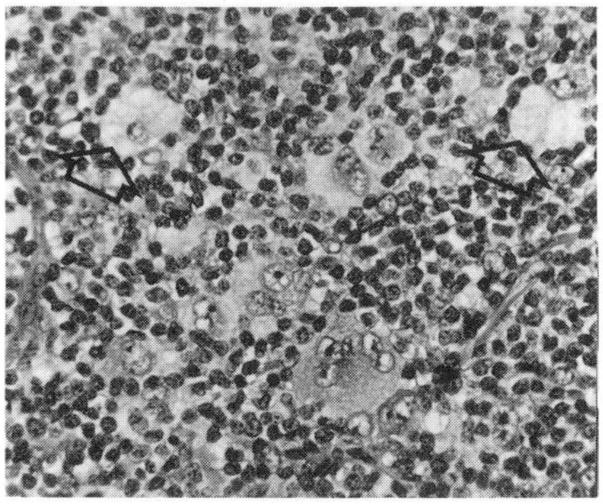

(c)

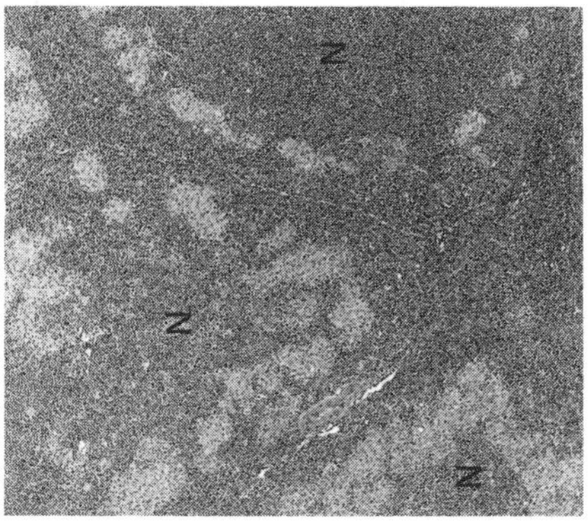

(d)

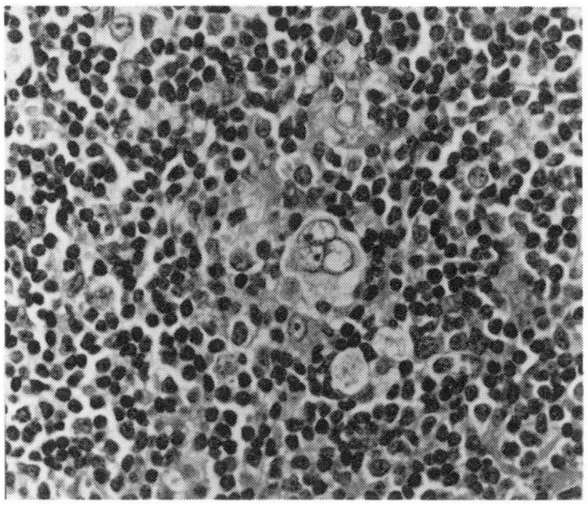

(e)

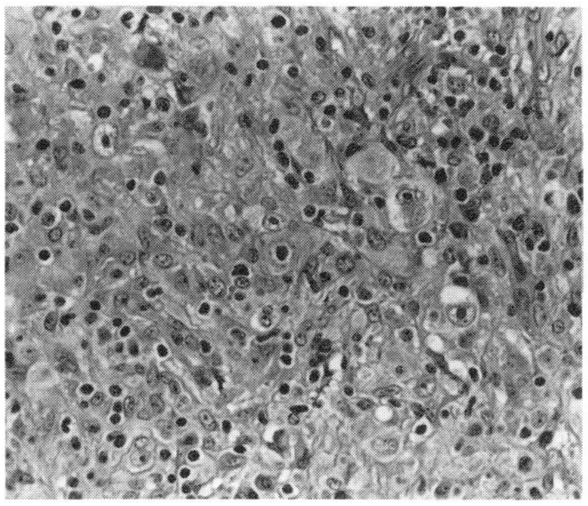

(f)

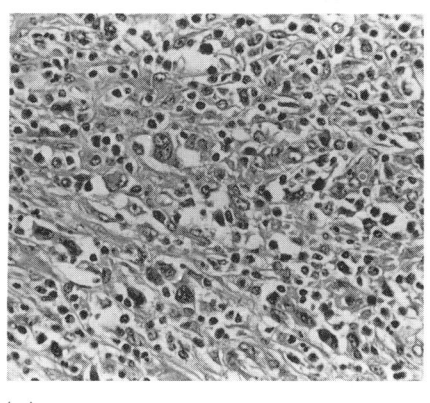

(g)

Fig. 3 (a) Mixed cellularity Hodgkin's disease showing frequent scattered Reed–Sternberg and mononuclear Hodgkin cells against a mainly lymphocytic background; eosinophils are inconspicuous in this field. The arrow indicates a classical binucleated mirror-image Reed–Sternberg cell (Haematoxylin and eosin (H + E) × 420). (b) Nodular-sclerosing Hodgkin's disease: cellular islands of Hodgkin's tissue bounded by dense collagenous bands. At this lower power lacunar cells appear as small clear spaces scattered amongst the background cells (H + E × 60). (c) Nodular-sclerosing Hodgkin's disease: high power to show several lacunar-type Reed–Sternberg cells with abundant cytoplasm and lobed nuclei. In this field only the cells arrowed have developed lacunae (H + E × 480). (d) Nodular- lymphocyte-predominant Hodgkin's disease: this low-power field includes part of three nodules (N) which, in this case, are outlined by unusually prominent clusters of pale-staining epithelioid histiocytes (H + E × 60). (e) Lymphocyte-predominant Hodgkin's disease: a Reed–Sternberg cell of L + H type occurring in a background of small lymphocytes (H + E × 540). (f) Lymphocyte-depleted Hodgkin's disease (reticular type): frequent large atypical cells including Reed–Sternberg cells with histiocytes and scanty lymphocytes in the background (H + E × 380). (g) Lymphocyte-depleted Hodgkin's disease (diffuse fibrous type): Reed–Sternberg cells and Hodgkin cells occurring against a background of stromal spindle cells and scattered lymphocytes (H + E × 480). (Photographs supplied by Martin Harris, Department of Pathology, Christie Hospital, Manchester.)

Mixed cellularity

This subtype is of variable appearance lacking sclerosis and containing more Reed–Sternberg cells than the lymphocyte-predominant type but fewer than the lymphocyte-depleted type. The reactive element consists of variable numbers of eosinophils, histiocytes, neutrophils, and lymphocytes.

Lymphocyte depletion

This subtype consists of two original groups proposed by Lukes and Butler (1966): diffuse fibrosis and reticular. The diffuse fibrosis group is characterized by a loose fibrosis and collagen banding is

not usually seen. There is general cellular depletion, especially of lymphocytes, but there are areas where Reed–Sternberg cells are numerous. In the reticular variant the Reed–Sternberg cells are prominent with a pleomorphic appearance showing bizarre nuclear shapes and giant nucleoli. Necrosis is common in this subtype. Lymphocyte depletion is the least common histological subtype (5 per cent or less of the total) although a greater proportion occurs in the elderly. It is also the group where there is most diagnostic difficulty and the histological appearances may be confused with lymphomas other than Hodgkin's disease. Patients with lymphocyte-depleted pathology have the most unfavourable outlook of all histological subtypes of Hodgkin's disease and are more likely to be of higher stage than other pathologies.

Patients with Hodgkin's disease are less likely to have extranodal involvement than patients with non-Hodgkin's lymphoma, but when the diagnosis is made by biopsy of such tissue the criteria are the same as for lymph nodes. Hodgkin's disease presenting in intestine, skin, and Waldeyer's ring is extremely rare and many of the reported cases are probably unacceptable by modern diagnostic criteria. If the diagnosis of Hodgkin's disease is already established by nodal biopsy, the criteria for diagnosis of extranodal involvement are less stringent. In this instance the presence of Reed–Sternberg cells is not essential and the identification of mononuclear Hodgkin cells in an appropriate cellular background is deemed to be sufficient (Rappaport *et al.* 1971).

Several studies have indicated that both clinical features and prognosis are correlated with histological type. An early study using the Lukes classification showed a relationship between survival and all six of his original subgroups. The 15 year survival was 43.5 per cent for patients with lymphocytic and histiocytic nodular, 27.5 per cent for lymphocytic and histiocytic diffuse, 15.4 per cent for nodular sclerosis, 10.3 per cent for mixed, 4.8 per cent for reticular, and 2.1 per cent for diffuse fibrosis (Lukes *et al.* 1966). This study involved United States Army cases from the Second World War and were mainly young adult males.

As treatment has improved, the association of histopathological subtype with other prognostic factors has become better understood and the relationship with prognosis has become less evident. There is an association between Rye histological subtype and pathological stage and in one large study 76 per cent of patients with lymphocyte predominance had stage I and II disease compared with 60 per cent of patients with nodular sclerosis, 44 per cent of patients with mixed cellularity, and only 19 per cent of patients with lymphocyte depletion (Deforges *et al.* 1989). When stage and age are taken into account and patients are treated using modern methods, most studies using appropriate multivariate analysis fail to show that the main histological subtypes are of independent prognostic importance. Further detailed histological classification may be of help in determining prognosis and the number of lymphocytes and fibroblasts and the amount of sclerosis have been reported to be independent prognostic factors for relapse-free survival (Colby *et al.* 1981). In this study cell-poor dense lamellar collagen imparted a good prognosis, whereas collagen-poor fibroblastic Hodgkin's disease carried a worse prognosis. An increase in lymphocyte infiltration was associated with improved relapse-free survival. A study of patients within the British National Lymphoma Group has suggested that features in the histology of patients with nodular sclerosing pathology can identify those with a poorer prognosis. Those with extensive and easily appreciated areas of lymphocyte depletion or containing numerous pleomorphic Hodgkin's cells were classified as the more malignant grade 2 variant of nodular sclerosis. A multivariate analysis showed that prognosis became worse from lymphocyte-predominant to nodular-sclerosis grade 1, nodular sclerosis grade 2, and mixed cellularity varieties of Hodgkin's disease (Haybittle *et al.* 1985). However, this study took no account of mediastinal bulk in the analysis and this could be important in view of the association between nodular sclerosis grade 2 and bulky mediastinal disease.

Histological assessment of the liver at presentation in patients with Hodgkin's disease has revealed a relatively low incidence of involvement overall but non-specific abnormalities are much more common. The most frequent abnormality is lymphocytic infiltration

of the portal tracts which is found in approximately half the patients. In addition there may be 'piecemeal necrosis' involving individual cells at the boundary between the infiltration and surrounding liver parenchyma (Skovsgaard *et al.* 1982). Pleomorphic infiltrates and epithelioid cell granulomas occur in approximately 10 per cent of cases (Sacks *et al.* 1978). There are no correlations between these non-specific changes and clinical characteristics, including prognosis. Epithelioid cell granulomas may also occur in the spleen, but they do not signify involvement by Hodgkin's disease and are not of prognostic significance.

Histological progression from a relatively favourable subtype of Hodgkin's disease to an unfavourable subtype may occur in patients suffering relapse. The features include a reduction in the number of lymphocytes and an increase in the number of atypical Hodgkin and Reed–Sternberg cells. However, a change to a less favourable histological subtype is uncommon and the histological appearances tend to be retained in the relapse biopsies (Colby and Warnke 1980). This is unlike the situation in non-Hodgkin's lymphoma where histological progression from a favourable to a less favourable histological subtype is more common.

The differential diagnosis of Hodgkin's disease includes benign conditions such as some forms of reactive follicular hyperplasia where, although the differentiation from follicular lymphoma and the nodular variety of lymphocyte predominant Hodgkin's disease is usually easily made, a small group of borderline cases may lead to diagnostic error. The nodal architecture is usually retained in reactive states. Progressive transformation of germinal centres may occur in reactive follicular hyperplasia with enlargement, blurring, and eventual loss of germinal centres. This phenomenon is difficult to distinguish from the nodular form of lymphocyte predominant Hodgkin's disease and the two conditions may occur in the same node. Infective conditions such as infectious mononucleosis, other viral infections associated with lymphadenopathy, and HIV infection may cause difficulty, as may histological changes in enlarged nodes in patients with toxoplasmosis and secondary syphilis, but serological investigation can be helpful.

Some patients with inflammatory disorders causing lymphadenopathy, including dermatopathic lymphadenopathy, allergic granulomatosis and autoimmune lymphadenitis, must also be distinguished from Hodgkin's disease. Lymphadenopathy associated with the use of hydantoin therapy for epilepsy may be difficult to distinguish from Hodgkin's disease but regression of the nodal disease after discontinuing medication is a regular feature. Certain forms of non-Hodgkin's lymphoma, such as T-cell lymphomas where Reed–Sternberg-like cells may occur, can also cause diagnostic difficulty.

IMMUNOLOGICAL DEFICIENCY: IMMUNOBIOLOGY; CELLULAR ORIGIN OF REED–STERNBERG CELLS AND MONONUCLEAR HODGKIN CELLS

Immune deficiency, disproportionate to the extent of disease or prior therapy, is a feature of Hodgkin's disease (Twomey *et al.* 1980; Ford *et al.* 1988). It is characterized by a defect in cell-mediated immunity and, whilst it has not been established whether it is causal or consequential of Hodgkin's disease, it is considered to be an integral part of the pathobiology of the disease, reflecting the nature of the Reed–Sternberg cell and the cellular microenvironment of the Hodgkin's disease 'lesion'.

Evidence for a cell-mediated immune defect has been obtained *in vivo* and *in vitro*. Thus, the susceptibility to infections characterized predominantly by a cell-mediated response, for example tuberculosis, fungal and protozoal infections, or 'opportunist infections', the poorly developed skin test response in the delayed hypersensitivity reaction to recall antigen, and the delayed and defective response to alloantigens in the *in vivo* lymphocyte transfer or tissue graft transfer attest to an *in vivo* cell-mediated immune deficit. *In vitro* peripheral blood lymphocytes from patients with Hodgkin's disease demonstrate impaired blastogenesis to mitogen and alloantigen and variable deficits of lymphokine production including deficient production of and response to interleukin-2, the growth factor for amplification of antigen-activated T-cells (thymus-derived lymphocytes responsible for effecting the cell-mediated immune response).

The defect in cell-mediated immune response appears to go beyond intrinsic T-lymphocyte hyporesponsiveness, however. Much *in vitro* evidence supports the concept of suppression of lymphocyte function through mechanisms involving monocytes or macrophages and also T-cell subset populations. Thus, the cell-mediated immunodeficiency of Hodgkin's disease, characterized as a progressive disorder of immunodepletion and immunoincompetence, would appear to be the final expression of an aberration of regulation at the afferent and efferent levels of the cellular immune response. Accessory cell function (macrophages and monocytes), possibly through interleukin-1 and also prostaglandin, influences T-cell function with resultant dysregulation of the normal T-cell response. In this milieu of aberrant production of soluble mediators of immune response and other related growth factors, it is possible to hypothesize that such products give rise to many of the clinico-pathological features of Hodgkin's disease; for example, pyrexia, the pleomorphic cellular nature of the histopathology, the fibroblast proliferation of nodular-sclerosing Hodgkin's disease, eosinophilia, the hyperactive bone-marrow commonly seen in symptomatic patients, the progressive lymphopenia characterizing histological progression of the disease, and the cell-mediated immunodeficiency state.

The observation and characterization of the defective cell-mediated immune response has paralleled attempts to define the nature of the malignant cell of Hodgkin's disease and the lineage of the Reed–Sternberg cell and mononuclear Hodgkin's cells. Even the use of the term 'the malignant cell' is controversial. Whilst none would argue that the disease demonstrates proliferation and metastasis and is fatal without effective therapy, it has not been possible to date to establish clonal growth reproducibly in an *in vitro* or *in vivo* environment or to define clonal origin by phenotypic, karyotypic, or genotypic criteria. Furthermore, unlike most other malignancies, the histopathology of the tumour is pleomorphic and the putative malignant cell (that is, the Reed–Sternberg cell), is the least commonly represented cell and as the disease grows in volume the tumour cell population demonstrates growth only in the same relative proportion to the presumed normal or reactive cellular component. Finally, the Reed–Sternberg cell appears to be the least mitotically active constituent of the Hodgkin's lesion.

Each of the principal cell types of lymphoreticular tissue has been a candidate for the origin of the Reed–Sternberg cell. The principal features in favour of a macrophage or monocyte origin include the cell size, the frequent but not uniform surface expression of Leu-MI (a monoclonal antibody characterizing monocytes and macrophages), the morphological similarity between interdigitating reticulum cells and Reed–Sternberg cells, and the occurrence of the earliest morphological evidence of Hodgkin's disease in

T-cell-dependent regions of lymphoid tissue where the interdigitating reticular cell(s) reside (for example, the paracortex of the lymph node and the periarteriolar sheath within the spleen). The possession of surface determinants for HLA DR and interleukin 2 (CD25) would be consistent with an immune accessory cell and would place the interdigitating reticular cell(s) in an ideal position with respect to a defect in cell-mediated immune response. The absence of degradative enzyme systems characteristic of macrophages (for example, esterases, phosphatases, etc.) would also be consistent with a relationship between the Reed–Sternberg cell and an immune-accessory cell (macrophage or monocyte) such as the interdigitating reticular cell(s). Somewhat similar arguments could be proposed for the dendritic reticulum cell, the immune-accessory macrophage or monocyte of the B lymphocyte region of the lymph node (the germinal follicle), given emerging evidence of a follicular origin for the subset of Hodgkin's disease; that is, the nodular lymphocyte predominant type.

Whilst the T lymphocyte would be an ideal candidate given the origin of the lesion in the T-cell zone and the cell-mediated immune defect, the most persuasive evidence, clonal T-cell receptor gene rearrangement, has, to date, been demonstrated in only a minor proportion of cases of Hodgkin's disease.

An origin from B lymphocytes had been considered less likely given the lack of demonstrable clonality by surface and cytoplasmic antibody studies and by immunoglobulin gene rearrangement analysis. However, a B-cell origin now appears distinctly possible for a subset of Hodgkin's disease based upon clonal immunoglobin rearrangement and Epstein–Barr virus genome incorporation within the genome of the Reed–Sternberg cell. Rarely, a patient may present with a composite lymphoma of Hodgkin's disease and a lymphoma (usually of B-cell type) in the same nodal tissue. This occurrence is more commonly associated with the nodular lymphocyte-predominant variant than with other subtypes and this, along with the immunophenotypic character of the atypical cells, has been cited as additional evidence for a B-cell origin of this variant.

To date, the reported studies have not settled the question of the origin of the Reed–Sternberg cell. The morphological, immunophenotypic, and genotypic studies suggest that at least one subset of Hodgkin's disease, the nodular variant of lymphocyte predominant disease, will have a B-lymphocyte lineage. Given the heterogeneity of the proposed lineage of Reed–Sternberg cells and the clinical and epidemiological differences in the natural history of Hodgkin's disease, it may be that the homogeneity implied by the term 'Hodgkin's disease' is artificial. It may well be that Hodgkin's disease is a spectrum of malignant diseases (lymphomas) with an origin from immunologically relevant cells of differing lineages resulting in a process of immunological dysregulation characterized by the pleomorphic cellular infiltrate that we identify histologically as Hodgkin's disease and manifest clinically by a cell-mediated immunodeficiency state. The correctness of this interpretation, or the identification of a cell of, as yet, uncharacterized lineage or a somatic-cell hybrid of mixed lineage as a cell of origin for the Reed–Sternberg cell, will await genomic studies at the single-cell level.

CLINICAL FEATURES
Clinical features at presentation

Nearly all patients with Hodgkin's disease present with painless lymphadenopathy. For the majority the apparent onset of the disease

Table 2 Involved sites of disease in untreated pathologically staged patients with Hodgkin's disease

Site		Percentage involved
Waldeyer's ring		1–2
Cervical nodes	Right side	50–60
	Left side	60–70
Axillary nodes	Right side	25–35
	Left side	30–35
Mediastinal nodes		50–60
Hilar nodes		15–35
Spleen		30–35
Liver		2–6
Para-aortic nodes		30–40
Iliac nodes		15–20
Mesenteric nodes		1–4
Inguinal nodes		8–15
Bone-marrow		1–4
Other extranodal sites (lung, bone, etc.)		10–12
Total extranodal		10–15

is in the cervical nodes. Spontaneous waxing and waning in nodal size is common. In approximately one-third of patients initial symptoms include fever, night sweats, pruritus, or weight loss, which may be profound. Occasionally there may be alcohol-induced pain or swelling in affected lymph nodes. A palpably enlarged spleen and liver is observed in approximately 10 and 5 per cent of patients, respectively. Axillary nodes are palpable in approximately 20 per cent of patients, but inguinal nodes are less commonly palpable at presentation (10–15 per cent).

The distribution of disease found in pathologically staged patients is shown in Table 2. In most patients, and typically in those with nodular sclerosis histology, the pattern of lymph node involvement is central (cervical, mediastinal, and para-aortic). For reasons which are not yet clear, certain chains of lymph nodes (mesenteric, hepatic hilar, hypogastric, presacral, epitrochlear, and popliteal) are seldom involved. Hodgkin's disease rarely involves Waldeyer's ring. Pulmonary hilar lymph nodes are clinically enlarged in approximately one-fifth of patients with mediastinal adenopathy, but the incidence is much higher in the presence of large mediastinal masses. Approximately 25 per cent of patients present with bulky mediastinal adenopathy, usually associated with multiple supradiaphragmatic nodal involvement and may have extension of tumour into the lung, pericardium, or chest wall. Systemic symptoms are also frequently associated with this type of presentation. Primary intrapulmonary Hodgkin's disease in the absence of intrathoracic adenopathy is rare.

Pleural effusions are common in Hodgkin's disease, complicating the clinical course of approximately 20 per cent of patients who are not cured. This complication can be produced either by lymphatic obstruction in the mediastinum or by tumour invasion of the pleura. Endobronchial disease may also occur but is rare at presentation. The pattern of disease at presentation varies with the histological subtype. Most patients with lymphocyte-predominant histology present with disease localized to peripheral sites, often in the upper cervical region whereas patients with lymphocyte-depleted histology frequently present with abdominal nodal involvement and often have extranodal disease. Most patients with nodular sclerosis histology present with supradiaphragmatic disease and mediastinal node involvement. Patients with mixed cellularity histology present with either upper torso disease or with lymphoma extended to both sides of the diaphragm without regional predilection.

In the majority of patients, the initial mode of spread occurs non-randomly and predictably via lymphatic channels to contiguous lymph node chains and other lymphatic structures. This observation forms the basis for prophylactic irradiation of adjacent nodal chains in patients with apparent localized disease. Tumour cells may also spread by recirculating through the lymphatic system and the blood stream. In addition, spread may occur by vascular invasion and histological evidence of this is seen in approximately 40 per cent of patients dying with Hodgkin's disease; the incidence is highest in lymphocyte-depleted and lowest in lymphocyte-predominant histology. Most extranodal sites manifest markedly greater vascular invasion, indicating that vascular spread may be an important factor in patients with extranodal disease and in those dying of Hodgkin's disease.

The incidence of clinically occult disease has been an important factor in influencing therapeutic strategy. Patients with lymphocyte-predominant or nodular-sclerosing histology and unilateral involvement of upper cervical nodes or adenopathy in the upper mediastinum without systemic symptoms have a low incidence of occult disease elsewhere. Upper para-aortic adenopathy (above L2) is an area which is not well defined using bipedal abdominal lymphangiography but is present in 10–20 per cent of cases and is most frequently observed in patients with nodular-sclerosing and mixed-cellularity histology. The spleen is involved, usually in association with adenopathy above and below the diaphragm, systemic symptoms, and mixed-cellularity or lymphocyte-depleted histological subtypes. Splenic involvement as the sole intra-abdominal site occurs in less than 10 per cent of patients with supradiaphragmatic Hodgkin's disease. Involvement of the liver is uncommon at presentation, occurring in only 1–6 per cent of patients. In almost all patients this occurs in the presence of widespread adenopathy and splenic involvement is almost invariably present. As with splenic infiltration, disease in the liver is most frequently encountered in patients with mixed-cellularity or lymphocyte-depleted histology and systemic symptoms. The diagnosis of liver involvement with Hodgkin's disease can be difficult because there is little correlation between liver size assessed clinically or radiologically and the presence of disease histologically. Liver function tests may be abnormal in the absence of histological involvement and imaging scans are insensitive and unreliable.

Infiltration of the bone-marrow tends to be focal and is almost always associated with extensive disease, systemic symptoms, and unfavourable histology. This is also the case for renal and lytic or sclerotic osseous involvement which is rare early in the course of disease. Very advanced intra-abdominal disease may be associated with ureteric obstruction or compression of the renal vein and very occasionally the nephrotic syndrome may occur. This is most commonly associated with immune complexes in the glomeruli and improves following treatment of the underlying Hodgkin's disease. It may also be due to renal vein thrombosis and, more rarely, to amyloid of the kidney.

Hodgkin's disease may involve the cerebral meninges and extradural deposits may be associated with spinal cord compression in the presence or absence of bony destruction. Fortunately, these complications are uncommon. Early recognition and treatment are the key to successful therapy, with the reversal of existing symptoms and the prevention of permanent neurological deficits. Early symptoms include central back pain with or without radicular pain or vertebral tenderness. Later symptoms include motor or sensory loss with abnormalities of micturition or bowel function. Radiological evaluation or magnetic resonance imaging is important to confirm the site and extent of involvement.

Other manifestations of Hodgkin's disease include anaemia, which is usually normochromic normocytic and associated with generalized disease. More rarely, a Coombs'-positive autoimmune haemolytic anaemia may occur. Skin manifestations include pruritus, ichthyosis, urticaria, erythema multiforme, necrotizing skin lesions, hyperpigmentation, and skin infiltration. A variety of paraneoplastic neurological syndromes have been associated with Hodgkin's disease but these are rare. Although uncommon, symptomatic hypercalcaemia may occur in patients presenting with Hodgkin's disease. This is usually associated with bony disease but may be associated with abnormalities of vitamin D metabolism.

Distribution of disease at autopsy

The pathological findings at autopsy have changed since a curative treatment approach has been widely applied. A distinct reduction in the extent of disease in patients treated after 1965 was reported from a 25 year experience at the National Cancer Institute in the United States (Grogan et al. 1982). Reduced involvement was the rule for most but not all organ sites, with a statistically significant reduction in abdominal involvement for both mixed-cellularity and lymphocyte-depleted histology and decreased lymphoreticular involvement for lymphocyte-predominant patients. This finding supports the view that treatment procedures established after 1965 reduced the spread of disease to extranodal organs. Lymphocyte-depleted histology was observed in a high percentage of patients, but precise histological subclassification is difficult in patients who have died following extensive treatment. In this situation there may be a relatively monomorphic histological appearance with numerous atypical mononuclear cells, few Reed—Sternberg cells or variants, and a paucity of inflammatory elements. This appearance, suggesting a non-Hodgkin's lymphoma, may be considered a treatment-altered form of Hodgkin's disease.

PATIENT EVALUATION, INVESTIGATION, AND STAGING

At the Workshop on the Staging of Hodgkin's Disease held at Ann Arbor, Michigan, in April 1971 an international panel of medical oncologists, radiotherapists, and pathologists agreed on a staging classification now known as the Ann Arbor Classification (Table 3) (Carbone et al. 1971). This classification provides a rational basis upon which curative treatment decisions can be made for patients at initial presentation.

A distinction is drawn between clinical stage (CS) and pathological stage (PS). Clinical stage is based on information derived from the initial biopsy, history, physical examination, laboratory tests, radiographic examinations, and radioisotopic scans. Pathological stage is based on additional macroscopic and microscopic evidence derived from laparotomy or laparoscopy, splenectomy, liver biopsy, marrow biopsy, and/or additional lymph node or other tissue biopsies. Each patient receives both a CS and a PS designation.

New features of prognostic importance have recently been recognized. For patients treated with radiotherapy alone prognosis correlates not only with the stage and the presence of symptoms as delineated in the Ann Arbor Classification but with other factors such as bulk of disease, number of involved nodal sites, and laboratory procedures which were not mentioned or considered optional in the Ann Arbor reports. New techniques for determining sites of disease such as computed tomographic (CT) scanning and magnetic resonance imaging (MRI) have since become available and have been introduced into routine staging, replacing others

Table 3 Ann Arbor Staging Classification

Stage	Definition
I	Involvement of a single extranodal site (I_E) or a single lymph node region (for example cervical, axillary, inguinal, mediastinal, hilar) or lymphoid structure such as spleen, thymus, or Waldeyer's ring
II	Involvement of two or more lymph node regions or lymph node structures on the same side of the diaphragm or localized involvement of an extranodal organ or site and of one or more lymph node regions on the same side of the diaphragm (II_E)
III	Involvement of lymph node regions or lymph node structures on both sides of the diaphragm
IV	Diffuse or disseminated involvement of one or more extranodal organs or tissues with or without associated lymph node involvement

recommended in the Ann Arbor report. For these reasons, a revision of the Ann Arbor scheme was carried out and modifications were recommended in the staging procedures within the framework of the Ann Arbor Classification (Cotswolds Report) (Lister et al. 1989).

Recommended pre-treatment evaluation

An adequate surgical biopsy should be undertaken. Where possible, a whole lymph node should be taken for pathological examination. Inguinal nodes should not be biopsied if equally suspicious peripheral nodes are present elsewhere. When the diagnosis of Hodgkin's disease is made from the biopsy of an extranodal site, a node biopsy confirmation of diagnosis is desirable unless the diagnosis is considered unequivocal. The diagnosis should always be based upon representative appropriately prepared material.

A detailed history must be obtained and a record made of the patients' age and gender, the presence or absence of unexplained fever and its duration, unexplained sweating (especially at night and its severity), unexplained weight loss (as a percentage of usual body weight) and rapidity of loss, and any pruritus with its extent and severity. These features are of prognostic importance. In addition, performance status, the presence of alcohol-induced pain, a family history of Hodgkin's disease, any history of immunosuppressive illness such as infection with human immunodeficiency viruses, or a previous history of malignancy together with any chemotherapy or radiotherapy should be documented.

A careful and complete physical examination must be performed by a physician experienced in the management of patients with Hodgkin's disease. Special attention must be directed to the areas where lymphadenopathy commonly occurs and the number of sites should be recorded. A measurement of the largest mass in each region must be made. Waldeyer's ring should be examined and the size of the liver and spleen in centimetres below the costal margin in the midclavicular line should be recorded.

Laboratory investigations should include a complete blood count with haemoglobin estimation, platelet count, white blood count, and differential. The absolute lymphocyte count has been reported to be of independent prognostic significance in some series and should be recorded. Any anaemia should be further investigated. The erythrocyte sedimentation rate (Westergren method) at 1 h should be measured. Biochemical assessment of liver, bone, and renal function should include measurements of serum alkaline phosphatase, aspartate aminotransferase, alanine aminotransferase, γ-glutamyl transaminase, lactate dehydrogenase, albumin, and calcium. Although these investigations may not necessarily

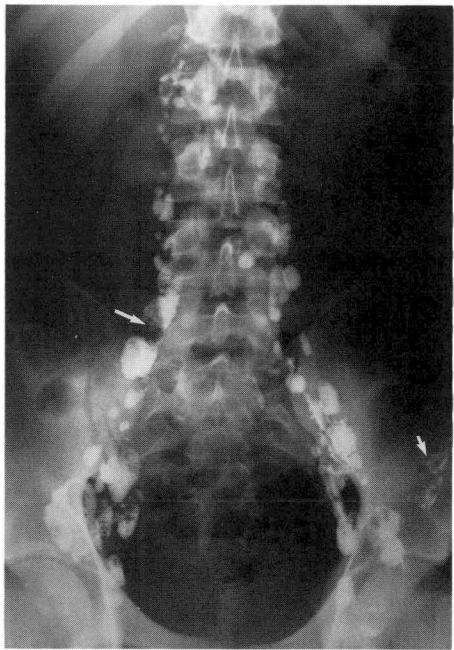

Fig. 4 Bipedal abdominal lymphangiogram showing enlarged nodes, some with filling defects (white arrow). Poor filling of the upper lumbar nodes together with stasis in the left iliac vessels and collateral circulation (white arrow) indicates more extensive involvement than can be appreciated on the lymphogram.

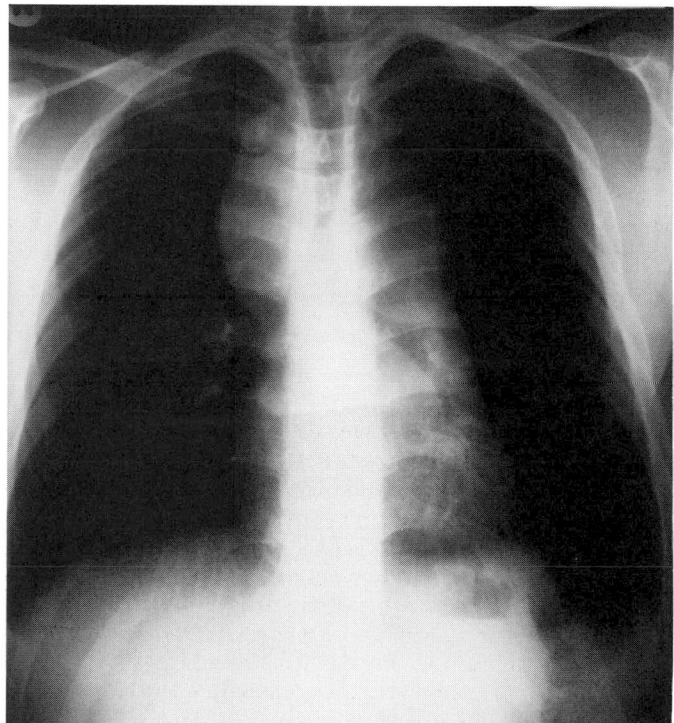

Fig. 5 Posteroanterior chest radiograph demonstrating mediastinal lymphadenopathy of paratracheal and prevascular distribution (superior and anterior mediastinum).

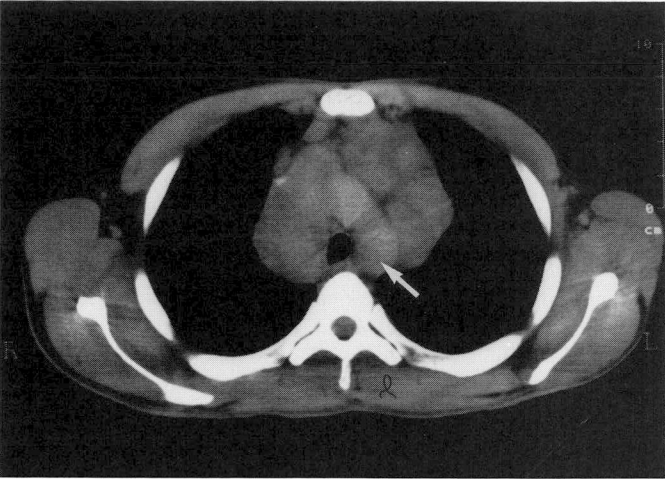

Fig. 6 The distribution and the effect on the trachea is better appreciated on the CT scan taken during contrast infusion (white arrow on aortic arch).

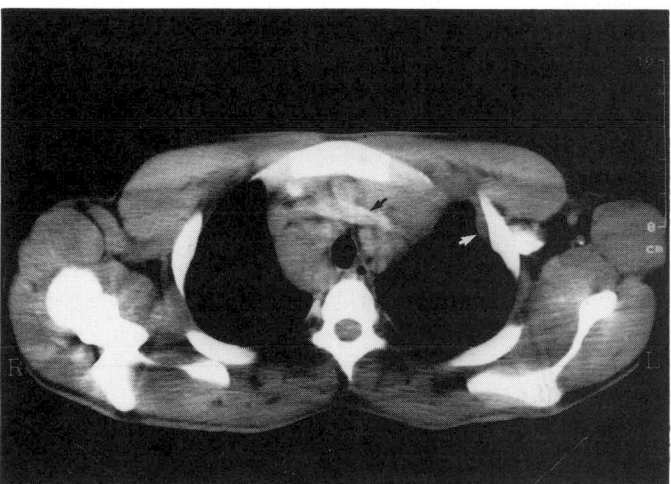

Fig. 7 At the level of the left innominate vein shown with intravenous contrast infusion (black arrow) there is pleural involvement (white arrow) visible on the CT scan which could not be appreciated on the chest radiographs.

contribute directly to staging, they may influence treatment modification and guide further investigations to other potential sites of disease.

Radiological investigations should include chest radiography with posteroanterior, 'penetrated' anteroposterior, and lateral views, CT of the thorax, abdomen, and pelvis, and bipedal lymphangiography (Figs 4–7). It may not be essential to have both abdominal CT and bipedal lymphangiography. Bipedal lymphangiography is an accurate diagnostic tool for the assessment of para-aortic, paracaval, and common iliac nodal disease in patients with Hodgkin's disease with a sensitivity of 85 per cent, specificity of 98 per cent, and accuracy of 95 per cent in these sites. The lymphatic vessels are delineated and the internal structure of the opacified node is shown by the storage pattern of the oily contrast material (Fig. 4). The contrast remains in the node for a variable period of time, allowing a dynamic assessment of lymph node changes with time using follow-up with plain abdominal radiography. Nodes involved by Hodgkin's disease are frequently enlarged with a reticular appearance and disruption of the normal granular storage pattern with filling defects. However, the nodes may not be enlarged yet show disruption of the storage pattern. Follow-up films at 2, 4, and 8 weeks have been recommended to determine any change in nodal size and any nodes remaining opacified over long periods should be considered with suspicion. Other factors which increase the index of suspicion include lymphatics remaining opacified after 24 h, lymphatics and collateral vessels taking an unusual course, nodes opacifying in unusual positions or numbers, nodes which are unusually dense, filling defects which look like 'expanding lesions', and nodes which show a disturbed reticular pattern (MacDonald 1982).

Unfortunately lymphography is poor in evaluating lymph nodes in the upper abdomen above the level of the second lumbar vertebra. Coeliac axis nodes are hardly ever visualized and this is a common site for Hodgkin's disease to be found at staging laparotomy. Portal, splenic hilar, and mesenteric nodes are never visualized. Other difficulties include risk of local infection and breathlessness associated with lipid microemboli in patients with large mediastinal masses or extensive retroperitoneal lymph node involvement. The technique may not be possible in patients with peripheral oedema.

CT has been accepted as an important technique in evaluating the presence of Hodgkin's disease in both the thorax and the abdomen (Crowther *et al.* 1979). CT scanning is capable of demonstrating additional mediastinal adenopathy not detected on plain radiographs and may show extension into extranodal tissues such as lung, pericardium, and chest wall (Figs 6 and 7). This information can be important in planning radiotherapy treatment fields and deciding whether chemotherapy should be used.

CT of the abdomen is helpful in evaluating upper abdominal nodal disease and can detect enlargement of coeliac, portal, and splenic hilar nodes. It is particularly useful in obese patients, since the retroperitoneal structures are better demonstrated in these patients because the surrounding fat has a low attenuation coefficient. Mesenteric adenopathy may also be detected but only when very large nodes are present, which is unusual in Hodgkin's disease. Although CT can detect enlarged nodes in the para-aortic, paracaval, and iliac areas, the investigation provides no useful information on lymph node architecture. Lymphography, however, can detect abnormalities in the structure of normal-sized nodes, but it is unwise to rely on this feature alone and if definite evidence of nodal involvement is required, histological ascertainment is necessary. The routine use of CT of the chest and abdomen may also be of value in assessing the bulk of the disease, which is one of the most important prognostic factors. Abdominal lymphography underestimates the bulk and extent of the disease within the abdomen.

In recent years CT scanning has become routine in the initial evaluation of Hodgkin's disease. Bipedal lymphangiography is being used less often. However, the techniques are complementary and ideally both should be used to evaluate the patient fully (Castellino *et al.* 1984).

Evaluation procedures considered necessary under certain conditions

Further imaging studies may be valuable in confirming clinical involvement at a given site. Patients with bone pain may have sclerotic, lytic, or mixed bony abnormality, but occasionally a periosteal reaction is all that can be seen using plain radiography. Usually bony lesions are found in the spine, pelvis, upper femora, and ribs, where they are often sclerotic in appearance. Technetium scanning may be helpful in documenting the distribution of bony disease and should be carried out in patients with bone pain or elevated levels of serum alkaline phosphatase. CT and MRI may be particularly helpful for suspicious lesions of bone. Focal lesions in the liver and spleen can be demonstrated by isotope scanning, ultrasonography, and CT, but these investigations are often

unreliable. MRI has also been used to advantage in this situation, but again is less reliable than laparotomy, splenectomy, and wedge biopsy of the liver with appropriate histological assessment. Intracranial disease is most effectively demonstrated by MRI and either MRI or CT have effectively replaced myelography for the definition of spinal extradural disease. CSF studies are very rarely of diagnostic value.

[67]Ga scanning can be useful in determining the extent of nodal involvement, particularly in the chest above the diaphragm (Fig. 8). The technique may also be of advantage in the reassessment of residual nodal abnormality at the end of therapy. Gallium scanning is of little value in assessing infradiaphragmatic disease with false-positive findings due to normal gallium accumulation in the liver, spleen, and faeces. Other imaging studies may be necessary to resolve the significance of symptoms or physical signs related to a particular ogan site.

Biopsy of specific sites to determine pathological involvement is of advantage in some situations. A bone-marrow aspirate with trephine biopsy should be carried out from at least one site for patients with CS III and IV or 'adverse feature' stage II disease. Radiographic techniques are of low sensitivity in detecting liver or splenic involvement, although CT can demonstrate space-occupying lesions which may be confirmed using ultrasonography or magnetic

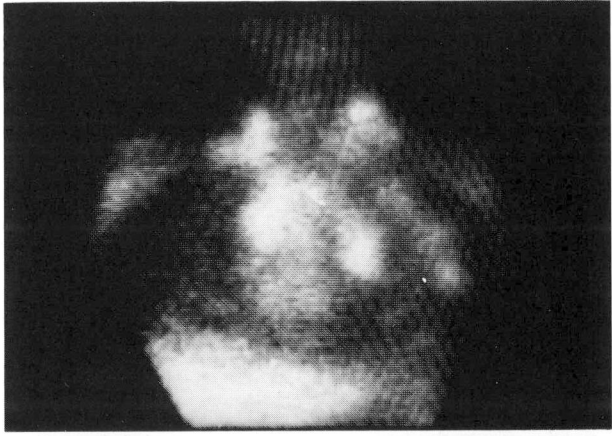

(a)

(b)

Fig. 8 (a) Gallium scan showing extensive areas of abnormal uptake involving both supraclavicular areas, left axilla, mediastinum, and left hilum; (b) normal scan of the same patient following chemotherapy. (Photographs supplied by R. J. Johnson, Department of Radiology, Christie Hospital, Manchester.)

resonance imaging. The latter technique is probably the most sensitive for detecting liver abnormalities, but if definite evidence of involvement is required to determine therapy then pathological confirmation may be required. Percutaneous needle biopsy of the liver is frequently negative even when disease is readily detectable using laparotomy. A percutaneous or laparoscopic liver biopsy can be helpful in patients with abnormal liver function or equivocally abnormal radiology of the liver. Histological proof of involvement is not always necessary in these circumstances, but if a positive result would alter the treatment approach then biopsy should be carried out. A guided bone biopsy using CT or a percutaneous open lung biopsy may be necessary under similar circumstances when evidence of involvement is otherwise equivocal.

Staging laparotomy

Staging laparotomy for Hodgkin's disease was introduced at Stanford in the United States to provide accurate information on the distribution of Hodgkin's disease within the abdomen and to help determine the best therapy for the individual patient. During the past 20–30 years the technique has provided a better understanding of the pathogenesis of Hodgkin's disease and has led to rational treatment decisions for pathologically staged patients. The decision whether or not to perform a staging laparotomy depends on weighing the consequences of its expected advantages in individualizing effective treatment with avoidance of unnecessary treatment and the disadvantage of the surgical procedure.

There is no evidence that laparotomy with splenectomy improves survival and the procedure can be associated with major surgical complications, delays in initiating therapy, and the subsequent risk of fulminating infection associated with immunodeficiency. The possibility of an increased risk of secondary leukaemia in splenectomized patients has also been raised (Van Leeuwen et al. 1987; Kaldor et al. 1990; Tura et al. 1993). For these reasons, oncologists from many centres have abandoned the use of staging laparotomy and make treatment decisions based on clinical staging methods. There is no evidence that this approach is inferior in terms of overall survival.

A series of 780 newly diagnosed patients from Toronto without routine staging laparotomy had an overall survival at 10 years of 69.6 per cent and a relapse-free survival of 48.9 per cent. The Stanford series in which staging laparotomy was used routinely showed a similar overall survival, although the relapse-free survival was significantly better (66.8 per cent at 10 years). However, comparisons between the centres are difficult and some selected patients in the Toronto series were submitted to a staging laparotomy. Other studies have attempted to address this issue and although no differences in survival have been demonstrated with or without staging laparotomy, there are difficulties in interpreting the data (Haybittle et al. 1985; Tubiana et al. 1989; Carde et al. 1993).

Patients with CS IIIB or IV disease are not candidates for staging laparotomy since combination chemotherapy is the treatment of choice and the results of laparotomy would not alter this decision. In addition, patients with bulky mediastinal disease who are to be treated by combined modality chemotherapy and radiotherapy should not be submitted to initial staging laparotomy since the surgery and any treatment delay could be hazardous.

If staging laparotomy is to be carried out, the technique should involve careful macroscopic examination of the abdominal contents and include biopsies of para-aortic and coeliac nodes, splenectomy with removal of splenic hilar nodes, a wedge biopsy and two needle biopsies of the liver, and a large iliac crest bone-marrow biopsy in selected cases. In addition, portal or iliac node biopsies should be considered. Table 4 shows the results in changing stage derived from six recent series and reflects the inaccuracy of clinical abdominal staging techniques (Moormeier et al. 1989). Abdominal CT scanning was only used in a small proportion of patients in these series, but would not be expected to alter the results significantly.

Anatomical staging criteria

Criteria for clinical staging

Lymph nodes are said to be involved if clinically enlarged and alternative pathology may be ruled out. Suspicious nodes should always be biopsied if treatment decisions are based on their involvement. Evidence of involvement is also provided by enlargement on plain radiography or CT. Textural abnormalities in addition to enlargement may provide evidence for involvement using lymphography.

Clinical evidence of splenic involvement includes unequivocal palpable splenomegaly or equivocal palpable splenomegaly with radiological confirmation of either enlargement or multiple focal defects. Radiological enlargement alone is insufficient for the diagnosis of splenic involvement. Clinical evidence of liver involvement includes multiple focal defects noted with at least two imaging techniques. Clinical evidence of lung involvement includes radiological evidence of parenchymal involvement in the absence of other likely causes such as infection. Evidence of bone involvement must be supported by plain radiographic changes or evidence from other imaging studies (for example, isotope scan, CT, or MRI). A spinal extradural deposit may be diagnosed on the basis of the clinical history and findings supported by plain radiograph, myelography, CT, and/or MRI. Intracranial involvement will rarely be diagnosed clinically at presentation but may be considered on the basis of a space-occupying lesion in the face of disease in additional extranodal sites. Clinical involvement of other extranodal sites may only be diagnosed if the site is contiguous or proximal to a known nodal site (that is, an E lesion).

Patients are classified as A (without) or B (with) symptoms of fever, sweats, and/or weight loss. The criteria for including a patient

Table 4 The effect of laparotomy on the stage of Hodgkin's disease

Clinical stage	Patient no.	Upstaged (%)	Downstaged (%)	Stage changed (%)
IA	352	25	0	25
IB	46	57	0	57
IIA	758	26	1	27
IIB	283	42	0	42
IIIA	296	9	34	43

After Moormeier et al. (1989).

in the B category consist of unexplained weight loss of more than 10 per cent of the body weight during the 6 months before initial staging investigation, unexplained, persistent, or recurrent fever with temperatures above 38°C during the previous month, and recurrent drenching night sweats during the previous month. The presence of any one of these symptoms is sufficient for including the patient in the B category. Although other symptoms may be associated with Hodgkin's disease, they are not classified as B symptoms, although some (such as severe pruritus) may prove to be of prognostic significance and should be recorded.

The presence of large amounts of bulky disease has been shown to indicate an unfavourable prognosis (Specht et al. 1988). For this reason it is important to measure the size of nodal masses. The bulk of palpable lymph nodes is defined as the largest dimension (in centimetres) of the single largest lymph node or conglomerate node mass in each region of involvement. A node or nodal mass must be 10 cm or greater to be classified as 'bulky'. In the abdomen the measurements are made using CT, MRI, ultrasonography, or lymphography. A mediastinal mass is defined as bulky on a 2 m plain abdominal chest radiograph when the maximum width is equal or greater than one-third of the internal transverse diameter of the thorax at the $T_{5/6}$ level. The subscript X may be used as a notation for bulk disease.

The Ann Arbor Staging Classification is shown in Table 3. For stage II disease the number of anatomical regions involved should be indicated by a subscript (for example, II_3). For the purposes of defining the number of anatomical regions, all nodal disease within the mediastinum is considered to be a single lymph node region. This includes prevascular, aortopulmonary, paratracheal, pretracheal, subcarinal, and posterior mediastinal subgroups. Hilar (broncho-pulmonary) nodes are considered to be outside the mediastinum and should be defined and recorded separately. Internal mammary nodes are part of the lymphatic system of the chest wall. They also drain the diaphragm. Paravertebral nodes, although in the posterior mediastinum, also drain the chest wall and diaphragm. Where possible these should be documented separately. Anterior extension of a mediastinal mass into the sternum or chest wall or extension to lung or pericardium should be recorded as extranodal extension. The staging notation and examples of staging are shown in Tables 5 and 6.

Involvement of extralymphatic tissue on one side of the diaphragm with limited direct extension from an extranodal site is classified as extranodal extension or E disease, with the expectation of a prognosis equivalent to that for treatment of nodal disease of the same anatomical extent when treated with radiation therapy to tumoricidal dose to all regions of involvement and their lymphatic drainage area. The E category may also include an apparently discrete single extranodal deposit consistent with extension from a regionally involved node. More extensive extranodal disease is designated as stage IV and multiple extranodal deposits or bilateral lung extension are not included in the E category. A single extranodal site as the only site of disease is classified as I_E; however, this is uncommon in Hodgkin's disease.

Criteria for pathological staging

Pathological staging depends on histological confirmation of specific sites of involvement, such as bone, bone-marrow, lung, liver, skin, etc. and involvement is designated by a subscript (that is, H=liver, M=bone-marrow, O=bone, L=lung, P=pleura, D=skin). The staging notation giving clinical examples incorporating modifications as recommended in the Cotswolds Report is shown in Tables 5 and 6.

Post-treatment evaluation

After completion of the planned therapy (or sooner if the outcome is unfavourable) response should be documented on the basis of the clinical situation and comparison of the results of laboratory procedures and imaging investigations which were abnormal at presentation, supplemented by tissue biopsy where appropriate.

The criteria for reporting response to therapy are as follows.

Complete remission (CR)

The patient has no clinical, radiological, or laboratory evidence of Hodgkin's disease. All abnormalities initially related to the presence of disease must have resolved. Changes consistent with the effects of previous therapy, such as radiation fibrosis, may be present.

Complete remission (unconfirmed/uncertain) (CR(u))

This category of response has been included to denote patients in whom remission status is unclear. The patient should be in normal health with no clinical evidence of Hodgkin's disease, but some radiological abnormality, not consistent with the effects of therapy persists at a site of previous disease. Implicit in this designation is considerable uncertainty about the significance of such abnormalities, since it is well known that abnormal widening of the mediastinum or architectural distortion of lymph node-bearing areas may persist for many years without therapy and without evidence of recurrent Hodgkin's disease. Attempts to resolve the dilemma of persistent disease versus residual anatomic distortion not indicative of Hodgkin's disease should include investigations such as radiological imaging, MRI, and gallium scanning. Within the bounds of acceptable morbidity, pathological examination may be appropriate, although the difficulties of 'sampling' artefact are acknowledged. Unusual or highly suspicious lesions should be rebiopsied. Persistent elevation of the erythrocyte sedimentation rate, while not diagnostic of active Hodgkin's disease, is an indication for very close surveillance since this has been shown to be an important prognostic factor for subsequent relapse in some series (Friedman et al. 1988).

Partial remission

The sum of the products of the largest perpendicular diameters of all measurable lesions should decrease by at least 50 per cent. There should also be an objective improvement in non-measurable but clinically evaluable malignant disease.

Progressive disease

The size of at least one measurable lesion should increase by 25 per cent or more or a new lesion should appear.

Anatomical staging criteria

Following completion of therapy, it is recommended that patients be seen at intervals of 2 or 3 months during the first and second year following therapy, at 4 month intervals in the third year, at 6 month intervals in the fourth and fifth years, and annually thereafter. The frequency and type of radiological studies should reflect the initial sites of disease. Appropriate investigation should accompany any concern about symptoms or signs of possible recurrent disease, but a full blood count, biochemical profile, and chest radiograph should be taken at each visit. An assessment of long-term complications of therapy should be undertaken at regular intervals and their presence or absence documented.

Table 5 Example 1

Stage at this level of information	Information		Stage at this level of information
CS II$_4$A	A 24 year old asymptomatic male presents with bilateral neck and axillary nodes; neck node biopsy reveals nodular-sclerosing Hodgkin's disease		CS II$_4$A
CS II$_{5X}$A	Chest radiograph shows 'bulky' mediastinal mass (greater than one-third transverse chest diameter at T$_{5/6}$) and right hilar nodal enlargement	Chest radiograph shows mediastinal mass (less than one-third transverse chest diameter at T$_{5/6}$)	CS II$_5$A
CS II$_{5X}$A	Liver function tests reveal elevated SAP but no other abnormalities	Liver function tests normal	CS II$_5$A
CS II$_{7XE}$A	Chest CT confirms mediastinal mass and identifies bilateral hilar nodes and extension into pericardium, sternum, and chest wall	Chest CT confirms mediastinal mass but shows no extranodal extension and no hilar involvement	CS II$_5$A
CS III$_{2XE}$A	Abdominal CT shows para-aortic, paracaval, and pelvic adenopathy; no abnormality of liver or spleen	Abdominal CT scan shows homogenous splenomegaly but the spleen is not clinically palpable and no other abnormalities are seen	CS II$_5$A
CS III$_{2XE}$A	Lymphography shows para-aortic, paracaval, and pelvic adenopathy	Lymphography normal	CS II$_5$A
CS III$_{2XE}$A	Bone-marrow aspirate and trephine negative	Bone-marrow aspirate and trephine negative	CS II$_5$A
CS III$_{2XE}$A	No further staging undertaken as patient is referred for chemotherapy	Following staging laparotomy, splenic disease with multiple nodules (two greater than 1 cm); splenic hilar and coeliac node contained disease	PS III$_1$A

SAP, serum alkaline phosphatase.

Table 6 Example 2

Stage at this level of information	Information		Stage at this level of information
CS II$_2$B	A 63-year-old male presents with bilateral neck nodes, profuse night sweats, fatigue, and weight loss of 15 kg (more than 10 per cent body weight) over past 3 months; neck node biopsy reveals mixed-cellularity Hodgkin's disease		CS II$_2$B
CS II$_4$B	Chest radiograph shows mediastinal mass (less than one-third transverse chest diameter at T$_{5/6}$) and right hilar nodal enlargement	Chest radiograph shows mediastinal, and bilateral hilar nodes and multiple discrete parenchymal/lung nodules	CS IVB$_L$
CS II$_4$B	SAP is 170 IU/l GGT is 120 IU/l LDH is 600 IU/l	SAP is 170 IU/l GGT is 120 IU/l LDH is 600 IU/l	CS IVB$_L$
CS II$_4$B	Chest CT shows nodal disease in mediastinal and right hilar regions; no extranodal extension	Chest CT shows nodal disease in mediastinum and hilar regions and multiple parenchymal nodules	CS IVB$_L$
CS IIIB	Abdominal CT shows para-aortic, paracaval, coeliac, and pelvic adenopathy; there is a 3 cm low density lesion in right lobe of liver	Abdominal CT scan shows para-aortic, paracaval, and pelvic adenopathy; multiple lesions (1–3 cm) are seen in liver	CS IVB$_L$
CS IIIB	Lymphography shows para-aortic, paracaval, and pelvic adenopathy	It is elected not to perform lymphography	CS IVB$_L$
CS IIIB	Abdominal ultrasound indicates that the liver lesion is cystic; no gallium uptake is seen in the liver, but is seen in the neck, mediastinum, retroperitoneum, and pelvis	Gallium uptake is seen in liver lesions; the areas of adenopathy are also visualized	CS IVB$_{LH}$
CS IIIB	Bone-marrow aspirate and trephine are negative	Bone-marrow shows evidence of Hodgkin's disease	PS IVB$_{LHM}$
	No further staging is undertaken and the patient is referred for chemotherapy		

SAP, serum alkaline phosphatase; GGT, gamma glutamyl transpeptidase; LDH, lactate dehydrogenase.

MANAGEMENT OF STAGE I AND II DISEASE

The incidence and mortality data for Hodgkin's disease for the past three decades in the Province of Ontario, Canada, is shown in Fig. 9. The figure illustrates the following points.

1. An unchanging incidence of 3 cases per 100 000 of the population.

2. An incidence to mortality ratio of 2:1 for the period up to approximately 1970, representing a cure rate of 50 per cent predominantly attributable to radiation therapy for patients with localized disease. During this period, chemotherapy was largely of palliative benefit.

3. An incidence to mortality ratio of 5:1 for the current period, representing a cure rate of 80 per cent attributable to the application of both radiation therapy and combination

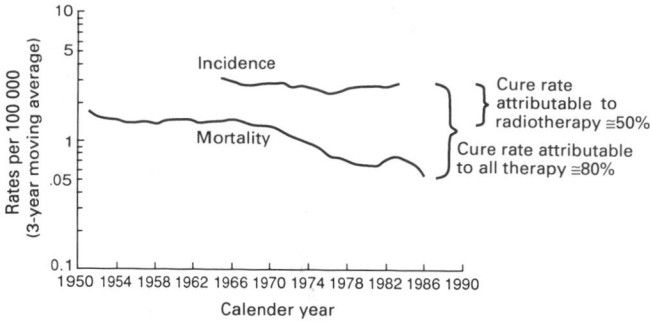

Fig. 9 Incidence and mortality rates for male and female patients with Hodgkin's disease in Ontario, Canada, 1950–1986. Rates are expressed per 100 000 of the population using a 3 year moving mean and are age-adjusted to the world standard population. (Data kindly provided by The Ontario Cancer Foundation.)

chemotherapy to patients with both localized and advanced disease.

During the past several decades, the curative role of radiation therapy for patients with localized disease has been amply demonstrated (Gilbert 1939; Peters 1950; Kaplan 1962). The period of intensive investigation during the past three decades to define disease more accurately has neither made radiation therapy more effective nor improved overall cure rates. However, it has increased our knowledge of the disease and maximized the curative potential of radiation therapy through selection of those with disease distributions most suitable for control by localized therapy. Fortuitously, the emergence of combination chemotherapy as a curative treatment modality coincident with more rigorous selection for radiation therapy has resulted in an improvement in cure rates for the total patient population rather than for any one subgroup selected through more intensive investigation.

The mortality rate shown in Fig. 9 identifies death from all causes. Over the past two decades the role of treatment as a contribution to cause of death has been increasingly recognized, with chemotherapy-induced leukaemogenesis and chemotherapy- and radiation therapy-induced solid second malignancies assuming an increasingly important contribution to mortality in survivors of Hodgkin's disease.

These four issues, the curative roles of radiation therapy and chemotherapy, the role and type of staging information required for management decisions, and the acute and chronic toxicities of therapy, are central to the definition of management strategy for patients with Hodgkin's disease. For patients with CS I and II disease, the management questions are as follows.

1. Which patient population and how selected is appropriate for treatment with radiation therapy alone?

2. What is the optimal form of therapy for those unsuitable for treatment with radiation therapy alone?

Selection of patients for radiation therapy alone

Supradiaphragmatic disease
Stage

In an unselected adult population of patients presenting with CS I and II Hodgkin's disease, approximately 90 per cent will have a supradiaphragmatic presentation, approximately 10 per cent will

have symptoms of night sweats, fever, or weight loss, over 50 per cent will have mediastinal adenopathy, and approximately 12–16 per cent will present with massive mediastinal disease with or without hilar node enlargement and/or pulmonary extension. Very few will be elderly or medically unfit for intensive investigation.

Several studies addressing the role of laparotomy and splenectomy in otherwise unselected patients with CS I and II disease have indicated the failure of clinical staging methods to define occult upper abdominal disease (Glatstein *et al.* 1969; Sutcliffe *et al.* 1976). Over time, the role of staging laparotomy has been re-examined (Kinsella and Glatstein 1983; Lacher 1983; Rosenberg 1988). However, the following conclusions have been drawn.

1. There is an upstaging rate from CS I and II to PS III and IV of approximately 25–30 per cent and a 'downstaging' rate of approximately 5 per cent in patients with CS III and IV disease.

2. The most common site of clinically occult upper abdominal disease is in the spleen, splenic hilar lymph nodes, and the coeliac axis lymph nodes.

3. For experienced observers, the sensitivity and specificity of lymphography in the interpretation of external iliac, common iliac, and para-aortic nodes to a superior limit approximating the second lumbar vertebral body is approximately 90 per cent.

4. Involvement of lymph nodes beyond the retroperitoneum (mesenteric, porta hepatis, internal iliac) is extremely unusual in the absence of gross intra-abdominal disease.

5. Liver involvement occurs in less than 5 per cent of patients with PS I and II disease and correlates with the presence and extent of splenic disease. Approximately 30 per cent of patients with CS I and II disease will have splenic disease; one-third of these will have extensive splenic disease (more than five nodules, >1 cm in diameter) and half of those with extensive splenic disease will have demonstrable liver involvement.

6. Bone-marrow involvement in asymptomatic patients with CS I and II disease is very rare.

Therefore in deciding on the role of stage as a determinant of treatment allocation, the following should be recognized.

1. Staging laparotomy remains the most accurate method of describing the anatomical extent of intra-abdominal disease, most appropriately defines patients with a high probability of cure with radiation therapy, and facilitates planning of upper abdominal radiation therapy fields.

2. Laparotomy staging requires commitment to quality assurance for the procedures of surgery, histopathology, and radiation therapy and carries with it not only the direct and indirect costs of the procedure but also a very small mortality rate and a significant morbidity rate approaching 15 per cent for all post-procedural complications.

3. A series of patients with PS I and II supradiaphragmatic disease is clearly a subset of a CS I and II patient population selected as follows:

   (a) exclusion of patients unsuitable for surgery through age or other medical conditions;

   (b) potential exclusion of patients with massive mediastinal disease who may be unsuitable for laparotomy either on medical grounds or by initial treatment preference for chemotherapy;

(c) exclusion of approximately 30 per cent of patients with proven intra-abdominal disease.

4. Whilst the laparotomy findings are unique for an individual patient, in large series findings with respect to probability of involvement, sites of involvement and distribution of disease are well characterized, uniform from centre to centre, and unlikely to change or further modify general views regarding patient management.

Prognostic factors other than stage

Although anatomical extent of disease, as defined in the Ann Arbor Classification, has been the discriminant of treatment mode, several other factors have emerged as independent determinants of survival and relapse following radiation therapy for stage I and II disease. They include the following.

1. Age: most investigators define a worse prognosis for the second age peak (age >40 years) (Vaughan Hudson *et al.* 1983; Sutcliffe *et al.* 1985; Tubiana *et al.* 1985).

2. Histology: a more favourable prognosis exists for lymphocyte-predominant and nodular-sclerosing as opposed to mixed-cellularity and lymphocyte-predominant histologies. Attention has also been drawn to additional prognostic discrimination within the nodular sclerosis subtype (types 1 and 2) (Bennett *et al.* 1983).

3. Symptoms: patients with B symptoms have a worse prognosis following radiation therapy alone than those who are asymptomatic (Crnkovich *et al.* 1987).

4. Number of involved sites (Peckham *et al.* 1975; Tubiana *et al.* 1989).

5. A raised erythrocyte sedimentation rate has been associated with a poorer prognosis (Tubiana *et al.* 1986).

6. Bulk of disease: the true rôle of tumour bulk as a prognostic determinant is difficult to define separately from issues relating to the site of bulky disease, most commonly in the mediastinum and the technical difficulties imposed upon radiation therapy planning in this site. Whilst it is clear that bulky mediastinal disease is predictive of intrathoracic failure following supradiaphragmatic irradiation, it is not at all clear that bulk in sites other than the mediastinum is prejudicial for local or loco-regional control following radiation to appropriate fields and at full tumouricidal dose, although some suggestion of a correlation between an increasing tumour bulk and decreasing local control with standard radiation doses has been made (Gunter-Seydel *et al.* 1967; Thar *et al.* 1979; Yarnold *et al.* 1982).

The rôle of these factors in addition to stage is well established and their ability to discriminate prognosis has been demonstrated (Tubiana *et al.* 1984c; Haybittle *et al.* 1985; Sutcliffe *et al.* 1985; Horwich *et al.* 1986; Gobbi *et al.* 1988). With respect to prognosis for patients with CS I and II disease, these factors are, in large part, surrogates for the presence of intra-abdominal disease (Table 7 (Tubiana *et al.* 1984c) and Table 8 (Brada *et al.* 1986)). The only defined factor with a predictive influence upon local control rate following radiation therapy is mediastinal bulk.

7. Mediastinal involvement: in general terms there is no prognostic significance as to the presence or absence of mediastinal adenopathy in CS I and II disease. Some investigators note that

Table 7 Results of laparotomy in patients from the favourable and unfavourable prognosis groups in the EORTC-H$_2$ trial

Subgroup	Percentage of positive laparotomy[a]		Extent of abdominal disease (percentage of patients with only one site involved)[b]	
CS I$_1$α	9/51 (18%)	14/76 (18%)	7/9	11/14 (78%)
CS II$_2$α	5/25 (20%)		4/5	
CS II$_3$	15/43 (35%)	24/66 (36%)	4/15	13/24 (54%)
CS I+II$_2$β	9/23 (39%)		6/9	

α, no symptoms (A) and erythrocyte sedimentation rate (ESR) <50 or symptoms (B) and ESR <30.
β, no symptoms (A) and ESR ≥50 or symptoms (B) and ESR ≥30.
I, one lymphatic area involved.
II$_2$, two lymphatic areas involved.
II$_3$, three or more lymphatic areas involved.
[a]p=0.02.
[b]p, not specified.
Reproduced with permission from Tubiana *et al.* (1984c).

Table 8 CS I and II Hodgkin's disease: prediction of risk of positive laparotomy based on age and sex

Sex	Age (years)	Predicted percentage[a] of positive laparotomies	Observed (PS III and IV, CS I and II)
Male	<19	62	18/24 (75%)
	20–39	31	28/90 (31%)
	>40	26	9/35 (26%)
Female	<19	34	4/21 (19%)
	20–39	13	7/48 (15%)
	>40	10	3/7 (43%)

[a]Derived from logistic regression analysis.
Reproduced with permission from Brada *et al.* (1985).

multiple sites of nodal involvement without mediastinal adenopathy are adverse (Tubiana *et al.* 1984a) and favour a higher probability of intra-abdominal disease. The importance of mediastinal disease is most apparent when the disease is 'bulky'. Definitions of 'bulky' have varied; above 7.5 cm diameter on a plain abdominal chest radiograph (Hagermeister *et al.* 1981), more than one-third of the transverse diameter of the chest on a plain abdominal chest radiograph (Hoppe *et al.* 1982; Mauch *et al.* 1988; Anderson *et al.* 1991). However, there is general unanimity that a large mediastinal mass is predictive of intrathoracic disease progression following standard supradiaphragmatic radiation fields.

Several factors probably account for the predominance of intrathoracic failure with standard mantle fields applied for large mediastinal masses, for example the association with anterior extension to the chest wall, the increased incidence of pulmonary hilar disease, extension to adjacent lung and pericardium, planning of conservative margins to radiation fields to 'spare' normal lung, and the use of 'shrinking fields' for disease that may change in size but not in anatomic position (pulmonary hilar nodes, extranodal extensions). What these factors have in common is the difficulty of including all known disease and lymphatic channels involved by contiguous or retrograde spread in a tumouricidal radiation field, given the necessity for restriction of an adequate volume of lung and heart to a level within radiation tolerance. Whilst direct proof of this proposition is lacking, it is supported by the change in recurrence patterns with whole thoracic radiation (Lee *et al.* 1981) or combined modality therapy supports it (Hoppe *et al.* 1982; Anderson *et al.* 1984).

Infradiaphragmatic disease

Infradiaphragmatic presentation accounts for 4–10 per cent of all patients with CS I and II disease. In general terms, various series have indicated a higher median age and a male predominance, but no major differences in the histological spectrum for patients with infradiaphragmatic disease (Krikorian *et al.* 1979, 1986; Barrett *et al.* 1981; Mauch *et al.* 1983; Dorreen *et al.* 1984; Lanzillo *et al.* 1985; Sutcliffe *et al.* 1985; Specht and Nissen 1988).

Patients with disease confined to the groin or ipsilateral pelvis with lymphogram-negative para-aortic nodes rarely have disease demonstrated in the spleen and upper abdomen. Conversely, patients with lymphogram-positive para-aortic nodes commonly have splenic and upper abdominal disease (Barrett *et al.* 1981; Dorreen *et al.* 1984).

Treatment approaches have varied from involved field radiation to combined modality therapy. No firm guidelines exist, given access to small numbers of patients treated with varying regimens over a 20 year period. However, the following points seem appropriate.

1. Asymptomatic patients with isolated inguinal or ipsilateral pelvic disease and no evidence of involvement of the para-aortic nodes by lymphography and CT are unlikely to change stage as a result of laparotomy and splenectomy and can achieve high relapse-free rates with extended field radiotherapy alone. Prophylactic supradiaphragmatic radiation is unnecessary.

2. Symptomatic patients and those with positive para-aortic nodes by lymphogram or CT criteria are likely to have more extensive disease defined by laparotomy, would have an unacceptably high relapse rate following radiation therapy to infradiaphragmatic fields, and are almost certainly treated optimally with a combined modality programme.

Most investigators have failed to demonstrate an inferior prognosis for patients with infradiaphragmatic disease. Specht and Nissen (1988), reporting the largest series to date, defined an inferior disease-free survival but no adverse overall survival for patients with infradiaphragmatic disease in multivariate analysis.

Radiation therapy for localized stage I and II Hodgkin's disease

Radiation dose

In 1966, Kaplan published a radiation dose–response curve for Hodgkin's disease indicating a continuous relationship between in-field control and tumour doses up to 40 Gy. Subsequent reanalysis of these data revealed a sigmoid response curve with a steep dose–control relationship between 15 and 30 Gy and no indication of increasing control rates at doses in excess of 35 Gy (Fletcher and Shukovsky 1975). These findings support earlier data using orthovoltage therapy with no in-field failures at doses in excess of 30 Gy (Jelliffe and Thomson 1955) and have in turn been confirmed by other investigators (Hanks *et al.* 1982; Schewe *et al.* 1988). In summary, the minimum tumour dose to any part of the radiation field should be no less than 30 Gy if in-field control rates are to exceed 95 per cent and there is no established therapeutic benefit to exceeding 40 Gy. Doses in excess of 40 Gy merely

increase morbidity. Although there has been a suggestion of a correlation between tumour dose and in-field control as a function of disease bulk (Thar *et al.* 1979; Yarnold *et al.* 1982; Gunter-Seydel *et al.* 1967), this view has not been supported by Schewe *et al.* (1988). As noted previously, this issue is clouded by the large numbers of patients with disease bulk in the mediastinum, a technically complex site for radiation therapy, compared with the small numbers with bulky disease in other anatomic regions.

It has also been proposed that radiation doses may be reduced for 'subclinical', 'microscopic', or prophylactic fields, and also when used in adjuvant mode following chemotherapy. There are no data to justify these claims; however, it is apparent that the sigmoid dose–response curve and the Patterns of Care Study would still predict in-field control rates of 90 per cent for doses of 25–30 Gy and more than 80 per cent control for doses in excess of 20 Gy (Hanks *et al.* 1982, 1983).

Radiotherapy fields

The principles of curative radiation therapy field planning emanate from the work of Finzi (1913), Gilbert (1939), Craft (1940), Peters (1950), and Kaplan (1962) and comprise the concept of homogeneous distribution of a tumoricidal dose to both areas of clinical involvement and the clinically negative lymph node areas adjacent to the primary site(s). Such large field planning requires consideration of the tolerances of normal tissues within the irradiated volume and the radiation volume. Dose and schedule are of equal importance in determining not only the likelihood of tumour control, but also the incidence and severity of acute and delayed treatment-related morbidity.

The radiation fields employed include the following (Fig. 10).

Involved field

Treatment of the involved area and the adjacent clinically negative nodes.

Extended field

All relevant nodal areas, both involved and non-involved, above the diaphragm (the 'mantle' field). Some publications include a para-aortic field with the mantle under the designation extended field (Collaborative Study 1984; Tubiana *et al.* 1984c; Farah *et al.* 1988). For infradiaphragmatic disease, the inverted Y field is employed with extension to cover the spleen or the splenic pedicle if splenectomy has been performed.

Total nodal irradiation

This implies a mantle field followed by an inverted Y field after a 3–4 week break to allow haematological recovery. The spleen or

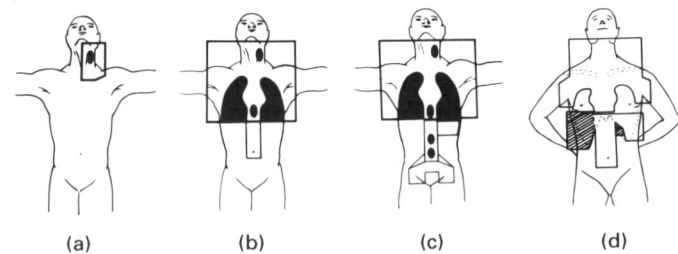

(a) (b) (c) (d)

Fig. 10 Radiation fields for the treatment of Hodgkin's disease: (a) involved field; (b) extended field; (c) total-nodal irradiation; (d) mantle plus upper abdomen (with or without liver and right kidney attenuator).

splenic pedicle should be within the abdominal radiation field. Prophylactic hepatic irradiation using doses attenuated to comply with liver tolerance may also be employed (Hoppe *et al.* 1980; Levitt *et al.* 1984). When abdominal fields are being applied prophylactically for patients with PS I and II supradiaphragmatic disease, the pelvic limbs of the inverted Y may be omitted to avoid haematological and gonadal morbidity. This field disposition is referred to as subtotal nodal-irradiation. Patients treated with irradiation alone for favourable supradiaphragmatic CS I and II disease (that is, without laparotomy and splenectomy) receive mantle irradiation followed by upper abdominal radiation fields which cover the spleen and retroperitoneum. An attenuated dose may be given to the liver and appropriate renal shielding is required.

Technical factors

The radiation therapy of Hodgkin's disease is complex for the following reasons:

(1) the requirement to treat a large target volume to a uniform tumoricidal dose;

(2) the limiting tolerance of critical normal structures within or in close proximity to the target volume;

(3) complicated irregularly shaped fields resulting from the spatial relationship between the target volume and adjacent normal tissues;

(4) large variation in external surface contour and internal tissue densities through the volume being irradiated.

Detailed consideration of the technical aspects of radiation therapy for Hodgkin's disease is available (Carmel and Kaplan 1976; Timothy *et al.* 1987). In brief, the principal issues are as follows.

Selection of treatment unit

Mantle and inverted Y fields are most appropriately treated by equally weighted parallel opposed fields if the most uniform dose distribution is to be achieved throughout the treatment volume. For adults, the patient thickness dictates the use of megavoltage equipment (^{60}Co or mid/high energy linear accelerator), with the depth dose characteristics of the photon beam increasing as a function of increasing photon energy. Skin sparing as a result of the increased depth in tissue to achieve maximum dose ('build-up') will be achieved with megavoltage beams. For high energy accelerators, the build-up depth of 2–3 cm may prejudice dose distribution to critical areas at superficial depth (for example, neck nodes). In this circumstance, bolus (tissue equivalent material) may be required over the relevant regions to bring a tumoricidal dose to more superficial tissues. The use of bolus may remove skin sparing and result in a dose-related acute skin reaction.

Treatment geometry

The treatment geometry is dependent upon the required field size, the desired penumbra width, and the treatment unit employed. To achieve a reliable, reproducible treatment each day, considerable attention is required to avoid minor changes in patient position that will be magnified into significant error given the distance between energy source, interposed beam-modifying devices, and the patient. Ideally, isocentric treatment units would be employed with the patient in the same position for both anterior and posterior fields. In practice, however, choice of available energy and limiting source to skin distance may necessitate the use of extended source to skin distance with fixed units and the patient in supine and prone positions for anterior and posterior fields.

Simulation

The setting-up of the patient in the treatment position within appropriate immobilization devices is essential if one is to establish that treatment is actually being directed to all relevant areas. All subsequent procedures are referenced to the simulation process and any inaccuracies in the set-up or determination of field outlines and shielding block design will be reproduced through the whole course of treatment. In the treatment position, patient thickness and missing tissue measurements can be made at a number of predetermined points of interest such that dose variation across the target volume can be established. Reference points, tattoos, etc., for positioning can be established. If the patient is being treated in supine and prone positions, the simulation procedure will be required for both anterior and posterior fields.

The importance of simulation and subsequent verification of the daily reproducibility of treatment has been amply demonstrated (Marks *et al.* 1974; Kinzie *et al.* 1983). In the Patterns of Care Study unacceptably high in-field and marginal recurrence rates were associated with radiation portals judged retrospectively to cover disease inadequately (Kinzie *et al.* 1983). In practice, recurrence due to inadequate planning constitutes a substantially greater problem than true in-field failure.

Treatment aids

Additional aids to establish accurate reproduction of patient position and uniform dose distribution throughout the target volume include immobilization devices, 'compensators' for missing tissue resulting from variation of external contour, shielding blocks to minimize radiation dose to critical normal tissues, and attenuators to deliver a modified dose to certain regions of limited tolerance.

Special consideration must be given to the 'junction' between supradiaphragmatic and infradiaphragmatic fields. Since the 'junction' is a region of dose uncertainty, it must not be placed in an area where there is concern regarding active disease. Junction construction will vary according to the use of isocentric or fixed units. Varying techniques are employed to ensure avoidance of overlapping fields at the junction with the attendant risk of spinal cord overdose, for example, a planned gap between fields, junction shields, and a 'moving' field border.

Treatment verification

Once the patient proceeds to therapy, it is essential that all therapy parameters, particularly those pertaining to the actual shape and location of the radiation fields, are verified with portal films taken in the position of actual treatment geometry with all treatment devices in place. The monitoring rate for the repetition of portal films throughout therapy should reflect the prevailing error rate within the treatment unit. Clearly, a technique with an unsatisfactory rate of reproducibility requires revision.

Treatment results of stage I and II Hodgkin's disease with radiation alone

CS I and II

The use of involved field radiation therapy for patients with CS I and II disease is associated with relapse rates exceeding 60 per cent. Virtually all recurrences occur distant to the irradiation field. Other than for highly specific circumstances, for example asymptomatic isolated high cervical or inguinal stage I disease, involved field radiation alone cannot be considered an effective treatment strategy because of the unacceptably high recurrence rate. Its use can only be sanctioned as part of a combined modality approach or where salvage of radiation failure by chemotherapy is considered an acceptable curative strategy for patients with early stage disease.

The use of extended field radiation, 'mantle' field, to treat CS I and II supradiaphragmatic disease is associated with a recurrence rate of 35–63 per cent (Rubin et al. 1974; Stoffel and Cox 1977; Timothy et al. 1978a; Tubiana et al. 1979; Liew et al. 1984; Sutcliffe et al. 1985). The majority of recurrences occur in nodal sites below the diaphragm, which should not be surprising given the 30 per cent probability of occult infradiaphragmatic disease in patients with CS I and II supradiaphragmatic presentations.

Recognizing the inherent risk of occult infradiaphragmatic disease, several groups have added abdominal radiation fields (inverted Y or upper abdominal fields) to the mantle field. In clinically staged patients, the abdominal fields must incorporate the entire spleen, splenic artery, coeliac axis, and retroperitoneal nodes. Where such techniques have been used, reduced recurrence rates of 17–35 per cent have been achieved (Rubin et al. 1974; Stoffel and Cox 1977; Tubiana et al. 1981; Sutcliffe et al. 1985).

PS I and II

The use of mantle fields in patients with a negative staging laparotomy has been associated with recurrence rates of 23–53 per cent (Stoffel and Cox 1977; Timothy et al. 1978a; Hagermeister et al. 1982; Liew et al. 1984; Anderson et al. 1984). These results reflect lack of selection by characteristics other than stage and the potential for sampling error in laparotomy, splenectomy, and lymph node mapping. Of particular relevance is the poor sampling in the region between the twelfth thoracic (coeliac axis level) and the second/third lumbar vertebral junction (inferior mesenteric artery). This region is not well characterized by lymphography, requires extensive dissection in the region of the duodenal loop and pancreas for node retrieval, and adds significantly to the time and morbidity of the procedure. Although the patterns of failure following mantle irradiation alone for supradiaphragmatic PS I and II disease are not well characterized, many groups feel that para-aortic and splenic pedicle radiation is required for such patients.

When supradiaphragmatic and infradiaphragmatic fields are employed for patients with supradiaphragmatic PS I and II disease, relapse rates of 15–34 per cent are achieved (Stoffel and Cos 1977; Wiernik et al. 1979; Tubiana et al. 1981; Hagermeister et al. 1982; Hoppe et al. 1982; Mauch et al. 1988; Farah et al. 1988; Nissen and Nordentoft 1982).

The above discussion begs three questions.

(1) Is there survival advantage following radiation according to CS or PS I and II?

(2) Historically, all series that compare equivalent approaches with radiation therapy for clinically staged as opposed to surgically staged patients demonstrate an inferior freedom from progression for the clinically staged group. This would not be unexpected given that the surgically staged group is a favourably selected subgroup of the entire population with stage I and II disease. Despite the higher relapse rate, there is no overall survival difference between clinically and surgically staged patients because of the effectiveness of chemotherapy in the salvage of patients recurring after radiation therapy (Bergsagel et al. 1982). Thus, survival cannot be the discriminant endpoint of the value of surgical versus clinical staging.

(3) Can equivalent control rates with irradiation be achieved in patients with CS I and II as in those with PS I and II disease?

The past decade has seen a considerable expansion of the factors determining outcome after radiation for localized Hodgkin's disease (see section above on radiotherapy fields). It is clear that heterogeneity within anatomic stage requires attention in designing optimal treatment strategy in addition to considerations relating to clinical versus pathological stage.

The H_2 study of the European Organization for Research and Treatment of Cancer (EORTC) addressed the issue of laparotomy or splenic irradiation in the patients with supradiaphragmatic CS I and II disease. All patients received mantle field and para-aortic irradiation with splenic irradiation in the non-laparotomy group. The aims of this randomized trial were to compare the therapeutic efficacy of splenic irradiation versus splenectomy and to assess the prognostic significance of the information provided by laparotomy. The survival and relapse-free survival rates were 79 and 77 per cent and 76 and 68 per cent for the splenectomy versus non-splenectomy groups, respectively (Tubiana et al. 1981). The subsequent H_5 study took into account additional information pertaining to initial prognostic indicators in patients with CS I and II disease. Favourable indicators included age below 40 years, lymphocyte-predominant and nodular-sclerosing histology, A symptoms and erythrocyte sedimentation rate below 50, B symptoms and erythrocyte sedimentation rate below 30, and CS I and II_2 (mediastinum). Unfavourable indicators were age over 40 years, mixed-cellularity and lymphocyte-depleted histology, A symptoms and erythrocyte sedimentation rate above 50, B symptoms and erythrocyte sedimentation rate above 30, and CS II_3 (non-mediastinal). Patients with favourable prognostic indicators proceeded to laparotomy. Retrospective analysis of the H_2 study indicated that the probability of a positive laparotomy in the favourable group would not exceed 18 per cent and 78 per cent of those who were positive would have only one site of involvement compared with 36 per cent and 54 per cent, respectively, for the unfavourable group (Tubiana et al. 1984c). Patients with negative laparotomy in the H_5 study, being a selected subset of the favourable group, were then randomized to mantle or mantle plus para-aortic irradiation. Patients with unfavourable indicators were not submitted to laparotomy and were randomized along with the laparotomy-positive favourable subgroup to receive total-nodal irradiation or combined modality therapy.

In the favourable subgroup of patients there was no difference in relapse-free survival or survival between mantle or mantle plus para-aortic irradiation. In the unfavourable group, disease-free survival was significantly lower in the total-nodal irradiation group although there was no significant survival difference.

In the most recent EORTC study, H_6, a randomization to laparotomy and splenectomy was undertaken in the favourable prognostic group. Those not undergoing laparotomy and splenectomy received mantle, para-aortic, and splenic irradiation. Those with a negative laparotomy received mantle irradiation (lymphocyte-predominant and nodular-sclerosing histology) or mantle plus para-aortic irradiation (mixed cellularity and lymphocyte predominant). Patients with a positive laparotomy and those with unfavourable prognostic indicators were randomized between a MOPP-based (nitrogen mustard, vincristine, prednisolone, and procarbazine) or an ABVD-based combined modality regimen. At 4 years of follow-up, relapse-free survival was approximately 10 per cent lower in the non-laparotomy group with favourable prognostic indicators (85 versus 75 per cent, $p=0.02$) although no survival difference was evident (93 versus 89 per cent). No significant differences are apparent in relapse-free or overall survival in the unfavourable group (Tubiana *et al.* 1989; Carde *et al.* 1993).

In summary, the EORTC group have evolved an approach to management of CS I and II Hodgkin's disease incorporating laparotomy and splenectomy in combination with a number of clinically derived prognostic factors at presentation. This approach has seen a reduction in the number of patients undergoing laparotomy and splenectomy, a rationalization of radiation fields, and a rationalization and reduction in the total number of patients receiving chemotherapy over the period of the H_1, H_2, and H_5 trials.

A similar approach identifying prognostic factors at presentation in CS I and II patients has been used by the Princess Margaret Hospital group in Toronto. Based upon analysis of outcome of 222 patients with supradiaphragmatic disease treated by radical irradiation alone during the period 1968–1977, age above 50 years, mixed-cellularity and lymphocyte-depleted histology, stage, and symptoms of disease were defined as adverse for relapse-free rate and survival. Bulky mediastinal disease was adverse for relapse-free rate only. Three groups of patients could be defined by relapse rate according to a multiparameter aggregation of prognostic factors (Sutcliffe *et al.*. 1985).

1. This group comprised 5.4 per cent of the patient population and was defined solely by isolated unilateral nodal stage IA disease (above the upper border of the thyroid cartilage). The relapse rate in this small group of patients was 8 per cent and was unrelated to irradiation field size (involved field or mantle field).

2. This group comprised 84.2 per cent of patients treated and was defined as follows:

   age <50, lymphocyte predominant+nodular sclerosing, CS IA, IB+IIB;
   age <50, mixed cellularity+lymphocyte depleted, CS IA, IIA;
   age >50, lymphocyte predominant+nodular sclerosing, CS IA, IIA.

   The overall relapse rate for group 2 was 34 per cent (63/187) and was 44 per cent for involved field, 32 per cent for mantle field, and 27 per cent for mantle plus upper retroperitoneal abdominal irradiation.

3. This group comprised 10.4 per cent of patients treated and was defined as follows:

   age <50, mixed cellularity+lymphocyte depleted, CS IB+IIB;
   age ≥50, lymphocyte predominant+nodular sclerosing, CS IB+IIB;
   age ≥50, mixed cellularity+lymphocyte depleted, CS IA, IIA, IB+IIB.

   The overall relapse rate for group 3 with radical irradiation alone was 74 per cent and was not influenced by irradiation field volume.

Clearly the implications of this multiparameter model of prognostic factors cannot be interpreted in the context of laparotomy findings as surgical staging was not performed on this series of patients. Interestingly, if the same model of prognostic factors is used for a surgically staged cohort of patients with supra-diaphragmatic Hodgkin's disease (Table 9), employing data from the MD Anderson Hospital, the probability of having abdominal

Table 9 Probability of abdominal disease in patients with CS I and II Hodgkin's disease using observed results of MD Anderson Hospital staging information applied to the Princess Margaret Hospital multiparameter prognostic factor matrix[a]

| Age | Histology | Stage | | |
		IA	IIA	IB+IIB
<50	LP+NS MC+LD		Group I+II 97/325[b] (30%)	
≥50	LP+NS MC+LD			Group III 21/30 (70%)

LP, lymphocyte predominant; NS, nodular sclerosing; MC, mixed cellularity; LD, lymphocyte depleted.
[a] See text for details.
[b] Number of patients with a positive laparotomy; number of patients with CS I+II disease in prognostic group.
Data supplied by Dr F. Hagermeister, MD Anderson Hospital, Texas.

disease would be 30 per cent (97/325) for patients in groups 1 and 2 and 70 per cent (21/30) for patients in group 3. Thus, as noted in Tables 7 and 8, multiparameter models based upon clinically derived prognostic factors predict predominantly for the presence of clinically occult intra-abdominal disease and thereby predict the probability of a satisfactory level of disease control with radiation alone.

In the Princess Margaret Hospital (1968–1977) analysis, radiation field allocation was not standardized and, as a result, a recommendation was made for the use of mantle plus upper abdominal radiation fields to include the spleen and a prophylactic dose to the liver for all patients in group 2 and for a combined modality approach for patients in group 3. The results of this policy at a median follow-up of 4 years is shown in Table 10. The recurrence rate for patients in group 2 treated with radical radiation is 16 per cent and that for patients receiving combined modality therapy is 23 per cent, with an overall relapse rate of 18 per cent (Princess Margaret Hospital, unpublished results).

The purpose of the Princess Margaret Hospital approach was to establish that upper abdominal recurrence in patients with supradiaphragmatic CS I and II disease could be prevented by upper abdominal radiation without undue morbidity and that long-term freedom from progression rates similar to those obtained for PS I and II could be achieved with radiation alone on the basis of selection by clinical presentation parameters. To that end, the Princess Margaret Hospital experience would suggest that a freedom from progression rate of the order of 80 per cent can be obtained by selection according to pre-treatment clinical attributes and that this selection process identifies a favourable subgroup comprising approximately 70 per cent of the total CS I and II patient population.

What are the implications in terms of treatment allocation (radiation therapy, chemotherapy) inherent in decision-making by clinical or surgical pathological criteria?

Given the uncertainty regarding involvement of the abdomen in one-third of patients with supradiaphragmatic CS I and II disease, there has been concern that fewer patients receive curative radiation therapy and more receive chemotherapy, either *ab initio* or for salvage, when treatment decisions are made according to clinical staging criteria. This issue can be addressed from a theoretical and practical viewpoint as shown in Table 11.

Using established probabilities for distribution of pathological stages following laparotomy and for relapse-free rates following radiation therapy, it can be predicted that of 100 patients with CS I and II disease, approximately 68 will be cured with radiation

Table 10 Relapse rates for CS I and II supradiaphragmatic Hodgkin's disease according to a multiparameter clinical prognostic factor model[a] and therapy, 1982–1988

| Therapy | Prognostic group | | | Total |
	Group 1	Group 2	Group 3	
Radical irradiation	2/17[b] (12%)	29/183 (16%)	5/7 (70%)	36/207 (17%)
Chemotherapy and irradiation	—	18/79 (23%)	2/11 (18%)	20/90 (22%)
Total	2/17 (12%)	47/262 (18%)	7/18 (39%)	56/297 (19%)

[a] See text.
[b] Number with disease progression number treated.
Princess Margaret Hospital (unpublished results).

Table 11 Management of 100 patients with supradiaphragmatic CS I and II Hodgkin's disease

PS (following laparotomy)	Number	Primary therapy	Salvage chemotherapy (for relapse)
IA IIB	70	Radiation	14 (20%)
IIIA	20	Radiation	8 (40%)
IIIB IV	10	Chemotherapy	

Total requiring chemotherapy, 32 per cent.

therapy alone and 32 will require chemotherapy either for initial management or for relapse following radiation. The latter figure is probably conservative as it does not take bulky mediastinal presentation into account; it is likely that 10 per cent of patients with CS I and II would have bulky mediastinal disease and would be treated with a combined modality approach.

Based upon the 1968–1977 analysis at Princess Margaret Hospital, the relapse-free rate following radical irradiation for CS I and II disease was 64 per cent (Sutcliffe *et al.* 1985), a cure rate with irradiation not dissimilar to the theoretical 68 per cent derived above. For the more recent 1978–1986 period, representing current management strategy, the proportion of patients receiving chemotherapy as the primary combined modality or for salvage of radiation failure is 37 per cent of the total CS I and II cohort. This figure is compatible with the theoretical prediction and also with the value of 43 per cent observed in the H_5 EORTC trial (Tubiana *et al.* 1986).

Selection of patients for combined modality therapy

Selection criteria

In the previous section, the effectiveness of radiation therapy for patients with stage I and II Hodgkin's disease has been described. However, within stage I and II, subgroups of patients can be identified in whom the risk of relapse with radiation therapy alone is unacceptably high. The decision to advocate combined modality therapy or chemotherapy for such patients requires that some dimension be placed upon 'unacceptably high'. 'Acceptable' relapse-free rates ranging from 65 (Glatstein 1984) to 80 per cent (Tubiana *et al.* 1984c) have been quoted for radiation therapy alone. Some justification for these figures can also be derived from a realistic expectation of outcome with chemotherapy alone, a 95 per cent complete remission rate, and a 75 per cent relapse-free rate giving rise to a freedom from progression rate slightly in excess of 70 per cent. Therefore it would seem reasonable to advocate that a relapse risk in excess of 30 per cent with radiation alone would justify consideration of combined modality therapy or chemotherapy alone.

This proposition presupposes that freedom from disease progression with initial therapy is the goal of management and that any progression is considered unacceptable. This view must be tempered by the failure of initial combined modality therapy approaches to modify overall survival compared with the use of chemotherapy for salvage following disease progression after radiation therapy. Therefore the issue depends on a relapse-free rate considered 'acceptable' with radiation alone balanced against the morbidity of an initial approach using chemotherapy with or without irradiation (Horwich and Peckham 1987). The identification of patients with a high risk of relapse with radiation alone by clinical criteria at presentation allows the use of chemotherapy with the least additional morbidity. Several groups have formulated the definition of high-risk groups based upon multiparameter aggregation of independent adverse prognostic factors: age, histology, stage including symptoms, erythrocyte sedimentation rate, mediastinal mass, number of involved sites (Tubiana *et al.* 1984c, 1985, 1989; Haybittle *et al.* 1985; Sutcliffe *et al.* 1985; Brada *et al.* 1986). The approach to combined modality therapy for patients with infradiaphragmatic presentation and large mediastinal masses has been discussed in earlier sections.

Rationale for combined modality therapy

Studies employing combined modality therapy have uniformly demonstrated improved freedom from progression rates compared with radiation alone, although no survival advantage has been evident.

The apparent benefits of the addition of chemotherapy to radiation might include the following:

(1) increased cell kill within the irradiated volume;

(2) tumour volume reduction rendering certain patients eligible for radiation therapy through reduction/avoidance of radiation to critical normal structure, for example large mediastinal masses;

(3) elimination of subclinical disease beyond the tumoricidal radiation volume; that is, under shielding blocks, at field margins and in non-irradiated areas beyond the field.

There is no evidence for a synergistic effect of radiation and chemotherapy within the irradiated volume. Indeed, in-field control rates with irradiation alone exceed 95 per cent provided that correct dose and field size issues are observed (see earlier). It is most likely that the benefits of the addition of chemotherapy represent 'spatial collaboration' between the two therapies, with chemotherapy addressing the problem of subclinical disease in areas of insufficient radiation dose or in areas beyond the radiation field. It should be noted that the majority of prognostic factors are surrogates for more extensive subclinical disease and do not predict for the outcome of local disease treated by radiation therapy other than for disease bulk in the mediastinum. In this circumstance subclinical intrathoracic disease beyond the radiation portals is the most likely source of failure following radiation.

Issues in combined therapy

Treatment schedule

Most experience with combined modality therapy derives from initial radiotherapy followed by chemotherapy. However, much of the rationale for combined modality therapy favours the initial use of chemotherapy followed by radiation, that is, chemotherapy is used to reduce the tumour volume to facilitate radiation or for elimination of subclinical disease beyond the tumouricidal radiation volume. Thus in most circumstances where combined modality therapy is favoured on the basis of inadequate control rates with irradiation alone, chemotherapy is addressing adverse prognostic parameters that correlate largely with extent of subclinical disease. In addition to these pragmatic considerations, which cannot be validated in terms of survival, the toxicity of chemotherapy immediately following irradiation may be more substantial (Yarnold et al. 1982; Duchesne et al. 1983).

Number of cycles and chemotherapy regimen

The success of combination chemotherapy regimens in advanced Hodgkin's disease has derived from the use of a number of induction cycles (commonly six), followed by two additional cycles to consolidate complete remission. The application of fewer cycles of chemotherapy when used in combination with radiation for lesser stages of disease has been adopted largely in the belief that chemotherapy of less duration or intensity is satisfactory for control of subclinical disease, for example occult intra-abdominal disease in patients with stage I and II disease or subclinical intrathoracic disease in patients with large mediastinal masses, pulmonary hilar, or extranodal extensions of disease. There is no direct proof that this hypothesis is correct. In practice, the use of fewer cycles of chemotherapy with radiation in patients with stage I and II disease has resulted in excellent relapse-free and overall survival rates (Hagermeister et al. 1981; Ferma et al. 1984; Zittoun et al. 1985). However, the use of fewer cycles of chemotherapy must also be considered in terms of the extent of radiation fields given, since most of the benefit accruing from chemotherapy is derived from control of disease beyond the radiation field.

The use of fewer cycles of chemotherapy in patients with early stage disease is also supported by the wish to reduce chemotherapy-related morbidity, particularly the impact upon gonadal function and induction of second malignancy. With two cycles of the MOPP regimen, a lesser impact upon the male germinal epithelium has been noted (da Cunha et al. 1983). The impact of a planned reduction in the number of cycles of MOPP on second malignancy rates is unclear; however, a recent retrospective study suggests a relationship between the cumulative amount of alkylating agent exposure and leukaemogenesis (Kaldor et al. 1990).

Although the ABVD regimen has a much lesser impact upon gonadal function (Viviani et al. 1985) and leukaemogenesis (Valagussa et al. 1986) and has been shown to be highly effective with radiation in a combined modality approach in early stages of disease (Santoro et al. 1987), the wish to avoid acute morbidity has stimulated interest in alternative regimens designed to minimize both short- and long-term side-effects. The VBM regimen (vinblastine, bleomycin, and methotrexate) in combination with radiation has been demonstrated to produce control rates in favourable Hodgkin's disease (PS I, IIA, and IIIA) that are the equivalent in historical comparison with MOPP and radiation (Horning et al. 1988). A modification of the ABVD regimen, EBVP (epirubicin, bleomycin, vinblastine, and prednisone), has been used in combined modality management of patients with stage I and IIIA disease with preliminary indications of its effectiveness (Zittoun et al. 1987).

Extent and dose of irradiation

The use of extended fields has clearly been shown to be appropriate for optimal control of localized Hodgkin's disease by irradiation alone. The addition of chemotherapy to involved field radiation has established relapse-free rates equivalent (Hoppe et al. 1982) or superior (Coltman et al. 1982) to extended field irradiation. Control rates with extended field radiation and chemotherapy have generally established superior relapse-free rates compared with radiation alone (see next section); however, recent studies indicate that involved field techniques as part of combined modality therapy provide equivalent benefit to extended field techniques (Horning et al. 1988).

Results of combined modality therapy for stage I and II disease

Several randomized and non-randomized studies indicate the superiority of combined modality therapy compared with irradiation alone in terms of relapse-free survival. However, there is uniform agreement that neither approach confers an overall survival advantage. In randomized studies in patients with PS I and II disease, quoted relapse-free survival rates for patients treated with extended field radiation alone range from 68 to 89 per cent compared with 81–94 per cent for the combined modality approach (Wiernik et al. 1979; Coltman et al. 1982; Hoppe et al. 1982; Hagermeister et al. 1982; Nissen and Nordentoft 1982; Anderson et al. 1984). It should be noted in these reports that randomization between treatment allocation was by stage alone and not by other prognostic factors, except for the exclusion of patients with massive mediastinal disease, advanced age, or compromised medical fitness for whom staging laparotomy was contraindicated. In the Stanford randomized study, which failed to define relapse-free survival advantage for those receiving combined modality treatment, a clear relapse-free survival difference was available for the subpopulation with bulky mediastinal disease; 45 versus 81 per cent with combined modality therapy (Hoppe et al. 1982). Non-randomized studies have been in accord with the above results, for example disease-free survival rates of 84 per cent at 10 years (Lagarde et al. 1988) and 85 per cent at 5 years (Baysogolov and Shakhtarina 1987).

In patients with unfavourable presentation of clinically localized disease, relapse-free survival rates of 76 versus 87 per cent were obtained with total-nodal irradiation and combined modality therapy (TNI+MOPP) in the EORTC H_5 study (Tubiana et al. 1984c; Carde et al. 1988, 1993). The unfavourable subgroup of PS I and II disease at MD Anderson Hospital (large mediastinal mass, any mediastinal disease with hilar adenopathy, B symptoms, large pelvic or abdominal disease) have a freedom from progression rate of 78 per cent at 4 years, with two cycles of MOPP therapy and radiation, a result equivalent to that achieved with radiation alone for favourable PS I and II disease (Hagermeister 1988).

In summary, no overall survival advantage accrues from combined modality therapy for stage I and II disease. Combined modality therapy results in higher relapse-free rates compared with radiation alone for unselected patients with stage I and II disease (Nissen and Nordentoft 1982; Anderson et al. 1990). However, with optimal selection with stage I and II according to multiple prognostic parameters, the incremental gain in relapse-free rate for combined modality therapy relative to radiation therapy must be balanced against the acute and long-term side-effects of combined therapy. A significant advantage in relapse-free rate exists for the subset with unfavourable presentation of localized disease. For this subgroup, the principal question now is the choice of optimal chemotherapy regimen and treatment schedule to achieve highest control rates with minimum morbidity.

The impressive results of combination chemotherapy for advanced and recurrent Hodgkin's disease have raised the issue of using chemotherapy alone for patients with localized disease. The initial reports reflect selection preference for chemotherapy by virtue of limited access to radiation therapy, incidental medical problems, and patient preference and are limited to a small number of patients treated. In four studies, high complete remission rates are reported with relapse rates of 8–30 per cent (Ziegler *et al.* 1972; Olweny *et al.* 1978; Lauria *et al.* 1979; Bubman *et al.* 1986). The experience of Colonna and Andrieu (1985) in a series of 21 patients in Algeria was less favourable; a complete remission rate of approximately 45 per cent and a relapse rate of 20 per cent. In this report, patients were clinically staged and a high proportion (75 per cent) were symptomatic, suggesting a cohort with an adverse prognosis.

Three studies have addressed random allocation of patients (IB and IIIA, O'Dwyer *et al.* (1985); I and II, Pavlovsky *et al.* (1988); I and IIA, Cimino *et al.* (1989)) to chemotherapy or combined modality or radiation alone. In the Grupo Argentino de Tratamiento de la Leucemia Agudo (GATLA) study, patients with clinical stage I and II disease were randomized between CVPP (cyclophosphamide, vinblastine, procarbazine, and prednisone) and CVPP plus involved field radiation. No survival difference was noted. There was a significant difference in disease-free survival between the two arms in favour of CVPP plus radiation (62 versus 71 per cent at 5 years). In the favourable group (below 45 years, no more than two nodal areas, no bulky disease), no difference in survival or disease-free survival was apparent at 84 months of follow-up. Patients in the unfavourable subgroup had improved disease-free survival (75 versus 34 per cent) and overall survival (84 versus 66 per cent) when treated with combined modality therapy (Pavlovsky *et al.* 1988). No difference in survival or relapse-free rate is apparent in the randomized study comparing chemotherapy alone with radiotherapy or combined modality therapy in patients with IB and IIIA disease (O'Dwyer *et al.* 1985; Longo *et al.* 1987). Cimino *et al.* (1989) reported no difference in overall survival and disease-free survival for patients with PS I and IIA disease randomized between MOPP chemotherapy and extended field radiotherapy at a median follow-up of 60 months. An inferior, albeit not statistically significant, actuarial survival probability was noted for patients relapsing after MOPP (45 per cent) compared with relapse following radiation (76 per cent).

These studies clearly indicate the effectiveness of chemotherapy in early stage Hodgkin's disease. For selected populations, unavailability of radiation therapy, paediatric patients, limited access to reliable staging methods, unsuitability for radical wide-field irradiation, chemotherapy alone provides an effective alternative. For those with unfavourable localized disease, the GATLA study would suggest the superiority of combined modality therapy compared with chemotherapy alone. For the majority of adult patients with favourable localized disease there is, as yet, no strong indication to withdraw from appropriate staging and radiation therapy until such time as equally effective systemic therapy with lesser acute and long-term side-effects than radiation therapy is available.

MANAGEMENT OF STAGE IIIA DISEASE

Stage IIIA according to the Ann Arbor Classification describes asymptomatic nodal disease on both sides of the diaphragm. Involvement of the spleen (S+) and disease extension contiguous with lymph nodes (E lesion) are both encompassed within Stage IIIA. Historically, the localization of disease to lymph node sites has favoured the use of irradiation as primary therapy. In practice, however, relapse-free survival rates following radiation therapy vary from 88 to 32 per cent. Such variability necessitates a re-examination of the stage IIIA concept, particularly with respect to prognostic factors for localized disease (see previous section) and also for heterogeneity of anatomical distribution of disease within the abdomen. In principle, it is necessary to resolve 'what amount and distribution of disease in stage IIIA can be satisfactorily treated with radiation alone and what presentations necessitate the use of chemotherapy or combined modality therapy'.

The first factor in selection is the distinction of pathological versus clinical stage IIIA disease. Non-invasive evaluation of the spleen is highly unreliable; palpability and size bear a poor correlation with histological involvement until such time as the spleen exceeds 500 g; that is, approximately three to four times normal size. Whilst CT has expanded the evaluation and interpretation of the upper abdomen, the definition of splenic nodules or liver deposits is relatively rare. As with the spleen, enlargement of the lymph nodes may be associated with reactive changes rather than involvement by Hodgkin's disease. Lymphography provides a reliable interpretation of retroperitoneal and pelvic adenopathy from the external iliac to superior mesenteric artery level (approximately the level of the interspace of the first and second lumbar vertebrae). Opacification of retroperitoneal lymph nodes above this level is variable or does not occur with pedal dye injection, thus coeliac axis, peripancreatic, splenic hilar, porta hepatic, and mesenteric nodes cannot be evaluated by lymphography. In practice, therefore, an accurate evaluation of the upper abdomen by staging laparotomy with splenectomy is required.

The issue of upper abdominal versus lower abdominal disease has been approached by Desser *et al.* (1977). Following staging laparotomy and splenectomy, patients were subclassified according to PS $IIIA_1$ (disease above the superior mesenteric artery (splenic, splenic hilar, coeliac, and porta hepatis)) and PS $IIIA_2$ (involvement of para-aortic, pelvic, and mesenteric nodes). A further distinction, PS $IIIA_3$ (pelvic disease), has been reported by the MD Anderson group (Hagermeister and Fuller 1988).

The subclassification of abdominal disease by Desser *et al.* (1977) has been expanded by consideration of the extent of splenic involvement. Patients with extensive splenic involvement, usually defined as the least five gross splenic nodules, clearly have an inferior prognosis following radiation alone (Hoppe *et al.* 1982; Stein *et al.* 1982). In addition, those with extensive splenic involvement and intra-abdominal lymphadenopathy have very low relapse-free survival rates with radiation (Levi and Wiernik 1977; Stein *et al.* 1982). The particular significance of splenic disease appears to be its predictive role for failure beyond the radiation field; that is, in the unirradiated pelvis in the series of Tubiana *et al.* (1981) and in extralymphatic sites in other series (Prosnitz *et al.* 1978; Mauch *et al.* 1979; Hoppe *et al.* 1982; Stein *et al.* 1982). The correlation of extensive splenic disease and liver disease has also been noted.

Bearing these issues in mind, the following points can be considered.

1. Radiation alone for CS IIIA disease; relapse-free survival rates of 15–71 per cent have been quoted using total-body irradiation—while 15 per cent (Prosnitz *et al.* 1978), 36 per cent (Peckham *et al.* 1975), 37 per cent (unpublished results; Princess Margaret Hospital, 1984), and 71 per cent (BNLI 1976) have been reported using total nodal irradiation;

2. Radiation alone for PS IIIA disease; relapse-free survival rates of 40 per cent (Hellman and Mauch 1982), 57 per cent (Hoppe *et al.* 1982), 77 per cent (Peckham *et al.* 1975), 77.5 per cent (BNLI 1976), and 74 per cent (Timothy *et al.* 1980);

3. Radiation alone for PS IIIA$_1$ disease; relapse-free survival rates of 50 per cent (Prosnitz *et al.* 1978), 53 per cent (Hellman and Mauch 1982), 59 per cent (Hoppe *et al.* 1982), 60 per cent (Stein *et al.* 1982), and 75 per cent (Timothy *et al.* 1980);

4. Radiation alone for PS IIIA$_2$ disease; relapse-free survival rates of 14 per cent (Hellman and Mauch 1982), 19 per cent (Stein *et al.* 1982), 25 per cent (Prosnitz *et al.* 1978), 63 per cent (Hoppe *et al.* 1982), and 75 per cent (Timothy *et al.* 1980);

5. Radiation alone for PS IIIA disease with extensive splenic involvement; relapse-free survival rates of 36 per cent (Hoppe *et al.* 1982), 41 per cent (Stein *et al.* 1982), and 7 per cent for patients with PS IIIA$_2$ disease with extensive splenic involvement (Stein *et al.* 1982).

Given these results with radiation alone, it is logical to question whether superior results would be achieved with combination chemotherapy. As in the discussion with stage I and II disease, the issue is not one of overall survival, given that survival rates are equivalent whether one uses chemotherapy as initial therapy or for management of relapse following radiation, but rather the greatest therapeutic gain with the least amount of therapy and the least toxicity.

Following chemotherapy, with or without irradiation, for stage IIIA disease, relapse-free survival rates of 53–100 per cent have been quoted. For patients with PS IIIA disease, relapse-free survival rates commonly exceed 75 per cent (Hoppe *et al.* 1982; Stein *et al.* 1982; Crowther *et al.* 1984; Hagermeister and Fuller 1988). The series from the MD Anderson group is notable in that the chemotherapy comprised two cycles of MOPP followed by sequential irradiation to mantle, upper abdominal, and pelvic fields (Hagermeister and Fuller 1988). No additional benefit of routine radiation to previous areas of disease following definitive chemotherapy (six cycles of MVPP) was defined in the Manchester series where both patient groups (MVPP alone versus MVPP and radiation therapy) had comparable survival (85 per cent) and relapse-free survival (80 per cent) rates at 5 years (Crowther *et al.* 1984).

The question of superiority of total-nodal irradiation versus chemotherapy for stage IIIA disease has been addressed in one randomized study. Superiority of radiation therapy was demonstrated, but was largely based upon a low complete remission rate in the chemotherapy group. Relapse rates were equivalent (BNLI 1976). In practice, it is no longer appropriate to consider optimal management of patients with stage IIIA disease in the context of randomization to irradiation or chemotherapy. Subsequent examination of patterns of failure after radiation therapy in clinically and pathologically staged patients has defined a host of factors to interpret the heterogeneity of outcome and these should be considered in the allocation of preferred therapy. These factors are summarized in Table 12.

Table 12 Factors influencing treatment allocation in stage IIIA Hodgkin's disease

Radiation therapy	Chemotherapy
Favourable prognostic factors	Unfavourable prognostic factors
PS IIIA	CS IIIA
PS IIIA$_1$	PS IIIA$_2$
Minimal splenic involvement	Extensive splenic involvement

ACUTE AND DELAYED SIDE-EFFECTS OF RADIATION

Radiation produces its beneficial effects by energy deposition within the malignant cell with subsequent destruction of the cell's ability to divide and proliferate. For tumour control, a dose–response relationship exists whereby a certain probability of local tumour sterilization will accrue provided that a certain minimum dose is achieved. In principle, it matters little how quickly this dose is achieved in the tumour; however, it matters considerably how this dose is achieved in surrounding normal tissues within the tumour volume. The 'breaking up' of the required total dose into daily treatments that permit continued viability and function of normal tissues is known as 'fractionation'; the total dose and fractionation bear a clear relationship to tumour control and normal tissue 'tolerance'. Even with radiation schedules that are within tissue tolerance, acute, predominantly epithelial, injury may occur. Such injury is generally either reversible or manageable without organ compromise. When tissue tolerances are exceeded, irreversible acute and delayed side-effects may be anticipated.

Acute side-effects

Acute side-effects include clinical features occurring concurrently or within 6–8 weeks of completion of radiation therapy and mainly involve tissues with a high cell-renewal fraction.

The majority of patients note fatigue and lassitude as a major accompaniment of therapy. Nausea is common and may require control with appropriate medication. The combination of anorexia, nausea, and emesis contribute to fatigue and not uncommonly result in weight loss of 2–7 kg during and shortly after therapy. Attention to rest, avoidance of stress, minimization of travelling, antinauseant medication, nutrition, and hydration is important.

A further contributor to the anorexia–weight loss syndrome is dysphagia, mucositis, altered taste perception, and xerostomia. The upper border of the mantle radiation field abuts on the floor of the oral cavity and encompasses the submandibular, sublingual, a portion of the parotid, and the minor salivary glands in the oral mucosa of the floor of the mouth. During radiation, taste perception is altered and saliva becomes thick and viscid. The resulting salivary gland dysfunction may remain for many months as manageable xerostomia. This has implications for dental health; dental hygiene and more frequent dental supervision are required to avoid accelerated dental caries. The common practice of applying posterior cervical spinal cord shields during therapy to minimize l'Hermitte's syndrome also serves to reduce the severity of the oesophageal reaction. Laryngeal mucositis is often perceived as a mild change of voice character with excessive 'clearing of the throat'. Whilst this may be minimized with anterior larynx shielding during therapy, it is important that the radiation dose to adjacent adenopathy is not compromised given that the laryngeal reaction to full dose mantle therapy is without significant long-term effect.

The use of megavoltage irradiation results in 'skin sparing' unless the build-up characteristics of the radiation are altered by external material applied to the skin ('bolus') to achieve dose homogeneity. Therefore, skin reaction is usually minimal and most commonly confined to the lateral aspects of the neck and the axillae. Mild erythema with subsequent mild hyperpigmentation and dry desquamation are all that should be expected, given no surface-applied bolus. Skin care during irradiation is important with avoidance of abrasion, wet shaving, topically applied perfumes, or scented deodorants. Patients should be encouraged to use mild soap with gentle towel drying. Sun exposure to the irradiated area should be avoided during therapy and for 3–4 months therafter. Beard hair and occipital hair up to the superior nuchal line (that is, within the irradiation field), are lost during therapy and grow back 2–3 months later. Fatigue, anorexia, nausea, emesis, and weight loss are common with infradiaphragmatic irradiation, as with supradiaphragmatic irradiation. The principal additional side-effect is gastrointestinal in the form of transient borborygmi, flatulence, 'cramps', and diarrhoea. During abdominal irradiation, the mucosal lining of the small bowel is dysfunctional; the bowel symptoms may be alleviated by avoidance of milk or milk products to minimize lactose intolerance and by the use of agents to reduce bowel motility.

Although mantle irradiation will cause cellular depletion of bone-marrow within the irradiation field, redistribution of haemopoiesis and continued function of non-irradiated marrow ensure that there is little impairment of peripheral blood counts. It is rare to require any haematopoietic support or delay in therapy due to blood count suppression. Subsequent upper abdominal fields or, more significantly, total-nodal irradiation results in more blood count suppression. Prior chemotherapy clearly influences haemological tolerance to radiation and may necessitate haemopoietic support or treatment modifications.

Fortunately, the dose fractionation scheme for control of Hodgkin's disease by irradiation is such that acute side-effects are virtually always manageable on an out-patient basis and do not result in long-term tissue injury.

Delayed side-effects

Delayed radiation effects occur months to years after therapy and are characterized by tissue or organ dysfunction caused by non-repairable injury to slowly proliferating tissue cells or the impairment of the tissue stroma with reduced vascularity. Such injury is usually permanent.

Mantle field irradiation necessitates that certain parts of the lung parenchyma are taken to levels exceeding tolerance. The areas affected are the lung apices and the paramediastinal lung. Lung morbidity is rarely clinically important, although it may be manifest as a dry irritating cough. Less commonly and only when larger volumes of lung are irradiated or lung tolerance is modified by pre-existing conditions or the use of chemotherapy prior or concurrent with irradiation (commonly bleomycin or adriamycin), does clinical dyspnoea and reduced exercise tolerance result. However, the impact of lung irradiation is commonly seen on chest radiographs as apical and paramediastinal fibrosis. Radiation fields that cover the spleen will also result in fibrosis of that portion of the left lower lobe within the irradiation field.

l'Hermitte's phenomenon, a 'tingling' or electric-shock-like sensation with neck flexion, occurs in a minority of patients with mantle field irradiation. It is presumed to be due to a transient demyelination following oligodendrocyte injury in the spinal cord. It commonly occurs 2–4 months after mantle field irradiation and

may last up to 9 months post-therapy. Posterior cervical cord shielding may be used to minimize the incidence of l'Hermitte's phenomenon. The doses used to control Hodgkin's disease are within spinal cord tolerance; however, assiduous attention to detail is required when field functions are constructed to avoid overlap of radiation dose from adjacent radiation fields over the spinal cord.

Delayed bowel complications are unusual. Prior laparotomy is recognized to predispose to adhesions and a small reoperation rate for relief of obstruction. Peptic ulceration is uncommon and has been recorded less commonly in those receiving radiation based upon clinical as opposed to pathological stage (Hayat 1984).

Cardiac damage is rare with mantle field irradiation provided that the technique respects dose, dose distribution, fractionation, and the volume of heart irradiated. The important issues are as follows:

(1) avoidance of low energy megavoltage equipment at short SSD;

(2) the use of equally weighted anterior and posterior fields;

(3) treating both anterior and posterior fields daily to achieve a midplane dose based upon a daily fraction size of 175 cGy;

(4) establishing a homogeneous dose distribution without significant 'hot spots' in vital tissues;

(5) restricting the volume of heart irradiated to the full tumour dose.

Radiation injury to the heart is most commonly manifest as a pericarditis and/or effusion (Stewart and Fajardo 1971; Kagan et al. 1972). This may progress to constrictive pericarditis requiring pericardiectomy. Myocardial fibrosis may also occur (Fajardo et al. 1968; Ruckdeschel et al. 1975; Kaplan 1980). A more recent concern, though less well documented, is the potential impact of mantle irradiation upon coronary artery integrity, given that long-term survivors following modern mantle irradiation are now accumulating in large numbers and reports of ischaemic heart disease are appearing.

Renal injury due to irradiation should not occur other than in the circumstances of planned upper abdominal irradiation in clinically staged patients. The upper third or half of the left kidney will be irradiated to above-tolerance levels in this circumstance. This will be apparent on renal imaging but is without impact upon biochemical function and blood pressure (LeBourgeois et al. 1979).

In the adult, no impact of radiation upon skeletal growth or function is apparent. This contrasts with the situation in childhood where growth and symmetry are important considerations in the choice and design of radiation fields. Osteonecrosis of the femoral heads is estimated to occur in approximately 2 per cent of patients treated for Hodgkin's disease (Sweet et al. 1976; Timothy et al. 1978b; Mould and Adam 1983). It may also involve the humeral heads. Radiological changes occur 6–24 months prior to the onset of symptoms. More recently, MRI has proved effective in imaging the early changes of osteonecrosis. The relationship of chemotherapy, steroids, radiation, and mechanical stress to the incidence and severity of osteonecrosis of the femoral head is unclear.

Radiation may have profound effects upon gonadal function (Sutcliffe 1987). The effects are dose dependent and the principal determinant, for both males and females, is the distance of the gonad from the edge of the therapeutic radiation field (Fig. 11). Other factors (for example, beam energy and treatment volume) are relevant but of lesser significance. In both sexes, the distance from the mantle field border to the gonad is such that the scatter dose is of the order of 1 per cent of the tumour dose; that is, 35 cGy delivered over 20 treatment days. This dose is of no significance

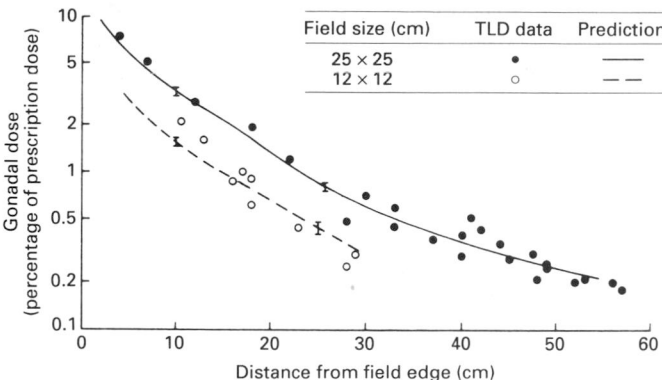

Fig. 11 Comparison of the scatter dose to the unshielded testes obtained with thermoluminescent dosimeters (TLDs) on patients (open and closed circles) and prediction from mock human phantoms (full and with broken lines). Data apply to opposed field treatment with 6 meV photons at a depth of 0.25 cm below the skin surface. (Reproduced from Shapiro *et al.* 1985, with permission.)

in terms of germinal epithelial or hormonal dysfunction of testes or ovary. Abdominal radiation fields pose much greater concern owing to the proximity to the gonad. Upper abdominal fields with a lower border at the level of the fourth lumbar vertebra result in a scatter dose of 4–5 per cent to the ovary; that is, 130–150 cGy over 20 treatments. This dose has little impact upon cyclic ovarian function. The testis dose in this circumstance is in the 2 per cent range (that is, 70 cGy in 20 treatments), which could result in transient oligospermia without long-term treatment sequelae. Pelvic radiation, inverted Y field, or total-nodal irradiation would result in exposure of the ovary to the full tumour dose with consequent radiation-induced ovarian ablation in the pre-menopausal patient. This situation can be resolved only by avoidance of radiation or by relocation of the ovaries. Transposition oophoropexy to the midline position behind the cervix with full shielding (anterior and posterior) will reduce the dose to the ovary to 550–1000 cGY over 20 treatments. This is compatible with continuing cyclical function at the lower end of the range, but is more likely to induce artificial menopause in the range above 800 cGy (Ray *et al.* 1970; Thomas *et al.* 1976). Relocation of the ovaries to a lateral position on the iliac crests or the lateral abdominal wall may result in a reduction of ovarian dose by a factor of three to four compared with central translocation (Sharma *et al.* 1981). Clearly, oophoropexy, in terms of requirement and site, is a subject that requires the input of patient, radiotherapist, and gynaecologist if the most privileged site with respect to the radiation beam is to be achieved. Loss of cyclic ovarian function due to therapy results in infertility and artificial menopause, a situation that should be corrected in the pre-menopausal woman by exogenous hormonal replacement therapy, unless medically contraindicated, not only to correct the functional and psychological sequelae of hormonal deprivation but also to protect against the long-term risks of excessive bone demineralization and premature atherosclerosis.

Inverted Y radiation in the male may result in a testis dose from 5 to 100 per cent of the tumour dose depending on the geometrical relationship of the testis to the inguinofemoral limbs of the radiation field. Even a dose of 5 per cent of the tumour dose is significant in terms of transient azoospermia and any higher dose carries a distinct possibility of prolonged azoospermia. Doses to the testis in excess of 250 cGy over 20 treatments (7–8 per cent) may result in permanent loss of the germinal epithelium, although hormonal function will not be compromised. In the male, the use of such radiation fields must be accompanied by external testicular shielding and/or germ cell cryopreservation. The use of appropriately designed external scrotal shields can reduce the scatter dose to the testes by a factor of 50–75 per cent; that is, a shielded testicular dose of 50–100 cGy over 20 treatments. Whilst this dose may cause transient oligospermia, historical evidence would suggest that prolonged injury is unlikely (Sandeman 1966; Speiser *et al.* 1973; Hahn *et al.* 1976; Slanina *et al.* 1977).

Irradiation with the mantle field results in exposure of the thyroid gland to the full tumour dose. Estimates of thyroid dysfunction range from 17 to 64 per cent for compensated biochemical hypothyroidism and 4–25 per cent for clinical or biochemical hypothyroidism (Fuks *et al.* 1996; Slanina *et al.* 1977; Schimpff *et al.* 1980; Smith *et al.* 1981; Tamura *et al.* 1981). These ranges are 70–80 per cent and 8–27 per cent, respectively, for patients receiving both radiation and chemotherapy (Schimpff *et al.* 1980; Sutcliffe *et al.* 1981). Chemotherapy alone appears to have much less impact. The rôle of exogenous iodine-based imaging as a goitrogen predisposing to the relatively high level of thyroid dysfunction has been recognized. Although overt clinical hypothyroidism is uncommon, awareness of the high frequency of latent and compensated biochemical hypothyroidism and the concern of chronic stimulation of an irradiated gland by elevated thyroid-stimulating hormone (TSH) levels justifies regular surveillance of thyroid biochemistry and replacement therapy in the presence of sustained elevated TSH levels.

MANAGEMENT OF ADVANCED HODGKIN'S DISEASE

Chemotherapy of Hodgkin's disease represents one of the undisputed successes of modern cancer treatment. The administration of properly designed drug regimens, either alone or combined with radiotherapy, has dramatically changed the prognosis in the intermediate and advanced stages with an increase in the cure rate from 50 per cent in an era before effective systemic therapy to 80 per cent with current chemotherapeutic programmes (Fig. 9).

The central issues involving modern chemotherapy of Hodgkin's disease include the following:

(1) an optimal multidrug chemotherapy programme with or without alternating drug regimens;

(2) the rôle of chemotherapy in the management of early disease;

(3) the rôle of combined chemotherapy; radiotherapy in patients with advanced disease;

(4) the optimal salvage regimen after primary treatment failure including the place of high-dose chemotherapy with autologous stem cell transplantation;

(5) whether less aggressive, but equally effective, therapies can decrease the frequency or magnitude of treatment-related side-effects.

Optimal chemotherapy regimens

Nitrogen mustard as a single agent was reported to have activity in patients with advanced Hodgkin's disease in 1946. Subsequently, complete response rates for a number of single agents were defined: nitrogen mustard (13 per cent), cyclophosphamide (12 per cent), procarbazine (38 per cent), vincristine (36 per cent),

Table 13 MOPP and ABVD regimens

Combination	Dose (mg/m^2) and route	Days of treatment	Frequency
MOPP[a]			Q 28 D
Nitrogen mustard	6 IV	1 & 8	
Vincristine (Oncovin)	1.4 IV	1 & 8	
Procarbazine	100 orally	1–14	
Prednisolone[b]	40 orally	1–14	
ABVD			Q 28 D
Doxorubicin (Adriamycin)	25 IV	1 & 15	
Bleomycin	10 IV	1 & 15	
Vinblastine	6 IV	1 & 15	
Dacarbazine	375 IV	1 & 15	

Q, four times daily; D, days.

[a] MVPP, vinblastine (6 mg/m^2) is substituted for vincristine and the regimen is delivered Q 42 D; ChlVPP, chlorambucil (6 mg/m^2 orally, days 1–14) is substituted for nitrogen mustard and vinblastine (6 mg/m^2 for vincristine).

[b] On cycles 1, 4, and 7 (MOPP). Every cycle in MVPP.

vinblastine (30 per cent), and chlorambucil (16 per cent). A combination of two active agents, vinblastine and chlorambucil, resulted in a complete response rate of 63 per cent with a mean response duration of 7.5 months (Lacher and Durant 1965).

For the past two decades, the standard drug regimen has been the MOPP programme, as designed in United States or its British variant MVPP where vinblastine is substituted for vincristine (Table 13). Administered for as many cycles as required to achieve complete tumour remission plus two additional cycles as consolidation (minimum six cycles), both drug regimens yield a superimposable treatment outcome (Longo et al. 1986; Wagstaff et al. 1988). In particular, in advanced Hodgkin's disease (stages IIB, III, and IV) the overall complete remission rate ranges from 70 to 80 per cent and 60–65 per cent of initial complete responders remain alive and continuously relapse free for 20 or more years from starting chemotherapy.

Analysis of prognostic factors influencing remission rate, relapse rate, and survival have been performed by several investigators following the use of either MOPP or MOPP-like therapy (reviewed by Selby et al. 1987). Adverse factors include the following.

1. Any prior chemotherapy.

2. Age greater than 40 years.

3. Systemic symptoms.

4. Stage IV disease.

5. Tumour burden defined by either multiple extranodal sites of disease or gross disease in one or more anatomic regions, a factor predictive for local relapse.

6. Certain extranodal sites; liver and pleural involvement were adverse for survival in the National Cancer Institute series, whilst bone-marrow involvement was adverse in the Stanford analysis.

7. Total lymphocyte count (Wagstaff et al. 1988).

8. Dose intensity of chemotherapy regimen; identified in terms of delivered dose of nitrogen mustard or vincristine, dose and schedule deviation, and mean three-cycle rate of drug delivery and the doses of nitrogen mustard, vincristine, and procarbazine

administered. Dose intensity remains important but somewhat controversial and its interpretation is confounded by retrospective versus prospective evaluation, its independent contribution in relation to other prognostic variables, and the role of other factors such as bone-marrow tolerance, bone-marrow involvement, individual drug pharmacokinetics, and patient compliance. In addition, the comparable outcome with the MOPP and MVPP regimens, despite dissimilar dose intensity due to 4 versus 6 week cycles respectively, is difficult to reconcile. However, the reported analyses are consistent with the premise that optimal therapy involves administration of maximally tolerated drug doses within the scheduled time course of the regimen.

9. Performance status.

10. Serum lactate dehydrogenase.

Several investigators have addressed the role of maintenance therapy following achievement of complete remission. No significant benefit has been demonstrated following maintenance programmes incorporating intermittent administration of MOPP, BCNU, two-drug (vinblastine plus procarbazine) versus four-drug (MVPP), BCVPP (BCNU, cyclophosphamide, vinblastine, procarbazine, prednisone), or Bacillus Calmette–Guérin immunotherapy (Selby et al. 1987).

Various modifications to the MOPP regimen have been employed to test increased effectiveness and greater tolerance. These include substitution of vinblastine for vincristine to reduce neurotoxicity, substitution of BCNU, chlorambucil, or cyclophosphamide for nitrogen mustard, and alteration of cycle periodicity to 6 weeks to enhance haematological tolerance. The ChlVPP regimen, employing chlorambucil, vinblastine, procarbazine, and prednisolone, minimizes peripheral neuropathy, nausea and emesis, and marrow toxicity whilst maximizing compliance in an ambulatory setting (Dady et al. 1982; McKendrick et al. 1989). Additional agents, bleomycin and BCNU, have also been added to the basic four-drug regimen. With some allowances for case mix, there is general consensus that neither substitutions nor single drug additions to the basic four-drug regimen result in improved effectiveness. Such modifications enhance tolerance and reduce acute treatment-related side-effects although their impact upon gonadal function and subsequent second malignant tumours is similar.

The search for less toxic regimens to reduce sterility and the incidence of secondary myelodysplasia or acute myelogenous leukaemia prompted the design of ABVD (Table 13) at the Milan Cancer Institute. ABVD is composed of drugs not contained in the MOPP, MVPP, or ChlVPP programmes and has therefore provided an alternative combination programme for Hodgkin's disease resistant to the MOPP regimen (Bonadonna 1982; Santoro et al. 1982). Through prospective randomized trials, ABVD was found to be as effective as MOPP (if not superior in patients with systemic B symptoms) and non-cross-resistant to MOPP when used as a salvage programme. These clinical observations resulted in the decision to include ABVD in an alternating programme with MOPP (Table 14) first in the treatment of stage IV and subsequently in the management of stage IIB and IIX and stage IIIA and IIIB disease (Bonadonna 1982; Bonadonna et al. 1986; Santoro et al. 1986). Table 15 shows the consistency of findings related to the superiority of MOPP/ABVD delivered using different sequences (that is, MM/AA or hybrid monthly programme, that is, MA/MA) in stage IV Hodgkin's disease (Bonadonna et al. 1989). It is also important to point out that the same results were achieved by decreasing the

Table 14 MHPP hybrid combinations

ChlVPP/EVA (Manchester/Barts regimen)
Chlorambucil 10 mg/m² orally, days 1–7
Vinblastine 10 mg/m² IV, day 1
Procarbazine 150 mg/m² orally, days 1–7
Prednisolone 50 mg/m² orally, days 1–7
Vincristine 2 mg/m² IV, day 8
Doxorubicin 50 mg/m² IV, day 8
Etoposide 200 mg/m² IV, day 8

MA/MA (Milan regimen)
Nitrogen mustard 6 mg/m² IV, day 1
Vincristine (oncovin) 1.4 mg/m² IV, day 1
Procarbazine 100 mg/m² orally, days 1–7
Prednisone 40 mg/m², days 1–14
Doxorubicin 25 mg/m² IV, day 15
Bleomycin 10 mg/m² IV, day 15
Vinblastine 6 mg/m² IV, day 15
Dacarbazine 375 mg/m² IV, day 15
Repeat every 28–35 days

MOPP/ABV (Vancouver regimen)
Nitrogen mustard 6 mg/m², day 1
Vincristine (Oncovin) 1.4 mg/m², day 1
Procarbazine 100 mg/m², days 1–7
Prednisone 40 mg/m², days 1–14
Doxorubicin 35 mg/m², day 8
Vinblastine 6 mg/m², day 8
Bleomycin 10 mg/m², day 8
Repeat every 28 days

Table 15 Five year results with alternating and hybrid regimens in stage IV Hodgkin's disease

	First study		Second study	
	MOPP (43)	MOPP/ABVD (45)	MM/AA (28)	MA/MA (28)
Complete remission (%)	74	89	86	89
Freedom from progression (%)	40	66	66	71
Relapse-free survival (%)	50	74	73	75

From Bonadonna *et al.* (1989).

has shown an advantage for the Vancouver Hybrid (MOPP/ABVD) over six to eight cycles of MOPP followed by three cycles of ABVD. A study from the UK has confirmed the advantage of a doxorubicin-containing combination over MVPP (Radford *et al.* 1993). MVPP was compared with ChVPP/EVA hybrid therapy (Table 14) with patients in the hybrid arm and showed a better 5 year progression-free survival (80 versus 65 per cent, *p*=0.005). There was also a trend towards improved survival in the hybrid arm of the trial (80 versus 70 per cent at 5 years, *p*=0.13).

The rôle of combined chemotherapy and radiation is unclear in advanced Hodgkin's disease. The precedents for the use of adjuvant radiation therapy are to be found in the failure analysis of the MOPP data, wherein the majority of patients relapse in sites of previous disease and single sites of recurrence are present in 50 per cent of those in relapse. In addition, several single-arm studies of combined modality therapy purport to demonstrate both feasibility and effectiveness when compared with chemotherapy alone. To date, however, no randomized study has demonstrated a survival advantage for combined modality treatment for patients with advanced Hodgkin's disease (Rosenberg *et al.* 1978; Bloomfield *et al.* 1982).

The rôle of adjuvant radiation therapy, whilst controversial in relation to the MOPP regimen, will now require re-evaluation in the light of 'patterns of failure' analysis with doxorubicin-containing regimens and in the context of prospective randomized studies. However, radiation therapy appears indicated for areas of initial bulky lymphoma.

Salvage treatment after chemotherapy failure

Although the MOPP regimen or its variants yield complete remission rates of 60–80 per cent, 20–40 per cent of patients with advanced disease fail to remit with primary therapy and 30–40 per cent relapse from a state of remission. Thus, additional therapy is necessary for approximately 50 per cent of all patients with advanced disease.

Retreatment with MOPP or derivatives results in a second complete remission rate of approximately 50 per cent, with a median duration of second complete remission of 21 months and a median survival of greater than 60 months for remitters and 31 months for non-remitters (Fisher *et al.* 1979). In this series the most significant prognostic factor defining response and survival was the duration of first remission, with an adverse outcome being associated with a first remission duration of less than 12 months.

This standard treatment of recurrence was revised following the demonstration that a variety of agents other than those contained in the MOPP regimen had significant single-agent activity. Subsequently, new combination regimens have been devised and tested formally in the circumstance of primary induction failure or

number of treatment cycles from 12 to eight in the new prospective study. Thus, the administration of two equally effective and non-cross-resistant regimens has been shown to be superior to MOPP alone in stage IV Hodgkin's disease either in patients previously untreated or relapsing in extranodal sites after primary subtotal-nodal irradiation. In both alternating and hybrid programmes the total number of treatment cycles should comprise two cycles following achievement of complete remission (commonly six to eight cycles) delivered at full dose and schedule where possible.

Treatment with doxorubicin (adriamycin)-containing regimens were also successfully tested in advanced Hodgkin's disease by Canadian investigators (Klimo and Connors 1988) through the delivery of a hybrid regimen (Table 14) without dacarbazine (MOPP/ABV) to avoid or limit severe vomiting. The American cooperative group, Cancer and Acute Leukaemia Group B (CALGB) recently reported the results of a randomized controlled trial of MOPP, ABVD, and MOPP/ABVD (Canellos *et al.* 1992). This study concluded that ABVD therapy for 6–8 months was as effective as 12 months of MOPP/ABVD and that both were superior to MOPP alone. ABVD was less myelotoxic than MOPP or MOPP/ABVD. Although overall survival was not significantly different for the three regimens, complete remission and failure-free survival rates were significantly better for ABVD and MOPP/ABVD compared with MOPP (82, 83, and 67 per cent for complete response and 61, 65, and 50 per cent for failure-free survival, respectively). In the context of equivalent or superior efficacy of the ABVD regimen compared with MOPP-based regimens, the lesser gonadal toxicity and the apparent lack of increased risk of induction of acute myeloid leukaemia or myelodysplasia compared with MOPP, the ABVD regimen would appear to be the primary chemotherapy regimen for patients with previously untreated advanced Hodgkin's disease or disease recurrent after radiation therapy. Glick *et al.* (1991) reporting for the intergroup in the USA relapse following MOPP. This latter distinction has proved to be of prognostic importance: the outcome with alternative regimens is less satisfactory in patients who are primarily 'MOPP resistant' compared with those who progress following prior demonstration of 'MOPP-sensitive' disease.

Several regimens have proved 'non-cross-resistant' with remission rates of up to 60 per cent in patients with progressive disease following MOPP therapy (Canellos *et al.* 1987; Sutcliffe and Timothy 1987; Bonadonna *et al.* 1988). The most notable and most frequently used combination has been the ABVD regimen (Bonadonna 1982; Viviani *et al.* 1990).

Considerable heterogeneity exists in the reported response and survival parameters following second-line chemotherapy regimens. Much of this heterogeneity is attributable to differences in 'case mix' within various clinical reports. Important variables include age, performance status, response to prior chemotherapy, extent of previous chemotherapy, presence of symptoms, nodal versus extranodal disease progression, and number of extranodal sites. In the most favourable circumstance (patients initially sensitive to MOPP and relapsing later than 12 months after completing therapy) second-line regimens such as MOPP, ABVD, or hybrid/alternating programmes are associated with remission rates in excess of 60 per cent, of which more than 60 per cent appear durable (Viviani *et al.* 1990). However, in overall terms, second remission rates of 25–60 per cent with progression rates exceeding 50 per cent over a 2 year period following second-line therapy imply potential long-term survival rates of 10–30 per cent for this group of patients. Accordingly, considerable effort has been expended to define better salvage therapy, particularly for those patients who fail to remit or who relapse within a 1 year period following exposure to MOPP and doxorubicin-containing regimens either in sequence or in combination. For such patients high-dose chemotherapy with autologous bone-marrow rescue has now become the generally accepted salvage strategy (Canellos *et al.* 1988). The rationale underlying this approach is the use of dose intensification for tumour control with reversal of treatment-induced bone-marrow failure by reinfusion of autologous marrow obtained prior to high-dose therapy. Certain criteria require consideration with respect to eligibility and feasibility of high-dose chemotherapy.

1. Age: patients over 60 years of age have a higher complication rate.

2. Performance status: those with poor performance status or with significant cardiac, pulmonary, or renal dysfunction have a low tolerance to intensive approaches.

3. Chemosensitive disease: for the majority of patients there is demonstrable chemosensitivity despite failure to achieve complete remission or relapse following eight-drug therapy (MOPP/ABVD). The use of an alternative regimen to achieve disease control prior to high-dose chemotherapy is commonly used as the indicator of chemosensitivity. Those totally refractory to alternative chemotherapy are unlikely to benefit from high-dose chemotherapy. The early introduction of high-dose chemotherapy with autologous bone-marrow rescue into salvage management of high-risk patients is justified by the wish to exploit remaining chemosensitivity by avoiding undue exposure to multiple alternative regimens of limited efficacy and attendant risk of developing refractory disease.

4. Absence of bone-marrow involvement: clearly, reinfusion of 'involved' marrow is to be avoided. Fortunately, bone-marrow involvement is a relatively uncommon circumstance even in a patient population selected for salvage therapy.

5. Absence of significant treatment-induced organ system failure other than bone-marrow failure.

6. Viral carriers: HIV or hepatitis virus.

Chemotherapy to 'debulk' disease and establish chemosensitivity commonly precedes high-dose chemotherapy with autologous bone-marrow rescue. Complete remission before intensive therapy, although advantageous, is not essential for long-term survival.

Several regimens have been applied as high-dose chemotherapy, for example multiple agents such as cyclophosphamide, etoposide, BCNU and cytosine arabinoside (BACT) or melphalan combinations (BEAM), melphalan and etoposide, or melphalan as a single agent (reviewed by Canellos *et al.* 1988) or high-dose sequential chemotherapy as used at the Milan Cancer Institute (cyclophosphamide, methotrexate with leucovorin, etoposide, mitoxantrone, and melphalan). Local or locoregional radiation may also be employed to achieve tumour control before or following high dose chemotherapy, although many patients will be precluded due to previous therapeutic radiation exposure. For similar reasons, total-body irradiation is less commonly a component of the conditioning regimen and in reality there is little rationale for the incorporation of low-dose systemic radiation therapy into the conditioning protocol for patients with Hodgkin's disease.

In the past, high-dose chemotherapy with autologous marrow rescue carried an acute treatment-related mortality rate of 5–30 per cent, with early deaths being principally due to infection during the period of marrow aplasia or to poor performance of the engrafted marrow. Prolonged hospitalization (4–8 weeks in the absence of major complications), blood product support growth factor, and antibiotic and antifungal therapy are essential components of the procedure and total parenteral nutrition may be necessary depending upon the choice of conditioning regimen. Today the use of peripheral blood progenitor cell rescue with haemopoietic growth factors has reduced the risk of high-dose chemotherapy by augmenting neutrophil and platelet recovery and has resulted in a reduction in the period required in hospital compared with rescue using autologous bone-marrow (Siena *et al.* 1988; Gianni *et al.* 1989; Sheridan *et al.* 1992). This is a practical procedure for those centres where expertise and experience is available and a recent report has indicated that haemopoietic progenitor cells mobilized using a haemopoietic growth factor, collected from the blood using a single apheresis, can be used for successful reconstitution (Pettengell *et al.* 1993). The advantage of this approach is now well documented and peripheral blood progenitor cells transfusions are replacing the use of autologous bone-marrow rescue.

High-dose chemotherapy with autologous stem cell rescue results in a complete remission rate of approximately 50 per cent, an actuarial relapse-free survival rate of 40–80 per cent, and an overall actuarial survival rate of 35–70 per cent based on current series with median follow-up periods of 3 years or more (Carella *et al.* 1988; Gianni *et al.* 1989*a,b*; Gribben *et al.* 1989; Jagannath *et al.* 1989; Phillips *et al.* 1989). These results cannot be compared directly with those obtained using conventional salvage regimens since the patient population submitted to high-dose therapy with autologous stem cell rescue is a selected subgroup. Furthermore, the heterogeneity in reported results of high-dose therapy with autologous haemopoietic rescue reflects the increasing selection for this treatment through the definition of good-risk and poor-risk populations based upon prognostic factor analysis.

Several issues remain to be defined regarding optimization of high-dose therapy with rescue for patients with Hodgkin's disease:

(1) appropriate patient selection;

(2) optimum timing of high-dose therapy in the management of Hodgkin's disease;

(3) optimum high-dose chemotherapy regimen;

(4) the rôle of radiation;

(5) time sequence relationship of chemotherapy and radiation;

(6) rôle of peripheral blood progenitor cell rescue with one or more haemopoietic growth factors.

CHEMOTHERAPY SIDE-EFFECTS

The side-effects of chemotherapy are related to the individual drugs included in each combination. Vomiting may be frequent and protracted following ABVD and can be severe for a few hours following the mustine injection in the MOPP or MVPP combinations. Repeated episodes of vomiting may lead to anticipatory symptoms on entering the hospital environment or follow events which remind the patient about chemotherapy. In order to reduce the incidence of vomiting dacarbazine has been omitted from the hybrid regimen used by Canadian investigators and chlorambucil has been substituted for mustine in the ChlVPP regimen devised by British investigators. The latter regimen is practically devoid of vomiting. Fortunately, chemotherapy-induced emesis has been largely ameliorated through the use of 5-HT_3 (serotonin)-antagonist anti-emetics, for example ondansetron. The substitution of vinblastine for vincristine in the MVPP and ChlVPP regimens has almost eliminated the incidence of peripheral neuropathy, and these regimens are not usually associated with alopecia. Myelosuppression is more severe following the use of drug regimens containing alkylating agents and procarbazine compared with ABVD, but in most patients the fall in blood granulocyte and platelet counts is reversible within 2 weeks of the last dose of chemotherapy. If these counts are low at the time further therapy is due, it is preferable to delay chemotherapy for a few days rather than reduce the optimal dose of alkylating agent, vinblastine, or adriamycin. Growth factors, for example G-CSF, may be used to maintain peripheral white cell counts such that schedule deviation or dose reduction are avoided.

Late complications following intensive chemotherapy have become more evident as greater numbers of patients are followed in the clinic for longer periods of time. Drug therapy for Hodgkin's disease has been shown to be associated with cardiac, pulmonary, and gonadal dysfunction and an increase in the frequency of second malignancies. Some of these late side-effects are potentially life-threatening. Thus, although the benefits of modern chemotherapy outweigh the risks for the patient population as a whole, there is a continuing need to devise new more effective, yet less toxic, drug combinations and schedules.

Cardiac dysfunction

Of the various chemotherapeutic agents used in the treatment of Hodgkin's disease, the anthracyclines have the greatest potential for cardiotoxicity. The incidence of clinically apparent chronic cardiomyopathy is clearly dose related but is less than 2 per cent with cumulative doses of doxorubicin below 450 mg/m². The most important additional risk factor for the development of cardiomyopathy is prior mediastinal irradiation. However, none of the patients in Milan subjected to primary ABVD (cumulative dose of doxorubicin equal to 300 mg/m² in six cycles) followed by

radiotherapy revealed symptoms or signs of cardiomyopathy. The prognosis of symptomatic cardiomyopathy is poor with a mortality approaching 50 per cent. Cyclophosphamide when given in high dose associated with bone-marrow rescue may occasionally cause a fatal haemorrhagic myocarditis.

Pulmonary dysfunction

The drug with the greatest potential for pulmonary fibrosis is bleomycin. The toxicity is related to cumulative dose with an incidence of less than 5 per cent in patients receiving up to 200 mg/m² as in the ABVD or hybrid regimens. The incidence may be higher when ABVD is given following mediastinal irradiation. The clinical presentation includes dyspnoea, dry cough, low-grade fever, and basal crepitations with interstitial infiltrates seen on the chest radiograph. An open-lung biopsy may be required to distinguish bleomycin toxicity from other causes of interstitial pneumonia such as *Pneumocystis carinii*. Histological changes include interstitial and alveolar oedema with an acute inflammatory infiltrate and hyaline membrane formation in addition to the interstitial fibrosis suggestive of chronic toxicity. Apart from prompt discontinuation of bleomycin, there is no effective therapy known to minimize the extent of fibrosis. When a combined modality treatment approach is used, it is deemed advisable to administer chemotherapy before irradiation and the dose of irradiation should be lower than that required when radiotherapy is given alone as primary treatment.

Nitrosourea derivatives such as carmustine (BCNU) and lomustine (CCNU) have potential for dose-related pulmonary fibrosis particularly when high doses are used in intensive regimens, but the frequency of this complication at the dosage normally utilized in the regimens for Hodgkin's disease is very low (less than 2 per cent).

Skeletal complications

Avascular necrosis of bone is an uncommon complication of chemotherapy involving steroids. The cumulative incidence ranges from 1.5 to 3 per cent, and symptoms may appear from 8 to 70 months after initiation of therapy. The risk is increased in patients who have previously received irradiation to the site of the affected bone. Avascular necrosis most commonly occurs in the femoral head, but the humeral head may be affected. The complication is bilateral in more than half the cases. Radionuclide bone scans may be helpful in diagnosing avascular necrosis in the presence of a normal plain radiograph. MRI is the most definitive investigation yielding the earliest and most discriminating diagnostic information. Bony changes may remain stable or progress to the point of extensive osseous destruction with oesteoarthritis and bony collapse. Approximately half the patients will require surgery for joint replacement.

Gonadal and sexual dysfunction

Preservation of normal reproductive function has become an important goal in the modern treatment of Hodgkin's disease since many patients are young and the potential for cure is high. Defects in spermatogenesis have been documented in approximately one-third of males with Hodgkin's disease prior to chemotherapy, particularly in advanced stages and in the presence of systemic symptoms. This raises questions concerning the advantage of semen cryopreservation (Vigersky *et al.* 1982; Bookman and Longo 1986), although this has been of value for some patients. Numerous studies have documented that the prolonged administration of alkylating agents, procarbazine, or nitrosourea derivatives, particularly in combination, have profound effects on spermatogenesis and ovarian function (Whitehead *et al.* 1982, 1983; Viviani *et al.* 1985; Waxman *et al.* 1987). Azoospermia or severe oligospermia occurs in almost all male patients treated with MOPP, MVPP, or ChlVPP. Recovery of spermatogenesis may occur in 10–20 per cent of patients, but is usually partial and may be delayed up to 10 years or more. Recovery is greater in patients less than 30 years old and is inversely related to the duration and total dose of chemotherapy. Testicular biopsy shows atrophy, while levels of follicle-stimulating hormone (FSH) and luteinizing hormone (LH) are increased in the serum.

Sterility is less common in adult females than in males, probably because the germ cell proliferation rate is low in the ovary and the organ is less sensitive to cytotoxic drugs than the testis. The incidence of prolonged amenorrhoea, indicating premature ovarian failure, is dependent upon the age of the patient at the time of treatment, with an incidence of approximately 20 per cent for patients less than 30 years old compared with approximately 85 per cent after the age of 30 years. Ovarian failure is progressive from 1 to 10 years after chemotherapy and may be associated with an early menopause. Re-establishment of menstruation and the possibility of pregnancy in a treated woman is also related to age and cumulative drug exposure. However, pregnancy may occur even in the presence of partial ovarian failure characterized by high serum gonadotrophin and low serum oestradiol levels. The administration of oestrogen and progesterone during chemotherapy does not protect from drug-induced ovarian failure, but hormone replacement therapy is of definite benefit in the symptomatic patient with premature ovarian failure following chemotherapy (Whitehead *et al.* 1983). The administration of a gonadotrophin-releasing hormone analogue, such as buserelin, is also ineffective in conserving fertility in both sexes (Waxman *et al.* 1987). Despite its limitations, sperm storage before chemotherapy is started remains important in retaining the possibility of a male patient fathering a child.

Regimens which do not contain alkylating agents, procarbazine, or nitrosourea derivatives, such as ABVD, produce only transient impairment of spermatogenesis and ovarian function. These regimens are preferred in patients who wish to preserve fertility. When MOPP is alternated with ABVD the recovery of spermatogenesis is approximately 50 per cent.

Libido tends to decrease after both the diagnosis of Hodgkin's disease and treatment with chemotherapy, regardless of the drug combination used. Although decreased libido and sexual activity are common during intensive chemotherapy, these return to normal in the majority of patients after completion of treatment. Before starting chemotherapy, advice should be given to patients concerning possible changes in sexual behaviour during treatment and the high incidence of permanent infertility following treatment (Whitehead *et al.* 1982).

Second malignancy

One of the most serious consequences of successful curative therapy for Hodgkin's disease is the emergence of second malignancies, many of which are fatal. Most common among these are acute myeloid leukaemia, myelodysplastic syndromes, and diffuse high grade lymphoma. In patients treated with MOPP, MVPP, ChlVPP, or other drug combinations containing alkylating agents, procarbazine, or nitrosourea derivates, the risk of developing acute myeloid leukaemia within 10 years is 1.4–11.5 per cent (Table 16).

Table 16 Frequency of secondary leukaemia at 10–15 years in three major series with Hodgkin's disease

Research centre	Total patients	Radiotherapy alone (%)	Chemotherapy alone (%)	MOPP +RT (%)	Salvage MOPP (%)
National Cancer Institute, USA	473	0	2.0	6.0	9.0
Stanford University, USA	1507	0.6	11.5	4.9	1.8
Milan Cancer Institute	1329	0	1.4	9.5	17.7

RT, radiotherapy.

The risk is increased in patients more than 40 years old at the time of systemic treatment and when combined modality treatment is used, especially if salvage MOPP is delivered after radiation therapy (over 15 per cent). The overall risk of developing non-Hodgkin's lymphoma is approximately 2 per cent and many of these are B-cell high-grade malignancies associated with the presence of the Epstein–Barr virus genome. The risk of developing a secondary solid tumour, unlike the increased incidence of acute myeloid leukaemia, continues to increase beyond 10 years with approximately two-thirds of the tumours occurring in the radiation field. The incidence of these tumours is also greater in the older patients. The selection of drugs for combination therapy is important. Published data suggest that ABVD is associated with a lower risk of developing acute myeloid leukaemia than for patients treated with MOPP, but the accrual of more data from patients who receive alternative drug regimens is essential in assessing the relative carcinogenicity of the treatment modalities. Drug combinations without alkylating agents, procarbazine, or nitrosourea, such as ABVD or VBM (vinblastine, bleomycin, methotrexate) as utilized at Stanford University in the United States, should be considered in order to reduce the incidence of secondary acute myeloid leukaemia.

PSYCHOLOGICAL PROBLEMS ASSOCIATED WITH THE DIAGNOSIS AND TREATMENT OF HODGKIN'S DISEASE

The period following diagnosis is a time of considerable emotional distress for patients with Hodgkin's disease. The major concern is the implication of the tumour on future health and life expectancy. Both retrospective and prospective studies have shown substantial psychiatric morbidity with Hodgkin's disease and the incidence of symptoms of depression appears similar to that of patients following traumatic events such as mastectomy or myocardial infarction. However, there have been reports of a lower incidence of symptoms of anxiety, perhaps because of the better prognosis for patients with Hodgkin's disease (Devlen *et al.* 1987*a,b*). Approximately one-third of patients are extremely anxious or significantly depressed at the time of diagnosis or during the months preceding this. Although the overall incidence of psychological morbidity diminishes once a full explanation of their disease has been given and treatment started, some morbidity persists and patients remain at risk of developing psychiatric illness for a year or more after diagnosis. In a series of patients from Edinburgh, 26 per cent were found to have significant depression or anxiety 4–6 months after diagnosis

(Lloyd *et al.* 1984) and in a series from Manchester 76 out of 120 patients developed psychiatric morbidity over a 15 month period with 39 experiencing a depressive illness or anxiety state and a further 37 experiencing borderline depression or anxiety (Devlen *et al.* 1978*b*). The mean duration of a depressive illness or anxiety state in the latter series was approximately 4 months and although many patients' symptoms resolved without formal treatment a substantial proportion required psychiatric intervention.

Most patients with malignant disease wish to know the nature and severity of their condition and a frank discussion of these problems with patients with Hodgkin's disease can give reassurance since the majority have an excellent prognosis. The patients show unanimous approval of being told the diagnosis and the nature of their disease. Most of the emotional problems can be contained if an open approach to communication is adopted.

Both radiotherapy and chemotherapy are associated with substantial psychological disturbances and emotional distress. Traditionally, most patients treated with chemotherapy experienced some degree of nausea and vomiting and approximately half developed a conditioned response to mustine-based combination chemotherapy. Some were nauseated and vomited at the sight or smell of the clinic; others experienced nausea and vomited when they saw their injection or thought about treatment or were reminded of it by a doctor, relative, or friend. Conditioned responses were usually firmly developed by the fourth or fifth cycle of treatment. Prevailing anti-emetic therapy and relaxation exercises were of value in reducing these symptoms, and it was important to recognize and treat these patients before conditioning became firmly established (Marrow 1982; Redd and Andrykowski 1982). The introduction of serotonin-antagonist anti-emetics, for example ondansetron, has been a dramatic advance in emesis control and has largely removed the concerns of nausea, emesis, and anticipatory emesis from current chemotherapy administration.

Although most patients return quickly to normal social activities, other patients reduce their activities and take a more passive role, particularly during their treatment. A substantial proportion of patients in the Manchester series had employment problems, with 21 of the 86 patients who were in regular employment before they became ill staying off work from 6 to 11 months and 16 being off work for 12 months or more (Devlen 1987*b*). A study from Stanford also reported a high incidence of employment problems with 42 per cent of long-term survivors having employment difficulties (Fobair *et al.* 1986).

A further problem of concern has been the report of subjective memory impairment in patients receiving combination chemotherapy (MVPP) (Devlen 1987*b*). In this study patients reported difficulty in recalling simple facts such as their home telephone number. The patients who reported memory impairment tended to be older, but this feature was a problem for a few patients in their twenties. The symptoms were not explained by the presence of an affective disorder. Despite these complaints, however, formal memory scales failed to confirm impairment of short-term memory.

The high incidence of sexual difficulties is an important problem in patients treated for Hodgkin's disease and decreased libido and sexual activity may continue for several years after therapy has been completed (Chapman *et al.* 1979, 1981). Approximately one-third of patients with advanced Hodgkin's disease have evidence of sexual dysfunction before treatment and this proportion increases following treatment. These effects have important consequences for the patients, their friends, and their families. Explanation of likely problems and counselling for symptomatic patients is important since patients may not relate their alteration in sexual activity to their disease or treatment.

HODGKIN'S DISEASE AND PREGNANCY

Cancer is estimated to complicate one in every 1000 pregnancies. The most common malignancies affecting women of child-bearing age are carcinoma of the breast, cervix, leukaemia, lymphoma (most commonly Hodgkin's disease), and malignant melanoma.

Decision-making for the pregnant patient with Hodgkin's disease necessitates an appreciation of the natural history of untreated and treated disease, the preferences and priorities of the parents, an advocacy position for the fetus, and a knowledge of the implications of investigation and treatment during the course of the pregnancy. To a certain extent the issues can be approached on a factual basis; however, decisions will always be individualized, given that they generally represent a compromise conditioned by the emotional and social connotations of a pregnancy complicated by cancer and the necessity of exposing the fetus to the implications of maternal therapy (Sutcliffe 1985; Allen and Nisker 1986*a,b*; Doll *et al.* 1988).

Given the high cure rates resulting from current therapy for Hodgkin's disease, decisions will rarely compromise maternal outcome even if planned delays in the initiation of therapy or reduction in supradiaphragmatic radiation field size are employed to minimize fetal exposure to therapy. Thus, a successful outcome for the mother without compromise of curative potential is generally afforded a high priority.

There is no indication that the natural history of Hodgkin's disease is modified by pregnancy, nor that the pregnancy is adversely affected by the presence of Hodgkin's disease independent of investigation and therapy. Reports of placental involvement of malignancy or of metastasis to the fetus are exceptionally rare (Rothman *et al.* 1973). The rarity of metastasis to the fetus is believed to be due in part to the 'barrier' effect imposed by the placenta and also to the development of immune competence by the fetus with rejection of a histo-incompatible tumour graft.

Staging of Hodgkin's disease in pregnancy poses a problem since much of the definition of disease extent is based upon radiological imaging or radionuclide scanning. Thus, other than history, physical examination, biopsy, blood count, and biochemistry, the only non-radiological procedures are ultrasound or MRI. The fetal exposure from commonly employed imaging procedures would range from less than 10^{-5} Sv for a chest radiograph to $10^{-2}-3\times10^{-2}$ Sv for a lymphogram or CT examination of the abdomen and pelvis. Such exposure, although minor in the context of elective investigation and therapy, would be inappropriate during pregnancy and should be avoided. Therefore management decisions should either be based on limited clinical staging, with acceptance of the need for additional staging and therapy after completion of pregnancy, or should be based upon accurate information according to established practice following termination of pregnancy. Staging laparotomy is rarely considered as part of the staging procedure, even during a planned termination procedure, given the increased vascularity and increased operative morbidity associated with abdominal surgery during pregnancy.

Radiation exposure during pregnancy has been studied in the mouse and the rat. Anecdotal data exist for humans such that the implications of exposure can be approached from both a theoretical and practical standpoint. Two issues are of importance: gestational age at the time of exposure and fetal dose.

Animal and human data indicate that radiation exposure during the first trimester results in structural and developmental anomalies in liveborn offspring or spontaneous abortion. This would be consistent with interference in the period of organogenesis and resultant fetal defects include cataracts, genital and skeletal abnormalities, pigmentary degeneration of the retina, microphthalmus, mental retardation, microcephaly, and stunted growth. The impact upon neurological development extends at least to week 20 of gestation. Radiation exposure in the second and third trimester is not associated with structural defects, although it is probable that growth retardation and/or organ atrophy might be associated with significant exposure. In animals, a significant dose during the period of organogenesis may be in the 0.1–0.15 Gy range. In humans it is clear that exposure in excess of 2.5 Gy results in severe anomalies up to week 20 of pregnancy.

In addition, data from the atomic fall-out in Japan suggest a linear relationship between exposure and incidence of severe mental retardation with no apparent threshold below which no deleterious effects were apparent. In practice, therefore, no radiation exposure can be considered 'safe' and any exposure must either be avoided or minimized. Such contraints clearly preclude the use of wide-field supradiaphragmatic (mantle) or abdominal fields to full tumour dose. Experience has indicated, however, that limited supradiaphragmatic irradiation fields treated to doses sufficient to control adenopathy may be administered without apparent fetal damage. Such a treatment approach clearly requires considerable attention to detail and the necessity of re-examining the overall treatment plan following completion of pregnancy. In addition, although the exposure may not be associated with immediate structural or developmental consequences, the implications for late genetic and somatic effects remain a concern.

Cytotoxic chemotherapy is strongly contra-indicated during the first trimester of pregnancy. Exposure, particularly to antimetabolites or alkylating agents, carries a high risk of fetal malformation. Much anecdotal experience with cytotoxic therapy has been accrued during the second and third trimester of pregnancy. A wide range of agents, given singly or in combination, have been administered for Hodgkin's disease, non-Hodgkin's lymphoma, and acute leukaemia. The experience to date would imply that such exposure does not result in structural malformation. Despite the lack of apparent malformation associated with second and third trimester exposure, it should not be construed that chemotherapy is without risk. Intrauterine growth retardation is a common finding in neonates experiencing chemotherapy during pregnancy and there remains a paucity of literature defining long-term follow-up implications of intrauterine chemotherapy exposure; that is, fertility and somatic and genetic effects.

Therapy for cancer during pregnancy gives rise to additional problems: increased nutritional requirements, control of emesis, candidiasis, constipation, attention to dental care, and management of cytopenias. Delivery should be planned according to the usual obstetric protocols and should be scheduled to avoid therapy-induced cytopenias. The neonate must be examined for structural defects, evidence of intrauterine growth retardation, adrenal or thyroid dysfunction, and cytopenias consequent upon cytotoxic therapy. The treatment plan for the mother must also be re-examined following delivery to ensure that any compromises in staging and therapy that have occurred are addressed appropriately. The decision to breast-feed is largely contingent upon the continuing requirement for maternal investigation or therapy, given that many drugs can be transferred in breast milk.

In summary, the management of the pregnant patient with Hodgkin's disease is dependent on several factors. In practice, in early pregnancy the decision is usually one of limited radiation therapy for those with asymptomatic localized disease with a re-evaluation of therapy after delivery or of termination of pregnancy for the patient with symptomatic or advanced disease. After week 20, an expectant policy without intervention is commonly practised for the asymptomatic patient with a planned induction of labour when fetal maturity is established. If therapy is required after week 20, cytotoxic therapy can be administered under appropriate supervision. The optimum regimen is unknown, but there are good theoretical reasons for avoiding alkylating agents and chronic oral chemotherapy.

Delivery should be planned such that the fetus be delivered at an appropriate level of maturity with the minimum exposure to therapy and at a time of adequate maternal blood counts.

REFERENCES

Abdulaziz Z, Mason DY, Stein H, Gatter KC, Nash JRG (1983). An immunohistological study of the cellular constituents of Hodgkin's disease using a monoclonal antibody panel. *Histopathology*, 8:1–25.
Allen HH, Nisker JA (eds) (1986a). *Cancer in pregnancy*. Futura, New York.
Allen HH, Nisker JA (1986b). *Cancer Bulletin*, 38:277–314.
Anderson H, et al. (1984). A randomized study of adjuvant chemotherapy after mantle radiotherapy in supradiaphragmatic Hodgkin's disease PS IA–IIB. A report from the Manchester Lymphoma Group. *British Journal of Cancer*, 49:695–702.
Anderson H, Crowther D, Deakin DP, Ryders WDJ, Radford JA (1990). A randomised study of adjuvant MVPP chemotherapy after mantle radiotherapy in PS IA–IIB Hodgkin's disease. *Annals of Oncology*, 2(Suppl. 2):49–54.
Armstrong AA, et al. (1993). Association of Epstein–Barr virus with pediatric Hodgkin's disease. *American Journal of Pathology*, 142(6):1683–8.
Barrett A, Gregor A, McElwain TJ, Peckham MJ (1981). Infradiaphragmatic presentation of Hodgkin's disease. *Clinical Radiology*, 32:221–4.
Baysogolov GD, Shakhtarina SV (1987). The efficiency of different combined treatment programs (combination chemotherapy–radiotherapy) used for stage I–II Hodgkin's disease. *Radiotherapy and Oncology*, 8:113–22.
Bennett MH, MacLennan KA, Easterling MJ, Vaughan-Hudson B, Jelliffe AM, Vaughan-Hudson G (1983). The prognostic significance of cellular subtypes in nodular sclerosing Hodgkin's disease: an analysis of 271 non-laparotomised cases. *British Journal of Haematology*, 44:347–58.
Bergsagel DE, et al. (1982). Results of treating Hodgkin's disease without a policy of laparotomy staging. *Cancer Treatment Reports*, 66:835–46.
Bloomfield CD, et al. (1982). Chemotherapy and combined modality therapy for Hodgkin's disease: a report on Cancer and Leukemia Group B studies. *Cancer Treatment Reports*, 66:835–46.
BNLI (British National Lymphoma Investigation) (1976). Initial treatment of stage IIIA Hodgkin's disease. *Lancet*, ii:991–5.
Bonadonna G (1982). Chemotherapy strategies to improve the control of Hodgkin's disease. The Richard and Hinda Rosenthal Foundation Award Lecture. *Cancer Research*, 42:4309–20.
Bonadonna G (1990). Does chemotherapy fulfil its expectations in cancer treatment? *Annals of Oncology*, 1:11–21.
Bonadonna G, Valagussa P (1990). Influence of clinical trials on current treatment strategy for Hodgkin's disease. *International Journal of Radiation Oncology—Biology—Physics*, 19:209–18.
Bonadonna G, Valagussa P, Santoro A (1986). Alternating non-cross-resistant combination chemotherapy or MOPP in stage IV Hodgkin's disease. A report of 8-year results. *Annals of Internal Medicine*, 104:739–46.
Bonadonna G, Santoro A, Viviani S, Valagussa P (1988). Treatment strategies for Hodgkin's disease. *Seminars in Hematology* 25(Suppl. 2):51–7.
Bonadonna G, Valagussa P, Santor A, Viviani S, Bonfante V, Banfi A (1989). Hodgkin's disease: the Milan Cancer Institute experience with MOPP and ABVD. *Recent Results in Cancer Research*, 117:169–74.
Bookman MA, Longo DL (1986). Concomitant illness in patients treated for Hodgkin's disease. *Cancer Treatment Reviews*, 13:77–11.

Borg-Grech A, Radford JA, Crowther D, Swindell R, Harris M (1989). A comparative study of the nodular and diffuse variants of lymphocyte predominant Hodgkin's disease. *Journal of Clinical Oncology*, 9:1–7.

Brada M, Easton DF, Horwich A, Peckham MJ (1986). Clinical presentation as a predictor of laparotomy findings in supradiaphragmatic stage I and II Hodgkin's disease. *Radiotherapy and Oncology*, 5:15–22.

Bubman I, Kirchhoff LV, Moroka H, de Bellis N (1986). Treatment of Hodgkin's disease stages I and II with chemotherapy alone. *Medical and Pediatric Oncology*, 14:208–10.

Canellos GP, Selby P, McElwain TJ (1987). Alternative combinations and new approaches: chemotherapy for Hodgkin's disease. In *Hodgkin's disease* (ed. P Selby and TJ McElwain), pp. 285–300. Blackwell, Oxford.

Canellos GP, Nadler L, Takvorian T (1988). Autologous bone marrow transplantation in the treatment of malignant lymphoma and Hodgkin's disease. *Seminars in Hematology*, 25(Suppl. 2):58–65.

Canellos GP, et al. (1992) Chemotherapy of advanced Hodgkin's disease with MOPP, ABVD or MOPP alternating with ABVD. *New England Journal of Medicine*, 327:1478–84.

Carbone PP, Kaplan HS, Musshoff K, Smithers DW, Tubiana M (1971). Report of the Committee on Hodgkin's Disease Staging Classification. *Cancer Research*, 31:1860–1.

Carde P, et al. (1988). Comparison of total nodal irradiation versus combined sequence of mantle irradiation with mechlorethanine, vincristine, procarbazine and prednisolone in clinical stages I and II Hodgkin's disease. Experience of the European Organization for Research and Treatment of Cancer. *National Institute of Cancer Monograph*, 6:303–10.

Carde P, et al. (1993). Clinical staging versus laparotomy and combined modality with MOPP versus ABVD in early stage Hodgkin's disease: the H6 twin randomised trials from the European Organisation for Research and Treatment of Cancer Lymphoma Cooperative Group. *Journal of Clinical Oncology*, 11:2258–72.

Carella AM, et al. (1988). High-dose chemotherapy with autologous bone marrow transplantation in 50 advanced resistant Hodgkin's disease patients: an Italian Study Group Report. *Journal of Clinical Oncology*, 6:1411–16.

Carmel RJ, Kaplan HS (1976). Mantle irradiation and Hodgkin's disease. *Cancer*, 37:2813–15.

Castellino RA, Hoppe RT, Blank N, Young SW, Neumann C, Rosenberg SA, Kaplan HS (1984). Computed tomography, lymphography and staging laparotomy. *American Journal of Roentgenology*, 143:37–41.

Chapman RM, Sutcliffe SB, Malpas JS (1979). Cytotoxic-induced ovarian failure in Hodgkin's disease II. Effects on sexual function. *Journal of the American Medical Association*, 242:1882–4.

Chapman RM, Sutcliffe SB, Malpas JS (1981). Male gonadal dysfunction in Hodgkin's disease. A prospective study. *Journal of the American Medical Association*, 245:1323–8.

Chittal SM, et al. (1988). Monoclonal antibodies in the diagnosis of Hodgkin's disease. The search for a rationale panel. *American Journal of Surgical Pathology*, 12:9–21.

Cimino G, et al. (1989). MOPP chemotherapy versus extended-field radiotherapy in the management of pathological stages I–IIA Hodgkin's disease. *Journal of Clinical Oncology*, 7:732–7.

Cohen BM, Smetana HF, Miller RW (1964). Hodgkin's disease: long survival in a study of 388 World War II army cases. *Cancer*, 17:856–66.

Colby TV, Warnke RA (1980). The histology of the initial relapse of Hodgkin's disease. *Cancer*, 45:289–92.

Colby TV, Hoppe RT, Warnke RA (1981). Hodgkin's disease: a clinicopathologic study of 659 cases. *Cancer*, 49:1848–85.

Collaborative Study (1984). Radiotherapy of stage I and II Hodgkin's disease. *Cancer*, 54:1928–42.

Colonna P, Andrieu J-M (1985). MOPP chemotherapy alone: a suitable treatment for early stage of Hodgkin's disease? *Lancet*, i:1224.

Coltman CA Jr, Fuller LM, Fisher R, Frei E (1979). Extended field radiotherapy versus involved field radiotherapy plus MOPP in stage I and II Hodgkin's disease. In *Adjuvant therapy of cancer II* (ed. SG Jones and SE Salmon), pp. 129–36. Grune and Stratton, New York.

Coltman CA, Myers JW, Motague E, Fuller LA, Grozea PN, DePersio EJ, Dixon DO (1982). The role of combined radiotherapy and chemotherapy in the primary management of Hodgkin's disease. South West Oncology Group studies. In *Malignant lymphomas* (ed. SA Rosenberg and HS Kaplan), pp. 523–35. Academic Press, New York.

Correa P, O'Conor GT (1971). Epidemiologic patterns of Hodgkin's disease. *International Journal of Cancer*, 8:192–201.

Craft CB (1940). Results with roentgen ray therapy in Hodgkin's disease. *Bulletin of the Staff Meetings of the University of Minnesota Hospital*, 11:391–409.

Crnkovich MJ, Leopold K, Hoppe RT, Mauch PM (1987) Stage I and IIB Hodgkin's disease: the combined experience at Stanford University and the Joint Centre for Radiation Therapy. *Journal of Clinical Oncology*, 7:1041–9.

Crowther D, Blackledge G, Best JK (1979). The role of computed tomography of the abdomen in the diagnosis and staging of patients with lymphoma. *Clinics in Haematology*, 8:567.

Crowther D, et al. (1984). A randomized study comparing chemotherapy alone with chemotherapy followed by radiotherapy in patients with pathologically staged IIIA Hodgkin's disease. *Journal of Clinical Oncology*, 2:892–7.

da Cunha MF, Meistorch ML, Saad MF (1983). Impact of treatment for Hodgkin's disease on the reproductive functions of adult patients. *Cancer Bulletin*, 35:233–8.

Dady PJ, McElwain TJ, Austin DE, Barrett A, Peckham MJ (1982). Five years' experience with ChlVPP: effective low-toxicity combination chemotherapy for Hodgkin's disease. *British Journal of Cancer*, 45:851–9.

Deforges JF, Rutherford CJ, Piro A (1989). Hodgkin's disease. *New England Journal of Medicine*, 301:1212–22.

Desser RK, et al. (1977). Prognostic classification of Hodgkin's disease in pathologic stage III, based on anatomic consideration. *Blood*, 49:883–93.

Devlen J, Maguire P, Phillips P, Crowther D, Chambers H (1987a). Psychological problems associated with diagnosis and treatment of lymphomas. I. Retrospective study. *British Medical Journal*, 295:953–4.

Devlen J, Maguire P, Phillips P, Crowther D (1987b). Psychological problems associated with diagnosis and treatment of lymphomas. II. Prospective study. *British Medical Journal*, 295:955–7.

Doll DC, Ringenberg S, Yarbro JW (1988). Management of cancer during pregnancy. *Archives of Internal Medicine*, 148:2058–64.

Dorreen MS, Wrigley PFM, Jones AC, Shand WS, Stansfield AG, Lister TA (1984). The management of localized infradiaphragmatic Hodgkin's disease. Experience of a rare clinical presentation at St. Bartholomew's Hospital. *Hematological Oncology*, 2:349–57.

Drexler HA, Amlot PL, Minowda J (1987). Hodgkin's disease—derived cell lines: conflicting clues for the origin of Hodgkin's disease. *Leukaemia*, 1:629–37.

Duchesnse G, Peckham MJ (1983). Chemotherapy and radiotherapy in advanced testicular non-seminoma. (2) Results of treatment. *Radiation Oncology*, 1:207–15.

Fajardo LF, Stewart JR, Cohn KE (1968). Morphology of radiation-induced heart disease. *Archives of Pathology*, 86:512–19.

Farah R, et al. (1988). Extended mantle radiation therapy of pathological stage I and II Hodgkin's disease. *Journal of Clinical Oncology*, 6:1047–52.

Ferma C, Teiller F, D'Agay MF, Gisselbrecht C, Marty M, Boiron M (1984). Combined modality in Hodgkin's disease comparison of six versus three courses of MOPP with clinical and surgical restaging. *Cancer*, 54:2324–29.

Finzi NS (1913). Treatment of internal disease. Lymphadenoma. In *Radium threapeutics*, Vol. 84. Oxford Medical Publications.

Fisher RI, DeVita VT Jr, Hubbard SP, Simon R, Young RC (1979). Prolonged disease-free survival in Hodgkin's disease with MOPP induction after first relapse. *Annals of Internal Medicine*, 90:761–3.

Fletcher GH, Shukovsky LJ (1975). The interplay of radio curability and the tolerance in the irradiation of human cancers. *Journal of Radio Electrolysis*, 56:383–400.

Fobair P, Hoppe RJ, Bloom J, Cox R, Varghese A, Spiegel D (1986). Psychological problems among survivors of Hodgkin's disease. *Journal of Clinical Oncology*, 4:805–14.

Ford RJ Jr, Mehta SR, Sharma S (1988). Immunobiology of Hodgkin's disease and non Hodgkin's lymphomas. In *Hodgkin's disease and non Hodgkin's lymphoma in adults and children* (ed. L Fuller, FB Hagermeister, MP Sullivan, and WS Velasquez), pp. 47–62. Raven Press, New York.

Friedman S, Henry-Amar M, Cossett JM, Carde P, Hayat M, Dupony N, Tubiana M (1988). Evolution of erythrocyte sedimentation rate as predictor of early relapse in post therapy early stage Hodgkin's disease. *Journal of Clinical Oncology*, 6:596–602.

Fuks Z, Glatstein E, Marsa GW, Bagshaw MA, Kaplan HS (1976). Long term effects of external radiation on the pituitary and thyroid glands. *Cancer*, 37:1152–61.

Gianni AM, Siena S, Bregni M, Tarella C, Stern AC, Pileri A, Bonadonna G (1989b). Granulocyte-macrophage colony-stimulating factor to harvest circulating haemopoietic stem cells for autotransplantation. *Lancet*, ii:580–4.

Gilbert R (1939). Radiotherapy in Hodgkin's disease (malignant granulomatosis): anatomic and clinical foundations; governing principles; results. *American Journal of Roentgenology*, 41:198–241.

Glatstein E, Guerney JM, Rosenberg SA, Kaplan HS (1969). The value of laparotomy and splenectomy in the staging of Hodgkin's disease. *Cancer*, 24:708–18.

Glick J, et al. (1991). A randomised phase III trial of MOPP/ABV hybrid vs sequential MOPP–ABVD in advanced Hodgkin's disease: preliminary results of the Intergroup Trial (Meeting abstract). *Proceedings of the Annual Meeting of the American Society of Clinical Oncology*, 10, abstract 941.

Gobbi PG, et al. (1988). Hodgkin's disease prognosis: a directly predictive equation. *Lancet*, i:675–9.

Gribben JG, Linch DC, Singer CRJ, McMillan AK, Jarrett M, Goldstone AH (1989). Successful treatment of refractory Hodgkin's disease by high-dose combination chemotherapy and autologous bone marrow transplantation. *Blood*, 73:340–4.

Grogan TM, et al. (1982). Changing patterns of Hodgkin's disease at autopsy: a 25-year experience at the National Cancer Institute 1953–1978. *Cancer Treatment Reports*, 66:653.

Grufferman S, Delzell E (1984). Epidemiology of Hodgkin's disease. *Epidemiologic Reviews*, 6:76–106.

Grufferman S, Cole P, Smith PG, Lukes RJ (1977). Hodgkin's disease in siblings. *New England Journal of Medicine*, 296:248–50.

Gunter-Seydel H, Bloedorn FG, Wisenberg MJ (1967). Time–dose–volume relationship in Hodgkin's disease. *Radiology*, 89:919–22.

Hagermeister FB (1988). Prognostic factors in decision-making in the clinical management of Hodgkin's disease. *Hematological Oncology*, 6:257–69.

Hagermeister FB, Fuller LM (1988). Stage III Hodgkin's disease. In *Hodgkin's disease and the other lymphomas in adults and children* (ed. LM Fuller, FB Hagermeister, M Sullivan, and WS Velasquez), pp. 230–40. Raven Press, New York.

Hall PA, d'Ardenne AJ, Stansfield AG (1988). Paraffin section immuno-histochemistry II Hodgkin's disease and large cell anaplastic (Ki-1) lymphoma. *Histopathology*, 8:1–25.

Hanks RE, Kinzie JJ, Herring DF, Kramer S (1982). Patterns of care outcome studies in Hodgkin's disease: results of the national practice and implications for management. *Cancer Treatment Reports*, 66:805–8.

Hanks RE, Kinzie JJ, White RL, Herring DF, Kramer S (1983). Patterns of care outcome studies results of the national practice in Hodgkin's disease. *Cancer*, 51:569–73.

Haybittle JL, et al. (1985). Review of British National Lymphoma Investigation studies of Hodgkin's disease and development of prognostic index. *Lancet*, i:967.

Hayat M (1984). Long term followup of patients with clinical stages I, II Hodgkin's disease; comparison of initial splenectomy and spleen irradiation. *Proceedings of the Second International Conference on Malignant Lymphoma, Lugano, 1984*, Abstract 25.

Hellman S, Mauch P (1982). Role of radiation therapy in the treatment of Hodgkin's disease. *Cancer Treatment Reports*, 66:915–23.

Herbst H, Stein H, Niedobitek G (1993). Epstein–Barr virus and CD30+ malignant lymphomas. *Critical Reviews in Oncology*, 4(2):191–239.

Hoppe RT, Rosenberg SA, Kaplan HS, Cox RS (1980). Prognostic factors in pathological stage IIA Hodgkin's disease. *Cancer*, 46:1240–6.

Hoppe RT, Coleman CN, Cox RS, Rosenberg SA, Kaplan HS (1982). The management of stage I–II Hodgkin's disease with irradiation alone or combined modality therapy: the Stanford experience. *Blood*, 59:455–6.

Horning SJ, Hoppe RT, Hancock SL, Rosenberg SA (1988). Vinblastine, bleomycin and methotrexate: an effective adjuvant in favourable Hodgkin's disease. *Journal of Clinical Oncology*, 6:1822–31.

Hors J, et al. (1980). HLA genotypes in familial Hodgkin's disease: excess of HLA identical affected SIBS. *European Journal of Cancer*, 16:809–15.

Horwich A, Peckham MJ (1987). Combined chemotherapy and radiotherapy in the management of adult Hodgkin's disease: indications and results. In *Hodgkin's disease* (ed. P Selby and TJ McElwain), pp. 250–68. Blackwell, Oxford.

Horwich A, Easton D, Nogueira-Costa R, Liew KH, Colman M, Peckham MJ (1986). An analysis of prognostic factors in early stage Hodgkin's disease. *Radiotherapy and Oncology*, 7(2):95–106.

Jagannath S, et al. (1989). Prognostic factors for response and survival after high-dose cyclophosphamide, carmustine, and etoposide with autologous bone marrow transplantation for relapsed Hodgkin's disease. *Journal of Clinical Oncology*, 7:179–85.

Jarrett RF, et al. (1991). Detection of Epstein–Barr virus genomes in Hodgkin's disease: relation to age. *Journal of Clinical Pathology*, 44:844–8.

Jelliffe AM, Thomson AD (1955). The prognosis in Hodgkin's disease. *British Journal of Cancer*, 9:21–8.

Kagan AR, Haferman M, Hamilton M, Pierce R, Morton D, Johnson R (1972). Etiology, diagnosis and management of pericardial effusion after irradiation. *Radiologia Clinica et Biologica*, 41:171–82.

Kaldor JM, et al. (1990). Leukaemia following chemotherapy for ovarian cancer. *New England Journal of Mecicine*, 322(1):52–3.

Kaplan HS (1962). The radical radiotherapy of regionally localized Hodgkin's disease. *Radiology*, 78:553–61.

Kaplan HS (1991). Evidence for a tumoricidal dose level in the radiotherapy of Hodgkin's disease. *Cancer Research*, 26:1221–4.

Kaplan HS (1980). *Hodgkin's disease* (2nd edn), pp. 412–41. Harvard University Press, Cambridge, MA.

Keller AR, Kaplan HS, Lukes RJ, Rappaport H (1968). Correlation of histopathology with other prognostic indicators in Hodgkin's disease. *Cancer*, 22:487.

Kinsella TJ, Glatstein E (1982). Staging laparotomy and splenectomy for Hodgkin's disease: current status. *Cancer Investigation*, 1:87–91.

Kinzie JJ, Hanks GE, Maclean CJ, Kramer S (1983). Patterns of care study: Hodgkin's disease relapse rates and adequacy of portals. *Cancer*, 52:2223–6.

Klimo P, Connors JM (1988). An update of the Vancouver experience in the management of advanced Hodgkin's disease treated with the MOPP/ABV hybrid program. *Seminars in Hematology*, 25:23–40.

Krikorian JG, Portlock CS, Rosenberg SA, Kaplan HS (1979). Hodgkin's disease stage I and II occurring below the diaphragm. *Cancer*, 43:1866–71.

Krikorian JG, Portlock CS, Mauch PM (1986). Hodgkin's disease presenting below the diaphragm: a review. *Journal of Clinical Oncology*, 4:1551–62.

Lacher MJ (1983). Routine staging laparotomy for patients with Hodgkin's disease is no longer necessary. *Cancer Investigation*, 1:93–9.

Lacher MU, Durant JR (1965). Combined vinblastine and chlorambucil therapy of Hodgkin's disease. *Annals of Internal Medicine*, 62:468–76.

Lagarde P, Eghbali H, Bonichon F, De Mascarel I, Chuvergene J, Hoerni B (1988). Brief chemotherapy associated with extended field radiotherapy in Hodgkin's disease. Long term results in a series of 102 patients with clinical stages I-IIIA. *European Journal of Cancer and Clinical Oncology*, 24:1191–8.

Lanzillo JH, Moylan DJ, Mohiuddin M, Kramer S (1985). Radiotherapy of stage I and II Hodgkin's disease with inguinal presentation. *Radiology*, 154:213–15.

Lauria F, Baccarini M, Fiacchini M, Mazza P, Tura S (1979). Combination chemotherapy in stage I or II Hodgkin's disease. *Lancet*, ii:1072–3.

LeBourgeois JP, Meignan M, Parmentier C, Tubiana M (1979). Renal consequences of irradiation of the spleen in lymphoma patients. *British Journal of Radiology*, 52:56–60.

Lee CKK, Bloomfield CD, Goldman AI, Nesbit MC, Levitt SH (1981). The therapeutic utility of lung irradiation for Hodgkin's disease patients with large mediastinal masses. *International Journal of Radiation Oncology—Biology—Physics*, 7:151–4.

LeShan L, Marvin S, Lyerly O (1959). Some evidence of a relationship between Hodgkin's disease and intelligence. *Archives of General Psychiatry*, 1:477–9

Levi JA, Wiernik PH (1977). The therapeutic implications of splenic involvement in stage IIIA Hodgkin's disease. *Cancer*, 39:2158–65.

Levitt SH, Lee CK, Bloomfield CD (1984). Radical radiation therapy in the treatment of laparotomy staged Hodgkin's disease patients. *International Journal of Radiation Oncology—Biology—Physics*, 10:265–74.

Liew KH, Easton D, Horwich A, Barrett A, Peckham MJ (1984). Bulky mediastinal Hodgkin's disease, management and prognosis. *Haematological Oncology*, 2:45–9.

Lister TA, *et al.* (1989). Report of a committee convened to discuss the evaluation and staging of patients with Hodgkin's disease (Cotswolds Meeting). *Journal of Clinical Oncology*, 7:1630–6.

Lloyd GG, Parker AC, Ludlam CA, Maguire RI (1984) Emotional impact of diagnosis and early treatment of lymphomas. *Journal of Psychosomatic Research*, 28:157–62.

Longo DL, *et al.* (1986). Twenty years of MOPP therapy for Hodgkin's disease. *Journal of Clinical Oncology*, 4:1295–1306.

Longo D, Glatstein E, Young R, Duffey P, Hubbard S, DeVita VT Jr (1987) Randomized trial of MOPP chemotherapy (CT) vs subtotal nodal radiation therapy (RT) in patients (PT) with laparotomy-documented early stage Hodgkin's disease (HD). *Proceedings of the American Society of Clinical Oncology*, 6:A812 (abstract).

Lukes RJ, Butler JJ (1966). The pathology of Hodgkin's disease. *Cancer Research*, 24:1063–81.

Lukes RJ, Craven LF, Hall TC, Rappaport H, Ruben P (1966). Report of the nomenclature of Hodgkin's disease. *Cancer Research*, 26:1311.

MacDonald JS (1982). Lymphography in lymph node disease. In *The lymphatics: surgery, lymphography and diseases of the chyle and lymph systems* (ed. JB Kinmonth), pp. 327–70. Edward Arnold, London.

McKendrick JJ, Mead GM, Sweetenham J, Jones DH, Williams CJ, Ryall R, Whitehouse JM (1989). ChlVPP chemotherapy in advanced Hodgkin's disease. *European Journal of Cancer and Clinical Oncology*, 25:557–62.

MacMahon B (1966). Epidemiology of Hodgkin's disease. *Cancer Research*, 26:1189–1200.

Marks JE, Haus AG, Sutton HG, Griem ML (1974). Localization error in the radiotherapy of Hodgkin's disease and malignant lymphoma with extended mantle fields. *Cancer*, 34:83–90.

Mason TJ, Fraumeni JF (1974). Hodgkin's disease among Japanese Americans. *Lancet*, i:215.

Mauch P, Goodman R, Rosenthal DS, Botnick L, Piro AJ, Hellman S (1979). An evaluation of total nodal irradiation as treatment for stage IIIA Hodgkin's disease. *Cancer*, 43:1255–61.

Mauch P, Greenberg H, Lewin A, Cassady JR, Weichselbaum R, Hellman S (1983). Prognostic factors in patients with subdiaphragmatic Hodgkin's disease. *Hematological Oncology*, 1:205–14.

Mauch P, *et al.* (1988). Stage IA and IIA supradiaphragmatic Hodgkin's disease: prognostic factors in surgically staged patients treated with mantle and para-aortic irradiation. *Journal of Clinical Oncology*, 6:1576–83.

Moormeier JA, Williams SF, Golomb HM (1989). The staging of Hodgkin's disease. *Hematology Clinics of North America*, 3(2):237–51.

Morrow GR (1982). Prevalence and correlates of anticipatory nausea and vomiting in chemotherapy patients. *Journal of the National Cancer Institute*, 68:585–8.

Mould JJ, Adam NM (1983). The problem of avascular necrosis of bone in patients treated for Hodgkin's disease. *Clinical Radiology*, 34:231–6.

Mueller N, *et al.* (1989). Hodgkin's disease and Epstein–Barr virus altered antibody pattern before diagnosis. *New England Journal of Medicine*, 320:689–95.

Nissen NI, Nordentoft AM (1982). Radiotherapy versus combined modality treatment of stage I and II Hodgkin's disease. *Cancer Treatment Reports*, 66:799–803.

O'Dwyer PJ, Wiernik PH, Stewart MB, Slawson RG (1985). Treatment of early stage Hodgkin's disease: a randomized trial of radiotherapy plus chemotherapy versus chemotherapy alone. *Developments in Oncology*, 32:329–36.

Olweny CLM, Katongole-Mbidde E, Kiine C, Lwange SK, Magrath I, Ziegler JL (1978). Childhood Hodgkin's disease in Uganda: a ten year experience. *Cancer*, 42:787–92.

Pavlovsky S, *et al.* (1988). Randomized trial of chemotherapy versus chemotherapy plus radiotherapy for stage I-II Hodgkin's disease. *Journal of the National Cancer Institute*, 80:1466–73.

Peckham MJ, Ford HT, McElwain TJ, Harmer CL, Atkinson K, Austin DE (1975). The results of radiotherapy for Hodgkin's disease. *British Journal of Cancer*, 32:391–400.

Peters MV (1950). A study of survivals in Hodgkin's disease treated radiologically. *American Journal of Roentgenology*, 63:299–311.

Peters MV, Middlemiss KCH (1958). A study of Hodgkin's disease treated by irradiation. *American Journal of Roentgenology*, 79:114–21.

Pettengell R, *et al.* (1993). Peripheral blood progenitor cell transplantation in lymphoma and leukaemia using a single apheresis. *Blood*, 82:3770–7.

Phillips CL, *et al.* (1989). Treatment of progressive Hodgkin's disease with intensive chemoradiotherapy and autologous bone marrow transplantation. *Blood*, 73:2086–92.

Pinkus GS, Said JW (1985). Hodgkin's disease, lymphocyte predominant type, nodular—a distinct entity? Unique staining profile for L and H variants of Reed–Sternberg cells defined by monoclonal antibodies or leucocyte common antigen, granulocyte-specific antigen and B cell-specific antigen. *American Journal of Pathology*, 118:1–6.

Poppema S, Kaiserling E, Lennert K (1979). Nodular paragranuloma and progressively transformed germinal centres. Ultrastructural and immuno-histological findings. *Virchows Archive B. Cell Pathology*, 31:211–25.

Prosnitz LR, Montalvo RL, Fischer DB (1978). Treatment of stage IIIA Hodgkin's disease: is radiotherapy alone adequate? *International Journal of Radiation Oncology—Biology—Physics*, 4:781–7.

Radford JA, *et al.* (1993). MVPP versus a seven drug hybrid regimen in Hodgkin's disease (HD); results of a randomised trial. *Proceedings of the Fifth International Conference on Malignant Lymphoma*, June 1993, Lugano. Abstract 61, p. 51.

Rappaport H, Berard CW, Butler JJ, Dorfman RF, Lukes RJ, Thomas LB (1971). Report of the Committee of Histopathological Criteria Contributing to the Staging of Hodgkin's Disease. *Cancer Research*, 31:1864–5.

Ray GR, Trueblood HW, Enright LP, Kaplan HS, Nelson TS (1970). Oophoropexy: a means of preserving ovarian function following pelvic megavoltage radiotherapy for Hodgkin's disease. *Radiology*, 96:175–80.

Razis DV, Diamond HD, Craver LF (1959). Familial Hodgkin's disease. Its significance and implications. *Annals of Internal Medicine*, 51:933–71.

Redd WH, Andrykowski MA (1982). Behavioural intervention in cancer treatment: controlling aversion reaction to chemotherapy. *Journal of Consulting and Clinical Psychology*, 50:1018–29.

Regula DP, Hoppe RT, Weiss LM (1988). Nodular and diffuse types of lymphocyte predominance, Hodgkin's disease. *New England Journal of Medicine*, 318:214–19.

Richards MA, *et al.* (1986). EVA treatment for recurrence of unresponsive Hodgkin's disease. *Cancer Chemotherapy and Pharmacology*, 18:51–3.

Robertson SJ, *et al.* (1987). Familial Hodgkin's disease. A clinical and laboratory investigation. *Cancer*, 59:1314.

Rose M (1981). *Curator of the dead. Thomas Hodgkin (1798–1866)*. Peter Owen, London.

Rosenberg SA (1988). Exploratory laparotomy and splenectomy for Hodgkin's disease. A commentary. *Journal of Clinical Oncology*, 6:574.

Rosenberg SA, Kaplan HS, Glatstein EJ, Porlock CS (1978). Combined modality therapy of Hodgkin's disease. A report of the Stanford trials. *Cancer*, 42:991–1000.

Rothman LA, Cohen CJ, Astarloa J (1973). Placental and fetal involvement by maternal malignancy: a report of rectal carcinoma and review of the literature. *American Journal of Obstetrics and Gynecology*, 116:1023–34.

Rubin P, Keys H, Mayer E, Antemann R (1974). Nodal recurrences following radical radiation therapy in Hodgkin's disease. *American Journal of Roentgenology Radium Therapy and Nuclear Medicine*, 120:536–658.

Ruckdeschel JG, Chang P, Martin RG, Byhardt RW, O'Connell MJ, Sutherland JC, Wiernik PH (1975). Radiation-related pericardial effusions in patients with Hodgkin's disease. *Medicine*, 54:245–59.

Sacks EL, Donaldson SS, Gordon J, Dorfman RF (1978). Epithelial granulomas associated with Hodgkin's disease. *Cancer*, 41:562–7.

Sandeman TF (1966). The effects of X irradiation on male human fertility. *British Journal of Radiology*, 39:901–7.

Santoro A, Bonfante V, Bonadonna G (1982). Salvage chemotherapy with ABVD in MOPP-resistant Hodgkin's disease. *Annals of Internal Medicine*, 96:139–44.

Santoro A, Viviani S, Villareal CJR, Bonfante V, Delfino A, Valagussa P, Bonadonna G (1986). Salvage chemotherapy in Hodgkin's disease irradiation failures: supriority of doxorubicin-containing regimens over MOPP. *Cancer Treatment Reports*, 7:344–8.

Santoro A, *et al.* (1987) Long-term results of combined chemotherapy–radiotherapy approach in Hodgkin's disease: superiority of ABVD plus radiotherapy versus MOPP plus radiotherapy. *Journal of Clinical Oncology*, 5(1):27–37.

Schewe KL, Reavis J, Kun LE, Cox JD (1988). Total dose, fraction size, and tumor volume in the local control of Hodgkin's disease. *International Journal of Radiation Oncology—Biology—Physics*, **15**:25–8.

Schimpff SC, Diggs CH, Wiswell JG, Salvatore PC, Wiernik PH (1980). Radiation-related thyroid dysfunction: implications for the treatment of Hodgkin's disease. *Annals of International Medicine*, **92**:91–8

Selby P, McElwain TJ, Canellos G (1987). Chemotherapy for Hodgkin's disease. In *Hodgkin's disease* (ed. P Selby and TJ McElwain), pp. 269–85. Blackwell, Oxford.

Sharma SC, Williamson JF, Khan FM, Lee CK (1981). Measurement and calculation of ovary and fetus dose in extended field radiotherapy for 10 MV X rays. *International Journal of Radiation Oncology—Biology—Physics*, **7**:843–6.

Sheridan WP, *et al.* (1992). Effect of peripheral blood progenitor cells mobilised by G-CSF (filgrastim) on platelet recovery after high-dose chemotherapy. *Lancet*, **339**:640.

Siena S, *et al.* (1991). Flow cytometry for clinical estimation of circulating haematopoietic progenitors for autologous transplantation in cancer patients. *Blood*, **77**:400.

Skovsgaard T, Brinckmeyer LM, Vesterager L, Thiede T, Nissen NI (1981). The liver in Hodgkin's disease—I Histopathologic findings. *European Journal of Cancer and Clinical Oncology*, **18**:429–35.

Slanina J, Musshoff K, Rahner R, Stiasny P (1977). Long-term effects in irradiated patients with Hodgkin's disease. *International Journal of Radiation Oncology—Biology—Physics*, **2**:1–19.

Smith RE Jr, Adler RA, Clark P, Brinck-Johnsen T, Tulloh ME, Colton T (1981). Thyroid function after mantle irradiation in Hodgkin's disease. *Journal of the American Medical Association*, **245**:46–9.

Specht L, Nissen NI (1988). Hodgkin's disease stages I and II with infra-diaphragmatic presentation: a rate and prognostically unfavourable combination. *European Journal of Haematology*, **40**:396–402.

Specht L, Nordentoft AM, Cold S, Clausen NT, Nissen NI (1988). Tumour burden as the most important prognostic factor in early stage Hodgkin's disease. *Cancer*, **61**:1719.

Speiser B, Rubin P, Casarett G (1973). Aspermia following lower truncal irradiation in Hodgkin's disease. *Cancer*, **82**:692–8.

Stein RS, *et al.* (1982). Anatomic substages of stage IIIA Hodgkin's disease: follow up of a collaborative study. *Cancer Treatment Reports*, **66**:733–41.

Stein H, Hansmann ML, Lennert K, Brandtzaeg P, Gatter KC, Mason DY (1988). Reed–Sternberg and Hodgkin's cells in lymphocyte predominant Hodgkin's disease of nodular subtype contains J chains. *American Journal of Clinical Pathology*, **12**:9–21.

Stewart JR, Fajardo LF (1971). Dose response in human and experimental radiation-induced heart disease. *Radiology*, **99**:403–8.

Stoffel TJ, Cox JD (1977). Hodgkin's disease stage I and II. A comparison between two different treatment policies. *Cancer*, **40**:90–7

Sutcliffe SB (1985). Treatment of neoplastic disease during pregnancy: maternal and fetal effects. *Clinical and Investigative Medicine*, **8**:333–8.

Sutcliffe SB (1987). Infertility and gonadal function in Hodgkin's disease. In *Hodgkin's disease* (ed. P Selby and TJ McElwain), pp. 339–60. Blackwell, Oxford.

Sutcliffe SB, Timothy AR (1987). Treatment of Hodgkin's disease. *Baillière's Clinical Haematology*, **1.1**:109–40.

Sutcliffe SB, Wrigley PFM, Smyth JF, Webb JAW, Tucker AK, Beard MEJ, *et al.* (1976). Intensive investigation in management of Hodgkin's disease. *British Medical Journal*, **11**:1343–7.

Sutcliffe SB, Chapman R, Wrigley PFM (1981). Cyclical combination chemotherapy and thyroid function in patients with advanced Hodgkin's disease. *Medical and Pediatric Oncology*, **9**:439–48.

Sutcliffe SB, *et al.* (1985). Prognostic groups in the management of localized Hodgkin's disease. *Journal of Clinical Oncology*, **3**(3):393–401.

Sweet DL, Rooth DG, Desser MD, Miller JN, Ultmann JE (1976). Avascular necrosis of the femoral head with combination therapy. *Annals of Internal Medicine*, **85**:67–8

Tamura K, Shimaoka K, Friedman M (1981). Thyroid abnormalities associated with treatment of malignant lymphoma. *Cancer*, **47**:2704–11.

Thar TL, Million RR, Hausner RJ, McKetty MHB (1979). Hodgkin's disease, stage I and II, relationship of recurrence to size of disease, radiation dose and number of sites unsolved. *Cancer*, **43**:1101–5.

Thomas PRM, Winstanly D, Peckham MJ, Austin DE, Murray MAF, Jacobs HS (1976). Reproductive and endocrine function in patients with Hodgkin's disease: effects of oophorepexy and irradiation. *British Journal of Cancer*, **33**:226–31.

Timothy AR, Sutcliffe SB, Stansfeld AG, Wrigley PFM, Jones AE (1978*a*). Radiotherapy in the treatment of Hodgkin's disease. *British Medical Journal*, i:1246–9.

Timothy AR, Tucker AK, Park WM, Cannell LN (1978*b*). Osteonecrosis in Hodgkin's disease. *British Journal of Radiology*, **51**:328–33.

Timothy AR, Sutcliffe SB, Lister TA, Wrigley PFM, Jones AE (1980). The management of stage IIIA Hodgkin's disease. *International Journal of Radiation Oncology—Biology—Physics*, **6**:135–42.

Timothy AR, Van Dyk J, Sutcliffe SB (1987). Radiation therapy for Hodgkin's disease. In *Hodgkin's disease* (ed. P. Selby and TJ McElwain), pp. 181–249. Blackwell, Oxford.

Tiwari JL, Terasaki PI (1985). Hodgkin's disease. In *HLA and disease associations*, pp. 314–20. Springer, New York.

Tubiana M, Henry-Amar M, Hayat M, Breur K, van der Werf-Messing B, Burgers M (1979). Long-term results of the EORTC randomised study of irradiation and vinblastine in clinical stages I and II of Hodgkin's disease. *European Journal of Cancer*, **17**:355–63.

Tubiana M, Hayat M, Henry-Amar M, Breur K, van der Werf-Messing B, Burgers M (1981). Five-year results of the EORTC randomised study of splenectomy and spleen irradiation in clinical stages I and II of Hodgkin's disease. *European Journal of Cancer*, **17**:355–63.

Tubiana M, *et al.* (1984*a*). Prognostic significance of the number of involved areas in the early stages of Hodgkin's disease. *Cancer*, **54**:885–94.

Tubiana M, Henry-Amar M, Burgers M, van der Werf-Messing B, Hayat M. (1984*b*). Prognostic significance of erythrocyte sedimentation rate in clinical stages I–II of Hodgkin's disease. *Journal of Clinical Oncology*, **2**:194–200.

Tubiana M, *et al.* (1984*c*). The EORTC treatment of early stage Hodgkin's disease: the role of radiotherapy. *International Journal of Radiation Oncology—Biology—Physics*, **10**:197–210.

Tubiana M, *et al.* (1985). A multivariate analysis of prognostic factors in early stage Hodgkin's disease. *International Journal of Radiation Oncology—Biology—Physics*, **11**:23–30.

Tubiana M, Cosset JM, Carde P, Amiel JL (1986). The contribution of clinical trials to the treatment of patients with early stages of Hodgkin's disease. *Drugs Experimental and Clinical Research*, **12**:105–12.

Tubiana M, *et al.* (1989). Toward comprehensive management tailored to prognostic factors of patients with clinical stages I and II in Hodgkin's disease. The EORTC lymphoma group controlled clinical trials: 1964–1987. *Journal of Clinical Oncology*, **1**:47–56.

Tura S, Fiacchinni M, Zinzani PL, Brusamolino E, Gobbi PG (1993). Splenectomy and the increasing risk of secondary acute leukaemia in Hodgkin's disease. *Journal of Clinical Oncology*, **11**(5):925–30.

Twomey JJ, Laughter AH, Rice L, Ford R (1980). Spectrum of immunodeficiencies with Hodgkin's disease. *Journal of Clinical Oncology*, **66**:629–37.

University of Texas, M.D. Anderson Hospital and Tumour Institute at Houston (1986). *Cancer Bulletin*, **38**(6).

Valagussa P, Santoro A, Fossate-Bellani F, Banti A, Bonadonna G (1986). Second acute leukemia and other malignancies following treatment for Hodgkin's disease. *Journal of Clinical Oncology*, **4**:830–7.

Van Leeuwen FE, Somers R, Hart AAM (1987). Splenectomy in Hodgkin's disease and second leukaemias. *Lancet*, ii:210–11.

Vaughan-Hudson B, MacLennan KA, Easterling MJ, Jelliffe AM, Vaughan-Hudson G, Haybittle JL (1983). The prognostic significance of age in Hodgkin's disease. Examination of 1500 patients. *Clinical Radiology*, **34**:503–4.

Vianna NJ, Greenwold P, Davies JNP (1971). Extended epidemic of Hodgkin's disease in high school students. *Lancet*, i:1209–11.

Vigersky RA, Chapman RM, Berenberg J, Glass AR (1982). Testicular dysfunction in untreated Hodgkin's disease. *Journal of the American Medical Association*, **73**:482–5.

Viviani S, Santoro A, Ragni G, Bonfante V, Bestetti O, Bonadonna G (1985). Gonadal toxicity after combination chemotherapy for Hodgkin's disease. *European Journal of Cancer and Clinical Oncology*, **21**:601–5.

Viviani S, Santoro A, Negretti E, Bonfante V, Valagussa P, Bonadonna G (1990). Salvage chemotherapy in Hodgkin's disease. Results in patients relapsing after twelve months from first complete remission. *Annals of Oncology*, **1**(2):123–7.

Wagstaff J, Gregory WM, Swindell R, Crowther D, Lister TA (1988). Prognostic factors for survival in stage IIIB and IV Hodgkin's disease: a multicentre analysis comparing two specialist treatment centres. *British Journal of Cancer*, **58**:487–92.

Watanabe S, Brown C, Young J (1986). Cumulative incidence rates for Hodgkin's disease and other haematologic malignancies with special reference to age-related carcinogenesis. *Japanese Journal of Cancer Research*, **77**:743–74.

Waxman JH, *et al.* (1987). Failure to preserve fertility in patients with Hodgkin's disease. *Cancer Chemotherapy and Pharmacology*, **19**:159–62.

Weiss LM, Movahed LA, Warnke RA, Sklar J (1989). Detection of Epstein–Barr viral genomes in Reed Sternberg cells of Hodgkin's disease. *New England Journal of Medicine*, **320**:502–6.

Whitehead E, Shalet SM, Blackledge G, Todd I, Crowther D, Beardwell CG (1982). The effects of Hodgkin's disease and combination chemotherapy on gonadal function in the adult male. *Cancer*, **49**:418–22.

Whitehead E, Shalet SM, Blackledge G, Todd I, Crowther D, Beardwell CG (1983). The effect of combination chemotherapy on ovarian function in women treated for Hodgkin's disease. *Cancer*, **52**:988–93.

Wiernik PH, Gustafson J, Schimpff SC, Diggs C (1979). Combined modality treatment of Hodgkin's disease confined to lymph nodes. *American Journal of Medicine*, **67**:183–93.

Yarnold JR, Jelliffe AM, Vaughan-Hudson G (1982). Patterns of relapse following radiotherapy for Hodgkin's disease. *Clinical Radiology*, **33**:137–40.

Ziegler JL, Fass L, Bluming AZ, Magrath IT, Templeton AC (1972). Chemotherapy of childhood Hodgkin's disease in Uganda. *Lancet*, **ii**:679–82.

Zittoun R, *et al.* (1985). Extended versus unsolved field irradiation combined with MOPP chemotherapy in early clinical stages of Hodgkin's disease. *Journal of Clinical Oncology*, **3**:207–14.

Zittoun R, *et al.* (1987). Association d'epirubicine, bleomycine, vinblastine et prednisolone (EBVP) avant radiotherapie dans les stades localises de la maladie de Hodgkin. Essai de phase II. *Bulletin du Cancer*, **74**:151–7.

12.6.3 Hodgkin's disease in children

JAMES S. MALPAS

INTRODUCTION

Hodgkin's disease is uncommon in children and forms only approximately 5 per cent of childhood malignancy. The disease differs from that seen in adults in a number of ways, for it is frequently less advanced at presentation, is less often symptomatic, and is almost invariably highly responsive to treatment. So successful is management that both investigation and treatment have tended to become less aggressive recently in order to spare the child the unwanted long-term toxic effects that may be produced. The situation is very similar to that now seen in long-term management of Wilms' tumour. Treatment strategies to reduce the risk of second malignant neoplasms and damage to various organs, such as the ovary and testes, thyroid, lungs, and heart, must now be a first priority.

EPIDEMIOLOGY

Hodgkin's disease is not a common tumour in childhood. It is exceedingly rare before the age of 5, but after that there is a steady increase in incidence. If it is considered that in most populations there is an incidence of new cases of childhood cancer of 100–150 cases per million children per year, then the age-standardized rates of Hodgkin's disease in 23 population-based series from America, Asia, and Europe are not only low but very variable. The age-standardized rates given in Fig. 1 show the variation from 1–10 per million (Parkin *et al.* 1988).

The highest rates are seen in two groups of children: those in Costa Rica and the Hispanics of Los Angeles. This high rate is not seen in all Hispanic children—the rates for Puerto Rico are similar to those for White children. The second-highest rate is seen in the

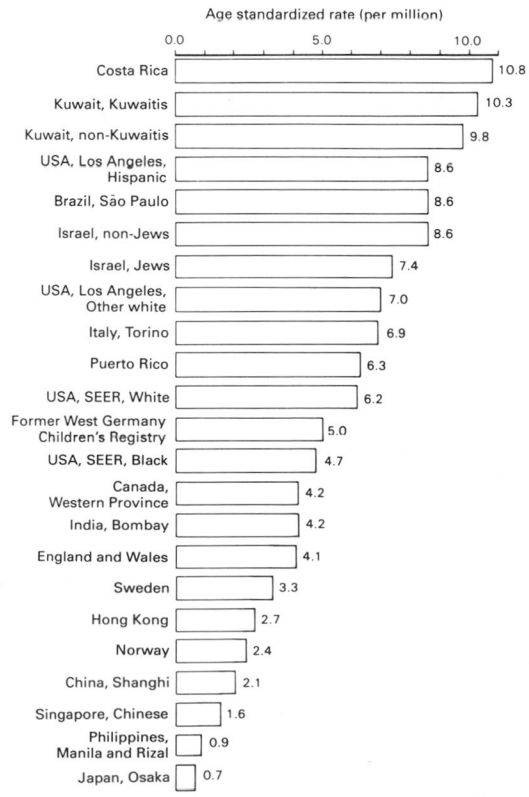

Age standardized rate (per million)

Costa Rica	10.8
Kuwait, Kuwaitis	10.3
Kuwait, non-Kuwaitis	9.8
USA, Los Angeles, Hispanic	8.6
Brazil, São Paulo	8.6
Israel, non-Jews	8.6
Israel, Jews	7.4
USA, Los Angeles, Other white	7.0
Italy, Torino	6.9
Puerto Rico	6.3
USA, SEER, White	6.2
Former West Germany Children's Registry	5.0
USA, SEER, Black	4.7
Canada, Western Province	4.2
India, Bombay	4.2
England and Wales	4.1
Sweden	3.3
Hong Kong	2.7
Norway	2.4
China, Shanghi	2.1
Singapore, Chinese	1.6
Philippines, Manila and Rizal	0.9
Japan, Osaka	0.7

Fig. 1 Age-standardized rate for the incidence of Hodgkin's disease in childhood in different nationalities.

Table 1 Annual incidence of childhood malignancy in various populations per 10^6

Lymphoma	Manchester Children's Tumour Registry	US White	US Black	Japan	Australia	Sweden
Non-Hodgkin's lymphoma	4.6	6.3	6.4	3.8	7.2	8.5
Hodgkin's disease	3.7	5.8	6.0	0.5	6.2	3.2
Total leukaemia and lymphoma	41.4	44.4	39.1	47.4	43.6	37.1

After Birch (1983).

Middle East. The incidence is high for both Kuwaitis and non-Kuwaitis in that area and high values are also noted in Turkish children. In the White Caucasian populations of North America and Europe, the incidence is higher in the warmer southern-most countries and lower in Canada and Scandinavia (Parkin *et al.* 1988).

The worldwide total incidence of lymphoid malignancies including Hodgkin's disease, non-Hodgkin's lymphoma, and acute lymphoblastic leukaemia, remains fairly constant (Table 1) (Birch 1983). Thus, while there is a low incidence of lymphoma in Japan, the incidence of lymphatic leukaemia brings the total to 47 per million of the population, similar to that for the total incidence in the United States.

In these countries, Hodgkin's disease (as well as non-Hodgkin's lymphoma and acute leukaemia) is more common in males than in females. In Western nations, the ratio is approximately 2:1, although this varies. Robinson *et al.* (1984) found a ratio of 2.3:1 in British children; Padmalatha *et al.* (1982) recorded a 1.5:1 ratio, but they had more patients in the adolescent range. Jacobs *et al.* (1984), reporting a 10 year experience in South Africa, described one of the highest male to female ratios at 4.4:1, but their patients were of mixed ancestral stock. As puberty approaches the ratio gradually decreases and in late adolescence it achieves the almost equal distribution seen in adults, particularly in developed countries. This pattern of increasing incidence with age is not seen over the whole world. If the incidence is examined in the three quinquennia of childhood (0–4 years, 5–9 years, and 10–14 years), there is a peak of incidence in the 5–9 years age group for series from the developing countries.

The incidence of Hodgkin's disease in children living in towns resembles that of developed countries, with a relatively late onset, while in urban areas the disease is seen more frequently in the 5–9 years age group (Hirayama *et al.* 1980).

There has been a 3-fold increase in the incidence of Hodgkin's disease in Connecticut, United States, in both sexes aged 15–19 years and in females aged 10–14 years over the period 1935–1979 (Van Hoff *et al.* 1988). This increase has been reported in the United States, Eastern Europe, and Japan (Breslow and Langholz 1983).

A number of problems are posed by the epidemiology of Hodgkin's disease. The greater number of males affected, the variation in the geographical distribution, and the persistent increase in incidence have no explanation at the present time. If an infective agent were responsible, increasing incidence should affect both sexes equally. The difference between the urban and rural incidence and the geographical differences would argue for an environmental factor.

PATHOLOGY IN CHILDREN

The same major types of lymph node pathologies are seen in children as in adults. Reed–Sternberg cells and large mononuclear Hodgkin cells are found in childhood and adolescent nodes affected by the disease (Fig. 2). There is considerable variation in the cellular

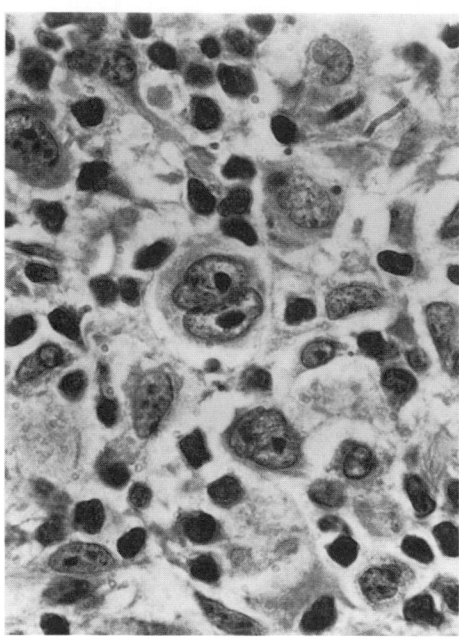

Fig. 2 Photograph showing classical binucleate giant cells of the Reed–Sternberg variety in a lymph node from a child with Hodgkin's disease.

background which defines lymphocytic predominance, nodular sclerosing, mixed cellularity, or lymphocyte depleted of the Rye classification. In children these subgroups vary with age, geographical area, and over the course of several years.

Histopathology and age

In a retrospective study White *et al.* (1983) compared histology in 125 young people aged 1–20 years. They found that in the age range 1–6 years, 21 per cent had lymphocyte predominance Hodgkin's disease compared with only 6 per cent in the 7–20 year old group. No lymphocyte depleted histology was seen in the under 6 years group, but a 5 per cent incidence occurred over this age. Nodular sclerosing Hodgkin's disease was seen in both groups, but was more common in the older children, with an incidence of 75 per cent compared with 50 per cent. In a study of 212 children presenting in Bombay, Dinshaw *et al.* (1989) again found no lymphocyte depleted disease in patients under 4 years old, but the incidence rose to 14 per cent in the 10–14 years age group. Nodular sclerosing Hodgkin's disease doubles its frequency from 6 per 96 children aged 5–9 years to 12 per 98 children aged 10–14 years. Lymphocyte predominance and mixed cellularity histology remained approximately equal. In the Surveillance, Epidemiology and End Results (SEER) programme, it was noted that the highest percentage of nodular sclerosing was 65 per cent in White children and the

Table 2   Distribution of histopathological subgroups in Hodgkin's disease in children

	Butler (1969)	Strum et al. (1970)	Teillet et al. (1969)	Chaves et al. (1973)	Poppema et al. (1980)	Norris et al. (1975)	Padmalatha et al. (1982)
No. of patients	58	35	56	14	278	116	89
Age range (years)	4–15	3–10	2–15	5–10	2.8–15	2.5–15	4–20
Lymphocyte predominance (%)	10	17.2	21.5	21.4	23	19	9
Nodular sclerosing (%)	40	62.8	12.5	7.2	38	58	65
Mixed cellularity (%)	34	2.8	53.5	64.0	33.5	21	22
Lymphocyte depleted (%)	12	0	12.5	7.2	4.7	3	1
Unclassified	4	11.3	–	–	–	–	2

After Padmalatha et al. (1982).

lowest incidence was in Hispanics. Conversely, Hispanics had a higher incidence of histology associated with poor prognosis (mixed cellularity and lymphocyte depleted) (Spitz et al. 1986).

Histopathology and geographical site

It has been found that the incidence of Hodgkin's disease in children varies considerably with the area being studied and this is reflected in the type of histopathology. Padmalatha et al. (1982) compared the histopathological subtypes seen in children with Hodgkin's disease in series in the West, the Middle East, the Indian subcontinent, and the Third World. The values are given in Table 2. Children with Hodgkin's disease in the Middle East show a much higher proportion of mixed cellularity and lymphocyte depleted histology than children in the West.

Biology of Hodgkin's disease

No animal model systems are available for testing hypotheses, but Schaadt et al. (1980) have been able to establish cell lines and more recently have successfully cultured cells over a considerable period of time. Previous work in this area was hampered by the difficulty of knowing the origin of the cells grown in culture and there was a question as to whether the cells were actually derived from patients with established Hodgkin's disease. It has been shown (Stein et al. 1982) that Hodgkin and Reed–Sternberg cells consistently express high levels of CD30 antigen. Antibodies can be raised against this antigen, which enables them to be recognized in human tissues. More recently Epstein–Barr virus (EBV) genomes and gene products have been detected in a high proportion of cells expressing CD30+ antigen and, in particular, the Reed–Sternberg cell of Hodgkin's disease. Herbst et al. (1993) conclude that EBV is a prime candidate for the causation of CD30+ lymphomas, including Hodgkin's disease.

CLINICAL PRESENTATION

Hodgkin's disease may be very variable in its presentation in children. In Western clinical practice the majority of children will be relatively well on presentation, with few having fever, sweats, or weight loss of more than 10 per cent. The commonest presentation is an enlarged lymph node in the neck. The node may be noticed by the parents or child and may fluctuate in size when it first presents. Treatment with antibiotics may coincide with regression and give a false sense of security. The gland enlargement is not usually painful, but pain may be present on occasions. Axillary and inguinal lymph node enlargement is much less common in children and relatively few will have either hepatomegaly or splenomegaly at presentation. Lymphadenopathy was the presenting feature in 72 out of 80 children (90 per cent) studied by Robinson et al. (1984) and cervical or supraclavicular lymph nodes occurred in 51 (63 per cent). Thirteen children (16 per cent) had splenomegaly and seven (8 per cent) had hepatomegaly. Only 17 (21 per cent) presented with symptoms of sweating, fever, or weight loss of more than 20 per cent (the so-called B symptoms). Pruritus is relatively uncommon in children. This frequency of symptoms was seen in other series (Parker et al. 1976; White et al. 1983), although in the latter study the older children showed B symptoms more than twice as often as the younger children. Increasing age correlates with presentation at a more advanced stage and an increasing proportion of bad prognostic histology.

The recognition of the classical lymphadenopathy associated with Hodgkin's disease should present no clinical difficulty when an orderly examination of the superficial lymph node sites is carried out. More difficult is the occurrence of lymph node enlargement in the post-nasal space, though a history of nasal obstruction, snoring, or nasal discharge may give an indication. Mediastinal lymph node enlargement may produce symptoms of mediastinal obstruction with breathlessness, dysphagia, facial oedema (particularly in the morning), and exacerbation of the symptoms when the arms are raised above the head or the patient lies down, but physical signs of mediastinal obstruction are often difficult to demonstrate. Occasionally the mediastinal dullness may be widened on percussion and d'Espine's sign or bronchial breathing, heard low over the back posteriorly may be a help. Plain posteroanterior radiographs, with lateral views, are usually sufficient to diagnose the presence of a mediastinal mass. In children, it must not be forgotten that a mass in the anterior mediastinum may be a thymus and other conditions that should be considered are the presence of cysts, ductus arteriosus aneurysms, intrathoracic liver, and, very rarely, neuromas or malignant thyroid tumours. Ultrasound may be very helpful in differentiating here, but it must be remembered that nodular sclerosing Hodgkin's disease may develop cystic spaces.

Differential diagnosis

Enlarged lymph nodes are commonly found in children. This is not surprising, because lymphoid tissue rapidly increases, reaching adult proportions by age 6 years. It exceeds the amount found in adults until puberty, when lymphoid tissue starts to decline. Therefore, lymph node enlargement is common in children and may be prominent even after quite trivial infection.

Acute bacterial infections of the pharynx, tonsils, and middle ear with staphylococci and streptococci should present no difficulty. In children of Asian origin, tuberculous infection must be considered. Viral infections include infectious mononucleosis due to Epstein–Barr virus, a recent contretemps with a cat in which the child has been bitten or scratched should suggest cat scratch disease, and lymph node enlargement is common in varicella or rubella. Protozoal and fungal infections such as toxoplasma, toxocara, or histoplasmosis are relatively rare in Britain.

In children on long-term anticonvulsant therapy, especially phenytoin, large lymph nodes with the consistency of those seen in Hodgkin's disease are not uncommon. The cause is obscure. Sarcoidosis and sinus histiocytosis with massive lymphadenopathy will usually only be diagnosied on biopsy.

Other neoplastic conditions seen in children which need to be considered in the differential diagnosis are of course non-Hodgkin's lymphoma, acute lymphoblastic leukaemia, neuroblastoma appearing as a late manifestation of disease, and the non-neoplastic Langerhans cell histiocytosis.

INVESTIGATION

Haematology

A blood examination including haemoglobin, total white-cell count, differential platelet count, and erythrocyte sedimentation rate should be carried out. In the early stages of the disease, particularly in children, anaemia or perturbation of the white count is unusual. Anaemia in Hodgkin's disease is not necessarily due to bone-marrow infiltration, but may be due to haemodilution, mild chronic red cell destruction, or occasionally a frank Coombs-positive haemolytic anaemia (Wrigley et al. 1973). Bone-marrow examination is rarely helpful. Aspirates virtually never show Hodgkin's pathology. Bone-marrow trephine is the only procedure likely to be helpful. Robinson et al. (1984), in reviewing 72 marrow trephines, found only one unequivocally positive and in that patient the stage was not altered as the child already had liver involvement. In a study of the erythrocyte sedimentation rate, comparing levels of copper and the copper-binding protein caeruloplasmin, Margerison and Mann (1985) found elevated levels of the erythrocyte sedimentation rate in some children with Hodgkin's disease. They concluded that the erythrocyte sedimentation rate was as sensitive as and much more easily performed than the other tests and that it correlated well with disease activity.

Biochemistry

Abnormalities in liver function tests may be seen in Hodgkin's disease in the absence of liver infiltration. The alkaline phosphatase may be raised, but it is important to note that in children this is likely to be due to the raised isoenzyme associated with bone growth and does not necessarily imply liver involvement. Table 3 shows that a high level of alkaline phosphatase is seen throughout childhood, but rapidly falls during the middle teens to the adult range of values. Occasionally a raised uric acid level is seen and hypercalcaemia is also rare.

Table 3 Serum alkaline phosphatase in children and adults

	International units
Infant	50–155
Child	20–150
Adult	20–70

⁔lson (1987).

Renal function is usually normal, but it should always be investigated as some drugs used in therapy may be excreted by the kidneys and it would be advisable to know if there is any renal impairment.

Radiology

Radiology is essential for delineating the extent of disease, monitoring the course and response to therapy, and detecting early recurrence. This is just as true in children as in adults, but there are some difficulties in the radiological assessment of children. The complete radiological assessment of the child should include radiology of the post-nasal space, since the majority of children present with disease in the cervical region, making it important to assess involvement of Waldeyer's ring clinically and radiologically. However, many pre-pubertal children have adenoidal enlargement and when in doubt the masses should be biopsied.

Children presenting particularly with nodular sclerosing pathology are likely to have mediastinal gland enlargement. Mediastinal shadowing may be seen in normal children and is due to thymic enlargement. The shape and size of the thymic mass, with waviness of the lateral border and a sail-like configuration, enable it to be recognized. CT scanning has proved to be of great value in children, often detecting mediastinal abnormality in the presence of a normal chest radiograph (Cohen et al. 1986).

Because it is non-invasive, abdominal CT scanning has been extensively employed in children. Young children may need to be sedated during the procedure. The lack of mesenteric and retroperitoneal fat in children decreases the contrast between tissues and may produce false-positive and false-negative results. The investigation may need to be supplemented by lymphangiography. The success of this tedious and difficult investigation is frequently a measure of the frequency with which a department employs the technique. A skilled operator who is practised in its performance in children will obtain adequate lymphograms in a high percentage of cases (Filler et al. 1975).

Accuracy of interpretation is varied in children. False-positive results were reported in more than one in four investigations in some series. Lymphangiography is contraindicated in children with bronchial asthma or a large mediastinal mass.

Ultrasound

Ultrasound in children has not been of the same value as CT scanning, but it has been useful as a non-invasive and simple method of determining resolution in the size of tumour mass. Occasionally it has been helpful in detecting nodular infiltration in the liver or spleen, but its value depends on the sophistication of the equipment and the skill of the operator.

Radioisotope scanning

Radioisotope imaging has a limited role in investigating childhood Hodgkin's disease. The main use now would appear to be in addressing the difficult problem of residual mediastinal or abdominal lymphadenopathy after chemotherapy and/or radiotherapy. It is not uncommon for a child to be left with definite mediastinal shadowing, for example and apart from biopsy there is no way except for follow-up of knowing whether this represents active disease. Weiner et al. (1989) found ⁶⁷Ga scans to be an accurate test for defining complete remission in a study of 46 children. In seven of these children with a positive CT scan but a negative ⁶⁷Ga scan, biopsy of the mediastinal mass was negative for Hodgkin's disease in all cases.

Staging laparotomy

The decision to use radiotherapy alone for treating Hodgkin's disease requires lymphangiography and laparotomy for accurate delineation of disease. This approach has been adopted at some time by nearly all units involved in the management of childhood Hodgkin's disease (Lanzkowsky *et al.* 1976; Wilimas *et al.* 1980; Malpas 1982; Schneeberger and Girvan 1988). In a review by Green *et al.* (1983) of 272 children treated at seven institutions, there was an upgrading to pathological stage III in approximately one-third of stage I and stage II patients. In Stanford and Boston, almost half the children considered to be clinical stage III patients were surgically downstaged (Filler *et al.* 1975; Schneeberger and Girvan 1988). However, the alterations in staging following pathological staging accorded closely with those seen in adults. With its proven ability to produce more accurate staging of disease, why has laparotomy become a matter of controversy in children?

With experience, it is evident that splenectomy probably confers a lifelong susceptibility to severe overwhelming bacterial infections with capsulated organisms. These infections may be rapid and fatal. An early review by Chilcote *et al.* (1976) suggested that septicaemia and meningitis occurred in 18 out of 200 children with Hodgkin's disease who had been splenectomized. Eight children died, giving a mortality of 4 per cent. Green *et al.* (1979), reviewing the experience in Buffalo, New York State, recorded an incidence of 16.6 per cent in children who had had splenectomy compared with 6.2 per cent in those who had not. Wilimas *et al.* (1980), in a series of 30 splenectomized children, noted that one died from pneumococcal sepsis, giving a 3 per cent overall mortality. In the series examined by Robinson *et al.* (1984), bacterial infection was seen in nine episodes in five patients who had had splenectomy, and in four episodes in three patients who had not (Table 4). The incidence is strikingly different and statistically significant. Susceptibility to virus infection was not seen. Many of the children reported in these series were on prophylactic penicillin (although, of course, compliance cannot be assessed).

Protagonists of laparotomy consider that the intensity of chemotherapy is responsible for the high infection rate and mortality (Green *et al.* 1979; Donaldson and Kaplan 1982) and they suggest that with the increasing tendency to reduce the amount of treatment given, these infections should no longer be seen. Furthermore, the use of prophylactic penicillin and pneumococcal vaccines will further reduce mortality, especially if vaccination is given before splenectomy. However, doubts have been cast on the value of vaccination (Donaldson *et al.* 1981). Despite these measures, deaths are still occurring in splenectomized Hodgkin's patients and in a condition where in the early stages long-term survival is now reaching a figure of 90–95 per cent, a 4 or 5 per cent mortality from a staging procedure is not acceptable.

Rosenberg (1988) has commented that there appears to be an association between splenectomy and the occurrence of second acute leukaemia in children. Meadows *et al.* (1989) have noted an increase in second malignancy in children subjected to splenectomy.

A novel means of trying to avoid the long-term consequences of splenectomy is to undertake partial splenectomy. This is done when the spleen at laparotomy appears to be normal in size and exhibits no nodules. The inferior splenic vessels are ligated and the discoloured lower portion of the spleen is removed, with haemostasis being achieved by electrocoagulation and by oversewing and applying a mentum to the cut surface. Experience with this procedure is limited and the questions that need to be answered are about the number and frequency of false-negative results and whether the amount of splenic tissue left does protect the patient from sepsis. At the present time no definite statement can be made about the efficacy of this procedure (Hoekstra and Kamps 1989). The greatest influence leading to the avoidance of laparotomy and splenectomy is the feeling that both extensive radiotherapy and intensive chemotherapy are unnecessary in children. If modified lower doses of radiotherapy or indeed no radiotherapy at all can be combined with lower doses of effective non-toxic chemotherapy regimens, why subject the child to a potentially hazardous staging manoeuvre? The balance of therapeutic options will be considered in more detail under Therapy. Finally, it should be mentioned that laparotomy is not without its immediate risks in that there is an incidence of adhesion formation and consequent intestinal obstruction.

STAGING SYSTEM

The Ann Arbor system is generally accepted as applicable to children and is widely used (Carbone *et al.* 1971) (Table 5).

The absence or presence of fever, night sweats, and/or unexplained loss of 10 per cent or more of the body weight in the 6 months preceding admission are denoted by the suffix letters A or B, respectively. Whilst generally understood, there has been debate about the suffix E and for practical purposes this can be

Table 4 Risk of bacterial infection in children with Hodgkin's disease

	Splenectomy	No splenectomy
	27	53
No. of episodes	9	4
No. of children	5	3
Risk of infection	0.33	0.08

After Robinson (1984).

Table 5 Ann Arbor staging classification of Hodgkin's disease

Stage I	Involvement of a single lymph node region (I) or of a single extralymphatic organ or site (IE)
Stage II	Involvement of two or more lymph node regions on the same side of the diaphragm (II) or localized involvement of an extralymphatic organ or site and of one or more lymph node regions on the same side of the diaphragm (IIE)
Stage III	Involvement of lymph node regions on both sides of the diaphragm (III), which may also be accompanied by localized involvement of an extralymphatic organ or site (IIIE) or by involvement of the spleen (IIIS) or both (IIISE)
Stage IV	Diffuse or disseminated involvement of one or more extralymphatic organs or tissues with or without associated lymph node enlargement

Each stage is subdivided into A and B categories

A	No systemic symptoms
B	Unexplained weight loss greater than 10 per cent of the body weight in the previous 6 months and/or unexplained fever with temperatures above 38 °C and/or night sweats

defined as that the additional local involvement is not so large that it cannot be encompassed by a radiotherapy field.

Subsequently tumour bulk has been a factor and this has been shown to be of prognostic significance. For example, mediastinal masses over one-third of the maximal thoracic diameter are considered to be unfavourable, with a liability to increased relapse rate (Mauch *et al.* 1983; Dorreen *et al.* 1984; Robinson *et al.* 1984). The influence of mediastinal masses greater than one-third of the chest width and of tumour mass above 10 cm and their deleterious effect on prognosis, has been recognized in the Cotswold Classification (Lister and Crowther 1990), which adds an extra suffix X for these features.

TREATMENT

It is important at the outset to define the population being discussed when considering treatment options. In early Hodgkin's disease the rate of response is so high and the freedom from recurrence so great in children, adolescents, and adults that the treatment employed is now more likely to be determined by the side-effects, particularly in the long-term and it is therefore important to distinguish these three age groups. The factors influencing decisions in children, where growth and development are at a high priority, are obviously different from those in the adolescent, who has virtually finished growing and the adult. The adolescent, who is at the beginning of sexual activity, marriage, and parenthood, will need different consideration compared with the adult who has completed a family. Consideration of the type of regimen and its likelihood of producing a second malignant neoplasm will be necessary in all three age groups.

At one time, on no very good evidence, it was said that children with Hodgkin's disease did less well than adults (Strum and Rappaport 1970; Young *et al.* 1973). This has now been proved incorrect and probably the reverse is true. Treatment of children largely reflected that used in adults until fairly recently. Radiotherapy has been used to treat children since the 1920s, with improved survival in children and adults where extended field irradiation was used (Gilbert 1939; Peters 1955; Kaplan 1962).

Single-agent chemotherapy was shown to be effective in inducing a response even in disseminated Hodgkin's disease and successive single agents such as nitrogen mustard, vinblastine, cyclophosphamide, and procarbazine became available in the late 1940s and 1950s. Although approximately half the patients had complete or good partial responses, long-term survival was still less than 10 per cent. The use of chlorambucil and vinblastine together (Lacher and Durant 1965) and, subsequently, four drugs (nitrogen mustard, vincristine, prednisolone, and procarbazine (MOPP)) by DeVita *et al.* (1970), introduced a new era in the management of disseminated Hodgkin's disease.

Treatment with radiotherapy

Initial therapy for Hodgkin's disease should be planned with curative intent. Age, stage of disease, amount of tumour present, and complications of therapy must be considered. Radiotherapy may be the treatment of choice in some young people. Many people would agree that adolescents or young adults who are fully grown and who have disease at an early stage are best treated with high dose extended-field radiotherapy using megavoltage irradiation from a linear accelerator. A good case can also be made for treating solitary high neck presentation of favourable histology disease, such as lymphocyte proliferative histology or solitary axillary or inguinal node disease, with high-dose involved-field irradiation.

Experience with involved- and extended-field irradiation in younger children is available. Involved-field irradiation was used by Jereb *et al.* (1984) to treat 57 children with pathological stage I and IIA disease. At median follow-up of just 4 years, there was a relapse-free survival of 71 per cent and survival of 96 per cent from successful salvage. Other series have shown extension to other sites in nearly 50 per cent after involved-field irradiation (Hagemeister *et al.* 1982; Russell *et al.* 1984; Rosenberg 1988). With the exceptions quoted above of solitary high cervical or small local single lymph node sites of good histological type, involved-field irradiation must be considered to have failed.

Extended-field irradiation, however, has a good reputation for producing long-term disease-free survival. Mauch *et al.* (1983) reported on 50 children with pathological stage IA and IIA disease followed for a median of over 5 years, who had a relapse-free survival of 88 per cent and a survival with salvage of 96 per cent. Jenkin and Berry (1980) reported a 57 per cent relapse-free survival and 89 per cent overall survival during a similar period of follow-up. Mauch *et al.* (1983) and Dearth *et al.* (1980) showed that a prime factor in relapse was the presence of significant mediastinal Hodgkin's disease in these children. In the Mayo Clinic series, only 50 per cent of children with mediastinal lymph node enlargement achieved disease-free survival, compared with 95 per cent who had clear chest radiographs.

Subsequent follow-up of children subjected to high-dose extended-field radiotherapy has demonstrated a significant and unacceptable reduction in crown–rump length, contraction of the upper thoracic region with shortening of the clavicles, and loss of tissue mass (Fig. 3). More recently, deterioration of pulmonary function, decreased cardiac function, and abnormality of thyroid function have been well documented in a study of 34 children with a median follow-up of 27.5 months (Mefferd *et al.* 1989).

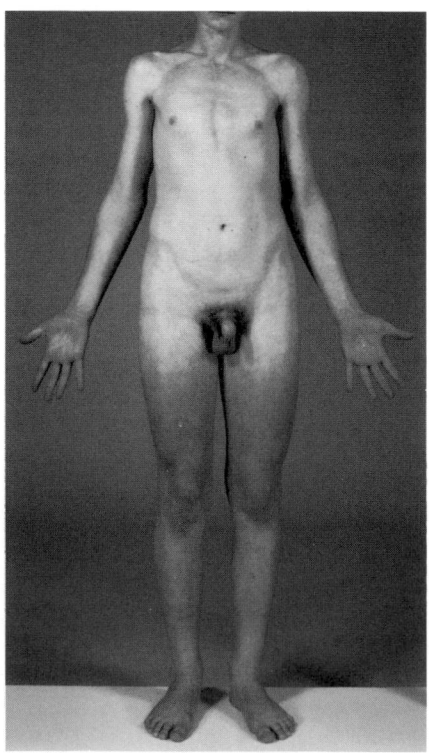

Fig. 3 Illustration of a child treated with mantle irradiation some 10 years previously, resulting in failure of development of the upper thorax and shortening of the clavicles.

In the early 1970s, Probert and Parker (1975) demonstrated that application of 2500 cGy to the spinal column during total node irradiation resulted in significantly less truncal shortening than in those patients treated with the standard 3000–3500 cGy or more. The possibility of combining this radiotherapy dose with chemotherapy could therefore be entertained and will be discussed later.

Chemotherapy

The principles of treatment with chemotherapy have been developed in the management of adult Hodgkin's disease and are equally applicable to children. There is no evidence that children respond less well, nor that the side-effects are more severe. A list of single agents that have been used in children is given in Table 6. It has been shown that single-agent chemotherapy should not be given in adults and this is equally true in children. Combination therapies are curative and, although there is a temptation to spare children the unpleasant immediate side-effects, it must be resisted. A series of effective combinations of proven value is given in Table 7.

A series of effective regimens has been introduced in the last decade or more, including MVPP (Nicholson *et al.* 1970), ABVD (Bonadonna *et al.* 1975), and chlorambucil VPP (Dady *et al.* 1982) (see Table 7 for acronyms).

Studies of combination chemotherapy in children in the late 1970s and early 1980s showed that even with extensive disease a high rate of response and long-term disease-free survival could be achieved (Table 8). Although the individual series are small, cumulative results show a complete response rate of 80 per cent, with a 60 per cent chance of disease-free survival of 9–108 months. The success of these treatments has encouraged the use of chemotherapy alone for all stages of disease. The first reports by Ziegler *et al.* (1972), updated by Olweny *et al.* (1978), recorded the use of MOPP in Ugandan children. Ekert and Waters (1983) reported the use of MOPP chemotherapy in 18 children, 10 of whom had stage I or stage II disease. Six courses were given to eight of the stage I or II patients. Those remaining stage I and II patients and the stage III and IV patients had seven to 12 courses. Complete remission was obtained in 17 of the 18 children. There has been one relapse and one death in complete remission. Actuarial disease-free survival with a median follow-up of 28 months was 80 per cent and survival was 92 per cent. In a follow-up of this very interesting study, Ekert (1989) has now treated 34 children in this manner. The subsequent

Table 6 Effective chemotherapeutic agents in Hodgkin's disease

Alkylating agents
  Nitrogen mustard
  Chlorambucil
  Cyclophosphamide
  Nitrosoureas CCNU and BCNU
  Ifosfamide
Vinca alkaloids
  Vincristine (Oncovin)
  Vinblastine
  Vindesine
Antibiotic antitumour agents
  Doxorubicin
  Bleomycin
Other agents
  Procarbazine
  Imidazole carboxamide (DTIC)
  Etoposide
Methyl glycosaminoglycan

Table 7 Combination chemotherapy for Hodgkin's disease in children

Study	Dose	Route	Frequency
MOPP (Young *et al.* 1973)			
HN$_2$	6 mg/m^2	IV	Days 1 and 8
Vincristine	1.0–1.4 mg/m^2	IV	Days 1 and 8
Procarbazine	100 mg/m^2/day	PO	Days 1–14
Prednisone	40 mg/m^2/day	PO	Days 1–14
14 day cycles separated by 14 day rest periods. Usually 6 cycles. Prednisolone in 1st and 4th cycles only			
MVPP (Nicholson *et al.* 1970)			
HN$_2$	6 mg/m^2	IV	Days 1 and 8
Vinblastine	6 mg/m^2	IV	Days 1 and 8
Procarbazine	100 mg/m^2	PO	Days 1–14
Prednisolone	4 mg/m^2	PO	Days 1–14
14 day cycles separated by 28 day rest periods. Usually 6 or more cycles. Prednisolone given in all cycles			
ABVD (Bonnadonna 1975)			
Adriamycin	25 mg/m^2	IV	Days 1 and 14
Bleomycin	10 mg/m^2	IV	Days 1 and 14
Vinblastine	6 mg/m^2	IV	Days 1 and 14
DTIC	150 mg/m^2	IV	Days 1–5
14 day cycle and 14 day rest periods			
Chl.VPP (Dady *et al.* 1982)			
Chlorambucil	6 mg/m^2/day	PO	Days 1–14
Procarbazine	100 mg/m^2/day	PO	Days 1–14
Prednisolone	40 mg/day	PO	Days 1–14[a]
Vinblastine	6 mg/m^2	IV	Days 1 and 8
14 day cycles with a 14 day rest period			

[a]Reduced appropriately in children.

Table 8 Treatment of advanced Hodgkin's disease in children by combination chemotherapy only

Regimen	No. of children	Response (CR)	Disease-free survival (months)		Authors
MOPP	17	9	6/9	9–66	Young *et al.* (1973)
ChlVPP or MOPP	10	8	7/10	–36	Smith *et al.* (1977)
MOPP	24	25	15/24	12–84	Ziegler *et al.* (1972)
MOPP	8	7	7/8	12–96	Ekert *et al.* (1983)
MOPP	7	5	4/7	72–108	Mauch *et al.* (1983)
Total	66	54 (80%)	39 (59%)	9–108	

16 children have been clinically staged. Some six patients have received ABVD rather than MOPP. Survival for the chemotherapy group as a whole is 88 per cent, with a median follow-up of 52 months and disease-free survival is 83 per cent. Two deaths occurred in stage I patients, one dying from acute graft versus host disease after transfusion. Another patient developed a T-cell acute lymphoblastic leukaemia but has subsequently gone into remission. Jacobs *et al.* (1984), reporting from South Africa on 27 children treated with nitrogen mustard, vinblastine, vincristine, procarbazine, and prednisolone, reported 100 per cent complete remission in the 11 stage I and II patients and a 68 per cent complete remission in the 16 stage III and IV patients. None of the stage I and II patients has relapsed at a median follow-up of 9.5 years. Although the results appear satisfactory, it has to be admitted that these are small selective series and long-term follow-up is lacking. There is increasing

concern that a high incidence of infertility is seen, particularly in the boys, with these programmes which include alkylating agents and procarbazine and there is evidence that this form of chemotherapy is associated with the later development of second malignant neoplasms, in particular acute myelogenous leukaemia (Behrendt *et al.* 1987; Meadows *et al.* 1989).

A search for chemotherapy that might be as effective, but gives a lower incidence of later complications, is being undertaken. The VEEP programme, comprising vinblastine, etoposide, epidaunorubicin and prednisolone, has been used by a British co-operative group. Although a satisfactorily high initial complete response rate of 95 per cent in previously untreated patients was achieved, the number of early relapses, which produced a relapse-free rate of only 67 per cent at 3 years, was unacceptable and this programme is being abandoned (O'Brien *et al.* 1992).

At the present time, the anthracycline-based regimen ABVD appears to have a good response rate, a low relapse rate, and preservation of fertility (Santoro *et al.* 1987), but the long-term effect of anthracyclines on cardiac function is a cause for concern (Lipschultz *et al.* 1991).

Combined modality therapy

The effectiveness of combining radiotherapy and chemotherapy in the treatment of adult patients, together with the pressure to reduce the morbidity from the full therapeutic dose of each modality, has been responsible for a number of series in which chemotherapy has been used in conjunction with radiotherapy in children.

One of the first centres to adopt this approach was St Jude's Children's Research Hospital (Wilimas *et al.* 1980). In reviewing their long-term results in 54 patients at all stages treated with either a mantle or an inverted Y field together with vincristine or cyclophosphamide or with additional procarbazine in later stages, it was found that 38 out of 57 evaluable patients (70 per cent) were in continuous complete remission for 71–130 months. Although laparotomy was included in their staging programme, only one patient was lost from sepsis; a second child died of acute myeloblastic leukaemia. The most striking morbidity was still growth retardation. Jenkin *et al.* (1982) abandoned staging laparotomy, but treated children with low-dose extended-field radiotherapy and MOPP. A complete remission rate of 82 per cent was achieved in 57 patients. Two children died of viral infections. No bacterial infectious deaths occurred and 5 year relapse-free and overall survival rates of 82 per cent and 92 per cent respectively were obtained.

Robinson *et al.* (1984) used chlorambucil, vinblastine, procarbazine, and prednisolone with involved-field radiotherapy in such a way as to tailor the intensity of treatment to the increasing burden of disease. A complete remission rate of 95 per cent was achieved in 80 children and disease-free and overall survival rates at 5 years were 92 per cent and 95 per cent, respectively. Relapses and deaths were almost entirely confined to pubertal girls with mediastinal disease of nodular sclerotic histology. One patient died of pseudomonas septicaemia during the neutropenic phase of the final course of chlorambucil VPP. There have been no major growth abnormalities and at nearly 5 years of follow-up no acute leukaemia has occurred. In all boys tested for fertility so far, complete azoospermia has been noted. Cramer and Andrieu (1985) achieved similar results in 72 children and adolescents, using a similar approach but MOPP chemotherapy. Seventy out of 72 patients achieved a complete remission and the actuarial probabilities for disease-free survival and survival were 87.6 per cent and 91.6 per cent, respectively. Bone growth was not impaired significantly, but

two of these children developed acute myeloblastic leukaemia. More recently, in a very large series of 506 German children under the age of 16 years and employing laparotomy for pathological staging, Schellong and co-workers (Schellong *et al.* 1988; Schellong 1989) have used involved-field radiotherapy, given together with two, four, or six courses of chemotherapy, depending on the stage of disease. The event-free survival for the entire group is 96 per cent at 5 years, 99 per cent for stage I and IIA, 96 per cent for stage IIB and IIIA, and 90 per cent for stage IIIB and IV. In a follow-up of the first group of 170 patients, in whom a complete response rate of 98.8 per cent was achieved, Schellong (1989) reported that seven patients died in complete remission in the 5–17 months after the start of therapy, three with pneumonia, two with septicaemia, one with varicella, and one with a graft versus host reaction to a granulocyte transfusion. All these patients had advanced disease. Ten patients had relapsed by early 1987. No second malignancies have been seen so far. Excellent results have recently been reported using low-dose involved radiotherapy with six cycles of MOPP/ABVD. At a maximum follow-up of 10 years, 96 per cent of 63 children with all stages of Hodgkin's disease were reported cured by Donaldson *et al.* (1993).

Two philosophies emerge quite clearly from these approaches to therapy in children: the first is the use of intensive staging, including laparotomy, followed by extended-field radiotherapy alone or involved-field irradiation with combination chemotherapy; the second is the use of clinical staging only, with involved-field radiotherapy and chemotherapy titrated to the severity of the disease. Randomized studies are never likely to be conducted, so that a comparison of the two approaches, reported by Donaldson *et al.* (1989), is of interest.

The results of treating 171 children with stage I and II Hodgkin's disease at Stanford University Medical Center Children's Hospital in the United States and at St Bartholomew's Hospital, London and the Hospital for Sick Children, Great Ormond Street, London, are detailed. The Stanford approach uses pathological staging, followed by extended-field radiotherapy alone or involved-field irradiation with combination chemotherapy. In the London series, clinical staging, followed by involved or regional field radiotherapy, was given. The two groups of children were remarkably similar. Relapse among the children with stage I disease was more frequent in the London group. However, it is important to note that the survival rate of the two centres at 10 years is exactly the same, at 91 per cent. Analysis of the freedom from relapse in the two groups shows a trend for better results at Stanford (90 per cent), compared with 83 per cent in London, but this was not statistically significant (*p*=0.185). There was remarkably little serious morbidity, with few late effects in either series. There was one fatal bacterial infection in each group, but no fatal viral infections. In the Stanford series there were three malignant tumours which were fatal: a retroperitoneal sarcoma, a gastric carcinoma, and a boy with a thyroid carcinoma and acute lymphoblastic leukaemia. In the London series, a case of myelodysplasia occurred; there was a case of fatal malignant fibrous histiocytoma at the edge of the irradiation field and in another child a thyroid carcinoma was successfully treated and the child is still alive. It is notable that no acute myelogenous leukaemia was seen in either series.

In conclusion, the lessons emerging would seem to be that treatment needs to be individualized. Localized minimal disease of good histological type, patients with massive mediastinal tumours, and extensive bulky disease at numerous sites will need to be addressed separately. Combined modality therapy with or without intensive initial assessment, including laparotomy, produces equally successful long-term results. The emergence of a second generation of combination chemotherapy, which is equally effective but without the risk of second malignant tumours, is now the goal.

Salvage therapy

Excellent response can be expected when children relapse after radiotherapy used as primary treatment. Jereb *et al.* (1984) used low-dose radiotherapy to previously irradiated sites and chemotherapy and were able to produce complete responses in over 90 per cent of the children. Similar results have been found by Mauch *et al.* (1983) and Lange and Littman (1983). Children who have had long remissions on combination chemotherapy and who have relapsed at nodal sites, will usually respond again to a combination chemotherapy containing alkylating agents. Early recurrence, especially at extranodal sites, is much more difficult to treat.

More recent studies in adults have indicated that response and survival rates after MOPP, MVPP, and ABVD are poor, with most patients relapsing. Anthracycline-containing regimens have not been helpful. Methyl GAG, ifosfamide, methotrexate, and etoposide (MIME) has been reported by Hagemeister *et al.* (1987) to give a complete remission rate of 23 per cent and a partial response rate of 40 per cent in a series of 47 patients. Patients with nodal disease alone did best and fared significantly better than those patients with extranodal disease. Even so, long-term results have been unsatisfactory and high-dose chemotherapy using high-dose melphalan supported by allogeneic or autologous bone-marrow transplantation is now being explored.

Most of the literature concerning this difficult clinical situation is related to adult patients. In a recent study of 160 children treated by combined modality therapy at St Bartholomew's Hospital and the Royal Marsden Hospital, London, James *et al.* (1992) found that 35 children (22 per cent) either did not achieve complete remission or subsequently relapsed. The actuarial survival following initial relapse or failure of primary treatment was 60 per cent at 5 years, falling to 45 per cent at 10 years. More than 50 per cent of patients requiring salvage therapy presented within 2 years and only three further relapses occurred after 3 years. It was very evident that patients with drug-resistant aggressive disease who relapsed early, died quickly and this group is best treated by intensive therapy. The second group that did badly were those with indolent relapsing disease who had prolonged survival, but in whom the remissions that were induced were never durable. In these children salvage therapy with high-dose chemotherapy with or without total-body irradiation, supported by bone-marrow transplantation or peripheral blood progenitor cells, appears to offer a possible form of treatment. Anecdotal evidence from a few children with Hodgkin's disease suggests this is possible, but the small numbers and short follow-up make it difficult to form any conclusions at the present time.

COMPLICATIONS OF MANAGEMENT

The main influence on the treatment policies described has been the effect on growth in children. The younger the child, the more severe the effects have been. Although the chief effect has been on bone growth and quite specific changes have followed certain radiation fields, loss of soft tissue has also been a consequence. Wilimas *et al.* (1980), in an assessment of the St Jude programme, recorded growth retardation as a major consequence of chemotherapy combined with mantle and inverted Y radiotherapy. Nearly all the 34 patients assessed, who had been exposed to both types of radiation field in the course of their treatment, were in less than the third percentile for both height and crown–rump lengths. This is confirmed by the experience at Boston, where Mauch *et al.* (1983) reported on similar children and radiation fields, showing that three out of 42 children were more than one standard deviation below the mean height when treated at 9–12 years; however, 19 of the children who were in the 3–16 age range at the time of their treatment with radiotherapy were between one and three standard deviations below the mean sitting height.

There is a need for studies on children treated with combined modality therapy, but the clinical impression is that these children are far more normal in appearance and the soft tissue wasting is also not so apparent.

Table 9 Second neoplasms in survivors of Hodgkin's disease in childhood

Author	Institution	No. of patients treated	Median follow-up (years)	Second malignancies
Radiotherapy treated patients				
Sullivan	MD Anderson	260	?	1 AML, 2 non-Hodgkin's lymphoma 4 thyroid carcinoma 4 sarcomas 1 glioma
Tan	Memorial	108	6	1 AML
Mauch	Joint Center–Harvard	83	5.5	1 AML, 1 sarcoma
Donaldson	Stanford	63	>10	1 thyroid carcinoma
Chemotherapy treated patients				
Olweny	Uganda	48	5	1 non-Hodgkin's lymphoma
Jacobs	South Africa–Capetown	27	7	1 AML
Combined modality patients				
Jenkin	Toronto	110	4.3	2 AML
Donaldson	Stanford	55	7.5	3 AML
Wilimas	St Jude	54	7.5	1 AML
Robinson	St Bartholomew's and Royal Marsden Hospitals	80	4.8	None
Donaldson	Stanford	66	>5	1 non-Hodgkin's lymphoma, 1 AML 2 sarcoma

After Pao and Kun (1989).
AML, acute myeloblastic leukaemia.

Second malignant neoplasms

The most outstanding concern is the occurrence of second malignant neoplasms, particularly leukaemia. Review of large series in children with sufficient length of follow-up shows that the incidence is small, but follow-up is still relatively short and it is possible that the maximum incidence has not yet been reached.

Pao and Kun (1989) have collated the large series available and Table 9 is taken from their summary. It is notable that 11 out of 28 children (nearly 40 per cent) with a second malignant neoplasm had acute myeloblastic leukaemia (AML). There is evidence that the incidence of acute myeloblastic leukaemia is related to alkylating agents. A close correlation was seen with the total quantity of alkylating agent administered: the incidence for high doses was considerably greater than that for low or intermediate doses (Bjergaard *et al.* 1987). In three of the series (Wilimas *et al.* 1980; Lange and Littman 1983; Robinson *et al.* 1984), where combination chemotherapy has been given and where sufficient time for second malignant neoplasms to occur has elapsed, the planned use of chemotherapy in close proximity to radiotherapy has not produced a high incidence of malignant disease.

There is now a need for a second generation of effective chemotherapy combinations that exclude alkylating agents and probably procarbazine.

Endocrine dysfunction

Endocrine dysfunction occurs primarily in the thyroid and gonads after radiation to fields including these sites or after chemotherapy. Biochemical evidence of thyroid dysfunction is seen following mantle irradiation. Elevated levels of thyroid stimulating hormone (TSH) and low levels of thyroxine are seen. Shalet *et al.* (1977) and Mauch *et al.* (1983) reported elevated TSH levels in approximately two-thirds of patients, while T_4 levels were abnormal in very few. Evidence of clinical hypothyroidism is rare: Mauch *et al.* (1983) reported one case and Wilimas *et al.* (1980) found none, but Lange and Littman (1980) found six out of 66 children and adolescents with overt hypothyroidism. In a large series from Stanford, Donaldson and Kaplan (1982) recorded approximately one-third of their patients showing evidence of hypothyroidism as recovering spontaneously.

Gonadal dysfunction has been documented in both adult males and females by Chapman *et al.* (1979) and Waxman *et al.* (1982) and the effects of MOPP chemotherapy on adolescent Ugandan boys with Hodgkin's disease have been described by Sherins *et al.* (1978). In these boys, gynaecomastia, germinal aplasia, increased follicle-stimulating hormone and luteinizing hormone, and decreased serum testosterone developed after MOPP. In most series there are relatively few children who have been investigated for fertility. The number is now growing and in boys treated with regimens containing alkylating agents the finding is that all have either azoospermia or severe oligospermia and recovery is rare (Donaldson and Kaplan 1982; Robinson *et al.* 1984; Shafford *et al.* 1993).

The outlook for girls is better. Donaldson and Kaplan (1982) record that 88 per cent of girls treated with chemotherapy have retained their menses and 12 of them have had 13 pregnancies. Robinson *et al.* (1984) noted that two girls given many courses of chlorambucil VPP had had normal offspring. It would seem that the advice to girls should be to have their families as soon as possible, as an early menopause is likely.

Psychosocial complications

The psychosocial status of large series of survivors of Hodgkin's disease, some of whom were children at the time of their treatment, is recorded in studies by Fabair *et al.* (1986) and that of children and adolescents is reported by Wasserman *et al.* (1987). Among the latter, most retained bad memories of their treatment and its side-effects, but, despite losing schooling, their education levels exceeded those of sex-, age-, and state-matched populations. The major problem they have to face is discrimination in employment and in obtaining health and life insurance. It is worth noting that, in Great Britain, continuous disease-free survival for 10 years after treatment for Hodgkin's disease now enables the subject to be assessed at the normal rates for life insurance.

CONCLUSION

The goal of certain cure of Hodgkin's disease in children is being approached. This is a major advance in what amounts to one professional lifetime. Further attempts will need to be made to find an effective treatment for the small numbers that are either proving non-responders or who relapse early and persistently. A second generation of effective multidrug chemotherapy that is devoid of potential for producing second malignant neoplasms and gonadal damage is needed. Until then, the most effective approach is low-dose in-field radiotherapy combined with chemotherapy, followed by careful assessment and follow-up.

REFERENCES

Behrendt H, van Bunningen BNFM, van Leeuwen EF (1987). Treatment of Hodgkin's disease in children with or without radiotherapy. *Cancer*, **59**:1870–3.

Birch JM (1983). Epidemiology of paediatric cancer. In *Paediatric oncology — recent results in cancer research* (ed. W Duncan), pp. 1–10. Springer-Verlag, Berlin

Bjergaard J, *et al.* (1987). Risk of therapy related leukaemia and preleukaemia after Hodgkin's disease. *Lancet*, **ii**:83–7.

Bonadonna G, Zucali R, Monfardini S, Delena M, Uslenghi C (1975). Combination chemotherapy of Hodgkin's disease with adriamycin, bleomycin, vinblastine and imidazole carboxamide versus MOPP. *Cancer*, **36**:252–9.

Breslow NE, Langholz B (1983). Childhood cancer incidence: geographic and temporal variations. *International Journal of Cancer*, **32**:703–16.

Carbone PP, Kaplan HS, Musshoff K, Smithers DW, Tubiana M (1971). Report of the Committee on Hodgkin's Disease Staging Classification. *Cancer Research*, **31**:1860–1.

Chapman RM, Sutcliffe SB, Malpas JS (1979). Cytotoxic induced ovarian failure in women with Hodgkin's disease. *Journal of the American Medical Association*, **242**:1877–81.

Chilcote RR, Baehner RL, Hammond D (1976). Septicaemia and meningitis in children splenectomised for Hodgkin's disease. *New England Journal of Medicine*, **295**:798–800.

Cohen MD, Siddiqui A, Weetman R (1986). Hodgkin's disease and non-Hodgkin's lymphoma in children. Utilization of radiological modalities. *Radiology*, **158**:499–505.

Cramer P, Andrieu J (1985). Hodgkin's disease in childhood and adolescence. Results of chemotherapy-radiotherapy in clinical stages IA–IIB. *Journal of Clinical Oncology*, **3**:1495–1502.

Dady PJ, McElwain TJ, Austin DE, Barrett A, Peckham MJ (1982). Five years experience with ChlVPP. Effective low toxicity combination chemotherapy for treatment of Hodgkin's disease. *British Journal of Cancer*, **45**:851–9.

Dearth JC, Gilchrist GS, Borget EO, Telander RL, Cupps RE (1980). Management of stage I–III Hodgkin's disease in children. *Journal of Pediatrics*, **96**:829–36.

DeVita VT, Serpik AA, Carbone PP (1970). Combination chemotherapy in the treatment of advanced Hodgkin's disease. *Annals of Internal Medicine*, **73**:891–5.

Dinshaw KA, *et al.* (1989). Hodgkin's disease in Indian children. In *Hodgkin's disease in children: controversies and current practice* (ed. WA Kamps, GB Humphrey, and S Poppema), pp. 233–40. Kluwer, Boston.

Donaldson SS, Kaplan HS (1982). Complications of treatment of Hodgkin's disease in children. *Cancer Treatment Reports*, **66**:977–89.

Donaldson SS, Vosti KL, Berberich FR, Cox RS, Kaplan HS, Schiffman G (1981). Response to pneumococcal vaccine among children with Hodgkin's disease. *Reviews of Infectious Diseases (Supplement)*, 3:5133–43.

Donaldson SS, Whitaker SJ, Plowman PN, Link MP, Malpas JS (1990). Stage I–II pediatric Hodgkin's disease: long-term follow-up demonstrates equivalent survival rates following different management schemes. *Journal of Clinical Oncology*, 8:1128–37.

Donaldson SS, Hunger SP, Link MP (1993). Abstract. *Medical and Pediatric Oncology*, 21:543.

Dorreen MS, Wrigley PFM, Laidlow JM (1984). The management of stage II supradiphragmatic Hodgkin's disease at St Bartholomew's Hospital. A retrospective review of 114 previously untreated cases over 14 years. *Cancer*, 54:2882–8.

Ekert H (1989). Treatment of childhood Hodgkin's disease with chemotherapy alone: experiences from the Royal Children's Hospital, Melbourne. In *Hodgkin's disease in children: controversies and current practice* (ed. WA Kamps, GB Humphrey, and S. Poppema), pp. 241–6. Kluwer, Boston.

Ekert H, Waters KD (1983). Results of treatment of 18 children with Hodgkin's disease with MOPP chemotherapy as the only treatment modality. *Medical and Pediatric Oncology*, 11:322–6.

Fabair P, Hoppe RT, Bloom J, Cox R, Varghese A, Spiegel D (1986). Psychosocial problems among survivors of Hodgkin's disease. *Journal of Clinical Oncology*, 4:805–14.

Filler RM, Jaffe N, Cassady JR, Traggis DG, Vawter GF (1975). Experience with clinical and operative staging of Hodgkin's disease in children. *Journal of Pediatric Surgery*, 10:321–8.

Gilbert R (1939). Radiotherapy in Hodgkin's disease (malignant granulomatosis)—anatomic and clinical foundations: governing principles. *American Journal of Roentgenology*, 41:198–241.

Green DM, et al. (1979). The incidence of post-splenectomy sepsis and herpes zoster in children and adolescents with Hodgkin's disease. *Medical and Pediatric Oncology*, 7:284–97.

Green D, et al. (1983). Staging laparotomy and splenectomy in children and adolescents with Hodgkin's disease. *Cancer Treatment Reviews*, 10:23–38.

Hagemeister FB, Fuller LM, Sullivan JA (1982). Treatment of patients with stage I and II non-mediastinal Hodgkin's disease. *Cancer*, 50:2307–13.

Hagemeister FB, et al. (1987). MIME chemotherapy (methyl-GAG, ifosfamide, methotrexate, etoposide) as treatment for recurrent Hodgkin's disease. *Journal of Clinical Oncology*, 5:556–61.

Herbst H, Stein H, Niedobitek G (1993). Epstein–Barr virus and CD30+ malignant lymphoma. *Critical Review in Oncogenesis*, 4:191–239.

Hirayama T, Waterhouse JAH, Fraumeni JF (1980). Cancer risks by site—Hodgkin's disease. In *UICC Technical Report Series* No. 41 (ed. T Hirayama, JAH Waterhouse, and JF Fraumeni), p. 198. International Union Against Cancer, Geneva.

Hoekstra HJ, Kamps WA (1989). Indications for staging laparotomy and partial splenectomy. In *Hodgkin's disease in children: controversies and current practice* (ed. WA Kamps, GB Humphrey, and S. Poppema), p. 121. Kluwer, Boston.

Jacobs P, King HS, Karabos C, Hartley P, Werner D (1984). Hodgkin's disease in children. A ten-year experience in South Africa. *Cancer*, 53:210–13.

James ND, et al. (1992). Outcome of children with resistant and relapsed Hodgkin's disease. *British Journal of Cancer*, 66:1155–8.

Jenkin RDT, Berry MP (1980). Hodgkin's disease in children. *Seminars in Oncology*, 7:202–11.

Jenkin RDT, et al. (1982). Hodgkin's disease in children: treatment results with MOPP and low-dose extended field irradiation. *Cancer Treatment Reports*, 66:949–59.

Jereb B, Tan C, Bretsky S, Shaoquin H, Exelby P (1984). Involved field (IF) irradiation with or without chemotherapy in the management of children with Hodgkin's disedase. *Medical and Pediatric Oncology*, 12:325–32.

Kaplan HS (1962). The radical radiotherapy of regionally-localised Hodgkin's disease. *Radiology*, 78:553–61.

Lacher MJ, Durant JR (1965). Combination vinblastine and chlorambucil therapy of Hodgkin's disease. *Annals of Internal Medicine*, 62:469–76.

Lang G, Littman P (1983). Management of Hodgkin's disease in children and adolescents. *Cancer*, 51:1371–7.

Lanzkowsky P, Shende A, Karayalcin G, Aral I (1976). Staging laparotomy and splenectomy: treatment and complications of Hodgkin's disease in children. *American Journal of Hematology*, 1:393–404.

Lipschultz SE, Colan SD, Gelber RD, Perez-Atayde AR, Sallan SE, Sanders SP (1991). Late cardiac effects of doxorubicin therapy for acute lymphoblastic leukaemia in childhood. *New England Journal of Medicine*, 324:808–15.

Lister TA, Crowther D (1990). Staging for Hodgkin's disease. *Seminars in Oncology*, 17:696–703.

Malpas JS (1982). Lymphomas in children. *Seminars in Hematology*, 19:301–14.

Margerison AC, Mann JR (1985). Serum copper, serum ceruloplasmin, and erythrocyte sedimentation rate measurements in children with Hodgkin's disease, non-Hodgkin's lymphoma and non-malignant lymphadenopathy. *Cancer*, 55:5501–6.

Mauch PM, Weinstein H, Botnick L, Belli J, Cassady JR (1983). An evaluation of long-term survival and treatment complications in children with Hodgkin's disease. *Cancer*, 51:925–32.

Meadows AT, et al. (1989). Second malignant neoplasms following childhood Hodgkin's disease: treatment and splenectomy as risk factors. *Medical and Pediatric Oncology*, 17:477.

Mefferd JM, Donaldson SS, Link MP (1989). Pediatric Hodgkin's disease: pulmonary, cardiac and thyroid function following combined modality therapy. *International Journal of Radiation Oncology—Biology—Physics*, 16:679–85.

Nelson WE (1987). In *Textbook of paediatrics* (ed. RE Behrman, VC Vaughan, and WE Nelson), p. 1552. Saunders, Philadelphia.

Nicholson WM, et al. (1970). Combination chemotherapy in generalized Hodgkin's disease. *British Medical Journal*, 3:7–10.

O'Brien MER, et al. (1992). 'VEEP' in children with Hodgkin's disease—a regimen to decrease late sequelae. *British Journal of Cancer*, 65:756–60.

Olweny CLM, Katongole-Mbidde E, Kiire C, Lwanga SK, Magrath I, Ziegler JL (1978). Childhood Hodgkin's disease in Uganda. *Cancer*, 42:787–92.

Padmalatha C, Ganick DJ, Hafez G-R, Gilbert EF (1982). Hodgkin's disease and non-Hodgkin's lymphoma in children and young adults: a clinicopathologic study of 127 cases. *Medical and Pediatric Oncology*, 10:175–84.

Pao WJ, Kun LE (1989). Hodgkin's disease in children. *Hematology and Oncology Clinics of North America*, 3:345–65.

Parker BR, Castellino RA, Kaplan HS (1976). Pediatric Hodgkin's disease I. *Cancer*, 37:2430–5.

Parkin DM, Stiller CA, Draper GJ, Bieber CA (1988). The International incidence of childhood cancer. *International Journal of Cancer*, 42:511–20.

Peters MV (1955). A study of survival in Hodgkin's disease treated radiologically. *American Journal of Roentgenology*, 63:299–311.

Probert JC, Parker BR (1975). The effects of radiation therapy on bone growth. *Radiology*, 114:155–62.

Robinson R, Kingston JE, Noguera Costa R, Malpas JS, Barrett A, McElwain TJ (1984). Chemotherapy and irradiation in childhood Hodgkin's disease. *Archives of Disease in Childhood*, 59:1162–9.

Rosenberg SA (1988). Exploratory laparotomy and splenectomy for Hodgkin's disease. A commentary (editorial). *Journal of Clinical Oncology*, 6:574–5.

Russell KJ, Donaldson SS, Cox RS, Kaplan HS (1984). Childhood Hodgkin's disease: patterns of relapse. *Journal of Clinical Oncology*, 2:80–7.

Santoro A, et al. (1987). Long term results of combined chemotherapy–radiotherapy approach in Hodgkin's disease, superiority of ABVD versus MOPP plus radiotherapy. *Journal of Clinical Oncology*, 5:27–37.

Schaadt M, Diehl V, Stein H, Fonatch S, Kirchner H (1980). Two neoplastic cell lines with unique features derived from Hodgkin's disease. *International Journal of Cancer*, 26:723–31.

Schellong GM (1989). The German Co-Operative Therapy Studies. An approach to minimise treatment modalities and invasive staging procedures. In *Hodgkin's disease in children: controversies and current practice* (ed. WA Kamps, GB Humphrey, and S. Poppema), p. 277. Kluwer, Boston.

Schellong G, Bramswig JH, Schwarze EW, Wannenmacher M (1988). An approach to reduce treatment and invasive staging in childhood Hodgkin's disease: the sequence of the German DAL multicenter studies. *Bulletin du Cancer*, 74:41–51.

Schneeberger AL, Girvan DP (1988). Staging laparotomy for Hodgkin's disease in children. *Journal of Pediatric Surgery*, 23:714–17.

Shafford EA, et al. (1993). Testicular function following the treatment for Hodgkin's disease in childhood. *British Journal of Cancer*, 68:1199–204.

Shalet SM, Rosenstock JD, Beardwell CG, Pearson D, Jones PH (1977). Thyroid dysfunction following external irradiation to the neck for Hodgkin's disease in childhood. *Clinical Radiology*, **28**:511–15.

Sherins RJ, Olweny CLM, Ziegler JL (1978). Gynaecomastia and gonadal dysfunction in adolescent boys treated with combination chemotherapy for Hodgkin's disease. *New England Journal of Medicine*, **299**:12–16.

Spitz MR, Sider JG, Johnson CC, Butler JJ, Pollack ES, Newell GR (1986). Ethnic patterns of Hodgkin's disease incidence among children and adolescents in the United States 1973–1982. *Journal of the National Cancer Institute*, **76**:235–9.

Stein H, *et al.* (1982). Identification of Hodgkin and Sternberg–Reed cells as a unique cell type derived from a newly-detected small cell population. *International Journal of Cancer*, **30**:445–59.

Strum SB, Rappaport H (1970). Hodgkin's disease in the first decade of life. *Pediatrics*, **46**:748–59.

Van Hoff J, Schymura MJ, Curwen MGM (1988). Trends in the incidence of childhood and adolescent cancer in Connecticut. *Medical and Pediatric Oncology*, **16**:78–87.

Wasserman AL, Thompson EI, Wilimas JA, Fairclough DL (1987). The

psychological status of survivors of childhood/adolescent Hodgkin's disease. *American Journal of Diseases of Childhood*, **141**:626–31.

Waxman JH, *et al.* (1982). Gonadal function in Hodgkin's disease: long term follow up of chemotherapy. *British Medical Journal*, **285**:1612–13.

Weiner M, Leventhal B, Brecher M, Marcus R, Ternberg J (1989). Gallium 67 scans as an adjunct to clinical restaging in pediatric patients with Hodgkin's disease. *Proceedings of the American Society of Clinical Oncology*, **8**:278 (abstract 1085).

White L, Siegel SE, McCourt BA, Stone SM, Isaacs H, Higgin GR (1983). Patterns of Hodgkin's disease at diagnosis in young children. *American Journal of Pediatric Hematology and Oncology*, **5**:251–7.

Wilimas J, Thompson E, Smith KL (1980). Long-term results of treatment of children and adolescents with Hodgkin's disease. *Cancer*, **46**:2123–5.

Wrigley PFM, Hamilton-Fairley G, Matthias JQ (1973). Anaemia and bone marrow involvement in Hodgkin's disease. In *Hodgkin's disease* (ed. D Smithers), pp. 154–63. Churchill-Livingstone, Edinburgh.

Young RC, DeVita VT, Johnson RE (1973). Hodgkin's disease in childhood. *Blood*, **42**:163–74.

Ziegler JL, Bluming AZ, Fass L, Magrath IT, Templeton AC (1972). Chemotherapy of childhood Hodgkin's disease in Uganda. *Lancet*, **ii**:679–80.

12.7.1 The pathology and biology of non-Hodgkin's lymphoma

PETER G. ISAACSON

INTRODUCTION

The term 'non-Hodgkin's lymphoma' is a rather clumsy negative definition, referring as it does to those neoplasms of the lymphoreticular system other than Hodgkin's disease. Although, therefore, the unqualified term 'lymphoma' refers to both Hodgkin's disease as well as non-Hodgkin's lymphoma, for the purposes of brevity this term will be used throughout this chapter, unless otherwise qualified, as indicative of non-Hodgkin's lymphoma. Lymphomas are by definition malignant; although some may be slow growing and clinically indolent, benign lymphomas are not described. The lymphoreticular system includes lymphoid organs such as the lymph nodes, spleen, and thymus, and foci within certain non-lymphoid organs such as the gut, in which lymphocytes are aggregated in an organized fashion. The organization of the lymphocytes is dictated by the reticulin framework and the distribution of blood vessels and lymphatics. Specific accessory cells, most of which are part of the mononuclear/phagocyte system, are integral components of the lymphoreticular system and, rarely, themselves give rise to lymphomas.

Most lymphomas arise in lymph nodes and these are collectively known as nodal lymphomas. Extranodal lymphomas, as their name implies, arise in components of the lymphoreticular system other than lymph nodes, either in lymphoid organs such as the spleen, thymus, or tonsils, in organs that have a lymphoid component, such as the gut, or, less frequently in sites where no native lymphoid tissue is recognized, such as the brain. Although accounting for a minority of lymphomas this minority can be substantial, amounting to 40 per cent in some series (Freeman *et al.* 1972).

The histology, cytology, and biology of lymphoma closely mimic that of normal lymphoid cells and, therefore, an appreciation of the

normal structure and function of lymphoid tissue and of lymphocyte ontogeny is essential for understanding the pathology and biology of lymphomas. As most studies of normal human lymphoid tissue have been aimed at peripheral lymph nodes, where most lymphomas arise, these will be described in some detail here. The properties of extranodal lymphoid tissue are broadly similar, but there are differences that are important in relation to extranodal lymphomas and these will be described before the discussion of extranodal lymphomas.

THE NORMAL LYMPH NODE

As part of the mononuclear/phagocyte system, lymph nodes are strategically placed to serve as filters of the lymph draining from a wide area and to perform the function of immune surveillance. Antigens in the lymph are carried to the nodes, where they are processed by specialized accessory cells that present them to large concentrations of effector cells; that is, the lymphocytes. Although concentrated in the lymph nodes, lymphocytes are constantly recirculating, thus increasing the chances of an encounter with their specific antigen both in lymph nodes and in the body generally.

Histology

The overall structure of the lymph nodes is shown diagramatically in Fig. 1. The lymph node is surrounded by a thin, fibrous capsule from which fibrous trabeculae penetrate the parenchyma, forming an extracellular matrix of collagen fibres. This matrix is probably an important factor in assisting the directional movement of lymphocytes and other cells within the node. The capsule is penetrated by afferent lymphatics, which communicate with the

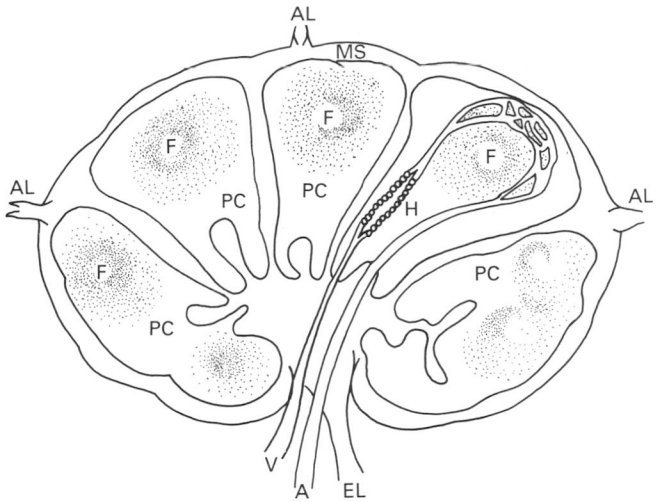

Fig. 1 Diagrammatic representation of a section through a lymph node. AL, afferent lymphatics; MS, marginal sinus; F, follicles; PC, paracortex; H, high endothelial venue; V, vein; A, artery; EL, efferent lymphatics.

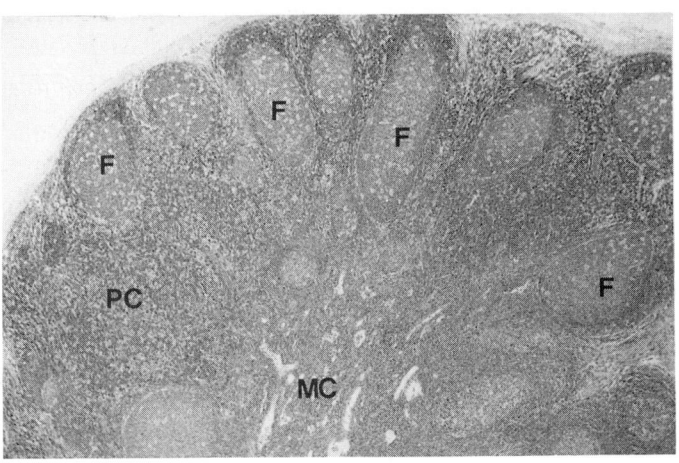

Fig. 2 Low-power photomicrograph of a reactive lymph node; compare with Fig. 1. F, follicles; PC, paracortex; MC, medullary cords.

marginal sinus. From the marginal sinus, cortical sinuses branch off into the node as an arborizing network before being gathered into the large medullary sinuses, which in turn enter the single efferent lymphatic vessel. The sinuses are lined by specialized endothelial cells, which are phagocytic and are traversed by fine collagen bands, which are also covered by these cells. Large numbers of phagocytic macrophages are present within the sinuses, which reinforce their filtering function. The blood supply of the lymph node is usually via a single artery that enters the node at the hilum, forming an arcade of smaller vessels before dividing into arterioles, which then supply the rich capillary network permeating throughout the node. The capillaries drain into the highly characteristic postcapillary venules, also called high endothelial venules after their plump, tall endothelium. These specialized blood vessels, which play an important role in lymphocyte traffic, lose their high endothelium as they enter larger veins in the lymph node medulla, which in turn fuse together at the hilum of the node. The different cells that make up lymphoid tissues are conveniently described in three groups, which, to a certain extent, are situated in different regions of the lymph node. These are the B-cells, T-cells, and accessory cells.

Most of the lymph node B-cells are present in the cortex, where they are concentrated in follicles (Fig. 2). In unstimulated or resting

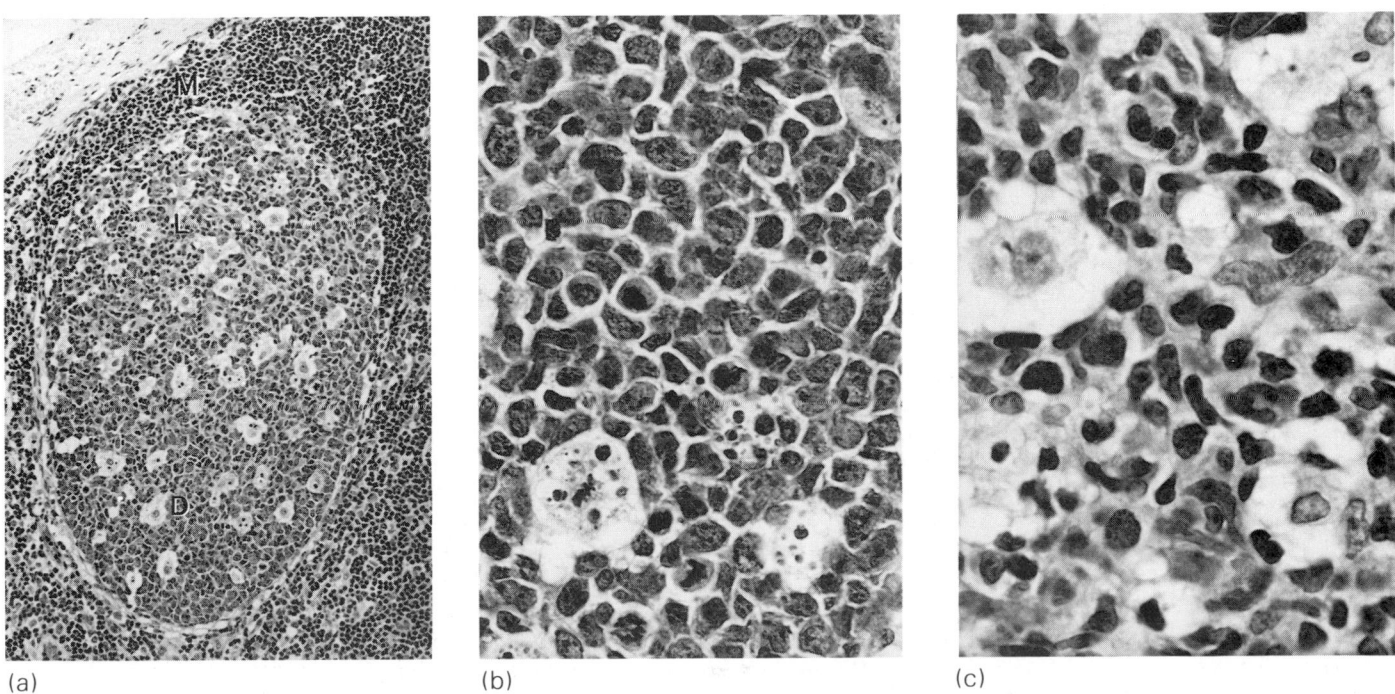

(a) (b) (c)

Fig. 3 (a) B-cell follicle showing follicle centre composed of a dark zone (D) populated by centroblasts and a light zone (L) populated by centrocytes. Tingible-body macrophages are distributed throughout the follicle centre. The follicle centre is surrounded by a mantle (M) of small lymphocytes. (b, c) High-powered detail of dark zone and light zone, respectively, showing centroblasts in the former and centrocytes in the latter together with tingible-body macrophages.

nodes, the follicles (known as primary follicles) are inconspicuous and consist of aggregates of small lymphocytes without a centre. In reactive nodes, however, the follicles (known as secondary follicles) are prominent structures consisting of a zone of small lymphocytes, the mantle zone, partially surrounding a follicle centre. The follicle centre (Fig. 3) is populated principally by two types of cell, the centroblast and centrocyte. Centroblasts are large, actively dividing cells with round nuclei and tend to be grouped together at the pole of the follicle furthest from the lymph node capsule. Centrocytes are smaller than centroblasts and contain irregularly shaped (cleaved) nuclei. Macrophages are a conspicuous component of follicle centres and characteristically contain phago-cytosed nuclear debris. The follicle centre also contains a population of cells known as dendritic reticulum cells (follicular dendritic cells). These can hardly be seen with the light microscope unless special techniques are used, but can be easily identified in electron micrographs. The nucleus and cytoplasm of dendritic reticulum cells are small and inconspicuous, but what distinguishes them is the interlacing network formed by their fine processes. Scattered B-cells are found outside follicles, presumably as part of the trafficking population, but the other site where cells of B lineage concentrate is in the medulla of the node. Here the medullary cords contain large numbers of plasma cells, which are the immunoglobulin-secreting B-cells.

The lymphoid tissue between the B-cell follicles and impinging on the medulla is known as the paracortex (Fig. 4) and it is here that the T-cells are found. These T-cells are not cytologically distinctive, appearing simply as small lymphocytes. The paracortex (Fig. 4) is distinguished by the presence of high endothelial venules, from which both B and T lymphocytes leave the blood after adhering to specific molecules on the specialized endothelium. Larger, transformed or blast cells, which may be either B- or T-cell derived, can be seen in the paracortex. Also present in the paracortex is a population of specialized macrophages known as interdigitating reticulum cells. As their name implies, these cells 'interdigitate' with the T lymphocytes around them via long, delicate processes.

The non-lymphoid cells in lymph nodes are known as accessory cells; they include sinus macrophages and the 'tingible body' macrophages in follicle centres (see Fig. 3), named for the phagocytosed nuclear fragments within their cytoplasm and paracortical interdigitating reticulum (see Fig. 4), whose role is one of antigen presentation to surrounding T-cells. There is no agreement about the origin of dendritic reticulum cells (follicular dendritic cells), although some workers believe that these, too, are bone-marrow derived. Their processes are heavily coated with antigen/antibody complexes and in forming a dense network amidst the B-cells of the follicle centre it would appear that dendritic reticulum cells are concerned with presentation of antigen to B-cells. Other accessory cells in lymph nodes include those of the granulocyte series, mast cells, and natural killer cells.

Immunocytochemistry of lymph nodes

Our knowledge of the different cell types in lymphoid tissue has been greatly enhanced by newly developed techniques whereby the phenotype of morphologically similar cells can be discriminated using polyclonal or monoclonal antibodies that react with distinctive molecules on the cell membrane or in the cytoplasm. This is accomplished by conjugating the antibodies to a label, usually an enzyme such as horseradish peroxidase or alkaline phosphatase, which can be rendered visible under normal light. A great variety of antibodies is now available that recognize antigenic determinants specific for the different lymphoid cells described above. Indeed, so many of these antibodies have been produced that it has become necessary to convene special international meetings or 'workshops', for the specific purpose of grouping closely similar antibodies together; as a result of these workshops an international classification of antibodies that recognize lymphoreticular cells has been formulated. Each group or 'cluster' of antibodies that recognizes the same or a closely similar antigen indicative of a certain type of cell differentiation receives a number. Hence, for example, the designation CD3 (cluster of differentiation 3) has been agreed for all those antibodies that recognize a certain molecule present on almost all T-cells. Not all antibodies in common use have necessarily been clustered and until sufficient numbers of other antibodies with similar specificity are produced, they retain their proprietary names. As well as antibodies that recognize molecules which are an integral part of the cell, antibodies to the different types of immunoglobulin secreted by B-cells are particularly useful in the study of

Table 1 Antibodies most commonly used for immunohistochemical analysis of lymphomas

Antibody	Specificity	Application in:	
		Paraffin sections	Frozen sections
Anti-immunoglobulin:			
Anti-IgG	γ heavy chain	+	+
Anti-IgM	μ heavy chain	+	+
Anti-IgA	α heavy chain	+	+
Anti-IgD	δ heavy chain	−	+
Anti-$\varkappa$ light chain	$\varkappa$ light chain	+	+
Anti-λ light chain	λ light chain	+	+
CD3	T-cells	+	+
CD4	T-helper/inducer cells	−	+
CD5[A]	T-cells, some B-cells	−	+
CD8	T-suppressor/cytotoxic cells	−	+
CD15	Granulocyte antigen	+	+
CD19	B-cells	−	+
CD20	B-cells	+	+
CD30	Activation antigen (ki-1)	+	+
CD45	Leucocyte common antigen	+	+
CD45RA	T-cells	+	+
Ki67	Proliferating cells	−	+

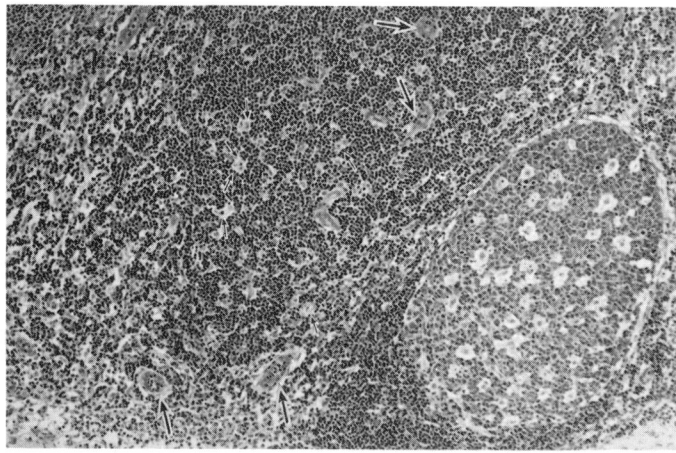

Fig. 4 Paracortex adjacent to a B-cell follicle at right. The paracortex consists of small lymphocytes (T-cells). Interspersed, clear-staining, interdigitating reticulum cells (small arrows) are scattered through the paracortex and high endothelial venules (heavy arrows) are prominent.

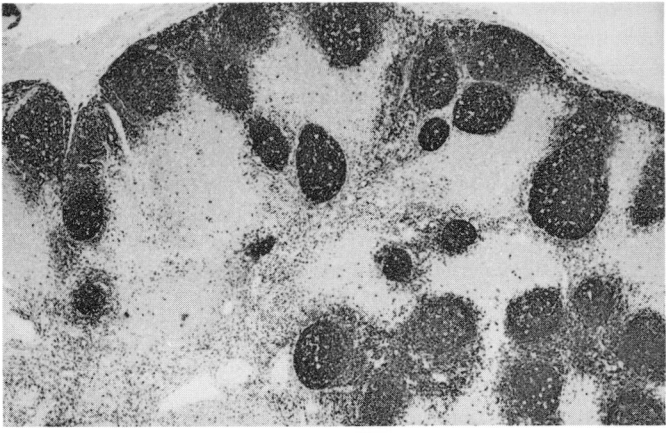

(a)

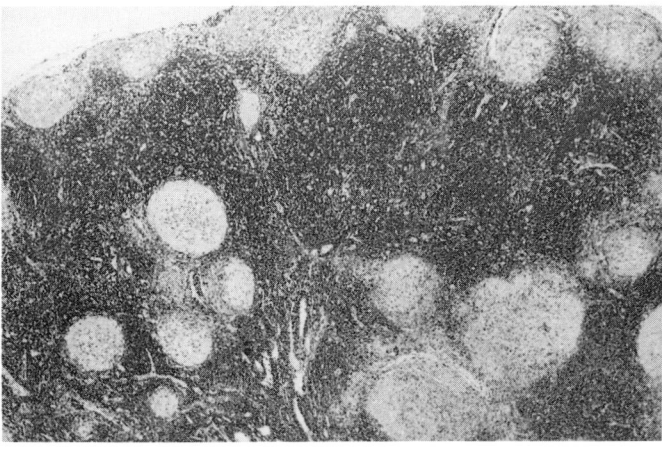

(b)

Fig. 5 Lymph node stained (a) with monoclonal antibody to B-cells and (b) with monoclonal antibody to T-cells. The B-cell areas, follicle centres, and mantle zones stain positively in (a) and scattered B-cells can be seen in the paracortex. Note that the paracortex in (b) consists principally of T-cells and that there are scattered T-cells within the follicles.

lymphorecticular tissue. A list of the most commonly used antibodies and their specificity is given in Table 1.

By using antibodies that recognize all B-cells (pan-B antibodies) and all T-cells (pan-T antibodies), the detailed distribution of these cells in the normal lymph node can be mapped (Fig. 5). The B- and T-cell populations can then further be subdivided with appropriate antibodies. The immunoglobulin expressed by each B-cell is of either $\varkappa$ or λ light-chain isotype, thus mixed or polytypic light-chain expression by a population of B-cells is indicative of polyclonal proliferation. B-cell neoplasms on the other hand are, by definition, monoclonal and therefore express only one type of light chain, a property known as light-chain restriction. The different subsets of T-cells can also be recognized with appropriate antibodies, but it is important to bear in mind that the expression of T-cell subset antigens does not have the same meaning with regard to clonality as that of $\varkappa$ and λ light chains by B-cells. The accessory cells in lymphoid tissue can also be distinguished immunocytochemically.

The relation of lymph node structure to function

Given the intimate relation that exists in lymph nodes between lymphatic sinuses carrying antigens, accessory cells capable of presenting the antigens, and lymphocytes whose function it is to respond to antigens, it is clear that the reason for the complexity of the structure of lymph nodes is to ensure effective immune responses to the antigens delivered to them. The interrelated functions of lymphoreticular cells are, however, so complex that it is impossible to establish with certainty the precise pathways that lead to the formation of antibody-producing B-cells and immunocompetent T-cells. For this reason, too, the mechanism of follicle-centre formation and the exact function of these structures remains poorly understood; nevertheless, there is a wealth of experimental data from which it is worth attempting to construct an outline of the functional and structural changes that occur in lymph nodes exposed to antigen.

Antigen arrives at a lymph node in the afferent lymphatics and in the process of diffusing through the sinuses and across their walls into the parenchyma is modified by macrophages and sinusoidal endothelium. The antigen then encounters B and T lymphocytes, which are constantly recirculating through the node, entering it across the high endothelium of the postcapillary venules and leaving via the efferent lymphatics. There appear to be specific receptors on the high endothelium to which lymphocytes bind, together with mechanisms for guiding them between the endothelial cells into the lymph node parenchyma. Differences in the receptors may be responsible for the selection of different lymphocyte populations depending on the particular anatomical site of the lymph node. Antigen-presenting cells, including interdigitating reticulum cells, then cooperate with lymphocytes that have entered the node and these undergo transformation into large, nucleolated cells (blasts), which are capable of further division into immunologically effective T-cells, antibody-secreting plasma cells, or memory cells of either T- or B-cell lineage. When secreted antibody encounters more antigen, the resulting antigen/antibody complexes are trapped by dendritic reticulum cells within primary B-cell follicles. These complexes are highly immunogenic and result in transformation of the B-cells, with the formation of the follicle centres that characterize secondary follicles. These B-cells are rapidly dividing and leave the follicle either as plasma-cell precursors or as memory cells. In this rapidly dividing population many cells die and it is their remnants that are phagocytosed by the intrafollicular (tingible body) macrophages. Exposure of a lymph node to antigens that react with T-cells (most viruses, for example) results in paracortical hyperplasia, while antigens to which B-cells are sensitive (pyogenic bacteria, for example) cause follicular hyperplasia. A lymph node draining a site of infection is usually exposed to many antigens and will therefore show generalized hyperplasia.

LYMPHOCYTE CIRCULATION AND HOMING

Both B and T lymphocytes are in a constant state of circulation and recirculation through the lymph nodes, spleen, bone-marrow, and other lymphoid aggregates. The lymphocytes gain access to these various concentrations of lymphoid tissue from the blood and after a variable time either themselves or their progeny leave these tissues in the efferent lymphatics, enter the thoracic duct and, hence, the circulation once more. The entry of lymphocytes into the efferent lymphatics is an orderly process that appears to be at least in part dependent on their place in the ontogenetic pathway. It is now clear that this and other factors also have a significant effect on the sites at which particular lymphocytes preferentially leave the circulation; some 'home' to most, if not all, lymphoid tissues while others are more selective. Neoplastic lymphoid cells share many of the characteristics of normal lymphocytes so that the mechanisms whereby lymphocytes enter and leave lymphoid tissue have an important bearing on the behaviour of lymphomas. This is perhaps best illustrated by the striking difference in behaviour between superficially similar low-grade lymphomas of the gastrointestinal tract, which rarely involve the marrow and those of the peripheral lymph nodes, which frequently do so. The mechanisms of lymphocyte homing are only beginning to be understood: they appear to be mediated by specific receptors (adhesion molecules) on the lymphocytes themselves and other receptors, known as addressins, on the high endothelial cells of the postcapillary venules; binding of the adhesion molecules to the addressin being the necessary step before entry of the lymphocyte into the tissue can occur (Pals *et al.* 1989).

LYMPHOCYTE ONTOGENY

Lymphocytes share a common bone-marrow stem cell with the myeloid, erythroid, and monocyte series. Lymphocyte ontogeny, however, unlike that of other bone-marrow-derived cells, is extremely complex and controversial. A simplified scheme is shown in Fig. 6. Although the general direction of lymphocyte differentiation is straightforward enough (that is, from B lymphoblast to plasma cell and T (thymic) lymphoblast to peripheral T-cell), a multitude of morphologically and phenotypically distinct cells appears as part of this process and these cells are echoed in and help to characterize, different subtypes of lymphoma. Such cells may be found at more than one point in the ontogenetic pathway along which, to make matters more complicated, there are numerous diversions and interconnections. Lymphocyte differentiation, unlike that in the myeloid and erythroid series, is difficult to assess, particularly as the size, shape, and nuclear characteristics of the cells are not always reliable indicators of their position in the ontogenetic pathway. The histopathology of lymphomas bears a direct relation to lymphocyte ontogeny and this relation is relied on to a considerable extent as a basis for the classification of these tumours. Lymphomas can be

thought of as a monoclonal expansion reflecting a limited range of the ontogenetic pathway, which can vary (depending on the type of disease) from a single cell (as is thought to be the case in Burkitt's lymphoma) to multiple cell types as in some follicular lymphomas. Thus, the use of the term 'histogenesis', which implies derivation from a single cell, is inappropriate when discussing lymphomas, which should rather be defined in terms of cell compartments. The histological appearances of lymphomas are further complicated by the large numbers of accessory cells that can accumulate within them, sometimes outnumbering the neoplastic population.

THE DIAGNOSIS OF LYMPHOMA IN THE HISTOPATHOLOGY LABORATORY

A precise histopathological diagnosis is central to the clinical management of lymphoma. As the classification of lymphoma into different clinicopathological entities has progressed, so have the demands for greater and greater precision on the part of the histopathologist. To meet these demands the range of histopathological techniques has broadened beyond that applied in the routine laboratory and today extends to include modern molecular techniques not generally thought of as 'histopathological' in nature. The aims of these techniques are really 3-fold: firstly, to allow accurate and reproducible demonstration of the morphological characteristics of the lymphoma; secondly, to establish the phenotype of the constituent cells; and, thirdly, especially in those cases where morphology is not entirely characteristic, to show that the lymphoproliferation is monoclonal. It should be stressed that the successful application of these techniques is entirely dependent on carefully excised fresh tissue reaching the laboratory as soon as possible after its removal. Full cooperation between oncologist, surgeon, and pathologist is required to ensure this and it is particularly important that the pathologist should be aware that a lymph node is to be excised, so that he or she can prepare for its

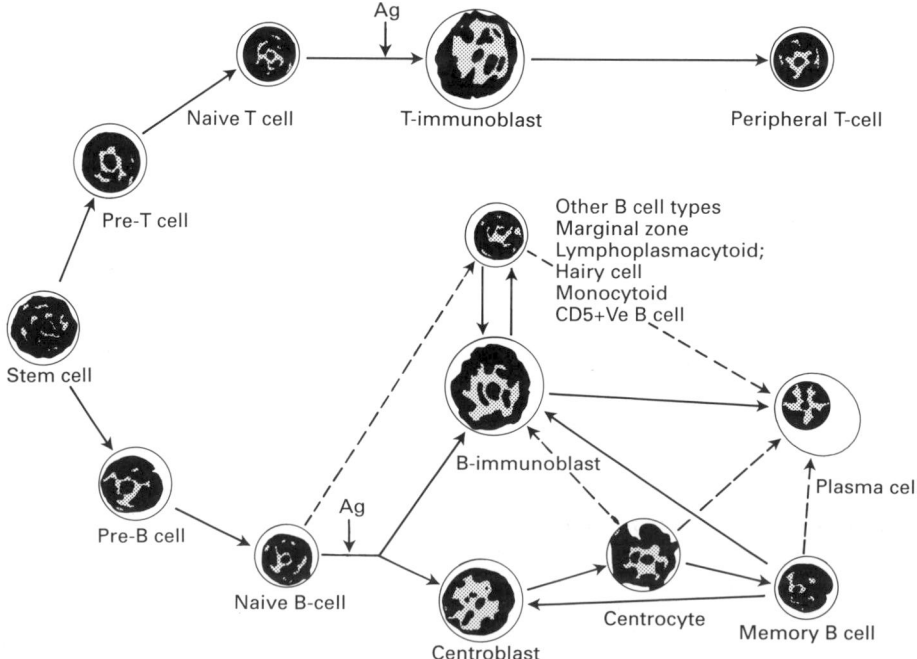

Fig. 6 Simplified schematic diagram of T- and B-lymphocyte ontogeny. Note the complex interrelations of different B-cell types. T-cell ontogeny is almost certainly more complex than illustrated here. Ag, antigen.

correct handling in the laboratory. If facilities for the full analysis of lymphoma are not available locally, fresh tissue can be transported as slices in tissue-culture fluid, where it will remain in satisfactory condition at room temperature for at least 24 h. The diagnostic techniques in current use can be summarized as follows.

1. Routine histology. This remains the mainstay in the diagnosis of lymphoreticular disease. One or more 2–3 mm blocks are taken across the equator of the node and placed in fixative for an optimum period. The nature of the fixative varies from laboratory to laboratory. After routine processing, 3–4 μm sections are cut and stained with haematoxylin and eosin. A variety of special stains can then be applied as required. To an increasing extent immunohistochemical techniques can be used on routinely processed tissue.

2. Frozen tissue. Blocks of the node are snap frozen, usually in liquid nitrogen. Frozen sections prepared from this tissue are used for immunohistochemistry and frozen tissue is also used for the extraction of DNA suitable for Southern blot analysis (see (8) below).

3. Electron microscopy. Small (1 mm cubes) fragments of the node are placed in an appropriate fixative.

4. Touch preparations. The cut surface of the lymph node is lightly touched on a glass slide or several slides. This type of preparation is suitable for studying detailed cytological features and for histochemical techniques.

5. Cell suspension. A small fragment of the node is gently teased apart into tissue-culture fluid. These cells can be separated in different ways, for example according to their density and used for phenotypic studies or to establish short- or long-term cultures, either of which is suitable for chromsome analysis (karyotyping).

6. Immunohistochemistry. Reference has already been made to this important technique by which cell surface and cytoplasmic antigens can be demonstrated, allowing an accurate determination of the phenotype of the tumour under study. The technique is applicable to fixed or frozen tissue sections, depending on the particular antigen being demonstrated (Isaacson and Wright 1986; Norton and Isaacson 1989a,b). It can also be applied to cell suspensions. In most cases a limited range of antibodies (see Table 1) will establish the phenotype of the lymphoma satisfactorily and in B-cell lymphomas the demonstration of light-chain restriction is a satisfactory indicator of monoclonality. Immunohistochemistry is of no value in determining clonality in T-cell lesions, as the different T-cell subsets do not reflect cell lineage, but an abnormal T-cell phenotype is considered strong evidence for a neoplastic lesion (Hastrup et al. 1989). The antibodies Ki67 and CD30 are important in the analysis of lymphomas. Ki67 recognizes a proliferation nuclear antigen and the 'score' of Ki67-positive cells has clinical relevance (Hall et al. 1988). The antibody CD30 recognizes an activation antigen that characterizes certain lymphomas including the Reed–Sternberg cells of Hodgkin's disease (Schwab et al. 1982).

7. Cytogenetics. Non-random chromosomal abnormalities can be demonstrated in most cases of lymphoma (Kristofferson et al. 1987), but in only a few instances are these indicative of a specific type and in these (Burkitt's lymphoma and follicular lymphoma) the histological appearance is more specific. Nevertheless, given the example of the leukaemias, it is likely that the role of cytogenetics in the diagnosis of lymphoma will grow. The technique requires expertise of a high order.

8. Molecular biology. The role of molecular biology in the study of lymphoma has expanded dramatically and at least one molecular technique, that of Southern blotting, has become an important part of the diagnostic repertoire. By using this it is possible, in most instances, to show unequivocally whether a lymphoproliferative lesion is monoclonal (that is, neoplastic) or not. In B-cell lymphomas, demonstration of light-chain restriction by immunohistochemical means is a reliable indicator of monoclonality (see above), but successful immunostaining of light chains is technically demanding and subject to a variety of artefacts. In T-cell lesions, immunohistochemistry is of no value in this respect and monoclonality can only be established by molecular techniques.

The Southern blotting technique (Southern 1975) as it is applied to lymphomas can be summarized as follows. The immunoglobulin gene exists as part of the germline in every cell in the body, but as each lymphocyte becomes an effector cell, the gene is uniquely rearranged by a complex process so that it transcribes a unique immunoglobulin specific for a certain antigen that is produced only by that cell and the clone derived from it. In any lymphoproliferative lesion there will be multiple copies of the germ-line immunoglobulin gene contained in the non-lymphoid tissue and, if the lesion is reactive (that is, polyclonal), a multitude of differently rearranged immunoglobulin genes; in neoplastic (that is, monoclonal) lesions, however, in addition to the germ-line genes there will be multiple copies of an identically rearranged immunoglobulin gene. By using specific restriction enzymes the DNA extracted from lymphoproliferative lesions can be cut at predictable sites that include the immunoglobulin gene. This digested extract is then subjected to electrophoresis in agarose gel, which results in separation of the DNA fragments according to their molecular weight. When multiple copies of identically rearranged genes are present in the DNA extract the digested fragments have the same molecular weight and will concentrate to form a band in the gel, as will the fragments from the multiple copies of the germ-line gene that are always

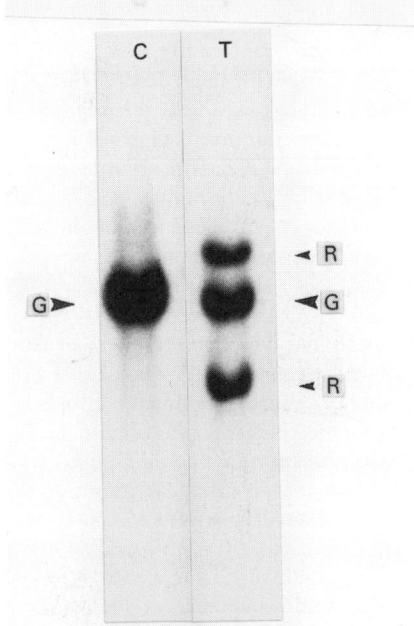

Fig. 7 Southern blot of placental DNA (channel C) and DNA from a B-cell lymphoma (channel T) probed for the J_H heavy-chain immunoglobulin gene. Note heavy staining of the germ-line (G) gene in both control and tumour as well as rearrangement (R) of both alleles of this gene in the lymphoma.

present. The DNA fragments from the multitude of immunoglobulin genes with different rearrangements present in polyclonal lesions all move to a slightly different position in the gel, resulting in an unconcentrated distribution along the electrophoretic pathway. The electrophoretic pattern is then transferred to a nylon membrane by the blotting process originally described by Southern (hence, the name of the technique), where the distribution of the DNA fragments can be demonstrated using radiolabelled DNA probes that hybridize to the immunoglobulin gene. The T-cell receptor gene behaves in the same way as the immunoglobulin gene, therefore, provided appropriate probes that hybridize with this gene are used, monoclonal rearrangements of this gene can be demonstrated in T-cell lymphomas as distinct from reactive conditions. Typical results of this technique are shown in Fig. 7.

THE CLASSIFICATION OF NON-HODGKIN'S LYMPHOMAS

To the early pathologists the histological appearances of all non-Hodgkin's lymphomas were alike, consisting of replacement of the normal lymph-node architecture by sheets of small, dark-staining cells. However, it was clear that not all cases behaved alike and pathologists were increasingly asked by their clinical colleagues to attempt to predict the natural course of the individual case, as, even without treatment, the survival of patients with non-Hodgkin's lymphoma varied from a few months to many years. As more effective means of therapy were developed and therapeutic successes with Hodgkin's disease (itself diagnosed on histological grounds) began to emerge, the demand for more meaningful histological diagnosis of non-Hodgkin's lymphoma grew to a clamour. In response to this, the first clinically relevant histological classification of the non-Hodgkin's lymphomas was formulated by Rappaport (1966).

The Rappaport classification broadly speaking divided lymphomas into those composed of small cells and large cells, each of which could be further subdivided into those with a follicular (or nodular) pattern and those that were diffuse. The follicular and small-celled tumours were biologically less aggressive; a better survival could, therefore, be expected and, importantly, less potent and therefore less toxic therapy was suitable for these cases. The converse applied to cases with a diffuse pattern, especially if composed of large cells.

As histological techniques improved, allowing finer discrimination between cells, so more detailed classification emerged. In parallel with these improvements it was becoming possible to identify the phenotype of the lymphoma cells using immunological techniques. It soon became evident that the lymphoma cells were closely related to normal lymph node cells and that most (50 per cent or more) non-Hodgkin's lymphoma were derived from B-cells of the follicle centre. It was also clear, however, that there was an alarmingly large variety of lymphoreticular neoplasms. A whole host of soundly based classifications sprung up, causing so much confusion that a series of special international meetings was convened to decide on a single, clinically relevant classification that could be used throughout the world. The result was the so-called Working Formulation for Clinical Use (National Cancer Institute 1982). It was stressed at the time that this 'formulation', although based on histopathological appearances, was not a substitute for a satisfactory pathological classification, but its rapid acceptance as such by pathologists in the United States has meant that that is indeed what it has become.

The working formulation uses imprecise, 'collective' morphological terms such as 'large cell', which results in different clinicopathological entities being included together; as new entities are described they merely become absorbed into this inflexible system. A more serious

Table 2 Updated Kiel classification of non-Hodgkin's lymphomas

B-cell lymphomas	T-cell lymphomas
Low grade	Low grade
Lymphocytic: chronic lymphocytic and prolymphocytic leukaemia; hairy cell leukaemia	Lymphocytic: chronic lymphocytic and prolymphocytic leukaemia
	Small, cerebriform cell: mycosis fungoides, Sézary's syndrome
Lymphoplasmacytic/cytoid (immunocytoma)	Lymphoepithelioid (Lennert's lymphoma)
Plasmacytic	Angioimmunoblastic (AILD)
Centroblastic/centrocytic: follicular±diffuse diffuse	T zone
Centrocytic	Pleomorphic, small cell (HTLV-1±)
High grade	High grade
Centroblastic	Pleomorphic, medium and large cell (HTLV-1±)
Immunoblastic	Immunoblastic (HTLV-1±)
Large cell anaplastic (Ki-1+)	Large cell anaplastic (Ki1+)
Burkitt's lymphoma	
Lymphoblastic	Lymphoblastic
Rare types	Rare types

criticism is the absence of any immunological basis for the formulation, in particular, its failure to take into account any of the vast amount of immunologically based, phenotypic data now available. Pathologists and clinicians using this formulation will remain isolated from many of the new developments in lymphoma research, much of which is clinically relevant. In particular, as evidence for the different behaviour of T- and B-cell lymphomas emerges (Brown et al. 1989), the working formulation will become increasingly unsatisfactory.

For these reasons, European pathologists, led by the prestigious German group from Kiel, have preferred to use the Kiel classification. This classification (Stansfeld et al. 1988) has now been updated (Table 2) to include many of the newly described entities alluded to above and an attempt, not always successful, has been made to classify the extremely heterogeneous T-cell lymphomas. In the Kiel classification, the terms 'high grade' and 'low grade' strictly refer to the histological and cytological characteristics of the lymphoma and not to the clinical behaviour or prognosis. While in the B-cell tumours the clinical behaviour usually reflects the histological grade, this is not necessarily the case in the T-cell lymphomas.

It should be noted that the various classifications referred to above were based largely on an analysis of nodal lymphomas. Not all extranodal lymphomas sit easily in these schemes and, importantly, may not exhibit the type of clinical behaviour suggested by their placing in the classifications. In this chapter the updated Kiel classification will be used when discussing nodal lymphomas and those extranodal lymphomas where it is relevant.

B-CELL NON-HODGKIN'S LYMPHOMAS

The majority of non-Hodgkin's lymphomas are of B-cell phenotype. This is often obvious from the morphological features of the lymphoma, which, for example, may show follicle formation or the cytological features of B-cells including centrocytes, centroblasts, or plasma cells. While in most instances it is not difficult to discriminate between a neoplastic and a reactive B-cell proliferation, at times this can be extremely difficult. Immunocytochemistry is particularly helpful in this respect because demonstration of light-chain restriction indicates a monoclonal B-cell proliferation. B-cell lymphomas, especially those showing differentiation into plasma cells, may secrete this light-chain-restricted immunoglobulin in amounts sufficient for detection in the circulation or, as light chains, in the urine. Thus, careful analysis of plasma or urine proteins can be a useful adjunct to the diagnosis and in following the response to treatment. On occasion, for technical reasons or because of an admixture of polyclonal B-cells in the lymphoma it is impossible to use immunocytochemistry to demonstrate light-chain restriction. Evidence for a monoclonal B-cell proliferation can then be obtained by analysing the tumour DNA for clonal immunoglobulin-gene rearrangements, using Southern blotting.

Low-grade B-cell lymphomas

The lymphomas included in this category share a number of features in common. The designation 'low grade' implies that they are composed of small lymphoid cells with dense nuclei in which the nucleoli are indistinct. Cell turnover as indicated by the number of mitotic figures and the Ki67 scores is low. In most but not all of these tumours the lineage of the neoplastic cells can be directly related to a normal cell population and the lymphoma behaves accordingly. Thus, these low-grade B-cell lymphomas disseminate widely, reflecting normal B-cell circulation and the bone-marrow, an important site through which B-cells circulate, is nearly always involved. Again, like their normal counterparts, the low-grade cells can transform into blast forms, resulting in a lymphoma of high-grade histology characterized by rapid growth; that is, a so-called secondary high-grade B-cell lymphoma. Clinically these lymphomas are characterized by slow but relentless progression. There is initially a good response to chemotherapy but 'cures' are rare. Again, as a reflection of the function of the equivalent normal cell lineage, immunological abnormalities often associated with the production of abnormal antibodies are common features of this group of lymphomas.

Malignant lymphoma, lymphocytic

This type of lymphoma is composed of small lymphocytes morphologically similar to those that form the mantle zone of the B-cell follicle in normal lymph nodes (Fig. 8). Most cases are

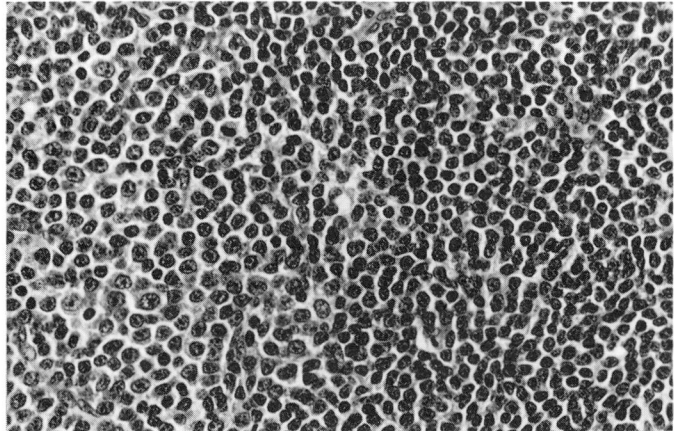

Fig. 8 Malignant lymphoma, lymphocytic showing a uniform population of small lymphocytes. On the left the cells are slightly bigger and nucleoli can be seen in their nuclei. This is a proliferation centre.

associated with chronic lymphocytic leukaemia, but in a minority the disease is confined to the lymph nodes at presentation. It is one of the most common types of lymphoma, characteristically occurring in adults past middle age. Lymphadenopathy is usually generalized and the bone-marrow is almost always involved. Malignant lymphoma, lymphocytic is a slowly progressive disease and many patients die of other causes unrelated to the disease itself or from complications resulting from impaired immunity, which is commonly present. Death directly attributable to the lymphoma usually follows transformation into a tumour of much higher grade; this is sometimes known as Richter's syndrome.

Included in the category of malignant lymphoma, lymphocytic is the rare condition known as hairy cell leukaemia. The lymph nodes are not usually significantly enlarged in this disease and so are seldom biopsied, but when they are the biopsy shows a diffuse infiltrate of small cells with clear cytoplasm and rather featureless nuclei. Infiltration of the spleen, liver, and bone-marrow results in a more distinctive picture caused by dilation of blood-filled sinuses lined by neoplastic hairy cells.

Malignant lymphoma, lymphoplasmacytic

This type of lymphoma is closely similar to the lymphocytic, from which it is distinguished by differentiation of a proportion of the small lymphocytes into plasma cells (lymphoplasmacytic) or cells with some plasma cell features (lymphoplasmacytoid). Malignant lymphoma, lymphoplasmacytic is much less common than the lymphocytic, but occurs in patients of the same age group, who also often present with chronic lymphocytic leukaemia. Presentation with isolated or generalized lymphadenopathy, without leukaemia, is more frequent than in malignant lymphoma, lymphocytic, however. Some cases present with a hyperviscosity syndrome (Waldenström's macro-globulinaemia) caused by secretion of large amounts of immuno-globulin (usually IgM) by the tumour. The prognosis of malignant lymphoma, lymphoplasmacytic/cytoid is highly variable, but overall is slightly worse than that of malignant lymphoma, lymphocytic.

Rarely a lymph node may show infiltration by a pure population of mature plasma cells. This condition is known as malignant lymphoma, plasmacytic, or extramedullary plasmacytoma to distinguish it from the much more common plasma cell neoplasm, multiple myeloma. The disease is often confined to a single lymph node, but even in these circumstances, a paraprotein may be present in the peripheral blood. Malignant lymphoma, plasmacytic is usually an extremely indolent disease and may be cured by a simple excision of the involved node. However, progression with eventual bone-marrow involvement, even after a long disease-free interval, sometimes occurs.

Malignant lymphoma, centroblastic/centrocytic

This is the most common type of non-Hodgkin's lymphoma in Western countries, accounting for approximately 50 per cent of cases. The follicles in this tumour are neoplastic equivalents of the normal B-cell follicles of reactive lymph nodes (Fig. 9). It is characteristically a tumour of late adult life and, although it can occur in young adults, childhood cases are extremely rare. Malignant lymphoma, centroblastic/centrocytic (**cb/cc**) usually presents as a group of enlarged lymph nodes or, less commonly, as generalized lymphadenopathy. Peripheral blood involvement, when it occurs, represents 'spill over' of cells from the lymph nodes rather than a primary phenomenon and is uncommon. Even when malignant lymphoma, cb/cc presents in a single group of nodes, it has usually already disseminated and trephine biopsy of the bone-marrow shows

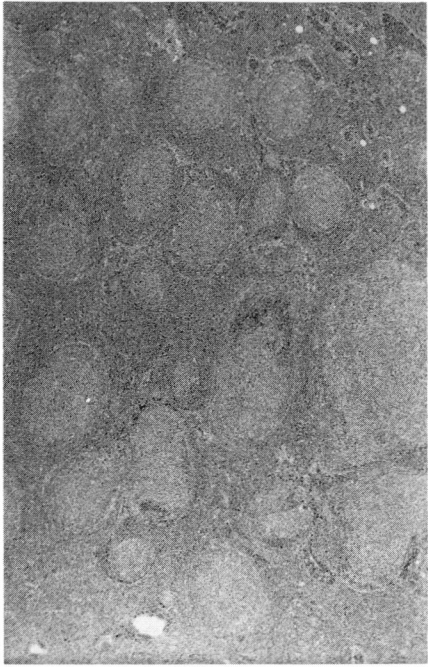

(a)

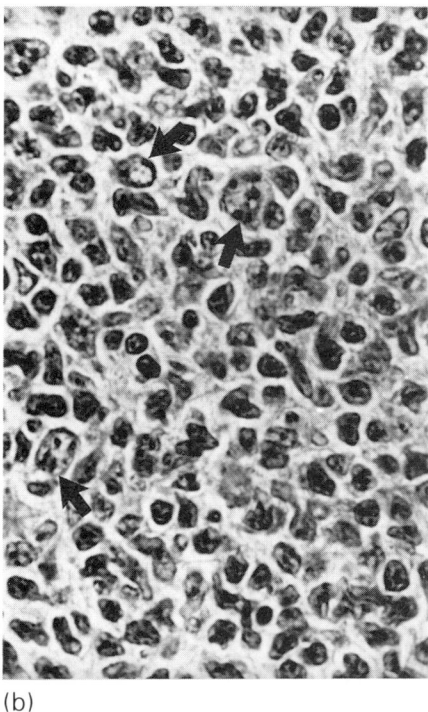

(b)

Fig. 9 Malignant lymphoma, centroblastic centrocytic, follicular: (a) shows replacement of the node by multiple follicles; in (b) the high-power view of these follicles shows predominantly centrocytes with scattered centroblasts (arrows).

involvement. The clinical course is usually a long one, punctuated by numerous therapeutically induced remissions followed by recurrences. The histological appearance of the tumour tends to alter during the course of the disease, gradually moving towards that of a higher-grade lymphoma, both cytologically and with the assumption of a diffuse growth pattern.

The close similarity between the follicles of malignant lymphoma, cb/cc and benign reactive hyperplasia can lead to considerable difficulty in the differential diagnosis between them. This has led to the formulation of detailed histological criteria characteristics, but never diagnostic, of either condition (Stansfeld 1985). The advent of immunocytochemistry has greatly simplified matters in that the B-cells of the neoplastic follicle will show light-chain restriction as opposed to those of the reactive follicle, which will express both $\varkappa$ and λ light chains (Norton and Isaacson 1987).

Cytogenetic studies of these follicular lymphomas have shown a translocation involving chromosomes 14 and 18, t(14; 18) (Yunis *et al.* 1982). This translocation results in the juxtaposition of the candidate proto-oncogene *bcl-2* located at 18q21 with the immunoglobulin heavy-chain locus at 14q32. By using chromosome-18 DNA probes flanking or within the *bcl-2* gene, rearrangements of the gene representing t(14; 18) translocations can be detected in up to 90 per cent of follicular lymphomas (Weiss *et al.* 1987). These gene rearrangements can also be detected in up to 28 per cent of diffuse, large B-cell lymphomas, especially those arising in a setting of follicular lymphoma (Weiss *et al.* 1987; Aisenberg *et al.* 1988).

Malignant lymphoma, centrocytic

Malignant lymphoma, centrocytic (Tolkdsdorf *et al.* 1980), while retaining its name, is no longer thought to be of the same lineage as the follicle-centre centrocyte. The centrocytic type occurs with approximately the same frequency as malignant lymphoma, lymphoplasmacytic and similarly may present with a leukaemic blood picture or with lymphadenopathy alone, the latter being much more common. It can also present as a primary lymphoma of the spleen or the gastrointestinal tract, as will be discussed in later sections of this chapter. Although grouped with the low-grade lymphomas, the centrocytic type carries a graver prognosis than the other B-cell tumours described above, including cb/cc. The initial response to treatment is often gratifying, but relapse with death due to dissemination of lymphoma is the rule.

The cells that comprise this type of lymphoma are cytologically indistinguishable from the centrocytes found in reactive follicle centres and this explains the name chosen for this tumour when it was first described. At that time it was thought that it was indeed a neoplasm of follicle-centre cells, but subsequent immunophenotypic and genetic studies have shown important differences between the tumour cell and its supposed benign equivalent.

Unlike follicle-centre centrocytes, which express surface (S) IgM, but not SIgD and express the CD10 but not the CD5 antigen, the cells of malignant lymphoma, centrocytic express both SIgM and D (of single light-chain type) and CD5 but not CD10 antigen. Centrocytic lymphomas are further characterized by the translocation t(11; 14), which involves the *bcl-1* gene (Weisenberger *et al.* 1989).

A number of different terms are used to define this category of lymphoma in the United States. These include 'diffuse small cleaved-cell lymphoma', 'intermediate-cell lymphoma' and 'mantle-zone lymphoma', the last being used most commonly (Weisenberger *et al.* 1987). While it is true that mantle zoning is a feature of some cases of centrocytic lymphoma, this is by no means always the case; furthermore, mantle zoning can be seen in other types of lymphoma. The suggestion that the normal equivalent of the CD5+ B-cell of centrocytic lymphoma can be found in the mantle zone is not sustainable; with the exception of fetal tissue, CD5 B-cells have not been identified convincingly in normal lymphoid tissue.

High-grade B-cell lymphomas

The term 'high grade' denotes a lymphoma composed of large cells with large nuclei and prominent nucleoli. These lymphomas have a higher turnover rate as indicated by Ki67 scores considerably higher than those of the low-grade tumours (Hall *et al.* 1988). High-grade B-cell lymphomas are usually localized at presentation and spread more in the manner of malignant tumours in general rather than 'disseminating' along the pathway of lymphocyte circulation as occurs in the low-grade tumours. These features are consistent with a cell lineage of transformed or 'blast' forms of lymphocytes. Lymphocyte transformation is a local phenomenon and the resulting blast cells do not ordinarily circulate. Because of their rapid growth, high-grade lymphomas often form bulky growths and behave as highly malignant neoplasms that can be fatal within a relatively short time when compared to the low-grade B-cell lymphomas. However, in the absence of the inherent tendency to circulate present in the low-grade lymphomas, high-grade lymphoma is more amenable to 'cure'.

Malignant lymphoma centroblastic

Malignant lymphoma, centroblastic is a tumour of adults and accounts for approximately 5 per cent of non-Hodgkin's lymphomas. The most usual presentation is one of regional lymphadenopathy, although the tumour may have already spread to the bone-marrow and spleen; peripheral blood involvement is rare.

This high-grade lymphoma is composed of a diffuse infiltrate of cells, the majority of which are morphologically identical or closely similar to centroblasts as described in the reactive follicle centre. Subtypes of centroblastic lymphomas are described in which the morphology is more variable (Hui *et al.* 1988). Centroblastic features may be present from the time that the tumour is diagnosed, in which case it is termed a primary centroblastic lymphoma or result from transformation of a cb/cc lymphoma, when it is called secondary centroblastic lymphoma. Immunocytochemistry is useful in confirming the B-cell nature of these lymphomas and in demonstrating light-chain restriction in the immunoglobulin that is synthesized by the centroblasts, sometimes in surprisingly high amounts.

Malignant lymphoma, immunoblastic (B-cell type)

This type of lymphoma (Fig. 10) is the most common high-grade lymphoma. The term 'immunoblast' refers to a large cell with abundant cytoplasm and a large, prominent, and often central nucleolus. A lymphoma may be immunoblastic from the outset or may evolve as a result of transformation of either lymphocytic (Richter's syndrome), lymphoplasmacytic, cb/cc, or centroblastic types. Whether it arises *de novo*, or following transformation of a lymphoma of lower grade, malignant lymphoma, immunoblastic carries a grave prognosis, worse than any of the other high-grade B-cell lymphomas.

Malignant lymphoma, Burkitt type

This entity was first reported by Burkitt (1959) as a tumour arising primarily in the jaws of African children that tends also to involve the retroperitoneum and the viscera, especially the kidneys and, in girls, the ovaries. This disorder, now known as endemic Burkitt's lymphoma, is also seen in other tropical countries where there is a high incidence of malaria such as Papua New Guinea. The Epstein–Barr virus (**EBV**) is thought to be implicated in the aetiology of endemic Burkitt's lymphoma. The virus can immortalize

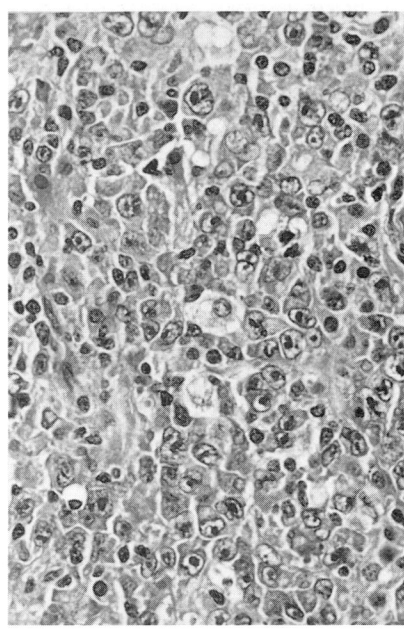

Fig. 10 Malignant lymphoma, immunoblastic. The cells in this high-grade B-cell lymphoma are characterized by large nuclei with prominent central nucleoli.

B-cells in culture and there is evidence of past infection in all cases of endemic Burkitt's lymphoma. Furthermore, viral genome has been shown to be incorporated into the nuclei of the tumour cells themselves. As infection with EBV (the cause of infectious mononucleosis) is so common, some other factor must be operating in Burkitt's lymphoma. It is thought that the combination of malaria, which may depress immunity and exposure to the virus in infancy rather than in young adulthood is important. Lymph node involvement in endemic Burkitt's lymphoma, while it occurs, is insignificant compared to extranodal disease of the jaws, retro-peritoneum, and viscera (Wright 1964). In approximately 90 per cent of cases of endemic Burkitt's lymphoma an abnormal karyotype, t(8; 14), is present in the malignant cells. This involves translocation of the c-*myc* oncogene from chromosome 8 to immunoglobulin heavy-chain gene locus on chromosome 22. In the remaining 10 per cent of cases, similar translocations involving c-*myc* and the light-chain loci occur.

Malignant lymphoma histologically indistinguishable from Burkitt's lymphoma occurs as a non-endemic tumour throughout the world. Again, it is children who are principally affected, but in non-endemic Burkitt's lymphoma the pattern of the disease is quite different, with a higher incidence of lymph node, gastrointestinal, and bone-marrow involvement (Wright 1966); jaw tumours are comparatively rare. The majority of cases of non-endemic Burkitt's lymphoma do not show incorporation of EBV genome into the tumour cell nuclei. The same karyotypic abnormalities are, however, present.

Burkitt's lymphoma is characterized by a diffuse monomorphic infiltrate of medium-sized, round, blast cells. A rapid rate of cell division is evident from the numerous mitotic figures present and the high turnover of cells results in much cell death. In response to this there are large numbers of phagocytic macrophages in the tumour, many of which have engulfed the debris of dead tumour cells. These macrophages, with their pale-staining cytoplasm, scattered among the tumour cells which have dark blue-staining nuclei, produce the well-described 'starry sky' effect. The extreme monomorphism of Burkitt's lymphoma and lack of any differentiation of the tumour cells suggest that the cells have been 'frozen' at a certain stage of maturation, perhaps, in the case of the endemic form, due to the effects of the EBV. There is considerable debate as to the lineage of Burkitt's lymphoma. Most workers favour a follicle-centre (centroblast) lineage, but it has to be said that these tumours bear no resemblance to centroblastic or other follicle centre cell lymphomas. Peripheral blood involvement may occur as spill-over phenomenon and should not be confused with B-cell lymphoblastic leukaemia (see below).

The designation 'Burkitt-like' is used for a type of lymphoma that resembles Burkitt's lymphoma but does not quite meet the stringent histological criteria for that diagnosis. The clinical setting may be similar but there is not the same histological monomorphism. These lymphomas show evidence of a broader cell lineage with different degrees of differentiation resulting in irregularity of nuclear size and shape and accumulation of cytoplasmic immunoglobulin in some cells. This is an ill-defined group of tumours at present.

Malignant lymphoma, lymphoblastic (B-cell type)

Patients with B-cell lymphoblastic lymphoma are usually, but not always, children and either have or soon develop acute lymphoblastic leukaemia (ALL). This type of leukaemia is known as 'common' ALL (C-ALL), a term coined before the advent of monoclonal antibodies and DNA analysis that established the B-cell phenotype of the cells. In some cases, nodal or extranodal (non-leukaemic) disease is the principal or sole manifestation. The small blast cells of lymphoblastic lymphoma tend to infiltrate in a non-destructive manner along the natural tissue planes, thus in lymph nodes there is preservation of the basic architecture.

Malignant lymphoma, large-cell anaplastic (Ki1) positive

This type of lymphoma is rarely of B-cell phenotype and is considered as a group below, together with T-cell lymphomas of similar type.

Malignant lymphoma unclassified

Inevitably, when dealing with a disease as complex as non-Hodgkin's lymphoma there will be cases that do not fit into any of the categories described above, even though it is possible to phenotype them as of B-cell lineage. As experience accumulates, these cases will either be recognized as variants of established conditions or new categories will be formulated.

NON-HODGKIN'S LYMPHOMA OF T-CELL TYPE

Introduction

T-cell lymphomas are much less common than those of B-cell origin, comprising 10–15 per cent of all non-Hodgkin's lymphomas in Europe and North America. In Japan, however, close to 40 per cent are T-cell derived, this being a reflection of the prevalence of the human T-cell lymphotrophic virus (HTLV-1) in that country. T-cell lymphomas can be divided into two main groups, those arising from early T-cell precursors, either prethymic or thymic and those arising from mature T-cells, the so-called peripheral T-cell lymphomas. The former group, known as the T-lymphoblastic lymphomas, are well characterized, but the peripheral T-cell lymphomas remain a challenge to the diagnostic histopathologist, immunologist, and clinician. Some entities, such as the cutaneous lymphomas consisting of small cerebriform cells, are well defined,

but any classification of the remainder can only be tentative, particularly with respect to their clinical behaviour, which is only beginning to be understood. It is important to understand that the terms high and low grade in the updated Kiel classification refer to histological rather than clinical properties of the neoplasms. The morphology of T-cell lymphomas is highly variable and the tumours tend to change their morphology in an unpredictable way, often defying classification. Furthermore, unlike B-cell lymphomas, there is no convenient method of establishing clonality immunocytochemically. Although some T-cell lymphomas show restriction of their phenotype, this is not consistent and is no reflection of clonality. Others may show an abnormal distribution of T-cell markers or deletion of certain antigens, features which are themselves a strong indication of malignancy (Hastrup et al. 1989). Distinguishing between reactive and neoplastic T-cell proliferation depends to a large extent on the demonstration of T-cell antigens on cells judged to be malignant on morphological grounds or, more specifically, on the demonstration of clonal T-cell receptor gene rearrangements using the Southern blotting technique on DNA extracted from the fresh tissue. It is now becoming clear that T-cell lymphomas behave differently from the B-cell tumours (Armitage et al. 1989) and that it is, therefore, important to distinguish them by immunohistochemical or other methods.

In considering the T-cell lymphomas the modified Kiel classification, which is based on that of Suchi et al. (1987), will be followed, except that the HTLV-associated tumours will be discussed as a group rather than in separate high- and low-grade categories. It is still too early to assess the full clinical relevance of this classification, but it represents a beginning of the task of evolving a clinical strategy for these tumours.

Malignant lymphoma, lymphocytic

Almost all cases of this type of lymphoma are accompanied by T-cell lymphocytic leukaemia and are, therefore, essentially haematological disorders. The leukaemia can be subclassified into different entities according to both morphology and phenotype and these differ somewhat in their clinical behaviour. The lymph nodes show infiltration by small lymphocytes, which usually have more nuclear irregularity than the cells of B-cell lymphocytic lymphoma.

Malignant lymphoma, small cerebriform cell (mycosis fungoides; Sezary's syndrome)

This is the only strictly extranodal lymphoma that is included in the Kiel classification and as such will be considered in the section on cutaneous lymphomas later in this chapter.

Malignant lymphoma, lymphoepithelioid type (Lennert's lymphoma)

Lennert's lymphoma (Patsouris et al. 1988) usually presents with regional lymphadenopathy, commonly accompanied by tonsillar involvement. Although classified as low grade the prognosis of Lennert's lymphoma is less favourable than that of low-grade B-cell lymphomas and it is considered by some as a clinically high-grade tumour (Spier et al. 1988). The lymph node is replaced by a mixed cell infiltrate in which small T-cells predominate. A variable number of larger neoplastic T-cells that may resemble Reed–Sternberg cells is present and the characteristic feature is the presence of numerous clusters of epithelioid cells (Fig. 11). These features lead to a great difficulty in the diagnosis and differential diagnosis of Lennert's lymphoma and careful immunocytochemistry or DNA analysis are often indicated.

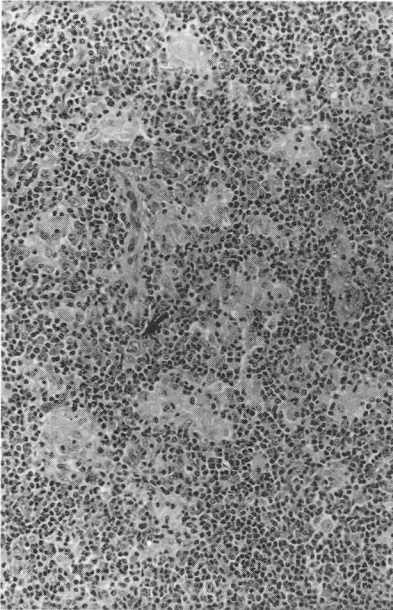

Fig. 11 Lennert's lymphoma. There is an infiltrate of small- to medium-sized T-cells and occasional large transformed cells (arrow). Numerous clusters of epithelioid histiocytes are present.

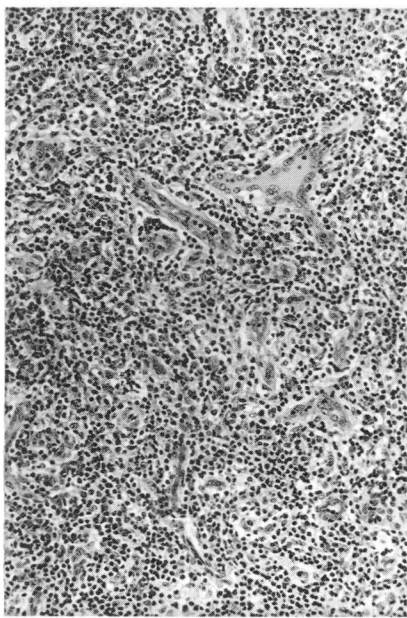

Fig. 12 T-cell lymphoma of AILD type. There are numerous branching high endothelial venules intersecting the T-cell infiltrate.

Malignant lymphoma, angioimmunoblastic

The condition angioimmunoblastic lymphadenopathy with dysproteinaemia (**AILD**) was first described in 1975 (Frizzera *et al.* 1975) and was thought to be a non-neoplastic disease that either resolved spontaneously, caused death due to the associated immunodeficiency, or was complicated by the evolution of lymphoma. Careful studies of large numbers of cases, together with DNA analysis, have shown that most if not all cases of AILD are, in fact, T-cell lymphomas (Feller *et al.* 1988). The clinical presentation is usually acute, with generalized lymphadenopathy, a skin rash, hepatosplenomegaly, and severe constitutional symptoms. Hyperglobulinaemia and associated autoimmune phenomena are characteristic. Response to treatment is initially good, but long-term survival is poor. Feller *et al.* (1988) have shown that a subgroup of AILD lymphoma, in which there is immunoglobulin as well as T-cell receptor gene rearrangement, carries a worse prognosis.

The most striking histological feature (Fig. 12) is the network of proliferating high endothelial venules, leading to the impression that the whole node consists of paracortical tissue. The T-cells between these venules are small to medium sized with intermingled blast forms and clusters of large cells, which often have clear cytoplasm. Numerous plasma cells are characteristically present. B-cell follicles are absent or seen only as small atrophic structures, but immunohistochemistry shows that large sheets of dendritic reticulum cells are present.

Malignant lymphoma, T-zone type

The infiltrate in this type of T-cell lymphoma is very similar to the AILD type, except for the presence of numerous, well-preserved, and often hyperplastic, B-cell follicles. Thus, in some cases, unless careful attention is given to the 'paracortex', the lymphoma may be confused with lymph node hyperplasia. T-zone lymphoma may progress into a diffuse high-grade lymphoma or become indistinguishable from AILD lymphoma.

Malignant lymphoma, pleomorphic (HTLV-1 positive or negative)

In the updated Kiel classification this group of T-cell lymphomas is divided into large and small cell variants, but, although there is some evidence that those composed of smaller cells have a better prognosis, the group is more conveniently subdivided into those cases in which there is evidence of infection with HTLV-1 and those in which there is not.

The retrovirus HTLV-1 was first isolated from a cell line derived from an American patient with a T-cell lymphoma. A similar virus, called adult T-cell lymphoma virus, was identified in south-western Japan as the agent responsible for an endemic form of T-cell lymphoma/leukaemia. It was later established that these two agents were identical (Gallo 1985). T-cell lymphoma/leukaemia is also endemic in certain areas in the Caribbean and cases have been reported from the United States and Europe. In endemic areas many more people are infected with the virus, as shown by antibody studies, than have lymphoma; in some patients the virus produces a chronic, grumbling illness that may later be complicated by lymphoma. The virus preferentially infects CD4+ T-cells, resulting in transformation and the evolution of 'immortal' cell lines that overexpress interleukin-2 receptors (**IL-2R**) and IL-2 itself. This uncontrolled polyclonal T-cell proliferation then becomes monoclonal. The mechanism appears to be that the transactivating (*tat*) gene product of HTLV acts on the enhancer sequences of both the *IL-2* and *IL-2R* genes.

T-cell lymphoma caused by HTLV is often, but not always, accompanied by leukaemia. The disease affects adults, usually of late middle age and the typical presentation is with generalized lymphadenopathy, splenomegaly, and a skin rash resembling that of mycosis fungoides. Hypercalcaemia is common and there may be profound hypogammaglobulinaemia together with defective cell-mediated immunity. The prognosis is grave, with a median survival of only a few months. Less commonly there is a chronic course with slow evolution through a pre-lymphomatous phase to lymphoma involving primarily the skin, producing only mild symptoms and no hypercalcaemia.

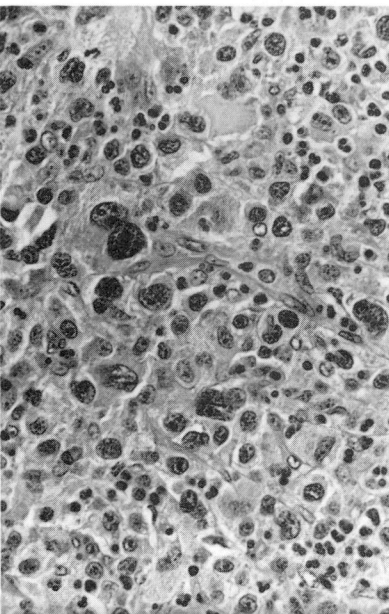

Fig. 13   High grade pleomorphic T-cell lymphoma (HTLV +).

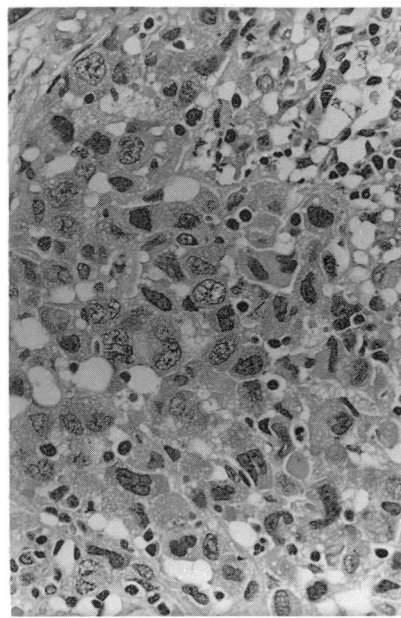

Fig. 14   Malignant lymphoma of large cell anaplastic (CD30 +) type. Note the almost syncitial growth of large pleomorphic cells with finely granular cytoplasm.

The lymph nodes typically show replacement by medium-sized to large cells with pleomorphic nuclei (Fig. 13). These features are reflected in the leukaemic cells in the peripheral blood, where the picture is characteristic. Immunohistochemistry shows that the cells are consistently CD4+, CD8−, and CD7−. In the low-grade cases, which usually run a chronic course, the cells are much smaller but nevertheless show considerable nuclear irregularity and pleomorphism.

HTLV–negative cases of pleomorphic T-cell lymphoma are marginally less aggressive than the virus-positive cases. They are less frequently accompanied by leukaemia and are seldom associated with hypercalcaemia. Most cases share the same phenotype as HTLV-positive lymphoma, but CD8 and CD7 antigen expression is more frequent.

Malignant lymphoma, immunoblastic (T-cell)

These tumours consist of large cells containing large, round nuclei with prominent nucleoli. The cells are uniform in size, unlike the pleomorphic variants described above. A minority of the cases are HTLV-1 positive.

Malignant lymphoma, anaplastic large cell (Ki-1 positive)

This histologically and clinically distinctive T-cell lymphoma (Stein et al. 1985) is characterized by expression of the Ki1 (CD30) antigen (Schwab et al. 1982). Many T-cell (and B-cell) lymphomas contain some large, activated cells that are CD30+ and CD30− lymphomas, especially T-cell lymphomas; many become CD30+ when they transform to a higher grade. The cells of large cell anaplastic T-cell lymphomas are, however, uniformly positive with CD30 from the outset. In comparison to the other high-grade T-cell lymphomas this tumour occurs in patients of a slightly younger age group, many cases having been described in children (Schnitzer et al. 1988) and has a slightly better prognosis especially if treated at an early stage.

Anaplastic large cell T-cell lymphoma is composed of very large cells with pale-staining cytoplasm and bizarre pleomorphic nuclei (Fig. 14). The tumour cells tend to infiltrate lymph node sinuses and not infrequently show phagocytosis of red cells and other

particles. Because of these features, cases were often misdiagnosed as examples of metastatic carcinoma or malignant histiocytosis in the past. The tumour cells are very variable in their expression of T-cell antigens, often failing to express many or even all T-cell markers, while a minority of cases demonstrate a B-cell phenotype. Genotypic analysis gives similar results, with the majority showing T-cell receptor gene rearrangement, a minority Ig gene rearrangement, or no evidence of either gene rearrangement (Herbst et al. 1989). All cases, however, express CD30 antigen. Karyotypic analysis suggests that a breakpoint on chromosome 5 may be a consistent finding in these lymphomas (Fischer et al. 1988).

Malignant lymphoma, lymphoblastic

This tumour occurs predominantly in children and adolescents and is often associated with T-cell acute lymphoblastic leukaemia (T-ALL). Lymphadenopathy with or without a mediastinal (thymic) mass is the common presenting feature. The pattern of infiltration is similar to that of B-cell lymphoblastic lymphoma.

Malignant lymphoma of T-cells, unclassified

The classification of T-cell lymphoma given above is, with few exceptions, such as the cerebriform cell type, only tentative at the present time. Many cases defy classification and, typically, T-cell lymphomas can change their histological appearances in sequential biopsies taken within a short time and even appear different in two biopsies taken at the same time.

Malignant lymphoma of rare and unusual types

Malignant lymphoma, histiocytic

Malignant tumours of tissue macrophages (histiocytes) were undoubtedly much overdiagnosed in the past; many of these cases were, in fact, examples of peripheral T-cell lymphoma, especially of the large cell anaplastic (CD30+) variety. Such neoplasms do occur, however, either as a disseminated malignancy throughout the monocyte/macrophage system, so-called malignant histiocytosis or as a localized tumour usually in lymph nodes. Stringent immunocytochemical requirements must be fulfilled before a diagnosis of true histiocytic malignancy is made. The malignant cells should react with one or more of the established, macrophage-specific, monoclonal antibodies and in most cases can be shown to synthesize lysozyme. Particular care must be taken to ensure that reactive macrophages, which may be present in huge numbers in both B- and T-cell lymphomas, especially the latter, are not mistaken for the tumour cell population.

PRIMARY EXTRANODAL NON-HODGKIN'S LYMPHOMA

Provided a careful distinction is made between those lymphomas that arise in the lymph nodes and involve extranodal sites secondarily and those that arise primarily from extranodal lymphoid tissue or other non-lymphoid tissues, it is clear that a significant proportion of non-Hodgkin's lymphomas, up to 40 per cent in some series (Freeman *et al.* 1972), may be truly extranodal in origin; primary extranodal Hodgkin's disease is, on the other hand, vanishingly rare.

The association of immunodeficiency and extranodal lymphoma

There is an increased incidence of lymphoma in both congenital and acquired immunodeficiency states and a steadily rising incidence of lymphoma associated with acquired immunodeficiency following therapeutic immunosuppression for organ transplantation and the acquired immune deficiency syndrome (**AIDS**). The great majority of these are extranodal high-grade B-cell lymphomas. They are often multifocal and the gut is the most common primary site, followed by the brain, which, for some reason, is a frequent primary site for American but not British patients with AIDS. The lymphomas frequently show evidence of integration of EBV in their genomes and current thinking has it that immunodeficiency results in unopposed action of the virus causing polyclonal B-cell proliferation that finally becomes monoclonal (Frizzera *et al.* 1980; Locker and Nalesnik 1989).

Lymphomas of mucosa-associated lymphoid tissue (MALT)

The majority of extranodal lymphomas arise in the gastrointestinal tract, which is not surprising as it contains more lymphoid tissue than the lymph nodes and spleen combined. This lymphoid tissue, known as gut-associated lymphoid tissue (**GALT**), has morphological and functional characteristics that are different from those of peripheral lymph nodes and this appears to account for certain histological and clinical differences between the nodal lymphomas and primary gastrointestinal lymphoma. Similar lymphoid tissue is found at other mucosal sites and, together with GALT, this is collectively known as mucosa-associated lymphoid tissue (**MALT**). Lymphomas arising from MALT in different organs share many clinicopathological features and are conveniently considered as a group that, in addition to primary gastrointestinal lymphoma, includes lymphomas of the lung, salivary gland, and thyroid (Isaacson and Spencer 1987). Extranodal lymphomas can, however, arise from any site in the body, whether or not lymphoid tissue is a natural component. The incidence of extranodal lymphoma shows considerable geographical variation, but everywhere accounts for a substantial proportion of lymphoma cases. Where previously it was thought that the clinicopathological characteristics of the well-studied nodal lymphomas could simply be extended to extranodal disease, this is clearly no longer the case, as has been well shown by recent studies of those lymphomas arising from MALT.

The structure and function of MALT

The highest, and most accessible, concentrations of MALT are to be found in the gastrointestinal tract (GALT) so that it is not surprising that in both man and experimental animals it is GALT that has been most extensively studied. The tendency, which may not be altogether justified, is to use GALT as a prototype for the properties of MALT as a whole. In man, mucosal lymphoid nodules are present throughout the small and large intestine, with the highest concentrations forming Peyer's patches in the terminal ileum. These nodules (Fig. 15) consist of B-cell follicles surrounded by a broad zone of B-cells known as the marginal zone (Spencer *et al.* 1985*a*,*b*). The marginal zone can be found in any lymphoid tissue, but is best developed in the spleen and Peyer's patches. Marginal-zone cells infiltrate the epithelium covering Peyer's patches, the so-called dome epithelium, where they are present as intraepithelial B-cells contrasting with the more common intraepithelial T-cells present in the remainder of the epithelium. The largest B-cell compartment in the gut consists of the plasma cells of the lamina propria, which are present throughout the intestine. The T-cell component of GALT consists of three compartments: the first resembles in every way the paracortex of lymph nodes and is situated in the mucosal lymphoid nodules (Peyer's patches) between the B-cell areas and abutting the muscularis mucosae, the second consists of the predominantly CD4+ T-cells of the lamina propria, and the third comprises the intraepithelial T-cells, a heterogeneous but predominantly CD8+ population. There are no afferent lymphatics in GALT and the efferent lymphatics drain into the mesenteric lymph nodes, which in turn drain into the thoracic duct.

Antigen enters Peyer's patches from the lumen of the gut, crossing the dome epithelium by an active process that involves specialized epithelial cells, the M-cells. By a mechanism that is not entirely understood, but which possibly involves specialized T-cells, antigenic stimulation of GALT B-cells results predominantly in

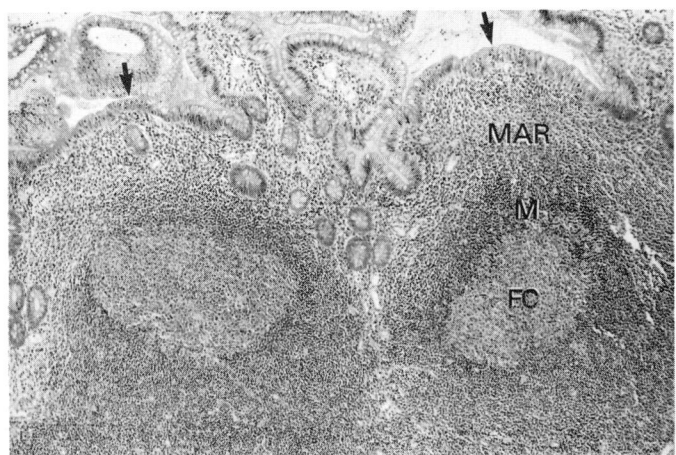

Fig. 15 Peyer's patches of human terminal ileum. These consist of a follicle centre (FC), mantle zone (MZ), and a broad marginal zone (MAR). A small focus of intraepithelial B-cells is present in the dome epithelium (arrows).

IGA-synthesizing blasts. These leave the Peyer's patches and pass through the mesenteric nodes into the thoracic duct and, hence, into the circulation. Thence, by 'homing' mechanisms discussed earlier, the cells return to the lamina propria of the gut as plasma cells or memory B-cells. Exactly at what stage transformation from blast to plasma cell or memory B-cell occurs is not clear.

Much less is known about the functional aspects of GALT T-cells. The paracortex-like areas in Peyer's patches and the T-cells of the lamina propria appear to be the seat of conventional T-cell responses to luminal antigens and there is some evidence that GALT-derived T-cells home to the gut in the same way as B-cells. The role of intraepithelial T-cells is much more obscure, but they too appear to be a gut-committed population.

The concepts of mucosa-derived lymphocytes specifically homing back to the mucosae are largely derived from animal experiments. Such experiments have also led to the suggestion that there is a common mucosal immune system in which lymphocytes from one mucosal site may home to another, but not to peripheral lymphoid tissue. It should be pointed out, however, that there are considerable interspecies differences in mucosal immunity and that data derived from animal experiments may not necessarily hold true in man. In this respect the mucosal lymphomas, in the way they parody normal lymphoid structure and function, may constitute a valid human 'experiment'.

B-cell lymphomas of MALT

A group of low-grade, B-cell, extranodal lymphomas has been identified whose histological features resemble closely those of MALT. This includes lymphomas of the gastrointestinal tract, lung, salivary gland, and thyroid (Isaacson and Spencer 1987). The clinical features of these lymphomas are similar and differ significantly from those of nodal, low-grade, B-cell lymphomas. These include a long history, associated autoimmune disease, good response to surgical excision, and a favourable prognosis. Transformation to high-grade lymphoma may occur and results in loss of many of the histological hallmarks of MALT lymphoma. Whether these secondary high-grade lymphomas or, indeed, primary high-grade lymphomas that arise in MALT, also have a better prognosis than their nodal counterparts is less certain, but appears to be the case.

There is, as yet, no satisfactory explanation for the indolent clinical behaviour of MALT lymphomas. The lineage of the tumour cells is clearly an important factor and needs to be conclusively established. Preferential homing of the tumour cells to the gut and other mucosae may be an important factor and there is some evidence to suggest that differentiation into non-tumourogenic plasma cells may occur when the lymphoma cells enter the circulation (Spencer et al. 1990).

Although MALT lymphomas form a distinctive group, not all lymphomas of mucosal organs are of MALT type. It is, therefore, more appropriate to consider the MALT lymphomas grouped together with other types of lymphoma, according to their organ of origin.

As with MALT itself, it is the gastrointestinal lymphomas of MALT that have been best characterized and serve as a prototype for the other members of the group. They will, therefore, be described in greatest detail in the following section.

PRIMARY GASTROINTESTINAL LYMPHOMA

Primary gastrointestinal lymphoma accounts for the majority of extranodal lymphomas. As can be seen from the provisional

Table 3 Primary gastrointestinal lymphoma

B-cell
  Lymphomas of MALT-type
    Low-grade B-cell lymphoma of MALT
    High-grade B-cell lymphoma of MALT with or without evidence of a low-grade component
    Immunoproliferative small-intestinal disease (IPSID), low grade and/or high grade
    (Plasmacytoma)
  Lymphomatous polyposis (centrocytic lymphoma)
  Burkitt's and Burkitt-like lymphoma
  Other types

T-cell
  Enteropathy-associated T-cell lymphoma
  Other types

classification of these tumours given in Table 3, not all cases fall into the MALT category, but they are, in any case, best discussed collectively. There is marked geographical variation in the incidence of gastrointestinal lymphoma and the disease is particularly common in the Middle East (Al-Bahrani et al. 1983). There is evidence that the incidence of primary gastric lymphoma is rising in Western countries (Hayes and Dunn 1989).

Low-grade B-cell lymphoma of MALT

In Western countries this type of lymphoma occurs most commonly as a primary gastric tumour; in the Middle East, both gastric and intestinal forms are common. Primary low-grade gastric lymphoma occurs predominantly in individuals over 50 years of age, but an increasing number of cases are being reported in younger patients in their 30s or less (Isaacson et al. 1986). The sex incidence is equal. The symptoms are usually those of upper abdominal dyspepsia; severe abdominal pain with the finding of a mass is rare. Endoscopy reveals features of non-specific gastritis or a peptic ulcer, the presence of a mass again being unusual. Unless a histological diagnosis is made early, repeated endoscopic examinations often follow intermittently successful treatment for gastritis or peptic ulcer. Staging procedures rarely reveal any extra-abdominal spread and when, as in most instances, the disease is confined to the gastric wall the prognosis is excellent (Weingrad et al. 1982). Much less is known about the clinical features of low-grade B-cell lymphoma of the intestine, which is rare in the West, but data from the Middle East suggests that it too carries a good prognosis (Cammoun et al. 1989).

The histological features of low-grade, B-cell, gastrointestinal lymphoma of MALT are closely similar to those of MALT itself (Fig. 16) (Isaacson and Spencer 1987). Reactive, non-neoplastic follicles are an integral component and beyond their mantle zones there is an infiltrate of cells bearing a resemblance to centrocytes, the so-called centrocyte-like cells. These cells, which also resemble marginal-zone B-cells, invade the epithelium of individual mucosal glands to form the characteristic lymphoepithelial lesions. Plasma cell differentiation occurs in approximately one-third of cases, usually in a band-like distribution beneath the surface epithelium and scattered transformed blasts are often present. A peculiar feature of these lymphomas is the tendency of the centrocyte-like cells to invade and selectively replace the reactive follicles, leading to an appearance that may be confused with true follicular lymphoma (Myhre and Isaacson 1987; Isaacson et al. 1991). The favourable prognosis of low-grade, B-cell, MALT lymphoma, when compared

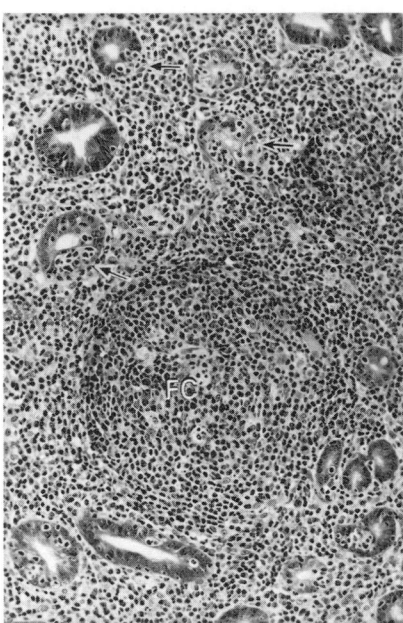

Fig. 16 Low grade B-cell gastric lymphoma of MALT. Note follicle centre (FC) with CCL infiltrate above forming lymphoepithelial lesions (arrows). Compared with Fig. 15.

to that of low-grade B-cell lymphomas of peripheral lymph nodes, had led to doubt as to their truly malignant nature and given rise to the term 'pseudolymphoma'. Immunohistochemistry, by demonstrating light-chain restriction, allows clear separation between reactive and neoplastic B-cell proliferation, obviating the need for the term pseudolymphoma (Spencer *et al.* 1989).

The precise lineage of the centrocyte-like cells in MALT lymphomas has not yet been established with certainty. Preferential localization of these cells around B-cell follicles, their tendency to infiltrate epithelium, and their cytological features suggest a marginal-zone B-cell lineage and this is, to a certain extent, supported by their immunohistochemical phenotype (Spencer *et al.* 1986). Molecular studies have shown that rearrangement of the *bcl2* candidate oncogene, a feature of up to 95 per cent of follicle centre-cell lymphomas, is not present in MALT lymphomas despite the presence of a follicular pattern in many cases. This is strong evidence against a follicle centre-cell lineage (Pan *et al.* 1989).

High-grade B-cell lymphoma of MALT

The majority of primary gastrointestinal lymphomas are histologically high grade. As indicated above, a variable number of transformed blast cells are present in low-grade MALT lymphomas. Sometimes these occur in significant numbers, resulting in a mixed high- and low-grade picture; if aggregated sheets of blasts are present, then the tumour is considered to be high grade (Chan *et al.* 1990). In many cases, however, there is no evidence of low-grade foci. The cytological features of the high-grade cells resemble those of centroblasts in all cases, whether or not a low-grade component is detected and there are no other features, including the immunophenotype, that usefully characterizes them. Thus, although there is circumstantial evidence similar to that linking high- and low-grade, follicle centre-cell, nodal lymphomas, that high-grade primary gastrointestinal lymphomas are of the same lineage as the low-grade MALT lyphomas, there is no conclusive proof that this is the case.

The high-grade lymphomas tend to form large, bulky masses, resulting in clinical features much more like those of gastrointestinal carcinoma. Although their local stage tends to be more advanced than that of the low-grade tumours, extra-abdominal spread is once more a late phenomenon and response to therapy, which is closely related to stage, is good (Weingrad *et al.* 1982). Although not completely characterized, the prognosis of these high-grade lymphomas appears to be better than that of their nodal counterparts, which is another argument in favour of a MALT-related lineage.

Immunoproliferative small-intestinal disease (IPSID)

This type of gastrointestinal MALT lymphoma, sometimes called Mediterranean lymphoma, occurs almost exclusively in the Middle East (Khojasteh *et al.* 1983). Cases have also been reported from the Cape area of South Africa and sporadically from elsewhere. The lymphoma occurs typically in the upper small intestine of young adults, is characterized by malabsorption, and has a prolonged course. IPSID is distinguished from other MALT lymphomas by its epidemiological features, its restriction, with few exceptions, to the small intestine, and the extreme degree of plasma cell differentiation in the tumour, which otherwise is histologically a typical low-grade MALT lymphoma (Isaacson *et al.* 1989). These plasma cells synthesize an abnormal α heavy chain without a light chain and in two-thirds of cases this can be detected in the blood as a paraprotein giving rise to the term α-chain disease. Perhaps the most curious feature of all is the response of a proportion of cases of early-stage IPSID to broad-spectrum antibiotics. Just how complete this response can be is not entirely clear, as with prolonged natural history of the disease, follow-up must extend over many years before definitive conclusions can be drawn. Like other MALT lymphomas, IPSID remains localized to the abdomen until late in its course when transformation into a high-grade lymphoma occurs.

Plasmacytoma

There are case reports of solitary plasmacytomas occurring throughout the gastrointestinal tract from the oesophagus to the rectum. These tumours have a favourable outlook and are possibly examples of MALT lymphoma with extreme plasma cell differentiation.

Lymphomatous polyposis

This uncommon type of primary gastrointestinal lymphoma does not share the features of MALT. It is characterized by multiple lymphomatous polyps involving long segments of the gut and/or stomach (Isaacson *et al.* 1983). The ileocaecal area is most commonly involved and the tumours tend to be largest there. Unlike MALT lymphoma, lymphomatous polyposis is an aggressive condition that rapidly disseminates to the bone-marrow, blood, and peripheral lymph nodes. The histological features and immunophenotype are identical to those of centrocytic lymphoma. However, biopsies of the more localized examples of this condition may be readily confused with MALT lymphoma; CD5 positivity of the cells and the absence of lymphoepithelial lesions are important discriminating features.

Burkitt's and Burkitt-like lymphoma

Classical African Burkitt's lymphoma is a tumour arising predominantly in the jaws of children, as described above. While other viscera are often secondarily involved, this only rarely includes the gut. In the Middle East, lymphoma histologically indistinguishable from Burkitt's lymphoma and showing the same association with EBV occurs commonly as a primary tumour in children (Al-Bahrani *et al.* 1986). In the West, primary gastrointestinal lymphoma is rare in children, but when it occurs it is most usually in the ileocaecal region and is histologically identical or closely similar to classical Burkitt's lymphoma. Like the MALT lymphomas, these lymphomas remain confined to the abdomen for prolonged periods, but they show none of the other MALT features.

Other types of B-cell lymphoma

Other B-cell lymphomas, including malignant lymphoma, cb/cc, and lymphocytic, may arise in the gut but are uncommon.

Primary T-cell gastrointestinal lymphoma

Primary T-cell gastrointestinal lymphomas are uncommon. While there are many case reports of T-cell lymphomas of varying histological type, there is only one defined clinicopathological entity in this group, namely enteropathy-associated T-cell lymphoma.

Enteropathy-associated T-cell lymphoma (EATL)

This type of lymphoma may complicate coeliac disease (gluten-sensitive enteropathy) of long standing but more usually follows a short history of adult coeliac disease (Isaacson and Wright 1978). In a proportion of cases there is no history of coeliac disease, but the jejunal mucosa shows crypt hyperplasia and villous atrophy when the tumour is excised. Recent evidence has suggested that failure to adhere to a gluten-free diet may predispose coeliacs to develop lymphoma (Holmes *et al.* 1989). There may be a long prodromal period with severe malabsorption not responding to gluten withdrawal. This is sometimes associated with non-specific small-intestinal mucosal ulceration, a condition known as ulcerative jejunitis. Although these ulcers are not obviously lymphomatous, careful searching often reveals an associated focus of lymphoma elsewhere in the intestine or in the base of one or more ulcers. The lymphoma frequently causes an acute abdominal emergency and is often multicentric, but may present as a single, large mass anywhere in the small intestine or, less commonly, in the large bowel or even the stomach. Extra-abdominal dissemination to the bone marrow, lung, skin, and lymph nodes is common and may have already occurred by the time the lymphoma is diagnosed, leading in some cases to a presentation with extra-abdominal manifestations.

The histology of EATL spans the full range of that described in T-cell lymphoma, both between cases and within any individual case. At one extreme the cells may be small and monomorphic while at the other the tumour has all the characteristics of a large-cell, anaplastic (CD30+), T-cell lymphoma. A heavy infiltrate of eosinophils is often present.

Certain features of EATL are consistent with it being a malignancy of a GALT-committed T-cell. Thus, the lymphoma clearly originates in the intestinal mucosa, where it may remain for prolonged periods and surgical excision sometimes effects long remissions or even 'cures'. The presence, in some cases, of intraepithelial tumour cells together with expression of the HML-1 antigen (Spencer *et al.* 1988), which is preferentially expressed by intraepithelial T-cells, support the suggestion that the cell lineage in EATL is that of the intraepithelial T-cell.

CUTANEOUS LYMPHOMAS

The skin is the second most common site of extranodal lymphoma after the gastrointestinal tract. The clinical behaviour of cutaneous lymphomas of both B- and T-cell types has much in common with those of the gut, suggesting that there are populations of lymphocytes whose function relates particularly to the skin and whose properties include specific homing to the skin. The analogy to MALT is strong, but no organized skin-associated lymphoid tissue (SALT) can be demonstrated in normal skin.

Small cerebriform T-cell cutaneous lymphoma

Perhaps because it was the first T-cell lymphoma to be recognized, this is the only extranodal lymphoma that has been included as a separate entity in all the modern classifications. In many ways it serves as a model to show that extranodal lymphomas have distinctive histological and clinical features that justify their separation from nodal tumours. The cerebriform T-cell is named for its nucleus, which has a strikingly irregular, folded appearance best seen in electron micrographs. These cells, sometimes known as Lutzner's cells, are seen in two clinically distinct lymphomas, both of which selectively involve the skin, namely mycosis fungoides and Sézary's syndrome.

Mycosis fungoides

This is a slowly evolving, cutaneous T-cell lymphoma, which over a number of years (up to 20 or more), passes through so-called pre-mycotic, infiltrative, and tumour phases. The first two are characterized, respectively, by flat, slightly reddened, and rough patches on the skin and by slightly thickened, violaceous patches. In the third stage, large, ulcerating plaques of tumour appear. Eventually the lymph nodes are involved and the tumour may transform into a high-grade T-cell lymphoma.

Histologically the skin shows infiltration of the upper dermis by cerebriform cells accompanied by variable numbers of reactive macrophages, eosinophils, and other cells (Fig. 17). The dermis is infiltrated by cerebriform cells either singly or in clusters forming so-called Pautrier's microabscesses.

Lymphadenopathy is common in patients with mycosis fungoides and may be due to dermatopathic lymphadenopathy or lymphomatous involvement. It may be impossible to differentiate between the two

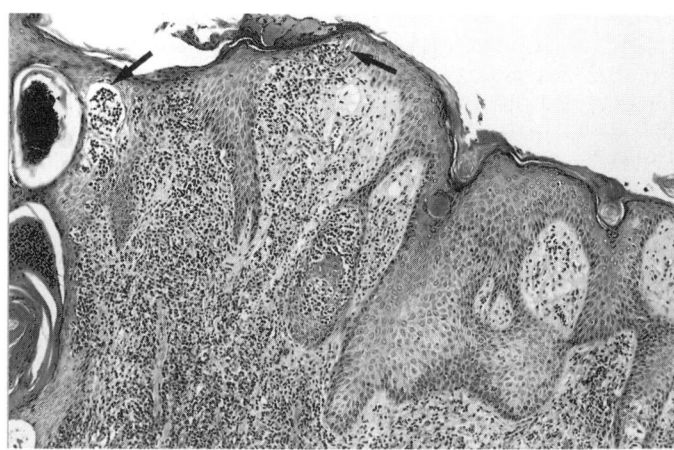

Fig. 17 Cerebriform T-cell lymphoma of skin (mycosis fungoides). A T-cell infiltrate hugs the epidermis which it invades and focally forms cell clusters known as Pautrier's microabscesses.

on histological grounds alone and analysis of the lymph node DNA for T-cell-receptor β-chain rearrangements frequently indicates the presence of tumour despite negative histological findings. The cerebriform cells in mycosis fungoides are, with very few exceptions, CD3+, CD4+, and CD8−.

Sézary's syndrome

In this disease, patients present with diffuse reddening of the skin, alopecia, and a leukaemic blood picture due to circulating cerebriform cells. Sézary's syndrome is, in effect, a leukaemic form of mycosis fungoides, but in contrast to other leukaemias, bone-marrow involvement is uncommon. The histological appearances of the skin are similar to those of mycosis fungoides.

Lymphomatoid papulosis and allied conditions

The three cutaneous lymphoproliferative conditions, that is, pityriasis lichenoides et variolaformis acuta (PLEVA), lymphomatoid papulosis, and regressing atypical histiocytosis, are related skin eruptions that usually remain localized to the skin, but which may after an indeterminate time (very many years in some instances) evolve into a generalized T-cell lymphoma. Genotypic studies have shown evidence of monoclonality in all three diseases (Weiss *et al.* 1986, 1987; Headington *et al.* 1987) and they are probably best regarded as extremely indolent forms of T-cell lymphoma.

Other cutaneous T-cell lymphomas

A proportion of cutaneous T-cell lymphomas present as dermal tumours and run an aggressive course. Many of these infiltrate the dermis in an angiocentric pattern and are further characterized by large foci of necrosis.

Cutaneous B-cell lymphomas

Primary B-cell lymphomas of the skin are much less frequent than T-cell tumours. They may be low or high grade. Like most of the T-cell lymphomas they characteristically remain localized to the skin for long periods, recurring in the skin, often at another site, after excision, radiotherapy, or spontaneous regression. This pattern of behaviour is strongly suggestive of specific B-cell homing to the skin.

PULMONARY LYMPHOMA

MALT is present in the lung as lymphoid nodules in the bronchi (BALT). Low-grade, B-cell, pulmonary lymphoma usually presents as an incidental finding of radiographic opacity. Sjögren's syndrome and diffuse interstitial pneumonia of the lymphoid type are associated in a proportion of cases (Hansen *et al.* 1989). Pulmonary lymphoma is particularly slow growing and many cases have been designated as 'pseudolymphoma' for this reason. However, unequivocal light-chain restriction and Ig gene rearrangement can be demonstrated in the cases. Indolent clinical behaviour is characteristic of primary B-cell pulmonary lymphoma. Local progression, dissemination of low-grade lymphoma, and transformation into a high-grade lymphoma can all occur. The histological features are entirely typical of a low-grade B-cell lymphoma of MALT with reactive follicles surrounded by centrocyte-like cells, which form lymphoepithelial lesions (Fig. 18) (Addis *et al.* 1988). High-grade B-cell lymphomas may occur in the lung and their relation to the low-grade MALT lymphoma is similar to that in the gastrointestinal tract.

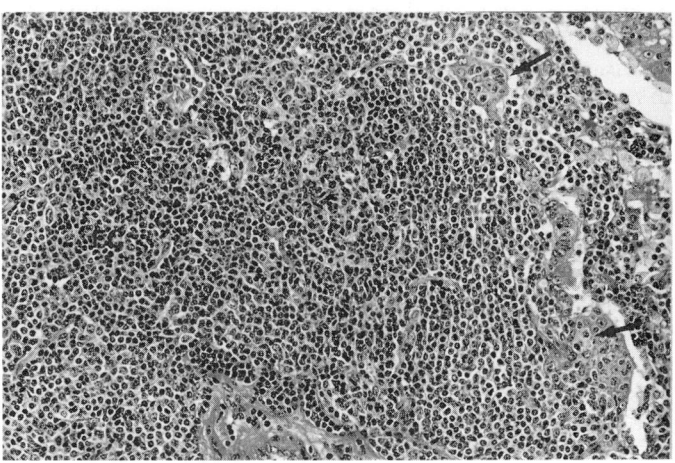

Fig. 18 MALT lymphoma of lung showing a follicle centre (FC) with surrounding CCL cells forming lymphoepithelial lesions with bronchiolar epithelium (arrows). Compare with Figs 16, 19, and 20.

T-cell lymphomas may also occur as primary lung tumours. Previously known as lymphomatoid granulomatosis, these T-cell lymphomas may be low or high grade and display an angiocentric pattern of infiltration.

SALIVARY GLAND LYMPHOMA

MALT is not an integral component of the parenchyma of the parotid gland, the most common site of salivary gland lymphoma. However, the lymphoid infiltrate that characterizes Sjögren's syndrome and allied conditions (collectively known as myoepithelial sialadenitis or **MESA**) effectively results in the acquisition of MALT by the salivary gland, with lymphoid nodules underlying dilated ducts showing all the features of Peyer's patches as described above (Hyjek *et al.* 1988). The majority of cases of salivary gland lymphoma arise in a setting of Sjögren's syndrome. The tumour is slow growing and may remain localized to the parotid for many years before dissemination or transformation to a high-grade lesion occurs. The histological features are the same as those of the other MALT lymphomas (Fig. 19). It can be difficult to decide on histological grounds alone just when lymphoma has supervened on MESA and immunohistochemistry with genotypic analysis may be necessary.

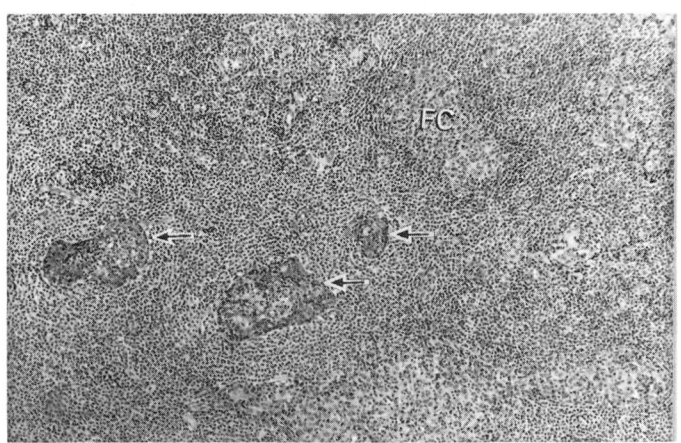

Fig. 19 MALT lymphoma of salivary gland showing follicle centre (FC) with surrounding CCL cells forming lymphoepithelial lesions (arrows). Compare with Figs 16, 18, and 20.

THYROID GLAND LYMPHOMA

This is a rare tumour that almost invariably occurs in the setting of Hashimoto's thyroiditis. There is no native MALT in the thyroid, which can only be considered a mucosal organ with reference to its embryological origin from the foregut. As in MESA the lymphoid infiltrate in Hashimoto's thyroiditis closely resembles MALT and the low-grade B-cell lymphoma is histologically identical with the other MALT lymphomas (Fig. 20) (Hyjek and Isaacson 1988). Especially prominent are the lymphoepithelial lesions formed by centrocyte-like cells invading thyroid acini. The clinical behaviour of thyroid lymphoma is the same as that of the other MALT lymphomas.

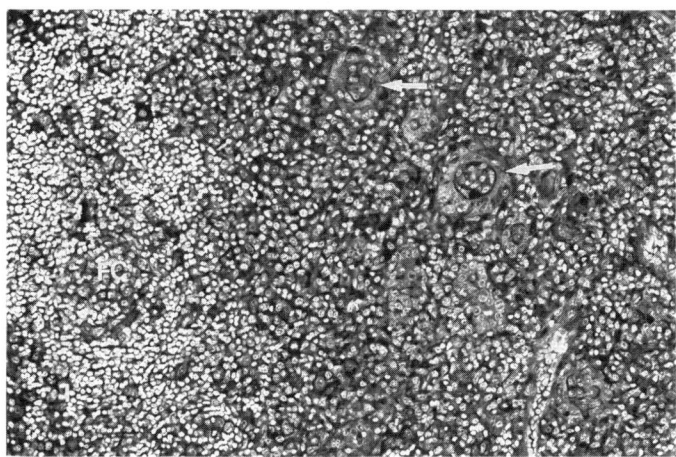

Fig. 20 MALT lymphoma of thyroid showing follicle centre (FC) surrounded by infiltrate of centrocyte-like (CCL) cells forming lymphoepithelial lesions with thyroid acini (arrows). Compare with Figs 16, 18, and 19.

LYMPHOMAS OF WALDEYER'S RING, NASOPHARYNX, AND NOSE

In its relation to the pharyngeal epithelium and its lack of afferent lymphatics the tonsil resembles GALT, but its overall structure, lack of prominent marginal zones, and the predominance of IgG rather than IgA secretion by its resident plasma cells are more characteristic of peripheral lymph nodes. This mixed picture is reflected in the lymphomas that arise in the tonsil. Thus, among low-grade lymphomas, primary follicular (cb/cc) lymphoma is quite common in the tonsil in contrast to the gut, where it is very rare. Lymphoplasmacytic lymphoma and centrocytic lymphoma also arise in the tonsil. Lymphoma of MALT type has been observed in the tonsil, but is uncommon. High-grade B-cell lymphomas account for 70–90 per cent of primary tonsillar lymphomas (Saul *et al.* 1986). There is an association between B-cell lymphoma of Waldeyer's ring and gastrointestinal lymphoma (Ree *et al.* 1980).

B-cell lymphomas of the nasopharynx and nose are less common and tend to be of high-grade histological appearances. Plasmacytoma is a fairly common nasal tumour and also occurs in the upper respiratory tract, where it carries a favourable prognosis.

T-cell lymphomas of the nasopharynx

This special category of extranodal lymphoma was poorly recognized in the past when it went by various names, the most common of which was 'lethal midline granuloma'. As this name suggests the condition often behaves as a locally destructive inflammatory lesion from which generalized T-cell lymphoma evolves in some instances (Chan *et al.* 1987). There are parallels in the behaviour of this tumour with primary angiocentric T-cell lymphoma of the lung.

LYMPHOMA OF THE THYMUS

T-lymphoblastic lymphoma is the most common thymic non-Hodgkin's lymphoma and is usually accompanied by acute lymphocytic leukaemia, which dominates the clinical picture. Peripheral T-cell lymphoma is exceedingly rare in the thymus.

Primary, high-grade, B-cell lymphoma of the mediastinum almost certainly arises in the thymus (Addis and Isaacson 1987). It is a clinicopathologically distinct tumour that can run an aggressive course. Histologically this lymphoma may show packeting of the cells in a carcinoma-like pattern and is often accompanied by considerable sclerosis. It is conceivable that the lymphoma is of the same lineage as the recently identified, native thymic B-cell population (Isaacson *et al.* 1987).

PRIMARY SPLENIC LYMPHOMA

Given the mass of lymphoid tissue in the spleen and its central role in B-cell immunity, together with its focal position in the circulation of B-cells, it is not surprising that it is so frequently involved by lymphoma. This involvement is almost always secondary, however and primary splenic lymphoma, which may be of any histological type, is rare.

PRIMARY LYMPHOMA OF BONE

The bone-marrow is the site of the genesis of lymphocytes and also an important site through which lymphocytes recirculate. Discounting acute and chronic lymphocytic leukaemias and myeloma, lymphomas of bone, presenting as a bone tumour that presumably arises as a solitary focus in the marrow, is very rare. Bone lymphoma is usually of high-grade B-cell type.

CEREBRAL LYMPHOMA

The incidence of primary cerebral lymphoma is increasing dramatically to the point where it is now amongst the more common primary cerebral tumours (Eby *et al.* 1988). This increase is not accounted for by those lymphomas occurring in association with immunosuppressive states (including AIDS), which have also increased independently. There is no native lymphoid tissue in the brain and the cell lineage of cerebral lymphomas, almost all of which are high-grade B-cell tumours, is unknown.

LYMPHOMA OF THE ORBIT

Low-grade B-cell lymphomas of the orbit, lacrimal gland, and eyelid are a collective group with similar clinicopathological features. These lymphomas are either lymphocytic or lymphoplasmacytic, while a proportion show the features of low-grade B-cell lymphoma of MALT (Medeiros and Harris 1989). The indolent clinical behaviour of some of these lymphomas is again very similar to that of MALT lymphomas and in the past has led to the use of the term 'pseudo-lymphoma' for some cases. However, approximately 50 per cent of cases disseminate to involve the bone-marrow and peripheral lymph nodes. At present there is no correlation between detailed histological findings and clinical behaviour.

LYMPHOMA OF THE TESTIS

Primary lymphoma accounts for 5 per cent of all testicular tumours but is the most frequent testicular tumour in patients over 50 years of age. These are invariably high-grade B-cell (centroblastic) lymphomas with a distinctive peritubular pattern of infiltration of the testis (Wilkins *et al.* 1989).

LYMPHOMA OF THE BREAST

Primary breast lymphomas surprisingly do not show either the histological or clinical features of MALT lymphoma. They are almost always B-cell lymphomas and their histological features embrace those of low- and high-grade lymphoma as detailed in the Kiel classification. Their clinical behaviour is similar to nodal lymphoma of equivalent type.

OTHER EXTRANODAL LYMPHOMAS

Primary lymphomas have been reported arising in almost every organ and soft tissue. Most of these are B-cell lymphomas, but, because of their rarity, there is little collective information on their clinicopathological characteristics.

REFERENCES

Addis BJ, Isaacson PG (1987). Large cell lymphoma of the mediastinum: a B cell tumour of probable thymic origin. *Histopathology*, **10**:379–90.

Addis B, Hyjek E, Isaacson PG (1988). Primary pulmonary lymphoma: a reappraisal of its histogenesis and its relationship to pseudolymphoma and interstitial pneumonia. *Histopathology*, **13**:1–17.

Aisenberg AC, Krontiris TG, Mak TW, Wilkes BM (1988). Rearrangement of the gene for the beta chain of the T cell receptor in T cell chronic lymphocytic leukaemia and related disorders. *New England Journal of Medicine*, **313**:529–33.

Al-Bahrani ZR, Al-Mondhiry H, Bakir F, Al-Saleem T (1983). Clinical and pathological subtypes of primary intestinal lymphoma. Experience with 132 patients over a 14 year period. *Cancer*, **52**:1666–72.

Al-Bahrani Z, Al-Mondhiry H, Al-Saleem T, Zaini S (1986). Primary intestinal lymphoma in Iraqi children. *Oncology*, **43**:243–50.

Armitage JO, *et al.* (1989). Peripheral T cell lymphoma. *Cancer*, **63**:158–63.

Brown DC, Heryet A, Gatter KC, Mason DY (1989). The prognostic significance of immunophenotype in high-grade non-Hodgkin's lymphoma. *Histopathology*, **14**:621–7.

Burkitt D (1959). Sarcoma involving jaws in African children. *British Journal of Surgery*, **46**:218–33.

Cammoun M, Jaafoura H, Tabbane F, Halphen M, Tufrali Group (1989). Immunoproliferative small intestinal disease without alpha-chain disease: a pathological study. *Gastroenterology*, **96**:750–63.

Chan JKC, Ng CS, Lau WH, Lo STH (1987). Most nasal/nasopharyngeal lymphomas are peripheral T cell neoplasms. *American Journal of Surgical Pathology*, **11**:418–29.

Chan JKC, Ng CS, Isaacson PG (1990). Relationship between high grade lymphoma and low grade B cell mucosa-associated lymphoid tissue lymphoma (MALToma) of the stomach. *American Journal of Pathology*.

Eby NL, Grufferman S, Flannelly CM, Schold SC, Vogel FS, Burger PC (1988). Increasing incidence of primary brain lymphoma in the US. *Cancer*, **62**:2461–5.

Feller AC, *et al.* (1988). Clonal gene rearrangement patterns correlate with immunophenotype and clinical parameters in patients with angioimmunoblastic lymphadenopathy. *American Journal of Surgical Pathology*, **133**:549–56.

Fischer P, *et al.* (1988). A Ki-1 (CD30)-positive human cell line (Karpas 299) established from a high-grade non-Hodgkin's lymphoma, showing a 2;5 translocation and rearrangement of the T cell receptor β-chain gene. *Blood*, **72**:234.

Freeman C, Berg JW, Cutler SJ (1972). Occurrence and prognosis of extranodal lymphomas. *Cancer*, **29**:252–60.

Frizzera G, Moran EM, Rappaport H (1975). Angio-immunoblastic lymphadenopathy with dysproteinaemia. *Lancet*, i:1070–3.

Frizzera G, Rosai J, Dehner LP, Spector BD, Kersey J (1980). Lymphoreticular disorders in primary immunodeficiencies. New findings based on an up-to-date histologic classification of 35 cases. *Cancer*, **46**:692–9.

Gallo RC (1985). Human T cell leukaemia (lymphotropic) retroviruses and their causative role in T cell malignancies and acquired immune deficiency syndrome. *Cancer*, **55**:2317–23.

Hall PA, Richards MA, Gregory WM, d'Ardenne AJ, Lister TA, Stansfeld AG (1988). The prognostic value of Ki67 immunostaining in non-Hodgkin's lymphoma. *Journal of Pathology*, **154**:223–5.

Hansen LA, Prakash UBS, Colby TV (1989). Pulmonary lymphoma in Sjögren's syndrome. *Mayo Clinic Proceedings*, **64**:920–31.

Hastrup N, Ralfkiaer E, Pallesen G (1989). Aberrant phenotypes in peripheral T cell lymphomas. *Journal of Clinical Pathology*, **42**:398–402.

Hayes J, Dunn E (1989). Has the incidence of primary gastric lymphoma increased? *Cancer*, **63**:2073–6.

Headington JT, Roth MS, Schnitzer B (1987). Regressing atypical histiocytosis: a review and critical appraisal. *Seminars in Diagnostic Pathology*, **4**:28–37.

Herbst H, *et al.* (1989). Immunoglobulin and T cell receptor gene rearrangements in Hodgkin's disease and Ki-1 positive anaplastic large cell lymphoma: dissociation between phenotype and genotype. *Leukaemia Research*, **13**:103–16.

Holmes GKT, Prior P, Lane MR, Pope D, Allan RN (1989). Malignancy in coeliac disease—effect of a gluten free diet. *Gut*, **30**:333–8.

Hui PK, Feller AC, Lennert K (1988). High-grade non-Hodgkin's lymphoma of B cell type. I. Histopathology. *Histopathology*, **12**:127–43.

Hyjek E, Isaacson PG (1988). Primary B cell lymphoma of the thyroid and its relationship to Hashimoto's thyroiditis. *Human Pathology*, **19**:1315–26.

Hyjek E, Smith WJ, Isaacson PG (1988). Primary B cell lymphoma of salivary gland and its relationship to myoepithelial sialadenitis. *Human Pathology*, **19**:766–76.

Isaacson PG, Spencer J (1987). Malignant lymphoma of mucosa-associated lymphoid tissue. *Histopathology*, **11**:445–62.

Isaacson PG, Wright DH (1978). Intestinal lymphoma associated with malabsorption. *Lancet*, i:67–70.

Isaacson PG, Wright DH (1986). Immunocytochemistry of lymphoreticular tumours. In *Immunocytochemistry. Practical applications in pathology and biology* (ed. JM Polack and S van Noorden), p. 249. Bristol.

Isaacson PG, MacLennan KA, Subbuswamy SG (1983). Multiple lymphomatous polyposis of the gastrointestinal tract. *Histopathology*, **8**:641–56.

Isaacson PG, Spencer J, Finn T (1986). Primary B cell gastric lymphoma. *Human Pathology*, **17**:72–82.

Isaacson PG, Norton AJ, Addis BJ (1987). The human thymus contains a novel population of B lymphocytes. *Lancet*, ii:1488–91.

Isaacson PG, Dogan A, Price SK, Spencer J (1989). Immunoproliferative small-intestinal disease: an immunohistochemical study. *American Journal of Surgical Pathology*, **13**:1023–33.

Isaacson PG, Wotherspoon AC, Disst P (1991). Follicular colonization in B-cell lymphoma of mucosa associated lymphoid tissue. *American Journal of Surgical Pathology*, **15**:819–28.

Khojasteh A, Haghshenass M, Haghighi P (1983). Immunoproliferative small intestinal disease. A 'third-world lesion'. *New England Journal of Medicine*, **308**:1401–5.

Kristoffersson U, Heim S, Olsson H, Akerman M, Mitelman F (1987). Relationship between cytogenetic findings and histopathology in non-Hodgkin lymphoma. *Acta Pathologica Microbiologica et Immunologica Scandinavica (A)*, **95**:1–5.

Locker J, Nalesnik M (1989). Molecular genetic analysis of lymphoid tumours arising after organ transplantation. *American Journal of Pathology*, **135**:977–87.

Medeiros LJ, Harris NL (1989). Lymphoid infiltrates of the orbit and conjunctiva: a morphological and immunophenotypic study of 99 cases. *American Journal of Surgical Pathology*, **13**:459–71.

Myhre MJ, Isaacson PG (1987). Primary B cell gastric lymphoma—a reassessment of its histogenesis. *Journal of Pathology*, **152**:1–11.

National Cancer Institute (1982). The non-Hodgkin's lymphoma pathological classification project. National Cancer Institute sponsored study of lymphomas: summary and description of a Working Formulation of clinical usage. *Cancer*, **49**:2112–35.

Norton AJ, Isaacson PG (1987). Detailed phenotypic analysis of B cell lymphoma using a panel of antibodies reactive in routinely fixed wax-embedded tissue. *American Journal of Pathology*, **128**:225–40.

Norton AJ, Isaacson PG (1989*a*). Invited review—lymphoma phenotyping in formalin-fixed and paraffin wax-embedded tissues. I. Range of antibodies and staining patterns. *Histopathology*, **14**:437–46.

Norton AJ, Isaacson PG (1989*b*). Invited review—lymphoma phenotyping in formalin-fixed and paraffin wax-embedded tissues. II. Profiles of reactivity in the various tumour types. *Histopathology*, **14**:557–9.

Pals ST, Horst E, Scheper RJ, Meijer CJLM (1989). Mechanisms of human lymphocyte migration and their role in the pathogenesis of disease. *Immunological Reviews*, **108**:111–33.

Pan L, Diss TC, Cunningham D, Isaacson PG (1989). The *bcl-2* gene in primary B cell lymphomas of mucosa associated lymphoid tissue (MALT). *American Journal of Pathology*, **135**:7–11.

Patsouris E, Noël H, Lennert K (1988). Histological and immunohistological findings in lymphoepithelioid cell lymphoma (Lennert's lymphoma). *American Journal of Surgical Pathology*, **12**:341–50.

Rappaport H (1966). Tumours of the haematopoietic system. In *Atlas of tumour pathology*, Section 3, Fascicle 8. US Armed Forces Institute of Pathology, Washington DC.

Ree HJ (1980). Malignant lymphoma of Waldeyer's ring following gastrointestinal lymphoma. *Cancer*, **46**:1528–35.

Saul SH, Kapadia SB (1986). Secondary lymphoma of Waldeyer's ring: natural history and association with prior extranodal disease. *American Journal of Otolaryngology*, **7**:34–41.

Schnitzer B, Roth MS, Hyder DM, Ginsberg D (1988). Ki-1 lymphomas in children. *Cancer*, **61**:1213–21.

Schwab V, *et al.* (1982). Production of monoclonal antibody specific for Hodgkin and Reed–Sternberg cells of Hodgkin's disease and a subset of normal lymphoid cells. *Nature*, **299**:65–7.

Southern EM (1975). Detection of specific sequences among DNA fragments separated by gel electrophoresis. *Journal of Molecular Biology*, **98**:503–10.

Spencer J, Finn T, Isaacson PG (1985*a*). Gut associated lymphoid tissue: a morphological and immunocytochemical study of the human appendix. *Gut*, **26**:672–9.

Spencer J, Finn T, Pulford KAF, Mason DY, Isaacson PG (1985*b*). The human gut contains a novel population of B lymphocytes which resemble marginal zone cells. *Clinical and Experimental Immunology*, **62**:607–10.

Spencer J, Finn T, Isaacson PG (1986). Human Peyer's patches: an immunohistochemical study. *Gut*, **27**:405–10.

Spencer J, *et al.* (1988). Enteropathy associated T cell lymphoma (malignant histiocytosis of the intestine) is recognized by a monoclonal antibody (HML1) that defines a membrane molecule on human mucosal lymphocytes. *American Journal Pathology*, **132**:1–5.

Spencer J, Smith WJ, Diss TC, Isaacson PG (1989). Primary B cell gastric lymphoma and 'pseudolymphoma': a genotypic analysis. *American Journal of Pathology*, **135**:557–64.

Spencer J, Diss TC, Isaacson PG (1990). A study of the properties of low grade mucosal B cell lymphoma using a monoclonal antibody specific for the tumour immunoglobulin. *Journal of Pathology*, **160**:231–8.

Spier CM, Lippman SM, Miller TP, Grogan TM (1988). Lennert's lymphoma. A clinicopathologic study with emphasis of phenotype and its relationship to survival. *Cancer*, **61**:517–24.

Stansfeld AG (ed.) (1985). *Lymph node biopsy interpretation*, pp. 228–76. Churchill Livingstone, Edinburgh.

Stansfeld AG, *et al.* (1988). Updated Kiel classification for lymphomas. *Lancet*, i:292–3.

Stein H, *et al.* (1985). The expression of the Hodgkin's disease associated antigen Ki-1 in reactive and neoplastic lymphoid tissue. *Blood*, **65**:848–58.

Suchi T, *et al.* (1987). Histopathology and immunohistochemistry of peripheral T cell lymphomas: a proposal for their classification. *Journal of Clinical Pathology*, **40**:995–1015.

Tolksdorf G, Stein H, Kennert K (1980). Morphological and immunological definition of a malignant lymphoma derived from germinal-centre cells with cleaved nuclei (centrocytes). *British Journal of Cancer*, **41**:168–82.

Weingrad DN, Decosse JJ, Sherlock P, Straus D, Lieberman PH, Flippa DA (1982). Primary gastrointestinal lymphoma: a 30-year review. *Cancer*, **49**:1258–65.

Weisenburger DD, Linder J, Daley DT, Armitage JO (1987). Intermediate lymphocytic lymphoma: an immunohistologic study with comparison to other lymphocytic lymphomas. *Human Pathology*, **18**:781–90.

Weisenburger DD, Sanger WG, Armitage JO, Purtilo DT (1989). Intermediate lymphocytic lymphoma: immunophenotypic and cytogenetic findings. *Blood*, **69**:1617–21.

Weiss LM, Wood GS, Trela M, Warnke RA, Sklar J (1986). Clonal T cell populations in lymphomatoid papulosis. Evidence of a lymphoproliferative origin for a clinically benign disease. *New England Journal of Medicine*, **315**:475–9.

Weiss LM, Warnke RA, Sklar J, Cleary ML (1987). Molecular analysis of the t(14:18) chromosomal translocation in malignant lymphomas. *New England Journal of Medicine*, **317**:1185–9.

Wilkins BS, Williamson JMS, O'Brien CJO (1989). A morphological and immunohistological study of testicular lymphomas. *Histopathology*, **15**:147–56.

Wright DH (1964). Burkitt's tumour: a post mortem study of 50 cases. *British Journal of Surgery*, **51**:245–51.

Wright DH (1966). Burkitt's tumour in England: a comparison with childhood lymphosarcoma. *International Journal of Cancer*, **1**:503–14.

Yunis JJ, Oken MM, Kaplan ME, Ensrud KM, Howe RR, Theologides A (1982). Distinctive chromosomal abnormalities in histologic subtypes of non-Hodgkin's lymphoma. *New England Journal of Medicine*, **307**:1231–6.

12.7.2 Non-Hodgkin's lymphoma in adults

FRANCO CAVALLI AND JACQUES BERNIER

The relevant data on incidence and epidemiology of the non-Hodgkin's lymphomas are presented in the previous chapter. Their incidence appears to be increasing each year, at least in the West (Devasa *et al.* 1987). The reasons are not entirely clear, although there is the possibility of some contribution from patients infected with human immunodeficiency virus (HIV). Lymphomas with T-cell immunological markers represent less than 15 per cent of the cases in the West, while they account for approximately half of the non-Hodgkin's lymphomas in Japan (Broder and Bunn 1980). In this chapter we will first discuss lymphomas of B-cell origin and summarize their T-cell counterpart separately at the end.

Non-Hodgkin's lymphomas occur in all age groups. Among patients with the 10 major subtypes, however, the age ranges are somewhat more limited. Table 1 lists the age range, median age,

Table 1 Working formulation of non-Hodgkin's lymphoma

	Age range (years)	Median age (years)	Frequency (%)	Sex ratio (M : F)
A Small lymphocytic	26–79	60.5	4	1.2–1
B Follicular, small cleaved cell	3–87	54.3	23	1.3–1
C Follicular, mixed	26–99	56.1	8	0.8–1
D Follicular, large cell	16–82	55.4	4	1.8–1
E Diffuse, small cleaved cell	10–91	57.9	7	2.0–1
F Diffuse, mixed	22–90	58.0	7	1.1–1
G Diffuse, large cell	10–88	56.8	20	1.0–1
H Immunoblastic	10–81	51.3	8	1.5–1
I Lymphoblastic	11–90	16.9	4	1.9–1
J Diffuse, small non-cleaved	3–90	29.8	5	2.6–1

frequency, and sex ratio of these subtypes according to the international working formulation of non-Hodgkin's lymphomas (The Non-Hodgkin's Lymphoma Pathologic Classification 1982).

The non-Hodgkin's lymphomas are a heterogeneous group of neoplasms that originate in lymphoreticular cells. The most indolent may cause few or no problems for up to 10–15 years without therapy. In contrast, without intensive treatment, the high-grade lymphomas are usually fatal within a few months. However, even this high-grade subgroup displays considerable diversity of behaviour. Clinicians must bear in mind the marked heterogeneity of this group of diseases and when choosing an appropriate treatment its clinical course must always be regarded as the main parameter. These neoplasms are highly responsive to therapy and can often be cured. Their heterogeneity, however, reduces the value of generalized statements and mandates a careful analysis of the different subtypes and of the influencing prognostic factors.

PRESENTATION AND CLINICAL FEATURES

When confronted with the diagnosis of a non-Hodgkin's lymphoma, the clinician should always recall that regardless of the classification used, there is considerable variation of opinion among expert pathologists (The Non-Hodgkin's Lymphoma Pathologic Classification 1982; Jones *et al.* 1985). A further complication is the fact that up to one-third of patients with lyphomas have divergent histologies in the same or different biopsy sites, and survival in such cases is reported to be intermediate between the two patterns (Fisher *et al.* 1981).

The presence of a more blastic diffuse large-cell lymphoma in patients with a follicular presentation has long been recognized at post-mortem (Gall and Mallory 1942). More recently, conversion during life to a high-grade non-Hodgkin's lyphoma has been documented in at least one-third of all rebiopsied cases: the frequency of this transformation is related to the duration of follow-up, but not to the treatment received (Hubbard *et al.* 1982; Acker *et al.* 1983). In studies carried out at Stanford, the actuarial risk of histological conversion was approximately 60 per cent at 8 years (Rosenberg 1985). Documented histological conversion has often been associated with a more aggressive clinical behaviour of the lymphoma and a median survival of less than 1 year.

Both the Working Formulation (The Non-Hodgkin's Lymphoma Pathologic Classification 1982) and the Rappaport classification (Rappaport *et al.* 1956) will be used to describe the different subtypes. Table 2 presents a comparison of the two schemes (see also Table 14 for an updated version of the Kiel classification, which has been widely used in different European countries). After 10

years the Working Formulation is showing many weaknesses (for example, it is not applicable for T-cell malignancies, subtype E is too heterogeneous in nature, and the distinction of subtypes is based primarily on survival curves) and a further refinement can be expected in the near future.

Small lymphocytic lymphoma (diffuse, well-differentiated, lymphocytic)

Small lymphocytic lymphoma constitutes approximately 4 per cent of the malignant lymphomas. The malignant lymphocytes are morphologically and immunologically similar to the neoplastic cells of chronic lymphocytic leukaemia; it is often asserted that small lymphocytic lymphoma is a solid tumour counterpart and that with time patients with small lymphocytic lymphoma may progress to chronic lymphoctyic leukaemia. The distinction between these two conditions is, therefore, based on relatively arbitrary clinical criteria. Approximately 20 per cent of small lymphocytic lymphomas present with plasmacytoid features, which have been related to a prognosis similar to (Morrison *et al.* 1989) or worse than that of small lymphocytic lymphomas without these features (Richards *et al.* 1989). A variable percentage of patients with plasmacytoid features secrete immunoglobulins of IgM and other classes in the serum (Morrison *et al.* 1989). When a high macroglobulin level is detected early, Waldenström's macroglobulinaemia is usually diagnosed (Pangalis *et al.* 1977). Some small lymphocytic lymphomas show a pseudofollicular architecture, a feature associated with a prolonged survival (Morrison *et al.* 1989). The small lymphocytic subtype may sometimes be confused with the so-called 'mantle-zone lymphoma', which represents a follicular variant of intermediate lymphocytic lymphoma (Weisenburger *et al.* 1982). Of all of the non-Hodgkin's lymphomas, the small lymphocytic subtype, which is very rare in young adults, is the one that most frequently affects the oldest age group (see Table 1). Most patients present with a symptomatic lymphadenopathy: the bone-marrow is involved in the majority of cases, with frequent infiltration in the liver, skin, mucous membranes, and other sites. Chylous pleural effusions may result from paravertebral lymph node masses.

In general, the prognosis of small lymphocytic lymphoma is good, with median survival from 6 to 10 years. Patients may present with or develop B symptoms; the presence or absence of systemic symptoms is the only clinicopathological feature that predicts a short survival (Morrison *et al.* 1989), while the prognostic value of other parameters (such as age, anaemia, and mitotic rate) remains controversial.

Follicular (nodular) lymphomas

Follicular lymphomas are those in which the neoplastic cells form circumscribed aggregates that morphologically resemble germinal centres. The nodular pattern may be present throughout the tumour or it may be manifested only in a portion of the lymphoma: the degree of nodularity appears to have a significant prognostic implication (Ezdinli *et al.* 1987). More than 80 per cent of follicular lymphomas carry the t(14;18) (q32;q21) chromosomal translocation (Price *et al.* 1991). This translocation is also found in slightly less than one-third of diffuse large cell lymphomas, suggesting in these cases a pathogenetical relationship to follicular lymphomas. The translocation results in juxtaposition of the *bcl-2* gene on chromosome 18 with the immunoglobulin heavy-chain locus on chromosome 14 (Bakshi *et al.* 1985). The break-points on both derivative chromosomes fall within well-defined areas and this

Table 2 A working formulation of non-Hodgkin's lymphoma and comparison to the Rappaport classification

Working Formulation	Rappaport classification
Low grade	
A Malignant lymphoma, small lymphocytic	Diffuse, well-differentiated, lymphocytic
Consistent with chronic lymphocytic leukaemia	
Plasmacytoid	
B Malignant lymphoma, follicular, predominantly small cleaved cell	Nodular, poorly differentiated, lymphocytic
Diffuse areas	
Sclerosis	
C Malignant lymphoma, follicular mixed, small cleaved and large cell	Nodular, mixed, lymphocytic, histiocytic
Diffuse areas	
Sclerosis	
Intermediate grade	
D Malignant lymphoma, follicular, predominantly large cell	Nodular, histiocytic
Diffuse areas	
Sclerosis	
E Malignant lymphoma, diffuse small cleaved cell	Diffuse, poorly differentiated, lymphocytic
F Malignant lymphoma, diffuse mixed, small and large cell sclerosis	Diffuse, mixed, lymphocytic–histiocytic
Epithelioid cell components	
G Malignant lymphoma, diffuse	Diffuse, histiocytic
Large cell	
Cleaved cell	
Non-cleaved cell	
Sclerosis	
High grade	
H Malignant lymphoma, large cell, immunoblastic	Diffuse, histiocytic
Plasmacytoid	
Clear cell	
Polymorphous	
Epithelioid cell component	
I Malignant lymphoma, lymphoblastic	Diffuse, lymphoblastic
Convoluted cell	
Non-convoluted cell	
J Malignant lymphoma, small non-cleaved cell	Diffuse, undifferentiated
Burkitt's	
Follicular areas	

clustering can be exploited for detection of the translocation by the polymerase chain reaction. However, the clinical relevance of this finding has still to be ascertained. The detection of occasional low levels of t(14;18) in benign reactive lymphoid hyperplasia (Limpens *et al.* 1990) and the persistence of cells bearing the translocation in the blood of patients in long-lasting remissions (Price *et al.* 1991) cast some doubts on the pathogenic rôle of this abnormality.

The three subtypes of the follicular lymphomas are mainly distinguishable by their percentage of large cells: less than 5 per cent in the follicular lymphoma with small cleaved cells (Working Formulation subtype B), greater than 15 per cent in the follicular lymphoma with predominantly large cells (Working Formulation subtype D), and an intermediate percentage in the mixed subtype (Working Formulation subtype C) (Mann and Bérard 1982). Follicular lymphomas are somewhat less frequent in Europe (15–25 per cent of all non-Hodgkin's lymphomas) than in the United States, where they comprise at least one-third of the lymphomas (Rosenberg 1985; Gallagher and Lister 1987). The more important prognostic factors are the presence of B symptoms, hepatomegaly, splenomegaly, and the level of anaemia and lactate dehydrogenase, while age and bulkiness of disease are of less importance (Gallagher and Lister 1987). Among the three subtypes, the follicular lymphoma with predominantly large cells (Working Formulation subtype D) carries a shorter survival than the two other variants, which have very similar natural courses (Simon *et al.* 1988).

Follicular, small cleaved cell lymphoma (nodular lymphocytic poorly differentiated)

Follicular, small cleaved cell lymphoma is the most common type of follicular lymphoma, accounting for approximately 60 per cent of the cases. It is a disease of adults with a median age of approximately 55 years, generally presenting with a symptomatic lymphadenopathy, which may wax and wane for years. This type of lymphoma is the one that most frequently undergoes spontaneous regression (Horning and Rosenberg 1984): these patients will usually have a recurrence of the disease, but they represent a subset with a very good prognosis. The initial lymphadenopathy, in contrast to most other lymphomas, is often found in the inguinal, axillary, high cervical, or mesenteric lymph nodes. Abnormalities in the chest radiograph are uncommon at onset, but bone-marrow involvement is present in at least 50 per cent of patients. These patients usually have no peripheral blood abnormalities; however, monoclonal populations of lymphocytes, identical to those found in involved lymph nodes, are often present in the peripheral blood, even in localized disease. It is not yet clear whether the presence of the circulating abnormal clone should alter the clinical stage or treatment approach in an individual patient.

The overall prognosis of patients with follicular, small cleaved, cell lymphoma is good, with an expected median survival of 8–10 years (Simon *et al.* 1988). Generally, the evolution is characterized by a slow progression to a stage at which B symptoms and/or local problems resulting from the enlarged lymph nodes will develop. It should be remembered, however, that in a significant proportion of these patients the lymphoma will convert to a more aggressive type, in 5–7 years after diagnosis (Acker *et al.* 1983). Therefore, in the event of any rapid progression of the disease, a new biopsy is mandatory.

Follicular, mixed small cleaved in large-cell lymphoma (nodular mixed lymphoma)

This form of follicular lymphoma (Working Formulation subtype C) represents approximately one-third of the follicular lymphomas. At onset only one-third of the cases will have an involved bone-marrow, and therefore approximately 30 per cent will have stage I to stage II disease (only 15 per cent in follicular, small cleaved cell lymphoma). This slightly more favourable presentation is balanced by a course which, in some instances, may be less indolent than that of follicular, small cleaved cell lymphoma. The final survival curves for these two variants are very similar (Simon *et al.* 1988).

Follicular, predominantly large-cell lymphoma (nodular histiocytic lymphoma)

Follicular, predominantly large-cell lymphomas (Working Formulation subtype D) represent only 10 per cent of all nodular lymphomas. At presentation one-third of the cases will be at stage I to II (similar to follicular, mixed lymphoma), but this is the only follicular subtype with a survival curve which is clearly worse than that of the other variants (Simon *et al.* 1988). The clinical picture is either of an isolated, rapidly enlarging lymph node or it is indistinguishable from that of the diffuse lymphomas.

Diffuse intermediately differentiated lymphocytic lymphoma

Diffuse intermediately differentiated lymphocytic lymphoma is a rare entity, not included in the Working Formulation, whose clinical features and median survival are quite similar to those of the other indolent lymphomas (Jaffe *et al.* 1987). It is related to mantle-zone lymphoma, which has a faintly follicular growth pattern: recently, it has been proposed that both entities should be designated mantle-zone lymphomas (Banks *et al.* 1992). This lymphoma is associated with a distinct cytogenetic abnormality t(11;14) (q13;q32) which can often be documented by *bcl-1* rearrangement (Banks *et al.* 1992).

Diffuse aggressive lymphomas

These lymphomas represent a group that shares a destructive histological growth pattern and many clinical features. They are most common in adults but occur in all age groups and present in both nodal (65 per cent) and extranodal (35 per cent) sites. Their prognosis is dire unless a sustained complete remission can be induced by intensive chemotherapy (median survival without treatment 6–24 months). If a complete remission can be achieved, the chance of a cure is good, in contrast to the prognosis of indolent lymphomas, which have a continuous relapse rate over time (Simon *et al.* 1988). Immunologically, diffuse lymphomas are heterogeneous and are composed of morphologically transformed B (85 per cent) and T (15 per cent) lymphocytes. In less than 5 per cent of cases only can true histiocytic markers be demonstrated. The prognostic significance of different immunological subtypes remains controversial

(Lippman *et al.* 1988; Shimoyama *et al.* 1988; Cheng *et al.* 1989; Coiffier *et al.* 1990; Kwak *et al.* 1991). T-cell lymphomas will be discussed at the end of this chapter.

Diffuse, small cleaved cell lymphoma (diffuse poorly differentiated lymphoma)

Diffuse, small cleaved cell lymphomas (Working Formulation subtype E) are composed of lymphoid cells that are similar to the small cleaved lymphocytes of follicular lymphomas. This tumour is equivalent to diffuse centrocytic lymphoma in the Kiel classification (see Table 14). This subtype shares many features with indolent lymphomas: they occur much more frequently in older patients, are monoclonal B-cell tumours, and a sustained complete remission is generally not seen. Clinically, histologically, and cytogenetically, these lymphomas are closely related to the mantle-zone lymphoma (Medeiros *et al.* 1990; Banks *et al.* 1992). However, as demonstrated by long-term follow-up (Simon *et al.* 1988) the end results are rather poor and an appropriate therapeutic strategy for this subtype has still to be devised.

Diffuse mixed small- and large-cell lymphoma (diffuse mixed lymphoma)

In approximately two-thirds of the cases the neoplastic cells of diffuse mixed lymphomas are cytologically identical to those of follicular mixed lymphomas and are immunologically of B-cell origin. These patients have an age distribution and a clinical presentation similar to those with nodular lymphomas. However, the natural history of diffuse mixed lymphoma is more aggressive and is otherwise similar to that of large-cell lymphomas. In approximately one-third of diffuse mixed lymphomas the cells do not resemble those of nodular lymphomas but appear instead to be a pleomorphic mixture of large and small atypical lymphoid cells. In the majority of such cases the malignant cells have been shown to bear markers of mature T lymphocytes. These peripheral T-cell lymphomas will be discussed separately; at present, however, it appears that clinically they should be approached in the same manner as other diffuse aggressive lymphomas (Kwak *et al.* 1991).

Diffuse large-cell lymphoma (diffuse histiocytic lymphoma)

The subtype designated as diffuse, large cell type in the Working Formulation (subtype G) corresponds most closely to the diffuse histiocytic lymphoma of Rappaport. It is a relatively aggressive lymphoma with a wide spectrum of clinical presentations. It occurs in all age groups, with a median age somewhat younger than for the indolent subtypes. More than any other subtypes, large-cell lymphomas present in extranodal sites, the most common localization being the gastrointestinal tract. However, almost any tissue may be the primary site of this lymphoma. Overall, almost half of the patients have a relatively localized extent of stage I and II disease, however, the lymphoma usually progresses rapidly, often locally.

Diffuse large-cell immunoblastic lymphoma (diffuse histiocytic lymphoma)

This category comprises all of the diffuse histiocytic lymphomas in the Rappaport scheme which do not have the cytological features of large follicular centre cells (De Vita *et al.* 1989). Different subtypes of B- or T-cell origin are described, in varying proportions depending on the series: overall no clear-cut differences among them have been documented. Both categories (Working Formulation subtypes G and H) are generally incorporated into the category of the 'diffuse, large-cell lymphomas'. This has also been the general rule for the therapeutic approach.

Lymphoblastic lymphoma (diffuse lymphoblastic lymphoma)

Lymphoblastic lymphoma (Working Formulation subtype I) is a very aggressive neoplasm, more common in males than in females and mainly affecting children and young adults (median age 16 years). The cellular morphololology of lymphoblastic lymphoma is indistinguishable from that seen in many patients with acute lymphoblastic leukaemia (ALL), particularly those with T-ALL. The major clinical characteristics distinguishing lymphoblastic lymphoma from acute lymphoblastic leukaemia are the extent of bone-marrow involvement and the lymph node enlargement. Patients with lymphoblastic lymphoma do not usually present with a leukaemic blood picture (50 per cent do have bone-marrow involvement at onset), but the majority have bulky tumour masses, especially in the anterior mediastinum. These intrathoracic tumours probably arise in the thymus and may produce life-threatening problems. Progression to acute lymphoblastic leukaemia is a frequent phenomenon in these patients. The presence of the enzyme TdT is a ubiquitous feature of all lymphoblastic malignancies. The cells in 85 per cent of cases have T-cell surface markers and share many characteristics with the cells of T-ALL (Cossman et al. 1983). In up to 10 per cent of cases the neoplastic cells demonstrate a phenotype similar to that of pre-B-cell acute lymphoblastic leukaemia: these cases tend not to present with mediastinal disease but isolated lytic bone lesions have been reported (Cossman et al. 1983). Management of lymphoblastic lymphoma (to be discussed later) has generally been based on the treatment of acute lymphoblastic leukaemia treatment: it must take into account the tendency to spread early to bone-marrow and to the meninges.

Diffuse, small non-cleaved cell lymphoma (diffuse undifferentiated lymphoma)

The most aggressive subtype of non-Hodgkin's lymphomas in the Working Formulation are diffuse, small non-cleaved cell types, both Burkitt's and non-Burkitt's. The Burkitt's type has a more uniform cytology and occurs in a younger age group and will therefore be discussed in the appropriate chapter. The non-Burkitt's type shows a greater degree of nuclear pleomorphism than is considered acceptable for Burkitt's lymphoma and presents most often in adults at a median age of 34 years. In contrast to Burkitt's lymphoma, which is always a B-cell neoplasm, in 5–10 per cent of cases the other variant shows a major T-cell phenotype. The two variants are the form of lymphoma most frequently seen in association with HIV infection.

Special entities

T-cell lymphomas, as well as special clinical situations, will be discussed later.

Mediterranean lymphoma

Most common among North Africans and Sephardic Jews, this neoplasm is associated with the finding of the α heavy chain of immunoglobulin as a monoclonal secretory product. Most cases of this disease correspond in the terminology of the Working Formulation to the immunoblastic lymphoma. Approximately 40 per cent of the patients will, however, present with a submucosal intestinal infiltration with relatively major plasma cells. This entity,

which has also been called immunoproliferative small intestinal disease, can have a benign or a malignant course (Salem et al. 1985).

Angioimmunoblastic lymphadenopathy

Angioimmunoblastic lymphadenopathy, first described in 1975, was initially thought to be a hyperimmune disorder (Frizzera et al. 1975). Although the disease is progressive and most often fatal (median survival 16 months), morphologically the cells do not look malignant. However, approximately 50 per cent of patients will develop overt lymphomas. Whether chemotherapy can prevent this progression is controversial. Initially angioimmunoblastic lymphadenopathy was considered to be a disorder of the B-cell system; however, more recently it has been shown to be a peripheral T-cell lymphoma (Stein et al. 1991).

Histiocytic sarcoma or 'true histiocytic lymphoma'

This still poorly defined entity represents the end-point of a spectrum of neoplasms which reflect different stages of maturation in the monocyte series. These also include acute monocytic leukaemia and malignant histiocytosis. Since they correspond to cells at the stage of the fixed-tissue histiocyte, histiocytic sarcomas are generally localized, relatively small tumours (Jaffe 1985). In addition to the reticuloendothelial system, common sites of involvement are skin and bone, with skin lesions in particular having been reported to have an indolent clinical course, sometimes with spontaneous regression. The usual treatment of choice is radiotherapy; the merits of chemotherapy remain controversial.

Mediastinal large-cell lymphoma with sclerosis

Different study series of the so-called mediastinal diffuse large-cell lymphoma with sclerosis, a new entity with a poor prognosis, have recently been reported (Perrone et al. 1986; Möller et al. 1987; Bertini et al. 1991). This primary mediastinal tumour occurs in young adults (median age 25 years), predominantly female, and responds only partially to aggressive chemotherapy; tumours tend to recur with an extensive involvement of the retroperitoneal space and abdominal organs. In most of the series the median survival is less than 1 year: this poor prognosis has recently been challenged by authors describing a series of 30 patients (Jacobson et al. 1988). The tumours are highly proliferative, have a diffuse growth pattern with a well-manifested sclerosis, and are composed of clear cells of various sizes. Immunologically they have been characterized as corresponding to the terminal steps of B-cell differentiation (Ig$^-$, CD19$^+$, CD20$^+$, CD21$^-$). However, at present it remains unclear whether this lymphoma really represents a distinct entity (Lister 1991a).

DIAGNOSTIC EVALUATION AND STAGING

The standard staging system used for non-Hodgkin's lymphomas is the same as that proposed for Hodgkin's disease at the Ann Arbor conference in 1971. Currently, however, there is considerable scepticism about the usefulness of this classification in non-Hodgkin's lymphomas. For some of the subtypes, in particular the low-grade lymphomas, widespread stage III or IV disease is very common without necessarily conferring an ominous prognosis. Moreover, in follicular lymphomas, stage II has a prognosis which is similar to that of stage IV disease (Simon et al. 1988). In addition, certain prognostic factors of particular importance in non-Hodgkin's lymphomas, such as the bulk of the lymphoma mass at presentation

Table 3 Clinical features of the lymphomas (modified from De Vita *et al.* 1989)

Hodgkin's disease	Lymphocytic lymphoma
Lymph node disease tends to be in axial lymph nodes	Lymph node disease tends to be non-contiguous
Epitrochlear nodes, Waldeyer's ring, testicular, and gastrointestinal sites uncommon	More common involvement of epitrochlear nodes, Waldeyer's ring, testes, and gastrointestinal tract
Mediastinal presentation in 50 per cent of patients	Mediastinal presentation less common (≈ 25 per cent)
Abdominal nodal involvement uncommon in asymptomatic but common in older patients or when fever or night sweats are present	Abdominal lymph node involvement common
Commonly localized; contiguous nodal disease	Rarely localized nodal disease ($\approx 10–15$ per cent)
Bone-marrow involvement uncommon	Bone-marrow involvement common
Liver involvement uncommon; when present, spleen usually involved	Liver commonly involved in follicular lymphoma, rare in diffuse lymphoma

or the relevance of certain sites of involvement (mediastinum, bone marrow, CNS), cannot be encompassed within the Ann Arbor staging system.

It is important that all physicians treating lymphomas realize that there are some clinical features which are basically different in Hodgkin's disease and non-Hodgkin's lymphomas. Table 3 summarizes the most important of these differences. Basically the spread of non-Hodgkin's lymphomas tends to be non-contiguous, while Hodgkin's disease tends to evolve along a more predictable axis.

Involvement of Waldeyer's ring occurs in less than 1 per cent of patients with Hodgkin's disease, but is identified in 15–30 per cent of patients with non-Hodgkin's lymphoma, especially in adult patients with intermediate and high-grade subtypes. The area should therefore be carefully examined by direct and indirect techniques. The association between Waldeyer's ring and gastrointestinal lymphomas has been noted by many observers. There might be a co-existence of lesions in the two regions as well as localized relapse in the gastrointestinal tract following successful initial therapy of the disease presenting in Waldeyer's ring (Gospodarowicz *et al.* 1987). The reverse situation, that is, late relapse in the Waldeyer's ring after the successful treatment of gastrointestinal lymphomas, has also been observed but more rarely (Gospodarowicz *et al.* 1987). In all cases of involvement of the Waldeyer's ring, upper gastrointestinal contrast studies or a gastroscopy are strongly advised. Correlations between other sites, though less frequent than the one between Waldeyer's ring and the gastrointestinal tract, should be borne in mind: primary lesions in bone or skin are frequently associated with involvement of regional nodes and primary lymphoma of the testes may present with extension to regional pelvic or para-aortic nodes (De Vita *et al.* 1989).

Required evaluation procedures

These procedures are summarized in Table 4. Patients should always be questioned about when the lymph node enlargement was first noted and the rate of tumour growth. In indolent lymphomas, mainly in the follicular, small cleaved variant, there will frequently be a waxing and waning of the size of the nodes, often over a long period of time.

Depending on the sites involved, the physician should then plan an adequate surgical biopsy and make certain that the material is reviewed by an experienced pathologist. In places where the necessary technology is available, the biopsy material should also be processed for immunophenotyping and for molecular techniques (gene rearrangements and specific chromosomal abnormalities). The latter may be useful in the detection of minimal disease and/or in the assessment of certain clinical symptoms (for example, cytologically negative pleural effusion) (Dorey *et al.* 1989).

Table 4 Staging non-Hodgkin's lymphomas: required evaluation procedures

1 Adequate surgical biopsy, reviewed by an experienced pathologist
2 A detailed history recording the rate of growth and presence of symptoms
3 A detailed physical evaluation; special attention to all node-bearing areas including Waldeyer's ring
4 Laboratory procedures
  a Complete blood count, including sedimentation rate
  b Lactate dehydrogenase, serum calcium, uric acid, electrophoresis, alkaline phosphatase
  c Evaluation of renal and liver function
5 Radiological studies
  a Chest radiograph (postero-anterior and lateral)
  b Abdominal–pelvic CT
6 Bilateral bone-marrow needle biopsies
7 If possible, immunophenotyping and molecular analyses of biopsies, search for monoclonal population in peripheral blood

Correlation between peripheral blood values and marrow involvement in the disease is poor: abnormalities in blood counts are found in only one-third of patients with bone-marrow infiltration. Conversely, approximately half of the patients with non-specific abnormalities in the peripheral blood values will be free of marrow involvement. Bone-marrow involvement is common in certain subtypes, either at onset or during the course of the disease. Table 5 summarizes its frequency at presentation in the 10 subtypes of the working formulation. An adequate bone-marrow biopsy (ideally performed bilaterally together with marrow smears) is required to demonstrate involvement of the disease, since this may be focal, especially early in the course of the disease. Perhaps in future magnetic resonance imaging (**MRI**) will reveal some of the marrow lesions which go undetected at initial bone-marrow biopsy (Shields *et al.* 1987). Immunophenotyping and/or molecular techniques may also be helpful in evaluating bone-marrow and peripheral blood (Smith *et al.* 1984; Brada *et al.* 1987).

Enlargement of the mediastinal lymph nodes is the abnormality most commonly revealed by radiograph in non-Hodgkin's

Table 5 Non-Hodgkin's lymphoma bone-marrow involvement (according to Simon *et al.* 1988)

Small lymphocytic	71
Follicular, small cleaved cell	51
Follicular, mixed	30
Follicular, large cell	34
Diffuse, small cleaved cell	32
Diffuse, mixed	14
Diffuse, large cell	10
Immunoblastic	12
Lymphoblastic	50
Diffuse, small non-cleaved	14

lymphomas: chest radiograph results are positive in approximately one-quarter of the patients. Full lung tomograms and/or CT scans are usually not necessary, in view of the scarcity of parenchymal disease in patients with normal chest radiographs (Reznek and Richards 1987). In contrast to Hodgkin's disease, the non-Hodgkin's lymphomas frequently involve the mesenteric lymph nodes and other abdominal lymph nodes outside the para-aortic chain (Rezneck and Richards 1987). Enlargement of these lymph nodes may be responsible for the initial symptoms of the disease. Numerous studies have assessed the overall efficacy of bipedal lymphography and computer tomography in the evaluation of abdominal lymph nodes in non-Hodgkin's lymphomas (reviewed by Rezneck and Richards 1987). Contrary to the situation in the staging of Hodgkin's disease, computer tomography is the primary method for the abdominal staging in patients with non-Hodgkin's lymphoma. Abdominal ultrasonography may be useful primarily for the continuous, regular evaluation of retroperitoneal lymphadenopathy, mainly in low-grade lymphomas and the related potential problems with the renal collecting system: renal problems may arise for purely mechanical reasons but can also be due to lymphomatous infiltration. Though primary kidney lymphomas are very rare, in an autopsy series lymphomatous involvement was shown in up to 30 per cent of patients who had lymphoma elsewhere (Rezneck and Richards 1987).

Optional evaluation procedures

Optional evaluation procedures encompass all diagnostic measures necessary to evaluate adequately disease involvement at special sites (summarized in Table 6). Approximately 50 per cent of patients will present with extranodal involvement (Anderson et al. 1982). This may occur at any given site, very rarely at several, while, on the other hand, a lymphomatous involvement occurs particularly often in certain regions.

The gastrointestinal tract is the most common primary site of extranodal lymphoma (List et al. 1988). Involvement there occurs much more frequently than is clinically appreciated, as is demonstrated by autopsy series. Abdominal pain is the most common complaint of patients with gastrointestinal lymphoma. Other features at initial presentation vary with the site of disease. Frank gastrointestinal bleeding is more frequently observed in patients with gastric (30 per cent) or large bowel lymphoma (30 per cent), whereas diarrhoea and visceral perforation are very rare when the primary is located in the stomach and more common with bowel lymphomas (40 per cent). Symptoms of visceral obstruction are generally limited to patients with small bowel primaries (30 per cent). An advanced stage of disease (stages IIIE and IV) is detectable in three-quarters of patients with low-grade lymphomas, while this is true only for 40 per cent of patients with higher grades of neoplasia (List et al. 1988).

Table 6   Staging non-Hodgkin's lymphomas: optional procedures

1   CT scan of the chest, if routine chest radiograph is abnormal or suspect
2   Abnormal ultrasonogram, upper and/or lower gastrointestinal contrast studies
       to investigate special situations
3   Plain bone radiographs of symptomatic areas
4   Head or spinal CT for neurological symptoms
5   Cerebrospinal fluid examination in patients at risk

Possible ancillary procedures:
   Magnetic resonance imaging (experimental)
   ^{67}Ga scanning
   Bone scan

All patients who have gastrointestinal symptoms or an important involvement of the mesenteric lymph nodes should have barium studies of the entire gastrointestinal tract. Endoscopy may be required to clarify the significance of prominent gastric rugae or ulceration. Gastrointestinal lymphomas confront the treating physician with special therapeutic problems and these will be discussed later.

Bone lesions are more common in patients with diffuse aggressive lymphomas than in those with the follicular type. Routine radiographic studies of bone have largely been replaced by bone scanning.

Primary CNS lymphoma accounts for approximately 2 per cent of brain tumours and 2 per cent of all lymphomas, even when their incidence is augmented by immunodepressed patients (that is, increased in conjunction with the AIDS epidemic) (Formenti and Levine 1989). CNS lymphoma appears on CT scan as a lesion of relatively greater density which uniformly enhances with contrast, usually homogeneously. The most common symptoms are headache, mental changes, and symptoms of increased intracerebral pressure. The cerebrospinal fluid usually has a high protein level but no cytologically malignant cells. More common is a secondary involvement of the CNS: this is reported in 7–9 per cent of the cases in the literature (Recht et al. 1988). As systemic chemotherapy regimens have become more successful, the meninges have emerged as one of the sites of relapses, especially for patients with lymphoblastic and diffuse, small non-cleaved (Burkitt's and non-Burkitt's) lymphomas. But all patients with intermediate- or high-grade lymphomas (with the exception of follicular, large and diffuse, small cleaved) seem to be at a certain risk of developing a meningeal involvement. It appears, however, that unlike patients with T-lymphoblastic lymphomas, those with peripheral T-cell lymphomas do not have a propensity to CNS disease (Liang et al. 1989). The following clinical factors (in decreasing order) predict for a higher risk of development of secondary CNS involvement: positive bone-marrow, involvement of the nasal or orbital region, bulky retroperitoneal disease, and young age (Liang et al. 1989). All patients at risk should have cerebrospinal fluid examination at the onset of the disease and during the course of the illness, if symptoms or clinical findings become suggestive. Even though hard data are still unavailable, there is a consensus at many centres that modern chemotherapy regimens, which include different types of CNS prophylaxis, lead to a decreased incidence of secondary CNS involvement.

The rôle of magnetic resonance imaging (MRI) in the staging procedure for lymphomas is still experimental, since only limited data are available (Rezneck and Richards 1987). MRI seems to be equivalent to CT in the evaluation of abdominal nodes, while inconsistent results were reported for the evaluation of liver involvement (Richards et al. 1986; Nyman et al. 1987). In the past ^{67}Ga scanning has yielded disappointing results. However, with technical improvement it is possible that this technique will, in future, add supportive information to that obtained from other tests.

The incidence of lymphoma involvement of the liver in patients who present with non-Hodgkin's lymphomas ranges from 20 to 40 per cent (Veronesi et al. 1974). The lymphoma yield increases as the size and number of biopsy specimens increase, which in turn is correlated with the aggressiveness of the staging procedure. Liver involvement is much more frequent in patients with follicular or diffuse, small cleaved cell lymphomas than in those with diffuse, large-cell lymphoma. Laparoscopy with multiple liver biopsies or even staging laparotomy, might be required, but only if a precise definition of liver and other abdominal involvement (not demonstrable otherwise) has obvious relevance for treatment planning. This is clearly not the case for most patients: without invasive procedures, most will have a demonstrated stage III or IV disease and even in the remaining cases, either a 'wait-and-see' policy or a treatment plan with chemotherapy will be advisable. The essential rôle of laparotomy remains that of a diagnostic tool in patients with unclear abdominal masses.

Restaging and follow-up

Accurate monitoring of the response to therapy is clearly vital for deciding whether to continue or to stop treatment. Imaging plays an important part in assessing the response; however, a study that evaluated laparotomy as a restaging tool showed that CT scans, lymphograms, and gallium scans can overpredict for residual disease (Fuks et al. 1982). A National Cancer Institute study of re-exploration of residual abdominal masses showed that in most patients with aggressive lymphomas who have otherwise completely responded to a carefully administered chemotherapy, stable residual abdominal masses can be closely followed clinically without surgical exploration (Surbone et al. 1988). A similar approach may also be justified in the case of persistently enlarged mediastinal nodes (Rezneck and Richards 1987). It was reported recently in a large series of patients that approximately one-quarter of those otherwise in complete remission will show persistence of fibronecrotic or radiological masses after the completion of treatment (Coiffier et al. 1989). Therefore, the consistent definition of complete remission is difficult in these patients. In such situations, perhaps in the future a new technological version of ^{67}Ga scanning will prove helpful (Lister et al. 1989).

Traditionally, recommendations for the follow-up of patients after curative therapy have been arbitrary and this applies also to lymphoma. To date, only one study has systematically evaluated the value of follow-up procedures in patients with aggressive lymphoma who achieved a complete remission (Weeks et al. 1991). This report demonstrates the uselessness of most follow-up procedures: of the screening tests performed, only lactate dehydrogenase testing was successful in detecting preclinical relapse, with a sensitivity of 42 per cent and specificity of 85 per cent for impending symptomatic relapse. Clearly, more work will be needed in future to devise a sensible and meaningful system of follow-up: this will have to screen with a frequency appropriate to a patient's risk of relapse and limit aggressive screening to those high-risk patients eligible for potentially curative salvage therapy.

TREATMENT OF NON-HODGKIN'S LYMPHOMAS
General considerations

The management of patients with non-Hodgkin's lymphomas is primarily influenced by the tumour type and extent as well as by the physiological status of the patient.

The influence of tumour histology on the natural course of this disease became evident as early as 1956 with the introduction of the Rappaport classification (Rappaport et al. 1956). Currently, the Working Formulation F subdivides lymphomas into three grades of malignancy: low, intermediate, and high grade. However, there are some entities that are not included in the working formulation and for a few subtypes (for example, diffuse, small cleaved) the clinical course is at variance with the assumed grade of malignancy. To solve these problems a practical schema was developed (De Vita

Table 7 National Cancer Institute clinical schema for non-Hodgkin's lymphoma

Indolent (median survival measured in years)
    Small lymphocytic
    Follicular, small cleaved cell
    Follicular, mixed
    Diffuse, small cleaved cells
    Diffuse, intermediately differentiated (or mantle zone)
    Cutaneous T-cell

Aggressive (median survival measured in months)
    Follicular, large cell
    Diffuse, mixed
    Diffuse, large cell
    Diffuse, immunoblastic
    Other peripheral T-cell

Highly aggressive (median survival measured in weeks)
    Diffuse, small non-cleaved cell (Burkitt's)
    Diffuse, small non-cleaved cell (non-Burkitt's)
    Lymphoblastic
    Adult T-cell leukaemia/lymphoma

et al. 1989). This schema divides the lymphomas into three groups: indolent lymphomas, whose mean natural history is measured in years, aggressive lymphomas, whose mean natural history is measured in months, and highly aggressive lymphomas, whose mean natural history is measured in weeks. This schema is presented in Table 7.

The second important determinant in the choice of treatment is the extent of disease, together with the related prognostic factors. Patients with stages I or II indolent lymphoma constitute only 10–15 per cent of those with this B-cell neoplasm: radiation therapy is usually recommended for such patients since it may be curative. Prognostic factors influencing the outcome of radiotherapy are histological subtype, age, number and localization of involved sites, and tumour bulk (Bush and Gospodarowicz 1982; Sutcliffe et al. 1985). In stages III and IV, the treatment of choice for indolent lymphoma is still controversial and will be discussed later in greater depth. Overall survival in indolent lymphoma correlates with gender (poorer for men), number of extranodal sites, lymph node size, and degree of bone-marrow involvement (Bastion et al. 1991; Romaguerra et al. 1991). Classical histological parameters, such as percentage of large cells and/or diffuse areas, play only a limited prognostic rôle (Bastion et al. 1991).

In determination of the treatment approach for aggressive lymphomas, prognostic factors should play a central rôle. The factors generally accepted as being associated with a poor prognosis include older age, low performance status, B-cell symptoms, an abdominal mass more than 10 cm in diameter, three or more extranodal sites of disease, bone-marrow involvement, a serum lactate dehydrogenase level over 500 IU/ml, and transformation from a previous low-grade histology (Table 8). Discrepancies among different series and the recognition of the importance of prognostic factors (which were somewhat underestimated in the chemotherapy enthusiasm of the recent past), led very recently to an overview analysis of more than 3000 patients with diffuse mixed, large-cell, or immunoblastic lymphoma treated with intensive chemotherapy between 1982 and 1987 (Shipp et al. 1992). In a multivariate analysis, five features were independently associated with survival: age, stage, number of extranodal sites, performance status, and serum lactate dehydrogenase levels. The patients could be divided into four groups with decreasing complete remission rates and shortened survivals (best group 73 per cent, worst group 26 per cent 5 year survival). This model

Table 8 Factors associated with poor prognosis in aggressive lymphomas

1 Generally accepted
  Poor performance status
  Presence of B symptoms
  $\geqslant 3$ extranodal sites
  Abdominal mass > 10 cm in diameter
  Bone-marrow involvement
  LDH > 500 IU/ml
  Transformation from low-grade histology

2 Probably important
  Age > 60 years
  Slow response
  High proliferation measured by Ki-67

3 Possibly important
  T-cell immunophenotype

LDH, lactate dehydrogenase.

has been called the International Index and could, perhaps, in future replace the Ann Arbor staging system for aggressive lymphoma.

Three recent reports suggest a better cure rate in patients with lymphomas who respond more rapidly to chemotherapy (Armitage and Cheson 1988). While there is little doubt that actual dose intensity plays a prognostic rôle, its exact importance remains to be determined (Kwak *et al.* 1990; Longo 1990). The prognostic significance of different immunophenotypes remains more controversial (Kwak *et al.* 1991).

The final determinant of the treatment approach in individual patients with lymphoma is the physiological status, which in turn is closely related to age. Since toxicities are nearly always dose related and predictable, skilled oncologists should always be able to devise drug dosages that can be administered safely. It has been our practice to administer the first cycle of drugs to older patients at two-thirds of full dose, with subsequent modification of the treatment according to tolerance. Serious underlying medical problems may further complicate the choice of therapy. Certain drugs must be omitted in the presence of serious organ failures: bleomycin in pulmonary diseases, methotrexate, bleomycin, and cisplatin in case of renal failure, and anthracyclines in the presence of a severe cardiomyopathy or severe hepatic dysfunction. Other drugs should be used only with great caution in special situations: vinca alkaloids in the presence of impaired liver function (not lymphoma-related), etoposide (VP-16) in cases of impaired renal function, and high-dose cytarabine (cytosine arabinoside, ara-C) in older patients. The special therapeutic problems that occur in the setting of an underlying immunodeficiency and in general with AIDS patients will be discussed in another chapter.

The natural history of the highly aggressive lymphoma (Table 7) is so short that almost all patients have disseminated disease at onset and there is no strong evidence that clinical staging should have any influence on approach to treatment, which is universally high-dose combination chemotherapy.

Treatment of indolent lymphomas

The indolent non-Hodgkin's lymphomas represent a heterogeneous group of malignancies with similar natural histories. Table 7 summarizes the subtypes which are considered as indolent in the schema proposed by the National Cancer Institute (De Vita *et al.* 1989).

In early stages most series will include patients with predominantly follicular small cleaved cell and follicular mixed lymphoma, since the other low-grade histological variants are rarely localized. However, patients with advanced stages of diffuse, small lymphocytic lymphoma, diffuse, small cleaved, and mantle-zone lymphoma are probably concealed within larger studies of the more common indolent lymphoma types and their disease will therefore be considered to be similar.

The optimal management of patients with indolent lymphoma still presents a substantial clinical challenge despite the high rate of response to modern radiotherapy and chemotherapy. In evaluating therapeutic responses one should remember that spontaneous regressions occur in up to 25 per cent of these lymphomas, mainly in the follicular, small cleaved cell subtype (Rosenberg 1985). The problem remains of how best to identify those patients with localized disease for whom radiotherapy would be the treatment of choice and how or when to treat most of those who present with disseminated disease which, although not immediately life-threatening, will nevertheless be fatal for many within 10 years of diagnosis.

Only 10–15 per cent of patients with indolent lymphoma present with stage I or stage II disease. In general, radiation therapy is recommended for this minority and is particularly indicated for patients less than 40 years of age, a group with an 80 per cent probability of remaining disease-free 10 or more years after adequate staging and irradiation (Rosenberg 1985). In supradiaphragmatic disease, radiation therapy can be limited to involved±first-echelon-uninvolved fields. Alternatively, a 'mini-mantle' (that is, a mantle without mediastinum) can be used, since the incidence of relapses in the mediastinum is negligible if this region is not primarily involved. With the latter technique, the lower margin of the field is set at the inferior portion of the heads of the clavicles. Doses generally ranging from 30 to 40 Gy have been shown to be important in determining the therapeutic outcome (Tubiana *et al.* 1986). In infradiaphragmatic stage I disease, the treatment can encompass involved±first-echelon-uninvolved fields or alternatively an inverted Y field. If radiotherapy is chosen for infradiaphragmatic stage II patients, fields usually encompass the whole abdomen up to 25 Gy, with the kidneys and liver shielded after 15 Gy. In some centres an additional boost of 15 Gy is applied to an inverted Y field. Since approximately two-thirds of relapses seen in patients who receive limited-field radiation occur in untreated lymph nodes (Lawrence *et al.* 1988), it has been suggested that clinically staged patients should receive total nodal radiation (Tubiana *et al.* 1986). However, a prospective study comparing total nodal radiation to extended fields radiotherapy in stage II patients did not confirm superiority for the former technique (Carde *et al.* 1984).

At present there is no rôle for combination chemotherapy in the management of early-stage indolent lymphoma since three randomized studies failed to demonstrate a superiority for chemotherapy plus radiation treatment over radiation therapy alone (Gallagher and Lister 1987).

The precise treatment of choice remains undetermined for patients with advanced (stage III/IV) and with 'unfavourable' (bulky, multiple sites) stage II indolent lymphoma. Most patients will respond to single-agent and combination chemotherapy, radiation therapy, and combined modality approaches. The latter strategy foresees the use of so-called 'iceberg radiotherapy' in a dose of 30 Gy to the initially involved areas, mostly in the presence of bulky masses or in the case of poor tumour regression after three courses of chemotherapy (Tubiana *et al.* 1986). By and large, long-term results are similar with all modalities; responses are not durable and, ultimately, almost all patients will relapse. The median duration of first remission averages 3 years (Lister 1991*b*). Whether the long survival (more than 10 years) of patients achieving a complete remission or a very good partial remission with the first treatment is therapy-related or only indicates a favourable subset of patients (like the ones showing spontaneous regressions) selected out by treatment, remains to be ascertained (Lister 1991*b*).

One study conducted at the National Cancer Institute suggested that patients with advanced follicular mixed disease treated with C-MOPP (cyclophosphamide, nitrogen mustard, vincristine, procarbazine, prednisone) may be cured, even though some patients relapsed up to 8 years after the diagnosis (De Vita *et al.* 1989). However, these results are inconsistent with the findings in another randomized trial (Glick *et al.* 1981) and even with a more realistic evaluation of the same trial (Simon *et al.* 1988). It remains to be seen whether even more intensive combination of chemotherapies will confer a survival advantage to some patients with indolent lymphomas.

The group at Stanford has chosen a more conservative approach; as early as 1979 they reported their experience with the management of 44 selected patients with low-grade non-Hodgkin's lymphomas without initial therapy (Portlock and Rosenberg 1979). The number of patients has now expanded and the results have been updated many times (Rosenberg 1985). The group shows a median survival of 11 years, with a collective median time to therapy requirement of 3 years. In this respect, however, histological subtypes differ significantly. The median times to therapy requirement for the three groups are 17, 48, and 72 months for the follicular, mixed, follicular, small cleaved cell, and small lymphocytic subtypes, respectively (Rosenberg 1985). Among the patients for whom a 'wait-and-see' policy was possible were those without B symptoms, a slow disease course, and an absence of symptoms related to occlusion/compression due to bulky tumour masses. This experience of the Stanford group has profoundly influenced the treatment approach of many centres. Our current policy dictates an initial abstention of therapy in most patients with indolent lymphomas (it remains unclear whether such a policy can be applied to patients with diffuse, small cleaved lymphomas) who fit into the previously mentioned criteria (absence of B symptoms, slow disease course, absence of mechanically induced symptoms, and absence of disease-related abnormalities in the peripheral blood values). In such cases a strict policy of regular follow-up is mandatory, particularly in the presence of a follicular, mixed subtype. If there is any indication for therapeutic intervention, the exact modality will be determined according to the nature of the problem. In case of mechanical problems due to enlarged lymph nodes, iceberg radiotherapy or combination chemotherapy may be chosen. Otherwise we prefer single-agent treatment with chlorambucil (generally 10 mg total daily dose, 2 weeks on, 2 weeks off). Combination chemotherapy usually achieves the expected result much quicker than does single-agent treatment (for a complete remission of up to 6 months in contrast to up to 12 months, respectively). It should be borne in mind, that successive retreatments (after a therapy-free period) with single-agent chemotherapy will generally lead to successive responses in a high percentage of cases (Gallagher *et al.* 1986).

An alternative approach, as yet only inadequately investigated, would consist in the exploration of the possible advantage of intensifying chemotherapy only in those patients who had shown a prompt and complete response to single-agent treatment.

Future prospects

The current lack of a curative approach to treatment of indolent lymphomas clearly shows the need for further studies. This is especially true for young patients whose disease may, but does not necessarily, have a less favourable prognosis. These patients have a poor prognosis, particularly if their disease is not responsive to

single-agent alkylating therapy, with a median survival of only 2 years (Gallagher and Lister 1987). The use of high-dose cyclophosphamide and total-body irradiation is being actively investigated in these and other patients with a poor prognosis (Spinolo 1992), as consolidation for those in remission after conventional therapy for relapse (Gallagher and Lister 1987; Rohatiner *et al.* 1991). The availability of monoclonal antibodies to B-cell antigens on the surface of the lymphoma cells makes support of the procedure possible with autologous bone-marrow treated with antibody and complement for lysing residual cells (Pedrazzini *et al.* 1989).

Other biological treatment alternatives are currently under investigation. The immunomodulator α-interferon has shown antitumour activity against indolent lymphomas (Cavalli 1988). Since α-interferon has shown *in vitro* synergy with a number of chemotherapeutic agents, clinical trials are now in progress to establish the optimal rôle of this drug (alone or in combination) in the treatment plan for indolent lymphomas. Perhaps α-interferon will be more effective in the maintenance than in the induction phase. Treatment with tumour-specific anti-idiotype monoclonal antibodies has also had a limited success (Levy *et al.* 1985) and these antibodies have recently been combined with α-interferon (Brown *et al.* 1989). Many studies using different monoclonal antibodies, alone or conjugated with a wide variety of substances, are currently under way. Particularly interesting are those of the CAMPATH-1 family of antibodies, which recognize an abundant glycoprotein expressed on virtually all human lymphocytes (Dyer *et al.* 1989) and those with radiolabelled antibodies (Press *et al.* 1989).

More recently, two purine analogues, fludarabine and 2-chloro-deoxyadenosine, have shown very promising results in the treatment of indolent lymphoma (Hochster *et al.* 1992; Kay *et al.* 1992); however, more data are needed to assess their exact merits properly.

Treatment of localized aggressive lymphomas

The aggressive lymphomas include follicular large cell, diffuse large-cell, diffuse mixed, and diffuse immunoblastic lymphomas. Historically, radiation therapy has been used as the primary treatment for patients with localized aggressive lymphomas. While 35–40 Gy are sufficient to achieve local control in patients with follicular lymphoma, 45–50 Gy (depending on the tumour bulk) are necessary in the presence of aggressive lymphoma (Tubiana *et al.* 1986). Even with adequate dosage, approximately 15 per cent of the patients will develop in-field relapses (Bush and Gospodarowicz 1982; Tubiana 1984). As might have been anticipated, better results have been obtained with radiotherapy in pathologically staged patients than in clinically staged limited disease (Honegger and Cavalli 1984). Studies with clinically staged patients report 5 year survival rates of 60–65 per cent for stage I or IE patients, but only 25 per cent for stage II or IIE patients. However, most stage I patients whose staging includes laparotomy can be cured by radiotherapy alone (Kaminski *et al.* 1986).

However, involved-field radiation therapy alone is insufficient for most clinical early-stage patients, in whom exploratory laparotomy is not justified. The Stanford group made an effort to improve on the outcome by delivering treatment to both sides of the diaphragm. The 5 year survival rate (39 per cent for involved fields, 50 per cent for extended fields, and 60 per cent for total nodal irradiation) did not show a statistically significant difference, but suggested in a limited group of patients a trend favouring the more extended radiation therapy (Jacobs and Hoppe 1985). Interestingly, the majority of relapses were observed in untreated regions and extranodal sites. Later, the same group demonstrated that involved-field radiation therapy combined with CHOP (cyclo-phosphamide, doxorubicin, vincristine, prednisone) gives results comparable to those achieved with total nodal irradiation (Kaminski *et al.* 1986). Various investigators have attempted to improve on the results obtained with radiation therapy alone by adding combination chemotherapy in clinically staged patients. Two randomized trials demonstrated a significantly superior disease-free survival with radiation therapy followed by CVP (cyclophosphamide, vincristine, prednisone) (Honegger and Cavalli 1984). However, the tendency now is to begin with chemotherapy and to follow it later with adjuvant radiotherapy: this approach should avert failures due to early dissemination. One such programme, three cycles of CHOP followed by involved-field radiation in 78 patients in stage I to II (without poor prognostic factors) aggressive lymphoma, achieved a response rate of 99 per cent and a long-term survival of 85 per cent (Connors *et al.* 1987). Only by future prospective trials will it be possible to define the precise rôle of this radiotherapy given as consolidation. An interim evaluation of such a study would favour the combined modality approach at least in stage II patients (O'Connell *et al.* 1986). Currently, there is renewed interest in the scheduling of the combination of radiation therapy and cytotoxic treatment, particularly with respect to the so-called 'interdigitated alternating regimens' (Cosset *et al.* 1985). In one such trial carried out in patients with bulky, stage I to II diffuse non-Hodgkin's lymphomas, eight monthly courses of chemotherapy were alternated with two or three courses of radiotherapy, given at a dose of 15 Gy after the second and the third cycles of chemotherapy (Cosset *et al.* 1991). With survival and freedom from progression rates at 5 years of 69 and 65 per cent, respectively, the results of the Villejuif study are markedly better than those reported in the previous European Organization for Research and Treatment of Cancer (EORTC) study (Carde *et al.* 1984).

There is only a little information on the use of combination chemotherapy alone in patients with early-stage aggressive lymphoma (Honegger and Cavalli 1984). For the time being we recommend that patients with localized aggressive lymphoma be clinically staged. Patients with fewer than three sites of disease and no bulky masses should receive CHOP for three to six cycles, followed by (or alternated with) involved-field radiation therapy. Patients with any factor associated with poor prognosis (see Table 8) should be managed similarly to patients with advanced-stage disease.

Treatment of advanced-stage aggressive lymphomas

Today most clinicians define all patients with Ann Arbor stage III or IV, as well as those with stage II and one or more of the poor prognostic factors summarized in Table 8, as patients with advanced-stage aggressive lymphomas. For these patients the most effective treatment is chemotherapy. Radiotherapy alone was shown in the 1970s to be insufficient to control this disease (Glatstein *et al.* 1976). The British National Lymphoma Investigation Report later confirmed that results achieved with CHOP were superior to those obtained with total-body irradiation (British National Lymphoma Investigation Report 1981).

In the past decade some centres have also used consolidation radiotherapy to sites of bulky disease in order to reduce relapse rates after chemotherapy alone (Tubiana *et al.* 1986). However, recent results indicate that patients with advanced-stage bulky disease do not consistently relapse in sites of prior bulky disease, at least if they are treated with modern aggressive chemotherapy (Shipp *et al.* 1989). This group of patients is therefore unlikely to benefit from

adjuvant radiation therapy administered after completion of combination chemotherapy: this was confirmed recently in a German multicentre study (Engelhard *et al.* 1991).

Numerous combination chemotherapy regimens have been developed for patients with non-Hodgkin's lymphomas and their historical development has clarified the principles on which treatment for aggressive lymphoma must be based (see Table 13). The initial experience with three-drug regimens of the CVP type (cyclophosphamide, vincristine, and prednisone), though producing high response rates, failed to provide adequate long-term control of the disease. The first significant improvement in treatment outcome came with the use of MOPP (nitrogen mustard, vincristine, procarbazine, prednisone) and C-MOPP, which induced complete remission in approximately 45 per cent of advanced-stage patients and, surprisingly at that time, most patients achieving complete remission were shown to remain disease-free (De Vita *et al.* 1975). Unquestionably, one of the success stories of modern oncology has been the development of curative chemotherapy for patients with advanced-stage aggressive lymphoma. The first major attempt to improve upon these early efforts involved the addition of Adriamycin® into combinations with other active agents, forming regimens such as CHOP and BACOP (bleomycin, doxorubicin, cyclophosphamide, vincristine, prednisone). The Southwest Oncology Group has shown that CHOP is curative in 30 per cent of patients with large cell lymphoma: these results are important, since they were achieved in a non-selected population and confirmed by 12 years of follow-up (Coltman *et al.* 1986). A long-term follow-up is indeed necessary, since it has been shown lately that relapses may occur up to 7 years after completion of chemotherapy (Coltman *et al.* 1986).

Nowadays regimens such as CHOP, BACOP, and C-MOPP are generally referred to as first-generation treatments. Except for BACOP, these combinations were administered as intermittent chemotherapies with long treatment-free intervals (2–3 weeks). A rapid tumour proliferation between chemotherapy courses was soon recognized as a factor predisposing to induction failure. Moreover, the development of CNS disease, particularly if bone-marrow or retroperitoneal lymph nodes were involved, became increasingly frequent (Honegger and Cavalli 1984). Therefore, more intensive chemotherapy regimens have been devised, generally by eliminating

Table 9 Treatment of aggressive lymphomas: first generation of combination chemotherapy

C-MOPP	
Cyclophosphamide	650 mg/m² i.v., days 1 and 8
Vincristine	1.4 mg/m² i.v., days 1 and 8
Procarbazine	100 mg/m² p.o. days 1–10
Prednisone	40 mg/m² p.o. days 1–14
CHOP	
Cyclophosphamide	750 mg/m² i.v., day 1
Doxorubicin	50 mg/m² i.v., day 1
Oncovin (vincristine)	1.4 mg/m² i.v. (max. 2 mg), day 1
Prednisone	100 mg p.o., days 1–5 (repeat every 2–3 weeks)
BACOP	
Bleomycin	5 mg/m² i.v., days 15 and 21
Doxorubicin	25 mg/m² i.v., days 1 and 8
Cyclophosphamide	650 mg/m² i.v., days 1 and 8
Oncovin (vincristine)	1.4 mg/m² i.v., days 1 and 8
Prednisone	60 mg/m² p.o., days 15 and 29 (repeat monthly)

Abbreviations: i.v., intravenously; max., maximum; p.o., *per os*.

or shortening therapy-free intervals and using drugs active against putative localizations in the CNS (Table 9). Other drugs were added to the earlier combinations. Because of its pronounced antitumour activity in non-Hodgkin's lymphoma, the podophillotoxine derivative, VP-16 (etoposide) has frequently been employed (Cavalli 1985) and bleomycin (sometimes with vincristine) was often added during bone-marrow recovery. Methotrexate and cytosine arabinoside have also been recently incorporated into newer regimens. These two drugs, as well as procarbazine, penetrate the blood–brain barrier and may provide protection to the central nervous system. These regimens (M-BACOD, COP-BLAM, ProMACE–MOPP) are nowadays referred to as 'second-generation' treatments (Table 10).

A further strategic element was incorporated into the ProMACE–MOPP flexible sequences. The ProMACE would be delivered for a flexible number of cycles, based on the rate of tumour response. Patients whose rates of response slowed in response to ProMACE were switched for their next cycle to MOPP chemotherapy, which contained three drugs to which their tumours had not been exposed (Fisher *et al.* 1983).

The dominant idea guiding the design of the newer third-generation chemotherapy regimens is the Goldie–Coldman hypothesis (Goldie and Coldman 1984). According to that hypothesis a larger fraction of patients with diffuse aggressive lymphomas could be cured if the patients were exposed to the largest possible number of active agents at full dose as early as possible in the treatment course.

There are now different third-generation treatment protocols (Table 11): their major focus, in addition to the principle of the rapid alternation of different drugs, is on the search for modifications of doses and schedules to augment dose intensity. In COP–BLAM III, bleomycin and vincristine are given as a continuous infusion, which was not the case in the original COP–BLAM (Coleman *et al.* 1988). MACOP-B consists of six drugs, each given at a rather high dosage (Connors and Klimo 1988): later on methotrexate was substituted with VP-16, resulting in VACOP-B (O'Reilly *et al.* 1991). While MACOP-B emphasizes dose intensity, the European scheme F-MACHOP consists of seven drugs administered sequentially within the first 3 days of a 3-week cycle (Amadori *et al.* 1985), consistent with the perceived importance of early exposure to as many drugs as possible. The National Cancer Institute regimen ProMACE–CytaBOM consists of the rotation of eight drugs and attempts to incorporate all of the strategic ideas of the third-generation protocols (Longo *et al.* 1987). An intermediate step between second- and third-generation protocols is represented by the French protocol LNH-80 (Coiffier *et al.* 1986), which has achieved one of the highest percentages of long-term survival (see Table 12). Recently the same group reported results with the LNH-84 regimen which represented a slight modification of the previous treatment (Coiffier *et al.* 1989). In the latter study, the data on the treatment of 737 patients were accrued in a multicentre protocol and by and large the results confirm those obtained with the LNH-80 regimen in 100 patients. This French report suggests, for the first time, that similar results with modern aggressive chemotherapy can be achieved in selected institutions and multicentre trials.

One of the possible drawbacks of this third-generation regimen is the possibility that, at least in an important proportion of patients (for example, the older ones), some drugs will be underdosed, because of the many cytotoxic agents used concomitantly. One British trial using a similar strategic approach showed that reduction of the Adriamycin® dosage to 20–25 mg/m² will significantly impair the long-term results (Smith *et al.* 1989). Furthermore, one

Table 10 Treatment of aggressive non-Hodgkin's lymphoma: second-generation chemotherapy

	Day 1	Day 8	Day 15	Days 16–28
ProMACE–MOPP flexitherapy				No therapy
Cyclophosphamide 650 mg/m² i.v.	x	x		
Doxorubicin 25 mg/m² i.v.	x	x		
Etoposide 120 mg/m² i.v.	x	x		
Methotrexate 1.5 mg/m² i.v.			x with leucovorin rescue	
Prednisone 60 mg/m² p.o.	x ————— x			

Flexible number of cycles until complete response or decreased rate of response, then switch to:

	Day 1	Day 8	Day 14	Days 15–28
				No therapy
Nitrogen mustard 6 mg/m² i.v.	x	x		
Vincristine 1.4 mg/m² i.v.	x	x		
Procarbazine 100 mg/m² p.o.	x ————— x			
Prednisone 60 mg/m² p.o.	x ————— x			

Same number of cycles as ProMACE, then restart ProMACE

	Day 1	Day 8	Day 15	Day 16–21
M-BACOD				No therapy
Cyclophosphamide 600 mg/m² i.v.	x			
Doxorubicin 45 mg/m² i.v.	x			
Vincristine 1 mg/m² i.v.	x			
Bleomycin 4 mg/m² i.v.	x			
Methotrexate 200 mg/m² i.v.		x rescue x with leucovorin rescue		
Dexamethasone 6 mg/m² p.o.	xxxxx			

	Day 1	Day 10	Day 14	Days 15–21
COP–BLAM				No therapy
Cyclophosphamide 400 mg/m² i.v.	x			
Doxorubicin 40 mg/m² i.v.	x			
Vincristine 1 mg/m² i.v.	x			
Procarbazine 100 mg/m² p.o.	x —— x			
Prednisone 40 mg/m²	x —— x			
Bleomycin 15 mg i.v.			x	

Abbreviations: i.v., intravenously; p.o., *per os.*

key drug in some combinations (etoposide, VP-16) is given in a suboptimal manner (weekly), while it is well known that the antitumour activity of this drug is schedule-dependent and more pronounced when used over many consecutive days than when administered weekly (Cavalli 1982).

Which is the best treatment for aggressive lymphomas?

The rapid development during the past decade of the numerous regimens of combination chemotherapy and the many methodological differences in the reported series have created a certain degree of confusion, even for specialists. This topic was recently summarized in an excellent review (Armitage and Cheson 1988). Even if in a randomized trial a marginal superiority of ProMACE–CytaBOM over ProMACE–MOPP was reported (Longo *et al.* 1991), we can assume that no one of the newer regimens is clearly superior to the others (Dana *et al.* 1990; Miller *et al.* 1990; Weick *et al.* 1991). Moreover, very recently the preliminary results of an American intergroup study comparing CHOP to M-BACOD, MACOP-B, and ProMACE–CytaBOM in almost 1200 patients have shown no

Table 11   Treatment of aggressive non-Hodgkin's lymphoma: third-generation chemotherapy

	Day 1	Day 2	Day 3	Day 4	Day 5
COP–BLAM III					
Cycle A					
Vincristine 1 mg/m²/day infusion	x ---------- x				
Bleomycin 7.5 mg/m² i.v. bolus, then 7.5 mg/m²/day infusion	x --- x				
Cyclophosphamide 350 mg/m² i.v.	x				
Doxorubicin 35 mg/m² i.v.	x				
Prednisone 40 mg/m² p.o.	x	x	x	x	x
Procarbazine 100 mg/m² p.o.	x	x	x	x	x

Cycle B

Like cycle A without bleomycin and without day 2 of vincristine infusion

Week	1	3	7	10	13	16	19	22	25	28	31	34
Cycle	A	B	A	B	A	B	A	B	A	B	A	B

	Day 1	Day 8	Day 14	Day 15–21
ProMACE–CytaBOM				No therapy
Cyclophosphamide 650 mg/m² i.v.	x			
Doxorubicin 25 mg/m² i.v.	x			
Etoposide 120 mg/m² i.v.	x			
Cytarabine 300 mg/m² i.v.		x		
Bleomycin 5 mg/m² i.v.		x		
Vincristine 1.4 mg/m² i.v.		x		
Methotrexate 120 mg/m² i.v.		x with leucovorin rescue		
Prednisone 60 mg/m² p.o.	x --- x			
Co-trimoxazole 2 p.o. b.i.d. throughout six cycles of therapy				

Week	1	2	3	4	5	6	7	8	9	10	11	12
MACOP–B												
Cyclophosphamide 350 mg/m²	x		x		x		x		x		x	
Doxorubicin 50 mg/m² i.v.	x		x		x		x		x		x	
Vincristine 1.4 mg/m² i.v.		x		x		x		x		x		x
Methotrexate 400 mg/m² i.v.[a]		x				x				x		
Bleomycin 10 mg/m² i.v.				x				x				x
Prednisone 75 mg/m² p.o. o.d.	x --- taper											
Co-trimoxazole 2 p.o. b.i.d.	x --- x											
PACE–BOM												
Cyclophosphamide 300 mg/m² i.v.	x		x		x		x		x		x	
Doxorubicin 35 mg/m² i.v.	x		x		x		x		x		x	
Etoposide 150 mg/m² i.v.	x		x		x		x		x		x	
Vincristine 1.4 mg/m² i.v.		x		x		x		x		x		x
Bleomycin 10 mg/m² i.v.				x				x				x
Methotrexate 100 mg/m² i.v.		x				x				x		
Prednisone 50 mg/m²	x --- x											
Co-trimoxazole 2 p.o. b.i.d.	x --- x											

[a]With leucovorin rescue.

Abbreviations: b.i.d., twice a day; i.v., intravenously; o.d., *omni die*; p.o., *per os*.

difference among the four treatment arms (Fisher *et al.* 1993). While obviously disappointing, these data and the definite reappraisal of the importance of prognostic factors in determining the outcome of first-line treatment indicate that in the years to come further clinical research will have to concentrate on the development of different treatments for various subgroups of patients with aggressive lymphoma. One retrospective analysis has already shown that in patients with 'low-risk aggressive lymphomas' (as defined by age, tumour bulk, and lactate dehydrogenase level), regimens of the first generation can be curative in a high percentage of cases (Jagannath *et al.* 1985). Different groups are currently working on elaborate prognostic models for predicting survival (Coiffier and Lepage 1989; Velasquez *et al.* 1989). These endeavours have already led to the proposition of an International Index, a prognostic system which

could, in the years to come, replace the Ann Arbor classification for aggressive lymphoma (Shipp *et al.* 1992).

We therefore feel that the future lies with the development of different treatment protocols for different risk groups of patients ('risk-adapted chemotherapy'). This is particularly necessary in view of the significant toxicity of the newer regimens, which have shown a percentage of toxic death varying between 2 and 10 per cent. Clearly, not all patients with aggressive lymphomas need to be exposed to this degree of toxicity. On the contrary, many cases with one or more unfavourable prognostic factors could be treated quite aggressively from the very beginning, for example by autologous bone-marrow transplantation (Gianni and Bonadonna 1989). The principles involved in the curative treatment of aggressive lymphomas are summarized in Table 13.

Table 12 Prospect for long-term survival from more recent treatment programmes for diffuse aggressive lymphoma (modified from De Vita *et al.* 1989)

Regimen	Complete responses (CR)		Relapse rate (RR)		Potential for long-term survival[a] CR×(1−RR)
ProMACE/MOPP					
flexitherapy	60/75	(80%)	21/60	(35%)	52%
M-BACOD	59/86	(70%)	15/59	(25%)	52%
COP–BLAM	24/33	(73%)	4/24	(17%)	61%
LNH–80	84/97	(87%)	18/24	(21%)	68%
COP–BLAM III	43/51	(84%)	4/43	(9%)	76%
MACOP-B	104/125	(84%)	23/104	(21%)	66%
ProMACE–CytaBOM	80/95	(84%)	20/80	(25%)	63%
LNH-84	NS/560	(75%)	NS	(25%)	67%

[a]Due to differences in follow-up and methodology, these data probably overestimate long-term results.
NS, not stated.

Table 13 Principles for the curative treatment of aggressive lymphomas (from Armitage and Cheson 1988)

1 Treatment must achieve a high rate of complete remissions
2 Cure must be accomplished with front-line therapy
3 Drugs must be delivered at curative doses
4 Rapidity of achieving a complete response may be related to the chance for a cure
5 Prolonged treatment is unnecessary
6 Curative therapy is toxic

Treatment of highly aggressive lymphomas

The highly aggressive lymphomas include diffuse, small non-cleaved cell lymphomas (Burkitt's and non-Burkitt's), lymphoblastic lymphoma, and adult T-cell leukaemia–lymphoma. The latter form is discussed in another chapter of this book.

We believe that diffuse, small non-cleaved cell non-Burkitt's lymphomas in adults should be treated in a manner similar to the one used in children with Burkitt's lymphoma. Appropriate treatment strategies are discussed in the following chapter. However, other strategies have been proposed, for example to use treatment designed for acute lymphoblastic leukaemia (Strauss *et al.* 1991) or high-intensity, brief-duration chemotherapy (McMaster *et al.* 1991). Overall, approximately one-half of adults with small non-cleaved cell lymphomas appear to be curable with intensive chemotherapy.

Lymphoblastic lymphoma (Working Formulation subtype I) is a very aggressive neoplasm, known to be rapidly progressive, with frequent involvement of the mediastinum and dissemination to the bone-marrow and CNS. Aggressive chemotherapy with different regimens, based generally on the strategy for acute lymphoblastic leukaemia, with due attention paid to cerebrospinal fluid prophylaxis, has produced a 90 per cent complete remission rate, with 50 per cent of the patients being probable long-term survivors (Bertino 1983; Coleman *et al.* 1986). Whether the results can be further improved with more aggressive approaches (for example, autologous bone marrow transplantation), remains to be shown (Santini *et al.* 1991). Patients with highly aggressive lymphomas are the ones most prone to develop metabolic disturbances, such as lactic acidosis, acute tumour lysis syndrome, and hyperuricaemia. These complications will be discussed later.

Salvage treatment of aggressive lymphomas

Until a few years ago patients with aggressive lymphoma who relapsed or failed to achieve complete response had a life expectancy of 3–4 months. First attempts to modify this natural history were initiated at the MD Anderson, Houston, with the combination of iphosphamide, etoposide, and methotrexate, to which methyl-GAG (methyl glyoxal bisguanylhydrazone; mitoguazone; MIME) was later added: complete remission rates in the order of 24–37 per cent were reported, but long-term remission remained a rare event (Cabanillas *et al.* 1987). Later on, better results were reported from the same investigators with cisplatin in combination with high-dose cytarabine (cytosine arabinoside; ara-C) and dexamethasone (DHAP) (Velasquez *et al.* 1988) and, even more so, with the further addition of etoposide (V-16) (Cabanillas *et al.* 1988; Velasquez *et al.* 1992) and the final development of an alternating regimen MINE–ESHAP (Rodriguez *et al.* 1992). Another, less-aggressive regimen called CEPP-B was developed at Stanford (Chao *et al.* 1990) and should be considered when the therapeutic aim is palliation only, while MINE–ESHAP should be envisaged in patients where a curative approach is still possible.

High-dose chemotherapy followed by autologous bone-marrow transplantation has recently been more often investigated as a potentially curative salvage strategy for refractory or relapsing lymphoma (Pedrazzini *et al.* 1989). The relative merit of this approach continues to be controversial (Rosenberg 1987): recently, the preliminary results of a randomized French study have indicated that autologous bone-marrow transplantation may be equivalent to a more 'standard' consolidation chemotherapy in patients in first remission (Haioun *et al.* 1992). It also remains unclear whether autologous bone-marrow transplantation is a more powerful salvage tool than, for example MINE–ESHAP.

What is clear from the available data is that patients who are not in complete remission at the beginning of the preparative regimen fare less well than those who have responded to conventional chemotherapy and are disease free (or nearly so) at that time. Furthermore, it is now evident that the procedure is not indicated in patients who have disease refractory to conventional salvage treatment (Pedrazzini *et al.* 1989). It is still unclear whether variations on the standard preparative regimen or bone-marrow purging can have a significant impact on outcome.

Treatment of lymphomas in special sites and special situations

Neoplastic involvement of the gastrointestinal tract is the most common primary site of extranodal lymphoma (List *et al.* 1988). In fact, primary gastrointestinal lymphoma accounts for at least 15 per cent of all non-Hodgkin's lymphoma and the incidence, mainly for gastric lymphoma (Severson and Scott 1990) is rapidly increasing. The primary lesion is in the stomach, in approximately 60 per cent of cases in the small bowel and the remaining 10–12 per cent of cases present in the large bowel. Approximately three-quarters of the patients will show an intermediate- or high-grade histology. Primary T-cell lymphomas in the gastrointestinal tract are exceedingly rare and are generally accompanied by clinically evident enteropathies.

The optimal management of patients with primary gastrointestinal lymphoma remains unclear, since there have been no randomized prospective therapeutic trials. The rapidly evolving understanding of the biology of these lymphomas (*Lancet* 1992) has added to the uncertainty and has even led recently to a proposal for a separate histological classification (Isaacson 1988). Lymphoproliferative lesions of the gastrointestinal tract (but also of lung, salivary gland, and thyroid) have been something of an enigma. Some low-grade lesions were called 'pseudolymphoma' because of their benign behaviour. Likewise, many of the clearly high-grade lymphomas seemed to behave more favourably than comparable lymph node lesions (Gospodarowicz et al. 1987; Isaacson 1991). The use of refined immunocytochemistry, coupled with molecular biology, has helped to define mucosa-associated lymphoid tissue (MALT) lymphomas as a specific biological entity, including lesions previously called pseudolymphoma (Isaacson 1991). The low-grade mucosa-associated lymphoid tissue lymphomas are of particular interest since they do not show the bcl-2 gene rearrangement typical of follicular lymphoma and tend to remain localized, only rarely involving bone-marrow (Pan et al. 1989).

On the other hand, the presence of gastrointestinal involvement represents an adverse prognostic factor (List et al. 1988), primarily because of complications such as perforation and/or bleeding, which tend to occur spontaneously or at the beginning of radio- or chemotherapy.

The concomitant occurrence of a biologically more favourable variant with the possibility of life-threatening complications explains why therapeutic results have varied according to different series (List et al. 1988; De Vita et al. 1989; Salles et al. 1991). More recently the analysis of 91 patients with aggressive gastrointestinal lymphoma treated with intensive chemotherapy within a randomized trial (LNH-84), encompassing more than 700 patients, has shown that the therapeutic outcome is comparable to that of similar stages without primary gastrointestinal involvement (Salles et al. 1991).

Debulking or radical surgery has generally been advocated as the first therapeutic measure (List et al. 1988; Shepherd et al. 1988). In at least two series, patients with complete resection of gastrointestinal lymphoma showed virtually no relapses after adjuvant chemotherapy (Shepherd et al. 1988). Lately, however, the rôle of surgery (at least in gastric lymphoma) has been questioned (Salles et al. 1991). Both a chemotherapy-only (Gobbi et al. 1990; Maor et al. 1990) and a more elaborate, endoscopy-based approach (Taal et al. 1989), which includes radiochemotherapy but no surgery, have been proposed.

In conclusion, we can say that currently the best approach has still to be determined. The physician with limited experience should therefore consult in each given case with a specialized centre. If this is not possible, then limited surgery and a careful start of chemotherapy, with close monitoring of the patient, are advisable.

Primary CNS lymphoma accounts for approximately 2 per cent of brain tumours and 2 per cent of all lymphomas, even when their incidence is increased in immunodepressed patients. They are somewhat less responsive to radiation therapy than those primaries in other sites, and the median survival is 12–24 months (Formenti and Levine 1989). Nevertheless, the main treatment modality remains whole-brain irradiation to approximately 40 Gy, with a boost to the primary lesion of approximately 10–15 Gy. Most relapses are in the CNS. Recently, there have been scattered reports about the use of systemic combination chemotherapy, with or without radiation therapy (Formenti and Levine 1989). It is still not yet clear whether systemic chemotherapy can add anything to the dismal results of radiation therapy alone: at the Royal Marsden Hospital, there were indeed no significant differences in overall survival between the patients treated with radiotherapy alone and those receiving initial chemotherapy (Brada et al. 1990). Probably chemotherapies more adapted to the biology of CNS lymphoma will have to be devised in order to obtain meaningful results.

Secondary involvement of the CNS is more common: this is reported in 7–9 per cent of cases (Recht et al. 1988). The generally advocated treatment is to administer methotrexate, cytosine arabinoside, and steroids into the canal or by way of an Ommaya reservoir. Methotrexate ($10 \, \text{mg/m}^2$; supplemented, if necessary, by leucovorin, since its application may cause prolonged low-level shedding of methotrexate in the blood) and cytosine arabinoside ($50 \, \text{mg/m}^2$) should be applied twice weekly until cytological normalization of the cerebrospinal fluid and weekly thereafter for six applications; a monthly maintenance is then generally added for 1 year. The treatment is basically similar to the therapeutic approach to leukaemic meningiosis and is often supplemented by a concurrent cranial irradiation. It is well known that meningial lymphoma can be eradicated, but generally the outlook is a function of the inability to control the systemic disease.

Orbital lymphomas are rare and can usually be managed with excellent local control by radiation therapy. Most primary lymphomas of bone have been treated by local therapy, usually radiation. Surgery has been used less commonly and sometimes both radiation and surgery have been used. Recent studies at the National Cancer Institute reported that bone involvement was present in more than one-quarter of 95 young patients with non-Hodgkin's lymphoma; however, in two patients this involvement was limited to a single bone only (Haddy et al. 1988). Even if this series is biased concerning the referral pattern, bone involvement is evidently more common than previously suspected in young patients with non-Hodgkin's lymphoma. However, bone involvement in itself does not appear to signal a poor prognosis; rather, it is usually an expression of extensive disease. In the National Cancer Institute series it did not appear that radiotherapy would improve the results of chemotherapy. Thus, exclusion of radiotherapy from the treatment of young persons with bone lymphoma is now regarded as possible and would lessen the high rate of late sequelae of this treatment.

Nearly 30 per cent of all non-Hodgkin's lymphomas will present in elderly patients (> 70 years of age) and approximately 10 per cent will be diagnosed in patients older than 80 years. The optimal treatment of non-Hodgkin's lymphoma in elderly patients is controversial, mainly because most published series actually consist of selected cases. Almost 15 cases were reported recently in a retrospective analysis carried out by the EORTC in 13 institutions (Tirelli et al. 1988). No differences were reported in the prevalence of high- and intermediate-grade subtypes and stage III/IV between patients younger and older than 70 years. Approximately half of the treating physicians used a 'conservative' policy, for example one or two cytotoxic drugs or local-field radiotherapy. There was a significantly higher prevalence of severe and slight toxicity in elderly patients treated with aggressive regimens at doses conventionally used in younger patients. However, only prospective clinical trials will be able to define the optimal treatment for elderly patients with non-Hodgkin's lymphoma.

It has been our practice to administer the first cycle of drugs to older patients at one-half to two-thirds of full dose, with subsequent modification of the treatment according to tolerance. First-generation regimens or, if anthracyclines cannot be tolerated, combinations similar to CEPP (B) (Chao et al. 1990) have been our first chemotherapeutic choice.

AIDS-related lymphomas are discussed in another chapter. Their outlook, because of the underlying disease and complications due to infections, remains poor, even though the first promising long-term results have been reported recently (Strauss et al. 1991).

Complications at the start of treatment

Lactic acidosis is an oncological emergency which arises rarely in patients with aggressive lymphoma who have extensive involvement of the liver: the normal liver is capable of metabolizing lactate efficiently, even under conditions of maximal extrahepatic production. Most patients reported in the literature to have this condition have died of it; however, immediate treatment with bicarbonate or dialysis and the prompt institution of modern systemic chemotherapy may lead to resolution of the lactic acidosis (Vandermolen et al. 1988).

Hyperurecaemia and the acute tumour lysis syndrome are related more to the beginning of chemotherapy, since this treatment induces massive lysis of the rapidly dividing cells, which results in release into the blood of large quantities of cellular products. Hyperurecaemia can usually be easily controlled with allopurinol and forced diuresis, supplemented if necessary with alkalinization. In cases of pre-existent elevated uric acid level in the serum and/or in all cases at high risk (important tumour bulk, massively elevated lactate dehydrogenase and aggressive histology) these measures should be instituted 24–36 h prior to the beginning of chemotherapy.

The acute tumour lysis syndrome is a more severe condition, which may occur on the first day after the start of treatment for acute lymphoblastic leukaemia and highly aggressive lymphomas (Cohen et al. 1980). It is characterized by hyperkalaemia but mainly by a severe hyperphosphataemia, which generally appears 24–48 h before the development of renal failure, usually due to calcium phosphate deposits in the kidneys. Because this latter process may be favoured by an alkaline urine, alkalization should not be used in patients at risk of developing this syndrome. Preventive measures would include control of hyperurecaemia (but without alkalinization), establishment of the correct state of hydration with an abundant diuresis at neutral pH, and daily monitoring of serum electrolytes, calcium, and phosphorus. However, renal failure can occur despite maximal pre-treatment prophylactic care, in which case the rapid institution of dialysis is mandatory. Whether phosphorus chelators are effective in the control of this syndrome remains to be proven.

T-CELL LYMPHOMAS

Since the Rappaport and Working Formulations were not developed specifically for classifying T-cell malignancies, some T-cell malignancies appear in these classifications and others do not. The Kiel classification, initially published in 1974 (Gérard-Marchand et al. 1974) has been recently updated to incorporate information derived from newer immunological and molecular biological techniques (Stansfeld et al. 1988). Table 14 summarizes this updated Kiel classification which is designed to encompass most T-cell malignancies.

The most immature T-cell malignancies are the lymphoblastic lymphomas and the T-cell acute lymphoblastic leukaemias. The malignant cells in these disorders have pre-thymic markers; lymphoblastic lymphoma was discussed in the previous section of this chapter.

Post-thymic or mature T-cell malignancies represent a broad spectrum of clinicopathological entities (Jaffe 1984), some of which have not yet been precisely defined. The term 'peripheral T-cell lymphoma' has been used generically to describe non-Hodgkin's lymphoma with a mature T-cell phenotype. It should be remembered that TdT activity is negative in mature T-cell tumours and that phenotypic markers cannot be used to demonstrate clonality, which has to be shown by methods used in molecular biology (T-cell receptor gene rearrangements). Table 15 summarizes the currently used classification of post-thymic T-cell malignancies. T-cell chronic lymphocytic leukaemias and mycosis fungoides/Sézary's syndrome (the two latter forms are also called cutaneous T-cell lymphomas) for the most part represent low-grade malignant lymphoid proliferations which find their clinical counterparts in the B-cell system in chronic lymphocytic leukaemia, small lymphocytic lymphomas, and most follicular lymphomas. These disorders have an indolent clinical course and can be controlled by therapy: in general, however, they cannot be cured and pursue a relentless clinical course. In contrast, the peripheral T-cell lymphomas and adult T-cell leukaemia/lymphoma are aggressive lymphoid malignancies. While most therapeutic strategies have been unsuccessful in adult T-cell leukaemia/lymphoma, better results have been obtained in peripheral T-cell lymphomas. The potential for long-term remission and possible cure appears similar to that seen in aggressive lymphomas of B-cell type. The angiocentric immunoproliferative lesions represent a broad clinical spectrum, ranging from low- to high-grade lymphoproliferative lesions and share with the follicular lymphomas a tendency to undergo histological and clinical progression with time. While the mature B-cell lymphomas relate well to different developmental and functional B-cell subsets, there has been less success in relating the post-thymic T-cell malignancies to distinct T-cell subpopulations

Table 14 Upated Kiel classification of non-Hodgkin's lymphomas (Stansfeld 1988)

B-cell lymphomas	T-cell lymphomas
Low grade	Low grade
Lymphocytic–chronic lymphocytic and prolymphocytic leukaemia; hairy cell leukaemia	Lymphocytic–chronic lymphocytic and prolymphocytic leukaemia
Lymphoplasmacytic/cytoid (LP immunocytoma)	Small, cerebriform cell; mycosis fungoides, Sézary's syndrome
Plasmacytic	Lymphoepithelioid (Lennert's lymphoma)
Centroblastic/centrocytic	Angioimmunoblastic (AILD, LgX)
Follicular±diffuse	T zone
Diffuse	Pleomorphic, small cell (HTVL-1±)
Centrocytic	
High grade	High grade
Centroblastic	Pleomorphic, medium and large cell (HTLV-1±)
Immunoblastic	Immunoblastic (HTLV-1±)
Large cell anaplastic (Ki-1+)	Large cell anaplastic (Ki-1+)
Burkitt's lymphoma	Lymphoblastic
Lymphoblastic	
Rare types	Rare types

Table 15 Classification of post-thymic T-cell malignancies (Jaffe 1984)

I   T-cell chronic lymphocytic leukaemia
    Helper
    Suppressor
    Prolymphocytic
II   Mycosis fungoides/Sézary's syndrome
III   Peripheral T-cell lymphomas
    Subtypes and/or related terms
      Node-based T-cell lymphoma
      T zone lymphoma
      AILD-like T-cell lymphoma
      Lymphoepithelioid cell (Lennert's) lymphoma
      Multilobated T-cell lymphoma
IV   Adult T-cell leukaemia/lymphoma
    (HTLV-associated disease)
V   Angiocentric immunoproliferative lesions
    (Lymphomatoid granulomatosis)
    (Polymorphic reticulosis)

(Jaffe 1984). T-cell lymphomas represent approximately half of all non-Hodgkin's lymphomas in Japan, but account for only approximately 5 per cent of all lymphomas in the West.

We will now discuss separately cutaneous T-cell lymphomas and peripheral T-cell lymphomas.

Cutaneous T-cell lymphomas

Mycosis fungoides and Sézary's syndrome are collectively referred to as the cutaneous T-cell lymphomas because of the universal infiltration of the skin by malignant T lymphocytes (Broder and Bunn 1980). The aetiology of cutaneous T-cell lymphomas is unknown, but recently a family history of atopic dermatitis has been suggested as a significant risk factor. While the clinical and histopathological features of the cutaneous lesions were well described in the period between 1806, when the original case was reported and 1939, when Sézary's syndrome was described, the lymphomatous nature of the malignant cells was not proven until 1970. The cells were subsequently shown to have both functional and phenotypic properties of the helper subset of T lymphocytes (Haynes et al. 1981). Initially, cutaneous T-cell lymphoma was thought to involve only the skin. Infiltration of lymph nodes and other organs, which generally occurred late in the natural history, was usually ascribed to the development of a second malignant process. Pathological studies in the 1970s demonstrated that extracutaneous lesions were frequent in autopsied cases (approximately 75 per cent) and were always related to the initial cutaneous lymphoma (Rappaport and Thomas 1972); they were not second neoplasms. More recent studies demonstrated that unsuspected malignant cells were almost universally present in extracutaneous sites (peripheral blood, lymph nodes, and/or visceral organs) by the time a diagnosis was established (Broder and Bunn 1980).

Most patients experience periods of months to years (mean 5–10 years) of transitory and non-specific cutaneous manifestations before establishment of a diagnosis of cutaneous T-cell lymphoma. This pre-mycotic phase, during which the most common symptom is itching, is often misdiagnosed. As the disease progresses, the exzematous patches gradually develop into indurated plaques: at this stage the disease frequently begins to progress more rapidly and the cutaneous involvement becomes more generalized. The plaques can grow not only in their surface dimensions, but also in thickness, gradually producing tumours which can be elevated a few centimetres.

Another common cutaneous variant of cutaneous T-cell lymphoma is the generalized erythroderma variant. Patients with erythroderma who have evidence of more than 5 per cent of circulating malignant convoluted atypical mononuclear (Sézary) cells have the so-called Sézary syndrome. Recent studies showed that when carefully staged, almost all patients with erythroderma and a variable percentage of patients with plaque-tumour will have some circulating Sézary cells (Bunn et al. 1980). Patients with high percentages of circulating Sézary cells have a shorter survival than those with lower percentages (Vonderheid et al. 1985).

The clinical course of cutaneous T-cell lymphoma is generally indolent but in occasional patients becomes fulminant, similarly to the observations in B-cell lymphoma. It has been shown recently that biopsies from patients with accelerating disease can reveal cytological transformation from previously observed small, convoluted lymphocytes to large cells that are similar to cells seen in large-cell lymphoma (Dmitrovsky et al. 1987). In one such series involving 150 patients with cutaneous T-cell lymphoma, who were treated from 1976 to 1984, cytological transformation was identified in 12 individuals (Dmitrovsky et al. 1987). The median time from diagnosis of cutaneous T-cell lymphoma to cytological transformation was slightly less than 2 years and the median survival after transformation was only 2 months.

The most commonly used staging classification system was proposed in 1979 and is summarized in Table 16 (Bunn and Lamberg 1979). Prognostically, patients can be divided into three groups. Patients with stage I or IIE (approximately 50 per cent of all cases) have a 90 per cent 5 year survival. Stage IIB, III, or IVA patients (approximately 40 per cent) have a median survival of approximately 5 years. Median survival for stage IVB patients (approximately 10 per cent of cases) is approximately 2 years (Bunn and Lamberg 1979).

A simplified classification system was recently suggested (Kaye et al. 1987). In this proposal patients could be divided into three prognostic categories: low risk, disease limited to skin without tumours, intermediate risk, cutaneous tumours or pathological node involvement, and high risk, erythroderma or visceral invasion.

Therapy of cutaneous T-cell lymphomas

There are four therapeutic modalities with proven effectiveness in patients with cutaneous T-cell lymphomas. These include topical chemotherapy with nitrogen mustard, PUVA (psoralen with ultraviolet light A), and whole-body electron beam therapy and systemic chemotherapy. Topical treatments are effective, although their impact on survival is still debatable.

Even if different series cannot be easily compared, the results of all three topical modalities seem by and large to be similar, although electron-beam therapy appears to be somewhat more effective (Broder and Bunn 1980). However, this therapy requires close attention to dosimetry to avert significant side-effects. Nitrogen mustard is particularly useful in patients with early cutaneous stages, while PUVA therapy is highly effective in clearing up skin lesions; approximately 60 per cent of treated patients in all D stages will achieve complete remission. However, a serious long-term complication of PUVA therapy is the development of secondary cutaneous malignancies; this modality should therefore not be used in early-stage disease. New uses of PUVA, such as, for instance, the extracorporeal treatment with ultraviolet light of peripheral blood cells containing psoralen or a combination of PUVA with α-interferon (Kuzel et al. 1990) are currently being investigated.

The treatment of choice for patients with skin-only disease without erythroderma or skin tumour is still topical nitrogen

Table 16 Cutaneous T-cell lymphoma workshop, staging classification (Bunn and Lamberg 1979)

T_1	Limited plaques ($<10\%$ body)	N_0	No adenopathy; histology negative	M_0	No involvement
T_2	Generalized plaques	N_1	Adenopathy; histology negative	M_1	Visceral involvement
N_3	Cutaneous tumours	N_2	No adenopathy; histology positive		
T_4	Generalized erythroderma	N_3	Adenopathy; histology positive		

Stage I   Limited (IA) or generalized plaques (IB) without adenopathy or histological involvement of lymph nodes or viscera ($T_1N_0M_0$ or $T_2N_0M_0$)

Stage II   Limited or generalized plaques with adenopathy (IIA) or cutaneous tumours with or without adenopathy (IIB); without histological involvement of lymph nodes or viscera ($T_{1-2}N_1M_0T_2N_{0-1}M_0$)

Stage III   Generalized erythroderma with or without adenopathy; without histological involvement of lymph nodes or viscera ($T_4N_{0-1}M_0$)

Stage IV   Histological involvement of lymph nodes (IVA) or viscera (IVB) with any skin lesion and with or without adenopathy ($T_{1-4}N_{2-3}M_0$ for IVA; $T_{1-4}N_{0-3}M_1$ for IVB)

mustard. At Stanford, patients with limited plaque had a 51 per cent complete response rate and those with generalized plaque a 26 per cent complete response rate (Hoppe *et al.* 1987). Forty per cent of the complete responders with limited plaque and 60 per cent of those with generalized plaque later relapsed, but most responded to subsequent treatments, including repeated courses of topical nitrogen mustard. It has also been shown that patients developing a cutaneous hypersensitivity to the aqueous preparation of nitrogen mustard will tolerate and respond to the ointment-based preparations (Hoppe *et al.* 1987).

Systemic chemotherapy offers the most direct way of attacking widely disseminated extracutaneous disease, but unfortunately this modality has proven to be non-curative. Objective responses that produce palliation of symptoms are frequent, in the order of 70 per cent. The most active agents include methotrexate, alkylating agents, etoposide and cisplatin. Different combinations including the previously listed agents have not been proven clearly superior to single-agent therapy (Broder and Bunn 1980).

Combined modality treatments have been evaluated in a few trials (Broder and Bunn 1980). The addition of topical nitrogen mustard either to chemotherapy or to irradiation is a reasonable approach, but is still non-curative and the results are controversial.

Recently, the combination of total skin electron-beam irradiation and systemic chemotherapy has been advocated for patients with tumour-stage cutaneous T-cell lymphoma (Hallahan *et al.* 1988). However, the results of a recently terminated trial are disappointing (Kaye *et al.* 1989). In this study 103 patients with all stages of disease were randomly assigned to receive either combination therapy, consisting of 3000 Gy of electron-beam radiation to the skin combined with cyclophosphamide, vincristine, doxorubicin, and etoposide or sequential topical treatment. After a median follow-up of 75 months, there were no significant differences between the treatment groups, while combined therapy produced considerable toxicity.

Different biological treatments have been evaluated in recent years in the treatment of cutaneous T-cell lymphoma. Clinical studies with heterologous antithymocyte globulin demonstrated an antitumour response, but severe toxicities prevented sustained therapy (Bunn *et al.* 1985). Recombinant interferons were shown to be active in the treatment of cutaneous T-cell lymphoma, with response rates of approximately 50 per cent for patients with advanced disease and 90 per cent for early-stage untreated patients (Cavalli 1988). Various other modalities, including monoclonal antibodies, retinoids, and deoxycoformycin, are still being investigated.

In conclusion, therapy for cutaneous T-cell lymphoma remains somewhat of an enigma, as described by two recent authoritative editorials (Young 1989; Jones 1990). Therefore, no straightforward guidance can be given, but the treating physician should always consult with a multidisciplinary team able to provide sufficient practical experience.

Peripheral T-cell lymphoma

A peripheral T-cell lymphoma is generally diagnosed when a patient with non-Hodgkin's lymphoma has a T-cell immunophenotype but has neither a lymphoblastic lymphoma nor a cutaneous T-cell lymphoma. Peripheral T-cell lymphoma represents the most common type of T-cell lymphoma in the West. It exhibits a variety of histological appearances, which formerly were usually classified within the diffuse mixed or immunoblastic categories of the Working Formulation. In the Rappaport system, 16 per cent of these lymphomas were classified as poorly differentiated lymphocytic, 40 per cent as mixed, and approximately the same percentage as histiocytic lymphomas (Jaffe 1984). Two series encompassing 63 and 184 cases of peripheral T-cell lymphoma were recently reported (Coiffier *et al.* 1988; Armitage *et al.* 1989). In the larger series (Armitage *et al.* 1989), the median age of the patients was 57 years and 59 per cent were male. Approximately 7 per cent of the patients had prior histories of various autoimmune disorders, whereas 19 per cent had prior diagnosis of a lymphoproliferative disease. The tumours were histologically composed of large cells (43 per cent), mixed large and small cells (40 per cent), and small cells (17 per cent). The stages at diagnosis were I (7 per cent), II (21 per cent), III (22 per cent), and IV (50 per cent), while B-cell symptoms were present in 57 per cent of the cases. The most frequent sites of extranodal involvement were bone-marrow (35 per cent), skin (13 per cent), and lung (11 per cent). Fifty per cent of the patients treated with a multiagent chemotherapy regimen with proven curative potential in B-cell lymphomas achieved complete remission and the actuarial 4 year survival was 45 per cent. However, the 4 year disease-free survival in patients with stage IV disease was only 10 per cent. In the other series (Coiffier *et al.* 1988), patients showing a CD4 phenotype seemed to have a better prognosis than those with other phenotypes. Variables associated with long survival were localized disease, absence of bulky tumour masses and of B-cell symptoms, and fewer than two extranodal sites of disease (Coiffier *et al.* 1988). In many respects, patients with peripheral T-cell lymphoma are similar to patients who present with various aggressive B-cell lymphomas. However, therapeutic results by stage seem to be somewhat inferior (especially in stage IV disease) to those achieved in patients with B-cell lymphomas. However, at present, data are too scanty and results from prospective therapeutic trials which might clarify these initial observations are still awaited. However, the results of a Japanese prospective trial comparing vincristine, cyclophosphamide, prednisolone, and doxorubicin (VEPA)±methotrexate (VEPA/M) in 81 patients with advanced

T-cell lymphoma/leukaemia showed that the results in patients with peripheral T-cell lymphoma were comparable to results in those with advanced B-cell lymphoma (Shimoyama *et al.* 1988). However, in that trial only 19 patients had peripheral T-cell lymphoma. However, it must be pointed out once again that the prognostic significance of different immunological subtypes is still controversial (Lippman *et al.* 1988; Cheng *et al.* 1989; Coiffier *et al.* 1990). It is probable that a new staging system for T-cell lymphomas will have to be established when the ongoing prospective studies with extensive chemotherapy are completed and their results make it possible to identify patients with high, low, and intermediate probabilities of cure (Bunn 1988).

REFERENCES

Acker B, *et al.* (1983). Histologic conversion in the non-Hodgkin's lymphomas. *Journal of Clinical Oncology*, 1:11–16.

Amadori S, *et al.* (1985). Treatment of diffuse aggressive non Hodgkin's lymphomas with an intensive multi-drug regimen including high-dose cytosine arabinoside (F-MACHOP). *Seminars in Oncology*, 12:218–26.

Anderson T, *et al.* (1982). Malignant lymphoma. I. The histology and staging of 473 patients at the National Cancer Institute. *Cancer*, 50:2699–707.

Armitage JO, Cheson BD (1988). Interpretation of clinical trials in diffuse large-cell lymphoma. *Journal of Clinical Oncology*, 6:1335–47.

Armitage JO, *et al.* (1989). Peripheral T-cell lymphoma. *Cancer*, 6:158–63.

Bakshi A, *et al.* (1985). Cloning the chromosomal breakpoint of t(14;18) human lymphomas: clustering around JH on chromosome 14 and near a transcriptional unit on 18. *Cell*, 41:899–906.

Banks PM, *et al.* (1992). Mantle cell lymphoma: a proposal for unification of morphologic, immunologic and molecular data. *American Journal of Surgical Pathology*, 16:120–3.

Bastion Y, *et al.* (1991). Follicular lymphomas: assessment of prognostic factors in 127 patients followed for 10 years. *Annals of Oncology*, 2 (Suppl. 2):123–9.

Bertini M, *et al.* (1991). Large B-cell lymphoma with sclerosis treated with MACOP-B. *Annals of Oncology*, 2:733–7.

Bertino JR (1983). Long-term remissions in lymphoblastic lymphoma. (Editorial.) *Journal of Clinical Oncology*, 1:515.

Brada M, *et al.* (1990). Management of primary cerebral lymphoma with initial chemotherapy: preliminary results and comparison with patients treated with radiotherapy alone. *International Journal of Radiation Oncology — Biology — Physics*, 18:787–92.

Brada M, *et al.* (1987). Circulating lymphoma cells in patients with B and T non-Hodgkin's lymphoma detected by immunoglobulin and T-cell receptor gene rearrangement. *British Journal of Cancer*, 56:147–54.

British National Lymphoma Investigation Report (1981). A prospective comparison of combination chemotherapy with total body irradiation in the treatment of advanced Non-Hodgkin's lymphomas. *Clinical Oncology*, 7:193–200.

Broder S, Bunn PA Jr (1980). Neoplasms of T-cell origin: immunological aspects and therapy. *Seminars in Oncology*, 7:310–31.

Brown SL, *et al.* (1989). Treatment of B-cell lymphomas with anti-idiotype antibodies alone and in combination with alpha interferon. *Blood*, 73:651–61.

Bunn PA (1988). Diagnostic factors in intermediate and high-grade lymphomas: pathologic, immunologic, and clinical. (Editorial.) *Journal of Clinical Oncology*, 7:1073–5.

Bunn PA, Lamberg SI (1979). Report of the Committee on Staging and Classification of Cutaneous T-cell lymphoma: *Cancer Treatment Reports*, 63:725–8.

Bunn PA, *et al.* (1980). Prospective staging evaluation of patients with T-cell lymphoma. Demonstration of high frequency of extracutaneous dissemination. *Annals of International Medicine*, 93:223–30.

Bunn PA, *et al.* (1985). Treatment of cutaneous T-cell lymphomas with biologic response modifiers: recombinant leukocyte α-interferon and T101 monoclonal antibody. In *Malignant lymphomas and Hodgkin disease: experimental and therapeutic advances* (ed. F Cavalli, G Bonadonna, and M Rozencweig), pp. 579–90. Martinus Nijhoff, Boston.

Bush RS, Gospodarowicz M (1982) The place of radiation therapy in the management of patients with localized non-Hodgkin's lymphoma. In *Malignant lymphoma* (ed. VA Rosenberg and HS Kaplan), p. 485. Academic Press, Orlando.

Cabanillas F, *et al.* (1987). MIME combination chemotherapy for refractory or recurrent lymphomas. *Journal of Clinical Oncology*, 5:407–11.

Cabanillas F, *et al.* (1988). Results of recent salvage chemotherapy regimens for lymphoma and Hodgkin's disease. *Seminars in Hematology*, 25:47–50.

Carde P, *et al.* (1984). Combined radiotherapy–chemotherapy for early stages of non-Hodgkin's lymphoma: the 1975–1980 EORTC controlled lymphoma trial. *Radiotherapy and Oncology*, 2:301–12.

Cavalli F (1982). VP16-213 (etoposide). A critical review of its activity. *Cancer Chemotherapy and Pharmacology*, 7:81–5.

Cavalli F (1985). VP-16 in the treatment of malignant lymphomas: a report from the Swiss Group for Clinical Cancer Research (SAKK). *Seminars in Oncology*, XII (Suppl. 2):33–6.

Cavalli F (1988). Alpha-interferon in the treatment of malignant lymphoma. *British Journal of Clinical Practice*, 42 (Suppl. 62):16–21.

Chao NJ, Rosenberg SA, Horning SJ (1990). CEPP (B), an effective and well tolerated regimen in poor-risk, aggressive non-Hodgkin's lymphoma. *Blood*, 7:1293–8.

Cheng Ann-Lii, *et al.* (1989). Direct comparisons of peripheral T-cell lymphoma with diffuse B-cell lymphoma of comparable histological grades—should peripheral T-cell lymphoma be considered separately? *Journal of Clinical Oncology*, 7:725–31.

Cohen LF, *et al.* (1980). Acute tumor lysis syndrome. *American Journal of Medicine*, 68:486–91.

Coiffier B, Lepage E (1989). Prognosis of aggressive lymphomas: a study of five prognostic models with patients included in the LNH-84 regimen. *Blood*, 74:558–64.

Coiffier B, *et al.* (1986). Intensive and sequential combination chemotherapy for aggressive malignant lymphomas (protocol LNH-80). *Journal of Clinical Oncology*, 4:147–53.

Coiffier B, *et al.* (1988). T-cell lymphomas: immunologic, histologic, clinical and therapeutic analysis of 63 cases. *Journal of Clinical Oncology*, 6:1584–9.

Coiffier B, *et al.* (1989). LNH-84 regimen: a multicenter study of intensive chemotherapy in 737 patients with aggressive malignant lymphoma. *Journal of Clinical Oncology*, 7:1018–26.

Coiffier B, *et al.* (1990). Peripheral T-cell lymphomas have a worse prognosis than B-cell lymphomas: a prospective study of 361 immunophenotyped patients treated with the LNH-84 regimen. *Annals of Oncology*, 1:45–50.

Coleman CN, *et al.* (1986). Treatment of lymphoblastic lymphoma in adults. *Journal of Clinical Oncology*, 4:1628–37.

Coleman M, *et al.* (1988). The COP-BAM programs: evolving chemotherapy concepts in large-cell lymphoma. *Seminars in Hematology*, 25:23–33.

Coltman CA Jr, *et al.* (1986). CHOP is curative in thirty percent of patients with large cell lymphoma: a twelve-year Southwest Oncology Group follow-up. Advances in cancer chemotherapy. Update on treatment for diffuse large cell lymphoma. In *Proceedings of the symposiums held November 14–17 1985*, Marco Island, Florida (ed. AT Skarin), pp. 71–82. John Wiley, New York.

Connors JM, Klimo P (1988). MACOP-B chemotherapy for malignant lymphomas and related conditions: 1987 update and additional observations. *Seminars in Hematology*, 25 (Suppl. 2):41–6.

Connors JM, *et al.* (1987). Brief chemotherapy and involved field radiation therapy for limited-stage, histologically aggressive lymphoma. *Annals of International Medicine*, 107:25–30.

Cosset JM, *et al.* (1985). An alternating chemotherapy and radiotherapy combination for non-Hodgkin's lymphomas of unfavourable histologies: feasibility and preliminary results. *Radiotherapy and Oncology*, 3:133–8.

Cosset JM, *et al.* (1991). Alternating chemotherapy and radiotherapy combination for bulky stage I and II intermediate and high grade non-Hodgkin lymphoma: an update. *Radiotherapy and Oncology*, 20:30–7.

Cossman J, *et al.* (1983). Diversity of immunologic phenotypes of lymphoblastic lymphoma. *Cancer Research*, 43:4486–91.

Cowan RA, *et al.* (1989). Prognostic factors in high and intermediate grade non-Hodgkin's lymphoma. *British Journal of Cancer*, 59:276–82.

Dana BW, *et al.* (1990). m-BACOD treatment for intermediate- and high-grade malignant lymphomas: a SWOG phase II trial. *Journal of Clinical Oncology*, 8:1155–62.

Devesa SS, *et al.* (1987). Cancer incidence and mortality trends among whites in the United States, 1974–84. *Journal of the National Cancer Institute*, **79**:701–15.

De Vita VT Jr, *et al.* (1975). Advanced diffuse histocytic lymphoma, a potentially curable disease. *Lancet*, 1:248–50.

De Vita VT, *et al.* (1989). Lymphocytic lymphomas. In *Cancer, principle and practice of oncology* (3rd edn) (ed. VT De Vita, S Hellmann, and SA Rosenberg), pp. 1741–98. Lippincott, Philadelphia.

Dmitrovsky E, *et al.* (1987). Cytologic transformation in cutaneous T cell lymphoma: a clinicopathologic entity associated with poor prognosis. *Journal of Clinical Oncology*, 5:208–15.

Dorey EL, *et al.* (1989). Assessment of bone marrow infiltration in B-cell non-Hodgkin's lymphoma (NHL). *British Journal of Cancer*, **59**:772–4.

Dyer MJS, *et al.* (1989). Effect of CAMPATH-1 antibodies *in vivo* in patients with lymphoid malignancies: influence of antibody isotype. *Blood*, **73**:1431–9.

Engelhard M, *et al.* (1991). Prospective multicenter trial for the response-adapted treatment of high-grade non-Hodgkin's lymphoma: updated results of the COP-BLAM/IMVP-16 protocol with randomized adjuvant radiotherapy. *Annals of Oncology*, **2** (Suppl. 2):177–80.

Ezdinli EZ, *et al.* (1987). Effect of the degree of nodularity on the survival of patients with nodular lymphomas. *Journal of Clinical Oncology*, 5:413–18.

Fisher RI, *et al.* (1981). Natural history of malignant lymphomas with divergent histologies at staging evaluation. *Cancer*, **47**:2022–5.

Fisher RI, *et al.* (1993). Comparison of a standard regimen (CHOP) with three intensive chemotherapy regimens for advanced non-Hodgkin's lymphoma. *New England Journal of Medicine*, **328**:1002–6.

Fisher RT, *et al.* (1983). Diffuse aggressive lymphomas: increased survival after alternating flexible sequences of ProMACE and MOPP chemotherapy. *Annals of Internal Medicine*, **98**:304–5.

Formenti SC, Levine AM (1989). Primary central nervous system lymphomas. In *Cancer chemotherapy: concepts, clinical investigations and therapeutic advances* (ed. FM Muggia), pp. 213–30. Kluwer Academic, Boston.

Frizzera G, Moran EM, Rappaport H (1975). Angioblastic lymphadenopathy: diagnosis and clinical course. *American Journal of Medicine*, **59**:803–8.

Fuks JZ, Aisner J, Wiernik PH (1982). Restaging laparotomy in the management of non-Hodgkin's lymphomas. *Medical and Pediatric Oncology*, **10**:429–36.

Gall EA, Mallory TB (1942). Malignant lymphoma: a clinicopathologic survey of 618 cases. *American Journal of Pathology*, **18**:381–429.

Gallagher CD, Lister TA (1987). Follicular non-Hodgkin's lymphomas. In *Baillière's clinical haematology, the lymphomas* (ed. TD McElwain and TA Lister), Vol. 1, pp. 141–55. Baillière Tindall, London.

Gallagher CJ, *et al.* (1986). Follicular lymphoma: prognostic factors for response and survival. *Journal of Clinical Oncology*, **4**:1470–80.

Gérard-Marchand R, *et al.* (1974). Classification of non-Hodgkin's lymphoma. *Lancet*, 2:406–8.

Gianni AM, Bonadonna G (1989). High-dose chemo-radiotherapy for sensitive tumors: is sequential better than concurrent drug delivery? *European Journal of Cancer and Clinical Oncology*, **25**:1027–30.

Glatstein E, *et al.* (1976). Non-Hodgkin's lymphoma stage III: is total lymphoid irradiation appropriate treatment? *Cancer*, **37**:2806–12.

Glick JH, *et al.* (1981). Nodular mixed lymphoma: results of a randomized trial failing to confirm prolonged disease-free survival with COPP chemotherapy. *Blood*, **58**:920–5.

Gobbi PG, *et al.* (1990). The role of surgery in the multimodal treatment of primary gastric non-Hodgkin's lymphomas. *Cancer*, **65**:2528–36.

Goldie JH, Coldman AJ (1984). The genetic origin of drug resistance in neoplasms: implications for systemic therapy. *Cancer Research*, **44**:3643–8.

Gospodarowicz MK, *et al.* (1987). Patterns of disease in localized extranodal lymphomas. *Journal of Clinical Oncology*, 5:875–80.

Haddy TB, *et al.* (1988). Bone involvement in young patients with non-Hodgkin's lymphoma: efficacy of chemotherapy without local radiotherapy. *Blood*, **72**:1141–7.

Haioun C, *et al.* (1992). Autologous bone marrow transplantation vs sequential chemotherapy in first complete remission aggressive lymphoma: an interim analysis. *Proceedings of the American Society of Clinical Oncology*, **11**:316.

Hallahan DE, *et al.* (1988). Combined modality therapy for tumor stage mycosis fungoides: results of a 10-year follow-up. *Journal of Clinical Oncology*, 6:1177–83.

Haynes BF, *et al.* (1981). Phenotypic characterization of cutaneous T-cell lymphoma. *New England Journal of Medicine*, **304**:1319–23.

Hochster HS, *et al.* (1992). Activity of Fludarabine in previously treated non-Hodgkin's low-grade lymphoma: results of an ECOG study. *Journal of Clinical Oncology*, **10**:28–32.

Honegger HP, Cavalli F (1984). Current status and perspectives in the treatment of non-Hodgkin's lymphomas. *European Journal of Cancer and Clinical Oncology*, **20**:305–14.

Hoppe RT, *et al.* (1987). Mycosis fungoides: management with topical nitrogen mustard. *Journal of Clinical Oncology*, 5:1796–803.

Horning SJ, Rosenberg SA (1984). Survival, spontaneous regression and histologic transformation in initially untreated non-Hodgkin's lymphomas of low grade. *New England Journal of Medicine*, **311**:1471–5.

Hubbard SM, *et al.* (1982). Histologic progression in non-Hodgkin's lymphoma. *Blood*, **59**:258–64.

Isaacson PG (1988). A proposal for a classification of primary gastrointestinal lymphomas. *Lancet*, 2:1149.

Isaacson PG (1991). Recent advances in the biology of lymphomas. *European Journal of Cancer*, **27**:795–802.

Jacobs C, Hoppe TR (1985). Non Hodgkin's lymphomas of head and neck extranodal sites. *International Journal of Radiation Oncology—Biology—Physics*, **11**:357–64.

Jacobson JO, *et al.* (1988). Mediastinal large cell lymphoma. An uncommon subset of adult lymphoma curable with combined modality therapy. *Cancer*, **62**:1893–8.

Jaffe ES (1984). Pathologic and clinical spectrum of post-thymic T-cell malignancies. *Cancer Investigation*, 2:413–26.

Jaffe ES (1985). Malignant histiocytosis and true histiocytic lymphomas. In *Surgical pathology of lymph nodes and related organs* (ed. ES Jaffe), pp. 381–411. W. B. Saunders, Philadelphia.

Jaffe ES, Bookman MA, Longo DL (1987). Lymphoctyic lymphoma of intermediate differentiation—mantle-zone lymphoma: a distinct subtype of B-cell lymphoma. *Human Pathology*, **18**:877–87.

Jagannath S, *et al.* (1985). Stage IV diffuse large-cell lymphoma: a long-term analysis. *Journal of Clinical Oncology*, 3:39–47.

Jones SE (1990). Enigma of therapy for cutaneous T-cell lymphoma. (Editorial.) *Journal of the National Cancer Institute*, **82**:169–70.

Jones SE, *et al.* (1985). Chemotherapy with cyclophosphamide, doxorubicin, vincristine and prednisolone alone or with levamisole or levamisole plus BC6 for malignant lymphoma. A Southwest Oncology Group Study. *Journal of Clinical Oncology*, 3:1318–24.

Kaminski MS, *et al.* (1986). Factors predicting survival in adults with stage I and II large-cell lymphoma treated with primary radiation therapy. *Annals of Internal Medicine*, **104**:747–56.

Kay AC, *et al.* (1992). 2-Chlorodeoxyadenosine treatment of low-grade lymphomas. *Journal of Clinical Oncology*, **10**:371–7.

Kaye FJ, *et al.* (1989). A randomized trial comparing combination electron-beam radiation and chemotherapy with topical therapy in the initial treatment of mycosis fungoides. *New England Journal of Medicine*, **321**:1784–90.

Kaye S, *et al.* (1987). Three prognostic groups in patients with mycosis fungoides. *Proceedings of the American Society of Clinical Oncology*, **6**:791.

Kuzel TM, *et al.* (1990). Interferon alfa-2a combined with phototherapy in the treatment of cutaneous T-cell lymphoma. *Journal of the National Cancer Institute*, **82**:203–7.

Kwak LW, *et al.* (1990). Prognostic significance of actual dose intensity in diffuse large-cell lymphoma: results of a tree-structured survival analysis. *Journal of Clinical Oncology*, **8**:963–77.

Kwak LW, *et al.* (1991). Similar outcome of treatment of B-cell and T-cell diffused large-cell lymphomas: the Stanford experience. *Journal of Clinical Oncology*, **9**:1426–31.

Lancet (1991). Primary gut lymphomas. (Editorial.) *Lancet*, **337**:1384–5.

Laurence J, *et al.* (1982). Combination chemotherapy of advanced diffuse histocytic lymphoma with the six-drug COP-BLAM regimen. *Annals of Internal Medicine*, **97**:190–5.

Lawrence TS, *et al.* (1988). Retrospective analysis of stage I and II indolent lymphomas at the National Cancer Institute. *International Journal of Radiation Oncology—Biology—Physics*, **14**:417–27.

Levy R, *et al.* (1985). The immunobiology of B-cell lymphoma. Studies with anti-idiotype antibodies. In *Malignant lymphomas and Hodgkin's disease: experimental and therapeutic advances* (ed. F Cavalli, G Bonadonna, and M Rozencweig), pp. 549–56. Martinus Nijhoff, Boston.

Liang RHS, *et al.* (1989). Central nervous system involvement in non-Hodgkin's lymphoma. *European Journal of Cancer and Clinical Oncology*, 25:703–10.

Limpens J, *et al.* (1990). Translocation t(14;18) in benign B-lymphocytes. *Blood*, 76:9.

Lippman SC, *et al.* (1988). Prognostic significance of the immunotype in diffuse large-cell lymphoma: a comparative study of the T-cell and B-cell phenotype. *Blood*, 72:436–41.

List AF, *et al.* (1988). Non-Hodgkin's lymphoma of the gastrointestinal tract: an analysis of clinical and pathologic features affecting outcome. *Journal of Clinical Oncology*, 6:1125–33.

Lister TA (1991*a*). Sclerosing B-cell lymphoma of the mediastinum: entity or non-entity? *Annals of Oncology*, 2:707–8.

Lister TA (1991*b*). The management of follicular lymphoma. *Annals of Oncology*, 2 (Suppl. 2):131–5.

Lister TA, *et al.* (1989). Report of a committee convened to discuss the evaluation and staging of patients with Hodgkin's disease. *Journal of Clinical Oncology*, 7:1630–6.

Longo DL (1990) Chemotherapy for advanced aggressive lymphoma: more is better . . . Isn't it? *Journal of Clinical Oncology*, 8:952–5.

Longo DL, *et al.* (1984). Prolonged initial remission in patients with nodular mixed lymphoma. *Annals of Internal Medicine*, 100:651–6.

Longo DL, *et al.* (1991). Superiority of ProMACE-CytaBOM over ProMACE-MOPP in the treatment of advanced diffuse aggressive lymphoma: results of a prospective randomized trial. *Journal of Clinical Oncology*, 9:25–38.

McMaster ML, *et al.* (1991). Effective treatment of small-non-cleaved-cell lymphoma with high-intensity, brief-duration chemotherapy. *Journal of Clinical Oncology*, 9:941–6.

Mann RB, Bérar CW (1982). Criteria for the cytologic subclassification of follicular lymphomas: a proposed alternative method. *Hematological Oncology*, 1:187–96.

Maor MH, *et al.* (1990). Stomach conservation in stage I E and II E gastric non-Hodgkin's lymphoma. *Journal of Clinical Oncology*, 8:266–71.

Medeiros LJ, *et al.* (1989). Numbers of host "helper" T cells and proliferating cells predict survival in diffuse small-cell lymphomas. *Journal of Clinical Oncology*, 7:1009–17.

Medeiros LJ, *et al.* (1990). Association of bcl-1 rearrangements with lymphocytic lymphoma of intermediate differentiation. *Blood*, 76:2086–90.

Miller TP, *et al.* (1990). Unfavourable histologies of non-Hodgkin's lymphoma treated with ProMACE-CytaBOM: a groupwide SWOG study. *Journal of Clinical Oncology*, 8:1951–8.

Möller P, *et al.* (1987). Mediastinal lymphoma of clear cell type is a tumor corresponding to terminal steps of B cell differentiation. *Blood*, 69:1087–95.

Morrison WH, *et al.* (1989). Small lymphocytic lymphoma. *Journal of Clinical Oncology*, 7:598–606.

Nyman R, *et al.* (1987). Magnetic resonance imaging, chest radiography, computed tomography and ultrasonography in malignant lymphoma. *Acta Radiologica*, 28:253–62.

O'Connell MJ, *et al.* (1986). Chemotherapy (CT) followed by consolidation radiation therapy (RT) for treatment of stage II non-Hodgkin's lymphoma (NHL). An ECOG combined modality trial. *Proceedings of the American Society of Clinical Oncology*, 191:748.

O'Reilly SE, *et al.* (1991). MACOP-B and VACOP-B in diffuse large-cell lymphomas and MAPP/ABV in non-Hodgkin's disease. *Annals of Oncology*, 2 (Suppl. 1):17–23.

Pan L, *et al.* (1989). The bcl-2 gene in primary B-cell lymphoma of mucosa-associated lymphoid tissue (MALT). *American Journal of Pathology*, 135:7–11.

Pangalis GA, Nathwani BN, Rappaport H (1977). Malignant lymphoma, well differentiated lymphocytic: its relationship with chronic lymphocytic leukemia and macroglobulinemia of Waldenström. *Cancer*, 39:999–1010.

Pedrazzini A, Freedman AS, Nadler IM (1989). Autologous bone-marrow transplantation in non-Hodgkin's lymphomas. *Biochimica et Biophysica Acta*, 989:11–24.

Perrone T, Frizzera G, Rosai J (1986). Mediastinal diffuse large-cell lymphoma with sclerosis. A clinicopathologic study of 60 cases. *American Journal of Surgical Pathology*, 10:176.

Portlock CS, Rosenberg SA. No initial therapy for stage III and IV non-Hodgkin's lymphoma of favorable histologic types. *Annals of Internal Medicine*, 90:10–13.

Press OW, *et al.* (1989). Treatment of refractory non-Hodgkin's lymphoma with radiolabeled MB-1 (anti-CD37) antibody. *Journal of Clinical Oncology*, 7:1027–38.

Price CGA, *et al.* (1991). The significance of circulating cells carrying t(14;18) in long remission from follicular lymphoma. *Journal of Clinical Oncology*, 9:1527–32.

Rappaport H, Thomas LB (1972). Mycosis fungoides: the pathology of extracutaneous involvement. *Cancer*, 34:1198–229.

Rappaport H, Winter WJ, Hicks EB (1956). Follicular lymphoma—a reevaluation of its position in the scheme of malignant lymphoma, based on a survey of 253 cases. *Cancer*, 9:792–821.

Recht L, *et al.* (1988). Central nervous system metastasis from non-Hodgkin lymphomas, treatment and prophylaxis. *American Journal of Medicine*, 84:425–35.

Reznek RH, Richards MA (1987). The radiology of lymphoma. In *Baillière's clinical haematology* (ed. TD McElwain and TA Lister), Vol. 1, pp. 77–107. Baillière Tindall, London.

Richards MA, *et al.* (1986). Detection of spread of malignant lymphoma to the liver by low field strength magnetic resonance imaging. *British Medical Journal*, 293:1126–8.

Richards MA, *et al.* (1989). Lymphoplasmacytoid and small cell centrocytic non-Hodgkin's lymphoma—a retrospective analysis from St Bartholomew's hospital 1972–1986. *Hematological Oncology*, 7:19–35.

Rodriguez MA, *et al.* (1992). MINE-ESHAP, a novel and effective salvage combination for lymphoma. *Proceedings of the American Society of Clinical Oncology*, 11:327.

Rohatiner AZS, *et al.* (1991). Myeloablative therapy with autologous bone marrow transplantation as consolidation of remission in patients with follicular lymphoma. *Annals of Oncology*, 2 (Suppl. 2):147–51.

Romaguera JE, *et al.* (1991). Multivariate analysis of prognostic factors in stage IV follicular low-grade lymphoma: a risk model. *Journal of Clinical Oncology*, 9:762–9.

Rosenberg SA (1985). The low-grade non-Hodgkin's lymphomas: challenges and opportunities. *Journal of Clinical Oncology*, 3:299–310.

Rosenberg SA (1987). Autologous bone marrow transplantation in non-Hodgkin's lymphoma. (Editorial.) *New England Journal of Medicine*, 316:541–2.

Salem P, *et al.* (1985). Immunoproliferative small intestinal disease. In *Malignant lymphomas and Hodgkin's disease: experimental and therapeutic advances* (ed. F Cavalli, G Bonadonna, and M Rozencweig), pp. 269–72. Martinus Nijhoff.

Salles G, *et al.* (1991). Aggressive primary gastrointestinal lymphomas: review of 91 patients treated with the LNH-84 regimen. A study of the Groupe d'étude des lymphomes agressifs. *American Journal of Medicine*, 90:77–84.

Santini G, *et al.* (1991). Autologous bone marrow transplantation for advanced stage adult lymphoblastic lymphoma in first complete remission. *Annals of Oncology*, 2 (Suppl. 2):181–5.

Severson RK, Scott D (1990). Increasing incidence of primary gastric lymphoma. *Cancer*, 66:1283–7.

Shepherd FA, *et al.* (1988). Chemotherapy following surgery for stages IE and IIE non-Hodgkin's lymphoma of the gastrointestinal tract. *Journal of Clinical Oncology*, 6:253–60.

Shields AF, *et al.* (1987). The detection of bone marrow involvement by lymphoma using magnetic resonance imaging. *Journal of Clinical Oncology*, 5:225–30.

Shimoyama M, *et al.* (1988). Major prognostic factors of adult patients with advanced T-cell lymphoma/leukemia. *Journal of Clinical Oncology*, 6:1088–97.

Shipp MA, *et al.* (1989). Patterns of relapse in large-cell lymphoma patients with bulk disease: implications for the use of adjuvant radiotherapy. *Journal of Clinical Oncology*, 7:613–18.

Shipp M, *et al.* (1992). Development of a predictive model for aggressive lymphoma: the international NHL prognostic factors project. *Proceedings of the American Society of Clinical Oncology*, 11:319.

Simon R, *et al.* (1988). The Non-Hodgkin Lymphoma Pathologic Classification Project. Long-term follow-up of 1153 patients with non-Hodgkin lymphomas. *Annals of Internal Medicine*, 109:939–45.

Skarin AT, *et al.* (1983). Improved prognosis of diffuse histiocytic and undifferentiated lymphoma by use of high-dose metotrexate alternating with standard agents (M-BACOD). *Journal of Clinical Oncology*, 1:91–8.

Smith BR, *et al.* (1984). Circulating monoclonal B lymphocytes in non-Hodgkin's lymphoma. *New England Journal of Medicine*, 311:1476–81.

Smith DB, *et al.* (1989). EMOP/CA chemotherapy for the treatment of aggressive non-Hodgkin's lymphomas. *European Journal of Cancer and Clinical Oncology*, 25:991–4.

Spinolo JA, *et al.* (1992). Therapy of relapsed or refractory low-grade follicular lymphomas: factors associated with complete remission, survival and time to treatment failure. *Annals of Oncology*, 3:227–32.

Stansfeld AE, *et al.* (1988). Updated Kiel classification for lymphomas. *Lancet*, 1:292–3, 603.

Stein H, *et al.* (1991). Peripheral T-cell lymphomas. *Annals of Oncology*, 2 (Suppl. 2):163–70.

Strauss DJ, *et al.* (1991). Small-non-cleaved-cell lymphoma in American adults: results with treatment designed for acute lymphoblastic leukaemia. *American Journal of Medicine*, 90:328–37.

Sutcliffe SB, *et al.* (1985). Role of radiation therapy in localized non-Hodgkin's lymphoma. *Radiotherapy and Oncology*, 4:211–23.

Surbone A (1988). Residual abdominal masses in aggressive non-Hodgkin's lymphoma after combination chemotherapy: significance and management. *Journal of Clinical Oncology*, 6:1832–7.

Taal BG, *et al.* (1989). Primary non-Hodgkin's lymphoma of the stomach: changing aspects and therapeutic choices. *European Journal of Cancer and Clinical Oncology*, 25:439–50.

The Non-Hodgkin's Lymphoma Pathologic Classification (1982). Project National Cancer Institute sponsored study of classification of non-Hodgkin's lymphomas. *Cancer*, 49:2347–57.

Tirelli U, *et al.* (1988). Non-Hodgkin's lymphomas in 137 patients aged 70 years or older: a retrospective European Organization for Research and Treatment of Cancer Lymphoma Group Study. *Journal of Clinical Oncology*, 6:1708–13.

Tubiana M, *et al.* (1986). Prognostic factors in non-Hodgkin's lymphoma. *International Journal of Radiation Oncology — Biology — Physics*, 12:503–14.

VanderMolen LA, Swain S, Longo DL (1988). Lactic acidosis in lymphoma: prompt resolution of acidosis with therapy directed at the lymphoma. *Journal of the National Cancer Institute*, 80:1077–8.

Velasquez WS, *et al.* (1988). Effective salvage therapy for lymphoma with cisplatin in combination with high-dose ara-C and dexamethasone (DHAP). *Blood*, 71:117–22.

Velasquez WS, *et al.* (1989). Risk classification as the basis for clinical staging of diffuse large-cell lymphoma derived from 10-year survival data. *Blood*, 74:551–7.

Velasquez W, *et al.* (1992). E-SHAP, an effective treatment for refractory and relapsing lymphoma. A long follow-up. *Proceedings of the American Society of Clinical Oncology*, 11:326.

Veronesi U, *et al.* (1974). The value of staging laparotomy in non-Hodgkin's lymphomas. *Cancer*, 33:446–52.

Vonderheid EC, *et al.* (1977). Topical chemotherapy and immunotherapy of mycosis fungoides: intermediate-term results. *Archives of Dermatology*, 113:454–62.

Vonderheid EC, *et al.* (1985). Diagnostic and prognostic significance of Sezary cells in peripheral blood smears from patients with cutaneous T-cell lymphoma. *Blood*, 66:358–66.

Vose JM, *et al.* (1988). The importance of age in survival of patients treated with chemotherapy for aggressive non-Hodgkin's lymphoma. *Journal of Clinical Oncology*, 6:1838–44.

Weeks JC, *et al.* (1991). Value of follow-up procedures in patients with large-cell lymphoma who achieve a complete remission. *Journal of Clinical Oncology*, 9:1196–203.

Weick JK, *et al.* (1991). Combination chemotherapy of intermediate-grade and high-grade non-Hodgkin's lymphoma with MACOP-B: a SWOG study. *Journal of Clinical Oncology*, 9:748–53.

Weisenburger DD, Kim H, Rappaport H (1982). Mantle-zone lymphoma: a follicular variant of intermediate lymphocytic lymphoma. *Cancer*, 49:1429–38.

Young RC (1989). Mycosis fungoides. The therapeutic search continues. (Editorial.) *New England Journal of Medicine*, 321:1822–3.

12.7.3 Non-Hodgkin's lymphomas in children

IAN MAGRATH

DEFINITIONS

The word 'lymphoma' was first used by Virchow to indicate a tumour arising *de novo* in lymph nodes (Magrath 1990), but, like many terms currently in widespread use, it was coined long before there was any real comprehension of the biology of the tumours we now know by this name. A more modern definition of a lymphoma is a neoplasm which presents as a solid tumour and arises from the cells of the lymphoreticular or immune system. Thus, the group of tumours commonly referred to as the non-Hodgkin's lymphomas nearly always arise from lymphocytes or their precursors. While for many years it was thought that a common form of lymphoma arose from histiocytes (Rappaport's 'diffuse histiocytic lymphoma'), this has been shown more recently to be erroneous, such cells being of lymphoid origin. The histiocytoses and malignant myeloma are not usually included among the lymphomas, a convention arising from earlier concepts (that is, they did not appear to arise in lymph nodes and rarely formed large masses) rather than modern rational taxonomy. However, a small number of solid tumours believed to arise in histiocytes are still referred to as lymphomas (that is, 'true' histiocytic lymphomas, to distinguish them from lymphomas of lymphoid origin that morphologically resemble histiocytes), although in the current biological era it would be logical to consider lymphomas as neoplasms that arise exclusively in the lymphocyte lineage.

Lymphoma versus leukaemia

A much more frequent area of confusion is the dividing line between lymphoma and leukaemia. This arises because the cytology of many of the extramedullary lymphoid tumours of childhood is indistinguishable from that of classical acute lymphoblastic leukaemia cells. At the present time there is no general agreement on this issue, which, although essentially of semantic origin, has implications for therapy since treatment approaches are quite often different for leukaemias and lymphomas. Some (perhaps harping back to the original connotation of the word 'leukemia', again coined by Virchow (Magrath 1990)) consider that leukaemia should only be diagnosed in the presence of neoplastic cells in the peripheral blood. Clearly, such a definition is quite inadequate, since a proportion of patients with otherwise typical leukaemia, including extensive involvement of the bone-marrow, may present without detectable peripheral blood involvement. Others, particularly paediatric oncologists, use an arbitrary numerical definition to distinguish between leukaemia and lymphoma, namely the percentage of blast cells in the bone-marrow aspirate. While different authors have used different criteria, a widely used numerical definition of leukaemia is that more than 25 per cent of the nucleated cells aspirated from a bone-marrow should be blast cells (Murphy 1977). Conversely, patients must have less than 25 per cent of blast cells in an aspirate to fall within the definition of lymphoma. Unfortunately, such a definition leaves much to be desired, since it is subject to both spatial and temporal sampling differences such that, depending on the adequacy or timing of sampling the same patient could be considered to be suffering from either leukaemia or lymphoma.

While the propensity of a given disease to involve the bone-marrow must ultimately arise from the biological characteristics of the component cells (for example, the possession of appropriate cell surface receptors), from a clinical perspective the most important question is whether bone-marrow involvement defines patient groups who, based on empirical experience, ought to receive different treatment regimens. As will become apparent, data available at present suggest that it is the cell type rather than the presence or absence of marrow involvement that should be the primary determinant of therapy.

MAJOR FORMS OF NON-HODGKIN'S LYMPHOMA IN CHILDHOOD

The spectrum of malignant non-Hodgkin's lymphomas in children differs considerably from that in adults. This is probably primarily a consequence of differences between children and adults with regard to the absolute number of lymphoid cells able to serve as targets for the pathogenetic events which result in a specific lymphoid neoplasm (Magrath 1981). Qualitative or quantitative differences in exposure to environmental factors between adults and children may also be relevant. Such factors, for example, could influence the number of target cells. Doubtless, the latent period required between the transformational event and the clinical manifestation of a particular tumour type also influences the earliest age of occurrence of a given tumour.

Based on the predominant cell types in childhood and adult lymphomas, it has been hypothesized that malignant transformation leading to childhood lymphomas occurs predominantly in lymphocyte precursors (that is, cells undergoing primary or antigen-independent differentiation), whereas malignant transformation leading to adult lymphomas occurs predominantly in cells participating in an immune response (that is, undergoing secondary or antigen-dependent differentiation) (Magrath 1981, 1982).

Lymphocyte precursors make up a higher proportion of lymphoid cells in children (note, for example, the relative size of the thymus) such that neoplasms of such cells are simply numerically more likely to arise in children. However, precursor cells do persist in adults, so that it is not surprising that a small proportion of adult lymphomas are apparently identical, at histological and biological levels, with the predominant childhood lymphomas. In contrast, the diseases which account for the bulk of adult lymphomas, primarily those classified as low grade according to the National Cancer Institute Formulation are essentially unknown in young children and are rare in older children and young adults (National Cancer Institute 1982). This may well be a consequence of the long 'latent period' of such diseases.

Childhood non-Hodgkin's lymphomas fall into three main categories, which have relatively uniform histomorphological, immunophenotypic, cytogenetic, and clinical features. While there is overlap with regard to each of these parameters, when all are taken into account readily discernible clinicopathological entities can be identified (Table 1). In the National Cancer Institute Formulation the three major histological subtypes are designated as small non-cleaved cell lymphomas, lymphoblastic lymphomas, and large cell lymphomas. Although each of these categories can be further subdivided, whether on the basis of histology, immunophenotyping, cytogenetics, or molecular genetics, it remains to be demonstrated that such subdivision has a significant impact upon treatment decisions.

Histopathology

The histological classification of lymphomas, including those that comprise the major childhood lymphomas, can be confusing, since a number of different histological classification schemes are in use (Bennett *et al.* 1974; Dorfman 1975; Lennert *et al.* 1975; Lukes and Collins 1975; Mathé *et al.* 1976; National Cancer Institute 1982). In this chapter, the National Cancer Institute Formulation will be used, but the equivalent terms in several other classification schemes are shown in Table 2. It is necessary to be aware that the same term may be used in different classification schemes in quite different ways. For example, the term lymphoblastic lymphoma in the Kiel (Lennert *et al.* 1975) and British Lymphoma (Bennett *et al.* 1974) classification schemes includes small non-cleaved lymphomas, whereas such lymphomas are considered as quite separate from the lymphoblastic lymphomas in other classification schemes.

The majority of the non-Hodgkin's lymphomas of childhood are diffuse lymphomas of high grade (in the nomenclature of the National Cancer Institute Formulation), although some large cell lymphomas (large non-cleaved or large cleaved), particularly those occurring in adolescents and young adults, may conform to the histological definition of intermediate grade. Such lymphomas are relatively uncommon in children, accounting for approximately half

Table 1 Predominant characteristics of the three major categories of childhood non-Hodgkin's lymphoma

Histology (formulation)	Immunophenotype	Most frequent disease sites	Primary marrow involvement[a]
Small non-cleaved cell	B (SIg+,TdT−)	Abdominal	L3 'ALL'
Lymphoblastic	T or Pre-B (SIg−,TdT+)	Mediastinal	L1 or L2 ALL
Large cell	T or B (SIg+ or SIg−, TdT−)	Variable	

ALL, acute lymphoblastic leukaemia.
[a]Alternative designation. Frequently the diagnosis of leukaemia as opposed to lymphoma is made when there are greater than 25 per cent of blast cells in the bone-marrow.

Table 2 Comparison of terminology in different classification schemes

Classification scheme	Indistinguishable from ALL	Indistinguishable or similar to BL	Large lymphoid cells[a]
Rappaport	Lymphoblastic lymphoma (convoluted or non-convoluted)	Undifferentiated lymphoma, Burkitt or non-Burkitt	Histiocytic lymphoma
Lukes and Collins	ML of convoluted lymphocytes (T-cell)	ML of small non-cleaved follicle centre cells (T- or B-cell)	ML of large follicle centre cells Immunoblastic sarcoma Histiocytic
Kiel	ML lymphoblastic, convoluted, and unclassified types	ML lymphoblastic, Burkitt type	ML centroblastic ML immunoblastic
British National Lymphoma	Lymphocytic poorly differentiated (lymphoblast); convoluted cell, mediastinal lymphoma	Lymphocytic poorly differentiated (lymphoblast); Burkitt's tumours, non-Burkitt's tumours	Undifferentiated large cell (large lymphoid cell) Histiocytic cell (mononuclear phagocytic cell)
World Health Organization	Diffuse lymphosarcoma, lymphoblastic	Diffuse lymphosarcoma, Burkitt's tumour	Diffuse lymphosarcoma, immunoblastic Reticulosarcoma
Working formulation	ML lymphoblastic convoluted and non-convoluted	ML small non-cleaved cell	ML large cells ML immunooblastic

ALL, acute lymphoblastic leukaemia; BL, Burkitt's lymphoma; ML, malignant lymphoma.
[a]Includes a recently defined entity, not included in any of the classification schemes: anaplastic large-cell (CD30+) lymphomas.

the large-cell lymphomas, with the other half being immunoblastic or anaplastic large-cell lymphomas.

Lymphoma cells tend to efface the architecture of lymphoid tissue, although when there is partial involvement of a lymph node or lymphoid organ there may be preservation of the normal architecture, including the presence of germinal follicles in some areas. The cells of lymphoblastic lymphoma tend to 'stream' into the medulla and uninvolved portions of the lymph node, as do the lymphoblasts of classical acute lymphoblastic leukaemia. In non-lymphoid tissue, the neoplastic cells usually infiltrate between the normal cells, collagen, or muscle fibres of involved tissues, but appear to do little damage to them so that full recovery of function of the normal tissue is the rule if complete remission can be achieved.

Small non-cleaved cell lymphomas can be divided into Burkitt's and non-Burkitt's variants. The former is indistinguishable from African Burkitt's lymphoma, while the latter is more pleomorphic and/or more of the cells contain a single large nucleolus. In childhood, there are no known clinical, immunophenotypic, karyotypic, or molecular features which correspond to this histological subdivision, which is often difficult to make reproducibly (Grogan *et al.* 1982; Wilson *et al.* 1987). In adults more than 40 years old, however, a proportion of small non-cleaved cell lymphomas, as many as 50 per cent, bear 14;18 translocations (Blood 1987), as do the majority of follicular lymphomas. In this circumstance, the small non-cleaved cell lymphoma could represent malignant progression of a low-grade lymphoma, possibly clinically undetected prior to the progression. Indeed, the transformation of follicular lymphomas into undifferentiated 'Burkitt-like' lymphomas, frequently containing the chromosomal translocations normally observed in small non-cleaved cell (Burkitt's) lymphomas as well as 14;18 translocations, has been reported (Pegoraro *et al.* 1984; Aventin *et al.* 1990).

Small non-cleaved lymphoma cells (Fig. 1) have a high nuclear to cytoplasmic ratio, although in cytological preparations not quite as high as in lymphoblastic lymphomas. The nucleus is round or oval and has an 'open' nuclear chromatin pattern (that is, giving the appearance of being able to see through the network of chromatin), a feature which contrasts with the appearance of the chromatin in lymphoblastic lymphomas. There are multiple (usually

two to five) readily discernible nucleoli. Occasional cells may have only a single central nucleolus, but if such cells are frequent, many pathologists would diagnose small non-cleaved cell lymphoma of non-Burkitt's type. The rim of cytoplasm is very basophilic (staining intensely with methyl green pyronine) because of the high RNA content and usually contains lipid vacuoles (which stain with lipid stains such as oil red O). The cells are frequently interspersed with macrophages (so-called 'tingible body macrophages') in which nuclear debris is discernible and which give rise to the frequently quoted 'starry sky' appearance. This pattern is not pathognomonic and may be seen in any rapidly proliferating tumour.

Lymphoblastic lymphomas are indistinguishable histologically and cytologically from the lymphoblasts of acute lymphoblastic leukaemia (Fig. 2). The cells are usually quite uniform in appearance, with a high nuclear to cytoplasmic ratio, frequently even higher than that of the small non-cleaved cell lymphomas, although there is variation in the quantity of cytoplasm from one tumour to another (similar to the L1 and L2 designations of acute lymphoblastic leukaemia). A variable percentage of the cells may contain irregularly shaped or linear patterned nuclei, a result of nuclear convolutions (the linear patterns are sometimes likened to the imprint of a crow's foot). These nuclear convolutions are not present in all cells or even in all lymphoblastic lymphomas, but they impressed Lukes and Collins (1975) sufficiently to lead to their term of 'convoluted T-cell lymphoma'. The nuclear chromatin is finely stippled (often referred to as 'dusty') and although multiple nucleoli are present, they are difficult to discern.

The distinction between lymphoblastic lymphoma and acute lymphoblastic leukaemia depends entirely upon whether or not the bone-marrow is involved and most paediatric oncologists still use the arbitrary distinction already referred to, in which patients in whom more than 25 per cent of the nucleated cells in the bone-marrow are blasts are said to have acute lymphoblastic leukaemia rather than lymphoblastic lymphoma.

Large-cell lymphomas have a significantly greater quantity of cytoplasm than either the small non-cleaved cell lymphomas or lymphoblastic lymphomas and represent a heterogeneous mixture of tumours at both the histological and the biological level. The cytoplasm may vary in appearance from deeply basophilic to amphophilic or even eosinophilic and the cells may have a significant

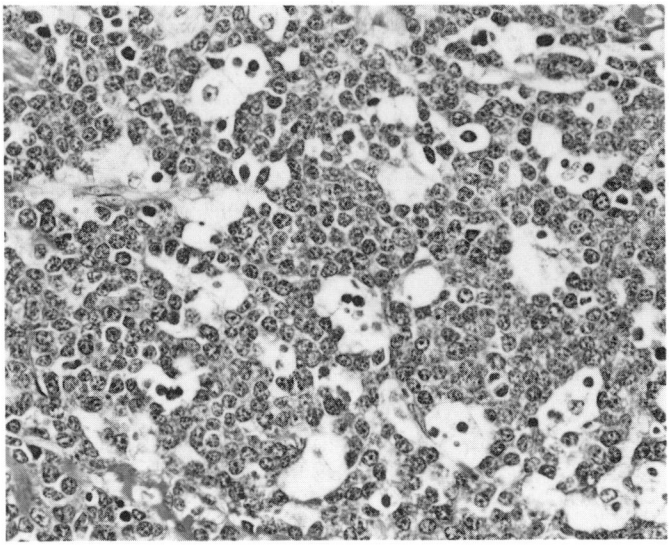

(a)

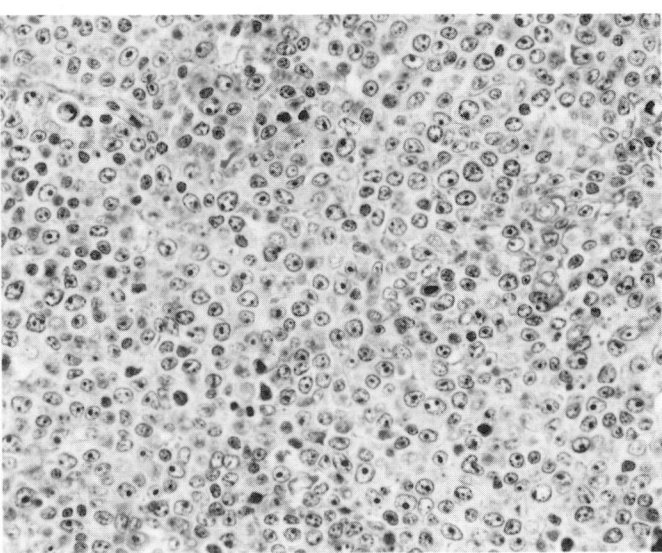

(b)

Fig. 1 Histological appearance of small non-cleaved (undifferentiated) lymphomas: (a) Burkitt's lymphoma; (b) non-Burkitt's lymphoma. The latter tumour was not diagnosed as Burkitt's lymphoma largely because of the frequent single large nucleoli. (Courtesy of Dr J. Cossman.)

degree of polymorphism. In a recent study carried out by the Pediatric Oncology Group in the United States (Nathwani *et al.* 1987) large cell lymphomas were classified according to both the National Cancer Institute Formulation (National Cancer Institute 1982) and the Lukes and Collins (1975) classification. Two major categories emerged from this analysis: large cleaved cell or non-cleaved cell lymphomas (referring to the presence of a nuclear cleft perceptible on light microscopy) (Fig. 3), which probably arise from cells in the germinal centres of secondary lymphoid follicles and are therefore of B-cell origin and immunoblastic lymphomas. The latter, which accounted for 40 of the 72 tumours studied (56 per cent), were further subdivided into plasmacytoid, clear cell, and polymorphous types. The plasmacytoid type corresponds to Lukes

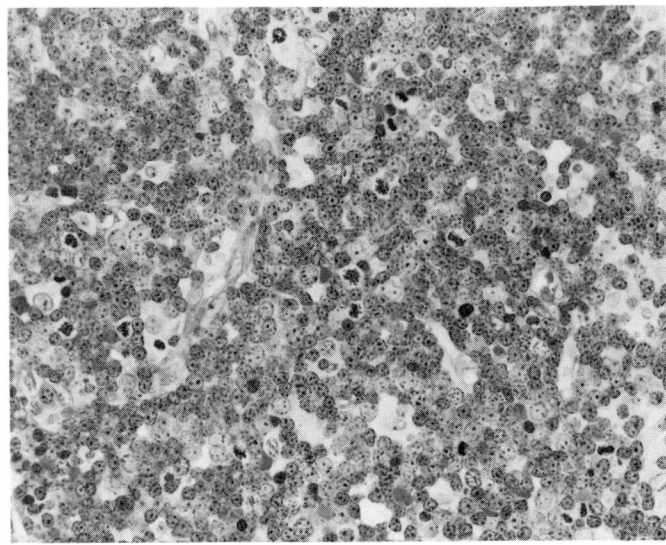

Fig. 2 Histological appearance of a lymphoblastic lymphoma. (Courtesy of Dr J. Cossman.)

and Collins' immunoblastic lymphoma of B-cell origin, while the other types appear to correspond to immunoblastic lymphoma of T-cell origin (Kadin *et al.* 1986) (Fig. 3). Occasionally the polymorphous appearance leads to a diagnosis of mixed cell lymphoma. Recently, a proportion of immunoblastic lymphomas have been recognized as expressing the Ki-1 (CD30) antigen on their surface (see below) and have been dubbed 'anaplastic large cell lymphomas' (Kaudewitz *et al.* 1989). These probably account for a majority of the clear cell and polymorphous types described in the Pediatric Oncology Group study.

A small and rather uncertain number of large cell tumours are probably of true histiocytic or tissue macrophage origin (van der Valk *et al.* 1984; Roholl *et al.* 1988) and the differentiation of such tumours from the histiocytoses becomes arbitrary and based more on semantics than biology. Tumours of true histiocytic origin are composed of cells with large nuclei and abundant dark blue cytoplasm and can be differentiated from lymphoid tumours by the

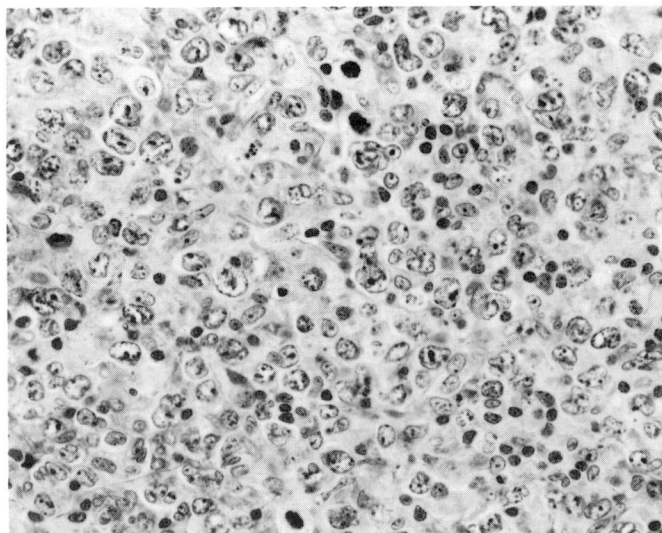

Fig. 3 Histological appearance of diffuse large-cell lymphomas. (Courtesy of Dr J. Cossman and Dr M. Kadin.)

presence of tumour cell erythrophagocytosis and diffuse cytoplasmic staining for non-specific esterases (Fig. 3). Staining for α-naphthyl acetate or butyrate esterases or the use, where available, of isoelectric focusing, which can distinguish monocyte/histiocyte esterases from those of other cell types, are currently the best available means of identifying tumours of true histiocytic origin (Koh *et al.* 1980; Thomas *et al.* 1984; van der Valk *et al.* 1984). Recently, however, several monoclonal antibodies, which may prove to be of value in defining cells of histiocytic origin, have been described (Roholl *et al.* 1988).

Lymphomas occurring in patients with immunodeficiency syndromes are usually classified as large-cell or immunoblastic lymphomas, but are frequently pleomorphic and may resemble small non-cleaved cell lymphomas or express marked lymphoplasmacytoid differentiation (Cotelingam *et al.* 1985; Magrath and Kadin 1990). Difficulty may be encountered in deciding when a neoplasm has arisen, since many such patients have preceding lymphadenopathy which may fluctuate in degree. Usually, however, the clinical setting is sufficient to alert the oncologist to the possibility of the development of a potentially fatal lymphoproliferative syndrome or true lymphoma.

Assignment of a tumour to one of the three major histological categories of non-Hodgkin's lymphoma is sufficient to permit the choice of an appropriate treatment regimen at the present time, but these categories are not homogeneous even when morphology alone is used as the discriminant. Each category can be subdivided on the basis of morphology (particularly small non-cleaved cell and large cell), immunophenotype, or genotype (particularly lymphoblastic and large cell). The differentiation of subtypes of small non-cleaved cell lymphoma on the basis of differences in the break-points of the chromosomes involved in the non-random chromosomal translocations associated with these tumours has also been reported (Pellici *et al.* 1986*b*; Neri *et al.* 1988; Shiramizu *et al.* 1991; Gutiérrez *et al.* 1992). These subdivisions are discussed below.

Histomorphology is largely a subjective discipline and consequently, when used as the only diagnostic modality, entails the acceptance of an inherent imprecision with regard to the delineation of the border between one lymphoid neoplasm and another (Wilson *et al.* 1984) and indeed a precise border may not exist (Sigaux *et al.* 1984). This problem is increased dramatically when the preparation of the biopsy sample is less than optimal, for example when there is crush artefact or inadequate fixation. Occasionally, there may even be difficulty in determining that a given neoplasm is a lymphoma, although differentiation, by a skilled pathologist, from non-lymphoid tumours is not usually difficult with well-prepared tissue sections. The tumours most likely to be confused with lymphomas are often referred to as 'small blue round cell tumours'. These include Ewing's sarcoma, peripheral neuroectodermal tumours, neuroblastoma, and rhabdomyosarcoma, particularly of the more undifferentiated kind. Anaplastic large-cell lymphomas which express the Ki-1 (CD30) antigen were, until the recent recognition of this tumour, quite frequently confused with anaplastic carcinomas or amelanotic melanomas (Kaudewitz *et al.* 1989; Magrath and Kadin 1990) and may provide a particular challenge to the pathologist.

Perhaps the most reproducible histological distinction among the childhood lymphomas is that between lymphoblastic lymphoma and all other non-Hodgkin's lymphomas, often collectively referred to as non-lymphoblastic lymphomas and often assumed, for the purposes of treatment, to consist entirely of lymphomas of B-cell origin. 'B-cell lymphoma' in paediatric oncology is therefore usually

considered to be synonymous with 'non-lymphoblastic lymphoma'. This distinction corresponds to differences in the expression of terminal deoxyribonucleotide transferose (TdT) and differences in clinical behaviour and, although simplistic from a biological perspective, it is perfectly adequate to determine optimal treatment with the treatment protocols used at present. On occasion, difficulty may arise in distinguishing between subcategories of small non-cleaved lymphomas (Burkitt's and non-Burkitt's) and between small non-cleaved cell and large-cell lymphomas, quite probably because there is no precise demarcation between them (Sigaux *et al.* 1984; Wilson *et al.* 1987). This is consistent with the observation that a proportion of large-cell lymphomas bear the same chromosomal translocations as the small non-cleaved cell lymphomas and are clearly similar, or identical, at a pathogenetic level. HIV-associated lymphomas in children appear to be particularly heterogeneous, and although small non-cleaved and immunoblastic histologies are recognized, variant histomorphological forms are common and histologic type and genotype are not always consistent. There are no histological correlates of the different immunophenotypic variants of lymphoblastic lymphoma or of lymphoblastic lymphoma versus acute lymphoblastic leukaemia.

Suspicion that the tumour may not be a non-Hodgkin's lymphoma should be raised whenever the pathologist is unable to classify the tumour further into one of the major histological types described, but even in the hands of the most skilled haematopathologist a small percentage of non-Hodgkin's lymphomas may not be further classifiable. Tumours occurring in immunodeficient hosts may give particular difficulties in this regard.

CELLULAR ORIGINS: IMMUNOPHENOTYPE AND IMMUNOGENOTYPE

The B-cell lymphomas of childhood include the histological categories of small non-cleaved cell lymphoma, which are exclusively of B-cell phenotype and a proportion of the large cell lymphomas (perhaps half) (Table 3). Large-cell lymphomas are heterogeneous with regard to immunophenotype as well as histology. While some are closely related to the small non-cleaved cell lymphomas, others are almost certainly the neoplastic counterparts of activated lymphocytes. The major categories are (a) those which arise from lymphoid germinal follicle centre cells and are therefore invariably of B-cell origin (Jaffe and Cossman 1985); the large cleaved and non-cleaved lymphomas and somewhat more mature immunoblastic lymphomas and (b) those that arise from perifollicular activated lymphocytes; the anaplastic Ki-1 (CD30) positive lymphomas (Stein *et al.* 1985). The latter are of either T (more commonly) or B phenotype.

The lymphoblastic lymphomas are generally of T-cell origin, but a small proportion have the same immunophenotype as pre-B acute lymphoblastic leukaemia (Table 3).

Table 3 Correspondence between histology and immunophenotype

Histology	Phenotype
Lymphoblastic	Immature T-cell (thymocyte)
	Precursor B-cell
Small non-cleaved	B-cell
Large cell	
Large follicle centre cell	B-cell
Immunoblastic	B-cell or T-cell
Anaplastic large cell	T-cell, B-cell, null cell

The lineage of lymphoid neoplasms is determined by the examination of immunophenotype by means of monoclonal antibodies (now usually referred to in terms of the cluster of differentiation (CD) group to which they have been assigned), which react with lineage-specific or lineage-associated antigens expressed at the cell surface or in the cytoplasm and/or genotype, in which there is rearrangement, and sometimes expression of the antigen receptor genes (immunoglobulin heavy and light chains, T-cell receptor delta, gamma, alpha, and beta genes) (Croce et al. 1985; Le Beau et al. 1985; Murre et al. 1985). Rearrangement refers to an alteration in the size of a specific restriction fragment brought about by an alteration of the germ-line structure of the antigen receptor loci. This occurs because the variable and constant regions of these molecules are separated in the genome and must be juxtaposed during lymphocyte differentiation in order to produce a functional gene (Alt et al. 1986). The process of assembly, or genetic recombination, results in the generation of antigen receptor diversity and since each cell contains a unique rearrangement the determination of the presence and size of a rearranged restriction fragment by Southern blotting provides a clonal marker of the neoplasm which may be of value in diagnosis or follow-up (Kneba et al. 1986; Minden and Mak 1986; Williams et al. 1987; Sigaux 1988). The antigen receptor genes rearrange in an ordered sequence during normal differentiation: mu, kappa, and lambda for immunoglobulin genes (Korsmeyer et al. 1981) and delta, gamma, beta, and alpha for T-cell receptor genes (Siu et al. 1984; Royer et al. 1985; Haars et al. 1986; Chien et al. 1987a,b). The development of the polymerase chain reaction, a technique permitting the amplification of a fragment of DNA specified by 3' and 5' primer oligodeoxynucleotides, has enormously increased the sensitivity of detection of a specific genetic rearrangement such as that which occurs during antigen receptor gene assembly.

Small non-cleaved cell lymphomas

The small non-cleaved cell lymphomas probably arise as a consequence of malignant transformation of cells of the B-cell lineage which are undergoing rearrangement of their immunoglobulin genes (Magrath 1985, 1990; Magrath et al. 1992). Thus, the B-cell lymphomas of childhood express surface immunoglobulin, almost exclusively of the IgM class associated with either kappa or lambda light chain, and B-cell-specific antigens including CD19 and CD20, as well as non-lineage-specific antigens such as CD24 (Benjamin et al. 1982; Foon and Todd 1986; Sondlund et al. 1986; Young et al. 1986; Magrath et al. 1992). Some of these tumours also express a protein, CD21 (or CR2), which can bind both a complement subcomponent (Col 3) and Epstein–Barr virus, these sites being detected by the monoclonal antibodies B2 and HB5, respectively (Magrath et al. 1980). HLA-DR antigens are also invariably present (Avila et al. 1987) and since the cells express surface immunoglobulin and therefore, by definition, are true B-cells that have completed their immunoglobulin rearrangements, they do not contain the enzyme TdT (Braziel et al. 1983). TdT is an enzyme which is present in cells undergoing antigen receptor gene rearrangements (Desiderio et al. 1984; Kunkel et al. 1986). The lack of TdT provides an objective correlate of the histological distinction of small non-cleaved cell lymphomas from lymphoblastic lymphomas (of both pre-B and T immunophenotypes), which are nearly always TdT positive (see below).

Small non-cleaved cell lymphomas nearly always express the common acute lymphoblastic leukaemia antigen, CD10, which is present on the surface of both precursor B-cells and a fraction of the more mature follicle centre cells. There are no reported phenotypic differences at the level of cell surface markers between large cell lymphomas of B-cell type and small non-cleaved cell lymphomas, although it is likely that this is simply a consequence of the lack of sufficiently detailed studies. Differences at a phenotypic level, however, have been described between equatorial (endemic) and North American (sporadic) small non-cleaved cell (Burkitt's) lymphomas. Sporadic tumours, for example, secrete IgM (often detectable as a serum monoclonal band on protein electrophoresis (Magrath et al. 1980)), whereas endemic tumours appear not to (Magrath et al. 1983). A number of differences have been described between cell lines derived from endemic and sporadic tumours. For example, there seems to be a reciprocal relationship between reactivity with the antibody CD23 (Tü1), which is present on mantle zone cells and CD10. Cell lines derived from endemic tumours express more CD23 and less CD10 antigen than sporadic tumours, which usually lack detectable CD23 expression but nearly always express CD10 antigen (Favrot et al. 1984).

While these differences in the phenotypes of cell lines suggest that the immunophenotype of endemic tumours differs from that of sporadic tumours, recent work has indicated that the phenotype of endemic cell lines often undergoes a change shortly after explantation. The cell lines tend to lose CD10 expression and begin to express a number of activation antigens at the cell surface, including CD23, Ki-67, and leucocyte adhesion molecules. Such changes are associated with the onset of the expression of several of the Epstein–Barr virus latent genes (EBNAs 2–6) and appear to be induced by these genes (Rowe et al. 1986, 1987). Thus, it is possible that the tumour cells in vivo differ little between endemic and sporadic tumours, but that the differences observed in the cell lines (that is, in explanted tumour cells), are caused by the difference in Epstein–Barr virus association. These differences in EBV association, however, suggest that the endemic and sporadic varieties of the small non-cleaved cell lymphomas may have different cellular origins or pathogenesis, or both, a suggestion that is supported by differences in the precise locations of the break-points in the chromosomes involved in the specific translocations associated with these tumours (Pellici et al. 1986b; Neri et al. 1988; Shiramizu 1990; Gutiérrez et al. 1992). This topic is discussed further below.

The protein detected by the monoclonal antibodies T1 and leu 1 (CD5), which is expressed by most T-cells but only by a subclass of B-cells (those which give rise to chronic lymphocytic leukaemia and lymphomas derived from B follicular mantle zone cells) (Casali et al. 1987; Cohen and Jaffe 1990), is not expressed on B-cell lymphomas of children (Cohen and Jaffe 1990). All small non-cleaved cell lymphomas have clonally rearranged immunoglobulin genes at both heavy and light chain loci, although one of the rearrangements is a consequence of the chromosomal translocation rather than the physiological rearrangement of an immunoglobulin gene. This provides a marker of the malignant clone, which could be exploited in the detection of minimal disease following treatment. These tumours, unlike the precursor B leukaemias of childhood, never have rearranged T-cell receptor genes.

Lymphoblastic lymphomas

Lymphoblastic lymphoma, in addition to its distinctive histology, differs from all other lymphomas by virtue of the almost invariable presence of the enzyme TdT (Braziel et al. 1983). Only a small percentage (some 5 per cent) of lymphoblastic lymphomas of the most mature stage of thymic differentiation fail to express this enzyme (Grogan *et al.* 1986; Morabito *et al.* 1987). TdT participates in the generation of diversity in antigen receptor genes of both T- and B-cells by catalysing the insertion of random nucleotides (N regions) into some of the component polypeptide chains of the antigen receptor molecule during the process of receptor gene rearrangements (Desiderio *et al.* 1984; Kunkel *et al.* 1986). Therefore, its presence indicates that the cell type is immature and is close to the point in the differentiation pathway at which antigen receptor genes are rearranged. This may be of importance in understanding the pathogenesis of the childhood lymphoid neoplasms, since many of them are associated with chromosomal translocations which may be mediated by the same enzymes that are responsible for the physiological recombination of variable- and constant-region gene segments of antigen receptor molecules (Finger *et al.* 1986; Haluska *et al.* 1986). Differentiation beyond this stage and loss of TdT may occur in some neoplasms after the translocation has occurred.

The majority of lymphoblastic lymphomas arise from T-cell precursors undergoing differentiation in the thymus (Magrath 1982; Foon and Todd 1986; Sandlund and Magrath 1990) and, thus, express T-cell markers whose patterns correspond to those observed on T-cells undergoing intrathymic differentiation, the major stages of which are usually designated as early, intermediate, and late (Fig. 4) (Reinherz and Schlossman 1980; Reinherz *et al.* 1980; Casten *et al.* 1985; Blue and Schlossman 1986). The glycoprotein gp 40, recognized by the monoclonal antibodies 4H9, 3A1, or WT1 (CD7) (Haynes 1981*a,b*; Link *et al.* 1983*b*; Vodinelich *et al.* 1983) is a particularly valuable marker of the early T-cell lineage and although this antigen is absent from some more mature T-cell neoplasms, it is present on essentially all immature T-cell malignancies; that is, lymphoblastic lymphomas and leukaemias of T-cell type. Additional antigens expressed at the surface of T-cell lymphoblastic lymphomas predominantly reflect an intermediate (CD7, CD5, CD2, CD1, CD4, and CD8) or late (CD7, CD2, CD3, and either CD4 or CD8) thymocyte phenotype, although atypical patterns are quite frequently observed (Bernard *et al.* 1981; Bernard

and Boumsell 1982; Roper *et al.* 1983). CD2, the protein responsible for the binding of sheep erythrocytes by T-cells, is usually present on lymphoblastic lymphoma cells although it may not be expressed by the earliest cells of the T lineage (usually referred to as pre-T-cells). However, such cells frequently express common acute lymphoblastic leukaemia antigen (CD10) and HLA-DR antigen (Thiel *et al.* 1989), although these antigens are not commonly detected on lymphoblastic lymphomas. CD3, a heterodimer which is expressed in concert with the antigen receptor itself to form the antigen receptor complex (Meuer *et al.* 1983; Hood and Hunkapillar 1985), may be present in the cytoplasm of immature T-cells, even though it is not expressed at the surface (van Dongen *et al.* 1988; Janossy *et al.* 1989). This is of practical importance in determining the differentiation status of a T-cell tumour, since whether or not CD3 antigen expression is considered to be consistent with a more or less mature phenotype depends upon whether the technique used to detect it was directed towards surface or cytoplasmic antigens. CD1 is an antigen which is only expressed on intermediate thymocytes, while CD4 and CD8 are expressed on the same cell in intermediate thymocytes but are expressed separately on more mature cells of helper and suppressor (or cytotoxic) phenotypes, respectively. All the antigen receptor molecules are present in the cytoplasm prior to expression at the cell surface in concert with the CD3 protein (Royer *et al.* 1984, 1985; Bertness *et al.* 1985; Haars *et al.* 1986; Dyer 1989; Falini *et al.* 1989).

In Europe and the United States a significantly higher proportion of T-cell acute lymphoblastic leukaemias than lymphoblastic lymphomas express early thymocyte markers and usually lack surface CD1, CD3, CD8, and CD4 (Reinherz *et al.* 1979; Bernard *et al.* 1981; Roper *et al.* 1983; Thiel *et al.* 1989). In one series, for example, the proportions of early, intermediate, and late thymocyte phenotypes in T-cell acute leukaemia were 34, 43, and 23 per cent, respectively, whereas the proportions in lymphoblastic lymphoma were 6, 62, and 32 per cent (Crist *et al.* 1988). The proportion of the most immature neoplasms was almost certainly underestimated in this series because only E-rosette positive cases were included,

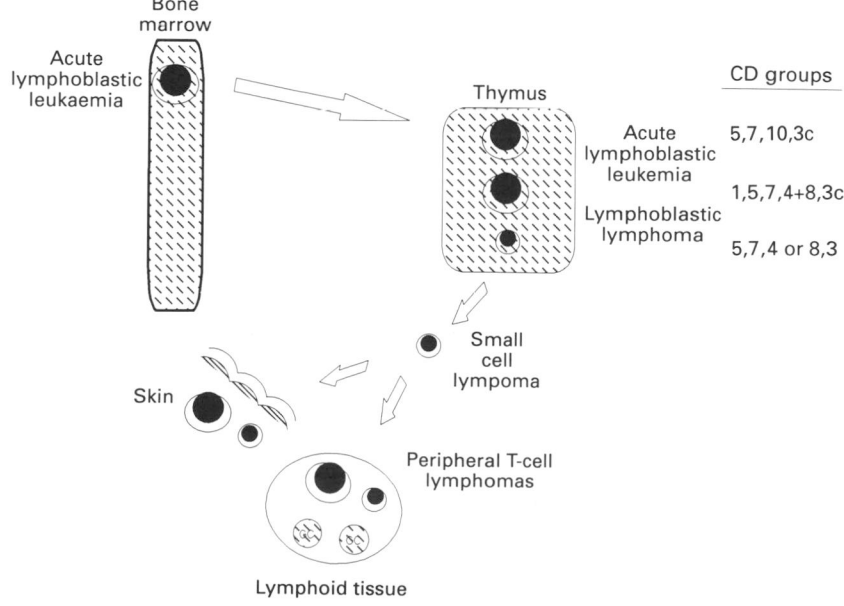

Fig. 4 Differentiation pathway of T-cells. Pre-T-cells originate from stem cells in the bone-marrow and migrate to the thymus where they undergo differentiation prior to migrating to secondary lymphoid organs as mature T-cells. The expression of surface antigens (CD groups) in the three levels of intrathymic differentiation are shown, as are the T-cell differentiation compartments which correspond to the predominant immunophenotypes of T-cell acute lymphoblastic leukemia and T-cell lymphoblastic lymphoma.

yet it is well accepted that in a proportion of T-cell cases, usually referred to as pre-T-cell disease, the cells do not form E rosettes and usually fail to express the CD2 antigen.

It cannot be assumed that the pattern of expression of thymocyte differentiation antigens on T-lineage lymphoblastic neoplasms will be similar throughout the world. Recently, for example, in a series of T-cell acute lymphoblastic leukaemias from Egypt (where the proportion of T-cell leukaemias in children was approximately 50 per cent (Kamel et al. 1989)), the phenotype was predominantly that of intermediate (58.1 per cent) or late (16.1 per cent) thymocytes (Kamel et al. 1990). Thus, the presence of bone-marrow involvement is probably a poor discriminant between early- and late-stage T-cell lymphoblastic neoplasms, although there is little doubt that pre-T neoplasms more often present as leukaemia. Further, as would be expected, the likelihood of a mediastinal mass is greatest in the intermediate group and least in the most mature and immature groups (Crist et al. 1988; Thiel et al. 1989).

T-cell lymphoblastic lymphomas have clonal rearrangements of their T-cell receptor genes which correlate with their degree of differentiation. Examination of T-cell acute lymphoblastic leukaemia or lymphoblastic lymphoma has shown that the most immature neoplasms (pre-T) usually have a clonal rearrangement of a T delta gene without rearrangement of other T-cell receptor genes (Asou et al. 1989; Dyer 1989; Yumura et al. 1989). Such tumours sometimes express T delta transcripts. Rarely, in pre-T neoplasms, all the T-cell receptor genes are in the germ-line configuration. T-cell neoplasms of intermediate maturity (cytoplasmic CD3) have rearrangements of T delta, T gamma, and T beta, and some may have biallelic deletion of T delta, which indicates alpha rearrangement since the delta locus lies within the T alpha locus. The more mature lymphoblastic neoplasms (expressing surface CD3 with either CD4 or CD8) have T gamma and T beta rearrangements with biallelic deletion of T delta (Foroni et al. 1987; Ha et al. 1987; Asou et al. 1989; Dyer 1989; Yumura et al. 1989). This pattern is similar to that of the peripheral T-cell lymphomas and is sometimes accompanied by expression of T alpha/beta transcripts (Yumura et al. 1989). In T-cell neoplasms, the second constant gamma region is usually rearranged and the first deleted (80 per cent of cases), but in the remaining 20 per cent of cases the first constant region is rearranged (Knowles 1989). Some 10 per cent of T-cell lymphoblastic neoplasms have rearrangements of immunoglobulin receptor genes (Bertness et al. 1985; Murre et al. 1985; Pellici et al. 1985; Ha et al. 1987; Tkachuk et al. 1988; Dyer 1989; Ito et al. 1989; Kimura and Kikuchi 1989; Kimura et al. 1989).

Infrequently, lymphoblastic lymphomas express the phenotype of precursor B-cells as seen in acute lymphoblastic leukaemia; B4 and HLA-DR, usually with common acute lymphoblastic leukaemia antigen but without surface immunoglobulin (Bernard et al. 1982; Cossman et al. 1983; Link et al. 1983a; Grogan et al. 1986). Such tumours have a rearrangement of at least a heavy chain gene and may, like acute lymphoblastic leukaemia, have a rearrangement of a light chain gene. Of considerable interest is the pattern of rearrangement of T-cell receptor genes in such cases. Rearrangements or deletions of the T delta gene are found in 70–100 per cent and only a slightly lower proportion of rearrangements of T gamma are found. Some 10 per cent have rearrangements of T beta (Bertness et al. 1985; Pellici et al. 1985) and some even have biallelic deletion of T delta, indicating T alpha rearrangement (Ha et al. 1987; Asou et al. 1989; Dyer 1989; Yumura et al. 1989). This could be due to an origin of these neoplasms in an uncommitted precursor cell. However, the lack of T-cell immunological markers in such tumours argues against this and

supports the alternative hypothesis that rearrangement of antigen receptor genes occurs in these tumours because the cell type is one in which the recombinases which catalyse such events remain active for at least some period of time after malignant transformation (Ha et al. 1987; Dyer 1989).

Recently, lymphoblastic lymphoma was described in which the phenotype was that of natural killer cells (Sheibani et al. 1987).

Large-cell lymphomas

The heterogeneous cellular origin of the large-cell lymphomas is reflected in the diversity of immunophenotypes (Lennert et al. 1975; Csako et al. 1982; Foon and Todd 1986; Ferguson et al. 1987; Magrath and Kadin 1990). The large-cell lymphomas of follicular centre cell origin (large cleaved and non-cleaved cell lymphomas) express, as expected, B-cell antigens including CD19, CD20, and CD24 surface immunoglobulin. However, (SIg) may be absent in up to one-third of these tumours (Magrath and Kadin 1990), a finding which is consistent with the observation that a proportion of large rapidly proliferating cells in normal germinal centres cells fails to express SIg (MacLennan et al. 1985; MacLennan and Gray 1986). It has been proposed that the temporary absence of SIg occurs during the process of somatic mutation of immunoglobulin gene variable regions. Mutated immunoglobulins are subsequently expressed on the cell surface and cells bearing immunoglobulins with the highest affinity for antigen are selected by virtue of the greater likelihood that they will bind and be activated by antigen (MacLennan and Gray 1986). If this sequence of events is correct, large cell lymphomas of this type may have a particular propensity to mutate their V-region genes, a characteristic which should be definable. In any event, it appears highly probable that lymphomas with the characteristics of large follicle centre cells are the neoplastic counterpart of antigen-stimulated B lymphocytes. In children, lymphomas with a true follicular pattern are extremely rare (a very small number have been described in older teenagers and young adults) (Frizzera and Murphy 1979) and large cell lymphomas arising in germinal follicles appear to do so de novo rather than in a follicular lymphoma undergoing histological transformation, a mechanism which occurs quite frequently in adults.

The characteristics of B-cell immunoblastic lymphomas have not been well defined, but some, at least, express more mature antigens, such as CD38 (T10) and PCA-1, that are usually expressed on plasma cells. Such cells may also lose antigens such as CD19, CD20, CD21, and CD24, and even surface immunoglobulin.

Some or all B-cell lymphomas arising in the thymus may originate in a unique B-cell subpopulation that was recently detected in the thymic medulla. Such cells, which have been characterized immunophenotypically, tend to cluster round Hassall's corpuscles and insinuate between epithelial cells (Christensson et al. 1988; Hofmann et al. 1988a,b; Kupper et al. 1989). These cells also stain strongly with antibodies of CD19, CD20, and CD22, and many express surface IgM, but they do not react with antibodies of CD21 and CD35, both of which stain mantle zone and follicle centre cells. To date, thymic B-cell tumours have not been sufficiently characterized to determine whether they are phenotypically similar to thymic B cells.

Some large cell lymphomas, particularly the clear cell and polymorphous immunoblastic types, express T-cell markers, most commonly CD4, CD2, and CD5 and a few express antigens characteristic of monocyte/histiocytes, although α-1-antitrypsin, α-1-antichymotrypsin, and lysozyme are probably not as reliable markers of a histiocytic origin as was originally thought (Magrath and Kadin 1990). Promising new monoclonal antibodies thought to be specific for this lineage have been described, the specificity of which awaits more extensive studies (Roholl *et al.* 1988). It seems likely that ultimately a panel of monoclonal antibodies will be established that are able to discriminate, by virtue of the pattern of reactivity, between different subtypes of large-cell lymphoma.

Recently, a group of large-cell lymphomas reactive with the monoclonal antibody Ki-1 (CD30) has been identified (Stein *et al.* 1985; Agnarsson and Kadin 1988; Kaudewitz *et al.* 1989). Many tumours which would formerly have been classified as malignant histiocytosis, true histiocytic lymphoma, or anaplastic carcinoma have been shown to be large lymphoid cell neoplasms which express CD30. This group of anaplastic large-cell lymphomas encompasses the groups classified morphologically as clear cell or polymorphous immunoblastic lymphoma in the United States.

Lymphomas which express CD30 characteristically involve the paracortical and peripheral sinus regions of the lymph nodes and are believed to arise from large activated lymphoid cells (of both B and T phenotype) which occur immediately adjacent to follicle centres (Stein *et al.* 1985; Kaudewitz *et al.* 1989). It has been suggested that, whereas both virgin B-cells (that is, cells which have not previously encountered antigen) and memory B-cells undergo initial activation by antigen presented by dendritic cells in the perifollicular area, only memory cells (undergoing a second or subsequent cycle of activation) can subsequently enter the germinal follicle under normal circumstances (Lortan *et al.* 1987). Whether CD30 positive lymphomas of B-cell origin arise from cells undergoing primary or secondary immune activation is not clear, but if the above hypothesis is correct CD30 cells can be considered to be the neoplastic counterparts of cells undergoing an earlier phase of activation than those within germinal follicles. It is apparent, however, that the majority (70–80 per cent) of CD30 lymphomas are of T-cell origin and represent antigen-activated T-cells (that is, are peripheral T-cell lymphomas). Such tumours clearly differ from T-cell lymphoblastic lymphoma, a tumour of thymocytes undergoing antigen-independent differentiation (Bernard *et al.* 1981; Feller *et al.* 1986; Grogan *et al.* 1986; Weiss *et al.* 1986; Sheibani *et al.* 1987; Kaneko *et al.* 1989; Sandlund and Magrath 1990). However, as is also the case with CD30 lymphomas of B-cell origin, surface markers clearly identifying the cell lineage are frequently absent in CD30 lymphomas. In such cases, molecular genetics (that is, the demonstration of rearrangements of either immunoglobulin or T-cell receptor genes), may provide the only method of identifying the cell lineage. Those with T-cell phenotype tend to have clonal rearrangements of the T beta receptor, with biallelic deletion of T delta, indicating T alpha rearrangement (Agnarsson and Kadin 1988; Dyer 1989; Magrath and Kadin 1990). Finally, some CD30 lymphomas have a mixed B- and T-cell phenotype, the significance of which is not clear (Magrath and Kadin 1990). It is possible that only one of these components is malignant.

The cellular origins of large-cell lymphomas which do not express T- or B-cell characteristics have not been determined with precision, although some may be of true histiocytic origin (van der Valk *et al.* 1984).

CYTOGENETICS AND MOLECULAR PATHOLOGY

A large body of evidence, collected in recent years, strongly supports the probability that tumorigenesis is the result of genetic changes which occur in specific target cells. In non-Hodgkin's lymphomas a number of non-random cytogenetic abnormalities have been identified and in non-Hodgkin's lymphomas of childhood these are predominantly reciprocal chromosomal translocations (Table 4). A general feature is the presence of an antigen receptor gene, either an immunoglobulin or T-cell receptor gene depending upon the cell lineage, at one of the locations of the two necessary chromosomal break-points. There is good indirect evidence that the translocations are sometimes mediated by the same enzymes which normally mediate the approximation of the variable to constant regions of antigen receptor genes. Such genes are composed of discontinuous elements prior to differentiation and the enzymes required to accomplish the approximation of the components of the complete functional receptor gene, by cutting and religating the DNA strand at appropriate signal sequences, are present in the precursor cells in which such rearrangements normally occur. Clearly, this enzymatic apparatus provides a potential means of effecting chromosomal translocation and provides circumstantial evidence, supported by the observed presence of the required signal sequences close to translocation break-points (Finger *et al.* 1986; Haluska *et al.* 1986; Magrath 1990), that the translocations occur in immature cells. This does not necessarily mean, however, that the predominant neoplastic cell conforms to the phenotype of the cell in which the chromosomal translocation occurred; some degree of differentiation may occur prior to manifestation of the malignant clone as a neoplasm.

The detection of non-random chromosomal translocations in the small non-cleaved cell lymphomas (Zech *et al.* 1976) has been of paramount importance in providing impetus to the development of an understanding of the pathogenesis of these tumours. The molecular characterization of the chromosomal translocations has provided the foundation for the development of a detailed hypothesis to account for the pathogenesis of these tumours and has led to the realization that even within an apparently homogeneous phenotype there may be pathological heterogeneity at a molecular genetic level.

The relevance to the clinician of this new ability to subcategorize at a molecular level remains to be determined, but there is no doubt that molecular abnormalities provide highly specific, even unique, markers of tumour cells. It is possible that particular genetic abnormalities may correlate with prognosis, permitting refinement of therapy for genetically defined subgroups. More immediately exploitable, however, is the new ability to enhance dramatically the sensitivity and specificity of the detection of residual tumour cells (for example, in patients with bone-marrow involvement) made possible by molecular markers. Already, some of the specific chromosomal translocations associated with lymphoid neoplasia can be detected by polymerase chain reactions (Stetlet *et al.* 1988;

Table 4 Correspondence between histology and cytogenetics

Histology	Reported cytogenetic abnormalities
Lymphoblastic	t(8;14)(q24;q11), t(11;14)(p15;q11), t(10;14)(q24;q11), t(1;14), t(9;17), t(7;15)
Small non-cleaved[a]	t(8;14)(q24;q32), t(8;22)(q24;q11) t(2;8)(p13;q24)
Large cell	
Large follicle centre cell Immunoblastic	t(14;18)(q32;q21)
Anaplastic large cell	t(2;5), t(9;14)

[a]Small non-cleaved cell lymphomas in older individuals sometimes possess t(14;18), or t(8;14) as well as t(14;18)

Cunningham *et al.* 1989; Ngan *et al.* 1989; Shiramizu and Magrath 1990), for the fragment of DNA containing the juxtaposition of the involved chromosomes can be enormously amplified by the use of synthetic oligonucleotides complementary to sequences on either side of the chromosomal juxtaposition. This technique permits the detection of minuscule numbers of tumour cells admixed with normal cells and may therefore be used to improve the definition of complete remission or to detect relapse before it is apparent by other methods. Finally, improved understanding of pathogenesis could eventually lead to the development of new approaches to treatment which are directed towards the abnormal biochemistry of the neoplastic cell (Magrath 1989). Indeed, a means of specifically inhibiting the growth of a subset of small non-cleaved cell lymphoma cell lines *in vitro* was recently reported; this method is based upon the use of antisense oligodeoxyribonucleotides directed towards abnormal species of messenger RNA which are present only in the tumour cells and not in normal cells (McManaway *et al.* 1990).

Small non-cleaved cell lymphomas

The small non-cleaved cell lymphomas bear characteristic non-random chromosomal translocations which are predominantly between chromosomes 8 and 14 (some 80 per cent of tumours) (Zech *et al.* 1976) and less often between chromosomes 8 and 2 or 8 and 22 (Bernheim *et al.* 1981) (Fig. 5). The recognition of these translocations led to crucially important insights into the pathogenesis of this disease, since the break-point on chromosome 8 coincides with the location of a proto-oncogene (c-*myc* on band q24) (Dalla-Favera *et al.* 1982; Taub *et al.* 1982), while the break-point on the other partner chromosome is in an immunoglobulin chain locus; either that of the heavy chains (chromosome 14, band q32) or that of one of the light chains (chromosome 22, band q11 or chromosome 2, band p11/p12, the loci of lambda and kappa genes, respectively) (Croce *et al.* 1979; McBride *et al.* 1982;

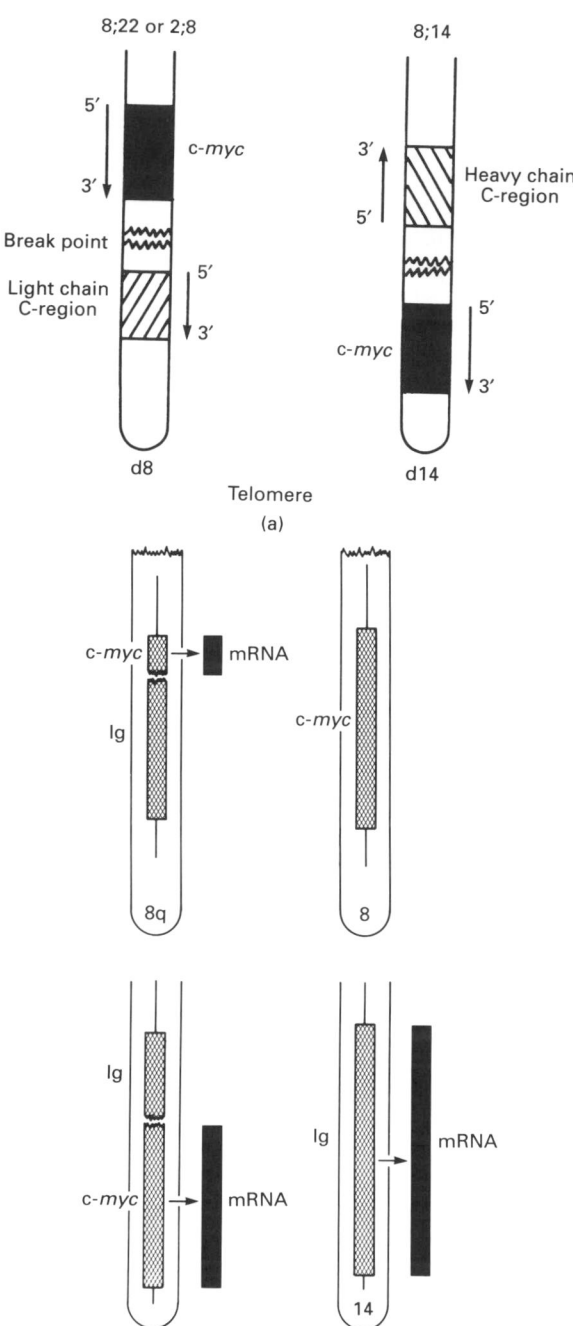

Fig. 6 (a) Juxtaposition of the c-*myc* and immunoglobulin genes brought about by the specific chromosomal translocations in small non-cleaved cell lymphomas (Burkitt's lymphoma). The opposite transcriptional orientation of the genes in the 8;14 translocation (arrows) should be noted. Only the derivative chromosomes which contain c-*myc* (d8 in variant translocations and d14 in 8;14 translocations) are shown. (b) Normal and derivative chromosomes 8 and 14 in small non-cleaved cell lymphomas, showing that c-*myc* is expressed only from the derivative chromosome d14 while immunoglobulin is expressed from the normal chromosome 14. Occasionally, a small transcript derived from the first exon of c-*myc* remaining on the derivative chromosome 8 (when the break-point transects the gene) can be detected.

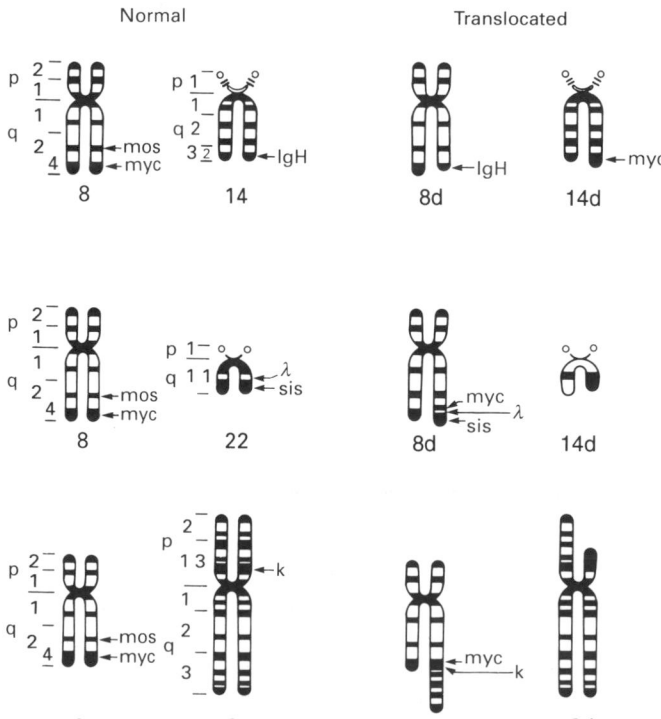

Fig. 5 The chromosomal translocations occurring in small non-cleaved cell lymphomas. Normal chromosomes and relevant gene locations are shown on the left and the consequences of the translocations on the right.

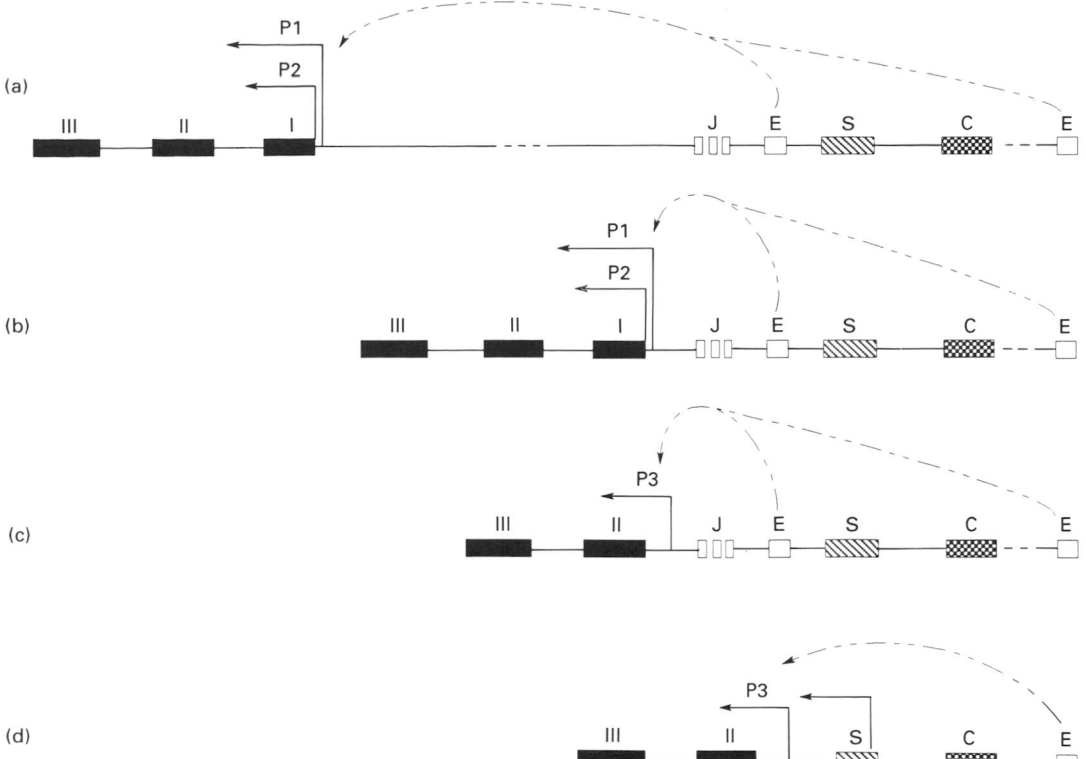

Fig. 7 Diagrammatic depiction of some of the possible molecular consequences of the 8;14 translocations in small non-cleaved cell lymphomas. Enhancer regions (E) of the immunoglobulin locus that can increase transcription from promoters P1, P2, and P3 are shown, as are the three c-*myc* exons (I, II, and III) and the joining (J), switch (S), and constant (C) regions of the immunoglobulin mu locus. Dotted lines show the locations of a considerable stretch of intervening DNA. Dotted arrows show the potential influence of enhancers in the immunoglobulin region. It is probable that these enhancers cause expression of c-*myc* when it comes to lie on the same chromosome by virtue of the translocation. (a) This may apply even when the break-point is far upstream of c-*myc*, as in the majority of endemic tumours. One or other of the enhancers, depending upon the break-point on chromosome 14, may be influential when the break-point is (b) in the immediate 5′ region or (c) and (d) intron of c-*myc*. In these cases, the normal c-*myc* regulatory region, and even the normal promoters (P1 and P2), are damaged or completely separated from c-*myc*. When the break-point is in the c-*myc* first intron, transcripts initiate from the remaining part of the intron in a region that has been called P3. (d) Transcripts may also initiate from within the switch region.

Malcolm *et al*. 1982; Rappold *et al*. 1984). In 8;14 translocations, the c-*myc* gene is translocated from chromosome 8 to the heavy chain locus on chromosome 14, while in the so-called 'variant' translocations, involving immunoglobulin light chains, a part of the constant immunoglobulin locus is translocated to chromosome 8, distal to the c-*myc* gene (Dalla-Favera *et al*. 1982; Taub *et al*. 1982; Magrath 1990). The common feature of all three translocations is the juxtaposition of the c-*myc* gene to immunoglobulin constant region sequences, whether of heavy or light chain origin (Fig. 6). There is little doubt that the expression of the c-*myc* gene, whose own regulatory regions are damaged or even deleted during the process of chromosomal translocation, becomes subordinate to the influence of the immunoglobulin gene regulatory sequences which now lie adjacent to it on the same chromosome (Fig. 7). Thus, the c-*myc* gene (it is always the gene involved in the translocation that is expressed) is regulated as if it were an immunoglobulin gene and, since immunoglobulin genes are constantly expressed in B-cells, the c-*myc* gene remains switched on even when it ought not to be expressed. The product of c-*myc* is known to be necessary for cellular proliferation (Armelin *et al*. 1984; Kelly and Siebenlist 1985, 1986, 1988; Kelly and Underwood 1987) and therefore it is highly likely that it is the inappropriate expression of c-*myc*, occasioned by the translocation, that maintains the cell in a proliferative state.

A reasonable hypothesis to account for the pathogenesis of the small non-cleaved cell lymphomas is depicted in Fig. 8. It is

postulated that the chromosomal translocation occurs in a proliferating cell, in an immature B cell during or shortly after the process of immunoglobulin gene rearrangement. An alternative, that may apply to a proportion of tumours, is that the chromosomal translocation occurs in temporal proximity to heavy chain class switching (Magrath 1990). However, the localization of the break-point to an immunoglobulin switch region does not necessarily indicate that the cell in which the translocation occurred was the equivalent of an activated lymphocyte about to undergo class switching, since the switch region is clearly susceptible to chromosome breakage even in pro-B cells (Altiok *et al*. 1989) and heavy chain class switching has been described in pre-B-cells (Radbruch *et al*. 1986; Magrath 1990). Nevertheless, it appears highly probable that at whatever stage of B-cell differentiation the translocation occurs, the continuous expression of the c-*myc* gene occasioned by it prevents the cell from entering a resting phase, the appropriate state for a cell which has generated an antigen receptor and thus is ready to participate in a primary or possibly secondary immune response (Magrath 1990). Hence, it has been hypothesized that a small non-cleaved cell lymphoma becomes manifest only at that point in B-cell differentiation when the cell would normally enter a resting phase and, as such, the tumour is the malignant counterpart of a resting B-cell (Magrath 1990).

It has been demonstrated that in small non-cleaved cell lymphomas the break-point location on chromosome 8 varies with

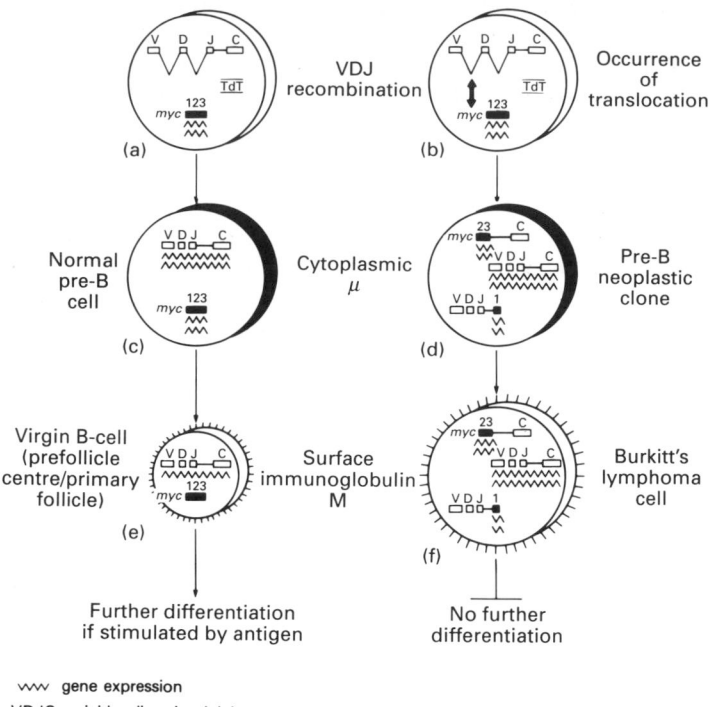

ww gene expression
VDJC variable, diversity, joining and constant immunoglobulin gene regions

Fig. 8 Hypothetical schemata depicting the timing and consequence of an 8;14 translocation in a B-cell precursor. Normally (vertical series on left), immunoglobulin gene rearrangements take place in precursor cells and result in a functional, that is, expressed immunoglobulin gene, first detectable at the pre-B-cell stage in which cytoplasmic mu chains are detectable. Subsequently, as the cell matures into a virgin (that is, unstimulated by antigen) B-cell, with surface immunoglobulin (antigen receptor), c-*myc* expression is down-regulated and the cell enters a resting phase. If a translocation occurs around the time of rearrangement of immunoglobulin genes (vertical series on right), the cell cannot down-regulate c-*myc* expression and remains in a proliferative mode.

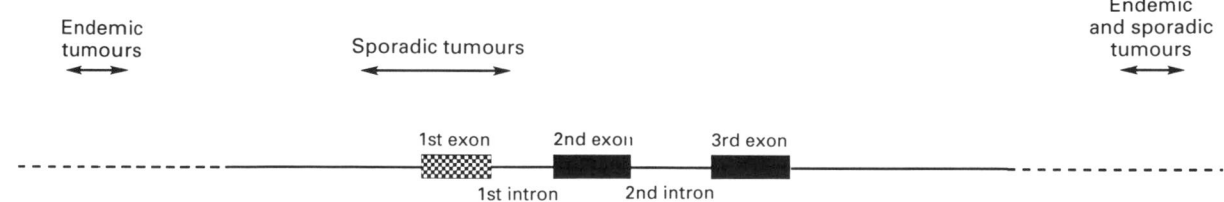

Fig. 9 Differences in break-point location in small non-cleaved cell lymphomas. In endemic tumours the break-point is usually far upstream of the gene; in sporadic tumours it is within or close to the gene. Both these break-points arise in the context of 8;14 translocations. The first exon contains coding sequences for the 64 kDa protein product of c-*myc*. In the variant translocations, regardless of geographical origin, the break-point is a variable distance downstream of c-*myc*.

the geographical origin of the tumour (Fig. 9) (Pellici *et al.* 1986*b*; Neri *et al.* 1988; Magrath 1990; Shiramizu *et al.* 1991; Gutiérrez *et al.* 1992). In endemic (equatorial African) lymphomas the break-point is usually a variable, but is often considerable distance upstream of the gene. In this circumstance, however, there are mutations in the first exon or intron of the c-*myc* gene, the consequence of which is not known, but which are likely to participate in the deregulation of the gene. In sporadic (North American) tumours the break-point is usually within the gene or in its immediate upstream flanking sequences, a region which is known to contain sequences involved in the regulation of c-*myc* expression (Magrath 1990). In fact, regulation of transcription has been shown to be influenced by sequences both upstream of the gene and within the 5' region of the gene itself (Hay *et al.* 1987; Lang *et al.* 1988; Kingston 1989). Thus, in the endemic tumours there are mutations in the c-*myc* regulatory sequence, while in the sporadic tumours the regulatory sequences are partly or wholly lost.

The molecular differences between endemic and sporadic tumours are not absolute, however, and some 10–25 per cent of tumours do not conform to the more usual pattern for the region (Shiramizu *et al.* 1991). Despite this, these observations are consistent with the probability that the cell in which the translocation occurs differs, presumably with respect to its level of differentiation, in the majority of endemic tumours versus the majority of sporadic tumours. This permits the further speculation that environmental factors (for example, holoendemic malaria in endemic regions of Africa) may influence the proportion of that specific cell type which is susceptible to the kind of chromosomal translocation (characterized by the break-point location on chromosome 8) that is predominant in the region. There is also some evidence that the break-point location correlates with the presence of Epstein–Barr virus DNA, which is present in the majority of endemic tumours but in a minority (approximately 20 per cent) of sporadic tumours, suggesting that this virus may have a pathogenic role in some tumours, but not others, depending upon the precise break-point location and the degree or type of damage to the regulatory region of the gene (Magrath 1990). The association of Epstein–Barr virus DNA with the small non-cleaved cell lymphomas is discussed further below.

Lymphoblastic lymphomas

Although non-random chromosomal abnormalities have been found in lymphoblastic lymphomas, unlike the small non-cleaved cell lymphomas, there is not a single translocation or class of translocations involving a single oncogene that is present in the majority of tumours. The translocations that have been described, however, usually involve chromosomal regions relevant to T-cell differentiation, including, in most cases, the T-cell antigen receptor genes (particularly the T alpha/T delta locus situated on chromosome 14q11) (Barker et al. 1985; Croce et al. 1985; Jones et al. 1985; Kristofferson et al. 1985; Levine et al. 1985; Dube et al. 1986; Finger et al. 1986; Le Beau and Rowley 1986; Le Beau et al. 1986; McKeithan et al. 1986; Mathieu-Mahul et al. 1986; Smith et al. 1986). To date, translocations between chromosomes 14(q11) and 11(p13/15) have been most often observed (in both leukaemia and lymphoma), but 1;14, 8;14, and 10;14 translocations have also been described, with the break-point on chromosome 14 being in the T alpha/T delta locus. These findings strongly suggest that the rearrangement of genetic material occurred during the process of cell differentiation close to the time when rearrangements of T-cell receptor gene subunits normally occur. As with B-cell tumours, the enzymes which mediate the chromosomal translocations may be responsible for physiological gene rearrangement (Finger et al. 1986). This has been well substantiated in the case of the most common molecular abnormality of immature T-cell neoplasms, a deletion present on chromosome 1 in which the tal-1/scl gene is disrupted (Aplan et al. 1992).

Additional insight into the pathogenetic mechanisms relevant to T-cell lymphoblastic neoplasia has been gained by molecular cloning of the translocation break-points. In two cell lines which contain 8;14 (q24;q11) translocations, for example, the T alpha constant region has been shown to be translocated from its location in chromosome 14 (the break-point being in the J region of the T alpha gene) to a point distal to c-myc on chromosome 8 (McKeithan et al. 1986; Mathieu-Mahul et al. 1986). This type of translocation is analogous to the variant translocations observed in small non-cleaved lymphomas and may result in deregulation of c-myc. The break-point on chromosome 11 in the 11;14 (p15;q11) translocation is between the genes for insulin and the insulin-like growth factor. The latter gene is translocated to chromosome 14, an observation that could be relevant to the cause of neoplastic growth (Le Beau et al. 1986). The 10;14 translocation, reported in four T-cell lymphoblastic neoplasms, results from chromosomal breaks in the q11 band (T alpha) on chromosome 14 and band q24 on chromosome 10, which includes the gene coding for TdT (Dube et al. 1986).

Chromosomal translocations which do not involve the antigen receptor loci have also been described in lymphoblastic lymphomas. These include a 9;17 translocation (Kaneko et al. 1988) and a 7;15 translocation (Biegel et al. 1988). The latter was described in a pre-B lymphoblastic lymphoma presenting as an isolated bone lesion. Another translocation involved in pre-B leukaemia is the 1;19 translocation in which a fusion gene involving two transcription factors, E2A and pbx is formed (Kamps et al. 1990). Little additional information is currently available on the spectrum of cytogenetic abnormalities in the non-T-cell lymphoblastic lymphomas.

To what extent these various translocations are associated with specific clinical presentations (for example, lymphoma versus leukaemia) remains unclear at present, but it is highly probable that they are relevant to pathogenesis.

Large-cell lymphomas

Consistent cytogenetic abnormalities have also not been observed in the large-cell lymphomas, but the most frequent in the childhood age group are identical with those observed in the small non-cleaved cell lymphomas, namely 8;14 and variant translocations (Bloomfield et al. 1983; Le Beau and Rowley 1986; Kato et al. 1987). These tumours have not been sufficiently analysed at a molecular level and the similarity or differences between small non-cleaved cell lymphomas and large-cell lymphomas with 8;14 chromosomal translocations remain to be determined. The 14;18 translocations, which occur in follicular lymphomas and some large-cell lymphomas in adults (Tsujimoto et al. 1984; Bakhshi et al. 1985) have not been described in children. This is not unexpected in view of the absence of true follicular lymphomas in children.

Recently, a 2;5 translocation was described in anaplastic large-cell lymphomas of either B or T phenotype (Fischer et al. 1988; Kaneko et al. 1989; Mason et al. 1990).

EPIDEMIOLOGY AND PATHOGENESIS

Lymphomas constitute approximately 10 per cent of all childhood cancers in the more developed countries, being third in relative frequency after acute leukaemias and brain tumours. In the United States, between 1973 and 1982, lymphomas constituted 12.6 per cent of all cancers in White children less than 15 years old; non-Hodgkin's lymphomas accounted for 7 per cent and Hodgkin's disease for the remaining 5.6 per cent (Young et al. 1986). During these same years, the mean annual incidence of non-Hodgkin's lymphomas was 9.1 per million White children. In Black children, lymphomas constituted 9 per cent of all neoplasms, with non-Hodgkin's lymphomas accounting for 4 per cent and the mean annual incidence of non-Hodgkin's lymphoma was 4.6 per million. Thus, taking into account all races, non-Hodgkin's lymphomas have a slightly higher incidence than Hodgkin's disease in children less than 15 years old. In older children Hodgkin's disease is more frequent than the non-Hodgkin's lymphomas (Table 5). However, the incidence and relative frequency of non-Hodgkin's lymphomas varies in different world regions (Table 6).

Unlike Hodgkin's disease, which has a bimodal incidence curve, the incidence of non-Hodgkin's lymphomas increases steadily with age throughout life and children below the age of 16 years account for only approximately 3 per cent of all patients with non-Hodgkin's

Table 5 Actual number of lymphoma cases diagnosed between 1973 and 1977 (Caucasian males and females, United States)

Age group	Hodgkin's lymphomas	Non-Hodgkin's lymphomas
<5	6 (0.2%)	39 (0.5%)
5–9	30 (1.1%)	63 (0.8%)
10–14	119 (4.3%)	86 (1.0%)
15–19	300 (11%)	79 (1.0%)
>20	2301 (83%)	7828 (97%)
All ages	2756	8095

Table 6   Mean annual incidence of selected childhood (< 15 years) neoplasms in selected registries[a]

	200/202[b]	204[c]	191/92[d]	All sites
Sao Paulo (1978)				
Males	10.3	8.4	14.9	93.7
Females	6.3	9.6	9.7	64.4
Bombay (1978–1982)				
Males	3.4	5.1	2.8	25.4
Females	1.0	3.0	2.3	15.9
Shanghai (1978–1982)				
Males	3.5	7.7	5.5	33.8
Females	1.7	7.3	4.5	29.9
Osaka (1979–1982)				
Males	4.9	8.4	11.9	54.1
Females	3.7	7.2	8.7	39.8
Finland (1977–1981)				
Males	6.3	15	19.2	64.9
Females	1.8	14.1	14.9	46.5
Scotland (1978–1982)				
Males	3.8	13.3	7.6	57.4
Females	2.2	10.6	9.2	49.6
Michigan (1978–1982)				
White males	5.0	12.5	6.8	42.0
White females	1.7	10.8	7.7	40.5
Black males	1.8	3.7	9.7	32.1
Black females	1.4	5.2	4.6	30.3

[a]Data taken from *Cancer incidence in five continents* (1987).
[b]200, lymphosarcoma; 202, other reticuloses.
[c]204, lymphoid leukaemia.
[d]191–192, brain and nervous system.

lymphomas (Young *et al.* 1986). Non-Hodgkin's lymphomas have a higher incidence in males than females; the male to female ratio is 2 or 3 to 1.

Geographical differences in lymphoid neoplasms in children

Childhood lymphomas occur throughout the world, although the relative frequency of non-Hodgkin's lymphoma varies quite markedly from country to country (West 1984). In equatorial Africa, for example, approximately 50 per cent of childhood cancers are lymphomas; this markedly increased frequency is the consequence of the very high incidence of small non-cleaved cell lymphoma (Burkitt's lymphoma) in this region (Magrath 1985). Both lymphoblastic and large-cell lymphomas also occur in equatorial Africa, probably with a similar incidence to that in the more developed countries, although accurate figures are not available. In Europe and the United States approximately one-third of childhood lymphomas are lymphoblastic lymphomas, half are small non-cleaved cell lymphomas (including Burkitt's lymphoma), approximately 15 per cent are large-cell lymphomas, and the remainder are unclassified.

Interestingly, there are a number of clinical and biological differences between endemic and sporadic small non-cleaved lymphomas (Table 7) which correlate with the molecular differences outlined above. It is probable that these are different diseases, although closely related and histologically identical (Magrath 1984, 1985, 1990). African Burkitt's lymphoma was originally recognized because of the high frequency of the characteristic jaw tumours (Burkitt 1958), but this is not a site of predilection in patients outside Africa. Abdominal involvement, however, is common in both endemic and sporadic varieties. One of Burkitt's major contributions was to demonstrate the remarkable geographical distribution of the endemic tumour in equatorial Africa and subsequently to show that the apparent limits of its distribution were climatically determined (Burkitt 1970*a*). This observation led to the hypothesis that a vectored virus could be of pathogenetic importance and prompted a search for associated viruses, which resulted in the discovery of Epstein–Barr virus in the cells of a cell line derived from a Burkitt lymphoma (Epstein *et al.* 1964). However, although 95 per cent of endemic tumours carry Epstein–Barr virus genomes in their cell nuclei, this is true for only some 15–30 per cent of North American tumours (Magrath 1985). Moreover, this difference does not simply reflect exposure to Epstein–Barr virus, since the majority of patients with endemic and therefore mostly Epstein–Barr virus negative tumours have antibodies to Epstein–Barr virus regardless of their country of origin (Epstein *et al.* 1962; Levine *et al.* 1982).

It is still not clear whether Epstein–Barr virus infection simply predisposes to the development of African Burkitt's lymphoma (and presumably those sporadic tumours which contain Epstein–Barr virus sequences) or whether Epstein–Barr virus is, in such cases, an essential component of pathogenesis. It has been shown, however, that Epstein–Barr virus infection occurs at an early age in Africans (almost the entire population has been infected by the age of 3 years) compared with individuals in more developed countries, where primary infection frequently occurs in late adolescence or early adulthood (Henle and Henle 1979). It seems probable that the B-cell mitogenic effect of Epstein–Barr virus both increases the size of certain B- or pre-B-cell populations, perhaps those that are already increased in young children compared with adults and causes individual cell clones to remain in a proliferative state, both of which may increase the likelihood of the development of the genetic

Table 7   Differences between endemic and sporadic Burkitt's lymphoma

	Endemic	Sporadic
Mean annual incidence (children below 16 years)	10 per 100 000	0.2 per 100 000
Distribution	Climatically dependent	Not climatically dependent
Association with Epstein–Barr virus[a]	95%	20%
Chromosome 8 break-points	Upstream of c-*myc*	Within c-*myc*
Immunophenotype	Surface IgM	Surface IgM
	No IGM secretion	Secretion of IgM
Common sites of tumour	Jaw	Abdomen
	Abdomen	Bone-marrow
	Orbit	Nasopharynx
	Paraspinal	Lymph nodes
Response of recurrent tumour including central nervous system	Good	Poor

[a]Presence of Epstein–Barr viral DNA in tumour cells

abnormalities which cause Burkitt's lymphoma. An alternative hypothesis, that Epstein–Barr virus immortalizes cells which already contain a specific translocation, has been proposed (Lenoir and Bornkamm 1988), although direct evidence supporting either of these hypotheses is lacking.

Recently, the discovery that the pattern of expression of Epstein–Barr virus latent genes differs in Burkitt's lymphoma compared with Epstein–Barr virus-transformed B-cells provides support, if indirect, for the possibility that Epstein–Barr virus has a direct role in malignant transformation or at least, in maintenance of the malignant phenotype (Magrath 1990). The Epstein–Barr virus latent genes are predominantly nuclear proteins and are responsible for B-cell transformation, but some of them are also expressed at the cell surface and, in the context of HLA class I antigens, result in the generation of an immune response against Epstein–Barr virus infected cells (Wallace *et al.* 1987; Magrath 1990). This accounts for the self-limited nature of Epstein–Barr virus associated infectious mononucleosis. Clearly, the expression of such antigens is incompatible with a malignant phenotype in an immunologically normal host and it is therefore of considerable interest that such antigens appear not to be expressed in Epstein–Barr virus-associated Burkitt's lymphoma (Rowe *et al.* 1986, 1987; Magrath 1990). Because the normal pattern of expression of Epstein–Barr virus latent genes would be a liability rather than an asset to a tumour cell in an immunologically competent host and because only a small number of cells in the body are infected with Epstein–Barr virus, it is surprising that Epstein–Barr virus is associated with Burkitt's lymphoma at all. This, in itself, suggests that Epstein–Barr virus does indeed have a direct role in pathogenesis in at least a fraction of tumours, particularly that fraction that occurs in equatorial Africa.

While there are quite considerable differences at molecular and clinical levels between endemic and sporadic small non-cleaved cell lymphomas, it is likely that the subtypes are not exclusive to specific geographical regions. Thus, the small proportion of Epstein–Barr virus negative tumours in equatorial Africa may represent the low level of sporadic tumours that occurs everywhere in the world. It is also possible that the endemic form of the disease occurs at lower frequency outside Africa. This possibility is supported by the occurrence of typically African jaw tumours in a fraction of patients with small non-cleaved cell lymphomas in other parts of the world, including Japan, South Africa, Turkey, and northern Brazil (Abe and Sato 1981; Wood *et al.* 1988; Hesseling *et al.* 1989; Magrath 1991).

There may be yet a third variety of Burkitt's lymphoma, which is characterized by a high rate of Epstein–Barr virus association and a low frequency of jaw tumours. In North Africa, for example, where jaw tumours are rare, more than 85 per cent of cases are Epstein–Barr virus associated (Lenoir and Bornkamm 1988) and a similar clinical pattern is observed in the Middle East (Anaissie *et al.* 1985; Madanat *et al.* 1986) (Table 8). In South America Burkitt's lymphoma has an intermediate frequency of Epstein–Barr virus association as well as an intermediate chromosomal break-point location on chromosome 8 (Gutiérrez *et al.* 1992). Further work is required in many parts of the world to determine the validity of this preliminary classification of Burkitt's lymphoma and to determine the relative proportions of different subtypes in various world regions and their relationship, if any, to different levels of socio-economic development.

Although the dependence of Burkitt's lymphoma on climatic factors led to the discovery of Epstein–Barr virus, this virus is ubiquitous and therefore its presence in African Burkitt's lymphoma

Table 8 Subtypes of Burkitt's lymphoma based on frequency of jaw tumours and Epstein–Barr virus association

World region	Frequency of jaw tumour	Epstein–Barr virus association
Equatorial Africa	High (60%)	High (95%)
North Africa	Low (<15%)	High (85%)
Europe/N.America/ Australasia	Low (<15%)	Low (~20%)
South America	Low (<15%)	Intermediate (~50%)

is unlikely to explain the geographical distribution of this condition. However, the region of high incidence corresponds to the distribution of holoendemic malaria (Burkitt's lymphoma also occurs at high frequency in New Guinea, another holoendemic malarial region), which may also predispose to the development of the tumour, since malaria, like Epstein–Barr virus, is a B-cell mitogen which increases the proportion of precursor B-cells in the bone-marrows of infected mice (Osmond *et al.* 1990) and also causes T-cell suppression. In fact, malaria impairs the ability of the immune system to regulate Epstein–Barr virus-infected cells (Moss *et al.* 1983; Whittle *et al.* 1984), so that the combination of early infection by Epstein–Barr virus and malaria may be sufficient to increase markedly the risk of the development of Burkitt's lymphoma in holoendemic malarial regions such as Africa and New Guinea (Fig. 10).

Little epidemiological information is available with regard to the other varieties of childhood non-Hodgkin's lymphoma, although both lymphoblastic and large cell lymphomas clearly occur throughout the world. Preliminary information indicates that

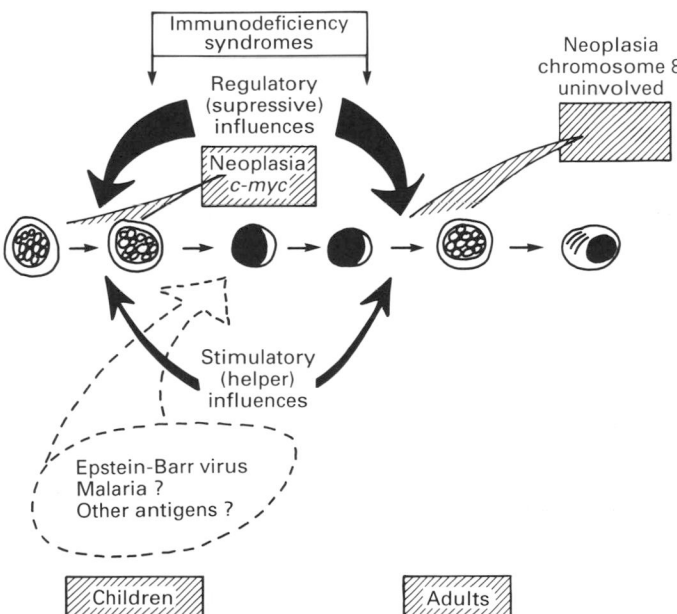

Fig. 10 Diagrammatic depiction of presumptive mechanisms whereby immunodeficiency and environmental factors predispose to the development of B-cell neoplasia. Cells undergoing differentiation in the B-cell lineage are shown in a horizontal direction. Alteration in the proportions of various B-cell precursors results from either inherited or acquired immunodeficiency or environmental factors such as malaria. The probability of the development of a translocation is thereby increased. In contrast with childhood lymphomas, the majority of adult lymphomas occur in activated B-cells, rather than B-cell precursors, and do not involve chromosome 8.

lymphoblastic lymphomas are considerably more common than undifferentiated tumours in some countries (for example, India), although caution must be exercised in interpreting figures since the distinction from acute lymphoblastic leukaemia is not always made in the same way in different parts of the world. It also seems likely that there are several subtypes of lymphoblastic lymphoma (based on immunophenotype and cytogenetics) which are likely to vary in frequency in different world regions. No virus association has yet been observed in lymphoblastic lymphoma.

The incidence of the large-cell lymphomas of childhood on a worldwide basis is unknown at present.

Pre-lymphomatous states

Since lymphomas arise from the constituent cells of the immune system, it is not surprising that disorders associated with abnormal regulation of lymphocytes are associated with an increased incidence of non-Hodgkin's lymphomas. This is probably a consequence of alterations in the size and self-renewal potential of selected lymphoid subpopulations. Epstein–Barr virus also appears to be important in the pathogenesis of lymphomas in immunodeficiency states, since a majority of these lymphomas and lymphoproliferative syndromes contain Epstein–Barr virus genomes (Hanto *et al.* 1981; Saemundsen *et al.* 1981; Purtilo 1984; Shearer *et al.* 1985; Subar *et al.* 1988; Magrath 1989; Seibel *et al.* 1989; Filipovich *et al.* 1990). One possible explanation of this is that defective T-cell regulation permits the expansion of Epstein–Barr virus-infected clones of B-cells which would normally be tightly controlled, but which, owing to the influence of viral genes, have a selective advantage over uninfected cells. Such cell clones would then be at increased risk of developing a genetic change capable of causing neoplastic behaviour (Table 9). In such patients, however, the borderland between lymphoproliferation, which is not neoplastic and true neoplasia is not easy to discern and is perhaps to some extent a semantic debate. Some families, for example, carry a sex-linked disorder known as X-linked lymphoproliferative syndrome which is characterized by the occurrence of aplastic anaemia, fatal infectious mononucleosis, and malignant non-Hodgkin's lymphomas (Purtilo 1984). Whether or not patients succumb to fatal infectious mononucleosis or lymphoma presumably reflects the degree to which immune reactivity against Epstein–Barr virus infection is impaired. Individuals with essentially no ability to regulate the proliferation of Epstein–Barr virus-infected cells die as a consequence of primary Epstein–Barr virus infection, whereas those with some ability to control Epstein–Barr virus-infected cells may simply be at increased risk for a B-cell lymphoma because of an enlarged pool of Epstein–Barr virus-infected B-cells and consequent increased risk of the development of a genetic abnormality leading to a clonal lymphoma (Magrath 1989; Seibel *et al.* 1989).

Surprisingly, in patients with AIDS, the incidence of Epstein–Barr virus associated polyclonal lymphoproliferation appears to be low. Prior to the development of monoclonal lymphomas, however, B-cell hyperplasia involving the expansion of a small number of

clones has been described (Pelicci *et al.* 1986*a*) and it is possible that malignant transformation occurs in one of these expanded clones. Some of the lymphomas which develop in adults (there is much less information in children) have the histology of small non-cleaved cell lymphoma and also carry the same chromosomal abnormalities (with break-point locations similar to those in sporadic lymphomas) (Chaganti *et al.* 1983; Whang-Peng *et al.* 1984; Pelicci *et al.* 1986; Subar *et al.* 1988). However, immunoblastic lymphomas increase in incidence with age. These tumours are more heterogeneous, but are often associated with Epstein–Barr virus. The Epstein–Barr virus association of small non-cleaved cell lymphomas is similar to that in non-HIV infected patients. HIV is believed to have only an indirect role, since it is not present in the tumour cells themselves.

In children, the genetically determined immunodeficiency syndromes with the greatest risk of lymphoma development are ataxia telangiectasia, Wiscott–Aldrich syndrome, common variable immunodeficiency disease, severe combined immunodeficiency syndrome, and X-linked lymphoproliferative syndrome (Filipovich *et al.* 1984, 1990; Purtilo 1987; Seibel *et al.* 1989). The estimated risk of non-Hodgkin's lymphoma in these syndromes is between 1 (severe combined immunodeficiency virus) and 35 per cent (X-linked lymphoproliferative syndrome). Some 12–14 per cent of patients with Wiskott–Aldrich syndrome develop non-Hodgkin's lymphomas. Other genetically determined immunodeficiency syndromes are associated with a much lower risk of lymphoma development. It is possible that in some of these syndromes the decreased ability to repair DNA and predisposition to chromosomal abnormalities (for example, ataxia telangiectasia, Bloom's syndrome, and xeroderma pigmentosum) also plays a rôle in the induction of lymphomas (Magrath 1982; Filipovich *et al.* 1984, 1990; Seibel *et al.* 1989).

Transplant recipients are also at risk of developing non-Hodgkin's lymphomas as a consequence of iatrogenic immunosuppression (lymphomas have been described in renal, heart, and bone-marrow recipients) (Saemundsen *et al.* 1981; Purtilo 1984; Seibel *et al.* 1989; Filipovich *et al.* 1990). In some series as many as 25 per cent of renal or cardiac allograft recipients have developed non-Hodgkin's lymphomas after 1 year.

Other types of pre-lymphomatous states or conditions associated with a predisposition to lymphoma development, such as alpha heavy chain disease (Salem 1985), angio-immunoblastic lymphadenopathy (Watanabe *et al.* 1986), and various forms of autoimmune disease, including Sjögren's syndrome, rheumatoid arthritis, and the angiocentric immunoproliferative lesions (Costa and Delacretaz 1986; Chan *et al.* 1988; Lipford *et al.* 1988; Cohen and Jaffe 1990), are rarely observed in children. Similarly, infection with the retrovirus (HTLV-I) which predisposes to a peripheral T-cell malignancy in adults, occurring predominantly in Japan, the Caribbean, and Africa, is very uncommon in children. The possibility, however, that an as yet unknown virus is causally implicated in the pathogenesis of one or more of the childhood lymphomas cannot be excluded.

Drugs and radiation as predisposing factors

Evidence that radiation induces lymphoma is scanty. Unlike leukaemia, there was no early lymphoma peak in exposed young persons among atomic bomb survivors in Nagasaki and Hiroshima and although there appeared to be slightly increased prevalence rates of lymphoma in individuals who received more than 2 Gy in Nagasaki and those exposed to more than 1 Gy in Hiroshima, there

Table 9 Lymphoproliferative syndromes in immunodeficient individuals

Morphology	Clonality	Cytogenetics	Epstein–Barr virus association
B immunoblastic	Polyclonal	Normal	Always
B immunoblastic/ small non-cleaved	Monoclonal	Abnormal	Sometimes

Monoclonal tumours may evolve from polyclonal lymphoproliferative processes.

was no significant trend for increased incidence with increased dose during the period 1950–1978 (Finch 1984). The relative risk during this same period for individuals exposed to greater than 2 Gy was 1.6, with wide confidence intervals. The majority of the lymphomas in the exposed groups were non-Hodgkin's lymphomas of large-cell type.

While a 4–5-fold increased risk of lymphoma development has been observed in American radiologists and uranium workers exposed during the 1950s and a 2-fold increase in the risk of lymphoma development for patients irradiated for ankylosing spondylitis for at least 6 years, there is little evidence for a lymphomagenetic effect of the once practised thymus gland irradiation in children (Finch 1984).

Patients with Hodgkin's disease treated with combined modality therapy are at increased risk of developing non-Hodgkin's lymphoma, perhaps 4–5 per cent of all patients so treated will develop non-Hodgkin's lymphoma within 10 years (Meadows et al. 1985; Valagussa et al. 1986; Barriga et al. 1990). The precise risk for children with Hodgkin's disease treated with either chemotherapy alone or combined modality therapy has not been determined because of small numbers of treated patients compared with adults.

Apart from immunosuppressive drugs used in transplant recipients, information regarding the capacity of other drugs to induce lymphoma is limited. Hydantoin derivatives are known to cause pseudolymphomas that regress with cessation of therapy, but there are reports of the development of lymphomas in long-term recipients of these drugs (Nadler et al. 1984). Unfortunately, no accurate figures are available regarding the size of this risk, but in view of the widespread use of these compounds it is likely to be very low. Various organic solvents, including dioxins and benzene and chemical sprays used in agriculture, have been incriminated in the aetiology of non-Hodgkin's lymphomas, but there is no evidence that they represent significant factors in the occurrence of childhood lymphomas (Nadler et al. 1984).

CLINICAL PRESENTATIONS AND SITES OF INVOLVEMENT

For the most part, patients with non-Hodgkin's lymphoma present with a limited number of syndromes, most of which correlate very well with cell type. Childhood lymphomas are much more often extranodal than are adult lymphomas, the most frequently involved sites being intra-abdominal (especially B-cell lymphomas) and intrathoracic (T-cell lymphomas).

Small non-cleaved cell lymphoma

Almost all patients with small non-cleaved lymphomas (in the United States and Europe) present with abdominal tumour (Magrath 1985; Magrath and Sariban 1985) which gives rise to abdominal pain or swelling, sometimes with a symptom complex caused by intussusception, a change in bowel habits, nausea and vomiting, evidence of gastrointestinal bleeding, or, rarely, intestinal perforation (Meyers et al. 1985). Presentation with a right iliac fossa mass is common, occurring in 25 per cent of patients in the National Cancer Institute series (Janus et al. 1984) (some 40 per cent of patients overall had tumour at this site) and can be confused with acute appendicitis or an inflammatory appendiceal mass. Frequently at surgery there are multiple enlarged mesenteric lymph nodes, which may or may not contain microscopically visible tumour and multiple peritoneal plaques of tumour may be observed.

Involvement of retroperitoneal structures, including kidneys and pancreas, is second only to bowel and mesentery involvement, while liver and splenic involvement are seen somewhat less frequently. Ovarian involvement is quite common in females.

Jaw involvement, involving multiple jaw quadrants in a high proportion of cases, is the most frequent site of involvement in patients with Burkitt's lymphoma in equatorial Africa, although it is very much age dependent, occurring particularly in young children (Burkitt 1970b). In an early series collected by Burkitt, 70 per cent of children below 5 years with Burkitt's lymphoma had jaw involvement as compared with 25 per cent of patients above 14 years (Burkitt 1970b). In very young children, orbital involvement is often present in patients who do not have jaw tumours, although at least some of these orbital tumours arise in the maxilla. Maxillary tumours are twice as frequent as mandibular tumours in endemic Burkitt's lymphoma. Jaw involvement in sporadic small non-cleaved cell lymphomas occurs in approximately 15–20 per cent of patients at presentation and is not age related (Sariban et al. 1984). Abdominal involvement is also frequent in endemic Burkitt's lymphoma, being present in just over half the patients, but involvement of the right iliac fossa (appendiceal/cecal region) is uncommon (Burkitt 1970c; Magrath 1985). A comparison of sites of disease at presentation in endemic (Ugandan) and sporadic (United States) small non-cleaved lymphomas is shown in Table 10. In addition to the differences in jaw involvement, there are striking differences in the frequency of involvement of the bone-marrow (higher in sporadic disease) and the central nervous system including spinal epidural disease (higher in endemic disease). Isolated lymphadenopathy (usually cervical) is also more common in sporadic than endemic disease, while abdominal tumour involves the bowel wall less often and presentation with a right iliac fossa mass is quite uncommon in endemic disease. Involvement of the mesentery and omentum and the ovary in females are very frequent in Africa.

Patients with small non-cleaved cell lymphomas in North Africa, the Middle East, and South America appear to have a spectrum of organ involvement which more closely approximates that of the sporadic disease rather than the endemic form (most obviously a low frequency of jaw involvement) (Burkitt 1970b; Ladjadj et al. 1984; Lenoir et al. 1984; Sariban et al. 1984; Magrath 1991). However, higher percentages of patients with jaw tumours have

Table 10 Disease sites at presentation in endemic and sporadic small non-cleaved cell lymphomas

	Percentage of patients with involvement[a]	
	Endemic	Sporadic
Abdomen (all)	58	91
Pleural effusion	3	19
Bone-marrow	7	20
Peripheral nodes	9	13
Bone	8	9
CSF/CNS	19	14
Paraspinal	17	2
Testis	2	6
Pharynx	0	10
Jaw	58	7
Mediastinum	<1	3
Orbit	11	1
Miscellaneous[b]	17	15

CSF/CNS, cerebrospinal fluid/central nervous system.
[a]Many patients had multiple sites of disease.
[b]Includes thyroid, breast, skin, shoulder, and thigh.

been reported in some Asian countries, South Africa (where both Whites and non-Whites appear to have as high a frequency of jaw tumours as in the endemic form of the disease), Turkey, Japan, and equatorial Brazil (Abe and Sato 1981; Wood *et al.* 1988; Hesseling *et al.* 1989; Magrath 1991). In the endemic region of Africa itself, the percentage of patients with jaw tumours appears to be inversely proportional to the incidence of the disease. In addition, the median age of patients tends to be higher in lower incidence areas such as highlands or arid regions (Kitinya and Lauren 1982).

Bone-marrow involvement is perhaps more common in sporadic small non–cleaved cell lymphomas than had previously been thought. At presentation, marrow involvement occurs in some 20 per cent of patients (Magrath and Ziegler 1980; Magrath and Sariban 1985), but there is evidence from *in vitro* culture and karyotyping of microscopically uninvolved bone-marrow that occult involvement occurs in approximately another 20 per cent of patients (Benjamin *et al.* 1983). Further, some patients present with a clinical syndrome consistent with leukaemia without any solid lymphomatous masses, apart from lymphadenopathy and hepatosplenomegaly, a disease usually referred to as L3 acute lymphoblastic leukaemia (after the French–American–British classification) acute B-cell leukaemia, or Burkitt's cell leukaemia (although it has become clear that not all leukaemias which conform to the criteria of L3 morphology express surface immunoglobulin and have 8;14 translocations) (Mangan *et al.* 1985). L3 leukaemia neoplasms constitute 2–5 per cent of most large series of patients with acute lymphoblastic leukaemia and, thus, has a similar incidence (perhaps 1–2 per million children less than 16 years old) to small non-cleaved cell lymphomas which present more typically as a lymphoma. Viewed from this perspective, bone-marrow involvement occurs at presentation in approximately two-thirds of patients in the United States and Europe with small non-cleaved cell neoplasms!

In African patients with Burkitt's lymphoma bone-marrow involvement occurs in only approximately 8 per cent of patients at presentation, but there are no estimates of the proportion of patients who have occult bone-marrow involvement, nor is the frequency of L3 acute lymphoblastic leukaemia known in Africa. The rarity of marrow involvement at relapse in African patients, even after multiple relapse, but the very high frequency of marrow involvement at relapse in North American patients (perhaps 90 per cent of patients) further confirms the tendency for sporadic, but not endemic, small non-cleaved cell lymphomas to involve the bone-marrow in the United States to a much greater degree than in Africa.

Involvement of the central nervous system occurs occasionally at presentation in patients with small non-cleaved cell lymphoma. It is significantly more common in the presence of bone-marrow disease (Magrath and Ziegler 1980; Sariban *et al.* 1983) and approximately two-thirds of patients with bone-marrow disease may have simultaneous central nervous system involvement. Meningeal infiltration, detected because of symptoms of raised intracranial pressure (uncommon) or on routine examination of the spinal fluid, is the commonest manifestation of central nervous system involvement. Cranial nerve infiltration, intracerebral disease, paraspinal disease, or some combination of these may also be present, the most frequently observed combination being meningeal and cranial nerve involvement (Magrath *et al.* 1974; Ziegler and Magrath 1974; Sariban *et al.* 1983). The presence of intracerebral disease at the time of presentation is very rare. Any cranial nerve can be involved, but the ophthalmic nerves and the facial nerve are more often affected. Very rarely the optic nerve can be infiltrated, giving rise to blindness. Central nervous system involvement, particularly paraspinal, is distinctly more common in patients with

endemic Burkitt's lymphoma. Paraplegia occurs, for example, in some 15 per cent of equatorial African patients at the time of presentation (Magrath and Sariban 1985; Magrath 1991), while cerebral spinal fluid malignant pleocytosis or cranial nerve involvement is seen in approximately one-third of patients.

Almost any organ or tissue of the body is involved on occasion, including endocrine and salivary glands, bones, skin, pleurae, pharynx, pericardium, breast, testis, and, rarely, mediastinum.

Lymphoblastic lymphomas

Patients with lymphoblastic lymphomas most commonly present with intrathoracic tumour, particularly a mediastinal mass (50–70 per cent of patients), frequently associated with pleural effusions. Symptoms may include pain, dysphagia, dyspnoea, or swelling of the neck, face, and upper limbs from superior vena caval obstruction. Inferior vena caval obstruction is also occasionally seen in such patients, from compression of the vein as it traverses the diaphragm, but it is rarely symptomatic. If patients with intrathoracic tumour have lymphadenopathy (which occurs in 50–80 per cent of all patients), it is likely to be above the diaphragm, in the neck, the supraclavicular regions, or the axillae. Pericardial tumour or effusion, sometimes with significant cardiac tamponade, can occur. Abdominal involvement is quite uncommon and almost never massive, being more likely to be detected simply as hepatic or splenic enlargement or retroperitoneal masses (including renal involvement) detected with special imaging techniques. Generalized peripheral lymphadenopathy is occasionally seen, but should raise suspicions of bone-marrow involvement. These and other 'peripheral' sites of disease, including bone, testis, nasopharynx, and skin, are not usually associated with a large mediastinal mass and may be composed of cells of a more mature phenotype.

In lymphoblastic lymphoma it is difficult to give a figure of the frequency of bone-marrow involvement since this depends entirely upon the definition of this disease. In the United States and the United Kingdom, T-cell acute lymphoblastic leukaemia accounts for some 15 per cent of all cases of acute lymphoblastic leukaemia and this form of T-cell acute lymphoblastic neoplasia is significantly more common than lymphoblastic lymphoma when the latter is diagnosed on the usual basis of having less than 25 per cent of blasts in the bone-marrow. In earlier series of patients with lymphoblastic lymphoma with a poor prognosis, bone-marrow involvement occurred at some point in the course of the disease in excess of 50 per cent of cases (Aur *et al.* 1971; Wanatabe *et al.* 1973).

Central nervous system involvement occurs in a small proportion of patients with lymphoblastic lymphoma at presentation. Its clinical manifestations are identical to those described for the small non-cleaved cell lymphomas.

Large-cell lymphomas

Unlike the lymphoblastic and small non-cleaved lymphomas of childhood, the clinical features of large-cell lymphomas with the exception of anaplastic large-cell lymphomas are not particularly characteristic. These tumours may arise in almost any tissue, both nodal and extranodal (for example, peripheral lymph nodes, Waldeyer's ring, bone, testis) and may involve the pharynx, abdomen (bowel, mesentery, and retroperitoneum), or mediastinum. Large-cell lymphomas account for essentially all the non-lymphoblastic non-Hodgkin's lymphomas arising in the mediastinum and almost all of them have immunoblastic histology (20 out of 24 in a recently published study) (Harousseau *et al.* 1982; Levitt *et al.* 1982; Waldron *et al.* 1985; Addis and Isaacson 1986; Jacobson *et al.* 1988; Willett *et al.* 1988; Lamarre *et al.* 1989; Wurtz *et al.* 1989). Based on histology alone, it would appear that approximately half the immunoblastic tumours arising in the mediastinum are of T-cell origin (peripheral T-cell lymphomas) and half are of B-cell origin. Lymph node involvement is also common in large-cell lymphoma, particularly when developing in a patient with an underlying immunodeficiency disorder. Sometimes there is fluctuating lymphadenopathy, which may be associated with fever and weight loss and often skin involvement. This form of presentation is particularly common in Ki-1 (CD30)-positive anaplastic large-cell lymphomas (Kaudewitz *et al.* 1989).

Immunoblastic lymphomas arising in patients with immunodeficiency also involve the brain much more frequently than spontaneously arising lymphomas. This is reminiscent of the ability of Epstein–Barr virus transformed lymphoblastoid cell lines to grow progressively in the brains of nude mice, but not in the subcutaneous tissues (Schaadt *et al.* 1979) and suggests that advantage is taken of an immunologically privileged site for a cell type that would not necessarily be neoplastic outside the central nervous system. Like other childhood lymphomas, large-cell lymphomas may also involve the meninges, producing malignant pleocytosis, cranial nerves, bone-marrow, and single or multiple bones. They also occur more often in 'atypical sites', such as muscle, lung parenchyma, and other soft tissues (particularly anaplastic large-cell lymphomas), as compared with small non-cleaved cell lymphomas and lymphoblastic lymphomas. This is an additional reason why some large-cell tumours have been misdiagnosed in the past, since such sites of involvement are not usually equated with lymphomas. Other unusual features including vascular (arterial and venous) obstruction have been observed.

DIAGNOSIS

The diagnosis of a patient with suspected non-Hodgkin's lymphoma must be confirmed by biopsy. In patients with small non-cleaved cell lymphoma this frequently entails laparotomy, at which time a fraction of patients (approximately 25 per cent) are shown to have completely resectable tumours (Janus *et al.* 1984). In patients with lymphoblastic lymphoma, lymph node biopsy, aspiration of pleural fluid, or needle biopsy of the mediastinum (if there is no evidence of tumour elsewhere) may be preferable to open or mediastinoscopic biopsy of a large mediastinal mass in view of the increased risk of surgery in such patients. Patients with a significant degree of airway obstruction are at high risk for serious morbidity and even fatality (from cardiac arrest) if anaesthetized (Piro *et al.* 1976; Halpern *et al.* 1983; Carabell and Goodman 1985; Aguado *et al.* 1986; Ruz *et al.* 1986; Delalande *et al.* 1987; Price and Hecker 1987) and it should be borne in mind that the degree of airway obstruction may increase in the supine position because of the influence of gravity on the mass. Superior vena caval obstruction may be associated with an increased degree of bleeding from the mass at the time of surgery. If tracheal intubation is performed, it may be difficult to extubate the patient until considerable reduction in the mediastinal mass has been achieved. The practice of initiating emergency radiation before establishing a diagnosis is not recommended, since the optimal treatment approach to tumours with different histologies varies markedly and irradiation is not considered a primary component of therapy. In experienced hands and with awareness of the risks of anaesthesia, it is rare indeed that a diagnostic procedure, whether operative or a fine-needle aspirate under local anaesthetic (Westcott 1981), cannot be rapidly and safely performed (Ferguson *et al.* 1987).

Histology remains the primary mode of diagnosis, but it is important to supplement this, wherever possible, with immunophenotyping, karyotyping, and genotyping, which provide additional objective reassurance of the diagnosis and in difficult cases may clearly indicate that the tumour is lymphoid in origin. To date, no antigen expressed exclusively on a tumour cell (excepting idiotypes) has been identified, so that all surface markers utilized will also be present on at least some populations of normal cells. However, the presence of a uniform population of cells expressing a phenotype that is unexpected for the tissue of origin provides strong corroborative evidence of malignancy. For example, CD10 should not normally be found on peripheral blood cells and CD1 is not normally found on peripheral blood cells or bone-marrow cells. Clonality of a lymphoid proliferative process, which in the B lineage can be determined, for all practical purposes, on the basis of the expression of a single light chain type or more definitively as also is the case for tumours of the T-cell lineage, by the demonstration of clonal rearrangement of an antigen receptor gene on a Southern blot (Korsmeyer *et al.* 1981; Bertness *et al.* 1985; Pellici *et al.* 1985), is strongly suggestive, but not conclusive, proof of a neoplastic process. Occasionally, monoclonal lymphoproliferative processes are benign (witness benign monoclonal gammopathy), while lymphoproliferation occurring in allograft recipients, histologically consistent with malignant lymphoma, is frequently polyclonal (Hanto *et al.* 1981; Cleary *et al.* 1988; Seibel *et al.* 1990; Filipovich *et al.* 1990). This is to some extent a semantic debate, since absolute criteria for the diagnosis of a malignant non-Hodgkin's lymphoma in such patients have not been agreed upon and polyclonal lymphoproliferation can certainly be fatal.

The presence of the leucocyte common antigen (Battifora and Trowbridge 1983), which is not present on non-haematological neoplasms, provides sufficient confirmation of a lymphoid cell population, but it is rare that insufficient tumour tissue is available for addional testing to be performed, particularly since immunophenotyping can be done on cytocentrifuge preparations, imprints, or smears of cells which require very little material. Some monoclonal antibodies also work well on formalin-fixed tissue. Similar material can also be used for *in situ* hybridization using nucleic acid probes (DNA or RNA) for genes, such as immunoglobulin or T-cell receptor genes, expressed only in lymphoid cells. Confirmation of a T- or B-cell phenotype or genotype provides irrefutable evidence of a lymphoid origin. Some immunoblastic lymphomas may not express T or B surface markers, but such tumours usually express the CD30 antigen and a lymphoid origin can be confirmed by genotyping by Southern blot (Alt *et al.* 1986). Such investigations are also possible by using polymerase chain reactions.

The presence of TdT is a very useful criterion, both for the identification of lymphoid cells and also for the further delineation of subtype, since only acute lymphoblastic leukaemias and lymphoblastic lymphomas of both B- and T-cell phenotype express this enzyme (Braziel *et al.* 1983) and under normal circumstances TdT-positive cells are found only in the bone-marrow in very small numbers (Janossy *et al.* 1979).

Tumours which lack all evidence of lymphoid markers could be 'true' histiocytic lymphomas. Non-specific esterases and sometimes the presence of the T_6 (CD1) antigen (expressed on Langerhans cells) or other monocyte antigens, as well as erythrophagocytosis, may be demonstrable in this case. Electron microscopy, which can also provide definitive evidence of a lymphoid origin (Vezzoni *et al.* 1984), can also be useful to confirm that a tumour is not of lymphoid origin (for example, ultrastructural evidence of neural differentiation or muscle differentiation may be provided).

Karyotyping can provide specific information only when one of the specific translocations described above is detected, although the presence of cytogenetic abnormalities is strongly suggestive of a neoplastic process. In the absence of karyotyping information, the presence of one of the specific chromosomal translocations associated with Burkitt's lymphoma, for example, can be inferred by the detection of a molecular rearrangement or specific mutation of the c-*myc* oncogene by means of a Southern blot or single strand conformational polymorphism assay followed by sequencing. One or other of these structural alterations in c-*myc* is present in all Burkitt's lymphomas (Pellici *et al.* 1986).

It seems likely that in the near future there will be an increase in the use of the highly sensitive polymerase chain reaction described above. In utilizing this technique to demonstrate the presence of a chromosomal translocation diagnostic of a specific tumour, the limiting factor becomes the tissue sampling itself. This contrasts with Southern blotting, where a clone of cells must comprise some 5 per cent of the population before it can be reproducibly detected. It seems highly likely that the polymerase chain reaction will permit the detection of very low levels of bone-marrow involvement and may also lead to the successful detection of tumour cells in the peripheral blood, even in the absence of microscopically evident bone-marrow involvement (Hu *et al.* 1985). The examination of cerebrospinal fluid by polymerase chain reaction may also reveal unsuspected cerebrospinal fluid involvement, but the possibility of false-positive results because of contamination by blood may limit the value of this use of the test. In addition, the clinical significance of the presence of small numbers of tumour cells in bone-marrow or cerebrospinal fluid will need to be evaluated empirically.

At present serum studies cannot provide diagnostic information for lymphomas, but may provide evidence of a non-lymphoid origin when, for example, there are high levels of serum or urinary catechol amines or their metabolites or in the presence of other tumour markers such as α-fetoprotein, carcinoembryonic antigen, or polyamines (Desser *et al.* 1983). A germ cell tumour in a young

man, for example, may sometimes be mistaken for a malignant lymphoma. Lactate dehydrogenase elevations are non-specific, although usually elevated in the B-cell lymphomas (Magrath *et al.* 1980, 1984; Csako *et al.* 1982). Other molecules may be present in greater than normal amounts in patients with lymphoma, for example, soluble interleukin-2 receptor (SIL-2-R) (Wagner *et al.* 1987; Pui *et al.* 1988) and beta 2-microglobulin (Hagberg *et al.* 1983). However, their non-specificity (they may also be elevated in a number of benign lymphoid hyperplasias) detracts from their use in diagnosis.

STAGING SYSTEMS AND STAGING PROCEDURES

Staging systems in childhood non-Hodgkin's lymphoma primarily reflect tumour volume, although tumour volume was not the basis for the formulation of such staging systems so that the individual stages do not form a linear progression with respect to increasing volume. There are several systems in common use, but only the most widely used, those of St Jude and the National Cancer Institute, will be described here. The former system is modified from the staging classification for Hodgkin's disease proposed at Ann Arbor, Michigan. It is applicable to all histological types of childhood lymphoma and separates patients with limited stage disease (stage I or II, with one or two masses on one side of the diaphragm or resected intra-abdominal disease) from those with extensive intrathoracic or intra-abdominal disease (stage III) (the meaning of the term 'extensive' is not defined). Patients with bone-marrow infiltration with greater than 5 per cent and less than 25 per cent tumour cells seen on aspirate and patients with involvement of the central nervous system are separated into the worst prognostic group (stage IV) (Table 11). The system used at the National Cancer Institute was originally devised as a staging system for African patients with Burkitt's lymphoma and reflects the rarity of marrow involvement and the high curability (approximately 50 per cent) of patients with central nervous system disease in Ugandan patients in whom, unlike American patients, CNS disease is often

Table 11 Staging systems for childhood non-Hodgkin's lymphoma

Staging system	Stage	Definition
St Jude (non-Hodgkin's lymphoma)	I	Single tumour (extranodal) Single anatomical area (nodal) Excluding mediastinum or abdomen
	II	Single tumour (extranodal) with regional node involvement Primary gastrointestinal tumour with or without involvement of associated mesenteric nodes only, grossly completely resected On same side of diaphragm (a) Two or more nodal areas (b) Two single (extranodal) tumours with or without regional node involvement
	III	On both sides of the diaphragm (a) Two single tumours (extranodal) (b) Two or more nodal areas All primary intrathoracic tumours (mediastinal, pleural, thymic) All extensive primary intra-abdominal disease All primary paraspinal or epidural tumours regardless of other sites
	IV	Any of the above with initial central nervous system or bone-marrow involvement (<25%)
Uganda Cancer Institute (Burkitt's lymphoma)	A	Single extra-abdominal tumour
	AR	Completely resected intra-abdominal tumour without extra-abdominal tumour
	B	Multiple extra-abdominal tumours
	C	Intra-abdominal tumour with or without a single jaw tumour
	D	Intra-abdominal tumour with extra-abdominal sites other than a single jaw tumour

unaccompanied by extensive systemic disease (Haddy *et al.* 1991; Magrath 1991). Therefore, this scheme should not be applied to patients with lymphoblastic lymphoma, nor is it optimal for patients with sporadic small non-cleaved lymphomas. It is useful in so far as it separates patients with tumour confined to the abdomen from patients with more extensive disease and provides a separate stage for patients with essentially completely resected intra-abdominal tumour.

Staging laparotomy is not advocated in patients with non-Hodgkin's lymphoma since chemotherapy is the primary therapeutic modality. Moreover, abdominal involvement is so frequently present in non-lymphoblastic lymphomas (in over 90 per cent) that a high proportion of patients will have had a laparotomy in order to make the diagnosis. In contrast, abdominal involvement is sufficiently uncommon in lymphoblastic lymphomas that laparotomy would be unlikely to reveal tumour.

Staging procedures are designed to determine the sites of disease, extent of involvement, and, where relevant, to evaluate the degree of anatomical compromise of vital structures. Since the primary treatment modality for all stages is chemotherapy, it is not important, unless this would influence the choice of regimen, for example in patients with apparently limited disease, to undertake extensive staging procedures to determine whether there are unsuspected sites of disease. However, because of the rapidity of tumour growth it is important to expedite staging procedures, for delay may permit a significant increase in tumour burden and a theoretical worsening of prognosis. Thus, a series of routine staging procedures should be conducted which can be completed within a day or at most two and which provide a sufficiently comprehensive picture of the sites and extent of disease to determine appropriate therapy (where this is dependent upon sites or extent of disease) and to estimate prognosis. The first component of staging is, of course, the clinical examination, supplemented where appropriate by special procedures such as endoscopic examinations, for example for pharyngeal tumour or upper gastrointestinal bleeding.

Modern imaging methods, including ultrasonography and CT provide adequate means of evaluating disease sites (Shawker *et al.* 1979; Krudy *et al.* 1981; Magrath and Wilson 1990). Ultrasonography has advantages over CT scanning when retroperitoneal fat is minimal (for example, in small children). In general, patients with small non-cleaved cell lymphomas should be routinely evaluated with abdominal CT or ultrasound examination, while patients with lymphoblastic lymphomas should have a CT scan of the thorax. Where resources permit and in patients with large cell lymphomas both thorax and abdomen should be routinely evaluated. A head CT is useful in the evaluation of patients with head and neck disease, especially where there is pharyngeal or sinus involvement, but otherwise is not normally indicated. Gallium scanning provides a useful whole-body screen, particularly for small non-cleaved cell lymphomas which avidly take up the isotope (Harwood *et al.* 1987; Magrath and Wilson 1990) and is also useful for following response (Kaplan 1990). A lymphangiogram is much less useful than in Hodgkin's disease because of the high frequency of extranodal tumour and is infrequently performed. A bone scan is the most sensitive means of detecting bony involvement, but may add nothing to a gallium scan in this regard, at least for the small non-cleaved cell lymphomas. Radionuclide liver and spleen scans also appear to add little to modern CT and ultrasound images and the role of magnetic resonance imaging (MRI) and positron emission tomography is not sufficiently well defined for these imaging techniques to be used routinely. The value of MRI in detecting patchy bone-marrow involvement and intracerebral tumour

undetectable by CT scanning appears to warrant use of this modality where such information is desired or there is a sufficiently high index of suspicion of disease in these sites (Magrath and Wilson 1990). In general, contrast studies of the bowel are not performed in children once the diagnosis of lymphoma has been established. Such studies are time-consuming, uncomfortable, provide little additional information of relevance to treatment, and may carry a risk of bowel perforation in some patients. Contrast radiography may be required, however, in the evaluation of a child presenting with abdominal pain. The value of plain radiography in evaluating specific sites of disease (for example, bone and sinus involvement) and sometimes following progress should not be overlooked.

Peripheral blood, bone-marrow, and cerebrospinal fluid examination are an essential part of staging, although when prophylactic intrathecal drug administration is simultaneously initiated with systemic therapy, the first cerebrospinal fluid examination can be carried out at this time. Bilateral bone-marrow aspirates and biopsies are necessary if the rate of detection of marrow involvement is to be maximized (Haddy *et al.* 1989). Other biopsy procedures (including liver biopsy) are not usually performed unless there are special indications.

Abnormal liver function tests may suggest hepatic involvement, and renal function tests (including assessment of urine output) and measurement of serum uric acid level are essential for determining the presence of uric acid nephropathy as well as the likelihood of the development of a tumour lysis syndrome (see below). Renal function tests are not usually helpful in assessing the presence of renal involvement because of the high likelihood of uric acid nephropathy in patients with very extensive disease. An acceptable list of staging investigations is shown in Table 12.

Although clinical examination and imaging studies are essential for the determination of the sites of disease, quantitative biochemical or immunochemical assays of molecules present in serum, including lactate dehydrogenase, IL-2, and β-microglobulin, may provide simpler and more objective measurements that correlate with tumour volume (Magrath *et al.* 1980, 1984; Wagner *et al.* 1987). For this reason they are particularly valuable in comparing the mean tumour burdens of one series of patients with another. Such measurements should be included in the evaluation of the patient

Table 12 Investigations required for accurate staging

Physical examination

Complete blood count
Liver and renal serum chemistries
Serum lactic dehydrogenase
Serum uric acid
Serum lactate (optional)
Serum IL-2-R (optional)

Chest radiography
Chest CT scan (particularly if chest radiography abnormal or suspiciously abnormal)
Abdominal ultrasonography (include liver/spleen, kidneys, abdomen, pelvis)
⁶⁷Ga scan
Abdominal CT scan (can be waived if ultrasound and gallium tests performed)
Bone scan (optional or if gallium suggests bone involvement)
MRI (research, but may be particularly useful for brain and marrow evaluation)

Bone-marrow examination
Cerebrospinal fluid examination

at initial presentation and, with time, may become an accepted component of stage.

MANAGEMENT
General considerations

The management of a child with non-Hodgkin's lymphoma can be conceptualized as consisting of three parts (Table 13). The most immediate consideration is the need for emergency management, a situation which arises more often in these tumours, which have very high growth fractions and doubling times. Burkitt's lymphoma in Africa, for example, has been estimated to have a potential doubling time as short as 24 h and cutaneous tumours have been observed to double in volume in 3 days (Iverson *et al.* 1972). Life-threatening complications may develop as a consequence of the physical encroachment of tumour masses on vital structures or the sheer volume of tumour present. Airway obstruction may result from pharyngeal or mediastinal masses, superior vena caval obstruction, and limitation of pulmonary volume from intrathoracic masses or massive pleural effusions, cardiac tamponade or arrhythmias from pericardiac tumour or pericardial effusion, paraplegia from epidural tumour, raised intracranial pressure and neurological deficits from intracranial lymphoma, and gastrointestinal bleeding, obstruction of the bowel or renal outflow tract, inferior vena cava, or lymphatic drainage from intra-abdominal tumour. Severe pain may result simply from rapid expansion of tumour growing within a confined space, including the abdomen (particularly when there is massive ascites), breasts, brain, or a limb compartment (uncommon). While venous obstruction of the great veins is relatively common, obstruction of peripheral veins or arteries is rare, but not unknown (for example, from tumour in the popliteal fossa) and occasionally peripheral neuropathy can result from compression of nerves by a mass or from direct infiltration of nerves, particularly nerve roots in the brachial and sacral plexuses (which may also give rise to pain).

Involvement of the bone-marrow can cause anaemia, neutropenia, with a consequent risk of infection, or thrombocytopenia and a risk of bleeding. Large tumour volumes, in addition to the risk of compression of adjacent structures, impose a biochemical burden on the body, particularly the kidney and may give rise to electrolyte or biochemical abnormalities of serious consequence. Rarely, because of the production by tumour cells of molecules with hormone-like activities, hypoglycaemia or hypocalcaemia may lead to a medical emergency. Fever, weight loss, and night sweats are occasionally caused by the tumour itself, rather than by infection, particularly in the case of anaplastic large-cell lymphoma.

Table 13 Evaluation of the child with suspected non-Hodgkin's lymphoma

1. Identify and address problems requiring emergency management
   Airway obstruction or other respiratory compromise
   Cardiac tamponade or arrythmia
   Raised intracranial pressure, paraparesis, etc.
   Superior or inferior caval obstruction
   Renal obstruction or metabolic nephropathy
   Other biochemical abnormalities
   Gastrointestinal obstruction
   Gastrointestinal bleeding
   Thrombocytopenia or neutropenia with fever
2. Confirm diagnosis
3. Initiate specific chemotherapy as rapidly as possible after emergency problems have been controlled

Because of the differences in the patterns of presentation of different types of lymphoma, there is a corresponding tendency for the pattern of complications to be contingent upon histology. Thus, compression of intrathoracic structures is much more likely with lymphoblastic lymphoma than with small non-cleaved lymphoma, while the reverse applies to intra-abdominal complications. Large cell lymphomas, however, may occur in either chest or abdomen and are also more likely to involve limbs than the other major histological types of non-Hodgkin's lymphoma. In addition, because the doubling time of the small non-cleaved lymphomas tends, on average, to be shorter and possibly because of biochemical differences, these tumours are more likely than others to present with electrolyte or biochemical abnormalities.

While immediate interventionary measures may be required in some circumstances (for example, tracheotomy, establishment of diuresis, or haemodialysis), it must be emphasized that all these complications can ultimately be dealt with only by reduction of tumour bulk, so that the initiation of specific therapy as rapidly as possible must always be a primary goal. Inordinate delays serve only to compound the problem. Only the management of the more frequent complications encountered at presentation or those more specific to childhood non-Hodgkin's lymphomas will be described here.

Management of the complications of intrathoracic lymphoma

The most serious complications of mediastinal masses are airway obstruction and cardiac tamponade. Superior vena cava obstruction is not a life-threatening complication, *per se*, although it is often associated with airway obstruction, such that in its presence a careful assessment of airway competence should be made. While clinical symptoms and signs are present with severe airway obstruction, narrowing of the trachea or major bronchi can occur without significant compromise of breathing while at rest. The best way of assessing competence of the major airways is to perform a CT scan of the chest (and neck if indicated).

Superior vena cava obstruction from a wide range of tumours has been traditionally treated with radiation therapy, but in highly chemotherapy-responsive tumours such as lymphoblastic lymphoma irradiation increases toxicity without therapeutic gain. In the event that no symptomatic improvement (or worsening) is observed within a few days of the initiation of specific chemotherapy in patients with large mediastinal masses and serious respiratory compromise, mediastinal irradiation can be considered, but this circumstance is rare indeed and augurs poorly for the long-term outcome. If radiation therapy must be used, relatively low-dose therapy, for example to a total of 1200 cGy, is preferable since radiation does not improve the long-term outcome but may decrease marrow tolerance to chemotherapy and will increase the risk of pulmonary and cardiac toxicity, especially in the presence of anthracyclines.

Cardiac tamponade from pericardial tumour or pericardial effusion is best managed by the rapid institution of specific therapy coupled to pericardial paracentesis, where considered necessary. The insertion of a catheter, suitable for continuous drainage, into the pericardial sac may be appropriate if the reaccumulation of fluid is rapid, but other measures, such as the construction of a pleuropericardial window or pericardiodesis with sclerosing agents, are not recommended because the problem will normally be resolved as soon as tumour regression has been accomplished. Similar considerations apply to the management of massive pleural effusions.

Rarely, antiarrhythmic drugs may be required because of myocardial infiltration or compression.

Management of the complications of intra-abdominal lymphoma

Massive intra-abdominal lymphoma is nearly always of B-cell type and histologically is most often diagnosed as small non-cleaved cell lymphoma. Obstruction of the bowel, ureters, inferior vena cava, or other retroperitoneal veins and lymphatics and intraluminal bleeding or perforation of the bowel from tumour necrosis are the most frequently encountered complications. Intestinal obstruction is most commonly due to intussusception resultant upon the intraluminal projection of a small tumour mass. The latter is a relatively common presentation of non-Hodgkin's lymphoma in children and leads to laparotomy, which both establishes the diagnosis and, in a proportion of patients, also leads to the removal of all apparent tumour, thus adding therapeutic advantage. In patients with gastrointestinal bleeding, surgical intervention should be considered prior to specific treatment since tumour necrosis following chemotherapy is likely to worsen the bleeding considerably. Ureteric obstruction (rarely, urethral obstruction) complicates the management of hyperuricaemia and the acute tumour lysis syndrome, since in both circumstances the major treatment strategy is the establishment of a profound diuresis. While some have used ureteric stents or nephrostomy, such measures are potentially hazardous, since the risk of a perforation of a ureter during placement of a stent or leakage of urine from a nephrostomy (particularly if the tumour is in close proximity) are significant. Haemodialysis until uric acid, electrolytes, urea, and creatinine are approximately normal, followed by immediate initiation of specific chemotherapy and subsequent dialysis as indicated by serum chemistries, is probably a safer course of action.

Venous obstruction within the abdomen is a potential problem from two perspectives. Firstly, intraluminal thrombosis may be present, necessitating consideration of anticoagulation or physical containment of thrombus to prevent pulmonary embolus. Anticoagulation can be hazardous because of the accompanying risk of gastrointestinal bleeding from involvement of the bowel or the presence of thrombocytopenia from bone-marrow involvement or chemotherapy. In addition, anticoagulation by oral drugs is difficult to control when potentially hepatotoxic chemotherapeutic agents (for example, methotrexate) are to be administered, limiting the choice of anticoagulant therapy to heparin. In patients with intra-abdominal lymphoma and venous thrombosis, therefore, anticoagulation is generally not indicated and a preferable means of preventing pulmonary embolus (which is certainly a significant risk) is the emergency placement of an intraluminal device below the renal veins in the inferior vena cava, for example a Hunter–Session balloon or filter (umbrella).

The second problem, which results from intra-abdominal venous or lymphatic obstruction is that the adequate establishment of a diuresis, to deal with associated hyperuricaemia or to avoid the consequences of the tumour lysis syndrome after the initiation of chemotherapy, is hampered by the tendency of fluid to accumulate in the lower limbs. This problem is dealt with in the next section.

Hyperuricaemia and the acute tumour lysis syndrome

The extremely high growth fraction and cell turnover rate of the childhood lymphomas (greater in B-cell than in T-cell neoplasms

(Braylan *et al.* 1978; Murphy *et al.* 1979), while possibly accounting for their high sensitivity to chemotherapy, also leads to the potential for the development of renal complications resulting from the increased solute burden on the kidneys. The likelihood that uric acid nephropathy will occur prior to the commencement of chemotherapy or of the development, immediately after chemotherapy, of the biochemical abnormalities leading ultimately to renal failure (the so-called 'acute tumour lysis syndrome') (Fig. 11), correlates directly with the tumour burden (Cohen *et al.* 1980; Tsokos *et al.* 1981). This syndrome does not occur in patients with completely resected disease.

Whereas it is important to initiate specific therapy as soon as possible, the initiation of chemotherapy in the presence of a markedly elevated uric acid and impaired urinary output would be highly likely to result in the death of the patient, probably from profound hyperkalaemia (Arsenau *et al.* 1973). Therefore, the biochemical abnormalities must be corrected before the initiation of specific therapy. This period of biochemical correction should not exceed 24–48 h at most. Reduction of serum uric acid to normal levels can usually be accomplished within this time by alkaline diuresis and allopurinol administration in all except patients with additional renal compromise, such as ureteric obstruction or, less commonly, massive involvement of the kidneys by tumour. In such circumstances there may be no other alternative than to institute haemodialysis prior to chemotherapy. In this case, chemotherapy should be commenced after the completion of a period of haemodialysis when biochemical parameters are close to normal. Since further dialysis is unlikely to be required for at least a few hours, the possibility of rapidly removing drugs (for example, cyclophosphamide) by dialysis is, in this way, minimized.

In all patients with a high tumour burden it is imperative to maintain a high urine flow (as much as $250 \, cm^3/m^2/h$ in the patients at highest risk) for the first few days after the initiation of chemotherapy to ensure that the high solute burden created by tumour lysis (primarily consisting of phosphates and oxypurines)

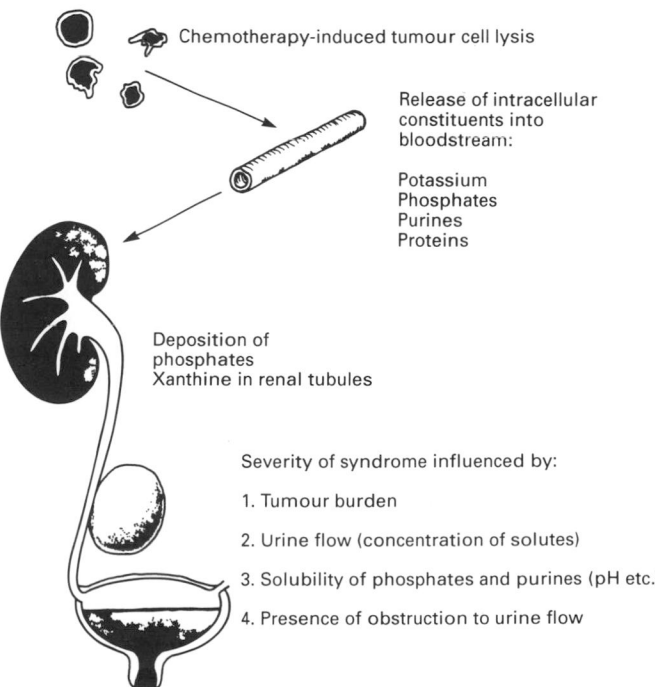

Chemotherapy-induced tumour cell lysis

Release of intracellular constituents into bloodstream:

Potassium
Phosphates
Purines
Proteins

Deposition of phosphates
Xanthine in renal tubules

Severity of syndrome influenced by:

1. Tumour burden

2. Urine flow (concentration of solutes)

3. Solubility of phosphates and purines (pH etc.)

4. Presence of obstruction to urine flow

Fig. 11 Pathogenesis of the tumour cell lysis syndrome and factors which predispose to it.

is accommodated without the onset of hyperkalaemia or acute renal failure. The latter complication is most likely to result from the intratubular deposition of oxypurines and phosphates, a consequence of exceeding their solubility in urine. Because of the relatively poor solubility of phosphates in alkaline urine, it is preferable to maintain the urine pH at about 7 and not to administer bicarbonate during chemotherapy. At this pH, uric acid is some 10–12 times more soluble (solubility is approximately 150 mg/l at pH 5) and xanthine more than twice as soluble (solubility at pH 5 is approximately 50 mg/l) than at pH 5. The solubility of hypoxanthine differs little at either pH (140–150 mg/l). Allopurinol should be given at high dosage (for example, 10 mg/kg), a dose which will ensure that a significant proportion of purine metabolites is excreted as xanthine and hypoxanthine. It is not advisable to prevent uric acid production completely because uric acid is more than ten times more soluble in urine than xanthine and slightly more soluble than hypoxanthine. Therefore, the objective of allopurinol therapy is to increase the total amount of oxypurine that can be excreted in a given volume of urine rather than to prevent uric acid formation.

The acute tumour lysis syndrome was originally recognized because of sudden death occurring as a consequence of hyperkalaemia, which may occur within hours of the initiation of therapy (Arsenau et al. 1973). Therefore, it is important to avoid potassium supplements shortly before and during the first few days of therapy, except in exceptional circumstances. Ideally the patient should be mildly hypokalaemic prior to the commencement of chemotherapy. Hyperkalaemia is most unlikely to occur in the presence of a high urine output and in fact urine flow is the key to the management of the tumour lysis syndrome. As long as a high urine flow can be maintained, other interventions are unlikely to be needed. If this is not the case, rapid progression of biochemical abnormalities will occur, necessitating urgent haemodialysis.

Hypocalcaemia, a consequence of hyperphosphataemia, should not be treated unless symptomatic and intravenous calcium chloride should be given with great caution, if at all, because of the risk of extraosseous calcification in the presence of a high serum phosphate level. Systemic alkalinity increases the possibility of symptomatic hypocalcaemia, including tetany and this is another reason that alkalinization of the urine is recommended only prior to chemotherapy and not during therapy. Rarely, haemodialysis may be required for symptomatic hypocalcaemia.

A problem which can considerably complicate the management of the tumour lysis syndrome is a tendency for fluids to collect in a third space, including serous effusions (more often ascites, but frequently complicated by pleural effusions) or even limb oedema from venous and/or lymphatic obstruction. In such patients vigorous hydration is complicated by weight gain and an inappropriately low urine flow. This situation can usually be managed by the judicious use of diuretics. Vascular pressure monitoring, for example central venous pressure or, preferably, pulmonary wedge venous pressure, is extremely helpful in managing complicated cases of this kind and if an acceptable urine output cannot be maintained under these circumstances, there is no alternative but to haemodialyse. Because of the amount and type of monitoring required, it is preferable to manage patients at high risk for the acute tumour lysis syndrome in a critical care unit.

Management of neurological emergencies

The primary neurological emergencies encountered include paraplegia, cranial nerve palsies, meningeal disease, and intracerebral tumour. Whereas radiation would at one time have been considered

appropriate therapy for each of these problems, this is no longer necessarily the case. There is no reason to presume that tumour will respond more rapidly to radiation than to chemotherapy. In fact, the reverse is usually the case for the small non-cleaved cell lymphomas. Reversal of neurological complications has been observed frequently in African Burkitt's lymphoma (Magrath 1991), when chemotherapy alone has been used and there would appear to be little justification for the use of radiotherapy in the case of the small non-cleaved cell lymphomas, particularly in view of the increase in toxicity that will occur as a consequence. Similar considerations apply to other histologies, although the data are less clear cut and it is likely that many oncologists will feel uncomfortable in refraining from radiation in situations where it has traditionally been administered.

In the small non-cleaved cell lymphomas, there is also no evidence that irradiation is of value in the presence of cerebrospinal fluid malignant pleocytosis (Sariban et al. 1983; Haddy et al. 1991), but the rôle of this modality in the presence of meningeal disease for patients with other histologies is unclear. Radiation is less and less used for the prevention or treatment of CNS disease in view of the efficacy of intrathecally administered drugs and high-dose systemic infusions of S-phase specific agents (Ara-C and methotrexate). Cranial irradiation would normally be given to patients with intracerebral disease because of the possibility of poor penetration of drugs. However, cranial irradiation in association with chemotherapy, particularly systemic and intrathecal methotrexate, is associated with a significant increase in neurotoxicity including leucoencephalopathy (Duffner et al. 1985; Glass et al. 1986; Rejou et al. 1989; Chessells et al. 1990).

Specific therapy: relative rôles of the three major treatment modalities

The primary therapeutic modality for the non-Hodgkin's lymphomas of childhood is chemotherapy, regardless of stage or sites of disease. Justified on the grounds that the non-Hodgkin's lymphomas are generalized diseases, this statement is firmly rooted in empirical clinical experience. Since, for much of the present century, the only effective therapy was radiation (a rare exception being an occasional cure after surgical resection of a small intra-abdominal tumour, for example one that has caused early symptomatology because of small bowel intussusception) there remains, in some quarters, a reluctance to abandon this modality, particularly in patients with limited disease in whom cures have been obtained with radiation alone (sometimes with the addition of single-agent therapy and surgery) (Aur 1971; Glatstein et al. 1974; Nelson et al. 1977). However, the mean survival in a combined analysis of eight published series of children with localized non-Hodgkin's lymphoma, a total of 370 patients, treated with radiation, surgery, and single-agent therapy was 18 per cent (Jenkin et al. 1984). Yet in similar patients treated with combination drug therapy with or without radiation, the cure rate is usually in excess of 90 per cent (Müller-Weihrich et al. 1984; Gadner et al. 1986; Murphy et al. 1986, 1989). Moreover, a randomized trial conducted in the United States has shown no therapeutic advantage, but a significant toxic cost, to the addition of radiation to chemotherapy in patients with localized disease (Link et al. 1990). In patients with extensive disease, radiotherapy can, at best, serve only an ancillary role, for example for testicular involvement (Haddy et al. 1988) or intracerebral tumour. There is no evidence for a beneficial role of irradiating sites of bulk disease; indeed, available data suggest that, as in limited disease, this results in increased toxicity without therapeutic gain (Murphy and Hustu 1980).

While few randomized clinical trials have addressed this point, the excellent results that are now being obtained in all childhood lymphomas with regimens that do not include radiation argue against the need for such studies. In fact, on occasion, randomized trials may even be misleading. For example, several studies have shown that very good overall results in the treatment of lymphoblastic lymphoma involving the mediastinum can be obtained without mediastinal irradiation (Magrath et al. 1984; Camitta et al. 1985; Müller-Weihrich et al. 1985; Gadner et al. 1986). One randomized trial, conducted in the United Kingdom, appears to support the opposite view; however, survival in the group treated without mediastinal irradiation was extremely poor (18 per cent), while survival in patients who received irradiation (over 60 per cent) was no better than that obtained in other trials in which radiation was not used (Mott et al. 1984). Despite this result, therefore, there seems to be no cogent reason for routine irradiation of the mediastinum where effective chemotherapy is given, even in the presence of superior vena caval obstruction (Barriga et al. 1990). In fact, the potential for added toxicity such as oesophagitis and pericarditis, especially if adriamycin, which enhances radiation damage, is included in the treatment regimen, argues against the use of routine mediastinal irradiation for lymphoblastic lymphoma.

Unlike radiation, surgery may have a limited and well-defined role in the childhood non-Hodgkin's lymphomas. Patients with bulky abdominal disease in whom tumour can be completely resected prior to chemotherapy have an excellent prognosis, which, in the past, appeared to be markedly better than that of patients with unresected abdominal disease (Magrath et al. 1974; Janus et al. 1984). However, a prospective randomized study designed to evaluate the rôle of surgery in patients in whom resection of all overt disease is a feasible option has not been carried out. Such a study would be extremely difficult to design in an ethical fashion. In addition, the recent improvement in the outcome of treatment in patients with extensive disease must also be considered, for this suggests that many patients in whom surgery is feasible, because of limited disease, would also enjoy a good prognosis if treated with chemotherapy alone. In practice, this is not as important an issue as might at first appear, for in a high proportion of patients with resectable disease laparotomy is necessary to establish the diagnosis and complete surgical resection may entail a minimal additional risk as well as minimal long-term consequences to the patient. Sometimes surgery may have additional benefits, including the prevention of gastrointestinal bleeding, bowel perforation, and, in rare patients with a large but resectable tumour burden (for example, massive ovarian enlargement), the acute tumour lysis syndrome. Thus, a decision regarding surgery need only be made in a small group of patients in whom a diagnosis has already been made and the sole site is potentially resectable abdominal disease. In such patients it may be reasonable to attempt resection if the chances of success are considered high and the possibility of late consequences of surgery, particularly if chemotherapy could be delayed, considered low.

At the present time, the differentiation between lymphoblastic lymphomas and all other lymphomas is widely used as a useful means of categorizing patients for therapeutic decisions. Most experienced paediatric oncologists treat all non-lymphoblastic lymphomas with regimens used for the therapy of small non-cleaved cell lymphomas. While good results have been obtained with large cell lymphomas treated with protocols used for either lymphoblastic or non-lymphoblastic lymphomas, the heterogeneity of this group

of tumours leaves open the possibility that good and poor risk patients may eventually be defined for a given regimen within this broad histological category (Anderson et al. 1983; Weinstein et al. 1984; Sullivan et al. 1985a; Magrath et al. 1990; Murphy and Magrath 1991).

Principles of chemotherapy of non-Hodgkin's lymphomas

All the childhood non-Hodgkin's lymphomas respond to a wide range of chemotherapeutic agents, no doubt due, in part, to their high growth fraction. This is exemplified by single-agent activities originally obtained in patients with African Burkitt's lymphoma (Table 14). A comparison of early trials using single agents with the results currently obtained with combination chemotherapy leaves no doubt that drug combinations are essential in all these diseases if cures are to be obtained (Burkitt 1967; Arsenau et al. 1975; Wollner et al. 1976; Ziegler 1977; Magrath 1985), but the optimal drug combination and sequence (that is, that which results in the least toxicity and which has the shortest duration), has yet to be determined, although impressive results are currently being reported in pilot studies and by the major paediatric oncology cooperative groups.

In the B-cell lymphomas (small non-cleaved cell lymphomas and most large cell lymphomas) the recent trend, which has resulted in progressively improved results, has been towards the use of short-duration intensive therapy with an emphasis on the repetitive use of alkylating agents (particularly cyclophosphamide) in combination with other drugs (particularly high-dose methotrexate). In order to minimize the possibility of tumour regrowth between cycles, sequential treatment cycles are begun as soon as possible. This tactic has been supported both by the results of empirical trials (Gadner et al. 1976; Murphy and Magrath 1991) and by the suggestion in one protocol (77-04) that the actual dose intensity $(mg/m^2/week)$ of the first two cycles of therapy, but not subsequent cycles, is positively associated with event-free survival (Magrath et al. 1990). The latter analysis suggests that an optimal dose (that which results in the maximal dose intensity) of a small number of highly active agents for only three or four cycles of therapy is likely to give

Table 14 Single-agent activity in African Burkitt's lymphoma[a]

Drug	No.	CR	R	% R
Cyclophosphamide	163	43	132	81
Nitrogen mustard	61	10	44	72
Melphalan	26	8	16	61
Chlorambucil	12	3	10	83
Procarbazine	6	0	0	0
Orthomerphalan	14	?	14	100
BCNU (bischloroethylnitrosourea)	5	0	4	80
Vincristine	21	10	17	81
Vinblastine	2	0	0	—
Methotrexate	45	11	26	58
6-Mercaptopurine	3	0	0	—
Cytosine arabinoside	3	2	2	—
Epipodophyllotoxin	2	2	2	—
Actinomycin D	4	1	4	—
Terephthalanilide	18	1	14	78

No., number of patients tested.
CR, complete response.
R, complete and partial responses.
% R, percentage of patients responding.
[a]See Magrath et al. (1980).

excellent results. The concept of optimal dose implies that the level of toxicity will also be acceptable, since unacceptable toxicity will result in delays in the initiation of therapy cycles and, hence, a reduction in dose intensity. This concept further implies that the use of a large number of drugs is not necessarily beneficial since the employment of less active agents could well result in the lowering of the dose intensity of more active agents. While this may not necessarily result in a worse outcome, the net therapeutic value of the additional agents may be small, while they may add to toxicity or late effects.

In extensive lymphoblastic lymphomas the most widely used therapy today is based on treatment protocols designed for acute lymphoblastic leukaemia, in which alkylating agent therapy has a minor rôle and therapy is prolonged, often for as long as 1.5–3 years (Anderson et al. 1983), although recent trials suggest that regimens containing more alkylating agent may be equally effective (Magrath et al. 1984; Hvizdala 1988). Whether such long durations of therapy are necessary for patients with extensive lymphoblastic lymphoma remains an unanswered question, but patients with limited disease have an excellent prognosis when treated for approximately 6 months (Link et al. 1990).

Optimal therapy for anaplastic large cell (Ki-1-positive) lymphomas is poorly defined in view of the recent recognition of these tumours. Successful therapeutic results in patients with large cell lymphomas not otherwise classified, as well as anaplastic large cell lymphomas, have been reported with stratagems based on treatment designed for either acute lymphoblastic leukaemia or B-cell lymphomas (Anderson and Jenkin 1983; Weinstein et al. 1984; Sullivan et al. 1985a; Murphy and Magrath 1991).

In all types of paediatric non-Hodgkin's lymphomas, prophylaxis against spread of tumour to the central nervous system is an essential component of therapy, the only possible exception to this being patients with minimal disease (for example, completely resected intra-abdominal disease) in whom central nervous system spread is a rare (though not completely unknown) event. Intrathecal therapy with either methotrexate alone or methotrexate and Ara-C is usually the mainstay of such prophylaxis, supplemented, particularly in patients with extensive disease, by intravenous infusions of S-phase specific agents such as methotrexate. Radiation of the cranium or craniospinal axis has never been shown to have an advantage over chemotherapeutic central nervous system prophylactic therapy and in some studies it has been shown to be ineffective (Olweny et al. 1977; Gasparini et al. 1981). Moreover, it is associated with significant toxicity, including intellectual impairment (Harten et al. 1984; Rowland et al. 1984; Duffner et al. 1985; Clayton et al. 1987; Said et al. 1989), which is likely to be greater in patients who receive high-dose infusions of Ara-C or methotrexate. Thus, few would advocate cranial radiation as routine prophylaxis against central nervous system spread in the paediatric lymphomas.

In view of the success of some salvage regimens of very high intensity, even when only a single therapy cycle is used in conjunction with bone-marrow transplantation, it has been questioned as to whether such an approach used after the induction of remission might provide an effective stratagem for high-risk patients regardless of histology. The disadvantages of this approach are the limited availability of matched allogeneic donors, the theoretical risk of reinfusion of the patient's own tumour cells if autologous marrow is used, and the specialized facilities and staff required to conduct such an intensive and potentially toxic treatment approach optimally. Further, results in recent years of more standard chemotherapy regimens, even in patients in the highest risk categories (bone-marrow and central nervous system involvement

at presentation) have improved to the point that marrow transplant regimens as part of primary therapy would appear to be unnecessary (Murphy and Magrath 1991).

CHEMOTHERAPY REGIMENS
Chemotherapy of small non-cleaved cell lymphomas

It has clearly been shown in several different studies that treatment protocols based upon the principles shown to be effective for acute lymphoblastic leukaemia, such as the LSA_2L_2, the BFM (Berlin–Frankfurt–Münster) 1976–1981, or the APO (adriamycin–prednisone–oncovin) regimens, are suboptimal for the treatment of small non-cleaved cell lymphomas (Anderson et al. 1983; Weinstein et al. 1984; Müller-Weihrich et al. 1985). Even patients who present with a leukaemic syndrome, but have a true B-cell acute leukaemia (that is, a small non-cleaved cell neoplasm in the leukaemic phase) have a poor prognosis with conventional therapy for acute lymphoblastic leukaemia and have a much better prognosis when treated with a protocol designed for small non-cleaved cell lymphoma (Murphy and Magrath 1991).

Several protocols utilizing cyclical cyclophosphamide combinations coupled with intermediate or high-dose methotrexate (Figs 12–16), have been shown to be highly effective for all patients with non-lymphoblastic lymphomas, although patients with bone-marrow and/or central nervous system involvement at presentation have generally had a poor prognosis. With these protocols, overall survival rates of 50–75 per cent have been reported (Table 15) (Anderson et al. 1983; Magrath et al. 1984; Müller-Weihrich et al. 1985, 1987; Gadner et al. 1986; Murphy et al. 1986; Patte et al. 1986; Murphy and Magrath 1991; Patte et al. 1991). Because of differences in the patient populations with regard to age (for example, the median age of the National Cancer Institute protocol is twice that of the French Society of Paediatric Oncology (SFOP) and BFM protocols), tumour burden, etc. (recognized and unrecognized), it is not clear that any one of these protocols is better than another. For the purposes of comparing such series, a more useful indicator than stage might be a more direct measure of tumour burden such as lactic dehydrogenase (LDH) or SIL-2R. For example, Fig. 17 shows a comparison of the results of the Total Therapy B and 77-04 protocols by LDH. When compared in this way, the results are remarkably similar, although the overall results of the Total B Therapy appeared to be better. Particular emphasis is currently being placed upon improvement of the treatment results in patients with very extensive tumour, particularly those with bone-marrow and cerebrospinal fluid involvement. The results of recent protocols in the United States, France, and Germany, focusing on such patients, appear to be excellent (that is, in the range of 70–90 per cent disease-free survival) (Murphy and Magrath 1991) and there is little doubt that this represents genuine improvement.

All reported successful protocols include cyclophosphamide in doses of at least 1 g/m^2 and either high- or intermediate-dose methotrexate as well as intrathecal methotrexate and, often, intrathecal Ara-C. Most also include an anthracycline (exceptions are the early Children's Cancer Study Group COMP protocol (Anderson et al. 1983) and a protocol used at the MD Anderson Hospital (Sullivan and Ramirez 1985)). The addition of daunomycin to the COMP protocol has been examined in a randomized study conducted by the Children's Cancer Study Group. Preliminary results do not demonstrate a difference between the two arms of this study, although the result can only be applied to the relatively

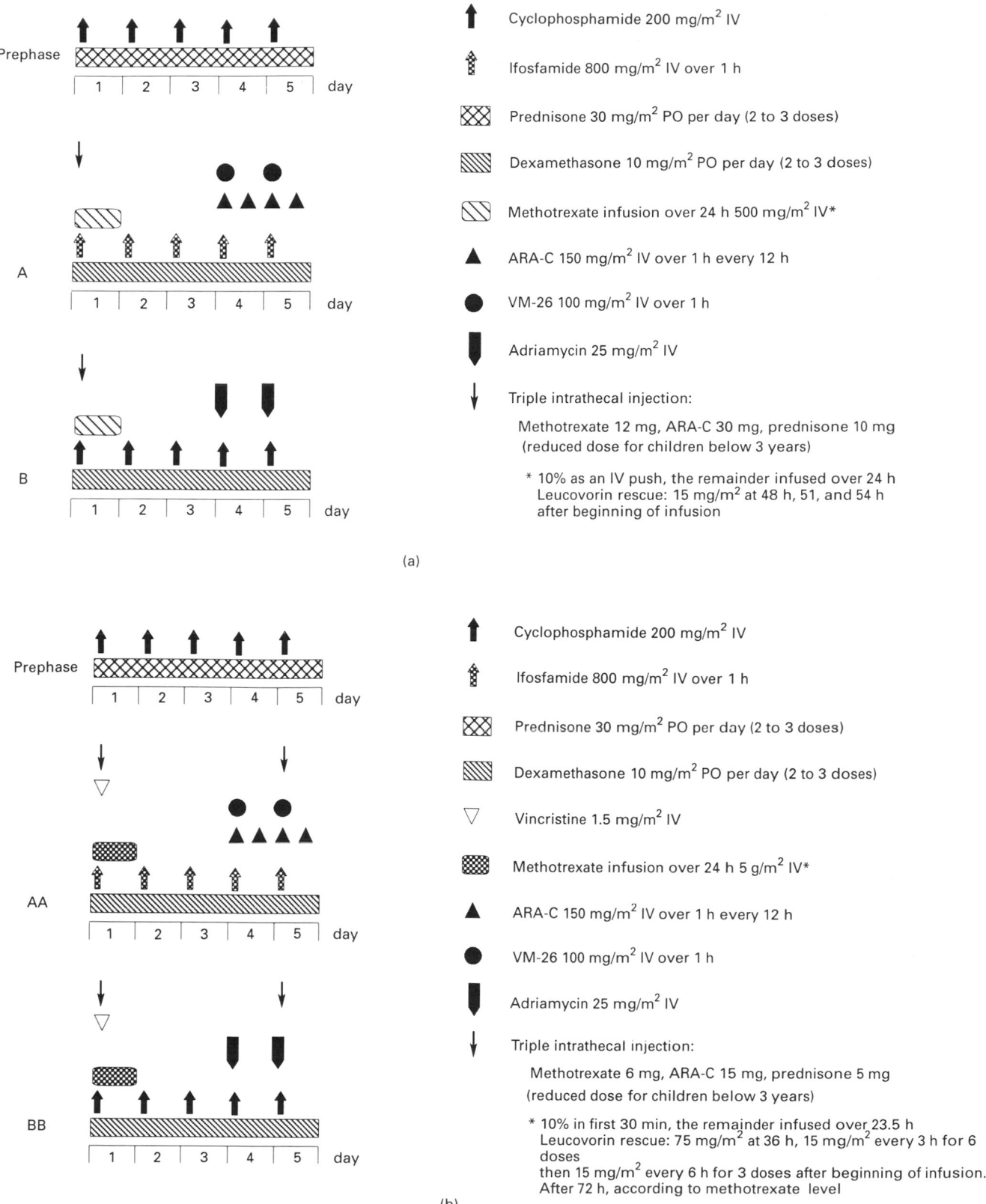

Fig. 12 The BFM protocol 86 for B-cell lymphomas. The schema for administration of initial cytoreductive therapy (V), (a) blocks A and B, for patients without bone-marrow involvement and (b) blocks AA and BB for patients with bone-marrow involvement are shown. A total of four therapy cycles, two each of A and B or AA and BB, are administered after the pre-phase. This protocol is a successor to the 83 protocol and differs primarily with regard to the substitution of ifosfamide for cyclophosphamide in blocks A and AA, the addition of dexamethazone to all blocks, the addition of vincristine to blocks AA and BB, triple intrathecal drugs instead of methotrexate, and changes in the doses of VM26 and Ara-C. Over three hundred children have been treated with excellent results, but at the time of preparation, data have only been presented orally. (Published with the permission of Dr H. Rhiem.)

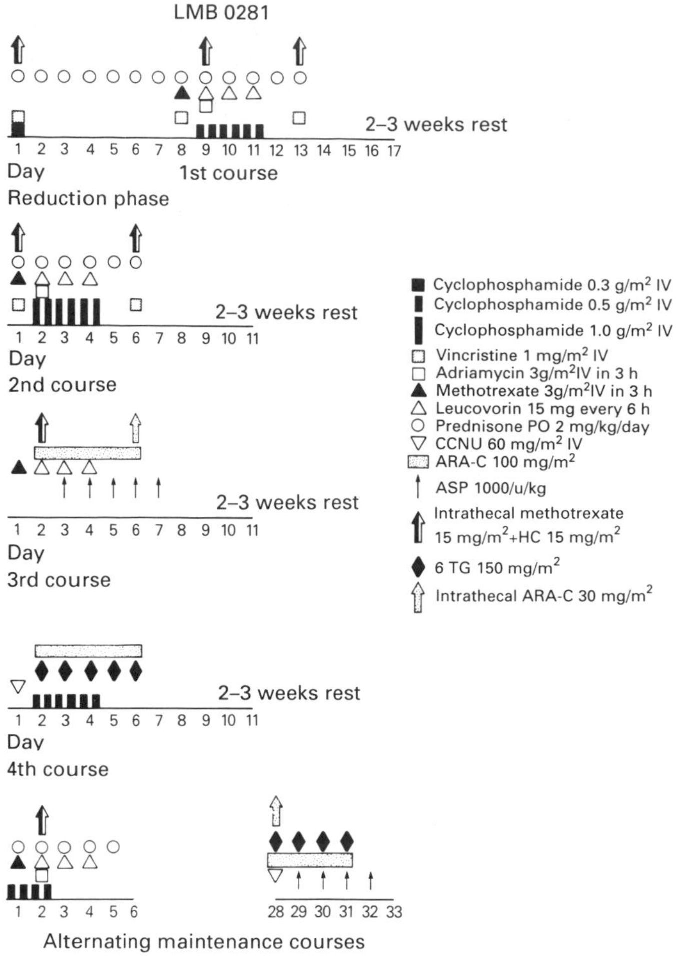

LMB 0281

Day
1st course
Reduction phase

2–3 weeks rest

Day
2nd course

2–3 weeks rest

Day
3rd course

2–3 weeks rest

Day
4th course

2–3 weeks rest

Alternating maintenance courses

■ Cyclophosphamide 0.3 g/m² IV
▮ Cyclophosphamide 0.5 g/m² IV
▮ Cyclophosphamide 1.0 g/m² IV
□ Vincristine 1 mg/m² IV
▢ Adriamycin 3g/m²IV in 3 h
▲ Methotrexate 3g/m²IV in 3 h
△ Leucovorin 15 mg every 6 h
○ Prednisone PO 2 mg/kg/day
▽ CCNU 60 mg/m² IV
▨ ARA-C 100 mg/m²
↑ ASP 1000/u/kg
⇑ Intrathecal methotrexate
  15 mg/m²+HC 15 mg/m²
◆ 6 TG 150 mg/m²
⇧ Intrathecal ARA-C 30 mg/m²

Day
Induction

Day
Induction

Day
Maintenance

Repeat every 28 days

■ Cyclophosphamide 1.2 gm/m² IV (induction), 1.0 g/m²
  (maintenance)
▨ Vincristine 2.0 mg/m² IV (induction),
  1.5 mg/m² (maintenance), maximum 2.0 mg
▲ Methotrexate 300 mg/m² IV (60% push, 40% 4 h infusion)
○ Prednisone 60 mg/m² PO (maximum 60 mg) in 4 divided doses
↑ Intrathecal methotrexate 6.25 mg/m² Omit first maintenance
  cycle

Total duration 18 months from day 1

Fig. 13 The LMB-02 protocol of the SFOP for stage I and II B-cell lymphomas (large nasopharyngeal primaries in stage II are included). Cyclophosphamide is given at the doses shown daily in two fractions. Maintenance courses are given monthly. During maintenance Ara-C is given as two subcutaneous fractions, otherwise it is given as a continuous intravenous infusion. Schema prepared from information in Patte *et al.* (1986).

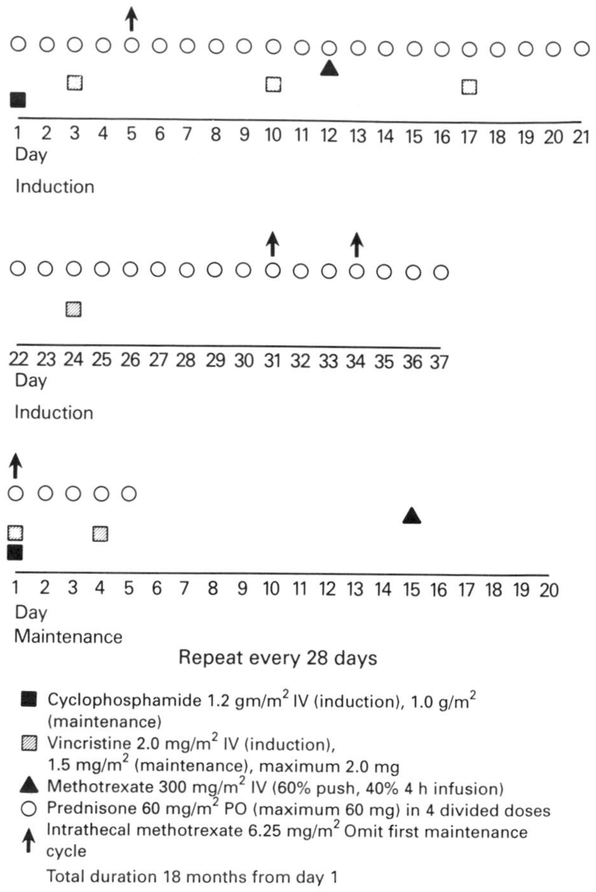

Fig. 14 The COMP protocol used by the CCG. This protocol includes radiation to sites of bulk disease. Schema prepared according to information provided by Anderson *et al.* (1983).

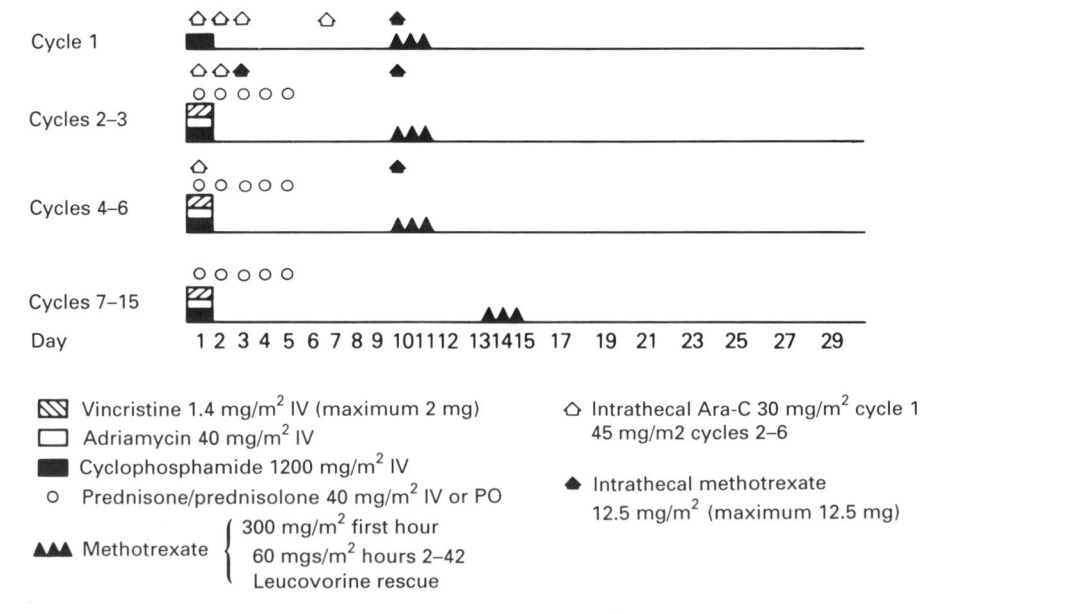

Cycle 1

Cycles 2–3

Cycles 4–6

Cycles 7–15

Day   1 2 3 4 5 6 7 8 9 101112 131415 17 19 21 23 25 27 29

▧ Vincristine 1.4 mg/m² IV (maximum 2 mg)
□ Adriamycin 40 mg/m² IV
■ Cyclophosphamide 1200 mg/m² IV
○ Prednisone/prednisolone 40 mg/m² IV or PO
▲▲▲ Methotrexate { 300 mg/m² first hour
                   60 mgs/m² hours 2–42
                   Leucovorine rescue

△ Intrathecal Ara-C 30 mg/m² cycle 1
  45 mg/m2 cycles 2–6

◆ Intrathecal methotrexate
  12.5 mg/m² (maximum 12.5 mg)

Cycles commence as soon as granulocytes are over 1500/mm³ (or day 28 cycles 7–15)

Fig. 15 The 7704 protocol of the National Cancer Institute. Radiation is not routinely included.

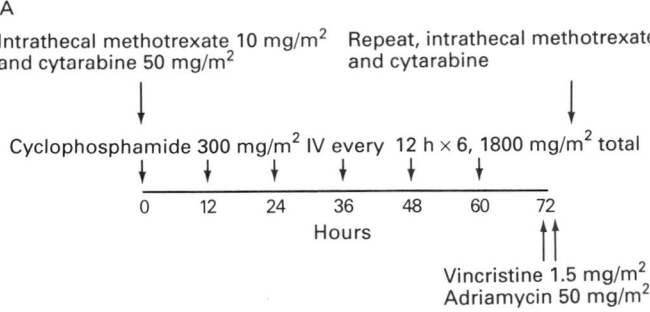

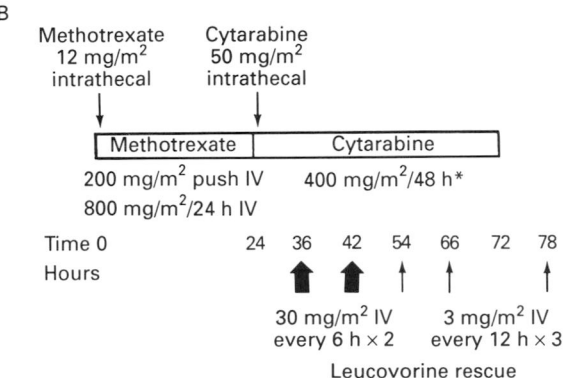

*Escalate succeeding courses:

800 mg/m²/48 h
1600 mg/m²/48 h
3200 mg/m²/48 h

Fig. 16 The Total Therapy B protocol used at St Jude Hospital. Successive cycles (A followed by B) are given as soon as haemopoietic recovery (18–21 days) has occurred to a total of four cycles each of A and B, 5–6 months is required for completion. In succeeding courses after the first, the second IT treatment in cycle A is omitted and the B infusion dose of Ara-C in cycle B is escalated to a total of 3200 mg/m². (Reproduced with permission from Murphy et al. (1986).)

small amount of daunomycin used in this protocol (G. Reaman, personal communication). Additional drugs included in regimens used for high-risk patients include epipodophyllotoxins, high-dose Ara-C, cisplatin and ifosfamide (Murphy and Magrath 1991; Gasparini et al. 1993).

Evaluation of the results of treatment is considerably assisted in the small non-cleaved cell lymphomas because relapse essentially never occurs beyond a year after the initiation of therapy. Thus, patients who remain in their first disease-free remission at this time can be considered cured or to have achieved 'long-term' disease-free survival. The term 'event-free survival' used below implies freedom from progression, so that patients who do not achieve disease-free status rather than only patients who achieve complete remission are included in survival curves of this kind.

Patients with limited disease, that is, localized or completely resected intra-abdominal disease (stages I and II, St Jude and stages A and AR, National Cancer Institute) have an excellent prognosis (at least a 90 per cent cure rate with the most effective current regimens). The primary therapeutic question in such patients is how little treatment can be given without reducing the currently achievable excellent survival rates. There is good evidence that only a few months of therapy with an appropriate combination regimen is necessary. For example, the Children's Cancer Study Group conducted a randomized clinical trial in such patients that demonstrated that 6 months is not inferior to 18 months of therapy (Meadows et al. 1989). In the former National Cancer Institute protocol 77-04 only six cycles of therapy were routinely given for stage I/II or A/AR patients (Magrath et al. 1984) and although the long-term survival rate in patients with completely resected abdominal disease or a single extra-abdominal mass was 85 per cent in this study, a number of patients with very extensive, but resected, intra-abdominal disease were included. When such patients are excluded from the group of patients with limited disease, the results are in excess of 90 per cent long-term survival. Retrospective analysis of received dose intensity of the National Cancer Institute 77-04 protocol and the results obtained by Sullivan and Ramirez (1985) suggest that it may be possible to treat such patients with

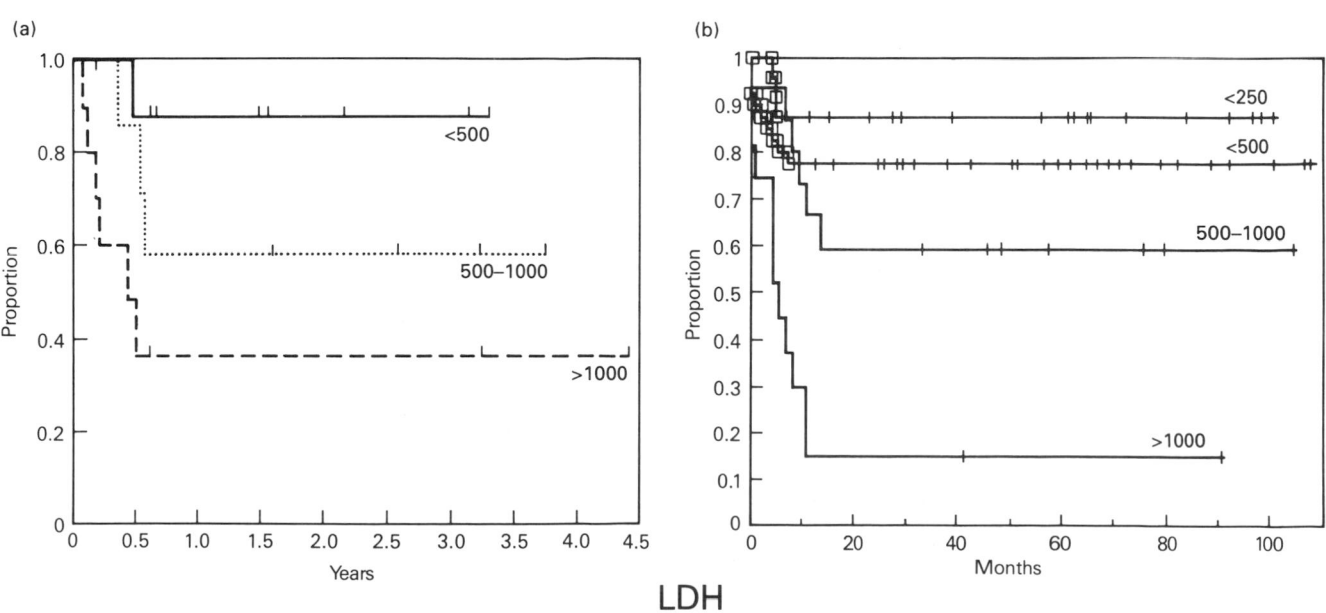

Fig. 17 Comparison of (a) Total Therapy B protocol from St Jude with (b) the 77-04 protocol when failure-free survival is plotted according to the lactic dehydrogenase level. (Reproduced with permission from Murphy et al. (1986).)

Table 15 Failure-free survival rates in childhood non-Hodgkin's lymphoma

Protocol	Stage[a]	No of patients	Failure-free survival (%)	Median follow-up (months)	Reference
Lymphoblastic lymphoma					
LSA$_2$L$_2$ (POG-7615)	I–III	29	55[b]	48	Sullivan et al. (1985)
	IV <25%	12	58	48	
	IV >25%	8	13	48	
LSA$_2$L$_2$ (CCG-551)	III	24	78[b]	>18	Anderson et al. (1983)
	IV[c]	7	71	>18	
BMF 75/81[d]	III/IV[c]	42	78	>48	Müller-Weihrich et al. (1987)
NCI 7704[e]	III	12	70	48	Magrath et al. (1984)
	IV[f]	6	16	48	
Non-lymphoblastic lymphoma					
COMP (CCG-551)	III	32	62	>18	Anderson et al. (1983)
	IV	6	33	>18	
NCI 7704[e]	III	38	60	48	Magrath et al. (1984)
	IV	9	28	48	
BMF 81/86[g]	III	75	73	21	Müller-Weihrich et al. (1987)
	IV	15	57[h]	21	
LMB-0281	III	167	80	38	Patte et al. (1991)
	IV	34	68[h]	38	
LMB-84[i]	III	126	74	2–14	Patte et al. (1986)
	IV[j]	34	65	2–14	
Total B	III	17	81	24	Murphy et al. (1986)
	IV	12	17	24	

[a]St Jude staging system except that stage IV includes patients with any degree of bone-marrow involvement unless otherwise stated
[b]At 24 months (actuarial estimate).
[c]Less than 25 per cent blasts in the bone-marrow.
[d]Non B-cell.
[e]Updated information
[f]All except two patients had less than 25 per cent blasts in the marrow. The surviving patient had central nervous system disease without bone-marrow involvement.
[g]Combined trials BFM 81/83 and 83/86.
[h]Includes patients with acute B-cell leukaemia.
[i]Patients with central nervous system disease are not included. There is a randomization between five and eight cycles of therapy. Preliminary information shows no difference between the two arms.
[j]Excluding patients with central nervous system disease.

cyclophosphamide and methotrexate alone for as few as two or three cycles without detriment to the results (Fig. 18) and currently patients with limited disease receive only three cycles of therapy at the National Cancer Institute, taking approximately 9 weeks to deliver. This approach is supported by the results of other empirical clinical trials. In the BFM protocols 81/83 and 83/86 (Fig. 12), for example, patients with limited disease received only 8 weeks and 6 weeks of therapy, respectively, yet achieved survival in excess of 90 per cent (Müller-Weihrich et al. 1984, 1985; Gadner et al. 1986). Thus, while the optimal duration of a treatment protocol also depends upon its component drugs and schedule, there seems little doubt that therapy durations of longer than two or three cycles (requiring 6–10 weeks for delivery) are excessive for patients with limited disease treated when reasonably intensive cyclophosphamide/methotrexate-containing regimens are used.

Because limited disease was one of the few circumstances in which radiation therapy has been curative in the past, albeit in little more than a third of patients, some paediatric oncologists have been reluctant to abandon this modality in such patients. This prompted the Pediatric Oncology Group to conduct a randomized study in which the role of radiation in the therapy of patients with localized tumour was examined (Link et al. 1990). The results demonstrated no difference in event-free survival between the two study arms and were similar to those obtained in protocols which included local irradiation, such as the first Children's Cancer Study Group trial

and the BFM 81/83 trial (Anderson et al. 1983; Müller-Weihrich 1985), as well as those that did not, including the SFOP, National Cancer Institute and later BFM trials (Magrath et al. 1984; Müller-Weihrich et al. 1985; Murphy et al. 1986; Patte et al. 1986, 1991). On the basis of these results it must now be concluded that in patients with limited disease radiation adds no therapeutic benefit to a well-designed chemotherapy protocol but does have a toxic cost.

Until recently, patients with extensive disease have had a significantly worse prognosis than patients with localized disease. For example, patients with unresectable abdominal disease without bone-marrow or central nervous system involvement (the majority of patients) have an expectancy of cure which is between 60 and 80 per cent in all major protocols reported prior to 1986 (Magrath et al. 1984; Müller-Weihrich et al. 1985; Gadner et al. 1986; Murphy et al. 1986; Patte et al. 1986) and 80–90 per cent in protocols reported since 1986 (Patte et al. 1991; Riehm, personal communication) (see Table 15). Until very recently, patients with bone-marrow involvement have tended to have a poor prognosis, ranging between 10 and 40 per cent prolonged survival in most reported studies (Magrath et al. 1984; Müller-Weihrich et al. 1985; Gadner et al. 1986; Murphy et al. 1986). In the SFOP LMB-0281 protocol (Fig. 13) 16 out of 21 (76 per cent) patients with bone-marrow disease (but without central nervous system involvement) achieved long-term survival (Patte et al. 1986; Vannier et al. 1988). No difference was apparent between patients with less or more than

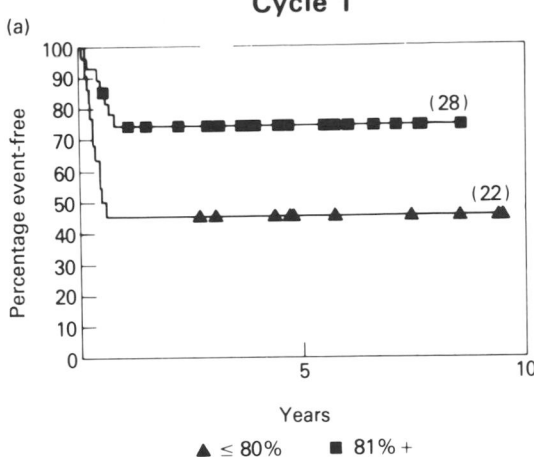

Cycle 1

(a)

▲ ≤ 80%   ■ 81% +

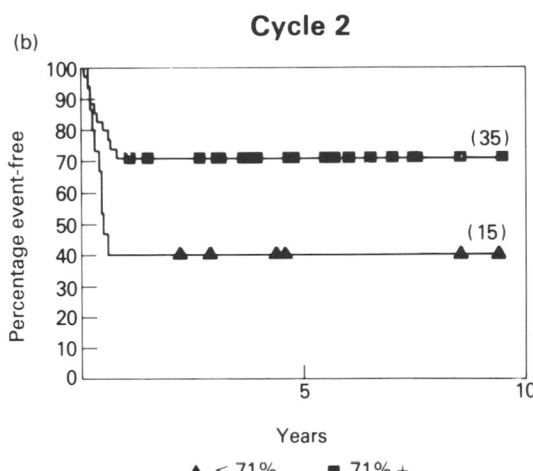

Cycle 2

(b)

▲ ≤ 71%   ■ 71% +

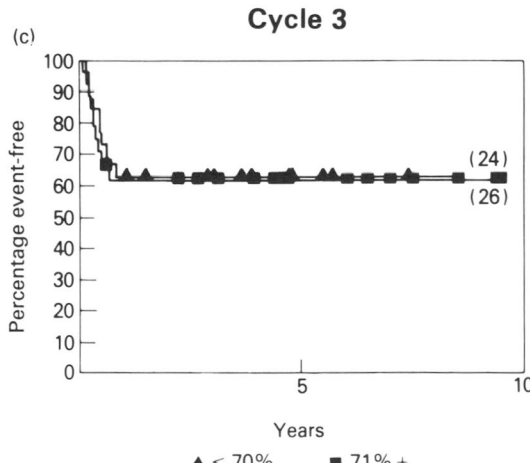

Cycle 3

(c)

▲ ≤ 70%   ■ 71% +

Fig. 18 Received dose intensity of methotrexate and cyclophosphamide combined as a function of event-free survival in protocol 77-04. A highly significant difference between patients with higher dose intensities was observed in cycles 1 ($p_2 = 0.022$) and 2 ($p_2 = 0.028$), but not in subsequent cycles.

25 per cent of tumour cells in the bone-marrow, although patients with central nervous system disease had a poor prognosis (19 per cent disease free at 2 years).

Using the same protocol, investigators in Lyon also obtained excellent results, but reported that patients with extensive

multiorgan involvement in the abdomen (often with additional disease outside the abdomen) had a poor outcome; less than 40 per cent achieved long-term disease-free survival (Philip *et al.* 1987). This is consistent with observations that tumour burden is one of the most important prognostic determinants (Magrath *et al.* 1980, 1984) and also suggests that many patients with bone-marrow disease have a lower tumour burden than some patients with extensive abdominal disease. Thus, the apparent advantage of the LMB-02 protocol could reflect differences in the patient series rather than a superior drug regimen.

It is also possible that patients with central nervous system disease have a worse prognosis, not because of the difficulty of treatment, although the limitation in the number of drugs that either cross the blood–brain barrier or can be given intrathecally certainly poses a problem in this regard, but because it is associated with extensive systemic disease. For example, it has been reported that in patients with equally extensive tumour burdens, as measured by the serum LDH level, the outcome of treatment is similar regardless of whether the central nervous system is involved or not (Sariban *et al.* 1983). This hypothesis, although contrary to popular dogma, is supported by the fact that in African patients with Burkitt's lymphoma, in whom central nervous system disease is much more often associated with limited systemic disease, a relatively high proportion (approximately 50 per cent) can be cured when treated with intrathecal and systemic chemotherapy, even when central nervous system disease presents as localized recurrence (Ziegler *et al.* 1979; Magrath 1991).

In view of these considerations, the approach advocated by some, following the induction of remission in patients with central nervous system disease at presentation with an autologous bone-marrow transplant, makes sense, although the advantage over more conventional therapy has not been shown and there is no evidence that the regimens used in autologous bone-marrow transplantation are superior to those used without transplantation; indeed, the reverse could be true (Philip *et al.* 1987). Most investigators have chosen to explore the benefit of adding agents to more conventional regimens. Ifosfamide and epipodophyllotoxin, both agents that have been shown to be effective in patients with recurrent disease (Gentet *et al.* 1990; Magrath *et al.* 1991) (Ara-C and VM26 have for long been incorporated into the BFM protocols (Müller-Weihrich *et al.* 1984, 1985)), and the use of additional infusions of high-dose S-phase specific agents (Murphy and Magrath 1991) appear to have resulted in improved survival rates (Patte *et al.* 1991). Both high-dose methotrexate and Ara-C are active in children with relapsed B-cell lymphomas and are effective against central nervous system disease (Jones and Ettinger 1985; Murphy and Magrath 1991), so that their use in patients with extensive disease, including central nervous system involvement is logical. Recent results reported by SFOP support the approach for increasing the dose of methotrexate to 8 g/m² and adding high dose Ara-C to the LMB-02 protocol has resulted in improvement in the outcome of patients with central nervous system disease (a 72 per cent event-free survival rate was recently reported in a small group of patients), whether or not the bone marrow is involved (Murphy and Magrath 1991).

The most recently reported regimens appear to have resulted in improvements in overall survival to 80–90 per cent such that focus is shifting from obtaining higher cure rates to maintaining presently high cure rates but reducing the toxic costs. The recent regimens may include components that are unnecessary and add to toxicity without contributing therapeutic benefit. This may well apply to the central nervous system irradiation used in the SFOP protocol, for some toxicity was encountered in the short-term and the combination of high-dose Ara-C and methotrexate with cranial irradiation could well give rise to serious long-term neurological or psychological sequelae. Even in the recently reported Pediatric Oncology Group protocol, in which radiation was not included, an unacceptably high degree of neurotoxicity (20–30 per cent) was encountered (Murphy and Magrath 1991). In this regard, the observation that the activation of Ara-C to Ara-CTP by kinases is saturable, particularly the first step which is catalysed by deoxycytidine kinase, is relevant to the optimal dose of Ara-C. Too high an infusion rate will have no advantage but a distinct disadvantage with respect to toxicity.

Putting aside these considerations of toxicity and optimalization of regimens, the most recent results in children with small non-cleaved cell lymphomas convey the exciting message that the majority of such patients, including those with stage IV disease, can now be cured by application of a small number of intensive therapy cycles coupled with effective central nervous system prophylaxis.

Chemotherapy of lymphoblastic lymphomas

The most widely used chemotherapy regimens for lymphoblastic lymphoma are based upon protocols designed for acute lymphoblastic leukaemia (Pichler et al. 1982; Anderson et al. 1983; Duque-Hammershaimb et al. 1983; Weinstein et al. 1983; Bogusawska et al. 1984; Sullivan et al. 1985a), but not all such protocols are equally satisfactory. The St Jude Study VIII protocol,

for example, produced very poor results in lymphoblastic lymphoma, with only 10 per cent of patients surviving at 2 years (Murphy 1977). Much more successful protocols are the German BFM protocols 75/81 and 81/83 (Fig. 19) (Müller-Weihrich et al. 1985), intensive protocols which have produced some of the best results in the world for acute lymphoblastic leukaemia and are equally successful regardless of the phenotype of the leukaemic cells and the LSA_2L_2 protocol (Fig. 20) designed at the Memorial Sloan-Kettering Cancer Research Institute (Wollner et al. 1976; Anderson et al. 1983; Sullivan et al. 1985a). Patients with lymphoblastic lymphoma treated with either protocol have an overall expected long-term survival of 60–80 per cent for extensive disease and 90 per cent or more with limited disease.

These protocols are presumably more effective than the St Jude Study VIII because they contain additional drugs. It seems probable that anthracyclines are an important component of drug regimens designed for the treatment of lymphoblastic lymphoma, since the majority of effective regimens reported to date have included either adriamycin or daunorubicin, while the unsuccessful Study VIII did not. However, it may be possible to substitute alternative drugs for anthracyclines. For example, a report from St Jude, in which Ara-C and VM-26 were added to a standard acute lymphoblastic leukaemia regimen, described a predicted disease-free survival at 4 years of 73 per cent (Dahl et al. 1985). The 23 patients in the study had a median follow-up of 30 months and clearly further follow-up and additional patients will need to be treated before this protocol can be considered an alternative to standard therapy

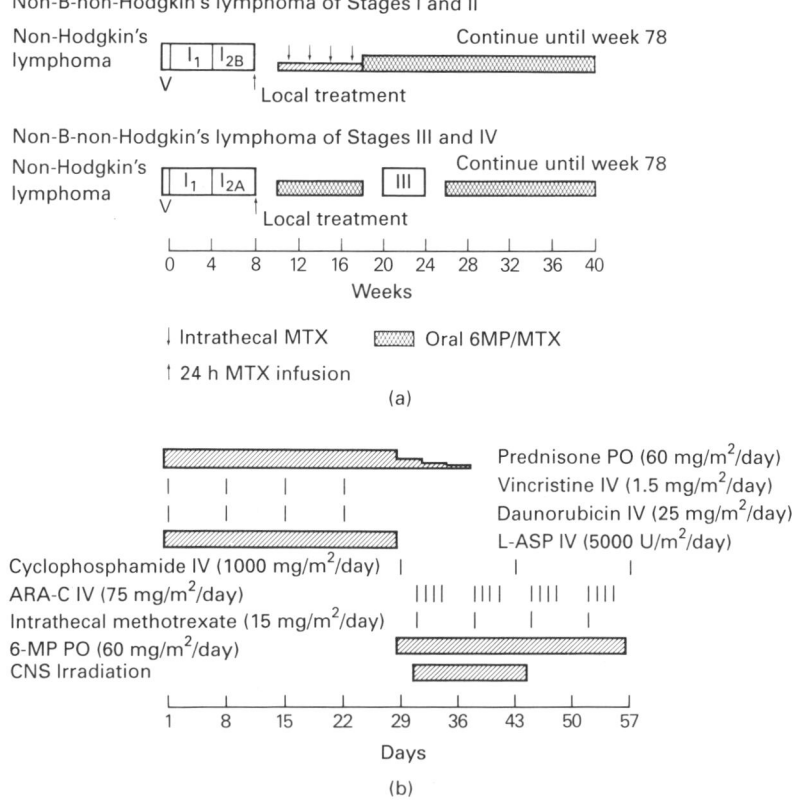

Fig. 19 (a) The BFM therapy schema (BFM NHL 1981/3) for patients with lymphoblastic (non-B) lymphomas: V, cytoreductive phase with cyclophosphamide and prednisone; I, protocol I (subscripts designate protocol phase; central nervous system irradiation is given during phase 2A only); III, Protocol III, reinduction therapy similar to protocol I; down arrows, intrathecal methotrexate (under 1 year, 6 mg; 1–2 years, 8 mg; 2–3 years, 10 mg; over 3 years, 12 mg) up arrows, 24 h infusion of MTX (500 mg/m²) with leucovorine rescue after 48 h; shaded area, oral 6-MP and MTX (thymic tumours were only irradiated in the presence of residual tumour after protocol I). (b) Schema of protocol I. (Reproduced with permission from Müller-Weihrich et al. (1985).)

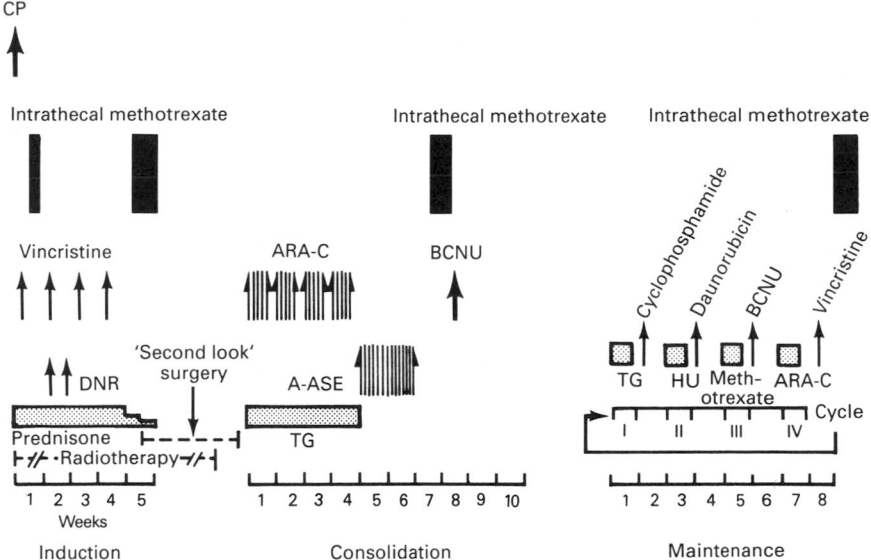

Fig. 20 LSA$_2$L$_2$ protocol: this figure shows the modified version used by the Pediatric Oncology Group (originally Southwestern Oncology Group). (Reproduced with permission from Sullivan *et al.* (1985*a*).)

approaches. Some protocols, for example the successful BFM protocols, already include both VM26 and an anthracycline.

Based on the results of the Children's Cancer Study Group randomized study, in which it was shown that the COMP regimen (cyclophosphamide, vincristine, methotrexate, and prednisone) was less effective for lymphoblastic lymphoma than the LSA$_2$L$_2$ regimen (Fig. 21) (Anderson *et al.* 1983), it has been widely accepted that patients with lymphoblastic lymphomas do poorly unless treated with an acute lymphoblastic leukaemia-like regimen. However, NCI Protocol 77-04, (Magrath *et al.* 1984) appears to provide equally effective therapy for patients with lymphoblastic lymphoma without bone-marrow involvement, although the number of patients studied is small (21). A second protocol which includes repeated doses of cyclophosphamide (A-COP) has also been shown by the Pediatric Oncology Group to be as successful, in their hands, as LSA$_2$L$_2$ (Hvizdala *et al.* 1988).

Other important issues which have been little studied include the duration of therapy and the impact of bone-marrow involvement on treatment results. Clearly, in some protocols, for example the BFM protocols in which excellent results are also obtained in patients with T-cell acute lymphoblastic leukaemia, the presence of bone-marrow involvement does not appear to be a prognostic factor. When patients are treated according to other protocols, however, bone-marrow involvement at presentation appears to be indicative of a poor outcome (Magrath *et al.* 1984), even when the protocol is designed for acute lymphoblastic leukaemia (Weinstein *et al.* 1983).

Patients with lymphoblastic lymphoma who have not relapsed after some 30 months from the start of treatment have a very high probability of remaining in complete remission and therefore it is reasonable to consider patients with a complete remission duration of 3 years or more as cured.

Patients with limited disease (stage I or II in the St Jude system) have an excellent long-term survival; approximately 90 per cent in all recent protocols. In the Children's Cancer Study Group study, early results seemed to indicate that the COMP and LSA$_2$L$_2$ regimens were equally effective. More recent analysis suggests a slight survival advantage for LSA$_2$L$_2$ (Meadows *et al.* 1989). As

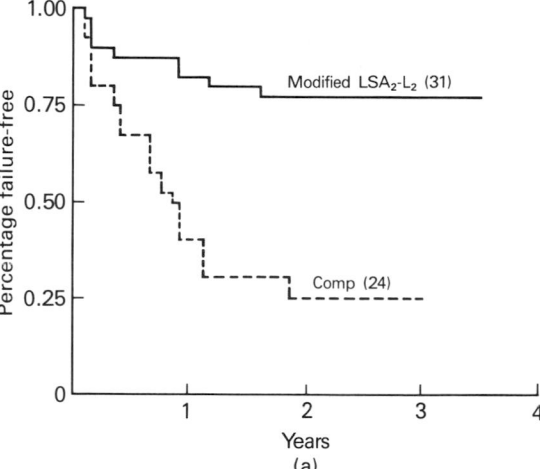

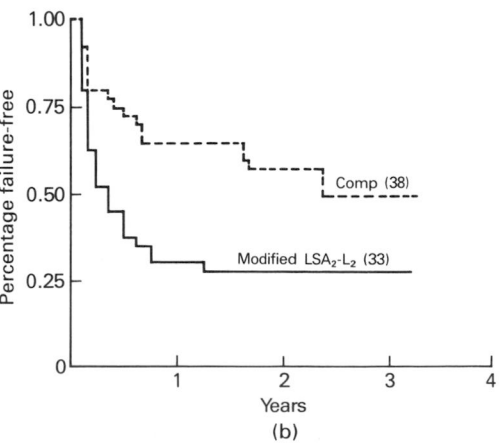

Fig. 21 Failure-free survival of patients with (a) extensive lymphoblastic lymphoma and (b) non-lymphoblastic lymphoma treated according to the LSA$_2$L$_2$ and COMP protocols. (Reproduced with permission from Anderson *et al.* (1983).)

is the case for the small non-cleaved cell lymphomas, radiation appears to add toxicity but has no survival advantage compared with chemotherapy alone in these patients (Link *et al.* 1990). From the results of these trials, it appears that most patients with limited lymphoblastic lymphoma can be effectively treated with approximately 8 months of therapy.

Patients with extensive disease can be divided into two major categories: those with extensive intrathoracic tumour, including a mediastinal mass, with or without pleural effusion and regional lymphadenopathy and those who have widely disseminated disease usually, but not always, including bone-marrow involvement but with a small or no mediastinal mass. From a biological perspective, it would seem likely that the more disseminated disease is likely to correspond to more mature neoplasms in which the normal counterpart cells would have already left the thymus (Pui *et al.* 1990). However, in a small series of Pediatric Oncology Group patients treated with the LSA_2L_2 or A-COP protocols there was no evidence that the thymocyte differentiation stage had any influence on prognosis (Pui *et al.* 1990), although differences in prognosis have been observed in relationship to the presence or absence of bone-marrow involvement. However, such differences are protocol dependent (Weinstein *et al.* 1983; Magrath *et al.* 1984).

In a recent Pediatric Oncology Group trial, the therapeutic results in patients with leukaemia and lymphoma (separated according to the 25 per cent criterion of bone-marrow blasts) were similar when treated with LSA_2L_2 or, in the case of some of the lymphoma patients, with A-COP+ (adriamycin, cyclophosphamide, onvovin, and prednisone). Event-free survival was approximately 40 per cent at 4 years for both groups (Pui *et al.* 1990). Within the T-cell acute lymphoblastic leukaemia patients a higher white count was associated with a worse prognosis and in patients with lymphoblastic lymphoma LSA_2L_2 appeared to be less effective for patients with a mediastinal mass (Sullivan *et al.* 1985a). In the Children's Cancer Study Group study of a very similar LSA_2L_2 regimen, the results were apparently better: patients with extensive disease had an event-free survival of 70 per cent at years, regardless of the presence of bone-marrow involvement (although only one of 11 patients had more than 25 per cent blast cells in the marrow). In this series the outcome in patients with mediastinal masses was not reported separately. In a small series treated with the 77-04 protocol patients with a mediastinal mass had an event-free survival of 70 per cent, but all of five patients with bone-marrow involvement (greater than 25 per cent blasts) relapsed.

It would seem appropriate at present to treat patients with bone-marrow involvement with an intensive protocol designed for acute lymphoblastic leukaemia, such as the BFM 81/83 protocol or the French version of LSA_2L_2 in which ten courses of high-dose methotrexate were given. Approximately 80 per cent of patients can be expected to achieve long-term disease-free survival with such regimens (Müller-Weihrich *et al.* 1985). Not all protocols designed initially for the treatment of patients with acute lymphoblastic lymphoma are equally effective; patients with bone-marrow involvement treated with the APO protocol, for example, had a poor prognosis (Weinstein *et al.* 1983; Camitta *et al.* 1985). Patients without bone-marrow involvement may be effectively treated with protocols based upon repeated alkylating agent therapy such as 77-04. All protocols for patients with lymphoblastic lymphoma should include effective prophylactic therapy against central nervous system spread.

The optimal duration of therapy for lymphoblastic lymphoma remains undetermined, but there is evidence that 18 months' therapy is sufficient for patients with a mediastinal mass without marrow involvement (Magrath *et al.* 1984). Shorter durations have not been assessed.

Chemotherapy of large-cell lymphomas

Most paediatric oncologists treat large-cell lymphomas in children in the same way as small non-cleaved cell lymphomas. However, unlike the small non-cleaved cell lymphomas, results obtained with protocols designed for the treatment of acute lymphoblastic leukaemia are not necessarily inferior (Weinstein *et al.* 1984; Sullivan *et al.* 1985a). With the APO regimen, 76 per cent of a series of patients were estimated to be alive and disease free at 6 years (Weinstein *et al.* 1984). Using the LSA_2L_2 protocol, the Children's Cancer Study Group reported a failure-free survival rate of 44 per cent at 3 years (an almost identical result to that obtained with COMP) (Anderson *et al.* 1983) in patients with extensive disease, while the Pediatric Oncology Group reported a 5 year failure-free survival of 57 per cent, with 55 per cent of 24 patients with St Jude stage III disease predicted to survive disease free beyond 3 years (Sullivan *et al.* 1985a). For patients with mediastinal large-cell lymphoma, the Pediatric Oncology Group reported that 55 per cent of 22 patients were alive and free of disease at 2 years (Bunin *et al.* 1986). The main disadvantage of the LSA_2L_2 regimens is its much longer duration.

Protocols designed for the treatment of lymphoma rather than leukaemia are at least as effective in the treatment of patients with large-cell lymphomas and have the advantage of a much shorter duration of therapy. In a retrospective analysis of 25 patients with non-lymphoblastic lymphomas of the mediastinum, 20 of which were immunoblastic and two large non-cleaved lymphomas, 18 were treated with a variety of 'lymphoma' regimens consisting predominantly of CHOP (cyclophosphamide, adriamycin, oncovin, and prednisone). Twelve of these patients achieved continuous complete remission (median remission duration for the study was 42 months) (Bunin *et al.* 1986). Similarly, in a Pediatric Oncology Group trial in which patients with non-lymphoblastic lymphomas (except Burkitt's lymphoma) were treated with the A-COP+ regimen 76 per cent of patients were disease free at 2 years (Hvizdala *et al.* 1983). There were no apparent differences in prognosis among the histological subtypes.

While it can be argued that the heterogeneity of the large-cell lymphomas may be obscuring possible differences in the response to different treatment regimens among subgroups, this finding also appears to apply specifically to the anaplastic large-cell lymphomas when considered separately. Recently, two groups, a combined Austrian–German consortium and the University of Bologna, reported their findings in small series of patients with this disease (Murphy and Magrath 1991). Eleven of the Austrian–German patients were originally diagnosed as malignant histiocytosis, 18 were included in the BFM 'B-cell lymphoma protocols', and eight were identified *per primam*. The 13 patients studied in Bologna were identified among 78 non-Hodgkin's patients. While all anaplastic large-cell lymphomas expressed the Ki-1 (CD30) antigen, these patients included three immunophenotypes: T (the majority), B (the minority), and null, possibly histiocytic (rare patients). In these studies, the Italian group used LSA_2L_2 and local radiation, a protocol shown by the Children's Cancer Study Group to be inadequate for the treatment of small non-cleaved cell (undifferentiated) lymphomas, and observed 73 per cent disease-free survival at 5 years, while the Austrian–German group used BFM B-cell lymphoma protocols with similar results. In view of the apparent similarity of results obtained with these protocols, it would seem appropriate to use that which has the shorter duration.

There seems no cogent reason to explore the efficacy in children of the specific treatment regimens used in large-cell lymphomas in adults, such as proMACE-CYTABOM, M/m-BACOD, COP-BLAM, and MACOB-B. Overall results are not superior to those that have been achieved in children with non-lymphoblastic lymphomas, and in some of these protocols high-grade lymphomas (including immunoblastic lymphomas) tend to have a worse prognosis although the basic strategies and drugs used are similar to those used in childhood B-cell lymphomas.

The role of local irradiation has not been specifically explored in the large-cell lymphomas of childhood and practice in this regard has differed among protocols. In all, however, there is no definite evidence that local irradiation has any benefit and it would appear that it would be appropriate to reserve this modality for patients in whom there is residual local disease after an appropriate induction regimen. All protocols should include effective intrathecal prophylactic therapy.

Treatment of lymphomas arising in immunosuppressed patients

A particularly difficult problem is the management of patients with an underlying immunodeficiency syndrome in whom a lymphoma develops. Because the cause and degree of immunosuppression and the type of lymphoma as well as the degree of spread, differ so markedly, the treatment of such patients must be individualized. Some patients may have localized intracerebral disease, while others may have widely disseminated disease. Some patients have polyclonal cytogenetically normal lymphoproliferations, others have quite classical small non-cleaved cell lymphomas (particularly patients with HIV infection), and still others have atypical large-cell lymphomas.

Where immunosuppression is iatrogenic, cessation of immunosuppressive drug or anti-T-cell monoclonal antibody therapy may sometimes permit tumour regression to occur. In patients with karyotypically abnormal monoclonal proliferations, the intensity of chemotherapy must take into account the degree of immunosuppression of the patient. Intensive chemotherapy in a severely immunosuppressed invidiual may simply hasten the occurrence of a fatal infectious process. With localized disease, particularly if lymphoma is confined to the central nervous system, it may be more appropriate to treat such patients with radiation alone, although normally systemic chemotherapy would also be given in this situation. If the process is disseminated, a compromise regimen that offers the patient a small chance of survival may be chosen. However, patients without a history of repeated serious infections should be treated with an intensive modern protocol since long-term survival is possible. In all these patients, it must be borne in mind that the prognosis includes that of the underlying disease.

Recent results with α-interferon in patients with an Epstein–Barr virus associated polyclonal lymphoproliferative process show promise (Shapiro et al. 1988; Shapiro 1990) and further exploration of the value of a wide range of lymphokines in severely immunosuppressed patients with this kind of lymphoproliferative syndrome is appropriate in view of the markedly increased risks of conventional combination chemotherapy regimens. However, in the face of clear progression cytotoxic therapy should not be withheld from a patient on the grounds that his or her disease is polyclonal or cytogenetically normal.

TREATMENT OF RECURRENT NON-HODGKIN'S LYMPHOMA

In general, patients with recurrent disease after modern intensive chemotherapy have a very low chance of survival if retreated with conventional therapy. Such patients should be considered candidates for massive chemotherapy, with or without bone-marrow transplantation.

Some relapse protocols have met with a degree of success, notably the very intensive BACT protocol, consisting of a single cycle of BCNU (bischloronitrosourea), high-dose cyclophosphamide, 6-thioguanine, and Ara-C daily for 4 days. This drug combination has been used primarily in relapsed Burkitt's lymphoma, originally at the National Cancer Institute, Bethesda (Appelbaum et al. 1978) and subsequently at the Centre Léon Bérard, Lyon, France (Philip et al. 1986a,b). In the National Cancer Institute trial, half the patients received autologous bone-marrow that had previously been cryopreserved after intensive therapy, but even those who did not receive bone-marrow rescue recovered bone-marrow function. Thus, if total-body irradiation is not used as part of the regimen, spontaneous bone-marrow recovery occurs even without marrow transplantation. In the National Cancer Institute study four out of 19 patients achieved long-term survival (8–14 years disease free), while similar results were obtained in France, where autologous bone-marrow transplantation was used following the BACT regimen or a derivative protocol, BEAM, which incorporates VP16 and melphalan (Philip et al. 1986b; Cross et al. 1987). However, the BACT regimen is associated with severe toxicity, including the possibility of acute myocardial necrosis. Four patients died from this complication in the National Cancer Institute study.

A successful outcome of intensive salvage therapy can be predicted according to the previous response to treatment. Patients with relapse responsive to conventional approaches have a much better prognosis with high-dose therapy, with relapse-free survival which may approach 50 per cent. Patients with tumour totally resistant to conventional therapy have an extremely poor prognosis, with no survivors after 9 months (Cabanillas et al. 1990). Patients with a partial response to primary treatment (that is, with residual disease, but not progressive disease) appear to have a good prognosis, although the definition of this group of patients, unless biopsy is performed, is subjective. In interpreting these results it should be remembered that patients with marrow involvement at the time of relapse are not usually considered for autologous bone-marrow transplantation, so that the above results have been obtained in a selected subgroup and do not reflect the results that are likely to be obtained when all relapsed patients are included.

Another group of patients that appears to do well with high-dose salvage therapy including autologous bone-marrow transplantation is that in which isolated central nervous system relapse occurs. In one series of 19 such patients 47 per cent were reported to achieve long-term survival (Cabanillas et al. 1990). However, some patients with isolated central nervous system relapse have also achieved long-term survival when treated with conventional systemic therapy and intrathecal chemotherapy (Sariban et al. 1983). A question which may be legitimately asked is whether the autologous bone-marrow transplantation and total-body irradiation is really necessary. Autologous bone-marrow transplantation always carries the risk of reinfusion of malignant cells and, although considerable effort has been put into purging bone-marrow with drugs or monoclonal antibodies (Favrot and Philip 1990), a definite advantage to such procedures has not yet been demonstrated. Autologous bone-marrow transplantation performed with and without total-body irradiation seems to give similar results except that there is more toxicity with total-body irradiation (Philip *et al.* 1986*a*; Cabanillas *et al.* 1990). This introduces the possibility of using massive therapy without the need for autologous bone-marrow transplantation (as in the earliest National Cancer Institute BACT protocol). Drugs such as high dose Ara-C and VP16 may have an important rôle in such protocols in the future. High-dose Ara-C and ifosfamide are known to be active in relapsed patients (Jones and Ettinger 1985; Lie and Sirdahl 1985) and a combination regimen of high-dose Ara-C, VP16, and ifosfamide for patients with relapsed non-lymphoblastic lymphomas has also shown a significant complete response rate (Magrath *et al.* 1991).

Allogeneic bone-marrow transplantation, usually following high-dose cyclophosphamide and total-body irradiation, has also been explored in relapsed patients with non-Hodgkin's lymphoma and overall results are quite similar to the autologous bone-marrow transplantation experience with patients with progressive disease at the time of transplant doing poorly (Appelbaum *et al.* 1985; Chopra *et al.* 1992).

LONG-TERM COMPLICATIONS OF THERAPY

The long-term complications of the treatment of non-Hodgkin's lymphoma in children have become less of a problem as treatment has been refined. The potentially serious consequences of radiation therapy on growth and development, including psychological development in patients undergoing cranial irradiation (Meadows *et al.* 1981; Moss *et al.* 1981; Robison *et al.* 1984; Rowland *et al.* 1984), have almost ceased to exist as this modality has played a smaller and smaller rôle in overall therapeutic strategies, including prophylactic therapy against central nervous system spread. The trend towards shorter therapy durations in the small non-cleaved lymphomas will further reduce the likelihood or seriousness of long-term complications. Perhaps the three most serious potential problems which are common to all patients are impaired reproductive function, the risk of second malignancies, and the psychological consequences of life-threatening illness.

Reproductive function is normally severely impaired in males undergoing chemotherapy, particularly when alkylating agents are used, but the consequences of treatment in this regard appear to be much less in the prepubertal patient, although azoospermia may still occur (Sullivan *et al.* 1985*b*). In women treated prior to the age of 20 years who do not receive abdominal irradiation reproductive function later in life appears to be normal (Hall and Green 1983) and regimens based on acute leukaemia therapy appear to be relatively benign with regard to reproductive function, even in males (Pasqualini *et al.* 1983).

In contrast with the situation in Hodgkin's disease and the solid tumours of children, second malignancies have not been a significant problem in the majority of studies reporting upon this complication in patients with non-Hodgkin's lymphomas (Meadows *et al.* 1985), although it is highly probable that the incidence of this complication will vary with the specific protocol being used. This may be the explanation for the recent report from the United Kingdom in which an incidence of 8.6 per cent of second malignancies was described (Ingram *et al.* 1987).

FUTURE CONSIDERATIONS

The treatment of non-Hodgkin's lymphomas in children has improved greatly in the last 15 years. The best reported results

Table 16 Future trends in the treatment of childhood non-Hodgkin's lymphoma

Optimalization of current regimens with regard to drugs, schedule, and duration of therapy

Evaluation of rôle of colony-stimulating factors in ameliorating toxicity and increasing dose intensity

Exploration of totally novel approaches in which tumour specificity is increased, for example by using the presence of viral genomes or molecular genetic abnormalities as targets for therapeutic endeavours

indicate that perhaps 80–90 per cent of all such patients can be cured when treated optimally. This result has largely been achieved by the use of intensive combination drug therapy and prophylactic therapy directed against the development of central nervous system involvement. Yet there is an ever present challenge to improve the results of treatment even further and to lessen its toxicity and inconvenience (Table 16). In this regard, we are likely to see the increasing use of cloned colony-stimulating factors such as G-CSF, GM-CSF and IL-3 to lessen toxicity and increase dose intensity.

Particularly exciting is the new knowledge of the molecular genetic and resultant biochemical abnormalities which underly the pathogenesis of the lymphoid neoplasms, an area of research which is particularly advanced with respect to the small non-cleaved cell lymphomas (Magrath 1990). This information will soon be utilized in the development of improved diagnostic techniques and identification of prognostic subgroups. It may even prove possible to develop highly specific treatment approaches directed against those very abnormalities which are responsible for the manifestation of the disease as a neoplastic process. Therefore, such therapy will be truly tumour specific with promise of minimal toxicity. There are few neoplasms in which this could be contemplated at the present time, but the large and increasing body of data concerning the molecular genetic abnormalities of the small non-cleaved cell lymphomas, consequent upon the specific chromosomal translocations associated with these tumours, provides one of the best opportunities of examining this approach. This possibility has already been given credibility by the recent demonstration of specific inhibition of abnormal c-*myc* (the oncogene which is abnormally expressed in these tumours) messenger RNAs present only in tumour cells by an antisense oligonucleotide (that is, a molecule with a sequence complementary to the c-*myc* messenger RNA whose translation is prevented when bound by the antisense molecule) (McManaway *et al.* 1990). Thus, it is clearly possible to use the molecular abnormalities which actually give rise to neoplastic behaviour as targets for therapeutic endeavours.

Other kinds of targeting, for example with anti-idiotypic or other monoclonal antibodies, perhaps coupled to drug, toxin, or radionuclide, are less distant possibilities, but it is rather disappointing that such approaches have been under study for a number of years and yet there are few tangible results (Myers *et al.* 1984; Hertler *et al.* 1987). The rôle of such approaches in the therapy of non-Hodgkin's lymphomas is likely to take years to define.

Finally, the use of biological response modifiers still has promise as a treatment approach, possibly combined with conventional therapy, but there have been few studies in this area with the childhood lymphomas (Ochs *et al.* 1986). None the less, the major progress which has been made in understanding the regulation of normal and neoplastic growth in lymphoid cells in recent years provides promise that, ultimately, this information will be of value in the development of novel therapeutic approaches.

These considerations justify increased effort directed towards the understanding of the pathogenesis of the childhood non-Hodgkin's lymphomas. If such studies also lead to the identification of specific individuals at high risk of developing lymphomas, for example because of the inheritance pattern of variant or abnormal alleles of relevant genes, this may permit the possibility of the ultimate intervention, prevention, to be entertained.

REFERENCES

Abe K, Sato T (1981). Burkitt's lymphoma in Japan: clinicopathological features of twenty-two patients. *Tohoku Journal of Experimental Medicine*, **134**:289–93.

Addis BJ, Isaacson PG (1986). Large cell lymphoma of the mediastinum: a B-cell tumour of probable thymic origin. *Histopathology*, **10**:379–90.

Agnarsson BA, Kadin ME (1988). Ki-1 positive large cell lymphoma. A morphologic and immunologic study of 19 cases. *American Journal of Surgical Pathology*, **12**:264–74.

Aguado GE, Jimenez DP, Pajuelo DA, Ontanilla LA, Lopez CJA (1986). Anesthesia management in tumors of the anterior mediastinum. Apropos of a case. *Revista Española de Anestesiologia y Reanimacion*, **33**:268–70 (in Spanish).

Alt FW, Blackwell TK, Depinho RA, Reith MG, Yancopoulos GD (1986). Regulation of genome rearrangement events during lymphoctye differentiation. *Immunological Reviews*, **89**:5–30.

Altiok E, et al. (1989). Epstein–Barr virus-transformed pro-B cells are prone to illegitimate recombination between the switch region of the mu chain gene and other chromosomes. *Proceedings of the National Academy of Sciences of the USA*, **86**:6333–7.

Anaissie E, Geha S, Allam C, Jabbour J, Khalyl M, Salem PT (1985). Burkitt's lymphoma in the Middle East. A study of 34 cases. *Cancer*, **56**(10):2539.

Anderson JR, Jenkin RDT (1983). Treatment of childhood non-Hodgkin's lymphoma. *New England Journal of Medicine*, **309**:311 (letter).

Anderson JR, et al. (1983). The results of a randomized therapeutic trial comparing a 4-drug regimen (COMP) with a 10-drug regimen (LSA2-L2). *New England Journal of Medicine*, **308**:559–65.

Aplan PD, Lombardi DP, Reaman GH, Sather HN, Hammond GD, Kirsch I (1992). Involvement of putative hemopoietic transcription factor SCL in T-cell acute lymphoblastic leukaemia. *Blood*, **79**:1327–33.

Appelbaum FR, et al. (1978). Prolonged complete remission following high dose chemotherapy of Burkitt's lymphoma in relapse. *Cancer*, **41**:1059.

Appelbaum F, et al. (1985). Treatment of malignant lymphoma in one hundred patients with chemoradiotherapy and marrow transplantation. *Experimental Hematology*, **13**:321 (abstract).

Armelin HA, et al. (1984). Functional role for c-*myc* in mitogenic response to platelet-derived growth factor. *Nature, London*, **310**:655–60.

Arseneau JC, Bagley CM, Anderson T, Canellos GP (1973). Hyperkalemia, a sequel to chemotherapy of Burkitt's lymphoma. *Lancet*, i:10–14.

Arseneau JC, Canellos GP, Banks PM, Berard CW, Gralnick HR, De Vita VT (1975). American Burkitt's lymphoma—a clinicopathological study of 30 cases. I. Clinical factors relating to long term survival. *American Journal of Medicine*, **58**:314–21.

Asou N, Hattori T, Matsuoka M, Kawano F, Takatsuki KT (1984). Rearrangements of T-cell antigen receptor delta chain gene in hematologic neoplasms. *Blood*, **74**:2707–12.

Aur RJ, Hustu HO, Simone JV, Pratt CB, Pinkel D (1971). Therapy of localized and regional lymphosarcoma of childhood. *Cancer*, **27**:1328–31.

Aventin A, et al. (1990). Variant t(2;18) translocation in a Burkitt conversion of follicular lymphoma. *British Journal of Haematology*, **74**:367–9.

Avila CJ, Torsteinsdottir S, Ehlin HB, Lenoir G, Klein G, Klein E, Masucci MG (1987). Paired Epstein–Barr virus (EBV)-negative and EBV-converted Burkitt lymphoma lines: stimulatory capacity in allogeneic mixed lymphocyte cultures. *International Journal of Cancer*, **40**:691–7.

Bakhshi AJJP, Goldman P, Wright JJ, McBride OW, Epstein AL, Korsmeyer SJ (1985). Cloning the chromosomal breakpoint of t(18;14)* bearing human lymphomas clustering around JH on chromosome 14 and near a transcriptional unit on 18. *Cell*, **41**:899–906.

Barker PE, Royer HD, Ruddle FH, Reinherz EL (1985). Regional location of T cell receptor gene Ti alpha on human chromosome 14. *Journal of Experimental Medicine*, **162**:387–92.

Barriga P, Wilson W, Magrath IT (1990). Complications of management. In *The non-Hodgkin's lymphomas* (ed. IT Magrath). Arnold, London.

Battifora H, Trowbridge IS (1983). A monoclonal antibody useful for the differential diagnosis between malignant lymphoma and non-hematopoietic neoplasms. *Cancer*, **51**:816–21.

Benjamin D, et al. (1982). Immunoglobulin secretion by cell lines derived from African and American undifferentiated lymphomas of Burkitt's and non-Burkitt's type. *Journal of Immunology*, **129**:1336.

Benjamin D, Magrath IT, Douglass EC, Corash LM (1983). Derivation of lymphoma cell lines from microscopically normal bone marrow in patients with undifferentiated lymphomas; evidence of occult bone marrow involvement. *Blood*, **61**:1017–19.

Bennett MH, Farrer-Brown G, Henry K, Jeliffe AM (1974). Classification of non-Hodgkin's lymphomas. *Lancet*, i:1295.

Bernard A, Boumsell L (1982). Cell-surface heterogeneity of human T-cell malignancies. *Progress in Cancer Research and Therapy*, **21**:93.

Bernard A, et al. (1981). Cell surface characterization of malignant T cells from lymphoblastic lymphoma using monoclonal antibodies: evidence for a phenotypic difference between malignant T cells from patients with acute lymphoblastic leukemia and lymphoblastic lymphoma. *Blood*, **57**:1105.

Bernard A, et al. (1982). Non-T, non-B lymphomas are rare in childhood and associated with cutaneous tumor. *Blood*, **59**:549.

Bernheim A, Berger R, Lenoir G (1981). Cytogenetic studies on African Burkitt's lymphoma cell lines; t(8;14), t(2;8) and t(8;22) translocations. *Cancer Genetics and Cytogenetics*, **3**:307.

Bertness V, et al. (1985). T-cell receptor gene rearrangements as clinical markers of human T-cell lymphomas. *New England Journal of Medicine*, **313**:534.

Biegel JA, Belasco JB, Emanuel BS (1988). A unique chromosome translocation, t(7;15), in a pediatric patient with pre-B-cell lymphoma presenting as a primary tumor of bone. *Cancer Genetics and Cytogenetics*, **36**:211–15.

Blood Fifth International Workshop on Chromosomes in Leukemia–Lymphoma. *Blood*, **70**:1554–64.

Bloomfield CD, Arthur DC, Frizzera G, Levine EG, Peterson BA, Gajl PKJ (1983). Non-random chromosome abnormalities in lymphoma. *Cancer Research*, **43**:2975–84.

Blue ML, Schlossman SF (1986). Biology of the T cell. *Progress in Clinical and Biological Research*, **224**:11–20.

Bogusawska JJ, et al. (1984). Evaluation of the LSA2L2 protocol for treatment of childhood non-Hodgkin's lymphoma: a report from the Polish Children's Leukemia/Lymphoma Study Group. *American Journal of Pediatric Hematology and Oncology*, **6**:363.

Braylan RCFBT, et al. (1978). Cell volumes and DNA distributions of normal and neoplastic human lymphoid cells. *Cancer*, **41**:201–9.

Braziel RM, et al. (1983). Terminal deoxynucleotidyl transferase in non-Hodgkin's lymphoma. *American Journal of Clinical Pathology*, **80**:655–9.

Bunin NJ, et al. (1986). Mediastinal nonlymphoblastic lymphomas in children: a clinicopathologic study. *Journal of Clinical Oncology*, **4**:154–9.

Burkitt D (1958). A sarcoma involving the jaws in African Children. *British Journal of Surgery*, **46**:218–23.

Burkitt D (1967). Long term remissions following one and two dose chemotherapy for African lymphoma. *Cancer*, **20**:756–9.

Burkitt DP (1970a). Geographical distribution. In *Burkitt's lymphoma* (ed. DP Burkitt and DH Wright), pp. 186–97. Livingstone, Edinburgh.

Burkitt DP (1970b). General features and facial tumours. In *Burkitt's lymphoma* (ed. DP Burkitt and DH Wright), pp. 6–15. Livingstone, Edinburgh.

Burkitt DP (1970c). Lesions outside the jaws. In *Burkitt's lymphoma* (ed. DP Burkitt and DH Wright), pp. 16–22. Livingstone, Edinburgh.

Cabanillas F, Jagannath S, Philip T (1990). Management of recurrent or refractory non-Hodgkin's lymphomas. *The non-Hodgkin's lymphomas* (ed. IT Magrath). Arnold, London.

Camitta BM, Lauer SJ, Casper JT, Kirchner PA, Kun LE, Oechler HW, Adair SE (1985). Effectiveness of a six-drug regimen (APO) without local irradiation for treatment of mediastinal lymphoblastic lymphoma in children. *Cancer*, **56**:738–41.

Cancer Incidence in Five Continents, Vol. V. International Agency for Research on Cancer, Lyon, 1987.

Carabell SC, Goodman RL (1985). Oncologic emergencies: superior vena cava syndrome. In *Cancer—principles and practice of oncology* (2nd edn) (ed. VT De Vita Jr, S Hellman, and SA Rosenberg), pp. 1855–60. Lippincott, Philadelphia.

Casali P, Burastero SE, Nakamura M, Inghirami G, Notkins AL (1987). Human lymphocytes making rheumatoid factor and antibody to ssDNA belong to Leu-1+ B-cell subset. *Science*, **236**:77–81.

Casten LA, *et al.* (1985). Anti-immunoglobulin augments the B-cell antigen presentation function independently of internalization of receptor-antigen complex. *Proceedings of the National Academy of Sciences of the USA*, **82**:5890–4.

Chaganti RSK, *et al.* (1983). Specific translocations characterize Burkitt's like lymphoma of homosexual men with the acquired immunodeficiency syndrome. *Blood*, **61**:1269–72.

Chan JK, Ng CS, Ngan KC, Hui PK, Lo ST, Lau WH (1988). Angiocentric T-cell lymphoma of the skin. An aggressive lymphoma distinct from mycosis fungoides. *American Journal of Surgical Pathology*, **12**:861–76.

Chessells JM, Cox TC, Kendall B, Cavanagh NP, Jannoun L, Richards S (1990). Neurotoxicity in lymphoblastic leukaemia: comparison of oral and intramuscular methotrexate and two doses of radiation. *Archives of Disease in Childhood*, **65**:416–22.

Chien Y, Iwashima M, Kaplan KB, Elliot JF, Davies MM (1987*a*). New T cell receptor gene located within the alpha locus and expressed early in T cell differentiation. *Nature, London*, **327**:677–82.

Chien Y, Iwashima M, Wettstein DA, Kaplan KB, Elliot JF, Born W, Davis MM (1987*b*). T cell receptor delta gene rearrangements in early thymocytes. *Nature, London*, **330**:722–7.

Chopra R, *et al.* (1992). Autologous versus allogeneic bone marrow transplantation for non-Hodgkins lymphoma: a case controlled analysis of the European Bone Marrow Transplant Group Registry data. *Journal of Clinical Oncology*, **10**:1690–5.

Christensson B, Biberfeld P, Matell G (1988). B-cell compartment in the thymus of patients with myasthenia gravis and control subjects. *Annals of the New York Academy of Science*, **540**:293–7.

Clayton PE, Shalet SM, Price DA, Surtees RA, Pearson D (1987). The role of growth hormone in stunted head growth after cranial irradiation. *Pediatric Research*, **22**:402–4.

Cleary ML, Nalesnik MA, Shearer WI, Sklar J (1988). Clonal analysis of transplant associated lymphoproliferations based on the structure of the genomic termini of the Epstein Barr virus. *Blood*, **72**:349–52.

Cohen PJ, Jaffe ES (1990). Histopathology and immunophenotyping. In *The non-Hodgkin's lymphomas* (ed. IT Magrath), pp. 49–76. Arnold, London.

Cohen LF, Balow JE, Magrath IT (1980). Acute tumor lysis syndrome: a review of 37 patients with Burkitt's lymphoma. *American Journal of Medicine*, **68**:486–91.

Cossman J, Chused TM, Fisher RI, Magrath I, Bollum F, Jaffe ES (1983). Diversity of immunological phenotypes of lymphoblastic lymphoma. *Cancer Research*, **43**:4486–90.

Costa J, Delacretaz F (1986). The midline granuloma syndrome. *Pathology Annual*, **21**(1):159–71.

Cotelingam JD, *et al.* (1985). Malignant lymphoma in patients with the Wiskott–Aldrich syndrome. *Cancer Investigation*, **3**:515–22.

Crist WM, *et al.* (1988). Clinical features and outcome in childhood T-cell leukemia-lymphoma according to stage of thymocyte differentiation: a Pediatric Oncology Group study. *Blood*, **72**:1891–7.

Croce CM, Shander M, Martinis J, Cicurel L, D'Ancona GG, Dolby TW, Koprowski H (1979). Chromosomal location of the genes for human immunoglobulin heavy chains. *Proceedings of the National Academy of Sciences of the USA*, **76**:3416–19.

Croce CM, *et al.* (1985). Gene for alpha-chain of human T-cell receptor: location on chromosome 14 region involved in T-cell neoplasms. *Science*, **227**:1044–7.

Cross S, *et al.* (1987). Regulation of the human interleukin-2 receptor alpha chain promoter. Activation of a nonfunctional promoter by the transactivator gene of HTLV I. *Cell*, **49**:47–56.

Csako G, Magrath IT, Elin R (1982). Serum total and isoenzyme lactate dehydrogenase activity in American Burkitt's lymphoma. *American Journal of Clinical Pathology*, **78**:712–17.

Cunningham D, Hickish T, Rosin RD, Sauven P, Baron JH, Farrell PJ, Isaacson P (1989). Polymerase chain reaction for detection of dissemination in gastric lymphoma. *Lancet*, i:695–7.

Dahl GV, *et al.* (1985). A novel treatment of childhood lymphoblastic non-Hodgkin's lymphoma: early and intermittent use of temposide plus cytarabine. *Blood*, **66**:1110–14.

Dalla-Favera R, *et al.* (1982). Human c-*myc* oncogene is located on the region of chromosome 8 that is translocated in Burkitt lymphoma cells. *Proceedings of the National Academy of Sciences of the USA*, **79**:7824.

Delalande JP, Abgrall JF, Le Gall G (1987). Post-anaesthesia respiratory distress caused by mediastinal lymphoblastic lymphoma. A new case. *Presse Medicale*, **16**:400 (in French).

Desiderio SV, *et al.* (1984). Insertion of N regions into heavy-chain genes is correlated with expression of terminal deoxytransferase in B cells. *Nature, London*, **311**:752.

Desser H, Walder R, Klaring W, Lutz D. (1983). Polyamines and histamine in serum from patients with hematological disease. *Advances in Polyamine Research*, **4**:49–58.

Dorfman RF (1975). The non-Hodgkin's lymphomas. In *The reticuloendothelial system* (ed. J Rebuck, CW Berard, and MR Abell), p. 262. Williams and Wilkins, Baltimore.

Dube ID, Raimondi SC, Pi D, Kalousek DK (1986). A new translocation, t(10;14)(q24;q11), in T cell neoplasia. *Blood*, **67**:1181–4.

Duffner PK, Cohen ME, Thomas PR, Lansky SB (1985). The long-term effects of cranial irradiation on the central nervous system. *Cancer*, **56**:1841–6.

Duque-Hammershaimb L, Wollner N, Miller D (1983). LSA2L2 protocol treatment of stage IV non-Hodgkin's lymphoma in children with partial and extensive bone marrow involvement. *Cancer*, **52**:39–43.

Dyer MJ (1989). T-cell receptor delta/alpha rearrangements in lymphoid neoplasms. *Blood*, **74**(3):1073–83.

Epstein MA, Achong BG, Barr YM (1964). Virus particles in cultured lymphoblasts from Burkitt's lymphoma. *Lancet*, i:702–3.

Falini B, *et al.* (1989). Distribution of T cells bearing different forms of the T cell receptor gamma/delta in normal and pathological human tissues. *Journal of Immunology*, **143**:2480.

Favrot M, Philip T (1990). Bone marrow purging. In *New approaches to cancer treatment* (ed. IT Magrath), pp. 343–57. Springer Verlag, Heidelberg.

Favrot MC, *et al.* (1984). Distinct reactivity of Burkitt's lymphoma cell lines with eight monoclonal antibodies correlated with the ethic origin. *Journal of the National Cancer Institute*, **73**:841–7.

Feller AC, Parwaresch MR, Stein H, Ziegler A, Herbst H, Lennert K (1986). Immunophenotyping of T-lymphoblastic lymphoma/leukaemia: correlation with normal T-cell maturation. *Leukaemia Research*, **10**:1025–31.

Ferguson MK, Lee E, Skinner DB, Little AG (1987). Selective operative approach for diagnosis and treatment of anterior mediastinal masses. *Annals of Thoracic Surgery*, **44**:583–6.

Filipovitch AH, *et al.* (1984). Lymphomas in persons with naturally occurring immunodeficiency disorders. In *Pathogenesis of leukemias and lymphomas: environmental influences* (ed. IT Magrath, G O'Conor, and B Ramot), pp. 225–34. Raven Press, New York.

Filipovich AH, Shapiro R, Robinson L, Mertens A, Frizzera G (1990). Lymphoproliferative disorders associated with immunodeficiency. In *The non-Hodgkin's lymphomas* (ed. IT Magrath), pp. 136–54. Arnold, London.

Finch S (1984). Ionizing radiation and drugs in the pathogenesis of lymphoid neoplasia. In *Pathogenesis of leukemias and lymphomas: environmental influences* (ed. IT Magrath, G O'Conor, and B Ramot), pp. 207–23. Raven Press, New York.

Finger LR, *et al.* (1986). A common mechanism of chromosomal translocation in T and B cell neoplasia. *Science*, **234**:982–5.

Fischer P, Nacheva E, Mason DY, Sherrington PD, Hoyle C, Hayhoe FGJ, Karpas A (1988). A Ki-1 (CD30)-positive human cell line (Karpas 299) established from a high-grade non-Hodgkin's lymphoma showing a 2;5 translocation and rearrangement of the T cell receptor beta-chain. *Blood*, **72**:234–40.

Foon KA, Todd RF (1986). Immunologic classification of leukemia and lymphoma. *Blood*, **68**:1–31.

Foroni L, *et al.* (1987). Alpha, beta and gamma T-cell receptor genes: rearrangements correlate with haematological phenotype in T cell leukaemias. *British Journal of Haematology*, **67**:307–18.

Frizzera G, Murphy SB (1979). Follicular (nodular) lymphoma in childhood: a rare clinical–pathological entity. Report of eight cases from four cancer centers. *Cancer*, 44:2218–35.

Gadner H, Müller-Weihrich S, Riehm H (1986). Treatment strategies in malignant non-Hodgkin lymphomas in childhood. *Onkologie*, 9:126.

Gasparini M, Lombardi F, Bellani FF, Gianni G, Pilotti S, Rilke F (1981). Childhood non-Hodgkin's lymphoma: long-term results of an intensive chemotherapy regimen. *Cancer*, 48:1508–12.

Gasparini M, *et al.* (1993). Curability of advanced Burkitt's lymphoma in children by intensive short-term chemotherapy. *European Journal of Cancer*, 29A:692–8.

Gentet JC, *et al.* (1990). Phase II study of cytarabine and etoposide in children with refractory or relapsed non-Hodgkin's lymphoma: a study of the French Society of Pediatric Oncology. *Journal of Clinical Oncology*, 8:661–5.

Glass JP, Lee YY, Bruner J, Fields WS (1986). Treatment-related leukoencephalopathy. A study of three cases and literature review. *Medicine (Baltimore)*, 65:154–62.

Glatstein E, *et al.* (1974). Non-Hodgkin's lymphoma VI. Results of treatment in childhood. *Cancer*, 34:204.

Grogan TM, Warnke RA, Kaplan K (1982). A comparative study of Burkitt's and non-Burkitt's 'undifferentiated' malignant lymphoma: immunologic, cytochemical, ultrastructural, cytologic, histopathologic, clinical and cell culture features. *Cancer*, 49:1817–28.

Grogan T, *et al.* (1986). Immunologic complexity of lymphoblastic lymphoma. *Diagnostic Immunology*, 4:81–8.

Gutiérrez M, *et al.* (1992). Molecular epidemiology of Burkitt's lymphoma from South America: differences in break-point locations and EBV association. *Blood*, 79:3236–66.

Ha KK, Yumura K, Hara J, Ishihara S, Yabuuchi HT (1987). Concomitant rearrangements of T, cell beta and gamma chain genes in childhood T lineage leukemia/lymphoma. *Leukemia Research*, 11:739–45.

Haars R, Kronenberg M, Gallatin WM, Weissman IL, Owel FL, Hood L (1986). Rearrangement and expression of T cell antigen receptor and gamma genes during thymic development. *Journal of Experimental Medicine*, 164:1–24.

Haddy TB, Sandlund JT, Magrath IT (1988). Testicular involvement in young patients with non-Hodgkin's lymphoma. *American Journal of Pediatric Hematology and Oncology*, 10:224–9.

Haddy TB, Parker RI, Magrath IT (1989). Bone marrow involvement in young patients with non-Hodgkin's lymphoma: the importance of multiple bone marrow samples for accurate staging. *Medical and Pediatric Oncology*, 17:418–23.

Haddy TB, Adde MA, Magrath IT (1991). Central nervous system involvement in small non cleaved cell lymphoma: is CNS disease *per se* a poor prognostic sign? *Journal of Clinical Oncology*, 9:1973–83.

Hagberg H, Killander A, Simonsson B (1983). Serum β2-microglobulin in malignant lymphoma. *Cancer*, 51:2220–5.

Hall BH, Green DM (1983). Sexual and reproductive function following treatment during childhood and adolescence for cancer. *Proceedings of the Annual Meeting of the American Society of Clinical Oncology*, 2:C-272.

Halpern S, Chatten J, Meadows AT (1983). Anterior mediastinal masses: anesthesia hazards and other problems. *Clinical and Laboratory Observations*, 102:407–10.

Haluska FG, *et al.* (1986). The t(8;14) translocation occurring in B-cell malignancies results from mistakes in V-D-J joining. *Nature, London*, 324:158.

Hanto DW, *et al.* (1981). Clinical spectrum of lymphoproliferative disorders in renal transplant recipients and evidence for the role of Epstein–Barr virus. *Cancer Research*, 41:4253–61.

Harousseau JL, Tricot G, Gisselbrecht C, Asselain B, Flandrin G (1982). Mediastinal lymphomas in adults. A clinical and histological study of 30 cases. *Nouvelle Presse Medicale*, 11:1393–6 (in French).

Harten G, Stephani U, Henze G, Langermann HJ, Riehm H, Hanefeld F (1984). Slight impairment of psychomotor skills in children after treatment of acute lymphoblastic leukemia. *European Journal of Paediatrics*, 142:189–97.

Harwood SJ, Carroll RG, Anderson M, Friedman BI, Zangara LM, Brunette AK, Kline R (1987). SPECT gallium scanning for lymphoma and infection. *Clinical Nuclear Medicine*, 12:694–702.

Hay N, Bishop JM, Levens D (1987). Regulatory elements that modulate expression of human c-*myc*. *Genes and Development*, 1:659–71.

Haynes BF (1981*a*). Differentiation pathways of human lymphocytes; use of monoclonal antibodies and malignant T cells as investigative probes. *Immunobiology*, 159:14.

Haynes BF (1981*b*). Human T lymphocyte antigens as defined by monoclonal antibodies. *Immunological Reviews*, 57:127–61.

Henle W, Henle G (1979). Seroepidemiology of the virus. In *The Epstein Barr virus* (ed. MA Epstein and BG Achong), pp. 61–78. Springer, New York.

Hertler A, *et al.* (1987). Intrathecal administration of WT1 ricin a chain immunotoxin (meeting abstract). *Proceedings of the American Society of Clinical Oncology*, 6:A989.

Hesseling P, Wood RE, Nortje CJ, Mouton S (1989). African Burkitt's lymphoma in the Cape Province of South Africa and in Namibia. *Oral Surgery, Oral Medicine, Oral Pathology*, 68:162–6.

Hofmann WJ, Momburg F, Moller P (1988*a*). Thymic medullary cells expressing B lymphocyte antigens. *Human Pathology*, 19:1280–7.

Hofmann WJ, Momburg F, Moller P, Otto HF (1988*b*). Intra- and extrathymic B cells in physiologic and pathologic conditions. Immunohistochemical study on normal thymus and lymphofollicular hyperplasia of the thymus. *Archiv*, 412:431–42.

Hood LKM, Hunkapillar T (1985). T cell antigen receptors and the immunoglobulin supergene family. *Cell*, 40:225–9.

Hu ETM, *et al.* (1985). Detection of B-cell lymphoma in peripheral blood by DNA hybridisation. *Lancet*, ii:1092–5.

Hvizdala E, *et al.* (1983). Histology and stage related response to therapy in children with non-Hodgkin's lymphoma. *Blood*, 62 (Suppl. 1):213a.

Hvizdala EV, *et al.* (1988). Lymphoblastic lymphoma in children—a randomized trial comparing LSA2-L2 with the A-COP+ therapeutic regimen: a Pediatric Oncology Group Study. *Journal of Clinical Oncology*, 6:26–33.

Ingram L, Mott MG, Mann JR, Raafat F, Darbyshire PJ, Morris JPH (1987). Second malignancies in children treated for non-Hodgkin's lymphoma and T-cell leukaemia with the UKCCSG regimens. *British Journal of Cancer*, 55:463–6.

Ito K, *et al.* (1989). TI: T cell receptor delta chain gene rearrangement in acute unclassified leukemia. *Rinsho Ketsueki*, 30:2024–8.

Iverson U, *et al.* (1972). Cell kinetics of African cases of Burkitt's lymphoma. A preliminary report. *European Journal of Cancer*, 8:305–10.

Jacobson JO, Aisenberg AC, Lamarre L, Willett CG, Linggood RM, Miketic LM, Harris NL (1988). Mediastinal large cell lymphoma. An uncommon subset of adult lymphoma curable with combined modality therapy. *Cancer*, 62:1893–8.

Jaffe ES, Cossman J (1985). Immunodiagnosis of lymphoid and mononuclear phagocytic neoplasms. *Developments in Oncology*, 34:83–115.

Janossy G, *et al.* (1979). Terminal transferase positive human bone marrow cells exhibit the antigenic phenotype of common acute lymphoblastic leukemia. *Journal of Immunology*, 123:1525–9.

Janossy G, Coustan SE, Campana D (1989). The reliability of cytoplasmic CD3 and CD22 antigen expression in the immunodiagnosis of acute leukemia: study of 500 cases. *Leukemia*, 3:170–81.

Janus C, Edwards BK, Sariban E, Magrath IT (1984). Surgical resection and limited chemotherapy for abdominal undifferentiated lymphomas. *Cancer Treatment Reports*, 68:599–605.

Jenkin RD, *et al.* (1984). The treatment of localized non-Hodgkin's lymphoma in children: a report from the Children's Cancer Study Group. *Journal of Clinical Oncology*, 2:88–97.

Jones GR, Ettinger LJ (1985). Continuous infusion of high-dose cytosine arabinoside for treatment of childhood acute leukemia and non-Hodgkin's lymphoma in relapse. *Seminars in Oncology*, 12 (Suppl. 3):150.

Jones C, Morse HG, Kao FT, Carbone A, Palmer E (1985). Human T-cell receptor alpha-chain genes: location on chromosome 14. *Science*, 228:83–5.

Kadin ME, *et al.* (1986). Childhood Ki-1 lymphoma presenting with skin lesions and peripheral lymphadenopathy. *Blood*, 68:1042–9.

Kamel AM, Assem MM, Jaffe E, Magrath I, Aboul EM, Hindawy D (1989). Immunological phenotypic pattern of acute lymphoblastic leukaemia in Egypt. *Leukemia Research*, 13:519–25.

Kamel A, Ghaleb FM, Assem MM, Hindawy DS, Jaffe ES, Magrath IT (1990). Phenotypic analysis of T cell leukemia in Egypt. *Leukemia Research*, 14(7):601–9.

Kamps MP, Murre C, Sun X-H, Baltimore D (1990). A new homeobox gene contributes the DNA binding domain of the t(1;19) translocation protein in pre-B ALL. *Cell*, **60**:547–55.

Kaneko Y, *et al.* (1988). A novel translocation, t(9;17)(q34;q23), in aggressive childhood lymphoblastic lymphoma. *Leukemia*, **2**:745–8.

Kaneko Y, *et al.* (1989). A novel translocation, t(2;5)(p23;q35), in childhood phagocytic large T-cell lymphoma mimicking malignant histiocytosis. *Blood*, **73**:806–13.

Kaneko Y, Frizzera G, Shikano T, Kobayashi H, Maseki N, Sakurai M (1989). Chromosomal and immunophenotypic patterns in T cell acute lymphoblastic leukemia (T ALL) and lymphoblastic lymphoma (LBL). *Leukemia*, **3**:886–92.

Kaplan WD (1990). Residual mass and negative gallium scintigraphy in treated lymphoma: when is the gallium scan really negative? *Journal of Nuclear Medicine*, **31**:369–71.

Kato A, *et al.* (1987). A variant Burkitt-type translocation (2p−;8q+) in a patient with diffuse large cell lymphoma. *Cancer Genetics and Cytogenetics*, **24**:225–9.

Kaudewitz P, *et al.* (1989). Primary and secondary cutaneous Ki-1+ (CD30+) anaplastic large cell lymphomas. Morphologic, immunohistologic, and clinical characteristics. *American Journal of Pathology*, **135**:359–67.

Kelly K, Siebenlist U (1985). The role of c-*myc* in the proliferation of normal and neoplastic cells. *Journal of Clinical Immunology*, **5**:65–77.

Kelly K, Siebenlist U (1986). The regulation and expression of c-*myc* in normal and malignant cells. *Annual Reviews of Immunology*, **4**:317–38.

Kelly K, Siebenlist U (1988). Mitogenic activation of normal T cells leads to increased initiation of transcription in the c-*myc* locus. *Journal of Biological Chemistry*, **263**:4828–31.

Kelly K, Underwood B (1987). Cell growth associated regulation of c-*myc* and c-*fos* in normal human T cells. *Advances in Experimental Medicine and Biology*, **213**:241–7.

Kimura N, Kikuchi M (1989). Analysis of T-cell receptor delta chain gene in hematological malignancies. *Nippon Ketsueki Gakkai Zasshi*, **52**:1471–8.

Kimura N, *et al.* (1989). Rearrangement of T-cell receptor delta chain gene as a marker of lineage a clonality in T-cell lymphoproliferative disorders. *Cancer Research*, **49**(16):4488–92.

Kingston RE (1989). Transcription control and differentiation: the HLH family c-*myc* and C/EBP. *Current Opinions in Cell Biology*, **1**:1081–7.

Kitinya JN, Lauren PA (1982). Burkitt's lymphoma on Mount Kilimanjaro and in the inland regions of North Tanzania. *East African Medical Journal*, **59**:256–60.

Klein G, Klein E (1985). Evolution of tumors and the impact of molecular oncology. *Nature, London*, **315**:190–5.

Kneba M, Krieger G, Brocke U, Bolz I, Kronke M (1986). Rearrangements of immunoglobulin and T-cell-antigen receptor genes as diagnostic markers in lymphatic neoplasms. *Onkologie*, **9**:6–9 (in German).

Knowles DM (1989). Immunophenotypic and antigen receptor gene rearrangement analysis in T cell neoplasia. *American Journal of Pathology*, **134**:761–85.

Koh SJ, Vargas GF, Caces JN, Johnson WW (1980). Malignant 'histiocytic' lymphoma in childhood. *American Journal of Clinical Pathology*, **74**:417–26.

Korsmeyer SJ, *et al.* (1981). Developmental hierarchy of immunoglobulin gene rearrangements in human leukemic pre-B-cells. *Proceedings of the National Academy of Sciences of the USA*, **78**:7096–100.

Kristoffersson U, Heim S, Heldrup J (1985). Cytogenetic studies of childhood non-Hodgkin lymphomas. *Hereditas*, **3**:77.

Krudy AD, Dunnick NR, Magrath IT, Shawker TH, Doppman JL, Spiegel R (1981). CT of American Burkitt's lymphoma. *American Journal of Radiology*, **136**:747–54.

Kunkel TA, Gopinathan KP, Dube DK, Snow ET, Loeb LA (1986). Rearrangements of DNA mediated by terminal transferase. *Proceedings of the National Academy of Sciences of the USA*, **83**:1867–71.

Kupper H, Ziermann S, Fiebig H, Vogt S, Heidrich L (1989). Secondary follicles in the thymus. Immunohistologic characterization of B lymphocytes using monoclonal antibodies. *Zentralblatt für Allgemeine Pathologie und Pathologische Anatomie*, **135**:269–75.

Ladjadj Y, *et al.* (1984). Abdominal Burkitt-type lymphomas in Algeria. *British Journal of Cancer*, **49**:503–12.

Lamarre L, Jacobson JO, Aisenberg AC, Harris NL (1989). Primary large cell lymphoma of the mediastinum. A histologic and immunophenotypic study of 29 cases. *American Journal of Surgical Pathology*, **13**:730–9.

Lang JC, Whitelaw B, Talbot S, Wilkie NM (1988). Transcriptional regulation of the human c-*myc* gene. *British Journal of Cancer Supplement*, **9**:62–6.

Le Beau MM, Rowley JD (1986). Chromosomal abnormalities in leukemia and lymphoma; clinical and biological significance. *Advances in Human Genetics*, **15**:1–54.

Le Beau MM, *et al.* (1985). Chromosomal localization of the human T cell receptor beta-chain genes. *Cell*, **41**:335.

Le Beau MM, *et al.* (1986). T-cell receptor alpha-chain gene is split in a human T-cell leukemia cell line with a t(11;14) (p15;q11). *Proceedings of the National Academy of Sciences of the USA*, **83**:9744–8.

Lennert K, Mohri N, Stein H, Kaiserling E (1975). The histopathology of malignant lymphoma. *British Journal of Haematology*, **31**:193.

Lenoir GM, Bornkamm GW (1988). Burkitt's lymphoma, a human cancer model for the study of the multistep development of cancer; proposal of a new scenario. In *Advances in viral oncology*, **7**:173–206.

Lenoir GM, Philip T, Sohier R (1984). Burkitt-type lymphoma: EBV association and cytogenetic markers in cases from various geographic locations. In *Pathogenesis of leukemias and lymphomas. Environmental influences* (ed. IT Magrath, G O'Conor, and B Ramot), pp. 283–95. Arnold, London.

Levine PH, *et al.* (1982). The American Burkitt's lymphoma registry; eight years experience. *Cancer*, **49**:1016–22.

Levine EG, *et al.* (1985). There are differences in cytogenetic abnormalities among histologic subtypes of the non-Hodgkin's lymphomas. *Blood*, **66**:1414.

Levitt LJ, Aisenberg AC, Harris NL, Linggood RM, Poppema S (1982). Primary non-Hodgkin's lymphoma of the mediastinum. *Cancer*, **50**:2486–92.

Lie SO, Sirdahl S (1985). High-dose cytosine arabinoside in the treatment of childhood malignancies. *Seminars in Oncology*, **12** (Suppl. 3):1605.

Link MP, *et al.* (1983a). Cutaneous lymphoblastic lymphoma with pre-B markers. *Blood*, **61**:838.

Link M, *et al.* (1983b). A single monoclonal antibody identifies T-cell lineage of childhood lymphoid malignancies. *Blood*, **62**:722.

Link MP, Donaldson SS, Berard CW, Shuster JJ, Murphy SB (1990). Results of treatment of childhood localized non-Hodgkin's lymphoma with combination chemotherapy with or without radiotherapy. *New England Journal of Medicine*, **322**:1169–74.

Lipford EH Jr, Margolick JB, Longo DL, Fauci AS, Jaffe ES (1988). Angiocentric immunoproliferative lesions: a clinicopathologic spectrum of post-thymic T-cell proliferations. *Blood*, **72**:1674–81.

Lortan JE, Roobottom CA, Oldfield S, MacLennan IC (1987). Newly produced virgin B cells migrate to secondary lymphoid organs but their capacity to enter follicles is restricted. *European Journal of Immunology*, **17**:1311–16.

Lukes RJ, Collins RD (1975). New approaches to the classification of the lymphomata. *British Journal of Cancer*, **31** (Suppl. II):1–28.

McBride OW, Hieter PA, Hollis GF, Swan D, Otey MC, Leder P (1982). Chromosomal location of human kappa and lambda immunoglobulin light chain constant region genes. *Journal of Experimental Medicine*, **155**:1480–90.

McKeithan TW, *et al.* (1986). Molecular cloning of the breakpoint junction of a human chromosomal 8;14 translocation involving the T cell receptor alpha-chain gene and sequences on the 3' side of MYC. *Proceedings of the National Academy of Sciences of the USA*, **83**:6636–40.

MacLennan IC, Gray D (1986). Antigen-driven selection of virgin and memory B cells. *Immunological Reviews*, **91**:61–85.

MacLennan IC, Bazin H, Chassoux D, Gray D, Lortan J (1985). Comparative analysis of the development of B cells in marginal zones and follicles. *Advances in Experimental Medicine and Biology*, **186**:139–44.

McManaway ME, *et al.* (1990). Special inhibition of proliferation of a subset of Burkitt's lymphoma cell lines by a c-*myc* intron antisense oligodeoxynucleotide. *Lancet*, **335**:807–11.

Madanat FF, Amr SS, Tarawneh MS, el Khateeb MS, Marar BT (1986). Burkitt's lymphoma in Jordanian children: epidemiological and clinical study. *Journal of Tropical Medicine and Hygiene*, **89**:189–91.

Magrath IT (1981). Lymphocyte differentiation pathways—an essential basis for the comprehension of lymphoid neoplasia. *Journal of National Cancer Institute*, **67**:501–14.

Magrath IT (1982). Malignant lymphomas. In *Cancer in the young* (ed. AS Levine), pp. 473–574. Masson, New York.

Magrath IT (1984). Biological features of pediatric non-Hodgkin's lymphoma. In *Hodgkin's disease and non-Hodgkin's lymphoma. New perspectives in immunotherapy, diagnosis and treatment* (ed. RJ Ford, L Fuller, and FB Hagermeister), pp. 201–12. Raven Press, New York.

Magrath IT (1985). Burkitt's lymphoma as a human tumour model: new concepts in etiology and pathogen. In *Pediatric hematology and oncology reviews* (ed. C Pochedly), pp. 1–51. Praeger, Westport, CT.

Magrath I (1989a). Infectious mononucleosis and malignant neoplasia. In *Infectious mononucleosis* (2nd edn) (ed. D Schlossberg), pp. 142–93. Springer, New York.

Magrath IT (1989b). Prospects for the development of antineoplastic therapy based on molecular pathology. In *New directions in cancer treatment* (ed. IT Magrath), pp. 399–427. Springer, Heidelberg.

Magrath IT (1990a). Historical perspective: the origins of modern concepts of biology and management. In *The non-Hodgkin's lymphomas* (ed. IT Magrath), pp. 15–28. Arnold, London.

Magrath IT (1990b). The pathogenesis of Burkitt's lymphoma. In *Advances in cancer research. The pathogenesis of Burkitt's lymphoma* (ed. G Van de Woude and G Klein), pp. 133–270. Academic Press, San Diego.

Magrath IT (1990c). Small non-cleaved cell lymphomas. In *The non-Hodgkin's lymphomas* (ed. IT Magrath), pp. 256–78. Arnold, London.

Magrath IT (1991). African Burkitt's lymphoma. *American Journal of Pediatric Hematology and Oncology*, **13**:222–46.

Magrath IT, Kadin M (1990). Large cell lymphomas in children. In *The non-Hodgkin's lymphomas* (ed. IT Magrath), pp. 279–92. Arnold, London.

Magrath IT, Sariban E (1985). Clinical features of Burkitt's lymphoma in the USA. In *Burkitt's lymphoma—a human cancer model*, pp. 119–27. IARC Publications, Lyon.

Magrath IT, Wilson W (1990). Clinical presentation and staging. In *The non-Hodgkin's lymphomas* (ed. IT Magrath), pp. 180–99. Arnold, London.

Magrath IT, Ziegler JL (1980). Bone marrow involvement in Burkitt's lymphoma and its relationship to acute B-cell leukemia. *Leukemia Research*, **4**:33–59.

Magrath IT, et al. (1974). Surgical reduction of tumour bulk in management of abdominal Burkitt's lymphoma. *British Medical Journal*, **2**:308.

Magrath IT, Mugerwa J, Bailey I, Olweny C, Kiryabwire Y (1974). Intracerebral Burkitt's lymphoma: pathology clinical features and treatment. *Quarterly Journal of Medicine*, **43**:489–508.

Magrath IT, et al. (1980). Characterization of lymphoma derived cell lines: comparison of cell lines positive and negative for Epstein–Barr virus nuclear antigen II surface markers. *Journal of the National Cancer Institute*, **64**:477–83.

Magrath IT, Lee YJ, Anderson T, Henle W, Ziegler J, Simon R, Schen P (1980). Prognostic factors in Burkitt's lymphoma: importance of total tumor burden. *Cancer*, **45**:1507–15.

Magrath I, Benjamin D, Papadopoulos N (1983). Serum monoclonal immunoglobulin bands in undifferentiated lymphomas of Burkitt and non-Burkitt types. *Blood*, **61**:726–31.

Magrath IT, et al. (1984). An effective therapy for both undifferentiated (including Burkitt's) lymphomas and lymphoblastic lymphomas in children and young adults. *Blood*, **63**:1102–11.

Magrath IT, Adde M, Sandlund J, Jain V (1991). Phase II studies of ifosfamide in pediatric non-Hodgkin's lymphomas. *Hematological Oncology*, **9**:267–74.

Magrath IT, Jain V, Jaffe E (1992). The pathology of Burkitt's lymphoma. In *Neoplastic pathology*, pp. 749–72. Williams & Wilkins, Baltimore.

Malcolm S, Barton P, Murphy C, Ferguson SMA, Bentley DL, Rabbitts TH (1982). Localization of human immunoglobulin kappa light chain variable region genes to the short arm of chromosome 2 by *in situ* hybridization. *Proceedings of the National Academy of Sciences of the USA*, **79**:4957–61.

Mangan KF, et al. (1985). Acute lymphoblastic leukemia of Burkitt's type (L-3 ALL) lacking surface immunoglobulin and the 8;14 translocation. *American Journal of Clinical Pathology*, **83**:121–6.

Mason DY, et al. (1990). CD30-positive large cell lymphomas ('Ki-1 lymphoma') are associated with a chromosomal translocation involving 5q35. *British Journal of Haematology*, **74**:161–8.

Mathé G, Rappaport H, O'Conor GT, Torloni H (1976). *Histological and cytological typing of neoplastic diseases of the haemopoietic and lymphoid tissues*. World Health Organization, Geneva.

Mathieu-Mahul D, et al. (1986). A t(8;14)(q24;q11) translocation in a T-cell leukemia (L1-ALL) with c-*myc* and TCR-alpha chain locus rearrangements. *International Journal of Cancer*, **38**:835–40.

Meadows AT, Gordon J, Massari DJ, Littman P, Fergusson J, Moss K (1981). Declines in IQ scores and cognitive dysfunctions in children with acute lymphocytic leukaemia treated with cranial irradiation. *Lancet*, **ii**:1015–18.

Meadows AT, et al. (1985). Second malignant neoplasms in children: an update from the late effects study group. *Journal of Clinical Oncology*, **3**:532–8.

Meadows AT, et al. (1989). Similar efficacy of 6 and 18 months of therapy with four drugs (COMP) for localized non-Hodgkin's lymphoma of children: a report from the Childrens Cancer Study Group. *Journal of Clinical Oncology*, **7**:92–9.

Meuer SCAO, et al. (1983). Evidence for the T3-associated 90K heterodimer as the T cell antigen receptor. *Nature, London*, **303**:808–10.

Meyers PA, Potter VP, Wollner N, Exelby P (1985). Bowel perforation during initial treatment for childhood non-Hodgkin's lymphoma. *Cancer*, **56**:259–61.

Minden MD, Mak TW (1986). The structure of the T cell antigen receptor genes in normal and malignant T cells. *Blood*, **68**:327–36.

Morabito F, Prasthofer EF, Pullen DJ, Mahoney D, Downing JR, Crist WM, Grossi CED (1987). Analysis of surface antigen profile, TdT expression, and T cell receptor gene rearrangement for maturational staging of leukemic T cells: a pediatric oncology group study. *Leukemia*, **1**:514–17.

Moss HA, Nannis ED, Poplack DG (1981). The effects of prophylactic treatment of the central nervous system on the intellectual functioning of children with acute lymphocytic leukemia. *American Journal of Medicine*, **71**:47–52.

Moss DJ, et al. (1983). A comparison of Epstein–Barr virus-specific T-cell immunity in malaria-endemic and nonendemic regions of Papua New Guinea. *International Journal of Cancer*, **31**:727–32.

Mott MG, et al. (1984). Adjuvant low dose radiation in childhood T cell leukaemia/lymphoma (A report from the United Kingdom children's cancer study group-UKC). *British Journal of Cancer*, **50**:457.

Müller–Weihrich S, et al. (1984). Childhood B-cell lymphomas and leukemias. Improvement of prognosis by a therapy developed for B-neoplasms by the BFM study group. *Onkologie*, **7**:205.

Müller–Weihrich S, Henze G, Odenwald E, et al. (1985). BFM trials for childhood non-Hodgkin's lymphomas. In *Malignant lymphomas and Hodgkin's disease: experimental and therapeutic advances* (ed. F Cavalli, G Bonadonna, and M Rozencweig), p. 633–42. Martinus Nijhoff Publishing, Boston.

Müller–Weihrich S, et al. (1987). B-type non-Hodgkin's lymphomas and leukemia: the BFM study group experience. In *Proceedings of the 3rd International Conference on Malignant Lymphoma* (ed. F Cavalli, G Bonadonna, and M Rozencweig), Abstract 43.

Murphy S (1977). The management of childhood non-Hodgkin's lymphoma. *Cancer Treatment Reports*, **61**:1161.

Murphy SB, Hustu HO (1980). A randomised trial of combined modality therapy of childhood non-Hodgkin's lymphoma. *Cancer*, **45**:630–7.

Murphy SB, Magrath IT (1991). Workshop on pediatric lymphomas: current results and prospects. *Annals of Oncology*, **2** (Suppl. 2):219–23.

Murphy SB, et al. (1979). Correlation of tumor cell kinetic studies with surface marker results in childhood non-Hodgkins lymphoma. *Cancer Research*, **39**:1534–8.

Murphy S, et al. (1986). Results of treatment of advanced stage Burkitt's lymphoma and B-cell, (SIg+) acute lymphoblastic leukemia with high-dose fractionated cyclophosphamide and coordinated high-dose methotrexate and cytarabine. *Journal of Clinical Oncology*, **4**:1732.

Murphy SB, Fairclough DL, Hutchison RE, Berard CW (1989). Non-Hodgkin's lymphomas of childhood: an analysis of the histology, staging, and response to treatment of 338 cases at a single institution. *Journal of Clinical Oncology*, **7**:186–93.

Murre C, et al. (1985). Human gamma-chain genes are rearranged in leukaemic T cells and map to the short arm of chromosome 7. *Nature, London*, **316**:549–52.

Myers CD, et al. (1984). An immunotoxin with therapeutic potential in T cell leukemia: WT1-ricin A. *Blood*, **63**:1178–85.

Nadler LM, et al. (1984). B cell origin of non-T cell acute lymphoblastic leukemia. A model for discrete stages of neoplastic and normal pre-B cell differentiation. *Journal of Clinical Investigation*, **74**:332.

Nathwani BN, et al. (1987). A morphologic study of childhood lymphoma of the diffuse 'histiocytic' type. The Pediatric Oncology Group experience. *Cancer*, **59**:1138–42.

National Cancer Institute (1982). National Cancer Institute sponsored study of the classifications of non-Hodgkin's lymphomas. Summary and description of a working formulation for clinical usage. *Cancer*, **49**:2112–35.

Nelson DF, *et al.* (1977). The role of radiation therapy in localized resectable intestinal non-Hodgkin's lymphoma in children. *Cancer*, **39**:89–97.

Neri A, Barriga F, Knowles DM, Magrath IT, Dalla FR (1988). Different regions of the immunoglobulin heavy-chain locus are involved in chromosomal translocations in distinct pathogenetic forms of Burkitt lymphoma. *Proceedings of the National Academy of Sciences of the USA*, **85**:2748–52.

Ngan BY, Nourse I, Cleary ML (1989). Detection of chromosomal translocation t(14;18) within the minor cluster region of bc1-2 by polymerase chain reaction and direct genomic sequencing of the enzymatically amplified DNA in follicular lymphomas. *Blood*, **73**:1759–62.

Ochs J, *et al.* (1986). Phase I–II study of recombinant alpha-2 interferon against advanced leukemia and lymphoma in children. *Journal of Clinical Oncology*, **4**:883–7.

Olweny CLM, *et al.* (1977). Cerebrospinal irradiation of Burkitt's lymphoma. *Acta Radiologica, Therapy, Physics, Biology*, **12**:225–31.

Osmond DG, Priddle S, Rico-Vargas S (1990). Proliferation of B cell precursors in bone marrow of pristane-conditioned and melanic-infected mice: implications for B cell oncogenesis. *Current Topics in Microbiology and Immunology*, **166**:149–57.

Pasqualini T, *et al.* (1983). Evaluation of testicular function following long-term treatment for acute lymphoblastic leukemia. *American Journal of Pediatric Hematology and Oncology*, **5**:11–20.

Patte C, *et al.* (1986). Improved survival rate in children with stage III and IV B cell non-Hodgkin's lymphoma and leukemia using multi-agent chemotherapy: results of a study of 114 children from the French Pediatric Oncology Society. *Journal of Clinical Oncology*, **4**:1219.

Patte C, *et al.* (1991). High survival rate in advanced stage B cell lymphomas and leukemias without CNS involvement with a short intensive poly-chemotherapy: results from the French Pediatric Oncology Society of a randomized trial of 216 children. *Journal of Clinical Oncology*, **9**:123–32.

Pegoraro L, *et al.* (1984). A 14;18 and an 8;14 chromosome translocation in a cell line derived from an acute B-cell leukemia. *Proceedings of the National Academy of Sciences of the USA*, **81**:7166–70.

Pellici PG, Knowles DM, Dalla-Favera R (1985). Lymphoid tumors displaying rearrangements of both immunoglobulin and T cell receptor genes. *Journal of Experimental Medicine*, **162**:1015–24.

Pellici PG, *et al.* (1986*a*). Multiple monoclonal B cell expansions and c-*myc* oncogene rearrangements in acquired immune deficiency syndrome related lymphoproliferative disorders. Implications for lymphomagenesis. *Journal of Experimental Medicine*, **164**:2049–60.

Pellici PG, *et al.* (1986*b*). Chromosomal breakpoints and structural alterations of the c-*myc* locus differ in endemic sporadic forms of Burkitt lymphoma. *Proceedings of the National Academy of Sciences of the USA*, **83**:2984.

Philip T, *et al.* (1986*a*). The role of massive therapy with autologous bone marrow transplantation in Burkitt's lymphoma. *Clinics in Haematology*, **15**:205.

Philip T, *et al.* (1986*b*). Massive therapy and autologous bone marrow transplantation in pediatric and young adults with Burkitt's lymphoma (30 courses on 28 patients: a 4-year experience). *European Journal of Cancer and Clinical Oncology*, **22**:1015–27.

Philip T, *et al.* (1987). Effective multiagent chemotherapy in children with advanced B-cell lymphoma: who remains the high risk patient? *British Journal of Haematology*, **65**:159–64.

Pichler E, *et al.* (1982). Results of LSA2-L2 therapy in 26 children with non-Hodgkin's lymphoma. *Cancer*, **50**:2740–6.

Piro AJ, Weiss DR, Hellman S (1976). Mediastinal Hodgkin's disease: a possible danger for intubational anaesthesia. Intubation danger in Hodgkin's disease. *International Journal of Radiation Oncology—Biology—Physics*, **1**:415–19.

Price SL, Hecker BR (1987). Pulmonary oedema following airway obstruction in a patient with Hodgkin's disease. *British Journal of Anaesthesia*, **59**:518–21.

Pui CH, *et al.* (1988). Serum interleukin 2 receptor levels in childhood acute lymphoblastic leukemia. *Blood*, **71**:1135–7.

Pui CH, *et al.* (1990). Heterogeneity of presenting features and their relation to treatment outcome in 120 children with T-cell acute lymphoblastic leukemia. *Blood*, **75**:174–9.

Purtilo D (1984). Immunoregulatory defects and Epstein–Barr virus-associated lymphoid disorders. In *Pathogenesis of leukemias and lymphomas. Environmental influences* (ed. IT Magrath, G O'Conor, and B Ramot), pp. 235–57. Raven Press, New York.

Purtilo DT (1987). Epstein–Barr virus: the spectrum of its manifestations in human beings. *Southern Medical Journal*, **80**:943–7.

Radbruch A, Burger C, Klein S, Muller W (1986). Control of immunoglobulin class switch recombination. *Immunological Reviews*, **89**:69–83.

Rappold GA, *et al.* (1984). c-*myc* and immunoglobulin kappa light chain constant genes are on the 8q+ chromosome of three Burkitt lymphoma lines with t(2;8) translocations. *EMBO Journal*, **3**:2951.

Reinherz EL, Schlossman SF (1980). The differentiation and function of human T lymphocytes. *Cell*, **19**:821–7.

Reinherz EL, Nadler LM, Sallan SE, Schlossman SF (1979). Subset derivation of T-cell acute lymphoblastic leukemia in man. *Journal of Clinical Investigation*, **64**:392–7.

Reinherz EL, Kung PC, Goldstein G, Levey RH, Schlossman S (1980). Discrete stages of human intrathymic differentiation; analysis of normal thymocytes and leukemic lymphoblasts of T-cell lineage. *Proceedings of the National Academy of Sciences in the USA*, **77**:1588–92.

Rejou F, Khatib N, Bourbotte M, Margueritte G, Jean R (1989). Isolated cerebral calcifications after prophylactic treatment of cerebromeningeal involvement of acute lymphoblastic leukemia: relation of psycho-intellectual sequelae. *Pediatrie*, **44**:405–11 (in French).

Robison LL, Nesbit ME Jr, Sather HN, Meadows AT, Ortega JA, Hammond GD (1984). Factors associated with IQ scores in long-term survivors of childhood acute lymphoblastic leukemia. *American Journal of Pediatric Hematology and Oncology*, **6**:115–21.

Roholl PJ, *et al.* (1988). Immunologic marker analysis of normal and malignant histiocytes. A comparative study of monoclonal antibodies for diagnostic purposes. *American Journal of Clinical Pathology*, **89**:187–94.

Roper M, *et al.* (1983). Monoclonal antibody characterization of surface antigens in childhood T-cell malignancies. *Blood*, **61**:830.

Rowe DT, Rowe M, Evan GI, Wallace LE, Farrell PJ, Rickinson AB (1986). Restricted expression of EBV latent genes and T-lymphocyte-detected membra antigen in Burkitt's lymphoma cells. *EMBO Journal*, **5**:2599–607.

Rowe M, Rowe DT, Gregory CD, Young LS, Farrell PJ, Rupani H, Rickinson AB (1987). Differences in B cell growth phenotype reflect novel patterns of Epstein–Barr virus latent gene expression in Burkitt's lymphoma cells. *EMBO Journal*, **6**:2743–51.

Rowland JH, *et al.* (1984). Effects of different forms of central nervous system prophylaxis on neuropsychologic function in childhood leukemia. *Journal of Clinical Oncology*, **2**:1327–35.

Royer HD, *et al.* (1984). Genes encoding the Tiβ subunit of the antigen/MHC receptor undergo rearrangement during intrathymic ontogeny prior to surface T3-Ti expression. *Cell*, **39**:261–6.

Royer HD, *et al.* (1985). Genes encoding the T-cell receptor alpha and beta subunits are transcribed in an ordered manner during intrathymic ontogeny. *Proceedings of the National Academy of Sciences of the USA*, **82**:5510–14.

Ruz OA, Alemany EF, Ruiz F, de Mesa L, Galan CA, Bahamonde LC (1986). Sudden death during anesthesia in a patient with a tumor of the mediastinum. *Revista Española de Anesesiologica y Reanimacion*, **33**:443–5 (in Spanish).

Saemundsen AK, *et al.* (1981). Documentation of Epstein–Barr virus infection in immunodeficient patients with life-threatening lymphoproliferative diseases by Epstein–Barr virus complementary RNA/DNA and viral DNA/RNA hybridization. *Cancer Research*, **41**:4237–42.

Said JA, Waters BG, Cousens P, Stevens MM (1989). Neuropsychological sequelae of central nervous system prophylaxis in survivors of childhood acute lymphoblastic leukemia. *Journal of Consulting and Clinical Psychology*, **57**:251–6.

Salem P, *et al.* (1985). Immunoproliferative small intestinal disease. *Developments in Oncology*, **32**:9–77.

Sandlund J, Magrath IT (1990). Lymphoblastic lymphomas. In *The non-Hodgkin's lymphomas* (ed. IT Magrath), pp. 240–55. Edward Arnold, London.

Sandlund JT, Kiwanuka J, Marti GE, Goldschmidts G, Magrath IT (1986). Characterization of Burkitt's lymphoma cell lines with monoclonal antibodies using an ELISA technique. In *Proceedings of the 2nd International Congress of Human Leukocyte Antigens*, Vol. 2, *Leukocyte typing* (ed. EL Reinherz, BF Hayes, LM Nadler, and ID Bernstein), pp. 403–19. Springer, New York.

Sariban E, Janus C, Edwards B, Magrath IT (1983). Central nervous system involvement in American Burkitt's lymphoma. *Journal of Clinical Oncology*, 11:677–81.

Sariban E, Donahue A, Magrath IT (1984). Jaw involvement in American Burkitt's lymphoma. *Cancer*, 53:141–6.

Schaadt M, Kirchner H, Fonatsch C, Diehl V (1979). Intracranial heterotransplantation of human hematopoietic cells in nude mice. *International Journal of Cancer*, 23:751–61.

Seibel NL, Cossman J, Magrath IT (1989). In *Principles and practice of pediatric oncology*. *Lymphoproliferative disorders* (ed. PA Pizzo and D Poplack), pp. 477–90. JB Lippincott, New York.

Shapiro RS, Chauvenet A, McGuire W, Pearson A, Craft AW, McGlave P, Filipovich A (1988). Treatment of B-cell lymphoproliferative disorders with interferon alfa and intravenous gamma globulin. *New England Journal of Medicine*, 318:1334.

Shapiro RS (1990). Epstein–Barr virus-associated B-cell lymphoproliferative disorders in immunodeficiency: meeting the challenge (comment). *Journal of Clinical Oncology*, 8:371–3.

Shawker TH, Dunnick NR, Head GL, Magrath IT (1979). Ultrasound evaluation of American Burkitt's lymphoma. *Journal of Clinical Ultrasound*, 7:279–83.

Shearer WT, et al. (1985). Epstein–Barr virus-associated B-cell proliferations of diverse clonal origins after bone marrow transplantation in a 12-year-old patient with severe combined immunodeficiency. *New England Journal of Medicine*, 312:1151–9.

Sheibani K, et al. (1987). Antigenically defined subgroups of lymphoblastic lymphoma. Relationship to clinical presentation and biologic behavior. *Cancer*, 60:183–90.

Sheibani K, et al. (1987). Lymphoblastic lymphoma expressing natural killer cell-associated antigens: a clinicopathologic study of six cases. *Leukemia Research*, 11:371–7.

Shiramizu B, Magrath IT (1990). Localization of breakpoints by polymerase chain reactions in Burkitt's lymphoma with 8;14 translocations. *Blood*, 75:1848–52.

Shiramizu B, et al. (1991). Patterns of chromosomal breakpoint locations in Burkitt's lymphoma: relevance to geography and EBV association. *Blood*, 77:1516–26.

Sigaux F (1988). Detection of residual disease: analysis of the gene arrangement of immunoglobulins and T-cell antigen receptors. *Pathologie Biologie*, 36:87–90 (in French).

Sigaux F, et al. (1984). Malignant lymphomas with band 8q24 chromosome abnormality: a morphologic continuum extending from Burkitt's to immunoblastic lymphoma. *British Journal of Haematology*, 57:393–405.

Siu G, et al. (1984). The structure, rearrangement and expression of d beta gene segments of the jurine T-cell antigen receptor. *Nature, London*, 311:344–50.

Smith SD, Morgan R, Link MP, McFall P, Hecht F (1986). Cytogenetic and immunophenotypic analysis of cell lines established from patients with T cell leukemia/lymphoma. *Blood*, 67:650–6.

Stein H, et al. (1985). The expression of the Hodgkin's disease associated antigen Ki-1 in reactive and neoplastic lymphoid tissue: evidence that Reed–Sternberg cells and histiocytic malignancies are derived from activated lymphoid cells. *Blood*, 66:848–58.

Stetlet SM, Raffeld M, Cohen P, Cossman J (1988). Detection of occult follicular lymphoma by specific DNA amplification. *Blood*, 72:1822–5.

Subar M, Neri A, Inghirami G, Knowles DM, Dalla FR (1988). Frequent c-*myc* oncogene activation and infrequent presence of Epstein–Barr virus genome in AIDS-associated lymphoma. *Blood*, 72:667–71.

Sullivan M, Ramirez I (1985). Curability of Burkitt's lymphoma with high-dose cyclophosphamide-high dose methotrexate therapy and intrathecal chemoprophylaxis. *Journal of Clinical Oncology*, 3:627–36.

Sullivan MP, et al. (1985a). Pediatric Oncology Group experience with modified LSA2-L2 therapy in 107 children with non-Hodgkin's lymphoma (Burkitt's lymphoma excluded). *Cancer*, 55:323–36.

Sullivan MP, et al. (1985b). Male reproductive functions in long-term survivors of childhood cancer; assessment by sperm count analysis (sca) (abstract). *Proceedings of the Annual Meeting of the American Association for Cancer Research*, 26:182.

Taub R, et al. (1982). Translocation of the c-*myc* gene into the immunoglobulin heavy chain locus in human Burkitt lymphoma and murine plasmacytoma cells. *Proceedings of the National Academy of Sciences of the USA*, 79:7837.

Thiel E, et al. (1989). Prethymic phenotype and genotype of pre-T (CD7+/ER−)-cell leukemia and its clinical significance within adult acute lymphoblastic leukemia. *Blood*, 73:1247–58.

Thomas P, Said JW, Rosenfelt FP, Heifetz LJ (1984). True histiocytic lymphoma: an immunohistochemical and ultrastructural study of two cases. *American Journal of Clinical Pathology*, 81:243–8.

Tkachuk DC, Griesser H, Takihara Y, Champagne E, Minden M, Feller ACK, Mak TW (1988). Rearrangement of T-cell delta locus in lymphoproliferative disorders. *Blood*, 72(1):353–7.

Tsokos GE, Balow JE, Siegel RJ (1981). Renal and metabolic complications of undifferentiated and lymphoblastic lymphomas. *Medicine*, 60:218.

Tsujimoto YFLR, Yunis J, Nowell PC, Croce C (1984). Cloning the chromosome breakpoint of neoplastic B cells with the t(14;18) chromosome translocation. *Science*, 226:1097–9.

Valagussa P, Santoro A, Fossati BF, Banfi A, Bonadonna G (1986). Second acute leukemia and other malignancies following treatment for Hodgkin's disease. *Journal of Clinical Oncology*, 4:830–7.

van der Valk P, et al. (1984). Histiocytic sarcoma (true histiocytic lymphoma); a clinicopathological study of 20 cases. *Histopathology*, 8:105–23.

van Dongen JJ, et al. (1988). Cytoplasmic expression of the CD3 antigen as a diagnostic marker for immature T-cell malignancies. *Blood*, 71:603–12.

Vannier JP, et al. (1988). Treatment of extensive B-cell lymphoma in children: studies of the French Pediatric Oncology Society. *Bulletin du Cancer*, 75:61–8.

Vezzoni P, et al. (1984). Multienzymatic analyses of human malignant lymphomas. Correlation of enzymatic data with pathologic and ultrastructural findings in Burkitt's and lymphoblastic lymphomas. *Cancer*, 54:489–99.

Vodinelich L, Tax W, Bai Y, Pegram S, Capel P, Greaves MF (1983). A monoclonal antibody (WT1) for detecting leukemias of T-cell precursors (T-ALL). *Blood*, 62:1108–13.

Wagner DK, Kiwanuka J, Edwards BK, Rubin LA, Nelson DL, Magrath IT (1987). Soluble interleukin-2 receptor levels in patients with undifferentiated and lymphoblastic lymphomas: correlation with survival. *Journal of Clinical Oncology*, 5:1262–74.

Waldron JA Jr, Dohring EJ, Farber LR (1985). Primary large cell lymphomas of the mediastinum: an analysis of 20 cases. *Seminars in Diagnosis and Pathology*, 2:281–95.

Wallace LE, Young LS, Rowe M, Rowe D, Rickinson AB (1987). Epstein–Barr virus, specific T cell recognition of B cell transformants expressing different EBNA 2 antigens. *International Journal of Cancer*, 39:373–9.

Wanatabe A, Sullivan MP, Sutow WW, Willow JR (1973). Meningeal and bone marrow involvement in children. *American Journal of Diseases in Childhood*, 125:57–61.

Watanabe S, et al. (1986). Immunoblastic lymphadenopathy, angioimmunoblastic lymphadenopathy, and IBL-like T-cell lymphoma. A spectrum of T-cell neoplasia. *Cancer*, 58:2224–32.

Weiss LM, Bindl JM, Picozzi VJ, Link MP, Warnke RA (1986). Lymphoblastic lymphoma: an immunophenotype study of 26 cases with comparison to T cell acute lymphoblastic leukemia. *Blood*, 67:474–8.

West R (1984). Childhood cancer mortality: international comparisons 1955–1974. World Health Statistics, 37:98.

Westcott JL (1981). Percutaneous needle aspiration of hilar and mediastinal masses. *Radiology*, 141:323–9.

Whang-Peng J, Lee EC, Sieverts H, Magrath IT (1984). Burkitt's lymphoma in AIDS: a cytogenetic study. *Blood*, 63:818–22.

Whittle HC, et al. (1984). T-cell control of Epstein–Barr virus infected B-cells is lost during *P. falciparum* malaria. *Nature, London*, 312:449–50.

Willett CG, et al. (1988). Three-dimensional volumetric assessment of response to treatment: stage I and II diffuse large cell lymphoma of the mediastinum. *Radiotherapy and Oncology*, 12:193–8.

Williams ME, et al. (1987). Immunoglobulin and T cell receptor gene rearrangements in human lymphoma a leukemia. *Blood*, 69:79–86.

Wilson JF, et al. (1984). Studies on the pathology of non-Hodgkin's lymphoma of child. I: the role of routine histopathology as a prognostic factor. A report from the children's cancer study group. *Cancer*, 53:169–75.

Wilson JF, et al. (1987). The pathology of non-Hodgkin's lymphoma of childhood: II. Reproducibility and relevance of the histologic classification of 'undifferentiated' lymphomas (Burkitt's versus non-Burkitt's). *Human Pathology*, **18**:1008–14.

Wollner N, *et al.* (1976). Non-Hodgkin's lymphoma in children; a comparative study of two modalities of therapy. *Cancer*, **37**:123.

Wood RE, Nortje CJ, Hesseling P, Mouton S (1988). Involvement of the maxillofacial region in African Burkitt's lymphoma in the Cape Province and Namibia. *Dentomaxillofacial Radiology*, **17**:57–60.

Wurtz A, Chambon JP, Fenaux P, Bauters F, Gosselin B (1989). Large B cell lymphoma of the mediastinum. Six cases. *Annales de Chirurgie*, **43**:165–70.

Weinstein HJ, Cassady JR, Levey R (1983). Long-term results of the APO protocol (vincristine, doxorubicin [adriamycin], and prednisone) for treatment of mediastinal lymphoblastic lymphoma. *Journal of Clinical Oncology*, **1**:537–41.

Weinstein HJ, Lack EE, Cassady JR (1984). APO therapy for malignant lymphoma of large cell 'histiocytic' type of childhood; analysis of treatment results for 29 patients. *Blood*, **64**:422.

Young JL, Ries LG, Silverberg E, Horm JW, Miller RW (1980). Cancer incidence, survival and mortality for children younger than age 15 years. *Cancer*, **58**:598–602.

Yumura YK, *et al.* (1989). Analysis of molecular events in leukemic cells arrested at an early stage of T-cell differentiation. *Blood*, **74**:2103–11.

Zech L, *et al.* (1976). Characteristic chromosomal abnormalities in biopsies and lymphoid-cell lines from patients with Burkitt and non-Burkitt lymphomas. *International Journal of Cancer*, **17**:47.

Ziegler JL (1977). Treatment results of 54 American patients with Burkitt's lymphoma are similar to the African experience. *New England Journal of Medicine*, **297**:75–80.

Ziegler JL, Magrath IT (1974). Burkitt's lymphoma. In *Pathobiology annual*, pp. 129–42. Appleton Century Crofts, New York.

Ziegler J, Magrath IT, Olweny CLM (1979). Cure of Burkitt's lymphoma: 10 year follow-up of 157 Ugandan patients. *Lancet*, ii:936–8.

12.8 Myeloma and other plasma cell malignancies

P. SELBY AND MARTIN GORE

INTRODUCTION

The first case of multiple myeloma was recognized by William MacIntyre who described many of the clinical features of the disease and those properties of urine when it is heated and cooled that are so characteristic. The sample of urine was sent to Henry Bence Jones who analysed it in more detail and the morphology of the malignant cells found in the bone-marrow of this patient were described by John Dalrymple. All three published their findings: Dalrymple in 1846 and Bence Jones in 1847, but it was not until 1850 that MacIntyre published his clinical description. John Clamp, in a remarkable piece of historical investigation, not only clearly laid out the sequence of these events but was also able to uncover the name and personal details of the first patient; he was Thomas McBean, a 45 year old married grocer who had 'numerous offspring' and lived in Devonshire Street, London and who had recently spent a holiday in Scotland (Clamp 1967)! The term multiple myeloma dates from 1873 and was introduced by von Rustizky (Riches and Hobbs 1988).

EPIDEMIOLOGY AND AETIOLOGY

Multiple myeloma and plasmacytoma are among the more common haemopoietic cancers in England and Wales. They account for approximately 20 per cent of such cancers and some 1 per cent of all cancers (Cuzick and De Stavola 1988). Figure 1 shows the age relationship of the incidence of multiple myeloma in males and females in England and Wales together with the absolute number of case registrations in each age group (Office of Population Census and Surveys 1986). The figure illustrates the outstanding features of the descriptive epidemiology of multiple myeloma, namely a rapid increase in incidence with increasing age and a moderate excess at all ages in males. It is very rare in childhood (Bernstein *et al.* 1985). It should be noted that the absolute number of new case registrations in each year falls sharply for ages above 70 years and

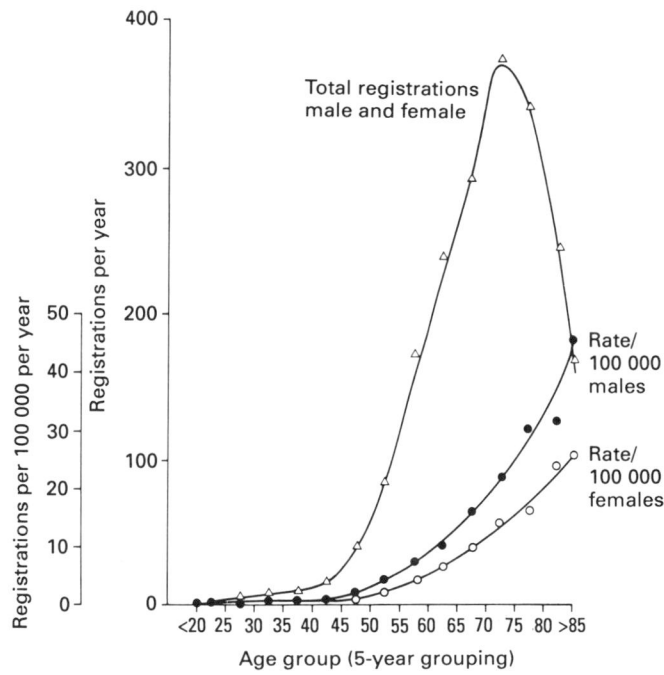

Fig. 1 Epidemiology of multiple myeloma

that almost half of the newly registered patients are less than 65 years old.

The recorded incidence of myeloma has been increasing in many countries (Cuzick *et al.* 1983). However, studies in stable populations with high diagnostic standards for this disease, such as those in Malmo, Sweden, suggest that the real increase in incidence may be quite small and that the reported increases are in part due to increasing diagnostic accuracy (Turesson *et al.* 1984). The incidence of the disease in the age group 20–44 years in the United Kingdom is stable with no evidence of the fall seen in many common epithelial tumours in this age group (Doll 1990).

Geographical and racial differences play an important part in the incidence of myeloma. The disease is much commoner in Black populations than in Caucasians and has a low incidence in Chinese. Data on age-standardized and cumulative incidence rates for multiple myeloma collected from worldwide cancer registries report incidence rates (standardized to the age group 35–64 years) between 0.6 per 100 000 per year in Chinese males and 13 per 100 000 for Black Americans. The highest reported rate of 20.5 per 100 000 is in non-Maori New Zealand Pacific Polynesian Islanders. The high rates of myeloma among Black populations and the low rates in Chinese appear to be retained after migration to new countries suggesting, perhaps, an inherited rather than environmental explanation for the racial differences (Cuzick 1986; Delamore 1986). Where comparisons are available, rates tend to be higher in urban than in rural populations (Muir *et al.* 1987), although this may in part be due to inaccurate registration of death (Nandakumar *et al.* 1986).

Extensive epidemiological studies have been carried out to identify risk factors associated with multiple myeloma. The data suggest associations with farming, agricultural employment, a variety of chemicals including asbestos, arsenic, cutting oils, heavy metals, petrochemicals, leather, and wood dust and those materials associated with plastic and rubber manufacture. The data for an association with farming occupations is the strongest, but remains unexplained (Gallagher *et al.* 1983; Cuzick 1986; Pearce *et al.* 1986; Cuzick and De Stavola 1988; Greenberg and Weiss 1993).

An association with radiation exposure is seen in survivors of the Second World War atomic bombs as well as in occupationally and therapeutically exposed groups (Ichimaru *et al.* 1982). There is a significant excess of myeloma among servicemen who attended the United Kingdom atmospheric nuclear weapons tests in the 1950s and 1960s (Darby *et al.* 1988).

It is attractive to speculate that myeloma may, in some part, be either initiated or promoted by chronic antigenic stimulation. High levels of polyclonal immunoglobulins in Black populations and anecdotal cases of specificity of the paraprotein for a known antigen provide some support for this view but it remains unproven.

The evidence for a familial basis to the genesis of multiple myeloma is not clear. Over 37 families with two or more affected members have been reported, but case-control studies have not demonstrated that the family members of patients with multiple myeloma are at significantly increased risk of developing the disease (Bourguet *et al.* 1985). In one case-control study, a family history of other haemopoietic malignancies was associated with multiple myeloma. Certain HLA types are reported to be increased among myeloma cases and benign paraproteinemias are reported to be increased in families of myeloma patients (Bourguet *et al.* 1985).

DEFINITION

To make the diagnosis of multiple myeloma at least two of the following characteristics should be present.

1. Monoclonal immunoglobulin (paraprotein) in blood and/or urine. These paraproteins may be the complete immunoglobulin or light chain molecules or fragments of either. The immunoglobulin isotype is IgG in 53 per cent of cases, IgA in 22 per cent, light chain only (Bence Jones myeloma) in 22 per cent, IgD in 1.5 per cent, IgM in 0.5 per cent, IgE in less than 0.01 per cent, and non-secretory myeloma in less than 0.01 per cent (Hobbs 1971).

2. Bone-marrow infiltration by malignant plasma cells which may be large and immature.

3. Osteolytic bone lesions.

PARAPROTEINAEMIA

The term 'monoclonal gammopathy' or 'paraproteinaemia' describes the presence of a homogenous immunoglobulin in the serum which is detected as a discrete band when serum proteins are separated electrophoretically in a solid medium such as filter paper, cellulose acetate membrane, or agarose.

Paraproteins are associated with myeloma, macroglobulinaemia, amyloidosis, and B-cell malignancies (B-cell lymphoma), but they may also appear in the serum of patients with inflammatory and immunological disorders. In addition, they are also associated in a non-causal way with non-B-cell malignancies and with vascular and other diseases.

The term 'benign paraproteinaemia' denotes the presence of monoclonal proteins in persons without evidence of multiple myeloma, macroglobulinaemia, amyloidosis, or other B-cell malignancies such as B-cell lymphoma (Kohn 1974). Thus, it includes those patients with inflammatory or immunological conditions where there may be a relationship between the paraprotein and the disease. More recently the term 'monoclonal gammopathy of undetermined significance' has been suggested (Kyle 1984) and it is now the preferred term. In 1837 consecutive patients presenting at the Mayo Clinic in 1984, 72 per cent had monoclonal gammopathy of undetermined significance, 13 per cent had myeloma, 7 per cent had primary amyloidosis, 6 per cent had lymphoma, and 2 per cent had Waldenström's macroglobulinaemia (Kyle 1985). The range of diagnoses within the monoclonal gammopathy of undetermined significance group is shown in Table 1.

The incidence of paraproteinaemia in patients without evidence of myeloma, macroglobulinaemia, amyloidosis, or other B-cell malignancy depends on the sensitivity of the test used and the age of the group that is screened. With conventional paper electrophoretic techniques, the incidence of paraproteinaemia in a population over the age of 25 years is 1 per cent (Axelsson *et al.* 1966). However, when agarose is used as the support medium the incidence in this population rises to 5 per cent (Papadopoulos *et al.* 1982). The relationship between age and incidence was shown very clearly by Kohn and Srivastava (1972) in their study of 9420 blood donors aged between 20 and 62 years. The incidence of paraproteinaemia was 0.06 per cent between 20 and 30 years and then rose almost exponentially with each decade to 0.6 per cent

Table 1 Frequency of diseases associated with monoclonal gammopathy without evidence of myeloma, macroglobulinaemia, amyloidosis, and other B-cell malignancy

No disease detected	26%
Cardio/cerebrovascular diseases	13%
Inflammatory diseases	11%
Malignant neoplasms	7%
Connective tissue diseases	6%
Neurological diseases	6%
Haematological diseases	4%
Endocrine diseases	4%
Other diseases (benign tumours, psychoneurosis, peptic ulcers, etc.)	23%

Reproduced from Kyle (1984), with permission.

between the ages of 60 and 62 years. A number of studies have looked at the incidence of paraproteinaemia over the age of 70 years and it has been found to be approximately 3 per cent (Axelsson *et al.* 1966; Hallen 1966; Kyle *et al.* 1972).

A working definition of monoclonal gammopathy of undetermined significance is that patients have a monoclonal gammopathy with a serum paraprotein concentration usually below 30 g/l, less than 5 per cent plasma cells of normal morphology in the bone-marrow aspirate, and no renal failure, anaemia, or bone lesions. Occasionally patients may have small amounts of Bence Jones proteinuria and mild immunoparesis; that is, reduction in normal immunoglobulins. The characteristic feature of monoclonal gammopathy of undetermined significance is that the concentration of the paraprotein remains stable. Patients with a paraprotein concentration above 30 g/l and more than 5 per cent plasmacytosis in the bone-marrow have myeloma and if there is no renal failure, bone lesions, or anaemia and the gammopathy remains stable then patients have 'smouldering myeloma'. Patients with smouldering myeloma remain stable for many years. Their plasma cells have a low labelling index and do not require treatment. An important differentiating feature between smouldering myeloma and monoclonal gammopathy of undetermined significance is that in the latter the bone-marrow should not be infiltrated by more than 5 per cent plasma cells and these should be of normal morphology. In both monoclonal gammopathy of undetermined significance and smouldering myeloma the plasma cells in bone-marrow include a clonal population when stained by immunocytochemical methods for light chain and heavy chain isotypes.

There has always been some debate as to the temporal definition of benign monoclonal gammopathy and arbitrary definitions such as stable paraprotein for 3 or 5 years have been suggested. However, it has now been shown that patients can develop myeloma anywhere from 2 to 21 years after the original recognition of a monoclonal gammopathy of undetermined significance with a median onset of myeloma at 9.6 years (Kyle 1989) and therefore they need to be followed up indefinitely. The cumulative probability of developing myeloma, macroglobulinaemia, amyloidosis, or another B-cell malignancy after the original recognition of a monoclonal gammopathy of undetermined significance is 16 per cent at 10 years and 30 per cent at 15 years (Kyle 1984). Kyle has now followed 241 patients for long periods (median follow-up 19 years). In this unique experience, 36 cases of myeloma, seven of macroglobulinaemia, seven of primary amyloidosis, and three of lymphoma have developed (Kyle 1989). Recently, it has been shown that 40 per cent of patients with asymptomatic myeloma or MGUS may have abnormalities on magnetic resonance imaging of the spine (Alexanian and Dimopoulos 1994), although there is still no evidence that treatment should be instituted in response to this finding alone.

In 2–10 per cent of patients with paraproteinaemia more than one band is found on electrophoresis (Gore *et al.* 1979; Nilsson *et al.* 1986). The clinical findings and disease associations are the same as for single-band paraproteinaemias. Occasionally paraproteinaemia may be transient in that an M band appears and then disappears completely over a period of weeks or months. This occurs in association with infection, particularly in children with immunodeficiency diseases and in adults with liver disease, cytomegalovirus infection, and a variety of malignancies. Transient paraproteinaemia also sometimes occurs in patients undergoing intensive chemotherapy and bone-marrow transplantation; in this situation several bands are visualized on the electrophoretic strip and this is known as an oligoclonal pattern.

LABORATORY INVESTIGATION OF PARAPROTEINAEMIA

The investigation of a patient with paraproteinaemia involves the identification and quantitation of the paraprotein, followed by an attempt to confirm or exclude the presence of a B-cell malignancy. Once these conditions have been excluded, a careful search should be made for non-malignant diseases which may have a possible causal relationship with the paraprotein. These include amyloid, connective diseases, papular mucinosis, pyoderma gangrenosa, autoimmune disease, liver disease, and peripheral neuropathy. The association between paraproteinaemia and any other condition is incidental and does not require further investigation.

Blood is collected in a plain tube with no anticoagulant; haemolysis should be avoided. The serum is separated and stored at 4°C with azide. An early morning urine sample must always accompany the serum, and it should be noted that 'dip-stick' testing for albumin may be negative in the presence of Bence Jones

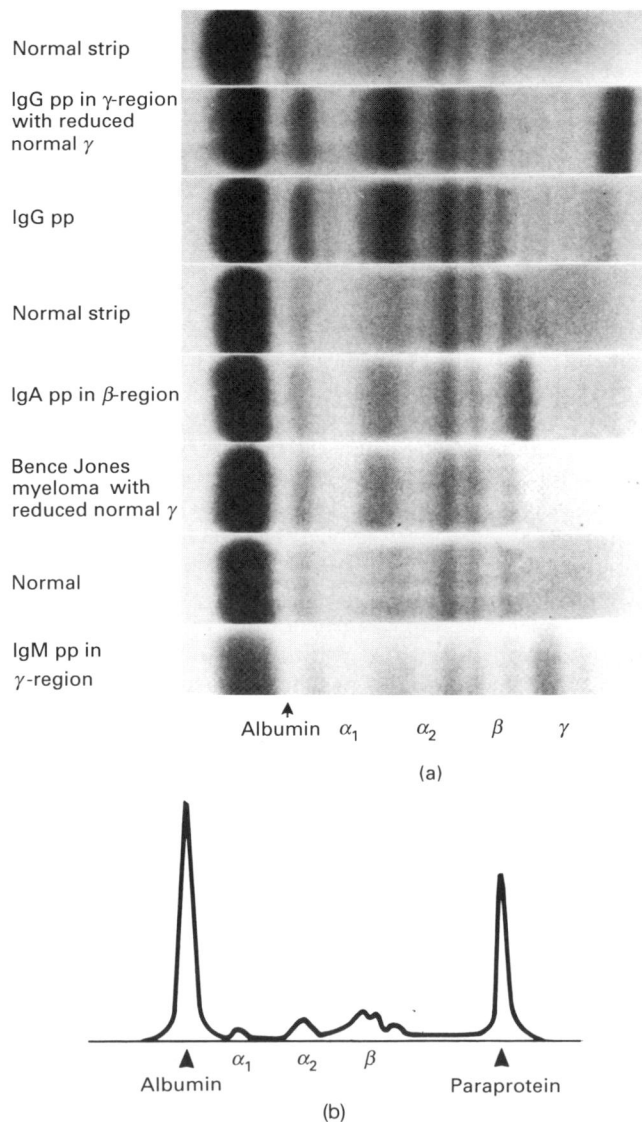

(a)

(b)

Fig. 2 (a) Protein electrophoresis: normals and paraproteins. (b) Photodensitometry of a protein electrophoretic strip showing a paraprotein in the γ-region and reduction of normal immunoglobulins; that is, reduced γ-region. pp, paraprotein.

proteinuria. Proteins in the serum and urine are separated electrophoretically using either cellulose acetate membrane or an agarose gel as the support medium. Separation takes approximately 30–40 min with either of these methods and the bands are visualized using a protein stain such as Ponceau S or Coomassie blue. In order to identify the class and isotype of the paraprotein, immunofixation is the recommended method. In this technique several aliquots from the same sample are loaded on adjacent tracks and the proteins are separated as before, but this time the support medium is not stained for protein but each track is incubated with a different antiheavy chain or antilight chain antiserum. In this way the paraprotein will be precipitated by its appropriate antiserum. The support medium is washed to remove the non-precipitated proteins and stained as before; the paraprotein–antiserum complex is thus visualized (reviewed by Riches and Hobbs 1988).

The level at which serum paraproteins can be detected varies with the separation and visualization technique used. Electrophoresis on paper and other carriers can detect 2–5 g/l. High voltage zone electrophoresis on agar or cellulose acetate membrane detects 0.1 g/l. Immunofixation detects 0.05 g/l and immunoblotting can detect paraprotein levels as low as 0.5–1 mg/l (Radl 1985). Similarly, the staining technique used can alter the sensitivity of the assay so that proteins are more likely to be detected if silver or gold stains are used rather than Coomassie blue or Ponceau S.

Patients with cryoglobulinaemia, cryofibrinogenaemia, or IgM paraproteins which are cold agglutinins cause a special problem of sample collection. Where this situation is suspected, serum samples should be collected from patients using pre-warmed syringes and tubes and the blood should be allowed to clot at 37°C. Patients who are being investigated for suspected heavy chain disease present a problem of protein identification in that specific antiserum to γ, α, and μ heavy chains are required.

Table 2 suggests clinical situations when a paraprotein should be sought by serum electrophoresis and Table 3 sets out a schema for investigating patients presenting with paraproteinaemia.

Table 2 Indications for serum electrophoresis

Symptoms	Fatigue
	Back pain
	Recurrent infections
Clinical syndromes	Peripheral neuropathy
	Carpal tunnel syndrome
	Cardiac failure
	Nephrotic syndrome
	Orthostatic hypotension
	Malabsorption
Haematology	Anaemia
	Raised erythrocyte sedimentation rate
Biochemistry	Abnormal renal function
	Raised calcium
	Bence Jones proteinaemia
	Hypogammaglobulinaemia
Radiology	Osteoporosis
	Osteolytic lesions(s)
	Fracture

Adapted from Kyle and Griepp (1988).

Table 3 Schema for investigating patients with paraproteinaemia

Stage 1 Exclude myeloma, Waldenström's macroglobulinaemia, heavy chain disease
    FBC, ESR
    U & Es, calcium
    Serum immunoglobulins
    Serum and urine electrophoresis with immunofixation
    Bone-marrow aspirate and trephine with immunohistochemistry
      (light chain restriction)
      (NB Bone-marrow examination or skeletal survey with a
      biopsy of any lytic lesions may be the only way of diagnosing
      non-secretory myeloma)

Stage 2 Exclude other B-cell malignancies
    Lymph adenopathy (clinical examination, CT scan): B-cell
      lymphoma
    Castleman's disease, angio-immunoblastic lymphadenopathy
    Bone-marrow examination: CLL, hairy cell leukaemia

Stage 3 Exclude causally associated diseases (liver disease)

FBC, full blood count.
ESR, erythrocyte sedimentation rate.
U & Es, urea and electrolytes.
CLL, chronic lymphoblastic leukaemia.

BONE-MARROW MORPHOLOGY

Neoplastic proliferation of plasma cells is visible in smears from bone-marrow aspirates or in bone-marrow trephine sections. This infiltrative process may be either diffuse or focal and the spread of the disease through a bone is usually uneven. The proportion of plasma cells in normal bone-marrow is usually said to be less than 4 per cent of nucleated cells (Hayhoe et al. 1986) although a working level of 5 per cent is often used to a normal level (Gore et al. 1989). However, in reactive plasmacytosis of bone-marrow the proportion of plasma cells may exceed 30 per cent (Bartl 1988), emphasizing how difficult it is to put firm diagnostic criteria on plasma cell infiltration figures alone.

In bone-marrow trephines typical features which suggest a diagnosis of myeloma are diffuse or band infiltration together with nodules of more than five or six plasma cells, fibrosis, and abnormal plasma cell morphology.

Marrow cytology in multiple myeloma may involve homogeneous or heterogeneous plasma cells and considerable variation can exist in size, shape, basophilia, and nuclear maturity (Hayhoe et al. 1986). When immunoglobulin accumulates towards the periphery of the cell and the preparation is stained with Romanowsky dye, a pink staining reaction occurs which is referred to as 'flaming cells' and is particularly, but not exclusively, associated with myeloma occasionally being seen in reactive states. Dense spherical accumulations of immunoglobulin may occur in the cytoplasm (Russell bodies). Binucleate plasma cells are commonly seen.

Although marrow morphology and cytochemistry can contribute to the diagnosis of multiple myeloma, more weight is currently placed on the use of immunocytochemistry with antisera to heavy and light chain components. With marrow infiltration a monoclonal proliferation is demonstrated by the clone reacting with antisera directed against one light chain type and only one heavy chain type. Evidence of monoclonality is thus useful in support of the diagnosis although, again, it is not diagnostic of multiple myeloma. More recently in situ hybridization for immunoglobulin messenger RNA has been shown to be an alternative way of demonstrating clonal proliferation (Akhtar et al. 1989).

BONE DISEASE

Bone disease is a major feature of myeloma. In adults skeletal turnover is mainly accounted for by the process of remodelling. This remodelling takes place in a series of phases which consist of osteoclast activation, osteoclast-mediated bone resorption, the movement of mononuclear cells off the resorption cavity, and, finally, the movement of osteoblasts into this site. The osteoblasts then synthesize an osteoid matrix which undergoes mineralization and completes remodelling. The attraction of osteoblasts into the sites of remodelling is termed 'coupling' and is probably under the control of the mononuclear cells that are found deep within the resorption cavities.

In myeloma, bone resorption is characteristically increased owing to the inappropriate activation of osteoclasts by a number of chemical mediators without concomitant stimulation of osteoblasts. This results in an 'uncoupling' of bone turnover. Thus, bone is resorbed without osteoblasts being attracted into the resorption cavities and no remodelling occurs (Kanis et al. 1988). The situation is made worse by the destruction of trabecular elements with the appearance of large gaps in bone and further impairment of new bone formation, since osteoblasts can normally only remodel and form osteoid on pre-existing bone surfaces.

The precise mechanisms responsible for increased bone resorption are not fully understood in myeloma, but it appears that myeloma cells produce an osteoclast-stimulating factor with biological properties similar to those of osteoclast-activating factor, a lymphokine that is produced by phytohaemoglutanin-activated peripheral blood lymphocytes. A number of lymphokines have bone-resorbing activity. These include interleukin-1, tumour necrosis factor alpha, and lymphotoxin/tumour necrosis factor beta (Gowen et al. 1983, 1986; Bertolini et al. 1986), though it has been suggested that the most likely candidate in patients with myeloma is lymphotoxin (Garrett et al. 1987).

IMMUNODEFICIENCY IN MULTIPLE MYELOMA

Myeloma patients are immunosuppressed and are particularly susceptible to bacterial as opposed to viral or fungal infections. Up to 43 per cent of patients have a serious problem with bacterial infection (Cohen and Rundles 1975). Commonly, patients have pulmonary and genitourinary tract infections. Staphylococcus aureus and Streptococcus pneumoniae are the most frequently encountered in the former site and Escherichia, Pseudomonas, Proteus, and Klebsiella species in the latter.

The causes of this immunodeficiency are complex and multifactorial but mainly involve abnormalities of immunoglobulin production. The immunosuppression is of an unusual type: patients are hypogammaglobulinaemic and demonstrate an impairment of the primary immune response, while the secondary immune response and cellular immunity remain relatively well preserved in untreated patients (Pruzanski et al. 1980; Ullrich and Zolla-Pazner 1982).

Some studies have shown that peripheral blood lymphocytes from patients fail to produce normal immunoglobulins and cannot proliferate in response to mitogens. This suggests that in patients with myeloma there may be a lack of normal B cells (Zolla-Pazner 1980). Furthermore, circulating mononuclear cells from patients can suppress lymphocytes from healthy subjects responding to pokeweed mitogen (Knapp and Baumgartner 1978; Paglieroni and MacKenzie 1980). The possibility that suppressor cells have a role

in humoral immunosuppression in myeloma has been known for some time (Broder et al. 1975). For instance, not only is macrophage function impaired by an inability to handle or present antigen normally, but in vitro studies suggest that suppressor macrophages are induced by a factor secreted by malignant plasma cells. These suppressor macrophages in turn secrete a factor termed 'plasmacytoma-induced macrophage substance' which inhibits B-cell proliferation and antibody production (Kennard and Zolla-Pazner 1980). MacKenzie et al. (1987) have also suggested that the humoral immunosuppression seen in myeloma is mediated through a cellular mechanism, namely the CD5+ B-cell which is present in the peripheral blood and spleen of patients with myeloma. They have postulated that this cell produces a 10–15 kDa protein which is responsible for the immunosuppression.

Pilarski (1989) has shown numerous defects in T- and B-cell lineages in patients with myeloma. In both these lineages there appears to be an arrest in differentiation and as a result an accumulation of precursor cells and it is suggested that this arrest may be mediated through anti-immunoglobulin-specific autoimmune T-cells. A maturation arrest of B-cells would of course result in cessation of immunoglobulin synthesis by memory B-cells and impair the response to either newly or frequently encountered pathogens.

Other abnormalities in the immune system that have been described are defects in cytotoxic T-lymphocyte and LAK-cell generation activity (Massaia et al. 1988, 1989), peripheral blood B-cell hyporesponsiveness to growth factors such as B-cell growth factor and interleukin (IL) 4, and impaired IL-6-mediated B-cell differentiation to staphylococcal A (Ford et al. 1989). Finally, it has been shown that T-cells bearing Fc receptors produce immunoglobulin-binding factors which bind to the surface immunoglobulin of B-cells and suppress immunoglobulin production. The mechanism probably involves the activation of protein kinase C, the suppression of immunoglobulin gene transcription, and the suppression of the c-myc gene (Roman et al. 1988).

Isotype suppression is a common finding in multiple myeloma. Leonard et al. (1979) first noted the reduction of kappa light-chain-bearing cells in the lamina propria of the gut of patients with kappa myeloma and similarly a loss of lambda cells in lambda myeloma. Similar observations were made for light-chain-expressing cells in the peripheral blood of myeloma patients (Wearne et al. 1984). This suppression presumably represents intact feedback onto the lymphocyte populations from the circulating paraprotein, although the mechanism in vivo is unclear. The presence of isotypic suppression is associated with stable disease, a good prognosis, and the achievement of a plateau after chemotherapy (Joshua 1988), while it is lost with disease progression.

CELL BIOLOGY
Clonal growth

Although myeloma includes a proliferation of monoclonal plasma cells which secrete a paraprotein of a single isotype and idiotype, the make-up of the whole malignant cell population is quite complex. The availability of antibodies which recognize unique determinants in the variable regions of the paraproteins (anti-idiotype) allows some analysis of the myeloma clone. In the circulation of a myeloma patient lymphocytes bearing the unique idiotype of that patient's paraprotein can be found and this may also be shown on pre-B-lymphocytes, presumably precursor cells. The presence of peripheral blood lymphocytes and active proliferation of such cells is associated with the activity of the disease and tends to parallel the proliferative rate of marrow myeloma cells (Boccadoro et al. 1983).

The malignant cells within a myeloma population may express a range of antigens normally associated with cells of other haemopoietic lineages including the common acute lymphoblastic leukaemia antigen and megakaryocytic, myeloid, and erythroid surface markers (see below and Epstein et al. 1990). This may indicate that myeloma originates within primitive haemopoietic stem cells or that myeloma cell gene expression is disordered with inappropriate lineage markers being synthesized. Molecular techniques confirm the presence of B-cell populations of progenitor cells within the myeloma clone (Billadeau et al. 1993).

Disease evolution is a common feature of multiple myeloma with a progressive increase in growth rate and clinical aggression. Myeloma protein production may fall during terminal phases. The development of acute myeloid leukaemia may represent further dedifferentiation and lineage non-specificity, although drug carcinogenesis is an alternative explanation.

Growth factors

A number of cytokines, including IL-1, IL-2, BCGF-1 (B-cell growth factor), and most notably IL-6, have been shown to be in vitro growth factors for myeloma (Kawano et al. 1988). However, the data are not entirely consistent and there are a number of controversies in this area. The precise rôle of these growth factors remains unresolved. For instance, there is evidence that IL-6 is not produced by myeloma cells and this would suggest that myeloma is under paracrine rather than autocrine control (Klein et al. 1989). Berenson et al. (1989) have found that the production of tumour necrosis factor, IL-1, and IL-6 is higher in patients with myeloma than in those with benign monoclonal gammopathy or in normal controls. Indirect evidence that IL-6 may have significance in vivo has been presented by Klein and Bataille (1989) who have shown that raised IL-6 levels are associated with the aggressiveness of the disease: significant serum IL-6 levels were detected in only 3 per cent of patients with monoclonal gammopathy of undetermined significance but in 41 per cent of those with overt myeloma, 60 per cent of those with fulminating myeloma, and 100 per cent of those with plasma cell leukaemia. It is also possible that myeloma cell growth is not under the control of any of the currently recognized growth factors but is regulated by cellular mechanisms involving T-lymphocytes (Deicher and Peest 1989).

Other growth factors can influence the proliferation of myeloma cells in vitro including insulin and insulin-like growth factors (Freund et al. 1993).

This is an area of major clinical relevance as it may allow new treatment strategies, such as antireceptor or antigrowth factor antibodies, to be developed.

Phenotype

Haemopoietic stem cells give rise to B-cells in the bone-marrow and these, in turn, mature into plasma cells. This maturation is antigen driven and during the process a variety of cell surface markers are gained and lost. Thus, mature B-lymphocytes express CD19 (B4), CD20 (B1), CD23, CD24, CD37, CD39, and CDw40, but these antigens are lost as the B-lymphocyte matures into a plasma cell and the antigens CD38 and PCA1 appear on the cell surface (Zola 1987).

A number of markers that are not normally present on the surface of plasma cells have been described as being present on myeloma cells: these include myelomonocytic markers (Grogan et al. 1989), natural killer cell markers (Van Camp et al. 1989), follicle centre B-cell markers (Franklin et al. 1989), and the common acute lymphoblastic leukaemia antigen which is found in approximately 55 per cent of patients with myeloma (Epstein et al. 1988). In general, most pan-B antigens are lost from the surface of myeloma cells (Jackson et al. 1988). Progesterone and oestrogen receptors have also been found on the surface of myeloma cells (Danel et al. 1988) and the presence of cytokeratins could result in diagnostic confusion (Wotherspoon et al. 1989). Cell adhesion molecules including intercellular adhesion molecules (ICAM), CD44, and fibronectin receptors are expressed on myeloma cells and may play a rôle in localizing the cells to the marrow (Kawano et al. 1993; Van Riet and Van Camp 1993).

There are no absolutely specific myeloma-associated antigens on the surface of myeloma cells, although a number of groups are working on this and attempting to develop methods to eliminate neoplastic cells from bone-marrow prior to high-dose chemotherapy and autologous bone-marrow transplantation. These methods employ a variety of antibodies, often in combination and a variety of techniques including complement lysis, immunoabsorption, immunotoxin, and magnetic beads have all been used (Shimazaki et al. 1988; Stone et al. 1988; Bontadini et al. 1989; Tabilio et al. 1989).

Millar et al. (1988, 1989) have demonstrated that there exist at least two morphologically distinct types of myeloma cell in culture, large plasmacytoid cells and smaller lymphoplasmacytoid cells and this finding is not only of significance in terms of defining lineage hierarchies but may also give a lead to the reasons for the emergence of drug-resistant disease.

Genotype

Typically the proportion of myeloma cells in DNA synthesis is low and so few mitoses are available for karyotypic analysis. However, numerous karyotypic and molecular abnormalities have been described in the genome of myeloma cell lines and myeloma cells from patients. The abnormalities described are numerous and varied and no consistent abnormality has been found that would allow the development of a unified theory of the oncogenic mechanisms responsible for myeloma. The multiplicity of karyotypic abnormalities is in keeping with a disease which has a long time course, allowing many acquired genetic changes and changes in karyotype to take place. Some of these alterations might be related to treatment (Clark et al. 1989).

Approximately 80 per cent of patients with myeloma show hyperdiploidy, the DNA content of myeloma cells is 10–15 per cent higher than that of normal diploid cells, and the RNA content is four to six times that of normal peripheral blood lymphocytes (Barlogie et al. 1988). This latter increase is a reflection of the large commitment to protein production in the form of immunoglobulin synthesis of these cells. On conventional analysis, 24–46 per cent of patients show karyotypic abnormalities (Dewald et al. 1985; Gould et al. 1988; Lisse et al. 1988; Nishida et al. 1989). These include structural alterations, additions, and losses. Abnormalities have been described on virtually every chromosome, but are commonly seen on chromosomes 1, 3, 6, 7, 8, 11, and 14 (Barlogie et al. 1988; Durie 1988a; Weh et al. 1993). Specifically, translocations involving chromosome 8 and in particular 8;14 translocations which are common for other B-cell malignancies, have been described by a number of authors. Gould et al. (1988) suggested that these 8;14 translocations were associated with IgA myeloma and they also described other clinical correlates, namely an association between hypodiploidy and Bence Jones myeloma or drug resistance. Other links between karyotype and clinical behaviour have been suggested, including deletions of the long arm of chromosome 6 with lytic bone disease (Durie *et al.* 1986*a*). Mutations of p53 tumour suppressor gene are uncommon in myeloma in patients, although common in cell lines (Willems *et al.* 1993).

Molecular studies have also identified a number of abnormalities involving several oncogenes including c-*myc*, H-*ras*, n-*ras*, and *bcl-1* (Selvanayagam *et al.* 1987, 1988; Ernst *et al.* 1988; Hollis *et al.* 1988; Greil *et al.* 1989; Neri *et al.* 1989). The involvement of c-*myc* is of interest since this occurs in other lymphoid malignancies and it is present on chromosome 8 which is, as we have already mentioned, one of the most commonly abnormal chromosomes in myeloma cells. Several different mechanisms of c-*myc* oncogene activation have been demonstrated in myeloma; these include gene amplification, 8;14 translocations, and enhanced transcription of the c-*myc* gene. Indeed, increased levels of myc and ras proteins have been found in myeloma cells (Tsuchiya *et al.* 1988) and elevated p^{21}, a *ras* gene product, has been claimed to indicate a shortened survival time for myeloma patients. A point mutation of *myc* oncogene has been described.

A recent development has been the finding of rearrangements of the T-cell receptor and immunoglobulin genes in some patients with myeloma (Berenson and Lichtenstein 1989; Zaccaria *et al.* 1989). The rearrangement of immunoglobulin genes would be anticipated in a B-cell malignancy. Clonal rearrangement of T-cell receptor genes was found in 35 per cent of cases in one study (Lee *et al.* 1987) and is unexpected.

In vitro culture

A number of tissue culture systems have been described for growing myeloma cells *in vitro* (Park 1971; Hamburger and Salmon 1977). A drawback of many systems has been the possible contamination of the culture by other haemopoietic cells. Two methods have been described to circumvent this problem: Izaguirre *et al.* (1980) depleted the marrow of T-cells prior to culture and Millar *et al.* (1988) used a heavily irradiated 'feeder' layer which prevented the outgrowth of normal haemopoietic cells. All these techniques result in short-term cultures of up to 3 weeks, but a method has been developed that allows myeloma cells with proliferative capacity to be grown in long-term culture (Takahasi *et al.* 1985).

Culture systems have been used for *in vitro* drug sensitivity assays (Durie *et al.* 1983; Peest *et al.* 1986), as correlates with prognosis (Takahasi *et al.* 1985), to study the growth requirements of myeloma cells (Klein and Bataille 1989) and to examine lineage hierarchies in myeloma and their relationship to clinical status (Maitland *et al.* 1990).

Recently, a model of myeloma growth in severe combined immunodeficiency mice (SCID) has been described and may be a useful means of reflecting treatment effects (Bellamy *et al.* 1993; Huang *et al.* 1993).

Drug resistance

In vitro drug sensitivity testing has not fulfilled its early promise and there is still no place for its routine use in clinical practice. Myeloma is one area where much attention has been paid to the causes of drug resistance, in particular in relation to the multiple-drug-resistant phenotype mdr-1. mdr-1 is associated with the presence of a 180 kDa cell membrane protein known as p-glycoprotein

and it is suggested that this protein is involved in the active transport of drugs out of the cell with a resulting reduction of intracellular drug concentrations. This phenotype has been found in drug-resistant myeloma cell lines and in myeloma cells from patients and it appears that resistance can be overcome by the addition of the calcium channel blocker verapamil (Dalton *et al.* 1989*a*). However, not all groups have found that the 'verapamil effect' is associated with the presence of p180 (Millar *et al.* 1989). The relationship between p-glycoprotein, drug resistance, and its reversal by calcium channel blockers is the subject of active study at present.

As previously mentioned, Millar *et al.* (1989) have recently demonstrated two morphologically distinct cell types, small lymphoplasmacytoid and large plasmacytoid cells, in their culture system. These two cell types have differing chemosensitivities, with the former being more chemoresistant. These small lymphoplasmacytoid cells may be selected out in more advanced disease, particularly after chemotherapy and the inherent resistance of these cells may explain the development of drug-resistant disease in patients.

Molecular mechanisms

Unlike some lymphomas and leukaemias, the precise molecular mechanisms which cause the formation and progression of myeloma are still unclear. DNA rearrangements reminiscent of non-Hodgkin's lymphomas occur but are infrequent. They presumably result from recombination errors during immunoglobulin gene rearrangement and may bring oncogenes into transcriptionally active sites of the genome. The control of gene expression in myeloma is abnormal, with inappropriate expression of lineage specific antigens, but we do not know why. Expression of c-myc protein correlates with prognosis and grade of myeloma cells and may be useful clinically (Skopelitou *et al.* 1993).

The clarification of the molecular mechanisms of myeloma will include showing abnormal expression of cellular genes as a result of rearrangement, mutation, or amplification and also a probable contribution from a deletion of tumour suppressor genes. Although this will be a lengthy task, the necessary experimental techniques to unravel these puzzles are now available.

CLINICAL FEATURES

Multiple myeloma has a very characteristic presentation and course. The principal presenting features are shown in Table 4 (Kyle 1975; Selby 1987). The majority of patients present with bone pain which usually affects the back and ribs and less often the limbs. It is usually worse with movement.

The diagnosis will be suggested by clinical features and the initial investigations listed in Table 3. A full investigation scheme is given in Table 5. Final confirmation of the diagnosis is only possible with the results of serum protein electrophoresis and immunofixation, radiological skeletal survey, and bone-marrow examination.

The full clinical picture of myeloma, both at presentation and during its clinical course, is a complex of bone destruction leading to bone pain or fracture with hypercalcaemia, infection due to immune deficiency, marrow failure leading to anaemia and, less commonly, thrombocytopenia and renal failure due to hypercalcaemia, direct damage from paraprotein or precipitation of light chain in tubules, amyloid in some patients, and the effects of infection in others. The pathogenesis of the major clinical features of myeloma is quite well understood and is summarized in Fig. 3. These clinical features in varying proportions, together with deposits

Table 4 Presenting features of multiple myeloma

Bone pain	68%
Bacterial infection	12%
Herpes zoster	2%
Fever due to disease	1%
Bleeding	7%
Weakness and fatigue	66%

Table 5 Investigations for patients with multiple myeloma

Full blood count[a] and erythrocyte sedimentation rate
Urea[a], creatinine[a], electrolytes, anion gap, uric acid
Calcium and alkaline phosphatase[a]
Glomerular filtration rate (creatinine or EDTA clearance)
Bone-marrow aspirate and trephine biopsy[a]; immunofluorescent staining in
    special cases
Protein electrophoresis of serum and urine[a]
Immunoelectrophoresis or immunofixation of serum or urine to type t
    paraprotein[a]
Immunoglobulin levels[a]
Skeletal survey (at least skull and axial bones[a])
β_2-Microglobulin[a]
Plasma viscosity

EDTA, ethylenediaminetetraacetic acid.
[a]Essential tests.

of plasmacytomata, hyperviscosity, and biochemical disturbances, will dominate the clinical course of most myeloma patients.

Bone disease

The cellular proliferation of myeloma cells within the cavity of bones in the axial skeleton produces the bone pain and destruction which dominates the clinical picture of myeloma. The pain arises in weight-bearing bones and it is uncommon for patients with lytic disease in the skull to complain of headache. Although bone pain may be gradual in onset, pathological fractures are frequent and are usually indicated by the sudden onset of local tenderness and pain. Trauma precipitating fracture may be very minor, as with other pathological fractures. The loss of height due to collapse of vertebrae and kyphosis are common. Bone lesions are radiologically osteolytic in

almost all cases. Less than 2 per cent of patients have osteosclerotic lesions and these may occasionally be associated with the syndrome of polyneuropathy and endocrine abnormality, known by the acronym POEMS syndrome (Solomons 1982).

Infections

Susceptibility to infection is a prominent feature of multiple myeloma and the mechanisms responsible for the failure of the immune response are complex and are discussed above. A biphasic pattern of infection is seen with pneumococcus, haemophilus, and streptococcus being most frequent during the first year of the illness and with staphylococcus and Gram-negative bacilli becoming more frequent later in the illness. These latter organisms are frequent causes of death in patients managed with conventional therapy. The prominence of pneumococcal infection presumably reflects the important rôle of humoral immunity in the defence against that organism. Although cellular immunity is usually regarded as intact in the untreated patient, multiple episodes of herpes zoster are described and generalized vaccinia was well recognized in the days of smallpox vaccination.

The most important element in the management of infection of myeloma patients is prompt diagnosis and treatment, but prophylactic long-acting penicillins and the use of prophylactic gammaglobulin in high doses have their advocates.

Patients with plasma cell tumours should not be vaccinated with live organisms.

Anaemia

Although the haemoglobin value at presentation will be less than 12 g/l in over half of myeloma patients (Kyle 1975), severe symptomatic anaemia is less frequent, occurring in approximately 15 per cent of patients. This is usually due to the severity of the myeloma, although alternative causes such as chronic blood loss, haemolysis, and folate or vitamin B12 deficiency should be considered and may be more common in myeloma patients than in the general population (Bergsagel and Riker 1985).

Adequate specific therapy will usually correct anaemia in responding patients. Transfusions will maintain adequate control in others. A novel approach which appears effective is the use of

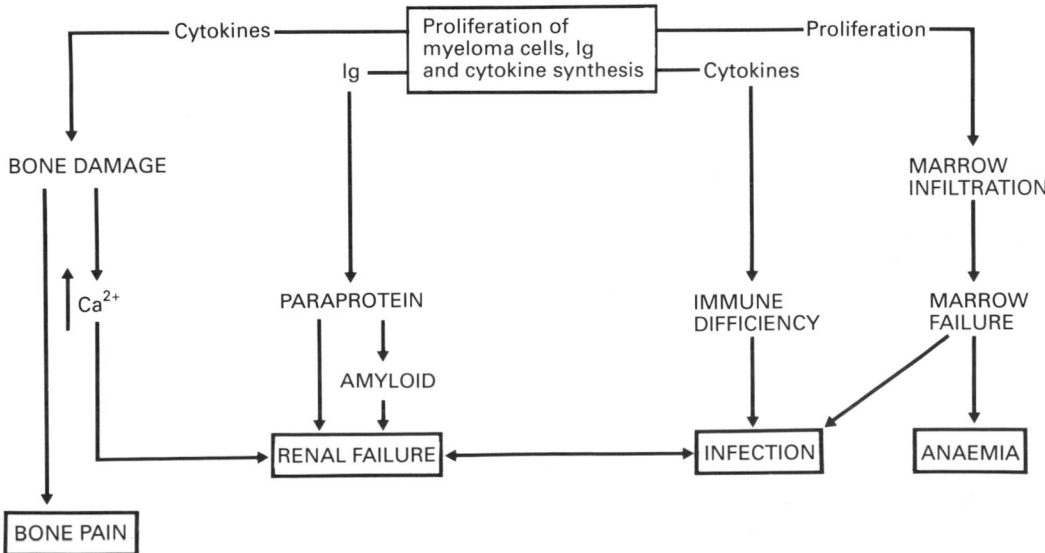

Fig. 3 The mechanisms underlying the clinical features of myeloma.

recombinant erythropoietin (Ludwig *et al.* 1990), but the indications for this new and expensive treatment are still unclear.

Hypercalcaemia

Approximately one-third of patients will be hypercalcaemic at presentation and approximately half of these will have symptoms on close questioning. A further 30–40 per cent of patients will become hypercalcaemic during the course of their illness. Symptoms including nausea, vomiting, polyuria, polydipsia, constipation, or mental confusion are quite characteristic and routine measurement of serum calcium at presentation is mandatory. Hypercalcaemia is the result of bone resorption by osteoclasts activated by osteoclast activating factors and is possibly also due to increased renal absorption of calcium secondary to the circulation of a factor stimulating proximal tubular adenylate cyclase.

Characteristically, despite hypercalcaemia and radiological bone destruction, the serum alkaline phosphatase is not usually raised because of the lack of osteoblastic bone regeneration. Although this widely taught observation is often true, moderate elevations of alkaline phosphatase are in fact not unusual.

Renal failure

Fifty per cent of myeloma patients will develop some form of renal impairment at some point of their illness (Kyle 1975; Bergsagel and Riker 1985). The specific renal lesions of multiple myeloma are the formation of intratubular casts of myeloma protein and its diffuse precipitation in renal tissue. However, many other factors will contribute to the development of renal failure in myeloma patients, including infection, hypercalcaemia, hyperuricaemia, direct plasma cell infiltration of the kidneys, dehydration, antibiotic therapy, and amyloidosis.

Free light chains (Bence Jones proteins) are inherently nephrotoxic to a variable extent. λ light chains tend to be more nephrotoxic than ϰ light chains. Normally light chains are filtered and reabsorbed and are catabolized by renal tubular cells and the basis of the nephrotoxic effects of light chains is not clearly understood.

Early renal lesions are principally due to failure of renal tubular reabsorption of electrolytes, amino acids, and glucose. Cast formation by light chains, complete immunoglobulin molecules, or other plasma proteins only occurs late in the process when the glomerular filtration rate has fallen and some renal tubules have ceased to function. Non-amyloid paraprotein deposition also occurs in glomeruli and blood vessels. Amyloid or non-amyloid deposition in glomeruli will lead to a non-specific proteinuria, whereas myeloma cast formation is more likely to be attended by a major light chain leak into the urine.

The clinical syndromes associated with myeloma kidney damage are varied. Most common is the gradual onset of chronic renal failure although acute failure with underlying chronic failure can occur. An acute episode of hypercalcaemia or infection is frequently the cause of rapid deterioration of renal function. Heavy proteinuria is common, but florid nephrotic syndrome is not common in our experience and is usually associated with amyloidosis.

The clinical course of renal impairment is variable. Acute episodes of renal failure are reversible and appropriate management is discussed below. Even the clinical syndrome of chronic renal failure can be improved by intensive treatment with hydration and reduction of the myeloma cell mass by specific chemotherapy. Nevertheless, the most important aspect of the management of renal failure in myeloma is preventative by the maintenance of a high fluid throughput and avoidance of the factors discussed earlier predisposing to renal failure (Medical Research Council 1984).

Bleeding

An abnormal tendency to bleed is apparent in 15–30 per cent of patients with myeloma or macroglobulinaemia and presents a clinical problem in perhaps 5 per cent. Thrombocytopenia is not usually severe unless it is treatment induced, but impairment of platelet function may contribute more to the bleeding predisposition. Coagulation abnormalities are described, including reduced levels of one or more coagulation factors or inhibition of coagulation factors by a variety of paraprotein. Inhibition of fibrinogen aggregation is said to be the commonest coagulation abnormality in patients with myeloma when this is specifically sought (Delamore 1986), possibly as a result of the binding of myeloma protein to fibrin during clotting.

Haemorrhagic complications are also seen as a result of amyloid deposition in blood vessels, producing the classic periorbital lesions, and haemorrhage is one of the major features of hyperviscosity.

Hyperviscosity and hyperuricaemia

Waldenström described hyperviscosity in association with macroglobulinaemia almost 50 years ago, but the hyperviscosity syndrome is much less frequent in patients with myeloma occurring in only 5–10 per cent of cases (Pruzanski and Watt 1972; Chandey *et al.* 1981). It is associated with hypervolaemia and there is a close correlation between serum gammaglobulin concentration and plasma volume (Bergsagel and Riker 1985).

The clinical hyperviscosity/hypervolaemia syndrome includes a predisposition to bleeding, particularly from mucosal services, dilatation, and segmentation of retinal and conjunctival veins. A range of central nervous system disturbances are seen, characterized by headache, drowsiness, weakness, and confusion which may progress to epileptic fits, paralysis, and coma. Distension of peripheral blood vessels can lead to cardiac failure. The clinical outcome of differing degrees of increased plasma viscosity is hard to predict. Most patients with a relative plasma viscosity below 4 are not symptomatic. Above that level, symptoms become more frequent and with relative viscosities above 8 most patients will have symptoms.

Apart from its striking association with macroglobulinaemia, hyperviscosity is also reported to be more frequent in IgA paraproteinaemia probably because of the tendency of IgA paraprotein to polymerize. Among IgG myelomas paraproteins of the IgG3 subclass are said to be more associated with hyperviscosity.

Clinical evidence of hyperviscosity should be managed as a medical emergency by plasmapheresis. Specific therapy to control the underlying disease should follow immediately.

Soft tissue lesions

Although the clinical course of myeloma is dominated by bony plasmacytomas, extramedullary disease is frequent at post-mortem and can be significant during the clinical course of the illness. Extramedullary plasmacytomas may either be isolated, in which case three-quarters of the tumours appear in the paranasal sinuses, nasopharynx, or tonsils, or they may be part of generalized myelomatosis. Extramedullary infiltration of subcutaneous tissues, lung, pleura, brain, heart, and almost every other organ have been described in a few cases (Whittaker 1986). Extradural deposits occur with resultant cord compression, and in this situation lesions at several levels can be encountered.

Neurological features

Disorders of the central and peripheral nervous system can play a prominent part in the clinical presentation and course of multiple myeloma. Non-specific higher cerebral dysfunction can result from hypercalcaemia, hyperviscosity, anaemia, or uraemia, and require urgent treatment.

Spinal cord or nerve root compression, myelomatous meningitis, and peripheral neuropathy can occur. Cerebral plasmacytoma is a rare but recognized feature of the disease. Spinal cord and nerve route compression now occur in approximately 10 per cent of myeloma patients and this probably represents a decreased incidence compared with the figure of one-third quoted in the early 1960s (reviewed by Bergsagel and Riker 1985). A spinal or rib plasmacytoma can invade into the spinal canal, causing compression of the cord in association with a paraspinal mass. The onset of clinical symptoms of cord compression can result from extension of the extradural mass or from collapse of a vertebra. Intramedullary myeloma is very rare. Progressive back pain, sensory disturbance, weakness, and disturbance of micturition are usually seen, but sudden onset of paraplegia may occur.

Any neurological symptoms in the legs, particularly when associated with back pain in myeloma, must be regarded as evidence of cord compression until proven otherwise by investigation by myelography, CT scanning, or magnetic resonance imaging. Our experience suggests that magnetic resonance imaging has advantages over the alternatives. It is non-invasive and can show the whole cord in sagittal section. This detects multiple levels of compression and delineates associated soft tissue masses (Joffe *et al.* 1988). Diagnostic laminectomy is rarely necessary.

Meningeal myelomatosis with malignant plasma cells in the cerebrospinal fluid is a rare finding of ominous prognosis, usually associated with rapidly progressive widespread myeloma.

Distal sensorimotor polyneuropathy is usually due to infiltration of the nerves by amyloid or plasma cells, but can also occasionally occur as a paraneoplastic phenomenon in less than 1 per cent of patients. The onset of this latter type of peripheral neuropathy is usually insidious, the distribution is symmetrical and distal, sometimes it is associated with painful dysaesthesia, and the cerebrospinal fluid protein is usually elevated. Patients tend to be young (mean age 50 years), male, and have solitary bony plasmacytomas. Osteosclerotic lesions are found more frequently in these patients (22 per cent). The mechanism of this remote effect of the myeloma tumour on peripheral nerves is not clear, although it has been suggested that the nerve sheath may carry antigenic determinants for the myeloma protein (Bergsagel and Riker 1985). A syndrome involving myeloma and peripheral neuropathy has been reported from Japan. It is known by the acronym POEMS and includes the following features: osteosclerotic myeloma, peripheral neuropathy, endocrine disturbances such as diabetes mellitus and gynaecomastia, and skin changes including hyperpigmentation and hyperhydrosis (Solomons 1982).

Cryoglobulins

Some 5 per cent of myeloma proteins can precipitate in the cold (Kyle 1975) but this does not usually result in clinical problems. Occasionally cryoglobulinaemia in myelomatosis can produce

vascular problems, leg ulcers, Raynaud's phenomenon, and renal, central nervous system, and gastrointestinal disorders. Biopsies will usually show a vasculitis affecting vessels in the involved organ. In severe cases peripheral gangrene, renal failure, severe purpura, or gastrointestinal perforation can result and vigorous treatment of the underlying myeloma as well as avoidance of exposure to cold is indicated.

Incidental biochemical findings

1. Hyponatremia and a low anion gap. Cationic proteins can lead to an artefactual hyponatremia associated with retention of chloride and bicarbonate leading to a low anion gap. These findings do not in themselves require any treatment.

2. Spurious hypercalcaemia. Binding of calcium to paraprotein can lead to elevated serum calcium in the absence of symptoms and may not require specific treatment.

3. Hyperlipidaemia. Binding of high- and low-density lipo-proteins to paraprotein has been described and can lead to the clinical syndrome of xanthomatosis and marked serum lipidemia.

4. Raised serum copper. Paraproteins binding copper have been described, leading to copper deposition in the cornea and visual impairment in rare cases.

5. Hyperuricaemia. Hyperuricaemia results from increased cell turnover and decreased renal excretion of urate and could theoretically be a factor in the development of renal failure. Prophylactic allopurinol is widely recommended at the time of initiating treatment.

PROGNOSTIC FACTORS AND STAGING SYSTEMS

The approach to the myeloma patient in order to judge prognosis appropriately and choose the correct management has evolved steadily over the last decade. Basic clinical information such as the patient's age and sex, renal function, haemoglobin, performance status, extent of bone lesions, serum calcium, serum albumin, uric acid, and probably the extent and nature of bone-marrow infiltration have all been evaluated as prognostic factors and some of these factors are undoubtedly useful. A number of the factors have been integrated to generate a staging system such as that of Durie and Salmon (1975a, b, c) (Table 6) and the Medical Research Council (1980a, b, c) (Table 7). More recently, the powerful prognostic significance of serum β_2-microglobulin has become clear and is widely used. Similarly, more sophisticated analysis of the tumour to reveal its cellular DNA content, karyotype, and molecular make-up are being applied to staging systems.

In assessing the appropriate current approach to prognosis and staging, it is worth emphasizing that prognostic factors should not be expected invariably to be consistent between centres or studies. The significance of a factor may vary according to the treatment given to patients and may be expected to change with time. The value of a staging system for a particular purpose may alter as clinical management changes. For instance, where treatment policies are allocated according to stage and are successful, a poor prognosis group treated in a new way may have an outcome comparable to a good prognosis group treated in a standard way. The prognostic power of the staging system will therefore disappear on subsequent analysis. Failure to appreciate some of these considerations has generated considerable confusion around the staging of multiple myeloma.

Table 6 Salmon and Durie staging system

| Cell mass category | | High (stage III) | Low (stage I) | Intermediate (stage II) |
Requirements		One of A, B, C, D	All of A, B, C, D	
Haemoglobin (pre-transfusion) (g%)	A	< 8.5	> 10	
Serum calcium (mg%)	B	> 12	Normal	Neither
M-component	C	IgG > 7 g%	IgG < 5 g%	I or III
		IgA > 5 g%	IgA < 3 g%	
		BJ > 12 g/day	BJ < 4 g/day	
Bone lesions on skeletal survey	D	Advanced lytic disease	None/solitary lesion	

Table 7 Medical Research Council staging system

		Poor prognosis (stage III) A, C or B, C	Good prognosis (stage I) All of A, B, C	Intermediate (stage II) Not in I or III
Blood urea concentration (mM)	A	> 10	≤ 8	Not in I or III
Haemoglobin (g/l)	B	≤ 75	> 100	Not in I or III
Performance status	C	Restricted activity	Minimal symptoms or asymptomatic	Not in I or III

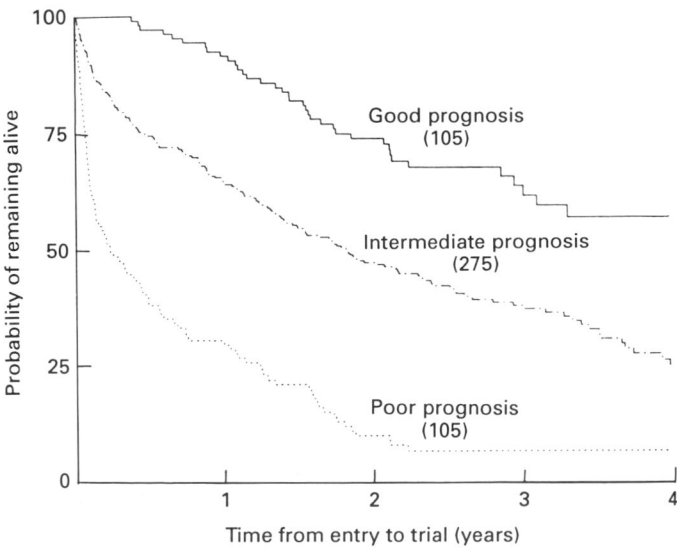

Fig. 4 Survival of patients with multiple myeloma separated by the Medical Research Council staging system (Table 7). (Reproduced with permission from the *British Journal of Cancer*.)

The features of patients with multiple myeloma which have been examined as prognostic factors include the following.

1. Performance status, renal function, and haemoglobin level. These all emerged from the Medical Research Council's studies in the early 1980s (Medical Research Council 1980*a*, *b*, *c*) and are the basis of the staging system shown in Table 7. These simple measurements separate patients into separate prognostic groups quite reliably (Fig. 4), and because they are made easily and early in the diagnostic work up of a myeloma patient, this system remains clinically valuable.

2. Features of bone damage. The extent of bone lesions and the presence of hypercalcaemia might be expected to reflect the aggressiveness of the disease. On this basis the extent of bone disease and the measurement of serum calcium are important elements in the staging system according to Salmon and Durie (1975) (Table 6). In fact, studies by the Medical Research Council and others suggests that the extent of skeletal disease is not a powerful prognostic

variable and most of its influence is reflected by measurements of performance status (Kelsey and Delamore 1986). In perhaps the largest study to address this question, Kelly *et al.* (1988) have analysed 1500 patients in Medical Research Council and Southwest Oncology Group trials and found that the presence of osteolytic bone lesions was significantly associated with a poor prognosis but the effect was only small. Since osteolytic bone lesions are only relatively weakly associated with prognosis and are to be found in well over half the patients with multiple myeloma, then they should not be a major element in an ideal staging system.

3. Age, sex, and race. No consistent association is found between sex or race and prognosis in multiple myeloma. The effects of age on outcome are relatively small. Kelly *et al.* (1988) found that age was of prognostic significance in some clinical trials but not in others, probably reflecting the influence of the therapy chosen.

4. β_2 Microglobulin. β_2-Microglobulin is a polypeptide that forms part of the extracellular portion of mixed histocompatibility complex class I molecules. It is non-covalently bound to those portions of the mixed histocompatibility complex that are encoded by the mixed histocompatibility complex gene and β_2-microglobulin itself is encoded by genes outside this area. It is released into the blood as cell turnover and serum levels are elevated in a number of conditions and rises with falling glomerular filtration rate. Norfolk *et al.* (1980) suggested that β_2-microglobulin might be valuable in assessing the prognosis of myeloma patients and that it correlated with myeloma cell mass stage and serum creatinine. Extensive subsequent evaluations have confirmed the prognostic power of β_2-microglobulin and this is illustrated by the data from the Medical Research Council IV myelomatosis trial (Fig. 5). Its prognostic power was clearly recently confirmed by the Southwest Oncology Group (Durie *et al.* 1990). Serum β_2-microglobulin is the single most important prognostic variable in multiple myeloma at present and although other factors continue to contribute information on multivariate analysis their contribution is relatively small.

5. Paraprotein type and level. There are claims that the level of paraprotein correlates with a poor prognosis and this was incorporated into the staging system devised by Durie and Salmon (1975). However, the association is in fact weak or absent in a number of studies. Similarly, there is no significant difference

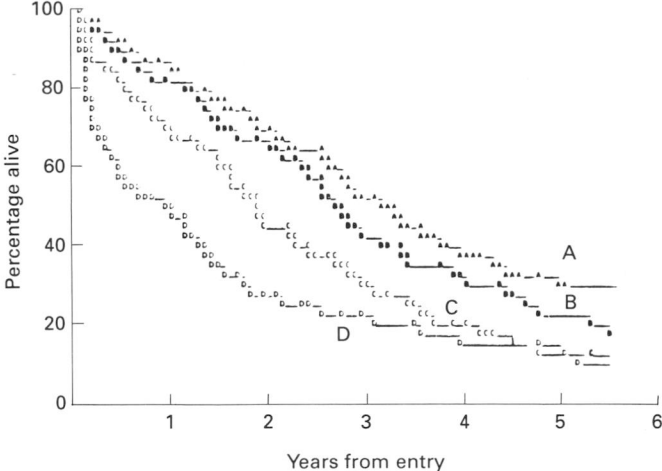

Fig. 5 Survival of patients with multiple myeloma separated by β_2-microglobulin concentration at diagnosis: A, <4 mg/l; B, 4–6 mg/l; C, 6–10 mg/l; D, >10 mg/l. (Reproduced with permission from *Haematological Oncology.*)

Ludwig *et al.* 1991), lactic dehydrogenase (Dimopoulos *et al.* 1991), and thymidine kinase activity (Brown *et al.* 1993).

10. Response to therapy. Within any prognostic subgroup, patients who require chemotherapy and who respond to it live longer than those who do not. However, the speed of response has a complex influence and rapid tumour regression may be associated with a shorter survival perhaps because it is a feature of rapidly proliferating tumours. Certainly in the Medical Research Council IV myelomatosis trial of conventional oral chemotherapy, fast responders did worse than slow responders (MacLennan *et al.* 1988). These comments are probably not relevant to more recent developments in intensive chemotherapy.

In conclusion, on prognostic features and staging we hold the view that a new approach to the staging of multiple myeloma is required. This needs to consider β_2-microglobulin and simple features such as performance status, renal function, and haemoglobin. In future, tumour proliferation indices may become more important. The system of Durie and Salmon (1975) is inadequate not only because of the emphasis it places upon bone lesions and paraprotein levels, which are relatively weak prognostic variables, but also because it fails to divide patients evenly between stages. The system devised by the Medical Research Council has clinical utility but fails to pay attention to modern knowledge of important prognostic variables. In any clinical trial a careful description of the prognostic characteristics of the patient population is required and this must include sex, age, performance status, serum β_2-microglobulin, haemoglobin, renal function, and albumin, as a minimum. Although data on bone disease and paraprotein should be collected, it is probably not necessary to include these in staging and they may be more important for the establishment of routine methods of estimating tumour kinetics.

TREATMENT

Principles of management

In approaching the management of a patient with myeloma, careful consideration should be given to a number of questions.

1. Does the patient require supportive care to control symptoms and to minimize the risks of the major complications of the disease?

2. Is specific treatment indicated?

3. How should the response to treatment be assessed and documented?

4. What is the best available current choice of systemic treatment for each category of patient?

Supportive care

Discussion of the management of patients with myeloma tends to focus upon specific measures to reduce the tumour bulk. However, the most immediate clinical decisions focus upon non-specific measures aimed at maintaining patient well-being, correcting metabolic abnormalities, maintaining renal function, and treating or preventing infectious complications.

Pain control and fractures

In the management of multiple myeloma, pain control will usually represent the first problem for the physician. It is one of the most

between IgG and IgA myeloma, although patients with light chain only myeloma appear to do consistently worse than those with a serum paraprotein. Rare subtypes of paraprotein (IgD and IgE) are not sufficiently frequent to allow formal analysis, but the impression from the literature is that they are associated with a relatively poor prognosis.

6. Bone-marrow infiltration. The extent and type of bone-marrow infiltration has not been systematically examined in all studies. However, the work of Bartl and colleagues (Bartl 1988) is outstanding in this respect for the quality of the samples examined and the size of the studies. When cell morphology, pattern of marrow infiltration, and extent of marrow infiltration were all analysed meticulously in over 1000 patients, it was found that this method can be used to distinguish multiple myeloma from reactive plasmacytosis and that multiple myeloma can be classified according to grades of malignancy on the basis of marrow morphology. Furthermore, these appearances are a powerful prognostic variable. These studies are of considerable biological interest and importance, but the difficulties experienced by many groups in obtaining data of this quality probably means that this approach will not be routinely applied in the investigation and staging of multiple myeloma.

7. Tumour kinetics. The tumour proliferation kinetics as expressed by the labelling index can now be measured relatively simply either by thymidine incorporation or by the identification of the incorporation of bromodeoxyuradine using monoclonal antibodies. This measurement appears to be of prognostic significance independent of β_2-microglobulin (Kyle 1988; Pileri *et al.* 1989; Greip *et al.* 1993).

8. Cell biological features. The value of estimating DNA content, RNA content, oncogene activation, cytokine production, cell membrane features such as p180 glycoprotein, and the presence of specific cluster differentiation antigens remains of interest and requires further evaluation (Barlogie *et al.* 1988).

9. Others. Biological features of the disease which have prognostic significance, possibly independently of the clinical features of the disease, include interleukin-6 (Bataille *et al.* 1989;

challenging areas of pain control because of the severity of bone pain and the relationship of this pain to movement. Patients may be pain free at rest but severely limited on any movement and their analgesic requirements are therefore closely related to their mobility. A careful clinical assessment will often reveal valuable clues such as clinical evidence of nerve entrapment or pathological fractures which can be amenable to local measures. However, opiate analgesics remain the mainstay of pain control. They may be usefully supplemented by non-steroidal anti-inflammatory drugs. Sudden exacerbation of pain may indicate pathological fracture, but can occur in myeloma without any radiological evidence of pathological fracture. In the latter circumstances, these episodes may be self-limiting and presumably result from fractures not visible on radiographs or perhaps from subperiosteal haemorrhages. These short-lived exacerbations in pain are not necessarily associated with progression of the underlying disease. Large lytic lesions in long bones should be pinned to avoid fractures.

Hypercalcaemia and osteolysis

Fractures can occur in any weight-bearing bone or in the ribs. Fixation is desirable to minimize pain, speed mobilization, and avoid non-union and should be attempted in all fit patients. Rib fractures are usually managed with analgesia and the patient is kept mobile. In rare instances, flail chests occur and these are usually associated with end-stage disease. When flail chest is found at presentation, energetic treatment of the myeloma and intensive supportive care can result in rapid healing sufficient to maintain respiration.

Treatment of hypercalcaemia must begin with careful correction of dehydration and maintenance of a high fluid throughput of 3–6 l of normal saline per day with careful monitoring of fluid balance and serum electrolytes. The use of loop diuretics will help to maintain fluid output in the rehydrated patient and increase calcium loss in the urine.

A number of specific agents have been used for the treatment of hypercalcaemia due to multiple myeloma, including corticosteroids and calcitonin which inhibit bone resorption, intravenous phosphate, and mithromycin, but their use has now been generally superseded by biphosphonates (diphosphonates). These structural analogues of pyrophosphate, the natural regulator of bone mineral precipitation and dissolution, are molecules characterized by phosphate–carbon–phosphate bonds as compared with the phosphate–oxygen–phosphate bonds of pyrophosphate. They are resistant to pyrophosphatase and manipulation of the molecular structure allows separation of their inhibitory effects on bone mineralization from their effects upon bone dissolution. The newer biphosphonates such as clodronate, administered orally and pamidronate (APD), administered intravenously will promptly inhibit bone resorption at doses which have little effect on bone mineralization.

At present biphosphonates are most widely used by slow intravenous infusion in the form of APD because they suffer from poor bioavailability and cause gastric irritation. Their effect upon the hypercalcaemia of malignancy is clear and frequently dramatic. A dose of 30 mg of APD infused over 1–8 h will restore normocalcaemia in the majority of patients. It remains unclear whether larger doses given over a prolonged period will be required for severe and resistant hypercalcaemia, but some studies suggest that there may be a dose–response relationship. APD is remarkably free from side-effects and normocalcaemia may be sustained for 3–4 weeks after a single treatment. Many patients whose disease may be resistant to specific chemotherapy can be maintained in good health with normocalcaemia by intermittent administration of APD every 1–6 weeks depending on careful monitoring of the serum calcium. There are few data on the use of APD in renal failure and caution is advised. However, in our experience it can be safely used with a prolonged (8 h) infusion time.

Several attempts have been made to reduce the incidence of hypercalcaemia and fracture by inhibiting the development of osteolysis. Earlier measures included attempts to produce fluorosis using sodium fluoride and some encouragement was obtained. However, randomized trials failed to show patient benefit and long-term fluoride therapy produced retinal damage. The early use of diphosphonates seemed to reduce the incidence of bone pain and radiological progression. However, there appeared to be an increased risk of acute leukaemia in some patients (Malpas 1986). Current efforts for the prevention of osteolysis focus on the newer diphosphonates. Oral clodronate given in the long-term is an effective way of reducing the incidence of hypercalcaemia and possibly reducing bone pain and skeletal metastases in patients with breast cancer, and long-term studies in multiple myeloma are presently being carried out (reviewed by Morton and Howell (1988)). Early results are encouraging (Merlini et al. 1990) and trials continue.

Renal failure

Even in patients with apparently normal renal function, the maintenance of a fluid intake of at least 3 l/day is an important determinant of outcome (Cooper et al. 1984).

Patients who present with or develop renal failure are managed according to the underlying pathology and the status of their multiple myeloma. Close cooperation between the oncologist and the renal physician is essential in the care of these patients. Precipitating factors such as hypercalcaemia, dehydration, infection, and hyperuricaemia should be sought. Unless it has reached the stage of known drug resistance, the underlying myeloma should be treated early and energetically. Renal function should be improved and supported. The choice of the appropriate techniques for supporting renal failure will be greatly influenced by the patient's overall medical state.

For patients who are not in oliguric renal failure, rehydration and forced diuresis with saline and frusemide can improve renal function considerably. If the underlying myeloma responds to chemotherapy, in a proportion of patients renal function will improve and often normalize (see Johnson et al. 1990). However, in approximately one-third of patients who present with severe renal failure there is little improvement with rehydration and, when renal biopsies are performed, classical features of myeloma kidney are apparent. The presence of casts is closely associated with irreversible renal failure (Johnson et al. 1990). Although slight and slow improvement occurs, most of the deficit in renal function in these patients will be irreversible.

Plasmapheresis has been used to speed up the reduction of myeloma protein in patients with renal failure. The theoretical advantage of reducing toxic myeloma proteins is clear, but the clinical advantages remain less clear (Johnson et al. 1990). One controlled trial of plasmapheresis in 29 patients with severe renal failure and Bence Jones proteinuria was reported to show significant benefit to improve both renal function and survival (Zucchelli et al. 1988), and this approach deserves further evaluation.

In patients nearing the end of their disease with drug-resistant myeloma and intractable renal failure, dialysis is not indicated. However, at presentation when the prognosis of the myeloma and of renal failure may be uncertain, dialysis should be employed as in any other case of acute or chronic renal failure. Patients with irreversible renal damage may respond well to treatment of their myeloma and then enter a stable clinical phase. In such patients chronic dialysis can be carried out satisfactorily with a reasonable quality of life. Haemodialysis and chronic ambulatory peritoneal dialysis appear equally effective, but with both these approaches infection is commoner in myeloma patients than in others. Patients treated using these approaches have survived for several years and the outcome is largely determined by their underlying myeloma (Iggo *et al.* 1989).

In patients with renal failure the choice of specific chemotherapy must be made with care. Melphalan is excreted via the kidneys and doses must be adjusted according to the level of renal failure. Cyclophosphamide is activated in the liver and is mainly metabolized; therefore it may be given safely at normal doses such as 500 mg/m^2/week intravenously.

In our experience and that of Aitchison *et al.* (1990) vincristine and adriamycin by continuous infusion together with high-dose steroids can be given easily and safely in patients with even the severest renal failure because these drugs are cleared principally through the liver. This regimen is therefore particularly suited for the initial management of patients with renal failure and can be started whilst active measures to correct renal failure are still ongoing. A presentation of myeloma with severe renal failure which limits the use of other drugs is an indication for the use of the vincristine–adriamycin–high-dose steroid regimens (for example, VAMP discussed below).

Hyperviscosity

Hyperviscosity with hypervolaemia is immediately life-threatening and should be treated by plasmapheresis using a cell-separator system which will prove effective and occasionally life-saving. This process has now become quite routine in most centres and plasma rich in paraprotein can be removed and readily replaced by plasma protein fraction in the order of 3 l. The procedure will take no more than 2 h and the patient's improvement is rapid.

Hyperuricaemia

The rapid turnover of proliferating cells can result in hyperuricaemia in many malignant conditions, particularly aggressive lymphoma and acute leukaemia. In myeloma the relatively slow rate of cellular proliferation and the common use of relatively non-toxic chemotherapy regimens means that treatment-induced hyperuricaemia is uncommon. However, hyperuricaemia may already exist in patients with pre-existing renal failure and the addition of antimyeloma treatment can precipitate uric acid nephropathy. For this reason routine prophylactic allopurinol is indicated and in patients with a high uric acid in whom treatment has to be instituted immediately intravenous allopurinol and a diuresis with alkaline saline is indicated.

Allopurinol is routinely indicated in patients who receive high-dose and intensive chemotherapy for multiple myeloma.

Indications for systemic treatment

Specific treatment with chemotherapy or biological therapy is not indicated in the treatment of all patients with paraproteinaemia or even all patients with multiple myeloma. Patients with monoclonal gammopathy of uncertain significance and those with smouldering myeloma should not receive specific treatment but should simply be followed carefully for evidence of disease progression. Indications for treatment would then be the development of symptoms or unequivocal evidence of progression with rising paraprotein or increasing marrow infiltration. The development of bone lesions, anaemia or renal failure, or progressive rising gammopathy takes the patient out of the diagnostic category 'smouldering myeloma' and specific treatment should be used.

In a prospective trial of patients with asymptomatic multiple myeloma, Hjorth *et al.* (1993) showed no advantage of early over deferred treatment.

In our view, once it is decided that specific chemotherapy is indicated, treatment should be selected in order to have the maximum chance of producing regression or complete remission of the disease. There is no evidence supporting the use of simple oral therapy such as melphalan in patients, particularly young patients, who are relatively fit at presentation. This may prejudice the effectiveness of subsequent therapy and reduce the patient's chance of remission.

Assessment of response

Once patients start on chemotherapy the most important principle of management is detailed monitoring of response. Patients whose paraprotein is stable or rising on therapy are not benefiting from treatment and that particular treatment should be stopped and altered. It is never acceptable to start a patient on a specific treatment and continue that treatment in the absence of evidence of response. If the patient's disease is stable 3 months after starting treatment, it should be stopped or altered. In most cases the stability is a feature of the disease and is not maintained by the treatment. Once a patient has responded to treatment and there is no further change in the paraprotein level, that is, the patient has entered a 'plateau' phase (defined below), then treatment should again be discontinued and the patient observed carefully.

Specific criteria for assessing response, particularly in clinical trials, have been suggested by a number of groups. The Leukaemia–Myeloma Task Force of the National Cancer Institute has published a set of response criteria (Chronic Leukaemia–Myeloma Task Force 1973) (Table 8). This principally involves a 50 per cent reduction in the serum or urinary paraprotein to define a remission. The Southwest Oncology Group introduced a greater degree of sophistication by taking account of the different catabolic rates of immunoglobulins at different serum concentrations. This 'synthetic

Table 8 Leukaemia–Myeloma Task Force response criteria

A drug which produces changes satisfying one or more of the following criteria can be said to have produced an objective effect on a direct manifestation of myeloma

1. Palpable (or radiography visualized) plasmacytomas: there should be reduction of 50 per cent or more in the product of the two largest diameters

2. Serum myeloma protein: a significant decrease, for example a fall to 50 per cent or less, of the pre-study value

3. Urinary myeloma protein: a significant decrease. If the pre-study value is greater than 1.0 g/24 h, there should be a fall to 50 per cent of this value or less; if the pre-study value is between 0.5 and 1.0 g/24 h there should be a fall to less than 0.1 g/24 h. This manifestation of the disease may not be a reliable indicator of response to therapy if the pre-study value is less than 0.5 g/24 h or if there is evidence of advancing renal insufficiency with increasing blood urea nitrogen

4. Definite radiographic evidence of skeletal healing

Table 9 Southwest Oncology Group myeloma response criteria

A Responsive patients who satisfy all the following criteria are considered to have achieved definite objective improvement.

1. A sustained decrease in the synthesis index of serum M protein to 25 per cent or less of the pre-treatment value and to less than 25 g/l on at least two measurements separated by 4 weeks. For IgA and Ig³M proteins the synthetic index is the same as the serum concentration. For IgG M proteins of subclasses 1, 2, and 4, the synthetic index must be estimated using a nomogram

2. A sustained decrease in 24 h urine globulin to 10 per cent or less of the pre-treatment value, and to less than 0.2 g/24 h on at least two occasions separated by 4 weeks

3. In all responsive patients the size and number of lytic skull lesions must not increase and the serum of calcium must remain normal. Correction of anaemia (hematocrit > 27 vol. %) and hypoalbuminemia (> 3.0 g/dl) is required if they are considered to be secondary to myeloma. With equivocal data (for example, non-secretors, or light chain producers for whom the pre-treatment urine collection was lost), the following support the conclusion that an objective response has occurred

4. Recalcification of lytic skull lesions

5. Significant increments in depressed normal immunoglobulins (for example, increments > 200 ml/l IgM, > 400 mg/l IgA, and > 4000 mg/l IgG)

B Improved patients show a decline in the serum M protein synthesis rate to less than 50 per cent, but not less than 25 per cent, of the pre-treatment value

C Unresponsive patients fail to satisfy the criteria for responsive or improved patients

index' of serum paraprotein can be read from simple nomograms or derived from a pocket calculator and is a more useful indicator of changes in the underlying myeloma cell number. However, the system is relatively clumsy and is not routinely used (Alexanian et al. 1972) (Table 9).

The Medical Research Council has introduced the assessment of the plateau phase. This depends not only upon a reduction in myeloma protein but also upon the attainment of a treatment-related plateau, that is, a state where the serum paraprotein or urinary light chain levels are stable or undetectable for 6 months and where the patient has no symptoms or minimal symptoms and is not transfusion dependent. Their results are therefore expressed in terms of the proportion of patients who experience complete loss of paraprotein and urinary light chain, the proportion who obtain an objective response short of this, and the proportion who achieve either stable disease or a plateau phase (MacLennan et al. 1988).

The Royal Marsden Group (Selby et al. 1987; Gore et al. 1989) have concentrated on establishing criteria to be regarded as complete remission for multiple myeloma. In their most recently stated criteria (Gore et al. 1989) complete remission was defined as follows:

(1) no paraprotein measurable by scanning densitometry of serum proteins separated on cellulose acetate membrane by electrophoresis and stained with Ponceau S;

(2) no detectable Bence Jones proteinuria on electrophoresis on neat urine stained with colloidal gold;

(3) 5 per cent or fewer plasma cells of normal morphology on bone aspiration;

(4) criteria (1)–(3) must persist for at least 3 months.

Patients were regarded as having achieved partial remission if there was a 50 per cent decrease in measurable paraprotein or bone-marrow infiltration which was sustained for 1 month or more.

There is still no consensus about the ideal way of assessing response in the management of myeloma. Indeed, the association between response to treatment and prolonged survival has been questioned (Palmer et al. 1987). Certainly we cannot assume at present that attaining complete remission will be associated with very prolonged survival and there was no difference in median survival between complete remission and partial remission patients in the Royal Marsden Group's first treatment series of high-dose melphalan therapy (Selby et al. 1987). Careful documentation of change in paraprotein, clinical state, and the stability of paraprotein is necessary. If the goal of developments in treatment is ultimately the cure of the disease, then it seems likely that attaining a substantial number of complete remissions will be an essential milestone along that road.

Specific treatment

Once a decision is taken to use specific treatment with either chemotherapy or, more recently, biological therapy for multiple myeloma, the choice of treatment remains wide and can encompass a single simple out-patient oral chemotherapy, a more intensive combination chemotherapy, the combination of chemotherapy with interferon, or the use of very intensive high-dose intravenous treatments sometimes with autologous or allogeneic bone-marrow transplantation and usually given with intensive supportive care to in-patients.

Chemotherapy

The development of the chemotherapy for multiple myeloma began in the 1950s with the early use of single alkylating agents, principally melphalan and cyclophosphamide. Before their introduction no specific therapy was available and the prognosis for patients with multiple myeloma was poor with median survival times in a number of studies ranging from 3.5 to 11.5 months (Love 1986).

Melphalan was introduced into clinical practice in the late 1950s and was used orally in various regimens as the standard therapy for multiple myeloma until well into the 1970s. Only some dosage regimens have taken account of the critically important variable oral absorption of melphalan between patients (Alberts et al. 1979). Unless this is considered, patients tend to be undertreated and it is appropriate with melphalan given orally to increase the dose until mild myelosuppression is seen, thus demonstrating adequate absorption. Either melphalan or single-agent cyclophosphamide chemotherapy will yield responses in a substantial proportion of myeloma patients. Although the literature contains reports of response rates varying between 19 and 80 per cent, most authorities would now expect a response in approximately 50 per cent of patients treated with these drugs. There is no difference in response rate or survival between melphalan or cyclophosphamide in conventional dosage (Medical Research Council 1980a, b). The median survival of patients treated with single alkylating agents is between 24 and 36 months in most studies and represents a substantial improval over the natural history of the disease. Although single-agent melphalan has been superseded for many myeloma patients, it remains the historical gold standard.

The addition of prednisolone to treatment with melphalan is common practice, but its role is still unclear. Moderate doses of prednisolone (40 mg daily) as a single agent will produce objective improvement in many myeloma patients, but in an early randomized trial survival was not prolonged. A series of trials subsequently evaluated the addition of prednisolone to melphalan and there was no consistent evidence of prolonged survival, although response rates did appear to be increased. Improvement in patient well-being and greater drug tolerance were probably the strongest arguments for including prednisolone with melphalan in the treatment of multiple myeloma.

Work with mouse models and some clinical experience (Bergsagel *et al.* 1972, 1975) suggested that alkylating agents were not always cross-resistant in multiple myeloma and this led to the concept of combination chemotherapy with multiple alkylating agents. Between 1979 and 1987 a series of prospective randomized trials were carried out by groups in North America and Europe in which combination chemotherapy including cyclophosphamide, melphalan, BCNU, and methyl CCNU, together with vincristine and prednisolone in some cases, were evaluated in various combinations and compared with melphalan+prednisolone. These studies have been summarized by Bergsagel (1988) and Simes (1986). The analysis of Bergsagel (1988) incorporates data from nine randomized prospective trials, and that by Simes (1986) uses data from 12 trials. Bergsagel's (1988) observations are elegantly summarized in Fig. 6 and we have updated the collected literature in Table 10. In this analysis the range of median survivals for melphalan+prednisolone or for drug combinations are plotted and listed and are seen to overlap substantially. Bergsagel's (1988) conclusion is that there is no

consistent advantage to the use of combination chemotherapy. Simes (1986) performed a meta-analysis of 12 studies and concluded that among all registered randomized prospective trials when meta-analysed there was a marginal advantage in favour of combination chemotherapy ($p=0.06$ for all patients; $p=0.03$ for poor risk patients) but the estimated magnitude of benefit was small. Both these analyses included data from the Southwest Oncology Group's trial 7704 (Salmon *et al.* 1983) as the only individual trial showing a survival benefit for combination chemotherapy and if this trial were to be excluded from the Simes (1986) meta-analysis it seems unlikely that any significant advantage from combination chemotherapy would be shown. If this trial is excluded from consideration and attention is focused only on the combinations of multiple alkylating agents, it can be seen that no single trial shows a statistically significant survival advantage in favour of combination chemotherapy, that a meta-analysis fails to show such an advantage, and that Bergsagel's (1988) plot of the accumulated data illustrates clearly the extent to which the results overlap. The conclusion from the published work is that combination chemotherapy with alkylating agents does not produce a useful improvement in patient survival. This is supported by a meta analysis of all trials (Gregory *et al.* 1992).

More recently, combination chemotherapy for multiple myeloma has included drugs other than alkylating agents and, in particular, adriamycin (Salmon *et al.* 1983; Durie 1986*b*; MacLennan *et al.* 1988). Three trials are now mature: the Medical Research Council V myelomatosis trial in which melphalan+prednisolone was compared with a combination of adriamycin, BCNU, cyclophosphamide, and melphalan (ABCM) and the Southwest Oncology Group protocols 7927/28 and 7704/05 in which the use of alternating combination chemotherapy including vincristine, adriamycin, cyclophosphamide, BCNU, and prednisolone was compared with more conventional therapy including melphalan+prednisolone. A trial from Sweden (Hjorth *et al.* 1990) has a rather shorter follow-up. The Southwest Oncology Group and Medical Research Council trials (Fig. 7) suggest a survival advantage for the use of adriamycin-based combination chemotherapy for multiple myeloma (Durie 1988*b*; MacLennan *et al.* 1988; MacLennan *et al.* 1992). An overview of the trials has suggested, in preliminary analysis, that their results are comparable when they are balanced for appropriate prognostic variables (Kelly *et al.* 1988). The Swedish trial is negative (Hjorth *et al.* 1990). Although there is undoubtedly greater subjective toxicity with the combination chemotherapy during the treatment phase, on balance the improved chance of achieving a

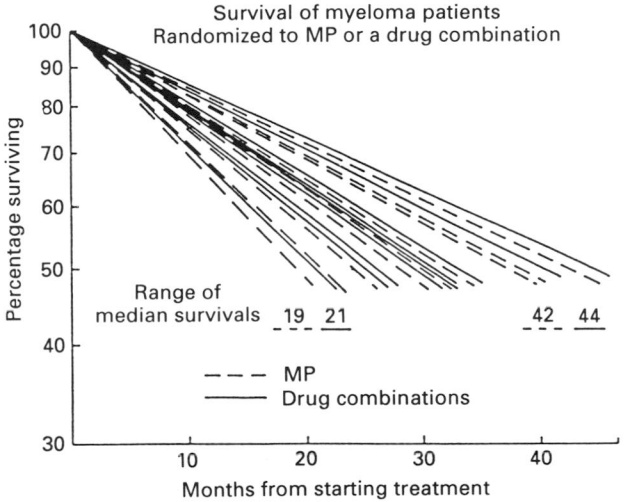

Fig. 6 Melphalan + prednisolone (MP) versus combination treatments for multiple myeloma. (Reproduced with permission from *Haematological Oncology*.)

Table 10 Randomized trials: melphalan+prednisolone versus combination chemotherapy

	Number of patients	Combination	Response rate MP/Comb (%)	Median survival MP/Comb (months)	Survival benefit (Comb vs MP)
Bergsagel *et al.* (1979)	299	BCMP	40/39	28/31	NS
Abramson *et al.* (1982)	188	BCP	43/50	19/25	NS
Salmon *et al.* (1983)	239	VMCP–VB/CAP	32/53	24/40	$p<0.02$
Alexanian and Driecar (1984)	105	VCP–M/A	53/57	37/26	NS
Hansen *et al.* (1985)	64	VBCMP	45/58	21/21	NS
Kildahl-Anderson *et al.* (1986)	67	VMCMP	67/74	32/33	NS
Oken *et al.* (1987)	431	VBCMP	51/72	30/31	NS
Pavlowsky *et al.* (1988)	260	VCMECMP	33/44	42/44	NS
Pavlowsky *et al.* (1988)	150	MECP	40/40	38/30	NS
MacLennan *et al.* (1988)	627	ABCM	50/60	21/28	$p<0.0004$

MP, melphalan+prednisolone; Comb, combination therapy; B, BCNU; C, cyclophosphamide; M, melphalan; P, prednisone; V, vincristine; A, adriamycin; ME, methyl CCNU; NS, not significant.

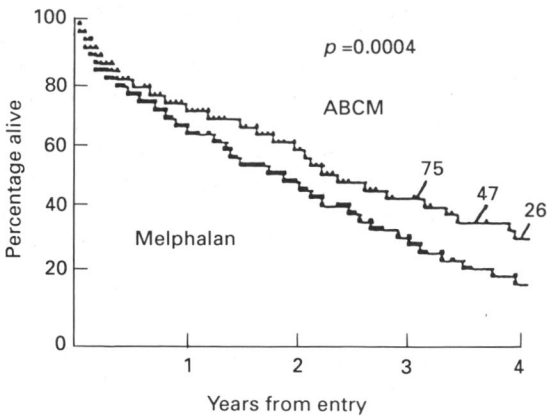

Fig. 7 Survival of patients with multiple myeloma treated with combination chemotherapy (ABCM) or melphalan in the Medical Research Council V myelomatosis trial (MacLennan *et al.* 1988). (Reproduced with permission from *Haematological Oncology*.)

period of good quality of life, with all treatment suspended, that is available to patients in, for instance, the ABCM arm of the Medical Research Council V myelomatosis trial seems to justify the cautious use of this combination in many patients, although in Medical Research Council V the age of the patient was a significant factor affecting outcome and the benefits of ABCM therapy were only seen in patients under 65 years (Fig. 7). This may be limited to patients with poor prognostic features (MacLennan *et al.* 1992).

Radiation therapy

Radiotherapy is valuable in the management of multiple myeloma (Mill and Griffith 1980; Rostem 1988). The principal roles are as follows.

1. Palliation of bone pain by local irradiation to moderate dose. Relief of pain due to progressive myeloma deposits is usually achieved by doses of 20–24 Gy and single large fractions of 8 Gy may be useful for this purpose.

2. Radical treatment of solitary plasmacytoma (see below).

3. Local treatment of myeloma deposits which are placed to cause actual or likely morbidity such as spinal cord compression or facial deformity. For these, radiation may be valuable as an adjunct to systemic treatment or as the main treatment for drug-resistant disease.

4. Treatment of pathological fractures after fixation.

5. Wide-field, for example, hemibody, irradiation as a palliative treatment of widespread painful bony metastases.

6. As part of intensive chemoradiotherapy with bone-marrow transplantation (see below).

Recommendations for conventional therapy

Where possible, it is appropriate to include patients with multiple myeloma in prospective randomized trials which are seeking to improve our knowledge of the biology and treatment of this disease. Indeed, there is evidence from population-based studies in Finland that the overall outcome for multiple myeloma is improved by wide usage of formal treatment protocols in trials (Karjalainen and Palva 1989). Where either patient or physician are unwilling to participate

in these approaches, a convention for choice of specific treatment can be suggested.

Patients over the age of 65 years for whom systemic treatment is indicated can be treated with oral melphalan+prednisolone. They should receive treatment until they enter a plateau phase but no chemotherapy thereafter until there is evidence of disease progression. There are several different ways of delivering oral melphalan, but we feel that care is needed to allow for variable absorption and myelosuppression. We recommend that patients should receive melphalan 9 mg/m^2 in the morning daily for 4 days with 100 mg of prednisolone in the morning for 4 days. The melphalan should be given at least 30 min before breakfast and the blood count should be repeated weekly and the drug repeated every 4–6 weeks. When an effective dose has been administered, the leucocyte and platelet counts will fall and recover by the fourth to sixth week. If no significant fall in leucocyte or platelet count is observed, then the melphalan dose can be increased by 2 mg/day until a leucocyte nadir of less than 2×10^9/l and more than 1×10^9/l is achieved.

Patients under the age of 65 years, particularly those with poor prognostic features, should receive adriamycin containing combinations such as ABCM (MacLennan *et al.* 1988, 1992) and again they should be treated to plateau, but there is no indication for maintenance chemotherapy (Medical Research Council 1985).

If patients fail to respond to these approaches or if they relapse, one of the newer developments in treatment discussed below should be considered. Secondary chemotherapy with conventional drugs is usually unsuccessful, although patients with long remissions (>1 year) may respond to second-line therapy with the same or similar drugs after their primary treatment. Second remissions are usually short.

Current developments in the treatment of multiple myeloma

Although it is clear that patients benefit from chemotherapy in multiple myeloma and of the order of 50 per cent will respond with a median survival of 2–3 years, the result of alkylating agent therapy or adriamycin-based combination chemotherapy remain unsatisfactory. This has resulted in a series of new developments in the treatment of multiple myeloma which now appear promising.

High-dose melphalan, bone-marrow transplantation and peripheral blood stem cell support

In experimental systems high doses of alkylating agents such as melphalan lead to increased tumour cell kill with a decreased risk of acquired drug resistance. These observations led, in 1981, to the initiation of studies of a single large intravenous dose of melphalan for the treatment of multiple myeloma (McElwain and Powles 1983). These initial encouraging results led to a larger evaluation of this treatment at the Royal Marsden Hospital (Selby *et al.* 1987). Melphalan was given at a dose of 140 mg/m^2 on a single occasion to previously untreated patients with multiple myeloma and this resulted in an overall response rate of 78 per cent in a group of 41 patients. The treatment was associated with prolonged myelosuppression with a median time to recover to 1×10^6 white cells/l of 28 days. This myelosuppression was associated with a significant infection risk and there were eight early deaths mainly due to infection and bleeding among the first 41 patients treated in this study. However, in addition to the very high response rate, the efficacy of the treatment was encouraging and 27 per cent of patients achieved a complete remission defined as a normal bone-marrow morphology and unmeasurable myeloma protein by electrophoresis. The median duration of complete and partial remissions was 19 months, but relapses have been seen in all the patients.

With high-dose melphalan given in this way to patients who had had previous chemotherapy, the response rate was again high but these remissions were of short duration and the majority of patients had relapsed within 6 months (Selby *et al.* 1987). This is similar with all of the myeloablative treatments developed so far and their value in patients with resistant or refractory disease is doubtful (Gobbi *et al.* 1989; Jagannath *et al.* 1990; Alexanian *et al.* 1994).

In a subsequent study melphalan was given at a dose of 140 mg/m^2 with the addition of high doses of methyl prednisolone (1 g/m^2 intravenously daily for 5 days). In this study the response rate and complete remission rate were maintained in a group of 22 patients and myelosuppression and other toxicities were identical. Most importantly there was a fall in the early death rate due to treatment-related complications as a result of improved patient selection and improved medical supportive measures during the period of myelosuppression (Selby *et al.* 1985).

In an effort to improve on the results of high-dose melphalan a programme was developed which aimed to allow further increased doses of melphalan with autologous bone-marrow transplantation. Patients were initially treated with infusioned combination chemotherapy with vincristine and adriamycin and methyl prednisolone according to a regimen known as VAMP (see below). This was well tolerated subjectively and results in a high response rate (70 per cent) with clearance of bone-marrow to less than 30 per cent infiltration in over half the patients (56 per cent). Patients were then treated with melphalan 200 mg/m^2 and autologous bone-marrow grafting was performed. This shortens the period of myelosuppression to a median of 21 days and the overall complete remission rate of the programme involving VAMP followed by high-dose melphalan with ABMT is now 25/50; that is, 50 per cent (Gore *et al.* 1989). The high initial complete remission rate and overall survival figures are encouraging (Fig. 8). Although long follow-up is incomplete, the results are sufficiently encouraging (Cunningham *et al.* 1994) to justify a prospective randomized trial currently being carried out by the Medical Research Council in the UK (Johnson and Selby 1994).

Other groups have sought to develop the intensive chemotherapy of myeloma in new directions. The addition of total-body irradiation to high-dose melphalan together with autologous bone-marrow transplantation has resulted in high partial response rates, but as yet no clear evidence of an advantage to the use of total-body irradiation or of a cured population of patients (Barlogie *et al.* 1989). Such studies are continuing, and the application of developments in haemopoietic growth factors and peripheral blood stem cell (PBSC) harvests may increase the safety and convenience of this approach (To *et al.* 1990, 1992). The value of PBSC may lie mainly in reducing the period of aplasia (Reiffers *et al.* 1989; Jagannath *et al.* 1990). Peripheral blood probably contains myeloma precursors (Dreyfus *et al.* 1993; Johnson and Selby 1994) and studies of marrow purging *ex vivo* have not yet shown benefits (Anderson *et al.* 1993, Reece *et al.* 1993).

Allogenic bone marrow transplantation has not been widely used in the treatment of multiple myeloma because the incidence and morbidity of graft versus host disease is high among older patients. In the collected experience of the European Bone Marrow Transplantation Cooperative Group (Gahrton *et al.* 1991) encouraging results were reported. As techniques for allogeneic transplantation improve and control of graft versus host disease increases there may be wider applications for this technique in selected patients. At present, although there are undoubtedly some good results with long remissions in some patients, the techniques are still being developed and patient selection, ideal regimens, and timing of treatment remain to be determined (Buckner *et al.* 1989; McElwain *et al.* 1989; Tura *et al.* 1989; Gahrton *et al.* 1991).

The status of myeloablative treatments for multiple myeloma is still uncertain and requires the completion of randomized controlled trials. An interim analysis of the French trial (IFM−90) recently showed advantages of intensive treatment in response rates but not survival (unpublished) and is not conclusive.

Infused chemotherapy with high-dose steroids

Alexanian and colleagues from the MD Anderson Hospital in Texas have developed a novel approach to the chemotherapy of multiple myeloma. They initially confirmed that high doses of glucocorticoid steroids were capable of producing remission in patients whose disease was refractory to alkylating agent therapy. The addition of adriamycin and vincristine given as a continuous infusion over 4 days to high-dose steroids using initially prednisolone and later dexamethasone resulted in a regimen capable of producing useful responses in patients with resistant myeloma. Sixty-five per cent of patients relapsing after previous chemotherapy and 32 per cent of patients refractory to first-line treatment responded to the VAD regimen (vincristine and adriamycin with high-dose dexamethasone). High-dose dexamethasone alone was found to be as effective as the combination in refractory patients (Alexanian *et al.* 1983, 1986; Barlogie *et al.* 1984). The use of methyl prednisolone as an alternative to dexamethasone in the VAMP regimen was shown to be effective in previously treated multiple myeloma (Forgeson *et al.* 1988) with a 36 per cent response rate and a median duration of remission of 11 months in previously treated patients. Weekly low-dose cyclophosphamide can be added to the VAMP regimen with moderate toxicity and a response rate of 61 per cent in a highly selected group of previously treated patients (Forgeson *et al.* 1988).

Both the VAD and the VAMP regimens have been used in the primary therapy of patients with multiple myeloma (Alexanian *et al.* 1990). VAMP results in a high response rate of 70 per cent, but follow-up information is not available because these patients have been subsequently treated with high-dose melphalan therapy (see above). VAD will also result in a rapid and high response rate with a reported median duration of remission of 18 months (Samson *et al.* 1989; Salmon and Crowley 1992). However, disappointing

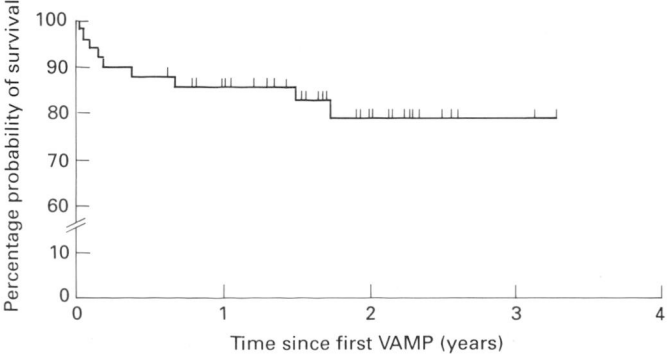

Fig. 8 Survival of patients with multiple myeloma treated with VAMP chemotherapy followed by high-dose melphalan (Gore *et al.* 1989). (Reproduced with permission from the *Lancet.*)

complete remission rates and overall survival have been seen so far when VAD or related regimens are used alone (Barlogie *et al.* 1989).

Vincristine–adriamycin infused chemotherapy with high-dose steroids is certainly an active regimen in the treatment of myeloma and some specific indications are emerging. The regimen is very useful in patients with renal failure because the drugs are principally cleared by the liver. It may be useful as a preparation for autologous bone-marrow grafting and in this case has the advantage that alkylating agents, which are the mainstay of intensive therapy, are not part of the VAMP regimen and, hence, the possibility of acquired resistance may be avoided. In patients relapsing from alkylating-agent-based therapy VAMP or VAD can produce useful palliation, but there is little evidence of long-term remission in this context.

Interferon

When interferons became available for clinical evaluation multiple myeloma was one of the cancers first treated, with initial encouragement in small patient numbers (Mellstedt *et al.* 1979). Subsequent studies have confirmed that α-interferons are capable of producing regression in multiple myeloma that is resistant to alkylating agent therapy, but the proportion of patients benefiting is lower than that initially observed. Response rates of the order of 20 per cent are to be expected (for reviews see Mellstedt (1988) and Mandelli *et al.* 1990). Remissions rarely last for more than 6 months when interferon is used in this way. There is no definite association between a subtype of multiple myeloma and responsiveness to interferon and no clear indication that any particular type of α-interferon (lymphoblastoid interferon, α-interferon 2a, α-interferon 2b) is superior to any other. The optimal dose is not known, but subcutaneous injections of 10 MU on alternate days are commonly employed. The place of interferon as a primary therapy for multiple myeloma was defined in a randomized prospective trial performed by the Myeloma Group of Central Sweden (Mellstedt 1988). In a comparison with melphalan+prednisolone chemotherapy a response rate for natural α-interferon of 14 per cent was observed compared with a response rate for melphalan+prednisolone of 44 per cent, a difference which favours melphalan+prednisolone both clinically and statistically. In a subsequent ongoing trial interferon was added to melphalan+prednisolone for primary therapy with a suggestion of an improved response rate for the combination (Mellstedt 1988).

Current research on the application of interferon in the management of multiple myeloma has concentrated on two directions. The first has been the addition of interferon to existing chemotherapy and the second the use of interferon to maintain responses induced by conventional chemotherapy.

Mandelli and colleagues from an Italian myeloma research group have investigated the role of interferon as a maintenance treatment in patients responding to conventional induction chemotherapy (Mandelli *et al.* 1990). One hundred and one patients with symptomatic multiple myeloma who had had a substantial objective response or disease stabilization after 12 cycles of induction chemotherapy were randomly assigned to receive recombinant α-interferon 2b as maintenance therapy at a dose of 3 MU/m² three times weekly or no further treatment. In the most recent analysis there was a highly significant prolongation of response in patients receiving α-interferon (Fig. 9) and a strong trend towards prolonged survival in the interferon maintenance group. This important study has significant implications for the management of multiple myeloma and ongoing studies, not yet published in detail, appear to support

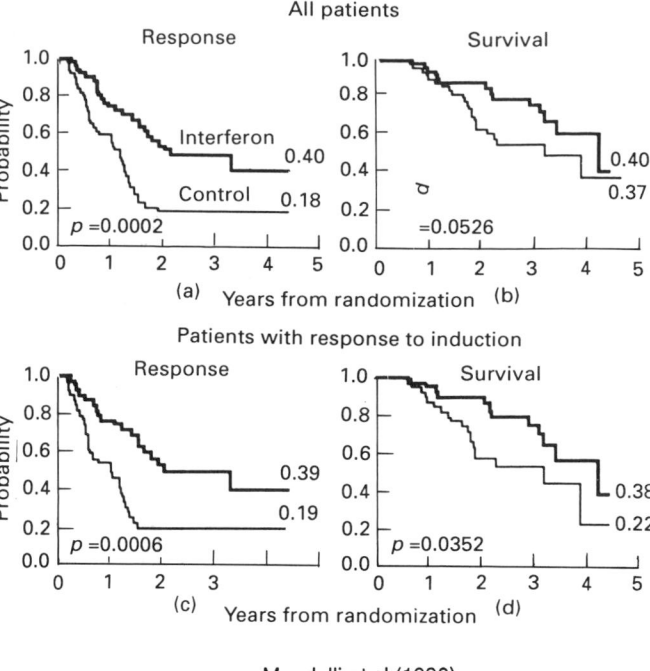

Fig. 9 Probability of continuing response or survival in patients treated with chemotherapy and then randomized to interferon or control. (Mandelli *et al.* 1990). (Reproduced with permission from the *New England Journal of Medicine*.)

its validity. High response rates are now achievable by a range of approaches and if these can be prolonged by relatively simple treatment like low-dose maintenance interferon then the prospects of significant improvements in the outcome for myeloma patients must be greatly improved. Certainly, current studies suggest that initial cytoreduction followed by maintenance interferon and result in impressive results (Cunningham *et al.* 1993; Fermand *et al.* 1993). The mechanism of action of interferon in this context requires clarification and measures to reduce the morbidity of prolonged interferon, principally fatigue, require investigation.

The combination of α-interferon with other antineoplastic treatments is suggested by evidence of synergism in experimental systems (Bonnem 1987). These encouraging laboratory studies have led to extensive evaluation in the clinic in pilot studies (see Bonnem 1987) and in prospective randomized comparative trials discussed above (Mellstedt 1988). The addition of α-interferon to combination chemotherapy has been explored and in recent reports the Eastern Cooperative Oncology Group have reported encouraging results. In a regimen consisting of 2 years of treatment with alternating 3 week cycles of vincristine, BCNU, melphalan, cyclophosphamide, and prednisolone with α-interferon 2, 5 MU/m² subcutaneously three times a week, has resulted in an overall response rate of 80 per cent together with a 30 per cent complete remission rate. Such a high response rate, including a substantial complete remission rate, is only otherwise achieved by very intensive chemotherapy regimens and the results of further follow-up of these studies and a randomized comparative trial from this group must be awaited with interest (Oken *et al.* 1990, 1992). Others have confirmed the high response rates with combination chemotherapy plus interferon, but survival advantages are still not proven (Scheithauer *et al.* 1989). Recent trials have been somewhat disappointing. Cancer and Leukaemia Group B showed no advantage of interferon added to melphalan and prednisolone (Cooper *et al.* 1993) and the Central

Swedish Group only showed advantages in some subgroups (Osterborg *et al.* 1993). Ludwig *et al.* (1991) showed a small survival advantage.

Other new approaches

As biological knowledge increases, new approaches are emerging. Interleukin-6 is an important promoter of myeloma growth and this leads to studies of anti-IL-6 antibodies (Klein *et al.* 1991) and down-regulators of IL-6 receptors (Sidell *et al.* 1991; Porter *et al.* 1993). The importance of multidrug resistance (MDR) expression in myeloma may be considerable and early trials of MDR inhibitors are in progress (Dalton *et al.* 1989*b*; Epstein *et al.* 1989; Sonneveld *et al.* 1992; Grogan *et al.* 1993; Cornellissen *et al.* 1994). Gene therapy strategies are being considered in multiple myeloma (Shu *et al.* 1993). These could include the expression of genetic constructs which cause immunomodulation or activate prodrugs. Their place even as experimental treatments remains to be found.

Recommendations for new approaches

Physicians caring for patients with multiple myeloma are now faced with a number of treatment choices which appear attractive for their patients and which may represent significant advances over those conventionally employed. Firm data indicating appropriate routine indication of these approaches are yet to be acquired, but many myeloma patients, particularly younger ones, may wish to consider the option of intensive treatment with autologous bone-marrow transplantation, combinations of biological therapy with chemotherapy, or the use of maintenance biological therapy. Most of these treatments should only be employed in the context of a properly conducted prospective clinical study or a comparative randomized trial. Outside these situations patients should only be treated with any of these approaches if they are fully informed of options and wish to consider a novel approach.

AMYLOIDOSIS

The term amyloid was originally used to describe a normal plant constituent which reacted with iodine and sulphuric acid (Schleiden 1838), but the first description of what we now called amyloid was given by Rokitansky (1842) when he described a waxy infiltration of the liver in patients with tuberculosis, syphilis, or osteomyelitis. Virchow was the first to use the term amyloid to refer to this material. The word literally means starch-like and Virchow used the word because the material reacted with iodine and therefore he thought that it was largely composed of carbohydrate (Virchow 1854). We now know that the material that makes up amyloid is largely composed of protein but the word continues to be used.

Amyloid is characterized by the deposition of insoluble persistent material that binds Congo red dye. It is largely composed of polymerized abnormal autologous protein subunits which are derived either from locally produced material or from circulating serum proteins. These subunits make up the amyloid fibrils which are then associated with sulphated glycosaminoglycans and a normal circulating glycoprotein (serum amyloid P component). These three elements together make up amyloid deposits.

Previously it was thought that all amyloid fibrils had a β-pleated secondary structure in which segments of polypeptide chains lay side by side and that it was this structure that made the material so resistant to *in vivo* protein catabolism. Recently it has been suggested that in at least some amyloid proteins the fibrils are composed of a stack of globular subunits, each of which contains only some β-structure (Turnell *et al.* 1986). This, together with the finding that once amyloid fibrils have been extracted from tissues they are relatively easily cleaved by proteolysis *in vitro* (Skogen and Natvig 1981), suggests that the persistence of amyloid *in vivo* is the result of complex mechanisms rather than the deposition of an intrinsically non-biodegradable substance. A number of different forms of amyloid fibrils exist and their characteristic protein subunits depend on their origin and, thus, on the cause. The origins of some are known, for instance pre-albumin in hereditary amyloidosis, β_2-microglobulin in patients with amyloidosis secondary to chronic haemodialysis, and of course immunoglobulin light chain, particularly λ light chain, in patients with myeloma. Amyloidosis is thus classified according to cause and fibril type: AL fibrils are associated with primary amyloidosis and myeloma, AA fibrils with secondary (reactive) amyloidosis (infection, inflammation, neoplasia), AF fibrils with familial amyloidosis, and ASc, AE, AL, and AD fibrils are all found in different forms of the localized amyloidosis (Pepys 1988).

The clinical features of amyloidosis associated with plasma cell malignancies are very similar to those of primary amyloidosis and patients develop peripheral neuropathy, cardiomyopathy, gastrointestinal involvement with macroglossia and dysphagia, purpura, and renal, skin, lung, and liver involvement. Approximately 10 per cent of patients with myeloma develop amyloidosis and it is more common with patients who have λ Bence Jones myeloma. Males are more often affected than females and the majority of patients are over 40 years. It should be remembered that abnormalities of immunoglobulins are common in patients with primary idiopathic amyloidosis, where half the patients either have hyper- or hypogammaglobulinaemia and nearly 90 per cent of patients demonstrate a serum or urine monoclonal spike on electrophoresis. Rectal biopsy is the commonest way of making the diagnosis and is positive in 73–98 per cent of cases (Kyle and Greipp 1983). Alternatively, subcutaneous fat can be aspirated or an affected organ biopsied, but there is the risk of haemorrhage. Sections are stained with Congo red and the presence of apple-green birefrigence under polarized light is diagnostic. There are as yet no non-invasive methods of making the diagnosis.

Treatment of amyloidosis is extremely difficult, although there are reports of amyloidosis improving if the underlying cause improves. The median survival for patients with amyloidosis is 12–15 months, but is 4–5 months for patients with amyloidosis associated with myeloma. Survival is very dependent on the presenting feature and there is a subset of patients who survive for 2 years. Therapy is very disappointing and a number of treatments have been tried including colchicine, dimethylsulphoxide, vitamin C, cytotoxic drugs such as cyclophosphamide, chlorambucil, and melphalan in low or high doses, and prednisolone in combination chemotherapy with adriamycin, melphalan, cyclophosphamide, and carmustine. Response rates are low and there is little evidence to suggest that any of these treatments has any impact on survival.

SOLITARY PLASMACYTOMA

Although plasmacytoma formation may be part of disseminated multiple myeloma, the occurrence of solitary plasmacytoma in bone or extramedullary sites is well recognized and can generate particular clinical and management problems. Extramedullary plasmacytoma appears to have a different natural history from plasmacytoma of bone.

Extramedullary plasmacytoma

Extramedullary lesions are usually solitary and occur in the upper airways and the nasopharyngeal space and nasal sinuses. They account for 3 per cent of all tumours of the nasal cavity and paranasal sinuses (Whittaker 1986).

There is a preponderance of male patients and the median age at presentation is approximately 60 years. In a cumulative series of 334 cases compiled from the literature, 79 per cent were in upper airways with other cases described in lymph nodes, spleen, skin and subcutaneous tissues, gastrointestinal tract, thyroid, and testes. The diagnosis is usually made by examination of a biopsy from the upper airways and this can be confirmed by immunocytochemistry for immunoglobulin production.

Spread from extramedullary plasmacytoma can occur in almost 50 per cent of cases and this usually develops in bone but, unlike multiple myeloma, tends to remain circumscribed even within bone with no particular predilection for the axial skeleton. Lymph nodes and sub-cutaneous deposits are seen and occasional visceral deposits in the liver, lung, and gastrointestinal tract are described. Localized extramedullary plasmacytoma uncommonly produces a paraprotein. Paraproteins in serum or urine are more frequently associated with widespread disease.

The treatment of choice for localized extramedullary plasmacytoma is radiotherapy. Although the optimal dose is not clear, many centres are using doses of 40–50 Gy. The literature suggests that 70 per cent of patients with extramedullary plasmacytoma are free of progression 10 years after adequate local therapy (Wiltshaw 1976; Whittaker 1986). If the disease becomes disseminated, then chemotherapy regimens comparable to those used in multiple myeloma are appropriate.

Solitary plasmacytoma of bone

Solitary bony plasmacytoma presents most frequently in men with a median age of 52 years. The spine is the commonest site followed by the pelvis and femur. Histological confirmation of a plasma cell tumour without evidence of spread on radiography of bones, marrow aspirate, and trephine and a serum paraprotein which disappears after local treatment are the criteria of diagnosis. The incidence of serum or urine paraprotein depends on the method of investigation, but up to 50 per cent of patients are reported to have paraprotein detectable with modern methods.

Although the natural history of solitary plasmacytoma of bone appears to be longer than that of multiple myeloma (Wiltshaw 1976; Whittaker 1986), the majority of patients will ultimately develop disseminated disease which will be clinically similar to that of multiple myeloma and the prognosis is considerably worse than that of extramedullary plasmacytoma, with only 20 per cent of patients alive after 10 years.

Initial treatment of solitary plasmacytoma of bone may be with radiotherapy if no other lesions are detected and this can produce local control. When the disease recurs or disseminates, then chemotherapy as for multiple myeloma is appropriate.

When patients appear to have a solitary plasmacytoma, it is suggested that investigations should include magnetic resonance imaging of the spine (Alexanian and Dimopoulos 1994) which may show dissemination.

PLASMA CELL LEUKAEMIA AND ACUTE MYELOID LEUKAEMIA

Plasma cell leukaemia, which can be defined as more than 2×10^9 plasma cells/l, occurs in less than 5 per cent of cases of multiple

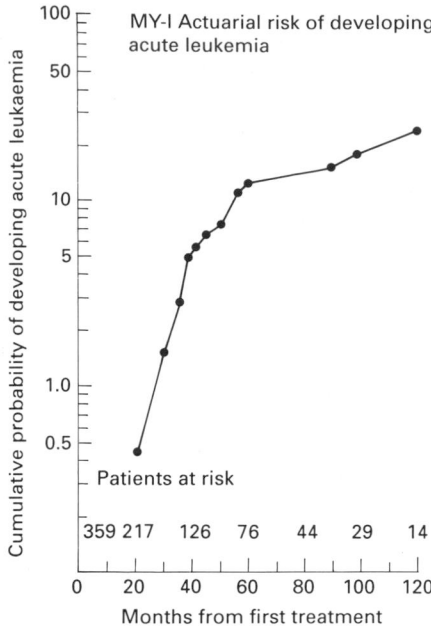

Fig. 10 Risk of developing acute leukaemia following treatment for multiple myeloma (Bergsagel 1988). (Reproduced with permission from *Haematological Oncology*.)

myeloma. It can occur at presentation as a distinct clinical entity or in the terminal phases of otherwise typical multiple myeloma. The clinical picture is aggressive with marrow failure a more prominent clinical feature than in typical multiple myeloma. Attempts at treatment with conventional chemotherapy are usually disappointing, with very few patients surviving beyond 6 months.

The incidence of non-plasma cell acute leukaemia is increased in myeloma patients. In a series of 364 myeloma patients treated with alkylating agents in a Canadian series, the first case of acute leukaemia was detected after 9 months of treatment and thereafter the actuarial risk of developing the condition increased rapidly to 14 per cent at 16 months, reaching 25 per cent at 10 years among the very small number of surviving patients (Bergsagel *et al.* 1979) (Fig. 10). This striking association may be due to a biological link between myeloid leukaemia and myeloma suggesting the origin from a common primitive stem cell or, in part, the influence of leukaemogenic alkylating agent therapy (Cuzick *et al.* 1987). The relatively early onset of acute leukaemia in myeloma patients distinguishes it from Hodgkin's disease and ovarian cancer and there is evidence of the occurrence of acute leukaemia in untreated patients with myeloma, macroglobulinaemia and monoclonal gammopathy of unknown significance, and amyloidosis (Bergsagel 1988). Indeed, there are reports of patients with plasma cell leukaemia whose plasma cells manifest cell surface markers normally associated with myeloid cells (Bergsagel 1988). However, there appears to be an association between the dose and choice of alkylating agent employed prior to the onset on acute leukaemia (Cuzick *et al.* 1987) which would suggest at least some role for leukaemogenic drug treatment.

WALDENSTRÖM'S MACROGLOBULINAEMIA

Macroglobulinaemia is both clinically and pathologically distinct from multiple myeloma. Patients present with anaemia, lymphadenopathy, and hepatosplenomegaly, usually without evidence of destructive bone disease. Hyperviscosity syndrome, with its attendant bleeding and visual manifestations, occurs in approximately 20 per cent of patients and is said to be associated with a worse survival (Kyle and Garton 1987). The mean age at diagnosis is 65 years with an approximately equal sex prevalence (Salmon and Cassady 1989).

The diagnosis is made from a typical clinical picture in association with an IgM paraprotein of more than 3 g/l and marrow infiltration with lymphocytes or plasma cells. The presence of an IgM paraprotein is not in itself diagnostic of Waldenström's macroglobulinaemia since they are also found in other B-cell tumours and very occasionally in cases with a clinical picture of multiple myeloma (<1 per cent). In fact, Waldenström's macroglobulinaemia accounts for only 17 per cent of all cases of macroglobulinaemia (Kyle and Garton 1987).

Apart from the clinical features mentioned above, patients may present or develop peripheral neuropathy. The neuropathy may be of mild sensory-motor type or purely sensory; it may also occur in association with cryoglobulinaemia and mononeuritis multiplex. Occasionally a demyelinating condition is encountered and these cases are associated with x light chains and IgM deposition in the myelin sheaths (Kelly 1987). Renal failure is uncommon, probably reflecting the low incidence of Bence Jones protein excretion.

The treatment of macroglobulinaemia is similar to that for other indolent B-cell tumours such as follicular non-Hodgkin's lymphoma or chronic lymphatic leukaemia. Oral alkylating agents, particularly chlorambucil, are generally used with or without steroids and plasmapheresis is often needed initially where there is evidence of hyperviscosity or to maintain chemoresistant patients. Occasionally patients attain worthwhile remissions from adriamycin containing combinations including the vincristine+adriamycin infusion regimens with high-dose steroids. Systemic chemotherapy is continued until serum IgM levels plateau, at which point it is discontinued and the patient observed. Complete remission is uncommon, but median survival is approximated at 5−6 years although some may survive for 10−15 years (Kyle and Garton 1987).

ACKNOWLEDGEMENTS

The authors would like to acknowledge warmly their debts to the late Professor Tim McElwain and to Professor Daniel Bergsagel who introduced them to and guided their work on the management and study of these diseases and to Nicole Goldman who patiently typed the manuscript.

REFERENCES

Abramson N, Lurie P, Mietlowski WL, Schilling A, Bennett J, Horton J (1982). Phase III study of intermittent carmustine (BCNU), cyclophosphamide and prednisone versus melphalan and prednisone in multiple myeloma. *Cancer Treatment Reports*, 66:1273−7.

Aitchison RG, Reilly IA, Morgan AG, Russell NH (1990). Vincristine, adriamycin and high dose steroids in myeloma complicated by renal failure. *British Journal of Cancer*, 61(5):765−6.

Akhtar N, Ruprai A, Pringle JH, Lauder I, Durrant ST (1989). *In situ* hybridization detection of light chain mRNA in routine bone marrow trephines from patients with suspected myeloma. *British Journal of Haematology*, 73:296−301.

Alberts DS, Chang SY, Chen HS (1979). Oral melphalan kinetics. *Clinical Pharmacology and Therapy*, 26:737−45.

Alexanian R, Dimopoulos M (1994). The treatment of multiple myeloma. *Drug Therapy*, 330, 484−9.

Alexanian R, Driecar R (1984). Chemotherapy for multiple myeloma. *Cancer*, 53:583−8.

Alexanian R, Yap BS, Bodey GP (1983). Prednisolone pulse therapy for refractory myeloma. *Blood*, 62:572−7.

Alexanian R, Barlogie B, Dixon D (1986). High dose glucocorticoid treatment of resistant myeloma. *Annals of Internal Medicine*, 105:8.

Alexanian R, Barlogie B, Tucker S (1990). VAD based regimens as primary treatments for multiple myeloma. *American Journal of Haematology*, 33(2):86−9.

Alexanian R, Dimopoulos M, Smith T, Delasalle K, Barlogie B, Champlin R (1994). Limited value of myeloablative therapy for late multiple myeloma. *Blood*, 83:512−16.

Anderson KC, *et al.* (1993). Monoclonal antibody-purged bone marrow transplantation therapy for multiple myeloma. *Blood*, 82:2568−76.

Axelsson U, Bachmann R, Hallen J (1966). Frequency of pathological proteins (M-components) in 6995 sera from an adult population. *Acta Medica Scandinavica*, 179:235−47.

Barlogie B, Smith L, Alexanian R (1984). Effective treatment of advanced multiple myeloma refractory to alkylating agents. *New England Journal of Medicine*, 310:1353−6.

Barlogie B, Epstein J, Alexanian R (1988). Genotypic and phenotypic characteristics of multiple myeloma. *Haematological Oncology*, 6:99−103.

Barlogie B, Epstein J, Selvassayagam P, Alexanian R (1989). Plasma cell myeloma—new biological insights and advances in therapy. *Blood*, 73:865−79.

Bartl R (1988). Histologic classification and staging of multiple myeloma. *Haematological Oncology*, 6:107−15.

Bataille R, Jourdan M, Zhang XG, Klein B (1989). Serum levels of interleukin 6, a potent myeloma cell growth factor, as a reflect of disease severity in plasma cell dyscrasias. *Journal of Clinical Investigation*, 84:2008−11.

Bellamy WT, *et al.* (1993). An *in vivo* model of human multidrug-resistant multiple myeloma in SCID mice. *American Journal of Pathology*, 142:691−8.

Berenson J, Lichtenstein A (1989). Clonal rearrangement of the beta-T cell receptor gene in multiple myeloma. *Leukaemia*, 3(2):133−6.

Berenson JR, Adelman D, Norman D, Castle S, Chang MP, Lichtenstein A (1989). Cytokine production by bone marrow cells and serum levels in patients with multiple myeloma. *Proceedings of the Second International Conference on Myeloma, Houston, Texas, 1989*, p. 10. Schering Plough, Bury St Edmunds, UK.

Bergsagel DE (1988). Chemotherapy of myeloma: drug combinations versus single agents, an overview and comments on acute leukaemia in myeloma. *Haematological Oncology*, 6:159−66.

Bergsagel DE, Riker WD (1985). Plasma cell neoplasms. In *Cancer: principles and practice of oncology* (ed. VT De Vita, S Hellman, and SA Rosenberg), pp. 1753−95. Lippincott, Philadelphia.

Bergsagel DE, Cowan DH, Hasselback R (1972). Plasma cell myeloma: response of melphalan-resistant patients to high dose cyclophosphamide. *Canadian Medical Association Journal*, 107:851−5.

Bergsagel DE, Ogawa M, Librach SL (1975). Mouse myeloma. A model for studies of cell kinetics. *Archives of Internal Medicine*, 135:109−13.

Bergsagel DE, Bailey AJ, Langley GR, MacDonald RN, White DF, Miller AB (1979). The chemotherapy of plasma cell myeloma and the incidence of acute leukaemia. *New England Journal of Medicine*, 301:743−8.

Bernstein SC, Perez-Atayde AR, Weinstein HJ (1985). Multiple myeloma in a child. *Cancer*, 56:2143−7.

Bertolini DR, Nedwin GE, Bringman TS, Smith DD, Munday GR (1986). Stimulation of bone resorption and inhibition of bone formation *in vitro* by human tumour necrosis factors. *Nature, London*, 319:516−18.

Billadeau P, Ahmann G, Greipp P, Van Ness B (1993). The bone marrow of multiple myeloma patients contains B cell populations at different stages of differentiation that are clonally related to the malignant plasma cell. *Journal of Experimental Medicine*, 178:1023−31.

Boccadora M, Gararoth P, Fossati G, Massaia M, Pileri A, Durie BGM (1983). Kinetics of circulating B lymphocytes in human myeloma. *Blood*, 61:812−14.

Bonnem E (1987). Alpha interferon: combinations with other anti-neoplastic modalities. *Seminars in Oncology*, 14:48−60.

Bontadini A, *et al.* (1989). Comparison between immunotoxin and immunoabsorption purging in multiple myeloma. *Proceedings of the Second International Conference on Multiple Myeloma, Houston, Texas, 1989*, p. 33. Schering Plough, Bury St Edmunds, UK.

Bourguet C, Grufferman S, Delzell E, Delong ER, Cohen HJ (1985). Multiple myeloma and a family history of cancer. *Cancer*, 56:2133−9.

Broder S, *et al.* (1975). Impaired synthesis of polyclonal (non-paraprotein) immunoglobulins by circulating lymphocytes from patients with multiple myeloma. *New England Journal of Medicine*, **293**:887−92.

Brown RD, Joshua DE, Nelson M, Gibson J, Dunn J, McLennan IC (1993). Serum thymidine kinase as a prognostic indicator for patients with multiple myeloma: results from the MRC(UK) V trial. *British Journal of Haematology*, **84**:238−41.

Buckner CD, *et al.* (1989). Marrow transplantation for malignant plasma cell disorders: summary of the Seattle experience. *European Journal of Haematology Supplement*, **51**:186−90.

Chronic Leukaemia Myeloma Task Force (1973). Proposed guidelines for protocol studies II. Plasma cell myeloma. *National Cancer Institute Cancer Chemotherapy Reports*, **3**(4):145−58.

Clamp JR (1967). Some aspects of the first recorded case of multiple myeloma. *Lancet*, **ii**:1354−6.

Clark RE, Geddes AD, Whittaker JA, Jacobs A (1989). Differences in bone marrow cytogenetic characteristics between treated and untreated myeloma. *European Journal of Cancer/Clinical Oncology*, **25** (12):1789−93.

Cohen HJ, Rundles W (1975). Managing the complications of plasma cell myeloma. *Archives of Internal Medicine*, **135**:177−84.

Cooper EH, Forbes MA, Crockson RA, MacLennan ICM (1984). Proximal renal tubular function in myelomatosis: observations in the fourth Medical Research Council trial. *Journal of Clinical Pathology*, **37**:852−8.

Cooper MR, *et al.* (1993). A randomized clinical trial comparing melphalan/prednisolone with or without interferon alfa-2b in newly diagnosed patients with multiple myeloma: a cancer and leukemia group B study. *Journal of Clinical Oncology*, **11**:155−60.

Cornelissen JJ, *et al.* (1994). MDR-1 expression and response to vincristine, doxorubicin, and dexamethasone chemotherapy in multple myeloma refractory to alkylating agents. *Journal of Clinical Oncology*, **12**:115−19.

Cunningham C, *et al.* (1994). High-dose melphalan and autologous bone marrow transplantation as consolidation in previously untreated myeloma. *Journal of Clinical Oncology*, **12**:759−63.

Cunningham D, *et al.* (1993). A randomised trial of maintenance therapy with intron-A following high dose melphalan and ABMT in myeloma. *ASCO Abstracts*, **12**:364.

Cuzick J (1986). Epidemiology of multiple myeloma. In *Multiple myeloma and other paraproteinaemias* (ed. IW Delamore), pp. 46−56. Churchill Livingstone, Edinburgh.

Cuzick J, De Stavola B (1988). Multiple myeloma—a case control study. *British Journal of Cancer*, **57**:516−20.

Cuzick J, Velez R, Doll R (1983). International variations and temporal trends in mortality from multiple myeloma. *International Journal of Cancer*, **32**:13−19.

Cuzick J, Erskine S, Edelman D, Galton DAG (1987). A comparison of the incidence of the myelodysplastic syndrome and acute leukaemia following melphalan and cyclophosphamide for myelomatosis. A report to the Medical Research Council's working party on leukaemia in adults. *British Journal of Cancer*, **55**:523−9.

Dalton WS, *et al.* (1989a). Drug-resistance in multiple myeloma and non-Hodgkin's lymphoma: detection of P-glycoprotein and potential circumvention by addition of verapamil to chemotherapy. *Journal of Clinical Oncology*, **7**:415−24.

Dalton WS, *et al.* (1989b). Immunohistochemical detection and quantitation of P-glycoprotein in multiple drug-resistant human myeloma cells: association with level of drug resistance and drug accumulation. *Blood*, **73**:747−52.

Danel L, *et al.* (1988). Estrogen and progesterone receptors in some human myeloma cell lines and murine hybridomas. *Journal of Steroid Biochemistry*, **30** (1−6):363−7.

Darby SC, *et al.* (1988). A summary of mortality and incidence of cancer in men from the United Kingdom who participated in the United Kingdom's atmospheric nuclear weapon tests and experimental programmes. *British Medical Journal*, **296**:332−8.

Deicher M, Peest D (1989). *In vitro* growth of human myeloma cells: regulation by autologous T cells. *Proceedings of the Second International Conference on Myeloma, Houston, Texas, 1989,* p. 13. Schering Plough, Bury St Edmunds, UK.

Delamore IW (1986). *Multiple myeloma and other paraproteinaemias.* Churchill Livingstone, Edinburgh.

Dewald GW, Kyle RA, Hicks GA, Greipp PR (1985). The clinical significance of cytogenetic studies in 100 patients with multiple myeloma, plasma cell leukaemia, or amyloidosis. *Blood*, **66**:380−90.

Dimopoulos MA, Barlogie B, Smith TL, Alexanian R (1991). High serum lactate dehydrogenase level as a marker for drug resistance and short survival in multiple myeloma. *Annals of Internal Medicine*, **115**:931−5.

Doll R (1990). Are we winning the fight against cancer? *European Journal of Cancer*, **26**(4):500−8.

Dreyfus F, Melle J, Quarre MC, Pillier C (1993). Contamination of peripheral blood by monoclonal B cells following treatment of multiple myeloma by high-dose chemotherapy. *British Journal of Haematology*, **85**:411−12.

Durie BGM (1988a). The biology of multiple myeloma. *Haematological Oncology*, **6**:77−81.

Durie BGM (1988b). Chemotherapy of myeloma: Southwest Oncology Group studies. *Haematological Oncology*, **6**:141−4.

Durie BGM, Salmon SE (1975). A clinical staging system for multiple myeloma. *Cancer*, **36**:842−5.

Durie BGM, Young LA, Salmon SE (1983). Human myeloma *in vitro* colony growth: interrelationships between drug sensitivity, cell kinetics and patient survival duration. *Blood*, **61**(5):929−34.

Durie BGM, Baum V, Vela V, Mundy G (1986a). Abnormalities of chromosome 6q and osteoclast activating factor production in multiple myeloma. *Blood*, **68**:208−10.

Durie BGM, *et al.* (1986b). Improved survival duration with combination chemotherapy induction for multiple myeloma: a Southwest Oncology Group Study. *Journal of Clinical Oncology*, **4**:1227−37.

Durie BGM, Stock-Novack D, Salmon SE, Finley P, Beckord J, Crowley J, Coltman CA (1990). Prognostic value of pretreatment serum beta 2 microglobulin in myeloma: a Southwest Oncology Group Study. *Blood*, **74**(4):823−30.

Epstein J, Barlogie B, Katzmann J, Alexanian R (1988). Phenotypic heterogeneity in aneuploid multiple myeloma indicates pre-B cell involvement. *Blood*, **71**(4):861−5.

Epstein J, Xiao HQ, Oba BK (1989). P-Glycoprotein expression in plasma-cell myeloma is associated with resistance to VAD. *Blood*, **74**:913−17.

Epstein J, Xias Huiqing, Xiao-Yan He (1990). Markers of multiple haemopoetic-cell lineages in multiple myeloma. *New England Journal of Medicine*, **322**:664−8.

Ernst TJ, Gazdar A, Ritz J, Shipp MA (1988). Identification of a second transforming gene, ras^n, in a human multiple myeloma line with a rearranged c-*myc* allele. *Blood*, **72**(4):1163−7.

Fermand JP, Chevret S, Ravaud P, Divine M, Leblond V, Dreyfus F, Marriette X, Brouet JC (1993). High-dose chemoradiotherapy and autologous blood stem cell transplantation in multiple myeloma: results of a phase II trial involving 63 patients. *Blood*, **82**:2005−9.

Ford RJ, Silva M, Mehta S, Alexanian R (1989). Studies on B cell growth and differentiation in multiple myeloma *Proceedings of the Second International Conference on Myeloma, Houston, Texas*, p. 6. Schering Plough, Bury St Edmunds, UK.

Forgeson G, Selby P, Lakhani S, Zulian G, Viner C, Maitland J, McElwain TJ (1988). Infused vincristine and adriamycin with high dose methylprednisolone (VAMP) in advanced previously treated multiple myeloma patients. *British Journal of Cancer*, **58**:469−73.

Franklin IM, Hamilton MS, Ball J, Ling NR (1989). The phenotype of neoplastic plasma cells suggests that the progenitor cell of myeloma may be a follicle centre B-cell. *Proceedings of the Second International Conference on Multiple Myeloma, Houston, 1989*, p. 3. Schering Plough, Bury St Edmunds, UK.

Freund GG, Kulas DT, Mooney RA (1993). Insulin and IGF-1 increase mitogenesis and glucose metabolism in the multiple myeloma cell line RPMI 8226. *Journal of Immunology*, **151**:1811−20.

Gahrton G, *et al.* (1991). Allogeneic bone marrow transplantation in multiple myeloma. *New England Journal of Medicine*, **325**:1267−73.

Gallagher RP, Spinelli JJ, Elwood JM, Skippen JK (1983). Allergies and agricultural exposure as risk factors for multiple myeloma. *British Journal of Cancer*, **48**:853−7.

Garrett IR, *et al.* (1987). Production of lymphotoxin, a bone resorbing cytokine by cultured human myeloma cells. *New England Journal of Medicine*, **317**:526−32.

Gobbi M, *et al.* (1989). Autologous bone marrow transplantation with immunotoxin-purged marrow for advanced multiple myeloma. *European Journal of Haematology*, **43** (Suppl. 51):176−81.

Gore ME, Riches PG, Kohn J (1979). Identification of the paraproteins and clinical significance of more than one paraprotein in serum of 56 patients. *Journal of Clinical Pathology*, **32**:313–17.

Gore ME, et al. (1989). Intensive treatment of multiple myeloma and criteria for complete response. *Lancet*, **ii**:879–82.

Gould J, Alexanian R, Goodacre A, Pathak S, Hecht B, Barlogie B (1988). Plasma cell karyotype in multiple myeloma. *Blood*, **71**(2):453–6.

Gowen M, Wood DD, Ihrie EJ, McGuire MKB, Russell RGG (1983). An interleukin-1 like factor stimulates bone resorption *in vitro*. *Nature, London*, **306**:378–80.

Gowen M, Nedwin G, Mundy GR (1986). Preferential inhibition of cytokine-stimulated bone resorption by recombinant interferon gamma. *Journal of Bone and Mineral Research*, **1**:469–74.

Gregory WM, Richards MA, Malpas JS (1992). Combination chemotherapy versus melphalan and prednisolone in the treatment of multiple myeloma: an overview of published trials. *Journal of Clinical Oncology*, **10**:334–42.

Greil R, Fasching B, Huber H (1989). C-*myc* oncogene in multiple myeloma: mRNA and protein analysis on the single cell level. *Proceedings of the Second International Conference on Multiple Myeloma, Houston, Texas, 1989*, p. 13. Schering Plough, Bury St Edmunds, UK.

Greenberg RS, Weiss NS (1993). A case–control study of multiple myeloma and occupation. *American Journal of Industrial Medicine*, **23**:629–39.

Greipp PR, Lust JA, O'Fallon WM, Katzmann JA, Witzig TE, Kyle RA (1993). Plasma cell labeling index and beta-2-microglobulin predict survival independent of thymidine kinase and C-reactive protein in multiple myeloma. *Blood*, **81**:3382–7.

Grogan TM, Durie BG, Spier CM, Richter L, Vela E (1989). Myelomonocytic antigen positive multiple myeloma. *Blood*, **73**(3):763–9.

Grogan TM, et al. (1993). P-Glycoprotein expression in human plasma cell myeloma: correlation with prior chemotherapy. *Blood*, **81**:490–5.

Hallen J (1966). Discrete gammaglobulin (M–) components in serum: clinical study of 150 subjects without myelomatosis. *Acta Medica Scandinavica (Supplement)*, **462**:1–127.

Hamburger AW, Salmon SE (1977). Primary bioassay of human myeloma stem cells. *Journal of Clinical Investigation*, **60**:846–54.

Hansen OP, Clausen NT, Drivsholm A, Laursen B (1985). Phase II study of intermittent 5-drug regimen (VBCMP) versus intermittent 3-drug regimen (VMP) versus intermittent melphalan and prednisolone (MP) in myelomatosis. *Scandinavian Journal of Haematology*, **35**:518–24.

Hayhoe FGJ, Swirsky DM, Bevan PC (1986). In *Morphological aspects in multiple myeloma and other paraproteinaemias* (ed. IW Delamore), pp. 75–102. Churchill Livingstone, Edinburgh.

Hjorth M, Hellquist L, Holmberg E, Magnusson B, Rodjer S, Westin J (1990). Initial treatment in multiple myeloma: no advantage of multidrug chemotherapy over melphalan-prednisolone. The Myeloma Group of Western Sweden. *British Journal of Haematology*, **74** (2):185–91.

Hjorth M, Hellquist L, Holmberg E, Magnusson B, Rodjer S, Westin J (1993). Initial versus deferred melphalan-prednisone therapy for asymptomatic multiple myeloma stage 1—a randomized study. *European Journal of Haematology*, **50**:95–102.

Hobbs JR (1971). Immunoglobulins in clinical chemistry. *Advances in Clinical Chemistry*, **14**:219–317.

Hollis GF, Gazdar AF, Bertness V, Kirsch IR (1988). Complex translocation disrupts c-myc regulation in a human plasma cell myeloma. *Molecular and Cellular Biology*, **8** (1):124–9.

Huang YW, Richardson JA, Tong AW, Zhang BQ, Stone MJ, Vitetta ES (1993). Disseminated growth of a human multiple myeloma cell line in mice with severe combined immunodeficiency disease. *Cancer Research*, **53**:1392–6.

Ichimaru M, Ishimaru T, Mikami M, Matsunaga M (1982). Multiple myeloma among atomic bomb survivors in Hiroshima and Nagasaki 1950–1976. *Journal of the National Cancer Institute*, **69**:323–8.

Iggo N, Palmer AB, Severn A, Trafford JA, Mufti GJ, Taube D, Parsons V (1989). Chronic dialysis in patients with multiple myeloma and renal failure: a worthwhile treatment. *Quarterly Journal of Medicine*, **73** (270):903–10.

Izaguirre CA, Minden MD, Howatson AF, McCulloch EA (1980). Colony formation by normal and malignant human B-lymphocytes. *British Journal of Cancer*, **42**:430–7.

Jackson N, Ling NR, Ball J, Bromidge E, Nathan PD, Franklin IM (1988). An analysis of myeloma plasma cell phenotype using antibodies defined at the Third International Workshop on Human Leucocyte Differentiation Antigens. *Clinical Experimental Immunology*, **72**:351–6.

Jagannath S, et al. (1990). Autologous bone marrow transplantation in multiple myeloma: identification of prognostic factors. *Blood*, **76**:1860–6.

Jagannath S, Vesole DH, Glenn L, Crowley J, Barlogie B (1992). Low-risk intensive therapy for multiple myeloma with combined autologous bone marrow and blood stem cell support. *Blood*, **80**:1666–72.

Joffe JK, Williams MP, Cherryman GR, Gore M, McElwain TJ, Selby P (1988). Magnetic resonance imaging in multiple myeloma. *Lancet*, **i**:1162–3.

Johnson WJ, Kyle RA, Pineda AA, O'Brien PC, Holley KE (1990). Treatment of renal failure associated with multiple myeloma. Plasmapheresis, hemodialysis and chemotherapy. *Archives of Internal Medicine*, **150** (4):863–9.

Joshua DE (1988). Host tumour interactions and immune regulation of disease activity. *Haematological Oncology*, **6**:83–8.

Kanis JA, McClosket EV, Thavarajah M, Evans D, Hamidy NAT, Preston E, Greaves M (1988). Calcium metabolism and myeloma and the treatment of hypercalcaemia. *Haematological Oncology*, **6**:115–17.

Karjalainen S, Palva I (1989). Do treatment protocols improve end results? A study of survival of patients with multiple myeloma in Finland. *British Medical Journal*, **299** (6707):1069–72.

Kawano M, et al. (1988). Autocrine generation and requirement of BSF-2/IL-6. *Nature, London*, **332**:83.

Kawano MM, et al. (1993). Identification of immature and mature myeloma cells in the bone marrow of human myelomas. *Blood*, **82**:564–70.

Kelsey PR, Delamore IW (1986). Prognostic features in multiple myeloma. In *Multiple myeloma and other proteinaemias* (ed. IW Delamore), pp. 137–43. Churchill Livingstone, Edinburgh.

Kelly JJ (1987). Polyneuropathies associated with plasma cell dyscrasias. *Seminars in Neurology*, **7**:30–7.

Kelly KA, Durie B, MacLennan IC (1988). Prognostic factors and staging systems for multiple myeloma. *Haematological Oncology*, **6**:131–41.

Kennard J, Zolla-Panzer S (1980). Origin and function of suppressor macrophages in myeloma. *Journal of Immunology*, **124**:268–73.

Kildahl-Andersen O, et al. (1986). Multiple myeloma in central Norway 1981–1982: a randomized clinical trial of 5-drug combination therapy versus standard therapy. *Scandinavian Journal of Haematology*, **37**:243–8.

Klein B, Bataille R (1989). Autocrine and paracrine myeloma cell growth factor (MCGF). *Proceedings of the Second International Conference on Multiple Myeloma, Houston, 1989*, p. 143. Schering Plough, Bury St Edmunds, UK.

Klein B, et al. (1989). Paracrine rather than autocrine regulation of myeloma-cell growth and differentiation by interleukin-6. *Blood*, **73**(2):517–26.

Klein B, et al. (1991). Murine anti-interleukin-6 monoclonal antibody therapy for a patient with plasma cell leukemia. *Blood*, **78**:1198–204.

Knapp W, Baumgartner G (1978). Monocyte-mediated suppression of human B lymphocyte differentiation *in vitro*. *Journal of Immunology*, **121**:1177–83.

Kohn J (1974). Benign paraproteinaemias. *Journal of Clinical Pathology (Supplement)*, **28**:77–82.

Kohn J, Srivastava PC (1972). Paraproteinaemia in blood donors and the aged: benign and malignant. *Protides of Biological Fluids*, **19**:257–61.

Kyle R (1975). Multiple myeloma. Review of 869 cases. *Mayo Clinic Proceedings*, **50**:29–40.

Kyle RA (1984). 'Benign' monoclonal gammopathy: a misnomer? *Journal of the American Medical Association*, **251**(14):1849–54.

Kyle RA (1988). Prognostic factors in multiple myeloma. *Haematological Oncology*, **6**:125–31.

Kyle R (1989). Monoclonal gammopathy of undetermined significance and smouldering multiple myeloma. *European Journal of Haematology (Supplement)*, **51**:70–5.

Kyle RA, Garton JP (1987). The spectrum of IgM monoclonal gammopathy in 430 cases. *Mayo Clinic Proceedings*, **62**:719–31.

Kyle RA, Greipp PR (1983). Amyloidosis (AL): clinical and laboratory features in 229 cases. *Mayo Clinic Proceedings*, **58**:665–83.

Kyle RA, Griepp PA (1988). Plasma cell dyserasias: current status. *CRC Critical Reviews in Oncology/Haematology*, **8**:93–152.

Kyle RA, Finkelstein S, Elveback LR, Kurland LT (1972). Incidence of monoclonal proteins in a Minnesota community with a cluster of multiple myeloma. *Blood*, **40**:719–24.

Lee M, Selvanayagam P, Alexanian R, Stass S, Barlogie B (1987). Rearrangement of T cell receptor genes in multiple myeloma. *Proceedings of the American Association of Cancer Research*, **706**: (Abstract).

Leonard RCE, MacLennan ICM, Smart Y, Van Heyan RI, Cusich P. (1979). Light chain isotype associated suppression of normal plasma cell numbers in patients with multiple myeloma. *International Journal of Cancer*, **24**:385–93.

Lisse IM, Drivsholm A, Christoffersen P (1988). Occurrence and type of chromosomal abnormalities in consecutive malignant monoclonal gammopathies: correlation with survival. *Cancer Genetics and Cytogenetics*, **35**:27–36.

Love EM (1986). The chemotherapy of multiple myeloma. In *Multiple myeloma and other proteinaemias* (ed. IW Delamore), pp. 373–5. Churchill Livingstone, Edinburgh.

Ludwig H, Fritz E, Kotzmann H, Hocker P, Gisslinger H, Barnas U (1990). Erythropoietin treatment of anaemia associated with multiple myeloma. *New England Journal of Medicine*, **322**(24):1693–9.

Ludwig H, *et al.* (1991). Interferon alfa-2b with VMCP compared to VMCP alone for induction and interferon alfa-2b compared to controls for remission maintenance in multiple myeloma: interim results. *European Journal of Cancer*, **27** (Suppl. 4):40–5.

Ludwig H, Nachbaur DM, Fritz E, Krainer M, Huber H (1991). Interleukin-6 is a prognostic factor in multiple myeloma. *Blood*, **77**:2794–5.

McElwain TJ, Powles RL (1983). High dose intravenous melphalan for plasma-cell leukaemia and myeloma. *Lancet*, **ii**:822–4.

McElwain TJ, Selby PJ, Gore ME, Viner C, Meldrum M, Millar BC, Malpas JS (1989). High-dose chemotherapy and autologous bone marrow transplantation for myeloma. *European Journal of Haematology Supplement*, **51**:152–6.

MacKenzie MR, Paglieroni TG, Warner NL (1987). Multiple myeloma: an immunologic profile. IV. The EA rosette-forming cell is a leu-1 positive immunoregulatory B cell. *Journal of Immunology*, **139**:24–8.

MacLennan ICM, Kelly K, Crockson RA, Cooper EH (1988). Results of the MRC myelomatosis trials for patients entered since 1980. *Haematological Oncology*, **6**:145–59.

MacLennan IC, Chapman C, Dunn J, Kelly K (1992). Combined chemotherapy with ABCM versus melphalan for treatment of myelomatosis. The Medical Research Council Working Party for Leukaemia in Adults. *Lancet*, **339**:200–5.

Maitland JA, Millar BC, Bell JBG, Montes A, Treleaven J, Gore ME, McElwain TJ (1990). Evidence that multiple myeloma may be regulated by homeostatic control mechanisms: correlation of changes in the number of clonogenic myeloma cells *in vitro* with clinical response. *British Journal of Cancer*, **61**:429–33.

Malpas JS (1986). Clinical management of myeloma. In *Multiple myeloma and other proteinaemias* (ed. IW Delamore), pp. 339–53. Churchill Livingstone, Edinburgh.

Mandelli F, *et al.* (1990). Maintenance treatment with recombinant interferon alpha 2b in patients with multiple myeloma responding to conventional induction chemotherapy. *New England Journal of Medicine*, **322**:1430–4.

Massaia M, Dianzani U, Bianchi A, Camponi A, Boccadoro M, Pileri A (1988). Defective generation of alloreactive cytotoxic T lymphocytes (CTL) in human monoclonal gammopathies. *Clinical Experimental Immunology*, **73**(2):214–18.

Massaia M, Bianchi A, Dianzani U, Camponi A, Attisano C, Boccadoro M, Pileri A (1989). Defective IL2 induction of LAK cells in blood T lymphocytes from monoclonal gammopathies. *Proceedings of the Second International Conference on Multiple Myeloma, Houston, Texas, 1989*, p. 157. Schering Plough, Bury St Edmunds, UK.

Medical Research Council Working Party on Leukaemia in Adults (1980*a*). Report on the second myelomatosis trial after five years of follow up. *British Journal of Cancer*, **42**:813–22.

Medical Research Council Working Party on Leukaemia in Adults (1980*b*). Treatment comparisons in the III MRC myelomatosis trial. *British Journal of Cancer*, **42**:823–30.

Medical Research Council Working Party on Leukaemia in Adults (1980*c*). Prognostic features in the III MRC myelomatosis trial. *British Journal of Cancer*, **42**:831–40.

Medical Research Council Working Party on Leukaemia in Adults (1984). Analysis and management of renal failure in the IV MRC myelomatosis trial. *British Medical Journal*, **288**:1411–16.

Medical Research Council Working Party on Leukaemia in Adults (1985). Objective evaluation of the role of vincristine in induction and maintenance therapy for myelomatosis. *British Journal of Cancer*, **52**:153–8.

Mellstedt H (1988). Treatment of multiple myeloma with natural alpha interferon. *Haematological Oncology*, **6**:187–92.

Mellstedt H, Bjorkholm M, Johansson B (1979). Interferon therapy in myelomatosis. *Lancet*, **i**:245–8.

Merlini G, *et al.* (1990). Long-term effects of parental dichloromethylene biphosphonate (CL2MBP) on bone disease of myeloma patients treated with chemotherapy. *Haematological Oncology*, **8**(1):23–30.

Mill WB, Griffith R (1980). The role of radiation therapy in the treatment of plasma cell tumours. *Cancer*, **45**:647–52.

Millar BC, Bell JBG, Lakhani A, Ayliffe MJ, Selby PJ, McElwain TJ (1988). A simple method of culturing myeloma cells from human bone marrow aspirates and peripheral blood *in vitro*. *British Journal of Haematology*, **69**:197–203.

Millar BC, Bell JBG, Maitland JA, Zuiable A, Gore ME, Selby PJ, McElwain TJ (1989). *In vitro* studies of ways to overcome resistance to VAMP-high dose melphalan in the treatment of multiple myeloma. *British Journal of Haematology*, **71**:213–22.

Morton AR, Howell A (1988). Biphosphonates and bone metastases. *British Journal of Cancer*, **58**:556–8.

Muir C, Waterhouse J, Mack R, Powell J, Whelan S (1987). *Cancer incidence in five continents* pp. 920–2. International Agency for Research on Cancer, Lyons.

Nandakumar A, Armstrong BK, De Klerk B (1986). Multiple myeloma in Western Australia: a case control study in relation to occupation, father's occupation, socioeconomic status and country of birth. *International Journal of Cancer*, **37**:223–6.

Neri A, Baldini L, Ferrero D, Murphy JP, Cro L, Tarella C, Dalla-Favera R (1989). Analysis of *ras* gene mutations in multiple myeloma. *Proceedings of the Second International Conference on Multiple Myeloma, Houston, Texas, 1989*, p. 11. Schering Plough, Bury St Edmunds, UK.

Nilsson T, Borberg B, Rudolphi O, Jacobsson L (1986). Double gammopathies: incidence and clinical course of 20 patients. *Scandinavian Journal of Haematology*, **36**:103–6.

Nishida K, Taniwaki M, Misawa S, Abe T (1989). Non-random rearrangement of chromosome 14 at band q32.33 in human lymphoid malignancies with mature B-cell phenotype. *Cancer Research*, **49**(5):1275–81.

Norfolk D, Child JA, Cooper EH, Kerrish S, Milford Ward A (1980). Serum β_2 microglobulin in myelomatosis; potential value in stratification and monitoring. *British Journal of Cancer*, **42**:510–15.

Office of Population Census and Surveys (1986). *Series MB1, No 15*. HMSO, London.

Oken MM, Tslatis A, Abramson N, Glick J (1987). Evaluation of intensive (VBMVP) vs standard (MP) therapy for multiple myeloma. *Proceedings of the American Society of Clinical Oncology*, **6**:203 (abstr. 802).

Oken MM, Kyle RA, Grippe PR, Kay NE, Tsiatis A, O'Connell MJ (1990). Chemotherapy plus interferon in the treatment of multiple myeloma. *Proceedings of the American Society of Clinical Oncology*, **9**:288.

Oken MM, Kyle RA, Greipp PR, Kay NE, Tsiatis A, O'Connell MJ (1992). Possible survival benefit with chemotherapy plus interferon (rIFNα2) in the treatment of multiple myeloma. *ASCO Abstracts*, **11**:358.

Osterborg A, *et al.* (1993). Natural interferon-α in combination with melphalan/prednisone versus melphalan/prednisone in the treatment of multiple myeloma stages II and III: a randomized study from the Myeloma Group of Central Sweden. *Blood*, **81**:1428–34.

Paglieroni T, MacKenzie MR (1980). Multiple myeloma: an immunologic profile. III. Cytotoxic and suppressive effects of the EA rosette-forming cell. *Journal of Immunology*, **124**:2563–70.

Palmer M, Belch A, Brox L, Pollock E, Cocks M (1987). Are the current criteria for response useful in the management of multiple myeloma? *Journal of Clinical Oncology*, **5**:1373–7.

Papadopoulos NM, Elin RJ, Wilson DM (1982). Incidence of gamma-globulin banding in a healthy population by high resolution electrophoresis. *Clinical Chemistry*, **28**:707–8.

Park CH (1971). Studies of the growth characteristics of myeloma *in vitro*, pp. 31–61. Doctoral thesis, University of Toronto.

Pavlowsky S, et al. (1988). An update of two randomized trials in previously untreated multiple myeloma comparing melphalan-prednisolone versus three and five drug combinations: a GATLA study. Journal of Clinical Oncology, 6:769–75.

Pearce NE, Smith AH, Howard JK, Shepperd RA, Giles HJ, Teague CA (1986). Case control study of multiple myeloma and farming. British Journal of Cancer, 54:493–500.

Peest D, Bartels B, Dallmann I, Schedel I, Deicher H (1986). Cytostatic drug sensitivity test for human multiple myeloma, measuring monoclonal immunoglobulin produced by bone marrow cells in vitro. Cancer Chemotherapy and Pharmacology, 17:69–74.

Pepys MB (1988). Amyloidosis: some recent developments. Quarterly Journal of Medicine, 67 (257):283–98.

Pilarski LM (1989). Development arrest in both T and B cell lineages underlies immune deficiency in patients with multple myeloma. Proceedings of the Second International Workshop on Myeloma, Houston, Texas, 1989, p. 3. Schering Plough, Bury St Edmunds, UK.

Pileri A, Ferrero D, Massaia M, Dianzani U, Boccadoro M (1989). Advances in biology of multiple myeloma: cell kinetics, molecular biology and immunology. European Journal of Haematology Supplement, 51:30–4.

Portier M, Zhang XG, Caron E, Lu ZY, Bataille R, Klein B (1993). Gamma-interferon in multiple myeloma: inhibition of interleukin-6-dependent myeloma cell growth and downregulation of IL-6 receptor expression in vitro. Blood, 81:3076–82.

Pruzanski W, Watt JG (1972). Serum viscosity and hyperviscosity syndrome in IgG multiple myeloma. Annals of Internal Medicine, 77:853–60.

Pruzanski W, Gidon MS, Roy A (1980). Suppression of polyclonal immunoglobulins in multiple myeloma: relationship to the staging and other manifestations at diagnosis. Clinical Immunology and Immunopathology, 17:280–6.

Radl J (1985). Four major categories of monoclonal gammopathies: introductory remarks. In Monoclonal gammopathies: clinical significance and basic mechanisms (ed. J Radl, W Hijmans, and B Van Camp), p. 3. Eurage, Rijswijk.

Reece DE, et al. (1993). Treatment of multiple myeloma with intensive chemotherapy followed by autologous BMT using marrow purged with 4-hydroperoxycyclophosphamide. Bone Marrow Transplantation, 11:139–46.

Reiffers J, Marit G, Boiron JM (1989). Autologous blood stem cell transplantation in high-risk multiple myeloma. British Journal of Haematology, 72:296–7.

Riches PG, Hobbs JR (1988). Laboratory investigation of paraproteinaemia. Journal of Clinical Pathology, 41:776–85.

Rokitansky K (1842). Handbuch der Pathologischen Anatomie, 311 (384):424.

Roman S, Moore JS, Darby C, Muller S, Hoover RG (1988). Modulation of Ig gene expression by Ig binding factors: suppression of α-H chain and −2-L chain mRNA accumulation in MOPC-315 by IgA-binding factor. Journal of Immunology, 140:3622–30.

Rostem A (1988). Radiation therapy of myeloma. Haematological Oncology, 6:201–3.

Salmon SE, Cassady JR (1989). Plasma cell neoplasms in cancer. In Principles and practice of oncology (ed. VT De Vita, S Hellman, and SA Rosenberg), pp. 1853–95. Lippincott, Philadelphia.

Salmon SE, Crowley J (1992). Impact of glucocorticoids and interferon on outcome in multiple myeloma. ASCO Abstracts, 11:316.

Salmon SE, Haut A, Bonnet JD, Amare M, Weick JK, Durie GM, Dixon DO (1983). Alternating combination chemotherapy and levamisole improves survival in multiple myeloma: a Southwest Oncology Group study. Journal of Clinical Oncology, 1:453–61.

Samson D, et al. (1989). Infusion of vincristine and doxorubicin with oral dexamethasone as first-line therapy for multiple myeloma. Lancet, ii (8668):882–5.

Schleiden MJ (1838). Einige Bermerkungen uber den vegetabilischen Faserstoff und sein Verhaltnis zum Starkemehl. Series 2. Annalen der Physik, 43:391.

Selby P (1987). Multiple myeloma and related diseases. Medicine International, 38:1664–7.

Selby P, Ayliffe M, Behrens J, McElwain TJ (1985). High dose treatment with melphalan and methylprednisolone for multiple myeloma. In Monoclonal gammopathies. Clinical significance and basic mechanisms. Topics in ageing research in Europe 5 (ed. J Radl, W Hijmans, and B Van Camp), pp. 151–5. European Organisation for Research on Ageing, Rekjavik.

Selby PJ, et al. (1987). Multiple myeloma treated with high dose intravenous melphalan. British Journal of Haematology, 66:55–62.

Scheithauer W, Cortelezzi A, Fritz E, Kuhrer I, Polli E, Baldini L, Ludwig H (1989). Combined alpha-2c-interferon/VMCP polychemotherapy versus VMCP polychemotherapy as induction therapy in multiple myeloma. Journal of Biological Response Modifiers, 8 (2):109–15.

Selvanayagam P, Goodacre A, Strong L, Saunders GF, Barlogie B (1987). Alterations of bcl-1 oncogene in human multiple myeloma. Proceedings of the American Association of Cancer Research, 28:76.

Selvanayagam P, et al. (1988). Alteration and abnormal expression of the c-myc oncogene in human multiple myeloma. Blood, 71 (1):30–5.

Shimazaki C, et al. (1988). Elimination of myeloma cells from bone marrow by using monoclonal antibodies and magnetic immunobeads. Blood, 72 (4):1248–54.

Shu L, Qi CF, Schlom J, Kashmiri SV (1993). Secretion of a single-gene-encoded immunoglobulin from myeloma cells. Proceedings of the National Academy of Sciences USA, 90:7995–9.

Sidell N, Taga T, Hirano T, Kishimoto T, Saxon A (1991). Retinoic acid-induced growth inhibition of a human myeloma cell line via downregulation of IL-6 receptors. Journal of Immunology, 146:3809–14.

Simes RJ (1986). Publication bias; the case for an international registry of clinical trials. Journal of Clinical Oncology, 4:1529–41.

Skogen B, Natvig JB (1981). Degradation of amyloid proteins by different serine proteases. Scandinavian Journal of Immunology, 14:389–96.

Skopelitou A, Hadjiyannakis M, Tsenga A, Theocharis S, Alexopoulou V, Kittas C, Agnantis N (1993). Expression of C-myc p62 oncoprotein in multiple myeloma: an immunohistochemical study of 180 cases. Anticancer Research, 13:1091–5.

Solomons REB (1982). Plasma cell dyscrasias with polyneuropathy, organomegaly, endocrinopathy, monoclonal gammopathy and skin changes: the POEMS syndrome. Journal of the Royal Society of Medicine, 74:553–5.

Sonneveld P, et al. (1992). Modulation of multidrug-resistant multiple myeloma by cyclosporin. Lancet, 340:255–9.

Stone MA, Tong AW, Fay JW, Lee JC (1988). Selective depletion of human myeloma clonogenic stem cells from bone marrow cell preparations by a plasma-cell reactive antibody and complement. Cancer Detection and Prevention, 12:621–35.

Tabilio A, Carotti A, Aversa F, Falzetti F, Latini P, Grignani F, Martelli MF (1989). Immunological purging of bone marrow in multiple myeloma: preliminary results. Proceedings of the Second International Conference on Multiple Myeloma, Houston, 1989, p. 31. Schering Plough, Bury St Edmunds, UK.

Takahashi T, et al. (1985). Colony growth and self renewal of plasma cell precursors in multiple myeloma. Journal of Clinical Oncology, 3(12):1613–23.

To LB, et al. (1990). Single high doses of cyclophosphamide enable the collection of high numbers of hemopoietic stem cells from the peripheral blood. Experimental Hematology, 18(5):442–7.

To LB, et al. (1992). Comparison of haematological recovery times and supportive care requirements of autologous recovery phase peripheral blood stem cell transplants, autologous bone marrow transplants and allogeneic bone marrow transplants. Bone Marrow Transplantation, 9:277–84.

Tsuchiya H, Epstein J, Selvanayagam P, Dedman JR, Gallick G, Alexanian R, Barlogie B (1988). Correlated flow cytometric analysis of H-ras p21 and nuclear DNA in multiple myeloma. Blood, 72(2):796–800.

Tura S, et al. (1989). High-dose chemotherapy and allogenic bone marrow transplantation in multiple myeloma. European Journal of Haematology Supplement, 51:191–5.

Turesson I, Zettervall O, Cuzick J, Waldenström JG, Velez R (1984). Comparison of trends in the incidence of multiple myeloma in Malmo Sweden and other countries 1950–1979. New England Journal of Medicine, 310:421–4.

Turnell W, Sarra R, Baum JO, Caspi D, Baltz ML, Pepys MB (1986). X ray scattering and diffraction by wet gels of AA amyloid fibrils. Molecular Biological Medicine, 3:409–24.

Ullrich S, Zolla-Pazner S (1982). Immunoregulatory circuits in myeloma. Clinics in Haematology, 11(1):87–111.

Van Camp B, et al. (1989). Plasma cells in multiple myeloma and related disorders express a natural killer cell associated (Leu-19; NKH-1) antigen. Proceedings of the Second International Conference on Multiple Myeloma, Houston, Texas, 1989, p. 5. Schering Plough, Bury St Edmunds, UK.

Van Riet I, Van Camp B (1993). The involvement of adhesion molecules in the biology of multiple myeloma. *Leukemia and Lymphoma*, **9**: 441–52.

Virchow R (1854). Über eine im Gehirn und Ruckenmark des Menschen aufgefundene Substanz mit der chemischen Reaction der Cellulose. *Virchows Archiv für Pathologische Anatomie*, **6**:135–8.

Wearne A, Joshua DE, Kronenberg DE (1984). Light chain isotype associated suppression of surface immunoglobulin expression on peripheral blood lymphocytes in myeloma during plateau phase. *British Journal of Haematology*, **58**:483–9.

Weh HJ, *et al.* (1993). Karyotype in multiple myeloma and plasma cell leukaemia. *European Journal of Cancer*, **29A**:1269–73.

Whittaker JA (1986). Solitary plasmacytoma. In *Multiple myeloma and other paraproteinaemias* (ed. IW Delamore), pp. 193–204. Churchill Livingstone, Edinburgh.

Willems PM, Kuypers AW, Meijerink JP, Holdrinet RS, Mensink EJ (1993). Sporadic mutations of the p53 gene in multiple myeloma and no evidence for germline mutations in three familial multiple myeloma pedigrees. *Leukemia*, 7:986–91.

Wiltshaw E (1976). The natural history of extra medullary plasmacytoma and its relation to solitary myeloma of bone and myelomatosis. *Medicine*, 55:217–38.

Wotherspoon AC, Norton AJ, Isaacson PG (1989). Immunoreactive cytokeratins in plasmacytomas. *Histopathology*, **14**(2):141–50.

Zaccaria A, Tassinari A, Saglio G, Guerrasio A, Tura S (1989). Immunoglobulin gene rearrangements in human multiple myeloma. *Proceedings of the International Conference on Multiple Myeloma, Bologna, 1989*, p. 9.

Zola H (1987). The surface antigens of human B lymphocytes. *Immunology Today*, 8(10):308–15.

Zolla-Pazner S (1980). Immunodeficiency induced by plasma cell tumours: comparison of findings in human and murine hosts. In *Progress in myeloma* (ed. M Potter), pp. 171–84. Elsevier/North-Holland, New York.

Zucchelli P, Pasquali S, Cagnoli L, Ferrari G (1988). Controlled plasma exchange trial in acute renal failure due to multiple myeloma. *Kidney International*, 33:1175–80.

12.9   Histiocyte disorders

JON PRITCHARD AND M. MALONE

GENERAL INTRODUCTION

Histiocytes (from the Greek ιστός, tissue, κύτταρο, cells) are derived from a common bone-marrow stem cell (Katz *et al.* 1979; Reid *et al.* 1990) and share structural and functional features that identify them as members of one cell family. There are two major groups of histiocytes: phagocytic (antigen-processing) cells and dendritic (antigen-presenting) cells, which are usually non-phagocytic. Phagocytic cells can be subgrouped into circulating monocytes and 'fixed' histiocytes in specific tissues, for example tingible body follicular cells and sinusoidal histiocytes (in lymph nodes), alveolar macrophages (lung), Kupffer cells (liver), osteoclasts, and microglial cells. The dendritic cells include interdigitating reticulum cells and dendritic reticulum cells, both found in spleen and lymph nodes and Langerhans cells, found almost exclusively in the skin and draining lymph nodes and the bronchial epithelium.

The function of dendritic cells is to prepare antigens for presentation to phagocytic cells: interdigitating reticulum cells and Langerhans cells both present antigen to T lymphocytes whilst dendritic reticulum cells present to B-cells. Phagocytic cells ingest soluble and particulate antigenic material prior to processing and disposal. Phagocytic and dendritic cells are distinguished from each other by their anatomical location, morphological differences, especially the presence or absence of phagocytosis, high (phagocytic cells) or low (dendritic cells) concentrations of lysozomal enzymes, and presence (dendritic cells) or absence (phagocytic cells) of class II major histocompatibility complex (MHC) antigens. Subsets of histiocytes can be distinguished by other features, for example only dendritic reticulum cells express complement receptors and only interdigitating reticulum cells and Langerhans cells are positive for S100 protein (Jaffe 1988). Langerhans cells have two specific features which help distinguish them from other histiocytes: they express the CD1a (T$_6$) antigen and they contain an ultrastructural body known as the Birbeck granule (Murphy 1985).

The terminology used to describe the histiocyte system and the associated lymphoid cells is confusing. The old term 'reticuloendothelial system' was imprecise and was replaced by 'mononuclear phagocytic system'. At the time that this description was introduced the crucial functional significance of dendritic cells, which are not phagocytic, was not appreciated and the term is now falling into disuse. Recently the term 'mononuclear phagocyte and immunoregulatory effector system' (M-PIRE) has been proposed (Foucar and Foucar 1990) but has not yet gained general acceptance.

Disorders of histiocytes are rare and their pathogenesis is poorly understood. Because histiocytes are common components of 'reactive' processes, it is not even clear, in most of the disorders, whether the histiocyte is primarily at fault or merely an 'involved bystander'. In an attempt to order thinking about pathogenetic mechanisms, the Histiocyte Society (Writing Group of Histiocyte Society 1987) has proposed the following classification.

Class I: Langerhans cell histiocytosis

Class II: histiocytosis of mononuclear cells other than Langerhans cells

Class III: malignant histiocytosis, either of Langerhans cells or of other types of histiocytes

These guidelines provide the most useful working formula proposed to date and, in this chapter, are used as a framework for classification. Two points should be noted, however: the classification is based on histiocyte disorders in children, in whom they occur more frequently than in adults and the two commonest groups (classes I and II) are not cancers. That they feature at all in a textbook on oncology may seem an anomaly but, because of the space-occupying, systemic, and invasive–destructive characteristics of the lesions, patients are often referred to oncologists and radiotherapists for management advice.

LANGERHANS CELL HISTIOCYTOSIS. CLASS I OF THE HISTIOCYTE SOCIETY CLASSIFICATION

Introduction and summary

In 1850, Paul Langerhans, who also identified the pancreatic islets, first described an argyrophilic cell at the dermal–epidermal junction of the skin. Because of their staining characteristics and because they bore short 'processes', he mistakenly supposed that these cells had a neural function. A century later Langerhans cells were correctly classified as immunoregulatory cells and it soon became clear that they were a critical component of cell-mediated immune regulation in the skin.

Langerhans cell histiocytosis (LCH) used to be known as 'Histiocytosis X' (Lichtenstein 1953), but was renamed in 1985 by the Histiocyte Society (Writing Group of Histiocyte Society 1987) because the new term identified the pathognomonic lesional cell; the 'LCH cell' (McLelland et al. 1987). The term LCH embraces the whole clinical spectrum of the disorder, from single bone lesions (eosinophilic granuloma) in otherwise well patients to widespread multisystem disease in very sick infants (Letterer–Siwe disease), with a wide variety of intermediate forms including the Hand–Schüller–Christian triad. Most parts of the body can be affected, though involvement of cardiac/skeletal muscle, kidney, gonads, and peripheral nerve has not yet been recorded. It is now regarded as a reactive disorder, not a malignancy. There is no official staging system but patients are grouped into those with single (organ) system and multisystem involvement.

Treatment is empirical. Many lesions heal spontaneously. Steroids (oral or intralesional), vinca alkaloids (vincristine or vinblastine), and etoposide (VP16) are active and are often used. Alkylating agents, combination chemotherapy, and radiation therapy are best avoided, especially in children. Almost all patients with single-system LCH recover without sequelae. Amongst those with multisystem disease, mortality is still 10–20 per cent and over 50 per cent of survivors have chronic morbidity. The main obstacles to progress are that the aetiology and pathogenesis of LCH are still conjectural (hence the arbitrary treatment) and the rarity of the disorder hampers basic research.

Incidence, demographics, and aetiology

The incidence is unknown because, unlike cancers, notification is not obligatory. In the United Kingdom between 30 and 60 cases per annum are recorded by children's tumour registries, but the figures are almost certainly an underestimate because bone disease and skin involvement in particular may be asymptomatic and/or misdiagnosed, patients are referred to a variety of organ specialists, and adult cases are not taken into account.

There is no evidence that LCH is a 'new' disease, because there is fairly good documentation of cases in the eighteenth century. The disease has been recorded in all races from all five continents with no hard evidence, as yet, of geographical clustering. There are a number of possible explanations for the observation that boys are more commonly affected than girls (ratio 1.5–2 : 1). One of the most attractive is that, in a disease with an immunological component, an X-linked gene is involved.

In the early 1980s, it was thought that LCH might be a primary immunological disorder (Osband et al. 1981), but the B- and T-cell function abnormalities demonstrable in LCH patients are now regarded as secondary rather than primary (McLelland et al. 1987).

Viral involvement in the aetiology of LCH has been repeatedly proposed, but there have been no comprehensive serological or molecular probe studies and therefore no direct supportive evidence for this theory. Proponents of the viral theory point out that LCH might represent the rare outcome of a common viral infection, perhaps via a secondary autoimmune process, a chronic infection by a rare virus, or a consequence of an unconventional virus, for example a prion. Interestingly, a condition indistinguishable from LCH sometimes occurs in patients before or after a second diagnosis of acute lymphoblastic leukaemia or lymphoma. In addition, the histopathological appearances of LCH can be seen adjacent to 'true' lymphoma (usually non-Hodgkin's lymphoma) in lymph node biopsies and epithelial malignancies. The presence of this LCH-like lesion makes no obvious difference to the behaviour of the lymphoma. Smoking markedly increases the number of Langerhans cells in bronchial epithelium. Compared with other organs, lung involvement is relatively common in adults, especially in smokers. As yet, no study of the consequences of passive smoking by children with LCH has been reported. These clues are all fascinating, but the reality is that the aetiology of LCH is still unknown.

Clinically, LCH does not behave as a malignancy; for instance, there is a high rate of spontaneous remission. The bland histopathological appearances also support this contention. More direct scientific evidence is provided by the demonstration that CD-1-positive cells, isolated from LCH lesions in six patients, had a normal (euploid) DNA content (McLelland et al. 1989). However, there are reports of lesional aneuploidy in individual cases, and recent evidence of monoclonality is LCH tissue, probably in CD1a-positive cells (Willman et al. 1993; Yu et al. 1994) has thrown open the debate about the aetiology of LCH. Some patients do, perhaps, have a true Langerhans cell malignancy.

Histopathology

The Writing Group of the Histiocyte Society (1987) has defined objective criteria for the diagnosis of LCH (Table 1), but histopathological appearances differ depending upon the site of the biopsy and the time from diagnosis (Favara and Jaffe 1987). Early in the course of the disease lesions are usually cellular, locally destructive, and feature aggregates of pathological Langerhans cells (LCH cells). LCH cells have homogeneous pink cytoplasm and lobulated nuclei, many with a longitudinal groove resulting in a 'coffee-bean' appearance. The number of eosinophils, ordinary histiocytes (macrophages), and lymphocytes is variable. Multinucleate giant cells, resembling osteoclasts but lacking markers for Langerhans cells, are frequently encountered. Occasionally, lesions consist of eosinophils, much necrosis, and few LCH cells. A striking feature of the infiltrate (Fig. 1) is its tendency to home towards and destroy

Table 1 Histopathological diagnosis of Langerhans cell histiocytosis

Presumptive diagnosis	H&E findings consistent with LCH
Diagnosis	H&E findings consistent with LCH plus two or more of the following: positive stain for ATPase, S-100 protein, or α-D-mannosidase, or characteristic binding of the lectin peanut agglutinin (PNA)
Definitive diagnosis	H&E findings consistent with LCH plus identification of Birbeck granules in lesional cells by electron microscopy or demonstration of CD1 determinants on the surface of lesional cells

H&E, haematoxylin and eosin.
Reproduced from Writing Group of Histiocyte Society (1987), with permission.

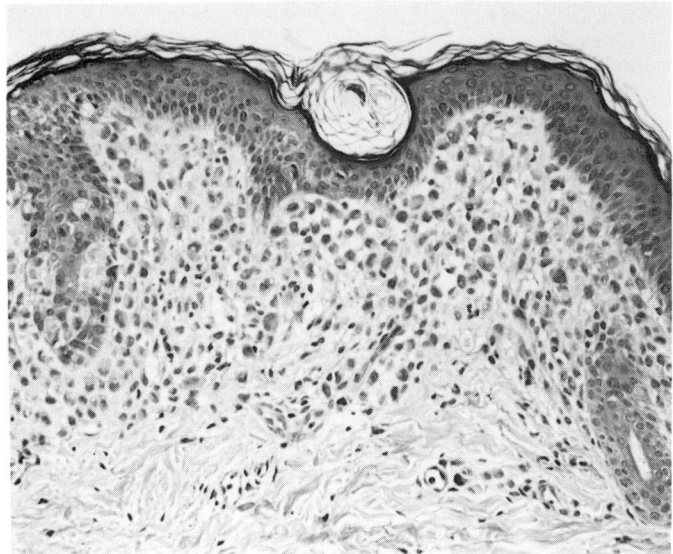

Fig. 1 LCH of the skin. Note the close proximity of the infiltrate to the epidermis and the mixed nature of the infiltrate.

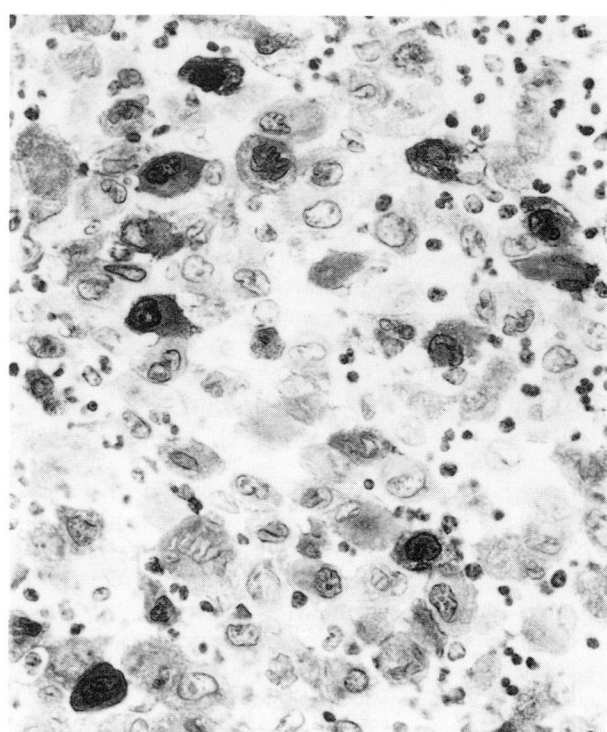

Fig. 2 Immunostaining of LCH cells for S100 protein. Note the variable degree of staining and that only a proportion of the cells are positive.

epithelial cells in skin, lung, and liver. Recent data, indicating that many LCH cells stain positively with the so-called proliferating cell nuclear antigen (PNCA) and the proliferation marker Ki-51, suggest that the cells divide within the tissues that they infiltrate rather than simply 'homing' there (Hage *et al.* 1993). Many LCH cells are also Ki67 positive. Later in the course of the disease lesions become less cellular and contain fewer LCH cells, more macrophages, and more fibrosis. In long-standing disease, LCH cells may no longer be demonstrable. Postnecrotic fibrosis is common in some organs, for example lung, liver, and bone-marrow.

Immunohistochemical studies are of great importance. Some markers are relatively resistant to processing and therefore are detectable in formalin-fixed paraffin-embedded tissue. A definitive diagnosis can be reached on this material by using antibodies to S100 protein and peanut lectin, in addition to electron microscopy. Approximately 60 per cent of LCH cells show cytoplasmic staining for S100 protein (Fig. 2). Peanut lectin is a more sensitive marker for skin involvement; a membrane halo is most characteristic, but some LCH cells also show a paranuclear dot. Macrophage determinants such as Mac 387, EBM 11, KP1, or KiM6 indicate that ordinary monocytes and macrophages, including giant cells, are also present within the infiltrate but LCH cells are negative. Reports of the use of macrophage enzyme markers (for example, lysozyme, α-1-antitrypsin, and α-antichymotrypsin) give conflicting views. Therefore, immunochemical studies of this disorder require careful interpretation.

Studies of frozen tissue are also strongly recommended (see Appendix). LCH cells stain positively with anti-CD1 and anti-CD4 antibodies. Histochemical staining shows positivity for ATPase and (on specially prepared specimens) for α-D-mannosidase (Elleder 1977).

Birbeck granules are trilaminar structures (Fig. 3) that probably represent infoldings of the cell membrane and are pathognomonic of normal or pathological Langerhans cells. Some granules have expanded ends, giving them a 'tennis racquet' shape. Birbeck granules are resistant to formalin and paraffin embedding but are much easier to demonstrate in some affected tissues, for example lung and skin, than in others, for example liver or spleen (Favara and Jaffe 1987).

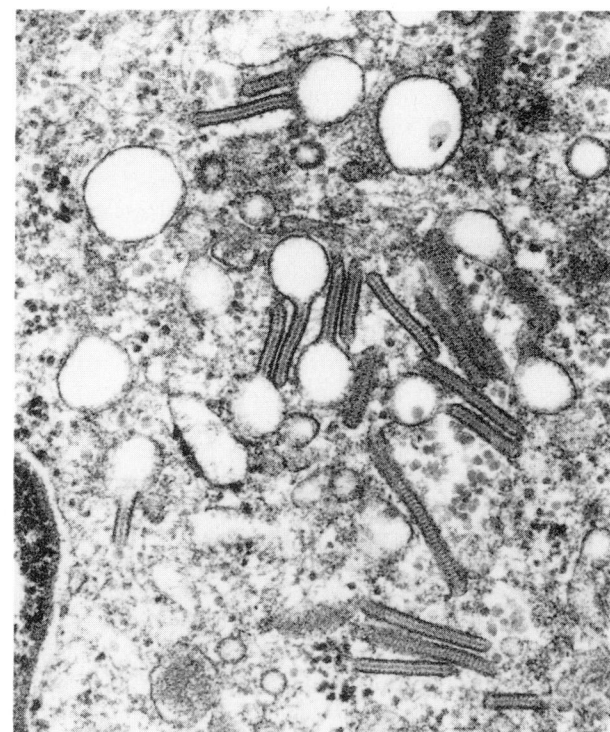

Fig. 3 Birbeck granules showing trilaminar rods and vesicular swellings giving a 'tennis racquet' appearance.

The histopathological differential diagnosis depends on the organ affected by the disease process. In skin, the main differential diagnosis is from juvenile xanthogranuloma. Definitive LCH cell markers (CD1 and Birbeck granules) are not found in juvenile xanthogranuloma, but Touton giant cells are pathognomonic in that condition and immunostaining shows that all cells in the infiltrate are positive for monocyte/macrophage markers. However, lesions similar to juvenile xanthogranuloma can occasionally be seen in the skin of patients with LCH.

In bone, the main differential diagnosis in the early phase of LCH is chronic osteomyelitis. The presence of plasma cells (extremely uncommon in LCH) may provide a clue. Immunostaining for S100 protein (which survives decalcification) may help identify LCH cells. Fibrosis is common in bone-marrow involved by LCH, even at an early stage of disease; occasionally, fibrosis is so severe that primary myelofibrosis (a myeloproliferative disorder) may be suspected.

In the lung, differential diagnosis is from a granulomatous response to infection or desquamative interstitial pneumonia. Opportunistic infection should always be considered whenever 'histiocytosis' is found and excluded by appropriate stains. Positive identification of LCH cells is the mainstay of diagnosis. Normal alveolar macrophages are positive for macrophage markers and some may be S100 positive. This immunostain is therefore not a reliable means of differentiating between LCH and desquamative interstitial pneumonia, but peanut lectin is much more specific for LCH cells and electron microscopy shows Birbeck granules. In the late stage of LCH the lung may be so fibrotic and lacking in LCH cells that the distinction from fibrosing alveolitis is impossible.

In the lymph node, the differential diagnosis includes dermatopathic lymphadenopathy and Rosai–Dorfman disease (sinus histiocytosis with massive lymphadenopathy). The paracortical accumulation of cells in dermatopathic lymphadenopathy helps distinguish it from LCH, which is primarily a sinusoidal disease. The morphology of the histiocytes in sinus histiocytosis with massive lymphadenopathy is different from LCH. S100 protein can be demonstrated in all three conditions, but peanut lectin and CD1 positivity and the presence of Birbeck granules confirm the diagnosis of LCH.

In liver, the infiltrate is centred on bile ducts. Secondary changes, particularly cholestasis and bile duct proliferation, may be marked. Early in the disease process, immunostaining for S100 protein may help identify LCH cells but Birbeck granules are hard to find. Early in its course and in chronic disease, liver histology may be indistinguishable from primary sclerosing cholangitis.

Biology and functional pathology

It is still not clear whether LCH cells or another cell population initiate the disease process, but LCH cells almost certainly play a major part in the damage to various organs caused by it. Inappropriate cytokine production can lead to tissue damage. For instance, normal Langerhans cells and probably LCH cells, produce interleukin(IL)-1 which stimulates T-cells to produce IL-2. T-cells are then provoked to produce interferon, leading in turn to the production by macrophages of more IL-1 (McLelland et al. 1987). Increased production of IL-6, an eosinophilotactic cytokine, could explain the presence of large numbers of eosinophils in LCH lesions.

The primary abnormality in LCH could vary: in some cases secretion of the cytokine could be qualitatively or quantitatively abnormal, whilst in others expression of cytokine receptors may be inappropriately regulated. Other soluble factors such as prostaglandins, known to be secreted by LCH cells, are probably also implicated in tissue damage, for example in the bone lysis seen in LCH (Arenzana-Seisdedos et al. (1986)). It is attractive to think of LCH as a cytokine disease and in situ techniques for cytokine mRNA and protein detection are now available to start to investigate this possibility.

Clinical features

LCH can present in the newborn period and in the elderly, but the peak age is approximately 2–4 years. In 75 per cent of patients presenting to children's hospitals, two or more organs are involved at presentation (multisystem disease); in the remainder only one organ or organ system is involved (single-system disease). Sites of disease presentation vary enormously and so symptoms vary also. Presenting symptoms in children, in order of frequency, are skin rash (approximately 50 per cent), recurrent aural discharge (20–25 per cent), and bone pain, scalp swelling, proptosis, failure to thrive, breathlessness, lymphadenopathy, abdominal distension from hepatosplenomegaly, and spinal cord compression (all below 20 per cent). The actual frequency of organ system involvement may be different because involvement is often subclinical. Twenty to thirty per cent of affected children grow poorly (Fig. 4). The cause is often multifactorial, resulting from the chronic production of 'catabolic' cytokines, loss of height of affected vertebrae, corticosteroid therapy, and growth hormone deficiency in some cases (Komp 1981). Clinical features in adults are also varied, but there is a higher proportion of patients with pulmonary involvement, probably provoked by smoking (Hance et al. 1986).

Individual organ systems are now discussed in alphabetical order.

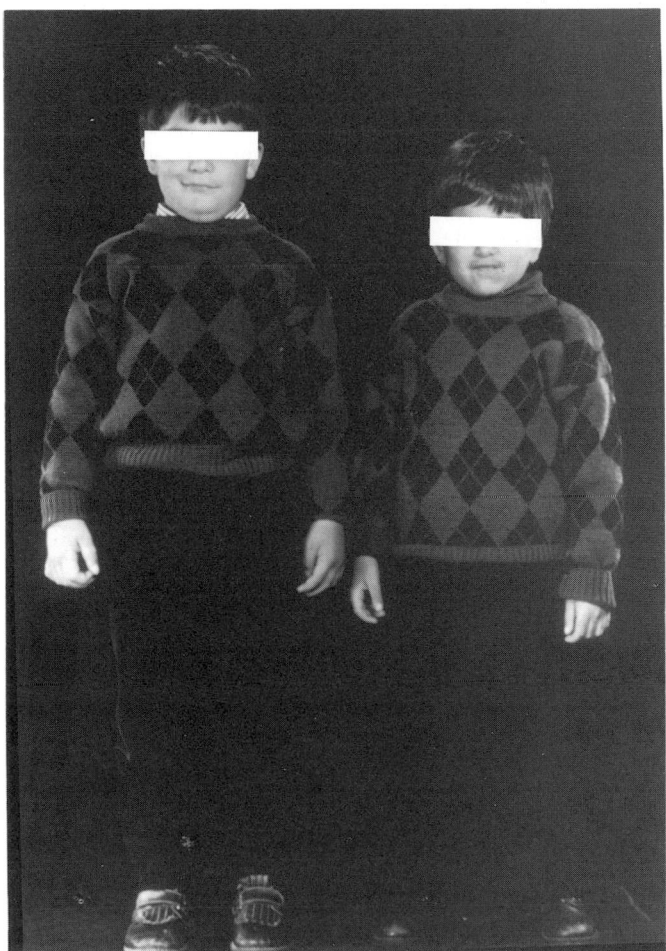

Fig. 4 Eight year old boy with lifelong multisystem LCH, with his healthy six year old brother. The patient's short stature was due to partial growth hormone deficiency and chronic disease; he also had partial diabetes insipidus and a chronic scalp rash. (Reproduced with parents' permission.)

Blood and bone-marrow

In most patients the blood count is either normal or shows evidence of a mild anaemia of chronic disorders. Peripheral blood monocytosis is rare and may be due to complicating infection. Although their precursor cells are derived from bone-marrow, there has been no unequivocal demonstration of LCH cells circulating in the blood (Katz *et al.* 1979). The ratio of CD4 to CD8 lymphocytes in peripheral blood is high, owing to a deficiency of CD8+ cells. In remission, the ratio returns to normal.

There are no consistent abnormalities of standard B- and T-lymphocyte function tests, though serum immunoglobulin levels can be raised (McLelland *et al.* 1987). Pancytopenia, of varying severity, occurs in 5–10 per cent of patients. In some patients low blood counts are clearly due to marrow failure, secondary to heavy marrow infiltration by LCH cells. In other patients, however, the marrow appears normal and pancytopenia is due to consumption of formed blood products by the phagocytic histiocytes that accumulate in LCH lesions in various parts of the body but particularly in spleen, lymph nodes, and liver. The degree of bone-marrow infiltration varies. Most patients have no detectable involvement, whilst a few have near-total replacement by LCH cells. Marrow trephines are more sensitive than aspirates, though special techniques, especially α-D-mannosidose staining, may reveal LCH cells in marrows reported negative by conventional staining.

Bones

Any bone may be affected but, whereas involvement of the small bones of the hand and foot is rare, for unknown reasons involvement of the bones of the skull is common (Fig. 5). Lesions are typically osteolytic, though in many patients lesions of various 'ages' can be seen simultaneously. Those that are healing have a sclerotic margin. In young children, in particular there may be a florid periosteal reaction closely mimicking malignancy (Fig. 6) and in others the whole bone may be involved (Fig. 7). Less than half of all bone lesions are painful. Invasion into adjacent tissues, particularly the skull vault and orbits, leads to contiguous soft tissue swellings. Occasionally, one of these soft tissue extensions of a bony lesion may rupture, liberating large amounts of pus-like necrotic material. Pathological fractures are unusual and may provoke healing.

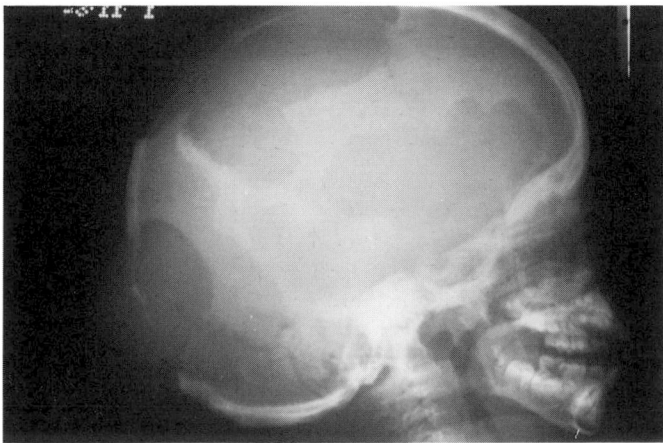

Fig. 5 LCH: large multiple destructive lesions in the skull vault of a 2 year old child.

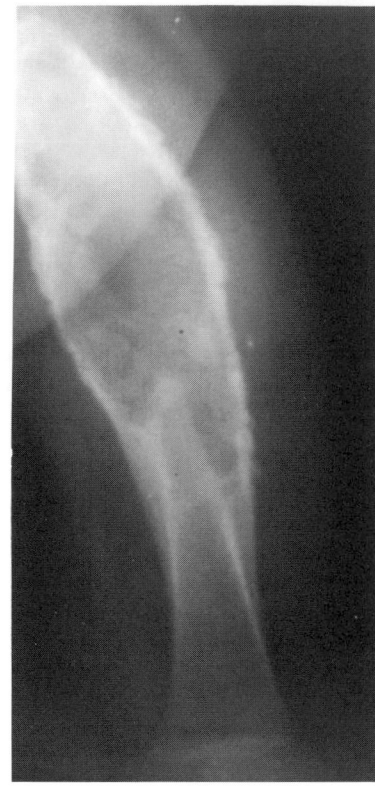 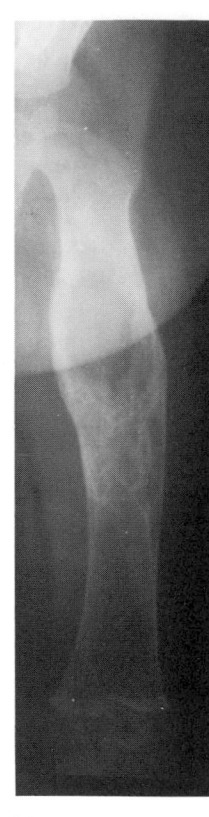

(a)   (b)

Fig. 6 Extensive lytic lesion, biopsy proven as LCH, in the left femur of a 6 month old boy: (a) at diagnosis and (b) 1 year later after spontaneous healing.

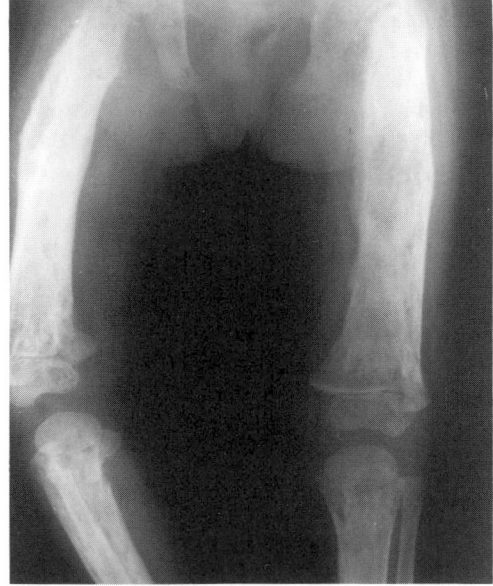

Fig. 7 Diffuse bony involvement in a 3 year old boy. He is in complete remission 7 years after these photographs were taken.

Brain and pituitary

Diabetes insipidus is a well-known complication of LCH affecting 10–50 per cent of patients. Approximately half have diabetes insipidus at presentation and the others develop it up to 4–5 years after onset (Dunger *et al.* 1989). Involvement of the anterior pituitary is less common, but probably affects approximately 10 per cent of patients overall. Growth hormone deficiency is the most common manifestation, but other anterior pituitary hormones can be affected and some patients develop panhypopituitarism. Rarely, patients develop a hypothalamic syndrome with hyperphagia, temperature dysregulation, and mood swings. Magnetic resonance imaging (MRI), now the method of choice or contrast-enhanced CT scanning shows a space-occupying lesion in the pituitary gland, the pituitary stalk, or the hypothalamus of up to 50 per cent of patients with pituitary dysfunction (Fig. 8). Autopsy data confirm direct infiltration by LCH cells. Why LCH cells so commonly 'home' into the hypothalamic–pituitary axis is unknown, but other parts of the central nervous system can sometimes be affected. Some patients with chronic LCH develop cerebellar dysfunction with ataxia, incoordination and white matter changes best detected with MRI (Fig. 9) (Rosenfield *et al.* 1990). It is not clear whether this lesion is due to active or burnt-out LCH, nor whether in its early stages the process is responsive to any form of therapy. Space-occupying lesions in the cerebral hemispheres have also been reported.

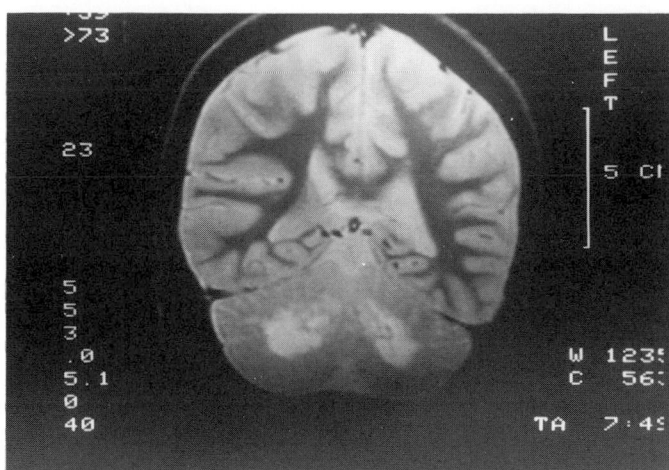

Fig. 9 Magnetic resonance brain scan in a child who developed ataxia 7–8 years after diagnosis of multisystem LCH. There is symmetrical increased signal in the white matter of the cerebellar hemispheres.

Ears

Aural discharge can be the result of either otitis externa, due to involvement of the skin in the external auditory canal or disease spread from the mastoid into the middle ear (Irving *et al.* 1993). The process is usually painless, but troublesome chronic aural discharge is common with accompanying partial deafness. Secondary bacterial infection is common and usually responds to topical antibiotics.

Eyes

Intraocular structures are hardly ever involved by LCH but orbital involvement is common (20–30 per cent of all patients) (Moore *et al.* 1981). Proptosis is usually due to soft tissue extension from a lytic lesion in the orbital wall. Ptosis, papilloedema, palsy of nerve VII, and optic atrophy can occur. Occasionally optic nerve function may be so compromised that emergency treatment (with intralesional steroids or radiotherapy) is needed.

Liver and spleen

Liver and spleen may be directly involved by LCH, with enlargement of either or both organs. When the liver is severely affected, there is jaundice and other evidence of liver failure such as hypoalbuminaemia and prolongation of coagulation times owing to decreased synthesis of clotting factors. The liver enzymes (alanine aminotransferase (ALT), aspartate aminotransferase (AST), and alkaline phosphatase (APT)) are rarely elevated, however. In chronic disease, periportal fibrosis (see Histopathology section) may lead to a condition radiologically indistinguishable from sclerosing cholangitis with biliary stasis and obstructive jaundice (Leblanc *et al.* 1981). In these instances, splenic enlargement may be due to portal hypertension. The incidence of hypersplenism is uncertain, because many patients with pancytopenia have both marrow involvement and splenomegaly.

Lungs and airways

Respiratory symptoms are commoner in adults than in children (Basset *et al.* 1978). Very rarely the upper airway, for example the trachea, may be involved, but lung involvement occurs in approximately 20–30 per cent of all patients (40 per cent of those with multisystem disease). Respiratory function testing reveals a restrictive defect; small 'stiff' lungs with reduced lung volumes (Ha *et al.* 1991). Functional abnormalities may precede radiological change. On plain chest radiographs the earliest radiological changes seem nodular, but CT scanning has shown that these lesions are in fact small cysts which either regress or coalesce as the disease progresses and lung tissue is destroyed. Rupture of a cyst into the pleural cavity often causes spontaneous pneumothorax. In sick patients with LCH great care must be taken to rule out opportunistic

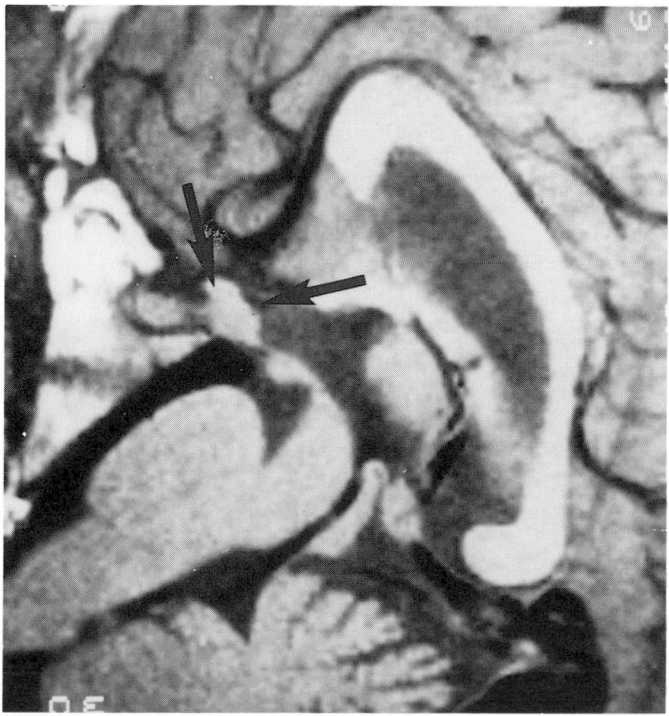

Fig. 8 Magnetic resonance imaging of base of brain in patient with Langerhans cell histiocytosis and diabetes insipidus. The arrow indicates the irregular thickening of the pituitary stalk; the normal 'bright signal' in the posterior pituitary gland (T_1-weighted sequence) is absent.

infection, such as *Pneumocystis carinii*, cytomegalovirus, or measles, particularly in patients receiving immunosuppressive therapy. Lung involvement does not seem to worsen the prognosis for patients with LCH (Ha *et al.* 1991).

Lymph nodes

The exact incidence of node involvement is difficult to establish but it is usually painless and rarely causes other symptoms. Sometimes, massive adenopathy can cause airway obstruction. Occasionally, suppuration, mimicking infection, occurs (Sacks *et al.* 1986). In some patients chronic draining sinuses develop, particularly in the neck.

Mouth and gastrointestinal tract

Early oral involvement manifests as granularity or thickening of the gingival or palatal mucosa and affects 30–40 per cent of patients (Sigala *et al.* 1972). More extensive involvement causes painful ulceration, prone to secondary infection. Exceptionally a palatal fistula can develop. Premature eruption of teeth, following gingival infiltration, is quite common and almost diagnostic. Loss of the dental lamina dura is a typical radiological feature. In severe cases, gum retraction and erosion of alveoli may cause loosening of the teeth.

There has been no systematic study of small or large bowel involvement or function in LCH. The small bowel can be affected, causing malabsorption or blood loss (Egeler *et al.* 1990). It is surprising that colonic and rectal involvement have been reported only recently: diarrhoea, with or without blood and mucus, is the presenting feature. The anal canal and perianal area are commonly affected as part of regional skin involvement (Fig. 10). Rarely, the pancreas can be infiltrated (Yu *et al.* 1993).

Pituitary gland

See Brain and pituitary section.

Skin

Infiltration by LCH has a characteristic distribution with a predeliction for the midline of the trunk, especially the lower dorsal region (Fig. 11) as well as the intertriginous regions (that is, groin, napkin area including vulva, and perianal region) and the scalp and postauricular areas (Fig. 12). There is often a history of cradle cap from early life. These features may previously have led to a mistaken diagnosis of seborrhoeic eczema.

Individual lesions are 1–5 mm brownish-pink maculopapules. In patients with apparently normal skin, these lesions should be sought diligently, especially on the trunk. At one time a condition affecting infants and known as 'self-healing reticulocytosis' (Hashimoto–Pritzker syndrome) (Hashimoto *et al.* 1982), which often

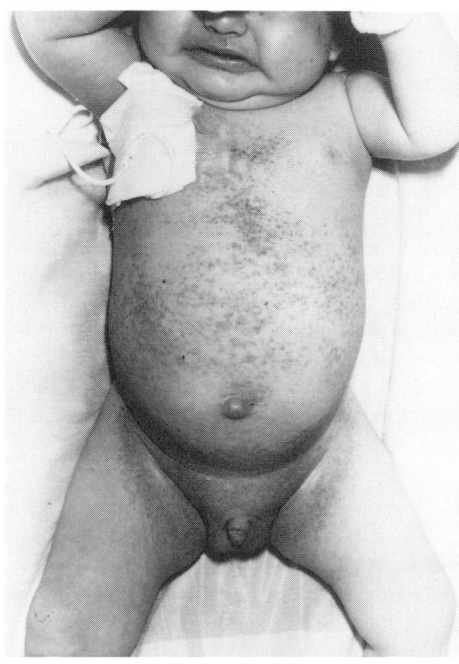

Fig. 11 Extensive skin involvement in a 1 year old boy with severe multisystem LCH. The rash is especially severe in the groins with excoriation. Some of the trunk lesions are haemorrhagic. The child also had hepatosplenomegaly and pancytopenia.

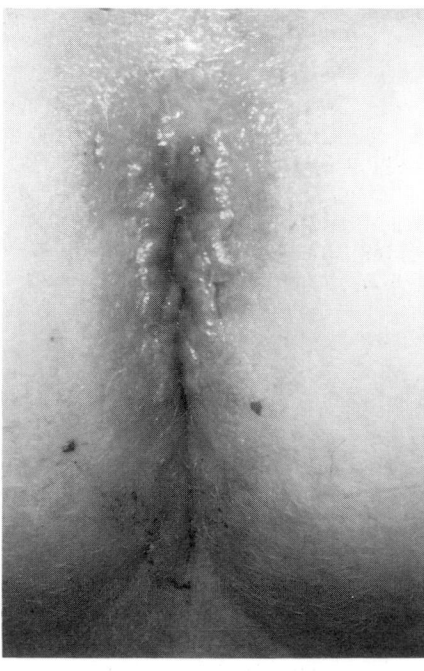

Fig. 10 Perianal changes in LCH; the process extended inside the anal canal.

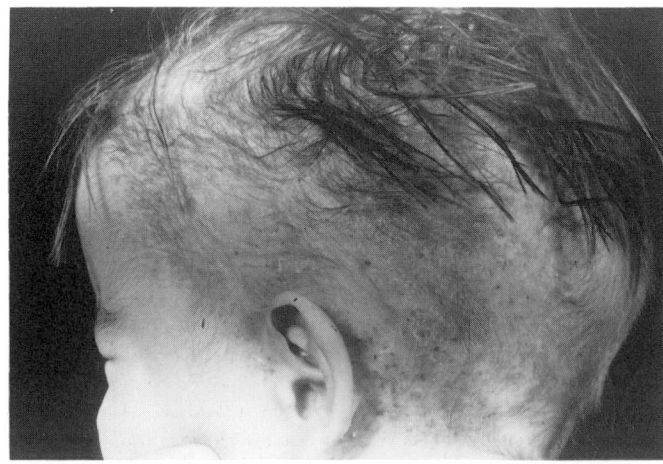

Fig. 12 Seborrhoeic distribution of rash in a 3 year old boy with multisystem LCH. Scalp and post-auricular involvement are characteristic. There was also otitis externa with aural discharge.

involves the soles and palms, was thought to be a separate entity. Although the infiltrate is deep in the dermis, as opposed to the dermoepidermal junction, the condition is believed to be part of the LCH disease spectrum. Skin involvement may be isolated and then often resolves spontaneously. In severely affected patients, the rash can be confluent (Fig. 11) with ulceration in moist intertriginous areas. When the platelet count is less than $20\times10^9/l$ the rash may be haemorrhagic. Large nodular lesions, which can ulcerate, also occur. In chronic disease, xanthelasma are sometimes found and may contain LCH cells.

Other organs

Muscles, including the heart, endocrine glands (excepting the pituitary), kidneys, and gonads are the only organs that regularly seem to escape involvement.

Differential diagnosis

Delay in diagnosis is more commonly the result of failure to think of LCH as a possibility than of difficulty in distinguishing it from other conditions. For instance, a patient with a chronic draining ear may be misdiagnosed as having chronic otitis media and skin involvement may be mistaken for seborrhoeic dermatitis. Once the diagnosis is considered, it is a relatively simple matter to confirm it by biopsy as long as there is adherence to strict histological criteria. In sick patients with multisystem involvement, the differential diagnosis includes acute leukaemia, chronic myeloproliferative disorders, storage disorders, and Rosai–Dorfman disease. In children with skin disease, various forms of xanthogranuloma should be excluded.

Investigation and grouping/staging

The following recommendations for investigations of newly diagnosed patients have been made by the Histiocyte Society (Broadbent *et al.* 1989): full blood count, including differential white cell count, liver function tests (ALT, AST, APT, bilirubin, total serum protein, and serum albumin), coagulation studies (prothrombin time, partial thromboplastin time, and fibrinogen), chest radiographs (posteroanterior and lateral), skeletal radiograph survey (which is more sensitive in LCH than isotope bone scan), and urine osmolality after overnight water deprivation. Other tests need only be carried out for specific indications as follows: bone marrow aspirate and trephine for anaemia, leucopenia, or thrombocytopenia, pulmonary function tests for abnormal chest radiograph or respiratory symptoms, small bowel meal or biopsy for unexplained chronic diarrhoea or failure to thrive, liver biopsy for liver dysfunction, including hypoproteinaemia not due to protein-losing enteropathy, contrast-enhanced CT of brain/hypothalamic–pituitary axis for hormonal, visual, or neurological abnormalities, panoramic dental radiography or mandible and maxilla plus orodental surgical consultation for oral involvement, endocrine evaluation, including measurement of serum AVP level, for short stature, growth failure, diabetes insipidus, hypothalamic syndrome, galactorrhoea, or precocious/delayed puberty, and ear, nose, and throat consultation and audiogram for aural discharge and deafness.

Immunological evaluation, including quantitation of serum immunoglobulins and T-cell subset numbers and function, are of research interest and not essential for diagnosis as long as the definitive histological criteria of the Histiocyte Society are applied.

A number of elaborate staging systems have been devised. The Lahey system (Lahey 1962) is the best known, but neither this system nor others have been generally accepted. Although objective criteria in a staging system may facilitate comparison of treatment results between centres, it is not clear that assignation of a 'stage' is helpful in determining management of a particular patient or in assessing prognosis. In practice, 'organ failure' seems to be a more important prognostic factor than 'organ involvement' (Lahey 1962; Broadbent and Pritchard 1985). Pancytopenia and liver failure are particularly ominous.

Management

General principles

There is no definitive treatment for LCH. Through the decades, treatment fashions have followed contemporary theory. Until the 1950s, treatment was with anti-infective agents and a wide variety of other measures, including vitamins and vaccines (Komp 1987). Steroids and ACTH came into fashion in the 1950s and in the 1960s responses to antimetabolites (for example, methotrexate) directed patients into the hands of oncologists who tried different cytotoxic agents, often in combination, without an increase in response rate (Pritchard 1979). In the early 1980s, LCH was thought to be a primary immunodeficiency and an uncontrolled trial of crude thymic extract (Osband *et al.* 1981) created much interest. Although a randomized trial was never performed, this form of therapy became unpopular when it was shown that many of the immunological abnormalities were secondary effects of the disease. At present, a conservative management philosophy prevails (Broadbent and Pritchard 1985; McLelland *et al.* 1990), with corticosteroids, vinca alkaloids, and epipodophyllotoxins as the backbone of treatment.

The pathogenesis of LCH is still unknown and so the approach to treatment is empirical and not rational. However, empirical measures have been moderately effective. Aggressive chemotherapy, because of its immediate and delayed toxicity, is contraindicated and the aim of the therapist should be to suppress symptoms of the disease, as in conditions like rheumatoid arthritis, rather than achieve complete remission, as in treating cancer. In North America and continental Europe, systemic treatment is used at a lower threshold than in the United Kingdom. During the 1980s systemic therapy was used in the United Kingdom only if there were systemic symptoms, failure to thrive, fever, disability, or discomfort, or organ failure (Broadbent and Pritchard 1985; McLelland *et al.* 1990). Since 1991, most countries have participated in a randomized trial, organized by the Histiocyte Society and known as LCH 1, which is described in more detail below.

Therapeutic mesaures are best divided into those used to treat specific organ systems and systemic measures.

Local treatment

Most bone lesions resolve spontaneously, but if there is pain or if the function of a vital organ (for example, the optic nerve or spinal cord) is threatened, intralesional corticosteroid injections (50–100 mg hydrocortisone (Solucortef®)) can be used. Sometimes localized troublesome soft tissue lesions are best managed in a similar way. Because of the risk of radiation-induced malignancy, radiotherapy should only be used when a disease site is inaccessible to the injecting needle and the dose should not exceed 10 Gy (Cassady 1987).

The symptoms of diabetes insipidus are completely reversed by intranasal administration of DDAVP (a synthetic form of antidiuretic hormone) at a dose of 5 μg twice or thrice daily. If diabetes insipidus is partial, it is worth trying therapy with etoposide (VP16, see below) as temporary reversal of the condition has been reported. There is controversy about the efficacy of radiotherapy, but most centres feel that it now has no value in the management of diabetes insipidus. Growth hormone deficiency is treated with daily growth hormone injections under the direction of an endocrinologist.

There are a number of measures that can help to control skin disease. Potassium permanganate soaks are helpful in the topical management of ulcerated skin. Using coco oil, followed by washing with a keratolytic shampoo, can be helpful in the removal of crusted scalp lesions and is followed by applications of topical steroid lotion to inflamed areas. Topical 20 per cent nitrogen mustard in aqueous solutions can be very effective where other methods have failed (Sheehan et al. 1991), but expert dermatological advice is needed. Corticosteroid eardrops can reduce the volume of aural discharge when the external or middle ear are affected and antibiotics are indicated when there is secondary infection. If gingival involvement is severe, surgical curettage can be helpful and may also reduce the incidence of later dental complications.

Patients with lung involvement who are immunosuppressed are best treated with cotrimoxazole (septrin) as prophylaxis against *P. carinii*. Pleurodesis may be needed for recurrent pneumothorax.

Systemic treatment

Spontaneous resolution of LCH occurs in 10–20 per cent of patients and so, unless indications for systemic therapy (see above) are present, an initial period of observation is worthwhile (Broadbent and Pritchard 1985). Treatment with cytotoxic agents dates back to the days when LCH was thought to be a malignancy, but combination chemotherapy gives no better results than single- or double-agent therapy (Pritchard 1979). Corticosteroids, vinca alkaloids (vinblastine and vincristine), and etoposide (VP16) (Ceci et al. 1988) are the most useful agents. Methotrexate and 6-mercaptopurine are also used by some centres, but agents likely to cause serious late complications (for example, alkylating agents and anthracyclines) are now contraindicated. Initial treatment is usually with corticosteroids (prednisolone, 2 mg/kg for 4 weeks, tailing off during the next 4–6 weeks) with or without vinblastine (6 mg/m^2 weekly) or etoposide (150 mg/m^2 IV or 300 mg/m^2 oral, both daily for 3 days every 3 weeks). Response rates are in the region of 60–70 per cent with no regimen yet shown to be superior to another.

In 1991, the Histiocyte Society started the first ever randomized clinical trial in LCH. Each patient receives an initial pulse of intravenous methylprednisolone and is then randomized to receive either etoposide or vinblastine for a total of 6 months. A formal comparison is considered important because of a suggestion that patients treated with etoposide may be less prone to chronic sequelae, particularly diabetes insipidus, than those treated with vinblastine. However, there is some concern that etoposide may be mutagenic and cause acute non-lymphoblastic leukaemia. The optimum duration of therapy is also unknown; a priority in future comparative clinical trials is to determine whether patients treated with maintenance chemotherapy have a more favourable outcome.

Other experimental treatments include immunostimulation using α-interferon (Jakobson et al. 1987), immune suppression using cyclosporin A with or without antithymocyte globulin (Mahmoud et al. 1991), or bone-marrow transplantation (Stoll et al. 1990; Greinix et al. 1992). Cyclosporin A seems to be the most promising alternative therapy. 'Targeted' therapy, using an anti-CD1a murine monoclonal antibody has also been proposed (Kelly and Pritchard 1994).

Response and outcome

Prognosis for patients with single system LCH is uniformly good. Progression to multisystem involvement is rare and survival is close to 100 per cent. Residual manifestations, usually bone lesions, resolve over 1–5 years (McLelland et al. 1990).

Patients with multisystem LCH have a better prognosis than many textbooks and reviews suggest. Overall mortality is 10–20 per cent. Invariably, those who die have presented with or develop organ failure. Of the remainder, 30–40 per cent of patients enter sustained clinical remission and 50–60 per cent enter a chronic disease phase, with involvement of new 'organ systems' in some cases. During this phase, problems include short stature, chronic discharging ears, deafness, lymph node 'suppuration', recurrent pneumothorax, dental and orthopaedic problems, diabetes insipidus, growth hormone deficiency, and ataxia.

In many patients, chronic sequelae resolve slowly but completely; however some can be seriously handicapped. Proptosis, unsightly scalp swellings, and smelly aural discharge alone or in combination, can stigmatize the child and lead to rejection by peers. Chronically sick children and their parents need the time, consideration, and support of their doctors and nurses to try to minimize the social consequences of their illness. A special effort should be made to give detailed information to the child's teachers and the school health service so that misunderstandings can be avoided and the child allowed to take part in as many normal school activities as possible.

HISTIOCYTOSIS OF 'ORDINARY' (PHAGOCYTIC) HISTIOCYTES. CLASS II OF THE HISTIOCYTE SOCIETY CLASSIFICATION

Haemophagocytic lymphohistiocytosis

Introduction and summary

Haemophagocytic lymphohistiocytosis (HLH) is a multisystem disorder, more common in children but also seen in adults, in which there is activation or proliferation or both, of phagocytic histiocytes, chiefly in the spleen, liver, bone-marrow, skin, lymph nodes, and central nervous system. The infiltrate also contains many lymphocytes. Haemophagocytosis is usually evident. The incidence of HLH (approximately 1 : 50 000) is similar in boys and girls, but this figure may be an underestimate because the disease is almost certainly underdiagnosed. HLH is considered to be a reactive disorder and not malignant. Although the exact aetiology is unknown, 30–50 per cent of all paediatric cases have a genetic basis with autosomal recessive inheritance. In other patients, including adults, the disease is sporadic although infection (especially viral infection) appears to precipitate it.

In decreasing order of frequency, presenting features are fever, hepatosplenomegaly, lymphadenopathy, and central nervous system abnormalities including altered consciousness, fits, and meningism. Hypertriglyceridaemia, coagulopathy, and a decrease in natural killer cells are characteristic blood findings. Etoposide (VP16) is often used for initial treatment and most patients respond. Corticosteroids are also used for their anti-inflammatory action and intrathecal methotrexate often leads to remission of central nervous system disease. In a few patients, response to this triple therapy is sustained, but in most cases the disease reappears between 3 months and 2 years from diagnosis. Second and third remissions are usually shorter than the first and most patients eventually die from organ failure and complicating infection. Because there appears to be an underlying genetic defect manifest in bone-marrow stem cells, a number of centres have recently carried out bone-marrow transplantation from histocompatible siblings, mismatched related donors, or matched unrelated donors, following conditioning by combinations of cytotoxic drugs and antibodies such as anti-lymphocyte functional antigen 1 (LFA1). Complete and sustained remissions can be achieved, but it is too early to say whether this treatment is actually curative.

Attempts to identify the gene (or genes) for HLH have so far been unsuccessful. Success would not only be an important finding for basic science but would also provide a crucial tool for identification of predisposed children in families with the inherited form of disease.

Nomenclature, incidence, and demographic findings

In 1952, Farquhar and Claireaux identified an inherited condition, characterized by hepatosplenomegaly, fever and pancytopenia which they named familial haemophagocytic reticulosis. Confusingly, other terms such as lymphohistiocytic reticulosis, haemophagocytic reticulosis, and familial reticuloendotheliosis were later used by other authors to describe the same condition. In 1979, Risdall and his colleagues in Minneapolis (Risdall *et al.* 1979) described patients with a similar clinical condition which appeared to be provoked by viruses. Their term virus-associated haemophagocytic syndrome was gradually replaced by the term infection-associated haemophagocytic syndrome (IAHS) when it was realized that microorganisms other than viruses could also provoke the disorder. During the early 1980s it was thought that familial haemophagocytic reticulosis and infection-associated haemophagocytic syndrome could be distinguished by the presence or absence of a family history, age of onset, and microbiological/serological studies. Histopathologically, however, there is no real difference between the two conditions; therefore, at least until reliable discriminating tests are available, the general term haemophagocytic lymphohistiocytosis (HLH) has been introduced.

A survey in Sweden covering the period 1971–1986 and including autopsy data (Henter *et al.* 1991*a*) suggested that the incidence of HLH was 1 : 50 000, but this may be an underestimate because the diagnosis is sometimes not even considered, haemophagocytosis is a common accompaniment of other processes, for example malignancy or other metabolic disorders, leading to misdiagnosis, and haemophagocytosis may be hard to identify in some patients. The incidence is rather higher in parts of the world, for example the Middle East, where inbreeding is a common cultural feature. The male to female incidence ratio is approximately 1 : 1 and the disease has been reported in every continent and in almost every ethnic group (Janka 1983). In familial cases, inheritance is autosomal recessive (Gencik *et al.* 1984). The gene frequency, based on the Hardy–Weinberg calculation and taking consanguinity into account, is between 0.5 and 1 per cent.

Aetiology and pathogenesis

In 30–50 per cent of patients there is a clear-cut family history, often with parental consanguinity. Analysis of multiple pedigrees shows a clear-cut autosomal recessive pattern of inheritance (Gencik *et al.* 1984). Obligate gene carriers seem to have no clinical abnormality. In many other cases the disease appears to be precipitated by infection, especially virus infection (Risdall *et al.* 1979). Organisms reported as implicated in the pathogenesis of HLH include Epstein–Barr virus, cytomegalovirus, rubella, HIV, *Toxoplasma gondii*, *Brucella* sp., and *Mycobacterium tuberculosis*.

Coagulopathy and lipid abnormalities, seen in many patients at diagnosis, are not found in remission and are therefore probably secondary manifestations. No primary metabolic defect has been identified, although isolated instances of hereditary fructosaemia and a hepatic ganglioside abnormality have been reported. An increase in circulating soluble IL-2 receptors has been identified in a few patients but not yet confirmed in large series. A recent interesting finding (Arico *et al.* 1988) is that in some patients there is a functional deficiency of natural killer cells in the parents and some siblings. This study is as close as any to the identification of a test for HLH predisposition, but is not reliable enough as a test for carrier status. The location of the gene is unknown and so no linked DNA probes are available at present.

The histopathological appearances suggest a reactive process with cytokines secreted by both histiocyte and lymphocyte populations as important mediators. Preliminary studies have suggested that IL-1, IL-2, γ-interferon, and tumour necrosis factor may all be involved. The network of cytokines secreted by immunoregulatory cells is extremely complex but techniques, especially *in situ* methods, will soon be available to investigate disorders like HLH.

Pathology

Whatever the aetiology of HLH, the histopathological findings in spleen, lymph node, and bone-marrow (the organs usually sampled) are alike. The infiltrates consist of bland-looking histiocytes with round nuclei and ample cytoplasm, often with easily detected haemophagocytosis and many lymphocytes. Enzyme stains are unhelpful in differential diagnosis, although there is often positive staining for lysozyme. In some patients demonstration of haemophagocytosis is difficult and repeated sampling may be needed.

Many patients with HLH are sick and have thrombocytopenia as well as coagulopathy. Biopsy may therefore be a hazardous undertaking and clinician and pathologist should discuss the pros and cons of different biopsy sites prior to the procedure. Less than 50 per cent of patients with HLH have enlarged lymph nodes and so node biopsy, though relatively safe, does not have a particularly high yield. Involved lymph nodes show sinus histiocytosis with haemophagocytosis. Bone-marrow is readily accessible but haemophagocytosis can be seen in patients with other diseases such

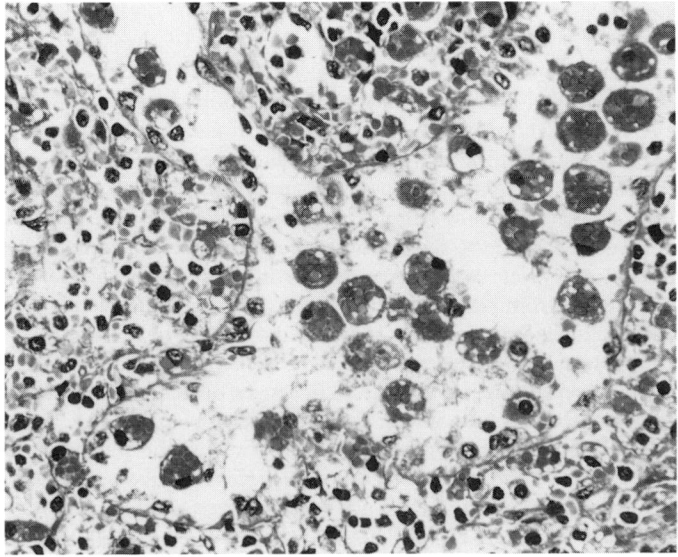

Fig. 13 Marked haemophagocytosis by splenic histiocytes in HLH.

as infections, malignancy, and collagen vascular disorders. Despite the hazards, liver and spleen (Fig. 13) may be the best organs to biopsy; recently, splenic fine-needle puncture has been advocated as being safe and effective. Liver biopsy can sometimes be safely performed with appropriate blood product support.

Histological changes in the liver can be subtle. The architecture is undisturbed and the hepatocytes look normal, but the portal tracts usually show a mild infiltrate of reactive lymphocytes (resembling chronic persistent hepatitis). Kupffer cells are prominent and, when examined carefully, may show evidence of haemophagocytosis. Some pathologists have described a mild fibrosis, extending from the central vein, together with subendothelial infiltration by reactive lymphocytes, which they consider virtually pathognomonic of HLH, but this observation is not universally accepted.

Clinical features

In paediatric series (Janka 1983) 50–60 per cent of patients develop initial symptoms during the first year of life, usually between 4 and 6 months of age. The remaining patients present throughout childhood and the disease also, very rarely, occurs in adults. The most common clinical findings, in decreasing order of frequency, are fever (90–95 per cent of patients), hepatomegaly (90 per cent), splenomegaly (80–85 per cent), neurological symptoms (30–40 per cent), and rash and node involvement (both 20 per cent) (W. Hirst et al., unpublished data). Fever is fluctuant, reaching peaks of 38.5–40°C. Hepatosplenomegaly is easily detected and usually progressive. Skin rash is usually described as maculopapular, is most prominent on the trunk, and is sometimes difficult to distinguish from rashes associated with viraemia. Neurological symptoms include alteration of consciousness, headache, meningism, increased intracranial pressure (with bulging fontanelle in infants), convulsions, cranial nerve palsies, and visual loss. Occasionally, central nervous system abnormalities may be the only initial manifestation of the disease. Less frequent findings include tachypnoea, jaundice, peripheral oedema (usually secondary to hypoalbuminaemia), purpura or bleeding, and muscle wasting. Disease activity may vary, with apparent spontaneous improvement for some days or weeks, but exacerbations are increasingly severe and, left untreated, patients die with organ failure, bleeding, infection complicating neutropenia, and/or progressive neurological deterioration.

Investigations

Mandatory investigations in a suspected case of HLH include full blood count with differential, coagulation studies including plasma fibrinogen level, plasma electrolytes, liver function tests including serum albumin, plasma triglycerides, and cerebrospinal fluid cell count with differential, and cytofuge preparation. Tests of natural killer cell function are helpful but not available in most centres. Infective agents, especially viruses, should be sought serologically and by appropriate microscopic and culture studies. The differential diagnosis is from infection, malignancy (both acute leukaemia and some solid tumour cells can show haemophagocytosis), and other histiocyte syndromes. Strict adherence to diagnostic guidelines for HLH, recently suggested by the Histiocyte Society (Henter et al. 1991b), should reduce the risk of misdiagnosis.

Thrombocytopenia and anaemia are usually the most severe elements of pancytopenia and transfusion dependence is common, particularly at diagnosis. The plasma fibrinogen level is often very low and evidence of disseminated intravascular coagulation (DIC) is unusual. Atypical lymphocytes may be found in the peripheral blood film. Serum transaminases are increased, particularly in jaundiced patients. Pleocytosis of the cerebrospinal fluid (10–1000 cells/mm^3) is seen in 50–70 per cent of patients. Cytofuge preparations show histiocytes (sometimes exhibiting phagocytosis), lymphocytes, and polymorphs in varying proportions. CT brain scans have been reported to show progressive brain atrophy with multiple hyperdense areas in the cortex. Neopterin levels in the cerebrospinal fluid may be a useful 'marker' for central nervous system involvement in HLH, particularly the familial form (Howells et al. 1990).

The most common plasma lipid abnormality is hypertriglyceridaemia with an increase in very low-density lipoproteins (VLDLs) and a decrease in high-density lipoproteins (HDLs) (Henter et al., in press). Serum ferritin, which can be elevated during active disease, platelet count, and serum IL-2 receptor levels (Komp et al. 1989) have been suggested as disease markers for HLH, but there is as yet no evidence that these measurements are more valuable than direct clinical observation.

Treatment

Until the 1980s, no effective treatment was available though brief remissions were obtained with a variety of cytotoxic regimens. Claims of 'cure' with combination chemotherapy were more likely the consequence of spontaneous remission of disease. In the early 1980s, etoposide (VP16) was shown to be an effective agent in HLH as well as in other types of histiocytosis and in monocytic leukaemia (Ambruso et al. 1980; Alverado et al. 1986). In 1985 Fischer and colleagues (Fischer et al. 1985) suggested that the combination of etoposide, corticosteroids, and intrathecal methotrexate, followed by cranial irradiation, produced good medium-term remissions. This triple regimen (minus cranial irradiation which does not seem appropriate in the very young child) was used in other centres between 1985 and 1990, with similar results, but with longer follow-up it was clear that most patients relapsed and subsequently died of their disease (W. Hirst et al., unpublished).

Though the pathogenesis of the disorder is not understood, it is clear that the target cell is bone-marrow derived. The disease process can apparently be suppressed by chemotherapy, but usually returns, perhaps because of an inborn metabolic error, as yet unidentified. A logical consequence was to attempt marrow ablation followed by bone-marrow transplantation and this procedure has been carried out by several European and North American centres. Various marrow-ablation regimens include etoposide, busulfan, and cyclophosphamide together with monoclonal antibodies such as CAMPATH IG, IGG2b, anti-LFA1, and cyclosporin to prevent graft versus host disease (GVHD), but as yet none has been shown to be superior to the others. As with all marrow-ablative treatments, there is a treatment associated mortality of 5–15 per cent, but marrow ablation can be achieved. After graft take, complete remission of HLH is often seen. In some patients there has been evidence of partial autologous marrow reconstitution, resulting in a chimeric state. Sustained remissions of duration up to 5 years are now being reported, but follow-up is too short to be sure that this treatment is truly curative. In patients without a bone-marrow donor, cyclosporin A seems promising as an agent for maintaining remissions induced by chemotherapy.

Other treatments should also be considered. Complicating infection should constantly be sought and appropriately treated with antimicrobials, intravenous immunoglobulin may be helpful when thrombocytopenia is severe, and, when no bone-marrow donor can be found, repeated plasma exchange may induce a temporary remission (Ladisch et al. 1982).

HLH is severe and usually fatal. Because of its rarity, it is best to refer patients to a specialized paediatric or adult haematology–oncology centre. At the very least, their advice on the best contemporary management should be sought.

Future prospects

In HLH, remission can be achieved with etoposide-based regimens, but it eventually proves fatal in most patients. In familial disease, where a genetic (and presumably irreversible) abnormality exists in the monocyte/histiocyte lineage, bone-marrow ablation and transplantation is a logical approach. Over the next few years, attention must be focused on devising a marrow-ablative and GVHD-suppressing regimen with acceptable immediate toxicity. By the time that the genetic defect is identified (see below), gene therapy should be a feasible proposition. The faulty gene could be introduced into a fraction of an infant's own bone-marrow and, after ablation of the child's remaining bone-marrow by high-dose chemotherapy, retransfused. The main caveat of this approach is that the abnormal gene might also be expressed, with unpredictable consequences, in non-haemopoietic tissues in later childhood but, given the problems of post-transplant GVHD, especially when the marrow donor is not a sibling, the approach seems well worth investigating.

Treatment is one thing but, in view of the high mortality of HLH, prevention is better. Discovery of restriction fragment length polymorphisms linked to the autosomal recessive gene and ultimately cloned DNA sequences corresponding to the gene itself will provide an opportunity for early post-natal prediction of susceptibility. Therapy might be more effective in predisposed healthy infants before the onset of widespread overt disease. The probes could also be used prenatally and the option of pregnancy termination offered to parents with a child or children already affected by HLH.

The recently established International HLH Registry (Dr Maurizio Arico, IRCCS Policlinico, S. Miteo, 1-27100 Pavia, Italy) provides a database for clinical information and a source of pathological material for basic research. It is still uncertain whether a subset of T-lymphocytes or of histiocytes is the primary offender in HLH but, whatever the pathway, there is no doubt that there is intense activation of monocytes and macrophages in these diseases. The consequent release of inflammatory cytokines is almost certainly responsible for much of the organ damage, so that HLH, like LCH, is probably a cytokine disease. Studies of IL-1, IL-6, γ-interferon, and tumour necrosis factor, in particular, both in serum and *in situ*, may provide critical leads in unravelling the pathogenetic process. The reported natural killer cell defect also needs further detailed study.

Rosai–Dorfman disease (sinus histiocytosis with massive lymphadenopathy)

Introduction and summary

This curious chronic reactive disorder was first reported in 1969 by two pathologists in the United States (Rosai and Dorfman 1969). A fuller clinicopathological description appeared in 1972 (Rosai and Dorfman 1972). The subcapsular sinus of affected lymph nodes and the interfollicular areas are grossly distended by massive accumulations of bland-looking non-Langerhans cell histiocytes, many showing lymphocytophagocytosis. There are also other inflammatory cells and perinodal fibrosis. Apart from lymph nodes, a wide variety of tissues including the central nervous system can also be affected. Aetiology is unknown and immune disturbances are likely to be a secondary feature in some patients. Peak age is approximately 20 years and males are more commonly affected than females. Complete spontaneous resolution can occur, although the disease lasts longer than a year in most patients. There is no standard treatment but response to corticosteroids, chemotherapy, and radiotherapy are well documented. Survival is probably well over 90 per cent, but disease-related fatalities have been recorded.

Case reports abound in the literature, but the most reliable information on this disorder is derived from a Sinus Histiocytosis with Massive Lymphadenopathy Registry, collated in New Haven, Connecticut, USA, by Professor Rosai and his colleagues (Rosai 1990). This section draws extensively on those data (Foucar *et al.* 1990) though, as the Registry is not population based, it can only indicate trends.

Epidemiology and demographics

Sinus histiocytosis with massive lymphadenopathy (SHML) has been recorded worldwide (Foucar *et al.* 1990). Many of the early reports were in Black individuals and the disease does seem to be commoner in populations with low socio-economic status. Occasional clusters of cases have been recorded, particularly in Black Africa. As with most histiocyte disorders, males are affected more commonly than females. Two pairs of affected identical twins are recorded. The peak age of onset is approximately 20 years, but the disease has been recorded in the newborn and the elderly.

Biology and aetiology

The lesional histiocytes have the characteristics of activated macrophages (Eisen *et al.* 1990). They express monocyte/macrophage-associated surface epitopes (for example, EBM 11, HAM-56, and Leu M3 (CD14)) as well as antigens associated with phagocytosis (for example, the Fc receptor of IgG and the C3 receptor) and lysosomal enzymes (for example, lysosyme and α-1-antitrypsin). Antigens generally characteristic of cell activation, for example CD11 (transferrin receptor) and CD25 (IL-2 receptor), are also found. This cell profile suggests derivation from recently circulating blood monocytes. Clinical characteristics, histopathology, and biological features all suggest a reactive disorder, but the aetiology of SHML is still unknown. There are interesting, though inconsistent, associations with various laboratory abnormalities, for example hypergammaglobulinaemia, antibodies to antinuclear and rheumatoid factors and red blood cell antigens, raised Epstein–Barr virus titres, and a possible clinical assocation with polyarthritis, glomerulonephritis, asthma, and juvenile diabetes mellitus. Four patients had concurrent non-Hodgkin's lymphoma and another developed LCH. Though Epstein–Barr virus titres are raised in some patients, no common pathogen has been identified and no consistent immunological abnormality recorded.

Histopathology

The sinuses and interfollicular areas of affected lymph nodes are engorged, often massively, with histiocytes (Fig. 14). The histiocytes have round or oval vesicular nuclei, most with a single small nucleolus and abundant pale or clear cytoplasm with indistinct margins. The cytoplasm of many of the cells contains well-preserved lymphocytes (lymphocytophagocytosis) (Fig. 15) and the distended sinuses often contain numerous plasma cells. The infiltrate in extranodal sites is similar.

Immunohistochemical studies can provide important confirmatory information. The histiocytic cells express the following markers: S100 protein, pan-macrophage antigens such as EBM/11, HAM

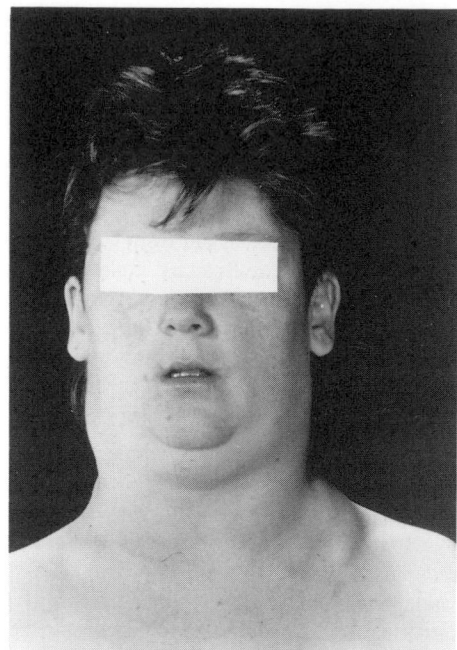

Fig. 14 Rosai–Dorfman disease (SHML): 10 year old girl with massive cervical lymphadenopathy, characteristic of this condition. She also had skin and small bowel involvement.

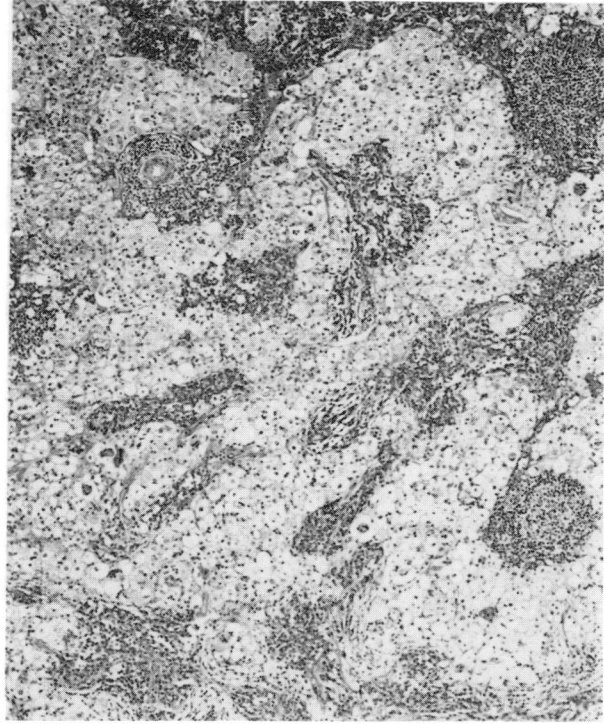

Fig. 15 Low-power view of a lymph node involved by SHML.

56, and Leu-M3, antigens functionally associated with phagocytosis (Fc receptor for IgG, complement receptor 3), antigens functionally associated with lysosomal activity (lysozyme, α_1-antichymotrypsin and α_1-antitrypsin), antigens associated with early inflammation (Mac 387), antigens commonly found on monocytes but not tissue macrophages (OKM5, Leu-M1), and activation antigens (Ki-1 and receptors for transferrin and IL-2). These data indicate that the

SHML cell is a member of the histiocyte family and although its exact origin is still uncertain, S100 protein positivity supports a potential relationship of SHML cells to the dendritic cell family (Hage *et al.* 1993). In addition, however, the cells express macrophage and monocyte markers. Perhaps the cells are true functionally activated macrophages which have recently arisen from circulating monocytes.

Clinical features

The characteristic presentation of SHML (>85 per cent of patients) (Foucar *et al.* 1990) is with bilateral massive cervical node enlargement (Fig. 16). Many patients are systemically well, but some have fever and have lost weight. Node enlargement is usually painless; besides cervical nodes, inguinal (25 per cent of patients), axillary (20–25 per cent), and mediastinal (15 per cent) nodes can also be involved. A few patients have no nodal enlargement and extranodal involvement is commoner than generally supposed. In descending order of frequency, the following organs have been affected: nasal/paranasal tissues (10–15 per cent of all cases), orbits and eyelids, bones, salivary glands, and skin (all 5–10 per cent), and central nervous system, mouth (especially palate), lower respiratory tract, optic lobe, larynx, liver, tonsil, breast, gastrointestinal tract, heart, thyroid, thymus, and middle ear (all <5 per cent). Skin lesions are described as 'xanthomatous', may be red–brown in colour, and are commoner in Whites than Blacks, perhaps because they are more easily seen. Bone lesions are lytic and resemble those in LCH patients. Approximately half the patients with central nervous system disease do not have detectable peripheral nodal involvement. Interestingly, neither splenic nor bone-marrow involvement has been described.

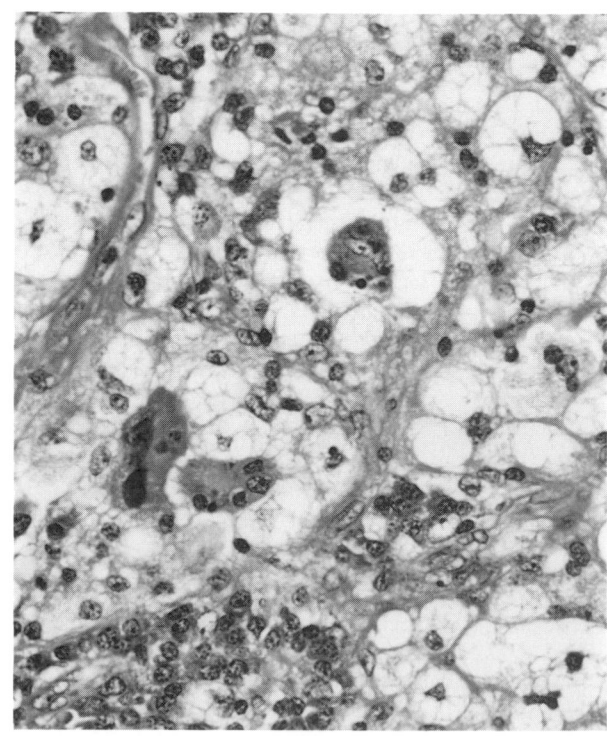

Fig. 16 Histiocytes in SHML. Note the bland nuclei, clear granular (eosinophilic) cytoplasm, indistinct cell margins, and lymphocyto-phagocytosis (lymph node biopsy from patient shown in Fig. 14).

Investigations

These patients do not have pancytopenia (Foucar *et al.* 1990). The most common haematological abnormality is a mild 'anaemia of chronic disorders'. Total white cell count and differential and platelet count are usually normal, but 30–40 per cent of patients have a neutrophil leucocytosis. In over 90 per cent the erythrocyte sedimentation rate is elevated, sometimes greatly.

Evidence of immune dysregulation is common. The total γ-globulin level is elevated in over 90 per cent of patients (IgG > 90 per cent, IgA 60–80 per cent, and IgM 40–50 per cent). Tests for rheumatoid factor and antinuclear antibodies can be positive and the ratio of CD4 to CD8 in circulating lymphocytes is often inverted. There are no other consistent laboratory abnormalities.

Differential diagnosis

Lymphoma or nasopharyngeal carcinoma with cervical node secondaries are often suspected, particularly in patients with systemic symptoms, but are excluded by lymph node biopsy findings. The main diagnostic problem lies in the distinction between SHML and major reactive adenopathy, characterized by severe sinus hyperplasia (sinus catarrh). However, histopathological findings, particularly the presence of lymphocytophagocytosis and the pattern of S100 staining, are usually diagnostic.

Natural history and prognostic factors

SHML is a chronic disease, lasting well over a year in most patients (Foucar *et al.* 1990). In 20 per cent it eventually resolves completely and in 50–60 per cent it improves but persists. Though it is known to progress in the remainder (15–20 per cent), only four deaths directly due to the disease itself have been documented. In other patients, associated conditions (for example, autoimmune haemolytic anaemia) have been fatal, but the exact cause of death is often not recorded. Extranodal involvement, even of the central nervous system, does not *per se* lessen the chance of survival but, according to Registry data, immunological abnormalities, involvement of kidney, lower respiratory tract, or liver, and disseminated nodal disease are adverse prognostic features (Foucar *et al.* 1990).

Treatment and results

As the cause is unknown, there is no specific treatment. Even the Registry provides no long-term follow-up, but it is reasonable to assume that, in most cases, the disease burns itself out. Therefore, as in LCH, a period of observation is usually justified unless constitutional symptoms are marked, there are pressure symptoms (usually upper airway) or, more arguably, if 'adverse prognostic features' (see previous section) are present. Some patients demand intervention for cosmetic reasons.

Responses to corticosteroid therapy, radiation therapy, and both single and multiagent cytotoxic regimens have been recorded (Komp 1990). By normal cancer criteria, response rates are probably no higher than 20–30 per cent, but any improvement can significantly relieve symptoms. Because of their unpleasant or unwanted immediate and delayed side-effects, alkylating agents, combination chemotherapy, and radiation therapy are best avoided, particularly in young patients and there is no justification for prolonged courses of steroids. Prednisolone can be used to overcome crises (suggested starting dose 2 mg/kg daily for 4 weeks) and then tailed off and discontinued. It is crucial to remember that SHML is not cancer and should not be treated as such; at the outset, it is worth considering referring these patients to a specialist, for example a rheumatologist, skilled in the management of chronic relapsing non–malignant disorders.

Other class II histiocytoses

The Histiocyte Society classification (Writing Group of Histiocyte Society 1987) includes a number of conditions, for example juvenile xanthogranuloma, reticulohistiocytoma, and xanthoma disseminatum, that, histopathologically, contain large numbers of histiocytes (reviewed by Chu 1991). However, in these conditions, the histiocyte may be more the culprit cell than in storage disorders and so their inclusion seems somewhat arbitrary. Most of the conditions are skin based and, clinically, can be mistaken for LCH. It is particularly noteworthy that involvement of the posterior pituitary gland, causing diabetes insipidus, has been recorded in xanthoma disseminatum (Altman and Winkelmann 1962). Here, careful histopathological studies must be performed to distinguish the two conditions (Gianotti and Caputo 1985; Favara 1990).

Some histiocytoses defy classification in the current Histiocyte Society system, for instance, cases with lesional cells that have the markers of ordinary histiocytes but the morphology of dendritic cells (Favara 1990). Future studies will perhaps help clarify whether other entities do exist and, if so, how they dovetail into the current Histiocyte Society classification.

MALIGNANT HISTIOCYTOSIS. CLASS III OF HISTIOCYTE SOCIETY CLASSIFICATION

Introduction and summary

Over 50 years ago, Bodley Scott and Robb–Smith described four adults and reviewed six others with fever, weight loss, generalized adenopathy, hepatosplenomegaly with jaundice, and pancytopenia (Bodley Scott and Robb–Smith 1939). They attributed the pathological findings to a 'systematized proliferation of erythrophagocytic histiocytes and their precursors', but regarded the disease as distinct from leukaemia and Hodgkin's disease and introduced the descriptive term 'histiocytic medullary reticulosis'. In 1966, Rappaport suggested the alternative term 'malignant histiocytosis' because he believed that the disorder represented a primary malignancy of histiocytic cells (Rappaport 1966) and this rubric gradually replaced 'histiocytic medullary reticulosis'. The Histiocyte Society classification distinguishes between malignant histiocytosis and 'true histiocytic lymphoma' on the rather arbitrary basis that the latter are 'tumoural processes rather than lesions of poorly cohesive cellularity' (Writing Group of Histiocyte Society 1987).

As a clinicopathological entity, malignant histiocytosis certainly exists, but it is much less common than previously supposed. In the past, haemophagocytic disorders, particularly those provoked by infection and large cell lymphomas were often mistakenly described as malignant histiocytosis, but recent histopathological review, using up-to-date immunohistochemical, cytogenetic, and molecular techniques, has revealed the correct diagnosis (Bucsky *et al.* 1989). In these circumstances it is difficult to be certain of the typical clinical and laboratory features of malignant histiocytosis, but clinical presentation is probably similar to lymphoma and leukaemia with central nervous system involvement in some patients. Complete remission and long-term survival can be achieved with combination chemotherapy including central nervous system directed therapy.

Epidemiology and demography

Malignant histiocytosis has been described in all continents and all races. Because of the uncertainty of previous diagnoses, exact incidence is uncertain, but it has been estimated that the ratio of patients with malignant histiocytosis to patients with malignant lymphoma is less than 1 : 200 (Ralfkiaer *et al.* 1990).

Aetiology and biology

No predisposing factors are known. 'Malignant histiocytosis' has been diagnosed in immunosuppressed patients, but in these circumstances an infection-provoked reactive haemophagocytic syndrome is much more likely.

True malignant histiocytosis cells express cytoplasmic enzymes and membrane markers indicating their derivation from the histiocyte/monocyte lineage (Ralfkiaer *et al.* 1990). Some haemato-pathologists feel that there are differences in the antigenic cell profile of malignant histiocytosis cells compared with cells of acute monocytic leukaemia, but there have been a few case reports of malignant histiocytosis evolving into M5 acute non-lymphoblastic leukaemia, suggesting that malignant histiocytosis is the solid end of a spectrum of histiomonocytic malignancy (Chong *et al.* 1980). Recently, Morgan *et al.* (1986) have described a translocation (t(2;5)(p23;q35)) in three cases of 'malignant histiocytosis'. However, others claim that the same translocation can be found in other rare entities such as the phagocytic large T-cell lymphoma (Kaneko *et al.* 1989) and so it may not be as specific as first supposed. In addition, expression of the c-*fms* and N-*myc* oncogenes, which lie on either side of the t(2;5)(p23;q35) translocation, seems to be unaltered. As in other forms of haemolymphopoietic malignancy, karyotypic studies are now mandatory. As soon as informative specific DNA probes are identified, the same will apply to molecular studies.

Histopathology

Malignant histiocytosis must be differentiated histopathologically from the much commoner Ki-1-positive anaplastic large cell lymphoma (usually of T-cell type, but occasionally B-cell or null cell) (Bucsky *et al.* 1989; Kaneko *et al.* 1989; Ralfkiaer *et al.* 1990), 'reactive' haemophagocytic disorders, atypical Hodgkin's disease, and 'sarcoma' of the interdigitating reticulum cell. Malignant histiocytosis and Ki-1-positive anaplastic large cell lymphoma cannot be distinguished on purely morphological grounds, as both are composed of large anaplastic cells with pleomorphic nuclei, bizarre mitoses, ample amounts of cytoplasm, and easily demonstrable phagocytosis.

To establish a diagnosis of malignant histiocytosis fresh or frozen tissue (see Appendix) should show no evidence of immunoglobulin or T-cell receptor gene rearrangement. In addition, tumour cells should be negative, on immunostaining, for T- and B-cell markers and positive for specific monoclonal macrophage-associated antigens. More recently, monoclonal macrophage markers such as Mac 387, KP1, and Ki-M6 (the last two recognize epitopes of the CD68 antigen) can be used on paraffin-embedded tissue. Lysozyme can usually be demonstrated in the tumour cells, but the test is not completely reliable and other macrophage/histiocyte markers such as α-1-antitrypsin are expressed too variably to be of diagnostic use.

Clinical features and differential diagnosis

It should again be stressed that the rarity of 'true' malignant histiocytosis (Kaneko *et al.* 1989; Ralfkiaer *et al.* 1990) makes it difficult to be sure of the typical features of this disease. Fever and fluctuating generalized adenopathy seem to be frequent early signs; in some cases the nodes are said to be tender. In established malignant histiocytosis, adenopathy can be marked, although not massive and the liver and spleen are usually enlarged. Generalized or focal central nervous system abnormalities and skin rash are also common. Pancytopenia is usually severe, with complicating infection, bruising and purpura, and transfusion dependency. Bone pain due to bone erosion is sometimes seen. Other visceral organs, for example, the lungs, can be involved.

Malignant histiocytosis has to be differentiated from the haemophagocytic lymphohistiocytoses (both genetic and sporadic) and from acute and chronic leukaemia and malignant lymphoma, including Hodgkin's disease. Haemophagoctyosis in bone-marrow or lymph nodes can be a feature of a number of malignancies including acute leukaemia and neuroblastoma.

Natural history and treatment

Without treatment the disease rapidly progresses and leads to failure of bone-marrow and liver and of other organs. Occasionally central nervous system involvement may be the dominant clinical feature. The impact of chemotherapy in reported adult (Lampert *et al.* 1978) and paediatric (Zucker *et al.* 1980; Brugieres *et al.* 1989) series of 'malignant histiocytosis' has to be treated very cautiously. As stressed in preceding sections, it is not at all clear how many cases of true malignant histiocytosis have been successfully treated.

Combination chemotherapy can induce complete remissions and central nervous system-directed therapy (central nervous system prophylaxis), in the form of cranial irradiation and intrathecal methotrexate, has been used by some groups. The most widely reported chemotherapy regimen is CHOP (cyclophosphamide, doxorubicin (hydroxydaunorubicin), oncovin (vincristine) and prednisolone) which is reported to induce complete remission in approximately 50 per cent of cases (Lampert *et al.* 1978; Zucker *et al.* 1980; Brugieres *et al.* 1989). Usually complete remission is sustained for many years and these patients are probably cured of their disease. Other regimens have been tried but none has been shown to be superior to CHOP. Logically, however, regimens most active in acute non-lymphoblastic leukaemia should also be most effective in malignant histiocytosis. Marrow-ablative chemoradiotherapy with bone-marrow transplant has been reported in a few instances, but it is by no means clear that this toxic procedure is essential for cure. The Histiocyte Society has set up a Malignant Histiocytosis Registry for paediatric cases of malignant histiocytosis. It is hoped that the Registry will also collate adult cases so that, in the future, more specific treatment recommendations can be made.

GENERAL CONCLUSIONS AND FUTURE PROSPECTS

There is still a fair amount of inspired guesswork as far as the pathophysiology of the histiocyte disorders is concerned, but as knowledge increases there is bound to be a shift in perspectives and consequently changes in the Histiocyte Society's classification. LCH and HLH are probably not malignant disorders, but if, as anticipated, they are shown to be disorders of cytokine dysregulation, reclassification (according to the cytokine primarily involved) may be preferred. It is also possible that the primary defect in these diseases resides in cells other than the histiocytes themselves. Malignant histiocytosis, though extremely rare, does seem to constitute a real entity. Cytogenetic and molecular probe studies should help determine whether, at the molecular level, one or more fundamental abnormalities can cause the malignant histiocytosis and whether or not malignant histiocytosis and M5 ANNL are or are not part of the same disease spectrum.

With greater understanding of pathophysiology, current arbitrary management policies, for LCH and HLH in particular, should eventually be replaced by rational treatments. Until recently, progress was painfully slow because the rarity of the disorders provokes little research. The formation of the Histiocyte Society and the establishment of regular research symposia (the Nikolas Symposia), focusing on the histiocytoses has already generated much research momentum. It is hoped that the pathogenesis of these diseases will soon be much better understood and treatment rationalized. Membership of the Histiocyte Society is open to any student of these disorders.*

APPENDIX

Handling of pathological specimens

The histopathological features of histiocyte syndromes overlap considerably and differential diagnosis can be difficult. Therefore detailed discussion with the pathologist and full provision of clinical information is necessary before a biopsy is undertaken. Collaboration between surgeon and pathologist is also necessary if material is to reach the laboratory in an optimum state for processing.

Ideally, fresh specimens should be taken immediately to the laboratory where the pathologist can divide the tissue and use some for virology and microbiology if necessary. Some material should then be snap-frozen and stored at −70°C and some fixed in formalin and routinely processed. Immunostaining for S100 protein, peanut agglutinin, and Mac 387, as well as electron microscopy, can be carried out on paraffin sections. The snap-frozen material can be used for immunostaining for CD1 and CD4 and tested for α-D-mannosidase.

REFERENCES

Altman J, Winkelmann RK (1962). Xanthoma disseminatum. *Archives of Dermatology*, 86:582–96.

Alvarado CS, Buchanan GR, Kim TH, Zaatari G, Sartain P, Ragab AH (1986). Use of VP-16-213 in the treatment of familial erythrophagocytyic lymphohistiocytosis. *Cancer*, 57:1097–1100.

Ambruso DR, Hays T, Zwartjes WJ, Tubergen DG, Favara BE (1980). Successful treatment of lymphohistiocytic reticulosis with phagocytosis with epipodophyllotoxin VP16-213. *Cancer*, 45:2516–20.

Arenzana-Seisdedos F, Barbey S, Virelizier JL, Kornprobst M, Nezelof C (1986). Histiocytosis X. Purified (T6⁺) cells from bone granuloma produce interleukin 1 and prostaglandin E₂ in culture. *Journal of Clinical Investigation*, 77:326–9.

Arico M, Nebpoli L, Maccario R, Montagana D, Bonetti F, Caselli D, Bargio GR (1988). Natural cytotoxicity impairment in familial haemophagocyte lymphohistiocytosis. *Archives of Disease in Childhood*, 63:292–6.

Basset F, *et al.* (1978). Pulmonary histiocytosis X. *American Review of Respiratory Diseases*, 118:811–20.

Bodley Scott R, Robb-Smith AHT (1939). Histiocytic medullary reticulosis. *Lancet*, ii:194–8.

Broadbent V, Pritchard J (1985). Histiocytosis X—current controversies. *Archives of Disease in Childhood*, 60:605–7.

Broadbent V, Gadner H, Komp DM, Ladisch S (The Clinical Writing Group of the Histiocyte Society) (1989). Histiocytosis syndromes in children: II. Approach to the clinical and laboratory evaluation of children with Langerhans cell histiocytosis. *Medical and Pediatric Oncology*, 17:492–5.

Brugieres L, *et al.* (1989). Malignant histiocytosis: therapeutic results in 27 children treated with a single polychemotherapy regimen. *Medical and Pediatric Oncology*, 17:193–6.

Bucksky P, *et al.* (1989). Zur frage der definition der malignen histiozytose und des grobzelligen anaplatischen (Ki-1) lymphoms im kindesalter. *Klinische Pädiatrie*, 201:233–6.

Cassady JR (1987). Current role of radiation therapy in the management of histiocytosis-X. *Hematology and Oncology Clinics of North America*, 1:123–9.

Ceci A, *et al.* (1988). Etoposide in recurrent childhood Langerhans' cell histiocytosis: an Italian co-operative study. *Cancer*, 62:2528–31.

Chong SKF, Marshall WC, Pritchard J (1980). Malignant histiocytosis in children from the Eastern Mediterranean. *Medical and Pediatric Oncology*, 8:403–4 (letter).

Chu AC (1991). The histiocytoses. In *The texbook of dermatology* (ed. J Wilkinson, J Burton, R Champion, and A Ebling). Blackwell, Oxford.

Dunger DB, Broadbent V, Yeomans E, Seckl JR, Lightman SR, Grant DB, Pritchard J (1989). The frequency and natural history of diabetes insipidus in children with Langerhans cell histioctyosis. *New England Journal of Medicine*, 321:1157–62.

Egeler RM, Schipper MEI, Heymans HSA (1990). Gastrointestinal involvement in Langerhans' cell histiocytosis (histiocytosis X): a clinical report of three cases. *European Journal of Pediatrics*, 149 (5):325–9.

Eisen RN, Buckley PJ, Rosai J (1990). Immunophenotypic characterisation of sinus histiocytosis with massive lymphadenopathy (Rosai–Dorfman disease). *Seminars in Diagnosis and Pathology*, 7:74–82.

Elleder M, Povysil C, Rozkovcova J, Cihula J (1977). α-D-Mannosidase activity in histiocytosis X. *Virchows Archiv, B Cell Pathology*, 26:139–45.

Farquhar J, Claireaux A (1952). Familial haemophagocyte reticulosis. *Archives of Disease in Childhood*, 27:519–25.

Favara BE (1990). Histiocytosis syndromes. Classification, diagnostic features and current concepts. *Leukemia and Lymphoma*, 2:141–50.

Favara B, Jaffé R (1987). Pathology of Langerhans cell histiocytosis. *Hematology and Oncology Clinics of North America*, 1:75–98.

Fischer A, Virelizier JL, Arenzana-Seisdedos F, Perez N, Nezelof C, Griscelli C (1985). Treatment of four patients with erythrophagocytic lymphohistiocytosis by a combination of epipodophyllotoxin, steroids, intrathecal methotrexate and cranial irradiation. *Pediatrics*, 76:263–8.

Foucar K, Foucar E (1990). The mononuclear phagocyte and immunoregulatory effector (M-PIRE) system: evolving concepts. *Seminars in Diagnosis and Pathology*, 7:4–18.

Foucar E, Rosai J, Dorfman RF (1990). Sinus histiocytosis with massive lymphadenopathy (Rosai–Dorfman disease): review of the entity. *Seminars in Diagnosis and Pathology*, 7:19–73.

Gencik A, Signer E, Muller HJ (1984). Genetic analysis of familial erythrophagocytic lymphohistiocytosis. *European Journal of Pediatrics*, 142:248–52.

Gianotti F, Caputo R (1985). Histiocytic syndromes: a review. *Journal of the American Academy of Dermatology*, 13:383–404.

Greinix HT, Storb R, Sanders JE, Petersen FB (1992). Marrow transplantation for treatment of multisystem progressive Langerhans cell histiocytosis. *Bone Marrow Transplantation*, 10:39–44.

Ha SY, Helms P, Fletcher M, Broadbent V, Pritchard J (1992). Lung involvement in Langerhans' cell histiocytosis—prevalence, clinical features and outcome. *Pediatrics*, 89:466–9.

Hage C, Willman CL, Favara BE, Isaacson PG (1993). Langerhans cell histiocytosis (histiocytosis X): immunophenotype and growth fraction. *Human Pathology*, 24:840–5.

Hance AJ, *et al.* (1986). Smoking and interstitial lung disease. The effect of cigarette smoking on the incidence of pulmonary histiocytosis X and sarcoidosis. *Annals of New York Academy of Sciences*, 465:643–56.

Hashimoto K, Griffin D, Kohsbaki M (1982). Self-healing reticulohistiocytosis: A clinical, histologic, and ultrastructural study of the fourth case in the literature. *Cancer*, 49:331–7.

---

*Details from the Secretariat of the Histiocyte Society, c/o Histiocytosis Association of America, 609 New York Road, Glassboro', NJ 08028, USA.

Henter J-I, Elinder G, Söder O, Öst Å (1991a). Incidence in Sweden and clinical features of familial hemophagocytic lymphohistiocytosis. *Acta Paediatrica Scandinavica.*

Henter J-I, Elinder G, Öst Å, for the Histiocyte Society (1991b). Diagnostic guidelines for hemophagocytic lymphohistiocytosis. *Seminars in Oncology,* **18**:29–33.

Howells DW, Strobel S, Smith I, Levinsky RJ, Hyland K (1990). Central nervous system involvement in the erythrophagocytic disorders of infancy: the role of CSF neopterins in their differential diagnosis and clinical management. *Pediatric Research,* **28**:116–19.

Irving RM, Broadbent V, Jones NS (1993). Langerhans cell histiocytosis in childhood: management of head and neck manifestations. *Laryngoscope.*

Jaffe ES (1988). Histiocytoses of lymph nodes: biology and differential diagnosis. *Seminars in Diagnosis and Pathology,* **5**:376–90.

Jakobson AM, Kreuger A, Hagberg H, Sundstrom C (1987). Treatment of Langerhans cell histiocytosis with alpha-interferon. *Lancet,* **ii**:1520–1.

Janka GE (1983). Familial hemophagocytic lymphohistiocytosis. *European Journal of Pediatrics,* **140**:221–30.

Kaneko Y, *et al.* (1989). A novel translocation t(2;5) (p23;q35) in childhood phagoctyic large T-cell lymphoma mimicking malignant histiocytosis. *Blood,* **73**:806–13.

Katz SI, Tamaki K, Sachs DH (1979). Epidermal Langerhans cells are derived from cells originating in bone marrow. *Nature, London,* **282**:324–6.

Kelly KM, Pritchard JL (1994). Monoclonal antibody therapy in Langerhans cell histiocytosis: feasible and reasonable? *British Journal of Cancer.* (In press).

Komp DM (1981). Long-term sequelae of histiocytosis X. *American Journal of Pediatric Hematology and Oncology,* **3**:165–8.

Komp DM (1987). Historical perspectives of Langerhans cell histiocytosis. *Hematology and Oncology Clinics of North America,* **1**:9–21.

Komp DM (1990). The treatment of sinus histiocytosis with massive lymphadenopathy (Rosai–Dorfman disease). *Seminars in Diagnosis and Pathology,* **7**:83–6.

Komp DM, McNamara J, Buckley P (1989). Elevated soluble interleukin-2 receptor in childhood hemophagocytic histioctyic syndromes. *Blood,* **73**: 2128–32.

Ladisch S, Ho W, Matheson D, Pilkington R, Hartman G (1982). Immunologic and clinical effects of repeated blood exchange in familial erythrophagocytic lymphohistiocytosis. *Blood,* **60**:814–21.

Lahey ME (1962). Prognosis in reticuloendotheliosis in children. *Journal of Pediatrics,* **60**:664–8.

Lampert IA, Catovsky D, Bergier N (1978). Malignant histiocytosis. A clinico-pathological study of 12 cases. *British Journal of Haematology,* **40**:65–77.

Leblanc A, Hadchouel M, Jehan P, Odièvre M, Alagille D (1981). Obstructive jaundice in children with histiocytosis X. *Gastroenterology,* **80**:134–9.

Lichtenstein L (1953). Integration of eosinophilic granuloma of bone, Letterer–Siwe disease and Schuller–Christian disease as related manifestations of a single nosologic entity. *Archives of Pathology,* **56**:84–102.

McLelland J, Pritchard J, Chu AC (1987). Histiocytosis X. Current controversies. *Hematology and Oncology Clinics of North America,* **1**:147–62.

McLelland J, Newton JA, Malone M, Camplejohn RS, Chu AC (1989). A flow cytometric study of Langerhans cell histiocytosis. *British Journal of Dermatology,* **120**:485–91.

McLelland J, Broadbent V, Yeomans E, Malone M, Pritchard J (1990). Langerhans cell histiocytosis: the case for conservative treatment. *Archives of Disease in Childhood,* **65**:301–3.

Mahmoud HM, Wang WC, Murphy SB (1991). Cyclosporine therapy for advanced Langerhans cell histiocytosis. *Blood,* **77**:721–5.

Moore AT, Pritchard J, Taylor DSI (1981). Histiocytosis X: an ophthalmological review. *British Journal of Ophthalmology,* **69**:7–14.

Morgan R, Hecht BK, Sandberg AA, Hecht F, Smith SD (1986). Chromosome 5q35 breakpoint in malignant histiocytosis. *New England Journal of Medicine,* **314**:1322 (letter).

Murphy GF (1985). Cell membrane glycoproteins and Langerhans cells. *Human Pathology,* **16**:103–12.

Osband ME, *et al.* (1981). Demonstration of abnormal immunity, T-cell histamine H2-receptor deficiency, and successful treatment with thymic extract. *New England Journal of Medicine,* **304**:146–53.

Pritchard J (1979). Histiocytosis X: natural history and management in childhood. *Clinical and Experimental Dermatology,* **4**:421–33.

Ralfkiaer E, Delsol G, O'Connor NTJ, Bradtzaeg P, Brousset P, Vejlsgaard GL, Mason DY (1990). Malignant lymphomas of true histiocytic origin. A clinical, histological, immunophenotypic and genotypic study. *Journal of Pathology,* **160**:9–17.

Rappaport H (1966). Tumours of the hematopoietic system. In *Atlas of tumour pathology,* Section III, Fascicle 8, pp. 48–88. Armed Forces Institute of Pathology, Washington.

Reid CDL, Fryer PR, Clifford C, Kirk A, Tikerpae J, Knight SC (1990). Identification of hematopoietic progenitors of macrophages and dendritic Langerhans cells (DL-CFU) in human bone marrow and peripheral blood. *Blood,* **76**:1139–49.

Risdall RJ, McKenna RW, Nesbit ME, Krivit W, Balfour HH Jr, Simmons RL (1979). Virus-associated haemophagocytic syndrome. *Cancer,* **44**:993–1002.

Rosai J (1990). SHML Registry. *Seminars in Diagnosis and Pathology,* **7**:3.

Rosai J, Dorfman RF (1969). Sinus histiocytosis with massive lymphadenopathy; a newly-recognised benign clinico-pathological entity. *Archives of Pathology,* **87**:63–70.

Rosai J, Dorfman RF (1972). Sinus histiocytosis with massive lymphadenopathy. A pseudolymphomatous benign disorder. *Cancer,* **30**:1174–88.

Rosenfield NS, Abrahams J, Komp D (1990). Brain MR in patients with Langerhans cell histiocytosis: findings and enhancement with Gd-DTPA. *Pediatric Radiology,* **20**:433–6.

Sacks SH, Hall I, Ragge N, Pritchard J (1986). Chronic dermal sinuses as a manifestation of histiocytosis X. *British Medical Journal,* **292**:1097–8.

Sheehan MP, Atherton DJ, Broadbent V, Pritchard J (1991). Topical nitrogen mustard an effective treatment for cutaneous Langerhans cell histiocytosis. *Journal of Pediatrics,* **119**:317–21.

Sigala JL, Silverman S Jr, Brody A, Kushner JH (1972). Dental involvement in histiocytosis X. *Oral Surgery,* **33**:42–8.

Stoll M, Freund M, Schmid H, Dercher H, Riehm M, Poliwoda H, Link H (1990). Allogeneic bone marrow transplantation for Langerhans cell histiocytosis. *Cancer,* **66**:284–8.

Willman CA, *et al.* (1993). Langerhans cell histiocytosis: a spectrum of clonal neoplastic and polyclonal reactive disorders. *Blood,* **82**:121 (abstract).

Writing Group of Histiocyte Society (1987). Histiocytosis syndromes in children. *Lancet,* **i**:208–9.

Yu RCH, Attra A, Quinn CM, Krausz T, Chu AC (1993). Multisystem Langerhans cell histiocytosis with pancreatic involvement. *Gut,* **34**:520–2.

Yu R, Chu CE, Bulwela, Chu AC (1994). Langerhans cell histiocytosis: a clonal proliferation of Langerhans cells. *Lancet.* (In press.)

Zucker JM, Caillaux JM, Vanel D, Gerard-Marchant R (1980). Malignant histiocytosis in childhood. Clinical study and therapeutic results in 22 cases. *Cancer,* **45**:2821–9.

12.10 Neoplastic complications of AIDS

SILVIO MONFARDINI

INTRODUCTION

The acquired immunodeficiency syndrome (AIDS) was first reported in 1981 as a combined epidemic of Pneumocystis pneumonia and Kaposi's sarcoma (Brice *et al.* 1988; Biggar 1992). In subsequent years many investigators in the United States and in Europe also reported patients with non-Hodgkin's lymphomas and several other tumours among the population at risk for AIDS (Ahmed *et al.* 1987; Beral *et al.* 1991). After Kaposi's sarcoma and non-Hodgkin's lymphomas, cervical cancer and Hodgkin's disease were found to be the most frequent neoplasms in patients with HIV infection (Biggar 1990; Levin *et al.* 1993; Reynolds *et al.* 1993), while in the United States a prevalence of squamous head and neck carcinomas and cloacogenic carcinomas of the rectum was initially reported among the other solid tumours. Between them, there are some rare cancers reported in HIV-positive patients that include testicular, cervical, and lung carcinomas (Monfardini *et al.* 1989*a*; Biggar 1990).

AIDS has emerged as the most important epidemic disease infection of our time. By the middle of 1990 nearly 270 000 cases have been reported worldwide (WHO 1990). The number of cases officially reported to the World Health Organization (WHO) represents probably one-third of the real total. Delay in reporting, under-reporting, and inadequate means of diagnosis almost certainly contribute to this gross underestimation. In the absence of major and rapid progress in therapy, most patients with AIDS will die in the next few years, many with malignant tumours. However, since many more persons have already been infected with the aetiological agent of AIDS (that is, the human immunodeficiency virus (HIV)), it has been calculated that, over the next decade, more than a million people will enter a state of immunodeficiency which will place them at risk of opportunistic diseases including some malignancies (Biggar 1990).

The identification of the human T-lymphotropic retrovirus represents one of the most significant steps in AIDS research (Gallo *et al.* 1984; Montagnier *et al.* 1984). HIV may infect many human cells, including those in the brain, but is able to recognize the T4 lymphocyte surface marker and has a strong affinity for this subset of lymphocytes. The selective cytopathic effect of HIV on T4 lymphocytes results in an imbalance in the usual ratio of T4 to T8 cells, with a decline in lymphocyte recognition and response to antigen. As the response to antigen by T lymphocytes is a prime initiator of the immune response, the lack of cellular immune response explains the increased susceptibility to opportunistic infections and neoplasms which an intact immune system will ordinarily resist.

HIV can cause a wide spectrum of clinical conditions ranging from asymptomatic state to severe chronic infections and cachexia. To encompass patients with AIDS and with less severe HIV infection status the Centers for Disease Control classification scheme (Table 1) is particularly useful even for clinical oncologists (Centers

for Disease Control 1986). The term AIDS has been used to describe the more serious manifestations of the disorder such as severe opportunistic infections or neoplasms. At present the diagnosis of AIDS is based on detection of antibodies to HIV or other serological evidence of exposure to the virus (such as viral p24 antigen, virus production, or reverse transcriptase activity), in combination with defects of cellular immunity (such as T-lymphocyte abnormalities) and the presence of the infectious or neoplastic complication mentioned above. The diagnosis of AIDS can also be made if HIV serology or other HIV markers are unknown when a disease index of AIDS with immunological deficit is present (Centers for Disease Control 1987).

The term persistent generalized lymphadenopathy has been adopted to denote a relatively healthy group of patients with lymphadenopathy found at two or more extrainguinal sites for 3

Table 1 Centers for Disease Control classification scheme for HIV infection

Group I	Acute HIV infection
Group II	Asymptomatic HIV infection
Group III	Persistent generalized lymphadenopathy: lymphadenopathy (>1 cm diameter) at two or more extrainguinal sites lasting more than 3 months without another condition to explain the findings
Group IV	Other HIV disease

Subgroup A	Constitutional disease: one or more of fever for >1 month, 10% weight loss, or diarrhoea lasting <1 month, with no other condition to explain the findings
Subgroup B	Neurological disease: one or more of dementia, myelopathy, or peripheral neuropathy, with no other condition to explain the findings
Subgroup C	Secondary infectious diseases
C1	One of the specified symptomatic or invasive diseases which define AIDS: *Pneumocystis carinii* pneumonia, chronic cryptosporidiosis, toxoplasmosis, extraintestinal strongyloidiasis, isoporiasis, candidiasis (oesophageal, bronchial, or pulmonary), cryptococcosis, histoplasmosis, *Mycobacterium avium* complex or *Myobacterium kansasii*, cytomegalovirus, chronic monocutaneous or disseminated herpes simplex infection, or progressive multifocal leucoencephalopathy
C2	Symptomatic or invasive disease with one of the following: oral hairy leucoplakia, multidermatomal herpes zoster, recurrent *Salmonella* bacteraemia, nocardiosis, tuberculosis, or oral candidiasis
Subgroup D	Secondary cancers: diagnosis of one of Kaposi's sarcoma, non-Hodgkin's lymphoma (small non-cleaved lymphoma or immunoblastic sarcoma), or primary lymphoma of the brain, all known to be associated with HIV infection
Subgroup E	Other conditions in HIV infection: a variety of clinical findings which may be attributable to HIV disease, including chronic lymphoid interstitial pneumonitis, constitutional symptoms not in subgroup IVA, patients with infectious diseases not in subgroup IVC, and patients with neoplasms not in subgroup IVD.

Adapted from Centers for Disease Control (1986).

Supported by a grant of the III Project AIDS. Istituto Superiore di Sanità (Italian Ministry of Health).

or more months, while the term AIDS-related complex has generally been used for patients with weight loss, fever, night sweats, or infections not included in the AIDS definition (Centers for Disease Control 1986).

Dealing with neoplasms in AIDS means not only antineoplastic treatment but also management of opportunistic infections and attempts at antiretroviral therapy of HIV. In fact, the first sign of underlying HIV infection may be the appearance of an opportunistic infection. This is often present atypically in HIV-infected patients, frequently in the form of disseminated disease and characterized by a high density of organisms. Conventional treatments are often inadequate since these infections tend to persist in HIV patients and usually require long-term suppressive therapy. Typically, the infections may be viral, bacterial, protozoan, or fungal in origin (Kovacs and Masur 1988).

While the diagnostic and therapeutic approaches to life-threatening opportunistic infections have been constantly improving and much information on the subject is now available (Glatt et al. 1988; Klein 1989), to date only two agents, zidovudine (azidothymidine, AZT) and didanosine (dideoxy hosine, DDI) have been definitely shown to alter the usually rapidly fatal course of AIDS (Fischl 1989; Kahn et al. 1992).

With this brief background, we can now turn our attention to the oncological aspects of AIDS.

EPIDEMIC KAPOSI'S SARCOMA

Introduction

The most frequently encountered neoplasm in HIV-positive patients is an aggressive variant of Kaposi's sarcoma. This tumour was first described by the Hungarian dermatologist Moritz Kaposi over 100 years ago in an article entitled 'Idiopathic multiple pigmented sarcoma of the skin' (Kaposi 1972). The classical form of Kaposi's sarcoma is rare and affects elderly patients of predominant Mediterranean or Jewish origin living in the United States and Europe. The lesions usually start with a reddish nodule on the lower extremity. The disease is generally indolent. In 1950 an African variant was described; in equatorial Africa this form is endemic and relatively frequent (3–9 per cent of all neoplasms). This variant is usually more aggressive than the classical Kaposi's sarcoma with multiple localizations.

Kaposi's sarcoma in HIV-positive patients, which has been defined as epidemic Kaposi's sarcoma, develops predominantly in homosexual men and to a much less extent in other risk groups such as intravenous drug users, haemophiliacs, polytransfused heterosexuals, and children of infected parents. The incidence of this neoplasm in patients with AIDS ranges from 3 to 46 per cent for the various risk groups (Harwood et al. 1979; de Jarlais et al. 1984; Safai et al. 1985; Groopman 1987; Krigel and Friedman-Kien 1988).

Kaposi's sarcoma has also been reported in organ transplant recipients treated with immunosuppressive agents (Harwood et al. 1979) and in patients treated with alkylating agents for multiple myeloma (Kapadia and Krause 1977).

Incidence and epidemiology

More than 70 per cent of all cases of epidemic Kaposi's sarcoma in the United States have been reported in homosexual or bisexual men (de Jarlais et al. 1984; Safai et al. 1985; Groopman 1987; Krigel and Friedman-Kien 1988). After an initial rapid increase, the proportion of epidemic Kaposi's sarcoma steadily declined from nearly half in 1981 to 15 per cent in 1986 in the USA (Biggar 1992) and from 38 per cent in 1983 to 14 per cent in 1991 in Europe (Serraino 1992). In Italy, where 66 per cent of AIDS patients are intravenous drug users and only 15 per cent are homosexual men, out of 9792 cases of AIDS reported up to June 1991 (Ministero della Sanità, Centro Operativo AIDS, personal communication) only 9 per cent had epidemic Kaposi's sarcoma (Vaccher et al. 1989a). In the other risk groups epidemic Kaposi's sarcoma has been described in 16 per cent of intravenous drug users with AIDS and in approximately 3 per cent of haemophiliacs and polytransfused heterosexuals with AIDS in the United States (Harwood et al. 1979; de Jarlais et al. 1984; Safai et al. 1985; Groopman 1987; Krigel and Friedman-Kien 1988). In Italy 30 per cent of epidemic Kaposi's sarcoma has been described in homosexual men, 9 per cent in heterosexuals, 9 per cent in intravenous drug users and homosexual men, 3 per cent in intravenous drug users, and 3 per cent in haemophiliacs and polytransfused heterosexuals (Ministero della Sanità, Centro Operativo AIDS, personal communication). Approximately 1 per cent of paediatric patients, whose parents had or were at risk of AIDS, have developed epidemic Kaposi's sarcoma in the United States (Krigel and Friedman-Kien 1988). Epidemic Kaposi's sarcoma has been described, in Central Africa, as well as in the United States and Western Europe.

Aetiology and pathogenesis

The nature of the Kaposi's sarcoma malignant cell is controversial but is generally linked to an endothelial origin. This has been suggested by the presence of the factor VIII, which is a histochemical marker of the cells of endothelial tissue, in the cellular components of the tumour (Jaffe 1977; Flotte et al. 1984).

Kaposi's sarcoma appears to be a sexually transmitted disease, independent of HIV, as demonstrated by epidemiologic patterns. A relationship between history of oral–faecal contact and subsequent development of Kaposi's sarcoma has been demonstrated (Beral et al. 1992). Cytomegalovirus has been associated with both the classical and the epidemic form of Kaposi's sarcoma. Elevated serological titres to cytomegalovirus have been found in patients with both forms. Cytomegalovirus viral DNA sequences were detected in biopsy specimens of neoplastic cells from Kaposi's sarcoma (Giraldo et al. 1980; Giraldo and Beth 1986). These data, together with the fact that cytomegalovirus infection is sexually transmitted and hyperendemic among homosexual men, has suggested a causal relationship with epidemic Kaposi's sarcoma. However, cytomegalovirus is associated with all forms of Kaposi's sarcoma and therefore cannot be considered characteristic of epidemic Kaposi's sarcoma. At the present time it is not yet established whether cytomegalovirus plays a significant role as a co-factor or simply represents an opportunistic infection.

Another co-factor associated with epidemic Kaposi's sarcoma is the presence of the antigen DR5 in the major histocompatibility system HLA. This has been observed in 60 per cent of males with both epidemic and classical Kaposi's sarcoma, but only in 20–24 per cent of control groups, indicating that the presence of this antigen increases many-fold the risk of development of Kaposi's sarcoma. HLA Dr2 has also been reported with higher frequency in these patients (Pollack et al. 1983). Other co-factors probably include repeated exposure to antigenic stimuli for example, the recreational use of nitrates as inhalants which act as immunodepressants. In this general scenario it should be noted that HIV per se plays an important role as a producer of immunodepression.

Recent studies showed that HIV regulatory proteins and some cytokines may be operative in the pathogenesis of Kaposi's sarcoma. Expression of the HIV-tat gene may initiate the process of cell transformation, as demonstrated by Vogel *et al.* (1988). Moreover, CD4 cells chronically infected by HIV produce Oncostatin M, a cytokine which, both directly and indirectly via induction of interleukin-6 (IL-6), serves as a major growth factor for Kaposi's sarcoma (Gallo *et al.* 1984; Nakamura *et al.* 1988; Miles *et al.* 1992). The full pathogenesis of epidemic Kaposi's sarcoma may thus involve a complex interplay of genetic factors, immunocompromise, and additional factors, such as unidentified sexually transmitted organism(s) and/or HIV-tat protein, the latter of which may initiate transformation by altering the expression of certain receptors on the Kaposi's sarcoma cell. In this setting, for Kaposi's sarcoma a cascade of other cytokines derived from HIV-infected mononuclear cells may also be associated with increased growth of Kaposi's sarcoma (Molina *et al.* 1989; Huang *et al.* 1992).

Pathology

The histopathology of all the clinical variants of Kaposi's sarcoma is similar. Differences in the histological description have been related to the progression of lesions from patches and plaques to nodules. The histological description of the initial lesions (patch or plaque stage) shows only minor changes such as an increase in the number of bizarre dilated vascular spaces lined with endothelial cells (Safai *et al.* 1985) and irregular vessels (Fig. 1). In the dermis there is a perivascular mononuclear cell infiltrate of lymphocytes and plasma cells. An increased number of spindle-shaped cells are present and extravasated erithrocytes and siderophages are often found in the cellular spaces between the spindle cells (Fig. 2). In the more advanced lesions (nodular), the endothelial component is reduced and compressed by bundles of spindle-shaped cells. Slit-like or irregular vascular spaces have been described. The inflammatory cells are absent at this point.

The lymph nodes involved contain multiple small foci of Kaposi's sarcoma tumours in the capsular and sinusoid regions (Fig. 3). The disseminated Kaposi's sarcoma lesions in visceral organs are proximate and associated with organ vessels.

Diagnostic aspects

The classical variant of Kaposi's sarcoma presents in older men (50–80 years) of Mediterranean or Jewish origin and is usually confined to the extremities with lymphoedema. The course is indolent, visceral involvement occurs late, and the median survival ranges from 10 to 15 years.

The African variant of Kaposi's sarcoma affects young adult black men and is characterized by aggressive tumours with localized nodular and indolent lesions or invasive lesions with slow but

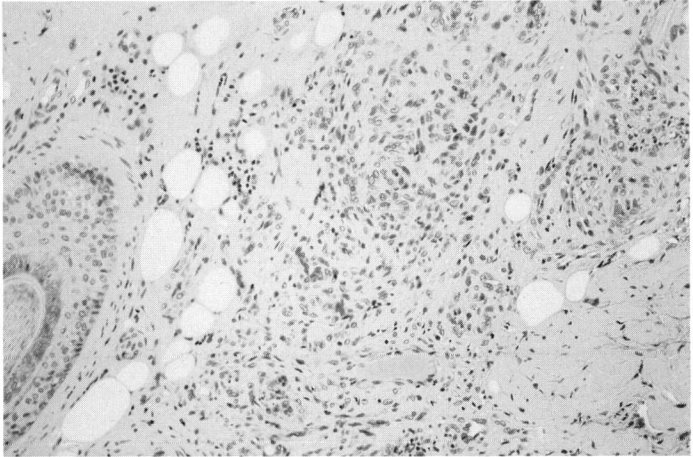

Fig. 1 Skin infiltration by 'early' Kaposi's sarcoma: several bizarre atypical cells with dilated vascular spaces can be seen.

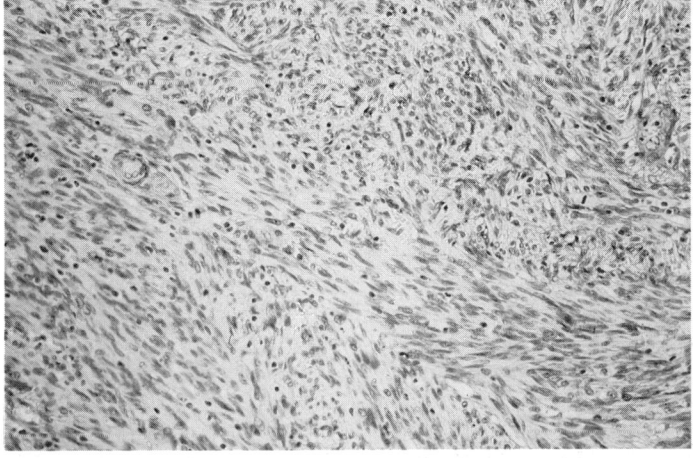

Fig. 2 Kaposi's sarcoma with sarcomatous pattern lesions of spindle-shaped neoplastic cells.

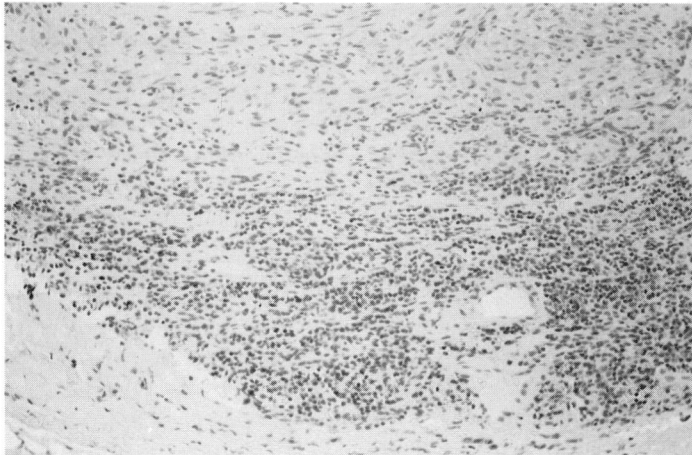

Fig. 3 Lymph node with capsular infiltration by Kaposi's sarcoma.

progressive development (median survival 5–8 years). In African children Kaposi's sarcoma rarely involves the skin, but is characterized by rapidly progressive disease (median survival 5–8 years).

The renal transplant variant affects patients after immuno-suppressive treatment. The disease can then be localized and indolent or rapidly progressive and may improve when immuno-suppressive therapy is interrupted. In approximately one-third of cases death is attributable to Kaposi's sarcoma progression.

The epidemic variant of Kaposi's sarcoma affects HIV-positive patients, predominantly homosexual men and to a lesser extent intravenous drug users. It presents with disseminated cutaneous lesions, often with lymph node and visceral involvement (gastrointestinal tract and lungs). After 2 years survival is more than 80 per cent in patients without opportunistic infections and less than 20 per cent in patients with opportunistic infections.

The majority of patients who initially present with the multiple cutaneous lesions of epidemic Kaposi's sarcoma are usually free of systemic symptoms, but systemic manifestations such as weight loss and fever (AIDS-related complex) may be present simultaneously or even precede the appearance of tumour lesions by several months. Kaposi's lesions in patients may be quite subtle at onset.

Clinicians caring for persons at high risk of AIDS should consider any new skin lesions with suspicion. Skin biopsy is then indicated for evaluation of any new suspicious dermatological lesion in HIV-positive patients. The initial lesions may occur anywhere on the integument or in the oropharynx, lymph nodes, and visceral organs. In epidemic Kaposi's sarcoma there is no clear predilection for initial involvement of the lower extremities, but widespread lesions at onset frequently involve skin, oral mucosa, lymph nodes, and visceral organs such as the gastrointestinal tract and lung.

Skin lesions of Kaposi's sarcoma occur as flat or raised plaques with dimensions ranging from a few millimetres to 2–3 cm and colour from blue–purple to red–brown (Safai *et al.* 1985). The majority of patients present with skin lesions; however, the clinician should remember that approximately 10 per cent of patients present with enlarged lymph nodes only and no skin lesions. In these cases only a biopsy will disclose whether one is dealing with epidemic Kaposi's sarcoma, persistent generalized lymphadenopathy, or lymph-nodal mycobacteria infection. Approximately 5 per cent of patients present with only oral or gastrointestinal Kaposi's sarcoma without cutaneous or lymph node involvement. Lesions from Kaposi's sarcoma have been observed at autopsy in all organs

Table 2 Sites and organs of involvement in 197 patients with Kaposi's sarcoma

Sites and organs	No. of patients	Percentage
Skin alone	86	44
Skin + other	86	44
Lymph node alone	5	3
Lymph node + other	27	14
GI tract alone	10	5
GI tract + other	69	35
Lung alone	3	2
Lung + other	14	7
Tonsil + other	4	2
Liver + other	3	2
Penis + other	5	3
Others	16[a]	8

[a]Conjunctiva, 4; bronchi, 3; kidney, 2; pleura, 2; pericardium, 1; adrenal gland, 1; nasopharynx, 1; larynx, 1; gum, 1.

including brain, pancreas, heart, and blood vessels. These lesions remain generally asymptomatic, although in some cases patients present with bowel obstruction. In contrast with involvement of other lesions, lung involvement is generally asymptomatic. It can be associated with mediastinal or hilar adenopathies and may show an appearance of interstitial pneumonia. Bronchial biopsy or sputum cytology are generally inadequate for diagnosis. The most useful diagnostic procedures are mediastinoscopy or open-lung biopsy. Epidemic Kaposi's sarcoma with lung involvement may present with fever and shortness of breath. The presumptive first diagnosis may be that of *Pneumocystis carinii*. Table 2 shows the initial sites of involvement of 197 Italian patients with epidemic Kaposi's sarcoma. In addition to skin, the most frequent locations were the gastrointestinal tract, lymph nodes, and lungs. Only 13 per cent of patients had oral involvement. Figures 4–7 show the main clinical pictures of Kaposi's sarcoma at physical examination (skin and oral cavity).

Eventually almost all patients with epidemic Kaposi's sarcoma develop aggressive disease. Progression often consists in the appearance of numerous lesions, with lymph node and gastro-intestinal tract involvement. In addition to epidemic Kaposi's sarcoma lesions, systemic manifestations may be present simultaneously or even precede the appearance of the tumour lesion by several months and include persistent and unexplained weight loss, diarrhoea, malaise, and fatigue. Persistent progressive viral

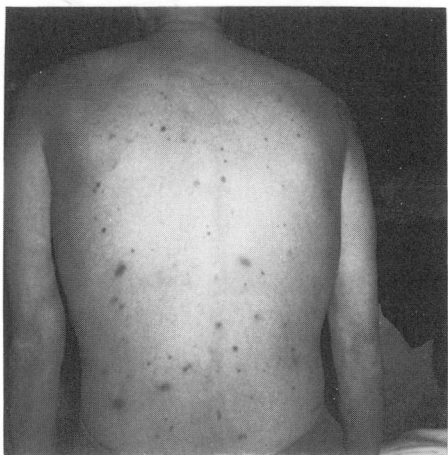

Fig. 4   Dorsal skin lesions.

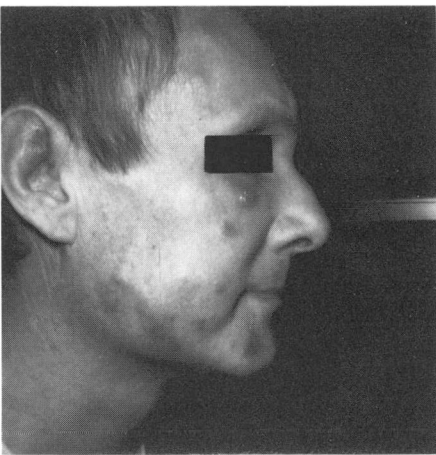

Fig. 5   Skin lesions of the face.

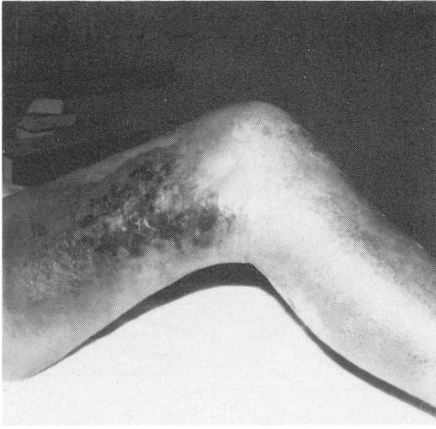

Fig. 6   Extensive skin and soft tissue involvement in the leg.

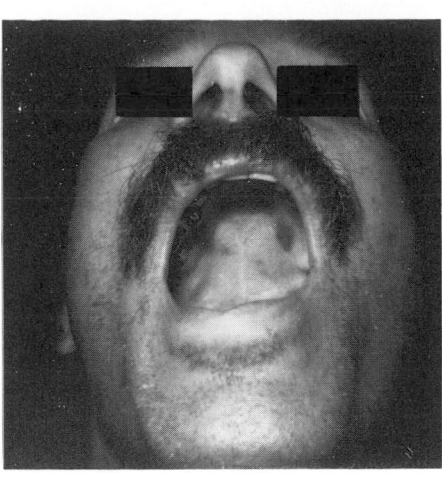

Fig. 7   Lesions of the oral mucosa.

patients with epidemic Kaposi's sarcoma have a marked reduction in the number of the T–helper lymphocytes and an inversion of the ratio of T-helper to T-suppressor lymphocytes. Leucopenia and mild anaemia are common in patients with epidemic Kaposi's sarcoma; other laboratory abnormalities characteristic of AIDS are described elsewhere in this text.

Staging

Various staging classifications for epidemic Kaposi's sarcoma have been proposed to account for the variation in the disease presentation and to facilitate following the progression of the disease and evaluating the response to therapy. The most widely used staging classification is that of Kriegel *et al.* (1988) of New York University. Stage I represents cutaneous locally indolent Kaposi's sarcoma, stage II represents cutaneous locally aggressive disease, stage III defines generalized cutaneous and/or lymph node involvement and/or minimal gastrointestinal disease, and stage IV represents the presence of visceral disease. A means that there are no systemic signs such as symptoms and B means that systemic signs such as 10 per cent weight loss or fever higher than 42.4 °C orally are present, unrelated to an identifiable source of infection and lasting for more than 2 weeks. According to this classification, the majority of patients in the United States and Europe present with stage III or stage IV disease; only a minority have stage I and stage II (Safai *et al.* 1985). Approximately one-quarter of patients have B symptoms. This form of staging classification, originally described by Kriegel *et al.* (1988), is mainly based on the extent of disease but does not account for other factors that may influence survival in AIDS patients with epidemic Kaposi's sarcoma such as the presence of opportunistic infections, severity of immunosuppression, and anatomical site at initial presentation. A recent staging classification including all these factors has been proposed by Krown *et al.* (1989) (Table 3) and judged as worthy of immediate clinical use (Volberding 1989).

The examination required to determine disease extent in Kaposi's sarcoma should include a complete physical examination, rectal and oral cavity examination, a CT scan of the abdomen in order to evaluate the lymph nodes, spleen, and liver, gastroscopy and colon endoscopy, and chest radiography. However, the value of determining the full extent of the disease in epidemic Kaposi's sarcoma has been questioned by some authors (Groopman 1986). According to this opinion, full staging of Kaposi's sarcoma is not

disease such as genital herpes simplex infections, severe opportunistic infections, and cytomegalovirus enteritis are also common complications observed in patients with AIDS and epidemic Kaposi's sarcoma (Safai *et al.* 1985). The course of epidemic Kaposi's sarcoma may also be complicated by the occurrence of non-Hodgkin's lymphomas. The great majority of

Table 3 Recommended staging classification (Krown et al. 1989)

	Good risk (0) (all the following)	Poor risk (1) (any of the following)
Tumour (T)	Confined to skin and/or lymph nodes and/or minimal oral disease[a]	Tumour-associated oedema or ulceration Extensive oral KS Gastrointestinal KS KS in other non-nodal viscera
Immune system (1)	CD4 cells >200 per μl	CD4 cells <200 per μl
Systemic illness (S)	No history of OI or thrush No B symptoms[b] Performance status >70 (Karnowsky)	History of OI and/or thrush B symptoms present Performance status <70 Other HIV-related illness (for example, neurological disease, lymphoma)

KS, Kaposi's sarcoma; OI, opportunistic infections.
[a]Minimal oral disease in non-nodular KS confined to the palate.
[b]B symptoms are unexplained fever, night sweats, >10% involuntary weight loss, or diarrhoea persisting for more than 2 weeks.

required in all circumstances but only if indicated by symptom findings on physical examination or laboratory investigation. However, it is clear that the determination and accurate documentation (for example, photographs) of the extent of the disease is essential for the evaluation of possible new active drugs.

Natural history

Epidemic Kaposi's sarcoma may remain asymptomatic for 6–12 months in patients with AIDS not presenting with systemic B symptoms (fever, sweat, weight loss, and diarrhoea). Some patients may develop rapidly progressive Kaposi's sarcoma with multifocal appearance of lesions over the integument and mucosal cavities. Such patients often have visceral involvement and involvement of the conjunctiva and orbit. The median survival of AIDS patients with Kaposi's sarcoma is 18–24 months in most case series. The most important prognostic indicators for length of survival are clinical: the survival ranges of patients without B symptoms at a lower tumour stage with lack of prior opportunistic infections and high CD4 cell numbers are improved by 6–8 months. No difference in clinical presentation and evolution between homosexual men and intravenous drug users has been described so far. A small subset of asymptomatic patients with Kaposi's sarcoma appear to have a plateau in the survival curve at 2 years; however, this finding which is based on actuarial analysis, may not be sustained over a longer period of follow-up.

Therapy

Epidemic Kaposi's sarcoma may cause severe functional impairment (difficulty in walking, difficulty with eating) or may lead to psychological stress because of cosmetic disfiguration, but only in rare instances (extensive pulmonary involvement) does tumour progression from epidemic Kaposi's sarcoma lead to death. In fact, it has never been demonstrated that either local or systemic treatment of epidemic Kaposi's sarcoma alters the ultimate course of the disease. However, treatment may produce a disappearance or reduction of specific skin lesions or be successful in controlling

symptoms associated with mucosal or visceral lesions. Despite some temporary palliation, none of the existing modalities of treatment such as surgery, radiation therapy, or systemic treatment has been found to alter the development of new lesions substantially or has led to an increased survival or improvement of the underlying immunodeficiency. Some lesions of Kaposi's sarcoma can be treated by surgical excision, electro desiccation, or intralesional injection of vinblastine, vincristine, and α-interferon. However, surgery is usually used in order to make a diagnosis. Kaposi's sarcoma is generally very responsive to radiation therapy. Good palliation can be obtained with doses in the range of 2000 cGy (Hill 1987). Good functional and cosmetic results can only be obtained in localized cutaneous lesions and some rare but painful bone lesions; however, possible control of visceral lesions can be achieved in cases of oesophagus, stomach, anorectal, and lung involvement. Most of the experience of radiation therapy has been obtained in cutaneous lesions of epidemic Kaposi's sarcoma. Oral and pharingeal lesions are equally radiosensitive but successful control is less frequent.

Chemotherapy

The initial attempts at evaluating the effect of chemotherapy and the management of epidemic Kaposi's sarcoma were based on the experience gained with the classical African Kaposi's sarcoma variants. In classical Kaposi's sarcoma response rates of 90–95 per cent have been observed with vinblastine, although the duration of the response seldom lasted for more than 1 year and a positive effect on survival has never been documented. The chemosensitivity of Kaposi's sarcoma has also been well demonstrated in the African variant treated with bleomycin, BCNU, actinomycin D, and dacarbazine (Safai et al. 1985; Volberding 1987).

The initial chemotherapy trials of epidemic Kaposi's sarcoma relied on single agents such as vinblastine or etoposide (Volberding 1987). These preliminary trials led to the development of combination chemotherapy regimens including doxorubicin, bleomycin, vincristine, and vinblastine. Table 4 shows the results of single- and multi-agent chemotherapy in epidemic Kaposi's sarcoma. Overall, single-agent chemotherapy controls epidemic Kaposi's sarcoma in approximately 30 per cent of patients, while combination chemotherapy produces responses in approximately 80 per cent. Immunosuppression is a major problem in patients treated with cytotoxic chemotherapy. Because of immunodepression patients with epidemic Kaposi's sarcoma may develop opportunistic infections. Therefore, many clinicians have been reluctant to use cytotoxic chemotherapy. This difficulty has been based on the

Table 4 Single- and multiple-agent chemotherapy of epidemic Kaposi's sarcoma

Reference	Drug	Overall response rate (%)
Volberding et al. (1985)	VCR	26
Mintzer et al. (1985)	VLB	61
Wernz et al. (1986)	BLM	77
Laubenstein et al. (1984)	VP16	76
Bakker et al. (1988)	VP16	0
Gill et al. (1991)	ADM	53
Kaplan and Volberding (1986)	VLB+VCR	43
Wernz et al. (1986)	VLB+BLM	62
Laubenstein (1984)	ADM+BLM+VLB	86
Gill et al. (1991)	ADM+BLM+VCR	88
Minor (1988)	VLB+VCR+methotrexate	81

VCR, vincristine; VLB, vinblastine; BLM, bleomycin; ADM, adriamycin.

assumption that such treatment will increase the immunosuppression, thus accelerating the development of opportunistic infections. However, at present it is recommended that patients with rapidly progressive disease should be treated with combination chemotherapy, particularly if there is visceral involvement. Single-agent chemotherapy has not been shown to be consistently superior to combination chemotherapy. What is gained in overall efficacy tends to be lost in toxicity and vice versa.

Biological response modifiers

Although cytotoxic chemotherapy is effective in Kaposi's sarcoma, it may further compromise immune responses in patients with AIDS. For this reason biological response modifiers such as interferons have been widely studied. Many studies have confirmed the efficacy of high doses of recombinant α_2-interferon, generally from 18 to 54 million units/day intramuscularly followed by a maintenance regimen three times a week (Kaplan and Volberding 1986; Groopman 1987a; Bakker et al. 1988; Gill et al. 1988, 1991; Minor 1988; Groopman and Scadden 1989). The percentage of response to recombinant interferon in patients without opportunistic infections ranges from 30 to 50 per cent. However, if the patients have a history of opportunistic infections and/or B symptoms, the percentage of response is lowered to 20 per cent. A randomized study has shown that low doses are followed by a decrease in the number of objective responses (Abrams and Volberding 1987; Groopman 1987a). Responses to α-interferon are observed after 3–4 weeks of treatment but they do not usually last for more than 12 months (Safai et al. 1985; Groopman 1987a). Many patients receiving treatment with α-interferon present toxic signs consisting of fever, headache, muscular pain, anorexia, and weakness. Transient elevation of hepatic transaminases and bone-marrow depression is often observed. In general, treatment with α-interferon is well tolerated, but no decrease in the incidence of opportunistic infections has been observed. Interferon probably acts through direct cytotoxicity, but detailed studies of T-cell subsites, lymphocyte proliferation to antigen and mitogen, and natural killer cell activity have failed to demonstrate an immunopotentiating effect (Mitsuyasu and Groopman 1984). Combination of α-interferon with cytotoxic chemotherapy has shown no benefit compared with either agent alone (Courderc et al. 1987; Krown 1987). Encouraging results have been obtained with a combination of α-interferon and AZT (Krown et al. 1990; Fischl et al. 1991). Using daily doses of 8–10 million units of α-interferon with 500 mg of zidovudine, antiretroviral synergy has been demonstrated. Response rates were somewhat improved over those achieved with higher doses of α-interferon alone and equivalent response rates (approximately 30 per cent) were documented in patients with poor prognostic factors. Toxicity of the combination regimen included neutropenia, anaemia, and elevated liver enzymes.

Other biological response modifiers, such as interleukin-2 (IL-2) and γ-interferon, have been used in an attempt to reverse the underlying immunodepression, but so far no positive data have been reported (Krigel et al. 1985; Parker et al. 1988).

Guidelines for therapy

Since it is not yet known whether therapy in early epidemic Kaposi's sarcoma has a positive influence on survival, observation for 4–8 weeks in patients without rapidly progressive disease is indicated. Every therapy should be weighed considering that death is attributable to Kaposi's sarcoma tumour progression in only a few instances. Since optimum treatment of all stages and of the various

clinical presentations of epidemic Kaposi's sarcoma is still in an early phase of development, patients should be treated according to study protocols whenever possible. This is particularly advisable for patients who are also receiving AZT for their HIV infection because of the possible overlapping myelotoxicity of this agent with antiproliferative agents. Even if a patient is not entered in a well-established treatment protocol some general recommendations should be followed.

1. Localized Kaposi's sarcoma may be treated with surgery or radiation therapy.

2. Early stage indolent epidemic Kaposi's sarcoma may receive no treatment.

3. Indolent disseminated Kaposi's sarcoma can be treated with single-agent chemotherapy or with interferons plus AZT.

4. Aggressive disseminated Kaposi's sarcoma or Kaposi's sarcoma with systemic B symptoms can be treated with combination chemotherapy; specific organ dysfunction (for example, pulmonary disease) requires cytoreductive therapy.

5. Painful lesions, tumour-associated oedema, and cosmetic disfiguration require palliative radiotherapy or chemotherapy.

NON-HODGKIN'S LYMPHOMAS
Incidence and epidemiology

The incidence of non-Hodgkin's lymphomas among persons at risk of AIDS in the United States has significantly increased since the beginning of the AIDS epidemic in 1984 (Biggar et al. 1987, 1989; Kristal et al. 1988; Bernstein et al. 1989; Biggar 1992). The risk of developing non-Hodgkin's lymphomas among intravenous drug users of New York is 6–18 times greater than that of the general population of the same age not at risk of AIDS. In the same area the risk of developing non-Hodgkin's lymphomas among young single males increased by a factor of 2–6 compared with the years 1973–1976 and in Los Angeles the number of cases of non-Hodgkin's lymphomas diagnosed in single men doubled in the period 1983–1985 compared with the period 1980–1982 (Kristal et al. 1988). Single male does not equal homosexual male, but the majority of young homosexual men fall into this group. In the city of San Francisco the incidence of non-Hodgkin's lymphomas among homosexual men in 1984 was three times that in the years before the AIDS epidemic (Biggar et al. 1987). Non-Hodgkin's lymphomas in HIV-positive patients have also been reported in Europe, mainly in France and Italy, but no epidemiological data are available at present to determine whether increases in the incidence have also taken place. Recent studies showed that the estimated risk of lymphoma developing in a patient with symptomatic HIV infection has ranged between 1 and 2 per cent per year (Rabkin et al. 1992) to as high as 10 and 29 per cent in 3 years after institution of antiretroviral therapy, with didanosine and zidovudine, respectively (Pluda et al. 1993). HIV-infected patients are now living longer due to advances in antiretroviral therapy and treatment or prophylaxis against opportunistic infections, but because of their immuno-deficiency they are vulnerable to cancers, especially NHL. The majority of cases consists of high-grade non-Hodgkin's lymphomas with the B phenotype; the most common histologies are Burkitt's lymphoma and otherwise unspecified 'undifferentiated' lymphoma. Taking into account these as well as other epidemiological data, the Centers for Disease Control, Atlanta, produced a third definition of AIDS in the summer of 1987. According to this definition, in addition to primary central nervous system non-Hodgkin's lymphomas, intermediate- and high-grade non-Hodgkin's lymphoma with the B phenotype or a non-B non-T phenotype which develops in HIV-positive patients even in absence of Kaposi's sarcoma is considered diagnostic of AIDS (Centers for Disease Control 1987). In the United States non-Hodgkin's lymphomas represent 4–10 per cent of all AIDS cases (Levine 1987), while in Europe they represented 2.5 and 2.9 per cent of all cases reported to the WHO in 1988 and 1989, respectively (WHO 1988a, 1989a). According to the principal available reports, 20–61 per cent of patients with AIDS-related non-Hodgkin's lymphomas in the United States and 33–40 per cent of patients in Europe have a preceding diagnosis of AIDS at onset of the lymphoma because of opportunistic infection and/or Kaposi's sarcoma (Ziegler et al. 1984; Lowenthal et al. 1986; Knowles et al. 1988; Levine et al. 1988; Markowitz et al. 1988, Kaplan et al. 1989).

The median age is 35–40 years and the risk group affected in the majority of case series is homosexual men (Ziegler et al. 1984; Lowenthal et al. 1986; Andrieu et al. 1988a; Knowles et al. 1988; Levine et al. 1988; Markowitz et al. 1988; Kaplan et al. 1989; Monfardini et al. 1990). However, in some countries such as Italy and Spain, where the majority of AIDS patients are intravenous drug users, the largest group affected by non-Hodgkin's lymphomas is not of homosexual men but intravenous drug users. In the HIV-positive population the ratio of Hodgkin's disease to non-Hodgkin's lymphoma, which favours Hodgkin's disease up to the age of 30 years, is reversed with respect to the general population of the same young age owing to the marked increase of non-Hodgkin's lymphomas.

Pathogenesis

The study of the factors involved in the development of HIV-associated non-Hodgkin's lymphomas may represent a useful model for the interpretation of pathogenesis of other non-Hodgkin's lymphomas. As with epidemic Kaposi's sarcoma, immunodepression caused by this virus is probably the principal predisposing factor for the development of the lymphoma (Penn 1978, 1981; Spector et al. 1978). A correlation with a herpes virus infection, particularly the Epstein–Barr virus, is quite possible for the B-cell type lymphomas which represent the majority of HIV-associated non-Hodgkin's lymphomas (Klein 1975; List et al. 1987). A relationship between Epstein–Barr virus and the Burkitt lymphoma and nasopharyngeal carcinoma has been known for some time. Seroepidemiological studies indicate that at least 90 per cent of the world population is infected by this virus (Essex 1984) which targets B lymphocytes and epithelial cells. B-Lymphocyte infection mediated by virus receptors located on the cell surface causes polyclonal proliferation of B-cells in vitro (Rosen et al. 1977) and in vivo (Robinson et al. 1980). In a healthy subject the B-cell proliferation is probably blocked by cell-mediated immunity of the host in which the virus remains in a latent form in a small number of lymphocytes. In a subject with immunodepression, such as that due to HIV, the proliferation of B lymphocytes probably persists indefinitely and might result in the development of malignant clones. It is easy to envisage that high polyclonal B-cell proliferation might favour the appearance of chromosomal translocation which 'activates' some oncogenes with the consequent development of cellular clones which are initially multiple (oligoclonal) and then single (monoclonal), thus determining the appearance of the transformed clone (List et al. 1987). A characteristic reciprocal translocation between chromosomes 8 and 14 (t8; 14), 8 and 22 (t8; 22), and 8 and 2

(t8; 2) has been documented in both endemic and sporadic Burkitt's lymphoma. The breaking point is situated in the band q24 of chromosome B which is the locus of the c-*myc* gene. The active transcription of the c-*myc* gene determined by the chromosomal translocation in the proximity of loci which codify for the immunoglobulin (in chromosome 14 the genes for the heavy chains and in chromosome 22 those for the light K of the immunoglobulin) determines the successive development of the malignant clone (Klein 1975; dalla Fevera et al. 1982; List et al. 1987). The Epstein–Barr virus genom has been documented in 98 per cent of patients with endemic Burkitt's lymphoma and in 20–50 per cent of patients with the sporadic form (Ernberg and Altiok 1988). The rôle of Epstein–Barr virus in the genesis of HIV-associated lymphomas is supported by the following data.

1. In the majority of HIV-positive patients there are signs of an active Epstein–Barr virus infection which might be attributed to a reactivation of the previous infection (liberation of virions from the oropharyngeal epithelium, increase of the antibody titres anti-Epstein–Barr virus, and increase of circulating virus-infected B lymphocytes (Rosen et al. 1977).

2. The immunological defence mechanisms of patients with AIDS or AIDS-related complex cannot control the Epstein–Barr virus infection (Robinson et al. 1980). According to the majority of authors, the B-cell polyclonal proliferation which is characteristic of HIV-infected subjects is mainly attributable to the Epstein–Barr virus infection in association with the HIV immunodeficiency.

3. An oligoclonal proliferation of B lymphocytes has been documented in the lymph nodes of some patients with persistent generalized lymphadenopathy and with HIV-related non-Hodgkin's lymphomas (Pelicci et al. 1986).

4. The Epstein–Barr virus genome and/or the presence of nuclear antigens of the virus have been documented in 28–58 per cent of HIV-related lymphomas, usually the Burkitt type and to a lesser extent immunoblastic lymphoma (Rosen et al. 1977). Such positivity is intermediate between that reported in the endemic form and that seen in the sporadic form of Burkitt's lymphoma.

5. A characteristic chromosomal translocation t8; 14 (11 cases) and t8; 22 (four cases) has been documented in many associated lymphomas (93 per cent) with cytogenic analysis (Magrath et al. 1983; Ernberg and Altiok 1988; Palmer et al. 1989).

6. c-*myc* rearrangements have been documented in HIV-related non-Hodgkin's lymphomas (Pelicci et al. 1986).

Recent studies showed that HIV may induce the production of cytokines, which may induce B-cell proliferation (Nakajima et al. 1989).

In conclusion, it is probable that the full pathogenesis of lymphoma in the setting of HIV infection may involve multiple factors, including underlying immunosuppression, chronic B-cell proliferation (due to HIV, cytokine release, and/or Epstein–Barr virus), chromosomal abnormality, and subsequent dysregulation of c-*myc* and/or other oncogenes.

Pathology

The majority of HIV-associated non-Hodgkin's lymphomas are high-grade lymphomas with the B phenotype. This includes small non-cleaved cells, Burkitt or Burkitt-like lymphomas, and

Table 5 Principal case series of HIV-related non-Hodgkin's lymphomas in the United States

Reference	No. of patients	Risk group	Clinicopathological characteristics
Ziegler et al. (1984)	90	Homosexual men	High grade 62%, intermediate 29% Stages III–IV 58% Extranodal sites 98% (CNS, bone-marrow, GI tract, mucocutaneous sites) Median survival 6 months
di Carlo et al. (1986)	29	Homosexual men (28) Polytransfused heterosexuals (1)	High grade 28%, intermediate 45% Extranodal sites 90% Phenotype B Median survival 6 months for intermediate and 3 months for high grade
Ioachim et al. (1987)	31	Homosexual men (3) Polytransfused heterosexuals (1)	High grade 97% Extranodal sites 48% (CNS, GI tract, heart, testis, bladder, kidney) Low response rate to therapy
Levine et al. (1988)	62	Homosexual men (59)	High grade 87% Stage IV 63% Extranodal sites: CNS 32% GI tract 26%, bone-marrow 25% Median survival <1 year Opportunistic infections after intensive CT
Markowitz et al. (1988)	8	Homosexual men (5) IVDUs (3)	Stage IV 100% Severe cytopenia after conventional doses of CT Short survival
Knowles et al. (1988)	89	Homosexual men IVDUs (17)	High grade 69% Stage III–IV 53% Extranodal sites 87% (GI tract, CNS, liver) Phenotype B, polyclonality Median survival 5 months
Kaplan et al. (1989)	84	Homosexual men (78) IVDUs (4) Heterosexuals (2)	High grade 77% Stage III–IV 82% Extranodal sites (bone-marrow 31%, liver 26%, CNS 12%) Median survival <4.3 months
Egert and Beckstead (1988)	31	Homosexual men (31)	High grade 98% Stage I 68% (CNS 43%) Phenotype B
Lowenthal et al. (1986)	43	Homosexual men (41) IVDUs (2) Homosexual IVDU (1)	Intermediate, high grade 93% Stage IV 49% Extranodal sites 65% (bone-marrow 46%, CNS 40%, lung 25%) Median survival 6 months

IVDUs, intravenous drug users; CNS, central nervous system; GI, gastrointestinal.

immunoblastic lymphomas. The prevalence of high-grade histotypes ranges from 60 to 98 per cent in the principal American case series (Table 5) and 75–100 per cent in the European case series (Table 6). For comparison with the histological subgroups of the other non-HIV-related lymphomas it should be mentioned here that, out of 1175 cases of non-Hodgkin's lymphomas including American and European cases examined by a panel of pathologists and used to define the better known Working Formulation, high-grade lymphomas comprised 20 per cent (Lukes et al. 1978). The experience of the California University group published in 1978 showed similar results in 425 cases of non-Hodgkin's lymphomas (National Cancer Institute 1982). High-grade lymphomas were present in 86 per cent of the case series reported by the Italian Cooperative Group on AIDS-related tumours (Monfardini et al. 1990). HIV-associated, low-grade non-Hodgkin's lymphomas did not constitute more than 7–10 per cent of the cases mentioned above. Sporadic T-cell non-Hodgkin's lymphomas have been reported in HIV-positive patients (Kobayashi et al. 1984; Howard

and McVerry 1987; Presant et al. 1987). These lymphomas are typically high-grade and paradoxically some of them show a T-helper phenotype.

Diagnostic aspects

The clinicopathological characteristics and the natural history of HIV-related non-Hodgkin's lymphomas are quite different from those of non-Hodgkin's lymphomas of the general population (Tables 7–9). Most intermediate and high-grade non-Hodgkin's lymphomas in seropositive patients present at an advanced stage with more frequent involvement of unusual extranodal sites such as the small bowel, rectum, skin, heart, ureter, central nervous system, bone-marrow, etc., than in non-Hodgkin's lymphomas diagnosed in the normal population. Disease confined to the lymph nodes is rare, in contrast with non-Hodgkin's lymphomas of the general population where over 60 per cent of cases have a lymph-nodal presentation. HIV-related non-Hodgkin's lymphomas at onset

Table 6 Literature review of HIV-related non-Hodgkin's lymphomas in Europe

Reference	No. of patients	Risk group	Clinicopathological characteristics
Raphael *et al.* (1986)	16	?	Immunoblastic lymphoma, 69% Burkitt's lymphoma (CNS, bone-marrow, mucosa)
			Median survival 9 months
Skinhoj *et al.* (1987)	3	Homosexual men (2)	High grade 3/3
		Haemophiliacs (1)	Stage III–IV 3/3
Jara *et al.* (1987)	5	Homosexual men ?	High grade 5/5
		IVDUs ?	Stage III–IV 5/5
			Reduced response rate to therapy
Huhn and Serke (1988)	16	Homosexual men?	Intermediate–high grade
		IVDUs ?	Stage II–IV 100%
			Extranodal sites 81% (CNS 38%, liver 31%, bone-marrow 31%)
			Phenotype B
Andrieu *et al.* (1988*a*)	92	Homosexual men (65)	High grade 96%
		IVDUs (8)	Stage III–IV 52%
		Heterosexuals (8)	RC after CT+RT 37%
		Polytransfused heterosexuals (4)	High mortality 54%
		Homosexual+IVDUs (4)	
		Unknown (8)	
Schmid (1987)	17	?	?
Oksenhendler *et al.* (1989)	53	Homosexual men ?	High grade 100%
		IVDUs ?	Stage III–IV 58%
Monfardini *et al.* (1990)	150	IVDUs (96)	High grade 73%
		Homosexual men (31)	Stage III–IV 66%
		Others (23)	

IVDUs, intravenous drug users; CNS, central nervous system.

present an advanced stage (Ann Arbor stages III and IV) in 53–100 per cent of cases with extranodal site involvement in 31–98 per cent of patients (Ziegler *et al.* 1984; Ioachim *et al.* 1987; Levine 1987; Oksenhendler *et al.* 1989; Monfardini *et al.* 1990). The central nervous system is the most involved organ either as the only site of disease or in association with other localizations (Ziegler *et al.* 1984; Monfardini *et al.* 1990). Primary central nervous system lymphomas represent only 0.3–1.6 per cent of all non-Hodgkin's lymphomas in the general population while, in contrast, HIV-related non-Hodgkin's lymphomas present with an incidence ranging from 3 to 36 per cent in the various case series previously reported. Central nervous system lymphoma appears as a single or multiple lesion which is located preferably in the white paraventricular matter, the ganglia of the base, the talamus, the corpus callosus, or the cerebral vermes (Snider *et al.* 1983). From a morphological point of view this is similar to the non-Hodgkin's lymphomas which develop in other sites, but the most frequently represented type is the immunoblastic lymphoma. Distinguishing between lymphomatous central nervous system involvement and opportunistic infections within the central nervous system is extremely difficult on purely clinical criteria in the absence of biopsy. The clinical and radiological characteristics are quite often similar. However, invasive diagnostic procedures such as stereotactic biopsy or open-sky biopsy after craniotomy may present practical problems in patients with poor performance status and in bad general condition. This consideration explains why a high number of cases of central nervous system involvement from non-Hodgkin's lymphomas are diagnosed only at autopsy (Gill *et al.* 1985). Bone-marrow is the second most involved site after central nervous system and is affected in 21–46 per cent of patients. The degree of bone-marrow infiltration may vary, with consequent variability of cytopenia in the pepripheral blood which may be absent in some cases.

Gastrointestinal tract involvement develops in 7–39 per cent of cases. All gastrointestinal segments can be affected by the lymphoma; in some patients extended involvement from the oesophagus to the anus has been documented radiographically and then at autopsy (Ziegler *et al.* 1984; Lowenthal *et al.* 1986). One characteristic of American case series is the presence of bulky rectal disease alone at onset or together with widespread disease in homosexual patients (Ziegler *et al.* 1984; Burkes *et al.* 1986; Levine 1987; Knowles *et al.* 1988; Levine *et al.* 1988; Morrison *et al.* 1989). This observation has been quite rare in the Italian case series where most of the patients are intravenous drug users (Monfardini *et al.* 1988). Among the unusual extranodal sites, cardiac lesions should be noted. The clinical presentation may be indistinguishable from myocardial infarction and the best diagnostic procedure is echocardiography.

In a third of cases the onset of lymphomas is preceded by persistent generalized lymphadenopathy. Enlargement of pre-existent lymph nodes requires a biopsy to exclude the suspicion of development of malignant lymphoma. Ideally, staging procedures in HIV-related lymphomas should be superimposed on those used for the general population of non-Hodgkin's lymphomas. Although poor performance status and bad general condition may be an obstacle to a thorough staging assessment, bone-marrow biopsy, chest radiography, CT scan of thorax and abdomen, gastrointestinal tract radiography, ear, nose, and throat examination, and lumbar puncture are recommended in all instances.

Therapy and prognosis

Primary central nervous system involvement and the presence of proceeding or concomitant opportunistic infections at diagnosis represent the main unfavourable prognostic factors in HIV-related

Table 7 HIV-associated solid tumours: literature review

Tumour type	No. of patients	Group at risk	HIV disease	Clinicopathological characteristics	Reference[a]
Anal cancer (squamous cell, cloacogenic)	>100	Homosexual men	?	Young age High prevalence in patients with anal condylomata Association with HPV16 infection	1–8
Oral cancer (squamous cell)	>100	Homosexual men	?	Young age	8–12
Testicular cancer (Embryonal cell, seminoma, embryonal mixed)	58	Homosexual men IVDUs ARC AIDS	Only HIV+ PGL	Aggressive (course two cases)	9–15
Cervical cancer (squamous cell)	56	IVDUs Heterosexuals Polytransfused heterosexuals	?	Young age TIS 33/56 T1 22/56 T4 1/56	8, 14, 16–19
Lung cancer (SCLC, non-SCLC, mesothelioma)	16	Homosexual men IVDUs Polytranfused heterosexual	Only HIV+ PGL ARC AIDS	Young age	6, 8, 10, 14, 20
CNS cancer (glioblastoma medulloblastoma)	6	IVDUs	ARC	None	8, 10
Colon cancer (adenocarcinoma)	5	IVDUs Heterosexuals Homosexual men	Only HIV+ PGL AIDS	Young age (two cases)	8, 10, 14, 21
Pancreatic cancer (adenocarcinoma)	2	IVDUs	Only HIV+	None	8, 14
Oesophagus carcinoma (squamous cell)	3	Heterosexuals Haemophiliacs	AIDS	None	22, 23

SCLC, small cell lung cancer; CNS, central nervous system; IVDUs, intravenous drug users; ARC, aids-related complex; PGL, persistent generalized lymphadenopathy.
[a]Key to references: 1, Austin (1982); 2, Peters and Mack (1983); 3, Sonnabend et al. (1983); 4, Frazer et al. (1986); 5, Scholefield et al. (1987); 6, Lake-Lewin and Arkel (1988); 7, Crombleholme (1989); 8, Vaccher et al. (1989b); 9, Tessler and Catanese (1987); 10, Gastaut et al. (1988); 11, Schmid (1988); 12, Sansone et al. (1989); 13, Damstrup et al. (1989); 14, Monfardini et al. (1989b); 15, Palmer et al. (1989); 16, Byrne et al. (1988); 17, Crocchiolo et al. (1988); 18, Provencher et al. (1988); 19, Spurrett et al. (1988); 20, Hoffken et al. (1988); 21, Cappell et al. (1988); 22, Frager et al. (1988); 23, Nakamura et al. (1988).

Table 8 HIV-associated solid tumours: literature review

Tumour type	No. of patients	Group at risk	HIV disease	Clinicopathological characteristics	Reference[a]
Malignant melanoma	5	IVDUs Homosexual men Homosexual IVDU	ARC AIDS	Associated with HD or epidemic KS (two cases)	1–3
Skin cancer (squamous cell)	3	Homosexual men Haemophiliacs	ARC AIDS	Metastatic basal cell cancer (two cases) Multiple squamous cell cancer	3, 4
Carcinoid tumour	2	IVDUs	ARC	Unusual site (tonsil one case)	3, 5
Rhabdomyosarcoma of probable galls	1	Daughters of Haitians	AIDS	Lymphoproliferative disorder associated with EBV infection	3
Fibrosarcoma of liver	1	African children	AIDS	Young age (8 years)	3
Breast cancer	1	?	?	None	6
Bone tumour	1	Homosexual man	Only HIV+	Metastatic disease	??
Renal cancer (adenocarcinoma)	1	Unknown	Only HIV+	Associated with epidemic KS	7
Thyroid carcinoma (adenocarcinoma)	1	IVDU	Only HIV+	None	7
Thymoma	1	IVDU	Only HIV+	None	7

IVDUs, intravenous drug users; ARC, AIDS-related complex; HD, Hodgkin's disease; KS, Kaposi's sarcoma; EBV, Epstein–Barr virus.
[a]Key to references: 1, Gastaut et al. (1988); 2, Schmid (1988); 3, Vaccher et al. (1989b); 4, Overly and Jakubek (1987); 5, Weitberg et al. (1986); 6, Lake-Lewin and Arkel (1988); 7, Monfardini et al. (1989b).

Table 9 HIV-associated haematological malignancies: literature review

Tumour type	No. of patients	Group at risk	HIV disease	Clinicopathological characteristics	Reference[a]
B-cell acute lymphoblastic leukaemia	14	Homosexual men IVDUs Heterosexuals	Only HIV+ PGL ARC AIDS	ALL L3	1–5
Acute non-lymphoblastic leukaemia	3	Homosexual men IVDUs	PGL AIDS	Young age	6
Chronic lymphocitic leukaemia	9	Homosexual men IVDUs	ARC AIDS ?	Young age	6
Chronic myeloid leukaemia	1	Heterosexuals	?	None	6
Multiple myeloma	8	Homosexual men IVDUs	?	Young age	6

IVDUs, intravenous drug user; PGL, persistent generalized lymphadenopathy; ARC, AIDS-related complex.
[a]Key to references: 1, Flanagan *et al.* (1988); 2, List (1988); 3, Milpied *et al.* (1988); 4, Gold *et al.* (1989); 5, Monfardini *et al.* (1989*b*); 6, Vaccher *et al.* (1989*b*); 7, Berman *et al.* (1985); 8, Keyserlingk *et al.* (1988).

lymphomas (Ziegler *et al.* 1984). In general, the response to the various combination chemotherapy regimens is inferior to that obtained with the same combination in the general population of patients with non-Hodgkin's lymphomas of the same cell subtype. In the case series described by Ziegler *et al.* (1984), who reported results obtained with various combination chemotherapy regimens (CHOP, Pro-MACE/MOPP, and M-BACOD) with or without radiation therapy, complete remissions did not exceed 53 per cent, relapses were 54 per cent, and median survival was only 6 months. Comparable results in terms of response and survival have been reported by Lowenthal *et al.* (1986) with the same combination chemotherapy regimens. In these series patients achieved a 50 per cent complete remission rate; however, 41 per cent relapsed after a median of 4 months (range 3–7 months). The complete remission rate with M-BACOD regimen in the series reported by Gill *et al.* (1987*a*) was 54 per cent (seven out of 13 patients); however, the median survival did not exceed 11 months. Using the new combination chemotherapy regimen COMET-A (cyclophosphamide, vincristine, methotrexate, VP16, and IT methotrexate) Kaplan *et al.* (1989) obtained complete remission in 58 per cent of cases with a relapse rate of 31 per cent. These data are superior to those obtained with conventional chemotherapy. In this case series, unfavourable prognostic factors for survival were a low value of CD4 lymphocytes in the presence of opportunistic infections, low Karnowsky performance status, and the administration of a high dose of cyclophosphamide (more than 1 g/m^2). The results and opinions of the various authors on the intensity of treatment of AIDS-related non-Hodgkin's lymphomas are conflicting. In principle, since the majority of patients have high-grade histology, intensive combination chemotherapy should be administered. However, whether high- or low-dose chemotherapy should be used in immunocompromised patients with bone-marrow impairment due to HIV infection is often a real therapeutic dilemma.

Levine *et al.* (1991) postulated that 'less might be better' and evaluated a low-dose modification of the M-BACOD regimen. The complete remission rate with this combination chemotherapy was 46 per cent, with a median duration of survival for all patients of 5.6 months. However, patients with history of prior AIDS had a lower complete remission rate (25 per cent). Despite the low doses of chemotherapy, approximately 60 per cent of patients experienced nadir granulocyte counts less than $1000/\text{mm}^3$. On the other hand,

Gisselbrecht *et al.* (1993) employed the intensive LNH-84 regimen in 141 patients without previous history of opportunistic infections and with good performance status, noting a complete remission rate of 63 per cent and a median survival of 9 months. A less intensive regimen administered with concomitant zidovudine to a group of 37 patients with poor prognostic factors (active opportunistic infections and poor PS) resulted in a complete remission rate of 16 per cent and median survival of only 3.5 months (Tirelli *et al.* 1992). It is thus apparent that future trials must stratify patients into good or poor prognostic categories in order to ascertain the optimal regimens for each group.

In an attempt to improve on the haematological toxicity profile, Kaplan *et al.* (1991) used granulocyte–macrophage colony-stimulating factor (GM-CSF) with the CHOP regimen. In this study GM-CSF was associated with higher nadir granulocyte counts and fewer chemotherapy cycles complicated by neutropenia and fever, when compared with CHOP given without concomitant GM-CSF. Serum HIV p-24 antigen levels increased during the third week of chemotherapy with GM-CSF, although its clinical significance could not be determined. Some differences between the natural history of the infectious complications of HIV infection in intravenous drug users and homosexual men (Burnerstone *et al.* 1988) have suggested that intravenous drug addiction may limit the intensity of treatment of AIDS-related non-Hodgkin's lymphoma. An analysis has been conducted by the Italian Cooperative Group on AIDS-related lymphomas based on the assumption that intravenous drug users could engage in behaviour that acts as a co-factor for the development of serious infections and also delay medical treatment until symptoms caused by non-Hodgkin's lymphomas were evident. The conclusion of this analysis was that intravenous drug use in non-Hodgkin's lymphomas should not be considered a limitation *per se* on the type or intensity of treatment. In this case series the overall median survival was 3.7 months for intravenous drug users and 3.6 months for homosexual men (Monfardini *et al.* 1990).

Since central nervous system is the most frequent site of relapse, cranial radiotherapy and prophylactic intrathecal administration of methotrexate is suggested in all patients. However, as yet there is no evidence that cranial prophylaxis in HIV-related non-Hodgkin's lymphomas decreases the incidence of this complication (Gill *et al.* 1987*a,b*). The prognosis for these patients is grim and overall survival is less than 1 year.

In summary the main problems of therapy for non-Hodgkin's lymphomas are as follows.

1. The presence of antecedent or concomitant opportunistic infections is an obstacle to full dose administration of cancer chemotherapy.

2. Reduced bone-marrow reserve due to possible non-Hodgkin's lymphomas involvement, HIV infection, opportunistic infections from cytomegalovirus or *Mycobacterium avium*, or treatment with AZT may render the optimum dose administration of antitumour drugs impossible.

3. Decreased treatment tolerance has a negative effect on both the intensity and duration of treatment.

In the future a possible decrease in the haematological toxicity after chemotherapy will be provided by the use of granulocyte colony-stimulating factor (G-CSF), that is not associated as GM-CSF with the potential stimulation of HIV replication (Perno *et al.* 1992). It is conceivable that this will allow an increase in intensity and a longer duration of treatment. Certainly, antiretroviral drugs need to be associated with combination chemotherapy in order to improve HIV-induced immunodepression. Zidovudine, itself associated with myelosuppression, may be very difficult to administer with combination chemotherapy. However, the simultaneous use of didanosine is an area of great interest.

In order to improve the response to therapy and survival in these patients future studies should also aim at correlating treatment tolerance to the type of infection. For example, it is easy to envisage that the endocarditis, bacterial pneumonia, and chronic liver insufficiency peculiar to intravenous drug users (Burnerstone *et al.* 1988) could further complicate the administration of antracycline and bleomycin as well as other antitumour drugs in this risk group but not in homosexual men.

OTHER TUMOURS IN HIV-POSITIVE PATIENTS
Hodgkin's disease

Hodgkin's disease is one of the most frequent neoplasms reported in patients with HIV infection after epidemic Kaposi's sarcoma and non-Hodgkin's lymphomas (Lowenthal *et al.* 1986; Raphael *et al.* 1986; Salahuddin *et al.* 1986; Huhn and Serke 1988; Knowles *et al.* 1988; Schmid 1988; Kaplan *et al.* 1989; Oksenhendler *et al.* 1989). Since Hodgkin's disease occurs typically in young adults it is not clear whether the cases described in the literature represent a true increase in the incidence of the disease or are merely a coincidence. Reports of possible increased incidence are quite recent (Bernstein *et al.* 1989) and need further confirmation since they refer only to New York State. The cases of Hodgkin's disease diagnosed in single men of this state in the period 1977–1985 doubled in 1985 compared with the pre-AIDS era (1973–1976).

Pathogenesis

The pathogenesis of Hodgkin's disease is less well known than that of non-Hodgkin's lymphomas. The existence of abnormalities of T lymphocytes, which remain even after the eradication of Hodgkin's disease in patients in the general population, has been known for a long time. The immunodeficiency due to HIV could increase the susceptibility to pathogens involved in the pathogenesis of Hodgkin's disease, but the immunodeficiency associated with Hodgkin's disease could also lead to increased susceptibility to HIV

(Safai *et al.* 1987). The rôle of the Epstein–Barr virus in the pathogenesis of Hodgkin's disease is the subject of controversy. Recent studies have documented the presence of the Epstein–Barr virus genome in clonal and episomal form in the Redstenberg cells of ten out of 12 lymph-nodal biopsies of patients with HIV and associated Hodgkin's disease (Crombleholme *et al.* 1989). Further information is required to understand the meaning of this association.

Pathology

Hodgkin's disease in HIV-positive patients was first described in the United States. Unusual sites such as skin, central nervous system, rectum, and bronchial tree have been described in North American case series. Another characteristic of American case series is the atypical diffusion of the lymphoma with non-contiguous lymph-nodal involvement. As far as the histology is concerned, the common characteristic of American and European series is the absence of lymphocytic predominance; in the majority of cases reported, the predominant histological type is mixed cellularity (Robert and Schneiderman 1984; Moore and Cook 1985; Scheib and Siegel 1985; Baer *et al.* 1986; Desablens *et al.* 1986; Mitsuyasu *et al.* 1986; Prior *et al.* 1986; Schoeppel *et al.* 1986; Temple and Andes 1986; Unger and Strauchen 1986; Alfonso *et al.* 1987; Bello *et al.* 1987; Colburn *et al.* 1987; de Luca *et al.* 1987; Góngora-Biachi *et al.* 1987; Kaplan *et al.* 1987; Palomera *et al.* 1987; Picard *et al.* 1987; Andrieu *et al.* 1988*b*; Brice *et al.* 1988; Devars du Mayne *et al.* 1988; Dimopolou *et al.* 1988; Gallagher and Meschter 1988; Gold *et al.* 1988; Keyserlingk *et al.* 1988; Socie *et al.* 1988; del Rio *et al.* 1989; de Mascarel *et al.* 1989; Lozano-Molero *et al.* 1989; Schurmann *et al.* 1989).

Diagnostic aspects

In all principal case series it is evident that the natural history of the disease in these subjects differs from that in the general population. In the United States 88 cases of Hodgkin's disease in HIV-positive patients have been described, mainly homosexual men (Robert and Schneiderman 1984; Moore and Cook 1985; Scheib and Siegel 1985; Baer *et al.* 1986; Mitsuyasu *et al.* 1986; Prior *et al.* 1986; Schoeppel *et al.* 1986; Temple and Andes 1986; Unger and Strauchen 1986; Colburn *et al.* 1987; de Luca *et al.* 1987; Góngova-Biachi *et al.* 1987; Kaplan *et al.* 1987; Gallagher and Meschter 1988; Gold *et al.* 1988; del Rio *et al.* 1989), in Europe outside Italy 65 cases have been described (Desablens *et al.* 1986; Alfonso *et al.* 1987; Bello *et al.* 1987; Palomera *et al.* 1987; Picard *et al.* 1987; Andrieu *et al.* 1988*b*; Brice *et al.* 1988; Devars du Mayne *et al.* 1988; Dimopolou *et al.* 1988; Keyserlingk *et al.* 1988; Socie *et al.* 1988; de Mascarel *et al.* 1989; Lozano-Molero *et al.* 1989; Schurmann *et al.* 1989), and in Italy 92 cases have been described (Tirelli *et al.* 1992). At diagnosis Hodgkin's disease presents in the advanced stage in 80 and 86 per cent of cases in the European and American series, respectively. In addition to unusual sites, a predominant characteristic of the American series is the atypical diffusion of the lymphoma which consists, for example, in the involvement of lung without concomitant mediastinal adenopathy and bone-marrow involvement in the absence of hepatosplenic disease. Massive extranodal involvement (bone, liver, spleen) with modest lymph-nodal disease at clinical staging is also frequent. So far, atypical presentation and diffusion has been less frequent in Europe. Hodgkin's disease in HIV-positive patients may occur in the asymptomatic phase of the HIV infection in 28–31 per cent of cases. Persistent generalized lymphadenopathy is present in approximately 28 per cent of European and American patients and in most cases lymph-nodal involvement from persistent generalized lymphadenopathy is difficult to distinguish clinically from Hodgkin's disease. AIDS-related complex is present at diagnosis of Hodgkin's disease in approximately 20 per cent of patients and AIDS itself is present in approximately the same percentage of cases.

Staging procedures

Appropriate staging is fundamental in the normal Hodgkin's disease population to plan the therapeutic approach. In HIV-positive patients with Hodgkin's disease bone-marrow biopsy should be performed in all instances, not only to detect possible bone-marrow involvement but also to determine whether there is impairment of bone-marrow reserve owing to the HIV infection. Lymphangiograms and abdominal CT scans should take differential diagnosis into account with enlargement of retroperitoneal lymph nodes from persistent generalized lymphadenopathy. Laparosplenectomy should be considered only in selected cases at clinical stages I and II, in the absence of systemic symptoms and opportunistic infections and with CD4 > 400/mm^3.

Therapy and prognosis

Haematological tolerance after conventional doses of combination chemotherapy (ABVD, MOPP, MOPP alternating with ABVD) is generally reduced even when the disease occurs in an early phase of the HIV infection. The complete remission rate after combination chemotherapy in patients with Hodgkin's disease and HIV infection ranges from 50 to 60 per cent; however, the median duration of complete response is short. The common characteristic of patients reported in the American and European case series is the aggressive course of the lymphoma which is often complicated by the occurrence of opportunistic infections and/or Kaposi's sarcoma. In the case series reported by Schoeppel et al. (1986) this complication occurred in 42 per cent of patients independent of the type of therapy used. Survival of this group of patients after the appearance of this complication ranged from 1 to 6 months. The median survival of HIV-positive patients with Hodgkin's disease is definitely less than that of subjects with Hodgkin's disease in the general population. In the majority of case series the median survival does not exceed 16 months. There are few data concerning radiation therapy in the treatment of Hodgkin's disease in HIV-positive patients since the number in the initial stages (I and II) is quite low.

Conclusions

The majority of HIV-positive patients with Hodgkin's disease in the United States is represented by homosexual men, whereas in European countries, where the majority of AIDS cases occur in intravenous drug users, Hodgkin's disease has been most frequently described in this risk group. The diagnosis of Hodgkin's disease in HIV-positive patients may not be easy, since in approximately half the patients the first manifestation is an increase in the size of a pre-existent adenopathy due to persistent generalized lymphadenopathy. Another problem is the difficulty in discriminating the B symptoms from those of HIV and opportunistic infections.

The optimum therapy of HIV-infected patients with Hodgkin's disease is not well codified. Aggressive combination chemotherapy is not well tolerated because of bone-marrow depression due to HIV infection and to AIDS therapy such as AZT. This explains the difficulty in completing antitumour chemotherapy. It is not clear whether intensive chemotherapy administration may favour the

occurrence of opportunistic infections and/or Kaposi's sarcoma with a more rapid evolution towards full-blown AIDS.

Solid tumours and other haematological neoplasms associated with the HIV infection

Neoplasms different from Kaposi's sarcoma and malignant lymphomas have been described in approximately 5 per cent of patients with AIDS. Invasive cervical cancer in HIV-infected women became an AIDS-defining condition on 1 January 1993 (CDC 1993). Several studies have found an increased prevalence of cervical dysplasia and in situ carcinoma among HIV-infected women (Alhashimi et al. 1985; Weitberg et al. 1986; Flanagan et al. 1988; List 1988; Milpied et al. 1988; Cavanna et al. 1989; Schafer et al. 1991; Laga et al. 1992). In a study on 310 HIV-infected women attending methadone maintenance and sexually transmitted disease clinics in the United States, cervical displasia was confirmed by biopsy and/or colposcopy in approximately 22 per cent, a prevalence rate ten times greater than that found among HIV-negative women attending family planning clinics (Sadeghi et al. 1988). Invasive cervical cancer is preventable by the proper recognition and treatment of cervical dysplasia. The addition of invasive cervical cancer to the list of AIDS-indicator diseases emphasizes the importance of integrating gynaecologic care into medical services for HIV-infected women.

While gynaecologic examination and Pap smears have been advised for HIV-infected women every 6–12 months, the Pap smears may be falsely negative. This was evidenced by a recent study of 241 women with normal Pap smears, who received follow-up evaluations every 4 months. Cervical intraepithelial neoplasia developed within 24 months in 28 per cent of HPV-positive women versus only 3 per cent of HPV-negative women over the same time period (Koutsky et al. 1992). The natural history of cervical disease appears more distinct in HIV-infected than in HIV-negative women, behaving in a more aggressive manner, with rapid evolution of disease, poorer responses to therapy, and increased risk of relapse (Maiam et al. 1990; Matorras et al. 1991). Among other neoplasms, there is a prevalence of squamous head and neck carcinoma and cloacogenic carcinomas of the rectum which were first reported in the United States (Conant et al. 1982; Alhashimi et al. 1985; Tessler and Catanese 1987; Crocchiolo et al. 1988; Gastaut et al. 1988; Kahn et al. 1988; Schmid 1988; Spurrett et al. 1988; Damstrup et al. 1989; Monfardini et al. 1989; Palmer et al. 1989; Sansone et al. 1989). However, neoplastic manifestations which occur in HIV-positive patients have not yet been studied in detail. Tables 7–9 provide a review of the literature describing cases of solid tumours and haematological malignancies (excluding Kaposi's sarcoma and malignant lymphoma) diagnosed in HIV-positive patients. A 2–3-fold increase in squamous carcinoma of the oral cavity and anorectal cloacogenic squamous carcinoma has been reported in HIV-positive patients compared with the normal male population of the same age (Alhashimi et al. 1985; Tessler and Catanese 1987; Crocchiolo et al. 1988; Gastaut et al. 1988; Kahn et al. 1988; Schmid 1988; Spurrett et al. 1988; Damstrup et al. 1989; Monfardini et al. 1989; Palmer et al. 1989; Sansone et al. 1989). These tumours are more frequent among homosexual men. A possible relationship with a viral origin (papilloma virus or herpes virus type II), similar to condilomas and carcinoma of the uterine cervix which has the same embryogenesis as the cloacogenic carcinoma, has been suggested (Sansone et al. 1989).

It is well known that numerous studies have documented an aetiological role of papilloma virus in the pathogenesis of condilomas and neoplasms of the genital tract. The infection from herpes simplex virus type II has been proposed as a promoter of the carcinogenesis in a uterine cervix already infected with papilloma virus. Presumably sexual habits play a fundamental role in the pathogenesis of carcinoma of the uterine cervix as well as in the neoplasms of the oral and anorectal mucosa, since this factor favours transmissions of oncogenic viruses as well as HIV. The immunodepression caused by HIV probably provides favourable conditions for viral replication and the development of this neoplasm at a young age. Other solid tumours, in particular germinal carcinomas of the testicle, lung cell carcinoma at a young age, and melanoma, have been reported in HIV-positive patients (Alhashimi et al. 1985; Tessler and Catanese 1987; Gastaut et al. 1988; Hoffken et al. 1988; Lake-Lewin and Arkel 1988; Schmid 1988; Damstrup et al. 1989; Monfardini et al. 1989b; Palmer et al. 1989; Sansone et al. 1989). A viral aetiology has been suggested for tumours of these types. In the case of embryonal carcinoma of the testicle a real increase in the incidence in the HIV population cannot be hypothesized with certainty because this tumour is typical of young age.

Case reports of B-phenotype acute lymphoblastic leukaemia as well as chronic lymphocytic leukaemia and multiple myeloma in HIV-positive patients are not surprising (Berman et al. 1985; Flanagan et al. 1988; Milpied et al. 1988; Gold et al. 1989; Voelkerding et al. 1989). During the polyclonal B-cell proliferation induced by the HIV infection a chromosomal rearrangement responsible for the development of the neoplastic clone may appear. Recently, Schneider and Picker (1985) have reported a myelo-dysplasia or pre-leukaemic picture in eight patients with AIDS. A probable multiple aetiology including immunological mechanisms, opportunistic infections, pharmacological therapy, and direct HIV action on the bone-marrow cannot be excluded. However, there are few data documenting a relationship between HIV infection and myelodysplasia and/or acute myeloid leukaemia (up to now only three cases with acute myeloblastic leukaemia have been reported). In conclusion, at the present time it might be premature to conclude that the population at risk for AIDS will not be at risk of tumours other than those which have been considered as diagnostic of AIDS. The number of tumours other than malignant lymphomas, Kaposi's sarcoma, and cervical cancer are now probably underestimated because their association with HIV infection is not diagnostic of AIDS and therefore their incidence is not reported to the central health authorities.

Even if the information currently available does not indicate a significant increase in the incidence of these malignancies among HIV-infected patients, clinical oncologists should be aware of a possible association between malignant tumours other than Kaposi's sarcoma, non-Hodgkin's lymphomas, and cervical cancer and HIV infection. Furthermore, they should consider performing HIV antibody testing on patients who have malignant tumours with unusual clinicopathological features, particularly when they occur in young people.

CONCLUSIONS

The problem of AIDS-related tumours deserves attention not only from a clinical point of view but also with respect to the possible progress achievable in understanding the aetiology and pathogenesis of neoplastic complications of these tumours and other human tumours which may be virus related.

It has been known for decades that some animal leukaemias and lymphomas can be induced by retroviruses. Experimental oncologists have been studying retroviruses extensively since they allow an understanding of unique biological processes such as the reverse flow of genetic information from RNA to DNA through reverse transcription, have provided biological models for the study of DNA recombination, and have facilitated both the identification of a large number of cellular oncogenes and the formulation of unifying models for the induction and progression of neoplastic diseases (Broder 1990; Lazo and Tsichlis 1990). One of the leading groups in this field at the National Cancer Institute made the major effort which led to the discovery and characterization of the virus responsible for AIDS.

However, while viral oncologists have made a major contribution to the understanding of the origin of AIDS, medical oncologists, primarily in the United States, have been fully involved in patient care and clinical research since the beginning of the epidemic. Should this happen in Europe as well? We believe that there are a number of reasons which render medical oncologists particularly suitable for following patients with AIDS and its neoplastic complications. Internists dealing with cancer are regularly confronted with patients in whom the incurable course of the disease will eventually lead to death. Dealing with this problem requires a particular strength of character and gentleness of mind in order not to abandon the patient and to provide him or her with all possible comfort and palliation of symptoms.

Medical oncologists have been described by an outside observer as needing to be peculiar types in the sense that they have to be satisfied with little success. While being frustrated by many therapeutic failures, at the same time they have devoted themselves to years of clinical research (Monfardini 1980).

Exactly the same psychological attitude is required towards the AIDS problem and an equal persistence in clinical research, where 'building brick by brick until the job is done' is necessary (both cancer and AIDS therapy). An overall philosophy is then required, for both patient care and clinical research. However, apart from these important considerations, since cancer patients can be immuno-depressed by chemotherapy and in some instances by their disease, medical oncologists were routinely treating patients with opportunistic infections long before the emergence of the AIDS epidemic.

The first drug that has so been demonstrated to be of use against AIDS, that is, AZT, was initially synthesized as an anticancer agent (Fischl 1989). The long experience in drug development and in phase I and II studies in oncology is another skill that can be also used in patients with AIDS. Furthermore, the need of a new methodology for rapid drug development in AIDS will probably have a positive effect on new drug development in the oncological field (Broder 1987, 1990). The final reason for the involvement of medical oncologists in neoplastic complications of AIDS is quite obvious: proper antitumour chemotherapy can be prescribed and administered only if they have full charge of patients in oncological wards. Too often in Europe seropositive patients with non-Hodgkin's lymphomas or Kaposi's sarcoma are treated by infectious disease specialists only. This situation can only be temporary, since the number of non-Hodgkin's lymphomas in HIV patients, particularly those treated with AZT, will increase substantially in the next decade, imposing a substantial health care burden (Gail et al. 1991).

ACKNOWLEDGEMENTS

The author wishes to thank Dr Emanuela Vaccher for critical revision of the manuscript and Dr Antonino Carbone for kindly providing the illustrations of the histology of Kaposi's sarcoma.

REFERENCES

Abrams DI, Volberding PA (1987). Alpha interferon therapy of AIDS-associated Kaposi's sarcoma. *Seminars in Oncology*, **14** (2, Suppl. 2):43–7.

Ahmed T, *et al.* (1987). Malignant lymphomas in a population at risk for acquired immunodeficiency syndrome. *Cancer*, **60**:719–23.

Alfonso GP, *et al.* (1987). Hodgkin's disease in HIV infected patients. *Proceedings of the European Conference of Clinical Oncology (ECCO 4)*, Madrid, 1–4 November 1987, Abstract 1051.

Alhashimi MM, Krasnow SH, Johnston-Early A, Cohen MM (1985). Squamous cell carcinoma of the epiglottis in a homosexual man at risk for AIDS. *Journal of the American Medical Association*, **253** (16):2366.

Andrieu JM, *et al.* (1988a). HIV-associated non-Hodgkin's lymphoma (NHL) in France. *Proceedings of the 13th Congress of the European Society of Medical Oncology (ESMO)*, Lugano, 30 October–1 November 1988, Abstract 55, C9.

Andrieu JM, *et al.* (1988b). HIV associated Hodgkin's disease in France. *Proceedings of the 13th Congress of the European Society of Medical Oncology (ESMO)*, Lugano, 30 October–1 November 1988, Abstract 24P, C6.

Austin DF (1982). Etiological clues from descriptive epidemiology: squamous cell carcinoma of the rectum and anus. *NCI Monographs*, **62**:89–90.

Baer DM, Anderson ET, Wilkinson LS (1986). Acquired immune deficiency syndrome in homosexual men with Hodgkin's disease. Three case reports. *American Journal of Medicine*, **80**:738–40.

Bakker PJ, Danner SA, Lange JM, Veenhof KH (1988). Etoposide for epidemic Kaposi's sarcoma: a phase II study. *European Journal of Cancer and Clinical Oncology*, **24** (6):1047–8.

Becker WB, *et al.* (1989). New T-lymphotropic human herpes viruses. *Lancet*, i:41.

Bello JL, Magallon M, Villar JM (1987). Hodgkin disease in haemophilia. *Annals of Internal Medicine*, **107** (2):257.

Beral V, Jaffe H, Weiss R (1991). Cancer surveys: cancer HIV and AIDS. *European Journal of Cancer*, **27**:1057–8.

Beral V, *et al.* (1992). Risk of Kaposi's sarcoma and sexual practices associated with faecal contact in homosexual or bisexual men with AIDS. *Lancet*, 632–5.

Berman M, *et al.* (1985). Burkitt cell acute lymphoblastic leukemia with partial expression of T-cell markers and subclonal abnormalities in a man with AIDS. *Cancer Genetics and Cytogenetics*, **16** (4):341–7.

Bernheim A, Berger R (1988). Cytogenetic studies of Burkitt lymphoma–leukemia in patients with acquired immunodeficiency syndrome. *Cancer Genetics and Cytogenetics*, **32** (1):67–74.

Bernstein L, Levin D, Menck H, Ross RK (1989). AIDS-related secular trends in cancer in Los Angeles county men: a comparison by marital status. *Cancer Research*, **49** (2):466–70.

Biggar RJ (1990). Cancer in acquired immunodeficiency syndrome: an epidemiological assessment. *Seminars in Oncology*, **17** (3):251–60.

Biggar R, Rabkin S (1992). The epidemiology of acquired immunodeficiency syndrome-related lymphoma. *Current Opinions in Oncology*, **4**:883–93.

Biggar RJ, Horm J, Goedert J, Melbye M (1987). Cancer in a group at risk of acquired immunodeficiency syndrome (AIDS) through 1984. *American Journal of Epidemiology*, **126** (4):578–86.

Biggar RJ, Burnett W, Mikl J, Nasca P (1989). Cancer among New York men at risk of acquired immunodeficiency syndrome. *International Journal of Cancer*, **43** (6):979–85.

Birx DL, Redfield RR, Tosato G (1986). Defective regulation of Epstein–Barr virus infection in patients with acquired immunodeficiency syndrome (AIDS) or AIDS-related disorders. *New England Journal of Medicine*, **314** (14):874–9.

Blumenfeld W, Egbert BM, Sagebiel RW (1985). Differential diagnosis of Kaposi's sarcoma. *Archives of Pathology and Laboratory Medicine*, **109** (2):123–7.

Brice P, *et al.* (1988). Maladie de Hodgkin chez deux femmes séropositives pour le virus de l'immunodéficience humaine. *Presse Medicale*, **17** (41):2201.

Broder S (1987). Identification of therapies against the retroviruses 569–574. Development therapeutics and the acquired immunodeficiency syndrome. *Annals of Internal Medicine*, **106**:568–81.

Broder S (1990). The interrelationship between acquired immunodeficiency syndrome and cancer research. *Seminars in Oncology*, **17** (3):375–8.

Burkes RL, *et al.* (1986). Rectal lymphoma in homosexual men. *Archives of Internal Medicine*, **146** (5):913–15.

Burnerstone RL, *et al.* (1988). A larger spectrum of severe HIV-1-related disease intravenous drug users in New York City. *Science*, **242**:916–19.

Byrne M, Taylor-Robinson D, Harris JRW (1988). Cervical dysplasia and HIV infection. *Lancet*, i:239.

Cappell MS, Yao F, Cho KC (1988). Colonic adenocarcinoma associated with the acquired immune deficiency syndrome. *Cancer*, **62** (3):616–19.

Cavanna L, *et al.* (1989). Carcinoma of the esophagus in a hemophiliac infected with the human immunodeficiency virus. *Haematologica*, **74**:411.

Centers for Disease Control (1986). Classification system for human T-lymphotropic virus type III/lymphadenopathy-associated virus infections. *Morbidity and Mortality Weekly Report*, **35** (20):334–9.

Centers for Disease Control (1987). Revision of the CDC surveillance case definition for acquired immunodeficiency syndrome. *Morbidity and Mortality Weekly Report*, **36** (Suppl. 1):15–155.

Centers for Disease Control (1993). Revised classification system for HIV infection and expanded surveillance case definition for AIDS among adolescents and adults. *Morbidity and Mortality Weekly Report*, **41**:1–18.

Colburn D, *et al.* (1987). Fulminant lymphocyte-depleted Hodgkin's disease in a homosexual man with HIV infection. *New York State Journal of Medicine*, **87** (10):570–1.

Conant MA, *et al.* (1982). Squamous cell carcinoma in sexual partner of Kaposi's sarcoma patient. *Lancet*, i:286.

Couderc LJ, *et al.* (1987). Treatment of AIDS-related Kaposi's sarcoma (KS/AIDS) by alpha-2-recombinant interferon and bleomycin. *Third International Conference on AIDS*, Washington, 1–7 June 1987, Abstract TP216.

Crocchiolo P, *et al.* (1988). Cervical dysplasia and HIV infection. *Lancet*, i:238.

Crombleholme T, Schecter W, Wilson W (1989). Anal carcinoma: changes in incidence, natural history and treatment: a 26 year review of the UCSF-SFGH experience. *Proceedings of the Annual Meeting of the American Society of Clinical Oncology*, San Francisco, 21–23 May 1989, Vol. 8, Abstract 13,4.

dalla Favera R, *et al.* (1982). Human c-*myc* oncogene is located on the region of chromosome 8 that is translocated in Burkitt's lymphoma cells. *Proceedings of the National Academy of Sciences USA*, **79** (24):7824–7.

Damstrup L, Daugaard G, Gerstoft J, Rrth M (1989). Effects of antineoplastic treatment of HIV-positive patients with testicular cancer. *European Journal of Cancer and Clinical Oncology*, **25** (6):983–6.

de Jarlais DC, *et al.* (1984). Kaposi's sarcoma among four different AIDS risk groups. *New England Journal of Medicine*, **310** (17):1119.

de Luca RR, Needleman SW, Schiffer CA (1987). Hodgkin's disease in HTLV-III positive patients. *Proceedings of the Annual Meeting of the American Society of Clinical Oncology*, Atlanta, 17–19 May 1987, Vol. 6, Abstract 12.

de Mascarel A, Merlio JP, Laborie V, Lacut JY (1989). Hodgkin's disease and malignant lymphoma in acquired immunodeficiency syndrome. *Archives in Pathology and Laboratory Medicine*, **113** (4):328.

del Rio C, Guarner JS, Carr D, Hendrix LE (1989). Lymphomas in patients with HIV infection. *Proceedings of the 5th International Conference on AIDS*, Montreal, 4–9 June 1987, Abstract MPBP 290, 270.

Desablens B, Piprot-Choffat C, Jaisson F, Daniel P (1986). Maladie de Hodgkin chez un homosexuel ayant une serólogie LAV positive. *Presse Medicale*, **15** (23):1099–1100.

Devars du Mayne JF, Teillet-Thiebaud F, Pulick M, Courtois F (1988). Seropositivity to HIV in Hodgkin's disease. *Lancet*, ii:1024.

di Carlo EF, *et al.* (1986). Malignant lymphomas and the acquired immunodeficiency syndrome. Evaluation of 30 cases using a working formulation. *Archives of Pathology and Laboratory Medicine*, **110** (11):1012–16.

Dimopoulou I, Dimopoulos AM, Tassopoulos N, Kalafatas P (1988). Nouvelle observation de maladie de Hodgkin chez un sujet ayant une séropositivité pour le virus de l'immunodéficience humaine. *Presse Medicale*, **17** (38):2037–8.

Egert DA, Beckstead JH (1988). Malignant lymphomas in the acquired immunodeficiency syndrome. Additional evidence for a B-cell origin. *Archives in Pathology and Laboratory Medicine*, **112** (6):602–6.

Ernberg I, Altiok E (1988). The role of Epstein–Barr virus in lymphomas of HIV-carriers. *Acta Pathologica, Microbiologica et Immunologica Scandinavica*, **8** (Suppl.):58–61.

Errante D, *et al.* (1989). Morbo di Hodgkin correlato all'HIV nei tossicodipendenti. *VII Riunione Nazionale di Oncologia Sperimentale e Clinica*, Genova, 19–22 November 1989, Abstract 319, 103.

Essex M (1984). Viral etiology for naturally occurring leukemias and lymphomas. In *Pathogenesis of leukemias and lymphomas: environmental influences* (ed. I Magrater), p. 315. Raven Press, New York.

Fauci AS, *et al.* (1984). Acquired immunodeficiency syndrome: epidemiologic, clinical, immunologic and therapeutic considerations. *Annals of Internal Medicine*, **100** (1):92–106.

Fischl AM (1989). State of antiretroviral therapy with zidovudine. *AIDS*, **3** (Suppl. 1):137–43.

Fischl M, *et al.* (1991). A phase I study of recombinant human interferon-α_{2a} or human lymphoblastoid interferon-α_{nl} and concomitant zidovudine in patients with AIDS-related Kaposi's sarcoma. *Journal of AIDS*, **4**:1–10.

Flanagan P, Chowdhury V, Costello C (1988). HIV-associated B-cell ALL. *British Journal of Haematology*, **69** (2):287.

Flotte TJ, Hatcher VA, Friedman-Kien AE (1984). Factor VIII-related antigen in Kaposi's sarcoma in young homosexual men. *Archives of Dermatology*, **120** (2):180–2.

Frager ND, *et al.* (1988). Squamous cell carcinoma of the esophagus in patients with acquired immunodeficiency syndrome. *Gastrointestinal Radiology*, **13** (4):358–60.

Frazer IH, *et al.* (1986). Association between anorectal dysplasia, human papillomavirus and human immunodeficiency virus infection in homosexual men. *Lancet*, **ii**:657–60.

Gail MH, *et al.* (1991). Projections on the incidence of non-Hodgkin's lymphoma related to acquired immunodeficiency syndrome. *Journal of the National Cancer Institute*, **89** (10):695–701.

Gallagher JG, Meschter SC (1988). Hodgkin's disease and non-Hodgkin's lymphoma in an adult with acquired immunodeficiency syndrome. *Proceedings of the Third International Symposium on Immunobiology in Clinical Oncology*, Abstract 161, 343.

Gallo RC, *et al.* (1984). Frequent detection and isolation of cytopathic retroviruses (HTLV-III) from patients with AIDS and at risk for AIDS. *Science*, **224**:500–3.

Gastaut JA, *et al.* (1988). Rare tumours in HIV+ patients. *Proceedings of the 4th International Conference on AIDS*, Stockholm, 13–16 June 1988, Abstract 7618.

Gill PS, *et al.* (1985). Primary central nervous system lymphoma in homosexual men. Clinical, immunologic, and pathologic features. *American Journal of Medicine*, **78** (5):742–8.

Gill PS, *et al.* (1987a). AIDS-related malignant lymphoma: results of prospective treatment trials. *Journal of Clinical Oncology* **5** (9):1322–8.

Gill PS, *et al.* (1987b). Malignant non-Hodgkin's lymphomas (NHL) in patients with HIV infection. *Proceedings of the Third International Conference on Malignant Lymphoma*, Lugano, 10–13 June 1987, Abstract 57, 49.

Gill P, *et al.* (1988). Randomized trial of ABV (adriamycin, bleomycin, vincristine) vs A in advanced Kaposi's sarcoma (KS). Preliminary results. *Proceedings of the Annual Meeting of the American Society of Clinical Oncology (ASCO)*, 22–24 May 1988, Vol. 7, Abstract 11.

Gill PS, *et al.* (1991). Systemic treatment of AIDS-related Kaposi's sarcoma: results of a randomized trial. *American Journal of Medicine*, **90** (4):427–33.

Giraldo G, Beth E (1986). The involvement of cytomegalovirus in acquired immunodeficiency syndrome and Kaposi's sarcoma. *Progress in Allergy*, **37**:319–31.

Giraldo G, Beth E, Huang ES (1980). Kaposi's sarcoma and its relationship to cytomegalovirus (CMNV). III, CMV DNA and CMV-early antigens in Kaposi's sarcoma. *International Journal of Cancer*, **26** (1):23–9.

Gisselbrecht C, *et al.* (1993). Human immunodeficiency virus-related lymphoma treatment with intensive combination chemotherapy. *American Journal of Medicine*, **95**:843–7.

Glatt AE, Chirgwin K, Landesman SH (1988). Current concepts. Treatment of infections associated with human immunodeficiency virus. *New England Journal of Medicine*, **318** (22):1439–48.

Gold JE, Jiménez E, Zalusky R (1988). Human immunodeficiency virus-related lymphoreticular malignancies and peripheral neurologic disease. A report of four cases. *Cancer*, **61** (11):2318–24.

Gold JE, Castella A, Zalusky R (1989). B-cell acute lymphocytic leukemia in HIV-antibody-positive patients. *American Journal of Hematology*, **32** (3):200–4.

Góngora-Biachi RA, González-Martínez P, Bastarrachea-Ortiz J (1987). Hodgkin's disease as the initial manifestation of acquired immunodeficiency syndrome. *Annals of Internal Medicine*, **107** (1):112.

Gottlieb MS, *et al.* (1981). *Pneumocystis carinii* pneumonia and mucosal candidiasis in previously healthy homosexual men. Evidence of a new acquired cellular immunodeficiency. *New England Journal of Medicine*, **305**(24):1425–31.

Groopman JE (1986). Therapy of epidemic Kaposi's sarcoma. *Seminars in Hematology*, **23** (3, Suppl. 1):14–9.

Groopman JE (1987a). Biology and therapy of epidemic Kaposi's sarcoma. *Cancer*, **59** (3, Suppl.):633–7.

Groopman JE (1987b). Neoplasms in acquired immune deficiency syndrome: the multidisciplinary approach to treatment. *Seminars in Oncology*, **14** (2, Suppl. 3):1–6.

Groopman JE, Scadden DT (1989). Interferon therapy for Kaposi's sarcoma associated with the acquired immunodeficiency syndrome (AIDS). *Annals of Internal Medicine*, **110** (5):335–7.

Hartshorn KL, *et al.* (1987). Synergistic inhibition of human immunodeficiency virus in vitro by azidothymidine and recombinant alpha A interferon. *Antimicrobial Agents and Chemotherapy*, **31** (2):168–72.

Harwood AR, *et al.* (1979). Kaposi's sarcoma in recipients of renal transplants. *American Journal of Medicine*, **67** (5):759–65.

Hill DR (1987). The role of radiotherapy for epidemic Kaposi's sarcoma. *Seminars in Oncology*, **14** (2, Suppl. 3):19–22.

Hoffken G, *et al.* (1988). Neoplasms as cause of pulmonary infiltrates in HIV-antibody-positives. *Fourth International Conference on AIDS*, Stockholm, 13–16 June 1988, Abstract 7616.

Howard MR, McVerry BA (1987). T-cell lymphoma in a haemophiliac positive for antibody to HIV. *British Journal of Haematology*, **67** (1):115.

Huang YQ, *et al.* (1992). Fibroblast growth factor 6 gene expression in AIDS-associated Kaposi's sarcoma. *Lancet*, **339**:1110–11.

Huhn D, Serke M (1988). Malignant lymphomas and HIV infection. *Recent Results in Cancer Research*, **112**:63–8.

Ioachim NL, Cooper MC, Hellmann GC (1987). Lymphomas associated with the acquired immune deficiency syndrome (AIDS): a study of 35 cases. *Cancer Detection and Prevention*, **1** (Suppl. 1):557–65.

Jaffe EA (1977). Endothelial cells and the biology of factor VIII. *New England Journal of Medicine*, **296** (7):337–83.

Jara C, *et al.* (1987). Presentation of 7 patients with human immunodeficiency virus infection and associated neoplasms. *Proceedings of the Fourth European Conference on Clinical Oncology (ECCO 4)*, Madrid, 1–4 November 1987, Abstract 1000, 261.

Kahn J, *et al.* (1988). Incidence of malignancies in men of San Francisco General Hospital during the HIV epidemic. *Proceedings of the Fourth International Conference on AIDS*, Stockholm, 13–16 June 1987, Abstract 7613, 328.

Kahn JO, *et al.* (1992). A controlled trial comparing continued zidovudine with didanosine in human immunodeficiency virus infection. *New England Journal of Medicine*, **327**:581–7.

Kapadia SB, Krause JR (1977). Kaposi's sarcoma after long-term alkylating agent therapy for multiple myeloma. *Southern Medical Journal*, **70** (8):1011–13.

Kaplan LD, Volberding PA (1986). Treatment of Kaposi's sarcoma in acquired immunodeficiency syndrome with an alternating vincristine–vinblastine regimen. *Cancer Treatment Reports*, **70** (9):1121–2.

Kaplan LD, *et al.* (1987). Clinical course and epidemiology of Hodgkin's disease (HD) in homosexual men in San Francisco. *Proceedings of the Third International Conference on AIDS*, Washington, 1–5 June 1987, Vol. 9.

Kaplan LD, *et al.* (1989). AIDS-associated non-Hodgkin's lymphoma in San Francisco. *Journal of the American Medical Association*, **261** (5):719–24.

Kaplan LD, *et al.* (1991). Clinical and virologic effects of recombinant human granulocyte–macrophage colony-stimulating factor in patients receiving chemotherapy for human immunodeficiency virus-associated non-Hodgkin's lymphoma: results of a randomized trial. *Journal of Clinical Oncology*, **9**:929–40.

Kaposi M (1972). Idiopathisches multiple pigment sarcoma der Haut. *Archiv für Dermatologie und Syphilis*, **4**:465.

Keyserlingk H, *et al.* (1988). Atypical presentation of Hodgkin's disease in a patient at risk for the acquired immunodeficiency syndrome. *Cancer Detection and Prevention*, **12** (1–6):243–8.

Klein G (1975). The Epstein–Barr virus and neoplasms. *New England Journal of Medicine*, **293** (26):1353–7.

Klein RS (1989). Prophylaxis of opportunistic infections in individuals infected with HIV. *AIDS*, **3** (Suppl. 1):S161–73.

Knowles DM, *et al.* (1988). Lymphoid neoplasia associated with the acquired immunodeficiency virus (AIDS). The New York University Medical Center experience with 105 patients (1981–1986). *Annals of Internal Medicine*, **108** (5):744–53.

Kobayashi M, *et al.* (1984). HTLV-positive T-lymphoma/leukemia in an AIDS patient. *Lancet*, i:1361–2.

Koutsky LA, *et al.* (1992). A cohort study of the risk of cervical intraepithelial neoplasia grade 2 or 3 in relation to papillomavirus infection. *New England Journal of Medicine*, 327:1272–8.

Kovacs JA, Masur H (1988). Opportunistic infections. In *AIDS. Etiology, diagnosis, treatment and prevention* (2nd edn) (ed. VT de Vita, S Hellman, and S Rosenberg). JB Lippincott, Philadelphia, PA.

Krigel RL, Friedman-Kien AE (1988). Kaposi's sarcoma in AIDS: diagnosis and treatment. In *AIDS. Etiology, diagnosis, treatment and prevention* (2nd edn) (ed. VT de Vita, S Hellman, and S Rosenberg), pp. 245–61. JB Lippincott, Philadelphia, PA.

Krigel RL, *et al.* (1985). Therapeutic trial of interferon-gamma in patients with epidemic Kaposi's sarcoma. *Journal of Biological Response Modifiers*, 4 (4):358–64.

Kristal AR, Nasca PC, Burnett WS, Mikl J (1988). Changes in the epidemiology of non-Hodgkin's lymphoma associated with epidemic human immunodeficiency virus (HIV) infection. *American Journal of Epidemiology*, 128(4):711–18.

Krown SE (1987). The role of interferon in the therapy of epidemic Kaposi's sarcoma. *Seminars in Oncology*, 14 (2, Suppl. 3):27–33.

Krown S, Metroka C, Wernz JC (1989). Kaposi's sarcoma in the acquired immunodeficiency syndrome: a proposal for uniform evaluation, response and staging criteria. *Journal of Clinical Oncology*, 7(9):1201–7.

Krown SE, *et al.* (1990). Interferon-A with zidovudine: safety, tolerance, and clinical and virologic effects in patients with Kaposi's sarcoma associated with the acquired immunodeficiency syndrome (AIDS). *Annals of Internal Medicine*, 112(11):812–21.

Laga M, *et al.* (1992). Genital papillomavirus infection and cervical dysplasia—opportunistic complications of HIV infection. *International Journal of Cancer*, 50:45–8.

Lake-Lewin D, Arkel YS (1988). Spectrum of malignancies in HIV positive individuals. *Proceedings of the Annual Meeting of the American Society of Clinical Oncology (ASCO)*, New Orleans, 22–24 May 1988, Vol. 7, Abstract 20, 5.

Laubenstein LJ, *et al.* (1984). Treatment of epidemic Kaposi's sarcoma with etoposide or a combination of doxorubicin, bleomycin, and vinblastine. *Journal of Clinical Oncology*, 2(10):1115–20.

Lazo PA, Tsichlis PN (1990). Biology and pathogenesis of retroviruses. *Seminars in Oncology*, 17(3):269–94.

Levine AM (1987). Non-Hodgkin's lymphomas and other malignancies in the acquired immune deficiency syndrome. *Seminars in Oncology*, 14 (2, Suppl. 3):34–9.

Levine AM (1993). AIDS-related malignancies: the emerging epidemic. *Journal of the National Cancer Institute*, 85(17):1382–97.

Levine A, *et al.* (1988). AIDS related non-Hodgkin's lymphoma: clinical, immunologic and pathologic characteristics in 68 patients from one institution. *Fourth International Conference on AIDS*, Stockholm, 13–16 June 1988, Abstract 7609, 327.

Levine AM, *et al.* (1991). Low-dose chemotherapy with central nervous system prophylaxis and zidovudine maintenance in AIDS-related lymphoma. *Journal of the American Medical Association*, 266,84:8.

List AF (1988). Metastatic giant-cell tumour in a man positive for HIV. *New England Journal of Medicine*, 318(8):517.

List AF, Greco FA, Vogler LB (1987). Lymphoproliferative disease in immunocompromised hosts: the role of Epstein–Barr virus. *Journal of Clinical Oncology*, 5(10):1673–89.

Lowenthal DA, *et al.* (1986). AIDS-related lymphoid neoplasia. The Memorial Hospital Experience. *Cancer*, 61(11):2325–37.

Lozano-Molero M, *et al.* (1989). Malignant lymphomas (non-Hodgkin's disease) associated with HIV infection by the human immunodeficiency virus. Study of 9 cases. *Medica Clinica, Barcelona*, 92(8):302.

Lukes RJ, *et al.* (1978). Immunologic approach to non-Hodgkin lymphomas and related leukemias. Analysis of the results of multiparameter studies of 425 cases. *Seminars in Hematology*, 15(4):332–51.

Magrath I, *et al.* (1983). Synthesis of kappa light chains by cell lines containing an 8:22 chromosomal translocation derived from a male homosexual with Burkitt lymphoma. *Science*, 222:1094–8.

Markowitz M, *et al.* (1988). HIV-related lymphoma. A recent experience. *Fourth International Conference on AIDS*, Stockholm, 13–16 June 1987, Abstract 7607, 326.

Miles SA, *et al.* (1992). Oncostatin M as a potent mitogen for AIDS-Kaposi's sarcoma-derived cells. *Science*, 255:1432–4.

Milpied N, Bourchis JH, Garand R, Harousseau JL (1988). B-cell ALL in anti-HIV positive patient: achievement of a complete response with aggressive chemotherapy. *British Journal of Haematology*, 70(4):501–2.

Minor DR (1988). Vimblastine–methotrexate–vincristine chemotherapy for epidemic Kaposi's sarcoma. *Proceedings of the Annual Meeting of the American Society of Clinical Oncology (ASCO)*, New Orleans, 22–24 May 1988, Vol. 7, Abstract 16, 4.

Mintzer DM, Real FX, Jovino L, Krown SE (1985). Treatment of Kaposi's sarcoma and thrombocytopenia with vincristine in patients with the acquired immunodeficiency syndrome. *Annals of Internal Medicine*, 102(2):200–2.

Mitsuyasu RT, Groopman JE (1984). Biology and therapy of Kaposi's sarcoma. *Seminars in Oncology*, 11(1):53–9.

Mitsuyasu RT, Colman MF, Sun NC (1986). Simultaneous occurrence of Hodgkin's disease and Kaposi's sarcoma in a patient with the acquired immunodeficiency syndrome. *American Journal of Medicine*, 8(5):954–8.

Molina JM, *et al.* (1989). Production of tumour necrosis factor alpha and interleukin 1 β by monocytic cells infected with human immunodeficiency virus. *Journal of Clinical Investigation*, 84:733–7.

Monfardini S (1980). The continuing care of terminal cancer patients. In *When to stop anticancer treatment* (ed. RG Twycross and V Ventafridda), pp. 13–18. Pergamon Press, Oxford.

Monfardini S, *et al.* (1988). Malignant lymphomas in patients with or at risk for AIDS in Italy. *Journal of the National Cancer Institute*, 80(11): 855–60.

Monfardini S, *et al.* (1989a). Unusual malignant tumours in 49 patients with HIV infection. *AIDS*, 3(7):449–52.

Monfardini S, *et al.* (1989b). Rare HIV-related tumours in intravenous drug abusers (IVDA) consist mainly in testicular, cervical and pulmonary rather than oral and anorectal carcinomas. *Proceedings of the Annual Meeting of the American Association of Clinical Oncology*, San Francisco, 21–23 May 1989, Vol. 8, Abstract 19, 5.

Monfardini S, *et al.* (1990). AIDS-associated non-Hodgkin's lymphomas in Italy: intravenous drug users vs homosexual men. *Annals of Oncology*, 1:203–11.

Montagnier L, *et al.* (1984). A new type of retrovirus isolated from patients presenting with lymphadenopathy and AIDS: structural and antigenic relatedness with equine infectious anemia virus. *Annales de Virologie*, 135E:119–34.

Moore GE, Cook DD (1985). AIDS in association with malignant melanoma and Hodgkin's disease. *Journal of Clinical Oncology*, 3(10):1437.

Morrison JG, Scharfenberg JC, Timmcke AE (1989). Perianal lymphoma as a manifestation of the acquired immune deficiency syndrome. Report of a case. *Diseases of the Colon and Rectum*, 32(6):521–3.

Nakajima K, *et al.* (1989). Induction of IL6 (B-cell stimulatory factor-2/IFN-β 2) production by human immunodeficiency virus. *Journal of Immunology*, 142:531.

Nakamura S, *et al.* (1988). Kaposi's sarcoma cells: long-term culture with growth factor from retrovirus-infected CD4+ T cells. *Science*, 242:426–30.

National Cancer Institute (1982). Sponsored study of classifications of non-Hodgkin's lymphomas: summary and description of a working formulation for clinical usage. *Cancer*, 49(10):2112–35.

Oksenhendler E, Molina TH, Gisselbrecht C (1989). Non-Hodgkin's lymphomas (NHL) and human immunodeficiency virus (HIV) infection. *Proceedings of the Third International Symposium on Immunobiology in Clinical Oncology*, Nice, Abstract 342, 235.

Overly WL, Jakubek DJ (1987). Multiple squamous cell carcinomas and human immunodeficiency virus infection. *Annals of Internal Medicine*, 106(2):334.

Palmer MC, Mador DR, Venner PM (1989). Testicular seminoma associated with the acquired immunodeficiency syndrome related complex: 2 case reports. *Journal of Urology*, 142(1):128–30.

Palomera L, Martin M, García Diez I, Gutiérrez MT (1987). Linfoma de Hodgkin y anticuerpos anti-HIV positívos. *Revista Clínica Espanola*, 181(4):230–1.

Parker B, *et al.* (1988). Phase II study of Betaseron in Kaposi's sarcoma. *Proceedings of the Annual Meeting of the American Society of Clinical Oncology*, New Orleans, 22–24 May 1988, Vol. 7, Abstract 13, 4.

Pelicci PG, *et al.* (1986). Multiple monoclonal B-cell expansions and c-*myc* oncogene rearrangements in acquired immune deficiency syndrome-related lymphoproliferative disorders. Implications for lymphomagenesis. *Journal of Experimental Medicine*, 164:2049.

Penn I (1978). Tumors arising in organ transplant recipients. *Advances in Cancer Research*, 28:31–61.

Penn I (1981). Depressed immunity and the development of cancer. *Clinical and Experimental Immunology*, 46(3):459–74.

Perno CF, *et al.* (1992). Effects of bone marrow stimulatory cytokines on human immunodeficiency virus replication and the antiviral activity of dideoxynucleosides in cultures of monocyte/macrophages. *Blood*, 80(4):995–1003.

Peters K, Mack TM (1983). Patterns of anal carcinoma by gender and marital status in Los Angeles county. *British Journal of Cancer*, 48:624.

Picard O, *et al.* (1987). Rectal Hodgkin disease and the acquired immunodeficiency syndrome. *Annals of Internal Medicine*, 106(5):775.

Pluda J, *et al.* (1993). Parameters affecting the development of non-Hodgkin's lymphoma in patients with severe human immunodeficiency virus infection receiving antiretroviral therapy. *Journal of Clinical Oncology*, 11:1099–107.

Pollack MS, Safai B, Dupont B (1983). HLA-Dr5 and Dr2 are susceptibility factors for acquired immunodeficiency syndrome with Kaposi's sarcoma in different ethnic populations. *Disease Markers*, 1:135.

Presant CA, *et al.* (1987). Human immunodeficiency virus-associated T-cell lymphoblastic lymphoma in AIDS. *Cancer*, 60(7):1459–61.

Prior E, *et al.* (1986). Hodgkin's disease in homosexual men. An AIDS-related phenomenon? *American Journal of Medicine*, 81(6):1085–8.

Provencher D, *et al.* (1988). HIV status and positive Papanicolau screening: identification of a high-risk population. *Gynecological Oncology*, 31(1):184–90.

Rabkin C, *et al.* (1992). Incidence of lymphomas and other cancers in HIV-infected and HIV-uninfected patients with hemophilia. *Journal of the American Medical Association*, 267:1090–4.

Raphael M, *et al.* (1986). Les lymphomes et le SIDA. *Annals of Pathology*, 6:278.

Reynolds P, *et al.* (1993). The spectrum of acquired immunodeficiency syndrome (AIDS)-associated malignancies in San Francisco, 1980–1987. *American Journal of Epidemiology*, 137:19–30.

Robert NJ, Schneiderman H (1984). Hodgkin's disease and the acquired immunodeficiency syndrome. *Annals of Internal Medicine*, 101(1):142–3.

Robinson JE, *et al.* (1980). Diffuse polyclonal B-cell lymphoma during primary infection with Epstein–Barr virus. *New England Journal of Medicine*, 302(23):1293–7.

Rosen A, *et al.* (1977). Polyclonal immunoglobulin production after Epstein–Barr infection of human lymphocytes *in vitro*. *Nature, London*, 267:52–4.

Sadeghi SB, Sadeghi A, Roboy SJ (1988). Prevalence of dysplasia and cancer of the cervix in a nationwide planned parenthood population. *Cancer*, 61:2359–61.

Safai B, *et al.* (1985). The natural history of Kaposi's sarcoma in the acquired immunodeficiency syndrome. *Annals of Internal Medicine*, 103(5):774–50.

Safai B, Lynfield R, Lowenthal DA, Koziner B (1987). High frequency of Epstein–Barr virus in HIV-positive patients with Hodgkin's disease. *Lancet*, i:1458.

Salahuddin SZ, *et al.* (1986). Isolation of a new virus, HBLV, in patients with lymphoproliferative disorders. *Science*, 234:596–601.

Sansone R, *et al.* (1989). Testicular cancer in HIV infected subjects. *Proceedings of the Third International Symposium on Immunobiology and Clinical Oncology*, Nice, Abstract 363, 168.

Schafer A, *et al.* (1991). The increased frequency of cervical dysplasia–neoplasia in women infected with the human immunodeficiency virus is related to the degree of immunosuppression. *American Journal Obstetrics and Gynecology*, 164:593–9.

Scheib RG, Siegel RS (1985). Atypical Hodgkin's disease and the acquired immunodeficiency syndrome. *Annals of Internal Medicine*, 102(4):554.

Schmid L (1987). AIDS-related neoplasia in Switzerland. *Proceedings of the European Conference of Clinical Oncology (ECCO 4)*, Madrid, 1–4 November 1987, Abstract 1000.

Schmid L (1988). AIDS-related neoplasias in Switzerland. *Recent Results in Cancer Research*, 112:69–74.

Schoeppel SL, *et al.* (1986). Hodgkin's disease (HD) in homosexual men: the San Francisco bay area experience. *Proceedings of the Annual Meeting of the American Society of Clinical Oncology*, 5, Abstract 9, 3.

Scholefield JH, *et al.* (1987). Anal and cervical intrahepithelial neoplasia possible parallel (Comments). *Lancet*, ii:765–9.

Schurmann D, *et al.* (1989). Malignant lymphomas in HIV infected patients: clinical and pathological features. *Proceedings of the Fifth International Conference on AIDS*, Montreal, 4–9 June 1989, Abstract WBO 20, 206.

Serraino D, *et al.* (1992). The epidemiology of acquired immunodeficiency virus infection receiving anti retroviral therapy. *Annals of Oncology*, 3: 595–603.

Skinhoj P, Ersbll J, Nissen NI (1987). Human immunodeficiency virus (HIV) associated non-Hodgkin's lymphomas in Denmark: report of three cases. *European Journal of Haematology*, 39(1):71–4.

Snider WD, Simpson DM, Aronyk KE, Nielsen SL (1983). Primary lymphoma of the nervous system associated with acquired immunodeficiency syndrome. *New England Journal of Medicine*, 308(1):45.

Socie G, *et al.* (1988). Problemes therapeutiques chez deux patients atteints de maladie de Hodgkin avec serologique HIV 1 positive. *Bulletin du Cancer*, 75(2):229–32.

Sonnabend J, Witkin SS, Purtilo DT (1983). Acquired immunodeficiency syndrome, opportunistic infections and malignancies in male homosexuals. An hypothesis of etiologic factors in pathogenesis. *Journal of the American Medical Association*, 249(17):2370–4.

Spector BD, Perry GS, Kersey JH (1978). Genetically determined immunodeficiency diseases (GDID) and malignancy: report from the Immunodeficiency Cancer Registry. *Clinical Immunology and Immunopathology*, 11(1):12–29.

Spurrett B, Shelley Jones D, Stewart G (1988). Cervical dysplasia and HIV infection. *Lancet*, i:237.

Temple JJ, Andes WA (1986). AIDS and Hodgkin's disease. *Lancet*, ii:454–5.

Tessler AN, Catanese A (1987). AIDS and germ cell tumors of testis. *Urology*, 30(3):203–4.

Tirelli U, *et al.* (1992*a*). Prospective study with combined low-dose chemotherapy and zidovudine in 37 patients with poor prognosis AIDS-related non-Hodgkin's lymphoma. *Annals of Oncology*, 3:843–7.

Tirelli U, *et al.* (1992*b*). Hodgkin's disease in 92 patients with HIV infection: the Italian experience. *Annals of Oncology*, 3 (Suppl. 4):569–72.

Uccini S, *et al.* (1989). High frequency of Epstein–Barr virus in HIV-positive patients with Hodgkin's disease. *Lancet*, i:1458.

Unger PD, Strauchen JA (1986). Hodgkin's disease in AIDS complex patients. Report of four cases and tissue immunologic marker studies. *Cancer*, 58(4):821–5.

Vaccher E, *et al.* (1989*a*). Centoventuno casi di sarcoma Kaposi epidemico (SKE) in Italia. *VII Riunione Nazionale di Oncologia Sperimentale e Clinica*, Genova, 19–22 November 1989, Abstract 12, 11.

Vaccher E, *et al.* (1989*b*). Complicazioni neoplastiche dell' AIDS. *Nuovi Argomenti di Medicina*, 5(7/8):368.

Voelkerding KV, *et al.* (1989). Plasma cell malignancy in the acquired immune deficiency syndrome. *American Journal of Clinical Pathology*, 92(2): 222–8.

Vogel J, *et al.* (1988). The HIV *tat* gene induces dermal lesions resembling Kaposi's sarcoma in transgenic mice. *Nature*, 335:606–11.

Volberding PA (1987). The role of chemotherapy for epidemic Kaposi's sarcoma. *Seminars in Oncology*, 14 (2, Suppl. 3):23–6.

Volberding PA (1989). Moving towards a uniform staging for human immunodeficiency virus-associated Kaposi's sarcoma. *Journal of Clinical Oncology*, 7(9):1184–5.

Volberding PA, *et al.* (1985). Vinblastine therapy for Kaposi's sarcoma in the acquired immune deficiency syndrome. *Annals of Internal Medicine*, 103(3):335–8.

Weitberg AB, Mayer K, Miller ME, Mikolich DJ (1986). Dysplastic carcinoid tumor and AIDS-related complex. *New England Journal of Medicine*, 314(22):1455.

Wernz J, *et al.* (1986). Chemotherapy and assessment of response in epidemic Kaposi's sarcoma (EKS) with bleomycin (B)/velban (V). *Proceedings of the Annual Meeting of the American Society of Clinical Oncology (ASCO)*, Los Angeles, 4–6 May 1986, Vol. 5, Abstract 15, 4.

WHO (1988). Acquired immunodeficiency syndrome (AIDS). Situation in WHO region as of 31 March 1988. *Weekly Epidemiological Record*, 63:201.

WHO (1989). Acquired immunodeficiency syndrome (AIDS). Situation in WHO region as of 31 March 1989. *Weekly Epidemiological Record*, 64:221.

WHO (1990). Acquired immunodeficiency syndrome (AIDS). Data as of 31 July 1990. *Weekly Epidemiological Record*, 65:237–44.

Yarchoan R, Pluda JM, Perno FC, *et al.* (1991). Antiretroviral therapy of human immunodeficiency virus infection: current strategies and challenges for the future. *Blood*, 78 (4):859–84.

Ziegler JL, Beckstead AJ, Volberding PA, *et al.* (1984). Non-Hodgkin's lymphomas in 90 homosexual men. Relation to generalized lymphadenopathy and the acquired immunodeficiency syndrome. *New England Journal of Medicine*, 311 (9):565–70.

Zur Hausen H (1982). Human genital cancer: synergism between two virus infections or synergism and initiating events? *Lancet*, ii:1370–2.

Section 13
Bone tumours and soft tissue sarcomas

13.1 Sarcoma of the soft tissues

HERMAN D. SUIT, CEES. J. VAN GROENINGEN, HENRY J. MANKIN, AND
ANDREW E. ROSENBERG

Sarcomas of soft tissues encompass the broad array of malignant tumours that arise in the mesenchymal soft tissues at all anatomical sites. This also includes malignant tumours developing from the peripheral nerves, despite their ectodermal origin; soft tissue lymphomas are not considered under this heading. Sarcomas of the parenchymatous organs and the hollow viscera are discussed elsewhere.

This is an uncommon group of tumours but, even so, includes a rich collection of histological types. The sarcomas are designated in most instances according to the probable line of differentiation, that is, fibrosarcoma, liposarcoma, leiomyosarcoma, rhabdomyosarcoma, angiosarcoma, etc. For others, the label is descriptive of the histological pattern, that is, synovial sarcoma, alveolar sarcoma of soft parts, epithelioid sarcoma, clear cell sarcoma of soft tissues, etc. The appearance of synovial sarcoma is in some cases suggestive of synovial tissue. However, these tumours are rarely seen to arise in, or even to involve directly, synovial tissue; the lining of the joints is involved only in the exceptional patient. Pertinent to this point is the report of a synovial sarcoma developing in the tongue; a diagnosis was supported by the demonstration of the t(X;18) chromosomal translocation (Bridge et al. 1988).

Although any of these tumours may appear at any anatomical site, there are sharp differences in site distribution among the various histological types, for example epithelioid sarcomas are predominantly seen in the distal part of the upper extremities and in the superficial tissues thereof and synovial sarcomas are uncommon in the head and neck region.

GENERAL COMMENTS

Epidemiology

Sarcomas of the soft tissues are uncommon. In the United States they comprise 0.55 per cent of the newly diagnosed cancers per year (American Cancer Society 1989), excluding epithelial cancers of the skin and carcinomas in situ. Understanding of the natural history and response to therapy of soft tissue sarcomas has progressed more slowly than for many other tumours because of their rarity. This is readily appreciated by noting that there were estimated to be 5600 new cases of sarcomas of the soft tissues in 1989 as compared with 143 000 cases of adenocarcinoma of the breast. The 5600 patients with sarcoma had lesions of numerous histological types distributed at most anatomical sites. In contrast, the 143 000 tumours of the breast were of one anatomical site and of relatively similar histological type. Despite these facts, substantial progress is being made, due, in part, to the tendency for patients with sarcoma to be managed by a small number of referral centres and the shift away from ablative surgical procedures toward more conservative but more complex, multidisciplinary approaches.

There are no demonstrated important racial or sex factors in these tumours. The male : female ratio is 1 : 1.1 in the Massachusetts General Hospital (MGH) series and the American Joint Committee on Cancer (AJC) series (Russell et al. 1977).

Aetiology

Genetic factors are increasingly recognized as of importance in oncogenesis and also in the growth and progression of the tumour. One or more oncogenes (activation or deletion) are likely to participate in the development of these sarcomas. There is good evidence for the involvement of the retinoblastoma (*Rb*) gene in the development of some sarcomas (Dryja et al. 1986; Friend et al. 1987); the case for the *Rb* gene is strong in osteosarcoma. There are now reports that provide evidence for participation of the *ras* gene in human rhabdomyosarcoma (Chardin et al. 1985), fibrosarcoma (Brown et al. 1987), and of *myc* expression in human rhabdomyosarcoma.

There is growing evidence of distinct chromosomal abnormalities in the sarcomas, which is a further and powerful indication of the genetic aspect to these tumours. For example, there is a translocation t(X;18) in nearly all instances of synovial sarcoma (Turc-Carel et al. 1986a). This is a helpful diagnostic feature and can aid in classifying a poorly differentiated tumour as a synovial sarcoma (Karakousis et al. 1987). There is also a specific abnormality in the myxoid liposarcoma (Smith et al. 1987; Turc-Carel et al. 1986b), namely t(12;16)(q13;p11). In Ewing's sarcoma there has been extensive documentation since 1983 of a reciprocal translocation t(11;12)(q24;12); with this change being recognized in approximately 90 per cent of these sarcomas (Aurias et al. 1983; Sandberg et al. 1988).

There is a hereditary tendency for certain benign and malignant tumours of the soft tissues (Strong 1977; Rowley 1983; Littlefield 1984). This may be especially evident in certain disease syndromes. An example is the high frequency of desmoid tumours among patients with familial polyposis (McAdam et al. 1970). Other examples include retinoblastoma (Jensen and Miller 1971), von Recklinghausen's disease (Fraumeni 1973), and the multiple endocrine neoplasia syndrome (Pizzo et al. 1985).

Radiation is well recognized as capable of inducing sarcoma of bone and soft tissue. The frequency of this increases with dose and with the post-radiation observation period (Hatfield and Schulz 1970; Kim et al. 1978; Sadove et al. 1981; Robinson et al. 1988). This is mainly a complication of high-dose treatment (for example, more than 60–70 Gy) and is only rarely seen after low doses (less than 40 Gy given in 2 Gy fractions). However, we have seen two patients presenting with a sarcoma of soft tissue many years after radiation for seminoma at other centres (the treatment records were not available). The actuarial frequency of sarcoma 15–20 years later is approximately 0.5 per cent for radiation of normal bone and soft tissue in the adult treated with radiation alone to full doses, without chemotherapy. The frequency is higher after treatment in childhood, especially with radiation and chemotherapy, with the frequency possibly being as high as 20 per cent (Strong et al. 1979).

Chemotherapeutic agents are likewise associated with risks of inducing sarcoma. For example, there are two reports that describe the appearance of osteosarcoma in children treated for leukaemia by drugs alone (Gohotsar *et al.* 1986; Shaw *et al.* 1988). Tucker *et al.* (1987) analysed the late sequelae in 9170 patients who survived for long periods after treatment for malignant disease as children. They concluded that chemotherapy alone was an independent risk factor.

These facts about the oncogenic potential of radiation and chemotherapy make it incumbent upon the physician to treat only to the extent essential. The radiation oncologist should employ all means feasible of excluding from the treatment volume tissues not suspected of being involved by tumour. Similarly, the drug dosage should be enough to control the disease, but not excessive. Fortunately, some clinical data indicate that the highly protracted courses are not necessarily more effective than the more abbreviated ones, particularly in regimens featuring alkylating agents. Hence, the shorter courses of many of the current protocols should mean less late toxicity.

Exposure to certain industrial chemicals may be followed by the appearance of sarcomas. For example, there is a clear association between exposure to vinyl chloride and hepatic angiosarcoma (Locker *et al.* 1979). Phenoxyacetic acid (Hardell and Eriksson 1988) and arsenic (Roth 1957; Lander *et al.* 1975) have also been strongly implicated as inducing agents for hepatic sarcomas in man.

Sarcomas of soft tissue may follow massive and rather protracted oedema (Stewart and Treves 1948; Taswell *et al.* 1962). Chronic irritation secondary to foreign bodies may be a factor in the induction of sarcomas. We have observed one patient in whom a fibrosarcoma appeared 15 years after the insertion of a plastic tube through the scalp for control of hydrocephalus.

Trauma is rarely accepted as a factor in the development of these tumours, with the exception of desmoid or aggressive fibromatosis. In an occasional patient there is a convincing history of major trauma to the affected site many months before the appearance of local symptoms of tumour. The more usual history is of a traumatic incident shortly before the patient became aware of the mass, suggesting that the trauma merely brought the mass to the patient's attention.

Natural history

The patient with a soft tissue sarcoma most often presents with a painless lump of only a few weeks' or months' duration. There are, of course, patients who present with symptoms secondary to the effects of pressure or direct invasion by the tumour, for example pain due to effects on peripheral nerves or bone, oedema due to the partial or complete obstruction of blood or lymphatic vessels, impaired respiratory, gastrointestinal, or genitourinary function, and anaemia secondary to sequestration of blood in a large tumour. At diagnosis some 90 per cent of patients do not have demonstrable metastatic tumour. Rydholm *et al.* (1984) made a study of all patients who developed a sarcoma of the soft tissues of the locomotor system during the period 1964–1978 in the Southern district of the Swedish National Cancer Registry. There was a total of 278 patients, 19 of whom had identifiable metastatic sarcoma at the time of diagnosis (6.8 per cent). Further, in nearly all of the remaining patients with localized disease (237/259 or 91.5 per cent), definitive treatment could be offered. During the follow-up period, 24 of the 237 patients treated definitively died of intercurrent disease and had no clinically evident tumour at death.

Sarcomas grow by direct local extension, infiltrating adjacent tissues and structures. Generally, soft tissue sarcomas extend along tissue planes and do not traverse or violate major fascial planes or bone. The local extensions may not be continuous but show skip

Table 1 Distribution (percentages) or sarcomas of soft tissues according to anatomical site

	MGH[a]	MDAH[b]	AJC[c]	ACS[d]
No. of patients	471	300	1215	4550
Site				
Lower extremity, foot	45.0	45	40	46.4
Upper extremity	18.9	21	13	13.1
Head and neck	10.6	9	15	8.9
Torso	13.0	18	18	17.9
Retroperitoneum	12.5	7	13	12.5
Other				1.3

[a] Massachusetts General Hospital.
[b] MD Anderson Hospital (Lindberg *et al.* 1981).
[c] American Joint Commission Task Force (Russell *et al.* 1977).
[d] American College of Surgeons (Lawrence *et al.* 1987).

areas. These skips are, with few exceptions, small. Sarcomas may also spread to regional lymph nodes. This is infrequent except for rhabdomyosarcoma and epithelioid sarcoma. Spread to distant sites is, however, a common development, especially for the large and high-grade sarcomas (see below). The most common site of metastatic tumour is the lung. In the study of Rydholm *et al.* (1984), 76 of the 237 treated patients developed metastatic tumour, with the lung being the first site of involvement in 62 (82 per cent). In the series of patients treated at the National Cancer Institute of the United States of America (NCI), the first metastasis (isolated) was in the lung in 70 per cent of patients with sarcomas of an extremity. For all sites the figure was 52 per cent of 107 patients who developed metastases in a total population of 307 (Potter *et al.* 1985).

In the AJC series, 84 per cent of the patients were 15 or more years of age (Russell 1977). In the MGH series of 543 patients, some 12–15 per cent were in each decade of life from the third to the eighth. The sixth decade had the peak incidence (26 per cent) in the NCI series (Potter *et al.* 1985).

The distribution of sarcomas of soft tissues according to anatomical site is presented in Table 1. Sarcomas of soft tissues are seen most frequently in the lower extremities (buttock/groin/thigh/leg regions), some 40–46 per cent of all sarcomas. The next most common sites are the upper extremity and torso, at approximately 13–21 and 14–19 per cent, respectively.

Patient management: a team approach

The optimal management of patients with sarcomas of the soft tissues is by a group of physicians who are primarily interested in this category of tumour. They should be responsible for the management from the diagnostic evaluation and biopsy through to the physiotherapy/rehabilitation and follow-up examinations. This, of course, means that these patients should be in the hands of a group at a major cancer treatment centre where substantial numbers of such patients are cared for each year (Rydholm *et al.* 1983). Not all activities need to be conducted at the centre but the sarcoma team should devise the strategy and participate in the management. The team should include diagnostic radiologists, pathologists, surgeons (orthopaedic and general), medical and paediatric oncologists, and radiation oncologists. The best circumstances would be expected in a centre where there is active clinical and laboratory research on sarcomas; that is, scientists involved in research on their molecular biology, cytogenetics, immunobiology, proliferation kinetics, radiation biology, pharmacology, and other aspects. Interaction between clinical and laboratory groups is likely to accelerate the advances in the care of these patients.

PATIENT ASSESSMENT

History

The history should include an estimate of the duration of symptoms and their character and severity. This information is helpful in deciding on the probable rate of growth and, hence, the need to expedite diagnosis and treatment. In addition, the history is of value in assessing the likelihood of involvement of nerves, vessels, and muscle groups. When there have been prior diagnostic or therapeutic procedures, full details need to be obtained, along with the written records. Because of the increasing evidence of a genetic role in the development of soft tissue sarcomas, the history should include information as to the health status and cause of death of the patient's parents, siblings, children, and grandparents.

Physical examination

In addition to a complete general physical examination there must, of course, be meticulous examination of the site of the primary tumour and the regional lymph nodes. Points of special importance include location (superficial or deep to the fascia), attachment to the deep structures (for example, bone), whether a single mass or a multiple nodular tumour, involvement of skin, vessels (pulse, oedema), and nerves, muscle and joint function (range of motion, gait, strength, etc.), and location, length, status of any surgical wound and drain wound. Although metastasis to the regional lymph nodes is unlikely, they have to be examined carefully because there will be an occasional positive finding. This is particularly so for the patients with grade 2–3 and T_2 sarcomas. An analysis of the MGH experience found that involvement of the regional nodes as the first metastasis or present at diagnosis occurred in 0/63 grade 1, 2/118 grade 2, and 17/142 grade 3 sarcomas (Mazeron and Suit 1987). Of the 17 patients who had grade 3 sarcomas, 16 were T_2 or larger than 5 cm. Hence, special attention needs be given to examination of the regional nodes in the stage II–IIIB patients. As mentioned earlier, rhabdomyosarcoma and epithelioid sarcoma are the histological types most likely to metastasize to the regional nodes.

Radiographic evaluation

Assessment of the location, size, and pattern of local extension of the primary tumour must include a comprehensive radiographic study; contrast-enhanced computerized tomography (**CT**) and/or magnetic resonance imaging (**MRI**) (including T_2-weighted sequences) are now considered essential for an adequate evaluation in patients with M_0 disease. Examples of these studies on representative patients are shown in Figs 1 and 2. In most instances the T_2 MRI images yield better definition of the margins and the patterns of extent, especially for lesions of extremities, than the CT images. Additionally, the availability of coronal and sagittal views in addition to the standard transverse sections of the CT scans makes the MRI more attractive to the clinician. The clinician should correlate the clinical and radiographic studies in collaboration with the radiologist. This can be valuable in examining for transgression of major fascial planes, displacement of nerves and vessels, and invasion of bone. Arteriograms are now limited to those situations where there may be a problem at planned surgery owing to vascular invasion. Bone scans are judged to be of minor value. A positive scan cannot be

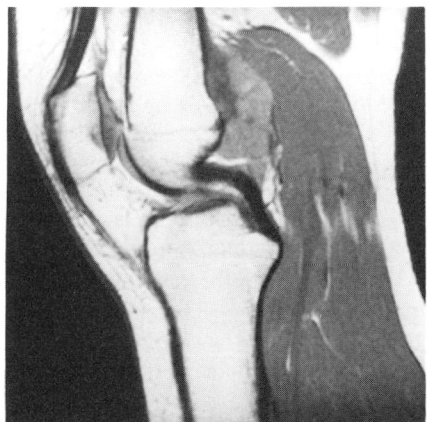

(a)

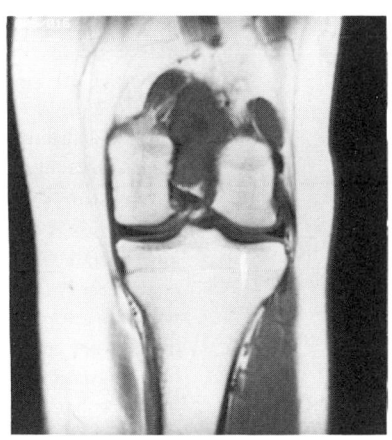

(b)

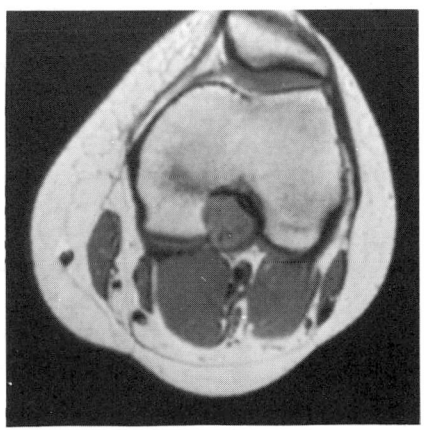

(c)

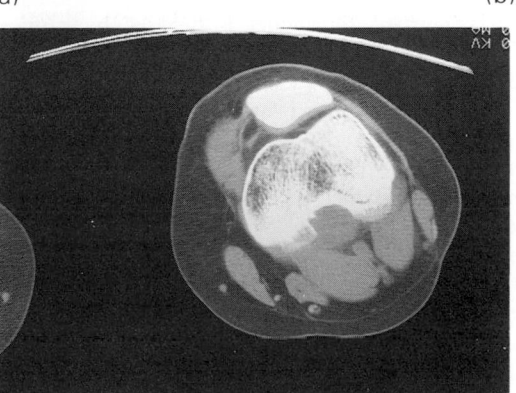

(d)

Fig. 1 The clear cell sarcoma arising in the intercondylar space of a 24-year-old woman is illustrated by the series of MRI and CT images. (a) T_2 sagittal cut showing the lesion extending into the popliteal space and that it is adjacent to the posterior joint capsule. (b) Coronal section showing the proximity of tumour to bone; there is no radiographic evidence of invasion of bone. (c) Transverse section through the condyles. The tumour does approach the vessel but is not invading the vessel; the nerve is, of course, more posteriorly and, hence, not a problem. (d) CT section through the condyles, similar to that in (c); note the less satisfactory display of the vessel.

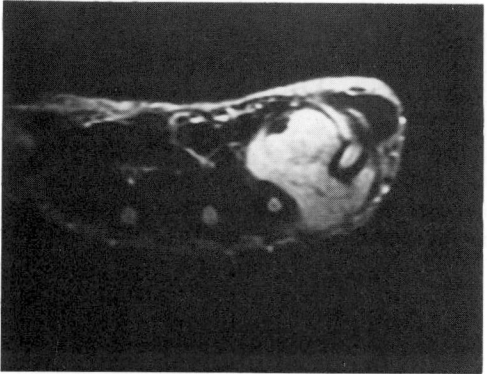

(a)

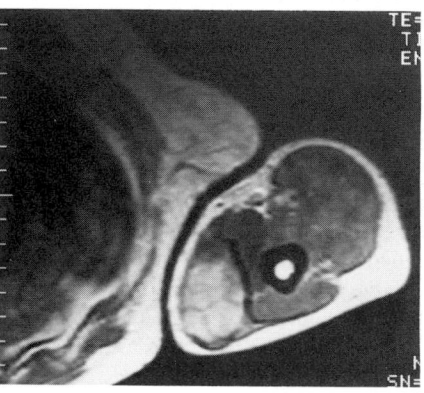

(b)

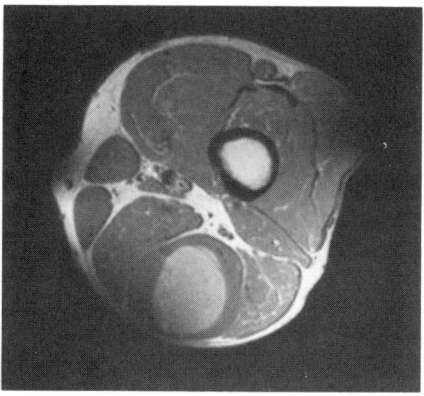

(c)

Fig. 2 (a) This T_2-weighted image demonstrates an alveolar rhabdomyosarcoma (Group III) of the left hypothenar eminence. (b) A grade 3 malignant fibrohistiocytoma of the triceps muscles is well demonstrated by the T_2-weighted image. (c) A grade 2 myxoid liposarcoma in the belly of the semi-membranous muscle of mid-portion of the posterior thigh is shown in this T_2 study.

accepted as proof of bone invasion. That requires radiographic evidence of destruction of cortical bone. The 'positive' bone scan often merely reflects an increased blood flow locally due to the tumour mass and may be seen in patients with intact bone. The examination for metastatic disease in the lung is based on CT. That metastatic disease is overlooked in an important proportion of patients by lesser examinations has been well documented (Peuchot and Libshitz 1987).

Biopsy

The definitive diagnosis of soft tissue sarcoma is based on the histopathological study of a biopsy sample. The purpose of the biopsy is to obtain enough tissue to determine the histological type and grade of the lesion. Soft tissue sarcomas pose some of the greatest diagnostic challenges to anatomical pathologists. Their confusing appearances all too often result in seemingly incompatible diagnoses of, for example various non-neoplastic processes (such as nodular fasciatis and myositis ossificans) vs high-grade sarcomas (malignant fibrohistiocytoma, extraskeletal osteosarcoma). In addition, soft tissue sarcomas are notorious for mimicking carcinomas, melanomas, and lymphomas. Standard light microscopy of soft tissue tumours is no longer enough for the diagnostic evaluation of the biopsy specimen. Additional studies may be very important in establishing the most likely histological diagnosis and grade; they include histochemistry, immunohistochemistry, electron microscopy, flow cytometry, and molecular genetics (Baumal *et al.* 1984; du Bolay 1985; Roholl *et al.* 1985; Kreicksbergs *et al.* 1987; Leyvraz and Costa 1988; Matsuno *et al.* 1988). The biopsy is a critical step in patient management. It is difficult, requires mature judgement, and should be carefully planned and reviewed with the other members of the staging team. Further, the biopsy should be done by a senior member of the team that will have responsibility for the patient's management. The plan must allow not only for the biopsy itself but all subsequent potential surgical and radiation treatments. A well-planned biopsy should be appropriately placed, with a short incision and meticulous attention paid to haemostasis. Ecchymosis around the biopsy site can be assumed to mean spread of tumour cells over the same area in which erythrocytes have spread. Extensive areas of ecchymosis make the planning of radiation therapy or surgery much more difficult. For lesions on the extremities, the biopsy should be in the long axis. Regrettably, it is not rare to see patients whose biopsy was so placed as either to preclude or make very difficult subsequent surgical resection and the preparation of flaps (Mankin *et al.* 1982). A transverse incision on an extremity is a serious problem and almost invariably complicates any subsequent surgical procedure.

Most surgical oncologists believe that an incisional rather than an excisional biopsy is the most effective method of obtaining an appropriate tissue sample (Mankin *et al.* 1982; Simon 1982). The exception is the small (2–3 cm) tumour in the superficial tissues, which is appropriately removed as an excisional biopsy. This is the usual story in patients whose tumour has the clinical appearance of benignancy. The rationale for the incisional approach to most lesions suspected of being soft tissue sarcoma is that there is greater potential for contamination of tissue planes over a wide area with excisional biopsy.

The use of a pneumatic tourniquet is debated by surgical oncologists and many do not use these devices during either biopsy or definitive resection. The theoretical objection (never proven!) is related to the damming effect of the tourniquet during manipulation of the tumour and the resultant shedding of cells. When the tourniquet is released it is postulated that the clumped cells may have a greater chance of surviving in the lungs and establishing metastatic tumour.

Whether or not a tourniquet is used, the surgeon should strive for careful haemostasis and a dry field at the time of closure of the biopsy site. Closure should be done in layers. Many surgeons do not drain the site. If a drain is warranted, its exit site should be adjacent to and in a linear alignment with one end of the biopsy incision, as it too will have to be resected with the specimen at definitive surgery. Placing the drain site far from the wound may make a subsequent resection impossible (Mankin *et al.* 1982).

Tissue should be sent for a frozen sectioning during the biopsy to be certain that pathological tissue has been obtained and that a definitive diagnosis is likely to be made on the paraffin sections. It is prudent to make a microbiological culture of the wound, even when the lesion is clearly a sarcoma. Representative portions of the tissue specimen should be fixed in formalin or another standard fixative for paraffin bedding, in glutaraldehyde for electron microscopy, fresh frozen for immunohistochemistry, and used fresh for flow cytometry and cytogenetic analysis.

Although we do not favour the approach, a definitive diagnosis of soft tissue sarcoma can be obtained by needle biopsy without the difficulties and inconvenience of a surgical procedure or the necessity of other than local anaesthesia. Numerous devices are available for such procedures, but the most frequently used is a Tru-cut® biopsy needle, with which sufficient tissue can be obtained to make not only histological slides but other studies as well, provided several cores are obtained (Kissin *et al.* 1986). The procedure should, in most instances, be under CT guidance. The needle tract may be seeded with tumour and, hence, will require resection with the specimen at definitive surgery. The biopsy is usually done under local anaesthesia as an out-patient. Aspiration biopsy with a thin needle provides cells for cytodiagnosis and some centres have claimed excellent results with this less invasive technique (Miralles *et al.* 1986; Akerman and Rydholm 1987).

In recent years, diagnostic radiologists have developed a technique for needle biopsy during CT visualization, which enhances the success of the procedure (Bland *et al.* 1987). A fine needle is used to obtain an aspirate of cells for cytodiagnosis; a tissue core may be obtained with a Tru-cut® device. This technique is especially valuable for deeply placed lesions, those adjacent to vital structures, or those in which the biopsy site is likely to bleed excessively. Needle biopsy techniques are deemed of value in the confirmation of metastatic or recurrent tumour, even in those centres that rely on incisional biopsies for the primary diagnosis.

PATHOLOGY

The histopathological evaluation of the material should be by a pathologist who is interested in and experienced with soft tissue sarcomas. The optimal classification and grading of each soft

tissue tumour should improve our understanding of the natural history and responses to the various treatment strategies in this diverse group of tumours. There is much optimism that using the available battery of immunohistochemical stains will produce a large advance in the designation of the histological type for each sarcoma. The distribution of histological types reported for several large series is presented in Table 2. The large range of frequencies of the different histological types among the listed cancer centres is in part due to differences in referral patterns, but also reflects difficulties and uncertainties in type definitions. Note that the frequencies reported for fibrosarcoma range from 2 to 19 per cent, while for liposarcoma the range is 9.4–30.3 per cent. There is a definite need for additional criteria in the designation of the histopathological type of sarcoma. In the review of the diagnoses of 240 soft tissue sarcomas accessioned from 1981 to 1986 by the Scandinavian Sarcoma Group, 61 were reclassified as to type (Alvegard and Berg 1989). This finding supports the earlier report by the Southwest Oncology Group (Presant *et al.* 1986).

At present, the most widely employed classification system is the Enzinger and Weiss (1988) modification of the World Health Organization formulation. In their system, soft tissue tumours, including non-neoplastic, tumour-like lesions, are categorized into three broad divisions: (i) tumours that differentiate along cell or tissue lines having normal counterparts, such as fat, vessels, smooth muscle, nerve, and cartilage, (ii) tumours whose line of differentiation has no normal counterpart, and (iii) tumours so poorly differentiated that they defy classification. In the experience of most centres nearly all sarcomas are placed into the first two categories. The system is clearly complex, with 60 different types of sarcomas and some 100 benign tumour types. This inevitably leads to differences between pathologists as to the diagnosis of an individual tumour. The diagnoses have, until the recent past, been based almost exclusively upon standard, haematoxylin and eosin stains. Greater objectivity in diagnosis may be obtained with immunohistochemical techniques; these are likely to be of substantial value in the designation of the cell of origin (Enzinger and Weiss 1988). As an example, the stain for desmin is particularly valuable in identification of tumour cells demonstrating myogenic differentiation, such as in rhabdo- and leiomyosarcoma. Positive stains for the S-100 protein indicate Schwann cell differentiation. The cytokeratin stain can be of value in the distinction between synovial sarcoma and epithelial sarcoma vs fibrosarcoma. Tumours with endothelial differentiation

Table 2 Distribution (percentages) of sarcomas of soft tissues according to histological type

	MGH[a]	AJC[b]	SSG[c]	Lund[d]	MDAH[e]	NCI[f]	Memorial[g]	ACS[h]
No. patients	471	1215	240	229	300	307	423	3457[i]
Fibrosarcoma	17.2	19.0	4.6	14	13.6	18.2	14.2	6.6
Liposarcoma	17.6	18.2	10.4	15	13.6	9.4	30.3	17.7
Malignant fibrohistiocytoma	15.9	10.5	35.8	24	20.0	22.8	13.2	25.9
Unclassified	9.3	10.0		8	6.0			5.4
Leiomyosarcoma	8.7	6.5	10.0	12	5.3	11.4	3.9	14.8
Neurosarcoma	7.2	4.9	5.0	10	20.0		9.2	4.0
Synovial sarcoma	6.6	6.9	14.2	9	8.0	19.5	14.9	3.6
Rhabdomyosarcoma	4.0	19.2		3	5.6			
Other	13.6	4.6	20.0	13	7.7	18.6	14.4	22.7

[a] Massachusetts General Hospital.
[b] American Joint Commission Task Force (Russell *et al.* 1977).
[c] Scandinavian Sarcoma Group (Alvegaard and Berg 1989).
[d] Rhydholm *et al.* (1984).
[e] MD Anderson Hospital (Lindberg *et al.* 1981).
[f] National Cancer Institute (US) (Potter *et al.* 1985).
[g] Memorial Sloan Kettering Institute (NYC) (Collin *et al.* 1987).
[h] American College of Surgeons (Lawrence *et al.* 1987).
[i] For the period 1983–1984.

Table 3 Five year actuarial probability of distant metastasis in patients with local control as a function of tumour size and grade in MGH series

Size (mm)	Grade 1		Grades 2 and 3	
	No. of patients	DM	No. of patients	DM
< 25	7	0	24	8 (2)
26–50	12	0	47	19 (9)
51–100	18	6 (1)	98	44 (43)
101–150	7	0	35	55 (19)
151–200	4	25 (1)	19	71 (13)
> 200	4	0	10	90 (9)
Total	52	6	233	41 (96)

DM, distant metastasis, expressed as percentage with actual number in parentheses.

may be identified by stains for factor VIII. As data accumulate from centres using immunohistochemical procedures and electron microscopy, there will almost certainly be much higher diagnostic concordance between pathologists. More meaningful statements about the dependence of prognosis on histopathological type for each strata of histological grade and tumour size can then be made.

Designation of histopathological grade is clearly important, as stage depends primarily upon grade. Hence, grade is judged to be the single most important clinical or pathological prognostic variable. The pathologist evaluates all of the histological and cytological features of the tumour in designating grade. The principal ones are cellular and nuclear pleomorphism and atypism, mitotic activity, presence of necrosis, degree of differentiation, abundance of stroma, and the extent of cellularity. Mitotic figures alone are not sufficient for definition of grade. Designation of grade is, of course, subjective to an important extent. Trojani et al. (1984) have developed a system for grading based on a weighting of numerical scores given to mitotic figures, differentiation, and necrosis. This approach apparently yields a higher level of agreement between pathologists (Coindre et al. 1986). A study by the Scandinavian Sarcoma Group on archival material provides evidence that DNA aneuploidy is an independent indicator of prognosis (T. A. Alvegaard, unpublished). Efforts are being made to develop objective measures of cell proliferative activity and potential for distant metastasis. One of these is the staining of cells by the monoclonal antibody Ki67, which reacts with a nuclear antigen present on cells actively cycling. Ki67-negative cells are in the G_0 phase of the cell cycle. A report from Osaka provides evidence that the proportion of Ki67-positive cells in soft tissue sarcoma is a prognostic indicator, based on a study of 34 patients (Ueda et al. 1989).

Frequency of distant metastasis is related to tumour size as well as grade. The importance of size to frequency of metastasis for grade 1 and grade 2–3 lesions is shown in Table 3 for patients who have locally controlled disease. Very few patients developed metastatic disease from a grade 1 sarcoma. For sarcomas of grade 2 and 3, however, there was a rapid increase in frequency of distant metastasis with size. Approximately 8 per cent of patients develop metastases by 5 years for tumours of 25 mm or less, whilst some 90 per cent do so for sarcomas of 200 mm or larger. The time to metastasis and to local regrowth are also inversely related to grade. In the Rydholm study (1984) the median times for development of distant metastasis in patients with grade 1–2, grade 3, and grade 4 sarcomas were 27, 22, and 12 months, respectively. The comparable times for local regrowth were 18, 13, and 6 months.

Ruka (1986) has proposed as a prognostic index the ratio of diameter (cm) to symptom duration (months). In his analysis of the outcome of 153 adult patients treated in Warsaw, there was a negative correlation between the ratio and survival. The prognostic value of grade and size is important to planning future clinical studies because assessments of the efficacy of new methods of treatment must be based on relatively homogeneous groups of patients. As a minimum, tumours should be of similar size and grade. In the not too distant future one hopes there will be enough data for the relation between probability of distant metastasis and size as a function of grade to be defined for each of the major histopathological varieties.

STAGING OF SARCOMAS OF SOFT TISSUES

The two important prognostic factors for development of distant metastasis are therefore histological grade and tumour size. Very good rates of local control are now being achieved at virtually all of the sarcoma centres (approximately 90 per cent at 5 years). Hence, serious interest in the staging system concerns its usefulness in prediction of distant failure in patients who have local control. We use the AJC/UICC (Union Internationale Contre le Cancer) staging system (American Joint Committee 1988) as it is based primarily on grade (G) and size (T) and, secondarily, on the involvement of regional nodes (N) and the appearance of distant disease (M). The system is simple in concept and is quite easy to use and is presented in outline form in Table 4. It is used for all sarcomas of soft tissues with the exception of the rhabdomyosarcomas of childhood for which a separate system is still being used. Sarcomas that are grade 1, 2, or 3 are stage I, II, and III, respectively. Each tumour is assigned a grade on the basis of its individual histopathological features. Thus, no tumour is graded merely because of its basic histopathological type, for example a synovial or angiosarcoma may be a G_1 or G_3; this contrasts with the earlier version of the AJC system in which all synovial and angiosarcomas were assigned to G_3 and, hence, to stage III. The present protocol means that the occasional patient with a low-grade tumour in those categories would not be overtreated. Each stage is subdivided into an A and B group according to size: $\leqslant 5$ cm and > 5 cm, respectively. Histologically confirmed involvement of regional lymph node(s) means stage IVA. Clinical or radiographic evidence of distant metastatic disease places the patient in Stage IVB. Thus, a grade 2 sarcoma of 6.5 cm diameter (G_2, T_2) without regional nodes (N_0) and a negative examination for metastatic tumour (M_0) would be Stage IIB.

This staging protocol has an important advantage over the Enneking system (Enneking et al. 1980) in that the emphasis is placed on tumour size and not location within or without the boundaries of an anatomical compartment. Local control is frequently achieved for both the intra- and extracompartmental sarcomas with multimodality treatment strategies. The particular requirement now is to use the staging system that best predicts the probability of distant metastasis. In the Enneking system, a patient with 15 cm G_3 sarcoma that is within an anatomical compartment in the thigh would be staged as IIA, whilst the patient whose G_2 sarcoma was 1.5 cm and located in the wrist (extracompartmental) would be staged as IIB (stages I and II are low G_1 and high grades G_2–G_3, respectively). The local control of both of these tumours by current treatment methods would be good. However, the probability of developing a distant metastasis would be high in the

Table 4 AJC/UICC staging system for sarcoma of soft tissues (American Joint Committee 1988)

G Histological grade of malignancy
  G_1 Low, well differentiated
  G_2 Moderately well differentiated
  G_{3-4} Poorly differentiated

T Primary tumour
  T_1 Tumour 5 cm or less
  T_2 Tumour greater than 5 cm in greatest dimension

N Regional lymph nodes
  N_0 No histologically verified metastases to regional lymph nodes
  N_1 Histologically verified regional lymph node metastasis

M Distant metastasis
  M_0 No distant metastasis
  M_1 Distant metastasis

Stage I
  Stage IA: $G_1T_1N_0M_0$ Grade 1 tumour 5 cm or less with no regional lymph node or distant metastasis
  Stage IB: $G_1T_2N_0M_0$ Grade 1 tumour greater than 5 cm with no regional lymph node or distant metastasis

Stage II
  Stage IIA: $G_2T_1N_0M_0$ Grade 2 tumour 5 cm or less with no regional lymph node or distant metastases
  Stage IIB: $G_2T_2N_0M_0$ Grade 2 tumour greater than 5 cm with no regional lymph node or distant metastasis

Stage III
  Stage IIIA: $G_{3-4}T_1N_0M_0$ Grade 3 tumour 5 cm or less with no regional lymph node or distant metastasis
  Stage IIIB: $G_{3-4}T_2N_0M_0$ Grade 3 tumour greater than 5 cm with no regional lymph node or distant metastasis

Stage IV
  Stage IVA: $G_{1-4}T_{1-2}N_1M_0$ Tumour of any grade or size with histologically verified metastasis to regional lymph nodes, but no distant metastasis
  Stage IVB: $G_{1-4}T_{1-2}N_{0-1}M_1$ Clinically diagnosed distant metastasis

former (>0.5) but low (<0.1) in the latter patient. The probability of metastasis in patients whose primary tumour has been treated successfully is substantially dependent on size (see Table 3). There is no good evidence that the probability of distant metastasis in patients with local control depends upon site when the data are stratified according to size. In the example above, the patient with the small tumour but the highest stage in that system would in most centres be accepted for the most intensive treatment protocol, including high-dose chemotherapy. This would in our judgement constitute overtreatment. As discussed below, patients with such small tumours have good prognosis for local and distant control and we would not recommend adjuvant chemotherapy.

MANAGEMENT STRATEGIES FOR THE PRIMARY SOFT TISSUE SARCOMA

The options for the successful management of the primary lesion are radical compartmental resection, amputation, radiation combined with conservative surgery (the radiation being given pre- or post-operatively or intraoperatively), systemic or intra–arterial chemotherapy plus radiation plus wide resection, or radical resection with radiation for the patients whose specimen has narrow histological margins. For patients who cannot be operated on, radiation alone in high doses ($\geqslant 70$ Gy in 7 weeks) yields less satisfactory but still entirely useful rates of local control. This variability in treatment methods has developed over the past two decades as progressively more studies have demonstrated effective options to radical wide-field surgery or compartmental resection. Radical surgical procedures do yield high rates of local control, but at the price of greater loss of grossly normal tissue, function, and cosmesis. Regrettably, there are no data on the relative efficacy of these diverse methods functionally and cosmetically. This should be addressed in future clinical studies. The question of concern to the patient is: for a probability of local control of 0.9, which procedure gives the best functional and cosmetic result? Undoubtedly the answer will not be simplistic and all embracing, but one which considers the site and size of the tumour, prior surgery, and the status of the tissue (age, obesity, nutrient perfusion, medical disease—for example, insulin-requiring diabetes—etc.).

Tables 5 and 6 present, in summary form, data on local failure from various centres using different methods of treatment. The results are in the range 5–15 per cent; these include varying times of follow-up, actuarial 5 year, and simple percentages of local control.

Table 5 Patterns of failure in patients treated by radical resection or amputation alone

Centre	No. of patients	Follow–up (years)	LF	LF+DM[a]	DM
Memorial Hospital	297	5–24	46	8	100
University of Florida	54	2–19	3	6	12
Göteborg	97	3–23	6	15	31
National Cancer Institute (USA)	16	1–7	0	0	3
Pooled data	464	1–24	55 (12.3%)	29 (6.5%)	146 (31.5%)

[a]LF, local failure; DM, distant metastasis.
From: Suit (1983).

Table 6 Local failure rate in patients with sarcoma of soft tissue treated by radiation and surgery (±chemotherapy)

Centre	No. of patients	Local failure (%)	Reference
MGH[a]:			
Post-operative	144	14.0	H. D. Suit et al. (unpublished)
Pre-operative	114	9.0	H. D. Suit et al. (unpublished)
IGR[b]	89	14.0	Abbatucci et al. (1986)
RPMI[c]	53	14.0	Karakousis et al. (1986)
MDAH[d]			
Post-operative	253	20.9	Lindberg et al. (1981)
Pre-operative	110	10.0	Barkley et al. (1988)
NCI[e]	128	10.0	Potter et al. (1986)
UCSF[f]	29	10.0	Leibel et al. (1982)
University of Florida	19	5.0	Enneking and McAuliffe (1985)
Memorial (implant)	74	7.0	Brennan et al. (1987)

[a]MGH, Massachusetts General Hospital; [b]IGR, Institut Gustav Roussay; [c]RPMI, Roswell Park Memorial Institute; [d]MDAH, M. D. Anderson Hospital; [e]NCI, National Cancer Institute (USA); [f]UCSF, University of California at San Francisco.

Surgery alone

The surgical management of soft tissue tumours is based on well-known principles of cancer surgery. The extent and nature of the procedure should only be planned after the staging information is complete (including the results of the biopsy) and after consultation with the radiation oncologists and medical oncologists of the team.

The extent of and potential disability associated with the procedures for resection of soft tissue tumours vary according to the anatomical site and the desired amount of grossly normal tissue to be sacrificed (the 'margin'). If the procedures are considered generically, both amputation and resection can be described according to the margin obtained. Four types of procedure are described (Enneking *et al.* 1980; Rydholm and Rooser 1987; Lawrence 1988; Bell *et al.* 1989). The clinically important margin is the most narrow one.

The first of these procedures, the intralesional, is, as the name implies, within the tumour and by definition leaves gross tumour in the bed. An amputation can be intralesional. This procedure is rarely indicated, but may be appropriate for certain benign lesions or as a 'debulking' in palliative treatment. Local recurrence is almost invariable after intralesional procedures for malignant lesions.

Marginal resection means that the margin is in the compressed soft tissue capsule surrounding the lesion. The 'reactive zone' around rapidly growing malignant tumours of soft tissue establishes a plane that allows the tumour to be 'shelled out' and involves little sacrifice of normal tissue and, hence, minimal disability. The difficulty with this approach for sarcomas or even desmoid tumours is that the compressed reactive zone contains not only small numbers of tumour cells but possibly satellite or daughter nodules. Marginal resections should be reserved for selected patients whose lesions are also to be treated by radiation given pre- or post-operatively (see below).

The third category of procedure is wide resection; this is the standard for amputation or resection of high-grade soft tissue (and bone) tumours. As the term implies, a cuff of grossly normal tissue surrounds the lesion and the reactive zone is removed with the gross lesion. The resection remains within the anatomical compartment in which the tumour arises and as such may leave microscopic tumour extensions along vessels or nerve trunks. If done correctly, however, the likelihood of a local recurrence after a wide resection (with more than 1 cm of histologically proven negative margin) is low and is reduced further if the tumour bed is irradiated.

A further procedure, known as radical and infrequently used today, is resection of the entire compartment in which the tumour arises. Hence, a lesion of the anterior compartment of the thigh treated by a radical procedure would require either a hip disarticulation or a resection of the entire quadriceps muscle mass.

The surgical resection should include the biopsy wound or track. Surgery should be done under tourniquet if there is a threat of major blood loss (see above for the theoretical objections to the use of a pneumatic tourniquet).

The resection plan is based on the clinical findings and the outcome of imaging, with the surgery done to achieve the predetermined margin. The specimen should be examined in the operating room by the pathologist and the tumour margins marked with ink. The orientation of the specimen should be recorded and important landmarks noted. If the gross margins are close, frozen sections should be taken of the resection margin of the tumour bed to help in deciding whether further resection is warranted. After resection or amputation, meticulous care should be taken to achieve haemostasis and secure closure over drains. Both drainage and antibiotics should be continued for a reasonable length of time. If pre-operative radiation has been given or if post-operative radiation is contemplated, the sutures should be left in for longer than usual. Rehabilitation is facilitated by appropriate exercises and mobilization techniques.

The resected specimen must be studied with care both grossly and microscopically. At MGH the entire tumour is examined microscopically if smaller than 5 cm in its greatest dimension and at least one section per cm if larger than 5 cm. Attention and sampling should be directed to variation in colour, texture, and consistency; these may guide the experienced eye to areas of higher-grade tumour.

Results of surgery alone from several sarcoma centres are given in Table 5 above. The overall rate of local failure is approximately 5–20 per cent. In patients whose surgical specimens were proven to have histologically negative margins the local failure rate was 5 per cent (6/122) in the series of Simon and Enneking (1976) and Markhede *et al.* (1982). In strong contrast the local failure rate was 89 per cent (24/27) among those with positive margins within an overall rate of 20 per cent. In the report of the phase III trial of radical surgery alone or combined with adjuvant doxurubicin from the Scandinavian Sarcoma Group, the local failure rate in the patients with proven negative margins was 8 per cent (Alvegard *et al.* 1989). There were local failures in 16 of 73 patients treated by surgery alone at the Memorial Hospital in the control arm of their phase III trial of intraoperative brachytherapy (Brennan *et al.* 1987).

When adjuvant radiation or chemotherapy are added to the protocol, special attention to details of surgical technique is essential as there is an increased potential for delayed wound healing. If radiation has been given pre-operatively, the surgery should be done 2.5–3 weeks later. Wound treatment during the operative procedure should be especially gentle, as the irradiated skin and soft tissues will be less forgiving than their normal counterparts. The incision should be carefully planned to avoid unusual configurations, sharp angulations, or closure under tension. Attention should be directed to saving some of the underlying muscle and particularly the deep fascia, as this will aid healing. Wound closure should in general be in layers, with placement of viable muscle layers over the resection bed where feasible.

If, at the time of planning the procedure or at completion of resection, the viability of the skin and subjacent soft tissues is judged to be in peril, a reconstructive surgical procedure should be considered. If this is a realistic option, primary healing should be markedly enhanced. Techniques or procedures often used include broad-based skin and soft tissue flaps (more frequently used over the back and buttocks), gastrocnemius, soleus, rectus, latissimus dorsi, and pectoralis major flaps (in which the viable and usually non-irradiated muscle on a neurovascular pedicle is lifted from its insertion or origin, positioned in the wound, and subsequently covered with a split-skin graft), and free pedicle flaps, principally using the latissimus dorsi muscle transplanted on a vascular pedicle anastomosed to a local artery and vein. That last procedure may or may not include a surface layer of skin, but more commonly includes a split-skin graft cover. The free flap is the most complex of the skin coverages, takes the longest (sometimes up to 8 h more surgery), and, as it opens up a new operative field, increases (at least theoretically) the hazard of transplantation of tumour cells (but this would not be a problem in patients who had received pre-operative radiation). Nevertheless, for selected wounds in some anatomical sites this procedure is of great value in providing skin coverage and inducing rapid functional recovery in a setting that would almost surely have failed to heal if more conventional closures had been employed. Regardless of the method used to achieve a good wound closure without tension, the wound site must be drained so as to avoid fluid collection in a dead space. Irradiated wounds, or those in patients on aggressive chemotherapeutic regimens, often produce sterile serosanguineous fluid, which is poorly resorbed and may persist for days or even weeks after surgery. An appropriately positioned and monitored drain(s) minimizes the fluid collections. The sides of the wound have to be in contact for healing to occur. In addition to the drains, this process may be aided by a pressure dressing; we often use a Robert Jones dressing. The extremity should be put at rest so that the sides of the wound can begin the bonding necessary for healing. Exercises should be started as soon as this has been achieved. Too early a start of an exercise programme can lead to poor healing or wound dehiscence. After large resections near joints, a delay of several weeks before starting any but a little movement may be a valuable aid to healing.

For radiation or chemotherapy given after surgery, a delay of some 2 weeks before the start of treatment is advisable. Sutures should remain in place until the radiation treatment is over (sometimes as long as 6 weeks or more). During such treatment, careful attention needs to be paid to signs of incipient wound breakdown, infection, or fluid accumulation. Ultrasonography or CT are valuable in detecting fluid accumulations. At times, repeated aspirations, firm dressings, and rest of the part can facilitate control of the 'seroma'.

The same risk factors that make wound healing problematical at any site after surgery alone compound the problem in the patient receiving multimodality therapy. The elderly patient with poor peripheral blood supply or the diabetic both run a greater risk of wound breakdown, infection, or delayed healing. Patients who are obese have an added risk of difficulties with wound closure and skin necrosis. Those patients who have been on medications such as corticosteroids and chemotherapeutic agents or have some form of connective tissue disorder, may present major problems as a result of poor wound healing. Patients with severe problems in these categories and large sarcomas (in relation to the size of the affected part) may be candidates for a primary amputation. This may actually be the more conservative approach to the problem, with greater likelihood of a rapid return to function than the more complex (and probably more complicated) limb-sparing procedure.

Radiation alone

For the patient who is medically inoperable or absolutely refuses the recommended surgery, radiation alone or combined with chemotherapy can be offered with the potential of permanent local control, although at a definitely lower probability than with the combination of surgery and radiation. Our position is that surgery should, if at all feasible, be part of the treatment to maximize the likelihood of local control.

In those patients for whom radiation is to be used alone, the plan must be carefully designed so as to permit doses of 70 Gy or more. This means excluding as much non-target tissue from the treatment volume as is technically feasible. For this, rigid immobilization, use of multiple fields, wedges, compensators, treatment of two fields or more per day, frequent portal films, dose uniformity (±5 per cent), and reducing field (volume) techniques should be used in order to give the indicated dose and keep the late tissue changes within tolerable limits. That eradication of soft tissue sarcoma can be achieved by radiation alone has long been established. For instance, Cade (1951) reported that six of 22 patients so treated were alive and well 5 years after treatment. Some of the earlier publications on this aspect of treatment have been reviewed by del

Regato (1963); for further data, see Windeyer *et al.* (1966), McNeer *et al.* (1968), and Lindberg (1980). An analysis of the experience of the MGH showed that useful rates of local control were obtained only in patients receiving the equivalent of 65 Gy or more (Tepper and Suit 1985) to the smaller lesions. Local control of the large tumours required doses of more than 70 Gy. The late changes were severe as the doses were high and the treatment volumes were large.

Rationale for combining radiation and surgery

The essential rationale is that the sarcoma infiltrates the normal-appearing tissue adjacent to the evident lesion. Thus, removal of the gross lesion by a simple excision (only a narrow margin) is followed by local recurrence in some 70–90 per cent of patients. Simple resection was therefore replaced by radical resection so that the surgical specimen would include a wide margin of apparently normal tissue around the tumour. This reduced the rate of local failure to approximately 25–30 per cent. More recently, with the advent of compartmental resections, that rate is down to 5–20 per cent in those patients accepted for such surgery, as shown in Table 5 above. Radiation at moderate dosage (60–65 Gy) should be effective in eradicating the microscopic extensions beyond the gross lesion. That is, a moderate radiation dose and relatively conservative surgery would accomplish the same as the expansion

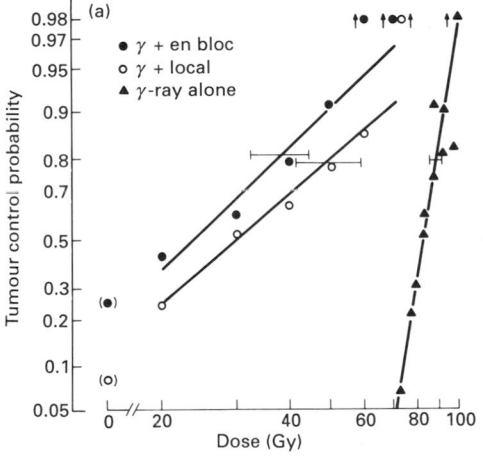

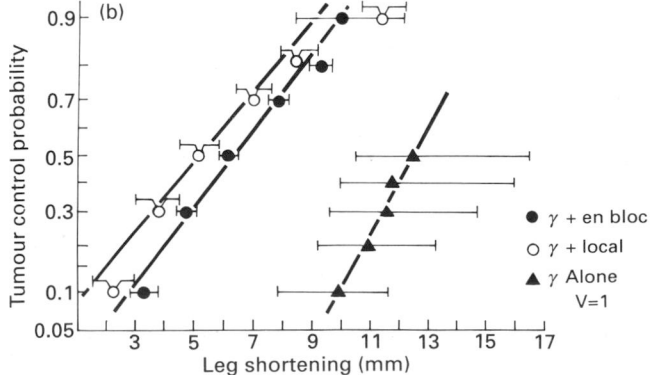

Fig. 3 (a) FSalI (a spontaneous fibrosarcoma of the C3H mouse studied as early-generation isotransplants) were irradiated at 8 mm diameter by single doses. Dose–response curves for local control following radiation alone (▲), radiation and then local (○) or *en bloc* (●) resection. (b) Tumour control–leg shortening relation for the 8-mm FSalI.

from simple to radical surgery. This appears to have been accomplished in a number of centres (see Table 6).

A major question is the appropriate surgical margin in planning the surgery and the radiation dosage. Here, mention should be made of the results of a study based on the spontaneous fibrosarcoma, FSaII, in the $C3H_f$/Sed mouse, grown as early-generation iso-transplants in the animal's leg (Todoroki and Suit 1985). Complete dose—response assays were made as shown in Fig. 3(a), for radiation given alone or pre-operatively for marginal excision, radical excision, or amputation. There was a major shift of the dose—response curve to the left when radiation was combined with simple excision. The extension of the surgery to radical resection caused only a minor further displacement of the curve. The plot of leg shortening vs the probability of tumour control demonstrates that the least damage for a specified control rate was achieved by radiation combined with relatively simple surgery (Fig. 3(b)).

Results of treatment by radiation and surgery

The results of the treatment of 317 consecutive patients with sarcoma of soft tissue by combination of radiation and relatively conservative surgery at MGH (1971–1986) are presented in Tables 7–10. The dosages used in these patients have been 64–68 Gy given in 1.8–2.0 Gy fractions and five fractions per week (a small number of patients have been treated on a BID schedule (2 fractions/day) and are included in the analyses given here). For details of dosage and technique see the section on technique below. Tables 8–10 give the current status and 5 year actuarial data for local control and disease-free survival in patients treated by post-operative (167) or by pre-operative (150) radiation. The rates of local control (5 years) for the post- and pre-operative groups were 85 and 89 per cent, respectively. The rate for locally successful treatment at the MGH has been marginally higher more recently. For example, in the period 1981–1985, rates of local control were 92 per cent for patients treated post-operatively (57 patients) or pre-operatively (73 patients). There is evidence of an advantage for pre-operative radiation, especially for larger lesions: rates of local control for lesions of 151–200 mm and those larger than 200 mm were 54 and 67 per cent for post-operative and 76 and 100 per cent for pre-operative radiation (Table 10). These results argue for consideration of the pre-operative approach in patients with sarcomas larger than 5 cm in diameter. Barkley *et al.* (1988) have reported 11 local failures in 110 patients treated pre-operatively at the M. D. Anderson Hospital, Houston, Texas. This 10 per cent compares favourably with their reported 20 per cent for post-operative radiation shown in Table 6.

Table 7 Current status and 5 year actuarial results in 317 patients treated by conservative surgery and radiation according to stage at MGH

Stages	No. of patients	NED	LF±DM	DM	ID	5-ALC (%)	OS (%)
IA	20	19	0	0	1	100	100
B	35	29	3	1	2	91	93
IIA	51	34	6	8	3	85	95
B	86	41	9	33	3	86	68
IIIA	37	27	3	4	3	90	87
B	85	29	11	40	5	81	48
IVA	3	3	0	0	0	100	100
Total	317	182	32	86	17	87	75

NED, no evident disease; LF, local failure; DM, distant metastasis; ID, dead of intercurrent disease; 5-ALC, 5 year actuarial (local control); OS, overall survival.

Table 8 Current status and 5 year actuarial results in 167 patients treated by surgery and post-operative radiation according to stage at MGH

Stages	No. of patients	NED	LF±DM	DM	ID	5-ALC (%)	OS (%)
IA	16	15	0	0	1	100	100
B	21	18	1	0	2	95	94
IIA	34	22	5	4	3	85	93
B	33	15	7	9	2	74	73
IIIA	29	21	1	4	3	96	87
B	33	11	7	15	0	71	46
IVA	1	1	0	0		100	100
Total	167	103	21	32	11	85	79

Abbreviations as in Table 7.

Table 9 Current status and 5 year actuarial results in 150 patients treated by pre-operative radiation and conservative surgery according to stage at MGH

Stages	No. of patients	NED	LF±DM	DM	ID	5-ALC (%)	OS (%)
IA	4	4	0	0	0	100	100
B	14	11	2	1	0	85	92
IIA	17	12	1	4	0	87	100
B	53	26	11	24	1	95	64
IIIA	8	6	2	0	0	72	88
B	52	18	4	25	5	90	49
IVA	2	2	0	0	0	100	100
Total	150	79	11	54	6	89	69

Abbreviations as in Table 7.

Table 10 Five year actuarial local control results according to size (MGH data)

Size (mm)	Post-operative No. of patients	LC (%)	Pre-operative No. of patients	LC (%)
<25	24	88	10	82
26–49	51	91	15	83
50–100	68	84	61	92
101–150	14	92	29	100
151–200	7	54	23	76
>200	3	67	12	100
Total	167	85	150	89

LC, local control.

Rates of local control and disease-free survival were high for patients with small sarcomas (≤ 5 cm); stages IA, IIA, or IIIA. For stages IIB and IIIB, local control was higher for the patients treated pre-operatively; 95 and 90 per cent, as compared with 74 and 71 per cent for post-operative irradiation. Disease-free survival was low for patients with stages IIB and IIIB tumours, regardless of the method of local treatment, because of the high frequency of distant metastasis. Barkley *et al.* (1988) also reported a negative correlation between survival and size and grade of sarcoma. Of 13 patients whose sarcomas were smaller than 5 cm the survival at 66 months was 90 per cent. For patients whose sarcomas were 5–15 cm the survival was approximately 60 per cent, but only 45 per cent for the patients with sarcomas larger than 15 cm.

Both in the MGH and the M. D. Anderson series pre-operative radiation there have been difficulties with delay of wound healing. This has especially been a problem for the elderly and obese patients with large sarcomas in the proximal thigh. Intensive efforts should be made to fill (at least in part) the defect produced by the resection by use of vascularized muscle flaps, careful monitoring of fluid accumulation in the wound, and rather longer periods of bed-rest post-operatively. Nearly all of these difficult cases do heal and achieve good function. However, five of the MGH patients did come to amputation because of poor wound healing. The overall functional results are judged to be good and to be improving as care of the wound becomes more intensive. Delays in wound healing are also seen in patients treated by surgery alone (Arbeit *et al.* 1987; Skibber *et al.* 1987). When such delays occur in patients scheduled for post-operative radiation, the residual tumour may grossly recur before treatment can be started. This has been observed several times for high-grade lesions.

The results described above for pre- or post-operative radiation are not unique, as shown by the data presented in Table 6 from several centres. Rates of local failure range from 5 to 20 per cent in a total experience with almost 1000 patients. Surgery varied from simple local excision or marginal resection to radical resection.

Further resection of the tumour bed

In planning treatment for a patient who has had a resection of sarcoma by a surgeon who is not an oncological surgeon and/or one who has not had the benefit of pre-operative CT or MRI, serious consideration should be given to a further resection. Radiation may be given either pre-operatively or post-operatively depending on the particular circumstances and/or the interests of the group looking after the patient. This recommendation is based on the findings in a number of series. For example, Giuliano and Eilber (1985) reported that approximately half of the patients referred to their group at UCLA after excision had macroscopically evident tumour in the further resection specimen. Of 11 patients treated at MGH by pre-operative radiation and re-excision, local control has been achieved in all 11 (H. D. Suit *et al.*, unpublished).

Intra-arterial doxorubicin and radiation

Treatment by the combination of intra-arterial doxorubicin, radiation, and then resection has been studied in a large number of patients by Eilber *et al.* (1988*a*) (see Table 11). In the period 1972–1976, 63 patients were treated surgically (amputation in 33 per cent) or by excision plus radiation; the local recurrence rate was 22 per cent. They then began a programme of doxorubicin 30 mg per day ×3 (intra-arterially) followed by radiation (3.5 Gy × 10) and then resection. This was subsequently changed to 3.5 Gy × 5 and more recently 3.5 Gy × 8 so as to decrease treatment-related morbidity. Sequential results are impressive in showing rates of local recurrence of 5–12 per cent. The proportion of patients who had amputation was below 5 per cent. Good results (one local failure in 30 patients; short follow-up) have been reported from another centre with this approach (Denton *et al.* 1984). F. Eilber (unpublished) has data from a trial of intra-arterial vs intravenous doxorubicin and finds comparable results, that is, no advantage in local control for the intra-arterial route.

Fast-neutron and negative-pion radiation therapy

Several centres have reported results of local control from fast-neutron irradiation of inoperable sarcomas of soft tissue that indicate a gain. Pickering *et al.* (1987) treated 50 patients with palpable soft tissue sarcomas (primary or recurrent after photon treatment)

Table 11 Results of treatment of patients with sarcoma of soft tissue by intra-arterial doxorubicin, radiation, and resection

Period	No. of patients	Doxorubicin	Radiation	Local failure (%)	Amputation (%)
1972–76	63	–	±	22	33
1974–84	77	+	3.5 Gy×10	5	4
1981–84	137	+	3.5 Gy×5	12	5
1984–87	97	+	3.5 Gy×8	5	2

Reproduced from: Eilber *et al.* (1988*b*), with permission.

by 7.5 MV fast neutrons alone and achieved a local control rate of approximately 50 per cent. A similar rate was reported by Schmitt *et al.* (1987) for fast-neutron treatment following incomplete resection. Franke and Schmidt (1987) reported four local failures in 17 patients treated for gross disease. The number of patients treated was small and they did not judge that there was an evident advantage of fast-neutron over photon therapy. For a review of this method of treatment, see Laramore *et al.* (1989). Negative-pion therapy has been reported to be highly effective against sarcomas of the retroperitoneal tissues by R. H. Greiner *et al.* (unpublished) at the Paul Scherer Institute, Switzerland. This appears to constitute a real gain for patients with these formidable tumours. They attribute their fine results to the better dose distribution rather than the effects of the high linear-energy transfer radiations.

Proton-beam therapy

A small series of patients has been treated at MGH by proton-beam techniques for their sarcomas in the paraspinal tissues and those that overlay the hip, elbow, shoulder, and wrist joints. The treatment was conservative surgery and post-operative radiation (approximately 65 Gy). In all instances, the sensitive underlying structures (spinal cord and joints) have not exhibited signs of radiation damage (H. D. Suit *et al.*, unpublished data). There has been local control in 7/8 patients with paraspinal lesions and all of the other cases. The entire basis for interest in the use of proton beams is in the superior dose distributions that can readily be achieved for many anatomical sites. This means that the dose to the target can be increased or that the dose to sensitive structures can be sharply reduced or virtually eliminated.

Intraoperative electron-beam therapy (IORT)

This technique employs a remarkably simple and direct approach to irradiation of tumours: after surgical exposure of the tumour site, the overlying and/or immediately adjacent sensitive structures are packed out of the beam path and the electron cone applied directly to the surface of the tumour site; the radiation is then given in a large, single dose, for example 10–20 Gy. In most applications, IORT is given as a boost or supplemental dose to conventionally fractionated radiation. Thus, the patient may receive 50 Gy as 25 fractions of 2 Gy over a period of 5 weeks. This is followed in some 2–3 weeks by surgical resection and an IORT dose of 10–20 Gy to the tumour bed. In 10 patients with retroperitoneal sarcoma treated at MGH by 40–50 Gy, grossly complete resection, and an IORT boost dose of 10–20 Gy, nine have local control (C. G. Willett, unpublished data). One concern is the sensitivity of major nerves to the combined treatment of 50 Gy over 5 weeks followed by the single dose of 10–20 Gy intraoperatively. There has been a larger test of this class of treatment by Kinsella *et al.* (1988) in the treatment of patients with retroperitoneal sarcomas by resection and IORT. The test cases experienced less symptomatic damage to the intestines than those given post-operative external-beam radiotherapy. There was not, however, a clear benefit in terms of tumour control.

Radiation sensitizers

There has for some 30 years been interest in pyrimidine analogues as sensitizers of mammalian cells to ionizing radiations. Special attention has been given to bromodeoxyuridine and iododeoxyuridine. These halogenated pyrimidines are incorporated into the DNA molecule competitively against thymidine. The resultant fraudulent DNA molecule is much more susceptible to breakage by radiation than are normal DNA molecules. Sensitization depends on the extent of replacement of thymidine by the analogues. The effect is to reduce both the shoulder and the slope of the cell survival curve. Despite disappointing results when tested against squamous cell carcinomas of the mouth and oropharynx and high-grade gliomas, some impressive results are now being reported from tests with locally far advanced soft tissue sarcomas. In a study by Kinsella and Glatstein (1987) this strategy yielded complete regression in 22/29 patients whose soft tissue sarcomas were judged to be inoperable. There is further research into this approach on the timing and duration of the drug infusion, dose, and the severity of the photosensitization of the skin and eyes after the drug administration.

Hyperfractionation and accelerated treatment

There is extensive testing of both of these approaches in the treatment of patients with tumours at other anatomical sites, especially in the head and neck region, but as yet little to be said on their efficacy against soft tissue sarcomas.

Hyperthermia and radiation therapy

There is an attractive rationale for the use of hyperthermia and radiation in the management of patients with large soft tissue sarcomas. Firstly, a substantial heat differential would be expected between tumour and the surrounding normal tissue for a uniform and constant power input because of the less satisfactory blood flow through the tumour. Secondly, the metabolically deprived region of the sarcoma (low pH, hypoxia, non-cycling cells) would be more sensitive to the heat than the adjacent normal tissues. It is these deprived regions that would be the least responsive to radiation given alone. Thirdly, the heated tumour cells (higher temperatures than the nearby normal cells) would be sensitized to the radiations. Fourthly, S-phase cells are the most sensitive to heat damage, the reverse of the situation for radiation killing. There is insufficient experience upon which to judge the efficacy of hyperthermia. Leopold et al. (1989) have reported on their preliminary experience: with radiation followed in 30–60 min by hyperthermia (42°C for around 60 min for one or two treatments per week) there were more severe histological changes in the heat-treated tumours.

Techniques of radiation therapy

The success of the conservative (combined) approach in the management of the primary sarcoma of soft tissue has been so high that primary amputation for such sarcomas arising on the extremities is done only in rather special circumstances. The functional and cosmetic results of the conservative procedure depend upon the size and anatomical location of the tumour, the magnitude of the surgical procedure, the extent to which muscles, tendons, or nerves must be sacrificed, the status of the normal tissues, radiation dosage, and the volume of normal tissue irradiated.

The principal concept in devising a technique for radiation therapy is to define the target volume and to estimate the distribution of clonogen number throughout that volume. Virtually all modern techniques for radiation treatment feature reduction of the volume as treatment progresses so as to distribute dose in accord with the likely distribution of clonogens. The treatment policy at the MGH is to consider that 50 Gy delivered in 5–5.5 weeks should be the minimum dose to tissues suspected of subclinical involvement. The treatment volume is reduced once or twice. Total doses of approximately 65 Gy are given to the tumour bed for radiation combined with surgery. For pre-operative radiation, the treatment plan has been to give 50 Gy in 5–5.5 weeks, then a rest period of 2.5–3 weeks, then conservative resection; a boost dose of 15–18 Gy directed to the tumour bed is given intraoperatively by brachytherapy or post-operatively with small fields directed towards the tumour bed. For the latter, 15 Gy may be given as 10 Gy to a volume of tissue slightly larger than that of the residual tumour bed and a final 5 Gy to the tumour bed itself, as defined by clips placed at surgery.

Radiation given post-operatively is started approximately 10–20 days after surgery (sufficient time to allow for a good start toward wound healing). After the resection of large tumours there may be a need to wait 3–4 weeks so that the 'seroma' will have been resorbed almost completely. The initial volume must include all tissues suspected of involvement as well as those handled during the surgical procedure, including the site of the drain tube. Here, the radiation dose is 50–54 Gy to the initial volume and then, through two subsequent treatment volumes, the final dose is 65–66 Gy. This assumes that the surgical procedure removes all gross disease. If gross disease remains, the patient is considered

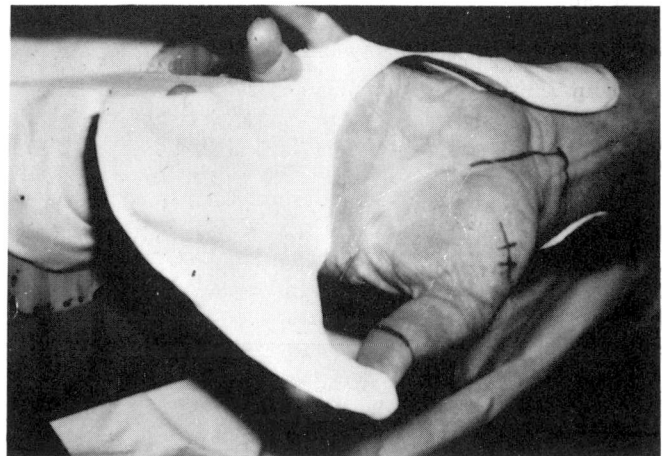

Fig. 4 An immobilization device for treatment of a sarcoma of the thenar eminence. The device must be designed to achieve secure immobilization of the part to be treated and reproducible positioning of the target in relation to the beam in each treatment session. The hand is not a particularly difficult part for immobilization provided there is sufficient 'cut-out' for its irradiation without intervening material, thus achieve skin sparing when this is intended. In the example shown here the beam was from a ^{60}Co unit, which does realize good skin sparing and with a minimum depth of D_{max}. A narrow strip of bolus (5 mm thick and 5–6 mm wide) is applied over the scar for the first 50 Gy).

as treated by radiation alone and the dose is 70–75 Gy, if judged tolerable, with an appropriate field-reduction technique.

The treatment should be carefully planned so that the tissues being irradiated are only those judged to be at risk. This means that the target volume should be defined on each CT section throughout the volume of concern and that there should be close collaboration between the physicist and the physician to devise an array of beams, beam energies, beam quality (photons, electrons, and even protons), and beam modifiers (wedge filters, compensators, etc.), to achieve the maximum concentration of radiation dose within the defined target volumes. In practical terms, this means that two or more fields are used, with at least two fields being treated each day.

To achieve the dose distribution as planned, the patient and the affected part need to be immobilized throughout each treatment. An immobilization device for treatment of a sarcoma of the hand is illustrated in Fig. 4. Individualized immobilization devices or systems for each patient are important aids to the accurate placement of the treatment volume.

Figure 5 is an example of the point that the treatment plan for the patient with soft tissue sarcoma often requires complex technical efforts. The dose distribution achieved in this patient with a sarcoma of the dorsum of the foot was based upon a plantar 25 MeV and a dorsal ^{60}Co beam. This provided a relatively low dose to the sensitive plantar tissues.

The extent of grossly normal tissue to be included in the treatment volume is not based on analyses of data for this point, but rather 'clinical experience and judgement'. The portion of failures in the MGH series that are marginal has been extremely low. The practice at the MGH has been to allow the following margins (in the long axis of an extremity): approximately 5 cm for small, grade 1 sarcomas, 5–10 cm for large grade 1 and small grade 2–3, and 10–15 cm for large grade 2–3. These numbers must be taken as guidelines only. Fascial membranes and bones are relatively strong barriers to tumour spread. For example, for a sarcoma near bone, only the adjacent cortex need be included in the target volume (provided the bony cortex is intact radiographically). Lesions in the anterior compartment of the arm or leg do not frequently transgress the interosseous membrane. Hence, treatment margins can be only a few centimetres in the transverse plane as distinct from the long axis. This is illustrated in Fig. 6, which presents clinical pictures, transverse CT, treatment plan, resected specimen, and follow-up photograph of a patient with a locally advanced sarcoma of the anterior compartment of the leg. In this example, the tumour had ulcerated through the biopsy scar and probably was displacing the interosseous membrane posteriorly. For treatment of this patient a wedge pair was used; this provided ample coverage of the anterior compartment and a margin of tissue posterior to the interosseous membrane. The resected specimen had only a thin margin. The wound did heal uneventfully. The patient has had a painless and oedema-free leg for 5 years; he is free of tumour and of any significant morbidity.

In treating sarcoma of an extremity, a good functional result demands that only a portion of the cross-section of the extremity be irradiated to any worthwhile dose level. Thus, some essentially unirradiated tissue must be left in order to provide a reasonable lymphatic drainage. If there has been a very large tumour with wide resection, there probably will be persistent oedema requiring (in the leg) use of a pressure-type stocking, even though the radiation treatment volume did not cover the entirety of the cross-section of the limb.

Although external-beam techniques are employed in the vast majority of radiation treatments, an effective alternative is

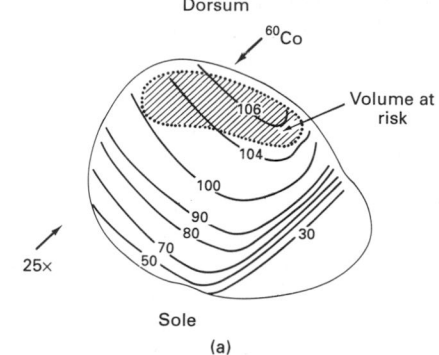

(a)

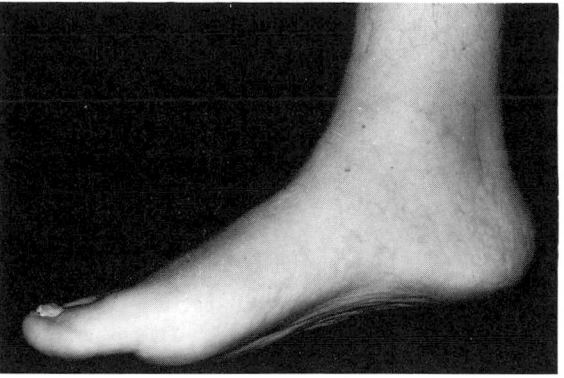

(b)

Fig. 5 (a) Dose distribution for the post-operative treatment of an 8 cm grade 3 sarcoma of the dorsum of the right foot of a 28-year-old man. The tumour had infiltrated the tissue spaces between the metatarsal bones and was thus not completely resected. The plan was a dorsal ^{60}Co and a plantar 25 MeV photon field; the result was an effective sparing of the sole of the foot, the dose being greater than 50 per cent and the dose to the target tissues being approximately 100 per cent. The final dose (one-field reduction) was 70 Gy in 35 fractions in 51 days. (b) The patient has enjoyed a fine result; at 4 years the sole looks normal and the foot is near normal in function for a sedentary life-style. The patient works regularly and successfully as a stockbroker. He cannot participate in outdoor athletic activities without discomfort.

brachytherapy. This approach has been used in combination with surgery for the entire radiation treatment or for boost dose. The group at Memorial Hospital (Brennan *et al.* 1987) have reported that results for local control from their trial of resection alone vs resection plus interstitial therapy are 78 vs 93 per cent. Other reports of brachytherapy for sarcoma include Mills and Hering (1981), Gerbaulet *et al.* (1985), and Curran *et al.* (1988).

The combination of radiation and chemotherapy has, in our experience, required reduction in the total radiation dose. For combination chemotherapy protocols featuring doxorubicin we reduce the total dose by 10–12 per cent and do not give radiation concurrently with doxorubicin. Two or three days are allowed between the doxoribicin and the radiation. For treatment given on a BID protocol, we reduce the total dose by approximately 10 per cent.

Desmoid tumours

Radiation may useful in the treatment of several benign but locally aggressive neoplasms. Amongst these, the most important for the

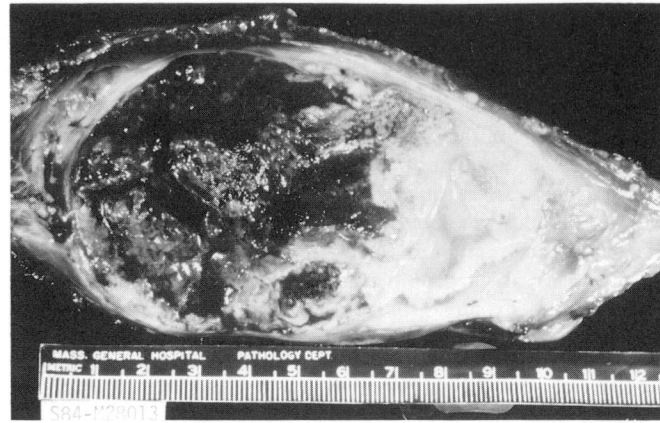

(a)

(b)

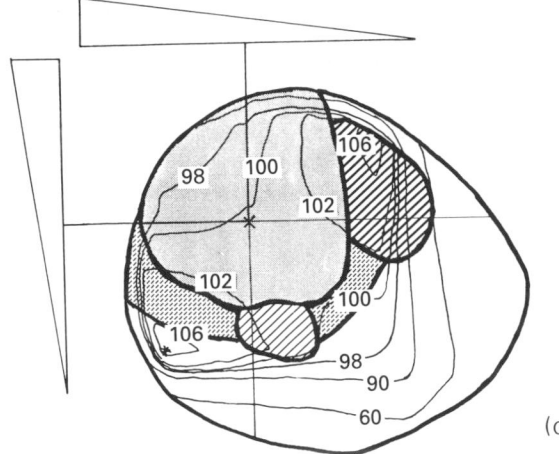

(c)

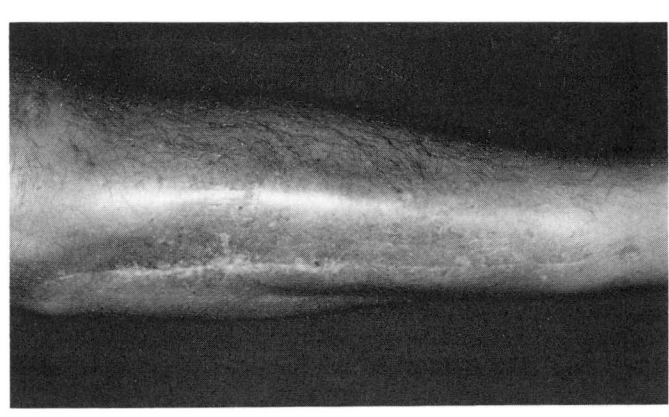

(d)

Fig. 6 This grade 3 15 × 8 × 6 cm fibrosarcoma was growing through the incision biopsy scar of a 63-year-old man when first seen at MGH at 6 weeks post-biopsy (panel (a)). The tumour filled the anterior compartment of the right leg. The treatment was 46 Gy pre-operatively, followed 4 weeks later by a marginal resection, and then a post-operative boost dose of 12 Gy for a total dose of 58 Gy given in 29 fractions of 2 Gy over a total of 89 days (radiation was given as two fractions per day, with 4 h between fractions). The resected specimen is shown in panel (b); there was a margin of less than 5 mm. The dose distribution is presented in panel (c); the angled wedge pair achieved generous coverage of the anterior compartment and a margin posterior to the interosseous membrane. The appearance of the treated part at 5 years is illustrated in panel (d). The result has been quite satisfactory in that there is no oedema or pain and he walks well and without prosthesis or an external support device. The exclusion of the bulk of the posterior compartment from the high-dose volume was an essential feature of this treatment plan.

radiation oncologist are the desmoid tumours. Desmoid tumours are also called aggressive fibromatoses. These tumours do not have the capacity to metastasize but they may grow in a relentless manner and destroy local structures. They are not, however, necessarily progressive and, hence, should not be viewed as true sarcomas. There are occasional instances of spontaneous regression of tumours. Desmoids do not necessarily regrow after resection with pathologically positive margins. Further, there are accounts of the occasional desmoid tumour regressing after treatment with agents such as anti-oestrogens or indomethacin.

Desmoid tumours were first described as tumours in the anterior abdominal wall in women post-partum. These were thought to be secondary to the chronic trauma of stretching during pregnancy. They are now known to arise at all anatomical sites, the most common being the torso and extremities. The aetiology of desmoids is not known, but they have been associated with trauma. They may be genetically associated with several diseases, most prominently Gardner's syndrome.

The desmoid tumours should be treated by surgical resection with a relatively wide margin as they are widely infiltrating; this usually achieves permanent eradication. Surgery may not be a

feasible option: the lesion may be unresectable for technical reasons, located where resection would produce serious complications, or the patient may refuse the recommended operation. In these circumstances, radiation offers an entirely credible alternative to radical surgery. Of 12 patients whose desmoid tumours were treated by radiation alone at the MGH (Miralbell *et al.* 1990), 10 are controlled locally (three lesions are partially regressed and stabilized, at 28, 50, and 93 months). A number of other centres have reported comparable results (Greenberg *et al.* 1981; Liebel *et al.* 1983; Keus and Bartelink 1986). Doses in the range of 55–60 Gy given over 6–8 weeks appear to achieve permanent eradication of desmoid tumours in 80 per cent or more of patients. There is little evidence to suggest that higher doses would be of clinical benefit. Further, the response rate shows minimal dependency on the size of the lesion.

The policy at the MGH is not to recommend radiation in patients who have had grossly complete resection of their *primary* desmoid but with microscopically positive margins provided that: (i) the patient is judged likely to adhere to a rigid follow-up protocol with examination at 3-monthly intervals for 36 months and (ii) were the lesion to recur, the case would be expected to be salvaged. Recent analysis of the MGH experience in 21 patients with primary desmoids is that the actuarial frequency of local control at 5 years is 74 per cent in patients who had positive surgical margins but grossly complete resection and were then only observed. The four failures have been salvaged. Five out of five patients whose resection was grossly incomplete had local recurrences. This conservative surveillance policy means that a worthwhile proportion of patients whose primary surgical resection leaves positive margins can be spared the long-term sequelae of radiation. Recurrent desmoid tumours have proven their aggresiveness and should be treated definitively.

Surgical treatment of metastatic sarcoma

As mentioned in the introductory section, the lung is by far the most common site of involvement by metastatic sarcoma. The frequency of distant metastasis is a complex function of the size, grade, and histopathological type of sarcoma. The appearance of metastatic sarcoma in the lung does not mean that there is no prospect for prolonged survival. Provided there is only a small number of lesions and the patient is fit there should be a prompt surgical attack. In nearly all instances the surgery should be combined with an intensive chemotherapy protocol (see below). There are several reports of long-term survival rates of 20–25 per cent after surgical resection of the pulmonary deposits, for example Beattie (1984) and Roth et al. (1985).

CHEMOTHERAPY

Chemotherapy for soft tissue sarcomas is as yet of limited proven value, although it has been increasingly used for patients with such tumours during the past decade. In advanced-stage soft tissue sarcoma, patients experienced response rates of up to 40–50 per cent following tolerable doses of several of the multiagent chemotherapeutic protocols. Rarely, a patient with metastatic disease may be cured by drugs alone. The role of chemotherapy as an adjuvant to surgery and/or radiation therapy is under active clinical investigation.

Chemotherapy in advanced disease

Single-agent chemotherapy

Several antineoplastic agents have established antitumour activity in soft tissue sarcomas, albeit rather modest. The most extensively studied and probably the most effective drug is doxorubicin or adriamycin (Bonadonna et al. 1975), with response rates of 15–35 per cent in patients not previously exposed to chemotherapy (Verwey et al. 1985; Borden et al. 1987). A dose–response relation has been suggested for doxorubicin: higher response rates are seen after 60–70 mg/m^2 than 50 mg/m^2 for drug given on a 3-week schedule (O'Bryan et al. 1977; Schoenfeld et al. 1982). A major limitation for doxorubicin given every 3–4 weeks to total dose levels of over 550 mg/m^2 is the risk of cardiotoxity. This risk and/or the severity of damage appear to be lessened by continuous infusion over 4 days (Legha et al. 1982; Baker et al. 1987a,b). The relative efficacy of bolus vs continuous infusion is not established. Moreover, important practical problems occur in continuous-infusion chemotherapy.

A second drug with a clear activity in soft tissue sarcoma is ifosfamide. Objective response rates are comparable to those with doxorubicin (Czownicki and Utracka-Hutka 1977; Klein et al. 1983; Antman et al. 1985, 1989; Wiltshaw et al. 1986; Bramwell et al. 1987; Legha et al. 1989). Ifosfamide is usually given at a dose of 5–10 g/m^2 per course, either in a daily×3–5 schedule or as a 24 h infusion at 3-weekly intervals. No particular schedule has proven

advantage. The high doses of ifosfamide result in the urinary excretion of considerable amounts of the metabolite acrolein, a substance toxic for the epithelial surface of the urinary tract. Cystitis can be reduced or avoided by giving mesna or N-acetyl cysteine. That ifosfamide is more active than the parent drug cyclophosphamide has been shown by the European Organization for Research on Treatment of Cancer (EORTC) Soft Tissue and Bone Sarcoma Group in a randomized phase II trial (Bramwell et al. 1987). Ifosfamide was given at a dose of 5 g/m^2, while cyclophosphamide was given at a dose of 1.5 g/m^2. The third drug of interest in this disease with a modest activity as a single agent is decarbazine (DTIC). In a study by Gottlieb et al. (1976), a response rate of 17 per cent was observed in 53 patients, while in a study of the EORTC (Buesa et al. 1987) the same result was achieved in 43 patients.

Most of the other commercially available antineoplastic agents have been without useful effect or were studied in too few patients to draw meaningful conclusions. This holds for methotrexate (high dose) (Isacoff et al. 1978; Von Hoff et al. 1978; Ambinder et al. 1979; Frei et al. 1979; Karakousis et al. 1980; Vaughn et al. 1984), methotrexate (standard dose) (Andrews and Wilson 1967; Buesa et al. 1984), bleomycin (Amato et al. 1985), actinomycin D (Golbey et al. 1968), 5-fluorouracil (Gold et al. 1959), vincristine (Selawry et al. 1968; Korbitzs et al. 1969), etoposide (Radice et al. 1979; Welt et al. 1983; Dombernowksy et al. 1987), cisplatin (Bramwell et al. 1979; Karakousis et al. 1979; Samson et al. 1979), cyclophosphamide (Bergsagel and Levin 1960; Bramwell et al. 1987), and mitomycin C (Van Oosterom et al. 1985). Unsatisfactory response rates were found for a number of experimental agents as well. Table 12 lists the results for a range of drugs tested singly against sarcoma of soft tissues.

There has been a relatively large number of trials on analogues of doxorubicin in the search for less toxicity (heart and marrow) but with retained antitumour effectiveness. Only one, epirubicin, apparently has antitumour activity comparable to that of the parent drug (Mouridsen et al. 1987) and with a toxicity profile, especially with respect to myelosuppression, clearly in favour of the analogue. Other analogues of doxorubicin were either ineffective or have been studied mainly in patients resistant to doxorubicin, a situation in which not much can be expected of the drug studied.

Combination chemotherapy

Analogous to the development in the chemotherapy against other types of solid tumour, combination chemotherapy has been studied extensively in soft tissue sarcoma. Results of the first doxorubicin-based combination chemotherapy trial were reported by Gottlieb et al. (1972). In that trial, 234 patients with metastatic soft tissue sarcoma were treated with doxorubicin and dacarbazine. A total objective response rate of 34 per cent was observed (9 per cent complete response and 25 per cent partial response). Since this publication, numerous studies on combination chemotherapy have been made in advanced soft tissue sarcoma. The majority of the combination chemotherapy regimens have been based on doxorubicin. The combination of doxorubicin and dacarbazine (ADIC) has also been studied by other investigators; however, lower response rates were usually observed. In an attempt to improve the results, other drugs have been added to the ADIC combination. When either cyclophosphamide (Blum et al. 1980; Benjamin et al. 1981; Ikeda et al. 1984) or vincristine (Gottlieb et al. 1975; Creagan et al. 1977) were incorporated into the ADIC regimen, no significant increase in response was achieved. Although neither cyclophosphamide or

Table 12 Phase II studies of experimental drugs in advanced soft tissue sarcomas

Drug	No. of patients	Response rate (%)	Reference
Gallium nitrate	31	6	Saiki et al. (1982)
Mitoxantrone	61	2	Bull et al. (1985)
Aziridinylbenzoquinone	39	3	Zidar et al. (1985)
Dibromodulcitol	45	2	Borden et al. (1982)
ICRF-159	37	3	Borden et al. (1982)
Maytansine	47	0	Borden et al. (1982)
VP-16	26	0	Welt et al. (1983)
VP-16	26	4	Dombernowsky et al. (1987)
Metoprine	46	9	Magill et al. (1982)
Lonidamine	21	5	Wissel et al. (1984)
Vindesine	15	7	Yap et al. (1983)
Vinblastine	15	0	Yap et al. (1983)
Bisantrene	17	0	Cowan et al. (1986)
PALA	20	5	Kurzrock et al. (1984)
PALA	27	4	Bramwell et al. (1982)
Chlorozotocin	29	14	Presant and Bartolucci (1984)
Chlorozotocin	17	0	Mouridsen et al. (1981)
Chlorozotocin	37	0	Amato et al. (1985)
Elleptinium	19	0	Somers et al. (1985)
Methyl-GAG	18	0	Sordillo et al. (1985)
Piperazinedione	19	5	Thigpen et al. (1985)
MGBG	36	3	Amato et al. (1985)
Bruceantin	34	0	Amato et al. (1985)
Diaziaquone	31	0	Chan et al. (1986)
Homoharringtonine	16	0	Ajani et al. (1986)
TGU	19	0	Rouesse et al. (1987)
Fludarabine	20	0	Zalupski et al. (1987)
Trimetrexate	20	15	Quirt et al. (1988)
Piritrexim	24	4	Carabasi et al. (1988)

Table 13 Treatment results of combination of the most active drugs in advanced soft tissue sarcoma

Drugs	No. of patients	Response rate (%)	Reference
DX+ifosfamide	50	36	Wiltshaw et al. (1986)
DX+ifosfamide	178	35	Schuette et al. (1987), Bramwell et al. (1988b)
DX+ifosfamide	42	36	Loehrer et al. (1989)
epiDX+ifosfamide	36	36	Frustaci et al. (1989)
epiDX+DTIC	19	47	Lopez et al. (1987)
DX+ifosfamide+DTIC	97	47	Elias et al. (1989)

DX, doxorubicin; epiDX, epirubicin; DTIC, dacarbazine.

vincristine can be considered very effective drugs in soft tissue sarcoma, they were nevertheless placed in an extensively studied combination chemotherapy regimen consisting of cyclophosphamide, vincristine, doxorubicin, and dacarbazine, better known as **CYVADIC**. A number of groups reported response rates for this combination varying from 33 to 50 per cent (Benjamin et al. 1976; Yat et al. 1980; Pfeffer et al. 1984; Bui et al. 1985; Choi et al. 1985). Adding other drugs such as actinomycin D, methyl CCNU, or streptozotocin to regimens based on doxorubicin has been largely ineffective (Chang and Wiernik 1976; Rivkin et al. 1980; Lopez et al. 1984). Although cisplatin as a single agent is not an effective drug in soft tissue sarcomas, a number of investigators have conducted clinical trials with regimens based on this drug (Cormier et al. 1980; Biernbaum et al. 1981; Klippstein et al. 1984; Edmonson et al. 1985; Piver et al. 1986). However, most of these schedules included doxorubicin as well, thus assessment of the role of cisplatin is obscured. The reported response rates varied between 25 and 50 per cent. Comparable remarks can be made for combination chemotherapy regimens which include methotrexate (Subramanian and Wiltshaw 1978; Presant et al. 1981; Lynch et al. 1982). More recently, combinations of the active drugs doxorubicin (or epirubicin), ifosfamide, and dacarbazine (Table 13) have shown consistently higher response rates (35–47 per cent) than the above mentioned other combination chemotherapy regimens.

An important observation in almost all of the clinical trials made on soft tissue sarcomas is the low rate of complete remissions, usually less than 10 per cent. This stresses the relatively modest effect of chemotherapy against these tumours, as it is judged that only drugs/protocols that achieve a complete response rate of greater than 10 per cent will provide a major benefit.

Table 14 shows the results of the most important phase III trials. There are five studies in which single-agent doxorubicin has been compared to different combination chemotherapy regimens (Schoenfeld et al. 1982; Omura et al. 1983; Muss et al. 1985; Borden et al. 1987; Santoro et al. 1988). In only two studies (Omura et al. 1983; Borden et al. 1987) was a higher response rate reported for the combination arm as compared with doxorubicin alone. However, these differences are rather small. The large EORTC trial failed to show that either the combination of doxorubicin with ifosfamide or CYVADIC was significantly superior to doxorubicin alone. Further, complete remissions were not observed more frequently in the combination regimens. The other randomized trials listed in Table 14 studied different combinations or schedules of administration. Baker et al. (1987b) showed that continuous infusion of doxorubicin and dacarbazine was as effective as bolus administration and that congestive heart failure was less frequent after the continuous infusion schedule. Pinedo et al. (1984) observed a significantly higher response rate with CYVADIC than when the four drugs were used in an alternating fashion. At present, it has to be concluded that combination chemotherapy is not proven superior to the best available single agent, doxorubicin. Whether the potency of the combination of the three most effective drugs (doxorubicin, ifosfamide, and dacarbazine) will be adequate to change this picture is currently being tested.

Based on the positive dose–response relation for chemotherapeutic agents, attempts to increase bone-marrow tolerance by combining haemopoietic growth factors (granulocyte colony-stimulating factor or granulocyte–macrophage colony-stimulating factor) with higher drug doses are being evaluated (Antman et al. 1988; Vadhan-Raj et al. 1989). It is to be hoped that this approach will lead to a better therapeutic index; initial results appear to be encouraging. For example, Antman et al. (1988) added granulocyte–macrophage colony-stimulating factor to the combination of doxorubicin, ifosfamide, and dacarbazine and observed an objective remission rate of 79 per cent in 14 patients. Further study of this promising new method should define its role in the therapy of soft tissue sarcomas.

How should today's patient with metastatic or recurrent soft tissue sarcoma be approached. If the disease is reasonably localized and the patient in good condition, surgical resection of the metastatic focus should be considered, if technically feasible or radiation in conjunction with an appropriate chemotherapy protocol. Obviously, for the great majority of cases chemotherapy is palliative rather than curative. Whenever possible, patients should be entered into clinical trials designed to define the efficacy of treatment. Outside of protocols, patients of younger age and in good performance status should be considered for intensive combination chemotherapy

Table 14 Randomized chemotherapy trials in advanced soft tissue sarcoma

Treatment	No. of patients	Response rate			Reference
		CR	PR	Total	
DX	80	6	10	16	Omura et al. (1983)
DX/DTIC	66	11	13	24	
DX	50	2	17	19	Muss et al. (1985)
DX/CTX	54	4	16	20	
DX/DTIC/CTX/VCR	71	20	18	38	Pinedo et al. (1984)
DX/DTIC–CTX/VCR	74	5	9	14	
DX (cycles at 3-week intervals)	93	6	13	19	Borden et al. (1987)
DX (weekly cycles)	92	4	12	16	
DX/DTIC	95	6	24	30	
DX/CTX/VCR/DTIC	221	14	38	52	Benjamin et al. (1976)
DX/CTX/VCR/ACD	224	12	28	40	
DX	66	6	21	27	Schoenfeld et al. (1982)
DX/CTX/VCR	70	4	15	19	
CTX/VCR/ACD	64	2	9	11	
DX/DTIC	79	14	18	32	Baker et al. (1987a)
DX/DTIC/CTX	95	13	22	35	
DX/DTIC/ACD	98	9	15	24	
DX/DTIC bolus	135	7	12	19	Baker et al. (1987b)
DX/DTIC c.i.	143	10	8	18	
DX	146	4	21	25	Santoro et al. (1988)
DX/IFOSFAMIDE	144	6	19	25	
DX/VCR/CTX/DTIC	131	6	21	27	

CR, complete remission; PR, partial remission; DX, doxorubicin; DTIC, dacarbazine; CTX, cyclophosphamide; VCR, vincristine; ACD, actinomycin D.

protocols. At the time of writing, the combination including doxorubicin, ifosfamide, and dacarbazine seems the most effective with regard to response rates. However, as mentioned earlier, one should realize that combination chemotherapy has not been proved to be more effective than single-agent treatment. Older patients or patients in a less good general condition are probably better candidates for treatment with a single agent, preferably doxorubicin. The rate of progression of the disease and/or the presence or absence of symptomatic disease may also be of importance when considering the use of chemotherapy. These latter characteristics are important because it has not been well established that chemotherapy enhances median survival, which is stated to be between 9 months and 1 year in most studies. Thus, the most realistic goal to be achieved with the available drugs is the palliation of symptomatic disease. Knowledge of certain prognostic factors may also play a role in the decision of whether to give or not to give chemotherapy. The most important prognostic factor for response appears to be the performance status (Verwey et al. 1989). No consensus exists with respect to other possible prognostic factors such as age, sex, and histological type of the tumour.

In patients with acquired or primary resistance to 'standard' chemotherapy, experimental drugs or new therapies may be tried.

Chemotherapy for occult metastatic sarcoma of soft tissues

Despite achievement of local control and good functional status of their stage M_0 soft tissue sarcomas, some 30–50 per cent of patients have occult metastatic tumour and ultimately fail. This constitutes a powerful challenge to develop systemic treatment that can eliminate the microscopic metastases. The need for such treatment is well recognized and has been the subject of much clinical investigation. The principal problem is the absence of really effective drugs and not the low frequency of the tumours. Despite

being even less common, the efficacy of adjuvant chemotherapy is well established and regularly used against Ewing's sarcoma, osteosarcoma, and rhabdomyosarcoma. Today, there is no clinically proven value for chemotherapy of soft tissue sarcoma in the adjuvant setting. There are, however, strong indications of small benefit. There needs to be further studies on the timing of the chemotherapy relative to the treatment of the primary lesion and the testing of new combinations of agents.

Phase III trials

Because of modest effectiveness of the presently available chemotherapeutic agents against soft tissue sarcoma, assessment of the value of adjuvant chemotherapy has to be based upon prospective, phase III trials. A number of these have been completed and are discussed here. Summary results are presented in Table 15. Because of the efficacy of doxorubicin against established metastatic tumour, several studies have used it alone. The number of patients in all these trials is low, few having more than 100 patients randomized to each arm. Only the study at Bologna found a statistically significant difference with respect to relapse-free survival ($p < 0.02$) and overall survival ($p < 0.05$) in favour of the patients who received chemotherapy (Gherlinzoni et al. 1986; Picci et al. 1988). However, the control arm of that study had an unusually poor result. The other studies with single-agent doxorubicin were all negative. Of note, in the study of Eilber et al. (1988b), patients in both arms received pre-operative intra-arterial doxorubicin, which may have influenced the results.

The EORTC Soft Tissue and Bone Sarcoma Group randomized 468 patients to no treatment or eight courses of CYVADIC (Bramwell et al. 1985, 1988a). CYVADIC was given over 3 days every 4 weeks starting within 13 weeks of definitive surgery. No significant differences were observed in either relapse-free or overall survival. However, the rate of local recurrence was significantly

Table 15 Phase III clinical trials of adjuvant chemotherapy against soft tissue sarcoma

Treatment	No. of patients	Median follow-up (months)	Survival (%) Overall	Relapse free	Reference
DX	77	40	75	62	Alvegard *et al.* (1989)
Control	77		70	56	
DX	33	36	88	68	Gherlinzoni *et al.* (1986)
Control	44		68	42	Picci *et al.* (1988)
DX	37	49	68	74	Wilson *et al.* (1986)
Control	38		68	62	
DX	56	28	85	58	Eilber *et al.* (1988*b*)
Control	63		80	54	
DX	32	20	82	67	Antman *et al.* (1987)
Control	32		89	67	
Randomized studies of adjuvant combination chemotherapy versus no treatment					
DX/CTX/HD-MTX	39	85	82	75	Chang *et al.* (1988)
Control	28		60	54	
DX/CTX/HD-MTX	17	35	68	77	Glenn *et al.* (1985)
Control	14		58	49	
VCR/CTX/ACD alternating with VCR/DX/DTIC	30	64	90	ns	Edmonson *et al.* (1984)
Control	31		77	ns	
VCR/DX/CTX/ACD	20	120	65	54	Benjamin *et al.* (1987)
Control	23		–	35	
CTX/VCR/DX/DTIC	178	44	74	67	Bramwell *et al.* (1985)
Control	196		68	52	Bramwell *et al.* (1988*a*)
CTX/VCR/DX/DTIC	31	40	83	65	Bui *et al.* (1989)
Control	28		43	34	

DX, doxorubicin; CTX, cyclophosphamide; HD-MTX, high-dose methotrexate; VCR, vincristine; ACD, actinomycin D; DTIC, dacarbazine; ns, not stated.

lower in the chemotherapy group for the non-extremity tumours ($p=0.003$), but not for the sarcomas of extremities ($p=0.38$). Furthermore, the EORTC study confirmed that the size and histological grade were independent prognostic factors with respect to survival (see above). The data from M. D. Anderson Hospital (Benjamin *et al.* 1987) and the NCI (Chang *et al.* 1988) also showed a significantly reduced rate of local recurrence favouring the chemotherapy arm. The study from Bordeaux (Bui *et al.* 1989) gave an advantage for chemotherapy, viz 83 vs 43 per cent ($p=0.002$) for overall survival and 65 vs 34 per cent ($p=0.003$) for relapse-free survival; these results have only been published in abstract form and come from small numbers of patients. With such small numbers the danger of an imbalance in prognostic factors between the treatment arms is likely to exist. Before these data can be accepted as realistic, the results have to be confirmed in a larger study.

At present, it must be concluded from these data that adjuvant chemotherapy does not have an established role in the overall treatment of soft tissue sarcomas. Currently, several groups are studying this question by further clinical trials.

BIOLOGICAL-RESPONSE MODIFIERS

Experience with biological-response modifiers is as yet very limited in soft tissue sarcoma. A few preliminary reports have been published on interferons (Harris *et al.* 1986; Edmonson *et al.* 1987). These studies were on a total of 36 patients, of whom the majority had received extensive prior chemotherapy. Only one partial response was observed in a patient with fibrosarcoma. Data on interleukin-2 are even more sparse. In the study of Rosenberg *et al.* (1987) no responses were seen in six patients. Interleukin-2 has also been given intra-arterially into the liver for the treatment of leiomyosarcoma metastatic to liver in six patients (Salem *et al.* 1989); only one minor response was observed. Biological-response modifiers as applied at

present appear not to play a major role in the treatment of soft tissue sarcoma.

PROGNOSTIC FACTORS

At present, there are no practical means of predicting the response of a soft tissue sarcoma in an individual patient. It is to be hoped that further developments in the testing of response of tissue *in vitro* will prove to be a powerful predictive tool.

REFERENCES

Abbatucci JS, *et al.* (1986). Local control and survival in soft tissue sarcomas of the limbs, trunk walls and head and neck: a study of 113 cases. *International Journal of Radiation Oncology—Biology—Physics*, 12:579–86.

Ajani JA, *et al.* (1986). Phase II studies of homoharringtonine in patients with advanced malignant melanomas, sarcoma, and head and neck, breast and colorectal carcinomas. *Cancer Treatment Reports*, 70:375–9.

Akerman M, Rydholm A (1987). Aspiration cytology of lipomatous tumors: a 10 year experience at an orthopedic oncology center. *Diagnostic Cytopathology*, 3:295–302.

Alvegard TA, Berg NO (1989). Histopathology peer review of high-grade soft tissue sarcoma: the Scandinavian Sarcoma Group experience. *Journal of Clinical Oncology*, 7:1845–51.

Alvegard TA, *et al.* (1989). Adjuvant chemotherapy with doxorubicin in high grade soft tissue sarcoma: a randomized trial of the Scandinavian Sarcoma Group. *Journal of Clinical Oncology*, 7:1504–13.

Amato DA, *et al.* (1985). Evaluation of bleomycin, chlorozotocin, MGBG, and bruceantin in patients with advanced soft tissue sarcoma, bone sarcoma, or mesothelioma. *Investigation of New Drugs*, 3:397–401.

Ambinder EP, *et al.* (1979). High-dose methotrexate followed by citrovorum factor reversal in patients with advanced cancer. *Cancer*, 43:1177–82.

American Cancer Society (1989). Cancer statistics. *Ca—a Cancer Journal for Clinicians*, 39:12–13.

American Joint Committee on Cancer (1988). *Manual for staging of cancer* (3rd edn). Lippincott, Philadelphia.

Andrews N, Wilson W (1967). Phase II study of methotrexate (NSC 740) in solid tumors. *Cancer Chemotherapy Reports*, **51**:471–4.

Antman KM, *et al.* (1985). Phase II trial of ifosfamide with mesna in previously treated metastatic sarcoma. *Cancer Treatment Reports*, **69**:499–504.

Antman K, *et al.* (1987). Preliminary results of a randomized intergroup soft tissue sarcoma adjuvant trial of doxorubicin versus observation. In *Adjuvant therapy of cancer*, Vol. V (ed. VS Salmon), p. 725. Grune & Stratton, Philadelphia.

Antman KH, Griffin JD, Elias A (1988). Effect of recombinant human granulocyte–macrophage colony-stimulating factor on chemotherapy-induced myelosuppression. *New England Journal of Medicine*, **319**:593–8.

Antman KH, *et al.* (1989). Response to ifosfamide and mesna: 124 previously treated patients with metastatic or unresectable sarcoma. *Journal of Clinical Oncology*, **7**:126–31.

Arbeit JM, Hilaris BS, Brennan MF (1987). Wound complications in the multimodality treatment of extremity and superficial truncal sarcomas. *Journal of Clinical Oncology*, **5**:480–8.

Aurias A, *et al.* (1983). Translocation of chromosome 22 in Ewing's sarcoma. An analysis of 4 fresh tumors. *New England Journal of Medicine*, **309**: 469–7.

Baker LH, *et al.* (1987a). Combination chemotherapy using adriamycin, DTIC, cyclophosphamide, and actinomycin D for advanced soft tissue sarcoma: a randomized comparative trial—a phase III Southwest Oncology Group study. *Journal of Clinical Oncology*, **5**:851–61.

Baker LH, *et al.* (1987b). SWOG 8024: combined modality therapy for disseminated soft tissue sarcoma, phase III. *Proceedings of the American Society of Clinical Oncology*, **6**:138.

Barkley HT, Martin RG, Romsdahl MM, Lindberg R, Zagard GK (1988). Treatment of soft tissue sarcomas by preoperative irradiation and conservative surgical resection. *International Journal of Radiation Oncology—Biology—Physics*, **14**:693–9.

Baumal R, Kahn HJ, Bailey D, Phillips MJ, Hanna W (1984). The value of immunohistochemistry in increasing diagnostic precision of undifferentiated tumours by the surgical pathologist. *Histochemistry Journal*, **16**:1061–70.

Beattie EJ (1984). Surgical treatment of pulmonary metastases. *Cancer*, **54**:2729–31.

Bell RS, *et al.* (1989). The surgical margin in soft tissue sarcoma. *Journal of Bone and Joint Surgery*, **71A**:370–5.

Benjamin RS, *et al.* (1976). CYVADIC vs CYVADACT—a randomized trial of cyclophosphamide, vincristine, and adriamycin plus either dacarbazine or actinomycin-D in metastatic sarcomas. *Proceedings of the American Association of Cancer Research*, **17**:256.

Benjamin R, *et al.* (1981). Combination chemotherapy for sarcomas with cyclophosphamide and continuous infusion adriamycin and dacarbazine (CI-CYA-DIC) with surgical intensification. *Proceedings of the American Society of Clinical Oncology*, **22**:526.

Benjamin RS, *et al.* (1987). The importance of combination chemotherapy for adjuvant treatment of high risk patients with soft tissue sarcomas of the extremities. In *Adjuvant treatment of cancer*, Vol. 5 (ed. VS Salmon), pp. 735–44. Grune & Stratton, New York.

Bergsagel DE, Levin WC (1960). A prelusive clinical trial of cyclophosphamide. *Cancer Chemotherapy Reports*, **8**:120–34.

Biernbaum W, *et al.* (1981). Chemotherapeutische behandlungmoglichkeiten bei fortgeschrittenen Sarkomen. *Deutsche Medizin Wochenschrift*, **106**:1181–5.

Bland KI, McCoy DM, Kinard RE, Copeland EM III (1987). Application of magnetic resonance imaging and computerized tomography as an adjunct to the surgical management of soft tissue sarcomas. *Annals of Surgery*, **205**:473–81.

Blum R, *et al.* (1980). Successful treatment of metastatic sarcomas with cyclophosphamide, adriamycin, and DTIC (CAD). *Cancer*, **46**:1722–6.

Bonadonna G, *et al.* (1975). Adriamycin (NSC-12312-7) studies at the Instituto Nazionale Tumori. *Cancer Chemotherapy Reports*, **6**:231–45.

Borden EC, *et al.* (1982). Phase II evaluation of dibromodulcitol, ICRF-159, and maytansine for sarcomas. *American Journal of Clinical Oncology (CTT)*, **5**:417–20.

Borden EC, *et al.* (1987). Randomized comparison of three adriamycin regimens for treatment of metastatic soft tissue sarcomas. *Journal of Clinical Oncology*, **5**:840–50.

Bramwell VHC, *et al.* (1979). EORTC phase II study of cisplatin in CYVADIC-resistant soft tissue sarcoma. *European Journal of Cancer*, **15**:1511–13.

Bramwell V, *et al.* (1982). N-(Phosphonacetyl)-L-aspartate (PALA) in advanced soft tissue sarcoma: a phase II trial of the EORTC Soft Tissue Sarcoma Group. *European Journal of Cancer and Clinical Oncology*, **18**:81–4.

Bramwell VHC, *et al.* (1985). European experience of adjuvant chemotherapy for soft tissue sarcomas: preliminary report of a randomized trial of cyclophosphamide, vincristine, doxuribicin, and dacarbazine. *Cancer Treatment Symposium*, **3**:99–108.

Bramwell VHC, *et al.* (1987). Cyclophosphamide versus ifosfamide: final report of a randomized phase II trial in adult soft tissue sarcomas. *European Journal of Cancer and Clinical Oncology*, **23**:311–21.

Bramwell VHC, *et al.* (1988a). European experience of adjuvant chemotherapy for soft tissue sarcoma: an interim report of a randomized trial of CYVADIC versus control. In *Recent concepts in sarcoma treatment* (ed. JR Ryan and LO Baker), pp. 157–64. Kluwer, Dordrecht.

Bramwell VHC, *et al.* (1988b). Review of the clinical trials activity of the Soft Tissue and Bone Sarcoma Group of the European Organization for Research and Treatment of Cancer. *Seminars in Surgical Oncology*, **4**:45–52.

Brennan MF, *et al.* (1987). Local recurrence in adult soft-tissue sarcoma. A randomized trial of brachytherapy. *Archives of Surgery*, **122**:1289–93.

Bridge JA, *et al.* (1988). Translocation t(X;18) in orofacial synovial sarcoma. *Cancer*, **62**:935–7.

Brown R, Marshall CJ, Pennie SG, Hall A (1984). Mechanism of activation of an N-*ras* gene in the human fibrosarcoma cell line HT1080. *EMBO Journal*, **3**:1321–6.

Buesa JM, *et al.* (1984). Treatment of advanced soft tissue sarcomas with low-dose methotrexate: a phase II trial by the European Organization for Research on Treatment of Cancer (EORTC) Soft Tissue and Bone Sarcoma Group. *Cancer Treatment Reports*, **68**:683–4.

Buesa J, *et al.* (1987). High-dose DTIC in advanced soft tissue sarcoma of the adult: a phase II study of the EORTC Soft Tissue and Bone Sarcoma Group. *Proceedings ECCO*, **4**:235.

Bui NB, *et al.* (1985). Analysis of a series of sixty soft tissue sarcomas in adults treated with a cyclophosphamide–vincristine–adriamycin–dacarbazine (CYVADIC) combination. *Cancer Chemotherapy and Pharmacology*, **15**:82–5.

Bui NB, *et al.* (1989). First results of a prospective randomized study of CYVADIC adjuvant chemotherapy in adults with operable high risk soft tissue sarcoma. *Proceedings of the American Society of Clinical Oncology*, **8**:318.

Bull FE, *et al.* (1985). Phase II trial of mitoxantrone in advanced sarcomas: a Southwest Oncology Group Study. *Cancer Treatment Reports*, **69**:231–3.

Cade S (1951). Soft tissue tumours: their natural history and treatment (Section of Surgery, President's address). *Proceedings of the Royal Society of Medicine*, **44**:19–36.

Carabasi MM, *et al.* (1988). A phase II trial of oral piritrexim for advanced sarcomas in adults. *Proceedings of the American Society of Clinical Oncology*, **7**:276.

Chan C, *et al.* (1986). Phase II trial of diaziquone in anthracycline-resistant adult soft tissue and bone sarcoma patients: a Southeastern Cancer Study Group trial. *Cancer Treatment Reports*, **70**:427–8.

Chang AE, *et al.* (1988). Adjuvant chemotherapy for patients with high grade soft tissue sarcomas of the extremity. *Journal of Clinical Oncology*, **6**:1491–500.

Chang P, Wiernik PH (1976). Combination chemotherapy with adriamycin and streptozotocin. *Clinical Pharmacology and Therapeutics*, **20**:606–10.

Chardin P, Yermian P, Madaule P, Tavitian A (1985). N-*ras* gene activation in the RD human rhabdomyosarcoma cell line. *International Journal of Cancer*, **35**:647–52.

Choi TK, Ng A, Wong J (1985). Doxorubicin, dacarbazine, vincristine, and cyclophosphamide in the treatment of advanced gastrointestinal leiomyosarcoma. *Cancer Treatment Reports*, **69**:443–4.

Coindre JM, *et al.* (1986). Reproducibility of a histopathologic grading system for adult soft tissue sarcoma. *Cancer*, **58**:306–9.

Collin C, Godbold J, Hajdu S, Brennan M (1987). Localized extremity soft tissue sarcoma: an analysis of factors affecting survival. *Journal of Clinical Oncology*, **5**:601–12.

Cormier WJ, Hahn RG, Edmonson JH (1980). Phase II study in advanced sarcoma: randomized trial of pyrazofurin vs combination cyclophosphamide, doxorubicin, and *cis*-dichlorodiammineplatinum (II) (CAP). *Cancer Treatment Reports*, **64**:655–8.

Cowan JD, Gehan E, Rivkin SE, Jones SE (1986). Phase II trial of bisantrene in patients with advanced sarcomas: a Southwest Oncology Group study. *Cancer Treatment Reports*, **70**:685–6.

Creagan ET, *et al.* (1977). A clinical trial of adriamycin (NSC 123127) in advanced sarcomas. *Oncology*, **34**:90–1.

Curran WJ, Littman P, Raney RB (1988). Interstitial radiation therapy in the treatment of childhood soft-tissue sarcomas. *International Journal of Radiation Oncology—Biology—Physics*, **14**:169–74.

Czownicki A, Utracka-Hutka B (1977). Contribution to the treatment of malignant tumors with ifosfamide. In *Proceedings of the International Holoxan Symposium* (ed. H Burkert and HC Voigt), pp. 109–11. Asta-Werke, Düsseldorf.

del Regato J (1963). Radiotherapy of soft-tissue sarcoma. *Journal of the American Medical Association*, **185**:216–18.

Denton JW, *et al.* (1984). Pre-operative regional chemotherapy and rapid fraction irradiation for sarcomas of the soft tissue and bone. *Surgery Gynecology Obstetrics*, **158**:545–51.

Dombernowsky P, *et al.* (1987). VP-16 in advanced soft tissue sarcoma: a phase II study of the EORTC Soft Tissue and Bone Sarcoma Group. *European Journal of Cancer and Clinical Oncology*, **23**:579–80.

Dryja TP, *et al.* (1986). Chromosome 13 homozygosity in osteosarcoma without retinoblastoma. *American Journal of Human Genetics*, **38**:59–66.

du Bolay CE (1985). Immunohistochemistry of soft tissue tumours: a review. *Journal of Pathology*, **146**:77–94.

Edmonson JH, *et al.* (1984). Randomized study of systemic chemotherapy following complete excision of non-osseous sarcomas. *Journal of Clinical Oncology*, **2**:1390–6.

Edmonson JH, *et al.* (1985). Phase II study of a combination of mitomycin, doxorubicin and cisplatin in advanced sarcomas. *Cancer Chemotherapy and Pharmacology*, **15**:181–2.

Edmonson JH, *et al.* (1987). Phase II study of recombinant gamma-interferon in patients with advanced non-osseous sarcomas. *Cancer Treatment Reports*, **71**:211–13.

Eilber FR, *et al.* (1984). Limb salvage for skeletal and soft tissue sarcomas. *Cancer*, **53**:2579–84.

Eilber FR, Giuliano A, Huth J, Mirra J, Rosen G, Morton D (1988*a*). Neoadjuvant chemotherapy, radiation, and limited surgery for high grade soft tissue sarcoma of the extremity. In *Recent concepts in sarcoma treatment*. (*Proceedings of International Symposium of Sarcomas*, Tarpon Springs, FL, 1987) (ed. JR Ryan and LH Baker), pp. 115–22. Kluwer, Dordrecht.

Eilber FR, *et al.* (1988*b*). A randomized prospective trial using postoperative adjuvant chemotherapy (adriamycin) in high-grade extremity soft tissue sarcoma. *American Journal of Clinical Oncology (CCT)*, **11**:39–45.

Elias A, *et al.* (1989). Response to mesna, doxorubicin, ifosfamide, and dacarbazine in 108 patients with matastatic or unresectable sarcoma and no prior therapy. *Clinical Journal of Oncology*, **7**:1208–16.

Enneking WF, McAuliffe JA (1985). Adjunctive preoperative radiation therapy in treatment of soft tissue sarcomas: a preliminary report. *Cancer Treatment Symposia*, **3**:37–42.

Enneking WF, Spanier SS, Goodman MA (1980). Current concepts review: the surgical staging of musculoskeletal sarcoma. *Journal of Bone and Joint Surgery*, **62A**:1027–30.

Enzinger F, Weiss S (1988). *Soft tissue tumors* (2nd edn). Mosby, St Louis.

Franke HD, Schmidt R (1987). Clinical results after therapy with fast neutrons (DT, 14 MeV) since 1976 in Hamburg-Eppendorf. In *Progress in radio-oncology III* (*Proceedings of the Third Meeting on Progress in Radio-Oncology*, Vienna, 1986) (ed. KH Karcher), International Club for Radio-Oncologists, Vienna.

Fraumeni JF (1973). Genetic factors in the etiology of cancer. In *Cancer medicine* (ed. JF Holland and EM Frei), pp. 7–15. Lea & Febiger, Philadelphia.

Frei E, *et al.* (1979). High-dose methotrexate with leucovorin rescue: rationale and spectrum of antitumor activity. *American Journal of Medicine*, **68**:370–5.

Friend SH, *et al.* (1987). Deletions of a DNA sequence in retinoblastomas and mesenchymal tumors: organization of the sequence and its encoded protein. *Proceedings of the National Academy of Science USA*, **84**:9059–63.

Frustaci S, *et al.* (1989). Full doses of ifosfamide and epirubicin in advanced soft tissue sarcomas. *Proceedings of the American Society of Clinical Oncology*, **8**:319.

Gerbaulet A, Panis X, Flamant F, Chassagne D (1985). Iridium afterloading curietherapy in the treatment of pediatric malignancies. *Cancer*, **56**:1274–9.

Gherlinzoni F, *et al.* (1986). A randomized trial for the treatment of high grade soft tissue sarcomas of the extremities: preliminary observation. *Journal of Clinical Oncology*, **4**:552–8.

Giuliano AE, Eilber FR (1985). The rationale for planned reoperation after unplanned total excision of soft-tissue sarcomas. *Journal of Clinical Oncology*, **3**:1344–8.

Glenn J, *et al.* (1985). A randomized prospective trial of adjuvant chemotherapy in adults with soft tissue sarcomas of the head and neck, breast and trunk. *Cancer*, **55**:1206–14.

Gohotsar D, Borges A, Shettz P (1986). Osteogenic sarcoma developing after successful therapy of acute lymphocytic leukemia. *American Journal of Pediatric Hematology and Oncology*, **8**:259–60.

Golbey R, Li MC, Kaufman RF (1968). Actinomycin in the treatment of soft part sarcomas. (Abstr.) James Ewing Society Scientific Program.

Gold G, *et al.* (1959). A clinical study of 5-fluorouracil. *Cancer*, **19**:935–9.

Gottlieb JA, *et al.* (1972). Chemotherapy of sarcomas with a combination of adriamycin and dimethyl triazeno imidazole carboxamide. *Cancer*, **30**:1632–8.

Gottlieb JA, *et al.* (1975). Adriamycin (NSC-123127) used alone and in combination for soft tissue and bony sarcomas. *Cancer Chemotherapy Reports*, **6**:271–82.

Gottlieb JA, *et al.* (1976). Role of DTIC (NSC-45338) in the chemotherapy of sarcomas. *Cancer Treatment Reports*, **60**:199–203.

Greenberg J, *et al.* (1981). Radiation therapy in the treatment of aggressive fibromatoses. *International Journal of Radiation Oncology—Biology—Physics*, **7**:305–10.

Hardell L, Eriksson M (1988). The association between soft tissue sarcomas and exposure to phenoxyacetic acids: a new case reference study. *Cancer*, **62**:652–6.

Harris J, *et al.* (1986). Treatment of soft tissue sarcoma with fibroblast interferon (beta-interferon): an American Cancer Society/Illinois Cancer Council study. *Cancer Treatment Reports*, **70**:293–4.

Hatfield PM, Schulz MD (1970). Post irradiation sarcoma: including 5 cases after X-ray therapy for breast carcinoma. *Radiology*, **96**:593–602.

Ikeda K, *et al.* (1984). A combination chemotherapy with adriamycin, cyclophosphamide and DTIC (ACD) for advanced adult soft part sarcoma. *Gan To Kagaku Ryoho*, **11**:235–9.

Isacoff WH, *et al.* (1978). Phase II clinical trial with high-dose methotrexate therapy and citrovorum factor rescue. *Cancer Treatment Reports*, **62**:1295–304.

Jensen RD, Miller RW (1971). Retinoblastoma: epidemiologic characteristics. *New England Journal of Medicine*, **285**:307.

Karakousis CP, Hoterman OA, Holyoke ED (1979). Cisdichlorodiamineplatinum (II) in metastatic soft tissue sarcomas. *Cancer Treatment Reports*, **63**:2071–5.

Karakousis CP, Rao U, Carlson M (1980). High-dose methotrexate as secondary chemotherapy in metastatic soft-tissue sarcomas. *Cancer*, **46**:1345–8.

Karakousis CP, Emrich LJ, Rao U, Krishnamsetty RM (1986). Feasibility of limb salvage and survival in soft tissue sarcomas. *Cancer*, **56**:484–91.

Karakousis CP, *et al.* (1987). Chromosomal changes in soft tissue sarcomas: a new diagnostic parameter. *Archives of Surgery*, **122**:1257–60.

Keus R, Bartelink H (1986). The role of radiotherapy in the treatment of desmoid tumors. *Radiotherapy and Oncology*, **7**:1–5.

Kim JH, *et al.* (1978). Radiation induced soft tissue sarcoma and bone sarcoma. *Radiology*, **129**:501–8.

Kinsella TJ, Glatstein E (1987). Clinical experience with intravenous radiosensitizers in unresectable sarcomas. *Cancer*, **59**:908–9.

Kinsella TJ, *et al.* (1988). Preliminary results of a randomized study of adjuvant radiation therapy in resectable adult retroperitoneal soft tissue sarcomas. *Journal of Clinical Oncology*, **6**:18–25.

Kissin MW, Fisher C, Carter RL, Horton LW, Westbury G (1986). Value of Tru-cut biopsy in the diagnosis of soft tissue tumours. *British Journal of Surgery*, **73**:742–6.

Klein HO, *et al.* (1983). High-dose ifosfamide and mesna as continuous infusion over five days: a phase I/II trial. *Cancer Treatment Reviews*, **10**:167–73.

Klippstein TH, *et al.* (1984). High-dose adriamycin (ADM) and *cis*-platinum (DDP) in advanced soft-tissue sarcomas and invasive thymomas: a pilot study. *Cancer Chemotherapy and Pharmacology*, **13**:78–81.

Korbitzs BC, *et al.* (1969). Low doses of vincristine (NSC-67574) for malignant diasease. *Cancer Chemotherapy Reports*, **53**:249–54.

Kreicbergs A, Tibukait B, Willems J, Bauer HCF (1987). Flow DNA analysis of soft tissue tumors. *Cancer*, **59**:128–33.

Kurzrock R, *et al.* (1984). Phase III evaluation of PALA in patients with refractory metastatic sarcomas. *American Journal of Clinical Oncology*, **7**:305–7.

Lander JJ, Stanley RJ, Summer HEW (1975). Angiosarcoma of the liver associated with Fowler's solution. *Gastroenterology*, **68**:1562–4.

Laramore GE, *et al.* (1989). Fast neutron radiotherapy for sarcomas of soft tissue, bone, and cartilage. *American Journal of Clinical Oncology*, **12**:320–6.

Lawrence W, Jr (1988). Concepts in limb-sparing treatment of adult soft tissue sarcomas. *Seminars in Surgical Oncology*, **4**:73–7.

Lawrence W Jr, *et al.* (1987). Adult soft tissue sarcomas. A pattern of care survey of the American College of Surgeons. *Annals of Surgery*, **205**: 349–59.

Legha S, *et al.* (1982). Reduction of doxorubicin cardiotoxicity by prolonged continuous intravenous infusion. *Annals of Internal Medicine*, **96**:133–9.

Legha S, *et al.* (1989). Role of ifosamide in the treatment of refractory sarcomas and an evaluation of *n*-acetylcysteine (NAC) as an uroprotector. *Proceedings of the American Society of Clinical Oncology*, **8**:322.

Leibel SA, Tranbaugh RF, Wara WM, Beckstead JH, Bovill EG, Phillips TL (1982). Soft tissue sarcomas of the extremities. *Cancer*, **50**:1076–83.

Leibel SA, *et al.* (1983). Desmoid tumors: local control and patterns of relapse following radiation therapy. *International Journal of Radiation Oncology—Biology—Physics*, **9**:1167–71.

Leopold KA, Harrelson J, Prosnitz L, Samulski TV, Dewhirst MW, Oleson JR (1989). Preoperative hyperthermia and radiation for soft tissue sarcomas: advantage of two vs one hyperthermia treatment per week. *International Journal of Radiation Oncology—Biology—Physics*, **16**:107–15.

Leyvraz S, Costa J (1988). Histological diagnosis and grading of soft tissue sarcomas. *Seminars of Surgical Oncology*, **4**:3–6.

Lindberg RD (1980). Soft tissue sarcoma. In *Textbook of radiotherapy* (ed. GH Fletcher), pp. 922–42. Lea & Febiger, Philadelphia.

Lindberg RD, Martin RG, Romsdahl MM, Barkley HT (1981). Conservative surgery and post-operative radiotherapy in 300 adults with soft tissue sarcomas. *Cancer*, **47**:2391–7.

Littlefield JW (1984). Genes, chromosomes and cancer. *Journal of Pediatrics*, **104**:489–94.

Locker GY, *et al.* (1979). The clinical features of hepatic angiosarcoma: a report of four cases and a review of the English literature. *Medicine*, **58**:48–64.

Loehrer PJ, *et al.* (1989). Ifosamide plus doxorubicin in metastatic adult sarcomas: a multi-institutional phase II trial. *Journal of Clinical Oncology*, **7**:1655–9.

Lopez M, *et al.* (1984). Alternating combination chemotherapy of advanced soft tissue sarcomas in adults. *American Journal of Clinical Oncology*, **7**:539–42.

Lopez M, *et al.* (1987). Epirubicin and DTIC (EDIC) in the treatment of advanced soft tissue sarcomas. *Proceedings of the American Society of Clinical Oncology*, **6**:134.

Lynch G, *et al.* (1982). Combination chemotherapy of advanced sarcomas with Cyomad. *Cancer*, **50**:1724–7.

McAdam WAF, Goligher JC (1970). The occurrence of desmoids in patients with familial polyposis coli. *British Journal of Surgery*, **57**:618–31.

McNeer GP, *et al.* (1968). Effectiveness of radiation therapy in management of sarcoma of soft somatic tissues. *Cancer*, **22**:391–7.

Magill GB, *et al.* (1982). Phase II trial of Metoprine (DDMP) in pretreated adults with advanced soft tissue sarcomas. *Proceedings of the American Society of Clinical Oncology*, **1**:22.

Mankin HJ, Lange TA, Spanier SS (1982). The hazards of the biopsy in patients with malignant primary bone and soft tissue tumors. *Journal of Bone and Joint Surgery*, **64A**:1121–7.

Markhede G, Angervall L, Stener B (1982). A multivariate analysis of the prognosis after surgical treatment of malignant soft tissue tumors. *Cancer*, **49**:1721–33.

Matsuno T, Gebhardt MC, Schiller AL, Rosenberg AE, Mankin HJ (1988). The use of flow cytometry as a diagnostic aid in the management of soft-tissue tumors. *Journal of Bone and Joint Surgery*, **70A**:751–9.

Mazeron JJ, Suit HD (1987). Lymph nodes as sites of metastases from sarcomas of soft tissue. *Cancer*, **60**:1800–8.

Mills EED, Hering ER (1981). Management of soft tissue tumours by limited surgery combined with tumour bed irradiation using brachytherapy and supplementary teletherapy. *British Journal of Radiology*, **54**:312–17.

Miralbell R, Suit HD, Mankin HJ, Zuckerberg LR, Stracher MA, Rosenberg AE (1990). Fibromatoses: from postsurgical surveillance to combined surgery and radiation therapy. *International Journal of Radiation Oncology—Biology—Physics*, **18**:535–40.

Miralles TG, Gosalbez F, Menendez P, Astudillo A, Torre C, Buesa J (1986). Fine needle aspiration cytology of soft tissue lesions. *Acta Cytologia*, **30**:671–8.

Mouridsen HT, *et al.* (1981). Treatment of advanced soft tissue sarcomas with chlorozotocin. A phase II trial of the EORTC Soft Tissue and Bone Sarcoma Group. *Cancer Treatment Reports*, **81**:509–11.

Mouridsen HT, *et al.* (1987). Adriamycin versus epirubicin in advanced soft tissue sarcomas: a randomized phase II/phase III study of the EORTC Soft Tissue and Bone Sarcoma Group. *European Journal of Cancer and Clinical Oncology*, **23**:1477–83.

Muss HB, *et al.* (1985). Treatment of recurrent or advanced uterine sarcoma—a randomized trial of doxorubicin versus doxorubicin and cyclophosphamide (a phase III trial of the Gynecologic Oncology Group). *Cancer*, **55**:1648–53.

Nardeux PC, Daya-Grosjean L, Landin RM, Andeol Y, Suarez HG (1987). A c-*ras*-Ki oncogene is activated, amplified and overexpressed in a human osteosarcoma cell line. *Biochemic Biophysics Research Communications*, **146**:395–402.

O'Bryan RM, *et al.* (1977). Dose response evaluation of adriamycin in human neoplasia. *Cancer*, **39**:1940–8.

Omura GA, *et al.* (1983). A randomized study of adriamycin with and without dimethyl trazenoimidazole carboxamide in advanced uterine sarcomas. *Cancer*, **52**:626–32.

Peuchot M, Libshitz HI (1987). Pulmonary metastatic disease: radiologic–surgical correlation. *Radiology*, **164**:719–22.

Pfeffer MR, Sulkes A, Biran S (1984). Treatment of advanced soft tissue sarcomas with a modified CYVADIC protocol. *Oncology*, **41**:308–13.

Picci P, *et al.* (1988). Results of a randomized trial for the treatment of localized soft tissue tumors of the extremities in adult patients. In *Recent concepts in sarcoma treatment* (ed. JR Ryan and LO Baker), pp. 144–8. Kluwer, Dordrecht.

Pickering DG, Stewart JS, Rampling R, Errington RD, Stamp G, Chia Y (1987). Fast neutron therapy for soft tissue sarcoma. *International Journal of Radiation Oncology—Biology—Physics*, **13**:1489–95.

Pinedo HM, *et al.* (1984). CYVADIC in advanced soft tissue sarcoma: a randomized study comparing two schedules. A study of the EORTC Soft Tissue and Bone Sarcoma Group. *Cancer*, **53**:1825–32.

Piver MS, Shashikant BL, Patsner B (1986). *Cis*-diamminedichloroplatinum plus dimethyltriazenoimidazole as second- and third-line chemotherapy for sarcomas of the female pelvis. *Gynecologic Oncology*, **23**:371–5.

Pizzo PA, Miser JS, Cassady JR, Filler RM (1985). Solid tumors of childhood. In *Cancer: principles & practice of oncology* (2nd edn) (ed. VT DeVita, S Hellman, and SA Rosenberg), pp. 1511–89. Lippincott, Philadelphia.

Potter DA, *et al.* (1985). Patterns of recurrence in patients with high-grade soft-tissue sarcomas. *Journal of Clinical Oncology*, **3**:353–66.

Potter DA, *et al.* (1986). High-grade soft tissue sarcomas of the extremities. *Cancer*, **58**:190–205.

Presant CA, Bartolucci AA (1984). Phase II evaluation of chlorozotocin in metastatic sarcomas. *Medical Pediatric Oncology*, **12**:25–7.

Presant CA, *et al.* (1981). Metastatic sarcomas: chemotherapy with adriamycin, cyclophosphamide, and methotrexate alternating with actinomycin D, DTIC, and vincristine. *Cancer*, **47**:457–65.

Present CA, *et al.* (1986). Soft tissue and bone sarcomas histopathology peer review: the frequency of disagreement in diagnosis and the need for second pathological opinions. Southeastern Cancer Study Group Experience. *Journal of Clinical Oncology*, **4**:1658–61.

Quirt I, *et al.* (1988). A phase 2 study of trimetrexate in metastatic soft tissue sarcoma. *Proceedings of the American Society of Clinical Oncology*, **7**:275.

Radice PA, Bunn PA Jr, Ihde DC (1979). Therapeutic trials with VP-16 and VM-26. *Cancer Treatment Reports*, **63**:1231–9.

Rivkin SE, *et al.* (1980). Methyl-CCNU and adriamycin for patients with metastatic sarcomas: a Southwest Oncology Group Study. *Cancer*, **46**: 446–51.

Robinson E, Neugut AI, Wylie P (1988). Clinical aspects of postirradiation sarcomas. *Journal of the National Cancer Institute*, **80**:233–40.

Roholl PJ, DeJong AS, Ramaekers FC (1985). Application of markers in the diagnosis of soft tissue tumours. *Histopathology*, **9**:1019–35.

Rosenberg SA, *et al.* (1987). A progress report on the treatment of 157 patients with advanced cancer using lymphokine-activated killer cells and interleukin-2 or high-dose interleukin-2 alone. *New England Journal of Medicine*, 316:890–7.

Roth F (1957). The sequelae of chronic arsenic poisoning in Moselle vintners. *German Medicine Monthly*, 2:172–5.

Roth JA, *et al.* (1985). Differing determinants of prognosis following resection of pulmonary metastases from osteogeneic and soft tissue sarcoma patients. *Cancer*, 55:1361–6.

Rouesse JG, *et al.* (1987). Phase II study of 1,2,4-triglycidyl urasol (TGU) in advanced soft tissue sarcoma: a trial of the EORTC Soft Tissue and Bone Sarcoma Cooperative Group. *European Journal of Cancer and Clinical Oncology*, 23:1413–14.

Rowley JD (1983). Human oncogene locations and chromosome observations. *Nature*, 301:290–1.

Ruka W (1986). The test for selection of 'high risk' patients with soft tissue sarcomas prior initial treatment. *Nowotwory*, XXXVI:104–13.

Russell WO, *et al.* (1977). A clinical and pathological staging system for soft tissue sarcomas. *Cancer*, 40:1562–70.

Rydholm A, Rooser B (1987). Surgical margins for soft tissue sarcoma. *Journal of Bone and Joint Surgery*, 69A:1074–8.

Rydholm A, Berg NO, Persson BM, Akerman M (1983). Treatment of soft-tissue sarcoma should be centralised. *Acta Orthopaedica Scandanavica*, 54:333–9.

Rydholm A, *et al.* (1984). Prognosis for soft-tissue sarcoma in the locomotor system. *Acta Pathologica Microbiologica et Immunologica Scandinavica (A)*, 92:375–86.

Sadove AM, *et al.* (1981). Radiation carcinogenesis in man: new primary neoplasms in fields of prior therapeutic radiation. *Cancer*, 48:1139–43.

Saiki JH, *et al.* (1982). Gallium nitrate in advanced soft tissue and bone sarcomas: a Southwest Oncology Group study. *Cancer Treatment Reports*, 66:1673–4.

Salem P, *et al.* (1989). Arterial infusion of interleukin-2 for treatment of hepatic metastases from GI leiomyosarcoma: predisposition to hypersensitivity to iodine-containing media. *Proceedings of the American Society of Clinical Oncology*, 8:322.

Samson MK, Baker LH, Benjamin RS (1979). Cisdichlorodiamineplatinum (II) in advanced soft tissue and bone sarcomas. A Southwest Oncology Group study. *Cancer Treatment Reports*, 63:2027–8.

Sandberg AA, Turc-Carel C, Gemmell RM (1988). Chromosomes in solid tumors and beyond. *Cancer Research*, 48:1049–59.

Santoro A, *et al.* (1988). A randomized EORTC study in advanced soft tissue sarcomas: ADM vs ADM-IFX vs CYVADIC. *Proceedings of the European Conference on Clinical Oncology*, 5:34–8.

Schmitt G, Furst G, von Essen CF, Scherrer (1987). Neutron and neutron-boost irradiation of soft tissues sarcomas. In *Progress in radio-oncology III* (*Proceedings of the Third Meeting on Progress in Radio-Oncology*, Vienna, 1986) (ed. KH Karcher), pp. 175–83. International Club for Radio-Oncologists, Vienna.

Schoenfeld D, *et al.* (1982). A comparison of adriamycin versus vincristine and adriamycin, and cyclophosphamide versus vincristine, actinomycin D and cyclophosphamide for advanced sarcoma. *Cancer*, 50:2757–62.

Schuette J, *et al.* (1987). Adriamycin and ifosfamide, a new effective combination in advanced soft tissue sarcoma; preliminary report of a phase II study of the EORTC Soft Tissue and Bone Sarcoma Group. *Proceedings of the European Conference on Clinical Oncology*, 4:232.

Selawry OS, Holland JF, Wolman Y (1968). Effect of vincristine (NSC-67574) on malignant solid tumors in children. *Cancer Chemotherapy Reports*, 52:497–9.

Shaw PJ, Bergen M, Stevens M (1988). Osteogenic sarcoma following acute lymphoblastic leukemia. *American Journal of Pediatric Hematology/Oncology*, 10:81–2.

Simon MA (1982). Biopsy of musculoskeletal tumors. *Journal of Bone and Joint Surgery*, 64A:1253–7.

Simon MA, Enneking WF (1976). The management of soft tissue sarcomas of the extremities. *Journal of Bone and Joint Surgery*, 58A:317.

Skibber JM, *et al.* (1987). Limb-sparing surgery for soft tissue sarcomas: wound related morbidity in patients undergoing wide local excision. *Surgery*, 102:447–52.

Smith S, Reeves BR, Wong L (1987). Translocation t(12;16) in a case of myxoid liposarcoma. *Cancer Genetics and Cytogenetics*, 26:185–6.

Somers R, *et al.* (1985). Phase II study of Elleptinium in metastatic soft tissue sarcoma. *European Journal of Cancer and Clinical Oncology*, 21:591–3.

Sordillo PP, Magill GB, Welt S (1985). Phase II trial of methylglyoxal-bis-guanylhydrazone (methyl-GAG) in patients with soft tissue sarcomas. *American Journal of Clinical Oncology (CTT)*, 8:316–18.

Stewart FW, Treves N (1948). Lymphangiosarcoma in post mastectomy lymphedema: a report of six cases of elephantiasis chirurgica. *Cancer*, 1:64–81.

Strong LC (1977). Genetic considerations in pediatric oncology. In *Clinical pediatric oncology* (ed. WW Sutow, *et al.*), pp. 16–32. Mosby, St Louis.

Strong LC, *et al.* (1979). Risk of radiation-related subsequent malignant tumors in survivors of Ewing's sarcoma. *Journal of National Cancer Institute*, 62:1401–6.

Subramanian S, Wiltshaw E (1978). Chemotherapy of sarcoma—a comparison of three regimes. *Lancet*, i:683–6.

Suit HD (1983). Patterns of failure after treatment of sarcoma of soft tissue by radical surgery or by conservative surgery and radiation. (Workshop of patterns of failure after treatment for cancer). *Cancer treatment symposia*, Vol. 2, pp. 241–250. US Government Printing Office, Washington DC.

Taswell HF, Soule EH, Coventry MG (1962). Lymphangiosarcoma arising in chronic lymphedematous extremities. *Journal of Bone and Joint Surgery*, 44:277–94.

Tepper JE, Wood WC, Suit HD (1989). Intra-operative radiation therapy of soft tissue sarcomas. In *Intraoperative radiation therapy* (ed. RR Dobelbower and M Abe), pp. 275–8. CRC Press, Boca Raton, FL.

Thigpen JT, *et al.* (1985). Phase II trial of piperazinedione in patients with advanced or recurrent uterine sarcoma: a Gynecologic Oncology Group study. *American Journal of Clinical Oncology (CT)*, 8:350–2.

Todoroki T, Suit HD (1985). Therapeutic advantage in pre-operative single dose radiation combined with conservative and radical surgery in different size murine fibrosarcomas. *Journal of Surgical Oncology*, 29:207–15.

Trojani M, *et al.* (1984). Soft tissue sarcomas of adults. Study of pathological prognostic variables and definition of a histopathological grading system. *International Journal of Cancer*, 33:37–42.

Tucker MA, *et al.* (1987). For the Late Effects Study Group. Bone sarcomas linked to radiotherapy and chemotherapy in children. *New England Journal of Medicine*, 317:588–93.

Turc-Carel C, *et al.* (1986a). Translocation X;18 in synovial sarcoma. *Cancer Genetics and Cytogenetics*, 22:93–4.

Turc-Carel C, *et al.* (1986b). Cytogenetic studies of adipose tissue tumors: II. Recurrent reciprocal translocation t(12/16)(q13;p11) in myxoid liposarcomas. *Cancer Genetics and Cytogenetics*, 23:291–300.

Ueda A, *et al.* (1989). Prognostic significance of Ki-67 reactivity in soft tissue sarcomas. *Cancer*, 63:1607–11.

Vadhan-Raj S, *et al.* (1989). Effects of recombinant human granulocyte–macrophage colony-stimulating factor (GM-CSF) on chemotherapy-induced myelosuppression in patients with sarcoma. *Proceedings of the American Society of Clinical Oncology*, 8:322.

Van Oosterom AT, Santoro A, Bramwell V (1985). Mitomycin C (MMC) in advanced soft tissue sarcoma: a phase II study of the EORTC Soft Tissue and Bone Sarcoma Group. *European Journal of Cancer and Clinical Oncology*, 21:459–61.

Vaughn C, *et al.* (1984). High-dose methotrexate with leucovorin recue plus vincristine in advanced sarcoma: a Southwest Oncology Group study. *Cancer Treatment Reports*, 68:409–10.

Verwey J, van Oosterom AT, Pinedo HM (1985). Melanomas, soft tissue and bone sarcomas. *European Journal of Cancer and Clinical Oncology*, 4 (Suppl.):75–85.

Verwey J, van Groeningen CJ, Pinedo HM (1989). Chemotherapy in advanced soft tissue sarcomas. In *Treatment of soft tissue sarcomas* (ed. HM Pinedo and J Verwey), pp. 75–92. Kluwer, Dordrecht.

Von Hoff DD, *et al.* (1978). 'Single'-agent activity of high-dose methotrexate therapy with citrovorum factor rescue. *Cancer Treatment Reports*, 62:233–5.

Welt S, *et al.* (1983). Phase II trial of VP-16-213 in adults with advanced soft tissue sarcomas. *Proceedings of the American Society of Clinical Oncology*, 2:234.

Wilson RE, *et al.* (1986). Doxorubicin chemotherapy in the treatment of soft tissue sarcoma: combined results of two randomized trials. *Archives of Surgery*, 121:1354–9.

Wiltshaw E, *et al.* (1986). Ifosfamide plus mesna with and without adriamycin in soft tissue sarcoma. *Cancer Chemotherapy and Pharmacology*, **18** (Suppl. 2):S10–12.

Windeyer B, Dische S, Mansfield CM (1966). The place of radiotherapy in the management of fibrosarcoma of the soft tissues. *Clinical Radiology*, **17**:32–40.

Wissel P, *et al.* (1984). Phase II trial of lonidamine (1,-2,4-dichlorophenyl)-1H-indazol-3-carbollytic acid) (LON) in advanced soft tissue sarcomas. *Proceedings of the American Society of Clinical Oncology*, **3**:258.

Yap B, *et al.* (1980). Cyclophosphamide, vincristine, adriamycin, and DTIC (CYVADIC) combination chemotherapy for the treatment of advanced sarcomas. *Cancer Treatment Reports*, **64**:93–8.

Yap BS, *et al.* (1983). A randomized study of continuous infusion vindesine versus vinblastine in adults with refractory metastatic sarcomas. *American Journal of Clinical Oncology* (*CTT*), **6**:235–8.

Zalupski M, Pazdur R, Samson M, Baker L (1987). Phase II clinical evaluation of fludarabine in soft tissue and osteosarcomas. *Proceedings of the American Society of Clinical Oncology*, **6**:135.

Zidar B, *et al.* (1985). A phase II study of aziridinylbenzoquinone (AZQ) in advanced soft tissue and bony sarcoma. A Southwest Oncology Group (SWOG) study. *Proceedings of the American Society of Clinical Oncology*, **4**:130.

13.2 Malignant mesenchymal tumours in childhood

F. FLAMANT, JEAN-LOUIS HABRAND, MARIE JOSÉ LACOMBE, AND Y. REVILLON

INTRODUCTION

Malignant mesenchymal tumours or soft tissue sarcomas are extremely varied. The most frequent and well known is rhabdomyosarcoma, and details regarding clinical and therapeutic aspects of this tumour will be given together with results of treatment. Other malignant mesenchymal tumours are frequently similar to the adult forms in terms of histopathology, but differences have been noted in the evolution of some of them in childhood. A description of these differences will be given, without reiterating information already provided in the chapter on adult sarcomas. Fifteen per cent of childhood malignant mesenchymal tumours remain unclassified: neither electron microscopy nor immunological markers have been able to determine the exact nature of these sarcomas which are ostensibly diverse.

In the past, the treatment of these tumours was mainly wide extensive surgery followed by radiotherapy in the event of incomplete excision. Very few patients survived and most of those who were cured suffered unpleasant sequelae due essentially to the type of surgery or extended radiotherapeutic fields (endocrine disorders, cosmetic and functional sequelae, etc.). In the case of rhabdomyosarcoma the administration of polychemotherapy associated with surgery and radiotherapy has resulted in a dramatic increase in the survival rate. The question addressed by the International Society of Paediatric Oncology (SIOP) studies is that of ascertaining whether it is possible, by administering chemotherapy initially, to attenuate the aggressiveness of local treatment in rhabdomyosarcoma patients who are good responders.

The efficacy of chemotherapy in other malignant mesenchymal tumours (non-rhabdomyosarcomal malignant mesenchymal tumour) has yet to be determined.

DEFINITION OF MALIGNANT MESENCHYMAL TUMOURS

Malignant mesenchymal tumours develop outside the epithelial and skeletal structures. They include tumours which derive from the mesoderm, smooth and striated muscle cells, fibroblasts, endothelial and perivascular cells, fat storage cells, elements related to synovial structures, and Schwann cells.

CLASSIFICATION AND PATHOLOGY OF MALIGNANT MESENCHYMAL TUMOURS IN CHILDHOOD

Classification

Current classifications are based on histogenesis and the nomenclature is derived from the type of tissue produced by the tumour. For example, the rhabdomyosarcoma tends to reproduce the stages of differentiation of striated muscles, the liposarcoma gives rise to adipose differentiation, etc. This system of classification separates different lesions into a large number of entities according to tumour differentiation. Well-differentiated tumours are easy to identify; however, identification becomes more difficult as differentiation decreases and certain forms of this neoplasm remain unclassified. The terms 'round cell' sarcoma, 'small cell' sarcoma, 'fusiform cell' sarcoma, and pleomorphic sarcoma are often used. These are general terms which combine different histological types.

The majority of malignant mesenchymal tumours (70 per cent) are striated cell tumours, that is, embryonal rhabdomyosarcomas. The other types of tumour are far less frequent. They can be classified into tumours of known or unknown/uncertain histogenesis. Tumours of known histogenesis (excluding rhabdomyosarcoma) are fibrosarcoma, synovial sarcoma, leiomyosarcoma, malignant Schwannoma and neuroepithelioma, liposarcoma, haemangiopericytoma, and mesenchymal chondrosarcoma. Tumours of unknown or uncertain histogenesis are embryonal sarcoma, fibrohistiocytic tumour, extra-osseous Ewing's sarcoma, epithelioid sarcoma, clear cell sarcoma, other exceptional tumours, and unclassified sarcomas.

Pathology

Rhabdomyosarcoma

The morphological diagnosis is generally based on three characteristics.

1. Myoid differentiation. At its worst, myoid differentiation is represented by rounded or discretely oval myoblastic cells with eosinophilic cytoplasm and a more or less nucleolated excentric nucleus. At its best, differentiation is represented by elongated or fusiform elements with or without double striation (rarely observed).

2. Architecture. The architecture is loose, dense, or alveolar. In the loose form the tumour cells are dispersed within a myxoid and oedematous stroma. In the more dense forms the cells are juxtaposed with relatively little stroma. Finally, in the alveolar forms, the cells are found grouped together and surrounded by fibrous bands of varying thickness. Inside these alveolar structures the cells appear to be either 'attached' to the peripheral fibrosis or 'free' within the alveolar cavity.

3. Cytology. Cells can be polymorphous with the association of rounded and fusiform elements of varying differentiation. Sometimes the major part of the tumour is composed of poorly differentiated rounded cells, while other tumours are essentially composed of fusiform cells.

Several classifications have been proposed based on these elements. The SIOP classification (Cailland *et al.* 1989) distinguishes five types of rhabdomyosarcoma: loose botryoid rhabdomyosarcoma, loose non-botryoid rhabdomyosarcoma, poorly differentiated dense rhabdomyosarcoma, well-differentiated dense rhabdomyosarcoma, and alveolar rhabdomyosarcoma. Loose botryoid rhabdomyosarcoma often shows well-differentiated neoplastic elements and the cells tend to congregate under the epithelium (cambium layer) of the

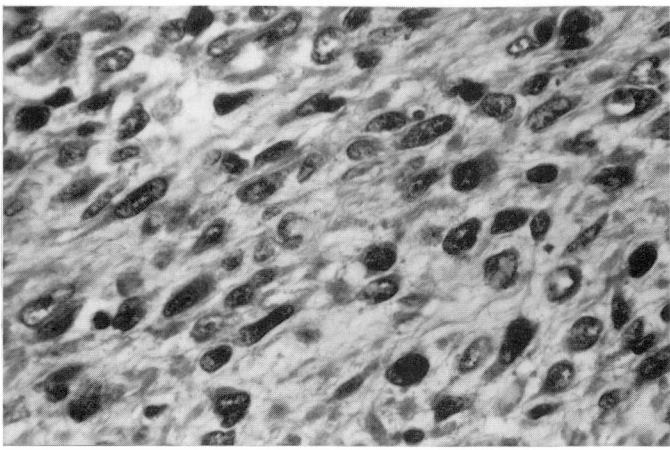

Fig. 2 Loose non-botryoid rhabdomyosarcoma.

organ concerned (Fig. 1). The main sites of this type of rhabdomyosarcoma are the bladder, the auditory canal, the vagina, and the bile ducts. Loose non-botryoid rhabdomyosarcoma lacks the characteristic cambium layer and is usually poorly differentiated (Fig. 2).

Poorly differentiated and well-differentiated dense rhabdomyosarcoma can only be distinguished in terms of the degree of differentiation (Figs 3 and 4). Alveolar or Riopelle-type rhabdomyosarcoma is characterized by the architecture described above. The mere presence of this characteristic is ample evidence for diagnosis. In this type of rhabdomyosarcoma, multinucleated elements exist and the tumour cells are often rounded and poorly differentiated (Riopelle and Theriault 1956) (Fig. 5). Enzinger's classification differentiates botryoid from alveolar forms. The other forms are grouped under the term embryonal rhabdomyosarcoma. Pleomorphic rhabdomyosarcoma and adult forms are rare in childhood (Enzinger and Weiss 1983).

An international classification, yet to be published, was described in 1989 by the pathologists of the American Intergroup Rhabdomyosarcoma Study (IRS), SIOP, and German and Italian groups during a workshop organized by SIOP. This classification identifies three subgroups of rhabdomyosarcoma according to prognosis in a univariate analysis.

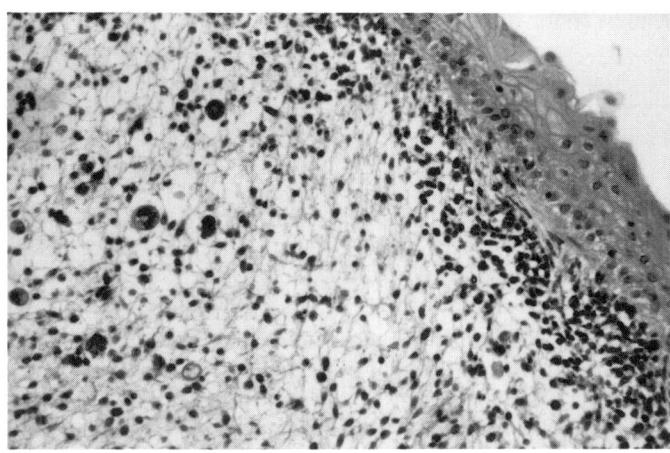

Fig. 1 Loose botryoid rhabdomyosarcoma.

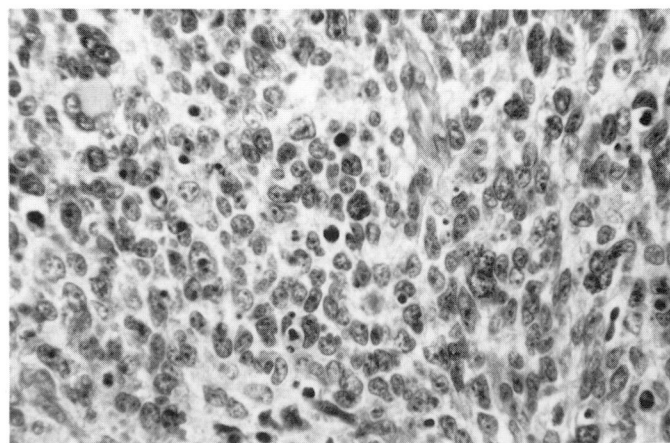

Fig. 3 Dense poorly differentiated rhabdomyosarcoma.

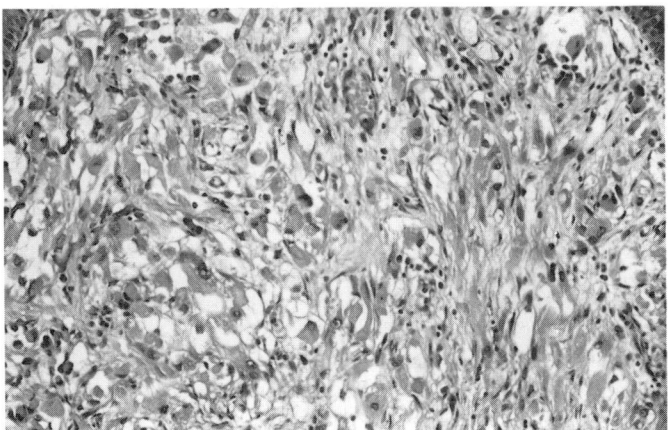

Fig. 4 Dense well-differentiated rhabdomyosarcoma.

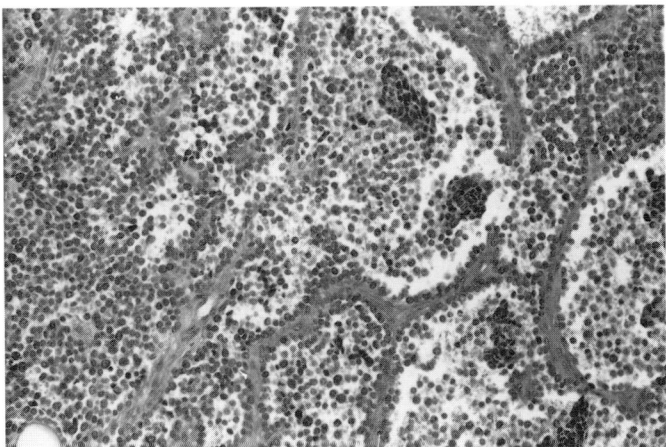

Fig. 5 Alveolar (Riopelle) rhabdomyosarcoma.

1. Good prognosis: botryoid and leiomyomatoid forms.

2. Intermediate prognosis: all embryonal forms.

3. Poor prognosis: alveolar type including a particular form designated 'solid alveolar type'.

This new definition of rhabdomyosarcoma does not include embryonal sarcomas without myoblastic differentiation or extra-osseous Ewing's sarcomas.

Some difficulties arise in the diagnosis of these tumours. The first is related to the quality and quantity of the tissue specimen. These tumours are fragile and modifications caused by sampling, staining, and fixation can render diagnosis impossible. The amount of tissue can also be a limiting factor, particularly after needle biopsy. In the case of loose botryoid rhabdomyosarcoma, the main problem is that of inflammatory reactions. Cells with myoid differentiation and the presence of a cambium layer should be sought. It can be extremely difficult to distinguish between poorly differentiated loose rhabdomyosarcoma and other 'round cell' tumours such as malignant non-Hodgkin's lymphoma (monomorphism and well-circumscribed rounded cells). Ewing's sarcoma (chromatin and architecture), and neuroepithelioma (presence of rosette structures).

In some very fusiform rhabdomyosarcoma (usually found in paratesticular sites) the appearance can evoke a leiomyosarcoma (the leiomyomatoid form). Zones which are characteristic of rhabdomyo-sarcoma and double striations should be sought. Techniques other than conventional histology may help to resolve these diagnostic problems. Imprint cytology using the May–Grunwald–Giemsa stain is a simple technique which should be performed for all childhood tumours. The method respects cytological features quite well and is particularly useful in differential diagnosis with malignant non-Hodgkin's lymphoma.

Immunocytochemical techniques using fixed sections of frozen specimens or cytological preparations (imprint or cytocentrifugation) permit the identification of substances which are more or less specific. Several antibodies can be used in rhabdomyosarcoma to detect the presence of desmin (intermediate filament of smooth and striated muscle cells), myoglobin (specific for striated muscle), myosin, actin, creatinin kinase, and enolase. The presence of these substances is related to the degree of differentiation. Their detection can be useful in poorly differentiated forms when morphological diagnosis is difficult. Caution is required here as normal residual muscle cells can be positive.

Other malignant mesenchymal tumours (non-rhabdomyosarcomal malignant mesenchymal tumours)

It is sometimes difficult to determine the precise pathological features of non-rhabdomyosarcomal malignant mesenchymal tumours and their classification is frequently modified. Many difficulties are encountered in diagnosis and are generally related to poor tumour differentiation. Therefore, flawless tissue specimens are essential and biopsies must be repeated frequently to achieve as accurate a diagnosis as possible. An inevitable consequence of these difficulties is that a large proportion of sarcomas remain unclassified (10–15 per cent depending on the series).

Immunocytochemical studies have been encouraging and may improve diagnostic accuracy. Unfortunately, not very many substances are currently available and those that exist are of poor specificity. We have mentioned the specificity of desmin and myoglobin in rhabdomyosarcoma. Cytokeratin may prove to be useful in synovial sarcomas but this study has remained somewhat inconclusive with regard to monophasic fusiform forms. The presence of S-100 protein has been reported in both malignant Schwannomas and clear cell sarcomas. The presence of vimentin points to a mesenchymal tumour but does not specify which type. Factor VIII is present in vascular tumours. Enolase of neural origin is present in neuroepitheliomas, but also appears in certain Ewing's soft tissue sarcomas and in the recently identified neuroectodermic tumours. Finally, many tumours remain negative after immunocyto-chemical studies. It is hoped that a better knowledge of the biology of mesenchymal tissues will result in the identification of more specific and reliable substances for the diagnosis of soft tissue tumours.

Electron microscopy, although promising at the outset, has provided a limited contribution to diagnosis. At present, cytogenetic studies and the study of oncogenes offer possibilities of improving the understanding of these tumours.

Tumours of known histogenesis

Fibrosarcoma

As in the adult forms, fibrosarcomas are composed of fusiform cells and have a fasciculated architecture. The bundles are usually elongated and occasionally have a 'herring-bone' appearance. Varying amounts of collagen are present. Nuclei are oval with frayed edges and the cytoplasm is sparse and poorly limited. Extremely atypical cells are infrequent. Differential diagnosis from embryonal rhabdomyosarcoma is rarely difficult. In contrast, the differential diagnosis of some cellular forms of fibromatosis can prove to be enigmatic. The term 'aggressive fibromatosis' was proposed to describe a particular type of fibromatosis. Enzinger and Weiss (1983) believe that this cellular form should have been classified among fibrosarcomas encountered in infants which have a different prognosis from fibrosarcomas found in children aged more than 1 year (see final section of this chapter). The other types of fibromatosis (fibrous hamartoma, fibromatosis of the sternocleidomastoideus muscle, digital fibromatosis, infantile myofibromatosis, and desmoid fibromatosis) have lower cellularity and are rich in collagen. Although their identification requires care, diagnosis is not too difficult. Fibrosarcoma must also be distinguished from other 'fusiform cell' (spindle cell) sarcomas with a poor degree of differentiation: leiomyosarcoma, malignant Schwannoma, monophasic synovial sarcomas, and certain fibrohistiocytic tumours.

Synovial sarcoma

The diagnosis of the biphasic form of synovial sarcoma is relatively simple owing to the association of an epithelial and a fusiform component. Problems arise for forms where the epithelial characteristic is not so distinct and differentiation of the purely fusiform type from fibrosarcomas is very difficult.

Neuroepithelioma

The characteristics of this tumour are similar to the adult form: in difficult cases, differential diagnosis from rhabdomyosarcoma is possible with immunological markers (enolase is positive). It is classified by some authors as a primitive neuroectodermic tumour. The Askin tumour which arises in the thoracic site should be classified under neuroepithelioma.

Other tumours

Hemangiopericytoma, which occurs in the first year of life, can have the same appearance as adult forms with mitoses and intravascular invasion, but these features are not malignant at this age. The differential diagnosis from certain forms of synovial sarcoma, mesenchymal chondrosarcoma, and malignant fibrohistiocytoma is often difficult.

Leiomyosarcoma is rare in children and must be differentiated from some types of rhabdomyosarcoma with fusiform (spindle) cells. The presence of myoblastic cells in rhabdomyosarcoma determines the diagnosis.

Malignant Schwannoma, liposarcoma, mesenchymal chrondrosarcoma (Louvet et al. 1981), and angiosarcoma (very rare) have no pathological difference from the same tumour in adults.

Tumours of unknown or uncertain histogenesis

Embryonal sarcoma is an undifferentiated tumour with fusiform or staired elements and a loose or fasciculated architecture. No myoid differentiation can be discerned. In the past, it was classified by the IRS in the rhabdomyosarcoma group.

Malignant histiocytofibroma (Abdul Karim et al. 1985; Bertoni et al. 1985) has no distinctive feature in children, as is the case with alveolar sarcoma, clear cell sarcoma of the tendons, and aponeuroses (Pavlidis et al. 1984).

Extra-osseous Ewing's sarcoma is part of the group of tumours with small round cells. A controversy persists regarding a distinction between extra-osseous Ewing's sarcoma and neuroepithelioma.

Other rare tumours seen in children include rhabdoid tumour, which is similar to the adult form, undifferentiated sarcoma of the liver (Ruymann et al. 1988), infantile pigmented neuroectodermic tumour (Dehner et al. 1979), comprising melanocytic features, immature elements of the neuroblastic type, and fusiform cells, and malignant ectomesenchymoma with ganglioneural and myoblastic cells.

AETIOLOGY, EPIDEMIOLOGY, INCIDENCE, AGE, AND SEX

The only information available to date concerns patients with rhabdomyosarcoma. The aetiology of rhabdomyosarcoma is unknown but various associations have been observed.

Associations with congenital malformations have been observed in 32 per cent of cases in an IRS study (115 patients) (Ruymann et al. 1988). Malformations were found in the genitourinary tract (8.7 per cent), the central nervous system (8 per cent), the digestive system (5.2 per cent), and the cardiovascular system (4.3 per cent). Other anomalies were an accessory spleen (4.3 per cent), musculoskeletal malformation (0.87 per cent), and hemihypertrophia (0.87 per cent). Rhabdomyosarcoma has been described in some syndromes where a malformation is associated with a predisposition to develop certain tumours: Wiedemann–Beckwith syndrome (Wiedemann 1983), Recklinghausen syndrome (Meckeen et al. 1978), Rubinstein–Taybi syndrome (Sobel and Woerner 1978), and Gorlin syndrome (Schweisguth et al. 1968; Beddis et al. 1983).

The likelihood of a familial predisposition in some cases was first suggested by Li and Fraumeni (1969, 1982) and confirmed in a more recent publication (Li et al. 1988). Eight to nine per cent of children with soft tissue sarcomas are from families in which the predisposition to develop malignant tumours is inherited as an autosomal dominant pattern. Tumours which belong to this category are breast cancers, osteosarcomas, melanomas, adrenal cortical carcinoma, brain tumours, and perhaps acute lymphocytic leukaemia. Individuals belonging to these families are characterized by the precocity of the first tumour and the frequent development of second malignancies. The presence of three tumours in the same family is required before the term Li–Fraumeni syndrome can be used. The locus of the gene(s) for this inherited cancer syndrome is located on the short arm of chromosome 17 (Malkin et al. 1990).

Birch et al. (1985) demonstrated from the Manchester Children's Tumour Registry that there is a high risk of breast cancer in mothers of male children with embryonal rhabdomyosarcoma of the genitourinary tract who are below the age of 24 months at diagnosis. A high risk for mothers was also associated with late age at first full-term pregnancy (27 years or more) and with an age of 31 years of age or over at birth of a child with rhabdomyosarcoma (Birch 1990).

Incidence, age, and sex

Rhabdomyosarcoma represents 70 per cent of all malignant mesenchymal tumours in children and 5 per cent of all malignant solid tumours. The median age for rhabdomyosarcoma is 5 years in the SIOP series (range from birth to 18 years), but some cases can be seen later in young adults.

The median age for non-rhabdomyosarcomal malignant mesenchymal tumours is 8 years and most of these tumours occur during pre-adolescence. Distribution by gender shows a higher incidence of rhabdomyosarcoma among males (sex ratio 1.7 in the SIOP series). The difference between the sexes for non-rhabdomyosarcomal malignant mesenchymal tumours is not so marked.

CYTOGENETICS AND MOLECULAR BIOLOGY

A few cytogenetic studies have been performed. Forty-five rhabdomyosarcomas with 15 specimens of the alveolar type were analysed. The most frequent anomaly was the t(2;13) translocation found in the alveolar rhabdomyosarcomas (Turc-Carel et al. 1986; Douglas et al. 1987; Lai et al. 1987; Lizard-Nalol et al. 1987; Wang Wuu et al. 1988). The break-off points of this translocation were in zone 13q14, where the retinoblastoma gene is situated and in an area which is implicated in some haemopathies.

The comparison of the constitutional and tumour genotype has revealed an absence of heterozygosity in the short arm of chromosome 11, suggesting that this chromosome has a locus where the recessive mutations confer a predisposition for this disease (Reik and Surani 1989). Some recent studies have shown that the lost allele is of maternal origin, although the mechanism is unknown (Reik and Surani 1989). The 11p13 zone implicated in the absence of this allele gene is similar to the deletion observed in Wiedemann–Beckwith disease and breast cancer, where a possible association with rhabdomyosarcoma has been suggested.

STAGING CLASSIFICATION

Until 1987, several staging systems were used throughout the world for rhabdomyosarcoma and other malignant mesenchymal tumours in children: the TNM–UICC staging system used by SIOP (UICC 1983) and at Stanford (Pedrick et al. 1986), the IRS grouping system (Lawrence et al. 1987), the system used at St Jude's Children's Hospital (Pratt et al. 1972) and at the Royal Marsden Hospital (Kingston et al. 1983), and the system used by the Memorial Sloan Kettering Center (Ghavimi et al. 1975). Consequently, comparison of the results of studies from different institutions and cooperative groups was difficult. The only pre-therapeutic staging system is the TNM–UICC system. The others are post-surgical systems, with the most commonly used being the IRS. (The other post-surgical staging systems contain only minor differences from the IRS version.) In 1987 SIOP organized an international workshop with the aim of harmonizing the definition of stage of disease, primary sites, and relevant end-points and standardizing statistical methods for reporting results. Indeed, the pre-surgical TNM–UICC staging system and the post-surgical IRS grouping system are based on divergent criteria and are not easily interchangeable. The TNM classification is shown in Table 1.

Table 1 SIOP–UICC soft tissue sarcoma clinical staging system: TNM classification

Stage	Description	
I	T_1	Tumour confined to the organ or tissue of origin
	N_0	No evidence of regional lymph node involvement
	M_0	No evidence of distant metastasis
II	T_2	Tumour involving one or more contiguous organs or tissues or with adjacent malignant effusion
	N_0	
	M_0	
III	Any T	
	N_1	Evidence of regional lymph node involvement
	M_0	
IV	Any T	
	Any N	
	M_1	Evidence of distant metastasis

Table 2 pTNM post-surgical histopathological classification

pT   Primary tumour
    pT_0 No evidence of tumour found on histological examination of specimen
    pT_1 Tumour limited to organ or tissue of origin; excision complete and margins histologically free
    pT_2 Tumour with invasion beyond the organ or tissue of origin; excision complete and margins histologically free
    pT_3 Tumour with or without invasion beyond the organ or tissue of origin; excision incomplete
        pT_{3a} Evidence of microscopic residual tumour
        pT_{3b} Evidence of macroscopic residual tumour
        pT_{3c} Adjacent malignant effusion regardless of the size
        pT_{3x} Extent of invasion cannot be assessed

The reliability of the two systems which were based on patient characteristics abstracted from medical records was comparable and satisfactory. However, the IRS grouping system which takes into account a treatment modality, namely surgery, is dependent on the surgeon, the institution, and the current prevalent concepts regarding treatment.

The TNM system, which offers the best description of the initial extent of the disease, was adopted by both the European and American participants and henceforth will be used alone or in conjunction with their own classification. In addition to the TNM pre-treatment staging system, there exists the post-surgical pathological TNM classification (pTNM), which takes into account the quality of the resection after primary surgery; it serves as a complement to therapeutic guidelines (Table 2). For example a localized tumour (T_1, N_0, M_0) which has been completely removed at initial surgery with margins free of tumour will be classified as T_1, N_0, M_0, pT_1.

RHABDOMYOSARCOMA

Clinical features and diagnosis

The symptoms at presentation depend on the site of the tumour and the extent of invasion. Rhabdomyosarcoma can arise wherever mesenchymal tissue is present. No area is spared, not even the brain where some cases of primary tumours have been reported (Bradford et al. 1985). Rhabdomyosarcoma progresses rapidly, invading neighbouring organs and bone by contiguity. Progression via lymphatic drainage is also possible, particularly in sites such as the extremities or the genitourinary tract. Spread to the meninges by contiguity is frequent, with lesions in head and neck sites close to the meninges (see Table 3). Distant metastases generally occur in the lungs, bones, and bone-marrow via the blood stream (Ruymann et al. 1984). Therefore, the initial work-up should include the following.

1. Chest radiography (a CT scan of the lung is not necessary except in the event of a suspicious chest radiograph).

2. A bone survey or a technetium bone scan.

3. A cytological examination of the bone-marrow.

If the site is a limb then a CT scan of the brain is to be recommended because of the likelihood (although rare) of initial asymptomatic brain metastases. In parameningeal head and neck sites (Table 3), a lumbar puncture is required in order to determine whether myoblastic cells are present in the cerebrospinal fluid (even though this is rare at the outset).

Table 3 Grouping of sites adopted by the international workshop of 1986[a]

Orbit (without involvement of parameningeal sites or bone destruction)
Head and neck: non-parameningeal sites
Head and neck: parameningeal sites[b] (including other site with extension to a parameningeal site)
Genitourinary tract
  (a) Bladder, prostate
  (b) Paratestis, vagina, uterus
Limbs
Other sites

[a]For details in each group, use the international topographic code (Donaldson *et al.* 1986).
[b]Parameningeal sites: nasopharynx, nasal cavity, paranasal sinus, middle ear mastoid, and pterygoid fossa.

Local invasion is determined using adapted radiological techniques, that is, ordinary radiography, ultrasound, and CT scan according to the site of the tumour. The application of magnetic resonance imaging has not yet been explored. For sites such as the limbs and genitourinary tract, particular attention must be given to an assessment of lymph node involvement; lymphangiography of the limbs is often replaced by a CT scan of the pelvis although neither of these two techniques has proved to be superior.

A grouping of sites was adopted at an international level in 1988 and is used here. The relative incidence rate per site is given in Table 4. Approximately half of all rhabdomyosarcomas occur in the head and neck, including the orbit. The next most frequent sites are the genitourinary tract followed by the limbs.

Rhabdomyosarcoma of the orbit or eyelids

These rhabdomyosarcomas can be identified from their symptoms, the extent of progression, and the particular problems they engender. They occur at all ages, developing from the motor muscles of the eye or from the eyelids and rapidly leading to ocular symptoms, for example exophthalmia, ocular deviation, and occasionally paraocular tumour (Fig. 6). The diagnosis is based on CT scan images which indicate opacity within the orbit (Fig. 7). Rhabdomyosarcoma is the most frequent malignant tumour in this area. The differential diagnosis must eliminate angioma, lymphosarcoma, and malignant germinal tumour (exceptional). Osseous tumours of the orbit (Ewing's sarcoma, neuroblastoma metastasis, or histiocytosis X) can clinically simulate an intra-orbital tumour when soft tissues are chiefly involved. Therefore, a biopsy is essential in the absence of biological markers. When possible the surgical approach is lateral, but in general a neurosurgical approach is required.

The extent of tumour invasion is determined by CT scan. Spread is towards the nasal cavities, with the inevitable destruction of the

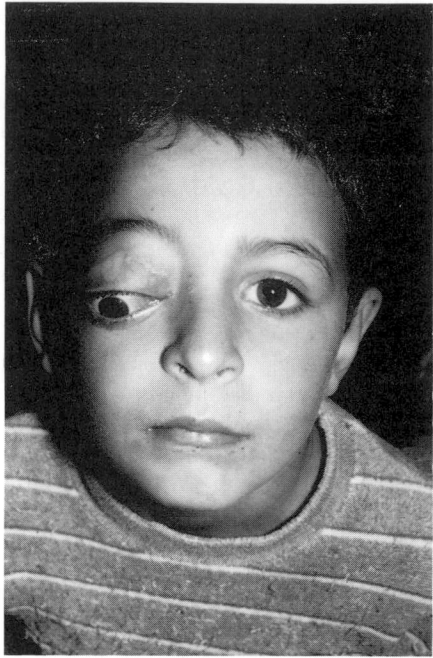

Fig. 6 Orbital rhabdomyosarcoma in a 7 year old boy.

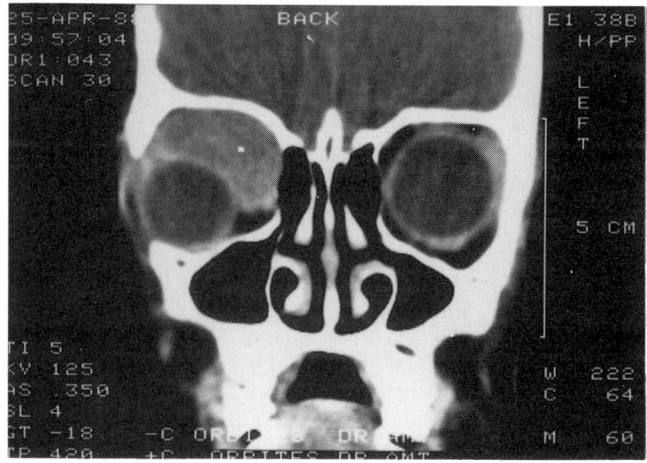

Fig. 7 CT scan of the orbital rhabdomyosarcoma in Fig. 6.

naso-orbital wall or to the upper wall of the maxillary sinus. Intracranial invasion is rare. When an orbital rhabdomyosarcoma extends to a parameningeal site (Table 3), it is considered to belong to a meningeal site, particularly from a treatment point of view.

Rhabdomyosarcoma of the head and neck

These tumours represent 29 per cent of the rhabdomyosarcoma cases in the SIOP 84–88 series. Head and neck sites are divided into non-parameningeal and parameningeal sites because of a difference in tumour development in the patients in these two groups which is mainly due to a possible extension to the meninges in the latter group. Table 4 lists the parameningeal and non-parameningeal sites and the number of patients included in each site in the SIOP 84–88 study.

The first symptoms depend on the site and extension of the tumour. Diagnosis of parameningeal tumours is often made later

Table 4 Relative incidence rate per site of head and neck sites in all stages (SIOP 1984–1988 study)

Non-parameningeal sites (total 30)	Oral cavity	10
	Face	8
	Parotid area	7
	Neck	5
Parameningeal sites (total 51)	Paranasal sinuses	16
	Nasopharynx	15
	Middle ear	12
	Pterygoid fossa	2

than diagnosis of non-parameningeal tumours which are found in more superficial sites.

Parameningeal sites

At the outset, a nasopharyngeal rhabdomyosarcoma has symptoms commonly found in children such as rhinorrhoea, nasal obstruction, nasal voice, and serous otorrhoea due to the occlusion or involvement of the eustachian tube. These symptoms are misleading. The physician should pay more attention to unilaterality and the fact that they persist relatively longer than most common infections in children. Dissemination to lymph nodes is possible (posterior cervical chains). Other signs appear later and are due to tumour invasion of other sites. They include cranial nerve palsies linked to local compression (VII) or intracranial spread (VI, X, XI, and XII) and deglutition or respiratory disorders. Anteriosuperior extension results in an exophthalmia which may be mistaken for a primitive orbital illness.

CT scanning performed at axial and frontal angles can lead to the firm diagnosis of a suspected rhabdomyosarcoma. Images of the base of the skull are required to determine intracranial invasion. Clinical features and imaging allow the diagnosis of nasopharyngeal angiofibroma to be excluded. This must be confirmed before the biopsy because of risks of haemorrhage. Angiofibromas occur during adolescence and have a regular circular non-ulcerated appearance. Bone involvement at the base of the skull and intracranial invasion is common. Arteriography is required to confirm diagnosis and the embolization of vascular pedicles prior to surgery, the first therapeutic modality employed. Differential diagnosis is from other non-neoplastic lesions such as choanal polyps and hypertrophia of the adenoid vegetations. Pathological examination after adenoidectomy can rectify the diagnosis. Other malignant tumours which arise in this area are non-Hodgkin's lymphoma and undifferentiated carcinoma of the nasopharyngeal type. The presence of bulky lymph nodes in a patient close to adolescence may point to a lymphoma or undifferentiated carcinoma of nasopharyngeal type, just as the ethnic origin of the patient can be of guidance in the latter. Bone destruction, cranial nerve palsies and youth unanimously point to rhabdomyosarcoma. A rhabdomyosarcoma which involves the brain with several palsies may be erroneously diagnosed as a brainstem tumour. Clinical examination of the nasopharynx is difficult in children and requires general anaesthesia for patients under the age of 7 years. It enables the physician to ascertain the local appearance of the tumour and the extent of spread and to perform multiple deep biopsies.

Rhabdomyosarcoma of the sinus cavities of the face can develop in the nasal or ethmoidal cavities and has common symptoms such as rhinorrhoea, haemorrhage, and nasal obstruction. Again, attention should be paid to the unilaterality of the symptoms and their persistence after antibiotic treatment. The other symptoms result from tumour extension to the orbit with ocular deviation and diplopia and to the subcutaneous tissue of the face with inflammation of the nasogenial area and the internal canthus. Anosmia or anopsia caused by the extension of the chiasma of an ethmoidal tumour are rarely the first symptoms. Clinical examination of the nasal cavity guides the physician towards a malignant tumour if an ulcerated haemorrhagic mass is present; a benign small polyp may be the only clinical manifestation but a biopsy is always necessary. In the ethmoidal sinus, differential diagnosis from allergic polyps, ethmoiditis, and ethmoidal mucocoele is straightforward. The diagnosis of an aesthesioneuroblastoma is sometimes difficult, even for pathologists. If the rhabdomyosarcoma arises in the maxillary sinus, the cheek is tumified and the lesion is often diagnosed as a dental abscess

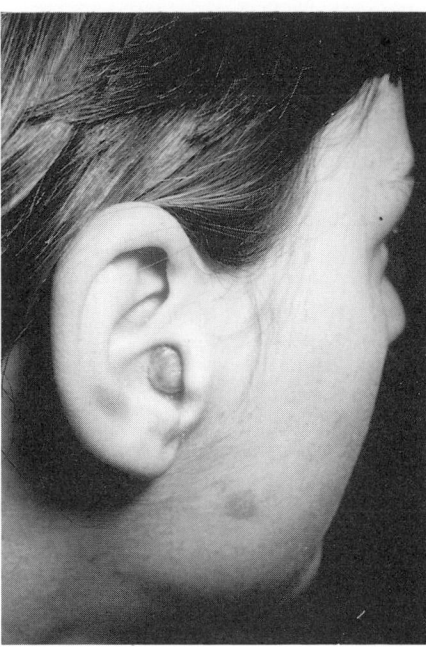

Fig. 8 Middle ear rhabdomyosarcoma in a 12 year old girl.

long before invasion of the palate, the gums, or even the orbit is seen. The biopsy needs to be intrabuccal (Caldwell–Luc). Diagnosis of osteodysplasia, which causes bone wall deformation without any apparent destruction, can be difficult. Fibrosarcomas may occur at these sites.

The most difficult site for early diagnosis is the pterygoid fossa. The tumour has very few symptoms at onset and is often bulky when diagnosed from a trismus, nerve palsy (VII, XII, V), sensitive nerve injury (V), or gum tumefaction. The tumour spreads rapidly to the base of the skull and there is often intracranial invasion at diagnosis.

The middle ear is one of the frequent sites of head and neck rhabdomyosarcoma. Clinical signs are infection, such as a purulent leaking of the ear, with or without fever. The examination will reveal a polyp in the conduit (Fig. 8) which must always be biopsied. In the absence of invasion or unequivocal clinical evidence of malignant disease (facial palsy, mastoid and parotid tumefaction, trismus, etc.) diagnosis is generally difficult, even for pathologists and errors are not rare. CT scanning must be performed systematically for it delineates bone destruction which occurs very early in the development of the disease at this site. Apart from infections, only histiocytosis X can be invoked in the differential diagnosis because it has similar clinical and radiological features as rhabdomyosarcoma when only the middle ear is involved.

Non-parameningeal sites

In the oropharynx, rhabdomyosarcoma can develop in the tonsils, in the soft palate, and at the base of the tongue. It is easily detected during the clinical examination performed for dysphagia or otalgia. The complete examination frequently has to be performed under general anaesthesia in order to visualize and palpate the tumour and its limits and to perform the biopsy. CT scanning cannot provide any assistance at this site; only a profile radiograph of the neck with barium sulphate opacification is useful. Differential diagnosis is from retropharyngeal and tonsil abscesses, which arise in an infectious context and non-Hodgkin's lymphoma.

The parotid area is considered a non-parameningeal site when there is no tumour invasion of the pterygoid fossa. Initially, parotid tumefaction is considered viral or infectious, even in the presence of facial palsy. The consistency of the tumefaction, resistance to antibiotics, and facial palsy will result in a request for a CT scan as it will indicate the degree and depth of invasion and the destruction of the maxillary bone, which are unequivocal signs of malignancy. An endobuccal biopsy can be performed in the event of pharyngeal invasion. If this is not possible, the surgical approach is necessary in order to avoid the facial nerve. The differential diagnosis is from non-Hodgkin's lymphoma and adenocarcinoma. With the surgical approach, benign tumours (for example, pleomorphic adenoma) can be removed by parotidectomy. Rhabdomyosarcoma is also found in the oral cavity (tongue, gums, etc.), soft tissues of the face (jaw, nose fold, etc.), and submaxillary glands, with or without lymph node spread. The differential diagnosis is from fibroblastic sarcoma, non-Hodgkin's lymphoma, and fibromatosis. Adenocarcinoma and mucoepidermoid carcinoma of the maxillary glands are exceptional in children. Rhabdomyosarcoma can also develop in the soft tissues of the neck and in the larynx (exceptional).

Rhabdomyosarcoma of the genitourinary tract

These tumours have been divided into specific groups because of a difference in prognosis: bladder and prostate rhabdomyosarcoma and paratesticular, vaginal, and uterine rhabdomyosarcoma.

Bladder and prostate rhabdomyosarcoma

Bladder rhabdomyosarcoma is more frequent in males than in females. It develops almost exclusively at the neck of the bladder (trigona) and involves the prostate gland. Some authors have made a distinction between rhabdomyosarcoma originating in the bladder or initially in the prostate with a difference in prognosis, but currently it is impossible to distinguish them without initial surgery. The tumours are generally large and affect both organs.

The first clinical signs are urinary; that is, dysuria, pollakiuria, and, above all, episodes of partial or complete urinary retention. In the absence of a palpable pelvic tumour, a rectal touch will reveal a firm tumour in the region of the neck of the bladder. Intravenous urography (Fig. 9) is increasingly being supplanted by CT scanning or ultrasonography. These techniques indicate the tumour mass, its local extension, and its influence on the upper urinary tract and kidneys where hydronephrosis can occur. Renal insufficiency only occurs at a late stage and in the presence of a massive tumour. A biopsy is essential to confirm the diagnosis, although errors may occur such as vesical polyps (very rare in childhood) and, exceptionally, benign bladder tumours. The biopsy specimen can generally be obtained by endoscopy but must occasionally be repeated as the pathological diagnosis can be difficult if the specimen is too superficial. If this approach is not feasible, a cystotomy will be necessary despite the risk of dissemination at this level. The transrectal approach is dangerous owing to the risk of cross-infection from intestinal germs in patients who generally require immediate chemotherapeutic treatment.

Girls are also prone to develop rhabdomyosarcoma of the bladder, although less frequently than boys. Local extension is rapid and towards the region of the vagina. Initial clinical manifestation may be a visible bud on the vulva or urinary disorders similar to those in boys.

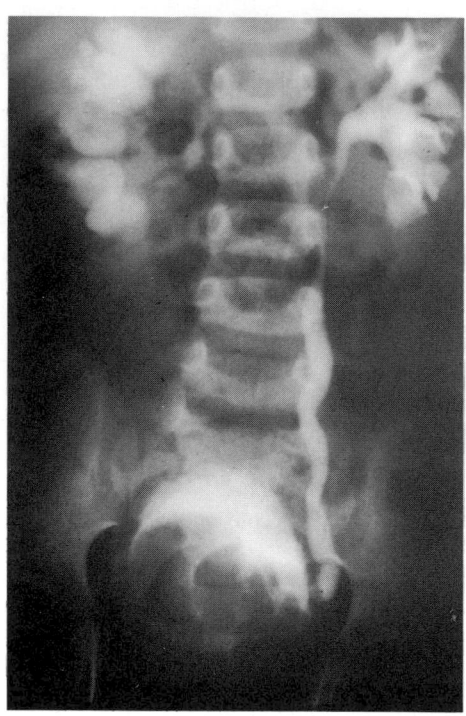

Fig. 9 Intravenous urography of bladder rhabdomyosarcoma.

Paratesticular rhabdomyosarcoma

Paratesticular rhabdomyosarcoma is revealed by scrotal swelling, although hydrocoele can be associated with the tumour. The scrotum is opaque under transillumination.

Surgery is prescribed by the scrotal approach, given the risk of intrascrotal dissemination. An orchidectomy should be performed by a high inguinal approach where the cord is cut as high as possible in the inguinal canal. A pathological examination of the cord and the scrotum is mandatory to determine the degree of extension. The rhabdomyosarcoma must be distinguished from a testicular germinal tumour which usually secretes α-fetoprotein and, thus, can be diagnosed prior to orchidectomy. The surgical approach is the same for both tumours. The evaluation of tumour invasion involves ultrasonography or CT scanning of the lumbar aortic region to detect lymph node invasion. Although the IRS holds the opposite opinion (Raney et al. 1978), we do not consider systematic lymphadenectomy to be strictly required (Olive et al. 1984).

Rhabdomyosarcoma of the vagina

Rhabdomyosarcoma of the vagina usually occurs during the first few years of life. Its clinical manifestation is a tumorous bud on the vulva or genital bleeding (Fig. 10). It is rarely perceived by rectal touch, unless bulky, because the buds are soft. Benign tumours of the vagina are rare. Differential diagnosis is mainly from germinal tumours which secrete α-fetoprotein. Surface buds are easily biopsied and usually only require local anaesthesia. Systematic examination of the vagina while the patient is under general anaesthesia is recommended in order to determine the seat of the tumour and its clinical extension (vagina, cervix, parameters).

Pelvic and/or lymph node invasion will be revealed by CT scanning. In rare cases rhabdomyosarcoma can also be intrauterine and tumour invasion proceeds via the cervix to the vagina. This particular localization occurs in older pubescent children (Hays et al. 1985). In adolescents, the differential diagnosis is from clear cell

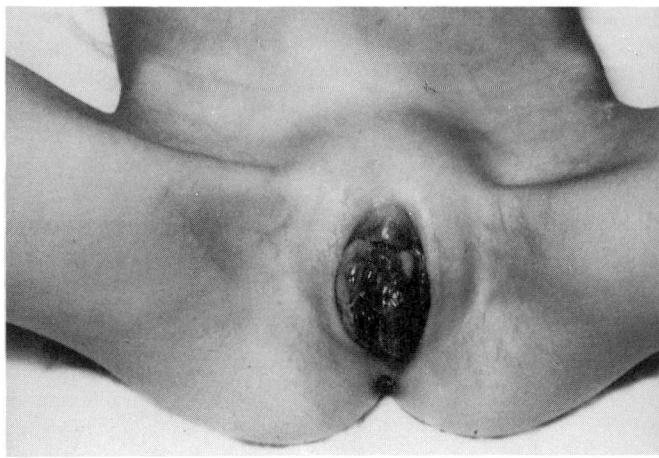

Fig. 10 Vaginal rhabdomyosarcoma: late diagnosis in a North African girl.

adenocarcinoma linked to maternally ingested diethylstilboestrol during pregnancy, although the minimum age for the disease will increase as this drug ceases to be administered to pregnant women (in 1988 the minimum age was 14 years). This type of tumour will undoubtedly be eradicated in children in the future.

Rhabdomyosarcoma of the extremities

The legs are mainly affected, with the emergence of a painless tumour embedded in a muscle. Any tumefaction of a limb which is not rapidly resorbed must be biopsied. A tentative diagnosis of haematoma or lipoma is inadequate. Lymph node involvement often occurs in this localization and can be the first clinical sign. Intrapelvic lymph node spread should be investigated thoroughly by means of CT scanning or pedal lymphangiography.

Other sites

Other sites are diverse and include the abdominal or thoracic wall (paravertebral tumours can lead to intraspinal extension and medullary compression), mediastinum, retroperitoneal space, abdomen, bile ducts, liver, pelvis, and perineum.

Initial medullary involvement gives rise to a specific clinical picture with an alteration in the patient's general condition: anaemia, fever, joint or bone pains, and occasionally subcutaneous nodules, mainly in the breast in females. It may evoke leukaemia or acute rheumatic arthritis (Rodary *et al.* 1988). The primary tumour may be small and undetected. Medullary invasion is due to myoblastic extra-haemopoietic cells; the main victims are older children with rhabdomyosarcoma of the limbs and the alveolar pathological form. Hypercalcaemia and a syndrome of disseminated intravascular coagulation can be associated and require urgent treatment (Leblanc *et al.* 1984).

Prognostic factors

Prognostic factors found in a multivariate analysis in the 1975–1984 SIOP study (Rodary *et al.* 1988) are, in order of importance, site, stage, and sex. Histological subgroups were not found to have a prognostic value. A univariate analysis performed using the new international pathological classification on the 200 IRS cases reviewed for this work found the prognostic values for the three subgroups given earlier.

Sites are classified into three groups of increasing severity: orbit, paratesticular, and vagina–vulva have the best prognosis and parameningeal head and neck and intra-abdominal tumours have the worst prognosis; all others are of intermediate prognosis.

Stage I disease is better than stages II and III which in turn are better than stage IV.

Lymph node involvement (stage III) was not considered prognostic in this multivariate analysis. Therefore, the survival rate of stage III patients is worse than that of stage II patients if only this factor is considered (univariate analysis), as in the recent 1984–1988 SIOP study.

Rhabdomyosarcoma is less frequent in girls than in boys but disease progression is less favourable, independently of other prognostic factors in the SIOP study (1975–1984).

Treatment

Surgery, radiotherapy, and chemotherapy are associated in the treatment of rhabdomyosarcoma. The aim of surgery and radiotherapy is to obtain local eradication of the tumour, while chemotherapy acts locally and systemically in order to prevent the emergence of metastatic disease.

Surgery

Surgery was the first treatment modality used in rhabdomyosarcoma and only 8 per cent of all patients were cured (Johnson 1975), except for patients with an orbital localization where exenteration achieved a survival rate of approximately 50 per cent. Since the introduction of chemotherapy, the role of surgery has changed. The initial removal of the tumour must still be performed, if possible with a conservative surgical approach, for instance in the case of small easily accessible tumours (limbs, walls, etc.). The quality of the surgical resection must be substantiated by careful histological examination of margins so as to determine the post-surgical stage and, hence, decide on the complementary treatment required. In other cases, only a biopsy is essential initially.

Secondary surgery following chemotherapy and/or radiotherapy is indicated in two instances: if the tumour has not responded, then extensive, wide, and often mutilating surgery is imperative; if the tumour responds, then surgery is used to ensure that treatment has resulted in its resorption. As in the case of initial surgery, complementary treatment will depend directly on the findings of the pathological examination of specimens acquired through secondary surgery.

Radiotherapy

Radiotherapy was employed as soon as high-energy machines permitted high doses to be delivered to large volumes. It was recommended as a complement to surgery when incomplete and for large inoperable tumours such as rhabdomyosarcoma of the head and neck. In these latter cases few patients were cured owing to the rapidity of tumour growth. The rate of survival was only 15–20 per cent despite doses of 45–50 Gy (Donaldson *et al.* 1973; Flamant *et al.* 1985).

The current knowledge regarding radiotherapy can be summarized as follows. When associated with chemotherapy, radiotherapy achieves local control in 75–90 per cent of cases. A wide margin around the tumour volume must be allowed. The results of the IRS studies seem to indicate that doses greater than 50 Gy with external-beam irradiation are not necessary and that 40–50 Gy should be adequate depending on the age of the patient.

Parameningeal rhabdomyosarcoma localizations had a very poor prognosis in the IRS I study because of the risk of secondary meningeal spread (Scable *et al.* 1987). Irradiation of the whole cerebrospinal axis at 30 Gy with a total of 45–50 Gy to the primary tumour combined with intrathecal chemotherapy has greatly increased the 2 year survival of such patients in the IRS II study. Therefore, the progress in survival is probably due more to the irradiation of a more precise tumour volume with wider margins than to irradiation of the entire cerebrospinal axis. Intrathecal chemotherapy has never demonstrated its activity and will undoubtedly be abandoned in the future for patients with parameningeal rhabdomyosarcoma. Irradiation is generally performed using an external ^{60}Co source or linear accelerators (photons or electrons for superficial tumours).

Interstitial brachytherapy using ^{192}Ir within the tumour bed or implanted by means of intracavitary moulds is effective for specific indications, for example accessible tumours of small volume (5 cm or less). This technique has the advantage of delivering a high continuous dose to the tumour while the neighbouring healthy tissue is spared. It is used for particular localizations such as the vagina or trunk walls. Good cooperation between surgeons, clinicians, and brachytherapist is a prerequisite for correctly coordinated treatment (Gerbaulet *et al.* 1985).

The capacity of radiotherapy to achieve local control must be considered against the background of long-term sequelae engendered by this form of treatment. Sequelae are extremely severe in children cured of rhabdomyosarcoma because of the high doses received, the extent of the irradiated volume, and the critical organs often included (eyes, ears, endocrine glands, bladder, etc.). The risk of second tumours at the sites of irradiation should not be neglected. At present, efforts in the SIOP studies are directed towards the suppression of radiotherapy or, failing that, a reduction of the irradiated volume. Novel approaches to the timing of the delivery of ionizing radiation (for example, fractionation, acceleration) may bring about an attenuation in sequelae while maintaining efficacy.

The indication of radiotherapy depends on the extent of tumour invasion. It has been shown in the IRS I study (Tefft *et al.* 1978) that patients who have had a complete removal of localized tumour (histopathologically verified) do not require local radiotherapy, provided that they are treated with a course of actinomycin D, cyclophosphamide, and vincristine for 2 years. Large tumours with regional extension are traditionally treated with chemotherapy and radiotherapy.

SIOP conducted a randomized trial on TNM stage II and stage III tumours. The aim of this trial was to determine whether it was feasible, for patients whose tumours respond well to initial chemotherapy, to treat only the residual tumour, rather than the initial tumour volume, by means of surgery or radiotherapy. No difference was found in the survival rate between the group which received initial chemotherapy and that which received initial radiotherapy or extensive surgery. Moreover, 50 per cent of the patients who received initial chemotherapy were free of sequelae. However, the study lacks statistical significance because of the small number of patients included (Flamant *et al.* 1985).

Chemotherapy

The drugs known to be effective in fighting rhabdomyosarcoma are vincristine, cyclophosphamide, actinomycin D, adriamycin, cisplatinum in association with VP 16 or adriamycin, and ifosfamide in various combinations. The choice of drugs, their association, and the length of treatment is dependent on the extent of tumour invasion. At present, the most frequently used combinations are vincristine, actinomycin D, and cyclophosphamide (VAC) or ifosfamide, vincristine, and actinomycin D (IVA). In the 1984–1988 SIOP study the percentage of complete remissions achieved with IVA on visible tumour was 58 per cent compared with 25 per cent obtained in the SIOP trial (Flamant *et al.* 1985) using VAC alternating with vincristine plus adriamycin.

The efficacy of chemotherapy in preventing metastases in localized stages of the disease appears to have been demonstrated in the trial conducted by the Children's Cancer Study Group (Heyn *et al.* 1974). Indeed, 82 per cent of the patients (aged 14–17 years) were alive 2 years after having been administered actinomycin D and vincristine for 2 years compared with 47 per cent of those (aged 7–15 years) who had not been administered chemotherapy. All these patients had initially undergone complete surgical removal of tumour and local irradiation. However, the difference was not statistically significant.

The study conducted at the Institut Gustave-Roussy (Flamant and Hill 1984) was based on historical comparisons and showed no difference in survival between patients with localized tumours treated with or without chemotherapy. However, the usefulness of chemotherapy following complete surgical removal of a localized tumour is universally accepted.

The same study showed that the rate of cure among patients with advanced rhabdomyosarcoma (stages II and III) of the head and neck or genitourinary sites had drastically improved since the introduction of combination chemotherapeutic regimens containing vincristine, actinomycin D, and cyclophosphamide, with or without adriamycin and associated with extensive surgery or radiotherapy. No modification in the survival curve was noted for patients with rhabdomyosarcoma of the limbs.

Therapeutic strategy and results

Two therapeutic problems are caused by rhabdomyosarcoma in children. Firstly, we need to increase the percentage of patients cured, which is currently approximately 70 per cent at 3 years for the entire group but is extremely low in some subgroups of sites.

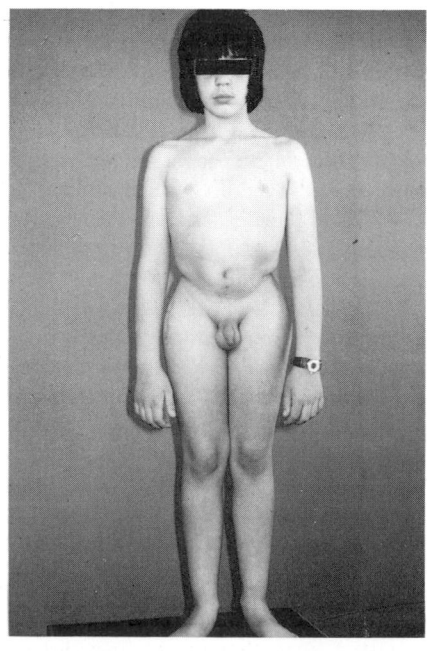

Fig. 11 Iliac bone and upper femur sequelae 4 years after 45 Gy radiotherapy in a 5 year old boy with bladder rhabdomyosarcoma.

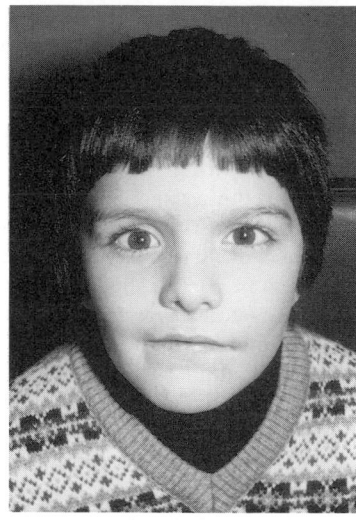

Fig. 12 A 12 year old boy irradiated (45 Gy) for maxillary sinus rhabdomyosarcoma at the age of 4 years: atrophy of half the face

Secondly, we wish to achieve cure with the minimum of sequelae. As has been seen, radiotherapy is an integral part of the therapeutic strategy but is chiefly responsible for the severe sequelae which occur, particularly in young patients. Indeed, the majority of rhabdomyosarcoma patients are young (the median age at diagnosis is 5 years in European studies).

These sequelae depend on the age, site, and extension of the primary tumour. Radiotherapy of large fields may include critical organs such as the hypophysis, thyroid, ovaries, testis, eyes, ears, bladder, and brain. Extensive major surgery, such as pelvectomy or enucleation, can also lead to unpleasant sequelae in some cases. Sequelae due to surgery are immediately visible; sequelae due to radiotherapy are gradual and can only be judged after puberty; that is, 10–15 years after treatment (Figs 11 and 12). Furthermore, second tumours can occur in irradiated fields, in particular osteosarcoma or chrondrosarcoma. Cure and the avoidance of major sequelae are the two basic objectives which underlie treatment planning.

The results of the treatment of such rare tumours are of interest if the patients are treated within the context of trials based on a protocol. During the last 15 years two large coordinated study groups have been set up: the IRS in the United States and the SIOP rhabdomyosarcoma group in Europe. Study groups on rhabdomyosarcoma have also been set up in Germany and Italy.

The differences between the groups are not so much the results in terms of survival but the different concepts in the European and American studies. The IRS group continues to consider radiotherapy as a crucial integral part of the treatment required to achieve local control, except for tumours which are totally removed with free margins at initial surgery. Chemotherapy is administered together with radiotherapy to facilitate local control and prevent distant metastases. The primary goal of the IRS studies is to obtain a cure rate of 90 per cent for all patients. As cure is the main objective, sequelae are not taken into account initially but a reduction in the aggressiveness of treatment is subsequently considered in some categories of patients with good prognosis.

European studies attempt to tailor treatment according to risk factors, inasmuch as these factors can be determined at diagnosis. The aim is to cure patients by minimizing as far as possible any foreseeable therapeutic sequelae and thereby risking failure in some instances. Initial chemotherapy in incompletely resected or inoperable primary tumours is included in the treatment strategy with the aim of reducing or dispensing with local treatment (either

extensive major surgery and/or radiotherapy with large fields) for good responders to chemotherapy. The German group has found a particular relationship between a rapid response to initial chemotherapy and outcome. This was not found in the SIOP 1984–1988 study.

In this study patients were treated as follows: patients with stage I pT_1 disease (that is, with a tumour which was completely removed initially), received three courses of IVA chemotherapy (Table 5). Patients with an incompletely removed tumour or an inoperable tumour (stage I, pT_{3a}, pT_{3b}, or pT_{3c}) or a locoregional tumour with or without lymph node involvement (stages II or III) received initial chemotherapy with an IVA combination regimen. If complete remission was obtained, if possible confirmed by surgery, patients did not receive radiotherapy (except for those with parameningeal tumours aged 5 years or over) but completed the courses of chemotherapy (six to ten courses in all). Poor responders or non-responders to chemotherapy received radiotherapy after a second-line drug combination (cisplatin plus adriamycin). For patients with parameningeal lesions aged 5 years or more, systematic irradiation was delivered after two courses of chemotherapy to obviate secondary meningeal spread. The whole brain was irradiated in the event of intracranial extension at diagnosis.

The overall 3 year crude survival rate is 66 per cent (standard error, 0.04) (Fig. 13) for the 288 patients from various countries (France, The Netherlands, Belgium, and Argentina). In the previous study (SIOP 1975–1984 study), a plateau was reached after only 5 years of follow-up. There is a consistent difference (Fig. 14) between the event-free and crude survival curves for stage I, II, and III patients. This difference is due in part to the underlying objective of the SIOP study. A higher percentage of relapses are accepted than in the IRS study by minimizing the primary treatment, with the hope of curing through secondary treatment a reasonable percentage of patients who relapse (the IRS III study has the same crude survival rate but the event-free survival rate is better because patients initially received intensive treatment). In

Table 5 IVA chemotherapy (SIOP 1984–1988 study)

Ifosfamide	3 g/m^2	Days 1 and 2
Vincristine	1–5 mg/m^2	Days 1–8 (maximum 2 mg per injection)
Actinomycin D	900 μg/m^2	Days 1 and 2 (maximum 1000 μg per injection)

Course every 21 days.

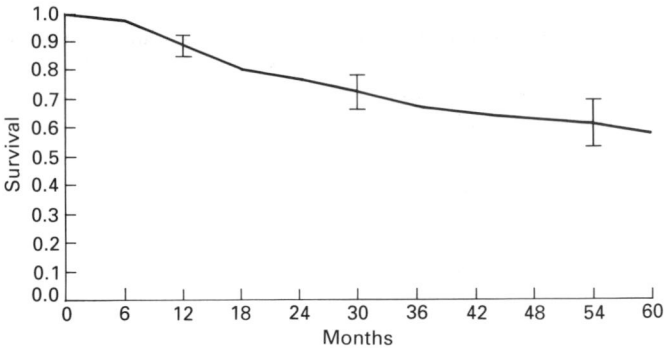

Fig. 13 Crude survival curve for rhabdomyosarcoma patients (all stages) in the SIOP 1984–1988 study.

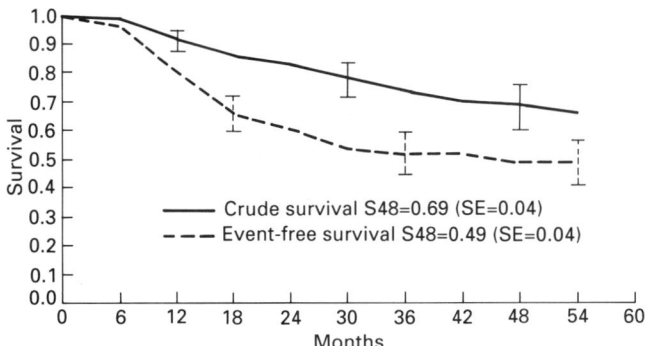

Fig. 14 Crude and event-free survival curves for rhabdomyosarcoma patients in the SIOP 1984–1988 study (stages I, II, and III).

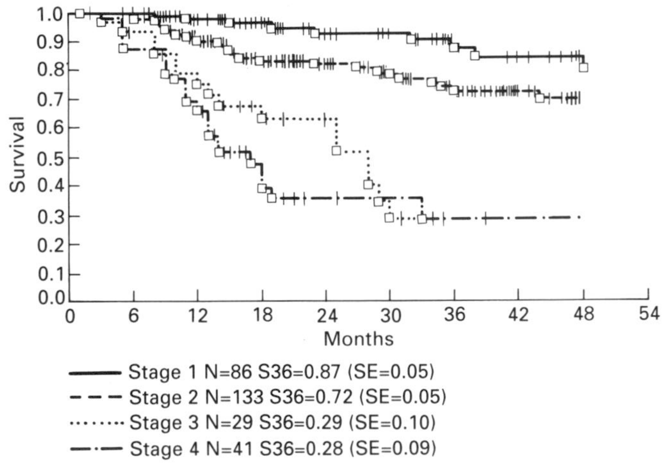

```
── Stage 1  N=86  S36=0.87 (SE=0.05)
─ ─ Stage 2  N=133 S36=0.72 (SE=0.05)
···· Stage 3  N=29  S36=0.29 (SE=0.10)
─·─ Stage 4  N=41  S36=0.28 (SE=0.09)
```

Fig. 15 Crude survival of rhabdomyosarcoma patients according to stage.

contrast, the majority of patients in first complete remission in the SIOP study will have no or minimal sequelae. The difference between the two curves shows the percentage of patients in second complete remission. Figure 15 shows the crude survival according to stage. It is important to note that the survival of patients with metastatic disease or lymph node involvement at diagnosis is very poor compared with that of stage I and II patients. The survival curves also differ according to the site considered. As mentioned earlier, tumours of the orbit, vagina, and paratesticular area have reasonable chances of being cured (3 year crude survival rate of 90 per cent), while the group comprising sites such as thoracic and

abdominal walls, the abdomen, the mediastinum, the parvertebral area, the liver, etc., has a less favourable outcome as is the case with parameningeal sites (3 year crude survival rate of approximately 50 per cent). A third SIOP study was initiated in 1989 and a new IRS study began in 1990. The aim of the IRS study is to enhance the efficacy of chemotherapy by comparing IVA and the conventional VAC combination. During recent years the IRS group has studied the ifosfamide plus VP 16 combination in a phase II trial, which has yielded a good percentage of responses (Miser *et al.* 1987). Radiotherapy will continue to be part of the treatment except for stage I pT$_1$ tumours; conventional and hyperfractionation schedules will be compared.

The SIOP 1989 study has an increased number of participating centres and includes the United Kingdom rhabdomyosarcoma group. The aim is still to isolate the good responders to chemotherapy in order to reduce their local treatment with more aggressive chemotherapy by shortening the number of courses required (IVA with 9 g/m^2 of ifosfamide). The experience of the German group has been taken into account and local treatment will be performed sooner than in the SIOP 1984 study for patients who do not respond rapidly to chemotherapy. New radiotherapeutic modalities will also be tested (accelerated hyperfractionation).

Chemotherapy has been reduced and alkylating agents eliminated for patients with stage I pT$_1$ tumours. For severe cases with metastatic disease and lymph node involvement the new European Intergroup Study has a different first-line chemotherapy regimen alternating carboplatin and epirubicin, IVA, ifosfamide, and VP 16 associated with local treatment by surgery and/or radiotherapy.

Radiotherapy is not given systematically to patients of less than 3 years of age with parameningeal tumours (again to avoid severe sequelae) as is the case for patients of other age groups, but only when complete remission has not been achieved with initial chemotherapy. In these patients chemotherapy will be intensified according to the stage IV protocol.

Since the international workshop organized by the SIOP, it has become possible to employ the same pre-treatment staging, the same criteria of evaluation, the same pathological subgroups, and the same grouping of sites. The ability to compare the results of four multicentric studies is a major step forward. By pooling small groups of patients in joint studies it will be possible to obtain a much larger number of patients. The three European groups have been working on a cooperative study on patients with metastatic disease since January 1989 and it is hoped that it will be the start of a future collaborative study of all stages.

NON-RHABDOMYOSARCOMAL MALIGNANT MESENCHYMAL TUMOURS

These tumours represent 30 per cent of malignant mesenchymal tumours in the SIOP series if embryonal sarcomas are included. (In previous IRS series they were included in rhabdomyosarcoma but this is no longer the case.) Eighty per cent of these non-rhabdomyosarcomal malignant mesenchymal tumours in children have been classified, but with difficulty and changes in category after further histopathological analysis are very frequent. Despite immunological studies, 20 per cent of these tumours remain unclassified. Non-rhabdomyosarcomal malignant mesenchymal tumours show some clinical differences from rhabdomyosarcoma. They are more localized than rhabdomyosarcoma (stage I, 41 versus 30 per cent). The site distribution is also different with two preponderant sites: the extremities (30 per cent) and 'other sites' (40 per cent).

Faced with a multitude of pathological diagnoses and frequent changes in classification (even between rhabdomyosarcoma and non-rhabdomyosarcomal malignant mesenchymal tumours), SIOP decided to incorporate non-rhabdomyosarcomal malignant mesenchymal tumours in the same treatment strategy as rhabdomyosarcoma. In particular, they were to receive the same chemotherapy protocol. However, surgery has a major role to play in both children and adults and initial complete conservative surgery is recommended when feasible. As yet, the efficacy of adjuvant chemotherapy is difficult to evaluate (Horowitz *et al.* 1986).

With regard to the response to initial chemotherapy, Horowitz *et al.* (1986) reported two responses in nine patients. In the SIOP 1984 study of malignant mesenchymal tumours (unpublished) the response to initial chemotherapy could only be evaluated in 45 patients with macroscopic tumours. Seventy per cent of responses (complete response plus partial response) were obtained with IVA. In 46 per cent of patients who were non-responders or who had a partial response, the use of primary chemotherapy did not obviate the need for extensive local treatment.

It was not possible to provide results according to pathological subtypes, except for embryonal sarcomas which responded to initial chemotherapy in the same way as rhabdomyosarcoma and synovial sarcomas which did regress in some instances under initial chemotherapy. For these non-rhabdomyosarcomal malignant mesenchymal tumours primary surgery must be performed if the tumour is in stage I. In other cases secondary surgery after chemotherapy should not be delayed for more than 3 months.

Some non-rhabdomyosarcomal malignant mesenchymal tumours show specific characteristics in children.

Fibrosarcomas

In children aged over 1 year fibrosarcomas are similar to those found in adult patients with local recurrences and late pulmonary metastases. A particular form has been identified in infants and designated 'infantile fibrosarcoma'. It is either congenital or occurs during the first year of life and generally has a favourable course, although there is a likelihood of local recurrence. Conservative surgery is the treatment of choice when feasible. If not, chemotherapy of the type used to treat rhabdomyosarcoma has been shown to be efficient in some cases (Grier *et al.* 1985).

Although these tumours are known to have a good prognosis in infants, distant metastases occurred in two cases in the Institut Gustave-Roussy series and led to a fatal outcome (Salloum *et al.* 1990).

Synovial sarcoma

Male children are the most affected by synovial sarcoma (sex ratio 3.7). Its site of predilection is usually, but not always, close to a joint. Its intra-articular origin has never been established. Twenty-one cases were treated at the Institut Gustave-Roussy between 1963 and 1983 (unpublished). Lymph node involvement at the outset is exceptional in children; thus systematic lymphadenectomy performed in adults is not required in children and the inevitable sequelae can be avoided. The biphasic pathological form appears to have a better prognosis than the monophasic form (survival rates of 84 per cent versus 25 per cent). The 5 year event-free survival is 75 per cent. Local control was achieved either through initial complete surgery or by microscopic incomplete surgery followed by radiotherapy (mean dose delivered 45 Gy). In three out of eight cases with macroscopic tumour, local control was achieved by initial chemotherapy followed by conservative surgery and supplemented by radiotherapy. Extensive major surgery such as amputation should be avoided initially.

Neuroepithelioma

Neuroepithelioma, peripheral primitive neuroectodermic tumour, the Askin tumour, and extra-osseous Ewing's sarcoma are often confused and controversies persist regarding diagnosis. It is hoped that in the future, with the contribution of cytogenetic studies and molecular biology, differentiation of these tumours will be facilitated (Marina *et al.* 1989). SIOP has now proposed a uniform approach to the treatment of all these tumours in an attempt to clarify a potential relationship between them. They are all treated as part of the malignant mesenchymal tumour group and not as Ewing's sarcoma or neuroblastoma.

Haemangiopericytoma

Like fibrosarcoma, haemangiopericytoma shows similar behaviour in adults and children over the age of 1 year. However, even with malignant pathological features, it has a favourable outcome in children. Complete surgery is the only treatment at this age.

Embryonal sarcoma

Embryonal sarcoma is specific to childhood. It is treated like rhabdomyosarcoma and responds to initial chemotherapy. It is not possible to determine whether this tumour has a particular evolution.

Infantile pigmented neuroectodermic tumour

This tumour has been described as benign, but it is possible to observe local relapse or metastases. It is extremely rare and is treated by initial surgery if possible. Its response to chemotherapy is unknown.

Summary

If we group together all these non-rhabdomyosarcomal malignant mesenchymal tumours which have different prognoses, the 4 year crude survival rate is 72 per cent and the crude and event-free survival rates for stages I–II and III are 73 and 61 per cent, respectively in the SIOP 1984–1988 study of malignant mesenchymal tumours (Figs 16 and 17).

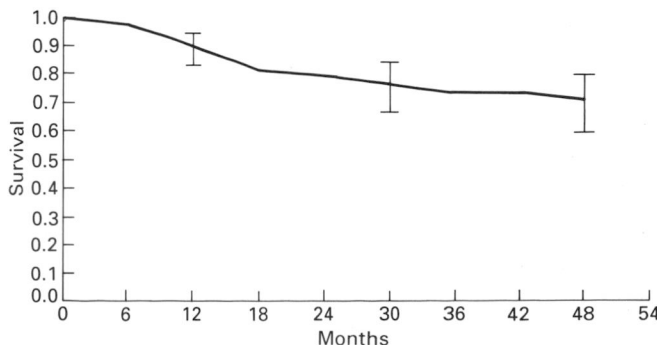

Fig. 16 Crude survival curve of non-rhabdomyosarcomal malignant mesenchymal tumour patients (SIOP 1984–1988 study).

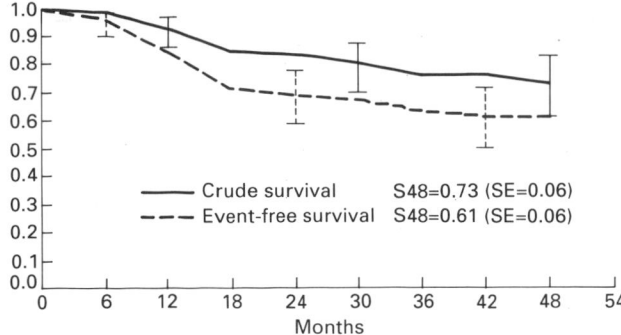

Fig. 17 Crude survival and event-free survival curves of non-rhabdomyosarcomal malignant mesenchymal tumour patients in stages I, II, and III.

Rhabdomyosarcomas are the predominant soft tissue sarcomas found in children. A considerable improvement in survival rates has been seen in the last decade, but much remains to be achieved, in particular for bulky tumours with very poor prognosis. The therapeutic strategy currently combines chemotherapy, surgery, and radiotherapy. European studies have attempted to select groups of patients who are good responders to chemotherapy in order to attenuate local treatment, in particular radiotherapy which is well known for its capacity to generate severe sequelae. There is no doubt that cure is the essential objective when treating the children, but they must also be allowed to have a good quality of life during their childhood and future adult life.

REFERENCES

Abdul-Karim FW, *et al.* (1985). Malignant histocytofibroma of jaws. *Cancer*, 56:1590–6.

Beddis IR, *et al.* (1983). Nasopharyngeal rhabdomyosarcoma and Gorlin's noevoid basal cell carcinoma syndrome. *Medical and Pediatric Oncology*, 11:178–9.

Bertoni F, *et al.* (1985). Malignant fibrohistiocytoma of soft tissue. *Cancer*, 56:356–67.

Birch JM, *et al.* (1985). Excess risk of breast cancer in the mothers of children with soft tissue sarcomas. *British Journal of Cancer*, 49:325–31.

Birch JM, *et al.* (1990). Identification of factors associated with high-risk in the mothers of children with soft tissue sarcomas. *Journal of Clinical Oncology*, 8:583–90.

Bradford R, *et al.* (1985). Primary of the central nervous system case report. *Neurosurgery*, 17:101–4.

Caillaud JM, *et al.* (1989). Histopathological classification of childhood rhabdomyosarcomas: a report from the International Society of Pediatric Oncology Pathology Panel. *Medical and Pediatric Oncology*, 17:391–400.

Dehner LP, *et al.* (1979). Malignant melanotic neuroectodermal tumor of infancy. *Cancer*, 43:1389–1410.

Donaldson SS, *et al.* (1973). Rhabdomyosarcoma of the head and neck in children. Treatment by surgery, irradiation and chemotherapy. *Cancer*, 31:26–35.

Donaldson S, *et al.* (1986). *Pediatric Hematology and Oncology*, 3:249–58.

Douglas E, *et al.* (1987). A specific chromosomal abnormality in rhabdomyosarcoma. *Cytogenetics and Cell Genetics*, 45:148–55.

Enzinger FM, Weiss SW (1983). *Soft tissue tumours.* CV Mosby, St Louis, MO.

Flamant F, Hill C (1984). The improvement in survival associated with combined chemotherapy in childhood rhabdomyosarcoma. A historical comparison of 345 patients treated in the same center. *Cancer*, 53:2417–21.

Flamant F, *et al.* (1985). Primary chemotherapy in the treatment of rhabdomyosarcoma in children: trial of the International Society of Pediatric Oncology. Preliminary results. *Radiotherapy and Oncology*, 3:227–36.

Gerbaulet A, *et al.* (1985). Iridium after loading curietherapy in the treatment of pediatric malignancies. *Cancer*, 56:1274–9.

Ghavimi F, *et al.* (1975). Multidisciplinary treatment of embryonal rhabdomyosarcoma in children. *Cancer*, 35:677–86.

Grier HE, *et al.* (1985). Chemotherapy for inoperable infantile fibrosarcoma. *Cancer*, 56:1507–10.

Hays DM, *et al.* (1985). Sarcoma of the vagina and uterus. IRS study. *Journal of Pediatric Surgery*, 20:718–24.

Heyn RM, *et al.* (1974). The role of combined chemotherapy in the treatment of rhabdomyosarcoma in children. *Cancer*, 34:2128–42.

Horowitz ME, *et al.* (1986). Therapy for childhood soft-tissue sarcomas other than rhabdomyosarcoma: a review of 62 cases treated at a single institution. *Journal of Clinical Oncology*, 4:559–64.

Johnson DG (1975). Trends in surgery for childhood rhabdomyosarcoma. *Cancer*, 35:916–20.

Kingston JE, *et al.* (1983). Childhood rhabdomyosarcoma: experience of the children's solid tumour group. *British Journal of Cancer*, 48:195–207.

Lawrence W, *et al.* (1987). Prognostic significance of staging factors of the UICC staging system in childhood rhabdomyosarcoma: a report from the Intergroup Rhabdomyosarcoma Study (IRS II). *Journal of Clinical Oncology*, 5:46–54.

Lai JC, *et al.* (1987). Translocation (2, 13) (q37, q14) in rhabdomyosarcoma: a new case. *Cancer Genetics and Cytogenetics*, 25:371–2.

Leblanc A, *et al.* (1984). Hypercalcemia preferentially occurs in unusual forms of childhood non-Hodgkin's lymphoma rhabdomyosarcoma and Wilms' tumor. *Cancer*, 54:2132–6.

Li FP, Fraumeni JF (1969). Soft tissue sarcoma, breast cancer and other neoplasms: a familial syndrome? *Annals of Internal Medicine*, 71:747–53.

Li FP, Fraumeni JF (1982). Prospective study of a family cancer syndrome. *Journal of American Medical Association*, 247:2692–4.

Li FP, *et al.* (1988). A cancer family syndrome in twenty four kindreds. *Cancer Research*, 48:5358–62.

Lizard-Nalol S, *et al.* (1987). Translocation (2, 13) (q37, q14) in alveolar rhabdomyosarcoma: a new case. *Cancer Genetics and Cytogenetics*, 25:373–4.

Louvet C, *et al.* (1981). Extraskeletal mesenchymal chondrosarcoma: case report and review of the literature. *Journal of Clinical Oncology*, 3:858–63.

Mackeen EA, *et al.* (1978). Rhabdomyosarcoma complicating multiple neurofibromatosis. *Journal of Pediatrics*, 93:992–3.

Malkin D, *et al.* (1990). Germ-line p53 mutations in a familial syndrome of breast cancer, sarcomas and other neoplasms. *Science*, 250:1233–8.

Marina NM, *et al.* (1989). Peripheral primitive neuroectodermal tumor (peripheral neuroepithelioma) in children. A review of the St Jude experience and controversies in diagnosis and management. *Cancer*, 64:1952–60.

Miser JS, *et al.* (1987). Ifosfamide with mesna uroprotection and etoposide: an effective regimen in the treatment of recurrent sarcomas and other tumors of childhood and young adults. *Journal of Clinical Oncology*, 5:1191–8.

Olive D, *et al.* (1984). Paraaortic lymphadenectomy is not necessary in the treatment of localized paratesticular rhabdomyosarcoma. *Cancer*, 54:1283–7.

Pavlidis NA, *et al.* (1984). Clear-cell sarcoma of tendons and aponeuroses. A clinicopathologic study. *Cancer*, 54:1412–17.

Pedrick TJ, *et al.* (1986). Rhabdomyosarcoma: the Stanford experience using a TNM staging system. *Journal of Clinical Oncology*, 4:370–8.

Pratt CB, *et al.* (1972). Coordinated treatment of childhood rhabdomyosarcoma with surgery, radiotherapy and combination chemotherapy. *Cancer Research*, 32:606–10.

Raney AB, *et al.* (1978). Paratesticular rhabdomyosarcoma in childhood. *Cancer*, 42:729–36.

Reik W, Surani AM (1989). Genomic imprinting and embryonal tumors. *Nature, London*, 338:112–13.

Riopelle JL, Theriault JP (1956). Sur une forme méconnue de sarcomes des parties molles: le rhabdomyosarcome alvéolaire. *Annales d'Anatomie Pathologique*, 1:88–92.

Rodary C, *et al.* (1988). Prognostic factors in 281 children with non metastatic rhabdomyosarcoma (RMS) at diagnosis. *Medical and Pediatric Oncology*, 16:71–7.

Ruymann FB, *et al.* (1984). Bone marrow metastases at diagnosis in children and adolescents with rhabdomyosarcoma. *Cancer*, 53:368–73.

Ruymann FB, *et al.* (1988). Congenital anomalies associated with rhabdomyosarcoma: an autopsy study of 115 cases. A report from the Intergroup Rhabdomyosarcoma Study Committee. *Medical Pediatric Oncology*, 16:33–9.

Salloum E, *et al.* (1990). Poor prognosis infantile fibrosarcoma with pathological features of malignant fibrous histiocytoma after local recurrence. *Medical and Pediatric Oncology.*

Scable HJ, *et al.* (1987). Chromosomal localisation of the human rhabdomyosarcoma locus by mitotic recombination mapping. *Nature, London,* **329**:345–7.

Schweisguth O, *et al.* (1968). Basal cell naevus syndrome: association with congenital rhabdomyosarcoma. *Archives Francaises de Pédiatrie,* **25**:1083–93.

Sobel RA, Woerner S (1978). Rubinstein–Taybi syndrome and nasopharyngeal rhabdomyosarcoma. *Journal of Pediatrics,* **92**:851–2.

Tefft M, *et al.* (1978). Incidence of meningeal involvement by rhabdomyosarcoma of the head and neck in children. A report of the Intergroup Rhabdomyosarcoma Study. *Cancer,* **42**:253–8.

Turc-Carel C, *et al.* (1968). Consistent chromosomal translocation in alveolar rhabdomyosarcoma. *Cancer Genetics and Cytogenetics,* **19**:361–2.

UICC (1983). *TNM: Classification des tumeurs principales de l'enfant,* pp. 23–8. UICC, Geneva.

Wiedemann MR (1983). Tumors and hemihypertrophy associated with Beckwith–Wiedemann syndrome. *European Journal of Pediatrics,* **17**:141–29.

13.3 Ewing's sarcoma

HERBERT F. JÜRGENS, ROLF SAUER, W. WINKELMANN, AND ULRICH GÖBEL

Ewing's sarcoma is the second most common malignant bone tumour in children and adolescents. It is histologically characterized by a uniform pattern of small cells with round nuclei but without distinct cytoplasmic borders of prominent nucleoli (Campanacci 1990; Huvos 1991). Following a long period of a solely light-microscopic definition of Ewing's sarcoma as the classical round cell sarcoma of bone, the use of immunocytochemistry and cytogenetics has provided new tools which allow a more exact definition (Turc-Carel *et al.* 1983; Whang-Peng *et al.* 1984; Schmidt *et al.* 1987; Schmidt and Harms 1990). Ten to 15 per cent of

primary malignant bone tumours fall into the category of Ewing's sarcoma (Larsson and Lorentzon 1974; Huvos 1991). The mean annual incidence approximates 0.6 per million population (Price and Jeffree 1977).

Ewing's sarcoma is rarely seen in children below 5 years of age or adults over the age of 30 years; the peak incidence is between 10 and 15 years. The male to female ratio is approximately 1.5 : 1, although it varies with age and is lower in children and higher in adolescents (Fig. 1) (Glass and Fraumeni 1970). The Black and Chinese populations are less affected (Glass and Fraumeni 1970; Li *et al.* 1980; Huvos 1991).

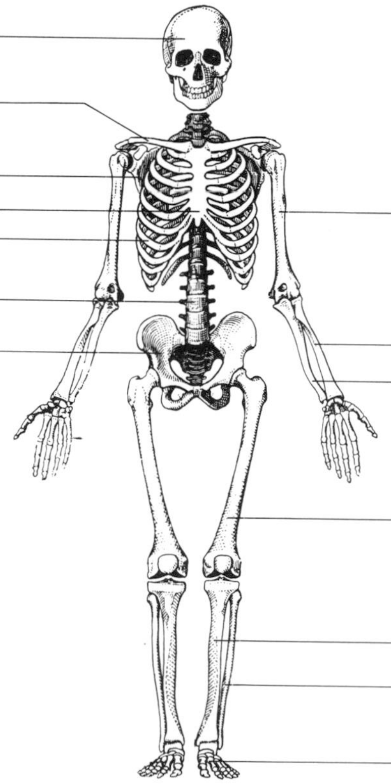

PATHOLOGY

Ewing's sarcoma originates in the intramedullary cavity and rapidly breaks through the cortex, producing a soft tissue component of varying consistency (Campanacci 1990; Huvos 1991). On histological examination, Ewing's sarcoma is characterized by a structureless array of small hyperchromatic cells (Salzer-Kuntschik 1976; Remagen and Salzer-Kuntschik 1981; Campanacci 1990; Huvos 1991) and in 90 per cent of cases glycogen can be demonstrated using the periodic acid–Schiff reagent and diastase reactions (Schajowicz 1959). A large cell variant of Ewing's sarcoma has been described and is believed to be associated with a poorer prognosis (Llombart-Bosch *et al.* 1978; Nascimento 1980).

To allow distinction from other small cell sarcomas, routine pathological examination is generally accompanied by immunohisto-chemistry (Schmidt *et al.* 1987; Schmidt and Harms 1990) and cytogenetic studies (Turc-Carel *et al.* 1983; Whang-Peng *et al.* 1984).

Cytogenetic analyses have revealed a consistent chromosomal translocation t(11;22) (q24;q12) in most cell lines derived from Ewing's sarcoma (Turc-Carel *et al.* 1983). The same chromosomal translocation has also been reported in peripheral neuroepitheliomas (Whang-Peng *et al.* 1984), reflecting the close relationship between these two tumours.

CLINICAL FEATURES AND DIAGNOSTIC PROCEDURES

The most common presentation is increasing persistent pain and swelling of the affected area, possibly with impairment of function. Slight to moderate fever may occur and is more likely in patients

Skull (1.5)
Clavicle (2)
Scapula (6)
Sternum (0.5)
Rib (10)
Vertebra (8)
Pelvis (8)
Humerus (7)
Radius (1)
Ulna (2)
Femur (19)
Tibia (10)
Fibula (11)
Foot (2)

Fig. 1 Skeletal distribution (per cent) of 300 consecutive patients with primary Ewing's sarcoma entered into the CESS trials (1981–1990).

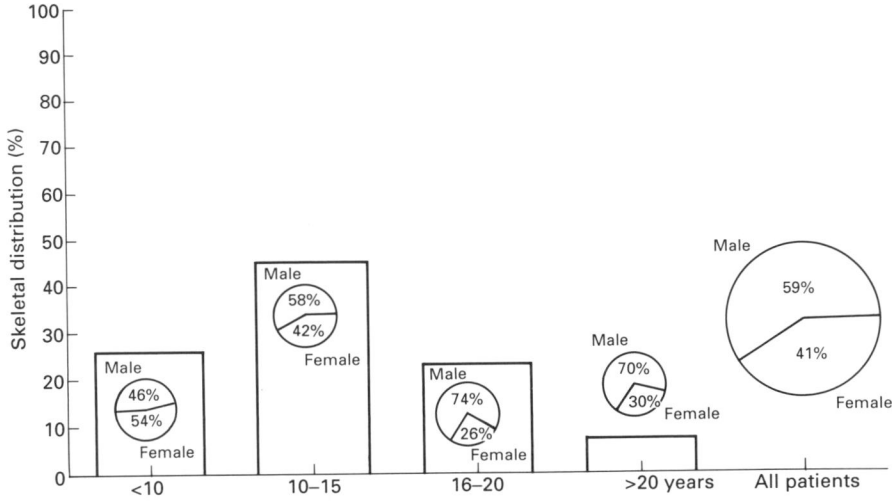

Fig. 2 Age and sex distribution of 300 consecutive patients with Ewing's sarcoma entered into the CESS trials (1981–1990).

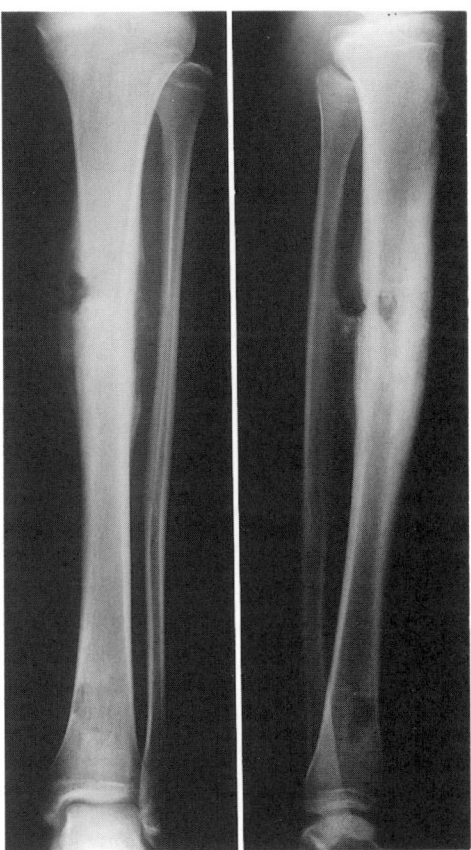

Fig. 3 Tibial Ewing's sarcoma with medullary bone destruction and periostal lamellation in a 15 year old girl.

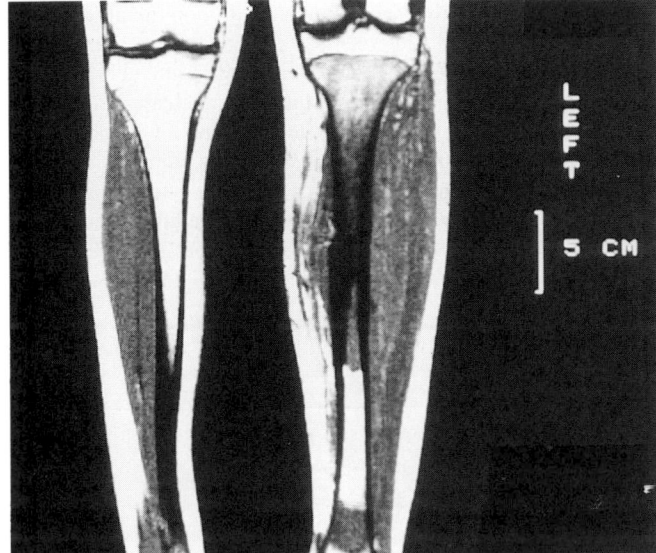

Fig. 4 MRI of tibial Ewing's sarcoma in a 15 year old girl, showing the tumour extension within the medullary cavity (radiograph shown in Fig. 3).

with advanced or metastatic disease (Dahlin 1978; Huvos 1991). The pelvis, femur, tibia, and fibula account for approximately 60 per cent of all primary sites; the remaining 40 per cent are distributed throughout the skeletal system (Fig. 1). In long bones Ewing's sarcoma usually originates from the intramedullary cavity of the diaphysis, either centrally or towards the end (Dahlin 1978; Campanacci 1990; Huvos 1991), which provides a distinction from osteogenic sarcoma.

The initial diagnostic procedure usually includes a conventional radiograph where Ewing's sarcoma typically appears as patchy 'moth-eaten' bone destruction with poorly defined margins and a parallel 'onion-skin' periostal lamellation with a varying degree of soft tissue extension of tumour (Fig. 3) (Vohra 1967; Campanacci 1990; Huvos 1991). The conventional radiographic diagnosis is complemented by CT scans and/or magnetic resonance imaging (**MRI**), with the latter being particularly helpful in outlining the exact intramedullary extension of the tumour (Fig. 4) (Bohndorf *et al.* 1986). A whole-body radionuclide bone scan is required to determine the extent of the primary tumour within the affected bone and also to detect other sites of bony involvement within the skeleton. To detect or rule out lung metastases, posteroanterior and lateral chest radiographs are needed, preferably complemented by full chest tomography and/or CT scan of the chest. Bone-marrow aspiration and/or biopsy, preferably obtained from several sites, are required to detect diffuse bone-marrow contamination (Rosen 1976).

Approximately 20 per cent of patients present with detectable metastases (Hayes *et al.* 1987; Wessalowski *et al.* 1988). Of these, approximately 50 per cent have lung metastases and approximately

40 per cent have multiple bone involvement and/or diffuse bone-marrow contamination. Lymphatic spread is seen in less than 10 per cent of cases. Involvement of the central nervous system, as either meningeal spread or parenchymal metastases, is extremely uncommon at initial presentation, but may occur in advanced disease (Kulick and Mones 1970; Mehta and Hendrickson 1974).

Laboratory studies usually show a moderately elevated erythrocyte sedimentation rate and may reveal some degree of anaemia and leucocytosis. Elevated serum lactate dehydrogenase (LDH) is believed to be of poor prognostic significance (Dahlin 1978; Glaubiger et al. 1981), probably because of its correlation with tumour burden (Miser et al. 1989). In some patients neurone-specific enolase is elevated in the serum, possibly more so in patients with small cell sarcomas with neural differentiation (Marangos and Polak 1986). Its relationship to prognosis has yet to be determined.

However typical the radiographic or magnetic resonance image may be, these findings cannot be considered pathognomonic, even in patients in the typical age group. Histological confirmation is required in all cases, both to confirm the suspected diagnosis and to distinguish between the various subcategories of small cell sarcomas (Feldmann 1977; Schmidt et al. 1987; Schmidt and Harms 1990).

DIFFERENTIAL DIAGNOSIS

The most important clinical differential diagnosis in Ewing's sarcoma is from osteomyelitis (Huvos 1991), where the radiological appearance may be very similar. In addition, Ewing's sarcoma of bone may become secondarily infected. A further complication is that these patients may present with fever and leucocytosis without active infection being present (Coley and Higinbotham 1953).

Ewing's sarcoma must be distinguished from other small round cell sarcomas on histological examination (Miser et al. 1989). Myxoid changes and cross-striations together with the typical ultrastructural appearance of thin or thick microfilaments arranged in z-bands lead to the diagnosis of rhabdomyosarcoma (Schmidt et al. 1987; Schmidt and Harms 1990). On immunocytochemistry, myogenous markers such as desmin, myoglobin, and myosin are usually positive and help to support this diagnosis (Miser et al. 1989). In children younger than 5 years of age, the classical differential diagnosis is neuroblastoma (Berthold et al. 1982). This differential diagnosis is confirmed when the 24 h urinary catecholamine secretion is increased and histological examination reveals the presence of intercellular neurofibrillary matrix or when neurosecretory granules are seen on electron microscopy (Schmidt et al. 1987). On immunocytochemistry, positive reactions with neural markers such as neurone-specific enolase and S100 are characteristic for neuroblastoma (Schmidt et al. 1987; Schmidt and Harms 1990). However, the presence of neural markers is also characteristic of the neural variant of Ewing's sarcoma, termed malignant peripheral neuroectodermal tumour (Jaffe et al. 1984; Schmidt et al. 1987, 1989; Miser et al. 1989). This entity was first described by Askin et al. (1979) as a typical osseous sarcoma of the chest wall and is referred to as Askin's tumour (Israel et al. 1989). Both classical Ewing's sarcoma and its neurally differentiated counterpart share the characteristic chromosomal translocation t(11;22), reflecting the close biological relationship between these tumours (Israel et al. 1989; Miser et al. 1989). The observation that some Ewing's sarcoma cell lines in culture express neural characteristics supports the hypothesis that both categories may reflect different stages of differentiation of the same malignancy (van Valen and Jürgens 1991).

The presence of extracellular matrix, particularly tumour osteoid, may lead to the diagnosis of small cell osteosarcoma (Sim et al. 1979). If cartilage is present, the diagnosis of mesenchymal chondrosarcoma can be made (Huvos et al. 1983). Finally, primary lymphoma of bone should be mentioned, although the absence of disseminated lymph node disease and visceral, meningeal, or bone-marrow involvement is not typical of non-Hodgkin's lymphomas occurring in childhood (Miser et al. 1989). Monoclonal antibodies against lymphoid markers are helpful in making this diagnosis and in subcategorization.

Rarely, Ewing's sarcoma may present solely as a soft tissue tumour, when it is referred to as extraskeletal Ewing's sarcoma (Angervall and Enzinger 1975; Meister and Gokel 1975). Distinction from primitive rhabdomyosarcoma, neuroblastoma, or lymphoma is usually possible using histochemistry, immunochemistry and electron microscopy (Angervall and Enzinger 1975; Wigger et al. 1977; Meister and Gokel 1978; Rose et al. 1983). However, the major differential diagnosis remains Ewing's sarcoma of bone with extensive soft tissue extension and an imperceptible intraosseous component (Angervall and Enzinger 1975). The predominant site of initial presentation is the trunk. Unlike Ewing's sarcoma of bone, there is no predominance in boys. The same rules as for Ewing's sarcoma of bone apply for the diagnostic approach to and systemic treatment of extraskeletal Ewing's sarcoma (Soule et al. 1978; Kinsella et al. 1983b). There appears to be a higher risk of lymphatic spread and, therefore, local therapy, particularly with radiation, has to be planned according to the principles applied to embryonal rhabdomyosarcoma (Soule et al. 1978).

MANAGEMENT

Ewing's sarcoma is a rapidly disseminating malignancy. Prior to the era of effective systemic treatment, over 90 per cent of patients died from systemic, pulmonary, and/or multiple bone metastases within 2–5 years (Falk and Alpert 1967; Philips and Higinbotham 1967). However, James Ewing had already observed that this form of sarcoma was sensitive to radiotherapy, which is a distinction from osteosarcoma (Ewing 1921, 1939).

Radiotherapy

Conventionally, because of its radiosensitivity, radiotherapy plays a major role in obtaining local control in Ewing's sarcoma (Perez et al. 1977; Chan et al. 1979; Razek et al. 1980; Donaldson 1981). However, the widespread adoption of systemic chemotherapy, which has resulted in prolonged disease-free survival, has drawn attention to local failure following radiation (Rosen et al. 1981a; Donaldson and Hendrickson 1983; Jürgens et al. 1985, 1988a). Consequently, there has been a re-examination of the role of surgery for local control (Kotz et al. 1977; Pritchard 1980). Owing to its variability in presentation and the diversity of radiation techniques applied, an exact assessment of the risk of local failure following radiation is difficult (Kinsella et al. 1984; Dunst et al. 1988). However, evidence is accumulating that the probability of cure with radiotherapy is associated with limited tumour bulk and chemosensitivity as measured clinically by tumour regression during initial chemotherapy (Göbel et al. 1987; Sauer et al. 1987). Therefore at present surgery appears to be indicated for patients with bulky primaries or with slow response to chemotherapy (Pritchard 1981; Winkelmann and Jürgens 1989).

Whenever a partial bone resection is considered for debulking of the tumour mass, post-operative radiation is required for control of microscopic or gross residual disease (Bacci et al. 1982; Jürgens et al. 1988a). However, when primary chemotherapy is used, this procedure may have to be adapted to the surgical margins and also to the histological evaluation of response to chemotherapy. Post-operative radiation would thus be omitted in patients with major surgical resections according to the Enneking criteria (Enneking 1987), at least in those with a good histological response to primary chemotherapy (Dunst *et al.* 1988; Jürgens *et al.* 1988*b*). The development of unambiguous guidelines for the role of post-operative radiotherapy following resections is currently the subject of ongoing clinical trials (Jürgens *et al.* 1988*b*; Hayes *et al.* 1989).

Appropriate radiotherapy portals must allow treatment of the entire bone with an additional boost to the region of visualized bulky disease (Tefft *et al.* 1977). Treatment planning has to be based upon the extent of the initial tumour (Razek *et al.* 1980; Jürgens *et al.* 1988*a*). The first Intergroup Ewing's Sarcoma Study (**IESS I**) showed that radiotherapy volumes failing to include the entire bone or with a less than 5 cm margin to the gross disease, are associated with an unacceptably high local failure rate (Perez *et al.* 1977; 1981*a*,*b*; Tefft *et al.* 1977; Razek *et al.* 1980). In a German cooperative trial, it has become evident that the use of limited portals following impressive tumour shrinkage under initial chemotherapy was also associated with an increased risk of local recurrences, particularly in larger tumours (Sauer *et al.* 1984, 1987; Dunst *et al.* 1988; Jürgens *et al.* 1988*a*). However, this has not been confirmed by other groups (Hayes *et al.* 1989) and, hence, the question as to whether the amount of radiation administered can be adjusted according to the histological response of the primary is still under investigation. In no case, however, is chemotherapy alone sufficient to control gross disease (Rosen *et al.* 1978; Thomas *et al.* 1984).

Well-defined radiotherapy dose–response rates for Ewing's sarcoma are lacking (Kinsella *et al.* 1984; Thomas *et al.* 1984). Previously recommended doses of 60–65 Gy have been questioned in view of the effectiveness of combination chemotherapy. Most investigators consider doses above 50 Gy combined with chemotherapy as the treatment of choice (Tepper *et al.* 1980; Thomas *et al.* 1984; Dunst *et al.* 1988). Recent data suggest that the definitive dose of radiation should be related to tumour size, unless surgery is considered to be the treatment of choice for larger tumours (Mendenhall *et al.* 1983; Marcus and Million 1984; Göbel *et al.* 1987; Dunst *et al.* 1988).

Conventional techniques involve fractional doses of 1.5–2.0 Gy/day on 5 days per week avoiding joints and epiphyses whenever possible. Conventional fractionation requires avoidance of known radiation sensitizers, such as adriamycin and actinomycin D, during radiotherapy. Alternative schedules of fractionation, such as hyperfractionation with 1.6 Gy twice daily, are currently under investigation for their impact on local control and acute or late complications (Dunst *et al.* 1988; Jürgens *et al.* 1988*b*). In growing children inclusion of the epiphysis may result in unacceptable functional deficits due to length discrepancies of the extremities. In many instances this may be a reason for advocating surgery as the treatment of choice (Lewis *et al.* 1977; Jentzsch *et al.* 1981; Gonzales-Gonzales and Breur 1983; Kinsella *et al.* 1983*a*).

Surgery

Problems related to the effectiveness of radiotherapy in controlling the primary lesion and to late side-effects and complications have made it necessary to reconsider the role of surgery in the treatment of the primary lesion (Kotz *et al.* 1971; Pritchard 1980, 1981; Rosen *et al.* 1981). Local recurrence rates vary as a function of the primary site and tumour size in the range of 5–50 per cent (Pritchard 1981; Göbel *et al.* 1987; Jürgens *et al.* 1988*a*). The highest local control rates following radiotherapy are observed in patients with small primaries, particularly in the distal part of the extremities. Local control rates obtained with radiation in lesions of the proximal parts

of the extremities or the trunk, which are usually deeper located and of larger size, are lower. Tumour bulk appears to have more influence than site on the local control achieved by radiation (Göbel *et al.* 1987; Jürgens *et al.* 1988*a*). The reported number of local recurrences may be artificially low since local sites are often not assessed at the time of systemic metastatic disease (Kinsella *et al.* 1984). True local control rates can only be established by histological assessment of the primary lesion as the first site of relapse (Rosen *et al.* 1978). Situations where surgical resections are preferable to radiation are listed in Table 1.

Ewing's sarcoma of the pelvis requires special attention since this site is associated with a particularly poor prognosis (Pritchard 1981; Li *et al.* 1983) (Fig. 5). Only rarely is the pelvic lesion small and primarily resectable. Most pelvic tumours are large with an extensive soft tissue mass invading the pelvic cavity (Göbel *et al.* 1979).

Table 1 Indications for surgery as local treatment in Ewing's sarcoma

1. Expendable bone
2. Pathological fracture
3. Distal extremity in growing children
4. Bulky primary
5. Poor response to initial chemotherapy

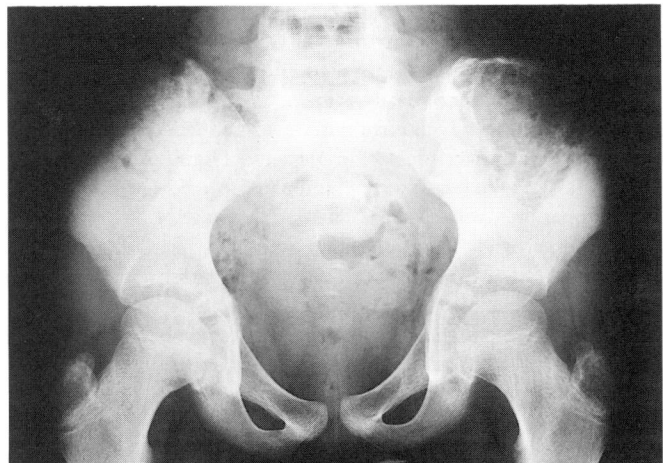

(a)

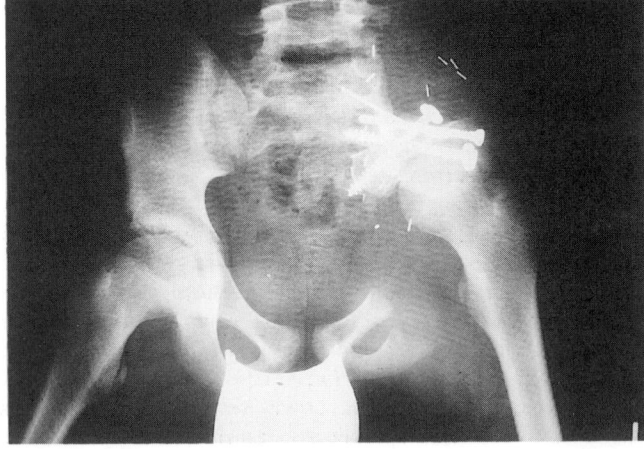

(b)

Fig. 5 Ewing's sarcoma of the left iliac bone (a) at diagnosis and (b) following surgery in a 10 year old girl.

However, there is good evidence that the prognosis of extensive pelvic lesions can be improved when the residual intraosseous disease is resected following tumour shrinkage induced by initial chemotherapy (Winkelmann and Jürgens 1989). Again, radiotherapy following resection is the treatment of choice. Whether radiotherapy can occasionally be omitted depending on surgical margins and response to chemotherapy is the subject of ongoing trials (Dunst et al. 1988).

Chemotherapy

Single-drug data demonstrate the chemosensitivity of Ewing's sarcoma. Alkylating agents such as cyclophosphamide (Samuels and Howe 1967; Rosen et al. 1974), nitrogen mustard, chlorambucil, and ifosfamide (Jürgens et al. 1989a,b) are particularly effective. Other agents studied include vincristine, actinomycin D, 5-fluorouracil, mithramycin (Seeber et al. 1974), and, in particular, adriamycin (Oldham and Pomeroy 1972).

The improved long-term disease-free survival rates above 50 per cent now being reported are the result of intensive combination multicycle chemotherapy regimens (Razek et al. 1980; Gasparini et al. 1981; Rosen et al. 1981a; Jürgens et al. 1985). The results of IESS I have convincingly shown the superiority of a four-drug regimen (vincristine, actinomycin D, cyclophosphamide, and adriamycin (VACA)) over a three-drug regimen (vincristine, actinomycin D, and cyclophosphamide (VAC)) in terms of disease-free survival (74 per cent versus 54 per cent) and the effectiveness of local control (96 per cent versus 86 per cent) (Perez et al. 1977; Razek et al. 1980; Nesbit et al. 1981, 1990). Results from the Memorial Sloan Kettering Cancer Center confirmed the effectiveness of the four-drug regimen and provided evidence that the use of these four effective agents in combination rather than sequentially further improved the results (Rosen et al. 1981b).

Recently, the impact of treatment intensity was shown by the analysis of the results of the Second Intergroup Ewing's Sarcoma Study (IESS II) where high dose intermittent chemotherapy was compared with moderate dose continuous chemotherapy. A significant benefit of the more intensive regimen was observed, with 68 per cent disease-free survival at 5 years compared with 48 per cent for the moderate regimen (Burgert et al. 1990). The first cooperative Ewing's sarcoma study of the German Society of Pediatric Oncology (CESS 81) has shown the prognostic significance of tumour burden at diagnosis and the histological response to initial chemotherapy and has also stressed the impact of surgery on the probability of local control (Göbel et al. 1987; Sauer et al. 1987; Jürgens et al. 1988a). Therefore in a follow-up study (CESS 86) patients with large primaries (tumour volume greater than 100 ml) received a more intense chemotherapy regimen where conventional doses of cyclophosphamide (1200 mg/m^2 body surface area/course) were replaced by high doses of ifosfamide (6000 mg/m^2 body surface area/course) in combination with the other agents (Dunst et al. 1988; Jürgens et al. 1988b). The results show a significant benefit for the high risk patients given the more intense regimen (Jürgens et al. 1988b, 1991), again emphasizing the impact of treatment intensity on disease-free survival.

The combination of ifosfamide and etoposide was recently shown to be highly effective in patients who had failed previous chemotherapy and was subsequently incorporated into first-line chemotherapy regimens (Miser et al. 1987).

In view of the increasing understanding of mechanisms of chemotherapy resistance (Goldie and Coldman 1979; DeVita 1983), for example P-glycoprotein-mediated resistance against anthracyclines and vinca alkaloids (Gerlach et al. 1987), it may be necessary in the future to focus attention on tailoring chemotherapy to the biology of the individual tumour. Because of the impact of treatment intensity on disease-free survival, the use of growth factors to ameliorate chemotherapy-induced myelodepression may also be of benefit, allowing safer administration of higher doses of chemotherapy over a shorter time period (Andreeff and Welte 1989).

METASTATIC DISEASE

Approximately 20 per cent of patients presenting with Ewing's sarcoma are known to have detectable metastatic disease at diagnosis (Hayes et al. 1987; Wessalowski et al. 1988). The prognosis for these patients is poor compared with those with primary tumours only and no detectable metastases (Glaubiger et al. 1980), but seems better for patients with pulmonary metastases only than for those with multiple bone lesions (Caparros et al. 1981; Wessalowski et al. 1988). Treatments indicated include combination chemotherapy, as outlined for patients with primary Ewing's sarcoma and, if pulmonary disease is present, radiation to both lungs in doses of 14–20 Gy depending on age in 1.5 Gy fractions daily on 5 days per week. In the case of multiple bone lesions all involved areas require local treatment. However, it may not be possible to irradiate the entire bone at all sites affected as this may exceed the chemotherapy tolerance limits (Pilepich et al. 1981; Vietti et al. 1981; Wessalowski et al. 1988). Survival in patients with multiple bone lesions at diagnosis has been very poor despite initial response to both intense systemic and local treatment. Survival of these patients 2 years after diagnosis is less than 10 per cent and is comparable with the prognosis of patients with disseminated neuroblastoma (Glaubiger et al. 1980; Wessalowski et al. 1988). Recently, encouraging results have been reported with autologous or allogeneic bone-marrow transplantation, particularly when performed in first remission (Pinkerton et al. 1986; Craft 1987). Conditioning regimens containing total body irradiation seem superior to those with chemotherapeutic conditioning alone. However, current experience is too sparse to allow definite conclusions to be drawn (Burdach et al. 1991). Consolidation with a 'megatherapy' conditioning regimen followed by bone-marrow transplantation is aimed solely at controlling residual microscopic systemic disease. It is essential to obtain local control of bulky disease prior to such a procedure, since the results of bone-marrow transplantation performed in partial remission are discouraging (Craft 1987).

Survival in patients who develop metastatic disease either during or after therapy is poor and second remissions are usually short lived (Craft 1987; Jürgens et al. 1988a). Exceptions may be related to the intensity of primary treatment (Hayes et al. 1989). Attempts are being made to increase salvage with the use of bone-marrow transplantation following intensive conditioning regimens (Burdach et al. 1993). This might be of value, in chemoresponsive relapses although results in patients with resistant disease have been disappointing so far (Craft 1987).

PROGNOSTIC FACTORS

Disease-free survival rates of 50 per cent or more necessitate a recognition of patients' characteristics related to prognosis, since knowledge of these factors may have important implications for tailoring treatment. Factors related to prognosis are listed in Table 2. The site of primary disease, serum LDH levels at diagnosis, and sex are usually recognized as prognostic discriminators for patients with Ewing's sarcoma (Pomeroy and Johnson 1975; Gehan

Table 2 Factors influencing prognosis in Ewing's sarcoma

Factor	Favourable	Unfavourable	Reference
Sex	Female	Male	Pomeroy and Johnson (1975), Gehan *et al.* (1981)
Serum LDH	Normal	Elevated	Glaubiger *et al.* (1981)
Size	<8 cm	>8 cm	Marcus and Million (1984), Hayes *et al.* (1989)
Volume	<100 ml	>100 ml	Göbel *et al.* (1987), Jürgens *et al.* (1988a)
Primary metastases	–	+	Glaubiger *et al.* (1981)
Histology	Small cell	Large cell	Nascimento (1980)
Histological response to chemotherapy	>90% necrosis	<90% necrosis	Jürgens *et al.* (1988a)
Chemotherapy	Four-drug	Three-drug	Nesbit *et al.* (1981, 1990)
Chemotherapy	High intensity	Moderate intensity	Jürgens *et al.* (1988b), Burgert *et al.* (1990)
Local therapy	Surgery	Radiotherapy	Bacci *et al.* (1989)

et al. 1981; Glaubiger *et al.* 1981). It must be stressed that prognostic factors are treatment dependent and may also be interrelated. A Cox regression analysis of the CESS 81 trial has identified tumour volume and histological response to initial chemotherapy as the major predictors of prognosis (Jürgens *et al.* 1988a). High serum LDH levels are also associated with large tumour burden and this may explain the prognostic significance of this factor (Pomeroy and Johnson 1975; Glaubiger *et al.* 1981). Morphological characteristics such as the large cell variant are associated with poor prognosis (Nascimento 1980). The extent to which the expression of immuno-chemically detectable markers offers the possibility of improved prognostic discrimination is yet to be determined (Schmidt *et al.* 1987; Schmidt and Harms 1990). Above all, the presence of visible metastases at the time of initial diagnosis is the most significant prognostic factor (Glaubiger *et al.* 1981). Hence, the importance of staging at the time of diagnosis cannot be overstressed, since such patients may benefit from treatment intensification such as irradiation to both lungs in the case of pulmonary metastases or bone-marrow transplantation in first remission for patients with multifocal and/or disseminated disease (Craft 1987; Burdach *et al.* 1993).

CONCLUSIONS

Since Ewing's sarcoma is fundamentally a systemic disease, a combination of safe local control and effective systemic combination chemotherapy has been able to improve the disease-free survival rates from approximately 10 per cent with local therapy only to 50–70 per cent. Future work should include careful analyses of patterns of failure and tailoring of the treatment approach to prognostic subgroups of patients. There is evidence that high dose ifosfamide with mesna uroprotection is more effective than cyclophosphamide in conventional doses as first-line treatment, at least for poor prognostic subgroups (Jürgens *et al.* 1988b; 1991). However, the risk of long-term renal toxicity of high cumulative doses of ifosfamide must be weighed against its benefits (Patterson and Khojasteh 1989; Skinner *et al.* 1989). Ewing's sarcoma cell lines respond *in vitro* to a combination of tumour necrosis factor α and γ-interferon (van Valen *et al.* 1990), suggesting a possible field of application for biological response modifiers. Finally, since bone-marrow transplantation is of benefit for patients with disseminated bone disease, it may also be of value in poor prognostic subgroups

of patients with pulmonary disease (Pinkerton *et al.* 1986; Craft 1987; Burdach *et al.* 1993).

REFERENCES

Andreeff M, Welte K (1989). Hematopoietic colony-stimulating factors. *Seminars in Oncology*, **16**:211–29.

Angervall L, Enzinger FM (1975). Extraskeletal neoplasm resembling Ewing's sarcoma. *Cancer*, **36**:240–51.

Askin FB, *et al.* (1979). Malignant small cell tumor of the thoracopulmonary region in childhood. *Cancer*, **43**:2438–51.

Bacci G, *et al.* (1982). The treatment of localized Ewing's sarcoma: experience at the Istituto Ortopedico Rizzoli in 163 cases treated with and without adjuvant chemotherapy. *Cancer*, **49**:1561–70.

Bacci G, *et al.* (1989). Long-term results in 144 localized Ewing's sarcoma patients treated with combined therapy. *Cancer*, **63**:1477–86.

Berthold F, *et al.* (1982). Ultrastructural, biochemical and cell-culture studies of a presumed extraskeletal Ewing's sarcoma with special reference to differential diagnosis from neuroblastoma. *Journal of Cancer Research and Clinical Oncology*, **103**:293–304.

Bohndorf K, *et al.* (1986). Magnetic resonance imaging of primary tumours and tumour-like lesions of bone. *Skeletal Radiology*, **15**:511–17.

Burdach S, *et al.* (1993). Myeloablative radiochemotherapy and hematopoietic stem-cell rescue in poor-prognosis Ewing's sarcoma. *Journal of Clinical Oncology*, **11**:1482–8.

Burgert EO, *et al.* (1990). Multimodal therapy for the management of nonpelvic localized Ewing's sarcoma of bone: Intergroup Study IESS-II. *Journal of Clinical Oncology*, **8**:1514–24.

Campanacci M (1990). Ewing's sarcoma. In: *Bone and soft tissue tumors* (ed. M Campanacci), pp. 509–38. Springer, Vienna.

Caparros B, Rosen G, McCormack B (1981). Treatment of metastatic Ewing's sarcoma with combination (comb) chemotherapy and delayed bilateral pulmonary irradiation (bpi). *Proceedings AACR/ASCO*, **22**:412, abstract C-312.

Chan RC, *et al.* (1979). Management and results of localized Ewing's sarcoma. *Cancer*, **43**:1001–6.

Coley BL, Higinbotham NL (1953). *Tumors of bone. A roentgenographic atlas.* Hoeber, New York.

Craft AW (1987). Chemotherapy of Ewing's sarcoma. *Baillière's Clinical Oncology*, **1**:205–21.

Dahlin DC (1978). *Bone tumors, general aspects and data on 6221 cases*, pp. 274–87. Thomas, Springfield.

DeVita VT (1983). The relationship between tumor mass and resistance to chemotherapy. *Cancer*, **51**:1209–20.

Donaldson SS (1981). A story of continuing success—radiotherapy for Ewing's sarcoma. *International Journal of Radiation Oncology—Biology—Physics*, **7**:279–81.

Donaldson SS, Hendrickson MR (1983). Patterns of failure in childhood solid tumors: Wilms' tumor, neuroblastoma and rhabdomyosarcoma. *Cancer Treatment Symposia*, **2**:267–83.

Dunst J, *et al.* (1988). Radiotherapie beim Ewing-Sarkom: Aktuelle Ergebnisse der GPO Studien CESS 81 und CESS 86. *Klinische Pädiatrie*, **200**:261–6.

Enneking WF (1987). A system of staging musculoskeletal neoplasms. *Baillière's Clinical Oncology*, **1**:97–110.

Ewing J (1921). Diffuse endothelioma of bone. *Proceedings of the New York Pathology Society*, **21**:17–24.

Ewing J (1939). A review of the classification of bone tumors. *Surgery, Gynecology and Obstetrics*, **68**:971–6.

Falk S, Alpert M (1967). Five-year survival of patients with Ewing's sarcoma. *Surgery, Gynecology and Obstetrics*, **124**:319–24.

Feldmann F (1977). Round cell lesions of bone. In *Diagnostic radiology* (ed. AR Margulis and CA Gooding), pp. 437–54. CV Mosby, St Louis.

Gasparini M, Lombardi F, Gianni C, Fossati-Bellani F (1981). Localized Ewing sarcoma: results of integrated therapy and analysis of failure. *European Journal of Cancer and Clinical Oncology*, **17**:1205–9.

Gehan EA, *et al.* (1981). Prognostic factors in children with Ewing's sarcoma. *National Cancer Institute Monographs*, **56**:273–8.

Gerlach JH, *et al.* (1987). P-Glycoprotein in human sarcoma: evidence for multidrug resistance. *Journal of Clinical Oncology*, **5**:1452–60.

Glass AG, Fraumeni JF, Jr (1970). Epidemiology of bone cancer in children. *Journal of the National Cancer Institute*, 44:187–99.

Glaubiger DL, *et al.* (1980). Determination of prognostic factors and their influence on therapeutic results in patients with Ewing's sarcoma. *Cancer*, 45:2213–19.

Glaubiger DL, Makuch RW, Schwarz J (1981). Influence of prognostic factors on survival in Ewing's sarcoma. *National Cancer Institute Monograph*, 56:285–8.

Göbel U, Salzer M, Remy R, Sekera J (1979). Resektion eines primär inoperablen Ewing-Sarkom des Beckens. *Klinische Pädiatrie*, 191:234–8.

Göbel V, *et al.* (1987). Prognostic significance of tumor volume in localized Ewing's sarcoma of bone in children and adolescents. *Journal of Cancer Research and Clinical Oncology*, 113:187–91.

Goldie JH, Coldman AJ (1979). A mathematical model for relating the drug sensitivity of tumors to their spontaneous mutation rate. *Cancer Treatment Reports*, 63:1727–33.

Gonzales-Gonzales D, Breur K (1983). Clinical data from irradiated growing long bones in children. *International Journal of Radiation Oncology—Biology—Physics*, 9:841–6.

Hayes FA, *et al.* (1987). Metastatic Ewing's sarcoma: remission induction and survival. *Journal of Clinical Oncology*, 5:1199–204.

Hayes FA, *et al.* (1989). Therapy for localized Ewing's sarcoma of bone. *Journal of Clinical Oncology*, 7:208–13.

Huvos AG, Rosen G, Dobska M, Marcove RC (1983). Mesenchymal chondrosarcoma. *Cancer*, 51:1230–7.

Huvos AG (1991). Ewing's sarcoma. In: *Bone tumors. Diagnosis, treatment and prognosis* (ed. AG Huvos), pp. 523–52. WB Saunders, Philadelphia.

Israel MA, Miser JS, Triche TJ, Kinsella T (1989). Neuroepithelial tumors. In: *Principles and practice of pediatric oncology* (ed. PA Pizzo and DG Poplack), pp. 623–34. J B Lippincott, Philadelphia.

Jaffe R, *et al.* (1984). Neuroendocrine tumor of bone: its distinction from Ewing's sarcoma. *Laboratory Investigation*, 50:5.

Jentzsch K, *et al.* (1981). Leg function after radiotherapy for Ewing's sarcoma. *Cancer*, 47:1267–78.

Jürgens H, *et al.* (1985). Die cooperative Ewing-Sarkom Studie CESS 81 der GPO—Analyse nach 4 Jahren. *Klinische Pädiatrie*, 197:225–32.

Jürgens H, *et al.* (1988*a*). Multidisciplinary treatment of primary Ewing's sarcoma of bone. A 6-year experience of a European Cooperative Trial. *Cancer*, 61:23–32.

Jürgens H, *et al.* (1988*b*). Die GPO cooperativen Ewing-Sarkom Studien CESS 81/86: Bericht nach 6 1/2 Jahren. *Klinische Pädiatrie*, 200:243–52.

Jürgens H, Treuner J, Winkler K, Göbel U (1989*a*). Ifosfamide in pediatric malignancies. *Seminars in Oncology*, 16:46–50.

Jürgens H, *et al.* (1989*b*). High-dose ifosfamide with mesna uroprotection in Ewing's sarcoma. *Cancer Chemotherapy and Pharmacology*, 24 (Suppl.):S40–4.

Jürgens H, *et al.* (1991). Improved survival in Ewing's sarcoma with response based local therapy and intense chemotherapy. *Proceedings ASCO*, 10, 316, abstract 1112.

Kinsella TJ, Loeffler JS, Fraass BA, Tepper J (1983*a*). Extremity preservation by combined-modality therapy in sarcomas of the hand and foot: an analysis of local control, disease-free survival and functional results. *International Journal of Radiation Oncology—Biology—Physics*, 9:1115–19.

Kinsella TJ, *et al.* (1983*b*). Extraskeletal Ewing's sarcoma: results of combined-modality treatment. *American Journal of Clinical Oncology*, 1:489–95.

Kinsella TJ, *et al.* (1984). Local treatment of Ewing's sarcoma: radiation therapy versus surgery. *Cancer Treatment Reports*, 68:695–701.

Kotz R, Kogelnik HD, Salzer-Kuntschik M, Lechner G (1977). Problems of local recurrence in patients with Ewing's sarcoma. *Österreich Zeitschrift für Onkologie*, 4:7–12.

Kulick A, Mones J (1970). The neurological complications of Ewing's sarcoma: incidence of neurologic involvement and value of radiotherapy. *Mount Sinai Journal of Medicine, New York*, 37:40–59.

Larsson SE, Lorentzon R (1974). The geographic variation of the incidence of malignant primary bone tumors in Sweden. *Journal of Bone and Joint Surgery A*, 56:592–600.

Lewis RJ, Marcove RC, Rosen G (1977). Ewing's sarcoma—functional effects of radiation therapy. *Journal of Bone and Joint Surgery*, 59A:325–31.

Li FP, *et al.* (1980). Rarity of Ewing's sarcoma in China. *Lancet*, i:1255.

Li WK, *et al.* (1983). Pelvic Ewing's sarcoma. Advances in treatment. *Journal of Bone and Joint Surgery*, 65A:738–47.

Llombart-Bosch A, Blache R, Peydro-Olaya A (1978). Ultrastructural study of 28 cases of Ewing's sarcoma: typical and atypical forms. *Cancer*, 41:1362–73.

Marangos PJ, Polak JM (1986). Neuron-specific enolase (NSE) as a marker for neuroendocrine tumors. In: *Markers of human neuroectodermal tumors* (ed. GEJ Stahl and CWM van Veelen), pp. 109–17. CRC Press, Boca Raton, FL.

Marcus RB, Million RR (1984). The effect of primary tumor size on the prognosis of Ewing's sarcoma. *International Journal of Radiation Oncology—Biology—Physics*, 10:88.

Mehta Y, Hendrickson R (1974). CNS involvement in Ewing's sarcoma. *Cancer*, 33:859–62.

Meister P, Gokel JM (1978). Extraskeletal Ewing's sarcoma. *Virchows Archiv A*, 378:173–9.

Mendenhall CM, *et al.* (1983). The prognostic significance of soft tissue extension in Ewing's sarcoma. *Cancer*, 51:913–17.

Miser JS, *et al.* (1987). Ifosfamide with mesna uroprotection and etoposide: an effective regimen in the treatment of recurrent sarcomas and other tumors of children and young adults. *Journal of Clinical Oncology*, 5:1191–8.

Miser JS, Triche TJ, Pritchard DJ, Kinsella T (1989). Ewing's sarcoma and the nonrhabdomyosarcoma soft tissue sarcomas of childhood. In: *Principles and practice of pediatric oncology* (ed. PA Pizzo and DG Poplack), pp. 659–88. JB Lippincott, Philadelphia.

Nascimento AG (1980). A clinicopathologic study of 20 cases of large-cell (atypical) Ewing's sarcoma of bone. *American Journal of Surgical Pathology*, 4:29–36.

Nesbit ME, *et al.* (1981). Multimodal therapy for the management of non-metastatic Ewing's sarcoma of bone: an intergroup study. *National Cancer Institute Monographs*, 56:255–62.

Nesbit ME, *et al.* (1990). Multimodal therapy for the management of primary nonmetastatic Ewing's sarcoma of bone: a long-term follow-up of the First Intergroup Study. *Journal of Clinical Oncology*, 8:1664–74.

Oldham RK, Pomeroy TC (1972). Treatment of Ewing's sarcoma with adriamycin (NSC-123, 127). *Cancer Chemotherapy Reports*, 56:635–9.

Patterson WP, Khojasteh A (1989). Ifosfamide-induced renal tubular defects. *Cancer*, 63:649–51.

Perez CA, *et al.* (1977). Analysis of local tumor control in Ewing's sarcoma. Preliminary results of a cooperative intergroup study. *Cancer*, 40:2864–73.

Perez CA, *et al.* (1981*a*). Radiation therapy in the multimodal management of Ewing's sarcoma of bone: report of the Intergroup Ewing's Sarcoma Study. *National Cancer Institute Monographs*, 56:263–71.

Perez CA, *et al.* (1981*b*). The role of radiation therapy in the management of non-metastatic Ewing's sarcoma of bone. Report of the intergroup Ewing's sarcoma study. *Journal of Radiation Oncology—Biology—Physics*, 7:141–9.

Philips RF, Higinbotham NL (1967). The curability of Ewing's endothelioma of bone in children. *Journal of Pediatrics*, 70:391–7.

Pilepich MV, *et al.* (1981). Radiotherapy and combination chemotherapy in advanced Ewing's sarcoma—Intergroup Study. *Cancer*, 47:1930–6.

Pinkerton R, *et al.* (1986). Autologous bone marrow transplantation in paediatric solid tumors. *Clinics in Hematology*, 15:187–203.

Pomeroy TC, Johnson RE (1975). Prognostic factors for survival in Ewing's sarcoma. *American Journal of Roentgenology*, 123:598–606.

Price CHG, Jeffree GM (1977). Incidence of bone sarcomas in SW England, 1946–74, in relation to age, sex, tumor site and histology. *British Journal of Cancer*, 36:511–22.

Pritchard DJ (1980). Indications for surgical treatment of localized Ewing's sarcoma of bone. *Clinical Orthopaedics*, 153:39–43.

Pritchard DJ (1981). Surgical experience in the management of Ewing's sarcoma of bone. *National Cancer Institute Monographs*, 56:169–71.

Razek A, *et al.* (1980). Intergroup Ewing's sarcoma study. Local control related to radiation dose, volume and site of primary lesion in Ewing's sarcoma. *Cancer*, 46:516–21.

Remagen W, Salzer-Kuntschik M (1981). Zur histopathologischen Problematik und Diagnose des Ewing-Sarkoms. *Klinische Pädiatrie*, 193:171–4.

Rose JS, Hermann G, Mendelson DS, Ambinder EP (1983). Extraskeletal Ewing's sarcoma with computed tomography correlation. *Skeletal Radiology*, 9:234–7.

Rosen G (1976). Management of malignant bone tumors in children and adolescents. *Pediatric Clinics of North America*, 23:183–213.

Rosen G, *et al.* (1974). Disease-free survival in children with Ewing's sarcoma treated with radiation therapy and adjuvant four-drug sequential chemotherapy. *Cancer*, 33:384–93.

Rosen G, *et al.* (1978). Curability of Ewing's sarcoma and considerations for future therapeutic trials. *Cancer*, 41:888–99.

Rosen G, *et al.* (1981*a*). Ewing's sarcoma: ten year experience with adjuvant chemotherapy. *Cancer*, 47:2204–13.

Rosen G, *et al.* (1981*b*). Combination chemotherapy (T-6) in the multidisciplinary treatment of Ewing's sarcoma. *National Cancer Institute Monographs*, 56:289–99.

Salzer-Kuntschik M (1976). Cytologic und cytochemical behavior in primary malignant bone tumors. In: *Malignant bone tumors* (ed. E Grundmann), pp. 145–56. Springer, Berlin.

Samuels ML, Howe CD (1967). Cyclophosphamide in the management of Ewing's sarcoma. *Cancer*, 20:961–6.

Sauer R, *et al.* (1984). Ewing-Sarkom: Lokalrezidive in Abhängigkeit von der Primärtherapie. *Verh Dtsch Krebs Ges*, 5:801–4.

Sauer R, *et al.* (1987). Prognostic factors in the treatment of Ewing's sarcoma. *Radiotherapy and Oncology*, 10:101–10.

Schajowicz F (1959). Ewing's sarcoma and reticulum cell sarcoma of bone. With special reference to the histochemical demonstration of glycogen as an aid to differential diagnosis. *Journal of Bone and Joint Surgery*, 41A:349–56.

Schmidt D, Harms D (1990). The applicability of immunohistochemistry in the diagnosis and differential diagnosis of malignant soft tissue tumors. A reevaluation based on the material of the Kiel Pediatric Tumor Registry. *Klinische Pädiatrie*, 202:224–9.

Schmidt D, Harms D, Pilon VA (1987). Small-cell pediatric tumors: histology, immunohistochemistry and electron microscopy. *Clinics in Laboratory Medicine*, 7:63–89.

Schmidt D, Harms D, Jürgens H (1989). Maligne periphere neuroektodermale Tumoren. Histologische und immunhistochemische Befunde an 41 Fällen. *Zentralblatt für Allgemeine Pathologie und Pathologische Anatomie*, 135:257–67.

Seeber S, *et al.* (1974). Fortschritte in der Therapie des Ewing-Sarkoms. *Deutsche Medizinische Wochenschrift*, 99:883–7.

Sim FH, Unni KK, Beabout JW, Dahlin DC (1979). Osteosarcoma with small cells simulating Ewing's sarcoma. *Journal of Bone and Joint Surgery*, 61A(2):207–15.

Skinner R, *et al.* (1989). Hypophosphataemic rickets after ifosfamide treatment in children. *British Medical Journal*, 298:1560–1.

Soule EH, Newton W Jr, Moon TE, Tefft M (1978). Extraskeletal Ewing's sarcoma: a preliminary review of 26 cases encountered in the Intergroup Rhabdomyosarcoma Study. *Cancer*, 42:259–64.

Tefft M, Chabora B, Rosen G (1977). Radiation in bone sarcomas. *Cancer*, 39:806–16.

Tepper J, *et al.* (1980). Local control of Ewing's sarcoma of bone with radiotherapy and combination chemotherapy. *Cancer*, 46:1969–73.

Thomas PR, *et al.* (1984). The management of Ewing's sarcoma: role of radiotherapy in local tumor control. *Cancer Treatment Reports*, 68:703–10.

Turc-Carel C, *et al.* (1983). Translocation chromosomique (11;22) dans les lignées cellulaires de sarcomas d'Ewing. *Comptes Rendus Hebdomadaires des Séances de l'Academie des Sciences*, 296:1101–3.

van Valen F, Winkelmann W, Jürgens H (1992). Expression of functional Y_2 receptors for neuropeptide in human Ewing's sarcoma cell lines in culture. *Journal of Cancer Research and Clinical Oncology*, 118:529–36.

van Valen F, Winkelmann W, Burdach S, Göbel U, Jürgens H (1993). Interferon γ and tumour necrosis factor α induce a synergistic antiproliferative response in human Ewing's sarcoma cels *in vitro*. *Journal of Cancer Research and Clinical Oncology*, 119:615–21.

Vietti TJ, *et al.* (1981). Multimodal therapy in metastatic Ewing's sarcoma: an Intergroup Study. *National Cancer Institute Monographs*, 56:279–84.

Vohra BG (1967). Roentgen manifestations in Ewing's sarcoma. A study of 156 cases. *Cancer*, 20:727–33.

Wessalowski R, *et al.* (1988). Behandlungsergebnisse beim primär metastasierten Ewing-Sarkom: eine retrospektive Analyse von 48 Patienten. *Klinische Pädiatrie*, 200:253–60.

Whang-Peng J, *et al.* (1984). Chromosome translocation in peripheral neuroepithelioma. *New England Journal of Medicine*, 311:584–5.

Wigger HJ, Salazar GH, Blanc WA (1977). Extraskeletal Ewing's sarcoma. An ultrastructural study. *Archives of Pathology and Laboratory Medicine*, 101:446–9.

Winkelmann W, Jürgens H (1989). Lokalkontrolle beim Ewing-Sarkom. Vergleichende Ergebnisse nach intraläsionaler, marginaler bzw. Tumorresektion im Gesunden. *Zeitschrift für Orthopädie*, 127:424–6.

13.4   Osteosarcoma

R. SOUHAMI AND STEPHEN R. CANNON

INTRODUCTION

The period from 1970 to the present has seen considerable advances in the management of osteosarcoma in children and young adults. Combination chemotherapy has improved the cure rate and limb conservation surgery has improved so that many patients are now spared amputation. The intertwining of intensive chemotherapy and complex surgery means that effective management can now only

We are very grateful to Dr Jean Pringle of the Department of Morbid Anatomy, Royal National Orthopaedic Hospital, Stanmore, UK, for supplying the photomicrographs in this chapter.

be undertaken in centres skilled in dealing with the numerous problems of diagnosis, investigation, and management.

INCIDENCE AND AETIOLOGY

The age and sex incidence for primary osteosarcoma is shown in Fig. 1. There is a 1.5–2.0×male preponderance and the period of greatest risk is 10–14 years for girls and 15–18 for boys. After 20 years of age the incidence falls but rises after 40, owing to post-radiation and Paget's sarcomas (Fig. 2). The classification of the sarcomas arising in later life is not clearly established so the true incidence of osteosarcoma is not well defined at this age. In juvenile osteosarcoma

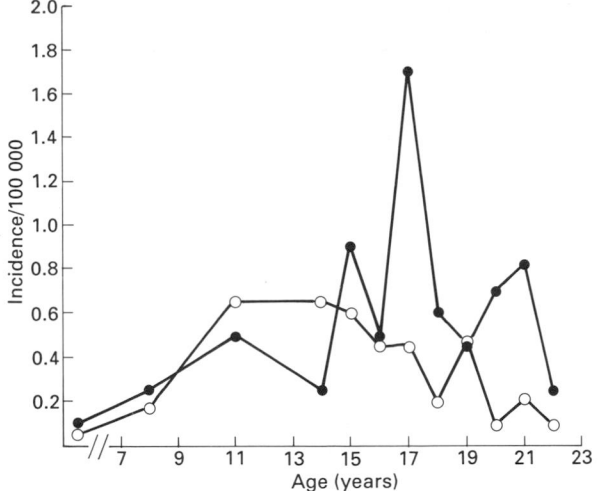

Fig. 1 Age-related incidence of primary osteosarcoma: open circles, females; closed circles, males.

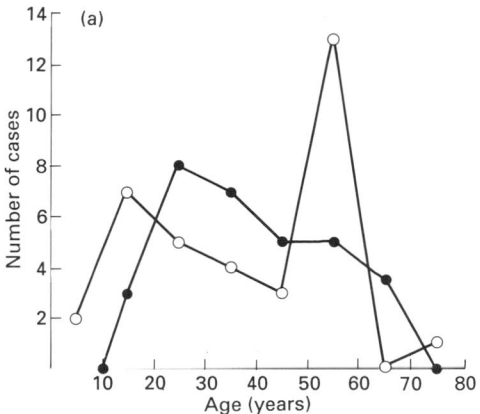

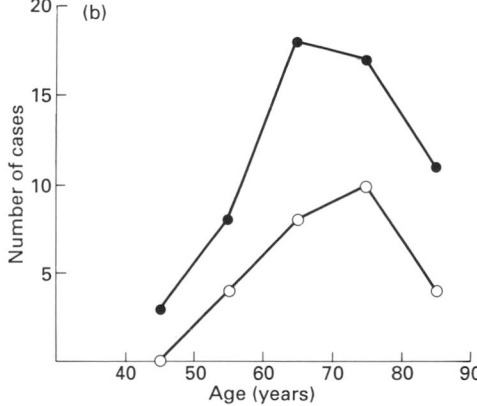

Fig. 2 Age at diagnosis of (a) radiation-induced bone sarcomas and (b) Paget's sarcoma: open circles, females; closed circles, males (data taken from several series).

there is a tendency for tumours in the humerus to arise earlier than those in the femur and for those in the axial skeleton to be later.

Genetic causes

The age of onset of osteosarcoma, its occurrence at sites of maximum velocity of bone growth, and its occurrence in Paget's disease suggest that rapid bone growth is a predisposing factor in

causation. The tumour is equally common in Black and White Americans (Polednak 1985), but with a tendency to occur more often in the upper tibia in Blacks (Huvos *et al.* 1983). The Li–Fraumeni syndrome is a cancer family syndrome in which the occurrence of a bone or soft tissue sarcoma in a young adult is accompanied by an increased incidence of cancer in first-degree relatives (Li *et al.* 1988). The associated cancers are of breast, brain, adrenal cortex, and leukaemia. Germ-line mutations of the *p53* gene have been found in these families (Malkin *et al.* 1990). In sporadic osteosarcoma germ-line mutations are sometimes found (Malkin *et al.* 1992). Screening of children with cancer who have a suggestive family history will also reveal germ-line *p53* mutation in approximately 30 per cent of cases (Brugières *et al.* 1993). In sporadic osteosarcoma, mutation of *p53* and loss of heterozygosity is a frequent finding in the tumour cells. In the germ-line mutations codons 248 and 282 are especially likely to be affected. The substitution of tryptophan for arginine which results, prevents the activity of the *p53* protein as a regulator of the cell cycle.

Osteosarcomas occur with increased frequency in retinoblastoma survivors at a latent interval of approximately 10 years. Hereditary retinoblastoma is associated with absence or inactivation of one allele of a gene localized to q14 on chromosome 13 (Ward *et al.* 1984). Absence or inactivation of the remaining gene may be a feature of retinoblastoma and osteosarcoma (Friend *et al.* 1986). Orbital radiation predisposes to osteosarcoma in the radiation field but tumours also arise at distant sites. One estimate suggests that the overall incidence of osteosarcoma is increased 500-fold in patients with the inherited form of retinoblastoma. There is no increase in bone sarcoma in first- or second-degree relatives of patients with retinoblastoma. A loss of heterozygosity on chromosome 13 in tumour cells has now been reported in osteosarcoma (Toguchida *et al.* 1988), with a recessive mutation in the retinoblastoma gene. The same group (Toguchida *et al.* 1989) has extended its studies and has shown that 76 per cent of cases of osteosarcoma show loss of heterozygosity on chromosome 17 in a wide region of the chromosome but especially in the 17p13 region. Osteosarcoma also arises in osteogenesis imperfecta and Maffucci's syndrome (enchondromas, cutaneous haemangiomata, and skin pigmentation). A rare familial disease of osteosarcoma and erythroid macrocytosis has been described (Mulvihill *et al.* 1977).

Radiation

The occurrence of osteosarcoma in the women who painted luminous dials on watches and instruments was a remarkable demonstration of the connection between radioactivity and bone cancer (Souhami 1987). At the time when the dial factories were established (1917–1924) there was no public suspicion of the dangerous effects of radium. The factory conditions were deplorable. In 1924 the first reports of aseptic bone necrosis appeared and in 1929 the first cases of osteosarcoma. Many cases of osteosarcoma appeared during the next 20 years, long after the factories had been closed. Autoradiographs of long bones (remote from the site of ingestion) showed dense radioactivity deposited in Haversian systems and trabeculae. Careful follow-up at the Centre for Human Radiobiology, Argonne, France, has indicated a 40 year risk of developing osteosarcoma of approximately 75 per cent in those ingesting more than 750 μCi and 30 per cent with lower intakes (Polednak 1978).

Bone sarcomas also develop after external-beam radiation (Weatherby *et al.* 1981). Not all of these are typical osteosarcomas, a fibrohistiocytomatous appearance being common. The age distribution is shown in Fig. 2(a). The increased frequency in women aged 45–60 years relates in part to chest-wall radiation for breast cancer. The tumours typically arise in the axial skeleton, which has sites likely to be included in a radiation field. The mean radiation dose is 45 Gy to a previously normal bone and the mean latent period is 10.5 years (range 40–30). Sarcoma may arise after irradiation of a previous malignant bone tumour such as Ewing's sarcoma (Strong *et al.* 1979) or of a benign bone lesion such as aneurysmal bone cyst. The position is more complex with irradiated giant cell tumours, as they have malignant potential at the outset. Bone sarcomas are a recognized complication of irradiation used in the treatment of childhood cancer. Many (25 per cent) arise in patients treated for retinoblastoma, with Ewing's tumour the other common primary tumour. The tumours may be typical osteosarcoma, malignant fibrous histiocytoma, or chondrosarcoma (Newton *et al.* 1991). The concomitant use of anthracyclines may diminish the latent period. Estimates of incidence in children treated for cancer vary widely. Draper *et al.* (1986) report a cumulative incidence of 4.2 per cent at 18 years for reginoblastoma (6.2 per cent for hereditary cases). Abrahamson *et al.* (1984) reported an excess risk of 20 per cent at 20 years for retinoblastoma patients.

Paget's sarcoma

In 1889 Paget reported five cases of sarcoma arising in osteitis deformans. Many reviews of the relation between sarcoma and Paget's disease have appeared since that time (Haibach *et al.* 1985). The true frequency of transformation is unknown, as Paget's disease is common and often asymptomatic. The frequency is probably approximately 1 in 500 cases of Paget's disease per year or 0.4/100 000 population over the age of 40 (Price and Goldie 1969). The sites of sarcomatous change do not entirely reflect the distribution of Paget's disease, as vertebral Paget's is common and sarcomas very rare at this site. The tumours are commonly osteosarcoma or fibrosarcoma, although other types (such as lymphoma) have been reported.

In summary, known aetiological factors in osteosarcoma indicate that rapid bone growth (during adolescence and in Paget's disease), genetic predisposition, and ionizing radiation are all causative factors in what is presumably a multistep oncogenesis.

CLASSIFICATION AND PATHOLOGY

A pathological and clinical classification is shown in Table 1. It cannot be stressed too strongly that a skilled bone tumour pathologist is required to make a correct diagnosis. Because the tumours are very rare it is essential that the biopsy be reviewed by those familiar with

Table 1 Classification of osteosarcoma

1. High-grade central osteosarcoma
   Osteoblastic
   Chondroblastic
   Fibroblastic
   Osteoclast-rich
   Telangiectatic
   Small cell
2. Periosteal osteosarcoma
3. Parosteal osteosarcoma
4. Low-grade central osteosarcoma
5. Osteoblastoma-like osteosarcoma
6. Paget's osteosarcoma
7. Post-irradiation osteosarcoma

the radiological and pathological appearances of primary bone cancer before definitive treatment is planned (Fig. 3). Mistakes are common. The pathologist and radiologist will often need to confer in order to assess all the diagnostic evidence before arriving at a final diagnosis.

High-grade central osteosarcoma

The tumour usually arises in the metaphysis of long bones in adolescence. The distal femur is the most common site, followed by proximal tibia and proximal humerus. The tumour begins in the medulla and, as it grows, it infiltrates the cortical bone, penetrating beneath the periosteum. The periosteum confines the tumour and on fine-detail radiographs the tumour bone can be seen under the periosteum (Fig. 4). As the tumour grows the periosteum is lifted off the bone and forms reactive bone (which, at the point where it touches normal bone, is termed Codman's triangle). Finally, the tumour extends through the periosteum into the soft tissues and, ultimately, the skin. At this stage periarticular structures such as major nerves and blood vessels will be invaded. The adjacent joint is invaded at a later stage. High-grade osteosarcomas may, rarely, arise in a juxtacortical site and must be distinguished from periosteal and parosteal osteosarcoma (see below).

Histologically the common or mixed type shows fibroblastic, osteoblastic, and chondroblastic areas. The tumour is derived from osteoblasts and the malignant cells can be shown to contain intracytoplasmic alkaline phosphatase if frozen sections or cytological preparations are examined. Examples of the main histological types are shown in Fig. 3. In the osteoblastic form there is copious tumour osteoid and numerous tumour osteoblasts, which may be very pleomorphic. The radiograph shows corresponding sclerosis. Chondroblastic variants may be mistaken for chondrosarcoma. There are islands of malignant chondroid but the tumour cells can be shown to contain alkaline phosphatase. It is distinguished from periosteal osteosarcoma by its location and grade. Telangiectatic tumours contain numerous spaces filled with blood. In these cases, tumour bone formation may be infrequent and a mistaken diagnosis of aneurysmal bone cyst made (although the radiographic appearances are usually quite dissimilar). Osteoclast-rich variants are unusual and contain large numbers of giant cells (which are not tumour cells). The mononuclear tumour cells are often pleomorphic and produce alkaline phosphatase (Sanerkin 1980). A mistaken diagnosis of osteoclastoma may be made and the radiographic appearances must be considered in arriving at a diagnosis. Small-cell osteosarcomas are unusual and may be difficult to distinguish from Ewing's sarcoma, lymphoma, and spindle cell sarcomas. The cells are closely packed with a variable amount of cytoplasm. Mitoses are numerous.

Periosteal osteosarcoma

This rare tumour, first described by Unni *et al.* (1976), usually occurs on the proximal tibia and has a mainly chondroid histological appearance. The chondroid may be well differentiated in parts but peripheral areas of the tumour are more pleomorphic. The tumour cells contain alkaline phosphatase. Delicate osteoid may be seen. Juxtacortical chondrosarcoma is often a difficult differential diagnosis in a small sample that has not been stained for alkaline phosphatase. Occasionally it maybe difficult to distinguish periosteal osteosarcoma from the superficial part of a high-grade chondroblastic osteosarcoma, although the latter shows a higher-grade histology. The clinical and radiological features may help.

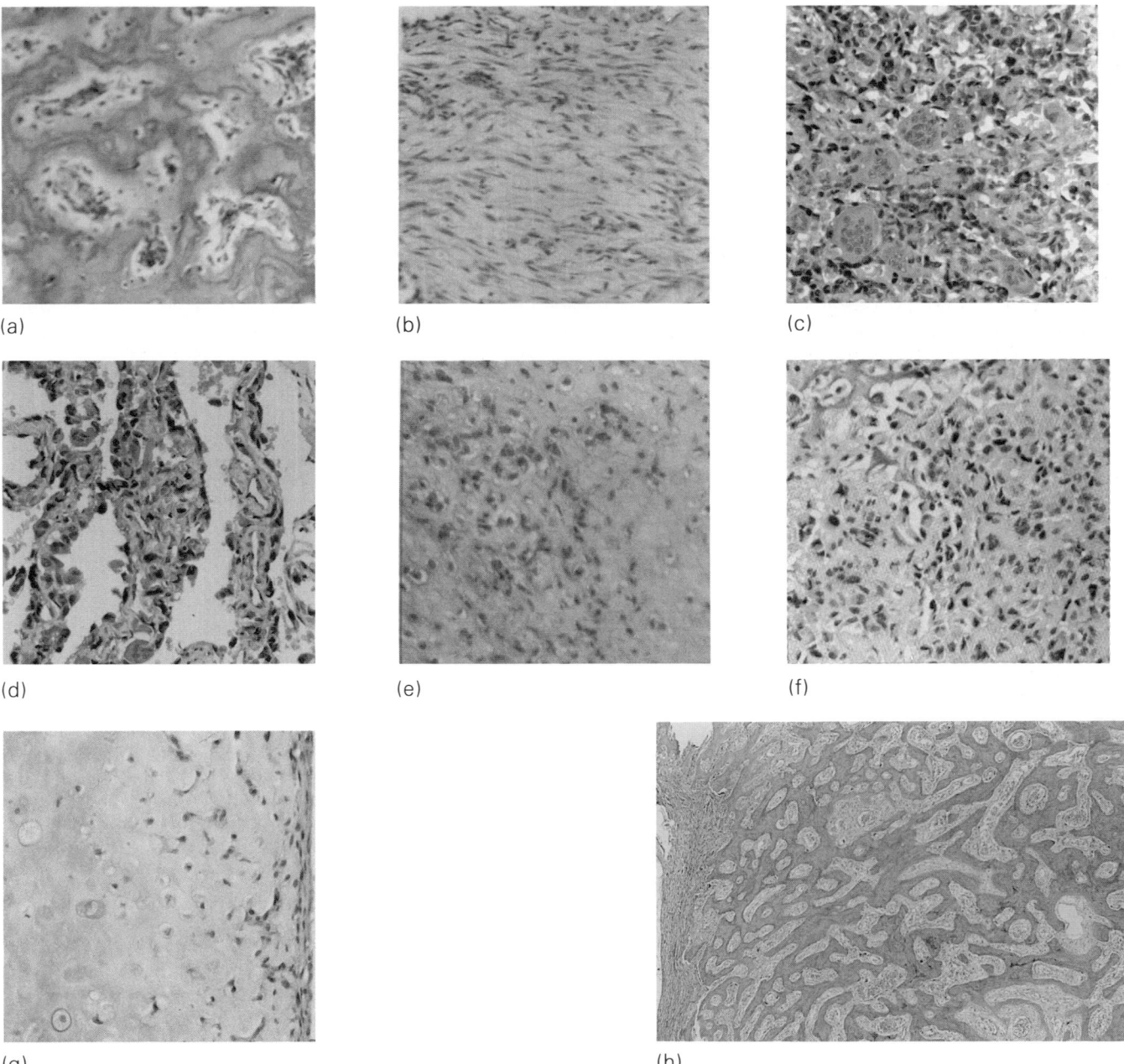

Fig. 3 Pathological appearances of osteosarcoma. (a) Osteoblastic type, (b) fibroblastic type, (c) giant cell-rich type, (d) telangiectatic type, (e) chondroblastic type, (f) mixed cell type, (g) periosteal type, and (h) parosteal type.

Parosteal osteosarcoma

This is a slow-growing tumour occurring later in life than central osteosarcoma. It may be erroneously diagnosed as a benign lesion such as chondroma or fibrous dysplasia, unless the radiological and pathological appearances are assessed together. The tumour is on the outer cortex wrapped round the bone. There is a spindle cell stroma with well-differentiated cartilage and tumour bone formation originating in the spindle cell areas. Areas of more high-grade tumour may be found and, although pulmonary metastases are uncommon, they seem to occur more frequently in tumours containing high-grade areas and in later cases where the central bone has been invaded by the tumour. Transformation to a high-grade osteosarcoma can also occur.

Osteoblastoma-like osteosarcoma

These rare tumours have also been called malignant or aggressive osteoblastoma. They tend to occur in the axial skeleton and consist of numerous osteoblasts, osteoid, and osteoclasts. The tumour recurs locally repeatedly. Pulmonary metastases can occasionally occur, although this is uncommon. Death is usually due to local extension of the tumour, particularly when the primary is in the spine or ribs.

Paget's osteosarcoma

These tumours always arise in an area of bone affected by Paget's disease. They may show appearances of osteosarcoma, malignant fibrous histiocytoma, sarcomas with many giant cells, or

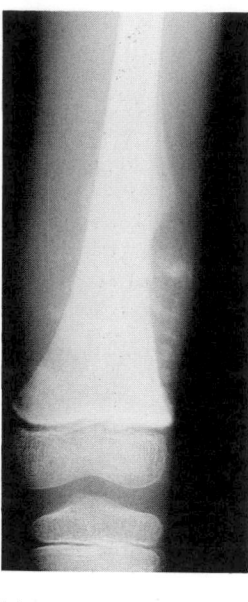
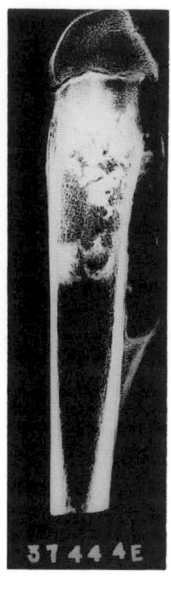
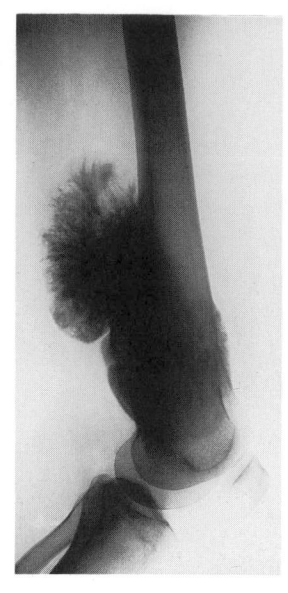
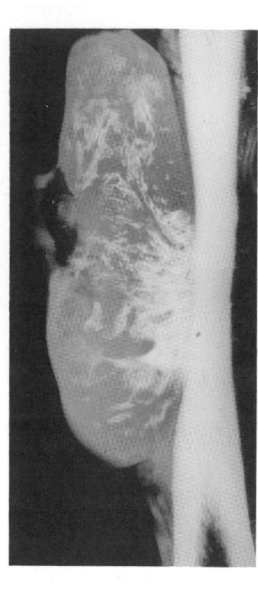

(a)　　　　　　　　　(b)　　　　　　　　(c)　　　　　　　(d)　　　　　　　(e)

Fig. 4 (a) Radiograph of high-grade central osteosarcoma of femur. The cortex has been eroded and tumour bone formation is visible in the soft tissues. The tumour has extended into the centre of the femur. (b) Radiograph of central osteosarcoma of femur. The tumour has caused dense sclerosis of bone, which stops at the epiphysis. A Codman's triangle is clearly seen, with 'sunray' spicules of tumour bone in the soft tissues. (c) Fine-detail resection specimen of osteosarcoma of humerus. The tumour stops at the epiphysis. The dense sclerosis in the tumour is clearly shown, as is the Codman's triangle. (d) Lateral radiograph of distal femur showing dense bone wrapping around the distal metaphysis typical of a parosteal osteosarcoma. (e) Fine-detail radiograph of resected specimen of a periosteal osteosarcoma. The origin of the tumour from the periosteum is well illustrated. The vast majority of the tumour is non-ossified.

undifferentiated sarcoma. The features are no different from these tumours when not in association with Paget's disease.

Post-radiation sarcoma

These tumours are high-grade sarcomas. Osteosarcoma, malignant fibrous histiocytoma, and fibrosarcoma are the most common histological appearances.

CLINICAL PRESENTATION

High-grade osteosarcoma typically occurs in an adolescent or young adult. The first symptom is usually pain, which may be present for many months before diagnosis. Occasionally an injury at school may intensify or start the pain and after a period of fruitless treatment with analgesics or physiotherapy a radiograph leads to the diagnosis of a tumour. Typically the pain is worse at night and this feature is an indication for further investigation. The rarity of the tumour leads to delay. In the United Kingdom a new case of osteosarcoma would present to an average family practitioner in a period of time twice the length of his or her working life. Swelling is noticed at some stage and this is usually appreciated as a more serious symptom and leads to investigation. Constitutional symptoms of weight loss and occasionally fever are sinister, usually indicating aggressive disease that is metastatic.

The tumour usually affects the distal femur, upper tibia, or proximal humerus. Axial skeletal lesions occur in somewhat older patients and account for approximately 10 per cent of all tumours (Dahlin 1978). In the pelvis the tumours may reach a considerable size before diagnosis. In middle-aged or elderly people the tumour is more likely to have arisen in a previously abnormal bone, for example the site of previous radiation or Paget's disease. Particular clinical problems arise (discussed below) when the sarcoma occurs

in the mandible or vertebral column. Occasionally there is a pathological fracture at presentation, which presents considerable problems for subsequent surgical management.

On physical examination there is usually swelling and limitation of movement. Particular points to record are the extent of the palpable swelling, its maximum circumference, and evidence of invasion of adjacent tissues, in particular the skin, muscle, and neurovascular bundle. At the knee the tumour may extend down to the joint. An effusion may be present but does not always denote involvement of the joint cavity. The popliteal artery and nerve should be examined and assessment made of attachment to the mass of tumour. At the shoulder the innermost aspect of the tumour should be determined. Large tumours extend into the axilla and, thence, to the chest wall. In the axilla the tumour may involve blood vessels and nerves.

Symptoms and signs from metastases are uncommon at presentation. Bone metastases may cause pain; chest-wall pain, breathlessness, and pleural effusion may be presenting features of pulmonary metastasis. Pulmonary metastases from osteosarcoma have the curious attribute of sometimes causing a pneumothorax, which may be present at diagnosis. This may be due to the typically subpleural position of osteosarcoma lung metastases (see Fig. 6(c)).

INVESTIGATION
Plain radiography

The orthodox radiograph provides a two-dimensional image of a three-dimensional structure and osteogenic sarcoma may be reflected as lytic or blastic areas depending upon the amount of new bone formation (Fig. 4(a) and (b)). Classically the tumour occurs in the metaphyses of a long bone, usually in the second decade of life. Frequently the tumour has breached the cortex and elevated the periosteum so that a Codman's triangle is present. Formation of tumour bone perpendicular to the cortical margin (sunburst) may also be present. Neither of these radiological appearances are, however, pathognomonic for osteosarcoma. The manner in which the radiological appearances are produced is well demonstrated by fine-detail radiographs taken from thin, longitudinal sections of resection specimens (Fig. 4c).

The plain radiographs usually indicate rapid growth of the tumour according to the classification of Lodwick *et al.* (1980). In this classification a permeative pattern of bone lysis indicates the most rapid tumour growth. Plain films can indicate the site most likely to provide representative material for a histological diagnosis and, therefore, guide the surgeon to the suitable area for biopsy.

Isotope scanning

Radionuclide bone scanning is a highly sensitive indicator of osteoblastic activity in bone, but is non-specific. It is valuable in the demonstration of multiple bone lesions and intrapulmonary metastases; soft tissue extension may also be demonstrated. Classically in osteosarcoma a scan is produced with intense activity and irregular outlines (Murray 1980). There is a tendency to overestimate the extent of intramedullary tumour involvement (Fig. 5).

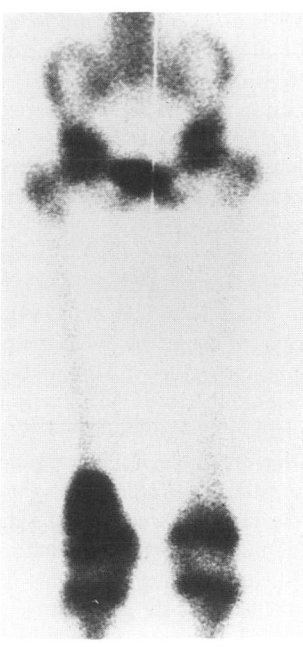

Fig. 5 An isotope bone scan in a 14-year-old patient with osteosarcoma of the right knee. The tumour is seen to extend up the femoral shaft. The increased uptake around the joints is at the site of the growing epiphyses.

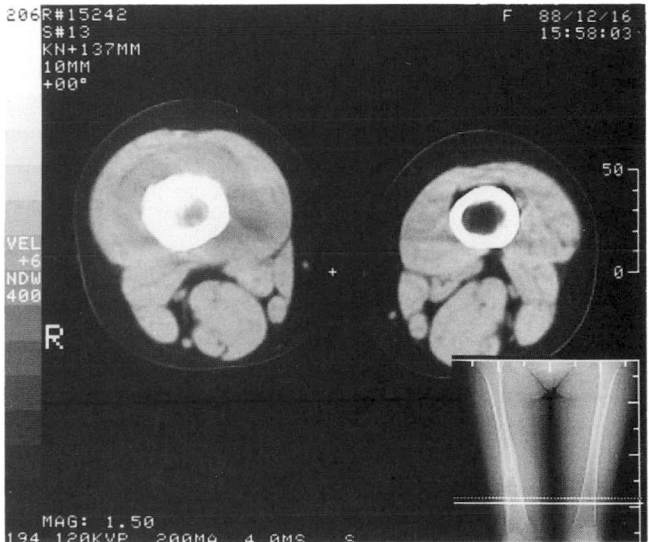

(a)

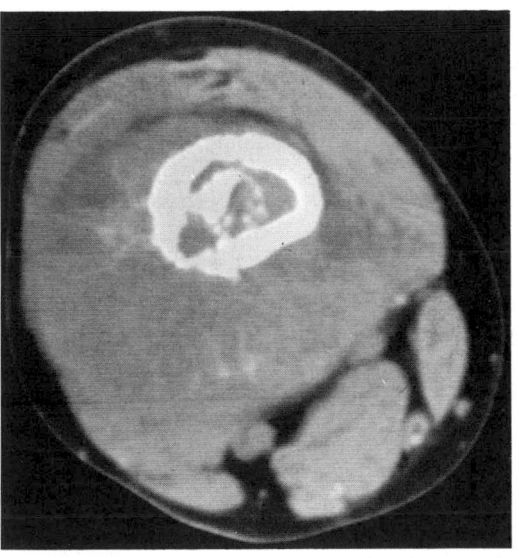

(b)

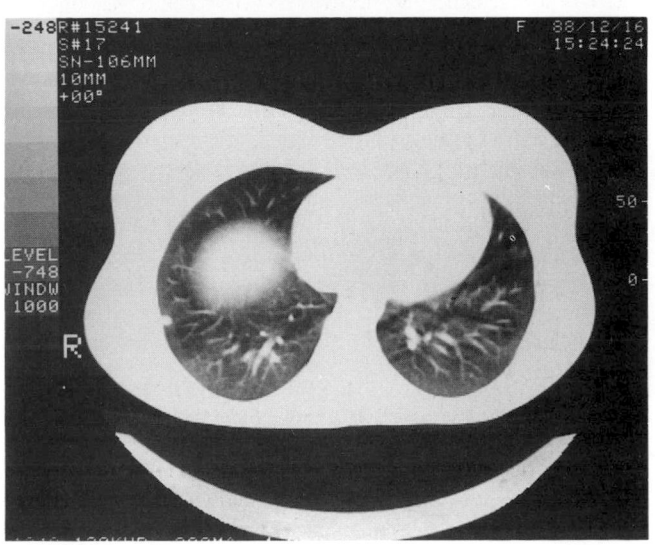

(c)

Fig. 6 (a) CT scan of osteosarcoma of right femur. The bone shows dense sclerosis extending into the medulla. The surface of the bone is irregular. A large soft tissue mass surrounds the bone anteriorly and laterally with normal muscle overlying it. (b) CT scan of osteosarcoma of femur. The cortical bone is thinned and eroded. Tumour bone formation is seen in the large soft tissue mass that extends posteriorly and laterally to the subcutaneous fat. (c) CT scan of the thorax in a patient with osteosarcoma. The chest radiograph was normal. A single metastasis is seen behind the right diaphragm in a typical subpleural position.

Computerized tomography

Computerized tomography (CT) is a valuable non-invasive investigation. It not only determines the intramedullary extension of the tumour but may indicate the presence of any extraosseous (extracompartmental) extension of the neoplasm (Fig. 6(a) and (b)). When used in conjunction with contrast medium it may outline the relations of the tumour to large vessels and may indicate the diagnosis by the presence of mineralization of the tumour matrix. CT scanning of the lungs is important in the establishment of accurate staging. Typically the metastases are found in a subpleural position (Fig. 6(c)). In spite of the greater sensitivity of the technique, the proportion of patients with normal chest radiographs at presentation who are shown to have metastases on CT scanning is only 10–15 per cent (Cohen *et al.* 1982).

Magnetic resonance imaging

Magnetic resonance imaging (MRI) is probably now the most sensitive single method for assessing medullary involvement by tumour (Zimmer

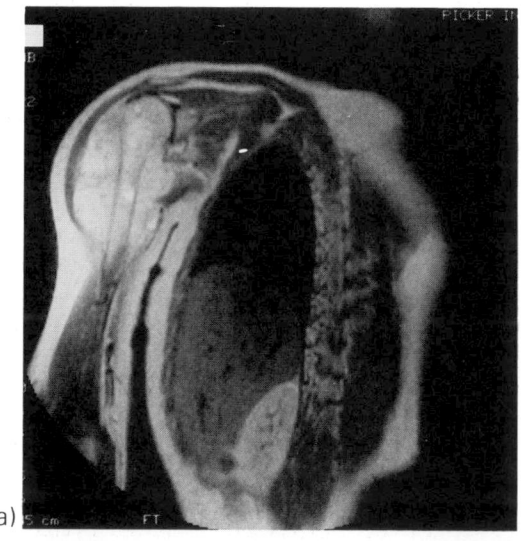

(a)

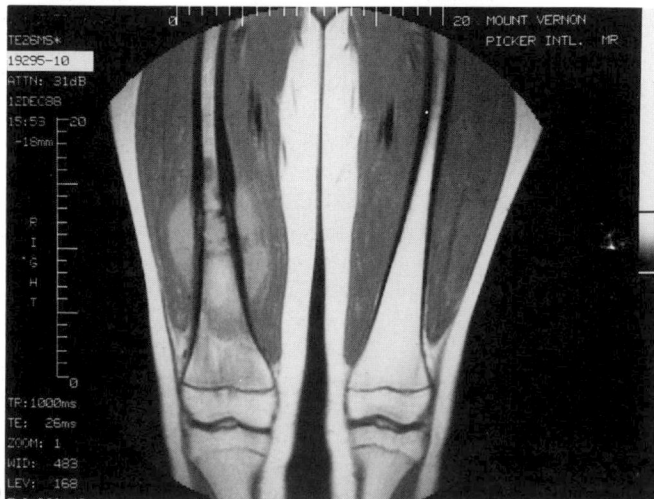

(b)

Fig. 7 (a) MRI scan of osteosarcoma of right humerus. The extent of the soft tissue component is clearly shown. (b) MRI scan of osteosarcoma of right femur. The extent of the intramedullary component is demonstrated and the soft tissue mass, displacing muscle, is clearly shown.

et al. 1985). Both CT and MRI can demonstrate the presence of extraosseous soft tissue extension (Fig. 7(a) and (b)) and in most circumstances MRI is superior to CT in differentiating tumour from adjoining muscle (Aisen *et al.* 1986; Bohndorf *et al.* 1986). There may be, however, considerable difficulty in differentiating between tumour and peripheral oedema in highly malignant tumours. MRI can be useful in delineating a response to treatment by radiotherapy or chemotherapy by reduction in tumoural mass and restoration of the normal MRI signal (Dooms *et al.* 1985).

The increasing sensitivity of staging investigations has been proposed as an explanation for the apparent increase of survival in adjuvant chemotherapy trials in recent years (Simon 1984). In studies made before 1970 patients were staged on the basis of a single chest radiograph or whole-lung tomography. More patients will now be shown to have metastases, either pulmonary or bony, by the sophisticated methods available.

Despite the increasing sophistication of radiological investigations the radiologist may only be able to offer a differential diagnosis. Included in these possibilities are stress fracture, chronic osteomyelitis, ectopic ossification and other highly malignant tumours that may induce reactive bone formation, such as Ewing's tumour. The ultimate diagnosis therefore rests in the hands of the histopathologist, but it is important that any histological interpretation is taken in conjunction with the radiological findings.

BIOPSY TECHNIQUES

Biopsy of the lesion is essential in the diagnosis and staging of osteogenic sarcoma (Mankin *et al.* 1982*b*). Most commonly, biopsy is by an open technique and ideally the biopsy tract should be as small as possible and go directly to bone. Post-operatively, haemostasis at the operation site is mandatory and the wound should be closed with a subcuticular suture. A rapid histological diagnosis can be made using imprint techniques (Pringle 1987), as unfixed tumour cells will show staining positive for alkaline phosphatase. It must be remembered when definitive surgery is done that the complete biopsy tract must be removed *en bloc* with the tumour. Failure to do so significantly increases the risk of local recurrence (Cannon and Dyson 1988). The surgeon performing the open biopsy should therefore consider the planning of the definitive resection and site the approach correctly.

Percutaneous needle biopsy using a Jamshidi or similar needle is often sufficient to give a diagnosis. Again, the needle tract should be removed *en bloc* at the definitive tumour resection. The analysis of such small amounts of biopsy material requires histological expertise of the highest calibre and is not recommended if this is not available.

Mankin *et al.* (1982*b*), in a large study, concluded that the incidence of significant problems in patient management produced by inappropriate biopsy techniques was 20 per cent and that the incidence of wound healing complications related to the biopsy was similar. They considered that 8 per cent of biopsies produced a significant adverse effect on the prognosis of the patient and that 5 per cent led to an unnecessary amputation. Errors in diagnosis leading to inadequate treatment occur twice as frequently when the biopsy is done in the referring hospital as when done at the definitive centre.

STAGING NOTATIONS

Despite the recognition that staging is valuable in both treatment planning and evaluation of treatments there is no universally accepted staging system in osteosarcoma. The surgical staging

Table 2 Surgical staging system of Enneking

Stage	Grade		Site	Metastases
I	A	Low (G_1)	Intracompartmental (T_1)	None (M_0)
	B	Low (G_1)	Extracompartmental (T_2)	None (M_0)
II	A	High (G_2)	Intracompartmental (T_1)	None (M_0)
	B	High (G_2)	Extracompartmental (T_2)	None (M_0)
III	A	Low (G_1)	Intra- or extra- (T_1–T_2)	Regional or distant (M_1)
	B	High (G_2)	Intra- or extra- (T_1–T_2)	Regional or distant (M_1)

system proposed by Enneking (Enneking *et al.* 1980*b*) is easy to use clinically, although it suffers from significant oversimplification. The system takes account of three basic features that are of recognized prognostic importance. These are the histological grade of the tumour, its location, and the presence or absence of regional or distal metastases. The histological grade is classified as either low grade (G_1) or high grade (G_2). This grading system does not completely match purely histological grading schemes, but in essence low-grade lesions will be the equivalent of Broders grade 1 and some 2s, while high-grade lesions would all be Broders 2, 3, and 4 (Broders 1964). As regards location, lesions are divided into those occurring in a specific compartment (T_1) and those that are extracompartmental in nature (T_2). The term 'compartments' is defined as 'an anatomic structure bounded by natural barriers to tumour extension'. In osteosarcoma a whole bone is considered a compartment, as is a functional muscle group bounded by major fascial septa. Tumours spreading beyond these compartments or involving the neurovascular structures are classified as extracompartmental. Some anatomical locations, such as the popliteal fossa, axilla, and paraspinal areas, are considered to be extracompartmental by definition.

Metastases occur most frequently in the lungs. They may occasionally occur in bone but are rare in local lymph nodes. The minority of patients who exhibit multiple skeletal metastases may or may not have associated pulmonary lesions and the prognosis is invariably poor. Multiple bony lesions are sometimes considered as examples of multicentric primary tumours, although usually one lesion has the radiological features of a primary lesion and the others have characteristics of secondary, intramedullary deposits (Ross 1964). Metastases occurring in the bone in which the primary tumour has initially developed may be true metastases or so-called 'skip' lesions. Skip lesions (a seemingly isolated area of tumour in the same bone) were originally thought to occur in approximately 25 per cent of cases of osteosarcoma (Enneking and Kagan 1975), but the true incidence is probably much lower (Lewis and Lotz 1974). Skip lesions may represent intramedullary or transepiphyseal spread of the primary growth where continuity with the main tumour is not demonstrated. Other skip lesions may be blood-borne bone metastases.

From the three variables outlined above a surgical staging system is constructed, as illustrated in Table 2.

SURGICAL TREATMENT

Amputation of the limb was once the only surgical treatment available in osteosarcoma. It usually took the form of a forequarter amputation in proximal humeral lesions, distal femoral amputation in proximal tibial lesions, and a high femoral amputation or disarticulation of the hip for distal femoral lesions (Pack *et al.* 1942; Sweetnam 1973). In 1955 the poor outcome of patients with osteosarcoma treated by amputation alone led Cade to advocate interval amputation. The local tumour was treated by radiotherapy, amputation only being done if the patient was free of metastases

some 6 months later. In the late 1970s, encouraged by techniques of limb salvage in benign and low-grade malignant lesions, many surgeons began to extend these techniques to osteogenic sarcoma. Initially such surgery was associated with rates of local recurrence in the order of 20 per cent but, with clearer definition of tumour extent, pre-operative staging, and appropriate selection of patients, this has now fallen to approximately 5 per cent (Marcove 1977; Marcove and Rosen 1979; Rosen *et al.* 1979).

The clear definition of tumour extent, particularly in the intramedullary area, is of utmost importance if local resection is to be done. MRI appears to be highly sensitive at delineating the intramedullary extent of the tumour and a level of bony resection at a distance of 5 cm is the usual point of division. The decision between amputation and local resection often cannot be made until the moment of surgery. Gross neurovascular or skin involvement is usually evident by clinical and staging investigations, although occasionally soft tissue extent may be difficult to elucidate clearly. Amputation is usually the only surgical treatment where there is extensive neurovascular involvement or skin invasion or in most cases where there is pathological fracture. Occasionally, patients with pathological fracture show such a complete response to pre-operative chemotherapy that limb preservation is possible, although the risk of local recurrence is higher (Jaffe *et al.* 1987).

Similarly, pre-operative chemotherapy will sometimes render a tumour involving vessels and nerves amenable to local resection rather than amputation. However, the converse can also be true: a large lesion, which may be on the borderline of resectability, may be resistant to chemotherapy. Pre-operative treatment may allow the lesion to progress to one only treatable by amputation. Great vigilance is therefore required by surgeon and chemotherapist alike.

Tumour clearance is confirmed intraoperatively by pathological or cytological examination of a marrow biopsy at the resection site. Doubtful areas in the soft tissues or adjacent to vessels or nerves can be examined at the time of resection by imprint or frozen-section techniques.

The incidence of local recurrence is higher if the biopsy scar is not excised, but in the absence of gross macroscopic invasion of the biopsy tract this is rarely an indication by itself for amputation. In the United States, metaphyseal lesions are often removed by means of an extraarticular resection of the adjacent joint, as penetration of the joint by osteosarcoma is considered to be frequent (Simon and Bos 1980; Simon and Hecht 1982). In Europe intra-articular resection appears to be preferred. After successful local resection of a tumour, reconstruction of the limb is usually required to provide stability. Occasionally, particularly in lesions around the pelvis and shoulder girdle, no reconstruction is feasible and the remaining distal limb is left to flail (Marcove *et al.* 1977).

Modified amputation is rarely used in the United Kingdom. The modified amputations of Sauerbruch and the Van Nes procedure allow the use of smaller artificial limbs than does straightforward amputation, but result in significant physical deformity (Van Nes 1948). In the United Kingdom it is considered that this procedure places considerable psychological strain on the patient by its physical appearance, particularly as the patient already faces the diagnosis of osteosarcoma. At best the reversed ankle joint offers 60° of movement from a fixed flexion position of some 30°. We must, however, acknowledge that the technique has wide popularity, particularly in Germany (Winkler *et al.* 1986). Autogenous bone grafting is rarely used after local resection of osteosarcoma because of the large defects involved and the long recovery time required. Grafts may be used in conjunction with large metallic implants. Large cancellous and cortical grafts, including transposition of the fibula, are commonly used; repair of these is retarded both by concomitant local radiation and systemic chemotherapy. However, 90 per cent of patients with segmental defects reconstructed in such a manner eventually regain functional stability of the extremity (Enneking *et al.* 1980*a*). The implantation of a vascularized cortical or fibula autograft anastomosed by microvascular techniques is an attractive proposition but its role is still to be confirmed. Occasionally, autoclaved or irradiated autograft can be used to reconstruct a defect (Smith and Simon 1975). This is rarely feasible in osteosarcoma, as the damage done to the bony structure is usually too great to allow for this reconstruction.

Mankin *et al.* (1982*a*) have renewed the interest in osteoarticular and intercalary allograft methods of reconstruction. Such techniques are not new and there are a number of previous reports (Lexer 1925; Ottolenghi 1966; Nilsonne 1969; Volkov 1970). The fate of any allograft will range from apparently complete incorporation and repair to total rejection and rapid resorption. The response is unpredictable. Even in successful allografts the repair period is extremely lengthy and there is a high incidence of complications (Mankin *et al.* 1975). Where an osteoarticular allograft is used the cartilage transplant in the joint may be necrotic. Any damage is repaired by fibrocartilage, which is prone to early degeneration. The long-term outlook for the joint is poor and there is now a trend to replace the resected joint and metaphysis with a composite prosthesis and allograft (Mankin *et al.* 1988). This combination allows strong attachment of the surrounding musculature to the allograft, which is a problem in prosthetic replacement.

The use of prosthetic materials to bridge large defects was first reported in the United States (Moore and Bohlman 1943). Since 1950 the method has been used and developed at the Royal National Orthopaedic Hospital in the United Kingdom and other centres. Burrows *et al.* (1975) first reported the use of prostheses to achieve limb salvage. The technique requires a custom-made prosthesis manufactured from measurement radiographs of low magnification

whilst the patient undergoes pre-operative chemotherapy (Fig. 8a and b). Alternatively, a modular system piecing the parts of the endoprosthesis together during the course of the operation can be used (Campanacci *et al.* 1983). The main attraction of using a prosthesis is the speed of rehabilitation. Patients undergoing reconstruction of whole or part of the femur and tibia have been able to bear weight completely in the immediate post-operative period. Two major problems remain. First, infection is common with all prosthetic surgery, particularly if the patient is immunosuppressed; secondly, the reattachment of muscle groups to the prosthesis requires further development.

In children with high growth potential it is feasible to construct a growing type of prosthesis. On one side the metal prosthesis slides out with growth of the preserved epiphyseal plate from a central polythene sleeve inserted into the diaphysis, whilst the other side of the joint requires insertion of C-rings of increasing depths, so committing the child to further open surgery whilst growth continues (Fig. 8(c)).

Functional assessment after reconstruction of a limb remains a highly complex problem, particularly as there is little international agreement on which variables are of importance. Enneking (1987) has proposed a system that assesses reconstruction about the knee in terms of range of movement, pain, stability, strength, and emotional acceptance. Complications are also recorded. Final ratings are excellent, good, fair, and poor. It is sufficiently flexible to allow some comparison between differing techniques of reconstruction. Similar grading systems based on radiological findings are now being developed.

Bradish *et al.* (1987) have analysed the clinical function of distal femoral and knee joint prosthetic reconstructions at between 5 and 18 years after insertion; 80 per cent of patients had good or excellent results and only 13 per cent were considered to have a poor outcome, related to either infection or local recurrence. Similar results can be achieved with upper femoral and hip replacement.

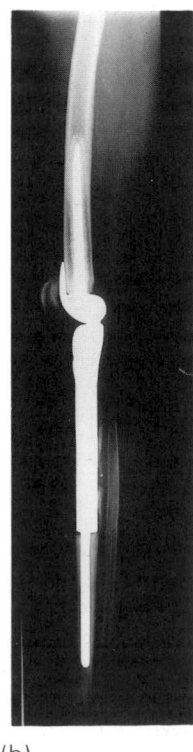

(a)   (b)   (c)

Fig. 8 (a) Photograph of the composite parts of a custom-made prosthesis: a medullary stem for cementation into the marrow cavity, a more bulky section to replace the resected diaphysis and metaphysis, and a constrained knee joint. (b) Radiograph of custom-made prosthesis in place after resection of an upper tibial osteosarcoma. (c) A prosthesis with a 'growing' mechanism. Here, on the resected side, the prosthesis may be opened at an open operation and the length maintained by a C-ring. On the non-resected side of the joint, further growth from the epiphysial plate may elevate the prosthesis from an uncemented polyethylene intramedullary tube.

Upper humeral and upper tibial replacements remain less satisfactory, owing to the difficulties of soft tissue attachment.

SURGERY OF SPECIAL SITES

Pelvis

Lesions in the pelvis often attain considerable size before diagnosis and radiographic interpretation by itself may be confusing. Both MRI and measurement CT scans are essential in the pre-operative assessment of pelvic osteosarcoma. A rectal examination is also essential to assess involvement of intrapelvic organs. Where local resection is feasible, there remains considerable debate as to the correct method of reconstruction. Lesions arising within the infra-acetabular position of the pelvis are not usually reconstructed. When the acetabular region has been resected, either an excision arthroplasty may be left or an iliofemoral arthrodesis can be done. A more attractive alternative, with shorter rehabilitation periods, would be the use of a 'saddle prosthesis' or a hemipelvic replacement (Fig. 9). Such devices require considerable sparing of a segment of upper ilium. Solitary ilial lesions can usually be reconstructed with bone grafting across the defect above a spared acetabulum, but where the whole ilium and acetabulum have to be removed, reconstruction must be either by a pseudarthrosis or unsightly ischiofemoral arthrodesis. The delay in diagnosis may, however, lead to wide intrapelvic or buttock involvement. The surgical option in this situation remains hind-quarter amputation, which, given a poor prognosis for survival, may be a poor option to gain local control.

Spine and sacrum

Osteosarcoma of the spine is extremely rare and is usually seen in the older patient in association with Paget's disease or after previous irradiation. Presentation may briefly be as mechanical dysfunction but neurological sequelae rapidly ensue. Surgical clearance is rarely possible, although marginal excision may be feasible. Tumours arising in the sacrum may be ablated but with subsequent

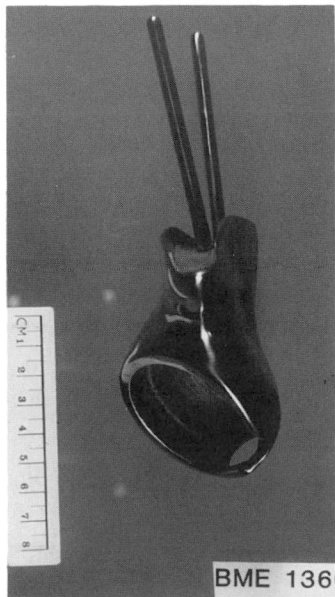

Fig. 9 Prosthesis for replacement of the hemipelvis. Divergent pins may be cemented or 'push-fit' into the residual ilium. A polyethylene cup is cemented into the cavity.

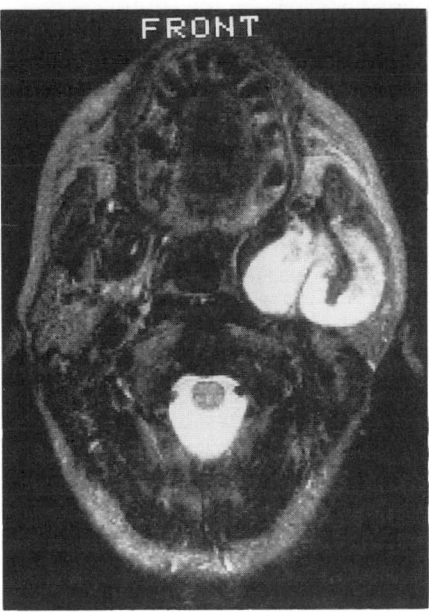

Fig. 10 Osteosarcoma of vertical ramus of the left mandible. This MRI scan shows the extent of the soft tissue component. The tumour extended vertically to the base of the skull.

neurological loss. The bladder and anal canal are innervated and continence preserved by bilateral supply from nerve roots S2, S3, and S4. Unilateral ablation appears not to affect continence significantly, but retention of the S2 root would be preferable. Where the nerve roots are affected bilaterally, both S2 roots must be preserved for normal sphincter function to be retained.

Jaw

Osteosarcoma may rarely affect the jaw, predominantly afflicting young adult males with an older age range of 20–40. Swelling and pain are the common presenting complaints and the body of the mandible, antrum, and the alveolar ridge of the maxilla are the most frequent sites of involvement. The most common histological type is chondroblastic and this is associated with the best survival rates. The tumour tends to be better differentiated than at other sites. Wide excision is difficult but is the only treatment likely to produce local control. The tumour may extend up to the base of the skull when it arises from the vertical ramus of the mandible (Fig. 10). Marginal surgery combined with radiotherapy gives poor results, most patients dying from uncontrolled local disease rather than metastases. The rôle of pre-operative chemotherapy is uncertain but it may help to reduce the tumour mass, so making radical excisional and reconstructive surgery possible. Metastasis may occur and is a further indication for chemotherapy, although local control remains the major problem.

CHEMOTHERAPY OF HIGH-GRADE OSTEOSARCOMA

Before the introduction of chemotherapy in the early 1970s the prognosis of osteosarcoma in childhood and young adults was predictably bad. Up to 80 per cent of patients developed pulmonary metastases after amputation, 50 per cent of these appeared in the first 6 months, and the great majority of patients developing metastases died within 3 years (Dahlin and Coventry 1967; Jeffree *et al.* 1975). The 5 year survival rate was approximately 20 per cent

Table 3 Single-agent response rates in metastatic osteosarcoma

Drug	Overall response (%)
High-dose methotrexate with folinic acid	25
Ifosfamide	24
Doxorubicin	21
Cisplatin	18
Mitomycin C	14
Melphalan	16
Cyclophosphamide	14
Actinomycin D	8

Data are approximate, being pooled from many sources.

(Friedman and Carter 1972). These depressing results led to an exploration of the use of chemotherapy as an adjunct to surgery, as it was clear that metastatic disease was present at the time of diagnosis in the great majority of patients. When used as single agents in metastatic disease, cytotoxic drugs have not shown great activity. Doxorubicin, ifosfamide, high-dose methotrexate, and cisplatin are the most effective agents (Table 3). The use of high-dose methotrexate, as compared with the drug in lower doses, has never been formally validated (Grem et al. 1988), but it seems unlikely that this will be regarded as a priority in investigation. High-dose methotrexate was one of the first agents to be shown to be active (Jaffe 1972) and has been incorporated into most adjuvant protocols. Doxorubicin has been shown to produce regression in approximately 25 per cent of patients with metastases (Cortes et al. 1972; Pratt and Shanks 1974) and cisplatin in 15–20 per cent (Gasparini et al. 1985; Pratt et al. 1985). The response rates may be higher for the primary tumours, but pre-operative chemotherapy (see below) is almost always with drugs in combination and direct comparisons cannot be made.

Single agents have been used for treatment of primary femoral tumours by the intra-arterial route (Benjamin 1989). The drugs most commonly used are cisplatin (Mavligit 1981) and high-dose methotrexate (Jaffe et al. 1985) and doxorubicin (Eckhardt et al. 1985). Responses occur in 50–70 per cent of patients but it is not clear if limb salvage or survival are superior to those achieved by intravenous combination chemotherapy. Cisplatin is the drug that

may have most to offer by the intra-arterial route as it is not vesicant and can be given at high dose. A randomization between intra-arterial and intravenous cisplatin is being made by the West German/Austrian group. Stephens et al. (1987) reported excellent responses in seven of eight large sarcomas (including three osteosarcomas) in the shoulder, pelvis, and thigh using intra-arterial doxorubicin and cisplatin. In selected cases, intra-arterial therapy may offer a higher response rate and a greater chance of less radical surgery, but the indications for its use are not clearly defined at present.

Numerous drug combinations have been assessed in treated and untreated metastatic disease. The most effective of these have contained cisplatin, doxorubicin, and high-dose methotrexate–citrovorum factor either as a two- or three-drug regimen; response rates of the order of 35–50 per cent have been obtained, although often based on rather small numbers (Table 4).

These results encouraged the use of chemotherapy as an adjuvant to surgery. Uncontrolled trials began in the early 1970s with high-dose methotrexate–citrovorum factor as the main agent used after amputation. Early reports (Jaffe et al. 1974) were encouraging and greeted enthusiastically. Later reports were less impressive (Rosenberg 1979). In a series of uncontrolled studies, Rosen and his co-workers at the Memorial Sloan Kettering Hospital explored the use of combination chemotherapy as an adjuvant to surgery (Rosen et al. 1979, 1982a,b). Two year survival in excess of 80 per cent was achieved. However, Taylor et al. (1985) suggested that survival of non-metastatic cases was improving even without chemotherapy, partly as a result of case selection and more successful detection of metastases. A small, randomized trial of high-dose methotrexate against no treatment did not show any advantage for chemotherapy (Edmonson et al. 1984). A summary of results from these uncontrolled studies of adjuvant chemotherapy is given in Table 5.

This controversy led to two randomized trials of post-surgical adjuvant chemotherapy compared with no immediate treatment (chemotherapy being given at the first sign of metastasis). The ethical problems attending these trials were formidable (Lange and Levin 1982). The study of the Paediatric Oncology Group (POG) (Link et al. 1986) showed a clear relapse-free survival advantage

Table 4 Response rates to combination chemotherapy in metastatic osteosarcoma

Drugs	No. of patients	Overall response (%)	Reference
Cyclophosphamide/doxorubicin/dacarbazine	29	24	Benjamin et al. (1978)
Cisplatin/vincristine/high-dose methotrexate	29	28	Morgan et al. (1974)
Dacarbazine/doxorubicin	20	35	Rosen et al. (1982b)
Dacarbazine/doxorubicin	19	26	Pratt et al. (1985)
Cyclophosphamide/doxorubicin/actinomycin D	20	25	Benjamin et al. (1978)

Studies including more than 15 patients.

Table 5 Relapse-free survival with adjuvant chemotherapy in uncontrolled trials

Drugs	No. of patients	Relapse-free survival (%)	Reference
Doxorubicin/vincristine/high-dose methotrexate	57	62	Eckardt et al. (1985)
Doxorubicin/cyclophosphamide/high-dose methotrexate	51	51	Pratt et al. (1984)
Vincristine/high-dose methotrexate	39	38	Rosenberg et al. (1979)
T4/5 (multidrug protocol)	52	48	Rosen et al. (1983)
T7 (multidrug protocol)	54	80	Rosen et al. (1983)
T10 (multidrug protocol)	79	92	Rosen et al. (1983)
Interferon	33	58	Strander et al. (1979)

Studies with more than 30 patients.

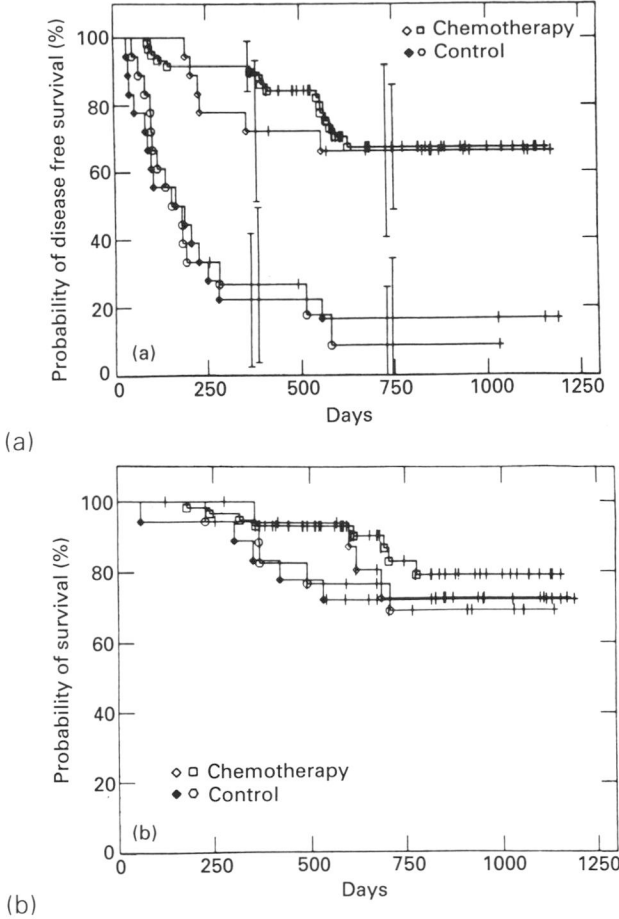

(a)

(b)

Fig. 11 (a) Disease-free survival and (b) overall survival in patients randomized to receive immediate or delayed chemotherapy for operable osteosarcoma. Diamond symbols represent randomized patients, open squares and circles are non-randomized patients. (Data from Link *et al.* (1986) with permission.)

for the patients treated with chemotherapy, although there was no survival advantage at the time of the report (Fig. 11). The difference in the two arms led to the trial being stopped with only 36 patients randomized. Long-term survival data are awaited. A further trial (Eckhardt *et al.* 1985) has also shown an advantage for adjuvant chemotherapy. In this small study all patients received pre-operative intra-arterial chemotherapy with doxorubicin but were then randomized to further chemotherapy or no further treatment post-operatively. A more recent, multivariate, retrospective analysis using data from several centres has failed to show the effect of chemotherapy as a prognostic factor (Taylor *et al.* 1989), but the limitations of this approach do not counterbalance the findings from prospective randomized trials.

Taken as a whole the data strongly support the use of adjuvant chemotherapy in improving relapse-free survival. The effect on overall survival is more difficult to judge. In this context the West German/Austrian 'COSS' (Cooperative Osteosarcoma Study) studies of adjuvant chemotherapy in childhood cases have shown a 5 year survival of 60 per cent, which, for a national study, is an impressive result (Winkler *et al.* 1988). Similar data have been obtained from the European Osteosarcoma Intergroup (**EOI**) trial (Bramwell *et al.* 1992), who have achieved a 60 per cent 3.5 year survival in a randomized trial with 220 unselected patients. Neither the EOI nor COSS studies were

comparing chemotherapy with controls but these data represent multicentre results that are quite different from the experiences of the early 1970s and from adjuvant studies using low-dose chemotherapy (Medical Research Council (**MRC**) 1986).

In the last 10 years there has been considerable interest in the use of chemotherapy before surgery; induction or 'neo-adjuvant' chemotherapy. This stems from the work of Rosen and his collaborators (Rosen *et al.* 1979), who pointed out several potential advantages in using chemotherapy as the first treatment. Chief among these are the following: the introduction of chemotherapy allows early control of micrometastases, the response of the primary tumour can be assessed, shrinkage of the primary tumour facilitates conservative resection and may diminish local recurrence, and it allows time for preparation of custom-made prostheses. The disadvantage of initial chemotherapy is that assessment of tumour response is not always easy and, in non-responding patients, metastases may occur that were not previously present. Growth of the primary in the face of chemotherapy may necessitate amputation instead of the conservative surgery that might have previously been possible. Vigilance and experience is therefore required during this initial phase of chemotherapy. At present there are no certain methods of objectively assessing response during the pre-operative treatment. Reduction in pain and swelling are useful signs. A fall in alkaline phosphatase is suggestive. Plain radiography is not usually helpful but CT scanning may be (Mail *et al.* 1985). The use of MRI is being investigated by several groups but its rôle is as yet undefined.

There are a few studies that have made a direct comparison of the duration and composition of chemotherapy (Table 6). Bacci *et al.* (1986) tested two regimens of methotrexate in a randomized trial. All patients received doxorubicin and vincristine but were randomized to receive methotrexate 2000 mg/m^2 over 15 min with folinic acid rescue at 24 h or 200 mg/m^2 over 6 h with folinic acid rescue at 12 h. No significant difference in response or survival was observed. However, in a subsequent study (Picci *et al.* 1987), high-dose methotrexate (7.5 g/m^2) was superior to 750 mg/m^2. In the study of the United Kingdom MRC (1986) the alternation of methotrexate in moderate dose with doxorubicin did not alter survival compared with doxorubicin alone. In the COSS-80 study (Winkler *et al.* 1984), cisplatin and BCD (bleomycin, cyclophosphamide, and dactinomycin) were equally effective (or ineffective) when added to doxorubicin, high-dose methotrexate, and vincristine. In the **CALGB** (Cancer and Acute Leukaemia Group B) study (Cortes and Holland 1981), doxorubicin appeared to be associated with slightly worse results when high-dose methotrexate was added, but the study was very small. The EOI trial used intensive chemotherapy lasting only 17 weeks and the two drug combination of cisplatin and doxorubicin achieved results comparable with the POG and COSS studies using the T10-based (multidrug) protocols of up to 44 weeks' duration (Bramwell *et al.* 1988). A randomized comparison of the 17 week cisplatin/doxorubicin protocol and a 44 week T10 protocol (modified to include pre-operative doxorubicin) by the EOI has now been completed and the results are awaited. The same group is also assessing more intensive treatments containing ifosfamide in patients with metastatic disease. This drug has shown promising activity in osteosarcoma (see Table 3). The more recent experience of the West German/Austrian trial COSS-82 (Winkler *et al.* 1988) suggests that it is an error to reserve active agents such as doxorubicin and cisplatin for those post-operative patients whose tumours show little histological response to chemotherapy. A better strategy appears to be to use the most effective agents early.

In demonstrating improvements in survival even as large as 15 per cent over current results, trials needing hundreds of patients

Table 6 Randomized comparisons of adjuvant chemotherapy regimens

Regimens	No. of patients	Relapse-free survival (%)	Difference	Reference
1 (a) Vincristine/high-dose methotrexate	99	27	No	MRC (1986)
(b) Doxorubicin/vincristine/high-dose methotrexate	95	27		
2 (a) High-dose methotrexate/doxorubicin/vincristine	50	50	No	Bacci et al. (1986)
(b) Low-dose methotrexate/doxorubicin/vincristine	56	55		
3 (a) BCD[a]+ doxorubicin/vincristine/high-dose methotrexate	59	77	No	Winkler et al. (1984)
(b) Cisplatin+doxorubicin/vincristine/high-dose methotrexate	49	73		
4 (a) Doxorubicin	51	52	Yes	Cortes and Holland (1981)
(b) Doxorubicin/high-dose methotrexate	38	40	Doxorubicin > Doxorubicin/high-dose methotrexate	

[a]BCD, bleomycin, cyclophosphamide, and actinomycin D in combination.

are essential. Smaller trials are more likely than not to miss a difference and are thus misleading. National and international collaboration will be necessary to make progress.

Responding tumours show considerable necrosis induced by the chemotherapy (Fig. 12). Rosen et al. (1982a) pointed out that patients showing a poor histological response had a worse prognosis than those showing extensive necrosis. This finding has been confirmed by others but an objective scoring system has not yet been described and it is by no means clear that changing chemotherapy in non-responders can alter the prognosis. The practical value of assessing necrosis is therefore questionable at present, except as an indication of response rate (and therefore effectiveness) to a particular chemotherapy regimen. The correlation of survival with tumour response has been observed in many cancers, but it cannot be assumed that improvement is due to the response since both response and survival might be related to other factors such as tumour size or histological type. Multivariate analysis on very large numbers of patients treated on defined protocols is needed to assess the independent contribution of tumour response to prognosis.

TREATMENT OF METASTATIC DISEASE

CT scanning has shown that 10–15 per cent of patients with normal chest radiographs have detectable pulmonary metastases at presentation (Cohen et al. 1982). In the remainder, 35–40 per cent will relapse after adjuvant chemotherapy, usually in the chest. Although, in the latter group, prevention of relapse remains the primary objective, the treatment of pulmonary metastases is a major problem. Bone metastases, usually detected by isotope scan, are an uncommon presenting feature (and, as mentioned previously, are sometimes difficult to distinguish from multiple primary tumours). They are more frequent on relapse, occurring in 20 per cent of patients and usually in the context of very advanced disease. Metastases in skin and brain occur occasionally. Liver and lymph node metastases are rare.

Pulmonary metastases

If patients present with pulmonary metastases the prognosis is poor but, if the metastases are few in number, respond to chemotherapy, and are resectable, cure is possible. Overall, 10–15 per cent of patients presenting with pulmonary metastases can be cured. It seems probable that, in addition to eliminating pulmonary metastases, chemotherapy may, in some patients, reduce their number and delay their appearance. Cure may then be achieved by metastectomy. Several studies have reported on the prognosis of patients undergoing pulmonary metastectomy. In one such study (Goorin et al. 1984), 11 out of 26 patients operated upon were long-term survivors. However, only 26 out of 32 relapsing in the lung were considered operable. Several studies have confirmed the observation that approximately 30 per cent of patients who relapse in the chest will be long-term survivors after surgery. In a detailed analysis of 59 patients from St Jude Hospital (Meyer et al. 1987), several factors were predictive of long-term survival following metastectomy. Patients with more than five or six nodules removed at the first thoracotomy had a very poor survival, as did those whose first thoracotomy did not result in complete removal of all metastases, although some of these patients became long survivors after a second thoracotomy. Patients with bilateral metastases had a worse prognosis and there were few female survivors. In a multivariate analysis, male sex and fewer than five metastases were predictive of long survival. In analyses of patients from the National Cancer Institute, prognosis was worse in those with a short (less than 6 months) treatment-free interval, numerous metastases (more than

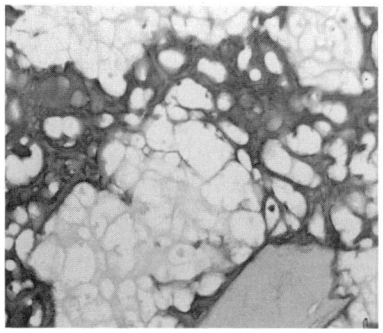

(a)

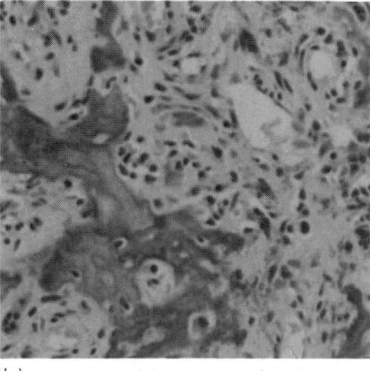

(b)

Fig. 12 (a) Good response to chemotherapy. Necrotic, partially-resorbed pre-existing bone surrounded by acellular and mineralized tumour. (b) Poor response to chemotherapy. A cellular osteosarcoma with little evidence of any chemotherapeutic effect.

three), and, of course, unresectable lesions (Putnam *et al.* 1983; Roth *et al.* 1984). Burgers *et al.* (1980) and Spanos *et al.* (1976) showed a worse survival when the disease-free interval was short. This accords with common sense, as such patients have, by definition, metastases that have been poorly controlled by chemotherapy. The study of Han *et al.* (1981) confirmed this finding.

In recommending guidelines it should be remembered that the above studies are retrospective and small in size, often including patients from before the era of intensive chemotherapy and CT scanning. Large-scale trials with homogeneous treatment will provide more reliable data on prognosis after pulmonary relapse. There is some evidence that some patients will relapse and die as long as 6 years after thoracotomy (Burk *et al.* 1991). Meanwhile the following approach seems reasonable. Thoracotomy should be considered in patients whose primary tumour is controlled or removed, who do not have bone metastases, and whose CT scans indicate that there is a reasonable likelihood of complete removal. Smaller numbers of metastases (less than five or six) appearing late after chemotherapy has ceased are likely to be associated with a better prognosis. Metastases occurring during chemotherapy or shortly after are likely to be associated with a bad outlook. In such patients further chemotherapy can be considered before thoractomy, though it is unlikely to be successful if intensive multiagent treatment has been given previously, even if different drugs are to be used. The value of chemotherapy or whole-lung irradiation after complete resection is unknown and awaits definition in patients relapsing from defined protocols of treatment in large-scale trials.

TREATMENT OF SPECIAL FORMS OF OSTEOSARCOMA

Axial skeletal lesions

The surgery of osteosarcoma in the pelvis, spine, sacrum, and mandible has been considered earlier. At all these sites, initial chemotherapy may help to reduce the size of the tumour before resection. Tumours of the mandible have a low potential for metastasis. The chemotherapy usually used is as for classical central osteosarcoma. The prognosis is determined by the size and resectability of the lesion. In unresectable, locally recurrent or incompletely excised lesions, radiotherapy may delay disease progression if given in a high dose (50–55 Gy).

Telangiectatic osteosarcoma

These are usually large, destructive, metaphyseal tumours that constitute approximately 10 per cent of all cases of osteosarcoma (Huvos *et al.* 1982). Bone radiographs show a lytic lesion without associated sclerosis. They are often associated with pathological fracture, and were thought to have a bad prognosis and usually to be metastatic at presentation or shortly after. Huvos *et al.* (1982) reported that the prognosis for this type was not as adverse as previously thought if adjuvant chemotherapy was given. Chawla *et al.* (1985) showed that five out of eight patients treated with intra-arterial cisplatin and intravenous dacarbazine and doxorubicin showed greater than 95 per cent tumour necrosis. Rosen *et al.* (1986) reported 'good' histopathological responses in 11 out of 16 patients who had pre-operative chemotherapy using the T10 programme and survival comparable with other forms of the disease. The tumours are therefore responsive in the same way as other forms of osteosarcoma and are treated in the same way.

Small-cell osteosarcoma

This variant of osteosarcoma is mentioned because it may be a source of diagnostic uncertainty. It was first reported by Sim *et al.* (1979). It is a high-grade tumour composed of small cells resembling Ewing's sarcoma, lymphoma, or spindle cells. The cells are closely packed with variable cytoplasm and numerous mitoses. Tests for common leucocyte antigen are negative, distinguishing the tumour from lymphoma. The cells may contain cytoplasmic glycogen according to Ayala *et al.* (1989), but the distinction from Ewing's sarcoma then becomes very uncertain, although tumour osteoid should be present for the diagnosis to be entertained and the tumour cells can be shown to produce alkaline phosphatase. Clinically the distribution and age range of the tumour is not different from other types. In the report of Ayala *et al.* (1989) the prognosis appeared quite poor, with 14/27 patients dead in 2 years and a poor response of distant metastasis to chemotherapy.

Parosteal and periosteal osteosarcoma

The histological appearances of these tumours have been described earlier.

Parosteal osteosarcoma

This tends to arise a decade later than classical osteosarcoma. The lesion arises on the surface of the metaphyseal area of the bone (Fig. 4(d)). It matures into a bulky mass of mature bone, which tends to displace rather than invade surrounding structures. With time it tends to wrap itself around the underlying bone. The radiological appearance is of a dense lesion of mature bone, which may exhibit a number of fibrous septa. Occasionally signs of medullary invasion may be evident. Parosteal osteosarcoma is of low-grade malignancy and, even at a later stage when the tumour has permeated the underlying cortex and extended into the medulla, it is still amenable to local resection and prosthetic replacement. The low risk of metastases means that adjuvant chemotherapy is not usually indicated. Occasionally, at a later stage, recurrent or primary tumours dedifferentiate into a high-grade and rapidly growing osteosarcoma (Wold *et al.* 1984). Treatment is then as for classical osteosarcoma, including the use of chemotherapy. The risk of this transition, and of metastatic spread in a few cases of parosteal osteosarcoma, may relate to areas of more high-grade activity that can occasionally be found on detailed histological examination of the tumour.

Periosteal osteosarcoma (Fig. 4(c))

This is another variant which may arise on the outer aspect of bone. Again a tumour of young adults, it is located on the metaphyseal region of a long bone. Radiographically it is usually radiolucent surrounded by Codman-like triangles of spicules of bone. The lesion may nestle in a defect in the cortex, which it does not invade until late in its course. The lesion is often of relatively high grade with a risk of local recurrence if excision is marginal. Metastases do occur but the value of chemotherapy is not known with certainty. Periosteal osteosarcoma is also amenable to local excision of the proximal tibia (its usual site). Endoprosthetic or other reconstruction may not be necessary, but such patients will need to have protected weight bearing in cast braces for 12 weeks or more post-operatively while the area of resection reforms.

Post-radiation and Paget's osteosarcoma

These tumours are defined as occurring in a previously normal bone within the irradiation field but usually include osteosarcoma occurring after Ewing's sarcoma. The incidence in patients with breast cancer is approximately 0.05 per cent. These tumours are often of high histological grade and the distinction from other forms of spindle cell sarcoma such as malignant fibrous histiocytoma may be difficult. The mainstay of treatment is surgical resection, but the lesions often occur in the axial skeleton (the site of previous irradiation or Paget's disease), which may make resection difficult. The tumours are usually highly malignant, with pulmonary metastases occurring early (Robinson *et al.* 1988). Little is known of their chemosensitivity but in Paget's sarcoma the age of the patient will often preclude intensive drug therapy. The overall prognosis is poor for radiation and Paget's sarcoma (Huvos 1986). Early diagnosis and radical resection are essential.

Osteosarcoma during pregnancy

Rarely the tumour may be diagnosed during pregnancy or a patient may become pregnant shortly after treatment is completed. There is no evidence that pregnancy worsens the prognosis of osteosarcoma as judged by matching cases with historical controls in the era before chemotherapy (Huvos *et al.* 1985). In modern practice the necessity for early chemotherapy means that a termination should be advised if the patient is in the first trimester and early delivery is advisable in the third trimester (Simon *et al.* 1984).

Osteosarcoma in the elderly

Osteosarcoma may occur in elderly people, even in bones that are not the site of Paget's disease or previous irradiation. In an analysis of 101 patients over the age of 60 (approximately 10 per cent of all cases), Huvos (1986) found that 58 of the skeletal tumours arose in a bone with Paget's disease and six arose at an irradiated site. The fibrohistiocytomatous and osteoblastic variants were the most frequent (55 per cent of cases). The distribution of involved bones was quite different from the juvenile form, with many more axial skeletal tumours. Median survival was only 1 year for the Paget's-associated tumours, with 4 per cent 5 year survival and was 18 months for the primary (*de novo*) tumours, with 30 per cent 5 year survival. Treatment can present formidable problems due to tumour location and the difficulty in giving chemotherapy of sufficient intensity to this population. Indeed, Huvos (1986) could find no evidence of improved survival in the period after 1974.

REFERENCES

Abrahamson DH, Ellsworth RM, Zimmerman LE (1976). Non-ocular cancer in retinoblastoma survivors. *Transactions of the Academy of Ophthalmology and Otolaryngology*, 81:454–7.

Abrahamson DH, *et al.* (1984). Second non-ocular tumors in retinoblastoma survivors. Are they radiation induced? *Ophthalmology*, 91:1351–5.

Aisen AM, Martel W, Braunstein EM, McMillin KI, Phillips WJ, Kling TF (1986). MR and CT evaluation of primary bone and soft tissue tumours. *American Journal of Roentgenology*, 146:749–56.

Ayala AG, *et al.* (1989). Small cell osteosarcoma: a clinicopathologic study of 27 cases. *Cancer*, 64:2162–73.

Bacci G, *et al.* (1986). Adriamycin/methotrexate high dose versus adriamycin/methotrexate moderate dose as adjuvant chemotherapy for osteosarcoma of the extremities: a randomized study. *Journal of Cancer and Oncology*, 22:1337–45.

Benjamin RS (1989). Regional chemotherapy for osteosarcoma. *Seminars in Oncology*, 16:323–7.

Benjamin RS, *et al.* (1978). Chemotherapy of metastatic osteosarcoma — studies by the M. D. Anderson Hospital and the Southwest Oncology Group. *Cancer Treatment Reports*, 62:237–8.

Bohndorf K, Reiser M, Lochner B, Feaux de Lacroix W, Steinbrich W (1986). Magnetic resonance imaging of primary tumours and tumour-like lesions of bone. *Skeletal Radiology*, 15:511–17.

Bradish CF, Kemp HBS, Scales JT, Wilson JN (1987). Distal femoral replacement by custom-made prostheses. *Journal of Bone and Joint Surgery*, 69B:276–84.

Bramwell V, *et al.* (1988). Preliminary report of the first European Osteosarcoma Intergroup Study. *American Association of Clinical Oncology* (Abstract).

Bramwell VHC, *et al.* (1992). A comparison of two short intensive adjuvant chemotherapy regimens in operable osteosarcoma of limbs in children and young adults: the first study of the European Osteosarcoma Intergroup. *Journal of Clinical Oncology*, 10:1579–91.

Broders AC (1964). The microscopic grading of cancer. In *Treatment of cancer and allied diseases* (ed. GT Pack and IM Arrel). Hoeber, New York.

Burgers JHV, *et al.* (1980). Role of metastatectomy without chemotherapy in the management of osteosarcoma in children. *Cancer*, 45:1664–8.

Burk CD, Belasco JB, O'Neil JA, Lange B (1991). Pulmonary metastases and bone sarcoma. Surgical removal of lesions appearing after adjuvant chemotherapy. *Clinical Orthopaedics*, 262:88–92.

Burrows JHF, Wilson JN, Scales JT (1975). Excision of tumours of humerus and femur with restoration by internal prosthesis. *Journal of Bone and Joint Surgery*, 57B, 353–9.

Campannacci M, Cappanna R, Cervellati C, Guerra A, Calderoni P (1983). Modular rotary endoprosthesis of the proximal humerus. In *Tumour prostheses for bone and joint reconstruction* (ed. E Chao and J Ivins). Thieme-Stratton, New York.

Cannonn SR, Dyson PHP (1987). The relationship of the location of open biopsy of maligant bone tumours to local recurrence after resection and prosthetic replacement. *Journal of Bone and Joint Surgery*, 69B:492.

Chawla SP, *et al.* (1985). High rates of complete remission limb salvage and prolonged survival in telangiectactic osteosarcoma after pre-operative chemotherapy with intra-arterial cisplatinum and systemic adriamycin. *Proceedings of the American Society of Clinical Oncology*, 4:152.

Cohen M, *et al.* (1982). Lung CT for detection of metastases: solid tissue neoplasms in children. *American Journal of Radiology*, 139:895–8.

Cortes EP, Holland JF (1981). Adjuvant chemotherapy for primary osteogenic sarcoma. *Surgical Clinics of North America*, 61:1391–404.

Cortes EP, Holland JF, Wang JJ, Sinks LF (1972). Doxorubicin in disseminated osteosarcoma. *Journal of the American Medical Association*, 221:1132–8.

Dahlin DC (1978). Osteosarcoma of bone and a consideration of prognostic variables. *Cancer Treatment Reports*, 62:189–92.

Dahlin DC, Coventry MB (1967). Osteogenic sarcoma: a study of 600 cases. *Journal of Bone and Joint Surgery*, 49:101–10.

Dooms GC, Hricak H, Sollitto RA, Higgins CB (1985). Lipomatous tumours and tumours with fatty component: MR imaging potential and comparison of MR and CT results. *Radiology*, 157:479–83.

Draper GJ, Sanders BM, Kingston JE (1986). Second primary neoplasms in children with retinoblastoma. *British Journal of Cancer*, 53:661–71.

Eckhardt JJ, *et al.* (1985). Management of stage IIB osteogenic sarcoma: experience at the University of California. *Los Angeles Cancer Treatment Symposia*, 3:117–30.

Edmonson JH, *et al.* (1984). A controlled pilot study of high-dose methotrexate as post-surgical adjuvant treatment for primary osteosarcoma. *Journal of Clinical Oncology*, 2:152–6.

Enneking WF (1987). *International symposium on limb salvage in musculoskeletal oncology, 1985.* Churchill Livingstone, Edinburgh.

Enneking WF, Kagan A (1975). 'Skip' metastases in osteosarcoma. *Cancer*, 36:2192–205.

Enneking WF, Eady SL, Burchardt HL (1980a). Autogenous cortical bone grafts in the reconstruction of segmental skeletal defects. *Journal of Bone and Joint Surgery*, 62A:1039–58.

Enneking WF, Spanier SS, Goodman MA (1980b). A system for the surgical staging of musculoskeletal sarcoma. *Clinical Orthopaedics and Related Research*, 153:106–20.

Friedman MA, Carter SK (1972). The therapy of osteogenic sarcoma: current status and thoughts for the future. *Journal of Surgical Oncology*, 4:482–510.

Friend SH, *et al.* (1986). A human DNA segment with properties of the gene that predisposes to retinoblastoma and osteosarcoma. *Nature*, 323:643–6.

Gasparini M, *et al.* (1985). Phase II study of cisplatin in advanced osteogenic sarcoma. *Cancer Treatment Reports*, 69:211–13.

Goorin AM, et al. (1984). Prognostic significance of complete surgical resection of pulmonary metastases in patients with osteogenic sarcoma: analysis of 32 patients. *Journal of Clinical Oncology*, 2:425–31.

Grem JL, King SA, Wittes RE, Leyland-Jones B (1988). The role of methotrexate in osteosarcoma. *Journal of the National Cancer Institute*, 80:626–56.

Haibach H, Carrell C, Dittrich FJ (1985). Neoplasms arising in Paget's disease of bone: a study of 82 cases. *American Journal of Clinical Pathology*, 83:594–600.

Han M-T, et al. (1981). Aggressive thoracotomy for pulmonary metastatic osteogenic sarcoma in children and young adolescents. *Journal of Pediatric Surgery*, 16:928–33.

Huvos AG (1986). Osteogenic sarcoma of bones and soft tissues in older persons. A clinicopathologic analysis of 117 patients older than 60 years. *Cancer*, 57:1442–9.

Huvos AG, et al. (1982). Telangiectatic osteosarcoma: a clinico-pathologic study of 124 cases. *Cancer*, 49:1679–89.

Huvos AG, Butler A, Betsky SS (1983). Osteogenic sarcoma in the American black. *Cancer*, 52:1959–65.

Huvos AG, Butler A, Betsky SS (1985). Osteogenic sarcoma in pregnant women. Prognosis, therapeutic implications and literature review. *Cancer*, 56:2326–31.

Jaffe N (1972). Recent advances in the chemotherapy of metastatic osteosarcoma. *Cancer*, 30:1627–31.

Jaffe N, Frei E, Traggis D, Bishop Y (1974). Adjuvant methotrexate and citrivorum factor treatment of osteogenic sarcoma. *New England Journal of Medicine*, 291:994–7.

Jaffe N, et al. (1985). Comparison of intra-arterial *cis*-diammine dichloroplatinum II with high dose methotrexate and citrovorum factor rescue in the treatment of primary osteosarcoma. *Journal of Clinical Oncology*, 3:101.

Jaffe N, et al. (1987). Pathologic fracture in osteosarcoma. Impact of chemotherapy on primary tumour and survival. *Cancer*, 59:701–9.

Jeffree GM, Price CHG, Sissons HA (1975). The metastatic patterns of osteosarcoma. *British Journal of Cancer*, 32:87–107.

Kotz R, Salzer M (1982). Rotation-plasty for childhood osteosarcoma of the distal part of the femur. *Journal of Bone and Joint Surgery*, 64A:959–69.

Lange B, Levin AS (1982). Is it ethical not to conduct a prospectively controlled trial of adjuvant chemotherapy in osteosarcoma? *Cancer Treatment Reports*, 66:1699–704.

Lewis RJ, Lotz MJ (1974). Medullary extension of osteosarcoma. *Cancer*, 33:371.

Lexer E (1925). Joint transplantations and arthroplasty. *Surgery, Gynaecology and Obstetrics*, 40:782.

Link MP, et al. (1986). The effect of adjuvant chemotherapy on relapse-free survival in patients with osteosarcoma of the extremity. *New England Journal of Medicine*, 134:1600–6.

Lodwick GS, Wilson AJ, Farrell C, Virtama P, Dittrich F (1980). Determining growth rates of focal lesions of bone from radiographs. *Radiology*, 134:577–83.

Mail JT, Cohen MD, Mirkin LD, Provisor AJ (1985). Response of osteosarcoma to pre-operative intravenous high dose methotrexate therapy: CT evaluation. *American Journal of Radiology*, 144:89–94.

Mankin H, Fogelson F, Thrasher A (1975). Massive allograft transplantation for bone tumours. *Journal of Bone and Joint Surgery*, 57A:1171.

Mankin HJ, Deppelt SH, Sullivan TR, Tomford WW (1982a). Osteoarticular and intercalary allograft transplantation in the management of malignant tumours of bone. *Cancer*, 50:613–30.

Mankin HJ, Lange TA, Spanier SS (1982b). The hazards of biopsy in patients with malignant primary bone and soft tissue tumours. *Journal of Bone and Joint Surgery*, 64A:1121.

Marcove RS (1977). En bloc resection for osteogenic sarcoma. *Cancer Journal of Surgery*, 20:521.

Marcove RS, Rosen G (1979). *En bloc* resections for osteogenic sarcoma. *Bulletin of the New York Academy of Medicine*, 55:44.

Marcove RS, Lewis MM, Huvos AG (1977). *En bloc* upper humeral interscapulothoracic resection: the Tikhoff–Linberg procedure. *Clinical Orthopaedics*, 124:219.

Mavligit GM (1981). Intra-arterial cisplatin for patients with inoperable skeletal tumors. *Cancer*, 48:1.

Medical Research Council (1986). A trial of chemotherapy in osteosarcoma. (A report to the Medical Research Council by their Working Party on Bone Sarcoma.) *British Journal of Cancer*, 53:513–18.

Meyer WH, et al. (1987). Thoracotomy for pulmonary metastatic osteosarcoma. An analysis of prognostic indicators of survival. *Cancer*, 59:374–9.

Moore AT, Bohlmann HR (1943). Metal hip joint, a case report. *Journal of Bone and Joint Surgery*, 25:688–92.

Morgan E, et al. (1984). Treatment of patients with metastatic osteogenic sarcoma: a report from the Children's Cancer Study Group. *Cancer Treatment Reports*, 68:661–4.

Mulvihill JJ, Gralnick HR, Whang-Peng J, Leventhal BE (1977). Multiple childhood osteosarcomas in an American Indian family with erythroid macrocytosis and skeletal anomalies. *Cancer*, 40:3113–22.

Murray IP (1980). Bone scanning in the child and young adult. Part 1. *Skeletal Radiology*, 5:1–14.

Newton WA, et al. (1991). Bone sarcomas as second malignant neoplasms following childhood cancer. *Cancer*, 67:193–201.

Nilsonne U (1969). Homologous joint transplantation in man. *Acta Orthopaedica Scandinavica*, 40:429–47.

Ottolenghi CE (1966). Massive osteoarticular bone grafts. Transplant of the whole femur. *Journal of Bone and Joint Surgery*, 48B:646–59.

Pack GT, McNeer G, Coley BL (1942). Interscapulo-thoracic amputation for malignant tumours of the upper extremity. A report of 31 consecutive cases. *Surgery, Gynecology, Obstetrics*, 74:161.

Picci P, et al. (1987). Neoadjuvant chemotherapy for localised osteosarcoma of the extremities. In *Adjuvant therapy of cancer V* (ed. SE Salmon), pp. 711–17. Grune & Stratton, Philadelphia.

Polednak AP (1978). Bone cancer among female radium dial workers. Latency periods and incidence rates by time after exposure. *Journal of the National Cancer Institute*, 60:77–82.

Polednak AP (1985). Primary bone cancer in blacks and whites in New York State. *Cancer*, 55:2883–90.

Pratt CB, Shanks EC (1974). Doxorubicin in treatment of malignant solid tumours in children. *American Journal of Diseases of Children*, 127:534–6.

Pratt CB, et al. (1984). Results of adjuvant chemotherapy for 77 patients with osteosarcoma of an extremity 1973–1981. *Proceedings of the American Society of Clinical Oncology*, 3:257.

Pratt CB, et al. (1985). Treatment of unresectable or metastatic osteosarcoma with cisplatin or cisplatin–doxorubicin. *Cancer*, 56:1930–3.

Price CHG, Goldie W (1969). Paget's sarcoma of bone. A study of 80 cases from the Bristol and Leeds Bone Tumour Registries. *Journal of Bone and Joint Surgery*, 51B:205–24.

Pringle JAS (1987). Pathology of bone tumours. *Baillière's Clinical Oncology*, 1(1):21–63.

Putnam JB, Roth JA, Wesley MN, Johnston MN, Johnston MR, Rosenberg SA (1983). Survival following aggressive resection of pulmonary metastases from osteogenic sarcoma: analysis of prognostic factors. *Annals of Thoracic Surgery*, 36:516–23.

Robinson E, Neught AI, Wylie P (1988). Clinical aspects of postirradiation sarcoma. *Journal of the National Cancer Institute*, 80: 233–40.

Rosen G, Marcove RC, Caparros R, Nirenberg A, Kosloff C, Huvos AG (1979). Primary osteogenic sarcoma. The rationale for preoperative chemotherapy and delayed surgery. *Cancer*, 43:163–77.

Rosen G, et al. (1982a). Preoperative chemotherapy for osteogenic sarcoma: selection of postoperative adjuvant chemotherapy based on the response of the primary tumour to preoperative chemotherapy. *Cancer*, 49:1221–30.

Rosen G, et al. (1982b). Cisplatin–adriamycin combination chemotherapy in evaluable osteosarcoma. *Proceedings of the American Society of Clinical Oncology*, 1:173.

Rosen G, et al. (1983). Primary osteogenic sarcoma: eight year experience with adjuvant chemotherapy. *Journal of Cancer Research and Clinical Oncology*, 106:55–67.

Rosen G, Huvos AG, Marcove R, Nirenberg A (1986). Telangiectatic osteogenic sarcoma. *Clinical Orthopaedics*, 207:164–73.

Rosenberg SA, et al. (1979). Treatment of osteogenic sarcoma. 1. Effect of adjuvant high-dose methotrexate after amputation. *Cancer Treatment Reports*, 63:739–75.

Ross, FGM (1964). Osteogenic sarcoma. *British Journal of Radiology*, 37:259–76.

Roth JA, Putnam JB, Wesley MN, Rosenberg SA (1984). Differing determinants of prognosis following resection of pulmonary metastases from osteogenic and soft tissue sarcoma patients. *Cancer*, 55:1361–6.

Sanerkin NG (1980). Definitions of osteosarcoma, chondrosarcoma and fibrosarcoma of bone. *Cancer*, **46**:178–85.

Sim FH, Unni KK, Beabout JW, Dahlin DC (1979). Osteosarcoma with small cells simulating Ewing's tumor. *Journal of Bone and Joint Surgery*, **61A**:207–15.

Simon MA (1982). Current concepts review biopsy of musculoskeletal tumours. *Journal of Bone and Joint Surgery*, **64A**:1253.

Simon MA, Bos GD (1980). Epiphyseal extension of metaphyseal osteosarcoma in skeletally immature individuals. *Journal of Bone and Joint Surgery*, **62A**:195–204.

Simon MA (1984). Causes of increased survival of patients with osteosarcoma. Current controversies. *Journal of Bone and Joint Surgery*, **66A**:306–9.

Simon MA, Hecht JD (1982). Invasion of joints by primary bone sarcomas in adults. *Cancer*, **50**:1649–55.

Simon MA, Phillips WA, Bonfiglio M (1984). Pregnancy and aggressive or malignant bone tumors. *Cancer*, **53**:564–9.

Smith WS, Simon MA (1975). Segmental resection for chondrosarcoma. *Journal of Bone and Joint Surgery*, **57A**:1097–103.

Souhami RL (1987). Incidence and aetiology of malignant primary bone tumours. In *Bone tumours* (ed. RL Souhami), *Baillière's Clinical Oncology*, Vol. 1, No. 1, pp. 1–20. London.

Spanos PK, Payne WS, Ivins JC, Pritchard DJ (1976). Pulmonary resection for metastatic osteogenic sarcoma. *Journal of Bone and Joint Surgery*, **58**:624–8.

Stephens FO, Tattersall MHN, Marsden W, Waugh RC, Green D, McCarthy SW (1987). Regional chemotherapy with the use of cisplatin and doxorubicin as primary treatment for advanced sarcomas in shoulder, pelvis and thigh. *Cancer*, **60**:724–35.

Strander H, *et al.* (1979). Adjuvant inteferon treatment of osteosarcoma. *Recent Results in Cancer Research*, **68**:40–4.

Strong LC, Henderson J, Osbourne BM, Satow WW (1979). Risk of radiation-related subsequent malignant tumours in survivors of Ewing's sarcoma. *Journal of the National Cancer Institute*, **62**:1401–5.

Sweetnam R (1973). Amputation in osteosarcoma. *Journal of Bone and Joint Surgery*, **55B**:189.

Taylor WF, *et al.* (1989). Trends and variability in survival among patients with osteosarcoma: a 7 year update. *Mayo Clinic Proceedings*, **60**:91–104.

Taylor WF, Ivins JC, Unni KK, Beabout JW, Cjolenzer HJ, Black LE (1989). Prognostic variables in osteosarcoma: a multi-institutional study. *Journal of the National Cancer Institute*, **81**:21–31.

Toguchida J, *et al.* (1988). Chromosomal reorganization for the expression of recessive mutation of retinoblastoma susceptibility gene in the development of osteosarcoma. *Cancer Research*, **48**:3939–43.

Toguchida J, *et al.* (1989). Assignment of common allele cross in osteosarcoma to the subregion 17p13. *Cancer Research*, **49**:6247–51.

Unni KK, Dahlin DC, Beabout JW (1976). Periosteal osteogenic sarcoma. *Cancer*, **37**:2476–85.

Van Nes CP (1948). Transplantation of the tibia and fibula to replace the femur following resection. *Journal of Bone and Joint Surgery*, **30A**:854–8.

Volkov M (1970). Allotransplantation of joints. *Journal of Bone and Joint Surgery*, **52B**:49–53.

Ward PS, *et al.* (1984). Location of the retinoblastoma susceptibility gene(s) and the human esterase D locus. *Journal of Medical Genetics*, **21**:92–5.

Weatherby RP, Dahlin DC, Ivins JC (1981). Post-radiation sarcoma of bone: review of 78 Mayo clinic cases. *Mayo Clinic Proceedings*, **56**:294–306.

Winkler K, Bielack S (1988). Chemotherapy of osteosarcoma. *Seminars in Orthopaedics*, **3**:48–58.

Winkler K, *et al.* (1984). Neoadjuvant chemotherapy for osteogenic sarcoma: results of a cooperative German/Austrian study. *Journal of Clinical Oncology*, **2**:617–24.

Winkler K, *et al.* (1986). Einfluß des Lokalchirurgischen Vorgehens auf die Inzidenz von Metastasen nach Neoadjuvanten Chemotherapie des Osteosarcoms. *Zeitschrift für Orthopädie*, **124**:22–9.

Winkler K, *et al.* (1988). Neoadjuvant chemotherapy of osteosarcoma: results of a randomized cooperative trial (Coss-82) with salvage chemotherapy based on histological tumour response. *Journal of Clinical Oncology*, **6**:329–37.

Wold LE, Unni KK, Beabout JW (1984). Dedifferentiated parosteal osteosarcoma. *Journal of Bone and Joint Surgery*, **66A**:53–9.

Zimmer WD, *et al.* (1985). Bone tumours: magnetic resonance imaging versus computed tomography. *Radiology*, **155**:709–18.

13.5 Malignant bone tumours other than osteosarcoma and Ewing's sarcoma

PAOLO CASALI AND ARMANDO SANTORO

Most malignant bone tumours (Table 1) other than osteosarcoma and Ewing's sarcoma are rare. However, chondrosarcoma has an intermediate incidence between these two tumours.

From the epidemiological point of view, rare malignant bone tumours differ from osteosarcoma and Ewing's sarcoma in that they arise after skeletal maturity. Whereas osteosarcoma has its peak incidence in the second decade of life, they tend to affect the middle-aged adult in the third to fifth decade, although younger people may also be affected.

Rare bone tumours often resemble osteosarcoma in clinical behaviour and biological aggressiveness. However, while osteosarcoma is usually a high-grade neoplasm and Ewing's sarcoma is always a high-grade malignancy with a systemic attitude, rare bone tumours vary widely even within the same histological type. In fact, most histological types are further divided into grades I–III.

Pathological diagnosis may be difficult. Differential diagnosis against osteosarcoma is based on the absence of tumour osteoid

Table 1 Histotypes included in bone tumours

Osteosarcoma
Chondrosarcoma
Ewing's sarcoma
Giant cell tumour
Malignant fibrous histiocytoma
Fibrosarcoma
Adamantinoma
Haemangioendothelioma, angiosarcoma, and malignant haemangiopericytoma
Chordoma
Neuroectodermal bone tumour
Other tumours (liposarcoma, neurogenic sarcoma, etc.)

production and alkaline phosphatase content (Sanerkin 1980*a*). In the case of malignancies such as chondrosarcoma or fibrosarcoma of bone, osteosarcoma (that is, chondroblastic osteosarcoma and fibroblastic osteosarcoma, respectively) will not be diagnosed if tumour osteoid is undetectable. Similarly, a biopsy specimen from the soft tissue component of a primary osteosarcoma may be indistinguishable from a specimen from a primary soft tissue sarcoma. For example, a soft tissue biopsy specimen from an osteosarcoma like the malignant fibrous histiocytoma subtype is indistinguishable from a malignant fibrous histiocytoma of soft tissues. Therefore it follows that differentiation requires consideration of the radiographic findings (whether neoplastic bone formation is present) and/or evaluation of a suitable osseous specimen (whether foci of osteoid production are present, since the periosteal zone may contain reactive osteoid).

Clinical presentation is similar to all bone tumours in terms of bone pain, swelling, and functional impotence. The site of origin may suggest the diagnosis (Moser 1987). Osteosarcoma typically arises from the metaphysis of long bones and Ewing's sarcoma arises from the diaphysis. Tumours such as malignant fibrous histiocytoma and fibrosarcoma tend to affect the same regions as affected by osteosarcoma, with the knee frequently being involved. Likewise, chondrosarcoma is detectable at the metaphysis of long bones, but a truncal origin is frequent. Giant-cell tumour typically affects the metaphysis to the epiphysis. Adamantinoma classically arises from the cortical region of the diaphysis (particularly the tibia). Chordoma has a preferential site of origin along the spinal column, particularly at its extremities.

Radiographic aspects should be described, as is usual for bone lesions, in terms of margins, periosteal reaction, and matrix (Moser 1987). Margins will be of the malignant type, that is, ill-defined, except for the less malignant giant cell tumour which tends to present as a well-demarcated lesion. The most malignant lesions may display a pattern of clusters of multiple lesions (moth-eaten and permeative destruction rather than the solitary lesion pattern). Periosteal reaction reflects the biological aggressiveness of the neoplasm and therefore will be found in the most malignant tumours. The pattern usually shows an interrupted or spiculated reaction or both. The appearance of the matrix usually differs from the homogeneous mineralization seen with osteosarcoma. Chondrosarcoma usually displays a pattern of discrete mineralization due to its mineralized cartilagineous matrix. Tumours which do not produce osteoid or cartilage will present as lesions without a mineralized matrix. Such lytic lesions must be differentiated from osteolytic osteosarcoma, lytic bone metastases, lymphoma, plasmocytoma, multiple myeloma, and bone cysts.

Series of rare bone tumours are usually small and it is not easy to draw conclusions with regard to standard treatment. Therefore cases should be properly recorded and series should be reported after accurate diagnosis and follow-up of each patient. Grading provides information concerning the biological aggressiveness of the tumour (Unni and Dahlin 1984) and can help to tailor treatment to the individual case, even in the absence of adequate published information on the given histotype. Low-grade tumours generally pose problems of local relapse, whereas high-grade forms tend to grow faster, have a higher potential to metastasize, and therefore possess a worse prognosis.

Surgery is the preferred treatment in all these tumours, with application of the same basic principles as used for osteosarcoma. Inadequate surgery should always be avoided. In low-grade tumours less destructive surgery (limited excision, cryosurgery, etc.) may be undertaken in selected cases. High-grade tumours should be treated as an osteosarcoma, with the same criteria for limb-sparing surgery applicable to both indications and techniques (Kemp 1987). Pre-operative evaluation using CT scanning and magnetic resonance imaging (MRI) provide useful information from surgical planning.

Lung CT scan and whole-bone scans should always be performed during pre-operative staging.

Sarcomas are generally considered to be radioresistant. Therefore radiotherapy cannot usually substitute for surgery (Spooner 1987). However, it plays a useful rôle, particularly in some histotypes, at least in a palliative setting. Likewise, it should be used as an adjuvant to surgery whenever the latter has not been completely satisfactory. It should also be employed in those cases where surgery is technically impossible. Good long-term results have been reported in patients with malignancies such as chondrosarcoma and chordoma. It is possible that fast neutron radiotherapy may improve the results achievable with radiotherapy in both high-grade tumours with hypoxic zones and low-grade tumours with slow growth (Laramore et al. 1989).

Chemotherapy shows definite activity in some histological types (Earl 1987). In general terms, high-grade tumours are more likely to respond to chemotherapy than their low-grade counterparts. Since such neoplasms are also more likely to disseminate systemically, adjuvant chemotherapy is of potential interest and has been found to be of value in malignant fibrous histiocytoma. Primary (neoadjuvant) chemotherapy (that is, prior to primary surgery) is of increasing interest. A potential advantage of administering chemotherapy prior to surgery is that it is possible to determine whether an individual tumour is sensitive to the chemotherapy being employed. However, it is not clear whether this approach results in improved local control or more prolonged survival. None the less, in some cases it can make conservative surgery easier. Obviously, the routine role of adjuvant and neoadjuvant chemotherapy will be difficult to determine until more data from published series are available. However, large randomized studies are difficult to perform in such rare malignancies. Therefore, with regard to the high-grade tumours, clinicians are justified in judiciously applying the same approaches as followed in osteosarcoma and entering their patients into clinical trials whenever possible.

The choice of individual chemotherapeutic agents is also difficult because of the lack of properly conducted clinical trials. However, agents which are active against both osteosarcoma and soft tissue sarcomas, such as adriamycin and ifosfamide, are indicated. The effectiveness of high doses of methotrexate and cisplatin, which are specifically active against osteosarcoma but inactive against soft tissue sarcomas, has been established in malignant fibrous histiocytoma of bone.

Limited metastatic disease of the lungs is amenable to metastasectomy (possibly combined with chemotherapy). More widely disseminated metastatic disease can be managed with palliative chemotherapy and/or radiotherapy depending on the extent of disease and the site of major involvement.

The prognosis of these patients is governed largely by the therapeutic options available, which are usually related to the location and extent of the primary tumour and by the histological grade of the tumour. The preferred therapy for these rare tumours is still surgery. As far as adjuvant and neoadjuvant chemotherapy is concerned, reference should be made to experience in osteosarcoma with regard to the high-grade histological types.

CHONDROSARCOMA

Chondrosarcoma is a relatively frequent round cell bone neoplasm of the middle-aged and elderly. It encompasses a series of widely differing tumours in clinical behaviour, ranging from slowly growing non-metastasizing malignancies to high-grade types. These tumours were described as a separate entity by Keiller in 1925 and Phemister in 1930.

Chondrosarcoma is the second most common bone tumour, accounting for some 20 per cent of bone malignant neoplasms. It has its peak incidence in the fourth to sixth decade of life and occurs twice as frequently in males as in females. The majority of chondrosarcomas (90 per cent) are primary in origin but 10 per cent arise in pre-existing enchondromas.

Macroscopically, chondrosarcoma presents as a lobulated translucent mass of gelatinous consistency. The tumour may develop within the bone-marrow or protrude outside the bone, often giving rise to bulky masses. The histological appearance may closely resemble benign chondromas. The identification of cellular anaplasia is essential to the diagnosis. Three grades of malignancy, which correlate with the prognosis, can be distinguished (Evans *et al.* 1977). Grading is founded on the mitotic rate and other cytological features (Sanerkin 1980*b*). Globally, low-grade forms predominate (Unni and Dahlin 1984). The majority of chondrosarcomas can be classified into central or peripheral, according to the site of origin within the bone. The following rare histological types have been recognized.

Dedifferentiated chondrosarcoma (10 per cent of all chondrosarcomas) displays areas of undifferentiated non-chondroid large spindle cell mesenchymal tissue (resembling fibrosarcoma, osteosarcoma, malignant fibrous histiocytoma, or rhabdomyosarcoma) co-existing with other areas of well-differentiated chondroid tissue (Johnson *et al.* 1986). This aspect may be established after repeated relapses due to progressive dedifferentiation or differentiation of the two separate clones (Tètu *et al.* 1986). Dedifferentiated chondrosarcoma is one of the most malignant bone tumours, with the outcome being determined by the more malignant component.

Mesenchymal chondrosarcoma is a high-grade metastasizing neoplasm (Nakashima *et al.* 1986), often involving the ribs or jaw. Variously differentiated chondroid tissue is found together with areas of small anaplastic cells often distributed in a perivascular fashion. Although prolonged in some cases, the natural history is malignant, with a high metastatic potential. Mesenchymal chondrosarcoma may also present with a similar picture to soft tissue sarcomas, typically with calcification detectable on radiographs.

Clear cell chondrosarcoma is characterized by the presence of distinct clear cells with abundant cytoplasm (Unni *et al.* 1976). It tends to behave as a low-grade slowly growing lesion which rarely metastasizes, but is likely to recur if inadequately excised.

The clinical presentation is dependent upon the site of the tumour. The pelvis is the most frequently affected site, followed by the femur, the humerus, and other bones. Central chondrosarcomas usually present with pain, which is an important indicator of active malignant disease. Peripheral chondrosarcomas generally present as large masses which are less frequently painful. Radiology shows destruction of the medullary portion of bone and the cartilagineous mass often contains areas of discrete calcification which may be stippled, flocculent, or form rings and arcs. Diagnosis requires an adequate incisional biopsy from a non-necrotic area of tumour. Metastases most frequently involve the lungs, with metastases to bone, lymph nodes (rare in classical chondrosarcoma but more frequent in mesenchymal chondrosarcoma), skin, and soft tissues occurring less often.

Surgery is the treatment of choice whenever technically feasible. Mesenchymal chondrosarcoma has been reported to respond to adriamycin, bleomycin, actinomycin D, cyclophosphamide, and ifosfamide, but not to methotrexate (Huvos *et al.* 1983). Results with chemotherapy in classical chondrosarcoma are less conclusive (Earl 1987). Attempts to improve evaluation of chemotherapy and to test it in adjuvant settings may be worthwhile, particularly

in high-grade chondrosarcomas such as the mesenchymal and dedifferentiated types. Contrary to previous beliefs, chondrosarcoma seems quite sensitive to radiotherapy (Harwood *et al.* 1980). The latter should be resorted to whenever locoregional disease is not amenable to surgery and after a less than radical surgical excision. Radiotherapy alone or in combination with chemotherapy may provide some chances of cure in patients who are not amenable to surgery but who have only local disease (McNaney *et al.* 1982).

One of the most important prognostic factors is the grade of the primary tumour. Ten year survivals have been reported as 83, 64, and 29 per cent for grades I, II, and III chondrosarcomas, respectively (Evans *et al.* 1977). A significant difference in overall survival has been demonstrated between grades I and II tumours, which are more frequent and grade III tumours. Peripheral tumours tend to be of a lower grade than central tumours. Grade I tumours do not seem to metastasize even after repeated recurrences, while grade II tumours metastasize in a minority of cases and grade III metastasize in most cases. In one series the metastatic risk was 5 per cent for low-grade lesions, 14 per cent for medium-grade lesions, and 75 per cent for high-grade lesions (Sanerkin and Gallagher 1979). The feasibility of a radical surgical resection has been demonstrated to be a fundamental prognostic criterion. Unfortunately, chondrosarcomas often present as gross unresectable masses and, even when surgery is adequate, recurrences may occur several years after primary therapy. Some patients have been reported as surviving for many years even in the presence of uncontrolled local tumour.

MALIGNANT FIBROUS HISTIOCYTOMA

Since its first description by O'Brien (1964), malignant fibrous histiocytoma has become the most frequently diagnosed histological subtype of soft tissue sarcomas. Its bone counterpart was first described as a distinct entity by Feldman and Norman (1972), and since then several hundred cases have been reported (Dahlin *et al.* 1977; Capanna *et al.* 1984). Malignant fibrous histiocytoma of bone is a usually high-grade spindle cell bone tumour.

Malignant fibrous histiocytoma of bone accounts for approximately 5 per cent of all bone tumours. The peak incidence of the disease is in the fifth decade, but it may occur at any age. Females seem to be preferentially affected in the second decade rather than in middle age. The male to female ratio is 1.7 : 1.

Pathologically, malignant fibrous histiocytoma of bone resembles malignant fibrous histiocytoma of soft tissues. A mixture of spindle cells together with histiocytic-like cells and giant cells gives rise to the typical storiform arrangement. This tumour must be differentiated from malignant fibrous histiocytoma of soft tissues and the malignant fibrous histiocytoma subtype of osteosarcoma. The former is diagnosed whenever the tumour arises from soft tissues and only secondarily infiltrates the bone. The latter is distinguishable on a pathological basis (Mirra 1980; Ballance *et al.* 1988) by osteoid production or the presence of bony structures which are lacking in malignant fibrous histiocytoma of bone.

The clinical presentation resembles other bone tumours with a history of variable duration. The long bones seem the most frequent site of origin. The region of the knee represents a site of predilection as is seen with osteosarcoma. Alkaline phosphatase levels are usually normal but may be elevated. The radiographic aspect of the tumour is one of a neoplastic lytic lesion with ill-defined margins, possibly with cortical perforation, periosteal reaction, and extraosseous growth. Clinically as well as pathologically, malignant fibrous histiocytoma of bone behaves as a high-grade sarcoma.

Traditionally, primary treatment has been surgical in many of the published cases. None the less, chemotherapy has been utilized increasingly in the recent past and its effectiveness has been reported (Bassett and Weiss 1978; Shuman et al. 1982; Urban et al. 1983; den Heeten et al. 1985). Its effect on the disease has been demonstrated through pathological data on response available in the neoadjuvant setting. Several cases of complete pathological response (no viable cells, Rosen grade IV type of regression) have been described. These responses were obtained with drugs proved to be active in osteosarcoma, such as adriamycin, high-dose methotrexate, and cisplatin. The latter two agents are not active in soft tissue sarcomas, which suggests that, from a clinical point of view, malignant fibrous histiocytoma bears a greater resemblance to osteosarcoma than to its soft tissue counterpart.

The natural history of the disease is one of an aggressive neoplasm with a potential to recur locally and to metastasize rapidly to lungs and bone (Capanna et al. 1984). Lymph node metastases are more common than in osteosarcoma (Spanier et al. 1975), but they remain an infrequent observation. The long-term survival from reported series is of the order of 35 per cent. Although adequate surgery is critical, death from systemic dissemination is all too frequent. As is the case in osteosarcoma, chemotherapy is very likely to alter the course of the disease significantly (Weiner et al. 1983; Chawla et al. 1984). A combined modality approach using adjuvant or neoadjuvant chemotherapy together with surgery seems advisable in view of the demonstrated chemosensitivity of the disease, its clinical aggressiveness, its high-grade attitude, and the relatively unfavourable prognosis after surgery alone.

FIBROSARCOMA

Fibrosarcoma of bone was first distinguished from fibrosarcoma of soft tissues with bony involvement by MacDonald and Budd (1943). Fibrosarcoma is a spindle cell bone tumour of either high- or low-grade malignancy.

Fibrosarcoma accounts for less than 5 per cent of bone tumours and the incidence has decreased after recognition of malignant fibrous histiocytoma as a distinct entity. Peak incidence is around the fourth decade and there is a slight predilection for females. Distribution by site does not differ in essence from osteosarcoma, with the distal femur most frequently involved. Fibrosarcoma may grow within an irradiated area, as well as in a previous osteoclastoma, in Paget's disease, in fibrous dysplasia, or in bone infarcts (Dahlin and Ivins 1969).

Pathologically, fibrosarcoma often presents as a high-grade fibroblastic tumour, but low-grade cases may occur and are more frequent than in osteosarcoma and malignant fibrous histiocytoma of bone. Distinction from fibroblastic osteosarcoma rests on the lack of osteoid production, while the lack of cellular pleomorphism helps distinguish it from malignant fibrous histiocytoma of bone. Medullary (central) fibrosarcoma has been distinguished from periostal (peripheral) fibrosarcoma (Bertoni et al. 1984). The former arises from the medullary or cortical parts of the bone, while the latter has its origin in the periostium. The existence of the periostal fibrosarcoma has been denied by some authors, who claim that it is a soft tissue fibrosarcoma secondarily infiltrating bone tissue.

Clinically, osteolysis is the prominent radiographic sign, while symptoms are not specific. Several months and even years may pass between the beginning of symptoms and the diagnosis.

Surgical extirpation with radical intent is the treatment of choice. Grading of the tumour should be taken into account, since a wide excision seems to guarantee local control in low-grade tumours. Periosteal lesions are more often of low grade. However, limb-sparing surgery should be attempted even in high-grade lesions whenever feasible. Insufficient data are available on chemotherapy, which might be assumed to be active in high-grade lesions (Earl 1987). The value of an integrated approach to locoregional disease, as in osteosarcoma and malignant fibrous histiocytoma, is currently under investigation. Radiotherapy plays only a palliative role.

Long-term follow-up of these patients is important because metastases may appear 5 years or more after the diagnosis. Low-grade tumours have a better prognosis, with an 83 per cent survival at 10 years compared with 34 per cent for high-grade lesions (Bertoni et al. 1984). The site of origin also provides prognostic information, with periosteal tumours having better prognosis than medullary lesions while soft tissue extension worsens prognosis. In general terms the natural history of fibrosarcoma resembles that of osteosarcoma, but it tends to have a slower evolution with a delayed metastatic potential (Huvos and Higginbotham 1975).

BONE TUMOURS OF VASCULAR ORIGIN

The terms haemangioendothelioma and angiosarcoma have been used as synonyms or distinguished from each other (Thomas 1942; Unni et al. 1971), while haemangiopericytoma has usually been regarded as a separate entity. Haemangio-endothelioma can be considered as a well-differentiated vascular tumour and angiosarcoma as its more anaplastic and highly metastasizing counterpart.

Haemangioendothelioma

Haemangioendothelioma has been described as a locally aggressive non-metastasizing tumour. Therefore, it can be regarded as a rare low-grade tumour of vascular origin. All age groups can be afflicted and there is a predilection for men. Pathologically it presents as a haemorrhagic soft tumour, with histological evidence of neoplastic vascular tissue. The lesion may be multicentric in origin. The radiographic appearance is that of an osteolytic lesion, sometimes with a honeycomb pattern.

Treatment is adequate surgery. Local recurrence or, occasionally, the appearance of a new lesion is a potential problem, with metastases being rare.

Haemangiopericytoma

Haemangiopericytoma of bone was first described by Stout (1956). It is a low- or high-grade spindle cell tumour. In 1988 a review of the literature (Tang et al. 1988) included only 45 cases. Therefore the incidence is extremely low. In the Mayo Clinic series it was 0.1 per cent of malignant bone tumours. Peak incidence seems to be around 40–50 years and the male to female ratio is 1.8 : 1.

Pathologically, the neoplasm closely resembles soft tissue haemangiopericytoma. A grading system has been proposed which distinguishes three grades of malignancy according to cytological features and the number of mitoses.

Diagnosis may be preceded by a long history, which can date back for many years. The pelvis and the lower limbs are the most frequent sites of disease. The soft radiographic appearance is of an osteolytic bone lesion. Soft tissue extension may be present, as well as periosteal reaction.

Surgery is the standard treatment according to the same criteria as used in osteosarcoma. Chemotherapy and radiotherapy have been used, but their effectiveness is difficult to assess from the published studies. Local recurrences are frequent, occurring in 50 per cent or more of cases, as are distant metastases to lungs and bone. Metastases may occur after many years (up to 26 years). The long-term disease-free survival rate is approximately 30 per cent.

Angiosarcoma

Angiosarcoma of bone is very rare and it accounts for less than 0.5 per cent of malignant bone tumours. It is a high-grade sarcoma, with an aggressive metastasizing potential. It corresponds to high-grade haemangioendothelial sarcomas. Clinical features and radiographic aspect resemble other vascular tumours, but reflect the more aggressive behaviour of this tumour.

Treatment is surgical, but prognosis is strongly influenced by the rapid occurrence of distant metastases in a high proportion of cases. Vascularity may make surgery difficult. Radiotherapy seems effective (Chow *et al.* 1970) and this would prompt the use of combined approaches utilizing radiotherapy and possibly chemotherapy as an adjuvant to surgery (Earl 1987).

GIANT CELL TUMOUR OF BONE

Giant cell tumour of bone (osteoclastoma) accounts for 5–10 per cent of all bone tumours. Criteria for diagnosis and grading were detailed by Jaffe *et al.* (1940), while recognition of the tumour dates back to 1818. Osteoclastoma, which is basically a tumour prone to local recurrence, can be regarded as intermediate between a benign and a malignant lesion. However, metastases are possible, particularly in atypical cases with features of frank malignancy. They have also been reported in apparently benign lesions (Jewell and Bush 1964). The third to fifth decades are most affected, with a slight propensity for females to develop the disease (Dahlin *et al.* 1970).

The pathological aspect is one of stromal cells, both spindle and round, with multinucleate giant cells distributed among them. The neoplastic population is found within the stromal cells, displaying a variable number of mitoses. A grading system for giant cell tumour was proposed by Jaffe *et al.* (1940) and modified by Sanerkin (1980c). Giant cell tumours are usually grade I and grade II lesions with no atypical stromal cells and with some degree of atypism. The presence of increasing features of malignancy (abnormal mitoses and/or vascular permeation) has been categorized as grade II$^+$. Frankly sarcomatous tumours (grade III) have been reported to make up between 5 and 30 per cent of cases in various series and must be regarded as malignant and therefore potentially metastasizing.

The most frequent site of origin is the knee, with the long bones being typically affected eccentrically at the epiphysis with extension to the metaphysis (Nascimento *et al.* 1979). Radiologically, the lesion is an osteolytic with relatively well-defined margins, without osteoid formation, and with scarce perilesional reaction (Moser 1987). Giant cell tumours may be multifocal in origin. Therefore a skeletal global evaluation should be performed in every patient. The lungs should be investigated because of the possibility of lung metastases in even apparently low-grade and less malignant histotypes.

Surgery is curative in most cases, provided that it can be adequate (Campanacci *et al.* 1987). Cryosurgery, wide excision, or radical resection can be used according to the site of origin and tumour extension. Radiotherapy cannot substitute for surgery, but may be indicated (at doses of 40–50 Gy) whenever surgery is not feasible (Chen *et al.* 1986; Spooner 1987). Radiotherapy has been associated with a high rate of malignant transformation. No data are available on the effectiveness of chemotherapy. Metastasectomy should be considered for patients with lung metastases.

Grading is a useful prognostic factor with regard to the metastatic potential, whilst the probability of local recurrence is related more to the adequacy of primary surgery (Sanerkin 1980c). The recurrence rate has been reported to be as high as 62 per cent and as low as 23 per cent in published series (Dahlin *et al.* 1970; Larsson *et al.* 1975; Sanerkin 1980c).

CHORDOMA

Chordoma is a rare tumour, often diagnosed late because of initial lack of symptoms. It is assumed to arise from rests of the notochord along the spine. The name was applied by Muller, in 1958, to small non-neoplastic foci of heterotopic notochordal tissue. Chordoma are usually malignant tumours of low grade and therefore are slow growing and locally aggressive. Chordoma has an incidence of approximately 2 per cent of all malignant bone tumours. It is rarely diagnosed in patients under the age of 30 years and is more common in males than in females.

Pathologically, neoplastic cells may display various aspects of the maturation of the notochord, from spindle fibrosarcoma-like cells to epithelial-like elements. Mucus production may be impressive and cells may be arranged in aggregates floating within the mucus. Vacuoles of mucus may be detected within the cytoplasm. The presence of chondroid cells gives rise to the so-called chondroid chordoma, which tends to be less aggressive and therefore to result in more prolonged survivals. Benign chordomas make up less than 5 per cent of cases. Pathological distinction may not be simple and only the clinical findings may help establish the process as being benign in nature (with lack of invasion of surrounding organs).

Clinically, chordomas arise from the sacrum in 50 per cent of cases and from the base of the skull in 35 per cent (Mindell 1981; Rich *et al.* 1985; Azzarelli *et al.* 1988). The remaining 15 per cent of cases develop elsewhere in the spinal column; that is, away from the two ends. Clinical presentation will depend on the site of origin. Low back pain and bowel and urinary disturbances are frequent in sacral lesions, while various neurological signs (such as diplopia, etc.) may occur according to the localization of the disease. Symptoms may date from a long time before the diagnosis is made, a feature resulting from the slow growth of chordomas, particularly the chondroid variety. Pain may be a major problem in the advanced phase.

Surgery is the mainstay of treatment, provided that it is technically feasible (Chetiyawardana 1984). Fear of neurological damage secondary to surgery must be balanced against the certainty of such damage after disease progression and the lack of valid therapeutic alternatives. Bowel, bladder, and sexual dysfunction, along with pelvic instability, may complicate surgery of sacral chordomas, but may be minimal after high (S1–S2) resections. Radiotherapy has been employed in diverse instances (Cummings *et al.* 1983; Rich *et al.* 1985). It may be useful for palliation in advanced disease, with doses of more than 60 Gy being given in such cases. Partial relief of pain is very likely to be achieved in this way. In localized disease, radiotherapy must be resorted to when surgery is impossible due to the tumour localization, as is the case in many tumours occurring in the cranial region of the spine. Some cases of long-term disease-free survival after radiotherapy alone have been reported. Radiotherapy must also be employed after an incomplete or marginal surgical excision. Pre-operative radiotherapy may be attempted in those cases in which a radical surgical approach would be allowed by some reduction of the mass. So far, post-operative routine radiotherapy in cases of adequate surgical excision has not proved to be of help, but represents the standard approach in some institutions (Azzarelli *et al.* 1988). No definite evidence is available with regard to the efficacy of chemotherapy.

The natural history is mainly related to the locoregional growth of such tumours and death often results from the local consequences of the disease. The duration of such growth may be exceedingly long. After local relapse or in the presence of gross local tumour, chordomas may metastasize to the lungs, the spine, other viscera, and the soft tissues. Surgery is able to cure some patients provided that adequate free margins are achieved. In other cases long-term survival may be obtained due to the slow growth displayed by the tumour. Radiation therapy and repeated excisions may be of significant help in this regard; the administration of adequate doses of radiotherapy, possibly in conjunction with surgery, may result in long-term remission in selected cases.

ADAMANTINOMA

Adamantinoma of long bones is a very rare bone tumour first described by Fisher in 1913 as originating from the tibia. A few dozen patients have been described in the published literature. It is a low-grade malignant tumour of the long bones of uncertain histogenesis, but possibly of epithelial origin (Rosai *et al.* 1969). Incidence is less than 1 per cent of malignant bone tumours, with a slight predilection for males. Females may have an earlier peak incidence than males; the affected ages are generally from 10 to 50 years, with the second and third decades being most affected.

Pathologically, the lesion presents as a well-circumscribed mass, both solid and cystic. Histologically, there is a mixture of spindle cells forming a fibrous stroma and islands of epithelial-like cells (with basal or squamous cell appearance), possibly lining cystic spaces. Fibrous dysplasia-like zones can be found. The picture resembles ameloblastoma of the maxilla and mandible. The biphasic aspect (epithelial and stromal) also parallels synovial sarcoma (Huvos and Marcove 1975). Differential diagnosis from metastatic carcinoma may be difficult because of the expression of epithelial markers (Pringle 1987).

Clinically, 90 per cent of cases involve the tibia, generally in the two lower-thirds of the diaphysis (Unni *et al.* 1974; Huvos and Marcove 1975). However, other long bones may be affected and multifocality may occur. The diagnosis may be made many years after the beginning of symptoms because of the slow growth of the tumour. Radiologically, the lesion is lytic and well defined, generally without great periosteal reaction or soft tissue extension. Malignancy is of low grade and metastases (to lungs, bones, and lymph nodes) occur late in the natural history of the disease (affecting 15–20 per cent of patients).

Treatment is surgical, possibly with limb-sparing approaches. Potential multifocality of the tumour should be remembered. The incidence of local recurrences tends to be high. The tumour is radioresistant and no data are available about chemotherapy.

NEUROECTODERMAL TUMOUR OF BONE

Intraosseous neuroectodermal tumour was first described by Jaffe *et al.* (1984). It can be classified within the primitive neuroectodermal tumours of the peripheral type. Peripheral neuroepithelioma of soft tissues and possibly Ewing's sarcoma of bone or soft tissues can be classified under the same heading (Dehner 1986). Neuroectodermal tumour of bone is likely to share the same clinical behaviour with such round blue small-cell neoplasms. Therefore, it seems reasonable to use the same therapeutic approaches in these patients, combining chemotherapy, radiotherapy, and surgery.

HAEMATOLOGICAL PRIMARY BONE TUMOURS

Haematological malignancies may affect the skeleton secondarily or may present as primary bone lesions. Obviously, treatment follows the same criteria as for non-osseous presentations. Therefore, the reader is referred to the relevant chapters in this textbook. However, solitary plasmocytoma and primary bone non-Hodgkin's lymphoma are briefly reviewed below.

Solitary plasmocytoma of bone (Woodruff *et al.* 1979; Chak *et al.* 1987) is diagnosed whenever a histologically proved bone lesion is not accompanied by other bone lesions in a complete skeletal radiographic survey and by bone-marrow involvement in a marrow aspirate. A paraprotein may be present and should disappear after treating the solitary lesion. The axial skeleton is affected in most cases. Solitary plasmocytoma can be regarded as an early multiple myeloma, as suggested by the peak incidence occurring a decade earlier (mean 50 years) than multiple myeloma. Radiotherapy at doses of approximately 40 Gy is usually administered as the only treatment. The combination of radiotherapy and chemotherapy (for example, melphalan plus prednisone) has never been proved to be superior to radiotherapy alone. Treatment does not prevent the disease from progressing to overt multiple myeloma in most cases, usually within 3 years. Multiple myeloma is treated with chemotherapy. Radiotherapy is employed in a palliative analgesic fashion whenever necessary.

Primary lymphoma of bone is rare, accounting for 5 per cent of bone tumours and 5 per cent of extranodal lymphomas. The former designation was reticulum cell sarcoma. Sites of origin are widely distributed. Lymphomas of bone are usually non-Hodgkin's lymphomas, generally of intermediate or high grade of malignancy. The subgroup is often the large cell diffuse type (G) of the Working Formulation, corresponding to the diffuse histiocytic type of the Rappaport classification and the centroblastic type of the Kiel classification. Basically, treatment should follow the same principles as for nodal non-Hodgkin's lymphomas of the same subgroups. Therefore, the disease should also be staged following the same indications as for more conventional presentations of non-Hodgkin's lymphoma. Stage I and stage II intermediate- and high-grade non-Hodgkin's lymphomas are generally treated with chemotherapy plus radiotherapy. A CHOP or CHOP-like regimen is of choice, while radiotherapy is usually administered at doses of 40–45 Gy. Stage III and stage IV intermediate- and high-grade non-Hodgkin's lymphomas are currently treated with more or less intensive chemotherapeutic regimens (CHOP-like or 'third-generation' regimens). Radiotherapy to bone lesions tends to be combined with chemotherapy. Less aggressive approaches are used in low-grade non-Hodgkin's lymphomas.

REFERENCES

Azzarelli A, *et al.* (1988). Chordoma: natural history and treatment results in 33 cases. *Journal of Surgical Oncology*, **37**:181–91.

Ballance WA, *et al.* (1988). Osteogenic sarcoma. Malignant fibrous histiocytoma subtype. *Cancer*, **62**:763–71.

Basset WB, Weiss RB (1978). Prolonged complete remission in malignant fibrous histiocytoma treated with chemotherapy. *Cancer Treatment Reports*, **62**:1405.

Bertoni F, *et al.* (1984). Primary central (medullary) fibrosarcoma of bone. *Seminars in Design Pathology*, 1:185–98.

Campanacci M, *et al.* (1987). Giant cell tumour of bone. *Journal of Bone and Joint Surgery*, **69A**:106–14.

Capanna R, *et al.* (1984). Malignant fibrous histiocytoma of bone. The experience of the Rizzoli Institute: report of 90 cases. *Cancer*, **54**:177–87.

Chak LY, *et al.* (1987). Solitary plasmocytoma of bone: treatment, progression, and survival. *Journal of Clinical Oncology*, **5**:1811–15.

Chawla SP, *et al.* (1984). Adjuvant chemotherapy of primary malignant fibrous histiocytoma of bone: prolongation of disease free and overall survival. In *Adjuvant therapy of cancer* IV (ed. SE Jones and SE Salmon). Grune & Stratton, Tucson, AZ.

Chen ZX, *et al.* (1986). Radiation therapy of giant cell tumour of bone: analysis of 35 patients. *International Journal of Radiation — Oncology — Biology — Physics*, **12**:329–34.

Chetiyawardana AD (1984). Chordoma: results of treatment. *Clinical Radiology*, **35**:159–61.

Chow RW, Wilson CB, Olsen ER (1970). Angiosarcoma of the skull. Report of a case and review of the literature. *Cancer*, **25**:902–6.

Cummings BJ, Hodson ID, Bush RS (1983). Chordoma: the results of megavoltage radiation therapy. *International Journal of Radiology — Oncology — Biology — Physics*, **9**:633–42.

Dahlin DC, Ivins JC (1969). Fibrosarcoma of bone. A study of 114 cases. *Cancer*, **23**:35–41.

Dahlin DC, Cupps RE, Johnson EW (1970). Giant cell tumor: a study of 195 cases. *Cancer*, **25**:1061–70

Dahlin DC, Unni KK, Matsuno T (1977). Malignant (fibrous) histiocytoma of bone — fact or fancy? *Cancer*, **39**:1508–16.

Dehner LP (1986). Peripheral and central primitive neuroectodermal tumors. A nosologic concept seeking a consensus. *Archives of Laboratory Medicine*, **110**:997–1005.

den Heeten GJ, *et al.* (1985). Treatment of malignant fibrous histiocytoma of bone. A plea for primary chemotherapy. *Cancer*, **56**:37–40.

Earl HM (1987). Chemotherapy of rare malignant bone tumours. *Baillière's Clinical Oncology*, **1**:223–41.

Evans HL, Ayala AG, Romsdhal MM (1977). Prognostic factors in chondrosarcoma of bone. A clinicopathologic analysis with emphasis on histologic grading. *Cancer*, **40**:818–31.

Feldman F, Norman D (1972). Intra- and extraosseous malignant histiocytoma (malignant fibrous xanthoma). *Radiology*, **104**:497–508.

Harwood AR, Krojbich JI, Fornasier VL (1980). Radiotherapy of chondrosarcoma of bone. *Cancer*, **45**:2769–77.

Huvos AG, Higginbotham NL (1975). Primary fibrosarcoma of bone — a clinical pathologic study of 130 patients. *Cancer*, **35**:837–47.

Huvos AG, Marcove RC (1975). Adamantinoma of long bones: a clinicopathological study of fourteen cases with vascular origin suggested. *Journal of Bone and Joint Surgery*, **57A**:148–54.

Huvos AG, *et al.* (1983). Mesenchymal chondrosarcoma. A clinicopathologic analysis of 35 patients with emphasis on treatment. *Cancer*, **51**:1230–7.

Jaffe HL, Lichtenstein L, Portis PB (1940). Giant-cell tumor of bone: its pathologic appearance, grading, supposed variants and treatment. *Archives of Pathology*, **30**:993–1031.

Jaffe R, *et al.* (1984). The neuroectodermal tumor of bone. *American Journal of Surgical Pathology*, **8**:885–98.

Jewell JH, Bush LF (1964). 'Benign' giant-cell tumor of bone with a solitary pulmonary metastasis. *Journal of Bone and Joint Surgery*, **46A**:848–52.

Johnson S, *et al.* (1986). Chondrosarcoma with additional mesenchymal component (dedifferentiated chondrosarcoma). I. A clinicopathologic study of 26 cases. *Cancer*, **58**:278–86.

Kemp H (1987). Limb conservation surgery for osteosarcoma and other primary bone tumours. *Baillière's Clinical Oncology*, **1**:111–36.

Laramore GE, *et al.* (1989). Fast neutron radiotherapy for sarcomas of soft tissue, bone, and cartilage. *American Journal of Clinical Oncology*, **12**:320–6.

Larsson S-E, Lorentzon R, Boquist L (1975). Giant cell tumor of bone. A demographic, clinical and histopathological study of all cases recorded in the Swedish Cancer Registry for the years 1958 through 1968. *Journal of Bone and Joint Surgery*, **57A**:167.

McNaney D, *et al.* (1982). Fifteen year radiotherapy experience with chondrosarcoma of bone. *International Journal of Radiation — Oncology — Biology — Physics*, **8**:187–90.

Mindell ER (1981). Current concepts review: chordoma. *Journal of Bone and Joint Surgery*, **63**:501–5.

Mirra JM (1980). *Bone tumours: diagnosis and treatment*. JB Lippincott, Philadelphia.

Moser RP (1987). An approach to primary bone tumors. *Radiologic Clinics of North America*, **25**:1049–93.

Nakashima Y, *et al.* (1986). Mesenchymal chondrosarcoma of bone and soft tissue. A review of 111 cases. *Cancer*, **57**:2444–53.

Nascimento AG, Huvos AG, Marcove RC (1979). Primary malignant giant cell tumor of bone. A study of eight cases and review of the literature. *Cancer*, **44**:1393–1402.

Pringle JAS (1987). Pathology of bone tumours. *Baillière's Clinical Oncology*, **1**:21–63.

Rich TA, *et al.* (1985). Clinical and pathologic review of 48 cases of chordoma. *Cancer*, **56**:182–7.

Rosai J (1969). Adamantinoma of the tibia: electron microscopic evidence of its epithelial origin. *American Journal of Clinical Pathology*, **51**:786–92.

Sanerkin NG (1980a). Definitions of osteosarcoma, chondrosarcoma, and fibrosarcoma of bone. *Cancer*, **46**:178–85.

Sanerkin NG (1980b). The diagnosis and grading of chondrosarcoma and fibrosarcoma of bone: a combined cytologic and histologic approach. *Cancer*, **45**:582–94.

Sanerkin NG (1980c). Malignancy, aggressiveness, and recurrence in giant cell tumour of bone. *Cancer*, **46**:1641–9.

Sanerkin NG, Gallagher P (1979). A review of the behaviour of chondrosarcoma of bone. *Journal of Bone and Joint Surgery*, **61B**:395–400.

Shuman LS, *et al.* (1982). Intra-arterial chemotherapy of malignant fibrous histiocytoma of the pelvis. *Radiology*, **142**:343–6.

Spanier SS, Enneking WF, Enriquez P (1975). Primary malignant fibrous histiocytoma of bone. *Cancer*, **36**:2084–98.

Spooner D (1987). The role of radiotherapy in the management of primary bone tumours. *Baillière's Clinical Oncology*, **1**:243–59.

Stout AP (1956). Tumours featuring pericytes: glomus tumor and hemangiopericytoma. *Laboratory Investigation*, **5**:213–23.

Tang JSH, *et al.* (1988). Hemangiopericytoma of bone. *Cancer*, **62**:848–59.

Têtu B, *et al.* (1986). Chondrosarcoma with additional mesenchymal component (dedifferentiated chondrosarcoma). II. An immuno-histochemical and electron microscopic study. *Cancer*, **58**:287–98.

Thomas A (1942). Vascular tumors of bone: pathological and clinical study of 27 cases. *Surgery, Gynecology and Obstetrics*, **74**:777–95.

Unni KK, Dahlin DC (1984). Grading of bone tumors. *Seminars in Design Pathology*, **1**:165–72.

Unni KK, *et al.* (1971). Hemangioma, hemangio-pericytoma and hemangioendothelioma (angiosarcoma) of bone. *Cancer*, **27**:1403–14.

Unni KK, *et al.* (1974). Adamantinoma of long bones. *Cancer*, **34**:1796–1805.

Unni KK, Dahlin DC, Beabout JW (1976). Chondrosarcoma: clear cell variant. A report of sixteen cases. *Journal of Bone and Joint Surgery*, **58A**:676–83.

Urban C, *et al.* (1983). Chemotherapy of malignant fibrous histiocytoma of bone: a report of five cases. *Cancer*, **51**:795–802.

Weiner M, *et al.* (1983). Adjuvant chemotherapy of malignant fibrous histiocytoma of bone. *Cancer*, **51**:25–9.

Woodruff RK, Malpas JS, White FE (1979). Solitary plasmocytoma. II: solitary plasmocytoma of bone. *Cancer*, **43**:2344–7.

Section 14
Paediatric tumours

14.1 The molecular pathology of childhood tumours

JOHN K. COWELL

INTRODUCTION

Histopathological analysis of the majority of children's tumours reveals an embryonic-like organization. This suggests an arrest in development whereby the normal differentiation signals are overridden, resulting in continued, uncontrollable division of embryonic cells. Tumour cells usually express specific genes, which may identify the stage of development at which this arrest occurred. Although usually committed to a particular pathway of differentiation, they are still relatively undifferentiated. As most tissues are fully differentiated at or soon after birth, the mutations responsible for the initiation of tumorigenesis probably occur during embryogenesis. Once the cells are fully differentiated they can no longer be part of the pool of potential tumour precursor cells. What is not clear is the stage during embryogenesis, the 'window of differentiation', in which cancer-causing mutations are effective. After initiation, tumours go through repeated rounds of clonal evolution where better adapted cells, as a result of genetic reorganization, gain growth advantages and eventually dominate the tumour. Progression therefore continues at different rates, is characterized by secondary genetic changes, and accounts for variation in the time of presentation.

Several embryonal tumours show familial aggregation, implying a genetic predisposition. Although rare, it has generally been the analysis of these patients that has led to the precise detection of the predisposing mutation. In particular, the study of retinoblastoma established many of the precedents for the analysis of other children's cancers.

RETINOBLASTOMA

Biology

Retinoblastoma is the most common intraocular tumour in children, with a mean worldwide incidence of approximately 1 : 20 000 live births. Histopathological inspection reveals a relatively undifferentiated mass of cells structurally similar to immature precursor retinal cells, although, in some retinoblastomas, differentiated structures such as pseudorosettes can be seen (Ts'o et al. 1969). The structural organization of retinoblastoma is consistent with a group of cells that has failed to respond to the normal signals of differentiation and has continued to divide uncontrollably. As the normal retina is always fully differentiated at birth it is clear that retinoblastomas originate during embryonic development, although the 'window of development' in which these events are initiated is uncertain.

Genetics

There are both familial and sporadic forms of retinoblastoma (Vogel 1979). In the approximately 10–20 per cent of cases with a positive family history, the retinoblastoma phenotype segregates as an autosomal dominant. Thus, offspring of individuals carrying the retinoblastoma gene have a 50 : 50 chance of inheriting it. In 10 per cent of cases, individuals inherit the defective gene but do not develop the tumour, that is, 'incomplete penetrance'. Thus, it is the predisposition to tumour development that is inherited and, at the cellular level, the mutation behaves in a recessive manner. This suggestion is further supported by the observation that, in gene carriers, not all retinal cells develop into cancers. It has also been reported that retinoblastomas can apparently regress spontaneously. In these cases a small scar is left on the retina, characteristic of that seen after successful treatment of the tumours. Where there are examples of non-penetrance this family pattern could be due to the inheritance of an unbalanced chromosome abnormality (Strong et al. 1981) or that one of the parents is a tissue mosaic and transmits the gene through the germ-line.

Clearly, if retinoblastoma is a recessive trait, a second mutation is required in the homologous normal gene. Knudson (1971) formulated a 'two-hit' hypothesis for retinoblastoma which contended that only two genetic events were required for tumour initiation. In the hereditary form the first 'hit' is inherited. The second mutational event is random but occurs with a relatively high frequency, which is why, in hereditary cases, tumours are usually bilateral and multifocal. As only a single additional mutation is required, hereditary tumours appear at an earlier age (mean, 10 months) than sporadic tumours. In non-familial cases both hits occur as sporadic, random events. The chance of the same pair of genes in the same retinal precursor cell experiencing two mutational events is very low, so sporadic tumours are usually unilateral, unifocal, and appear later in infancy (mean, 18 months). Carriers of the predisposing gene are at a significantly higher risk than the general population of developing second, non-ocular tumours. These second tumours usually occur in mesenchymal tissues; 66 per cent are osteosarcomas and soft tissue sarcomas (Abramson et al. 1984). Therapeutic radiotherapy accelerates (causes) a majority of these tumours but more than one-third develop in unirradiated tissue. It would appear, therefore, that a gene essential to the normal retinal development also plays a part in bone and muscle development during puberty.

Early detection of retinoblastoma in familial cases is relatively straightforward because 'at risk' individuals can be identified and screened from birth by ophthalmoscopy. The children of bilaterally affected individuals, together with those with a proven family history, are screened regularly during the first 5 years of life.

13q– syndrome

Some patients with retinoblastoma have other congenital abnormalities, notably mental retardation and particular dysmorphic features (Motegi et al. 1983). These patients invariably carry a constitutional chromosome abnormality, most usually a deletion from the long arm of chromosome 13. Larger deletions are associated with more severe congenital abnormalities. Usually the only phenotypic consequence of smaller deletions is retinoblastoma. Chromosome region 13q14 is always involved indicating the location of the retinoblastoma gene (Sparkes *et al.* 1984; Cowell *et al.* 1989). Deletions are the most common chromosome abnormality in patients with retinoblastoma but translocations have also been reported (Turleau *et al.* 1985). Usually these rearrangements involve break-points in region 13q14, presumably constituting the first hit. In translocations also involving the X chromosome, however, the chromosome 13 break-points were not always in 13q14 (Hida *et al.* 1980). In these cases, which were always in females, it is assumed that the spreading of X chromosome inactivation during development extended to the relocated chromosome 13 and included the retinoblastoma predisposition gene (Ejima *et al.* 1982). Rather than structural mutation within the predisposition gene, this functional inactivation constituted the first 'hit'.

The esterase-D gene lies in 13q14 and is also deleted in even the smallest 13q deletions (Sparkes *et al.* 1980). Cells from these patients show only 50 per cent of normal enzyme activity. This assay has been used in population screening programmes (Cowell *et al.* 1986, 1989). Of the 18 detected in our study, eight small deletions were only identified after quantitation of esterase-D. At least half of these patients with deletion only developed unilateral tumours, apparently in contradiction of Knudson's hypothesis. It appears that some deletions are associated with a lower than average penetrance, possibly due to the lethal consequences of other gene mutations within the deletion (Dryja *et al.* 1984). Small deletions can be transmitted from parent to child (Cowell *et al.* 1988).

The esterase-D gene has two electrophoretic variants, type 1 and type 2, which are separable by starch-gel electrophoresis (Hopkinson *et al.* 1973). This protein polymorphism, although rare, has been used in linkage analysis in retinoblastoma families and Sparkes *et al.* (1983) were able to demonstrate that the hereditary, non-deletion form of *RB* (the retinoblastoma gene) was also located in region 13q14. There have been no reported cases, to date, of recombination between these two genes.

Chromosome analysis of tumour cells

Chromosome analysis of tumour cells can often be overinterpreted, as they represent highly evolved cells arising from successive clonal evolution during which time advantageous rearrangements leading to tumour progression have occurred. Given this caveat, the presence of consistent chromosome abnormalities may reflect important events in tumorigenesis. The involvement of genetic changes in region 13q14 in sporadic tumours was first implied from the analysis of chromosome abnormalities in cells prepared directly from tumours or in cell lines. Although early reports suggested frequent involvement of 13q in cytogenetic abnormalities in retinoblastoma cells, detailed subsequent analysis of many more tumours failed to confirm this (Squire *et al.* 1985). In the course of these studies it became clear that chromosomes 1 and 6 (Table 1) were also frequently involved in structural abnormalities (Squire *et al.* 1985).

Homozygosity

Knudson's hypothesis (Knudson 1971) predicts that the retino-blastoma phenotype is recessive at the cellular level. Both copies of the gene, therefore, have to be inactivated for tumour initiation. Deletions, translocations, or point mutations may result in loss of function of the *RB* gene. Loss of alleles in the tumours from some individuals has been shown using chromosome 13-specific DNA probes (Cavenee *et al.* 1983; Godbout *et al.* 1983; Dryja *et al.* 1984). By analysing flanking markers, Cavenee *et al.* (1983) provided formal proof for mitotic recombination and non-dysjunction as mechanisms

Table 1 Summary of consistent karyotypic changes in tumour and constitutional cells reported in patients with childhood solid tumours

Tumour type	Constitutional[a]	Tumour[b]	Homozygosity[c]
Retinoblastoma	del(13q)	del(17p)	13q
	t(X;13)	iso(6p)	
	t(A;13)	trisomy-1q	
		del(13q)	
Wilms' tumour	del(11p)	trisomy 1q	11p
	t(A;11)	del(11p)	
		16q−	
Neuroblastoma	t(A;1)	del(1p)	1p, 14q, 17p
Rhabdomyosarcoma	None	t(2;13)(q35;q14)	11p
		t(2;8)(q35;q13)	
		t(2;5)(q35;q31)	
Ewing's sarcoma	None	t(11;22)(q24;q12)	
Childhood brain tumours	None	1p abnormalities	10q
		iso(17q)	

[a] A, autosomal: the autosome involved in these predisposing rearrangements may vary; the position of the invariant break-point indicates the site of the predisposition gene.
[b] Only consistent chromosome abnormalities are shown.
[c] Although allele loss is consistently found for the chromosomes indicated, many of the human chromosomes have still to be analysed in these tumours.

for the generation of homozygosity in tumour cells. In all cases it was assumed that the chromosome region containing the normal *RB* gene was lost with duplication of the mutant allele. Later this was confirmed by showing that, in familial retinoblastoma, the chromosome transmitted from the affected parent was retained in the tumour in the affected offspring (Cavenee *et al.* 1985).

Isolation of the retinoblastoma gene

Chromosome 13-specific DNA sequences have been isolated at random and mapped along the length of the chromosome. Lalande *et al.* (1984) identified a sequence H3−8, which mapped to the critical region of 13q14 and, using this probe, Friend *et al.* (1986) subsequently isolated a gene sequence, *4.7R*. mRNA transcripts of this sequence were either absent from tumour cells or were smaller than normal, indicating deletions (Fung *et al.* 1987; Lee *et al.* 1987). The *RB1* gene is 4757 bp long and spans approximately 200 kb of genomic DNA (Friend *et al.* 1986; Bookstein *et al.* 1988). Complete sequencing of the gene has identified 27 exons, the majority of which are only 50−150 bp long.

Abnormal gene expression in tumours provided strong evidence for the authenticity of the *RB1* gene, but did predisposing mutations also involve this gene? One patient with retinoblastoma carried a constitutional reciprocal translocation between chromosomes 1 and 13. Somatic cell hybrids, which retained the derivative t(13;1) chromosome (Mitchell and Cowell 1989) were analysed using DNA probes from the 5' and 3' end of the genomic sequence. The 13q14 break-point of the translocation was shown to lie in the middle of the *RB1* genomic sequence. Cavenee and colleagues (Higgins *et al.* 1989) reported several other translocations from retinoblastoma patients with break-points interrupting the *RB1* gene. Dunn *et al.* (1988) were able to demonstrate more subtle abnormalities in predisposed individuals by using RNAse protection methods.

Studies using specific antibodies against the retinoblastoma gene product (see below) have shown that even though transcription occurs in some tumours, translation did not; no detectable gene product was found in tumour cells (Whyte *et al.* 1988). The availability of the complete *RB1* gene sequence means that it is now possible to analyse mutations in tumours and predisposed individuals to produce a more complete picture of the nature of the genetic events leading to the inactivation of the gene (Yandell *et al.* 1989). Eventually the molecular pathology of retinoblastoma should be as complete as, say, that of the thalassaemias.

RB *mutations in other tumours*

As discussed earlier, patients with retinoblastoma are at a significantly higher risk of development of second malignancies. Hansen *et al.* (1985) analysed cells from three osteosarcomas from patients with bilateral retinoblastoma and showed that all of them had lost heterozygosity for region 13q14. Toguchida *et al.* (1988) showed loss of heterozygosity for chromosome 13 markers in 64 per cent (19/30) of osteosarcomas. This observation has been interpreted as indicating a common aetiology in these tumours. Structural abnormalities of the retinoblastoma gene in osteosarcoma were reported by Friend *et al.* (1987), who also studied tumours from other sites often associated with secondary neoplasms in retinoblastoma patients. Abnormalities involving the *RB1* gene have also been demonstrated in a variety of other tumours such as small cell lung cancer (Harbour *et al.* 1988), bladder cancer (Horowitz *et al.* 1989), and breast cancer (T'ang *et al.* 1989). What precise role *RB1* plays in the development of these tumours remains to be seen, although it is likely to be related more to progression than initiation as mutations in this gene only confer predisposition to a narrow range of malignancies.

The retinoblastoma protein

Sequencing of the *RB1* cDNA (Friend *et al.* 1987; Lee *et al.* 1987) predicted the amino acid sequence of its product. No motifs common to classes of genes whose products localize to the cell membrane or ATP-binding domains, for example were detected, neither was there any structural homology with known oncogenes or developmental regulator genes such as homeoboxes. More recently, Whyte *et al.* (1988) demonstrated that the retinoblastoma gene product binds to the early protein, E1A, of adenovirus. DNA tumour viruses encode a set of proteins capable of overriding normal regulation of cellular growth. E1A regulates gene expression, can immortalize cells on its own, and activate transcription of other early viral and cellular genes (see Berk (1986) for a review). E1A has also been shown to associate with the *RB1* protein, possibly mediating some of its pathophysiological effects. It has been suggested that retinoblastoma is a component of a pathway allowing cells to respond to developmental signals. By blocking this pathway, E1A prevents growth inhibition. The *RB* protein has also been shown to bind to other oncogene products from transforming viruses such as large-T antigen from SV40 (de Caprio *et al.* 1988) and the E7 transforming protein from human papilloma virus-16 (Dyson *et al.* 1989), suggesting that its binding of oncogene transforming proteins may be a common feature. The retinoblastoma protein has both phosphorylated and hypophosphorylated forms. Phosphorylation accompanies entry into the cell cycle (see Cowell (1991) for a review). It appears, therefore, that the hypophosphorylated form prevents entry into S-phase and phosphorylation effectively inactivates the protein. By binding oncogene proteins such as large-T the protein is also effectively inactivated allowing cells to divide.

WILMS' TUMOUR

Wilms' tumour is a kidney tumour affecting 1 : 10 000 children each year and accounting for approximately 6 per cent of all children's tumours. Although often considered a hereditary tumour (Knudson and Strong 1972), the genetic component is not as obvious as in

retinoblastoma. In a recent survey in the United Kingdom only 4 per cent of cases were bilateral and less than 1 per cent were familial (J. Pritchard, personal communication). In a few cases, Wilms' tumour is associated with aniridia; that is, congenital absence of irises. There are sporadic and hereditary forms of aniridia. Only sporadic cases of aniridia are associated with Wilms' tumour (Miller *et al.* 1964); the syndrome is referred to as the aniridia–Wilms' tumour association (AWTA). Many of these children (Riccardi *et al.* 1978) also have mental retardation and/or abnormal genitalia, that is, the **AGR** triad (for *A*niridia, *G*onadal dysplasia, *R*etardation) and this confers a 50 per cent risk to the individual for the development of Wilms' tumour (Narahara *et al.* 1984). Chromosome analysis in these patients reveals a constitutional deletion on the short arm of chromosome 11. Although the extent of the deletion varies from patient to patient, all or part of region 11p13 is missing. In the smallest deletion there is no mental retardation or gonadal dysplasia. These observations place the aniridia and Wilms' genes in the same subregion of 11p13.

Turleau *et al.* (1984*b*) described a Wilms' tumour patient with mental retardation and gonadal dysplasia but no aniridia and a deletion of region 11p12–p13. The break-point was in the distal part of band p13, placing the aniridia locus distal to the Wilms' locus. The 11p13 deletion can also be transmitted by carriers of balanced translocations (Hittner *et al.* 1979; Yunis and Ramsay 1980). The inheritance of the unbalanced form of this rearrangement leads to the Wilms' AGR phenotype. Only 52 per cent of patients with this deletion develop a tumour, suggesting that the 'second hit' occurs more rarely than in retinoblastoma. Alternatively, more than one gene may be important in tumorigenesis (see below). Wilms' tumour is not the only malignancy associated with deletion of region 11p13. Andersen *et al.* (1978) reported one AGR patient, a girl, who developed bilateral gonadoblastoma at the age of 21 months. Kidneys and gonads are all of mesodermal origin and derive from embryologically adjacent sites involving the mesonephros. These observations imply either that genes in 11p13 may act in a pleiotropic fashion and affect the development of a number of different tissues or that several genes are involved.

The presence of other genes in 11p13 important in genitourinary development was suggested by the presence of a translocation, t(2;11)(p11;p13) in a stillborn with Potter's syndrome (Porteous *et al.* 1987), which is characterized by kidney agenesis. The break-point site in 11p in this case was shown to be different from that of the Wilms' tumour locus (Compton *et al.* 1988) but suggests a possible 'cluster' of genes controlling kidney development in this region.

Several Wilms' tumour families have now been reported (Grundy *et al.* 1988; Huff *et al.* 1988) in whom it was possible to carry out linkage analysis using probes from the short arm of chromosome 11. The unanimous finding was that the Wilms' tumour phenotype in these families was not linked to 11p DNA markers. Although the familial incidence of Wilms' tumour (much less than 1 per cent) is even lower than that of 11p− deletions, it is clear that there may be other genes associated with predisposition to Wilms' tumour.

Chromosome analysis in Wilms' tumour cells

Chromosome analysis of Wilms' tumours has shown the same overall pattern as in retinoblastoma. Thus, although aberrations involving the short arm of chromosome 11 are the most frequently observed single abnormality (Table 1), the majority of tumours have two normal copies of chromosome 11 (Douglass *et al.* 1985; Slater 1986; Solis *et al.* 1988). Abnormalities of chromosome 1q are also frequently observed.

Loss of heterozygosity

The loss of chromosome 11 alleles in Wilms' tumours was demonstrated by several groups (Fearon *et al.* 1984; Koufos *et al.* 1984; Orkin *et al.* 1984). Homozygosity can result from mitotic recombination, non-dysjunction, or chromosome deletion. The frequency in Wilms' tumour is much lower than that seen for retinoblastoma, at approximately 30 per cent. A rather higher (40 per cent) frequency of allele loss in the distal part of chromosome 11p15 has been reported (Mannens *et al.* 1988; Reeve *et al.* 1989; Wadey *et al.* 1990) and in some cases the loss of alleles is restricted to that site.

Loss of heterozygosity on the short arm of chromosome 11 has since been reported in several laboratories (Dao *et al.* 1987; Schroeder *et al.* 1987; Mannens *et al.* 1988; Williams *et al.* 1989; Wadey *et al.* 1990). Schroeder *et al.* (1987) showed that the paternally derived allele was retained in five out of five tumours; others have confirmed this observation (Reeve *et al.* 1984; Mannens *et al.* 1988; Williams *et al.* 1989).

Wilkins (1988) proposed a theory of genomic imprinting to try to explain these observations. According to Comings (1973), inactivation of a diploid pair of regulatory genes that normally suppress function of a transforming gene would be required to release cells from normal growth controls. It also appears, in many cases, that the maternal genome largely determines embryonic development (see Solter (1988) for a review) and that expression of some genes differs depending on their maternal or paternal origin. Wilkins (1988) suggested that the transforming gene for Wilms' tumour is on chromosome 11 but only active on the paternal chromosomes, the maternal allele having been inactivated by genomic imprinting. Thus, only the paternal transforming gene would respond to the absence of the suppressing gene product and expression of the transforming gene would only occur if the paternal chromosome is retained. The exact mechanism of genomic imprinting is still unclear but one possibility is that gene inactivation could result from selective methylation of genes. Williams *et al.* (1989) claimed a reduction in the degree of methylation of the HRAS locus in Wilms' tumours compared with normal tissues from the same patients. Our own studies show that in Wilms' tumours the degree of methylation appears to be reduced, but not eliminated, for most loci along the length of chromosome 11p.

Beckwith–Wiedemann syndrome

Beckwith–Wiedemann syndrome is a state of somatic overgrowth (Beckwith 1963; Wiedemann 1964) with a complex phenotype. One feature of this syndrome is that there is often an associated predisposition to the development of rare childhood tumours, most usually Wilms' tumour but also hepatoblastoma, rhabdomyosarcoma, adrenal carcinoma, pancreatoblastoma, and non-Hodgkin's lymphoma (Wiedemann 1983). In rare cases, patients with this syndrome have constitutional chromosome abnormalities involving the distal tip of the short arm of chromosome 11 (Waziri *et al.* 1983; Turleau *et al.* 1984a; Henry *et al.* 1989). Linkage in the familial form of Beckwith–Wiedemann syndrome (Koufos *et al.* 1989; Ping *et al.* 1989) also implicates region 11p15 in the syndrome's aetiology. In some patients, combinations of these tumours have been reported, suggesting a common aetiological event arising as a result of a mutation at the same locus. Koufos *et al.* (1986) analysed three hepatoblastomas and showed that in two there was a loss of heterozygosity for chromosome-11 markers, whilst in a third tumour heterozygosity was retained. There were similar findings in two

rhabdomyosarcomas. Scrable *et al.* (1987) have shown that loss of heterozygosity in embryonal rhabdomyosarcomas was restricted to the distal half of the short arm of chromosome 11 and mitotic recombination mapping suggests that the predisposition locus is in the 11p15.5–pter region. Markers from other chromosomes were the same in tumour and normal tissues.

Molecular analysis of 11p13

Molecular cloning strategies, similar to that described for retinoblastoma, have been designed to try to identify the Wilms' predisposition gene. They mostly involve random mapping strategies of chromosome 11-specific DNA sequences, isolated from a variety of chromosome-specific DNA libraries (Davis *et al.* 1988; Lewis *et al.* 1988; Gessler *et al.* 1989; Rose *et al.* 1990).

Porteous and colleagues have used chromosome-mediated gene transfer to make libraries (Porteous *et al.* 1987) enriched for 11p sequences. The EJ bladder cell line contains an activated Ha-*ras* gene that can transform mouse 3T3 cells in DNA transfection experiments. A candidate gene (*WT33*) has now been isolated from the 11p13 region (Call *et al.* 1990; Gessler *et al.* 1990). This candidate gene was shown to have a 'zinc-finger' motif, a feature associated with DNA-binding function, which raises the possibility that it may regulate the expression of other genes. *WT33* is also only expressed in fetal kidney, the gonads, and the spleen. The specific localization to the kidney and the gonads might have been expected because of their common embryological origin. Why expression is also found in the spleen is not clear. Specifically, Pritchard-Jones *et al.* (1991) have shown that expression of *WT33* occurs in cells making the transition from mesenchymal to epithelial cells and is only maintained during that transition. This highly temporal pattern of expression of *WT33* supports the view that it plays an important part in differentiation. The next step is to determine whether structural abnormalities of this gene, implicating it in tumorigenesis, can be detected in tumour cells. Homozygous deletions of *WT33* have been reported in a small percentage of tumours (Gessler *et al.* 1991) involving the whole gene and we have now detected a partial deletion of this gene involving only the 3' end (Cowell *et al.* 1991), which is reminiscent of observations with the retinoblastoma gene (Friend *et al.* 1986). Ultimately it will require the correction of the malignant phenotype in tumour cells to confirm the authenticity of *WT33* as the Wilms' tumour gene.

NEUROBLASTOMA

Neuroblastoma arises from primitive neural-crest cells and is the most common neoplasm diagnosed in infancy. There have been a few reported cases of familial neuroblastoma, although, as for Wilms' tumour, they are rare. To date the only indication as to the location of the predisposition gene for neuroblastoma comes from chromosome analysis of tumour cells. In the majority of cases, abnormalities involving the short arm of chromosome 1 have been reported, specifically region 1p31–36. Family pedigrees have not, so far, been suitable for linkage analysis. Homozygosity studies have implicated 1p in advanced-stage tumours (Fong *et al.* 1989), although chromosome 14q also frequently shows allele loss. Cytological evidence for gene amplification in the form of double minutes and homogeneously staining regions have been frequently reported in neuroblastoma (Cowell 1982) and represent amplification of the N-*myc* oncogene, which is often associated with translocation from the normal position on chromosome 2 to the p31–p36 region of chromosome 1.

It has been suggested that N-*myc* amplification is an indication of advanced-stage disease in neuroblastoma (Brodeur *et al.* 1984; Seeger *et al.* 1985; Kaneko *et al.* 1987), although amplification appears to be more related to the capacity for progression than to a particular stage. For tumours in which cells have only a single copy of N-*myc* at diagnosis, 94 per cent had progression-free survival and generally did better after therapy, regardless of stage. In contrast, 50 per cent of tumours with elevated N-*myc*, regardless of stage, go on to metastasize and kill the patient. Seeger *et al.* (1985) also noted that, whilst stage IV and stage IVS disease are both widely disseminated at diagnosis, the better prognosis IVS tumours did not show amplification of N-*myc*, whereas stage IV disease did. Thus, N-*myc* amplification is a reasonable indicator of poor prognosis, identifying one-half of cases. A better prognostic indicator, however, was reported to be the presence of abnormalities involving the short arm (p) of chromosome 1 (Christiansen and Lampert 1988). In their study, 83 per cent of poor-prognosis patients had 1p abnormalities, whereas only 33 per cent of those tested had N-*myc* amplification. This observation was in contrast with that of Kaneko *et al.* (1987), who found that 60–70 per cent of poor-prognosis tumours had both 1p abnormalities and elevated N-*myc*. The significance of these observations remains to be determined but it is clear that molecular pathology of this kind is providing better indications for prognosis.

ONCOGENES IN CANCER

It will be clear from the preceding discussion that loss of function of a particular gene is important in the development of predisposition syndromes for childhood cancer. By implication, therefore, the presence of these genes promotes normal development in the appropriate tissue. This observation has led them to be defined as 'anti-oncogenes', 'recessive cancer genes', and 'tumour suppressor genes'. There is, however, another class of cancer genes that apparently acts in a dominant manner: the cellular oncogenes. These oncogenes on their own cannot transform primary cells but in combination they can (Land *et al.* 1983). As oncogenes are the mutated forms of normal cellular genes, proto-oncogenes, a simple model predicts that, because they only control a limited subset of the cellular regulation mechanism controlling growth, their successive mutation forms the basis of multistep carcinogenesis. The *ras* genes, for example control cytoplasmic processes, whereas the *myc* oncogenes specify nuclear proteins; *myc* induces pre-malignant phenotypes, which makes these cells responsive to transformation by *ras* oncogenes (Weinberg 1989). Direct involvement of these genes in human cancer came from the observation that oncogenes were frequently located near to the break-point in chromosome translocations consistently found in some tumours. Thus, C-*myc* is relocated next to the various immunoglobulin genes in Burkitt's lymphoma and the c-*abl* oncogene is relocated in the Philadelphia translocation in chronic myeloid leukaemia to a genetic locus known as *bcr* (break-point cluster region). This genetic fusion results in a chimeric protein containing the functional part of c-*abl*, which is now more robust than the normal gene (Bishop 1987). The consequences of the *myc* relocation in Burkitt's lymphoma are still controversial but it is possible that the inappropriate temporal expression of *myc* contributes to tumorigenicity. Alternatively, either regulatory controls of *myc* may be damaged, resulting in inappropriate levels of expression or damage to the *myc* gene by translocation may result in the production of a more stable mRNA.

OTHER CANCER PREDISPOSITION SYNDROMES

The location of cancer predisposition genes can only be assigned unequivocally through linkage analysis. Although constitutional chromosome abnormalities usually imply that the break-points interrupt the critical gene, this may not always be the case because substantial deletions may also be associated with these rearrangements. The development of somatic homozygosity for particular regions of chromosomes directs attention to potential sites but cannot be used reliably to pinpoint cancer genes as many chromosomes may show loss of alleles in the same tumour and are seen only in advanced tumours and therefore, are more likely associated with tumour progression than with tumorigenesis. Tumour chromosome analysis can give a misleading impression of the site of predisposition genes; although consistent abnormalities may be noted, they may have no relevance to tumorigenicity. Given this caveat there is fragmentary information about a variety of other childhood tumours, which is reviewed below. For many of these tumours there are rare cases of familial aggregations but insufficient for linkage studies. Relatively poor survival of patients with these cancers has been a contributing factor.

Medulloblastoma is the most common malignant primary brain tumour of children and arises from primitive cells in the neuroepithelium. There have been a few cytogenetic studies but, although chromosome 1q is implicated, no clear pattern emerges (Bigner *et al.* 1988; Griffin *et al.* 1989). In Ewing's sarcoma, a primary sarcoma of osseous and non-osseous origin, chromosome analysis has shown a consistent translocation between chromosomes 11 and 22, t(11;22)(q23;q12), in tumour cells (see Griffin *et al.* 1986). It is hard to interpret the importance of these rearrangements as it appears that the exact position of the break-points is variable. There has also been a consistent rearrangement recorded in rhabdomyosarcomas, t(2;13)(q35;q14), where the consistent break-point is on chromosome 2 (Douglass *et al.* 1987).

SUMMARY

The analysis of childhood embryonal tumours offers a unique opportunity to study not only the cancer phenotype but also, possibly, genes that are important in normal embryonic development. To date only the retinoblastoma predisposition gene and a candidate for the Wilms' tumour gene have been isolated, although it seems likely that others will soon follow. The availability of these genes will mean that mutations in individual patients can be characterized in the tumours. The demonstration of a mutation in constitutional cells defines the patient as a gene carrier. As patterns emerge it may be that particular mutations will be associated with a particular course of the disease, thereby allowing predictions to be made about invasiveness, prognosis, and susceptibility to other tumours, for example. If these objectives are realized then this type of molecular pathology will become increasingly important but will depend on the careful collection and processing of tumour and normal tissue from each patient.

REFERENCES

Abramson DH, Ellsworth RM, Kitchin FD, Tung G (1984). Second nonocular tumours in retinoblastoma survivors. Are they radiation-induced? *Ophthalmology*, **91**:1351–5.

Andersen S, *et al.* (1978). Aniridia, cateract and gonadoblastoma in a mentally retarded girl with deletion of chromosome 11. *Ophthalmologica*, **176**:171–7.

Beckwith JP (1963). Extreme cytomegaly of the adrenal fetal cortex, omphalocele hyperplasia of kidneys and pancreas, and Leydig-cell hyperplasia: another syndrome? *Western Society of Pediatric Research*, Los Angeles, November 11th.

Berk AJ (1986). Adenovirus promoters and E1A transaction. *Annual Review of Genetics*, 20:45–79.

Bigner SH, Mark J, Friedman HS, Biegel JA, Bigner DD (1988). Structural chromosomal abnormalities in human medullablastoma. *Cancer Genetics and Cytogenetics*, 30:91–101.

Bishop JM (1987). The molecular genetics of cancer. *Science*, 235:305–11.

Bookstein R, *et al.* (1988). Human retinoblastoma susceptibility gene: genomic organization and analysis of heterozygous intragenic deletion mutants. *Proceedings of the National Academy of Sciences USA*, 85:2210–14.

Brodeur GM, Seeger RC, Schwab M, Varmus HE, Bishop JM (1984). Amplification of N-*myc* in untreated human neuroblastomas correlates with advanced disease stage. *Science*, 224:1121–4.

Call KM, *et al.* (1990). Isolation and characterisation of a zinc finger polypeptide gene at the human chromosome 11 Wilms' tumour locus. *Cell*, 60:509–520.

Cavenee WK, *et al.* (1983). Expression of recessive alleles by chromosomal mechanisms in retinoblastoma. *Nature*, 305:779–84.

Cavenee WK, *et al.* (1985). Genetic origin of mutations predisposing to retinoblastoma. *Science*, 228:501–3.

Christiansen H, Lampert F (1988). Tumour karyotype discriminates between good and bad prognostic outcome in neuroblastoma. *British Journal of Cancer*, 57:121–6.

Comings DE (1973). A general theory of carcinogenesis. *Proceedings of the National Academy of Sciences USA*, 70:3324–8.

Compton DA, Weil MM, Jones C, Riccardi VM, Strong LC, Saunders GF (1988). Long range physical map of the Wilms' tumour–aniridia region on human chromosome 11. *Cell*, 55:827–36.

Cowell JK (1982). Double minutes and homogeneously staining regions: gene amplification in mammalian cells. *Annual Review of Genetics*, 16:21–59.

Cowell JK (1991). The nuclear oncoproteins RB and p53. *Seminars in Cancer Biology*.

Cowell JK, Rutland P, Jay M, Hungerford J (1986). Deletions of the esterase-D locus from a survey of 200 retinoblastoma patients. *Human Genetics*, 72:164–7.

Cowell JK, Rutland P, Hungerford J, Jay M (1988). Deletion of chromosome region 13q14 is transmissible and does not always predispose to retinoblastoma. *Human Genetics*, 80:43–5.

Cowell JK, Hungerford J, Rutland P, Jay M (1989). Genetic and cytogenetic analysis of patients showing reduced esterase-D levels and mental retardation from a survey of 500 individuals with retinoblastoma. *Ophthalmic Pediatrics and Genetics*, 110:117–27.

Cowell JK, Wadey RB, Haber DA, Call KM, Housman DE, Pritchard J (1991). Structural rearrangements of the *WT1* gene in Wilms' tumour cells. *Oncogene*.

Dao DD, *et al.* (1987). Genetic mechanisms of tumour-specific loss of 11p DNA sequences in Wilms' tumour. *American Journal of Human Genetics*, 41:202–17.

Davis LM, *et al.* (1988). Two anonymous DNA segments distinguish the Wilms' tumour and aniridia loci. *Science*, 241:840–2.

De Caprio JA, *et al.* (1988). SV40 large tumor antigen forms a specific complex with the product of the retinoblastoma susceptibility gene. *Cell*, 54:275–83.

Douglass EC, Wilimas JA, Green AA, Look AT (1985). Abnormalities of chromosome 1 and 11 in Wilms' tumour. *Cancer Genetics and Cytogenetics*, 14:331–8.

Douglass E, *et al.* (1987). A specific chromosomal abnormality in rhabdomyosarcoma. *Cytogenetics and Cell Genetics*, 45:148–55.

Dryja TP, *et al.* (1984). Homozygosity of chromosome 13 in retinoblastoma. *New England Journal of Medicine*, 310:550–3.

Dunn JM, Phillips RA, Becker A, Gallie BL (1988). Identification of germline and somatic mutations affecting the retinoblastoma gene. *Science*, 241:1797–800.

Dyson N, Howley PM, Munger K, Harlow E (1989). The human papilloma virus-16 E7 oncoprotein is able to bind to the retinoblastoma gene product. *Science*, 243:934–6.

Ejima Y, *et al.* (1982). Possible inactivation of part of chromosome 13 due to 13qXp translocation associated with retinoblastoma. *Clinical Genetics*, 21:357–61.

Fearon ER, Vogelstein B, Feinberg AP (1984). Somatic deletion and duplication of genes on chromosome 11 in Wilms' tumours. *Nature*, 309:176–8.

Fong C-T, *et al.* (1989). Loss of heterozygosity for the short arm of chromosome 1 in human neuroblastomas: correlation with N-*myc* amplification. *Proceedings of the National Academy of Sciences USA*, 86:3753–7.

Friend SH, *et al.* (1986). A human DNA segment with properties of the gene that predisposes to retinoblastoma and osteosarcoma. *Nature*, 323:643–6.

Friend SH, *et al.* (1987). Deletions of a DNA sequence in retinoblastomas and mesenchymal tumors: organization of the sequence and its encoded protein. *Proceedings of the National Academy of Sciences USA*, 84:9059–63.

Fung YT, Murphree AL, T'Ang A, Qian J, Hinrichs SH, Benedict WF (1987). Structural evidence for the authenticity of the human retinoblastoma gene. *Science*, 236:1657–61.

Gessler M, *et al.* (1989). A deletion map of the WAGR region on chromosome 11. *American Journal of Human Genetics*, 44:486–95.

Gessler M, Poustka A, Cavenee W, Neve RL, Orkin SH, Bruns GAP (1990). Homozygous deletion in Wilms' tumours of a zinc-finger gene identified by chromosome jumping. *Nature*, 343:774–8.

Godbout R, Dryja TP, Squire J, Gallie BL, Phillips RA (1983). Somatic inactivation of genes on chromosome 13 is a common event in retinoblastoma. *Nature*, 304:451–3.

Griffin CA, *et al.* (1986). Comparison of constitutional and tumor-associated 11;22 translocations: non-identical breakpoints on chromosomes 11 and 22. *Proceedings of the National Academy of Sciences USA*, 83:6122–6.

Griffin CA, Hawkins AL, Packer RJ, Rorke LB, Emanuel BS (1989). Chromosome abnormalities in pediatric brain tumours. *Cancer Research*, 40:175–9.

Grundy P, Koufos A, Morgan K, Li FP, Meadows AT, Cavenee WK (1988). Familial predisposition to Wilms' tumour does not map to the short arm of chromosome 11. *Nature*, 326:375–6.

Hansen MF, *et al.* (1985). Osteosarcoma and retinoblastoma: a shared chromosomal mechanism revealing recessive predisposition. *Proceedings of the National Academy of Sciences USA*, 82:6216–20.

Harbour JW, Lai S-L, Whang-Peng J, Gazdar AF, Minna J, Kaye FJ (1988). Abnormalities in structure and expression of the human retinoblastoma gene in SCLC. *Science*, 241:353–7.

Henry I, *et al.* (1989). Molecular definition of the 11p15.5 region involved in Beckwith–Wiedemann syndrome and probability in predisposition to adrenocortical carcinoma. *Human Genetics*, 81:273–7.

Hida T, Kinoshita Y, Matsumoto R, Suzuki N, Tanaka H (1980). Bilateral retinoblastoma with 13qXp translocation. *Journal of Paediatric Ophthalmology and Strabismus*, 17:144–6.

Higgins MJ, Hansen MF, Cavenee WK, Lalande M (1989). Molecular detection of chromosomal translocations that disrupt the putative retinoblastoma susceptibility locus. *Molecular and Cellular Biology*, 9:1–5.

Hittner HM, Riccardi VM, Francke U (1979). Aniridia caused by a heritable chromosome 11-deletion. *Ophthalmologica*, 86:1173–83.

Hopkinson DA, Mestriner MA, Cortner J, Harris H (1973). Esterase-D: a new human polymorphism. *Annals of Human Genetics*, 37:119–37.

Horowitz JM, *et al.* (1989). Point mutational inactivation of the retinoblastoma antioncogene. *Science*, 243:937–40.

Huff V, Compton DA, Chao L-Y, Strong LC, Geiser CF, Saunders GF (1988). Lack of linkage of familial Wilms' tumour to chromosomal band 11p13. *Nature*, 336:377–8.

Kaneko Y, *et al.* (1987). Different karyotypic patterns in early and advanced stage neuroblastomas. *Cancer Research*, 47:311–18.

Knudson AG (1971). Mutation and cancer: statistical study of retinoblastoma. *Proceedings of the National Academy of Sciences USA*, 68:820–3.

Knudson AG, Strong LC (1972) Mutation and cancer: a model for Wilms' tumour of the kidney. *Journal of the National Cancer Institute*, 40:313–24.

Koufos A, *et al.* (1984). Loss of alleles at loci on human chromosome 11 during genesis of Wilms' tumour. *Nature*, 309:170–2.

Koufos A, Hansen MF, Copeland NG, Jenkins MA, Lampkin BC, Cavenee WK (1986). Loss of heterozygosity in 3 embryonal tumours suggests a common pathogenetic mechanism. *Nature*, 316:330–4.

Koufos A, *et al.* (1989). Familial Wiedemann–Beckwith syndrome and a second Wilms' tumour locus both map to 11p15.5. *American Journal of Human Genetics*, 44:711–19.

Lalande M, Dryja TP, Schreck RR, Shipley J, Flint A, Latt SA (1984). Isolation of human chromosome 13-specific DNA sequences cloned from flow sorted chromosomes and potentially linked to the retinoblastoma locus. *Cancer Genetics and Cytogenetics*, **13**:283–95.

Land H, Parada LF, Weinberg RA (1983). Tumorigenic conversion of primary embryo fibroblasts requires at least two cooperating oncogenes. *Nature*, **300**:596–602.

Lee WH, Bookstein R, Hong F, Young L, Shew JY, Lee EP (1987). Human retinoblastoma susceptibility gene: cloning, identification and sequence. *Science*, **235**:1394–9.

Lewis WH, *et al.* (1988). Homozygous deletion of a DNA marker from chromosome 11 in sporadic Wilms' tumour. *Genomics*, **3**:25–31.

Mannens M, *et al.* (1988). Molecular nature of genetic changes resulting in loss of heterozygosity of chromosome 11 in Wilms' tumours. *Human Genetics*, **81**:41–8.

Miller RW, Fraumeni JR, Manning MD (1964). Association of Wilms' tumour with aniridia, hemihypertrophy, and other congenital malformations. *New England Journal of Medicine*, **27**:922–7.

Mitchell CD, Cowell JK (1989). Predisposition to retinoblastoma due to a translocation within the *4.7R* locus. *Oncogene*, **4**:253–7.

Motegi T, *et al.* (1983). A recognizable pattern of the midface of retinoblastoma patients with interstitial deletion of 13q. *Human Genetics*, **64**:160–2.

Narahara K, *et al.* (1984). Regional mapping of catalase and Wilms' tumour–aniridia, genitourinary abnormalities, and mental retardation triad loci to the chromosome segment 11p1305–p1306. *Human Genetics*, **66**:181–5.

Orkin SH, Goldman DS, Sallan SE (1984). Development of homozygosity for chromosome 11p markers in Wilms' tumour. *Nature*, **309**:172–4.

Ping AJ, Reeve AE, Law DJ, Young MR, Boehnke M, Feinberg AP (1989). Genetic linkage of Beckwith–Wiedemann syndrome to 11p15. *American Journal of Human Genetics*, **44**:720–3.

Porteous DJ, *et al.* (1987). *HRAS-1* selected chromosome transfer generates markers that co-localise aniridia- and genitourinary dysplasia-associated translocation breakpoints and the Wilms' tumour gene within band 11p13. *Proceedings of the National Academy of Sciences USA*, **84**:5355–9.

Pritchard-Jones K, *et al.* (1991). The candidate Wilms' tumour gene is involved in genitourinary development. *Nature*, **346**:194–7.

Reeve AE, Housiaux PJ, Gardner RJM, Chewings WE, Grindley RM, Millow LJ (1984). Loss of a harvey *ras* allele in sporadic Wilms' tumour. *Nature*, **309**:174–6.

Reeve AE, Sih SA, Raizis AM, Feinberg AP (1989). Loss of alleleic heterozygosity at a second locus on chromosome 11 in sporadic Wilms' tumour cells. *Molecular Cell Biology*, **9**:1799–803.

Riccardi VM, Sujansky E, Smith AC, Francke U (1978). Chromosome imbalance in the aniridia–Wilms' tumour association: 11p interstitial deletion. *Pediatrics*, **61**:604–10.

Rose EA, *et al.* (1990). Complete physical map of the WAGR region of 11p13 localizes a candidate Wilms' tumour gene. *Cell*, **60**:495–508.

Schroeder WT, *et al.* (1987). Non-random loss of maternal chromosome 11 alleles in Wilms' tumours. *American Journal of Human Genetics*, **40**:413–20.

Scrable HJ, Witte DP, Lampkin BC, Cavenee WK (1987). Chromosomal localisation of the human rhabdomyosarcoma locus by mitotic recombination mapping. *Nature*, **329**:645–7.

Seeger RC, *et al.* (1985). Association of multiple copies of the N-*myc* oncogene with rapid progression of neuroblastomas. *New England Journal of Medicine*, **311**:1111–16.

Slater RM (1986). The cytogenetics of Wilms' tumour. *Cancer Genetics and Cytogenetics*, **19**:37–41.

Solis V, Pritchard J, Cowell JK (1988). Cytogenetics of Wilms' tumours. *Cancer Genetics and Cytogenetics*, **34**:223–34.

Solter D (1988). Differential imprinting and expression of maternal and paternal genomes. *Annual Review of Genetics*, **22**:127–46.

Sparkes RS, *et al.* (1980). Regional assignment of genes for human esterase D and retinoblastoma to chromosome band 13q14. *Science*, **208**:1042–4.

Sparkes RS, *et al.* (1983). Gene for hereditary retinoblastoma assigned to human chromosome 13 by linkage to esterase-D. *Science*, **217**:971–3.

Sparkes RS, Sparkes MC, Kalina RE, Pagon RA, Salk DJ, Disteche CM (1984). Separation of the retinoblastoma and esterase D loci in a patient with sporadic retinoblastoma and del(13)(q14.1q22.3). *Human Genetics*, **68**:258–9.

Squire J, Gallie BL, Phillips RA (1985). A detailed analysis of chromosomal changes in heritable and non-heritable retinoblastoma. *Human Genetics*, **70**:291–301.

Strong LC, Riccardi VM, Ferrel RE, Sparkes RS (1981). Familial retinoblastoma and chromosome 13 deletion transmitted via an insertional translocation. *Science*, **213**:1501–3.

T'Ang A, *et al.* (1989). Genomic organization of the human retinoblastoma gene. *Oncogene*, **4**:401–7.

Toguchida J, *et al.* (1988). Chromosomal reorganization for the expression of recessive mutation of retinoblastoma susceptibility gene in the development of osteosarcoma. *Cancer Research*, **48**:3939–43.

Ts'o MO, Fine BS, Zimmerman LE (1969). The Flexner–Wintersteiner rosette in retinoblastoma. *Archives of Pathology*, **88**:664–71.

Turleau C, De Grouchy J, Chavin-Colin F, Martelli H, Voyer M, Charlas R (1984*a*). Trisomy 11p15 and Beckwith–Wiedemann syndrome. A report of two cases. *Human Genetics*, **67**:219–21.

Turleau C, DeGrouchy J, Nihoul-Fekete C, Dufier JL, Chavin-Colin F, Junien C (1984*b*). Del 11p13/nephroblastoma without aniridia. *Human Genetics*, **67**:455–6.

Turleau C, *et al.* (1985). Cytogenetic forms of retinoblastoma: their incidence in a survey of 66 patients. *Cancer Genetics and Cytogenetics*, **16**:321–34.

Vogel W (1979). The genetics of retinoblastoma. *Human Genetics*, **52**:1–54.

Wadey RB, Pal NP, Buckle B, Yeomans E, Pritchard J, Cowell JK (1990). Loss of heterozygosity in Wilms' tumour involves two distinct regions of chromosome 11. *Oncogene*.

Waziri M, Patil SR, Hanson JW, Bartley JA (1983). Abnormality of chromosome 11 in patients with features of Beckwith–Wiedemann syndrome. *Journal of Pediatrics*, **102**:873–6.

Whyte P, *et al.* (1988). Association between an oncogene and an anti-oncogene: the adenovirus E1A proteins bind to the retinoblastoma gene product. *Nature*, **334**:124–9.

Wiedemann HR (1964). Complexe malformatif familial avec hernieombilicle et macroglossie; un syndrome nouveau? *Journal de Genetique Humaine*, **13**:223–32.

Wiedemann HR (1983). Tumours and hemihypertrophy associated with Wiedemann–Beckwith syndrome. *European Journal of Pediatrics*, **141**:129.

Weinberg RA (1989). Oncogenes, antioncogenes, and the molecular bases of multistep carcinogenesis. *Cancer Research*, **49**:3713–21.

Wilkins RJ (1988). Genomic imprinting and carcinogenesis. *Lancet*, i:329–30.

Williams JC, Brown KW, Mott MG, Maitland NJ (1989). Maternal allele loss in Wilms' tumour. *Lancet*, i:283–4.

Yandell DW, *et al.* (1989). Oncogenic point mutations in the human retinoblastoma gene: their application to genetic counseling. *New England Journal of Medicine*, **321**:1689–95.

Yunis JJ, Ramsay KC (1980). Familial occurrence of the aniridia–Wilms' tumour syndrome with deletion 11p13–14.1. *Journal of Pediatrics*, **96**:1027–30.

14.2   Neuroblastoma

BORGHILD ROALD AND JACQUES NINANE

INTRODUCTION

Neuroblastoma is a malignant tumour of the autonomic nervous system, derived from the embryonic neural crest. It is one of the most common and most malignant neoplasms of childhood and is seen only rarely in adults. In contrast with the majority of childhood malignancies, neuroblastoma has not shown a significant improvement in prognosis following the introduction of high dose chemotherapy. The prognosis for a child with high stage neuroblastoma is still usually poor although, thanks to intensive chemotherapy, the number of long-term survivors has increased somewhat over the past decade.

Even though great efforts have been put into the study of the neoplasm through the years, neuroblastoma is still an enigmatic tumour. It is usually highly malignant and lethal, but nevertheless appears to show the most frequent spontaneous regression rate among human malignancies. Disturbance of the normal maturation of stem cells seems to be an important factor in at least a fraction of neuroblastomas. The intrinsic mechanism and stimulus for maturation or disappearance of the neuroblastoma tumour cells remain unknown.

The highly variable clinical behaviour has made the handling of the individual patient difficult. In addition, the increasing understanding of the biology of this malignancy makes neuroblastoma a real challenge.

INCIDENCE AND AGE INCIDENCE

Neuroblastoma accounts for 5–10 per cent of all cancers observed in patients up to the age of 15. It is essentially a tumour of infancy and early childhood. It is the most common solid tumour in the neonatal period and can be well established and widely disseminated at birth. In most series 85 per cent of the children are less than 5 years old and 35 per cent are less than 1.5 years old at the time of diagnosis. The mean age at diagnosis is 2 years. Approximately 15 per cent of cancer deaths in children are due to neuroblastoma. Males and females are affected equally. There is a small but important and possibly underestimated hereditary association.

PATHOLOGY

Neuroblastoma was first described by Virchow in 1865 as a glioma. In 1891 Marchand linked the tumour to the sympathetic nervous system and the term neuroblastoma was proposed by Wright in 1910.

Histopathology

Macroscopically, the tumour may appear well defined, encapsulated, and lobulated. In other neuroblastomas the border towards the surrounding structures may be vaguely defined. The cut surface may appear reddish and soft with foci of yellow necrosis, calcification, and haemorrhage. The calcifications can be seen radiographically and are a diagnostic criterion for neuroblastoma. However, some tumours are partly or completely firm and white. Microscopically, the tumours of the neuroblastoma group show a complex picture. They consist of a spectrum of histological patterns ranging from undifferentiated tumours, composed solely of cells similar to those found in the embryonal neural crest, through tumours with increasing signs of differentiation (eosinophilic fibrillary material separating the tumour cells, sometimes with rosette formation and sometimes including larger cells with abundant eosinophilic cytoplasm and well-defined nucleoli) to tumours consisting only of differentiated structures such as nerve fibres and ganglion cells.

The general nomenclature reflects this changing degree of differentiation. The tumour is called a neuroblastoma when it is composed solely or mostly of undifferentiated small round hyperchromatic cells without nucleoli, sometimes with a background of fine fibrillary structures. Ganglioneuroblastoma contains a mixture of mature or maturing ganglion cells, fibrils, and undifferentiated neuroblasts. In some tumours there may be a tendency for maturation towards bundles of nerve structures and fibrous connective tissue in the periphery. Ganglioneuroma is a tumour consisting entirely of mature and maturing ganglion cells and nerve fibres. The microscopic picture may be diverse and may vary within the tumour. Usually, however, the tumour will fit into one of the categories without major difficulty (Fig. 1).

Within a ganglioneuroblastoma there may be areas of undifferentiated neuroblastoma (sometimes referred to as 'composite' ganglioneuroblastomas). Maturation of undifferentiated neuroblastomas has been seen clinically, as well as experimentally, in cell lines.

Various histopathological classification systems have been proposed, focusing mainly on the degree of cellular differentiation. There is a correlation between increasing neural differentiation and a less aggressive clinical behaviour. The grading systems of Beckwith and Martin (1968) and Hughes *et al.* (1974) have been most widely used.

Additional morphological elements were included in the grading systems in the age-linked classification of Shimada *et al.* (1984), who introduced a so-called MK index (MKI). MKI is the sum of cells undergoing either mitosis or karyorrhexis among 5000 tumour cells in randomly selected fields and is subgrouped into low (<2 per cent), intermediate (2–4 per cent), and high (>4 per cent). The classification also focused on the amount of Schwannian stroma (fibrovascular septa, fibrous tissue, and nerve bundles) and tumour cell differentiation. Using the Shimada system, the tumours are first assigned to stroma-rich or stroma-poor groups, defined according to the amount of Schwannian stroma. MKI is the parameter that will determine the prognostic grouping in infants younger than 1.5 years with stroma-poor tumours; a high MKI will put the patient in the poor prognosis group. For patients between 1.5 and 5 years, a lack of differentiation in the tumour cells or MKI at intermediate or high level accounts for a poor prognosis. Children over the age of 5 years are put directly into the unfavourable group.

A striking correlation with prognosis was found, with 84 per cent of surviving patients in the favourable stroma-poor group versus

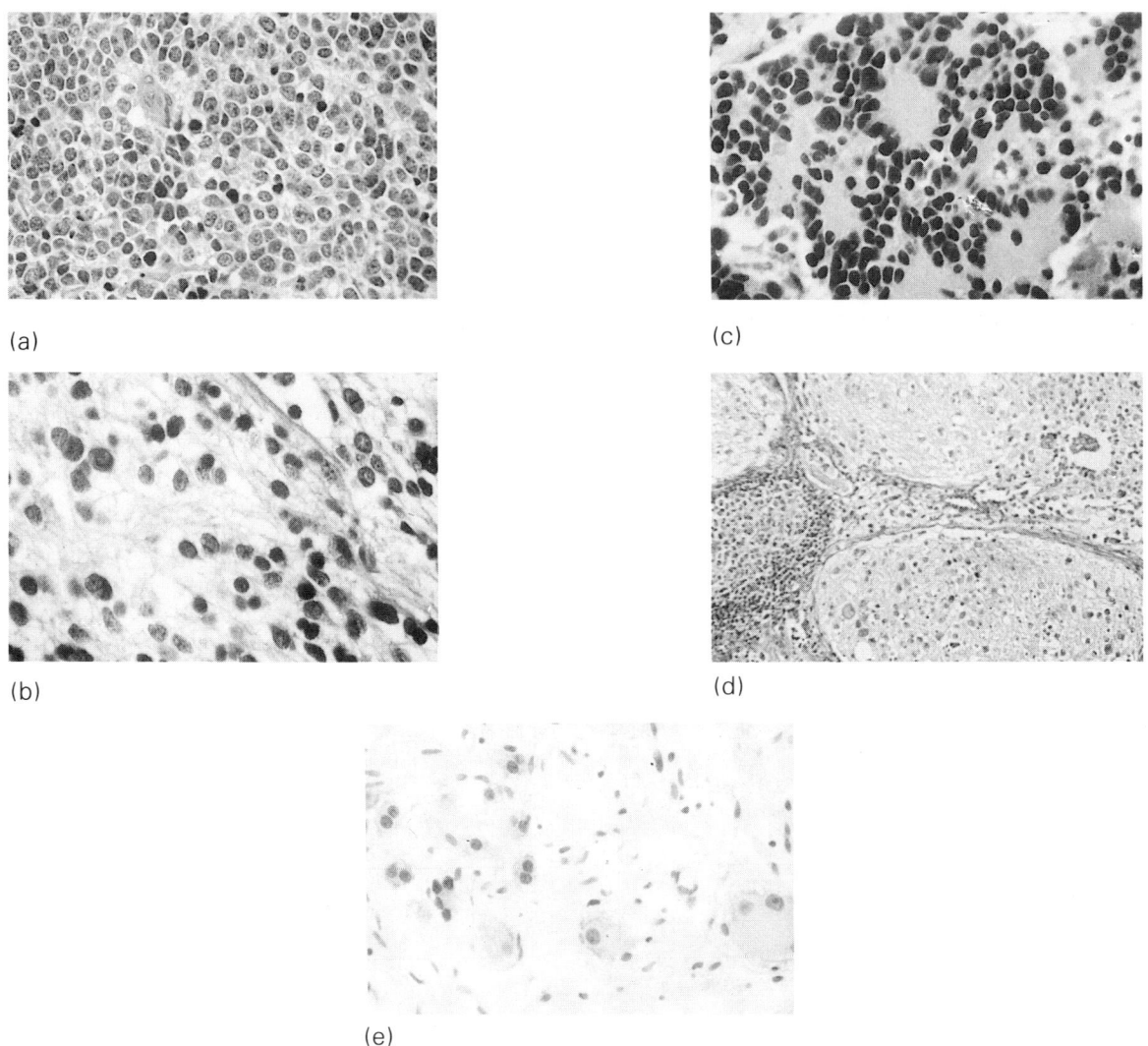

Fig. 1 The histopathology of the group of neuroblastoma tumours: (a) primitive neuroblastoma, the typical small round blue-celled malignant tumour of childhood (160×); (b) neuroblastoma with typical fine fibrillary background between dense hyperchromatic tumour cell nuclei (160×); (c) Homer–Wright rosettes (160×); (d) ganglioneuroblastoma with admixture of mature and undifferentiated tumour cells, with dividing septa of fibrovascular stroma with Schwann cells (note the lymphoid focus in the stromal system in the lower left part) (40×); (e) ganglioneuroma consisting of differentiated cells and structures only (160×).

4.5 per cent in the unfavourable stroma-poor group (2 year survival), showing that this new criterion really adds new prognostic information. Other investigations have confirmed that this classification identifies groups of patients at high risk.

The only stroma-rich tumour belonging to the poor prognosis group is the so-called nodular stroma-rich type (survival <20 per cent), consistent with composite ganglioneuroblastoma. The stroma-rich tumours without such distinct undifferentiated nodules had a 2 year survival of 90 per cent.

Immunohistochemistry

The diagnosis of small cell tumours may be difficult on the basis of purely morphological criteria, particularly when the biopsies are small (throughcut or pistol biopsies). Immunological techniques, identifying more or less cell-specific antigens, have proved to be a valuable adjunct in the diagnosis of neuroblastoma. This is true both for the primary lesion and in the often difficult diagnosis of bone-marrow involvement. A number of polyclonal antisera and monoclonal antibodies reacting with neuroblastoma cells have been reported (Fig. 2). Many of these antibody-defined antigens are shared with haematopoietic cells, fetal neural tissue, or various normal tissues. In fact, none has proved to be selectively reactive with neuroblastoma cells. Moreover, not all neuroblastomas express all antigens. Despite this, the antibodies can be of decisive diagnostic help when used as a part of a selected panel. In addition to diagnostic procedures on cell suspensions and tissue sections, such monoclonal antibodies have been used in imaging studies and purging procedures prior to autologous bone-marrow transplantation.

An increasing number of markers are commercially available and can even be used on paraffin-embedded and formaldehyde-fixed tissues. However, some of them require enzyme pre-treatment of the tissue sections and certain antigens are

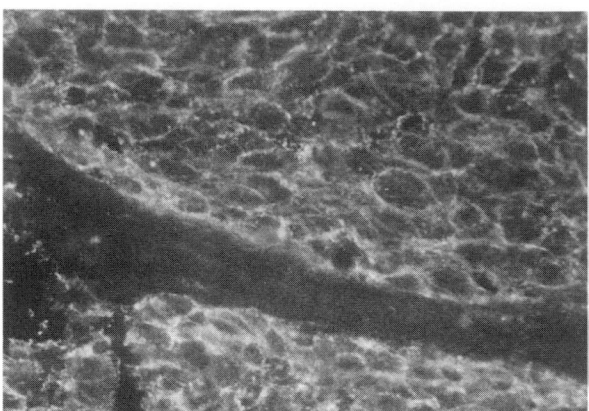

Fig. 2 Immunofluorescence staining of undifferentiated neuroblastoma with monoclonal antibody to neuroblastoma cells, NCAM (160×).

only detectable in native cells, ethanol-fixed tissues, or frozen sections. Therefore, the panel of antibodies employed will vary and must be tested in the individual laboratory prior to their diagnostic use.

In addition to antibodies and neuroblastoma markers such as NCAM, neuron-specific enolase, neurofilament, S-100 protein, and synaptophysin, the group of markers in a diagnostic panel for immunohistochemistry should include leucocyte markers and intermediate filament markers for cytokeratin (epithelial cells), desmine (muscle cells), and vimentin (mesenchymal cells) to exclude leukaemia/lymphoma, Wilms' tumour and hepatoblastoma, rhabdomyosarcoma, Ewing's sarcoma, and neuroectodermal tumours. In contrast with neuroblastoma, the tumour cells in Ewing's sarcoma and primitive neuroectodermal tumours are positive for vimentin.

Electron microscopy

The ultrastructural features of neuroblastoma cells have been well documented and consist of neuritic cytoplasmic processes with filaments, microtubules, and cytoplasmatic neurosecretory granules. The presence of neurosecretory granules is more diagnostic for neuroblastoma than the neuritic processes.

The neurosecretory granules are small (50–200 nm) spherical membrane-bound units with an electron-dense core. Their number has been reported to correlate with the biochemical pattern of catecholamine metabolites in the tumours. They are the sites of conversion of dopamine to noradrenalin and also the storage sites of noradrenalin.

Tissue culture

Tissue culture studies may also be helpful in the diagnosis of neuroblastoma. Neuroblasts, even from undifferentiated neuroblastomas, will grow readily in suitable media and form branching fibrillary processes.

As an adjunct to the establishment of a diagnosis of neuroblastoma, electron microscopy and tissue culture studies were more important prior to the era of immunohistochemistry.

SPECIAL TUMOUR VARIANTS
Neuroblastoma *in situ*

Minute foci of primitive neuroblasts are routinely found in the adrenal glands of neonates. Beckwith and Perrin (1963) reported as neuroblastoma *in situ* small nodules in the adrenal glands, histologically indistinguishable from neuroblastoma, in necropsy specimens from infants (less than 3 months) dying of unrelated causes. The incidence of these lesions was 40 times higher than that of clinical neuroblastoma. These findings have been used as evidence to prove that most neuroblastomas spontaneously regress or mature into benign lesions. Alternatively it has been postulated that many *in situ* neuroblastomas are normal developmental remnants rather than true neoplasms.

Esthesioneuroblastoma

Olfactory neuroblastoma (also known as esthesioneuroblastoma, esthesioblastoma) is a malignant neoplasm originating in the olfactory apparatus. The lesions arise in the nose and may obliterate the ethmoid sinus as a fleshy pinkish-grey tumour, histologically and ultrastructurally resembling a neuroblastoma. However, this tumour is not derived from the neural crest, but from neuroepithelial elements in the roof of the nasal cavity. The tumour has been reported in patients from 3 to 79 years (mean 50 years), possibly reflecting the continuous proliferation of the neuronal aspect of sensory epithelium. The histopathological pattern does not predict the clinical outcome. Neurosecretory granules have been seen ultrastructurally but serum catecholamines are not elevated.

Primitive neuroectodermal tumours

The number of tumours derived from the primitive neural crest is probably higher than previously recognized. These tumours resemble neuroblastomas histologically. At times the tumour is clearly associated with an identifiable nerve. The tumours are found in a variety of anatomical locations. Generally, there is no elevation of catecholamine metabolites. A distinct cytogenetic translocation t(11;22) and the lack of N-*myc* amplification are diagnostic for these tumours.

BIOLOGY
DNA ploidy

Numerous cytometric studies in a wide variety of neoplasms have reported an association between abnormal DNA content and aggressive tumour behaviour, with poor prognosis for the patient regardless of treatment. Acute lymphoblastic leukaemia and neuroblastoma are two important exceptions to this pattern. In neuroblastoma a hyperdiploid (near triploid) DNA content of the malignant cells apparently predicts a better response to chemotherapy than diploidy. This seems to be of particular importance in infants (Look *et al.* 1984) and in children below the age of 1.5 years.

Cytogenetics

The most characteristic cytogenetic abnormality in human neuroblastoma is a deletion at the short arm of chromosome 1, between 1p32 and 1pter. This deletion is present in 70–85 per cent of neuroblastoma tumours and cell lines, suggesting that this is an important neuroblastoma locus. Genes that have been identified as important for hereditary cancers and at least some of their non-hereditary counterparts seem to cause cancer when both copies are defective or lost.

Homogeneously staining regions and the presence of small chromosome fragments without centrosomes (double minutes) are other characteristic karyotypic aberrations seen in neuroblastoma tumour cells and neuroblastoma cell lines. It has been suggested that double minutes either form from or are breakdown products of homogeneously staining regions. These regions are not restricted to any specific chromosome, but have been shown in 18 different chromosomes in human neuroblastomas. Moreover, homogeneously staining regions and double minutes are not specific for neuroblastoma, but have been found in other paediatric malignancies including rhabdomyosarcoma, Ewing's sarcoma, and retinoblastoma.

N-*myc* oncogene

Homogeneously staining regions and double minutes have been shown to be the site of gene amplification. *In situ* hybridization studies have shown that in neuroblastoma the amplified gene is N-*myc*, an oncogene with partial homology to the *myc* oncogene. The N-*myc* gene is normally found on chromosome 2(2p 23–24). Amplification of the N-*myc* oncogene in high stage neuroblastoma has been shown to be of prognostic importance. Patients with a high number of genomic N-*myc* copies appear to relapse faster after multimodal chemotherapy than those with a single copy of the gene (Seeger *et al.* 1985).

CLINICAL FEATURES

Symptoms, signs, and differential diagnosis

The initial symptoms of neuroblastoma are frequently non-specific. They may mimic a wide variety of more common paediatric conditions. A growing infiltrative tumour in the thorax, abdomen, or pelvis may invade and compress surrounding structures. At times pain from widespread metastasis to the bones and bone-marrow dominates the picture, while the primary tumour itself can be small and difficult to find.

The condition may present during the early weeks of life and may even be apparent at birth. In infants, the first sign is usually a rapidly enlarging liver, sometimes accompanied by skin nodules and bone-marrow involvement. The infant is unwell and compression of lungs and abdominal viscera causes feeding difficulties accompanied by vomiting, weight loss, dyspnoea, and failure to thrive. The important differential diagnosis is hepatoblastoma.

Tumours growing through the intravertebral foramina and compressing the spinal cord (dumb-bell tumours) may present with neurological symptoms such as flaccid paralysis of the legs or urinary dysfunction with distention of the bladder.

The metabolic effect of the tumour can cause systemic symptoms. The high level of the catecholamines and sometimes vasoactive intestinal peptides produced by neuroblastoma can result in bouts of sweating and pallor associated with diarrhoea and hypertension. These rare symptoms are probably unrelated to the site and size of the tumour and regress after successful treatment.

Neuroblastoma is frequently a systemic disease at the time of diagnosis. The signs and symptoms can be confused with those of leukaemia, consisting of anaemia and mucosal or skin haemorrhage due to pancytopenia caused by bone-marrow infiltration with neuroblastoma cells.

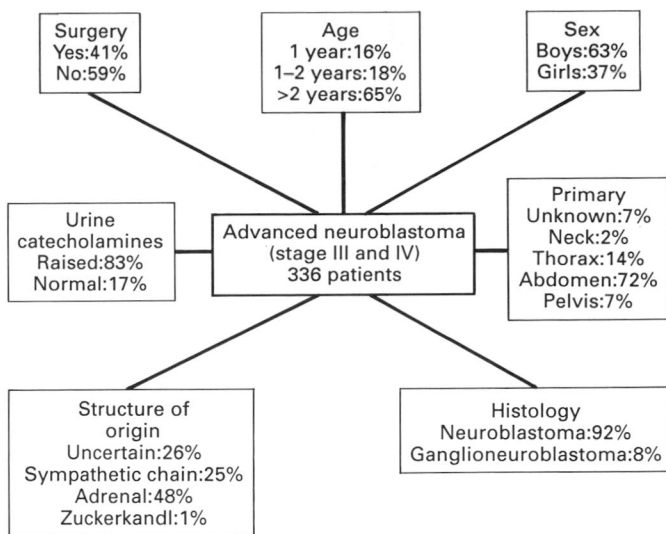

Fig. 3 Characteristics of 336 children with advanced neuroblastoma (Evans stages III and IV).

Table 1 Neuroblastoma: primary sites and frequency

Abdominal/retroperitoneal	45%–70%
Adrenal	27%–36%
Extra adrenal	18%–41%
Thorax/mediastinum	15%
Head and neck	7%
Other	10%
Unknown	7%

Finally, the tumour may be discovered by a routine clinical examination. Figure 3 shows the characteristics at presentation of 336 patients with unresectable tumour or metastatic disease diagnosed in a 10 year period (Ninane 1987).

Sites of involvement

Cells from the neural crest normally migrate throughout the body along well-defined routes and accumulate at precise positions. Because of the wide distribution of neural crest cells throughout the trunk, neuroblastomas can develop in a variety of sites. They are most frequently found close to the autonomic chain, mainly in the adrenal gland and in various paraspinal locations. The most common sites and the frequency of their involvement by neuroblastomas are summarized in Table 1. In general, the majority of cases originate in the upper retroperitoneal area. On rare occasions, neuroblastomas can also be found in the cerebrum. At times a primary site cannot be identified.

INVESTIGATION AND MANAGEMENT STRATEGY

The conventional diagnostic methods are numerous and cumbersome for the child and its family. They include skeletal survey and bone scan, abdominal ultrasound, CT scan of the pelvis, abdomen, and mediastinum, tumour biopsies, bone-marrow aspirates and biopsies (at least two), and 24 h urine collection for measurement of catecholamines and catecholamine metabolite levels. These investigations are not only conducted for diagnostic purposes but are also repeated at the end of pre-operative chemotherapy and for months and years during the follow-up period. In order to improve the quality of life for these children it is desirable to replace these techniques by simpler ones. New methods such as I-131-MIBG, magnetic resonance imaging, and *in vivo* radio-immunodection are useful advances but may sometimes miss primary tumours and some metastases, particularly following chemotherapy.

Tumour markers

There is no ideal neuroblastoma marker. Four markers, detectable in blood or urine, have been reported to give valuable diagnostic or prognostic information: catecholamines, neurone-specific enolase, ferritin, and gangliosides. In institutions with good clinical research facilities all these markers should ideally be examined at the same time.

Neuroblastoma cells secrete large amounts of one or more catecholamines, as well as their metabolites (Fig. 4). For practical purposes, vanillylmandelic acid and homovanillic acid are most widely measured in the diagnosis and follow-up of children with neuroblastoma. Conflicting results have been reported concerning the correlation of vanillylmandelic acid and homovanillic acid levels in pre-treatment urines and prognosis of neuroblastoma patients. In cases of 'non-secreting' tumours, less frequently measured metabolites may be useful in establishing the diagnosis.

Most authors still recommend the classical methodology where a 24 h urine collection is necessary. Recently, random urinary homovanillic acid and vanillylmandelic acid levels have been shown to be adequate in the diagnosis of neuroblastoma. Moreover, sequential determinations of random homovanillic acid and vanillylmandelic acid levels were also helpful in the follow-up of these patients. In view of data from Tuchman *et al.* (1987), random sampling of urine for sequential determination of homovanillic acid and vanillylmandelic acid is probably the best test if one considers both its sensitivity and specificity and the comfort of the child.

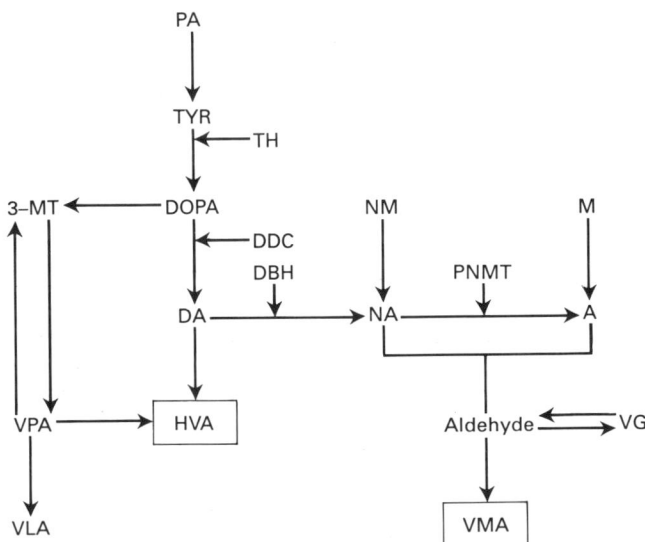

Fig. 4 Metabolism of catecholamines. Enzymes: TH (tyrosine hydrolase), DDC (dopadecarboxylase), PNMT (phenylethanolamine-*N*-methyl transferase), DBH (dopamine-β-hydroxylase). Catecholamines, metabolites, and precursors: PA (phenylalanine), TYR (tyrosine), DOPA (3,4-dihydroxylphenylalanine), DA (dopamine), NA (noradrenalin), A (adrenalin), VMA (vanillylmandelicacid), HVA (homovanillic acid), NM (normetanephrine), M (metanephrine), MT(3-methoxytyramine), VLA (vanillactic acid), VPA (vanillpuric acid), VG (vanilglycol).

Although high serum neurone-specific enolase levels are suggestive of neuroblastoma, increased levels can also be seen in children with other malignancies such as Wilms' tumour, Ewing's sarcoma, non-Hodgkin's lymphoma, soft tissue sarcoma, and the acute leukaemias. Thus, caution should be exercised in using neurone-specific enolase as a diagnostic test in children with malignancies. In addition the test is not particularly sensitive. Raised serum neurone-specific enolase levels can be found in all stages of neuroblastoma at diagnosis. In general, the degree of elevation is related to prognosis with a high level being indicative of a poor outcome. It is interesting to observe that patients with 4S neuroblastoma (see section on Staging), which generally presents with a large tumour burden but has a particularly favourable prognosis, usually have lower levels of neurone-specific enolase than children with stage 4 disease of equivalent tumour bulk. This is further confirmation that the biological characteristics of 4S neuroblastoma are quite different from the other types of this disease. It remains to be determined whether serial neurone-specific enolase measurements are of more value than repeated catecholamine estimation in monitoring the course of the disease.

Children with advanced neuroblastoma frequently present with an increased level of ferritin in serum. The levels usually decrease during treatment and may return to normal values when the patients are in clinical remission. There is evidence that tumour cells are at least partially responsible for the increased amounts of serum ferritin in patients with neuroblastoma.

Gangliosides, which are glucosphingolipids containing sialic acid, are mainly detected in the cell surface membrane and are shed or released *in vitro* by a variety of cells, particularly tumour cells. Elevated concentrations of disialoganglioside G2 to more than 50 times the normal level have been demonstrated in the serum of children with active neuroblastoma. Sequential determination of circulating G2 reveals that plasma levels diminish in children responding to therapy and reappear in patients in relapse. In contrast, circulating G2 has not been detected in the plasma of children with ganglioneuroblastoma or ganglioneuroma.

STAGING CLASSIFICATION

Three major staging systems are used for neuroblastoma throughout the world:

(1) the system utilized by the Children's Cancer Study Group (CCSG) and many others (Evans *et al.* 1971);

(2) the system used by St Jude Children's Research Hospital (SJCRH) and the Pediatric Oncology Group (POG) (Hayes *et al.* 1983);

(3) the TNM system proposed by the International Union Against Cancer (UICC-TNM 1987).

Modifications of these systems are employed by the Italian Cooperative Working Group, the Malignant Tumour Committee of the Japanese Society of Paediatric Surgeons, and others. In general, the various staging systems give comparable results in distinguishing low stage patients with good prognosis from high stage patients with poor prognosis. However, some of the differences between these staging systems are substantial, particularly when applied to individual patients. Thus, the results of different groups cannot be readily compared. Points of disagreement include (1) the prognostic significance of the tumour crossing midline, (2) the prognostic importance of ipsilateral and/or contralateral lymph node involvement, and (3) the importance of resectability of the primary tumour.

Table 2 Staging

The CCSG staging system (Evans et al. 1971)

Stage I	Tumour confined to the organ or structure of origin
Stage II	Tumour extending in continuity beyond the organ or structure of origin but not crossing the midline; regional lymph nodes on the ipsilateral side may be involved
Stage III	Tumour extending in continuity beyond the midline; regional lymph nodes may be involved bilaterally
Stage IV	Remote disease involving the skeleton, organs, soft tissue, and distant lymph nodes groups.
Stage IV-S	(Special category) Patients who would otherwise be stage I or stage II but who have remote disease confined to liver, skin, or bone-marrow, and who have no radiographic evidence of bone metastases on complete skeletal survey

The TNM classification (UICC-TNM 1987)

Stage I	T1	N0	M0
Stage II	T2	N0	M0
Stage III	T1T2	N1	M0
	T3	Any N	M0
Stage IV A	T1T2T3	Any N	M1
Stage IV B	T4	Any N	Any M

Primary tumour (T)

T0	No evidence of primary tumour
T1	Single tumour, diameter < 5 cm
T2	Single tumour, diameter > 5 cm but < 10 cm
T3	Single tumour, diameter > 10 cm
T4	Multiple simultaneous tumours
Tx	Minimum requirements to assess the tumour cannot be met

Regional lymph nodes (N)

N0	No evidence of lymph node involvement
N1	Regional lymph node involvement
Nx	Minimum requirements to assess the regional lymph nodes cannot be met

Distant metastases (M)

M0	No evidence of distant metastases
M1	Evidence of distant metastases
Mx	Minimum requirements to assess distant metastases cannot be met

INSS: International Staging System for Neuroblastoma (Brodeur et al. 1988)

Stage 1	Localized tumour confined to the area of origin; complete gross excision, with or without microscopic residual disease; identifiable ipsilateral and contralateral lymph nodes negative macroscopically
Stage 2a	Unilateral tumour with incomplete gross excision; identifiable ipsilateral and contralateral lymph nodes negative microscopically
Stage 2b	Unilateral tumour with complete or incomplete gross excision; positive ipsilateral regional lymph nodes; contralateral lymph nodes negative microscopically
Stage 3	Tumour infiltrating across the midline with or without regional lymph node involvement or unilateral tumour with contralateral regional lymph node involvement or midline tumour with bilateral regional lymph node involvement
Stage 4	Dissemination of tumour to distant lymph nodes, bone, bone-marrow, liver, and/or other organs (except as defined in stage 4S)
Stage 4S	Localized primary tumour as defined for stages 1 or 2 with dissemination limited to liver, skin, and/or bone-marrow

of the Japanese Society of Paediatric Surgeons, and others. In general, the various staging systems give comparable results in distinguishing low stage patients with good prognosis from high stage patients with poor prognosis. However, some of the differences between these staging systems are substantial, particularly when applied to individual patients. Thus, the results of different groups cannot be readily compared. Points of disagreement include (1) the prognostic significance of the tumour crossing midline, (2) the prognostic importance of ipsilateral and/or contralateral lymph node involvement, and (3) the importance of resectability of the primary tumour.

Agreement on the definition of stage with regard to these and other issues has been achieved (Brodeur et al. 1988). This new staging system, known as the International Neuroblastoma Staging System (INSS) will facilitate comparisons of different studies if it is widely adopted. For comparison, Table 2 shows the CCSG, TNM, and INSS staging for neuroblastoma patients.

PROGNOSTIC FACTORS

The age at diagnosis is still the single most important factor forecasting the prognosis for a child with neuroblastoma. Children under the age of 1.5 years at diagnosis have a much better prognosis than those who are older. Other important prognostic factors at the time of diagnosis include the extent of disease spread (stage) and the primary site of the tumour. The prognosis for children with ISSN stage 1 and stage 4S disease is better than for those with more advanced disease. Retroperitoneal and particularly adrenal neoplasms are associated with the poorest prognosis, while thoracic neoplasms usually have the most favourable outcome. Signs of histopathological differentiation within the tumour is a favourable prognostic feature. However, the most unpredictable poorly differentiated neoplasms, the neuroblastomas, account for the majority of tumours. The age-linked classification of Shimada et al. (1984), with the focus on mitosis and karyorrhexis, gives valuable prognostic information. The composite ganglioneuroblastomas containing compact areas or foci of neuroblastoma within an otherwise maturing neoplasm retain the ability to metastasize as a neuroblastoma. Thus, they should be considered as a group of potentially more dangerous neoplasms than the diffuse form of ganglioneuroblastoma. The differentiated ganglioneuroma is a benign neoplasm and does not metastasize.

Flow cytometric studies of tumour cell DNA content may help to identify a specific group of triploid (near diploid) tumours in small children that seem to respond better to therapy. Molecular biology studies of oncogene amplification have shown that amplification of the N-*myc* oncogene is an important and independent factor, forecasting a very poor prognosis and rapidly fatal clinical course for the child with neuroblastoma.

Biochemical profiles, particularly increased secretion of catecholamines and their metabolites, are important in the diagnosis and follow-up of neuroblastoma patients. Increased serum neurone-specific enolase and ferritin levels can be found in all stages of neuroblastoma at diagnosis, as well as in other paediatric malignancies and, thus, have lesser diagnostic importance. In a neuroblastoma patient, however, a low neurone-specific enolase level predicts a good prognosis and a high level predicts a poor outcome. Ferritin is seldom raised in sera from children with stages I and II neuroblastoma, but is abnormally raised in some patients with stages III and IV disease when it indicates a significantly poorer prognosis. Ganglioside concentration in plasma seems to be a good indicator for the child's response to therapy and to relapses.

Mass screening for neuroblastoma

The treatment of advanced stages of neuroblastoma in older children is a major problem. The majority of these children will die of their tumour. In contrast, approximately 80 per cent of babies under 1 year are probably curable. Since 1973 a successful mass screening for neuroblastoma has been organized in Kyoto, Japan, including approximately 70 per cent of the births in the area. At 6–7 months of age the children are tested for urinary catecholamines. A follow-up of 25 children with neuroblastoma detected by screening of almost half a million infants showed that 23 (92 per cent) of these patients were free from disease, after a medium follow-up time of more than 3 years (Sawada 1986). However, the Japanese screening material consists of a higher number of neuroblastomas in prognostically favourable stages and it is unclear whether or not such screening will improve the outcome for the neuroblastoma patients with poor prognosis. Nevertheless, there is a tendency to embark on similar screening programmes in other parts of the world.

MANAGEMENT AND RESULTS OF TREATMENT

Localized neuroblastoma

The definition of localized neuroblastoma is not as obvious as it might seem. It is here referred to the new INSS stages 1, 2a, and 2b.

Stage 1 tumours are often discovered by chance; only the homolateral Claude Bernard Horner syndrome associated with a cervical tumour is symptomatic. Surgery alone is curative for stage 1 tumours. Furthermore, it will permit a precise histological diagnosis and confirmation of the stage. Nevertheless, long-term follow-up of these children is necessary to make sure that there is no local recurrence of the disease or distant metastases.

Stage 2a tumours are curable by surgery involving an approach identical in all respects to that for stage 1. The persistence of malignant tissue after surgery is probably not an indication for adjuvant therapy in the other forms of stage 2a disease. The only exception is the 'dumb-bell' form of paravertebral neuroblastoma, in which case adjuvant chemo- or radiotherapy may be given. However, there is no evidence that this unusual form of neuroblastoma needs a different therapeutic approach. In contrast, surgical treatment should be followed by chemotherapy in children with stage 2b tumours, according to their ages. Chemotherapy is not needed in children under 6 months, as their youth is an independent favourable prognostic factor. The advantage of youth diminishes between 6 months and 1 year, warranting 'conventional' chemotherapy (vincristine and cyclophosphamide) of short duration. The prognosis for children over 1 year of age with stage 2b is between that of stage 2/2a and advanced neuroblastoma. Thus, more intensive chemotherapy is necessary.

Advanced neuroblastoma

Treating advanced neuroblastoma is a real challenge. Unlike other childhood tumours, such as Wilms' tumour and soft tissue sarcomas, the introduction of conventional chemotherapy has had little impact on survival in children with stages 3 or 4 neuroblastomas. This is a paradox, as neuroblastoma cells are particularly sensitive to chemotherapy and radiotherapy. However, responders invariably relapse with local recurrences or distant metastases.

The 'conventional' treatment for neuroblastoma consisted of various vincristine–cyclophosphamide combinations and adriamycin. Cyclophosphamide and, to a lesser extent, vincristine are active

Table 3 Recent published combination chemotherapies in advanced neuroblastoma

OPEC (Shafford et al. 1984)		
Vincristine	1.5 mg/m²	day 1
Cyclophosphamide	600 mg/m²	day 1
Cisplatinum	60 mg/m²	day 2
Teniposide (VM-26)	150 mg/m²	day 4
(6–10 courses, repeated every 3 weeks)		
CADO (Hartmann et al. 1987)		
Vincristine	1.5 mg/m²	days 1 and 5
Cyclophosphamide	300 mg/m²	days 1–5
Doxorubicin	60 mg/m²	day 5
(6–8 courses, repeated every 3 weeks)		
PE-CADO (Bernhard et al. 1987)		
Vincristine	1.5 mg/m²	days 1 and 5
Cyclophosphamide	300 mg/m²	days 1–5
Doxorubicin	60 mg/m²	day 5
Cisplatinum	100 mg/m²	day 21
Teniposide (VM-26)	150 mg/m²	day 23
(3–4 courses, repeated every 3 weeks)		

against neuroblastoma when used singly. When combined, they induce responses in a larger number of cases. Some children with neuroblastoma resistant to the vincristine–cyclophosphamide combination may respond to adriamycin alone.

In order to increase the response rate in patients with advanced neuroblastoma, new therapeutic regimens have been designed. Almost all of them include cisplatinum and an epipodophyllotoxin (VM-26 teniposide or VP-16 etoposide). Three combination chemotherapy regimens are summarized in Table 3. It is crucial that the same definition of response is given to patients treated with pre-operative chemotherapy (Brodeur et al. 1988). The rate of good partial response or complete response with these regimens is between 50 and 60 per cent in stages 3 and 4 patients. However, the relapse rate is still high even in good responders and complete responders, particularly in children more than 1 year old.

Megatherapy with bone-marrow rescue

Because of high relapse rate, several 'megatherapy' and 'consolidation therapy' regimens have been designed, aiming to increase the number of long-term survivors. For several reasons it is difficult to compare the results of the various regimens (Table 4). The clinical status of the children at the time of consolidation treatment as well as the type of 'megatherapy' differs in the various studies. However, despite patient heterogeneity and methodological differences in the treatment administered, three important points can be made.

1. The patients who received megatherapy after complete response or good partial response survived longer than those who were treated in relapse.

2. At 2 years, high dose melphalan administered as single-drug therapy yielded comparable results to those of intensive multiple chemotherapy, even if the latter was combined with total body irradiation.

3. Mortality due to treatment was lower in the European Neuroblastoma Study Group (ENSG) study.

High dose therapy given as consolidation treatment to children with advanced neuroblastomas in complete or good partial response increases their 2 year survival rate significantly, although the toxicity

Table 4 Megatherapy and bone-marrow rescue

Cooperative groups	ENSG-1[a]	LMCE[b]	IGR[c]	CCSG[d]
No. of children	30	37	26	47
Stage	III–IV	V	III–IV	IV
Status	CR/GPR	CR/GPR	CR/GPR/PR	REL (28) CR/GPR/PR (19)
Randomization	Yes	No	No	No
Megatherapy	HDM	TBI+VCR+ HDM	HDM (15) HDM+BCNU +VM-26	TBI+HDM+ other drugs
Bone-marrow rescue	AMT	ABMT (35) BMT (2)	ABMT	ABMT (26) BMT (21)
Ex-vitro treatment of bone-marrow	No	MoAB	ASTA-Z (11)	NO
2 year survival	54%	44%	?	25%
Toxic deaths	2 (7%)	7 (19%)	3 (12%)	15 (32%)

Cooperative groups: ENSG, European Neuroblastoma Study Group; LMCE, Lyon, Marseille, Paris, Curie, East of France; IGR, Institut Gustave Roussy; CCSG, Children's Cancer Study Group.
Status at the time of megatherapy: CR, complete response; GPR, good partial response; PR, partial response; REL, relapse.
Megatherapy: HDM, high dose melphalan; TBI, total body irradiation; VCR, vincristine; BCNU, carmustine; VM-26, teniposide.
Bone-marrow rescue: ABMT, autologous bone-marrow transplantation; BMT, allogeneic bone-marrow transplantation.
Ex vivo treatment of bone-marrow cells: ASTA-Z, mafosfamide; MoAB, monoclonal antibodies.
[a]Pritchard et al. 1986
[b]Philip et al. 1987
[c]Hartmann et al. 1985
[d]D'Angio et al. 1985.

of the treatment cannot be discounted. The value of purging the marrow of residual malignant cells when it appears cytologically and histologically normal remains to be demonstrated.

The place of surgery

Previously, only children with localized disease were subjected to surgery. At present, even children with advanced localized or metastatic diseases are treated surgically. Metastases may be cleared by chemotherapy, leaving only a small primary tumour to be excised. These operations are frequently very difficult, but complete or near-complete excision is now possible for the majority of patients.

The place of radiotherapy

Theoretically, external-beam radiotherapy can be used in residual tumours. However, some tumours may recur even in the field of radiotherapy. Moreover, the long-term side-effects of radiotherapy given to small children are now very well recognized.

Two specific types of radiotherapy treatment are used for neuroblastoma patients. As part of the ablative regimen in poor prognosis patients, prior to bone-marrow transplantation total body irradiation is used. Secondly, radionucleotide treatment with MIBG labelled with ^{131}I has been successfully used as targeted

radiotherapy in the diagnosis and treatment of neuroblastoma. The immediate results are quite impressive.

Even if the 2 year disease-free survival of children with advanced neuroblastoma has increased over the past decade as a result of intensive treatment, it is still far too low. Therefore other types of treatment should be explored in addition to chemotherapy, preferably in children with no evidence of clinical disease after consolidation therapy: 'targeting' with MIBG or monoclonal antibodies and adoptive immunotherapy with tumour necrosis factor or lymphokine-activated killer cells and different 'maturating agents' (retinoids).

REFERENCES

Beckwith JB, Martin RF (1968). Observations on the histopathology of neuroblastomas. *Journal of Pediatric Surgery*, 3:106–10.

Beckwith JB, Perrin EV (1963). *In situ* neuroblastoma: a contribution to the natural history of neural crest tumours. *American Journal of Pathology*, 43:1089–104.

Bernhard JL, et al. (1987). Sequential cisplatin/VM-26 and vincristine/ cyclophosphamide/doxorubicin in metastatic neuroblastoma: an effective alternating non-cross resistant regimen? *Journal of Clinical Oncology*, 5:1952–9.

Brodeur GM, et al. (1988). International criteria for diagnosis, staging and response to treatment in patients with neuroblastoma. *Journal of Clinical Oncology*, 6:1874–81.

D'Angio GJ, et al. (1985). Metastatic neuroblastoma managed by supralethal therapy and bone marrow reconstitution. Results of a four-institutions Children's Cancer Study Group pilot study. In: *Advances in neuroblastoma research* (ed. AE Evans, GJ D'Angio, and RD Seeger), pp. 557–63. Liss, New York.

Evans AE, D'Angio GJ, Randolph J (1971). A proposed staging for children with neuroblastoma. Children's Cancer Study Group A. *Cancer*, 27:374–8.

Gilbert F, et al. (1984). Human neuroblastomas and abnormalities of chromosome 1. *Cancer Research*, 44:5444–9.

Hartmann O, Kalifa C, Beujean F (1985). Treatment of advanced neuroblastoma with two consecutive high-dose chemotherapy regimens and ABMT. In: *Advances in neuroblastoma research* (ed. AE Evans, GJ D'Angio, and RD Seeger), pp. 565–8. Liss, New York.

Hartmann O, et al. (1987). Repeated high-dose chemotherapy followed by purged autologous bone marrow transplantation as consolidation therapy in metastatic neuroblastoma. *Journal of Clinical Oncology*, 5:1205–11.

Hayes F, et al. (1983). Surgicopathologic staging of neuroblastoma: prognostic significance of regional lymph node metastases. *Journal of Pediatrics*, 102:59–62.

Hughes M, Marsden HB, Palmer MK (1974). Histologic patterns of neuroblastoma related to prognosis and clinical staging. *Cancer*, 34:1706–11.

Labrosse EM, et al. (1976). Catecholamine metabolism in neuroblastoma. *Journal of the National Cancer Institute*, 57:633–8.

Look AT, et al. (1984). Cellular DNA content as a predictor of response to chemotherapy in infants with unresectable neuroblastoma. *New England Journal of Medicine*, 311:231–5.

Ninane J (1987). Childhood neuroblastoma: diagnostic and therapeutic strategy. Thesis.

Philip T, et al. (1987). High-dose chemoradiotherapy with bone marrow transplantation as consolidation treatment in neuroblastoma: an unselected group of stage IV patients over 1 year of age. *Journal of Clinical Oncology*, 5:266–72.

Pritchard J, Germond FN, Jones D (1986). High dose melphalan (HDM) of value in treatment of advanced neuroblastoma (AN): preliminary review results of a randomized trial by the European Neuroblastoma Study Group (ENSG). *Proceedings of the American Society of Clinical Oncology, 1986*, **205**.

Sawada T (1986). Outcome of 25 neuroblastoma revealed by screening in Japan (Letter). *Lancet*, i:377.

Seeger RC, *et al.* (1985). Association of multiple copies of the N-*myc* oncogene with rapid progression of neuroblastomas. *New England Journal of Medicine*, **313**:1111–16.

Shafford E, Rogers D, Pritchard J (1984). Advanced neuroblastoma: improved response rate using a multiagent regimen (OPEC) including sequential cisplatin and VM-26. *Journal of Clinical Oncology*, **2**:742–7.

Shimada H, *et al.* (1984). Histopathologic prognostic factors in neuroblastic tumours. Definition of subtypes of ganglio-neuroblastoma and an age-linked classification of neuroblastomas. *Journal of the National Cancer Institute*, **73**:405–9.

Tuchman M, Ramnaraine M, Woods W, Krivit W (1987). Three years of experience with random urinary homovanillic and vanillylmandelic acid levels in the diagnosis of neuroblastoma. *Pediatrics*, **79**:203–5.

UICC-TNM (1987). *Classification of malignant tumours*, 4th edn. Springer Verlag, Berlin.

14.3   Retinoblastoma

JUDITH E. KINGSTON AND JOHN HUNGERFORD

Retinoblastoma, the most common intraocular tumour of childhood, has been heralded as the prototypical hereditary neoplasm that provides a model for the study of the origin of cancer (Knudson 1978). It can occur in two forms, a genetic or hereditary variant, which is usually multifocal and a non-genetic, non-hereditary variant, which is unifocal. Patients with the genetic form of the disease have an increased susceptibility to the subsequent development of other malignant tumours (Draper *et al.* 1986). The principal aims of the clinician looking after a child with retinoblastoma are, firstly, to save the life of the child and, secondly, to preserve vision. Achievement of these aims involves close collaboration between the ophthalmic surgeon, paediatric oncologist, and radiotherapist. When retinoblastoma remains confined to the eye, it has one of the best survival rates of all childhood cancers but once spread outside the globe occurs, the prognosis for survival is dismal. Management of the child with metastatic disease remains a considerable challenge to all concerned. Early diagnosis is, therefore, of paramount importance and identification of gene carriers is likely to make a significant contribution to prognosis.

EPIDEMIOLOGY

In the White (Caucasian) population, retinoblastoma accounts for between 2.5 and 4 per cent of all cancers in children under the age of 15 years (Parkin *et al.* 1988). The annual incidence of retinoblastoma in that population is between 3 and 5 per million children under the age of 15 years, equivalent to approximately 1 in every 20 000 live births. There is evidence that the incidence is higher (5.1–7.6 per million children) in the Black populations of the United States and Africa and in Brazil (Parkin *et al.* 1988). It appears that the high incidence in some areas reflects an increased incidence of the unilateral (non-genetic) form of retinoblastoma, which suggests that there may be an environmental factor leading to the increased prevalence in these areas. There is no significant variation between the sexes. Seventy-five per cent of cases are diagnosed before the age of 3 years and less than 5 per cent after the age of 5 years. The peak incidence of age at diagnosis for children with unilateral disease is between 24 and 29 months, and during the first 6 months for children with bilateral disease (Sanders *et al.* 1988). In the United Kingdom there are between 40 and 50 new cases of retinoblastoma a year, of which approximately one-third have bilateral and two-thirds unilateral disease. There is no definite evidence that the incidence of retinoblastoma is increasing, although a small increase might be anticipated secondary to the improved survival rate of patients with the hereditary or genetic form of the disease.

AETIOLOGY

The aetiology of retinoblastoma is unknown. Knudson (1971) proposed a two-mutation hypothesis to explain the observed clinical differences between the genetic and non-genetic forms. He suggested that two independent events are required for a cell to acquire the potential to develop into a retinoblastoma. His hypothesis was based primarily on epidemiological data which indicated that children with the genetic form of retinoblastoma developed tumours at an earlier age than those with the non-genetic form. He proposed that in children with the genetic form, loss or mutation of one allele of the retinoblastoma predisposition gene occurs pre-zygotically in the germ cell line and is present in every retinal cell, while the second event affects a somatic retinal cell. In children with the non-genetic, unifocal form of the disease, both events occur sequentially in a somatic retinal cell. The need for two additional events in the appropriate somatic cell, rather than one, is the reason why tumours tend to appear later in the non-genetic cases. Knudson also proposed that the number of tumours acquired by a gene carrier seems to be a matter of chance since it follows a Poisson distribution with a mean number of three tumours per person. The number of gene carriers who do not develop a tumour is unknown, but is estimated to be in the order of 5 per cent. Knudson noted that most of the genetic cases result from a new germ cell mutation, probably arising as a result of spontaneous mutations at a 'background' rate. Two studies (Dryja *et al.* 1989; Zhu *et al.* 1989) have now suggested that new germ-line mutations are more frequently derived from the paternal allele, suggesting that germ-line mutations may occur more frequently during spermatogenesis rather than oogenesis.

GENETICS

Knudson *et al.* (1976) suggested that the mutations leading to retinoblastoma involved chromosome 13 sub-band q14 and that the defect in the gene could be caused by either microscopic or submicroscopic change. He proposed that retinoblastoma probably occurs as a result of two mutational events at the same gene site in homologous chromosomes and that in the genetic form of retinoblastoma the first of these mutations is inherited. Murphree and

Benedict (1984) suggested that the development of retino-blastoma is controlled by a 'suppressor' or regulating gene, sometimes referred to as an 'anti-oncogene'. This gene is recessive at the cellular level, as inactivation or loss of both of its homologous alleles appears to be necessary for the development of retinoblastoma. Dryja *et al.* (1984) using polymorphic DNA probes were able to demonstrate homozygosity for large portions of chromosome 13q in retinoblastoma tissue *in vivo*.

The human retinoblastoma susceptibility gene was first identified by Friend *et al.* (1986) and subsequently cloned by Lee *et al.* (1987a). The gene transcript is encoded in 27 exons dispersed over approximately 200 kb of genomic DNA (Hong *et al.* 1989; McGee *et al.* 1989). The gene product has been characterized as a 105–110 kDa nuclear phosphoprotein with DNA-binding activity (Lee *et al.* 1987b; Mihara *et al.* 1989).

The retinoblastoma gene is closely linked to the locus for esterase-D, a gene dose-dependent human polymorphic enzyme also assigned to 13q14 (Sparkes *et al.* 1983). The retinoblastoma susceptibility gene has been implicated in the development of other tumours including osteosarcoma (Benedict *et al.* 1988), small cell carcinoma of the lung (Harbour *et al.* 1988), bladder cancer (Horowitz *et al.* 1989), breast cancer (Lee *et al.* 1988), and various soft tissue sarcomas (Weichselbaum *et al.* 1988; Reissmann *et al.* 1989).

Cytogenetic studies

In a small proportion of patients with retinoblastoma, routine karyotyping reveals a deletion or translocation involving chromosome 13. The association of retinoblastoma with deletion of part of a D-group chromosome in a child with bilateral retinoblastoma and developmental delay was first described by Lele *et al.* (1963). Characteristic clinical features of the so-called D-deletion syndrome include mental retardation, developmental delay, facial dysmorphism, and retinoblastoma. Details of the facial dysmorphism, which involves the mid-face and is manifested by bushy eyebrows, broad nasal bridge, bulbous tip of the nose, long philtrum, and thin upper lip, were outlined by Motegi *et al.* (1983). These features, particularly the degree of mental retardation, are variable in expression. Routine karyotypic analysis and identification of a D-deletion in babies presenting with congenital dysmorphism or failure to thrive can lead to the diagnosis of retinoblastoma at an early stage, when the tumour is likely to be amenable to conservative therapy (Seidman *et al.* 1987; Kingston *et al.* 1990).

Approximately 5 per cent of patients with retinoblastoma carry a constitutional deletion on the long arm of chromosome 13 (Cowell *et al.* 1986). However, with more sophisticated, high-resolution banding techniques, a deletion can be demonstrated in blood lymphocytes in approximately 10 per cent of patients with retinoblastoma (Turleau and De Gruchy 1987). In 1989, Lemieux *et al.* demonstrated a homozygotic deletion in region 13q14 in retinoblastoma cells in primary culture in a patient with a normal constitutional karyotype, thereby providing the first cytogenetic evidence of the two somatic mutations considered essential to inactivate the retinoblastoma gene and allow tumour development. With the use of these more sophisticated banding techniques, the proportion of cases in which abnormalities of chromosome 13 can be demonstrated is likely to increase.

Genetic counselling

An essential part of the initial assessment of a child with retinoblastoma should include a careful examination of both parents' eyes for the presence of spontaneously regressed retinoblastoma. Approximately 40 per cent of children with retinoblastoma have the genetic form of the disease. In 10–15 per cent of patients there is a known family history of retinoblastoma, whilst the remainder have either bilateral or unilateral, multifocal disease and therefore have the genetic form of the disease as a result of a new mutation.

The retinoblastoma gene has a high degree of penetrance, of the order of 80–100 per cent (Vogel 1979), so that the risk of retinoblastoma in the offspring of patients with the genetic form of the disease is 40–50 per cent. The sporadic, unilateral case is usually a spontaneous mutation but there is a small chance that one of the parents may be an unaffected gene carrier. Draper *et al.* (1992), using follow-up data from a national registry including nearly 1600 cases of retinoblastoma estimated that the overall risk of retinoblastoma developing in the offspring of a sporadic case is approximately 1 per cent, considerably lower than the previously accepted figure of 5 per cent. If normal parents have an affected child with bilateral disease, the risk to subsequent children is very small, probably not more than 2 per cent and is only approximately 1 per cent if the first child has unilateral disease. Nussbaum and Puck (1976) have devised mathematical formulae for more complicated situations.

Yandell *et al.* (1989) have described a method, using a sensitive technique of primer-directed enzymatic amplification followed by DNA sequence analysis, to identify mutations as small as a single nucleotide in patients with retinoblastoma and no family history of the disease. By applying this technique to both tumour and normal somatic cells from the same patient, they were able to identify which patients carried new germ cell mutations and, thus, were able to distinguish between the hereditary and the non-hereditary form of retinoblastoma.

All patients with the genetic form of retinoblastoma have an increased risk of developing second primary malignancies (Meadows *et al.* 1985; Draper *et al.* 1986). There also appears to be an increased risk of osteosarcoma in unaffected gene carriers (Francois 1977) and a generally increased risk of cancer in relatives of patients with retinoblastoma (Fedrick and Baldwin 1978; Strong *et al.* 1984; Sanders *et al.* 1989).

HISTOPATHOLOGY

The name 'retinoblastoma' was first suggested by Verhoeff (1922) to describe an intraocular tumour developing in the cells of the fetal neuroretina. Retinoblastoma, like medulloblastoma and neuro-blastoma, is a tumour of neuroepithelial origin and may be classified as one of the primitive neuroectodermal tumours (**PNET**) of childhood. It appears to arise from retinal precursor cells and the tumour cells bear certain structural similarities to retinal photo-receptor and amacrine cells. Retinoblastoma is characterized by a rapid growth pattern and as a consequence may outgrow its blood supply with resulting necrosis. Calcification occurs in the necrotic areas and is a common feature of large retinoblastomas.

Classically, two patterns of macroscopic growth have been described: (i) endophytic, in which the tumour grows towards the centre of the eye, breaking through the inner layers of the retina into the vitreous cavity and (ii) exophytic, in which the tumour grows predominantly from the outer layers of the retina, away from the centre of the eye and towards the subretinal space. Large tumours with an exophytic growth pattern may cause detachment of the retina from the choroid with subsequent accumulation of fluid in the subretinal space. Both endophytic and exophytic growth patterns may be present in the same eye and neither pattern is significant in terms of prognosis. A third type of growth pattern, diffuse infiltrating retinoblastoma, is also recognized and is found in 1–2 per cent of enucleated eyes, usually in older patients (Morgan 1971). When retinoblastoma cells break off from the main tumour mass they grow independently as spheroidal aggregates, a process known as seeding. Seeding may occur into either the vitreous or the subretinal space. Subretinal seeds may invade the retinal pigment epithelium and from there cross Bruch's membrane into the choroid. The rich vascularity of the choroid predisposes to haematogenous spread of the tumour.

The Flexner–Wintersteiner rosette is the characteristic morphological form of differentiation found in retinoblastoma and appears to represent an attempt to differentiate into photoreceptor cells. The undifferentiated cells in retinoblastoma are similar to those seen in other PNETs and are small cells with large basophilic nuclei of variable morphology, scant cytoplasm, and containing few organelles (Sang and Albert 1982). Immunohistochemical studies using an antibody to neurone-specific enolase (NSE) have demonstrated that many retinoblastomas stain positively for this glycolytic enzyme (Kyritis et al. 1984). Positivity to antibodies against glial fibrillary acidic protein has also been reported in retinoblastoma but may possibly be due to reactive astrocytes as it is thought that glial differentiation is a rare event in retinoblastoma (Hermann et al. 1989). The product of the N-myc oncogene has been described in both retinoblastoma cell lines (Seshadri et al. 1988) and in primary retinoblastomas (Yokoyama et al. 1989) and these investigators suggest that the amount of the N-myc gene product may be inversely correlated with the differentiation of retinoblastoma cells and may relate to prognosis. However, this remains to be proven.

Following enucleation of an eye containing retinoblastoma, it is important for the pathologist to establish the extent of optic nerve invasion; that is, whether the involvement is prelaminar, retrolaminar, or to the resection margin itself. Tumour at the resection margin is an indication for orbital irradiation. It is also necessary to assess the degree of choroidal invasion, that is, whether the tumour involves just the superficial layers or is more extensive, involving greater than half the thickness of the choroid. This latter finding is likely to indicate an increased risk of metastatic spread. The degree of choroidal invasion is often related to the extent of invasion of the optic nerve (Rootman et al. 1978).

In some patients who are known to carry the retinoblastoma gene, non-progressive retinal lesions can be observed. Controversy surrounds the aetiology of these lesions. Some workers consider that they represent spontaneous regression of a previously malignant retinoblastoma (Steward et al. 1956), similar to the phenomenon that has been observed in some infants with neuroblastoma. An alternative explanation, proposed by Gallie et al. (1982), is that the lesions are benign hyperplastic nodules or 'retinomas', which have developed from a mutation in relatively mature retinoblasts. The former hypothesis could explain the phenomenon of late onset of retinoblastoma, which has been described in a small number of patients and which could be due to reactivation of a previously spontaneously arrested growth.

CLINICAL PRESENTATION

In developed countries, retinoblastoma usually presents with disease confined to the eye. The most common presentation is an abnormal

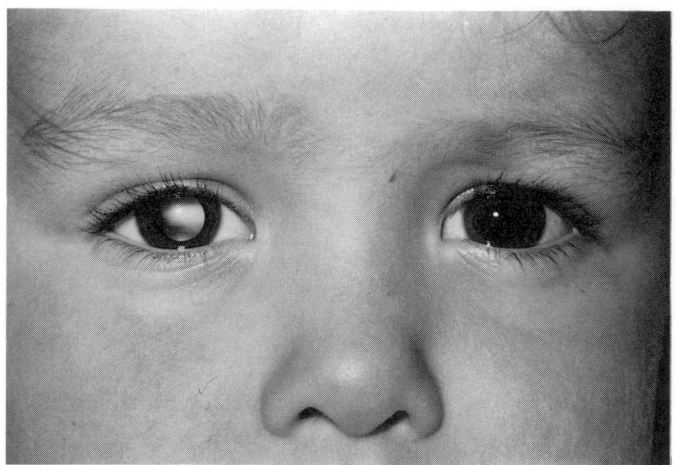

Fig. 1 Right-sided leucocoria as the presenting sign in a 2-year-old boy with retinoblastoma.

or white reflex from the pupil, termed leucocoria (Fig. 1). It indicates a large tumour, which has usually grown from the periphery before disturbing vision. The second most common presentation is a squint, usually reflecting a tumour situated at or near the macula that disturbs central vision at an earlier stage causing strabismus before leucocoria is apparent. Occasionally, children with bilateral disease can present with deteriorating vision; if the tumour is very large and/or bleeding occurs, the child can present with a painful, red, or enlarged eye with secondary glaucoma. A very small proportion of children may present to their general paediatrician with failure to thrive or abnormal facies and routine cytogenetic analysis reveals a deletion of chromosome 13. Subsequent ophthalmological assessment may then lead to the detection of retinoblastoma. Very occasionally, retinoblastoma can present with a pseudohypopyon with tumour cells in the anterior chamber or with a secondary cataract.

Extraocular extension occurs late in the course of the disease and, although not an uncommon finding at presentation in Africa and the Indian subcontinent, is rare in Western and developed countries.

DIAGNOSIS AND STAGING

The diagnosis of retinoblastoma is made clinically by ophthalmoscopic examination. To establish the full extent of the intraocular disease it is advisable to conduct the examination under general anaesthesia with the pupil fully dilated and with indirect ophthalmoscopy, including scleral indentation, to examine the pre-equatorial retina. The characteristic appearance of retinoblastoma is of an elevated white mass, sometimes with a large feeder vessel (Fig. 2) The tumour may be unifocal or multifocal; in tumours with an exophytic growth pattern, detachment of part or all of the retina may be observed. The intraocular pressure should be measured and the presence or absence of rubeosis noted. The differential diagnosis includes Coats' disease, toxocariasis, persistent hyperplastic primary vitreous, retrolental fibroplasia, endophthalmitis, and hamartomata. Coats' disease can usually be excluded by two dimensional B-scan ultrasonography, which, in retinoblastoma, demonstrates a solid mass with calcification, not seen in Coats' disease. Calcification within the tumour can also be demonstrated by computerized tomographic (CT) scanning (Fig. 3) and in a study by Arrigg et al. (1983), 83 per cent of tumours had evidence of calcification on CT scan. They also suggested that in patients under the age of

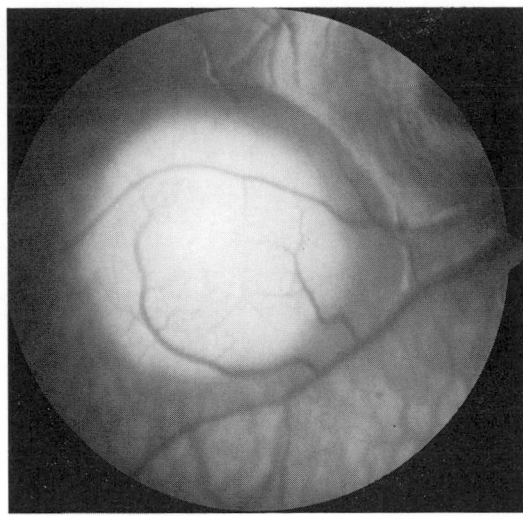

Fig. 2 Ocular fundus photograph of an early retinoblastoma confined to the retina.

3 years in whom the diagnosis of retinoblastoma is suspected, the presence of calcification on CT is virtually diagnostic. CT scanning is also useful in demonstrating extraocular extension of the tumour and as a baseline to exclude ectopic intracranial retinoblastoma. In some centres in Europe and America, magnetic resonance imaging has also been used to try and identify extraocular disease (Schulman *et al.* 1986) and may facilitate identification of intracranial extension of tumour.

Systemic staging investigations are probably unnecessary in children with small intraocular tumours (Pratt *et al.* 1989). However, for children with large retinal tumours requiring enucleation in whom adverse histological factors, such as extensive choroidal or optic nerve involvement, are identified, staging investigations should include cytological examination of the cerebrospinal fluid, bone-marrow aspirate, and technetium bone scanning, in addition to ultrasonography of the eye and CT scanning of the head and orbits. All children should have blood taken for cytogenetic analysis and estimation of esterase-D to exclude the possibility of a deletion of chromosome 13 (Cowell *et al.* 1987).

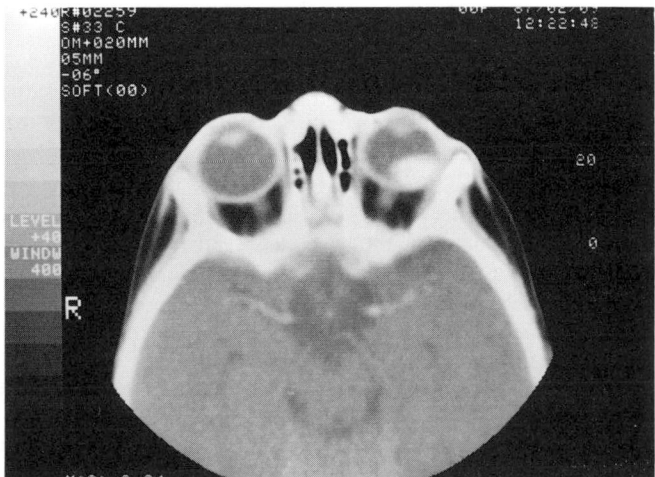

Fig. 3 CT scan of orbital region showing calcification in a retinoblastoma of the left eye.

Table 1 Reese–Ellsworth classification of retinoblastoma

Group I Very favourable
(a) Solitary tumour, less than 4 disc diameters[a] in size, at or behind the equator
(b) Multiple tumours, none over 4 disc diameters in size, all at or behind the equator

Group II Favourable
(a) Solitary tumour, 4–10 disc diameters in size, at or behind the equator
(b) Multiple tumours, 4–10 disc diameters in size, behind the equator

Group III Doubtful
(a) Any lesion anterior to the equator
(b) Solitary tumours larger than 10 disc diameters in size, behind the equator

Group IV Unfavourable
(a) Multiple tumours, some larger than 10 disc diameters
(b) Any lesion extending anteriorly to the ora serrata

Group V Very unfavourable
(a) Massive tumours involving over half the retina
(b) Vitreous seeding

[a] 1 disc diameter=1.5 mm.

Staging classification

There is no satisfactory staging system for the overall management of retinoblastoma. The classification in general use over the past three decades has been that defined by Reese and Ellsworth (1963) (Table 1). This was intended as a classification relating to the prognosis for retaining an eye with retinoblastoma and was not designed as a staging system with regard to prognosis for survival. In 1972, Pratt at the St Jude Children's Research Centre proposed a classification system based on histological and clinical features at diagnosis to provide a guide to prognosis and treatment.

TREATMENT

The aim of the clinician looking after a child with retinoblastoma is to preserve vision without compromising survival. The choice of treatment is determined by the number, location, and size of the tumours; in bilateral disease, each eye is treated on its own merit. In severe bilateral disease, conservative management may be advised for both eyes, even when the visual outlook is poor, providing there is no risk to the life of the child from metastatic spread.

Focal methods

Photocoagulation

Tumours up to 4 mm in diameter and confined to the retina can be treated by indirect xenon-arc photocoagulation and this method is most applicable to lesions posterior to the equator of the eye. A powerful beam of light is focused accurately on the retina around the base of the tumour by means of an ophthalmoscopic attachment. The tumour is encircled by burns in healthy retina and regression depends on interruption of the blood supply to the tumour (Fig. 4). Several treatments may be necessary and should be continued until a flat white scar remains. This method of therapy is not suitable for tumours very close to the optic disc on the temporal side or near to the macula because of possible damage to the macula or to the papillomacular bundle of nerve fibres that runs from the macula to the optic nerve. Direct xenon-arc photocoagulation of retinoblastoma should be avoided because viable tumour cells may be released into the vitreous by small explosions and lead to late vitreous recurrence.

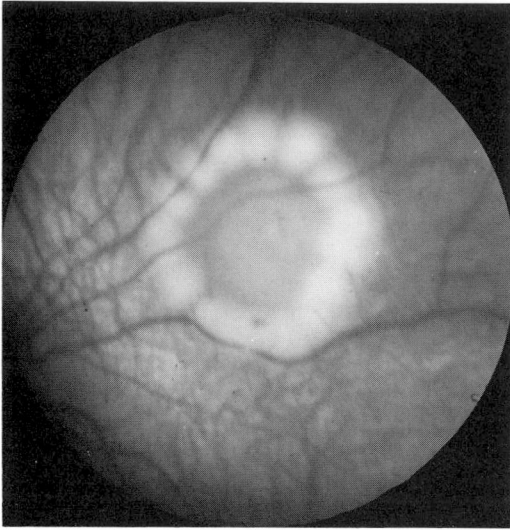

Fig. 4 Fundus photograph showing correct placement of indirect photocoagulation burns around a small retinoblastoma.

Cryotherapy

Tumours up to 7 mm in diameter can be treated by triple-freeze cryotherapy. Small lesions anterior to the equator are difficult to visualize with the direct ophthalmoscope supplied with most photocoagulators and are best treated with a cryoprobe. The correct positioning of the cryoprobe over the external surface of the tumour is ascertained by indirect ophthalmoscopy and the tumour is then treated by a triple 'freeze–thaw' method (Fig. 5). It is important to allow complete thawing to take place before refreezing. The treatment may be applied through the conjunctiva for anterior lesions. When radiation-induced lens opacities are present, making photocoagulation difficult by direct ophthalmoscopy, the conjunctival sac may be opened and cryotherapy applied to posterior lesions. As with xenon-arc photocoagulation, it may be necessary to repeat cryotherapy on several occasions over several weeks.

Both photocoagulation and cryotherapy can be used for small foci of residual active disease after external-beam irradiation.

Radiotherapy

Retinoblastoma is a highly radiosensitive tumour and fortunately the retina itself is relatively radioresistant. The successful treatment of retinoblastoma with X-rays was first reported in 1903. Subsequently, Foster Moore and Scott (1929) in London and Martin and Reese (1936) in New York confirmed that ionizing radiation could effectively destroy retinoblastoma. Radiotherapy in the form of radon-seed brachytherapy for the treatment of retinoblastoma was first developed at St Bartholomew's Hospital in London (Foster Moore 1931). From a study of the histological sections of eyes treated with radon seeds, Stallard (1936) determined that a dose of 35 Gy was lethal to retinoblastoma cells. Subsequently, in 1948, surface applicators were designed and have remained the primary treatment for certain localized tumours.

Scleral-plaque therapy

Tumours up to 10 mm in diameter may be treated using a radioactive scleral-surface applicator such as an iodine, ruthenium, or cobalt plaque. The original surface applicators used γ emission from the decay of ^{60}Co. These have the disadvantage that they

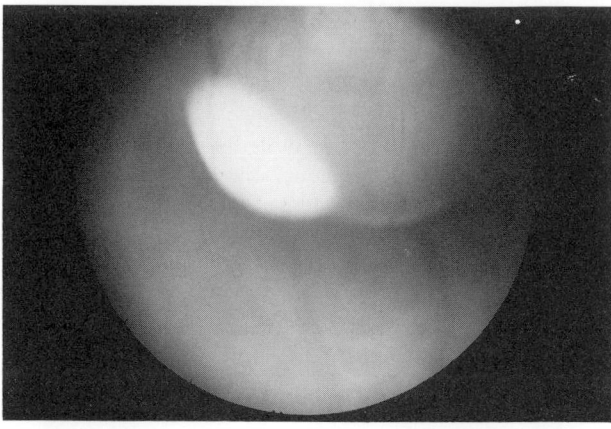

(a)

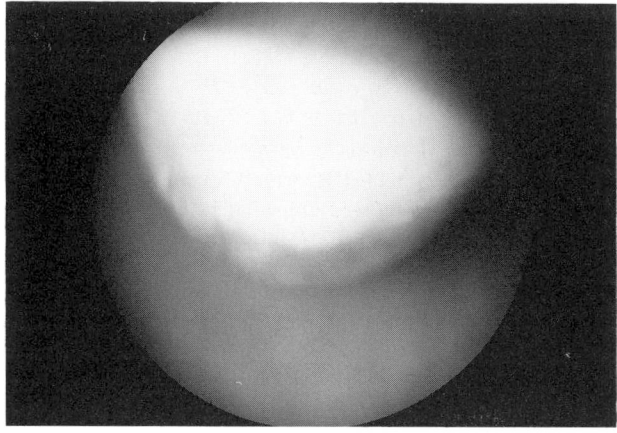

(b)

Fig. 5 Fundus photographs showing (a) the eye wall indented by a cryotherapy probe correctly located under a small retinoblastoma and (b) the same tumour during freezing. Note that the ice ball extends throughout the tumour and into the vitreous overlying it.

cannot be shielded on their external surface and therefore deliver a significant dose of radiation to the orbital bones and to the surgeon inserting and removing the plaque. Their advantage is that they can be used repeatedly because of their long half-life of 5.2 years. ^{125}I plaques have the advantage of a lower emission energy, thus reducing the dose to the surrounding tissues, but the disadvantage of a shorter half-life of 60 days and therefore the necessity for regular replacement.

Each form of applicator is available in a range of sizes and each has an inner radius of curvature corresponding to that of the eye. An applicator of appropriate size is sutured directly over the base of the tumour under general anaesthetic and removed once the recommended dose has been delivered. The technique is the same as that employed in the treatment of ocular melanoma but the dose delivered to the apex of the tumour need not exceed 40 Gy. The base of the tumour will receive a much higher dose, which may result in vascular occlusion. For this reason, surface applicators should not be used for treating tumours near the optic disc or macula. However, single lesions situated away from the disc and macula are eminently suitable for treatment with a surface applicator and two applicators can be applied simultaneously where the fields do not overlap. Residual or recurrent disease after external-beam radiotherapy can be treated by a surface applicator, although radiation retinopathy may develop in the areas of retina that have been irradiated twice and result in late vitreous haemorrhage.

External-beam radiotherapy

External-beam radiotherapy is indicated when any single tumour is larger than 10 mm in diameter, when more than two scleral plaques would be required to treat multiple tumours less than 10 mm in diameter, when retinal detachment or vitreous seeding is present, and in cases where the tumour is adjacent to the optic disc or macula. Depending on the location of the tumour and on the presence or absence of vitreous seeding or retinal detachment, either a whole-eye or a 'lens sparing' approach is used. For patients with anterior lesions, vitreous seedlings, or a retinal detachment extending to the ora serrata, a whole-eye approach is necessary, but means that these patients will have late morbidity affecting the lens and anterior segment with the development of cataract and the 'dry eye' syndrome, respectively.

At St Bartholomew's Hospital, when a whole-eye approach is deemed necessary, treatment is given via an anterior field when the other eye is in place. However, when the contralateral eye has been enucleated a lateral beam is preferred, as the exit dose will then traverse less critical tissues. When both eyes require whole-eye, external-beam irradiation, parallel opposed portals are chosen. The tumour dose, usually prescribed at a depth of 2 cm, calculated to be the back of the eye, is 40 Gy given in 20 fractions over 28 days, treatment being administered every weekday. When there are multiple vitreous seedlings the dose is increased to 44 Gy in 22 fractions. All radiotherapy is done with megavoltage photon apparatus using either a linear accelerator or telecobalt machine.

For children with posteriorly situated tumours, a lens-sparing technique, first developed at Utrecht University (Schipper 1983) and subsequently modified (Harnett et al. 1987), is preferred. This technique allows screening of the lens and anterior chamber. A contact lens fitted to the cornea of the infant provides a fixed reference point from which all measurements can be made (Fig. 6). This point is connected accurately to a linear accelerator, the beam of which is split to minimize beam divergence and using an extended collimator, produces an anterior beam edge almost free of penumbra and divergence. The distance from the front of the cornea to the back of the lens can be ascertained by ultrasound. A special, individually cast, head shell is made for each child, greatly aiding immobilization and facilitating a repeated, highly accurate set-up each day. Planning marks on the shell also help to check the child's position. A lateral beam encompasses the retina up to the back of the lens and, where the other eye is still in place, is appropriately angled at 40° to avoid an exit dose to the contralateral eye (Harnett et al. 1987). This approach is recommended for posteriorly situated

tumours without vitreous seeding, particularly for lesions situated critically on the temporal side of the optic disc. It is especially appropriate for solitary lesions in relatively older children in whom the likelihood of further tumours developing is small. However, it can also be used in younger children in whom anterior tumours may subsequently develop, as these are usually amenable to cryotherapy.

With scleral-plaque or external-beam irradiation, response to treatment is assessed at approximately 4 weeks after completion of therapy (Fig. 7). Various patterns of tumour regression can be observed. The two common ones are type I or 'cottage cheese' due to calcium deposition and type II or 'fish flesh', in which a homogeneous, avascular mass with an annulus of atrophic pigment around the base is observed. In this situation, the expertise of an experienced ophthalmologist, familiar with the different regression patterns, is essential. If the tumour does not show complete regression it is usually possible to treat residual disease by focal methods such as cryotherapy.

Enucleation

Enucleation is recommended when the tumour involves more than half the retina, where there is involvement of the optic nerve, when there is evidence of glaucoma, and when no useful vision is likely to be retained with conservative therapies. Enucleation is occasionally required after failure of conservative methods. In a series of 516 children with retinoblastoma seen in the ocular oncology units at St Bartholomew's and Moorfields Eye Hospitals during the period 1970–1989, 80 per cent of the children with unilateral retinoblastoma have had the affected eye enucleated, whilst 72 per cent of the bilateral cases have had one eye removed and 12 per cent have had both eyes removed.

Enucleation is not an easy procedure, particularly in very young infants and the most important aspect of the operation is to excise as much as possible of the orbital portion of the optic nerve with the eye. When retinoblastoma cells are found at the cut end of the optic nerve, full staging investigations should be undertaken and a course of orbital radiotherapy given without delay.

Chemotherapy

The role of chemotherapy in the management of retinoblastoma remains controversial, although its value in extraocular disease is not disputed. A multi-institutional study carried out by the Children's Cancer Study Group and the Pediatric Oncology Group in America (Wolff et al. 1981) failed to show a benefit for adjuvant chemotherapy in children with unilateral, Reese–Ellsworth group V retinoblastoma undergoing enucleation as primary treatment. Nevertheless, a small proportion of children with tumours

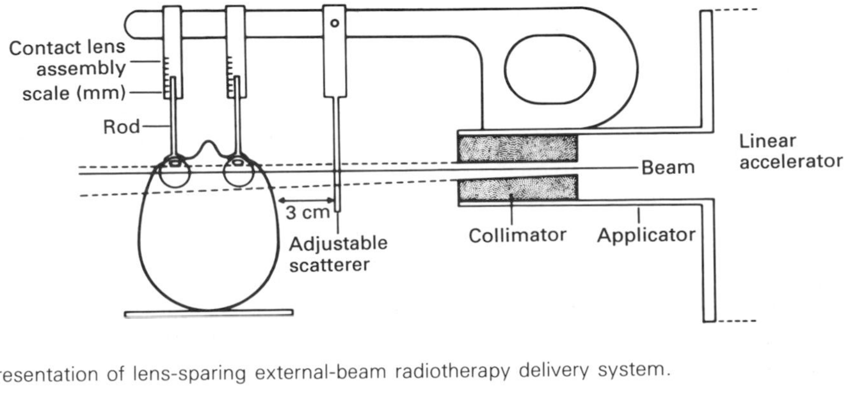

Fig. 6 Diagrammatic representation of lens-sparing external-beam radiotherapy delivery system.

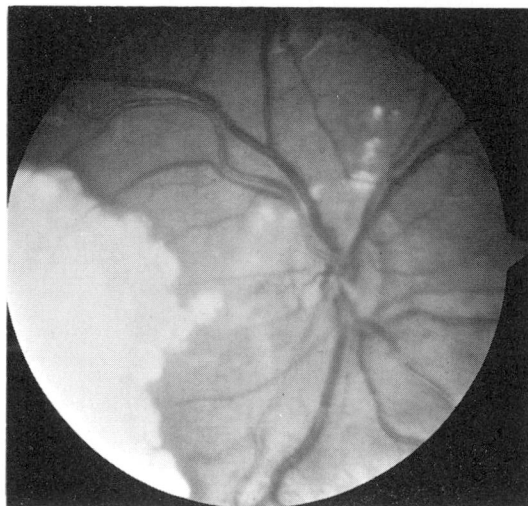

(a)

(b)

Fig. 7 (a) Pre-treatment fundus photograph showing a large retinoblastoma immediately temporal to the optic disc. (b) The appearance of the tumour 1 month after completion of lens-sparing external-beam radiotherapy. The tumour has regressed and has shrunk away from the optic disc.

apparently confined to the eye develop metastatic disease after enucleation. It is obviously important to try to identify the children potentially at risk of this complication, because it is in this group of patients that the use of adjuvant chemotherapy is likely to have a beneficial effect. Clinical and histological factors reportedly associated with an increased risk of metastatic disease include optic nerve length of less than 5 mm removed at enucleation (Rubin *et al.* 1985), extensive choroidal invasion in the presence of retrolaminar optic nerve invasion (McCartney *et al.* 1988), and extension of tumour to the cut end of the optic nerve (Stannard *et al.* 1979; Kopelman *et al.* 1987). The current indications for the use of chemotherapy at St Bartholomew's Hospital are outlined in Table 2. Prospective multi-institutional trials with patients staged by a common staging classification according to potentially predictive prognostic factors may provide a rationale for the role of chemotherapy as an adjuvant.

Table 2 Indications for chemotherapy (St Bartholomew's Hospital)

Extra ocular disease
(a) Orbital relapse
(b) Metastatic spread
(c) Ectopic intracranial retinoblastoma

Adjuvant therapy following enucleation in patients with poor prognostic histological features
(a) Cut end of optic nerve invasion
(b) Extensive choroidal invasion associated with retrolaminar invasion of the optic nerve
(c) Scleral invasion

Salvage therapy in child with recurrent disease in an only eye following failure of external beam irradiation

Primary therapy
(a) In combination with external beam irradiation in child with extensive bilateral disease in an attempt to improve visual outcome
(b) In child with small bulk unilateral disease to enable conservative treatment of the eye by scleral plaque or other focal method

The published record on chemotherapy in metastatic disease is remarkable if only for the dearth of single-agent data. In one of the few reported studies that attempted to look at the response of metastatic disease to single-agent therapy, Lonsdale *et al.* (1968) showed that cyclophosphamide produced the best therapeutic effect (with a response rate of 47 per cent), while vincristine appeared to achieve a lesser response (16 per cent). Pratt *et al.* (1985) at St Jude Children's Research Hospital confirmed that the best responses could be achieved with the alkylating agents cyclophosphamide and ifosfamide. Pratt's studies on two-drug therapy showed superior results for the combination of cyclophosphamide and vincristine. In view of the similarity of retinoblastoma to other neuroectodermal tumours such as neuroblastoma, multidrug combinations containing platinum have been used and have been shown successful in achieving remissions in children with extraocular disease (Kingston *et al.* 1987*a*).

Laboratory and clinical research projects are essential to develop and test new agents. The human tumour clonogenic assay established by Hamburger and Salmon (1977) has been used to test the chemosensitivity profiles of primary and cultured human retinoblastoma cells (Inomata and Kaneko 1987; Chan *et al.* 1989). A xenograft model with heterotransplantation of human retinoblastoma cells into the anterior chamber of the nude mouse eye has been developed by White *et al.* (1989) for testing chemotherapeutic agents. Using this model, they showed that a new agent, diaziquone, was more effective than cyclophosphamide and other conventional agents against a retinoblastoma xenograft cell line.

PROGNOSIS

The 3 year survival rate for children with retinoblastoma in Great Britain is nearly 90 per cent (Sanders *et al.* 1988). These results have been achieved by the judicious use of surgery, radiotherapy, and focal methods of treatment such as cryotherapy and photocoagulation. During the period 1960–1987, 702 children with retinoblastoma were seen in the ocular oncology units at St Bartholomew's and Moorfields Eye Hospitals. The actuarial overall 5 year survival rate for all patients was 87 per cent. The corresponding survival for these patients by laterality of the tumour is shown in Fig. 8. This shows that children with unilateral retinoblastoma surviving for 5 years from diagnosis can be

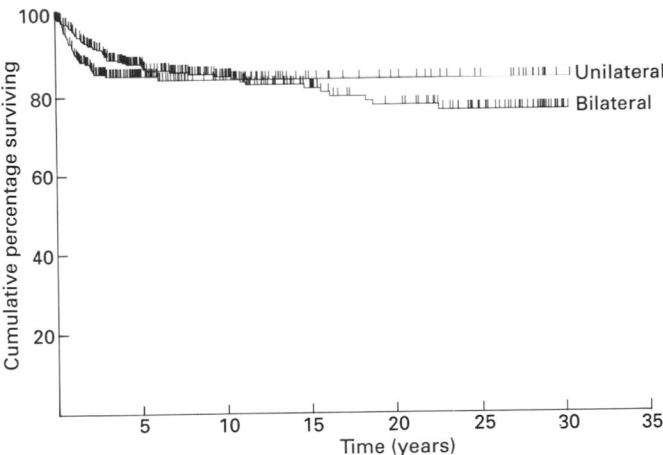

Fig. 8 Effect of laterality on survival in retinoblastoma; St Bartholomew's and Moorfields Eye Hospitals 1960–1987.

considered cured. This is not the case for patients with bilateral disease in whom the continuing attrition is due to deaths from ectopic intracranial retinoblastoma and second tumours.

Histological factors also affect prognosis in children with large tumours undergoing enucleation. Most workers have shown poor survival rates for patients with invasion of the cut end of the optic nerve and heavy choroidal involvement (see above) (Stannard *et al.* 1979; Rubin *et al.* 1985), although the effect of choroidal invasion remains controversial (Redler and Ellsworth 1973; Kopelman *et al.* 1987). Multivariate analysis of our data revealed two groups with a particularly poor prognosis; children with retinolaminar extension and heavy choroidal invasion, for whom the 5 year survival was only 31 per cent and children with extensive invasion of both the choroid and the cut end of the optic nerve, for whom the 5 year survival rate was 25 per cent.

The prognosis for vision depends on the size and location of the tumours within the eye. Migdal (1983), reporting a series of 116 patients with bilateral disease treated at St Bartholomew's and Moorfields Eye Hospitals, found that 50 per cent of patients achieved a final acuity of 6/12 or better in one eye at the age of 8 years. Tumours involving the macula always lead to poor central visual acuity and in a series reported from Stanford by Egbert *et al.* (1978), this was the most common cause of reduced visual acuity.

ORBITAL RECURRENCE

In most series the median interval from diagnosis of intraocular retinoblastoma to the development of an orbital recurrence is less than 8 months. It is commonly manifested clinically by poor fitting of the ocular prosthesis or the development of an obvious lump in the socket (Fig. 9). An orbital relapse is associated with a poor prognosis for survival, because in many cases extraorbital spread is detected at the time of the orbital recurrence or develops shortly afterwards.

In a series of 16 children with an orbital recurrence reported by Hungerford *et al.* (1987), 15 of the children died, with a median survival of only 14 months from diagnosis of recurrence. Death resulted either from intracranial spread or from the development of distant metastatic disease. The one long-term survivor had been treated with adjuvant chemotherapy in addition to orbital radiotherapy and surgery. In a subsequent report from the same institution (Goble *et al.* 1990), five children with an isolated orbital recurrence were successfully salvaged with combined treatment

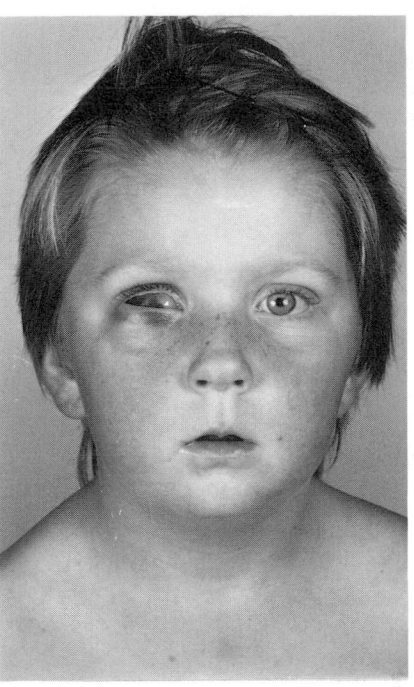

Fig. 9 Orbital recurrence of retinoblastoma: a lump appeared in the enucleated socket 3 months after removal of the right eye.

including 'lumpectomy', multiagent systemic chemotherapy, and orbital radiotherapy. Adjuvant chemotherapy would therefore appear to play an essential part in the management of a child with an orbital relapse.

Factors predisposing to the development of an orbital recurrence include invasion of the cut end of the optic nerve and an intraocular biopsy undertaken for diagnostic purposes (Stevenson *et al.* 1989). To reduce the risk of an orbital recurrence, radiotherapy to the orbit should always be advised when there is evidence of invasion of the cut end of the optic nerve and in the presence of extrascleral extension.

ECTOPIC INTRACRANIAL RETINOBLASTOMA

The problem of ectopic non-metastatic retinoblastoma was first recognized by Jacobiec *et al.* (1977). In 1980, Bader *et al.* used the term 'trilateral' retinoblastoma to describe the clinical syndrome of bilateral retinoblastoma with an ectopic midline intracranial tumour. In a subsequent paper (Bader *et al.* 1982), it was suggested that the development of an ectopic midline neuroblastic tumour in a patient with bilateral retinoblastoma represented an additional focus of multicentric retinoblastoma rather than a second primary tumour. Attention was drawn to the ontogenesis of the pineal gland, likening the human pineal to a third eye. Bader postulated that the retinoblastoma gene confers an increased susceptibility to the development of neuroblastic tumours, which, although usually presenting in the retina, can occur in other intracranial sites, particularly in sites of photoreceptor origin.

The child with ectopic intracranial retinoblastoma usually presents either with symptoms and signs of raised intracranial pressure due to secondary hydrocephalus or, when the lesion arises in the suprasellar region, with symptoms of diabetes insipidus. The finding of a discrete, calcified, midline mass, most commonly in the pineal region, on CT head scanning (Fig. 10) in a child with the genetic form of retinoblastoma is sufficient for diagnosis.

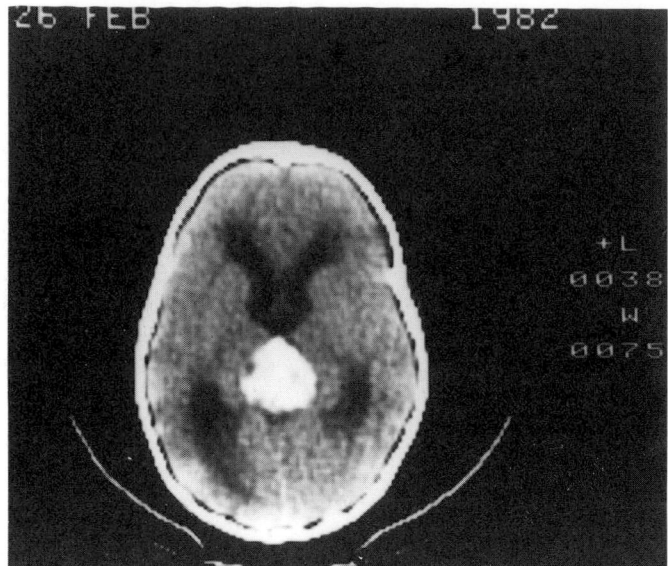

Fig. 10 Characteristic CT head scan appearances of child with ectopic intracranial retinoblastoma, showing a calcified mass in the pineal region and secondary hydrocephalus.

In a series of 12 children with ectopic intracranial retinoblastoma reported by Kingston *et al.* (1985), the median interval from the initial diagnosis of intraocular retinoblastoma to the development of an isolated intracranial lesion was 34 months (range 4–70 months). All 12 children died, with a median survival of 8 months. The major cause of death in these patients was the development of spinal metastases. One subsequent child treated in our institution with a combination of intensive chemotherapy and radiotherapy, including a stereotactic gold-grain implant, survived for 5 years before succumbing from spinal metastases. The poor prognosis for survival of children with ectopic intracranial retinoblastoma has been observed in other series (Bader *et al.* 1982; Holladay *et al.* 1991).

METASTATIC DISEASE

Metastatic disease usually manifests itself within a year of diagnosis. Spread can occur by a number of routes: by direct extension through the sclera into the orbital tissues, by direct extension along the optic nerve into the central nervous system, through the blood vessels of the choroid, and via the lymphatics of the conjunctiva and lid. Haematogenous spread most frequently leads to metastases in bones, bone–marrow, and brain. Lymphatic spread commonly involves the preauricular and submandibular nodes and may be the cause of the subcutaneous deposits seen around the orbit and on the scalp. The patterns of metastatic spread have been reviewed by MacKay *et al.* (1984).

The child with metastatic retinoblastoma usually shows a good initial response to chemotherapy but, unfortunately, these responses are often not sustained, with subsequent early relapse and death (White 1983; Kingston *et al.* 1987*a*). However, although in the past, metastatic disease has usually been associated with a fatal outcome, an increasing number of reports now appearing in the literature are of long-term survival following metastatic retinoblastoma achieved by the use of intensive chemotherapy (Petersen *et al.* 1987; Saleh *et al.* 1988).

COMPLICATIONS OF TREATMENT

As the outcome with regard to survival from retinoblastoma is so good, attention must be paid to the quality of life of these survivors, in particular the quality of vision. Radiation-induced complications in the eye, described in detail by MacFaul and Bedford (1970), include cataract formation, decrease of corneal sensitivity, reduced or absent lacrimal secretion, vitreous haemorrhage, microaneurysms, and diffuse changes in pigmentary epithelium.

The risk of cataract development is related both to the dose of radiation given and to the technique of radiotherapy. Schipper's (1983) study suggests that the threshold dose for a detectable lens opacity in humans is probably in the region of 10–20 Gy fractionated over 5 weeks, a higher dose than indicated in earlier reports. The time to the development of a detectable lens opacity is variable and dose dependent. In children given 40 Gy by a whole-eye approach, significant lens opacities usually develop at 18–24 months after irradiation.

Radiation damage to the lacrimal gland may result in decreased or absent lacrimal secretion with consequent drying of the surface of the eye; when this happens the surface of the cornea becomes rough and filaments can be seen in the epithelium of the cornea and conjunctiva, leading to the 'dry eye' syndrome, which is accompanied by considerable ocular discomfort. New radiotherapy techniques to spare the lens and anterior chamber, as outlined above, have been successful in preventing cataract formation and the 'dry eye' syndrome.

Retinal vascular injury is a more serious complication and is likely to occur in eyes that need treatment with further courses of radiation for recurrent disease. Retinal vascular injury does not usually occur with radiation doses up to 45 Gy when the total dose is divided between at least 15 fractions. With doses of 50–60 Gy, the risk of retinopathy and vitreous haemorrhage increases; with doses greater than 65 Gy, the risk of retinal damage and optic atrophy is substantial (Shukovsky and Fletcher 1972). There is some evidence that giving chemotherapy in addition to radiotherapy may increase the risk of radiation complications in the eye (Chan and Shukovsky 1976).

Abnormalities of orbital bone growth may occur after both enucleation and radiotherapy. There is a significant reduction in growth of the orbit after enucleation (Osborne *et al.* 1974) and both bone and soft tissue growth is retarded by radiotherapy, which may lead to asymmetry of the orbits when only one orbit is irradiated.

SECOND TUMOURS

It is now well recognized that patients with the genetic form of retinoblastoma have a significant risk of developing a second, histologically distinct, primary neoplasm (Abramson *et al.* 1976; Meadows *et al.* 1980; Draper *et al.* 1986). Patients with the non-genetic form of retinoblastoma do not appear to have an increased risk of developing second tumours. Estimates of the risk in patients with genetic retinoblastoma have ranged from 8.4 per cent at 18 years (Draper *et al.* 1986) to 90 per cent at 30 years (Abramson *et al.* 1984). In the former study, the incidence of second tumours in patients with the genetic form of retinoblastoma who had been irradiated was much greater than the incidence in patients with the non-genetic form who received radiation. In a series of 215 patients with bilateral retinoblastoma reported by Roarty *et al.* (1988), the cumulative incidence was 35.1 per cent for the 137 patients who received radiation therapy compared with an incidence rate of 5.8 per cent for the 78 patients who were not irradiated. There is thus some evidence from these data that patients with the genetic form of retinoblastoma may be particularly sensitive to the carcinogenic effect of radiation. It has been proposed that radiation-induced tumours may result from deletion of tissue-specific regulatory genes (Weichselbaum *et al.* 1989). Nevertheless, although many sarcomas in patients with retinoblastoma develop within the radiation field and are, therefore, attributed to radiotherapy, similar numbers occur outside the radiation field and also in patients not treated with radiation (Abramson *et al.* 1979).

Osteosarcoma is the most common second malignancy occurring after retinoblastoma (Meadows *et al.* 1980; Draper *et al.* 1986). Other common second malignancies reported include soft tissue sarcomas, mainly fibrosarcoma and leiomyosarcoma, central nervous tumours, malignant melanoma, and acute leukaemia (Kingston *et al.* 1987*b*). Tucker *et al.* (1987) suggested that the risk of bone tumours following retinoblastoma was approximately 1000 times the rate in the normal population. Hawkins *et al.* (1987) reported a relative risk of 415 for the development of a malignant bone tumour after genetic retinoblastoma and a relative risk of 130 for the development of a soft tissue sarcoma.

Aggressive management of the second primary tumour with combined therapy can achieve long-term remissions (Smith *et al.* 1989).

THE FUTURE

Retinoblastoma is a rare neoplasm and optimal management can only be achieved by concentrating expertise in a limited number of centres where there can be close collaboration between the ophthalmic surgeon, radiotherapist, and paediatric oncologist working with the back-up help of geneticists, experienced pathologists, and nursing staff. Fortunately, recognition of the need for specialist centres is increasing and influencing referral patterns.

The prognosis for survival for a child with retinoblastoma is excellent, with an actuarial survival at 5 years in excess of 85 per cent. Late deaths are mostly due to second malignancies rather than to the retinoblastoma itself. Considerable advances in the treatment of retinoblastoma have been made over the past two decades and the majority of children now retain useful vision. New techniques of radiotherapy have been introduced to reduce radiation damage to the normal structures of the eye and there is scope for further refinement. Effective chemotherapy is now available to prevent the spread of retinoblastoma outside the eye and localized extraocular disease can now be cured by the combined use of chemotherapy and radiotherapy. New agents and the exploration of megatherapy techniques supported by bone marrow transplantation are needed for the unfortunate child who develops metastatic disease. For children with visual impairment, progress in the electronics industry is producing devices to help them achieve their full potential in education, career, and life-style.

Close surveillance of all children with a family history of retinoblastoma leads to earlier diagnosis and increases the chance of successful treatment. Recognition of the retinoblastoma gene and the technology to identify point mutations within it mean that antenatal diagnosis can be offered to an increasing number of patients. These advances at the molecular level will help to determine whether a new mutation is of somatic or germinal origin and thereby identify gene carriers. They will also contribute to our understanding of the aetiological factors responsible for tumorigenesis in retinoblastoma.

REFERENCES

Abramson DH, Ellsworth RM, Zimmerman LE (1976). Nonocular cancer in retinoblastoma survivors. *Transactions of the American Academy of Ophthalmology and Otolaryngology*, 81:454–7.

Abramson DH, Ronner HJ, Ellsworth RM (1979). Second tumors in nonirradiated bilateral retinoblastoma. *American Journal of Ophthalmology*, 87:624–7.

Abramson DH, Ellsworth RM, Kitchin D, Tung G (1984). Second nonocular tumors in retinoblastoma survivors. Are they radiation induced? *Ophthalmology*, 91:1351–5.

Arrigg PG, Hedges TR, Char DH (1983). Computed tomography in the diagnosis of retinoblastoma. *British Journal of Ophthalmology*, 67:588–91.

Bader JL, Miller RW, Meadows AT, Zimmerman LE, Champion LAA, Voute PA (1980). Trilateral retinoblastoma. *Lancet*, ii:582–3.

Bader JL, et al. (1982). Bilateral retinoblastoma with ectopic intracranial retinoblastoma: trilateral retinoblastoma. *Cancer Genetics and Cytogenetics*, 5:203–13.

Benedict WF, Fung Y-KT, Murphree AL (1988). The gene responsible for the development of retinoblastoma and osteosarcoma. *Cancer*, 62:1691–4.

Chan HS, Canton MD, Gallie BL (1989). Chemosensitivity and multidrug resistance to antineoplastic drugs in retinoblastoma cell lines. *Anticancer Research*, 9:469–74.

Chan RC, Shukovsky LJ (1976). Effects of irradiation on the eye. *Radiology*, 120:673–5.

Cowell JK, Rutland P, Jay M, Hungerford JL (1986). Deletions of the esterase-D locus from a survey of 200 retinoblastoma patients. *Human Genetics*, 72:164–7.

Cowell JK, Thompson E, Rutland P (1987). The need to screen all retinoblastoma patients for esterase D activity: detection of submicroscopic chromosome deletions. *Archives of Disease in Childhood*, 62:8–11.

Draper GJ, Sanders BM, Kingston JE (1986). Second primary neoplasms in patients with retinoblastoma. *British Journal of Cancer*, 53:661–71.

Draper GJ, Sanders BM, Brownhill PA, Hawkins MM (1992). Patterns of risk of hereditary retinoblastoma and applications to genetic counselling. *British Journal of Cancer*, 66:211–19.

Dryja TP, et al. (1984). Homozygosity of chromosome 13 in retinoblastoma. *New England Journal of Medicine*, 310:550–3.

Dryja TP, Mukai S, Petersen R, Rapaport JM, Walton D, Yandell DW (1989). Parental origin of mutations of the retinoblastoma gene. *Nature*, 339:556–8.

Egbert PR, et al. (1978). Visual results and ocular complications following radiotherapy for retinoblastoma. *Archives of Ophthalmology*, 97:1826–30.

Fedrick J, Baldwin JA (1978). Incidence of cancer in relatives of children with retinoblastoma. *British Medical Journal*, 1:83–4.

Foster Moore R (1931). Retinal gliomata treated by radon seeds. *British Journal of Ophthalmology*, 15:673–96.

Foster Moore R, Scott RS (1929). Clinical and pathological report of bilateral glioma retinae. *Proceedings of the Royal Society of Medicine*, 22:951–62.

Francois J (1977). Retinoblastoma and osteogenic sarcoma. *Ophthalmologica*, 175:185–91.

Friend SH, et al. (1986). A human DNA segment with properties of the gene that predisposes to retinoblastoma and osteosarcoma. *Nature*, 323:643–6.

Gallie BL, Ellsworth RM, Abramson DH, Phillips RA (1982). Retinoma: spontaneous regression of retinoblastoma or benign manifestation of the mutation? *British Journal of Cancer*, 45:513–21.

Goble RR, McKenzie J, Kingston JE, Plowman PN, Hungerford JL (1990). Orbital recurrence of retinoblastoma successfully treated by combined therapy. *British Journal of Ophthalmology*, 74:97–8.

Hamburger AW, Salmon SE (1977). Primary bioassay of human tumor stem cells. *Science*, 197:461–3.

Harbour JW, Lai S-L, Whang-Peng J, Gazdar AF, Minna JD, Kaye FJ (1988). Abnormalities in structure and expression of the human retinoblastoma gene in SCLC. *Science*, 241:353–7.

Harnett AN, et al. (1987). Modern lateral external beam (lens sparing) radiotherapy for retinoblastoma. *Ophthalmic Paediatrics and Genetics*, 8:53–61.

Hawkins MM, Draper GJ, Kingston JE (1987). Incidence of second primary tumours among childhood cancer survivors. *British Journal of Cancer*, 56:339–47.

Hermann MM, *et al.* (1989). Neuroblastic differentiation potential of the human retinoblastoma cell lines Y-79 and WERI-Rb1 maintained in organ culture system: an immunohistochemical, electron microscopic, and biochemical study. *American Journal of Pathology*, 134:115–32.

Holladay DA, Holladay A, Montobello JF, Redmond KP (1991). Clinical presentation, treatment and outcome of trilateral retinoblastoma. *Cancer*, 67:710–15.

Hong FD, *et al.* (1989). Structure of the human retinoblastoma gene. *Proceedings of the National Academy of Sciences USA*, 86:5502–6.

Horowitz JM, *et al.* (1989). Point mutational inactivation of the retinoblastoma antioncogene. *Science*, 243:937–40.

Hungerford JL, Kingston JE, Plowman PN (1987). Orbital recurrence of retinoblastoma. *Ophthalmic Paediatrics and Genetics*, 8:63–8.

Inomata M, Kaneko A (1987). Chemosensitivity profiles of primary and cultured human retinoblastoma cells in a human tumor clonogenic assay. *Japanese Journal of Cancer Research*, 78:858–68.

Jacobiec FA, Tso MOM, Zimmerman LE, Danis P (1977). Retinoblastoma and intracranial malignancy. *Cancer*, 39:2048–58.

Kingston JE, Hungerford JL, Plowman PN (1985). Ectopic intracranial retinoblastoma in childhood. *British Journal of Ophthalmology*, 69:742–8.

Kingston JE, Hungerford JL, Plowman PN (1987a). Chemotherapy in metastatic retinoblastoma. *Ophthalmic Paediatrics and Genetics*, 8:69–72.

Kingston JE, Hawkins MM, Draper GJ, Marsden HB, Kinnier Wilson LM (1987b). Patterns of multiple primary tumours in patients treated for cancer during childhood. *British Journal of Cancer*, 56:331–8.

Kingston JE, Clark J, Santos H, Jones D, Hungerford JL (1990). Failure to thrive leading to early detection of retinoblastoma. *Pediatric Hematology and Oncology*, 208:191–5.

Knudson AG (1971). Mutation and cancer: statistical study of retinoblastoma. *Proceedings of the National Academy of Sciences USA*, 68:820–3.

Knudson AG (1978). Retinoblastoma: a prototypic hereditary neoplasm. *Seminars in Oncology*, 5:57–60.

Knudson AG, Meadows AT, Nichols WW, Hill R (1976). Chromosomal deletion and retinoblastoma. *New England Journal of Medicine*, 295:1120–3.

Kopelman JE, McLean IW, Rosenberg SH (1987). Multivariate analysis of risk factors for metastasis in retinoblastoma treated by enucleation. *Ophthalmology*, 94:371–7.

Kyritisis AP, Tsokos M, Triche TJ, Chader GJ (1984). Retinoblastoma—origin from a primitive neuroectodermal cell? *Nature*, 307:471–3.

Lee EY-HP, To H, Shew J-Y, Bookstein R, Scully P, Lee W-H (1988). Inactivation of the retinoblastoma susceptibility gene in human breast cancers. *Science*, 241:218–21.

Lee W-H, Bookstein R, Hong FD, Young LJ, Shew J-Y, Lee EY-HP (1987a). Human retinoblastoma susceptibility gene: cloning, identification and sequence. *Science*, 235:1394–9.

Lee W-H, *et al.* (1987b). The retinoblastoma susceptibility gene encodes a nuclear phosphoprotein associated with DNA binding activity. *Nature*, 329:642–5.

Lele KP, Penrose LS, Stallard HB (1963). Chromosome deletion in a case of retinoblastoma. *Annals of Human Genetics*, 27:171–4.

Lemieux N, Milot J, Barsoum-Homsy M, Michaud J, Leung T-K, Richer C-L (1989). First cytogenetic evidence of homozygosity for the retinoblastoma deletion in chromosome 13. *Cancer Genetics and Cytogenetics*, 43:73–8.

Lonsdale P, *et al.* (1968). Chemotherapeutic trials in patients with metastatic retinoblastoma. *Cancer Chemotherapy Reports*, 52:631–4.

McCartney ACE, Olver JM, Kingston JE, Hungerford JL (1988). Forty years of retinoblastoma; into the fifth age. *Eye*, Suppl. 2, S13–18.

MacFaul PA, Bedford MA (1970). Ocular complications after therapeutic irradiation. *British Journal of Ophthalmology*, 54:237–47.

McGee TL, Yandell DW, Dryja TP (1989). Structure and partial genomic sequence of the human retinoblastoma susceptibility gene. *Gene*, 80:119–28.

MacKay CJ, Abramson DH, Ellsworth RM (1984). Metastatic patterns of retinoblastoma. *Archives of Ophthalmology*, 102:391–6.

Martin H, Reese AB (1936). Treatment of retinal gliomas by the fractionated or divided principle of roentgen radiation. *Archives of Ophthalmology*, 16:733–61.

Meadows AT, *et al.* (1980). Bone sarcoma as a second malignant neoplasm in children. *Cancer*, 46:2603–6.

Meadows AT, *et al.* (1985). Second malignant neoplasms in children: an update from the Late Effects Study Group. *Journal of Clinical Oncology*, 3:532–8.

Migdal C (1983). Bilateral retinoblastoma: the prognosis for vision. *British Journal of Ophthalmology*, 67:592–5.

Mihara K, *et al.* (1989). Cell cycle-dependent regulation of phosphorylation of the human retinoblastoma gene product. *Science*, 246:1300–3.

Morgan G (1971). Diffuse infiltrating retinoblastoma. *British Journal of Ophthalmology*, 55:600–6.

Motegi T, *et al.* (1983). A recognizable pattern of the mid-face of retinoblastoma patients with interstitial deletion of 13q. *Human Genetics*, 64:160–2.

Murphree AL, Benedict WF (1984). Retinoblastoma: clues to human oncogenesis. *Science*, 223:1028–33.

Nussbaum R, Puck J (1976). Recurrence risks for retinoblastoma: a model for autosomal dominant disorders with complex inheritance. *Journal of Pediatric Ophthalmology*, 13:89–98.

Osborne D, Hadden OB, Deeming LW (1974). Orbital growth after childhood enucleation. *American Journal of Ophthalmology*, 77:756–9.

Parkin DM, Stiller CA, Draper GJ, Bieber CA (1988). The international incidence of childhood cancer. *International Journal of Cancer*, 42:511–20.

Petersen RA, Friend SH, Albert DM (1987). Prolonged survival of a child with metastatic retinoblastoma. *Journal of Pediatric Ophthalmology and Strabismus*, 24:247–8.

Pratt CB (1972). Management of malignant solid tumors in children. *Pediatric Clinics of North America*, 19:1141–55.

Pratt CB, Crom DB, Howarth C (1985). The use of chemotherapy for extraocular retinoblastoma. *Medical and Pediatric Oncology*, 13:330–3.

Pratt CB, Meyer D, Chenaille P, Crom DB (1989). The use of bone marrow aspirations and lumbar punctures at the time of diagnosis of retinoblastoma. *Journal of Clinical Oncology*, 7:140–3.

Redler LD, Ellsworth RM (1973). Prognostic importance of choroidal invasion in retinoblastoma. *Archives of Ophthalmology*, 11:106–14.

Reese AB, Ellsworth RM (1963). The evaluation and current concept of retinoblastoma therapy. *Transactions of the American Academy of Ophthalmology and Otolaryngology*, 67:164–72.

Reissmann PT, Simon MA, Lee WH, Slamon DJ (1989). Studies of the retinoblastoma gene in human sarcomas. *Oncogene*, 4:839–43.

Roarty JD, McLean IW, Zimmerman LE (1988). Incidence of second neoplasms in patients with bilateral retinoblastoma. *Ophthalmology*, 95:1583–7.

Rootman J, Ellsworth RM, Hofbauer J, Kitchen D (1978). Orbital extension of retinoblastoma: a clinicopathological study. *Canadian Journal of Ophthalmology*, 13:72–80.

Rubin CM, *et al.* (1985). Intraocular retinoblastoma group V: an analysis of prognostic factors. *Journal of Clinical Oncology*, 3:680–5.

Saleh RA, Gross S, Cassano W, Gee A (1988). Metastatic retinoblastoma successfully treated with immunomagnetic purged autologous bone marrow transplantation. *Cancer*, 62:2301–3.

Sanders B, Draper GJ, Kingston JE (1988). Retinoblastoma in Great Britain 1969–80: incidence, treatment and survival. *British Journal of Ophthalmology*, 72:576–83.

Sanders BM, Jay M, Draper GJ, Roberts EM (1989). Non-ocular cancer in relatives of retinoblastoma patients. *British Journal of Cancer*, 60:358–65.

Sang DN, Albert DM (1982). Retinoblastoma: clinical and histopathologic features. *Human Pathology*, 13:133–47.

Schipper J (1983). An accurate and simple method for megavoltage radiation therapy of retinoblastoma. *Radiotherapy and Oncology*, 1:31–41.

Schulman JA, *et al.* (1986). The use of magnetic resonance imaging in the evaluation of retinoblastoma. *Journal of Pediatric Ophthalmology and Strabismus*, 23:144–7.

Seidman DJ, Shields JA, Augsburger JJ, Nelson LB, Lee M-L, Sciorra LJ (1987). Early diagnosis of retinoblastoma based on dysmorphic features and karyotype analysis. *Ophthalmology*, 94:663–6.

Seshadri R, Matthews C, Norris MD, Brian MJ (1988). N-*myc* amplified in retinoblastoma cell line FMC-RB1. *Cancer Genetics and Cytogenetics*, 33:25–7.

Shukovsky LJ, Fletcher GH (1972). Retinal and optic nerve complications in a high dose irradiation technique of ethmoid sinus and nasal cavity. *Radiology*, 104:629–34.

Smith LM, Donaldson SS, Egbert PR, Link MP, Bagshaw MA (1989). Aggressive management of second primary tumors in survivors of hereditary retinoblastoma. *International Journal of Radiation Oncology—Biology—Physics*, 17:499–505.

Sparkes RS, *et al.* (1983). Gene for hereditary retinoblastoma assigned to human chromosome 13 by linkage to esterase-D. *Science*, **219**:971–3.

Stallard HB (1936). Glioma retinae treated by radon seeds. *British Medical Journal*, **2**:962–4.

Stannard C, Lipper S, Sealy R, Sevel D (1979). Retinoblastoma: correlation of invasion of the optic nerve and choroid with prognosis and metastases. *British Journal of Ophthalmology*, **63**:560–70.

Stevenson KE, Hungerford JL, Garner A (1989). Local extraocular extension of retinoblastoma following intraocular surgery. *British Journal of Ophthalmology*, **73**:739–42.

Steward JK, Smith JLS, Arnold EL (1956). Spontaneous regression of retinoblastoma. *British Journal of Ophthalmology*, **40**:449–61.

Strong LC, *et al.* (1984). Cancer mortality in relatives of retinoblastoma patients. *Journal of the National Cancer Institute*, **73**:303–11.

Tucker MA, *et al.* (1987). Bone sarcomas linked to radiotherapy and chemotherapy in children. *New England Journal of Medicine*, **317**:588–93.

Turleau C, De Gruchy J (1987). Constitutional karyotypes in retinoblastoma. *Ophthalmic Paediatric Genetics*, **8**:11–17.

Verhoeff FH (1922). *Archives of Ophthalmology*, **51**:120.

Vogel F (1979). Genetics of retinoblastoma. *Human Genetics*, **52**:1–54.

Weichselbaum RR, Beckett M, Diamond A (1988). Some retinoblastomas, osteosarcomas, and soft tissue sarcomas may share a common aetiology. *Proceedings of the National Academy of Sciences USA*, **85**:2106–9.

Weichselbaum RR, Beckett MA, Diamond AA (1989). An important step in radiation carcinogenesis may be inactivation of cellular genes. *International Journal of Radiation Oncology—Biology—Physics*, **16**:277–82.

White L (1983). The role of chemotherapy in the treatment of retinoblastoma. *Retina*, **3**:194–9.

White L, Szirth B, Benedict WF (1979). Evaluation of response to chemotherapy in retinoblastoma heterotransplanted to the eyes of nude mice. *Cancer Chemotherapy and Pharmacology*, **23**:63–7.

Wolff JA, Boesel CP, Dyment PG (1981). Treatment of retinoblastoma: a preliminary report. *International Congress Series*, **570**:364–8.

Yandell DW, *et al.* (1989). Oncogenic point mutations in the human retinoblastoma gene: their application to genetic counseling. *New England Journal of Medicine*, **321**:1689–95.

Yokoyama T, Tsukahara T, Nakagawa C, Kikuchi T, Minoda K, Shimatake H (1989). The N-*myc* gene product in primary retinoblastomas. *Cancer*, **63**:2134–8.

Zhu XP, *et al.* (1989). Preferential germline mutation of the paternal allele in retinoblastoma. *Nature*, **340**:312–13.

14.4 Wilms' tumour

CHRISTOPHER D. MITCHELL

INTRODUCTION AND DEFINITION

Wilms' tumour, the most common genitourinary malignancy of childhood, is a triphasic embryonal malignancy, consisting of varying proportions of blastema, stroma, and epithelium. It develops from proliferation of the metanephric blastema, possibly in the absence of normal stimulation from the metanephric ducts, to produce differentiated tubules and glomeruli. Although the specific histological appearance was described by Max Wilms in 1899, the eponym is now loosely applied to virtually any malignant tumour arising in the kidney in childhood, some of which are pathologically, clinically, and probably genetically distinct. Recent developments in molecular biology have been applied to the molecular pathology underlying the development of Wilms' tumour in an attempt to isolate the gene whose mutation is responsible for its initiation. This work is now at an exciting stage and, although more complex than the equivalent analysis of retinoblastoma, an understanding of the genetic basis of Wilms' tumour is close at hand.

EPIDEMIOLOGY

The annual incidence of Wilms' tumour is approximately eight per million children under the age of 15 years. There are both racial and regional variations in incidence, so that the previously held view that the incidence of Wilms' tumour was constant throughout the world (the 'index' tumour) is not correct (Parkin *et al.* 1988). The risk of developing Wilms' tumour is approximately 1 in 10 000 live births. The tumour accounts for approximately 8 per cent of childhood malignancies so, in incidence, it ranks fifth among the solid tumours of childhood, below central nervous system tumours, lymphoma, neuroblastoma, and soft tissue sarcoma. The tumour

occurs with equal frequency in boys and girls, with a peak incidence in the third year. Although very rare in the neononatal period (Hrabovsky *et al.* 1986), over three-quarters of Wilms' tumour patients are under 4 years of age and at least 90 per cent are less than 7 years old at diagnosis (Breslow and Beckwith 1982; J. Barnes, personal communication, see Fig. 1). A few cases are

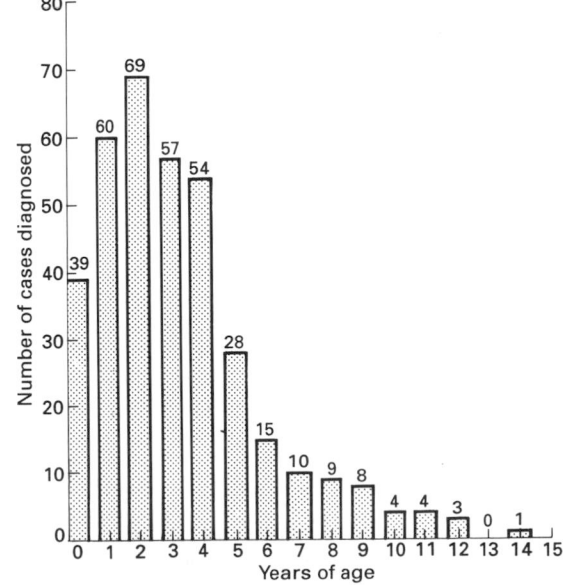

Fig. 1 Proportion of Wilms' tumour cases diagnosed per year of life (United Kingdom Children's Cancer Study Group data, 361 cases, the absolute number of cases for each year is given at the top of each bar).

diagnosed in the neonatal period and a very few after the age of 11 years.

Despite speculation to the contrary, the incidence of familial Wilms' tumour is extremely low. The United Kingdom Children's Cancer Study Group (UKCCSG) has only one family exhibiting clear-cut Mendelian dominant inheritance on record; three patients out of 670 (J. Barnes, personal communication). The first national Wilms' tumour study, in North America, reported 20 patients (1 per cent) with one or more relatives affected by Wilms' tumour. However, in only one case had a parent been affected and in seven had a sibling been affected (Breslow and Beckwith 1982). Only one patient developed bilateral tumours. The vast majority of Wilms' tumours are, therefore, sporadic. However, in view of the 'two-mutation' hypothesis advanced by Knudson (1971), it is interesting to note that the mean age of onset of bilateral Wilms' tumour is significantly younger than that for unilateral tumours (Breslow and Beckwith 1982). One implication of this finding is that bilateral cases may have inherited a predisposing germ-line mutation from an unaffected parent, a situation paralleled in retinoblastoma where up to 40 per cent of cases are familial and where transmission of predisposing germ-line mutations has been confirmed (Dunn et al. 1988; Zhu et al. 1989).

A variety of congenital abnormalities, most frequently genitourinary anomalies, hemihypertrophy, and aniridia, are associated with Wilms' tumour. Other associations include Beckwith–Wiedemann syndrome (Wiedemann 1964; Beckwith 1969) and the Drash syndrome (Drash et al. 1970). The incidence of these anomalies in Wilms' tumour patients is shown in Table 1.

Aniridia may be familial (two-thirds of cases) or sporadic (one-third of cases) (McKusick 1986). Wilms' tumour is associated exclusively with the sporadic form. The incidence of aniridia in the general population is approximately 1 : 50 000, while in contrast the incidence among children with Wilms' tumour has been reported to be as high as 1 in 73 (Miller et al. 1964), a 700-fold excess risk. When aniridia, genitourinary anomalies, and mental retardation occur together, the syndrome is known as the AGR triad (Riccardi et al. 1978; Franke et al. 1979). This group of patients has approximately a 50 per cent risk of developing Wilms' tumour (Narahara et al. 1984).

Drash syndrome (Drash et al. 1970) is of interest because of the concurrence of Wilms' tumour with another congenital renal abnormality, in this case the presence of a congenital nephrotic syndrome associated with specific histology typified by diffuse mesangial sclerosis (Habib et al. 1985). It is now clear that the classical syndrome should be expanded to include children of both sexes on the basis of renal histology and not limited to those with male pseudohermaphroditism as originally described. Indeed, the genital appearances may be very variable. An XY karyotype may be seen in a patient with phenotypically normal female genitalia, as may varying degrees of intersex. Normal females with XX karyotypes, but in whom the histology and presence of Wilms' tumour support the diagnosis of Drash syndrome have also been reported (Jadresic et al. 1988). The reason for these patients' predisposition to Wilms' tumour has not been elucidated, but might be the result of submicroscopic chromosomal deletion involving a number of genes important in genitourinary development. These patients progress into end-stage renal failure which makes the management of any co-existing Wilms' tumour considerably more complex. These problems are discussed further in the section on treatment.

BIOLOGY

Embryology

Understanding of the complexities of histological classification of childhood renal tumours and of the genetic processes at work during renal development is aided by knowledge of the embryology of the kidney.

Three successive renal systems, the first two of which are vestigial, develop in man (Fitzgerald 1978). The first is the pronephros which, save for the caudal end of the pronephric duct, disappears at approximately 30 days of gestation. The second vestigial system, the mesonephros, appears as the pronephros regresses. Renal tubules are formed in intermediate mesoderm in the thoracolumbar region and are invaginated by capillary tufts developing in situ. The distal ends of the tubules open into the persisting, caudal end of the pronephric duct, now referred to as the mesonephric duct. The final renal system arises as the ureteric bud develops from the dorsal aspect of the mesonephric duct, close to its point of entry into the cloaca. The bud extends into the intermediate mesoderm behind the lower end of the mesonephros and this stalk then acquires a lumen, forming a ureter. The lumen invades the advancing bud and at its cephalic end dilates to form a renal pelvis. Adjacent cells in the intermediate mesoderm then multiply to form a metanephric 'cap' of blastema, which invests the invaginated ureteric bud around the pelvis. The cells of the ureteric bud divide, forming in turn first the major and minor calyces, then the collecting tubules, and finally the nephrons. This wave of differentiation spreads outwards into the metanephric cap. Contact between blastema and ducts seems critical to this orderly succession of events.

Genetics

For an account of the genetic basis of Wilms' tumorigenesis please see Chapter 14.1.

CLINICAL FEATURES

The majority of children with Wilms' tumour are well and present only because of the detection of an abdominal mass by a parent or other relative. The differential diagnoses are, therefore, all causes of an abdominal mass in childhood, but particularly those causing renal enlargement. Clinical distinction of a Wilms' tumour from many of the other causes of an abdominal mass, particularly masses of renal origin, may be difficult and possible only by diagnostic imaging procedures. Other symptoms such as abdominal pain, haematuria, and fever may occur (Ledlie et al. 1970), as

Table 1 Incidence of associated anomalies in Wilms' tumour patients

All genitourinary abnormalities	2.6%
(Cryptorchidism	1.3%)
Hemihypertrophy	2.5%
Aniridia	0.68%
Beckwith–Wiedemann syndrome	0.21%

Table 2 Frequency of presenting symptoms

Abdominal mass	74%
Pain	44%
Fever	1%

noted in Table 2, but generally the contrast with the clinical picture of abdominal neuroblastoma, the major differential diagnosis, is very marked. Physical examination should include a search for the stigmata of the various associated conditions, such as hemihypertrophy, Beckwith–Wiedemann syndrome, genital abnormalities, and aniridia. Hypertension, which may arise as a result of excessive renin production, vascular compression by the tumour, or, rarely, as part of pre-existing renal disease, occurs in some patients and may be sufficiently severe to require treatment. Therefore, the blood pressure must be measured. Examination of the abdomen reveals the presence of a smooth rounded or lobulated mass arising in the loin. It may be possible to feel the attached normal kidney. The mass is usually ballotable and does not move with respiration, thus allowing distinction from liver or spleen. Previously held views that abdominal examination should not be repeated for fear of tumour rupture or tumour emboli are unfounded. Any metastases present at diagnosis, usually pulmonary, will only very rarely be detected by clinical examination.

Rarely, a patient may present with signs of inferior vena caval obstruction, due to obstruction of this vessel by extensive tumour thrombus. A more common manifestation of tumour thrombus is that of a varicocele, usually on the left side, as a result of obstruction of the left testicular vein by thrombus in the left renal vein, into which the testicular vein drains.

INVESTIGATIONS

The objectives of investigation in this context are to confirm the diagnosis, delineate the extent of the tumour, determine that the contralateral kidney functions, discover the presence of any metastases, and ensure that the child is fit to undergo anaesthesia and surgery.

A blood count may detect anaemia resulting from haemorrhage into the tumour. There may also be thrombocytosis in response to haemorrhage. Urinalysis, particularly for protein, and measurement of serum electrolytes, urea, and creatinine should detect any gross abnormalities of renal function. A serum α-fetoprotein can help distinguish a Wilms' tumour invading the liver from a hepatoblastoma or hepatocellular carcinoma, as in the former case it will be normal, but in the latter two cases it will be elevated. A vanillylmandelic acid estimation is essential to exclude neuroblastoma, especially in hypertensive children, if immediate surgery is contemplated. No imaging investigation can exclude the presence of a neuroblastoma with complete accuracy and some neuroblastomas are intrarenal. There are two reasons for taking care to exclude the diagnosis of neuroblastoma. First, immediate surgery may not be appropriate if the tumour is a neuroblastoma and, secondly, catecholamine-secreting tumours pose particular problems for the use of anaesthetics, which should be recognized pre-operatively.

An abdominal ultrasound scan is the imaging investigation of choice for determining the organ of origin of the mass, the extent of any spread within the abdomen, the patency of the inferior vena cava, and detection of any involved lymph nodes. It is important that the contralateral kidney is shown to function prior to surgery. Conventionally this has been by intravenous urography, which is available in virtually all centres, can delineate the inferior vena cava (although not distinguish compression from invasion), and provides good images for any subsequent radiotherapy planning. A $^{99}Tc^m$ dimercaptosuccinic acid scan is an alternative, but facilities for this investigation are probably more limited. Some radiologists and urologists hold the view that normal renal size and indices of renal function are sufficient to exclude a non-functioning contralateral kidney. Those centres carrying out computed axial tomographic (CT) scanning of the chest may use the excretion of contrast at the end of that examination as an indication of function of the contralateral kidney. Non-function of the contralateral kidney is a clear contraindication to primary nephrectomy. Suggestions for the management of such patients are given in the section on treatment.

Postero-anterior and lateral chest X-rays are mandatory in the exclusion of pulmonary metastases. The place of CT scanning for the detection of pulmonary metastases in Wilms' tumour is not yet resolved. It seems reasonable to use the most sensitive technique in the search for metastatic disease, but it is not clear that an increase in sensitivity for detecting pulmonary metastases significantly improves the outcome. A preliminary study at the Hospital for Sick Children in London suggests that only a very small proportion of patients have metastases detected by CT that are invisible with conventional radiography. Conversely a North American study found X-ray-negative/CT-scan-positive pulmonary disease in 11/124 children (Wilimas et al. 1988), but there was no significant difference in the relapse rate when X-ray-positive and X-ray-negative/CT-positive patients were compared.

Post-operatively, other imaging investigations are indicated as a result of specific histological findings. A $^{99}Tc^m$ bone scan is indicated after the diagnosis of the so-called 'bone-metastasizing renal tumour' (also called a clear cell sarcoma). A radiological skeletal survey in addition is unnecessary. In rhabdoid Wilms' tumour a CT scan of the head should be performed to exclude the presence of an intracranial second tumour (Bonnin et al. 1984).

PROGNOSTIC FEATURES

It is important to acknowledge that prognostic factors arise as an artefact of treatment regimens. If treatment was uniformly successful or a disease uniformly fatal there would be no prognostic factors. In Wilms' tumour the recognition of prognostic factors has allowed the stratification of treatment, with intensive treatment directed to patients with 'bad-risk' disease and the refinement of treatment for patients with 'good-risk' disease. The most important prognostic factors in Wilms' tumour are histological appearance and stage (Breslow et al. 1978, 1985, 1986), features first delineated by the series of National Wilms' Tumour Studies conducted in North America.

Pathology

Two broad groups of patients may be recognized on the basis of histological appearances. By far the larger group consists of the 'favourable' histologies, with the 'unfavourable' histologies forming the second group (reviewed by Beckwith 1986). Table 3 gives the incidences of histological subtypes in the first Wilms' tumour study (UKW1) run by the UKCCSG (J. Barnes, personal communication).

Table 3 Distribution of histological subtypes

Favourable histology	88%
Bone metastasizing	4%
Pleomorphic	4%
Rhabdoid	4%

Favourable histology

The major proportion of the favourable histology group consists of those patients with classical triphasic tumours, in which epithelial, blastemal, and stromal elements are all present. There is debate about the origin of the stromal elements in Wilms' tumour which may represent a component of the tumour, but may represent normal vascular and connective tissue, proliferating because of the influence of neighbouring malignant cells. The occasional presence of undifferentiated sarcomatous stroma weighs against the latter suggestion. The presence of such sarcomatous stroma is not itself an unfavourable feature. Some triphasic tumours may exhibit rhabdomyoblastic differentiation, so that the cells resemble fetal rhabdomyoblast, often with cross-striations. This appearance is not unfavourable and it must not be confused with the 'malignant rhabdoid tumour of the kidney' which is an unfavourable variant. Another form of triphasic Wilms' tumour which may not have such a favourable outlook has infiltrating tongues of tumour growing in vessels (M. Malone and A. Risdon, personal communication). At present this observation appears restricted to stage I (see below) tumours. The monomorphous epithelial variant, usually seen in children under 1 year of age, is easily recognized as it appears to consist entirely of primitive tubules. This appearance has a very favourable outlook.

Unfavourable histology

Anaplasia is an unfavourable feature occasionally observed in triphasic tumours and is characterized here by the presence of large (>4×normal) hyperchromatic nuclei, an increased nuclear : cytoplasmic ratio, and abnormal (for example, tripolar) mitoses. Anaplasia in Wilms' tumour is often a patchy, focal change which may escape notice unless a deliberate search is made, including widespread sampling, with blocks cut every centimetre across the widest diameter of the tumour. The appearances are often best recognized by scanning the slide at low power. Anaplasia is the only unfavourable form of histology seen in Wilms' tumour developing in the setting of one of the predisposing syndromes such as aniridia. The significance of anaplasia is complicated by the finding in National Wilms' Tumour Studies that for stage I patients, only diffuse anaplasia is associated with an unfavourable prognosis and that stage I patients with focal anaplasia have as good an outcome as stage I patients with atypical favourable histology.

The major unfavourable histological types are probably distinct renal tumours, rather than true variants of Wilms' tumour. The bone-metastasizing renal tumour of childhood was first reported by Kidd in 1970 and subsequently separately identified by Marsden and Lawler (1978) and by Beckwith and Palmer (1978), as a distinctive neoplasm with a particular propensity for skeletal metastases and aggressive clinical behaviour. The incidence of bone metastasis reported was 76 per cent of 38 cases in the British series and 17 per cent of 75 cases in the American series. In the third National Wilms' Tumour Study, bone-metastasizing renal tumour of childhood comprised nearly 6 per cent of cases, making it the most frequent form of 'unfavourable' histology. The age distribution of bone-metastasizing renal tumours of childhood is similar to that of Wilms' tumour. There appears to be a distinct male preponderance in both American and British series, although not as great as originally suggested by Marsden. There have been no reports of bone-metastasizing renal tumour of childhood occurring in a patient with a Wilms' tumour-associated condition such as sporadic aniridia.

The other unfavourable type of histology is the malignant rhabdoid tumour of the kidney, first recognized by Beckwith and Palmer in their report from the first National Wilms' Tumour Study (1978). It is the least common of the unfavourable entities and comprises only 2 per cent of patients entered in the National Wilms' Tumour Studies. The age distribution is markedly different to that of Wilms' tumour, with nearly half the patients being diagnosed in the first year of life (reviewed by Weeks et al. 1989). In addition, there is an association with second primary tumours of different histology (usually primitive neuroectodermal tumours) arising in the midline of the posterior intracranial fossa (Bonnin et al. 1984). The intracranial tumour may precede or follow the renal tumour. Hypercalcaemia has been reported in a number of cases of malignant rhabdoid tumours (Rousseau-Merck et al. 1982; Mitchell et al. 1985), but may also occur in congenital mesoblastic nephroma.

Ploidy

Ploidy refers to the number of chromosomes within a cell and in Wilms' tumour may be studied by measuring the DNA content of a sample of tumour cells using standard flow cytometric techniques. Douglass et al. (1986) studied 48 cases of Wilms' tumour seen at the St Jude Children's Research Hospital, all of whom were treated uniformly according to disease stage by National Wilms' Tumour Studies protocols. A DNA content of 1.0 represents a diploid chromosome complement. A hyperdiploid DNA content of 1.7–3.2 characterized 9/10 tumours with anaplasia. Tumours of favourable histology and 1/10 tumours with anaplasia had a DNA content of 1.0–1.4. Karyotypic analysis of the anaplastic tumours showed that, in some cases, complex chromosomal rearrangements, including translocations, were present. Patients whose tumours contained complex rearrangements fared less well than those with tumours of diploid DNA content or those with hyperdiploid tumours but in which complex chromosomal rearrangements were absent. The authors suggested that the emergence of drug resistance during treatment is related to chromosomal instability of the malignant clone and that such instability is reflected by hyperdiploidy and the presence of complex chromosomal rearrangements. These results require verification in a prospective controlled trial, but may allow for further stratification of treatment.

Other histological variants and renal tumours

Congenital mesoblastic nephroma is a rare distinctive tumour of the infantile kidney, with a characteristically benign outcome. This tumour was first recognized as a distinct entity by Bolande et al. (1967) (reviewed by Bolande 1973). There have been reports of local recurrences and metastases but in only one of these cases was the patient under 3 months of age and in that case resection had been incomplete. Other recurrences have occurred in patients over 3 months of age in whom the histology revealed dense cellularity and numerous mitotic figures. In addition, vascular invasion and tumour rupture have also been associated with an unfavourable outcome. Fortunately the majority of congenital mesoblastic nephromas are recognized in the early weeks of life, when the chances of recurrence are minimal provided adequate margins of resection are ensured.

A review of 290 patients with Wilms' tumour treated at St Jude Children's Hospital (Fernandes *et al.* 1988) showed that three patients had histology compatible with the diagnosis of 'teratoid Wilms' tumour', a term which has been used to describe a tumour in which the classical triphasic histology is present but where diverse cell types and tissues are represented (Variend *et al.* 1984). These tumours must be distinguished from true intrarenal teratomas in which the tumour is of intrarenal origin but shows evidence of non-renal differentiation only. Beckwith (1986) considers that intrarenal teratomas, teratoid Wilms' tumour, and classical Wilms' tumour form a continuum. Two of the patients described by Fernandes had bilateral tumours extending into the renal pelvis, causing ureteral obstruction and renal failure. Beckwith (1986) has also suggested that botryoid growth into the renal pelvis is evidence of the tumours' origin from intralobar (deep) nephroblastomatosis, that intralobar nephroblastomatosis is an early defect in nephrogenesis, and that tumours derived from it are more likely to include diverse cell types and tissues at diagnosis (see below).

Renal cell carcinoma is rare in childhood. Raney *et al.* (1983) reviewed 20 cases and found that most presented with pain and haematuria. Half the patients died of metastatic disease at a median of 1 year from diagnosis. There was a strong correlation between survival and stage (using the National Wilms' Tumour Studies staging system), but age was also an important factor: 6/6 aged less than 11 years survived, compared with only 4/11 over the age of 11. Radiotherapy and chemotherapy had little influence on the outcome. Adequate surgical resection appeared to be the only effective form of treatment. Occasionally, in contrast to adults, renal cell carcinoma in childhood can be chemoresponsive, and non-resectable tumours can become resectable. The usual regimen in these few cases has been CVA (cyclophosphamide, vincristine, Adriamycin®).

Nephroblastomatosis

Nephroblastomatosis, first described by Hou and Holman (1961) is defined as the persistence of metanephric blastema or its incompletely differentiated derivatives beyond the 36th week of gestation. It is a rare incidental discovery in childhood autopsies, but is seen more commonly in association with Wilms' tumour, with a frequency of 15–30 per cent. It is also seen in a number of other genetic conditions associated with Wilms' tumour, but in the absence of malignancy (reviewed by Bove and McAdams 1985; Beckwith 1986). These findings have led to the suggestion that nephroblastomatosis is a precursor of Wilms' tumour, a view supported by the finding of a chromosome 11p deletion in nephroblastomatosis tissue from a patient with a normal somatic karyotype (Heidemann *et al.* 1986). Another school of thought proposes that the lesions represent a developmental anomaly which may be related to the genesis of Wilms' tumour, but which is neither a precursor of, nor a predisposition to, tumour development. Beckwith (1986) has proposed a classification of nephroblastomatosis into intralobar (deep), perilobar (superficial), mixed, and a rare panlobar form.

The most common form of nephroblastomatosis occurs as multiple small nodules lying superficially in the subcapsular cortex. Occasionally a continuous subcapsular layer may be formed which can result in clinically detectable renal enlargement. The lesions of superficial perilobar nephroblastomatosis tend to enlarge with age and to become well differentiated and well defined. Proliferative nodules of monophasic embryonal epithelium may also be seen, with rosetting or a more differentiated tubular or papillary pattern and prominent mitotic activity. Such lesions can be

Table 4 National Wilms' Tumour Studies 3, staging system

I	Tumour limited to the kidney and completely excised. Surface of renal capsule intact; no tumour rupture; no residual tumour apparent beyond margin of excision
II	Tumour extends beyond kidney but is completely excised; regional extension of tumour; vessel infiltration; tumour biopsy or local spillage of tumour confined to flank. No residual tumour apparent at or beyond margins of excision
III	Residual non-haematogenous tumour confined to the abdomen. Lymph node involvement of hilum, periaortic chains or beyond; diffuse peritoneal contamination by tumour spillage; peritoneal implant tumour extends beyond resection margins, either microscopically or macroscopically; tumour not completely removable because of local infiltration into vital structures
IV	Deposits, beyond stage III lung, liver, bone, brain
V	Bilateral renal involvement at diagnosis

indistinguishable from Wilms' tumour, hence the name of Wilms' tumourlets. The intralobar or deep form of nephroblastomatosis (Machin and McCaughey 1984) is usually a solitary nodule consisting of tubules and blastema. The association with Wilms' tumour is clear as the lesion is seldom recognized in the absence of a tumour. In these circumstances the tumours are often multifocal or bilateral and are usually predominantly stromal or blastemal with minimal epithelial differentiation. The rarest form of nephroblastomatosis is panlobar, which is bilateral and involves the whole renal parenchyma apart from the medullopelvic area. This variety of nephroblastomatosis has not been associated with Wilms' tumour, probably because of limited survival.

In those patients whose tumours are judged to be 'unresectable', initial pathological diagnosis may depend on percutaneous Tru-Cut® biopsy specimens. There is concern that such specimens may not provide a representative sample of the tumour and may fail to reveal unfavourable features such as anaplasia. Subsequent pre-operative treatment may then mask the unfavourable features in the eventually resected specimen and result in undertreatment of the patient. No unfavourable features were found in 23 samples in a review of 26 pre-treatment trucut samples nor in the eventual associated resection specimens (J. Pritchard, personal communication). In one case anaplasia was present both in the biopsy and resection specimens. However, in two cases, anaplasia was present in the resection specimen but not in the biopsy. This small study shows that it is possible to diagnose Wilms' tumour successfully on biopsy samples and suggests that unfavourable features will not be eradicated by pre-operative chemotherapy. It does, however, demonstrate that unfavourable features may not be detected by percutaneous biopsy and illustrates that the results from such samples must be interpreted with care.

Staging systems

Several staging systems have been used for Wilms' tumour, evolving as successive studies have redefined the criteria for each stage. The major contribution to these systems has been from the United States National Wilms' Tumour Studies. The group system used in the first National Wilms' Tumour Studies and the stage system used in the third of these studies are summarized in Table 4. The grouping system for the first and second National Wilms' Tumour Studies defined group I as those tumours limited to the kidney, the capsule intact, no rupture during removal, and no residual tumour beyond the line of resection. Group II tumours were defined as those extending beyond the kidney, but completely resected. Thus, the tumour could penetrate beyond the pseudocapsule into perirenal soft tissue, periaortic lymph nodes, or renal vessels, provided no residual tumour was present beyond the line of resection. Group III tumours included all those tumours with residual non-haematogenous spread, confined within the abdomen. This group included those tumours biopsied or ruptured before or during surgery, implants on peritoneal surfaces, lymph nodes beyond the periaortic chains, and those tumours not resectable because of local invasion into vital structures. Group IV tumours comprised all cases of haematogenous spread and group V were those cases with simultaneous or metachronous bilateral tumours. Changes in the groups following the first trial followed the realization that there existed a group of tumours with variant histologies ('unfavourable histology') that conferred a worse outcome (Beckwith and Palmer 1978), as did the presence of involved lymph nodes (Breslow *et al.* 1985). The patients with an unfavourable histology had such a poor survival, regardless of stage, that subsequently they were treated with the most intensive regimen. The presence of involved lymph nodes up-graded patients from group II to group III, so that they received radiotherapy and more intensive chemotherapy. In the third National Wilms' Tumour Study the groups were renamed 'stages', and the stages were redefined on the basis of information acquired during the first two studies. Stage I was unchanged. Stage II was redefined to include patients previously in group II, but in addition those in whom biopsy had been performed or in whom rupture of the tumour had occurred, provided the spill was confined to the flank. Following the second National Wilms' Tumour Study, it was noted that local spillage at operation or renal vein invasion had not adversely affected outcome. These patients were down-graded from stage III to stage II, with a concomitant reduction in therapy. Because of its adverse prognostic import, lymph node involvement at the hilus or periaortic chain was up-graded from group II to stage III. Stages IV and V were unchanged. Studies performed by the United Kingdom Children's Cancer Study Group (UKCCSG) have confirmed the validity of these staging systems.

In general, age and stage are directly correlated, with infants rarely having stage IV tumours, whereas approximately 40 per cent of children over the age of 6 years have stage IV disease (Lennox *et al.* 1979; J. Barnes, personal communication).

Wilms' tumour in adults

The incidence of Wilms' tumour in the adult is difficult to determine, since many cases are aggregated with renal cell carcinoma. Approximately 200 cases of adult Wilms' tumour have been reported in the literature, with the majority faring badly. Byrd *et al.* (1982) reviewed those patients over 16 years of age who had been enrolled in National Wilms' Tumour Studies. The median age at presentation was 25 years and the commonest presenting symptom was pain. The commonest signs were an abdominal mass and haematuria. No patient had bilateral disease, but there was a higher proportion of patients with higher-stage disease, compared to children. Despite treatment according to National Wilms' Tumour Studies recommendations, the actuarial overall survival was only 24 per cent at 3 years. Despite improvements in treatment in childhood, Wilms' tumour in the adult remains an unfavourable disease.

TREATMENT
Surgical considerations

Despite advances in chemotherapy, surgical resection remains the fundamental treatment of Wilms' tumour. According to the strategy

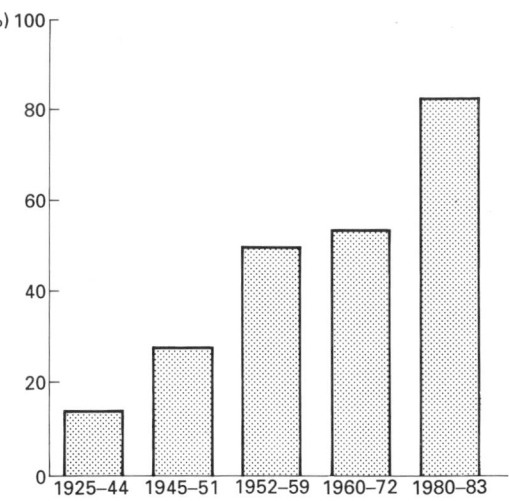

Fig. 2 Absolute 3 year survival for patients seen at the Hospital for Sick Children, London, during the time periods specified.

adopted by the National Wilms' Tumour Studies and the United Kingdom Children's Cancer Study Group, the information gained by histopathological study of the resected specimen directs the rational use of subsequent therapy.

Prior to the development of adjuvant chemotherapy, the results of purely operative treatment of Wilms' tumour reflected the risks of major abdominal surgery on small children and the systemic nature of cancer, in that those patients who survived surgery had a high chance of developing metastases. Much of the early improvement in outcome was due to improved surgical and anaesthetic techniques, development of intravenous fluid therapy, and blood transfusion. Thus, in a review from a single North American centre, survival rose from 14.9 per cent with operative mortality of 23 per cent in the period 1914–1930, to a survival of 47 per cent with no operative mortality in the period 1940–1947 (Gross and Neuhauser 1950). Similar results from a single British centre are shown in Fig. 2 (Williams 1972; Bond 1975; J. Pritchard, personal communication).

It is essential that surgery for Wilms' tumour starts with a generous transverse abdominal incision, so that subsequent examination of the abdominal cavity can be thorough and to ease the manipulation of the tumour during its removal. It is important that both kidneys are properly inspected before any excisional surgery starts. The contralateral kidney must be mobilized and both anterior and posterior surfaces inspected carefully for the presence of previously undetected tumour. The remainder of the abdominal cavity must then be examined. If the contralateral kidney and remainder of the abdominal cavity is normal and the tumour is resectable, the operation then proceeds with the mobilization of surrounding structures, disturbing the tumour as little as possible at this stage. The ureter is dissected free, transected, and a plane of cleavage developed towards the renal pelvis and its associated vessels. The vein, which lies anterior to the artery, is mobilized so that the artery can be tied first. The vein is then tied and the tumour mobilized. Finally, the tumour with associated tissue is removed *en bloc* with care to avoid rupture and contamination of the abdominal cavity. Para-aortic lymph nodes are then biopsied, especially if they are enlarged.

The three major contraindications to surgery are:

(1) the presence of bilateral disease;

(2) a large 'fixed' tumour;

(3) hepatic invasion.

In general 'heroic' surgery is not appropriate, as chemotherapy shrinks tumours very effectively, sparing the child a radical operation with its attendant risks. Particular problems may arise with very large tumours overlying the major blood vessels. Care is needed to avoid the inadvertent ligation of contralateral renal vessels, superior mesenteric artery, or even the aorta and inferior vena cava. The presence of tumour thrombus in the renal vein or inferior vena cava is usually revealed by the pre-operative ultrasound scan, but occasionally it is only discovered intraoperatively. In these circumstances the inferior vena cava should be mobilized so that control can be established above and below the thrombus, prior to attempted removal.

Bilateral tumours provide a particular challenge and here the key is 'conservation of nephrons'. Initial surgery in these circumstances is limited to establishing the histological diagnosis, either by open or closed (Tru-Cut®) biopsy. Both kidneys should be biopsied since the histology of the tumours can differ and can be nephroblastomatosis. Chemotherapy is then instituted. Once a maximal response has been obtained, the operative procedure is usually bilateral partial nephrectomy. If these procedures will not result in clearance of the residual tumour with preservation of adequate renal function, then 'bench surgery' has been advocated. Here, the kidney is removed and residual tumour resected. The kidney is then reimplanted. In the presence of unilateral Wilms' tumour, but with extensive nephroblastomatosis in the contralateral kidney, there is a possibility of a subsequent metachronous tumour. It has been suggested that surgery in these patients should also be conservative (Heidemann et al. 1985). Similar approaches to those outlined for bilateral tumours may be useful in such patients.

Resection of bilateral tumours with preservation of renal function may be impossible in a few children and it may be necessary to carry out bilateral nephrectomies with subsequent renal transplantation after a period of dialysis. This strategy, though, is one of last resort and should not be contemplated until conventional therapies have clearly failed.

'Second-look' surgery, when a definitive operation is performed some period after an initial open biopsy poses no particular problems save for obtaining adequate mobilization of a *previously* mobilized kidney to permit full inspection.

Specific post-operative measures include close monitoring of urine output for 48 h and adequate pain relief using either a morphine infusion or an epidural anaesthetic. Paralytic ileus, as a consequence of mobilization of the bowel, may be accentuated by treatment with vincristine, but this is a rare complication.

Chemotherapy considerations

Stratification of therapy, based on the extent of the primary tumour, presence of involved lymph nodes or metastases, and the extent of any tumour spillage at operation is the key to rational use of chemotherapy. Reduction in therapy for 'good-risk' patients and more intensive therapy for 'bad-risk' patients results in fewer adverse effects of treatment in the former group, while achieving good survival in the latter. The treatment of Wilms' tumour should only be undertaken in recognized paediatric oncology centres, which will invariably be members of large cooperative groups. Specific details

of drug dosage and timing will not be given in this review, since they will be available to appropriate centres.

The first National Wilms' Tumour Study was the first concerted attempt to analyse post-operative chemotherapy and radiotherapy in a systematic fashion (D'Angio et al. 1976). The first National Wilms' Tumour Study and its successors (D'Angio et al. 1981, 1989) have been instrumental in devising prognostic stages and in their revision, as has already been noted. Equally important has been the steady progress in delineating optimal treatment within the various disease stages. The major findings in the National Wilms' Tumour Study series are summarized in Table 5. At the conclusion of the third National Wilms' Tumour Study, therapy had been significantly reduced for stage I patients, who appear to need only 10 weeks of adjuvant chemotherapy and not to need radiotherapy. In stage II patients, by using a more intensive regimen of vincristine and actinomycin D, neither Adriamycin®, with its associated cardiotoxicity, nor radiotherapy are required. For stage III disease, the intensive two-drug regimen is as effective as the three-drug regimen and it has been possible to reduce radiotherapy from 20 to 10 Gy. The addition of cyclophosphamide to Adriamycin®, actinomycin D, and vincristine does not enhance the survival of patients in stage IV or those with an unfavourable histology. The use of Adriamycin® appears specifically to improve the outlook for patients with bone-metastasizing renal tumour. Strategies for malignant rhabdoid tumour of the kidney probably ought to be quite different for those used for the other renal tumours of childhood (D'Angio et al. 1989).

The UKCCSG has built its study in part on the results of the National Wilms' Tumour Studies and also on United Kingdom Medical Research Council trials (Lennox et al. 1979; Morris-Jones et al. 1987). A major difference between UKCCSG and National Wilms' Tumour studies is that the former enrols all patients, even those deemed initially to have surgically unresectable tumours, whereas initial resectability is a criterion for entry into the latter.

In the UKW1 trial, stage I patients treated for 10 weeks with vincristine at weekly intervals, followed by five 3-weekly doses

Table 5 Summary of the results of the National Wilms' Tumour Studies

NWTS1

Group I   Patients < 2 years do not require radiotherapy

Group II/III   Actinomycin D plus vincristine is better than either alone

Group IV   Pre-operative vincristine is of no benefit

Other findings   Unfavourable histology and lymph-node involvement are adverse factors

NWTS 2

Stage I   No patients benefit from radiotherapy, regardless of age. Six months of VCR and AMD is as good as 15 months

Stages II, III, IV   Addition of Adriamycin® to VCR and AMD improves survival

Other findings   Stages II and III have the same survival. Local spillage and invasion of the renal vein do not affect the outcome

NWTS 3

Stage I   10 weeks' therapy with AMD/VCR are as effective as 6 months' therapy

Stage II   Intensive VCR/AMD is as effective as three drugs. Addition of radiotherapy does not enhance survival

Stage III   Intensive VCR/AMD is as effective as three drugs. A dose of 10 Gy is as effective as one of 20 Gy

Other findings   Addition of cyclophosphamide to VCR/AMD/ADR does not improve survival

Abbreviations: ADR, Adriamycin®; AMD, actinomycin D; NWTS, National Wilms' Tumour Study; VCR, vincristine.

had a survival of 96 per cent at 6 years, suggesting that actinomycin D can be avoided in these patients. In the current UKW2 trial, therapy for favourable-histology stage I patients has been reduced further to 10 doses of vincristine at weekly intervals, without diminution of survival. In contrast to this successful reduction in therapy, however, both event-free and overall survivals of stage IV favourable-histology patients in UKW1 are inferior to those of patients in the second and third National Wilms' Tumour Studies (event-free survival of 53 versus 76.6 per cent at 5 years). Since the chemotherapy regimens used are similar, it may be instructive to search for other reasons for this discrepancy. Apart from the possible effect of patient selection noted above, the main differences between the two studies are the longer duration of therapy in the National Wilms' Tumour Studies (15 versus 12 months) and the uniform use of whole-lung irradiation in the third National Wilms' Tumour Study.

Like the National Wilms' Tumour Studies, the recognition of unfavourable histologies and the adverse impact of lymph node metastases has led to the use of more aggressive therapy for these patients, with an improvement in their overall survival, so that the current 2 year disease-free survival of patients in stage I to III with unfavourable histology is approximately 50 per cent.

Unlike the American or British studies, the cooperative European studies run by the International Society of Paediatric Oncology (SIOP) have concentrated on the use of pre-operative therapies in an effort to reduce surgical morbidity, particularly tumour rupture. In the first SIOP study (SIOP 1) patients were randomized either to immediate surgery or to pre-operative radiotherapy (20 Gy) (Lemerle et al. 1976). The frequency of tumour spillage at operation was significantly reduced in the radiotherapy group. Although there was no difference in the overall survival, recurrence-free survival was better in the rupture-free group. SIOP 2 was a non-randomized observational study in which some patients had immediate surgery, at the discretion of the investigator, usually because the tumour was thought to be suitable for primary resection. Other patients received pre-operative treatment of 20 Gy radiation and five doses of actinomycin D. Again, a reduced incidence of tumour rupture was found in the group treated pre-operatively. SIOP 5 (Lemerle et al. 1983) compared pre-operative chemoradiotherapy as used in SIOP 2 with chemotherapy alone, consisting in this instance of two 5-day courses of actinomycin D and four weekly doses of vincristine. There were no significant differences in recurrence-free or overall survivals or in the frequency of tumour spillage, indicating equal efficacy of chemotherapy and chemoradiotherapy regimens. Comparison of the chemotherapy arm of SIOP 5 with the immediate surgery arm of SIOP 1 demonstrated that an additional benefit for the former group was the lower stage disease found at the time of operation. Thus, the proportion of stage I patients arose from 22 to 48 per cent, with concomitant falls in the proportion of patients with stage II node-negative tumours (45–32 per cent) and stage II node-positive or stage III tumours (33–19 per cent). In SIOP 6, in which all patients received pre-operative chemotherapy, it was found that stage II node-negative tumours did not benefit from post-operative radiotherapy. Extrapolating from these results, it would appear that, using the SIOP approach, approximately 80 per cent of patients would not need radiotherapy and would still achieve a survival rate of 88–92 per cent; in the third National Wilms' Tumour Study 70 per cent of patients with favourable histology, non-metastatic tumours did not require radiotherapy (D'Angio 1983), with comparable survival rates.

Radiotherapy considerations

Radiotherapy is now used less frequently and in lower doses in the treatment of Wilms' tumour because of its harmful effects on growing normal tissue. The general trend has been to reduce the dose delivered, as successive trials have indicated that dose reduction does not compromise cure rates.

The radiation dose originally recommended varied from 18 to 24 Gy in children over 40 months, delivered through parallel opposed megavoltage photon portals, with daily treatment fractions of up to 2 Gy. For patients in groups I and II the irradiation portal covered the kidney and associated tumour as defined on the pre-operative intravenous urogram. The other border came across the midline medially to encompass the whole of the vertebral bodies but not the contralateral normal kidney. Group III patients and those in groups I and II with intraoperative tumour spillage were treated with whole-abdominal radiation, from the domes of the diaphragm to the pelvic floor and to the lateral reflections of the peritoneum. The recommended doses were 25 Gy in 3 weeks for children under 4 years and 35 Gy in 4 weeks to those over 4 years, delivered in 1.5 Gy daily fractions with shielding of the contralateral kidney and liver so that their dosage did not exceed 15 Gy and 30 Gy, respectively. Analysis of the results of this trial suggested that whole-abdominal radiation was not necessary if tumour spillage was restricted to the flank. The local recurrence rate was only 12 per cent.

Initially it was considered that radiotherapy had been instrumental in producing this low rate (Tefft et al. 1976), but later it became clear that there was no difference in local or distant relapse rates dependent on radiation dosage (D'Angio et al. 1978). The second National Wilms' Tumour Study showed that omission of radiotherapy in all stage I patients was safe. Data from the third such study showed that radiotherapy was not needed for stage II disease. In stage III disease relapse-free and overall survival were similar whether the patients received 10 or 20 Gy or whether they received two or three drugs. However, there was a trend for a more favourable result with three drugs. In addition, the three-drug regimen was associated with fewer abdominal relapses (four versus 11).

Although none of these differences achieved statistical significance, the National Wilms' Tumour Study committee advocates the three-drug regimen together with the lower radiation dose. In making this choice they gave the following reasons: there were fewer abdominal relapses with this regimen, a lower radiation dose should lead to fewer disturbances of musculoskeletal growth, and no increase in cardiac problems, which might be expected in patients receiving Adriamycin®, has been recorded in National Wilms' Tumour Study patients surviving more than 5 years. The current study, the fourth National Wilms' Tumour Study, is exploring the possibility of using a reduced dose to the renal bed to 10 Gy in conjunction with three-drug chemotherapy in favourable-histology stage III patients (D'Angio et al. 1989).

Special problems

Management of stage V (bilateral) Wilms' tumour

Cooperative studies have not, in general, addressed the problem of managing stage V Wilms' tumour patients, although there is widespread agreement on the general principles to be followed. The majority of stage V tumours occur in younger children and, with the exception of the anaplastic variant, will be of favourable histology. As noted above, surgical management is based on the principle of 'conservation of nephrons'. Thus, initial surgery is limited to biopsy of the tumours so as to confirm the diagnosis, with definitive surgery delayed until an optimal response to chemotherapy has been obtained. Following diagnostic biopsy, stage V patients start chemotherapy, usually using vincristine, actinomycin D, and Adriamycin®. Regular clinical and radiological assessment during chemotherapy provide a measure of response. The relative degree of tumour regression in each kidney may be judged from an abdominal CT scan. Dimercaptosuccinic acid scanning indicates the relative degree of function in each kidney. These two investigations provide both anatomical and functional information and pre-operative decisions about timing and type of definitive surgical intervention can be made with some precision.

Wilms' tumour in patient with single kidneys

Very occasionally, Wilms' tumour will be found in a patient with a single functioning kidney. The management of these patients should follow the guidelines for patients with bilateral tumours, since preservation of normal, functioning renal tissue is critical. Thus, initial chemotherapy with careful monitoring of the response and careful timing of definitive surgery will provide the most favourable result. Immediate nephrectomy followed by dialysis, chemotherapy, and subsequent transplantation would be an option, but one fraught with many additional problems, so it is best avoided if at all possible.

Wilms' tumour in patients with pre-existing renal disease

In these patients, variations in management willl be dictated by the type and prognosis of the pre-existing renal disease. Where there is likely to be inexorable progression to end-stage renal failure, there seems little virtue in delaying surgical removal of the tumour and associated kidney. If necessary, dialysis can be instituted to supplement residual renal function. Timing of subsequent transplantation is more difficult, but to avoid the complexity of simultaneous cancer chemotherapy and transplantation immunosuppression, it seems better to delay transplantation until chemotherapy has been completed and sufficient time has elapsed so that recurrence of malignancy is unlikely. In practice, this period would be approximately 2 years from completion of chemotherapy.

Recurrence of Wilms' tumour in the transplanted kidney is extremely unlikely, since Wilms' tumorigenesis is due to local, rather than to systemic factors. Similarly, there are no grounds on which to modify immunosuppression after transplantation.

FOLLOW-UP AND SCREENING INVESTIGATIONS

The place of repeated 'screening' investigations in patients with conditions associated with or predisposing to Wilms' tumour has not been resolved. Often the physicians taking care of such patients are not primarily oncologists and may not recognize all of the issues involved when making a decision to initiate screening investigations. Some physicians propose that repeated screening will permit earlier detection of clinically occult tumours and so lead to an improvement in outcome. Others note that tumours may be clinically detectable only a few weeks after apparently normal screening, usually by ultrasound.

There are two separate issues to consider. First, what is the evidence that screening of presymptomatic, predisposed children will lead to earlier detection of tumours? Secondly, will detection of presymptomatic tumours result in a reduction of mortality or a reduction of morbidity (as less therapy would be necessary for lower-stage disease)? Palmer and Evans (1983) reviewed nine Wilms' tumour patients with aniridia, who had been subjected to routine screening intravenous urography in an attempt to diagnose their tumours presymptomatically. An unsuspected tumour was detected in only one patient. It was concluded that intravenous urography was an inefficient method for screening and suggested that ultrasonography might be more efficient. While there is less morbidity than with intravenous urography, there has been no published evidence that ultrasonography is more useful in this context than intravenous urography. Furthermore, it is very unlikely that presymptomatic detection will reduce mortality. The most important prognostic factor is histology and the two groups of unfavourable histology do not occur in any of the predisposing conditions. As stage is, in part, linked to histology (that is, unfavourable histologies tend to be a worse stage at diagnosis), it seems unlikely that morbidity would be much influenced either. Thus, the weight of evidence is that presymptomatic screening by any currently available method is insensitive and is unlikely to influence the subsequent course of therapy or outcome. It is even possible that in such circumstances the 'normal' scan may provide false reassurance and so delay diagnosis. It seems more sensible to explain to parents that the child has a condition which may predispose to Wilms' tumour, to teach them to examine the child's abdomen, and to encourage them to seek medical advice if they are at all concerned. Routine screening investigations are not warranted.

During and after therapy, investigation is aimed at detecting early local or distant relapses, so that the appropriate treatment may be instituted. Generally, local relapses are less frequent than pulmonary relapse. Chest radiographs (postero-anterior and lateral) should be obtained regularly during treatment and continued after cessation of treatment for the period when relapse is most likely to occur. Pulmonary relapse may be clinically undetectable until quite advanced, whereas local (abdominal) relapses are usually more overt. Typically, therefore, chest radiographs would be obtained every 9 weeks during treatment, then every 2 months for the first year and every 3 months for the second year after completing treatment. Stage IV patients should continue chest radiographs every 3 months for a further year. Screening for local relapse need not be so frequent and abdominal ultrasonography at completion of treatment and then every 6 months for 2 years is adequate. Other sites of relapse are rare, even, despite its name, in bone-metastasizing renal tumour (pulmonary metastases are the commonest site of metastatic recurrence). Thus, patients with bone-metastasizing renal tumour warrant radionucleide bone scans, if at all, only at 6-monthly intervals for 2 years. A suggested system for follow-up investigations is outlined in Table 6.

Table 6 Follow-up investigations

During treatment
    Chest X-ray (postero-anterior and lateral): every 9 weeks
    Abdominal ultrasound: every 18 weeks
    (Bone scan in bone-metastasizing renal tumour at 3, 6, and 12 months from start of therapy)

Off treatment
    Chest X-ray (postero-anterior and lateral)
    Abdominal ultrasound: 6-monthly for 2 years
    (Bone scan in bone-metastasizing renal tumour cases: 6-monthly for 2 years)

PATTERNS AND TREATMENT OF RELAPSE

The most frequent site of relapse overall is the lungs. In the second and third National Wilms' Tumour Studies this site accounted for 58 per cent of all cases. Abdominal relapse accounted for a further 29 per cent of cases (Grundy *et al.* 1989). These results differ from those of the first National Wilms' Tumour Study, where 74 per cent of relapses were pulmonary and only 18 per cent were abdominal (Sutow *et al.* 1982). This difference is not accounted for by the cessation of radiotherapy for stage I and II patients, since the relapse rates at each site were identical in irradiated and non-irradiated patients. It may reflect a greater efficacy of chemotherapy on pulmonary micrometastases compared to those in other sites. In the SIOP 5 study, 54 per cent of all relapses were isolated pulmonary events, the remainder being in other or multiple sites (Lemerle *et al.* 1983). Sixteen per cent of all relapses involved the abdomen, but only in association with other sites. Isolated pulmonary relapse accounted for 41 per cent of all relapses in the UKW1 study, with abdominal relapses accounting for 24 per cent, the remaining 35 per cent being patients with multiple simultaneous sites of relapse (R. Pinkerton, personal communication).

Both British and American studies (Grundy *et al.* 1989; Groot-Loonen *et al.* 1990) have identified prognostic factors which identify an increased probability of salvage of relapsed patients. Favourable-histology tumours that recurred only in the lungs or in the abdomen where radiotherapy had not been included in the primary treatment or that occurred more than 12 months from diagnosis were associated with a more favourable outcome. Patients with relapsed, unfavourable-histology tumours had poor survival regardless of the site or timing of relapse. Breslow *et al.* (1986) had previously noted that patients with hepatic metastases, developing either during or after therapy, had a particularly poor outcome.

Retrieval therapy is in part dictated by the therapies previously used. Initial surgery may not be necessary for unirradiated favourable-histology abdominal recurrences when radiotherapy and further chemotherapy can be given, an important consideration if the tumour appears to be unresectable. If not previously used, radiotherapy is indicated for multiple pulmonary relapses and is used in conjunction with salvage chemotherapy. Apart from the three standard agents vincristine, actinomycin D, and Adriamycin®, other agents which may be useful in relapse include iphosphamide or VP-16 (etoposide) (Groot-Loonen *et al.* 1990).

PROGNOSIS

With the use of modern anaesthetic and surgical techniques and the rational application of combination chemotherapy, the majority of patients with Wilms' tumour will be cured. In part this is because most patients will present with favourable-histology low-stage disease, but there have been genuine advances in chemotherapy. The overall survival from the SIOP 5 trial was 86 per cent at 3 years, with a relapse-free survival of 71 per cent. Results for the better arm for each stage of the third National Wilms' Tumour Study and for the UKW1 study are shown in Table 7. Thus, the vast majority of Wilms' tumour patients are cured, many with minimal short- or long-term morbidity. In comparing the results of National Wilms' Tumour Studies with UKCCSG or SIOP studies, it is important to remember that patients enrolled in the former are 'selected' on the basis of initial surgical resectability, whereas the latter include patients initially deemed inoperable.

Table 7 Results of National Wilms' Tumour (NWTS) and UKW1 Studies

	Relapse-free survival	Overall
NWTS 3 Five-year results		
Favourable histology		
Stage I	90.5	96.1 (10 weeks of A+V)
Stage II	88.9	94.6 (15 months of A+V+Ad)
Stage III	80.6	88.6 (A+V±Ad, +10 Gy)
Stage IV	76.6	81.4
UKW1 Six-year results		
Favourable histology		
Stage I	88	96
Stage II	85	92
Stage III	82	83
Stage IV	53	64
Stage V	73	80
Unfavourable histology		
Stage I	79	90
Stage II	67	67
Stage III	44	60
Stage IV	0	0
Stage V	50	50

Abbreviations: A, actinomycin D; Ad, Adriamycin®; V, vincristine.

FUTURE PROSPECTS

Progress on the genetic basis of Wilms' tumour may allow redefinition of the entity of Wilms' tumour, with a clear demonstration that the bone-metastasizing renal tumours and malignant rhabdoid tumours of the kidney arise by distinct genetic events. Molecular characterization of secondary mutations within tumours may define groups of varying prognosis and so lead to a further rationalization of therapy.

The two continuing clinical challenges in Wilms' tumour are to refine therapy in the good-prognosis patients so that treatment-related morbidity and mortality is negated and to improve therapy for poor-prognosis and relapsing patients, so that their survival improves. Stage I favourable-histology patients already receive minimal treatment, but the recognition of very favourable histological patterns may define a group of patients who need no adjuvant chemotherapy. Pre-operative chemotherapy may provide a route to the overall reduction of chemotherapy and obviation of radiotherapy in the intermediate stages of favourable-histology disease. Improvements in results for patients with unfavourable histology await the development of novel strategies.

REFERENCES

Beckwith JB (1963). Extreme cytomegaly of the fetal adrenal cortex, omphalocele, hyperplasia of the kidneys and pancreas, and Leydig cell hyperplasia: another syndrome? *Western Society for Pediatric Research*, November 11.

Beckwith JB (1969). Macroglossia, omphalocoele, adrenal cytomegaly gigontism and hyperplastic visceromegaly. In: *Birth defects*, Vol. 5 (ed. D Bergsma, VA McKusick, JG Hall, and CI Scott). Original article series, Stratton Intercon, New York.

Beckwith JB (1986). Wilms' tumor and other renal tumors of childhood. In *Pathology of neoplasia in children and adolescents* (ed. M Finegold), pp. 313–32. WB Saunders, Philadelphia.

Beckwith JB, Palmer NF (1978). Histopathology and prognosis of Wilms' tumour: results from the first National Wilms' tumour study. *Cancer*, **41**:1937–48.

Bolande RP (1973). Congenital mesoblastic nephroma of infancy. *Perspectives of Pediatric Pathology*, **1**:227–50.

Bolande RP, Brough AJ, Izant RJ (1967). Congenital mesoblastic nephroma of infancy. *Pediatrics*, **40**:272–8.

Bond JV (1975). Prognosis and treatment of Wilms' tumour at Great Ormond Street Hospital for Sick Children, 1960–72. *Cancer*, **36**:1202–7.

Bonnin JM, Rubinstein LJ, Palmer NF, Beckwith JB (1984). The association of embryonal tumours originating in the kidney and in the brain. A report of seven cases. *Cancer*, **54**:2137–46.

Bove KE, McAdams AJ (1985). The nephroblastomatosis complex and its relationship to Wilms' tumour: a clinicopathologic treatise. *Perspectives in Pediatric Pathology*, **3**:185–222.

Breslow NE, Beckwith JB (1982). Epidemiological features of Wilms' tumor: results of the National Wilms' Tumour Study. *Journal of the National Cancer Institute*, **68**:429–36.

Breslow NE, Palmer NF, Hill LR, Buring J, D'Angio JD (1978). Prognostic factors for patients without metastases at diagnosis. Results of the National Wilms' Tumour Study. *Cancer*, **41**:1577–89.

Breslow NE, *et al.* (1985). Prognostic factors for Wilms' tumor patients with non-metastatic disease at diagnosis. Results of the second National Wilms' Tumor Study. *Journal of Clinical Oncology*, **3**:521–31.

Breslow NE, *et al.* (1986). Clinicopathologic features and prognosis for Wilms' tumour patients with metastases at diagnosis. *Cancer*, **58**:2501–11.

Byrd RL, Evans AE, D'Angio GJ (1982). Adult Wilms' tumor: effect of combined therapy on survival. *Journal of Urology*, **127**:648–51.

D'Angio GJ (1983). SIOP and the management of Wilms' tumour. *Journal of Clinical Oncology*, **1**:595–6.

D'Angio GJ, *et al.* (1976). The treatment of Wilms' tumour. Results of the first National Wilms' Tumour Study. *Cancer*, **38**:633–46.

D'Angio GJ, *et al.* (1978). Radiation therapy of Wilms' tumour. Results according to dose, field, post-operative timing and histology. *International Journal of Radiation Oncology — Biology — Physics*, **4**:769–80.

D'Angio GJ, *et al.* (1981). The treatment of Wilms' tumour: results of the second National Wilms' Tumor Study. *Cancer*, **47**:2302–11.

D'Angio GJ, *et al.* (1989). The treatment of Wilms' tumor. Results of the third National Wilms' Tumor Study. *Cancer*, **64**:349–60.

Douglass EC, *et al.* (1986). Hyperdiploidy and chromosomal rearrangements define the anaplastic variant of Wilms' tumor. *Journal of Clinical Oncology*, **4**:975–81.

Drash A, Sherman F, Hartman WH, Blizzard RM (1970). A syndrome of pseudohermaphroditism, Wilms' tumour, hypertension, and degenerative renal disease. *Journal of Pediatrics*, **76**:585–93.

Dunn JM, Phillips RA, Becker A, Gallie BL (1988). Identification of germline and somatic mutations affecting the retinoblastoma gene. *Science*, **241**:1797–800.

Fernandes ET, Parham DM, Ribeiro RC, Douglass EC, Kumar APM, Wilimas J (1988). Teratoid Wilms' tumor: the St Jude Experience. *Journal of Pediatric Surgery*, **23**:1131–4.

Fitzgerald JHT (1978). *Human embryology: a regional approach*, pp. 1–205. Harper and Rowe, London.

Francke U, Holmes LB, Atkins L, Riccardi VM (1979). Aniridia–Wilms' tumor association: evidence for a specific relation of 11q13. *Cytogenetics and Cell Genetics*, **24**:185–92.

Groot-Loonen JJ, Pinkerton CR, Morris-Jones P, Pritchard J (1990). How curable is Wilms' tumour after relapse? Salvage chemotherapy after United Kingdom Children's Cancer Study Group neuroblastoma study 1. *Archives of Disease in Childhood*, **65**:968–70.

Gross RE, Neuhauser EBD (1950). Treatment of mixed tumours of the kidney in childhood. *Pediatrics*, **6**:843–50.

Grundy P, Breslow N, Green DM, Sharples K, Evans AE, D'Angio GJ (1989). Prognostic factors for children with recurrent Wilms' tumour: results from the second and third National Wilms' Tumour Study. *Journal of Clinical Oncology*, **7**:638–47.

Habib R, *et al.* (1985). The nephropathy associated with male pseudohermaphroditism and Wilms' tumour (Drash syndrome): a distinctive glomerular lesion—report of 10 cases. *Clinical Nephrology*, **24**:269–78.

Heidemann RL, Haase GM, Foley CL, Wilson HL, Bailey WC (1985). Nephroblastomatosis and Wilms' tumor: clinical experience and management of seven patients. *Cancer*, **555**:1446–51.

Heidemann RL, McGavran L, Waldstein G (1986). Nephroblastomatosis and deletion of 11p. The potential etiologic relationship to subsequent Wilms' tumour. *American Journal of Pediatric Hematology and Oncology*, **8**:231–4.

Hou LT, Holman RL (1961). Bilateral nephroblastomatosis in a premature infant. *Journal of Pathology and Bacteriology*, **82**:249–55.

Hrabovsky EE, Othrsen HB, deLorimier A, Kelalis P, Beckwith JB, Takashima J (1986). Wilms' tumor in the neonate: a report from the national Wilms' tumor study. *Journal of Pediatric Surgery*, **21**:385–7.

Jadresic L, Dillon MJ, Grant DB, Pritchard J, Barratt TM (1988). The nephropathy associated with male pseudohermaphroditism and nephroblastoma. *Pediatric Nephrology*, **2**:C149 (abstract).

Kidd JM (1970). Exclusion of certain renal neoplasms from the category of Wilms' tumour. *American Journal of Pathology*, **59**:16.

Knudson AG (1971). Mutation and cancer: statistical study of retinoblastoma. *Proceedings of the National Academy of Science USA*, **68**:820–3.

Ledlie EM, Mynors LS, Draper GJ, Gorbach PD (1970). Natural history and treatment of Wilms' tumour: an analysis of 335 cases occurring in England and Wales, 1962–1966. *British Medical Journal*, **4**:195–200.

Lemerle J, *et al.* (1976). Preoperative versus post-operative radiotherapy, single versus multiple courses of actinomycin D in the treatment of Wilms' tumors. Preliminary results of a controlled clinical trial conducted by the International Society of Pediatric Oncology (SIOP). *Cancer*, **38**:647–54.

Lemerle J, *et al.* (1983). Effectiveness of preoperative chemotherapy in Wilms' tumour: results of an International Society of Pediatric Oncology (SIOP) clinical trial. *Journal of Clinical Oncology*, **1**:604–10.

Lennox EL, Stiller CA, Morris-Jones PH, Kinnier-Wilson LM (1979). Nephroblastoma: treatment during 1970–73 and the effect on survival of inclusion in the first MRC trial. *British Medical Journal*, **2**:567–9.

Machin GA, McCaughey WTE (1984). A new precursor lesion of Wilms' tumour (nephroblastoma): intralobar multifocal nephroblastomatosis. *Histopathology*, **8**:35–53.

McKusick VA (1986). *Mendelian inheritance in man* (7th edn). Johns Hopkins University Press, Baltimore, MD.

Marsden HB, Lawler W (1978). Bone-metastasising renal tumour of childhood. *British Journal of Cancer*, **38**:437–41.

Miller RW, Fraumeni JF, Manning MD (1964). Association of Wilms' tumour with aniridia, hemihypertrophy and other congenital malformations. *New England Journal of Medicine*, **270**:922–7.

Mitchell CD, Harvey W, Gordon D, Womer RB, Dillon MJ, Pritchard J (1985). Rhabdoid Wilms' tumour and prostaglandin-mediated hypercalcaemia. *European Paediatric Haematology and Oncology*, **2**:153–7.

Morris-Jones P, Marsden HB, Pearson D, Barnes J (1987). *MRC second nephroblastoma trial, 1974–78: long-term results*. Abstract 121, SIOP Proceedings, Jerusalem.

Narahara K, Kikkawa K, Kimura S, Kimoto H, Ogata M, Kasai M, Matsuoka K (1984). Regional mapping of catalase and Wilms' tumour–aniridia genitourinary abnormalities and mental retardation tried loci to the chromosome segment 11p13.05–p13.06. *Human Genetics*, **66**:181–5.

Palmer N, Evans AE (1983). The association of aniridia and Wilms' tumour: methods of surveillance and diagnosis. *Medical and Pediatric Oncology*, **11**:73–5.

Parkin DM, Stiller CA, Draper GJ (1988). The international incidence of childhood cancer. *International Journal of Cancer*, **42**:511–20.

Pritchard J, *et al.* (1988). *Preliminary results of the first United Kingdom Childrens Study Group Wilms' tumour study (UKW1)*. Abstract 107, SIOP Proceedings, Trondheim.

Raney RB, Palmer N, Sutow WW, Baum E, Ayala A (1983). Renal-cell carcinoma in children. *Medical and Pediatric Oncology*, **11**:91–8.

Riccardi VM, Sujansky E, Smith AC, Francke U (1978). Chromosomal imbalance in the aniridia–Wilms' tumor association: 11p interstitial deletion. *Paediatrics*, **61**:604–10.

Rousseau-Merck MF, *et al.* (1982). An original hypercalcemic infantile renal tumour without bone metastasis: heterotransplantation to nude mice. *Cancer*, **50**:85–93.

Sutow WW, Breslow NE, Palmer NF, D'Angio GJ, Takashima J (1982). Prognosis in children with Wilms' tumor metastases prior to or following diagnosis. Results from the first Wilms' tumor study. *American Journal of Clinical Oncology*, **5**:339–47.

Tefft M, D'Angio GJ, Grant W (1976). Post-operative radiation therapy for residual Wilms' tumor. Review of group III patients in the National Wilms' Tumor Study. *Cancer*, **37**:2768–72.

Variend S, Spicer RD, MacKinnon AC (1984). Teratoid Wilms' tumour. *Cancer*, 53:1936–42.

Weeks DA, Beckwith JB, Mierau GW, Luckey DW (1989). Rhabdoid tumour of the kidney. A report of 111 cases from the National Wilms' Tumour Study Center. *American Journal of Surgical Pathology*, 13:439–58.

Wiedemann NR (1964). Complexe malformatif familial avec hernie ombilicale et macroglossie: un "syndrome nouveau"? *Journeau de Genetique Humaine*, 13:223–32.

Wilimas JA, Douglass EC, Magill HL, Fitch S, Hustu HO (1988). Significance of pulmonary computed tomography at diagnosis in Wilms' tumour. *Journal of Clinical Oncology*, 6:1144–6.

Williams IG (1972). *Tumours of childhood—a clinical treatise*, pp. 103–4. Heinemann, London.

Wilms M (1899). *Die Mischgeschwulste der Nieren*, pp. 1–90. Arthur Georgi, Leipzig.

Zhu Z, et al. (1989). Preferential germline mutation of the paternal allele in retinoblastoma. *Nature*, 340:312–13.

14.5   Germ cell tumours of childhood

JILLIAN R. MANN

INCIDENCE, EPIDEMIOLOGY, AND AETIOLOGY

Incidence

In the United Kingdom the incidence of malignant germ cell tumours is approximately 2.7 per 10^6 person years (Birch *et al.* 1988) and is increasing (Birch *et al.* 1982; Mann and Stiller 1993). Germ cell tumours may be benign, malignant, or have both benign and malignant components. Benign tumours are more frequent, but their incidence is known less precisely than is that for malignant germ cell tumours, as their notification to tumour registries is incomplete.

In a review of several large paediatric series which included benign and malignant tumours, the sacrococcygeal site was the most common, accounting for 41 per cent of cases, followed by the ovary (29 per cent), testis (7 per cent), mediastinum/pericardium (6 per cent), intracranium (5 per cent), retroperitoneum (4 per cent), neck (3 per cent), and head, stomach, uterus/vagina, spinal cord, bladder/prostate, liver, and umbilical cord (all less than 1 per cent) (Dehner 1986). A different incidence pattern is evident if only malignant germ cell tumours are considered. For example, in a British study open to children with only malignant germ cell tumours (except intracranial) the primary sites were testis (61 cases), ovary (29), sacrococcygeal (21), vagina/uterus (3), prostate (1), retroperitoneum (2), thorax/mediastinum (5), abdomen (2), bile duct (1), and lip (1) (Mann *et al.* 1989).

Some tumours present at birth, when they are generally histologically benign, but may be large enough to obstruct delivery. These congenital teratomas are most often found in the sacrococcygeal/presacral site, but may also present in the head and neck or, more rarely, elsewhere. If they are incompletely resected, malignant recurrence may take place months or years later. Sacrococcygeal/presacral tumours first presenting beyond the neonatal period are usually malignant but may also contain benign elements.

Age and sex

Sacrococcygeal/presacral tumours occur much more often in girls than boys and generally present before the age of 4 years. Malignant germ cell tumours in the ovary tend to present in the latter part of the first decade or in the second decade, whereas those in the testis, vagina, uterus, and prostate generally present before the age of 5 years (Mann *et al.* 1989). Ethnic differences exist; Li and Fraumeni (1972) noted low mortality rates from testicular tumours in Black children, whereas pineal teratomas are approximately twice as common in Japan as in Western countries (Wakai *et al.* 1980).

Aetiology

Some germ cell tumours are genetically determined. For example, gonadoblastoma and malignant germ cell tumours often develop in the gonads of individuals with intersex states. Those with dysgenetic gonads and a Y chromosome are particularly at risk (Taylor *et al.* 1966; Mann *et al.* 1983). Mediastinal germ cell tumours have been described in Klinefelter's syndrome. Tumours of the ovary and testis may be familial and so may sacrococcygeal/presacral tumours (often occurring with hereditary sacral agenesis, meningocoele, and other pelvic malformations). A variety of other malformations also have an excess incidence in children with germ cell tumours (Fraumeni *et al.* 1973; Marsden *et al.* 1981; Johnston *et al.* 1986). Boys with undescended testes have an increased risk of developing testicular germ cell tumours (Li and Fraumeni 1972). There is an association between malignant germ cell tumours and certain haematological malignances especially monocytic leukaemia (Dement *et al.* 1985; Nicols *et al.* 1985; Beasley *et al.* 1987; Waters *et al.* 1987; Mann *et al.* 1989).

Increasing teratoma rates in adults (OPCS 1986) suggest possible environmental causes in some patients and these could also be responsible for the increasing incidence in children (Birch *et al.* 1982; Mann and Stiller 1993), possibly due to parental exposure to chemicals and dusts (Johnston *et al.* 1986).

An excess of twins, both among patients with teratomas and their families, has been noted and it has been suggested that germ cell tumours may arise as an abortive attempt at twinning or as a result of fetus–fetus interaction leading to the disappearance of one twin (Rogers 1976).

PATHOLOGY

Embryology

Germ cells first appear in the extraembryonic yolk sac of the 4-week-old embryo and probably arise from the yolk sac endoderm. During the sixth week of gestation they migrate into the embryo through the midline dorsal mesentery to the genital ridge in the retroperitoneum, where the gonads develop and later descend to the scrotum or pelvis (Fig. 1). Aberrant germ cell migration may lead to the accumulation of germ cells in the presacral/sacrococcygeal area, mediastinum, retroperitoneum, vagina, prostate, liver, nasopharynx, or pineal. Subsequently these may proliferate to form benign or malignant germ cell tumours.

Teilum's theory of the origin of the various germ cell tumour types (Teilum 1976) states that the primitive germ cell is capable of producing either of two tumour cell types, germinoma (seminoma or dysgerminoma) and embryonal carcinoma and only the latter has the potential to differentiate into the other cell types (Fig. 2).

Histology

There are a number of histological classifications (Marsden *et al.* 1981; Mostofi *et al.* 1985) but Dehner's (Table 1) has proved suitable in the paediatric context (Dehner 1986).

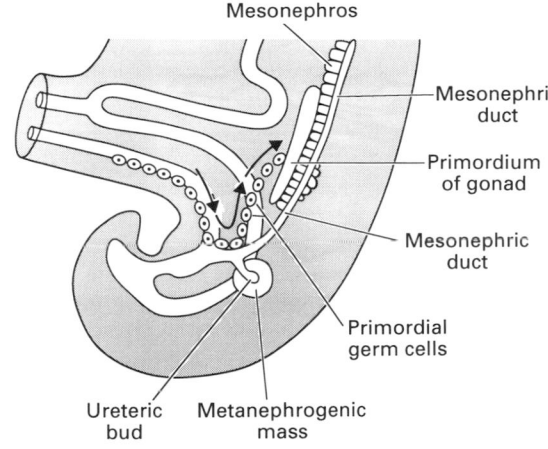

Fig. 1 A sketch of a 5-week-old embryo, illustrating the migration of primordial germ cells (after an illustration by Glen Reid in Moore 1977).

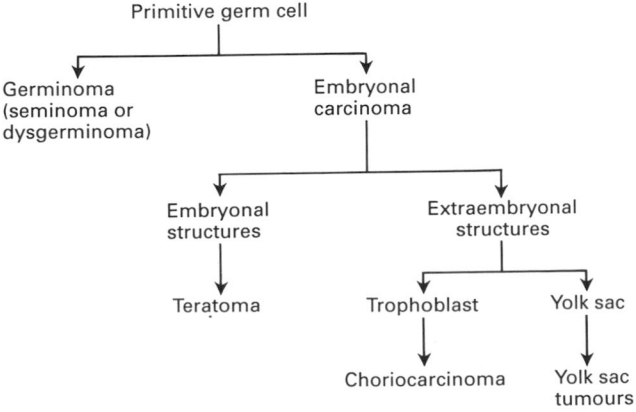

Fig. 2 The origin of the various germ cell tumour types (Teilum 1976).

Table 1 Working classification of germ cell tumours in childhood (after Dehner 1986)

I	Germinomas	
	A Non-invasive: intratubular (*in situ*) germ cell neoplasm	
	B Invasive: seminoma, dysgerminoma, germinoma	
II	Teratoma	
	A Polydermal	
	1 Mature (benign)	
	2 Immature	
	a Indeterminant biological behaviour	
	b Malignant	
	B Monodermal	
III	Embryonal carcinoma, adult type	
IV	Endodermal sinus tumour (infantile type of embryonal carcinoma or yolk sac tumour)	
V	Choriocarcinoma	
VI	Gonadoblastoma	
	A Pure	
	B With invasive component	
VII	Malignant germ cell tumour of mixed histological pattern	

Germinoma

This is known as seminoma when it occurs in the testis (seldom seen in children) and as dysgerminoma when it arises in the ovary. At extragonadal sites, such as the pineal or mediastinum, it is known simply as germinoma. The tumour is often found in combination with other germ cell tumour types and is the most frequent malignant germ cell tumour occurring in dysgenetic gonads. The pre-invasive or *in situ* stage is referred to as intratubular germ cell neoplasm (IA in Dehner's classification).

Teratoma

Entirely benign (mature) teratomas contain only differentiating or mature tissues from ectoderm, endoderm, and/or mesoderm, but in some tumours both benign and immature or malignant, germ cell tumour elements are present together. Dehner (1986) subclassified the immature teratomas into a group with indeterminant biological behaviour and a malignant group. However, Kooijman (1988) recommended that the teratoma group should be subclassified as shown in Table 2. This distinction may be important because the immature teratomas, especially grades 1 and 2, are considerably less aggressive than the malignant germ cell tumours (Dehner's types I, III, IV, V, and VII) and can often be cured by surgery alone, although close follow-up is required. In the British terminology mature teratomas are known as teratoma differentiated

Table 2 Subclassification of the teratoma group (Kooijman 1988)

A	Mature (benign)
B	Immature, grades 1–3[a]
	Grade 1 Immature tissue in one low-power field
	Grade 2 Immature tissue comprising more than one and less than four low-power fields
	Grade 3 Immature teratoma in more than four low-power fields
C	Mature or immature teratoma combined with malignant germ cell tumour (germinoma, endodermal sinus tumour, embryonal carcinoma, or choriocarcinoma)

[a]Grading as described by Thurlbeck and Scully (1960).

(TD) while the term malignant teratoma intermediate (MTI) is used to describe a subgroup (which usually occurs in adults) of the American immature teratoma group (Pugh and Cameron 1976).

Embryonal carcinoma, adult type

This is one of the most common types of non-seminomatous germ cell tumour of the testis in young adults and occurs at other sites, but is seldom seen in children. In the British terminology it is known as malignant teratoma undifferentiated (MTU).

Endodermal sinus tumour

(Infantile type of embryonal carcinoma, yolk sac tumour, Teilum tumour, orchioblastoma, adenocarcinoma of the infant testis.) This is the commonest malignant germ cell tumour of childhood. In a recent British series 97 of the 126 patients had yolk sac tumours, five had germinomas, 11 had immature teratomas, and 13 had mixed malignant germ cell tumours (Mann et al. 1989). Yolk sac tumours arise in the infant testis, the ovary, sacrococcygeal region, vagina, uterus, prostate, abdomen, liver, retroperitoneum, thorax, and pineal/third ventricle. When congenital benign tumours have been incompletely removed, yolk sac tumour recurrence may follow months or years later. There are four histological patterns, pseudopapillary, reticular, polyvesicular vitelline, and solid. The pseudopapillary type usually contains Schiller–Duval bodies which are often associated with intra- and extracellular eosinophilic hyaline bodies containing α-fetoprotein.

Choriocarcinoma

(Malignant teratoma trophoblastic in the British terminology: MTT.) Pure gonadal or extragonadal choriocarcinoma is rare in children. More often it is found as a component of mixed malignant germ cell tumours. It produces human chorionic gonadotrophin which may cause precocious puberty. The region of the pineal gland/third ventricle, the anterior mediastinum, and the gonads are the principal sites of pure non-gestational choriocarcinoma. Girls of reproductive age may develop gestational trophoblastic choriocarcinoma and, very rarely, neonates present with visceral metastases derived from placental primary tumours.

Gonadoblastoma

This is a benign tumour which almost invariably arises in dysgenetic gonads. Affected individuals are usually of 46XY karyotype, although they may be phenotypically female or have 46XY/45XO mosaicism. Other intersex conditions, especially those having a Y chromosome, predispose to this tumour, which is often associated with malignant germ cell tumours especially germinoma, in the same or the contralateral dysgenetic gonad. Therefore, prophylactic gonadectomy is usually desirable in patients with XY karyotypes and gonadal dysgenesis.

Malignant germ cell tumours of mixed histological pattern

Any of the malignant germ cell tumour types may occur together in the same tumour with or without benign (mature) elements. In childhood mixed tumours are most frequently seen in the ovarian and sacrococcygeal sites.

BIOLOGY
Genetics

By studies of the karyotype of germ cell tumours and the degree of homo- or heterogeneity of enzymes with known polymorphism within the tumour and normal tissues, it has been shown that in benign ovarian teratomas, which all had a normal 46XX karyotype but no polymorphism for specific enzymes, the tumours had arisen from post-meiotic cells (Linder et al. 1975). Failure of meiosis I or II or duplication of a mature ovum, were the mechanisms suggested by other workers (Parrington et al. 1985) who found normal diploid female constitution except in one teratoma which had trisomy 7 and 8, possibly indicating pre-malignant change.

In malignant testicular teratomas of adults, however, all tumours have possessed a Y chromosome, indicating a pre-meiotic origin, but they are also usually aneuploid. The genome may be duplicated in many areas, but parts of it are also lost, particularly regions on the short arm of chromosome 1 (Parrington et al. 1985). Flow cytometry has confirmed that a high percentage of malignant testicular teratomas in adults are aneuploid; 64 per cent in a series reported by Quirke et al. (1985) who postulated that differentiated teratomas should be diploid, but that the level of aneuploidy increases in malignant teratoma undifferentiated and malignant teratoma intermediate, to be almost 100 per cent in yolk sac and trophoblastic tumours.

Of potential clinical value in the management of residual mature teratoma after intensive chemotherapy for malignant germ cell tumours is the assessment by flow cytometry of the DNA index of residual tumour, compared with the original primary. That residual tumours with deceptively benign histology may have malignant potential can be demonstrated by the finding of aneuploidy (Oosterhuis et al. 1985).

Flow cytometric assays for the c-myc oncogene indicate that this method may have prognostic value (Sikora et al. 1985) as it has in the management of neuroblastoma.

An isochromosome of the short arm of chromosome 12 (designated i(12p)) was originally detected in four seminomas (Atkin and Baker 1982). Subsequent work in 24 adult males with testicular or extragonadal germ cell tumours revealed i(12p) in all cases and in all histologic cell types. Also, i(12p) was present in an acute leukaemia of the same clonal origin as a mediastinal germ cell tumour which was present in the same patient (Bosl et al. 1989), thus suggesting a common cell lineage.

Tumour markers
Immunohistochemistry

Immunohistochemical detection of α-fetoprotein and the β-subunit of human chorionic gonadotrophin are of established value in aiding the histological diagnosis of germ cell and trophoblastic tumours, respectively (Palmer et al. 1976; Kurman et al. 1977). Cells positive for α-fetoprotein were present in 74 per cent of yolk sac tumours, 33 per cent of embryonal carcinomas (adult type), and 42 per cent of teratomas, but not in pure choriocarcinomas or seminomas/dysgerminomas in one study (Niehans et al. 1988). All choriocarcinomas showed strong syncytiotrophoblastic reactivity for human chorionic gonadotrophin and some embryonal carcinomas (adult type) and germinomas (seminomas) contained human chorionic gonadotrophin-positive cells. Placental alkaline phosphatase was another sensitive marker (positive in 87 per cent of germinomas, 86 per cent of adult-type embryonal carcinoma, 53 per cent of yolk sac tumours, and 54 per cent of choriocarcinomas). However, neurone-specific enolase positivity was demonstrated in 84 per cent of germinomas, 81 per cent of adult-type embryonal carcinomas, 68 per cent of yolk sac tumours, and 46 per cent of choriocarcinomas, calling into question the specificity of this enzyme.

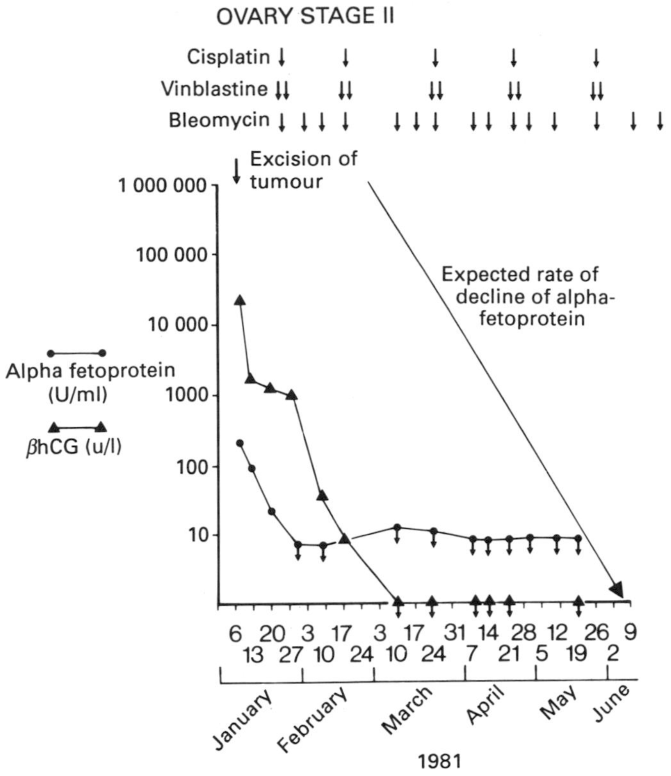

OVARY STAGE II

Cisplatin ↓   ↓   ↓   ↓   ↓
Vinblastine ↓↓   ↓↓   ↓↓   ↓↓   ↓↓
Bleomycin ↓ ↓ ↓ ↓   ↓ ↓ ↓   ↓↓ ↓ ↓ ↓   ↓   ↓ ↓

Fig. 3 Decline of α-fetoprotein and human chorionic gonadotrophin levels in a girl with stage II ovarian mixed germ cell tumour treated by incomplete excision and PVB (cisplatin, vinblastine, bleomycin) chemotherapy.

Serum markers

α-Fetoprotein

α-Fetoprotein is an α-1 globulin which resembles albumen and is the principal serum protein of the fetus. At first it is produced by the yolk sac and later by the fetal liver and gastrointestinal tract. Synthesis of α-fetoprotein reaches a peak around the thirteenth week of gestation, when serum levels of 3–4 mg/ml (approximately 3 000 000 international units/ml) are found (Elwood and Elwood 1980). The level then decreases progressively to approximately 50 μg/ml (42 000 IU/ml) at birth and then falls exponentially to reach adult levels of less than 12 ng/ml (10 IU/ml) during the second 6 months of life (Tsuchida 1978; Wu et al. 1981). Sensitive radioimmunoassay is required to detect normal adult and childhood levels.

Serum α-fetoprotein was elevated in all 94 children with yolk sac tumours who were tested in the United Kingdom Children's Cancer Study Group's (UKCCSG's) studies (Mann et al. 1989), in seven of 11 children with immature teratoma, and 12 of 13 with mixed malignant germ cell tumours. Unexpectedly, levels were also found to be elevated in two out of five children with apparently pure germinomas, although it was impossible to examine the whole of these large tumours to exclude totally the presence of other elements. In adults and children the half-life of α-fetoprotein is approximately 5 days; in 27 UKCCSG patients cured by orchidectomy of stage I testicular yolk sac tumours it was 4.98 days (Huddart et al. 1990). Successful treatment, whether by surgery or chemotherapy, is reflected by α-fetoprotein levels falling at the appropriate rate for its half-life (Fig. 3). However, in infants the half-life is longer (Tsuchida et al. 1978; Wu et al. 1981) because the liver continues to produce some α-fetoprotein during the first months of life. Interpretation of serial α-fetoprotein levels in infants must take this into account. Also, α-fetoprotein levels may be raised

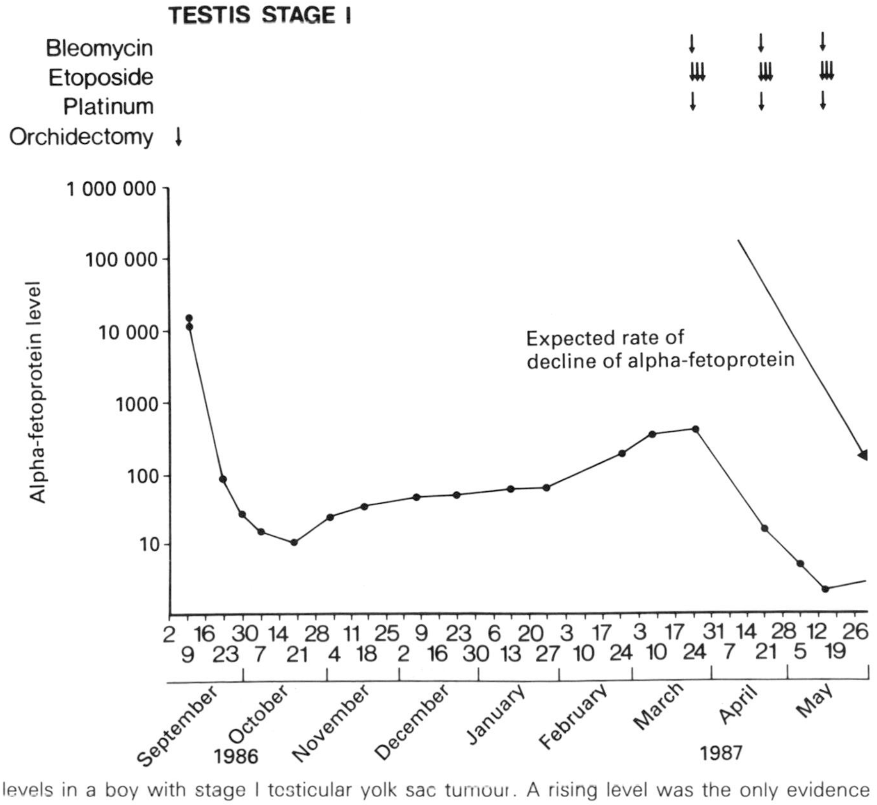

TESTIS STAGE I

Bleomycin   ↓   ↓   ↓
Etoposide   ↓↓↓ ↓↓↓ ↓↓↓
Platinum   ↓   ↓   ↓
Orchidectomy ↓

Fig. 4 α-Fetoprotein levels in a boy with stage I testicular yolk sac tumour. A rising level was the only evidence for recurrence, and a satisfactory decline followed BEP (bleomycin, VP-16, cisplatin) chemotherapy (Mann et al. 1989; reproduced by permission of the American Cancer Society, Inc., J. B. Lippincott Company).

in children with hepatomas, hepatitis, tyrosinosis, ataxia telangiectasia, Indian childhood cirrhosis, and certain other disorders (Mann *et al.* 1978).

Serial measurements of α-fetoprotein have proved valuable in the early detection of failed treatment, rising levels usually being the first or sometimes the only evidence for recurrence (Mann *et al.* 1989) and chemotherapy has been followed by appropriate decline in α-fetoprotein levels (Fig. 4).

β-Subunit of human chorionic gonadotrophin (β-HCG)

Human chorionic gonadotrophin is a glycoprotein produced by the placental trophoblast and its function is to maintain the successful implantation of the embryo. It is composed of two polypeptide chains, α and β, which resemble several pituitary hormones. Specific antibodies which recognize β-human chorionic gonadotrophin and which lack cross-reactivity with luteinizing-hormone, follicle stimulating hormone, and thyroid stimulating hormone permit measurement of β-human chorionic gonadotrophin by radio-immunoassay.

The value of serum β-human chorionic gonadotrophin levels in the diagnosis and follow-up of patients with gestational chorio-carcinoma, hydatidiform mole, and adults with non-gestational germ cell tumours is well established (Bagshawe *et al.* 1973; Bagshawe 1976). The half-life is shorter than for α-fetoprotein, in the order of 2–3 days.

Serum human chorionic gonadotrophin levels were elevated in four out of five children with germinomas, one out of six with immature teratomas, seven out of 56 with apparently pure yolk sac tumours (although it was impossible to exclude the presence of trophoblastic elements within these tumours), and seven out of 10 with malignant mixed germ cell tumours in the UKCCSG series (Mann *et al.* 1989). There were no patients with pure choriocarcinoma, although several of the mixed germ-cell tumours had a substantial component of choriocarcinoma, associated with raised human chorionic gonadotrophin levels. Serial monitoring of levels after successful treatment showed the expected decline (Fig. 3) and such monitoring should give early warning of recurrence in paediatric tumours producing human chorionic gonadotrophin, as it does in adults.

CLINICAL FEATURES

The presenting features, investigation, and management depend on the site of the primary tumour.

Gonadal sites

Testis

In over 1000 boys with testicular tumours reported by Weissbach *et al.* (1984), 71 per cent were germ cell tumours and 29 per cent were of other histological types. The germ cell tumours were malignant in 82 per cent of cases and benign (mature) in 18 per cent). Yolk sac tumours comprised 69 per cent of the malignant germ cell tumours, the remainder being seminoma, embryonal carcinoma, immature teratoma, or mixed malignant germ cell tumour. The yolk sac tumours occurred in infants and young boys, whereas seminoma and embryonal carcinoma were seen mainly in adolescents.

Testicular germ cell tumours are usually unilateral and cause a painless swelling of the organ. They may be confused with hydrocoele or hernia, which may also be present. A minority of

Table 3 WHO classification of ovarian tumours

Common 'epithelial' tumours
Sex cord–stromal tumours
Lipoid cell tumours
Germ cell tumours
Mixed germ cell and sex cord–stromal tumours
Soft tissue tumours not specific to ovary
Unclassified tumours
Secondary (metastatic) tumours
Tumour-like conditions

patients present with metastatic disease in retroperitoneal, mediastinal, or cervical lymph nodes, the lungs or bone, or with ascites, abdominal pain, or inguinal lymphadenopathy.

The differential diagnosis includes orchitis, epididymitis, or torsion, which, however, usually cause painful swelling and epididymal cyst. The other, non-germinal primary testicular tumours must also be considered, that is Sertoli cell and Leydig (interstitial) cell tumours. The former usually occur in infancy and may produce androgens or oestrogens. The latter occur throughout childhood and may produce androgens and present with gynaeco-mastia or precocious virilization. Both lymphoblastic leukaemia and non-Hodgkin's lymphoma may metastasize to the testis, causing testicular swelling. Paratesticular tumours, particularly rhabdomyosarcoma must also be included in the differential diagnosis, as well as metastases via a patent processus vaginalis, for example of abdominal neuroblastoma.

Ovary

The World Health Organization classification of ovarian tumours is summarized in Table 3 and is described in detail by Serov and Scully (1972).

Approximately 60 per cent of ovarian tumours in childhood are benign, the majority being mature teratomas and the remainder benign epithelial or mesenchymal tumours (Lindfors 1971). Among 172 malignant ovarian tumours diagnosed in British children during 1962–1978 (La Vecchia *et al.* 1983) 84 per cent were germ cell tumours (54 dysgerminomas, 36 malignant teratomas, 26 yolk sac tumours, four embryonal carcinomas, two pure choriocarcinomas, 20 mixed germ cell neoplasms, and three gonadoblastomas), 8 per cent were epithelial carcinomas (three serous or undifferentiated and 10 mucinous), 5 per cent were sex cord–stromal tumours (three granulosa cell, three Sertoli–Leydig, three unclassified), and 3 per cent were other miscellaneous tumours. In 7 per cent of cases the tumours were bilateral.

Abdominal pain, abdominal distension, fever, vomiting, vaginal bleeding, or amenorrhoea may draw attention to an ovarian tumour. If torsion occurs, the patient presents acutely with severe abdominal pain. Rarely, when the tumour is producing human chorionic gonadotrophin, premature breast enlargement, growth of pubic hair, and menarche may occur. Usually an abdominal mass is palpable but, particularly when no mass can be felt, appendicitis is the most important alternative diagnosis. Other conditions which must be considered include lymphoma, rhabdomyosarcoma and other malignancies, abdominal tuberculosis, and pregnancy.

Malignant ovarian germ cell tumours spread by direct extension to the Fallopian tubes and other pelvic structures and to the peritoneal cavity, causing ascites and/or solid intra-abdominal metastases. Lymphatic spread leads to enlargement of retroperitoneal, mediastinal, or cervical nodes and blood-borne spread results in metastases in lungs, liver, bones/bone-marrow, or brain. In most

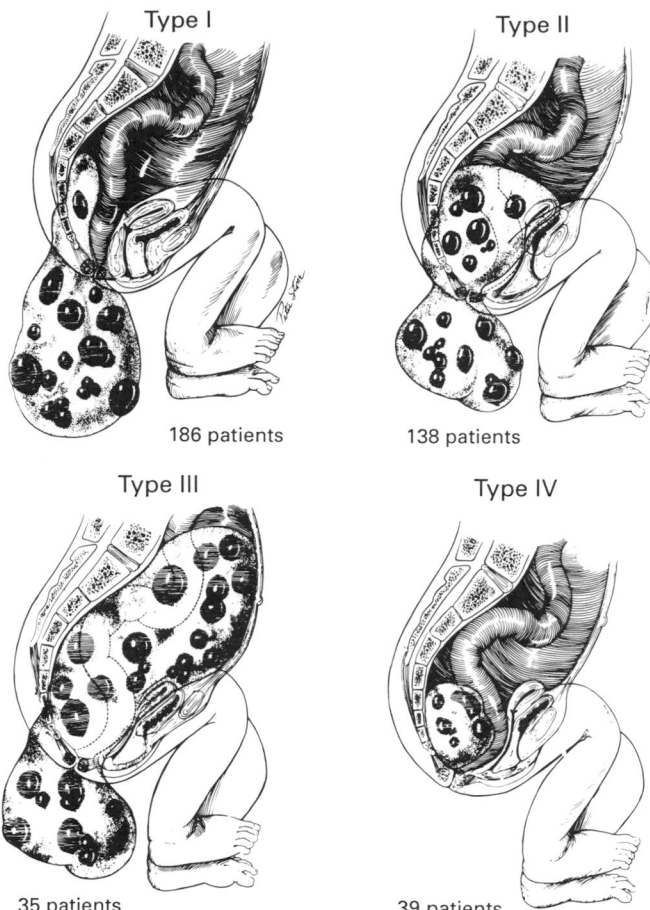

Type I   Type II

186 patients   138 patients

Type III   Type IV

35 patients   39 patients

Fig. 5 Location and frequency of 398 sacrococcygeal teratomas in infants and children (Altman *et al.* (1974); reproduced by permission of the *Journal of Pediatric Surgery*).

girls presenting with malignant ovarian germ cell tumours spread has occurred to the pelvis or abdomen and a few have distant metastases (Mann *et al.* 1989). Hydronephrosis may be present, caused by the large size of the primary tumour and/or large retroperitoneal nodes or because of pelvic tumour compressing the ureters.

Extragonadal sites

Sacrococcygeal/presacral

Sacrococcygeal/presacral teratomas have been grouped into four anatomical types (Fig. 5) (Altman *et al.* 1974). Type I (47 per cent) were predominantly external and least likely to be malignant, type II (34 per cent) were both external and intrapelvic, type III (9 per cent) were external, pelvic, and abdominal, and type IV (10 per cent) were entirely presacral. Teratomas diagnosed before 6 months of age were rarely malignant (2/119) whereas those diagnosed later were frequently malignant (26/40). Malignant recurrence, usually of yolk sac tumour, may present from a few months up to 3–4 years after incomplete excision of apparently benign sacrococcygeal/ presacral tumours.

Children with teratomas at these sites frequently have congenital anomalies of the vertebrae, genitourinary system, anus, or rectum (Fraumeni *et al.* 1973; Altman *et al.* 1974).

Types I, II, and III are easily diagnosed clinically, because of the visible mass, but type IV may not declare itself until it extends through the sciatic notch into the buttock or causes functional

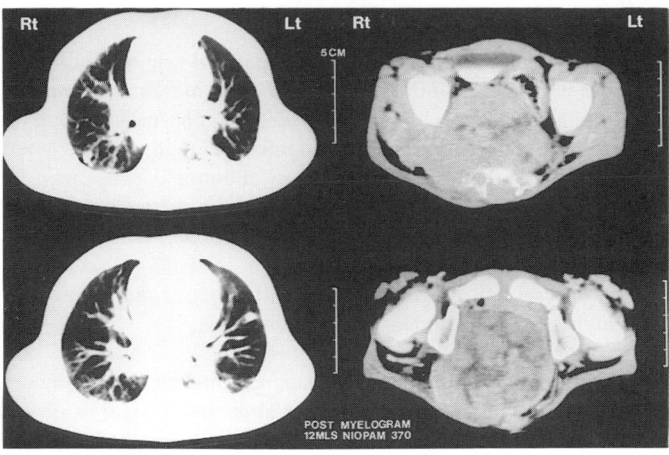

Fig. 6 CT scans of pelvis and thorax of a 20-month-old girl with stage IV presacral yolk sac tumour. Round metastases are shown in both lungs. Myelogram with CT scan showed destruction of the lower half of the sacrum and extension of tumour into the right buttock and filling the spinal canal to L5. The patient had partial paralysis of the legs and bladder but made a full recovery after BEP (bleomycin, VP-16, cisplatin) chemotherapy. Residual benign teratoma was subtotally excised 5 months later.

disability such as constipation, neuropathic bladder, or neurological deficits in the legs due to involvement of the lumbosacral plexus. Rectal examination then reveals a firm mass in the presacral region, which, if very large, may also be palpable per abdomen. Types II and III may also present with bowel and bladder symptoms or lower limb weakness, especially when malignant, due to involvement of the lumbosacral plexus or invasion of the spinal canal (Fig. 6).

The differential diagnosis of sacrococcygeal teratomas includes other skin-covered lesions of the caudal spine, such as meningocoele, lipoma, lipomeningocoele, pilonidal cyst, haemangioma, epidermal cyst, abscess, and bone tumours. Radiological investigations, including ultrasound or CT scan, will usually aid diagnosis by demonstrating, for example spina bifida or a cerebrospinal fluid-containing cyst, but biopsy should be undertaken in uncertain cases. Other presacral lesions to be considered include chordoma, duplication of the rectum, neuroblastoma (elevated urinary catecholamines or their metabolites are usually diagnostic), sarcomas, and other benign and malignant tumours.

Mediastinum/thorax

These are usually located in the anterior superior mediastinum, but also occur elsewhere in the thorax and may involve the pericardium. Benign, malignant, and mixed histological types occur (Lack *et al.* 1985). Symptoms include chest pain, cough, wheeze, and dyspnoea. Radiology, including CT scan, is required for diagnosis and may show calcification within the mass. Elevated serum markers may assist in distinguishing teratomas from other conditions which present with anterior mediastinal tumours in childhood, such as thymomas and thymic cysts, T-non-Hodgkin's lymphoma and T-acute lymphoblastic leukaemia, cystic hygroma/lymphangioma, and bronchial and enteric cysts. Neuroblastoma and ganglioneuroma must be distinguished from the rare teratomas that arise in the posterior mediastinum. Inflammatory lymphadenopathy, especially tuberculosis, must also be considered.

Retroperitoneum and abdomen

Aberrant germ cell migration is the presumed origin of germ cell tumours which arise in the retroperitoneum, mesentery, stomach, liver, and abdominal wall. They may be benign or malignant, all the latter being yolk sac tumours in the United Kingdom series (Mann *et al.* 1989). Patients present with an abdominal mass, pain, or gastrointestinal symptoms. Germ cell tumours in the retroperitoneum must be distinguished from Wilms' tumour, neuroblastoma, lymphoma, and rhabdomyosarcoma.

The differential diagnosis of the abdominal primaries includes lymphoma, mesothelioma, and tuberculosis and that of liver primaries includes primary hepatomas (hepatoblastoma and hepatocellular carcinoma), hepatic malignant mesenchymal tumours, cysts, haemangioma, hamartoma, and abscess (Mann *et al.* 1990).

Vagina, uterus, bladder, and prostate

These tumours are nearly all yolk sac tumours of young children. Vaginal and uterine primaries present with bloodstained vaginal discharge and polypoid tumour may appear at the vulva or be found during examination under anaesthetic. The principal differential diagnosis is rhabdomyosarcoma (sarcoma botryoides). Bladder and prostate primaries present with haematuria, retention of urine, and strangury, and must also be distinguished from rhabdomyosarcoma. Rarely, yolk sac tumours arise in the vulva and clitoris.

Head and neck

Germ cell tumours arising in the orbit, oral cavity, nasopharynx, face, and neck generally are present at birth and are histologically benign, but they may cause airways obstruction and be extremely difficult to remove. Incomplete removal may be complicated by subsequent malignant yolk sac tumour recurrence (Fig. 7).

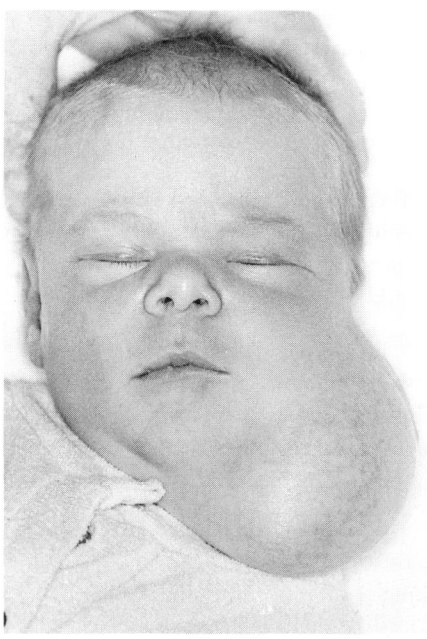

Fig. 7 Apparently mature (benign) teratoma in the neck and nasopharynx of a 3-day-old girl. The tumour was subtotally excised but yolk sac tumour recurred at the original site when she was 11 months old and has responded to chemotherapy with BEP (bleomycin, VP-16, cisplatin), JEB (carboplatin, VP-16, and bleomycin) and VAC (vincristine, actinomycin D, cyclophosphamide).

The differential diagnosis includes rhabdomyosarcoma, lymphoma, haemangioma, and lymphangioma/cystic hygroma.

Intracranial

Germ cell tumours arise in the suprasellar and pineal regions and should be distinguished from gliomas (astrocytoma and ependymoma), true pinealomas (pinealoblastoma and pinealocytoma), ganglioneuroma, and cysts. Improved neurosurgical techniques, such as CT-assisted stereotaxis, have allowed a policy of pre-treatment biopsy to be followed in certain centres and this has shown that the proportion of suprasellar and pineal tumours which are germ cell tumours is lower than previously supposed. In Philadelphia, 32 per cent of pineal and 24 per cent of suprasellar tumours were germ cell tumours and clinical parameters, CT findings, and cerebrospinal fluid markers (α-fetoprotein and human chorionic gonadotrophin) were unreliable in distinguishing germ cell tumours from other tumour types (Packer *et al.* 1984; Legido *et al.* 1989).

The principal symptoms of suprasellar tumours are diabetes insipidus and other signs of hypopituitarism (such as hypothyroidism, growth delay, and pubertal delay), diplopia, decreased visual acuity, and symptoms of raised intracranial pressure (headache and vomiting). Pineal tumours cause hydrocephalus and symptoms of raised intracranial pressure if they extend to obstruct the third ventricle and, if they compress the midbrain, they cause paralysis of vertical gaze, lid retraction, and Parinaud's syndrome. They may also cause hemiparesis, visual defects, incoordination, and movement disorders.

Cerebrospinal fluid examination may reveal malignant cells, as intracranial and spinal seeding occurs in approximately one-third of patients unless the whole CNS is irradiated. Rarely, intracranial germ cell tumours metastasize outside the CNS to the lung or bone or, via a ventriculoperitoneal shunt, to the abdomen.

INVESTIGATION AND MANAGEMENT STRATEGY

General considerations

While certain 'basic' investigations will usually be undertaken in all patients with germ cell tumours, such as blood count, biochemistry to assess renal and hepatic function, serum α-fetoprotein and human chorionic gonadotrophin, and chest X-ray, other tests required and the order in which they are done depend upon the site and anticipated natural history of the tumour. Thus, as the majority of congenital sacrococcygeal/presacral tumours are benign and surgically curable, pre-operative investigations are directed more towards defining the extent of the primary tumour for the surgeon than towards detecting metastatic disease. Also, in boys with testicular tumours, after the 'basic' investigations, surgical removal is usually the first step, with further staging procedures only if the tumour is malignant. The same applies to small, easily resected ovarian tumours. However, large ovarian tumours and germ cell tumours at other sites are often more appropriately managed by biopsy followed by staging investigations and then chemotherapy, with further surgery later if needed. In the case of intracranial tumours, the principal problem lies in obtaining a histological diagnosis, since many neurosurgeons are reluctant to undertake biopsy of, in particular, pineal tumours, although biopsy has been strongly advocated (Packer *et al.* 1984; Legido *et al.* 1989).

The attitude to staging procedures, especially those of an 'invasive' nature, such as lymphangiography and retroperitoneal node sampling, has been altered by two factors. First, most malignant germ cell tumours in childhood produce α-fetoprotein and therefore regular α-fetoprotein monitoring provides a sensitive measure of treatment success and of the presence of residual or recurrent disease (Mann *et al.* 1989; Huddart *et al.* 1990). Secondly, modern chemotherapy is producing high cure rates when given as part of initial therapy or for recurrence of stage I disease. Therefore, if 'non-invasive' staging procedures give normal results, after removal of the primary most therapists now rely on α-fetoprotein monitoring to detect residual or recurrent disease and have abandoned 'invasive' staging methods.

The effectiveness of chemotherapy has also altered the approach to surgery for malignant germ cell tumours, removal or debulking of the primary being undertaken only when this can be done without resection of major organs. Otherwise, biopsy followed by chemotherapy and later further surgery, if necessary, to remove residual disease, is the preferred approach. It is nearly always possible to preserve the uterus, vagina, other ovary (in ovarian tumours), and bladder, and other major organs.

Investigation/management strategy of tumours at specific sites

Testis

Figure 8 shows the management strategy used in Britain. Approximately two-thirds of boys with malignant germ cell tumours are cured by surgery alone, while the remainder require chemotherapy.

Radical orchidectomy via an inguinal incision and high ligation of the spermatic cord is recommended (Kaplan *et al.* 1988; Huddart *et al.* 1990). If high ligation has not been done and there is doubt whether the cut end was free of tumour, further excision of the cord should be undertaken. If the tumour is malignant, a CT scan of the chest and abdomen should be done to exclude metastases in the lungs, liver, or retroperitoneal or mediastinal nodes. Simultaneous intravenous urography may be valuable in demonstrating retroperitoneal nodes. Skeletal survey and/or a bone scan are recommended to exclude skeletal metastases and bone-marrow

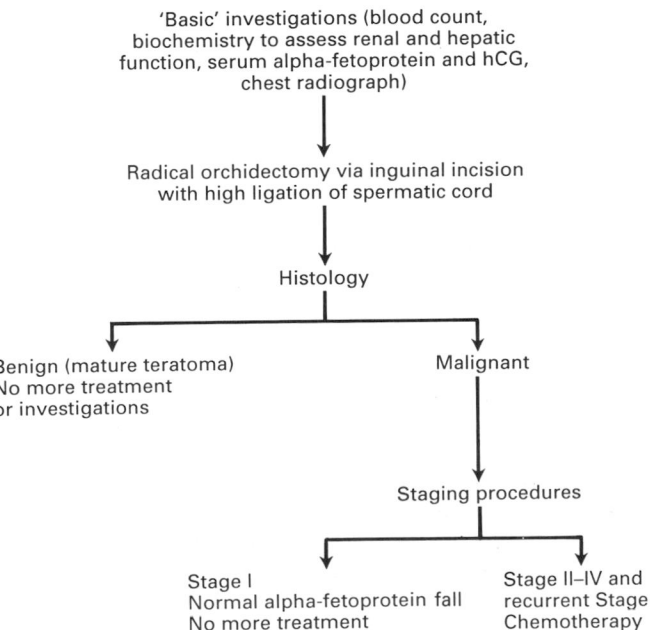

'Basic' investigations (blood count, biochemistry to assess renal and hepatic function, serum alpha-fetoprotein and hCG, chest radiograph)

↓

Radical orchidectomy via inguinal incision with high ligation of spermatic cord

↓

Histology

Benign (mature teratoma) No more treatment or investigations

Malignant

↓

Staging procedures

Stage I Normal alpha-fetoprotein fall No more treatment

Stage II–IV and recurrent Stage I Chemotherapy

Fig. 8 Management strategy for testicular germ cell tumours.

aspirate and trephine should be performed when there is evidence of metastatic disease elsewhere. A liver scan may be useful if liver metastases are suspected.

Lymphangiography is very difficult to perform and has not proved helpful in the management of young boys with malignant testicular germ cell tumours. Also, because of its potential morbidity, para-aortic lymph node biopsy, especially if bilateral, is generally considered not to be justified by the information obtained (Kaplan *et al.* 1988; Huddart *et al.* 1990).

Ovary

A suggested management strategy for ovarian germ cell tumours is shown in Fig. 9. Abdominal and pelvic ultrasound are useful preliminary investigations, but CT scan, preferably with simultaneous intravenous urography, is the preferred imaging technique for pre-operative assessment of the primary tumour and to demonstrate any compression of the ureters, hydronephrosis, ascites, intra-peritoneal metastases, liver deposits, or enlarged retroperitoneal nodes. Calcification in the tumour usually indicates mature (benign) teratoma. CT scan of the lungs should be performed in cases suspected to be malignant.

Some 10 per cent of girls with malignant 'ovarian' germ cell tumours have intersex states, in which the tumour arises in a dysgenetic gonad situated in an ovarian anatomical location (Mann *et al.* 1989). Therefore, the patient's karyotype should be determined and physical examination should seek evidence of intersex conditions, for example individuals with XY gonadal dysgenesis are phenotypic females with vagina and uterus, but generally fail to achieve normal breast development and menstruation.

At laparotomy the surgeon should assess the extent of the primary tumour and examine the pelvis, peritoneal cavity (including the diaphragm), liver, and retroperitoneal nodes for the presence of metastases. If removal of the primary and obvious metastases is possible without damage to other organs, resection should be undertaken. Otherwise, biopsy should be done. In girls with intersex states and a Y chromosome, whose tumour has arisen in a dysgenetic gonad, prophylactic removal of the other gonad should be undertaken. However, in normal 46XX females, surgery should be undertaken with preservation of the other ovary, the uterus, vagina, bladder, and other major organs. Biopsy of the other ovary is suggested, particularly if it appears abnormal, since some 10 per cent of ovarian tumours are bilateral.

After surgery, if histological examination of the tumour shows mature (benign) teratoma, no further investigations or treatment are required. If the tumour is a malignant or immature germ cell tumour, then staging procedures should include skeletal survey and/or bone scan, bone-marrow aspirate, and trephine when there is evidence of metastatic disease elsewhere and liver scan if necessary to confirm liver metastases.

The majority of girls with malignant ovarian germ cell tumours (including the immature group) have stage II to IV disease and, after staging investigations and surgical removal or biopsy of the tumour, they require chemotherapy. Some authors argue that as the rare patients with completely resected stage I dysgerminoma (Lucraft *et al.* 1980) and girls with stage I or even more advanced immature teratomas (Kooijman 1988) may be curable by surgery alone, chemotherapy should only be given to them for recurrence. Others (Gobel *et al.* 1993) have recommended chemotherapy for invasive immature teratomas should be assessed in a prospective study.

At the completion of chemotherapy, checking of α-fetoprotein levels and repeat CT scanning are recommended, with 'second look'

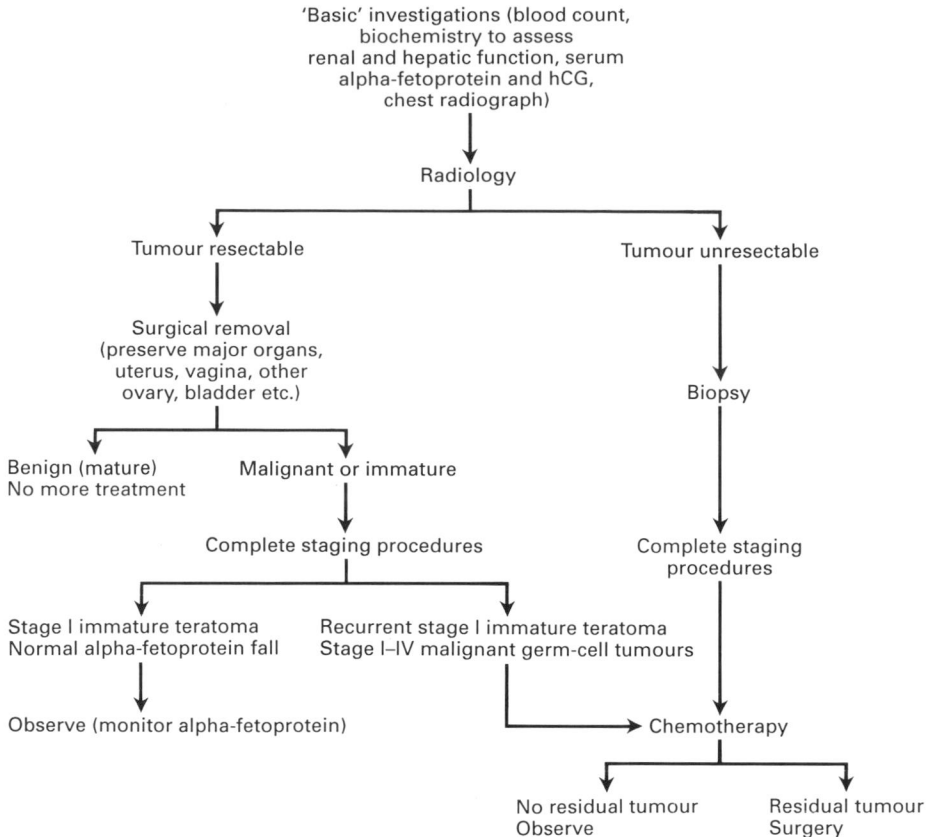

Fig. 9 Management strategy for ovarian germ cell tumours.

surgery to remove any residual tumour, which usually consists of mature elements only.

Sacrococcygeal/presacral site

In most infants with congenital tumours, which are usually mature (Altman *et al.* 1974), surgical excision is curative. The surgical approach may be sacrococcygeal or combined abdominal and sacrococcygeal or occasionally just transabdominal. Complete excision, which includes removal of the coccyx, is essential. Pre-operative imaging, preferably CT scan with simultaneous intravenous urography, is required to determine the extent of the primary tumour, but apart from the 'basic' investigations, other tests are not usually needed.

In sacrococcygeal/presacral tumours presenting after the neonatal period and for malignant recurrences of neonatal tumours, after the 'basic' investigations, CT scan of the primary tumour, preferably with simultaneous intravenous urography, CT scan of the abdomen and lungs, skeletal survey, and/or bone scan, and, if metastatic disease is present elsewhere, bone-marrow aspirate and trephine should be done. If imaging or neurological signs suggest intraspinal spread, myelography may be helpful. Most malignant sacrococcygeal/presacral tumours are unresectable or can be removed only with gross surgical morbidity. Therefore, biopsy and chemotherapy are preferred, with re-evaluation at the end of treatment and further surgery for residual tumour (strategy as for unresectable ovarian tumours, see Fig. 9).

Other sites (except intracranial)

A management strategy as for ovarian tumours (Fig. 9) is appropriate.

Intracranial tumours

CT scan or magnetic resonance imaging (MRI) reveals an isodense or hyperdense mass in the suprasellar or pineal region, sometimes containing cystic areas or calcification (Packer *et al.* 1984; Legido *et al.* 1989). After contrast, it tends to enhance heterogeneously. Examination of cerebrospinal fluid, usually obtained during surgery to the primary, may reveal malignant cells and elevated levels of α-fetoprotein or human chorionic gonadotrophin. Since cerebrospinal fluid metastases have been reported in approximately one-third of patients with suprasellar germinomas and in up to 10 per cent with pineal germinomas, when possible myelography or MRI of the spine is also done.

As the radiological features and cerebrospinal fluid markers do not reliably differentiate germ cell tumours from the other tumours which arise in these sites, a histological diagnosis is desirable before treatment is planned. Better neurosurgical techniques (CT-assisted stereotaxis) make biopsy and, in some patients, resection of tumour safer than hitherto (Kersh *et al.* 1988). Investigations to detect diabetes insipidus and other forms of hypopituitarism are needed in patients with suprasellar tumours, as well as evaluation of visual fields and acuity.

The optimal further management of intracranial germ cell tumours has not been established. They are radiosensitive tumours and, because of the risk of cerebrospinal fluid metastases, the whole of the neuroaxis is usually irradiated. High cure rates have been achieved following radiotherapy for pure germinomas, but the results have been less good for non-germinomas (Göbel *et al.* 1989; Hoffman *et al.* 1991; Sebag-Montefiore 1992). When a histological diagnosis cannot be obtained, a good response to radiotherapy may be considered to support a radiological diagnosis of germ cell tumour. Doses of 4000–5000 cGy are usually given to the primary site, with smaller doses to the rest of the brain and the spine.

There have been reports of small numbers of child and adult patients with metastatic and primary germ cell tumours of the brain who have been treated successfully with chemotherapy (Allen *et al.* 1985; Rustin *et al.* 1986; Kobayashi *et al.* 1989; Castaneda *et al.* 1990; Smith *et al.* 1991) or chemotherapy and radiotherapy (Lester *et al.* 1984; Allen *et al.* 1987; Deméocq *et al.* 1988; Göbel *et al.* 1992). Chemotherapy with lower radiotherapy doses therefore requires evaluation (Legido *et al.* 1989) as they may reduce the adverse long-term effects of neuroaxis irradiation. However, adults and children given over 5000 cGy to the primary tumour with spinal irradiation had higher survival rates than patients given smaller doses (Kersh *et al.* 1988). Some patients also require shunts to relieve hydrocephalus.

Monitoring the response to treatment using serum markers

The majority of childhood malignant germ cell tumours produce α-fetoprotein and serial measurements provide the most sensitive indicator of treatment success or failure. Pre-treatment and frequent (weekly) measurements after treatment are necessary to assess whether the half-life is consistent with cure. Once the α-fetoprotein level is normal for the child's age, monthly measurement is recommended. If α-fetoprotein levels rise again or do not fall to normal, residual disease must be suspected and may be confirmed by imaging. However, even if radiology fails to identify the

recurrence, rising levels are now considered to provide sufficient evidence for introducing chemotherapy (Mann *et al.* 1989).

Experience of the value of human chorionic gonadotrophin monitoring in paediatric practice is more limited but has been well established for adults (Bagshawe *et al.* 1973; Bagshawe 1976). Therefore, in children with tumours producing human chorionic gonadotrophin, monitoring as for α-fetoprotein is recommended.

Localization of malignant germ cell tumours by external scanning after injection of radiolabelled anti-α-fetoprotein

Sheep IgG antibody to α-fetoprotein labelled with ^{131}I has been used successfully to identify human germ cell tumours by emission scanning (Halsall *et al.* 1981). The technique may be valuable in demonstrating metastases not visualized by other means.

STAGING CLASSIFICATIONS

There is no universally agreed staging system for malignant germ cell tumours. Those used by the United Kingdom Children's Cancer Study Group for gonadal tumours are also used in adults, thus facilitating comparisons between treatment strategies and outcome in adults and children (Table 4).

Certain other staging systems for testicular germ cell tumour in children (Table 5) imply that retroperitoneal node dissection will have been done (Tsuji *et al.* 1973; Haas *et al.* 1983; Kaplan

Table 4 Staging systems used by the UK Children's Cancer Study Group

Testis (Peckham and McElwain 1976)		Ovary, uterus, vagina, prostate, sacrococcygeal/presacral sites (simplified FIGO system; Kottmeier 1971)		Other sites (Mann *et al.* 1989)	
I	Tumour confined to testis	I	Tumour confined to ovary, uterus, vagina, prostate, or sacrococcygeal/presacral area	I	Tumour confined to site of origin and resectable
II	Tumour confined to testis and retroperitoneal/abdominal lymph nodes	II	Tumour spread limited to the pelvis	II	Local spread
III	Supradiaphragmatic nodal disease (mediastinal and/or supraclavicular)	III	Tumour spread limited to the abdomen (excluding liver)	III	Extensive spread confined to one side of the diaphragm (excluding the liver)
IV	Extralymphatic spread (for example, to liver, lung, bone, brain, or skin)	IV	Tumour spread to liver or beyond the abdominal cavity	IV	Tumour spread to the liver, to both sides of the diaphragm, and/or to bones, bone-marrow, or brain

FIGO, Federation Internationale de Gynecologie Oncologique.

Table 5 Other staging systems for malignant testicular germ cell tumours in children

Academy of Pediatrics (Tsuji *et al.* 1973)		Kaplan *et al.* (1988)		German Society of Pediatric Oncology (Haas *et al.* 1983)	
I	Tumour confined to the testis, AFP levels normal within 1 month after orchidectomy: chest radiography and retroperitoneal imaging normal	I	Cancer limited to scrotum	I	Limited to scrotum
IIA	Similar to group I, but retroperitoneal node dissection reveals unsuspected nodal metastases	IIA	Persistently elevated AFP levels; without other evidence of metastatic disease or positive retroperitoneal nodes unsuspected by imaging tests	IIA	A single retroperitoneal metastasis of up to 2 cm diameter completely removable at operation
IIB	Retroperitoneal metastasis demonstrated on imaging studies, AFP levels persistently elevated	IIB	Bulky retroperitoneal disease demonstrated surgically or by imaging	IIB	A solitary metastasis of up to 5 cm diameter or more than one retroperitoneal metastases that can be removed at operation
III	Demonstrable metastases beyond the peritoneum	III	Metastatic disease outside the peritoneum	IIC	A retroperitoneal metastasis partially removed at operation and/or a large palpable abdominal mass
				III	Generalized disease

AFP, α-fetoprotein.

Table 6 Staging systems for malignant germ cell tumours in children

All sites (Brodeur *et al.* 1981)		Non-testicular, non-seminomatous (Göbel *et al.* 1988)		Sacrococcygeal/presacral (Raney *et al.* 1981)
I	Localized disease, completely resected, without microscopic disease in the resected margins or in the regional lymph nodes	A Patients with completely resected tumours	I	Grossly complete excision
		B Patients with incompletely resected tumours	II	Gross residual disease
II	Microscopic residual disease, capsular invasion, or microscopic lymph node involvement	C Patients with extensive tumours diagnosed by biopsy	III	Distant metastases
III	Gross residual disease (>2 cm) or cytological evidence of tumour cells in ascites or pleural fluid			
IV	Disseminated disease involving lung, liver, brain, bone, distant nodes, or other sites			

et al. 1988) but most therapists no longer considered this to be necessary.

For non-testicular or sacrococcygeal/presacral sites the systems of Göbel *et al.* (1987) and Raney *et al.* (1981) are simple but do not well describe disease bulk. That of Brodeur *et al.* (1981) has the advantages of being applicable both to gonadal and extragonadal sites and of relating to tumour bulk (Table 6).

Staging systems for ovarian (Kottmeier 1971) and testicular tumours (Peckham *et al.* 1979; Loehrer *et al.* 1988) in adults and the Union Internationale Contre le Cancer TNM system (1974), for example see Jacobs *et al.* (1979), are more detailed than are required in paediatric practice, although they have good precision.

DETAILS OF MANAGEMENT

General considerations

Treatment strategies in relation to the sites of origin, including some surgical details, have been outlined. However, it is important to stress that, even when there is metastatic disease, over 70 per cent of cases can be cured. Therefore, treatments are chosen with a view to preservation of function, avoidance of unnecessary surgical removal of organs (such as the bladder and uterus), and limitation of late effects from chemotherapy, so that the quality of life, including fertility, in survivors is good.

Chemotherapy

Historical background

Before the introduction of effective chemotherapy, some 60–75 per cent of boys with malignant testicular germ cell tumours were curable by surgery alone (Jeffs 1973; Brown and Langley 1976), but cures of metastatic disease were rare. Malignant ovarian tumours, being generally more advanced, were frequently fatal when treated by surgery, with or without radiotherapy (Brown and Langley 1976). Before chemotherapy, malignant sacrococcygeal teratomas were almost universally fatal (Bale *et al.* 1975).

During the 1970s there were reports of successful treatment of children with metastatic testicular (Young *et al.* 1970; Ise *et al.* 1976; Smith *et al.* 1977), ovarian (Smith *et al.* 1973; Wollner *et al.* 1976; Cangir *et al.* 1978; Slayton *et al.* 1978; Ungerleider *et al.* 1978), and sacrococcygeal tumours (Flamant and Pellerin, 1975), using various combinations of vicristine, actinomycin D, Adriamycin®, cyclophosphamide, and methotrexate, together with radiotherapy in some patients. However, vincristine, actinomycin, and cyclophosphamide (VAC)-based regimens were more successful in

limited than in advanced disease, for example VAC cured all eight girls with stage I and II ovarian tumours, but only six out of 37 with stage III, and one out of five stage IV cases treated by Cangir *et al.* (1978).

The combination of vinblastine, bleomycin, and cisplatin (PVB) that had proved successful in treating metastatic testicular tumours in young men (Einhorn and Donohue 1977) was reported to be too toxic for children (Exelby 1980) and deaths from bleomycin lung and renal toxicity have been recorded (Mann *et al.* 1989). Nevertheless, in 1983 Green *et al.* described the successful treatment of four children with pelvic yolk sac tumours who were given vincristine, cisplatin, and bleomycin followed by VAC and in 1984 Flamant *et al.* described a 63 per cent disease-free survival in 35 children with advanced ovarian, testicular, sacrococcygeal, thoracic, and abdominal non-seminomatous germ cell tumours given vincristine, actinomycin, cyclophosphamide, Adriamycin®, cisplatin, and bleomycin.

Recent studies

From America, the Children's Cancer Study Group has reported on 89 children with malignant germ cell tumours at all sites except testes and brain and excluding germinoma and immature teratoma histology, who were treated with vinblastine, bleomycin, cisplatin, cyclophosphamide, actinomycin, and Adriamycin® (Ablin *et al.* 1987). Those with residual disease at second-look surgery at 18 weeks received radiation therapy too. The disappointing progression-free survival rate at 5 years of 47 per cent might possibly be explained by the low doses of cyclophosphamide (600 mg/m^2) and cisplatin (60 mg/m^2) compared with those in certain other protocols (see below). At St Jude Children's Hospital, 51 children with gonadal and extragonadal primary tumours were given VAC or PVB, with cross-over to the alternate regimen if the response was incomplete, followed when necessary by further surgery and, for residual tumour after surgery, radiotherapy. Complete remissions were obtained in 46 per cent given VAC and 35 per cent given PVB, but 71 per cent overall survival was achieved (Etcubanas *et al.* 1987). Wollner *et al.* (1987) achieved a median survival at 5 years of 87 per cent in 64 children given various combinations of vincristine, vinblastine, Adriamycin®, actinomycin, cyclophosphamide, cisplatin, methotrexate, and bleomycin and also, in some patients, radiotherapy.

In Europe, French workers have reported 75 per cent survival in 82 patients with non-seminomatous germ cell tumours of sacrococcygeal, testicular, ovarian, vaginal, mediastinal, and other origins (Flamant *et al.* 1987). Stage I patients (25 cases) were treated by surgery alone unless serum markers did not return to normal. All other patients were given chemotherapy with actinomycin and cyclophosphamide alternating with vincristine, bleomycin, Adriamycin®, and cisplatin for 12 months. The doses of cyclophosphamide (300 mg/m^2 daily ×5) and cisplatin (100 mg/m^2) were substantially larger than those given in the Children's Cancer Study Group combination, possibly accounting for the better results. However, there were three iatrogenic deaths. Only three patients received radiotherapy. The first protocol (1985–1989) of the French Society of Pediatric Oncology (SFOP) was shorter, with vinblastine replacing vincristine and Adriamycin® omitted. The overall disease free survival was 74 per cent at 8 years, 85 per cent in gonadal and 54 per cent in extragonadal tumours (Baranzelli et al. 1993). In their current protocol (since 1990) for children with cerebral germ cell tumours the SFOP has been giving chemotherapy before radiotherapy. In localized germinomas the aim is to reduce radiation doses and fields in patients achieving a good response to drugs. In children with metastatic tumours and tumours producing α-fetoprotein/human chorionic gonadotrophin they hope to improve the outcome by giving intensive chemotherapy alone but, in patients

with incomplete response, whole-neuroaxis irradiation is given as well (Flamant, personal communication).

In Germany, treatment for non-testicular malignant germ cell tumours has been stratified according to histology, site, and stage, children with favourable histology receiving surgery alone for early stage disease, but also four courses of PVB or VAC for more advanced disease (Gobel et al. 1987). For most children with tumours of more malignant histology (yolk sac, choriocarcinoma, mixed tumours) four PVB courses, second-look surgery, and then four courses of etoposide, ifosfamide, and cisplatin were given. Radiotherapy was given only for dysgerminomas. In extensive and sacrococcygeal tumours, surgery was delayed until after four courses of chemotherapy. Disease-free rates of 87 per cent for 60 patients with mature teratomas and 83 per cent for 66 with highly malignant germ cell tumours were achieved, although there were two treatment-related deaths and three children developed bleomycin-induced pulmonary fibrosis.

In the subsequent (MAKE1 89) study, vinblastine was replaced by etoposide, resulting in a chemotherapeutic regimen of three

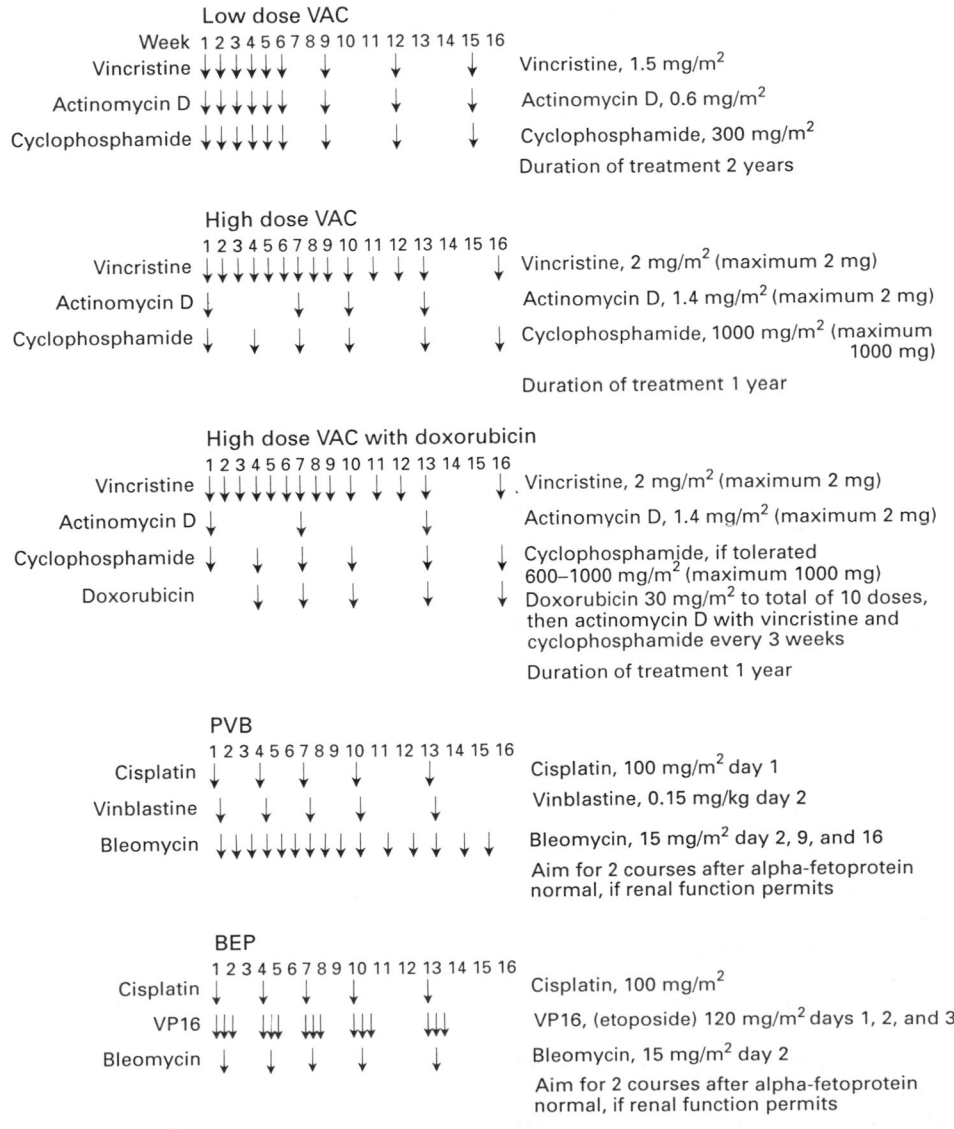

Fig. 10 Chemotherapy regimens which have been used for children with malignant germ cell tumours by the United Kingdom Children's Cancer Study Group (Mann et al. (1989); reproduced by permission of the American Cancer Society, Inc., J. B. Lippincott Company). In the current protocol carboplatin is used with VP-16 and bleomycin instead of cisplatin (see text).

to four courses of BEP and three to four courses of VIP. Total chemotherapy was reduced by 25 per cent and bleomycin dosage was also reduced or omitted. Event-free survival of 91 per cent was achieved in 47 patients with malignant non-germinomatous germ cell tumours (Göbel *et al.* 1993).

From 1979 to 1988, the United Kingdom Children's Cancer Study Group used the treatment strategies outlined in Figs 8 and 9 for children with malignant germ cell tumours (including dysgerminomas) at all sites, except intracranial (Mann *et al.* 1989). Five chemotherapy regimens were used (Fig. 10). The initial 'low-dose' VAC proved ineffective, actuarial survival at 5 years being only 8 per cent (12 patients). The VAC doses were therefore increased, with Adriamycin® added in some patients and a 5 year actuarial survival of 87 per cent was achieved in 17 patients (one iatrogenic death). PVB yielded poor results because of two deaths from bleomycin lung among nine children given this as their initial chemotherapy and in another child given PVB for recurrence. Severe renal toxicity was also seen in two children, and it was suspected that children may be more susceptible than adults to bleomycin lung damage, especially if excretion of the drug were impaired due to cisplatin-induced renal damage. Therefore, when another platinum-containing regimen (bleomycin, VP-16, cisplatin; BEP) was introduced, it was recommended that bleomycin be given only once per course. This proved successful, as no treatment-related deaths occurred in 33 children given BEP, 84 per cent of whom survived. However, significant toxicity was observed from the cisplatin, namely deafness in three children and impaired renal function in 13 (with a glomerular filtration rate of less than 40 ml/min/1.73 m^2 in only one). The overall results of the United Kingdom Children's Cancer Study Group were that 101 of 122 patients treated between 1979 and 1987 were alive, of whom 44 were cured by surgery alone (41 with testicular, two with ovarian, and one with a sacrococcygeal tumour) while the remaining 78 had chemotherapy (Mann *et al.* 1989). Radiotherapy was used in only eight patients. Excluding the 12 'low-dose' VAC cases, survival by site was as follows: testis (59 patients, 100 per cent), vagina, uterus, and prostate (four patients, 100 per cent), ovary (25 patients, 88 per cent), thorax (five patients, 40 per cent), and other (four patients, 67 per cent). Survival by stage was stage I (62, 97 per cent), stage II (14, 86 per cent), stage III (18, 83 per cent), and stage IV (16, 72 per cent). Survival rates were also analysed in cases whose histology had been reviewed and, excluding 'low-dose' VAC cases, were 99 per cent for 68 with yolk sac tumours, 75 per cent for eight with immature teratomas, 70 per cent for 11 with mixed tumours, and 50 per cent for four with germinomas.

Since 1989 in the UKCCSG protocols the cisplatin in the BEP combination has been replaced by carboplatin at a dose of 600 mg/m^2 or calculated using the formula carboplatin dose in mg=6×(glomerular filtration rate uncorrected for surface area+15×surface area) (Pinkerton *et al.* 1987). Courses are given every 3–4 weeks until tumour markers are normal and then, if possible, two more courses are given (the median number of BEP courses required had been five). Initial results have been encouraging and similar to those obtained with BEP but with less renal and ototoxicity (Oakhill 1993).

A study of the quality of life in 35 survivors of ovarian germ cell tumours treated by the United Kingdom Children's Cancer Study Group between 1979 and 1988 revealed that the policy of preserving gynaecological function had been fairly successful, all but five patients being potentially fertile (Mann and Stiller 1993).

Current challenges

Now that the majority of children with germ cell tumours can be cured, refinements of therapy are needed to increase the efficacy of treatment for the small proportion of patients for whom present treatments are unsuccessful. Studies to define prognostic factors based on site, stage, histology, or other features are needed so that high-risk patients can be identified and given more intensive treatment.

For the majority of curable cases, the trends are away from invasive investigations and damaging surgical procedures, with greater reliance on chemotherapy for extensive tumours. Surgery and chemotherapy protocols are being planned with a view to preserving function and reducing adverse long-term toxicities. To avoid the late effects of radiotherapy, especially in young children, chemotherapy is preferred, irradiation being reserved for residual disease after chemotherapy and surgery. Whether high-dose chemotherapy can replace radiotherapy or allow dose reductions, in children with intracranial germ cell tumours may be demonstrated by studies currently in progress (Balmaceda *et al.* 1993).

REFERENCES

Albin A, *et al.* (1987). Biologic characteristics and response to therapy in 89 patients with malignant germ cell tumors (MGCT): a Children's Cancer Group (CCG) study. *Medical and Pediatric Oncology*, 15:294.

Allen JC, Bosl G, Walker R (1985). Chemotherapy trials in recurrent primary intracranial germ cell tumours. *Journal of Neuro-Oncology*, 3:147–52.

Allen JC, Kim JH, Packer RJ (1987). Neoadjuval chemotherapy for newly diagnosed germ-cell tumors of the central nervous system. *Journal of Neurosurgery*, 67:65–70.

Altman RF, Randolph JG, Lilly JR (1974). Sacrococcygeal teratoma: American Academy of Pediatrics surgical section survey—1973. *Journal of Pediatric Surgery*, 9:389–98.

Atkin NB, Baker MC (1982). Specific chromosome change, i(12p) in testicular tumours? *Lancet*, 2:1349.

Bagshawe KD (1976). Risk and prognostic factors in trophoblastic neoplasia. *Cancer*, 38:1373–85.

Bagshawe KD, Wilson H, Dublon P, Smith A, Baldwin M, Kardana A (1973). Follow-up after hydatidiform mole. *Journal of Obstetrics and Gynaecology of the British Commonwealth*, 80:461–8.

Bale PM, Painter DM, Cohen D (1975). Teratomas in childhood. *Pathology*, 7:209–18.

Balmaceda C, Diez B, Villablanca J, Walker R, Finlay J (1993). Chemotherapy only strategy in primary central nervous system germ cell tumors (CNS GCT): results of an international study. Abstracts for the Tenth International Conference on Brain Tumour Research and Therapy, Norway, September 1993. *Journal of Neuro-Oncology*, 15 (Suppl.):3.

Baranzelli MC, Flamant F, Patte C, de Lumley L, Legall E, Lejars O (1993). Extracranial nonseminomatous germ cell tumors (TGMnS)—French Society of Pediatric Oncology experience (SFOP)/1985–89. Abstracts of SIOP XXV meeting, San Francisco, October 1993. *Medical and Pediatric Oncology*, 21:574.

Beasley SW, Tiedemann K, Howat A, Werther G, Auldist AW, Tuohy P (1987). Precocious puberty associated with malignant thoracic teratoma and malignant histiocytosis in a child with Klinefelter's syndrome. *Medical and Pediatric Oncology*, 15:277–80.

Birch JM, Marsden HB, Swindell R (1982). Pre-natal factors in the origin of germ cell tumours of childhood. *Carcinogenesis*, 1:75–80.

Birch JM, Marsden HB, Morris Jones PH, Pearson D, Blair V (1988). Improvements in survival from childhood cancer: results of a population based survey over 30 years. *British Medical Journal*, 296:1372–6.

Bosl GJ, *et al.* (1989). Isochromosome of chromosome 12: clinically useful marker for male germ cell tumors. *Journal of the National Cancer Institute*, 81:1874–8.

Brodeur GM, Howarth CB, Pratt CB, Caces J, Hustu HO (1981). Malignant germ cell tumors in 57 children and adolescents. *Cancer*, 48:1890–8.

Brown NJ, Langley FA (1976). Teratomas and other genital tumours. In *Tumours in children* (ed. HB Marsden and JK Steward), p. 383. Springer-Verlag, Berlin.

Cangir A, Smith J, van Eys J (1978). Improved prognosis in children with ovarian cancers following modified VAC (vincristine sulfate, dactinomycin and cyclophosphamide) chemotherapy. *Cancer*, 42:1234–8.

Castaneda VL, Parmley RT, Geiser CF, Saldivar VA, Mullins JK, Marlin AE (1990). Postoperative chemotherapy for primary intracranial germ cell tumor. *Medical and Pediatric Oncology*, 18:299–303.

Dehner LP (1986). Gonadal and extragonadal germ cell neoplasms—teratomas in childhood. In *Pathology of neoplasia in children and adolescents. Major problems in pathology* (ed. M Finegold and JL Benington), Vol. 18, pp. 282–312. WB Saunders, Philadelphia.

Dement SH, Eggleston JC, Spivak JL (1985). Association between mediastinal germ cell tumors and hematologic malignancies. *American Journal of Surgical Pathology*, 9:23–30.

Deméocq F, *et al.* (1988). Traitement des tumeurs germinales malignes intracraniennes de l'enfant. *La Presse Médical*, 17:2183–5.

Einhorn L, Donohue J (1977). Cisdiamminedichloroplatinum, vinblastine and bleomycin combination chemotherapy in disseminated testicular cancer. *Annals of Internal Medicine*, 87:293–8.

Elwood JM, Elwood JH (1980). *Epidemiology of anencephalus and spina bifida*, 255–67. Oxford University Press, Oxford.

Etcubanas E, *et al.* (1987). Clinical management of childhood malignant germ cell tumors. *Medical and Pediatric Oncology*, 15:305–6.

Exelby PR (1980). Testicular cancer in children. *Cancer*, 45:1803–9.

Flamant F, Pellerin D (1975). Teratomas in general and tumours of the reproductive organs. In *Cancer in children* (ed. HJG Bloom, J Lemerle, MK Neidhardt, and PA Voute), pp. 245–9. Springer-Verlag, Berlin.

Flamant F, Schwartz L, Delons E, Caillaud JM, Hartmann O, Lemerle J (1984). Non-seminomatous malignant germ cell tumors in children. Multidrug therapy in stages III and IV. *Cancer*, 54:1687–91.

Flamant F, Hartmann O, Kalifa C, Patte C, Caillaud JM, Lemerle J (1987). Review of a series of 82 non-seminomatous germ cell tumours (nsGCT) treated at the same center between 1978 and 1984. *Medical and Pediatric Oncology*, 15:307.

Fraumeni JF, Li FP, Dalager N (1973). Teratomas in children; epidemiologic features. *Journal of the National Cancer Institute*, 51:1425–30.

Göbel U, *et al.* (1987). Strategy and treatment results of a cooperative trial for non-testicular germ cell tumors (GCT's) of the German Society of Pediatric Oncology (GPO) (MAKEI 83/86). *Medical and Pediatric Oncology*, 15:306.

Göbel U, *et al.* (1989). Intracraniale Keimzelltumoren: analyse der Therapiestudie MAKE1 83/86 und Protokolländerungen für die Nachfolgestudie. *Klinische Pädiatrie*, 201:261–8.

Göbel U, *et al.* (1992a). Combined modality treatment of intracranial germ cell tumors (GCTs): first results of the therapy studies MAKE1 86 and 89. Abstracts of SIOP XXIV meeting, Hannover, October 1992. *Medical and Pediatric Oncology*, 20:417.

Göbel U, *et al.* (1992b). BEP/VIP bei Kindern und Jugendlichen mit malignen nichttestikulären Keimzelltumoren. *Klinische Pädiatrie*, 205:231–40.

Green DM, *et al.* (1983). The use of different induction and maintenance chemotherapy regimens for the treatment of advanced yolk-sac tumors. *Journal of Clinical Oncology*, 1:111–16.

Haas RJ, Bramswig J, Göbel U, Harms D, Janka G, Weisbach L (1983). Maligne hodentumoren bei kindern und jugendlichen: Konzept der kooperativen therapiestudie MAHO 82 der GPO. *Klinische Pädiatrie*, 195:196–200.

Halsall AK, *et al.* (1981). Localisation of malignant germ-cell tumours by external scanning after injection of radiolabelled anti-alpha-fetoprotein. *British Medical Journal*, 283:942–4.

Hoffman HJ, *et al.* (1991). Intracranial germ-cell tumors in children. *Journal of Neurosurgery*, 74:545–51.

Huddart SN, *et al.* (1990). The UK Children's Cancer Study Group: testicular malignant germ cell tumours 1979–1988. *Journal of Pediatric Surgery*, 25:406–10.

Ise T, Ohtsuki H, Matsumoto K, Sano R (1976). Management of malignant testicular tumors in children. *Cancer*, 37:1539–45.

Jacobs EM, Muggia FM, Rozencweig M (1979). Chemotherapy of testicular cancer: from palliation to curative adjuvant therapy. *Seminars in Oncology*, 6:3–13.

Jeffs RD (1973). In *Proceedings of the 17th Clinical Conference of the Ontario Cancer Research Foundation, Nov. 1972* (ed. JO Godden), pp. 66–77. Plenum, New York.

Johnston HE, *et al.* (1986). The Inter-Regional epidemiological study of childhood cancer (IRESCC): a case-control study in children with germ cell tumours. *Carcinogenesis*, 7:717–22.

Kaplan GW, Cromie WC, Kelalis PP, Silber I, Tank ES (1988). Prepubertal yolk sac testicular tumors—report of the Testicular Tumor Registry. *Journal of Urology*, 140:1109–12.

Kersh CR, *et al.* (1988). Primary central nervous system germ cell tumors. Effect of histologic confirmation on radiotherapy. *Cancer*, 61:2148–52.

Kobayashi T, Yoshida J, Ishiyama J, Noda S, Kito A, Kida Y (1989). Combination chemotherapy with cisplatin and etoposide for malignant intracranial germ cell tumors. *Journal of Neurosurgery*, 70:676–81.

Kooijman CD (1988). Immature teratomas in children. *Histopathology*, 12:491–502.

Kottmeier HL (1971). Classification and staging of malignant tumours in the female pelvis. *International Journal of Gynaecology and Obstetrics*, 9:172–80.

Kurman RJ, Scardino PT, McIntire KR, Waldmann TA, Jayadpour N (1977). Cellular localization of alphafetoprotein and human chorionic gonadotrophin in germ cell tumors of the testis using an indirect immunoperoxidase technique: a new approach to classification utilizing tumor markers. *Cancer*, 40:2136–51.

La Vecchia C, Morris HB, Draper GJ (1983). Malignant ovarian tumours in childhood in Britain, 1962–78. *British Journal of Cancer*, 48:363–74.

Lack EE, Weinstein HJ, Welch KJ (1985). Mediastinal germ cell tumors in childhood. A clinical and pathologic study of 21 cases. *Journal of Thoracic and Cardiovascular Surgery*, 89:826–35.

Legido A, *et al.* (1989). Suprasellar germinomas in childhood. *Cancer*, 63:340–4.

Lester SG, Morphis JG, Hornbach NB, Williams SD, Einhorn LH (1984). Brain metastases and testicular tumors: need for aggressive therapy. *Journal of Clinical Oncology*, 2:1397–403.

Li FP, Fraumeni JF (1972). Testicular cancers in children: epidemiologic characteristics. *Journal of the National Cancer Institute*, 48:1575–82.

Linder D, Kaiser-McCaw B, Hecht F (1975). Parthogenetic origin of benign ovarian teratomas. *New England Journal of Medicine*, 292:63–6.

Lindfors O (1971). Primary ovarian neoplasms in infants and children. A study of 81 cases diagnosed in Finland and Sweden. *Annales Chirurgiae et Gynaecologiae Fenniae*, 60 (Suppl. 177):1–66.

Loehrer PJ, Williams SD, Einhorn LH (1988). Testicular cancer; the quest continues. *Journal of the National Cancer Institute*, 17:1373–82.

Lucraft H, Mann JR, Pearson D (1980). Malignant ovarian tumours in children. In *Ovarian cancer* (ed. CE Newman, CHJ Ford, and JA Jordan), pp. 97–114. *Advances in the biosciences*, Vol. 26, Pergamon Press, Oxford.

Mann JR, *et al.* (1978). Clinical applications of serum carcinoembryonic antigen and alpha-fetoprotein levels in children with solid tumours. *Archives of Disease in Childhood*, 53:366–74.

Mann JR, *et al.* (1983). The X-linked recessive form of XY gonadal dysgenesis with a high incidence of gonadal germ cell tumours: clinical and genetic studies. *Journal of Medical Genetics*, 20:264–70.

Mann JR, Pearson D, Barrett A, Raafat F, Barnes JM, Wallendszus KR (1989). Results of the United Kingdom Children's Cancer Study Group's malignant germ cell tumor studies. *Cancer*, 63:1657–67.

Mann JR, *et al.* (1990). Malignant hepatic tumours in children: incidence, clinical features and aetiology. *Paediatric and Perinatal Epidemiology*, 4:220–33.

Mann JR, Stiller CA (1993). Changing patterns of incidence and survival in children with germ cell tumours (GCTs). In *Germ cell tumours III* (ed. WG Jones, P Harnden, and I Appleyard). *Advances in the biosciences*, Pergamon Press, Oxford. (In press.)

Marsden HB, Birch JM, Swindell R (1981). Germ cell tumours of childhood: a review of 137 cases. *Journal of Clinical Pathology*, 34:879–83.

Moore KL (1977). *The developing human* (2nd edn). WB Saunders, Philadelphia.

Mostofi FK, Sesterhenn IA, Davis CJ Jr (1985). World Health Organisation International Classification of germ cell tumours of the testes. In *Germ cell tumours II* (ed. WG Jones, A Milford Ward, and CK Anderson), pp. 1–23. *Advances in the biosciences*, Vol. 55. Pergamon Press, Oxford.

Nicols CR, Hoffman R, Einhorn LH, Williams SD, Wheeler LA, Garnick MB (1985). Hematologic malignancies associated with primary mediastinal germ-cell tumours. *Annals of Internal Medicine*, **102**:603–9.

Niehans GA, Manivel JC, Copland GT, Scheithauer BW, Wick MR (1988). Immuno–histochemistry of germ cell and trophoblastic neoplasms. *Cancer*, **62**:1113–23.

Oakhill A (1993). UKCCSG studies of paediatric germ cell tumours (GCTs). In *Germ cell tumours III* (ed. WG Jones, P Harnden, and I Appleyard). *Advances in the biosciences*. Pergamon Press, Oxford. (In press.)

Oosterhuis JW, *et al.* (1985). Karyotyping and DNA—flow cytometry of mature residual teratoma after intensive chemotherapy for disseminated non-seminomatous germ cell tumour of testis. In *Germ cell tumours II* (ed. WG Jones, A Milford Ward, and CK Anderson), pp. 55–6. *Advances in the biosciences*, Vol. 55. Pergamon Press, Oxford.

OPCS (Office of Population Censuses and Surveys) (1986). *Cancer statistics—registration 1982*. HMSO, London.

Packer RJ, *et al.* (1984). Pineal region tumors of childhood. *Pediatrics*, **74**:97–102.

Palmer PE, Safaii H, Wolfe JH (1976). Alpha-1-antitrypsin and alphafetoprotein: protein markers in endodermal sinus (yolk sac) tumors. *American Journal of Clinical Pathology*, **65**:575–82.

Parrington JM, West LF, Povey S (1985). Chromosome changes in germ cell tumours. In *Germ cell tumours II* (ed. WG Jones, A Milford Ward, and CK Anderson), pp. 61–7. *Advances in the biosciences*, Vol. 55. Pergamon Press, Oxford.

Peckham MJ, McElwain TJ (1976). The management of testicular tumours. In *Recent advances in urology II* (ed. WF Hendry), p. 324. Churchill Livingstone, Edinburgh.

Peckham MJ, McElwain TJ, Barrett A, Hendry WF (1979). Combined management of malignant teratoma of the testis. *Lancet*, **2**:267–70.

Pinkerton R, McElwain T, Horwich A, Pritchard J (1987). Carboplatin (JM8), VP16, bleomycin: (JEB) in children with malignant germ cell tumours (MGCT). *Medical and Pediatric Oncology*, **15**:296.

Pugh RCB, Cameron KM (1976). Teratoma. In *Pathology of the testis*, (ed. RCB Pugh), p. 199. Blackwell, Oxford.

Quirke P, Dyson JED, Sutton J, Anderson CK, Joslin CAF, Bird CC (1985). Assessment of germ cell tumours of testis by flow cytometry and histopathology. In *Germ cell tumours II* (ed. WG Jones, A Milford Ward, and CK Anderson), pp. 45–54. *Advances in the biosciences*, Vol. 55. Pergamon Press, Oxford.

Raney RB, *et al.* (1981). Treatment strategies for infants with malignant sacrococcygeal teratoma. *Journal of Pediatric Surgery*, **16** (4):573–7.

Rogers SC (1976). Anencephalus, spina bifida, twins and teratoma. *British Journal of Preventative and Social Medicine*, **30**:26–8.

Rustin GJS, Newlands ES, Bagshawe KD, Begent RHJ, Crawford SM (1986). Successful management of metastatic and primary germ cell tumors in the brain. *Cancer*, **57**:2108–13.

Sebag-Montefiore DJ, Douek E, Kingston JE, Plowman PN (1992). Intracranial germ cell tumours: I. Experience with platinum based chemotherapy and implications for curative chemoradiotherapy. *Clinical Oncology*, **4**:345–50.

Serov SF, Scully RE (1972). *Histological typing ovarian tumors*. International Histological Classification of Tumors No. 9 World Health Organisation, Geneva.

Sikora K, Evan G, Stewart J, Watson JV (1985). Detection of the c-myc oncogene product in testicular cancer. *British Journal of Cancer*, **52**:171–6.

Slayton RE, *et al.* (1978). Treatment of malignant ovarian germ cell tumors. Response to vincristine, dactinomycin and cyclophosphamide (Preliminary report). *Cancer*, **42**:390–8.

Smith DB, Newlands ES, Begent RHJ, Rustin GJS, Bagshawe KD (1991). Optimum management of pineal germ cell tumours. *Clinical Oncology*, **3**:96–9.

Smith IE, Eckstein HB, Kohn J, McElwain TJ (1977). Metastatic orchioblastoma: alpha 1-fetoprotein in diagnosis and combination chemotherapy in treatment: a case report. *British Journal of Urology*, **49**:427–30.

Smith JP, Rutledge F (1987). Malignant gynecologic tumors. In *Clinical pediatric oncology* (ed. WW Sutow, JJ Vietti, and DJ Fernbach), pp. 515–19. CV Mosby, St Louis.

Taylor H, Barter RH, Jacobson CB (1966). Neoplasms of dysgenetic gonads. *American Journal of Obstetrics and Gynecology*, **96**:816–23.

Teilum G (1976). *Special tumours of ovary and testis*. JB Lippincott, Copenhagen.

Thurlbeck WM, Scully RE (1960). Solid teratoma of ovary. A clinico-pathological analysis of 9 cases. *Cancer*, **13**:804–11.

Tsuchida Y, Endo Y, Saito S, Kaneko M, Shiraki K, Ohmi K (1978). Evaluation of alpha-fetoprotein in early infancy. *Journal of Pediatric Surgery*, **13**:155–6.

Tsuji I, Nakajima F, Nishida T, Nakanoya Y, Inoue K (1973). Testicular tumors in children. *Journal of Urology*, **110**:127–9.

Ungerleider RS, Donaldson SS, Warnke RA, Wilbur JR (1978). Endodermal sinus tumour. The Stanford experience and the first reported case arising in the vulva. *Cancer*, **41**:1627–34.

Union Internationale Contre le Cancer (1974). *TNM classification of malignant tumors*. UICC, Geneva.

Wakai S, *et al.* (1980). Teratoma in the pineal region in two brothers. *Journal of Neurosurgery*, **53**:239–43.

Waters KD, Tiedemann K, Ekert H (1987). Malignant germ cell tumours of childhood: the Melbourne experience. *Medical and Pediatric Oncology*, **15**:306–7.

Weissbach L, Altwein JE, Stiens R (1984). Germinal testicular tumours in childhood. *European Urology*, **10**:73–85.

Wollner N, Exelby PR, Woodruff JM, Cham WC, Murphy ML, Lewis JL (1976). Malignant ovarian tumors in childhood: prognosis in relation to initial therapy. *Cancer*, **37**:1953–64.

Wollner N, Luks E, Wachtel T, Ghavimi F (1987). Malignant germ cell tumors (MGCT) in children. Memorial Sloan-Kettering Cancer Center experience. *Medical and Pediatric Oncology*, **15**:306.

Wu JT, Book L, Sudar K (1981). Serum alphafetoprotein (AFP) levels in normal infants. *Pediatric Research*, **15**:50–2.

Young PG, Mount BF, Foote FW, Whitmore WF (1970). Embryonal adenocarcinoma in the pubertal testis. *Cancer*, **26**:1065–75.

14.6 Liver tumours

P. A. VOÛTE AND ROSS PINKERTON

INTRODUCTION

Primary tumours of the liver are comparatively rare in infancy and childhood and account for 0.5–2 per cent of all paediatric malignancies. However, 15 per cent of all abdominal tumours in childhood are primary liver tumours, approximately two-thirds of which are malignant. Benign tumours such as hamartomas and angiomas occur more frequently than malignant tumours, of which hepatoblastoma and hepatocellular carcinoma are the most commonly seen.

BENIGN TUMOURS

Unlike malignant tumours, benign tumours of the liver in children occur slightly more often in girls than in boys. The most common tumours are hamartomas and haemangioendotheliomas.

Hamartomas are usually confined to one lobe and may be pedunculated with characteristic multiple cellular differentiation. Haemangioendotheliomas may be uni- or multinodular and may reach a considerable size. They are composed of multiple vascular channels and resemble the haemangiomas of skin. Less commonly, adenoma, teratoma, and biliary cysts may occur.

MALIGNANT TUMOURS

Most cases of primary malignant liver tumours in children occur under the age of 2 years. There is some geographical variation in incidence, as these tumours are comparatively rare in Europe, whereas in Africa and, in particular, Southwest Asia, their occurrence is more common. Overall, there is a greater frequency in males, with a sex ratio of 1.4:1.

AETIOLOGY

Environmental factors may play a role in hepatoblastoma (Buckley et al. 1989). The known association between hepatoblastoma and the Beckwith–Wiedemann syndrome has indicated a role for abnormalities on chromosome 11 (Koufos et al. 1985). Loss of heterozygosity on 11p has been documented in tumour tissue. The increased incidence of hepatoblastoma in families with familial adenomatosis polypi also indicates a possible significance for abnormalities on chromosome 5q (Kingston et al. 1983). There is a need for further study of the molecular pathology of these tumours, emphasizing the importance of adequate initial biopsy samples at presentation.

As in adults, hepatocellular carcinoma may occur in association with hepatitis B. This association tends to reflect the incidence of hepatitis in the general population and its significance in Europe is unclear. Hepatocellular carcinoma may also be associated with inborn errors of metabolism, such as galactosaemia, tyrosinaemia, and Wilson's disease.

PATHOLOGY

Three main pathological subtypes of hepatoblastoma have been described: fetal, embryonal, and anaplastic. In the fetal type there is a monotonous pattern of cells resembling those seen in fetal liver; more poorly differentiated cells which are smaller and basophilic with prominent pleomorphism are described as the embryonal type. Finally, in the anaplastic type there are small cells with dark nuclei and scanty cytoplasm, lacking specific morphological features and in some cases resembling neuroblasts (Weinberg and Finegold 1986; Haas et al. 1989).

In all subtypes, osteoid tissue, immature mesenchyme, and haematopoietic foci may be found within the tumour tissue in addition to the hepatoblastoma cells. The tumours may also be very vascular.

Hepatocellular carcinoma is histologically similar to that seen in adults. It differs from hepatoblastoma by the presence of tumour cells larger than normal hepatocytes. There is considerable nuclear pleomorphism with prominent nucleoli. The fibrolamellar subtype is distinguished by broad fibrous septa.

CLINICAL FEATURES

Most patients present with abdominal distension or an abdominal mass. The latter is of variable consistency and usually readily palpable on initial presentation. Pain is an uncommon feature and anorexia, vomiting, anaemia, fever, or jaundice are usually signs associated with advanced malignant tumours. Hypovolaemic shock with haemoperitoneum occurs occasionally and is due to tumour rupture. Patients have been reported to develop osteopenia due to the tumour release of substances with an osteoclastic stimulating activity.

LABORATORY TESTS

Full blood count may reveal high levels of haemoglobin or platelet count caused by tumour production of erythropoietin or thrombopoietin-like substances (Nickerson et al. 1980). Serum cholesterol may be elevated.

α-Fetoprotein is present in the serum of 90 per cent of children with hepatoblastoma and approximately 60 per cent of those with hepatocellular carcinoma. The very rare intrahepatic malignant germ cell tumour will also present with a hepatic mass and raised α-fetoprotein. Healing liver after trauma or partial liver resection may be associated with moderately high levels of α-fetoprotein and these are also seen in cirrhotic liver.

Human chorionic gonadotropin may be detectable in the serum and urine of children with hepatoblastoma, who in some cases may show precocious puberty. This is not seen in hepatocellular carcinoma.

In some patients with hepatoblastoma cystathionine levels in the urine may be elevated, which can be a useful tumour marker.

DIAGNOSTIC IMAGING

The plain radiograph of the abdomen generally shows non-specific enlargement of the liver. Calcification is seldom seen at presentation but may occur with chemotherapy. Ultrasound is a useful first imaging technique to confirm the intrahepatic nature of the tumour and may exclude cystic lesions such as cholidocal cyst, biliary cysts, and liver abscesses. The ultrasound pattern, particularly with Doppler techniques, may be pathognomonic for a haemangioma.

Either CT scanning or magnetic resonance imaging (MRI) is essential to localize the tumour to the liver accurately and to define its precise anatomical position (Finn et al. 1990). The latter is of great importance in deciding the resectability of the tumour prior to or following chemotherapy. Intravenous contrast with CT scan will give characteristic patterns for a primary tumour or a vascular haemangioma. In some cases, however, a very vascular malignant tumour may be extremely difficult to distinguish on the basis of imaging alone. Occasionally serial aortography, coeliac arteriography, or subtraction arteriography of the liver and the tumour are necessary to establish its exact location and the relationship between the blood supply to liver and tumour. However, these may all be clear on a high quality MRI scan. Such accurate imaging is an important pre-operative investigation for both benign and malignant tumours. Liver scanning with various isotopes, such as ^{99}Tc, Rose Bengal ^{131}I, and ^{67}Ga, have been used to image primary liver tumours in the past, but these techniques are now rarely indicated.

The staging system for the International Society of Paediatric Oncology (SIOP) study is determined by the anatomical position on initial imaging (Fig. 1).

TREATMENT OF MALIGNANT TUMOURS

With the introduction of combination chemotherapy, which is highly effective, particularly in hepatoblastoma, the use of aggressive primary surgery is no longer appropriate. In the current SIOP study the sole indication for attempting initial resection is

Hepatoblastoma and hepatocellular carcinoma

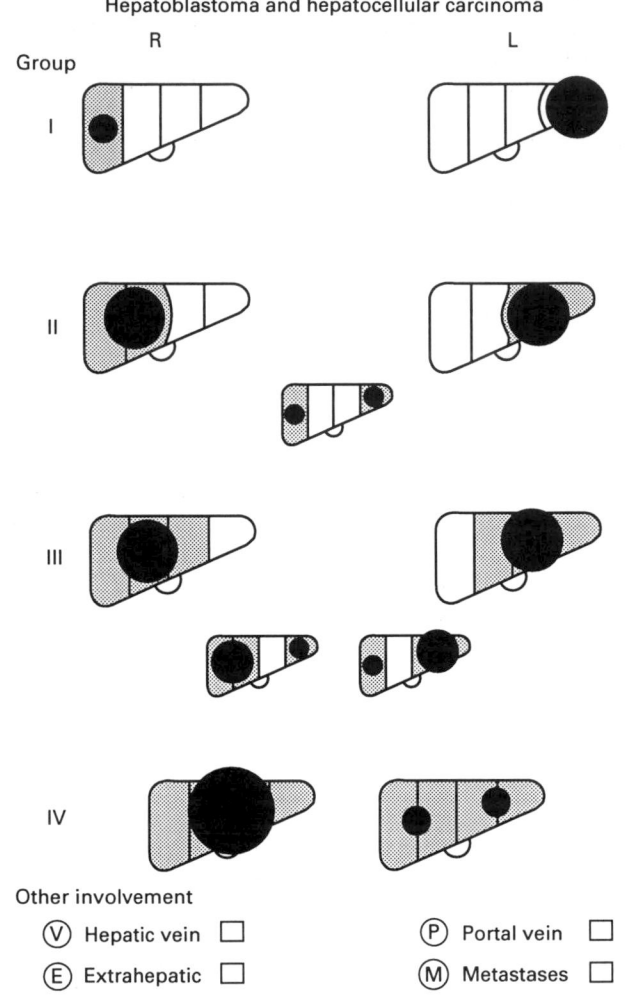

Fig. 1 SIOP pre-treatment grouping system describing extent of disease.

a small localized tumour where complete clearance with minimal risk is likely (Fig. 1).

The role of primary chemotherapy is to shrink the tumour, increasing the likelihood of complete resectability. The latter is usually a prerequisite to cure in these tumours, unlike a number of other paediatric solid tumours where local radiotherapy to microscopic residual disease is of proven benefit. Systemic chemotherapy also eliminates undetectable micrometastases, a common cause of relapse where surgery alone is used. Effective agents include vincristine, actinomycin D, cyclophosphamide, cisplatin, anthracyclines, and 5-fluorouracil. Although the results with regimens based on vincristine, actinomycin D and cyclophosphamide have been disappointing in the past, the introduction of cisplatin–doxorubicin combinations has had a dramatic effect on outcome (Quinn et al. 1985).

The most effective combinations currently under evaluation are cisplatin, vincristine, and 5-fluorouracil, as used by the American Paediatric Oncology Group (Douglass et al. 1993) and the combination of continuous infusion doxorubicin and cisplatin, as used by the American CCS Group (Ortega et al. 1991) and the SIOP Group (Pritchard et al. 1989). Using these regimens, patients with completely resected hepatoblastoma or microscopic residual disease following primary surgery achieve actuarial disease-free

survival rates of approximately 90 per cent and those with non-metastatic unresectable primary tumour achieve between 50 and 60 per cent. Provisional results from the SIOP regimen suggest that approximately 30–40 per cent of children with initial metastatic disease may be long-term survivors.

The outcome in patients with hepatocellular carcinoma is less encouraging, although the number of patients treated with these protocols is small. In one series using cisplatin and doxorubicin fewer than 20 per cent of patients with non-metastatic disease were long-term survivors. This reflected a failure to convert initially unresectable hepatocellular carcinoma to resectable masses.

SURGICAL THERAPY

As mentioned earlier, complete resection of the tumour is usually a prerequisite for cure. Recent improvements in imaging have enabled increased sophistication in planning surgery on the basis of anatomical features. It has been recognized that it is more accurate to treat the two lobes of the liver as separate independently functioning units. Additionally, the liver can be divided into two different anatomical segments which, starting with the caudate lobe, evolve in a left turning spiral around the central axis. It is possible to remove half the liver and one of the remaining segments with ultimate return of normal liver function (hemihepatectomy, segmentectomy, and extended hemihepatectomy).

Infants and children tolerate resection of up to 80 per cent of the liver, but careful anaesthetic and intraoperative supportive care is essential. It has been shown that the liver regenerates rapidly after resection and recovers its original volume within 6 months. Although no precise studies of liver regeneration in children have been reported, clinical experience suggests that this capacity is better in children than in adults. The size of the mass and the age of the patient should not be an obstacle to definitive surgery. The major limitations are the extension of tumour across the anatomical boundaries mentioned above.

An important technical improvement in the surgical treatment of liver tumours was the development of the ultrasonic dissector. This device uses ultrasonic vibration to separate tumour from surrounding tissue. The tumour tissue is removed immediately by a built-in suction system. This enables complete removal of tumour from around vessels without damaging the latter.

In general, patients are in good overall condition at the time of surgery, but it is important to correct any anaemia and exclude any coagulation defect pre-operatively. Superior vena caval cannulation is performed for monitoring central venous pressure and for infusing fluid during the operation. Since temporary occlusion of the inferior vena cava or its angulation due to traction of the liver often disturbs venous return from the lower half of the body to the heart, venous access through the saphenous route is inappropriate. Since the costal margin is soft and the abdominal wall is elastic in young people, the left paramedian or midline incision extending along the seventh right intercostal space with subperiosteal division of the cartilaginous costal margin, without thoracotomy, usually gives an adequate exposure. Controlled positive-pressure ventilation should prevent air embolism in the case of injury to the inferior vena cava. Prior to surgery it is also essential that adequate imaging of the inferior vena cava and hepatic vein exclude the presence of tumour or tumour-related thrombus, which would pose a risk of pulmonary emboli. Perioperatively, albumin levels should be monitored and hypoglycaemia detected early and corrected with intravenous glucose. Since clotting factors (prothrombin, factor V, and factor IX) decrease and fibrinolytic activity increases after liver resection, vitamin K and antiplasmin should be given to avoid bleeding. The altered metabolic function of the liver following resection is usually restored to normal within 2 weeks.

RADIOTHERAPY

Radiotherapy plays only a modest part in the treatment of liver tumours. Its role is generally reserved for the treatment of microscopic residual disease following surgery after primary chemotherapy. Recent reviews have failed to show any convincing benefit from this, but the question has never been addressed in a formal study. The limiting factor may be the total dose which can be delivered to a large area of the liver without toxicity to normal tissue (Habrand *et al.* 1992). However, most oncologists would recommend local irradiation in the above clinical setting, in the absence of any other effective treatment.

PATIENT FOLLOW-UP

The α-fetoprotein marker is an invaluable guide to tumour response with both hepatoblastoma and hepatocellular carcinoma (Matsumoto *et al.* 1974; Pritchard *et al.* 1982). The rate of fall usually indicates the effectiveness of chemotherapy, and if this fails to approach the normal half-life of α-fetoprotein (10–14 days), it is likely that the chemotherapy is suboptimal.

With complete resection of the tumour the α-fetoprotein should fall to normal and remain so during follow-up. Monthly checks of α-fetoprotein should be performed for the following 18–24 months and a persistent increase in α-fetoprotein is an indicator of disease recurrence.

MANAGEMENT OF INITIAL METASTATIC DISEASE

Intensive primary chemotherapy has improved the prognosis in these patients and in general attempted resection of the primary mass is reserved for those in whom the lung metastases have resolved, at least on plain radiographs. Aggressive surgery to pulmonary metastases has been recommended by some authors (Black *et al.* 1991), with long-term survival described in a small number of patients with persisting active lung nodules following primary chemotherapy. Elective lung irradiation is generally recommended for those who achieve a response to chemotherapy and in whom the primary tumour is completely resected.

FIBROLAMELLAR CARCINOMA

This rare subgroup of hepatocellular carcinoma usually affects adolescents or young adults and stands out by its lack of initial chemosensitivity (Craig *et al.* 1980). Unless this tumour is completely resected at presentation it is unlikely to be curable, although the precise response rate to modern platinum-based chemotherapy remains to be defined.

TREATMENT OF BENIGN TUMOURS

The commonest of these, the haemangioma or haemangio-epithelioma, are essentially surgical problems. In the neonate or small infant presenting with an asymptomatic tumour, a wait and watch policy may be appropriate. However, these tumours may be associated with consumptive coagulopathy or haemodynamic instability. In such cases, if the tumour is not resectable, low-dose radiotherapy may be used. In addition, steroid therapy may be beneficial and is the primary treatment of choice (Stanley *et al.* 1989).

Mesenchymal hamartomas may require early operation because of rapid enlargement resulting from fluid accumulation within the tumour. Operations for benign tumours of the liver are generally carried out to reduce local pressure effects and also to differentiate them from malignant tumours.

OTHER INTRAHEPATIC MALIGNANCIES

Unlike adult malignancies, metastatic liver tumours in children are comparatively rare. Focal deposits may occur in metastatic neuroblastoma and the diffuse infiltration in those with 4s disease is characteristic. Focal metastatic lesions are also seen with nephroblastoma and soft tissue or bone sarcomas. Diffuse or, in some cases, patchy infiltration occurs with leukaemias and lymphomas. The treatment of these lesions is as appropriate for the primary tumour. Surgery or radiotherapeutic intervention is rarely indicated.

REFERENCES

Black CT, Luck SR, Musemeche CA, Andrassy RJ (1991). Aggressive excision of pulmonary metastases is warranted in the management of childhood hepatic tumors. *Journal of Pediatric Surgery*, **26**:1082–6.

Buckley JD, Sather R, Ruccione K, Rogers PCJ, Haas JE, Henderson BE, Hammond GD (1989). A case-control study of risk factors for hepatoblastoma. A report from the Children's Cancer Study Group. *Cancer*, **64**:1169–76.

Craig JR, Peters RL, Edmondson HA, Omata M (1980). Fibrolamellar carcinoma of the liver: a tumor of adolescents and young adults with distinctive clinicopathologic features. *Cancer*, **46**:372–9.

Douglass EC, Reynolds M, Finegold M, Cantor AB, Glicksmann A (1993). Cisplatin, vincristine and fluorouracil therapy for hepatoblastoma: a Pediatric Oncology Group Study. *Journal of Clinical Oncology*, **11**:96–9.

Finn JP, *et al.* (1990). Primary malignant liver tumours in childhood: assessment of resectability with high-field MR and comparison with CT. *Paediatric Radiology*, **21**:34–8.

Haas JE, Muczynski KA, Krailo M, Ablin A, Land V, Vietti TJ, Hammond GD (1989). Histopathology and prognosis in childhood hepatoblastoma and hepatocarcinoma. *Cancer*, **64**:1082–95.

Habrand J-L, *et al.* (1992). Is there a place for radiation therapy in the management of hepatoblastomas and hepatocellular carcinomas in children? *International Journal of Radiation Oncology—Biology—Physics*, **23**:525–31.

Kingston JE, Herbert A, Draper GJ, Mann JR (1983). Association between hepatoblastoma and polyposis coli. *Archives of the Diseases of Childhood*, **58**:959–62.

Koufos A, *et al.* (1985). Loss of heterozygosity in three embryonal tumours suggests a common pathogenetic mechanism. *Nature, London*, **316**:330–4.

Matsumoto Y, Suzuki T, Ono H, Nakase A, Honjo I (1974). Response of alpha-fetoprotein to chemotherapy in patients with hepatomas. *Cancer*, **34**:1602–6.

Nickerson HJ, Silberman T, McDonald TP (1980). Hepatoblastoma, thrombocytosis and increased thrombopoietin. *Cancer*, **45**:315–17.

Ortega JA, *et al.* (1991). Effective treatment of unresectable or metastatic hepatoblastoma with cisplatin and continuous infusion doxorubicin chemotherapy: a report from the Children's Cancer Study Group. *Journal of Clinical Oncology*, 12:2167–76.

Pritchard J, *et al.* (1989). Cis-platinum, doxorubicin and surgery for advanced hepatoblastoma (Hbl): a real chance for cure? *ASCO Proceedings*, 1159:298.

Pritchard J, da Cunha A, Cornbleet MA, Carter CJ (1982). Alphafetoprotein monitoring of response to adriamycin in hepatoblastoma. *Journal of Pediatric Surgery*, 17:429–30.

Quinn JJ, Altman AJ, Robinson HT, Cooke RW, Hight DW, Foster JH (1985). Adriamycin and cisplatin for hepatoblastoma. *Cancer*, 56:1926–9.

Stanley P, Geer GD, Miller JH, Gilsanz V, Landing BH, Boechat IM (1989). Infantile hepatic hemangiomas. *Cancer*, 64:936–49.

Weinberg AG, Finegold MJ (1986). Primary hepatic tumors in childhood. In *Pathology of neoplasia in children and adolescents* (ed. M Finegold). WB Saunders, Philadelphia.

14.7 Rare tumours of childhood

DAVID A. WALKER

INTRODUCTION

The purpose of describing this diverse tumour category is to meet the needs of the clinician faced with the management of an unusual tumour. The definition of this category is complicated by the very nature of the task. It could be based upon the absolute incidence of the tumour. However, all cancer is rare in childhood. The tumours included in this chapter are those which are unusual in childhood and which are not rare variants of the common childhood tumour categories. The range of tumours described has been identified by literature review, by consultation with experienced clinical colleagues, and with the assistance of the Childhood Cancer Research Group registry (Tables 1 and 2). They have been grouped anatomically where possible or by tissue of origin.

The tumours described in this chapter are generally more common in the adult population. This difference in age-related incidence requires an explanation. The epithelial cancers (carcinomas) are the single largest group, accounting for 2 per cent of all childhood malignant disease registered by the Childhood Cancer Research Group (McWhirter *et al.* 1989) (Table 1). Their early presentation may simply represent the very beginning of a pattern of incidence increasing with age, well into adulthood, although there are alternative explanations for certain tumours. Thyroid cancer has been shown to develop in childhood after early thyroid irradiation and carcinoma of the colon may be secondary to an inherited predisposition as in familial adenomatous polyposis. Developmental factors may also play a part, as demonstrated by the age-related incidence peaks in adrenal carcinoma and nasopharyngeal carcinoma. These specific mechanisms may act alone or in combination with other unknown factors to accelerate oncogenesis.

Table 1 Carcinomas 1971–1990 in UK National Registry of Childhood Tumours (excluding skin, kidney, and liver)

ICD-9 classification	Site	Male	Female	0–4 years	5–9 years	10–14 years	Total	ASR	5 year % survival
142	Salivary glands	16	21	3	6	28	37	0.16	89
141, 143–145	Other mouth	3	9	0	6	6	12	0.05	92
146–149	Nasopharynx, etc.	44	30	3	13	58	74	0.31	53
150–154	Gastrointestinal	18	8	0	1	25	26	0.11	14
157	Pancreas	2	7	1	4	4	9	0.04	—
162	Bronchus, lung	4	6	1	1	8	10	0.04	50
	Malignant carcinoid	2	2	0	0	4	4	0.02	—
	Other	2	4	1	1	4	6	0.03	—
164.0	Thymus	7	6	1	5	7	13	0.06	8
174	Female breast	0	2	0	0	2	2	0.01	—
183	Ovary	0	18	1	3	14	18	0.08	72
180, 184	Other female genital	0	5	2	2	1	5	0.02	—
186	Testis	2	0	0	0	2	2	0.01	—
188	Bladder	7	2	0	2	7	9	0.04	—
190	Eye	0	3	0	0	3	3	0.01	—
193	Thyroid	34	77	2	19	90	111	0.46	98
194	Adrenal	10	36	27	10	9	46	0.2	28
195, 199	Ill-defined primary and unknown primary site	11	18	2	5	22	29	0.12	45

ASR, age standardized annual incidence per million, standardized to uniform age distribution.

Table 2 Selected rare malignant tumours 1971–1990 in UK National Registry of Childhood Tumours

ICD-O classification	Morphology	Male	Female	0–4 years	5–9 years	10–14 years	Total	ASR
8680/3 8693/3	Malignant paraganglioma	1	3	2	1	1	4	0.02
8940/3	Malignant mixed salivary gland tumours	2	3	0	0	5	5	0.02
—	Pancreaticoblastoma	3	0	3	0	0	3	0.01
8981/3	Pneumoblastoma	1	0	1	0	0	1	0.00
9050/3	Malignant mesothelioma	0	1	0	0	1	1	0.00
9150/3	Maligant haemangiopericytoma	8	7	4	3	8	15	0.06
—	Triton tumour	0	1	0	1	0	1	0.00
9580/3	Malignant granular cell tumour	2	1	0	3	0	3	0.01
—	Peripheral neuroectodermal tumour[a]	37	31	18	15	35	68	0.29
	Registrations (1981–1990)	30	27	17	12	28	57	0.53

ASR, age standardized annual incidence per million, standardized to uniform age distribution.
[a]Including Askin's tumour, soft tissue Ewing's sarcoma, and neuroepithelioma, outside the central nervous system.

HEAD AND NECK

Salivary carcinomas

Salivary tumours in childhood are most commonly benign pleomorphic adenomas. Carcinomas are the most common malignant tumours, occurring equally in both sexes and arising most frequently in the major salivary glands. Parotid gland tumours are more common than tumours of the submandibular and minor salivary glands. Muco-epidermoid carcinoma is by far the commonest histological subtype, followed by acinic cell carcinoma, adenoid cystic carcinoma, and adenocarcinoma (Shikhani and Johns 1988).

Clinical presentation and investigation

Clinical presentation is with a localized mass with or without facial pain and/or a facial palsy in parotid tumours (Fig. 1). Regional lymph nodes may be involved. Investigation with facial radiographs and CT scanning or magnetic resonance imaging (MRI) should be performed to define local tumour extension prior to surgery; a closed or incisional biopsy is not recommended. A search for distant metastases in the lungs and bones should be performed in high-grade tumours once the diagnosis has been confirmed histrologically.

Treatment

The primary aim of treatment is to achieve complete surgical excision. In the parotid gland, preservation of the facial nerve is desirable but may not be achievable. There is a high incidence of local recurrence in both benign and malignant tumours. Evidence of incomplete resection or disseminated tumour justifies consideration of repeat surgery or radiotherapy if the disease is localized. Chemotherapy should be considered if the disease is disseminated. Responses to chemotherapy have been reported with combinations of cisplatin (CDDP), doxorubin (DX), and 5-fluorouracil (Venook et al. 1987) or cyclophosphamide (CTX) (Belani et al. 1988) and justify further evaluation in children.

Angiofibroma

This tumour of adolescence occurs almost exclusively in males and suggests an endocrine component of growth control. The tumour, which is a mixed fibroblastic vascular tumour thought to be of mesenchymal origin (Taxy 1977), commonly arises in the nasopharynx or oropharynx and invades local surrounding hard and soft tissues. Metastases are very rare indeed. Direct spread intracranially as well as to the orbit, maxilla, and hard and soft palates has been reported. Presentation is usually with a unilateral facial swelling, obstructed nares, and recurrent epistaxis. Anterior or posterior rhinoscopy reveals a dark red glistening tumour, indicating extreme vascularity and justifying advice against biopsy. Treatment is mainly restricted to surgical resection, although some tumours are suitable for embolization. Local recurrence is possible. Diethylstilboestrol and radiation have been used, although short- and long-term side-effects limit the acceptability of these treatments.

Nasopharyngeal carcinoma

Nasopharyngeal carcinoma accounts for approximately one-third of nasopharyngeal neoplasms in this age group. Those that present in childhood are mainly undifferentiated carcinomas (type 3) or non-keratinizing carcinomas (type 2), according to the World Health Organization (WHO) classification.

Incidence

There is a marked variation in the incidence around the world ranging from one in 100 000 in European and American Caucasians to 25 in 100 000 in the population of Hong Kong. There is a bimodal

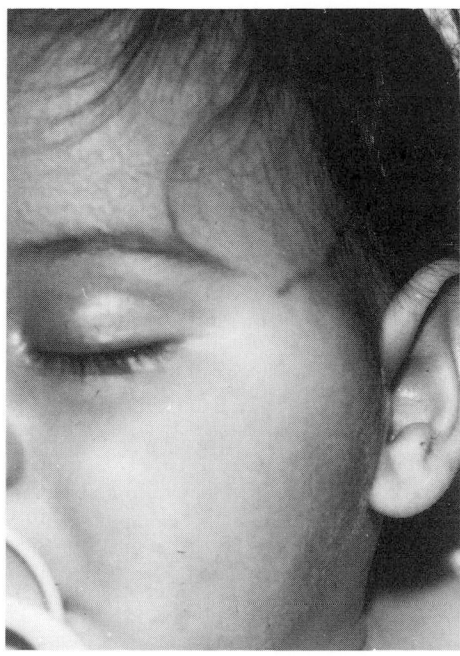

Fig. 1 Parotid gland carcinoma in a child.

age distribution with an early peak in adolescence and young adulthood in European and American Caucasians but not in Southeast Asians or North Africans. Nasopharyngeal carcinoma occurs more commonly in males, although this male preponderance is less marked in the younger age groups than it is later in adulthood (Gastpar *et al.* 1981).

Aetiology

The aetiology of these tumours is thought to be multifactorial with evidence for involvement of genetic, viral, and environmental factors. The marked variations in incidence between different population groups, together with evidence for family clustering and an association with specific HLA types (Gajwani *et al.* 1980), is suggestive of genetic predisposition to tumour formation. Evidence for a viral aetiology is strongly suggested by the established association between nasopharyngeal carcinoma and infection with the Epstein–Barr virus. The evidence for Epstein–Barr virus infection is supplied by seroepidemiological surveys, the demonstration of Epstein–Barr virus nuclear antigen in carcinoma cells, and the demonstration of antibodies to the Epstein–Barr viral capsid antigen in patients with nasopharyngeal carcinoma. Environmental factors such as exposure to environmental and dietary carcinogens are suspected but not proved.

Pathology

Histologically, types 2 and 3 nasopharyngeal carcinomas are accompanied by an inflammatory infiltrate of lymphocytes, oesinophils, and plasma cells, which explains their earlier name of 'lymphoepithelioma'. The tumours usually arise in the fossa of Rosenmüller and spread locally to the rest of pharynx and the base of the skull. They metastasize to cervical lymph nodes, bone, mediastinum, lungs, and liver.

Clinical presentation

The most common clinical presentation is with cervical lymphadenopathy; the primary tumour is often clinically undetectable in the nasopharynx. The main differential diagnosis is non-Hodgkin's lymphoma. Symptoms related to the primary tumour result from involvement of local structures and include hearing loss, a local mass, nasal obstruction, otitis media, epistaxis, and pain (Jereb *et al.* 1980). Disseminated tumour may produce symptoms related to the site of metastasis. Patients with disseminated disease may present with a paraneoplastic syndrome consisting of osteoarthropathy, clubbing, and bone or joint pain.

Tumour staging

Tumour evaluation should be directed at the delineation of the extent of the primary tumour, local lymph node involvement, and a search for distant metastases (Table 3). Indirect nasolaryngoscopy may not reveal a primary tumour. If not, blind biopsies may be taken. Imaging of the base of the skull with plain radiography and CT or MRI scans helps to define tumour size, site, and lymph node involvement, as well as local bony or central nervous system invasion. Cerebrospinal fluid cytology may be indicated if central nervous system invasion is suspected. Evidence of metastatic disease should be sought with radionuclide bone scanning and chest and abdominal imaging with CT, MRI, and/or ultrasound. The detection of Epstein–Barr virus genetic material may assist with diagnosis. Raised serum immunoglobin A (IgA) antibodies to the viral capsid antigen may be of prognostic value and has been used as a marker for relapse (Lynn *et al.* 1985). Five year survival rates of 50–60 per cent are reported for children treated with radiation and chemotherapy (Papavasiliou *et al.* 1977; Jenkin *et al.* 1981).

Table 3 Modified TNM classification of nasopharyngeal carcinoma

Primary tumour
- T_0 No evidence of tumour
- T_{is} Carcinoma *in situ*
- T_1 Tumour confined to nasopharyngeal mucosa or no tumour visible but biopsy positive
- T_2 Tumour extended to nasal fossa, oropharynx, or adjacent muscles or nerves below base of skull
- T_3 Tumour beyond T_2 limits and subclassified as follows
  - T_{3a} Bone involvement below base of skull
  - T_{3b} Involvement of base of skull
  - T_{3c} Involvement of cranial nerves
  - T_{3d} Involvement of orbit, laryngopharynx, or infratemporal fossa

Nodal tumour
- N_0 No clinically positive node
- N_1 Nodes wholly in upper cervical level above lower third of neck
- N_2 Nodes palpable in lower third of neck or supraclavicular area

Distant metastases
- M Distant metastases present

Stage grouping
- Stage A T_1, N_0
- Stage B T_1, N_1; T_2, N_0, or N_1
- Stage C T_3 any N or N_2 any T
- Stage D M_1

Source: Ho (1977).

Surgery

The curative role of surgical treatment is limited by the high incidence of early spread of the primary tumour at diagnosis. Surgical efforts are generally limited to biopsy and the treatment of otitis media prior to local radiotherapy. Successful treatment is dependent upon the use of radiotherapy and chemotherapy.

Radiation

Irradiation of the nasopharynx requires careful planning to treat the whole tumour volume, excluding adjacent uninvolved structures. Prescription of the radiation dosage should include the consideration of the growth potential of the tissues to be irradiated. Doses greater than 50 Gy have not been shown to be more effective in the younger age groups and so most therapists have avoided the 70 Gy doses advised in the adult population. Careful follow-up in cured patients is important in identifying sequelae of inner ear, hypothalamic, pituitary, and thyroid irradiation.

Chemotherapy

The high incidence of metastatic relapse favours aggressive systemic chemotherapy early in treatment. Whether it is appropriate to use chemotherapy only in those with more extensive disease is controversial (Pao *et al.* 1989). A number of combination chemotherapy regimes have been used with good responses. These include bleomycin, methotrexate, and CDDP (Tannock *et al.* 1987), DX and CTX with or without vincristine (Lobo-Sanahuja *et al.* 1986; Gasparini *et al.* 1988), and VCR, DX, 5-fluorouracil, and CTX (Kim *et al.* 1989). At The Hospital for Sick Children, Great Ormond Street, we have seen good responses to a combination of bleomycin (Bleo), etoposide (VP16), and CDDP (BEP).

Future directions

The value of Epstein–Barr virus antibody titres for prognosis and the monitoring of disease response in children requires evaluation.

The established value of chemotherapy in this disease justifies the exploration of high-dose treatment with marrow rescue in poor prognosis groups. Further exploration of treatment with biological response modifiers such as interferon seems justified by early reports (Dimery *et al.* 1989).

Laryngeal carcinoma

Laryngeal carcinoma occasionally occurs and is a recognized sequel to external-beam irradiation of juvenile laryngeal papillomatosis (Schnadig *et al.* 1986). Presentation is with cough, hoarseness, haemoptysis, stridor, and dysphagia. Diagnosis is made at microlaryngoscopy. Metastases to lung and bone occur only rarely.

Preservation of the larynx is a high priority and so laser surgery (partial or total laryngectomy with or without local irradiation) is employed. This approach is associated with an overall survival rate of approximately 60 per cent (Gindhart *et al.* 1980). The inhibition of laryngeal growth coupled with the increased risk of secondary laryngeal and thyroid malignancies after irradiation makes the investigation of chemotherapy in these tumours a high priority, although experience of such treatment approaches in adults is not good.

Thyroid cancer

The incidence of thyroid cancer in childhood and adolescence rises with age, although the female preponderance seen in adulthood is less marked. Neck irradiation in infancy and childhood has been established as a predisposing cause of its development (Barnes 1988) and excesses of environmental radiation have also been implicated (Sala *et al.* 1993).

Pathology

Most tumours are of the highly differentiated papillary type or the less differentiated follicular and 'mixed' types. Anaplastic tumours are virtually unknown. Metastases occur at presentation in up to 66 per cent of all thyroid cancers. They are found in local lymph nodes in 50–55 per cent of patients and in lungs in 8–10 per cent (Richardson *et al.* 1974; Merrick and Hansen 1989). Medullary cell tumours arise from the thyroid parafollicular C cells which secrete calcitonin. In childhood they account for up to 20 per cent of all thyroid cancers (McWhirter *et al.* 1989) and are associated with the multiple endocrine neoplasia syndrome type II.

Clinical presentation

In thyroid cancer, clinical presentation is invariably with neck swelling in a euthyroid patient. Medullary cell tumours in relatives of patients with multiple endocrine neoplasia syndrome type II may be detected by screening, early in childhood, with clinical examination, provocation of calcitonin release by the calcium–pentagastrin test, or thyroid scanning (Graham *et al.* 1987). Such patients have less advanced disease than those who present symptomatically (Bergholm *et al.* 1989).

Investigation

A scheme for planning investigation, treatment, and follow-up of thyroid tumours is shown in Fig. 2. A combination of colloid and ultrasound scanning can differentiate between multinodular goitre, 'hot' and 'cold' nodules, and cysts. Thyroid cancers and medullary cell tumours present as 'cold' non-cystic nodules. The use of fine-needle aspiration biopsy in experienced hands has become accepted practice for pre-operative diagnosis in adults. The value of serum thyroglobulin as a tumour marker is best assessed by measuring thyroglobulin levels after a week's treatment with thyroxine or tri-iodothyronine. Thyroglobulin is now accepted as a reliable tumour marker in differentiated thyroid cancers (Ryff-de Leche *et al.* 1986; Black *et al.* 1987; Kirk *et al.* 1992), although its sensitivity for detecting relapse may be influenced by whether the patient is euthyroid or hypothyroid on replacement therapy (Müller-Gartner and Schneider 1988). Elevated calcitonin at diagnosis is a marker of medullary cell tumour and can be used as a tumour marker during therapy.

Surgery

The extent of surgical resection in thyroid cancer has long been the subject of debate. The minimum accepted operation has become total lobectomy with isthmusectomy. Therefore, the indications for extension of resection to the contralateral lobe and local lymph nodes are the basis of the discussion. The risks of radical thyroidectomy are related to the increased risk of hypoparathyroidism and damage to the recurrent laryngeal nerve. The risks of partial thyroidectomy include incomplete tumour resection, increased difficulty of subsequent surgical procedures, and the complications of ablating large thyroid remnants with radio-iodine. The indolent nature of the disease, the high survival rate, and the efficacy of disease management with thyroglobulin, ^{131}I scanning, and ^{131}I therapy all point to a reduced need for radical neck surgery at presentation (Schroder *et al.* 1986; La Quaglia *et al.* 1988). However, total thyroidectomy is recommended for medullary cell tumours in view of the high incidence of multifocal tumours.

Radiotherapy

Therapy with ^{131}I is used for thyroid ablation and subsequently for the treatment of local residual disease and metastatic deposits. Repeated doses can be used. The influence of radio-iodine treatment on survival has not been tested in a randomized trial. The long-term side-effects of ^{131}I therapy in children are uncertain, but the implications of such treatment must be carefully considered for children with a high chance of long-term survival.

Chemotherapy

Thyroid tissue stimulation is reduced by suppression of thyroid-stimulating hormone with thyroxine or tri-iodothyronine. Cytotoxic chemotherapy has not been used in these tumours.

Prognosis

The indolent nature of the majority of papillary and follicular thyroid cancers is associated with a 5 year survival rate of more than 95 per cent (Table 1). Deaths have been reported up to 30 years after diagnosis (Schlumberger *et al.* 1987), and the standard mortality ratio in patients under 15 years of age at diagnosis has been calculated at 11.2 times that of normal controls (Tubiana *et al.* 1985). Prognostic variables include age at diagnosis, nodal invasion, and degree of tumour differentiation. DNA aneuploidy has been associated with increasing age and tumour malignancy, but was not of independent prognostic value in 125 adult patients (Joensuu *et al.* 1986). Survival rates for children with medullary cell carcinoma in the national registry show 93 and 87 per cent survival at 5 and 10 years, respectively.

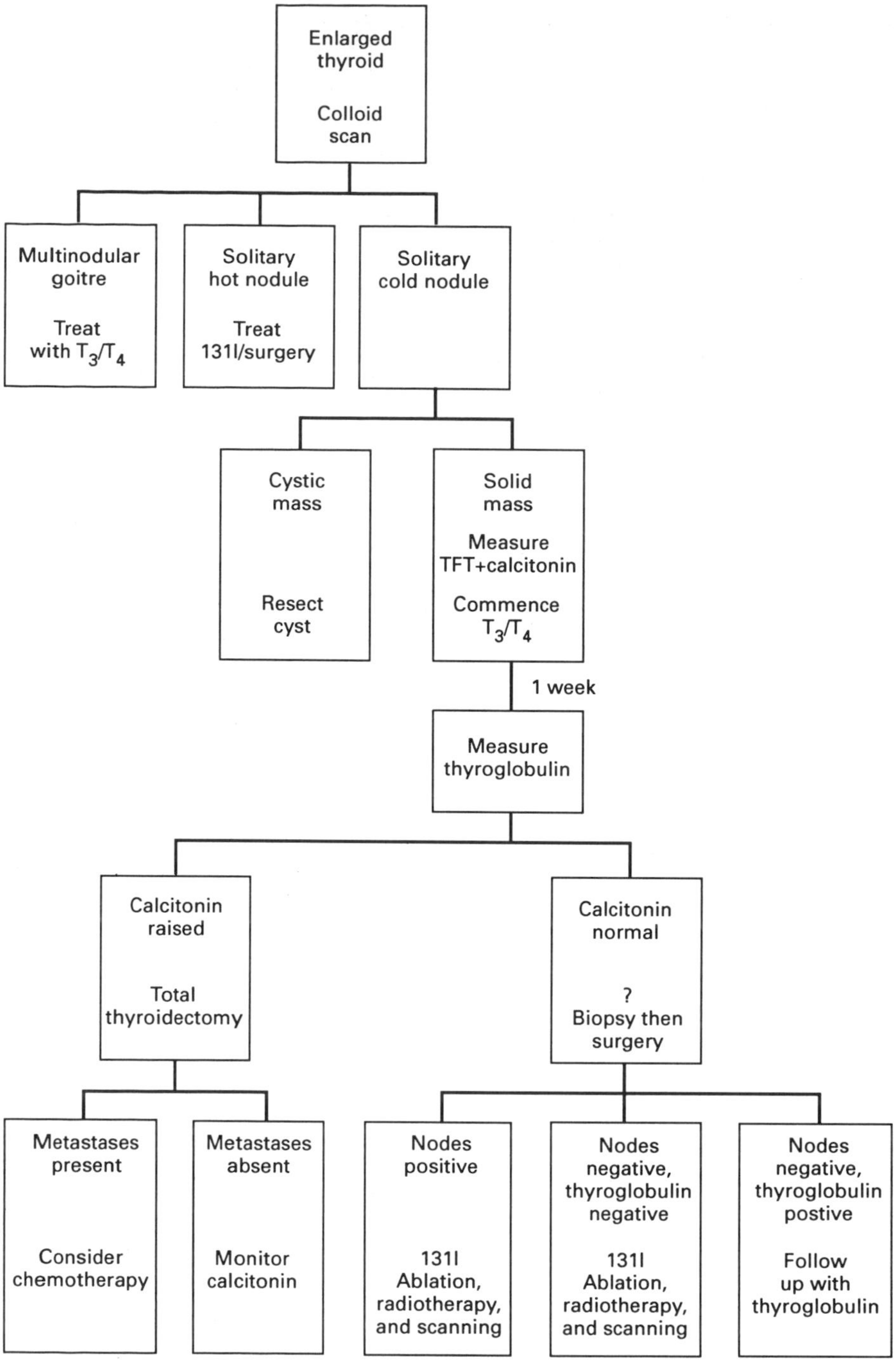

Fig. 2 Schema for investigation of a thyroid nodule in children.

Future directions

The use of fine-needle biopsy for diagnosis, where this expertise is available, should be evaluated in children. The role of DNA aneuploidy as an indicator of malignant potential in thyroid cancers of childhood requires further evaluation. Clinical follow-up with serum thyroglobulin as a tumour marker in localized papillary/follicular thyroid cancers is well established in adult practice. Its application during childhood may preclude the need for radio–ablation of the thyroid and routine ^{131}I scanning in some patients, thereby avoiding the risks of repeated radiation exposure

and the need for interruption of thyroid replacement therapy during critical periods of a child's development and education.

Ameloblastoma (adamantimoma)

These tumours arise most commonly in the mandible and maxilla, although they are occasionally reported in the long bones (Keeney *et al.* 1989). The facial presentation has been associated with enamel development of the teeth and primordial or dentigenous cysts (Keszler and Dopminguez 1986). Radiographs of the tumour reveal a solitary osteolytic lesion. The treatment of choice is local tumour excision. Radiotherapy has produced tumour responses however, the sensitivity to chemotherapy is unknown.

Granular cell tumour (myoblastoma)

Granular cell tumours are thought to arise from muscle-derived cells and/or Schwann cells. They occur at all ages and 7–25 per cent are multiple. In infancy and childhood they most commonly arise in the skin, tongue, and subcutaneous tissue of the head and neck; visceral lesions are rare (Cussen and MacMahon 1975; Rubenstein *et al.* 1987). Occasionally, tumours in adults may become malignant, although such an occurrence has not yet been reported in childhood. Clinical presentation is with subcutaneous or submucosal pruritic nodules with a smooth or scaly surface. Complete resection is needed to avoid local recurrence.

Chordoma

This rare tumour is thought to develop from remnants of the notochord and presents as a slow-growing locally invasive lobulated mass. It is more common in boys than girls and can arise anywhere within the axial skeleton. It is most common in the spheno-occipital and sacrococcygeal regions, but can occur in vertebrae and extra-axial sites such as the facial bones and sinuses. There is a tendency for childhood chordomas to invade intracranially and to be more aggressive. Metastatic spread occurs in approximately 10 per cent of patients as a late event, but is much lower in intracranial tumours (Reddy *et al.* 1981).

Tumours are often large, with a prolonged history of symptoms resulting from tumour invasion or pressure on local structures. Investigation with radiography, CT scans, and MRI defines the extent of the tumour. Treatment is with a combination of local excision and radiotherapy. The restrictions on wide surgical excision imposed by the tumour site lead to a high incidence of local recurrence and a poor prognosis. The use of high radiation doses, close to the limits of normal tissue tolerance, has produced measurable responses and perhaps prolongation of survival (Amendola *et al.* 1986). The use of chemotherapy has not been reported, but responses to radiotherapy might justify a trial of intensive chemotherapy in selected cases.

THORACIC TUMOURS
Primary lung and pleural tumours

Tumours of the lung and pleura are most commonly secondary deposits. The anatomical location of primary tumours dictates their clinical presentation and helps predict the probable tumour type.

Clinical presentation

In childhood and adolescence the majority of tumours are at the lung periphery and present with symptoms or signs of chest wall involvement such as chest and shoulder pain or Horner's syndrome. Centrally located tumours are more likely to present with signs of bronchial obstruction such as wheeze, recurrent infection, haemoptysis, or superior vena cava obstruction (Anderson *et al.* 1954).

Pathology

Rare pulmonary tumours include adenomas, carcinomas, and pleuropulmonary and chest wall tumours including pulmonary blastoma, neuroepithelioma (Askin's tumour), and malignant mesothelioma.

Investigation

Imaging with radiography, CT scanning, and MRI is necessary to delineate the number, site, and extent of the tumours. Where dissemination is likely, bone scanning is necessary to look for distant metastases.

Pulmonary 'adenomas'

This term covers a variety of slow-growing tumours with low malignant potential including carcinoid tumour, mucoepidermoid carcinoma, and cylindroma (Torres and Ryckman 1988). They most commonly occur in the main bronchi. Primary treatment of these tumours is by surgical resection.

Lung carcinoma

Carcinomas are well documented in childhood and occur in both sexes. Histologically they are most commonly undifferentiated bronchoepidermoid carcinomas or adenocarcinomas. Squamous carcinoma is exceptionally rare. Lung carcinomas in children are more commonly located peripherally. They are even more aggressive than in adults and may present at diagnosis with metastases (Anderson *et al.* 1954). Treatment has followed adult guidelines with resection of operable tumours. The use of chemotherapy in adults with small cell lung carcinoma now results in a significant prolongation of survival in the majority, but cure is achieved in less than 5 per cent (Viallet and Ihde 1989). In view of the greater chemoresponsiveness of most types of cancer in children, the use of such treatment should be explored, with CDDP and VP16 being a favoured regimen (Seifter and Ihde 1988). Radiotherapy has been used palliatively.

Pulmonary blastoma

This embryonic lung tumour is also seen in adults. It is found equally in both sexes. Histologically, mesenchymal elements are predominant. The epithelial elements described in the adult tumours are present less commonly in paediatric cases. Nearly a third of reported cases have been associated with lung cysts (Holland-Morritz and Heyn 1984). Metastasis is rare at presentation. Primary surgical resection is often complicated by local recurrence. Reports of chemotherapy are few and are not promising (Manivel *et al.* 1988).

Breast tumours

Malignant breast tumours in childhood are often less aggressive than their adult counterparts but they pose difficult management problems. Differentiating between premature thelarche, juvenile papillomatosis, fibroadenoma, and malignant tumours such as juvenile secretory carcinoma, fibro-, rhabdo-, and liposarcomas, and cystosarcoma phylloides requires surgical biopsy which may result in damage to the undeveloped breast tissue. Histological differential diagnosis is difficult in view of the variable appearance of the developing breast. However, *in situ* studies of oestrogen and progesterone receptors may help in identifying hormonally dependent and independent tissues (Ferguson *et al.* 1987). Fibroadenoma and juvenile papillomatosis are benign. Areas of secretory carcinoma have been reported within them, although the interpretation of such appearances should be approached with care (Mies and Rosen 1987). Imaging should include a search for metastases with CT scanning and MRI of the chest and bone scans.

Malignant tumours are most commonly juvenile secretory carcinomas for which conservative primary surgical resection is recommended, after which long disease-free periods have been observed with occasional late relapses. Undifferentiated carcinomas have been reported and have a much poorer prognosis, justifying an aggressive multimodality approach to treatment with surgery, chemotherapy, and radiotherapy. Radiation is used for localized unresectable disease in adolescents.

Thymoma

Thymoma is an epithelial tumour which can be encapsulated or locally invasive; metastatic spread is rare. Benign thymomas have been reported in childhood. In adults it is associated with systemic syndromes such as myasthenia gravis, pure red cell aplasia, and hypogammaglobulinaemia. Clinical presentation is often incidental upon chest radiography or with superior vena cava obstruction. CT scanning and MRI is necessary to delineate the extent of the tumour. Investigations to rule out other causes of anterior mediastinal masses, such as lymphoma, carcinoid tumour, and germ cell tumour, should be performed. Histological diagnosis may require electron microscopy and immunocytochemistry to identify the epithelial nature of the cells with certainty. Local excision may be followed by subsequent radiotherapy, if resection was incomplete. Tumour responses to a variety of platinum-containing regimens have been reported in adults (Dy *et al.* 1988) and require further evaluation.

Malignant mesothelioma

This tumour arises in the mesothelium of the pleura, pericardium, or peritoneum. Eighty cases have been reported in the world literature (Fraire *et al.* 1988).

Aetiology

The aetiological role of asbestos exposure is well documented in adults. Exposure to asbestos has only been demonstrated in a limited number of children with this tumour. If the same mechanism is involved in children, it would represent a shortened transformation time from mutagen exposure to tumour formation.

Pathology

The fibrous and sarcomatous histological subtypes are more common in childhood, whilst the epithelial subtypes are more common in adulthood. It is not possible to differentiate histologically between the malignant and benign tumours, but the majority (over 90 per cent) behave in a malignant way.

Clinical presentation

Pleural tumours present with signs and symptoms similar to other chest tumours. Peritoneal tumours present with abdominal distension and/or intestinal obstruction. These tumours spread over the mesothelial surface but do not penetrate deeply into tissues. Metastases are thought to be more common at presentation in children than in adults.

Treatment (malignant mesothelioma)

Successful treatment is dependent upon complete surgical resection. Responses to chemotherapy with CDDP and DX have been reported (MCG Stevens personal communication). In peritoneal mesothelioma, widespread dissemination of the tumour within the peritoneal cavity causes difficulty with tumour monitoring. We have had some success in the use of positron emission tomography (PET) in documenting tumour response to chemotherapy (M Hewitt personal communication). Radiotherapy is not considered an effective treatment.

ABDOMEN

Gastric carcinoma

Gastric carcinomas in children accounted for only 19 (3.8 per cent) of 501 cases in patients less than 30 years of age at diagnosis. They may be associated with features associated with ataxia telangiectasia and common variable immunodeficiency (Siegel *et al.* 1976; Conley *et al.* 1988). Clinical presentation is with weight loss, iron deficiency anaemia, and anorexia. Endoscopic or open biopsy will confirm the diagnosis. The tumours have a tendency to disseminate early and invade locally and so are usually unresectable. Radiotherapy is of little value. Promising results in adults have been reported with a variety of chemotherapy regimes, including fluorouracil, doxorubicin, and mitomycin (FAM), and CDDP alone and in combination with 5-fluorouracil, DX and VP16. Intraperitoneal CDDP has also been used to treat colonic spread (Cunningham 1989). Such treatment approaches require evaluation in children.

Colon and rectal carcinoma

Most of the 1 per cent of cases of large bowel malignancy which arise in patients less than 30 years of age are carcinomas (Anderson and Bergdahl 1978). Colon cancer is almost unheard of in infancy. The majority of reported cases occur during adolescence with boys affected twice as frequently as girls (Middelkamp and Haffner 1963). Histologically, the tumours are either mucus-secreting adenocarcinomas or poorly differentiated. Colonic polyps secondary to familial adenomatous polyposis predispose to the tumour (Miller *et al.* 1976). The association with ulcerative colitis is established, but carcinoma is unlikely to occur during childhood in view of the 10 year latent period between onset of inflammation and the increased risk of malignancy.

Clinical presentation is with rectal bleeding and abdominal pain with or without signs of intestinal obstruction. Diagnosis is made by biopsy at colonoscopy or laparotomy. Metastases should be looked for in the liver, lungs, and bone. Dukes' staging system is widely accepted and predicts for prognosis. Treatment requires tumour resection with hemicolectomy in tumours of the large bowel and a sphincter-sparing approach, if possible, in rectal tumours. Total colectomy should be considered if there is an associated predisposition such as familial adenomatous polyposis or ulcerative colitis. Childhood tumours seem to be more aggressive and more likely to spread through the peritoneum. Overall survival in childhood is 14–20 per cent (see Table 1) (La Quaglia *et al.* 1992). Recent work exploring the role of 5-fluorouracil given by infusion or in combination with folinic acid or IFN has shown improved response rates in adult patients, although there is significant toxicity (Cunningham 1989). Similar approaches should be considered in children.

Pancreatic tumours

Benign tumours of the pancreas in children are very rare and are either dermoid cysts or cystadenomas. Malignant tumours of the pancreas occur more commonly with an equal gender distribution (Kissane 1982). Standard classifications distinguished between pancreatic carcinoma, pancreaticoblastoma, and islet-cell tumours.

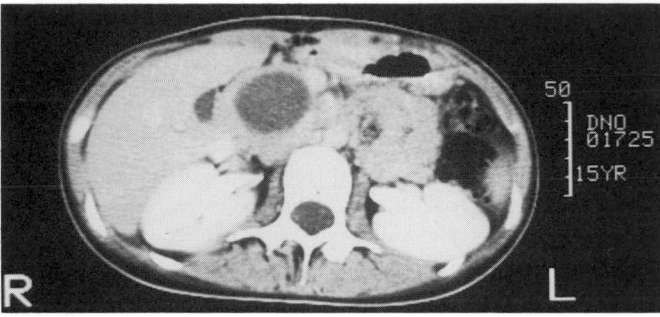

Fig. 3 CT scan showing pancreatic carcinoma.

A recent revised histological classification (Pysher *et al.* 1982) identifies four histological subtypes: (1) adenocarcinoma, (2) pleomorphic type with acinar differentiation, (3) solid and papillary type, and (4) islet-cell tumours. Pancreaticoblastomas are included in groups (2) and (3).

Clinical presentation

Clinical presentation is usually with an upper abdominal mass and pain. Rarely, there are also symptoms of disturbed exocrine pancreatic function (diarrhoea, weight loss), duodenal obstruction (vomiting, weight loss), or symptoms related to hormone secretion by the tumour such as gastric ulceration, hypoglycaemia, or diarrhoea.

Investigation

Tumour localization is best performed by ultrasound, CT scanning, and MRI (Fig. 3). A search for metastases in the liver, lungs, and bones should be undertaken. Endoscopic retrograde cholangio-pancreaticoduodenoscopy may be helpful in obtaining a cytological diagnosis. Surgical biopsy can be hazardous. Endocrine-secreting tumours may release a variety of peptides, including insulin, glucagon, somatomedins, ACTH, gastrin, and vasoactive intestinal peptide (VIP).

Treatment

Effective treatment depends upon complete tumour resection. The nature of the operative approach is dictated by the anatomical location of the tumour within the pancreas and the need for biliary diversion. Chemotherapy and radiotherapy may be considered in the event of unresectable or partially resected tumours and in adenocarcinoma, where the risk is of metastasis is high. A recent report of the successful use of pre-operative CDDP and 5-fluorouracil to improve operability is promising (Strauss *et al.* 1993). Streptozotocin, mitomycin C, DX and 5-fluorouracil have been used in adults (Smith and Schein 1979; Bukowski *et al.* 1982).

The extreme rarity of these tumours in childhood means that there is no standard method of management. Pysher *et al.* (1982) have recommended a 'wait and see' policy after surgery for the low-grade solid and papillary tumour types. The pleomorphic tumours (group 2) have a tendency to metastasize, perhaps justifying a more aggressive approach including chemotherapy. The endocrine disorders of islet cell tumours may also require specific management.

Adrenal carcinoma

Adrenal carcinoma is an unusual tumour in childhood since it is more common in girls than in boys (3–4:1 female to male) and has a bimodal age distribution, with peaks in the first 4 years and during adolescence. A 5 year survival rate of 24 per cent is reported by the CCRG (Table 1).

Aetiology

The aetiology of these tumours is unknown. However, their association with hemihypertrophy and brain neoplasms (Fraumeni and Miller 1967), together with association with cancer family syndromes (Hartley *et al.* 1987) and p53 germ-line mutations (Sameshima *et al.* 1992), are strongly suggestive of an inherited predisposition. The age distribution and a reported association with salt-losing adrenal hyperplasia (Bauman and Bauman 1982) suggest that endocrine mechanisms may play a part in tumour development.

Pathology

Differentiation between adenoma and carcinoma on histological grounds alone is difficult. Histological features of malignancy, including frequent mitoses, cellular pleomorphism, and vascular invasion, may be seen in both adenomas and carcinomas. Tumours of size less than 6 cm do well. Tumours of size greater than 6 cm (or 500 g in weight) are rarely cured by surgery alone (Neblett *et al.* 1987).

Clinical presentation

Clinical presentation may be with signs of virilization, cortisol excess, feminization, or a combination of these features. Less commonly, rapidly growing carcinomas present with abdominal pain, weight loss, and fever. Clinical examination reveals an abdominal mass but no evidence of endocrine disturbances.

Investigation

Endocrine investigations are directed at differentiating between an adrenal tumour, Cushing's disease, congenital adrenal hyperplasia, and premature adrenarche. The dexamethasone suppression test, measuring urinary 17-ketosteroid excretion, identifies the tumours by the failure of dexamethasone to suppress 17-ketosteroid production. Tumours are almost always independent of ACTH control and may be associated with markedly elevated basal urinary 17-ketosteroid production (more than 40 mg/24 h). Imaging with abdominal ultrasound, CT scans, and MRI will permit the definition of tumour size and local and distant spread. Vascular invasion of the inferior vena cava has been reported and its demonstration is important prior to attempts at surgical removal (Heijne and Venables 1987).

Treatment

Primary surgical removal has been the standard first treatment of choice. Great care is needed in the post-operative period to manage the rebound steroid deficiency that develops secondary to long-standing tumour suppression of ACTH secretion. Chemotherapy with mitotane (*o,p*'-DDD) has been used to control steroid side-effects and has been reported to reduce primary and secondary tumour size. However, most reports do not claim curative success with this treatment. Cytotoxic chemotherapy has generally been restricted to the treatment of relapse. Responses have been reported with combination regimes such as 5-fluorouracil, DX, and CDDP (Schlumberger *et al.* 1988), vincristine, *cis*-platinum, etoposide, and cyclophosphamide (OPEC) (Crock and Clark 1989), and etoposide and *cis*-platinum (VP-P) (Johnson and Greco 1986). Radiotherapy has been used to treat residual disease, but its efficacy is not established and a recent report of a second primary tumour within the radiation field is worrying (Squire *et al.* 1988).

Future directions

More precise methods of predicting the malignant potential of these tumours are needed. Tumour cytogenetics and studies of DNA ploidy seem worth investigating. Pre-operative chemotherapy of large invasive tumours might be considered in an attempt to alleviate difficulties encountered during surgery, thereby increasing the chances of complete resection. Trials of single agents are required.

PELVIS

Genital tract tumours

The majority of genital tract tumours in childhood are rhabdomyosarcomas or germ cell tumours. Carcinomas may occur throughout the genital tract in girls, whereas in boys they have only occasionally been reported in the testis (La Vecchia and Draper 1984).

Clear cell adenocarcinoma of the vagina and cervix

Aetiology

There is a long-established association between intrauterine exposure to diethylstilboestrol and an increased incidence of clear cell vaginal adenocarcinoma with vaginal adenosis (Greenwald et al. 1971; Herbst et al. 1971). Subsequent prospective screening of the 'at-risk' population established an association between intrauterine diethylstilboestrol exposure and vaginal and cervical adenosis, but not clear cell carcinoma as originally proposed (McFarlane et al. 1986). The use of diethylstilboestrol during pregnancy was widespread in the United States, but limited in the United Kingdom and was discontinued in 1971. Screening has been recommended for exposed children from the age of 14 years or from menarche (Emens 1984). Clinical presentation is with abnormal vaginal bleeding in the prepubertal and adolescent years.

Investigation and treatment

Diagnosis is by biopsy. A thorough vaginal examination and colposcopy examination is also required. The tumour is locally invasive and may metastasize to the lungs as well as local lymph nodes. Local treatment is dictated by the stage of the tumour at presentation. Interstitial or transvaginal radiotherapy is reserved for stage I tumours, thereby sparing the ovaries from ablative irradiation. More extensive disease has been treated by radical surgery followed by vaginal reconstruction or by external irradiation of the entire pelvis. Chemotherapy has not been explored except for the treatment of recurrent disease, but responses to CTX, melphalam (L-PAM), actinomycin D (ACD), and 5-fluorouracil have been reported (Cangir 1986; McWhirter et al. 1989).

Prognosis

Overall survival is approximately 80 per cent (stage I, 85 per cent; stage II, 70 per cent; stage III, 50 per cent; stage IV, 0 per cent) and older patients (over 19 years) fare better than younger patients (less than 15 years). The survival difference is attributable to the presence of tubulocystic differentiation, a 'favourable feature', in the older age group (Emens 1984). The extensive surgery or radiotherapy recommended in advanced stages has many long-term physical and psychological side-effects. Tumour shrinkage via early chemotherapy may permit less radical local treatment.

Tumours of the Fallopian tube

Malignant tumours of the Fallopian tubes in adolescence are extremely rare. Pure carcinomas and mixed Müllerian tumours have been reported. The latter are biphasic tumours containing both mesenchymal and carcinomatous elements (Spanos et al. 1984; Gatto et al. 1986). Conventional treatment approaches combine radical surgery and radiotherapy. Chemotherapy has rarely been used, but anecdotal reports of responses to chemotherapy with BEP in mixed Müllerian tumours justify further investigation in an attempt to reduce iatrogenic morbidity (Deppe et al. 1984).

Ovarian carcinoma

Adeno- or cystadenocarcinomas of the ovary account for less than 10 per cent of ovarian tumours in childhood (La Vecchia et al. 1983). The strong association between these tumours in adults and cancer families raises the possibility that the childhood presentation of this disease represents a more exaggerated predisposition.

Clinical presentation is with acute or chronic lower abdominal pain together with abdominal distension and a palpable mass. Ascites is commonly demonstrable. Pelvic and abdominal ultrasound is important for differentiating between solid and cystic masses. Most, but not all, cystic masses are benign (Thind et al. 1989). Surgery is recommended for solid, palpable, or calcified masses and for those associated with persistent fever to exclude appendix abscess. Where a tumour is suspected, unilateral oophorectomy with or without salpingectomy is recommended at surgery. Staging is performed at surgery according to the International Federation of Obstetrics and Gynecology system (FIGO). Serum CA 125, an epithelial carcinoma cell-line antigen, has been used to monitor tumour burden in adults; its role in children requires evaluation. Postoperative chemotherapy with combinations of CTX, hexamethylmelamine (HMM), CDDP, and DX have been used successfully in extensive disease (Raney et al. 1987). Second-look operations with random sampling of the peritoneum are necessary to monitor disease response. Abdominopelvic radiation may be used to treat the residual disease. Targeted radiotherapy with ^{131}I-labelled antibodies is being investigated in adults.

VASCULAR TUMOURS

Chemodectoma and glomus cell tumour

These are benign tumours developing in association with arteriovenous anastomoses in the subcutaneous tissue of the limbs with a predilection for the digits and nailbed. They may be hereditary (autosomal dominant) and multiple, occurring at any age from birth (Wood and Dimmick 1977). The solitary form rarely presents before adulthood. Clinical presentation is with a soft blue–black raised skin lesion which does not blanch on pressure and is often painful. Histologically, they are fatty lesions surrounded by glomus cells and fibrous tissue in association with muscular blood vessels. In patients with multiple tumours, treatment need only be offered if the lesion is symptomatic; local excision is successful.

Haemangiopericytoma

Haemangiopericytoma is a vascular tumour which can be benign or malignant. It may occur throughout the body (Fig. 4) and may present at any age from birth to old age (Jenkins 1987; van Baarlen et al. 1988). A review of 247 published cases demonstrated a relatively even distribution of tumour presentation throughout life,

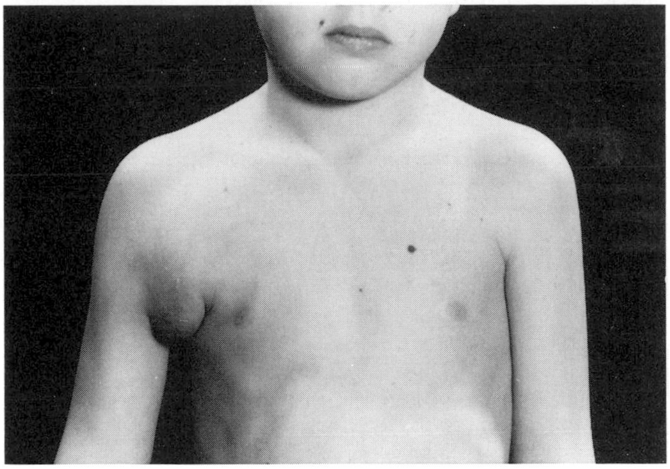

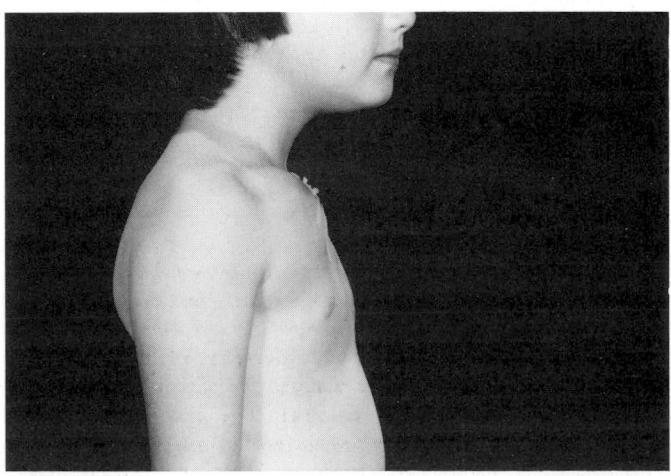

Fig. 4 Haemangiopericytoma.

with a peak in middle age (Backwinkel and Diddams 1970). Histologically, the tumour is composed of capillaries surrounded by elongated cells known as pericytes. Clinical presentation depends upon the tumour site; biopsy is essential for diagnosis. Tumour-associated hypoglycaemia has been reported in adults as a presenting feature and is thought to be secondary to the secretion of excessive quantities of insulin-like growth factors (Gorden *et al.* 1981).

Treatment is dependent upon the tumour site. Wide local excision has been the mainstay of treatment in adults, with a 50 per cent cure rate. However, the site of presentation seems to play a large part in the rate of local recurrence, with thoracic and mediastinal tumours recurring early (after less than a year) and central nervous system tumours having a high local recurrence rate later in the clinical course. The role of chemotherapy and radiotherapy has not been established, although well-documented responses to both modalities have been seen. Approaches to treatment similar to those used with rhabdomyosarcoma would seem appropriate in view of the sarcomatous nature of the tumour and the similar anatomical distribution.

PERIPHERAL MALIGNANT PRIMITIVE NEUROECTODERMAL TUMOURS

Malignant primitive neuroectodermal tumour or neuroepithelioma describes a collection of tumours thought to arise from the embryonic neural crest. They may arise in the nervous system or 'peripherally'. Peripheral malignant primitive neuroectodermal tumours are small round cell neoplasms with typical cytogenetic abnormalities t(11q:22q)(q24;q12) as well as histochemical, immunohistochemical, and electron microscopic features of neural crest origin. Whether they are developmentally related to primitive neuroectodermal tumours of the central nervous system is not clearly established. They may occur at almost any site within the trunk, limbs, or cervical region and up to 20 per cent may be metastatic at diagnosis (Kushner *et al.* 1991). A number of specific clinical entities have been described in this group of tumours including malignant primitive neuroectodermal tumour of bone, Askin's tumour (thoracopulmonary malignant primitive neuroectodermal tumour), malignant melanotic neuroectodermal tumour of infancy, and ectomesenchymoma (Dehner 1986).

Malignant primitive neuroectodermal tumour of bone and chest wall (Askin's tumour)

Jürgens *et al.* (1988) reported 42 patients with peripheral malignant primitive neuroectodermal tumours who were aged less than 23 years at diagnosis. The tumour was twice as common in boys than in girls and the median age at presentation was 15 years. Of these tumours, 24 were located in the thoracopulmonary region, six were in the abdomen and/or pelvis, four in the head and neck, and eight in the limbs; 74 per cent involved bone. A single congenital case has been described (Das *et al.* 1982). Of the 24 thoracopulmonary tumours reported by Jürgens *et al.* (1988), 15 were costal, five were vertebral, two were scapular, and two were sternal; 67 per cent were in boys and 33 per cent in girls.

Clinical presentation
Clinical presentation depends on the site of the tumour. Vanillylmandelic acid (VMA) excretion is generally not elevated. In the chest wall tumours, the external size of the mass is often misleading since there may be a large intrathoracic component invading the lung (Fig. 5).

Investigation
Tumour staging with radiography, CT and bone scanning, and bone-marrow aspirates should be performed to define the size and extent of the tumour and to look for evidence of metastatic spread to the bones, bone-marrow, or lung. The diagnosis is made by tumour biopsy, supported by immunocytochemical and electron microscopic appearances. Molecular studies may demonstrate a specific translocation t(11;22)(q24;q12) in tumour tissue.

Treatment
Treatment approaches to this tumour are not established. However, well-documented responses to both chemotherapy and radiotherapy have been reported. The effective chemotherapy agents include those commonly used to treat Ewing's tumour; that is, ifosfamide (ifos) or CTX, ACD, VCR, and DX. Local control of the primary with surgery and/or local radiotherapy is of paramount importance since local relapse is a common feature. The timing of tumour resection, if employed, is controversial. Some authors report

Fig. 5 Askin's tumour of the chest wall.

approaches with initial resection, whilst others report post-chemotherapy resection (Miser *et al.* 1987). At The Great Ormond Street Hospital for Sick Children we have used initial chemotherapy in an attempt to improve the chances of complete resection and to avoid the need for local high-dose radiotherapy. The presence of a pleural effusion at diagnosis poses a therapeutic dilemma in deciding on radiation fields, since whole-lung irradiation to therapeutic doses may be associated with a significant morbidity and a risk of mortality. With multimodality therapy, a 3 year survival rate of 50–60 per cent has been reported for those with localized disease. Those with metastatic disease at diagnosis have a worse prognosis (10–20 per cent).

Melanotic primitive neuroectodermal tumour of infancy (melanotic progonoma)

This malignant primitive neuroectodermal tumour is unusual in that it is made up of two populations of cells derived from the neural crest, neuroblasts and melanocytes. Ninety-five per cent of the tumours occur under the age of 1 year. Sites of origin include maxilla (69 per cent), skull (11 per cent), mandible (6 per cent), and brain (4 per cent), as well as a variety of other bony and soft tissues. It has a favourable prognosis, with a low malignant potential and low local recurrence risk (15 per cent) (Cutler *et al.* 1981).

Ectomesenchymoma (Triton tumour)

This is another tumour of neural crest tissue with heterologous cellular elements including ganglion cells, rhabdomyoblasts, melanocytes, Schwann cells, malignant fat cells, and cartilage elements (Karcioglu *et al.* 1977).

CONCLUSION

These rare tumours have been collected within a single chapter in order to promote interest in the registration of the rare tumour subtypes and to consider management approaches appropriate for children. Their rarity poses special problems as they form a group for which insufficient recent data are available to reach a 'best treatment consensus' and even national and international organizations have no established treatment protocols. The standard treatment approaches recommended have often evolved from adult practice, where surgery and radiotherapy are the mainstay of treatment, with chemotherapy being reserved for palliation at relapse. Such treatment approaches may cause unacceptable morbidity in the tissues of the growing child. The greater chemoresponsiveness of tumours in children when compared with the adult counterpart justifies a wider consideration of early high-dose chemotherapy in treatment planning. Such an approach offers the hope of improved cure rates with reduced morbidity.

REFERENCES

Few references published after 1990 are listed. The reader's attention is drawn to the proceedings of the XXIII meeting of the International Society of Paediatric Oncology (SIOP) where the focus of the meeting was on rare tumours of childhood. The abstracts are published in *Medical and Pediatric Oncology*, **19** (5), 1991.

Amendola BE, Amendola MA, Oliver E, McClatchey KD (1986). Chordoma: role of radiotherapy. *Radiology*, 158:839–43.
Anderson A, Bergdahl L (1978). Carcinoma of the colon in children: a report of six new cases and a review of the literature. *Journal of Pediatric Surgery*, 11:967–71.

Anderson AE, Bueghner HA, Yager I, Ziskind MM (1954). Brochogenic carcinoma in young men. *American Journal of Medicine*, March, 404–15.
Backwinkel KD, Diddams JA (1970). Hemangiopericytoma. *Cancer*, 25:896–901.
Barnes ND (1988). Effects of external irradiation on the thyroid gland in childhood. *Hormone Research*, 30:84–9.
Bauman A, Bauman CG (1982). Virilizing adrenocortical carcinoma. Development in a patient with salt-losing congenital adrenal hyperplasia. *Journal of the American Medical Association*, 248:3140–1.
Belani CP, Eisenberger MA, Gray WC (1988). Preliminary experience with chemotherapy in advanced salivary gland neoplasms. *Medical and Pediatric Oncology*, 16:197–202.
Bergholm U, *et al.* (1989). Clinical characteristics in sporadic and familial medullary thyroid carcinoma: a nationwide study of 249 patients in Sweden from 1959 through 1981. *Cancer*, 63:1196–204.
Black EG, Sheppard MC, Hoffenberg R (1987). Serial serum thyroglobulin measurements in the management of differentiated thyroid carcinoma. *Clinical Endocrinology*, 27:115–20.
Bukowski RM, Schacter LP, Groppe CW, Hewlett JS, Weick JK, Livingston RB (1982). Phase II trial of 5-fluorouracil, adriamycin, mitomycin C and streptozotocin (FAM-S) in pancreatic carcinoma. *Cancer*, 50:197–200.
Cangir A (1986). Malignant genital tract tumors in children. *Current Problems in Cancer*, 10(6):304–41.
Conley ME, Ziegler MM, Borden S, IV, Huff DS, Boyle JT (1988). Multifocal adenocarcinoma of the stomach in a child with common variable immunodeficiency. *Journal of Paediatric Gastroenterology and Nutrition*, 7:456–60.
Crock PA, Clark ACL (1989). Combination chemotherapy for adrenal carcinoma: response in a 5½-year-old male. *Medical and Pediatric Oncology*, 17:62–5.
Cunningham D (1989). Cytotoxic drugs for gastric and colorectal cancer. *British Medical Journal*, 299:1479–80.
Cussen LJ, MacMahon RA (1975). Congenital granular-cell myoblastoma. *Journal of Pediatric Surgery*, 10:249–53.
Cutler LS, Chaudhry AP, Topazian R (1981). Melanotic neuroectodermal tumor of infancy: an ultrastructural study, literature review, and re-evaluation. *Cancer*, 48:257–70.
Das L, Chang C-H, Cushing B (1982). Congenital primitive neuroectodermal tumor (neuroepithelioma) of the chest wall. *Medical and Pediatric Oncology*, 10:349–58.
Dehner LP (1986). Peripheral and central primitive neuro-ectodermal tumours. A nosologic concept seeking a consensus. *Archives of Pathology and Laboratory Medicine*, 110:97–105.
Deppe G, Zbella E, Friberg J, Thomas W (1984). Combination chemotherapy for mixed Müllerian tumor of the Fallopian tube. *Cancer*, 54:1517–20.
Dimery IW, Jacobs C, Tseng A, Saks S, Pearson G, Hong WK, Gutterman JU (1989). Recombinant interferon in the treatment of recurrent nasopharyngeal carcinoma. *Journal of Biological Response Modifiers*, 8:221–6.
Dy C, *et al.* (1988). Undifferentiated epithelial-rich invasive malignant thymoma: complete response to cisplatin, vinblastine, and bleomycin therapy. *Journal of Clinical Oncology*, 6:536–42.
Emens M (1984). Vaginal adenosis and diethylstilboestrol. *British Journal of Hospital Medicine* January, 42–8.
Ferguson TB, McCarthy KS, Filston HC (1987). Juvenile secretory carcinoma and juvenile papillomatosis: diagnosis and treatment. *Journal of Pediatric Surgery*, 22:637–9.
Fraire AE, Cooper S, Greenberg SD, Buffler P, Langston C (1988). Mesothelioma of childhood. *Cancer*, 62:838–47.
Fraumeni JF Jr, Miller RW (1967). Adrenocortical neoplasms with hemihypertrophy, brain tumors, and other disorders. *Journal of Pediatrics*, 70:129–38.
Gajwani BW, Devereaux JM, Beg JA (1980). Familial clustering of nasopharyngeal carcinoma. *Cancer*, 46:2325–7.
Gasparini M, Lombardi F, Rottoli L, Ballerini E, Morandi F (1988). Combined radiotherapy and chemotherapy in stage T_3 and T_4 nasopharyngeal carcinoma in children. *Journal of Clinical Oncology*, 6:491–6.
Gastpar H, Wilmes E, Wolf H (1981). Epidemiologic, etiologic, and immunologic aspects of nasopharyngeal carcinoma. *Journal of Medicine*, 12:257–84.
Gatto V, Selim MA, Lankerani M (1986). Primary carcinoma of the Fallopian tube in an adolescent. *Journal of Surgical Oncology*, 33:212–14.

Gindhart TD, Johnston WH, Chism SE, Dedo HH (1980). Carcinoma of the larynx in childhood. *Cancer*, **46**:1683–7.

Gorden P, Hendricks CM, Kahn CR, Roth J (1981). Hypoglycemia associated with non-islet-cell tumor and insulin-like growth factors. *New England Journal of Medicine*, **3**:1452–5.

Graham SM, Genel M, Touloukian RJ, Barwick KW, Gertner JM, Torony C (1987). Provocative testing for occult medullary carcinoma of the thyroid: findings in seven children with multiple endocrine neoplasia type IIa. *Journal of Pediatric Surgery*, **22**:501–3.

Greenwald P, Barlow JJ, Nasca PC (1971). Vaginal cancer after maternal treatment with synthetic estrogens. *New England Journal of Medicine*, **285**:390–2.

Hartley AL, Birch JM, Marsden HB, Reid H, Harris M, Blair V (1987). Adrenal cortical tumours: epidemiological and familial aspects. *Archives of Disease in Childhood*, **62**:683–9.

Heijne L, Venables HK (1987). Tumour spread to the inferior vena cava from an adrenal carcinoma. *Radiography*, **52**:78–80.

Herbst AL, Ulfelder H, Howard MD, Poskanzar DC (1971). Adenocarcinoma of the vagina: association of stilbestrol therapy with tumour appearance in young women. *New England Journal of Medicine*, **284**:878–81.

Ho JHC (1977). *Nasopharyngeal carcinoma: etiology and control*, pp. 99–113. International Agency for Research in Cancer, Lyon.

Holland-Morritz RM, Heyn RM (1984). Pulmonary blastoma associated with cystic lesions in children. *Medical and Pediatric Oncology*, **12**:85–8.

Jenkin RDT, Anderson JR, Jereb B, Thompson JC, Pyesmany A, Wara WM, Hammond D (1981). Nasopharyngeal carcinoma—a retrospective review of patients less than thirty years of age. A report from the Children's Cancer Study Group. *Cancer*, **47**:360–6.

Jenkins JJ III (1987). Congenital malignant hemangiopericytoma. *Pediatric Pathology*, **7**:119–22.

Jereb B, Huvos AG, Steinherz P, Abdurraham U (1980). Nasopharyngeal carcinoma in children: a review of 16 cases. *International Journal of Radiation Oncology—Biology—Physics*, **6**:487–91.

Joensuu H, Klemi P, Eerola E, Tuominen J (1986). Influence of cellular DNA content on survival in differentiated thyroid cancer. *Cancer*, **58**:2462–7.

Johnson DH, Greco FA (1986). Treatment of metastatic adrenal cortical carcinoma with cisplatin and etoposide (VP-16). *Cancer*, **58**:2198–202.

Jürgens H, *et al.* (1988). Malignant peripheral neuro-ectodermal tumours. A retrospective analysis of 42 patients. *Cancer*, **61**:349–57.

Karcioglu Z, Someren A, Mathes SJ (1977). Ectomesenchymoma. A malignant tumor of migratory neural crest (ectomesenchyme) remnants showing ganglionic, Schwannian, melaonocytic and rhabdomyoblastic differentiation. *Cancer*, **39**:2486–96.

Keeney GL, Unni KK, Beabout JW, Pritchard DJ (1989). Adamantimoma of long bones. A clinicopathological study of 85 cases. *Cancer*, **64**:730–7.

Keszler A, Dominguez FV (1986). Ameloblastoma in childhood. *Journal of Oral and Maxillofacial Surgery*, **44**:609–13.

Kim TH, *et al.* (1989). Adjuvant chemotherapy for advanced nasopharyngeal carcinoma in childhood. *Cancer*, **63**:1922–6.

Kirk JMW, Mort C, Grant D, Touzel RJ, Plowman N (1992). The usefulness of serum thyroglobulin in the follow-up of differentiated thyroid carcinoma. *Medical and Pediatric Oncology*, **20**:201–8.

Kissane JM (1982). Tumors of the exocrine pancreas in childhood. In *Cancer treatment and research* Vol. 8, *Pancreatic tumors in children* (ed. GB Humphrey, GB Grindley, LP Dehner, RT Acton, and TY Pysher), pp. 99–129. Nijhoff, The Hague.

Kushner BH, Hajdu SI, Gulati SC, Erlandson RA, Exelby PR, Lieberman PH (1991). Extracranial primitive neuroectodermal tumors. *Cancer*, **67**:1825–9.

La Quaglia MP, Corbally MT, Heller G, Exelby PR, Brennan MF (1988). Recurrence and morbidity in differentiated thyroid carcinoma in children. *Surgery*, **104**:1149–56.

La Quaglia MP, *et al.* (1992) Prognostic factors and outcome in patients 21 years and under with colorectal carcinoma. *Journal of Paediatric Surgery*, **27**:1085–90.

La Vecchia C, Morria HB, Draper GJ (1983). Malignant ovarian tumours in childhood in Britain 1962–78. *British Journal of Cancer*, **48**:363–74.

Lobo-Sanahuja F, Garcia I, Carranza A, Camacho A (1986). Treatment and outcome of undifferentiated carcinoma of the nasopharynx in childhood: a 13-year experience. *Medical and Pediatric Oncology*, **14**:6–11.

Lynn T-C, Tu S, Kanamura A (1985). Long term follow up of IgG and IgG antibodies against viral capsid antigen of Epstein–Barr virus in nasopharyngeal carcinoma. *Journal of Laryngology and Otology*, **99**:567–72.

McFarlane MJ, Feinstein ER, Horwitz RI (1986). Diethylstilbestrol and clear cell vaginal carcinoma. Reappraisal of the epidemiological evidence. *American Journal of Medicine*, **81**:855–63.

McWhirter WR, Stiller CA, Lennox EL (1989). Carcinomas in childhood. A registry-based study of incidence and survival. *Cancer*, **63**:2242–6.

Manivel JC, Priest JR, Watterson J, Steiner M, Woods WG, Wick MR, Dehner LP (1988). Pleuropulmonary blastoma: the so-called pulmonary blastoma of childhood. *Cancer*, **62**:1516–26.

Merrick Y, Hansen HS (1989). Thyroid cancer in children and adolescents in Denmark. *European Journal of Surgical Oncology*, **15**:49–53.

Middelkamp JN, Haffner H (1963). Carcinoma of the colon in children. *Pediatrics*, **32**:558–71.

Mies C, Rosen PP (1987). Juvenile fibroadenoma and atypical epithelial hyperplasia. *American Journal of Surgical Pathology*, **11**:184–90.

Miller MS, Costanza ME, Li FP, Stolbach L, Stone R, Nathanson L (1976). Familial colon cancer. *Cancer*, **37**:946–8.

Miser JS, *et al.* (1987). Treatment of peripheral neuroepithelioma in children and young adults. *Journal of Clinical Oncology*, **5**:1752–9.

Müller-Gärtner H-W, Schneider C (1988). Clinical evaluation of tumour characteristics predisposing serum thyroglobulin to be undetectable in patients with differentiated thyroid cancer. *Cancer*, **61**:976–81.

Neblett WW, Frexes-Steed M, Scott HW Jr (1987). Experience with adrenocortical neoplasms in childhood. *American Surgeon*, **53**:117–25.

Pao WJ, Douglass EC, Beckford NS, Kun LE (1989). *International Journal of Radiation Oncology—Biology—Physics*, **17**:299–305.

Papavasiliou C, Pavlatou M, Pappas J (1977). Nasopharyngeal cancer in patients under the age of thirty years. *Cancer*, **40**:2312–16.

Pysher T, Humphrey GB, Wilson SD, Schein PS, Donaldson SS, Bukowski RM, Kissane J (1982). Overview of childhood pancreatic tumors. In *Cancer treatment and research* Vol. 8, *Pancreatic tumours in children* (ed. GB Humphrey, GB Grindley, LP Dehner, RT Acton, and TJ Pysher), pp. 201–13. Nijhoff, The Hague.

Raney RB, Sinclair L, Uri A, Schnaufer L, Cooper A, Littman P (1987). Malignant ovarian tumours in children and adolescents. *Cancer*, **59**:1214–20.

Reddy EK, Mansfield CM, Hartman GV (1981). Chordoma. *International Journal of Radiation Oncology—Biology—Physics*, **7**:1709–11.

Richardson JE, Beaugie JM, Brown CL, Doniach I (1974). Thyroid cancer in young patients in Great Britain. *British Journal of Surgery*, **61**:85–9.

Rubenstein D, Shanker D, Finlayson L, Boxall L, Krafchik B (1987). Multiple cutaneous granular tumours in childhood. *Pediatric Dermatology*, **4**:94–7.

Ryff-de Leche A, Staub J-J, Kohler-Faden R, Müller-Brand J, Heitz PU (1986). Thyroglobulin production by malignant thyroid tumours. *Cancer*, **57**:1147–53.

Sala E, Olsen JH (1993). Thyroid cancer in the age group 0–19: time trends and temporal changes in radioactive fallout. *European Journal of Cancer*, **29A**:1443–5.

Sameshima Y, *et al.* (1992). Detection of novel germ-line p53 mutations in diverse-cancer-prone families identified by selecting patients with childhood adreno-cortical carcinoma. *Journal of National Cancer Institute*, **84**:703–7.

Schlumberger M, de Vathaire F, Travagli JP, Vassal G, Lemerle J, Parmentier C, Tubiana M (1987). Differentiated thyroid carcinoma in childhood: long term follow-up of 72 patients. *Journal of Clinical Endocrinology and Metabolism*, **65**:1088–94.

Schlumberger M, Ostronoff M, Bellaiche M, Rougier P, Droz J-P, Parmentier C (1988). 5-Fluorouracil, doxorubicin, and cisplatin regimen in adrenal cortical carcinoma. *Cancer*, **61**:1492–4.

Schnadig VJ, Clark WD, Clegg TJ, Yao CS (1986). Invasive papillomatosis and squamous carcinoma complicating juvenile laryngeal papillomatosis. *Archives of Otolaryngology and Head and Neck Surgery*, **112**:966–71.

Schroder DM, Chambers A, France CJ (1986). Operative strategy for thyroid cancer. Is total thyroidectomy worth the price? *Cancer*, **58**:2320–8.

Seifter EJ, Ihde DC (1988). Therapy of small cell lung cancer: a perspective on two decades of clinical research. *Seminars in Oncology*, **15**:278–99.

Shikhani AH, Johns ME (1988). Tumours of the major salivary glands in children. *Head and Neck Surgery*, **10**:257–63.

Siegel SE, Hays DM, Romansky S, Isaacs H (1976). Carcinoma of the stomach in childhood. *Cancer*, **38**:1781–4.

Smith FP, Schein PS (1979). Chemotherapy of pancreatic cancer. *Seminars in Oncology*, **6**:368–77.

Spanos WJ Jr, Wharton JT, Gomez L, Fletcher GH, Oswald MJ (1984). Malignant mixed Müllerian tumors of the uterus. *Cancer*, **53**:311–16.

Squire R, Bianchi A, Jakate SM (1988). Radiation-induced sarcoma of the breast in a female adolescent. *Cancer*, **60**:2444–7.

Strauss JF, Hirsch VJ, Rubey CN, Pollock M (1993). Resection of a solid and papillary epithelial neoplasm of the pancreas following treatment with *cis*-platinum and 5-fluorouracil: a case report. *Medical and Pediatric Oncology*, **21**:365–7.

Tannock I, Payne D, Cummings B, Hewitt K, Panzarella T and The Princess Margaret Hospital Head and Neck Cancer Group (1987). Sequential chemotherapy and radiation for nasopharyngeal cancer: absence of long term benefit despite a high rate of tumour response to chemotherapy. *Journal of Clinical Oncology*, **5**:629–34.

Taxy JB (1977). Juvenile nasopharyngeal angiofibroma. An ultrastructural study. *Cancer*, **39**:1044–54.

Thind CR, Carty HM, Pilling DW (1989). The role of ultrasound in the management of ovarian masses in children. *Clinical Radiology*, **40**:180–2.

Torres AM, Ryckman FC (1988). Childhood tracheobronchial mucoepidermoid carcinoma: a case report and review of the literature. *Journal of Pediatric Surgery*, **23**:367–70.

Tubiana M, *et al.* (1985). Long term results and prognostic factors in patients with differentiated thyroid cancer. *Cancer*, **55**:794–804.

van Baarlen J, Drogtrop AdP, Bax NMA (1988). Congential hemangiopericytoma. *Pediatric Pathology*, **8**:109–15.

Venook AP, Tseng A Jr, Meyers FJ, Silverberg I, Boles R, Fu KK, Jacobs CD (1987). Cisplatin, doxorubicin and 5-fluorouracil chemotherapy for salivary gland malignancies: a pilot study of the North California Oncology Group. *Journal of Clinical Oncology*, **5**:951–5.

Viallet J, Ihde DC (1989). Systemic therapy for small cell lung cancer: old themes replayed, new ones awaited. *Journal of Clinical Oncology*, **7**:985–7.

Wood WS, Dimmick JE (1977). Multiple infiltrating glomus tumours in children. *Cancer*, **40**:1680–5.

Section 15
Tumours of the central nervous system

15.1 Brain tumours in children

CLIFFORD C. BAILEY AND DAVID SPOONER

INTRODUCTION

A brain tumour in a child presents the greatest challenge to face the neurosurgeon, paediatric radiotherapist, and paediatric oncologist. The therapeutic team is faced with the problem of a neoplasm in the developing central nervous system (CNS) and must therefore devise therapeutic approaches which not only eradicate the neoplasm but which respect the immediate and long-term function of the CNS. Improved neurosurgical technique along with improved anaesthesia have, in recent years, made the 'total' removal of intracranial neoplasms in children a more frequently achieved goal, with improved survival rates. Radiotherapy remains the major treatment modality after surgery and is essential to achieve a cure in most of the malignant neoplasms. However, its rôle in the treatment of 'benign' neoplasms is controversial and over recent years the damaging effect of radiotherapy on the developing brain has become increasingly apparent. The effects are more marked in younger children and particularly in those under the age of 3 years at the time when they receive their radiotherapy. Therefore, new strategies need to be developed to improve survival in this age-group while avoiding the use of radiotherapy until after the full development of the brain has taken place. Chemotherapy has been explored increasingly in the therapy of brain tumours in children in the past decade. It is clear that many chemotherapeutic agents and multiagent schedules can produce significant tumour responses. It is the hope of all therapists working in this field that the next decade will see the translation of these responses into long-term cures.

INCIDENCE AND PREDISPOSING CONDITIONS

Brain tumour is the commonest non-haematological malignancy in childhood, with an incidence of 2.5 cases per 100 000 children per year. The tumours can occur from the neonatal period through into adult life; however, there is a peak incidence between the ages of 5 and 10 years. Males develop tumours slightly more frequently than females with a male : female ratio of 60 : 40. Brain tumours occur in children of all racial origins but are less common in Black populations (Davies 1973; Williams 1975).

The majority of children presenting with a primary intracranial neoplasm have no discernible predisposing factor. However, a small number of children will be found who have a hereditary neurocutaneous disorder. The most common of these is neuro-fibromatosis, but associations have been described with tuberous sclerosis and von Hippel—Lindau angiomatosis.

Medulloblastoma in childhood has been associated with the basal cell naevus syndrome. This is an inherited disorder characterized by cutaneous tumours, skeletal abnormalities, pitting of the skin of the hands and the feet, and central nervous system anomalies. Medulloblastoma may occasionally be the first manifestation of the disease. Tumour genesis in this syndrome may be associated with a defect in DNA synthesis and/or repair. It has been observed that there are familial clusters of patients with brain tumour. These may be associated with some of the above syndromes but, in addition,

increased incidences of brain tumours in children have been seen in members of cancer-prone families who have a variety of otherwise unrelated malignant diseases (Li *et al.* 1976). An increased incidence of brain tumour has also been described in children suffering from other primary neoplasms, including adrenocortical tumours, adenocarcinoma of the colon, acute leukaemia, hepatocellular carcinoma, and rhabdoid kidney tumours (Wriggleson *et al.* 1965; Fraumeni and Miller 1967).

Brain tumours are also reported in children with hereditary immunodeficiency syndromes, in particular, children with ataxia telangiectasia have developed medulloblastoma and glioma. This is a particularly important subset of children to recognize because of the great dangers associated with treating such children with radiotherapy.

It has been suggested (van de Wiel 1960) that brain tumours occur with increased frequency in children with major congenital defects of the spine and skull.

CLINICAL PRESENTATION

The clinical presentation of brain tumours in childhood depends on the age of the child and the position of the tumour. Seventy per cent of childhood brain tumours are situated in the posterior fossa and 30 per cent in the supratentorial regions.

The physical signs of a brain tumour in a child clearly depend on the position of the tumour. Tumours in the posterior fossa present with physical signs attributable to cerebellar infiltration and raised intracranial pressure. Infiltration or stretching of meninges in this area may give rise to neck stiffness or head tilt. Physical examination of the child will reveal ataxia which may affect predominantly the trunk or be lateralized to the limbs. Nystagmus is commonly present and a sixth nerve palsy may be demonstrable, this being a false localizing sign associated with a raised intracranial pressure. Examination of the optic fundi will reveal papilloedema and this may be associated with decreased visual acuity. In cases of severe raised intracranial pressure there will be lethargy, confusion, and ultimately progression to coma.

Tumours in the brainstem rarely give rise to raised intracranial pressure but present with physical signs attributable to infiltration in this area. There will usually therefore be a combination of cranial nerve palsy, long-tract signs, and ataxia. Children with brainstem tumours have sometimes presented with behavioural disturbance.

Tumours in the hypothalamic area have been associated with a variety of somatic symptoms. These include the symptoms of failure of the hypothalamic pituitary axis, with growth failure and diabetes insipidus. There may be delayed puberty or sexual precocity. The syndrome of failure to thrive, which has been called the diencephalic syndrome, is associated with a tumour in the anterior part of the hypothalamus and the child will be found to have growth failure despite an apparently adequate calorific intake. Visual loss due to involvement of the optic chiasm and the optic nerves is a frequent presenting sign.

INVESTIGATION AND MANAGEMENT

A plain radiograph of the skull should be taken in anteroposterior and lateral views. In the young infant this may reveal separation of the cranial sutures and in chronic raised intracranial pressure may show erosion of the dorsum of the cella tursica. Intracranial calcification may be seen in the supracellar region in cases of craniopharyngioma. Calcification in the cerebral hemispheres occasionally occurs with gliomas, ependymomas, and ogliodendrogliomas.

The electroencephalogram may occasionally be helpful in localizing a supratentorial tumour. However, in the vast majority of children's tumours situated in the posterior fossa it is of no value.

Computerized tomography (**CT**) scanning is the major diagnostic tool now used for the investigation of childhood brain tumours. A CT scan with intravenous injection of contrast to enhance abnormal tissue will be successful in delineating the vast majority of childhood tumours. Areas of difficulty lie in the detection of tumours in or around the base of the skull, in the brainstem, and, occasionally in a child who has difficulty in flexing the neck, there may be problems in delineating small tumours in the posterior fossa. In the follow-up of children who have had surgery for brain tumour the CT scan can be a useful diagnostic tool; however, its interpretation may be difficult. In the immediate post-operative period the occurrence of haematoma in the operative field and of surrounding oedema makes it impossible to assess the amount of residual tumour after surgery and scans for this purpose should be carried out within 3 days of the date of surgery, when these effects are minimal.

Myelography should be carried out as a post-operative investigation in children in whom the pathological diagnosis is one of medullo-blastoma, primitive neuroectodermal tumour, or ependymoblastoma. Between 10 and 20 per cent of chilren with these diagnoses will be demonstrated to have clinically silent intraspinal disease. In the recent International Society for Paediatric Oncology (**SIOP**) II study, 28 out of 186 children undergoing myelography in the post-operative period were demonstrated to have previously unsuspected intraspinal tumour deposits. In none of the children was myelography followed by any significant complication. Greater sensitivity can be obtained if the myelogram is combined with CT scanning of the spine.

Nuclear magnetic resonance imaging (**MRI**) seems to give greater sensitivity than CT scanning for the examination of the brain and spinal cord. The images obtained on MRI can be enhanced by the use of intravenous gadolinium, further increasing the sensitivity of the technique. This is particularly important if MRI is to be used to detect occult spinal disease, as early experience suggests that the sensitivity of MRI without gadolinium enhancement is less than that of CT myelography.

RADIOTHERAPY TECHNIQUE

The localization of megavoltage radiotherapy in the radical treatment of paediatric CNS tumours is a precise and careful art. It is dependent on the skill of mould-room technicians in making appropriate shells, radiation physicists in accurately determining dosimetry and careful localization of the tumour volume using the latest imaging techniques, and the natural history and the surgical findings for each individual tumour.

Craniospinal radiotherapy is commonly employed in the management of tumours which are likely to seed throughout the meninges, such as medulloblastoma, infratentorial ependymoblastoma, and primitive neuroectodermal tumour. A prone custom-made shell for each patient, made from lightweight plastic material using a mould injection technique, restrains the patient in an accurately reproduceable position. Care must be taken to include the whole of the meningeal system, yet sparing normal tissues. The lens is

particularly sensitive and lithium fluoride can be used in certain measurements to monitor the given dose. The junction of fields has to be calculated carefully to avoid under- or overdosage. This is particularly relevant when fields abut from different planes, for example the two lateral fields used to treat the whole brain join the direct spinal field at the vertebral level of C3. Some centres have overcome this problem by altering the level of this junction two or three times during a course of treatment.

It is no longer necessary to widen the spinal field at the cauda equina. In girls this practice caused ovarian failure without a demonstrable reduction in meningeal recurrence at this site.

A supine cast is used for patients who are receiving whole-brain radiotherapy only (for example, in the treatment of acute lymphoblastic leukaemia) or patients with anterior or superior primary tumours.

It has been suggested that in children under the age of 6 years, the central cribriform plate overlaps the upper third of the orbit and therefore cannot be totally included in two lateral fields if the orbits are to be shielded to reduce the dose to the lens (Williams 1987). Some centres have boosted the anterior central volume with a direct electron field (Hardy *et al.* 1978), but the clinical value of this remains to be demonstrated.

On combining whole-CNS radiotherapy with cytotoxic chemotherapy (in the treatment of medulloblastoma, for example), it is probably prudent to perform a full blood count at least at weekly intervals during the course of external-beam radiotherapy and every 2 weeks for 4 weeks afterwards. It would be unwise to proceed with radiotherapy if the platelet count falls below $40\times10^9/l$ or if neutrophil levels fall to below $1\times10^9/l$.

INFRATENTORIAL TUMOURS

Approximately 70 per cent of childhood brain tumours are situated in the infrantentorial region. Thirty per cent of these tumours will be cerebellar astrocytomas, a further 30 per cent medulloblastomas, approximately 15 per cent will be brainstem tumours, which are usually astrocytic lesions, 10 per cent of the tumours will be ependymomas, and the rest of the tumours in this region will be of miscellaneous mixed diagnoses.

Cerebellar astrocytoma

Cerebellar astrocytoma is one of the more favourable primary CNS paediatric malignancies. Its peak incidence occurs in children aged between 5 and 10 years. It is often a cystic space-occupying lesion with an associated mural nodule.

Histological subtypes are recognized: the commoner low-grade tumour, which tends to be circumscribed and slowly growing in the majority of cases (75 per cent 5 year disease-free survival) and the more diffuse higher-grade astrocytomas, with a poorer prognosis (30–40 per cent 5 year disease-free survival) (Gol and McKissock 1959). Complete surgical resection is possible in at least 65 per cent of tumours, which usually prove to be the low-grade circumscribed type. In completely resected tumours and tumours of grade I–II there is a very low risk of recurrence. However, in up to 35 per cent of tumours only a subtotal resection is possible. The established practice is to offer patients with subtotal resection or high-grade tumours local radiotherapy, using a prone shell and giving 4500–5000 cGy in 30 daily fractions over 6 weeks.

A prospective controlled trial of delayed versus immediate post-operative radiotherapy in these children has not been performed, because of the rarity of this tumour and its long natural history.

Therefore the clear contribution of immediate post-operative radiotherapy is unknown.

Locally recurrent disease can occur many years later and subsequent treatment will be palliative, whether surgery, re-irradiation, cytotoxic chemotherapy, or interstitial implantation.

Medulloblastoma

The medulloblastoma is a malignant tumour originating in the vermis of the cerebellum. Its histological origin is still uncertain. It may arise from the outer granular layer of the cerebellum, which is a cell layer developing from embryonal precursors in the area of the roof of the fourth ventricle. These cells migrate in a dorsolateral direction towards the surface of the cerebellum, where they form the matrix cells of the inner granular layer during the development of the cerebellum. During the first year of life the outer granular layer disappears, but it is possible that small groups of cells able to proliferate may remain. It is assumed that these cells may be the origin of medulloblastomas. An alternative view is that the medulloblastomas originate from undifferentiated cells in the subependymal region in the roof of the fourth ventricle. These cells have the ability to differentiate into neuronal and glial cells and they are found at all ages and in various areas of the brain, in particular in the area of the fourth ventricle, in the cerebellum, and in those parts of the pallidum, nucleus caudatus, and thalamus which are next to the ventricles. Medulloblastoma-like tumours found in these areas are described as primitive neuroectodermal tumours.

Histologically, medulloblastoma occurs in two common forms.

1. The so-called classical type of medulloblastoma, which consists of a tumour with densely packed oval or carrot-shaped cells with hyperchromatic nuclei and a thin rim of cytoplasm. Mitotic activity is usually present within the tumour, as are areas of necrosis, although these are usually in the form of single-cell necrosis rather than larger areas of necrotic tissue. Approximately one-third of cases of classical medulloblastoma show evidence of neurone differentiation, with the cells forming Homer–Wright rosettes. Immunohistochemical staining of the tumours gives further evidence for neuronal differentiation, with the presence of neurofilament protein and neurone-specific enolase being demonstrated. Glial differentiation can be seen in the occurrence of regular structures, with palisade formation of the nuclei of tumour cells and uni- or bipolar cell processes resembling spongioblasts. Staining for glial fibrillary acidic protein can be seen in approximately 50 per cent of the tumours.

2. The so-called desmoplastic variant. The desmoplastic medulloblastoma is commonly localized in the lateral parts of the cerebellar hemispheres and grows preferentially into the pia and arachnoid mater. It is characterized histologically by islands of light appearance which are free of reticulin within a tumour characterized by a dense net of connective tissue (Burger et al. 1987).

The tumour infiltrates into the adjacent cerebellar tissue and into the fourth ventricle. As the tumour progresses, the fourth ventricle is crossed and the brainstem may be invaded. Tumour cells may be exfoliated from the surface of the tumour and be disseminated through the cerebrospinal fluid pathways. Cells may be found in cerebrospinal fluid removed at operation and before mobilization of the tumour and if myelography is undertaken in the immediate post-operative period, deposits of tumour may be demonstrated in the spinal canal of up to 20 per cent of patients. The tumour may rarely metastasize outside the central nervous system, when the most common sites for metastases will be in bone and the lymph nodes. Occasional patients have been described in which a tumour has disseminated through cerebrospinal fluid shunt pathways and peritoneal seedlings have been formed. In the recent SIOP study of 364 children with medulloblastoma, 7 children developed extracranial metastases, of whom 5 had shunts in situ. In some patients who present with life-threatening raised intracranial pressure the placing of a cerebrospinal fluid shunt may be essential. However, it should be avoided in all other patients. It is usually possible to restore the cerebrospinal fluid pathway during the primary removal of the tumour. At surgery the goal should be to remove as much of the tumour as possible. Jenkin et al. (1990) suggested that the surgeons determination of total removal was a strong prognostic indicator. However, in neither the CCSG study (Evans et al. 1990) nor the SIOP II study was it shown to be an independent variable. Surgery alone can never be curative in medulloblastoma. Radiotherapy is necessary to eradicate the microscopic residual disease which is always present after the completion of surgery.

CHEMOTHERAPY OF BRAIN TUMOUR

Brain tumours present a particular challenge to the chemotherapist. These tumours have been shown to have marked heterogeneity within their structure. The cells within the brain tumour may differ morphologically and cytogenetically one from the other. Within different areas of the tumour the cytokinetic characteristics of the cells also vary. In the centre of tumours many cells will be in a resting phase, while towards the edge of a tumour far more cells will be involved in active division. Studies of the integrity of the blood–brain barrier in brain tumours have shown that in the central areas of the tumour the blood–brain barrier is disrupted while at the growing edge of the tumour, at the brain–tumour interface, the blood–brain barrier appears still to be intact. In early studies it was thought that for a chemotherapeutic agent to be effective in the treatment of a brain tumour it had to have the ability to cross the blood–brain barrier. This meant that the molecule had to be highly lipid-soluble, non-ionized, and had to have a demonstrated lack of protein binding. However, more recent work has demonstrated that blood-to-tissue transport is increased in the brain tumours (Vick et al. 1977) and, thus, water-soluble chemotherapeutic agents may well have a greater rôle in the therapy of these tumours than was originally supposed. Large numbers of drugs have been used as single-agent therapy against recurrent tumours. Agents showing activity include vincristine (Rosenstock et al. 1976), procarbazine (Edwards et al. 1980), etoposide (**VP-16**) (Tirelli et al. 1984), carmustine (**BCNU**) and lomustine (**CCNU**) (Wilson et al. 1976), cyclophosphamide (Edwards et al. 1980), cisplatin (Walker and Allen 1988), carboplatin (Allen et al. 1987a), methotrexate (Djerassi et al. 1985), and dibromolducitol (Levin et al. 1984).

In recent years several large cooperative trials have studied the efficacy of multiple chemotherapeutic agents as adjuvant chemotherapy in children following surgery and radiotherapy and these have begun to show survival advantages for those children receiving the chemotherapy. In an attempt to further capitalize on this advance, recent studies have been constructed in which chemotherapy is administered in the time interval between surgery and radiotherapy. The rationale of this manoeuvre is to take advantage of a time period in which the permeability of the tumour to the drug is at its greatest because of disruption of the blood–brain barrier and when the blood flow into the tumour is also maximal because of the tumour neovascularization, which will inevitably be reduced by the delivery of radiotherapy. In the future it may be possible for therapeutic strategies to be developed whereby chemotherapy is delivered to the patient as their primary therapy. This may have the advantage of reducing tumour size and enabling more complete removal of the tumour to be achieved at a subsequent neurosurgical operation.

Chemotherapeutic trials

Two major randomized studies of chemotherapy have been carried out in the treatment of medulloblastoma. The Children's Cancer Study Group (**CCSG**) followed a design in which all patients received the maximum possible surgical tumour removal, followed by radiation therapy to the cranium and spine with a boost to the tumour-bearing area in the posterior fossa. Upon completion of the radiotherapy, children were randomly assigned to receive no further therapy or to receive eight cycles of chemotherapy consisting of vincristine, lomustine, and prednisolone. The structure of the SIOP study was very similar to the CCSG study, the children being assigned on the completion of surgery and radiotherapy to receive either no further therapy or eight cycles of chemotherapy utilizing vincristine and lomustine. In the two studies, the 5 year relapse-free survival rate of the children randomized to treatment with surgery and radiation therapy alone was 49.4 per cent, whereas that for children receiving chemotherapy was 59.5 per cent and 56.3 per cent, respectively (Evans *et al.* 1990; Tait *et al.* 1990) (Fig. 1).

Retrospective analysis of the data in both studies revealed that a child with a small tumour which had been totally removed, who had no evidence of involvement in the brainstem and in whom there was no demonstrable evidence of dissemination of his tumour, fell into a 'good' prognostic group, whereas those children with less than total removal, brainstem involvement, or evidence of disease dissemination fell into the 'poor' prognostic group. When these groups were further analysed for the benefit or otherwise of chemotherapy, it became clear that children in the 'good' prognostic group derived little benefit from the receipt of chemotherapy, whereas those in the 'poor' prognostic group appeared to derive a greater benefit. As a result of these studies, both groups have now gone on to perform second studies, basing their therapeutic strategies upon division of the patients into 'good' and 'poor' prognostic groups. For 'good' prognosis patients, both study groups elected to address the same question: whether or not a reduction in the dose of radiotherapy given to the cranium and spine while maintaining the dose of radiation therapy administered to the posterior fossa could be made without jeopardizing disease-free survival and whether such a reduction would result in a reduction in late effects of radiation therapy on the developing brain. In addition, the SIOP group explored the question as to whether a pulse of chemotherapy given immediately following surgery and before radiotherapy would further enhance disease-free survival. The CCSG study was terminated because of an unacceptable rate of spinal relapse in the reduced rate arm, whilst the SIOP study showed an interaction between chemotherapy and reduced dose radiotherapy in which patients whose radiotherapy was (i) delayed by chemotherapy and (ii) reduced in dose to the 'prophylactic' fields did less well (Fig. 2). For 'poor' prognostic patients the CCSG study compares the disease-free survival outcome for patients treated with vincristine, lomustine, and prednisolone upon completion of surgery and radiotherapy with that obtained with two doses of the 'eight drugs in 1 day' chemotherapy schedule, as described by Pendergrass

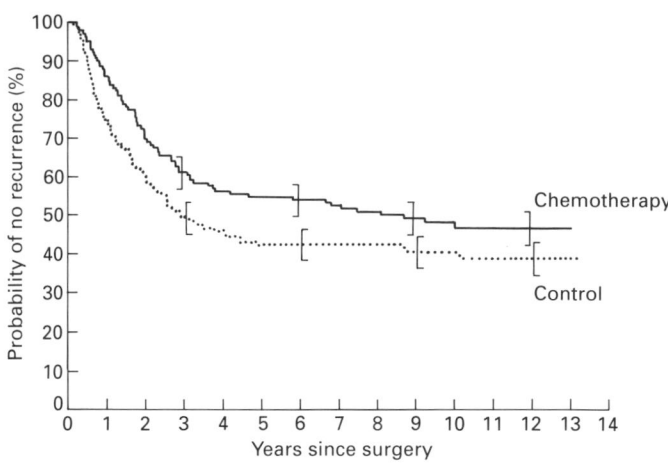

Fig. 1 SIOP I medullablastoma trial. Disease-free survival by treatment regime. Treatment outcome in 286 patients with biopsy proven medullablastoma treated with surgery and radiotherapy followed by chemotherapy with vincristine and CCNU or not treated.

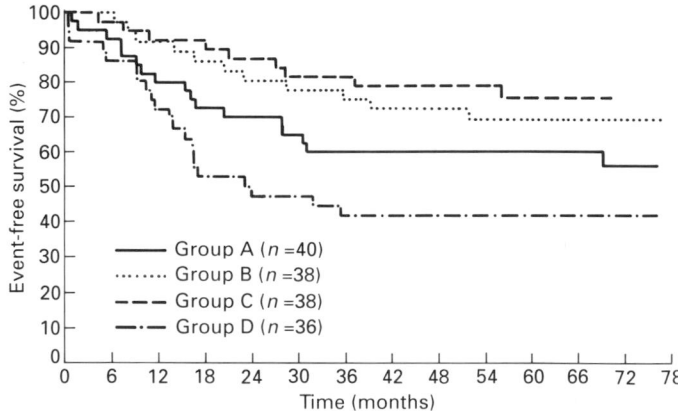

Fig. 2 SIOP I medullablastoma trial. Event-free survival for low-risk patients by randomly assigned therapy. Group A received standard radiotherapy alone, group B received reduced radiotherapy alone, group C received sandwich chemotherapy followed by standard radiotherapy, and group D received sandwich chemotherapy followed by reduced dose chemotherapy.

et al. (1987), administered before radiotherapy and a further six doses after radiotherapy. This study has not diminished any advantage of the 'eight i̅ i̅ chemotherapy over vincristine and CCNU.

Ependymoma

Ependymomas account for approximately 10 per cent of childhood brain tumours. They can originate throughout the CNS but occur most frequently in the fourth ventricular region. They occur most frequently in children under the age of 5 years (Kun *et al.* 1988). Ependymomas have been classified as being of low grade or benign nature in approximately 75 per cent of cases and of high-grade anaplastic malignant lesions in approximately 25 per cent of cases. However, this classification can be confused by the occurrence within a single tumour of areas of relative differentiation and areas of anaplasia. Some authorities therefore believe that all ependymomas should be regarded as having malignant potential.

The malignant tumours spread by seeding throughout the cerebrospinal fluid and an incidence of 12 per cent has been reported, largely associated with tumours of an anaplastic nature situated in the infratentorial area.

The therapeutic approach to ependymoma therefore parallels that of medulloblastoma. Initial therapy should be the surgical removal of the tumour and the surgeon should aim to remove all tumour tissue completely. Following surgery, radiation therapy should be given, at a dose of a minimum of 55 Gy to the tumour-bearing area. Controversy has surrounded the need for extended-field radiation therapy to cover the cerebrospinal fluid pathways. In patients in whom there is any evidence of anaplasia within the tumour or, and in particular, if the tumour is situated in the posterior fossa, it is recommended that whole-CNS radiation therapy is employed, whereas for differentiated tumours and tumours outside the posterior fossa involved-field radiation may be sufficient therapy. However, survival rates for children with ependymoma are poor. Historical series have shown a 5 year disease-free survival rate of approximately 20 per cent (Tomita *et al.* 1988). In an attempt to improve this, children with ependymoma have been included in chemotherapeutic trials primarily designed for children with medulloblastoma. However, the number of children with ependymoma in these studies has been small and the benefits of chemotherapy have not yet been demonstrated. Nevertheless, there does appear to be some justification for regarding the undifferentiated ependymoma as a primitive neuroectodermal tumour, with the same biological behavioural characteristics as a medulloblastoma. Large clinical trials are now underway in the United States and Europe in which all children with medulloblastoma, ependymoma, and classical primitive neuro-ectodermal tumours are entered into a single chemotherapeutic trial.

Brainstem gliomas

Brainstem gliomas constitute approximately 10 per cent of CNS tumours in children. The structure of the brainstem has, in the past, made biopsy of these lesions inadvisable and many reported series of these tumours therefore contain little histological information. However, information obtained at post-mortem suggests that the majority of these tumours are astrocytic in nature but vary in histological grading from the benign through to the highly malignant. The prognosis for a child with a brainstem tumour is determined by the feasibility of surgical removal of the tumour and its degree of malignancy. Tumours that grow exophytically to the brainstem and invade into the fourth ventricle are often of low-grade malignancy and may be amenable to surgical removal. These tumours usually present with signs of raised intracranial pressure rather than with cranial nerve palsies. In contrast, tumours which are intrinsic to the brainstem usually present with the classical combination of cranial nerve palsy and long tract signs. Two reviews, by Albright *et al.* (1986) and Stroink *et al.* (1986), showed that the presence of a cranial nerve palsy, the presence of mytotic activity in a biopsy specimen, and the presence of a hypodense tumour on pre-enhancement CT scan all heralded a poor prognosis.

SUPRATENTORIAL TUMOURS

Pineal tumours

Tumours of the pineal gland have been described with several patterns of histology. Most common are the pineal germ cell tumours, which may be germinomas or teratomas. The teratomas may be of a benign nature or may include immature tissues, particularly chorion carcinoma, endodermal sinus tumour, or embryonal carcinoma. Mixed cell types may occur in the one tumour. Primitive neuroectodermal tumours may also occur in the pineal gland, in which case they have been called pineoblastomas. Very rarely, children with retinoblastoma have been described in which a retinoblastoma-like tumour has also developed in the pineal gland, a so-called trilateral retinoblastoma. Patients with intracranial germ cell tumours can be diagnosed by CT scanning but may also produce tumour markers, for example β-human chorionic gonadotrophin (β-hCG), α-fetoprotein, or carcinoembryonic antigen. These markers may be elevated in both serum and cerebrospinal fluid and serve as diagnostic tools and as markers of tumour regression, remission, and progression.

Treatment of pineal tumours is directed towards the cell type of the tumour and tissue diagnosis is therefore of paramount importance. In recent years the development of stereotactic biopsy techniques has made the biopsy of tumours in the pineal region a safer technique and therefore attempts should be made to obtain biopsy material and, if possible, to undertake tumour removal. Following surgery, radiotherapy is the primary mode of treatment for germinomas and has been associated with cure rates of the order of 60–70 per cent (Jenkin *et al.* 1978). Pineal teratomas are relatively resistant to radiotherapy and, until recently, have carried a very poor prognosis. The demonstration that multidrug chemotherapy regimes were highly effective in the therapy of yolk sac tumours arising in extraneural tissues encouraged their use in pineal yolk sac tumours and recent reports have suggested that tumours in the pineal gland are equally sensitive to these regimes. Although the number of cases reported at the present time is relatively small, the data are sufficiently encouraging to suggest that this will be the treatment of choice for patients with pineal teratomas in the future. The drug regimes utilized include vinblastine, bleomycin, cyclophosphamide, and cisplatin (Allen *et al.* 1987*b*) or vincristine, methotrexate, bleomycin, and cisplatin (**PNOB**) and etoposide, actinomycin D, and cyclophosphamide (**ACE**) (Rustin *et al.* 1986).

Malignant astrocytoma

Malignant astrocytomas of grades III and IV situated in the posterior fossa or in the cerebral hemispheres have a poor prognosis. A maximal survival rate of 20 per cent can be expected for children with these tumours.

Prolonged survival may occur in those children in whom a surgical removal of the tumour is possible and who then receive radiation therapy to the tumour-bearing area. An improvement in survival may be obtained with the use of chemotherapy. However, at the present time only one large trial investigating this mode of therapy has been completed. The American Children's Cancer Study Group Trial randomized 942 children to receive or not chemotherapy with vincristine, lomustine, and prednisone following surgery and radiotherapy. In this study there was a marked survival advantage at 2 years and 5 years for those children who received the chemotherapy. The Children's Cancer Study Group has conducted a randomized study comparing children given the above chemotherapy with a group of children who received the 'eight drugs in 1 day' chemotherapy protocol. The study showed an overall survival at 5 years of 32 per cent with no difference demonstrated between vincristine/CCNU/prednisone and 8 : 1 chemotherapy. In the future advances may be made by the use of either new techniques in radiation therapy or simpler chemotherapeutic regimes, in which the known effective agents are given in dosage regimes which can be shown, on pharmacokinetic studies, to produce effective therapeutic levels within the CNS.

Chiasmatic/hypothalamic gliomas

Chiasmatic and hypothalamic gliomas in children are difficult tumours to assess and treat because of the variety of behaviours that they exhibit. Some tumours remain quiescent while others pursue slow but inexorable growth rates and can cause progressive visual and neurological deficits. These tumours are usually low-grade gliomas in nature but are situated such that surgical removal is never an achievable goal. Therapy has been directed towards protection of the visual pathways. An assessment should be made from the antecedent history of the rate of progression of the tumour and in those tumours which appear to be remaining quiescent or very slowly growing with no major threat to the visual pathway no further therapy may be needed. However, in those tumours for which progression can be documented and vision is at risk, radiotherapy will often halt the progression of the tumour.

Packer et al. (1988) pointed out that these tumours frequently become evident in young children and that radiotherapy to the local tumour site of such children may result in significant permanent intellectual and endocrinological sequelae. Despite the relatively low-grade nature of these tumours, this group has utilized a therapeutic regime of vincristine and actinomycin D with avoidance of radiotherapy until after the child's fifth birthday. Fifteen of 24 children so treated have remained free of progressive disease and have received no other therapy. Responses have also now been documented to a combination of vincristine and carboplatin.

Optic nerve glioma

Whether this tumour is truly a low-grade astrocytoma of the optic nerve or a benign hamartoma is controversial. It accounts for 1–5 per cent of all paediatric brain tumours and is strongly associated with neurofibromatosis (10–50 per cent). Eighty per cent of optic nerve gliomata occur in the first 5 years of childhood and, although they are usually of the low-grade juvenile pilocytic subtype, their extremely slow progress may cause an infiltrative nature to be overlooked.

The prognosis is best in younger children with anterior tumours affecting an optic nerve alone. The larger and more posterior situated tumours, especially those in the posterior aspect of the optic nerve chiasm are associated with a poorer prognosis (Borit and Richardson 1982). Late progression of tumours which may appear stationary either before or after treatment may be deceptive. A 5 year disease-free survival of 80 per cent has been quoted and 10 year disease-free survival of 50 per cent (McCulloch and Epstein 1985). Ten per cent of tumours are thought to transform to high-grade astrocytoma (Gjerris 1978).

The management is controversial. In very young children (under the age of 3 years) local radiotherapy is contraindicated. Anterior and focal abnormalities in front of the optic nerve may be watched, however, subtle alteration in the visual field is often difficult to assess prospectively (Hoyt and Baghdassarian 1969). Often the rôle of surgery is to biopsy these tumours; diffuse involvement of the chiasm excludes attempts at excision.

Local radiotherapy especially of chiasmal tumours, is indicated in children over the age of 3 years. Doses of 4500 cGy in 30 daily fractions over 6 weeks have improved or arrested visual loss, reduced proptosis, and reduced tumour masses (Horwich and Bloom 1985). The cost of this treatment may be impaired mental development,

Table 1 The incidence of spinal cord tumour (from De Sousa et al. 1979)

Malignant tumours	
Astrocytoma	11
Ependymoma	7
Sarcoma	11
Neuroblastoma	6
Teratoma	6
Total	41
Benign tumours	
Meningioma	3
Neurinoma	9
Epidermoid and dermoid cyst	8
Granulomata	4
Vascular malformation	8
Total	32

requiring special schooling in up to 25 per cent of patients and more than 25 per cent of patients will require growth hormone replacement. These tumours may respond to vincristine and carboplatin chemotherapy.

Craniopharyngioma

A relatively common space-occupying lesion (incidence 6–9 per cent), it is histologically a benign tumour of developmental origin yet, due to its suprasellar position, it is disabling and life-threatening. It often has an insidious presentation, with reduced visual function and endocrine abnormalities due to the proximity of the optic nerve and hypothalamus and the rôle of different treatment modalities is still controversial.

Developments in paediatric neurosurgery over the past decade, with the development of the Cavitron and the dissecting microscope and better pre-operative imaging, have enabled experienced paediatric neurosurgeons to select patients for radical surgery. The operative mortality has been reduced in the past two to three decades from 40 per cent to less than 5 per cent. Approximately one-third of patients will be suitable for radical surgery, giving a realistic chance of complete tumour removal without damaging the surrounding optic chiasm, pituitary stalk, third ventricle, and internal carotid arteries.

For the larger tumours, subtotal surgical removal with cyst drainage is often desirable and should be followed by external-beam radiotherapy. There is still controversy as to the optimal dose of external-beam radiotherapy, but high doses of 5000–5400 cGy in 180 cGy daily fractions have been suggested.

In a series of combined published data, complete resection alone has been shown to have a local control rate of 70 per cent, incomplete resection of 26 per cent, and incomplete resection plus post-operative radiotherapy of 75 per cent (Wen et al. 1989). The quality of life of patients is still poor. Only 25 per cent of patients with a craniopharyngioma will live a normal independent life, 50 per cent will have some mild but definite handicap, and 25 per cent will have significant and serious handicap with visual impairment, hemiparesis, and epilepsy and may be completely dependent.

Spinal cord tumour

Primary spinal cord tumours are extremely rare in childhood, accounting for less than 2 per cent of CNS malignancies. The largest published series is one of 81 cases, only half of which were malignant tumours (Table 1).

The development of nuclear magnetic resonance has facilitated the diagnosis and advanced neurosurgical techniques have facilitated surgical excision of these tumours. There are unsubstantiated claims for the value of complete surgical resection of astrocytoma of the spinal cord. The established management of spinal cord astrocytoma is safe surgery, often subtotal and then wide-field local radiotherapy. Often astrocytomas of the spinal cord are low-grade tumours that can present at an extremely late stage due to mistaken diagnosis.

THE TREATMENT OF BRAIN TUMOURS IN VERY YOUNG CHILDREN

Infants under the age of 2 years have a different pattern of physical signs of presentation, a different distribution of anatomical tumour location, a different distribution of histological tumour type, and a poorer prognosis than older children. The late effects of radiation therapy are also more pronounced in this group of children.

Dufner and Cohen (1985/6) reported that infants under the age of 6 months are more likely to have a supratentorially placed lesion than the usual infratentorial predominance. In the second 6 months of life the supratentorial and infratentorial tumours display an equal prominence and by the second year of life the more usual infratentorial predominance has been established. Children under 2 years of age are more likely to develop malignant tumours, particularly primitive neuroectodermal tumours and malignant astrocytomas, than older children. These tumours often achieve large size before diagnosis and this may be due to the fact that the skull of a young infant is well able to expand to accommodate the increasing tumour bulk, therefore the signs and symptoms of raised intracranial pressure may be significantly delayed. There is, in general, a low index of suspicion for intracranial neoplasm in infants. It therefore becomes easy to attribute symptomatology, such as vomiting or developmental delay, to other causes and this may contribute to a delay in diagnosis and an increase in the size of the primary tumour. The association of developmental delay or locomotor deficit with expanding head circumference is strongly suggestive of an intracranial mass lesion and this should be excluded in the diagnostic work-up.

The treatment of the relatively rare benign tumours in infancy, such as optic glioma and low-grade astrocytoma, should be conservative. Optic glioma should be followed carefully with the use of CT scanning and assessment of the visual pathway using visual evoked responses. These tumours may be extremely slow growing and no therapeutic intervention may be required. In tumours that do show progression, the standard treatment has been to use radiation therapy, but recent reports have suggested that these tumours may be sensitive to chemotherapy and, if this is confirmed, this would clearly be a preferable course of action to radiation therapy which, in these very small children, will inevitably be followed by a degree of intellectual loss and growth hormone deficiency. Benign astrocytomas should be removed surgically and then followed carefully without further therapeutic intervention. If the tumour recurs, it may be preferable to use a second surgical exploration and to avoid the use of radiotherapy until beyond the child's third birthday.

Malignant tumours are a very different proposition. These tumours are often very large, rapidly growing, and carry an extremely poor prognosis. Therapy has usually involved surgical exploration with the removal of as much tumour as possible, followed by radiation therapy. The well-known incidence of late effects of radiation therapy in these very young children has led traditionally to a dosage reduction of 20 per cent from the traditional radiotherapy doses. This, however, is an unsatisfactory compromise in that even with such a dose reduction late effects of radiation therapy are going to be seen and the dosage reduction may be a contributing factor in the failure to achieve tumour control which is the major cause of death in this group of patients. Reports from Van Eys et al. (1985) and Horowitz et al. (1988) have indicated that infant brain tumours are sensitive to combination chemotherapy and that the use of radiation therapy can be delayed until beyond the child's third birthday. Multi-institutional studies of this approach are currently being developed by the National Study Groups in the United States and by the International Society for Paediatric Oncology in Europe. In all of these studies it is hoped that brain tumours in very young infants can be controlled by the use of chemotherapy until at least the child's third birthday, when radiation therapy can be administered more safely. It may be possible to eliminate radiation therapy entirely from the therapeutic schedule of infants in whom a complete tumour response to chemotherapy is seen.

LATE EFFECTS

Survivors of childhood brain tumour may suffer from a variety of long-term handicaps. These may be the effects of brain damage caused by the tumour itself, by raised intracranial pressure, or by neurosurgical intervention. Or they may be caused by radiotherapy or by chemotherapy which the children were given in an attempt to prevent the recurrence of their tumours.

Children with severe neurological deficit in the immediate post-operative period have a poor prognosis for recovery of full neurological function. They may frequently be left with varying degrees of ataxia, with or without accompanying hemiparesis or hemiplegia. If raised intracranial pressure has been present for a significant length of time or if the tumour affected the optic chiasm, as in craniopharyngioma or optic glioma, then optic atrophy may develop with associated visual handicap. Strabismus following sixth nerve palsy may also become a chronic condition. Children with supratentorial lesions may continue to suffer from epileptic fits and need medication for this condition for many years.

Radiotherapy to the developing brain is associated with a consequent loss of intellectual function. The younger the child at the time when radiotherapy is received, the greater this loss is likely to be. When children suffering from cerebellar astrocytomas, which have been treated with radiotherapy, are compared with children suffering from medulloblastoma treated with radiotherapy also, the level of intellectual functioning of the children suffering from astrocytoma is found to be superior to that of the children suffering from medulloblastoma. The difference between the two sets of children is that the children with astrocytoma have only received radiotherapy to the posterior fossa whereas the children with medulloblastoma have received radiotherapy to the posterior fossa and 'prophylactic' radiotherapy to the rest of the cranium and spine. Therefore, it is presumably this prophylactic cranial field which is implicated in the subsequent loss of intellectual function. When intellectual loss is combined with physical handicap, the risk of scholastic failure is high. In a survey of the literature on 23 series of children surviving medulloblastoma in whom intellectual testing had been carried out, 41 per cent of the children reported were classified as suffering from moderate or severe handicap.

Various hormonal deficiencies have been described in children surviving brain tumours. Short stature may be the result of a variety of mechanisms in these children. A small number of children in whom there has been raised intracranial pressure, and/or who have received radiation therapy, will develop precocious puberty. In this condition, although the child's growth may appear to be satisfactory at the time, premature fusion of the epiphyses will take place and the ultimate prognosis for adult height is decreased. Children may also develop growth hormone deficiency. This may be due to a direct effect on the hypothalamic pituitary axis by the tumour or may be associated with radiation therapy to that area. A dose of 27–35 Gy delivered over 3 weeks has been shown to be sufficient to produce subnormal growth hormone responses to standard provocation tests in most patients within 2 years of therapy (Shalet 1989). These children should be treated with replacement growth hormone within 2 years of completing their radiation therapy, as there is evidence that the earlier that this replacement is commenced the better the prognosis for ultimate adult height.

Children with medulloblastomas and ependymomas will receive spinal radiation therapy as well as cranial radiation. Shalet has calculated that a dose of irradiation of between 27 and 35 Gy given over 22–27 days will appreciably impair spinal growth, with a loss of ultimate height of 9 cm if irradiation takes place at the age of 1 year and up to 5.5 cm if the radiation is given before 10 years of age. Thyroid dysfunction may also be seen in this group of patients receiving craniospinal irradiation, as the thyroid gland is included in the exit beam from the spinal field. The thyroid dysfunction may take the form of frank hypothyroidism or so-called compensated hypothyroidism, in which there is a normal thyroxine concentration but increased levels of thyroid stimulating hormone. In either case, thyroid hormone replacement therapy should be undertaken to be certain that the child is euthyroid.

The gonads may be affected by both radiation and cytotoxic therapy. In children receiving spinal radiation therapy and particularly where a spade-shaped field has been used to cover the lower end of the spinal column, both the ovaries and testicles may receive small doses of irradiation, sufficient to cause ovarian failure or oligospermia or aspermia. Many cytotoxic drugs, particularly the alkalating agents, are associated with gonadal damage. Children with brain tumours are frequently treated with either carmustine (**BCNU**) or lomustine (**CCNU**) and these children have been shown to have high incidences of primary gonadal dysfunction (Clayton *et al.* 1988, 1989). Children receiving therapy with carmustine have been reported to have developed progressive pulmonary fibrosis (Bailey *et al.* 1978). The group of patients from which this index patient was taken has now been followed over a period of 10 years, during which time all patients within the group have developed demonstrable pulmonary fibrosis and in several more patients this has had a fatal outcome.

Recent chemotherapeutic regimes have often included platinum compounds as a major part of the therapeutic combination. It is well known that these drugs are associated with hearing loss and, particularly, high-tone deafness. It has also been shown that radiation therapy to the middle ear, an area which is included in the radiation port for most posterior fossa tumours, potentiates this hearing loss and children treated with these drugs will therefore need to be assessed carefully for their auditory function.

REFERENCES

Albright AL, Guthkelch AN, Packer RJ, Price RA, Rourke LB (1986). Prognostic factors in brainstem gliomas. *Journal of Neurosurgery*, 65:751–5.

Allen JC, *et al.* (1987*a*). Carboplatin and recurrent childhood brain tumours. *Journal of Clinical Oncology*, 5:459–63.

Allen JC, Kim JH, Packer RJ (1987*b*). Neo-adjuvant chemotherapy for newly diagnosed germ cell tumours of the central nervous system. *Journal of Neurosurgery*, 67:65–70.

Bailey CC, Marsden HB, Morris-Jones P (1978). Pulmonary fibrosis following therapy with BCNU. *Cancer* 42:74–6.

Borit A, Richardson EP (1982). The biological and clinical behaviour of pilocytic astrocytomas of the optic pathways. *Brain*, 105:161–87.

Burger PC, Grahmann FC, Bliestle A, Klihues P (1987). Differentiation in the medulloblastoma: a histological and immunohistochemical study. *Acta Neuropathologica (Berlin)*, 73:115–23.

Clayton PE, Shalet SM, Price DA, Morris-Jones PH (1988). Testicular damage after chemotherapy for childhood brain tumours. *Journal of Pediatrics*, 112:922–6.

Clayton PE, Shalet SM, Price DA, Morris-Jones PH (1989). Ovarian function following chemotherapy for childhood brain tumours. *Journal of Pediatrics*, 17:92–6.

Davies JNP (1973). *Childhood tumours in Templeton AC. Tumours in a tropical country—a survey of Uganda 1964–1968*. Springer Verlag, New York.

De Sousa AL, *et al.* (1979). Intraspinal tumour in children. *Journal of Neurosurgery*, 51:437–45.

Djerassi I, Kim JS, Reggev A (1985). Response of astrocytoma to high dose methotrexate with citrovorum factor. *Cancer*, 55:2741–7.

Dufner PK, Cohen ME (1985/6). Treatment of brain tumours in babies and very young children. *Pediatric Nueroscience*, 12:304–10.

Edwards MS, Levin VA, Wilson CB (1980). Brain tumour chemotherapy as evaluation of agents in current use for phase II and III trials. *Cancer Treatment Reports*, 64:1179–205.

Evans AE, *et al.* (1990). The treatment of medulloblastoma. Results of a prospective randomized trial of radiation therapy with and without CCNU, vincristine and prednisolone. *Journal of Neurosurgery*, 72:572–82.

Fraumeni JF, Miller RW (1967). Adrenocortical neoplasms with hemi-hypertrophy, brain tumours and other disorders. *Journal of Pediatrics*, 70:129.

Gjerris F (1978). Clinical aspects and long-term prognosis in supra-tentorial tumours of infancy in childhood. *Acta Neurologica Scandinavica*, 57:445–70.

Gol A, McKissock W (1959). Cerebellous astrocytomas; a report on 98 verified cases. *Journal of Neurosurgery*, 16:287–96.

Hardy DJ, Hope-Stope HF, McKenzie LG, Schulz CL (1978). Recurrence of medulloblastoma after homogenous field radiotherapy. *Journal of Neurosurgery*, 49:434–40.

Horowitz ME, *et al.* (1988). Primary brain tumour in the very young child—post-operative chemotherapy in combined modality treatment. *Cancer*, 61:428–34.

Horwich A, Bloom HJG (1985). Optic gliomas; radiation therapy and prognosis. *International Journal of Radiation Oncology—Biology—Physics*, 11:1067.

Hoyt WF, Baghdassarian SA (1969). Optic gliomas of childhood. *British Journal of Ophthalmology*, 53:793–8.

Jenkin RDT, Simpson WJK, Keen CW (1978). Pineal and supracellar germinomas, results of radiation treatment. *Journal of Neurosurgery*, 48:99–107.

Jenkin D, *et al.* (1990). Posterior fossa medulloblastoma in childhood: treatment results and a proposal for a new staging system. *International Journal of Radiation Oncology—Biology—Physics*, 19:265–74.

Kun LE, Kovnar EH, Sanford RA (1988). Ependymomas in children. *Pediatric Neuroscience*, 14:57–63.

Levin VA (1984). Phase II evaluation of di-bromodulcitol in the treatment of medulloblastoma, ependymoma and malignant astrocytoma. *Journal of Neurosurgery*, 61:1063–8.

Li FP, Tucker MA, Fraumeni JF (1976) Childhood cancer in sibs. *Journal of Pediatrics*, 88:419.

McCulloch DS, Epstein F (1985). Optic pathway tumours, a review with proposals for clinical staging. *Cancer*, 56:1789–91.

Packer RJ, *et al.* (1988). Treatment of chiasmatic/hypothalamic gliomas of childhood with chemotherapy—an update. *Annals of Neurology*, 23:79–85.

Pendergrass TW, *et al.* (1987). Eight drugs in one day chemotherapy for brain tumours: experience in 107 children and rationale for pre-irradiation chemotherapy. *Journal of Clinical Oncology*, 5:1221–31.

Rosenstock J, Evans A, Schut L (1976). Response to vincristine of recurrent brain tumours in children. *Journal of Neurosurgery*, 45:135–40.

Rustin GJS, Newlands ES, Bagshaw KD, Begent Richard HJ, Crawford SM (1986). Successful management of metastatic and primary germ cell tumours in the brain. *Cancer*, 57:2108–13.

Shalet SM (1989). Endocrine consequences of treatment of malignant disease. *Archives of Diseases in Childhood*, 64:1635–41.

Stroink AR, Hoffman HJ, Hendrick EB, Humphries RP (1986). Diagnosis and management of paediatric brainstem gliomas. *Journal of Neurosurgery*, 65:45–50.

Tait DM, Thornton-Jones H, Bloom HJ, Lemerle J, Morris-Jones P (1990). Adjuvant chemotherapy for medulloblastoma: the first multi-centre control trial of the International Society of Paediatric Oncology (SIOP I). *European Journal of Cancer*, 26:464–9.

Tirelli V, D'Incalci M, Cavetta R (1984). Etoposide (VP 16–23) in malignant brain tumours: a phase II study. *Journal of Clinical Oncology*, 2:432–7.

Tomita T, McLone DG, Das L, Brand WN (1988). Benign ependymomas of the posterior fossa in childhood. *Pediatric Neuroscience*, 14:277–85.

Van de Wiel HJ (1960). *Inheritance of glioma, the genetics of cerebral glioma and its relation to status dysrhaphicus*. Elsevier, Amsterdam.

Van Eys J, et al. (1985). MOPP regimen as primary chemotherapy for brain tumours in infants. *Neurology and Oncology*, 3:237.

Vick NA, Khandekar JD, Bigner DD (1977). Chemotherapy of brain tumours. The blood barrier is not a factor. *Archives of Neurology*, 34:523–6.

Walker RW, Allen JC (1988). Cisplatin in the treatment of recurrent childhood primary brain tumours. *Journal of Clinical Oncology*, 6:62–6.

Wen BC, et al. (1989). A comparison of the role of surgery and radiation therapy in the management of craniopharyngioma. *International Journal of Radiation Oncology — Biology — Physics*, 16:17–24.

Williams AO (1975). Tumours of childhood in Ibadan, Nigeria. *Cancer*, 36:370.

Williams MV (1987). The cribriform plate; essentially site for meningeal leukaemia. *British Journal of Radiology*, 60:469–75.

Wilson C, et al. (1976). Single agent chemotherapy of brain tumours. *Archives of Neurology*, 33:739–44.

Wriggleson W, et al. (1965). Incidence of secondary primary tumours in children with cancer and leukaemia—a seven year survey of 150 consecutive autopsied cases. *Cancer*, 18:58.

15.2 Tumours of the brain and spinal cord in adults

MICHAEL BRADA AND D. G. T. THOMAS

EPIDEMIOLOGY

Primary intracranial neoplasms represent only 2–5 per cent of tumours and the age-adjusted incidence ranges from 5.9 to 12.6 per 100 000 population per year (Barker *et al.* 1976; Schoenberg 1982; Fogelholm *et al.* 1984; Velema and Percy 1987; Helseth *et al.* 1988). The apparent variation between different populations is most likely due to differences in the methods of data collection and case ascertainment (Schoenberg 1982). It is not the reflection of a true geographical variation except in cranial germinomas, which are commoner in Japan and China.

Gliomas constitute the largest histological group of primary brain tumours (35–75 per cent, depending on the rate of histological confirmation) with an age-adjusted incidence rate of 3–7 per 100 000. The prevalence of brain tumours (reported in the population of the United States) is 20.6 per 100 000 (Feldman *et al.* 1986). Although some studies have suggested an increasing incidence of glial tumours, this trend most likely represents more frequent diagnosis which has accompanied the introduction of computerized tomography (CT) scanning. Primary cerebral lymphoma, which only represents 1 per cent of primary intracranial tumours, has increased in incidence both in men and women of all ages and this preceded the onset of the acquired immune deficiency syndrome (AIDS) epidemic (Eby *et al.* 1988).

Age and sex distribution

The incidence of most glial and meningeal tumours in adults rises with age, with a peak at 65–75 years. The rate of increase is most marked in glioblastoma compared to other glial tumours (Velema and Percy 1987). Medulloblastomas, primitive neuroectodermal tumours, and pilocytic astrocytomas are mostly seen in children but also occur in adults at a reducing frequency (Zulch 1986). Pineal and suprasellar germ cell tumours have a specific age distribution with a peak incidence in children and young adults. There is a slight male predominance in glial tumours, with a male to female ratio of 1.2–1.5 : 1, while meningiomas are equally distributed between the sexes.

AETIOLOGY

Genetic predisposition

Although the majority of brain tumours are sporadic, a small proportion occur in association with familial conditions of autosomal dominant inheritance. Patients with type 1 neurofibromatosis (peripheral, von Recklinghausen's neurofibromatosis, NF1) have an increased incidence of primary intracranial tumours. Hospital-based population studies of clinically overt neurofibromatosis suggest a 10–15 per cent incidence of optic nerve glioma (Lewis *et al.* 1984; Listernick *et al.* 1989) and up to 2.5 per cent incidence of malignant astrocytoma. Neurofibromatosis is also associated with an increased risk of meningioma and other glial tumours such as ependymoma. The relative risk of malignant and benign CNS neoplasms on long-term follow up is 4 (2.8–5.6); gliomas account for 84 per cent of the histologically documented CNS tumours and of these 38 per cent are optic nerve and chiasmal gliomas and 13 per cent meningiomas (Sorensen *et al.* 1986). Central neurofibromatosis (NF2) characterized by bilateral acoustic neurofibroma is associated with the development of meningiomas which may be multiple.

Tuberous sclerosis is characterized by adenoma sebaceum, together with visceral and central nervous system lesions (most often cortical nodules; tubers). The classical tumours associated with tuberous sclerosis, spongioblastoma, giant cell astrocytoma, and 'ventricular tumour of tuberous sclerosis', are usually benign and most commonly occur at the foramen of Monro (Russell and Rubinstein 1989).

Patients with von Hippel–Lindau syndrome, which consists of multiple haemangioblastomas within the central nervous system, together with angiomas of the retina, may develop angioblastoma of the cerebellum. Von Hippel–Lindau syndrome is also associated with renal carcinoma (Russell and Rubinstein 1989).

Brain tumours have been described in patients with familial adenomatous polyposis and this association is named Turcot's syndrome. The majority are gliomas or medulloblastomas and usually present before the diagnosis of familial adenomatous polyposis (Kropilak *et al.* 1989). Medulloblastomas are also found in 3–5 per cent of cases of Gorlin's syndrome (Evans *et al.* 1991).

Radiation

Exposure to radiation in atomic bomb survivors, low-dose radiation in workers in nuclear plants (Smith and Douglas 1986), and in populations living near nuclear installations has not been shown to carry an increased risk of developing primary intracranial neoplasms. However, long-term studies of 11 000 children who received scalp irradiation as treatment for tinea capitis have revealed an increased incidence of brain tumours with a relative risk of 9.5 for meningiomas and 2.6 for gliomas for radiation doses of 1–2 Gy as well as a dose–response relationship (Ron *et al.* 1988). Exposure to dental X-rays has also been considered a risk factor.

Suspicion that radiation is one of the factors associated with the development of glioma derives from a number of reported cases of brain tumour in patients receiving radiotherapy for craniopharyngioma, pituitary adenoma, and medulloblastoma, and following cranial prophylaxis in acute lymphatic leukaemia. Although there is a suggestion of a common familial predisposition to CNS tumours and leukaemia (Farwell and Flannery 1984), there is a 20–22-fold excess risk of brain tumours in children receiving cranial irradiation for acute lymphatic leukaemia (Hawkins *et al.* 1987; Neglia *et al.* 1991). The review of reported cases of apparently radiation-induced second tumours suggests a median time to detection of glioma of 7 years, of sarcoma 10 years, and of meningioma 14 years with a very wide range (Brada *et al.* 1992). Meningiomas, sarcomas, and other glial tumours have been also reported following cranial irradiation for pituitary adenomas with a relative risk of second tumour of 9 and a 1.9 per cent cumulative risk of developing a second tumour over 20 years following radiotherapy.

Trauma

Head injury is often recalled as an event prior to the development of brain tumour. Although some case control studies have suggested a significant association with trauma, such reports may be influenced by a recall bias and studies of head-injury victims do not show an increased risk of brain tumours (Schoenberg 1982). There is no clear association between physical trauma and glioma, but meningioma may be related to a serious head injury 20 or more years before diagnosis (Preston-Martin *et al.* 1989).

Exposure to carcinogens

Brain tumours have been induced in animals by carcinogens, particularly aliphatic alkylating agents and polycyclic hydrocarbons.

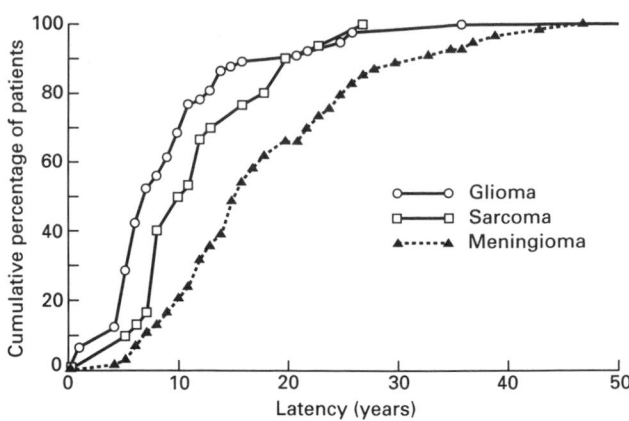

Fig. 1 Frequency distribution of presumed radiation-induced gliomas reported in the literature.

Exposure to chemicals during synthetic rubber manufacture, polyvinyl chloride production, and in the petrochemical industry has been suspected as carcinogenic in humans (Kessler and Brandt-Rauf 1987). Other occupational groups that may have an increased risk for brain tumours include farmers, chemists, vets, and workers in industries exposed to electromagnetic fields, although none of the associations is conclusively proven.

The development of tumours by transplacental exposure to carcinogens in rats stimulated research into perinatal exposure to chemicals, largely as presumed occupational exposure of parents. 'Hydrocarbon'-related occupations, agriculture, and metal-related and electrical jobs are potential risk factors, but they also remain unproven. Exposure to high-frequency electromagnetic radiation has also been postulated as a risk factor in perinatal as well as in adult life. The ubiquitous presence of such electromagnetic radiation makes the estimate of exposure difficult and the association is not clear.

Immune deficiency

Primary cerebral lymphoma has been described in association with immune deficiency following organ transplantation. Lymphoma in patients with acquired immune deficiency syndrome also has a predilection for the brain as well as other extranodal sites.

THE BIOLOGY OF BRAIN TUMOURS

Molecular genetics

Inherited predisposition to malignancy

Allele loss from chromosome 22, which is the location of the NF2 locus (chr.22, q11.1–q13.1) (Rouleau *et al.* 1987), has been detected in acoustic neuroma, neurofibroma, and meningioma of patients with NF2 (Seizinger *et al.* 1987*b*). Frequent loss of a part or the whole of chromosome 22 in sporadic meningioma at karyotype and molecular level (Seizinger *et al.* 1987*a*) suggests a common pathogenic mechanism in sporadic meningiomas and tumours associated with NF2.

Specific loss of alleles from the short arm of chromosome 3 detected in tumours from patients with von Hippel–Lindau (VHL) disease is also consistent with a recessive mechanism of tumour genesis involving the VHL gene on chromosome 3 (Tory *et al.* 1989).

Genetic changes in sporadic tumours

Abnormal karyotypes are frequently detected in glial tumours, particularly those of high-grade malignancy (Bigner *et al.* 1988; Jenkins *et al.* 1989). Non-random numerical changes most frequently involve gains of chromosome 7, loss of chromosome 10, and structural abnormalities of 9p and 19q, as well as the presence of double minute chromosomes (Bigner *et al.* 1988). Chromosomal changes observed in tumour biopsies are unstable and show alteration on culture; karyotypic abnormalities observed in cell lines may therefore not be representative of tumours *in vivo*.

Molecular genetic analyses have detected a loss of heterozygosity of chromosome 10 markers in the majority of high-grade tumours tested (James *et al.* 1988) and loss of sequences on the short arm of chromosome 17 in both low- and high-grade tumours (El-Azouzi *et al.* 1989; James *et al.* 1989). The chromosome 17 loci are distinct from the NF1 gene. These changes suggest the presence of potential tumour suppressor genes.

Glial tumours arise in the offspring of pregnant rats treated with *N*-ethyl-*N*-nitrosourea and the transformation is associated with the activation of the *neu* oncogene, tested by NIH 373 assay. The human homologue c-*erb* B is closely related to the epidermal growth factor receptor (EGF-R) and the amplification of the EGF-R gene and overexpression of the epidermal growth factor receptor has been reported in a proportion of human glial tumours. The presence of double minute chromosomes in glioma biopsies has been associated with the amplification of the EGF-R gene in 30–40 per cent of glial tumours (Libermann *et al.* 1985; Bigner *et al.* 1988) and in approximately 30 per cent of glioma cell lines. Amplification of the *gli* gene, a putative oncogene (on 12q), has only been demonstrated in two glioma cell lines.

The most frequent karyotypic abnormalities described in medulloblastoma involve chromosomes 1 and 17 (Bigner *et al.* 1988). Medulloblastoma shares many features in common with neuroblastoma, but amplification of the N-*myc* gene has not been demonstrated, although a proportion of cases overexpress this gene (Garson *et al.* 1989).

Frequent loss of chromosome 22 in sporadic meningioma led to molecular genetic studies which have demonstrated DNA deletions on chromosome 22, which is the site of DNA loss in NF2 (see above).

Cell kinetics

Cell kinetic parameters have been measured both in animal and human gliomas using [³H]thymidine labelling, 5-bromo-2'-deoxyuridine (BUdR) uptake, and Ki-67 antibody staining and the labelling indices determined by these techniques are similar. Malignant gliomas have labelling indices in the range of 1–20 per cent, with higher labelling indices for higher-grade tumours (Raghavan *et al.* 1988). There is considerable variation between tumours of the same histological type, partly due to cellular heterogeneity and partly due to problems of sampling. Medulloblastomas and metastatic tumours have labelling indices as high as 60 per cent. In low-grade gliomas, meningiomas, and pituitary adenomas the labelling index rarely exceeds 1 per cent, although it may be higher in meningiomas with malignant features and in recurrent meningiomas. The prognostic value of cell kinetic indices is not yet clear, although there is possible association between labelling index and survival or relapse-free interval (Hoshino *et al.* 1989).

Immunology

Although the brain has no lymphatic system, the microglia of the CNS possess a number of immunological functions. They express panmacrophage markers and are phagocytic in culture. They also express major histocompatibility complex class I and II antigens and secrete immune modulators such as interleukin-1, tumour necrosis factor-alpha, and γ-interferon (de Tribolet *et al.* 1984). In the normal brain, the blood–brain barrier limits the entry of immunoglobulin and lymphocytes into the brain substance. However, within the tumour the blood–tumour barrier is, to a large extent, permeable, allowing an interaction between the immune response of the host and tumour cells. Circulating lymphocytes may pass into the tumour and lymphocytic infiltration is commonly seen in histological examination of surgical biopsy material. The mononuclear cells in glioma have been mostly identified as T lymphocytes, with a predominance of the cytotoxic/suppressor subset. Natural killer cells, macrophages, and B lymphocytes have also been demonstrated. Tumour-infiltrating lymphocytes may, however, be inhibited by suppressor factors produced by glial tumour cells (Kuppner *et al.* 1988).

The surface antigens found on glioma cells are predominantly of neuroectodermal origin and are the same as those on fetal brain cells, melanomas, neuroblastomas, and some brain endothelial cells. Major histocompatibility complex class I antigens, particularly HLA-A and class II, particularly HLA-DR, are also expressed on glioma cells. These antigens are necessary for mitotic action of effector cells and for foreign antigen recognition and imply that immunological responses of these types could take place in brain tumours. Several normal brain antigens are also expressed by gliomas (Darling *et al.* 1981). Evidence of a humoral immune response to gliomas has been reported in a small fraction of patients with these tumours. Antiglioma antibody has also been demonstrated in the cerebrospinal fluid of some patients with gliomas (Mori *et al.* 1978). The presence of immune complexes in the sera of patients with glioma appears to have an unfavourable prognostic implication.

Brain tumours in experimental animals
Chemically and virally induced tumours
Brain tumours may be induced in rodents by direct application of polycyclic hydrocarbons to the brain. Intrauterine exposure to dimethylbenzanthracene can produce brain tumours in the fetus. The alkylating agents methyl- or ethylnitrosourea have been used extensively to induce experimental tumours in rats (Bigner and Swenberg 1977; Lantos and Pilkington 1979), both to study pathogenesis and to undertake treatment trials of radiation and chemotherapy.

Adeno- and papovaviruses (DNA viruses) have induced experimental tumours in animals. Simian virus (SV40) and related human strains of progressive multifocal leucoencephalopathy (PML) and Jakob–Creutzfeldt (JC) viruses can induce a wide variety of histological tumour types, including gliomas and medulloblastomas. Avian sarcoma virus (RNA virus) has been used to develop a standardized rodent model for studies of radiation and chemotherapy (Schold and Bigner 1983). It remains unclear whether the ability of oncogenic viruses to induce brain tumours experimentally in animals and to transform glia cells *in vitro* has parallels in the aetiology of naturally occurring brain tumours in man (Ibelgaufts 1982).

Transplantable tumours and human xenografts
Reproducible and reliable experimental brain tumour models have been developed using transplantation. Spontaneously arising or induced animal tumours have been transplanted intracerebrally or subcutaneously in syngeneic animals, as well as in animals of other strains or species (Pilkington and Lantos 1990). Xenografting of human gliomas intracerebrally and subcutaneously has also been achieved (Horten *et al.* 1981) with retention of the histological features of the human tumour.

Table 1 WHO classification of CNS tumours (after Zulch 1979; Provisional Revision of WHO Classification 1990)

I Tumours of neuroepithelial tissue
 A Astrocytic tumours
  1 Astrocytoma
   Variants: fibrillary, protoplasmic, gemistocytic, or mixed
  2 Anaplastic (malignant) astrocytoma
  3 Glioblastoma
   Variants:
    Giant cell glioblastoma
    Gliosarcoma
  4 Pilocytic astrocytoma
  5 Pleomorphic xanthoastrocytoma
  6 Subependymal giant cell astrocytoma
   (usually in association with tuberous sclerosis)

 B Oligodendroglial tumours
  1 Oligodendroglioma
  2 Anaplastic (malignant) oligodendroglioma

 C Ependymal tumours
  1 Ependymoma
   Variants: cellular, papillary, epithelial, clear cell, or mixed
  2 Anaplastic (malignant) ependymoma
  3 Myxopapillary ependymoma
  4 Subependymoma

 D Mixed gliomas
  1. Mixed oligo-astrocytoma
  2 Anaplastic (malignant) oligo-astrocytoma
  3 Others

 E Choroid plexus tumours
  1 Choroid plexus papilloma
  2 Choroid plexus carcinoma

 F Neuroepithelial tumours of uncertain origin
  1 Astroblastoma
  2 Polar spongioblastoma
  3 Gliomatosis cerebri

 G Neuronal and mixed neuronal–glial tumours
  1 Gangliocytoma
  2 Dysplastic gangliocytoma of cerebellum (Lhermitte–Duclos)
  3 Desmoplastic infantile ganglioglioma
  4 Dysembryoplastic neuroepithelial tumour
  5 Ganglioglioma
  6 Anaplastic (malignant) ganglioglioma
  7 Central neurocytoma
  8 Olfactory neuroblastoma (esthesioneuroblastoma)
   Variant: olfactory neuroepithelioma

 H Pineal tumours
  1 Pineocytoma
  2 Pineoblastoma
  3 Mixed pineocytoma/pineoblastoma

 I Embryonal tumours
  1 Medulloepithelioma
  2 Neuroblastoma
   Variant: ganglioneuroblastoma
  3 Ependymoblastoma
  4 Retinoblastoma
  5 Primitive neuroectodermal tumours (PNETs)
   with multipotent differentiation: neuronal, astrocytic,
   ependymal, muscle, melanotic, etc.
   a Medulloblastoma
    Variants: desmoplastic medulloblastoma,
     medullomyoblastoma, melanocytic medulloblastoma
   b Cerebral or spinal PNETs

II Tumours of cranial and spinal nerves
 A Schwannoma (neurilemoma, neurinoma)
  Variants:
  a Cellular
  b Plexiform
  c Melanotic

 B Neurofibroma
  a Circumscribed (solitary)
  b Plexiform
  c Mixed neurofibroma/schwannoma

 C Malignant peripheral nerve sheath tumour (MPNST)
  (neurogenic sarcoma, anaplastic neurofibroma, 'malignant
  schwannoma')
  Variants:
  a Epithelioid
  b MPNST with divergent mesenchymal and/or epithelial
   differentiation
  c Melanotic

III Tumours of the meninges
 A Tumours of meningothelial cells
  1 Meningioma
   Histological types:
    a Meningothelial (syncytial)
    b Transitional/mixed
    c Fibrous (fibroblastic)
    d Psammomatous
    e Angiomatous
    f Microcystic
    g Secretory
    h Clear cell
    i Chordoid
    j Lymphoplasmacytoid
    k Metaplastic variants (xanthomatous, myxoid, osseous,
     cartillagenous, etc.)
  2 Atypical meningioma
  3 Anaplastic (malignant) meningioma
   a Variants of 1 a–k (see above)
   b Papillary

 B Mesenchymal, non-meningothelial tumours
  Benign neoplasms
  1 Osteocartilagenous tumours
  2 Lipoma
  3 Fibrous histiocytoma
  4 Others
  Malignant neoplasms
  5 Mesenchymal chondrosarcoma
  6 Malignant fibrous histiocytoma
  7 Rhabdomyosarcoma
  8 Meningeal sarcomatosis
  9 Others

 C Primary melanocytic lesions
  1 Diffuse melanosis
  2 Melanocytoma
  3 Malignant melanoma
   Variant: meningeal melanomatosis

 D Tumours of uncertain origin
  1 Haemangiopericytoma
  2 Haemangioblastoma (capillary haemangioblastoma)

(*Continued*)

Table 1 (*Continued*)

IV Haemopoietic neoplasms
    1 Malignant lymphomas
    2 Plasmacytoma
    3 Granulocytic sarcoma
    4 Others

V Germ cell tumours
    1 Germinoma
    2 Teratoma
       a Embryonal carcinoma
       b Yolk sac tumour (endodermal sinus tumour)
       c Immature
       d Mature
       e Teratoma with malignant transformation
    3 Mixed germ cell tumours
    4 Choriocarcinoma

VI Cysts and tumour-like lesions
    A Rathke's cleft cyst
    B Epidermoid cyst
    C Dermoid cyst
    D Colloid cyst of the third ventricle
    E Enterogenous cyst
    F Neuroglial cyst
    G Other cysts
    H Lipoma
    I Granular cell tumour (choristoma, pitulcytoma)
    J Hypothalamic neuronal hamartoma
    K Nasal glial heterotopia

VII Tumours of the anterior pituitary
    A Pituitary adenoma
       (classification based on hormonal immunohistochemistry)
    B Pituitary carcinoma

VIII Malformations and local extensions of regional tumours
    A Craniopharyngioma
       a Adamantinous
       b Squamous papillary
    B Paraganglioma (chemodectoma)
    C Chordoma
       Variant: chondroid chordoma
    D Chondroma
    E Chondrosarcoma
    F Adenoid cystic carcinoma (cylindroma)
    G Others

IX Metastatic tumours

Table 2 Immunocytochemical markers used in the diagnosis of brain tumours (from Weller 1986)

Marker antigens	Cell type stained
Intermediate filaments	
Glial fibrillary acidic protein	Astrocytes, (ependymal cells)
Neurofilament proteins	Neurones and axons
Vimentin	Fetal brain and other tissues
Cell proteins and enzymes	
Neurone-specific enolase	Neurones
S-100 protein	Glia and Schwann cells
Carbonic anhydrase C	Choroid plexus; oligodendrocytes
Myelin basic protein	Myelin; oligodendrocytes in infants
Factor VIII-related antigen	Endothelial cells
Hormones	
Pituitary hormones	Anterior pituitary

Table 3 The comparative frequency (per cent) of different types of brain tumours (from 14 958 cases; Zimmerman 1969)

Glioma	38
Meningioma	16
Pituitary adenoma	8
Schwannoma	6
Craniopharyngioma	3
Haemangioblastoma	2
Metastases	12
Others	15

PATHOLOGY

Intracranial tumours have historically been classified according to the putative cell of origin and its stage of development. Many classifications have been derived from this concept and a number of them are in current use. Attempts at defining tumour behaviour by correlating histological and cellular features with clinical outcome have led to the concept of grading (Kernohan and Sayre 1952). The recently introduced WHO classification listed in Table 1 integrates features of both of these approaches. In addition to assigning tumour types according to the cell of origin, the lesions are graded. The most common brain tumour, glioma including glioblastoma, falls within the neuroepithelial tumours and the details of grading are described in the glioma section. The apparent complexity of this and other classifications is due to the inclusion of many rare tumours and their variants. The immunocytochemical markers used in the diagnosis of brain tumours are listed in Table 2. The comparative frequency of different tumour types presenting at a neurosurgical centre is shown in Table 3. It is not representative of the distribution of cases seen in an oncology centre.

The grading of degree of malignancy of brain tumours must be considered differently to most other neoplasms. Any intracranial space-occupying lesion can be fatal due to brain herniation and even small tumours at specific sites may be life-threatening. Most primary CNS tumours do not metastasize but expand and spread locally.

CLINICAL MANIFESTATIONS OF BRAIN TUMOURS

The presenting symptoms and signs of patients with cerebral tumours are due to raised intracranial pressure and to local or general brain dysfunction. The relative frequency of such symptoms in adult cerebral tumours is shown in Table 4 (McKeran and Thomas 1980). The clinical symptoms of raised intracranial pressure are headache, vomiting, and papilloedema, occasionally with transient visual obscuration leading to blindness. The headache

Table 4 Clinical features at diagnosis of cerebral glioma (653 patients, National Hospital, London, 1955–1975; modified from McKeran and Thomas 1980)

Symptoms	Frequency (%)	Signs	Frequency (%)
Headache	71	Hemiparesis	62
Epilepsy	54	Cranial nerve palsy	54
Mental change	52	Mental deterioration	53
Hemiparesis	43	Papilloedema	52
Vomiting	32	Hemianaesthesia	35
Dysphasia	27	Hemianopia	33
Impaired consciousness	25	Dysphasia	28
Visual failure	18	Visual failure	21
Hemianaesthesia	14		
Cranial nerve palsy	11		

is often bifrontal or occipital, although occasionally localized to the side of the tumour and is most noticeable in the morning. 'Hydrocephalic attacks' may exacerbate pain, particularly in patients with intraventricular tumours. The first symptom may be a change in conscious level, ranging from slight drowsiness to loss of consciousness. Generally, alteration of brain function causing mental deterioration and change in personality are insidious and slow in onset and may be more obvious to relatives than to the patient.

Epilepsy is a common feature of brain tumours (Table 4) as well as of other organic brain damage. Epilepsy of 'late onset' (after the age of 25 years), either focal or as generalized convulsions, is indicative of structural brain disease and merits further investigation. The presence of focal neurological symptoms or signs is strong clinical evidence of the presence and possible site of brain disease.

Specific clinical syndromes

Cerebral hemisphere tumours

Frontal lobe tumours commonly cause personality change together with impairment of intellectual function and epilepsy. An abnormal grasp reflex may be detected, with mild facial weakness and spastic hemiparesis as the more posterior frontal region is involved, as well as dysphasia if the dominant left hemisphere is affected. Involvement of the corpus callosum is often associated with dementia and incontinence. Temporal lobe tumours may be associated with hemiparesis, homonymous hemianopia, temporal lobe epilepsy, and dysphasia with dominant hemisphere tumour. Involvement of the parietal sensory cortex causes neglect of the contralateral side of the body and inattention. Right parietal lobe tumours cause diminished ability to orientate the body image and impaired left/right discrimination, in addition to possible motor impairment and receptive as well as expressive dysphasia in dominant hemisphere involvement. Occipital tumours may lead to homonymous hemianopia.

Midline and third ventricle region tumours

Gliomas in the optic chiasma or hypothalamus occurring in children or adolescents may impair growth or lead to precocious puberty and disturbances of temperature and appetite control as well as failure of vision. Interruption of cerebrospinal fluid circulation causes hydrocephalus, and with colloid cysts of the third ventricles this may be intermittent. Compression of the quadrigeminal plate, due to intrinsic tumours in the posterior part of the third ventricle and in the pineal region, leads to palsy of upward gaze, ptosis, and pupillary dilation (Parinaud's syndrome) in addition to hydrocephalus. Tumours affecting the thalamus and basal ganglia tend to cause contralateral motor and sensory deficit and occasional impairment of consciousness.

Posterior fossa tumours

Brainstem

Brainstem tumours cause low cranial nerve palsies associated with varying degrees of disturbance of long tract function and ataxia. Hydrocephalus is unusual.

Cerebellum and fourth ventricle

Tumours of the cerebellar hemispheres give rise to ataxia of the ipsilateral limbs associated with nystagmus. Obstructive hydrocephalus is common. Midline tumours around the fourth ventricle or in the cerebellar vermis cause trunkal ataxia.

Hydrocephalus may be associated with symptoms of neck stiffness due to the location of the tumour.

Cranial nerve tumours

Eighth nerve neurilemmoma, the most common of intrinsic nerve sheath tumours, usually presents with unilateral progressive deafness. It may not become symptomatic until the tumour has expanded into the cerebello-pontine angle, causing ataxia and involvement of the trigeminal and facial nerves. Neurilemmoma may rarely involve the trigeminal, glossopharyngeal, vagus, or hypoglossal nerves and these may also affect the cerebello-pontine angle.

Pituitary and suprasellar tumours

Non-functioning pituitary adenomas become symptomatic due to the involvement of the visual pathways (typically bitemporal hemianopia) or due to hypopituitarism. Spontaneous haemorrhage into such tumours (pituitary apoplexy) results in abrupt loss of vision with severe headache and impaired consciousness. Functioning pituitary adenomas present with specific endocrine disturbance.

The presenting features of craniopharyngioma are similar to those of non-functioning adenomas. Endocrine symptoms also include diabetes insipidus, failure to grow and attain puberty, or isolated hypothyroidism and hypoadrenalism. Hydrocephalus may be caused by obstruction of the ventricular system at the foramen of Monro and superior extension may lead to frontal lobe syndromes.

INVESTIGATIONS

Patients with features suggestive of a brain tumour should have a screening test to establish the presence of a lesion. This consists of a computerized tomography (CT) scan of the brain or magnetic resonance imaging (MRI). Additional non-invasive tests may include plain skull radiography, electroencephalogram (EEG), isotope scan, and psychometric evaluation, but are rarely necessary. Further tests help in accurate delineation of the tumour for surgery or radiation treatment and in subsequent follow-up.

CT scanning

CT scanning is widely available; the scanning time may be shorter than that for MRI and it is likely to continue as the primary investigation in patients with suspected brain tumours. The anatomical information provided by CT and MRI studies is similar. Localized swelling of the brain with associated peritumoural oedema and compression of the ventricular system, as well as midline shift, are features of supratentorial tumours, although MRI frequently reveals abnormality to a greater extent than is shown by CT (Fig. 2). On plain CT scan, meningiomas, lymphomas, and some metastases (such as melanoma) are usually hyperdense (Fig. 3), while gliomas, ependymomas, and most metastases are iso- or hypodense. They can still be recognized as tumour masses by contrasting them with surrounding low-density oedema. Tumour calcification is seen in approximately 10 per cent of gliomas and 50 per cent of oligodendrogliomas. Following injection of iodinated contrast, which demonstrates any alteration in the blood–brain barrier, the degree of contrast enhancement usually correlates with the degree of malignancy, particularly in gliomas. Over 85 per cent of high-grade gliomas, as well as meningiomas and metastases and only a minority of lower-grade tumours, show enhancement (Figs 3 and 4). Following intrathecal injection of contrast agents for myelography,

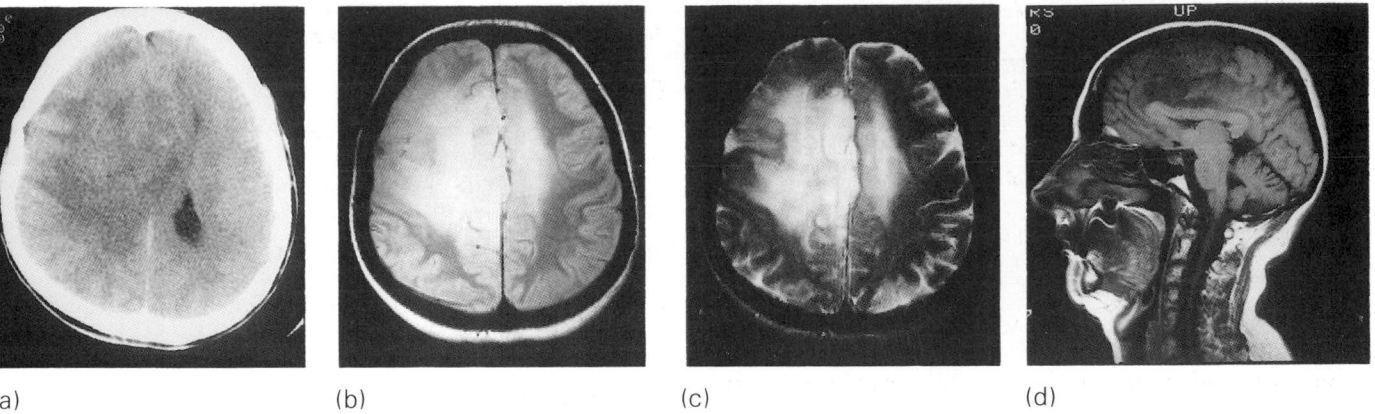

(a)　　　　　　　　(b)　　　　　　　　(c)　　　　　　　　(d)

Fig. 2　CT and MRI images of low-grade frontal/corpus callosum astrocytoma. (a) An axial CT scan showing mass effect and a low-density non-enhancing lesion without a clear margin. (b) and (c) Two axial MR images of different sequences, more clearly demonstrating an abnormal margin which represents either infiltrating tumour or oedema. (d) A sagittal T_1-weighted MR image demonstrating a pericallosal abnormality.

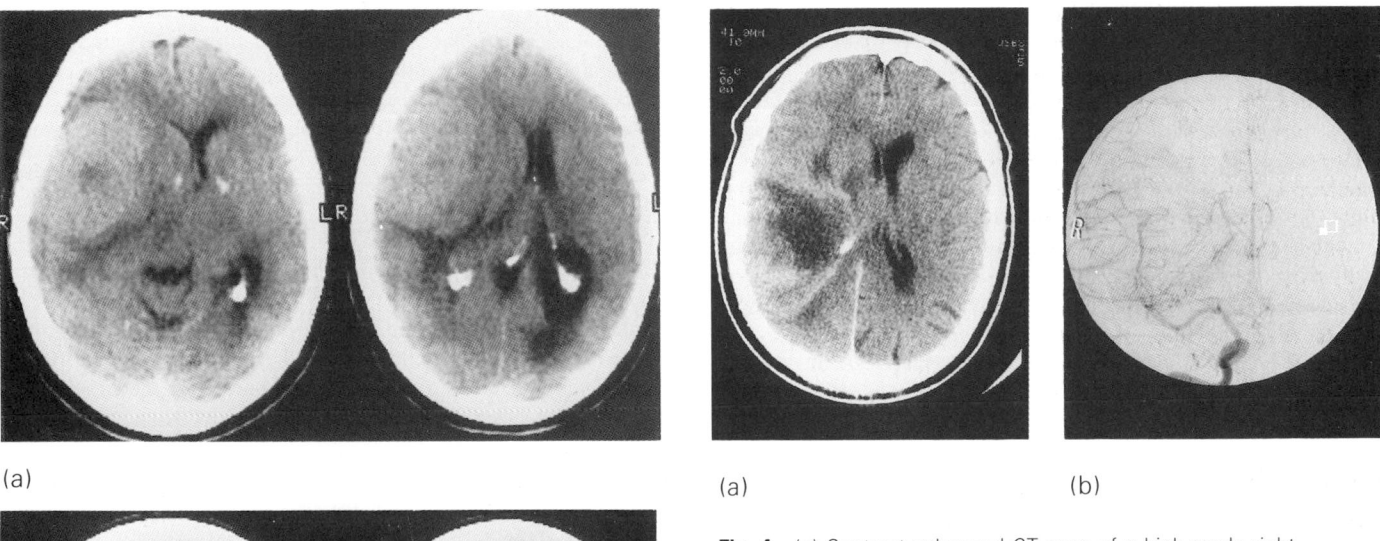

(a)

(b)

Fig. 3　A large sphenoid wing meningioma, showing (a) displacement of the brain by the extracerebral mass and (b) uniform contrast enhancement.

(a)　　　　　　　　(b)

Fig. 4　(a) Contrast-enhanced CT scan of a high-grade right temporoparietal glioma, showing a mass of inhomogeneous density with enhancement. (b) Anteroposterior projection of a right carotid angiogram (subtraction film), showing pathological tumour circulation.

distinguish from tumour and an interval CT may be required. Occasionally low-density regions associated with an encephalitic process, such as herpes simplex encephalitis, may be confused with low-grade tumours. A smooth enhancing ring of even thickness with low central attenuation suggests an abscess; tuberculomas may also mimic tumour appearance closely (Kendall 1980). The accuracy of CT in brain tumour diagnosis is in the region of 80 per cent. Ten per cent of benign lesions resemble glial tumours and 10 per cent of malignant gliomas have an atypical CT appearance suggestive of other pathology; histological diagnosis is therefore required in the majority of patients.

Magnetic resonance imaging (MRI)

MRI is concerned with the number and physical state of hydrogen nuclei/protons. In addition to the varying proton density, the physical state of the protons may be altered by changing magnetic variables and by obtaining data at different stages in the decay curves produced during this process. The application of a radiofrequency pulse and observation of the subsequent energy decay can be

computed tomography can image the cerebrospinal fluid spaces to provide additional information (Kendall 1980; Kingsley 1990).

The acute phase of cerebral infarction may occasionally demonstrate a mass effect of low attenuation which is difficult to

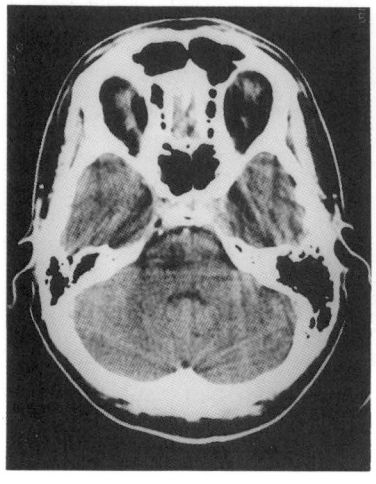

(a)

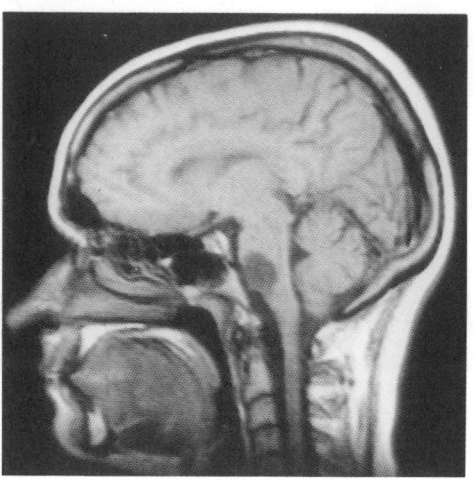

(b)

Fig. 5 Low-grade brainstem astrocytoma, poorly demonstrated (a) as a non-enhancing low-density region on axial CT, while clearly visible (b) on sagittal MRI.

measured for two time constants, T_1 and T_2. The T_1 decay curve gives a high signal (white image on a grey scale) when the decay is rapid and a low signal (black image) when it is slow.

Fat and haematomas have short T_1 decays and appear white on MRI, while most cerebral tumours and associated oedema have a higher water content, longer T_1 decays, and appear dark. Fluid and tissues with high water content, which contain relatively more mobile protons than are found in solid tissue, have a high signal on the T_2 decay curve. Thus, most tumours and associated cerebral oedema appear white in T_2-weighted MRI. The most commonly used sequences in the brain involve spin–echo, with variable repetition and echo times to bring out features of T_1, T_2, or proton density in particular pathological areas. The intravenous contrast agent gadolinium (Gd-DTPA) (Carr *et al.* 1981) is used similarly to contrast in CT scanning and may help in distinguishing between the tumour margin and the surrounding oedema.

In comparison with CT, MRI has better contrast discrimination (Fig. 5). Sagittal and coronal images can be produced more readily and in the posterior fossa or in the spinal canal the lack of a signal from bone obviates bone-induced artefacts (Fig. 5). Cerebrospinal fluid spaces, major blood vessels, and grey and white matter can all be visualized. Pathological changes such as haemorrhage can be diagnosed, although calcification and bone changes are seen less well than on CT. Demyelination, ischaemic areas, and low-grade gliomas, often not demonstrated by CT, are generally well shown by MRI. However, the characteristic capsule of a cerebral abscess, which can usually be distinguished on CT, may not be clearly visible on MRI.

Present evidence indicates that MRI is free of the hazards of ionizing radiation, although it is contraindicated in patients who may suffer from high magnetic fields, such as those with cardiac pacemakers and patients with metallic (and magnetic) aneurysmal clips. The aperture of the MR scanner is small and claustrophobia or the patient's physical size may restrict the investigation.

New developments in MR technology enable non-invasive MR angiography and the study of blood–brain barrier impairment. MR spectroscopy is an investigative tool to study biochemical changes in tumours and normal brain.

Cerebral angiography

Angiography is a supplementary rather than a screening procedure, which is occasionally useful for demonstrating the relationship of

a tumour to major vessels and in showing its blood supply (Fig. 4). A pathological circulation, with irregular tumour vessels and early draining veins, is frequently seen in high-grade gliomas and cerebral metastases; meningiomas show a characteristic tumour blush. In many cases the indications for angiography are to exclude vascular malformations or for planning the technical aspects of surgery.

Positron emission tomography (PET)

Radionuclides with a short half-life (^{15}O, ^{13}N, ^{18}F, and ^{11}C) and a longer half-life (^{82}Rb, ^{68}Ga, and ^{124}I) have been used in the PET studies of normal brain and brain tumours. PET can complement anatomical imaging methods and, because of the quantitative detection of tracers, it gives information on tissue biochemical and physiological processes, at present largely for research purposes. The currently measurable physiological parameters in the brain include regional blood flow and blood volume, blood–brain barrier permeability, oxygen and glucose metabolism and extraction, and amino acid metabolism (Brooks 1990). More recent studies include benzodiazepine receptor ligand and antibody binding and drug metabolism.

PET studies of glucose and oxygen metabolism have revealed high metabolic activity (particularly anaerobic glycolysis) of brain tumours and the uptake of fluorodeoxyglucose has been correlated with tumour grade (Di Chiro *et al.* 1982) and with prognosis (Alavi *et al.* 1988). The blood flow between tumours and in different regions of the same tumour varies greatly. High fluorodeoxyglucose uptake may help to distinguish recurrent tumour from necrosis and infarction, although tumour cells have been detected in areas of low activity assumed to be necrotic (Valk *et al.* 1988). Studies using amino acids, such as methionine, appear to demonstrate an anatomical boundary that corresponds more closely to pathological information (Bergstrom *et al.* 1983) than those given by CT or MRI. Studies of the functional properties of the blood–brain barrier, using ^{68}Ga-EDTA and ^{82}Rb, have demonstrated its disruption within primary and metastatic tumours and provide quantitative measurements of tissue permeability (Ott *et al.* 1990).

SURGERY OF INTRACRANIAL TUMOURS

Surgery for intracranial tumours should provide biopsy material for tissue diagnosis and, where possible, allow tumour resection to prolong survival and improve the patient's quality of life. The surgeon must review critically the pre-operative neuroradiological investigations in order to perform the procedure in the least invasive way and with minimal injury to normal brain and cranial nerve tissues. The operative approach entails opening the skull, most commonly in the cranial vault or in the occipital region. Transsphenoidal, translabyrinthine, and transclival approaches may be more appropriate for certain basal tumours. Where precise biopsy or resection is required, image-directed stereotactic methods can be employed which allow localization of intracranial lesions with millimetre accuracy.

Over the past 25 years, several technical advances have aided the neurosurgeon in the management of brain tumours. The control of cerebral oedema by osmotic diuretics and by glucocorticoids has reduced the number of emergency decompression operations and improved the operative mortality and morbidity. Advances in understanding of the neurophysiology of blood flow and raised intracranial pressure have led to remarkable improvements in anaesthetic technique for intracranial operations (Loh 1985). Improvements in surgical instrumentation have included the surgical microscope, which improves both magnification and illumination of the operative field, the ultrasonic tissue aspirator, and surgical lasers which, in selected cases, provide improved methods of tumour resection. Peroperative ultrasound improves tumour localization, as does the application of image-directed stereotactic surgery.

RADIOTHERAPY OF CNS TUMOURS

Radiation tolerance of the CNS

The adverse effects of radiation on the brain and spinal cord are classified clinically according to the time of appearance. Acute reactions occur during or immediately after a course of irradiation. Delayed reactions may be either 'early delayed', appearing a few weeks to a few months after radiotherapy or 'late delayed', starting months to years later (Sheline 1986). The time to response in irradiated normal tissue is determined mainly by the lifespan of mature cells, whilst tolerance is determined by the characteristics of stem cells; that is, their radiosensitivity, recovery potentials and capacity for proliferation. The biology of such normal tissue reactions, together with identification of target cell lineages within the CNS has been studied extensively in rodent models (van der Kogel 1991). The early delayed reaction is usually one of transient demyelination due to temporary depletion of oligodendroglia (Mastaglia *et al.* 1976). Late delayed damage results from the combination of oligodendroglial loss and endothelial damage, leading to demyelination and necrosis. In addition to the classical late radiation reaction, a less severe form of late damage may follow lower doses of radiation. This is recognized in children as cognitive impairment and is age related (Packer *et al.* 1989). A similar late effect is suspected in adults following high radiation doses (Hochberg and Slotnick 1980) or in association with chemotherapy (Twijnstra *et al.* 1987; Fleck *et al.* 1990; Lishner *et al.* 1990), with a contribution to such damage by the tumour itself.

The biologically effective dose (BED) formula based on the linear–quadratic model of radiation action aims to describe a range of fractionation schedules that is isoeffective for a particular end-point, for example normal tissue tolerance or tumour control probability. There is an implicit assumption that the isoeffect has a direct relationship to a certain level of cell inactivation or survival (*SF*). As the fraction of surviving cells associated with an isoeffect

is unknown it is customary to work in terms of a level of tissue effect, termed E.

$$\text{Effect } (E) = -\log_e(SF) = D(\alpha + \beta d)$$

$$E/\alpha = D\,[1 + d/(\alpha/\beta)] = \text{biologically effective dose (BED)}$$

BED is a measure of the effect (E) of a course of fractionated or continuous irradiation, having the units of dose (usually Gy). With appropriate reference dose values for tissue tolerance and an estimate of the α/β ratio, the BED formula provides a means of calculating isoeffective radiotherapy schedules appropriate to the CNS. Whilst estimates for the α/β ratio of both normal CNS tissue and tumours are available, such isoeffect calculations can only be used as a guide to the modification of clinical practice. In particular, schedules with multiple daily fractions or continuous low dose-rate treatments require estimates of repair half-times, which are not fully defined within the CNS.

Brain tolerance

The somnolence syndrome represents an early delayed radiation reaction in the brain and in adults is characterized by a transient period of exhaustion at 2 weeks and drowsiness, lethargy, and anorexia at 4–6 weeks, after irradiation. It has been reported in up to 80 per cent of children receiving 24 Gy as prophylactic cranial irradiation for acute lymphoblastic leukaemia and is less common following lower doses.

The results of late radiation damage to the brain are necrosis and demyelination. The dose-fractionation limits for brain necrosis are approximately 35 Gy in 10 fractions, 60 Gy in 35 fractions, and 70 Gy in 60 fractions (Sheline *et al.* 1980), although higher limits have also been reported, such as 60 Gy in 31 fractions (Marks *et al.* 1981) and 62 Gy in 30 fractions (Pezner and Achambeau 1981). The effects of lower doses of radiation on the developing brain in children are described elsewhere. Adult survivors of radical brain irradiation at or below the standard tolerance limits may develop neuropsychological sequelae (Hochberg and Slotnick 1980); these have also been described for lower doses of radiation when combined with chemotherapy (Twijnstra *et al.* 1987; Fleck *et al.* 1990; Lishner *et al.* 1990). Irradiation of the pituitary and hypothalamus may lead to pituitary failure and this is particularly recognized following radiotherapy of pituitary and suprasellar tumours.

Radiobiology of human brain tumours

Mechanisms determining clinical radioresistance in human glioma remain poorly understood. Cell lines derived from high-grade gliomas lie at an extreme of radioresistance *in vitro*, suggesting that at least part of the explanation of clinical failure may reside in the phenomenon of intrinsic cellular radioresistance. Mean SF_2 values obtained for human glioma at 0.6 (range 0.5–0.7), in comparison with mean SF_2 of 0.45 in human carcinomas (Taghian *et al.* 1992). Information on the relative radiosensitivity of other human brain tumours is limited due to difficulties in establishing representative cell lines. An estimation of the radiosensitivity of one well-characterized medulloblastoma, D283MED, revealed an SF_2 of 0.18, which lies in the range observed for highly radiocurable human tumours (McMillan 1993). Similarly, all human neuroblastomas cell lines examined exhibit extreme radiosensitivity *in vitro*, with typical SF_2 values of 0.15 (Holmes *et al.* 1990).

Radiotherapy technique

External-beam radiotherapy of intracranial tumours varies from high-precision focal irradiation through involved-field radiotherapy to whole-brain and craniospinal axis radiotherapy. The individual steps involved in the planning and delivery of radiotherapy are the same as those used at other sites. CT and MRI allow for accurate localization of the tumour, providing the margins can be visualized and assuming that they represent the true extent of the tumour. The precision of treatment planning and treatment delivery is helped by the use of immobilization devices. These can vary from mouth bites attached to the couch table to individually moulded plastic masks. With a correctly fitting mask, made by a two-step procedure of face impression and a positive plaster cast, relocalization is possible with an accuracy of approximately 3 mm. Other less labour-intensive devices, such as plastics mouldable at low temperatures, can be employed, but with reduced accuracy.

Whole-brain irradiation for palliative purposes may be carried out in a supine position without an immobilization device, while the need for cervical extension and matching to a spinal field as part of craniospinal axis irradiation requires precise positioning in a prone cast. Whole-brain irradiation in conditions of potential meningeal spread should include all limits of extension of the subarachnoid space (cribriform plate, optic nerves) and should extend beyond the margins of the middle cranial fossa. When forming part of craniospinal irradiation, the inferior limit of cervical extension is usually at the intervertebral disc space of C3–C4. The technique used for irradiation of a medulloblastoma is the same as that employed in children.

The site and size of the tumour within the cranial cavity determine the positioning of the patient. Frontal, anterior parietal, and central lesions are best treated in a supine position, while more posteriorly placed lesions are treated prone. The lateral position, technically suitable for more laterally placed central tumours (in the temporal lobe, for example) is rarely employed because of poor repositioning accuracy and the patient's discomfort.

Conventional planning utilizes images from CT and MRI. The target volume comprises the visualized tumour edge and a margin of suspected microscopic tumour spread. It also has to take into account the technical inaccuracy of planning, immobilization, and treatment delivery. The current margins beyond the rim of enhancement on CT scan vary from 2 to 5 cm for malignant brain tumours (for example, 3 cm for high-grade gliomas). In non-enhancing lesions the margin is usually 2 cm beyond the region of low density or a similar distance beyond the high signal-intensity area on T_2 sequences on MRI. The precise definition of tumour extent is operator dependent and should be based on pre-operative images. Conventional involved-field irradiation utilizes two or three fixed fields, while large, centrally placed tumours may best be treated by an opposing pair of fields. Pituitary adenoma and craniopharyngioma require smaller, usually 1 cm, margins and are treated either by three fixed treatment fields or by a rotation technique. In conventional partial brain irradiation, individually shaped shielding blocks may be employed to reduce the volume of normal brain irradiated and the use of shaped blocks along the scalp may reduce the risk of permanent alopecia.

Specialized radiotherapy techniques

Highly localized radiation can be given by stereotactic techniques using either brachytherapy or external-beam radiotherapy. Brachytherapy sources (^{192}Ir or ^{125}I, which has a superior dose distribution and simpler shielding requirements) are inserted into afterloading tubes positioned using stereotactic coordinates to ensure accurate localization. Doses up to 120 Gy (median 70 Gy) have been given over several days at 2–5 mm from the tumour margin to high-grade gliomas of small volumes (< 6 cm diameter) (Leibel et al. 1989; Gutin et al. 1991; Sieed and Gutin 1993), low-grade gliomas (Osterlag 1993), but ependymomas, pituitary adenomas, meningiomas, and chordomas have also been treated. Craniopharyngiomas and cystic astrocytomas have been treated by instillation of β-emitting colloidal [^{32}P] chromic phosphate, ^{198}Au, and ^{90}Y (Lunsford et al. 1985).

Stereotactic external-beam radiotherapy with a multiheaded cobalt unit (described as the 'gamma knife') was introduced in the 1950s by Leksell (1951). Although this technique of radiosurgery has been used principally in the treatment of cerebral arteriovenous malformations, a number of tumours, particularly acoustic neuromas (Norén and Leksell 1979), have also been treated. The high capital cost and limitation of field size (< 2 cm diameter) are the major drawbacks. Stereotactic external-beam radiotherapy with multiple non-coplanar arcs on a linear accelerator (Betti and Derechinsky 1983; Brada and Graham 1993) achieves a similar dose distribution. Stereotactic external-beam radiotherapy using multiple axes is only suitable for tumours of less than 5 cm diameter as the relative sparing of normal tissue diminishes with increasing target size (Graham et al. 1991). Non-spherical targets may be treated with static conformal beams (stereotactically guided conformal radiotherapy; Laing et al. 1993); treatment given as a single fraction with neurosurgical stereotactic frames which fix by pins to the skull vault is described as radiosurgery. The development of relocatable stereotactic frames which fix via the upper dentition (Gill et al. 1991; Graham et al. 1991) or the external auditory meati (Hariz et al. 1990) allows for fractionated radiotherapy described as stereotactic radiotherapy. This technique is likely to have an application in the administration of a localized high-dose boost following conventional external-beam irradiation of high-grade gliomas and in solitary brain metastases.

Heavy-particle accelerators deliver localized stereotactic radiotherapy without definite radiobiological advantages. The results are comparable to those of other stereotactic external-beam techniques, with response rates of up to 80 per cent in the treatment of arteriovenous malformations (Marks et al. 1988). The application of neutrons to the treatment of brain tumours has been largely abandoned because of the lack of clinically demonstrable therapeutic benefit (see below).

CHEMOTHERAPY

The response of intracranial tumours to chemotherapy depends, as at other sites, on drug delivery and the individual sensitivity of tumour cells. Factors influencing drug delivery to tumours include blood flow, permeability across capillaries and cell membranes, and the half-life of the drug. Cerebral capillary endothelial cells differ from endothelium at other sites by the presence of tight intercellular junctions which restrict the passage of material across the capillary wall and this is defined as the blood–brain barrier. The ability of a drug to cross the blood–brain barrier is determined by its molecular weight and lipophilicity (Levin et al. 1980), so water-soluble drugs of molecular weight more than 200 kDa penetrate poorly. Although drugs can be defined in terms of their brain capillary permeability (Table 5; Workman 1986), it is the transfer of drugs across the tumour endothelial membrane (blood–tumour barrier) which is of most relevance to drug delivery. The capillary

Table 5 Brain capillary permeability of chemotherapeutic agents (from Workman 1986)

High—intermediate	Low
BCNU	Adriamycin®
CCNU	Bleomycin
PCNU	Cyclophosphamide
Procarbazine	Chlorambucil
5-Fluorouracil	Melphalan
Dibromodulcitol	Methotrexate
AZQ	Vincristine
Hydroxyurea	Vinblastine
	Cisplatin
	Etoposide

Abbreviations: AZQ, diaziquone; BCNU, carmustine (bis-chloroethyl-nitrosourea); CCNU, lomustine; PCNU, 1-(2-chloroethyl)-3-(2.6-dioxo-1-piperidyl) nitrosourea.

permeability of brain tumour vasculature varies in different regions of the tumour as well as between tumours, even of the same histological type and the precise rôle of the blood—tumour barrier in determining chemoresponsiveness is not known.

The intrinsic cellular chemosensitivity of intracranial tumours relates to tumour histology. Germinomas, primitive neuro-ectodermal tumours, and primary cerebral lymphomas are chemoresponsive. Glial tumours have a relatively poor chemosensitivity as judged by clinical response rates (see below). *In vitro* studies of short-term cultures of glial tumours and glioma cell lines demonstrate heterogeneity in cellular composition which is also reflected in the varying chemoresponsiveness within subclones from the same tumour as well as between tumours of similar histology (Shapiro and Shapiro 1986). Predictive chemosensitivity testing of tumour cultures suggests a correlation between *in vitro* chemosensitivity and *in vivo* tumour control (Thomas *et al.* 1985).

Attempts at improving the results of chemotherapy in glial tumours have used techniques to improve drug delivery. This can be achieved by selecting drugs that penetrate the blood—brain barrier, by disruption of the blood—brain barrier or by increasing the drug concentration by high-dose systemic chemotherapy (with autologous bone-marrow transplant) and regional perfusion with intra-arterial chemotherapy. Attempts have also been made to introduce chemotherapeutic agents directly into the tumour by intralesional injection. None of these techniques has so far shown a benefit over conventional drug delivery.

MEDICAL MANAGEMENT

All patients with features of raised intracranial pressure and a significant neurological deficit should be treated initially with a short-term course of corticosteroids, such as dexamethasone 4 mg 6 hourly orally or parenterally. This should be given together with an H$_2$-antagonist (for example, ranitidine or cimetidine) to reduce the risk of gastric bleeding. In non-responding patients, high-dose steroids (up to 60—80 mg dexamethasone daily) may afford temporary benefit. Following debulking surgery the dose should be reduced rapidly and titrated against symptoms and should be discontinued where possible to avoid long-term effects, of which proximal myopathy is particularly disabling. Long-term anticonvulsant treatment is also recommended in patients presenting with epilepsy and for 1—2 years following neurosurgical intervention.

Many symptoms in patients with brain tumour are due to depression associated with the knowledge of the diagnosis of such serious consequence. Patients and their family and friends require intensive psychological support, both in hospital and in the community. In addition, patients should be offered intensive rehabilitation to overcome or to learn to cope with disability caused by the tumour and its treatment.

GLIOMAS

Gliomas are neuroepithelial tumours comprising astrocytomas, oligodendrogliomas, and ependymomas. Astrocytic tumours, which constitute 65—70 per cent of all gliomas, can be graded on the basis of histological features into grades I—IV (Kernohan and Sayre 1952) or into three grades described as astrocytoma, anaplastic astrocytoma, and glioblastoma (Burger 1986; Table 1).

Presentation and diagnosis

The presenting features fit into the pattern described for cerebral tumours. The diagnosis is established by imaging followed by histological verification of a surgical specimen. The tumour mass of high-grade gliomas is generally inhomogeneous on CT scan, with variable enhancement after intravenous contrast and extensive peritumoural oedema (Fig. 4). Low-grade gliomas tend to show low density on a CT scan without enhancement (Fig. 2), occasionally associated with calcification. Haemorrhagic presentation with haematoma is often difficult to distinguish from calcification on a CT scan, although these can be differentiated on MRI. Ependymomas do not have a typical CT appearance unless they involve white matter adjacent to the lateral ventricle. Oligodendrogliomas are more frequently calcified but this is not a pathognomonic feature.

High-grade astrocytomas

High-grade astrocytomas are the most common primary malignant brain tumours; their incidence increases with age, with a peak between 65 and 75 years. They are classified into anaplastic astrocytoma (grades III and IV) and glioblastoma (grade IV). In anaplastic astrocytoma increased cellularity and mitotic activity is associated with pleomorphism, focal necrosis, and endothelial hyperplasia. The presence of necrosis in the classification of Burger is indicative of a glioblastoma. Nevertheless, in anaplastic astrocytoma there are areas of recognizable astrocytic differentiation, while in glioblastoma the cells are more anaplastic and pleomorphic and necrosis, endothelial proliferation, and haemorrhage are common. On immunohistochemical staining, astrocytic neoplasms stain positively with glial fibrillary acidic protein (Table 2).

A major difficulty in the grading of astrocytomas is the high histological heterogeneity (Russell and Rubinstein 1989) which may lead to sampling error in small biopsy specimens. This is also reflected in a marked heterogeneity in karyotype. It is believed that the final grade and, consequently, the natural history, is determined by the most malignant portion of the tumour. Low-grade tumours are frequently found to become high grade at the time of recurrence. This may represent either tumour progression or the predominance of a more malignant clone within an initially heterogeneous tumour.

Treatment

Surgery

High-grade gliomas are diffusely invasive and cannot be removed completely even by radical resection. It is possible to recognize three levels of surgery: biopsy, partial removal, and more extensive resection in the form of lobectomy or subtotal macroscopic removal. Surgical practice varies widely, but typically approximately

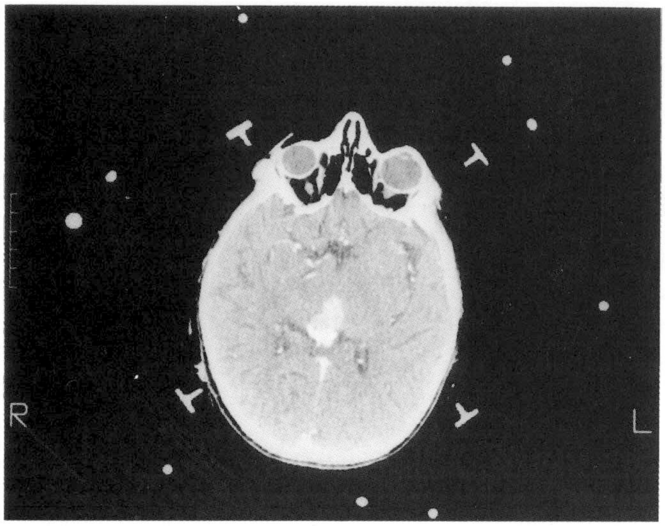

Fig. 6 Pre-operative CT scan with stereotactic apparatus in position for stereotactic biopsy of an enhancing pineal region tumour; histology showed the presence of a high-grade astrocytoma.

one-third of the patients will fall into each of the three categories (McKeran and Thomas 1980).

Biopsy may be performed either freehand or with image-directed stereotactic control (Fig. 6) through a skull burr-hole under local or general anaesthesia. The latter method is more time-consuming but carries lesser morbidity and is more accurate, with a higher success rate in establishing tissue diagnosis. Patients too old or disabled to undergo open surgery may have biopsy as the only procedure. Tumours that are deep and inaccessible, diffuse tumours, or multiple lesions should also be biopsied rather than being dealt with by open surgery.

Partial removal of a tumour is performed through a craniotomy in the skull vault and with the surgeon controlling resection so as to remain within the intrinsic tumour in order to minimize the risk to surrounding normal brain. More radical surgery consists of craniotomy associated with classical frontal, temporal, or occipital lobectomy or, alternatively, resection to an apparent demarcation zone between frank tumour and surrounding brain, often using the operative microscope to improve visualization. In patients with polar tumours within the frontal, temporal, or occipital lobe, craniotomy and extensive removal with lobectomy are indicated.

Gliomas are infiltrating tumours and have no defined plane of cleavage. Although a boundary to the tumour may appear macroscopically, there is invariably further microscopic infiltration. Kelly introduced a method of interactive image-directed stereotactic craniotomy (Kelly et al. 1982) which permits radical excision of gliomas up to the apparent tumour margin seen on scanning. The morbidity is less than that occurring in conventional craniotomy and debulking, but it is not yet established whether survival is improved by this type of resection. Photodynamic therapy has been investigated in an attempt to treat the tumour-infiltrated normal brain surrounding gliomas (Kaye et al. 1987). Laser light is used within the tumour cavity after extensive glioma resection to 'sterilize' the tumour bed by virtue of the differential increased sensitivity of tumour cells to light following the administration of photosensitizers.

In many reports extensive tumour resection is a factor associated with prolonged survival. There are no randomized studies addressing the question of the extent of resection and it is not clear whether undefined factors influencing tumour resectability or the tumour debulking itself determine the outcome. Although it is debatable whether tumour debulking improves survival, there is general agreement that it can provide good initial palliation.

Reoperation has a minor rôle in glioma management and is often reserved for small symptomatic and easily accessible tumours, largely as a palliative procedure. A repeat biopsy may be indicated to differentiate tumour recurrence from radiation necrosis, particularly following high-dose interstitial radiotherapy.

Radiotherapy

Radiotherapy has an established rôle in the management of patients with high-grade astrocytoma. In randomized studies it was shown to prolong survival (Walker et al. 1978; Kristiansen et al. 1981) and it improves the quality of life of those with responding tumours. Normal function prior to radiotherapy is usually maintained until tumour progression and functional deficits improve in one-third and stabilize in one-half of patients so affected (Nelson et al. 1986).

The traditional policy of whole-brain irradiation was based on pre-CT scanning experience of the spread of tumour beyond the suspected margin visualized surgically or by radioisotope imaging. Improved tumour imaging has allowed for a more localized delivery of radiation. Although there are no randomized studies comparing whole-brain with involved-field radiotherapy, the reported survival results of localized treatment as practised in individual centres are similar. A randomized study comparing whole-brain irradiation with treatment to the whole brain followed by a local boost to identical tumour doses has not demonstrated a survival difference (Shapiro et al. 1989).

In detailed pathological studies, tumour cells are frequently seen beyond the enhancing CT margin and occasionally beyond the region of suspected oedema (Burger et al. 1988). Localized radiotherapy may therefore frequently miss the suspected tumour (Halperin et al. 1989). However, the common experience of recurrence of a glioma at or near the primary tumour site (Hochberg and Pruitt 1980) or as an extension of the pre-existing residual mass, suggests that local treatment failure is due to poor control of the main tumour mass. Therefore, the current target volume is either whole-brain irradiation in the initial phase, treating to levels of 40–45 Gy, followed by a local boost confined to the tumour as visualized by CT or MRI with a 3–5 cm margin, or localized irradiation throughout. The optimal total dose is 55–60 Gy in doses of 1.7–2 Gy per fraction. The dose–response relationship, as suggested from sequential non-randomized studies up to a dose of 60 Gy (Walker et al. 1979), has been confirmed by a study comparing 45 Gy in 20 fractions with 60 Gy in 30 fractions (Bleehen and Stenning 1991). Radiation doses beyond 60 Gy to large target volumes have not demonstrated any further survival benefit (Chang et al. 1983). A policy of increasing the dose to a small target volume, such as can be achieved with high-precision stereotactic external-beam radiotherapy or with interstitial irradiation, is being tested in randomized trials. Despite the theoretical objection of extensive tumour infiltration, it may be of benefit in a selected group of patients with small, localized tumours.

Modification of standard radiotherapy

Unconventional fractionation

Attempts at improving tumour control have included accelerated fractionation and hyperfractionation; these studies are listed in Table 6. No clear survival benefit has been demonstrated for either

Table 6 Radiotherapy studies of altered fractionation

Study	Randomization[a]	Dose/fraction (Gy)	Treats/day	Total dose[c] (Gy)	Treatment time (weeks)	Survival advantage
Douglas and Worth (1982)	N[b]	1.0	3	45–60+10B	5	Yes
Shin et al. (1983)	R[b]	0.89	3	40+10B	4	Yes
Payne et al. (1982)	R	1.0	4	36–40	2	No
Fulton et al. (1984)	R	0.89	3	61.4	4.5	No
Keim et al. (1987)	N	1.6	3	60	2	No
Deutsch et al. (1989)	R	1.1	2	66	6	No

[a] R, randomized; [b], small number of patients; [c] B, boost; N, non-randomized; Treats, treatments.

approach. However, if accelerated schedules prove to be equally effective as conventional radiotherapy without increasing early or late toxicity, accelerated radiotherapy may be employed to shorten the overall treatment time, particularly in patients with poor overall prognosis. At present altered fractionation regimens have to be used with caution as they carry the potential risk of increased late damage to normal tissue. The survival of patients with high-grade astrocytoma is often too short for the full expression of late CNS injury and the potential late effects are not fully documented.

Radiation sensitizers and particle irradiation
Misonidazole and hyperbaric oxygen have failed to improve survival in patients with high-grade gliomas (Chang 1977; MRC Working Party 1983). The potential benefit of sensitization of proliferating tissues with halogenated pyrimidine analogues 5-bromo-2'-deoxyuridine (BUdR) and 5-iodo-2'-deoxyuridine (IUdR) remains to be demonstrated in clinical practice. Neutrons have been explored extensively, either alone or in combination with photons. Despite a high tumour sterilization rate, the incidence of normal tissue damage is high and randomized studies have not shown an improvement in survival (Duncan et al. 1986).

High-dose localized irradiation
With stereotactic technology and improved tumour localization it is possible to deliver high-dose focal irradiation, either with interstitial or stereotactic external-beam radiotherapy. Such techniques are limited to small volumes and to tumours within less functionally important regions of the brain. The radiation doses employed are well beyond the known radiation tolerance limits, but the more localized delivery minimizes the amount of radiation given to the normal brain. The reported median survival following interstitial radiotherapy with ^{125}I seeds to 50–120 Gy (median 70 Gy) in selected patients with recurrent supratentorial high-grade astrocytoma is beyond 50 weeks (Leibel et al. 1989). The treatment carries a high risk of necrosis which requires reoperation. Similar results are obtained with single-fraction radiosurgery or with fractionated stereotactic radiotherapy (Laing et al. 1993). At present high-dose localized irradiation is an effective palliative treatment in patients with small recurrent gliomas. The role in primary therapy remains to be defined.

Chemotherapy

Adjuvant chemotherapy
Many agents have been tested in randomized trials (Table 7) and such studies have been summarized by Kornblith and Walker (1988) and Stewart (1989). An overview analysis of randomized studies employing nitrosoureas in adjuvant protocols has shown a survival advantage of 9 per cent at 1 year and 3 per cent at 2 years (Stenning et al. 1987). Combination chemotherapy is not clearly superior to single agents, with the possible exception of lomustine (CCNU),

Table 7 Agents tested in randomized adjuvant chemotherapy trials for the treatment of high-grade astrocytomas

Single agents	Or in combination with
BCNU	HU, MPL
CCNU	PCZ, HU, PCZ+VCR, PCZ+VCR+MTX
MeCCNU	DTIC
PCZ	
MPL	
HU	
DBD	

Abbreviations: BCNU, carmustine (1,3-bis[2-chloroethyl]-1-nitrosourea); CCNU, lomustine; DBD, dibromodulcitol; DTIC, dacarbazine (5-[3,3-dimethyl-1-triazeno]imidazole-4-carboxamine); HU, hydroxyurea; MeCCNU, semustine (methyl-CCNU); MPL, methylprednisolone; MTX, methotrexate; PCZ, procarbazine; VCR, vincristine.

Table 8 Conventional chemotherapy regimens used in the treatment of gliomas

Single agent		
BCNU	80 mg/m² IV daily for 3 days or 200–240 mg/m² IV once	
		Repeated every 6 weeks
CCNU	100–130 mg/m² orally once	
		Repeated every 6 weeks
Combination (PCV)		
CCNU	100 mg/m² orally day 1 only	
Vincristine	1.4 mg/m² IV day 1 (or days 8 and 15)	
Procarbazine	60–100 mg/m² orally for 7–14 days	
		Repeated every 6 weeks

Abbreviatons: BCNU, carmustine (1,3-bis[2-chloroethyl]-1-nitrosourea); CCNU, lomustine; PCV, procarbazine, CCNV, vincristine.

vincristine, and procarbazine when compared to carmustine (BCNU) alone (Levin et al. 1990). At present, adjuvant chemotherapy should be given in the context of clinical trials. The potential remains that a subgroup of patients may benefit from adjuvant chemotherapy and it is important to pursue further prospective studies to define the clinical and biological parameters which will identify this group.

Chemotherapy in recurrent tumours
Nitrosoureas have been widely employed as single agents in recurrent astrocytomas and their overall effectiveness in terms of a response rate judged by CT and clinical criteria is 20–40 per cent. The chemoresponsiveness of recurrent tumours to various common single agents administered intravenously is poor (for example, complete and partial responses have been reported for etoposide (9 per cent), Adriamycin® (7 per cent), carboplatin (9 per cent), cisplatin (7 per cent)). Numerous phase 2 studies have been reviewed by Stewart (1989) and Dropcho and Mahaley (1990).

There are few randomized studies in recurrent disease comparing single agents or combinations and the high response rates reported for individual drugs in some studies may be due to patient selection and varying response criteria. The currently employed chemotherapy protocols are shown in Table 8.

Experimental chemotherapy approaches

A 30–50 per cent response rate to high-dose carmustine with autologous bone-marrow transplantation has been demonstrated in recurrent tumours. Adjuvant high-dose carmustine in doses of $600-800 \, mg/m^2$, combined with autologous bone-marrow transplantation, does not significantly improve survival when compared to matched controls (Mbidde et al. 1988), although there have been occasional unexpected long-term survivors. There are no randomized studies comparing conventional and high-dose treatment.

Intra-arterial injection increases the peak drug concentration during the first passage of a drug through the cerebral circulation. Carmustine has been the most widely employed agent for intra-arterial therapy. Although response rates are high, this treatment may result in symptomatic leucoencephalopathy and retinal damage unless the catheter is placed above the ophthalmic artery. Intra-arterial cisplatin, either alone or in combination with other agents (carmustine, etoposide) has also been used in phase 2 studies. High response rates have been reported, although a benefit over conventional administration is not clear (see Stewart 1989). A randomized Brain Tumor Cooperative Group (BTCG) study, comparing adjuvant intra-arterial and intravenous carmustine administration, demonstrated higher toxicity without a survival advantage for intra-arterial therapy (Shapiro et al. 1989).

Temporary disruption of the blood–brain barrier may be achieved by the infusion of a hyperosmolar saturated solution of 25 per cent mannitol into the carotid or vertebral arteries under general anaesthesia. This technique increases the delivery of water-soluble drugs to both the tumour and the normal brain. Although increasing cell kill it also significantly increases treatment toxicity and so far there is no definite clinical information to prove the additional effectiveness of this technique compared to conventional drug administration in the treatment of gliomas (Neuwelt et al. 1986).

Management of recurrent disease

Patients with recurrent high-grade glioma usually have large recurrent tumours with severe disability. Their prognosis is poor and further active treatment is rarely advisable. Occasional patients with small recurrences at easily accessible sites may be treated by reoperation (Moser 1988) and/or reirradiation with localized forms of therapy. Re-excision of a recurrent tumour, particularly following a short progression-free interval, is rarely indicated. Recurrent tumours are usually large and palliative chemotherapy remains the only active treatment option, with a 20–40 per cent probability of a short-term response often accompanied by symptomatic improvement. Chemotherapy does not have a curative rôle, although responding patients may have a prolonged period of survival. Cystic degeneration within the recurrent tumour may be aspirated and recurrent fluid reaccumulation treated with instillation of radioactive chromic phosphate to surface doses of 100–200 Gy.

Treatment recommendations and prognosis

The median survival of patients with high-grade astrocytomas is 40–50 weeks. Many well-conducted randomized studies have identified age (<40, 40–60, >60), performance status (Karnofsky <40, 40–70, >70), and histology (anaplastic astrocytoma vs glioblastoma multiforme) as the most important independent prognostic factors for survival, while the length of history, the presence of fits, and the extent of resection may also be of some prognostic significance (Shapiro 1986). The current treatment recommendation is biopsy or tumour debulking (so as to avoid any disabling neurological deficit) followed by radiotherapy, not only to prolong survival but also to improve the patient's quality of life. The benefit of chemotherapy remains controversial. The treatment has to be tailored to the patient's age and general condition and it may be appropriate not to offer treatment to severely disabled and elderly patients who have a short life expectation. Symptoms may be temporarily controlled with a reducing course of corticosteroids. Because of the devastating consequences of the diagnosis, the physical and mental disability, and the stress to the family and friends, sympathetic and intensive support should be provided by professionals within a neuro-oncology team.

Low-grade gliomas

Astrocytoma

Low-grade astrocytomas in adults primarily occur in the cerebral hemispheres and include the variants of astrocytoma shown in Table 1, grade I and grade II tumours, and the pilocytic astrocytoma. The fibrillary type of astrocytoma contains abundant fibres, while the protoplasmic type has cells with regular small nuclei and few or no glial fibres. Gemistocytic astrocytomas have large globular cells with eccentrically placed nuclei and eosinophilic cytoplasm containing glial fibres. Pilocytic astrocytomas have narrow, elliptical cell nuclei, with long fibrillary cell processes often containing eosinophilic Rosenthal fibres. The cells are generally oriented in parallel bundles and there is often calcification and microcyst formation. Cerebellar, third ventricle, and optic nerve gliomas are usually of this type and can be described as grade I. Although usually occurring in the posterior fossa in children, the adult variant has a similar indolent behaviour.

Oligodendroglioma

Oligodendrogliomas usually arise in frontal and, less frequently, temporal and parietal, lobes. They occur in all age-groups, with a peak incidence between 40 and 60 years. Although relatively indolent, they usually recur at the primary site and may display a tendency for subependymal spread, with an incidence of cerebrospinal fluid seeding of less than 5 per cent.

Oligodendrogliomas have a distinctive cellular morphology with large, round nuclei surrounded by clear cytoplasm, giving a 'halo' effect. The cells lie in a trabeculated honeycomb network of thin-walled vessels with frequent calcification. In the WHO grading system, these are usually rated grade II tumours, although anaplastic, high-grade forms with necrosis and vascular hyperplasia may occur, being classified as anaplastic oligodendroglioma. Mixed oligo-astrocytomas consist of both astrocytic and oligodendroglial cells, either mixed or combined as discrete areas of individual tumours.

Ependymoma

Ependymomas project from ependymal surfaces, most commonly the floor of the fourth ventricle and less frequently in the central canal of the spinal cord or the lateral and third ventricles and in the cerebello-pontine angle. They may also arise in the brain parenchyma. The most common cell type consists of uniform ependymal cells containing a specific organelle; the blepharoblast. The cells are oriented around vessels, giving a perivascular rosette appearance. There are a number of variants, such as papillary ependymoma which may resemble a choroid plexus papilloma. The subependymoma usually appears as a large mass occupying the ventricle or as a symptomatic small nodule. Myxopapillary ependymomas usually occur in the cauda equina region. Although most ependymomas are low-grade (grades I–II) tumours with occasional high-grade anaplastic variants, there is no uniform agreement on grading. Differentiation into low- and high-grade tumours has prognostic significance in some studies of intracranial and spinal tumours. The term ependymoblastoma is reserved for embryonal tumours of the primitive neuroectodermal tumour category (Table 1).

Treatment

Surgery

Low-grade gliomas, particularly astrocytomas and oligodendrogliomas, often diffusely involve the cerebral hemispheres and in many cases resection and debulking procedures carry unacceptable risks of neurological deficit. CT- or MRI-directed stereotactic biopsy has a low risk of serious morbidity and mortality (just over 1 per cent) with a 93 per cent chance of obtaining a definite histological diagnosis (Thomas and Nouby 1989). In children and young adults with pilocytic astrocytomas extensive surgical resection may be practical without causing unacceptable deficits.

Intrinsic low-grade glioma of the brainstem can be biopsied either by open surgery or by stereotactic means. In the presence of an exophytic component, open surgery may allow partial tumour removal. Posterior fossa exploration in cases of cerebellar astrocytoma usually reveals a tumour cyst with a small mural nodule of solid neoplasm. Generally, total removal can be achieved, but even following incomplete resection the recurrence rate is low. Ependymomas of the fourth ventricle are approached through an occipital craniectomy and should be resected as fully and safely as possible to reduce the tumour burden and to re-establish the flow of cerebrospinal fluid.

Radiotherapy chemotherapy, treatment recommendation and prognosis

Low-grade astrocytoma

The rôle of radiotherapy in the treatment of low-grade astrocytomas is controversial. Although retrospective studies of patients with incompletely excised tumours suggest a survival benefit for patients treated with post-operative irradiation (Leibel et al. 1975; Fazekas 1977), particularly with target doses exceeding 50 Gy (Shaw et al. 1989). The precise rôle of radiotherapy awaits the results of prospective randomized studies. Radiotherapy stabilizes or improves neurological deficit caused by the tumour and often reduces the frequency of convulsions which accompany the presentation of low-grade tumours and is currently recommended in inoperable or incompletely excised symptomatic tumours. The recommended radiation dose is 55–60 Gy at 1.6–1.8 Gy per fraction and the treatment should be restricted to the tumour and a surrounding margin of normal tissue. The extent of disease in these often unenhancing tumours is usually defined as the region of low density on CT and is better delineated with MRI. The target volumes are usually large and radiotherapy should be carried out cautiously with a protracted course of treatment, as many patients may survive beyond 5 years.

Like high-grade astrocytoma, histology, age, performance status, and the extent of resection are the most important prognostic factors.

The reported 5 and 10 year survival rates for patients with pilocytic astrocytoma are 85 and 79 per cent, respectively and for patients with ordinary astrocytomas and mixed oligoastrocytomas, 51 and 23 per cent, respectively (Shaw et al. 1989).

Oligodendroglioma

Retrospective studies reporting the use of radiotherapy in the treatment of pure oligodendroglioma show only a marginal survival benefit (Sheline et al. 1964; Lindegaard et al. 1987; Bullard et al. 1989). As in the case of low-grade astrocytoma, radiotherapy is effective as palliation and should be employed in patients with a neurological deficit due to the tumour so that stabilization and improvement can be achieved. The role of adjuvant radiotherapy following incomplete tumour excision is not clear. The recommended doses and techniques are the same as for low-grade astrocytoma. The median survival of patients with oligodendroglioma is similar to other low-grade gliomas (Lindegaard et al. 1987). Preliminary reports suggest effectiveness of chemotherapy in oligodendrogliomas, particularly the anaplastic variety.

Ependymoma

Despite the lack of formal comparison of surgery with and without radiotherapy, the use of post-operative irradiation in the treatment of intracranial ependymoma has become accepted as standard treatment. This is based on retrospective studies which demonstrate good long-term control following partial tumour excision and radiotherapy (Salazar 1983; Shaw et al. 1987; Vanuytsel et al. 1991). Recommendations on the extent of radiotherapy are based on the apparent pattern of spread. Ependymomas have a tendency for cerebrospinal fluid seeding, with a reported incidence of 5–10 per cent. The risk of seeding is higher with high-grade compared to low-grade tumours, in infratentorial compared to supratentorial location and in cases of uncontrolled disease at the primary site (Vanuytsel and Brada 1991). There is no clear evidence that spinal irradiation prevents isolated spinal metastases, particularly if the primary tumour remains uncontrolled. Our view is that ependymomas should be treated with local irradiation applied to the site of the tumour and the appropriate margin, regardless of tumour grade and site. The technique and doses used are the same as those employed for other low-grade gliomas. Other authors recommend whole-brain irradiation with cervical spine extension in high-grade supratentorial tumours and craniospinal irradiation in high-grade infratentorial tumours.

The overall 5 year survival of selected patients with cranial ependymomas is 50–60 per cent and progression-free survival is approximately 10 per cent less. The prognosis is related to the histological grade and in low-grade tumours to the extent of surgical resection. Nevertheless, 30 per cent of patients with incompletely excised ependymomas, particularly of low grade, remain alive without evidence of tumour progression at 5 years (Vanuystel et al. 1992).

Brainstem gliomas

Glial tumours may involve any of the structures from the thalamus and hypothalamus through the midbrain to the pons and medulla (Fig. 5). Brainstem tumours, particularly involving the pons, are more common in children. The prognosis of histologically verified gliomas is poor, with prolonged survival of less than 20 per cent (Grigsby et al. 1989) and the principles of management are identical to those involved in the treatment of children with brainstem glioma.

MEDULLOBLASTOMA

Medulloblastoma has a peak incidence in childhood and represents only 2–6 per cent of intracranial tumours in adults. It is considered to be a part of the spectrum of primitive neuroectodermal tumours, which include pineoblastoma, ependymoblastoma, and medulloblastoma. Histologically adult medulloblastoma is identical to the childhood variant and consists of densely cellular masses of small, oval or round cells of uniform appearance with frequent mitoses.

Tumours usually arise with similar frequency in the cerebellar vermis or the hemispheres and often invade the fourth ventricle, with occasional brainstem involvement. They may extend inferiorly through the foramen magnum. Through its tendency to penetrate the ependymal surface, medulloblastoma is associated with a high risk of seeding through the subarachnoid space.

Clinical presentation and diagnosis

Patients with medulloblastoma present with a combination of symptoms of raised intracranial pressure (usually due to hydrocephalus), cerebellar signs, and occasionally brainstem cranial nerve palsies. CT scan may demonstrate a hydrocephalus and a hyperdense and homogeneously enhancing posterior fossa mass with distortion of the fourth ventricle. The differential diagnosis lies between medulloblastoma, ependymoma and glioma, and solitary cerebellar metastasis. Lateral tumours may resemble meningioma. The addition of MRI improves the diagnostic accuracy and better delineates the tumour extension, particularly to the upper cervical cord. Medulloblastomas usually exhibit prolonged T_1 and T_2 relaxation times.

Following histological diagnosis, subsequent staging investigations should include cerebrospinal fluid cytology for the presence of malignant cells and a myelogram or spinal MRI to detect occult spinal seeding. The Chang staging system (Chang et al. 1969), based on the anatomical extent of disease, is a prognostic predictor in childhood medulloblastoma but its significance in adults is not clear.

Treatment

Surgery

Medulloblastoma is approached by posterior fossa craniectomy. The surgery is directed at obtaining as complete tumour removal as possible, while avoiding damage to the floor of the fourth ventricle. The resection is aimed not only at reducing the tumour burden but also at avoiding the requirement for cerebrospinal fluid drainage.

Radiotherapy

Post-operative radiotherapy is indicated in all patients regardless of the extent of tumour resection. The whole craniospinal axis should be irradiated and the principles of adequate craniospinal axis dose are the same as in childhood medullablastoma, the whole brain being exposed to 35 Gy in 19–21 fractions and the whole spine being exposed to 35 Gy in 20–25 fractions. The posterior fossa is boosted to a total dose of 55 Gy. Isolated spinal seeding should be treated with a radiotherapy boost to a small volume to the level of spinal cord tolerance.

Chemotherapy

The use of adjuvant chemotherapy in adult medulloblastoma has not been tested in a separate randomized trial. As the natural history of adult medulloblastoma is similar to that in children, similar indications for chemotherapy should be accepted (high risk with T_3 and T_4 and M_1–M_3—see below), although some authors recommend the use of adjuvant chemotherapy in all adults (Bloom and Bessell 1990). The regimens used are those tested in randomized trials in children (Evans et al. 1990; Tait et al. 1990). The conventional regimen consists of weekly vincristine ($1–1.5$ mg/m^2) during radiotherapy followed after a break of 1 month by lomustine (100 mg/m^2 orally) given every 6 weeks, with vincristine (1.4 mg/m^2 intravenously) on days 1, 8, and 15 of each cycle. More recent regimens under test in childhood medullablastoma contain carboplatin, cyclophosphamide, and etoposide and require evaluation in adults.

Prognosis

The extent of disease as defined by the Chang criteria is the most important prognostic indicator in children. This has not been demonstrated in adults. The most important prognostic factor for survival in adult patients with medulloblastoma is the extent of surgical excision. The overall results are similar to the results in children, with 5 and 10 year survival of 50–60 per cent (Bloom and Bessell 1990). Most patients who relapse do so at the primary site in the cerebellum. Isolated spinal recurrences are rare with craniospinal axis irradiation.

The prognosis of patients with metastatic medulloblastoma is poor. The commonest site of recurrence is either within the posterior fossa (over half of recurrences) or in other CNS sites. In up to 10 per cent of patients disease recurs outside the CNS, particularly in the bone-marrow and systemic spread may be seen in the absence of a ventricular shunt. Recurrent tumours frequently remain chemoresponsive, although they are rarely curable by chemotherapy. Active agents (apart from lomustine, vincristine, and procarbazine as used in adjuvant trials) include carboplatin, cisplatin, Adriamycin®, etoposide, cyclophosphamide, or melphalan. The best regimen at present is not defined.

PINEAL TUMOURS

Pineal tumours are rare, comprising up to 1 per cent of all intracranial neoplasms, although they are more common in Japan. They are classified as pineal germ cell tumours (germinoma or teratoma), pineal parenchymal tumours (pineoblastoma or pineocytoma), glial tumours (Fig. 6), and benign cysts. The respective frequencies are 61, 15, and 7 per cent (Bloom 1983). Germ cell tumours and pinealomas are most frequent between 15 and 25 years of age, with germinomas and teratomas showing a male predominance. Pineoblastomas are more frequent in childhood, while more differentiated pineocytomas occur from childhood through to adult life.

Pathology

The most frequent intracranial germ cell tumours are germinomas, which are histologically indistinguishable from testicular seminoma or ovarian dysgerminoma. They are composed of large spheroidal or polygonal cells and small cells resembling lymphocytes. Although they most frequently arise in the pineal body, they also occur in the suprasellar region. The tumours at both sites are identical histologically and in their behaviour. The tumour masses invade adjacent structures and may infiltrate the ventricular space, with a propensity for seeding through the cerebrospinal fluid. Pineoblastoma is a highly cellular tumour, histologically indistinguishable from medulloblastoma and can be included in the group of primitive neuroectodermal tumours. It is locally infiltrative and, like medulloblastoma, may spread through the cerebrospinal fluid. Pineocytoma is usually a circumscribed, less densely cellular tumour, composed of relatively mature cells of pineal parenchyma organized into lobules and occasionally containing neuronal and astrocytic components. Any type of glial tumour may be seen in the pineal region, as well as benign epidermoid and dermoid cysts.

Clinical presentation

Pineal tumours lie in close proximity to the third ventricle and the aqueduct and the commonest presentation is hydrocephalus, caused by occlusion of cerebrospinal fluid drainage. Other features reflect the involvement of adjacent structures, such as the midbrain, hypothalamus, and the brainstem. Compression of the quadrigeminal plate causes paresis of upward gaze and the pupils become unresponsive to light or accommodation (Parinaud's syndrome). Downward gaze paresis usually indicates further inferior tumour extension. Pineal germ cell tumours, like their systemic testicular counterparts, may secrete α-fetoprotein and human chorionic gonadotrophin into the cerebrospinal fluid and systemic circulation. The presence of α-fetoprotein is specific for teratoma, while human chorionic gonadotrophin levels may be elevated by either teratoma or germinoma.

Diagnosis and staging

Most pineal region tumours appear as enhancing masses of varying size in the pineal region, with possible hydrocephalus and distortion of surrounding structures. Although, typically, germinomas tend to be homogeneous, hyperdense, uniformly enhancing masses and teratomas more often cystic, enhancing tumours, the differentiation on the basis of diagnostic CT scans is often difficult and unreliable (Fig. 6). It is also difficult to differentiate germ cell tumours from glial tumours, although the latter have more infiltrating characteristics with an irregular enhancing edge. Pineoblastomas and pineocytomas have no specific radiological features.

Germinomas and pineoblastomas are highly radioresponsive and have been differentiated from other tumours of the pineal region by therapeutic 'diagnostic' testing, as a reduction in the size of the enhancing tumour mass following a limited dose of radiation.

In patients with undiagnosed pineal tumours and those with verified germ cell tumours, the blood and, if possible, the cerebrospinal fluid should be assayed for α-fetoprotein and human chorionic gonadotrophin. In addition to the diagnostic value, monitoring the levels provides a measure of disease activity following treatment and during subsequent follow-up. Cerebrospinal fluid cytology is mandatory in the absence of raised intracranial pressure and can indicate cerebrospinal fluid seeding. Myelography or spinal MRI are also indicated in germ cell tumours and pineoblastomas to examine the spinal subarachnoid space for the presence of occult metastases.

Surgery

Surgical management of pineal tumours remains controversial. It is possible to surgically remove teratoma, for example via a posterior transoccipital supracerebellar route, while germinoma and glioma cannot be effectively resected. CT- or MRI-directed stereotactic biopsy may be performed with acceptable low morbidity and in most cases will achieve a diagnosis to help with the decision about further treatment. A shunt procedure to relieve obstruction of the outlet of the third ventricle should be avoided if possible as functioning shunts may precipitate systemic seeding.

Radiotherapy

Histologically unverified pineal tumours

If the nature of the tumour remains in doubt, the pineal region can receive a therapeutic trial of radiotherapy to 20 Gy in 12 fractions to the tumour and appropriate margin, with pre- and post-treatment CT or MRI scan. A reduction in tumour size is accepted as evidence for germinoma or pineoblastoma and radiotherapy is continued either to the whole brain or to the craniospinal axis, reaching a total dose of 50–55 Gy to the pineal mass. The risk of spinal seeding of unverified tumours appears higher than in germinomas (Brada and Rajan 1990) and spinal irradiation is recommended. The results of this policy are excellent, with cure rates of 70–90 per cent.

Histologically verified germ cell tumours

In histologically verified germinoma, the treatment is usually given in two phases: 30 Gy to the whole brain and a 10–20 Gy boost using a three-field technique.

Radiotherapy policy in the treatment of teratomas has been identical to that of germinomas. However, the results are disappointing, with a 5 year cause-specific survival of 10–30 per cent (Bloom 1983; Dearnaley et al. 1990). There is a need to exploit new treatment strategies combining chemotherapy, radiotherapy, and post-treatment resection of residual pineal masses, which is akin to the policy in disseminated testicular tumours.

The unresolved issue in the treatment of CNS germinomas is the extent of irradiation which relates to the risk of spinal seeding. A summary of the reported literature suggests that the risk of developing spinal metastases is 13 per cent in histologically verified germinomas treated by whole-brain irradiation alone and that this is reduced to 5 per cent in patients treated with craniospinal radiotherapy (Brada and Rajan 1990). The current reasonable and safe practice therefore includes craniospinal irradiation to a dose of 30 Gy to the spinal cord (given in 20–25 fractions) in adults where the side-effects of spinal irradiation are acceptable. In children with incomplete spinal growth and in young women where the ovaries are in the exit beam of the spinal field, the decision is more debatable. Spinal irradiation should probably only be employed in the presence of positive cerebrospinal fluid cytology and occasionally following major surgical interference, when the risk of seeding may be higher. The treatment of verified germinoma with radiotherapy alone results in excellent cure rates, reaching a cause-specific survival probability of 100 per cent (Dearnaley et al. 1990).

The known radiation sensitivity of seminoma suggests that a dose of 30 Gy may be sufficient to control intracranial germinomas. The current policy of a dose of 50 Gy is based on retrospective studies reporting higher control rates of pineal tumours with doses over 50 Gy (Sung et al. 1978). Unfortunately these studies included a variety of pineal tumours and the minimum required dose for the control of pure germinomas is not known. The current trend is to reduce doses to the primary tumour volumes but the long-term results of this policy are not available.

Pineal parenchymal tumours

Pineoblastomas as PNET, are treated with radiotherapy along similar lines to the treatment of germinomas or medulloblastomas. Pineocytomas do not share the same radioresponsiveness, but following local radiotherapy to a dose of 55–60 Gy, prolonged survival and occasional cures have been reported (Disclafani *et al.* 1989).

Chemotherapy for germinoma and teratoma

Cisplatin–based chemotherapy (as used for treatment of testicular germ cell tumours) is effective in treating recurrent germ cell tumours by producing radiological and clinical responses (Dearnaley *et al.* 1990). It may be employed as the first line treatment in patients with extensive tumours at presentation and is being tested in single arm prospective studies. The routine use of chemotherapy in the treatment of verified intracranial germinomas is at present not justified, although in future studies the use of combined regimens may allow for a reduction in radiation dose (Allen *et al.* 1987).

Pineal and suprasellar non-seminomatous germ cell tumours should be treated with initial chemotherapy along similar lines to testicular teratomas. An optimum regimen has not yet been defined. This should be followed by craniospinal axis radiotherapy and resection of residual masses, where possible. Current results suggest improved survival, although this policy is not invariably curative.

Summary and treatment recommendations

Histological diagnosis should be attempted in the majority of patients presenting with pineal tumours. Raised serum/CSF markers are diagnostic. The primary treatment of pineal germinomas is radiotherapy, although chemotherapy may be employed in extensive tumours. In the presence of a positive cerebrospinal fluid cytology or with extensive tumours, the use of craniospinal irradiation is recommended and this also remains a reasonable option when the toxicity of spinal irradiation is acceptable. Cranial teratomas should be treated with initial systemic chemotherapy. Pineoblastomas are treated along similar lines to medulloblastomas, while pineocytomas should be treated with surgery and/or local radiotherapy only. Glial tumours in the pineal region are treated in the same way as gliomas at other sites.

PRIMARY CEREBRAL LYMPHOMA

Primary cerebral lymphoma is a non-Hodgkin's lymphoma localized to the CNS. It is a rare tumour with a reported frequency of 1 per cent of intracranial tumours (Zulch 1986) and it occurs in adults, particularly in the fourth and fifth decades. It is associated with immune deficiency, following organ transplantation and in AIDS, when it presents in a younger age group. The incidence of sporadic primary cerebral lymphoma appears to be rising (Eby *et al.* 1988).

Pathology

Primary cerebral lymphoma is a highly cellular tumour which is histologically identical to systemic non-Hodgkin's lymphoma of intermediate and high-grade histology (International Working Formulation). The predominant subtype is a diffuse, large-cell lymphoma. It is a B-cell neoplasm demonstrating light-chain restriction on immunohistochemistry and immunoglobulin gene rearrangement, although occasional rare cases of T-cell tumour have been reported. The typical microscopic pattern is of diffuse, highly cellular masses with perivascular cuffing and infiltration of the surrounding brain and ependymal and meningeal surfaces. The tumours have a tendency for subependymal and leptomeningeal spread and distant seeding, particularly through the cerebrospinal fluid. There is no specific site predilection. Ocular involvement, with infiltration of the vitreous and retina, has also been described.

Clinical presentation and diagnosis

The presentation is the same as that of other primary intracranial tumours, although clinical deterioration is often rapid with a median duration of symptoms of 3 months. Uveitis may precede or accompany other neurological features in 5–10 per cent of patients. CT findings are of single or multiple iso- or hyperdense masses, often with uniform enhancement and frequent evidence of subependymal spread. The features are not diagnostic and histological confirmation is required. An occasional indication of the histological nature of the tumour is the reduction in tumour size following treatment with corticosteroids. The MRI features are not pathognomonic and at present do not add to the CT findings unless the tumour is situated in the posterior fossa.

Subsequent staging should include cerebrospinal fluid cytology. Myelogram studies are not required unless spinal metastases are suspected on clinical grounds. In HIV-negative patients and in the absence of a preceding history of systemic non-Hodgkin's lymphoma, the likelihood of systemic lymphoma at presentation is very small and at present there is rarely a need for systemic lymphoma staging. Involvement of the CNS by metastatic lymphoma in the form of solid tumours is also rare.

Surgery

Extensive tumour excision is not warranted and in suspected cases biopsy is sufficient for diagnostic purposes. The rapid response to corticosteroids and radiation precludes the need for extensive debulking operations.

Radiotherapy

Radiotherapy has been, the mainstay of management. Radiation produces a radiological and a clinical response. It prolongs survival and usually produces functional improvement or stabilization of neurological deficit. However, a long-term cure with radiotherapy alone remains elusive. There are no controlled data on the optimum radiation parameters, but the widely accepted current practice is whole-brain irradiation to a dose of 40 Gy, followed by a boost to 15–20 Gy to the primary tumour site (with a margin) using 1.6–1.8 Gy per fraction. The rôle of spinal irradiation is unproven but is recommended in patients with a positive cerebrospinal fluid cytology. Such radiotherapy policy results in a median survival of 10–18 months (Hochberg and Miller 1988; Brada *et al.* 1990; Nelson *et al.* 1991). The majority of tumours recur within the CNS, either at the primary site or elsewhere in the brain or spinal cord, with occasional systemic relapses.

Chemotherapy

Primary cerebral lymphoma is responsive to a variety of chemotherapy regimens, such as high-dose methotrexate, CHOP (cyclophosphamide, doxorubicin, vincristine, prednisone), or MACOP-B (methotrexate, doxorubicin, cyclophosphamide, vincristine, prednisone, bleomycin). Combined regimens of chemotherapy and radiography are being exploited, but so far have not yielded convincingly superior survival results (Brada *et al.* 1990; DeAngelis *et al.* 1992). Attempts at improving the effectiveness of drugs include the use of high-dose chemotherapy and intracarotid infusion in combination with disruption of the blood–brain barrier with a suggestion of survival benefit (Neuwelt *et al.* 1991).

The independent prognostic factors for survival are age and neurological performance status and the aggressiveness of therapy should therefore be tailored to these. The present recommendation is primary chemotherapy followed by radiotherapy in suitable patients. The long-term survival results of 30–40 per cent are comparable to the results of chemotherapy in advanced systemic aggressive non-Hodgkin's lymphoma.

MENINGIOMA

Meningiomas comprise 10–19 per cent of intracranial tumours and occur most frequently in adults. They arise from dural sites where arachnoid villi are concentrated or from the tela choroidea. The particular sites of origin include the cerebral convexity and falx and less frequently the olfactory groove, sphenoid ridge and suprasellar region, posterior fossa, and tentorium. Most meningiomas are solitary lobulated masses, which remain encapsulated and attached to the dura while expanding into adjacent space (Fig. 3). Although the invasion of brain parenchyma by benign meningiomas is rare, the tumours may invade the adjacent skull, eliciting an osteoblastic reaction.

The majority of meningiomas are benign tumours consisting of sheets of polygonal cells with oval nuclei. The specific cellular shape and arrangement and the intercellular matrix allow differentiation into the various histological subtypes listed in Table 1. The differentiation of benign meningiomas into histological subgroups is of no prognostic significance, with the possible exception of the haemangiopericytic subtype which is considered to have a worse prognosis (Guthrie *et al.* 1989).

The criteria which indicate a more malignant nature of meningioma include an increased mitotic rate, the presence of necrosis and cellular atypia, and higher labelling indices (over 1 per cent) particularly in recurrent tumours. A more malignant nature of the tumour is also indicated by the tendency to recurrence, invasion of brain parenchyma, and a metastatic potential (Russell and Rubinstein 1989). Meningeal sarcoma, which is classified separately, shows typical features of spindle cell sarcoma and may occasionally arise within a more differentiated meningioma.

The higher incidence of meningiomas in women, the manifestation of tumours during pregnancy (Bickerstaff *et al.* 1958), and the association of meningiomas with breast and genital cancer (Schoenberg *et al.* 1975) have suggested oestrogen and progesterone dependency. Most of these tumours demonstrate a high concentration of progesterone receptors and few oestrogen receptors (Blankenstein *et al.* 1983). There is conflicting evidence on the *in vitro* responsiveness of meningiomas to antiprogesterone therapy and the clinical effectiveness of this treatment has not yet been fully demonstrated.

Clinical presentation

Vault meningiomas may present with focal deficits, due to disturbance of the underlying cortex, together with focal or generalized epilepsy. Meningiomas in the anterior part of the supratentorial compartment (from the cranial vault, the sagittal sinus, or falx) are relatively asymptomatic until a late stage. Deterioration of intellectual function and personality changes caused by such tumours may pass unnoticed until features of raised intracranial pressure appear.

Skull base subfrontal meningiomas of the olfactory groove cause anosmia and occasionally result in ipsilateral optic atrophy with contralateral papilloedema (Foster Kennedy syndrome). Suprasellar meningiomas may compress the optic chiasm and result in visual deficit. Clivus or foramen magnum region tumours impinge on the

lower cranial nerves, brainstem, and midbrain, with attendant focal deficit.

Meningiomas of the sphenoid ridge are relatively frequent and are often en plaque, causing hyperostosis of bone rather than a large intracranial mass effect. Such tumours in the inner or middle third of the sphenoid wing may lead to proptosis with involvement of the optic nerve and, later, oculomotor, trochlear, and abducent nerve palsies. Tumours of the outer third of the sphenoid wing impinge on the posterior frontal and temporal lobes. Meningiomas of the tentorium cerebelli may present with cerebellar ataxia or with epilepsy and hemianopia, due to irritation of the overlying occipital hemisphere.

The characteristic CT appearance of meningioma is of a well-defined extra-axial mass with attachment to the meningeal surface. It is usually uniformly hyperdense, showing homogeneous enhancement with intravenous contrast (Fig. 3). Occasional atypical features, such as cystic changes and extensive surrounding oedema, may cause difficulty in differentiation from intrinsic tumours. MRI can better delineate the tumours, particularly in the temporal and the posterior fossae. Plain radiology of the skull may demonstrate a characteristic hyperostotic reaction.

Surgery

Easily accessible tumours in the meninges of the skull vault of the subfrontal region or the anterior part of the falx can be totally resected, together with a surrounding rim of normal dura and associated infiltrated bone. If not possible, subtotal removal with diathermy of the dural attachment is carried out. Tumours of the sphenoid ridge and suprasellar region may be removed in their entirety, although occasionally residual tumour remains in the dural attachment or in the associated areas of bony involvement, particularly if the inner third of the sphenoid wing is involved. Meningiomas at other sites, such as the cerebello-pontine angle, the clivus, or the anterior part of the foramen magnum, are less readily accessible and their removal is associated with higher morbidity. Tumours which arise in the parasagittal or falcine region posteriorly in the intracranial compartment are also difficult to remove completely, because of their relationship with the sagittal sinus and important draining veins which cannot be sacrified. The morbidity and recurrence rates of meningiomas at these sites remain higher than for tumours elsewhere.

Simpson (1975) graded the extent of surgical removal into five categories:

(1) complete macroscopic removal of tumour and dural attachment together with any abnormal bone;

(2) complete macroscopic removal of tumour with diathermy coagulation of its dural attachment;

(3) complete macroscopic removal of intradural tumour without resection or coagulation of its dural attachment or of any extradural extensions;

(4) partial removal leaving intradural tumour *in situ*;

(5) simple decompression with biopsy.

The control rates are 91, 81, 71, and 56 per cent for resection grades 1, 2, 3, and 4, respectively. Mirimanoff *et al.* (1985) reported actuarial 5, 10, and 15 year recurrence-free rates of 93, 80, and 68 per cent, respectively, following total excision of meningioma, contrasting with the respective progression-free rates after incomplete removal of 63, 45, and 9 per cent. Ninety-six per cent of convexity meningiomas were totally removed, with a recurrence rate of only 3 per cent at 5 years; this compares with 28 per cent of sphenoid ridge tumours being totally removed, having a progression rate of 34 per cent at 5 years. Parasagittal and posterior fossa meningiomas, both difficult to excise completely, had a 5 year progression-free rate of 78 per cent.

Radiotherapy

The evidence for the effectiveness of radiotherapy is available from retrospective studies comparing partial excision alone with partial excision plus radiotherapy. The recurrence rate at 5 years following incomplete excision of benign meningioma is 30–40 per cent and this is halved with adjuvant radiotherapy (Barbaro et al. 1987; Taylor et al. 1988). Occasional patients with inoperable tumours have been treated with radiotherapy alone and the progression-free survival and overall survival of these patients at 5 years is reported to be over 50 per cent (Glaholm et al. 1990). The recommended technique is involved-field irradiation, where the target volume includes regions with potential residual tumour, as judged by pre-operative imaging and surgical findings and a 1–2 cm margin. This should be treated to 55–60 Gy in 1.7–2 Gy per fraction.

The prognosis in patients with malignant meningiomas is poor. Complete excision is rarely achieved because of infiltration of the underlying brain parenchyma. Post-operative radiotherapy is generally employed and its rôle is the same as that of radiotherapy in the treatment of extremity sarcomas. As these tumours are rare and comparative studies are not available, the precise rôle of radiotherapy is not clear.

Prognosis and treatment recommendations

Prognosis in patients with meningioma is determined by tumour histology, the extent of surgery, and neurological performance status at the time of presentation. Benign meningiomas should be treated by complete excision alone whenever possible. Post-operative radiotherapy is recommended in patients with incompletely excised tumours. Recurrence following apparently complete excision should be treated with further reoperation and radiotherapy. Atypical meningiomas and haemangiopericytic type of angioblastic meningioma have a prognosis that is intermediate between benign and malignant forms. Attempts at complete excision and adjuvant post-operative radiotherapy are indicated in all. Patients with malignant meningiomas have a poor prognosis despite extensive treatment with surgery and radiotherapy, with a median survival of 1–3 years (Glaholm et al. 1990). Although both surgery and radiotherapy are recommended, there is a need for new treatment strategies for this group of tumours.

CRANIOPHARYNGIOMA

Craniopharyngiomas are benign neoplasms arising from epithelial rests associated with Rathke's pouch in the sella or more frequently the suprasellar region. They represent 2–9 per cent of intracranial tumours. Approximately half of them occur in childhood, with a second, smaller peak of incidence at 50–60 years.

Pathology

Craniopharyngiomas are partly cystic and partly solid tumours. They often compress and adhere to one or more adjacent structures; the optic nerves and chiasma, the pituitary, hypothalamus, and the third ventricle. Histologically, they consist of bands of stratified squamous epithelium with few mitotic figures, supported by a connective tissue stroma. The epithelium shows degenerative changes, with cystic spaces filled with thick fluid containing cholesterol crystals and with calcium deposition in the 'keratoid' regions. The tumour capsule is surrounded by gliosis. Although the lesion is benign, small islands of epithelium may be seen outside the capsule and this probably represents epithelial budding rather than true invasion.

Clinical presentation and investigations

The primary location of the tumour and the rate of progression will determine the presenting clinical features, which include endocrine, visual, and mental disturbances, as well as features of raised intracranial pressure. The most frequent endocrine presentation in children is growth hormone deficiency with retardation of growth, although gonadotrophin, thyroid-stimulating hormone, and adrenocorticotrophic hormone deficiency and diabetes insipidus also occur. Pituitary involvement in adults frequently leads to hypopituitarism. Compression of the chiasma and optic nerve or optic tract results in visual field defects in 75–85 per cent of patients (Chen Wen et al. 1989; Rajan et al. 1993), most frequently presenting as bitemporal or homonymous hemianopia (Kennedy and Smith 1975) which may be unnoticed by the patient. Lesions extending upwards away from the visual pathway spare vision in up to 20 per cent of patients (Kennedy and Smith 1975). Raised intracranial pressure is usually due to hydrocephalus caused by the obstruction of cerebrospinal fluid flow at the foramen of Monro. Involvement of the hypothalamus and occasional tumour extension into the frontal lobes may lead to changes in personality and memory defects.

Calcified suprasellar lesions and sella enlargement are often seen on plain skull radiography. CT or MRI scans are frequently diagnostic and show a partly cystic and partly solid suprasellar mass with calcification in the cyst wall. Pituitary adenomas with cystic change and calcification can mimic this appearance, although other suprasellar lesions, which include aneurysms of the anterior part of the circle of Willis, suprasellar germinoma, optic chiasmal glioma, Langerhans' cell histiocytosis, and a variety of benign cysts, should be distinguished from craniopharyngioma by their radiological appearance. Angiography is recommended prior to craniotomy to document the relationship of vessels to the tumour, although coronal MRI images may also demonstrate the relationship of the tumour to the cavernous carotid arteries.

Treatment

The natural history of craniopharyngioma varies from a benign to a rapidly progressive and destructive tumour, causing damage to the surrounding structures. At presentation, tumours vary in size from small lesions in the sella or suprasellar region to large cysts extending into the brain parenchyma and third ventricle. The need for treatment depends on the degree of deficit and its rate of progression, as well as the age of the patient.

Surgery

The presence of hydrocephalus requires urgent surgical intervention by shunting or direct tumour decompression. Initial decompression may be achieved with a stereotactically guided cyst aspiration, although without further treatment fluid frequently reaccumulates. More radical tumour removal can be carried out through a transtemporal, subfrontal, or transseptal transsphenoidal route. The transtemporal approach is favoured, particularly for lesions lying in the region of the floor of the third ventricle. Although benign and encapsulated, the tumour is firmly adherent to surrounding neural structures, such as the hypothalamus and radical attempts at removal may lead to hypothalamic damage.

Although operative mortality has decreased and is less frequent in experienced hands and with the use of an operating microscope, severe post-operative morbidity is frequent (22–40 per cent) (Symon and Sprich 1985; Chen Wen et al. 1989) and includes endocrine deficiency, such as diabetes insipidus and hypopituitarism and more serious damage to the hypothalamus, with altered temperature control, a fluctuating level of consciousness, and late sequelae such as uncontrolled obesity.

Following complete resection the mean recurrence rate is 29 per cent and 5 and 10 year survivals 80 and 70 per cent, respectively (Brada and Thomas 1993). However, attempts at complete excision may be unsuccessful, particularly in large lesions and radical surgery should be avoided. Partial excision alone results in high recurrence rate (mean 73 per cent) and poor long-term survival.

Radiotherapy

The local tumour control and survival following conservative surgery and radiotherapy is superior to the results of radical surgery (Brada and Thomas 1993), with reduced operative mortality and less frequent post-treatment morbidity. Review of reported cases in the literature suggests a recurrence rate of 17 per cent with a 5 year survival of 80–100 per cent and a 10 year survival of 70–90 per cent (Brada and Thomas 1993) with limited morbidity.

The radiotherapy technique is similar to that used for pituitary adenoma, with three fixed fields (anterior and two wedged lateral fields) encompassing the tumour and a 1–2 cm margin. Because of the proximity of the optic chiasm and optic nerves, the dose and fractionation should be below the CNS tolerance level (see above) and the recommended dose is 50 Gy in 30–33 daily fractions, treating all fields daily. A dose–response relationship beyond 50 Gy has not been demonstrated.

The incidence of optic nerve damage is less than 1 per cent with total doses of 50 Gy or less and up to 1.8 Gy per fraction (Rajan et al. 1993). Panhypopituitarism due to the combination of tumour-induced damage, surgery, and radiation is frequent and occurs more commonly following radical excision when compared to limited surgery and radiation (Thomsett et al. 1980).

Cystic craniopharyngiomas have been treated with instillation of radioactive colloidal gold and, more recently, with [^{32}P] colloidal chromic phosphate, which can control the reaccumulation of cystic fluid following aspiration (Pollack et al. 1988).

Treatment recommendation and prognosis

The low morbidity and excellent long-term results of limited surgery followed by radiotherapy favour this approach in the majority. Ten year survival following such a policy is between 70 and 100 per cent and late effects are minimal. Total excision is best reserved for young children where radiotherapy may result in unacceptable late damage and for patients with recurrent tumours following radiotherapy. Radical surgery carries a significant mortality as well as long-term morbidity, even in experienced hands and the reported recurrence rate varies from 20 to 30 per cent of surviving patients (mean 29 per cent) following the apparent complete removal of the tumour (Amacher 1980; Danoff et al. 1983; Symon and Sprich 1985; Chen-Wel et al. 1989). The use of colloidal chromic phosphate is

at present reserved for patients with recurrent cystic craniopharyngioma requiring frequent aspirations.

PITUITARY ADENOMA

Pituitary tumours present in all age groups. Pituitary adenomas are slowly proliferating benign clonal tumours arising from the cells of the anterior pituitary. They present with a combination of features of endocrine syndromes of hypersecretion (prolactinoma, acromegaly, Cushing's syndrome, and rarely gonadotrophin or thyroxin hypersecretion), pituitary insufficiency, or due to enlarging mass causing compression of the visual apparatus.

Plain skull radiography may demonstrate enlargement of the sella. CT or MRI scans reveal iso- or hyperdense mass arising from the pituitary fossa which enhances with contrast. Prior to treatment, patients with suspected pituitary adenoma should have full endocrine and ophthalmological assessment. On subsequent follow-up these may provide a clinical measure of tumour control.

Surgery

The aim of surgery is tumour removal and decompression of the visual apparatus. Large pituitary adenomas with significant suprasellar extension causing visual disturbance are approached most commonly through a right frontal craniotomy with subfrontal retraction to expose the optic chiasm and the tumour. Occasionally a lateral approach with partial temporal lobe resection may be anatomically more favourable. Both pituitary adenomas and craniopharyngiomas may contain cyst fluid and aspiration of this prior to subtotal removal of the tumour by microdissection may be helpful. Where craniotomy is not indicated on account of the patient's age or general medical condition, it is possible to achieve satisfactory decompression of the optic chiasm by transsphenoidal surgery, even for relatively large tumours. Pituitary microadenomas (less than 1 cm in diameter and usually associated with endocrine syndromes) and intrasellar adenomas are best treated by a transsphenoidal route, which is associated with lower morbidity. In the early post-operative period, control of diabetes insipidus with desmopressin and adequate corticosteroid replacement are the most important requirements.

Radiotherapy

Radiotherapy is effective in producing long-term tumour control of pituitary adenoma and achieves control of excess pituitary hormone secretion. There is a delay in the normalization of hormone levels and the time to return to normal depends on the pre-treatment hormone level. Radiotherapy is recommended as adjuvant treatment following incomplete tumour excision, as primary treatment in patients not suitable for surgery, in patients with acromegaly and Cushing's disease where control is not obtained by surgery, and in Nelson's syndrome (see Section 16). The recommended dose for pituitary adenoma is 45 Gy in 25 fractions, using a three-field technique with the target volume localized to the pituitary mass and a 1 cm margin. The morbidity of this technique is low with 1–2 per cent risk of optic nerve damage and a 1 per cent risk of a second tumour in the first 10 years. A large proportion of patients require hormone replacement therapy due to progressive pituitary failure.

Medical treatment

The dopamine agonist, bromocriptine, is the mainstay of treatment of prolactinoma. It may also reduce growth hormone secretion in acromegaly. Somatostatin analogues are used in the treatment of acromegaly and may have an additional growth inhibitory effect.

Treatment recommendations and prognosis

The treatment of choice in non-secreting pituitary adenomas is limited surgical decompression (for example transphenoidal resection) followed by conventional fractionated external-beam radiotherapy. Surgery remains an effective means of decompression of the pituitary fossa and provides rapid relief of chiasmal and optic nerve compression and reduction in hormone secretion. Different degrees of resection of pituitary adenoma which do not achieve complete excision do not influence the long-term prognosis in terms of ultimate tumour control of non-secreting adenomas. The 10 and 20 year progression-free survivals of patients treated with conservative surgery and conventional external-beam radiotherapy are 94 and 88 per cent and for patients with non-functioning pituitary adenomas 97 and 92 per cent, respectively (Brada et al. 1993). The results of conservative surgery and radiotherapy reported from other centres range from 80 to 95 per cent 10 year progression-free survival.

Prolactinomas are treated initially with bromocriptine. This can be followed by local radiotherapy which provides lasting tumour and hormonal control. In the absence of satisfactory response to medical treatment tumours can be resected. Acromegaly is best treated with attempted complete tumour removal, usually by transphenoidal resection. Patients with persistently elevated growth hormone following surgery can be temporarily treated with bromocriptine or somatostatin analogues. Further persistent elevation is successfully treated with local radiotherapy although there is considerable delay in the normalization of growth hormone levels.

Cushing's syndrome may be initially treated with primary medical therapy. Following failure of medical treatment patients should undergo resection with radiotherapy reserved for failure of conventional treatment. Patients with ACTH-secreting pituitary adenoma treated by bilateral adrenalectomy are at risk of developing Nelson's syndrome and should receive prophylactic pituitary irradiation.

OPTIC NERVE GLIOMA

Because of the indolent natural history of low-grade glioma affecting the optic nerve and chiasm, the tumour may manifest in adults although it is predominantly a tumour of childhood. In 15–30 per cent of patients it is seen in association with neurofibromatosis.

The natural history of slow progression has led to controversy regarding the optimum management. Some tumours display aggressive behaviour, with involvement of the optic chiasm and local extension into the third ventricle and adjacent brain, particularly the hypothalamus and others remain confined to the chiasm with little change over long periods of time. Complete excision of the optic nerve or chiasmal tumour is rarely possible and surgical intervention is usually confined to biopsy to avoid the risk of visual impairment.

The results of radiotherapy in patients with progressive inoperable disease are excellent, with improvement or stabilization of the visual deficit. CT/MRI findings frequently stabilize and occasionally improve, suggesting that radiation prevents tumour progression. The currently recommended radiation dose is 50 Gy in 30–35 fractions, employing a three-field technique to a target volume carefully defined on the basis of CT and MRI. Following

radiotherapy, vision improves in 40–50 per cent of patients (Horwich and Bloom 1985; Flickinger et al. 1988). The overall 5 and 10 year progression-free and overall survivals range from 80 to 90 per cent (Horwich and Bloom 1985; Flickinger et al. 1988), with a suggestion of better prognosis in adults (Kovalic et al. 1990). Carboplatin-containing chemotherapy has been employed in children but its rôle in adults is not defined.

At present, radical radiotherapy along similar lines to the radiotherapy regime employed in children is the treatment of choice in optic nerve and chiasmal glioma, particularly in patients with clinical evidence of tumour progression.

SKULL TUMOURS

The most frequent site of primary bone tumours of the skull is the base of the cranium, with rare involvement of other regions. The commonest tumours are chordomas, chondromas, and chondrosarcomas, with occasional osteomas, giant cell tumours of the bone, and osteosarcomas. Base of skull (clivus) tumours present with symptoms of local bone destruction (usually pain) and gradually progressive features of brainstem or mid-brain damage from intracranial components. Tumours may also invade other surrounding structures, such as the sphenoid sinus, pituitary fossa, orbits, and nasopharynx, with attendant focal clinical features.

Chordomas are tumours involving the axial skeleton and are derived from the remnants of the primitive notochord. They form large masses of cartilaginous tumour composed of cohesive sheets, nests, and cords of cells (Russell and Rubinstein 1989). Despite their benign histological appearance, they have an infiltrative and invasive growth pattern.

Surgery is the primary treatment but the tumour site and extensive invasion of surrounding structures make complete excision difficult. Radiotherapy is essentially palliative and is effective in relieving pain. In inoperable and partially excised tumours it may produce temporary tumour control without long-term cure (Cummings et al. 1983; Fuller and Bloom 1988). The 5 year progression-free survival of patients treated with radiotherapy after incomplete resection or biopsy alone is 20–30 per cent (Fuller and Bloom 1988).

Chondromas and chondrosarcomas are rare tumours involving the skull base as well as the petrous temporal bone. They are histologically distinct but clinically pose the same problems as chondromas, namely the difficulty in achieving complete excision, the poorly defined rôle of adjuvant therapy, and ultimate failure at the primary site.

High-energy charged-particle radiation (protons and helium ions) has been employed in the treatment of skull-base chordomas and low-grade chondrosarcomas. Early results of selected patients with small tumours treated to high photon equivalent doses suggest 50–70 per cent tumour control rates at 5 years, although the technique carries a significant morbidity (Berson et al. 1988; Seymour-Austin et al. 1989).

Treatment recommendations

Surgery is the current treatment of choice, although it rarely achieves total tumour resection. With improved surgical techniques of skull base and lateral skull approaches, complete excision may become feasible in a larger proportion of patients. The rôle of adjuvant treatment is not defined. Radiotherapy is effective as palliation and should be given to patients with symptomatic recurrence to doses approaching CNS tolerance. Proton therapy is considered experimental at present.

NEURONAL TUMOURS

Gangliocytomas and gangliogliomas are tumours composed of mature gangliocytes supported by glial cells, which in gangliogliomas are mature glial tumour cells. They most frequently occur in children and young adults. Although they may arise in any part of the CNS, they have a predilection for the temporal lobe (Russell and Rubinstein 1989), presenting with temporal lobe epilepsy.

These tumours are characterized by a slow growth rate and, following surgery or combined surgery and radiotherapy, the 5 and 10 year survival is 80–90 per cent, even in the presence of histologically more malignant glial elements (Johannsson et al. 1981; Kalyan-Raman and Olivero 1987). The indolent behaviour and possible hamartomatous nature of these tumours would argue for a conservative treatment approach with limited surgery alone. Although frequently employed, the rôle of radiotherapy is not defined.

ACOUSTIC NEUROMA

Acoustic neuromas (schwannoma, neurilemmoma) are benign encapsulated tumours of the eighth cranial nerve, representing 8 per cent of intracranial tumours in surgical series, either as sporadic tumours or as part of neurofibromatosis (NF2). Similar tumours can occur on the fifth or ninth cranial nerves. Acoustic neuromas arise on the vestibular nerve at the fundus of the internal auditory meatus (70 per cent inferior vestibular nerve and 30 per cent superior vestibular nerve) and are graded according to local tumour extention and size. Histologically they are highly cellular, with interlacing bundles of spindle cells whose nuclei are often in parallel arrays, alternating with lesser-textured, often partially cystic, areas. In neurofibromatosis these often incorporate axons and Schwann cells.

Clinical presentation and diagnosis

Patients present with progressive unilateral deafness. Large tumours may involve the adjacent seventh nerve and trigeminal nerve, occasionally disturb cerebellar and brainstem functions, and may cause hydrocephalus. The tumour is visualized as an enhancing mass on CT scan; small intrameatal lesions can be shown on CT cisternography. MRI demonstrates small neuromas particularly well.

Treatment

Tumours may be resected by suboccipital, subtemporal, or translabyrinthine routes. Total surgical excision can usually be achieved, although there is a significant rate of complications, including facial paralysis and brainstem dysfunction. The likelihood of complete resection and the frequency of complications are related to tumour size (Symon et al. 1989).

Conventional radiotherapy has been employed rarely in the treatment of inaccessible or incompletely excised neuromas of the eighth and other cranial nerves. Although there is a suggestion of decreased local tumour progression with post-operative irradiation of incompletely excised tumours, the rôle of irradiation is not clear (Wallner et al. 1987, 1988). Stereotactic radiosurgery has been employed in the treatment of acoustic neuromas, with a reported success rate of 85 per cent defined as failure of tumour progression. With this technique the early preservation of hearing is comparable to that achieved with surgery, although there is continued progressive loss of hearing in a large proportion of patients (Norén et al. 1988). At present, surgical excision remains the treatment of choice, with radiosurgery reserved for those patients unsuitable for surgery.

CHOROID PLEXUS TUMOURS

Choroid plexus papilloma is an indolent, mostly benign tumour, representing 0.5 per cent of intracranial tumours in adults. It is a papillary tumour (grade I) arising in the fissure of the ventricular system and consisting of epithelial cells over a dense vascular core. The presence of a basement membrane and absence of glial cells distinguish it from a papillary variant of ependymoma. The tumours are found in the lateral ventricles, in the fourth ventricle, and rarely in the cerebello-pontine angle or in the third ventricle. They usually present with hydrocephalus and other features of intracranial lesion which are not diagnostic. Very rarely, benign papillomas may demonstrate metastatic lesions.

The treatment of choice in benign choroid plexus papilloma is surgery (Boyd and Steinbok 1987; McGirr et al. 1988). Recurrences following complete excision are rare and adjuvant treatment is not recommended. Following incomplete excision, radiotherapy has been employed with variable results (McGirr et al. 1988). It is recommended as routine treatment only in patients with gross macroscopic residual disease and in those with recurrent tumour and should be delivered by localized irradiation to doses of 50–55 Gy as for low-grade gliomas.

The presence of atypical histological features usually signifies more aggressive clinical behaviour. Choroid plexus carcinoma is a rare malignant variety, to be distinguished histologically from metastatic adenocarcinoma and ependymoma. Despite aggressive treatment with surgery and radiotherapy the prognosis is poor.

BRAIN METASTASES

Most malignant tumours are associated with the development of brain metastases, either by haematogenous spread from distant lesions or by direct extension from tumours adjacent to the cranial cavity. The most frequent presentation is of multiple lesions within the brain parenchyma or, less frequently, as single metastases, and in some tumours as meningeal disease. The risk of brain metastasis is particularly high in patients with small cell lung cancer, acute lymphatic leukaemia, in lymphoblastic and Burkitt's type lymphomas, and in patients with breast and non-small cell lung cancer.

Patients with brain metastases present with typical features of brain tumour. Confusional states and multiple neurological deficits are common. CT scan usually reveals multiple hyperdense, homogeneously enhancing masses surrounded by oedema, although 25 per cent of metastases are iso- or hypodense and approximately 20 per cent show only ring enhancement. Metastases other than melanoma usually have a reduced T_1 relaxation time on MRI. They enhance with gadolinium and the high sensitivity may allow for detection of subclinical metastases. Differential diagnosis of multiple enhancing lesions includes multiple abscesses, particularly in immunosuppressed patients, primary cerebral lymphoma, and rarely, other multifocal brain tumours. Primary intracranial tumours may be difficult to distinguish from solitary brain metastases. Approximately two-thirds of patients presenting with brain metastases have a known underlying primary tumour, usually with metastatic disease at other sites. In the absence of known malignant disease it is necessary to obtain histological diagnosis.

Treatment

The aim of therapy is palliation. Corticosteroids improve symptoms in up to 60 per cent of patients. This may be sufficient palliation in patients with extensive systemic metastatic disease. In patients with brain metastases and a reasonable expectation of life and in those who enjoy a good quality of life further treatment aimed at tumour control should be considered, provided systemic metastatic disease is not life-threatening and the tumours are relatively indolent.

Radiotherapy

Whole-brain irradiation provides effective palliation and can produce neurological improvement in 35–70 per cent of patients. Randomized studies by the Radiation Therapy Oncology Group compared various fractionation regimens (20 Gy in five fractions, 30 Gy in 10 and 15 fractions, 40 Gy in 15 and 20 fractions, and 50 Gy in 20 fractions) with no difference in survival, palliation, or the duration of neurological improvement between the schedules (Borgelt et al. 1980; Diener-West et al. 1989). Stratification by prognostic groups has also not identified subgroups which might benefit from more intensive treatments. The recommended treatment schedule should therefore be short, such as 20 Gy in five fractions given to the whole brain. Unconventional fractionation, particularly fewer treatments with large doses per fraction, may, on theoretical grounds, be considered beneficial in some tumours, such as melanoma. However, this approach does not result in improved survival (Carella et al. 1980) but such regimens require further testing in large prospective trials.

Stereotactic radiotherapy used either alone or in combination with whole-brain irradiation achieves local tumour control and survival similar to neurosurgical excision (Loeffler et al. 1990; Laing et al. 1993). It can be considered a non-invasive alternative to surgery in patients with solitary brain metastases.

Surgery

Stereotactic biopsy should be performed in the absence of histological diagnosis. Tumour excision is of proven survival benefit only in patients with solitary brain metastases (Patchell et al. 1990) and this should be followed by whole-brain irradiation which further improves intracranial tumour control (Smalley et al. 1987). Resection of isolated metastases is also more likely to improve neurological function when compared to radiotherapy alone (Patchell et al. 1990).

Chemotherapy

Systemic chemotherapy administered to patients with brain metastases of chemosensitive tumours, such as lymphoma, teratoma, small cell lung cancer, and breast cancer, can induce CT and clinical responses, particularly in previously untreated patients (Lee et al. 1989; Twelves et al. 1990). On present evidence, patients in systemic remission should receive a subsequent course of palliative radiotherapy, which is likely to prolong intracranial disease control.

Prognosis

The median survival of a large cohort of patients presenting with brain metastases is 4 months. The performance status, control of primary tumour, patient's age, and the extent of metastatic disease have been identified as independent prognostic factors for survival (Diener-West et al. 1989), allowing the separation of patients into prognostic groups. The reported median survival in patients with solitary brain metastases treated with combined surgery and radiotherapy ranges from 8 to 21 months and is particularly favourable in patients with minimal neurological impairment with brain metastases presenting more than 1 year after primary therapy (Smalley et al. 1987; Patchell et al. 1990).

SPINAL TUMOURS

The most frequent tumours affecting the spinal cord are secondary deposits which are usually extradural. The incidence of primary spinal cord tumours is low and ranges from 0.8 to 2.5 per 100 000 population (Fogelholm et al. 1984). In a large series of primary spinal cord tumours 29 per cent were schwannomas, 26 per cent meningiomas, and 22 per cent gliomas, of which ependymoma was the commonest (Slooff et al. 1964).

Clinical presentation

The main symptoms of spinal tumours are local pain at the site of the lesion and impairment of neurological function at and below the spinal level. Pain due to bone or spinal-root involvement, is localized to the level of the lesion and may predate other symptoms by months or years. It is usually worse at night and coughing or straining may exacerbate it and provoke paraesthesiae or temporary impairment of neurological function. Pain from intramedullary tumours is less severe.

Spinal compression by tumour causes segmental loss of power and tendon reflexes. Below this level it causes impairment of long-tract function, with loss of sensation of pain, temperature, vibration, and motor deficit (paraparesis or paraplegia) with hyper-reflexia and dysfunction in bladder and bowel sphincter control (usually urinary retention and constipation or incontinence). Laterally placed tumours may cause a Brown-Séquard syndrome.

Clinical features may indicate the level of spinal compression due to a tumour but confirmatory radiological investigations are essential. In adults the spinal cord segmental level differs from that of the bony vertebral level. Thus, below the level of the axis (C2) in the cervical and thoracic region the approximate segmental level of the cord can be obtained by adding two to the corresponding vertebral level. The spinal cord terminates at the conus medullaris at the level of L1–L2 lumbar vertebrae, so that the lumbar segments of the spinal cord lie at the T11–T12 vertebral levels, with the sacral spinal segments at the L1–L2 level. Below the conus the lumbar and sacral nerve roots form the cauda equina.

Specific syndromes

Spinal tumours may arise within the spinal theca (intradural), that is, in the substance of the cord (intramedullary) or in the subarachnoid space (extramedullary) or may lie outside the theca (extradural).

Intradural intramedullary tumours result in diffuse spinal cord swelling over several spinal segments, often in the cervical or upper thoracic region and are associated with cyst formation centrally in the spinal medulla. They initially result in loss of local function over several spinal segments, particularly involving crossing spinothalamic tract fibres, as well as pain and subsequent loss of neurological function below the level of the tumour. The cyst may give rise to a syringomyelic clinical picture, with a predominant loss of spinothalamic sensation and impaired tendon reflexes at the level of the tumour. A late but diagnostic feature of intrinsic spinal cord tumour is sacral sparing. Tumours in the conus or in the filum terminale cause cauda equina and conus involvement. The cauda equina syndrome typically presents with local pain (rectal or genital), backache, loss of sphincter tone and function, and later lower limb flaccid paralysis. Perianal sensory loss (saddle anaesthesia) is a frequent early sign.

Intradural extramedullary tumours (neurofibromas or rarely meningiomas) present with spinal root involvement, pain, and impaired neurological function due to spinal compression. In the cervical region combined intradural and extradural components are often found, while in the thoracic region tumours are sometimes wholly extradural. Large extraspinal components may present with a mass in the neck or mediastinum.

Angiomas or arteriovenous malformations of the spinal dura or of the spinal cord may present with a sudden onset of pain and loss of function due to spinal subarachnoid haemorrhage or with symptoms of progressive spinal compression associated with pain and fluctuating loss of function, particularly pronounced with exercise.

Extradural tumours, which are most frequently metastatic, present with pain and features of spinal cord compression which are dominated by motor impairment, initially as mild spastic paraparesis. This is accompanied by sphincter disturbance and ascending sensory loss, often starting as paraesthesiae.

Investigations

Plain radiographs

Plain radiographs of the spine may reveal features of metastatic disease such as pathological fracture and collapse of the vertebral body or erosion of the lamina or pedicle at the affected level. Intramedullary spinal tumours often cause widening of the bony spinal canal over several segments, sometimes with thinning of the laminae. Neurofibroma is frequently associated with erosion of the pedicle or widening of the intervertebral foramen, while large cervical or intrathoracic dumb-bell extensions of such tumours may appear as soft tissue shadows. More rarely, spinal meningiomas may cause bony erosion or areas of calcification. Associated spina bifida may be seen in cases of dermoid or lipoma.

Magnetic resonance imaging

MRI of the spinal cord shows, in a non-invasive way, many lesions that are difficult to demonstrate by other neuroradiological methods. As it becomes more widely and freely available it is likely to be the single most important investigation in the diagnosis of intradural spinal tumours and complementary to myelography and CT in the investigation of extradural lesions. At present it is the best technique for non-invasive delineation of the longitudinal extent of spinal lesions. Gadolinium is particularly useful in demonstrating enhancing intramedullary tumours.

CT scan

CT scan allows visualization of the spinal cord as well as the bony spinal canal and related soft tissues, particularly in cases of extradural spinal tumour (Fig. 7). CT myelography with residual intrathecal contrast from a spinal injection for myelography better delineates the position of intradural extramedullary tumours in relation to the cord and delayed scanning may help in identifying intramedullary cysts.

Myelography

Contrast material (usually water soluble) injected by lumbar or cervical puncture outlines the spinal subarachnoid space. Intradural and extradural tumours produce characteristic types of block to the flow of contrast (Fig. 7). Myelography may demonstrate abnormal vascular patterns due to angioma. At the time of myelography, cerebrospinal fluid samples should be obtained for biochemical and cytological diagnosis. In the presence of a spinal block the cerebrospinal fluid protein level is high, often in excess of 1000 mg/100 ml (normal <40 mg/100 ml).

Myelography in patients with spinal tumour may occasionally precipitate acute deterioration, leading to abrupt loss of neurological function. In this situation it is essential to proceed urgently to appropriate surgical treatment.

Spinal angiography

Angiography of the spinal arteries is essential in the definition of spinal and dural angiomas and may be helpful in cases of other

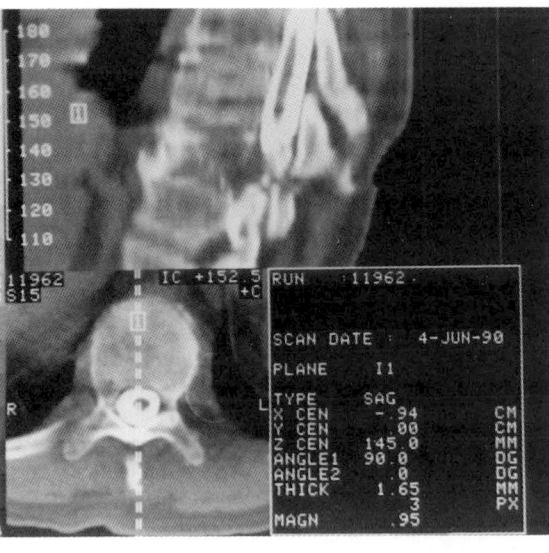

(a) (b)

Fig. 7 Metastatic carcinoma involving a thoracic vertebral body. (a) Myelogram in lateral projection, showing partial obstruction to the upward flow of contrast at the level of a collapsed vertebra. (b) CT myelogram with sagittal reconstruction from an axial image, showing the extent of bony infiltration and collapse in addition to spinal compression.

vascular spinal tumours (for example, haemangioblastoma). The procedure carries a small but significant neurological morbidity and it should be performed only when definitive further treatment with embolization or surgery is under consideration.

Treatment of spinal tumours

Surgery

The surgical approach to most spinal tumours is by posterior laminectomy performed at the level of the lesion as determined by clinical and neuroradiological findings. Lateral or anterior approaches to the spine, through the mouth, neck, chest, or abdomen may be indicated occasionally to provide a more direct route to the tumour, minimizing spinal cord retraction. This may require extensive bone removal and subsequent bone grafting or alternative internal fixation.

In neurofibroma and meningioma, the aim of surgery is complete tumour removal, which is usually possible through an exposure by posterior laminectomy and with opening of the spinal theca. The tumour is removed piecemeal with the minimum operative trauma to the spinal cord. The use of the operative microscope and of an ultrasonic surgical aspirator or laser may help in minimizing trauma to the normal tissue. Neurofibroma can usually be dissected from the normal nerve root, but occasionally it is necessary to sacrifice some rootlets.

Intrinsic spinal cord tumours are generally approached by posterior laminectomy and dural opening. Associated cyst fluid may be aspirated and further tumour removal ranges from biopsy to subtotal excision employing microneurosurgical techniques. Complete resection in the cervical and thoracic region is rarely possible, particularly in more malignant tumours, and attempts to achieve this may result in further neurological impairment.

Classically, the surgical treatment of acute spinal compression due to extradural metastatic tumour has been through posterior laminectomy with partial removal of the accessible extradural tumour. Where the metastatic deposit is favourably close, this achieves rapid decompression of the spinal cord, but the required resection of bone may increase spinal instability. In cases where the malignant tumour has invaded the body of the vertebra and caused collapse and compression anteriorly or where the main extradural deposit lies anterior to the spinal cord, it is more appropriate to consider anterior or lateral surgical approaches to the spine. The diseased vertebral body and extradural deposit may be removed directly, although the operation will be more major and usually necessitate spinal fusion with a bone graft, bone cement, or metallic internal fixation in order to achieve post-operative stability. This approach should be reserved for patients with good performance status and limited metastatic disease.

The results of surgical spinal cord decompression are often disappointing and an initial trial of treatment by radiotherapy as the primary modality may be indicated. Needle biopsy of bone or soft tissue under radiological control may be sufficient to obtain histological diagnosis.

Radiotherapy

Spinal cord tolerance

The dose–response curves for spinal cord damage are steep, suggesting that even small increments of dose beyond radiation tolerance will significantly increase the risk of myelopathy. Spinal cord radiation tolerance studies in primates using 2.2 Gy fractions estimated doses for 1 and 0.1 per cent myelopathy as 59 and 52 Gy,

respectively, which is close to clinical experience. Using clinically relevant fraction sizes between 1.2 and 2 Gy in rodent spinal cord irradiation, revealed a biexponential repair mechanism for sublethal damage with repair half-times of 0.7 and 4 h (Ang et al. 1992). Shortening the interfraction interval from 24 to 8 h decreases the spinal cord tolerance by approximately 15 per cent (Ang et al. 1992).

The dose limits of spinal cord tolerance in clinical radiotherapy are related to the number of fractions and total dose and to the length of cord treated. Data on cord sensitivity have been derived from irradiation of the neck and thoracic or upper abdominal structures where the cord is included in the target volume. Published clinical data are inadequate for valid statistical dose–response analyses and can only serve as a guide for 'best estimate'. Evaluating more than 1100 patients the risk of permanent neurological damage was very low for fractions of less than 2 Gy given once a day or 1.2 Gy given twice a day to a total dose of 55 Gy or less (Marcus and Million 1990). The estimated incidence of myelopathy at 45 Gy in 1.8–2 Gy fractions is most likely below 0.2 per cent. In conventional fraction schedules, the dose causing a 5 per cent incidence of myelopathy (TD_5) was estimated to be in the 57–61 Gy range and the dose for 50 per cent (TD_{50}) to be in the 68–73 Gy range (Schultheiss 1990). A clinical consensus proposed a somewhat lower TD_5 of 50 Gy for a treated length of 5–10 cm and 47 Gy for a length of 20 cm (Emami et al. 1991).

Spinal irradiation: technique

Palliative spinal irradiation, usually for extradural spinal cord compression, is given by a direct posterior field where the field width covers the suspected tumour extent by a minimum of 1–2 cm. The field length is determined by myelography or by MRI which gives a better delineation of tumour extent. Primary intramedullary tumours are treated by radical spinal irradiation to spinal cord tolerance doses. The target volume, ideally based on MRI should include the whole circumference of the spinal canal and tumour extension with a 1–2 cm margin. Treatment can be delivered either by a direct posterior field or through a planned volume of three or two wedged fields. The exit beam usually traverses sensitive structures such as the kidneys and the lungs and the chosen technique has to take into account their limits of radiation tolerance. In whole-spine irradiation as part of craniospinal axis radiotherapy the superior margin is matched to the cervical extension of the whole-brain field.

SPINAL EPENDYMOMAS

Spinal cord ependymomas present in all age-groups (median age 40 years). The tumour has a predilection for the cauda equina and conus medullaris, although it also occurs in the cervical, thoracic, and lumbar spinal cord. Multiple spinal ependymomas are associated with neurofibromatosis NF1. Low-grade tumours have a long natural history with only minimal progression over many years.

The tumours lie within the spinal cord and are initially demonstrated as spinal cord expansion. They are best seen on MRI with gadolinium enhancement; myelography and CT myelography show an expanded cord.

Ependymomas range from low- to high-grade tumours, although the former are more common. They consist of cellular masses of ependymal cells of varying cytological appearance and may contain blepharoblasts. The diagnostic feature in the more differentiated type is the presence of ependymal rosettes. The typical cauda equina tumour is a low-grade myxopapillary ependymoma arising from the conus medullaris or the filum terminale, although other histological types may be found at this site. A myxopapillary variant consists of cuboidal and low columnar cells with abundant, highly vascular collagenous stroma and hyaline and mucinous material. It is usually a well-defined fusiform mass, which may be closely attached to and infiltrate the roots of the cauda equina. Large masses may cause bone erosion. The risk of isolated brain seeding is approximately 6 per cent and is marginally more frequent in patients with high-grade tumours (Whitaker *et al.* 1991).

Treatment

Low-grade cauda equina and conus medullaris tumours can usually be completely excised and, provided the margins of resection are clear, further adjuvant therapy is not required.

Despite the advances in technology, the complete resection rate of intramedullary tumours is only 60 per cent (Peschel *et al.* 1983) and the radical attempts at tumour excision advocated by some authors (Cooper and Epstein 1985; McCormick *et al.* 1990) may result in unacceptable neurological deficits without known long-term survival benefit. Following less radical surgical procedures (partial excision or biopsy alone) and radiotherapy, a significant proportion of patients remain alive and free of tumour progression at 5 and 10 years (Whitaker *et al.* 1991). Irradiation is confined to the region of the tumour and the margin of potential spread. The use of more extensive irradiation, including brain and whole spinal cord, is not advocated.

Prognosis

The most important prognostic factors for tumour control and survival are tumour grade and, for low-grade ependymoma, the extent of resection (Whitaker *et al.* 1991). Complete excision of low-grade tumour (usually cauda equina ependymoma) is associated with a high cure rate. Patients with incompletely excised tumours treated with radical post-operative radiotherapy have a 5 and 10 year progression-free survival of 50–60 per cent, suggesting that radiotherapy may achieve long-term tumour control in half the patients with residual tumour.

SPINAL ASTROCYTOMA

Astrocytomas are rare spinal intramedullary tumours, representing 6–8 per cent of primary spinal neoplasms. Histologically they resemble intracranial glial tumours and range from low to high grade, although the former are more common. In addition to their tendency for local infiltration the tumours have a significant propensity for cerebrospinal fluid spread, as judged by a high incidence of cranial recurrences, particularly in high-grade tumours. The clinical presentation and diagnostic procedures are the same as those of other intramedullary spinal cord tumours. The rate of progression of neurological deficit is usually related to the tumour grade.

Treatment

The treatment guidelines are similar to those for spinal ependymoma, although the precise rôles of surgery and radiotherapy are less well defined because of the rarity of the tumour. The usual treatment is attempted excision or biopsy, followed by radiotherapy. The extent of resection should be limited to preserve useful neurological function. Although more radical attempts at excision are advocated by some authors, a survival advantage for this approach has not been demonstrated (Cohen *et al.* 1989).

The rationale for post-operative radiotherapy is equivalent to that for the treatment of intracranial gliomas. Neurological deficit due to tumour or surgery is rarely relieved by radiotherapy and patients with high-grade tumours have very poor prognosis (Linstadt *et al.* 1989; Huddart *et al.* 1993).

Prognosis

The prognostic factors are tumour grade and length of history. Intracranial recurrences occur in up to 50 per cent of patients with high-grade spinal astrocytomas and it is not clear whether this is reduced by prophylactic cranial irradiation.

METASTATIC SPINAL CORD TUMOURS

Metastatic tumours to the spine are usually extradural, arising from bone or surrounding soft tissue masses. Rarely, tumours may be intramedullary. The neurological deficit is the result of the combination of local cord oedema, ischaemia, and direct pressure (Ushio *et al.* 1977).

The aim of therapy is functional improvement and pain control. Survival depends usually on the extent of metastatic disease and the tumour type; the median survival is 4–10 months (Sørensen *et al.* 1990). The functional outcome of treatment is largely dependent on pre-treatment status and depends relatively little on the type of treatment (Gilbert *et al.* 1978; Sørensen *et al.* 1990). Although half the patients are able to walk after therapy, both surgery and radiotherapy have a high failure rate, even in patients who are initially mobile. Following complete paraplegia, recovery is rare (Table 9).

Treatment guidelines

Corticosteroids are the initial treatment in patients with suspected spinal cord compression. Treatment with higher doses than those given conventionally (dexamethasone 4 mg, 6 hourly) improves the functional outcome in studies of animal models (Delattre *et al.* 1989), but has not been demonstrated to benefit patients. The choice of subsequent treatment lies between surgery, radiotherapy, or both, although in patients with chemosensitive tumours chemotherapy may be the initial treatment. The decision depends on the patient's general condition, the treatment toxicity, and the tumour type.

Spinal cord compression by a tumour of unknown histology and primary site and the progression of signs despite radiotherapy are indications for surgery. Tumours with a poor response to radiotherapy (for example, melanoma, renal carcinoma, sarcoma) should also be considered for surgery first. Posterior cord compression is best relieved by decompressive laminectomy. Patients

Table 9 Outcome of treatment in relation to pre-treatment mobility and treatment modality in patients with metastatic spinal cord compression (modified from Findlay 1984)

Mobility at presentation	Per cent ambulant after treatment (number of patients)		
	Surgery	Surgery and radiotherapy	Radiotherapy alone
Ambulant	48 (81)	67 (240)	79 (126)
Paretic	31 (134)	35 (419)	42 (144)
Paraplegic	3 (40)	7 (163)	2 (45)

with limited metastatic disease and favourable overall prognosis, where the tumour is arising from the vertebral body, causing anterior compression, can be considered for anterior/lateral resection and stabilization.

Patients with highly radioresponsive tumours and those with common solid tumours, such as breast, lung, and prostatic carcinoma, should receive initial radiotherapy. Post-operative radiotherapy improves pain control and, in patients with limited metastatic disease, may reduce the risk of local recurrence. An optimal radiotherapy regimen has not been defined and in patients with a limited prognosis a dose of 20 Gy in five fractions by direct field is usually adequate. More radical treatment is reserved for solitary lesions such as plasmacytoma (40 Gy in 20 fractions). Chemotherapy can be used as the initial treatment in tumours such as teratoma or lymphoma as the functional outcome is not jeopardized by this approach (Eeles *et al.* 1990).

As the chance of recovering mobility is inversely related to the degree of initial impairment, it is important to detect spinal cord compression early, before any significant loss of function. Therefore, the key to successful treatment is early diagnosis. Radiotherapy for painful bony metastatic disease in the spine may occasionally prevent the evolution of myelopathy (Redmond *et al.* 1988).

REFERENCES

Alavi BJ, *et al.* (1988). Positron emission tomography in patients with glioma. A predictor of prognosis. *Cancer*, 62:1074–8.

Allen JC, Jim JH, Packer RJ (1987). Neoadjuvant chemotherapy for newly diagnosed germ cell tumours of the central nervous system. *Journal of Neurosurgery*, 67:65.

Amacher AL (1980). Craniopharyngioma: the controversy regarding radiotherapy. *Child's Brain*, 6:57–64.

Ang KK, *et al.* (1992). Impact of spinal cord repair kinetics on the practice of altered fractionation schedules. *Radiotherapy and Oncology*, 25:287–94.

Austin-Seymour M, *et al.* (1989). Fractionated proton radiation therapy of chordoma and low-grade chondrosarcoma of the base of the skull. *Journal of Neurosurgery*, 70:13–17.

Barbaro NM, Gutin PH, Wilson CB, Sheline GE, Boldrey EB, Wara WM (1987). Radiation therapy in the treatment of partially resected meningiomas. *Neurosurgery*, 20(4):525–8.

Barker DJP, Weller RO, Garfield JS (1976). Epidemiology of primary tumours of the brain and spinal cord: a regional survey in southern England. *Journal of Neurology, Neurosurgery and Psychiatry*, 39:290–6.

Bergstrom M, *et al.* (1983). Discrepancies in brain tumour extent as shown by computed tomography and positron emission tomography using (^{68}Ga)EDTA, (^{11}C)Glucose, and (^{11}C)Methionine. *Journal of Computer Assisted Tomography*, 7:1062–6.

Berson AM, *et al.* (1988). Charged particle irradiation of chordoma and chondrosarcoma of the base of skull and cervical spine: the Lawrence Berkeley Laboratory Experience. *International Journal of Radiation Oncology—Biology—Physics*, 15:559–65.

Betti OO, Derechinsky V (1983). Multiple beam stereotaxic irradiation. *Neurochirurgie*, 29:295–8.

Bickerstaff ER, Small JM, Guest IA (1958). The relapsing course of certain meningiomas in relation to pregnancy and menstruation. *Journal of Neurology, Neurosurgery and Psychiatry*, 21:89–91.

Bigner DD, Swenberg JA (1977). *Experimental tumors of the central nervous system.* Upjohn Company, Kalamazoo, MI.

Bigner SH, *et al.* (1988). Specific chromosomal abnormalities in malignant human gliomas. *Cancer Research*, 88:405–11.

Blankenstein MA, Blaauw G, Lamberts, SWJ Mulder E. (1983). Presence of progesterone receptors and absence of oestrogen receptors in human intracranial meningioma cytosols. *European Journal of Cancer and Clinical Oncology*, 19:365.

Bleehen NM, Stenning SP on behalf of the Medical Research Council Brain Tumour Working Party (1991). A Medical Research Council trial of two radiotherapy doses in the treatment of grades 3 and 4 astrocytoma. *British Journal of Cancer*, 64:769–74.

Bloom HJG (1983). Primary intracranial germ cell tumours. *Clinical Oncology*, 2:233–57.

Bloom HJG, Bessell EM (1990). Medulloblastoma in adults: a review of 47 patients treated between 1952 and 1981. *International Journal of Radiation Oncology—Biology—Physics*, 18:763–72.

Borgelt B, *et al.* (1980). The palliation of brain metastases: final results of the first two studies by the Radiation Therapy Oncology Group. *International Journal of Radiation Oncology—Biology—Physics*, 6:1–9.

Boyd MC, Steinbok P (1987). Choroid plexus tumor: problems in diagnosis and management. *Journal of Neurosurgery*, 66:800–5.

Brada M, Graham JD (1993). Stereotactic external beam radiotherapy. In *Stereotactic and image directed surgery of brain tumours* (ed. DGT Thomas), pp. 149–68. Churchill Livingstone, London.

Brada M, Rajan B (1990). Spinal seeding in cranial germinoma. *British Journal of Cancer*, 61:339–40.

Brada M, Thomas DGT (1993). Craniopharyngioma revisited. *International Journal of Radiation Oncology—Biology—Physics*, 27:471–5.

Brada M, Dearnaley D, Horwich A, Bloom HJG (1990). Management of primary cerebral lymphoma with initial chemotherapy: preliminary results and comparison with patients treated with radiotherapy alone. *International Journal of Radiation Oncology—Biology—Physics*, 18:787–92.

Brada M, *et al.* (1992). Risk of second brain tumour following conservative surgery and radiotherapy of pituitary adenoma. *British Medical Journal*, 304:1343–6.

Brada M, Rajan B, Traish D, Ashley S, Nussey S, Uttley D (1993). The long term efficacy of conservative surgery and radiotherapy in the control of pituitary adenomas. *Clinical Endocrinology*, 38:571–8.

Brooks DJ (1990). *In vivo* metabolism of human cerebral tumours. In *Neuro-oncology: primary malignant brain tumours* (ed. DGT Thomas), pp. 122–34. Edward Arnold, London.

Bullard DE, *et al.* (1987). Oligodendroglioma. An analysis of the value of radiation therapy. *Cancer*, 60:2179–88.

Burger PC (1986). Malignant astrocytic neoplasms: classification, pathologic anatomy, and response to treatment. *Seminars in Oncology*, 13:16–26.

Burger PC, Heinz ER, Shibata T, Kleihues P (1988). Topographic anatomy and CT correlations in the untreated glioblastoma multiforme. *Journal of Neurosurgery*, 68:698–704.

Carella RJ, Gelber R, Henrickson F, Berry HC, Cooper JS (1980). Value of radiation therapy in the management of patients with cerebral metastases from malignant melanoma. Radiation Therapy Oncology Group Brain Metastases Study I and II. *Cancer*, 45:679–83.

Carr DM, Brown J, Bydder GM (1981). Intravenous chelated gadolinium as a contrast agent in NMR imaging of cerebral tumours. *Lancet*, i:484–6.

Chang CH (1977). Hyperbaric oxygen and radiation therapy in the management of glioblastoma. In *Modern concepts in brain tumour therapy: laboratory and clinical investigations*. National Cancer Institute Monograph No. 46, p. 163. US Government Printing Office, Washington DC.

Chang CH, Honsepian EM, Herbert P (1969). An operative staging system and a megavoltage radiotherapeutic technique for cerebellar medulloblastoma. *Radiology*, 93:1351–9.

Chang CH, *et al.* (1983). Comparison of postoperative radiotherapy and combined postoperative radiotherapy and chemotherapy in the multidisciplinary management of malignant gliomas. *Cancer*, 52:997.

Chen Wen B, *et al.* (1989). A comparison of the roles of surgery and radiation therapy in the management of craniopharyngiomas. *International Journal of Radiation Oncology—Biology—Physics*, 16:17–24.

Cohen AR, Wisoff JH, Allen JC, Epstein F (1989). Malignant astrocytomas of the spinal cord. *Journal of Neurosurgery*, 70:50–4.

Cooper PR, Epstein, F (1985). Radical resection of intramedullary spinal cord tumors in adults. *Journal of Neurosurgery*, 63:492–9.

Cummings BJ, Hodson I, Bush RS (1983). Chordoma: the results of megavoltage radiation therapy. *International Journal of Radiation Oncology—Biology—Physics*, 9:633–42.

Danoff BF, Cowchock FS, Kramer S (1983). Childhood craniopharyngioma: survival, local control, endocrine and neurologic function following radiotherapy. *International Journal of Radiation Oncology—Biology—Physics*, 9:171–5.

Darling JL, Hoyle NR, Thomas DGT (1981). Self and non-self in the brain. *Immunology Today*, 2:176–8.

de Tribolet N, Harmon MF, Mach JP, Carrel S, Schreyer M (1984). Demonstration of HLA-DR antigens in normal brain. *Journal of Neurology, Neurosurgery and Psychiatry*, 47:417–18.

DeAngelis LM, Yahaloin J, Thales AT, Khan U (1992). Combined modality therapy for primary CNS lymphoma. *Journal of Clinical Oncology*, 10:635–43.

Dearnaley DP, A'Hearn R, Whitaker S, Bloom HJG (1990). Pineal and CNS germ cell tumours: Royal Marsden Hospital experience 1962–1987. *International Journal of Radiation Oncology—Biology—Physics*, 18:773–81.

Delattre JW, *et al.* (1989). A dose–response study of dexamethasone in a model of spinal cord compression caused by epidural tumor. *Journal of Neurosurgery*, 70:920–5.

Deutsch M, *et al.* (1989). Results of a randomised trial comparing BCNU plus radiotherapy, streptozotocin plus radiotherapy, BCNU plus hyperfractionated radiotherapy, and BCNU following misonidazole plus radiotherapy in the postoperative treatment of malignant glioma. *International Journal of Radiation Oncology—Biology—Physics*, 16:1389–96.

Di Chiro G, *et al.* (1982). Glucose utilization of cerebral gliomas measured by (^{18}F) fluorodeoxyglucose and positron emission tomography. *Neurology*, 32:1323–9.

Diener-West M, Dobbins TW, Phillips TL, Nelson DF (1989). Identification of an optimal subgroup for treatment evaluation of patients with brain metastases using RTOG study 7916. *International Journal of Radiation Oncology—Biology—Physics*, 16:669–73.

Disclafani A, Hudgins RJ, Edwards MSB, Wara W, Wilson CB, Levin VA (1989). Pineocytomas. *Cancer*, 63:302–4.

Douglas BG, Worth AJ (1982). Superfractionation in glioblastoma multiforme—results of a phase II study. *International Journal of Radiation Oncology—Biology—Physics*, 8:1787–94.

Dropcho EJ, Mahaley MS (1990). Chemotherapy for malignant gliomas in adults. Neuro oncology: primary malignant brain tumours. In *Contemporary medicine and public health* (ed. DG Thomas and J Hopkins), pp. 222–41. Johns Hopkins University Press, Baltimore.

Duncan W, *et al.* (1986). Report of a randomised pilot study of the treatment of patients with supratentorial gliomas using neutron irradiation. *British Journal of Radiology*, 59:373.

Eby N, *et al.* (1988). Increasing incidence of primary brain lymphoma in the US. *Cancer*, 62:2461–5.

Eeles RA, O'Brien P, Horwich A, Brada M (1991). Non-Hodgkin's lymphoma presenting with extradural spinal cord compression: Functional outcome and survival. *British Journal of Cancer*, 63:126–9.

El-Azouzi M, *et al.* (1989). Loss of distinct regions on the short arm of chromosome 17 associated with tumorigenesis of human astrocytomas. *Proceedings of the National Academy of Sciences USA*, 86:7186–90.

Emami B, *et al.* (1991). Tolerance of normal tissue to therapeutic irradiation. *International Journal of Radiation Oncology—Biology—Physics*, 21:109–22.

Evans AE, *et al.* (1990). The treatment of medulloblastoma: results of a prospective randomized trial of radiation therapy with and without CCNU, vincristine, and prednisone. *Journal of Neurosurgery*, 72:572–82.

Evans DGR, Farndon PA, Burnell LD, Rao Gatamaneni H, Birch JM (1991). Incidence of gorlin syndrome in 173 consecutive cases of medullablastoma. *British Journal of Cancer*, 64:959–61.

Farwell J, Flannery JT (1984). Cancer in relatives of children with central nervous system neoplasms. *New England Journal of Medicine*, 311:749–53.

Fazekas JT (1977). Treatment grades I and II brain astrocytomas. The role of radiotherapy. *International Journal of Radiation Oncology—Biology—Physics*, 2:661–6.

Feldman AR, Kessler L, Myers MH, Naughton MD (1986). The prevalence of cancer (estimated based on the Connecticut Tumor Registry). *New England Journal of Medicine*, 315:1394–8.

Findlay GFG (1984). Adverse effects of the management of malignant spinal cord compression. *Journal of Neurology, Neuroscience and Psychiatry*, 47:761–8.

Fleck JF, *et al.* (1990). Is prophylactic cranial irradiation indicated in small-cell lung cancer? *Journal of Clinical Oncology*, 8:209–14.

Flickinger JC, Torres C, Deutsch M (1988). Management of low-grade gliomas of the optic nerve and chiasm. *Cancer*, 61:635–42.

Fogelholm R, Uutela T, Murros K (1984). Epidemiology of central nervous system neoplasms. A regional survey in Central Finland. *Acta Neurologica Scandinavica*, 69:129–36.

Fuller DB, Bloom JG (1988). Radiotherapy for chordoma. *International Journal of Radiation Oncology—Biology—Physics*, 15:331–9.

Fulton DS, *et al.* (1984). Misonidazole combined with hyperfractionation in the management of malignant glioma. *International Journal of Radiation Oncology—Biology—Physics*, 10:1709–12.

Garson JA, Pemberton LF, Sheppard PW, Varndell M, Coakham HB, Kemshead JT (1989). N-*myc* gene expression and oncoprotein characterisation in medulloblastoma. *British Journal of Cancer*, 59:889–94.

Gilbert RW, Kim JH, Posner JB (1978). Epidural spinal cord compression from metastatic tumour: diagnosis and treatment. *Annals of Neurology*, 3:50–1.

Gill SS, Warrington AP, Thomas DGT, Brada M (1991). Relocatable frame for stereotactic external beam radiotherapy. *International Journal of Radiation Oncology—Biology—Physics*, 20:599–603.

Glaholm J, Bloom HJG, Crow JH (1990). The role of radiotherapy in the management of intracranial meningiomas. The Royal Marsden Hospital experience with 186 patients. *International Journal of Radiation Oncology—Biology—Physics*, 18:755–61.

Graham JD, Nahum AE, Brada M (1991a). A comparison of techniques for stereotactic radiotherapy by linear accelerator based on 3-dimensional dose distributions. *Radiotherapy and Oncology*, 22:29–35.

Graham JD, Warrington AP, Gill SS, Brada M (1991b). A non-invasive relocatable frame for fractionated radiotherapy and multiple imaging. *Radiotherapy and Oncology*, 21:60–2.

Grigsby PW, *et al.* (1989). Prognostic factors and results of therapy for adult thalamic and brainstem tumors. *Cancer*, 63:2124–9.

Guthrie BL, *et al.* (1989). Meningeal hemangiopericytoma: histopathological features, treatment, and long-term follow-up of 44 cases. *Neurosurgery*, 25:514–22.

Gutin PH, *et al.* (1991). External irradiation followed by interstitial high activity iodine-125 implant "boost" in the initial treatment of malignant gliomas. *International Journal of Radiation Biology—Oncology—Physics*, 21:601–6.

Halperin EC, Bentel G, Heinz ER, Burger PC (1989). Radiation therapy treatment planning in supratentorial glioblastoma multiforme: an analysis based on post mortem topographic anatomy with CT correlations. *International Journal of Radiation Oncology—Biology—Physics*, 17:1347–50.

Hariz MI, Henriksson R, Lofroth PO, Laitinen LV, Saterborg NE (1990). A non-invasive method for fractionated stereotactic irradiation of brain tumours with linear accelerator. *Radiotherapy and Oncology*, 17:57–72.

Hawkins MM, Draper GJ, Kingston JE (1987). Incidence of second primary tumours among childhood cancer survivors. *British Journal of Cancer*, 56:339–47.

Helseth A, Langmark F, Mork SU (1988). Neoplasms of the central nervous system in Norway. II Descriptive epidemiology of intracranial neoplasms 1955–1984. *APMIS*, 96:1066–74.

Hochberg FH, Miller DC (1988). Primary central nervous system lymphoma. *Journal of Neurosurgery*, 68:835–53.

Hochberg FH, Pruitt A (1980). Assumptions in the radiotherapy of glioblastoma. *Neurology*, 30:907–12.

Hochberg FH, Slotnick B (1980). Neuropsychologic impairment in astrocytoma survivors. *Neurology*, 30:172–7.

Holmes A, McMillan TJ, Peacock JH, Steel GG (1990). The radiation dose–effect in two human neuroblastoma cell lines. *British Journal of Cancer*, 62:791–5.

Horten BC, Baster GA, Shapiro WR (1981). Xenograft of human malignant glial tumors into brains of nude mice: a histopathological study. *Journal of Neuropathology and Experimental Neurology*, 40:493–511.

Horwich A, Bloom HJG (1985). Optic gliomas: radiation therapy and prognosis. *International Journal of Radiation Oncology—Biology—Physics*, 11:1067–79.

Hoshino T, Prados M, Wilson CB, Cho KG, Lee KS, Davis RL (1989). Prognostic implications of the bromodeoxyuridine labeling index of human gliomas. *Journal of Neurosurgery*, 71:335–41.

Huddart R, Traish D, Ashley S, Moore A, Brada M (1993). Management of spinal astrocytoma with conservative surgery and radiotherapy. *British Journal of Neurosurgery*, 7:473–81.

Ibelgaufts H (1982). Are human DNA tumour viruses involved in the pathogenesis of human neurogenic tumours? *Neurological Research*, 5:3–24.

James CD, *et al.* (1988). Clonal genomic alterations in glioma malignancy stages. *Cancer Research*, 48:5546–51.

James CD, Carblomn E, Nordenskjold M, Colins VP, Cavenee WK (1989). Mitotic recombination of chromosome 17 in astrocytomas. *Proceedings of the National Academy of Sciences USA*, 86:2858–62.

Jenkins RB, *et al.* (1989). A cytogenetic study of 53 human gliomas. *Cancer Genetics and Cytogenetics*, 39:253–79.

Johannsson JH, Rekate HL, Rosessmann U (1981). Gangliogliomas: pathological and clinical correlation. *Journal of Neurosurgery*, 54:58–63.

Kalyan-Raman UP, Olivero WC (1987). Ganglioglioma: a correlative clinicopathological and radiological study of ten surgically treated cases with follow-up. *Neurosurgery*, 20(3):428–33.

Kaye AH, Morstyn G, Brownbill D (1987). Adjuvant high-dose photoradiation therapy in the treatment of cerebral glioma: a phase 1–2 study. *Journal of Neurosurgery*, 67:500–5.

Keim H, Potthoff PC, Schmidt K, Schiebusch M, Neiss A, Trott KR (1987). Survival and quality of life after continuous accelerated radiotherapy of glioblastomas. *Radiotherapy and Oncology*, 9:21–6.

Kelly PJ, Alker GJ, Goerss S (1982). Computer-assisted stereotactic laser microsurgery for the treatment of intracranial neoplasms. *Neurosurgery*, 10:324–31.

Kendall BA (1980). Neuroradiology. In *Brain tumours: scientific basis, clinical investigation and current therapy*, (ed. D. G. T. Thomas and D. I. Graham), pp. 321–67. Butterworths, London.

Kennedy HB, Smith RJS (1975). Eye signs in craniopharyngioma. *British Journal of Ophthalmology*, 59:689–95.

Kernohan JW, Sayre GP (1952). *Tumours of the central nervous system*. Forces Institute of Pathology, Washington DC.

Kessler, E. and Brandt-Rauf, P. W (1987). Occupational cancers of the brain and bone. In *Occupational medicine – occupational cancer and carcinogenesis*, (ed. Paul W. Brandt-Rauf), pp. 155–63.

Kingsley DPE (1990). Neuroradiological imaging of brain tumours. In *Neuro-oncology primary malignant brain tumours*, (ed. D. G. T. Thomas), pp. 94–121. Edward Arnold, London.

Kornblith PL, Walker M (1988). Chemotherapy of malignant gliomas. *Journal of Neurosurgery*, 68:1–17.

Kovalic JJ, Grigsby PW, Shepard MJ, Fineberg BB, Thomas PR (1990). Radiation therapy for gliomas of the optic nerve and chiasm. *International Journal of Radiation Oncology—Biology—Physics*, 18: 927–32.

Kristiansen K, *et al.* (1981). Combined modality therapy of operated astrocytomas grade III and IV. Confirmation of the value of postoperative irradiation and lack of potentiation of bleomycin on survival time. *Cancer*, 47:649–52.

Kropilak M, *et al.* (1989). Brain tumors in familial adenomatous polyposis. *Diseases of the Colon and Rectum*, 32:778–82.

Kuppner MC, Harmon MF, Bodmer S, Fontana A, de Tribolet N (1988). The glioblastoma-derived T-cell supressor factor/transforming growth factor beta2 inhibits the generation of lymphokine activated killer (LAK) cells. *International Journal of Cancer*, 42:562–7.

Laing R, Bentley R, Nahum A, Warrington AP, Brada M (1993a). Stereotactic radiotherapy of irregular targets: a comparison between static conformal beams and non-coplanar arcs. *Radiotherapy and Oncology*, 28:241–6.

Laing RW, Warrington AP, Hines F, Graham JP, Brada M (1993b). Fractionated stereotactic external beam radiotherapy in the management of brain metastases. *European Journal of Cancer*, 29A:1387–90.

Laing RW, Warrington AP, Graham J, Britton J, Hines F, Brada M (1993c). Efficacy and toxicity of fractionated stereotactic radiotherapy in the treatment of recurrent gliomas (phase I/II study). *Radiotherapy and Oncology*, 27:22–30.

Lantos PL, Pilkington GJ (1979).The development of experimental brain tumours. A sequential light and electron microscope study of the subependymal plate. 1. Early lesions (abnormal cell clusters). *Acta Neuropathologica (Berlin)*, 45:167–75.

Lee JS, Murphy WK, Glisson BS, Dhingra HM, Holoye PY, Hong WK (1989). Primary chemotherapy of brain metastases in small cell lung cancer. *Journal of Clinical Oncology*, 7:916–22.

Leibel SA, *et al.* (1975). The role of radiation therapy in the treatment of astrocytomas. *Cancer*, 35:1551–7.

Leibel SA, *et al.* (1989). Survival and quality of life after interstitial implantation of removable high activity iodine-125 sources for the treatment of patients with recurrent malignant gliomas. *International Journal of Radiation Oncology—Biology—Physics*, 17:1129–39.

Leksell L (1951). The stereotaxic method of radiosurgery on the brain. *Acta Chirurgica Scandinavica*, 102:316–19.

Levin PS, Patlack CS, Landall HD (1980). Heuristic modeling of drug delivery to malignant tumors. *Journal of Pharmacokinetics and Biopharmaceutics*, 8:257–96.

Levin VA, *et al.* (1990). Superiority of post-radiotherapy adjuvant chemotherapy with CCNU, procarbazine, and vincristine (PCV) over BCNU for anaplastic gliomas: NCOG 6G61 final report. *International Journal of Radiation Oncology—Biology—Physics*, 18:321–4.

Lewis RA, *et al.* (1984). Von Recklinghausen neurofibromatosis. II. Incidence of optic gliomata. *Ophthalmology*, 91:929–35.

Libermann TA, *et al.* (1985). Amplification, enhanced expression and possible rearrangement of EFG receptor gene in primary human brain tumours of glial origin. *Nature*, 313:144–7.

Lindegaard KF, *et al.* (1987). Statistical analysis of clinicopathological features, radiotherapy and survival in 170 cases of oligodendroglioma. *Journal of Neurosurgery*, 67:224–30.

Linstadt DE, Wara WM, Leibel SA, Gutin PH, Wilson CB, Sheline GE (1989). Postoperative radiotherapy of primary spinal cord tumors. *International Journal of Radiation Oncology—Biology—Physics*, 16:1397–403.

Lishner M, *et al.* (1990). Late neurological complications after prophylactic cranial irradiation in patients with small-cell lung cancer: the Toronto Experience. *Journal of Clinical Oncology*, 8:215–21.

Listernick R, *et al.* (1989). Optic gliomas in children with neurofibromatosis type 1. *Journal of Pediatrics*, 114:788–92.

Loeffler J, *et al.* (1990). The treatment of recurrent brain metastases with stereotactic radiosurgery. *Journal of Clinical Oncology*, 8:576–82.

Loh L (1985). Anaesthesia and the maintenance of brain function. In *Neurosurgery, the scientific basis of clinical practice*, (ed. A Crockard, R Hayward, and JT Hoff), pp. 297–306. Blackwell, Oxford.

Lunsford LD, Gumerman L, Levine G (1985). Stereotactic intracavitary irradiation of cystic neoplasms of the brain. *Applied Neurophysiology*, 48: 146–50.

McCormick PC, Torres R, Post KD, Stein BM (1990). Intramedullary ependymoma of the spinal cord. *Journal of Neurosurgery*, 72: 523–32.

McGirr SJ, Ebersold MJ, Scheithauer BW, Quast LM, Shaw EG (1988). Choroid plexus papillomas: long-term follow-up results in a surgically treated series. *Journal of Neurosurgery*, 69:843–9.

McKeran RO, Thomas DGT (1980). The clinical study of gliomas. In *Brain tumours —scientific basis, clinical investigation and current therapy* (ed. DGT Thomas and DI Graham), pp. 194–230. Butterworths, Oxford.

McMillan TJ (1993). *In vitro* radiosensitivity of medulloblastoma cell lines. *Journal of Neuro-Oncology*, 15:91–2.

Marcus RB, Million RR (1990). The incidence of myelitis after irradiation of the cervical spinal cord. *International Journal of Radiation Oncology—Biology—Physics*, 19:3–8.

Marks JP, Baglan RJ, Prassad SC, Blank WF (1981). Cerebral radionecrosis: incidence and risk in relation to dose, time, fractionation and volume. *International Journal of Radiation Oncology—Biology—Physics*, 7:243–52.

Marks MP, *et al.* (1988). Intracranial vascular malformations: imaging of charged-particle radiosurgery. Part I Results of therapy. *Radiology*, 168: 447–55.

Mastaglia FL, *et al.* (1976). Effects of X-radiation of the spinal cord: an experimental study of the morphological changes in central nerve fibres. *Brain*, 99:101–2.

Mbidde EK, *et al.* (1988). High dose BCNU chemotherapy with autologous bone marrow transplantation and full dose radiotherapy for grade IV astrocytoma. *British Journal of Cancer*, 58:779–82.

Mirimanoff RO, Dosoretz DE, Linggood RM, Ojemann RG, Martuza RL (1985). Meningioma: analysis of recurrence and progression following neurosurgical resection. *Journal of Neurosurgery*, 62:18–23.

Mori T, Morimoto K, Ushio Y, Haykawa T, Mogami H, Sekiguchi K (1978). Radioimmunoassay of astroprotein (an astrocyte specific cerebroprotein) in cerebrospinal fluid and its clinical significance. *Neurologia Medico-chirurgia (Tokyo)*, **15**:23–5.

Moser RP (1988). Surgery for glioma relapse (factors that influence a favorable outcome) *Cancer*, **62**:381–90.

MRC Working Party (1983). A study of the effect of misonidazole in conjunction with radiotherapy for the treatment of grades 3 and 4 astrocytomas. A report from the MRC Working Party on misonidazole in gliomas. *British Journal of Radiology*, **56**:673.

Neglia, *et al.* (1992). Second neoplasm after acute lymphoblastic leukemia in childhood. *New England Journal of Medicine*, **325**:1330–6.

Nelson DF, Diener-West M, Horton J, Chang CM, Schoenfeld D, Nelson JS (1986). *Combined modality approach to treatment of malignant gliomas reevaluation of RTOG 7401/ECOG 1374 with longer-term follow-up. Interaction of radiation therapy and chemotherapy.* Williamsburg, VA.

Nelson DF, *et al.* (1991). Non-Hodgkin's lymphoma of the brain: can high dose, large volume radiation therapy improve survival? Report on a prospective trial by the Radiation Therapy Oncology Group (RTOG): RTOG 8315. *International Journal Radiation Oncology — Biology — Physics*, **23**:9–17.

Neuwelt EA, *et al.* (1986). Therapeutic efficacy of multiagent chemotherapy with drug delivery enhancement of blood-brain barrier modification. *Neurosurgery*, **19**:573–82.

Neuwelt EA, *et al.* (1991). Primary CNS lymphoma treated with osmotic blood–brain barrier disruption: prolonged survival and preservation of cognitive function. *Journal of Clinical Oncology*, **9**:1580–90.

Norén G, Leksell L (1979). Stereotactic treatment of acoustic tumours. In *Stereotactic cerebral irradiation* (ed. G Szikla), pp. 241–4. Elsevier/North-Holland, Amsterdam.

Norén G, Arndt J, Hindmarsh T, Hirsch A (1988). Stereotactic neurosurgical treatment of acoustic neuromas. In *Modern stereotactic surgery* (ed. LD Lunsford), pp. 481–90. Martinus Nijhoff, Boston.

Osterlag ChB (1993). Interstitial irradiation treatment of low grade gliomas. In *Stereotactic and image directed surgery of brain tumours* (ed. DGT Thomas), pp. 125–34. Churchill Livingstone, London.

Ott RJ, Brada M, Flower MA, Babich JW, Cherry S, Deehan B (1991). Measurements of blood–brain barrier permeability in patients undergoing radio-chemotherapy for primary cerebral lymphomas. *European Journal of Cancer*, **27**:1356–61.

Packer RJ, *et al.* (1989). A prospective study of cognitive function in children receiving whole-brain radiotherapy and chemotherapy: 2-year results. *Journal of Neurosurgery*, **70**:707–13.

Patchell RA, *et al.* (1990). A randomized trial of surgery in the treatment of single metastases to the brain. *New England Journal of Medicine*, **322**:494–500.

Paulus and Peiffer 1989

Payne DG, Simpson WJ, Keen C, Platts ME (1982). Malignant astrocytoma. Hyperfractionated and standard radiotherapy with chemotherapy in a randomised prospective clinical trial. *Cancer*, **50**:2301.

Peschel RE, Kapp DS, Cardinale F, Manuelidis EE (1983). Ependymomas of the spinal cord. *International Journal of Radiation Oncology — Biology — Physics*, **9**:1093–6.

Pezner RD, Achambeau JO (1981). Brain tolerance unit: a method to estimate risk of radiation brain injury for various dose schedules. *International Journal of Radiation Oncology — Biology — Physics*, **7**:397–402.

Pilkington GJ, Lantos PL (1990). Pathology of experimental brain tumours. In *Neuro-oncology. Primary malignant brain tumours* (ed. BGT Thomas), pp. 51–76. Edward Arnold, London.

Pollack IF, Lunsford LD, Slamovits TL, Gumerman LW, Levine G, Robinson AG (1988). Stereotaxic intracavitary irradiation for cystic craniopharyngiomas. *Journal of Neurosurgery*, **68**:227–33.

Preston-Martin S, Mack W, Henderson BE (1989). Risk factors of gliomas and meningiomas in males in Los Angeles County. *Cancer Research*, **49**:6137–43.

Raghavan R, Stewart PV, Weller RO (1988). Cell proliferation patterns in the diagnosis of astrocytomas, anaplastic astrocytomas and glioblastoma multiforme: A Ki-67 study. *Neuropathology and Applied Neurobiology*, **16**:123–33.

Rajan B, *et al.* (1993). Craniopharyngioma – long term results following limited surgery and radiotherapy. *Radiotherapy and Oncology*, **26**:1–10.

Redmond J, *et al.* (1988). Clinical usefulness of an algorithm for the early diagnosis of spinal metastatic disease. *Journal of Clinical Oncology*, **6**(1):154–7.

Rimm IJ, Li FC, Tarbell NJ, Winston KR, Sallan SE (1987). Brain tumours after cranial irradiation for childhood acute lymphoblastic leukemia. *Cancer*, **59**:1506–8.

Ron E, *et al.* (1988). Tumours of the brain and nervous system after radiotherapy in childhood. *New England Journal of Medicine*, **319**:1033–9.

Rouleau GA, *et al.* (1987). Genetic linkage of bilateral acoustic neurofibromatosis to a DNA marker on chromosome 22. *Nature*, **329**:246–8.

Russell DS, Rubinstein LJ (1989). *Pathology of tumours of the nervous system*, (5th edn). Edward Arnold, London.

Salazar CM (1983). A better understanding of CNS seeding and a brighter outlook for post-operatively irradiated patients with ependymomas. *International Journal of Radiation Oncology — Biology — Physics*, **9**:1231–4.

Schoenberg BS (1982). Nervous system. In *Cancer epidemiology and prevention* (ed. D Schottenfeld), pp. 968–83. Joseph F. Fraumeni, Jr.

Schoenberg BS, Christine BW, Whisnant JP (1975). Nervous system neoplasms and primary malignancies of other sites. The unique association between meningiomas and breast cancer. *Neurology*, **25**:705–12.

Schold SC, Bigner DD (1983). A review of animal brain tumour models that have been used for therapeutic studies. In *Oncology of the nervous system* (ed. MD Walker), pp. 31–6. Martinus Nijhoff, Boston.

Schultheiss TE, Stephens LC, Moor MH (1988). Analysis of the histopathology of radiation myelopathy. *International Journal of Radiation Oncology — Biology — Physics*, **14**:27–32.

Seizinger BR, De La Monte S, Atkins L, Gusella JF, Martuza RL (1987*a*). Molecular genetic approach to human meningioma: loss of genes on chromosome 22. *Proceedings of the National Academy of Sciences USA*, **84**:5419–23.

Seizinger BR, *et al.* (1987*b*). Common pathogenic mechanism for three tumour types in bilateral acoustic neurofibromatosis. *Science*, **236**:317–19.

Shapiro WR (1986). Therapy of adult malignant brain tumours: what have the clinical trials taught us? *Seminars in Oncology*, **13**:38–45.

Shapiro WR, Shapiro JR (1986). Principles of brain tumour chemotherapy. *Seminars in Oncology*, **13**:56–69.

Shapiro S, Mealey J, Sartorius C (1989). Radiation-induced intracranial malignant gliomas. *Journal of Neurosurgery*, **71**:77–82.

Shaw EG, *et al.* (1987). Postoperative radiotherapy of intracranial ependymoma in pediatric and adult patients. *International Journal of Radiation Oncology — Biology — Physics*, **13**:1457–62.

Shaw EG, *et al.* (1989). Postoperative radiotherapy of supratentorial low-grade gliomas. *International Journal of Radiation Oncology — Biology — Physics*, **16**:663–8.

Sheline GE (1986). Normal tissue tolerance and radiation therapy of gliomas of the adult brain. In *Tumours of the brain* (ed. NM Bleehen), pp. 141–60. Springer-Verlag, Berlin

Sheline GE, *et al.* (1964). Therapeutic consideration in tumours affecting the central nervous system: oligodendroglioma. *Radiology*, **82**:84–9.

Sheline GE, Wara W, Smith W (1980). Therapeutic irradiation and brain injury. *International Journal of Radiation Oncology — Biology — Physics*, **6**:1215–28.

Shin KH, Muller PJ, Geggie PHS (1983). Superfractionation radiation therapy in the treatment of malignant astrocytomas. *Cancer*, **52**:2040–3.

Simpson D (1975). The recurrence of intracranial meningiomas after surgical treatment. *Journal of Neurology Neuroscience and Psychiatry*, **20**:22–6.

Slooff JL, Kernohan JW, MacCarty OS (1964). *Primary intramedullary tumours of the spinal cord and folium terminate.* Saunders, Philadelphia.

Smalley SR, Schray MF, Laws ER Jr, O'Fallon JR (1987). Adjuvant radiation therapy after surgical resection of solitary brain metastasis: association with pattern of failure and survival. *International Journal of Radiation Oncology — Biology — Physics*, **13**:1611–16.

Smith PG, Douglas AJ (1986). Mortality of workers at the Sellafield plant of British Nuclear Fuels. *British Medical Journal*, **293**:845–54.

Sneed PK, Gutin PH (1993). Interstitial radiotherapy for high grade gliomas. In *Stereotactic and image directed surgery of brain tumours* (ed. DGT Thomas), pp. 135–47. Churchill Livingstone, London.

Sørensen PS, *et al.* (1990). Metastatic epidural spinal cord compression. *Cancer*, **65**:1502–8.

Sorensen SA, Mulvihill JJ, Nielsen A (1986). Long-term follow-up of von Recklinghausen neurofibromatosis. Survival and malignant neoplasms. *New England Journal of Medicine*, **314**:1010–15.

Stenning SP, Freedman LS, Bleehen NM (1987). An overview of published results from randomized studies of nitrosoureas in primary high grade malignant glioma. *British Journal of Cancer*, **56**:89–90.

Stewart DJ (1989). The role of chemotherapy in the treatment of gliomas in adults. *Cancer Treatment Reviews*, **16**:129–60.

Sung D, Harisiadis L, Chang CH (1978). Midline pineal tumors and suprasellar germinomas: highly curable by irradiation. *Radiology*, **128**:745–51.

Symon L, Sprich W (1985). Radical excision of craniopharyngioma (results in 20 patients). *Journal of Neurosurgery*, **62**:174–81.

Symon L, Bordi LT, Compton JS, Sabin H, Sayin E (1989). Acoustic neuroma: a review of 392 cases. *British Journal of Neurosurgery*, **3**:343–7.

Taghian A, *et al.* (1993). Intrinsic radiation sensitivity may not be the major determinant of the poor outcome of glioblastoma multiforme. *International Journal of Radiation Oncology — Biology — Physics*, **25**:243–9.

Tait DM, Thornton-Jones H, Bloom HJG, Lemerle J, Morris-Jones P (1990). Adjuvant chemotherapy for medulloblastoma: the first multi-centre controlled trial of the International Society of Paediatric Oncology (SIOP I). *European Journal of Cancer*, **26**:464–9.

Taylor BW, Marcus RB, Friedman WA, Ballinger WE, Million RR (1988). The meningioma controversy: postoperative radiation therapy. *International Journal of Radiation Oncology — Biology — Physics*, **15**:299–304.

Thomas DGT, Nouby RM (1989). Stereotactic technique: experience in 300 cases of CT-directed stereotactic surgery for lesion biopsy and aspiration of haematoma. *British Journal of Neurosurgery*, **3**:321–6.

Thomas DGT, *et al.* (1985). Assay of anticancer drugs in tissue culture: relationship of relapse free interval (RFI) and *in vitro* chemosensitivity in patients with malignant cerebral glioma. *British Journal of Cancer*, **51**:525–32.

Thomsett MJ, Conte FA, Kaplan SL, Grumbach MM (1980). Endocrine and neurologic outcome in childhood craniopharyngioma: review of effect of treatment in 42 patients. *Journal of Pediatrics*, **97**(5):728–35.

Tory K, *et al.* (1989). Specific genetic change in tumors associated with von Hippel-Lindau disease. *Journal of the National Cancer Institute*, **81**:1097–101.

Twelves CJ, *et al.* (1990). The response of cerebral metastases in small cell lung cancer to systemic chemotherapy. *British Journal of Cancer*, **61**:147–50.

Twijnstra A, *et al.* (1987). Neurotoxicity of prophylactic cranial irradiation in patients with small cell carcinoma of the lung. *European Journal of Cancer and Clinical Oncology*, **23**:983–6.

Ushio Y, Posner R, Posner JB, Shapiro WR (1977). Experimental spinal cord compression by epidural neoplasms. *Neurology*, **27**:422–9.

Valk PE, Budinger TF, Levin VA, Silver P, Gutin PH, Doyle WK (1988). PET of malignant brain tumours after interstitial radiotherapy: demonstration of metabolic activity and correlation with clinical outcome. *Journal of Neurosurgery*, **69**:830–8.

Van der Kogel AJ (1991). Central nervous system injury in small animal models. In *Radiation injury to the nervous system* (ed. PH Gutin, SA Leibel, and GE Sheline). Raven Press, New York.

Vanuytsel L, Brada M (1991). The role of prophylactic spinal irradiation in localised intracranial ependymoma. *International Journal of Radiation Oncology — Biology — Physics*, **21**:825–30.

Vanuytsel L, Bessell EM, Ashley S, Bloom HJG, Brada M (1992). Intracranial ependymoma: long term results of a policy of surgery and radiotherapy. *International Journal of Radiation Oncology — Biology — Physics*, **23**:313–19.

Velema JP, Percy CL (1987). Age curves of central nervous system tumour incidence in adults: variation of shape by histologic type. *Journal of the National Cancer Institute*, **79**:623–9.

Walk MD, *et al.* (1978). Evaluation of BCNU and/or radiotherapy in the treatment of anaplastic gliomas. A cooperative clinical trial. *Journal of Neurosurgery*, **49**:333–43.

Walker MD, Strike TA, Sheline GE (1979). An analysis of dose-effect relationship in the radiotherapy of malignant gliomas. *International Journal of Radiation Oncology — Biology — Physics*, **5**:1725.

Wallner KE, Sheline GE, Pitts LH, Wara WM, Davis RL, Boldrey E (1987). Efficacy of irradiation of incompletely excised acoustic neurilemomas. *Journal of Neurosurgery*, **67**:858–63.

Wallner KE, Pitts LH, Davis RL, Sheline GE (1988). Radiation therapy for the treatment of non-eighth nerve intracranial neurilemmoma. *International Journal of Radiation Oncology — Biology — Physics*, **14**:287–90.

Weller RO (1986). The immunopathology of brain tumours. In *Tumours of the brain* (ed. NM Bleehen), pp. 19–33. Springer Verlag, Berlin.

Whitaker SJ, Bessell ED, Ashley S, Bloom HJG, Bell BA, Brada M (1991). Postoperative radiotherapy in the management of spinal cord ependymomas. *Journal of Neurosurgery*, **74**:720–8.

Workman P (1986). The pharmacology of brain tumour chemotherapy. In *Tumours of the brain* (ed. NM Bleehen), pp. 183–200. Springer Verlag, Berlin.

Zimmerman HM (1969). Brain tumors: their incidence and classification in man and their experimental production. *Annals of the New York Academy of Sciences*, **159**:337–59.

Zulch KJ (1979). *Histological typing of tumours of the central nervous system*. World Health Organization, Geneva.

Zulch KJ (1986). *Brain tumours, their biology and pathology*. Springer-Verlag, New York.

Section 16
Endocrine tumours

16.1 Carcinoma of the thyroid

MAURICE TUBIANA AND MARTIN SCHLUMBERGER

INTRODUCTION

Clinically apparent thyroid cancer is an uncommon neoplasm, with an annual incidence ranging from 0.1 to 3.7 per 100 000 in males and from 0.4 to 9.6 per 100 000 in females (Young et al. 1981; Waterhouse et al. 1982). Occult papillary thyroid carcinoma is found at necropsy in 2–28 per cent of the thyroid glands (Sampson 1977), indicating that many of these occult carcinomas never become clinically detectable.

Although overall long-term survival is clearly among the best for human neoplasia, thyroid cancer and its treatment causes morbidity and mortality. Therefore, treatment must be influenced by consideration of prognostic variables (Tubiana et al. 1975, 1985a; Byar et al. 1979; Young et al. 1980; Fourquet et al. 1983; Bacourt et al. 1986; Hannequin et al. 1986; Kerr et al. 1986; McConahey et al. 1986; Tennvall et al. 1986; Hay et al. 1987; Mazzaferri 1987; Simpson et al. 1987; Cady et al. 1988; Schelfhout et al. 1988; Smith et al. 1988; Thoresen 1989). The long-term survival of patients with differentiated thyroid cancer has markedly increased in the past decades. Besides a better assessment of prognostic variables, the improved management results from techniques which were able to detect and delineate residual diseases, in particular, whole body scanning in the early 1960s and thyroglobulin assays in the late 1970s (Fig. 1).

AETIOLOGY

Thyroid tumours can be produced in animals by iodine deficiency, goitrigenic drugs, external irradiation, or radio-iodine. A common factor in all these experimental conditions is prolonged stimulation by thyroid-stimulating hormone (TSH). A sequence of reversible hyperplasia followed by irreversible adenomatous hyperplasia and in some cases by the subsequent development of follicular carcinoma has been noted (Schaller and Stevenson 1966).

The relationship between radiation and thyroid cancer is well established in humans, with almost 90 per cent of these carcinomas being papillary. The risk of developing a thyroid cancer increases with the dose of irradiation, is greater in females than in males, and is greater the younger the patient at the time of irradiation (Schneider 1986). The latent period may range from 10 to 35 or more years. There is no evidence that radiation-induced thyroid cancers exhibit unusual biological behaviour. Up to the present time, surveys have not found any evidence of subsequent increase of thyroid tumours following the use of radioactive iodine (^{131}I) in adults (Holm et al. 1989, 1991) for diagnostic or therapeutic purposes. However, a dramatic increase in the incidence of thyroid carcinoma has been recently reported in children from Belarus and the Ukraine, who were contaminated by radioactive iodine after the Chernobyl accident (Baverstock et al. 1992; Kazakov et al. 1992).

There is no convincing evidence of a primary TSH-related induction of thyroid tumours in humans. In fact, it is not certain that carcinomas occur with increased frequency in areas of endemic goitre. However, the incidences of papillary and follicular carcinomas are influenced by the iodine content of the diet, with papillary carcinomas being more frequent in areas where dietary iodine is high (Williams et al. 1977).

A familial occurrence of differentiated thyroid carcinoma has been reported (Staffer et al. 1986), but this was encountered in only 2.5 per cent of the families (M. Schlumberger, F. De Vathaire, C. Ceccarelli et al., submitted). An elevated frequency in differentiated thyroid carcinoma is observed in patients with colon polyposis and Cowden's disease. Thyroid carcinoma shows a female preponderance of 2–3:1. It occurs at any age, but the incidence of papillary carcinoma peaks during the third and fourth decades and that of follicular carcinoma peaks during the fourth and fifth decades. Less differentiated carcinoma occurs later than well differentiated carcinoma.

HISTOLOGY

Tumours of the thyroid can be divided into three main groups:

(1) tumours arising from the thyroid cells, that is, of follicular cell origin;

(2) medullary carcinoma arising from the parafollicular cells;

(3) primary thyroid lymphoma.

The WHO classification (Hedinger et al. 1989) subdivides malignant tumours of follicular cell origin into undifferentiated carcinoma and differentiated thyroid carcinoma, either papillary or follicular carcinoma. In this classification, follicular tumours are defined as tumours lacking the features of papillary carcinoma, whereas papillary tumours may contain follicles. Tumours arising from the thyroid cells are by far the most common and will be considered first.

Papillary carcinoma

Papillary carcinomas account for approximately two-thirds of thyroid carcinomas. Pure papillary tumours exhibit the same clinical behaviour as tumours with papillary and follicular components. The nuclei may show a number of characteristic changes. The existence of trabecular structures and the mitotic rate permit histological grading (Sakamoto et al. 1983; Hay et al. 1987; Schelfhout et al. 1988; Hedinger et al. 1989). Multicentricity ranges in frequency from 20 to 80 per cent, depending on the detail with which the thyroid is examined (Russell et al. 1963). Papillary carcinoma has a marked propensity for lymphatic invasion (Tubiana et al. 1985a; Noguchi and Murakami 1987), which may lead to contiguous lymphatic spread (Tubiana et al. 1975; Schlumberger et al. 1987b). Distant metastases occur mainly in lungs and less frequently in bones.

Follicular carcinoma

Microscopic morphology is extremely variable, ranging from follicles which look normal to solid cellular growth pattern. Neither architectural nor cytological atypicalities, nor mitotic activity, are reliable criteria of malignancy. In fact, the diagnosis of malignancy depends on the demonstration of vascular or capsular invasion. Widely invasive tumours and those with a trabecular pattern exhibit aggressive behaviour (Sakamoto *et al.* 1983; Tubiana *et al.* 1985*a*; Lang *et al.* 1986; Schlumberger *et al.* 1986; Schelfhout *et al.* 1988). Lymph node metastases are less frequent than in papillary carcinoma. The lungs and bones are the most frequent metastatic sites.

Thyroglobulin localization by immunochemistry is of value for the differential diagnosis of tumours with an atypical pattern (Boecker *et al.* 1980).

Undifferentiated (anaplastic) carcinoma

These rare tumours are partially or wholly composed of undifferentiated cells. The use of immunohistochemistry or electron microscopy may be necessary to confirm their epithelial origin and to exclude lymphoma. They occur predominantly in the elderly and appear to arise as a progression from differentiated carcinoma.

BIOLOGY
Hormonosynthesis

A low radio-iodine uptake and a low stable iodine content is observed in all differentiated thyroid cancers (Thomas-Morvan *et al.* 1974). The radio-iodine uptake is weakly correlated with stable iodine concentration, but, more interestingly, response to TSH stimulation is mostly observed in tumours with the highest iodine content. The distribution of iodine is extremely heterogeneous (Fragu and Larras-Regard 1986). The turnover rate of iodine is always far more rapid than in a normal thyroid gland, with a half-life of only 1–4 days (normal half-life, 100 days).

A large number of biochemical defects which may explain these findings have been described (Valenta 1974). An impairment in the iodine transport mechanism is always observed. The rate of organification is generally very low, particularly in less differentiated tumours. This may be due to a defect in enzymatic processes leading to oxidation and organification of iodine. Indeed, a majority of thyroid cancers have a very low peroxidase activity (Fragu and Nataf 1977). Thyroglobulin (Tg) is the main thyroid protein. Its concentration is always reduced in tumours and is very low in a large proportion of tumours (Thomas-Morvan *et al.* 1974; Valenta 1974; van Herle 1979). However, Tg can still be detected by immunochemistry in most thyroid carcinomas (Boecker *et al.* 1980). Because of the low Tg concentration, there is a high proportion of low molecular weight iodoproteins and hormone synthesis is low. However, the lack of Tg is not sufficient to account for the deficiency in iodine concentration. Conversely, the release of Tg in the blood is higher than in normal thyroid tissue (van Herle *et al.* 1979; Ashcraft and van Herle 1981; Schlumberger *et al.* 1981, 1988*b*; Pacini *et al.* 1985; Girelli *et al.* 1986; de Vathaire *et al.* 1988).

With regard to the structure of the Tg molecule in thyroid cancers (van Herle *et al.* 1979), the most consistent findings are its reduced content of sialic acid and its low rate of iodization. In a given tumour, the number of atoms of iodine per Tg molecule is extremely heterogenous. These defects may be related to abnormalities in the structure of Tg or to a defect in the peroxidase system (Fragu and Nataf 1977). When iodine is incorporated into Tg, synthesis proceeds at a rate which is comparable with that seen in thyroid glands with a similar mean number of iodine atoms per molecule of Tg (Thomas-Morvan *et al.* 1974). Nevertheless, most iodinated compounds released are not functional and metastatic lesions are usually not able to produce detectable amounts of T_3 and T_4 in the serum (Schlumberger *et al.* 1980).

Control mechanisms

The cells of most differentiated thyroid tumours possess TSH receptors. Their number varies with the histological type, the highest being found in follicular well-differentiated tumours and the lowest in less differentiated ones. Moreover, response to TSH stimulation, as assessed by adenyl-cyclase levels and radio-iodine uptake, varies for a given number of TSH receptors.

TSH stimulation increases radio-iodine uptake by all thyroid tissues able to pick up ^{131}I (Goldman *et al.* 1980; Schneider *et al.* 1981; Schlumberger *et al.* 1983) and also increases Tg release into the blood even by tumours unable to concentrate ^{131}I (Schlumberger *et al.* 1980; Schneider *et al.* 1981). This shows that all tumours are TSH dependent.

TSH also plays a major role in the control of thyroid cell proliferation, as shown in the *in vitro* culture of normal human thyroid cells (Roger *et al.* 1988). Suppressive therapy with T_4 decreases the recurrence rate, tumour progression, and death rate from thyroid cancer (Clark 1981; Mazzaferri 1987). Other factors, such as thyroid-stimulating immunoglobulins, may enhance thyroid cell proliferation (Filetti *et al.* 1988).

In summary, although it is known that a sizeable proportion of thyroid tumours develop the ability to concentrate iodine after prolonged stimulation by supranormal levels of TSH, there is currently no satisfactory way of predicting which particular tumour will do so. Histology, stable iodine concentration, and initial thyroid uptake remain the only indicators of iodine uptake.

Hormone synthesis requires both a complex enzymatic system and a strict structural organization. It is not surprising that several defects can impair this delicate process. The number and variety of defects observed in malignant cells leaves little hope of improving radio-iodine concentration by simple means.

Oncogenes

The study of the molecular defects which cause thyroid carcinoma is of great importance since the identification of the growth factors which are involved in tumour cell proliferation may lead to new approaches for treatment.

Clonal chromosomal abnormalities have been described recently, some involving chromosome 10 (Antonini *et al.* 1989). Genes of the *ras* family are frequently activated by a point mutation in both follicular and papillary tumours (Suarez *et al.* 1988, 1990; Lemoine *et al.* 1989). However, the activation of this oncogene is found at all stages from benign through well-differentiated to undifferentiated carcinoma. This suggests that it represents an early event and that this defect is not by itself sufficient for carcinogenesis. Therefore other cooperative molecular defects are being sought.

Gsp mutations were found in 8 per cent of hypofunctioning tumours (Suarez 1991). Activation of genes coding for the protein kinase receptor superfamily has been found in papillary carcinoma but not in adenomas or in follicular carcinomas. The activation of the *ret* oncogene by intrachromosomal rearrangement was found in 16 per cent of papillary carcinomas and was called PTC (Fusco *et al.* 1987; Donghi *et al.* 1989); the *trk* oncogene has been found to be activated with a lower frequency only in papillary carcinomas through a chromosomal rearrangement (Bongarzone *et al.* 1989). Overexpression of the *met*-HGF receptor was found in 70 per cent of papillary carcinomas and may be associated with a more aggressive behaviour (Di Renzo *et al.* 1992). Changes in c-*myc* and *fos* expression have been reported but no structural abnormality was found (Aasland *et al.* 1988; Terrier *et al.* 1988). Their overexpression is likely to be a consequence rather than a cause of malignant transformation as TSH stimulation of normal cells has been shown to activate the c-*myc* oncogene (Yamashita *et al.* 1986).

Point mutations inactivating the p53 gene were observed with a high frequency in poorly differentiated and anaplastic thyroid carcinomas, but not in well-differentiated thyroid carcinomas (Ito *et al.* 1992). There is some evidence of autocrine growth factor production such as IGF-1 in follicular adenoma (Williams *et al.* 1989) and transforming growth factor alpha (TGF-α) in papillary carcinoma. TGF-α is capable of binding to the epidermal growth factor receptor which is expressed by both malignant and normal thyroid cells.

DIAGNOSIS

Palpable thyroid nodules are present in 4–7 per cent of the adult population. Most surgical series report a cancer incidence of 5–20 per cent in patients with no history of radiation exposure. Therefore, it is neither practical nor necessary to remove every nodule in order to exclude malignancy and investigations are directed to select for surgery those with an increased risk of malignancy (van Herle *et al.* 1979; Molitch *et al.* 1984; Rojeski and Gharib 1985; Krenning *et al.* 1988).

Most thyroid carcinomas present as an asymptomatic slow-growing nodule. Several clinical features may give rise to the clinical suspicion of malignancy. These include a history of external irradiation to the neck, young age, progressive although not sudden growth, hoarseness, adherence of the nodule to surrounding tissues, and cervical lymphadenopathy. These patients should be operated upon, as well as those with large nodules (>3 cm), irrespective of the results of diagnostic tests. In contrast, a long-standing familial goitre without a dominant mass is likely to be benign.

A thyroid scan with ^{99m}Tc or ^{123}I is suggestive of malignancy where there is a cold nodule. The prevalence of carcinoma in hot nodules is less than 1 per cent. When a cold nodule is solitary, needle aspiration or sonography should be performed to exclude a cyst. The risk of malignancy in a cyst is small (<4 per cent) and becomes practically negligible when the nodule shrinks completely after aspiration and does not reappear.

There is a good correlation between aspiration cytology and histology. The technique requires practice in obtaining samples and making the smear preparations and the skills of an expert cytologist. Technical failures occur in 5–10 per cent of patients, who should be considered candidates for surgery. On adequate smears, cytological results can be scored as negative, suspicious, or positive for malignant disease; these account for 60, 35 and 5 per cent, respectively of aspirations. A false-positive report of malignancy is rare but the rate of false negatives is 5–10 per cent. This is largely because of the difficulty in distinguishing cells from benign adenoma, atypical adenoma, and follicular carcinoma. Thus, a safe policy is to regard all such lesions as suspicious and advise surgical exploration.

Such a selective approach, that is, operating only on patients with suspicious or malignant nodules on the basis of clinical grounds and cytology, reduces the number of patients requiring surgery by a factor of 3. However, there is a significant risk of neglecting a cancer. In the absence of surgery, the patient is usually followed-up at 6 month intervals with or without suppressive therapy. Whether repeated cytology is warranted in benign nodules is still a matter of debate. However, an increase in the size of the mass should indicate surgery.

PROGNOSTIC FACTORS AND NATURAL HISTORY OF DIFFERENTIATED THYROID CARCINOMAS

Most differentiated thyroid carcinomas are extremely slow growing, with doubling times of more than 1 year and time courses extending over several decades. Some misconceptions concerning the course of thyroid cancer have arisen from studies with a mean follow-up of only 5–10 years. In this context the study of prognostic factors is of great clinical importance (Tubiana *et al.* 1975).

In patients without distant metastases at initial treatment (Tubiana *et al.* 1985a), total uncorrected survival (Fig. 1) was significantly lower than that of a reference population. These data, as well as others (Byar *et al.* 1979; Young *et al.* 1980; Fourquet 1983; Tubiana *et al.* 1985a; Bacourt *et al.* 1986; Hannequin *et al.* 1986; Kerr *et al.* 1986; McConahey *et al.* 1986; Tennvall *et al.* 1986;

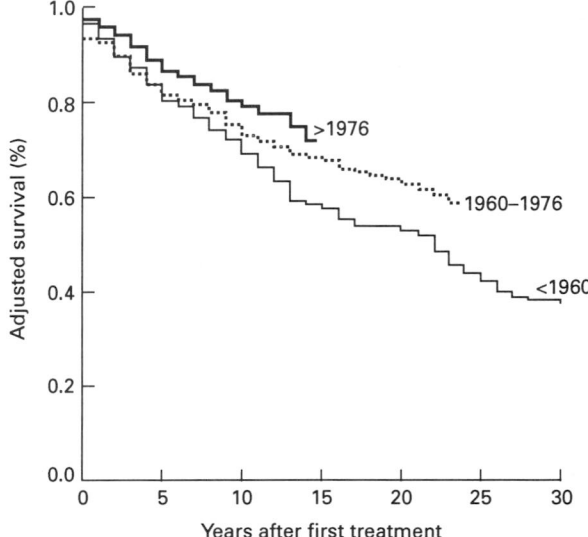

Fig. 1 Differentiated thyroid cancer: overall survival for three cohorts of patients treated at Villejuif from 1952 to 1960, 1960 to 1975, and after 1976 after adjustment for prognostic variables (2107 patients). The statistical difference between the three cohorts is highly significant before and after adjustment for the the two main prognostic variables (age and histology) ($s = p < 10^{-4}$). Each cohort comprises all patients with differentiated cancers (follicular well differentiated, follicular moderately differentiated and papillary) with or without clinically detectable distant metastases at initial treatment, whose clinical treatment was carried out at the Institut Gustave Roussy, Villejuif, during the corresponding period. In order to make the three cohorts comparable, the patients were adjusted for the main prognostic variables. From 1952 to 1988, the treatment was performed by a team under the same leadership of surgeons, radiotherapists, and nuclear medicine specialists. The main differences are related to the techniques used for the work-up of the patient. In 1960, a more effective technique for the whole-body scintigraphy was introduced (stimulation by TSH of thyroid tissue and administration of high activities of ^{131}I, up to 100 mCi). In 1976, routine serum thyroglobin assay was introduced. The scintigraphy technique greatly improved the delineation of tumour mass and therefore resulted in a more effective loco-regional treatment. The detection of residual metastatic tissue, by whole body scanning and, in 1976 by Tg assay, made earlier treatment of local relapse or distant metastases possible.

Hay *et al.* 1987; Mazzaferri 1987; Simpson *et al.* 1987; Cady and Rossi 1988; Schelfhout *et al.* 1988; Smith *et al.* 1988; Thoresen *et al.* 1989) indicate the fallacy of the statement that patients with differentiated thyroid carcinoma may die with, but not from their thyroid cancer. Recurrent disease is frequently seen and is associated with high mortality rates (Fig. 1). Survival in the presence of distant metastases is discussed below.

Prognostic factors have been identified by univariate analysis. Since all factors are closely interrelated, only multivariate analyses can identify their individual prognostic significance (Byar *et al.* 1979; Fourquet 1983; Tubiana *et al.* 1985a; Bacourt *et al.* 1986; Hannequin *et al.* 1986; Kerr *et al.* 1986; Tennvall *et al.* 1986; Hay *et al.* 1987; Simpson *et al.* 1987; Cady and Rossi 1988; Schelfhout *et al.* 1988; Thoresen *et al.* 1989). The variation in their respective prognostic influences between these studies may be due to differences in patient selection, staging, treatment, and duration of follow-up.

Multivariate analysis in differentiated thyroid carcinomas

Most reports consider as a group either patients with papillary and follicular cancer (Tubiana *et al.* 1985a; Bacourt *et al.* 1986; Tennvall *et al.* 1986; Cady and Rossi 1988; Schelfhout 1988; Thoresen *et al.* 1989) or all histological subtypes (Byar *et al.* 1979; Fourquet 1983; Kerr *et al.* 1986; Hay *et al.* 1987). In these studies age is found to be the most important prognostic determinant. Older patients have an increased cancer-related mortality. Disease mortality increases with age and increases sharply around 40 years (Fig. 2) (Tubiana *et al.* 1985a; Kerr *et al.* 1986; Simpson *et al.* 1987; Thoresen *et al.* 1989). In older patients, the probability of relapse is greater and the interval between initial treatment and relapse is shorter suggesting a more rapid growth rate (Tubiana *et al.* 1985a).

Although the long-term prognosis is favourable in children, the excess mortality caused by cancer is highly significant (Winship and Rosvoll 1970; Schlumberger *et al.* 1987b; Zimmerman *et al.* 1988).

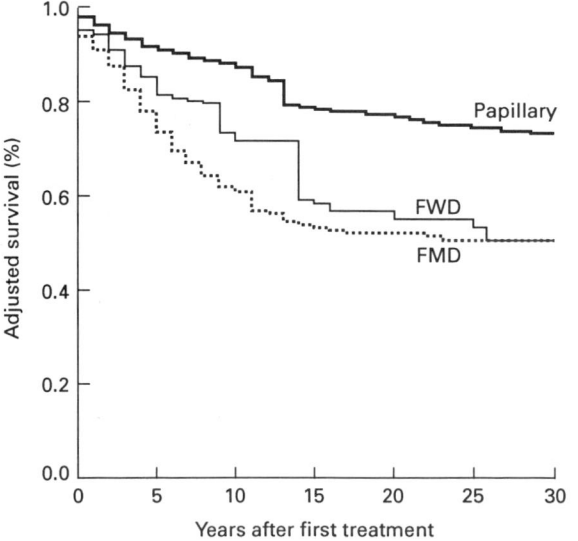

Fig. 2 Differentiated thyroid cancer (2107 patients). Survival according to age and after adjustment for histologic type and time period during which the patient was treated. In the young age group (<19 years) most deaths occur after more than 20 years of follow-up. They occur much sooner in older patients ($s = p < 10^{-4}$).

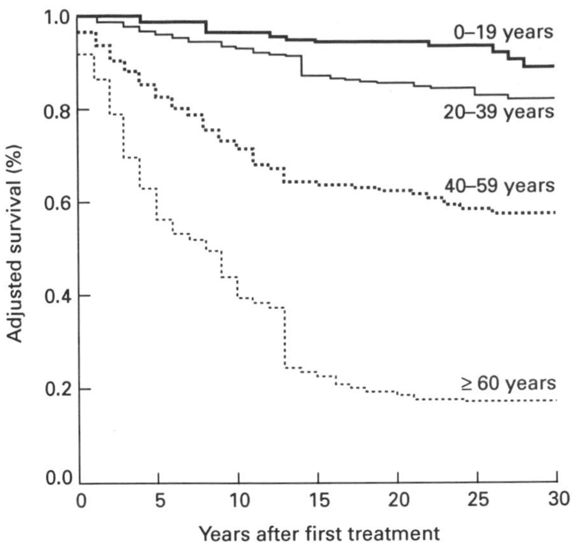

Fig. 3 Differentiated thyroid cancer (2107 patients). Influence on overall survival of histologic type (FWD, follicular well differentiated; FMD, follicular moderately differentiated). After adjustment for the two main other prognostic variables (age and time at which patients were treated) the difference remains highly significant. However, the difference between FMD and FWD decreases with time ($s = p < 10^{-4}$).

Moreover, the occurrence of metastases and the relapse rate were higher than in adults, in particular in children younger than 10 years at diagnosis. These data suggest that the same management should be used in both children and adults.

Histology provides highly significant prognostic information. Patients with papillary and follicular well-differentiated tumours have a similar prognosis, but those with less differentiated cancer fared worse (Fig. 3) (Tubiana *et al.* 1985a; Bacourt *et al.* 1986; Schelfhout *et al.* 1988).

Male sex is associated in some series with a higher risk of death and of relapse (Byar *et al.* 1979; Fourquet 1983; Tubiana *et al.* 1985a; Bacourt *et al.* 1986; Schelfhout *et al.* 1988), but the prognostic significance of gender is small.

Tumour stage and size is prognostically important. Although controversial, nodal status is found to be significant in some series, in particular for the risk of loco-regional recurrence and where involved nodes are palpable (Tubiana *et al.* 1985a; Hannequin *et al.* 1986; Kerr *et al.* 1986).

Some prognostic studies have considered papillary and follicular cancer separately. Papillary carcinoma has a prolonged course in most patients (McConahey *et al.* 1986; Mazzaferri 1987). However, high mortality rates may be seen in some subsets of patients. Four studies were conducted using multivariate analysis in patients with papillary carcinoma (Kerr *et al.* 1986; Tennvall *et al.* 1986; Hay *et al.* 1987; Simpson *et al.* 1987). Four variables were independently predictive for survival: age, histological grade, tumour extent, and tumour size.

Older patients and those with moderately differentiated papillary carcinoma have an increased mortality rate. Prognosis is altered by direct invasion of the primary tumour into the surrounding neck structures. In recent years, patients presenting with large inoperable tumour masses have been rare in developed countries. The risk of death increases with the size of the tumour. Patients with a small tumour of dimensions less than 1–2 cm have an excellent prognosis. The discovery of a tumour less than 1 cm in diameter in a gland

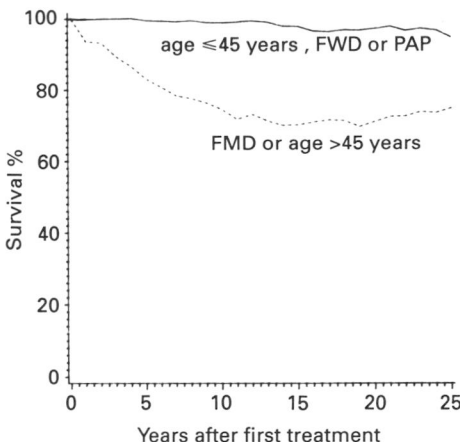

Fig. 4 Corrected survival of patient without initial distant metastasis according to high- or low-risk group (546 patients with follow-up longer than 20 years). Only the two main prognostic variables (age and histological type) were taken into account. Corrected survival was obtained by comparison with a reference French population of the same age and gender. A plateau does not mean that patients do not die from the cancer since there may be a balance between cancer-related deaths and a reduction in the number of deaths due to intercurrent diseases resulting from the careful follow-up of the patients. The late slight increase in survival observed in the high-risk group (follicular moderately differentiated and/or age greater than 45 years) shows that with time the latter phenomenon prevails.

removed for other clinical reasons warrants a long-term follow-up and L-thyroxine treatment, but not aggressive initial treatment.

These prognostic factors have allowed risk group classifications based on age and histology (Tubiana *et al.* 1985*a*) (Fig. 4) and scoring systems based on age, histology, sex, stage, and metastases (Byar *et al.* 1979) or age, metastasis, extent, and size (Cady and Rossi 1988) or age, grade, extent, and size (Hay *et al.* 1987). When these prognostic factors were used 86 per cent of the patients in one series were found to be in the low-risk group (Hay *et al.* 1987). Tumour cell DNA content may provide additional information with non-diploid tumours being associated with an increased risk of mortality (Bäckdahl *et al.* 1985; Hamming *et al.* 1988; Smith *et al.* 1988).

Disease-related mortality is higher in patients with follicular carcinoma than in those with papillary carcinoma (Young *et al.* 1980). Multivariate analyses have determined the prognostic importance of several variables (Tennvall *et al.* 1986; Kim and Leeper 1987; Simpson *et al.* 1987). Age, although significant, did not appear to be the most important variable. A highly significant difference in survival was observed between moderately differentiated follicular tumours and papillary or well-differentiated histological subtypes (Tubiana *et al.* 1985*a*) and the treatment–relapse and relapse–death intervals are shorter for those tumours than for other types. These data strongly suggest that moderately differentiated and well-differentiated follicular subtypes should be considered separately. Invasiveness is closely related to the grade of differentiation. Recurrence rates and mortality significantly increase when the lesion exhibits wide capsular and vascular invasion (Lang *et al.* 1986). Indeed, the data suggest that the marked improvement in survival which has been observed over the past decades (Fig. 1) was mostly due to

(1) detection and delineation of otherwise occult disease by only sensitive whole-body scan in 1963;

(2) after 1976 by both whole-body scan and thyroglobulin assays (Van Herle *et al.* 1973, 1979).

Mortality from large primary tumours is significantly greater than from small cancers, but a substantial number of patients with small follicular carcinoma die of their disease. The prognostic usefulness of tumour cell nuclear DNA content in follicular carcinoma is still controversial.

INITIAL TREATMENT

The treatment approach should be based on risk groups and the extent of disease. Prognostic factors and scoring systems may be of help in assessing an individual patient's risk of dying from cancer at the time of initial treatment (Tubiana *et al.* 1975, 1985*a*; Byar *et al.* 1979; Hay *et al.* 1987; Cady and Rossi 1988). The low-risk group includes young patients with favourable prognostic indicators. In this group, most recurrences are curable and long-term prognosis is excellent. The extent of surgical excision should be related to the extent of the disease. Frequently, when a macroscopically complete surgical excision of neoplastic tissue present in the neck has been performed, no further therapy is required. However, some still advocate total thyroidectomy and ablative radio-iodine treatment.

The high-risk group includes patients above the age of 45 with a large thyroid tumour or with capsular breach or with less differentiated thyroid carcinoma. In this group, the incidence of recurrence and death from cancer is high and treatment of the recurrence is often unsuccessful. Here, total ablation of the thyroid gland should be systematically performed by thyroidectomy followed by an ablative dose of ^{131}I.

It is worth noting that there is no evidence that the surgical protocol for lymph node dissection should be different for the two groups.

Surgery

The initial management of differentiated thyroid carcinoma is surgical. However, some differences in opinion still exist concerning the extent of surgical resection of both the thyroid gland and the lymph nodes (Lacour *et al.* 1977; Thompson *et al.* 1978; Clark 1982; Hay *et al.* 1987; Noguchi and Murakami 1987; Attie 1988; Cady and Rossi 1988; Grant *et al.* 1988).

An extracapsular lobectomy and isthmusectomy is the minimal surgical procedure, limiting damage to the parathyroid glands and recurrent laryngeal nerve. In fact, after total thyroidectomy recurrent laryngeal nerve injury occurs in 5 per cent of patients, but fortunately bilateral nerve injury is rare. The incidence of parathyroid insufficiency has decreased in recent years from 10–15 to less than 2 per cent. This is due, at least in part, to the use of modern techniques for staining and transplantation of the parathyroid glands (Elias *et al.* 1983).

Some authors advocate total or near total thyroidectomy (Thompson *et al.* 1978; Clark 1982; Attie 1988) in view of the high frequency of bilateral multicentricity (Russell *et al.* 1963) and the lower risk of local recurrence after bilateral resection than after lobectomy alone (Hay *et al.* 1987; Mazzaferri 1987; Grant *et al.* 1988). However, not all these foci are of clinical importance and the recurrences are treatable (Lacour *et al.* 1977; Thompson *et al.* 1978; Tubiana *et al.* 1985*a*; Hay *et al.* 1987; Grant *et al.* 1988). Furthermore, involvement of the contralateral lobe can be identified on frozen section, allowing surgery to be adapted to disease during the surgical procedure.

Knowledge of prognostic factors may dictate the extent of surgery. In fact, survival of patients with favourable prognostic indicators was similar following lobectomy or bilateral resection (Hay *et al.* 1987; Cady and Rossi 1988). Conversely, survival was improved with bilateral as opposed to unilateral resection in patients with unfavourable prognostic indicators (Hay *et al.* 1987; Grant *et al.* 1988). For these reasons, a total or near total thyroidectomy is performed only when its advantages outweigh its potential morbidity, that is, in case of multicentricity (which can be shown by frozen sections) or in the presence of unfavourable prognostic indicators. In these latter cases, an ablative dose of ^{131}I is administered post-operatively. Lobectomy and isthmusectomy are performed in patients with favourable prognostic indicators without clinical or histological evidence of multicentricity.

Microscopic lymph node involvement is found at histological examination in up to 90 per cent of the patients (Noguchi and Murakami 1987; Schlumberger *et al.* 1987*b*). The recurrent laryngeal nerve chain and the jugulocarotid chain are involved with the same frequency. Involvement of the ipsilateral recurrent laryngeal nerve chain is difficult to detect clinically or by radiological means. It may lead to mediastinal invasion and lung metastases. Therefore, it should be systematically dissected and when involved nodes are present the anterior superior mediastinum should also be dissected, eventually with a sternotomy. In patients with palpable lymph nodes, a modified neck dissection is recommended, sparing the sternocleidomastoid muscle, the internal jugular vein, and the spinal accessory nerve (Attie 1988). In the absence of palpable lymph nodes, arguments for a systematic modified neck dissection are controversial. Microscopic lymph node metastases expose patients to clinical relapse; however, these relapses can generally be treated successfully. The involvement of the lower third of the jugulocarotid chain on frozen sections has a high predictive value (> 80 per cent) upon the involvement of its upper two-thirds. Therefore, dissection of the lower third of the jugulocarotid chain should be preferred to involved lymph node excision or 'picking', as it appears to be a reliable indicator for a modified neck dissection (Lacour *et al.* 1977).

Other surgical procedures are required in a minority of patients. Tracheal resection and eventually tracheotomy and even more occasionally an oesophageal resection or an oesophagectomy, may be required where there is infiltration of these structures.

POST-OPERATIVE RADIO-IODINE THERAPY

The value of post-operative ^{131}I after total surgical removal of the neoplastic tissue is debatable. It may have two advantages. First, it allows the subsequent search by a whole-body scan of residual neoplastic tissue and increases the sensitivity of Tg measurement and of whole-body ^{131}I scan during the follow-up. Second, relapse rates were lower in patients systematically treated post-operatively with ^{131}I in some series (Maheshwari *et al.* 1981; Massin *et al.* 1984; Beierwaltes 1987; Mazzaferri 1987) but not in all. Indeed, in some subsets of patients, prognosis is so favourable after surgery alone that little further improvement is obtained by systematic ablation with ^{131}I (Tubiana *et al.* 1975, 1985*a*; McConahey *et al.* 1986; Cady and Rossi 1988). Similarly, the reasons usually given for not using ^{131}I are also unconvincing. After a single ablative dose of ^{131}I, the theoretical risk of leukaemia is very small (Hall *et al.* 1992) and the theoretical risk of genetic defect or infertility remains currently unproven (M. Schlumberger, F. De Vathaire, C. Ceccarelli *et al.*, submitted).

The present data do not justify routine administration of ^{131}I to all patients with a favourable prognosis, although an ablative dose of ^{131}I is justified in those with poor prognostic indicators because it will facilitate an early discovery of relapses. The ablative dose is given after adequate TSH stimulation. The use of 30 mCi of ^{131}I leads to successful ablation in only 60 per cent of cases (Kuni and Klingensmith 1980) and many authors advocate the routine use of 100 mCi.

In addition to its therapeutic effects, the administration of 100 mCi helps by total body ^{131}I scan to delineate or detect residual neoplastic tissue that may warrant further treatment, in particular in the mediastinum or the lungs. Therefore, a whole-body ^{131}I scan can be performed 5–7 days after each administration of 100 mCi (Tubiana and Mabille 1963; Pacini *et al.* 1987; Schlumberger *et al.* 1988*a*). However, it must be remembered that not all neoplastic tissue takes up ^{131}I.

EXTERNAL-BEAM IRRADIATION

Post-operative irradiation of residual tumours is indicated if no ^{131}I uptake is found in the tumour remnant (Tubiana *et al.* 1975, 1985*b*; Simpson *et al.* 1988). However, this should be performed only after an experienced surgeon believes that everything possible has been done, which may involve re-exploration of the neck. External irradiation is not warranted routinely following satisfactory tumour excision.

Patients are irradiated with telecobalt or megavoltage X-rays. The target volume should include the thyroid bed, the neck lymph nodes, and the upper part of the mediastinum. A dose of 50 Gy in 25 fractions is given to the tumour followed by 5–10 Gy boosts to areas of macroscopic tumour. Patients are irradiated with a direct anterior field shaped by lead blocks to protect the lungs and the larynx and with a posterior field limited to the upper mediastinum. Doses greater than 42 Gy to the thoracic spinal cord are avoided. The respective dose contributions of these two fields should be adapted according to the anteroposterior diameter of the upper thorax.

SUPPRESSIVE TREATMENT

L-Thyroxine (L-T$_4$) treatment is advocated for all patients with differentiated thyroid cancer (Clark 1981; Mazzaferri 1987) with the aim of suppressing TSH secretion without inducing thyrotoxicosis. Since the introduction of sensitive TSH (sTSH) assays, TSH suppression can be accurately monitored (Schlumberger *et al.* 1987*a*). The routine use of the thyrotrophin-releasing hormone (TRH) stimulation test can be avoided since there is a close correlation between the basal TSH and maximal TSH level after TRH stimulation.

Some authors have advocated the total suppression of TSH secretion, that is, an undetectable sTSH serum level, which agrees with the absence of response of TSH to TRH stimulation. When this is achieved, at least one-third of these patients have clinical or biochemical symptoms of thyrotoxicosis. Furthermore, there is no evidence that undetectable serum TSH levels have any advantage over low but detectable TSH levels. Therefore a decrease of sTSH level below 0.1 μU/ml has been advocated (Schlumberger *et al.* 1987*a*). When TSH is above 0.1 μU/ml, the daily dose of L-T$_4$ is increased by 25 μg and T$_4$, TSH, and Tg levels are remeasured 3 months later. The mean daily dose of L-T$_4$ used is 2.4 μg/kg body weight in adults, higher in children, and lower for patients over 65 years of age.

FOLLOW-UP

Long-term results in patients with metastatic thyroid carcinoma have shown that prognosis is strongly related to the total tumour burden at discovery of metastases (Samaan *et al.* 1985; Schlumberger *et al.* 1986). This should encourage the detection of metastases by the combined use of serum Tg measurement and of whole-body ^{131}I scan at an early stage when radiographs are still normal.

Most relapses occur within the first 5 years, but may also emerge after decades of apparent complete remission. Therefore, follow-up should be intensive during the first 2–3 years but should also be pursued throughout the patient's life.

CLINICAL EVALUATION

Neck recurrences are often discovered by palpation or ultrasonography, but prior external neck irradiation may hamper clinical examination. Thus, sonography, CT scan, or scintigraphy of the neck may be required and fine-needle aspiration is helpful in determining the nature of any abnormal mass.

The lungs and bones are the most frequent locations of distant metastases. Metastases in the brain, liver, or skin tend to appear late in patients who already have multiple bone or lung metastases. Clinical symptoms usually indicate large metastases; that is, macronodular lung metastases, pleural effusion, or bone abnormalities on radiographs (Schlumberger *et al.* 1986).

RADIOLOGICAL FINDINGS

Most patients with metastatic disease have elevated serum Tg before metastases are visible on chest radiographs. Therefore, the routine use of chest radiographs appears to be unnecessary. In patients with normal chest radiographs and diffuse radio-iodine uptake in the lungs, lung tomograms rarely detect micronodules whereas lung CT is much more sensitive. However, despite a diffuse uptake of ^{131}I in the lungs, CT scanning may reveal only a few peripheral micronodules (Piekarski *et al.* 1985).

Most bone metastases are osteolytic and therefore difficult to find on skeletal survey radiographs. ^{99m}Tc diphosphonate bone scans are more sensitive (de Groot and Reilly 1984; Tenenbaum *et al.* 1993) but may give false-negatives.

SERUM Tg MEASUREMENT

Tg is a reliable marker of differentiated thyroid carcinoma during follow-up (van Herle *et al.* 1973; Ashcraft and van Herle 1981; Schlumberger *et al.* 1981, 1986, 1988b; Pacini *et al.* 1985; Girelli *et al.* 1986; de Vathaire *et al.* 1988; Schlumberger *et al.* 1991a) and the contradictory results reported in some series appear to have been due to insufficient sensitivity or accuracy (van Herle *et al.* 1985; Feldt-Rasmussen and Schlumberger 1988). Endogenous anti-Tg antibodies are found in approximately 15 per cent of cancer patients. However, when immunoradiometric assays monoclonal antibodies are used, interferences are found in only 2–3 per cent of sera (Schlumberger *et al.* 1991a).

The serum Tg level is detectable in 90–100 per cent of patients with metastases during T_4 treatment (Ashcraft and van Herle 1981; Schlumberger *et al.* 1981, 1986; Pacini *et al.* 1985; Girelli *et al.* 1986). However, an increase in Tg levels may be relatively small in patients whose metastases are not visible on radiographs (Pacini *et al.* 1987; Schlumberger *et al.* 1988a) and in those with involvement of neck lymph nodes. Therefore, Tg measurement

must be sensitive enough to detect these low Tg levels reliably. This result also underlines the need for systematic lymph node dissection at initial treatment and thereafter for a systematic post-operative ^{131}I whole-body scan to search for foci of ectopic uptake.

Serum Tg may increase following TSH stimulation even in patients whose metastases do not pick up radio-iodine (Schlumberger *et al.* 1981; Schneider *et al.* 1981; Pacini *et al.* 1985; Girelli *et al.* 1986). Nevertheless, false-negative Tg measurements have occasionally been reported in this situation, but they may be due to technical problems in Tg assays.

False-positive Tg measurements appeared to be more frequent in patients without thyroid remnants. Tg was detected in 13 per cent of the patients with no other evidence of disease during T_4 treatment (Schlumberger *et al.* 1981; Pacini *et al.* 1987) and in a greater proportion following thyroid hormone withdrawal. However, the Tg level remains relatively low in most patients with no other evidence of disease, whereas it increases to significantly higher levels in patients with metastatic disease (Schlumberger *et al.* 1988b). Furthermore, when interpreting these results it should be remembered that thyroid cancer has a slow growth rate. Therefore, an increased Tg level may be detected long before metastases become detectable, in particular when they do not pick up radio-iodine.

During follow-up of patients with thyroid remnants, serum Tg measurement during T_4 treatment is less specific. However, no relapse was observed among patients without a detectable serum Tg and the probability of relapse was significantly correlated with Tg level. Therefore, Tg measurement during T_4 treatment is useful for detecting relapse and for avoiding 60 per cent of whole-body ^{131}I scans (de Vathaire *et al.* 1988); that is, in patients with low or undetectable Tg levels. The interpretation of an increase in Tg level following TSH stimulation is more difficult in these patients since Tg can be released by either normal thyroid remnants or neoplastic foci.

^{131}I WHOLE-BODY SCAN

As the efficacy of whole-body scans depends upon the ability of malignant tissue to take up radio-iodine, iodine overload should be avoided and stimulation by TSH is of critical importance (Tubiana and Mabille 1963). In practice, patients are taken off T_4 therapy and receive T_3 for 3 weeks as it has a shorter half-life. Thereafter T_3 is withdrawn for 14 days. T_3 withdrawal for more than 2 weeks is unnecessary and may be harmful (Goldman *et al.* 1980). Serum TSH level should be measured before the scan is performed because in some patients it is inadequate (Vagenakis *et al.* 1975). The availability of recombinant human TSH in the near future will probably allow the scanning of patients without withdrawal of thyroid hormone treatment (Braverman *et al.* 1992).

The ^{131}I dose generally used in testing is 2–5 mCi. The optimal scanning time is usually 72 h after the ^{131}I dose. The scintigram can be performed with either a rectilinear scanner or a gamma camera, but quantification of uptake is mandatory (Schlumberger *et al.* 1983, 1986).

A post-therapy whole-body ^{131}I scan is warranted in all patients treated with ^{131}I, as it may detect occult neoplastic uptake not shown after a diagnostic dose (Tubiana and Mabille 1963; Pacini *et al.* 1987; Schlumberger *et al.* 1988a) (Figs 5–7).

STRATEGY OF FOLLOW-UP

A strategy has been developed for the follow-up of patients without interference in the Tg assay (Schlumberger *et al.* 1988b). The

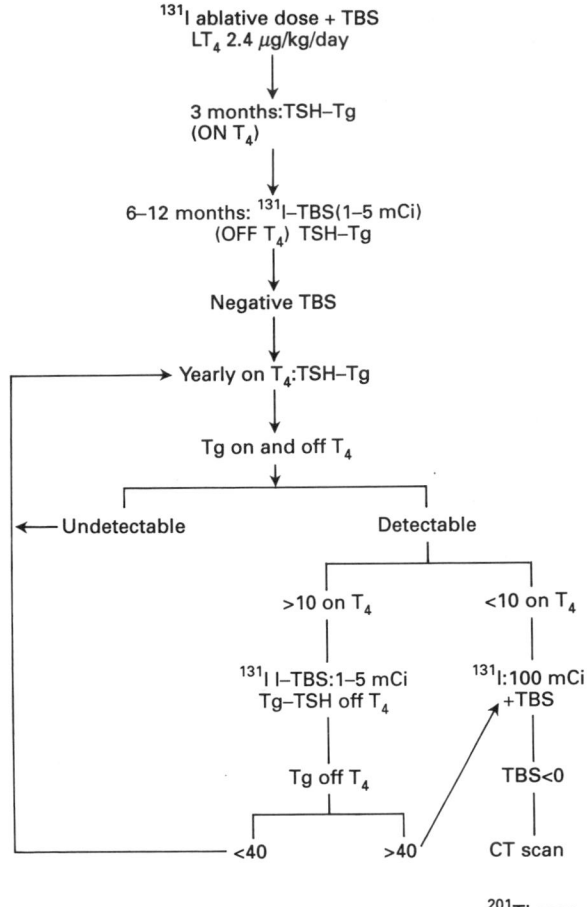

Fig. 5 Strategy of follow-up in thyroid cancer patients without thyroid remnants.

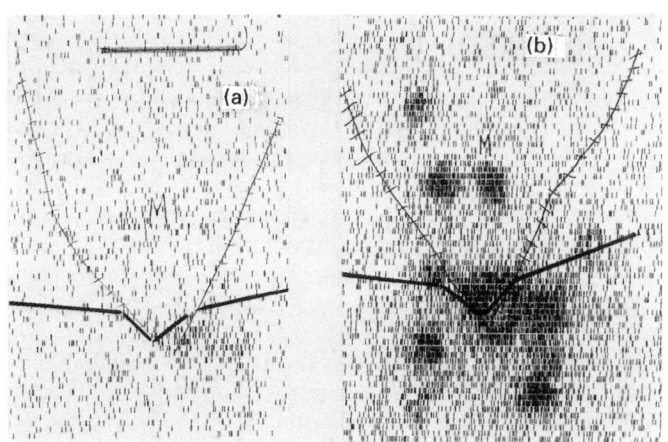

Fig. 6 ^{131}I scans performed after the administration of (a) 2 mCi and (b) 100 mCi. Uptake in lymph nodes behind the left sternoclavicular joint was seen after 2 mCi. After 100 mCi, this uptake was better visualized and uptake in the right oesotracheal groove was discovered. This patient was operated on and 12 lymph node metastases were found.

ablation of thyroid remnants increases the sensitivity of both Tg measurement and whole-body ^{131}I scan and is advocated in patients at high risk of developing relapses.

A whole-body ^{131}I scan is performed each year for 2 years after initial therapy. Thereafter, in patients with undetectable or low Tg

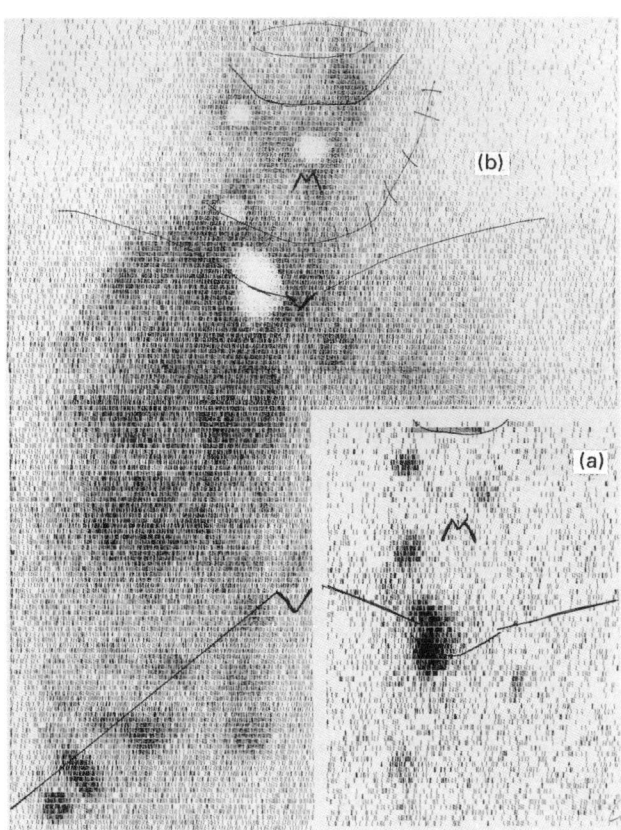

Fig. 7 ^{131}I scan performed after the administration of (a) 2 mCi and (b) 100 mCi. After the administration of 100 mCi, lung metastases were clearly demonstrated and uptake in the neck was 1.16 mCi. This ^{131}I whole-body scan clearly illustrates the progression of a papillary carcinoma along the oesotracheal groove and the mediastinum to the lungs.

levels after thyroid hormone withdrawal, follow-up is resumed with clinical evaluation, TSH measurements, and Tg measurements once a year while on T_4 therapy.

In patients without thyroid remnants, when the Tg level is detectable during T_4 treatment a whole-body ^{131}I scan and a chest radiograph are performed and Tg is measured again after thyroid hormone withdrawal. Patients with positive whole-body scans are treated with 100 mCi ^{131}I. In those patients with a negative whole-body ^{131}I scan, where Tg levels increased significantly after thyroid hormone withdrawal, additional attempts to localize thyroid tissue are made by neck ultrasound and neck and thorax CT scan. Administration of 100 mCi of ^{131}I with a whole-body scan 5 days later is particularly useful in these patients and permits the detection of unknown normal or neoplastic thyroid tissue which could subsequently be cured (Pacini *et al.* 1987; Schlumberger *et al.* 1988*a*).

Patients with thyroid remnants, whose Tg levels are elevated during T_4 treatment, are given 100 mCi of radio-iodine with a whole-body scan 5 days later.

^{201}Tl whole-body scans (Hoefnagl *et al.* 1986) appeared less reliable than whole-body ^{131}I scan for the routine follow-up. Venous sampling catheterization did not reveal any Tg concentration gradient in these patients, and scanning with the ^{133}I-labelled anti-Tg monoclonal antibody has not proved to be useful (Schlumberger *et al.* 1988*b*).

Since the routine use of the Tg assay was introduced, the number of total body ^{131}I scans performed has been reduced, but they are more effective because their indications are better defined. This allows an earlier discovery of relapse which should improve the long-term results of treatment (Schlumberger *et al.* 1986).

LOCAL RECURRENCE

Recurrent disease is associated with a high mortality rate (Tubiana *et al.* 1985*a*; Simpson *et al.* 1987; Smith *et al.* 1988). Survival after local recurrence was shorter among older patients, in those with less differentiated tumours and in those without ^{131}I uptake. Furthermore, a local recurrence often precedes or is associated with the appearance of distant metastases. Therefore, patients with recurrent disease should be assessed with a view to further treatment by all modalities.

The treatment of a local recurrence includes the administration of 100 mCi ^{131}I with a scan 5 days later which allows for a better delineation of known neoplastic tissue and sometimes the discovery of unsuspected neoplastic foci. Reoperation is then undertaken. Recurrences only rarely require extensive resection, but this may be warranted in some patients with extensive local disease without evidence of distant metastases. With the remaining ^{131}I activity, the patient is scanned again in order to ensure the completeness of surgical excision. External-beam radiotherapy to the neck is warranted in the absence of ^{131}I uptake, particularly in cases with a large recurrence or in whom surgical excision has been incomplete or dubious.

DISTANT METASTASES

Incidence

Metastases outside the neck occurred in 10–15 per cent of patients with differentiated thyroid cancer (Hoie *et al.* 1988; Ruegemer *et al.* 1988). Almost half the metastases were present initially, but in industrialized countries large neck masses and synchronous distant metastases have almost disappeared as presenting signs in recent years.

Methods of treatment

Surgery

Surgery should be considered on bone metastases in patients with orthopaedic or neurological complications. It should also be considered with a curative intent in patients with mediastinal involvement and in those with single or a few bone, lung, or cerebral metastases (Roy Camille *et al.* 1980).

Radio-iodine

^{131}I is the most frequently employed form of irradiation in the treatment of metastatic cancer. Only two-thirds of the patients take up iodine in their metastases (Schlumberger *et al.* 1986) and are amenable to therapy with ^{131}I. However, radio–iodine can eradicate small foci of neoplastic tissue but may not permanently eradicate large tumour deposits and therefore the addition of surgery or external irradiation may be warranted.

The treatment dose is 100–150 mCi in adults and 1 mCi/kg body weight in children. It is given after TSH stimulation (see above). A post-therapy scan is performed 5–7 days later and T_4 treatment is resumed. Other treatments with ^{131}I are given 3–6 months later until any residual uptake is ablated or adverse reactions are seen. There is no upper limit for the cumulative ^{131}I dose administered. The early discovery of metastases at a stage when they are not visible on radiographs, permits a reduction in the total dose of ^{131}I

necessary for cure and, hence, in body irradiation (Schlumberger *et al.* 1988*a*).

External-beam radiotherapy

External-beam radiotherapy is used for bone metastases not amenable to surgery, particularly when they are located in the vertebral column, near the base of skull or in sites where a pathological fracture would result in a serious disability (Tubiana *et al.* 1975, 1985*b*).

The importance of combining radio-iodine and external irradiation is often underestimated (Tubiana *et al.* 1975, 1985*b*). A positive relationship has been shown between the outcome of radio-iodine therapy and effective radiation dose (Muxon *et al.* 1983). This is related to both concentration and half-life. The range of concentration is quite variable, is often relatively low, and should be assessed *in vivo* (Schlumberger *et al.* 1986). The half-life is often short, ranging from 1 to 3 days in most metastases. Therefore, the dose delivered by ^{131}I is often relatively low.

Furthermore, with ^{131}I, the radiation dose is mostly delivered by β particles whose mean path is approximately 1 mm. Therefore, the dose received by a mass of iodine-concentrating tissue with a diameter of less than 1 mm could actually be much smaller than that calculated by the equations generally used which assume that sources are relatively large in size. Moreover, the minimal dose can be smaller because the distribution in neoplastic tissues is heterogeneous owing to the patchy distribution of radio-iodine.

Fortunately, external-beam radiotherapy can effectively complement radio-iodine, easily delivering 40 Gy to large volumes with little additional toxic effects. Moreover, treatment with radio-iodine is still possible after external-beam radiotherapy.

Chemotherapy

The only effective agent in patients with metastatic differentiated thyroid carcinoma is doxorubicin which has a response rate of 15–20 per cent. Responses were partial and lasted for only a few months. In two recent reports, doxorubicin was given in combination with cisplatin with similar response rates to that of doxorubicin alone but with greater toxicity (Shimaoka *et al.* 1985; Williams *et al.* 1986). The combination of doxorubicin and external-beam radiotherapy appeared to be effective in some patients with large tumour masses in the neck (Kim and Leeper 1987). Therefore, chemotherapy is used only to palliate patients with progressive metastases unable to take up radio-iodine or within phase II clinical trials.

Treatment results and prognostic factors

Overall survival rates from the time of detection of metastases were 54 per cent at 5 years, 37 per cent at 10 years, and 29 per cent at 15 years (Leeper 1973; Tubiana *et al.* 1975; Nemec *et al.* 1979; Massin *et al.* 1984; Samaan *et al.* 1985; Schlumberger *et al.* 1986; Beierwaltes 1987; Hoie *et al.* 1988; Ruegemer *et al.* 1988; Casara *et al.* 1993).

Multivariate analysis (Schlumberger *et al.* 1986) has shown that histology, age at the time of discovery of the metastases, ^{131}I uptake, and extent of the metastases have a significant impact on survival (Fig. 8). The paramount importance of an early discovery of distant metastases upon survival has been confirmed by two other multivariate analyses (Ruegemer *et al.* 1988; Casara *et al.* 1993). It appeared that bone metastases were associated with a poor prognosis when they were visible on radiographs, which is generally the case. Patients with metastases at the sternum or the base of the skull were more frequently cured than patients with skeletal

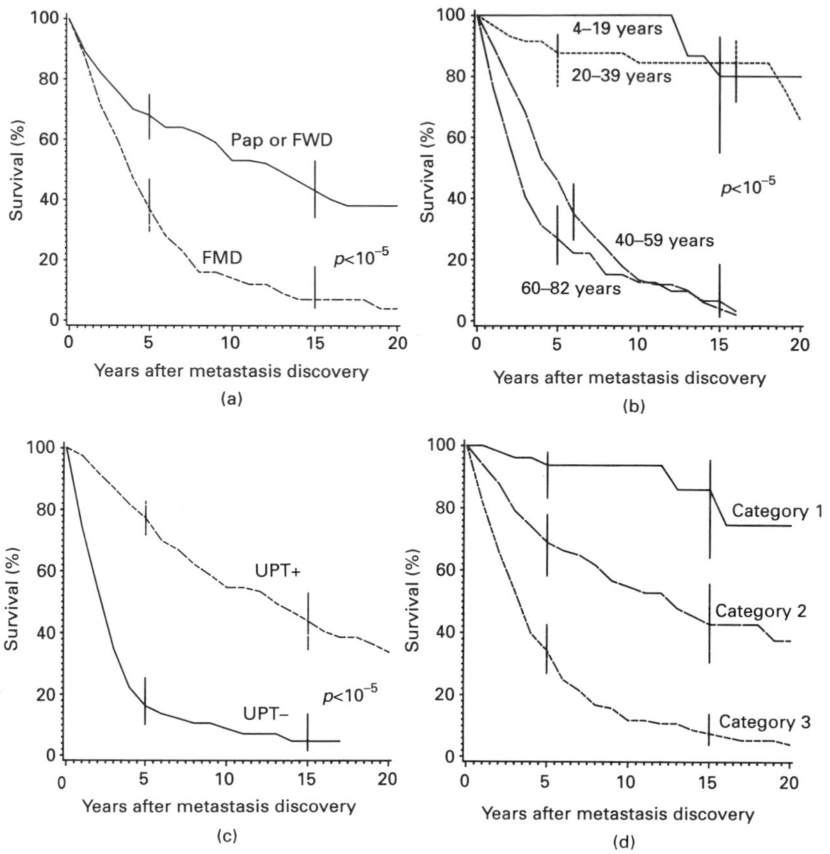

Fig. 8 (a) Survival of patients with distant metastases according to histology of the thyroid tumour; (b) survival of patients with distant metastases according to age at discovery of the metastases; (c) survival of patients with distant metastases according to radio-iodine uptake (upt +, presence of radio-iodine uptake in the metastases; upt −, absence of radio-iodine uptake in the metastases); (d) survival of patients with distant metastases according to the extent of disease at discovery of the metastases (category 1, metastases with normal radiographs; category 2, lung micronodules or single bone metastases with abnormal radiographs; category 3, lung macronodules or multiple bone metastases).

metastases in other locations (Tubiana *et al.* 1975) and this curability may be due to their relatively early detection (Schlumberger *et al.* 1986).

The better survival observed after ^{131}I treatment in patients with positive uptake cannot be explained by differences in growth rate despite the rare possibility of long-term survival without treatment (Leeper 1973; Nemec *et al.* 1979; Massin *et al.* 1984; Samaan *et al.* 1985; Schlumberger *et al.* 1986; Beierwaltes 1987). In fact, therapy with a thyroid hormone alone is insufficient for lung metastases, even when they are not visible on chest radiographs (Pacini *et al.* 1987; Schlumberger *et al.* 1988a). Conversely, to what has been claimed (Ruegemer *et al.* 1988), treatment of metastases with radio-iodine is highly effective both for remission and survival rates in patients with small metastases. Therefore, it should be undertaken as early as possible during the course of metastatic disease.

In conclusion, disseminated thyroid cancer can be cured in a significant proportion of patients. In others, durable palliation can be achieved and the presence of metastases may be compatible with prolonged survival. Furthermore, in most patients these treatments provide a good quality of life.

COMPLICATIONS OF TREATMENT WITH ^{131}I

Acute side-effects

Administration of therapeutic doses of ^{131}I causes remarkably few acute side-effects. Occasionally, patients complain of nausea and

transient sialadenitis has been observed but has rarely led to long-term xerostomia.

Leukaemogenesis

In large surveys, leukaemia occurred in approximately 1 per cent of the patients after multiple therapeutic doses of ^{131}I (Edmonds and Smith 1986; Schlumberger *et al.* 1986). Mild pancytopenia may occur in patients with bone metastases after extended fields of external radiotherapy and repeated treatments with ^{131}I. No significant excess of solid cancers and of leukaemias has been found in the Swedish series (Hall *et al.* 1991, 1992). However, the maximal cumulative doses of radio-iodine were not higher than 400 mCi. A slight excess of bladder cancer has been reported in patients treated with larger total ^{131}I doses (Edmonds and Smith 1986).

Genetic defects and infertility

Particular care must be taken to avoid the use of ^{131}I in pregnant women. The follow-up of patients treated with ^{131}I disclosed no apparent increase in the occurrence of infertility, miscarriages, birth defects, or malignancies (Winship and Rosvoll 1970; Sarkar *et al.* 1976; M. Schlumberger, F. de Vathaire, C. Ceccarelli *et al.*, submitted) in accordance with theoretical data. The only abnormality was a slight increase in the incidence of miscarriages in women who have been treated with radio-iodine during the year preceding conception (M. Schlumberger, F. De Vathaire, C. Ceccarelli et al., submitted). In fact, the dose to the ovaries is only 0.14 cGy per mCi administered. Therefore, there is no reason for disease-free patients to avoid pregnancy, but a 12 month interval is recommended after the last ^{131}I treatment and until a perfect control of the thyroid hormonal status has been achieved. Pregnancy does not appear to enhance tumour aggressiveness (Mazzaferri 1987).

Pulmonary fibrosis

In patients with diffuse long metastases, radiation fibrosis can be obviated when doses (<150 mCi) are administered at sufficiently large intervals (>3 months) (Schlumberger et al. 1986).

ANAPLASTIC CARCINOMA

Anaplastic or undifferentiated carcinomas are among the most aggressive human tumours. They frequently present as rapidly growing tumours with early infiltration into the surrounding tissue. They usually occur in elderly patients. Histologically, these tumours appear with highly malignant cells, often with frequent or atypical mitoses, amongst a dense fibrous stroma. The cells can appear spindle shaped or sometimes lie along strands of the fibrous stroma. Anaplastic carcinomas do not usually form papillary or follicular structures and do not contain amyloid. It is important to distinguish them from thyroid lymphoma. Undifferentiated carcinomas do not produce thyroglobulin and are not able to pick up radioactive iodine. TSH receptors are not found in their cell membranes. Their pathogenesis is unclear, although they frequently occur in patients with long-standing goitre. They make up approximately 10 per cent of all thyroid carcinomas. Clinically, they usually present as a rapidly enlarging thyroid gland which can cause stridor. On examination the thyroid gland is frequently 'woody' hard with tumour infiltrating locally. Biopsy is necessary as thyroid lymphoma can present similarly.

Prognosis is dismal as these tumours are highly malignant, invade locally and extensively, and metastasize rapidly, usually to the lungs. Rarely, they can present with symptoms and signs of metastatic disease. Survival is not effected by treatment with either radiotherapy or chemotherapy alone, and the tumour often grows even during treatment. Treatment is then usually palliative and directed to symptom control. Palliative external-beam radiotherapy combined with dexamethasone treatment can be used to relieve symptoms of tracheal compression, while chemotherapy can be used in an attempt to palliate metastatic disease. Doxorubicin is believed to be the most useful single agent, although clinical data are sparse. In most patients, death is caused by local tumour invasion. Median survival is estimated to be 2–6 months and only in exceptional cases does survival exceed 12 months (Tubiana et al. 1985b).

Combined therapy using external radiotherapy and doxorubicin (Shimaoka et al. 1985; Kim and Leeper 1987) or other drugs (Tallroth et al. 1987; Schlumberger et al. 1991b) has also been reported to be effective, mostly in patients who had undergone gross tumour resection and who had no distant metastases at the initiation of therapy. Five year survivals of 20–25 per cent have been claimed, but such early cases are rare.

MEDULLARY CARCINOMAS

Medullary carcinomas arise from the parafollicular cells and consist of solid masses of pleomorphic cells. Histological staining demonstrates the presence of amyloid. Up to 20 per cent of cases have a familial predisposition and may arise in patients with multiple endocrine neoplasia syndrome. Serum calcitonin can be raised and used as a marker of disease. They do not take up ^{131}I and management is therefore surgical with external-beam radiotherapy required for residual disease.

THYROID LYMPHOMA

Lymphoma of the thyroid gland accounts for approximately 5 per cent of all thyroid malignancy and usually presents as a fairly rapidly enlarging solitary nodule in elderly females. There is an association with pre-existing Hashimoto's thyroiditis and indeed this can make an accurate histological diagnosis important. Symptoms depend on speed of growth and position and include pain, tenderness, dysphasia, dysphagia, or hoarseness. Cervical lymphadenopathy may also be present. Histological diagnosis with biopsy is necessary to exclude an anaplastic carcinoma. Thyroid lymphomas are usually of high-grade non-Hodgkin's lymphomas, although low-grade non-Hodgkin's lymphoma and Hodgkin's disease do occur. Staging and management are the same as for nodal lymphoma. Staging investigations include CT scans of the neck, chest, and abdomen and bone-marrow aspiration and trephine. There is also an increased incidence of gastrointestinal lymphoma and investigation of the gastrointestinal tract may be indicated. Management of localized disease has involved local or regional irradiation with or without surgery. Local control is important if bulky disease is resected, but this is not always possible owing to local infiltration. Disseminated disease is treated with combination chemotherapy. Overall survival is similar, stage for stage, as nodal lymphoma.

REFERENCES

Aasland R, et al. (1988). Expression of oncogenes in thyroid tumors: coexpression of c-erb B2/neu and c-erb B. British Journal of Cancer, 57:358–63.

Antonini P, et al. (1989). Translocation t(7; 10) (q 35; q 21) in a differentiated papillary carcinoma of the thyroid. Cancer, Genetics and Cytogenetics, 41:139–44.

Ashcraft MW, van Herle AJ (1981). The comparative value of serum thyroglobulin measurements and iodine 131 total body scans in the follow-up study of patients with treated differentiated thyroid cancer. American Journal of Medicine, 71:806–14.

Attie JN (1988). Modified neck dissection in treatment of thyroid cancer: a safe procedure. European Journal of Cancer, 24:315–24.

Bäckdahl M, et al. (1985). Comparison of nuclear DNA content in primary and metastatic papillary thyroid carcinoma. Cancer Research, 45:2890–4.

Bacourt F, et al. (1986). Multifactorial study of prognostic factors in differentiated thyroid carcinoma and a re-evaluation of the importance of age. British Journal of Surgery, 73:274–7.

Baverstock K, et al. (1992). Thyroid cancer after Chernobyl. Nature, 359:21–2.

Beierwaltes WH (1987). Carcinoma of the thyroid. Radionuclide diagnosis, therapy and follow-up. Clinics in Oncology, 5:23–37.

Boecker W, et al. (1980). Immunohistochemical analysis of thyroglobulin synthesis in thyroid carcinomas. Virchows Archiv A, 385:187–200.

Bongarzone I, et al. (1989). High frequency of activation of tyrosine kinase oncogenes in human papillary thyroid carcinomas. Oncogene, 4:1457–62.

Braverman LE, Pratt BM, Ebner S, Longcope C (1992). Recombinant human thyrotropin stimulates thyroid function and radioactive iodine uptake in the rhesus monkey. Journal of Clinical Endocrinology and Metabolism, 74:1135–9.

Byar DP, et al. (1979). A prognostic index for thyroid carcinoma. A study of the EORTC thyroid cancer cooperative group. European Journal of Cancer, 15:1033–41.

Cady B, Rossi R (1988). An expanded view of risk-group definition in differentiated thyroid carcinoma. Surgery, 104:947–53.

Casara D, et al. (1993). Different features of pulmonary metastases in differentiated thyroid cancer: natural history and multivariate statistical analysis of prognostic variables. Journal of Nuclear Medicine, 34:1626–31.

Clark OH (1981). TSH suppression in the management of thyroid nodules and thyroid cancer. *World Journal of Surgery*, 5:39–47.

Clark OH (1982). Total thyroidectomy, the treatment of choice for patients with differentiated thyroid cancer. *Annals of Surgery*, 196:361–70.

de Groot LJ, Reilly M (1984). Use of isotope bone scans and skeletal survey X-rays in the follow-up of patients with thyroid carcinoma. *Journal of Endocrinological Investigation*, 7:175–7.

de Vathaire F, Blanchon S, Schlumberger M (1988). Thyroglobulin level helps to predict recurrence after lobo-isthmusectomy in patients with differentiated thyroid carcinoma. *Lancet*, i:52–3.

Di Renzo MF, *et al.* (1992). Overexpression of the c-*met*/HGF receptor in human thyroid carcinomas. *Oncogene*, 7:2549–53.

Donghi R, *et al.* (1989). The oncogene associated with human papillary thyroid carcinoma (PTC) is assigned to chromosome 10 q11-12 in the same region as multiple endocrino-neoplasia type 2A (MEN 2A). *Oncogene*, 4:521–3.

Edmonds CJ, Smith T (1986). The long term hazards of the treatment of thyroid cancer with radioiodine. *British Journal of Radiology*, 59:45–51.

Elias D, *et al.* (1983). Repérage des parathyroïdes par le bleu de méthylène au cours de la chirurgie thyroïdienne. *Presse Medicale*, 12:1229–31.

Feldt-Rasmussen U, Schlumberger M (1988). European interlaboratory comparison of serum thyroglobulin measurement. *Journal of Endocrinological Investigation*, 11:175–81.

Filetti S, *et al.* (1988). The role of thyroid-stimulating antibodies of Graves' disease in differentiated thyroid cancer. *New England Journal of Medicine*, 318:753–9.

Fourquet A, Asselain B, Joly J (1983). Cancer de la thyroïde. Analyse multidimensionnelle des facteurs pronostiques. *Annales d'Endocrinologie (Paris)*, 44:121–6.

Fragu P, Nataf BM (1977). Thyroid peroxidase activity in benign and malignant thyroid disorders. *Journal of Clinical Endocrinology and Metabolism*, 45:1089–96.

Fragu P, Larras-Regard E (1986). The ionic microscope enables the visualization of stable iodine within follicles of human thyroid gland. In *Frontiers in thyroidology* (ed. G Medeiros-Neto and E Gaitan), pp. 465–9. Plenum, New York.

Fusco A, *et al.* (1987). A new oncogene in human thyroid papillary carcinomas and their lymph-nodal metastases. *Nature, London*, 328:170–2.

Girelli ME, *et al.* (1986). Critical evaluation of serum thyroglobulin (Tg) levels during thyroid hormone suppression therapy versus Tg levels after hormone withdrawal and total body scan: results in 291 patients with thyroid cancer. *European Journal of Nuclear Medicine*, 11:333–5.

Goldman JM, Line BR, Aamodt RL, Robbins J. (1980). Influence of triiodothyronin withdrawal time on ^{131}I uptake post-thyroidectomy for thyroid cancer. *Journal of Clinical Endocrinology and Metabolism*, 50:734–9.

Grant CS, *et al.* (1988). Local recurrence in papillary thyroid carcinoma: is extent of surgical resection important. *Surgery*, 104:954–62.

Hall P, *et al.* (1991). Cancer risk in thyroid cancer patients. *British Journal of Cancer*, 64:159–63.

Hall P, *et al.* (1992). Leukaemia incidence after iodine 131 exposure. *Lancet*, 340:1–4.

Hamming JF, *et al.* (1988). Prognostic value of nuclear DNA content in papillary and follicular thyroid cancer. *World Journal of Surgery*, 12:503–8.

Hannequin P, Liehn JC, Delisle MJ (1986). Multifactorial analysis of survival in thyroid cancer: pitfalls of applying the results of published studies to another population. *Cancer*, 58:1749–55.

Hay ID, Grant CS, Taylor WF, McConahey WM (1987). Ipsilateral lobectomy versus bilateral lobar resection in papillary thyroid carcinoma: a retrospective analysis of surgical outcome using a novel prognostic scoring system. *Surgery*, 103:1088–95.

Hedinger C, Williams ED, Sobin LH (1989). The WHO histological classification of thyroid tumors: a commentary on the Second Edition. *Cancer*, 63:908–11.

Hoefnagel CA, Delprat CC, Marcuse HR, de Vijlder JJM (1986). Role of thallium-201 total body scintigraphy in follow-up of thyroid carcinoma. *Journal of Nuclear Medicine*, 27:1854–7.

Hoie J, Stenwig AE, Kullmann G, Lindegaard M (1988). Distant metastases in papillary thyroid cancer. A review of 91 patients. *Cancer*, 61:1–6.

Holm LE, *et al.* (1989). Cancer risk in a population examined with diagnostic doses of ^{131}I. *Journal of the National Cancer Institute*, 81:302–6.

Holm LE, *et al.* (1991). Cancer risk after iodine 131 therapy for hyperthyroidism. *Journal of the National Cancer Institute*, 83:1072–7.

Ito T, *et al.* (1992). Unique association of p53 mutations with undifferentiated but not differentiated carcinomas of the thyroid gland. *Cancer Research*, 52:1369–72.

Kazakov VS, Demidchik EP, Astakhova LN (1992). Thyroid cancer after Chernobyl. *Nature*, 359:21.

Kerr DJ, *et al.* (1986). Prognostic factors in thyroid tumours. *British Journal of Cancer*, 54:475–82.

Kim JH, Leeper RD (1987). Treatment of locally advanced thyroid carcinoma with combination doxorubicin and radiation therapy. *Cancer*, 60:2372–5.

Krenning EP, Ausema L, Bruining HA, Hennemann G (1988). Clinical and radio-diagnostic aspects in the evaluation of thyroid nodules with respect to thyroid cancer. *European Journal of Cancer*, 24:299–304.

Kuni CC, Klingensmith WC (1980). Failure of low doses of ^{131}I to ablate residual thyroid tissue following surgery for thyroid cancer. *Radiology*, 137:773–4.

Lacour J, *et al.* (1977). Surgical treatment of differentiated thyroid cancer at the Institut Gustave-Roussy. *Annales de Radiologie (Paris)*, 20:767–70.

Lang W, Choritz H, Hundeshagen H (1986). Risk factors in follicular thyroid carcinomas: a retrospective follow-up study covering a 14-year period with emphasis on morphological findings. *American Journal of Surgical Pathology*, 10:246–65.

Leeper RD (1973). The effect of ^{131}I therapy on survival of patients with metastatic papillary or follicular thyroid carcinoma. *Journal of Clinical Endocrinology and Metabolism*, 36:1143–52.

Lemoine NR, *et al.* (1989). High frequency of *ras* oncogene activation in all stages of human thyroid tumorigenesis. *Oncogene*, 4:159–64.

McConahey WM, *et al.* (1986). Papillary thyroid cancer treated at the Mayo Clinic, 1946 through 1970: initial manifestations, pathologic findings, therapy and outcome. *Mayo Clinic Proceedings*, 61:978–96.

Maheshwari YK, *et al.* (1981). ^{131}I therapy in differentiated thyroid carcinoma: MD Anderson Hospital experience. *Cancer*, 47:664–71.

Massin JP, *et al.* (1984). Pulmonary metastases in differentiated thyroid carcinoma. Study of 58 cases with implications for the primary tumor treatment. *Cancer*, 53:982–92.

Maxon HR, *et al.* (1983). Relation between effective radiation dose and outcome of radioiodine therapy for thyroid cancer. *New England Journal of Medicine*, 309:937–41.

Mazzaferri EL (1987). Papillary thyroid carcinoma: factors influencing prognosis and current therapy. *Seminars in Oncology*, 14:315–32.

Molitch ME, *et al.* (1984). The cold thyroid nodule: an analysis of diagnostic and therapeutic options. *Endocrine Reviews*, 5:185–99.

Nemec JV, Zamrazil V, Pohunkova D, Rohling S (1979). Radioiodine treatment of pulmonary metastases of differentiated thyroid cancer: results and prognostic factors. *Nuklearmedizin*, 18:86–90.

Noguchi S, Murakami N (1987). The value of lymph-node dissection in patients with differentiated thyroid cancer. *Surgical Clinics of North America*, 67:251–61.

Pacini F, *et al.* (1985). Diagnostic value of a single serum thyroglobulin determination on and off thyroid suppressive therapy in the follow-up of patients with differentiated thyroid cancer. *Clinical Endocrinology*, 23:405–11.

Pacini F, *et al.* (1987). Therapeutic doses of iodine-131 reveal undiagnosed metastases in thyroid cancer patients with detectable serum thyroglobulin levels. *Journal of Nuclear Medicine*, 28:1888–91.

Piekarski JD, *et al.* (1985). Chest computed tomography (CT) in patients with micronodular lung metastases of differentiated thyroid carcinoma. *International Journal of Radiation Oncology—Biology—Physics*, 11:1023–7.

Roger P, Taton M, van Sande J, Dumont JE (1988). Mitogenic effects of thyrotropin and adenosine 3¹,5¹-monophosphate in differentiated normal human thyroid cells *in vitro*. *Journal of Clinical Endocrinology and Metabolism*, 66:1158–65.

Rojeski MT, Gharib H (1985). Nodular thyroid disease: evaluation and management. *New England Journal of Medicine*, 313:428–36.

Roy Camille R, *et al.* (1980). Perspectives actuelles dans le traitement des métastases osseuses des cancers thyroïdiens. *Chirurgie (Paris)*, 106:32–6.

Ruegemer JJ, *et al.* (1988). Distant metastases in differentiated thyroid carcinoma: a multivariate analysis of prognostic variables. *Journal of Clinical Endocrinology and Metabolism*, 67:501–8.

Russell WO, Ibanez ML, Clark RL, White EC (1963). Thyroid carcinoma: classification, intraglandular dissemination and clinicopathologic study based upon whole organ sections of 80 glands. *Cancer*, **16**:1425–60.

Sakamoto A, Kasai N, Sugano H (1983). Poorly differentiated carcinoma of the thyroid, a clinicopathologic entity for a high risk group of papillary and follicular carcinomas. *Cancer*, **52**:1846–55.

Samaan NA, Schultz PN, Haynie TP, Ordonez NG (1985). Pulmonary metastasis of differentiated thyroid carcinoma: treatment results in 101 patients. *Journal of Clinical Endocrinology and Metabolism*, **60**:376–80.

Sampson RJ (1977). Prevalence and significance of occult thyroid cancer. In *Radiation associated thyroid carcinoma* (ed. LJ de Groot *et al.*), pp. 137–53. Grune and Stratton, New York.

Sarkar SD, Beierwaltes WH, Gill SP, Cowley BJ (1976). Subsequent fertility and birth histories of children and adolescents treated with ^{131}I for thyroid cancer. *Journal of Nuclear Medicine*, **17**:460–4.

Schaller RT, Stevenson JK (1966). Development of carcinoma of the thyroid in iodine-deficient mice. *Cancer*, **19**:1063–7.

Schelfhout LJDM, *et al.* (1988). Multivariate analysis of survival in differentiated thyroid cancer: the prognostic significance of the age factor. *European Journal of Cancer*, **24**:331–7.

Schlumberger M, *et al.* (1980). Circulating thyroglobulin and thyroid hormones in patients with metastases of differentiated thyroid carcinoma: relationship to serum thyrotropin levels. *Journal of Clinical Endocrinology and Metabolism*, **51**:513–9.

Schlumberger M, Fragu P, Parmentier C, Tubiana M (1981). Thyroglobulin assay in the follow-up of patients with differentiated thyroid carcinomas: comparison of its value in patients with or without normal residual tissue. *Acta Endocrinologica*, **98**:215–21.

Schlumberger M, *et al.* (1983). Relationship between thyrotropin stimulation and radioiodine uptake in lung metastases of differentiated thyroid carcinoma. *Journal of Clinical Endocrinology and Metabolism*, **57**:148–51.

Schlumberger M, *et al.* (1986). Long-term results of treatment of 283 patients with lung and bone metastases from differentiated thyroid carcinoma. *Journal of Clinical Endocrinology and Metabolism*, **63**:960–7.

Schlumberger M, *et al.* (1987a). Surveillance post-opératoire des épithéliomas thyroïdiens différenciés. Apport du dosage ultra sensible de la TSH. *Presse Medicale*, **16**:1791–3.

Schlumberger M, *et al.* (1987b). Differentiated thyroid carcinoma in childhood: long-term follow-up of 72 patients. *Journal of Clinical Endocrinology and Metabolism*, **65**:1088–94.

Schlumberger M, *et al.* (1988a). Detection and treatment of lung metastases of differentiated thyroid carcinoma in patients with normal chest X-ray. *Journal of Nuclear Medicine*, **29**:1790–4.

Schlumberger M, *et al.* (1988b). Follow-up of patients with differentiated thyroid carcinoma. Experience at Institut Gustave-Roussy, Villejuif. *European Journal of Cancer*, **24**:345–50.

Schlumberger M, *et al.* (1991a). A new Irma system for Tg measurement in the follow-up of thyroid cancer patients. *European Journal of Nuclear Medicine*, **18**:153–7.

Schlumberger M, *et al.* (1991b). Combination therapy for anaplastic giant cell thyroid carcinoma. *Cancer*, **67**:564–6.

Schneider AB (1986). Radiation induced thyroid cancer. In *Werner's The thyroid* (ed. SH Ingbar and LE Braverman), pp. 801–6. JB Lippincott, Philadelphia.

Schneider AB, Line BR, Goldman JM, Robbins J (1981). Sequential serum thyroglobulin determinations ^{131}I scans and ^{131}I uptakes after triiodothyronine withdrawal in patients with thyroid cancer. *Journal of Clinical Endocrinology and Metabolism*, **53**:1199–206.

Shimaoka K, *et al.* (1985). A randomized trial of doxorubicin versus doxorubicin plus cisplatin in patients with advanced thyroid carcinoma. *Cancer*, **56**:2155–60.

Simpson WJ, *et al.* (1987). Papillary and follicular thyroid cancer. Prognostic factors in 1578 patients. *American Journal of Medicine*, **83**:479–88.

Simpson WJ, *et al.* (1988). Papillary and follicular thyroid cancer: impact of treatment in 1578 patients. *International Journal of Radiation Oncology—Biology—Physics*, **14**:1063–75.

Smith SA, *et al.* (1988). Mortality from papillary thyroid carcinoma. A case–control study of 56 lethal cases. *Cancer*, **62**:1381–8.

Stoffer SS, *et al.* (1986). Familial papillary carcinoma of the thyroid. *American Journal of Medical Genetics*, **25**:775–82.

Suarez HG, *et al.* (1988). Detection of activated *ras* oncogenes in human thyroid carcinoma. *Oncogene*, **2**:403–6.

Suarez HG, *et al.* (1990). Presence of mutations in all three ras genes in human thyroid tumors. *Oncogene*, **5**:565–70.

Suarez HG, *et al.* (1991). Gsp mutations in human thyroid tumors. *Oncogene*, **6**:677–9.

Tallroth E, *et al.* (1987). Multimodality treatment in anaplastic giant cell thyroid carcinoma. *Cancer*, **60**:1428–31.

Tenenbaum F, *et al.* (1993). Usefulness of technetium-99m hydroxy methylene disphosphonate scans in localizing bone metastases of differentiated thyroid carcinoma (DTC). *European Journal of Nuclear Medicine*, **20**:1168–74.

Tennvall J, *et al.* (1986). Is the EORTC prognostic index of thyroid cancer valid in differentiated thyroid carcinoma? Retrospective multivariate analysis of differentiated thyroid carcinoma with long follow-up. *Cancer*, **57**:1405–14.

Terrier P, *et al.* (1988). Structure and expression of c-*myc* and c-*fos* proto-oncogenes in thyroid carcinoma. *British Journal of Cancer*, **57**:43–7.

Thomas-Morvan C, Nataf B, Tubiana M (1974). Thyroid proteins and hormone synthesis in human thyroid cancer. *Acta Endocrinologica*, **76**:651–69.

Thompson NW, Nishiyama RH, Harness JK (1978). Thyroid carcinoma: current controversies. *Current Problems in Surgery*, **25**:1–17.

Thoresen SO, *et al.* (1989). Survival and prognostic factors in differentiated thyroid cancer. A multivariate analysis of 1055 cases. *British Journal of Cancer*, **59**:231–5.

Tibiana M, Mabille JP (1963). L'iode radioactif et le cancer de la thyroïde—problèmes diagnostiques. *Journal of Radiology and Electrology* (*Paris*), **44**:179–86.

Tubiana M, *et al.* (1975). External radiotherapy and radioiodine in the treatment of 359 thyroid cancers. *British Journal of Radiology*, **48**:894–907.

Tubiana M, *et al.* (1985a). Long-term results and prognostic factors in patients with differentiated thyroid carcinoma. *Cancer*, **55**:794–804.

Tubiana M, *et al.* (1985b). External radiotherapy in thyroid cancers. *Cancer*, **55**:2062–71.

Vagenakis AG, *et al.* (1975). Recovery of pituitary thyrotropic function after withdrawal of prolonged thyroid-suppression therapy. *New England Journal of Medicine*, **293**:681–4.

Valenta LJ (1974). Biochemical parameters of the function of thyroid carcinoma. *Journal of Cancer*, **2**:172–9.

van Herle AJ, Uller RP, Matthews NL, Brown J (1973). Radioimmunoassay for measurement of thyroglobulin in human serum. *Journal of Clinical Investigation*, **52**:1320–7.

van Herle AJ, Vassart G, Dumont JE (1979). Control of thyroglobulin synthesis and secretion. *New England Journal of Medicine*, **301**:239–49, 307–14.

van Herle AJ, *et al.* (1982). The thyroid nodule. *Annals of Internal Medicine*, **96**:221–32.

van Herle AJ, van Herle IS, Greipel MA (1985). An international cooperative study evaluating serum thyroglobulin standards. *Journal of Clinical Endocrinology and Metabolism*, **60**:338–43.

Waterhouse J, Muir C, Shanmugaratnam K, Powell J (1982). Cancer incidence in five continents, Vol. 4. *IARC Scientific Publication*, **42**:760–1.

Williams DW, Williams ED, Wynford-Thomas D (1989). Evidence for autocrine production of IGF-1 in human thyroid adenomas. *Molecular and Cellular Endocrinology*, **61**:139–43.

Williams ED, Doniach I, Bjarnason PO, Mickie W (1977). Thyroid cancer in an iodide rich area. *Cancer*, **39**:215–22.

Williams SD, Birch R, Einhorn LH (1986). Phase II evaluation of doxorubicin plus cisplatin in advanced thyroid cancer: a Southeastern Cancer Study Group trial. *Cancer Treatment Reports*, **70**:405–7.

Winship T, Rosvoll RV (1970). Thyroid carcinoma in childhood: final report on a 20-year study. *Children's Hospital*, **26**:327–48.

Yamashita S, Ong J, Fagin JA, Melmed S (1986). Expression of the *myc* cellular proto-oncogene in human thyroid tissue. *Journal of Clinical Endocrinology and Metabolism*, **63**:1170–3.

Young JL, Percy CL, Asire AJ (1981). Surveillance, epidemiology, and end results: incidence and mortality data, 1973–77. *National Cancer Institute Monograph*, **57**, pp. 10–11. Bethesda MD: National Cancer Institute.

Young RL, Mazzaferri EL, Rahe AJ, Dorfman SG (1980). Pure follicular thyroid carcinoma: impact of therapy in 214 patients. *Journal of Nuclear Medicine*, **21**:733–7.

Zimmerman D, *et al.* (1988). Papillary thyroid carcinoma in children and adults: long-term follow-up of 1039 patients conservatively treated at one institution during three decades. *Surgery*, **104**:1157–66.

16.2   Medullary carcinoma of the thyroid

BRUCE A. J. PONDER

INTRODUCTION

Medullary carcinoma of the thyroid is an uncommon cancer which arises from the 'C'-cells, which produce calcitonin. Approximately 75 per cent of cases are probably non-hereditary, but the remaining 25 per cent occur as part of the dominantly inherited cancer syndrome multiple endocrine neoplasia, type 2 (MEN 2). In both hereditary and non-hereditary forms, surgery of the localized disease is the only curative treatment, although useful palliation may be gained with radiotherapy and, rarely, with chemotherapy. The best prospects for improved quality and duration of survival probably rest with more thorough attempts to evaluate and surgically remove local disease in the neck and mediastinum and with better recognition and screening of family members at risk from the heritable disease.

EPIDEMIOLOGY

The incidence of medullary carcinoma of the thyroid is approximately 1 per 1 000 000 population per year, (approximately 60–80 cases in the United Kingdom). Approximately 10 per cent of these will give a family history clearly suggestive of MEN 2; a further 10–15 per cent will be found to have evidence of familial involvement after further detailed investigation (Sizemore *et al.* 1977; Chong *et al.* 1985; Ponder *et al.* 1988*b*). A further unknown, but small, proportion of apparently isolated cases arises at new mutations. Overall, therefore, approximately 25 per cent of cases are of the heritable type.

It is important to bear in mind when reading the literature that the hereditary and non-hereditary forms are often not clearly distinguished. A young patient with no family history will probably be classified as non-hereditary, but could still have hereditary disease either because they have inherited the gene from a parent who did not develop clinically evident disease or because they are a new mutation to MEN 2. The description 'sporadic medullary carcinoma of the thyroid' should therefore be used with care: it is a practical usage which means 'having no evident family history, an isolated case'. It does not mean that the case is necessarily non-hereditary.

Non-hereditary medullary carcinoma of the thyroid

This presents at an older age than the hereditary disease, the peak incidence in several series occurs in patients in their fifties (Chong *et al.* 1975; Ponder *et al.* 1988*b*). The older an isolated case at presentation, the less likely it is to be MEN 2: but age is not an

Table 1   Clinical varieties of MEN 2

	MTC	Phaeochromocytoma	Parathyroid hyperplasia or adenoma	Other features
MEN 2A	+	+	+	Commonest form; no associated physical anomalies
MEN 2B	+	+	–	Less common; younger onset; associated developmental anomalies especially mucosal neuromas
MTC-only	+	–	–	Extensive families with MTC as only feature; late onset, indolent course

Abbreviations: 2A, type 2A; 2B, type 2B; MEN, multiple endocrine neoplasia; MTC, medullary carcinoma of the thyroid.

absolute criterion. The male : female ratio is approximately equal (Saad *et al.* 1984). Specific aetiological factors have not been identified.

Medullary carcinoma of the thyroid in the MEN 2 syndromes

MEN 2 shows an autosomal dominant pattern of inheritance and, like the other inherited cancer syndromes, it involves a specific and limited set of tissues. Three varieties of MEN 2 are distinguished on clinical grounds (Table 1). Current evidence suggests that at least two of these are due to mutation at the same or closely adjacent loci on chromosome 10.

MEN 2A

This is the most common form of MEN 2. Figure 1 gives the age–incidence curves for presentation with clinical disease and for detection by biochemical screening (Ponder *et al.* 1988*a*; Easton *et al.* 1989). Note that an estimated one-third of individuals who inherit the MEN 2A gene have not developed disease to an extent that leads them to seek medical help by the age of 70 years. This has implications for the recognition and management of families. It also raises the question of why this variability in expression of the mutant gene occurs. There is variation in age at onset within a single family, as well as between families (Easton *et al.* 1989).

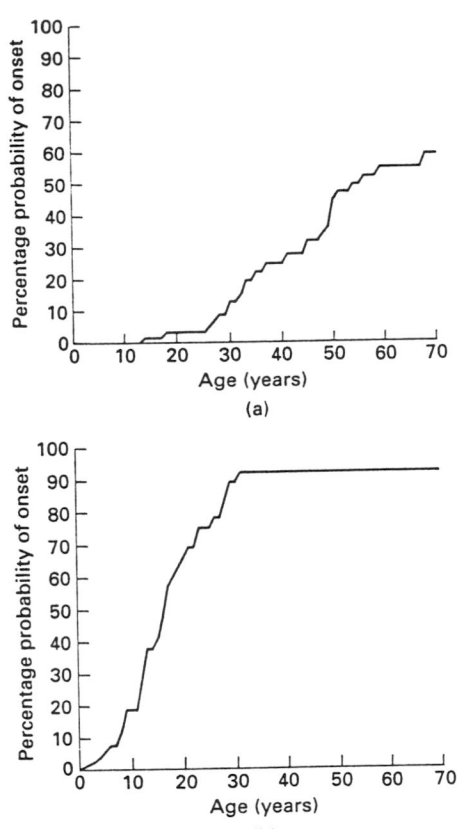

Fig. 1 Age-related probability of detection of disease in MEN 2A. Probability that an individual with the MEN 2A gene will (a) have presented to medical attention and (b) be detectable by a pentagastrin stimulation test (see text) by a given age. (Reproduced from Easton *et al.* (1989), by kind permission of University of Chicago Press.)

The variation cannot, therefore, be explained entirely by differences in the mutant forms of the MEN 2 gene in different families. Other modifying factors must be involved; but how much is due to interacting genes, to environment, or to chance is unknown. Neither the sex of the affected individual, nor the sex of the parent who transmitted the gene, have any evident effect. Prediction of the age at onset or severity of the disease in a given individual is currently not possible.

MEN 2 has been described in Caucasians, Negroes, Indians, and Asiatics. The incidence and behaviour of both hereditary and non-hereditary MTC is similar in Japanese and European populations.

MEN 2B

This accounts for approximately 5 per cent of MEN 2. Points of difference from MEN 2A (Gorlin *et al.* 1968; Carney *et al.* 1979; Dyck *et al.* 1979) include:

(1) associated developmental abnormalities in other tissues (Table 2);

(2) rare or absent parathyroid involvement (Carney *et al.* 1980);

(3) younger age at onset of tumours;

(4) possibly a more aggressive natural history of the thyroid tumours, though this is controversial (Norton *et al.* 1979; Kullberg and Nieuwenhuijzen-Kruseman 1987; Samaan *et al.* 1988);

Table 2 Features of MEN 2B and their recognition

Pathology	Recognition
Musculoskeletal abnormalities	
Marfanoid body build (no lens or palate, or cardiac abnormality)	Clinical features
Pes cavus	
Pectus excavatum	
Slipped femoral epiphysis	
Hypotonia, proximal muscle weakness (Dyck *et al.* 1979)	EMG consistent with chronic neurogenic atrophy
Neuromas of lips, anterolateral surface of tongue, conjunctiva	Typical facies; biopsy of nodule
Medullated corneal nerve fibres (Khalil and Lorenzetti 1980)	Slit-lamp examination
Ganglioneuromatosis of intestine (Carney *et al.* 1976) and other viscera	Constipation and diarrhoea; failure to thrive in childhood; barium studies, rectal biopsy

(5) low reproductive success due probably to a combination of impaired survival, low marriage rate, impotence due to neurological problems, and infertility, with the result that the majority of cases are apparently isolated new mutations to the hereditary disease.

MTC has been diagnosed at the age of 15 months in MEN 2B, but in other cases with undoubted MEN 2B phenotype, the thyroid tumour does not present until the third decade. In a review of the literature, Carney *et al.* (1979) found a mean age of presentation of MTC of 19 years, at which time 76 per cent of patients had involved lymph nodes.

MTC-only

A small number of very extensive pedigrees have been described in which medullary carcinoma of the thyroid (MTC) alone is inherited as an autosomal dominant trait with incomplete penetrance; there is no associated adrenal or parathyroid involvement. The medullary carcinoma of the thyroid presents, on average, later than in MEN 2A and is rarely, if ever, the cause of death (Farndon *et al.* 1986). The consistent pattern in such large families supports the separation of 'MTC-only' as a distinct clinical entity; genetic mapping has so far failed to show whether it is genetically distinct. In small families medullary carcinoma of the thyroid is often seen without evidence of adrenal tumour; other families are seen in which there are several individuals with medullary carcinoma of the thyroid but only one with phaeochromocytoma. This suggests that there may be a continuum of MEN 2A families with differing degrees of adrenal involvement and there is no clear dividing line for allocation of families between the categories MEN 2A or 'MTC-only'. Other than in the rare large 'MTC-only' families with no evidence at all of phaeochromocytoma, there is no clear evidence that medullary carcinoma of the thyroid has later onset or is less aggressive in families with few adrenal tumours (Easton *et al.* 1989). This problem may be resolved when the predisposing mutation in each family can be described at the DNA level.

PATHOLOGY
Gross

Medullary carcinoma of the thyroid is typically a circumscribed rounded tumour which occurs within the middle or upper third of the thyroid lobe, where the concentration of C-cells is greatest. Calcification of the primary tumour or of metastases is not uncommon. Multiple or bilateral foci of tumour are typical of MEN 2, where the inherited predisposition may result in several independent primaries.

Histology

A variety of cellular and morphological patterns are seen (Cance and Wells 1985). Tumours are typically composed of nests or trabeculae of cells, separated by septae of connective tissue, and often containing amyloid deposits. Distinct follicular structures may be seen within sheets of tumour cells. The cells may have a polygonal, spindle-shaped, or round cell morphology.

Because of the variable morphology, diagnosis should be confirmed with special stains. Amyloid positivity is strongly suggestive of medullary carcinoma of the thyroid, but cases of medullary carcinoma of the thyroid have been reported in which amyloid was lacking (Saad et al. 1984) and occasional non-MTC thyroid tumours are amyloid positive (Valenta et al. 1977). Calcitonin immunostaining is the best diagnostic criterion. However, less well differentiated tumours, especially metastases, may show weak or absent calcitonin staining. Heterogeneity of staining for calcitonin in the primary tumour or in metastases is reported to be associated with poor prognosis (Lippman et al. 1982).

Sikri et al. (1985) found 100 per cent of 25 medullary carcinomas of the thyroid to be positive for the Grimelius silver stain, for calcitonin gene-related peptide (an alternative RNA splice product of the calcitonin gene), and for the neuroendocrine marker chromogranin. A variable proportion of medullary carcinomas of the thyroid show at least some cells positive for somatostatin, gastrin-releasing peptide, adrenocorticotrophic hormone, bombesin, neurone-specific enolase, and other markers characteristic of APUD cells.

Carcinoembryonic antigen has been reported in C-cell hyperplasia and in medullary carcinoma of the thyroid (DeLellis et al. 1978) and, controversially, in normal C-cells (Lloyd et al. 1983). Serum calcitonin : carcinoembryonic antigen ratios may be related to the state of differentiation of the tumour cells (Mendelsohn et al. 1984) and have prognostic significance.

'Mixed' follicular and C-cell tumours have been reported. The evidence that they contain elements of thyroid follicular differentiation is based on morphology but also on thyroglobulin staining, while the C-cell component is identified by calcitonin staining. The suggestion that these 'mixed' tumours originate by 'entrapment' of normal follicular elements within a C-cell tumour is ruled out by the finding of 'mixed' metastases in cervical glands. The origin of these tumours remains in doubt. While some may represent anomalous differentiation in a subclone within a tumour of primary follicular or C-cell origin, it is probable that many arise from a cell of branchial pouch origin which has the capacity for follicular cell or parafollicular (C-cell) differentiation (Ljungberg and Nilsson 1983; Ljungberg et al. 1984).

Metastases

Medullary carcinoma of the thyroid disseminates by direct and lymphatic spread within the neck and upper mediastinum and by haematogenous spread to distant sites. The sites most commonly involved are liver, bone, and lung. It is important to note, in relation to screening, that metastasis is common once the primary tumour is above 1 cm in diameter.

BIOLOGY
Embryology of C-cells

The neural ectodermal origin of C-cells has been demonstrated by following the fate of neural crest grafts in chick—quail chimeras (in which the chick and quail cells are readily distinguished) (Le Douarin and Le Lièvre 1970) and by following the fate of neural crest cells labelled in vivo in mouse embryos (Pearse and Polak 1971). The C-cells migrate to the fourth pharyngeal pouch (in birds, the ultimobranchial body) and, thence, to the developing thyroid gland. Although some authors report calcitonin-staining cells in adjacent regions of the neck and mediastinum (for example, the thymus) proven primary C-cell tumours in these sites have not been described.

The other tissues which are involved in MEN 2 are also of neural ectodermal origin, with the exception of the parathyroid glands. The cause of the parathyroid involvement is yet to be explained. The lack of parathyroid abnormality in MEN 2B suggests that involvement of these glands in MEN 2 must have a genetic basis, rather than being a secondary result of the elevated calcitonin levels due to medullary carcinoma of the thyroid.

Genetics of MEN 2
The germ-line mutation

The predisposing gene for MEN 2A has been mapped by genetic linkage to the region near the centromere of chromosome 10 (Mathew et al. 1987; Simpson et al. 1987). At the time of writing, the gene itself has not been identified and the nature of the predisposing mutation is still unknown. In contrast to the situation in several others of the inherited cancer syndromes, no individual with MEN 2 has yet been found to have an inherited chromosomal deletion or translocation in the relevant chromosomal region. Reports of an abnormality of chromosome 20 in several MEN 2A families and individuals with MEN 2B remain unexplained (Babu et al. 1984). Linkage in the same families has excluded the predisposing gene from this region. Several genetic markers have been identified close to the MEN 2 locus on chromosome 10, which can already be used for genetic diagnosis and the management of families (Nakamura et al. 1989) (see below).

The evidence is strong that the gene for MEN 2B also maps to the same region of chromosome 10. It is likely, but not proven, that MEN 2B is due to a different mutation at the same locus as the mutation for MEN 2A. There are anecdotes of families in which a parent with MEN 2A has a child with the MEN 2B phenotype, which might suggest a 'progression' of the mutation, but the evidence for MEN 2B phenotype in these cases is usually based on facial appearance, which may not be reliable.

The evidence that the gene responsible for 'MTC-only' families also maps to chromosome 10 is still inconclusive.

Genetic events in tumour progression

The germ-line mutation on chromosome 10 is not, of course, sufficient alone for tumour formation. It is present in every cell, but only some cells progress to tumour. Several other events are needed, many of them involving mutation. Events which have been identified so far include losses of genes on chromosomes 1p, 13q, and 22, but interestingly not on chromosome 10 (Ponder et al. 1989) and mutation or increased expression of various oncogenes, of which the most consistently reported are Ha-ras and n-Myc. The same spectrum of changes is seen in both hereditary and non-hereditary medullary carcinoma of the thyroid and in phaeochromocytomas, which indicates that the biology of tumour development is similar in each case.

Relationship of genetic events to progression and prognosis

The timing of the genetic events in relation to the stages of tumour progression defined by pathology is not yet known. It has been suggested that n-*Myc* expression distinguishes hyperplastic from normal C-cells (Boultwood *et al.* 1988), but it is not known whether C-cell hyperplasia is a direct expression of the germ-line mutation or whether a further somatic mutation is needed for hyperplasia to develop, which would imply that each hyperplastic focus is clonal. The invasive and metastatic behaviour of medullary carcinoma of the thyroid contrasts with the generally benign behaviour of phaeochromocytoma, although the generic events so far identified in tumour progression are common to both.

Genetic instability in MEN 2

Several reports (including Wurster-Hill *et al.* 1986) have suggested that the normal fibroblasts or lymphocytes of carriers of the MEN 2 gene show evidence of genetic instability. Similar observations have been made in many other familial cancers. The effects are mostly slight and rather variable between laboratories. Their relevance to the biology of MEN 2 is still unclear. None is sufficiently discriminatory between gene carriers and normal subjects to be of clinical use.

Production of ectopic substances by tumours

Besides calcitonin, medullary carcinoma of the thyroid may synthesize a number of hormonal and non-hormonal substances. These include:

(1) polypeptide hormones: adrenocorticotrophic hormone, β-endorphin, somatostatin, vasoactive intestinal polypeptide;

(2) bioactive amines and enzymes: dopamine, dopadecarboxylase, histaminase, serotonin;

(3) miscellaneous: carcinoembryonic antigen, melanin, nerve growth factor, prostaglandins.

Their role in the clinical syndromes associated with medullary carcinoma of the thyroid is discussed below. None has proved to be a better tumour marker than calcitonin.

Culture of C-cells

C-cells may be grown in short-term culture, but no established lines of normal or hyperplastic C-cell origin have been reported. Several cell lines derived from human or rodent medullary carcinoma of the thyroid are available. Although aneuploid, these retain differentiated characteristics, in particular calcitonin secretion.

Animal models of medullary carcinoma of the thyroid

C-cell tumours occur with high frequency in several strains of rat, notably the WAG/Rij strain (Boorman and Hollander 1976). They are associated with a high incidence of other endocrine tumours and the incidence of tumours tends to be low in F$_1$ crosses between high- and low-incidence strains, contrary to what would

be expected if a single dominant gene were involved, so their relevance as models for the genetics of the human disease is unclear.

C-cell tumours have been induced in rats by combinations of radiation and vitamin D (Thurston and Williams 1982).

A syndrome apparently similar to MEN 2 occurs in some strains of cattle. Phaeochromocytoma and medullary carcinoma of the thyroid are seen. Of interest, medullary carcinoma of the thyroid develops only in bulls, suggesting that differences in calcium metabolism associated with lactation may protect the cows (Wilkie and Krook 1970; Ljungberg and Nilsson 1985).

C-cell hyperplasia

C-cell hyperplasia is characteristic of the hereditary forms of MEN 2 (Block *et al.* 1980). The recognition of C-cell hyperplasia in a thyroid resected from an apparently isolated case of medullary carcinoma of the thyroid is therefore of great importance because it implies familial disease and therefore the need to consider family screening (Wolfe and DeLellis 1981).

The recognition of C-cell hyperplasia is not, however, always straightforward. There appears to be a grey area between the extremes of physiological variation in C-cells and hyperplasia indicative of MEN 2. C-cells normally lie between the epithelium of the thyroid follicles and the basement membrane. The criteria of abnormality are

(1) increased numbers of C-cells;

(2) the arrangement of the C-cells in clusters or nodules;

(3) the position of the C-cells in relation to the follicle;

(4) cytological atypia.

A total of more than ten C-cells per low-power microscope field was originally proposed as a criterion for hyperplasia, but studies of autopsy thyroids from individuals without thyroid disease (Gibson *et al.* 1982; O'Toole *et al.* 1985) show that there is a great range in C-cell numbers in the normal population, with higher numbers in the elderly. A cut-off based only on numbers is unlikely to be diagnostic. Discrete nodules of C-cells, especially if they displace or are associated with degeneration of the follicular epithelium, are strongly suggestive of pathological hyperplasia, as is cytological atypia (Wolfe and DeLellis 1981; Gibson *et al.* 1982). Breach of the follicular basement membrane may be taken as the criterion of carcinoma, but in practice the distinction between C-cell hyperplasia and early carcinoma is hard to make and of little significance.

Because of the possible overlap with the normal appearance, C-cell hyperplasia on its own is rarely a completely reliable indicator of heritable disease in an otherwise isolated case; conversely, because of the uneven distribution of C-cells through the thyroid and the possibility of sampling errors, the absence of C-cell hyperplasia cannot completely exclude heritable disease.

CLINICAL FEATURES AND DIAGNOSIS

Medullary carcinoma of the thyroid may present clinically with

(1) local or metastatic tumour masses;

(2) the effects of biologically active substances secreted from the tumour;

(3) presentation of other components of the MEN 2 syndrome.

A few cases are incidental findings at thyroidectomy for other disease and an increasing proportion of familial cases are diagnosed by screening. By far the commonest presentation is a painless lump in the neck; the next most common is probably diarrhoea, due to an unidentified tumour product (Saad *et al.* 1984).

Tumour masses

Local disease presents in the thyroid, cervical lymph nodes, and mediastinum. The commonest sites of metastatic presentation are the liver and lung. The primary or the metastases may show radiological calcification.

Paraneoplastic syndromes

The commonest is the diarrhoea mentioned above, which is often an indication of a large tumour burden. A few patients present with Cushing's syndrome due to adrenocorticotrophic hormone secretion or episodes of flushing, for which the causative agent has not been identified. Any of the bioactive substances which may be secreted by a medullary carcinoma of the thyroid will produce their typical associated syndrome. Two families have been described in which MEN 2A was associated with localized amyloid of the skin (Gagel *et al.* 1989).

Presentation with other components of the MEN 2 syndrome

MEN 2A

Medullary carcinoma of the thyroid is the commonest clinical presentation, but occasional patients present first with phaeochromocytoma or with renal stones or hypercalcaemia due to parathyroid disease. In these cases, if the patient has MEN 2, a stimulated calcitonin screening test will almost certainly be positive (Gagel *et al.* 1988). The proportion of patients with MEN 2A who present with parathyroid adenoma or unilateral phaeochromocytoma is not sufficient to justify screening for medullary carcinoma of the thyroid in these patients unless there are other indications, for example a suggestive family history or multiple foci of parathyroid or adrenal hyperplasia.

MEN 2B

The clinical features of MEN 2B are listed in Table 2. The characteristic facial appearance, the neuromas of the distal third of the tongue, lips, and conjunctiva, the failure to thrive in infancy, and the constipation or diarrhoea and sometimes nausea and vomiting with pseudo-obstruction, caused by ganglioneuromatosis of the intestine should lead to the diagnosis at an early age, but many cases are missed or misdiagnosed. Failure to take food and the 'floppy baby' syndrome in the neonatal period, while of course not specific to MEN 2B, are common features. The characteristic facies is probably overdiagnosed and, if necessary, the diagnosis can be confirmed by biopsy of a mucosal neuroma or by slit-lamp examination for thickened corneal nerves. Suspicion of the diagnosis should also lead to biochemical testing for medullary carcinoma of the thyroid.

Differential diagnosis

Medullary carcinoma of the thyroid has only been widely recognized since the late 1960s and it is certain that many cases in the past have been missed. The differential diagnoses include lymphomas and anaplastic thyroid epithelial cancers. Staining for calcitonin and for amyloid will give the correct diagnosis in most cases.

INVESTIGATION AND MANAGEMENT

Screening for medullary carcinoma of the thyroid

Who should be screened?

Decisions in a known MEN 2 family

The decision to screen depends on

(1) the risk to the individuals themselves; but also

(2) on the implications of a positive or negative result for the rest of the family.

Thus, it may be justified to screen a 75 year old, not for their own risk, but to exclude the possibility that their descendants are at risk.

The risk calculation has two components:

(1) the 'prior genetic risk', which is determined by closeness of relationship to a known gene carrier;

(2) the 'conditional risk', which is a modification of the prior risk to take account of the survival of the individual thus far without evident disease.

A detailed account and worked example is given in Ponder *et al.* (1988*a*).

Decisions in the family of an apparently isolated case

Here the need is to estimate the probability that the patient has familial disease. The risk calculations have the same form as in a known family.

(1) The 'prior risk' is now the risk that a patient with medullary carcinoma of the thyroid presenting at a given age will have familial disease, regardless of the family history.

(2) The 'conditional risk' takes account of the family history: if this is positive, the final risk becomes 1, if negative, the final risk is less than the prior risk by an amount dependent on the ages and numbers of apparently unaffected relatives.

Table 3 Probability that a patient presenting with medullary carcinoma of the thyroid at a given age with no history of MEN 2 in the parents may yet have the hereditary form of the disease

| | | Age at which parents were apparently unaffected[a] | | | | |
		30,70	40,70	50,70	60,70	70,70
Age of	30	0.29	0.27	0.25	0.22	0.21
patient at	45	0.15	0.14	0.13	0.11	0.10
diagnosis	60	0.06	0.06	0.05	0.04	0.04
of MTC	70	0.03	0.03	0.02	0.02	0.02
(years)						

[a] The age at which the parents were known to have had no symptoms suggestive of MEN 2 modifies the risk ('30,70' means that one parent was known symptom-free aged 70 years, the other aged 30 years). For example, a patient diagnosed with medullary carcinoma of the thyroid (MTC) aged 30 years, whose parents are both well aged 70 years, and in whom there is no other family history, has a 21 per cent chance of having MEN 2. Note that C-cell hyperplasia is not taken into account in this table; nor is the possibility of new mutation (see text). The risk calculations and the assumptions on which they are based are given in Ponder *et al.* (1988*a*).

In practice, only the parents are usually considered. An explanation and worked example is given in Ponder *et al.* (1988*a*): illustrative risks are shown in Table 3. Note that a young 'sporadic' patient is still at significant risk of having hereditary disease. The presence or absence of C-cell hyperplasia in the thyroid specimen can also be taken into account, although the data are insufficient to do this in a quantitative way. The presence of C-cell hyperplasia is a strong indication to screen the family; but because of sampling problems, absence of C-cell hyperplasia should not carry much weight unless the thyroid has been systematically examined with unusual care.

The possibility of new mutation

Even if the risk calculations from family history are low, there is always the possibility that an isolated case of medullary carcinoma of the thyroid could be the start of a new family bearing this disease. The proportion of medullary carcinoma of the thyroid which falls into this category is not precisely known, but is probably less than 5 per cent. Even so, it may be wise to consider screening the children of any patient presenting with medullary carcinoma of the thyroid, especially those presenting young.

Screening procedure: general points

Family history; explanations

A careful family history is the first essential, with review of thyroid pathology for C-cell hyperplasia where the familial disease is in doubt.

The nature and purpose of screening should be carefully discussed with the family, and the time-scale for the results and the possibility of equivocal or wrong results explained. Non-specialist clinicians should consider referral to a clinical genetics centre.

Choice of screening test

All screening should be preceded by a simple clinical examination, to include palpation of the neck and measurement of blood pressure.

The simplest biochemical screen is a basal calcitonin level, but this is not sufficiently sensitive either to detect all medullary carcinoma of the thyroid at a stage when surgical cure is possible or to exclude the possibility that a family member is a gene carrier. A stimulated calcitonin test or genetic prediction using DNA markers is far preferable. In difficult circumstances, a basal calcitonin may be done first, as an unequivocal positive may be sufficient, but a negative must be interpreted with care.

Biochemical screening: stimulated calcitonin tests

Types of stimuli

A variety of stimuli have been proposed, but the principle of each is the same. The C-cells are induced to release their stored calcitonin into the circulation and the size of the calcitonin peak following the stimulus is a measure of the C-cell mass and, hence, of C-cell hyperplasia. The stimuli most commonly used are intravenous pentagastrin (Telenius-Berg *et al.* 1977; Wells *et al.* 1978*b*), intravenous calcium (Wells *et al.* 1978*b*) or ethanol (Dymling *et al.* 1976) by mouth. Procedures are given in Table 4.

Ethanol is easy to administer to most adults, but not children and one may feel more comfortable using it outside the hospital, for example at home in the case of an elderly family member whose MEN 2 status is needed to decide on family screening strategy. Although direct comparisons are few, there is an impression that ethanol gives a less marked peak than pentagastrin or calcium and,

Table 4 Procedure and stimuli for calcitonin tests

	Stimulus	Blood samples
Ethanol	50 ml whisky or vodka by mouth in 1–2 min	Immediately before; 5,10,15,30 min after
Pentagastrin	0.5 μg/kg body weight intravenously; dilute in 5–10 ml sterile saline and inject IV in 5–15 s	Immediately before; 1,2,5,10 minutes after
Calcium	2 mg/kg body weight of Ca^{2+} as 10 per cent calcium gluconate injected IV in 1 min	Immediately before; 1,2,5,10 min after
Calcium + pentagastrin	2 mg/kg body weight of Ca^{2+} as 10 per cent calcium gluconate IV in 1 min followed by 0.5 μg/kg pentagastrin IV in 5–15 s	Immediately before; 1,2,5,10 min after

Note: procedures used by different groups vary in detail from those given.
The subject need not be fasting, but only a light food intake and no alcohol in the hours before the test are advisable. The subject lies on a couch and a cannula is inserted in an arm vein. Blood is withdrawn for one or two baseline samples, the stimulus is given (pentagastrin or Ca^{2+} can be given through the same cannula), the cannula flushed with dilute heparin; and blood samples withdrawn at the times shown. The side-effects of pentagastrin and Ca^{2+} should be explained just before the test.
Each blood sample should be 5–10 ml, taken into a heparin tube pre-cooled in an ice bucket. The sample tubes are labelled and replaced on ice and centrifuged to separate plasma immediately the test is completed. Two or three 1 ml aliquots of plasma from each sample should be immediately frozen in dry ice and placed in a −70 °C freezer. One aliquot is sent (on dry ice) for assay; the others are kept in reserve in case the first samples are thawed in transit or the assay results require to be confirmed.

thus, a greater proportion of equivocal and false-negative results. If subjects are driving their own cars to and from the test, 50 ml of whisky on an empty stomach is not recommended.

Pentagastrin is the most widely used stimulus. Its advantages are that more data are available to aid interpretation of the results and it is probably more discriminatory than ethanol. Its disadvantages are that it causes unpleasant side-effects of tightness in the chest, tingling in the limbs, nausea, flushing, or stomach cramps, which, although tolerable in most subjects, are occasionally severe. These always subside within 2 min, usually less. Perhaps surprisingly, in my experience children tolerate pentagastrin better than adults and they much prefer it to ethanol.

Calcium infusion is gaining in popularity and may be as discriminatory as pentagastrin, with fewer side-effects. These consist of flushing or an unpleasant feeling of warmth and nausea.

When applied individually, both calcium and pentagastrin fail to detect some cases of C-cell hyperplasia which the other does detect; therefore many groups, especially in the United States, use a combination of both stimuli (Wells *et al.* 1978*b*). The side-effects are stated to be no worse and sensitivity may be increased. It is not, however, clear at what point the benefits of detecting C-cell hyperplasia at the earliest stages become outweighed by the risk of removing normal thyroids (Wells *et al.* 1978*a*; Brouwers-Smalbraak *et al.* 1986; Ponder *et al.* 1988*b*). Each centre must define its own range of normal by testing controls and by experience of the stimulation test in practice.

Wells *et al.* (1982*a*,*b*) have reported better discrimination in family members with borderline increases in peripheral blood calcitonin following repeating the stimulation test after catheterization of the thyroid vein. This procedure seems logical but in practice many centres have reported difficulty in obtaining useful results. The procedure has not become generally adopted.

Assay of plasma calcitonin

A number of conditions other than C-cell hyperplasia can cause elevation of the plasma calcitonin. These include pregnancy, the contraceptive pill, renal failure, liver disease, and various tumours, including lung, breast, and pancreatic islet cell tumours, hepatoma, and leukaemias. The elevations are slight and there should not be an increment in the stimulation tests. Age and sex influence plasma calcitonin levels (Deftos *et al.* 1980). The history of calcitonin radioimmunoassay has also been plagued by a variable number of 'false-positives' in most assays (Body and Heath 1984). For these reasons, it is wise

(1) not to accept a small elevation of basal calcitonin as indicating C-cell hyperplasia unless at least a 2-fold increment can be obtained on stimulation;

(2) to store duplicate aliquots of plasma for measurement in a different assay with different characteristics in case of doubt;

(3) to get to know the characteristics of the assay that you will use and discuss the interpretation of results with the assay team.

The problems may be less with the newer two-site assays.

Age and frequency of screening

The age-onset curve in Fig. 1 indicates that the first positives to pentagastrin screening in MEN 2A can be expected at or before 5 years of age and approximately 90 per cent of gene carriers are detected by age 30 years. Reported instances of conversion from negative to positive after 40 years of age are very rare. The time taken for C-cell hyperplasia to progress from first detection to medullary carcinoma of the thyroid not curable by surgery, which would determine the screening interval, is not known. A consensus screening strategy for MEN 2A might be pentagastrin or pentagastrin/Ca^{2+} stimulation yearly from age 5 years to the late teens (some clinicians, especially in the United States, start at age 2 years), then every 2 years until the late 20s, then every 3–5 years until age 40 years. For MEN 2B, there is no published consensus. In view of the sometimes early onset and aggressive tumour, screening for medullary carcinoma of the thyroid in the child of an MEN 2B patient should start in early childhood, probably at the age of 1 year. In cases with no family history, biochemical confirmation should be sought as soon as the phenotype is suspected.

Other components of the MEN 2 syndrome

Phaeochromocytoma

Screening usually consists of annual blood pressure measurement and plasma or urinary catecholamines. In MEN 2A, however, it is very uncommon for a family member who presents with symptoms from phaeochromocytoma not to have also an unequivocal abnormality on stimulated calcitonin screening (Gagel *et al.* 1988). Probably, therefore, screening for phaeochromocytoma is unnecessary as a routine until the calcitonin tests are abnormal. An exception should be made in cases at particular risk, for example women of child-bearing age and those about to undergo general anaesthesia.

Catecholamine measurements will miss some phaeochromocytomas and in family members diagnosed with medullary carcinoma of the thyroid, adrenal imaging by computerized tomography (CT) scan or ultrasound is advisable before thyroid surgery.

Parathyroid

It is sufficient to check that the plasma calcium is normal.

Special considerations in MEN 2B

The children of every case of MEN 2B are at 50 per cent risk and should be carefully assessed for the phenotype from birth. Pentagastrin or Ca^{2+} stimulation tests should probably begin at age 1 year, even if the child has no recognizable MEN 2B phenotype. Some experienced clinicians would regard an unequivocal MEN 2B phenotype or a positive DNA test in those families where this is possible, as an indication for thyroid surgery even in the absence of biochemical evidence: while I personally tend to support this view, it is controversial.

DNA screening

Although the MEN 2A gene itself has not been identified, prediction of the inheritance of the gene is possible in some families using DNA markers which are closely linked to the MEN 2 locus. Description of the principles is beyond the scope of this chapter but will be found in standard genetic texts. The accuracy of the prediction depends upon the marker used and the availability of sufficient family members to establish with confidence which chromosome in a given parent is carrying the MEN 2 gene. At present, the markers are sufficient to provide predictions of estimated accuracy 98 per cent or better in the children of two-thirds of families where the DNA of an affected parent and one other affected close relative is available to identify the MEN 2 chromosome (Ponder 1990). Accuracy will improve as new markers are found. It is important to realize that no prediction is possible for the children of an isolated case until the MEN 2 gene itself and the causative mutations are identified.

The steps to follow to obtain DNA testing for a family are as follows.

1. Take a full family history, including affected and unaffected individuals, their ages and screening status.

2. Send the history to the genetics laboratory and discuss with them the likelihood that DNA prediction will be possible and the blood samples required, before arranging to collect the blood.

3. Guided by information from the laboratory, warn the family of the probability that prediction will or will not be possible and the likely accuracy.

4. Collect the blood (usually 20 ml ethylenediaminetetraacetic acid (EDTA) anticoagulated) taking great care that each sample is correctly and unambiguously labelled.

The blood can either be sent to the laboratory at ambient temperature, to arrive within 4 days or frozen as whole blood by putting it into a $-20°$ or $-70°C$ freezer. It will keep for many months; longer at $-70°C$. There has not yet been time for experience to accumulate in the use of DNA results. A positive DNA prediction is a strong indication that the individual should be carefully followed by biochemical screening. Because of the very wide range of ages at clinical presentation of medullary carcinoma of the thyroid (Fig. 1), it will probably not be considered an indication for immediate surgery, unless borderline abnormal calcitonin results have already been obtained. A negative DNA prediction may possibly justify the exclusion of an individual from further biochemical screening: the level of risk which is acceptable is a matter for discussion between clinician and family. Risk estimates from biochemical screening and DNA testing may be

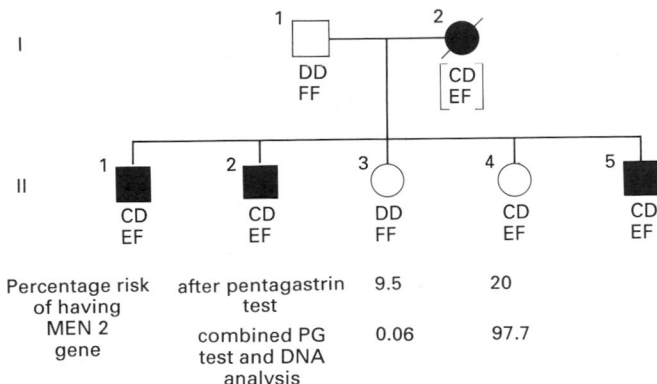

Percentage risk of having MEN 2 gene	after pentagastrin test	9.5	20
	combined PG test and DNA analysis	0.06	97.7

Fig. 2 Risk estimates in an MEN 2A family. ■, ○, Proven MEN 2; ◑, dead. C,D and E,F are alleles for genetic markers lying either side of the MEN 2 locus. II-3 and II-4 had normal pentagastrin-stimulated calcitonin values at ages 30 and 21 years, respectively. They each had a 50 per cent chance at birth of having inherited the MEN 2A gene; this probability is reduced to 9.5 and 20 per cent, respectively, by the normal pentagastrin tests (lower in II-3 than II-4 because she is older). The inheritance of the DNA markers indicates that II-3 has almost certainly inherited the normal chromosome 10 (bearing alleles D,F) from her mother and is thus at very low risk, but II-4 has inherited the (C,E) chromosome and probably therefore the MEN 2 gene.

combined (Fig. 2). This may be especially useful to determine a very low risk for the head of a branch of a family, so that the descendants in that branch can be excluded.

Investigation of a patient with known medullary carcinoma of the thyroid

Investigation of local disease

CT scanning

Computerized tomography is probably the most sensitive technique for the delineation of disease within the thyroid and in the neck and upper mediastinum. With iodide enhancement, C-cell nodules as small as 2–3 mm can be demonstrated within the thyroid. For this technique the patient is given two to three capsules of potassium iodide 180 mg (with a large glass of milk to minimize gastric irritation) 24 h before the scan. C-cell nodules appear as low–density areas.

Ultrasound

This is less sensitive, but occasionally useful (Schwerk *et al.* 1985).

Radionuclide scans

Although tumours can be demonstrated as cold areas on standard technetium pertechnetate scans of the thyroid, these have little value in the assessment of medullary carcinoma of the thyroid. Two new scanning agents are reported to show uptake in this disease. The most promising is pentavalent [99mTc]dimercaptosuccinic acid which in one series gave 95 per cent sensitivity of detection of bony and soft tissue lesions, without false-positives (Clarke *et al.* 1988). [131I]Metaiodobenzylguanidine was developed as an agent for imaging phaeochromocytoma, but has been shown to accumulate in tumours in some patients with medullary carcinoma of the thyroid. In the study of Clarke *et al.* (1988) only 12 per cent of lesions were imaged, which suggests that metaiodobenzylguanidine

does not have a primary diagnostic role, but in tumours which show uptake, it may have therapeutic potential. Occasional positives are obtained with 201Tl and [99mTc]methylenediphosphonate will image approximately 50 per cent of bony metastases from medullary carcinoma of the thyroid.

For the assessment of local disease in neck and mediastinum, therefore, dimercaptosuccinic acid seems likely to be a useful adjunct to CT scanning.

Selective venous catheterization

Transfemoral catheterization of the neck veins and selective sampling for calcitonin assay has been proposed as a logical means of locating small or diffuse deposits of residual disease, which are unlikely to show on scans, before secondary surgery. Although successful in the hands of the group that did the initial work (Wells *et al.* 1982a), informal and published reports suggest that others have found the technique either difficult to use or of uncertain value (for example, Rougier *et al.* 1983).

Investigation of metastatic disease

The common sites are liver, lung, and bone. Since there is no effective systemic treatment and the disease is often indolent, a detailed search for asymptomatic deposits may not be clinically justified. Knowledge of metastatic disease is useful

(1) if an attempt at cure by radical removal of local disease is contemplated;

(2) if there are symptoms that might be related to metastases;

(3) at sites at which complications might be foreseen and averted by early treatment, for example bone deposits in the femora;

(4) if objective evidence is needed to judge the response to therapy.

A large tumour burden and, hence, the probability of metastatic disease, is suggested by a very high level of calcitonin or carcinoembryonic antigen and by the symptom of diarrhoea.

Apart from the use of the scanning agents [99mTc]dimercaptosuccinic acid and possibly [131I]metaiodobenzylguanidine, the plan of investigation is similar to that for any other metastatic tumour.

Investigation for other components of MEN 2 syndrome

It is essential to remember the possibility that any new patient with medullary carcinoma of the thyroid may have MEN 2. Before proceeding to thyroid surgery one must exclude the possibility of concomitant phaeochromocytoma and of parathyroid hyperplasia or adenoma. Pre-operative diagnosis of medullary carcinoma of the thyroid by needle biopsy of a thyroid cold nodule may be very useful here. Even if adrenal or parathyroid involvement is not detected in the initial investigation, the possibility should be kept under review.

STAGING

The UICC and TNM classifications are shown in Table 5. They are almost never used in published reports, which suggests that they may not meet clinical needs. Two large published series are based instead on four 'clinical' stages, which take account of surgical and pathological information (Saad *et al.* 1984; Bergholm *et al.* 1989). These are

(1) tumour localized to the thyroid gland;

(2) tumour localized to the thyroid gland and movable cervical nodes;

Table 5 TNM staging of medullary thyroid carcinoma

Stage	I	T1	N0	M0
	II	T2	N0	M0
		T3	N0	M0
		T4	N0	M0
	III	Any T	N1	M0
	IV	Any T	Any N	M1

T1 Tumour 1 cm or less in greatest dimension, limited to the thyroid.
T2 Tumour more than 1 cm but not more than 4 cm in greatest dimension, limited to the thyroid.
T3 Tumour more than 4 cm in greatest dimension, limited to the thyroid.
T4 Tumour of any size extending beyond the thyroid capsule.
N0 No regional lymph node metastasis.
N1 Regional lymph node metastasis
   N1a Metastasis in ipsilateral cervical lymph node(s);
   N1b Metastasis in bilateral, midline, or contralateral cervical or mediastinal lymph node(s).

(3) direct local invasion and/or 'fixed' cervical nodes;

(4) distant metastases.

Other authors incorporate information about pre- or post-operative calcitonin levels (Wells *et al.* 1982*b*), which are almost certainly the best indication of tumour burden and a good basis for objective comparison. The objection that some of the most aggressive tumours are poorly differentiated and associated with a relatively low calcitonin is correct, but applies only to a few cases.

There is therefore no generally used staging system for medullary carcinoma of the thyroid. In cases detected by screening, the level of basal and stimulated calcitonin pre-operatively is probably the best staging criterion by which to assess the results of primary surgery. The level of basal and stimulated calcitonin post-operatively is the best measure of residual disease and, thus, the best short-term indicator of the probable success or otherwise of surgery in securing a long-term cure.

Staging based on a description of the extent of disease may correlate with prognosis, define groups of patients who may benefit from intervention, and stratify patients to assess the effects of that intervention. It does not take account of the rate of progression of the disease, which in medullary carcinoma of the thyroid may be extremely variable and is probably the strongest prognostic factor of all. The most complete staging of disease after thyroidectomy would therefore contain three elements:

(1) clinical/pathological evidence of spread;

(2) the level of basal or stimulated calcitonin;

(3) the rate of change of that level over the immediate past.

MANAGEMENT

Table 6 An outline of management once the diagnosis of medullary carcinoma of the thyroid is made

Diagnosis of MTC

Management of the family

(1) Is the family history positive?
  —If not, estimate the probability that the patient has a heritable disease even so (see text)
  —If family history is positive, construct an accurate family tree and estimate the risks to each member (see text)

Consider the possibility of genetic tests with DNA markers

(2) Contact clinical geneticist or endocrinologist if necessary to organize appropriate screening

Management of the patient

(1) Does the patient have MEN 2? Check:
  — MEN 2B phenotype
  — careful family history
  — CCH-immunostains of thyroid
  — urinary catecholamines/clinical evidence of phaeo
  — serum calcium

If positive:

probably
familial disease

(2) Was a total thyroidectomy done (if technically possible)?

If no, consider further surgery unless MEN 2 is very unlikely and post-op. CT is normal.

(3) Follow up with repeated clinical examination and plasma CT and serum CEA levels (approximately every 3 months at first; 6–12 months if stable)
  —normal basal CT and CEA: consider CT stimulation test to search for minimal residual disease if surgeon would reoperate (e.g. if only limited neck dissection so far)
  —elevated but stable CT/CEA, patient well: consider localizing tests before further surgery , especially if neck/mediastinum not fully explored at previous surgery. If no prospect of further surgery for local residual disease, do nothing.
  —rising CT or CEA: vigorous search for local disease for possible surgery/local radiotherapy. If disseminated disease, try [131I] MIBG uptake for possible therapy. Use chemotherapy with reluctance if clinical picture demands it.

Abbreviations: CCH, C-cell hyperplasia; CEA, carcinoembryonic antigen; CT, calcitonin; MEN, multiple endocrine neoplasia; MIBG, metaiodobenzylguanidine; phaeo., phaeochromocytoma; post-op., post-operative.

A flow chart for the management of a patient presenting with medullary carcinoma of the thyroid is given Table 6.

Surgical treatment

Surgery is the only proven curative treatment for medullary carcinoma of the thyroid. The proper extent of primary surgery is controversial. For all patients with this disease, total thyroidectomy is advised. This is because of the possibility of inherited (and, thus, bilateral) disease and of intrathyroidal metastasis. For all patients, even those detected only by stimulated calcitonin screening and without macroscopic tumour, dissection of the nodes in the central compartment of the neck is advisable, taking intraoperative frozen sections to look for metastases. Some surgeons advocate a more extensive dissection, extending into the lateral compartment of the neck, the mediastinum, and including removal of the thymus. Others extend the dissection only if there is gross or frozen-section evidence of node involvement (Russell et al. 1983).

Post-operatively, the patient must be followed with measurement of calcitonin and carcinoembryonic antigen. Early reoperation is advised if the levels show a rising trend and there is evidence or reasonable suspicion of resectable disease in the neck or mediastinum without distal metastases. More controversial is what to do if the calcitonin and/or carcinoembryonic antigen levels are elevated post-operatively, but stable. The decision will be influenced by the extent of primary surgery and the likely site and extent of residual disease, judged by calcitonin level and by clinical and radiological evidence. If primary surgery was limited, reoperation with dissection of the remaining nodes may be advisable (Block et al. 1978). Even if not curative, it may postpone distressing symptoms of local disease and surgery may be easier than at a later stage when the anatomy is distorted.

A particularly difficult case is that in which the evidence of residual disease is minimal, only detectable by raised levels of calcitonin after stimulation. Tisell et al. (1985) have claimed that a super-radical neck dissection may provide a chance of cure in these patients. The evidence for benefit so far is based on the conversion of a marginally raised calcitonin level to an undetectable level: a much longer follow-up period is needed to see whether this translates to cure. If this approach is to be taken, patients with undetectable basal calcitonin post-operatively must be followed at regular intervals with stimulation tests and action taken as soon as an abnormality is detected (since normal levels in this context are hard to define, in practice this means a rising calcitonin level). If the surgeon involved is not prepared to consider reoperation on such evidence, there is, of course, no point in subjecting the patient to the repeated tests.

Whenever technically feasible, surgery is the first line of treatment for local disease which is causing or about to cause symptoms.

Radiation therapy

External-beam radiation

Medullary carcinoma of the thyroid is generally poorly sensitive to radiation. In patients who have evidence of cervical node involvement and residual disease after surgery, there is evidence that radiation may reduce the risk of local recurrence over the next 10 years (Rougier et al. 1983). There are, however, disadvantages. Because of the high dose needed, many patients experience distressing long-term side-effects of cough and dryness and the scarring of the neck makes clinical assessment and reoperation difficult. The use and timing of radiation therapy in patients with known local residual disease is controversial, but a consensus is probably as follows.

1. There is no place for radiation as an adjuct to apparently successful primary surgery.

2. For a patient with clinical or biochemical evidence of residual disease, further surgery is the preferred treatment.

3. Radiotherapy should usually be reserved until there is either symptomatic local disease or clear evidence of progressing disease, not amenable to surgery.

4. In some instances, for example threatened tracheal or oesophageal compression, a combination of 'debulking' surgery and radiotherapy is likely to be appropriate.

5. Radiation is, of course, to be used for metastatic deposits, such as painful bony metastases, as in any other cancer.

Radio-iodine

Attempts have been made to use ^{131}I to ablate C-cells in the thyroid remnant following incomplete thyroidectomy for MEN 2 and, thus, prevent second tumours. These were apparently unsuccessful (Nieuwenhuijzen-Kruseman et al. 1984) and complete thyroidectomy is to be preferred.

[^{131}I] Metaiodobenzylguanidine (see above), a scanning agent, is taken up by a small number of medullary carcinomas of the thyroid. In cases where a systemic treatment is needed, it is worth testing uptake with a scanning dose and, if positive, considering therapy. Therapy has been successful in phaeochromocytoma and there are anecdotes of responses in medullary carcinoma of the thyroid.

Chemotherapy

Medullary carcinoma of the thyroid is generally unresponsive. Chemotherapy should therefore be reserved for patients with rapidly progressing or symptomatic disease, in whom other measures have failed.

In small series, responses have most often been reported with Adriamycin® and cisplatin (singly or together) and with etoposide (see Hoskin and Harmer 1987; Petursson 1988 for references). Some medullary carcinomas of the thyroid express oestrogen receptors and tamoxifen has been used as therapy with a few anecdotal reports of response.

Management of diarrhoea associated with medullary carcinoma of the thyroid

Diarrhoea is a common and distressing symptom, for which there is no universally satisfactory treatment. Standard remedies such as codeine phosphate should be tried first and then combined with other drugs. If these fail, surgical removal of bulk tumour may help. Nutmeg is often recommended (Cole et al. 1973) but is probably of limited use.

Management of phaeochromocytoma in MEN 2

Just as in medullary carcinoma of the thyroid, phaeochromocytoma in MEN 2 may be multifocal and bilateral. There continues to be considerable debate as to whether bilateral adrenalectomy should be performed as soon as the first phaeochromocytoma is detected or unilateral adrenalectomy with continued surveillance (Jansson *et al.* 1988). The argument for bilateral surgery is the risk of hypertensive crisis or malignancy as a result of an undetected second tumour. The argument against is the supposed difficulty of life following total compared with unilateral adrenalectomy and the supposed greater risk associated with illness or childbirth. Subtotal adrenalectomy with preservation of the cortex has also been proposed (Hamberger *et al.* 1987).

Adrenal or parathyroid autotransplants

Attempts have been made to circumvent the problems of adrenalectomy or parathyroidectomy by transplant of the patient's own adrenal cortical or parathyroid tissue to another site: usually the forearm muscles have been used (Mallette *et al.* 1987).

RESULTS OF TREATMENT
Success of screening

Historical comparisons indicate strongly that screening is successful in reducing morbidity and mortality in MEN 2 (Telenius-Berg *et al.* 1984; Gagel *et al.* 1988). Not surprisingly, randomized studies have not been undertaken, but family members detected by prospective screening have almost all maintained normal calcitonin levels after thyroidectomy, with follow-up of 10 years and more, suggesting long-term eradication of the disease.

Surgery

Surgery is the only means of cure. It is, however, controversial whether further exploration of the neck in a patient who has a persistent elevation of calcitonin following primary surgery, can ever provide a cure.

General

Non-hereditary medullary carcinoma of the thyroid is detected, on average, at a later stage than the hereditary disease. If age and extent of disease at presentation are taken into account, there is probably little difference in survival from medullary carcinoma of the thyroid between patients with hereditary and non-hereditary disease (Samaan *et al.* 1988). Overall 10 year survival figures reported by Samaan *et al.* (1988) were disease confined to thyroid gland, 90 per cent, involving local nodes, 70 per cent, nodes and soft tissue, 60 per cent, and distant metastases, 20 per cent. Many patients with hereditary and non-hereditary disease can live with metastatic tumours for many years with minimal or no symptoms. Treatment of such patients is probably meddlesome. Once the disease is clearly progressive, palliation can sometimes be obtained by combination of surgery and radiotherapy or chemotherapy, usually for a few weeks or months, but occasionally for longer, but death from metastatic disease is very probable. Rising carcinoembryonic antigen levels with stable or falling calcitonin levels may indicate an evolution of the tumour to a less well-differentiated state and are often associated with a particularly poor prognosis.

NOTE ADDED IN PROOF
Ret is the MEN 2 gene

The predisposing gene for the MEN 2 syndromes has been identified as *ret*, a member of the family of tyrosine kinase receptors (Mulligan *et al.* 1993). These receptor molecules comprise an extracellular domain, a transmembrane region, and an intracellular tyrosine kinase domain. Binding of specific ligand to the extracellular domain activates the receptor (usually by causing dimerization, although this has not yet been demonstrated in the case of *ret* in MEN 2), causing the kinase domain to catalyse the phosphorylation of tyrosine residues on itself and possibly other interacting proteins, which initiates an onward signalling cascade (Ullrich and Schlessinger 1990).

In the majority of families with MEN 2A and F-MTC, the mutations in *ret* affect one of several cysteine residues which lie in the extraellular domain of the protein, just outside the cell membrane. Most commonly, in MEN 2A, the mutations affect Cys634, the cysteine closest to the membrane. Each of the possible amino acid changes from cysteine has been seen. Interestingly, there seems to be a correlation between the precise mutation and the spectrum of tissues involved. In F-MTC families, the mutations are more likely to affect one of the cysteines further out from the cell membrane, whereas in MEN 2A families Cys634 is most often affected and Cys634 mutations which lead to substitution of cysteine by arginine are the most likely to be associated with parathyroid disease (Mulligan *et al.* 1994). In approximately 5 per cent of MEN 2A families (defined as MTC with either phaeochromocytoma or parathyroid disease) and in approximately 30 per cent of families in which MTC is the only tumour, the *ret* mutations have still not been found.

In MEN 2B, the mutations are quite distinct. Almost all are identical, a point mutation leading to the replacement of methionine by threonine at codon 918, in the catalytic core of the tyrosine kinase domain (Eng *et al.* 1994; Hofstra *et al.* 1994). Two apparently typical MEN 2B cases have been reported so far in which this mutation is not present.

Hirschsprung disease is associated with absence of the enteric autonomic ganglion plexus, in contrast to MEN 2B where there is hyperplasia of the plexus. The finding that predisposition in some families with Hirschsprung mapped by linkage to the MEN 2 region of chromosome 10 (Lyonnet *et al.* 1993) and the finding that transgenic mice in which *ret* had been inactivated developed a gut pathology resembling Hirschsprung (Schuchardt *et al.* 1994), suggested *ret* as a candidate gene for Hirschsprung as well. This has been confirmed by the finding of germ-line mutations in both the extracellular (Edery *et al.* 1994) and tyrosine kinase (Romeo *et al.* 1994) domains of *ret* in Hirschsprung families.

The functional consequences of these different *ret* mutations are still unclear (Mulligan *et al.* 1994). However, the deletion of one allele of *ret* in some cases of Hirschsprung disease suggests that loss of activity of one copy of the gene causes this phenotype. The contrasting hyperplasia of the enteric nervous system in MEN 2B and the apparent lack of mutations in the wild-type *ret* allele in MEN 2-related tumours, suggests that the mutations in F-MTC, MEN 2A, and MEN 2B may result in inappropriate activation of the *ret* gene.

Preliminary results from analysis of sporadic MTC tumour DNA and phaeochromocytomas suggest that mutations similar to that seen in MEN 2B are not uncommon, but that there are few, if any, mutations of the MEN 2A type. This suggests that the functional consequences of the MEN 2B tyrosine kinase mutation are more effective than are mutations of the type seen in MEN 2A, in driving tumour formation in somatic cells.

Clinical implications
Predictive testing in families

Prediction of the inheritance of the predisposing gene is now possible in the majority of families with classical MEN 2A or MEN

2B and in many families with MTC only, without the need for typing several family members to establish the inheritance of a linked genetic marker. Because the number of different mutations is quite small, mutation screening should be rapid; for several of the mutations, a simple restriction enzyme recognition site assay can be used instead of DNA sequencing (McMahon *et al.* 1994). It is not yet possible to predict with enough accuracy to be of clinical value the risk of either phaeos or parathyroid disease within a given family, nor the likely age at development or aggressiveness of the disease. Requests for DNA testing should be made through a clinical genetics laboratory.

The apparently sporadic case of MTC

The recognition of the potentially familial cases among those presenting with apparently sporadic disease is an important clinical problem. Screening of DNA from the blood of such cases is now recommended, as the finding of a typical MEN 2 mutation will provide strong evidence that this is a familial case and indicate the possibility of screening the rest of the family for the same mutation. Failure to find a mutation in the original case cannot, however, completely rule out inherited disease (though it can reduce the chances), because the mutations have still not been identified in some 30 per cent of familial cases.

REFERENCES

Babu VR, Van Dyke DL, Jackson CE (1984). Chromosome 10 deletion in human multiple endocrine neoplasia type 2A and 2B. A double-blind study. *Proceedings of the National Academy of Sciences USA*, 81:2525–8.

Bergholm W, *et al.* (1989). Clinical characteristics in sporadic and familial medullary thyroid carcinoma. *Cancer*, 63:1196–204.

Block MA, Jackson CE, Tashjian AH (1978). Management of occult medullary thyroid carcinoma. *Archives of Surgery*, 113:368–72.

Block MA, Jackson CE, Greenawald KA, Yott JB, Tashjian AH (1980). Clinical characteristics distinguishing hereditary from sporadic medullary thyroid carcinoma. *Archives of Surgery*, 115:142–8.

Body JJ, Heath H, III (1984). 'Nonspecific' increases in plasma immunoreactive calcitonin in healthy individuals: discrimination from medullary thyroid carcinoma by a new extraction technique. *Clinical Chemistry*, 30:511–14.

Boorman GA, Hollander CF (1976). Animal model: medullary carcinoma of the thyroid in the rat. *American Journal of Pathology*, 83:237–40.

Boultwood J, Wylie FS, Williams ED (1988). N-*myc* expression in neoplasia of human thyroid C cells. *Cancer Research*, 48:4073–7.

Brouwers-Smaalbraak GJ, Vasen HFA, Struyvenberg A, Nieuwenhuijzen-Kruseman AC, Helsloot MH, Lips CJM (1986). Multiple endocrine neoplasia type 2a (MEN-2A): natural history, screening and central registration. *Netherlands Journal of Medicine*, 29:111–17.

Cance WG, Wells SA (1985). Multiple endocrine neoplasia type IIa. *Current problems in surgery*, Vol. 22, pp. 7–56.

Carney JA, Go VLW, Sizemore GW, Hayles AB (1976). Alimentary-tract ganglioneuromatosis. A major component of the syndrome of multiple endocrine neoplasia, type 2B. *New England Journal of Medicine*, 295:1287–91.

Carney JA, Sizemore GW, Hayles AB (1979). C-cell disease of the thyroid in multiple endocrine neoplasia, type 2b. *Cancer*, 44:2173–83.

Carney JA, Roth SI, Heath H, III Sizemore GW, Hayles AB (1980). The parathyroid glands in multiple endocrine neoplasia type 2B. *American Journal of Pathology*, 99:387–98.

Chong GL, Beahrs OH, Sizemore GW (1975). Medullary carcinoma of the thyroid gland. *Cancer*, 35:695–704.

Clarke SEM, Lazaro CR, Wright P, Sampson C, Maisey MN (1988). Pentavalent [^{99m}Tc]DMSA, [^{131}I]MIBG, and [^{99m}Tc]msp—an evaluation of three imaging techniques in patients with medullary carcinoma of the thyroid. *Journal of Nuclear Medicine*, 29:33–8.

Cole BR, Giangiacomo J, Ingelfinger JR, Robson AM (1973). Nutmeg for diarrhoea of medullary thyroid carcinoma. *New England Journal of Medicine*, 289:108–9.

Deftos LJ, *et al.* (1980). Influence of age and sex on plasma calcitonin in human beings. *New England Journal of Medicine*, 302:1351–3.

DeLellis RA, Rule AH, Spiler I, Nathanson L, Tashjian AH Jr, Wolfe HJ (1978). Calcitonin and carcinoembryonic antigen as tumor markers in medullary thyroid carcinoma. *American Journal of Clinical Pathology*, 70:587–94.

Dyck PJ, Carney A, Sizemore GW, Okazaki H, Brimijoin WS, Lambert E (1979). Multiple endocrine neoplasia, type 2B: phenotype recognition. *Annals of Neurology*, 6:302–14.

Dymling JF, Ljungberg O, Hillyard CJ, Greenberg PB, Evans IMA, MacIntyre I (1976). Whisky: a new provocative test for calcitonin secretion. *Acta Endocrinologica*, 82:500–9.

Easton DF, *et al.* (1989). The clinical and screening age-at-onset distribution for the MEN 2 syndrome. *American Journal of Human Genetics*, 44:208–15.

Edery P, *et al.* (1994). Mutations of the RET proto-oncogene in Hirschsprung's disease. *Nature*, 367:378–80.

Eng C, *et al.* (1994). Point mutation within the tyrosine kinase domain of the RET proto-oncogene in multiple endocrine neoplasia type 2B and related sporadic tumours. *Human Molecular Genetics*, 3:237–41.

Farndon JR, Dilley WG, Baylin SB, Smallridge RC, Harrison TS, Wells SA (1986). Familial medullary thyroid carcinoma without associated endocrinopathies: a distinct clinical entity. *British Journal of Surgery*, 73:278–81.

Gagel RF, *et al.* (1988). The clinical outcome of prospective screening for multiple endocrine neoplasia type 2a. *New England Journal of Medicine*, 318:478–84.

Gagel RF, Levy ML, Donovan DT, Alford BR, Wheeler T, Tschen JA (1989). Multiple endocrine neoplasia type 2a associated with cutaneous lichen amyloidosis. *Annals of Internal Medicine*, 111:802–6.

Gibson WGH, Peng T-C, Croker BP (1982). Age-associated C-cell hyperplasia in the human thyroid. *American Journal of Pathology*, 106:388–93.

Gorlin RJ, Sedano HO, Vickers RA, Cervenka J (1968). Multiple mucosal neuromas, phaeochromocytoma and medullary carcinoma of the thyroid—a syndrome. *Cancer*, 22:293–9.

Hamberger B, Telenius-Berg M, Cedermark B, Grondal S, Hansson B, Werner S (1987). Subtotal adrenalectomy in multiple endocrine neoplasia type 2. *Henry Ford Hospital Medical Journal*, 35:127–8.

Hofstra RMW, *et al.* (1994). A mutation in the ret protooncogene associated with multiple endocrine neoplasia type 2B and sporadic medullary thyroid carcinoma. *Nature*, 367:375–6.

Hoskin PJ, Harmer CL (1987). Chemotherapy for thyroid cancer. *Radiotherapy and Oncology*, 10:187–94.

Jansson S, Tisell LE, Fjalling M, Lindberg S, Jacobson L, Zachrisson, BF (1988). Early diagnosis of and surgical strategy for adrenal medullary disease in MEN II gene carriers. *Surgery*, 103:11–18.

Khalil MK, Lorenzetti DWC (1980). Eye manifestations in medullary carcinoma of the thyroid. *British Journal of Ophthalmology*, 64:789–92.

Kullberg BJ, Nieuwenhuijzen-Kruseman AC (1987). Multiple endocrine neoplasia type 2b with a good prognosis. *Archives of Internal Medicine*, 147:1125–7.

Le Douarin N, Le Lièvre C (1970). Demonstration de l'origine neurale des cellules de poulet. *Comptes Rendus de l'Academie des Sciences Paris*, 270:2857–60.

Lippman SM, Mendelsohn G, Trump DL, Wells SA, Baylin SB (1982). The prognostic and biological significance of cellular heterogeneity in medullary thyroid carcinoma: a study of calcitonin, L-dopa decarboxylase, and histaminase. *Journal of Clinical Endocrinology and Metabolism*, 54:233–40.

Ljungberg O, Nilsson PO (1985). Hyperplastic and neoplastic changes in ultimobranchial remnants and in parafollicular (C) cells in bulls: a histologic and immunohistochemical study. *Veterinary Pathology*, 22:95–103.

Ljungberg O, Bondeson L, Bondeson A-G (1984). Differentiated thyroid carcinoma, intermediate type: a new tumour entity with features of follicular and parafollicular cell carcinoma. *Human Pathology*, 15:218–28.

Lloyd RV, Sisson JC, Marangos PJ (1983). Calcitonin, carcinoembryonic antigen and neuron-specific enolase in medullary thyroid carcinoma. *Cancer*, 51:2234–9.

Lyonnet S, *et al.* (1993). A gene for Hirschsprung's disease maps to the proximal long arm of chromosome 10. *Nature Genetics*, 4:346–50.

McMahon R, *et al.* (1994). Direct non radioactive detection of mutations in multiple endocrine neoplasia type 2A families. *Human Molecular Genetics*. (In press.)

Mallette LE, Blevins T, Jordan PM, Noon GP (1987). Autogenous parathyroid grafts for generalised primary parathyroid hyperplasia: contrasting outcome in sporadic hyperplasia versus multiple endocrine neoplasia type 1. *Surgery*, 101:738–45.

Mathew CGP, *et al.* (1987). A linked genetic marker for multiple endocrine neoplasia type 2a on chromosome 10. *Nature*, 328:527–8.

Mendelsohn G, Wells SA, Baylin SB (1984). Relationship of tissue carcinoembryonic antigen and calcitonin to tumor virulence in medullary thyroid carcinoma. *Cancer*, 54:657–62.

Mulligan LM, *et al.* (1993). Germ-line mutations of the RET proto-oncogene in multiple endocrine neoplasia type 2A. *Nature*, 363:458–60.

Mulligan LM, *et al.* (1994). Specific mutations of the ret proto-oncogene are related to disease phenotype in MEN 2A and FMTC. *Nature Genetics*, 6:70–4.

Nakamura Y, *et al.* (1989). Linked markers flanking the gene for multiple endocrine neoplasia type 2A. *Genomics*, 5:199–203.

Nieuwenhuijzen-Kruseman AC, Bussemaker JK, Frolich M (1984). Radioiodine in the treatment of hereditary medullary carcinoma of the thyroid. *Journal of Clinical Endocrinology and Metabolism*, 59:491–4.

Norton JA, Froome LC, Farrell RE, Wells SA (1979). Multiple endocrine neoplasia type IIb, the most aggressive form of medullary thyroid carcinoma. *Surgical Clinics of North America*, 59:109–18.

O'Toole K, Fenoglio-Preiser C, Pushparaj N (1985). Endocrine changes associated with the aging process. III. Effect of age on the number of calcitonin immunoreactive cells in the thyroid gland. *Human Pathology*, 16:991–1000.

Pearse AGE, Polak JM (1971). Cytochemical evidence for the neural crest origin of mammalian ultimobranchial C cells. *Histochemistry*, 27:96–102.

Petursson S (1988). Metastatic medullary thyroid carcinoma. Complete response to combination therapy with Dacarbazine and s-fluorouracil. *Cancer*, 62:1899–903.

Ponder BAJ (1990). Multiple endocrine neoplasia type 2: the search for the gene. *British Medical Journal*, 300:484–5.

Ponder BAJ, *et al.* (1988*a*). Risk estimation and screening of families of patients with medullary thyroid carcinoma. *Lancet*, i:397–400.

Ponder BAJ, *et al.* (1988*b*). Family screening in medullary thyroid carcinoma presenting without a family history. *Quarterly Journal of Medicine*, 252:299–308.

Ponder BAJ, *et al.* (1989). Genetic events in tumorigenesis in multiple endocrine neoplasia type 2. In *Cancer cells*, Vol. 7: *The molecular diagnosis of human cancer*, pp. 219–21. Cold Spring Harbor, New York.

Romeo G, *et al.* (1994). Point mutations affecting the tyrosine kinase domain of the ret protooncogene in Hirschsprungs disease. *Nature*, 367:377–8.

Rougier P, *et al.* (1983). Medullary thyroid carcinoma: prognostic factors and treatment. *International Journal of Radiation Oncology — Biology — Physics*, 9:161–9.

Russell CF, *et al.* (1983). The surgical management of medullary thyroid carcinoma. *Annals of Surgery*, 197:42–8.

Saad MF, *et al.* (1984). Medullary carcinoma of the thyroid: a study of the clinical features and prognostic factors in 161 patients. *Medicine (Baltimore)*, 63:319–42.

Samaan NA, Schultz PN, Hickey RC (1988). Medullary thyroid carcinoma: prognosis of familial versus sporadic disease and the role of radiotherapy. *Journal of Clinical Endocrinology and Metabolism*, 67:801–5.

Schuchardt A, *et al.* (1994). Defects in the kidney and enteric nervous system of mice lacking the tyrosine kinase receptor ret. *Nature*, 367:380–2.

Schwerk WB, Grun R, Wahl R (1985). Ultrasound diagnosis of C-cell carcinoma of the thyroid. *Cancer*, 55:624–30.

Sikri KL, *et al.* (1985). Medullary carcinoma of the thyroid: an immunocytochemical and histochemical study of 25 cases using 9 separate markers. *Cancer*, 56:2481–91.

Simpson NE, *et al.* (1987). Assignment of multiple endocrine neoplasia type 2A to chromosome 10 by linkage. *Nature*, 328:528–30.

Sizemore GW, Carney JA, Heath H, III (1977). Epidemiology of medullary carcinoma of the thyroid gland: a 5-year experience (1971–1976). *Surgical Clinics of North America*, 57:633–45.

Telenius-Berg M, *et al.* (1977). Screening for medullary carcinoma of the thyroid in families with Sipple's syndrome: evaluation of new stimulation tests. *European Journal of Clinical Investigation*, 7:7–16.

Telenius-Berg M, *et al.* (1984). Impact of screening on prognosis in the multiple endocrine neoplasia type 2 syndromes: natural history and treatment results in 105 patients. *Henry Ford Hospital Medical Journal*, 32:225–32.

Thurston V, Williams ED (1982). Experimental induction of C cell tumours of vitamin D_3. *Acta Endocrinologica*, 100:41–5.

Tissell L-E, Hansson G, Jansson S, Salander H (1985). Reoperation in the treatment of medullary thyroid carcinoma. *Surgery*, 99:60–6.

Ullrich A, Schlessinger J (1990). Signal transduction by receptors with tyrosine kinase activity. *Cell*, 61:203–12.

Valenta LJ, Michelbechet M, Mattson JC, Singer FR (1977). Microfollicular thyroid carcinoma and amyloid rich stroma, resembling medullary thyroid carcinoma. *Cancer*, 39:1573–86.

Wells SA, *et al.* (1978*a*). Medullary thyroid carcinoma: relationship of method of diagnosis to pathologic staging. *Annals of Surgery*, 188:377–83.

Wells SA, Baylin SB, Linehan WM, Farrell RE, Cox EB, Cooper CW (1978*b*). Provocative agents and the diagnosis of medullary carcinoma of the thyroid gland. *Annals of Surgery*, 188:139–41.

Wells SA, *et al.* (1982*a*). Thyroid venous catheterisation in the early diagnosis of familial medullary thyroid carcinoma. *Annals of Surgery*, 196:505–11.

Wells SA, Baylin SB, Leight GS, Dale JK, Dilley WG, Farndon JR (1982*b*). The importance of early diagnosis in patients with hereditary medullary thyroid carcinoma. *Annals of Surgery*, 195:595–9.

Wilkie BN, Krook L (1970). Ultimobranchial tumor of the thyroid and phaeochromocytoma in the bull. *Pathologica Vetinara*, 7:126–34.

Wolfe HJ, DeLellis RA (1981). Familial medullary thyroid carcinoma and c cell hyperplasia. *Clinical Endocrinology and Metabolism*, 10:351–65.

Wurster-Hill DH, Noll WW, Bircher LY, Devlin J, Schulz E (1986). A cytogenetic study of familial medullary carcinoma of the thyroid. *Cancer Research*, 46:2134–8.

16.3 Pituitary tumours

J. A. H. WASS AND MICHAEL BESSER

INTRODUCTION

Pituitary tumours account for approximately 10 per cent of clinically apparent intracranial neoplasms. Microadenomas (less than 10 mm in diameter) are found fortuitously in 25 per cent of pituitary glands at routine post-mortem examination (Costello 1936). Recent advances have improved the diagnosis and management of these tumours, including imaging of the pituitary by computed tomography and nuclear magnetic resonance, radioimmunoassay of circulating pituitary hormones, the advent of microsurgical techniques during transsphenoidal hypophysectomy, immunocytochemistry, refinement of techniques for administering external pituitary irradiation, and new drug therapies.

These tumours metastasize very rarely, but may be locally invasive into meninges and bone and may compromise sight and sometimes life. Morbidity is due to the mass effect and endocrine consequences, which may relate either to hypersecretion of an anterior pituitary hormone or hormones or hyposecretion of pituitary hormones, caused either by compression of the normal pituitary gland by a tumour or interference with the pituitary stalk blood vessels so that the chemical signals from the hypothalamus which normally control secretion from the pituitary fail to reach the gland. These effects may be prevented by early diagnosis and treatment. Successful treatment involves the careful use of surgical techniques, external pituitary irradiation, and drugs, either alone or in combination, individually matched to the type and size of the tumour. Obstacles to progress in the successful treatment of pituitary tumours are numerous. The aetiology is unknown. Because of their slow growth and the frequently insidious onset of related symptoms they are often diagnosed many years after onset and, although there is evidence that they are diagnosed earlier than they once were, late presentation and treatment remain significant problems. Because of local invasion at presentation, cure by surgical techniques alone is comparatively uncommon in the majority of large pituitary neoplasms. External pituitary irradiation requires careful planning in order to avoid complications, which can include hypopituitarism, optic nerve damage, and the late development of malignant tumours in the field of irradiation. Drugs which suppress the secretory products of these tumours are not always effective and may have side-effects.

CLASSIFICATION OF PITUITARY NEOPLASMS

Neoplasms of the pituitary (Table 1) may be divided into adenomas or carcinomas, which may be either functioning or non-functioning in terms of pituitary hormone production, craniopharyngiomas, other primary tumours, and metastatic malignancies. A number of parapituitary neoplasms occur (Table 2). However aggressive local invasion appears to be, the term pituitary carcinoma should not be used unless metastases within and separate or without the neuroaxis are found, and this is very rare.

Pituitary adenomas

Pituitary adenomas can be classified on the basis of their anatomical, histological, or functional characteristics. Anatomically, microadenomas are defined as tumours of less than 10 mm in diameter (the maximum diameter of the normal gland), and larger tumours are defined as macroadenomas.

From the histological point of view, pituitary tumours have classically been divided into acidophilic, basophilic, and chromophobe adenomas. This classification is unsatisfactory and inadequate for several reasons. First, the histological appearances are subjective. Secondly, chromophobe adenomas were originally thought to be non-functioning, but in fact often secrete peptide hormones and glycoproteins. Thirdly, this classification gives no information on hormone storage and structure—function relationships.

Table 1 Classification of pituitary neoplasms

Adenomas: functioning or apparently non-functioning
Carcinomas: functioning or apparently non-functioning
Craniopharyngiomas
Other pituitary tumours
Metastatic malignancies

Table 2 Hypothalamic and parapituitary neoplasms

Ganglioneuroma	Meningioma	Reticulosis
Astrocytoma	Chordoma	
	Pinealoma	
	Optic nerve glioma	
	Ependymoma	
	Dermoid cyst	
	Epidermoid cyst	
	Arteriovenous malformation	

The new classification of pituitary tumours is based upon immunocytological and ultrastructural features of the tumour cell. It is now possible to identify positively the five major cell types of the anterior pituitary: the lactotroph, producing prolactin, the somatotroph, producing growth hormone, the corticotroph, producing adrenocorticotrophic hormone, the thyrotroph, producing thyroid stimulating hormone, and the gonadotroph, producing luteinizing hormone and follicle-stimulating hormone. Similarly, adenomas which immunostain for these hormones but do not secrete them can be identified. Some adenomas are negative to immunostaining of all the anterior pituitary hormones (null cell adenomas) and a small percentage immunostain for more than one anterior pituitary hormone (plurihormonal adenomas). The relative incidence of these in surgical material is shown in Table 3. It will be seen that prolactin cell and null cell adenomas occur most commonly, followed by growth hormone cell adenomas. Glycoprotein hormones (luteinizing hormone, follicle-stimulating hormone and thyroid-stimulating hormone) are less commonly associated with adenoma formation.

Functional classification of pituitary adenomas

From the point of view of the practising clinician, it is perhaps best to start with the functional classification of pituitary adenomas and build into this the histological classification. We discuss these below in their order of frequency.

Pituitary tumours associated with hyperprolactinaemia

High prolactin levels cause amenorrhoea or oligomenorrhoea, galactorrhoea, and infertility in women in the reproductive phase of life and relative or absolute impotence in men. These tumours vary from microadenomas, which more commonly present in women, to macroadenomas, which may be very large and with extrasellar extension. Although prolactinomas occur less frequently in men, when they do they tend to be larger, present a mean of a decade later, and are more likely to be associated with compression effects. Patients with large prolactin-secreting pituitary tumours usually have levels of prolactin greater than 5000 mU/l (normal up to 360 mU/l). True prolactinomas are only occasionally associated with lower circulating prolactin levels, between 1500 and 5000 mU/l. Some large non-secreting pituitary tumours may also

Table 3 Pituitary adenomas and their relative incidence (per cent) in surgical material (Kovacs and Horvath 1987)

Prolactin cell (lactotroph) adenomas	28	
Null cell (non-functioning) adenomas	26	
Growth-hormone cell (somatotroph) adenomas	15	
Corticotroph cell adenomas	14	(45 silent)
Plurihormonal adenomas	12	
Gonadotroph cell adenomas	4	
Thyrotroph cell adenomas	1	

cause mild hyperprolactinaemia (below 5000 mU/l) by compressing the pituitary stalk and interfering with the passage of dopamine, the hypothalamic hormone that inhibits prolactin release from the anterior pituitary. These are now called pseudoprolactinomas. Intrasellar and suprasellar craniopharyngiomas, meningiomas, or any other parapituitary lesion, may have the same effect and cause a mild elevation in circulating prolactin. Mixed prolactin- and growth hormone-secreting tumours occur, so that some patients with hyperprolactinaemia may have the features of acromegaly.

Pituitary tumours associated with no elevation of circulating anterior pituitary hormones

These tumours present with pressure effects, that is, headache, field defects due to upward extension, third, fourth, or sixth cranial palsies due to lateral extension, or, rarely, cerebrospinal fluid rhinorrhoea due to inferior extension. They also present with the features of hypopituitarism, due to compression of the normal pituitary gland, hypothalamus, or the pituitary stalk and the latter may also result in mild hyperprolactinaemia. These tumours tend to be large. Non-functioning pituitary microadenomas are very rarely seen in clinical practice. Some silent, non-secreting adenomas are found occasionally to stain for adrenocorticotrophic hormone, the silent corticotroph adenoma. The reason for this paradox is unclear.

Pituitary tumours associated with high levels of circulating growth hormone

These tumours cause acromegaly and/or gigantism. Microadenomas are rare and the tumours are more commonly intrasellar or extrasellar macroadenomas. They tend to be more aggressive and rapidly enlarging in younger patients. Approximately 35 per cent of patients with acromegaly also have hyperprolactinaemia and this is due either to a plurihormonal tumour or a large somatotroph adenoma compressing the pituitary stalk. Between 1 and 2 per cent of patients with acromegaly have a large pituitary full of hyperplastic somatroph cells rather than a tumour, associated with elevated levels of growth hormone-releasing hormone. The growth hormone-releasing hormone may originate ectopically from a carcinoid tumour in either the pancreas or the lung.

Pituitary tumours associated with Cushing's syndrome

Cushing's disease may be associated with normal or elevated adrenocorticotrophic hormone levels, but in Nelson's syndrome (post-bilateral adrenalectomy enlargement of the pituitary and pigmentation) the level of adrenocorticotrophic hormone is invariably very elevated. Corticotroph adenomas tend to be small and are frequently microadenomas. Only rarely are they large and they may be highly invasive.

Pituitary tumours associated with high gonadotrophin(s)

Pituitary tumours may secrete follicle-stimulating hormone alone, which is more common than luteinizing hormone secretion alone or both luteinizing hormone and follicle-stimulating hormone. They usually present with space-occupying symptoms and are almost invariably very large tumours. In contrast to men with large pituitary tumours and hypopituitarism, men with these tumours have testes that are not atrophied. Otherwise, hypopituitarism is frequently present.

A tumour in the region of the pituitary with elevated immuno-reactive luteinizing hormone but normal levels of follicle-stimulating hormone may suggest human chorionic gonadotrophin production by a germinoma. Because of the similar structures of luteinizing hormone and human chorionic gonadotrophin the latter cross-reacts in some radioimmunoassays.

Pituitary tumours associated with thyrotoxicosis and high levels of thyroid-stimulating hormone

This is a rare cause of hyperthyroidism mediated by thyroid-stimulating hormone. The tumours are usually macroadenomas and may also secrete prolactin.

Pituitary carcinomas

Primary carcinomas of the anterior lobe are very rare indeed and originate in adenohypophyseal cells. Most frequently they are non-secreting, but they may secrete adrenocorticotrophic hormone, prolactin, or growth hormone.

Craniopharyngiomas

These tumours account for 3 per cent of all intracranial neoplasms and arise in the remnants of Rathke's pouch, which is the dorsally directed outgrowth of the stomatodeum. They are more frequently suprasellar than intrasellar.

More than 50 per cent are calcified, so they are readily discernible on plain skull radiographs. They may be solid or cystic and are usually benign. Recent observations have shown that the cyst fluid uniformly contains human chorionic gonadotrophin-β, and this may rarely get into the cerebrospinal fluid, where it is detectable by radioimmunoassay (Harris et al. 1988). These tumours present with hypopituitarism due to compression of the hypothalamus or, in the case of intrasellar tumours, the anterior pituitary. They most frequently present in children, but can occur throughout life. Suprasellar tumours may present with diabetes insipidus and some patients, because of pressure on the pituitary stalk, have mild hyperprolactinaemia (see above).

Other primary tumours of the pituitary

Sarcomas of the pituitary occur. These are very rare and may occasionally be seen after irradiation of the pituitary.

Metastatic malignancies

Secondary tumours of the pituitary and parapituitary region are infrequent and rarely recognized clinically. They occur most frequently in patients with primary tumours of the breast, but bronchial, prostatic, and colonic neoplasms may also metastasize here. Hypopituitarism is extremely rare and, in fact, metastases occur more frequently in the region of the hypothalamus than in the pituitary itself, presumably because of the high blood supply of this region of the brain. These suprasellar metastases may produce clinical hypopituitarism, including diabetes insipidus. At post-mortem, secondary tumour deposits are found in the hypophysis in approximately 1–3 per cent of all cancer patients. Histiocytosis X, leukaemia, and lymphoma tend to replace large parts of the posterior lobe, causing diabetes insipidus.

HYPOTHALAMIC AND PARAPITUITARY NEOPLASMS

These are shown in Table 2.

EPIDEMIOLOGY OF ANTERIOR PITUITARY TUMOURS

Most pituitary tumours have an equal sex incidence and occur most frequently between the ages of 30 and 50 years, exceptions being tumours that secrete prolactin and adrenocorticotrophic hormone, which are commoner in women. Approximately 10 per cent of pituitary tumours occur in young patients, causing delayed puberty; this will occur if the the patients are deficient in luteinizing hormone/follicle-stimulating hormone and also if the tumour secretes prolactin, because of the effect of prolactin centrally to inhibit the pulsatile release of the gonadotrophin secretion necessary for gonadal stimulation and peripherally to block the effects of gonadotrophins on the gonads. If tumours secreting growth hormone occur in the young before epiphyseal fusion, they cause gigantism. Pituitary tumours also occur in the elderly.

There are few data on the prevalence of pituitary tumours, but studies have been carried out on the prevalence of acromegaly (Alexander et al. 1980). Working in the Newcastle region of the United Kingdom, these workers found three new cases per million per year, with a prevalence of diagnosed cases of 40 per million.

AETIOLOGY OF ANTERIOR PITUITARY TUMOURS

The aetiology of pituitary tumours is largely unknown and it is probable that there are various causes for their development (Molitch 1987). All cell types in the pituitary can become neoplastic.

Hypothalamic abnormalities

In patients with acromegaly it is now well recognized that this condition can be associated, rarely, with hyperplasia of the somatotrophs in the absence of a localized pituitary tumour. Such an occurrence may be seen with excess secretion of growth hormone-releasing hormone as a result of a hypothalamic lesion, most frequently a hamartoma, but somatotroph hyperplasia is also seen with hypothalamic gangliocytomas producing growth hormone-releasing hormone.

In acromegaly, from the functional point of view, irrespective of the presence of a pituitary tumour, pulsatile growth hormone release, like that seen in normal subjects, persists and in some, abnormal growth hormone dynamics persist even after the removal of the somatotroph adenoma, implying that despite correction of high growth hormone levels, intrinsic hypothalamic disturbances continue to prevail.

There are, likewise, several lines of evidence that suggest that Cushing's disease can result from corticotroph overactivity secondary to accentuated hypothalamic drive. Furthermore, damage to hypothalamic neurones may cause prolactinomas in animals and adenomas secreting thyroid-stimulating hormone have been described in patients with prolonged primary hypothyroidism.

Pituitary abnormalities

However, a large amount of data suggests that pituitary tumours are primary abnormalities. In acromegaly, for example there is a relatively low rate of recurrence following complete removal of a growth hormone-secreting adenoma and somatotrophs surrounding the tumour are remarkably normal. In Cushing's disease there is a moderately high success rate for selective adenomectomy and, frequently, after complete removal of such a tumour, there is

prolonged dormancy of the normal corticotroph population suppressed by the previously elevated circulating corticosteroids, producing isolated deficiency of adrenocorticotrophic hormone in an otherwise normally functioning gland.

Other abnormalities

Genetic factors may play a role in some tumours, as in familial multiple endocrine neoplasia type 1 (MEN 1) where chromophobe or acidophil adenomas may constitute one of the neoplastic components. Recently a subset of growth hormone-secreting human pituitary tumours which carry somatic mutations of G-protein α-chains that inhibit GTPase activity in somatotroph cells have been described. The resulting activation of adenylate cyclase bypasses the normal requirement of the cell to be activated by growth hormone-releasing hormone and it is thus autonomous. Such an oncogenic mutation may promote tumour growth by producing autonomous activity of proteins that normally transmit proliferative signals initiated by extracellular factors.

The weighted evidence that exists suggests that for the majority of pituitary tumours there is a primary pituitary abnormality and it seems certain that in the future other types of pituitary tumour will be found to have oncogenic mutations which allow cells to bypass their normal requirements for trophic hormone stimulation.

PATHOLOGY OF PITUITARY TUMOURS

Growth and local invasion

An assessment of the invasiveness and extrasellar extension is of immense importance both from the surgical and the prognostic point of view and is frequently crucial in deciding the modality of therapy. Pituitary tumours have a remarkable propensity for local infiltration. The incidence of dural invasion visualized grossly may be as high as 40 per cent. It is even higher, amounting to 85 per cent when verified microscopically and there is a clear correlation between such histological evidence of dural invasion, tumour size, and the prognosis after surgical intervention. In the course of this invasion considerable bony erosion may take place. Suprasellar extension usually follows expansion of the sella and this is most frequently in the midline. This process is one of invagination and the neural tissues are pushed ahead of the tumour which remains confined by a capsule formed by the leptomeninges. Less frequently, suprasellar extensions of the adenoma may occur in a lateral direction into the posterior orbital surface of the frontal lobe or laterally into the medial aspect of the temporal lobe. More commonly, however, lateral encroachment upon one or both of the cavernous sinuses, when the dural capsule of the gland is often breached, may cause pressure on cranial nerves, which may be either surrounded or stretched by the adenoma. Least commonly, bony erosion of the floor of the pituitary fossa may occur, with extension of the tumour into the sphenoid sinus.

Histopathology of the pituitary

The epithelial cells of the anterior lobe are mostly arranged in groups or chords supported by delicate connective tissue and surrounded by a rich network of capillary sinusoids (Doniach 1977). In haematoxylin- and eosin-stained sections three cell types are recognizable: eosinophils containing cytoplasmic red granules, basophils containing bluish-red granules, and chromophobe cells. The introduction of Mallory's trichrome stain has made recognition of these three cell types much easier. In this method the acidophils stain with red (acidfuchsin)-stained granules, the basophils with blue (aniline)-stained granules, and the chromophobes with a grey-coloured cytoplasm. In the normal human pituitary there is a consistent arrangement of cell types, with the majority of acidophils grouped in the two posterolateral wings and the basophils lying predominantly in the median wedge and in the anterior and anterolateral portions of the gland. The application by Pearse of the periodic acid–Schiff method for demonstration of glycoprotein proved to be a significant advance. In the periodic acid–Schiff–orange G (pas-OG) technique, the basophils containing glycoprotein cytoplasmic granules colour magenta, the acidophils containing simple protein-containing cytoplasmic granules are stained yellow or orange, and the nuclei are stained black. This technique is free from the subjectiveness of the Mallory method.

It was recognized early on that the function of the acidophils is the secretion of growth hormone and prolactin. This was based on the evidence that tumours of acidophils are associated with acromegaly and that in pregnancy and lactation there is a marked proliferation and partial degranulation of the acidophils. The basophils secrete the glycoprotein hormones thyrotrophin (thyroid-stimulating hormone) and the gonadotrophins (follicle-stimulating hormone and luteinizing hormone), and adrenocorticotrophic hormone: fully processed adrenocorticotrophic hormone is a non-glycosylated polypeptide but its precursor is glycosylated.

More recently the application of immunocytochemical methods using purified human pituitary hormones as antigens and fluorescent labelling of antibody has confirmed the existence of separate growth hormone- and prolactin-secreting acidophils. Thyrotrophs and gonadotrophs, as well as corticotrophs, have similarly been identified (Table 4).

The electron microscope has further enlarged our knowledge of the normal human pituitary and demonstrates secretory granules very clearly. Although these vary in size within each cell, it is clear that the cells fall into subgroups according to mean granule diameter. Thyrotrophs contain the smallest granules and lactotrophs the largest. After prolactin, growth hormone cells contain the next largest granules and constitute the majority of cells in the posterolateral wings of the anterior human pituitary. The mean granule diameter of cells secreting thyroid-stimulating hormone is approximately 135 nm, that of prolactin cells, 550 nm, and in cells secreting growth hormone, 450 nm (Table 4).

Histology of pituitary tumours

A useful publication in this field is Kannan (1987).

Prolactin (lactotroph) adenomas

One notable feature of normal lactotrophs is the differential staining of these cells with prolactin antisera using immunoperoxidase techniques. Some cells are densely granulated with intense immunopositivity, reflected as diffuse brown deposits throughout the cytoplasm, while other lactotrophs are only sparsely immunopositive. Accordingly, prolactinomas can be densely granulated or sparsely granulated. The densely granulated prolactinoma represents the classic eosinophilic (acidophilic) adenoma in the conventional classification. The sparsely granulated prolactinoma is chromophobic and this is far more common. The cells of the sparsely granulated prolactinomas show ultrastructural signs of high secretory activity.

Null cell (non-functioning) adenomas

The tumour cells of the null cell adenoma fail to show immunopositivity with antisera to any of the adenohypophyseal hormones. These tumours appear chromophobic and pas-OG negative on conventional staining. Ultrastructurally the tumour cells show cytoplasmic secretory granules which characteristically fail to demonstrate immunopositivity for any of the known adenohypophyseal hormones, their subunits, or their precursors. These tumours represent the true chromophobe adenomas by the conventional classification and are much more common in older patients.

Growth hormone (somatotroph) adenomas

As with prolactinomas, growth hormone cell adenomas occur in both sparsely and densely granulated forms. Unlike the prolactinoma, however, the sparsely and densely granulated varieties occur with nearly equal frequency. Of these the appearance of the densely granulated variety bears a striking resemblance to normal somatotrophs. The cells stain with acid dye and represent the eosinophilic (acidophilic) adenoma in the conventional classification. By contrast, the sparsely granulated somatotroph adenoma represents the chromophobic variety but, with immunoperoxidase stains, growth hormone can be located in the sparse secretory granules. Clinically the sparsely granulated somatotroph adenomas tend to be more aggressive, cells show less differentiation, and the tumour is more invasive.

Corticotrophic adenomas

Classically, corticotrophic adenomas are small (usually less than 10 mm in diameter and often under 5 mm), readily stain basophilic, and are pas-OG positive. They are densely granular and demonstrate intense immunopositivity with adrenocorticotrophic hormone antisera. Less commonly, they appear chromophobic and are sparsely granulated. Such tumours tend to be larger and more aggressive in behaviour. Crooke cell change is present in those cells away from the tumour that secrete adrenocorticotrophic hormone. This appearance refers to enlargement of the cells, including the nuclei, with associated degranulation and is characteristically associated with elevated circulating glucocorticoids.

Table 4 Anterior pituitary cell types, staining reactions, and mean secretory granule diameter

| Cell type | Hormone produced | Staining reactions of cytoplasmic granules | | Mean granule diameter (nm) | Main distribution |
		Mallory	PAS OG		
Acidophil	Prolactin	Red	Yellow	550	Random
Acidophil	Growth hormone	Red	Yellow	450	Posterolateral
Basophil	ACTH	Blue	Red	360	Anterior median and anterolateral border
Basophil	LH, FSH	Blue	Red	200	Posterior median
Basophil	TSH	Blue	Red	135	Anterior median and anterolateral border

Abbreviations: ACTH, adrenocorticotrophic hormone; FSH, follicle-stimulating hormone; LH, luteinizing hormone; PAS OG, periodic acid–Schiff–orange G; TSH, thyroid-stimulating hormone.

A further group of corticotrophic adenomas is referred to as silent corticotroph tumours. These tumours may appear basophilic or chromophobic by conventional stains and contain secretory granules that demonstrate intense immunopositivity for adrenocortocotrophic hormone. They are not associated with adrenocorticotrophic hormone hypersecretion, and patients with these tumours do not have Cushing's disease. The reason for this paradox is unclear. Surprisingly, the corticotrophic cells in the normal pituitary away from the tumour also show Crooke cell changes, so in these circumstances these changes cannot be due to elevated corticosteroid levels.

Plurihormonal adenomas

True plurihormonal adenomas or mixed adenomas are bimorphous and bihormonal, containing two separate and distinct cell types. Immunostaining may identify both cell types co-existing side by side in the same tumour, with either dense or sparse granulation. These tumours commonly co-secrete both growth hormone and prolactin.

In addition to the true mixed cell adenoma, two other tumours are characterized by immunopositivity to both growth hormone and prolactin. These are the acidophil stem cell adenomas and the mammosomatotrophic adenomas. Acidophil stem cell adenomas are often aggressive tumours that originate in the common precursor cell, the acidophil stem cell, from which both the somatotrophs and the lactotrophs are derived. Remarkably, both growth hormone and prolactin are present in the same cells, which contain small sparsely distributed granules. Mammosomatotrophic adenomas are believed to be the mature counterparts of the acidophil stem cell adenoma. This is reflected by their slow growth, less aggressive behaviour, and tendency to show numerous densely staining granulated monomorphous cells.

Gonadotrophic adenomas

These are chromophobic and stain for follicle-stimulating hormone and luteinizing hormone. On electron microscopy, tumour cells of the gonadotrophic adenomas differ from normal gonadotrophs. Kovacs and Horvath (1987) have observed the presence of a unique honeycomb-like Golgi apparatus in gonadotrophic adenomas from females but not from males.

Thyrotrophic cell adenomas

Thyrotrophic adenoma cells contain fine granules that are immunopositive for thyroid-stimulating hormone. They appear chromophobic by conventional stains.

Pituitary carcinomas

The presence of cellular pleomorphism, mitotic figures, and even local invasion are not conclusive evidence of malignancy and an unequivocal diagnosis requires the demonstration of either deposits surviving and growing on the brain and spinal cord discontinuous from the pituitary or extraneuronal metastases. Some but not all authorities accept cerebrospinal dissemination in this grouping. The most common site of blood-borne metastases is the liver, with other sites including lymph nodes, lungs, bone, and myocardium.

Craniopharyngiomas

Craniopharyngiomas usually contain both solid and cystic portions. Solid tissue is smooth, firm, and grey or pink and the cysts are filled with a brownish-yellow, turbid, oil-like fluid containing suspended cholesterol crystals. Microscopically, craniopharyngiomas are well-differentiated tumours with sheets of squamous epithelial cells

separating cysts of various sizes. Gliosis around the tumour is often marked, consequent upon their tendency to infiltrate locally the surrounding neural tissues. The cyst fluid has recently been shown by radioimmunoassay to contain, consistently, human chorionic gonadotrophin-β (Harris et al. 1988) and immunostaining of the cells of the cyst wall can sometimes be shown. The presence of human chorionic gonadotrophin-β in the fluid can be of diagnostic value. It does not have the expected biological luteinizing hormone-like activity, probably because it is not fully glycosylated.

CLINICAL ASPECTS OF PITUITARY TUMOURS

Non-functioning pituitary tumours

Although described as non-functioning because there are no associated abnormalities of known circulating hormones, from the histological point of view these tumours frequently contain secretory granules which most often stain for the α-subunit common to the glycoprotein hormones luteinizing hormone, follicle-stimulating hormone, and thyroid-stimulating hormone. Because these tumours are unassociated with any clinical syndrome related to hormone excess, they most frequently present as large masses associated with local pressure effects. Rarely, because of bleeding into the pituitary tumour, they may present with the acute onset of headache associated with visual disturbance and meningism due to blood in the cerebrospinal fluid; that is, pituitary apoplexy.

Clinical features

Local pressure

Headache is the most frequent symptom, but it varies in location and severity. It may be due to stretching of the dura above the pituitary. If there is upward extension of the pituitary tumour, visual disturbances are the most typical abnormality. Usually, upper temporal field defects occur, but the exact abnormality depends on the position of the optic chiasma in relation to the tumour. A decrease in visual acuity may occur and it is therefore essential to test the fields of all patients with decreased visual acuity, as this may be the presenting feature of a pituitary tumour (Moore et al. 1986). With long-standing pressure on the chiasma, irreversible optic atrophy occurs.

Lateral extension of the tumour causes interference of the function of the third, fourth, or sixth cranial nerves, most frequently that of the third cranial nerve. Rarely, anterior pituitary tumours extend into the temporal lobe and present as epilepsy. Hypothalamic involvement may cause diabetes insipidus, but this is much more commonly seen in patients with craniopharyngioma than in those with non-functioning or, indeed, functioning anterior pituitary tumours. Obesity and sleep disturbances may occur, but are less common symptoms of hypothalamic disturbance. Cerebrospinal fluid rhinorrhoea is rare but pituitary tumours may erode the sphenoid bone and appear in the sphenoid sinus or post-nasal space.

Hormonal changes

These occur with great frequency in patients with pituitary tumours. Therefore, all cases need detailed endocrinological evaluation. The most common cause of hypopituitarism is a pituitary tumour in adults and a craniopharyngioma in children. In progressive hypopituitarism, there is usually a characteristic order in the development of trophic hormone deficiency. Usually growth hormone and luteinizing hormone secretions fail first, followed later by that of follicle-stimulating hormone, adrenocorticotrophic hormone and thyroid-stimulating hormone. Prolactin deficiency is rare, except in post-partum pituitary necrosis (Sheehan's syndrome). Diabetes insipidus is extremely uncommon in patients with anterior pituitary tumours, so much so that its presence in a new patient with a pituitary mass must raise doubts that the lesion is a primary anterior pituitary tumour.

Growth hormone deficiency causes short stature in children and sometimes, but not always, retarded bone development. There are a number of features of growth hormone deficiency in adults. These include impaired psychological well-being, increased abdominal adiposity, and reduced strength. In children, growth hormone deficiency is most commonly seen in association with craniopharyngioma.

Gonadotrophin deficiency occurs early in progressive hypopituitarism. If secretion of growth hormone is maintained, in adolescence there is normal or increased height due to delayed epiphyseal closure which causes a eunochoid habitus. In men with gonadotrophin deficiency, there is decreased libido, impotence, and a decrease in sperm count. Testicular size decreases and they may become soft. In addition, there is loss of pubic, axillary, and facial hair in both sexes. In women, a decrease in libido may occur and dyspareunia or amenorrhoea due to decreased oestrogen secretion is also seen. Infertility is common in both sexes. Prolactin deficiency is rare and most commonly pressure by a functionless tumour on the pituitary stalk results in elevation of circulating prolactin levels. Secretion of thyroid-stimulating hormone in children causes growth retardation. In adults, when hypothyroidism develops, the swelling of the subcutaneous tissue is less prominent in pituitary hypothyroidism than in the primary form of the disease. Secretion of adrenocorticotrophic hormone is associated with the features of hypoadrenalism, but in pituitary adrenocorticotrophic hormone deficiency there is also a pallor of the skin.

Deficiency of antidiuretic hormone causes diabetes insipidus. Cranial diabetes insipidus may occur after pituitary surgery. Its severity varies and between 4 and 10 l of dilute urine may be produced over 24 h. It may be particularly difficult to control if, in the presence of hypothalamic disease, the function of the thirst centre is also abnormal. Usually, post-operative diabetes insipidus spontaneously remits but this may take a few days, weeks, or over a year.

Rarely, patients with hypopituitarism may present in coma. Reasons for this include hypoglycaemia (which is in part related to the increased insulin sensitivity caused by growth hormone and cortisol deficiency), hypothyroidism, hypothermia, salt depletion, and water intoxication. Patients with hypopituitarism may have anaemia, although the pallor of their skin usually outweighs their degree of anaemia. They are usually of normal weight.

INVESTIGATION OF PATIENTS WITH PITUITARY DISEASE

Neuro–ophthalmological investigation

Neuro–ophthalmological examination, particularly formal perimetry, remains an essential part of the clinical evaluation of any patient with a pituitary tumour. Not only does such an examination aid the diagnosis, but serial examinations help to follow both the progress of the disorder and the effect of treatment. The level of visual function often determines the type and the timing of treatment. Visual fields should be tested by confrontation with a red pin or, more formally, using the Goldman apparatus (objects of differing light intensity). Eye movements should be fully assessed and the optic disc carefully examined in case of optic atrophy.

Radiological investigation

Plain skull radiography

A single anteroposterior and lateral skull radiograph should be obtained in all patients who are undergoing evaluation for sellar or parasellar lesions, in order to assess the size and configuration of the sella turcica and skull, any calcification in the sella and/or suprasellar region, and determination of the extent of the pneumatization of the sphenoid sinus, which may be important subsequently for the neurosurgeon.

Computerized tomography

Currently, either magnetic resonance imaging (MRI) or high-resolution computerized tomography (CT) of the sella turcica are the most valuable diagnostic radiological procedures available for evaluating pituitary and parapituitary tumours. One or the other is therefore recommended as a routine examination in all patients undergoing investigations for such lesions. For CT of pituitary tumours, several thin axial sections (1–1.5 mm apart), with and without contrast injection, are obtained and coronal and saggital computer images may be reconstructed to obtain saggital and coronal views of the pituitary. Some prefer direct coronal views rather than reconstructions; although more convenient, we find them much less satisfactory technically than reconstructions and, without the latter, sagittal views are unobtainable. Because the pituitary gland does not have a blood–brain barrier, opacification by intravenous contrast is virtually instantaneous. Unlike tumours, the gland enhances homogeneously. Differentiation of the cavernous sinuses can be achieved with rapid-sequence (dynamic) scanning. The reconstructions will often demonstrate the relationship of the pituitary mass to the optic chiasma.

Assessment of pituitary function

A useful reference for this topic is Wass and Besser (1989). It is essential to assess and correct anterior pituitary function before testing that of the posterior pituitary. This is because cortisol and thyroxine deficiency may decrease the symptoms of diabetes insipidus by decreasing the glomerular filtration rate.

Anterior pituitary function

Basal hormone levels of thyroxine, cortisol, prolactin, luteinizing hormone, follicle-stimulating hormone, thyroid-stimulating hormone, testosterone, or oestradiol should be assessed. It is then important to correlate the levels of the effector gland hormone (for example, thyroxine) with that of the trophic hormone (for example, thyroid-stimulating hormone). Thus, a low level of thyroxine in the presence of a low or normal serum thyroid-stimulating hormone implies hypothyroidism due to a central rather than an end-organ deficit. Similar reasoning can be used to assess whether luteinizing hormone deficiency is present by measuring both luteinizing hormone and testosterone or oestradiol levels.

The insulin hypoglycaemia test is the standard way of assessing adrenocorticotrophic hormone and growth hormone reserves and is safe if adequate precautions are taken. It should not be performed in patients with known ischaemic heart disease or epilepsy. Patients should not be left unattended and intravenous glucose and hydrocortisone should be at hand. The insulin is given intravenously in a dose of between 0.15 and 0.3 units per kilogram, depending on whether there is likely to be any insulin resistance (for example, the higher dose is used in patients with acromegaly or Cushing's syndrome). Adequate hypoglycaemia has to occur (< 2.2 mmol/l) and this should be accompanied by symptoms of neuroglycopenia, for example sweating and tachycardia. Throughout the test, glucose, cortisol, and growth hormone levels are measured; cortisol levels should rise to above 550 nmol/l and growth hormone levels to above 20 mU/l. If the growth hormone level does not rise, this implies growth hormone deficiency; however, if cortisol does not rise, this could be due to pituitary insufficiency or adrenal failure. This can best be differentiated either by measuring adrenocorticotrophic hormone levels, which are high in primary adrenal failure or by giving synthetic depot adrenocorticotrophic hormone intramuscularly and measuring the cortisol, which will respond to adrenocorticotrophic hormone if the atrophy is due to deficiency of the latter.

Thyrotrophin-releasing hormone (200 μg), luteinizing hormone-releasing hormone (100 μg), and corticotrophin-releasing hormone (CRH-41) (100 μg) may be given intravenously to assess the reserves of thyroid-stimulating hormone, luteinizing hormone, follicle-stimulating hormone, and adrenocorticotrophic hormone. However, these tests are not as useful in pituitary disease as had formerly been hoped and as much information can be obtained from measuring the basal concentrations of the hormones, as discussed above. Use of these releasing hormones merely assesses how much readily releasable hormone is present in the gland, not how much will be released physiologically. Often, hypothalamic mechanisms are impaired because of pressure on the stalk and portal vessels, so that physiological release does not occur despite adequate reserves of releasable hormone. Therefore, releasing hormone tests do not give clinically relevant information regarding whether or not hormone replacement is required.

If a patient is unable to have an insulin tolerance test, glucagon (1 mg subcutaneously) may be given as this stimulates both growth hormone and cortisol. However, it is not such a reliable stimulus of these two hormones as is insulin. The growth hormone reserve may also be tested by intravenous administration of arginine.

Posterior pituitary function

Posterior pituitary function is tested with a water deprivation test, prior to which other causes of polyuria, including diabetes mellitus, chronic renal failure, hypercalcaemia, and hypokalaemia, must be excluded, as these impair the efficiency of antidiuretic hormone. During water deprivation, it is important to ensure that the patient is not drinking. This is particularly so in patients with psychogenic polydipsia who have to be distinguished from patients with true diabetes insipidus. Water is withheld for 8 h by day and throughout the test urine and plasma osmolality are measured. In normal subjects the urine osmolality should rise above 600 mOsm/kg and there should be little rise in plasma osmolality. Certainly, it should not rise above 300 mOsm/kg. At the end of 8 h, intramuscular vasopressin (as desmopressin, DDAVP 2 μg), is given. If there has been no concentration of urine before this and the urine then concentrates, the diagnosis is clearly one of cranial diabetes insipidus. If, despite the administration of vasopressin, no concentration occurs, the diagnosis is one of nephrogenic diabetes insipidus. It is important to note that this dehydration test can cause a dangerous electrolyte disturbance in patients with severe diabetes insipidus. If the patient loses more than 3 per cent of their body weight, plasma osmolality should be measured immediately and if the plasma osmolality rises above 300 mOsm/kg, the test should be stopped and vasopression administered.

DIFFERENTIAL DIAGNOSIS OF ANTERIOR PITUITARY TUMOURS

The differential diagnosis revolves around conditions that cause sellar enlargement as shown on plain skull radiography (Table 5). Pituitary tumours (Table 1) and hypothalamic and parasellar tumours (Table 2) need to be considered. If the tumour is non-secretory, there will be no elevation in any of the anterior pituitary hormones, except possibly for an elevation in circulation prolactin because of stalk compression (< 5000 mU/l). Less commonly, metastatic disease, infiltrative disease, and secondary pituitary tumours need to be considered. If diabetes insipidus is a presenting feature, it is unlikely that an anterior pituitary tumour is responsible, and craniopharyngioma or pinealoma are more likely. Meningiomas are very vascular and enhance considerably after contrast. Chordomas usually show heavy calcification with extensive sellar destruction and on CT the tumour may extend behind the clivus. Germinomas occur posteriorly in the region of the pineal gland but also in the anterior hypothalamus above the pituitary and are often associated with raised levels of human chorionic gonadotrophin-β in the cerebrospinal fluid. Protrusion of an internal carotid artery aneurysm into the sella may cause asymmetric bone destruction. It is clearly important to recognize these pre-operatively. The definitive investigation is angiography. The empty sella syndrome, caused usually by arachnoid herniation into the sella, due to an inherent weakness in the diaphragma, is a frequent cause of sellar enlargement detected by plain skull radiography but it may also follow infarction of a pituitary tumour. It is usually seen in middle-aged females who

Table 5 Causes of enlarged sella turcica

Disorder	Plain skull radiograph	CT
Pituitary macroadenoma	Enlarged sella turcica often with erosion and destruction of the floor	Large contrast-enhancing lesion+suprasellar extension
Craniopharyngioma	Enlarged sella; suprasellar calcification in over 50 per cent	Intra- or suprasellar tumour often cystic, floccular or curvilinear calcification
Meningioma	Enlarged sella; hyperostosis of adjacent bone in 50 per cent	Parasellar location enhancement after contrast
Chordoma	Enlarged sella; heavy calcification; extensive sella destruction	
Germinoma	Enlarged sella	Suprasellar midline mass
Aneurysm of internal carotid artery	Enlarged sella	Dynamic CT scan may reveal aneurysm
Empty sella syndrome	Enlarged sella	Continuation of cerebrospinal fluid into the sella with pituitary stalk visible to floor
Pituitary apoplexy	Enlarged sella	Enlarged fossa; rim of pituitary at base of sella enhances
Hypophysitis	Enlarged sella	Suprasellar extension may be present

are often obese and hypertensive. There are often no symptoms and trophic hormone deficiency is rare. Hypophysitis is rare but can present as a mass lesion within the sella, associated with varying degrees of hypopituitarism as well as suprasellar extension. Lymphocytic hypophysitis shows a strong predilection for females. Pituitary cysts can occur within the pituitary gland. Most of these are developmental in origin and their major differential diagnosis is intrasellar craniopharyngioma.

MANAGEMENT OF ANTERIOR PITUITARY TUMOURS

Medical management of patients with pituitary tumours who are hypopituitary

Replacement therapy in hypopituitary patients

In patients who are adrenocorticotrophic hormone deficient, glucocorticoid replacement alone is necessary as mineralocorticoid secretion is not under pituitary control. It is now common practice to give hydrocortisone twice daily, on waking and in the early evening, usually in doses of 20 and 10 mg (total 30 mg per day). This drug is given in preference to cortisone acetate which is irregularly absorbed and has to be converted in the liver to hydrocortisone. It is possible to monitor the serum levels of cortisol on replacement therapy and this is important because the needs of individual patients vary considerably. In the presence of adrenocorticotrophic hormone deficiency, the patients should carry a steroid card in case of an emergency, as well as a bracelet such as that supplied by the MedicAlert organization.

In the presence of thyroid-stimulating hormone deficiency, thyroxine should be given in a dose of 0.05–0.2 mg daily. It is rarely necessary to exceed this dose. Adequate replacement is indicated by a serum triiodothyronine (T_3) in the upper part of the normal range. Growth hormone deficiency in children is treated by injections of biosynthetic human growth hormone. The requirement for growth hormone replacement in adults is currently under evaluation (Cuneo and Sontien 1992). Growth hormone-releasing hormone may also be used to induce the pituitary to secrete its own growth hormone (Ross et al. 1987).

It is important to treat gonadotrophin deficiency, as a long-term deficiency of sex steroids will lead to premature osteoporosis. In males, Sustanon® or Primoteston Depot®, mixtures of testosterone esters with an extended duration of action, may be given intramuscularly in doses of 500–750 mg every 3–4 weeks. This will provide adequate testosterone levels, which are unreliably obtained with oral testosterone preparations. In the female with gonadotrophin deficiency it is usual to give cyclical oestrogen and progestogen. A typical regimen is to give ethinyloestradiol, 10–30 μg daily, continuously and, during the first 14 days of each calendar month, medroxyprogesterone, 5 mg daily, to induce a withdrawal bleed.

Posterior pituitary replacement is best given with an analogue of vasopressin, although agents which stimulate vasopressin release or potentiate its action on the kidney are available for patients with partial vasopressin deficiency. The treatment of diabetes insipidus has been revolutionized by the development of a long-acting analogue of arginine vasopressin. The molecule has been modified so that no vasoconstriction occurs and the diuretic effect is preserved and prolonged. The drug, desmopressin (desamino-cys'D-arginine'8-vasopressin, DDAVP), may be given intranasally (10–20 μg) or intramuscularly (2 μg) once or twice daily, according to the needs of the patient. It is also effective orally in doses of 50–200 μg up to three times daily. In partial vasopressin deficiency, chlorpropamide, by increasing the sensitivity of the adrenal tubule to vasopressin, may result in a reduction in urine volume. The usual dose is between 100 and 350 mg daily. Clearly this may cause hypoglycaemia, particularly in the elderly, who should be warned to have some food before sleeping to prevent this.

Surgery

Transfrontal surgery has a greater morbidity and mortality than transsphenoidal surgery. The main indication for it is the decompression of the optic chiasma in patients with a large and inaccessible suprasellar extension (greater than 2–3 cm). Surgery using this route virtually never results in complete removal of the tumour and subsequent radiotherapy is necessary as 80 per cent of tumours will recur. However, provided they are sufficiently small, transsphenoidal surgery for pituitary tumours can completely remove them. This route can be used by some surgeons to remove tumours with extrasellar extensions of up to 2 cm. The technique clearly requires a great deal of expertise but is being increasingly widely applied. If it is possible to dissect the tumour from the rest of the pituitary and this is disputed by some neurosurgeons, it is not certain how often the tumour recurs and how often there is a long-term cure. Using this technique, hypopituitarism may develop and it is important to bear this possibility in mind when advising on treatment.

The operation of hypophysectomy rarely results in panhypopituitarism. This may be largely because the pars tuberalis around the stalk contains cells of the anterior pituitary. The transsphenoidal route has a low morbidity and mortality but is rarely curative in patients with lateral extensions or large suprasellar extensions. Complications such as cerebrospinal fluid rhinorrhoea, sinusitis, and meningitis occur but are uncommon. Diabetes insipidus may occur, but this is usually temporary and should be treated with intranasal or intramuscular desmopressin. Patients having hypophysectomies are usually given hydrocortisone cover in a 6 hourly dose of 100 mg intramuscularly. Once the patient has recovered consciousness and is eating this can be reduced to between 20 and 30 mg hydrocortisone given orally in divided doses. This should be continued until the post-operative assessment.

Post-operatively, visual fields improve if the chiasma has been successfully decompressed and this improvement continues for 6 months post-operatively.

Radiotherapy

Radiotherapy has been used for many years in the treatment of pituitary tumours (Jones 1991). Cobalt and proton sources, a linear accelerator, and intrasellar implants of ^{90}Y seeds have been used. Most experience has been gained using cobalt or, preferably, a linear accelerator. Using these methods, successful therapy requires careful planning and the assistance of a pre-radiotherapy CT scan. If conventional radiotherapy is given via three fields (one frontal and two temporal) in doses of no more than 200 cGy per session up to a total of a dose of 4500 cGy, the risks of optic chiasmal and hypothalamic damage are minimized. Hypopituitarism develops rarely and late, but the fact that it does means that after radiotherapy patients need yearly assessment of pituitary function. Less than 1 per cent of pituitary adenomas recur if external pituitary irradiation is given.

FUNCTIONING PITUITARY TUMOURS

Prolactinoma

In women, prolactinomas (Wass 1984*a*) tend to present earlier than in men. Furthermore in women they tend to be smaller at presentation. Therefore, local effects of a pituitary tumour secreting prolactin occur commonly in men. In these patients pituitary function may also be affected as described above.

Symptoms of hyperprolactinaemia

Any cause of hyperprolactinaemia may be associated with gonadal disturbances in both sexes. In women, amenorrhoea is the most frequently encountered disturbance of gonadal function. These patients do not ovulate and are therefore infertile. Some patients may have irregular menstrual cycles but polymenorrhoea may occur and a small proportion of patients have regular menstrual cycles associated with either anovulation or an inadequate luteal phase. In long-standing cases, there are symptoms of low oestrogen levels, including low libido, dyspareunia, and osteoporosis.

Galactorrhoea is present in approximately 30 per cent of patients with prolactinoma. Galactorrhoea is not, however, synonymous with hyperprolactinaemia. Indeed, 50 per cent of the patients with galactorrhoea have normal serum prolactin levels, so that this sign alone is a poor predictor of hyperprolactinaemia. In patients with hyperprolactinaemia, Montgomery tubercle hyperplasia may be present. A smaller proportion of patients also have acne, a greasy skin, and hirsutism because prolactin enhances adrenal androgen secretion.

In men, galactorrhoea is less frequent and gynaecomastia is a rare feature of hyperprolactinaemia. The most important symptom is impotence and this occurs in 80–90 per cent of these patients. Soft testes may eventually occur and testosterone levels, particularly in those patients who have long-standing hyperprolactinaemia, tend to fall. It is important to remember to consider hyperprolactinaemia as a cause of impotence.

Hypogonadism is caused by a number of different disturbances associated with hyperprolactinaemia. In females, high levels of prolactin interfere with the positive feedback of oestrogen on luteinizing hormone secretion and inhibit the essential pulsatile pattern of gonadotrophin secretion, thus, in part, accounting for anovulation. There is also a peripheral effect and high prolactin levels interfere with the action of gonadotrophins on the gonads. Lastly, hyperprolactinaemia may, in some, cause an elevation in adrenal androgens, accounting for the symptoms of acne, a greasy skin, and hirsutism.

Diagnosis of prolactinoma

The diagnosis is made by taking one or two basal, unstressed, blood samples for prolactin estimation. No dynamic tests are necessary. The differential diagnosis of raised prolactin levels is shown in Table 6. Once drugs and hypothyroidism have been excluded, hypothalamo–pituitary disease is by far the commonest cause of hyperprolactinaemia.

Investigations

Investigations should establish the degree of elevation of prolactin and residual pituitary function. As far as possible, an anatomical assessment should be made, involving assessment of the visual fields and the use of plain skull radiography and CT/MRI scanning with contrast.

Table 6 Causes of hyperprolactinaemia

Physiological: sleep, coitus, nipple stimulation, pregnancy, suckling, neonatal state

Prolactin-secreting pituitary tumours (secreted alone or in combination, for example, with GH or ACTH)

Hypothalamic disorders

Pituitary stalk section (for example, surgical or head injury)

Drugs

    Dopamine blockers: metoclopramide, sulpiride, pimozide, phenothiazines (for example, chlorpromazine), butyrophenones (for example, haloperidol)

    Dopamine depleting agents: resperine, methyldopa

    Miscellaneous: oestrogens (high-dose oral contraceptive), TRH

Hypothyroidism

Renal failure

Chest wall injury, for example, trauma, surgery, herpes zoster

Abbreviations: ACTH, adrenocorticotrophic hormone; GH, growth hormone; TRH, thyrotrophin-releasing hormone.

Management of prolactinoma

Before discussing the details of different treatments, it is important to have an idea of treatment goals (Wass 1984*a*). Successful treatment of a prolactinoma reduces prolactin levels to normal, removes the tumour mass with the preservation of anterior pituitary function, and does not cause significant side-effects, particularly hypopituitarism. If a pituitary tumour secreting prolactin is causing symptoms, it should be treated.

If it is decided to treat the pituitary tumour, three methods are available. First, medical treatment using dopamine agonists, secondly, surgical treatment using either the transsphenoidal or transcranial route, and, thirdly, external pituitary irradiation.

Medical treatment

Medical therapy has the major primary role in the treatment of small and large pituitary tumours secreting prolactin. It can be used either on its own as primary therapy or as an adjunct in the treatment of patients with large pituitary tumours whose levels of prolactin are not adequately normalized by surgery or pituitary irradiation.

There are a number of dopamine agonists but most experience in the medical management of prolactinomas has been gained with bromocriptine, an ergot alkaloid that works as a long-acting dopamine agonist. This drug suppresses prolactin because it stimulates dopamine receptors present on the prolactin-secreting cells of the pituitary tumour. It has been convention to administer bromocriptine two to three times daily. On doses of 2.5 mg every 8 h, prolactin levels become normal in the majority of patients. Recently it has been shown that the daily dose can be given altogether, once daily, with equal efficiency (Cicarelli *et al.* 1989). A small group of patients, usually with very large pituitary tumours or very high levels of prolactin, require higher doses of between 15 and 60 mg/day. As a result of lowering prolactin levels, galactorrhoea ceases and menstruation and ovulation return. In 80 per cent of patients this occurs within 2 months. In men, symptoms also improve rapidly and potency and libido return shortly after starting bromocriptine. In either sex, normal gonadal function fails to return only in the rare patient with persisting gonadotrophin deficiency.

A number of patients with prolactinoma desire fertility. Before treating these patients with bromocriptine, it is important to consider the risk of tumour enlargement during pregnancy, which may cause chiasmal compression and visual field defects. This has been reported to occur in 5 per cent of patients with microadenomas and 15 per cent with macroadenomas. In view of these risks, therefore, prior treatment with surgery or external pituitary irradiation is advisable in patients with macroadenomas. Worldwide experience with ovulation induction in hyperprolactinaemic women using bromocriptine indicates that the drug is not teratogenic. Hypopituitarism does not occur and, indeed, pituitary function may actually improve.

Bromocriptine must be administered carefully in order to avoid side-effects at the start of treatment. These consist of nausea, vomiting, and postural hypotension. They are usually avoided by beginning therapy with half a tablet (1.25 mg) last thing at night taken in bed during a snack. The patient then remains supine overnight. The tablets are always taken during food and the dose is increased every 3–7 days by 1.25 mg until the patient is taking 5 or 7.5 mg daily. Though any initiating side-effects are usually transient, there is a small group of patients who cannot tolerate bromocriptine because of nausea or persistent headache. Long-term side-effects on this dose of bromocriptine are rare and no serious side-effects have been reported in patients who have taken the drug continuously for up to 20 years.

There is good clinical and radiological evidence that pituitary tumour size may be decreased dramatically by drugs that stimulate dopamine receptors. Bromocriptine appears to reduce prolactin secretion by reducing exocytotic events. Prolonged therapy also decreases the prolactin content of prolactinomas, so an effect on synthesis is also apparent. Other workers have shown a decrease in DNA synthesis in rat prolactin-secreting tumours and the mitotic activity of prolactin-producing cells induced by oestrogens is also decreased by this drug.

Many groups have now demonstrated tumour size reduction on bromocriptine, either by improvement in visual field defects or by radiological means. Tumour shrinkage may commence rapidly, within a few days sometimes, with resolution of headaches, field defects, and ocular palsies, but the responses are sometimes delayed for several weeks. Residual pituitary function, if deficient before treatment, often returns to normal. Published trials suggest that 80 per cent of large prolactinomas with extrasellar extension decrease in size within approximately 3 months of treatment.

In view of these findings, in patients with prolactinoma presenting with large extrasellar extensions, it is appropriate to attempt to reduce the size of the pituitary gland medically in order to obviate the need for surgery or to make surgery easier. This should clearly be carried out under carefully controlled conditions, with regular visual acuity and visual field monitoring. If there is any deterioration in any of these parameters, surgery should be carried out forthwith. The same course of action should be followed if no improvement has occurred by the end of a 3 month trial period.

Catergoline, a drug with a much longer half-life than bromocriptine is effective at reducing prolactin levels to normal in 85 per cent in doses of between 0.25 mg every 2 weeks and 2 mg twice weekly.

Surgery

The results of bromocriptine therapy must be compared with those of surgery. Small tumours seem more amenable to successful surgery. However, medical treatment is effective in 95 per cent of this group of patients without surgery. The major risk of surgical treatment is hypopituitarism and this is particularly pertinent in young females desiring fertility. Recently, it has become clear that following successful surgery alone, a proportion of patients develop a recurrence of their pituitary tumour; 80 per cent of macroadenomas and 40 per cent of microadenomas by 5 years.

Radiotherapy

External pituitary irradiation (Tsagarakis *et al.* 1990) is also used in the treatment of prolactinoma. It is clear that it arrests tumour growth, prevents further enlargement subsequently during pregnancies, and gradually decreases the circulating levels of prolactin. It may take between 5 and 10 years to reduce prolactin levels to normal off bromocriptine. In some patients it is associated with the gradual development of hypopituitarism. Growth hormone deficiency occurs uniformly by 2 years but is of no consequence, luteinizing hormone/follicle-stimulating hormone deficiency occurs in over 50 per cent of patients but not for 8–14 years by which time their families are complete and hormone replacement is simple, and thyroid-stimulating hormone and adrenocorticotrophic hormone deficiencies are most common and occur later.

Treatment policy for prolactinomas

The choice of therapy depends on the size of the tumour, the presence of local complicating factors, the degree of elevation of serum prolactin, and the expertise that is locally available. In all but the largest tumours compressing local structures, medical treatment with bromocriptine should be attempted as first-time therapy. In a large proportion of patients this will suppress prolactin levels to normal without side-effects and will cause a resumption of normal gonadal function without risk of hypopituitarism.

Acromegaly

If growth hormone hypersecretion occurs before fusion of the epiphyses, gigantism results. If secretion occurs after fusion, the acromegaly syndrome develops, often over many years and this is much more common than gigantism.

Clinical features

As with non-functioning tumours, some symptoms of acromegaly result from the local effects of the pituitary tumour and others from the endocrine effects of interference with other normal pituitary functions by pressure of the tumour upon the uninvolved portion of the gland.

The clinical effects of excessive growth hormone are numerous (Wass 1984*b*). The first symptom is usually coarsening of the facial features and acral overgrowth is seen in all patients; both soft tissues and bones enlarge. These are recognized by the patient through a change in appearance and a need for larger rings, dentures, gloves, and shoes. The facial bones also enlarge; this is most striking in the mandible, where there is prognathism and increased interdental separation, but the supraorbital ridges and zygomatic bones also enlarge. Macroglossia also occurs. The dermal changes are the result of connective tissue proliferation and the accumulation of intercellular matrix. The deposition of hyaluronates leads to interstitial oedema and as the duration of acromegaly increases, regression is less and less complete because of progressive collagenation of the dermis.

A more reliable assessment may be made by measuring skin thickness on the dorsum of the hand, just behind the third metacarpal–phalangeal joint, using skin callipers or by measuring

ring size with a set of jeweller's rings. Serial measurements of this nature are particularly important in assessing the response to treatment. Increased sweating is extremely common and occurs in approximately 80 per cent of patients. Excessive pigmentation is sometimes seen in active acromegaly and acanthosis nigricans occurs rarely. Increased sebaceous activity has been noted, which causes greasy skin. In addition, hirsutism may be a troublesome symptom in women. In 40 per cent of patients there is a gain in weight. The ribs continue to elongate because of proliferation of the cartilage—bone junction. In long-standing cases, this leads to a deep, barrel chest. Cartilaginous proliferation of the larynx frequently results in a deep voice, which is resonant because of large sinuses.

In the cardiovascular system, hypertension occurs frequently and a diastolic pressure of 100 mmHg or more is approximately twice as common in acromegalics as in non-acromegalic controls. Occasional patients have a co-existent phaeochromocytoma or a Conn's tumour as part of a multiple endocrine disorder and acromegalics may have a disorder of the renin—angiotensin—aldosterone system; it is known that plasma volume, total body water, and exchangeable sodium are increased. In addition, cardiomyopathy may occur in association with acromegaly and it is possible that growth hormone has a myocardiopathic effect. However, few studies of heart muscle disease in acromegaly completely exclude all other causes of myocardial dysfunction, particularly coronary artery disease, which is commoner in these patients who may be hypertensive or diabetic. In the respiratory system, there is often thickening of the mucous membranes, sinusitis is frequent, and upper airway obstruction, possibly related to acromegaly of the larynx, occurs. Total lung capacity also increases and small airways narrowing occurs; these abnormalities relate to the duration of the acromegaly.

Myopathy may occur and peripheral neuropathy is also seen even in the absence of diabetes mellitus, so that paraesthesiae in the hands are not always due to carpal tunnel compression but this is the commonest cause. Narcolepsy has also been reported to occur more frequently in acromegaly, but daytime somnolence is still an infrequent feature of the disease. The aetiology of this disturbance is unknown; in some cases an obstructive apnoea syndrome may be present. Another important feature of acromegaly is arthritis. Early osteoarthritis, particularly of the weight-bearing joints, the hips and knees, may occur and a specific entity of acromegalic joint disease has been postulated, which involves striking overgrowth of the articular cartilage, sometimes associated with joint effusions.

A large number of female patients present with disturbances of the menstrual cycle and, most commonly, secondary amenorrhoea occurs. This may be due to decreased luteinizing hormone reserve as a result of a progressively enlarging pituitary tumour causing hypopituitarism. However, these patients are more commonly hyperprolactinaemic (27—35 per cent) and this is the most frequent cause of the menstrual disturbances and sometimes associated galactorrhoea. In men, loss of libido and potency are common and this, too, most frequently relates to associated hyperprolactinaemia. In association with this, the fertility of patients with acromegaly, both male and female, is decreased.

Diabetes mellitus may occur despite different criteria for the assessment of abnormal glucose tolerance and it is clear that altered carbohydrate metabolism is a common feature of pituitary tumours which secrete excessive growth hormone. This occurs because of the anti-insulin effects of growth hormone which potentiate insulin release and patients with acromegaly may have high insulin levels both at rest and after intravenous glucose. As β-cell exhaustion occurs in patients with long-term acromegaly, carbohydrate tolerance worsens and there is no insulin response to a glucose load.

Patients with persistent hypercalcaemia usually have multiple endocrine adenomas involving the pituitary and parathyroid glands but parathyroid hyperplasia may be seen. Hypercalciuria is seen in approximately 70 per cent of acromegalics. This is due to increased concentrations of 1,25-dihydroxy-vitamin D, which is known to rise during physiological states of increased calcium demand, including growth. Goitre, which is often multinodular, is also seen with increased frequency in patients with acromegaly.

Diagnosis of acromegaly

The chemical diagnosis of acromegaly is made by an oral glucose tolerance test (75 g), during which growth hormone levels fail to suppress to less than 1 mU/l. Single growth hormone values may be helpful in excluding the condition if lower than 1 mU/l but higher values are not diagnostic because of the effects of stress on growth hormone secretion and the pulsatility of its basal secretion in normal subjects.

Other causes of failure of suppression of growth hormone during a glucose tolerance test include anorexia nervosa, uncontrolled diabetes mellitus, and chronic renal and liver disease, in which there is probably abnormal insulin-like growth factor-1 feedback at the hypothalamus and pituitary as a consequence of poor nutrition or decreased hepatic production of this protein. Laron's syndrome, due to resistance of the actions of growth hormone and defective IGF-1 production, is associated with high growth hormone levels. These conditions are unlikely to be confused clinically with acromegaly.

Differential diagnosis

Few diseases present such a striking visual impact as long-standing acromegaly. Unmistakable as the somatic features of acromegaly are, occasionally the features of myxoedema may overlap. Pachydermoperiostitis is a disorder characterized by acropachy and thickening of the skin, particularly on the palmer and plantar aspects of hands and feet. Growth hormone levels are normal in this condition.

Investigations
Radiology

The majority of patients (99 per cent) have an abnormal skull radiograph, which shows either enlargement or asymmetry of the pituitary fossa. Visual fields and CT scanning of the pituitary should be carried out as described above. In addition to the abnormal pituitary fossa on plain skull radiograpy, the radiograph may show a thickened skull vault, enlarged sinuses, and a loss of angle of the mandible. Hand radiographs show a tufting of the terminal phalanges and a thickening of the joint spaces due to cartilaginous overgrowth. The thoracic spine may show wedging, which causes kyphosis and the lumbar spine may show posterior indentation and, in long-standing cases, new bone formation on the anterior aspect of each spine.

Biochemical investigations

Besides oral glucose tolerance tests, growth hormone levels should be assessed throughout the day, both to give an estimation of the degree of elevation of growth hormone and later to monitor the effects of treatment.

The remaining pituitary function should be assessed as described above.

Management of acromegaly

Acromegaly is a disease which approximately halves life expectancy (Wright *et al.* 1970). Increased mortality is due in part to cardiovascular and cerebrovascular causes related to hypertension and diabetes mellitus, as well as to respiratory causes. Therefore, it is important to treat acromegalics once the diagnosis has been made. The same objectives pertain as in the treatment of prolactinoma.

Definitive treatment usually involves transsphenoidal surgery and, if this is unsuccessful at normalizing growth hormone levels, external pituitary irradiation is given afterwards. The role of medical therapy is also important. It may be used before surgery to decrease the size of a large pituitary tumour; bromocriptine is particularly effective at decreasing the size of mixed growth hormone- and prolactin-secreting tumours and the long-acting somatostatin analogue, octreotide, may also decrease the size of pure growth hormone-secreting tumours pre-operatively. Post-operatively, medical treatment is used while waiting for the effects of external pituitary irradiation in those patients not completely cured by surgery.

Surgery

The best results follow surgery for small pituitary tumours with early diagnosis and prompt definitive therapy. In experienced hands up to 70 per cent of patients with microadenomas can expect to be cured by transsphenoidal surgery. Larger tumours and most particularly tumours which extend out of the sella turcica are cured by transsphenoidal surgery in less than 20 per cent of patients. Cure of acromegaly is strictly defined as reduction of circulating growth hormone levels to less than 1 mU/l at some time during the day. The incidence of hypopituitarism after surgery is much greater (25 per cent) if the tumour is large or extrasellar pre-operatively.

External pituitary irradiation

Several studies suggest that the response of growth hormone to pituitary irradiation is dependent on the pre-irradiation growth hormone concentration and the length of time after treatment. The main indication for radiotherapy is in those patients who fail to have their growth hormone levels normalized by a surgical procedure. Growth hormone levels continue to fall up to at least 15 years after external pituitary irradiation. If growth hormone levels are greater than 50 mU/l, the time taken for there to be a fall in the mean growth hormone level to less than 5 mU/l is longer (6 versus 4 years, for pre-treatment <50 mU/l and >50 mU/l, respectively). The major side-effect of radiotherapy in acromegaly, as in the treatment of other pituitary conditions, is the development of hypopituitarism. This continues to occur up to at least 12 years after radiotherapy, thus necessitating regular assessment of pituitary function after its administration.

Medical treatment of acromegaly

Medical treatment of acromegaly is given either using octreotide, a long-acting analogue of somatostatin or the dopamine agonist bromocriptine. Dopamine agonists raise growth hormone levels in normal subjects but, paradoxically, they lower the levels in patients with acromegaly. Bromocriptine suppresses growth hormone levels in the majority of patients (greater than 70 per cent of those studied). However, only rarely are growth hormone levels reduced to normal. Doses of between 10 and 60 mg a day (in four divided doses) are used. Prolactin levels fall to normal in all patients treated with bromocriptine.

Octreotide, an octapeptide analogue of somatostatin differing from the parent molecule by having a prolonged half-life of approximately 80 min, has the ability to suppress growth hormone in over 90 per cent of patients with acromegaly, for between 8 and 12 h (Battershill and Clissold 1989). It has to be administered subcutaneously three times daily. It has a preferential effect on growth hormone secretion but also suppresses insulin and although initially it may be associated with a mild worsening of glucose tolerance this is not a problem with long-term management because of the dramatic fall of growth hormone. Occasionally abdominal pain may be induced by the compound, but it appears to be more effective than bromocriptine at suppressing growth hormone levels, although prolactin levels are, in the majority of cases, unaffected. Because somatostatin has a number of other effects, including the inhibition of other gut peptides (including cholecystokinin), gallstones are seen with increased frequency in patients treated with this compound. Tumour shrinkage occurs in 50 per cent of patients treated.

Overall management of patients with acromegaly

Most acromegalics have either mixed growth hormone- and prolactin-secreting tumours (35 per cent) or pituitary lesions that secrete growth hormone alone. Clinical experience suggests that there is a spectrum of disease ranging from young patients, who often have very large tumours associated with very high levels of growth hormone which behave aggressively, to older patients at the other end of the spectrum, who have much smaller tumours and lower levels of growth hormone; these tend to progress more slowly. Earlier debates suggesting that all patients should be treated with only one modality are no longer tenable. Often all three modalities of treatment may be needed in a single patient, particularly the younger ones with aggressive tumours.

It is clear that surgery results in rapid fall in growth hormone levels but, equally, surgery is not always successful or permanent, particularly in patients with larger tumours in whom there is a significant incidence of surgically induced hypopituitarism and occasional recurrence.

External pituitary irradiation, although eventually effective in the majority, takes some time to work, and bromocriptine, although being extremely effective in some patients, only rarely reduces growth hormone levels to normal. Octreotide is more frequently effective. In the past the treatment depended on the local expertise. With more widely available surgery and radiotherapy, this should no longer be the case. Each patient's management has to be judged individually, usually treating with surgery first and, if only partially effective, then proceeding to radiotherapy, with medical treatment in the interim until growth hormone levels fall to normal. Regular assessment of residual pituitary function is essential.

Patients who are unwilling to undergo operation may be treated with radiotherapy together with octreotide; this is withdrawn at intervals to assess whether the radiotherapy has been fully effective. Medical treatment of acromegaly alone is rarely indicated, except in those patients who are too old or unwilling to undergo ablative therapy to the pituitary.

Cushing's syndrome

Cushing's syndrome is the name given to all conditions resulting from the sustained and inappropriate elevation of circulating free glucocorticoids. Cushing's disease is applied to that form of the syndrome caused by a pituitary adenoma secreting adrenocorticotrophic hormone. Clinically this has to be differentiated from other causes of Cushing's syndrome, which include adrenal tumours, either adenomas or carcinomas and ectopic adrenocorticotrophic hormone production. Recently it has been found that excess alcohol intake causes the clinical and biochemical disturbances of Cushing's syndrome. It is also obvious that adrenocorticotrophic hormone or steroids given in supraphysiological amounts have the same clinical effects. In total, pituitary-dependent Cushing's disease and adrenal tumours account for 70 per cent of patients with Cushing's syndrome, but it is probable that ectopic adrenocorticotrophic hormone secretion and alcohol-induced pseudo-Cushing's syndrome are underdiagnosed. Pituitary-dependent Cushing's disease causes bilateral adrenal hyperplasia, as does ectopic adrenocorticotrophic hormone production. The most usual cause of ectopic adrenocorticotrophic hormone production is a secretion of this hormone by an oat cell carcinoma of the lung. In contrast to patients with Cushing's disease, patients with oat cell carcinoma may not look cushingoid. They have usually developed the disease quickly and suffer most profoundly from both its metabolic effects and those of malignancy, particularly weight loss. However, other tumours are harder to diagnose as secreting ectopic adrenocorticotrophic hormone; these include bronchial carcinoid, thymoma, islet cell tumours of the pancreas, carcinoids of the pancreas, stomach, or ovary, medullary carcinoma of the thyroid, and phaeochromocytoma.

Adrenal tumours are comparatively easy to diagnose; 10 per cent of adults with Cushing's syndrome have these tumours, but in children adrenal carcinoma is the commonest cause of Cushing's syndrome.

Clinical features

The clinical features of a rounded, plethoric face and central obesity are classical. The thin arms and legs are, in part, attributed to the myopathy that occurs in all patients, as well as to protein wasting induced by high levels of glucocorticoid. Loss of libido, amenorrhoea, and galactorrhoea may occur, particularly if there is associated prolactin production by a pituitary tumour. Hirsutism and acne also occur. In patients with long-standing Cushing's syndrome, vertebral collapse occurs as a result of osteoporosis. Psychiatric manifestations, particularly depression, are seen in 40–50 per cent of patients with this syndrome. With ectopic adrenocorticotrophic hormone production, pigmentation may occur, particularly in the buccal mucosa, skin creases, and scars.

Differential diagnosis and investigation

There is no single test which is totally reliable in the diagnosis of Cushing's syndrome which may be difficult because intermittent, mild and atypical forms of the disease occur (Trainer and Grossman 1990).

Diagnosis occurs in two stages: first, that Cushing's syndrome exists and, secondly, the differential diagnosis of the cause. In Cushing's syndrome there is a loss of circadian rhythm so that sleeping adrenocorticotrophic hormone and cortisol levels are elevated at midnight. This may also occur during stress, so that it is usual not to test circadian rhythms until the patient has been in hospital for at least 48 h. There is no suppression of plasma cortisol after dexamethasone (0.5 mg 6 hourly for 48 h). This low-dose dexamethasone test is not completely reliable, but is more reliable than overnight dexamethasone tests. However, dexamethasone suppressibility may also be lost in patients with severe depression and physical stress. The most reliable test in the diagnosis of Cushing's syndrome is the insulin tolerance test. If there is no rise in cortisol in response to a fall in blood sugar to less than 2.2 mmol/l, it is highly likely that the patient has Cushing's

syndrome, as in depressed, simply obese, and stressed patients, the cortisol response to hypoglycaemia is preserved. In the differential diagnosis of Cushing's syndrome, the level of adrenocorticotrophic hormone is important. Clearly, it is undetectable in patients with adrenal adenoma or carcinoma.

The major diagnostic problem involves differentiating Cushing's syndrome due to ectopic adrenocorticotrophic hormone production by occult and often very small neoplasms (less than 5 mm) from Cushing's disease. Pituitary-dependent disease is suggested by adrenocorticotrophic hormone values of less than 200 pg/ml but, unfortunately, such levels may occur in some patients with carcinoid tumours secreting adrenocorticotrophic hormone. Cushing's disease is also suggested, if, when giving the patient dexamethasone 8 mg daily for 48 h (2 mg 6 hourly), there is greater than 50 per cent suppression of plasma cortisol. Unfortunately, some patients with ectopic adrenocorticotrophic hormone production may show such suppression and 10 per cent of patients with Cushing's disease fail to suppress. Ectopic adrenocorticotrophic hormone secretion is suggested by the presence of hypokalaemia, provided the patient is not taking diuretics.

More recently, the administration of corticotrophin-releasing hormone (CRH-41) has helped in the differential diagnosis of pituitary-dependent versus ectopic adrenocorticotrophic hormone secretion, in that patients with pituitary-dependent Cushing's disease have an exaggerated cortisol and adrenocorticotrophic hormone response to CRH-41 whereas most patients with ectopic adrenocorticotrophic hormone secretion do not respond to the administration of this compound.

Lastly, confirmation of pituitary-dependent Cushing's syndrome may be obtained by bilateral catheterization of the inferior petrosal veins draining the pituitary fossa and cavernous sinuses and monitoring of cortisol and adrenocorticotrophic hormone levels after the administration of corticotrophin-releasing hormone. In patients with Cushing's disease, secretion of adrenocorticotrophic hormone is detected after intravenous injection of corticotrophin releasing hormone and levels in the inferior petrosal sinus are higher than those detected in simultaneously taken peripheral venous samples.

Management of Cushing's disease
Surgery

It is now generally accepted that the cure rate of transsphenoidal pituitary surgery far exceeds every other available treatment option for Cushing's disease. Cure rates vary according to the criteria used. Adrenocorticotrophic hormone secretion from the normal pituitary will be completely suppressed by the high levels of glucocorticoid and this will persist when the adenoma is removed. The level of circulating cortisol should, therefore, be < 50 mU/l and carefully monitored post-operatively.

If these strict criteria are used, cure rates after the first attempt are between 50 and 60 per cent. Success rates drop significantly when the tumour is no longer confined to the sella (25–40 per cent). The overall success rate of transsphenoidal surgery in Cushing's disease is higher than that in acromegaly because the pituitary adenoma is usually small. If hypoadrenalism does not develop immediately after pituitary surgery, it is unlikely that the patient is cured. The transient hypoadrenal state caused by prolonged suppression of normal corticotrophs lasts for a variable amount of time, ranging from 3 months to many years. The morbidity of transsphenoidal surgery is low. Transient diabetes insipidus is the most frequent complication.

Reasons for failure of transsphenoidal surgery include the presence of corticotrophic hyperplasia, the presence of an invasive tumour, or erroneous diagnosis (most commonly missed condition is ectopic adrenocorticotrophic hormone secretion).

Pituitary irradiation

Pituitary irradiation using the standard technique described above is most frequently indicated after unsuccessful surgery. As with all pituitary hypersecretory syndromes, external pituitary irradiation may take some years to be effective and hypopituitarism may develop. Pituitary irradiation is particularly effective in the treatment of children with Cushing's disease.

Medical treatment

Medical treatment may be used as an adjunct to surgery and radiotherapy while the effects of radiotherapy are awaited or, alternatively, for the pre-operative treatment of patients very ill with Cushing's disease. Metyrapone, an 11β-hydroxylase inhibitor, inhibits the synthesis of cortisol. This is associated with only a small rise in adrenocorticotrophic hormone so that cortisol levels are reduced. This allows a significant improvement to occur in the patient's condition prior to surgery; this is particularly important if there are severe psychiatric manifestations of the disease or the patient is severely ill. Between 500 mg and 8 g daily may be used. Cortisol levels should be monitored during therapy with the aim of reducing the mean cortisol level (six samples taken from 09.00 to 21.00) to between 300 and 400 nmol/l, but it is vital to use a radioimmunoassay which does not cross-react with the pre-cortisol metabolites which rise to high levels.

Side-effects of metyrapone include worsening of hirsutism because of an associated rise in testosterone levels. If not carefully monitored, metyrapone may result in adrenal insufficiency.

Mitotane (o,p'DDD) is an adrenolytic agent which may be used together with metyrapone in patients not responding adequately to this drug alone. Between 2 and 4 g are administered daily. It has a slow onset of action, so careful monitoring of cortisol levels is necessary. Side-effects include adrenal insufficiency, hyper-cholesterolaemia, and cerebellar ataxia because of its incorporation into cerebellar neurones. Ketoconazide, 600–1200 mg daily is highly effective in lowering cortisol secretion by enzyme inhibition, but it also lowers androgen production.

Overall management

Cushing's disease presents on occasions a most difficult diagnostic problem. The correct differentiation of pituitary from ectopic adrenocorticotrophic hormone production can be one of the most challenging problems in clinical endocrinology. Once the correct diagnosis of pituitary-dependent Cushing's disease is arrived at, the correct treatment is transsphenoidal hypophysectomy. Because these tumours are usually basophil adenomas which are small in size and only rarely invasive chromophobe adenomas, the results of surgery are good; the best of all surgery performed for the pituitary hypersecretory syndromes. In patients not cured by transsphenoidal surgery, external pituitary irradiation should be recommended followed, until this has been successful, by metyrapone, ketoconazole, or mitotane. Only rarely is bilateral adrenalectomy indicated for patients who are not cured by the above treatment modality or those who have severe side-effects with medical treatment after radiotherapy.

CONCLUSION

Pituitary tumours occur frequently. They present with a wide number of differing symptoms and signs and, despite evidence that they are diagnosed earlier than they were, late diagnosis, with its potentially serious problem of blindness as well as irreversible changes in the heart in acromegaly and in the bones in Cushing's syndrome, remains a significant problem for general physicians and endocrinologists.

Treatment has been revolutionized in recent years. Often careful juxtaposition of all three main modalities of treatment, namely surgery, radiotherapy, and drugs, needs to be considered. We have a long way to go in order to improve the diagnosis and management of patients with pituitary tumours.

REFERENCES

Alexander L, Appleton D, Hall R, Ross WM, Wilkinson R (1980). Epidemiology of acromegaly in the Newcastle region. *Clinical Endocrinology*, 12:71–9.

Battershill PE, Clissold SP (1989). Octreotide, a review of its pharmacodynamic and pharmacokinetic properties, and therapeutic potential in conditions associated with excessive peptide secretion. *Drugs*, 38:658–702.

Cicarelli E, *et al.* (1987). Long-term treatment with oral single administration of bromocriptine in patients with hyperprolactinaemia. *Journal of Endocrinological Investigation*, 10:51–3.

Costello RT (1936). Subclinical adenoma of the pituitary gland. *American Journal of Pathology*, 12:205–16.

Doniach I (1977). Histopathology of the anterior pituitary. *Clinics in Endocrinology and Metabolism*, 6:21–52.

Harris PE, *et al.* (1988). Immunoreactive human chorionic gonadotrophin from the cyst fluid and CSF of patients with craniopharyngioma. *Clinical Endocrinology*, 29:503–8.

Jones AE (1991). Radiotherapy for pituitary tumours. *Clinical Endocrinology*, 35:379–97.

Kannan CR (1987). *The pituitary gland*, pp. 443–97. Plenum Medical, New York.

Kovacs K, Horvath E (1987). Pathology of pituitary tumours (1977). *Endocrinology and Metabolism Clinics of North America*, 16:529–51.

Molitch ME (1987). Pathogenesis of pituitary tumours. *Endocrinology and Metabolism Clinics of North America*, 16:503–27.

Moore KP, Wass JAH, Besser GM (1986). Late diagnosis of pituitary and parapituitary lesions causing visual failure. *British Medical Journal*, 293:609–10.

Ross RJM, *et al.* (1987). Treatment of growth hormone deficiency with growth hormone releasing hormone. *Lancet*, 1:5–8.

Trainer P, Grossman A (1990). The diagnosis and differential diagnosis of Cushing's syndrome. *Clinical Endocrinology*, 34:317–30.

Tsagarakis S, *et al.* (1990) Megavoltage pituitary irradiation in the management of prolactinomas: long term follow up. *Clinical Endocrinology*, 34:399–406.

Wass JAH (1984a). Prolactinomas. In *Advanced medicine* (ed. A Ferguson), pp. 282–92. Pitman, New York.

Wass JAH (1984b). Clinical presentation of acromegaly. In *Management of pituitary disease* (ed. PE Belchetz), pp. 123–40. Chapman and Hall, London.

Wass JAH, Besser GM (1989). Tests of pituitary function. In *Endocrinology* (2nd edn) (ed. LJ De Groot), pp. 492–502. W. B. Saunders, New York.

Wright AD, Hill DM, Lowy C, Russell-Fraser T (1970). Mortality and acromegaly. *Quarterly Journal of Medicine*, 39:1–16.

16.4   Adrenal tumours

ASHLEY GROSSMAN

ADRENOCORTICAL TUMOURS

Tumours arising from the adrenal cortex may be functioning or non-functioning, the latter being a not uncommon incidental finding on computerized tomography (**CT**) scanning. With increasing use of CT imaging, 1.6 per cent of tumours of the adrenal have been shown to be greater than 5 mm in diameter (Thompson and Cheung 1987). The majority of these are single cysts or non-functioning adenomas, while functioning tumours of the zona glomerulosa and fasciculata give rise to Conn's and Cushing's syndromes, respectively. Virilizing or feminizing tumours, probably arising from the zona reticularis, are extremely rare. In addition, CT imaging will not differentiate between tumours arising from the adrenal cortex and the adrenal medulla.

Cushing's syndrome

Pathology and biology

Cushing's syndrome is due to an adrenal adenoma in 10–30 per cent of cases and, like pituitary-dependent Cushing's syndrome (Cushing's disease), has a marked female preponderance of approximately 5 : 1. There is no clear evidence for any aetiological feature in its production, although recent work has indicated that certain of the peptides co-secreted with adrenocorticotrophic hormone from the common precursor pro-opiomelanocortin may be growth factors for the adrenal cortex. These include fragments cleaved from the N-terminus of adrenocorticotrophic hormone derived from pro-γ-melanocyte stimulating hormone. One model for this process is the rare condition of adrenal micronodular hyperplasia, where it appears that a basophil tumour, secreting adrenocorticotrophic hormone and its related peptides, progresses to semi-autonomous adrenal function, akin to tertiary hyperparathyroidism. However, any putative role for pituitary peptides in this progression must be initiating rather than sustaining, as such peptides eventually become undetectable in the circulation. Other growth factors, such as epidermal growth factor, may also be important (Reed and James 1989). Adrenal adenomas may occur at any age. Histologically, the tumours are usually small and encapsulated and typically consist of abundant cells of zona fasciculata type, with an admixture of more compact zona reticularis-type cells (Neville and O'Hare 1985; Fig. 1a).

Clinical features

The clinical features of Cushing's syndrome have been described elsewhere and there are no features that specifically define an adrenal adenoma. Benign adenomas are usually pure secretors of cortisol, but components of the syndrome apparently due to mineralocorticoid excess (hypertension, hypokalaemia) may also be present. We have also seen female patients presenting with virilization, so it is clear that such clinical factors alone do not point to the underlying pathology. However, the increasing pigmentation noted in some patients with the ectopic adrenocorticotrophic hormone syndrome is not seen.

Investigation

As in other cases of Cushing's syndrome, the principal diagnostic tests are the low- and high-dose dexamethasone suppression tests. In the low-dose test, dexamethasone 0.5 mg is given orally at intervals of exactly 6 h for 48 h, while with the high-dose test, 2 mg dexamethasone is used instead. The tests may be performed sequentially (Trainer and Grossman 1991). While the original description of Liddle involved the measurement of urinary steroid metabolites, we prefer to measure 09.00 h serum cortisol at the beginning and end of each test: in our laboratory a normal response to low-dose dexamethasone is an 09.00 h cortisol of less than 50 nmol/l, while 'normal' suppression by high dose is defined as a relative fall of 50 per cent or more. Patients with adrenal adenomas causing Cushing's syndrome show a failure of suppression by either test (Howlett et al. 1985). The differential diagnosis is usually between other causes of Cushing's syndrome. In Cushing's disease, 80 per cent of patients will demonstrate suppression by high-dose dexamethasone, while in the ectopic adrenocorticotrophic hormone syndrome a similar pattern of both low- and high-dose resistance is usually seen (Howlett et al. 1986). However, these may be readily differentiated from adrenal tumours by measurement of plasma adrenocorticotrophic hormone, which is persistently undetectable by conventional assays in all patients with adrenal adenomas. Patients with adrenal adenomas show no change in cortisol following administration of corticotrophin-releasing factor (CRF-41) (Grossman et al. 1988), but this is rarely necessary. We no longer use the metyrapone test (Howlett et al. 1986). Confirmation and localization of the tumour is by means of CT scanning (Fig. 2(a)). For the exceptionally rare patient with 'ectopic' adrenal adenomas, arising from nests of cells in the gonads, iodocholesterol isotope scans may be helpful.

Management

The treatment of choice is surgery, preferably by a thoracolumbar approach. Unless the cortisol hypersecretion is very mild, we prefer to lower the elevated levels with the 11-hydroxylase inhibitor metyrapone for several weeks, in order to render surgery more safe and expedite wound healing. In our assay, a mean daily cortisol of 150–300 nmol/l produces rapid resolution of the clinical stigmata, although there may be a transient exacerbation of virilization prior to operation. Post-operatively, it is essential to realize that the contralateral adrenal will be atrophic and may take from weeks to years to recover. It is therefore important to cover the surgical procedure with hydrocortisone 100 mg six-hourly for 2–3 days and thereafter maintain the patient on prednisolone. In our experience, prednisolone 5 mg in the morning and 2.5 mg in the evening (not enteric-coated, which is variably absorbed) is sufficient to keep the patient in good health and allow for gradual recovery of the hypothalamo–pituitary–adrenal axis. It is probable that the delay in recovery of the hypothalamo–pituitary–adrenal axis is either hypothalamic or pituitary, such that priming with adrenocorticotrophic hormone treatment to hasten adrenal responsiveness is rarely

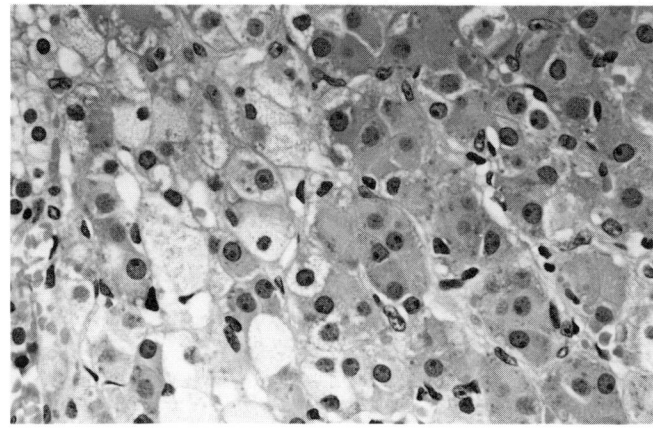

(a)

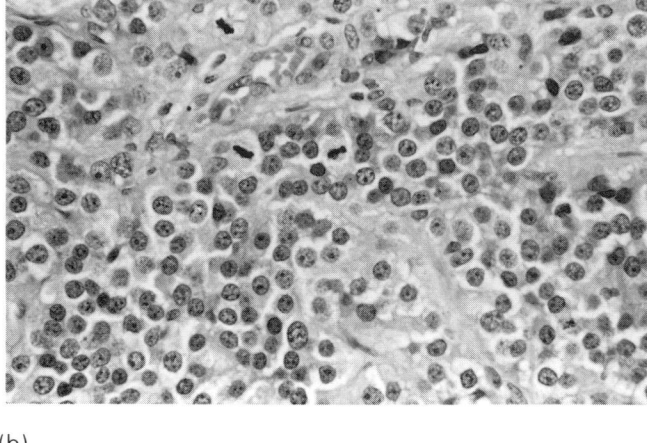

(b)

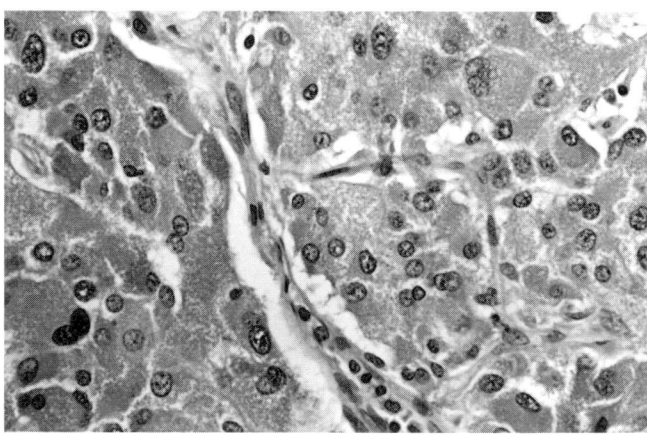

(c)

Fig. 1 High-power photomicrographs of three adrenal tumours. Each is stained with haematoxylin and eosin and is magnified ×400. (a) Adrenal adenoma causing Cushing's syndrome. Note the admixture of compact and other lipid-laden cells. The patient was cured by unilateral adrenalectomy. (b) Lymph node metastasis from an adrenal carcinoma causing Cushing's syndrome. There is nuclear pleomorphism with several mitoses in this section. In spite of metastatic disease at the time of diagnosis, the patient survived for 10 years on mitotane (o,p'DDD) therapy. (c) Adrenal phaeochromocytoma. The finely granular cytoplasm is indicative of plentiful chromaffin granules. All sections are reproduced with the permission of Mr P. Crocker and Professor I. Doniach.

effective. Until normalization of the hypothalamo–pituitary–adrenal axis is obtained, preferably demonstrated by a normal cortisol response to an insulin tolerance test, corticosteroid replacement should be increased during stress and full cover given during surgery. Appropriate diagnosis and surgical treatment of adrenal adenomas is associated with a cure rate of nearly 100 per cent and a normalized survival (Bertagna and Orth 1981).

Adrenal carcinoma

Approximately one-third of adrenal tumours associated with Cushing's syndrome are malignant, but this proportion is higher in childhood. The childhood and biochemical features are similar to those seen with benign adenomas, except that a variety of steroids in addition to cortisol may be secreted, especially androgens (for example, androstenedione, dehydroepiandrosterone-sulphate). Thus, virilization may be out of proportion to the severity of the Cushing's syndrome and other precursors, such as 11-deoxycortisol and deoxycorticosterone, may be present. Malignancy is also suggested by the size of the tumour: a mass greater than 100 g (approximately 6 cm in diameter) usually indicates an adrenal carcinoma and 50 per cent of these tumours may be palpable at presentation (Fig. 2(b)). Other features include evidence of local invasiveness and, most importantly, metastasis to bone, liver, lymph nodes, and lung. In cases of uncertainty, iodocholesterol isotope scanning tends to show little or no uptake in malignant tumours. Such tumours tend to show vascular invasion, nuclear pleomorphism, and plentiful mitoses (Fig. 1(b)). However, in the final analysis, malignancy may

only be definitively diagnosed by metastatic spread. We have seen one patient in whom an adrenal tumour was associated with cervical lymphadenopathy, but in whom the lymph node biopsy was equivocal; in this case, demonstration of the high cortisol concentration of the lymph node confirmed the diagnosis of metastatic disease and, hence, of adrenal carcinoma. The mainstay of treatment is with the adrenolytic drug o,p'DDD (mitotane). This is not only effective in lowering serum cortisol levels, albeit slowly over a period of weeks to months, but has direct tumoricidal properties (Bergenstal *et al.* 1960; Hutter and Kayhoe 1966). It has been reported that the drug is associated with dose-limiting side-effects, such as nausea and somnolence, but it has recently been realized that these are predominantly due to contamination with dichlorodiphenyl-trichloroethane (DDT). A pure form of o,p'DDD is available from Roussel Laboratories and, in our experience, in the majority of cases patients can receive up to 10 g daily without problems. However, tumour regression, as opposed to control of steroid excess, is usually limited to under 1 year (Gutierrez and Crooke 1980) and probably does not influence survival. Metyrapone can be used temporarily to obtain immediate normalization of cortisol levels although doses of 4–6 g daily may be necessary. When neither drug is effective, either separately or in combination, the antifungal agent ketoconazole (400–1200 mg daily in divided doses) may be added cautiously, although it may induce hepatitis (McCance *et al.* 1987; Sonino 1987). Untreated, the median survival in adrenocortical carcinomas is less than 3 months. Our current plan is to surgically debulk adrenal carcinomas as far as possible, and

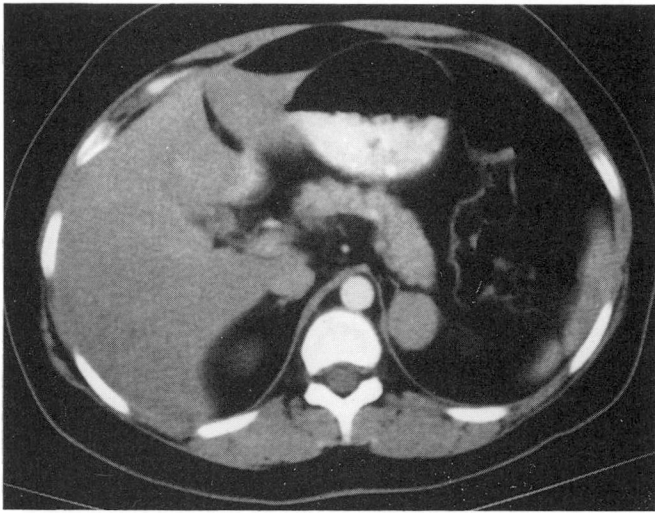

(a)

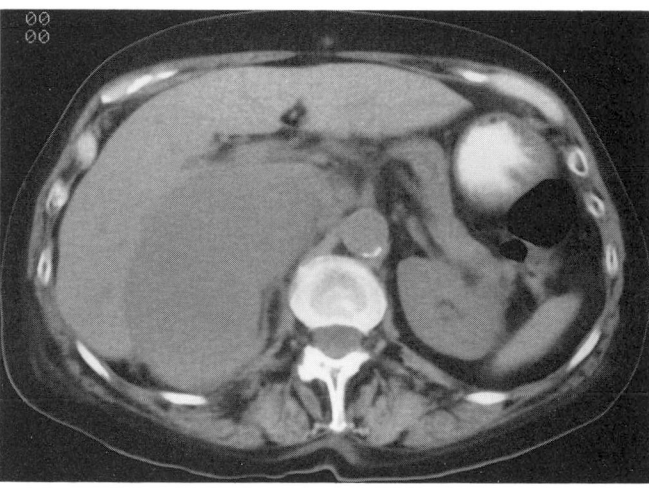

(b)

Fig. 2 CT scans of (a) a left-sided adrenal adenoma and (b) a massive right-sided adrenal carcinoma, both associated with the clinical and biochemical features of Cushing's syndrome.

then use as high a dose as possible of mitotane (up to 10 g daily) as a long-term chemotherapeutic agent. Radiotherapy to the tumour bed may also be used, although whether this is worthwhile, particularly with metastatic disease, is unclear. However, even with this combination of treatments, long-term survival is poor, with a 2 year survival of less than 50 per cent and a published 5 year survival of 31 per cent (Hajjar *et al.* 1975). Other chemotherapy regimes are of unproven value, as is suramin. More recently, the natural cotton seed derivative, gossypol, has been shown to induce partial responses in patients refractory to other forms of therapy (Flack *et al.* 1993) and clearly warrants further investigation.

Conn's syndrome

Aldosterone-producing adrenal adenomas are an uncommon cause of hypertension, but their ready accessibility and cure by surgery suggests that they should always be kept in mind as a curable form of hypertension. However, the differential diagnosis of a true adenoma as opposed to idiopathic hyperaldosteronism can be

extremely difficult and may tax even the most experienced workers in this field.

In spite of greatly varying claims, the current consensus is that approximately 1 per cent of unselected hypertensives have aldosteronism, some 75 per cent of these being due to an adrenal adenoma. The majority of the rest have idiopathic hyperaldosteronism, with only very exceptional patients having aldosterone-secreting adrenal carcinomas. There is an approximately 2 : 1 female : male incidence in adrenal adenomas, which may occur throughout life but congregate in the age range 30–50 years and have a slight tendency to occur preferentially on the left; by contrast, idiopathic hyperaldosteronism is seen predominantly in men in later life, usually over the age of 50 years. There are no known aetiopathological features (Neville and O'Hare 1982).

The typical Conn's tumour is a small (less than 4 g), well-encapsulated tumour, which may lie entirely within the adrenal cortex and is golden-yellow in colour. Microscopically, the tumours tend not to be homogeneous, with an admixture of lipid-laden, zona glomerulosa-type and zona fasciculata-type cells. As in adrenal tumours associated with other hypersecretory states, occasional tumours with abundant lipofuscin may appear as 'black adenomas'. Generally speaking, the heterogeneous nature of the cell population and some degree of nuclear and cellular pleomorphism, tends to distinguish aldosterone-secreting adenomas from non-functioning nodules.

Patients with Conn's syndrome classically present with the triad of hypertension, hypokalaemic alkalosis, and muscle weakness. However, the latter may only be apparent on direct questioning and it is therefore prudent to investigate any unmedicated patient with hypertension and hypokalaemia (plasma potassium less than 3.5 nmol/l in a fresh unhaemolysed sample). The hypokalaemia may also give rise to other symptoms and signs, including paraesthesiae and tetany and those secondary to nephrogenic diabetes insipidus. There are cases recorded of patients with Conn's syndrome and normokalaemia but it is certainly impractical to screen for these by means of aldosterone and renin measurements in large populations. Having established hypokalaemia, the second stage is to establish the presence of hyperaldosteronism: basal supine aldosterone and renin should be measured by a laboratory interested in such assays, as there are a variety of different renin assays (renin concentration, renin activity, etc.) which have specific methods of sample collection and storage. Normal ranges may also differ and are differentially affected by age, pregnancy, etc., according to the specific assay. In general, a very low or undetectable renin level demands further investigation. A normal plasma renin in the absence of treatment essentially excludes aldosteronism, regardless of the level of serum aldosterone; conversely, aldosterone levels may or may not be frankly elevated in proven Conn's syndrome. It is now well established that idiopathic hyperaldosteronism is part of the spectrum of 'low renin hypertension' and does not appear to be a disorder *sui generis*. It is therefore most important that it is differentiated from a Conn's adenoma, the primary therapy of which is surgical. A variety of stimulation and suppression tests have been devised, few of which are suitable for routine use (Drury 1985). Basal levels of potassium, renin, or aldosterone are poor discriminators, although a plasma potassium below 2.5 mmol/l is rare in idiopathic hyperaldosteronism. Perhaps the best biochemical test is the response of serum aldosterone to 4 h ambulation between the hours of 8 a.m. and 12 p.m.; ambulation produces a rise in aldosterone (by angiotension II) in normal subjects and in many patients with idiopathic hyperaldosteronism, while a fall is strongly suggestive of an adenoma (in Conn's adenomas, aldosterone appears to be partially under the control of circadian changes in adrenocorticotrophic hormone). There is also evidence that Conn's adenomas show specifically high levels of 18-hydroxy-corticosterone, but this assay is not generally available. Imaging by means of CT scanning is now the investigation of choice and, with the newer high-resolution machines, more than 90 per cent of Conn's adenomas are localized accurately. Initial encouraging results with isotope scanning have not been realized in larger studies, although increasing investigation of newer radionuclides, such as 6-iodomethyl 19-norcholesterol, may increase the sensitivity and specificity of this technique. Due to the small size of most Conn's adenomas, venography, arteriography, and ultrasound are rarely diagnostic. In most instances the aldosterone response to posture and the results of CT scanning are sufficient to identify an adenoma and allow the patient to proceed to surgery. Where there is a residual uncertainty, venous catheterization with sampling of both adrenal veins for aldosterone levels is a rapid diagnostic manoeuvre in experienced hands. This is best carried out transfemorally and should include the examination of simultaneous cortisol (or preferably catecholamine) samples to ensure placement within the adrenal veins (Drury 1985).

In terms of treatment, some authorities advise a 6–12 week course of spironolactone (200–400 mg daily) to demonstrate normalization of blood pressure and plasma potassium and, thus, confirm the diagnosis. However, it then remains unclear as to how to proceed when there is an obvious adenoma and only a poor response to spironolactone. We believe that such preparation is useful to replete body potassium stores and increase the safety of surgery, but would advise adenomectomy in all instances when there are no other contraindications. A flank approach is less traumatic than a midline incision and is generally appropriate as the tumours are small and intra-adrenal. However, bilateral adenomas have been reported. Post-operatively, the patient may require careful monitoring for the first few days for rebound hyperkalaemia. The extremely rare Conn's carcinoma may respond, at least temporarily, to mitotane (o,p'DDD).

Feminizing tumours

Just under 10 per cent of adrenal tumours are feminizing, producing oestrogenic steroids such as oestradiol, oestrone, and oestriol. The great majority (90 per cent) of such tumours are seen in the male, usually in those aged 25–45 years, but this may be an overestimate as signs of hyperoestrogenism are clearly more subtle in women than in men. Clinically, such tumours present in males with evidence of gynaecomastia and other evidence of hypogonadism, such as poor libido and potency, and genital atrophy; in females isosexual precocity may be seen in childhood, although regular menstruation will not be achieved. In elderly women there may be the acute onset of post-menopausal bleeding. The elevated levels of oestrogens are usually unresponsive to endocrine manipulation, such as adrenocorticotrophic hormone stimulation or dexamethasone suppression and may be associated with elevated levels of other steroids such as cortisol and 11-deoxycortisol.

Feminizing tumours of the adrenal are almost always malignant, with an equal preference for the left or right glands. The occasional benign adenoma tends to be reported in childhood. Pathologically, the tumours tend to show necrosis with occasional calcification and are usually relatively large (> 1 kg); over half may be palpable at presentation. As is the case for cortisol-producing tumours, there are few histological criteria which clearly differentiate benign from malignant lesions and the microscopic appearances bear little relation to the type of steroid produced. On the whole, adenomas are much

smaller than carcinomas, but the ultimate distinction is related to the presence of metastases, which may not be obvious at presentation. Thus, apart from small prepubertal tumours, all should be regarded as malignant, regardless of size or histology (Neville and O'Hare 1982, 1985).

The prognosis must be considered as poor, with little agreement as to the optimal therapy. It would be reasonable to attempt surgical debulking, possibly followed by radiotherapy to the tumour bed. There are few data available to suggest whether either non-specific cytotoxic chemotherapy or mitotane are useful options; where the excessive feminization is clinically problematic, tamoxifen may be cosmetically useful.

Virilizing tumours

Virilizing adrenal tumours may present at any age, but tend to be more common in childhood, with 75 per cent occurring in females. There is a slight preponderance in the left-hand gland (Neville and O'Hare 1982). Clinically, girls may present with virilization such as clitoromegaly, hirsutism, and accelerated growth, while in adults oligomenorrhoea and increased muscle mass is seen. We have found that deepening of the voice in adult women is a useful and ominous clinical sign.

The differential diagnosis is usually between congenital adrenal hyperplasia in young girls and the polycystic ovary syndrome in adult females. In congenital adrenal hyperplasia, the increased adrenal androgens are associated with an elevated plasma adrenocorticotrophic hormone and 17-α-OH-progesterone and all will suppress to within or below the normal range following the low-dose dexamethasone suppression test (see above). In women with the polycystic ovary syndrome, the virilization and menstrual irregularity almost always date from puberty and are progressive: in virilizing tumours, the onset is more acute and tends to follow normal menstruation. Androgens are also generally higher in adrenal tumours. In our experience, when there is residual uncertainty a venous catheter with sampling for the elevated androgen from the adrenal and ovarian veins is the investigation of choice, in association with CT scanning of adrenals and ultrasound scanning of the ovaries. Patients with the polycystic ovary syndrome have elevated levels of androgens arising from both adrenals and ovaries, although the relative proportions vary in individual patients.

In men, symptoms may be minimal, but boys may show isosexual precocity with a lack of the expected testicular enlargement.

Functionally, such tumours usually secrete a variety of adrenal androgens, particularly the so-called delta-5 steroids such as dehydroepiandrosterone-sulphate, as well as testosterone and androstenedione. A more mixed pattern, often combined with glucocorticoid and mineralocorticoid excess, is seen in the older patient with a malignant tumour. Steroid output is generally unresponsive to dexamethasone, a factor of importance in distinguishing these tumours from congenital adrenal hyperplasia and the polycystic ovary syndrome, but may occasionally rise in response to stimulation with adrenocorticotrophic hormone or human chorionic gonadotrophin.

Small lesions are more often benign than larger lesions, but the distinction is much less clear-cut than is the case for cortisol-producing adrenal tumours and even very large tumours may be functionally benign (Kirk *et al.* 1990). These tumours tend to be well encapsulated, with areas of necrosis and haemorrhage increasing with tumour size. Clear, lipid-laden cells are relatively uncommon, but individual cell necrosis (apoptosis) is frequent. The diagnosis of malignancy is extremely difficult, especially as mitotic figures are not often seen: capsular or vascular invasion may be a helpful pointer. Clinically, these tumours seem to occur along a spectrum of malignancy, with even clearly malignant tumours growing slowly and metastasizing late. Thus, prognosis and response to treatment are very difficult to quantitate in these rare tumours. Surgical debulking, with or without radiotherapy, is the first requirement, while mitotane has been reported to be useful on occasion. Signs and symptoms of virilization may also regress with cyproterone acetate (50–200 mg daily) in patients with residual or recurrent disease. However, it should be emphasized that, at present, there is no effective tumouricidal agent for malignant tumours.

ADRENOMEDULLARY TUMOURS

Tumours of the adrenal medulla are not especially rare and are important both in terms of their protean manifestations and their usually ready accessibility to cure if treated early. The prototypic tumour, the phaeochromocytoma, appears to arise from mature adrenomedullary tissue, but forms part of a continuum with other tumours derived from related neuroectoderm tissue, either mature or embryonal. Embryologically, sympathogonia are the most primitive cells and differentiate into either neuroblasts or phaeochromoblasts: the former develop further into sympathetic ganglion cells, the latter into mature phaeochromocytes, that is, normal adrenomedullary tissue. Tumours may develop at any of these stages, forming neuroblastomas, ganglioneuromas, and phaeochromocytomas. Neuroblastomas are tumours of early childhood and will not be further discussed here; phaeochromocytomas are the most common tumours of neural-crest origin developing in adult life and will be discussed in detail, while the much rarer ganglioneuroma will be touched on only briefly.

Phaeochromocytomas

Pathology and biology

Catecholamine-secreting tumours of the adrenal have exerted a continuing fascination over the medical imagination ever since the first one was removed from a patient by Charles Mayo in 1927. Recent work has suggested that nerve growth factor is involved in the normal growth and development of adrenomedullary tissue and changes in nerve growth factor or its receptor are particularly likely to be involved in the phaeochromocytomas associated with neurofibromatosis. In addition, extensive study of the immortalized adrenal tumour PC-12 has increased our knowledge of the biosynthetic pathways of such cells (Lindenbaum *et al.* 1988), although the presumptive derangement in autocrine or intracine regulation in phaeochromocytomas remains unclear.

Phaeochromocytomas have an approximate incidence of 1 : 100 000 patients/year, with an equal sex incidence and an age spread at diagnosis which includes every decade but peaks in the third to fifth decades. In selected groups the incidence is likely to be higher and may be approximately 0.1–0.5 per cent in hypertensives and 1 per cent in patients with neurofibromatosis. Autopsy studies have suggested that up to 85 per cent of patients are undiagnosed in life and in many of these the tumour is likely to have been a proximate cause of death (Beierwaltes 1985; Krane 1986). Commonly known as the '10 per cent tumour', some 10 per cent of phaeochromocytomas are bilateral and 10 per cent are malignant; 10–15 per cent are extra-adrenal, particularly in the organs of Zuckerkandl (around the aortic origin of the inferior mesenteric artery), pelvis, and bladder. A small minority of these extra-adrenal tumours, best referred to as functional paragangliomas, occur above the diaphragm in the

mediastinum, in the lungs, and around the carotid sheath. Bilateral tumours are common in the multiple endocrine neoplasia syndrome type 2 (MEN 2), when they may be associated with primary hyperparathyroidism and medullary carcinoma of the thyroid. In this situation the tumours may be preceded by adreno-medullary hyperplasia, with spread of medulla to the tail of the adrenal, but this should not otherwise be diagnosed. Phaeochromocytomas as a feature of MEN 2 or other syndromes such as neurofibromatosis, von Hippel–Lindau, Sturge–Weber, or Bourneville's disease may be more likely in children or young adults.

Phaeochromocytomas are usually benign adenomas, containing sheets of homogeneous cells which are frequently basophilic because of their neurosecretory granules (Fig. 1(c)). These cells are referred to as 'chromaffin' as they stain brown with conventional stains and may be further identified as containing reducing substances, the catecholamines, by appearing golden-yellow with dichromate. The granules contain dopamine, noradrenalin and adrenalin, ATP, large peptides of unknown function known as chromogranins, the enzyme dopamine-β-hydroxylase, and a whole variety of neuropeptides such as enkephalins (Yanase *et al.* 1987), endorphins, vasoactive intestinal polypeptide, CRF-41, and vasopressin. The function of these peptides is unclear, but they may either modulate the release of the catecholamines or modify their effects on end-organs. Pathophysiologically, certain of the clinical and biochemical features of phaeochromocytomas not readily ascribable to catecholamines (such as changes in bowel habit, flushing, hypercalcaemia) may be secondary to neuropeptide hypersecretion. Certainly, blockade of opiate receptors with naloxone in patients with phaeochromocytomas (Mannelli *et al.* 1986) or functional paragangliomas (Bouloux *et al.* 1986) enhances catecholamine release, suggesting the presence in tumour tissue of functioning inhibitory opiate receptors.

The enzyme mediating the conversion of noradrenalin to adrenalin, phenylethylamine-N-methyltransferase, is subject to induction by corticosteroids at high concentrations: as the adrenal medulla is downstream to the venous effluent of the adrenal cortex, phenylethylamine-N-methyltransferase is readily induced in the normal adrenal, producing a preferential synthesis of adrenalin, with adrenal vein ratios of adrenalin : noradrenalin of 4–10 : 1. However, in adrenomedullary tumours, growth of the tumour leads to a progressive decrease in local corticosteroid concentrations and, hence, a fall in the adrenalin : noradrenalin ratio. This is especially true in extra-adrenal tumours. Thus, in all but the smallest phaeochromocytomas there is a selective secretion of noradrenalin; this is particularly pertinent when measuring adrenal vein catecholamine levels in cases of suspected bilateral tumours (see below).

The 10 per cent of phaeochromocytomas which are malignant cannot be diagnosed with any certainty histologically. Furthermore, metastatic spread from malignant phaeochromocytomas must be differentiated from functional paragangliomas, especially when these are multifocal. It is therefore evident that the diagnosis of a malignant phaeochromocytoma must be made with considerable circumspection, although modern scanning techniques with agents such as metaiodobenzylguanidine (see below) suggest that these are less rare than previously considered.

Clinical features

The diverse ways in which these tumours may present are well described; patients with phaeochromocytomas may initially present themselves to any specialty. However, the great majority have symptoms of headache, palpitations, and sweating, which are often (but not always) paroxysmal, with a variable neuropsychiatric component of anxiety and occasionally psychosis or dementia. During attacks, which may be precipitated by certain foods, posture, or even, in the case of bladder phaeochromocytomas, micturition, pallor and hypertension are notable clinical signs. However, approximately 50 per cent of patients present with sustained rather than intermittent hypertension. Flushing is rarely a manifestation of a phaeochromocytoma and, when present, more commonly indicates some other ectopic humoral or carcinoid-type syndrome. These may occur together and there are documented cases of adrenal tumours secreting catecholamines, adrenocorticotrophic hormone, and even CRF-41 (Jessop et al. 1987); changes in bowel habit (Sackel 1985) and hypercalcaemia may also be associated. Patients may often appear hypermetabolic, thin, and agitated and clearly the differential diagnosis must include thyrotoxicosis. Phaeochromocytoma may be particularly difficult to diagnose during pregnancy, when changes in uterine position are liable to induce clinical paroxysms. The elevated catecholamines may give rise to hyperglycaemia and occasionally glycosuria and also lead to intense vasoconstriction. This, in turn, produces relative polycythaemia (absolute polycythaemia may also occur, secondary to ectopic secretion of an erythropoietin-like factor). The decrease in intravascular volume may produce dizziness as a manifestation of postural hypotension, which may be exacerbated by the injudicious use of β-blockers. Finally, the combination of meteoric hypertension plus grossly elevated catecholamines may be associated with a catecholamine myocarditis, which manifests as tachyarrhythmias or congestive cardiac failure. However, in spite of these features, it should be emphasized that the clinical examination is frequently not diagnostic and investigation is usually required on the basis of a suggestive personal or family history or other features of syndromes associated with phaeochromocytomas.

Investigation

The principal diagnostic considerations are 2-fold: to prove autonomous catecholamine secretion and then to demonstrate the source. The first of these criteria has proved most taxing to clinical science over the past 50 years. Measurement of urinary catecholamines and their metabolites has been the mainstay of diagnosis over this time, with improvements in biochemical and biophysical techniques gradually increasing the sensitivity and specificity of state-of-the-art assays. Unfortunately, these improvements in possible techniques have not been generally paralleled by their increased availability to the practising clinician, such that many physicians are still reliant on imprecise and outmoded biochemistry.

Vanillylmandelic acid is the final metabolite of the catecholamines and is usually assayed on a 24 h acidified urine collection by a spectrophotometric technique. The assay is simple and readily available, but false-positives may be seen in patients on a high vanillin diet: such foods include bananas, coffee, and nuts. More importantly, the false negative rate is 30–35 per cent (Bravo et al. 1979), rendering this test completely unsuitable for routine screening. Urinary metanephrines have a lower false-negative rate, especially if fractionated into normetanephrine and metanephrine, but this involves a difficult and time-consuming radioenzymatic assay. More recently, it has been suggested that urinary free noradrenalin, measured by means of gas chromatographic–mass spectrometric analysis, provides the best discriminant for the diagnosis of phaeochromocytoma (Duncan et al. 1988), with 100 per cent sensitivity and 98 per cent specificity. Unfortunately, the methodology is not readily available, but high-performance liquid chromatography with electrochemical detection may offer similar results with more easily accessible equipment and technology. In

our experience, the measurement of total urinary adrenalin and noradrenalin by this technique has produced no false-negatives in the diagnosis of phaeochromocytoma, although levels above the normal range may be seen in patients with acute debilitating non-endocrine illness (Ross et al. 1993). These patients may be discriminated from true phaeochromocytomas by means of post-suppression plasma catecholamine samples (see below).

In order to avoid the problems associated with urine collection (incomplete samples, home collection, and contamination), developments in assay technology have permitted the direct measurement of plasma catecholamines, originally by expensive and tedious radioenzymatic assays and more recently by high-pressure liquid chromatography with electrochemical detection. The disadvantages of these assays is that plasma levels may be normal between paraoxysms (false-negatives) or high due to anxiety and sympathetic overactivity (false-positives). The former are indeed problematic, but are fortunately rare; provocation tests with tyramaine (1 mg intravenously), glucagon (1 mg intravenously), histamine (0.025–0.05 mg intravenously), or naloxone (10 mg intravenously; Bouloux et al. 1986) may be used, but are not without risk and are now rarely necessary. The converse problem of physiological hypersecretion may be tackled by administration of either the ganglion blocker, pentolinium (2.5 mg intravenously) or clonidine (0.3 mg orally), which will suppress physiologically elevated catecholamine levels to within the normal range. Neither test is ideal (Burris and D'Angelo 1982; Taylor et al. 1986), but the pentolinium test at least has the advantage of rapidity and out-patient utility. Our current procedure is therefore to screen all suspected phaeochromocytomas for urinary catecholamines and to measure plasma catecholamine pre- and post-pentolinium in all cases where urine levels are borderline or high. With a suitably modified extraction technique (Ross et al. 1990), urine and plasma samples can be analysed sequentially with the same apparatus.

For tumour localization, and further confirmation of the diagnosis when the biochemistry is inconclusive, the imaging techniques of choice are currently CT and metaiodobenzylguanidine scanning. The former has a sensitivity approaching 80 per cent, but may miss very small or extra-adrenal lesions; where the suspicion of a phaeochromocytoma is high, most authorities would advise full-blockade before scanning with contrast (Fig. 3). The metaiodobenzylguanidine isotope scan makes use of the fact that metaiodobenzylguanidine is highly selectively taken up into adreno-medullary tissue and will demonstrate functional hyperactivity in phaeochromocytomas with a specificity of near 100 per cent (although some carcinoid tumours may also take up the isotope) and a sensitivity of 85–90 per cent (Shapiro et al. 1985; Fig. 4). The use of metaiodobenzylguanidine has also demonstrated the much increased prevalence of extra-adrenal tumours (38 per cent; Cheung et al. 1988), tumours which were probably not previously diagnosed in life. Drawbacks to metaiodobenzylguanidine are expense, poor resolution (better with the [123]I- than with the ^{131}I-labelled compound; Lynn et al. 1985), and the fact that quantitation is difficult. As the normal adrenal is not suppressed in the presence of a phaeochromocytoma, this renders the diagnosis of bilateral phaeochromocytomas particularly difficult. However, there is no doubt that the combined judicious use of CT and metaiodobenzyl-guanidine scanning will diagnose the vast majority of catecholamine-secreting tumours (Cheung et al. 1988). Further localization of extra-adrenal tumours may be obtained by selective venous catheterization with assay of plasma samples (Jones et al. 1979; Miller et al. 1983), while with bilateral adrenal tumours the noradrenalin : adrenalin ratio will be unity or greater in both adrenal

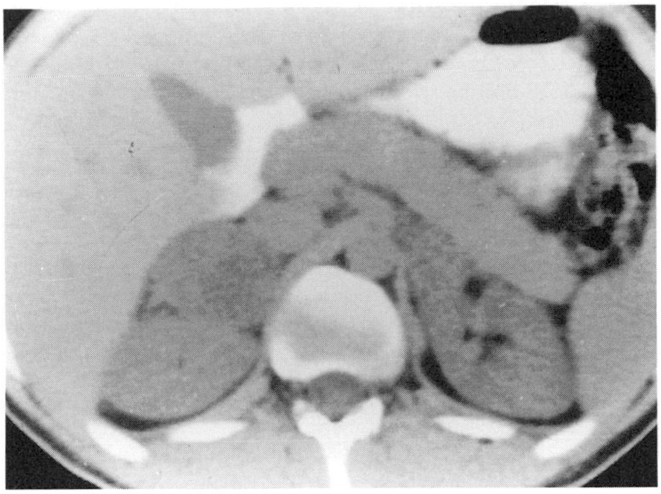

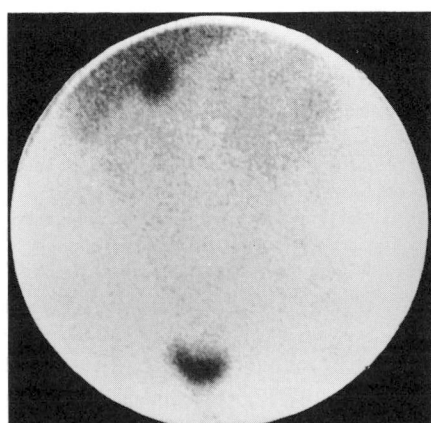

Fig. 3 CT scan of a large right-sided and smaller left-sided adrenal phaeochromocytoma. The presence of bilateral phaeochromocytomas was confirmed on adrenal vein catheterization for catecholamines and both tumours were removed from this patient with von Hippel–Lindau disease.

veins (Newbould *et al.* 1990). It is possible that magnetic resonance imaging (MRI) with gadolinium enhancement will localize more difficult cases, particularly if utilizing T_2-weighted images (Cockroft *et al.* 1987).

Management

All patients must be given full α-adrenoceptor blockade prior to any invasive investigation and particularly before surgery. We use phenoxybenzamine, 0.5 mg/kg in 200 ml N saline by intravenous infusion for 2 h, repeated daily to a total of three infusions, followed by oral phenoxybenzamine adjusted according to blood pressure (usually 40–80 mg daily in divided doses). Any marked fall in blood pressure is soon compensated for by volume expansion. Further addition of β-blockade with propranolol can be added as necessary. It has been suggested that the combined α/β-blocker labetalol is as effective, but we prefer to stay with a well-tried combination and labetalol may interfere with certain of the catecholamine determinations. Careful pre-operative tumour localization and good

Fig. 4 [^{123}I]Metaiodobenzylguanidine isotope scan of a patient with a single right-sided adrenal phaeochromocytoma. The excretion of the isotope by the bladder is shown, as well as hepatic uptake.

adrenoceptor blockade should render surgery completely safe, although nitroprusside should be available in the operating theatre and post-removal plasma expanders may be necessary. No particular surgical approach is mandatory, but for small adrenal tumours, especially on the left, a thoracolumbar approach may be preferred. Post-operatively, the blood pressure may remain elevated for several weeks following complete removal, possibly due to increased stores of catecholamines in normal sympathetic tissues. In a small proportion of patients it may remain elevated in the long term. Surgical mortality is now extremely low with adequate preparation and, thus, complete cure is the rule (Stenstrom *et al.* 1988).

Malignant phaeochromocytoma

While the vast majority of benign phaeochromocytomas are readily curable by surgery, the outlook for malignant tumours is much less sanguine. Principally diagnosed in terms of metastatic spread, these tumours are being seen more commonly since the advent of metaiodobenzylguanidine scanning (Shapiro *et al.* 1984). Blood-pressure control is usually obtained as above, with combined α- and β-blockade; in resistant cases, α-methylparatyrosine, which blocks the rate-limiting enzyme in catecholamine synthesis, tyrosine hydroxylase, can be useful. In long-term use, α-methylparatyrosine can cause parkinsonism. Malignant tumours more frequently have increased excretion of dopamine, which is a vasodilator and, thus, hypotensive, such that hypertension may, paradoxically, be less problematic in these patients (Tippett *et al.* 1986). There is no consensus as to definitive therapy aimed at the tumour, but limited success has been achieved with chemotherapy, including cyclophosphamide, doxorubicin, vincristine, and dacarbazine (Keiser *et al.* 1985). More recently, high-dose [^{131}I]metaiodobenzylguanidine has been used therapeutically and we have two patients who are presently alive more than 5 years after metaiodobenzylguanidine therapy for their malignant tumours (Bomanji *et al.* 1993). Dosage regimens have not been clearly established and are highly empirical, but this offers considerable promise for the future, although it should be emphasized that such therapy is mainly palliative and rarely curative. At present, the published figure for 5 year survival is a little less than 50 per cent, but many tumours run a slow and indolent course.

Ganglioneuromas

These are rare tumours arising from sympathetic ganglion cells, which may form a continuum with neuroblastomas and neuroepitheliomas. It seems likely that in the occasional long-term childhood survivor from neuroblastoma, the tumour has differentiated into the more mature and benign ganglioneuroma. There are few data regarding age or sex incidence, but the two cases we have seen recently were in a young woman and man in their second and third decades, respectively. Both patients were normotensive and asymptomatic and the abdominal mass was diagnosed by CT and metaiodobenzylguanidine scanning; urinary noradrenalin and dopamine were slightly elevated in the young woman. Both tumours were easily removed surgically and there is currently no evidence of metastatic disease. Thus, the limited evidence suggests that a CT mass which takes up metaiodobenzylguanidine but is associated with normal or minimally elevated urinary catecholamines may be a ganglioneuroma: we would still advise full adrenoceptor blockade (see above) before operative intervention.

CONCLUSIONS

In an unselected autopsy series, it has been shown that approximately 1 per cent of a previously normotensive population has functionless adrenal tumours greater than 8 mm in diameter and approximately the same proportion appears incidentally on CT scans performed for other reasons. As CT scanning becomes increasingly frequent in clinical investigation, it is obvious that the clinician will frequently be faced with the problem of patients with such 'incidentalomas' (Thompson and Cheung 1987). With small tumours of less than 3 cm diameter and in the absence of the clinical features of Cushing's syndrome, hypertension, virilization, or feminization, it is likely that the tumour is non-functioning and, therefore, clinically unimportant. The best diagnostic screen for Cushing's syndrome and a virilizing tumour is the low-dose dexamethasone suppression test, with measurement of serum cortisol and androgens, respectively. In the presence of hypertension, if plasma potassium and plasma or urinary catecholamines are normal *when the patient is hypertensive*, the hypertension is unlikely to be due to a phaeochromocytoma. However, as many phaeochromocytomas are only diagnosed at autopsy and 60 per cent of incidental adrenal masses are functional phaeochromocytomas, if there is any residual uncertainty, there should be a low threshold for a metaiodobenzylguanidine scan (Beierwaltes 1985). Adrenocortical carcinomas are almost always large at presentation, such that a small well-circumscribed lesion is rarely important. However, follow-up repeat CT or MR scanning at intervals is probably a reasonable safeguard.

REFERENCES

Beierwaltes WH (1985). A new method of identifying pheochromocytoma and proving that a "mass" is a "pheo". *Journal of Urology*, **134**:105.

Bergenstal DM, Hertz R, Lipsett MB, Moy RH (1960). Chemotherapy of adrenocortical cancer wth o,p'DDD. *Annals of Internal Medicine*, **53**:672–82.

Bertagna C, Orth DN (1981). Clinical and laboratory findings and results of therapy in 58 patients with adrenocortical tumours admitted to a single medical center (1951–1978). *American Journal of Medicine*, **71**:855–75.

Bomanji J, Britton KE, Ur E, Hawkins L, Grossman AB, Besser GM (1993). Treatment of malignant phaeochromocytoma, paraganglioma and carcinoid tumours with ^{131}I-metaiodobenzylguanidine. *Nuclear Medicine Communications*, **14**:856–61.

Bouloux PMG, Grossman A, Besser GM (1986). Naloxone provokes catecholamine release in phaeochromocytomas and paraganglioneuromas. *Clinical Endocrinology*, **24**:319–25.

Bravo EL, Tarazi RC, Gifford RW, Stewart BH (1979). Circulating and urinary catecholamines—diagnostic and pathophysiologic implications. *New England Journal of Medicine*, **301**:682–6.

Burris JF, D'Angelo LJ (1982). Complications of clonidine suppression test for pheochromocytoma. *New England Journal of Medicine*, **307**:756–7.

Cheung PSY, Thompson NW, Dmuchowski CF, Sisson JC (1988). Spectrum of pheochromocytoma in the ^{131}I-MIBG Era. *World Journal of Surgery*, **12**:546–51.

Cockroft JR, *et al.* (1987). Location of extra-adrenal catecholamine secreting tumours by selective venous sampling and nuclear magnetic resonance scanning. *Postgraduate Medical Journal*, **63**:451–4.

Drury PL (1985). Disorders of mineralocorticoid activity. *Clinics in Endocrinology and Metabolism*, **14**:175–202.

Duncan MW, Compton P, Lazarus L, Smythe GA (1988). Measurement of norepinephrine and 3,4-dihydroxyphenylglycol in urine and plasma for the diagnosis of pheochromocytoma. *New England Journal of Medicine*, **319**:136–42.

Flack MR, *et al.* (1993). Oral gossypol in the treatment of metastatic adrenal cancer. *Journal of Clinical Endocrinology and Metabolism*, **76**:1019–24.

Grossman AB, *et al.* (1988). CRF in the differential diagnosis of Cushing's syndrome: a comparison with the dexamethasone suppression test. *Clinical Endocrinology*, **29**:167–78.

Gutierrez ML, Crooke ST (1980). Mitotane (o,p'-DDD). *Cancer Treatment Reviews*, **7**:49–55.

Hajjar RA, Hickey RC, Samaan NA (1975). Adrenal cortical carcinoma. *Cancer*, **35**:549–54.

Howlett TA, Rees LH, Besser GM (1985). Cushing's syndrome. *Clinics in Endocrinology and Metabolism*, **14**:911–45.

Howlett TA, *et al.* (1986). Diagnosis and management of ACTH-dependent Cushing's syndrome: comparison of the features in ectopic and pituitary ACTH production. *Clinical Endocrinology*, **24**:699–713.

Hutter AM, Kayhoe DE (1966). Adrenal cortical carcinoma: results of treatment with o,p'DDD in 138 patients. *American Journal of Medicine*, **41**:581–92.

Jessop DS, *et al.* (1987). A phaeochromocytoma presenting with Cushing's syndrome associated with increased concentrations of circulating corticotrophin-releasing factor. *Journal of Endocrinology*, **113**:133–8.

Jones DH, Allison DJ, Hamilton CA, Reid JL (1979). Selective venous sampling in the diagnosis and localisation of phaeochromocytoma. *Clinical Endocrinology*, **10**:179–86.

Keiser HR, *et al.* (1985). Treatment of malignant pheochromocytoma with combination chemotherapy. *Hypertension*, **7**:18–24.

Kirk JMW, Perry LA, Kirby RS, Besser GM, Savage MO (1990). Female pseudohermaphroditism due to a maternal adrenocortical tumour. *Journal of Clinical Endocrinology and Metabolism*, **70**:1280–4.

Krane NK (1986). Clinically unsuspected pheochromocytomas. *Archives of Internal Medicine*, **146**:54–7.

Lindenbaum MH, *et al.* (1988). Transcriptional and post-transcriptional effects of nerve growth factor on expression of the three neurofilament subunits in PC-12 cells. *Journal of Biological Biochemistry*, **25**:5662–7.

Lynn MD, *et al.* (1985). Pheochromocytoma and the normal adrenal medulla: improved visualization with I-123 MIBG scintigraphy. *Radiology*, **156**:789–92.

McCance DR, *et al.* (1987). Clinical features with ketoconazole as a therapy for patients with Cushing's syndrome. *Clinical Endocrinology*, **27**:593–9.

Mannelli M, *et al.* (1986). Opioid modulation of normal and pathological human chromaffin tissue. *Journal of Clinical Endocrinology and Metabolism*, **62**:577–82.

Miller JL, Immelman EJ, Roman TE, Mervis B (1983). Phaeochromocytoma of the urinary bladder localised by selective venous sampling and computed tomography. *Postgraduate Medical Journal*, **59**:533–5.

Neville AM, O'Hare MJ (1982). *The human adrenal cortex*. Springer-Verlag, Berlin.

Neville AM, O'Hare MJ (1985). Histopathology of the human adrenal cortex. *Clinics in Endocrinology and Metabolism*, **14**:791–820.

Newbould EC, *et al.* (1991). The use of venous catheterisation in the diagnosis and localisation of unilateral and bilateral phaeochromocytomas. *Clinical Endocrinology*, **35**:55–9.

Reed MJ, James VHT (1989). Regulation of steroid synthesis and metabolism by growth factors. *Clinical Endocrinology*, **31**:511–25.

Ross GA, Newbould EC, Grossman A, Perrett D (1990). Analysis of plasma and urinary catecholamines using a single LC–EC system. *Journal of Pharmaceutical and Biomedical Analysis*, **8**:1039–43.

Ross GA, Newbould EC, Thomas J, Bouloux PMG, Besser GM, Perrett D, Grossman A (1993). Plasma and 24 h-urinary catecholamine concentrations in normal and patient populations. *Annals of Clinical Biochemistry*, **30**:38–44.

Sackel SG, Manson JE, Harawi SJ, Burakoff R (1985). Watery diarrhea syndrome due to an adrenal phaeochromocytoma secreting vasoactive intestinal polypeptide. *Digestive Diseases and Sciences*, **30**:1201–7.

Shapiro B, *et al.* (1984). Malignant phaeochromocytoma: clinical biochemical and scintigraphic characterization. *Clinical Endocrinology*, **20**:189–203.

Shapiro B, *et al.* (1985). Iodine-131 metaiodobenzylguanidine for the locating of suspected pheochromocytoma: experience in 400 cases. *Journal of Nuclear Medicine*, **26**:576–85.

Sonino N (1987). The use of ketoconazole as an inhibitor of steroid production. *New England Journal of Medicine*, **317**:812–18.

Stenstrom G, Ernest I, Tisell L-E (1988). Long-term results in 64 patients operated upon for pheochromocytoma. *Acta Medica Scandinavica*, **223**:345–52.

Taylor HC, Mayes D, Anton AH (1986). Clonidine suppression test for pheochromocytoma: examples of misleading results. *Journal of Clinical Endocrinology and Metabolism*, **63**:238–42.

Thompson NW, Cheung PSY (1978). Diagnosis and treatment of functioning and nonfunctioning adrenocortical neoplasms including incidentalomas. *Surgical Clinics of North America*, **67**:423–36.

Tippett PA, McEwan AJ, Ackery DM (1986). A re-evaluation of dopamine excretion in phaeochromocytoma. *Clinical Endocrinology*, **25**:401–10.

Trainer PJ, Grossman A (1991). The diagnosis and differential diagnosis of Cushing's syndrome. *Clinical Endocrinology*, **34**:317–30.

Yanase T, *et al.* (1987). Preproenkephalin A-derived opioid peptides and mRNA of preproenkephalin A in human pheochromocytomas. *Molecular and Cellular Endocrinology*, **51**:237–41.

16.5 Neuroendocrine gastroenteropancreatic tumours

DAVID WYNICK, JULIA M. POLAK, AND STEPHEN R. BLOOM

INTRODUCTION

Gastroenteropancreatic tumours are rare and usually slow growing. Many secrete a variety of peptides causing associated clinical syndromes. Symptoms are usually caused by the secreted peptides rather than by tumour bulk alone until an extremely late stage in the disease.

Tumour classification

Gastroenteropancreatic tumours are classified according to their secretory products and this appropriately imposes a functional rather than morphological categorization. However, some tumours may be clinically silent if the peptides they produce are not biologically active or if they secrete no peptides at all. Others may produce a number of peptides and, thus, the clinical presentation may be a mixed picture or one clinical syndrome may predominate.

Frequency

Gastroenteropancreatic tumours are rare (less than 1 per 100 000 of the population) and with the exception of carcinoid tumours are found most commonly in the pancreas. This apparent rarity may, in part, reflect a failure of diagnosis mainly because of relatively little knowledge about these lesions and past lack of appropriate laboratory diagnostic tests. Over the last decade, the techniques of radio-immunoassay and immunocytochemistry have greatly aided the detection and clinical management of the tumours, thus increasing the chances of cure or better palliation.

It is not known why some tumours, such as carcinoid, insulinoma, and gastrinoma, appear to be relatively common whilst others, such as glucagonoma, VIPoma, and somatostatinoma, are extremely rare.

Histology

The histological features of peptide-producing endocrine tumours of the gut and pancreas are often similar and in most instances the tumours are composed of round or polygonal cells with a clear finely granulated cytoplasm (Fig. 1). Connective tissue strands and blood vessels are often seen dividing the tumour, whereas necrotic and haemorrhagic areas are rarely seen. Mitotic activity may often vary but is usually minimal. With the development of more accurate diagnostic techniques, tumours with a mixed population of

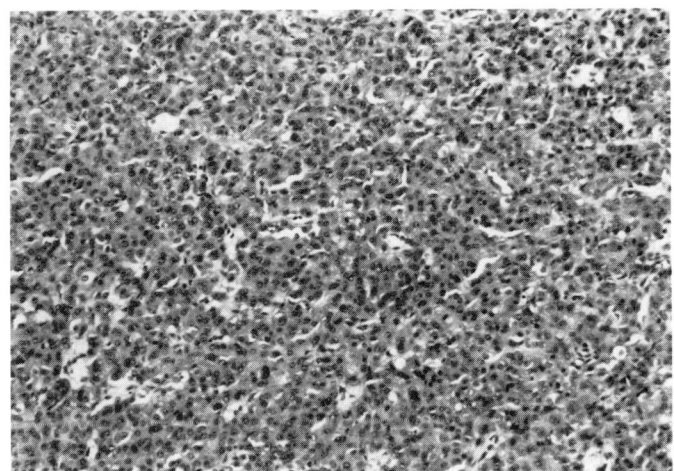

Fig. 1 Pancreatic tumour composed of sheets and cords of small round regular tumour cells with round nuclei (haematoxylin and eosin). Magnification 180×.

neoplastic cells and highly anaplastic cytological features can now be classified as being endocrine in origin.

Electron microscopy

The presence of electron-dense secretory granules with different characteristics which depend on the cell type is often diagnostic of secretory tumours and the morphology of the granules is frequently indicative of the peptide products stored in the tumour.

Histochemistry and immunocytochemistry

Different histochemical stains have been used to reveal the endocrine activity of neoplastic tissue. Among these, lead haematoxylin and particularly silver impregnation still represent reliable diagnostic methods. However, these techniques are sometimes difficult to interpret, particularly when tumour granulation is poor. Immunocytochemical techniques represent a major step forward in this respect. Using a wide variety of specific antibodies to many peptides, many of which are now available commercially (Fig. 2), it is possible to localize various peptides to neoplastic cells and to quantitate and characterize their chemical nature by such techniques as radio-immunoassay, chromatography, and *in situ* hybridization.

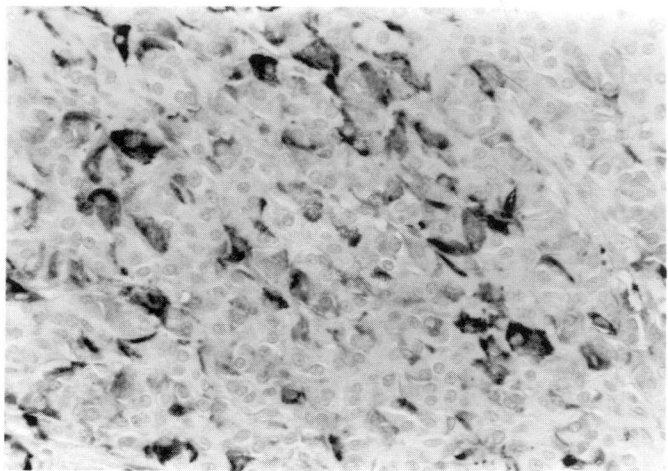

Fig. 2 Individual tumour cells with a positive reaction for vasoactive intestinal polypeptide. Magnification 500 × .

Radio-immunoassay

Measurement of a tumour product by radio-immunoassay is considered to be an important step in the diagnostic management of patients with endocrine tumours. The detection of abnormal levels of peptides in the blood stream is considered essential to the diagnosis in addition to the clinical syndrome. Nevertheless, the bioactivity of the tumour product is not always related to the amount as measured by the radio-immunoassay, since tumours may secrete a wide variety of peptides of heterogeneous molecular form, many of which are biologically inactive. Similarly, radio-immunoassay using a specific antibody may fail to detect a non-cross-reacting peptide despite the fact that it has comparable biological function; for example, insulin-like growth factors (IGF-1 and IGF-2) may cause hypoglycaemia and parathyroid hormone-related peptides may cause hypercalcaemia.

Tumour markers

Despite the number of gastroenteropancreatic syndromes, many of the tumours contain and secrete pancreatic polypeptide, 7B2, chromogranins, and the protein neurone-specific enolase which thus act as tumour markers charting the progress of the disease and its response to treatment.

Malignancy

With the exception of insulinomas, most pancreatic endocrine tumours are malignant although slow growing. With proper treatment patients may survive for years, even in the presence of hepatic metastases.

CLINICAL SYNDROMES

There are few signs and symptoms that are completely diagnostic of pancreatic endocrine tumours. The commonest symptoms are vague malaise, abdominal discomfort, weight loss, and diarrhoea. Clinical suspicion is usually raised when the commoner causes of these symptoms are excluded.

Plasma levels of various peptides may be raised in non-malignant conditions such as gastrin in achlorhydria and renal failure and glucagon in conditions such as hypoglycaemia. Care has to be exercised to exclude these common causes before making the diagnosis of a gastroenteropancreatic tumour.

Insulinoma

The islets of Langerhans are a cluster of endocrine cells distributed throughout the exocrine pancreas and represent approximately 1 per cent of its mass. Four types of cells (A, B, D, and PP) can be distinguished by their respective locations within the islets and by their size, shape, and hormone content. All four cell types may develop into gastroenteropancreatic tumours. Insulinoma, glucagonoma, and somatostatinoma are associated with distinct clinical syndromes; however, this is not the case with PP-secreting tumours.

Shortly after Banting and Best discovered insulin in 1922, they and their co-workers described hypoglycaemia associated with insulin excess. This led others to postulate that patients with spontaneous hypoglycaemia may suffer from insulin excess. This prediction was confirmed in 1927 when W. J. Mayo performed what was probably the first resection of a metastatic islet cell carcinoma of the pancreas in a physician with hypoglycaemic symptoms. Extracts from this tumour, when injected into rabbits, caused profound hypoglycaemia.

Clinical features

The incidence of insulinoma is approximately one per million of the population. Insulinomas have been reported in patients of all ages from the newborn to the very elderly. The peak incidence is between 40 and 60 years and the sex ratio is equal. All patients diagnosed as having an insulinoma should also be checked for other endocrine disturbances, since beta or non-beta cell adenomas may be associated with the other inherited endocrine neoplasias included in the multiple endocrine neoplasia type 1 (MEN-1) syndrome. Approximately 90 per cent of insulinomas are benign and the patient can be cured by their complete surgical removal.

Diagnosis

Since insulin is a potent hormone, clinical symptoms are noticed early when the tumours are still extremely small. The diagnosis should be suspected in any patient with recurrent hypoglycaemic attacks. Although the symptoms of hypoglycaemia are often easily discernible, they can manifest themselves in a bizarre fashion with a typical epileptic seizure or even neuropsychiatric symptoms mimicking temporal lobe epilepsy. The diagnosis requires hypoglycaemia and plasma insulin concentrations that are inappropriately elevated in relation to the hypoglycaemia.

Gastrinoma

Two patients with non-beta islet cell tumours of the pancreas believed to be producing a potent gastric secretagogue were reported in 1955. It was later shown that this tumour product was probably gastrin. It became apparent that patients with such tumours produced large volumes of gastric acid-rich secretions which could not be controlled by vagotomy.

Clinical features

Whilst gastrinoma is uncommon, it is not as rare as first believed. The diagnosis can now be made earlier in patients with ulcer or ulcer-like symptoms, as well as unexplained diarrhoea, with the advent of specific and routinely available radio-immunoassay. Approximately one-third of patients with the gastrinoma syndrome have MEN-1. At least 50 per cent of gastrinomas are malignant and 60–70 per cent of patients have metastases at the time of presentation.

Diagnosis

Elevated serum gastrin levels in the presence of high levels of free hydrochloric acid in the stomach are essential to the diagnosis of the gastrinoma. However, serum gastrin levels may also be elevated by gastric achlorhydria, pernicious anaemia, atrophic gastritis, renal failure, and raised serum calcium, emphasizing the need for basal and stimulated acid secretion studies in all patients in whom the diagnosis is suspected.

Glucagonoma

Clinical features

The first well-documented case of glucagon-secreting islet cell tumour was described in 1966 when a patient presented with diabetes mellitus, skin rash, and a pancreatic tumour. Mallinson *et al.* (1974) described the complete syndrome, reporting nine cases of dermatitis, diabetes mellitus, weight loss, anaemia, and an α-cell tumour of the pancreas.

The incidence is approximately one per 10–15 million of the population. Peak incidence is in the sixth decade of life and the syndrome has not been reported in children.

Patients present with the typical skin rash of necrolytic migratory erythema (Fig. 3), thus making glucagonoma the only pancreatic endocrine tumour that can be diagnosed with reasonable certainty on clinical grounds. Skin lesions usually start in the groin or the perioral area. Initially the lesions are flat and scaly; later they become raised and bullous and finally crust over. Healing results in hyperpigmentation and induration of the skin; in addition, most patients have atrophic glossitis. Low epidermal and dermal levels of amino acids and zinc are probably involved in the pathogenetic mechanisms causing the rash, since similar lesions occur in patients with advanced protein malabsorption and children suffering from the inherited condition of low plasma zinc acrodermatitis enteropathica.

Diagnosis

Most patients with a glucagonoma have mild to moderate glucose intolerance. Patients are best controlled with insulin, since many

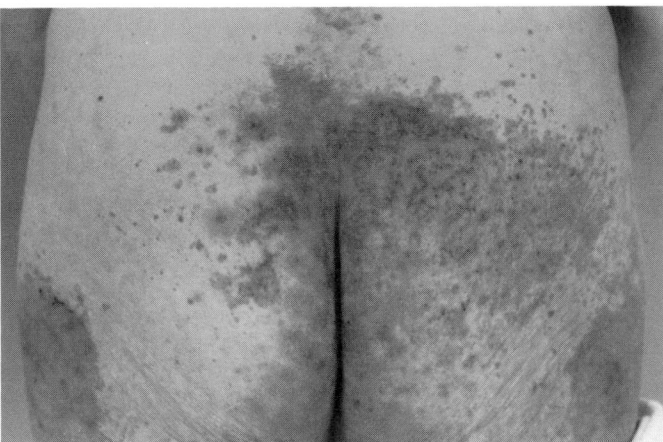

Fig. 3 Glucagonoma rash in a woman with a malignant pancreatic tumour and liver metastases.

of the tumours are partially responsive to the negative feedback of hypoglycaemia and therefore glucagon levels may be reduced if blood sugars are well controlled.

Severely depressed plasma levels of nearly all amino acids are a constant and reliable feature in patients with glucagonoma. Other associated features are normochromic normocytic anaemia, weight loss, and thromboembolic disease and it is this last feature that may often kill the patient. Anticoagulation is advised, although to date no large study has been published showing a true benefit in terms of a reduction in associated morbidity and mortality. The diagnosis is made on clinical grounds and from the finding of an elevated plasma pancreatic glucagon. However, it should be noted that renal or hepatic insufficiency, hypoglycaemia, and the use of the steroid danazol may all produce a raised glucagon.

All glucagonomas reported so far have been solitary and more than 90 per cent of patients present with metastases to the liver with very large tumour bulk. Asymptomatic tumours are usually small (0.4–2 cm) and benign. Symptoms only develop after the tumour has reached a large size and plasma glucagon levels have risen to high levels.

VIPoma syndrome

VIPomas are almost always malignant and, in the adult, pancreatic in origin. However, vasoactive intestinal peptide (VIP) may also be secreted, particularly in childhood, by ganglioneuroblastomas and phaeochromocytomas.

Clinical features

Patients usually present with intermittent or continuous watery diarrhoea, hypokalaemia, and achlorhydria (WDHA syndrome or the Verner–Morrison syndrome). Commonly, there is also dehydration, weakness, abdominal pain, and weight loss, but, unlike gastrinoma, steatorrhoea is absent. The severity of the hypokalaemia and metabolic acidosis is proportional to the frequency of the diarrhoea and not to plasma levels of VIP. Achlorhydria is present in approximately 50 per cent of cases because of suppression of gastric acid secretion by VIP, but it is not a diagnostic criterion. Less commonly, hypercalcaemia and hypophosphataemia may occur owing to association with the MEN-1 syndrome or direct secretion from the pancreatic tumour of parathyroid hormone (PTH) or a PTH-like peptide.

Diagnosis

There is now little doubt that VIP is not merely a marker but, along with a co-secreted peptide (peptide histidine valine) derived from the same precursor molecule, is the actual mediator of the VIPoma syndrome. The diagnosis of VIPoma is made when an appropriate clinical picture is seen in association with raised fasting VIP and peptide histidine valine levels. Multiple molecular forms of VIP and peptide histidine valine are found in both the plasma and tumour extracts of these patients and often a considerable proportion of the plasma immunoreactivity is of a larger molecular size.

Other peptides secreted by neuroendocrine tumours

As well as containing the α- and β- cells, the islet of Langerhans also contains two other cell types, the D-cells which produce somatostatin and the pancreatic polypeptide cells which produce pancreatic polypeptide (PP). Therefore, is is not surprising to find some pancreatic endocrine tumours producing large quantities of somatostatin and/or pancreatic polypeptide. In approximately half the cases of somatostatinomas the patients suffer no clinical symptoms; the rest usually present with diabetes mellitus, gallstones, and low acid output with some weight loss. These tumours are believed to be the slowest growing of all pancreatic neuroendocrine tumours, since patients who have had diabetes mellitus for as long as 25 years may then be found to have a somatostatinoma and return to euglycaemia with no abnormality of oral glucose tolerance after the tumour is resected. At presentation the tumour bulk may be considerable, making it difficult to completely resect.

While the somatostatinoma produces relatively mild clinical symptoms, the pancreatic tumour secreting pancreatic polypeptide produces none. Indeed, elevation of plasma pancreatic polypeptide is usually picked up as an incidental finding in patients suffering from excess production of one of the other pancreatic tumour hormones.

In approximately 10 per cent of VIPomas plasma neurotensin is also found to be elevated and one or two patients appear to have a 'pure neurotensinoma'. Depsite the fact that neurotensin physiologically causes increased secretions from the intestinal wall and in large doses encourages defecation, those patients with pure neurotensin-secreting tumours are asymptomatic. Thus, it seems that the effect of neurotensin is relatively weak or that down-regulation of receptors rapidly occurs in the presence of continuously elevated hormonal levels. A whole range of other peptides secreted by neuroendocrine pancreatic tumours with the appropriate clinical syndromes have been described in the literature. They include adrenocorticotrophic hormone, corticotrophin-releasing factor, calcitonin, and growth-hormone-releasing factor.

Carcinoid tumours

In 1909 the term *Karzinoid* was first used to describe a morphological distinct class of intestinal tumours that behaved less aggressively than the more common adenocarcinoma. The first clinical description of the carcinoid syndrome dates back to 1890 when Ransom described a patient with an ileal carcinoma and multiple metastases who experienced diarrhoea and dyspnoea induced by eating. Since then these tumours have been characterized by their argentaffin properties and Lembeck demonstrated the presence of serotonin in tumours in 1953. The rapid progress in immunohistochemical techniques during the last 15 years has allowed the determination of a large range of peptides stored within carcinoid tumours. However, most tumours are clinically silent and must therefore be classified according to morphological and biochemical characteristics rather than clinical features.

Carcinoid tumours are derived from the diffuse neuroendocrine system and characteristically demonstrate agentaffin and argyrophilic reactions. Carcinoid tumours are classified according to site of origin as foregut, midgut, and hindgut; endocrine tumours of the respiratory tract and pancreas are foregut carcinoids.

Approximately 85 per cent of the carcinoid tumours develop in the gastrointestinal tract, 10 per cent in the lung, mostly as bronchial carcinoids, and the rest in other organs such as the larynx, kidney, ovary, prostate, and skin. The most frequent location in the gastrointestinal tract is the appendix followed by the rectum and the ileum. The survival rate of patients with the carcinoid depends on the growth rate of the tumour and the presence of metastases at diagnosis. The main site of metastases are lymph nodes in the mesentery, liver, lung, and peritoneum. Five year survival depends entirely on the site of the primary tumour and is 99 per cent for carcinoids of the appendix regardless of stage and 75 per cent for

localized carcinoids of the small intestine, but only 54 per cent if all stages are considered.

Morphology

Carcinoid tumours are easily identified by light microscopy because of their uniform round cell nuclei and regular growth pattern. Foregut carcinoids exhibit a grimelius reaction, whereas almost all gut carcinoids also show an argentaffin reaction indicating that the cells contain 5-hydroxytryptamine (5-HT). Most of the classic syndromes related to the overproduction of gastrointestinal and pancreatic hormones originate from the bronchial system, pancreas, duodenum, or upper jejunum. Many of the foregut carcinoids contain peptide-producing cells. However, the amounts of hormones secreted are presumably so low that no clinical symptoms are produced and the increased hormone levels are often not detectable in the plasma. Similarly, a variety of gastrointestinal hormones and neuropeptides have been found in the gastric carcinoids, but rarely is there a corresponding endocrine disease present.

In contrast with the wide range of hormones found in foregut and hindgut tumours, midgut carcinoids contain a small variety of endocrine cells. They produce mainly 5-HT, substance P, and other tachykinins, which can be used as markers for these tumours.

Carcinoid syndrome

Although carcinoids have been known for nearly 100 years, the clinical symptoms of an endocrine disorder related to these tumours were described as recently as 1953. Despite the improved diagnostic methods now available, recognition of clinical syndromes related to hormone production by carcinoids is extremely rare. The clinical symptoms of the carcinoid syndrome are flushing, diarrhoea, abdominal pain, and cardiac lesions, followed by asthma and oedema. Episodic or permanent flushing is a clinical hallmark of the syndrome. Whilst the whole spectrum of symptoms was originally believed to be related to the production and secretion of 5-HT by the tumour metastases, it is now realized that, although 5-HT and its metabolites are often raised in such patients, the disease symptomatology cannot be due to 5-HT secretion alone. The exact pathogenesis of many of the symptoms of the carcinoid syndrome remains unexplained.

TUMOUR LOCALIZATION

Since in the carcinoid syndrome a reduction in tumour bulk may give many months, if not years, of disease-free life, tumour localization is extremely important. A combination of ultrasound, high-resolution CT scanning, and highly selective visceral angiography will localize between 85 and 92 per cent of pancreatic tumours (Fig. 4). If the patient has a clinical syndrome with elevated plasma levels of the appropriate hormone and yet localization is not possible, it is generally considered appropriate to repeat the localization tests every 2–3 years. Newer techniques of localization, including radio-isotope tags to specific antibodies and peptides such as long-acting somatostatin analogues, intraoperative ultrasound, and magnetic resonance image scanning, have yet to be fully evaluated.

TREATMENT

The treatment of gastroenteropancreatic tumours follows the same general principles as that of any other malignancy with certain additional considerations.

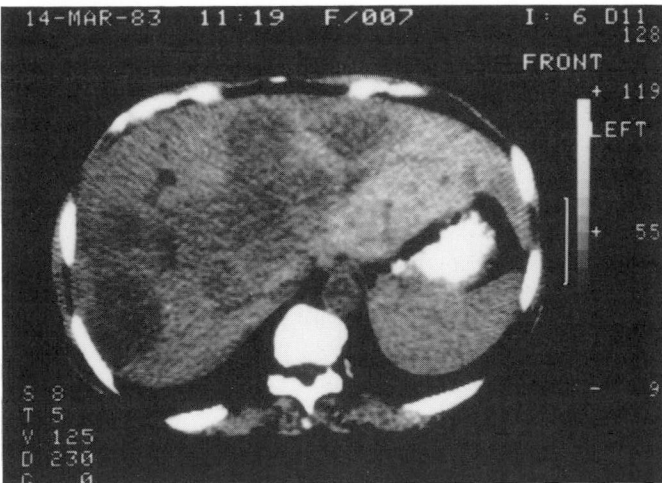

Fig. 4 Multiple liver metastases in a man with a pancreatic VIPoma and liver secondaries

1. The plasma level of the peptide secreted by tumour is a reliable index of tumour status and, hence, can be monitored after any treatment to assess the response.

2. Since the tumours themselves are slow growing, morbidity and even mortality are caused by the metabolic disturbance induced by the secreted peptide(s) rather than by tumour bulk alone.

Therefore, active treatment of such tumours and reduction of peptide secretion is worthwhile even when multiple metastases have occurred. Thus, long-term palliation may be achievable in many instances.

Surgery

Complete surgical excision is the only means of cure of such tumours. This is feasible in up to 90 per cent of insulinomas and may occasionally be appropriate for VIPoma and glucagonoma, although in such cases hepatic metastases usually occur even when laparotomy reveals a single lesion with no evidence of metastases 5 or even 10 years post-resection. As the majority of such gastroenteropancreatic tumours present with metastases, palliative surgery may be useful. This consists of debulking the primary tumour and the metastases since a decrease in tumour bulk will reduce peptide production and, hence, relieve symptoms.

Hepatic artery embolization

Good palliation may result from embolizing the hepatic artery supplying the liver metastases. This requires considerable expertise and the portal vein must be patent (Fig. 5) All patients become pyrexial and have striking increases in liver function test during the first post-embolization week. The median duration of response is 5 months (range 3–10 months). The procedure can be repeated a number of times when symptoms recur, provided that the portal vein remains patent.

Cytotoxic chemotherapy

Initial reports of chemotherapy in carcinoid (Moertel *et al.* 1980) using 5-fluorouracil and streptozotocin were encouraging, with a response rate for the islet cell carcinomas of 63 per cent compared with 25–30 per cent for the carcinoid. Subsequent studies using different dosage regimens of streptozotocin and

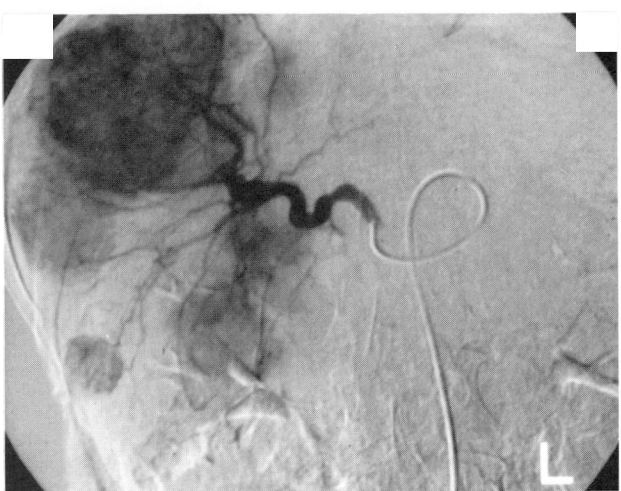

(a)

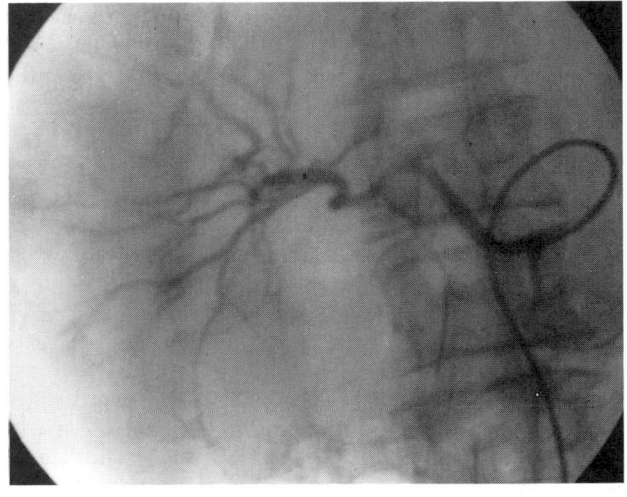

(b)

Fig. 5 Hepatic angiograms from a patient with multiple liver metastases: a pancreatic glucagonoma (a) before and (b) after hepatic artery embolization.

5-fluorouracil with or without the addition of vincristine or adriamycin have shown little improvement on these figures. VIPomas are particularly sensitive to chemotherapy with response rates as high as 80 per cent, but gastrinomas respond less well the figure being similar to that of the carcinoid syndrome. The median duration of palliation is 12–18 months. Various therapeutic regimes are currently being investigated. We use intravenous administration of 500 mg/m^2 streptozotocin and 400 mg/m^2 5-fluorouracil on alternate days for 10 days. This course is repeated every 2–3 months, with close monitoring of renal, hepatic, and bone-marrow function.

α-Recombinant interferon has been used predominantly by Oberg's group in Sweden (Oberg *et al.* 1986). Patients with the carcinoid syndrome were treated with daily doses of 3–6 million units. Ten of the 42 patients showed a response with a mean duration of 15 months; all ten patients showed a decrease in tumour markers but an objective reduction in tumour size was noted in only four of them. However, there were a considerable number of side-effects including influenza-like symptoms, bone-marrow depression, and liver fibrosis. It should also be remembered that hepatic

Somatostatin (SRIF)

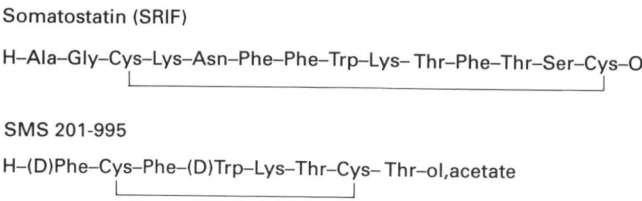

H–Ala–Gly–Cys–Lys–Asn–Phe–Phe–Trp–Lys– Thr–Phe–Thr–Ser–Cys–OH

SMS 201-995

H–(D)Phe–Cys–Phe–(D)Trp–Lys–Thr–Cys– Thr–ol,acetate

Fig. 6 Structures of somatostatin and its long-acting analogue octreotide (SMS 201–995).

metastases often undergo spontaneous necrosis, thus making any specific therapy difficult to evaluate.

Antisecretory therapy

Since somatostatin was first isolated more than a decade ago, it has been shown to be a potent inhibitor of peptide secretion in both the normal state and tumoral hypersecretion. However, the physiological half-life of somatostatin is only 3 min so that continuous intravenous administration is required. In 1982 a long-acting somatostatin analogue with a half-life of 113 min, which could be administered subcutaneously, was synthesized (Fig. 6). Antisecretory therapy with this analogue, octreotide (SMS 201–995), has now been used for over 10 years in both islet cell and carcinoid patients with good palliative results. The dose administered varied between 150 and 1500 μg per day. Over this time there has been no evidence of renal, hepatic, neurological, or haematological toxicity, although a mild deterioration in glucose tolerance, steatorrhoea, and the development of gallstones may be expected with long-term therapy.

Use of octreotide in the long-term treatment of pancreatic islet cell tumours has also been shown to be effective. Over the last 5 years we have treated seven patients with this analogue for up to 29 months (range 13–54 months). Treatment was initially very effective in all seven cases. Symptoms were improved or alleviated and the concentrations of tumour-related hormones were significantly reduced, although in no case did values return to normal (Fig. 7).

Worsening of symptoms and rising levels of tumour-related hormone concentrations occurred 5 months after the start of therapy and were initially reversed by increasing the dose of octreotide over a 6–12 month period to a maximum dose of 500 μg injected subcutaneously every 8 h. However, after 24 months at the maximum dosage symptoms recurred and were no longer responsive to a further increase in dosage of octreotide or other therapeutic measures.

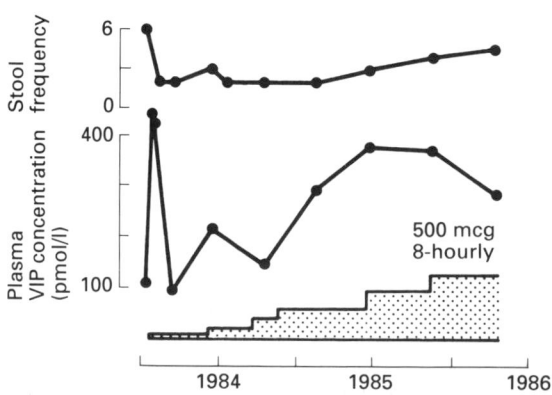

Fig. 7 Clinical progress of a patient with a VIPoma over 2.5 years, showing that increases in the dose of octreotide will suppress diarrhoea despite a rise of plasma VIP to pre-diagnosis levels.

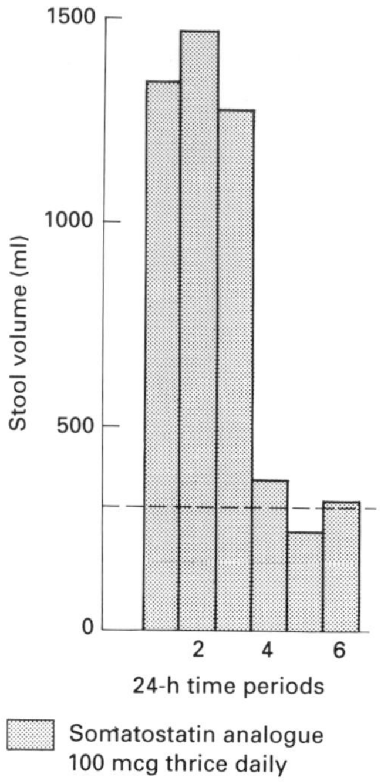

Fig. 8 Suppression of diarrhoea in a patient with the carcinoid syndrome using octreotide.

Therefore, it appears that a symptomatic response with good initial palliation is achieved for all gastroenteropancreatic tumours, but it decreases and eventually disappears. Death occurs within 6 months once this resistant phase of the illness has been reached.

Use of the analogue in the treatment of the carcinoid syndrome produces a prompt relief of flushing and diarrhoea (Fig. 8). More than 90 per cent of patients show a decrease in 24 h urine 5HIAA secretion. The mean duration of the biochemical response is 9 months (range 1–15 months).

Other treatments

Insulinoma

Dioxide is probably the most widely used drug when the tumour is inoperable or has not been located. Dioxide is a benzothiazide that raises blood sugar by directly inhibiting insulin release via α-adrenergic stimulation, enhancement of glycogenolysis, and by inhibition of cAMP phosphodiesterase. To prevent sodium retention it is usually given with a diuretic. Side-effects of dioxide include gastrointestinal irritation, hypertrichosis, and occasional hypotension if given intravenously.

Gastrinoma

Omeprazole, a substituted benzimidizole, is now in common usage. It is a non-competitive proton pump inhibitor and inhibits hydrogen potassium ATPase in the gastric mucosa. It is extremely effective in doses of 80–120 mg a day given orally and will reduce the basal acid output to less than 5 mmol/h within 48 h of therapy in almost all gastrinoma patients. More than 95 per cent of ulcers in gastrinoma patients will heal within 2 weeks on therapy and provided that treatment is maintained symptoms do not recur. The theoretical risk that permanent hypergastrinaemia may stimulate gastric carcinoids is not of relevance in gastrinoma where the gastrin is already grossly elevated.

Glucagonoma

In addition to specific chemotherapy, hepatic artery embolization, and the use of octreotide, other therapeutic measures include oral and topical zinc for the rash, amino acid supplementation, and blood transfusions.

VIPoma

Again, chemotherapy, hepatic artery embolization, and octreotide are the main treatment modalities. Other palliative measures include electrolyte support during an acute exacerbation. If these measures fail, high-dose steroids (40–60 mg prednisolone per day) may sometimes be effective in controlling symptoms and reducing plasma VIP, although this is generally a temporary effect and symptoms usually recur within 6 months.

Carcinoid syndrome

Parachlorophenylalanine has been shown to relieve diarrhoea and reduce urine 5-HIAA excretion. However, flushing is rarely helped. The side-effects of this agent are predominantly hypersensitivity reactions and psychiatric disturbances, making it unsuitable for long-term use although occasionally a patient derives great benefit from it for a number of years. 5-HT antagonists may also be of benefit. Cyproheptadine and, more recently, ketanserine are of some use; these are directed against the diarrhoea and other abdominal symptoms but are not usually helpful in preventing flushing.

SUMMARY

The increase in the availability of radio-immunoassay and histochemistry for a large range of regulatory peptides has led to the description of an increasing number of different tumour types and clinical syndromes. However, the peptide secretions from the tumours are frequently mixed. Most tumours, except insulinomas, are malignant and metastases at the time of diagnosis make a surgical cure rare. Effective treatment regimens with cytotoxic agents, hepatic artery embolization, and the recently developed long-acting somatostatin analogue octreotide have provided useful palliation in otherwise terminal cases, allowing the patient to return home with a much improved quality of life.

REFERENCES

Adrian TE, Uttenthal LO, William SJ, Bloom SR (1986). Secretion of pancreatic polypeptide in patients with pancreatic and endocrine tumours. New England Journal of Medicine, 315:287–91.

Ajani JA, Carrasco CH, Charnsangavej C, Samaan NA, Levin B, Wallace S (1988). Islet cell tumors metastatic to the liver: effective palliation by sequential hepatic artery embolization. Annals of Internal Medicine, 108(3):340–4.

Alison DM (1978). Therapeutic embolisation. British Journal of Hospital Medicine, 20:707–15.

Alison DM, Modlin IM, Jenkins WJ (1977). Treatment of carcinoid liver metastases by hepatic artery embolisation. Lancet, ii:1323–5.

Anderson JV, Bloom SR (1986). Neuroendocrine tumours of the gut: long-term therapy with the somatostatin analogue SMS 201-995. Scandinavian Journal of Gastroenterology, 21(Suppl. 119):115–28.

Axelrod L, Bush MA, Hirch HJ, Loss WH (1981). Malignant somatostatinoma; clinical features and metabolic studies. Journal of Clinical Endocrinology and Metabolism, 52:886–96.

Bauer W, et al. (1982). SMS 201-995: a very potent and selective octapeptide analogue of somatostatin with prolonged action. Life Sciences, 31:1133–41.

Blackburn AM, Bryant MG, Adrian TE, Bloom SR (1981). Pancreatic tumours produce neurotensin. Journal of Clinical Endocrinology and Metabolism, 52:820–2.

Boden G, et al. (1986). Treatment of inoperable glucagonoma with the long-acting somatostatin analogue SMS 201-995. New England Journal of Medicine, 314:1686–9.

Broder LE, Carter SK (1973). Pancreatic islet cell carcinoma. II. Results of therapy with streptozotocin in 52 patients. Annals of Internal Medicine, 79:108–18.

Davis Z, Moertel CG, McIlrath DC (1973). The malignant carcinoid syndrome. Surgery, Gynecology and Obstetrics, 137:P637–44.

Frame J, et al. (1988). A phase II trial of streptozotocin and adriamycin in advanced APUD tumors. American Journal of Clinical Oncology, 11(4):490–5.

Friessen SR (1982). Tumors of the endocrine pancreas. New England Journal of Medicine, 306:P580–90.

Galiber AK, et al. (1988). Localization of pancreatic insulinoma: comparison of pre- and intraoperative US with CT and angiography. Radiology, 166(2):405–8.

Hansen R, Helm J, Wilson JF, Wilson S (1988). Nonfunctioning islet cell carcinoma of the pancreas. Complete response to continuous 5-fluorouracil infusion. Cancer, 62(1):15–17.

Krejs GJ, et al. (1979). Somatostatinoma syndrome: biochemical, morphologic and clinical features. New England Journal of Medicine, 301:285–92.

Kvols LK, et al. (1986). Treatment of the malignant carcinoid syndrome. Evaluation of a long-acting somatostatin analogue. New England Journal of Medicine, 315:663–6.

Lamberts SW, et al. (1988). Development of resistance to a long-acting somatostatin analogue during treatment of two patients with metastatic endocrine pancreatic tumours. Acta Endocrinologica, 119(4):561–6.

Lee SM, Forbes A, Williams R (1988). Metastatic islet cell tumour with clinical manifestations of insulin and glucagon excess: successful treatment by hepatic artery embolization and chemotherapy. European Journal of Surgery and Oncology, 14(3):265–8.

Lokich J, Bothe A, O'Hara C, Fedamen D (1987). Metastatic islet cell tumour with ACTH, gastrin and glucagon secretion clinical and pathological studies with multiple therapies. Cancer, 59:P2053–8.

London NJ, et al. (1988). Localization of an occult impalpable insulinoma by intraoperative ultrasonography. Journal of the Royal Society of Medicine, 81(11):663–4.

McArthur KE, et al. (1985). Omeprazole: effective, convenient therapy for Zollinger–Ellison syndrome. Gastroenterology, 88:939–44.

McCarthy DE (1980). The place of surgery in the Zollinger Ellison syndrome. New England Journal of Medicine, 302:P1344–7.

Mallinson CN, et al. (1974). A glucagonoma syndrome. Lancet, ii:P1–5.

Moertel CG, Hanley JA, Johnson LA (1980). Streptozotocin alone compared with 5-flurouracil in treatment of advanced islet cell carcinoma. New England Journal of Medicine, 303:P1189–94.

Norheim I, et al. (1987). Malignant carcinoid tumours. Annals of Surgery, 206(2):P115–25.

Oberg K, Norheim I, Lundqvist G, Wide L (1986). Treatment of the carcinoid syndrome with SMS 201-995, a somatostatin analogue. Scandinavian Journal of Gastroenterology, 21:191–2.

Polak JM, Marangos PJ (1984). Neuron-specific enolase a marker for neuroendocrine cells. In Evolution and tumour pathology of the neuroendocrine system (ed. S. Falkmer, R. Hakanson, and F. Sundler). Elsevier, Amsterdam.

Polak JM, et al. (1976). Pancreatic polypeptide in insulinomas, gastrinomas, VIPomas and glucagonomas. Lancet, i:P328–30.

Rossi P, et al. (1989). Endocrine tumors of the pancreas. Radiological Clinics of North America, 27(1):129–61.

Stefanini P, Carboni M, Patrassi N, Basoli A (1974). Beta islet cell tumours of the pancreas. Result of a study of 1,067 cases. Surgery, 75(4):P597–609.

Suzuki H, et al. (1986). Product of pituitary protein 7B2 I-R by endocrine tumours and its possible diagnostic value. Journal of Clinical Endocrinology and Metabolism, 63:P758–65.

Sweet D (1984). A dermatosis specifically associated with a tumour of pancreatic alpha cells. British Journal of Dermatology, 90:P301–8.

Thompson GB, et al. (1988). Islet cell carcinomas of the pancreas: a twenty-year experience. Surgery, 104(6):1011–17.

Tjon A, et al. (1989). MR, CT ultrasound findings of metastatic vipoma in pancreas. Journal of Computer Assisted Tomography, 13(1).142–4.

Tomita T, et al. (1983). Pancreatic polypeptide secreting islet cell tumours: a study of three cases. American Journal of Pathology, 113:P134–42.

Verner JV, Morrison AB (1958). Islet cell tumour and a syndrome of refractory, watery diarrhoea and hypokalemia. *American Journal of Medicine*, **25**:P374–380.

Whipple AP, Franz VK (1935). Adenoma of islet cells with hyperinsulinism. *Annals of Surgery*, **101**:1299–335.

Wynick D, Williams SJ, Bloom SR (1988). Symptomatic secondary hormone syndromes in patients with established malignant pancreatic endocrine tumors. *New England Journal of Medicine*, **319**:599–604.

Wynick D, Anderson JV, Williams SJ, Bloom SR (1989). Resistance of metastatic pancreatic endocrine tumours after long term treatment with the somatostatin analogue octreotide (SMS 201-995). *Clinical Endocrinology*. **30**:134–6.

Yiangou Y, *et al.* (1987). Peptide–histidine–methionine-immunoreactivity in plasma and tissue from patients with VIP secreting tumours and watery diarrhoea. *Journal of Clinical Endocrinology and Metabolism*, **64**:P131–9.

Zollinger RM, Ellison EH (1955). Primary peptic ulceration of the jejunum associated with islet cell tumours of the pancreas. *Annals of Surgery*, **142**:P709–73.

Section 17
Tumours of unknown primary site

17 Tumours of unknown primary site

G. J. LINDEMAN AND MARTIN TATTERSALL

DEFINITION

Management of the patient who presents with metastatic cancer without an obvious primary site is a common problem in oncological practice. This situation is usually referred to as occult primary malignancy or cancer of unknown primary site. The definition of cancer of unknown primary site has varied from study to study and in early series the term referred to the primary tumour site remaining unknown despite autopsy. Several authors excluded tumours of epidermoid histology because of a more favourable prognosis with locoregional therapy (Osteen *et al.* 1978; Nystrom *et al.* 1979; Grosbach 1982). A pragmatic definition of cancer of unknown primary site is as follows:

(1) a biopsy-proven cancer which is inconsistent with a primary tumour at that site;

(2) the primary site remains occult despite thorough history, physical examination (which includes rectal, pelvic, and breast examination), urinalysis, and appropriate additional investigations (discussed below).

INCIDENCE

The entity of cancer of unknown primary site has only really been appreciated in the last 15 years. The incidence of cancer of unknown primary site depends on both the thoroughness of investigation and the population studied. Cancer of unknown primary site represents up to 15 per cent of new referrals in large, hospital-based oncology centres (Stewart *et al.* 1979; Markham 1982; Jordan and Shildt 1985; Altman and Cadman 1986). In developed countries, typically 5–6 per cent of all new cases of cancer present with cancer of unknown primary site. The incidence increases with age and is low below 40 years. It is the third most common cancer presentation in females over 70 years. The mean age of diagnosis is 60 years. The crude incidence rate is approximately 14–18 per 100 000 and the lifetime risk of developing cancer of unknown primary site is 1 in 56 for males and 1 in 77 for females. Cancer of unknown primary site is a common cause of cancer death. In Australia, for example, it is the fourth most common cause of cancer deaths in males and the third most common cause in females (Krementz *et al.* 1979; NSW Central Cancer Registry 1983; McCredie *et al.* 1988).

The increased risk of a concomitant unrelated malignancy in patients with cancer of unknown primary site has been observed in several studies. The incidence is approximately 7 per cent (Altman and Cadman 1986; Hamilton and Langlands 1987).

AETIOLOGY

Conceptually, cancer of unknown primary site can be considered to represent a heterogeneous cluster of tumours with a propensity for early dissemination compared with tumours which present as primary malignancies with or without apparent metastases. The process of early dissemination is reflected in autopsy studies, in which the primary site cannot be determined in 15–25 per cent of cases (Neumann and Nystrom 1982; Hamilton and Langlands 1987).

Localization of the primary tumour site may be difficult for several reasons. Diagnostic tools may be inadequate or sampling errors may occur. The primary may have been removed or sloughed from skin or a mucosal surface or undergone spontaneous regression (Holmes and Fouts 1970). The latter phenomenon has been best characterized in malignant melanoma (McGovern 1975). The primary tumour may remain microscopic because of a long doubling time during which there is rapid growth of metastatic lesions.

While cancers of unknown primary site are usually considered to represent a mixture of occult tumour types, they share two fundamental characteristics: an absent primary tumour and an unpredictable metastatic pattern which does not parallel that seen in metastatic tumours with a known primary site (see below). In addition, several cytogenic abnormalities have recently been demonstrated. Consistent deletion of the short arm of chromosome 1 was observed in eight cases of cancer of unknown primary site, despite apparently diverse phenotypic properties *in vitro*. Analysis of four of these patients also revealed duplication of 1q (in three cases), the presence of a homogeneously staining region (two cases), and evidence of gene amplification (Bell *et al.* 1989). Chromosome 1 abnormalities are generally associated with advanced malignancy (Atkin 1986). This suggests that cancers of unknown primary site rapidly develop malignant properties soon after transformation, as reflected in their rapid acquisition of a metastatic phenotype and abnormalities in chromosome 1. Further data are needed to confirm this proposition.

NATURAL HISTORY

The prognosis for patients with cancer of unknown primary site is poor, with median survival in most studies between 3 and 4 months. Fewer than 25 per cent of patients survive to 1 year and less than 10 per cent are alive at 5 years (Smith *et al.* 1967; Holmes and Fouts 1970; Richardson and Parker 1975). These figures do not appear to have changed in 60 years (Fig. 1).

As a generalization, intensive pursuit of the primary site and treatment does not greatly alter survival. This reflects the observations that the primary tumour may be difficult to find and that the majority of cancers of unknown primary site are refractory to currently available systemic treatment. However, there are subgroups of these cancers, somewhat ill defined, which carry a better prognosis and which are discussed below.

Pattern of metastatic involvement

As mentioned above, the biological behaviour of cancer of unknown primary site differs from cancers in which the primary site is known. This is most apparent when the patterns of metastases are compared; the sites of metastasis in patients with cancer of unknown primary site often differ from the usual pattern of metastasis (Nystrom

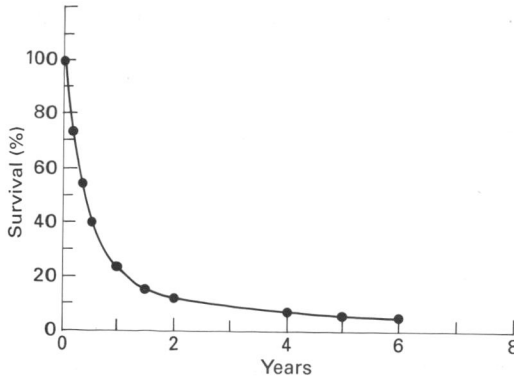

Fig. 1 Survival time from the diagnosis of cancer of unknown primary site. (Adapted from Altman and Cadman 1986.)

et al. 1977). For example, osseous metastases from a known primary lung cancer are approximately 10 times more common than when the primary is occult. Osseous metastases from pancreatic cancer are approximately three times more common when the primary is occult. Whereas patients with prostatic cancer commonly present with osseous metastases, this is less usual when the primary is occult. In the latter case unusual sites such as lung, liver, and brain are frequently involved. This differing pattern of metastasis between cancers of unknown primary site and known primary tumours further complicates the search for a primary site (Table 1).

Anatomical location of the primary

Extensive investigation may successfully establish the extent of metastatic disease, but does not necessarily localize the primary tumour. In the majority of cancers of unknown primary site, the primary tumour site remains unknown ante-mortem, despite investigation. An ante-mortem primary site is identified in 8–31 per cent of cases (Moertel *et al.* 1972; Didolkar *et al.* 1977; Osteen *et al.* 1978; Stewart *et al.* 1979; Nystrom *et al.* 1979; Neumann and Nystrom 1982; Gaber *et al.* 1983; Jordan and Shildt 1985). In our experience a primary tumour site is found ante-mortem in approximately 20 per cent of patients (Kirsten *et al.* 1987). In a considerable number of cases an isolated radiological diagnosis

proves to be a false-positive. Post-mortem review may also lead to a change in histological diagnosis. In a significant number of cases the primary tumour remains undiagnosed even after post-mortem. This is variously reported as occurring in 15–27 per cent of cases. These issues are discussed below.

Pursuing the location of the primary tumour site has theoretical merits: vigorous investigation may result in specific treatment, allow prediction and prevention of local complications, and be of prognostic benefit. Arguments against this approach include the high number of non-contributory investigations and the longer period in hospital that a patient must endure. Additionally, even when the primary tumour site is located, there is usually no effective treatment for the systemic disease and local symptoms may not arise. In general terms, localizing the primary is of little practical benefit as the length of survival is not increased when the primary tumour site is found. We believe that simple measures aimed at diagnosing treatable tumours are appropriate.

Table 2 lists the primary tumour sites identified (and includes autopsy data) in several series. Several common tumours such as breast and prostate cancer are relatively simple to detect and rarely present as a cancer of unknown primary site. This to some extent explains why the pattern of sites of primary malignancy in cancer of unknown primary site (when this can be established) is considerably different to the primary sites in patients with overt primary malignancies.

Table 3 groups the identified primary tumour sites in patients with cancer of unknown primary site by location above or below the diaphragm. The location of the primary is infradiaphragmatic in up to 75 per cent of cases (Nystrom *et al.* 1977; Nissenblatt 1981). The pancreas followed by the liver and colon are the most common primary sites. The remaining 25 per cent of cases have a supradiaphragmatic primary malignancy. A primary lung tumour accounts for most of the 25 per cent of cases metastatic from above the diaphragm.

Nystrom *et al.* (1977) devised a schema to predict whether the primary site was supradiaphragmatic or infradiaphragmatic, depending on the summation of scores ascribed to various metastatic sites at presentation. According to their findings, the occult primary is commonly on the same side of the diaphragm as its metastases.

Table 1 Pattern of metastatic involvement

| Primary site | Metastatic involvement for occult (CUP) and overt primary (%) | | | | | | | |
| | Bone | | Lung | | Liver | | Brain | |
	Occult	Overt	Occult	Overt	Occult	Overt	Occult	Overt
Lung	4	30–50	90	34	36	30–50	21	15–30
Breast	33	50–85	66	60	66	45–60	33	15–25
Thyroid	0	39	100	65	50	60	0	1
Pancreas	28	5–10	31	25–40	72	50–70	3	1–4
Liver	31	8	19	20	100	—	6	0
Colorectal	13	5–10	40	25–40	87	71	0	1
Gastric	9	5–10	18	20–30	36	35–50	9	1–4
Renal	66	30–50	77	50–75	33	35–40	0	7–8
Ovary	0	2–6	25	10	25	10–15	0	1
Prostate	25	50–75	75	13–53	50	13	25	2

CUP, cancer of unknown primary site.
Adapted from Nystrom *et al.* (1977).

Table 2 Distribution of primary tumour sites in cancer of unknown primary site

Site	Moertel *et al.* (1972) (*n*=162)	Osteen *et al.* (1978) (*n*=67)	Nystrom *et al.* (1979) (*n*=266)	Stewart *et al.* (1979) (*n*=87)	Hamilton and Langlands (1987) (*n*=287)	Kirsten *et al.* (1987) (*n*=286)
Pancreas	16	6	30	1	7	4
Lung	1	8	28	7	22	23
Liver	4	2	16	2	4	2
Colon/ rectum	5	5	15	5	5	8
Stomach	5	2	12	3	6	6
Kidney	2	2	9	2	1	6
Prostate	1	4	4	2	1	5
Ovary	0	5	4	4	3	11
Breast	2	3	3	0	1	10
Lymphoid tissue	0	4	0	0	0	2
Testis	0	0	0	2	0	2
Other	6	4	8	2	10	9
Total	42	55	129	30	60	88

Table 3 Infra- and supradiaphragmatic location of primary tumours

	Patients	Percentage
Above diaphragm		
Lung	28	11
Breast	3	3
Thyroid	2	<1
Parotid	1	<1
Below diaphragm		
Pancreas	30	11
Liver	16	6
Colorectal	15	6
Gastric	12	5
Renal	9	3
Ovary	4	2
Prostate	4	2
Adrenal	1	<1
Other	4	2
Undetermined	137	52
Total	266	100

Adapted from Nystrom *et al.* (1979).

PROGNOSTIC FACTORS

Several studies have examined favourable prognostic factors (Pasterz *et al.* 1986; Kirsten *et al.* 1987). A good performance status is probably the most important predictor of survival, while extensive weight loss and older age are adverse prognostic factors (Stewart *et al.* 1979). Patients with predominantly palpable lymphadenopathy (particularly high cervical and axillary), tend to have a more prolonged survival. Metastatic sites of progressively worse prognostic significance include lymph nodes, subcutaneous tissue, pulmonary and abdominal viscera (Stewart *et al.* 1979). Involvement of multiple different metastatic sites of disease is also associated with poorer survival and patients with squamous histology have a slightly longer median survival than those with undifferentiated carcinoma or adenocarcinoma (Altman and Cadman 1986). Tumour ploidy has not been demonstrated to be of prognostic value (Hedley *et al.* 1985). As emphasized earlier, establishing the primary tumour site during life does not necessarily affect median survival (Stewart *et al.* 1979). Patient survival as a group is unaffected by treatment.

Histological types

There is marked disparity in the reported relative frequencies of histological types of cancers of unknown primary site. The majority have adenocarcinoma or undifferentiated histology. Less frequently, squamous cell carcinoma, melanoma, sarcoma, and neuroendocrine tumours may present as cancer of unknown primary site. The proportion of squamous histology varies in the literature, depending particularly upon whether cancers of unknown primary site with high cervical lymphadenopathy at presentation are included (Table 4).

Optimal evaluation requires an experienced review of the biopsy specimen as this may provide the best clue to a treatable tumour. Histological misclassification can occur and rebiopsy for more and/or fresh tissue may be warranted. In three of the 16 patients who underwent autopsy in one series, the review diagnosis changed from adenocarcinoma to melanoma (one), potentially drug-sensitive Hodgkin's disease (one), and histiocytic lymphoma (one) (Stewart *et al.* 1979).

Open biopsy has been reported as being preferable to needle aspiration by some (MacKay and Ordonez 1982). Obtaining adequate material is important for thorough assessment, which may include special stains and electron microscopy. Nevertheless, fine-needle aspiration cytology often proves to be more expedient and has reduced the need for major procedures such as diagnostic laparotomy (Ng and Philips 1985). A cytological diagnosis of cancer can be achieved using fine-needle aspiration cytology in over 20 per cent of cancers of unknown primary site (Hamilton and Langlands 1987).

Thorough evaluation by histological, immunohistochemical, and, if possible, electron microscopy methods is vital. In well-differentiated tumours the tumour type (epithelial, mesenchymal, haematopoietic, or neuroectodermal) is usually apparent. Further stains can be helpful. Examples include mucin stains such as mucicarmine and alcian blue for adenocarcinoma and glycogen stains using the periodic acid–Schiff reagent procedure (diastase sensitive). Renal cell adenocarcinoma typically is rich in cytoplasmic glycogen, but other tumours such as germ cell, Ewing's sarcoma, or rhabdomyosarcoma may also contain this material. Diastase-resistant periodic acid–Schiff reagent staining indicates the presence of mucopolysaccharides (glycosaminoglycans) and suggests gastric origin in an adenocarcinoma (MacKay and Ordonez 1982).

Identifying the histogenesis of more poorly differentiated tumours can be difficult. Poorly differentiated carcinoma may easily be confused with lymphoma, seminoma, amelanotic melanoma, sarcoma, and epidermoid carcinoma (Kern and Abbott 1980). Immunohistochemical methods may assist in the evaluation (DeLellis and Dayal 1987). Examples include stains for keratin (epithelial), leucocyte common antigen (lymphoid cells) (Kurtin and Pinkus 1985), S-100 (neuroectodermal antigen, for example melanomas), prostate-specific antigen (prostatic cancer) (Tell *et al.* 1985), α-fetoprotein (for example, hepatoma, germ cell tumour) β-human chorionic gonadotrophin (for example, germ cell tumour), and thyroglobulin (thyroid cancer). The recognition of an undifferentiated germ cell tumour is particularly important, as discussed below. Positive stains are not absolutely specific and should be interpreted in the clinical context. Therefore, interaction between clinician and pathologist is vital. Examples of more common tissue markers which may be of use in the histological diagnosis of poorly differentiated cancer of unknown primary site are shown in Table 5.

Unfixed specimens for measurement of oestrogen receptor and other steroid or hormone receptor proteins may also indicate a breast or endometrial primary if the level is markedly raised. Increasingly, immunohistochemical stains for these receptors are being used.

Table 4 Frequency of histological subtypes of cancer of unknown primary site

	Patients	Percentage
Adenocarcinoma	223	36
Carcinoma	113	18
Undifferentiated carcinoma	108	18
Squamous cell carcinoma	50	8
Melanoma	40	7
Malignancy, type undetermined	83	13
Total	617	100

Adapted from Holmes and Fouts (1970).

Table 5 Tissue markers commonly used in poorly differentiated cancer of unknown primary site

Marker	Tumour type				
	Lymphoma	Carcinoma	Melanoma	Sarcoma	Germ cell
Cytokeratin[a]	–	+	–	–/+	–/+
CEA	–	+	–	–	–
EMA or HMFG	–	+	–	–	–
LCA	+	–	–	–	–
Vimentin	+	–	+	+	–
Desmin	–	–	–	–/+	–
S-100 protein	–	–/+	+	–/+	–
Placental alkaline phosphatase	–	–/+	–	–	+
HCG	–	–/+	–	–	–/+
AFP	–	–/+	–	–	–/+

CEA, carcinoembryonic antigen; EMA, epithelial membrane antigen; HMFG, human milk-fat globule-derived antigen; LCA, leucocyte common antigen; HCG, human chorionic gonadotrophin; AFP, α-fetoprotein.
[a]Sarcomas are cytokeratin negative with the exception of synovial and epithelioid sarcomas. Germ cell tumours, with the exception of seminomas, may be cytokeratin positive. Adapted from DeLellis and Dayal (1987).

Monoclonality in lymphoproliferative disorders can be established by demonstrating the presence of B- or T-cell lineage-specific gene rearrangements (immunoglobulin gene and T-cell receptor gene, respectively) or gene products (intracytoplasmic or surface immunoglobulin). This may be useful in differentiating a large cell lymphoma from poorly differentiated carcinoma.

In our experience immunocytochemical staining is diagnostically useful for prostate-specific antigen, β-human chorionic gonado-trophin, and α-fetoprotein, but organ site non-specific markers of histogenesis or cellular differentiation (for example, carcinoembryonic antigen, IgA secretory component, peanut lectin binding, epithelial membrane antigen, and keratin) show no correlation with identified primary sites and responsiveness to empirical chemotherapy or survival (Kirsten et al. 1987).

Electron microscopy can occasionally (10 per cent) be of benefit in determining the line of differentiation of cancer of unknown primary site not otherwise identified by light microscopy (Mackay and Ordonez 1982). Well-developed cell junctions (desmosomes) attached to intermediate filaments (tonofilaments) are seen in squamous cell tumours. Acinar spaces, tight junctions, and microacini (surface or intracytoplasmic) occur in adenocarcinomas. Irregularities or admixtures of these changes can make distinction difficult. For example, both types can undergo spindle cell transformation resembling sarcoma. Polyribosomes and absence of

junctions occur in diffuse histiocytic or undifferentiated lymphoma. Myofibrils, dilated rough endoplasmic reticulum, or extracellular osteoid occur in poorly differentiated sarcoma. Core granules and electron-dense secretory granules may be seen in poorly differentiated neuroendocrine tumours and premelanosomes may be seen in amelanotic melanomas (MacKay and Ordonez 1982; Herrera and Reimann 1984; Hanna and Kahn 1985; Hainsworth et al. 1988).

CLINICAL PRESENTATIONS

The clinical presentation of patients with metastatic cancer of unknown primary site can be broadly divided into six categories depending on the predominant site of metastatic involvement: lymphadenopathy, pulmonary, hepatic, or other abdominal presentations, osseous, and neurological involvement. The frequency of involvement of these sites has varied between published series and probably reflects differing referral patterns (Table 6). Additionally, it is likely that regional or racial differences alter the pattern of presentation. For example, consideration of an underlying nasopharyngeal carcinoma or hepatocellular carcinoma in geographical areas of high prevalence would clearly be important. Weight loss is a prominent sign in approximately 35 per cent of cases (Didolkar et al. 1977).

Investigations and management according to the pattern of presentation is the logical approach. In this context it is important to recall that the pattern of metastatic involvement in cancer of unknown primary site is not the same as that seen in patients with identified primary tumours (Nystrom et al. 1977, 1979).

Lymphadenopathy

The proportion of patients with cancers of unknown primary site of various histological types who present with predominant lymphadenopathy is variously reported between 14 and 49 per cent (Didolkar et al. 1977; Stewart et al. 1979). The site of lymphadenopathy is an important guide to investigations aimed at identifying the primary tumour site, to management, and to prognosis.

Axillary lymph node metastases

The prognosis for patients with cancer of unknown primary site presenting with axillary lymph node metastases is generally better than other presentations of cancer of unknown primary site, with occasional long-term survival (Kirsten et al. 1987). Patients are usually managed as if they had an occult breast primary (Westbrook and Gallagher 1971; Copeland and McBride 1973). In a series from

Table 6 Predominant site of presentation in cancer of unknown primary site

Predominant site	Series						
	Didolkar et al. (1977)[a]	Osteen et al. (1978)	Stewart et al. (1979)	Steckel et al. (1980)	Kirsten et al. (1987)	Hamilton and Langlands (1987)	Alberts et al. (1989)
Lymph node (%)	49	16	14	26	14	20	12
Pulmonary (%)	39	11	24	15	29	17	19
Hepatic (%)	12	19	17	11	18	18	30
Abdominopelvic (%)	11	—	18	17	15	14	22
Osseous (%)	21	27	6	16	16	18	7
Neurological (%)	—	9	8	7	8	8	2

[a]No statement of predominant site; figures given refer to percentage with site involved.

the M. D. Anderson Hospital, 18 out of 37 females with a malignant axillary node subsequently proved to have a breast primary. Negative mammography did not exclude breast cancer, as this investigation was normal in approximately 50 per cent of proven cases (Copeland and McBride 1973). Other studies have supported these observations (Feigenberg et al. 1976; Patel et al. 1981; Inglehart et al. 1982). Other possible primary sites, such as lung and ovarian cancer, should be considered. Appropriate investigations include mammography, pelvic examination, serum CA125 antigen, chest radiography, and sputum cytology. The oestrogen receptor status of the tumour may support the diagnosis. Tumour markers and, if possible, electron microscopy to exclude melanoma and lymphoma should also be carried out.

Most investigators recommend that female patients undergo at least an upper outer quadrant sector mastectomy with breast and axillary irradiation, with or without adjuvant systemic therapy, even if the tumour is oestrogen receptor negative.

Cervical and supraclavicular lymphadenopathy

Cervical adenopathy with cancer of unknown primary site represents a clinical entity which may be controlled by locoregional therapy. Patients are typically male, aged between 50 and 70 years, and tumour histology is squamous in 60–85 per cent of cases. Median survival of 3 years is reported as between 35 and 53 per cent after radical radiotherapy and/or surgery and reflects the site of occult primary which is in the head and neck in approximately 75 per cent of cases (Barrie et al. 1970; Jesse et al. 1973). Metastasis to high cervical nodes and squamous or anaplastic histology have a better prognosis; long-term survival with adenocarcinoma is rare. This entity is further discussed in the chapter on head and neck malignancy.

Supraclavicular node presentations are more likely to signify a more distant primary site and more distant dissemination and have a much poorer prognosis than high cervical presentation. Lung and breast primary sites should be excluded. The possibility of an atypical teratoma syndrome (discussed below) should be considered. Therefore, serum markers for α-fetoprotein and β-human chorionic gonadotrophin and immunoperoxidase staining of the tumour are important. Involvement of Virchow's node may reflect an abdominal primary with spread via the thoracic duct. Testing for faecal occult blood, gastroscopy, and colonoscopy are often carried out. However, pursuit of a primary gastrointestinal lesion may not alter prognosis or management.

Inguinal lymphadenopathy

Melanoma from an occult lower limb primary and lymphoma should be excluded (by immunoperoxidase and electron microscopy). Thorough examination of the perineum and lower extremities is important. In patients with undifferentiated or squamous metastases, cystoscopy and detailed gynaecological examination may disclose a cloacogenic primary. Further investigations are often unrewarding. Patients with inguinal lymphadenopathy from cancer of unknown primary site may achieve prolonged responses with radiotherapy (Guarischi et al. 1987).

Pulmonary metastases

Cancer of unknown primary site presenting with pulmonary (pleural, parenchymal, or malignant effusion) involvement occurs in 11–39 per cent of cases. Mesothelioma should be considered if the disease is largely pleural. In mesothelioma mucin stains are usually negative and the tumour is hyaluronidase sensitive. Special markers (for example, Leu M1) and electron microscopy may be of use. If a pleural-based cancer of unknown primary site is an adenocarcinoma, then pelvic ultrasound, serum CA125 antigen, and sputum cytology and/or bronchoscopy may be rewarding.

In patients with predominantly parenchymal disease, treatable subsets such as breast cancer, ovarian cancer, prostatic cancer, and atypical teratoma syndrome should be excluded. Appropriate investigations include serum α-fetoprotein, β-human chorionic gonadotrophin, prostate-specific antigen, sputum cytology, and bilateral mammography. Gastrointestinal assessment is rarely helpful. The metastatic deposit may mimic a lung primary. In this context it is not unusual for a pancreatic carcinoma to present with the initial diagnosis of primary carcinoma of the bronchus (Weber et al. 1973). A metastatic lesion is still most likely to have arisen from a lung primary (see above). This is particularly true of squamous lesions (Ringenberg 1985).

Hepatic metastases

Clinical presentation with cancer of unknown primary site involving the liver occurs in 12–19 per cent of cases. Only 65 per cent of these prove to have an adenocarcinoma (Nesbit et al. 1981). A biopsy to identify the histological type of metastatic disease should be the first investigation. Pancreatic imaging is often performed but may not be reliable. Once again, faecal occult blood and subsequent gastroscopy and colonoscopy may be considered, but there is little evidence that detection and resection of a primary lesion alters survival. Mammography and pelvic ultrasound and serum CA125 antigen are important investigations in females. Measurement of α-fetoprotein will assist in the identification of hepatocellular carcinoma and prostate-specific antigen should be measured in males. Carcinoembryonic antigen, which is not tumour site specific, is of little benefit.

Abdominal (non-hepatic) metastases

Between 11 and 18 per cent of patients with cancer of unknown primary site present with predominant abdominal signs. Examination of the gastrointestinal tract is carried out by some investigators. Laparotomy and debulking surgery in the absence of obstructive symptoms is of no value, except for occult ovarian cancer (Nesbit et al. 1981). In the presence of malignant ascites, mammography, pelvic ultrasound, and serum CA125 antigen are appropriate investigations. The CA125 antigen is a reasonable marker for ovarian and other Müllerian duct cancers but has not been evaluated in cancer of unknown primary site (Kabawat et al. 1983). However, it is not a useful marker of poorly differentiated or mucus-secreting ovarian carcinomas.

Peritoneal carcinomatosis in women may represent a distinctive subset of treatable cancer of unknown primary site. The clinical presentation closely resembles advanced ovarian cancer (Dalrymple et al. 1990). The natural history is relatively indolent compared with other cancers of unknown primary site, with a median survival of 12 months. Cytoreductive surgery probably benefits patients in terms of both survival and subsequent chemoresponsiveness. A subset of patients achieve a complete response to cisplatinum-based chemotherapy (Strnad et al. 1989).

An umbilical mass (Sister Mary Joseph's nodule) is usually metastatic, particularly if the tumour is an adenocarcinoma; primary umbilical tumours, usually epidermoid, are rare. The most common site of primary is gastric carcinoma, although other intra-abdominal or pelvic tumours occur (Key *et al.* 1976; Scarpa *et al.* 1979).

Osseous metastases

The frequency of osseous presentations of cancer of unknown primary site is between 6 and 27 per cent. However, bone scans are positive in almost 50 per cent of patients without skeletal symptoms and in 90 per cent of symptomatic patients (Gaber *et al.* 1983). The common associations between primary lung, breast, thyroid, prostate, and renal neoplasms and osseous metastases are less well defined in cancer of unknown primary site.

The radiological appearance may provide a clue to the occult primary tumour. Blastic lesions are common in prostatic carcinoma and can occur in Hodgkin's disease and in non-Hodgkin's lymphoma and ovarian, thyroid, carcinoid, and small cell lung cancer. Mixed blastic and lytic lesions are characteristic of breast cancer and can occur in squamous cancer. Pure lytic lesions are typical of myeloma, renal cancer, melanoma, and non-small cell lung cancer.

Mammography, chest radiography, sputum cytology, prostate-specific antigen, and serum immunoelectrophoresis are important investigations in excluding treatable disease.

Neurological presentations

Patients presenting with cancer of unknown primary site and cerebral metastases comprise less than 10 per cent of cases, since a chest radiograph may reveal lung cancer and breast cancer may be detected prior to craniotomy. Primary tumours most commonly responsible for cerebral cancer of unknown primary site include lung, melanoma, breast, pancreatic, and prostatic cancer. Gestational trophoblastic disease should be considered in females of reproductive age who present with a subarachnoid haemorrhage.

Spinal cord presentations are more frequent neurological manifestations of cancer of unknown primary site. High spinal cord lesions are said to originate most commonly from a lung or breast primary, while lower lesions arise in association with retroperitoneal lymphoma or prostatic malignancy. Occult melanoma should also be considered.

Oestrogen receptor measurements, immunoperoxidase stains, and electron microscopy may be diagnostic. Serum β-human chorionic gonadotrophin may indicate choriocarcinoma and, less frequently, a raised α-fetoprotein identifies the patient with a midline germ cell tumour.

Other less common presentations

Skin

Skin presentation of cancer of unknown primary site is rare since the primary tumours that commonly metastasize to skin tend to be easily detected. Moreover, cancer of unknown primary site with skin involvement often involves other metastatic sites so that the skin tumours are often overlooked (Ringenberg 1985). Possible primary sites include lung, melanoma, oral cavity, colon, and stomach.

Bone-marrow

Cancer of unknown primary site presenting as bone-marrow metastases is infrequently reported but may account for up to 12 per cent of cancers detected by bone-marrow biopsy (Singh *et al.* 1977). Patients tend to be elderly and present with bone pain or abdominal pain. Anaemia, thrombocytopenia, and a leuco-erythroblastic blood picture are common laboratory findings in these patients. Median survival in these patients tends to be very short (18 days in one series) (Ringenberg *et al.* 1986). Bone-marrow metastases most frequently arise from lung, breast, and prostate cancers (Anner and Drewinko 1977). Therefore, it is appropriate to evaluate patients with cancer of unknown primary site presenting in marrow with chest radiography, mammography, and prostate-specific antigen.

Pericardial effusion

Cancers of unknown primary site presenting with malignant pericardial effusion are usually adenocarcinomas. The primary site, when located, is often the lung (Fraser *et al.* 1980).

The extragonadal germ cell syndrome

Richardson *et al.* (1979) reported six young males with disseminated poorly differentiated carcinomas or adenocarcinomas whose tumours responded to platinum-based combination chemotherapy. They suggested the possibility of an unrecognized extragonadal germ cell tumour in these patients. Subsequent reports of complete tumour responses and long-term survival have been published. In a minority of these patients germ cell tumours were subsequently confirmed (Greco *et al.* 1982).

In the same year Fox *et al.* (1979) described a similar syndrome which they termed the 'atypical teratoma syndrome'. They reported five young men with undifferentiated carcinoma involving lung, mediastinum, and lymph nodes who responded to a germ cell chemotherapy protocol. Their response to treatment, serum or tumour markers, and histology review suggested a diagnosis of embryonal cell carcinoma.

Greco *et al.* (1986) subsequently reported 71 (prospectively identified) patients with advanced poorly differentiated cancer of unknown primary site with one or more features of the 'extragonadal germ cell syndrome', which they defined as follows:

(1) age less than 50 years;

(2) predominantly midline structures (mediastinal or retro-peritoneum), pulmonary nodules, or lymphadenopathy;

(3) elevated serum β-human chorionic gonadotrophin or α-fetoprotein;

(4) rapid tumour growth;

(5) very responsive to prior radiotherapy or chemotherapy.

No patients had histological evidence for a haematopoietic or germ cell tumour. Tumours were characteristically poorly differentiated and rapidly dividing, rather than being specifically germ cell in phenotype. Sixty-two patients received some form of intensive platinum-based chemotherapy and 38 (56 per cent) had a major tumour response; 15 patients (22 per cent) achieved a complete response, with nine of these remaining disease free for more than 3 years. There was a predominance of patients with lymph node involvement, particularly mediastinal and retroperitoneal and this was associated with a favourable outcome. Poorly differentiated carcinomas tended to have a higher response rate than poorly differentiated adenocarcinomas (Hainsworth *et al.* 1987). The Vanderbilt University group felt that at least some of the patients with dramatic tumour responses had histologically atypical extragonadal germ cell tumours and that patients with poorly differentiated carcinomas with predominant involvement of the mediastinum, retroperitoneum, and other lymph node areas should receive empirical cisplatinum-based combination chemotherapy.

Although the Vanderbilt University experience contrasts with the findings of several other groups, where response to chemotherapy has been poor (Mostofi and Price 1973; Jones *et al.* 1985; Logothetis *et al.* 1985), it may be appropriate to treat patients with features of the extragonadal germ cell syndrome with cisplatinum-based chemotherapy in the hope of achieving a major response and prolonged survival in a subgroup.

INVESTIGATIONS

Cost–benefit of investigations

The mean stay in hospital for patients with cancer of unknown primary site is longer than for patients in whom the primary is identified (25 versus 15 days) (Didolkar *et al.* 1977). Most of the excess time is spent in fruitless search for a primary tumour.

In a speculative review, Levine *et al.* (1985) contrasted the cost of an extensive search for a primary tumour with that of a limited search aimed at diagnosing a treatable tumour, with specific chemotherapy being given if the tumour was found and symptomatic treatment only if the primary remained undiagnosed. In 1985 it was calculated that a comprehensive search increased median 1 year survival from 11.0 to 11.5 per cent and that the additional costs in treating 1000 patients would range from two to eight million Canadian dollars depending on the treatment option.

Hamilton and Langlands (1987) reported reduced cost when investigations for cancer of unknown primary site were undertaken in an oncology unit compared with a general hospital unit. The mean numbers of investigations were 2.2 and 3.4, respectively. Significantly fewer speculative investigations unlikely to influence patient management were performed when the patient was managed in an oncology unit. They reviewed costs in financial terms and in terms of the test morbidity and compared these with the direct and indirect benefits achieved by investigations. Mammography, pelvic and testicular ultrasound, and CT, particularly head and abdominal, were found to be of value in diagnosing a treatable condition. Most gastrointestinal investigations such as barium studies and endoscopy were speculative and of little patient benefit.

Radiological procedures

Laboratory and radiological procedures directed at identifying the primary tumour or determining disease extent should only be carried out if patient management will benefit. Many studies reveal an extremely poor yield despite extensive investigations (Osteen *et al.* 1978; Stewart *et al.* 1979). Only 58 primary sites were identified by non-invasive investigations in 286 patients (20 per cent) in a recent series from our unit. A further 30 were identified at post-mortem (Kirsten *et al.* 1987). In an earlier series more primaries were identified by the development of new symptoms at follow-up than by intensive investigation at initial presentation (Stewart *et al.* 1979).

Nystrom *et al.* (1979) reviewed 266 cases of cancer of unknown primary site investigated between 1967 and 1974. Diagnostic work-up included upper and lower gastrointestinal tract barium studies, chest radiography, intravenous pyelography, liver scan, skeletal survey, and usually mammography in women. The primary site was established in 129 patients (48 per cent), usually at autopsy. A primary site was identified in only 22 out of 136 patients (16 per cent) who did not undergo autopsy.

In a significant number of cases autopsy failed to confirm primary or metastatic tumour involvement in the kidneys or gastrointestinal tract when prior radiographic procedures had suggested a primary (Nystrom *et al.* 1979). Therefore, barium meals and enemas have a high false-positive rate and very low (2–5 per cent) diagnostic yield (Didolkar *et al.* 1977; Osteen *et al.* 1978; Nystrom *et al.* 1979; Stewart *et al.* 1979). Routine performance of these tests appears inappropriate in terms of cost, time, patient discomfort, and yield, as the results are likely to be misleading. There may be some justification in performing such tests in the presence of symptoms or signs, as this may assist in palliation. Endoscopic procedures are also of infrequent direct benefit unless there are symptoms. The results of radiological investigations from several series are shown in Table 7.

Mammography may detect clinically occult breast carcinoma. Up to 13 per cent of women with disseminated cancer of unknown primary site have a mammographically detectable breast primary (Didolkar *et al.* 1977; Kirsten *et al.* 1987). Although the number of true-positives is small, they represent a treatable subset of patients.

Testicular and thyroid ultrasound tend to have a low diagnostic yield, but are clearly of potential benefit in diagnosing treatable tumours. Abdominal and pelvic ultrasound are rarely diagnostic, but they have the potential to identify ovarian malignancy (Hamilton and Langlands 1987).

Liver–spleen scanning is not helpful in patients with normal liver function tests (Osteen *et al.* 1978). We recommend that these or similar studies only be carried out in the presence of symptoms and if a positive finding would alter patient management. Gallium scanning has an established role in managing lymphoma and is generally of little use in cancer of unknown primary site. Bone scanning and plain radiography often provide useful information in the staging and active management of patients rather than in defining tumour extent. The high incidence of positive bone scans in cancer of unknown primary site was described above.

CT scanning, particularly of the abdomen and pelvis, may be of value in the work-up of selected cases of cancer of unknown primary site. In two series the primary site was identified in approximately one-third of cases (Karsell *et al.* 1982; McMillan *et al.* 1982). This represents a 3- to 4-fold improvement over earlier techniques. CT was clinically helpful in either the discovery or further definition of the extent of tumour in most of these cases. A pancreatic, renal, or pulmonary primary accounted for 21 of the 31 cases identified (Karsell *et al.* 1982). Chest CT has less diagnostic value. A coin lesion, malignant effusion, or hilar mass could be either the primary tumour or a metastasis. However, multiple nodules and infiltrative lesions tend to represent metastatic disease (Nystrom *et al.* 1979). Bronchoscopy may be warranted for suspicious perihilar lesions. In selected cases of cancer of unknown primary site, CT

Table 7 Radiological procedures in the investigation of cancer of unknown primary site

	Barium meal	Barium enema	IVP	Mammogram
Total patients tested	497	449	438	59
Positive	53	42	41	6
True-positive	28	22	15	6
False-positive	25	20	26	0

IVP, intravenous pyelography.
Data from Didolkar *et al.* (1977), Osteen *et al.* (1978), Nystrom *et al.* (1979), and Stewart *et al.* (1979).

is most cost effective as it assists in diagnosis, detection of early problems, and planning management.

Evaluation of the usefulness of newer modalities in the diagnosis and staging of cancer of unknown primary site, including magnetic resonance imaging, positron emission tomography, and monoclonal antibody scanning, is awaited.

MANAGEMENT

Selecting treatable subsets

Active systemic therapy is available in only 10–15 per cent of cancer of unknown primary site. Investigations should be primarily directed at identifying this group. Table 8 lists the majority of tumours for which effective systemic therapy is available. Secondly, investigations may identify a cancer for which there is no known effective therapy. This justifies a 'no treatment' policy and, thus, no treatment-related toxicity. Thirdly, investigations may lead to the prevention of a local complication. Examples include spinal cord compression, bowel obstruction, and pathological bone fracture.

A schema for the management of cancer of unknown primary site is outlined in Fig. 2. Such an approach should achieve a rapid ante-mortem identification of treatable cancers (Kirsten *et al.* 1987). The initial step should include a detailed histology review of adequate biopsy material with the assistance of special stains and electron microscopy. Serum tumour markers such as α-fetoprotein, β-human chorionic gonadotrophin, prostate-specific antigen, and CA125 may rapidly establish a treatable primary. Subsequent investigations by mammography and testicular and pelvic ultrasound may be appropriate and abdominal CT may play both a diagnostic and management role. Further investigations are unlikely to reveal a treatable primary cancer and should only be carried out if they will alter management.

Specific therapy

In a small number of cases the primary site is discovered after work-up and it is possible to institute specific therapy for that metastatic malignancy. In another small subset of patients it is appropriate to institute therapy specific for the most probable treatable neoplasm. Examples include axillary metastases in females, squamous cell cancer presenting in high cervical nodes, and patients suspected of having the atypical extragonadal germ cell syndrome. As described above, effective palliation and prolonged survival is possible in some of these patients.

Table 8 Treatable tumours which may present as cancer of unknown primary site

Cure possible
  Germ cell tumours
  Hodgkin's disease
  Non-Hodgkin's lymphoma
  Thyroid cancer
  Trophoblastic tumours

Effective palliation

Chemoresponsive (⩾50%)	Hormonal treatment
Breast cancer	Breast cancer
Gastric cancer	Endometrial cancer
Head and neck cancer	Prostatic cancer
Ovarian cancer	Thyroid cancer
Sarcomas	
Small cell (lung) cancer	

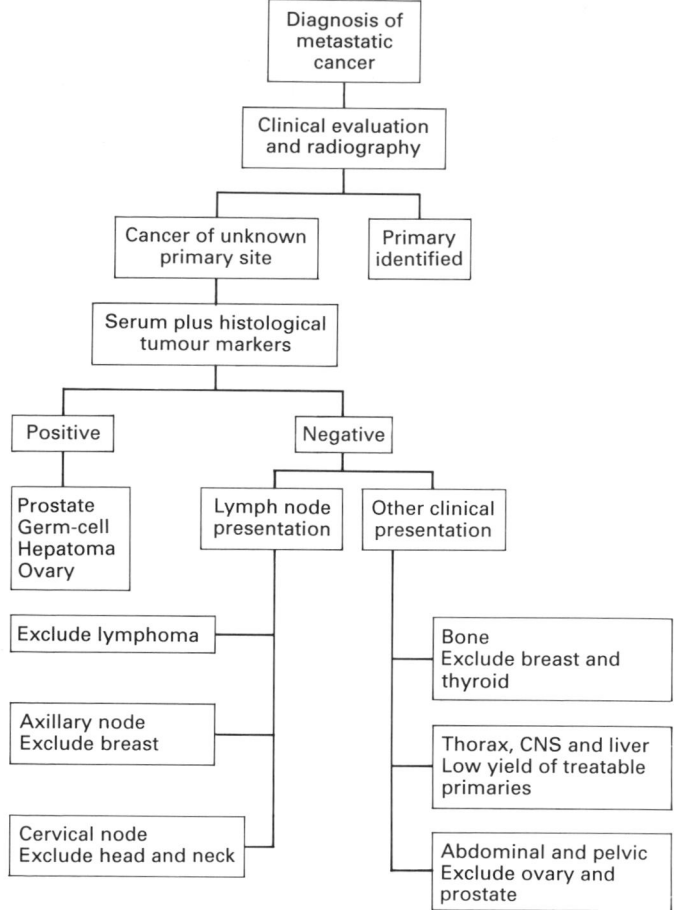

Fig. 2 Identification of treatable cancer of unknown primary site.

Most local metastases can be palliated with local radiotherapy. We believe that local metastases should only be treated when the patient becomes symptomatic or when the cancer of unknown primary site is thought to originate from a primary tumour for which effective curative or palliative therapy is available (see Table 8).

In the majority of cancer of unknown primary site the primary remains occult. Several trials of single-agent and combination chemotherapy are reported in the literature (Table 9). Tumour response rates are seldom greater than 20 per cent. Trials have generally not demonstrated a significant survival advantage using simple or intensive combination chemotherapy. The major obstacle facing effective therapy is that the majority of cancers of unknown primary site are derived from tumours which tend to be chemoresistant or in which the duration of response is short.

There have been several randomized trials of combination chemotherapy in symptomatic patients. However, no studies have contained a 'no treatment' arm. We have participated in two randomized trials, the first comparing cyclophosphamide, methotrexate, and 5-fluorouracil (CMF) with doxorubicin and mitomycin C (DMi) and the second comparing DMi with cisplatinum, vinblastine, and bleomycin (PVB) (Woods *et al.* 1980; Milliken *et al.* 1987). A tumour response occurred in one-third of patients treated with DM and PVB, but there was no demonstrable survival advantage in patients treated by chemotherapy. There was a trend towards better survival in patients treated with DMi compared with CMF, but this did not attain statistical significance.

Table 9 Chemotherapy trials in cancer of unknown primary site

Study	Patients	Regimen[a]	Response rate[b] (%)	Median survival	Comments
Randomized trials					
Woods et al. (1980)	47	DMi vs CMF	36 vs 4.5	18 vs 7 weeks	p=NS No difference in toxicity six responders survived > 2 years
Shildt et al. (1983)	36	F vs FAC	Nil	105 vs 95 days	Toxicity with FAC more common and severe
Milliken et al. (1987)	95	DMi vs PVB	42 vs 32	18 vs 25 weeks	p=NS Differing toxicities: haematologic/gastrointestinal Limited efficacy
Eagan et al. (1987)	55	MiA vs MiAP	7 vs 18.5	5.5 vs 4.6 months	p=NS Toxicity increased with cisplatin
Non-randomized trials					
Moertel et al. (1972)	162	F, Mi, or F.BCNU	12 PR	11 months (4 months overall)	
Didolkar et al. (1977)	130	COMN	6 PR	(6 months overall)	
Valentine et al. (1979)	14	CAF	14 PR		
Indupalli et al. (1981)	38	Various	21 PR	(31 weeks overall)	Adriamycin-containing treatments better response; longer median survival (but better prognostic factors)
Anderson et al. (1983)	20	VcAC	20 CR 30 PR	(8 months overall)	CRs alive at 13–39 months Karnofsky improved Toxicity minimal Resp vs NonResp: p=NS
Fiore et al. (1985)	42	VdD	3 CR 11 PR	>8 months Resp 6 months NonResp	Well tolerated
Jordan and Shildt (1985)	37	Various	8 PR	6 months (4 months overall)	Amelioration, not reflected in survival
Goldberg et al. (1986)	45	FAMi	9 CR 21 PR	>14 months (>10 months overall)	'Well tolerated' but three toxic deaths; seven patients survived >2 years
Pastertz et al. (1986)	70	FAC, FAM, or CyVcADIC	28 PR	16 months (7 months overall)	Significant toxicity No difference between regimens
Walach and Horn (1987)	21	COMF	29 CR 19 PR	Not stated	Well tolerated Response: CR 43 months, PR 8 months
Van der Gaast et al. (1988)	23	FAMi	14 PR	54+ weeks (33+ weeks overall)	Overall well tolerated FAMi not recommended
Alberts et al. (1989)	100	Various		(125 days overall)	Prognostic factors: nodal mass Good performance status
	61	FIVcBCNU	19 PR	286 days (107 days overall)	
Becouarn et al. (1989)	85	FAP.HMM	21 PR	12.5 months (7 months overall)	Limited efficacy in palliation Non-negligible toxicity
Treat et al. (1989)	19	m-FAMi	37 PR 47 SD	16 months 10 months (15 months overall)	Toxicity acceptable Response duration: PR 11 months, SD 6 months

NS, not significant.

[a] HMM, altretamine; B, bleomycin; BCNU, carmustine; C or Cy, cyclophosphamide; I or DIC, decarbazine; A or D, doxorubicin; F, 5-fluorouracil; M or m, methotrexate; Mi, mitomycin-C; N, mustard; P, cisplatin; V, vinblastine; Vc or O, vincristine; Vd, vindesine.

[b] RR, response rate; CR, complete response; PR, partial response; SD, stable disease; Resp, responders; NonResp, non-responders.

The Southwest Oncology Group compared 5-fluorouracil versus 5-fluorouracil plus doxorubicin and cyclophosphamide in 36 patients. There was no response in either group and no survival advantage for the most intensive and toxic regimen (Shildt et al. 1983).

Such results emphasize our view that at present management of patients with cancer of unknown primary site should consist of a rapid search directed at detecting a small subgroup of treatable tumours. More intensive and expensive investigations, described above, are usually unrewarding and unjustified. Patients in whom a treatable primary tumour cannot be demonstrated are unlikely to benefit significantly from current empirical chemotherapy schedules and ideally should only be treated in the context of a randomized trial.

REFERENCES

Alberts AS, Falkson G, Falkson HC, Van Der Merwe MP (1989). Treatment and prognosis of metastatic carcinoma of unknown primary: analysis of 100 patients *Medical and Pediatric Oncology*, 17:188–92.

Altman E, Cadman E (1986). An analysis of 1539 patients with cancer of unknown primary site. *Cancer*, 57:120–4.

Anderson H, et al. (1983). VAC (vincristine, adriamycin, cyclophosphamide) chemotherapy for metastatic carcinoma from an unknown primary site. European Journal of Cancer and Clinical Oncology, 19:49–52.

Anner RM, Drewinko B (1977). Frequency and significance of bone marrow involvement by metastatic solid tumours. Cancer, 39:1337–44.

Atkin NB (1986). Chromosome 1 aberrations in cancer. Cancer Genetics and Cytogenetics, 21:279–85.

Barrie JR, Knapper WH, Strong EW (1970). Cervical nodal metastases of unknown origin. American Journal of Surgery, 120:466–70.

Becouarn Y, Brunet R, Barbe-Gaston C (1989). Fluorouracil, doxorubicin, cisplatin and altretamine in the treatment of metastatic carcinoma of unknown primary. European Journal of Cancer and Clinical Oncology, 25:861–65.

Bell CW, Pathak S, Frost P (1989). Unknown primary tumors: establishment of cell lines, identification of chromosomal abnormalities and implications for a second type of tumour progression. Cancer Research, 49:4311–15.

Copeland EM, McBride CM (1973). Axillary metastases from unknown primary sites. Annals of Surgery, 178:25–7.

Dalrymple JC, et al. (1989). Extraovarian (peritoneal) serous papillary carcinoma: a clinicopathological study of 31 cases. Cancer, 64:110–15.

DeLellis RA, Dayal Y (1987). The role of immunohistochemistry in the diagnosis of poorly differentiated malignant neoplasms. Seminars in Oncology, 14:173–92.

Didolkar MS, Fanous N, Elias EG, Moore RH (1977). Metastatic carcinomas from occult primary tumours. Annals of Surgery, 186:625–30.

Eagan RT, et al. (1987). Lack of value for cisplatin added to mitomycin–doxorubicin combination chemotherapy for carcinoma of unknown primary site. American Journal of Clinical Oncology, 10:82–5

Feigenberg Z, Zer M, Dintsman M (1976). Axillary metastases from an unknown primary source: a diagnostic and therapeutic approach. Israel Journal of Medical Science, 12:1153–8.

Fiore JJ, et al. (1985). Adenocarcinoma of unknown primary origin: treatment with vindesine and doxorubicin. Cancer Treatment Reports, 69:591–4.

Fox RM, Woods RL, Tattersall MHN, McGovern VJ (1979). Undifferentiated carcinoma in young men: the atypical teratoma syndrome. Lancet, i:1316–18.

Fraser RS, Viloria JB, Wang N (1980). Cardiac tamponade as a presentation of extracardiac malignancy. Cancer, 45:1697–704.

Gaber AO, et al. (1983). Metastatic malignant disease of unknown origin. American Journal of Surgery, 145:493–7.

Goldberg RM, et al. (1986) 5-Fluorouracil, adriamycin and mitomycin in the treatment of adenocarcinoma of unknown primary. Journal of Clinical Oncology, 4:395–9.

Greco FA, Oldham RF, Fer MF (1982). The extragonadal germ cell cancer syndrome. Seminars in Oncology, 9:448–55.

Greco FA, Vaughn WK, Hainsworth JD (1986). Advanced poorly differentiated carcinoma of unknown primary site: recognition of a treatable syndrome. Annals of Internal Medicine, 104:547–53.

Grosbach AB (1982). Carcinoma of unknown primary site: a clinical enigma. Archives of Internal Medicine, 142:357–9.

Guarischi A, Keane TJ, Elhakim T (1987). Metastatic inguinal nodes from an unknown primary neoplasm: a review of 56 cases. Cancer, 59:572–7.

Hainsworth JD, Wright EP, Gray GF, Greco FA (1987). Poorly differentiated carcinoma of unknown primary site: correlation of light microscopic findings with response to cisplatin-based combination chemotherapy. Journal of Clinical Oncology, 5:1275–80.

Hainsworth JD, Johnson DH, Greco FA (1988). Poorly differentiated neuroendocrine carcinoma of unknown primary site: a newly recognized clinicopathologic entity. Annals of Internal Medicine, 109:364–71.

Hamilton CS, Langlands AO (1987). ACUPS (adenocarcinoma of unknown primary site): a clinical and cost benefit analysis. International Journal of Radiation Oncology — Biology — Physics, 13:1497–503.

Hanna WM, Kahn HJ (1985). The ultrastructure of metastatic adenocarcinoma in serous fluids: an aid in the identification of the primary site of the neoplasm. Acta Cytologica, 29:206–10.

Hedley DW, Leary JA, Kirsten F (1985). Metastatic adenocarcinoma of unknown primary site: abnormalities of cellular DNA content and survival. European Journal of Cancer and Clinical Oncology, 21:185–9.

Herrera GA, Reimann BE (1984). Electron microscopy in determining origin of metastatic adenocarcinoma. Southern Medical Journal, 77:1557–66.

Holmes FF, Fouts TL (1970) Metastatic cancer of unknown primary site. Cancer, 26:816–20.

Indupalli R, Bedikian AY, Bodey GP (1981). Adenocarcinoma of unknown primary origin: impact of chemotherapy on survival. Southern Medical Journal, 74:1431–5.

Inglehart JD, et al. (1982). An ultrastructural analysis of breast carcinoma presenting as isolated axillary adenopathy. Annals of Surgery, 196:8–13.

Jesse RH, Perez CA, Fletcher GH (1973). Cervical lymph node metastasis: unknown primary cancer. Cancer, 31:854–9.

Jones A, Farrow G, Richardson RL (1985) The extragonadal germ cell cancer syndrome—the Mayo Clinic experience. In Poorly differentiated neoplasms (ed. MF Fer, FA Greco, and RK Oldham), pp. 203–16. Grune & Stratton, Orlando, FL.

Jordan WE, Shildt A (1985). Adenocarcinoma of unknown primary site: the Brooke Army Medical Centre experience. Cancer, 55:857–60.

Kabawat SE, et al. (1983). Immunopathologic characterization of a monoclonal antibody that recognizes common surface antigens of human ovarian tumours of serous, endometrioid and clear cell types. American Journal of Clinical Pathology, 79:98–103.

Karsell PR, Sheedy PF, O'Connell MJ (1982). Computed tomography in search of cancer of unknown origin. Journal of the American Medical Association, 248:340–3.

Kern WH, Abbott M (1980). The determination of unknown primary sites based upon the histologic appearance of metastases. Surgery, Gynecology and Obstetrics, 151:73–6.

Key JD, Shephard DAE, Walters W (1976). Sister Mary Joseph's nodule and its relationship to diagnosis of carcinoma of the umbilicus. Minnesota Medicine, 59:561–6.

Kirsten F, et al. (1987). Metastatic adeno or undifferentiated carcinoma from an unknown primary site—natural history and guidelines for identification of treatable subsets. Quarterly Journal of Medicine, 62:143–61.

Krementz ET, Cerise EJ, Foster DS, Morgan LR (1979). Metastases of undetermined source. Current Problems in Cancer, 4:4–37.

Kurtin PJ, Pinkus GS (1985). Leukocyte common antigen: a diagnostic discriminant between hematopoietic and nonhematopoietic neoplasms in paraffin sections using monoclonal antibodies. Correlation with immunological studies and ultrastructural localization. Human Pathology, 16:353–65.

Levine MN, Drummond M, Labelle RJ (1985). Cost-effectiveness in the diagnosis and treatment of carcinoma of unknown primary origin. Canadian Medical Association Journal, 133:977–87.

Logothetis CJ, et al. (1985). Chemotherapy of extragonadal germ cell tumors. Journal of Clinical Oncology, 3:316–25.

McCredie M, Coates MS, Ford JM (1988). The changing incidence of cancer in adults in New South Wales. International Journal of Cancer, 42:667–71.

McGovern VJ (1975). Spontaneous regression of melanoma. Pathology, 7:91–9.

MacKay B, Ordonez NG (1982). The role of the pathologist in the evaluation of poorly differentiated tumours. Seminars in Oncology, 9:396–415.

McMillan JH, Levin E, Stephens RL (1982) Computed body tomography in the evaluation of metastatic adenocarcinoma from an unknown primary site. Radiology, 143:143–6.

Markham M (1982). Metastatic adenocarcinoma of unknown primary site: analysis of 245 patients seen at the Johns Hopkins Hospital from 1965–1979. Medical and Pediatric Oncology, 10:569–74.

Milliken ST, et al. (1987). Metastatic adenocarcinoma of unknown primary site. A randomized study of two combination chemotherapy regimens. European Journal of Cancer and Clinical Oncology, 23:1645–8.

Moertel CG, Reitemeier RJ, Schutt AJ, Hahn RG (1972). Treatment of the patient with adenocarcinoma of unknown origin. Cancer, 30:1469–72.

Mostofi FK, Price ED (1973). Tumors of the male genital system. In Atlas of tumor pathology, pp. 121–5, Fascicle 8. AFIP Tumor Fascicle Series 2, Washington, DC.

Nesbit RA, Tattersall MHN, Fox RM, Woods RL (1981). Presentation of unknown primary cancer with metastatic liver disease—management and natural history. Australian and New Zealand Journal of Medicine, 11:16–19.

Neumann KH, Nystrom JS (1982). Metastatic cancer of unknown origin: nonsquamous cell type. Seminars in Oncology, 9:427–34.

Ng A, Philips J (1985). Fine needle aspiration. Professional Information News Sheet. NSW Cancer Council.

Nissenblatt MJ (1981). The CUP syndrome (carcinoma unknown primary). *Cancer Treatment Review*, 8:211–24.

NSW Central Cancer Registry (1983). *Cancer in New South Wales. Incidence and mortality.* NSW Cancer Council: 64–5.

Nystrom JS, *et al.* (1977). Metastatic and histologic presentations in unknown primary cancer. *Seminars in Oncology*, 4:53–8.

Nystrom JS, *et al.* (1979). Identifying the primary site in metastatic cancer of unknown origin: inadequacy of roentgenographic procedures. *Journal of the American Medical Association*, 241:381–3.

Osteen RT, Kopf G, Wilson RE (1978). In pursuit of the unknown primary. *American Journal of Surgery*, 135:494–8.

Pasterz R, Savaraj N, Burgess M (1986). Prognostic factors in metastatic carcinoma of unknown primary. *Journal of Clinical Oncology*, 4:1652–7.

Patel J, *et al.* (1981). Axillary lymph node metastasis from an occult breast cancer. *Cancer*, 47:2923–7.

Richardson RG, Parker RG (1975). Metastases from undetected primary cancers—clinical experience at a radiation oncology center (medical information). *Western Journal of Medicine*, 123:337–9.

Richardson RL, *et al.* (1979). Extra-gonadal germ cell malignancy: value of tumor markers in metastatic carcinoma in young males. *Proceedings of the American Association for Cancer Research*, 20:204.

Ringenberg QS (1985). Tumors of unknown origin. *Medical and Pediatric Oncology*, 13:301–6.

Ringenberg QS, Doll DC, Yarbro JW, Perry MC (1986). Tumors of unknown origin in the bone marrow. *Archives of Internal Medicine*, 146:2027–8.

Scarpa FJ, Dineen JP, Boltax RS (1979). Visceral neoplasia presenting at the umbilicus. *Journal of Surgical Oncology*, 11:351–9.

Shildt RA, *et al.* (1983). Management of patients with metastatic adenocarcinoma of unknown origin: a Southwest Oncology Group Study. *Cancer Treatment Reports*, 67:77–9.

Singh G, Krause JR, Volker B (1977). Bone marrow examination for metastatic tumor: aspirate and biopsy. *Cancer*, 40:2317–21.

Smith PE, Krementz ET, Chapman W (1967) Metastatic cancer without a detectable primary site. *American Journal of Surgery*, 113:633–7.

Steckel RJ, Kagan AR (1980). Diagnostic persistance in working up metastatic cancer with an unknown primary site. *Diagnostic Radiology*, 134:367–9.

Stewart JF, Tattersall MHN, Woods RL, Fox RM (1979). Unknown primary adenocarcinoma: incidence of overinvestigation and natural history. *British Medical Journal*, 1:1530–3.

Strnad CM, *et al.* (1989). Peritoneal carcinomatosis of unknown primary site in women: a distinctive subset of adenocarcinoma. *Annals of Internal Medicine*, 111:213–17.

Tell DR, Khoury JM, Taylor HG, Veasey SP (1985). Atypical metastases from prostate cancer; clinical utility of the immunoperoxidase technique for prostate-specific antigen. *Journal of the American Medical Association*, 253:3574–5.

Treat J, *et al.* (1989). Phase II trial of methotrexate-FAM (m-FAM) in adenocarcinoma of unknown primary. *European Journal of Cancer and Clinical Oncology*, 25:1053–5.

Valentine J, Rosenthal S, Arseneau J (1979). Combination chemotherapy for adenocarcinoma of unknown origin. *Cancer Clinical Trials*, 2:265–8.

Van der Gaast A, Verweij J, Planting AST, Stoter G (1988). 5–Fluorouracil, doxorubicin and mitomycin C (FAM) combination chemotherapy for metastatic adenocarcinoma of unknown primary. *European Journal of Cancer and Clinical Oncology*, 24:765–8.

Walach N, Horn Y (1987). Combination chemotherapy in the treatment of adenocarcinoma of unknown primary origin. *Cancer Treatment Reports*, 71:605–7.

Weber P, Troger J, Ernst H (1973). Das pankreaskarzinom klinisch als zentrales Brouchuskarzinom maskiert. *Deutsche Medizinische Wochenschrift*, 98:1389–91.

Westbrook KG, Gallagher HS (1971). Breast carcinoma presenting as an axillary mass. *American Journal of Surgery*, 122:607–11.

Woods RL, *et al.* (1980). Metastatic adenocarcinomas of unknown primary site: a randomized study of two combination-chemotherapy regimens. *New England Journal of Medicine*, 303:87–9.

Section 18
Cancer in the elderly

18   Cancer in the elderly

DEREK RAGHAVAN, MICHAEL P. N. FINDLAY, AND E. B. McNEIL

INTRODUCTION

During the twentieth century, the proportion of the population older than 70 years has increased and is now approaching 15 per cent (Vestal 1978; WHO 1981). In contrast, nearly 30 per cent of health resources are consumed by this group. As the aged population is increasing and because the prevalence of malignancy rises with age, it is clear that the management of cancer in the elderly will occupy a much greater proportion of health expenditure in the future. Given that the active life expectancy of the elderly has increased, so that patients aged 65 and 70 years can expect an active life of more than 10 and 8 years, respectively (Katz et al. 1983; Fentiman et al. 1990), the potential benefits of a rational approach to cancer care in the elderly are self-evident. It will become increasingly important to define clearly the extent of clinical activity or aggression that should be employed in this group of patients, the level of health resources that should be expended in their care, and the philosophical and ethical considerations that will govern such approaches. Thus, it is timely to review the state of our knowledge regarding the biology of cancer in the aged and the biology of the aged with cancer and to apply this information to the resolution of these dilemmas.

BIOLOGY OF AGEING

The elderly undergo age-related changes in their physiology which may result in altered tolerance to disease and to the requirements of the management of illness. One of the most important physiological changes to occur with ageing is a diminution of physiological reserves, characterized by a generalized decline in the ability to respond to physiological insults and a slower recovery from them (Leventhal 1986). These alterations in physiology occur in the absence of disease and simply reflect the phenomenon of ageing, although they may be substantially exacerbated by intercurrent illness.

Cardiovascular system

Ageing may be associated with loss of cardiac muscle fibres from ischaemia or degenerative disorders or with ventricular hypertrophy. Of particular importance, cardiac output reduces by approximately 1 per cent each year between the ages of 25 and 80 years (Bender 1965). As a result, there is a reduction in the perfusion of the kidneys, liver, lungs, gastrointestinal tract, and skeletal muscle, although compensatory mechanisms retain blood flow to the brain and heart. Some studies suggest that the systolic blood pressure increases after the age of 65 years, although the diastolic pressure often falls (Bender 1965).

Renal function

Between the fourth and eighth decades, the kidneys lose approximately 20 per cent of their weight, with an associated reduction of glomerular number, number of functioning nephrons, and cortical volume (Hollenberg et al. 1974; McLachlan 1978). The renal blood flow is reduced to a greater extent than would be predicted solely on the basis of reduced cardiac output (Triggs and Nation 1975) and probably reflect glomerular sclerosis. The glomerular filtration rate consequently decreases with advancing age (Greenblatt et al. 1982). With increased age, the kidney is less able to concentrate urine maximally (Dontas et al. 1972) and the consequent increased flow of dilute urine may, in fact, decrease the contact time of potential tubular toxins (Hrushesky et al. 1974). Furthermore, in the elderly, a substantial decrease in lean muscle mass results in reduced creatinine excretion. This reduction and the decrease in creatinine clearance with ageing may not necessarily be reflected by a rise of serum creatinine, which may thus be a misleading index of renal function in the aged (Rowe et al. 1976).

Hepatic and gastrointestinal function

With increasing age, there is a reduction of up to 40 per cent in hepatic blood flow (Greenblatt et al. 1982). The liver mass also decreases, as does the ability to repair or replace damaged hepatocytes (Popper 1986). Hepatic enzyme activity may decrease with age, but such changes are unpredictable and are strongly influenced by intercurrent disease. For example, the functions of acetylation and conjugation do not usually change with age, whereas the function of the microsomal oxidative enzymes is reduced in the aged. Age-related changes are evident throughout the alimentary tract. Oesophageal peristalsis is impaired in old age (Khan et al. 1977). Furthermore, gastric emptying is slowed (Evans et al. 1981) and there is a reduction in gastric acid secretion and in the number of functional absorbing cells. The gastric emptying time rises and intestinal motility is reduced (Brocklehurst and Khan 1969). These factors may be compounded by changes in diet, excessive ingestion of antacids or laxatives, and the presence of intercurrent diseases such as congestive cardiac failure or cirrhosis. These changes are of particular importance in the absorption and metabolism of orally administered medications (see below).

Respiratory system

There are several age-related changes in pulmonary function which contribute to ventilation–perfusion mismatch and a consequent reduction in respiratory function. The vital capacity, $FEV_{1.0}$ and respiratory reserve decline because of decreases in compliance and alveolar septal loss (Brandsteller and Kazemi 1983). The composition of collagen changes, with the formation of more cross-links between its subunits, which may also account for some of the changes in the lung (Boucek et al. 1961). The pulmonary diffusing capacity decreases with age because of a loss of capillary segments in the lung, deranged ventilation–perfusion ratios, and a reduced cardiac output.

Haemopoiesis and immunity

The bone-marrow progressively involutes in distribution and cellularity with increasing age (Hartstock et al. 1965). Anaemia occurs more commonly in elderly males, although much of this may be due to a dilutional effect from the increasing proportion of extracellular fluid (Piomelli *et al.* 1962). However, it is generally believed that there is also a slight reduction in stem cell function with a consequent decline in the circulating haemoglobin level after 70 years of age (Lipschitz and Udupa 1986). Of greater importance is the reduction in reserve capacity with increased age, i.e. the inability of the marrow to respond as effectively to blood loss or other stresses. In the elderly, the neutrophil count and neutrophil function remain stable, but there is a reduction in the number of peripheral blood lymphocytes (Bender *et al.* 1986) which may contribute to the reduced immune function of the aged. In fact, there is an overall reduction of cell-mediated and humoral immune responses to foreign antigens in the aged, while the responses to self-antigens are increased (Schwab *et al.* 1989). The reduced cell-mediated immunity is partly a result of the thymic involution of ageing. There is also a reduction in febrile response (Gleckman and Hibert 1982) and in the antibody response to antigenic stimulation in the elderly (Ershler *et al.* 1984).

Nervous system

After the age of approximately 25 years, there is progressive loss of neuronal tissue in the central nervous system. As this increases, there are progressive changes in behavioural patterns and reductions in cognitive function. Although the consumption of glucose and oxygen is not reduced at rest in the aged brain, sensory stimulation results in smaller increments in metabolic activity with advancing age, suggesting a limited ability of the central nervous system to adapt to stress in old age (Rapaport 1986). In addition, there is a progressive reduction of peripheral neuronal function with increased age, a situation which is often compounded by intercurrent disorders such as depression, malnutrition, diabetes, or alcohol abuse.

Metabolic changes

A broad range of other biochemical and physiological changes occur as part of the ageing process. The ageing process is characterized by a slowing of protein synthesis and degradation, with an accumulation of altered proteins that may be a function of reduced transcriptional or translational accuracy (Tollefsbol and Cohen 1986). For example, there is an impairment in the induction of glucose-metabolizing enzymes with age, accompanied by increased peripheral insulin resistance. There are also age-related perturbations in the enzyme systems that control lipid metabolism and there may also be changes in the hepatic microsomal oxidative system with advancing age (Tollefsbol and Cohen 1986). There is a progressive reduction of lean body mass, with replacement by fat or adipose tissue with increasing age (Rossman 1977).

These issues may be compounded by the nutritional state of the patient. Malnutrition is a frequent concomitant of ageing for a range of reasons: poverty and depression are prevalent in this population, there is often a diminished sense of smell and taste and appreciation of food (Cohen and Gitman 1959; Schiffman *et al.* 1976), and intercurrent illness may alter the gastrointestinal absorption of various nutrients or even the requirements for such nutrients.

The physiological changes discussed above reflect the normal changes of ageing in the healthy individual. However, each of the organ systems can be further compromised by specific disorders, intercurrent disease, or cancer. For example, the prevalence of coronary artery disease increases with age, accounting for nearly 50 per cent of all deaths in the elderly. The normal age-related

Table 1 Age-specific incidence of common cancers in the elderly

| Type | Age-specific incidence (per 100 000 population in age group) | | | |
	65–69 years	70–74 years	75–79 years	80+ years
Male				
All sites	1530	2083	2526	3080
Lung	374	485	460	450
Prostate	221	378	558	788
Colon	119	187	235	307
Bladder	117	140	209	241
Rectum	106	111	122	185
Pancreas	48	82	83	105
Stomach	51	114	160	171
Oesophagus	37	33	49	21
Melanoma	58	71	67	87
Lymphoma[a]	34	53	52	56
Female				
All sites	936	1003	1198	1392
Breast	196	183	226	223
Colon	87	139	199	267
Lung	97	103	84	35
Rectum	47	53	70	80
Stomach	30	28	67	120
Pancreas	36	31	50	58
Bladder	35	35	41	47
Ovary	34	44	26	35
Melanoma	42	31	34	35
Uterus				
Body	38	43	41	40
Cervix	32	20	14	17

[a] Lymphoma, ICD 200 including lymphosarcoma and reticulum cell sarcoma.
Data from New South Wales Cancer Registry (1986).

changes in cardiac function can be exacerbated by coronary artery disease, cardiac arrhythmias, and cardiac valve disorders.

THE BIOLOGY OF CANCER IN THE ELDERLY

Epidemiological aspects

In Western society, more than 50 per cent of cancer occurs in only 15 per cent of the community; those over 65–70 years of age (Ries *et al.* 1983; Crawford and Cohen 1987). It has been estimated that a man aged 65 years has 50 times the probability of developing cancer in the next 5 years as a man aged 25 years (Peto *et al.* 1975).

As shown in Table 1, there is an illusion that cancer is predominantly a disease of late middle age and not of the elderly. However, if reduced population numbers over the age of 70 years are allowed for, it is clear that the absolute age-specific cancer incidence and mortality continue to rise as a function of age (Ries *et al.* 1983; Crawford and Cohen 1987).

Associations between cancer and ageing

The basis of the association between malignancy and ageing has been the subject of several authoritative reviews, although a clear resolution of the issue has not been achieved (Peto *et al.* 1975; Pitot 1977; Doll 1978; Anisimov 1987; Crawford and Cohen 1987). The possible reasons for the increased prevalence of cancer in the elderly may include any of the following: a longer potential duration of

Table 2 Correlation between age and stage at diagnosis

Site	Series		
	Holmes *et al.*	Goodwin *et al.*	Mor *et al.*
Bladder	Positive	Positive	—
Breast	Positive	Positive	Positive
Colon	—	—	—
Kidney	Positive	—	—
Lung	Negative	Negative	—
Melanoma	—	Positive	—
Ovary	Positive	Positive	—
Pancreas	—	Negative	—
Prostate	—	—	Positive
Rectum	—	Negative	—
Stomach	—	Negative	—
Thyroid	—	Positive	—
Uterus			
Body	Positive	Positive	Positive
Cervix	Positive	Positive	Positive

Positive correlation, increased tumour aggression in the elderly; negative correlation, reduced tumour aggression in the elderly.

exposure to carcinogens, a longer period for expression of outcome from such exposure, increased susceptibility of aged cells to the effects of carcinogens, a reduced ability to repair DNA, reduced host defences against malignancy, and programmed changes in the organism during ageing (as a function of gene expression) which increase the probability of development of cancer.

Tumour aggression and age

Another controversial issue is whether the activity or aggression of malignancy changes with age. Conflicting data have been produced from experimental models (Anisimov 1987; Kaesberg and Ershler 1989) and from clinical studies (Holmes and Hearne 1981; Lipschitz *et al.* 1985; Goodwin *et al.* 1986; Holmes 1989). In many animal tumours, an age advantage is seen in those that arise spontaneously, those which are weakly immunogenic, and those under endocrine control (Kaesberg and Ershler 1989). In the case of highly immunogenic tumours (for example, sarcomas induced by methylcholanthrene or by ultraviolet irradiation), older animals have a shorter survival.

The optimal index of tumour aggression in the elderly has not been defined. Potential parameters include stage at presentation, histological grade, survival, and distribution of malignancy at death. However, each of these can be strongly influenced by intercurrent factors. As shown in Table 2, some tumours are more advanced at presentation in the elderly. Whether this is a function of increased tumour aggressiveness or is simply a reflection of delayed clinical presentation in the elderly is not clear. Several other factors may influence survival in this context (Lipschitz *et al.* 1985; Mor *et al.* 1985; Holmes 1989): there may be differences in the biology of the tumour, the prevalence of intercurrent diseases, physical fitness and the ability to withstand treatment, biases among clinicians which influence the treatment actually prescribed, and available facilities for treatment.

Data culled from large series of autopsies contrast with those reported in Table 2. For example, in such studies cancers of bladder, breast, colorectum, kidney, lung, pancreas, prostate, and uterus have been documented to metastasize less often in the elderly (Suen *et al.* 1974; Saitoh *et al.* 1982; Ershler *et al.* 1983; O'Rourke *et al.*

1987). However, it should be noted that the apparent distribution of metastases at autopsy may also reflect the aggression of clinical management before death. For example, early referral for terminal care (without active intervention) in an elderly patient may be associated with early death from a primary bronchogenic malignancy with insufficient time to develop clinically or histologically evident metastases.

Histological evidence of tumour aggression or indolence *per se* does not generally appear to be a function of age (Lees and Park 1950; Holmes 1989). It has been suggested that indolent patterns of ovarian cancer may be more common in the young (Richardson *et al.* 1985), but that more aggressive, and less differentiated mammary carcinomas are a feature of the old (Schottenfeld and Robbins 1971; McCarty *et al.* 1983). In contrast, it has been reported that there is a trend towards reduced differentiation with increasing age for cancers of the lung, prostate, bladder, and colorectum (Holmes 1989). It is generally agreed that Hodgkin's disease is more aggressive in the elderly, based upon a more advanced pattern of presentation, a predominance of mixed cellularity histology, and the results of treatment (Lokich *et al.* 1974; Ries *et al.* 1983; Austin-Seymour *et al.* 1984; Kennedy *et al.* 1985). More recently, more sophisticated indices of tumour aggression have been assessed in the elderly, including the measurement of DNA content (Taylor *et al.* 1983; Nanus *et al.* 1989), as discussed below in the context of specific diseases.

When survival is considered as a parameter of tumour aggression, many of the factors noted above can cause artefacts in the outcome: death from intercurrent disease, selection factors of patients and treatment, inaccurate data from death certificates, and changing demographic patterns among the elderly. Although there is no real concordance of published data, it appears that, at least in the context of definitive surgery, there is no difference in outcome of care between young and old patients treated for bronchogenic or colonic cancer (Calabrese *et al.* 1973; Kirsh *et al.* 1976). In contrast, the surveillance, epidemiology, and end results (SEER) data show a decline in observed 5 year survival for all tumour sites and stages with increasing age in both sexes, although this situation is substantially different if deaths from intercurrent disease are excluded (Ries *et al.* 1983; Sondik *et al.* 1987). This issue is discussed further in the sections on specific diseases.

PROBLEMS OF ACTIVE TREATMENT OF CANCER IN THE ELDERLY

Surgical considerations

There are two major roles for surgical intervention in the elderly patient with cancer: the establishment of a diagnosis and the definitive or palliative treatment of the malignancy. A limited surgical procedure, by establishing the diagnosis quickly, may reduce the length of a hospital stay and its attendant morbidity, in contrast with a prolonged schedule of 'non-invasive' (but often morbid) investigations. The issues pertaining to the use of palliative or curative surgical approaches are discussed below in the context of specific cancers.

When approaching surgery for the elderly, it should not be forgotten that most patients in this population have a substantial fear of any such procedure and may entertain the misconception that surgery will cause cancer to spread (Stults 1983). Thus, care should be taken to explain the details of the planned procedure and to resolve such concerns with both the patient and the family.

Pre-operative assessment

Before surgery is undertaken, the clinical team must consider several issues: the anticipated life expectancy of the patient, the physiological status of the patient and ability to withstand the stress of the planned procedures, the influence of the surgical procedure on quality of life and life expectancy, the morbidity of the procedure, alternatives to surgery (for example, percutaneous bypass rather than surgical bypass of an obstruction, radiotherapy versus surgery to achieve local tumour control), the competence of the patient to give informed consent regarding the procedure and its implications, and the intellectual and physical ability of the patient to cope with sequelae of the surgery (for example, a colostomy or ileostomy).

It is clear that, in general, elective surgery can be performed safely on geriatric patients, provided that care is taken to manage their specific physiological problems (Bowles 1983; Patterson 1989). As discussed above, a range of changes occur with ageing, which contribute to a reduced ability of the elderly to withstand physiological or surgical stress (Cohen 1985). For example, Del Guerico and Cohn (1980) reported that only 13.5 per cent of a series of pre-operative patients aged at least 65 years had normal levels of physiological function and 23 per cent had abnormalities that could not be corrected before operation. Elective surgery is clearly preferable to an emergency procedure. A planned operation allows pre-operative assessment and correction of common medical problems in this age group (for example, cardiac failure, dehydration, hypertension, infection, or malnutrition) and attention to prophylactic manoeuvres to reduce intra- and post-operative complications (cessation of smoking for the pre-operative period, chest physiotherapy, bowel care).

The clinician evaluating such a patient should be experienced in the care of the aged to avoid common traps in management. For example, specific physical characteristics of the elderly must be recognized (Johnson 1987): lack of periorbital fat and reduced skin elasticity may be mistaken for dehydration, peripheral oedema may be due to vascular insufficiency or lymphatic obstruction, rather than cardiac failure, trivial cardiac murmurs may mistakenly be interpreted to represent significant valve lesions in the elderly, and cursory clinical examination may not reveal the subtle signs of dementia.

The most appropriate operation and anaesthetic should be planned. In general, a curative procedure should not be compromised solely because of the age of the patient. However, common sense and experience will dictate the ability of the patient to withstand radical surgery and the balance between the probable benefits and drawbacks of such a procedure. For example, there is a higher perioperative mortality rate among elderly patients with lung cancer who undergo pneumonectomy compared with those who undergo a lesser procedure such as lobectomy (Martini 1986). In that situation, the potential for cure from each procedure must be balanced by the risks of operative death. These considerations are of particular relevance in patients with smoking-related malignancies, particularly in the context of their increased cardiac and respiratory risk status.

In some instances, where cardiorespiratory function is of concern, local anaesthesia may offer a useful alternative although the patient must not be subjected to unnecessary pain or the discomfort of a prolonged procedure without appropriate sedation and analgesia.

Intraoperative care

Particular care must be taken in the intraoperative monitoring of an aged patient. Attention must be paid to replacement of fluids and blood products, with regard to both overload and under-replacement. Aged tissues (teeth, skin) are more liable to inadvertent trauma and particular care should be taken in the insertion of the endotracheal tube, positioning on the operating table, and insertion of cannulae. In major procedures or with an unusually frail patient, there should be facilities for continuous intraoperative monitoring of cardiorespiratory function (electrocardiography, blood oxygenation, etc.); in prolonged procedures, changes in electrolytes, renal function, blood glucose, haematological indices, and coagulation should be assessed serially. Pragmatic considerations, such as the cost-effectiveness of interventions, are also of importance; for example, intensive monitoring is usually not necessary for a simple biopsy in a fit elderly patient and many such procedures can be performed safely in a day-surgery unit with less disruption to the aged patient's routine.

Post-operative management

As with the other aspects of the surgical care of the geriatric patient, the principles of post-operative management simply reflect the practice of good general surgical care. A continuing awareness of the aged patient's diminished capacity to respond to stress is essential and there should be careful monitoring of the same indices that are assessed during the procedure. In addition, attention should be given to the provision of adequate analgesia to ensure that the patient is able to move freely and to perform the necessary breathing exercises. Care should be taken to avoid thromboembolism, with measures such as anticoagulation, the use of support stockings, etc. Attention must be directed to skin care, the avoidance of pressure sores, and active management of the operative wound.

The post-operative routine is important in the care of the elderly. A diurnal rhythm should be maintained and the potential loss of such a rhythm in prolonged admission to an intensive care facility should be avoided. The elderly are at particular risk of nocturnal disorientation in reduced light.

Palliative surgery

The importance of a simple surgical procedure in palliating an incurable locally advanced malignancy should not be forgotten. The elderly patient may benefit greatly, both in a reduction of symptoms and in the duration of hospitalization, from surgical resection or bypass of an obstructing gastrointestinal malignancy, the removal of a fungating skin cancer, or even surgical attention to a locally advanced breast cancer. As noted previously, consideration of appropriate alternatives is of great importance in this context; for example, it has been proposed that simple hormonal manipulation (tamoxifen, progestational drugs) may control a locally advanced breast cancer with less morbidity and equal efficacy to a surgical procedure (Gazet et al. 1988; Robertson et al. 1988).

Preventative surgery

Another suspect of the care of the elderly is the attention to pre-malignant and early malignant conditions. As noted previously, the aged are at particular risk of developing malignant degeneration of adenomatous polyps and changes in skin lesions (for example, solar keratosis, Hutchinson's melanotic freckle). Such conditions can often best be managed by early surgical resection, thus limiting the extent of requisite surgery and increasing the chances of cure. The issues of prevention and screening for malignancy in the elderly are reviewed elsewhere (Warnecke *et al.* 1983; Stults 1986).

Radiotherapy in the aged

Analogous to the practice of surgery in the aged, the optimal delivery of radiotherapy to such patients requires careful planning. The specific considerations vary widely, depending upon the organ to be treated. However, some general principles apply, although little has been published regarding the specific problems that pertain to radiotherapy in the elderly (Tudway 1962; Gunn 1980; Crocker and Prosnitz 1987). As noted above, elderly tissues (particularly skin and mucosal surfaces) are less resilient and are repaired less rapidly and, thus, the elderly patient will often tolerate standard treatment protocols less well (Gunn 1980; Cohen 1985; Crocker and Prosnitz 1987). This should be taken into consideration when planning the dosage, field size, and fractionation of radiotherapy of tumours arising in the oral cavity, larynx, lung, oesophagus, colorectum, and genitourinary tract. The probable gains in terms of potential for cure or long-term local control must be balanced against the toxicity of radical treatment doses. Conversely, the improvement in quality of life due to reduced fraction sizes and doses may be offset by a reduction in survival. For example, the technique of split-course irradiation (in which the planned dose is delivered in two parts, separated by a gap of 2–3 weeks to reduce toxicity) achieves a lower rate of local control in some forms of head and neck cancer (Parsons *et al.* 1980).

Other practical problems may require attention. The elderly patient with severe arthritis may experience substantial difficulty or pain when being positioned for radiotherapy, particularly when prone. Chronic airways limitation or cardiac failure, with associated orthopnoea, may also cause problems. The elderly male with severe prostatism or with an extensive pelvic malignancy may not be able to remain comfortably in the correct position for prolonged periods during definitive treatment.

Elderly patients suffering severe radiation-induced nausea or diarrhoea may develop substantial iatrogenic complications from antinauseant or antidiarrhoeal medications (discussed below in the context of chemotherapy).

The radiotherapy treatment bunker, often colourless and isolated, may present a frightening spectre to the elderly patient, particularly if he or she is confused or demented, and great care should be taken to explain the nature of treatment and to reassure the patient. In some instances, prophylactic gentle sedation may be used effectively to minimize the distress of the geriatric patient.

Pharmacology of anticancer drugs in the elderly

Many of the physiological changes of old age, discussed previously, may alter the pharmacological disposition of drugs, including cytotoxics. The prediction of these changes is complex for many reasons. Dose–response relationships may be different in the aged (Triggs and Nation 1975; Vestal 1978; Greenblatt *et al.* 1982; Ho and Triggs 1984). Moreover, it has been estimated that 80 per cent of such patients have one or more chronic disorders (WHO 1981) and that they are treated with a mean of 3–12 concomitant

Table 3 Examples of predisposing factors to toxicity of cytotoxic drugs in the elderly

Side-effect	Predisposing factors	Cytotoxic drugs potentially affected
Cardiac failure	Reduced cardiac output	Doxorubicin
	Ischaemic heart disease	Daunorubicin
	Cardiac valve disorder	Mitoxantrone
	Impaired hepatic function	Epirubicin
Pneumonitis	Reduced density of lung	Bleomycin
	Reduced renal function	
	Chronic bronchitis/airways limitation	
Myelosuppression	Reduced plasma protein binding	Methotrexate
	Reduced renal function	
	Reduced hepatic function	Doxorubicin Epirubicin Mitoxantrone
	Age-related changes in fat stores and marrow reserves	Nitrosoureas
Mucositis	Reduced renal function	Methotrexate
	Age-related changes in mucosae	Fluorouracil
	Reduced plasma protein binding	
	Reduced hepatic function	Doxorubicin Epirubicin
Peripheral neuropathy	Age-related changes in nerves	Vinca alkaloids
	Diabetes mellitus	Cisplatin
	Chronic alcohol abuse	
	Peripheral vascular disease	
Deafness	Noise-induced hearing loss	Cisplatin
	Age-related hearing loss[a]	
	Reduced renal function?	
Haemorrhagic cystitis	Prostatism	Cyclophosphamide[b]
Constipation	Age-related changes in nerves and bowel function	Vinca alkaloids

[a]No obvious increment noted in elderly patients with bladder cancer (Raghavan *et al.* 1988*b*).
[b]Theoretical consideration; not observed in a series of 60 cases treated with oral cyclophosphamide.

medications (Shaw 1982). As a result, the assessment of the pharmacology of drugs in the elderly will often be confounded by potential drug interactions. Furthermore, while the prevalence of adverse drug reactions has been shown to rise with age (Williamson 1979), the available data may be under-representative as the elderly (or their medical attendants) tend to report side-effects less reliably. The situation is further complicated by poor compliance with schedules of oral medication. Factors contributing to this problem include decreased memory/senile dementia, deafness or impaired vision, lack of social support, poverty, direct or incidental effects of the drugs themselves (including the complexity of some regimens), and depression.

The changes of organ function in the aged, as discussed above, may cause changes in absorption, distribution, and elimination of many drugs, as reviewed elsewhere (Triggs and Nation 1975; Greenblatt *et al.* 1982; Ho and Triggs 1984; Raghavan *et al.* 1988*a*). As many of the cytotoxic drugs have a relatively narrow therapeutic index, any factors that potentially alter the pharmacokinetics in the elderly may be of great importance with regard to efficacy and toxicity (Table 3).

Absorption

Most cytotoxics are administered parenterally, although cyclophosphamide, methotrexate, busulphan, etoposide, demethoxy-daunorubicin, and chlorambucil may be used orally and are thus subject to variable absorption. Perhaps of greater importance for this group of patients, many ancillary medications, such as analgesics, anti-emetics, laxatives, steroids, and folinic acid, are administered by mouth. The major factors that determine the bioavailability of most of these drugs include the absorption process itself and initial elimination (first-pass hepatic metabolism or degradation in the small bowel) (Cohen 1985). The age-related reduction in gastric acid secretion and in gastrointestinal motility affect the absorption of basic and poorly lipid soluble drugs in particular (Cohen 1985; Hutchins and Lipschitz 1987). The changes of hepatic blood flow can either increase or reduce bioavailability. The metabolic implications of metastases in the liver are variable and poorly understood.

Drug distribution

The distribution of a drug is a function of its relative lipid–water partition characteristics, the degree of binding to plasma proteins and other tissues, and the overall patterns of blood flow (Vestal 1978). Because of the reduction in lean body mass, increase in lipid composition of the body, and reduction of total body water, the distribution of lipid-soluble drugs (for example, diazepam, nitrosoureas) changes markedly in the elderly (Greenblatt et al. 1982). Similarly, plasma protein binding is reduced in the elderly, with a concomitant rise in the level of free drug. In patients with substantial third spaces (pleural effusions from malignancy or cardiac failure, ascites), the distribution of water-soluble drugs is further distorted and toxicity can be significantly increased.

Metabolism

Hepatic and extrahepatic enzyme systems contribute to the metabolism of most drugs. The rate of drug metabolism is influenced by the state of nutrition, the hepatic function, drug interactions, intercurrent diseases, smoking, and plasma protein levels (Ho and Triggs 1984; Cohen 1985). There are no simple indices of drug metabolism and standard liver function tests are an unreliable guide. This variability of function is a particular hazard for the use of antinauseants, analgesics, and sedatives in the elderly.

Excretion

The kidneys provide the major route of excretion for many cytotoxic drugs, including methotrexate, bleomycin, and cisplatin. If renal function is impaired, the drugs that are predominantly excreted by this route have prolonged half-lives, with increased plasma concentrations and the concomitant risk of increased toxicity. In elderly patients with tumours of the urothelium, the aetiology of the malignancy can be of particular importance. For example, the association of analgesic nephropathy, chronic renal failure, and multifocal bladder cancer, complicated by hydronephrosis or antecedent nephrectomy (Raghavan et al. 1988a), may have a significant influence on excretion of the drug. In the elderly patient,

the ability of a solitary kidney to compensate after nephrectomy is reduced by approximately 50 per cent.

Most other cytotoxics are excreted via the biliary tract and toxicity is thus dependent upon the changes in hepatic function outlined above. Chronic alcohol abuse and the presence of congestive cardiac failure, as well as the reduction in hepatic perfusion consequent upon the normal decline in cardiac output, are of particular importance in the elderly.

General applications

A general dictum, to a large extent unsupported by objective evidence, is that increased toxicity of chemotherapy is a function of advanced age, irrespective of the general physiological state of the patient. Early studies represented only small numbers of cases. For example, methotrexate was noted to cause increased haematological side-effects in the aged (Hansen et al. 1971). Similarly, bleomycin was said to be associated with increased lung damage in the elderly (Haas et al. 1976; Ginsberg and Comis 1982). However, Begg and Carbone (1983), in a detailed review of more than 5000 patients from studies by the Eastern Cooperative Oncology Group, noted that the extent and severity of side-effects were functions of the agents and doses employed, rather than being due to the ages of the patients. Although age-related toxicity occurred with methotrexate and methyl-CCNU, this did not appear to be the case for doxorubicin, cyclophosphamide, the vinca alkaloids, and mitomycin. Although this is an important study, it should not be forgotten that there may have been significant selection of patients as the data were obtained only from cases entered into randomized trials. Similarly, in selected elderly patients with bladder cancer (Raghavan et al. 1988b) and other malignancies (Hrushesky et al. 1974), the toxicity of cisplatin is not a function of age.

There have been conflicting views on the topic of dose modification in the elderly and the balance between reduced toxicity (from dose reduction) compared with the potential for reduced antitumour efficacy (Armitage and Potter 1984; Gelman and Taylor 1984; Kahn et al. 1984). This is discussed in detail in the context of specific malignancies.

Psychosocial factors

When planning active management of cancer in the elderly, whatever modality of treatment is intended, their unique psychosocial context must be considered if optimal care is to be achieved. A range of such factors can have an important impact on the presentation and management of cancer in elderly patients. In Western society, the older patient who develops cancer must face the dual social stigmata of advanced age and cancer (Holland and Massie 1987).

The ageing process itself is heavily influenced by a changing psychological profile in addition to physical change. In addition to changes in cognitive function, health behaviour and attitudes are likely to alter as a function of ageing (Yancik 1983); there is a greater acceptance of ill health, less awareness of current or evolving attitudes to optimal health care, changes in patterns of smoking and alcohol intake, and often a reduction in the level of personal interactions with medical attendants. Other important factors include a reduced level of social integration (fewer friends and relatives, reduced family or social support, fewer incentives, poverty), evolving physical weakness and problems with sight and hearing, and variable coping mechanisms. Changing patterns of acceptance of the elderly in society will often influence the quality, availability and use of health care for the aged.

Many of these factors influence the time of presentation with cancer; although the elderly receive medical attention more frequently than the young (and thus may benefit from earlier medical diagnosis), factors that contribute to delayed presentation include procrastination by the patient (due to misconceptions regarding outcome, greater acceptance of ill health, fear, poverty, etc.) and, in some cases, reluctance of the medical profession to seek out problems in elderly patients (Holland and Massie 1987). These issues must be taken into consideration when devising strategies for health in this group.

Despite this, the elderly often have a better psychosocial adaptation to established illness than do the young (Holland and Massie 1987). Using the Cancer Inventory of Problem Situations, a self-administered survey of physical and psychosocial problems associated with cancer, Ganz et al. (1985) compared 158 men aged 65 years or less with 82 men over the age of 65 years and showed that the older cohort had a similar spectrum of problems as their younger counterparts, despite a higher prevalence of chronic illness. However, the younger group experienced more psychosocial problems, particularly in coping with the health care environment, chemotherapy, and work-related problems.

When establishing a plan of active management, in addition to considering the balance between the toxicity of treatment and the consequent prognosis, such issues must be considered and incorporated into the programme of treatment. Although not the only health professional able to deal with the psychosocial context, the clinician should be able to muster the appropriate social resources (district nursing, occupational therapy, social work, psychogeriatric support, etc.) to ensure adequate resolution of these issues.

SPECIFIC EXAMPLES OF CANCER MANAGEMENT IN AGED PATIENTS

Lung cancer

Cancer of the lung is the most common cancer in males in Western society and the most common cause of cancer deaths in males and in females. Half of all lung cancers occur in patients aged 65 years or older (Ries et al. 1983) and 500 new cases are reported each year per 100 000 men aged 70 years or more. However, it is important to note that many of the patients treated in clinical trials represent a younger cohort (Simes 1985).

Screening for lung cancer

With increasing age, the relative proportion of squamous carcinoma increases, rising to nearly 50 per cent in patients older than 70 years, whereas the proportion of adenocarcinoma and small cell carcinoma falls with advancing age (Auerbach et al. 1975; Dodds et al. 1986; Teeter et al. 1987). This may be of particular importance in the context of programmes for early diagnosis, as it has been reported that squamous carcinoma is the subtype most likely to be detected at an early stage by screening (Early Lung Cancer Cooperative Study 1984). In fact, several studies have suggested that lung cancer presents earlier in the elderly (Holmes and Hearne 1981; Ershler et al. 1983; Goodwin et al. 1986). This could be explained by several reasons: less intensive staging in older patients, yielding the artefact of apparent early stage disease, more frequent visits to medical practitioners by the elderly, affording the opportunity of earlier

detection, and reduced biological aggression of lung cancer in the elderly. Whatever the reason, the apparent earlier presentation of lung cancer in the elderly may be an argument for screening programmes for this population group, especially in the context of the increasing age-specific incidence (O'Rourke and Crawford 1987). A curious contrast is the decline in 5 year survival figures with advanced age in population surveys of outcome (Ries et al. 1983), although this may be explained by a failure to treat elderly patients in an active fashion (Mor et al. 1985).

Diagnosis

The diagnosis of lung cancer is more difficult in the elderly as many of the symptoms mimic those of other diseases of the elderly, particularly in the context that lung cancer is a smoking-related disorder. Elderly smokers characteristically have chronic air-flow limitation or chronic bronchitis, the features of ischaemic heart disease, and may exhibit the more general age-related problems such as depression, malnutrition, dementia, and arthritis.

In the elderly patient, the general approach to the staging and investigation of lung cancer should be similar to that used in younger patients, with the exception that the physical infirmity or restriction of the older patient should be considered when planning a programme of tests. In general, the approach to investigation should also be governed by the potential influence on management; for example, careful staging is particularly important in the patient for whom thoracotomy and resection of tumour is under consideration (to avoid the risk of unnecessary surgery in a patient with established metastases).

In the general population, there is a major difference in approach to the management of small cell lung cancer and the non-small cell cancers. Thus, it is appropriate to discuss the management of lung cancer in the elderly in terms of these histological classifications.

Non-small cell lung cancer

In the general population, the best survival figures have been reported from centres with an aggressive approach to surgical resection of non-small cell carcinoma of the lung, although these results may be partly due to careful patient selection. Five year survival figures of 70–80 per cent for pathological stage $T_1N_0M_0$, 60–65 per cent for $T_2N_0M_0$, and more than 50 per cent for pathological stage II disease have been reported (Early Lung Cancer Cooperative Study 1984; Martini 1986). In elderly patients considered fit enough to undergo thoracotomy, there is no evidence that the operative mortality or 3–5 year survival figures are inferior for patients with pathological stages I or II non-small cell carcinoma of the lung when compared with the general population (Martini 1986; O'Rourke and Crawford 1987; Sherman and Guidot 1987). The results obtained in series of elderly patients undergoing thoracotomy are summarized in Table 4.

Radiotherapy is often used in elderly patients with non-small cell carcinoma of the lung, either with curative or palliative intent, depending upon the age and general health of the patient as well as the stage of the tumour. As it is often prescribed in patients who are not fit for operation or who refuse to undergo surgery, the results of treatment represent a selection bias. Furthermore, most reported series represent clinically rather than surgically staged tumours. In most series, the reported median survival is less than 12 months, with 3–5 year survival rates of only 10–20 per cent (Cox 1986; Perez 1986; Noordijk et al. 1988). The pattern of toxicity in the elderly is important and it should not be forgotten that the aged

Table 4 Thoracotomy for elderly patients with lung cancer

Series	Study period	Number of operations	Perioperative mortality	Five year survival[a] (%)
Ebner et al. (1985)	1978–1982	51	10	40
Ginsberg et al. (1983)	1979–1981	453	7	—
Martini (1986)	1973–1980	177	2	—
Sherman and Guidot (1987)	1977–1984	64	9	38
Yellin et al. (1981)	1979–1983	53	7	40

[a]Patients with predominantly stages I and II non-small cell lung cancer.

mucosa has a reduced capacity for repair and, hence, an increased risk of radiation-induced mucosal damage. In addition, radical schedules and doses of radiotherapy may cause increased parenchymal lung damage in view of age-related changes in the normal lung. In contrast, the pattern of side-effects is minimal in patients treated for peripheral non-small cell carcinoma of the lung with small irradiation fields (Noordijk et al. 1988). In patients with severe mucosal reactions, attention to hydration, mucosal candidiasis, and occasional prescription of systemic corticosteroids (while monitoring for diabetes mellitus) can be helpful. In general, we do not recommend topical or local anaesthetic preparations (for example, xylocaine solution) as they can exacerbate the local inflammatory reaction, although masking the pain.

In our view, age per se should not be an important determinant in the overall philosophy of management of early stage non-small cell lung cancer. If a patient is deemed fit for surgery, appropriate staging protocols should be effected and thoracotomy performed if the tumour is shown to be clinically localized. However, it is clear that patients over the age of 70 years have increased morbidity and perioperative mortality if pneumonectomy is performed and this should be avoided if possible (Martini 1986). In the patient who is not fit for thoracotomy, the judicious use of radiotherapy is appropriate, with clear guidelines being defined for the use of curative or palliative dose schedules.

For patients with advanced disease, particularly with metastases, age itself should be a much more important determinant of management. In the general population with advanced non-small cell carcinoma of the lung, there is only a limited impact from radiotherapy or chemotherapy survival, with median values of less than 12 months and only rare long-term survival (Simes 1985). Accordingly, as the potential for significant toxicity from radical radiotherapy or intensive chemotherapy rises with age (as discussed before), the potential cost–benefit ratio becomes less favourable. In our institution, we regard the use of chemotherapy for patients with non-small cell carcinoma of the lung as investigational and do not usually treat geriatric patients with chemotherapy, concentrating instead on symptom control, supportive care, and palliative radiotherapy (if appropriate). However, more recently, it has become clear that the combination of systemic chemotherapy with surgery or radiotherapy yields improved outcomes in patients with stage III disease and we are using this approach more often in otherwise healthy geriatric patients.

Small cell lung cancer

The incidence of small cell lung cancer reduces with increasing age, dropping from 22 per cent in the 40–49 year age group to 13 per cent in patients older than 80 years (Teeter et al. 1987). As for non-small cell carcinoma of the lung, the symptoms of small cell lung cancer often mimic those of intercurrent disease in the elderly. In this context, a relevant factor is the prevalence of intercurrent disease, which may reflect the relationship of small cell lung cancer to smoking. Clamon et al. (1982) have reported that 92 per cent of a series of elderly patients with small cell lung cancer had intercurrent medical disorders at presentation, including 58 per cent with cardiac disease and 25 per cent with second malignancies. In our experience (Table 5), 25 per cent of patients had ischaemic heart disease, 20 per cent had peripheral vascular disease, 18 per cent had chronic airways limitation, and 13 per cent had second malignancies (Findlay et al., unpublished data). Thus, many of this group of patients are less robust and consequently less able to withstand intensive treatment. Not surprisingly, the pattern of intercurrent disease is different from our experience with elderly patients with diffuse lymphoma or ovarian cancer, who have a lower prevalence of smoking (Table 5).

In contrast with non-small cell carcinoma of the lung in the elderly (with a greater tendency for a more localized extent of tumour), small cell lung cancer tends to metastasize early. Because of age-related exclusion criteria for entry into multicentre clinical trials, there are few reported series of patients treated intensively for small cell lung cancer. In younger patients, chemotherapy is regarded as the treatment of choice, irrespective of the extent of disease, with median survival figures of 12–18 months being reported for limited disease (with 3–5 year survival of 15–25 per cent) and 6–8 months for extensive disease. As shown in Table 6, the elderly appear to fare less well in this context. Reporting the experience of Cancer and Acute Leukemia Group B, Spiegelman et al. (1989) reported a higher death rate among elderly patients with limited disease, although there was no difference among those with extensive disease and no difference in response rates between age groups. In contrast, elderly patients with extensive disease had a worse prognosis in a three-arm comparison of combinations of etoposide, vincristine, doxorubicin, and cyclophosphamide (Hong et al. 1989).

Although advanced age does not appear to be associated with a significant reduction of response rate in most series (Maurer and Pajak 1981; Clamon et al. 1982; Spiegelman et al. 1989; Findlay et al., submitted for publication), it should also be noted that intensive chemotherapy for small cell lung cancer may not confer a major survival benefit to geriatric patients. In a retrospective non-randomized comparison, there was no clinically relevant difference in long-term survival between patients treated with intensive regimens (four to six cycles of vincristine, doxorubicin, cyclophosphamide) and those treated with low-dose or palliative chemotherapy schedules (Findlay et al., unpublished data). In contrast, Chahinian et al. (1989) demonstrated a reduced reponse rate but no difference in survival between patients aged more than 65 years versus the younger cohort.

Although there is no quantitative difference in the severity of iatrogenic myelosuppression between younger and older groups of patients with lung cancer (Begg and Carbone 1983; Dixon et al. 1984), the associated risk of pneumonia is greater in the elderly (Dixon et al. 1984) and other patterns of toxicity have also been reported to be more severe in the aged (Poplin et al. 1987).

We believe that fit geriatric patients without major intercurrent medical problems should be considered for treatment with moderately intensive schedules of chemotherapy for small cell lung cancer. We are currently assessing the impact of carboplatin-containing regimens in this context (Raghavan et al. 1990a). However, as outlined in Table 6, the potential benefits for the less

Table 5 Patterns of intercurrent disease in elderly patients with cancer: experience at Royal Prince Alfred Hospital, Sydney

Intercurrent disorder	Small cell lung cancer (%)	Non-Hodgkin's lymphoma (%)	Ovarian cancer (%)	Bladder cancer (%)
Cardiovascular				
Cardiac	25	37	20	20
Peripheral vascular	20	9	2	14
Hypertension	15	26	25	27
Respiratory				
Chronic airways limitation	18	9	11	20
Genitourinary				
Benign prostatic hyperplasia	3	6	NA	25
Analgesic nephropathy/renal calculi	?	?	2	14
Endocrine				
Diabetes mellitus[a]	3	9	4	7
Thyroid disease	?	?	7	7
Gastrointestinal				
Peptic ulcer	2	3	2	14
Diverticulitis	?	9	?	?
Musculoskeletal				
Arthritis	7	17	11	?
Other cancers	13	23	2	?

[a]From patient's past medical history (not biochemical screening).

Table 6 Chemotherapy for small cell lung cancer in the elderly

Series	Limited extent of disease			Extensive disease		
		Survival			Survival	
	Number	Median (months)	2 year (%)	Number	Median (months)	2 year (%)
Conventional regimens[a]						
Clamon et al. (1984)	7	8	0	13	10	0
Maurer and Pajak (1981)	15	9	0?	13	2	0
Poplin et al. (1987)	24	12	15?	25	7	0
Findlay et al. (unpublished data)	26	9	4	46	6	2
Carboplatin-based regimens[b]						
Raghavan et al. (1990a)	11	14	<10	15	11	7

[a]Based on cycles of cyclophosphamide, vincristine, doxorubicin±etoposide.
[b]Use of combination regimen, incorporating carboplatin and etoposide (D. Raghavan and J. F. Bishop, unpublished data).

robust subject are more limited and the accurate assessment of cost–benefit is critical in this situation. In the medically unfit geriatric patient, useful prolongation of survival and palliation of symptoms can be achieved with radiotherapy in the first instance, particularly as small cell lung cancer responds to lower doses of irradiation than non-small cell carcinoma of the lung.

Lymphomas

Hodgkin's disease

Hodgkin's disease has a bimodal age distribution. After an early peak in the third decade, the age-specific incidence increases from the fifth decade (Ries et al. 1983), with 20–25 per cent of all cases occurring in patients over the age of 60 years (Ries et al. 1983; Kennedy et al. 1985).

The pattern of presentation is similar to that of the general population, with the exception that the elderly tend to present more often with B symptoms and the features of advanced stage disease (Lokich et al. 1974; Austin-Seymour et al. 1984; Eghbali et al. 1984).

Consistent with the pattern of advanced presentation, the histological subtype of mixed cellularity, which is associated with a worse prognosis, is commonly found in the elderly (Austin-Seymour et al. 1984; Eghbali et al. 1984).

Patterns of investigation of Hodgkin's disease are often modified in the elderly. For example, the potential morbidity of the staging laparotomy in an elderly unfit patient has influenced clinicians to place greater reliance on non-invasive staging procedures. Austin-Seymour et al. (1984), reporting in the era before the routine use of computerized axial tomography and high-dose gallium scanning, noted longer disease-free and total survival in patients undergoing staging laparotomy compared with those who did not. However, this study did not address the confounding biases, such as prevalence of intercurrent disease and aggression of definitive treatment. There has also been controversy regarding the application and toxicity of lymphography in the elderly (Lokich et al. 1974; Austin-Seymour et al. 1984). At Royal Prince Alfred Hospital, Sydney, in all age groups with Hodgkin's disease, a lesser reliance has been placed on staging laparotomy and lymphography since the introduction of high-dose gallium scanning (Blackwell et al. 1986).

18 CANCER IN THE ELDERLY

Table 7 Hodgkin's disease in the elderly

Number	Stage	Treatment	Complete response (%)	Median survival (months)	Series
18	III–IV	MOPPr	67	39	Austin-Seymour *et al.* (1984)
9	II–IV	COPPr/MOPPr	?	27	Eghbali *et al.* (1984)
73	III–IV	MOPP	40	18	Peterson *et al.* (1982)

M, nitrogen mustard; O, vincristine (Oncovin); P, procarbazine; Pr, prednisone; C, cyclophosphamide.

Even when optimal staging and treatment are used for advanced stage Hodgkin's disease, the geriatric patient with Hodgkin's disease has a poorer outcome (Table 7). Disease-free and total 5 year survival rates of less than 40 per cent have been reported from series incorporating all stages of disease (Austin-Seymour *et al.* 1984; Eghbali *et al.* 1984; Kennedy *et al.* 1985). However, in a highly selected series of pathologically staged patients over the age of 60 years, workers at Stanford University reported an actuarial 14 year overall survival of 60 per cent, but with 80 per cent relapse-free survival (Austin-Seymour *et al.* 1984) (that is, a significant proportion of patients died of intercurrent disease) and these figures were more comparable with those obtained from patients of younger age. In contrast, Roach *et al.* (1990) have shown that age is an adverse independent prognostic factor in a multivariate analysis of patients relapsing after radiotherapy for stage I–II disease; patients older than 50 years suffered a higher incidence of relapse and of death from lymphoma.

In addition to the lower survival figures, elderly patients treated intensively for advanced disease have more severe patterns of toxicity, including myelosuppression and gastrointestinal problems (Peterson *et al.* 1982; Austin-Seymour *et al.* 1984). For example, in one study reported by the Cancer and Acute Leukemia Group B, severe or life-threatening myelosuppression was reported in only 14 per cent of patients less than 40 years of age compared with 33 per cent of those aged more than 60 years (Peterson *et al.* 1982). Similarly, neurotoxicity was more severe after administration of vinca alkaloids in the older patients.

An additional problem for the elderly patient with Hodgkin's disease is a 10-fold increased risk of developing second malignancies, both leukaemias and solid tumours (Valagussa *et al.* 1986; Van Leeuwen *et al.* 1989). However, it should not be forgotten that aged patients may also develop intercurrent malignancies before presentation (Table 5), independently of the nature of the malignancy or its treatment.

Despite these potential problems, sustained remissions can be achieved with the judicious use of radiotherapy for early stage disease or combination chemotherapy (for example, chlorambucil, vincristine or vinblastine, procarbazine, and prednisone) for elderly patients with advanced Hodgkin's disease (Table 7).

Non-Hodgkin's lymphoma

Analogous to Hodgkin's disease, the incidence of non-Hodgkin's lymphomas rises with age, with approximately 50 per cent occurring in patients aged 65 years or more (Ries *et al.* 1983; Newell *et al.* 1987). Many surveys have suggested that intermediate and high-grade lymphomas predominate in the elderly (Mead *et al.* 1984; Carbone *et al.* 1986), although this may be due to the referral biases of the centres reporting the data; that is, elderly patients with indolent non-Hodgkin's lymphoma were managed independently in the community. However, Barnes *et al.* (1987) have reported an increased proportion of diffuse histology among the elderly in a large

community survey from Yorkshire, United Kingdom. The correlation between age and histological subtype has been made more difficult by the profusion of systems of classification of non-Hodgkin's lymphoma and the lack of concordance between these systems (Patchefsky *et al.* 1974; Nathwani *et al.* 1978; Anderson *et al.* 1982; Newell *et al.* 1987).

Notwithstanding these problems, an increased stage of disease has been associated with advancing age, at least in cases of diffuse lymphoma (Foucar *et al.* 1983; Mead *et al.* 1984). Furthermore, there is a high prevalence (30–70 per cent) of extranodal disease in the elderly (Hancock *et al.* 1983; Mead *et al.* 1984; Findlay *et al.*, unpublished data), although Vose *et al.* (1988) did not show an increased prevalence in the aged.

Despite the potential for referral biases, the patterns of presentation in the elderly are similar to those of younger patients, although the diagnosis may be more difficult in the patient with subtle symptoms against a background of intercurrent disease. Few studies have documented the prevalence of intercurrent illness in elderly patients with non-Hodgkin's lymphoma (Mead *et al.* 1984; Hoerni *et al.* 1988). As outlined in Table 5, a range of intercurrent medical problems occur in this group, with the emphasis on chronic cardiovascular and lung diseases.

Because the pattern of spread of non-Hodgkin's lymphoma, in contrast with Hodgkin's disease, is not one of contiguity (with a sequential or ordered pattern), there is a lesser reliance on intensive staging and virtually no role for staging laparotomy in our view. Although this issue has not been addressed systematically in the elderly, Paryani *et al.* (1983), in a study of radiotherapy for patients with early stage nodular non-Hodgkin's lymphoma, postulated an apparent benefit in relapse-free survival, favouring patients who underwent staging laparotomy. However, a difference in total survival was not seen, the pathological staging probably contributed to the phenomenon of stage migration, and it is also possible that a major selection bias (in terms of physical fitness of the aged patients) favoured the group undergoing laparotomy.

Whether age is an independent prognostic determinant in elderly patients with lymphomas is the subject of controversy (Bloomfield *et al.* 1974; Paryani *et al.* 1983; Dixon *et al.* 1986; Gallagher *et al.* 1986; Jones *et al.* 1989). It has been reported that it is an important adverse prognostic factor in nodular lymphoma (Rudders *et al.* 1979; Paryani *et al.* 1983), although others have not found this, once other prognostic factors have been eliminated (Gallagher *et al.* 1986; McLaughlin *et al.* 1988). Paryani *et al.* (1983) reported a 5 year survival of 70 per cent for patients over the age of 40 years with stage I–II nodular lymphoma with favourable histology; they did not categorize deaths from lymphoma and deaths from intercurrent disease in the different age groupings for 10–15 year follow-up, perhaps explaining this discrepancy.

It appears that age is an independent prognostic factor in poor risk non-Hodgkin's lymphoma (Table 8), which may largely be predicated on the physical fitness and number of intercurrent disorders of the patients (Dixon *et al.* 1986; Kaminski *et al.* 1986),

2178

Table 8 Aggressive non-Hodgkin's lymphoma in the elderly: results of treatment

No.	Age (years) Median	Age (years) Range	Stage (%) I–II	Stage (%) III–IV	Treatment	Rx death (%)	Extranodal (%)	CR (%)	3+ year survival (%)	Series
41	75	(70–85)	8	92	T	2	?	32	21	Tirelli et al. (1988)
25	76	(70–86)	24	76	EP	0	?	48	a	Tirelli et al. (1988)
112	>60	(60–91)	28	72	CHP/BOP	7	56	61	34	Vose et al. (1988)
81	>65	(?)	0	100	CHOP	6	65	37	30	Dixon et al. (1986)
20	75	(70–94)	25	75	CHOP	25	>55	45	25	Armitage and Potter (1984)
21	75	(65–88)	30	70	CHOP etc.	?	?	57	40	Foucar et al. (1983)
38	75	(65–91)	40	60	CHOP etc.	8	70	42	11	Mead et al. (1984)
35	74	(70–89)	49	51	CHOP etc.	0[b]	33	60	20	Findlay et al. (unpublished data)

E, etoposide; T, teniposide; P, prednisone; CHOP, cyclophosphamide, doxorubicin, vincristine, and prednisone; CHP/BOP, cyclophosphamide, doxorubicin, prednisone, bleomycin, vincristine, and procarbazine; CR, complete response.
[a]Previously untreated cases, 24 per cent.
[b]Three lost to follow-up.

although not all series have found an impact from age *per se* (Bloomfield *et al.* 1974). Survival depends to a large extent on the level of intensity of treatment that can be administered safely and there is a risk of severe and lethal toxicity in geriatric patients treated with some of the intensive regimens at the doses used for younger patients (Tirelli *et al.* 1988).

In stage I and II intermediate and high-grade non-Hodgkin's lymphoma, Kaminski *et al.* (1986) reported a 30 per cent 5 year survival in patients over the age of 60 years compared with 63 per cent for patients aged 60 years or less. In this study, a higher prevalence of intercurrent deaths was documented in the elderly. Dixon *et al.* (1986), reporting the results of two studies by the Southwest Oncology Group, found a significant reduction in response rates and median survival in the elderly. These data may have reflected the impact of the protocol requirement of a 50 per cent dosage reduction in patients over the age of 65 years. However, in this study, 28 per cent of patients in the older age group actually received full-dose therapy, and still had inferior survival compared with the patients aged less than 65 years of age. Similarly, Armitage and Potter (1984) reported a series that included 20 patients aged 70 years or more in whom no dose reductions were initiated because of age. Although there was no difference in response rates between younger and older age groups, patients aged 70–94 years had a median survival of 13 months compared with a median survival of 41 months for patients aged 33–55 years. Once again, there was a statistically significant increase in early non-lymphoma deaths among the elderly, which may have reflected the statistically significantly increased treatment-related mortality. Klimo and Connors (1985) also reported an increased treatment-induced mortality rate in the elderly. Vose *et al.* (1988) documented a higher response rate among younger patients with diffuse large cell or immunoblastic non-Hodgkin's lymphoma, with equivalent toxicity in both groups; however, 5 year survival for patients over 60 years of age was only 34 per cent, compared with 62 per cent for the younger age group. When these figures were adjusted to reflect only deaths from lymphoma or treatment-related causes, there was no difference in survival between the younger and older groups. Similarly, Jones *et al.* (1989) found no significant difference in relapse-free survival between younger patients and those over the age of 65 years who were treated for diffuse large cell lymphoma with cyclophosphamide, doxorubicin, vincristine, and prednisone.

Thus, although the situation regarding the optimal management and prognosis for aggressive non-Hodgkin's lymphoma in the elderly

is not completely defined, most of the available evidence suggests that optimal results are obtained by using intensive treatment regimens for intermediate and high-grade disease, provided that patients are sufficiently robust to withstand the toxicity of treatment (Table 8).

Breast cancer

Breast cancer is the commonest invasive malignancy in women and its incidence increases with advancing age (Table 1). Nearly 40 per cent of women who develop breast cancer in Western society are over 65 years at diagnosis (Ries *et al.* 1983). However, age-related patterns of breast cancer incidence differ throughout the world: whereas the incidence rises after the menopause in Western countries, there is a decrease after the menopause in Asian women (MacMahon *et al.* 1973).

The impact of age on breast cancer

Much has been written on the changing biology of breast cancer with age (McCarty *et al.* 1983; Taylor *et al.* 1983; Rosen *et al.* 1985; Adami *et al.* 1986a; Host and Lund 1986; Cox 1987; Kurtz *et al.* 1990), but disagreement remains about the true impact of age in this context. Infiltrating duct carcinoma remains the commonest histological pattern, independent of age group. However, there are some differences in the histology of breast cancer, in that there is an increased prevalence of mucinous carcinoma in the elderly compared with an increased frequency of medullary and inflammatory patterns in the young (Rosen *et al.* 1985; Cox 1987). In most studies, it has been suggested that there is an increased level of differentiation in elderly breast cancer, an observation that is consistent with increased expression of oestrogen receptor activity (McCarty *et al.* 1983) and a reduction of thymidine labelling index (Meyer *et al.* 1986). Curiously, Taylor *et al.* (1983) have demonstrated increased DNA content in breast cancer in elderly patients, but without significant correlations between ploidy and histological type, tumour size, lymph node involvement, or oestrogen receptor content. It is not known whether the apparent increase in oestrogen receptor content with advancing age is due to reduced circulating oestrogens (occupying fewer binding sites) or to increased differentiation or some other property of ageing.

There is disagreement as to whether the disease in the elderly is more advanced or aggressive either at presentation or during its course. It has been reported that elderly patients have more advanced disease at diagnosis (Holmes and Hearne 1981; Goodwin *et al.* 1986), although others have shown that the apparent increase in distant metastases at presentation is offset by a reduction in regional disease so that equivalent numbers of young and old patients have only local involvement (Allen *et al.* 1986; Host and Lund 1986). In contrast, Suen *et al.* (1974), in an autopsy series, reported a lower propensity to distant metastasis in the elderly and Rosen *et al.* (1985) documented a higher prevalence of nodal metastases in a surgical series comparing very young and old patients. Mueller *et al.* (1978) reported an increased death rate among elderly patients with breast cancer (irrespective of deaths from intercurrent disease), whereas others have found no such difference (Herbsman *et al.* 1981; Rosen *et al.* 1985). As discussed previously, age-modified patterns of care in the elderly may influence the outcome when survival is used as an index of the malignancy of the disease. Several studies have shown that the level of activity or intensity of management in aged patients with breast cancer is substantially reduced (Mor *et al.* 1985; Allen *et al.* 1986; Samet *et al.* 1986; Greenfield *et al.* 1987). Nevertheless, the SEER study has shown comparable 5 year relative survival statistics among all age groups (Ries *et al.* 1983).

Screening for breast cancer

In view of the high incidence of breast cancer in elderly women and their possible predilection for advanced presentation (Holmes and Hearne 1983; Goodwin *et al.* 1986), theoretically this group would constitute an ideal population for the evaluation of screening or early diagnosis programmes. However, initial studies have suggested that the elderly have a marked resistance to participation in such programmes (Foster *et al.* 1978; Tabar *et al.* 1985). For example, in a randomized trial in Sweden, women aged 40 years or more were invited to undergo a programme of mammographic screening for breast cancer; nearly 90 per cent of women aged 40–49 years took an active part in two screening examinations, in contrast with less than 70 per cent of women aged 70–74 years (Tabar *et al.* 1985). Despite this, a statistically significant reduction in death rate from breast cancer was seen only in women over the age of 50 years, with no perceived survival benefit at the time of reporting for the younger women who participated in the screening programme. Of particular importance will be the completion of the evaluation of such screening programmes. If they are proved to yield a significant survival benefit, there will be a requirement for new educational methods to encourage the participation of the aged in such exercises. Despite the failure of elderly women to participate fully in the programmes discussed above, Carlile *et al.* (1983) have not found any age-related differences in participation in similar screening programmes provided that adequate and personalized education is provided, an observation that may be useful in planning a strategy of screening for the elderly.

Management of early stage breast cancer

As discussed elsewhere in this volume, a relatively standard approach to clinical staging of breast cancer, irrespective of age, may include careful physical examination, measurement of biochemical and haematological indices, and a series of tests including chest radiography, radionuclide bone scanning, and CAT of the abdomen (in some institutions). Prior to the establishment of a plan of management, a tissue diagnosis is required, usually from a fine-needle aspiration biopsy or excision of the putative lump. Thus, the

options for definitive treatment of clinically localized breast cancer in the elderly include the following:

(1) modified radical mastectomy;
(2) excision of the breast lump with radical radiotherapy;
(3) either of the above, with surgical node sampling;
(4) any of the above, with adjuvant hormonal therapy;
(5) 1–3 above, with adjuvant chemotherapy;
(6) other variants of mastectomy (radical, simple), with or without adjuvant radiotherapy, chemotherapy, or hormone therapy;
(7) hormone therapy alone.

The optimal treatment of localized breast cancer in aged patients has not yet been defined with respect to either the choice of modality or the use of combined treatment. As discussed previously, elderly patients tolerate elective cancer surgery well, particularly in the absence of major intercurrent illnesses (Herbsman *et al.* 1981; Bowles 1983; Patterson 1989). It is not clear whether a segmental resection or a simple mastectomy (with a lower attendant morbidity) offers benefits over a more radical procedure (Herbsman *et al.* 1981). In fact, the results of two randomized trials in the United Kingdom have suggested that surgery may not even be necessary as first-line treatment in such patients, with equivalent 3 year survival being afforded by initial treatment with tamoxifen (Gazet *et al.* 1988; Robertson *et al.* 1988). Although the surgery (local resection) in each study may not have been optimal, survival figures were comparable with those reported when more radical surgery was employed (Herbsman *et al.* 1981; Rosen *et al.* 1985). However, others have suggested that this approach may be associated with an unacceptable rate of relapse and progression as high as 60 per cent (Falk *et al.* 1989; Fentiman *et al.* 1990).

Although the traditional approach to local tumour control has required mastectomy, more recent trials have demonstrated that excision of the breast lump and radical radiotherapy, if practised in a specialized and experienced unit, yield equivalent results (Veronesi 1985). Whether simple mastectomy or radical radiotherapy yield less morbidity in the very old or frail patient has not been addressed in any randomized trials. However, in the context of such a fragile patient, the issue may only be of academic relevance, and it may be more prudent simply to treat with initial tamoxifen, as outlined above.

Several randomized trials have failed to show any significant impact on overall survival from the use of adjuvant chemotherapy in post-menopausal women, although Fisher *et al.* (1990) have recently proposed that a small but significant survival benefit may be obtained if doxorubicin and cyclophosphamide are added to the treatment of post-menopausal women with tamoxifen-responsive tumours; however, an analysis of outcome in patients over the age of 70 years has not been published.

Notwithstanding this controversy, it is clear that post-menopausal women with node-positive disease (stage II) have improved disease-free and/or total survival if treated with adjuvant tamoxifen, whether or not adjuvant radiotherapy is used, particularly if the duration of tamoxifen treatment exceeds 2 years (Nolvadex Adjuvant Trial Organisation 1985; Mouridsen *et al.* 1986; Early Breast Cancer Trialists' Collaborative Group 1988; Castiglione *et al.* 1990). However, this effect is somewhat reduced by the prevalence of deaths from intercurrent disease among aged patients with breast cancer (Castiglione *et al.* 1990).

At the meeting of the Early Breast Cancer Trialists' Collaborative Group in which an overview of randomized trials was constructed, clear evidence of improved recurrence-free and total survival was shown for post-menopausal women with node-positive breast cancer

CANCER IN THE ELDERLY

Table 9 Chemotherapy for metastatic breast cancer in the elderly

Number	Age range (years)	Treatment	Response rate (%)	Median survival (months)	Series
39	>60	CAF	56	?	Aisner *et al.* (1987)
38	>60	CMF	36	?	Aisner *et al.* (1987)
29	>60	CAFVP	58	?	Aisner *et al.* (1987)
28	>60	CAF	64	20	Cummings *et al.* (1985)
29	>60	CMFP	45	13	Cummings *et al.* (1985)
79	>66	CMF	?	22	Falkson *et al.* (1986)
92	>65	CMF	*c.* 44	*c.* 19	Gelman and Taylor (1984)

C, cyclophosphamide; A, doxorubicin (adriamycin); M, methotrexate; F, fluorouracil; P, prednisone.

treated with tamoxifen. Of importance, although the geriatric age group was not specifically evaluated prospectively, this retrospective analysis showed a significant benefit in women aged 70 years or more (Early Breast Cancer Trialists' Collaborative Group 1990). This analysis failed to reveal any significant benefit from adjuvant cytotoxic chemotherapy for the elderly, although the small numbers of treated patients and the probable selection bias may well have prejudiced this outcome.

Metastatic breast cancer

The general principles governing the management of metastatic breast cancer are not a function of age. For practical purposes, metastatic breast cancer is incurable with currently available treatment and the aim of management is to provide sustained palliation with minimal cost to the patient in terms of morbidity, inconvenience, and the other indices of quality of life. Although a detailed discussion of the hormonal or cytotoxic treatment of breast cancer is beyond the scope of this chapter, certain principles obtain. As post-menopausal breast cancer has a high prevalence of oestrogen and progesterone receptor positivity, there is a high chance of response to a range of hormonal manipulations in this context, including tamoxifen, progestational agents, and aminoglutethimide. If the tumour is resistant to hormone therapy, radiotherapy may be useful in controlling localized disease, particularly in the case of bone or brain metastases or in the presence of recurrence in the breast.

Alternatively, cytotoxic agents can be used effectively and without undue toxicity, provided that account is taken of the patient's general physical condition and such factors as renal and hepatic function. Gelman and Taylor (1984) have shown that the toxicity of the CMF regimen (cyclophosphamide, methotrexate, and fluorouracil) can be ameliorated by dose modification based upon renal function. Whether a significant reduction in antitumour efficacy occurs if doses are reduced in elderly patients with advanced malignancy remains the subject of controversy (Hryniuk and Bush 1984). As the metabolism of cyclophosphamide and fluorouracil is not predictably age dependent, another option is the routine prescription of folinic acid in the elderly patient, reducing the likelihood of myelosuppression or mucosal toxicity from methotrexate. Alternatively, less toxic analogues of conventional agents which have activity against breast cancer have been shown to have modest activity in this context, for example mitoxantrone (Stuart-Harris *et al.* 1987) and carboplatin (Canetta *et al.* 1990). The results of typical active management programmes for elderly patients with breast cancer are summarized in Table 9.

In our institution, unless an elderly patient is involved in a clinical trial, the standard approach to metastatic disease includes the use of hormonal manipulation as first-line therapy, with radiotherapy, second-line hormones, or cytotoxic agents being used judiciously as salvage therapy after the failure of initial treatment.

Gastrointestinal cancers

Analogous to the situation in younger age groups, the treatment of choice for most gastrointestinal malignancies is surgical resection, as discussed elsewhere in this volume. As gastrointestinal cancers occur predominantly in the elderly, much of the published information on their management reflects populations of patients with a significant proportion of the aged. However, specific features that pertain to the elderly are worthy of review.

Colorectal carcinoma

As shown in Table 1, approximately 60 per cent of colorectal malignancies occur in patients over the age of 65 years, with small differences in incidence between colon and rectum and no relationship to gender. Although the elderly are characteristically beset by chronic constipation, irregular bowel habit, and a tendency to delayed presentation, major surveys have not shown any difference in the extent of colorectal malignancy in the aged at diagnosis (Table 2). There is an approximately equal distribution of cases among localized, regional, and metastatic presentations in patients over the age of 65 years and in the younger group (Patterson 1983; Neilan 1987).

There are no specific features of presentation in the elderly, apart from the difficulties of rationalizing a non-specific constellation of symptoms and signs in a patient group with the features of ageing (Neilan 1987). Early diagnosis can be achieved by the inclusion of elderly groups in appropriate screening programmes, with clinical rectal examination, colonoscopy, and radiographic studies. No differences have been demonstrated of compliance or complications among the elderly in such studies (Winawer *et al.* 1983).

In general, there appears to be no reason for considering age *per se* as a major factor when defining a management plan for most elderly patients with non-metastatic colorectal cancer (Bader 1986; Payne *et al.* 1986). Prognosis is determined primarily by the stage of disease, rather than by the age of the patient (Payne *et al.* 1986). The 5 year survival is more than 80 per cent for Dukes' stage A, 60–70 per cent for Dukes' stage B, and 30–40 per cent for Dukes' stage C (Neilan 1987). The observed survival rates at 3 and 5 years for patients older than 75 years with colonic cancer (36 and 26 per cent, respectively) reported by the SEER study (Ries *et al.* 1983) were rather different from those of all ages (46 and 37 per cent); however, when deaths from intercurrent disease were taken into consideration, the relative survival rates in the older age group (49 and 45 per cent) were not significantly different from those of the total population (54 and 48 per cent), but

2181

were lower than those for patients aged less than 45 years (60 and 53 per cent). In contrast, in this study relative 3 and 5 year survival rates from rectal cancer in patients aged 75 years or more were 46 and 37 per cent compared with 55 and 46 per cent for the total population (and 60 and 50 per cent, respectively for patients less than 45 years old).

As noted previously, the clinical context must be evaluated, balancing the potential for cure or long-term survival against the morbidity of surgery. Operative risk must be assessed. For example, fit patients with no or one intercurrent condition have less than a 2 per cent chance of perioperative death after colectomy, irrespective of age (Boyd et al. 1980); in contrast, if two or more intercurrent conditions are present, the mortality rate rises from 8.6 per cent in patients aged 70 years or less to 16.2 per cent in older age groups (Boyd et al. 1980). As noted previously, the hazards of surgery can be reduced in an elective setting compared with emergency procedures (Patterson 1989). In the case of an elderly patient with significant intercurrent diseases (thus presenting a major surgical hazard), a more conservative approach to a localized lesion with diathermy or radiotherapy may yield equivalent results (Patterson 1983; Neilan 1987).

A more controversial issue is the use of adjuvant therapy after surgical resection of colorectal malignancy. Moertel et al. (1990) have recently proposed that adjuvant fluorouracil-based chemotherapy can reduce recurrence rates and improve survival in patients with resected Dukes' stage C carcinoma. In this study, the median age of patients was 61 years and no difference in survival was noted between patients aged less than 61 years and those in the older age group; however, toxicity profiles were not reported in these age groups. Whether the toxicity encountered in the elderly patients will be justified by a 20 per cent increase in 3 year survival remains to be seen and further studies of this type will be required to resolve the issue.

Metastatic colorectal cancer is usually an incurable disease and this must govern the decision-making process in the elderly. There is no rationale, at least in the context of survival of patients with metastatic colorectal cancer, for the early introduction of cytotoxic chemotherapy (Begg and Carbone 1983). In their review of more than 1200 patients with advanced colorectal cancer treated by the Eastern Cooperative Oncology Group, Begg and Carbone (1983) showed a median survival of less than 30 weeks, with age having no impact on survival. It is our practice to delay the use of chemotherapy in elderly patients until the development of tumour-related symptoms, as the progression of such disease can be quite variable and prolonged symptom-free periods are frequently encountered. Although it has been shown in large surveys that there is no specific increase in the overall morbidity of chemotherapy for elderly patients with advanced colon cancer when compared with younger counterparts (Begg and Carbone 1983), the modest gains achieved by chemotherapy (in the reduction of tumour-related symptoms) are often offset by a prolonged period in hospital, the cost for the patient and family, and subtle (often unrecorded) side-effects due to chemotherapy. This is compounded by the fact that conservative management with support and analgesics often yields equivalent palliation.

To date, randomized clinical trials have not shown improved survival when multiagent regimens are compared with single agents in any age group with bowel cancer. In the absence of a patient's involvement in a randomized clinical trial, our approach (in selected symptomatic patients) is to administer a trial of single-agent bolus doses of fluorouracil in a weekly low-dose schedule or in third-weekly doses, assessing objective response, amelioration of symptoms,

and level of toxicity. If apparent benefit is demonstrated in the absence of significant and unacceptable toxicity, chemotherapy is continued to secure palliation (usually a course of 3–4 months).

Upper gastrointestinal malignancies

A detailed discussion of the management of upper gastrointestinal cancer is beyond the scope of this chapter. However, in general terms, the principles of diagnosis and treatment of these conditions in the younger population groups apply to the elderly. In view of the prevalence of gastrointestinal malignancy with advancing age (Table 1), features such as dysphagia, abdominal pain, and unexplained weight loss should be assessed carefully. Biopsy and staging investigations will set the case into a clinical context and the potential for surgical resection and cure (or effective palliation) can be determined (Keppen 1987).

Aggressive surgical management of oesophageal cancer is associated with perioperative mortality rates as high as 30 per cent (Keppen 1987) and long-term survival is uncommon. To date, radical radiotherapy or combined radiotherapy–surgery protocols have not contributed a major improvement in outcome. The more aggressive combinations of chemotherapy and radiotherapy for oesophageal cancer should be regarded as investigational. In the elderly patient, simple surgical procedures, including the insertion of an oesophageal tube or the use of endoscopic laser therapy and appropriate use of analgesics and supportive techniques may provide useful palliation. For metastatic disease, combination chemotherapy remains investigational and there is no place for its routine application to geriatric patients in this context. Nevertheless, at Roswell Park Cancer Institute, we have treated patients aged 70–75 years safely with the combination of mitomycin, ifosfamide, mesna and cisplatin, achieving sustained responses in locally advanced and metastatic disease. Of particular importance, it should not be forgotten that the elderly gastrointestinal mucosa is less rapidly repaired and more sensitive to the toxicity of radical radiation doses or intensive chemotherapy regimens, especially infusional 5-fluorouracil.

Similarly, pancreatic cancer is frequently associated with a poor prognosis, independent of the nature of treatment (Ries et al. 1983). In the aged patient, it is of particular importance to emphasize quality of life rather than a fruitless expenditure of resources in aggressive treatment programmes. Of particular relevance, nerve blocks and effective analgesics may reduce symptoms dramatically. Occasionally, modest doses of fluorouracil (250–500 mg/m^2 intravenously every 3–4 weeks) can cause a reduction in the level of intractable pain, allowing a reduction in the dosage of narcotic analgesics.

Although the incidence of gastric cancer is declining, the elderly still constitute a high-risk group (Table 1). Prognosis is determined by the stage of the disease and the nature of the resection. It has been suggested that younger patients have a more aggressive disease with a concomitantly worse prognosis (Goodwin et al. 1986), although this is not supported by large surveys of outcome (Ries et al. 1983). Nanus et al. (1989) have reported a possible basis for a difference in behaviour of these tumours in the young and in the elderly in a study of ploidy of gastric cancers; they reported no diploid tumours in seven patients under the age of 45 years, in contrast with 50 per cent diploidy among 28 older patients. Patients without nodal involvement or direct extension will have a 5 year survival of more than 60 per cent if they can tolerate total or subtotal gastrectomy (Keppen 1987). Because of the extent of the operative approach and the requisite surgery, careful pre-operative assessment by a clinician experienced in geriatric surgery is essential and attention should be directed to such factors as intercurrent disease and nutritional status. However, it should not be forgotten that large population surveys have only shown a 6 per cent 5 year survival among patients aged 75 years or more, a figure which is still only 11 per cent if deaths from intercurrent disease are excluded (Ries et al. 1983).

In some instances, palliative subtotal gastrectomy or surgical bypass can usefully be applied to the elderly patient with significant symptoms (obstruction, pain, or haemorrhage). Similarly, endoscopic guided photocoagulation can effectively palliate obstructing or bleeding lesions (Fleischer and Sivak 1985). Although gastric cancer can be sensitive to radiotherapy, the effectiveness of this modality is limited by the tolerance of the gastric mucosa, particularly in an elderly patient.

Begg and Carbone (1983) showed no difference in response rate or toxicity between elderly patients treated for advanced gastric cancer and a younger cohort. Despite a range of reported response rates of 20–50 per cent, less than 10 per cent of patients survive 3 years and considerable caution should be exercised in the use of cytotoxics for this indication in the elderly. Of importance, randomized trials have failed to demonstrate a survival benefit of intensive combination chemotherapy regimens over the use of single agents (Keppen 1987).

Genitourinary cancer

A range of genitourinary malignancies occur in the elderly. Tumours arising in the kidney represent less than 2 per cent of malignancies in the geriatric population, with testicular neoplasms occurring even less commonly. A detailed discussion of the management of testicular tumours in the aged is beyond the scope of this chapter. However, it should be noted that the majority of such tumours in this age group are lymphomas or metastases, rather than tumours of germinal origin. These issues have been discussed in detail elsewhere (Hamilton and Horwich 1988).

Tumours of the kidney

There are no particular features to distinguish renal carcinomas in the elderly. They are commonly silent until advanced, although they may present with abdominal or flank pain, haematuria, or a range of non-specific symptoms. These tumours are notoriously resistant to treatment when advanced and cure is only achieved by surgical resection of early stage disease. As in the other malignancies discussed previously, a cost–benefit analysis should govern the approach to management in the elderly. Fit geriatric patients tolerate nephrectomy without undue complications and the solitary geriatric kidney can compensate adequately for the loss of the contralateral organ. As in younger patients, there is no proven role for adjuvant radiotherapy, chemotherapy, hormonal manipulation, or immune therapy in this context. In advanced renal carcinoma, aggressive management has little place in the aged patient and our emphasis is on palliation and support. The aged fare less well than younger patients. For example, Ries et al. (1983) have documented a 5 year disease-specific survival of only 39 per cent for patients over 75 years of age compared with 65 per cent for patients younger than 45 years. It is likely that this represents patterns of presentation in the elderly and conservatism of clinical practice, rather than being due to innate features of the disease in the elderly.

Occasionally, patients with a past history of analgesic nephropathy or the excessive intake of phenacetin-containing analgesics (see section on bladder cancer) develop transitional cell cancers of the upper urinary tract. These tumours are relatively sensitive to cytotoxic agents and there may be a limited role for their use in the otherwise healthy geriatric patient with advanced disease (Malden et al. 1988).

Prostate cancer

Prostate cancer, with a median age at presentation of 70 years, is the commonest malignancy in geriatric males (Ries et al. 1983; Silverberg 1987) and illustrates many of the previously discussed problems in diagnosis and management. Although it has been documented that more than 50 per cent of males over the age of 75 years harbour some form of prostatic cancer, many of these tumours are initially asymptomatic and incidental (so-called stage A1) and are merely documented at routine transurethral prostatic resection for benign hyperplasia or as the result of an autopsy study (Raghavan and Rogers 1990). However, up to 40 per cent of patients first present with metastases and a large proportion of the remainder will develop metastatic deposits during the course of the disease (Raghavan 1988).

The initial diagnosis can be quite difficult in the context that patients are elderly, with a range of intercurrent medical disorders that can mimic the features of early or advanced prostate cancer (Raghavan and Rogers 1990). Geriatric males characteristically have benign prostatic hyperplasia, which can mimic or mask the features of early prostate cancer. More advanced disease (for example, osseous metastases) can be masked by the features of chronic arthritis or Paget's disease of bone. To date, routine approaches to screening have not been of great benefit, probably because of the inaccuracy of clinical, biochemical, or ultrasonographic assessment of early disease and the confounding issue of the benign natural history of stage A1 cancer. In addition, the inadequate level of education for the at-risk elderly population has not fostered early presentation in response to the symptoms of early prostate cancer (Slack et al. 1986).

It has been reported that prostatic cancer runs a more indolent course in the very elderly (Cook and Watson 1968), although this has been the subject of considerable controversy. Smedley et al. (1983), in a study of nearly 600 cases, found no relationship between age and histological grade or survival. Adami et al. (1986b) reported a 10 per cent reduction in survival among patients aged less than 45 years or older than 75 years compared with patients in the 46–74 year age group. In contrast, Borek et al. (1990), reviewing nearly 5000 cases, noted that men over the age of 80 years had a statistically significant reduction in tumour differentiation and that this difference was maintained in patients presenting with localized disease or with regional spread but was not statistically significant in patients presenting with distant metastases. In a large population survey, Ries et al. (1983) reported 5 year survival rates of 45 per cent for patients under 45 years of age, 68 per cent for patients aged 46–74 years, and 56 per cent for patients older than 74 years (excluding deaths from intercurrent disease for all groups). This apparent paradox can be explained by the postulate that there are two distinct types of prostate cancer in the elderly: the relatively indolent pattern that presents as stage A1 disease and a more aggressive, less differentiated variant with a high mortality rate (Borek et al. 1990).

Decisions regarding the management of geriatric males with prostate cancer are strongly influenced by the general physical state of the patient. In early stage disease, if all age groups are considered, comparable long-term survival rates are obtained with radical radiotherapy or from cystoprostatectomy (Raghavan and Rogers

1990). Selected geriatric patients with stages A–C prostate cancer have been treated with radical radiotherapy (Green *et al.* 1985; Forman *et al.* 1986) and have sustained 5 year survival rates of 60–80 per cent, with high rates of local tumour control. Similar populations of elderly patients have been treated by radical prostatectomy (with or without pelvic lymphadenectomy) and have had comparable long-term survival (Zincke *et al.* 1981). To date, no randomized comparisons of treatment options in geriatric patients have been reported and, thus, direct comparisons are not possible.

The morbidity of each procedure can be substantial in the elderly and it is essential to define the cost–benefit ratio for such treatment in the individual case. Radical radiotherapy involves tumour doses of 65–70 Gy, which can be associated with significant toxicity to surrounding tissues including urethral stricture, radiation cystitis, diarrhoea, and pelvic or scrotal oedema (Green *et al.* 1985; Forman *et al.* 1986). Similarly, the morbidity of pelvic surgery, with the potential complications of a major operation, the possible loss of sphincter function and potency, or the development of pelvic or lower limb oedema (Narayan and Lange 1980; Zincke *et al.* 1981), is a major consideration in a geriatric patient.

The management of advanced disease must also be predicated on the physical and emotional resources of the patient. Bilateral orchidectomy yields objective response rates of 50–70 per cent, depending upon the criteria of evaluation (Raghavan and Rogers 1990) and we regard this to be the initial treatment of choice for advanced disease. Systemic oestrogens are associated with a significant risk of vascular complications and the analogues of luteinizing-hormone-releasing hormone are costly without providing added benefit over bilateral orchidectomy. Few geriatric patients have intercurrent medical problems that would contraindicate the modest toxicity of bilateral orchidectomy.

In patients who have relapsed after bilateral orchidectomy, there is no effective panacea, irrespective of age (Raghavan 1988). Subjective response rates of 35–40 per cent and objective response rates of 15–20 per cent have been recorded after treatment with aminoglutethimide, megestrol acetate, medroxyprogesterone acetate, and flutamide (Raghavan 1988). Cytotoxic chemotherapy has only a limited role in such patients (Raghavan 1988), although relatively gentle agents, such as mitoxantrone or oral cyclophosphamide, can achieve improved symptoms and objective response in elderly patients without undue toxicity (Raghavan *et al.* 1989).

Of particular importance, adequate control of symptoms must be provided, with particular attention to the problems of the aged. Often the aged patient will be reluctant or unable to report accurately the scope or intensity of pain or other symptoms. Certain problems are increased in the aged, for example great care must be taken to maintain a regular bowel habit in the elderly patient receiving narcotic analgesics. Age-related problems of drug metabolism and pharmacological interactions, as discussed previously (see also Table 3), must be taken into consideration when planning management (Raghavan *et al.* 1988a). The possible accumulation of narcotics and sedatives should be considered, as well as their potential to cause other side-effects. Effective management of pain in this situation can often require complex balancing of analgesics, stool softeners, sedatives, and other intercurrent medications; this can, in itself, cause the added problem of coping with complex directions and care must be taken to ensure compliance with the treatment by recruiting assistance from family or other sources of support. In fact, the optimal management of advanced prostate cancer in an elderly patient illustrates most of the principles reviewed and requires active collaboration of the oncologist, geriatrician, family practitioner, paramedical staff, and other sources of care and support.

Bladder cancer

As outlined in Table 1, bladder cancer is predominantly a disease of the elderly, with most cases occurring in males over the age of 60 years. The incidence of the disease is higher in industrialized countries; the aetiological factors include smoking, excessive intake of phenacetin-containing analgesics, and occupational exposure (Raghavan *et al.* 1990b). There are no specific features of presentation in the elderly, apart from the difficulty of making the diagnosis early in a population group (elderly males) who characteristically suffer from the symptoms of prostatism and urinary infection. It has been suggested that a haematuria diagnostic service will lead to the diagnosis of bladder cancer at an earlier stage and is associated with improved outcomes of treatment (Hendry 1988) and it seems likely that this approach could be of particular benefit to the elderly. As this disease is associated with cigarette smoking, industrial exposure, and phenacetin abuse, patients characteristically have a wide range of intercurrent medical disorders that complicate the process of diagnosis and management (Raghavan *et al.* 1988a,b).

There are two predominant patterns of bladder cancer. Superficial disease (restricted to the mucosa, submucosa, and lamina propria) occurs at first presentation in approximately 80 per cent of cases and is associated with a pattern of relapse and remission but with more than 70 per cent of patients surviving at least 5 years (Hendry 1988; Raghavan *et al.* 1990b). Invasive bladder cancer, which is found at presentation in approximately 20 per cent of cases, is usually associated with a worse prognosis, with less than 50 per cent of patients surviving 5 years (Hendry 1988; Raghavan *et al.* 1990b). Results from the SEER study have shown a relative 5 year survival of 58 per cent for all stages of disease among patients aged 75 years or older compared with more than 85 per cent for patients less than 55 years of age (Ries *et al.* 1983). However, it is not clear whether these data reflect differences in the extent of presenting disease in the respective age groups or in the aggression of management.

With respect to superficial bladder cancer, treatment is predicated on local tumour control which can be achieved by transurethral resection or diathermy, the use of cytotoxics administered topically into the bladder (intravesical chemotherapy), laser therapy, radiotherapy, or cystectomy, as reviewed in detail elsewhere (Hendry 1988; Raghavan *et al.* 1990b). As the morbidity of most of these approaches is modest, age *per se* is not a major consideration. When considering radiotherapy or cystectomy, the age-related issues discussed previously with respect to the morbidity and mortality of treatment will obtain. Occasionally, in the elderly patient with a long history of superficial bladder cancer that has been repeatedly treated by endoscopic resection or diathermy, the syndrome of 'malignant cystitis' will be unusually severe; debilitating urinary symptoms including dysuria, nocturia, frequency, haematuria, strangury, and perineal pain. These may prove to be intractable, and may necessitate either cystectomy with urinary diversion (in which the urinary outflow is diverted to a loop of bowel that is converted into an internal reservoir or brought to the skin and connected to a urinary collection bag) or urinary diversion alone. With the improvements in pelvic surgery and the increased fitness of the aged, more patients are able to undergo cystectomy safely in this context (Zincke 1982; Skinner *et al.* 1984; Hendry 1988).

The management of invasive or metastatic disease in the elderly is more difficult. Conventional approaches to invasive bladder cancer (defined on the basis of invasion at least of muscle in the bladder wall) include radical cystectomy with lymph node dissection or radical radiotherapy and, in some instances, the combination of radiotherapy and cystectomy (Raghavan *et al.* 1990*b*). In general, the very elderly tolerate these radical approaches less well than when simple cystectomy or palliative doses of irradiation are applied. Once again, a balance must be developed between the efficacy of tumour control and the morbidity of treatment. This is made more difficult by the lack of consensus regarding the prognostic implications of age for tumour-specific survival (Van der Werf Messing 1979; Batata *et al.* 1981; Bloom *et al.* 1982; Narayana *et al.* 1983; Gospodarowicz *et al.* 1989). In general, we believe that age itself is not a major consideration in the fit geriatric patient with bladder cancer who would otherwise have a prolonged life expectancy. Provided that appropriate precautions are taken, such patients will survive the necessary surgery or radical radiotherapy without undue complications.

More recently, cytotoxic chemotherapy has been introduced earlier into the management of invasive non-metastatic bladder cancer in an attempt to increase long-term survival. We have demonstrated that single agents, such as cisplatin, can be administered safely to fit elderly patients even in the presence of intercurrent diseases, provided that care is taken with hydration and follow-up (Raghavan *et al.* 1988*a,b*). Others have shown that combination chemotherapy can also be delivered in this context without toxic deaths, although the specific complications of treatment in the aged have not been reported (Zincke *et al.* 1988; Scher *et al.* 1989). However, to date, the use of cytotoxics in this context remains investigational for all age groups as no randomized trial has demonstrated a survival benefit from such treatment when compared with conventional management.

In the case of metastatic disease, despite response rates as high as 70 per cent, only 20 per cent of patients at best can expect to be cured by chemotherapy (Raghavan 1990). Thus, the use of chemotherapy in elderly patients with metastatic bladder cancer requires great caution, particularly if combination regimens are being considered. In most instances, we only use single-agent regimens (for example, cisplatin 80–100 mg/m² every 3 weeks; methotrexate 50–100 mg/m² intravenously every 2–3 weeks with folinic acid as needed) for aged patients with metastases. Only one randomized trial to date has demonstrated a superior antitumour activity of combination chemotherapy (the MVAC regimen (methotrexate, doxorubicin, vinblastine, cisplatin)) over single agents in the treatment of advanced bladder cancer (Loehrer *et al.* 1992), whereas four randomized studies have not shown any significant difference when outmoded combination regimens were compared with single-agent cisplatin (Raghavan 1990). However, all these studies have shown a significantly increased toxicity from the combination regimens. Of importance, Loehrer *et al.* (1992) showed that age *per se* was not an adverse prognostic factor in these patients.

FUTURE CONSIDERATIONS

By the end of the century, the problems of geriatric patients will dominate the pattern of care in internal medicine, with a large component of expenditure of resources being allocated to the management of cancer. The 'baby boomers', born in the period after the Second World War, will become the 'elder boomers', with a projected figure of 51.4 million in the United States by the year 2020 (Kennedy 1990). The management of the increasing population of geriatric patients, with an increased active life expectancy and an increased potential prevalence of malignancy,

will require careful planning. Adequate allocation of resources will be necessary, particularly as the costs of new treatment programmes are increasing and the proportional financial burdens on the young are likely to become insupportable.

In order to cope effectively with this problem, we must address these issues now. Large cooperative cancer trial groups should be encouraged to deal specifically with the management of common cancers in the elderly, emphasizing the cost–benefit ratio of the treatments under consideration. Patterns of response and toxicity must be defined with increasing precision to facilitate the modification of standard treatment approaches and the development of new management strategies for the unique characteristics of the aged. The specific problems of health screening in the elderly must be addressed and public health education campaigns should be tailored to the characteristics and whims of the elderly if they are to be effective. If these issues are not addressed now, we shall be faced with a problem of epidemic proportions in the early part of the next century and *we* will be the likely victims of a system that cannot cope with the onslaught.

REFERENCES

Adami H-O, *et al.* (1986*a*). The relation between survival and age at diagnosis in breast cancer. *New England Journal of Medicine*, 315:559–63.

Adami, H-O, Norlen BJ, Malker B, Meirik O (1986*b*). Long-term survival in prostatic carcinoma, with special reference to age as a prognostic factor. A nation-wide study. *Scandinavian Journal of Urology and Nephrology*, 20:107–12.

Aisner J, *et al.* (1987). Chemotherapy versus chemoimmunotherapy (CAF v. CAFVP v. CMF Each±MER) for metastatic carcinoma of the breast: a CALGB study. *Journal of Clinical Oncology*, 5:1523–33.

Allen C, Cox EB, Manton KG, Cohen HJ (1986). Breast cancer in the elderly. Current patterns of care. *Journal of the American Geriatric Society*, 34:637–42.

Anderson T, *et al.* (1982). Malignant lymphoma: 1. The histology and staging of 473 patients at the National Cancer Institute. *Cancer*, 50:2699–707.

Anisimov VN (1987). *Carcinogenesis and aging*, Vol. 1, pp. 1–47. CRC Press, Boca Raton, FL.

Armitage JO, Potter JF (1984). Aggressive chemotherapy for diffuse histiocytic lymphoma in the elderly: increased complications with advancing age. *Journal of the American Geriatric Society*, 32:269–73.

Auerbach O, Garfinkel L, Parks VR (1975). Histologic type of lung cancer in relation to smoking habits, year of diagnosis and site of metastases. *Chest*, 67:382–7.

Austin-Seymour MM, *et al.* (1984). Hodgkin's disease in patients over sixty years old. *Annals of Internal Medicine*, 100:13–18.

Bader TF (1986). Colorectal cancer in patients older than 75 years of age. *Diseases of Colon and Rectum*, 29:728–32.

Barnes N, *et al.* (1987). Variation in lymphoma incidence within Yorkshire Health Region. *British Journal of Cancer*, 55:81–4.

Batata MA, *et al.* (1981). Factors of prognostic and therapeutic significance in patients with bladder cancer. *International Journal of Radiation Oncology—Biology—Physics*, 7:575–9.

Begg CB, Carbone PP (1983). Clinical trials and drug toxicity in the elderly: the experience of Eastern Cooperative Oncology Group. *Cancer*, 52:1986–92.

Bender AD (1965) The effects of increasing age on the distribution of peripheral blood flow in man. *Journal of the American Geriatric Society*, 13:192–8.

Bender BS, *et al.* (1986). Absolute peripheral blood lymphocyte count and subsequent mortality of elderly men. *Journal of the American Geriatric Society*, 34:649–54.

Blackwell EA, *et al.* (1986). Early supra-diaphragmatic Hodgkin's disease: high dose gallium scanning obviates the need for staging laparotomy. *Cancer*, 58:883–5.

Bloom HJG, Hendry WF, Wallace DM, Skeet RG (1982). Treatment of T3 bladder cancer: controlled trial of preoperative radiotherapy and radical cystectomy versus radical radiotherapy. Second report and review. *British Journal of Urology*, 54:136–51.

Bloomfield CD, et al. (1974). Multivariate analysis of prognostic factors in the non-Hodgkin's malignant lymphomas. *Cancer*, **33**:870–9.

Borek D, Butcher D, Hassanein K, Holmes F (1990). Relationship of age to histologic grade in prostate cancer. *Prostate*, **16**:305–11.

Boucek RJ, Noble NL, Marks A (1961). Age and fibrous proteins of the human lung. *Gerontologia*, **5**:150.

Bowles LT (1983). Surgical essentials in the care of the elderly cancer patient. In *Perspectives on prevention and treatment of cancer in the elderly* (ed. R Yancik, et al.), pp. 57–61. Raven Press, New York.

Boyd JB, Bradford B, Watne AL (1980). Operative risk factors of colon resection in the elderly. *Annals of Surgery*, **192**:743–6.

Brandsteller RD, Kazemi H (1983). Aging and the respiratory system. *Medical Clinics of North America*, **67**:419–31.

Brocklehurst JC, Khan Y (1969). A study of fecal stasis in old age and use of Dorbamex in its prevention. *Gerontology Clinics*, **2**: 293–300.

Calabrese CT, Adam YG, Volk H (1973). Geriatric colon cancer. *American Journal of Surgery*, **125**:181–4.

Canetta R, Smaldone L, Bragman K, Rozencweig M. (1990). Clinical trials with carboplatin in other tumor types: adult and pediatric malignancies. In *Carboplatin: current perspectives and future directions* (ed. PA Bunn, Jr, R Canetta, RF Ozols, and M Rozencweig), pp. 345–52. Saunders, Philadelphia.

Carbone A, et al. (1986). Non-Hodgkin's lymphoma in the elderly. *Cancer*, **57**:2185–9.

Carlile T, Kopecky KJ, Hadaway EN (1983). Breast cancer screening in the elderly. In *Perspectives on prevention and treatment of cancer in the elderly* (ed. R Yancik, et al.), pp. 289–9. Raven Press, New York.

Castiglione M, Gelber RD, Goldhirsch A (1990). Adjuvant systemic therapy for breast cancer in the elderly: competing causes of mortality. *Journal of Clinical Oncology*, **8**:519–26.

Chahinian AP, et al. (1989). A randomized trial of anticoagulation with warfarin and of alternating chemotherapy in extensive small-cell lung cancer by Cancer and Leukemia Group B. *Journal of Clinical Oncology*, **7**:993–1002.

Clamon GH, Audeh MW, Pinnick S (1982). Small cell lung carcinoma in the elderly. *Journal of the American Geriatric Society*, **30**:299–302.

Cohen HJ (1985). Clinical aspects of cancer in the elderly. In *Interrelationship among aging, cancer and differentiation* (ed. B Pullman, POP Ts'o, and EL Schneider), pp. 15–21. Reidel, Dordrecht.

Cohen T, Gitman L (1959). Oral complaints and taste perception in the aged. *Journal of Gerontology*, **14**:294–8.

Cook GB, Watson FR (1968). A comparison by age of death rates due to prostate cancer alone. *Journal of Urology*, **100**:669–71.

Cox EB (1987). Breast cancer in the elderly. *Clinics in Geriatric Medicine*, **3**:695–713.

Cox JD (1986). Non-small cell lung cancer: role of radiation therapy. *Chest*, **89**:284S–8S.

Crawford J, Cohen HJ (1987). Relationship of cancer and aging. *Clinics in Geriatric Medicine*, **3**:419–31.

Crocker I, Prosnitz L (1987). Radiation therapy of the elderly. *Clinics in Geriatric Medicine*, **3**:473–81.

Cummings FJ, Gelman R, Horton J (1985). Comparison of CAF versus CMFP in metastatic breast cancer: analysis of prognostic factors. *Journal of Clinical Oncology*, **3**:932–40.

Del Guerico LRM, Cohn JD (1980). Monitoring operative risk in the elderly. *Journal of the American Medical Association*, **243**:1350–5.

Dixon CL, et al. (1984). Small cell bronchogenic carcinoma: factors associated with pneumonia during chemotherapy. *Journal of Clinical Oncology*, **2**: 201–6.

Dixon DO, et al. (1986). Effect of age on therapeutic outcome in advanced diffuse histiocytic lymphoma: the Southwest Oncology Group experience. *Journal of Clinical Oncology*, **4**:295–305.

Dodds L, Davis S, Polissar L (1986). A population based study of lung cancer incidence trends by histologic type, 1974–81. *Journal of the National Cancer Institute*, **76**:21–9.

Doll R (1978). An epidemiological perspective of the biology of cancer. *Cancer Research*, **38**:3573–83.

Dontas AS, Marketos S, Papanayiotou P (1972). Mechanisms of renal tubular defects in old age. *Postgraduate Medical Journal*, **48**:295.

Early Breast Cancer Trialists' Collaborative Group (1988). Effects of adjuvant tamoxifen and of cytotoxic therapy on mortality in early breast cancer. An overview of 61 randomized trials among 28,896 women. *New England Journal of Medicine*, **319**:1681–92.

Early Lung Cancer Cooperative Study (1984). Early lung cancer detection: summary and conclusions. *Annual Review of Respiratory Disease*, **130**:565–70.

Ebner H, Sudkamp N, Dragojevic D (1985). Selection and preoperative treatment of over-seventy-year-old patients undergoing thoracotomy. *Thoracic and Cardiovascular Surgery*, **33**:268–71.

Eghbali H, et al. (1984). Hodgkin's disease in the elderly: a series of 30 patients aged older than 70 years. *Cancer*, **53**:2191–3.

Ershler WB, Socinski MA, Greene CJ (1983). Bronchogenic cancer, metastases, and aging. *Journal of the American Geriatric Society*, **31**:673–6.

Ershler WB, Moore AL, Socinski MA (1984). Influenza and aging: age-related changes and the effects of thymosin on the antibody response to influenza vaccine. *Journal of Clinical Immunology*, **4**:445.

Evans MA, et al. (1981). Gastric emptying rate in the elderly: implications for drug therapy. *Journal of the American Geriatric Society*, **29**: 201–5.

Falk GL, Gwynne-Jones D, Gray JG (1989). Efficacy of tamoxifen on the primary treatment of operable breast cancer in the high risk patient. *Australia and New Zealand Journal of Surgery*, **59**: 543–5.

Falkson GS, Gelman RS, Pretorius FJ (1986). Age as a prognostic factor in recurrent breast cancer. *Journal of Clinical Oncology*, **4**:663–71.

Fentiman IS, et al. (1990). Cancer in the elderly: why so badly treated? *Lancet*, **335**:1020–2.

Findlay MPN, et al. (1991). Retrospective review of chemotherapy for small cell lung cancer in the elderly: does the end justify the means? *European Journal of Cancer*, **27**, 1597–601.

Fisher B, et al. (1990). Postoperative chemotherapy and tamoxifen compared with tamoxifen alone in the treatment of positive-node breast cancer patients aged 50 years and older with tumors responsive to tamoxifen: results from the National Surgical Adjuvant Breast and Bowel Project B-16. *Journal of Clinical Oncology*, **8**:1005–8.

Fleischer D, Sivak MB (1985). Endoscopic Nd:YAG laser treatment as palliation for esophage gastric cancer. *Gastroenterology*, **89**: 827–31.

Forman JD, et al. (1986). Carcinoma of the prostate in the elderly: the therapeutic ratio of definitive radiotherapy. *Journal of Urology*, **136**:1238–41.

Foster R, Jr, et al. (1978). Breast self-examination practices and breast-cancer stage. *New England Journal of Medicine*, **299**:265–70.

Foucar K, Armitage JO, Dick FR (1983). Malignant lymphoma, diffuse mixed small and large cell. A clinicopathologic study of 47 cases. *Cancer*, **51**:2090–9.

Gallagher CJ, et al. (1986). Follicular lymphoma: prognostic factors for response and survival. *Journal of Clinical Oncology*, **4**:1470–80.

Ganz PA, Schag CC, Heinrich RL (1985). The psychosocial impact of cancer on the elderly: a comparison with younger patients. *Journal of the American Geriatric Society*, **33**:429–35.

Gazet, J-C, et al. (1988). Prospective randomised trial of tamoxifen versus surgery in elderly patients with breast cancer. *Lancet*, **i**:679–81.

Gelman RS, Taylor SG (1984). CMF chemotherapy in women more than 65 years old with advanced breast cancer: the elimination of age trends in toxicity by using doses based on creatinine clearance. *Journal of Clinical Oncology*, **2**:1404–13.

Ginsberg RJ, Hill LD, Eagen RT (1983). Modern thirty-day operative mortality for surgical resection in lung cancer. *Journal of Thoracic and Cardiovascular Surgery*, **86**:654–8.

Ginsberg SL, Comis RL (1982). The pulmonary toxicity of antineoplastic agents. *Seminars in Oncology*, **9**:34–51.

Gleckman R, Hibert D (1982). Afebrile bacteremia. *Journal of the American Medical Association*, **248**:1478.

Goodwin JS, et al. (1986). Stage at diagnosis of cancer varies with the age of the patient. *Journal of the American Geriatric Society*, **34**:20–6.

Gospadarowicz MK, et al. (1989). Radical radiotherapy for muscle invasive transitional cell carcinoma of the bladder: failure analysis. *Journal of Urology*, **142**:1448–54.

Green N, Bodner H, Broth E (1985). Prostate cancer: experience with definitive irradiation in the aged. *Urology*, **25**:228–32.

Greenblatt DJ, Sellers EM, Shader RI (1982). Drug disposition in old age. *New England Journal of Medicine*, **306**:1081–8.

Greenfield S, Blanco DM, Elashoff RM, Ganz PA (1987). Patterns of care related to age of breast cancer patients. *Journal of the American Medical Association*, **257**:2766–70.

Gunn WG (1980). Radiation therapy for the aging patient. *A Cancer Journal for Clinicians*, **30**:337–47.

Haas CD, *et al.* (1976). Phase II evaluation of bleomycin: a Southwest Oncology Group study. *Cancer*, **38**:8–12.

Hamilton CR, Horwich A (1988). Rare tumours of the testis and paratesticular tissues. In *Textbook of uncommon cancer* (ed. CJ Williams, JC Krikorian, MR Green, and D. Raghavan), pp. 225–48. Wiley, Chichester.

Hancock BW, Aitken M, Ross CMF, Dunsmore IR (1983). Non-Hodgkin's lymphoma in Sheffield, 1971–1980. *Clinics in Oncology*, **9**:109–19.

Hansen HH, Selawry OS, Holland JF, McCall CB (1971). The variability of individual tolerance to methotrexate in cancer patients. *British Journal of Cancer*, **25**:298–305.

Hartstock RJ, Smith EB, Petty ES (1965). Normal variations with aging on the amount of hematopoietic tissue in bone marrow from the anterior iliac crest. *American Journal of Clinical Pathology*, **43**:326–31.

Hendry WF (1988). Diagnosis and management of primary bladder cancer: a British perspective. In *The management of bladder cancer* (ed. D Raghavan), pp. 69–93. Edward Arnold, London.

Herbsman H, *et al.* (1981). Survival following breast cancer surgery in the elderly. *Cancer*, **47**:2358–63.

Ho PC, Triggs EJ (1984). Drug therapy in the elderly. *Australia and New Zealand Journal of Medicine*, **14**:179–90.

Hoerni B, *et al.* (1988). Non-Hodgkin's malignant lymphomas in patients older than 80 years: 70 cases. *Cancer*, **61**:2057–9.

Holland JC, Massie MJ (1987). Psychosocial aspects of cancer in the elderly. *Clinics in Geriatric Medicine*, **3**:533–8.

Hollenberg NK, *et al.* (1974). Senescence and the renal vasculature in normal man. *Circulation Research*, **34**:309–16.

Holmes FF (1989). Clinical evidence for a change in tumor aggressiveness with age. *Seminars in Oncology*, **16**:34–40.

Holmes FF, Hearne E (1981). Cancer stage-to-age relationship: implications for cancer screening in the elderly. *Journal of the American Geriatric Society*, **29**:55–7.

Hong WK, *et al.* (1989). Etoposide combined with cyclophosphamide plus vincristine compared with doxorubicin plus cyclophosphamide plus vincristine and with high-dose cyclophosphamide plus vincristine in the treatment of small-cell carcinoma of the lung: a randomized trial of the Bristol Lung Cancer Study Group. *Journal of Clinical Oncology*, **7**:450–6.

Host H, Lund E (1986). Age as a prognostic factor in breast cancer. *Cancer*, **57**:2217–21.

Hrushesky, WJ, Shimp W, Kennedy BJ (1974). Lack of age-dependent cisplatin nephrotoxicity. *American Journal of Medicine*, **76**:579–84.

Hryniuk W, Bush H (1984). The importance of dose intensity in chemotherapy of metastatic breast cancer. *Journal of Clinical Oncology*, **2**:1281.

Hutchins LF, Lipschitz DA (1987). Cancer, clinical pharmacology and aging. *Clinics in Geriatric Medicine*, **3**:483–503.

Johnson JC (1987). Perioperative care in cancer surgery. *Clinics in Geriatric Medicine*, **3**:463–71.

Jones SE, Miller TP, Connors JM (1989). Long-term follow-up and analysis for prognostic factors for patients with limited-stage diffuse large-cell lymphoma treated with initial chemotherapy with or without adjuvant radiotherapy. *Journal of Clinical Oncology*, **7**:1186–91.

Kaesberg PR, Ershler WB (1989). The change in tumor aggressiveness with age: lessons from experimental animals. *Seminars in Oncology*, **16**:28–33.

Kahn SB, *et al.* (1984). Full dose versus attenuated dose daunorubicin, cytosine arabinoside, and 6-thioguanine in the treatment of acute non-lymphocytic leukaemia in the elderly. *Journal of Clinical Oncology*, **2**:865–70.

Kaminski MS, Coleman CN, Colby TV (1986). Factors predicting survival in adults with stage I and II large cell lymphoma treated with primary radiation therapy. *Annals of Internal Medicine*, **104**:747–56.

Katz S, *et al.* (1983). Active life expectancy. *New England Journal of Medicine*, **309**:1218–24.

Kennedy BJ (1990). Presidential address: aging and cancer. *Journal of Clinical Oncology*, **6**:1903–11.

Kennedy BJ, *et al.* (1985). National survey of patterns of care for Hodgkin's disease. *Cancer*, **56**:2547–56.

Keppen M (1987). Upper gastrointestinal malignancies in the elderly. *Clinics in Geriatric Medicine*, **3**:637–47.

Khan TA, *et al.* (1977). Esophageal motility in the elderly. *American Journal of Digestive Diseases*, **22**:1049–54.

Kirsh MM, *et al.* (1976). Major pulmonary resection for bronchogenic carcinoma in the elderly. *Annals of Thoracic Surgery*, **22**:369–73.

Klimo P, Connors JM (1985). MACOP-B chemotherapy for the treatment of diffuse large-cell lymphoma. *Annals of Internal Medicine*, **102**:596–602.

Kurtz JM, *et al.* (1990). Why are local recurrences after breast-conserving therapy more frequent in younger patients? *Journal of Clinical Oncology*, **8**:591–8.

Lees JC, Park WW (1950). The malignancy of cancer at different ages: a histological study. *British Journal of Cancer*, **3**:186–97.

Leventhal EA (1986). The dilemma of cancer in the elderly. In *Cancer and the elderly* (ed. JM Vaeth and J Meyer), pp. 1–13. Karger, Basel.

Lipschitz DA, Udupa KB (1986). Age and the hematopoietic system. *Journal of the American Geriatric Society*, **34**:448–54.

Lipschitz DA, *et al.* (1985). Cancer in the elderly: basic science and clinical aspects. *Annals of Internal Medicine*, **102**:218–28.

Loehrer PJ, Sr, *et al.* (1992). A randomized comparison of cisplatin alone or in combination with methotrexate, vinblastine, and doxorubicin in patients with metastatic urothelial carcinoma. A cooperative group study. *Journal of Clinical Oncology*, **10**, 1066–73.

Lokich JJ, Pinkus GS, Moloney WC (1974). Hodgkin's disease in the elderly. *Oncology*, **29**:484–500.

McCarty KS, *et al.* (1983). Relationship of age and menopausal status to estrogen receptor content in primary carcinoma of the breast. *Annals of Surgery*, **197**:123–7.

McLachlan MSF (1978). The ageing kidney. *Lancet*, **ii**:143–6.

McLaughlin P, *et al.* (1988). Stage I–II follicular lymphoma. Treatment results for 76 patients. *Cancer*, **58**:1596–602.

MacMahon B, Cole P, Brown J (1973). Etiology of human breast cancer: a review. *Journal of the National Cancer Institute*, **50**:21–42.

Malden LT, Raghavan D, Eisinger D, Pearson BS (1988). Cancer of the upper urothelial tract. In *The management of bladder cancer* (ed. D Raghavan), pp. 299–316. Edward Arnold, London.

Martini N (1986). Lung cancer in the elderly. In *Cancer and the elderly* (ed. JM Vaeth and J Meyer), pp. 125–32. Karger, Basel.

Maurer LH, Pajak TF (1981). Prognostic factors in small cell carcinoma of the lung: a Cancer and Leukemia Group B study. *Cancer Treatment Reports*, **65**:767–74.

Mead GM, *et al.* (1984). Poor prognosis non-Hodgkin's lymphoma in the elderly: clinical presentation and management. *Quarterly Journal of Medicine*, **211**:381–90.

Meyer JS, *et al.* (1986). Breast carcinoma cell kinetics, morphology, stage and host characteristics: a thymidine labeling study. *Laboratory Investigation*, **54**:41.

Moertel CG, *et al.* (1990). Levamisole and fluorouracil for adjuvant therapy of resected colon carcinoma. *New England Journal of Medicine*, **322**:352–8.

Mor V, *et al.* (1985). Relationship between age at diagnosis and treatments received by cancer patients. *Journal of the American Geriatric Society*, **33**:585–9.

Mouridsen HT, *et al.* (1986). Adjuvant tamoxifen in postmenopausal high-risk breast cancer patients: present status of Danish Breast Cancer Cooperative Group trials. *National Cancer Institute Monograph*, **1**:115–18.

Mueller CB, Ames F, Anderson GD (1978). Breast cancer in 3558 women: age as a significant determinant in the rate of dying and causes of death. *Surgery*, **83**:1223–32.

Nanus DM, *et al.* (1989). Flow cytometry as a predictive indicator in patients with operable gastric cancer. *Journal of Clinical Oncology*, **7**:1105–12.

Narayan P, Lange PH (1980). Current controversies in the management of carcinoma of the prostate. *Seminars in Oncology*, 460–7.

Narayana AS, Loening SA, Slymen DJ, Culp DA (1983). Bladder cancer: factors affecting survival. *Journal of Urology*, **130**:56–60.

Nathwani BN, Kim H, Rappaport H, Solomon J, Fox M (1978). Non-Hodgkin's lymphomas: a clinicopathologic study comparing two classifications. *Cancer*, **41**:303–25.

Neilan B (1987). Colorectal cancer. *Clinics in Geriatric Medicine*, **3**:625–35.

New South Wales Cancer Registry (1982). *Cancer, New South Wales, 1982*. Publication CCR 86–051. New South Wales Department of Health: 49–58.

Newell GR, Cabanillas FG, Hagemeister FJ, Butler JJ (1987). Incidence of lymphoma in the US classified by the Working Formulation. *Cancer*, **59**:857–61.

Nolvadex Adjuvant Trial Organisation (1985). Controlled trial of tamoxifen as single adjuvant agent in management of early breast cancer. *Lancet*, i:836–40.

Noordijk EM, Clement E vdP, Hermans J (1988). Radiotherapy as an alternative to surgery in elderly patients with resectable lung cancer. *Radiotherapy and Oncology*, 13:83–9.

O'Rourke MA, Crawford J (1987). Lung cancer in the elderly. *Clinics in Geriatric Medicine*, 3:595–623.

O'Rourke MA, et al. (1987) Age trends of lung cancer stage at diagnosis: implications for lung cancer screening in the elderly. *Journal of the American Medical Association*, 258:921–6.

Parsons J, Bova F, Million R (1980). A reevaluation of split-course technique for squamous cell carcinoma of the head and neck. *International Journal of Radiation Oncology — Biology — Physics*, 6:1645–52.

Paryani SB, et al. (1983). Analysis of non-Hodgkin's lymphomas with nodular and unfavourable histologies, stage I and II. *Cancer*, 52:2300–7.

Patchefsky AS, et al. (1974). Non-Hodgkin's lymphomas: a clinicopathologic study of 293 cases. *Cancer*, 34:1173–86.

Patterson WB (1983). Oncology perspective on colorectal cancer in the geriatric patient. In *Perspectives on prevention and treatment of cancer in the elderly* (ed. R Yancik, et al.), pp. 105–20. Raven Press, New York.

Patterson WB (1989). Surgical issues in geriatric oncology. *Seminars in Oncology*, 16:57–65.

Payne JE, Chapuis PH, Pheils MT (1986). Surgery for large bowel cancer in people aged 75 years and older. *Diseases of Colon and Rectum*, 29:733–7.

Perez CA (1986). Radiotherapy in lung cancer. *Chest*, 89:345S–6S.

Piomelli S, Nathan DG, Cummins JF, Gardner, FH (1962). The relationship of total red cell volume to total body water in octogenarian males. *Blood*, 19:89–98.

Peterson BA, et al. (1982). The effects of age on therapeutic response and survival in advanced Hodgkin's disease. *Cancer Treatment Reports*, 66:889–98.

Peto R, et al. (1975). Cancer and ageing in mice and men. *British Journal of Cancer*, 32:411–26.

Pitot HC (1977). Carcinogenesis and aging — two related phenomena? *American Journal of Pathology*, 87:444–72.

Poplin E, Thompson B, Whitacre M, Aisner J (1987). Small cell carcinoma of the lung: influence of age on treatment outcome. *Cancer Treatment Reports*, 71:291–6.

Popper H (1986). Aging and the liver. *Progress in Liver Diseases*, 8:659–83.

Raghavan D (1988). Non-hormone chemotherapy for prostate cancer: principles of treatment and application to the testing of new drugs. *Seminars in Oncology*, 15:371–89.

Raghavan D (1990). Chemotherapy for advanced bladder cancer: 'Mid-summer Night's Dream' or 'Much Ado About Nothing'? *British Journal of Cancer*, 62. (In press.)

Raghavan D, Rogers J (1990). Update in the management of prostate cancer. *Medical Journal of Australia*, 152:419–26.

Raghavan D, Grundy R, Malden LT (1988a). Cytotoxic chemotherapy in the elderly. In *The management of bladder cancer* (ed. D Raghavan), pp. 174–88. Edward Arnold, London.

Raghavan D, et al. (1988b). Pre-emptive (neo-adjuvant) chemotherapy prior to radical radiotherapy for fit septuagenarians with bladder cancer: age itself is not a contraindication. *British Journal of Urology*, 62:154–9.

Raghavan D, et al. (1989). Management of hormone-resistant prostate cancer: experience at Royal Prince Alfred Hospital. In *Systemic therapy for genitourinary cancers* (ed. DE Johnson, CJ Logothetis, and A Von Eschenbach), pp. 473–84. Year Book, Chicago.

Raghavan D, et al. (1990a). Carboplatin combination chemotherapy regimens for undifferentiated small cell lung cancer. In *Carboplatin: current perspectives and future directions* (ed. PA Bunn, R Canetta, RF Ozols, and M Rozencweig), pp. 235–41. WB Saunders, Philadelphia.

Raghavan D, et al. (1990b). Biology and management of bladder cancer. *New England Journal of Medicine*, 322:1129–38.

Rapaport SI (1986). Positron emission tomography in normal aging and Alzheimer's disease. *Gerontology*, 32:6–13.

Richardson GS, et al. (1985). Common epithelial cancer of the ovary. *New England Journal of Medicine*, 312:415–24.

Ries LG, Pollack ES, Young JL (1983). Cancer patient survival: surveillance, epidemiology, and end results. *Journal of the National Cancer Institute*, 70:693–707.

Roach M, et al. (1990). Prognostic factors for patients relapsing after radiotherapy for early-stage Hodgkin's disease. *Journal of Clinical Oncology*, 8:623–9.

Robertson JFR, et al. (1988). Comparison of mastectomy with tamoxifen for treating elderly patients with operable breast cancer. *British Medical Journal*, 297:511–14.

Rosen PP, Lesser ML, Kinne DW (1985). Breast carcinoma at the extremes of age: a comparison of patients younger than 35 years and older than 75 years. *Journal of Surgical Oncology*, 28:90–6.

Rossmann I (1977). Anatomic and body composition changes with aging. In *Handbook of the biology of aging* (ed. CF Finch and L Hayflick), p. 189. Van Nostrand Reinhold, New York.

Rowe JW, et al. (1976). The effect of age on creatinine clearance in man: a cross sectional and longitudinal study. *Journal of Gerontology*, 31:155–63.

Rudders RA, et al. (1979). Nodular non-Hodgkin's lymphoma (NHL): factors indicating prognosis and indicators for aggressive treatment. *Cancer*, 43:1643–51.

Saitoh H, Shiramizu T, Hida M (1982). Age changes in metastatic patterns in renal adenocarcinoma. *Cancer*, 50:1646–8.

Samet J, et al. (1986). Choice of cancer therapy varies with age of patient. *Journal of the American Medical Association*, 255:3385–90.

Scher HI, et al. (1989). Neo-adjuvant chemotherapy for invasive bladder cancer. Experience with the M-VAC regimen. *British Journal of Urology*, 64:250–6.

Schiffman SS, Moss J, Erickson RP (1976). Thresholds of food odors in the elderly. *Experimental Aging Research*, 2:389–98.

Schottenfeld D, Robbins FG (1971). Breast cancer in elderly women. *Geriatrics*, 26:121–31.

Schwab R, Walters CA, Weksler ME (1989). Host defence mechanisms and aging. *Seminars in Oncology*, 16:20–7.

Shaw PG (1982). Common pitfalls in geriatric drug prescribing. *Drugs*, 23: 324–8.

Sherman S, Guidot CE (1987). The feasibility of thoracotomy for lung cancer in the elderly. *Journal of the American Medical Association*, 258:927–30.

Silverberg E (1987). Statistical and epidemiologic data on urologic cancer. *Cancer*, 60:692–17.

Simes RJ (1985). Risk–benefit relationship in cancer clinical trials: the ECOG experience with non-small cell lung cancer. *Journal of Clinical Oncology*, 3:462–72.

Skinner EC, Lieskovsky G, Skinner DG (1984). Radical cystectomy in the elderly patient. *Journal of Urology*, 131:1065–8.

Slack NH, Lane WW, Priore RL, Murphy GP (1986). Prostatic cancer: treated at a categorical center, 1980–1983. *Urology*, 27:205–13.

Smedley HM, et al. (1983). Age and survival in prostatic carcinoma. *British Journal of Urology*, 55: 529–33.

Sondik EJ, Young JL, Horn JW (1987). *1986 Annual cancer statistics review*. NIH Publication 87–2789, Department of Health and Human Service, Bethesda, MD.

Spiegelman D, et al. (1989). Prognostic factors in small-cell carcinoma of the lung: an analysis of 1521 patients. *Journal of Clinical Oncology*, 7:344–54.

Stuart-Harris R, et al. (1987). Patient treatment preference in advanced breast cancer: a randomized cross-over study of doxorubicin and mitozantrone. *European Journal of Cancer and Clinical Oncology*, 23:557–61.

Stults BM (1983). Preventive cancer care for the elderly. In *Cancer and the elderly* (ed. JM Vaeth and J Meyer), pp. 182–91. Karger, Basel.

Suen KC, Lau LL, Yermakov V (1974). Cancer and old age. An autopsy study of 3535 patients over 65 years old. *Cancer*, 33:1164–8.

Tabar L, et al. (1985). Reduction in mortality from breast cancer after mass screening with mammography. Randomised trial from the Breast Cancer Screening Working Group of the Swedish National Board of Health and Welfare. *Lancet*, i:829–32.

Taylor IW, et al. (1983). The influence of age on the DNA ploidy levels of breast tumours. *European Journal of Cancer and Clinical Oncology*, 19:623–8.

Teeter SM, Holmes FF, McFarlane MJ (1987). Lung carcinoma in the elderly population: influence of histology on the inverse relationship of stage to age. *Cancer*, 60:1331–6.

Tirelli U, et al. (1988). Non-Hodgkin's lymphomas in 137 patients aged 70 years or older: a retrospective European Organisation for Research and Treatment of Cancer lymphoma group study. *Journal of Clinical Oncology*, 6:1708–13.

Tollefsbol TO, Cohen HJ (1986). Role of protein molecular and metabolic aberrations in aging, in the physiologic decline of the aged, and in age-associated diseases. *Journal of the American Geriatric Society*, 34:282–94.

Triggs EJ, Nation RLL (1975). Pharmacokinetics in the aged: a review. *Journal of Pharmacokinetics and Biopharmacology*, **3**:387–418.

Tudway R (1962). The age of the patient and tolerance to radiation. *British Journal of Radiology*, **35**:36–42.

Valagussa P, *et al.* (1986). Second acute leukaemia and other malignancies following treatment for Hodgkin's disease. *Journal of Clinical Oncology*, **4**:830–7.

Van der Werf Messing B (1979). Preoperative irradiation followed by cystectomy to treat carcinoma of the urinary bladder category T3NX, 0-4M0. *International Journal of Radiation Oncology—Biology—Physics*, **5**:394–401.

Van Leeuwen FE, *et al.* (1989). Increased risk of lung cancer, non-Hodgkin's lymphoma, and leukemia following Hodgkin's disease. *Journal of Clinical Oncology*, **7**:1046–58.

Veronesi U (1985). Randomized trials comparing conservation techniques with conventional surgery: an overview. In *Primary management of breast cancer: alternatives to mastectomy* (ed. JS Tobias and MJ Peckham), pp. 131–52. Edward Arnold, London.

Vestal RE (1978). Drug use in the elderly: a review of problems and special considerations. *Drugs*, **16**:358–82.

Vose JM, *et al.* (1988). The importance of age in survival of patients treated with chemotherapy for aggressive non-Hodgkin's lymphoma. *Journal of Clinical Oncology*, **6**:1838–44.

Warnecke RB, Havlicek PL, Manfredi C (1983). Awareness and use of screening by older-aged persons. In *Perspectives on prevention and treatment of cancer in the elderly* (ed. R Yancik, *et al.*), pp. 275–87. Raven Press, New York.

WHO (World Health Organization) (1981). Health care in the elderly: a report of the technical group on use of medicaments by the elderly. *Drugs*, **22**:279–94.

Williamson J (1979). Adverse reactions to prescribed drugs in the elderly. In *Drugs and the elderly: perspectives in geriatric clinical pharmacology* (ed. J Crooks and IH Stevenson), pp. 239–57. Macmillan, London.

Winawer SJ, Baldwin M, Herbert E, Sherlock P (1983). Screening experience with fecal occult blood testing as a function of age. In *Perspectives on prevention and treatment of cancer in the elderly* (ed. R Yancik, *et al.*), pp. 265–74. Raven Press, New York.

Yancik R (1983). Cancer and the life course. In *Perspectives on prevention and treatment of cancer in the elderly*, (ed. R Yancik, *et al.*), pp. 25–31. Raven Press, New York.

Yellin A, Hill RL, Lieberman Y (1981). Pulmonary resections in patients over 70 years of age. *Israel Journal of Medical Sciences*, **21**:833–40.

Zincke H (1982). Cystectomy and urinary diversion in patients eighty years old and older. *Urology*, **19**:139–45.

Zincke H, *et al.* (1981). Radical retropubic prostatectomy and pelvic lymphadenectomy for high-stage cancer of the prostate. *Cancer*, **47**:1901–10.

Zincke H, Sen SE, Hahn RG, Keating JP (1988). Neoadjuvant chemotherapy for locally advanced transitional cell carcinoma of the bladder: do local findings suggest a potential for salvage of the bladder? *Mayo Clinic Proceedings*, **63**:16–22.

Section 19
Medical and surgical complications of cancer

19.1 Acute emergencies in oncology: general overview

CHRISTOPHER G. A. PRICE AND PAT PRICE

INTRODUCTION

Acute oncological emergencies can be defined as complications of cancer or its treatment which threaten death or irreversible disability if appropriate management is delayed. Their growing importance stems from the increased complexity and potential toxicity of some treatments in common use, but is also a particular consequence of our ability to treat larger numbers of cancer patients effectively, whether with curative or palliative intent. This means that increasingly often reversal of the acute crisis is a goal worth striving for, rather than the denial of an opportunity for 'merciful release' from suffering.

Emergencies may be encountered at any one of three stages during the management of a patient with cancer.

1. *At presentation*, where successful treatment of an acute life-threatening event may permit subsequent delivery of definitive treatment for the underlying tumour. Ideal management of the emergency should compromise the proper investigation, staging, and treatment of the malignancy to a minimal degree. For example, an adequate biopsy of a mediastinal mass causing superior vena caval obstruction should be obtained, if at all possible, before corticosteroids or radiotherapy are commenced, since the subsequent management will differ appreciably depending on whether the diagnosis is, for example Hodgkin's disease, non-Hodgkin's lymphoma, or carcinoma. The opportunity to differentiate between these entities may be lost after treatment has been started and may not present itself again until a later stage in the patient's disease. In some instances reversal of the presenting emergency and stabilization of the patient's condition must precede definitive treatment. For example, relief of urinary obstruction and stabilization of renal function is necessary before administration of nephrotoxic chemotherapeutic agents such as cisplatinum. However, in many cases where the emergency arises as a consequence of the tumour, definitive treatment of the tumour is an essential component of the immediate management. For example, chemotherapy for acute leukaemia should not be delayed while attempts are made to correct septicaemia with antibiotics.

2. *In the course of treatment*, where the emergency may arise wholly or partly as a complication of therapy. Some complications of treatment, such as septicaemia consequent upon myelosuppressive chemotherapy, can be expected to occur in a proportion of treated patients and a management approach should be decided upon in advance. One of the chief aims should be to restart definitive therapy (possibly with modifications designed to obviate recurrence of complications) at the earliest opportunity.

3. *Later in the patient's disease* as a consequence of disease progression. Here, as elsewhere, a careful assessment of the context in which the crisis has occurred and of the patient's overall prognosis is of critical importance. The available options for treatment once the emergency has been controlled need to be reviewed fully at this stage. Clearly, it may be inappropriate to reverse a potentially terminal event where therapeutic measures are no longer available to halt the progress of the underlying tumour. However, full intensive care support will often be appropriate for a young patient with a tumour which is still potentially eradicable even at relapse, such as acute leukaemia, Hodgkin's disease, or teratoma. In some instances successful management of the emergency will significantly enhance the quality of life of the patient even though no definitive treatment exists for the underlying tumour. An example of this might be avoidance of paraplegia in a patient with advanced cancer through prompt treatment of spinal cord compression.

The most frequently encountered acute oncological emergencies are reviewed in this chapter. It is important to remember that unrelated acute medical conditions such as myocardial infarction or pneumonia may occur in patients with malignant disease. There may be a predisposition to these conditions consequent upon the relative debility and immunodeficiency of the cancer sufferer as well as the cumulative toxicity of cancer treatment. In general, the management is the same as that of the general population, allowing for the overall prognosis and condition of the individual patient.

CARDIOVASCULAR EMERGENCIES

Superior vena cava obstruction

The superior vena cava is susceptible to compression, as it is encased within the thorax and surrounded by hilar and peritracheal lymph nodes. It has a thin wall and the venous pressure is low. Obstruction of the superior vena cava is common and dangerous because, if unrelieved, it can result in raised intracranial pressure and eventually neurological damage or coma; venous thrombosis may develop, thus reducing the opportunity for symptoms to resolve even after appropriate therapy.

Malignant disease accounts for approximately 95 per cent of superior vena cava obstruction in adults (Lokich and Goodman 1975). Most cases are due to carcinoma of the bronchus or lymphoma. Less common causes are metastatic carcinoma from distant sites (for example, breast) or primary mediastinal tumours (for example, thymoma and germ cell tumour). Benign causes include thyroid goitre and superior mediastinal fibrosis.

The cardinal symptoms are a sensation of fullness in the neck, facial swelling, and headache; alteration in conciousness may occur. Hoarseness can result from laryngeal oedema. There may be other associated symptoms of mediastinal compression such as dyspnoea, cough, and dysphagia. The diagnosis is made on the clinical features of swelling in the face, neck, and arms and distension of the veins of the neck, arms, and upper trunk. Conjunctival oedema, proptosis, and papilloedema may be present. Urgent treatment should be initiated provided that a histological diagnosis of the underlying tumour has been made. If there is no evidence of disease outside the mediastinum, establishment of a histological diagnosis will require cytological examination of sputum or biopsy via bronchoscopy, mediastinoscopy, or thoracotomy.

Choice of treatment depends upon the diagnosis. Radiotherapy is used unless the tumour is highly chemosensitive (for example, small cell lung cancer or non-Hodgkin's lymphoma) where the appropriate chemotherapeutic regimen for the disease will relieve symptoms of superior vena cava obstruction equally rapidly and will also simultaneously treat distant sites of involvement. Radiotherapy doses in the region of 50–60 Gy are often required when the diagnosis is squamous carcinoma of the bronchus. Occasionally acute worsening of the syndrome may occur with radiotherapy and steroid cover may be required at the beginning of treatment. With either form of treatment, symptoms usually start to improve within 72 h. Davenport et al. (1978) found that 89 per cent of patients had objective evidence of response to radiotherapy within 14 days. Non-response suggests that venous thrombosis has occurred and anticoagulation should be considered.

Cardiac tamponade

Cardiac tamponade is a state of low cardiac output which results from reduced ventricular filling in diastole consequent upon raised intrapericardial pressure. Initially, reduction in stroke volume is compensated by a reflex increase in adrenergic tone with increased heart rate, myocardial contractility, and peripheral resistance. If these compensatory mechanisms are overwhelmed, peripheral hypoperfusion and eventually circulatory collapse will result.

Tamponade is a rare presentation of malignant disease. It is most commonly a complication of breast and lung carcinomas or lymphoma. In the context of malignancy it is usually caused by accumulation of fluid within the pericardial sac as a result of tumour deposits in the pericardium. Occasionally, the pericardium may be thickened and non-compliant ('constrictive') as a result of diffuse infiltration by tumour or radiation fibrosis. Tamponade secondary to radiation pericarditis has been reported to occur up to 20 years after radiotherapy (Applefeld et al. 1981).

There are few specific symptoms of tamponade before the onset of congestive cardiac failure. Precordial chest pain may be present. The physical signs are raised jugular venous pressure, narrow arterial pulse pressure, and pulsus paradoxus (a drop of more than 10 mmHg in arterial pressure during inspiration). Absence of this latter sign does not exclude the diagnosis. The important investigations are chest radiography, which will usually show a large globular heart (except in cases of pericardial infiltration or fibrosis) and echocardiography. The latter investigation will demonstrate the presence of pericardial effusion and help determine its functional significance. Occasionally, right heart catheterization may be required; the increased intrapericardial pressure will be reflected by an increase and equalization of pressures from the right atrium to the pulmonary capillary wedge during diastole.

While asymptomatic malignant pericardial effusions can be treated conservatively, once tamponade has developed decompression of the heart is required. This is usually achieved by pericardiocentesis performed under ECG or preferably ultrasound control. In experienced hands it is a safe procedure, although cardiac arrhythmias or haemorrhage may occur. Intracardiac pressures and cardiac output rapidly return to normal. An intrapericardial catheter can be left in place to prevent reaccumulation of fluid until definitive treatment is instituted.

Surgical approaches to the long-term prevention of tamponade include pericardiectomy, formation of a pleuropericardial window, and subxiphoid pericardiotomy. The first of these requires a thoracotomy and is largely reserved for malignant or radiation-induced constrictive pericarditis. Formation of a pleuropericardial window is safe and effective, although effusions can recur in 5–20 per cent of patients (Gregory et al. 1985). Subxiphoid pericardotomy is highly effective and, since it can be performed under local anaesthetic, can be used for initial decompression of tamponade as well as for longer-term control.

An alternative to these surgical manoeuvres is the instillation of sclerosant into the pericardial sac via the drainage catheter. As well as tetracycline, a variety of chemotherapeutic agents such as thiotepa and mustine have been used. There is no evidence to indicate a differential mode of action. Control of effusions with repeated instillation of tetracycline can be achieved in more than 80 per cent of patients (Shepherd et al. 1987).

External beam radiotherapy is effective in radiosensitive tumours. Doses below 35 Gy in daily fractions of up to 2 Gy have been used without causing radiation pancarditis. Time to response is delayed and so radiotherapy can only be used after initial relief of significant tamponade. Where effective chemotherapy exists for a given tumour, this should be instituted early, possibly obviating the need for other measures. Chemotherapy is usually the treatment of choice for lymphoma.

RESPIRATORY EMERGENCIES

Acute large airway obstruction

Primary carcinoma of the trachea is rare. Although patients with tumours of the oesophagus, lung, or thyroid may develop stenosis of the trachea, the trachea is relatively resistant to external compression and the symptoms of cough, stridor, and dyspnoea tend to develop slowly; the airway is rarely threatened acutely. However, rapid enlargement of the paratracheal lymph nodes can occur in some cases of Hodgkin's disease or non-Hodgkin's lymphoma and may be life-threatening. General anaesthesia, for example to facilitate a diagnostic biopsy procedure, should be used cautiously if there is external tracheal compression, since intubation can be unexpectedly difficult and post-operative removal of the endotracheal tube can be hazardous (Mackie and Watson 1984). Penetrated and lateral chest radiography and CT scan of the neck and upper chest are the best methods of demonstrating the site and extent of the obstructing lesion. Corticosteroids and either radiotherapy (most commonly) or chemotherapy (for non-Hodgkin's lymphoma and for Hodgkin's disease when there is bulky or widespread involvement) should be started without delay.

Obstruction of the right or left main bronchus will lead to emphysema, consolidation, or collapse of the underlying lung. Primary bronchogenic carcinoma is the most common cause, but pulmonary or hilar metastases can result in extrinsic compression. Radiotherapy is the usual treatment; lasers are sometimes used in the temporary relief of obstruction caused by intrabronchial lesions (Dumon et al. 1984) but recurrence is inevitable because this approach does not permit complete excision.

Pulmonary haemorrhage

Major intra-alveolar haemorrhage can occur in malignant disease as a consequence of thrombocytopenia, particularly in association with disseminated intravascular coagulation in which there is consumption of clotting factors. Overall this has been seen most commonly during treatment for acute promyelocytic leukaemia. Fungal pneumonia in pancytopenic patients can also result in diffuse pulmonary haemorrhage (Panos et al. 1988). Management depends upon maintaining adequate gas exchange, if necessary with

Table 1 Causes of respiratory failure in malignant disease

	Associated condition
Pneumonia	
Bacterial	Neutropenia
Pseudomonas	
Klebsiella	
Staphylococcus	
Pneumocystis carinii	Lymphoma/leukaemia
	Prolonged corticosteroids
	Transplantation
Fungi	
Aspergillus	Prolonged neutropenia
Candida	
Cytomegalovirus	Transplantation (allogeneic, particularly with graft versus host disease)
Malignant pulmonary infiltrates	
Lymphangitis carcinomatosis	
Leucostasis: AML, CML (blast crisis), ALL	
Other conditions	
Lymphoma	
Hodgkin's disease (late)	
Large airway obstruction	
Bronchial carcinoma	
Tracheal carcinoma	
Extrinsic compression	
Mediastinal tumour	
Pulmonary metastases	
Pulmonary fibrosis	
Drugs	
Busulphan	
Bleomycin	
Mitomycin C	
Nitrosoureas	
Interleukin-2	
Radiation	

AML, acute myeloid leukaemia.
CML, chronic lymphoblastic leukaemia.
ALL, acute lymphoblastic leukaemia.

Table 2 Factors influencing outcome for patients with haematological malignancies requiring intensive care for respiratory failure

Good prognostic features	Poor prognostic features
Stage of treatment: first remission induction	Stage of treatment: second or subsequent remission induction
APACHE II* score ≤ 25	APACHE II* score ≥ 30
Failure of ≤ 3 organ systems	Failure of ≥ 4 organ systems
Recovery of granulocyte count	Persistent leucopenia
Pneumonia not associated with septicaemic shock	Pneumonia associated with septicaemic shock
	Failure to respond to chemotherapy

*Acute Physiology and Chronic Health Evaluation II (Knaus et al. 1985).
Adapted from Lloyd-Thomas et al. (1988).

Respiratory failure may also be caused by infection, often with an opportunistic organism, as an indirect consequence of cancer or its treatment. Here full supportive measures up to and including mechanical ventilation should be considered, although requirement for ventilation during cancer management carries a poor prognosis (Lloyd-Thomas et al. 1988). Careful selection of circumstances when such an approach justifies the necessary allocation of resources and the potential distress to the patient and family is essential. Optimum management demands early recognition of clinical situations in which ventilation may be required and close cooperation between the oncologist and the intensive care team in the optimum management of the emergency. Causes of respiratory failure in the cancer patient are summarized in Table 1. Factors influencing the outcome for patients with haematological malignancies requiring mechanical ventilation for respiratory failure are listed in Table 2 (Lloyd-Thomas et al. 1988). Importantly, in paracytopenic patients in remission from curative malignancies such as lymphoma or teratoma, can develop respiratory failure from lung infiltration as their granulocyte count recovers. This is an important indication for full supportive care.

RENAL AND METABOLIC EMERGENCIES

Obstructive uropathy

Obstructive uropathy in malignant disease is most commonly the result of compression by tumour mass either at the level of the ureters or at the bladder outflow tract. The ureters are in close relation to the retroperitoneal lymphatics throughout their course and may be obstructed by secondary spread to this site from a variety of primary tumours, particularly carcinomas arising within the pelvis; that is, those of the cervix, prostate, bladder, corpus uteri, and colon. Unless there is pre-existing renal impairment, unilateral ureteric obstruction is frequently asymptomatic and does not lead to significant clinical or biochemical disturbance. Urgent correction is only required if both upper tracts are affected; decompression of the unilateral obstructed kidney will follow from successful treatment of the tumour and unless the obstruction is of long standing it is likely that function will recover. In contrast, significant bladder outflow obstruction will inevitably lead to bilateral hydronephrosis; this is a common complication of prostatic carcinoma but is also seen in carcinoma of the cervix. Occasionally, bilateral ureteric obstruction can develop as a result of post-radiation fibrosis.

mechanical ventilation, treatment of infection, and vigorous replacement of clotting factors and platelets.

Massive haemoptysis can also occur as a consequence of pulmonary vascular erosion or necrosis of a bronchogenic carcinoma. This distressing complication is seen most frequently with squamous tumours (Miller and McGregor 1980). Intubation may be necessary to prevent fatal aspiration. Chest radiography and bronchoscopy will help to define the site of the lesion. Iced saline bronchial lavage, arterial embolization, or coagulation of the bleeding site with a neodymium YAG laser are possible methods of achieving haemostasis without surgical intervention. Surgical resection is the treatment of choice for potentially operable tumours in patients with good performance status.

Respiratory failure

Respiratory failure may be the direct result of tumour progression, for example where there is extensive lung infiltration or lymphangitis carcinomatosa. Usually this occurs at a late stage in the disease when the clinical circumstances and overall prognosis dictate that emergency treatment is not appropriate.

The diagnosis should be considered in all cases of unexplained impairment of renal function in cancer patients. Most frequently this will be detected on biochemical monitoring. Unless there is bladder outflow obstruction, symptoms and signs may often be delayed until the onset of uraemia. At that stage there may be drowsiness, confusion, and nausea associated with signs of fluid imbalance, asterixis, and, in some cases, pericarditis. Hydronephrosis is best confirmed by ultrasonography; renal failure is a relative contraindication to intravenous pyelography. If necessary, the level of obstruction can be determined either by antegrade pyelography via a percutaneous nephrostomy or by CT scanning. The former approach is most commonly used since nephrostomy tubes can be left *in situ* to decompress the upper tracts percutaneously; renal function may then improve sufficiently to enable definitive management of the obstructing lesion to be undertaken. Longer-term drainage can be effected either by retrograde insertion of ureteric stents or by permanent urinary diversion, for example via an ileal conduit.

Bladder outflow obstruction can be relieved acutely by insertion of a urethral or suprapubic catheter. If the cause is carcinoma of the prostate, transurethral resection or endocrine manipulation with the anti-androgen cyproterone acetate, for example can provide effective control in the longer term.

Urate nephropathy and tumour lysis syndrome

Treatment of highly chemosensitive tumours such as testicular teratoma, acute leukaemia, and high grade non-Hodgkin's lymphoma (particularly Burkitt's lymphoma) can provoke an acute metabolic derangement through the rapid lysis of tumour cells; the 'tumour lysis syndrome'. The efflux of metabolites and electrolytes into the extracellular compartment can exceed the homeostatic capability of the kidneys, leading to hyperkalaemia, hyperphosphataemia, hypocalcaemia, and hyperuricaemia with the resultant risk of cardiac arrhythmias and renal failure. The type of tumour and volume of disease appear to be more important than the specific chemotherapy utilized (Slevin *et al.* 1981). Pre-existing renal impairment increases the risk. Optimal management, summarized in Table 3, depends upon prevention of the complication in patients at risk rather than treatment of the syndrome, once established. Adequate hydration should be ensured, usually via intravenous infusion. The xanthine inhibitor allopurinol should be started at least 12 h before chemotherapy, longer if there is pre-existing elevation of the serum urate (DeConti and Calabresi 1966). Allopurinol dosage should be reduced in renal failure and monitoring of plasma oxipurinol levels may be helpful (Simmonds *et al.* 1986). The urine should be alkalinized either with oral or intravenous sodium bicarbonate; this increases the solubility of uric acid crystals and so guards against their deposition in the renal collecting ducts.

Careful biochemical monitoring of the patient during the first 24–48 h after initiation of therapy is essential. More vigorous efforts may be necessary to prevent hyperkalaemia and uric acid deposition if serum creatinine and potassium continue to rise despite the above measures. Deteriorating renal function will result in acceleration of the general metabolic derangement which in turn leads to further renal damage. This cycle is difficult to disrupt without recourse to renal dialysis, which is necessary in a small proportion of cases.

Hypercalcaemia

Hypercalcaemia is a common metabolic complication of malignancy and may require urgent correction to prevent renal failure and the

Table 3 Management of tumour lysis syndrome

Initial prophylaxis in patients at risk
(1) Before starting chemotherapy measure
    Urea, creatinine
    Electrolytes
    Urate
(2) Start allopurinol (300 mg once daily) 12–24 h prior to chemotherapy
(3) Establish hydration
    Minimum 3 l/day
    Urine output $\geqslant 100$ ml/h
(4) Start chemotherapy if serum urate normal
(5) Monitor daily
    Electrolytes
    Urea, creatinine
    Calcium, phosphate
    Urate
Correction of metabolic derangement
(1) Alkalinize urine to pH $\geqslant 7$ (for example, substitute 1.4% bicarbonate solution for normal saline in fluid regimen)
(2) Correct hyperkalaemia with standard measures (for example, calcium resonium by mouth or by enema; dextrose and insulin infusion)
(3) Reduce allopurinol dosage if renal function impaired
(4) Discontinue urine alkalinization when uric acid falls within normal range
Consider dialysis if
(1) Renal function deteriorates
(2) Potassium > 6.5 mmol/l
    despite above measures

onset of coma. Lung cancer (particularly squamous tumours), breast cancer, and myeloma are the most common underlying primary tumours. There is an incomplete association with the presence of bony metastases. Mechanisms of hypercalcaemia in malignancy include elaboration of parathyroid hormone-like protein, osteoclast-activating cytokines, and prostaglandins by tumour cells. The symptoms include nausea, anorexia, lethargy, weakness, thirst, polyuria, and constipation. The most striking clinical feature is dehydration, which may be severe. The diagnosis is made by measuring the serum calcium level (corrected for serum albumin) but is occasionally overlooked in patients incorrectly assumed to be terminally ill. Hypercalcaemia leads to dehydration through a direct effect on the renal tubule, resulting in a reversible loss of concentrating ability analogous to that seen in nephrogenic diabetes insipidus. The primary component of therapy, vigorous rehydration with normal saline, restores intravascular volume and also inhibits the reabsorption of calcium in the proximal tubule. Frusemide is a useful adjunct to saline administration once rehydration has been achieved since it has an additional calciuric effect. Prednisolone is commonly used (1–2 mg/kg daily) although it is of limited efficacy in tumours which are not otherwise steroid responsive. It is most effective in the treatment of hypercalcaemia associated with multiple myeloma. Intravenous biphosphonates, which block bone resorption by osteoclasts, have rapidly become established as the treatment of choice in moderate to severe hypercalcaemia (Ralston *et al.* 1985). Etidronate (7.5 mg/kg daily for 3 days) or pamidronate (30–90 mg as a single infusion) will begin to lower the serum calcium within 24–48 h, reaching a nadir level after approximately 5 days. The effect may be sustained for up to 21 days and the response rate is approximately 80 per cent. A dose–response relationship has been demonstrated for pamidronate so that the initial dose should be tailored to the degree of hypercalcaemia (Thiebaud *et al.* 1988). There is preliminary evidence that, once serum calcium is normalized, regular use of oral biphosphonate may result in sustained normocalcaemia. Salmon calcitonin acts rapidly, but in comparison with the diphosphonates has the disadvantage that patients rapidly become refractory to its effects. Mithramycin, the cytotoxic antibiotic, is effective but is now rarely indicated since the development of less toxic alternatives.

GASTROINTESTINAL EMERGENCIES

Obstruction

Bowel obstruction as a result of malignant disease can occur at any level from the oesophagus to the rectum. The primary tumour may be the obstructing lesion; gastric or colonic obstruction for example, is usually caused by a carcinoma intrinsic to one of those sites. Small bowel obstruction, however, is usually the result of extrinsic compression from other primary tumours within the abdominal cavity or involvement in diffuse peritoneal carcinomatosis.

The patient may be acutely unwell as a consequence of intravascular volume depletion or, in the case of oesophageal or gastric obstruction, aspiration pneumonia. Immediate resuscitation depends upon replacement of fluids and bowel decompression by nasogastric drainage.

The site of obstruction is often apparent from the clinical features and appearances on a plain abdominal radiograph. In cases of oesophageal or gastric obstruction, barium swallow or gastroscopy will be required. Definitive management of obstruction depends upon the site and clinical circumstances. Surgery is usually required to resect or bypass the obstruction unless the overall prognosis, even in the short term, is very poor. Oesophageal tumours may be treated with radiotherapy and diffuse intra-abdominal spread of ovarian carcinoma may respond to chemotherapy. In the chronic partial obstruction frequently seen in advanced abdominal and pelvic malignancy, where the extent of the tumour often renders surgery inappropriate or non-feasible, supportive measures such as fluid replacement, anti-emetics, and stool-softening agents may be effective in limiting acute exacerbations and minimizing distress.

Perforation

Gastrointestinal cancers may perforate and so present as an emergency with an acute abdomen. Distinction from a benign cause will usually only be made at laparotomy.

Gastrointestinal non-Hodgkin's lymphoma is the tumour most often associated with bowel perforation (Lundy et al. 1975). In this condition spontaneous perforation at presentation is less common than that occurring after initiation of therapy (Weingrad et al. 1982). Response to lymphoma infiltrating the full thickness of the bowel wall can result in perforation at several sites simultaneously. The characteristic clinical features of intestinal perforation, that is, acute onset of abdominal pain and 'board-like' rigidity of the abdomen musculature, may be masked by the corticosteroids which will commonly have been given as part of the combination chemotherapy regimen. The diagnosis can be confirmed from the appearance of free gas under the diaphragm on plain abdominal radiographs. Management depends upon prompt surgical intervention. Since in this instance perforation indicates tumour response, the prognosis is often good provided that the acute emergency is dealt with effectively.

Haemorrhage

Gastrointestinal haemorrhage is common in patients with gastro-intestinal malignancy, but bleeding from the tumour itself is the cause in a minority of cases. Other causes include peptic ulceration, gastritis, and Mallory–Weiss tear. Mucositis consequent upon chemotherapy, radiotherapy, or fungal and viral infections may be contributory. Since bleeding from the tumour cannot be assumed, it is mandatory to establish the source of all significant haemorrhage in patients who are being managed actively for their disease.

Bleeding is the presenting symptom in up to 25 per cent of gastrointestinal lymphomas, possibly higher in cases involving the stomach (Fleming et al. 1982). Again, treatment can be hazardous. The initial period of 7–10 days after chemotherapy as the lymphoma starts to regress requires careful monitoring as severe haemorrhage can occur at this stage. Surgery is necessary in a proportion of cases, but transfusion and supportive management are preferable in the first instance, particularly in those patients with widespread infiltration for whom an operation, if required, may be technically difficult and involve extensive resection.

ACUTE NEUROLOGICAL EMERGENCIES

Spinal cord compression

Spinal cord compression occurs most frequently with tumours that characteristically metastasize to bone, where the mechanism of compression is extension of tumour from within the vertebral body into the epidural space, often in association with vertebral collapse. The most common primary sites are breast, lung, prostate, kidney, and myeloma. Lymphoma is also a frequent cause of cord compression, but here the mechanism is usually extension of paraspinal lymph nodes in the mediastinum or retroperitoneum through the intervertebral foramina.

Compression of the thoracic cord accounts for over two-thirds of all cases. Early diagnosis, when the symptoms may be mild and the clinical picture incomplete, is of primary importance since functional recovery is largely dependent on pre-treatment status. Fewer than 10 per cent of patients with established paraplegia from metastatic disease regain the ability to walk (Gilbert et al. 1978). Symptoms of compression include local or radicular pain, limb weakness, autonomic dysfunction (hesitancy or incontinence of urine and sluggish bowels), and sensory loss including ataxia. If the compression is below the base of the cord at the level of L1–L2, a cauda equina syndrome is seen with sciatic pain, sacral sensory impairment, urinary retention with overflow, and loss of anal sphincter tone. Back pain is often the crucial early symptom which should not be overlooked.

Careful neurological assessment is mandatory. Investigation should include plain radiography of the spine to demonstrate bony metastases, fracture, erosion of pedicles, or paraspinal mass, but may be normal in 15–20 per cent of cases. Myelography will define the site, limits, and extent of the compression and may indicate more than one lesion. Cisternal puncture should be performed when a complete block precludes visualization of the upper cord to exclude this latter possibility. Magnetic resonance imaging (**MRI**) is a useful and less invasive alternative if the facilities and expertise are available locally. MRI will also provide optimal imaging of an intramedullary spinal cord lesion (Modic et al. 1983). CT scanning will demonstrate an abnormality within a defined region of the cord but is unsuitable as a primary investigation in cases where the site of compression cannot be predicted accurately from the clinical and plain radiography findings.

Patients with suspected cord compression should be given corticosteroids to reduce oedema around the cord and preserve function until definitive treatment is started. Dexamethasone (4 mg six hourly) is usually given. Treatment of cord compression is either surgical decompression (usually via posterior laminectomy) or radiotherapy. Surgery is indicated if there is vertebral collapse causing mechanical compression, if the histology of the primary tumour is unknown, if the tumour has relapsed after radiotherapy, or if it is known to be radioresistant. Since surgical excision of the lesion is virtually always incomplete, post-operative radiotherapy should be given routinely. Chemotherapy is reserved for responsive tumours such as small cell lung cancer, non-Hodgkin's lymphoma, neuroblastoma, or myeloma where recently it has been used as the sole treatment modality in some centres (Sanderson *et al.* 1989; Sinoff and Blumsohn 1989).

Raised intracranial pressure

Primary or metastatic brain tumours may produce raised intracranial pressure through mass effect. There may be focal signs and symptoms determined by the site of the lesion as well as headache, vomiting, altered mental state, and papilloedema. Usually progression is sufficiently slow after the onset of symptoms to allow investigation with urgent CT scan before initiation of therapy, which depends upon corticosteroids (dexamethasone) and either surgery (for solitary lesions in sites amenable to operation) or radiotherapy. Sometimes, however, rapid enlargement of a tumour or intracranial haemorrhage can result in a rise in intracranial pressure sufficient to provoke a shift in brain substance with herniation through the foramen magnum (with posterior fossa lesions) or tentorial opening (with cerebral hemisphere lesions). Inappropriate lumbar puncture in a patient with raised intracranial pressure can produce the same effect. The clinical picture is of rapid neurological deterioration with loss of consciousness. Although the prognosis is poor, resuscitative measures, which should usually be started before imaging investigations can be performed, sometimes result in sufficient improvement to permit subsequent surgical procedures such as the insertion of a cerebrospinal fluid shunt or drainage of a subdural haematoma. Mannitol 20 per cent should be given intravenously in doses of up to $1-2$ g/kg together with intravenous dexamethasone. The former will create an osmotic gradient, temporarily reducing the volume of cerebrospinal fluid; it may need to be repeated, since the effect wears off after $4-6$ h. Intubation and mechanical hyperventilation to maintain a low arterial $p\mathrm{CO}_2$ ($3-4$ kPa) produces cerebral vasoconstriction and may also be helpful in reducing intracranial pressure.

Fits

Approximately $15-30$ per cent of patients with intracranial metastases will present with fits. Fits may be caused by intracranial haemorrhage, infection, or metabolic abnormalities such as hyponatraemia, for example as a result of inappropriate ADH secretion in small cell lung cancer. Management depends upon control of the acute episode if fits are repeated or continuous (status epilepticus), typically with a short-acting intravenous anticonvulsant such as diazepam. The diagnosis should then be established and any underlying metabolic abnormality corrected. Oral anticonvulsants should be commenced in patients with a structural lesion. Patients with intracranial tumours should be treated with dexamethasone and radiotherapy or surgery as appropriate. Long-term prophylaxis with regular oral anticonvulsant therapy will be required in most instances.

HAEMATOLOGICAL EMERGENCIES AND CONSEQUENCES OF MYELOSUPPRESSION

Haematological emergencies are most commonly associated with myeloproliferative and lymphoproliferative disorders, but haemorrhagic or cytopenic states can also complicate non-haematological malignancies. Myelotoxic chemotherapy and radiotherapy regimens are in common usage and iatrogenic neutropenic sepsis is by far the most frequently encountered emergency in current oncological practice.

Leucostasis

High numbers of circulating blasts in acute leukaemia or in blast crisis of chronic myeloid leukaemia may result in increased blood viscosity and leucostasis. The resultant capillary plugging may have severe clinical consequences (Lichtman and Rowe 1982). In the central nervous system there may be visual disturbance, drowsiness, and coma and irreversible damage may result from intracranial haemorrhage. Plugging of the pulmonary microvasculature leads to hypoxia due to interference with oxygen transport and eventually respiratory failure. The appearance of the chest radiographs may be unremarkable, but more commonly there will be diffuse interstitial shadowing due to capillary leak syndrome. There is no clear threshold level of circulating leukaemic blasts above which these features start to occur. The nature of the leukaemic cell is important, in that different cells affect the rheology of the blood differently. In general, higher levels of lymphoid blasts in lymphoblastic leukaemia can be tolerated than of myeloblasts in acute myeloid leukaemia, where counts in excess of 100×10^9/l will often be associated with symptoms. Leucostasis may be seen, albeit in the presence of high counts, in chronic myeloid leukaemia in the chronic phase, but is rarely a feature of chronic lymphocytic leukaemia. In this latter condition the lymphocytes are small and deformable and do not lead to capillary plugging even with counts in excess of 500×10^9/l (Gray *et al.* 1974). Treatment of leucostasis depends upon the rapid reduction of the leucocyte count and prompt initiation of specific therapy for the underlying leukaemia. Leucapheresis will bring about a transient reduction in the circulating leukaemic blast count of up to 50 per cent and if necessary this can be repeated daily until the count falls as a consequence of cytotoxic therapy. It should be appreciated that acute leukaemia presenting with a high circulating blast count has a poor prognosis and the clinical picture is often one of multiple organ failure. There is a high early mortality despite prompt initiation of treatment to reduce the leucocyte count (Lester *et al.* 1985).

Hyperviscosity

Symptomatic hyperviscosity syndrome complicates up to 50 per cent of IgM paraproteinaemias and occasional cases of IgG and IgA paraproteinaemia (less than 5 per cent). Headache, drowsiness, and visual disturbances are common central nervous system symptoms. Clinical signs may include dilation and tortuosity of retinal vessels, retinal haemorrhage, and papilloedema. There may be bruising, epistaxis, and bleeding from mucous membranes as a result of impairment of platelet function. Cardiac failure can result from expansion of plasma volume and increased vascular resistance. Diagnosis depends upon recognition of the clinical features in association with the diagnosis of paraproteinaemia and demonstration of raised plasma viscosity. Plasmapheresis will produce a rapid but temporary improvement in symptoms; several daily or alternate day treatments may be necessary to obtain a maximum reduction in plasma paraprotein. In most cases definitive cytotoxic therapy should be started concurrently. In some cases of Waldenström's macroglobulinaemia, particularly where hyperviscosity is associated with a low tumour burden and adequate bone-marrow reserve, plasmapheresis at regular intervals can be used as sole therapy.

Disseminated intravascular coagulation

Disseminated intravascular coagulation frequently complicates the presentation and initial treatment of acute promyelocytic leukaemia. Lysis of neoplastic promyelocytes results in the release of a procoagulant into the circulation (Gralnick and Abrell 1973). In this case active prophylactic and therapeutic measures are usually necessary if fatal haemorrhage is to be avoided. Mild disseminated intravascular coagulation is often present in association with a variety of other malignancies, but rarely requires active management beyond appropriate treatment for the underlying tumour. Occasionally acute disseminated intravascular coagulation requiring urgent correction is present with adenocarcinoma, particularly of the prostate, stomach, or pancreas. Disseminated intravascular coagulation presents as abnormal bleeding (demonstrable by prolonged partial thromboplastin and thrombin times), thrombocytopenia, reduction in fibrinogen level, and elevation of fibrin degradation products. Correction depends upon replacement of clotting factors by administration of fresh frozen plasma and platelet transfusion. Heparin infusions to prevent coagulation and the resultant clotting factor consumption are used widely, though their role remains controversial.

Thrombocytopenia

Thrombocytopenia may occur in association with disseminated intravascular coagulation (described above) in cases where the bone-marrow is suppressed or replaced by tumour or as a consequence of hypersplenism in haematological malignancy. Most commonly, however, it is a complication of myelosuppressive chemotherapy. Most regimens of moderate intensity for solid tumours, Hodgkin's disease, or non-Hodgkin's lymphoma do not result in symptomatic thrombocytopenia unless there is bone-marrow involvement (particularly in lymphoma) or other cause of reduced bone-marrow reserve. A period of severe thrombocytopenia is the expected consequence of induction therapy for acute leukaemia. Central nervous system or gastrointestinal haemorrhage are the potentially life-threatening complications of severe thrombocytopenia; bleeding from these sites is usually unheralded and optimum management depends upon prevention. Prophylactic support for therapy-related thrombocytopenia is usually given in the form of platelet transfusions to maintain a level above $15-20 \times 10^9/l$. Platelets should also be given if any bleeding, bruising, or purpura occur in the presence of higher counts and frequent careful clinical examination is mandatory in all patients with thrombocytopenia. Particular significance should be attached to retinal haemorrhages. Frequent transfusions may result in sensitization to a wide range of foreign antigens so that when transfusions are subsequently required, they are ineffective. This can be a significant problem in patients undergoing repeated courses of myelosuppressive therapy. The use of single-donor transfusions has been shown to delay the development of antibody (Sintnicholaas et al. 1981) and HLA-matched donor platelets may produce more favourable results than unmatched transfusions. Intravenous gammaglobulin may help in refractory cases (Schiffer et al. 1984).

Neutropenia

Neutropenia most commonly occurs as a consequence of chemotherapy, although occasional patients receiving radiotherapy become neutropenic, for example when a significant amount of bone-marrow is included in the radiation field. Some haematological malignancies, such as acute leukaemia and hairy cell leukaemia, are commonly associated with neutropenia at presentation. Neutropenia is best considered as a state of extreme vulnerability rather than an emergency in itself. The risk of infection relates to the degree of neutropenia, becoming significant at neutrophil counts of less than $1 \times 10^9/l$ and also to its duration. Host and environmental factors also contribute to the risk of development of certain categories of infection (Table 4). Many myelosuppressive chemotherapy regimens used in the treatment of chemosensitive tumours, such as lymphoma, small cell lung cancer or germ cell tumours, are associated with a brief period of mild to moderate neutropenia such that only a proportion of patients are predicted to develop infections during a course of treatment. Neutropenia under these circumstances is best managed at home, away from the risk of hospital-acquired infection. Patients must be instructed to attend hospital for immediate review if they become pyrexial or develop other symptoms suggestive of infection. In contrast, a severe prolonged neutrophil nadir usually accompanies intensive treatment regimens, such as those used for remission induction and consolidation in acute leukaemia. Here, development of infection can be predicted for most patients and monitoring of the period of neutropenia in hospital is preferable. A variety of prophylactic measures may be used to reduce the incidence and severity of infections in this group (Table 5). Autologous bone-marrow or peripheral blood stem-cell transplantation and haematopoietic growth factors are increasingly being used to reduce the period of neutropenia in treatment regimens of high intensity.

Table 4 Risk factors for treatment-related infections

Treatment-related factors
  Degree of myelosuppression
  Duration of myelosuppression
  High-dose corticosteroids
  Use of indwelling central venous catheters
  Invasive procedures, for example urinary catheterization, sigmoidoscopy
Host factors
  Disease-related immunodeficiency, for example hypogammaglobulinaemia in myeloma, CLL
  Chronic infections, for example diverticular disease, old tuberculosis
  Chronic immunodeficiency states, for example HIV infection
  Asymptomatic carriage of organisms, for example *Staphylococcus aureus*
  Seropositivity to latent viruses, for example *Herpes simplex*
  Seronegativity to common viruses, for example cytomegalovirus
Environmental factors
  Local pathogens, for example antibiotic-resistant bacteria, *Aspergillus*

CLL, chronic lymphoblastic leukaemia

Table 5 Prophylaxis against treatment-related infections

Host
General measures
Rigorous oral hygiene
Prophylaxis against specific organisms

Pneumocystis carinii	Co-trimoxazole, one tablet twice daily
Gram-negative organisms	Co-trimoxazole[a]
	Norfloxacin[b]
CMV	Use of CMV negative blood products

Environment
Cleanliness and personal hygiene (including staff and visitors)
Protected environment, for example side rooms, laminar flow cubicles

CMV, cytomegalovirus.
[a]Gurwith *et al.* (1979).
[b]Karp *et al.* (1987).

Fever in the neutropenic patient

The majority of patients who are severely neutropenic for more than a week will develop fever due to presumed or microbiologically confirmed infection. Infections in the presence of neutropenia frequently present without focal signs. Therefore fever should be assumed to indicate infection even if alternative explanations, such as transfusion or drug reaction (for example, bleomycin) are considered. Careful clinical examination and chest radiography should be performed and cultures taken from blood and any other potential site of infection such as throat, skin, or intravenous cannula insertion site. Untreated infective episodes in neutropenic patients can progress very rapidly to collapse and death, particularly if the causative organism is a Gram-negative bacterium such as *Escherichia coli*, *Pseudomonas*, or *Klebsiella*. Therefore, it is essential that such episodes are treated promptly with broad-spectrum antibiotics which give Gram-negative cover before culture results are available. Combinations of aminoglycoside and either a third- or fourth-generation cephalosporin (for example, cefotaxime or ceftazidime) or a broad-spectrum semi-synthetic penicillin (for example, piperacillin or azlocillin) are frequently used. If potential sources of infection include the skin or an indwelling central venous catheter, superior antistaphylococcal cover will be provided by the addition of, for example flucloxacillin or vancomycin. Sinus, dental, and perineal infections are frequently caused by anaerobic organisms and the use of metronidazole should be considered in those circumstances. Modification to the antibiotic regimen should be considered if the fever fails to lyse within 48 h of starting antibiotics. Fungal infections are frequently seen in association with prolonged periods of neutropenia and should be suspected in fevers refractory to broad-spectrum antibiotics. The empirical use of intravenous amphotericin should be considered early (Pizzo *et al.* 1982), as the response of fungal infections to treatment may be slow. No causative organism is identified in a significant proportion of cases.

MISCELLANEOUS EMERGENCIES AT CRITICAL SITES

Orbital and intraocular metastases

Ocular and orbital metastases may be unilateral or bilateral and jeopardize vision through their position. They most commonly arise from carcinoma of the breast. Choroidal deposits may damage the retina or may cause intraocular bleeding. Extraocular orbital deposits

can cause proptosis and ocular motor palsy and may threaten the optic nerve. Full external eye and retinal examination should be carried out and radiotherapy initiated urgently if permanent visual loss or nerve palsy is to be avoided. A dose of 30 Gy in 10 fractions can be given and response is generally satisfactory unless permanent damage has been done to the macula.

Bone pain and pathological fracture

Pain from bony metastases can be severe and immobilizing. Radiotherapy to relieve pain is often given as a matter of urgency. A prospective randomized trial (Price *et al.* 1986) showed no difference in analgesic effect or time of onset of pain relief between a single 8 Gy fraction and 30 Gy in 10 daily fractions. In many patients there is an analgesic effect within 24–48 h. The mechanism of the analgesic action of ionizing radiation is unknown, but does not appear to be wholly dependent on tumour shrinkage. Pathological fracture is a frequent complication of bony metastases, particularly when they are lytic or extensive. If long bones are involved, orthopaedic stabilization and fixation may be required. Radiotherapy is often given post-operatively.

Gynaecological haemorrhage

Vaginal bleeding is a complication of either cervical or endometrial carcinoma and can occasionally be massive and life-threatening. Vaginal packing can temporarily arrest the bleeding and external-beam radiotherapy can halt bleeding in 2–4 days. Occasionally, arterial ligation is required.

REFERENCES

Applefeld MM, *et al.* (1981). Delayed pericardial disease after radiotherapy. *American Journal of Cardiology*, **47**:210–13.

Davenport D, *et al.* (1978). Radiation therapy in the treatment of superior vena caval obstruction. *Cancer*, **42**:2600–3.

DeConti RC, Calebresi P (1966). Use of allopurinal for prevention and control of hyperuricaemia in patients with neoplastic disease. *New England Journal of Medicine*, **274**:481–86.

Dumon JF, *et al.* (1984). Treatment of tracheobronchial lesions by laser photoresection. *Chest*, **81**:278–84.

Fleming ID, Mitchell S, Dilawar RA (1982). The role of surgery in the management of gastric lymphoma. *Cancer*, **49**:1135–41.

Gilbert RW, Kim JH, Posner JB (1978). Epidural spinal cord compression from metastatic tumour: diagnosis and treatment. *Annals of Neurology*, **3**:40–51.

Gralnick H, Abrell E (1973). Studies of the procoagulant and fibrinolytic activity of promyelocytes in acute promyelocytic leukaemia. *British Journal of Haematology*, **24**:89–99.

Gray JL, Jacobs A, Block M (1974). Bone marrow and peripheral blood lymphocytosis in the prognosis of chronic lymphocytic leukemia. *Cancer*, **33**:1169–78.

Gregory JR, McMurtrey MJ, Mountain CF (1985). A surgical approach to the treatment of pericardial effusion in cancer patients. *American Journal of Clinical Oncology*, **8**:319–23.

Gurwith MJ, Brunton JL, Lank BA (1979). A prospective controlled investigation of prophylactic trimethoprim/sulfamethoxazole in hospitalized granulocytic patients. *American Journal of Medicine*, **66**:248–97.

Karp JE, *et al.* (1987). Oral norfloxacin for prevention of Gram-negative bacterial infections in patients with acute leukaemia and granulocytopenia. *Annals of Internal Medicine*, **106**:1–6.

Knaus WA, Draper EA, Wagner DP, Zimmerman JE (1985). APACHE II: a severity of disease classification system. *Critical Care Medicine*, **13**:818–29.

Lester TJ, Johnstone JW, Cuttner J (1985). Pulmonary leukostasis as the single worst prognostic factor in patients with acute myelocytic leukemia and hyperleukocytosis. *American Journal of Medicine*, **79**:43–8.

Lichtman MA, Rowe JM (1982). Hyperleukocytic leukemia: rheologic, clinical and therapeutic considerations. *Blood*, 60:279–83.

Lloyd-Thomas AR, Wright I, Lister A, Hinds CJ (1988). Prognosis of patients receiving intensive care for lifethreatening medical complications of haematological malignancy. *British Medical Journal*, 296:1025–9.

Lokich JJ, Goodman R (1975). Superior vena caval syndrome clinical management. *Journal of the American Medical Association*, 231:58–61.

Lundy J, et al. (1975). Spontaneous perforation of the gastrointestinal tract in patients with cancer. *American Journal of Gastroenterology*, 63:447–50.

Mackie AM, Watson CB (1984). Anaesthesia and mediastinal masses. A case report and review of the literature. *Anaesthesia*, 39(9):899–903.

Miller RR, McGregor DH (1980). Haemorrhage from carcinoma of the lung. *Cancer*, 46:200–5.

Modic MT, et al. (1983). Nuclear magnetic resonance imaging of the spine. *Radiology*, 148:757–62.

Panos RJ, et al. (1988). Factors associated with fatal haemoptysis in cancer patients. *Chest*, 94:1008–13.

Pizzo PA, Robichaud KT, Gill TA, Witebsky FB (1982). Empiric antibiotic and antifungal therapy for cancer patients with prolonged fever and granulocytopenia. *American Journal of Medicine*, 72:108–11.

Price P, et al. (1986). Prospective randomised trial of single and multifraction radiotherapy schedules in the treatment of painful bony metastases. *Radiotherapy and Oncology*, 6:247–55.

Ralston SH, et al. (1985). Comparison of aminohydroxypropylidene diphosphonate, mithramycin and corticosteroids/calcitonin in treatment of cancer associated hypercalcaemia. *Lancet*, ii:907–10.

Sanderson IR, Pritchard J, Marsh HT (1989). Chemotherapy as the initial treatment of spinal cord compression due to disseminated neuroblastoma. *Journal of Neurosurgery*, 70(5):688–90.

Schiffer CA, et al. (1984). High dose intravenous gammaglobulin in alloimmunized platelet transfusion recipients. *Blood*, 64:937–40.

Shepherd FA, et al. (1987). Medical management of malignant pericardial effusion by tetracycline sclerosis. *American Journal of Cardiology*, 60:1161–6.

Simmonds HA, Cameron JS, Morris GS, Davies PM (1986). Allopurinol in renal failure and the tumour lysis syndrome. *Clinica Chimica Acta*, 160:189–95.

Sinoff CL, Blumsohn A (1989). Spinal cord compression in myelomatosis: response to chemotherapy alone. *European Journal of Cancer and Clinical Oncology*, 25(2):197–200.

Sintnicholaas K, et al. (1981). Delayed alloimmunisation by random single donor platelet transfusions. *Lancet*, i:750–4.

Slevin ML, Bell R, Cotterill AM, Lister TA (1981). 'The tumour overkill syndrome': a potentially lethal complication of cancer chemotherapy. *Postgraduate Medical Journal*, 57:727–9.

Thiebaud D, Jaeger P, Jacquet AF, Burkhardt P (1988). Dose–response in the treatment of hypercalcaemia of malignancy by a single infusion of bisphosphonate AHPrBP. *Journal of Clinical Oncology*, 6:762–8.

Weingrad DN, et al. (1982). Primary gastrointestinal lymphoma. *Cancer*, 49:1258–65.

19.2 Metabolic disturbances

A. T. VAN OOSTEROM, LUC Y. DIRIX, AND RUUD VAN RIJSWIJK

Tumour- or treatment-related metabolic disturbances frequently occur in cancer patients. Examples are the occurrence of hypercalcaemia in patients with breast, non-small-cell lung, and head and neck cancer, electrolyte disorders associated with cisplatin and ifosfamide, and hyperglycaemia induced by corticosteroid-containing anti-emetic regimens. Awareness of the specific dysregulations common to certain malignancies or associated with cytotoxic or hormonal agents will allow early diagnosis and intervention in order to reduce the accompanying morbidity. In this chapter, the emphasis will be laid upon the clinical presentation, differential diagnosis, and practical guidelines for the management of these problems.

HYPERCALCAEMIA AND HYPOCALCAEMIA
Calcium homeostasis

Calcium is essential to man for both his biochemical and structural composition. Most of the calcium in the adult human is contained in the skeleton, and only 1 per cent is present in the extracellular fluid and soft tissues. Major gradients in calcium exist over cellular membranes and between intracellular compartments, and rapid transmembrane fluxes accompany biological processes such as neurotransmission and contractile phenomena. Many different enzyme systems are dependent upon calcium as a co-factor, for example the coagulation system, the complement system, and enzymes involved in intracellular transduction processes. These points highlight the importance of an efficient homeostatic system in order to control intra- and extracellular calcium concentrations.

Plasma calcium consists of three fractions: a protein-bound fraction (40 per cent), a diffusible but non-ionized fraction (10 per cent), and an ionized fraction (50 per cent). The majority of the protein-bound fraction is bound to albumin. Calcium binding to albumin is strongly pH dependent between pH 7 and 8. Acute acidosis decreases protein binding, resulting in an increase in free, ionized calcium, whereas alkalosis has the opposite effect. It is only this free calcium that is physiologically important. A reduction of free calcium, such as occurs during the hyperventilation syndrome, increases the sodium permeability of cell membranes and, hence, the excitability of muscle cells and is responsible for the spasms that may occur during the hyperventilation syndrome (Agus et al. 1982).

Serum calcium should always be given in relation to the existing serum albumin concentration. Total serum calcium concentration is decreased in the presence of hypoalbuminaemia, although the ionized calcium will be unchanged. Several formulae for correcting measured calcium to the existing serum protein or albumin concentration are available. It should be remembered that the total serum calcium is decreased by 0.2 mmol/l for every 10 g/l change in serum albumin below 46 g/l and increased with the same value at higher albumin levels (Berry et al. 1973). In complex situations, such as hypoalbuminaemia and acid–base disturbances, direct assessment of the ionized calcium concentration may be helpful.

The extracellular fluid calcium concentration is the result of the effect of three different endocrine effectors: parathyroid hormone (PTH), 1,25-dihydroxy-vitamin D (1,25[OH]$_2$D), and calcitonin. Three target organs are susceptible to the influence of these humoral mediators in order to regulate calcium concentration: the gastrointestinal tract, bone tissue, and the kidney. Under normal conditions 99 per cent of the body calcium content (1000 g) is present as skeletal calcium and this is as such not available for day-to-day electrolyte regulation (Mundy 1987). In normal adult life no net calcium uptake takes place and bone formation is balanced by continuous bone degradation. This balance in bone remodelling is often shifted towards increased bone degradation in patients with malignancy associated hypercalcaemia.

Dietary calcium intake averages 20 mmol/day (range 15−30 mmol/day) of which some 30−40 per cent is absorbed. The active part of this process is under the control of $1,25(OH)_2D$, the active metabolite of vitamin D. This implies a direct control by PTH of gastrointestinal absorption, as this hormone modulates the 1-hydroxylation of 25-hydroxyvitamin D in the kidney. Renal excretion is the only important way of removing excess calcium from the body and of maintaining extracellular calcium within the normal range. Normal adults filter approximately 270 mmol of calcium every day. Under these conditions urinary calcium excretion is 4−6 mmol/day, implying that 97 per cent of the filtered amount of calcium is being reabsorbed by the renal tubuli. The majority of this reabsorptive activity takes place in the more proximal portion of the nephron. Calcium reabsorption in the proximal convoluted tubule accounts for approximately 60 per cent of the filtered load. Reabsorption is enhanced by extracellular fluid contraction and diminished by extracellular fluid expansion. The thick ascending limb of Henle's loop reabsorbs some 20 per cent of the filtered load. In the distal convoluted tubule some 10 per cent more is reabsorbed and it is here that PTH increases calcium reabsorption independent of changes in sodium reabsorption or luminal potential. Acid−base status also influences renal calcium handling. Acidosis decreases serum calcium, increases calcium release from the bone, and produces calciuria by inhibiting tubular reabsorption. During alkalosis hypocalciuria occurs, mediated in part by increased PTH secretion.

The most important factor determining plasma calcium concentration is bone turnover. The balance between bone formation and bone accretion is the determining factor of the calcium flux into the circulation. The kidney has considerable, albeit finite capacity to protect against the occurrence of hypercalcaemia by increasing calcium excretion up to five times the normal amount; however, urinary excretion seldom exceeds 15 mmol/day. If the amount released from the bone is in excess of this, hypercalcaemia is likely to occur (Mundy 1988).

Primary hyperparathyroidism (PHPT) ranks equally with hypercalcaemia associated with malignant disease as a cause of hypercalcaemia and these two disorders are responsible for the majority of cases. In primary hyperparathyroidism an elevated PTH level exists in the presence of an increased plasma calcium concentration. PTH, by promoting the production of $1,25(OH)_2D$, indirectly stimulates gastrointestinal absorption of calcium. The effects of PTH on the renal tubular cells are mediated by adenylate cyclase activity which increases intracellular cyclic AMP concentration (Buckle 1974; Fitzpatrick and Bilezikian 1987). Hypercalcaemia in primary hyperparathyroidism is characterized by increased bone resorption and increased gastrointestinal calcium resorption due to high levels of $1,25(OH)_2D$, increased renal calcium absorption, increased levels of nephrogenous cyclic AMP, a reduction in tubular phosphate reabsorption, and moderately increased calciuria. In the majority of cases primary hyperparathyroidism is caused by a single adenoma in one of the parathyroid glands and the finding of diffuse enlargements of all four glands requires consideration of the multiple endocrine neoplasia syndrome, hyperparathyroidism being one of the features of the MEN-1 or MEN-2a syndrome.

Pathophysiology of malignancy-associated hypercalcaemia

In the hospital population an underlying malignancy is the most frequent cause of hypercalcaemia (Table 1). In a study on 7610 patients with different neoplasms, 1.5 per cent had hypercalcaemia (Blomqvist 1986). Breast, lung, head and neck, and kidney cancer are the leading causes among solid tumours (Table 2) (Fisken *et al.* 1980; Blomqvist 1986). The pathophysiology and the incidence of the hypercalcaemia, however, differs markedly according to the underlying malignancy. In bronchial carcinoma, hypercalcaemia is frequent in squamous cell carcinoma and its occurrence does not necessarily point to metastatic disease. In contrast, hypercalcaemia is rare in small cell anaplastic bronchial carcinoma. In patients with

Table 1 Aetiology of hypercalcaemia according to the major underlying mechanism

I. Increased bone resorption
    (a) Malignancy
    (b) Primary hyperparathyroidism
    (c) Immobilization
    (d) Hyperthyroidism
    (e) Vitamin A intoxication
    (f) Post-transplantation hypercalcaemia

II. Increased intestinal absorption
    (a) Vitamin D intoxication
    (b) Sarcoidosis
    (c) Granulomatous diseases
    (d) Milk-alkali syndrome
    (e) Idiopathic hypercalcaemia of infancy

III. Other causes
    (a) Recovery from acute renal failure
    (b) Familial hypocalciuric hypercalcaemia
    (c) Addison's disease
    (d) Phaeochromocytoma
    (e) Acromegaly
    (f) Thiazide diuretics
    (g) Lithium treatment

Table 2 Frequency distribution of underlying malignancies in 219 patients with malignancy-associated hypercalcaemia

Primary site	Number of cases
Lung	54
Breast	44
Ear, nose, or throat	15
Ureters, bladder, or urethra	15
Myeloma	14
Female genital tract	14
Oesophagus	13
Unknown primary	10
Lymphoma	9
Kidney	7
Large bowel	5
Thyroid	4
Prostate	3
Others	12

Data from Fisken *et al.* (1980).

breast cancer, hypercalcaemia invariably occurs in patients with bone metastases. Separate entities with a different pathophysiological mechanism are the hypercalcaemia in breast cancer patients in response to endocrine therapy, hypercalcaemia associated with multiple myeloma, and the rise in calcium in the human T-cell leukaemia/lymphoma.

Malignancy-associated hypercalcaemia with bone metastasis

The main source of calcium in this syndrome is the skeleton. In patients with bone metastasis a direct stimulating effect of tumour cells on osteoclasts results in a major inflow of calcium into the extracellular compartment. In patients with breast cancer, who account for 50 per cent of all patients with malignancy-associated hypercalcaemia, this is the principal mechanism for the emergence of hypercalcaemia. Most patients already have extensive skeletal disease and hypercalcaemia is very often a terminal event (Coleman and Rubens 1987). In many patients with breast cancer and skeletal metastasis an increased urinary calcium excretion and increased urinary calcium/creatinine ratio can be observed even in the absence of overt hypercalcaemia (Coleman and Rubens 1987). It is evident that kidney function plays a critical role in determining whether this will lead to hypercalcaemia. In 16 patients with breast carcinoma with lytic bone metastasis, who were treated with intravenous aminohydroxypropylidene (APD) bisphosphonate, four developed sclerosis of lytic areas (Morton *et al.* 1988). Bisphosphonates are potent inhibitors of osteoclasts, and since in bone metastasis both osteoclastic and osteoblastic activity are enhanced, the reduction of osteoclastic activity will result in sclerosis. This observation also argues in favour of the hypothesis that calcium release from bone in patients with skeletal metastasis is mainly mediated via the osteoclast or osteoclast-like multinucleated giant cells and is not only the result of a direct effect of the tumour cells on bone (Athanasou *et al.* 1989).

The factors responsible for the increased osteoclast activation have not been clearly identified. Production of prostaglandins of the E series have been implicated. *In vitro* studies show that breast carcinoma cells incubated with oestrogens produce an osteolytic factor and that this production can be inhibited by adding indomethacin (Valentin-Opran *et al.* 1985). Colony stimulating factors, including M-CSF and GM-CSF and other cytokines are other possible candidates. In studies with GM-CSF bone pain has been one of the most important side-effects; whether this is due to medullary expansion or to osteoclast stimulation is uncertain (Steward *et al.* 1989). In patients with bone metastasis of breast cancer and hypercalcaemia increases in nephrogenous cyclic AMP and gastrointestinal calcium absorption have not, however, been observed.

A specific condition is the often very sudden rise in serum calcium in patients with breast cancer treated with oestrogens or tamoxifen (Kennedy *et al.* 1973). In a series of 470 patients with metastatic breast cancer treated with tamoxifen, ten (2.3 per cent) developed hypercalcaemia (Legha *et al.* 1981). Hypercalcaemia occurred after a median period of 7 days (4–11 days). Patients with extensive lytic bone metastasis were more prone to this complication. The mechanism of this hypercalcaemia is probably due to the partial oestrogenic effect of tamoxifen, and its stimulatory effect on tumour cells (Valentin-Opran *et al.* 1985).

This type of hypercalcaemia should not lead to interruption of treatment, as it is often predictive of tumour response (Villalon *et al.* 1979). Patients with breast carcinoma and lytic bone metastasis should have a regular control of the serum calcium during the first 3 weeks after starting tamoxifen.

Malignancy-associated hypercalcaemia without bony metastasis

Although only a minority in comparison with the patients with bone metastasis and hypercalcaemia, this group has received major interest by both clinical researchers. This group has been termed paraneoplastic hypercalcaemia, pseudohyperparathyroidism, or, preferably, humoral hypercalcaemia of malignancy (HHM). Whereas a local destruction is relatively easy to conceive as the mechanism of bone resorption and subsequent calcium release into the extracellular compartment in patients with bone metastasis, this is not the case in this group of patients. None the less, increased bone resorption takes place in patients with humoral hypercalcaemia of malignancy and this is most certainly the basic mechanism of the emergence of hypercalcaemia. Some humoral factor is supposed to be produced by the tumour cells and released into the circulation. This factor would increase bone resorption and, thus, increase the daily renal calcium load, eventually leading to overt hypercalcaemia. On the biochemical level, hypercalcaemia in these patients is characterized by an increased calciuria, increased bone resorption, increased hydroxyprolinuria, often increased levels of nephrogenous cyclic AMP, and a decrease in the threshold of phosphate reabsorption in the kidney. The rôle of increased renal calcium reabsorption is still controversial (Mundy 1987; Mundy 1988).

Parathyroid hormone

In 1941, Albright suggested that humoral hypercalcaemia of malignancy was being caused by tumoural production of parathyroid hormone. Although many of the biochemical abnormaltiies seen in humoral hypercalcaemia of malignancy resemble those seen in primary hyperparathyroidism, it remains impossible to explain the many biochemical characteristics of humoral hypercalcaemia of malignancy exclusively on the basis of tumoural-related PTH production (Buckle 1974; Skrabanek *et al.* 1980). Osteoclastic bone resorption is much more prominent in patients with humoral hypercalcaemia of malignancy and the treatment with bisphos-phonates, agents that inhibit osteoclast-mediated bone resorption, is more efficient in humoral hypercalcaemia of malignancy than in primary hyperparathyroidism. The latter patients have increased levels of $1,25(OH)_2D$, whereas the majority of humoral hyper-calcaemia of malignancy patients have suppressed levels of the active vitamin D metabolite. Patients with primary hyperparathyroidism tend to be hyperchloraemic and mildly acidotic, whereas those with humoral hypercalcaemia of malignancy are more frequently alkalotic. In a biochemical comparison of 41 patients with humoral hypercalcaemia of malignancy and increased urinary cyclic AMP levels and 15 patients with primary hyperparathyroidism a similar increase in the production of renal cyclic AMP was observed, but urinary calcium excretion was higher in the humoral hypercalcaemia of malignancy group. $1,25(OH)_2D$ levels were much lower and PTH levels suppressed in humoral hypercalcaemia of malignancy (Stewart *et al.* 1980). Using Northern blot analysis of messenger RNAs extracted from human tumours associated with humoral hypercalcaemia of malignancy, Simpson *et al.* (1983) failed to detect parathyroid hormone transcript in any of the 13 human tumours that were investigated. Interestingly, in the patients with humoral hypercalcaemia of malignancy and increased urinary cyclic AMP, renal phosphate wasting was much more elevated than in those patients with humoral hypercalcaemia of malignancy and normal levels of urinary cyclic AMP. As a result of this biochemical analysis it can be concluded that patients in the high-cyclic AMP group have a circulating renotropic factor that resembles native parathyroid hormone on its ability to stimulate proximal-tubular adenylate cyclase and to inhibit proximal tubular phosphate reabsorption. However, the factor differs from native parathyroid hormone in its relative inability to stimulate distal-tubular calcium reabsorption, its inability to stimulate 25-vitamin D α-hydroxylase, and its diminished or absent reactivity with a variety of region-specific parathyroid-hormone antisera. Only in rare instances is increased parathyroid hormone production actually responsible for hypercalcaemia in patients with malignancies.

Parathyroid hormone-related protein

Although no clear evidence exists for the rôle of parathyroid hormone itself in the pathogenesis of humoral hypercalcaemia of malignancy, several biochemical characteristics suggested the presence of a humoral factor with functional properties resembling in part those of 'native' parathyroid hormone (Kukreja et al. 1980; Steward et al. 1988). The stimulating capacity of tumoral extracts of patients with humoral hypercalcaemia of malignancy on PHT-sensitivie adenylate cyclase in isolated renal cortical membranes has been reported (Strewler et al. 1987). This activity was competitively inhibited by PTH receptor antagonists but not by an antiserum directed against PTH itself. Elevated levels of this parathyroid hormone-like protein (PLP) have been found in a high proportion of patients with solid malignancies complicated by hypercalcaemia (Budayr et al. 1989). Prevalence of increased serum levels of PLP was highest among tumour types associated with humoral hypercalcaemia of malignancy, such as squamous cell and renal carcinomas, but a subset of patients with breast cancer metastatic to bone and myeloma also showed elevated PLP levels. Functionally, PLP can mimic the effects of PTH, such as stimulation of bone resorption, increased cyclic AMP excretion, decreased calcium excretion, and increased phosphorus excretion, probably by acting upon the PTH receptor. Structurally, the homology between PLP and PTH is limited. It has been suggested that PLP might be a fetal protein, promoting calcium transport across the placenta. However, many questions about the biology of PLP and the mechanisms involved in governing normal and abnormal PLP gene expression, are currently unresolved.

Prostaglandins

Tashjian (1972, 1973) suggested a rôle for prostaglandins of the E series in the pathogenesis of humoral hypercalcaemia of malignancy on the basis of their experimental model in mouse fibrosarcoma cells. In the study of Seyberth et al. (1975), the common urinary metabolite of PGE_1 and PGE_2 was found to be strikingly elevated in 12 out of 14 patients with solid tumours and hypercalcaemia. Treatment with indomethacin in six of these patients resulted in a marked decrease in urinary prostaglandin E-M excretion and some decrease of the hypercalcaemia. No clear statement was made by these authors concerning the site of increased prostaglandin production. Several case reports mention the usefulness of indomethacin in the treatment of hypercalcaemia. Many of these patients had renal cell carcinoma. Several other investigators failed, however, to observe a beneficial effect of these drugs. In view of the general physiological rôle of prostaglandins, it seems much more likely that their rôle is confined to that of a local mediator of bone resorption, rather than a tumoural product stimulating calcium release from bone.

Transforming growth factors

Transforming growth factor-α (TGF-α) is a 5.6 kDa single chain, polypeptide which shares considerable identity with epidermal growth factor (EGF) and competes with EGF for binding to the EGF receptor. Several studies in the rat Leydig cell tumour, which rapidly induces severe hypercalcaemia, have demonstrated the bone resorbing capacity of TGF-α and its blocking by neutralizing antibodies to the EGF receptor (Ibbotson et al. 1983). In an in vitro model for bone resorption both TGF-α and EGF stimulated bone resorption in neonatal mouse calvaria with TGF-α being the more potent of the two agents (Ibbotson et al. 1985; Stern et al. 1985). Fetal rat limb bone appeared less sensitive to the bone resorbing effects of TGF-α. Interestingly, the effect of TGF-α could be totally blocked by indomethacin in the calvaria model, but less efficiently in a limb bone model. Several human tumours associated with the emergence of humoral hypercalcaemia of malignancy are known to express TGF-α or one of its precursor molecules. The exact rôle of TGF-α in the pathogenesis of humoral hypercalcaemia of malignancy is still uncertain.

Transforming growth factor-β (TGF-β) has been the focus of recent investigations attempting to elucidate mediators of humoral hypercalcaemia of malignancy. It is a 25 kDa protein composed of two identical 112 amino acid polypeptide chains linked by disulphide bounds. With Northern blot analysis, its transcript has been localized in a wide variety of normal and transformed cells. Depending on the exposed cell type, TGF-β can have both stimulatory and inhibitory effects. TGF-β has also been shown to increase bone resorption in mouse calvaria, which can be blocked by indomethacin suggesting that prostaglandins act as second messengers of this effect. In a recent study with the SK-Luci-6 cell line, derived from a large-cell anaplastic lung tumour of a patient with humoral hypercalcaemia of malignancy, Linkhart et al. (1989) have shown that the mitogenic, the bone resorbing, and the TGF-β-like activity all showed co-elution, suggesting that these effects are all associated with the same polypeptide. This cell line did not produce TGF-α or PTH-related proteins. Because many, if not all, tumours produce transforming growth factors and transforming growth factors are capable of stimulating bone resorption, it is very likely that transforming growth factors contribute to the emergence of humoral hypercalcaemia of malignancy in some cases.

Other mediators

Granulocyte-macrophage-colony stimulating factor (GM-CSF) is one of an ever growing family of cytokines, with specific stimulatory and differentiating capacities on specific precursor cells of the bone-marrow. It could therefore potentially contribute to the differentiation of osteoclast cells. It should, however, be noted that in studies with GM-CSF no hypercalcaemia has as yet been observed (Steward et al. 1989). The sometimes observed association of leucocytosis and hypercalcaemia could lead to more insight into the interrelation between these two paraneoplastic conditions (Sato et al. 1986).

Multiple myeloma

Multiple myeloma is characterized by extensive lytic bone disease with moderate or even absent osteoblastic bone remodelling (Kanis *et al.* 1988). Hypercalcaemia and skeletal disease are major problems in patients with myelomatosis. Hypercalcaemia is a frequent complication in advanced disease. In myeloma bone resorption is characterized by activation of osteoclasts due to the production of osteoclastic activating factors (OAFs). Myeloma cells *in vitro* produce such factors in large amounts. The number of potential mediators that could fulfil the OAF role is abundant. Interleukin-1 is one of the most potent bone resorbing substances of B-cell origin. In 11 human cell lines of human myeloma, however, no spontaneous production of interleukin-1 was observed. Tumour necrosis factor-β (lymphotoxin, TNF-β), however, was produced by 10 out of the 11 cell lines (Bataille *et al.* 1989). TNF-β is also known to have osteolytic activity. It is now apparent that from all the major bone resorbing cytokines, TNF-β is the most probable candidate for mediating bone resorption in multiple myeloma (Mundy 1988). The bone resorbing activity of culture media from five cultured myeloma cell lines was inhibited by antibodies against lymphotoxin (Garret *et al.* 1987).

The often impaired renal function in multiple myeloma patients further increases the susceptibility of these patients for hypercalcaemia. PTH levels are suppressed in these cases and increased urinary calcium reabsorption is not present. Hypercalcaemia can even occur in patients with non-secreting myeloma (Chew and Playfer 1988).

Treatment with osteoclast inhibitors is probably most suited for patients with hypercalcaemia and multiple myeloma.

Lymphomas

In 1977 a rapidly fatal T-cell lymphoproliferative syndrome was described in adults born in the south-western Japanese archipelago. This syndrome was characterized by pleomorphic neoplastic T-cells, lymphadenopathy, splenomegaly, hepatomegaly, cutaneous infiltration, hypercalcaemia, and interstitial pulmonary infiltrates. In a study of the first ten patients identified with this syndrome in the United States, nine out of ten suffered from hypercalcaemia (Broder 1984). Gallo's group first identified the human type-C retrovirus HTLV-I as the cause of this disease. Patients with this T-cell proliferation and hypercalcaemia have evidence of increased osteoclast activation with increased bone turnover. In those cases where parathyroid hormone assays were performed, levels were appropriately low, suggesting normal parathyroid function. One of the cytokines resembling the OAFs of multiple myeloma, interleukin-1α, is one of the possible candidates for mediating osteolytic activity in these patients (Shirakawa *et al.* 1988).

In patients with Hodgkin's disease hypercalcaemia is rare. In a report on three patients with symptomatic hypercalcaemia without skeletal involvement and bulky abdominal disease, serum 1,25-dihydroxyvitamin D was found to be elevated in two and paralleled serum calcium in the third case (Jacobson *et al.* 1989). This is in accordance with earlier reports suggesting a similar mechanism of hypercalcaemia in Hodgkin's disease as in sarcoidosis. In spite of the elevated levels of the active vitamin D metabolite, another factor must be responsible for the increased bone resorption in Hodgkin's disease-associated hypercalcaemia.

Clinical manifestations of hypercalcaemia

The clinical manifestations of hypercalcaemia are dependent on the degree and rate of progression of hypercalcaemia and the underlying aetiology. Other associated diseases or metabolic abnormalities can influence clinical presentation. The clinical spectrum can vary from asymptomatic to deep coma.

The major clinical features can be grouped according to the four major target organs of hypercalcaemia.

Central nervous system

The neurological features of hypercalcaemia can be very subtle with only discrete changes in affect or mild headache. Delusions and changes in personality are most often present. Episodes of depression and memory impairment are sometimes very prominent in patients with extensive solid tumours, but although these symptoms can be explained otherwise, hypercalcaemia should always be excluded. Agitation or even frank psychosis can be seen, but in general severe hypercalcaemia is more often associated with decreased central nervous activity leading to stupor or coma. Focal or generalized seizures are rare. Muscular weakness is also a prominent feature, which can seem paradoxical from a physiological point of view, as calcium ions are responsible for the excitation–contraction coupling in all muscle cells.

Cardiovascular effects

Hypercalcaemia leads to a shortening of systolic time intervals, which is seen on the ECG as a shortening of the QT-interval. Major arrhythmias do not tend to occur with mild hypercalcaemia. At high levels of hypercalcaemia; that is, above 4 mmol/l, paradoxical slowing of conduction occurs with QT-time and PR-time prolongation. Different degrees of heartblock can occur and this may lead to ventricular fibrillation in patients with hypercalcaemia of rapid onset. Digitalis and all other anti-arrhythmic drugs should be used with great care in these patients. Hypertension is another manifestation of hypercalcaemia. The positive influence on peripheral vascular tone can be explained in part by a direct effect of increased ionized calcium, but an indirect effect on the renin–angiotensin axis has also been suggested.

Renal manifestations

One of the earliest clinical manifestations of hypercalcaemia is increased diuresis and thirst. Impairment of sodium reabsorption in the thick ascending limb of Henle's loop and in the distal tubules, leads to the loss of the medullary concentration gradient and the emergence of a nephrogenic, vasopressin-resistant form of diabetes insipidus. Calcium can inhibit adenylate cyclase and directly oppose the effects of antidiuretic hormone on the collecting ducts. This fluid loss will lead to a volume contraction, thus limiting the renal excretory capacity for calcium and aggravating the hypercalcaemia. Loss of tubular reabsorption will lead in a later phase to hypomagnesaemia, hypokalaemia, glycosuria, aminoaciduria, and hyperuricaemia. Although some degree of calcium phosphate precipitation occurs in the kidney, nephrolithiasis is very uncommon in comparison with patients suffering from primary hyperparathyroidism.

Gastrointestinal effects

Diminished motility in the gastrointestinal tract will lead to constipation and will contribute to anorexia, nausea, and vomiting. Calcium has a direct stimulatory effect on gastric acid secretion and an indirect effect via the stimulation of gastrin secretion. Duodenal ulcers are a frequent complication of hypercalcaemia.

Treatment of hypercalcaemia

Treatment of hypercalcaemia is aimed at increasing urinary calcium excretion, decreasing skeletal calcium release, decreasing gastrointestinal calcium uptake, or increasing the formation of calcium complexes.

Fluid repletion

The renal concentration defect and the neurological and gastrointestinal symptoms all lead to extracellular volume contraction, leading to further aggravation of the hypercalcaemia. The cornerstone of therapy is the institution of an aggressive intravenous fluid repletion with normal saline solution. A first litre of normal saline solution can be given over 1 h; generally 4–5 l of normal saline will be needed in the first 24 h. Careful monitoring of the patient's fluid balance is mandatory. In patients with severe cardiac or renal insufficiency a central venous line should be inserted early and central venous pressure can be used as a guide for fluid administration. This vigorous fluid re-expansion is effective in both ameliorating the symptoms and in increasing urinary calcium excretion. Frequent monitoring of serum potassium and magnesium are needed. The measurement of calcium excretion per unit of glomerular filtration, (CaE), is useful in predicting the effect on calcaemia (Hosking *et al.* 1981). Patients with moderate hypercalcaemia (that is, $\leqslant 3.2$ mmol/l) can be treated with saline infusions alone. If dehydration and reversible renal dysfunction are present, this type of therapy is most efficacious.

With aggressive fluid repletion, a fall in serum calcium of 0.5–0.75 mmol/l can be expected within 36 h in a majority of patients. The emergence of hypernatraemia and fluid overload remain major limitations.

Diuretics

The use of the loop diuretics, frusemide or ethacrynic acid, will inhibit renal tubular calcium reabsorption. Frusemide must be used in high doses (up to 100 mg intravenously given every 1 or 2 h) until serum calcium begins to drop (Suki *et al.* 1970). Frusemide (40 mg intravenously every 6 h) can be used once adequate rehydration with 2 l of normal saline over 2 h has been established. Careful management of fluid balance and serum electrolytes is essential if these high doses of potent diuretics are given. Serum electrolytes should be monitored every 8 h during the entire duration of the treatment with high-dose calciuretics.

Corticosteroids

Glucocorticosteroids lower serum calcium by decreasing gastro-intestinal calcium absorption, as well as by inhibiting osteoclastic bone resorption and increasing calciuria. In view of the possible role of prostaglandins and the different cytokines in the mediation of bone resorption, corticosteroids could work by inhibiting any of these factors. Their efficacy is well known in the treatment of hypercalcaemia associated with haematological malignancies, for example leukaemia, myeloma, lymphoma, and in breast cancer. In other solid tumours their efficacy is in general disappointing and unpredictable and is no longer routinely recommended (Percival *et al.* 1984), except for their combined use with calcitonin (Binstock *et al.* 1980).

Calcitonin

Calcitonin decreases serum calcium by inhibiting osteoclast bone resorption and renal calcium reabsorption (Hosking and Gilson 1984). Calcitonin has the major advantage of being without any serious side-effect and is able to induce a rapid decrease of serum calcium. It remains one of the main tools in the early treatment of severe, life-threatening hypercalcaemia. Its major disadvantage is the occurrence of an 'escape' phenomenon after 2–4 days. In combination with 60 mg of prednisolone this escape to treatment could be alleviated (Binstock *et al.* 1980).

Calcitonin can be given intravenously, intramuscularly, or subcutaneously. MRC 5–10 U/kg/24 h divided over four doses each in 250 ml normal saline to be given over 1 h may be recommended. A continuous infusion in 500 ml of normal saline over 6 h is reported to be equally efficient. As an alternative route 2–4 MRC U/kg can be given subcutaneously or intramuscularly every 12 h. Minor side-effects include some nausea and flushing; allergic phenomena occur rarely.

Mithramycin

This cytostatic antibiotic inhibits DNA-dependent RNA synthesis. It lowers serum calcium by inhibition of osteoclastic bone resorption. It can be given as a 4-hourly infusion in 1 l of 5 per cent glucose or as a bolus injection at a dose of 15–25 µg/kg body weight. It is a very efficient therapy, lowering serum calcium within 6–48 h. If no response has occurred by then a second dose can still be efficient. Relapse, however, frequently occurs (Ralston *et al.* 1985). Toxicity can be important, with bone-marrow suppression and liver and kidney toxicity as the most prominent features. Extravasation leads to severe ulceration and subsequent fibrosis.

Bisphosphonates

Bisphosphonates probably constitute the most efficient tool in the treatment of tumour related hypercalcaemia. These drugs are characterized by a P–C–P link and are analogues of pyrophosphate. Their primary mode of action is the inhibition of the action of osteoclasts on bone. Three different bisphosphonates are currently undergoing extensive clinical trials: dichloromethylene diphosphonate (C12MDP) (Siris *et al.* 1980), ethane-1-hydroxy-1-diphosphonate (EHDP), and, probably the most promising of the three, aminohydroxypropylidene diphosphonate (APD).

EHPD not only inhibits bone resorption but also interferes with bone mineralization leading to osteomalacia if used for longer periods. Oral administration is apparently ineffective; the intravenous dose is 500 mg/day (5–10 mg/kg).

The principal mode of action of APD is by inhibiting bone resorption and not by increasing calciuria (Van Breukelen *et al.* 1979). Dose–response studies have shown that a single intravenous dose of 15–45 mg administered in 500 ml of normal saline over 2 h is efficient (Ralston *et al.* 1988). In a study of hypercalcaemic patients with breast carcinoma 15 out of 23 become normocalcaemic after a single dose of less than 15 mg, whilst three patients needed a higher dose (Coleman and Rubens 1987). Other dose–response studies have confirmed these findings (Body *et al.* 1987). A clear fall in serum calcaemia occurs within 48 h after administration. Normalization of serum calcium usually takes from 2 to 5 days. Side-effects are mild and include nausea and diarrhoea, fever, and, with higher dosages (>3.0 mg/kg), hypotension (Body *et al.* 1987). In a comparative study between APD, mithramycin, and the corticosteroid–calcitonin combination, APD was the slowest acting in restoring serum calcium to normal levels, but its duration of action was the longest (Ralston *et al.* 1985). The combination of APD with calcitonin and mithramycin has been reported to be useful in refractory cases (Ralston *et al.* 1988).

Gallium nitrate

Gallium nitrate was originally developed as an anticancer agent. During early clinical trials it was found to possess hypocalcaemic properties (Warrell *et al.* 1984; Bockman *et al.* 1986; Guidon and Bockman 1990). The mechanism whereby gallium nitrate perturbs calcium homeostasis is incompletely understood. Elemental gallium has been shown to localize preferentially to bone and is known to make hydroxyapatite significantly less soluble to cell-mediated resorption (Anghileri 1971; Warrell *et al.* 1984; Cournot-Witmer *et al.* 1987; Repo *et al.* 1988; Bockman *et al.* 1990). Clinical treatment with gallium nitrate reduces parameters indicative of increased bone turnover such as urinary calcium and hydroxyproline excretion (Scher *et al.* 1987; Warrell *et al.* 1987) whilst also exerting a favourable effect on bone formation (Bockman *et al.* 1986; Guidon and Bockman 1990). Unlike mithramycin gallium nitrate does not, however, induce lethal effects on osteoclasts (Cournot-Witmer *et al.* 1987; Hall and Chambers 1990).

During sequential phase 2 studies gallium nitrate was found to be a safe and effective therapy for patients with moderate to severe cancer-related hypercalcaemia (Warrell *et al.* 1986, 1987, 1988). In a recent study (Warrell *et al.* 1991) gallium nitrate was compared in a randomized fashion with the bisphosphonate, etidronate. Normocalcaemia was obtained in 82 per cent of patients given gallium nitrate and in 43 per cent of editronate-treated subjects ($p < 0.001$). The latter figure is similar to that observed in other studies with bisphosphonates (Ritch *et al.* 1989). Furthermore, the median duration of normocalcaemia was significantly longer ($p = 0.043$) for those patients receiving gallium nitrate. Although gallium nitrate has been shown to produce renal toxicity when used as an anticancer agent there were no differences in mean daily serum creatinine levels in the two patients groups in this study. These data suggest that gallium nitrate may be the treatment of choice for patients with cancer-related hypercalcaemia.

Dialysis

In patients with renal failure, both haemo- and peritoneal dialysis are effective in lowering serum calcium. This can be particularly useful in the management of hypercalcaemia in the setting of multiple myeloma.

Antitumour treatment

Every therapy of hypercalcaemia can only be judged to be meaningful if it is accompanied with a general oncological treatment strategy, to prevent its recurrence.

Hypocalcaemia in malignancy

Introduction

Generally, the aetiology of hypocalcaemia can be traced back to some defect in either PTH or vitamin D function. Calcitonin, a hormone produced by the C-cells of the thyroid gland, has a calcium-lowering effect, but increased secretion of this hormone rarely results in hypocalcaemia. The discussion will be limited to hypocalcaemia where the cause is more or less specific to or frequently occurs in patients with cancer.

Aetiology of hypocalcaemia in cancer patients

Although in post-mortem studies malignant infiltration of the parathyroid glands in patients with widespread metastatic cancer has been reported to be as high as 5–15 per cent, clinical hypoparathyroidism is very rare in patients with cancer (Horwitz *et al.* 1972). Sporadic cases of hypoparathyroidism have been reported after external radiotherapy to the neck and mediastinum or high doses of radioactive iodine (^{131}I). Transient hypocalcaemia, occurring within a few days after total or subtotal thyroidectomy is not exceptional, but permanent hypoparathyroidism occurs in probably less than 1 per cent of patients.

One of the most frequent causes of hypocalcaemia in cancer patients is related to cisplatin (CDDP)-based chemotherapy. This type of hypocalcaemia is secondary to magnesium wasting resulting from renal tubular damage by CDDP and usually is accompanied by hypokalaemia. Other metabolic causes of hypocalcaemia are multiple citrated blood transfusions, hyperventilation, osteoblastic bone metastases (Hall *et al.* 1972), and oncogenic osteomalacia. Hypocalcaemia associated with the tumour lysis syndrome will be discussed below (Jaffe *et al.* 1972).

Clinical symptomatology

Clinical symptomatology consists of increased neuromuscular irritability. Early findings may be feelings of numbness or paraesthesia involving fingers, toes, and perioral region. Tetany of facial muscles in response to stimulation of the facial nerve (Chvostek's sign) and carpopedal spasm after inflation of a blood pressure cuff (Trousseau's sign) are classic signs of this increased irritability. Central nervous system abnormalities vary from grand to petit mal seizures, impairment of cognitive functions, and emotional disturbances. Extrapyramidal signs may occur. In severe or acute onset hypocalcaemia laryngospasm or bronchospasm may be life-threatening. Hypocalcaemia results in a moderate slowing of atrioventricular and intraventricular conduction during cardiac depolarization. Electrocardiographically, QT prolongation can be observed, thus increasing the vulnerable period for the emergence of Q on T extrasystoles. Certainly in the presence of hypo-magnesaemia and hypokalaemia this may lead to a special type of ventricular fibrillation, the so-called *torsades de pointe*. Isolated hypocalcaemia will rarely lead to arrhythmias.

Diagnosis and treatment

A decreased serum calcium after correction for existing serum albumin concentration will confirm the diagnosis. Measurement of ionized calcium may be helpful in complex situations, such as concurrent acid–base disturbances. Assessment of circulating parathyroid hormone, serum phosphate, and eventually vitamin D metabolites will lead to a diagnosis in the majority of cases.

Acute severe hypocalcaemia has to be treated with intravenous calcium administration. This can best be done with ECG monitoring, especially in digitalized patients who are sensitive to arrhythmias that may arise from temporary hypocalcaemia. Intravenous calcium salts exist in two forms: (1) calcium chloride 10 per cent containing 9 mmol of elemental calcium in ampoules of 10 ml or (2) calcium gluconate 10 per cent containing 2.25 mmol calcium in a 10 ml ampoule. Ampoules must be diluted with 50–100 ml of glucose solution 5 per cent. Solutions of more than 50 mmol/l (1 mmol per 20 ml) should be avoided as these are irritating to veins.

In patients with chronic hypocalcaemia due to hypopara-thyroidism, treatment is aimed at maintaining serum calcium levels in the low normal range. Oral calcium supplementation will consist of 2–4 g of elemental calcium in combination with a vitamin D metabolite. The biological potency of these metabolites differs widely, for example $1,25(OH)_2 D$ (rocalcitrol) is 1000 times more potent than ergocalciferol (vitamin D_2). In practice this means that virtually no extra oral calcium intake is needed with rocalcitrol (0.5–2.0 µg daily) and time needed to achieve normocalcaemia is shortened compared to that when ergocalciferol is used. Ergocalciferol is much cheaper and the daily dose is 750–3000 µg.

Osteogenic osteomalacia

Osteogenic osteomalacia is a tumour-associated form of osteomalacia characterized by renal wasting of phosphorus and markedly reduced levels of $1,25(OH)_2D_3$. Symptoms consist of bone pain, muscle weakness, and occasionally fractures of bone or gait disturbances. Biochemical alterations include hypophosphataemia with increased phosphaturia, increased alkaline phosphatase levels, low or undetectable $1,25(OH)_2D_3$ levels, and normal levels of 25(OH)D and PTH. Radiological appearance is that of osteomalacia. Histological examination of bone biopsies shows the presence of increased amounts of unmineralized osteoid covering the trabecular bone surface. There is no evidence of increased bone resorption.

Removal of the tumour leads to return of serum phosphate levels to normal within 1 week and the healing of bone lesions within months (Cotton and van Puffelen 1986).

Most frequently the syndrome has been found in association with benign or malignant tumours of mesenchymal origin (Cotton and van Puffelen 1986), but it has also been described in association with carcinoma of the prostate (Lyles et al. 1980), oat cell lung cancer (Tayler et al. 1984), and breast cancer (Agus 1983). The pathophysiology of the altered phosphate transport remains unclear, but the disappearance of all manifestations of the syndrome after removal of the tumour suggests the production of a humoral factor that may affect multiple functions of the proximal renal tubule, including inhibition of phosphate reabsorption and synthesis of $1,25(OH)_2$ vitamin D_3.

Transplantation of a haemangiopericytoma associated with osteomalacia in nude mice induced hyperphosphaturia, hypophosphataemia, and high serum alkaline phosphatase levels in tumour-bearing animals. Tumour extracts added to cultured mouse renal tubular cells resulted in decreased $1,25(OH)_2$ vitamin D formation (Miyauchi et al. 1988), again pointing to a humoral tumour-secreted factor.

Treatment preferably consists of removal of the tumour. However, when this is not feasible, administration of high-dose $1,25(OH)_2$ vitamin D_3 and moderate oral phosphate administration may heal bone lesions. A suggested regimen is 3 mg of $1,25(OH)_2$ vitamin D_3 and 2 mmol of phosphate daily (Leight 1990). It is important to be aware of this syndrome in prostatic cancer patients who present with hypophosphataemia and bone pains.

MAGNESIUM DISTURBANCES IN MALIGNANCY

Magnesium homeostasis

Magnesium is the fourth most abundant cation in the body and, after potassium, the second most abundant intracellular cation. Liver and muscle cells have an intracellular concentration around 7.5–10 mmol/l and red blood cell magnesium is 2.5 mmol/l. Serum magnesium ranges between 0.75 and 1.05 mmol/l, approximately 55 per cent being ionized, with 30 per cent being protein bound and 15 per cent complexed. Gastrointestinal absorption is probably entirely passive and is situated in the upper gastrointestinal tract.

An average diet will contain some 12.5 mmol, nearly 300 mg, of magnesium per day. Approximately 30–40 per cent of this will be absorbed; in stable conditions of magnesium balance nearly all of this will be found in the urine, with only minimal amounts (0.1 mmol) being eliminated in the stools. Extracellular fluid status, parathyroid hormone, and serum magnesium and calcium are the major factors determining tubular magnesium reabsorption.

Magnesium is a critical co-factor for various phosphokinases and phosphatases. Among these are the various ATPases regulating cellular calcium, hydrogen, sodium, and potassium pumps. Magnesium is also a co-factor in the phosphorylation of glucose and in the oxidative metabolism of mitochondria.

Aetiology and pathogenesis of hypomagnesaemia in cancer patients

Cisplatin

The occurrence of hypomagnesaemia and hypermagnesuria in 21 out of 37 patients treated with cisplatin was first described by Schilsky and Anderson (1979). This suggested a primary tubular lesion responsible for the increased urinary loss in the face of the hypomagnesaemia. Other studies have confirmed the finding, and this reversible complication may develop in 50 per cent of patients within 14 days of cisplatin administration. The cisplatin-induced renal wasting of magnesium increases with the applied cisplatin dose and is of concern in regimens using high-dose cisplatin administration. Simple supplementation with intravenous and later oral magnesium ameliorates hypomagnesaemia, but will not prevent the renal magnesium wasting (Willox et al. 1986). The hypomagnesaemia will frequently cause hypokalaemia and hypocalcaemia. These will not be corrected with calcium and potassium repletion, until the hypomagnesaemia itself has been corrected (Blachley and Hill 1981).

In most cases, hypomagnesaemia will resolve spontaneously after interruption of treatment; in a minority of cases, however, it can persist for long periods. In a study of six patients the hypomagnesaemia persisted for 2–6 years after PVB chemotherapy for testicular carcinoma. Interestingly these patients had hypocalciuria, that persisted even after intravenous correction of magnesium levels. Under 'normal' conditions, hypomagnesaemia would lead to an increased renal reabsorption of both calcium and magnesium. However, correction of hypomagnesaemia had no effect on the hypocalciuria (Mavichak et al. 1988).

The use of diuretics, volume expansion with saline infusion, and mannitol diuresis will further aggravate renal magnesium wasting. Carbenicillin and tinarcillin also cause a solute diuresis and thus increase magnesuria (Flombaum 1984). Aminoglycosides and amphotericin B can potentiate the cisplatin nephrotoxicity and increase renal magnesium wasting in these patients. If possible, the use of these potentially nephrotoxic agents should be avoided in patients receiving cisplatin.

Other causes

The syndrome of inappropriate antidiuretic hormone secretion and hyperaldosteronism, will cause renal magnesium wasting by increasing extracellular fluid volume. Hypercalcaemia will also lead to an increased urinary magnesium loss. Hypokalaemia can be caused by and also be the result of hypomagnesaemia.

Clinical manifestations

It is important to be aware of the consequences of other electrolyte deficiencies due to the function of magnesium on ion distribution pumps. The effects of magnesium deficiency on the appearance of hypocalcaemia has been discussed above. The interactions between potassium and magnesium are manifold and complicated. Hypomagnesaemia is accompanied by hypokalaemia in approximately 40 per cent of cases. Intracellular potassium depletion is often very pronounced, due to the effect on the sodium–potassium ATPase pump. Hypokalaemia refractory even to parenteral substitution should always raise the suspicion of underlying magnesium deficiency. Hypophosphataemia is also frequently associated with hypomagnesaemia.

Electrocardiographic abnormalities are difficult to define as in the majority of cases other electrolyte disturbances are present. Most important, however, is the QT interval prolongation as a reflection of slower diastolic depolarization. These patients are at risk for sudden death due to *torsade de pointe*-type ventricular fibrillation. The inhibition of the Na/K–ATPase pump by both hypomagnesaemia and digitalis, implies that this drug should never be used in conditions of hypomagnesaemia. Digitalis will also slow cardiac conduction with a resultant further increment in QT-interval (Commerford and Lloyd 1984).

Neuromuscular and central nervous symptomatology is comparable with those of hypocalcaemia. Seizures and even coma have been described in patients with cisplatin-induced hypomagnesaemia. Raynaud's phenomenon developed in 13 out of 30 patients treated with PVB for testicular cancer and the severity of prior hypomagnesaemia had a predictive value (Vogelzang et al. 1985).

HYPONATRAEMIA

Introduction

Sodium is the major cation in the plasma and extracellular fluid. The plasma sodium concentration (normal range 137–145 mmol/l) is regulated indirectly by alterations in total body water content. This is accomplished by sensors that either promote the uptake of water or the excretion of urine. Total body water constitutes approximately 60 per cent of the lean body weight in men and 50 per cent in women. Approximately 60 per cent of total body water is in the intracellular and 40 per cent in the extracellular compartment. Approximately one-quarter to one-fifth of the total extracellular fluid is contained in the plasma compartment. The distribution of total body water between the intracellular and extracellular compartment is governed by the osmolality of the fluids on both sides of the cell membrane. The osmolality of a solution is determined by the number of solute particles per kilogram of water. The major determinants of plasma (and extracellular fluid) osmolality are sodium salts, which account for 95 per cent of the plasma osmotic pressure, whereas glucose, potassium, and urea under normal circumstances play a minor rôle. Intracellularly, potassium salts are the major solutes. Plasma osmolality can be measured directly, or it can be estimated by the equation:

$$\text{plasma osmolality (mosmol/kg)} = 2 \times \text{sodium concentration (mmol/l)} + \text{glucose concentration (mmol/l)} + \text{urea concentration (mmol/l)}$$

The normal value of plasma osmolality varies between 285 and 295 mosm/l. Since the cell membrane is freely permeable to water, any gradient between intracellular and extracellular osmolality will result in a movement of water from the compartment with the lower to the one with the higher osmolality until equilibrium has been reached. However, this flow of water is not affected by changes in urea concentration, because urea can freely cross the cell membrane and its concentration inside and outside the cell will be the same. Only the 'effective osmolality' or tonicity will affect the distribution of total body water (Gennari 1984). Hence, the distribution of water between the intracellular and extracellular compartment will be primarily directed by the prevailing concentrations of sodium salts, potassium salts, and glucose (Rose 1986). Any decrease in plasma sodium concentration which is not compensated by the presence of other osmols, for example glucose or mannitol, will lower plasma osmolality, resulting in a shift of water from the extracellular to the intracellular compartment and cellular oedema. It is this cellular overhydration, especially of brain cells, that is responsible for symptomatic hyponatraemia.

The water balance of the body is regulated by a system of osmoreceptors, that affect the release of antidiuretic hormone (ADH) and feelings of thirst. The antidiuretic hormone arginine vasopressin (AVP) is a nonapeptide synthesized as part of a larger precursor molecule, AVP-neurophysin, in the neurones of the supraoptic and paraventricular nuclei of the hypothalamus. The vasopressin precursor gene comprises three exons coding for the three major protein components: AVP, neurophysin II and a C-terminal glycopeptide (Schmale et al. 1987). It is believed that the precursor molecule is cleaved to its constituents along the axonal transport towards the neurohypophysis. The synthesis of AVP is not restricted to the hypothalamic region. The presence of vasopressin and its associated neurophysin has been identified in many different peripheral organs, for example the ovaries, the uterus, the testis, the adrenal glands, the thymus, and both central and peripheral nervous tissue. The physiological implications of these observations are not obvious (Clements and Funder 1986), but a paracrine rôle for these peptides has been suggested. ADH promotes the back-diffusion of free water in the collecting tubules of the nephrons, thus decreasing urinary volume and increasing the concentration of urinary solutes. In healthy adults plasma ADH levels will be undetectable when plasma osmolality is below 280 mosmol/kg. In these circumstances, diuresis will be maximal, allowing the excretion of large amounts ($> 10 \, l/day$) of diluted urine (low urine osmolality and specific gravity). Within the physiological range of plasma osmolality plasma ADH concentration increases linearly with increases in osmolality and maximal antidiuresis is achieved with plasma ADH levels of 5 pmol/l, a level that is usually reached when plasma osmolality approaches 295 mosmol/kg. At this time a concentrated urine will be produced and urinary

Table 3 Conditions associated with hyponatraemia

Isotonic and hypertonic replacement hyponatraemia
   Presence of increased concentrations of glucose, mannitol, or other non-sodium solutes
Hypotonic hyponatraemia
   Hypervolaemic
      Cardiac failure, liver cirrhosis, inferior vena cava obstruction, nephrotic syndrome
   Hypovolaemic
      Diuretics, Addison's disease, salt-losing nephropathy, osmotic diuresis, diarrhoea, vomiting
   Euvolaemic
      SIADH, water intoxication, reset osmostat, hypothyroidism, glucocorticoid deficiency

volume may be as low as 20 ml/h. This corresponds with the activation of specialized receptors located in the supraoptic nucleus that induce thirst. The set point of these receptors is approximately 10–15 mosmol/kg above the set point of the osmoreceptors that influence the secretion of ADH (Robertson *et al.* 1982). The ADH–thirst system regulating water balance is closely connected to the volume regulatory system that is responsible for the maintenance of adequate tissue perfusion. The latter system is built up by baroreceptors located in the arterial wall, the atria, and the venous system and governs urinary sodium excretion. Effectors of this baroreceptor system, the renin–angiotensin II–aldosterone axis and atrial natriuretic peptide, modulate the sensitivity and the set point of the receptors governing the release of ADH (Robertson 1987). In addition to antidiuresis, ADH also exerts vasopressor effects and in some instances, such as cardiac failure or hypovolaemic shock, the secretion of ADH may be stimulated in order to maintain effective circulating volume although this might lead to hypotonicity (Gross *et al.* 1987). However, the discussion of hyponatraemia will be limited to those causes judged to be frequent and more or less specific for patients with malignant disease (Table 3).

Pathophysiology

Syndrome of inappropriate antidiuretic hormone secretion

The syndrome of inappropriate antidiuretic hormone secretion (SIADH) was first described by Schwartz and Bartter in two patients with bronchogenic carcinoma, who continued to produce hypotonic urine in the presence of serum hyponatraemia (Schwartz *et al.* 1957). The initial explanation for this syndrome was a suspected stimulation, by the primary tumour, on the neurohypophysis to secrete an excess of ADH. It took several years before the actual production of ADH by the tumour could be demonstrated (Amatruda *et al.* 1963). Afterwards *in vitro* cultures of cell lines producing ADH provided further insight into the syndrome (Pettengill *et al.* 1977).

AVP has a prime role in modulating urinary water excretion. In response to many stimuli, most of all from the osmoreceptors, AVP secretion will increase the permeability of the renal collecting system, thus allowing water reabsorption in relation to the prevailing interstitial concentration of the renal medulla. In the presence of a hypertonic medulla, AVP will cause the production of concentrated urine and thus result in a negative free water clearance. This condition is judged to be appropriate if it occurs in the presence of an increased serum osmolality (Robertson *et al.* 1982). Responses of the osmoreceptors and the ensuing AVP release are, amongst other factors, very dependent on the duration of this hypo-osmolality. Apart from the condition of underlying malignancy, a wide variety of stimuli other than osmolality, can influence ADH secretion and the response of the kidney to ADH. The basic abnormality underlying SIADH is a failure to suppress AVP secretion when plasma osmolality drops below the normal threshold value of 275–280 mosmol/kg.

Patients with SIADH produce a hypotonic urine, but the urinary volume is related to fluid intake. Serum sodium concentration can be as low as 105 mEq/l (De Troyer and Demanet 1976). Hypouricaemia is a frequent feature of SIADH of any type (Passamonte 1984; Decaux *et al.* 1985; Sorensen *et al.* 1988). Urinary salt loss can be normal in absolute terms, that is, in balance with the intake. Urinary sodium concentration is, however, nearly always in excess of 20 mEq/l. This increased loss of sodium with its negative free water clearance will lead to hyponatraemia when

Table 4 Differential diagnosis of SIADH

I. Malignancies
Small-cell lung cancer
Carcinoid tumours of the 'foregut' type (for example, bronchial carcinoids)
Hodgkin's disease and non-Hodgkin's lymphoma
Leukaemia
Ewing's sarcoma
Thymoma
Mesothelioma
Neuroblastoma
Nasopharyngeal carcinoma
Pancreatic, duodenal, prostatic carcinoma

II. Chest diseases
Infections: tuberculosis, pneumonia, lung abscess, aspergillosis
Cystic fibrosis
Acute respiratory failure, chronic obstructive airway disease
Pneumothorax
Positive pressure ventilation

III. Central nervous system disease
Trauma, subdural haematoma, subarachnoid haemorrhage
Infections: meningitis, encephalitis, brain abscess
Guillain-Barré syndrome
Cerebral thrombosis, sinus cavernosus thrombosis
Acute psychosis
Primary brain tumour
Brain metastases
Multiple sclerosis, acute intermittent porphyria, Wernicke's encephalopathy
Seizures

IV. Drug related
Vasopressin, oxytocin, desmopressin
Vincristine (Slater *et al.* 1969; Cutting 1971), vinblastine (Antony *et al.* 1980)
Cisplatin (Levin *et al.* 1982; Littlewood and Smith 1984; Porter 1985; Ritch 1988)
Cyclophosphamide (DeFronzo *et al.* 1973; Harlow *et al.* 1979), high-dose melphalan (Greenbaum-Lefkoe *et al.* 1985)
Somatostatin (Halma *et al.* 1987)
Thiazide diuretics, sulphonylureas
Phenothiazines, tricyclic antidepressants
Carbamazepine
Nicotine, ethanol
Clofibrate

V. Idiopathic

hypotonic fluids are taken in order to maintain euvolaemia. In patients with euvolaemic, hypotonic hyponatraemia and a urinary osmolality above 100 mosmol/kg, the diagnosis of SIADH is almost certain. In patients with a urinary osmolality below 100 mosmol/kg a dehydration test is the only diagnostic test to determine the presence of a reset osmostat (Vokes and Robertson 1988).

The tumour type most often associated with SIADH is small-cell carcinoma of bronchogenic or extrapulmonary origin, but the syndrome is not restricted to patients with malignancy (Table 4). Overt SIADH has been reported in 7–14 per cent of patients with small-cell carcinomas and the incidence was higher in patients with extensive compared to limited disease (20 versus 11 per cent) (Hainsworth *et al.* 1983; Lockton and Thatcher 1986). An abnormal response to water loading was found in up to 47 per cent of patients with small-cell lung cancer (Comis *et al.* 1980). Others have

Table 5 Aetiology of hypernatraemia

I. Loss of water in excess of sodium loss
  (a) Gastrointestinal: diarrhoea, vomiting, hypertonic enemas
(b) Renal
  Central and nephrogenous diabetes insipidus
  Osmotic diuresis, for example mannitol, IV contrast, glucose, calcium
  Chronic renal failure
(c) Skin: fever, heat stroke
(d) Lung: hyperventilation
(e) Other: impossibility or unavailability of fluids to drink

II. Excessive sodium intake or retention
  (a) Hyperaldosteronism
(b) Excessive sodium administration (oral or intravenous), for example, sodium bicarbonate, fresh frozen plasma

III. Essential hypernatraemia

Table 6 Aetiology of central diabetes inspidus

Post-hypophysectomy
Post-trauma
Primary tumours
  Craniopharyngioma
  Pinealoma
  Pituitary adenoma
Secondary tumours
  Breast carcinoma
  Bronchogenic carcinoma
  Leukaemia
  Lymphoma
Infections
Vascular disorders
Granulomas
Drug related
  Clonidine
  Phencyclidine
Idiopathic
Hereditary

confirmed this high prevalence of subclinical disturbed ADH secretion (Gilby *et al.* 1976). In patients with oat cell carcinoma and central nervous system metastasis the prevalence of SIADH is even higher (Lokich 1982). No clear significance regarding prognosis can be given to the presence or absence of SIADH in small cell carcinoma, unless brain metastasis is being diagnosed. The response of the SIADH to chemotherapeutic treatment is probably of greater prognostic value and the emergence of SIADH in a patient with oat cell carcinoma suggests systemic relapse or brain metastases.

Drug-related SIADH

A variety of chemotherapeutic drugs have been implicated in the aetiology of hyponatraemia due to SIADH. A well-known example is vincristine (Rosenthal and Kaufman 1974). The emergence of hyponatraemia was first reported in children with leukaemia, while case reports in adults confirmed the association of SIADH with vincristine therapy (Cutting 1971). Cyclophosphamide, its analogue ifosfamide, and melphalan have all been reported to cause severe

hyponatraemia due to SIADH (Harlow *et al.* 1979; Greenbaum-Lefkoe *et al.* 1985). Cisplatin is associated with renal tubular damage and may cause severe perturbations in electrolyte and water balance. Most prominent are urinary magnesium wasting and, eventually, hypokalaemia and hypocalcaemia, and hyponatraemia due to a salt-losing nephropathy (Hutchinson *et al.* 1988). Treatment with short-acting intravenous somatostatin can also produce severe hyponatraemia (Halma *et al.* 1987).

Symptomatology

Symptoms of acute hyponatraemia, occurring within 24 h, consist of headache, nausea, vomiting, mental changes such as lethargy, apathy, or agitation, seizures, coma, and ultimately cerebral anoxia and death. The symptomatology of hyponatraemia primarily results from cellular overhydration of brain cells and its severity is strongly dependent on the rapidity of onset and the degree of the hyponatraemia. Acute hyponatraemia may cause severe neurological symptoms, whereas a long-standing hyponatraemia may be asymptomatic. This is thought to be due to defence mechanisms of the brain against overhydration diverting excess interstitial fluid into the liquor (Melton and Nattie 1983) and lowering the intracellular osmotic pressure by extrusion of amino acids (Thurston *et al.* 1987).

Treatment

The treatment of hyponatraemia will differ depending on the underlying disorder, the presence of symptoms and the rapidity of its onset. Hypovolaemia, hypotension, and vomiting, if present, need correction. There are conflicting opinions, however, with regard to the administration of sodium. Correction of hyponatraemia will lead to movement of water out of the cells. The degree to which this occurs is dependent upon the duration of the hyponatraemia and the presence of specific adaptation mechanisms to hypo-osmolality in the brain. After 48 h the neurones have reconstituted their cellular osmolality by extruding osmotically active particles. If under these circumstances hypertonic saline is administered, a specific osmotic syndrome, known as pontine myelinolysis, may develop, characterized by seizures, limb paralysis, a persistent vegetative state, or even death (Tomlinson *et al.* 1976). To prevent this syndrome, the following guidelines have been developed with regard to the correction of hyponatraemia and the associated hypo-osmolality. Acute onset severe hyponatraemia should be treated promptly using hypertonic saline and frusemide, aiming at an increase of serum sodium of at least 1 mmol/h (Cluitmans and Meinders 1990). The rate of correction in patients who have a severe symptomatic hyponatraemia of a more chronic duration should be below 0.5 mmol/h, as severe morbidity and even mortality have been associated with a more aggressive approach (Sterns *et al.* 1986; Sterns 1987). In patients with asymptomatic severe hyponatraemia treatment must be directed at the prevention of a further decline of serum sodium and active intervention should be performed very carefully (Berl 1990). Treatment of patients with SIADH classically consists of fluid restriction to 500 ml/day. This will limit urinary volume and sodium loss and prevents the dilution of the extracellular volume due to hypotonic fluid intake. This therapy is often difficult to manage outside hospital. Democycline, a tetracycline derivative, in a dose up to 1200 mg/day, causes a form of transient nephrogenic diabetes insipidus and is superior to lithium (Forrest *et al.* 1978). The effect on hyponatraemia becomes apparent within 5–7 days and serum sodium will return to normal within 5–14 days.

Oral urea in a dose of 30 g will cause osmotic diuresis and alleviate the need for fluid restriction, but one of its major drawbacks is its bad taste. Loop diuretics such as frusemide and ethacrynic acid will increase diuresis and decrease the concentrating capacity of the kidney. Thiazide diuretics, on the contrary, will worsen the hyponatraemia in SIADH. For patients with an underlying malignancy as the cause of SIADH, treatment of the underlying neoplasm is the best and only lasting therapy.

HYPERNATRAEMIA IN MALIGNANCY

Introduction

Sodium is the major determinant of serum osmolality and tonicity. Rapid changes in serum sodium levels, will lead to parallel changes in tonicity and will cause water movement across cellular membranes. In the case of hypernatraemia this would result in cellular dehydration. Because sodium and water intake are very variable, a major feedback control mechanism exists to provide protection from too drastic changes in tonicity. This is the integration of the two major osmoregulatory systems. The first is the thirst centre in the hypothalamus with cortical extensions leading to increased fluid intake whenever tonicity threatens to increase; the second is neurohypophyseal antidiuretic hormone (ADH) secretion. When osmolality is less than 280 mosmol/kg, ADH is undetectable and urinary osmolality is less than 150 mosmol/kg. Once plasma osmolality rises above 280 mosmol/kg both plasma ADH and urinary osmolality rise sharply in a linear fashion. The mechanism of action of ADH is primarily mediated by stimulation of adenylate cyclase on the serosal surface of the epithelial cells of the renal collecting tubules. This will ultimately lead to an increased permeability of collecting tubular cells. The high tonicity in the renal medulla will force water out of the tubular lumen into the renal medulla. This will lead, in the presence of a high plasma ADH, to the excretion of a very concentrated urine with a 'negative' free water clearance. Thus, an excess of sodium to water will be lost from the body, in an attempt to counterbalance serum hyperosmolality. Due to the integrated action of thirst and ADH secretion, an increased intake of largely hypotonic solutes will lead to a further fall in serum osmolality (Vokes and Robertson 1988). Hypernatraemia is therefore infrequent in adult patients who are mentally alert and have access to water. Although other reasons can be responsible for the occurrence of hypernatraemia (Table 5) in patients with malignancy, attention here will be focused mainly on both central and nephrogenous diabetes insipidus (Table 6).

Pathophysiology

Diabetes insipidus

Central diabetes insipidus can result from either partial or complete deficiency of ADH secretion. The different anatomical parts of the osmostat, ADH-producing neurones, neurohypophysis, and their interconnections can be destroyed by any space-occupying lesion. Although primary tumours can be responsible for this syndrome, discussion here will be limited to secondary localizations. In a survey from the Mayo Clinic (Kimmel and O'Neill 1983), 14 out of 1000 consecutive newly diagnosed cases of diabetes insipidus were due to metastatic disease. In the majority of cases, diabetes insipidus emerges at a late stage of the disease. In the Mayo Clinic series, however, 11 out of a total of 25 patients with diabetes insipidus

as a complication of malignancy, presented with diabetes insipidus emerges at a late stage of the disease. In the Mayo Clinic series, however, 11 out of a total of 25 patients with diabetes insipidus as the initial manifestation of their malignancy. Three of these patients had myeloid leukaemia, two had a carcinoma of unknown primary, one patient had a breast carcinoma and two other patients suffered from small-cell lung cancer. Autopsy studies showed pituitary metastasis to be present in 1–27 per cent of patients with cancer, but this is only rarely translated into clinical symptomatology (Teears 1975).

Of the solid tumours, breast cancer and lung carcinoma are most frequently responsible for metastatic diabetes insipidus. A survey studied 39 cases of diabetes insipidus due to metastatic involvement in patients with breast carcinoma (Yap et al. 1979). All patients had widely metastatic disease at the time of diagnosis of diabetes insipidus. Many of them had either other CNS metastasis or meningeal carcinomatosis. Although in their cases diabetes insipidus was resistant to radiotherapy, they observed one patient who had a complete response of her lung and soft tissue metastasis and in whom the diabetes insipidus disappeared concurrently. Although lung cancer is complicated by a high incidence of CNS metastasis, diabetes insipidus is rare (Krol and Wood 1982).

Haematological malignancies of the leukaemia/lymphoma group are more frequently complicated with diabetes insipidus (Kornberg et al. 1980; Kimmel and O'Neill 1983; Badon et al. 1985; Juan et al. 1985; Smits et al. 1989). Diabetes insipidus can be caused both by direct infiltration, by vascular complications such as bleeding or infarction, or even due to extramedullary haematopoiesis.

Nephrogenic diabetes insipidus

Several diseases, metabolic abnormalities, and drugs can interfere with the normal capacity of the kidney to produce concentrated urine. Kidney infiltration by multiple myeloma as well as amyloidoses can lead to a decreased responsiveness of the kidney to ADH. Prolonged use of diuretics and mannitol can impair the build up of a significant osmotic gradient in the renal medulla. Colchicine, lithium carbonate, amphotericin B, and demeclocycline all lead to a decreased efficacy of ADH on the kidney. A patient with normal kidney function and metastatic leiomyosarcoma was reported to have a primary nephrogenic diabetes insipidus, in the absence of ADH antibodies (Feibush et al. 1980).

Clinical symptomatology

Clinical symptoms consist mainly of pronounced polyuria and polydipsia. Patients drink up to 15–20 l, often very cold drinks per day. This intact thirst mechanism, although often very bothersome, protects patients against more pronounced hypertonicity and the ensuing cellular dehydration. Symptoms due to hypertonicity are listed in Table 7.

Table 7 Symptoms due to hypertonicity

Muscular weakness
Restlessness, irritability, disorientation
Depression, lethargy
Low-grade fever
Intracranial bleeding
Convulsions
Stupor, coma

Diagnosis and treatment

Signs of dehydration, thirst, rapid weight loss, recent infusions and drugs, serum sodium and osmolality, urine volume, and osmolality often are enough to make a correct diagnosis of the pathophysiology of the hypernatraemia.

CT scan and MRI may assist in the diagnosis of metastatic diabetes insipidus. The brain is particularly vulnerable to cellular dehydration. This can lead to rupture of blood vessels connected to the calvarium. To protect itself from these harmful consequences, brain cells generate new intracellular solute, so-called 'idiogenic osmoles'. This takes some time to occur and it will not prevent severe brain dehydration in rapidly-emerging hypernatraemia. On the other hand treatment of a more subacute hypernatraemia with hypotonic fluids may lead to severe brain oedema. A discriminant time interval seems to be between 6 and 12 h, before these protective mechanisms come into action.

The fluid deficit can be estimated from the equation:

$$\text{Body weight} \times 0.65 = \frac{\text{Normal serum sodium} - \text{actual serum sodium}}{\text{Normal serum sodium}}$$

The fluid deficit can be repleted with glucose 5 per cent solutions in alternation with 0.45 per cent NaCl solution. The hypernatraemia should be corrected over 2–3 days. Too rapid correction can lead to brain oedema and should only be undertaken if rapid onset hypernatraemia is suspected and this occurs in the presence of neurological symptoms.

HYPERURICAEMIA

Introduction

Uric acid is the main end-product of the catabolic pathway of the purine bases adenine and guanine. Purines are part of many cellular components, such as DNA, RNA, and of nucleosides, being critical to cellular function, either as an energy source or as second messengers, such as ATP and GTP. Normal metabolism of purine bases leads to the formation of inosinic acid, which is converted to inosine by the enzyme 5'-nucleotidase or to adenylic acid or guanylic acid, both compounds being substrates for nucleic acid and deoxynucleic acid synthesis. Further catabolism of inosine leads to the formation of hypoxanthine, xanthine, and uric acid, successively. Normal serum urate concentrations vary between 0.24 and 0.48 mmol/l and are higher in men than in women. Increased levels are positively correlated with protein intake, alcohol consumption, weight, body mass, and social class. At physiological pH of 7.40 uric acid exists for 98 per cent of the time in its monovalent sodium salt. Serum is saturated with monosodium urate at a concentration of 0.42 mmol/l, but higher levels may remain stable in supersaturated solution for long periods of time and the majority of individuals with hyperuricaemia are asymptomatic. The total body pool of uric acid normally is around 200 mmol (1200 mg) (Boss and Seegmiller 1979). Approximately 60 per cent of the total body pool turns over every day. Two-thirds of the urate formed each day is excreted by the kidney and the remainder is eliminated via the gastrointestinal tract. Gut bacteria metabolize uric acid further to form carbon dioxide and ammonia.

The renal handling of uric acid consists of glomerular filtration, proximal renal tubular reabsorption, active tubular secretion, and post-secretory reabsorption. A variety of factors modify the final uric acid excretion. Expansion of the volume of the extracellular compartment will promote uric acid clearance, whilst volume contraction will have the opposite effect. Acidosis also reduces uric acid excretion, most probably by competitive interaction between different organic acids. Several drugs can influence any of these steps and lead to a change in uricaemia and uricosuria. Urinary pH markedly influences the solubility of uric acid. At pH 5.5 or less, uric acid is present in its free acidic form, whereas at higher pH more uric acid is present as urate. This change in ionization has dramatic consequences on solubility, being 20 mmol/l for the salt and 1.1 mmol/l for the acid (Seegmiller et al. 1963). In the distal portions of the nephron the high urinary concentration of uric acid and the low pH may lead to supersaturation of urine risking the formation of uric acid crystals. Hypoxanthine and xanthine, earlier products of the purine catabolism, are more soluble in an aqueous medium and the beneficial effect of allopurinol in patients with hyperuricaemia is explained by its inhibition of the further metabolism of these compounds to uric acid.

Pathophysiology

Hyperuricaemic nephropathy

Serum urate concentration depends on the balance between purine ingestion, endogenous purine metabolism, and urinary elimination. The mechanisms of hyperuricaemia and/or hyperuricosuria in malignancy are due to an increased production with the eventual aggravating presence of diminished renal excretory capacity, the hyperuricaemia being the consequence of increased cellular turnover. This may result in hyperuricaemic nephropathy and acute renal failure and, only rarely, in acute arthritis. Hyperuricaemic nephropathy is caused by intratubular precipitation of uric acid crystals in the urine oversaturated with uric acid. This form of acute renal failure may be part of the tumour lysis syndrome and occurs only, although not exclusively, after the institution of an effective treatment regimen in patients with haematological malignancies (Kjellstrand et al. 1974; Crittenden and Ackerman 1977). Sporadic cases have been reported in patients with solid tumours (Crittenden and Ackerman 1977). The uric acid load to be disposed of by the kidneys depends on the growth fraction of the tumour, the tumour burden, and the sensitivity of the tumour to the treatment (Tsokos et al. 1981). Some chemotherapeutic agents such as the folic acid antagonists interfere with purine metabolism at a stage before that of uric acid formation and their use more often leads to a decrease in uricosuria. Studies of uric acid metabolism in untreated patients with haematological malignancies disclosed that uricosuria is markedly increased in acute lymphoblastic leukaemia (ALL) and markedly so in acute myelocytic leukaemia and chronic granulocytic leukaemia (Lynch 1962). In ALL the hyperuricosuria has a direct correlation with the peripheral blood cell count. In patients with chronic lymphocytic leukaemia, a disease with a much slower cell turnover, uricosuria was found to be normal in most instances. Among the myeloproliferative disorders, idiopathic myelofibrosis is associated with the most profound hyperuricosuria, polycythaemia vera being the second one of this group. In multiple myeloma the frequent occurrence of impairment of renal function often leads to hyperuricaemia. In patients with solid tumours hyperuricaemia is virtually limited to patients suffering from fast growing and bulky tumours such as testicular teratomas.

Acute arthritis

Secondary gout refers to a condition in which hyperuricaemia is part of a known abnormality as a cause of uric acid overproduction. This most frequently occurs in patients with myeloproliferative disorders, but it is infrequent in patients with underlying non-haematological malignancies. The mechanism by which uric acid crystals invoke an acute inflammatory tissue response is far from clear, but it has been suggested that the release of interleukin-1 by activated macrophages may be responsible for many of the symptoms of acute gouty arthritis.

Clinical manifestations

The acute renal failure due to hyperuricaemic nephropathy is most often of the oliguric or anuric type. Patients usually present with symptoms of uraemia. Most often they have, at the time of diagnosis, an uricaemia in excess of 330 mmol/l. Sometimes flank pain suggestive of ureteral colic is present and voiding of concrement or haematuria may occur.

The onset of acute renal failure in a patient with cancer and an elevated serum uric acid should always lead to a suspicion of hyperuricaemic nephropathy. A positive diagnosis of uric acid-induced renal failure is however not straightforward once uraemia has already been established, as renal failure in itself will produce elevated uric acid levels. In this respect the clinical context of a therapy-sensitive malignancy with a large tumour load and the recent onset of chemo- and/or radiotherapy is important. Kjellstrand et al. (1974), however, described five patients out of a total of 16 patients with haematological malignancies who developed acute renal failure without prior treatment. Urine analysis may reveal the presence of uric acid crystals and the concentration of uric acid in the urine may exceed 25 mmol/l. A urinary uric acid to creatinine ratio above 0.66 is suggestive of hyperuricaemic nephropathy (Kelton et al. 1978), although a similar ratio may occur in acute renal failure due to infection (Tungsanga et al. 1984). Ultrasound examination of the kidney may show distension of the renal pelvis.

Treatment

With insights into the pathophysiology of this condition and the availability of allopurinol most cases of hyperuricaemic nephropathy can be prevented. Vigorous hydration is important in order to prevent dehydration with its associated impairment of uric acid excretion and to stimulate glomerular filtration. A standard infusion of 3–4 l over 24 h aiming at a urinary output of 100 ml/h is recommended to prevent urinary saturation with uric acid (Schilsky 1982) and urinary pH should be kept above 7.0 to improve its solubility. Frequent control of urinary pH should be performed at the bedside. Acetazolamide, a carboxyanhydrase inhibitor, will also lead to alkalinization of the urine and can be administered either orally at a dose of 500 mg twice daily or intravenously (2–3×250 mg). The presence of metabolic acidosis precludes the use of this drug.

Allopurinol and its major oxidation product oxipurinol are inhibitors of xanthine oxidase, the enzyme that catalyses the breakdown of hypoxanthine via xanthine to uric acid. Consequently, more hypoxanthine and xanthine is excreted in the urine and the formation of uric acid is reduced. This is beneficial, as hypoxanthine and xanthine have a higher solubility in aqueous media than uric acid. Allopurinol was originally developed in an attempt to inhibit the degradation of 6-mercaptopurine. Different trials in the mid-1960s established the rôle of allopurinol in the prevention of hyperuricaemia and hyperuricaemic nephropathy (Krakoff and Meyer 1965; DeConti and Calabresi 1966; Muggia et al. 1967). The usual starting dose is 300 mg daily. The long half-life of oxipurinol (18–30 h), makes multiple daily dosing unnecessary. After oral administration in hyperuricaemic patients, a decline in serum uric acid is observed within 24–48 h, although it can take up to 14 days before its maximal effect is reached. A dose–response relationship for allopurinol is present. Patients treated with doses up to 800 mg daily had a more rapid decline in serum uric acid levels compared to those who received 200 mg daily. Allopurinol and oxipurinol excretion is decreased in renal failure, necessitating dose adjustments depending on the prevailing creatinine clearance (Hande et al. 1984). The prolonged half-life of oxipurinol can lead to severe toxicity. Haemodialysis is an effective way of clearing oxipurinol (Kjellstrand et al. 1974). The use of uricosuric agents is not advisable in patients with an increased production. Inhibition of production constitutes a more rational approach.

Side-effects of allopurinol are fever, gastrointestinal discomfort, and dermatitis. Although skin rash is frequent, a generalized hypersensitivity reaction with toxic epidermolysis is a rare complication. Some drug interactions of allopurinol are relevant to patients with malignancy. The biological activity of azathioprine and 6-mercaptopurine is prolonged by allopurinol. Only one-quarter of the scheduled doses should be administered in the presence of allopurinol. Cyclophosphamide is also potentiated by allopurinol. Oral anticoagulants of the coumarin series also have a prolonged half-life, which often makes dose reduction of these drugs necessary.

Once hyperuricaemic nephropathy is present, allopurinol can at best impair further uric acid production, but whether it will reverse renal failure is doubtful (Watts et al. 1966). Other measures can be tried, such as mannitol diuresis and urinary alkalinization. Early use of haemodialysis is, however, the treatment of choice. Haemodialysis is 10–20 times more efficient than peritoneal dialysis in removing uric acid. A 6 h dialysis session reduces serum uric acid levels by 50 per cent (Kjellstrand et al. 1974). The ominous prognosis of this form of acute renal failure has changed dramatically for the better due to early institution of haemodialysis.

Treatment of gouty arthritis associated with malignancy is similar to primary gout. Non-steroidal anti-inflammatory agents are very effective in reducing the inflammatory component, whereas allopurinol is used if recurrent attacks occur. In these circumstances the dose of allopurinol is carefully adjusted to keep serum uric acid levels within the normal range.

TUMOUR LYSIS SYNDROME

Introduction

The tumour lysis syndrome is characterized by the development of hyperphosphataemia, hypocalcaemia, hyperuricaemia, hyperkalaemia, and renal failure, which typically occurs 1–2 days after the initiation of chemotherapy. The syndrome arises most frequently in association with the treatment of rapidly-growing non-Hodgkin's lymphomas and a large tumour load, in particular with Burkitt's lymphoma, with acute lymphoblastic leukaemia, and in some myeloproliferative syndromes, most notably with chronic myelocytic leukaemia in the accelerated phase (Arsenau et al. 1973; Fenneley et al. 1974; Meyers and Jowsey 1974; Muggia et al. 1974; Cohen et al. 1980; Tsokos et al. 1981; Cervantes et al. 1982; Vogler et al. 1983). More recently, tumour lysis syndrome has also been reported in patients with chronic lymphocytic leukaemia (List et al. 1990; McCroskey et al. 1990; Frame et al. 1992; Dann et al. 1993). It is less frequent in the treatment of solid tumours, but case reports have reported its occurrence in patients with breast cancer, small-cell lung cancer, and Merckel cell carcinoma (Vogelzang *et al.* 1983; Stark *et al.* 1987; Dirix *et al.* 1991).

Pathophysiology

Phosphate is the major intracellular anion in any cell, but in lymphoblasts the concentration of phosphorus is four times that of mature lymphocytes (Zusman *et al.* 1973). The massive tumour cell necrosis with release of phosphate will lead to an acute onset hyperphosphataemia, this being more severe in direct correlation with the prevailing serum creatinine. When the ion solubility product of phosphate × calcium concentration is exceeded, calcium phosphate will precipitate in extraskeletal tissues, including the kidney, with concomitant decrease of serum calcium. The risk occurs if the calcium × phosphate concentration reaches 4.6 mmol/l (Herbert LA *et al.* 1966). The nephrocalcinosis will compromise renal function, limiting further the excretory capacity for phosphate.

Hypocalcaemia has early been recognized as a feature of the tumour lysis syndrome (Jaffe *et al.* 1972). It has always been thought to be the consequence of the massive phosphate release into the extracellular compartment. This would be followed by extracellular calcium phosphate deposition (Cadman *et al.* 1977). Although this appears an adequate explanation for the acute hypocalcaemia, it seems insufficient to explain the often prolonged hypocalcaemia seen in this syndrome. The condition of massive rhabdomyolysis in emergency medicine closely resembles the tumour lysis syndrome. Just as in the tumour lysis syndrome, one would expect an augmented parathyroid hormone secretion both for increasing phosphate excretion and mobilizing calcium from the bone as a homeostatic protection against hypocalcaemia. In patients with rhabdomyolysis, PTH levels were appropriately elevated, but $1,25(OH)_2D$ levels were very low. It has been postulated that hyperphosphataemia leads to an altered hydroxylation of vitamin D by the proximal renal tubular cells. As mentioned previously, $1,25(OH)_2D$ has a potentiating rôle on the different effects of PTH. Interestingly, hypocalcaemia was reversed in a patient with the tumour lysis syndrome after treatment with $1,25(OH)_2D$ (Dunlay *et al.* 1989).

The release of intracellular potassium will rapidly lead to hyperkalaemia when renal function is impaired. This may be life-threatening, as the simultaneous occurrence of hypocalcaemia may increase the susceptibility to ventricular fibrillation and sudden death has been reported in patients with the tumour lysis syndrome. Intravenous calcium administration remains the most effective treatment for the electrophysiological abnormalities caused by the hyperkalaemia, even at the risk of causing some increment in calcium phosphate precipitation.

It has become more and more apparent that patients suffering from a wide variety of haematological malignancies have pre-existing, often subclinical renal abnormalities (Tsokos *et al.* 1981). Many patients who develop tumour lysis syndrome have elevated serum uric acid concentrations prior to treatment. This is another threat to renal function, as uric acid nephropathy will further increase potassium, uric acid, and phosphate concentration. Once this stage has been reached, dialysis is the only effective treatment.

Clinical manifestations

Clinical symptomatology is initially limited to non-specific complaints such as general weakness, anorexia, and vomiting. Later on muscle weakness and cramps, convulsions and mental disturbances, cardiac dysrhythmias, and, eventually, ventricular fibrillation and sudden death arise as a consequence of hyperkalaemia and hypocalcaemia. Renal failure is often of the anuric or oliguric form with rapidly increasing blood urea and creatinine levels.

Prevention and treatment

Pre-existing renal function impairment and hyperuricaemia, bulky disease, and increased LDH levels are risk factors for the development of tumour lysis syndrome. Preventive measures should include vigorous intravenous hydration with normal saline (4–5 l over 24 h) provided that kidney and cardiac function allow this. Allopurinol (300 mg/24 h) should be started 2–3 days prior to the initiation of chemotherapy in order to return serum uric acid levels to normal. Intensive hydration and allopurinol administration should be continued for 3–4 days after the start of chemotherapy. Urine alkalinization is efficient in promoting renal uric acid secretion. Urinary pH should be kept above 7 with administration of intravenous sodium bicarbonate, but too high pH values should be avoided as these are associated with an increased risk of phosphate precipitation. Measurement of urinary pH at every micturition and of serum electrolytes, calcium, magnesium, uric acid, and serum albumin at least daily is recommended. Close monitoring of fluid balance is essential, especially in patients with reduced cardiac reserve or renal function. The use of methotrexate under these circumstances may pose an increased risk for unanticipated toxicity due to diminished renal excretion. If, in spite of the above mentioned measures, severe metabolic disturbances emerge, early dialysis should be initiated (Table 8).

LACTIC ACIDOSIS

Introduction

At physiological pH lactic acid is completely dissociated into lactate and hydrogen ions and under normal conditions its concentration in venous blood is maintained between 0.6 and 1.2 mmol/l. Lactate is formed in the cytosol from pyruvate, which is an important intermediate component of glucose metabolism via the Embden Meyerhof pathway. The conversion of pyruvate to lactate is catalysed by lactic dehydrogenase and is affected by intracellular oxygenation and pH. The reaction kinetics are such that the concentration of lactate is approximately ten times higher than that of pyruvate. Most of the lactate is produced in muscles, erythrocytes, brain, skin, and renal medulla. The liver and renal cortex are the organs which remove lactate from the blood by utilizing it as a substrate for glyconeogenesis. This succession of events is called the Cori cycle (Fig. 1). Lactic acidosis arises when the buffer system of the blood is not capable of maintaining pH within the physiological limits of 7.36–7.42. During strong exercise or tissue hypoxia excess lactate is generated, but the large reserve capacity of the liver to extract lactate from the blood will usually prevent overt acidosis, unless utilization of lactate is also compromised. A reduction in hepatic blood flow to less than 30 per cent or severe hypoxia ($Pa_{O_2} < 6.2$ kPa) markedly depresses lactate uptake by the liver and more severe alterations may even lead to net lactate production. Lactate acidosis, therefore, results from both increased production and decreased utilization. Clinical experience has taught that lactic acidosis only occurs when the serum lactate exceeds 4–5 mmol/l.

Table 8 Criteria for haemodialysis in the tumour lysis syndrome[a]

Serum potassium >6 mmol/l
Serum uric acid >600 μmol/l
Serum creatinine >880 μmol/l
Serum phosphorus >3.22 mmol/l
Fluid overload
Symptomatic hypocalcaemia

[a]According to Cohen *et al.* (1980).

Pathophysiology

Lactic acidosis is commonly divided into types A and B, according to the presence or absence of tissue hypoxia (Table 9). Lactic acidosis may be suspected if the anion gap exceeds 18 mEq/l. The anion gap is the amount of anions that escape routine detection and is derived from the equation:

$$\text{anion gap} = [Na^+] + [K^+] - [Cl^-] - [HCO_3^-]$$

Proof of the presence of lactate acidoses will only be obtained by direct measurement of serum pH and lactate, as excess quantities of other organic anions, for example 3-hydroxybutyrate and acetoacetate, will also increase the anion gap. Elevated concentrations of the latter compounds are often present in diabetic ketoacidosis and starvation.

Type A lactic acidosis is the most common type of lactic acidosis, and may be accompanied by signs of tissue hypoxia or poor tissue perfusion. Examples are cardiorespiratory failure and septicaemia. Both increased production and decreased utilization of lactate are thought to be responsible for the hyperlactataemia in these circumstances. Incidentally, however, a type B lactic acidosis has been described in association with malignant disease. Most often this is observed in acute lymphoblastic leukaemia, acute myelocytic leukaemia, high-grade non-Hodgkin's lymphoma, and Hodgkin's disease (Cohen *et al.* 1980; Doolittle *et al.* 1988). Reports of the same phenomenon in patients with solid tumours are even scarcer; however, type B lactic acidosis has been reported in breast carcinoma, colon cancer, small-cell lung carcinoma, osteosarcoma, soft tissue sarcoma, and phaeochromocytoma (Medalle *et al.* 1971; Holroyde *et al.* 1975; Spechler *et al.* 1978; Nadiminti *et al.* 1980; Bornemann *et al.* 1986; Madias 1986). The pathophysiological derangements underlying this condition are incompletely understood, but the high glycolytic capacity of malignant tissue is probably important. Massive, near complete replacement of normal

Table 9 Aetiology of lactic acidosis

Type A: with tissue hypoxia	Type B: without tissue hypoxia
Cardiac failure	Sepsis
Respiratory failure with $Pa_{O_2} < 4.6$ kPa	Diabetes mellitus
Shock from any cause, for example septicaemia	Malignant disease
Severe anaemia	Liver failure
Strong muscular exercise	Drugs, for example biguanides
Generalized convulsions	Intoxications, for example ethanol, salicylates, paracetamol
	Catecholamine excess, for example phaeochromocytoma
	Inborn errors of carbohydrate metabolism

liver by metastatic infiltration was also present in the majority of patients (Sculier *et al.* 1983). Several metabolic studies in cancer patients have demonstrated increased glucose uptake and increased Cori cycle activity (Waterhouse 1974; Holroyde *et al.* 1975). In patients with phaeochromocytoma, lactic acidosis is probably caused by a combination of peripheral vasoconstriction, leading to some degree of tissue hypoxia, and the effects of catecholamines on intermediary metabolism (Bornemann *et al.* 1986). In patients with soft tissue tumours and paraneoplastic hypoglycaemia, the lactic acidosis observed may well be explained by the combination of reactive hypercatecholaemia and decreased liver function due to hypoglycaemia, the first stimulating lactate production and the second a decreased uptake of lactate (Medalle *et al.* 1971). The disappearance of severe lactic acidosis with successful chemotherapy in a patient with Hodgkin's disease lends further support to the concept of tumoural production of lactate (Nadiminti *et al.* 1980).

Symptomatology

Symptoms of lactic acidosis are heavily influenced by the underlying condition. General malaise, anorexia, vomiting, disorientation, cardiac instability, and hyperventilation are symptoms that should alert the clinician to the presence of acidosis. Hypobicarbonataemia and an increased anion gap further support the diagnosis. This should lead to a thorough search for any active infection or other causes of type A lactic acidosis. Only after exclusion of these more common causes of hyperlactataemia should tumour-associated hyperlactataemia be considered.

Treatment

Treatment of lactic acidosis should be directed towards the underlying aetiology. Lactic acidosis carries a poor prognosis and vigorous treatment is necessary, preventing tissue hypoxia and circulatory collapse. The rôle of bicarbonate administration, aimed at the reduction in the degree of acidosis and an improvement of cardiac function, is controversial, the only exception being the correction of acidosis accompanying cardiac arrest. Bicarbonate administration may adversely affect tissue oxygenation by diminishing arterial vasodilatation, oxygen delivery, myocardial contractility, and intracellular pH (Stacpoole *et al.* 1986; Cooper *et al.* 1990; Ritter *et al.* 1990). Sodium dichloroacetate ameliorates lactic acidosis by inhibiting lactate production and increasing lactate uptake in peripheral tissues and stimulates myocardial contractility. The potential advantage of this compound did not translate,

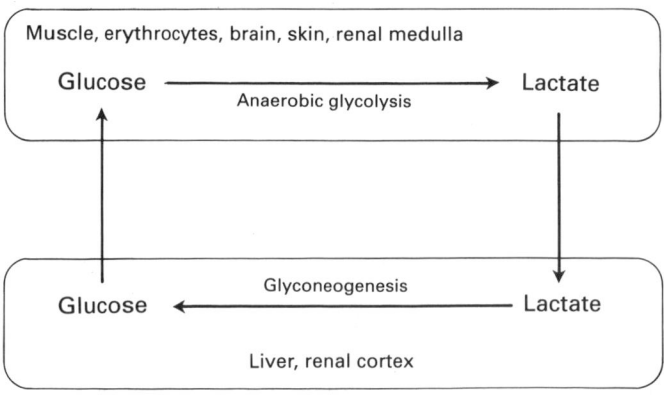

Fig. 1 The Cori cycle.

however, into improved survival of patients being treated with this agent in an intensive care setting (Stacpoole *et al.* 1992). In 'paraneoplastic' lactic acidosis bicarbonate administration may actually increase lactate concentration (Fraley *et al.* 1980). The explanation for this paradoxical effect may be that acidosis in itself inhibits lactate production. Only institution of antitumour directed treatment will have a long-lasting effect.

TUMOUR-ASSOCIATED HYPOGLYCAEMIA

Introduction

Tumour-associated hypoglycaemia (TAH) is a rare disorder in which low insulin levels are found in the presence of severe hypoglycaemia. Its occurrence has been described in non-β-cell tumours of mesenchymal, epithelial, or haematological origin (Table 10). Usually these tumours are slowly growing and bulky (> 1 kg) neoplasms located in the retroperitoneum, the abdomen, or the thorax (Kahn 1980). The tumour types most often associated with tumour-associated hypoglycaemia are fibrosarcoma, mesothelioma, haemangiopericytoma, malignant hepatoma, and adrenocortical carcinoma. Other causes of hypoglycaemia which must be excluded are pancreatic β-cell tumours, drugs (especially insulin, sulphonylureas, alcohol), heapatic, renal, and cardiac disease, sepsis, hormonal deficiencies (cortisol, growth hormone, glucagon), and congenital deficiencies of glycogenic enzymes.

Pathophysiology

Normally fasting blood glucose is maintained between 4 and 5 mmol/l and whenever the blood glucose falls below this level, the liver produces glucose either from glycogen stores or through new synthesis (glyconeogenesis). Hypoglycaemia during fasting may result from decreased production, increased utilization, or a combination. Any severe reduction of functioning liver parenchyma, for example fulminant hepatitis, advanced cirrhosis, or extensive involvement with hepatocellular carcinoma or metastasis, may diminish the synthetic capacity for glucose. Other causes of a decreased production of glucose are deficiency of hormones that stimulate hepatic glucose production such as glucagon, cortisol, and growth hormone, alcohol consumption, and inborn errors of glucose metabolism.

Table 10 Non-β-cell tumours associated with hypoglycaemia

Tumour		Incidence
Mesenchymal tumours		50%
Fibrosarcoma, mesothelioma, neurofibroma, leiomyosarcoma, rhabdomyosarcoma, haemangiopericytoma, spindle cell sarcoma		
Hepatocellular carcinoma		25%
Poorly differentiated (type A)	87%	
Moderately differentiated (type B)	13%	
Adrenocortical carcinoma		5–10%
Gastrointestinal carcinomas		5–10%
Pancreatic and biliary carcinoma		
Lymphomas		5–10%
Other tumours		
Kidney, anaplastic lung tumours, carcinoid, Wilms' tumour, phaeochromocytoma, ovarian carcinoma, neuroblastoma		

Table 11 Differential diagnosis of fasting hypoglycaemia

Disorder	Plasma insulin	C peptide
Insulinoma	↑	↑
Factitious hypoglycaemia		
Sulphonylurea drugs	↑	↑
Exogenous insulin	↑	↓
Low-affinity insulin antibodies	↑	↓
Tumour-associated hypoglycaemia	↓	↓

Glucose utilization is stimulated by insulin. When the blood glucose concentration decreases, insulin secretion is inhibited and when blood glucose levels are below 2.5 mmol/l, plasma insulin becomes undetectable. Circulating antibodies to insulin or the insulin-receptor have occasionally been associated with fasting hypoglycaemia in cancer patients (Braund *et al.* 1987; Walters *et al.* 1987; Redmon *et al.* 1992). Assessment of plasma concentrations of glucose, insulin, and C-peptide (which is co-secreted with endogenous insulin) during hypoglycaemia will usually enable a diagnosis of the underlying cause (Polonsky 1992). A low or undetectable insulin concentration when blood glucose is below 2.5 mmol/l will rule out an insulinoma and points to tumour-associated hypoglycaemia (Table 11).

Investigators have long been puzzled by the mechanism of extrapancreatic tumour-associated hypoglycaemia, as it has been calculated that increased glucose consumption by the tumour could not be the sole explanation (Unger 1966). The identification of insulin-like activity residing in the insulin-like growth factors (IGFs) has greatly contributed to the unravelling of the pathophysiology of this paraneoplastic phenomenon.

Both IGF-I and IGF-II show homology to proinsulin and their rôle in health and disease has been the subject of several reviews (LeRoith 1992; Macaulay 1992; Zapf 1993). IGF-I and IGF-II consist of 70 and 67 amino acid residues, respectively and both have a molecular weight of approximately 7.5 kDa. In the circulation, the IGFs are extensively bound to specific binding proteins (IGFBPs) and, consequently, plasma levels of free IGFs are low. The IGFBPs occur in two forms, a 50 and a 150 kDa complex. Binding of IGFs to IGFBP-3 generates a binary 50 kDa complex and the larger ternary complex is generated by binding of IGFBP-3 to an α-acid labile subunit (Fig. 2). Most of the IGFs in the circulation are bound to the ternary complex (the 'inactive' form), which retains IGFs in the circulation. Only free IGFs and the 50 kDa subunits may traverse the capillary wall, enter the intercellular space, and, thus, expose target tissues to the effects

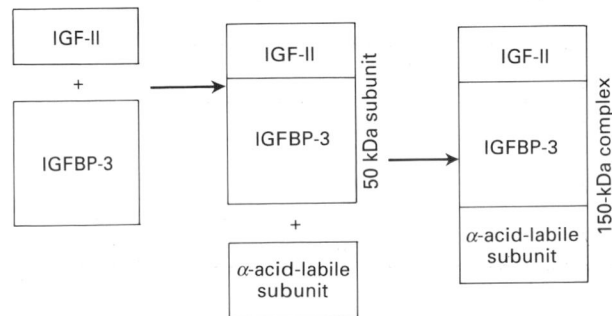

Fig. 2 Generation of the 150 kDa complex consisting of IGF-II, IGFBP-3, and α-subunit.

of IGFs. A feedback system between the IGFBPs, IGF-I, and growth hormone promotes the formation of the 150 kDa complex when plasma concentrations of IGF-I and growth hormone increase. IGF-I and IGF-II each have specific cellular membrane receptors. The receptor for IGF-I shares homology with the insulin receptor, but the IGF-II receptor has a different structure. IGF-II may also activate the receptors for IGF-I and insulin, but this will only occur if IGF-II is present at higher concentrations.

In tumour-associated hypoglycaemia, plasma concentrations of insulin, growth hormone, and IGF-I are decreased, whereas the concentration of IGF-II is normal or slightly elevated. Metabolic studies in tumour-associated hypoglycaemia using clamp techniques showed that the glucose output by the liver was considerably suppressed. After removal of the tumour, plasma levels of growth hormone, insulin, and IGF-I became normal and an increased expression of IGF-II mRNA in the resected material is well documented (Daughaday et al. 1988; Lowe et al. 1989; Schofield et al. 1989; Hoekman et al. 1994). These findings suggested that IGF-II was an important mediator of tumour-associated hypoglycaemia, but how IGF-II accomplished this became clear only after it was appreciated that differences between tumour IGF-II and normal IGF-II altered the affinity of tumour IGF-II to IGFBPs (Daughaday 1988). Normal IGF-II is synthesized as proIGF-II, which consists of IGF-II with a carboxy terminal extension of 89 amino acids, the E-domain (Rotwein 1991). During the processing of this proIGF-II stepwise cleavage of the E-domain yields immature IGF-II fragments that are bigger than normal IGF-II. The IGF-II secreted by tumours associated with tumour-associated hypoglycaemia appears to be in the incompletely processed and slightly modified form (Daughaday et al. 1993). These immature fragments are only incompletely recognized by IGF-II RIA, but possess biological activity. This 'big' IGF-II can still bind to smaller (< 50 kDa) binary complexes, but the generation of the larger 150 kDA ternary complex consisting of IGFBP-3 and the α-subunit is inhibited (Daughaday and Kapadia 1989; Zapf et al. 1992). Thus, in tumour-associated hypoglycaemia more IGF-II in the circulation appears in a form that facilitates access to the tissues. The increased concentration of free IGF-II may easily activate insulin receptors and suppress insulin, IGF-I, and growth hormone levels (Ron et al. 1989). The hypoglycaemia is thought to arise through interaction of 'big' IGF-II with the receptors of IGF-I and insulin, leading to stimulation of glucose uptake by muscles, fat, and, potentially, also by tumour cells, while glucose output by the liver is suppressed.

Symptomatology

Symptoms of hypoglycaemia usually occur when blood glucose is below 2.5 mmol/l, but the set point varies from person to person. In patients who have frequent hypoglycaemic attacks the set point before symptoms arise may become considerably lower, whereas the reverse is true for patients with poorly controlled diabetes mellitus. Symptomatology of tumour-associated hypoglycaemia is similar to that of insulinoma and many other causes of hypoglycaemia and consists of pallor, sweating, behavioural changes, drowsiness, seizures, and coma. The attacks in tumour-associated hypoglycaemia occur most often at night or at waking. The onset may be insidious and initially rapidly relieved by food or administration of glucose. Unlike patients with insulinoma, patients with tumour-associated hypoglycaemia frequently lose weight, despite their increased intake of food.

Treatment

The only effective treatment of tumour-associated hypoglycaemia is removal of the tumour. If this is not feasible, resection of the tumour bulk will alleviate the symptoms. Regular meals, divided over the day and at night, are recommended. When effective antitumour treatment becomes more problematic, the severity and frequency of the attacks will increase. Sometimes dexamethasone is temporarily beneficial, but eventually patients have to be kept on continuous intravenous administration of glucose. Unlike the situation in insulinoma, long-acting analogues of somatostatin are not particularly helpful (Joffe et al. 1988). However, alleviation of the hypoglycaemia has been noticed incidentally in patients being treated with growth hormone (Teale et al. 1992).

HYPERCORTISOLISM

Introduction

Symptomatic hypercortisolism (Cushing's syndrome) is a rare disorder. It mainly results from increased production of adrenocorticotrophic hormone (ACTH), either in pituitary or non-pituitary ('ectopic') tumours. Only in the minority of cases tumours from adrenal origin produce glucocorticoids autonomously (Table 12). In normal subjects cortisol is secreted in a circadian rhythm: levels peak early in the morning and are lowest around midnight. Ninety per cent of circulating cortisol is bound to cortisol binding globulin (CBG). The binding reaches saturation with cortisol concentrations of approximately 650 nmol/l. Unbound (free) cortisol is filtered by the glomerulus and urinary excretion of free cortisol will exponentially increase as the binding capacity of CBG is exceeded. As conventional plasma cortisol assays measure total cortisol, conditions associated with increased CBG content, for example oestrogen treatment, pregnancy, and oral contraceptive use, may falsely suggest hypercortisolism. However, the unbound, biologically active fraction will be normal and urinary-free cortisol concentration will not be elevated. Plasma cortisol has a double negative feedback on its own secretion by inhibiting hypothalamic secretion of corticotrophin-releasing hormone (CRH) and pituitary ACTH production.

ACTH is derived from a larger precursor molecule, pro-opiomelanocortin (POMC). Processing of POMC to smaller peptides yields pro-ACTH and β-lipotrophin (βLPH) and further

Table 12 Prevalence of the different aetiologies of Cushing's syndrome

ACTH dependent 79%	Pituitary 80%
	Ectopic 15%
	Indeterminate 5%
ACTH independent 21%	Adrenal adenoma 80%
	Adrenal carcinoma 20%

Data from Trainer and Grossman (1991).

cleavage leads to the formation of ACTH, melanocyte stimulating hormone, β-endorphin, and several related peptides (reviewed in White *et al.* (1990)). Under normal conditions the synthesis and release of ACTH at the pituitary level is regulated by CRH, arginine vasopressin (AVP), oxytocin, catecholamines, glucocorticoids, and a number of other hormones. These provide for the circadian rhythm of ACTH and the acute stress-related ACTH response, although the underlying regulatory mechanisms are incompletely understood. Transcription of the POMC gene, a process which is stimulated by CRH and inhibited by cortisol, occurs predominantly, but not exclusively, in the pituitary gland. Low level expression of the POMC gene has been found in a large variety of tissues, including adrenal, testis, spleen, kidney, ovary, lung, thyroid, liver, colon, and duodenum (DeBold *et al.* 1988). The size of the POMC mRNA isolated from these sources is usually significantly shorter than that in the pituitary and it is uncertain to what extent these POMC-derived products reach the circulation (White *et al.* 1990).

Pathophysiology

The pathophysiological mechanisms of Cushing's syndrome are summarized in Table 13. Several reviews have summarized the differences in clinical manifestations and molecular biology between pituitary adenomas versus ectopic ACTH-producing tumours (Gold 1979; White *et al.* 1990; White and Clark 1993). In pituitary corticotrophic adenomas circadian rhythmicity of ACTH secretion is usually absent, but ACTH release remains suppressible by exogenous corticosteroids and can be stimulated by CRH. POMC gene expression and transcription and the enzymatic processing of POMC are usually qualitatively unaltered (de Keyzer *et al.* 1985; Clark *et al.* 1989), the exception to this being some large aggressive pituitary tumours, which can present with the clinical features of ectopic ACTH syndrome (Hale *et al.* 1985). This contrasts with non-pituitary ACTH-producing tumours, in which POMC gene expression and the enzymatic cleavage of POMC are frequently altered (de Keyzer *et al.* 1985) and the response to exogenous steroids and CRH is absent or impaired.

It remains an enigma as to why tumours derived from non-endocrine tissues may become secretors of hormones such as ACTH, although it has become evident that many different types of tumours contain immunoreactive ACTH, β-endorphin, and other POMC-derived peptides (Bloomfield *et al.* 1977; DeBold *et al.* 1988). Apart from small quantities of the normal pituitary POMC mRNA transcript, many tumours also contain a larger species of POMC mRNA (DeKeyzer *et al.* 1985; Clark *et al.* 1989). In addition, short transcripts have been found, probably identical to the short transcripts found in normal tissues (DeBold *et al.* 1988). This indicates that many tumours apparently are able to synthesize POMC peptides, although only a minority of them give rise to symptoms of hormonal overproduction. Thus, it is unclear whether the 'ectopic' secretion of ACTH is merely inappropriate secretion

Table 13 Pathogenetic mechanisms of Cushing's syndrome

Cushing's disease (pituitary microadenoma secreting ACTH)
Ectopic ACTH production
Ectopic corticotrophin-releasing hormone (CRH) production
Adrenal adenoma and nodular adrenal hyperplasia
Adrenal carcinoma
Pseudo-Cushing's syndrome in alcoholism, obesity, or depression
Exogenous steroid treatment

Table 14 Distribution of underlying tumours in 51 patients with ectopic ACTH secretion

Type of cancer	Number of patients	
Bronchogenic carcinoma	15	
Small-cell		19
Large-cell		2
Adenocarcinoma		3
Squamous cell		1
Carcinoid tumours	8	
Bronchus		4
Thymus		1
Oesophagus		1
Stomach		1
Duodenum		1
Malignant thymoma	5	
Pancreatic islet cell carcinoma	3	
Medullary thyroid carcinoma	3	
Oesophageal oat cell carcinoma	3	
Squamous laryngeal carcinoma	1	
Phaeochromocytoma	1	
Plasmocytoma	1	
Small-cell, unknown primary	1	

Data from Imura (1980).

or truly ectopic. Tentatively it has been suggested that the tumour products transcribed from short POMC mRNA may not be in a form that can be secreted by the cell (White *et al.* 1990) or that high molecular weight ACTH precursor molecules have reduced bioactivity (Odell *et al.* 1991). While this could explain the presence of increased levels of ACTH precursors and βLPH in the blood of 50 per cent of patients with lung cancer without causing symptoms of Cushing's syndrome (Odell and Wolphsen 1978), many questions remain. Interestingly, ectopic ACTH syndrome may be confined to tumours capable of generating high amounts of a precursor transcript similar to that found in the pituitary, a phenomenon that seems to be restricted to an occasional tumour with features of neuroendocrine differentiation (Texier *et al.* 1991). The tumour types most commonly associated with ectopic ACTH secretion are small-cell lung cancer (SCLC) and bronchial carcinoids.

Epidemiological considerations

The overall incidence of ectopic ACTH-secreting tumours is low. Based on retrospective surveys ectopic ACTH secretion had been diagnosed in less than 5 per cent of patients with small-cell lung cancer (Shepherd *et al.* 1992; Delisle 1993). Similarly, only 15 cases of ectopic Cushing's syndrome associated with bronchial carcinoids were identified over a 40 year period during which a total of 626 patients were evaluated for bronchial carcinoid tumours (Limper *et al.* 1992). In only approximately half of the patients with small-cell lung cancer was Cushing's syndrome found at initial diagnosis; in the remainder this was associated with recurrent disease. The striking female preponderance of pituitary corticotrophic adenomas (male–female ratio 1:8) contrasts with the male preponderance of ectopic ACTH-producing tumours. This can be mainly attributed to the large proportion of small-cell lung cancer, which is more prevalent in males. Carcinoid tumours associated with ectopic secretion of ACTH may have an even higher male to female ratio (Findling and Tyrrell 1986). In children with Cushing's syndrome, adrenal tumours as the cause of hypercortisolism predominate.

Table 15 Clinical features of Cushing's syndrome. Frequency of classical symptoms versus symptoms in ectopic ACTH syndrome

Classical Cushing's syndrome[a]		Ectopic ACTH syndrome			
		Small-cell lung cancer[b]		Occult tumours[c]	
Symptom	(%)	Symptom	(%)	Symptom	(%)
Obesity	88	Peripheral oedema	83	Centripetal obesity	100
Moon face	75	Proximal myopathy	61	Proximal myopathy	100
Hypertension	74	Moon face	52	Moon face	100
Hirsutism	64	Truncal obesity	35	Polydipsia/polyuria	100
Muscle weakness	61	Hyperpigmentation	22	Mental disorders	100
Menstrual disorders	60	Psychosis	22	Hirsutism in women	100
Acne	45	Hypertension	22	Hypertension	70
Ecchymoses	42	Ecchymoses	17	Ecchymoses	50
Mental disorders	42	Hirsutism	4	Acne	50
Backache (osteoporosis)	40	Striae	4	Oedema	50
				Striae	40
				Pigmentation	30

Derived from data of: [a]Gold (1979); [b]Shepherd *et al.* (1992); [c]Howlett *et al.* (1986).

Symptomatology

Cushing's syndrome is a characteristic array of clinical features that gradually develop as a result of prolonged overproduction of cortisol. Consequently, classical symptoms of Cushing's syndrome may be absent in patients with ACTH-producing tumours associated with an aggressive clinical course, such as small-cell lung cancer (Table 15). In patients with slowly growing tumours, such as carcinoids, the clinical presentation may be much more complete due to the longer natural history of the underlying disease in comparison with bronchogenic carcinoma and symptoms of Cushing's syndrome may even precede the clinical diagnosis for many years in 'occult tumours', which usually prove to be small carcinoids (Findling and Tyrrell 1986). However, with the advent of CT scanning these 'occult tumours' are nowadays more often detected (White *et al.* 1982).

Metabolic abnormalities may be the only clue to the diagnosis of ectopic ACTH production. Hypokalaemia, proximal muscle weakness, weight loss, oedema, hypoglycaemia, mental disorders, and striking hyperpigmentation are often prominent features. Hypokalaemia, sometimes associated with metabolic alkalosis, is present in more than 90 per cent of patients with the ectopic ACTH syndrome, compared to an incidence of 10 per cent in Cushing's syndrome of other aetiologies (Howlett *et al.* 1986). Conventionally, hypokalaemic alkalosis in ectopic ACTH syndrome has been attributed to increased secretion of DOC or corticosterone. Alternatively, the hypokalaemia may be accounted for by a direct inhibitory influence of high circulating ACTH levels on 11β-hydroxysteroid dehydrogenase in the kidney. As a consequence, peripheral conversion of cortisol to cortisone decreases, resulting in a relatively increased level of cortisol in ectopic ACTH syndrome, compared to other causes of Cushing's syndrome. It was suggested that under these circumstances cortisol might act as a mineralocorticoid (Walker *et al.* 1992). Other metabolic disturbances, such as decreased glucose tolerance and overt diabetes mellitus, occur frequently in all causes of Cushing's syndrome and do not provide a diagnostic clue.

Diagnosis and treatment

A suggestive clinical presentation will usually be the stimulus for further investigation. The laboratory diagnosis of Cushing's syndrome requires the demonstration of sustained cortisol overproduction with at least a certain degree of autonomy. As an initial screening test measurement of the excretion of free cortisol in a 24 h urine sample is superior to urinary 17-keto- and 17-hydroxycorticosteroids. The test is not influenced by alterations in plasma CBG content, as the kidneys only filter unbound cortisol and smooth out the variations in cortisol during the day. In normal subjects urinary-free cortisol excretion is below 270 mmol/day (Blunt *et al.* 1990). The false-negative rate is approximately 5 per cent, but in 11 per cent of patients with proven Cushing's syndrome at least one (out of 4) sample was in the normal range (Nieman and Cutler 1990). Repeated sampling over 3 or 4 days will thus increase the sensitivity of the test and a normal result makes the diagnosis of Cushing's syndrome extremely unlikely. If the result is ambiguous, plasma cortisol measurements are indicated. Single plasma cortisol measurements are of little use, as cortisol values fluctuate during the day and are subject to stress-like conditions. Measured cortisol values may also be elevated in conditions associated with increases in CBG, while the free cortisol will be normal. Sampling of cortisol values at 9.00 a.m. and at midnight may reveal the absence of circadian rhythmicity, but in general dynamic tests have to be preferred. Dexamethasone, which does not cross-react in most radioimmunoassays for cortisol, is commonly used for the assessment of the integrity of the hypothalamic–pituitary–adrenal axis and in the differential diagnosis of Cushing's syndrome. A dose of 0.5–1 mg of dexamethasone administered to normal subjects at bedtime will suppress morning plasma cortisol levels to below 50 nmol/l, depending on laboratory conditions and can conveniently be performed in the out-patient clinic (Trainer and Grossman 1991). Reportedly, the 1 mg overnight dexamethasone suppression test has a false-negative rate of 2 per cent or less, but the false-positive rate is 12.5 per cent (Cronin *et al.* 1990). Plasma cortisol and urinary free cortisol measurements after administration of 2–8 mg dexamethasone for 48 h and cortisol measurements during deliberately invoked hypoglycaemia may be required to differentiate between Cushing's syndrome and other conditions mimicking this disorder, notably obesity, depression, and alcoholism and to distinguish Cushing's disease from the ectopic ACTH syndrome (Howlett *et al.* 1986; Blunt *et al.* 1990; Trainer and Grossman 1991).

Plasma ACTH measurements are most useful in differentiating adrenal overproduction of cortisol from other causes of Cushing's syndrome. In the absence of exogenous corticosteroid administration, a low or undetectable plasma ACTH concentration is a strong indication that the adrenals are the source of the increased cortisol production. Plasma ACTH levels are usually unhelpful in the differentiation between Cushing's syndrome of pituitary or ectopic origin. Circulating ACTH levels in patients with pituitary Cushing's syndrome may be within the normal laboratory range, although sequential sampling over several hours may reveal the occurrence of elevated concentrations (White *et al.* 1990). Greatly increased plasma ACTH levels have been described in the majority of patients with the ectopic ACTH syndrome, but they cannot be used to discriminate between patients with pituitary and non-pituitary tumours because ACTH concentrations do overlap with those found in pituitary hypercortisolism (Howlett *et al.* 1986; Trainer and Grossman 1991). Observations of tumoural production of CRH and only secondary increase in ACTH and cortisol makes the differential diagnosis even more challenging (Asa *et al.* 1984; Carey *et al.* 1984; Belsky *et al.* 1985). Moreover, co-secretion of other hormones, for example bombesin, calcitonin, antidiuretic hormone, and gastrin, may complicate the clinical presentation. The differentiation between pituitary and ectopic ACTH-producing tumours has been reported to be improved by measurement of circulating ACTH precursor molecules, which occur in increased concentrations in the blood of patients with the ectopic ACTH syndrome (Crossby *et al.* 1988; White *et al.* 1993).

While none of the tests appears fully capable of distinguishing the differing aetiologies of Cushing's syndrome, the clinical presentation and CT and NMR imaging procedures will usually provide additional information for establishing a diagnosis and treatment plan. NMR appears superior to CT scanning in localizing small pituitary adenomas (Kaye and Crapo 1990). CT scanning of the chest and abdomen is often helpful in localizing ectopic ACTH producing tumours and for detecting metastases. If results are indeterminate, selective venous sampling of ACTH and eventually other tumour products that have been identified on screening, could be considered.

Pituitary adenomas, adrenal tumours, and carcinoids are preferably treated with surgical resection. Ectopic ACTH syndrome associated with small-cell lung cancer must be treated with chemotherapy. Results of treatment are, however, poor. The median survival of these patients is less than that of patients with small-cell lung cancer without this syndrome due to a high incidence of infectious complications and gastrointestinal bleeding and ulceration (Shepherd *et al.* 1992; Delisle *et al.* 1993).

If tumour reduction is not feasible or the cause of hypercortisolism remains obscure, medical treatment is indicated. Mitotane, metyrapone, and ketoconazole have all been used to interfere with adrenal steroid production (Orth *et al.* 1971; Carey *et al.* 1973; Feldman 1986). Perhaps ketoconazole is the drug of choice, because its toxicity profile compares favourably with that of other compounds. Doses of 400–1200 mg will rapidly block corticosteroid synthesis in Cushing's disease, but in four patients with ectopic ACTH syndrome the effect was only temporary or incomplete (Tabarin *et al.* 1991).

ADRENAL CORTICAL FAILURE
Aetiology

Adrenocortical failure is a rare disorder in the general population, but may be more frequently encountered in a population consisting of cancer patients. The recognition of the syndrome is important because it affects a patient's well-being and may present as a life-threatening disease, yet proper treatment will reverse the condition rapidly. The clinical manifestations mainly result from deficiency of glucocorticoid and mineralocorticoid activity, although other hormone inadequacies may also be present. Both diseases of the adrenocortex and hypothalamic–pituitary disorders may lead to adrenocortical failure, the clinical presentation depending on the underlying cause and the rapidity of its onset. Acute pituitary insufficiency can result from sudden haemorrhage in a large pituitary tumour and constitutes a medical emergency (Cardoso and Petersen 1984; Onesti *et al.* 1990). Patients will experience severe headache, vomiting, and frequently acute visual field loss. Radiographs of the sella region, CT scanning, or NMR will reveal the presence of a mass lesion (Kyle *et al.* 1990). Treatment consists of immediate transsphenoidal decompression of the optic chiasma and institution of corticosteroid administration, after blood samples have been taken for hormonal assays. Chronic hypopituitarism may result from pituitary tumours, craniopharyngioma, autoimmune disease, amyloidosis, granulomatous disease, and extensive metastasis, causing either isolated ACTH deficiency or, more commonly, multiple alterations in the secretion of pituitary hormones (reviewed in Gaillard 1992). Acute adrenal insufficiency may result from adrenal haemorrhage, but more frequently the condition is precipitated by stress-like conditions, for example surgery or an intercurrent infection, in a patient in whom subclinical Addison's disease has been present. The differing aetiologies of adrenocortical failure are summarized in Table 16. A full discussion of the various autoimmune disorders and endocrine syndromes that may lead to adrenal insufficiency is beyond the scope of this chapter and will be found in endocrinological textbooks (Burke 1992). AIDS-related abnormalities of adrenocortical function are discussed in Dluhy (1990).

Table 16 Aetiology of adrenal cortical insufficiency

Autoimmune disease
    Adrenal cytoplasmic antibodies
    ACTH receptor blocking antibodies
Infection
    Tuberculosis, histoplasmosis, blastomycosis
    AIDS related
Bilateral adrenal metastases
    Lung and breast carcinoma, malignant melanoma
    Non-Hodgkin's lymphoma
Haemorrhage
    Anticoagulation (heparin)
    Post-operative
    Sepsis (Waterhouse-Friedrichsen syndrome)
Drugs interfering with steroidogenesis
    Imidazole derivates (ketoconazole, etomidate), metyrapone
    Aminogluthetimide, trilostane, RU486, *o,p*,DDD (mitotane)
    Suramin
    Medroxyprogesterone acetate
Recent corticosteroid withdrawal

The adrenal glands are a common site for metastases and at autopsy malignant infiltration of the adrenal glands has been found in 8.6–27 per cent of cases (Mor *et al.* 1985). The incidence of adrenal metastases is particularly high in breast cancer (58 per cent), malignant melanoma (50 per cent), lung carcinoma (42 per cent), and non-Hodgkin's lymphoma (25 per cent) (Kannan 1988). The general opinion is that these metastases rarely give rise to adrenocortical failure, unless more than 75–90 per cent of adrenocortical tissue has been destroyed. However, this does not take into account the limited adrenal reserve that may remain subclinical unless severe stress is induced. Several authors have reported that symptoms of adrenocortical failure in patients with bilateral adrenal metastases on CT scanning occurred at a higher than expected incidence and have recommended assessment of adrenocortical function in these circumstances (Seidenwurm *et al.* 1984; Gamelin *et al.* 1992).

Adrenal haemorrhage most frequently develops in association with heparin treatment (Dahlberg *et al.* 1990). Adrenal haemorrhage may complicate surgery or sepsis, but a provoking condition is not always clear. Typically the patient develops acute flank pain, fever, tachycardia, and hypotension, whereas laboratory investigations often reveal hyponatraemia. The diagnosis requires confirmation by the biochemical demonstration of adrenal insufficiency, while CT scans will show bilateral adrenal enlargement that shrinks with time (Siu *et al.* 1990).

A number of drugs being used for the treatment of cancer are associated with risk of adrenal failure. Aminoglutethimide was originally introduced as a 'medical adrenalectomy' for breast cancer patients (Hughes and Burley 1970), although inhibition of steroidogenesis most probably is not of clinical relevance at the presently used dosage of approximately 500 mg daily (Hoffken *et al.* 1986). Mitotane (o',p'-DDD) and suramin were considered for the treatment of adrenocortical carcinoma because of their ability to produce adrenal cortical necrosis (Gutierrez and Crooke 1980; Feuillan *et al.* 1987). Presently, suramin is being investigated for the treatment of prostate cancer. Similarly, high-dose ketoconazole (800–1200 mg) has been used for the treatment of prostate carcinoma and Cushing's syndrome after it was demonstrated that the drug could inhibit cytochrome P450-dependent steps in steroidogenesis (Feldman 1986). More recently the abrupt onset of adrenal failure after withdrawal of medroxyprogesterone acetate has been observed in breast cancer patients who had received treatment with this agent for more than 2 years (Hug *et al.* 1991). Temporary suppression of adrenocortical function should be considered in patients who receive high-dose corticosteroids, for example in anti-emetic regimens.

Symptomatology

In acute primary adrenocortical failure (Addisonian crisis) unexplained hypovolaemic shock, fever, and tachycardia may dominate the clinical presentation. Chronic adrenal failure usually presents with general weakness, fatigue, and (orthostatic) hypotension. Other symptoms include anorexia, nausea and vomiting, myalgias, and abdominal cramping. Hyperpigmentation in the White race is characterically present around recent scars and the creases of the palms of the hands; in all races patchy pigmentation on the buccal mucosa is seen. This ACTH-related hyperpigmentation is not a feature of secondary adrenal failure.

Laboratory diagnosis

In primary adrenal insufficiency the biochemical findings are related to glucocorticoid and mineralocorticoid deficiencies. Hyponatraemia,

hypovolaemia, elevated urea, and an increased urinary sodium concentration occur in more than 90 per cent of patients, whereas hyperkalaemia is present in approximately 60 per cent of cases. Occasionally mild hypercalcaemia and hypoglycaemia are observed (Kokko 1985). Inappropriately elevated ADH levels in glucocorticoid deficiency will impair free water excretion, but this will rapidly be corrected after glucocorticoid replacement therapy (Kamoi *et al.* 1993). In secondary adrenal failure mineralocorticoid activity is usually better preserved. Hyponatraemia is present, but patients appear water intoxicated and serum potassium levels are less often increased.

Confirmation of the diagnosis is obtained by assessment of free cortisol excretion in a 24 h urine collection and the demonstration of functional impairment of cortisol secretion in response to a test dose of 0.25 mg synthetic ACTH. Plasma ACTH levels will discriminate between primary and secondary adrenal failure, low levels being found in secondary failure.

Treatment

When adrenocortical failure is suspected in an emergency, 50–100 mg of hydrocortisone acetate should be administered intravenously, after blood has been taken for glucose, electrolyte, cortisol, and aldosterone assessments. Parenteral fluid administration should be carefully monitored because of the relative inability of these patients to excrete free water. Long-term treatment consists of replacement doses of corticosteroids, preferably hydrocortisone (20 mg in the morning and 10 mg in the evening). Alternatively, cortisone acetate (25 mg) or prednisone (5 mg in the morning and half of the same dose in the evening) may be used. Patients with primary adrenal failure will usually need exogenous substitution of mineralocorticoid activity. This is supplied with fludrocortisone (0.05–0.15 mg daily). While the recommended hydrocortisone dosages will usually suffice in uncomplicated adrenocortical failure, higher dosages may be required in patients treated with mitotane or suramin. Under conditions of stress, such as surgery and infections, dosages should be increased, for example hydrocortisone 50–100 mg orally or intravenously three times daily.

REFERENCES

Agus ZS (1983). Oncogenic hypophosphatemic osteomalacia. *Kidney International*, 24:113–23.

Agus ZA, Wasserstein A, Goldfarb S (1982). Disorders of calcium and magnesium homeostasis. *American Journal of Medicine*, 72:473–87.

Amatruda TT, *et al.* (1963). Carcinoma of the lung with inappropriate antidiuresis. Demonstration of antidiuretic-hormone-like activity in tumor extract. *New England Journal of Medicine*, 269:544–9.

Anghileri L (1971). Studies on the accumulation mechanisms of radioisotopes used in tumor scanning. *Strahlentherapie*, 456–62.

Antony A, Robinson WA, Roy C, Pelander W, Donohue R (1980). Inappropriate ADH secretion after high-dose vinblastine. *Journal of Urology*, 123:783–4.

Arseneau JC, Bagley CXM, Anderson T, Canellos GP (1973). Hyperkalaemia, a sequel to chemotherapy of Burkitt's lymphoma. *Lancet*, i:10–14.

Asa SL, *et al.* (1984). Cushing's disease associated with an intrasellar gangliocytoma producing corticotrophin-releasing factor. *Annals of Internal Medicine*, 101:789–93.

Athanasou NA, *et al.* (1989). The origin and nature of stromal osteoclast-like multinucleated giant cells in breast carcinoma: implications for tumour osteolysis and macrophage biology. *British Journal of Cancer*, 59:491–8.

Badon SJ, *et al.* (1985). Diabetes insipidus caused by extra medullary hematopoiesis. *American Journal of Clinical Pathology*, 83:509–12.

Bataille R, *et al.* (1989). Spontaneous secretion of tumor necrosis factor-beta by human myeloma cell lines. *Cancer*, 63:877–80.

Belsky JL, *et al.* (1985). Cushing's syndrome due to ectopic production of corticotropin-releasing factor. *Journal of Clinical Endocrinology and Metabolism*, **60**:496–500.

Berl T (1990). Treating hyponatraemia: what is all the controversy about? *Annals of Internal Medicine*, **113**:417–19.

Berry EM, *et al.* (1973). Variations in plasma calcium with induced changes in plasma specific gravity, total protein and albumin. *British Medical Journal*, **4**:640–3.

Binstock ML, Mundy GR (1980). Effect of calcitonin and glucocorticoids in combination on the hypercalcemia of malignancy. *Annals of Internal Medicine*, **93**:269–72.

Blachley JD, Hill JB (1981). Renal and electrolyte disturbances associated with cisplatin. *Annals of Internal Medicine*, **95**:628–32.

Blomqvist CP (1986). Malignant hypercalcaemia—a hospital survey. *Acta Medica Scandinavica*, **220**:455–63.

Bloomfield GA, *et al.* (1977). Lung tumours and ACTH production. *Clinical Endocrinology*, **6**:95–104.

Blunt SB, Sandler LM, Burrin JM, Joplin GF (1990). An evaluation of the distinction of ectopic and pituitary ACTH dependent Cushing's syndrome by clinical features, biochemical tests and radiological findings. *Quarterly Journal of Medicine*, **77**:1113–33.

Bockman RS (1980). Hypercalcemia in malignancy. *Clinics in Endocrinology and Metabolism*, **9**:317–33.

Bockman RS, *et al.* (1986). Gallium increases bone calcium and crystallite perfection of hydroxyapatite. *Calcified Tissue International*, **39**:376–81.

Bockman RS, *et al.* (1990). Gallium localization in bone: micron range resolution using synchrotron X-ray microscopy. *Proceedings of the National Academy of Sciences USA*, **87**:4149–53.

Body JJ, *et al.* (1987). Dose/response study of aminohydroxypropylidene bisphosphonate in tumor-associated hypercalcemia. *American Journal of Medicine*, **82**:957–63.

Bornemann M, Hill SC, Kid II GS (1986). Lactic acidosis in pheochromocytoma. *Annals of Internal Medicine*, **105**:880–2.

Boss GR, Seegmiller JE (1979). Hyperuricemia and gout. *New England Journal of Medicine*, **300**:1459–68.

Braund WJ, *et al.* (1987). Autoimmunity to insulin receptor and hypoglycaemia in patient with Hodgkin's disease. *Lancet*, **i**:237–40.

Broder S (1984). T-cell lymphoproliferative syndrome associated with human T-cell leukemia/lymphoma virus. *Annals of Internal Medicine*, **100**:543–57.

Buckle R (1974). Ectopic PTH syndrome, pseudohyperparathyroidism: hypercalcemia of malignancy. *Clinics in Endocrinology and Metabolism*, **3**:237–50.

Budayr AA, *et al.* (1989). Increased serum levels of a parathyroid hormone-like protein in malignancy-associated hypercalcemia. *Annals of Internal Medicine*, **111**:807–12.

Burke CW (1992). Primary adrenocortical failure. In *Clinical endocrinology* (ed. A Grossman), pp. 393–404. Blackwell, Oxford.

Cadman EC, Lundberg WB, Bertino JR (1977). Hyperphosphatemia and hypocalcemia accompanying rapid cell lysis in a patient with Burkitt's lymphoma and Burkitt cell leukemia. *American Journal of Medicine*, **62**:283–90.

Cardoso ER, Petersen EW (1984). Pituitary apoplexy: a review. *Neurosurgery*, **14**:363–73.

Carey RM, Orth DN, Hartmann W (1973). Malignant melanoma with ectopic production of adrenocorticotropic hormone: palliative treatment with inhibitors of adrenal steroid biosynthesis. *Journal of Clinical Endocrinology and Metabolism*, **36**:482–7.

Carey RM, *et al.* (1984). Ectopic secretion of corticotropin-releasing factor as a cause of Cushing's syndrome. *New England Journal of Medicine*, **311**:13–20.

Cervantes F, Ribera JM, Granena A, Montserrat E, Rozman C (1982). Tumour lysis syndrome with hypocalcemia in accelerated chronic granulocytic leukemia. *Acta Haematologica*, **68**:157–9.

Chew D, Playfer JR (1988). Hypercalcemia in a patient with non-secretory myeloma. *Postgraduate Medical Journal*, **64**:438–40.

Clark AJL, Lavender PM, Besser GM, Rees LH (1989). Pro-opiomelanocortin in ACTH-dependent Cushing's syndrome. *Journal of Molecular Endocrinology*, **2**:3–9.

Clements JA, Funder JW (1986). Arginine vasopressin (AVP) and AVP-like immunoreactivity in peripheral tissues. *Endocrine Reviews*, **7**:449–65.

Cluitmans FHM, Meinders AE (1990). Management of severe hyponatraemia: rapid or slow correction? *American Journal of Medicine*, **88**:161–6.

Cohen LF, Balow JE, Magrath IT, Poplack DG, Ziegler JL (1980). Acute tumor lysis syndrome. A review of 37 patients with Burkitt's lymphoma. *American Journal of Medicine*, **68**:486–91.

Coleman RE, Rubens RD (1987). 3-(Amino-1, 1-hydroxypropylidene) bisphosphonate (APD) for hypercalcaemia of breast cancer. *British Journal of Cancer*, **56**:465–9.

Coleman RE, Rubens RD (1987). The clinical course of bone metastases from breast cancer. *British Journal of Cancer*, **55**:61–6.

Comis RL, Miller M, Ginsberg SJ (1980). Abnormalities in water homeostasis in small cell anaplastic lung cancer. *Cancer*, **45**:2414–21.

Commerford PJ, Lloyd EA (1984). Arrhythmias in patients with drug toxicity, electrolyte, and endocrine disturbances. *Medical Clinics of North America*, **68**:1051–78.

Cooper DJ, Walley KR, Wiggs BR, Russell JA (1990). Bicarbonate does not improve hemodynamics in critically ill patients who have lactic acidosis. *Annals of Internal Medicine*, **112**:492–8.

Cotton GE, Van Puffelen P (1986). Hypophosphaemic osteomalacia secondary to neoplasia. *Journal of Bone and Joint Surgery*, **68A**:129–33.

Cournot-Witmer G, *et al.* (1987). Bone modeling in gallium nitrate-treated rats. *Calcified Tissue International*, **40**:270–5.

Crittenden DR, Ackerman GL (1977). Hypericemic acute renal failure in disseminated carcinoma. *Archives of Internal Medicine*, **137**:97–9.

Cronin C, Igoe D, Duffy MJ, Cunningham SK, McKenna TJ (1990). The overnight dexamethasone test is a worthwhile screening procedure. *Clinical Endocrinology (Oxford)*, **33**(1):27–33.

Crossby SR, Stewart MF, Ratcliffe JG, White A (1988). Direct measurement of the precursors of adrenocorticotropin in human plasma by two-site immunoradiometric assay. *Journal of Clinical Endocrinology and Metabolism*, **67**:1272–7.

Cutting HO (1971). Inappropriate secretion of antidiuretic hormone secondary to vincristine therapy. *American Journal of Medicine*, **51**:269–71.

Dahlberg PJ, Goellner MH, Pehling GB (1990). Adrenal insufficiency secondary to adrenal hemorrhage. Two case reports and a review of cases confirmed by computed tomography. *Archives of Internal Medicine*, **150**(4):905–9.

Dann EJ, Gillis S, Polliack A, Okon E, Rund D, Rachmilewitz EA (1993). Brief report: tumor lysis syndrome following treatment with 2-chlorodeoxyadenosine for refractory chronic lymphocytic leukemia. *New England Journal of Medicine*, **329**:1547–8.

Daughaday WH, *et al.* (1988). Synthesis and secretion of insulin-like growth factor II by a leiomyosarcoma with associated hypoglycaemia. *New England Journal of Medicine*, **319**:1434–40.

Daughaday WH, Trivedi B, Baxter RC (1993). Serum 'big insulin-like growth factor II' from patients with tumor hypoglycaemia lacks normal E-domain O-linked glycosylation, a possible determinant of normal propeptide processing. *Proceedings of the National Academy of Sciences USA*, **90**:5823–7.

Daughaday WH, Kapadia M (1989). Significance of abnormal serum binding of insulin-like growth factor II in the development of hypoglycaemia in patients with non-islet-cell tumors. *Proceedings of the National Academy of Sciences USA*, **86**:6778–82.

DeConti RC, Calabresi P (1966). Use of allopurinol for prevention and control of hyperuricemia in patients with neoplastic disease. *New England Journal of Medicine*, **274**:481–6.

De Keyzer Y, Beragna X, Lenne F, Girard F, Luton J-P, Kahn A (1985). Altered proopiomelanocortin gene expression in adrenocorticotropin-producing nonpituitary tumors. *Journal of Clinical Investigation*, **76**:1892–8.

De Troyer A, Demanet JC (1976). Clinical, biological and pathogenic features of the syndrome of inappropriate secretion of antidiuretic hormone. *Quarterly Journal of Medicine*, **180**:521–31.

DeBold CR, Menefee JK, Nicholson WE, Orth DN (1988). Proopiomelanocortin gene is expressed in many normal human tissues and in tumors not associated with ectopic adrenocorticotropin syndrome. *Molecular Endocrinology*, **2**:862–70.

Decaux G, *et al.* (1988). Mechanisms of hypouricemia in the syndrome of inappropriate secretion of antidiuretic hormone. *Nephron*, **39**:164–8.

DeFronzo RA, Braine H, Colvin M, Davis PJ (1973). Water intoxication in man after cyclophosphamide therapy: time course and relation to drug inactivation. *Annals of Internal Medicine*, **78**:861–9.

Delisle L, *et al.* (1993). Ectopic corticotropin syndrome and small-cell carcinoma of the lung. *Archives of Internal Medicine*, 153:746–52.

Dirix LY, Prove A, Becquart D, Wouters E, Vermeulen P, Van Oosterom A (1991). Tumour lysis syndrome in a patient with metastatic Merkel cell carcinoma. *Cancer*, 67(8):2207–10.

Dluhy RG (1990). The growing spectrum of HIV-related endocrine abnormalities. *Journal of Clinical Endocrinology and Metabolism*, 70:563–5.

Doolittle GC, Wurster MW, Rosenfeld GS, Bodensteiner DC (1988). Malignancy-induced lactic acidosis. *Southern Medical Journal*, 81:533–6.

Dunlay RW, Camp MA, Allon M, Fanti P, Malluche HH, Llach F (1989). Calcitriol in prolonged hypocalcemia due to tumor lysis syndrome. *Annals of Internal Medicine*, 110:162–4.

Feibusch J, Barbosa-Salvidar JL, Bernstein RS (1980). Tumor-associated nephrogenic diabetes insipidus. *Annals of Internal Medicine*, 92:797–8.

Feldman D (1986). Ketoconazole and other imidazole derivatives as inhibitors of steroidogenesis. *Endocrine Reviews*, 7:409–20.

Fenneley JJ, Smyth H, Muldowney FP (1974). Extreme hyperkalemia due to rapid lysis of leukemic cells. *Lancet*, i:27.

Feuillan P, *et al.* (1987). Effects of suramin on the function and structure of the adrenal cortex in the cynomolgus monkey. *Journal of Clinical Endocrinology and Metabolism*, 65:153–8.

Findling JW, Tyrrell JB (1986). Occult ectopic secretion of corticotropin. *Archives of Internal Medicine*, 146:929–33.

Fisken RA, Heath DA, Bold AM (1980). Hypercalcemia—a hospital survey. *Quarterly Journal of Medicine*, 196:405–18.

Fitzpatrick LA, Bilezikian JP (1987). Acute primary hyperparathyroidism. *American Journal of Medicine*, 82:275–82.

Flombaum CD (1984). Hypomagnesemia associated with cisplatin combination chemotherapy. *Archives of Internal Medicine*, 144:2336–7.

Forrest JN, *et al.* (1978). Superiority of democycline over lithium in the treatment of chronic syndrome of inappropriate secretion of antidiuretic hormone. *New England Journal of Medicine*, 298:173–7.

Fraley DS, *et al.* (1980). Stimulation of lactate production by administration of bicarbonate in a patient with a solid neoplasm and lactic acidosis. *New England Journal of Medicine*, 303:1100–2.

Frame JN, Dahut WL, Crowley S (1992). Fludarabine and acute tumor lysis syndrome in chronic lymphocytic leukemia. *New England Journal of Medicine*, 327:1396–7.

Gaillard RC (1992). Pituitary gland emergencies. *Baillière's Clinical Endocrinology and Metabolism*, 6:57–75.

Gamelin E, *et al.* (1992). Non-Hodgkin's lymphoma presenting with primary adrenal insufficiency. A disease with an underestimated frequency? *Cancer*, 69:2333–6.

Garret IR, *et al.* (1987). Production of lymphotoxin, a bone-resorbing cytokine, by cultured human myeloma cells. *New England Journal of Medicine*, 317:526–32.

Gennari FJ (1984). Serum osmolality. *New England Journal of Medicine*, 310:102–5.

Giaccone G, *et al.* (1985). Disorders of serum electrolytes and renal function in patients treated with *cis*-platinum on an out-patient basis. *European Journal of Cancer and Clinical Oncology*, 21:433–7.

Gilby ED, Bondy PK, Fosling M (1976). Impaired water excretion in oat cell lung cancer. *British Journal of Cancer*, 34:323–4.

Gold EM (1979). The Cushing syndrome: changing views of diagnosis and treatment. *Annals of Internal Medicine*, 90:829–44.

Graber ML, Schulman G (1986). Hypomagnesemic hypocalcemia independent of parathyroid hormone. *Annals of Internal Medicine*, 104:804–5.

Greenbaum-Lefkoe B, Rosenstock JG, Belasco JB, Rohrbaugh TM, Meadows AT (1985). Syndrome of inappropriate antidiuretic hormone secretion: a complication of high-dose intravenous melphalan. *Cancer*, 55:44–6.

Gross PA, Ketteler M, Hausmann C, Ritz E (1987). The charted and the uncharted waters of hyponatraemia. *Kidney International*, 32 (Suppl. 21):S67–S75.

Guidon PT, Bockman RS (1990). Gallium nitrate initiates expression of early and late genes responsible for bone formation. *Journal of Bone and Mineral Research*, S91 (abstr. Suppl. 2).

Gutierrez ML, Crooke ST (1980). Mitotane (*o,p'*-DDD). *Cancer Treatment Reports*, 7:49–55.

Hainsworth JD, Workman R, Greco A (1983). Management of the syndrome of inappropriate antidiuretic hormone secretion in small cell lung cancer. *Cancer*, 51:161–5.

Hale AC, *et al.* (1985). A case of pituitary-dependent Cushing's disease with clinical and biochemical features of the ectopic ACTH syndrome. *Clinical Endocrinology*, 22:479–88.

Hall TJ, Chambers TJ (1990). Gallium inhibits bone resorption by a direct effect on osteoclasts. *Bone and Mineral*, 8:211–16.

Hall TC, Griffiths CT, Petranek JR (1972). Hypocalcemia—an unusual metabolic complication of breast cancer. *New England Journal of Medicine*, 275:1474–7.

Halma C, Jansen JBMJ, Janssens AR, Griffioen G, Lamers CBHW (1987). Life-threatening water intoxication during somatostatin therapy. *Annals of Internal Medicine*, 107:518–20.

Hande KR, Noone RM, Stone WJ (1984). Severe allopurinol toxicity. *American Journal of Medicine*, 76:47–56.

Harlow PJ, DeClerck YA, Shore NA, Ortega JA, Carranza A, Heuser E (1979). A fatal case of inappropriate ADH secretion induced by cyclophosphamide therapy. *Cancer*, 44:896–8.

Herbert LA, Leman J, Petersen JR, Lennon EJ (1966). Studies of the mechanism by which phosphate infusion lowers serum calcium concentration. *Journal of Clinical Investigation*, 45:1886–94.

Hoekman K, *et al.* (1994). Tumour-induced hypoglycaemia: a case report. *Annals of Oncology*, 5:277–81.

Hoffken K, *et al.* (1986). Aminoglutethimide without hydrocortisone in the treatment of postmenopausal patients with advanced breast cancer. *Cancer Treatment Reports*, 70:1153–7.

Holroyde CP, *et al.* (1975). Altered glucose metabolism in metastatic carcinoma. *Cancer Research*, 35:3710–14.

Horwitz CA, *et al.* (1972). Secondary malignant tumors of the parathyroid glands: report of two cases with associated hypoparathyroidism. *American Journal of Medicine*, 52:797.

Hosking DJ, Gilson D (1984). Comparison of the renal and skeletal actions of calcitonin in the treatment of severe hypercalcaemia of malignancy. *Quarterly Journal of Medicine*, 211:359–68.

Hosking DJ, Cowley A, Bucknall CA (1981). Rehydration in the treatment of severe hypercalcaemia. *Quarterly Journal of Medicine*, 200:473–81.

Howlett TA, Drury PL, Doniach PI, Rees LH, Besser GM (1986). Diagnosis and management of ACTH-dependent Cushing's syndrome: comparison of the features in ectopic and pituitary ACTH production. *Clinical Endocrinology*, 24:699–713.

Hug V, Kau S, Hortobagyi GN, Jones L (1991). Adrenal failure in patients with breast carcinoma after long-term treatment of cyclic alternating oestrogen progesterone. *British Journal of Cancer*, 63:454–6.

Hughes SWM, Burley DM (1970). Aminoglutethimide. A 'side-effect' turned to therapeutic advantage. *Postgraduate Medical Journal*, 46:409–16.

Hutchinson FN, *et al.* (1988). Renal salt wasting in patients treated with cisplatin. *Annals of Internal Medicine*, 108:21–25.

Ibbotson KJ, *et al.* (1983). Tumor-derived growth factor increases bone resorption in a tumor associated with humoral hypercalcemia of malignancy. *Science*, 221:1292–4.

Ibbotson KJ, *et al.* (1985). Stimulation of bone resorption *in vitro* by synthetic transforming growth factor-alpha. *Science*, 228:1007–9.

Ikeda T, *et al.* (1988). Prostaglandin E-producing hepatocellular carcinoma with hypercalcemia. *Cancer*, 61:1813–14.

Imura H (1980). Ectopic hormone syndromes. *Clinics in Endocrinology and Metabolism*, 9:235–60.

Jacobson JO, *et al.* (1989). Humoral hypercalcemia in Hodgkin's disease. *Cancer*, 63:917–23.

Jaffe N, Kim BS, Vawther GF (1972). Hypocalcemia—a complication of childhood leukemia. *Cancer*, 29:392–8.

Joffe BI, *et al.* (1988). Evaluation of the synthetic somatostatin analogue SMS 201-995 in patients with hypoglycaemia associated with hepato-cellular carcinoma. *British Journal of Cancer*, 58:91–2.

Juan D, Hsu SD, Hunter J (1985). Case report of vasopressin-responsive diabetes insipidus associated with chronic myelogenous leukemia. *Cancer*, 56:1468–9.

Kabadi UM (1983). Osteomalacia associated with prostatic cancer and osteoblastic metastases. *Urology*, XXI:65–7.

Kahn CR (1980). The riddle of tumour hypoglycaemia revisited. *Clinics in Endocrinology and Metabolism*, 9:335–60.

Kamoi K, Tamura T, Tanaka K, Ishibashi M, Yamaji T (1993). Hyponatremia and osmoregulation of thirst and vasopressin secretion in patients with adrenal insufficiency. *Clinical Endocrinology and Metabolism*, 77:1584–8.

Kanis JA, et al. (1988). Calcium metabolism and myeloma and the treatment of hypercalcemia. *Hematology and Oncology*, 6:115–17.

Kannan CR (1988). *The adrenal gland*, pp. 31–96. Plenum, New York.

Kaye TB, Crapo L (1990). The Cushing's syndrome: an update on diagnostic tests. *Annals of Internal Medicine*, 112:434–44.

Kelton JG, Kelley WN, Holmes EW (1978). A rapid method for the diagnosis of acute uric acid nephropathy. *Archives of Internal Medicine*, 138:612–15.

Kennedy BJ, et al. (1973). Hypercalcemia, a complication of hormone therapy of advanced breast cancer. *Cancer Research*, 445–9.

Kimmel DW, O'Neill BP (1983). Systemic cancer presenting as diabetes insipidus. *Cancer*, 52:2355–8.

Kjellstrand CM, et al. (1974). Hyperuricemic acute renal failure. *Archives of Internal Medicine*, 144:349–59.

Kokko JP (1985). Primary acquired hypoaldosteronism. *Kidney International*, 27:690–702.

Kornberg A, et al. (1980). Acute lymphoblastic leukemia. Association with vasopressin-responsive diabetes insipidus. *Archives of Internal Medicine*, 140:1236.

Krakoff IH, Meyer RL (1965). Prevention of hyperuricemia in leukemia and lymphoma. *Journal of the American Medical Association*, 193:1–6.

Krol TC, Wood WS (1982). Bronchogenic carcinoma and diabetes insipidus: case report and review. *Cancer*, 49:596–9.

Kukreja SC, et al. (1973). Pheochromocytoma causing excessive parathyroid hormone production and hypercalcemia. *Annals of Internal Medicine*, 79:838–40.

Kukreja SC, et al. (1980). Elevated nephrogenous cyclic AMP with normal serum parathyroid hormone levels in patients with lung cancer. *Journal of Endocrinology and Metabolism*, 51:167–9.

Kyle CA, Laster RA, Burton EM, Sanford RA (1990). Subacute pituitary apoplexy: MR and CT appearance. *Journal of Computer Assisted Tomography*, 14:40–44.

Legha SS, et al. (1981). Tamoxifen-induced hypercalcemia in breast cancer. *Cancer*, 47:2803–6.

Leight E, Biro G, Lauger H-J (1990). Tumour-induced osteomalacia: pre- and postoperative biochemical findings. *Hormone and Metabolism Research*, 22:640–3.

LeRoith D, Clemmons D, Nissley P, Rechler MM (1992). Insulin-like growth factors in health and disease. *Annals of Internal Medicine*, 116:854–62.

Levin L, Sealy R, Barron J (1982). Syndrome of inappropriate antidiuretic hormone secretion following *cis*-dichlorodiammineplatinum II in a patient with malignant thymoma. *Cancer*, 50:2279–82.

Limper AH, Carpenter PC, Scheithauer B, Staats BA (1992). The Cushing syndrome induced by bronchial carcinoid tumors. *Annals of Internal Medicine*, 117:209–14.

Linkhart TA, et al. (1989). Copurification of osteolytic and transforming growth factor beta activities produced by human lung tumor cells associated with humoral hypercalcemia of malignancy. *Cancer Research*, 49:271–8.

List AF, Kummet TD, Adams JD, Chun HG (1990). Tumor lysis syndrome complicating treatment of chronic lymphocytic leukemia with fludarabine phosphate. *American Journal of Medicine*, 89:388–90.

Littlewood TJ, Smith AP (1984). Syndrome of inappropriate antidiuretic hormone secretion due to treatment of lung cancer with cisplatin. *Thorax*, 39:636–7.

Lockton JA, Thatcher NA (1986). A retrospective study of thirty-two patients with small cell bronchogenic carcinoma and inappropriate secretion of antidiuretic hormone. *Clinical Radiology*, 37:47–50.

Lokich JJ (1982). The frequency and clinical biology of the ectopic hormone syndromes of small cell carcinoma. *Cancer*, 50:2111–14.

Loehrer PJ, Einhorn LH (1984). Cisplatin. *Annals of Internal Medicine*, 100:704–13.

Lowe WL, et al. (1989). Insulin-like growth factor-II in nonislet cell tumours associated with hypoglycaemia: increased expression of messenger ribonucleic acid. *Journal of Clinical Endocrinology and Metabolism*, 69:1153–9.

Lufkin EG, Kao PC, Heath H III (1987). Parathyroid hormone radioimmunoassays in the differential diagnosis of hypercalcemia due to primary hyperparathyroidism or malignancy. *Annals of Internal Medicine*, 106:559–80.

Lyles KW, et al. (1980). Hypophosphatemic osteomalacia: association with prostatic carcinoma. *Annals of Internal Medicine*, 93:275–8.

Lynch EC (1962). Uric acid metabolism in proliferative disease of the marrow. *Archives of Internal Medicine*, 109:639–53.

Macaulay VM (1992). Insulin-like growth factors and cancer. *British Journal of Cancer*, 65:311–20.

Madias NE (1986). Lactic acidosis. *Kidney International*, 29:752–74.

Malden LT, Novak U, Burgess AW (1989). Expression of transforming growth factor alpha messenger RNA in the normal and neoplastic gastro-intestinal tract. *International Journal of Cancer*, 43:380–4.

Mangin M, et al. (1988). Identification of a cDNA encoding a parathyroid hormone-like peptide from a human tumor associated with humoral hypercalcemia of malignancy. *Proceedings of the National Academy of Sciences USA*, 85:597–601.

Martin TJ, Sura LJ (1989). Parathyroid hormone-related protein in hypercalcaemia of malignancy. *Clinical Endocrinology*, 31:631–47.

Mavichak V, et al. (1988). Renal magnesium wasting and hypocalciuria in chronic *cis*-platinum nephropathy in man. *Clinical Science*, 75:203–7.

McCroskey RD, Mosher DF, Spencer CD, Prendergast E, Longo WL (1990). Acute tumor lysis syndrome and treatment response in patients treated for refractory chronic lymphocytic leukemia with short-course, high-dose cytosine arabinoside, cisplatin, and etoposide. *Cancer*, 66:246–50.

McLellan EA, Reid SR, Lane PL (1984). Massive blood transfusion causing hypomagnesemia. *Critical Care Medicine*, 12:146–7.

Medalle R, Webb R, Waterhouse C (1971). Lactic acidosis and associated hypoglycemia. *Archives of Internal Medicine*, 128:273–8.

Melton JE, Nattie EE (1983). Brain and CSF water and ions during dilutional and isoosmotic hyponatraemia in the rat. *American Journal of Physiology*, 244:R724–R732.

Merendino JJ, et al. (1986). A parathyroid hormone-like protein from culture human keratinocytes. *Science*, 231:388–90.

Meyers AM, Jowsey J (1974). Hyperphosphatemia and hypocalcemia in neoplastic disorders. *New England Journal of Medicine*, 299:858–9.

Miller M, et al. (1970). Recognition of partial defects in antidiuretic hormone secretion. *Annals of Internal Medicine*, 73:721–9.

Miyauchi A, Fukase M, Tsutsumi M, Fujita T (1988). Hemangiopericytoma-induced osteomalacia: tumor transplantation in nude mice causes hypophosphatemia and tumor extracts inhibit renal 25-hydroxyvitamin D 1-hydroxylase activity. *Journal of Clinical Endocrinology and Metabolism*, 67(1):46–53.

Mor F, et al. (1985). Addison's disease due to metastases to the adrenal glands. *Postgraduate Medical Journal*, 61:637–9.

Morton AR, et al. (1988). Sclerosis of lytic bone metastasis after disodium aminohydroxypropilidene bisphosphonate (APD) in patients with breast carcinoma. *British Medical Journal*, 297:772–3.

Moseley JM, et al. (1987). Parathyroid hormone-related protein purified from a human lung cancer cell line. *Proceedings of the National Academy of Sciences USA*, 84:5048–52.

Muggia FM, Ball TJ, Ultmann JE (1967). Allopurinol in the treatment of neoplastic disease complicated by hyperuricemia. *Archives of Internal Medicine*, 120:12–18.

Muggia FM, Chia GA, Mickley DW (1974). Hyperphosphatemia and hypocalcemia in neoplastic disorders. *New England Journal of Medicine*, 299:857–8.

Mundy GR (1988). Hypercalcemia of malignancy revisited. *Journal of Clinical Investigation*, 82:1–6.

Mundy GR (1987). The hypercalcemia of malignancy. *Kidney International*, 31:142–55.

Nadiminti Y, et al. (1980). Lactic acidosis associated with Hodgkin's disease. Response to chemotherapy. *New England Journal of Medicine*, 303:15–17.

Nieman LK, Cutler GB (1990). The sensitivity of the urine free cortisol measurement as a screening test for Cushing's syndrome. *72nd annual meeting of The Endocrine Society (Atlanta) 1990*, abstract 822.

Odell WD (1991). Ectopic ACTH secretion: a misnomer. *Endocrinology and Metabolism Clinics of North America*, **20**:371–9.

Odell WD, Wolphsen AR (1978). Humoral syndromes associated with cancer. *Annual Reviews of Medicine*, **29**:379–406.

Olefsky J, *et al.* (1972). Tertiary hyperparathyroidism and apparent cure of vitamin-D-resistant rickets after removal of an ossifying mesenchymal tumor of the pharynx. *New England Journal of Medicine*, **286**:740–5.

Onesti ST, Wisniewski T, Post KD (1990). Clinical versus subclinical pituitary apoplexy: presentation, surgical management, and outcome in 21 patients. *Neurosurgery*, **26**:980–6.

Orth DN, Liddle GW (1971). Results of treatment in 108 patients with Cushing's syndrome. *New England Journal of Medicine*, **285**:243–7.

Passamonte PM (1984). Hypouricemia, inappropriate secretion of antidiuretic hormone, and small cell carcinoma of the lung. *Archives of Internal Medicine*, **144**:1569–70.

Percival RC, *et al.* (1984). Role of glucocorticoids in management of malignant hypercalcemia. *British Medical Journal*, **289**:287.

Pettengill OS, *et al.* (1977). Isolation and characterization of a hormone-producing cell line from human small cell anaplastic carcinoma of the lung. *Journal of the National Cancer Institute*, **58**:511–18.

Polonsky KS (1992). A practical approach to fasting hypoglycaemia. *New England Journal of Medicine*, **326**:1020–1.

Porter AT (1985). Syndrome of inappropriate antidiuretic hormone secretion during *cis*-dichlorodiammineplatinum therapy in a patient with ovarian carcinoma. *Gynecologic Oncology*, **21**:103–5.

Prestayko AW, *et al.* (1979). Cisplatin (*cis*-diamminedichloroplatinum II). *Cancer Treatment Reviews*, **6**:17–39.

Ralston SH, *et al.* (1986). Humoral hypercalcemia of malignancy: metabolic and histomorphometric studies during surgical management of the primary tumour. *Quarterly Journal of Medicine*, **227**:325–35.

Ralston SH, *et al.* (1988). Treatment of severe hypercalcaemia with mithramycin and aminohydroxypropylidene bisphophonate. *Lancet*, **ii**:277.

Ralston SH, *et al.* (1985). Comparison of aminohydroxypropylidene diphosphonate, mithramycin and corticosteroids/calcitonin in treatment of cancer-associated hypercalcaemia. *Lancet*, **ii**:907–10.

Ralston SH, *et al.* (1986). Treatment of cancer-associated hypercalcaemia with combined aminohydroxypropylidene diphosphonate and calcitonin. *British Medical Journal*, **292**:1549–60.

Redmon B, Pyzdrowski KL, Elson MK, Kay NE, Dalmasso AP, Nuttall FQ (1992). Brief report: hypoglycaemia due to a monoclonal insulin-binding antibody in multiple myeloma. *New England Journal of Medicine*, **326**:994–8.

Repo MA, *et al.* (1988). Effect of gallium on bone mineral properties. *Calcified Tissue International*, **43**:300–6.

Ritch PS (1988). Cis-dichlorodiammineplatinum II-induced syndrome of inappropriate secretion of antidiuretic hormone. *Cancer*, **61**:448–50.

Ritch P, *et al.* (1989). Pamidronate (APD) and etidronate disodium (EHDP) in hypercalcaemia of malignancy: preliminary report of comparative multicentre trial. In *The management of bone metastases and hypercalcaemia by osteoclast inhibition* (ed. RD Rubens), pp. 47–9. Hogrefe and Huber, London.

Ritter JM, Doktor HS, Benjamin N (1990). Paradoxical effect of bicarbonate on cytoplasmic pH. *Lancet*, **335**:1243–6.

Robertson GL (1987). Physiology of ADH secretion. *Kidney International*, **32** (Suppl. 21):S20–S26.

Robertson GL, Aycinena P, Zerbe RL (1982). Neurogenic disorders of osmoregulation. *American Journal of Medicine*, **72**:339–53.

Rodan SB, *et al.* (1985). Factors associated with humoral hypercalcemia of malignancy stimulate adenylate cyclase in osteoblastic cells. *Journal of Clinical Investigation*, **72**:1511–15.

Ron D, Powers AC, Pandian MR, Godine JE, Axelrod L (1989). Increased insulin-like growth factor II production and consequent suppression of growth hormone secretion: a dual mechanism for tumour-induced hypoglycaemia. *Journal of Clinical Endocrinology and Metabolism*, **68**:701–6.

Rose BD (1986). New approach to disturbances in the plasma sodium concentration. *American Journal of Medicine*, **81**:1033–40.

Rosenthal S, Kaufman S (1974). Vincristine neurotoxicity. *Annals of Internal Medicine*, **80**:733–7.

Rotwein P (1991). Structure, evolution, expression and regulation of insulin-like growth factors I and II. *Growth Factors*, **5**:3–18.

Sato K, *et al.* (1986). Production of bone-resorbing activity and colony-stimulating activity in vivo and in vitro by a human squamous cell carcinoma associated with hypercalcemia and leukocytosis. *Journal of Clinical Investigation*, **78**:145–54.

Scher HI, *et al.* (1987). Gallium nitrate in prostatic cancer: evaluation of antitumor activity and effects on bone turnover. *Cancer Treatment Reports*, **71**:887–93.

Schilsky RL, Anderson T (1979). Hypomagnesemia and renal magnesium wasting in patients receiving cisplatin. *Annals of Internal Medicine*, **90**:929–31.

Schilsky RL (1982). Renal and metabolic toxicities of cancer chemotherapy. *Seminars in Oncology*, **9**:75–83.

Schmale H, Fehr S, Richter D (1987). Vasopressin biosynthesis—from gene to peptide hormone. *Kidney International*, **32** (Suppl. 21):S8–S13.

Schofield PN, Connor H, Turner RC, Zapf J (1989). Tumour hypoglycaemia: raised tumour IGFII mRNA associated with reduced plasma somatomedins. *British Journal of Cancer*, **60**:661–3.

Schwartz WB, *et al.* (1957). Syndrome of renal sodium loss and hyponatraemia probably resulting from inappropriate secretion of antidiuretic hormone. *American Journal of Medicine*, **23**:529–42.

Sculier JP, Nicaise C, Klastersky J (1983). Lactic acidosis: a metabolic complication of extensive metastatic cancer. *European Journal of Cancer and Clinical Oncology*, **19**:597–601.

Seegmiller JE, Laster L, Howell RR (1963). Biochemistry of uric acid and its relation to gout. *New England Journal of Medicine*, **268**:712–16.

Seidenwurm DJ, Elmer EB, Kaplan LM, Williams EK, Morris DG, Hoffman AR (1984). Metastases to the adrenal glands and the development of Addison's disease. *Cancer*, **54**:552–7.

Seyberth HW, *et al.* (1975). Prostaglandins as mediators of hypercalcemia associated with certain types of cancer. *New England Journal of Medicine*, **293**:1278–83.

Shepherd FA, Laskey J, Evans WK, Goss PE, Johansen E, Khamsi F (1992). Cushing's syndrome associated with ectopic corticotropin production and small-cell lung cancer. *Journal of Clinical Oncology*, **10**:21–7.

Shirakawa F, *et al.* (1988). Production of bone-resorbing activity corresponding to interleukin-1α by adult T-cell leukemia cells in humans. *Cancer Research*, **48**:4284–7.

Simpson EL, *et al.* (1983). Absence of parathyroid hormone messenger RNA in non parathyroid tumors associated with hypercalcemia. *New England Journal of Medicine*, **309**:325–30.

Siris ES, *et al.* (1980). Effects of dichloromethylene diphosphonate on skeletal mobilization of calcium in multiple myeloma. *New England Journal of Medicine*, **302**:310–15.

Siu SCB, Kitzman DW, Sheedy PF II, Northcutt RC (1990). Adrenal insufficiency from bilateral hemorrhage. *Mayo Clinic Proceedings*, **65**:664–70.

Skrabanek P, McPartlin J, Powell D (1980). Tumor hypercalcemia and 'ectopic hyperparathyroidism'. *Medicine*, **59**:262–82.

Slater LM, Wainer RA, Serpick AA (1969). Vincristine neurotoxicity with hyponatraemia. *Cancer*, **23**(1):122–5.

Sleeboom HP, *et al.* (1983). Comparison of intravenous (5-amino-hydroxypropylidene)-1, 1-bisphosphonate and volume repletion in tumour-induced hypercalcemia. *Lancet*, **ii**:245.

Smits P, *et al.* (1989). Diabetes insipidus associated with leukemia. *The Netherlands Journal of Medicine*, **34**:264–9.

Sorensen JB, *et al.* (1988). Hypouricemia and urate excretion in small cell lung carcinoma patients with syndrome of inappropriate antidiuresis. *Acta Oncologica*, **27**:351–5.

Spechler SJ, *et al.* (1978). Lactic acidosis in oat cell carcinoma with extensive hepatic metastasis. *Archives of Internal Medicine*, **138**:1663–4.

Stacpoole PW, *et al.* and the dichloroacetate-lactic acidosis study group (1992). A controlled trial of dichloroacetate for treatment of lactic acidosis in adults. *New England Journal of Medicine*, **327**:1564–9.

Stark ME, Dyer MCD, Coonley CF (1987). Fatal acute tumor lysis syndrome with metastatic breast carcinoma. *Cancer*, **60**:762–4.

Stern PH, *et al.* (1985). Human transforming growth factor-alpha stimulates bone resorption in vitro. *Journal of Clinical Investigation*, **76**:2016–19.

Sterns RH (1987). Severe symptomatic hyponatremia: treatment and outcome. A study of 64 cases. *Annals of Internal Medicine*, **107**:656–64.

Sterns RH, Riggs JE, Schochet SS (1986). Osmotic demyelination syndrome following correction of hyponatremia. *New England Journal of Medicine*, **314**:1535–42.

Steward WP, *et al.* (1989). Recombinant human granulocyte macrophage (rhGM-CSF) given as daily short infusions—a phase I dose–toxicity study. *British Journal of Cancer*, **59**:142–5.

Stewart AF, Wu T, Gonmas D, Burtis WJ, Broadus AE (1987). N-terminal amino acid sequence of two novel tumor-derived adenylate cyclase-stimulating proteins: identification of parathyroid hormone-like and parathyroid hormone-unlike domains. *Biochemical and Biophysics Research Communications*, **146**:672–8.

Stewart AF, *et al.* (1980). Biochemical evaluation of patients with cancer-associated hypercalcemia. *New England Journal of Medicine*, **303**:1377–83.

Stewart AF, *et al.* (1988). Synthetic human parathyroid hormone-like protein stimulates bone resorption and causes hypercalcemia. *Journal of Clinical Investigation*, **81**:596–600.

Strewler GJ, *et al.* (1987). Parathyroid hormone like protein from human renal carcinoma cells. *Journal of Clinical Investigation*, **80**:1803–7.

Suki WN, *et al.* (1970). Acute treatment of hypercalcemia with furosemide. *New England Journal of Medicine*, **283**:836–40.

Sura LJ, *et al.* (1987). A parathyroid hormone-related protein implicated in malignant hypercalcemia: cloning and expression. *Science*, **237**:893–6.

Tabarin A, Navarranne A, Guérin J, Corcuff J-B, Parneix M, Roger P (1991). Use of ketoconazole in the treatment of Cushing's disease and ectopic ACTH syndrome. *Clinical Endocrinology*, **34**:63–9.

Tashjian AH Jr, *et al.* (1973). Successful treatment of hypercalcemia by indomethacin in mice bearing a prostaglandin-producing fibrosarcoma. *Prostaglandins*, **3**(4):515–24.

Tashjian AH Jr, *et al.* (1972). Evidence that the bone resorption-stimulating factor produced by mouse fibrosarcoma cells is prostaglandin E_2. A new model for the hypercalcemia of cancer. *Journal of Experimental Medicine*, **136**(6):1329–43.

Taylor HC, Fallon MD, Velasco ME (1984). Oncogenic osteomalacia and inappropriate antidiuretic hormone secretion due to oat-cell carcinoma. *Annals of Internal Medicine*, **101**:786–8.

Teale JD, Blum WF, Marks V (1992). Alleviation of non-islet cell tumour hypoglycaemia by growth hormone therapy is associated with changes in IGF binding protein-3. *Annals of Clinical Biochemistry*, **29**:314–23.

Teears RJ, Silverman EM (1975). Clincopathologic review of 88 cases of carcinoma metastatic to the pituitary gland. *Cancer*, **36**:216–20.

Texier P-L, *et al.* (1991). Proopiomelanocortin gene expression in normal and tumor human lung. *Journal of Clinical Endocrinology and Metabolism*, **73**:414–20.

Thurston JH, Hauhart RE, Nelson JS (1987). Adaptive decreases in amino acids (taurine in particular), creatinine and electrolytes prevent cerebral edema in chronically hyponatraemic mice. *Metabolic Brain Diseases*, **2**: 223–41.

Tomlinson BE, Pierides AM, Bradley WG (1976). Central pontine myelinolysis. *Quarterly Journal of Medicine*, **179**:373–86.

Trainer PJ, Grossman A (1991). The diagnosis and differential diagnosis of Cushing's syndrome. *Clinical Endocrinology*, **34**:317–30.

Tsokos GC, *et al.* (1981). Renal and metabolic complications of undifferentiated and lymphoblastic lymphomas. *Medicine*, **60**:218–29.

Tungsanga K, *et al.* (1984). Urine uric acid and urine creatinine ratio in acute renal failure. *Archives of Internal Medicine*, **144**:934–7.

Unger RH (1966). The riddle of tumor hypoglycaemia. *American Journal of Medicine*, **40**:325–30.

Valentin-Opran A, *et al.* (1985). Estrogens and antiestrogens stimulate release of bone resorbing activity by cultured human breast cancer cells. *Journal of Clinical Investigation*, **75**:726–31.

Van Breukelen FJM, Bijvoet CLM, Van Oosterom AT (1979). Inhibition of osteolytic bone lesions by (3-amino-1-hydroxypropylidene)-1, 1-bisphosphonate (A.P.D.). *Lancet*, i:803–5.

Villalon AH, *et al.* (1979). Hypercalcaemia after tamoxifen for breast cancer: a sign of tumour response. *British Medical Journal*, 1329–30.

Vogelzang NJ, Nelimark RA, Nath KA (1983). Tumor lysis syndrome after induction chemotherapy of small-cell bronchogenic carcinoma. *Journal of the American Medical Association*, **249**:513–14.

Vogelzang NJ, Torkelson JL, Kennedy BJ (1985). Hypomagnesemia, renal dysfunction, and Raynaud's phenomenon in patients treated with cisplatin, vinblastine, and bleomycin. *Cancer*, **56**:2765–70.

Vogler WR, Morris JG, Winton EF (1983). Acute tumor lysis in T-cell leukemia induced by amsacrine. *Archives of Internal Medicine*, **143**:165–6.

Vokes TJ, Robertson GL (1988). Disorders of antidiuretic hormone. *Endocrinology and Metabolism Clinics of North America*, **17**:281–99.

Walker BR, Campbell JC, Fraser R, Stewart PM, Edwards RW (1992). Mineralocorticoid excess and inhibition of 11β-hydroxysteroid dehydrogenase in patients with ectopic ACTH syndrome. *Clinical Endocrinology*, **37**:483–92.

Walters EG, Tavaré JM, Denton RM, Walters G (1987). Hypoglycaemia due to an insulin-receptor antibody in Hodgkin's disease. *Lancet*, i:241–3.

Warrell RP Jr, *et al.* (1984). Gallium nitrate inhibits calcium resorption from bone and is effective treatment for cancer-related hypercalcemia. *Journal of Clinical Investigation*, **73**:1487–90.

Warrell RP Jr, Alcock NW, Bockman RS (1987). Gallium nitrate inhibits accelerated bone turnover in patients with bone metastases. *Journal of Clinical Oncology*, **5**:292–8.

Warrell RP Jr, *et al.* (1986). Gallium nitrate for acute treatment of cancer-related hypercalcemia: clinicopharmacologic and dose–response analysis. *Cancer*, **46**:4208–12.

Warrell RP Jr, *et al.* (1987). Treatment of refractory hypercalcemia from parathyroid carcinoma with gallium nitrate. *Annals of Internal Medicine*, **107**:683–6.

Warrell RP Jr, *et al.* (1988). Gallium nitrate for acute treatment of cancer-related hypercalcemia: a randomized, double-blind comparison to calcitonin. *Annals of Internal Medicine*, **108**:66974.

Warrell RP Jr, Murphy WK, Schulman Ph, O'Dwyer PJ, Heller G (1991). A randomized double-blind study of gallium nitrate compared with etidronate for acute control of cancer-related hypercalcemia. *Journal of Clinical Oncology*, **9**:1467–75.

Waterhouse C (1974). Lactate metabolism in patients with cancer. *Cancer*, **33**:66–71.

Watts RWE, *et al.* (1966). Allopurinol and acute uric acid nephropathy. *British Medical Journal*, **1**:205–8.

White FE, White MC, Drury PL, Fry IK, Besser GM (1982). Value of computed tomography of the abdomen and chest in the investigation of Cushing's syndrome. *British Medical Journal*, **284**:771–4.

White A, Clark AJL (1993). The cellular and molecular basis of the ectopic ACTH syndrome. *Clinical Endocrinology*, **39**:131–41.

White A, Clark AJL, Stewart MF (1990). The synthesis of ACTH and related peptides by tumours. *Baillière's Clinical Endocrinology and Metabolism*, **4**:1–27.

Willox JC, *et al.* (1986). Effects of magnesium supplementation in testicular cancer patients receiving cis-platin: a randomised trial. *British Journal of Cancer*, **54**:19–23.

Yap HY, *et al.* (1979). Diabetes insipidus and breast cancer. *Archives of Internal Medicine*, **139**:1009–11.

Zapf J, Futo E, Peter M, Froesch ER (1992). Can 'big' insulin-like growth factor II in serum of tumor patients account for the development of extrapancreatic tumor hypoglycaemia? *Journal of Clinical Investigation*, **90**:2574–84.

Zapf J (1993). IGFs: function and clinical importance. 3. Role of insulin-like growth factor (IGF) II and IGF binding proteins in extrapancreatic tumour hypoglycaemia. *Journal of Internal Medicine*, **234**:543–52.

Zusman J, Brown DM, Nesbit ME (1973). Hyperphosphatemia, hyperphosphaturia and hypocalcemia in acute lymphoblastic leukemia. *New England Journal of Medicine*, **289**:1335–40.

19.3   Paraneoplastic syndromes

VALENTINE M. MACAULAY AND IAN E. SMITH

INTRODUCTION

Paraneoplastic syndromes are remote and often insidious effects of cancer, not mediated directly by local infiltration or metastatic spread. They occur in approximately 10 per cent of patients with cancer overall (Ihde 1987; Richardson and Johnson 1992), but their incidence varies markedly with different tumours (Table 1). These syndromes are important because (1) they may be the presenting feature of a treatable tumour, (2) they cause morbidity which may sometimes be treatable, (3) they may run parallel to the course of the cancer and act as markers of disease activity, and (4) research into their cause may shed light on similar diseases of unknown aetiology (for example, arthritis).

Underlying mechanisms

The causes of paraneoplastic disease are not fully understood, but in general two main mechanisms have been identified. The first is inappropriate secretion of hormones or growth factors, and the second is cross-reaction of antitumour antibodies with normal tissues.

Inappropriate hormone secretion occurs through excessive or unregulated secretion by the normal source of the hormone ('eutopic' secretion) or through synthesis by an organ or tissue not normally associated with that hormone ('ectopic' secretion). Ectopic production may reflect random gene derepression or tumour development from isolated neuroendocrine cells in non-endocrine tissues. Genes encoding ectopic hormones are structurally normal and are not amplified. With the possible exception of the gene encoding pro-opiomelanocortin they are transcribed normally from the conventional promoter (Clark 1988). However, tumours may produce multiple or abnormal forms of a hormone because of alternative or incomplete processing of the mRNA or peptide, differential glycosylation, or defective storage and/or release (Sorenson et al. 1985). Many cancer patients have inappropriately high circulating levels of a variety of peptides in the absence of a clinically evident paraneoplastic syndrome. This is often because incomplete processing by the tumour leads to secretion of a biologically inactive high molecular weight precursor (Odell 1989).

Clinical and experimental studies have used the following criteria to assess whether a given paraneoplastic syndrome is caused by inappropriate secretion of a hormone or growth factor by a specific tumour type (Orth 1987).

1. Association of specific tumour type(s) with an endocrine syndrome.

2. Association of tumour with inappropriately elevated levels of hormone in plasma or urine.

3. Failure to suppress elevated plasma/urine levels of hormone in response to normal homeostatic stimuli.

4. Fall in hormone level after effective antitumour treatment, in parallel with resolution of the paraneoplastic syndrome.

5. Arteriovenous step-up gradient across tumour capillary bed.

6. Immunoreactive hormone and hormone-specific mRNA detectable in tumour tissue, tumour explants, and cultured tumour cells in vitro but not detectable, or present at lower levels, in normal cells/tissues from which the tumour arose.

In addition to the endocrine syndromes, inappropriate secretion of hormones or growth factors is increasingly recognized as a probable cause of some paraneoplastic haematological and dermatological conditions, fever, and cachexia.

The second group of paraneoplastic syndromes are those caused by antitumour antibodies which cross-react with epitopes on normal tissues (Graus and Rene 1992; Zeballos and McPherson 1992). This is the probable cause of syndromes affecting the nervous system and some haematological conditions. Local or systemic release of tumour antigens, and subsequent antibody formation, may be more likely to occur in a rapidly-growing neoplasm with areas of necrosis (Kornguth et al. 1986). As an extension of this mechanism, immune complex formation between antitumour antibodies and cross-reacting normal cellular epitopes may be the cause of paraneoplastic glomerulonephritis and arthritis (Butler et al. 1987; Boulton-Jones 1988). However, antitumour antibodies or immune complexes may be found in the absence of a clinically evident paraneoplastic syndrome. Antineuronal antibody expression has been shown in a small proportion of normal controls and cancer patients without paraneoplastic syndromes (Kornguth et al. 1986; Grisold et al. 1987). Circulating immune complexes have been detected in 10–80 per cent of patients with lung cancer, breast cancer, and melanoma (Boulton-Jones 1988; Bukh et al. 1989). In order to cause a clinical paraneoplastic syndrome, the immune mediator must first gain access to the target, which in the case of the nervous system may require increased permeability of the blood–brain or blood–retinal barrier, and must interact with the target and impair its function. Thus the demonstration of antineuronal antibodies or immune complexes is not, in itself, sufficient evidence to implicate these in the pathogenesis of paraneoplastic syndromes. It is possible that some alternative agent causes neuronal damage, exposing epitopes which are usually hidden and thus non-immunogenic (Crofts et al. 1988). This would explain why these same epitopes fail to stimulate an immune response in the majority of normal subjects.

Criteria for assessing the role of immune mechanisms in the pathogenesis of clinical paraneoplastic syndromes include the following (Kornguth et al. 1986; Antel and Moumdjian 1989).

1. Clinical/epidemiological link between specific tumour(s) and defined paraneoplastic syndrome.

2. Patients with the tumour and paraneoplastic syndrome should have high-titre immunoglobulins which react with specific group(s) of neurons.

3. Evidence that a specific immune mechanism is active at the site of the lesion in patients but not in controls (that is, access to target).

4. Target neurons are reduced in numbers in patients with paraneoplastic syndromes (that is, immunoablation).

Table 1   Tumour associations of paraneoplastic syndromes

Tumour	Syndrome																				
	Endocrine				Neurological									Haematological						Skin	
	Cushing's	SIADH	HHM	Hypoglycaemia	Limbic Enceph.	PCD	CAR syndrome	OM	Necr. myelo.	SSN	PN	LEMS	PM/DM	AIHA	Erythrocytosis	TED	DIC	NBTE	MAHA	Ac. nigricans	Leser-Trélat
Head and neck	++	+	+++		+	+							+								+
Thymus	++	+			+	+						+			++					++	+
Breast	+++		+		++	+++	+	+	+		++	++	++		++	++	++		++	++	
SCLC	+++	+++	+++		+++	+++	++	++	++	+++	+++	+++	+++			++	++	+++	++	++	
Non-SCLC	++	+	++[a]		++	++	+	++	+	+++	++	+	++			++	+++	+++	++	++	
GI including pancreas	++	+	+	+	+	+	+		+		++	+	++			+++	+++	+++	+++	+++	+++
Hepatic				++											+++						
Renal			+++		+							+			+++						
Bladder		+	++		+			+					+								
Ovary	+	+	+		++	+++			+				++		+				+	++	
Prostate	+	+				+			+			+	+			+++	+++		+	+	
Hodgkin's		+			+	++		+	+		+++			++					+++		++
Non-Hodgkin's lymphoma		+				+		+	+			+		+++						+	+
Myeloma											+++										
Sarcomas		+		++				+			+									+	

For abbreviations see text.
+++ Well-described association.
++ Described association.
+ Isolated reports.
[a] Squamous carcinoma of oesophagus.

5. Evidence from passive transfer experiments that the same pathological and clinical features can be induced by specific immune mechanisms (autoantibodies extracted from patients' sera or antibodies raised experimentally against the same or similar antigenic determinants).

6. Clinical response to removing or lowering the titre of autoantibodies. There is less emphasis here than in the endocrine syndromes for the necessity to show a parallel clinical course. Some neurological syndromes do run parallel to the clinical course of the tumour (for example, Lambert–Eaton myasthenic syndrome). This is by no means invariable, probably due to persistence of immune-mediators even after effective treatment of the tumour, and the limited ability of neural tissue to repair damage.

In some cases, it has been possible to characterize the antigenic determinant(s) common to the tumour and the normal tissue target. Patients with small-cell lung cancer and paraneoplastic neurological involvement have circulating antineuronal antibodies (Grisold et al. 1987; Antel and Moumdjian 1989). Experimental studies have identified several antigens common to normal neurones and the small-cell lung cancer cells, which may act as autoantibody targets (Willison et al. 1986; Patel et al. 1989). HNK-1 is a mouse monoclonal antibody (MoAb) which recognizes a surface antigen on natural killer cells and myelin-associated glycoprotein (MAG; Schuller-Petrovic et al. 1983). This epitope is also present on surface glycoproteins on small-cell lung cancer cells, although the structural similarity between MAG and small-cell lung cancer glycoproteins is confined to carbohydrate determinants (Willison et al. 1986). Some experimentally raised small-cell lung cancer MoAbs have strong neural reactivity, so-called 'cluster 1' MoAbs (Souhami et al. 1987). These have been shown to react with murine fibroblasts transfected with a cDNA clone coding for human neural cell adhesion molecule (NCAM). Western blot analysis confirmed that NCAM is the antigen recognized by cluster 1 MoAbs (Patel et al. 1989).

The clinical relevance of these observations is supported by studies of IgM paraproteins synthesized by patients with monoclonal gammopathy associated with polyneuropathy. Most of these monoclonal IgM autoantibodies are directed against MAG and some also react with certain central nervous system (CNS) neurons. Immunoblotting experiments have demonstrated that human monoclonal anti-MAG IgM reacts with purified avian NCAM, suggesting that NCAM may be the putative antibody target in the clinical setting as well as experimentally (Steck et al. 1987).

Patients with paraneoplastic syndromes often have a protracted clinical course and small occult tumours which may be diagnosed only at post-mortem examination. Henson and Urich (1982) suggested that the cross-reacting antitumour antibodies which are responsible for some paraneoplastic syndromes may also keep the tumour in check in some way. Support for this concept comes from a retrospective post-mortem study of patients with small-cell lung cancer. Patients with clinical evidence of a paraneoplastic syndrome had significantly less CNS metastases at autopsy, and a significantly longer survival than patients without (10.5 versus 7.4 months) (de la Monte et al. 1984).

ENDOCRINE SYNDROMES

Inappropriate ACTH secretion (Cushing's syndrome)

Cushing's syndrome is due to inappropriate overproduction of adrenocorticotrophic hormone (ACTH) or cortisol. Ectopic production of ACTH by tumours was first recognized by Liddle et al. (1965). ACTH and other pituitary peptides are synthesized from a common high molecular weight precursor pro-opiomelanocortin (molecular weight, 31 kDa). This is cleaved to pro-ACTH (22 kDa) and then to ACTH 1–39 (Fig. 1(a)). Pro-opiomelanocortin is probably made in small amounts by most normal tissues, although only the pituitary has processing enzymes to generate bioactive ACTH. Similarly, many tumours probably synthesize pro-opiomelanocortin, though most lack the enzymes necessary to generate bioactive peptides. Immunoreactive ACTH is detectable in the plasma of 20–70 per cent of lung cancer patients and also in cell extracts of at least 50 per cent of small-cell lung cancer cell lines. Specific immunoradiometric assays indicate that most or all of this immunoreactivity is attributable to pro-opiomelanocortin or pro-ACTH, with little or no processing to ACTH 1–39. Pro-ACTH is bioactive and can therefore lead to clinical and/or biochemical features of Cushing's syndrome (Odell 1989; Stewart et al. 1989; Pierce 1993).

Several other neuropeptides are generated by cleavage of pro-opiomelanocortin (Fig. 1(a)). Some of these, including lipotrophin, β-endorphin and β- and γ-melanocyte-stimulating hormone (MSH) can be detected in the plasma of patients with ectopic ACTH secretion (Hale et al. 1986). Rarely, tumours may synthesize corticotrophin-releasing factor (CRF), which causes pituitary

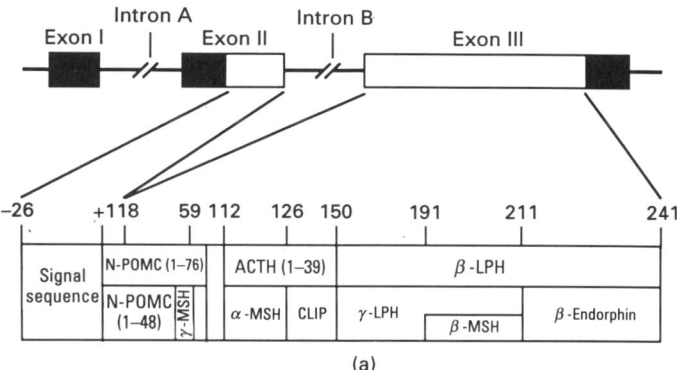

(a)

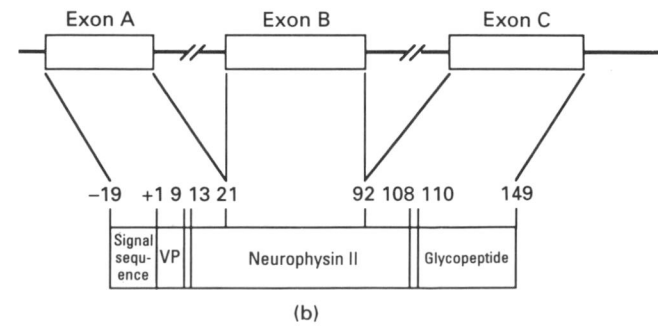

(b)

Fig. 1 (a) Diagramatic representation of the human pro-opiomelanocortin gene: N POMC, N-terminal pro-opiomelanocortin; LPH, lipotrophin; CLIP, corticotrophin-like intermediate peptide; MSH, melanocyte-stimulating hormone. Open and closed boxes indicate translated and untranslated regions respectively. Numbers refer to amino acid residues. Reproduced with permission from Grewal et al. (1989). (b) Diagrammatic representation of the vasopressin (VP) gene in Brattleboro rats. Reproduced with permission from Richter (1988).

hyperplasia, overproduction of pituitary ACTH 1–39, and adrenal hyperplasia. Five such patients have been described, including one with small cell prostatic carcinoma, one with medullary thyroid carcinoma, two with bronchial carcinoids, and one with phaeochromocytoma (Orth 1987). Most small-cell lung cancer tumours and cell lines synthesize bombesin which can act as or potentiate CRF, enhancing the secretion or effect of pituitary or tumour-derived ACTH (Stewart et al. 1987).

The clinical picture of ectopic ACTH production occurs most commonly in patients with lung cancer and in particular small-cell lung cancer. Fifty per cent of patients with small-cell lung cancer have elevated serum cortisols which do not suppress with dexamethasone (Odell 1989). However, the clinical syndrome is rare and is seen in only 3 per cent of small-cell lung cancer patients. There are some important differences from classical Cushing's syndrome. The illness is typically of rapid onset, with marked weakness due to proximal myopathy. Many patients show hyperpigmentation, and metabolic disturbance with hypokalaemic alkalosis and hyperglycaemia is a striking feature. The typical phenotypic changes of Cushing's syndrome (altered fat distribution, striae, spontaneous bruising) are less common because of the rapid onset (Howlett et al. 1986).

Cushing's syndrome can also be the presenting feature of a second group of tumours, including bronchial carcinoids and neuroendocrine tumours of the thymus, adrenal, and pancreas. Thymic tumours make up 10 per cent of cases of ectopic ACTH production and conversely 40 per cent of thymic carcinoids present with Cushing's syndrome (Farwell et al. 1988). These slow-growing tumours are often occult at the time of presentation and Cushing's syndrome here is more difficult to distinguish from pituitary-dependent ACTH secretion (Howlett et al. 1986). Table 2 describes the clinical features of these groups and the diagnostic tests used to distinguish them.

Ectopic hormone production by a tumour is ideally treated by specific antitumour treatment. If the tumour is not identifiable or effectively treatable, cortisol secretion can be abolished surgically by bilateral adrenalectomy or medically using metyrapone, mitotane, aminoglutethimide, octreotide, or ketoconazole. Aminoglutethimide, ketoconazole, and mitotane must be given with hydrocortisone to prevent hypoadrenalism (Farwell et al. 1988; Lamberts et al. 1988; Sheeler 1988). The prognosis in cases of ectopic ACTH production is usually very poor and most patients die soon after presentation, often with opportunistic infections (Dimopoulos et al. 1992). However, the group presenting with a slower onset and an occult neoplasm may have a good prognosis, and early diagnosis and tumour resection may be curative (Howlett et al. 1986).

The syndrome of inappropriate ADH secretion (SIADH)

Antidiuretic hormone (ADH), also known as arginine-vasopressin, is a nonapeptide synthesized in the hypothalamus as a precursor propressophysin (20 kDa), which is processed to arginine-vasopressin

Table 2   ACTH-dependent Cushing's syndrome: clinical features and diagnosis

		Ectopic ACTH production	
	Pituitary-dependent Cushing's disease	With signs of underlying neoplasm	With occult neoplasm
Tumour associations	Pituitary adenoma	SCLC, pancreas	Bronchial, thymic, pancreatic carcinoids adrenal, for example phaeochromocytoma, medullary carcinoid of thyroid
Onset	Slow—months/years	Rapid: weeks/months	Slow: 3 months to 4 years
Clinical features	Classical Cushing's syndrome	Muscle weakness, wasting, hyperpigmentation	Classical Cushing's syndrome
Plasma potassium	Low in 10% untreated patients (more if on K^+-losing diuretics)	Low, 2–3.2 mmol/l	Low, 2–3.2 mmol/l
Plasma bicarbonate	May be normal/high	High, >28 mmol/l	>28 mmol/l
Plasma cortisol (normal at 9 a.m., 200–700 nmol/l)	440–1100 nmol/l Loss diurnal rhythm	900–3650 nmol/l Loss diurnal rhythm	700–2400 nmol/l Loss diurnal rhythm
Urine-free control (normal, 24–108 μg/24 h)	Elevated	Elevated	Elevated
Plasma ACTH (normal at 9 a.m., 10–80 ng/l)	40–430 ng/l (ACTH 1–39)	400–2340 ng/l (high MW forms)	70–250 ng/l (high MW forms)
Low-dose dexamethasone test (0.5 mg 6 hourly for 48 h)	No suppression of plasma cortisol	No suppression	No suppression
High-dose dexamethasone test 2 mg 6 hourly for 48 h starting at 9 a.m.)	80–90% show normal suppression of urinary steroids by ⩾50% basal value on second day of test and 80% suppression of plasma cortisol by >50% at 48 h	No suppression	Suppression of urinary steroids in 30%, plasma cortisol in 10%
Metyrapone test (750 mg 4 hourly for 24 h starting at 9 a.m.)	Most show normal response—plasma ACTH and/or urinary 17-OGS increase by >100% basal levels	No response	60% show normal response
CRF test 100 μg IV at 9 a.m. (normal response—peak cortisol 430–820 nmol/l, 30–90 min after CRF)	75% show extensive rise in cortisol, >820 nmol/l	No response	No response

17-OGS, 17-oxogenic steroids. Data from Howlett et al. (1986); Case Records (1987); Carpenter (1988); Grossman et al. (1988); Lamberts et al. (1988); and Odell (1989).

(1 kDa) and neurophysin II (10 kDa) (Fig. 1(b)). Hypothalamic synthesis of oxytocin occurs in a similar way from a linked gene. Arginine-vasopressin is secreted by the posterior pituitary in response to hypovolaemia and inhibits water excretion across the distal renal tubule.

Schwartz et al. (1957) described two patients with small-cell lung cancer complicated by hyponatremia, hypervolaemia, and urine of inappropriately high osmolarity and sodium concentration. This was correctly thought to be due to ectopic arginine-vasopressin synthesis by the tumour. Plasma precursors of arginine-vasopressin and oxytocin have been shown to be elevated in the plasma of 65 per cent of patients with small-cell lung cancer and 20 per cent with non-SCLC. Almost 50 per cent of small-cell lung cancer patients with high arginine-vasopressin and neurophysin II had SIADH and all small-cell lung cancer patients with SIADH had elevated arginine-vasopressin and neurophysin II (Maurer et al. 1983). Arginine-vasopressin and neurophysin II have been found covalently linked in SCLC tumour tissue of patients with SIADH (Yamaji et al. 1981). A human small-cell lung cancer cell line has been shown to possess the genes for arginine-vasopressin and oxytocin and to produce significant amounts of propressophysin, but the oxytocin gene was not transcribed (Sausville et al. 1985). High levels of atrial natriuretic factor have been described in the setting of small-cell lung cancer with SIADH. Atrial natriuretic factor is a powerful natriuretic and vasodilator which causes increased glomerular filtration rate and blocks secretion and/or actions of renin, angiotensin II, and aldosterone. This may explain the conspicuous absence of arterial hypertension in SIADH (Cogan et al. 1986).

In SCLC, which accounts for 75 per cent of tumour-associated SIADH, the reported incidence has ranged from 1 per cent (patients with clinical manifestations) to 70 per cent (patients unable to excrete a standard water load). When strict diagnostic criteria (Table 3) are used, SIADH is present in approximately 10 per cent of patients with small-cell lung cancer (List et al. 1986). SIADH has been linked with extensive disease, propensity for CNS metastasis, and poor response to chemotherapy, but these findings were not confirmed in a recent study (List et al. 1986). Other causes of SIADH are listed in Table 4. In 80 per cent of patients serum sodium increases (>130 mmol/l) within 3 weeks of starting chemotherapy, often pre-dating clinical or radiological evidence of response. Arginine-vasopressin levels often take longer to fall to normal, possibly because of the effect on serum sodium of treatment for SIADH or the prolonged plasma clearance of arginine-vasopressin. Occasionally hyponatremia persists despite clinical remission. Patients who had SIADH at presentation often develop recurrent symptoms of hyponatremia at relapse (List et al. 1986).

Table 3 Diagnostic criteria for SIADH

Hyponatremia (Na$^+$ <130 mmol/l)
Serum hypo-osmolarity (<275 mmol/kg)
Urinary sodium >25 mmol/l
Urine osmolarity $>$ serum osmolarity
Normal plasma glucose
Normal serum albumin (>30 g/l)
Normal renal and thyroid function in a non-oedematous patient
Plasma ADH not suppressed (normally undetectable if Na$^+$ <130 mmol/l, serum osmolarity <270 mmol/l)

From List et al. (1986).

Table 4 Causes of SIADH

1 Ectopic VP production by tumours
 SCLC
  Carcinoma of pancreas
  Carcinoma of prostate
  Carcinoma of bladder
  Lymphomas (Hodgkin's, non-Hodgkin's)
  Thymoma
  Carcinoma of duodenum
  Mesothelioma
  Ewing's sarcoma
2 Non-neoplastic pulmonary disorders (? ectopic VP synthesis or enhancement of central VP release in response to reduction in left atrial filling)
  Infections
   Pneumonia—bacterial/viral
   Tuberculosis
   Lung abscess
   Empyema
   Aspergillosis
  Other
   Asthma
   Pneumothorax
   Positive pressure ventilation
   Cystic lesions
3 Central nervous system disorders (enhancing pituitary VP release)
  Trauma
  Infection
   Encephalitis (viral/bacterial)
   Meningitis (viral/bacterial)
   Brain abscess
  Vascular
   Cerebral infarction/haemorrhage
   Subdural or subarachnoid haematoma/haemorrhage
   Cavernous sinus thrombosis
  Brain tumours
  Other
   Systemic lupus erythematosus
   Acute psychosis
   Delirium tremens
   Guillain–Barré syndrome
   Acute intermittent porphyria
   Hydrocephalus
   Multiple sclerosis
4 Drugs
  Cytotoxics (vincas, cyclophosphamide, cis-platinum)
  Chlorpropamide
  Thiazides
  Carbamazepine
  Oxytocin
  Narcotics including morphine, haloperidol, phenothiazines
  Antidepressants (tricyclics, monoamine oxidase inhibitors)
  Clofibrate

VP, vasopressin; SCLC, small-cell lung cancer.
Modified from Robertson (1987) and Streeten et al. (1987).

The treatment of SIADH is fluid restriction (0.5–1 l/day) and the tetracycline antibiotic demeclocycline (150–300 mg, 6–8 hourly) which induces nephrogenic diabetes insipidus; that is, the distal tubule becomes refractory to the effect of ADH (Robertson 1987).

Hypercalcaemia

Hypercalcaemia is a common problem in patients with cancer, and is usually a late event with poor prognosis (Burtis et al. 1988). In

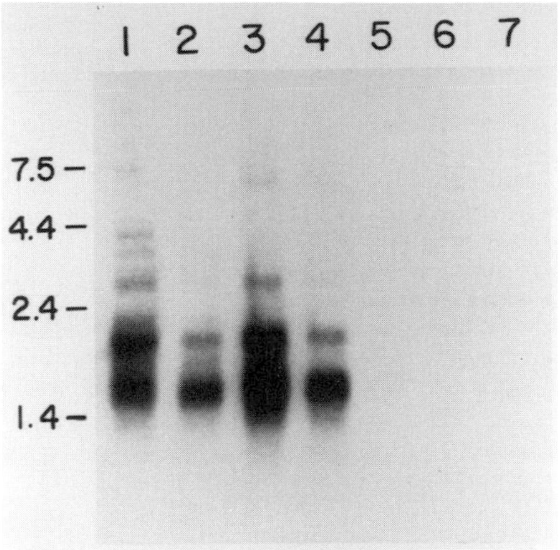

Fig. 2 Northern blot analysis of mRNAs from human renal carcinomas. Lanes 1–4 contain mRNAs from renal carcinomas associated with humoral hypercalcaemia of malignancy. These show two major hybridizing species of approximately 1.6 and 2.1 kb and several less abundant species of 3.2–4.2 kb. Lanes 5–7 contain mRNA from renal carcinomas that did not secrete PTH-like activity *in vitro* nor induce hypercalcaemia when grown as xenografts in nude mice. (Reproduced with permission from Ikeda *et al.* (1988).)

50 per cent of patients the main cause is metastatic invasion of bone (for example, from breast cancer) which is dealt with in Section 8 of this volume. Thirty per cent have solid tumours but without evidence of bone metastases (for example, squamous cancers of head and neck, lung, and oesophagus) and the final 20 per cent have haematological or lymphoid malignancy including in particular myeloma and non-Hodgkin's lymphoma.

Fuller Albright (1941) described a patient with carcinoma and a solitary bone metastasis associated with hypercalcaemia and hypophosphataemia. He postulated that the tumour was secreting parathyroid hormone (PTH) or a related peptide. Subsequently more such patients were described, with little or no bone involvement. This condition is known as the humoral hypercalcaemia of malignancy and early radio-immunoassays supported the idea that this was due to ectopic PTH secretion. However, in the 1970s improvements in PTH radio-immunoassay began to cast doubts on the idea that immunoreactive PTH in cancer patients was identical to authentic PTH. Intensive research in the last 10 years has shown that humoral hypercalcaemia of malignancy is due to tumour production of a PTH-like peptide released into the circulation, acting on the target organs of PTH to cause hypercalcaemia. This peptide has been termed humoral hypercalcaemia of malignancy factor or PTH-related protein (Martin *et al.* 1989). The main form has 141 amino acids and molecular weight 16–18 kDa, compared with PTH 1-84 which has molecular weight 9.6 kDa and PTH 1-34 (the active moiety) which has molecular weight 4.1 kDa. Significantly, the amino acid sequences from four human cancers (breast, renal, and two squamous lung cancers) were identical, as were predicted sequences derived from cDNAs from two different carcinomas, one renal and one squamous (Burtis *et al.* 1988). Eight of 13 N-terminal residues in PTH-related protein are homologous with PTH. Thereafter the sequences are completely different, explaining the lack of antigenic cross-reactivity. PTH-related protein cannot be inhibited by anti-PTH antisera, although

it is blocked by PTH antagonists, indicating that it acts via the PTH receptor (Mundy 1988). Synthetic PTH-related protein 1-34 stimulates bone resorption *in vitro*, activates PTH-sensitive adenylate cyclase in bone and kidney, and induces hypercalcaemia and hypophosphataemia when infused into rats (Burtis *et al.* 1988). Antibodies to this synthetic fragment suppress hypercalcaemia in animal models (Kukreja *et al.* 1988). Thus it seems very likely that PTH-related protein is responsible for humoral hypercalcaemia of malignancy (Rosol and Capen 1992) (Fig. 2). PTH-related protein is also synthesized by some benign tumours, normal keratinocytes, placenta, and fetal parathyroid. It may have a physiological function, possibly in maternal–fetal calcium transport (Care 1989; Martin *et al.* 1989).

PTH-related protein acts like PTH on kidney and bone, causing hypercalcaemia, hypophosphataemia due to lowering of the renal tubular phosphate threshold, increased renal cAMP excretion and increased osteoclastic bone resorption. Unlike PTH, PTH-related protein has no effect on intestinal calcium absorption or synthesis of 1-25 dihydroxyvitamin D (1,25 OHD_3). Patients with humoral hypercalcaemia of malignancy tend to have increased osteoclastic bone resorption and decreased osteoblastic bone formation compared with primary hyperparathyroidism (Burtis *et al.* 1988; Mundy 1988). Table 5 gives the clinical and biochemical features which distinguish hypercalcaemia due to bone metastases, humoral hypercalcaemia of malignancy, and primary hyperparathyroidism.

Two other groups of host- or tumour-derived factors contribute to bone resorption experimentally and probably also clinically: (1) cytokines produced by tumour cells or non-malignant host monocytes or macrophages and including IL-1, IL-6, tumour necrosis factor alpha (cachexin), and tumour necrosis factor beta (lymphotoxin); (2) tumour growth factors including transforming growth factors alpha and beta, epidermal growth factor, and platelet-derived growth factor. These may act via increased local production of prostaglandin E_2 (PGE_2) which stimulates local osteoclastic bone resorption. It is unclear how far this mechanism could account for systemic hypercalcaemia, since PGE_2 is very labile in the circulation and if calcium homeostasis were otherwise intact, the excess calcium liberated from bone would simply be excreted in the urine (Tashjian *et al.* 1982; Martin *et al.* 1989; Black *et al.* 1991).

Other disorders of calcium metabolism

There are two rarer disorders of calcium metabolism which occur in patients with cancer (Orth 1987). Tumour-induced osteomalacia has been described in approximately 50 cases, most with benign or, rarely, malignant mesenchymal tumours including haemangioma, haemangiopericytoma, fibroangioma, neuroma, and osteosarcoma. There are isolated reports in patients with cancer of the prostate and breast and with small-cell lung cancer. Patients complain of muscle weakness and bone pain, especially in the back. Investigations show hypophosphataemia (< 1.5 mmol/l), normal serum calcium, markedly elevated alkaline phosphatase, and low serum 1,25 OHD_3. There is profound hyperphosphaturia and sometimes also amino aciduria and glycosuria. These findings suggest a defect in the proximal renal tubule, presumed to be due to a humoral tumour-derived factor, the identity of which is at present unknown. If complete tumour resection is not possible, symptoms may be ameliorated by oral phosphate supplements and 1,25 OHD_3 (Orth 1987).

Hypocalcaemia is found in approximately 15 per cent of patients with bone metastases, particularly sclerotic metastases from breast,

Table 5 Differential diagnosis of hypercalcaemia

	Bone metastases	HHM	Primary hyperparathyroidism
Tumour association	Breast cancer Myeloma	Squamous carcinomas (head and neck, lung, oesophagus, vulva), renal adenocarcinoma, transitional cell carcinoma, ovarian and gynaecological malignances, occasionally breast cancer	Parathyroid hyperplasia or adenoma
Duration of hypercalcaemia	Short	Short, abrupt onset symptoms, particularly nausea and constipation	Long, slowly progressive
Other clinical features	Patients unwell ±symptoms/signs of tumour	Patients unwell ±symptoms/signs of tumour	Patients usually well ±bone keratopathy, renal calculi, hypertension, pruritis, osteitis fibrosa cystica
Biochemistry	Ca^{2+} >2.7 mmol/l P normal Albumin normal/low	Ca^{2+} >2.7 mmol/l P low Often mild hypokalaemic alkalosis Cl and albumin low	Ca^{2+} >2.7 mmol/l P low Chloride high Albumin normal
Urinary Ca^{2+}	Hypercalciuria +++	Hypercalciuria +++	Hypercalciuria +
Urinary P	Normal	High	High
Plasma 1,25-OHD$_3$ (normal, 20–65 ng/l)	Low	Low	High (PTH stimulates renal synthesis of this metabolite)
Plasma PTH	Low/undetectable	Low/undetectable	High
Renal cAMP excretion (normal, 0.5–2.5 nmol per 100 ml glomerular filtrate)	Low	High +++	High +
Bone scan	Multiple metastases	Normal/few metastases	Increased uptake in areas of demineralization/erosion (particularly calvarium, mandible, acromioclavicular, sternum, lateral humeral epicondyles, hands) and in 'brown tumours' (particularly long bones) ± late stage: extraskeletal uptake in areas of soft tissue calcification

+++ Marked abnormality.
+ Result abnormal but not markedly so.
HHM, humoral hypercalcaemia of malignancy.
Data from Boyd and Ladenson (1984), Mundy *et al.* (1984), Kim and Haynie (1987), Burtis *et al.* (1988), Mundy (1988), Heath (1989), and Martin *et al.* (1989).

prostate, or lung cancer. This is usually asymptomatic, but very rarely causes tetany.

Calcitonin is secreted eutopically by medullary carcinoma of the thyroid and ectopically by a wide variety of tumours. Serum immunoreactive calcitonin is elevated in 60 per cent of patients with small cell lung cancer, 15 per cent with non-small-cell lung cancer, and many patients with breast cancer and leukaemia. High levels are also found in some patients with tumours of the gastrointestinal tract, pancreas, kidney, hepatoma, lymphoma, melanoma, carcinoid tumours, and phaeochromocytoma (Milhaud 1985). Human small-cell lung cancer cells express calcitonin mRNA, which undergoes alternative processing to generate mRNAs encoding two different peptides, calcitonin and calcitonin gene-related peptide (Craig *et al.* 1985). However, there is no evidence that calcitonin mediates hypocalcaemia in patients with cancer (Orth 1987).

Tumour hypoglycaemia

Hypoglycaemia associated with non-islet cell tumours is a rare but interesting paraneoplastic complication which was first described by Doege (1930). Hypoglycaemia occurs typically in large slow-growing mesenchymal tumours of the thorax or retroperitoneum

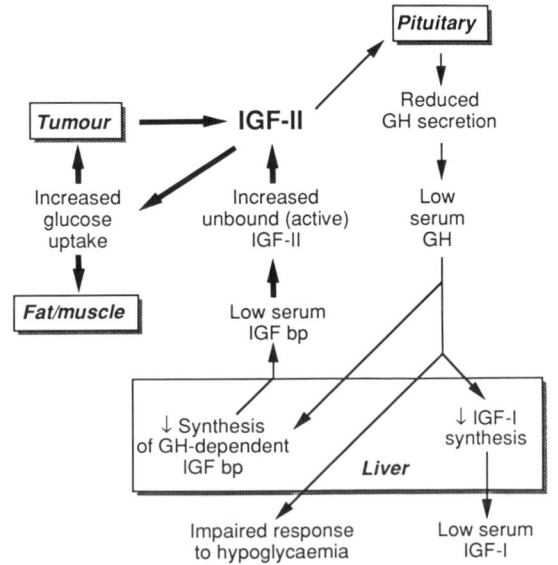

Fig. 3 Mechanisms of tumour hypoglycaemia: → stimulatory effect; → inhibitory effect; bp, binding protein; GH, growth hormone.

Table 6 Causes of gynaecomastia

Hypogonadism
  Testicular failure/damage
    Viral orchitis, trauma, castration, granulomatous diseases
  Secondary (pituitary/hypothalamic) hypogonadism
  Klinefelter's syndrome
Tumours
  Oestrogen-producing
    Adrenal carcinoma
    Leydig or Sertoli cell tumour of testis
    Hepatoma
  hCG-producing
    Teratoma
    Lung cancer especially adenocarcinoma
  Hypogonadism
    Pituitary tumours
Systemic diseases
  Refeeding after starvation
    Including recovery from any prolonged illness
    Renal failure after commencing dialysis
  Hepatic especially alcoholic cirrhosis
  Hyperthyroidism
Drugs
  Hormones: oestrogens, androgens, gonadotrophins
  Inhibitors of testosterone synthesis: ketoconazole, cytotoxics
  Inhibitors of testosterone action: spironolactone, cimetidine, marihuana, progestogens
  CNS mechanism, especially enhancing prolactin secretion: metoclopramide, domperidone, phenothiazines, amphetamines, tricyclic antidepressants, diazepam
  Refeeding mechanism: digoxin, isoniazid

Modified from Carlson (1980), Santen (1987), Wilson (1987), Coen *et al.* (1991), and Wilson (1991).

including sarcomas, mesotheliomas, and hemangiopericytomas (Axelrod and Ron 1988).

In contrast with islet cell tumours, this form of hypoglycaemia is not mediated by insulin. Recent studies have shown overexpression of insulin-like growth factor-II (IGF-II) mRNA in tumours of three patients with hypoglycaemia (fibrosarcoma, mesothelioma, thoracic leiomysarcoma) with high tumour and serum levels of immunoreactive IGF-II (Daughaday *et al.* 1988; Ron *et al.* 1989). Probable mechanisms of IGF-II-induced hypoglycaemia are shown in Fig. 3.

Ectopic gonadotrophin secretion

The pituitary hormones follicle-stimulating hormone and luteinizing hormone are heterodimers consisting of non-covalently bound glycosylated alpha and beta subunits. Placental human chorionic gonadotrophin (hCG) has the same structure. Gonadotrophins are secreted eutopically by pituitary and trophoblastic tumours. Expression of ectopic gonadotrophic heterodimers and/or subunits has been detected by radio-immunoassay and Northern analysis in patients' sera and tumour cell lines, including lung, breast, gastrointestinal, pancreatic, and cervical carcinomas, islet cell tumours, and hepatoma (Orth 1987; Cosgrove *et al.* 1989). The discrepancy between the apparent high incidence of circulating gonadotrophins and the rarity of associated clinical syndromes is probably due to secretion of inactive single subunits or differentially glycosylated heterodimers.

Precocious puberty has been described in children with hepatoblastoma and high hCG levels. Gynaecomastia in adult men is the commonest manifestation of ectopic hCG secretion and is usually bilateral and occasionally painful. Tumour-derived hCG leads to conversion within the tumour of circulating dehydroepiandrosterone to oestradiol, and it is probably this which acts on the breast to cause gynaecomastia. Gynaecomastia has many non-neoplastic causes (Table 6). The commonest cause of gynaecomastia and elevated β-hCG is a germ cell tumour of the testis or extragonadal site, or lung cancer, particularly adenocarcinoma. If no tumour is immediately apparent, patients should be carefully followed up as gynaecomastia may predate tumour diagnosis. Paraneoplastic gynaecomastia may respond to effective antitumour treatment, but reduction mammoplasty may be required to relieve pain or embarrassment (Orth 1987).

Thyrotoxicosis is a rare complication of extremely high circulating levels of hCG which occur in gestational trophoblastic tumours (Fierro and Freeman 1988). This syndrome is rare because hCG is a weak thyrotropin, and it is only the very high levels secreted by trophoblastic tumours which can cross-react to a significant degree with the thyroid-stimulating hormone receptor (Orth 1987).

Ectopic secretion of other hormones

Immunoreactive growth hormone has been detected in lung cancer of all histological subtypes, bronchial carcinoids, and gastric and endometrial carcinomas. It has been suggested that ectopic growth hormone secretion may be responsible for osteoarthropathy, but there is no clear evidence to support this. Carcinoid or pancreatic islet cell tumours may secrete growth-hormone-releasing hormone, which is a rare cause of acromegaly (<1 per cent of cases).

Thyrotrophin-releasing hormone has been detected in a few cases of lung cancer (small-cell lung cancer and adenocarcinoma) and melanoma, and low levels of somatostatin are secreted by small-cell lung cancer, lung adenocarcinoma, and bronchial, thymic, and duodenal carcinoids. Neither of these peptides is associated with clinical effects. Eutopic secretion of high levels of somatostatin by pancreatic somatostatinomas causes the systemic somatostatinoma syndrome characterized by diabetes mellitus, steatorrhoea, and cholelithiasis (Case Records 1989).

Gastrin-releasing peptide is synthesized by small-cell lung cancer, where it functions as an autocrine growth factor (Cuttitta *et al.* 1985) and also by other tumours including carcinoid, medullary carcinoma of the thyroid, and phaechromocytoma (Orth 1987; Clark 1988). Again, there is no clear clinical manifestation of gastrin-releasing peptide excess although the related peptide bombesin causes anorexia in experimental animals (Brown *et al.* 1977).

Human placental lactogen has been detected in the serum of 9 per cent of patients with non-trophoblastic non-gonadal tumours, most of whom had lung cancer. Some had gynaecomastia but none had galactorrhoea, possibly because circulating levels of human placental lactogen were low or in a high molecular weight biologically inactive form. High levels of bioactive prolactin have been found in only two patients, one with undifferentiated lung cancer and the other with renal carcinoma and galactorrhoea.

Ectopic renin production by extrarenal tumours has been described in two patients with lung cancer (one with small-cell lung cancer and one with adenocarcinoma), paraovarian carcinoma, and pancreatic adenocarcinoma. This causes hypokalaemic alkalosis and hypertension which can be controlled with captopril (Orth 1987).

NEUROLOGICAL SYNDROMES

Neurological paraneoplastic syndromes occur in approximately 7 per cent of patients with malignant disease, including 15 per cent

Table 7 Clinical features of neurological paraneoplastic syndromes

	Clinical features	References
Brain		
Encephalomyelitis		
(i) Limbic	Memory impairment, altered affect, confusion, dementia. CSF: raised protein, lymphocytes±oligoclonal banding; CT scan usually normal, MRI may be abnormal. Corticosteroids unhelpful; may remit with effective antitumour treatment	Brennan and Craddock (1983), Burton et al. (1988), Camara and Chelune (1987), McArdle and Milligen (1988), Case Records (1988b), Batson et al. (1992), Kalkman et al. (1993)
(ii) Brainstem	Ataxia, vertigo, nystagmus, diplopia, bulbar palsy	Henson and Urich (1982), Anderson et al. (1987)
(iii) Myelitis	Predominant anterior horn lesion: LMN signs in neck, arms, trunk, including respiratory muscles; sensory loss if DRG affected. Plasmapheresis, steroids unhelpful. May improve with intrathecal dexamethasone and systemic chemotherapy	Babikian et al. (1985), Dancey et al. (1988)
PCD	Subacute onset of bilateral cerebellar signs. Late diplopia, dementia. Brain CT normal initially, later shows cerebellar atrophy. Occasional response to plasmapheresis, steroids, antitumour treatment. NB: 50% of patients >40 years with acquired progressive cerebellar dysfunction turn out to have an underlying neoplasm	Henson and Urich (1982), Anderson et al. (1987), McLellan et al. (1988), Greenlee et al. (1992), Graus et al. (1992), Clouston et al. (1992), Hammack et al. (1992), Peterson et al. (1992)
CAR syndrome	Blurred vision, scotomata, impaired colour vision±episodic bizarre visual defects. Rapidly progressive painless loss of vision. Diagnostic triad: photosensitivity, ring scotomatous visual field loss, attenuated retinal arteriole calibre. May respond to immunosuppressive agents	Kornguth et al. (1986), Crofts et al. (1988), Thirkill et al. (1987), Jacobson et al. (1990)
OM	Opsoclonus, myoclonus. In children: ataxia, hypotonia±fits. May improve with steroids or ACTH but may have residual ataxia/intellectual impairment. In adults: vertigo, ataxia, dysarthria	Solomon and Chutorian (1968), Anderson et al. (1988), Case Records (1988a), Schor (1992)
CPM	Bulbar palsy, quadriparesis±impairment of higher function and conjugate gaze, nystagmus, extraocular palsies. CT: low density in central pons. Treatment: supportive, maintain normal electrolyte levels	Yufe et al. (1980)
Cord		
Necrotizing myelopathy	Back pain/nerve root pain herald acute ascending flaccid paraplegia with sensory impairment±brainstem, visual involvement. CSF: elevated protein, pleiocytosis. Myelography: slight swelling of cord. Treatment unhelpful	Henson and Urich (1982), Mandel (1989)
SSN	Loss of all modalities sensation, starts distally, moves proximally over few months. Sensory ataxia, pseudoathetosis	Henson and Urich (1982), Anderson (1987), Chad and Recht (1988)
SMN	Subacute progressive painless patchy weakness of LMN type legs>arms. Spares bulbar muscles	Schold et al. (1979)
Peripheral nerves		
Chronic inflammatory neuropathy		
(i) Progressive sensorimotor PN	May be motor/sensory/mixed. Distal, progressive. Affects touch, vibration, joint position sense	McLeod (1984); Valli et al. (1988)
Complicating monoclonal gammopathy	Anti-MAG paraprotein: affects extremities with weakness, ataxia, intention tremor	Steck et al. (1987)
	Anti-glycolipid: diasialosyl gangliosides: sensory demyelinating PN. Chondroitin-C: sensorimotor axonal PN. Anti-intermediate filament: demyelinating PN. Gangliosides GM or GD_{1b}: LMN syndrome	
(ii) Remitting/relapsing sensorimotor PN	Fluctuating course	Henson and Urich (1982), Mandel (1989)
Guillain–Barré syndrome	Weakness proximal >distal, areflexia, minimal/mild sensory loss. CSF protein raised, cells normal. May be acute, fulminant (quadriplegia, ventilator dependence ≤24 h) or more slowly progressive (days/weeks)	Henson (1986), Anderson et al. (1987), Chad and Recht (1988)
Autonomic neuropathy	Dry mouth, impaired sweating. Cardiovascular: postural hypotension, loss of beat to beat variation, failure of vasoconstrictive response to Valsalva. Gut: abdominal pain, altered bowel habit may precede tumour diagnosis by many months. X-rays show abnormal/decreased gut motility. Ocular: dry eyes, tonic ('Holmes–Adies') pupils. Genitourinary: impotence, failure of ejaculation, difficulty with micturition. May respond to antitumour treatment	Park et al. (1972), Vasudevan et al. (1981), Schuffler et al. (1983), Chinn et al. (1988), Khurana et al. (1988), Lennon et al. (1991)

Neuromuscular junction		
LEMS	Proximal weakness legs >arms±muscle aching, stiffness, ptosis. Spares extraocular and bulbar muscles. 50% have autonomic symptoms. Improves in parallel with response to antitumour treatment	Newsom-Davis (1988), Khurana *et al.* (1988), Chalk *et al.* (1990)
MG	Fatiguability, proximal limb weakness. Ptosis, diplopia, dysphagia, dysarthria. Symptoms worse in evening	Anderson *et al.* (1987), Chad and Recht (1988)
Muscle		
PM/DM	Subacute proximal muscle weakness[a], pain[a]±ptosis, dysphagia, respiratory muscle weakness. 50% have violacious rash on face, upper chest, hands±interstitial lung disease, cardiac involvement (usually asymptomatic). Raised ESR and creatine kinase[a], abnormal EMG[a], inflammation[a] on muscle biopsy	DeVere and Bradley (1975), Barnes (1976), Henson and Urich (1982), Chad and Recht (1988), Callen (1993)

LMN, lower motor neurone; DRG, dorsal root ganglion; for other abbreviations see text.
[a]Diagnostic criteria for PM.
See also reviews by Henson and Urich (1982), Henson (1986), Anderson *et al.* (1987), Chad and Recht (1988), Mandel (1989), Dalmau *et al.* (1992), and Graus and Rene (1992).

of patients with carcinomas of the lung or ovary (Croft and Wilkinson 1965). Most have proximal myopathy or mild peripheral neuropathy; the other neurological syndromes are rare, occurring in less than 1 per cent of patients (Anderson *et al.* 1987). Myasthenia gravis and Lambert–Eaton myasthenic syndrome, described in more detail below, are classic examples of neurological syndromes mediated by humoral immunity. There are clear associations with specific tumours: myasthenia gravis with thymoma and Lambert–Eaton myasthenic syndrome with small-cell lung cancer. Target-specific autoantibodies are almost invariably detected, both conditions improve in response to treatment designed to reduce antibody titres, and clinical and pathological features of each disease can be induced in passive transfer experiments (Antel and Moumdjian 1989). There is increasing evidence for an immune mechanism in other neurological syndromes, including encephalomyelitis/subacute sensory neuropathy, paraneoplastic cerebellar degeneration, cancer-associated retinopathy, and peripheral neuropathies associated with IgM paraproteinaemia (Anderson *et al.* 1987). The main syndromes are listed in Table 7 with references for further reading.

Syndromes involving the brain

Dementia

Acute impairment of higher function without specific localizing signs is almost always a manifestation of an organic confusional state. Common causes include drugs, infections, endocrine/metabolic disturbances, myocardial infarction, and pulmonary embolus. Subacute or chronic deterioration in cognitive function is the commonest cerebral abnormality in cancer patients, occurring in 33 per cent of those with paraneoplastic neurological involvement (Mandel 1989). If truly paraneoplastic, dementia is often associated with other neurological paraneoplastic syndromes and sometimes also with antineuronal antibodies (Anderson *et al.* 1988a). However, true paraneoplastic dementia is unusual and it is important to rule out direct tumour involvement or indirect effects of the tumour or its treatment (Henson and Urich 1982).

Encephalomyelopathies

Paraneoplastic encephalomyelopathic syndromes are characterized by common pathological features, with perivascular inflammation and selective neuronal degeneration and possibly also by common immune aetiology (Antel and Moumdjian 1989). Seventy-five

per cent of patients have lung cancer (mostly small-cell lung cancer); other associations include carcinomas of the breast, ovary, stomach, and uterus, and Hodgkin's disease (Henson and Urich 1982). Patients with paraneoplastic encephalomyelopathies and small-cell lung cancer have been shown to express autoantibodies directed against 35–40 kDa brain-specific neuronal nucleoprotein, which may have a role in neuron-specific RNA processing (Grisold *et al.* 1987; Antel and Moumdjian 1989; Szabo *et al.* 1991).

Pathological changes are found throughout the neuraxis late in the natural history of this disease. Early on the changes are often localized, resulting in defined clinical syndromes of limbic, cerebellar, or brainstem encephalitis, myelitis, or subacute sensory neuropathy (ganglioradiculitis). In general, these syndromes pursue a progressive course and patients rarely survive beyond 2 years. In the majority, death is directly related to the tumour, but in some the tumour remains occult and is diagnosed only at autopsy. These patients die because of neurological impairment, usually bulbar palsy (causing aspiration pneumonia), bulbospinal respiratory failure, or chronic gross neurological incapacity (Henson and Urich 1982).

Paraneoplastic cerebellar degeneration (PCD)

Paraneoplastic cerebellar involvement may be predominantly inflammatory ('cerebellar encephalitis') as described above or predominantly degenerative, a condition known as paraneoplastic cerebellar degeneration. These two syndromes may represent two stages in the same disease process (Henson and Urich 1982). Patients with paraneoplastic cerebellar degeneration have profound loss of Purkinje cells and degeneration of those Purkinje cells which remain, associated with circulating anti-Purkinje cell antibodies (Greenlee and Lipton 1986). Several cDNAs encoding antigens recognized by anti-Purkinje cell antibodies have been cloned. That identified by Dropcho *et al.* (1987) encoded a protein with sequence homology to α_2-macroglobulin and α_1-antitrypsin, which are acute phase proteins and protease inhibitors. It was suggested that antibody-mediated alteration in protease inhibitor activity could affect the turnover of pulmonary connective tissue matrix and thus modulate the tumour's propensity for local growth and metastasis (Kornguth 1989). Indeed patients with ovarian and other gynaecological cancers and anti-Purkinje cell antibodies had significantly smaller volume metastatic disease compared with a control group with equivalent stage and grade of disease (Hetzel *et al.* 1990). Later studies have identified zinc finger and leucine zipper domains, both well-characterized DNA binding motifs, as major epitopes of Purkinje cell autoantigens (Sato *et al.* 1991; Gress *et al.* 1992; Sakai *et al.* 1993). This suggests that antibody binding to the target proteins could alter the regulation of transcriptional activity in Purkinje cells (Sakai *et al.* 1993).

Paraneoplastic cerebellar degeneration may present during the clinical course of the cancer or predate the diagnosis by up to 3 years. Cerebellar signs proceed relentlessly; improvement has occasionally been reported with effective antitumour treatment but patients usually die within a few months (Anderson *et al.* 1987).

Visual paraneoplastic syndromes

Cancer-associated retinopathy (CAR syndrome)

Rapid loss of visual acuity or visual field was first described as a paraneoplastic syndrome in patients with small-cell lung cancer (Sawyer *et al.* 1976). There are approximately 20 case reports of CAR syndrome in small-cell lung cancer and isolated reports in other solid tumours. The serum of patients with small-cell lung cancer and CAR syndrome contains high titres of autoantibodies which react with both antigens on retinal ganglion cells and cultured small-cell lung cancer cells. The principal ocular autoantigen is recoverin, a 23 kDa protein expressed in photoreceptor cells (Thirkill *et al.* 1992). Visual symptoms usually precede diagnosis of the tumour and patients develop blurred vision, scotomata (often with bizarre episodic visual defects), and sometimes impaired colour vision; this is followed by rapidly progressive painless loss of vision (Anderson *et al.* 1987). Retinal arterioles are narrowed, and there are changes in vitreous cells and retinal pigment epithelium (Crofts *et al.* 1988). Electroretinography is abnormal, indicating widespread damage to rods and cones. Post-mortem examination has confirmed loss of rods and cones, together with loss of the outer nuclear layer of the retina (specifically the ganglion cells) and with IgG or IgM in the retinal ganglion layer. This suggests that antiretinal autoantibodies had been able to cross the blood–retinal barrier to gain access to the target cells (Kornguth *et al.* 1986).

Other visual syndromes

There are isolated reports of optic neuritis as the major manifestation of paraneoplastic encephalomyelitis in patients with lung cancer and non-Hodgkin's lymphoma (Anderson *et al.* 1987; Malik *et al.* 1992). However, this may be a chance association or related to meningeal metastases, which can be difficult to diagnose except at autopsy. Acquired night blindness has been described as a remote effect of cancer in a patient with malignant melanoma. Electroretinography showed impaired rod responses (Berson and Lessell 1988).

Opsoclonus–myoclonus (OM)

Opsoclonus occurs when there is loss of inhibitory control over ocular saccades, which are reflex or voluntary brief rapid conjugate eye movements necessary for fixation of the visual target on the fovea (Case Records 1988*a*). Opsoclonus is usually accompanied by ataxia, and myoclonus involving the trunk, limbs, head, diaphragm, larynx, pharynx, and palate (Anderson *et al.* 1987). The condition was first described in 1927 and has been recognized since 1968 as a remote effect of carcinoma, particularly neuroblastoma in children where it complicates 7 per cent of cases (Solomon and Chutorian 1968). Paraneoplastic opsoclonus–myoclonus has also been described in approximately 20 adults, of whom 11 had lung cancer (Anderson *et al.* 1987, 1988*b*). At least half the cases present up to a year before the diagnosis of malignancy and therefore opsoclonus–myoclonus is an important clue to the presence of a tumour. Pathological features are often absent even in the presence of severe neurological symptoms. Antineural antibodies have been detected in paraneoplastic opsoclonus–myoclonus, consistent with an immune aetiology (Budde-Steffen *et al.* 1988*a*).

Central pontine myelinolysis (CPM)

Symmetrical demyelination in the pons is associated in approximately 15 per cent of cases with underlying malignancy, including carcinoma of the pancreas, non-Hodgkin's lymphoma, leukaemia, and primary intracranial tumours. However, central pontine myelinolysis is most common in non-malignant conditions, including alcoholism, malnutrition, and pancreatitis, where it is precipitated by rapid correction of hyponatremia. The aetiology is unknown (Henson and Urich 1982; Mandel 1989).

Progressive multifocal leucoencephalopathy (PML)

This condition occurs particularly in immunocompromised patients, with an incidence of approximately 0.5 per cent in patients with Hodgkin's or non-Hodgkin's lymphoma and 2.5 per cent in chronic lymphatic leukaemia (Henson and Urich 1982). Progressive multifocal leucoencephalopathy is characterized by multiple foci of demyelination scattered throughout the brain and has traditionally been described as a paraneoplastic condition. In 1971 a papovavirus was cultured from brain tissue of a patient with this condition and most recently studied cases have been associated with the Jakob–Creutzfeldt papovavirus (Padgett *et al.* 1976). The virus attacks oligodendrocytes, causing demyelination in the CNS. Patients present with progressive lethargy, nausea, headache, and behavioural changes, often followed by hemiparesis and disorders of speech and vision including hemianopia. Late features include involuntary movements, fits, and coma. The CT scan is the definitive investigation, showing low attenuation areas in the white matter. There is no effective treatment, and most patients die within months of diagnosis (Henson and Urich 1982; Mandel 1989).

Spinal cord syndromes

The spinal cord is primarily involved in approximately 10 per cent of all paraneoplastic neurological syndromes (Croft and Wilkinson 1965).

Myelitis

Patients with paraneoplastic encephalomyelopathy may present with predominant cord involvement. Paraneoplastic myelitis is particularly associated with small-cell lung cancer and Hodgkin's disease. A patient with myelopathy and small-cell lung cancer was shown to have circulating antineuronal IgG antibodies which bound to a 52 kDa protein in normal human cord, cerebral grey matter, retina, and the patient's own tumour. There is intense inflammation and loss of neurons in the anterior and posterior horns, affecting either a few segments (usually cervical or lumbar) or the entire cord. Destruction of anterior horn cells often predominates, leading to degeneration of the anterior roots, with motor neuropathy and muscle atrophy (Babikian *et al.* 1985; Dancey *et al.* 1988). Neurological impairment may respond to intrathecal dexamethasone (Hughes *et al.* 1992).

Necrotizing myelopathy

This is a very rare complication of lymphoma, leukaemia, and lung cancer, especially small-cell lung cancer. There is patchy multifocal necrosis throughout the cord (particularly white matter of the posterior and lateral columns) or massive necrosis of the thoracic cord. The aetiology is unknown and there is no evidence of vascular occlusion or vasculitis (Henson and Urich 1982; Mandel 1989).

Motor neuron disease (MND)

An early study found a significant association between amyotrophic lateral sclerosis and malignancy (Norris and Engel 1965), but subsequent reviews have given conflicting opinions on this point (Anderson et al. 1987; Rosenfeld and Posner 1991). There is, however, an increased incidence of lymphoma in patients with amyotrophic lateral sclerosis and it has been suggested that both diseases could have a common viral aetiology (Jubelt 1992). In some patients with clinical features resembling motor neuron disease, motor neuron loss in the anterior horns is due to subacute motor neuronopathy or encephalomyelitis which usually has other clinical manifestations elsewhere in the neuraxis (Anderson et al. 1987).

Subacute sensory neuropathy (SSN)

Subacute sensory neuropathy, also known as ganglioradiculitis, was first recognized as a paraneoplastic syndrome by Denny-Brown (1948). There are only approximately 40 cases in the literature, two-thirds of whom had small-cell lung cancer. In most patients the neuropathy antedates tumour diagnosis, sometimes by many years and the tumour may be diagnosed only at post-mortem examination. The dorsal root ganglia are infiltrated by lymphocytes and macrophages, leading to loss of dorsal root ganglia neurons and secondary degeneration of the posterior nerve roots, peripheral sensory nerves, and posterior columns of the cord. Approximately 50 per cent of patients have evidence of paraneoplastic encephalomyelitis elsewhere in the cord and brain (Chalk et al. 1992). Patients with subacute sensory neuropathy and small-cell lung cancer have antineuronal antibodies which recognize basic nuclear protein(s) of molecular weight 35–38 kDa present in the neuronal nuclei of dorsal root ganglia, trigeminal ganglia, the CNS, and primary and metastatic small-cell lung cancer (Graus et al. 1985a, 1986). Thus, it seems likely that subacute sensory neuropathy represents an immunological reaction to an antigen shared by small-cell lung cancer and neuronal nuclei (Budde-Steffen et al. 1988b).

Subacute motor neuronopathy (SMN)

This very rare condition (reported in fewer than 15 patients) is associated with Hodgkin's disease and non-Hodgkin's lymphoma and is the motor counterpart of subacute sensory neuropathy. Unlike subacute sensory neuropathy, subacute motor neuropathy may be benign with remissions, independent of the activity of the lymphoma. The aetiology is unknown and there is no effective treatment (Schold et al. 1979; Anderson et al. 1987; Chad and Recht 1988).

Peripheral neuropathy (PN)

In contrast with the neuropathies described above where the key lesion is neuronal degeneration, paraneoplastic peripheral neuropathies are caused by axonal degeneration or demyelination. EMG is useful in pinpointing the anatomical site of the lesion and in differentiating axonal and demyelinating pathology. Symptomatic peripheral neuropathy occurs in approximately 1–2 per cent of patients with carcinoma, Hodgkin's disease, and myeloma (Henson and Urich 1982). However, asymptomatic EMG abnormalities are

much commoner and occur in 35–50 per cent of patients with lung cancer, 25 per cent of patients with Hodgkin's disease, and 13 per cent of patients with myeloma (Croft and Wilkinson 1969; Henson and Urich 1982). Previously undiagnosed cancer is a relatively rare cause of progressive peripheral neuropathy (Valli et al. 1988). In small-cell lung cancer there is an association between the development of peripheral neuropathy and the loss of more than 15 per cent of body weight (Hawley et al. 1980). There are many different classifications of peripheral neuropathy; in general progressive neuropathies are usually axonal and remitting/relapsing syndromes and Guillain–Barré syndrome are demyelinating (Table 7).

Chronic inflammatory neuropathy

This can be progressive due to axonal neuropathy in carcinoma and lymphoma, or remitting/relapsing due to demyelination in seminoma and non-Hodgkin's lymphoma (Valli et al. 1988; Mandel 1989). An autoimmune cause for chronic inflammatory neuropathy is supported by the finding that small-cell lung cancer cells express an antigen common to Schwann cells. A patient with small-cell lung cancer, subacute sensorimotor peripheral neuropathy, and myelopathy had a circulating IgG which bound to a 25 kDa protein present in peripheral nerve and the patient's tumour. Deposits of IgM, C3, and C1q have been found in the perineurium and endoneural capillaries of patients with paraneoplastic peripheral neuropathy but not in controls with cancer but no peripheral neuropathy, or peripheral neuropathy without cancer (Anderson et al. 1987).

Patients investigated for peripheral neuropathy are frequently found to have monoclonal gammopathy. Sensorimotor peripheral neuropathy occurs in 7–10 per cent of patients with Waldenström's macroglobulinaemia or benign IgM monoclonal gammopathy and also in plasmacytoma, multiple myeloma (less than 5 per cent of patients), and osteosclerotic myeloma. Autoantibody reactivity has been defined in over 70 per cent of cases of monoclonal IgM gammopathy and 50 per cent of these are anti-myelin-associated glycoprotein (anti-MAG). Most patients with anti-MAG IgM autoantibodies are elderly men, who present with a mixed motor–sensory peripheral neuropathy which progresses slowly over 10–20 years (Steck et al. 1987).

Guillain–Barré syndrome

Typical Guillain–Barré syndrome is a very uncommon paraneoplastic complication, but it has been reported in patients with Hodgkin's disease (Anderson et al. 1987).

Autonomic neuropathy

So-called pseudo-obstruction was first described by Ogilvie (1948) in a patient with carcinoma and metastases outside the gastrointestinal tract. This and other manifestations of autonomic neuropathy are particularly associated with small-cell lung cancer, but also occur in pancreatic cancer and pulmonary carcinoid (Thomas and Shields 1970; Chinn and Schuffler 1988). In the gastrointestinal tract there is a visceral neuropathy of the myenteric plexus, with infiltration by lymphocytes and plasma cells. Later there is widespread degeneration of axons and neurons, and glial proliferation in the myenteric plexus (Schuffler et al. 1983). Patients with small-cell lung cancer and intestinal pseudo-obstruction have been shown to have circulating IgG antibodies reactive with neurons of the myenteric and submucosal plexuses of the gastrointestinal tract (Lennon et al. 1991). Autonomic neuropathy also occurs in Lambert–Eaton myasthenic syndrome, mainly affecting

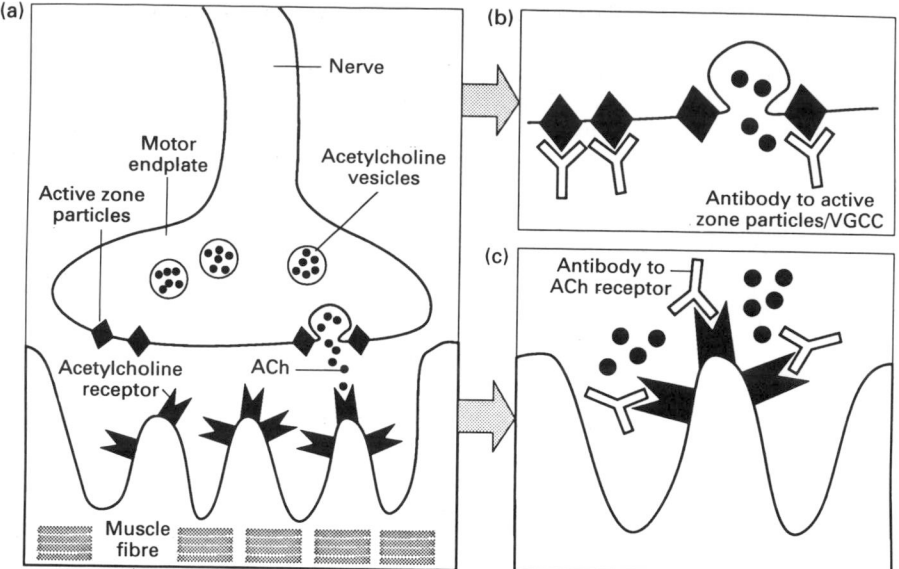

Fig. 4 Diagram of the neuromuscular junction. (a) Normal. The nerve impulse arriving at the motor end-plate causes calcium influx through voltage-gated calcium channels (VGCC), represented morphologically by orderly arrays of 10 nm particles clustered at active zones (acetylcholine (ACh) release sites). ACh vesicles undergo exocytosis, releasing ACh which diffuses across the neuromuscular junction and binds to ACh receptors on post-junctional membrane folds. Ion channels in the muscle membrane open, causing depolarization and muscle fibre contraction. (b) Lambert–Eaton myasthenic syndrome. IgG antibodies directed against VGCC cause disorganization and loss of active zone particles/VGCC, leading to reduction in ACh release. (c) Myasthenia gravis. IgG antibodies against the ACh receptor block binding of ACh to its receptor. They also increase the rate of turnover of ACh receptors and hence decrease the number of receptors expressed on the post-junctional membrane. Modified with permission from Male (1989).

parasympathetic (cholinergic) functions. Here the damage is probably mediated by autoantibodies against small-cell lung cancer antigens common to membranes of motor and autonomic nerve terminals (Khurana *et al.* 1988).

Mononeuritis and mononeuritis multiplex

Mononeuritis occurs in patients with carcinoma and lymphoma, as an isolated lesion or in the setting of an underlying symmetrical peripheral neuropathy, particularly in small-cell lung cancer. Paraneoplastic mononeuritis multiplex is due to vasculitis of the vasa nervorum of unknown cause (Rubinstein 1966; Henson and Urich 1982). Clinical and electrophysiological response to cyclophosphamide has been described (Oh *et al.* 1991).

Disorders of the neuromuscular junction

There are two important paraneoplastic disorders of the neuromuscular junction (Fig. 4). Lambert–Eaton myasthenic syndrome is a pre-synaptic disorder characterized by impaired release of acetylcholine. Myasthenia gravis is a post-synaptic disorder affecting the acetylcholine receptor.

Lambert–Eaton myasthenic syndrome (LEMS)

A myasthenic syndrome associated with lung cancer was first described in 1953. In 1956, Lambert and colleagues recognized the distinctive electrophysiological features of this condition, distinct from myasthenia gravis (Lambert *et al.* 1956). This is now recognized as a pre-synaptic disorder of peripheral cholinergic neurotransmission in which calcium-dependent acetylcholine release is reduced both in the resting state and in response to motor nerve stimulation (Newsom-Davis 1988). Half the patients with Lambert–Eaton myasthenic syndrome have small-cell lung cancer

and a few have other tumour types (see Table 1). The prevalence of Lambert–Eaton myasthenic syndrome among small-cell lung cancer patients is approximately 3 per cent (Elrington *et al.* 1991). In a third of patients Lambert–Eaton myasthenic syndrome occurs in the absence of detectable tumour, in association with autoimmune conditions such as rheumatoid arthritis, thyroid disease, and pernicious anaemia.

There is strong evidence for an autoimmune aetiology here. Circulating organ-specific autoantibodies (against thyroid, gastric parietal cells, or striated muscle) are detectable in approximately 50 per cent of Lambert–Eaton myasthenic syndrome patients without cancer and 28 per cent of those with cancer, compared with 17 per cent in controls. Lambert–Eaton myasthenic syndrome patients have a high incidence of the histocompatibility antigens HLA B8 and Dr3, which are associated with other organ-specific autoimmune diseases. Lambert–Eaton myasthenic syndrome patients with cancer have a significant reduction in helper–inducer (OKT4+) T-cell subsets and show clinical and electrophysiological improvement with daily plasma exchange. Finally, passive transfer of this condition has been accomplished: IgG from Lambert–Eaton myasthenic syndrome patients induces the pathological and EMG features of Lambert–Eaton myasthenic syndrome in mice. The clinical, ultrastructural, and electrophysiological features of Lambert–Eaton myasthenic syndrome are believed to be due to antibody-mediated loss of functional voltage-gated calcium channels (Anderson *et al.* 1987; Newsom-Davies 1988; Lang *et al.* 1990). Autoantibodies from a patient with this syndrome have been used to isolate a cDNA clone encoding a protein with a high degree of homology to the beta subunit of calcium channel complexes (Rosenfeld *et al.* 1993).

Lambert–Eaton myasthenic syndrome occurs in patients over the age of 45 years and is four times more common in men than women. The tumour usually presents soon after diagnosis of Lambert–Eaton myasthenic syndrome or within 2 years. Proximal muscle weakness occurs in all patients and is the presenting symptom in 60 per cent. This may be demonstrable clinically or conversely may be difficult to detect as strength is augmented during the course of maximal effort. Reflexes may be depressed or absent, but are similarly enhanced after voluntary muscle contraction. The diagnostic EMG feature is reduced amplitude of the compound muscle action potential evoked by supramaximal nerve stimulation, with enhancement (>200 per cent) immediately after 10–15 s maximal voluntary contraction or during high frequency nerve stimulation. There is minimal or no improvement after administration of the short-acting anticholinesterase edrophonium (Tensilon test), distinguishing Lambert–Eaton myasthenic syndrome from myasthenia gravis (Newsom-Davies 1988).

Corticosteroids and daily plasma exchange produce clinical and electrophysiological improvement. Oral 4-aminopyridine stimulates release of acetylcholine at the neuromuscular junction, probably by increasing calcium influx during depolarization. It crosses the blood–brain barrier and has significant CNS toxicity, causing confusion and fits. Oral 3,4-diaminopyridine improves motor and autonomic symptoms and electrophysiological abnormalities and appears to be less toxic (McEvoy *et al.* 1989). Most patients with small-cell lung cancer show improvement in Lambert–Eaton myasthenic syndrome in parallel with response of the tumour to combination chemotherapy (Jenkyn *et al.* 1980; Chalk *et al.* 1990).

Myasthenia gravis (MG)

Most patients with myasthenia gravis do not have an underlying neoplasm. However, approximately 10 per cent have a thymoma and 30 per cent of patients presenting wih thymoma have myasthenia gravis. There is no association with any other tumour type. Ninety per cent of patients with myasthenia gravis and thymoma have detectable anti-acetylcholine receptor antibodies which bind to receptors, increasing their turnover and blocking interaction with acetylcholine. There may also be damage to the post-synaptic part of the junction mediated by immune complexes and cell-mediated immunity. These lead to reduced acetylcholine receptor density and failure of neuromuscular transmission (Chad and Recht 1988). It is not clear how the thymus contributes to the pathogenesis of this disease. Autoantibodies with heterogeneous specificities for contractile elements of striated muscle are found in 80–90 per cent of patients with myasthenia gravis and thymoma (Williams *et al.* 1992). However, these antibodies have not been shown to react with the acetylcholine receptor or to impair neuromuscular transmission (Anderson *et al.* 1987).

Myasthenia gravis usually precedes diagnosis of thymoma. The diagnosis is confirmed by the Tensilon test which provokes a short-lived (2–10 min) increase in muscle strength. The EMG shows a decremental motor response to repetitive nerve stimulation. Tumour resection rarely improves the symptoms of myasthenia gravis and patients usually need treatment with long-acting anticholinesterases and steroids. Patients with myasthenia gravis and thymoma tend to be more difficult to manage than those with isolated myasthenia gravis and may require plasmapheresis for rapidly progressive or chronic profound weakness. Survival is shorter than if there is no associated thymoma and myasthenia gravis is the usual cause of death (Anderson *et al.* 1987; Chad and Recht 1988).

Syndromes involving muscle

Dermatomyositis (DM) and polymyositis (PM)

Dermatomyositis and polymyositis are acquired inflammatory myopathies which affect all ages (Chad and Recht 1988). Stertz

(1916) was the first to describe the association with carcinoma, but the strength of this association is unclear. It has been claimed that 10–25 per cent of patients with inflammatory myopathies develop carcinoma, but using strict diagnostic criteria (see Table 7) DeVere and Bradley (1975) found carcinoma in 8 per cent of patients with dermatomyositis or polymyositis. In patients over 40 years, cancer (especially of the breast, lung, stomach, or ovary) was found in 3 per cent of those with polymyositis and up to 40 per cent with dermatomyositis. More recent studies have found a lower incidence and have even questioned the existence of a clinically significant association (DeVere and Bradley 1975; Barnes 1976; Anderson *et al.* 1987).

Patients over 40 years who present with dermatomyositis should be investigated for occult malignancy, with physical examination including pelvic assessment, chest radiography, and stool analysis for occult blood. However, contrast studies of the gastrointestinal tract and CT scans of chest, abdomen, and pelvis have not increased the tumour yield (Chad and Recht 1988). Steroids are the generally recommended treatment, although there have been no controlled trials of their effects. Azothioprine has been used where steroids are ineffective or to spare the steroid dose. Polymyositis/dermatomyositis may remit with effective antitumour treatment and may worsen with progressive disease. However, inflammatory myopathies can fluctuate spontaneously and in general the clinical course of polymyositis/dermatomyositis does not run parallel to that of the tumour (Barnes 1976; Henson and Urich 1982).

Other paraneoplastic disorders of muscle

Polymyalgia rheumatica occurs in elderly patients who may commonly develop cancer, and it is not clear whether these two conditions are specifically associated. Myopathy may develop in patients with Cushing's syndrome, hypercalcaemia, hyponatremia, and, rarely, carcinoid syndrome. Carcinoid myopathy usually presents several years after the onset of carcinoid syndrome. It is thought to be due to myopathic effects of 5-hydroxytryptamine and usually responds to cyproheptadine.

Acute necrotizing myopathy has been the presenting feature in eight patients with cancer of the lung, stomach, colon, breast, or bladder. There was symmetrical muscle pain and weakness, initially of the limbs and later involving bulbar and respiratory muscles. Creatine kinase levels were elevated and the EMG showed myopathic changes. There was widespread necrosis of skeletal muscle with little or no inflammation. ACTH and corticosteroids were unhelpful, although one patient improved following mastectomy. However, most patients had a rapidly progressive course and died within 12 weeks.

Myotonia is a rare paraneoplastic complication of lung cancer and may also occur in polymyositis/dermatomyositis. It may remit spontaneously or in response to diphenylhydantoin (Anderson *et al.* 1987).

HAEMATOLOGICAL SYNDROMES
Syndromes affecting the formed elements
Red cell disorders

The anaemia of chronic disorders is one of the commonest paraneoplastic manifestations of cancer and accounts for approximately 15 per cent of total cases of anaemia (E. Beutler 1988). The cause may involve a block in the transfer of iron from macrophages to developing erythroblasts. Inflammation or tumours may induce granulocytes to synthesize lactoferrin which interferes with iron transport. There are conflicting data on possible impairment of erythropoeitin synthesis or erythroblast response to erythropoeitin. Thus, the anaemia is probably multifactorial and some of the effects may be mediated by cytokines such as interleukin-1 (IL-1) (Pippard and Hoffbrand 1989). Plasma iron and saturation of iron-binding protein are both low, but ferritin is high. The diagnosis is one of exclusion and it is important not to overlook correctable causes of anaemia, particularly iron deficiency, in which ferritin is low.

Two types of haemolytic anaemia occur as remote complications of cancer: autoimmune haemolytic anaemia, which is common in lymphoproliferative neoplasia, and microangiopathic haemolytic anaemia (see below). Autoimmune haemolytic anaemia may be of warm or cold antibody type (Gordon-Smith and Hows 1989). Warm autoimmune haemolytic anaemia is associated with B-cell chronic lymphoblastic leukaemia, low-grade B-cell non-Hodgkin's lymphoma, and Hodgkin's disease. The autoantibodies are usually polyclonal IgG, probably synthesized as a result of immune deregulation rather than antibody production by the malignant clone. The antibodies often react with membrane epitopes on all erythroctyes, but occasionally are of limited specificity. A few patients with warm autoimmune haemolytic anaemia develop thrombocytopenia due to platelet antibodies (Evans' syndrome), immune neutropenia, or pancytopenia. Serum autoantibody is detectable by the indirect antiglobulin test at 37°C. Cold autoimmune haemolytic anaemia is associated with B-cell lymphomas and chronic lymphoblastic leukaemia. The autoantibody is usually complement-fixing IgM, a monoclonal product of the malignant clone and is detected by agglutination of normal red cells at 4°C. These autoantibodies often have specific reactivity and unlike warm autoimmune haemolytic anaemia may be associated with intravascular haemolysis. Patients complain of purplish skin discoloration, especially in the extremities (acrocyanosis), because of stasis in the peripheral circulation caused by red cell agglutination.

Rarely, anaemia may be due to red cell aplasia, with failure of marrow erythropoiesis. A third to a half of patients with acquired pure red cell aplasia have a thymoma and may also have myasthenia gravis. Approximately 50 per cent of patients respond to thymectomy, but some relapse later (Gordon-Smith and Lewis 1989).

Erythrocytosis is diagnosed in the presence of raised haemoglobin, packed cell volume, and red cell mass (>55 per cent in men, 50 per cent in women). Erythrocytosis due to eutopic secretion of erythropoietin occurs in approximately 3 per cent of patients with renal cell carcinoma, although serum immunoreactive erythropoietin is elevated in up to 60 per cent of patients with this tumour, with no apparent haematological manifestations. This suggests that in the majority erythropoietin is secreted as an inactive precursor or there is a concurrent block in erythrocyte production (Laski and Vugrin 1987). Excessive erythropoietin production also causes erythrocytosis in 7–12 per cent of patients with hepatoma and 18 per cent with cerebellar haemangioblastomas. Erythrocytosis also occurs in benign renal tumours and cysts, Wilms' tumours, uterine fibroids, small-cell lung cancer, thymic or adrenal carcinoids, and phaeochromocytoma. Secretion of beta adrenergic agonists by phaeochromocytomas, androgenic steroids by adrenal or ovarian tumours, or prostaglandins by uterine fibroids may enhance normal erythropoietin secretion from the liver or kidney or increase the sensitivity to erythropoietin of responsive marrow precursor cells (Orth 1987; Lewis and Pearson 1989).

White cell disorders

Neutropenia in cancer patients is almost always due to marrow infiltration by malignant cells or the myelosuppressive effects of treatment, but a very few cases are autoimmune. Rarely, granulocytosis (neutrophils >7.5×10⁹/l) can be due to tumour cell production of haemopoeitic colony-stimulating factor(s). This has been reported in patients with squamous carcinomas of the lower jaw, lung, and thyroid (Saito et al. 1981; Kondo et al. 1983; Yoneda et al. 1991a). Granulocytosis was accompanied by hypercalcaemia, possibly due to tumour production of interleukins, TNF, or PTH-related protein. Xenografts from these tumours were grown in immune-deprived mice and were shown to cause granulocytosis and hypercalcaemia (Yoneda et al. 1991b).

Eosinophilia (eosinophils >440×10⁶/l) occurs in 5 per cent of patients with Hodgkin's disease and occasional patients with metastatic cancer. In Hodgkin's disease the eosinophil count may be as high as 20–40×10⁹/l, possibly due to excess production by the tumour cells of an eosinophil growth factor such as IL-5 (Lopez et al. 1986; Goldman 1989).

Platelet disorders

Thrombocytopenia in patients with cancer is usually due to treatment-induced myelosuppression, marrow infiltration, or disseminated intravascular coagulation (see below) with increased peripheral platelet destruction (Rickles and Edwards 1983). Idiopathic thrombocytopenia is a frequent complication of chronic lymphoblastic leukaemia and has also been reported in Hodgkin's disease and non-Hodgkin's lymphomas. Here it is associated with raised levels of platelet-associated IgG autoantibodies (Hardisty 1989). Idiopathic thrombocytopenia is a rare finding in solid tumours (lung, gut, ovary); thrombocytopenia here is more commonly due to bone-marrow involvement or microangiopathy (see below).

Thrombocytosis (platelets >400×10⁹/l) has been found in approximately 30 per cent of untreated cancer patients, especially those with Hodgkin's or non-Hodgkin's lymphoma and cancers of the lung, breast, and kidney. This secondary thrombocytosis is generally mild (platelet count 400–700×10⁹/l) and asymptomatic (Hardisty 1989). In renal cell carcinoma, thrombocytosis, leucocytosis and cachexia may be due to IL-6 production (Black et al. 1991; Tsukamoto et al. 1992).

Coagulopathy

In 1868 Armand Trousseau described the association of recurrent migratory thrombophlebitis and arterial thrombosis in cancer patients. Cancer coagulopathy may be initiated by factor X activators such as mucus and other products of solid tumours (Pineo et al. 1973) and by tissue-factor-like(thromboplastin-like) procoagulants produced by human promyelocytic leukaemia cells or reactive host granulocytes and monocytes (Rickles and Edwards 1983). These enter the circulation and trigger the coagulation cascade leading to intravascular deposition of fibrin and platelet aggregation, with resultant depletion of fibrinogen. There is localized secondary activation of the fibrinolytic pathway in an attempt to limit thrombus formation. Fibrin breaks down leading to elevation in fibrin degradation products (FDPs). These inhibit the action of thrombin and platelets by binding to the platelet membrane. Consumption of coagulation factors and platelets, together with the inhibitory actions of raised fibrin degradation products cause a generalized bleeding tendency. Overcompensation by increased synthesis of fibrinogen, clotting factors, and platelets may lead to a thrombotic tendency rather than a bleeding diathesis, although both may be present in the same patient. Fifty per cent of all cancer patients have some abnormality of clotting or fibrinolysis and this figure rises to over 90 per cent in patients with metastatic disease (Anonymous 1986). This is usually ayymptomatic, but up to 15 per cent have clinical manifestations with bleeding, thrombosis, or embolism. Several clinical syndromes have been described (Lesher 1993).

Thromboembolic disease (TED)

There is clinical evidence of thromboembolic disease in up to 10 per cent of cancer patients, presenting with deep venous thrombosis/pulmonary embolus or with migratory thrombophlebitis. The syndrome is classically associated with mucin-secreting tumours of the gastrointestinal tract, including primaries in the pancreas (18 per cent of all cancer-associated thromboembolic disease), stomach (17 per cent), colon (15 per cent), and lung cancer (25 per cent) (Rickles and Edwards 1983). Vitamin K antagonists such as warfarin are ineffective here and intravenous heparin should be used for at least 3–4 days. Continuous intravenous treatment may achieve the best control, but subcutaneous heparin may be substituted, aiming to keep the partial thromboplastin time at least one and a half times normal (Anonymous 1986). If effective anti-tumour treatment is available, it may be possible to stop heparin, but otherwise anticoagulation should be continued to avoid severe thromboembolism (Bell et al. 1985). Novel approaches to treatment include low molecular weight heparin(s) for long-term administration, or placement of a filter in the vena cava. Either of these may give better results than standard heparin treatment (Naschitz et al. 1993).

Disseminated intravascular coagulation (DIC)

Disseminated intravascular coagulation is characterized by inappropriate and excessive activation of haemostasis. Approximately 60 per cent of clinical cases of disseminated intravascular coagulation are associated with septicaemia. There are two common tumour associations. Most patients with acute promyelocytic leukaemia have disseminated intravascular coagulation, particularly following chemotherapy when rapid tumour cell kill leads to the release of procoagulant(s) from cytoplasmic granules. Secondly, disseminated intravascular coagulation may complicate mucin-secreting adenocarcinomas, especially cancer of the pancreas, lung, stomach, and prostate.

The main abnormalities in disseminated intravascular coagulation are a prolonged prothrombin time, low fibrinogen level (< 1.0 g/l, normal $1.5–4$ g/l), and thrombocytopenia of less than 100×10^9/l. Patients with acute disseminated intravascular coagulation usually have FDP levels above $100\ \mu g$/ml (normal $< 10\ \mu g$/ml). A low fibrinogen level (< 1 g/l) and a platelet count below 100×10^9/l are virtually diagnostic of disseminated intravascular coagulation, especially if associated with a generalized bleeding diathesis (Machin 1989).

Disseminated intravascular coagulation may be low grade and asymptomatic or overt and acute with bleeding and/or thrombosis. Asymptomatic patients with abnormal clotting tests probably need no treatment, although persistence of low-grade coagulopathy may be related to tumour progression. Fibrin forming around a primary tumour may inhibit metastasis, while fibrin formation at distant sites may favour implantation of blood-borne metastases. Aspirin, dipyridamole, and warfarin have been shown to inhibit the incidence of experimental metastases. In a small clinical study, patients with small-cell lung cancer treated with warfarin and combination chemotherapy had a significantly longer time to disease progression and median survival (50 versus 26 weeks) compared with those treated by chemotherapy alone (Rickles and Edwards 1983).

Overt disseminated intravascular coagulation occurs in 9–15 per cent of cancer patients and is manifest by bleeding or thrombosis. The most important aspects of treatment are effective antitumour therapy and treatment of infection. Bleeding should be treated with vigorous replacement therapy with fresh frozen plasma, cryoprecipitate (factor VIII), and platelets. The use of heparin is controversial; at low dose (100–200 units per hour intravenously) it may be beneficial in patients with acute promyelocytic leukaemia (Anonymous 1986).

Non-bacterial thrombotic endocarditis (NBTE)

Non-bacterial thrombotic endocarditis is found in approximately 1 per cent of patients dying of cancer. There are sterile platelet/fibrin vegetations on the mitral and/or aortic valves, which can be imaged using two-dimensional echocardiography. The common tumour associations are adenocarcinomas of the lung and gastrointestinal tract, especially the colon. Most patients have disseminated cancer and manifestations of disseminated intravascular coagulation or thromboembolic disease. They present with acute focal neurological symptoms or diffuse encephalopathy (Rosen and Armstrong 1973; Rogers et al. 1987).

Cerebrovascular disease

Cerebrovascular disease is detectable at autopsy in 15 per cent of patients with systemic (non-CNS) cancer. Haemorrhagic and ischaemic lesions occur with equal frequency and approximately half are symptomatic. Intracerebral haemorrhage is mainly due to bleeding into the tumour (especially melanoma and germ cell tumours) and coagulopathy, and less often to subdural/subarachnoid haemorrhage or hypertension. Subdural haematomata may occur supratentorially, or in the lumbar region following a lumbar puncture on a thrombocytopenic patient. Symptomatic cerebral infarction in cancer patients is usually due to non-bacterial thrombotic endocarditis or disseminated intravascular coagulation rather than arteriosclerosis. Rare causes include tumour embolism, usually from primary or secondary tumours involving the heart or lungs, or septic emboli, particularly with fungi in patients with haematological malignancies (Graus et al. 1985b). Primary cerebral venous thrombosis is usually due to direct tumour infiltration of veins or sinuses, but rarely can be a remote complication of acute leukaemia, lymphoma, breast cancer, and non-small-cell lung cancer (Hickey et al. 1982).

Cancer patients with cerebrovascular disease often present with diffuse encephalopathy rather than a typical acute 'stroke'. This is particularly true with disseminated intravascular coagulation, septic infarction, and subdural haematoma. However, some develop focal signs, often acute or subacute hemiparesis, and the differential diagnosis of a 'stroke' in patients with cancer includes brain metastases, cerebrovascular disease, septic or tumour emboli, and subacute bacterial endocarditis (Graus et al. 1985b; Rogers et al. 1987).

Microangiopathic haemolytic anaemia (MAHA)

Microangiopathic haemolytic anaemia occurs (1) with vascular tumours including giant haemangioma and haemangioendothelioma, (2) in association with disseminated intravascular coagulation complicating acute promyelocytic leukaemia or carcinoma, and (3) rarely in association with widespread metastatic carcinoma but without disseminated intravascular coagulation. Ninety per cent of patients with microangiopathic haemolytic anaemia have extensive metastatic involvement of lymph and blood vessels, particularly in the lungs. Intravascular tumour cells can damage red cells directly and can stimulate the formation of fibrin microthrombi which cause red cell fragmentation. Some tumour surface glycoproteins aggregate platelets, and those that do may be associated with limited metastatic potential. In a rat model, microangiopathic haemolytic anaemia can be induced by intravenous injection of Walker carcinosarcoma cells, leading to acute intravascular haemolysis (Murgo 1987).

Clinically, microangiopathic haemolytic anaemia is characterized by acute severe haemolytic anaemia, often accompanied by a bleeding diathesis. The peripheral blood film shows fragmented red cells, nucleated red cells, and a marked reticulocytosis. The total white count is often elevated, with a leucoerythroblastic picture. Up to 60 per cent of patients have marrow involvement by tumour cells, but uninvolved marrow shows erythroid hyperplasia and normal or increased megakaryocytes. Heparin and transfusions of blood and plasma may lead to transient improvement in coagulopathy, bleeding diathesis, and anaemia, but most patients die within a few weeks (Gordon et al. 1987; Murgo 1987).

PARANEOPLASTIC CONDITIONS OF THE SKIN

Pruritus

Pruritus is one of the commonest skin symptoms of patients with underlying tumours. It is a characteristic complaint (B symptom) in lymphomas and also occurs in patients with brain tumours where it may be associated with hyperkeratosis and vitiligo or hyperpigmentation (see below; Finlay 1988; Lober 1993).

Disorders of pigmentation

Hyperpigmentation

Generalized hyperpigmentation

Generalized increase in skin pigmentation can occur with adrenal insufficiency (which can be due to metastatic destruction of the adrenals), pituitary tumours, or ectopic production of MSH or related peptides such as ACTH or β-lipotrophin. Melanosis is the generalized pigmentation, typically slaty-grey, which occurs in patients with metastatic malignant melanoma. Its incidence has been estimated at up to 1 per cent of such patients, although most of these cases are very subtle. It may be due to the release into the general circulation of melanin or melanin precursors (Lerner 1992).

Acanthosis nigricans

The association of acanthosis nigricans with internal malignancy was first recognized by Darier in 1893. There are itchy brown hyperkeratotic plaques principally affecting the flexures including the axilla. Occasionally there is generalized skin thickening and hyperpigmentation (Finlay 1988). Acanthosis nigricans is associated with endocrine abnormalities (obesity, polycystic ovaries, acromegaly, hypothyroidism) and malignancies. In a review of tumour-associated cases, 73 per cent of patients had intra-abdominal tumours, with gastric adenocarcinoma making up 55 per cent of the total (Rigel and Jacobs 1980). Appearance of skin lesions may precede the diagnosis of malignancy by up to 16 years and yet when the tumour is diagnosed it is often found to be highly malignant, metastatic, and associated with a poor prognosis. 'Tripe palms' describes thickened velvety palms with pronounced dermatoglyphics which can occur with acanthosis nigricans, especially in patients with lung or gastric cancer (Cohen et al. 1989, 1993).

In the setting of endocrine abnormalities, acanthosis nigricans is clearly related to insulin resistance and all cases described have antibodies to the insulin receptor. High levels of circulating anti-insulin receptor antibodies have been found in a patient with a functioning metastatic phaeochromocytoma, acanthosis nigricans, and insulin-resistant diabetes mellitus. This suggests that insulin resistance may also be relevant to the pathogenesis in cases associated with malignancy (Matsuoka et al. 1987). In addition there is recent evidence implicating overexpression of transforming growth factor alpha by the tumour (Wilgenbus et al. 1992).

Vitiligo

Vitiligo is acquired depigmentation often affecting the face, neck, and hands. It is associated with autoimmune endocrine disorders such as thyroiditis and pernicious anaemia and also develops in approximately 20 per cent of patients with malignant melanoma. These patients tend to survive longer than predicted from the thickness of the primary tumour and the stage of disease. An immune mechanism may be responsible for both the depigmentation and the relatively good prognosis, but so far there is no evidence for specific antibodies or lymphocytes directed against normal and malignant melanocytes. Vitiligo-like depigmentation also occurs in patients with Hodgkin's disease, multiple myeloma, chronic lymphocytic leukaemia, and cutaneous T-cell lymphoma (Nordlund 1992).

The sign of Leser-Trélat

This sign describes the sudden appearance, or increase in the number and size, of seborrhoeic keratoses. There is a frequent association with pruritus and acanthosis nigricans. The sign is usually seen in patients with advanced metastatic malignancy, including gastric adenocarcinoma, other gut adenocarcinomas, breast cancer, squamous carcinomas, and lymphomas (Holdiness 1986). As with isolated acanthosis nigricans, this condition may be associated with overexpression of transforming growth factor alpha by the tumour and epidermal growth factor receptor by the target skin lesions (Ellis et al. 1987).

Conditions characterized by scaling or hypertrichosis

Acquired ichthyosis describes generalized scaliness of the skin, particularly of the face and trunk, due to thickening of the stratum corneum (Griffin and Massa 1993). Hodgkin's disease is the commonest cause and the skin abnormality usually appears weeks or months after other manifestations of the disease. Other tumour associations include non-Hodgkin's lymphoma, carcinomas of lung, breast, and cervix, Kaposi's sarcoma (with or without AIDS), mycosis fungoides, and soft tissue sarcoma, including one patient with a parallel course between the skin condition and the malignancy. Acquired ichthyosis can complicate non-malignant conditions, including sarcoidosis, systemic lupus erythematosus, and drugs such as clofazimine and nicotinic acid (Ebling et al. 1986; Dreizen et al. 1987; Finlay 1988).

Palmar and plantar hyperkeratosis (tylosis) is massive thickening of the skin of the palms and soles. It is inherited in an autosomal dominant fashion and can be isolated or associated with carcinoma,

Table 8 Paraneoplastic erythematous skin conditions

	Tumour associations	Rash	Other features	Treatment
Necrolytic migratory erythema	Glucagonoma syndrome: pancreatic islet alpha-cell tumour	Ring-like areas of erythema→ vesicles/bullae→burst→crust →scaling, hyperpigmentation on face, vulva±lower abdomen, thighs, limbs	Typical in middle-aged diabetic women; stomatitis, anaemia, weight loss, depression; serum glucagon, 1000– 5000 pg/ml (normal < 200 pg/ml)	?Long-acting somatostatin analogues
Erythema gyratum repens	Carcinoma of breast, lung	Parallel curving red bands with scaly edge 'wood-grain' pattern; move from day to day; trunk, limbs		Antitumour treatment
Sweet's syndrome	80% idiopathic, 20% malignancy especially AML; also lymphoma, CML, solid tumours (genitourinary, breast, rectal)	Painful red plaques: dermal neutrophil infiltrate; may become bullous/ulcerate; limbs, head, neck±oral mucosa	Fever, neutrophilia±myalgia/ arthralgia, proteinuria, conjunctivitis/iritis, pulmonary, hepatic infiltrates	Oral corticosteroids
Pyoderma gangrenosum	(i) Monoclonal gammopathy, myeloma, NHL	Painful ulcerating nodules/ vesicopustules; heal with scarring	Fever	Oral corticosteroids and antitumour treatment
	(ii) Leukaemia	Painful concentric superficial bullae with blue–grey halos	Fever	
Cutaneous histiocytosis	(i) Acute myelomonocytic leukaemia	Eruption of blue–red nodules		
	(ii) Leukaemia, multiple myeloma	Generalized plane xanthomata	Perivascular deposition of lipoprotein–Ig complexes, C_1 esterase inhibitor deficiency	Antitumour treatment

AML, acute myeloid leukaemia; CML, chronic myeloid leukaemia; NHL, non-Hodgkin's lymphoma.
Data from Elsborg and Glenthoj (1985), Champion (1986), Greaves (1986), Ryan and Wilkinson (1986), Cohen *et al.* (1988), Finlay (1988), Boyd *et al.* (1992), and Cohen and Kurzrock (1993).

especially of the oesophagus. However, the latter association is very rare and the discovery of hereditary tylosis is not in itself an indication for investigation for an underlying malignancy (Finlay 1988).

Bazex paraneoplastic acrokeratosis is erythematous scaly involvement of the hands, feet, ears, and bridge of the nose. It is particularly associated with squamous tumours of the laryngopharyngeal region, including metastatic squamous carcinoma in cervical lymph nodes without an identifiable primary (Wishart 1986; Richard and Giroux 1987). In more than half the cases, the cutaneous lesions precede tumour diagnosis by a year on average. In 90 per cent, the skin lesion runs parallel to the course of the tumour, with improvement in the cutaneous syndrome in response to effective antitumour treatment (Bolognia *et al.* 1991).

Acquired hypertrichosis is usually a side-effect of drugs including spironolactone, phenytoin, and minoxidil. 'Hypertrichosis lanuginosa acquisita' describes the acquired generalized growth of fair downy hair without signs of virilization. Rarely, it has been associated with an underlying carcinoma of the lung or colon (Jemec 1986; Hovenden 1993).

Calcinosis cutis

Dermal/subcutaneous deposition of calcium phosphate and carbonate can occur in association with bone destruction secondary to metastatic carcinoma, multiple myeloma, and leukaemia. This condition is characterized by the slow development of hard nodules under the skin, which ultimately ulcerate (Dreizen *et al.* 1987).

Erythematous conditions

There are several rare cutaneous markers of malignancy in which erythema is the main skin manifestation. These are summarized in Table 8.

Bullous conditions

A paraneoplastic variant of pemphigus has recently been described, associated with lymphoid malignancies, thymomas, and poorly differentiated sarcomas (Oursler *et al.* 1992). Bullous lesions occur on the skin and mucous membranes and there are characteristic histological features including epidermal acantholysis, suprabasal cleft formation, dyskeratotic keratinocytes, and epidermal inflammatory cells (Horn and Anhalt 1992). Patients have circulating autoantibodies to desmoplakins, polypeptide components of desmosomes (Oursler *et al.* 1992).

Pemphigoid occurs in elderly patients and may be associated with tumours simply by chance.

In dermatitis herpetiformis there are chronic intensely itchy vesicles over the elbows, knees and lumbosacral region. Most patients have a degree of villous atrophy on jejunal biopsy, although clinical malabsorption is rare. As with coeliac disease, dermatitis herpetiformis may be complicated by non-Hodgkin's lymphoma, particularly arising in the jejunum. Up to 12 years may separate the diagnosis of dermatitis herpetiformis from a subsequently diagnosed lymphoma. It is not yet clear whether a gluten-free diet will reduce the risk of malignancy in dermatitis herpetiformis (Finlay 1988; Ahmed and Hameed 1993).

Porphyria

Porphyria is a rare paraneoplastic complication of liver tumours. A clinical picture resembling porphyria cutania tarda (photosensitivity, increased skin fragility, hypertrichosis, and hyperpigmentation) has been described in approximately ten cases of malignant hepatoma and a few cases with liver metastases or benign hepatoma. Porphyrin fluorescence has been shown in a biopsy specimen of liver tumour but not normal hepatocytes or erythrocytes, suggesting porphyrin synthesis by the tumour. The definitive treatment is resection, but where complete resection is not feasible, local arterial perfusion with cytotoxic drugs may reduce tumour bulk and symptoms of porphyria (Finlay 1988).

Inherited skin conditions associated with increased risk of malignancy

Cowden's disease (multiple hamartoma syndrome) is a rare autosomal dominant condition characterized by multiple facial trichilemmomas (benign tumours arising from hair follicles), oral fibromas, and keratoses on the hands. There is a high incidence of tumours, both benign (fibrocystic disease of the breast, thyroid adenomas, meningiomas, lipomas, haemangiomas, neuromas, and multiple gut polyps) and malignant (especially cancers of the breast and thyroid). Torre's syndrome is also autosomal dominant and consists of multiple sebaceous gland tumours of the skin, which histologically may be benign adenomas, basal cell carcinomas, or squamous carcinomas. They present in patients over 40 years in association with tumours of the gastrointestinal tract (50 per cent of patients have colon cancer) and also with tumours of the genitourinary tract and non-Hodgkin's lymphoma. All tumours appear low grade and the mean survival after diagnosis of malignancy is 12 years (Finlay 1988). There are several other genetic disorders with a cutaneous component and increased risk of malignancy, including neurofibromatosis, ataxia telangiectasia, and the syndromes of Peutz–Jeghers, Gardner, and Werner (pangeria) (Roberts and Weismann 1986).

PARANEOPLASTIC RHEUMATIC DISORDERS

Paraneoplastic rheumatic disorders can present with predominant articular or systemic involvement (Butler et al. 1987; Brooks 1992).

Articular disorders

Hyperuricaemia occurs in myeloproliferative disorders, especially polycythaemia rubra vera where gout may be a presenting feature. Gout is a rare presenting complaint in patients subsequently found to have solid tumours, but may occur later in the setting of disseminated bulky tumour.

Patients with cancer may coincidentally also have arthritis. However, there is a specific association between carcinoma, particularly of lung, breast, or prostate, and a seronegative polyarthritis. Joint pain and swelling may antedate diagnosis of the tumour by up to 2 years. The condition may be clinically indistinguishable from rheumatoid arthritis but some patients have atypical features, including very acute onset, monoarticular or asymmetrical involvement, or unusual distribution favouring the lower limbs. Most patients lack circulating rheumatoid factor and radiological evidence of joint erosion. In some cases the arthritis

has clearly paralleled the clinical course of the tumour, with remission apparently induced by effective antitumour treatment and exacerbation of arthritis with tumour relapse. Apart from specific antitumour treatment, the joint symptoms should be treated with analgesics and anti-inflammatory drugs. Cancer arthritis is of unknown aetiology but could be due to antitumour antibodies cross-reacting with determinants expressed on normal cartilage. There is conflicting evidence that immune complexes, formed between tumour antigens and host antitumour antibodies, may be deposited within the joints in these patients (Butler et al. 1987).

Systemic disorders

Hypertrophic osteoarthropathy is characterized by finger clubbing, periosteal new bone formation, and arthropathy, ranging from mild arthralgia to a diffuse polyarthritis similar to rheumatoid arthritis (Benedek 1993). It occurs in 4–12 per cent of patients with primary lung cancer, particularly non-small-cell lung cancer (Table 9). However, finger clubbing is not associated with small cell lung cancer (Yacoub 1965), perhaps because of its short natural history. Patients with hypertrophic osteoarthropathy complain of pain and swelling particularly affecting the knees, ankles, wrists, metacarpophalangeal joints, and sometimes also the elbows and shoulders. Periostitis causes tenderness over the adjacent long bones, where radiographs show periostial shadowing due to new bone formation. The bone scan may show increased uptake over the shafts of affected bones before radiological abnormality is apparent. The pathogenesis of this condition is unclear but may relate to abnormal innervation of bone and joint microvasculature, a possibility supported by the rapid symptomatic response to vagotomy and atropine (Shneerson 1981). Other measures which reportedly cause symptomatic improvement include non-steroidal anti-inflammatory agents, corticosteroids, and intercostal nerve section. The symptoms, signs, radiographic, and radionuclide imaging abnormalities improve within 2–6 months of effective antitumour treatment (Ali et al. 1980; Vasudevan et al. 1981; Butler et al. 1987).

Reflex dystrophy syndrome, characterized by non-segmental pain in the extremities, trophic skin changes, vasomotor instability, and localized osteoporosis, has been described as a paraneoplastic effect

Table 9 Causes of clubbing

Malignancy
  Non-small-cell lung cancer
  Pulmonary metastases from extrathoracic tumours including renal carcinoma, melanoma, sarcomas
  Pleural mesothelioma
  Thoracic Hodgkin's disease
  Carcinoma of thyroid
  Malignant thymoma
  Nasopharyngeal carcinoma
  Oesophageal leiomyoma
Other
  Intrathoracic sepsis including tuberculosis, cystic fibrosis
  Congenital cyanotic heart disease
  Subacute bacterial endocarditis
  Inflammatory bowel disease
  Hepatic cirrhosis
  Thyroid acropathy

In the setting of malignant disease, clubbing may occur with other manifestations of hypertrophic osteoarthropathy (see text). Clubbing is rarely accompanied by periostitis in patients with cyanotic heart disease, cirrhosis of the liver, and inflammatory bowel disease. Data from Anonymous (1977) and Case Records (1978).

of tumours of the brain, lung, ovary, and breast (Michaels and Sorber 1984).

Rarely, patients with lymphoma, leukaemia, or myeloma may present with manifestations of systemic vasculitis, including erythema nodosum, Henoch–Schönlein purpura, cryoglobulinaemia, necrotizing vasculitis, or polyarteritis nodosa. Immune complex deposition seems a likely but unproven mechanism. However, circulating immune complexes are common in many types of cancer and paraneoplastic vasculitis is very rare (Butler et al. 1987).

Systemic lupus erythematosus is described in patients with thymoma. There are isolated reports of a lupus-like syndrome in non-Hodgkin's lymphoma, mesothelioma, and adenocarcinoma of breast or ovary.

Scleroderma/progressive systemic sclerosis may be accompanied by lung fibrosis, when there appears to be an increased risk of lung cancer. The commonest type is alveolar cell carcinoma, but all types of bronchial carcinoma have been described, as has mesothelioma. Scleroderma, with pain and stiffness of the fingers and sclerodactyly, may antedate the diagnosis of non-pulmonary tumours including carcinoma of the stomach, malignant melanoma, and carcinoid tumours. However, very few of these cases have been described and the association between scleroderma and malignancy may be fortuitous (Talbott and Barrocas 1979; Butler et al. 1987).

RENAL SYNDROMES

Rarely, extrarenal tumours can cause a paraneoplastic nephrotic syndrome. An association has been described between carcinomas, usually lung cancer, and membranous nephropathy. Hodgkin's disease is associated with minimal change nephropathy (Boulton-Jones 1988).

In patients with membranous nephropathy the renal biopsy shows discrete deposits of antigen and antibody along the subepithelial side of the glomerular basement membrane. In one patient with paraneoplastic membranous nephropathy and lung cancer, immunoglobulins eluted from the glomeruli were shown to bind tumour cells but not normal lung. In another patient with colonic cancer and membranous nephropathy, deposits of carcinoembryonic antigen were found along the glomerular basement membrane. The current thinking is that immune complexes are formed in situ: antigen is deposited in the glomerulus and fixed there by antibody (Boulton-Jones 1988). Paraneoplastic membranous nephropathy is commoner in men and carries a poor prognosis with a median survival of only 3 months from diagnosis. However, successful antitumour treatment may induce the nephropathy to remit (Norris 1993).

Approximately 40 patients with Hodgkin's disease and minimal change nephropathy have been reported. A few cases of minimal change nephropathy have been described in association with cancers of the lung and breast (Meyrier et al. 1992). The two conditions usually present simultaneously or within a few months of one another. There is a close temporal relationship with improvement in minimal change nephropathy and nephrotic syndrome in response to treatment, and exacerbation on relapse. Renal biopsy shows normal light microscopic appearance with no deposits of immunoglobulin or complement on the glomerular basement membrane. Electron microscopy shows fusion of epithelial foot processes which is a non-specific consequence of proteinuria. The pathogenesis of this condition is not known, but theories include a nephrotoxin produced by the tumour or by another cell population such as T-lymphocytes in response to the tumour (Boulton-Jones 1988).

AMYLOIDOSIS

Amyloidosis is characterized by extracellular deposition of fibrillary protein, and occurs in two groups of malignant diseases (Hawkins 1988; Tschen 1993).

Amyloid AL in monoclonal gammopathy

Amyloidosis complicates up to 15 per cent of cases of myeloma and approximately 5 per cent of cases of 'benign' monoclonal gammopathy. Amyloid is made up of two components, fibrillar and non-fibrillar. The fibrils in monoclonal gammopathy are AL fibrils which have been identified as light chains, hence AL standing for Amyloid Light chain. The light chains are nearly always lambda and may be whole molecules, fragments, or a mixture thereof, with molecular weights of 8–30 kDa.

AL amyloidosis typically affects patients over the age of 50 years and causes amyloid deposits in mesenchymal tissues, although it can affect any organ system, and renal and gut involvement are common. The clinical features of systemic amyloidosis are summarized in Table 10. The prognosis in AL amyloid complicating myeloma is poor with a median survival of only 5 months.

Amyloid AA in other malignancies

Amyloidosis occasionally complicates Hodgkin's disease, renal carcinoma, cancer of the lung, urogenital tract, and malignant melanoma, basal cell carcinoma, and hairy cell leukaemia. In these patients the fibrillar component of amyloid is AA protein. This 76 amino acid protein, with molecular weight 8 kDa, is derived from a circulating precursor serum amyloid A (SAA) which is an acute phase protein. Therefore AA amyloidosis is found in any condition associated with sustained elevation in circulating SAA levels, principally chronic infections, inflammation, and the tumours listed above. The non-fibrillar component is derived from serum amyloid P (SAP), as in other forms of amyloid.

The clinical picture is known as reactive systemic amyloidosis and is characterized by involvement of parenchymal organs, particularly liver, spleen, kidney, and adrenal. Patients may be asymptomatic from amyloidosis, but the commonest clinical presentation is with proteinuria, nephrotic syndrome, and hepatosplenomegaly. Infiltration of the gut is common and rectal biopsy is nearly always positive; 50–60 per cent have cardiac involvement, but this is often asymptomatic.

If specific antitumour treatment succeeds in lowering the circulating paraprotein or SAP, it may be possible to slow the rate of amyloid deposition. Unfortunately, there is no other effective treatment to stop the accumulation of fibrils or to encourage resorption of fibrils already laid down and the prognosis for patients with amyloidosis in the setting of malignant disease is very poor (Hawkins 1988).

CONSTITUTIONAL SYMPTOMS

Fever

Fever in cancer patients is most commonly due to infection, particularly in immunocompromised patients, but can be the presenting symptom of Hodgkin's disease, non-Hodgkin's lymphoma, renal cell carcinoma, and hepatoma. Fever may be mediated by constitutive production by tumour cells of IL-1, which is synthesized by Hodgkin's cell lines in vitro. IL-1 has also been detected by

Table 10 Clinical features of systemic amyloidosis

Organ system	Involvement characteristic of	Clinical features
Renal	AA	Proteinuria, nephrotic syndrome Renal failure Microcopic haematuria Hypertension Nephrogenic diabetes insipidus Renal tubular acidosis
Heart	AL	Restrictive cardiomyopathy Conductive disturbances, including heart block Angina, myocardial infarction Heart failure
Lungs	AL	Dyspnoea, haemoptysis, cough: diffuse or nodular pulmonary involvement Stridor if upper airway involved
Gut	AL AA	Macroglossia Diffuse infiltration and/or discrete masses anywhere in gut Often subclinical, occasionally symptomatic: dysphagia, GI bleeding, diarrhoea, constipation, malabsorption, perforation, obstruction Hepatic infiltration in 90%, hepatomegaly 50%, but LFTs usually normal Splenomegaly, hyposplenism
Skin	AL	Purpura, plaques, papules, nodules, alopecia, nail changes
Nervous system	AL	Peripheral or autonomic neuropathy in 10–20% AL Diagnosis: sural nerve biopsy
Joints	AL	Polyarthropathy similar to rheumatoid arthritis in 5% AL, especially kappa myeloma 'Shoulder pad' sign: glenohumeral infiltration 50% have subcutaneous nodules
Other	AL	Lymphadenopathy, goitre, Sicca syndrome; haemorrhage with normal clotting factors or factor IX or X deficiency

Modified from Hawkins (1988).

immunohistochemistry in 50 per cent of Hodgkin's disease biopsies, although there was poor correlation between the degree of staining and the presence of B symptoms (Ree *et al.* 1987). IL-1 mRNA has been detected in human non-Hodgkin's lymphoma cells and IL-1 pyrogenic bioactivity has been found in monocytic leukemia cells and non-Hodgkin's lymphoma cells. IL-1 enhances synthesis of PGE_2 from arachidonic acid in brain microvessel endothelium, leading to an increase in the hypothalamic temperature 'set point'. A similar mechanism is thought to mediate the febrile response to tumour necrosis factor and interferons. PGE_2 synthesis can be inhibited by blocking brain cyclo-oxygenase with non-steroidal anti-inflammatory drugs including aspirin and ibuprofen (Dinarello *et al.* 1988).

The diagnosis of tumour-associated fever is essentially one of exclusion and patients should be carefully evaluated for the possibility of infections. Tumour necrosis or haematomas may also cause fever. The best diagnostic test is the response of pyrexia to antitumour therapy. Corticosteroids suppress most types of fever but may be dangerous if infection has not been definitely excluded. Non-steroidal anti-inflammatory drugs such as indomethacin are also effective, alone or in combination with steroids (Tsavaris *et al.* 1990).

Cancer cachexia

Fifty per cent of cancer patients experience some weight loss, with 15 per cent losing more than 10 per cent of their pre-illness weight. Significant weight loss is of adverse prognostic significance. Patients with cancer may experience anorexia and weight loss due to identifiable complications of the tumour (oral ulceration, intestinal obstruction, abdominal distension, depression, anxiety) or its treatment. Patients with no clear cause for weight loss are said to have cancer cachexia, which is a complex metabolic syndrome probably resulting from an endogenous host response to the tumour. Apart from anorexia and severe weight loss, the syndrome is characterized by lethargy, muscle wasting, hypoproteinaemia, anaemia, glucose intolerance, and oedema. Most of the weight lost is fat and skeletal muscle, and it has been shown that patients who had lost 30 per cent of their pre-illness stable weight had lost over 70 per cent of body fat and skeletal muscle (Fearon 1988). The incidence of cancer cachexia varies with tumour type, stage, bulk, and performance status. Significant weight loss (> 10% pre-morbid weight) occurs in 80–90 per cent of patients with cancer of the pancreas or stomach and in 50–60 per cent of patients with lung or colon cancer.

There is some evidence to suggest abnormal appetite control in cancer patients, possibly related to changes in blood glucose, free fatty acid and amino acid kinetics, and sometimes also to changes in the neural or hormonal (insulin, glucagon, bombesin, cholecystokinin) regulation of the gastrointestinal tract. A further possibility is that decreased binding of tryptophan to albumin may increase 5-hydroxytryptamine synthesis or turnover, which is associated with anorexia in a rodent model. One-third of cancer patients have been shown to be hypermetabolic, possibly because of enhanced activity of energy-dependent metabolic cycles. There are inconsistent reports of increased protein turnover or increased Cori cycle activity in cancer patients with weight loss (Fearon 1988). The catabolic response to cancer is mediated, at least in part, by host production of cachectin (tumour necrosis factor alpha). *In vitro* treatment with cachectin has been shown to cause metabolic abnormalities including loss of cell lipid in adipocytes. Mice inoculated with Chinese hamster ovary cells transfected with cachectin developed a profound wasting syndrome in large part due to anorexia. Thus, cachectin/tumour necrosis factor may be responsible for both the suppression of appetite and the metabolic abnormalities which characterize cancer cachexia (B. Beutler 1988). Interferon-gamma and IL-1 and IL-6, acting either alone or in combination, can also produce the clinical and biochemical features of cancer cachexia (Nelson *et al.* 1994).

Cancer cachexia may respond to corticosteroids (prednisolone or dexamethasone) with an improvement in appetite and well-being in 40–80 per cent of patients. Other drugs reported to be helpful include metoclopramide, megestrol acetate, and tetrahydrocannabinol (Nelson *et al.* 1994).

REFERENCES

Ahmed AR, Hameed A (1993). Bullous pemphigoid and dermatitis herpetiformis. *Clinical Dermatology*, 11:47–52.

Albright F (1941). Case records of the Massachusetts General Hospital (case 27401). *New England Journal of Medicine*, 225:789–91.

Ali A, *et al.* (1980). Distribution of hypertrophic pulmonary osteoarthropathy. *American Journal of Radiology*, 134:771–80.

Anderson NE, Cunningham JM, Posner JB (1987). Autoimmune pathogenesis of paraneoplastic neurological syndromes. *CRC Critical Reviews in Neurobiology*, 3:245–99.

Anderson NE, *et al.* (1988*a*). The metabolic anatomy of paraneoplastic cerebellar degeneration. *Annals of Neurology*, 23:533–40.

Anderson NE, Budde-Steffen C, Rosenblum MK, Graus F, Ford D, Synek BJL, Posner JB (1986*b*). Opsoclonus, myoclonus, ataxia and encephalopathy in adults with cancer: a distinct paraneoplastic syndrome. *Medicine*, 67:100–9.

Anonymous (1977). Finger clubbing and hypertrophic pulmonary osteoarthropathy. Editorial. *British Medical Journal*, September.

Anonymous (1986). Haemostatic abnormalities and malignant disease. Editorial. *Lancet*, i:303–4.

Antel JP, Moumdjian R (1989). Paraneoplastic syndromes: a role for the immune system. *Journal of Neurology*, 236:1–3.

Axelrod L, Ron D (1988). Insulin-like growth factor II and the riddle of tumor-induced hypoglycemia. *New England Journal of Medicine*, 319:1477–9.

Babikian VL, *et al.* (1985). Paraneoplastic myelopathy: antibodies against protein in normal spinal cord and underlying neoplasm. *Lancet*, ii:49–50.

Barnes BE (1976). Dermatomyositis and malignancy. A review of the literature. *Annals of Internal Medicine*, 84:68–76.

Batson OA, Fantle DM, Stewart JA (1992). Paraneoplastic encephalomyelitis. Dramatic response to chemotherapy alone. *Cancer*, 69:1291–3.

Bell WR, *et al.* (1985). Trousseau's syndrome. Devastating coagulopathy in the absence of heparin. *American Journal of Medicine*, 79:423–9.

Benedek TG (1993). Paraneoplastic digital clubbing and hypertrophic osteoarthropathy. *Clinical Dermatology*, 11:53–9.

Berson EL, Lessell S (1988). Paraneoplastic night blindness with malignant melanoma. *American Journal of Ophthalmology*, 106:307–11.

Beutler B (1988). Cachexia: a fundamental mechanism. *Nutrition Reviews*, 46:369–73.

Beutler E (1988). The common anemias. *Journal of the American Medical Association*, 259:2433–7.

Black K, Garrett IR, Mundy GR (1991). Chinese hamster ovarian cells transfected with the murine interleukin-6 gene cause hypercalcaemia as well as cachexia, leukocytosis and thrombocytosis in tumor-bearing nude mice. *Endocrinology*, 128:2657–9.

Bolognia JL, Brewer YP, Cooper DL (1991). Bazek syndrome (acrokeratosis paraneoplastica). An analytical review. *Medicine (Baltimore)*, 70:269–80.

Boulton-Jones JM (1988). Renal complications of malignant disease. *Baillière's Clinical Oncology*, 2(2):347–73.

Boyd AS, Neldner KH, Menter A (1992). Erythema gyratum repens: a paraneoplastic eruption. *Journal of the American Academy of Dermatology*, 26:757–62.

Boyd JC, Ladenson JH (1984). Value of laboratory tests in the differential diagnosis of hypercalcaemia. *American Journal of Medicine*, 77:863–72.

Brennan LV, Craddock PR (1983). Limbic encephalopathy as a non-metastatic complication of oat cell lung cancer. *American Journal of Medicine*, 75:519–20.

Brooks PM (1992). Rheumatic manifestations of neoplasia. *Current Opinions in Rheumatology*, 4:90–3.

Brown M, Rivier J, Vale W (1977). Bombesin affects the central nervous system to produce hyperglycemia in rats. *Life Science*, 21:1729–34.

Budde-Steffen C, Anderson NE, Rosenblum MK, Ford D, Wray SH, Posner JB (1988*a*). An antineuronal autoantibody in paraneoplastic opsoclonus. *Annals of Neurology*, 23:528–31.

Budde-Steffen C, *et al.* (1988*b*). Expression of an antigen in small cell lung carcinoma lines detected by antibodies from patients with paraneoplastic dorsal root ganglionopathy. *Cancer Research*, 48:430–4.

Bukh A, *et al.* (1989). Human lung cancer—a comparative study of the levels of circulating immune complexes in pulmonary blood draining the tumor area and peripheral venous blood. *International Journal of Cancer*, 43:837–40.

Burtis, WJ, *et al.* (1988). Humoral hypercalcemia of malignancy. *Annals of Internal Medicine*, 108:454–6.

Burton GV, *et al.* (1988). Paraneoplastic limbic encephalopathy with testicular carcinoma. A reversible neurologic syndrome. *Cancer*, 62:2248–51.

Butler RC, Thompson JM, Keat ACS (1987). Paraneoplastic rheumatic disorders: a review. *Journal of the Royal Society of Medicine*, 80:168–72.

Callen JP (1993). Dermatomyositis and malignancy. *Clinical Dermatology*, 11:61–5.

Camara EG, Chelune GJ (1987). Paraneoplastic limbic encephalopathy. *Brain Behaviour and Immunity*, 1:349–55.

Care AD (1989). Development of endocrine pathways in the regulation of calcium homeostasis. *Baillière's Clinical Endocrinology and Metabolism*, 3:671–88.

Carlson HE (1980). Gynecomastia. Current concepts. *New England Journal of Medicine*, 303:795–9.

Carpenter PC (1988). Diagnostic evaluation of Cushing's syndrome. *Endocrinology and Metabolism Clinics of North America*, 17:455–72.

Case Records of the Massachusetts General Hospital (1978). Case 38. *New England Journal of Medicine*, 299:708–14.

Case Records of the Massachusetts General Hospital (1987). Case 52. *New England Journal of Medicine*, 317:1648–58.

Case Records of the Massachusetts General Hospital (1988*a*). Case 9. *New England Journal of Medicine*, 318:563–70.

Case Records of the Massachusetts General Hospital (1988*b*). Case 39. *New England Journal of Medicine*, 319:849–60.

Case Records of the Massachusetts General Hospital (1989). Case 15. *New England Journal of Medicine*, 320:996–1004.

Chad DA, Recht LD (1988). Neurological paraneoplastic syndromes. *Cancer Investigation*, 6:67–82.

Chalk CH, Murray NMF, Newsom-Davis J, O'Neill JH, Spiro SG (1990). Response of the Lambert–Eaton myasthenic syndrome to treatment of associated small-cell lung carcinoma. *Neurology*, 40:1552–6.

Chalk CH, Windebank AJ, Kimmel DW, McManis PG (1992). The distinctive clinical features of paraneoplastic sensory neuropathy. *Canadian Journal of Neurological Science*, 19:346–51.

Champion RH (1986) Disorders affecting small blood vessels: erythema and telangiectasia. In *Textbook of dermatology*, (4th edn), (ed. A Rook *et al.*), pp. 1081–97. Blackwell, Oxford.

Chinn JS, Schuffler MD (1988). Paraneoplastic visceral neuropathy as a cause of severe gastrointestinal motor dysfunction. *Gastroenterology*, 95:1279–86.

Clark AJL (1988) Ectopic hormone production. *Baillière's Clinical Endocrinology and Metabolism*, 2(4):967–86.

Clouston PD, Saper CB, Arbizu T, Johnston I, Lang B, Newsom-Davis J, Posner JB (1992). Paraneoplastic cerebellar degeneration. III. Cerebellar degeneration, cancer, and the Lambert–Eaton myasthenic syndrome. *Neurology*, 42:1994–50.

Coen P, et al. (1991). An aromatase-producing sex-cord tumor resulting in prepubertal gynecomastia. *New England Journal of Medicine*, 324:317–22.

Cogan E, et al. (1986). High plasma levels of atrial natriuretic factor in SIADH. *New England Journal of Medicine*, 314:1258–9.

Cohen PR, Kurzrock R (1993). Sweet's syndrome and cancer. *Clinical Dermatology*, 11:149–57.

Cohen PR, Talpaz M, Kurzrock R (1988). Malignancy-associated Sweet's syndrome: review of the world literature. *Journal of Clinical Oncology*, 6:1887–97.

Cohen PR, et al. (1989). Tripe palms and malignancy. *Journal of Clinical Oncology*, 7:669–78.

Cohen PR, Grossman ME, Silvers DN, Kurzrock R (1993). Tripe palms and cancer. *Clinical Dermatology*, 11:165–73.

Cosgrove DE, Campain JA, Cox GS (1989). Chorionic gonadotropin synthesis by human tumor cell lines: examination of subunit accumulation, steady-state levels of mRNA, and gene structure. *Biochemica et Biophysica Acta*, 1007:44–54.

Craig RK, et al. (1985). Differential expression of the human calcitonin CGRP gene in medullary thyroid and lung cancer cell lines. *Recent Results in Cancer Research*, 99:71.

Croft PB, Wilkinson MIP (1965). The incidence of carcinomatous neuromyopathy in patients with various types of carcinoma. *Brain*, 88:427–34.

Croft PB, Wilkinson MIP (1969). The course and prognosis in some types of carcinomatous neuromyopathy. *Brain*, 92:1–8.

Crofts JW, Bachynski BN, Odel JG (1988). Visual paraneoplastic syndrome associated with undifferentiated endometrial carcinoma. *Canadian Journal of Ophthalmology*, 23:128–32.

Cuttitta F, et al. (1985). Bombesin-like peptides can function as autocrine growth factors in human small cell lung cancer. *Nature, London*, 316:823–6.

Dalmau J, Graus F, Rosenblum MK, Posner JB (1992). Anti-Hu-associated paraneoplastic encephalomyelitis/sensory neuronopathy. A clinical study of 71 patients. *Medicine (Baltimore)*, 71:59–72.

Dancey RD, Hammond-Tooke GD, Lai K, Bezwoda WR (1988). Subacute myelopathy: an unusual paraneoplastic complication of Hodgkin's disease. *Medical and Pediatric Oncology*, 16:284–6.

Daughaday WH, et al. (1988). Synthesis and secretion of insulin-like growth factor II by a leiomyosarcoma with associated hypoglycemia. *New England Journal of Medicine*, 319:1434–40.

de la Monte S, Hutchins GM, Moore GW (1984). Paraneoplastic syndromes and constitutional symptoms in prediction of metastatic behaviour of small cell carcinoma of the lung. *American Journal of Medicine*, 77:851–7.

Denny-Brown D (1948). Primary sensory neuropathy with muscular changes associated with carcinoma. *Journal of Neurology, Neurosurgery and Psychiatry*, 11:73–87.

DeVere R, Bradley WG (1975). Polymyositis: its presentation, morbidity and mortality. *Brain*, 98:637–66.

Dimopoulos MA, Fernandez JF, Samaan NA, Holoye PY, Vassilopoulou-Sellin R (1992). Paraneoplastic Cushing's syndrome as an adverse prognostic factor in patients who die early with small cell lung cancer. *Cancer*, 69:66–71.

Dinarello CA, Cannon JG, Wolff SM (1988). New concepts on the pathogenesis of fever. *Reviews of Infectious Diseases*, 10:168–89.

Doege KW (1930). Fibro-sarcoma of the mediastinum. *Annals of Surgery*, 92:955–60.

Dreizen S, et al. (1987). External expressions of internal malignancy. *Postgraduate Medicine*, 82:91–100.

Dropcho EJ, Chen Y-T, Posner JB, Old LJ (1987). Cloning of a brain protein identified by autoantibodies from a patient with paraneoplastic cerebellar degeneration. *Proceedings of the National Academy of Sciences USA*, 84:4552–6.

Ebling FJG, Marks R, Rook A (1986). Disorders of keratinization. In *Textbook of dermatology*, (4th edn), (ed. A Rook et al.), pp. 1393–468. Blackwell, Oxford.

Ellis DL, et al. (1987). Melanoma, growth factors, acanthosis nigricans, the sign of Leser-Trélat and multiple acrochordons. A possible role for alpha-transforming growth factor in cutaneous paraneoplastic syndromes. *New England Journal of Medicine*, 317:1582–7.

Elrington GM, Murray NMF, Spiro SG, Newsom-Davis J (1991). Neurological paraneoplastic syndromes in patients with small cell lung cancer. A prospective survey of 150 patients. *Journal of Neurology, Neurosurgery and Psychiatry*, 54:764–7.

Elsborg L, Glenthoj A (1985). Effect of somatostatin in necrolytic migratory erythema and glucagonoma. *Acta Medica Sandinavica*, 218:245–9.

Farwell AP, Devlin JT, Stewart JA (1988). Total suppression of cortisol excretion by ketoconazole in the therapy of the ectopic adrenocorticotrophic hormone syndrome. *American Journal of Medicine*, 84:1063–6.

Fearon KCH (1988). Nutritional and gastrointestinal complications of malignant disease. *Baillière's Clinical Oncology*, 2(2):375–95.

Fierro V, Freeman JS (1988). Choriocarcinoma-induced thyrotoxicosis: report of a case and review of the literature. *Journal of the American Osteopathic Association*, 88:525–7.

Finlay AY (1988). Dermatological complications of malignant disease. *Baillière's Clinical Oncology*, 2(2):479–97.

Goldman JM (1989). Granulocytes, monocytes and their benign disorders. In *Postgraduate haematology* (ed. AV Hoffbrand and SM Lewis), pp. 294–324. Heinemann, London.

Gordon LI, Kwaan HC, Rossi EC (1987). Deleterious effects of platelet transfusions and recovery thrombocytosis in patients with thrombotic microangiopathy. *Seminars in Hematology*, 24:194–201.

Gordon-Smith EC, Hows J (1989). Acquired haemolytic anaemias. In *Postgraduate haematology* (ed. AV Hoffbrand and SM Lewis), pp. 183–207. Heinemann, London.

Gordon-Smith EC, Lewis SM (1989). Aplastic anaemia and other types of bone marrow failure. In *Postgraduate haematology* (ed. AV Hoffbrand and SM Lewis), pp. 83–120. Heinemann, London.

Graus F, Rene R (1992). Clinical and pathological advances on central nervous system paraneoplastic syndromes. *Reviews of Neurology Paris*, 148:496–501.

Graus F, Cordon-Cardo C, Posner JB (1985a). Neuronal antinuclear antibody in sensory neuropathy from lung cancer. *Neurology*, 35:538–43.

Graus F, Rogers LR, Posner JB (1985b). Cerebrovascular complications in patients with cancer. *Medicine*, 64:16–35.

Graus F, Elkon KB, Cordon-Cardo C, Posner JB (1986). Sensory neuropathy and small cell lung cancer. Antineuronal antibody that also reacts with the tumor. *American Journal of Medicine*, 80:45–52.

Graus F, Vega F, Delattre JY, Bonaventura I, Rene R, Arbaiza D, Tolosa E (1992). Plasmapheresis and antineoplastic treatment in CNS paraneoplastic syndromes with antineuronal autoantibodies. *Neurology*, 42:536–40.

Greaves MW (1986). Histiocytic proliferative disorders. In *Textbook of dermatology*, (4th edn), (ed. A Rook et al.), pp. 1699–711. Blackwell, Oxford.

Greenlee JE, Lipton HL (1986). Anticerebellar antibodies in serum and cerebrospinal fluid of patients with oat cell carcinoma of the lung and paraneoplastic cerebellar degeneration. *Annals of Neurology*, 19:82–5.

Greenlee JE, Brashear HR, Jaeckle KA, Geleris A, Jordan K (1992). Pursuing an occult carcinoma in a patient with subacute cerebellar degeneration and anticerebellar antibodies. Need for vigorous follow-up. *West Journal of Medicine*, 156:199–202.

Gress T, Baldini A, Rocchi M, Furneaux H, Posner JB, Siniscalco M (1992). *In situ* mapping of the gene coding for a leucine zipper DNA binding protein (CDR62) to 16p12–16p13.1. *Genomics*, 13:1340–2.

Grewal TS, Lowry PJ, Savva D (1989). Expression and partial purification of human pro-opiomelanocortin in *Escherichia coli*. *Journal of Molecular Endocrinology*, 3:105–12.

Griffin LJ, Massa MC (1993). Acquired ichthyosis and pityriasis rotunda. *Clinical Dermatology*, 11:27–32.

Grisold W, et al. (1987). Antineuronal antibodies in small cell lung carcinoma—a significance for paraneoplastic syndromes? *Acta Neuropathology*, 75:199–202.

Grossman AB, et al. (1988). CRF in the differential diagnosis of Cushing's syndrome: a comparison with the dexamethasone suppression test. *Clinical Endocrinology*, 29:167–78.

Hale AC, Besser GM, Rees LH (1986). Characterisation of pro-opiomelanocortin-derived peptides in pituitary and ectopic adrenocorticotrophin-secreting tumours. *Journal of Endocrinology*, 108:49–56.

Hammack J, Kotanides H, Rosenblum MK, Posner JB (1992). Paraneoplastic cerebellar degeneration. II. Clinical and immunologic findings in 21 patients with Hodgkin's disease. *Neurology*, 42:1938–43.

Hardisty RM (1989). Platelet disorders. In *Postgraduate haematology* (ed. AV Hoffbrand and SM Lewis), pp. 598–626. Heinemann, London.

Hawkins PN (1988). Amyloidosis. *Blood Reviews*, 2:270–80.

Hawley RJ, et al. (1980). The carcinomatous neuromyopathy of oat cell lung cancer. Annals of Neurology, 7:65–72.

Heath DA (1989). Hypercalcaemia in malignancy. British Medical Journal, 298:1468–9.

Henson RA (1986). Neurologic manifestations of paraneoplastic disorders. In Diseases of the nervous system, clinical neurobiology (ed. AK Asbury, GM McKhann, and WI McDonald), pp. 1436–47. WB Saunders, Philadelphia.

Henson RA, Urich H (ed.) (1982). Paraneoplastic disorders. In Cancer and the nervous system, pp. 309–621. Blackwell Scientific, Oxford.

Hetzel DJ, Stanhope CR, O'Neill BP, Lennon VA (1990). Gynecologic cancer in patients with subacute cerebellar degeneration predicted by anti-Purkinje cell antibodies and limited in metastatic volume. Mayo Clinic Proceedings, 65:1558–63.

Hickey WF, Garnick MB, Henderson IC, Dawson DM (1982). Primary cerebral venous thrombosis in patients with cancer—a rarely diagnosed paraneoplastic syndrome. American Journal of Medicine, 73:740–50.

Holdiness MR (1986). The sign of Leser-Trélat. International Journal of Dermatology, 25:564–72.

Horn TD, Anhalt GJ (1992). Histologic features of paraneoplastic pemphigus. Archives in Dermatology, 128:1091–5.

Hovenden AL (1993). Hypertrichosis lanuginosa acquisita associated with malignancy. Clinical Dermatology, 11:99–106.

Howlett TA, et al. (1986). Diagnosis and management of ACTH-dependent Cushing's syndrome: comparison of the features in ectopic and pituitary ACTH production. Clinical Endocrinology, 24:699–713.

Hughes M, Ahern V, Kefford R, Boyages J (1992). Paraneoplastic myelopathy at diagnosis in a patient with pathologic stage 1A Hodgkin's disease. Cancer, 70:1598–600.

Ihde DC (1987). Paraneoplastic syndromes. Hospital Practice, 22:105–24.

Ikeda K, et al. (1988). Identification of transcripts encoding a parathyroid hormone-like peptide in messenger RNAs from a variety of human and animal tumours associated with humoral hypercalcaemia of malignancy. Journal of Clinical Investigation, 81:2010–14.

Jacobson DM, Thirkill CE, Tipping SJ (1990) A clinical triad to diagnose paraneoplastic retinopathy. Annals of Neurology, 28:162–7.

Jemec GBE (1986). Hypertrichosis lanuginosa acquisita. Archives of Dermatology, 122:805–8.

Jenkyn LR, Brooks PL, Forcier J, Maurer LH, Ochoa J (1980). Remission of the Lambert–Eaton syndrome and small cell anaplastic carcinoma of the lung induced by chemotherapy and radiotherapy. Cancer, 46:1123–7.

Jubelt B (1992). Motor neuron diseases and viruses: poliovirus, retroviruses and lymphomas. Current Opinions in Neurology and Neurosurgery, 5:655–8.

Kalkman PH, Allan S, Birchall IW (1993). Magnetic resonance imaging of limbic encephalitis. Canadian Association of Radiology Journal, 44:121–4.

Khurana RK, Koski CL, Mayer RF (1988). Autonomic dysfunction in Lambert–Eaton myasthenic syndrome. Journal of Neurological Science, 85:77–86.

Kim EE, Haynie TP (1987). Nuclear diagnostic imaging. Practical clinical applications, pp. 134–5. Macmillan, New York.

Kondo Y, et al. (1983). Association of hypercalcaemia with tumors producing colony-stimulating factor(s). Cancer Research, 43:2368–74.

Kornguth SE (1989). Neuronal proteins and paraneoplastic syndromes. New England Journal of Medicine, 321:1607–8.

Kornguth SE, et al. (1986). Anti-neurofilament antibodies in the sera of patients with small cell carcinoma of the lung and with visual paraneoplastic syndrome. Cancer Research, 46:2588–95.

Kukreja SC, et al. (1988). Antibodies to parathyroid hormone-related protein lower serum calcium in athymic mouse models of malignancy associated hypercalcaemia due to human tumors. Journal of Clinical Investigation, 82:1798–1802.

Lambert EH, Eaton LM, Wrooke ED (1956). Defects of neuromuscular conduction associated with malignant neoplasms. American Journal of Physiology, 187:612–13.

Lamberts SWJ, et al. (1988). Successful treatment with SMS 201-995 of Cushing's syndrome caused by ectopic adrenocorticotropin secretion from a metastatic gastrin-secreting pancreatic islet cell carcinoma. Journal of Clinical Endocrinology, 67:1080–3.

Lang B, Vincent A, Newsom-Davis J (1990). Paraneoplastic myasthenia: autoantibodies to calcium channels shared by cancer cells and motor nerve terminals. Progress in Neuroendocrinimmunology, 3:83–9.

Laski ME, Vugrin D (1987). Paraneoplastic syndromes in hypernephroma. Seminars in Nephrology, 7:123–30.

Lennon VA, Sas DF, Busk MF, Scheithauer B, Malagelada JR, Camilleri M, Miller LJ (1991). Enteric neuronal autoantibodies in pseudoobstruction with small-cell lung carcinoma. Gastroenterology, 100:137–42.

Lerner AB (1992). The Seiji memorial lecture. Pigment stories: from vitiligo to melanomas and points in between. Pigment Cell Research, 2 (Suppl.):19–21.

Lesher JL (1993). Thrombophlebitis and thromboembolic problems in malignancy. Clinical Dermatology, 11:159–63.

Lewis SM, Pearson TC (1989). Non-leukaemic myeloproliferative disorders. In Postgraduate haematology, (ed. AV Hoffbrand and SM Lewis), pp. 530–59. Heinemann, London.

Liddle GW, et al. (1965). The ectopic ACTH syndrome. Cancer Research, 25:1057–61.

List AF, et al. (1986). The syndrome of inappropriate secretion of antidiuretic hormone (SIADH) in small cell lung cancer. Journal of Clinical Oncology, 4:1191–8.

Lober CW (1993). Pruritis and malignancy. Clinical Dermatology, 11:125–8.

Lopez AF, et al. (1986). An eosinophil-specific colony-stimulating factor with activity for human cells. Journal of Experimental Medicine, 163:1085–99.

McArdle JP, Millingen KS (1988). Case report. Limbic encephalitis associated with malignant thymoma. Pathology, 20:292–5.

McEvoy KM, et al. (1989). 3,4-Diaminopyridine in the treatment of Lambert–Eaton myasthenic syndrome. New England Journal of Medicine, 321:1567–71.

McLellan R, et al. (1988). Ovarian carcinoma and paraneoplastic cerebellar degeneration. Obstetrics and Gynecology, 72:922–4.

McLeod JG (1984). Carcinomatous neuropathy. In Peripheral neuropathy, Vol. II, (2nd edn), (ed. PJ Dyck, PK Thomas, EH Lambert, and R Bunge), p. 2180. WB Saunders, Philadelphia.

Machin SJ (1989). Acquired disorders of haemostasis. In Postgraduate haematology, (ed. AV Hoffbrand and SM Lewis), pp. 655–71. Heinemann, London.

Male DK (1989). Hypersensitivity—type II. In Immunology, (2nd edn), (ed. IM Roith, J Brostoff, and DK Male), pp. 20.1–10. Churchill Livingstone, Gower Medical, London.

Malik S, Furlan AJ, Sweeney PJ, Komorsky GS, Wong M (1992). Optic neuropathy: a rare paraneoplastic syndrome. Journal of Clinical Neuroophthalmology, 12:137–41.

Mandel S (1989). Paraneoplastic syndromes. How to recognise the remote neurologic effects of cancer. Postgraduate Medicine, 85: 141–52.

Martin TJ, et al. (1989). Parathyroid hormone-related protein: isolation, molecular cloning and mechanism of action. Recent Progress in Hormone Research, 45:467–506.

Matsuoka LY, et al. (1987). Antibodies against the insulin receptor in paraneoplastic acanthosis nigricans. American Journal of Medicine, 82:1253–6.

Maurer LH, et al. (1983). Human neurophysins in carcinoma of the lung: relation to histology, disease stage, response rate, survival and syndrome of inappropriate antidiuretic hormone secretion. Cancer Treatment Reports, 67:971–6.

Meyrier A, Delahousse M, Callard P, Rainfray M (1992). Minimal change nephrotic syndrome revealing solid tumors. Nephron, 61:220–3.

Michaels RM, Sorber JA (1984). Reflex sympathetic dystrophy as a probable paraneoplastic syndrome: case report and literature review. Arthritis and Rheumatism, 27: 1183–5.

Milhaud G (1985). Calcitonin in human malignancies. Recent Results in Cancer Research, 99:67–70.

Mundy GR (1988). Hypercalcemia of malignancy revisited. Journal of Clinical Investigation, 82:1–6.

Mundy GR, et al. (1984). Hypercalcaemia of cancer. Clinical implications and pathogenic mechanisms. New England Journal of Medicine, 310:1718–27.

Murgo AJ (1987). Thrombotic microangiopathy in the cancer patient including those induced by chemotherapeutic agents. Seminars in Hematology, 24:161–77.

Naschitz JE, Yeshurun D, Lev LM (1993). Thromboembolism in cancer. Changing trends. Cancer, 71:1384–90.

Nelson KA, Walsh D, Sheehan FA (1994). The cancer anorexia–cachexia syndrome. Journal of Clinical Oncology, 12:213–25.

Newsom-Davis J (1988). Lambert–Eaton myasthenic syndrome. A review. Monographs in Allergy, 25:116–24.

Nordlund JJ (1992). The significance of depigmentation. *Pigment Cell Research*, 2 (Suppl.):237–41.

Norris FH Jr, Engel WK (1965). Carcinomatous amyotrophic lateral sclerosis. In *The remote effects of cancer of the nervous system*, (ed. Lord Brain and FH Norris Jr), pp. 24–34. Grune & Stratton, New York.

Norris SH (1993). Paraneoplastic glomerulopathies. *Seminars in Nephrology*, 13:258–72.

Odell WD (1989). Paraendocrine syndromes of cancer. *Advances in Internal Medicine*, 34:325–52.

Oh SJ, Slaughter R, Harrell L (1991). Paraneoplastic vasculitic neuropathy: a treatable neuropathy. *Muscle Nerve*, 14:152–6.

Ogilvie H (1948). Large intestine colic due to sympathetic deprivation. *British Medical Journal*, 2:671–3.

Orth DN (1987). Ectopic hormone production. In *Endocrinology and metabolism*, (2nd edn.) (ed. P Felig, JD Baxter, AE Broadus, and LA Frohman), pp. 1692–735. McGraw-Hill, New York.

Oursler JR, Labib RS, Ariss-Abdo L, Burke T, O'Keefe EJ, Anhalt GJ (1992). Human autoantibodies against desmoplakins in paraneoplastic pemphigus. *Journal of Clinical Investigations*, 89:1775–82.

Padgett BL, Walker DL, ZuRhein GM, Hodach AE, Chou SM (1976). JC papovavirus in progressive multifocal leukencephalopathy. *Journal of Infectious Diseases*, 133:686–90.

Park DM, Johnson RH, Crean GP, Robinson JF (1972). Orthostatic hypotension in bronchial carcinoma. *British Medical Journal*, 3:510–11.

Patel K, *et al.* (1989). Neural cell adhesion molecule (NCAM) is the antigen recognised by monoclonal antibodies of similar specificity in small cell lung carcinoma and neuroblastoma. *International Journal of Cancer*, 44:573–8.

Peterson K, Rosenblum MK, Kotanides H, Posner JB (1992). Paraneoplastic cerebellar degeneration. I. A clinical analysis of 55 anti-Yo antibody-positive patients. *Neurology*, 42:1931–7.

Pierce ST (1993). Paraendocrine syndromes. *Current Opinions in Oncology*, 5:639–45.

Pineo GF, Regoeczi E, Hatton MWC, Brain MC (1973). The activation of coagulation by extracts of mucus: a possible pathway of intravascular coagulation accompanying adenocarcinomas. *Journal of Laboratory and Clinical Medicine*, 82:255–6.

Pippard MJ, Hoffbrand AV (1989). Iron. In *Postgraduate haematology*, (ed. AV Hoffbrand and SM Lewis), pp. 26–54. Heinemann, London.

Ree HJ, Crowley JP, Dinarello CA (1987). Anti-interleukin-I reactive cells in Hodgkin's disease. *Cancer*, 59:1717–20.

Richard M, Giroux J-M (1987). Acrokeratosis paraneoplastica (Bazex' syndrome). *Journal of the American Academy of Dermatology*, 16:178–83.

Richardson GE, Johnson BE (1992). Paraneoplastic syndromes in lung cancer. *Current Opinions in Oncology*, 4:323–33.

Richter D (1988). Molecular events in expression of vasopressin and oxytocin and their cognate receptors. *American Journal of Physiology*, 255:F207–19.

Rickles FR, Edwards RL (1983). Activation of blood coagulation in cancer: Trousseau's syndrome revisited. *Blood*, 62:14–31.

Rigel DS, Jacobs MI (1980). Malignant acanthosis nigricans: a review. *Journal of Dermatologic Surgery and Oncology*, 6:923–7.

Roberts SOB, Weisman K (1986). The skin in systemic disease. In *Textbook of dermatology*, (4th edn), (ed. A Rook, *et al.*), pp. 2343–74. Blackwell, Oxford.

Robertson GL (1987). The posterior pituitary. In *Endocrinology and metabolism*, (2nd edn), (ed. P Felig, JD Baxter, AE Broadus, LA Frohman), pp. 338–85. McGraw-Hill, New York.

Rogers LR, *et al.* (1987). Cerebral infarction from non-bacterial thrombotic endocarditis. *American Journal of Medicine*, 83:746–56.

Ron D, *et al.* (1989). Increased insulin-like growth factor II production and consequent suppression of growth hormone secretion: a dual mechanism for tumor-induced hypoglycemia. *Journal of Clinical Endocrinology and Metabolism*, 68:701–6.

Rosen P, Armstrong D (1973). Nonbacterial thrombotic endocarditis in patients with malignant neoplastic diseases. *American Journal of Medicine*, 54:23–9.

Rosenfeld MR, Posner JB (1991). Paraneoplastic motor neurone disease. *Advances in Neurology*, 56:445–59.

Rosenfeld MR, Wong E, Dalmau J, Manley G, Posner JB, Sher E, Furneaux HM (1993). Cloning and characterisation of a Lambert–Eaton myasthenic syndrome antigen. *Annals of Neurology*, 33:113–20.

Rosol TJ, Capen CC (1992). Mechanisms of cancer-induced hypercalcemia. *Laboratory Investigations*, 67:680–702.

Rubinstein MK (1966). Mononeuritis in association with malignancy. *Los Angeles Neurological Society Bulletin*, 31:157–63.

Ryan TJ, Wilkinson DS (1986). Cutaneous vasculitis: 'angiitis'. In *Textbook of dermatology*, (4th edn.), (ed. A Rook *et al.*), pp. 1121–85. Blackwell, Oxford.

Saito K, *et al.* (1981). Primary squamous cell carcinoma of the thyroid associated with marked leukocytosis and hypercalcaemia. *Cancer*, 48:2080–3.

Sakai K, Ogasawara T, Hirose G, Jaeckle KA, Greenlee JE (1993). Analysis of autoantibody binding to 52-kd paraneoplastic cerebellar degeneration-associated antigen expressed in recombinant proteins. *Annals of Neurology*, 33:373–80.

Santen RJ (1987). The testis. In *Endocrinology and metabolism*, (2nd edn), (ed. P Felig, JD Baxter, AE Broadus, and LA Frohman), pp. 821–905. McGraw-Hill, New York.

Sato S, *et al.* (1991). Antibody to a zinc finger protein in a patient with paraneoplastic cerebellar degeneration. *Biochemistry and Biophysics Research Communications*, 178:198–206.

Sausville E, Carney D, Battey J (1985). The human vasopressin gene is linked to the oxytocin gene and is selectively expressed in a cultured lung cancer cell line. *Journal of Biological Chemistry*, 260:10236–41.

Sawyer RA, *et al.* (1976). Blindness caused by photoreceptor degeneration as a remote effect of cancer. *American Journal of Ophthalmology*, 81:606–13.

Schold SC, Cho E-S, Somasundaram M, Posner JB (1979). Subacute motor neuronopathy: a remote effect of lymphoma. *Annals of Neurology*, 5:271–87.

Schor NE (1992). Nervous system dysfunction in children with paraneoplastic syndromes. *Journal of Child Neurology*, 7:253–8.

Schuffler MD, *et al.* (1983). Intestinal pseudo-obstruction as the presenting manifestation of small-cell carcinoma of the lung. *Annals of Internal Medicine*, 98:129–34.

Schuller-Petrovic S, *et al.* (1983). A shared antigenic determinant between natural killer cells and nervous tissue. *Nature, London*, 306:179–81.

Schwartz WB, *et al.* (1957). A syndrome of renal sodium loss and hyponatremia probably resulting from inappropriate secretion of antidiuretic hormone. *American Journal of Medicine*, 23:529–42.

Sheeler LR (1988). Cushing's syndrome—1988. *Cleveland Clinic Journal of Medicine*, 55:329–37.

Shneerson JM (1981). Digital clubbing and hypertrophic osteoarthropathy: the underlying mechanisms. *British Journal of Diseases of the Chest*, 75:113–31.

Solomon GE, Chutorian AM (1968). Opsoclonus and occult neuroblastoma. *New England Journal of Medicine*, 279:475–7.

Sorenson GD, Cate CC, Pettengill OS (1985). Regulation of hormone production in small cell carcinoma of the lung. *Recent Results in Cancer Research*, 99:143–56.

Souhami RL, Beverley PCL, Bobrow LG (1987). Antigens of small-cell lung cancer. First International Workshop. *Lancet*, ii:325–6.

Steck AJ, *et al.* (1987). Peripheral neuropathy associated with monoclonal IgM autoantibody. *Annals of Neurology*, 22:764–7.

Stertz G (1916). Polymyositis. *Berliner Klinischer Wochenschrift*, 53:489.

Stewart MF, White A, Ratcliffe JG (1987). Hormones in lung cancer. In *Human tumour markers*, (ed. F Cimino, GD Birkmayer, JV Klavins, E Pimental, and F Salvatore), pp. 675–94. Walter de Gruyter, New York.

Stewart MF, *et al.* (1989). Small cell lung cancer cell lines secrete predominantly ACTH precursor peptides not ACTH. *British Journal of Cancer*, 60:20–4.

Streeten DHP, Moses AM, Miller M (1987). Disorders of the neurophysins. In *Harrison's principles of internal medicine*, (11th edn), (ed. E Braunwald *et al.*), pp. 1722–32. McGraw-Hill, New York.

Szabo A, *et al.* (1991). HuD, a paraneoplastic encephalomyelitis antigen, contains RNA-binding domains and is homologous to Elav and Sex-lethal. *Cell*, 67:325–33.

Talbott JH, Barrocas M (1979). Progressive systemic sclerosis (PSS) and malignancy, pulmonary and non-pulmonary. *Medicine*, 58:182–207.

Tashjian AH Jr, *et al.* (1982). Platelet-derived growth factors stimulates bone resorption via a prostaglandin-mediated mechanism. *Endocrinology*, 111:118–24.

Thirkill CE, Roth AM, Keltner JL (1987). Cancer-associated retinopathy. *Archives of Ophthalmology*, 105:372–5.

Thirkill CE, Tait RC, Tyler NK, Roth AM, Keltner JL (1992). The cancer-associated retinopathy antigen is a recoverin-like protein. *Investigations in Ophthalmology and Vision Science*, 33:2768–72.

Thomas JP, Shields R (1970). Associated autonomic dysfunction and carcinoma of the pancreas. *British Medical Journal*, 4:32.

Trousseau A (1868). *Phlegmasia alba dolens*, pp. 695–727. Clinique Medicale de Hotel-Dieu de Paris. New Sydenham Society, London.

Tsavaris N, *et al.* (1990). A randomised trial of the effect of three non-steroid anti-inflammatory agents in ameliorating cancer-induced fever. *Journal of Internal Medicine*, 228:451–5.

Tschen JA (1993). Amyloidosis and neoplasia. *Clinical Dermatology*, 11:33–6.

Tsukamoto T, Kumamoto Y, Miyao N, Masumori N, Takahashi A, Yanase M (1992). Interleukin-6 in renal cell carcinoma. *Journal of Urology*, 148:1778–82.

Valli G, Strada O, Pirovano C (1988). Clinical and neurophysiologic features in paraneoplastic polyneuropathy. *Tumori*, 74:237–41.

Vasudevan CP, *et al.* (1981). Reversible autonomic neuropathy and hypertrophic osteoarthropathy in a patient with bronchogenic carcinoma. *Chest*, 79:479–81.

Wilgenbus K, Lentner A, Kuckelkorn R, Handt S, Mittermayer C (1992). Further evidence that acanthosis nigricans maligna is linked to enhanced secretion by the tumour of transforming growth factor alpha. *Archives of Dermatology Research*, 284:266–70.

Williams CL, Hay JE, Huiatt TW, Lennon VA (1992). Paraneoplastic IgG striational autoantibodies produced by clonal thymic B cells and in serum of patients with myasthenia gravis and thymoma react with titin. *Laboratory Investigations*, 66:331–6.

Willison HJ, Minna JD, Brady RO, Quarles RH (1986). Glycoconjugates in nervous tissue and small cell lung cancer share immunologically cross–reactive carbohydrate determinants. *Journal of Neuroimmunology*, 10:353–65.

Wilson JD (1991). Gynecomastia. A continuing diagnostic dilemma. *New England Journal of Medicine*, 324:334–5.

Wilson JP (1987). Endocrine disorders of the breast. In *Harrison's principles of internal medicine*, (11th edn), (ed. E Braunwald *et al.*), pp. 1837–40. McGraw-Hill, New York.

Wishart JM (1986). Bazex paraneoplastic acrokeratosis: a case report and response to Tigason. *British Journal of Dermatology*, 115:595–9.

Yacoub MH (1965). Relation between the histology of bronchial carcinoma and hypertrophic pulmonary osteoarthropathy. *Thorax*, 20:537–9.

Yamaji T, Ishibashi M, Katayama S (1981). Nature of the immunoreactive neurophysin in ectopic vasopressin-producing oat cell carcinomas of the lung. *Journal of Clinical Investigation*, 68:388–98.

Yoneda T, Nishimura R, Kato I, Ohmae M, Takita M, Sakuda M (1991a). Frequency of the hypercalcemia–leukocytosis syndrome in oral malignancies. *Cancer*, 68:617–22.

Yoneda T, *et al.* (1991b). Occurrence of hypercalcemia and leukocytosis with cachexia in a human squamous cell carcinoma of the maxilla in athymic nude mice: a novel experimental model of three concomitant paraneoplastic syndromes. *Journal of Clinical Oncology*, 9:468–77.

Yufe RS, Hyde ML, Terbrugge K (1980). Auditory evoked responses and computed tomography in central pontine myelinolisis. *Canadian Journal of Neurological Science*, 7:297–300.

Zeballos RS, McPherson RA (1992). Update of autoantibodies in neurologic disease. *Clinical Laboratory Medicine*, 12:61–83.

19.4 Immunological and haematological complications of cancer

P. L. AMLOT AND O. SMITH

IMMUNOLOGICAL COMPLICATIONS

Introduction

Immunosuppression is the almost invariable outcome of the many ways in which cancer can affect the immune response. First, cancer can alter immunity through direct physical invasion and replacement of normal lymphoid tissue (particularly evident in lymphomas, myelomas, and leukaemias) or through the production of humeral factors which interfere with immune function. Second, if the cancer is not controlled by treatment but grows and disseminates, the patient may become cachectic and malnourished which increases the severity of the immunodeficiency. Third, the integrity of mucosal or epidermal surfaces is often breached either directly by the cancer or indirectly because of surgical and medical intervention (e.g. operations, indwelling venous lines, intubation, etc.) which breaks down natural defence barriers to invasion by microorganisms. Fourth, all modes of cancer therapy impair immunity as a result of surgery and anaesthesia, radiotherapy, cytotoxic chemotherapy, corticosteroids, or antimicrobial chemotherapy. Fifth, pre-existing immunodeficiency may contribute to the development of cancer. Sixth, in association with immunodeficiency some patients make abnormal or autoimmune responses. Finally, the psychological characteristics and attitudes of patients have been correlated with their ability to survive with cancer. Immunological effector mechanisms have been invoked to explain why patients with beneficial attitudes towards their cancer may survive longer. Depression is the only psychological state which consistently produces immunological deficiency (Dorian and Garfinkel 1987) and a reactive depression to cancer may contribute in its turn to the cascade of immunosuppressive effects induced by this disease. In view of all these potentially immunosuppressive influences, it is hardly surprising that cancer patients are prone to common infections and occasional patients become infected with microorganisms that are not normally pathogenic. Indeed, serious and life-threatening infection occurs most often when the immunosuppressive effects are multiple, particularly where there is progressive tumour growth despite cytotoxic chemotherapy or radiotherapy. Infection is a major contributory cause of death in patients with cancer. The degree of immunodeficiency is most severe in patients with malignancies of the haemopoietic tissues (leukaemias) or lymphoid tissues (lymphomas and myelomas). The focus of this chapter will be the immunodeficiency or abnormal immune responses ensuing from cancer rather than the immunosuppression following cancer treatment which is dealt with elsewhere. Pre-existing immunodeficiency which predisposes to malignancy will be covered briefly, while psychological effects on immunity will not be addressed.

Cancer predisposing to immunodeficiency and infection

As a direct result of cancer or because of treatment given to patients with cancer a number of deficiencies in immune effector mechanisms may arise.

Granulocytopenia

A low granulocyte count is widely used as an indicator of acute susceptibility to bacterial infection. This can occur spontaneously in leukaemias and more rarely in other cancers, but overwhelmingly it follows cancer therapy particularly with cytotoxic drugs. Granulocytopenia predisposes the patient to a variety of bacterial infections. The commonly encountered infections are from Gram-negative aerobic organisms (*Escherichia coli*, *Pseudomonas aeruginosa*, *Klebsiella*, and *Proteus*), which usually arise from the patient's own gastrointestinal tract, mucosal flora, or cutaneous flora. Patients with granulocytopenia are also susceptible to certain types of fungi (*Candida albicans* and *Aspergillus*). Meningitis, when it occurs, usually arises from the patient's own enteric Gram-negative organisms of the types described above.

Neutrophil function is usually normal in untreated malignant disease and, although *in vitro* studies have occasionally shown decreased chemotaxis (McCormack *et al.* 1979), it is not of great clinical significance.

Lymphocytopenia and cell-mediated anergy

Although many sophisticated tests can be performed to examine lymphocyte function, the simple lymphocyte count is almost as good an index of susceptibility to infection as any other. Less attention is paid to the lymphocyte count in patient monitoring (compared with granulocytes) because of the variable and often prolonged delay between a fall in lymphocyte number and any evidence of infection. None the less, an individual with persistently low lymphocyte counts is more susceptible to viral, fungal, and opportunistic infection. In comparison with the total lymphocyte count, clinical testing of delayed cutaneous hypersensitivity has to be performed with a battery of recall delayed cutaneous hypersensitivity antigens if it is to be of any value in grading the strength of cell-mediated immunity and for monitoring it would have to be performed repeatedly. However, there are problems of interpretation and convenience when repeated delayed cutaneous hypersensitivity testing is performed. Lymphocyte subset determinations of helper T-cells (CD4) and cytotoxic/suppressor T-cells (CD8) have been of value in monitoring patients with the acquired immunodeficiency syndrome (AIDS) but have not been widely used in patients with cancer even though an inversion in the CD4 to CD8 ratio is often found.

Anergy to several antigens inducing delayed cutaneous hypersensitivity (for example, tuberculin, candida, trichophyton, mumps, and streptokinase–streptodornase) is associated with a greater risk of post-operative infection (Belghiti *et al.* 1978; Perramant *et al.* 1981). Anergy is often a manifestation of the patient's state of health, degree of cachexia, and the stage of malignant dissemination. Cellular immunity appears to be normal in the early stages of cancer and then becomes impaired as the cancer spreads. Impairment of cell-mediated immunity may appear early in the course of some cancers, for example Hodgkin's disease and later in others, but the trend is the same. Lymphocyte responses to phytohaemagglutinin in both cancer of the lung and Hodgkin's

disease become increasingly depressed as the cancer spreads, but the lymphocyte impairment is more marked in the latter (Fig. 1). In fact, immunity may be augmented in the early stages of cancer and then suppressed as the disease disseminates progressively. An animal model, using *Listeria monocytogenes* as an infective organism, showed augmented resistance to *Listeria* after implantation of a methylcholanthrene-induced tumour, but with progression of the tumour the resistance diminished and became subnormal (Nomoto *et al.* 1987).

The most severe expression of cellular immunodeficiency is in graft versus host disease (GVHD). Fatal graft versus host disease from transfusion with blood can occur in untreated patients with malignant disease. Although very rare, this is most likely to affect patients with leukaemias or lymphomas and only occasionally other cancers such as neuroblastoma (Kennedy and Ricketts 1986).

Bacterial and fungal infections

Patients with impaired cell-mediated immunity are particularly susceptible to infection by intracellular pathogens (*Listeria monocytogenes*, *Brucella*, and *Mycobacteria*), protozoa (*Pneumocystis carinii* and *Toxoplasma gondii*), fungi (*C. albicans*, *Nocardia asteroides*, *Aspergillus*, and *Cryptococcus*), and viral infections (herpes viruses, measles and vaccinia). *Salmonella*, *Pseudomonas aeruginosa*, and *Staphylococci* are also more frequent than would be expected (Klastersky 1985).

Pneumocystis carinii is a frequent and dangerous infection developing in the immunocompromised host. A revew at the Mayo clinic of 53 patients developing *P. carinii* illustrated its predilection for cancer: 28 per cent had leukaemia, 16 per cent had lymphoma, and 9 per cent had non-haematological malignancy, while the remainder had inflammatory diseases treated by corticosteroids. Over half these patients died within a month of admission to hospital (Peters and Prakash 1987). Patients treated with corticosteroids are prone not only to *P. carinii* but also to *C. albicans* and cytomegalovirus.

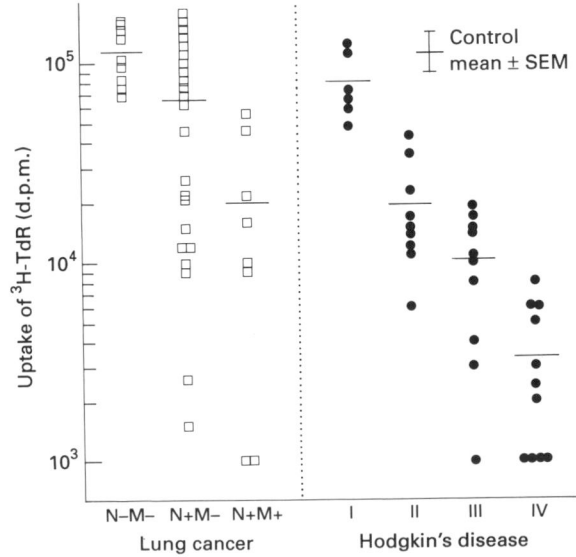

Fig. 1 Proliferation of lymphocytes in response to phytohaemagglutinin was measured by uptake of tritiated thymidine (^{3}H-TdR). Patients with lung cancer were subdivided into those with localized disease (N−M−), those with lymph node spread (N+M−), and those with distant metastases (N+M+). Patients with Hodgkin's disease were subdivided according to stage (Ann Arbor classification).

The diagnosis of toxoplasmosis is often missed in immunocompromised patients and most cases are diagnosed post-mortem. This is unfortunate because therapy with pyrimethamine and sulphonamide can be successful in approximately three-quarters of cases (Ruskin and Remington 1976). Tuberculosis occurs in approximately 1.5 per cent of all patients dying of cancer and shows florid growth with elongated and numerous bacteria in immunocompromised patients.

Fungi, usually originating in the lung and often with associated lung lesions, are the most common organisms infecting the central nervous system in anergic patients: *N. asteroides* causes brain abscesses, *Cryptococcus neoformans* causes meningitis, meningoencephalitis, and focal masses, *Candida* infecting the central nervous system can lead to multiple small abscesses, particularly when there is an associated neutropenia, but unlike the other fungal infections it usually arises from the gastrointestinal tract or infected cannulae, and *Aspergillus* causes abscesses, infarction, and focal meningitis (Escudier *et al.* 1986).

The presentation of certain infecting organisms will vary depending upon which effector arm of the immune system is impaired. Thus, systemic candidiasis is the more usual manifestation in granulocytopenic patients but it is often limited to oesophageal candidiasis in patients with cell-mediated immunodeficiency alone (Walsh *et al.* 1988). Although much more frequently seen in treated patients, candidal infection can be a presenting manifestation in patients with acute leukaemia or lymphoma (Cole *et al.* 1987). Hepatic candidiasis is a severe complication in such patients and is frequently fatal (34 per cent), which may prompt the use of more adventurous therapy with formulations such as lipsome-encapsulated amphotericin B (Haron *et al.* 1987).

Viral infections

Primary infection with herpes viruses (herpes simplex I, herpes simplex II, varicella-zoster, Epstein–Barr, or cytomegalovirus) leads to persistent infection of the host. Reactivation may occur because of impairment or deficiency of either specific cytotoxic T-cells (CD8+) or non-specific natural killer cells. It is debatable whether herpes simplex virus reactivated is increased in patients with depressed cell-mediated immunity, but patients with cell-mediated immunity are obviously more susceptible to viral warts and varicella-zoster virus (Morison 1975). Rarely, chronic herpes virus infections, accompanied by hypogammaglobulinaemia, can occur in areas of skin infiltrated by chronic lymphoblastic leukaemia or lymphoma (Meunier *et al.* 1986). Herpes zoster or shingles ensues from reactivation of varicella-zoster virus in 36 per cent of bone-marrow transplant patients, in 25 per cent of patients with Hodgkin's disease, where it will often affect X-irradiated dermatomes, and up to 50 per cent of Hodgkin's disease patients who have undergone splenectomy as well and in 5 per cent of leukaemic patients; subclinical reactivation, detected by antibody responses and proliferation to varicella-zoster virus *in vitro*, occurred as frequently as clinical involvement (Ljungman *et al.* 1986). Lesions from varicella-zoster virus may become generalized but visceral involvement is rare. Cytomegalovirus reactivation occurs in immunocompromised hosts. The presence of cytomegalovirus antibody has little significance and usually implies viral shedding which can continue for months. As immunosuppression becomes more severe, viral shedding can progress to cytomegalovirus dissemination and multiorgan infection (Betts and Hanshaw 1977). Interestingly, there is a close relationship to the HLA system and cytomegalovirus infection can trigger graft versus host disease in bone-marrow transplant transplants or allograft rejection in solid organ transplants.

Like adults, children with malignant disease are at high risk from varicella-zoster virus infection but they are particularly susceptible to measles. Interstitial pneumonitis due to measles is a severe and often fatal infection in children with cancer (Lemerle *et al.* 1976). Twenty-nine per cent of all deaths while in first remission from childhood acute lymphoblastic leukaemia were due to measles or its complications (Gray *et al.* 1987). Acyclovir and possibly interferon have helped greatly in treating herpes virus infections (Abb 1985). Acyclovir can shorten the infection, restrict dissemination, and accelerate healing of lesions if given within the first 3 days of infection and is superior to vidarabine (Shepp *et al.* 1986). Immune globulin can confer protection from varicella-zoster virus infections if given within the first 3 days of exposure. For prophylactic treatment of varicella-zoster virus there is an attenuated varicella vaccine (Oka strain) which induces an antibody response of more than 90 per cent. Side-effects include rashes and fever and these are increased in high-risk groups and can be severe in the immunocompromised (Katsushima *et al.* 1984). Live attenuated vaccine given to children in remission from leukaemia induced immunity in approximately 80 per cent of patients (Gershon *et al.* 1986).

It should be remembered that antibody-based tests for infection in immunocompromised patients may be unreliable because the patient may not be able to make an antibody response.

Immunotherapy

The interaction between the immune system and cancer has been highlighted by attempts to use immunostimulatory agents as a means of treating cancer or its associated immunodeficiency. The rationale of this approach was that correction of depressed cell-mediated immunity might not only protect individuals from opportunistic infections but also mobilize the immune system into attacking the cancer. More recent therapeutic modalities using cytokines, which are dealt with elsewhere, have had the same aims as the earlier attempts at immunotherapy, such as the injection of bacille Calmette–Guérin (BCG) or *Corynebacterium parvum*, which were given to patients with cancer in an attempt to augment immune responses in a non-specific manner. Both these bacteria can activate macrophages which are then capable of causing tumour cell destruction as a bystander effect. Injection of BCG at a remote site from the tumour is not effective (Zbar 1972). This mode of therapy has found a place in treating transitional cell cancers of the bladder because these are superficial and amenable to repeated instillation of BCG directly into the bladder (Morales *et al.* 1976). Use of these attenuated microorganisms in immunocompromised patients with malignant disease runs the risk of iatrogenic illness from persistent and disseminated BCG infection with hepatitis, activation of old tuberculosis, and possible hypersensitivity reactions (Aungst *et al.* 1975) or dysuria in bladder cancer (Lamm 1986). Disseminated BCG infection can be treated with antituberculous drugs. In certain instances the opposite to the intended effect can follow the use of immunomodulatory substances, such as BCG or even cytokines such as tumour necrosis factor, whereby metastasis of tumours is facilitated (Ishibashi *et al.* 1980). The whole concept of tumour-specific antigens as a means by which tumours can be treated through augmentation of the immune response to tumour-specific antigens has undergone a radical revision. It is now generally accepted that virally induced tumours are highly immunogenic and those associated with the Epstein–Barr virus in transplant patients can often be eliminated by simply stopping the immunosuppressive treatment given to the affected transplant patients. Animal experiments which gave rise to the hopes of eliminating cancer by augmenting the immune response were based largely on virally induced tumours or repeatedly passaged cell lines which became strongly immunogenic. Unfortunately, when spontaneously arising animal tumours were used for the same immunological experiments they were found to be resistant to rejection (Klein and Klein 1977). Potent immune responses, involving many effector mechanisms, directed towards viruses can explain tumour regressions which occasionally follow viral infections, such as measles, in patients with cancer. This is believed to come about because of the xenogenization of tumour cells by which cancer cells (as well as normal cells) become infected and express viral determinants which lead to their destruction by virus-specific cytotoxic T-cells. Corroboration for this clinically observed phenomenon has come from animal models (Zbar et al. 1983; von Hoegen et al. 1988).

The rare occurrence of spontaneous regression of cancers has been described. Over half of the 176 authenticated cases were restricted to renal carcinoma (18 per cent), neuroblastoma (16 per cent), malignant melanoma (11 per cent), and choriocarcinoma (11 per cent). Although speculative immunological reactions offered the best explanation for these regressions (Cole 1981), 40 per cent of all cases of spontaneous regression were associated with surgical trauma.

Splenectomy, functional asplenia, or hypogammaglobulinaemia

The loss of the spleen is infrequently followed by overwhelming post-splenectomy infections and the frequency of their occurrence is determined by the patient's age and the underlying disease process which led to the splenectomy. Splenectomy performed as part of the staging laparotomy for Hodgkin's disease precedes overwhelming post-splenectomy infections in 2–4 per cent of adults and 6–9 per cent of children. However, the same operation performed for patients with hypersplenism or idiopathic thrombocytopoenic purpura leads to a 5 and 14 per cent incidence of overwhelming post-splenectomy infections, respectively. Identical overwhelming infections may arise in patients with chronic leukaemias or lymphomas without splenectomy as a result of hypogammaglobulinaemia and/or functional asplenia. The pathogenesis of overwhelming post-splenectomy infections is linked to the loss of both the special phagocytic and antibody-producing properties of the spleen (Amlot and Hayes 1978).

The major pathogenic organisms in all these conditions, in the order of their frequency, are Streptococcus pneumoniae, Haemophilus influenzae, E. coli and P. aeruginosa. For patients with chronic leukaemias, P. aeruginosa replaces S. pneumoniae as the most frequent infecting organism (Mower et al. 1986). Most of these infections are readily treated with the penicillin group of antibiotics. Long-term prophylactic penicillin therapy should be used in splenectomized children and adults should be educated as to the dangers of splenectomy so that antibiotics can be used rapidly if a febrile or infective illness develops. Before elective splenectomy, patients may be immunized with Pneumovax to give protection against 80 per cent of all pathogenic strains of S. pneumoniae. Immunization against pneumococcal antigens should not lead to complacency. First the benefit of immunization for splenectomized patients has not been clearly established and, second, it will not protect at all against non-pneumococcal infections.

Hypogammaglobulinaemia occurring in chronic lymphocytic leukaemia and low-grade lymphomas which leads to recurrent infection should be treated with replacement intravenous or intra-muscular gammaglobulin. The dose and frequency should be adjusted to the individual aiming to maintain the serum IgG above 4 g/l.

Immunodeficiency predisposing to cancer

Cancer is more frequent in patients who are chronically immunodeficient (Table 1). Even with minor immunodeficiency states, such as the hyper IgE syndrome, lymphomas are more common (Gorin et al. 1989). Estimates of the relative risk of developing cancer are fairly consistent for the major different categories of immunodeficiency (60–100 times normal; see Table 1), but some calculate the risk as being much higher (up to 1000 times normal) in congenitally immunodeficient patients. This may be because the early onset of immunodeficiency increases the risk of developing cancer as a result of potentially oncogenic viruses to which no immunity exists. The risk of developing a lymphoma in all AIDS patients is 60 times normal, but it rises to 360 times normal for patients aged 20 years or less (Beral et al. 1991).

The frequency of cancer in specific immunodeficiency states is given in Table 2. The very high incidence of malignancy (mostly lymphomas) in ataxia–telangiectasia is attributed not so much to its mild immunodeficiency as to its associated susceptibility to chromosomal breakage and translocation which selectively involve genes of the immune system, namely the immunoglobulin genes at 2p12, 14q32, and 22q11 and the T-cell receptor genes at 7p13, 7q35, and 14q11 (Hecht and Hecht 1987). There is also an unusually high frequency of lymphoma (as the only malignancy) in the rare x-linked recessive lymphoproliferative syndrome. This

Table 1 Relative risk of cancer in immunodeficient patients compared with the general population

Immunodeficiency	Relative risk[a]
Congenital or primary	100–1000×
Transplant recipient	80×
AIDS	60×

[a]Age may play an important role (see text).
Source: Penn (1990) and Beral et al. (1991).

Table 2 Estimated frequency of cancer in specific immunodeficient states

Immunodeficiency	Frequency (%)
Congenital	
Selective IgA	1
XLA	4
SCID	9
Wiskott–Aldrich syndrome	14
Ataxia–telangiectasia	29
XLRLS	40
Acquired	
Common variable	11
Transplantation	
Kidney	1
Heart	2
Liver	2
Heart–lung	5
AIDS	
Lymphoma	3
Kaposi's sarcoma	16

XLA, x-linked agammaglobulinaemia; SCID, severe combined immunodeficiency; XLRLS, x-linked recessive lymphoproliferative syndrome.
Source: Kersey et al. (1974), Purtilo et al. (1978), Cunningham-Rundles et al. (1987), and Nalesnik et al. (1988).

condition is associated with a defective x gene controlling lymphoproliferation and the affected males suffer from a variety of abnormal responses to Epstein–Barr virus infection including hypogammaglobulinaemia or a rapidly fatal infectious mononucleosis or high-grade disseminated B-cell lymphoma.

Chronic immunosuppression associated with all forms of transplantation is associated with increased malignancy including allogenic bone-marrow grafts (Kersey *et al.* 1988).

Cancers arising in immunodeficiency are distinguished by a number of features.

Types of cancer

These cancers are not the common cancers seen in the general population (for example, lung, prostate, breast, colon, or uterine cervix) but consist predominantly of lymphomas. For example, 67 per cent of all cancers arising in congenital immunodeficiency are lymphomas compared with 8 per cent in 'normal' children. Other cancers arising more commonly in immunodeficiency are squamous cell carcinomas of the skin (particularly of the lip and vulva), Kaposi's and other sarcomas (Kaposi's sarcoma is strikingly prevalent in AIDS and particularly associated with sexual promiscuity), carcinoma of the kidney, and hepatobiliary tumours.

Characteristics of lymphomas in immunodeficiency

The lymphomas are usually high grade (immunoblastic). In AIDS there is a marked increase in lymphomas classified as 'Burkitt-like' (estimated as 1000 times the frequency in the general population).

Commonly, there is extranodal involvement (69 per cent compared with approximately 30 per cent normally). Primary brain lymphomas are common (28 per cent, which is 1000 times the normal risk). Two-thirds of brain lymphomas arising in immunodeficiency are primary and solitary tumours, unlike the brain lymphomas arising spontaneously in immunocompetent subjects which are more often associated with disease at other sites in the body and usually arise late in the course of the disease. Lymphomatous involvement of the allograft is common (18 per cent) in transplant patients.

Lymphomas are usually associated with evidence of Epstein–Barr virus infection and expression of EBNA (50 per cent of all lymphomas in AIDS and 80 per cent in transplant patients). For example, central nervous system lymphomas arising in immunocompromised patients were positive by *in situ* hybridization for Epstein–Barr virus (BAMH1V: 3.1 kb) whereas in central nervous system lymphomas from immunocompetent patients they were negative (Bashir *et al.* 1989). Patients may show evidence of chronic Epstein–Barr virus infection (Okano *et al.* 1986). Many immunodeficient patients with lymphoma have elevated IgG antibody titres to the viral capsid antigen and the early antigen and although IgA antibodies to both these antigens characterize nasopharyngeal carcinoma, these can be found in approximately 40 per cent of patients with chronic lymphoblastic leukaemia but at a 10-fold lower titre than for nasopharyngeal carcinoma (Dolken *et al.* 1986). Lymphoproliferation in acquired immunodeficiencies often shows progression from polyclonal to monoclonal phenotypes. Cessation of immunosuppressive therapy at the polyclonal stage in transplant patients often leads to a resolution of lymphoproliferative disease.

Time to development of cancer

The length of time between the onset of immunodeficiency and the diagnosis of cancer varies according to the type of cancer. This incubation time is based mostly on transplant statistics because of the clearly defined start of immunodeficiency when transplant immunosuppression begins. Examples are as follows.

1. Kaposi's sarcoma, 20 months.
2. Lymphoma, 33 months.
3. Carcinoma, 107 months.

However, the time to oncogenesis is affected by the intensity and duration of immunosuppression (see below).

Intensity of immunosuppression

Both the frequency and the speed of oncogenesis increase in proportion to the intensity of immunosuppression. Again, this is most evident from examination of transplantation data. The frequency of cancer differs according to the grafted organ and reflects the intensity of immunosuppressive therapy required to prevent graft rejection (Table 2). The prolonged use of excessive non-specific immunosuppression increases the risk of cancer. This was seen in early clinical studies of cyclosporin where it was combined with steroids and azathioprine at excessive dosage. Recently, the use of the monoclonal antibody OKT3 which suppresses virtually all T-cell function has been associated with a striking increase in lymphomas (overall 11 per cent). OKT3 at cumulative dosage above 75 mg has been associated with a further sharp rise (36 per cent) in lymphomagenesis (Swinnen *et al.* 1990). There is an uncommon syndrome called post-transplant lymphoproliferative disease which is reminiscent of x-linked recessive lymphoproliferative syndrome, with fever, renal failure, cytopenia, encephalopathy, exudative pharyngitis, lymphadenopathy, and immunoblastic-lymphoplastic infiltrates into kidneys, livers, and lymph nodes together with necrosis. It is fatal in the majority of cases (86 per cent) and has been seen more frequently (approximately 2 per cent) since the use of OKT3 for treatment of solid organ grafts, particularly where grafts from Epstein–Barr-virus positive donors are given to Epstein–Barr virus-negative recipients. This pattern is similar to the marked rise in infectious complications occurring when increasingly intensive cytotoxic therapy is given to patients with unresponsive lymphomas or Hodgkin's disease.

Treatment of cancers arising in immunodeficient patients is conventional, but may have to be modified because of the type of immunodeficiency or because of past therapy and bone-marrow suppression. Where possible, the immunosuppression must be reversed and this alone may prevent the development of lymphomas. Acyclovir reduces the morbidity of Epstein–Barr virus in normal individuals but not in patients with x-linked recessive lymphoproliferative syndrome in which there is an 85 per cent mortality from fulminant infectious mononucleosis, hypogammaglobulinaemia, or malignant lymphoma. Attempts to provide prophylaxis for x-linked recessive lymphoproliferative syndrome patients with immunoglobulin containing Epstein–Barr-specific antibodies are under way based on the observation that the syndrome does not occur while maternal antibodies are still present (Purtilo 1986). There is the prospect of an Epstein–Barr virus vaccine which has been used successfully to immunize tamarin cottontops against the development of lymphomas (Morgan *et al.* 1988).

Autoimmunity in cancer

Conceptually, there are three situations in which autoantibodies arise in cancer: (1) as a product of malignant B-cells, (2) because of dysregulation of normal or malignant T-cells, and (3) where immunogenic, degraded, or altered self-proteins are released by a tumour.

Autoantibodies produced by lymphomas

Coombs' positive warm antibody haemolytic anaemia occurs in 5–15 per cent and idiopathic thrombocytopenia in 5–10 per cent of chronic lymphocytic leukaemias and well-differentiated lymphocytic lymphomas (ML lymphocytic, Kiel) and a variety of haemolytic anaemias occur in Waldenström's macroglobulinaemia (ML lymphoplasmacytoid, Kiel). Until the recent identification of new lineage of B-cells it was difficult to understand why autoantibodies should occur in chronic lymphoblastic leukaemia more frequently than in other forms of lymphoma. The novel lineage of B-cells is known as the CD5+ B-cell because of its unusual expression of an antigen (CD5) normally present on T-cells. These CD5+ B-cells are increased in autoimmune diseases such as rheumatoid arthritis, have a natural propensity to produce autoantibodies, differentiate completely independently of other B-cells, and have chronic lymphoblastic leukaemia and lymphoplasmacytoid lymphomas, both of which express the CD5 antigen, as their malignant counterparts (Hardy *et al.* 1987; Lydyard *et al.* 1987). Small amounts of monoclonal paraprotein can be detected in the serum of chronic lymphoblastic leukaemia patients using sensitive techniques and obviously this can have a dramatic effect if the monoclonal paraprotein produced reacts with erythrocyte or platelet antigens. Far larger quantities of paraprotein are produced in lymphoplasmacytoid lymphomas (for example, Waldenström's lymphoma) where the hyperviscosity syndrome, impairment of coagulation or platelet function, neurological symptoms, cold sensitivity (cryoglobulins), haemolysis (cold agglutinins), or pseudohyponatraemia may occur. The incidence of lymphomas is increased in a number of autoimmune diseases such as Sjögren's syndrome and rheumatoid arthritis. Chronic T-cell immunodeficiency and Epstein–Barr virus infection may combine to cause this increased susceptibility (Weir *et al.* 1989).

T-cell dysregulation and T-cell lymphomas

Angio-immunoblastic lymphadenopathy with dysproteinaemia, normally a T-cell lymphoma, is characterized by hypergammaglobulinaemia, Coombs' positivity, and high titres of smooth muscle antibody (anti-intermediate filament) in 75 per cent of cases. These antibodies may relate to either the marked vascular endothelial proliferation in this disease or viral antigens cross-reacting with intermediate filaments because of the common viral infections which precede angio-immunoblastic lymphadenopathy with dysproteinaemia (Dellagi *et al.* 1984). The antibodies are polyclonal and consist of IgM, IgG, and IgA classes at titres of 1/64–1/512. They react with determinants shared by vimentin, desmin, and keratin. This multiple determinant reactivity or polyspecificity is characteristic of CD5+ B-cells and raises the question as to whether cytokines produced by the malignant T-cells stimulate their differentiation and antibody production.

Patients have been described with T-cell lymphocytic leukaemia, immunodeficiency, and hyper-IgM. The leukaemic T-cells had selective helper function for IgM, but suppressor function for IgG and IgA (Raziuddin *et al.* 1989).

Release of altered self-proteins

In the paraneoplastic syndromes, particularly those associated with small cell carcinoma of the lung and ovarian carcinoma, the distant effects of the tumour may be related to autoimmune phenomena. It is possible that the antibodies arise because of damaged neural antigens released systemically. Autoantibodies arising in paraneoplastic syndromes can react with the following.

1. Retinal antigens in the cancer-associated retinal syndromes which lead to visual loss (Thirkill *et al.* 1989).

2. Purkinje cells in cerebellar degeneration (Greenlee and Lipton 1986).

3. Neurofilaments with subacute sensory neuropathy (Graus *et al.* 1986).

4. Neuronal nuclear antigens in the Eaton–Lambert syndrome (Dropcho *et al.* 1989).

5. Epithelial antigens with pemphigus (Anhalt *et al.* 1990).

In most of these cases the autoantibody binds to both the tumour cells and the autoantigen and can be shown to be able to induce similar neurological damage in animals.

Pure red cell aplasia arises in some cases of thymoma and this rare event may occur because of an autoantibody reactive with erythroid precursors (CFU-E). An even rarer event has been described where neutropenia occurred in a patient with thymoma, hypogammaglobulinaemia, and absent B-cells due to an inhibitor of CFU-GM (Degos *et al.* 1982). Insulin receptor antibodies occur in the paraneoplastic syndrome acanthosis nigricans (Kahn *et al.* 1976).

HAEMATOLOGICAL COMPLICATIONS

Introduction

Primary haematological problems occasionally arise in patients with non-haematological malignancy. However, much more frequently the haematological abnormalities occur as a complication of malignant disease or its treatment. Disorders of erythrocyte, leucocyte, platelet, or coagulation will be dealt with in this chapter and particular attention will be paid to their aetiology and treatment.

Red cells

Anaemia occurs in more than half of cancer patients and is by far the commonest haematological manifestation. Symptoms related to anaemia, such as breathlessness or angina, are rarely presenting features except in elderly patients where a compromised cardiovascular system would be more susceptible to hypoxia. The aetiology of the anaemia can be multifactorial (Table 3) and it is important to identify all possible causes in order to initiate effective treatment.

Table 3 Causes of anaemia in patients with cancer

1. Anaemia of chronic disease
2. Blood loss
3. Haemolysis
   Non-immune (microangiopathic haemolytic)
   Immune (IgG/IgM±complement)
4. Acquired pure red cell aplasia
5. Haematinic deficiency
6. Anaemia secondary to marrow infiltration

Anaemia of chronic disease

Most patients with cancer will develop the anaemia of chronic disease at some stage in their illness. This is particularly true for those patients with solid tumours (Cartwright and Lee 1971; Bentley 1982; Lee 1983). The anaemia is usually mild (8–11 g/dl) and becomes apparent within 2 months of the symptomatic onset of the illness. The degree of anaemia generally reflects the extent of the malignancy. The peripheral blood characteristically shows normocytic or slightly microcytic and normochromic red cells and the reticulocyte count is inappropriately low for the degree of the anaemia, suggesting a degree of ineffective erythropoiesis. The diagnosis can be confirmed by the demonstration of abundant stainable iron in the bone-marrow together with a marked reduction in the number of iron-containing erythroblasts to 5–20 per cent compared with the normal 30–50 per cent. A low serum iron and a low iron-binding capacity (Samson 1983) are usually present. When there is a co-existing iron deficiency the diagnosis of the anaemia of chronic disease can prove difficult (see section on blood loss).

The pathogenesis of the anaemia of chronic disease remains to be fully elucidated. Evidently, there is an inadequate utilization of iron by developing erythroblasts. Reduced red cell lifespan and disordered red cell maturation contribute to the anaemia. The roles played by erythropoietin and interleukin 1 remain unclear. Since the anaemia is usually mild, blood tranfusions are rarely necessary. Treatment of the underlying disease often raises the haemoglobin concentration, but it should be remembered that it may be compounded by haematinic deficiency or blood loss.

Blood loss

Blood loss is the second most common cause of anaemia in patients with malignant disease. Chronic loss from ulcerating tumours of the gastrointestinal tract, lung, and renal carcinoma lead to iron deficiency. A microcytic hypochromic anaemia with associated poikilocytosis, 'pencil' cells, and target cells, as well as thrombocytosis, are seen on peripheral blood smear examination. It is important to distinguish between iron deficiency anaemia and anaemia of chronic disease as both may co-exist in the same patient. If iron deficiency anaemia is the main factor responsible for anaemia, it is eminently treatable with iron replacement.

In iron deficiency anaemia serum iron is low while total iron-binding capacity is high (Samson 1983). While serum ferritin levels correlate very well with iron stores in the marrow (Lipschitz et al. 1974), assessment of the latter is susceptible to considerable error (Bentley and William 1974). Ferritin, an acute phase protein, is usually elevated in malignant disease (Al-Ismail et al. 1979; Bentley 1982). A confident diagnosis of iron deficiency anaemia can be made when the serum ferritin is below 12 μg/l (Blake et al. 1980). If the patient has co-existing anaemia of chronic disease, a ferritin in the low normal range (13–100 μg/l) may exist with no stainable iron in the marrow (Bentley and William 1974; Baynes et al. 1987). Therefore, if the ferritin is in the low normal range in patients suspected to have anaemia of chronic disease, a therapeutic trial of oral ferrous sulphate 300 mg three times daily for 30 days is warranted.

Haemolytic anaemia

Non-immune: microangiopathic haemolytic anaemia

Microangiopathic haemolytic anaemia is a clinical syndrome characterized by intravascular haemolysis with fragmentation of red cells caused by their destruction as they pass through fibrin deposited in abnormal blood vessels. The pathological processes responsible for this condition include disseminated intravascular coagulopathy (DIC), platelet aggregation, and vasculitis. In malignant disease the fragmentation process can occur within abnormal vessels of the primary tumour or as a result of metastatic tumour thrombi. Chemotherapeutic agents such as mitomycin C alone or in combination with cisplatinum, bleomycin, and vincristine may also be responsible for triggering this type of intravascular haemolysis.

The anaemia is usually severe (Hb 7–9 g/dl) and develops over a short period of time. Fragmented red cells, thrombocytopenia, and reticulocytosis are seen on peripheral blood smear examination. A leucoerythroblastic blood picture (that is, circulating immature red and white cell precursors) usually indicates malignant metastases in the bone-marrow. Bone-marrow examination is indicated in the presence of a leucoerythroblastic blood film or severe thrombocytopenia. If the bone-marrow is clear of metastatic malignancy, hyperplasia of the erythroid series is usually found (Kressel et al. 1981). Other features of intravascular haemolysis are usually present including raised serum levels of lactate dehydrogenase and bilirubin, while haptoglobins are reduced and the direct Coombs' test is negative. Coagulation abnormalities are variable, but in most cases only minor aberrations of the prothrombin time, the partial thromboplastin time with kaolin, or the thrombin time occur. The urea and creatinine levels are usually elevated at some stage during the illness. The pathological process responsible for this renal insufficiency is fibrin deposition in blood vessels and endothelial proliferation in glomeruli and small arterioles, a histological picture which is not unlike that seen in proliferative arteriopathy. In mild cases the process can be reversed by treating the underlying disease. When progressive renal failure accompanies severe haemolysis the outlook is poor. Red cell and platelet transfusions may be required when the haemoglobin and platelet counts drop to dangerously low levels. It should be remembered that in these patients with renal failure red cell transfusions may cause pulmonary oedema together with further activation of the clotting cascade and escalation of the haemolytic process. Other therapeutic interventions, which have included corticosteroids, antiplatelet drugs, azathioprine, and plasma exchange, have generally been disappointing. If circulating immune complexes are present, the use of immunoperfusion filters with plasma exchange may be useful (Korek et al. 1986).

Immune haemolytic anaemia

Autoimmune haemolytic anaemia very rarely occurs in patients with solid tumours. Extravascular haemolysis occurs in the reticuloendothelial system (predominantly spleen) following red cell sensitization with IgG and/or IgM (cold agglutinins) plus complement. This complication has been reported in patients treated with chlorambucil, cyclophosphamide, melphalan, methotrexate, and cis-platinum (Doll and Weiss 1985).

The anaemia can be severe and has an insidious onset and jaundice with splenomegaly is usually present. Polychromasia, spherocytosis, and nucleated red cells are usually present in the peripheral blood, particularly when the autoantibody is IgG. If cold agglutinins are present, then red cell agglutination may be seen on the peripheral blood smear. Treatment of the underlying malignancy plus corticosteroids usually suppresses the haemolytic process. In refractory cases additional immunosuppressive therapy and elective spenectomy may prove effective.

Acquired pure red cell aplasia

Approximately 50 per cent of patients with acquired pure red cell aplasia have a thymoma; however, this complication only occurs in 5 per cent of patients with thymomas. Failure of erythropoiesis is characterized by anaemia and reticulocytopenia with reduction of red cell precursors, particularly later forms, in the bone-marrow. The aetiology is thought to be autoimmune (Anonymous 1982; Krantz 1984) and in some cases antibodies to erythroid precursors have been demonstrated (Marmont et al. 1975; Messner et al. 1981). Removal of the thymoma, which is usually benign, gives remission rates of 30–50 per cent (Roland 1964), but a significant number of these patients will relapse. Occasionally pure red cell aplasia can develop following thymectomy. Immunosuppression with corticosteroids, cyclophosphamide, and azathioprine have been used but are often disappointing and other agents that modulate the immune system should be considered; these include cyclosporin A, antilymphocyte globulin, and vincristine either alone or in combination. Plasma exchange is of value in some cases (Messner et al. 1981). Resistant cases may require regular red cell transfusions and iron chelation therapy.

Haematinic deficiency

Deficiency of folic acid and vitamin B_{12} frequently occurs in patients with cancer. Folate deficiency is the commoner of the two and usually results from a combination of reduced absorption, increased utilization (rapidly proliferating cells, prolonged cytotoxic therapy), and sometimes direct antagonism (methotrexate). Vitamin B_{12} deficiency mainly occurs in patients who have undergone gastric surgery (site of intrinsic factor production) or when malabsorption is present secondary to resection and/or bypass procedures involving the terminal ileum (site of vitamin B_{12} absorption). The haematological changes are identical for vitamin B_{12} or folate deficiency: megaloblastic anaemia with oval macrocytes and hypersegmented neutrophils (more than five nuclear lobes) are found in blood smears. The bone-marrow is hypercellular with megaloblastic erythroblasts, giant megakaryocytes, and many dying cells. Measurement of the serum vitamin B_{12} and red cell folate levels is the most satisfactory method of diagnosing each deficiency. Treatment is by regular intramuscular injection of vitamin B_{12} and/or oral folic acid.

Erythrocytosis

Erythrocytosis is characterized by an elevation in haemoglobin concentration, haematocrit, and total red cell volume. When it occurs in combination with malignancy, it is termed inappropriate erythrocytosis and in the majority of cases it is due to tumour production of erythropoietin or erythropoietin-like peptides. Other causes of polycythaemia, such as polychythaemia rubra vera, polycythaemia secondary to tissue hypoxia (appropriate erythrocytosis), and polycythaemia due to reduction in plasma volume, need to be excluded (Firkin et al. 1989). The tumours most commonly associated with inappropriate erythrocytosis include renal cell carcinoma (Damon et al. 1958) and primary liver cell cancer (Brownstein and Ballard 1966). Associations with cerebellar haemangioblastoma, phaeochromocytoma, adrenal adenoma, uterine myoma, and androgen-secreting ovarian tumours have also been reported (Modan 1971).

If the patient is symptomatic (from increased plasma volume/viscosity) and/or the haematocrit is greater than 0.55, venesection

Table 4 Causes of leucoerythroblastosis

Marrow infiltration
  Metastatic carcinoma
  Osteoporosis (myelosclerosis)
  Lymphoma (particularly Hodgkin's disease)
  Myelomatosis
Others
  Severe haemolysis
  Massive haemorrhage
  Megaloblastic anaemia
  Disseminated infection (particularly tuberculosis)
  Thrombotic thrombocytopenic purpura
  Burns
  Eclampsia

should be performed as this is the most direct and simple method of relieving symptoms. Regular venesections are usually required to control haemoglobin concentration and haematocrit values. Myelosuppressive agents, such as busulphan, hydroxyurea, and radioactive phosphorus, are used regularly in cases of polycythaemia rubra vera but only occasionally in patients with inappropriate erythrocytosis.

White cells

Granulocytosis is common in patients with malignant disease and is called a leukaemoid reaction when it is associated with myeloblasts and promyelocytes in the blood. The total granulocyte count can be as high as $100 \times 10^9/l$ and it is important to distinguish this from a primary myeloproliferative condition. Indicators of a primary myeloproliferative disorder include the presence of circulating immature white cell precursors, the presence of the Philadelphia chromosome, splenomegaly, and a low neutrophil alkaline phosphatase score (Goldman 1989). The mechanism of the leukaemoid reaction is unknown but may relate to tumour-secreting growth factors similar in biological activity to granulocyte–macrophage colony-stimulating factor and granulocyte colony-stimulating factor. The presence of a leukaemoid reaction is not synonymous with bone-marrow metastasis. Carcinomas that frequently metastasize to the bone-marrow include lung, breast, prostate, kidney, and gastrointestinal tract. Extensive metastases in the bone-marrow can cause various cytopenias which are usually associated with circulating myelocytes and nucleated red cells; a leucoerythroblastic picture. This term should not be confused with a leukaemoid reaction as leucoerythroblastosis occurs in many clinical settings (Table 4). Unfortunately, when associated with proven malignancy, leucoerythroblastosis usually indicates bone-marrow involvement. Phenotypic studies using monoclonal antibodies to epithelial antigens or cytokeratin can be helpful in identifying individual metastatic tumour cells in bone-marrow samples (Ghush et al. 1985).

Eosinophilia also occurs frequently in patients with malignancy. High eosinophil counts have been seen in peritoneal tumour metastasis, when necrosis occurs within a tumour or following abdominal radiotherapy. Hypersensitivity reactions to chemotherapeutic agents are also a cause of eosinophilia. While monocytosis is also occasionally seen in malignancy, basophilia and lymphocytosis are extremely rare. Patients with malignant disease who are leucopoenic are usually pancytopenic. Management of their bone-marrow failure is difficult. Anaemia can be controlled with regular red cell transfusions, but neutropenia and thrombocytopenia usually prove fatal. Infiltration of the bone-marrow with malignant cells precludes autologous bone-marrow transplantation (Anonymous 1987).

Platelets

Thrombocytopenia

Thrombocytopenia is a common complication of solid tumours. Its severity and duration are usually less than that seen in bone-marrow failure due to leukaemia or bone-marrow aplasia (Dutcher *et al.* 1984). Decreased production secondary to bone-marrow infiltration or myelotoxic drugs are the commonest cause of thrombocytopenia, but other mechanisms can operate which lead to increased platelet destruction (Table 5). The incidence of thrombocytopenia in cancer patients has increased over the past 10 years because of the more frequent use of myelotoxic chemo- or radiotherapeutic regimens. Generally, patients with solid tumours have enough marrow reserve following myelotoxic chemotherapy to maintain an adequate platelet count. Transient but significant thrombocytopenia ($10-30\times10^9/l$) lasting a few days does not warrant platelet transfusion unless there is active bleeding. Inappropriate use of blood products may expose the patient to unnecessary risks and waste scarce as well as expensive resources. Significant haemorrhage may be prevented by maintaining the platelet count above $20\times10^9/l$. The prophylactic use of platelet support is essential when bleeding has occurred or when there is further risk of bleeding (Table 6). Dilutional thrombocytopenia can occur after massive transfusions and requires extra platelet support. Infection, particularly Gram-negative bacteraemia, will increase platelet consumption. The mechanisms underlying this include subclinical or overt DIC, microangiopathic haemolytic anaemia, or splenomegaly. A history of peptic ulceration or mucositis following high dose chemo- or radiotherapy does not itself warrant platelet support. However, if active bleeding occurs without severe thrombocytopenia (platelets $>20\times10^9/l$), then it is prudent to administer platelets before a further fall in the platelet count and exacerbation of bleeding. Bleeding into the central nervous system usually has catastrophic results and therefore patients with primary or secondary brain tumours with moderately severe thrombocytopenia ($20-50\times10^9/l$) may deserve the use of prophylactic platelet support particularly if thrombocytopenia is secondary to treatment. All elective surgical procedures, even minor ones such as endoscopic investigation and insertion of Hickman catheters or long intravenous lines, should be covered by platelet transfusion during and after the procedure. Defects of platelet function can occur secondary to paraproteinaemia, uraemia, or drug therapy (melphalan, cytosine arabinoside). Platelet transfusion in this situation is often ineffective and treatment of the underlying disease offers the best approach for reversing the abnormality of platelet function.

The problems encountered following regular platelet transfusion in patients with primary bone-marrow failure (aplastic anaemia or acute leukaemia) who undergo myeloablative chemo- or radiotherapy and bone-marrow transplantation for their disease can occur in patients with solid tumours, but fortunately are rare. The most frequent are transfusion reactions (chilliness, fevers, rigors) reflecting sensitization of HLA, red cell antigens, or plasma proteins. Contamination with infectious agents (particularly bacteria), while rare, is another important cause of these symptoms. The use of antihistamines and corticosteroids prior to platelet transfusion in patients with troublesome side-effects is generally effective in

Table 5 Causes of thrombocytopenia in patients with cancer

1. Marrow infiltration with bone-marrow failure
2. Drugs (myelotoxic chemotherapy, heparin, interferon)
3. DIC
4. Microangiopathic haemolytic anaemia
5. Thrombotic thrombocytopenic purpura
6. Immune thrombocytopenic purpura (alloimune, idiopathic)
7. Post-transfusional purura/massive transfusion
8. Splenomegaly (sequestration)
9. Haematinic deficiency (B_{12} and folate)

Table 6 Situations that warrant prophylactic platelet transfusions in moderately severe thrombocytopenic patients ($20-50\times10^9/l$)

1. Potential bleeding sites (peptic ulcer, mucositis)
2. Elective surgical procedures (for example, endoscopy)
3. Concurrent infection (with associated coagulopathy)
4. Massive transfusion
5. Brain tumour (primary/secondary)

controlling symptoms. Alloimmunization against HLA class I antigens on platelet membranes occurs in approximately 70 per cent of patients receiving multiple platelet transfusions. Clinically this is characterized by a failure of the platelet count to rise after transfusion of platelet concentrates. In this situation patients can be considered refractory to random donor platelets unless conditions are present which are known to contribute to increased platelet utilization, such as DIC, microangiopathic haemolytic anaemia, splenomegaly, high fevers/infections, or haemorrhage. Screening for the presence of HLA antibodies in refractory patients allows for the possibility of collecting antigen-compatible platelets from appropriately matched donors. The use of white cell filters to remove contaminating white cells from red cell and platelet transfusions may help to prevent HLA sensitization. Transmission of infectious disease, particularly viruses, is still a problem associated with transfusion of blood products. Its incidence has been reduced by screening donors for antibodies to hepatitis B and HIV, but hepatitis C still remains a problem. The other main potential risk is graft versus host disease. This occurs when donor lymphocytes (present in the platelet or red cell transfusion) engraft in the recipient. It is extremely rare, only occurs in very immunocompromised patients, and is almost always fatal. It can be prevented by irradiating the blood products prior to transfusion.

Thrombocytosis

High platelet counts ($>400\times10^9/l$) are frequently seen in patients with non-haematological malignant conditions. The thrombocytosis is said to be 'reactive' despite the lack of metastatic deposits or increased numbers of megakaryocytes in the bone-marrow. The aetiology is unknown. Reactive thrombocytosis rarely requires therapeutic intervention, except for treatment of the underlying disease.

Coagulation

Hypercoagulability (thrombosis)

In the normal individual haemostasis is so finely controlled that haemorrhage is promptly arrested and inappropriate thrombosis does not occur. In cancer patients abnormalities of this process have been known since 1865 when Trousseau described the association of recurrent migratory thrombophlebitis and malignancy (Trousseau 1865). It has been estimated that 5–15 per cent of patients with malignancy develop thrombosis and patients with carcinoma of the pancreas have a 50 per cent chance of developing this complication (Brick 1978; Richles and Edwards 1983). Thromboembolic disease is second to infection as the commonest cause of death in patients with solid tumours (Ambrus et al. 1975). The pathogenetic mechanisms responsible for the hypercoagulable state are numerous (Sack et al. 1977; Brick 1978; Richles and Edwards 1983) and involve perturbations in the clotting cascade and fibrinolytic pathway as well as platelet activation. Laboratory findings include (1) shortening of the partial thromboplastin time, (2) elevated clotting factors (fibrinogen, V, VII, IX, and XI), (3) decreased antithrombin III levels, and (4) raised fibrin/fibrinogen degradation products and fibrinopeptide A. There is also increased fibrinogen and platelet turnover with accelerated fibrinolysis.

The diagnosis of the thrombosis is provisionally made by clinical examination and confirmed by venography, radiolabelled fibrinogen scanning, or plethysmography. Unexplained superficial migratory thrombophlebitis is a useful clinical sign suggesting the possibility of an occult malignancy, while the presence of both venous thrombosis and arterial emboli is highly suggestive of a mucin-secreting adenocarcinoma. The treatment of thrombosis in cancer patients can be very difficult. Most patients are resistant to currently used anticoagulants and unfortunately there is a high incidence of haemorrhage in those who are not resistant. Correction of the coagulopathy usually follows successful treatment of the underlying malignancy.

Thrombotic thrombocytopenic purpura

A syndrome similar to thrombotic thrombocytopenic purpura may develop in patients wth mucin-secreting adenocarcinoma or following treatment with mitomycin C. The condition is characterized by fever, microangiopathic haemolytic anaemia, thrombocytopenia, neurological disturbance, and renal abnormalities. Unlike DIC, there are no significant clotting abnormalities. The mainstay of treatment is plasma exchange or replacement with fresh frozen plasma, plasma protein fraction, and platelets. Suppression of platelet function using antiplatelet agents such as prostacyclin (PGI_2) is sometimes beneficial. Elimination of the triggering mechanisms (that is, treatment of the underlying carcinoma) is essential for the successful outcome.

Disseminated intravascular coagulopathy

DIC frequently occurs in patients with metastatic malignancy. It arises from inappropriate activation of the coagulation cascade with reduction in circulating clotting factors and platelets, leading to secondary fibrinolysis and formation of fibrin/fibrinogen degradation products which in turn act as anticoagulants.

There are two distinct forms of DIC. The chronic or subacute type is more common in patients with solid tumours; it results from slow activation of the haemostatic process and is said to be compensated. Most patients with chronic DIC do not bleed, but when bleeding occurs it is usually mild mucosal bleeding or slight bruising. In the acute form the coagulopathy is severe and uncompensated resulting in catastrophic bleeding from many sites and/or end-organ damage with microangiopathic haemolytic anaemia, oliguria, and renal failure. The severe type of DIC is

usually seen in patients with acute promyelocytic leukaemia or following surgery for prostatic carcinoma.

The diagnosis of acute DIC is established when there is prolongation of the thrombin time, hypofibrinogenaemia (fibrinogen < 1.0 g/l), and thrombocytopenia (platelet count $<100\times10^9$/l) in a patient who is bleeding. Universal agreement on many aspects of the management of acute DIC has not been reached (Machin 1989). What is agreed is that removal of the underlying triggering mechanism (that is, tumour or concurrent infection) is the main therapeutic aim to ensure a favourable outcome in patients with this acquired coagulopathy.

Coagulation miscellanea

Abnormalities of the fibrinolytic pathway are also seen in patients with malignant disease. The tumour most commonly associated is prostatic carcinoma, but sarcoma, carcinoma of the breast, thyroid, colon, and stomach may also activate fibrinolysis following secretion of plasminogen activators such as urokinase and other proteolytic enzymes. Both quantitative and qualitative abnormalities in the clotting factors are seen in patients with metastatic liver disease which is responsive to vitamin K administration. Drugs commonly used in patients with malignancy have also been implicated in haemostatic abnormalities. These include the anthracyclines (doxorubicin and daunorubicin), which promote primary fibrinolysis, actinomycin D, which is a vitamin K antagonist, and L-asparaginase which can cause production of abnormal fibrinogen.

Thromboembolic disease and haemostatic abnormalities occur frequently in patients with malignant disease. Fortunately, clinically significant thrombosis or haemorrhage affects very few. Subclinical coagulopathy is now being diagnosed more frequently with the availability of more sophisticated laboratory techniques, but whether this early detection will lead to a decrease in the incidence of severe coagulopathy remains to be seen.

Summary

Haematological complications which occur in patients with malignant disease are common. Anaemia occurs in over half the patients but rarely is allowed to cause significant morbidity. Life-threatening neutropenia following myelotoxic chemotherapy may prove less of a problem in future because of the clinical introduction of recombinant colony-stimulating factors. Bleeding secondary to coagulopathy and/or thrombocytopenia remains an important cause of mortality in this population. Further successful treatment of these complications may follow a more comprehensive understanding of the pathophysiological events leading to these haematological abnormalities.

REFERENCES

Abb J (1985). Prevention and therapy of herpes virus infections. *Zentralblat fur Bakteriologie und Mikrobiologie*, **180**:107–20.

Al-Ismail S, et al. (1979). Erythropoiesis in Hodgkin's disease. *British Journal of Cancer*, **40**:365–70.

Ambrus JL, Ambrus CM, Wink IB, Pickren JW (1975). Causes of death in cancer patients. *Journal of Medicine*, **6**:61–71.

Amlot PL, Hayes AE (1978). Impaired human antibody response to the thymus independent antigen, DNP-Ficoll, after splenectomy. *Lancet*, i:1008–100.

Anhalt GJ, et al. (1990). Paraneoplastic pemphigus. An autoimmune mucocutaneous disease associated with neoplasia. *New England Journal of Medicine*, **323**:1729–35.

Anonymous (1982). Editorial. Pure red cell aplasia. *Lancet*, ii:546–7.

Anonymous (1987). Editorial. Autologous bone marrow transplantation. *Lancet*, ii:303–4.

Aungst CW, Sokal JE, Jager BV (1975). Complications of BCG vaccination in neoplastic disease. *Annals of Internal Medicine*, 82:666–9.

Bashir RM, Harris NL, Hochberg FH, Singer RM (1989). Detection of Epstein–Barr virus in CNS lymphomas by *in-situ* hybridisation. *Neurology* 39:813–17.

Baynes RD, *et al.* (1987). Haematological and iron-related measurements in rheumatoid arthritis. *American Journal of Clinical Pathology*, 87:196–200.

Belghiti J, Champault G, Fabre, F, Patel JC (1978). Assessment of postoperative infective risk by delayed hypersensitivity tests. The influence of deficient nutrition and its correction. *Nouvelle Presse Medicale*, 7:3337–41.

Bentley DP (1982). Anaemia and chronic disease. *Clinical Haematology*, 11:465–79.

Bentley DP, William P (1974). Serum ferritin concentration as an index of storage iron in rheumatoid arthritis. *Journal of Clinical Pathology*, 27:286–9.

Beral V, Peterman T, Berkelman R, Jaffe H (1991). AIDS-associated non-Hodgkin lymphoma. *Lancet*, 337:805–9.

Betts RF, Hanshaw JB (1977). Cytomegalovirus in the compromised host. *Annual Review of Medicine*, 28:103–10.

Brick RL (1978). Alterations of haemostasis associated with malignancy: aetiology, pathophysiology, diagnosis and management. *Seminars in Thrombosis and Haemostasis*, 5:1–26.

Brownstein MH, Ballard HS (1966). Hepatoma associated with erythrocytosis: report of 11 cases. *American Journal of Medicine*, 40:204–10.

Cartwright GE, Lee GR (1971). Annotation: the anaemia of chronic disorders. *British Journal of Haematology*, 21:147–52.

Cole S, *et al.* (1987). *Candida* epiglottitis in an adult with acute nonlymphocytic leukaemia. *American Journal of Medicine*, 82:662–4.

Cole WH (1981). Efforts to explain spontaneous regression of cancer. *Journal of Surgical Oncology*, 17:201–9.

Cunningham-Rundles C, Siegal FP, Cunningham-Rundles S, Lieberman P (1987). Incidence of cancer in 98 patients with common varied immuno-deficiency. *Journal of Clinical Immunology*, 7:294–9.

Damon A, Hollut DA, Melicon MM, Ucon AC (1958). Polycythemia and renal cell carcinoma. *American Journal of Medicine*, 25:182–97.

Degos L, *et al.* (1982). Syndrome of neutrophil agranulocytosis, hypogammaglobulinaemia and thymoma. *Blood*, 60:968–72.

Dellagi K, Brouet J-C, Seligmann M (1984). Antivimentin autoantibodies in angioimmunoblastic lymphadenopathy. *New England Journal of Medicine*, 310:215–18.

Dolken G, *et al.* (1986). Increased incidence of IgA antibodies to the Epstein–Barr virus-associated viral capsid antigen and early antigens in patients with chronic lymphocytic leukaemia. *International Journal of Cancer*, 38:55–9.

Doll DC, Weiss RB (1985). Haemolytic anaemia associated with antineoplastic agents. *Cancer Treatment Reports*, 69:777–82.

Dorian B, Garfinkel PE (1987). Stress, immunity and illness—a review. *Psychological Medicine*, 17:393–407.

Dropcho EJ, Stanton C, Oh SJ (1989). Neuronal antinuclear antibodies in a patient with Lambert–Eaton myasthenic syndrome and small-cell lung carcinoma. *Neurology*, 39:249–51.

Dutcher JP, *et al.* (1984). Incidence of thrombocytopoenia and bleeding among patients with solid tumours. *Cancer*, 53:557–62.

Escudier E, Cordonnier C, Poirier J (1986). Infections of the CNS in malignant haemopathies. *Revue Neurologique de Paris*, 142:116–25.

Firkin F, Chesterman C, Pennington D, Davor R (ed.) (1989). Polycythemia, myelofibrosis. In *de Gruchy's clinical haematology in medical practice*, (5th edn), pp. 318–45. Blackwell, Oxford.

Gershon AA, Steinberg SP, Gelb L (1986). Live attenuated varicella vaccine use in immunocompromised children and adults. *Pediatrics*, 78:757–62.

Ghush AK, *et al.* (1985). Detection of metastatic tumour cells in routine bone marrow smears by immuno-alkaline phosphatase labelling with monoclonal antibodies. *British Journal of Haematology*, 61:21–30.

Goldman JM (1989). Granulocytes, monocytes and their benign disorders. In *Postgraduate haematology*, (ed. AV Hoffbrand and SM Lewis), pp. 294–324. Heinemann Medical Books, London.

Gorin LJ, *et al.* (1989). Burkitt's lymphoma developing in a 7-year-old boy with hyper-IgE syndrome. *Journal of Allergy and Clinical Immunology*, 83:5–10.

Graus F, Elkon KB, Cordon-Cardo C, Posner JB (1986). Sensory neuropathy and small cell lung cancer: antineuronal antibody that also reacts with the tumor. *American Journal of Medicine*, 80:45–52.

Gray MM, *et al.* (1987). Mortality and morbidity caused by measles in children with malignant disease attending four major treatment centres: a retrospective review. *British Medical Journal of Clinical Research*, 295:19–22.

Greenlee JE, Lipton HL (1986). Anticerebellar antibodies in serum and cerebrospinal fluid of a patient with oat cell carcinoma of the lung and paraneoplastic cerebellar degeneration. *Annals of Neurology*, 19:82–5.

Hardy RR, *et al.* (1987). Rheumatoid factor secretion from human Leu-1+ B cells. *Science*, 236:81–4.

Haron E, *et al.* (1987). Hepatic candidiasis: an increasing problem in immunocompromised patients. *American Journal of Medicine*, 83:17–26.

Hecht F, Hecht BK (1987). Chromosome changes connect immunodeficiency and cancer in ataxia-telangiectasia. *American Journal of Pediatric Hematology and Oncology*, 9:185–8.

Ishibashi T, *et al.* (1980). Distant metastasis facilitated by BCG: spread of tumour cells injected in the BCG-primed site. *British Journal of Cancer*, 41:553–61.

Kahn CR, *et al.* (1976). The syndromes of insulin resistance and acanthosis nigricans: insulin receptor disorders in man. *New England Journal of Medicine*, 294:739–45.

Katsushima N, Yazaki N, Sakamoto M (1984). Effect and follow up study on varicella vaccine. *Biken Journal*, 27:51–8.

Kennedy JS, Ricketts RR (1986). Fatal graft v host disease in a child with neuroblastoma following a blood transfusion. *Journal of Pediatric Surgery*, 21:1108–9.

Kersey JH, Spector BD, Good RA (1974). Cancer in children with primary immunodeficiency diseases. *Journal of Pediatrics*, 84:263–4.

Kersey JH, Shapiro RS, Filipovich AH (1988). Relationship of immunodeficiency to lymphoid malignancy. *Pediatric Infectious Diseases Journal*, 7:S10–12.

Klastersky J (1985). Infections in immunocompromised patients. *Clinical Therapy*, 8:90–9.

Klein G, Klein E (1977). Immune surveillance against virus-induced tumours and non-rejectability of spontaneous tumours; contrasting consequences of host versus tumor evolution. *Proceedings of the National Academy of Sciences USA*, 74:2121–5.

Korek S, *et al.* (1986) Treatment of cancer associated haemolytic uraemic syndrome with staphylococcal protein A immunoperfusion. *Journal of Clinical Oncology*, 4:210–15.

Krantz SB (1984). Pure red cell aplasia. In *Current therapy in haematology–oncology*, (ed. MC Brian, PB McCullock, and BC Decker). Ontario.

Kressel BR, *et al.* (1981). Microangiopathic haemolytic anaemia, thrombocytopoenia and renal failure in patients treated for adenocarcinoma. *Cancer*, 48:1738–45.

Lamm DL (1986). Complications of bacillus Calmette–Guérin immunotherapy in 1278 patients with bladder cancer. *Journal of Urology*, 135:272–4.

Lee GR (1983). The anaemia of chronic disease. *Seminars in Haematology*, 20:61–80.

Lemerle J, *et al.* (1976). Interstitial pneumopathies in children treated for malignant disease. *Archives Francaises de Pediatrie*, 33:569–98.

Lipschitz DH, Cook JD, Finch CA (1974). A clinical evaluation of serum ferritin as an index of iron stores. *New England Journal of Medicine*, 290:1213–16.

Ljungman P, *et al.* (1986) Clinical and subclinical reactivations of varicella–zoster virus in immunocompromised patients. *Journal of Infectious Diseases*, 153:840–7.

Lydyard PM, Youinou PY, Cooke A. (1987). CD-5-positive B cells in rheumatoid arthritis and chronic lymphocytic leukaemia. *Immunology Today*, 8:37.

McCormack RT, *et al.* (1979). Neutrophil function in lymphoreticular malignancy. *Cancer*, 44:920–6.

Machin SJ (1989). Acquired disorders of haemostasis. In *Postgraduate haematology*, (ed. AV Hoffbrand and SM Lewis). Heinemann Medical Books, London.

Marmont A, Peschle C, Sanguineti M, Condorelli M (1975). Pure red cell aplasia: response of three patients to cyclophosphamide and/or antilymphocyte globulin and demonstration of two types of serum IgG inhibitors to erythropoiesis. *Blood*, 45:247–61.

Messner HA, Fauser AA, Curtis JE, Dotten D (1981). Control of antibody mediated pure red cell aplasia by plasmapheresis. *New England Journal of Medicine*, 304:1334–8.

Meunier L, *et al.* (1986). Chronic herpes of the pyodermatitis vegetans type in chronic lymphoid leukaemia. *Annales de Dermatologie et Venereologie*, 113:1199–204.

Modan B (1971). *The polycythemic disorders*. Thomas, Springfield, IL.

Morales A, Eidinger D, Bruce AW (1976). Intracavitary bacillus Calmette–Guérin in the treatment of superficial bladder tumors. *Journal of Urology*, 116: 183–7.

Morgan AJ, *et al.* (1988). Prevention of Epstein–Barr (EB) virus induced lymphoma in cottontop tamarins by vaccination with the EB virus envelope glycoprotein gp340 incorporated into immune-stimulating complexes. *Journal of General Virology*, 69:2093–6.

Morison WL (1975). Viral warts, herpes simplex and herpes zoster in patients with secondary immune deficiencies and neoplasms. *British Journal of Dermatology*, 92:625–30.

Mower WR, Hawkins JA, Nelson EW (1986). Post splenectomy infection in patients with chronic leukaemia. *American Journal of Surgery*, 152: 583–6.

Nalesnik MA, Makowka L, Starzl TE (1988). The diagnosis and treatment of posttransplant lymphoproliferative disorders. *Current Problems in Surgery*, 25:371–472.

Nomoto K, *et al.* (1987). Augmented non-specific resistance and simultaneous impairment of specific immunity to *Listeria monocytogenes* in tumour bearing mice. *Journal of Clinical and Laboratory Immunology*, 24:75–9.

Okano M, *et al.* (1986). Epstein–Barr infection and oncogenesis in primary immunodeficiency. *AIDS Research*, 2:S115–19.

Penn I (1990). Cancers complicating organ transplantation. *New England Journal of Medicine*, 323:1767–9.

Perramant M, *et al.* (1981). Significance of skin tests in preoperative assessment. *Annales d'Anaesthiologie Francaise*, 22:279–84.

Peters SG, Prakash UB (1987). *Pneumocystis carinii* pneumonia. Review of 53 cases. *American Journal of Medicine*, 82:73–8.

Purtilo DT (1986). Prevention and treatment of Epstein–Barr virus (EBV)-associated lymphoproliferative diseases in immune deficient patients. *AIDS Research*, 2:S177–81.

Purtilo DT, Paquin L, Gindhart T (1978). Genetics of neoplasia—impact of ecogenetics on oncogenesis. *American Journal of Pathology*, 91:607–53.

Raziuddin S, Assaf HM, Teklu B (1989). T cell malignancy in Richter's syndrome presenting as hyper IgM. *European Journal of Immunology*, 19:469–74.

Richles FR, Edwards RL (1983). Activation of blood coagulation in cancer: Trousseau's syndrome revisited. *Blood*, 61:14–31.

Roland AS (1964). The syndrome of benign thymoma and primary agenerative anaemia: an analysis of 43 cases. *American Journal of Medical Science*, 247:719–31.

Ruskin J, Remington JS (1976). Toxoplasmosis in the immunocompromised host. *Annals of Internal Medicine*, 84:193–9.

Sack GH, Levin J, Bell WR (1977). Trousseau's syndrome and other manifestations of chronic disseminated coagulopathy in patients with myeloma: clinical, pathophysiologic and therapeutic features. *Medicine*, 56:1–37.

Samson D (1983). The anaemia of chronic disorders. *Postgraduate Medical Journal*, 59:543–50.

Shepp DH, Danderliker PS, Meyers JD (1986). Treatment of varicella–zoster virus infection in severely immunocompromised patients. A randomised comparison of acyclovir and vidarabine. *New England Journal of Medicine*, 314:208–12.

Swinnen LJ, *et al.* (1990). Increased incidence of lymphoproliferative disorders after immunosuppression with the monoclonal antibody OKT3 in cardiac-transplant patients. *New England Journal of Medicine*, 323:1723–8.

Thirkill CE, *et al.* (1989). Cancer-associated retinopathy (CAR syndrome) with antibodies reacting with retinal, optic-nerve and cancer cells. *New England Journal of Medicine*, 321:1589–94.

Trousseau A (1865). Phlegmasia alba dolens. In *Clinique Médicale de L'Hôtel Dieu de Paris*, (2nd edn). Baillière, Paris.

von Hoegen P, Weber E, Schirrmachr V (1988). Modification of tumour cells by a low dose of Newcastle disease virus. Augmentation of the tumor-specific T cell response in the absence of an anti-viral response. *European Journal of Immunology*, 18:1159–66.

Walsh TJ, Hamilton SR, Belitsos N (1988). Oesophageal candidiasis. Managing an increasingly prevalent infection. *Postgraduate Medicine*, 84:193–6.

Weir AB, Herrod HG, Lester EP, Holbert J (1989). Diffuse large-cell lymphoma of B-cell origin and deficient T cell function in a patient with rheumatoid arthritis. *Archives of Internal Medicine*, 149:1688–90.

Zbar B (1972). Tumor regression mediated by *Mycobacterium bovis* (strain BCG). *National Cancer Institute Monographs*, 35:341–4.

Zbar B, Nagai A, Terata N, Hovis J (1983). Tumour rejection mediated by an amphotrophic murine leukaemia virus. *Cancer Research*, 43:46–53.

19.5   Serous effusions

IAN S. FENTIMAN

INTRODUCTION

Serous effusions may signal either the onset or relapse of cancer and can produce severe yet reversible symptoms. Failure to give appropriate treatment results in prolonged morbidity and the need for multiple hospital admissions. Effective local procedures can rapidly improve the quality of life and may postpone the requirement for toxic systemic therapy. Nevertheless, a few patients will develop effusions as pre-terminal events and when possible these should be identified so that they are not overtreated.

In patients with pleural effusions and ascites the decision to treat and the technical details of the procedure are often left to the most inexperienced member of the oncological team. Involvement of senior staff in definitive therapy for effusions will lead to the improvement of results. A large body of evidence from clinical trials can be used to frame management schemes for patients with malignant pleural effusions. Treatments for ascites and pericardial effusions have not been subjected to randomized study but, despite this, guidelines can be suggested.

PATHOPHYSIOLOGY

Normal trans-serosal flux of fluid is from the parietal to the visceral surface; despite a diurnal flow of 5–10 l, the pleural space contains only 5–10 ml and the peritoneal cavity less than 100 ml (Black 1972). A balance is maintained with homeostatic mechanisms which

Table 1 Primary tumours of patients with proven malignant pleural effusions

Male	Percentage	Female	Percentage
Lung	49	Breast	37
Lymphoma/leukaemia	21	Genitourinary	21
Gastrointestinal	7	Lung	15
Genitourinary	6	Lymphoma/leukaemia	8
Melanoma	1	Gastrointestinal	4
Mesothelioma	1	Melanoma	3
Other	4	Other	2
Unknown	11	Unknown	9

Adapted from Johnston (1985).

Table 2 Cytological identification of malignant cells in patients with proven metastatic pleural effusions

Reference	n	Cytology negative	Cytology positive
Graham *et al.* (1953)	333	221 (66%)	112 (34%)
Hirsch *et al.* (1979)	117	54 (46%)	63 (54%)
Madrid *et al.* (1983)	118	39 (33%)	79 (67%)
Broghamer *et al.* (1984)	312	169 (54%)	143 (46%)
Martensson *et al.* (1985)	139	79 (57%)	60 (43%)
Total	1019	562 (55%)	457 (45%)

can cope with increases in fluid production resulting from exercise. Fluid enters the serosal space as a result of high hydrostatic pressure and capillary permeability of the parietal surface. Resorption occurs on the visceral surface which has a relatively large capillary network draining into the low pressure pulmonary or hepatic portal systems. Capillary permeability leads to small losses of protein into serous cavities and the larger molecules are absorbed by lymphatics. This maintains a low colloid osmotic pressure within the space so that egress of fluid is facilitated.

Either singly or jointly all four factors modulating fluid flux can be disturbed in patients with malignancy. The most common cause is change in capillary permeability arising from tumour deposits on the serosal surface. Obstruction of lymphatics resulting from either tumour or radiation can lead to a failure of absorption of protein which in turn increases the colloid osmotic pressure within the serous cavity (Fig. 1).

These causes lead to the production of an exudate (protein >3 g/100 ml). Rarely patients with malignancy may develop congestive cardiac failure leading to bilateral pleural effusions which are transudates (protein <3 g/100 ml). Similarly, transudates may occur in patients with hypoproteinaemia resulting from malignant cachexia.

PLEURAL EFFUSIONS

Aetiology

From an oncological rather than a general thoracic viewpoint, the commonest cause of malignant pleural effusions is lung cancer in males and breast cancer in females. A review of primary histology from patients with cytologically verified malignant pleural effusions is summarized in Table 1 (Johnston 1985).

Most commonly, these effusions result from increased production of fluid due to alteration in capillary permeability at the site of parietal pleural metastases. Under these circumstances pleural fluid will most likely contain malignant cells which may also be detectable on blind pleural biopsy. Patients with pulmonary metastases and visceral pleural involvement may also shed cells into the pleural fluid, but for those with lymphatic obstruction as a cause, malignant cells are least likely to be present.

Presenting features

The commonest symptom is dyspnoea, which may or may not be associated with dull or pleuritic pain. Often patients complain of an irritating dry cough. Not infrequently a patient will attribute the onset of symptoms to a viral infection from which recovery has been incomplete. The relationship of pulmonary infection to

precipitation of a pleural fluid collection in patients with metastatic malignancy has not been formally investigated.

Depending upon the volume of fluid there may be dullness to percussion over the lung base(s) with decreased breath sounds. Confirmation of clinical suspicion is by chest radiograph. A posteroanterior view will show basal opacity which shifts to lie inferiorly on the lateral decubitus view. Having verified that an effusion is present in a patient with known malignancy, further evaluation will be necessary to determine whether cancer relapse is responsible. This will be a reasonable assumption in a case where there is other evidence of recurrent disease, but poses more problems when the effusion is the first evidence of possible relapse and when non-malignant causes, such as cardiac failure, have been excluded by clinical examination.

DEFINITIVE DIAGNOSTIC PROCEDURES

Thoracentesis

In a patient with an isolated pleural effusion the first invasive step should be a diagnostic thoracentesis, taking a small volume of pleural fluid (10–20 ml) for cytological examination. This has been recommended recently by the American College of Physicians (Health and Public Policy Committee 1985). The only contraindications to this procedure are the presence of a clotting abnormality or a low platelet count which might predispose to production of a haemothorax.

Cytology

The colour of pleural fluid is variable but is most commonly yellow or amber with sanguinous effusions being infrequent. Very rarely those patients with thoracic duct infiltration will have a milky chylothorax. Even among those patients with proven malignant effusions, cytologically identifiable malignant cells will be present in approximately 50 per cent, as is shown in Table 2. Atypical cells were reported to be present in 12 per cent of such cases (Martensson *et al.* 1985). Because of the low specificity of cytology, other techniques have been used in an attempt to reduce the number of false-negative reports in patients with metastatic effusions.

Cell culture has been examined as an adjunct to cytology, but the results were not encouraging. Cell pellets from centrifuged effusions were cultured from 30 patients (Singh *et al.* 1978) and after 4–21 days the attached cells and supernatants were fixed and examined. Of the ten cases in which malignant cells were identified on original cytology, similar cells were detected in the culture supernatant of eight and in the monolayer in only six. No

Table 3 Carcinoembryonic antigen in serous effusions: numbers of patients with concentrations greater than 5 mg/ml

Reference	Benign		Malignant	
Klockars et al. (1980)	5/73	(7%)	19/41	(46%)
Martinez-Vea et al. (1982)	10/76	(13%)	14/30	(47%)
Wardman et al. (1984)	3/26	(12%)	26/70	(46%)
Pierucci et al. (1984)	17/67	(25%)	25/40	(63%)
Niwa et al. (1985)	6/33	(18%)	20/30	(66%)
Tamura et al. (1988)	4/39	(10%)	40/66	(60%)
Mezger et al. (1988)	4/30	(13%)	41/96	(43%)
	49/344	(14%)	185/360	(51%)

	Production	Absorption
Hydrostatic pressure		Mediastinal obstruction Cardiac tamponade Diffuse liver metastases
Colloid pressure	Hypoproteinaemia	Lymphatic obstruction
Capillary permeability	Serosal deposits	
Lymphatic absorption		Lymphatic infiltration

Fig. 1 Mechanisms of serous effusion in malignancy.

malignant cells were cultured from effusions originally deemed cytologically negative.

Karyotype

Another approach has been to study the chromosomes in effusion cells both by standard staining and by banding (Dewald et al. 1976). Among the 82 cases with malignant effusions, positive cytology was present in 65 per cent and chromosome abnormalities in 71 per cent. The combination of the two techniques had a specificity of 83 per cent. Karyotyping was of particular value in patients with leukaemias and lymphomas, where cytology was positive in only 31 per cent whereas chromosome abnormalities were detected in 85 per cent. An alternative cytogenetic approach was used by Hostmark et al. (1985) who examined the karyotype of cells in effusions with flow cytometry. Of 37 patients with malignant effusions, 13 contained malignant cells and of these nine were aneuploid and four diploid. Among the 24 cases where no malignant cells were seen cytologically, 21 contained diploid cells and three contained aneuploid cells. The accuracy of cytology was not improved by flow cytometry among patients with primary tumours of lung, breast, pancreas, and ovary.

Enzymes

The presence of malignant cells may be associated with detectable changes in the supernatant fluid including alteration of pH, enzymes, and glucose. However, these measures cannot be used as surrogates for the presence of malignant cells in effusions which are cytologically negative. Sahn et al. (1988) measured the pH of 60 effusions from patients with malignancy and divided them into a low pH group (pH <7.3), of which there were 20 and a group of 40 with normal pH (>7.3). Malignant cells were detected in 90 per cent of the low-pH group compared with 68 per cent of those with normal pH. In the former group significantly lower glucose concentrations and higher levels of lactate dehydrogenase were found. These findings were subsequently confirmed and it was also demonstrated that patients with more extensive intrapleural malignancy (assessed thoracoscopically) were more likely to have positive cytology and a low pH in the pleural effusion (Rodriguez-Panadero et al. 1989).

Elevated levels of salivary amylase have been found occasionally in pleural effusions and most of these cases had primary lung lesions (Kramer et al. 1989). The presence of pancreatic amylase in a pleural exudate suggests a diagnosis of either a pancreaticopleural fistula or, alternatively, a ruptured oesophagus. The unusual circumstances of salivary amylase in a pleural effusion of unknown cause is an indication for a CT scan of the chest.

Carcinoembryonic antigen

Since elevated levels of carcinoembryonic antigen have been found in patients with a variety of malignancies (Burtin 1978), many studies have measured carcinoembryonic antigen concentrations in serous effusions of both benign and malignant aetiology. Results of recent studies are summarized in Table 3, which shows that, when carcinoembryonic antigen levels of greater than 5 mg/ml are taken as positive, the test has a sensitivity of 51 per cent and a specificity of 86 per cent.

When carcinoembryonic antigen was measured in combination with other tumour markers such as α acid glycoprotein, α-fetoprotein, phosphohexose isomerase, and β_2-microglobulin, no clinically significant increase in discrimination between effusions of benign and malignant aetiology was found (Martinez-Vea et al. 1982). Similarly, putative markers such as ferritin, adenosine deaminase, and immunosuppressive acidic protein showed great overlap of levels in effusions of malignant and non-malignant causation (Tamura et al. 1988). Other tumour-associated antigens, including tissue polypeptide antigen and Ca125, were also of little value (Mezger et al. 1988).

Levels of hyaluronic acid in effusion fluid may be of some value in patients with suspected mesothelioma. Hyaluronic acid concentrations greater than 100 mg/ml were found in 73 per cent of patients with mesotheliomas, in 23 per cent of those with non-malignant effusions, and in none of the effusions secondary to other cancers (Pettersson et al. 1988).

Pleural biopsy

In patients with suspected malignant effusions, but in whom cytology was negative, attempts have been made to increase the diagnostic

Table 4 Positive blind pleural biopsies in patients with malignant effusions

Reference	n	
Samuels et al. (1958)	25/52	(48%)
Scerbo et al. (1971)	26/66	(39%)
Salyer et al. (1975)	53/95	(56%)
Frist et al. (1979)	16/44	(36%)
Winkelmann et al. (1984)	35/64	(55%)
Poe et al. (1984)	54/83	(65%)
Prakash et al. (1985)	123/281	(44%)
	332/685	(48%)

Table 5 Thoracoscopy in the diagnosis of malignant pleural effusion: proportion of malignant effusions in which the diagnosis was made thoracoscopically

Reference	n	
Lloyd (1953)	12/16	(75%)
Bloomberg (1970)	18/22	(82%)
DeCamp et al. (1973)	47/50	(94%)
Lewis et al. (1976)	21/22	(95%)
Boutin et al. (1980)	113/128	(88%)
Baumgartner (1980)	11/12	(92%)
Wu et al. (1989)	71/74	(96%)
	293/324	(90%)

yield by blind biopsy of the parietal pleura using either an Abram or a Cope needle. Because of the patchy nature of parietal nodules or the location of tumour on the visceral surface, the additional histological yield has been variable.

Results of pleural biopsies from patients with malignant effusions are shown in Table 4 which indicate an overall positivity rate of 48 per cent. It has been reported that, when parietal pleural biopsies were positive, 11 per cent of such cases had negative effusion cytology (Winkelmann et al. 1984). In one series, the combination of cytology and pleural biopsy yielded pathological proof of malignancy in 90 per cent of cases (Salyer et al. 1975).

The diagnostic yield of pleural biopsy can be increased slightly by altering the needle angle, thereby taking a larger area of parietal pleura (Raja et al. 1980). Repeated blind biopsies may again increase the rate of positivity, although there was no significant increase after three separate biopsies (Salyer et al. 1975). Because of the inexact nature of blind biopsy, the assessment of patients with suspected malignant effusions can be improved when thoracoscopy is included within the diagnostic work-up. This may also have therapeutic implications when pleurodesis is being considered.

Thoracoscopy

This procedure can be performed using either regional or general anaesthesia. In the majority of cases when patients are fit enough the latter should be considered, particularly if it is planned to proceed to a pleurodesis.

The diagnostic yield of thoracoscopy in patients with suspected malignant effusions is shown in Table 5. Overall, 90 per cent of such cases were correctly diagnosed by the procedure and in the majority a histological diagnosis was made. Exceptions would be patients with visceral pleural metastases in whom the thoracoscopist was reluctant to perform a biopsy because of risk of bronchopleural fistula formation. Morbidity from parietal pleural biopsy is minimal, although occasionally it may be necessary to apply diathermy to bleeding vessels.

Prognosis

Determination of the prognosis and, thus, the need for aggressive local therapy, can be difficult. There are wide ranges of survival for patients with particular primary tumours. The median survival after development of a pleural effusion in patients with breast cancer is 15 months (Fentiman et al. 1981). For patients with lung primaries, median survival is 6 months, falling to 3 months in those with gastric cancer (Yamada et al. 1983). Like breast cancer,

mesothelioma has a relatively prolonged survival of 18 months after presentation with an effusion (Martini et al. 1975).

Patients who have lymphoma and pleural effusions are treated by systemic rather than local therapy and their prognosis relates to the response of the effusion (Xaubet et al. 1985). Non-responders had a median survival of 6 months, compared with greater than 40 months for those whose effusion disappeared after systemic therapy.

It is an indication of the imprecision of prognostic factors that almost one in five of patients entered into clinical trials of different pleurodesis methods died within 2 months of treatment (Fentiman 1987). Until more reliable techniques of determining prognosis are found, whenever possible patients should be offered definitive treatment for malignant pleural effusion.

Direct approaches

Decortication of entrapped lung and stripping of parietal pleura will lead to a very successful pleurodesis (Martini et al. 1975). However, because of the associated mortality of 10 per cent and short-term morbidity, this approach should be reserved for patients who have had previous unsuccessful attempts or in whom a thoracotomy for a suspected operable lung lesion showed the disease to be unresectable and where an effusion was present.

External radiotherapy has been used to treat pleural effusions in patients with lung and breast cancer (Strober et al. 1973). Control of the effusion was achieved in 14 out of 17 patients, with relief of pain from parietal tumour. The technique can be time-consuming and may be contraindicated because of prior radiotherapy.

A direct drainage approach has been used whereby an implanted LeVeen or Denver shunt connects the pleural and peritoneal cavities (Dorsey and Cogordan 1984; Cimochowski et al. 1986; Little et al. 1988). Such shunts do not drain spontaneously because of the similar intrapleural and intraperitoneal pressures and patients have to compress the pump up to 80 times daily.

Although shunts carry the theoretical risk of transforming a malignant pleural effusion into a malignant peritoneal effusion, this has not been encountered. The need for regular pumping may cause problems in patients becoming incapacitated by other problems of metastatic malignancy.

Pleurodesis

Despite intensive efforts, there will be 5–10 per cent of patients with pleural effusions due to malignancy in whom proof of recurrence of disease cannot be obtained. Provided that other causes of effusions have been excluded by appropriate tests, if the patient is dyspnoeic, pleurodesis should be performed. The object of treatment is to achieve palliation as simply and effectively as possible without compromising the use of subsequent systemic therapy. Although hospital admission may be required at the time of pleurodesis, if this is successful it will substantially reduce subsequent hospital visits since repeated thoracenteses will be unnecessary. It is important that appropriate therapy is given at the time of first diagnosis. Unsuccessful pleurodesis will lead to loculation and pleural entrapment which can be difficult to treat by means other than pleurectomy.

Despite the existence of a plethora of agents which have been used and sometimes tested, they can be divided into four main groups: radioactive isotopes, cytotoxic agents, biological response modifiers, and sclerosants. Although there are theoretical reasons for particular approaches having a greater or lesser tumouricidal effect, the success of any of these techniques depends upon the ability of the agent to excite a pleural reaction whereby the parietal and visceral layers of pleura fuse. In order to achieve this, the pleural space needs to be drained of fluid and the parietal and visceral layers of pleurae must be apposed so that they are joined by the resulting inflammatory response engendered by the intracavitary agent. Even the most effective agents will not achieve pleural fusion in the presence of undrained effusions or where the lung has not re-expanded because of a persistent pneumothorax.

Assessment of response

The major problem in the interpretation of the results of studies using intracavitary agents is the absence of any agreed system of measuring response to treatment. A variety of methods have been used, ranging from subjective end-points such as relief of dyspnoea to objective measurements such as presence or absence of fluid on subsequent radiographs or the need for subsequent aspirations. Often no defined length of follow-up is given.

A simple system has been proposed which includes both an objective and a subjective element (Fentiman 1987). There are three categories, each based on chest radiography and symptoms. The post-aspirational chest radiograph is used as the baseline. The complete response category comprises those who have no recurrence of fluid from the time of pleurodesis until death or the date of the last follow-up. A minimum of 4 weeks should elapse between treatment and follow-up chest radiograph. Partial responders have recurrence of fluid but without a need for further treatment. The failure category means that there has been symptomatic reaccumulation of pleural fluid, confirmed by chest radiography.

Radioactive isotopes

Radioactive colloidal gold (^{198}Au) was first used as an intracavitary agent to treat metastatic pleural effusion by Hahn and Carothers (1950). The international results were reviewed after 10 years and it was shown that control of effusion occurred in approximately 50 per cent of treated cases (Card et al. 1960). ^{198}Au is predominantly a beta emitter and has a short half-life of 2.7 days, requiring an instilled dosage of 100–200 mCi. Chromic radiophosphate (^{32}P) has a half-life of 14 days, so that a dose of 10 mCi could be used. Jacobs (1958) reported a success rate of 61 per cent with ^{32}P, which was cheaper and safer to use than ^{198}Au.

Radioactive yttrium (^{90}Y), a pure beta emitter requiring only moderate shielding, was used to treat 20 patients with malignant pleural effusion (Austgen et al. 1984). When ^{90}Y was given at a dosage of 50 mCI, there was a decrease in effusion formation in 17 cases (85 per cent).

Seventeen patients were treated with intracavitary ^{131}I bound to human albumin (Kent and Moses 1951). Control was achieved in 71 per cent of cases. This approach is now being reconsidered, but using ^{131}I bound to monoclonal antibodies (Pectasides et al. 1986). A trial is under way to determine whether there is an additional benefit in terms of control, when a specific rather than a non-specific carrier for the ^{131}I is used.

Cytotoxic agents

The first cytotoxic drugs used in an intracavitary role were nitrogen mustard (mustine) and triethylene phosphoramide (thiotepa). Using mustine at a dosage of 0.4 mg/kg, Weisberger et al. (1955) reported that effusions were controlled in 18 out of 30 of cases (60 per cent). Of the subsequent larger series, Kinsey et al. (1964) achieved control

in 54 out of 62 cases (87 per cent) and Anderson in 42 out of 66 (64 per cent) (Anderson et al. 1974).

Intrapleural thiotepa was first used by Bateman et al. (1955) who treated 16 patients in this way, with control of the effusions in 12 cases (75 per cent) and decreased fluid production in one case. Anderson and Brincker (1968) reported control of effusion in 43 per cent of 42 cases treated with intracavitary thiotepa. In a large series of 138 patients, an objective response was recorded in 28 per cent and subjective improvement in an additional 25 per cent (Fracchia et al. 1970).

Subsequently, Suhrland et al. (1965) reported the use of intracavitary 5-fluorouracil with improvement in 66 per cent of 35 patients. Thereafter an increasing number of cytotoxics have been used for local treatment of pleural effusions, including bleomycin (Paladine et al. 1976), adriamycin (Tattersall et al. 1979), cytarabine and cis-platinum (Markman et al. 1985), and mitomycin C (Hagiwara et al. 1987).

Biological response modifiers

Using a rat ascites model tumour, it was found that intrapleural instillation of BCG, either before or after tumour injection, led to suppression of tumour development and prolongation of survival (Pimm et al. 1976). Intracavitary use in patients with malignant pleural effusions was less successful (Richman et al. 1981). At doses of 150–3000 μg a complete or partial response was seen in 46 per cent, with associated fever and pain. The response rate was not related to dosage.

The thymic hormone thymostimulin has been given intrapleurally to 12 patients with malignancy at a dosage of 140 mg (Rimoldi et al. 1984). There were no side-effects and complete remission of the effusion was seen in 75 per cent.

Corynebacterium parvum has been used at a dosage of 4–7 mg to achieve pleurodesis. A complete response was achieved in 92 per cent of patients, but the treatment carried toxicity so that pyrexia occurred in 61 per cent and chest pain in 41 per cent (Felletti and Ravazzoni 1983; McLeod et al. 1985; Ross et al. 1987; Casali et al. 1988). It was reported that a few cases had unexpectedly prolonged survival and it was postulated that systemic benefits might be obtained from intrapleural administration (McLeod et al. 1985). However, there was no evidence of any enhancement of local cell-mediated immunity as measured by the proportion of helper–inducer and suppression–cytotoxic T-cells or natural killer cells (Rossi et al. 1987).

Human leucocyte interferon (α-interferon) was administered intrapleurally to seven patients with metastatic breast cancer (Jereb et al. 1987). Although malignant cells disappeared from the pleural fluid in six cases, there was persistence of the effusion although no patient required subsequent drainage. Side-effects included chest pain and pyrexia.

β-Interferon was given as an intracavitary therapy to 32 patients with recurrent pleural effusion at a dosage of 5–20 MU (Rosso et al. 1988). Of the evaluable cases, a complete or partial remission was achieved in 38 per cent without any side-effects.

Sclerosants

The technique of talc poudrage was originally introduced by Bethune (1935) who used the procedure as a prelude to lobectomy. It was first used for the palliation of malignant effusions in 1958 (Chambers 1958) and has been reported to be almost invariably successful in preventing recurrence of effusions (Haupt et al. 1960;

Pearson and McGregor 1966; Jones 1969; Shedbalkar et al. 1971; Harley 1979; Weisberg 1981).

An alternative sclerosant approach is the use of quinacrine (mepacrine) which was originally used because it had a cytotoxic action in vitro (Gellhorn et al. 1961). Of 31 patients with pleural effusions, there was only one failure. However, subsequent work showed a lower success rate (48 per cent) with frequent pyrexia and pain after instillation (Ultmann et al. 1963). It was reported that two patients developed convulsions, one of whom died of status epilepticus, after intrapleural administration of quinacrine (Borda and Krant 1967).

Sodium hydroxide, which has been instilled as a 0.5 per cent solution in water with successful palliation in 21 cases (Rioseco 1980), is a very simple and inexpensive agent. However, there is little experience using this alkali technique. One of the most widely used sclerosants is tetracyline, the use of which was first reported by Rubinson and Bolooki (1972) with control of the effusion in ten out of 12 cases. Instillation of tetracycline (500 mg) can result in severe pleuritic pain, which is prevented by adding lignocaine (15 ml of 1 per cent solution) (Wallach 1978). More recent results suggest a lower rate of effusion control, so that overall the success rate in uncontrolled studies was 56 per cent (confidence interval (CI) 50–63) (Lees and Hoy 1979; Gravelyn et al. 1987).

Controlled trials of agents for pleurodesis

Representatives of each of the four classes of agents have been tested in prospective randomized trials. Only one study examined the use of a radioisotope and this compared intrapleural instillation of ^{32}P with drainage alone (Izbicki et al. 1975). There were 68 evaluable cases and control was achieved in 19 out of 31 (60 per cent) of those treated with ^{32}P and 16 out of 37 (34 per cent) of those who had drainage alone.

Three trials have examined the efficacy of mustine which has been compared with C. parvum, adriamycin/tetracycline, and talc (Millar et al. 1979; Kefford et al. 1980; Fentiman et al. 1983b). The overall success rate was 47 per cent (95 per cent CI, 43–54). One explanation for the relative inefficiency is the rapid transpleural flux, as witnessed by early production of nausea after instillation, so that there is insufficient retained drug within the pleural space to elicit an inflammatory response. The rapid hydrolysis of mustine in aqueous solution also limits its vesiccant effect.

Bleomycin has been used as an intracavitary agent in three trials (Hillerdal et al. 1986; Hamed et al. 1989; Ostrowski et al. 1989). With the exception of the trial performed by Ostrowski et al. (1989), it was found that less than half the patients treated had successful control of their effusions.

Thiotepa was tested against quinacrine and against drainage alone (Mejer et al. 1977). Control was achieved in only 27 per cent of those treated with thiotepa, in 11 per cent of those having drainage alone, and in 64 per cent of cases in which quinacrine was instilled. Only one published trial used intracavitary adriamycin and achieved a control rate of 80 per cent (Kefford et al. 1980). Recently, a trial in Hong Kong compared intracavitary mitomycin C and C. parvum (Yew et al. 1988). Thirty patients were treated and control of the effusion was achieved in only five out of 15 (33 per cent) of the cases in each group.

Corynebacterium parvum is the only biological agent which has been used in randomized trials of intracavitary therapy and five studies have been carried out (Millar et al. 1979; Leahy et al. 1985; Hillerdal et al. 1986; Yew et al. 1988; Ostrowski et al. 1989). The early trials were very promising and reported high control

Table 6 Ranking of success rates of agents used for pleurodesis in clinical trials

Agent	Percentage control (95% CI)
Talc	96 (93.5–98.5)
Quinacrine	82 (76–85)
C. parvum	72 (52–87)
Tetracycline	65 (58–72)
Mustine	48 (43–54)
Drainage alone	46 (38–54)
Bleomycin	39 (24–53)

rates, but more recently effusion control has been unexpectedly disappointing. Overall effusion control was achieved in 72 per cent of cases (95 per cent CI, 57–87).

Of the sclerosing agents, tetracycline has been the most extensively studied in controlled trials (Bayly et al. 1978; Kefford et al. 1980; Zaloznik et al. 1983; Leahy et al. 1985; Fentiman et al. 1986). The overall rate of control was 65 per cent (95 per cent CI, 58–72). Despite this low rate of success, tetracycline is still regarded by many as the ideal agent for pleurodesis. When tetracycline instillation was compared with dilute hydrocholoric acid, at a similar pH of 2.8, the latter had a very low success rate, suggesting that the mechanism of sclerosis is unrelated to the low pH of tetracycline solution (Zaloznik et al. 1983).

Three studies have tested intracavitary quinacrine (Mejer et al. 1977; Bayly et al. 1978; Stitska et al. 1979). The overall success rate was 82 per cent (95 per cent CI, 76–88). Stiksa et al. (1979) compared two methods of administering quinacrine, with and without an intercostal drain and achieved similar rates of control after repeated thoracentesis or continuous drainage.

There have been four trials of talc poudrage (Fentiman et al. 1983b, 1986; Sorensen et al. 1984; Hamed et al. 1989). The results mirror those from uncontrolled studies with a consistently high rate of effusion control in 96 per cent of cases (95 per cent CI, 93.5–98.5).

When agents are ranked in terms of success rates derived from clinical trials (Table 6), it is apparent that the best control of pleural effusions is obtained after talc poudrage. The majority of trials used simple rather than iodized talc. Thus, insufflations or simple talc should be regarded as the treatment of choice for patients with malignant pleural effusions who are fit enough for a general anaesthetic. It is possible to instil the agent under local anaesthesia, but it is better if the procedure is performed under general anaesthesia. This enables a complete drainage of pleural fluid and permits thoracoscopy to be performed, with the opportunity to biopsy pleural lesions and obtain tissue confirmation of relapse (Fentiman et al. 1982). However, it should be stressed that an experienced anaesthetist is required to administer the anaesthetic.

Plan of treatment

A scheme of management for patients with malignancy and who have developed effusions is shown in Fig. 2. For a patient with a symptomatic effusion, in whom no non-malignant cause is present, the decision to perform a talc pleurodesis should be made as soon as the effusion is symptomatic, irrespective of effusion cytology. The procedure, which may appear deceptively simple, needs to be performed by an experienced team. The effusion is drained to dryness and then 10–15 g of simple talc is insufflated. One intercostal drain is sufficient, provided that there have not been previously unsuccessful attempts at pleurodesis using inferior techniques.

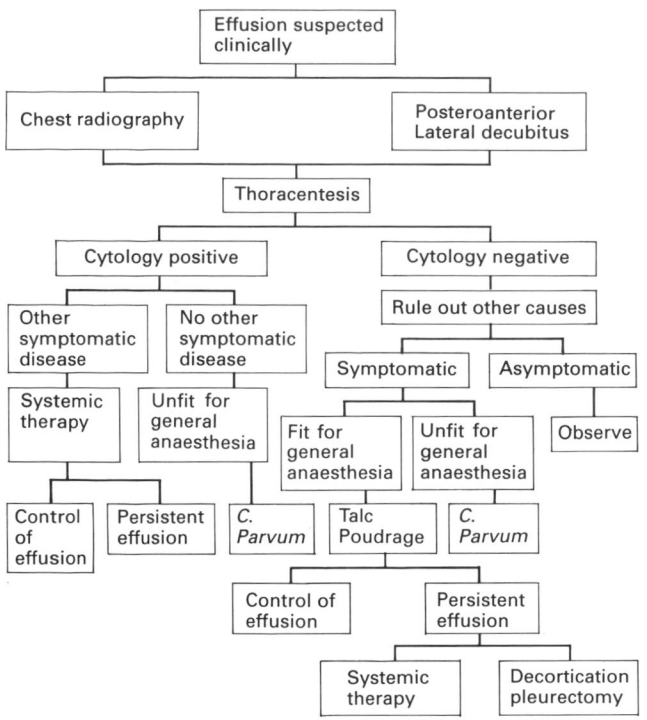

Fig. 2 Scheme of management for patients with cancer and pleural effusions.

Post-operatively the drain remains *in situ* for 5 days, with applied negative pressure and physiotherapy if there is a persistent pneumothorax. Premature drain removal may lead to further fluid accumulation so that the parietal and visceral pleural surfaces become separated. Retention of intercostal drains beyond 5 days leads to an increased risk of empyema.

Talc pleurodesis has an undeserved reputation for producing severe post-operative pain. Opiate analgesics may be required for 24 h post-operatively and, occasionally, prior to physiotherapy. Thereafter only moderate analgesics are required. Now that talc poudrage is becoming accepted as first-line therapy, it is important that better prognostic indices are developed in order that effective local treatment is given to those who will benefit and that simple palliation (thoracentesis) is used for patients in a terminal state.

PERICARDIAL EFFUSIONS

Aetiology

Excess fluid within the pericardial space of patients with cancer may arise either as a result of altered capillary permeability associated with visceral or parietal tumour nodules or, alternatively, from lymphatic obstruction due to infiltration of mediastinal lymphatics (Miller 1970). Additionally, the effusion may be non-neoplastic in origin from causes such as trauma, infection, or connective tissue disease. Finally, pericardial effusions may follow radiotherapy or be mimicked by the pericardial fibrosis resulting from such treatment.

In a series from the Sidney Farber Institute approximately 60 per cent of patients had malignant infiltration of the pericardium, 32 per cent had idiopathic pericarditis, and 10 per cent had radiation-induced effusions (Posner *et al.* 1981).

Presenting features

Some pericardial effusions are asymptomatic and are detected as a result of routine chest radiographs or echocardiogram. In other patients the effusion produces cardiac tamponade and presents as an acute medical emergency.

The commonest symptom in patients with pericardial effusions is dyspnoea on exertion, at night, or in the form of orthopnoea. A cough may be associated and chest pain may be present. In a large series of 66 cases, dyspnoea was present in 97 per cent, cough in 26 per cent, orthopnoea in 21 per cent, and chest pain in 18 per cent (Reitknecht *et al.* 1985).

The most frequent clinical signs are pulsus paradoxus (50 per cent), jugular venous distension (42 per cent), peripheral oedema (36 per cent), and hypotension (33 per cent). Heart sounds may be distant and a pericardial rub and hepatomegaly are present in up to one-quarter of cases. More rarely there may be splenomegaly, pleural effusions, a gallop rhythm, or rales. Patients with idiopathic effusions are more likely to be pyrexial and to have an associated pericardial friction rub (Posner *et al.* 1981). The key to diagnosis is a high index of suspicion in patients with malignancy whose condition suddenly deteriorates with shortness of breath and chest pain.

Investigations

A plain chest radiograph will show evidence of cardiomegaly, possibly with associated bilateral effusions. The simplest test to confirm that fluid is present is an echocardiogram, which if positive will show a pericardial echo distinct from the posterior cardiac border. More complex techniques include simultaneous cardiac and lung isotopic scans or a CT scan of the chest. Electrocardiographic changes are usually non-specific, showing low voltage activity and occasional T-wave abnormalities and alterations in the ST segment (Cham *et al.* 1975).

Pericardiocentesis

Confirmation of the presence of an effusion is by pericardial aspiration, which may be both diagnostic and therapeutic. The standard approach to the pericardium is subxiphoid. A 14 gauge needle is used and inserted midway between the xiphoid process and the left costal margin (Flannery *et al.* 1975). It is angled at 45° to the chest wall and aimed in the direction of the right sternoclavicular joint. Once the pericardial space has been entered, fluid is withdrawn, after which a fine catheter (5F) can be inserted in order to drain the cavity and, if necessary, to serve as a conduit for instillation of sclerosants. During the procedure, continuous ECG monitoring is used to give warning of the needle abutting

Table 7 Results of pericardiocentesis (with or without drainage) for malignant pericardial effusion

Reference	Method	Success rate
Flannery *et al.* (1975)	Tap	2/2
	Catheter drainage	4/4
Reynolds and Byrne (1977)	Tap	3/3
Posner *et al.* (1981)	Catheter drainage	4/9
Woll *et al.* (1987)	Tap	18/22
Buck *et al.* (1987)	Tap	1/4
		32/41 (78%)

Table 8 Results of intracavitary agents for control of malignant pericardial effusions

Reference	Agent	Success rate
Weisberger et al. (1955)	Mustine	3/3
Suhrland and Weisberger (1965)	Fluorouracil	3/3
Smith et al. (1974)	Mustine	0/1
	Thiotepa	2/4
	Quinacrine	2/2
Davies et al. (1984)	Tetracycline	30/32
		40/43

Table 9 Pericardial window formation and control of malignant pericardial effusions

Reference	Success rate
Hawkins et al. (1980)	17/17
Appelqvist et al. (1982)	3/3
Bitran et al. (1984)	4/4
Piehler et al. (1985)	13/16
Osuch et al. (1985)	12/12
Woll et al. (1987)	2/2
Buck et al. (1987)	10/10
	61/64 (95%)

against the ventricle and to avoid myocardial puncture with risk of ventricular fibrillation or haemorrhage.

Treatment

Pericardial aspirations may serve as definitive therapy for some patients. Series reporting results of aspiration alone, with or without catheter drainage, are summarized in Table 7. Overall, this relatively simple procedure achieved control of the effusion and prevented recurrence in 78 per cent of cases.

Because of the success of intrapleural agents in producing pleurodesis and thereby preventing recurrent pleural effusions, similar procedures have been used in patients with pericardial effusion. The results with a variety of agents are summarized in Table 8.

With the exception of the study by Davies et al. (1984), which indicated control of effusions by intracavitary tetracycline in 30 out of 32 cases (94 per cent), all the other reports comprised small numbers of cases. Overall control of the pericardial effusion was achieved in 93 per cent. Thus, there is, at best, only a small gain from intracavitary instillation of sclerosants in patients with malignant pericardial effusions and no evidence that there is subsequent difficulty in controlling effusions which do not respond to drainage alone.

Formation of pericardial window

This procedure may be performed as an emergency, if necessary under local anaesthesia, to achieve relief of tamponade and prevent recurrence of the pericardial effusion. Usually the surgical approach is subxiphoid, but a thoracic approach may be used in patients in whom pulmonary resection is contemplated. The xiphoid process is resected and the pericardium displayed after splitting the sternal attachment of the diaphragm. After insertion of stay sutures a 2 cm diameter pericardial window is made and one of the drains inserted into the pericardial cavity. These remain *in situ* until drainage of fluid has ceased, usually after 4–7 days.

Almost universally good results have been reported, as shown in Table 9. An overall control rate of 95 per cent was achieved. For those few patients in whom recurrent fluid develops or when pericardial fibrosis produces tamponade, a pericardectomy may be necessary, but this will be a rare event. Park et al. (1991) compared the results of pericardial window versus pericardiectomy and found similar survival rates, but significantly less post-operative morbidity in those treated by window formation.

Treatment scheme

Figure 3 is a suggested algorithm for the management of patients with malignant pericardial effusions. Unless the patient has non-life-threatening disease and has lymphoma where systemic therapy would be first-line treatment, a local approach should be used.

Among patients in whom effusion control cannot be achieved after two attempts at drainage, surgical formation of a pericardial window should be considered since this will almost invariably lead to control of symptoms and prevention of recurrence of pericardial fluid.

PERITONEAL EFFUSIONS

Aetiology

Malignant ascites commonly results from the presence of peritoneal metastatic nodules which both increase the production and inhibit the absorption of peritoneal fluid. This particularly follows ovarian carcinoma where it is the presenting feature of the disease in one-third of cases and occurs during the course of the disease in two-thirds (Lifshitz 1982). Alternatively, it may arise in the terminal stages of liver metastases from almost any primary source. The different causes have important prognostic implications: patients with breast cancer who have malignant ascites associated with hepatomegaly or jaundice may carry a poor prognosis (Fentiman et al. 1983a). Of such cases, 90 per cent were dead within 3 months of developing ascites.

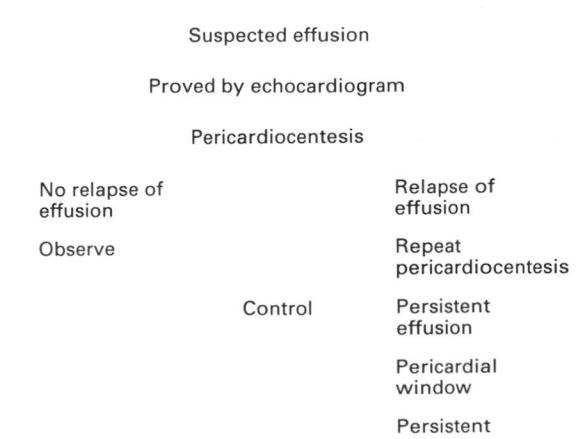

Fig. 3 Management scheme for patients with malignant pericardial effusions.

Diagnosis

The usual presenting symptom is abdominal swelling which is uncomfortable and may be associated with an unpleasant feeling of fullness and consequent diminution of appetite. Patients may also complain of weight gain, despite eating very little. Clinically the abdomen is tensely distended with a dull percussion note which may become tympanic in the flank on shifting the patient from a supine to a lateral position. The diagnosis may be backed up by an ultrasound and can be confirmed by needle aspiration. In a patient who has not relapsed previously and who has no other evidence of metastatic disease, proof that the ascites is malignant in origin may be more difficult. Cytological confirmation of the presence of malignant cells is possible in approximately 50 per cent of cases, but it can sometimes be difficult to distinguish between atypical mesothelium and malignant cells. As with pleural effusions, high levels of carcinoembryonic antigen may suggest a malignant aetiology. In a few patients, CT may show the presence of peritoneal metastases.

Treatment

First-line therapy in malignant ascites is medical, with surgical intervention being reserved for refractory cases. For those patients with other sites of metastatic disease, systemic cytotoxic or endocrine therapy will be required as this may in itself produce regression of ascites. If this does not achieve control or in patients with isolated ascites, diuretic therapy should be instituted to palliate the problem.

Unless the patient is severely distressed by massive ascites, aspiration of large volumes should be avoided since there will be rapid refilling and large losses of protein will occur.

Diuretic therapy

Just as with ascites of non-malignant origin, so it is possible in some cases to achieve control of malignant ascites with the appropriate use of diuretics. Seventeen patients with malignant ascites resulting from a variety of primaries were treated with spironolactone at an initial dosage of 150 mg daily, in divided doses, increasing by 50 mg if the weight loss was less than 0.5 kg daily (Greenway et al. 1982). Of these cases, two died within a week and control of the effusion was achieved in 13 out of 15 (87 per cent) of the others. Plasma renin levels were elevated in all cases in which this was measured and aldosterone levels were elevated in 60 per cent of these. In another study of patients with malignant ascites, frusemide was used at a dosage of 100 mg/24 h and control was achieved in four out of four cases (100 per cent) (Amiel et al. 1984).

Instillation of intraperitoneal agents

Because of the success of intracavitary isotopes, cytotoxics, sclerosants, and biological agents in controlling pleural effusions, they have been similarly employed in attempts to control malignant ascites. Bonte (1956) used ^{198}Au and achieved control in 22 out of 38 (58 per cent) of cases. In a series of 50 patients intracavitary thiotepa achieved control in 16 (32 per cent) (Andersen and Brincker 1968). A similar control rate of 35 per cent was reported for fluorouracil (Suhrland and Weisberger 1965), whereas intracavitary mustine achieved control in 75 per cent of cases (Weisberger et al. 1955).

Results of uncontrolled studies of intraperitoneal bleomycin are given in Table 10. Overall control occurred in 49 per cent of cases. Better results have been reported for intracavitary quinacrine as

Table 10 Intracavitary bleomycin in the control of malignant ascites

Reference	Success rate
Paladine et al. (1976)	4/11 (36%)
Bitran et al. (1984)	3/5 (60%)
Ostrowski (1982)	22/47 (47%)
Ostrowski (1986)	10/16 (63%)
	39/79 (49%)

Table 11 Intracavitary quinacrine in the control of malignant ascites

Reference	Success rate
Gellhorn et al. (1961)	3/10 (30%)
Ultmann et al. (1963)	9/12 (75%)
Rochlin (1964)	28/38 (74%)
Dollinger et al. (1967)	4/5 (80%)
	44/65 (68%)

Table 12 Uncontrolled studies of intracavitary biological agents for the control of malignant ascites

Reference	Agent	Rate of control
Webb et al. (1978)	C. parvum	4/5 (80%)
Currie et al. (1983)	C. parvum	7/11 (64%)
Torisu et al. (1983)	OK-432	76/134 (57%)

shown in Table 11, where an overall rate of control of 68 per cent was achieved.

Studies of biological agents used for malignant ascites are summarized in Table 12. Using C. parvum, control of ascites occurred in 80 per cent of cases (Webb et al. 1978). In a slightly larger series ascites was controlled in only 64 per cent of cases (Currie et al. 1983).

Intraperitoneal OK-432, an extract from Streptococcus pyogenes, was given to 134 Japanese patients with malignant ascites. The effusion disappeared in 76 (57 per cent) and was reduced in volume in a further eight (6 per cent) (Torisu et al. 1983). Recent work suggests that OK-432 attracts natural killer cells into the peritoneal cavity via a neutrophil-derived lymphocyte chemotactic factor (Hayashi and Torisu 1990).

Only one prospective randomized trial has evaluated the role of intracavitary agents in the control of ascites (Kefford et al. 1980). Three agents were compared—adriamycin, mustine, and tetracycline—and 15 patients were treated. A complete response was achieved in two out of four given adriamycin and in none of those given either mustine or tetracycline. A partial response to therapy was seen in two out of four receiving adriamycin, two out of eight given tetracyline, and none of those given tetracycline. Thus, none of the studies of intracavitary agents provide unequivocal proof that they are better than diuretics in achieving control of ascites.

Peritoneovenous shunts

These devices offer a mechanical approach to the long-term control of ascites without the protein loss associated with repeated paracenteses. They comprise a distal perforated cathether which is placed in the peritoneal cavity, a valve chamber, with or without

Table 13 Results of peritoneovenous shunts for malignant ascites

Reference	Success rate	
	LeVeen shunt	Denver shunt
Kudsk *et al.* (1978)	6/8 (75%)	
Straus *et al.* (1979)	27/35 (77%)	
Oosterlee (1980)	5/13 (38%)	7/8 (88%)
Lokich *et al.* (1980)	6/8 (75%)	
Vo *et al.* (1981)	4/7 (57%)	
Holman and Albo (1981)		5/6 (83%)
Gough (1982)	9/11 (82%)	
Souter *et al.* (1985)	5/16 (31%)	14/27 (52%)
	62/98 (63%)	26/41 (63%)

Table 14 Complications of peritoneovenous shunting for malignant ascites

Total cases	86	
Wound complications		
Leakage	1	(1%)
Pump failure		
Early thrombosis	8	(9%)
Late thrombosis	10	(12%)
Mechanical problems		
Axillary vein thrombosis	1	(1%)
Biological/functional		
Pyrexia	25	(29%)
Septicaemia	2	(2%)
DIC	6	(7%)
Renal failure	2	(2%)
Fluid overload	1	(1%)
Pulmonary embolism	1	(1%)
Pulmonary oedema	1	(1%)
Metastasis	2/18	(11%)
Long-term function	28	(33%)

DIC, disseminated intravascular coagulopathy.
Adapted from Vo *et al.* (1981).

a valve located subcutaneously just above the costal margin, and a proximal catheter which is tunnelled subcutaneously and placed via the external or internal jugular vein with its tip in the superior vena cava.

Originally, a Holster shunt was implanted to treat patients with both peritoneal and pleural effusions (Pollock 1978). Subsequently, LeVeen and Denver shunts have been employed and the results of series reporting their use are given in Table 13. Overall control was achieved in 63 per cent of patients treated with LeVeen shunts and in 63 per cent of those given Denver devices. The latter shunt carries the theoretical advantage of a compressible chamber associated with the valve which enables external compression to increase flow through the catheter and reduce blockage resulting from stasis of ascitic fluid. Despite similar rates of control the Denver shunt is being used more frequently. It has been reported that peritoneovenous shunts function for longer periods in patients with negative effusion cytology (Chueng and Raaf 1982). The median shunt survival time was 140 days in cases with cytologically negative effusion compared with only 26 days for those with positive effusion.

No randomized trials have compared shunts with diuretic therapy for patients with malignant effusions. However, a similar study was conducted in patients with massive ascites secondary to cirrhosis

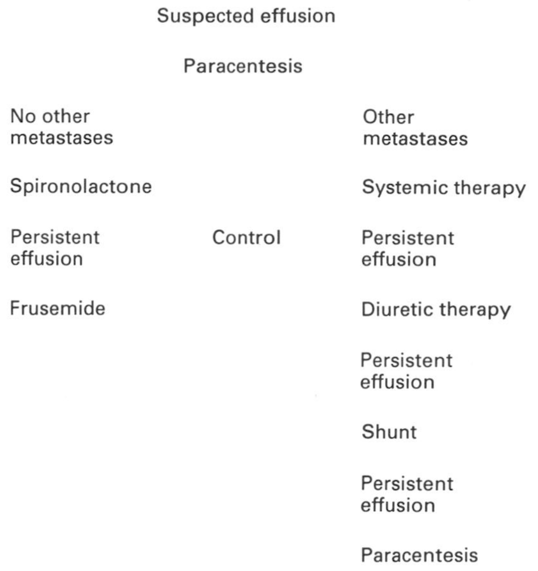

Fig. 4 Treatment plan for patients with malignant ascites.

(Wapnick *et al.* 1979). Seventeen matched pairs were treated by either medical or surgical therapy; the drug regime comprised a low salt diet followed by gradually escalating doses of spironolactone, subsequently supplemented in refractory cases with chorodiazide and frusemide. The group treated surgically had a LeVeen shunt inserted. In 12 out of 14 assessable pairs the surgical group achieved better control of ascites, had a shorter stay in hospital and survived for a longer period.

Despite the benefits of shunts, several problems can be associated with their use. The complications have been assigned to five categories: wound problems, mechanical pump problems, biological/functional metastasis, and long-term failure (Vo *et al.* 1981). These have been reviewed by Vo *et al.* (1981) and are summarized in Table 14. The commonest problem was pyrexia, followed by shunt failure in the medium term, that is, between 1 and 3 months after implantation. Disseminated intravascular coagulopathy due to probable activation of factor X in ascitic fluid is less common in patients with ascites of malignant origin than in those with cirrhosis.

Because malignant asacites is usually an end-stage of malignancy, intravenous perfusion of tumour containing ascitic fluid has not been found significantly to affect prognosis although shunt-related metastases have been reported.

Many of the problems associated with shunt placement are technical and relate to surgical technique so that problems diminish with increasing experience. Perioperative monitoring of the location of the shunt catheter tip can help to ensure that it is located in the superior vena cava and has not become unintentionally situated in the axillary vein.

Management scheme

Figure 4 is a suggested scheme for the management of patients with suspected malignant ascites. Unless cytotoxics are indicated for other symptomatic metastases, diuretic therapy should be given as first-line treatment. Only for the few patients with refractory ascites in whom it is anticipated that survival will be more than 3 months should a shunt be inserted. Many patients with malignant ascites are pre-terminal and require simple palliative procedures rather than aggressive therapy.

REFERENCES

Amiel SA, Blackburn AM, Rubens RD (1984). Intravenous infusion of frusemide as treatment for ascites in malignant disease. *British Medical Journal*, 288:1041.

Andersen AP, Brincker H (1968). Intracavitary thiotepa in malignant pleural and peritoneal effusions. *Acta Radiologica, Therapy, Physics, Biiology*, 7:369–78.

Anderson CB, Philpott GW, Ferguson TB (1974). The treatment of malignant pleural effusions. *Cancer*, 33:916–22.

Appleqvist P, Maamies T, Grohu P (1982). Emergency pericardiotomy as primary diagnostic and therapeutic procedure in malignant pericardial tamponade: report of three cases and a review of the literature. *Journal of Surgical Oncology*, 21:18–22.

Austgen M, *et al.* (1984). Palliative therapy of tumour-induced pleural effusion with ^{90}yttrium silicone. *European Journal of Respiratory Diseases*, 65:64–7.

Bateman JC, Moulton B, Larsen NJ (1955). Control of neoplastic effusion by phosphoramide chemotherapy. *Archives of Internal Medicine*, 95:713–19.

Baumgartner WA (1980). The use of thorascopy in the diagnosis of pleural disease. *Archives of Surgery*, 115:421.

Bayly TC, *et al.* (1978). Tetracycline and quinacrine in the control of malignant pleural effusions. A randomised trial. *Cancer*, 41:1188–92.

Bethune N (1935). Pleural poudrage. *Journal of Thoracic Surgery*, 4:251–61.

Bitran JD, Evans R, Brown C (1984). The management of cardiac tamponade in patients with breast cancer. *Journal of Surgical Oncology*, 27:42–4.

Black LF (1972). The pleural space and pleural fluid. *Mayo Clinic Proceedings*, 47:493–506.

Bloomberg AE (1970). Thoracoscopy in diagnosis of pleural effusions. *New York State Journal of Medicine*, 70:1974–7.

Bonte FJ, Storassli JP, Weisberger AS (1956). Comparative evaluation of radioactive gold and nitrogen mustard in the treatment of serous effusions of neoplastic origins. *Radiology*, 67:63–6.

Borda I, Krant M (1967). Convulsions following intrapleural administration of quinacrine hydrochloride. *Journal of the American Medical Association*, 201:173–4.

Boutin C, Cargnino P, Viallat JR (1980). Thoracoscopy in the early diagnosis of malignant pleural effusions. *Endoscopy*, 12:155–60.

Broghamer WL, Richardson ME, Faurest SE (1984). Malignancy-associated serosanguinous pleural effusions. *Acta Cytologica*, 28:46–50.

Buck M, *et al.* (1987). Pericardial effusion in women with breast cancer. *Cancer*, 60:263–9.

Burtin P, *et al.* (1978). Carcinoembryonic antigen. *Scandinavian Journal of Immunology*, (Suppl. 8):27–30.

Card RY, Cole DR, Henschke UK (1960). Summary of ten years of the use of radioactive colloids in intracavitary therapy. *Journal of Nuclear Medicine*, 1:195–8.

Casali A, *et al.* (1988). Treatment of malignant pleural effusion with intracavitary corynebacterium parvum. *Cancer*, 62:806–11.

Cham WC, *et al.* (1975). Radiation therapy of cardiac and pericardial metastases. *Radiology*, 114:701–4.

Chambers JS (1958). Palliative treatment of neoplastic pleural effusion with intercostal intubation and talc instillation. *Western Journal of Surgery, Obstetrics and Gynecology*, 66:26–8.

Cheung DK, Raaf JH (1982). Selection of patients with malignant ascites for a peritoneovenous shunt. *Cancer*, 50:1204–9.

Cimochoswki GE, *et al.* (1986). Pleuroperitoneal shunting for recalcitrant pleural effusions. *Journal of Thoracic and Cardiovascular Surgery*, 92:866–70.

Currie JL, *et al.* (1983). Intracavitary corynebacterium parvum for treatment of malignant effusions. *Gynecologic Oncology*, 16:14.

Davies S, Rambotti P, Grifnani F (1984). Intra-pericardial tetracycline sclerosis in the treatment of malignant pericardial effusion: an analysis of thirty-three cases. *Journal of Clinical Oncology*, 2:631–4.

DeCamp PT, Moseley PW, Scott ML, Haton HB (1973). Diagnostic thoracoscopy. *Annals of Thoracic Surgery*, 16:79–84.

Dewald G, Dines DE, Weiland LH, Gordon H (1976). Usefulness of chromosome examination in the diagnosis of malignant pleural effusions. *New England Journal of Medicine*, 295:1494–1500.

Dollinger MR, Krakoff IH, Karnofsky DA (1967). Quinacrine (Atabrine) in the treatment of neoplastic effusions. *Annals of Internal Medicine*, 66:249–57.

Dorsey JS, Cogordan JA (1984). Pleuroperitoneal shunt for intractable pleural effusion. *Canadian Journal of Surgery*, 27:598–9.

Felletti R, Ravazzoni C. (1983). Intrapleural corynebacterium parvum for malignant pleural effusions. *Thorax*, 38:22–4.

Fentiman IS (1987). Diagnosis and treatment of malignant pleural effusions. *Cancer Treatment Review*, 14:107–18.

Fentiman IS, Millis RR, Sexton S, Hayward JL (1981). Pleural effusion in breast cancer: a review of 105 cases. *Cancer*, 47:2087–92.

Fentiman IS, Rubens RD, Hayward JL (1982). The pattern of metastatic disease in patients with pleural effusions secondary to breast cancer. *British Journal of Surgery*, 69:193–4.

Fentiman IS, Rubens RD, Hayward JL (1983a). Ascites in breast cancer. *British Medical Journal*, 287:1023.

Fentiman IS, Rubens RD, Hayward JL (1983b). Control of pleural effusions in patients with breast cancer. A randomised trial. *Cancer*, 52:737–9.

Fentiman IS, Rubens RD, Hayward JL (1986). A comparison of intracavitary talc and tetracycline for the control of pleural effusions secondary to breast cancer. *European Journal of Cancer and Clinical Oncology*, 22:1079–81.

Flannery EP, Gregoratos G, Corder MP (1975). Pericardial effusions in patients with malignant disease. *Archives of Internal Medicine*, 135:976–7.

Fracchia AA, *et al.* (1970). Intrapleural chemotherapy for effusion from metastatic breast carcinoma. *Cancer*, 26:626–9.

Frist B, Kahan AV, Koss LG (1979). Comparison of the diagnostic values of biopsies of the pleura and cytologic evaluation of pleural fluids. *American Journal of Clinical Pathology*, 72:418–51.

Gellhorn A, *et al.* (1961). The use of Atabrine (quinacrine) in the control of recurrent neoplastic effusions. *Diseases of the Chest*, 39:165–76.

Gough IR (1982). Peritoneo-venous shunts for malignant ascites. *Australian and New Zealand Journal of Medicine*, 52:47–9.

Graham GG, McDonald JR, Clagett OT, Schmidt HW (1953). Examination of pleural fluid for carcinoma cells. *Journal of Thoracic Surgery*, 25:366–70.

Gravelyn TR, *et al.* (1987). Tetracycline pleurodesis for malignant pleural effusions. *Cancer*, 59:1973–7.

Greenway B, Johnson PJ, Williams R (1982). Control of malignant ascites with spironolactone. *British Journal of Surgery*, 69:441–2.

Hagiwara A, *et al.* (1987). Chemotherapy for carcinomatous peritonitis and pleuritis with MMC-CH, mitomycin C adsorbed on actuated carcon particles. *Cancer*, 59:245–51.

Hahn PF, Carothers EL (1950). Use of radioactive metallic gold in treatment of malignancies. *Nucleonics*, 6:54–62.

Hamed H, Fentiman IS, Chaudary MA, Rubens RD (1989). A trial comparing intracavitary bleomycin and talc for control of pleural effusions secondary to carcinoma of the breast. *British Journal of Surgery*, 76:1266–7.

Harley HRS (1979). Malignant pleural effusions and their treatment by intercostal talc pleurodesis. *British Journal of Diseases of the Chest*, 73:173–7.

Haupt GJ, *et al.* (1960). Treatment of malignant pleural effusions by talc poudrage. *Journal of the American Medical Association*, 172:918–21.

Hawkins JR, *et al.* (1980). Pericardial window for malignant pericardial effusion. *Annals of Thoracic Surgery*, 30:465–71.

Hayashi Y, Torisu M (1990). New approaches to management of malignant ascites with streptococcol preparation OK-432. III. OK-432 attracts natural killer cells through a chemotactic factor released from actuated neutrophils. *Surgery*, 107:74–84.

Health and Public Policy Committee. American College of Physicians (1985). Diagnostic thoracentesis and pleural biopsy in pleural effusion. *Annals of Internal Medicine*, 103:799–802.

Hillerdal G, *et al.* (1986). *Corynebacterium parvum* in malignant pleural effusion. A randomised prospective study. *European Journal of Respiratory Diseases*, 69:204–6.

Hirsch A, *et al.* (1979). Pleural effusion: laboratory tests in 300 cases. *Thorax*, 34:106–12.

Holman JM, Albo D (1981). Peritoneovenous shunts in patients with malignant ascites. *American Journal of Surgery*, 142:774–6.

Hostmark J, Viganander T, Skaarland E (1985). Characterisation of pleural effusions by flow-cytometric DNA analysis. *European Journal of Respiratory Diseases*, 66:315–19.

Izbicki R, Weyhing BT, Baker C (1975). Pleural effusion in cancer patients. A prospective randomised study of pleural drainage with the addition of radioactive phosphorus to the pleural space versus pleural drainage alone. *Cancer*, **36**:1511–18.

Jacobs ML (1958). Radioactive colloidal chronic phosphate to control pleural effusion and ascites. *Journal of the American Medical Association*, **166**:597–9.

Jereb B, *et al.* (1987). Intrapleural application of human leukocyte interferon (HLI) in breast cancer patients with ipsilateral pleural carcinomatosis. *Journal of Interferon Research*, **7**:357–63.

Johnston WW (1985). The malignant pleural effusion. A review of cytopathologic diagnosis of 584 effusions from 472 consecutive patients. *Cancer*, **58**:905–9.

Jones GR (1969). Treatment of recurrent malignant pleural effusion by iodized talc pleurodesis. *Thorax*, **24**:69–72.

Kefford RF, *et al.* (1980). Intracavitary adriamycin nitrogen mustard and tetracycline in the control of malignant effusions. *Medical Journal of Australia*, **2**:447–8.

Kent EM, Moses C (1951). Radioactive isotopes in the palliative management of carcinomatosis of the pleura. *Journal of Thoracic Surgery*, **22**:503–16.

Kinsey DL, Carter D, Klassen KP (1964). Simplified management of malignant pleural effusion. *Archives of Surgery*, **89**:389–92.

Klockars M, *et al.* (1980). Carcinoembryonic antigen in pleural effusions: a diagnostic and prognostic indicator. *European Journal of Cancer*, **16**:1149–52.

Kramer MR, Saldand MJ, Cepero RJ, Pitchenik AE (1989). High amylase levels in neoplasm-related pleural effusion. *Annals of Internal Medicine*, **110**:567–8.

Kudsk KA, *et al.* (1978). LeVeen shunts. *Lancet*, i:881.

Leahy BC, *et al.* (1985). Treatment of malignant pleural effusions with intrapleural *Corynebacterium parvum* or tetracycline. *European Journal of Respiratory Diseases*, **66**:50–4.

Lees AW, Hoy W (1979). Management of pleural effusions in breast cancer. *Chest*, **75**:51–3.

Lewis RJ, Kunderman PJ, Sister GF, Mackenzie JW (1976). Direct diagnostic thoracoscopy. *Annals of Thoracic Surgery*, **21**:536–9.

Lifshitz S (1982). Ascites, pathophysiology and control measures. *International Journal of Radiation—Oncology—Biology—Physics*, **8**:1423–6.

Little AG, *et al.* (1988). Pleuroperitoneal shunting. Alternative therapy for pleural effusions. *Annals of Surgery*, **208**:443–50.

Lloyd MS (1953). Thoracoscopy and biopsy in the diagnosis of pleurisy with effusion. *Quarterly Bulletin of Seaview Hospital*, **14**:128–33.

Lokich J, *et al.* (1980). Complications of peritoneovenous shunt for malignant ascites. *Treatment Reports*, **64**:305–9.

McLeod DT, *et al.* (1985). Further experience of *Corynebacterium parvum* in malignant pleural effusion. *Thorax*, **40**:515–18.

Madrid A, *et al.* (1983). Derrame pleural en pacientes con cancer. Revision de 118 cases. *Medica Chinica (Barcelona)*, **80**:823–5.

Markman M, *et al.* (1985). Cisplatin and cytarabine administered intrapleurally as treatment of malignant pleural effusions. *Medical and Pediatric Oncology*, **13**:191–3.

Martensson G, Petterson K, Thringer G (1985). Differentiation between malignant and non-malignant pleural effusion. *European Journal of Respiratory Diseases*, **67**:326–34.

Martinez-Vea A, *et al.* (1982). Diagnostic value of tumoral markers in serious effusions. *Cancer*, **50**:1783–8.

Martini N, Bains MS, Beattie EJ (1975). Indications for pleurectomy in malignant effusions. *Cancer*, **35**:734–8.

Mejer J, Mortensen KM, Hansen HH (1977). Mepacrine hydrochloride in the treatment of malignant pleural effusion. A controlled randomised trial. *Scandinavian Journal of Respiratory Diseases*, **58**:319–23.

Mezger J, *et al.* (1988). Tumour associated antigens in diagnosis of serous effusions. *Journal of Clinical Pathology*, **41**:633–43.

Millar JW, Hunter AM, Horne NW (1979). Intrapleural immunotherapy with *Corynebacterium parvum* in recurrent malignant pleural effusions. *Thorax*, **35**:856–8.

Miller AJ (1970). Some observations concerning pericardial effusions and their relationship to the venous and lymphatic circulation of the heart. *Lymphology*, **2**:76–8.

Niwa Y, Kishimoto H, Shimokata K (1985). Carcinomatous and tuberculous pleural effusions. *Chest*, **87**:351–5.

Oosterlee J (1980). Peritoneovenous shunting for ascites in cancer patients. *British Journal of Surgery*, **67**:663–6.

Ostrowski MJ (1986). An assessment, or long-term results, of controlling the reaccumulation of malignant effusions using intracavitary bleomycin. *Cancer*, **57**:721–7.

Ostrowski MJ, Halsall GM (1982). Intracavitary bleomycin in the management of malignant effusions: a multicenter study. *Cancer Treatment Reports*, **66**:1903–7.

Ostrowski MJ, *et al.* (1989). A randomised trial of intracavitary bleomycin and *Corynebacterium parvum* in the control of malignant pleural effusions. *Radiation Oncolog,y* **14**:19–26.

Osuch JR, Khandekar JD, Fry WA (1985). Emergency subxiphoid pericardial decompression for malignant pericardial effusion. *Annals of Surgery*, **51**:298–300.

Paladine W, *et al.* (1976). Intracavitary bleomycin in the management of malignant effusions. *Cancer*, **38**:1903–8.

Park JS, Rentschler R, Wilbury D (1991). Surgical management of pericardial effusions in patients with malignancies. *Cancer*, **67**:76–80.

Pearson FG, MacGregor DC (1966). Talc poudrage for malignant pleural effusion. *Journal of Thoracic and Cardiovascular Surgery*, **51**:732–8.

Pectasides D, *et al.* (1986). Antibody-guided irradiation of malignant pleural and pericardial effusion. *British Journal of Cancer*, **53**:727–32.

Pettersson T, Froseth B, Riska H, Klockars M (1988). Concentration of hyaluronic acid in pleural fluid as a diagnostic aid for malignant mesothelioma. *Chest*, **94**:1037–9.

Piehler JM, *et al.* (1985). Surgical management of effusive pericardial disease. *Journal of Thoracic and Cardiovascular Surgery*, **90**:506–16.

Pierucci G, Lucivero G, Amoruso C, Bonomo C (1984). Diagnostic value of carcinoembryonic antigen (CEA) assay in pleural effusions. *Tumori*, **70**:421–5.

Pimm MV, Hopper DG, Baldwin RW (1976). BCG treatment of malignant pleural effusions in the rat. *British Journal of Cancer*, **34**:368–73.

Poe RH, *et al.* (1984). Sensitivity, specificity, and predictive values of closed pleural biopsy. *Archives of Internal Medicine*, **144**:325–9.

Pollock AV (1978). The treatment of resistant malignant ascites by insertion of a peritoneo-atrial Hotter valve. *British Journal of Surgery*, **62**:104–7.

Posner MR, Cohen GI, Skarin AT (1981). Pericardial disease in patients with cancer. *American Journal of Medicine*, **71**:407–13.

Prakash UBS, Reiman HM (1985). Comparison of needle biopsy with cytologic analysis for the evaluation of pleural effusion: analysis of 414 cases. *Mayo Clinic Proceedings*, **60**:158–64.

Raja OG, Lalor AJ (1980). Modification to the technique of percutaneous pleural biopsy using Abram's needle. *British Journal of Diseases of the Chest*, **74**:285–6.

Reitknecht F, *et al.* (1985). Management of cardiac tamponade in patients with malignancy. *Journal of Surgical Oncology*, **30**:19–22.

Reynolds PM, Byrne MJ (1977). The treatment of malignant pericardial effusion in carcinoma of the breast. *Australian and New Zealand Journal of Medicine*, **7**:169–71.

Richman SP, *et al.* (1981). Administration of BCG cell wall skeleton into malignant effusions: toxic and therapeutic effects. *Cancer Treatment Reviews*, **65**:383–7.

Rimoldi R, *et al.* (1984). Thymostimulin in malignant pleural effusions. *International Journal of Tissue Reactions*, **6**:53–5.

Rioseco A (1980). More about NaOH in the management of malignant pleural effusions. *Chest*, **77**:813.

Rodriguez-Panadero F, Mejias JL (1989). Low glucose and pH levels in malignant pleural effusions. *American Review of Respiratory Disease*, **139**:663–7.

Rochlin DB, Smart CR, Wagner DE, Silva ARM (1964). The control of recurrent malignant effusions using quinacrine hydrochloride. *Surgical and Gynecological Obstetrics*, **118**:991–4.

Rossi GA, Felletti R, Balbi B (1987). Symptomatic treatment of recurrent malignant pleural effusion with intrapleurally administered *Corynebacaterium parvum*. *American Review of Respiratory Disease*, **135**:885–90.

Rosso R, *et al.* (1988). Intrapleural natural beta interferon in the treatment of malignant pleural effusions. *Oncology*, **45**:253–6.

Rubinson RM, Bolooki H (1972). Intrapleural tetracycline for control of malignant pleural effusion: a preliminary report. *Southern Medical Journal*, **65**:847–9.

Sahn SA, Good JT (1988). Pleural fluid pH in malignant effusions. Diagnostic, prognostic and therapeutic implications. *Annals of Internal Medicine*, **108**:345–9.

Salyer WR, Eggleston JC, Erozan YS (1975). Efficacy of pleural needle biopsy and pleural fluid cytopathology in the diagnosis of malignant neoplasm involving the pleura. *Chest*, **67**:536–9.

Samuels ML, Old JW, Howe CD (1958). Needle biopsy of the pleura; an evaluation in patients with pleural effusion of neoplastic origin. *Cancer*, 11:980–3.

Scerbo J, Keltz H, Stone DJ (1971). A prospective study of closed pleural biopsies. *Journal of The American Medical Association*, 218:377–80.

Shedbalkar AR, *et al.* (1971). Evaluation of talc pleural symphysis in management of malignant pleural effusion. *Journal of Thoracic and Cardiovascular Surgery*, 61:492–7.

Singh G, Dekker A, Ladoulis CT (1978). Tissue culture of cells in serous effusions. Evaluation as an adjunct to cytology. *Acta Cytologica*, 22:487–9.

Smith FE, Lane M, Hudgins PT (1974). Conservative management of malignant pericardial effusion. *Cancer*, 33:47–57.

Sorensen PG, Svendsen TL, Erik B (1984). Treatment of malignant pleural effusion with drainage, with and without instillation of talc. *European Journal of Respiratory Diseases*, 65:131–5.

Souter RG, *et al.* (1985). Surgical and pathologic complications associated with peritoneovenous shunts in management of malignant ascites. *Cancer*, 55:1973–8.

Stiksa G, Korsgaard R, Simonsson BG (1979). Treatment of recurrent pleural effusion by pleurodesis with quinacrine. Comparison between instillation by repeated thoracentesis and by tube drainage. *Scandinavian Journal of Respiratory Diseases*, 60:197–205.

Straus AK, Roseman DL, Shapiro TM (1978). Peritoneo-venous shunting in the management of malignant ascites. *Archives of Surgery*, 114:489–91.

Strober SJ, *et al.* (1973). Malignant pleural disease. A radiotherapeutic approach to the problem. *Journal of the American Medical Association*, 226:296–9.

Suhrland LG, Weisberger AS (1965). Intracavitary 5-fluorouracil in malignant effusions. *Archives of Internal Medicine*, 116:431–3.

Tamura S, *et al.* (1988). Tumor markers in pleural effusion diagnosis. *Cancer*, 61:298–302.

Tattersall MHN, *et al.* (1979). Intracavitary doxorubicin in malignant effusions. *Lancet*, i:390.

Torisu M, *et al.* (1983). New approach to management of malignant ascites with a streptococcal preparation OK-432. 1. Improvement of host immunity and prolongation of survival. *Surgery*, 93:357–64.

Ultmann JE, *et al.* (1963). The effect of quinacrine on neoplastic effusions and certain of their enzymes. *Cancer*, 16:283–8.

Vo NM, *et al.* (1981). Complications of peritoneovenous shunting for malignant ascites. A collective review. *Connecticut Medicine*, 45:1–4.

Wallach HW (1978). Intrapleural therapy with tetracycline and lidocaine for malignant pleural effusions. *Chest*, 73:246.

Wapnick S, Grosberg SJ, Evans MI (1979). Randomised prospective matched pair study comparing peritoneovenous shunt and conventional therapy in massive ascites. *British Journal of Surgery*, 66:667–70.

Wardman AG, Bowen M, Struthers CPC, Cooke NJ (1984). The diagnosis of pleural effusions—are cancer markers clinically helpful. *Medical and Pediatric Oncology*, 12:68–72.

Webb HE, Oaten SW, Pike CP (1978). Treatment of malignant ascitic and pleural effusions with *Corynebacterium parvum*. *British Medical Journal*, 1:338–40.

Weisberg D (1981). Talc pleurodesis: a controversial issue. *Poumon et le Coeur*, 37:291–4.

Weisberger AS, Levine B, Storaasli JP (1955). Use of nitrogen mustard in treatment of serous effusions of neoplastic origin. *Journal of the American Medical Association*, 159:1704–7.

Winkelmann M, Pfitzer P (1984). Blind pleural biopsy in combination with cytology of pleural effusions. *Acta Cytologica*, 25:373.

Woll PJ, Knight RK, Rubens RD (1987). Pericardial effusion complicating breast cancer. *Journal of the Royal Society of Medicine*, 80:490–1.

Wu M-H, Hsive R-H, Tseng K-H (1989). Thoracoscopy in the diagnosis of pleural effusions. *Japanese Journal of Clinical Oncology*, 19:116–19.

Xaubet A, Diumenjo MC, Maria A, *et al.* (1985). Characteristics and prognostic value of pleural effusions in non-Hodgkin's lymphomas. *European Journal of Respiratory Diseases*, 66:135–40.

Yamada S, Takeda T, Matsumoto K (1983). Prognostic analysis of malignant pleural and peritoneal effusion. *Cancer*, 51:136–140.

Yew WW, Chan SL, Kwan SYL (1988). Comparison of efficacy of mitomycin-C and Corynebacterium parvum in the management of malignant pleural effusion. *Chinese Medical Journal*, 101:737–9.

Zaloznik AJ, Oswald SG, Langin M (1983). Intrapleural tetracycline in malignant pleural effusions. A randomized study. *Cancer*, 51:752–5.

19.6   Spinal metastatic disease

ALISTAIR JENKINS AND GORDON FINDLAY

INTRODUCTION

Metastasis to the spine is an important and frequent complication of cancer. At autopsy, between 20 and 30 per cent of cancer patients are found to have spinal involvement and approximately 5 per cent have invasion of the extradural space (Barron *et al.* 1959; Sundaresan *et al.* 1986). Precise data are unavailable, but it is likely that, at some point in their disease, 5–10 per cent of patients develop symptomatic neurological manifestations of metastasis, including cord compression, nerve root compression, intraparenchymal metastasis, and meningeal carcinomatosis (Constans *et al.* 1983). Pain, often with spinal instability, is even more common. Although in the overwhelming majority the underlying disease must have a hopeless prognosis, it is of great importance to recognize that there is much that can be done to improve the lot of these unfortunate patients. Early active treatment, sometimes of an aggressiveness not normally considered in metastatic cancer, can restore function or prevent deterioration while providing valuable pain relief.

However, the optimum management of patients with malignant spinal cord compression remains a matter of some debate. The traditional approach of laminectomy followed by radiotherapy has fallen into disrepute as a blanket treatment. Although data from large prospective controlled trials are not available, retrospective analysis suggests that steroids and radiotherapy produce equally good functional results without the morbidity and mortality attached to laminectomy. However, more recent studies suggest that overall results may be improved by preceding radiotherapy with a careful choice of surgical approach, for example posterior or radical anterior (transthoracic/transabdominal), in specific cases. In this chapter the clinical features, diagnostic work-up, and management of this group of patients is described and the problem of meningeal carcinomatosis is discussed.

EPIDEMIOLOGY

The incidence of spinal neurological complications of cancer is probably of the order of 5–10 per cent (Constans *et al.* 1983), which

Table 1   Common primary sources of metastatic spinal cord compression

Primary site	Percentage	Primary site	Percentage
Lung	20	Sarcoma	7
Breast	15	Kidney	6
Lymphoma	10	Other genitourinary tract	3
Prostate	8	Thyroid	5
Myeloma	7	Digestive tract	4

agrees with the post-mortem finding of epidural invasion of tumour in 5 per cent of patients with cancer (Barron *et al.* 1959; Sundaresan *et al.* 1986). Metastasis is thus commoner than spinal injury as a cause of spinal compression, and metastasis from extraspinal solid tumours accounts for 30–80 per cent of spinal neoplasms with lymphoma and myeloma accounting for a further 10 per cent (Sundaresan *et al.* 1986). As the life expectancy of patients with cancer increases with advances in therapy, so the incidence of symptomatic spinal metastasis is likely to rise. The prevalence of spinal meningeal carcinomatosis is unknown, but there is growing awareness and recognition of this disease entity. Its true incidence is thought to be rising. The use of chemotherapy with poor blood–central nervous system (CNS) penetration can lead to control of disease elsewhere in the body together with development of meningeal metastases. With improving oncological care it is to be hoped that fewer cases of spinal metastasis will present too late for treatment.

Most studies of metastatic spinal disease show only a slight preponderance of male patients, although British series, such as that of Shaw *et al.* (1980), show a male to female ratio as high as 1.8 : 1. The reason for this is unclear, but differences in sex distributions in various tumour types or differing referral patterns may be partially responsible. The age range of patients with symptomatic spinal complications is very wide in most series, ranging from a few months to ages of 80–90 years. However, the condition is overwhelmingly more common in the fifth, sixth, and seventh decades, with 60–70 per cent of patients being over 50 years and 25–45 per cent being over 60 years (Wright 1963; Black 1979). This is in keeping with cancer statistics in general.

PATHOLOGY

The axial skeleton is a common site for bone metastasis, accounting for approximately 40 per cent of positive isotope bone scans in malignant disease. All extracranial malignancies can metastasize to the spine, although the tendency to do so varies between tumours. Thus, while the commonest primary site is breast in females (>50 per cent) and lung in males (>25 per cent), multiple myeloma, prostatic carcinoma, and renal carcinoma have the highest propensity for spinal metastasis (osteotropism; Bockman 1980). Approximately 10 per cent of patients with these primary tumours will be found at autopsy to have spinal involvement. Table 1 summarizes the most common causes of metastatic spinal compression (Wright 1963; Shaw *et al.* 1980; Sundaresan *et al.* 1985; Perrin and McBroom 1987).

In the case of meningeal carcinomatosis, the common sources include primary neuroectodermal tumour such as neuroblastoma, tumours of the haemopoietic system such as lymphoma, lung, breast, and gastrointestinal tumours, and melanoma. Of the carcinomas, adenocarcinoma has the highest propensity for meningeal spread, while bladder and lung tumours tend to have the shortest time

interval from onset to meningeal spread. The incidence of meningeal metastasis in lymphoma has risen enormously with effective therapy for peripheral disease; in some series (Evans *et al.* 1970) the incidence is as high as 50 per cent. This has led to the use of prophylactic adjuvant therapy to the CNS (Green *et al.* 1980).

In up to 50 per cent of patients, the site of the primary tumour is unknown at the time of diagnosis of spinal compression and it remains unknown following biopsy in 10–30 per cent (Shaw *et al.* 1980). Meningeal spread is usually manifest later in the disease and the primary has already been diagnosed in most cases. In patients with known primaries, the interval between the original diagnosis and the occurrence of symptomatic spinal disease is usually short, but it may be as long as 20 years in the case of more indolent tumours or those, such as breast carcinoma, with very variable activity.

Malignant tumours reach the spine principally by haematogenous spread. It is now thought more likely that the principal route is arterial rather than via the paravertebral and extradural venous plexuses as had been described by Batson (1940). Invasion by direct extension does occur, particularly from the lung and from retroperitoneal tumours such as renal carcinoma. Direct spread from lymphomas in mediastinal or retroperitoneal lymph nodes to the spinal canal is often by permeation through the intervertebral foramina. Spread via the cerebrospinal fluid pathways occurs in neuroectodermal tumours.

Any level of the spinal canal may be affected and the frequency of involvement of cervical, thoracic, and lumbosacral regions is approximately in proportion to their relative lengths (Torma 1957; Wright 1963). The cervical spine is perhaps rather less commonly affected (9–15 per cent), and lesions in the upper cervical spine (C1–C2) less often give rise to neurological problems by direct compression until gross instability occurs, as the spinal canal is wider at that level. Similarly, metastases to the lumbosacral spine (15–30 per cent) are more likely to cause local and radicular pain than neurological compromise, as the cord itself usually terminates around the first lumbar level in the adult. Spinal nerve roots may also be compressed or invaded by extraspinal tumour in the pelvis. The thoracic spine is most commonly involved (50–72 per cent), particularly in its middle part. Individual primary tumours show little preference regarding the segment to which they metastasize, although there appears to be a slight tendency for lung and breast tumours to favour the thoracic spine and colonic tumours to favour the lumbosacral spine. Meningeal spread from neuroectodermal tumours is found more commonly in the lumbar region, probably due to the effect of gravity. Tumours at the thoracolumbar junction have a higher tendency to produce instability because of the mechanical stresses in that region. In most patients, disease is confined to one (13 per cent) or more (72 per cent) contiguous vertebrae (Wright 1963; Constans *et al.* 1983) and approximately 15 per cent of patients will be found to have disease in more than one region of the spine.

When the vertebra itself is the site of metastasis, any combination of body, lamina, pedicle, or spinous process may be involved. The vertebral body is involved in 85 per cent of cases (Siegal and Siegal 1985). Both the dura mater and the intervertebral disc are resistant to tumour invasion, with disc invasion by tumour occurring in less than 0.5 per cent of patients. If radiology of spinal lesions reveals disc involvement, osteomyelitis is a much more likely diagnosis. Intradural metastatic tumour is similarly rare (1–4 per cent of all spinal secondaries) (Black 1979; Constans *et al.* 1983) and is seldom continuous with tumour outside the dura. Approximately one-third of these metastases will be intramedullary. Meningeal carcinomatosis, which is often asymptomatic, occurs in 4 per cent of cancer patients and is usually secondary to leukaemia or lymphoma. Solid tumours, in particular breast carcinoma, have also been implicated, while medulloblastomas may spread within the CNS in this way.

While some metastatic tumours are undoubtedly confined to the extradural space, increasing sophistication in imaging together with autopsy studies have shown that most (85 per cent) reach this area by direct spread from an adjacent vertebral body (Torma 1957; Arseni *et al.* 1959; Barron *et al.* 1959). Vertebral tumour may be osteolytic (71 per cent), osteoblastic (8 per cent), or mixed (21 per cent) (Constans *et al.* 1983). Osteoblastic lesions are primarily due to prostate cancer or lymphomas, while breast cancer metastases often present a mixed appearance.

There are several possible mechanisms leading to neurological compromise. Collapse of a vertebra due to tumour replacement gives rise to a focal kyphosis and kinking of the spinal cord, with extrusion of bone and tumour causing further compression. This may happen acutely and may cause radicular symptoms such as girdle pain by pressure of the collapsed bone on the segmental spinal nerves as they pass through the intervertebral foramina. Expansion of a bone lesion into the extradural space without vertebral collapse can cause progressive narrowing of the spinal canal with cord compression. Such masses may be anterior, posterior, lateral, or encircling. Direct or transforaminal extension from a paravertebral mass can occur, as can purely extradural metastasis. Invasion rather than compression of cord or nerve roots is rare (in contrast with parenchymal intracranial metastasis), although tumour cells may be seen within nerve roots on microscopy.

The spinal cord can adapt functionally to slow chronic compression and is often found to be greatly attenuated but with near-normal function in cases of meningioma, but it tolerates more rapid compression poorly. While the rate of compression in metastatic tumours varies, it is usually on a much faster time-scale than in the case of benign conditions and may declare itself over a matter of hours, making early diagnosis and appropriate referral a matter of great urgency. Extradural compression causes progressive distortion of the cord or cauda equina, followed by oedema with interruption of both arterial supply and venous drainage. If the pressure is unrelieved, infarction will occur. In patients surviving extradural compression resulting in permanent neurological dysfunction, subsequent post-mortem examination will show replacement of neural tissue by gliotic scarring.

The histology of spinal metastases, as with all metastatic deposits, varies according to the primary source. The degree of anaplasia often precludes the accurate localization of the primary site, although it will usually narrow the differential diagnosis. Immunohistochemistry, electron microscopy, and molecular techniques may aid diagnostic specificity. An accurate histological diagnosis is important for patients in whom cancer has not been known to be present previously because some tumour types, such as lymphoma, are curable and others, such as breast cancer, may be associated with very long patient survival when treated with the appropriate systemic therapy.

Post-mortem analysis of the CNS and particularly of spinal nerve roots, commonly shows micro-infiltration with tumour cells. These micrometastases are asymptomatic, but presumably it is the growth of such 'colonies' which leads to macroscopic intramedullary deposits with neurological symptoms. As expected in a malignant process, and in contrast with many cases of primary intramedullary tumour, these deposits are diffusely infiltrative and may develop areas of necrosis. Macroscopic intramedullary metastases are rare, and are

seen in 1–2 per cent of necropsy specimens (Chason *et al.* 1963; Costigan and Winkelman 1985; Grem *et al.* 1985; Winkelman *et al.* 1987) and are even more rarely symptomatic. Fifty per cent are from lung and approximately 15 per cent from breast primaries. The site of metastasis within the length of the cord is random. Occasionally only one segment will be affected, but more commonly disease will extend over several levels. Macroscopically, the cord is firm and shows a fusiform widening and microscopy may show it to be almost completely replaced by tumour with areas of infarction.

Meningeal carcinomatosis is rare and may arise either from seeding of primary or secondary tumour already present in the central nervous system or from other sites, presumably by blood spread. It is not an uncommon finding in medulloblastoma and care must be taken to prevent tumour spillage during operation for this condition. Other primary CNS tumours do not generally spread in this manner. The condition may also occur in the absence of macroscopic tumour. The characteristic findings are of a very high protein level in the cerebrospinal fluid, microscopy of which will usually show tumour cells. These are often bizarre or occur in clumps. The diagnosis is most often made fortuitously when cerebrospinal fluid is taken for other tests during the investigation of neurological symptoms which finally prove to be caused by this process. Nodular thickening of nerve roots is seen post-mortem and the roots may be matted together. There may be direct parenchymal invasion, with obliteration of leptomeningeal vessels.

PRESENTATION

In common with malignant disease in general, spinal metastasis does not present a stereotyped clinical picture. Onset may be very rapid and may precede other symptoms of malignancy or it may be insidious. Similarly the symptoms, even for a specific site in the spine, vary considerably between patients.

When a tumour mass is present, pain is almost invariable and is the initial symptom (although often disregarded) in 60–95 per cent of patients (Brice and McKissock 1965; Shapiro and Posner 1983). Cancer pain and musculoskeletal pain are not always easy to differentiate, particularly when the onset follows minor trauma. The relentless nature of the former, its failure to improve with rest and its tendency to dysaesthesia are pointers. Discomfort is often present at rest and increased by movement, coughing, or straining; marked exacerbation by minor flexion or rotation implies a degree of instability. Pain is usually localized to the site(s) of disease and may be elicited by gentle percussion over the area. It is caused by stimulation of pain receptors in the longitudinal ligaments, dura, or periosteum as the tumour expands. Radicular pain is less common and is due to compression of nerve roots by extradural tumour or bony collapse or to tumour infiltration of the roots themselves. Both local and radicular pain are useful in the clinical localization of affected level(s), and are usually more accurate than neurological evaluation.

It is extremely important in the management of patients with known cancer to be aware of the possible significance of axial or radicular pain and to have a low threshold for initiating investigation when these symptoms arise.

Of patients presenting *de novo* with spinal mass lesion, the majority have some degree of neurological impairment at the time of first examination. Despite increasing awareness of the problem, this is still the factor which prompts investigation in most cases. Indeed, by the time treatment is started up to 50 per cent of patients will no longer be able to walk and 10–30 per cent will be paraplegic (Shaw *et al.* 1980; Shapiro and Posner 1983).

Paraparesis with variable sensory symptoms is the most usual mode of presentation; quadriparesis is rarer because of the shorter length of cord which may be affected and because lesions in the cervical region tend to evolve more slowly, causing progressive pain, stiffness, and late deformity. Weakness is usually symmetrical and its onset may be rapid or slow; in over a quarter of patients with paraplegia, less than 48 h will have elapsed between the first motor symptoms and the completed lesion. A further 50–65 per cent will become paraplegic within 7 days and 10–20 per cent within a month (Constans *et al.* 1983). In cord compression of rapid onset, tone is usually flaccid, with the typical spasticity and reflex accentuation of the upper motor neuron lesion taking time to establish. Tone in cauda equina lesions generally remains flaccid.

Sensory change is seldom complained of as a first symptom, but is demonstrable in well over 50 per cent of patients at diagnosis (Black 1979; Shapiro and Posner 1983). It is usually symmetrical, but with lateral compression the Brown-Séquard syndrome may occur. In cauda equina compression sensory loss may be asymmetrical or patchy; compression of its lower extent will cause saddle anaesthesia. The upper level of sensory loss provides a guide for lesion localization but is often not conclusive; frequently sensory levels will be found to vary between left and right sides and the vertebral level of the lesion is often higher than predicted on sensory evidence. Although it is occasionally possible to differentiate anterior from posterior compression by the relative extent of spinothalamic and dorsal column sensory loss, in practice this is of little value as the definitive diagnosis must always be made on radiological grounds.

Loss of control of bladder and anal sphincters occurs late in the process of spinal compression, except in the case of lesions affecting the conus medullaris or sacral roots where it may arise in isolation (2–3 per cent). Retention of urine, often painless, is the first symptom, while constipation may be wrongly attributed to analgesics. Eventually, painless urinary retention wth overflow incontinence and incontinence of faeces will occur. In the early stages, a high residual urine volume (>150 ml) or a lax anal sphincter with reduced saddle sensation may be found in the asymptomatic patient. It is often only when bladder involvement becomes manifest that patients are referred to specialist centres. More than 50 per cent of patients will be found to have sphincter dysfunction at presentation (Black 1979). It must be emphasized that painless urinary retention is a neurosurgical emergency requiring immediate specialist assessment.

In the patient in whom malignancy has not previously been suspected, the differential diagnosis of malignant cord compression is theoretically fairly wide, but in practice the clinical presentation is often relatively typical. A middle-aged to elderly patient with back pain, bilateral leg weakness and sensory disturbance and possible loss of sphincter control must be assumed to have malignant cord compression and urgent diagnosis and treatment must be sought. This applies no less to patients who do not fit this syndrome exactly but in whom the suspicion of cord compression is raised; many studies have shown that the chances of successful preservation or restoration of mobility depend greatly on the extent of neurological compromise at the time of definitive treatment. Indeed, the goal of management should be to identify these patients before neurological deterioration has occurred, when pain is the only symptom.

Differential diagnoses include spinal infection, intervertebral disc herniation, spondylosis, Guillain–Barré syndrome, multiple sclerosis, compression by benign tumour or intrinsic primary cord tumour, non-metastatic carcinomatous neuropathy/myelopathy,

occlusion or haemorrhage affecting the anterior cerebral arteries, spinal subarachnoid, extradural, or subdural haemorrhage, spinal artery occlusion, and parasagittal cerebral lesions such as meningioma. Careful history, examination, and modern diagnostic methods will clarify the diagnosis in the majority of doubtful cases.

Neoplastic meningitis presents much more of a problem of diagnosis. There is diffuse or multifocal infiltration of the meninges with variable neurological involvement. Features may thus be related to any part or parts of the nervous system and may appear bizarre as they do not fit any recognizable neurological syndrome. Spinal nerve root signs, sensory or motor, are fairly common but are usually only noticed in the limbs where there is less overlap of root function. Cerebral manifestations, including dysphasia, fits, intellectual deterioration, and gait disturbance, may be present and may culminate in coma. Papilloedema or other cranial nerve abnormalities may be found. Careful clinical examination is required for the diagnosis to suggest itself. As malignant meningitis is usually a late manifestation of disease, the primary tumour site is usually known and indeed the diagnosis of this complication is most commonly made at autopsy.

INVESTIGATIONS

The establishment of a definitive diagnosis of metastatic tumour is a matter of some urgency, as results depend heavily on the neurological status of the patient at the time of starting treatment. It is not possible to predict which patients will extend their deficit quickly, and so referral to a specialist centre should be made as soon as the clinical diagnosis is made. In the acute case it is seldom worth delaying referral to search for a primary tumour source if this is not known or immediately apparent. Similarly, investigations should be started as soon as is feasible.

Mass lesions

Plain spinal radiographs should be obtained by the hospital clinician who first examines the patient. While attention should be centred on the level clinically judged to be involved, anteroposterior and lateral films of the whole spine should be obtained. These may show evidence of the involvement of vertebrae at other levels, with important implications for treatment and prognosis. Plain radiographs will not normally demonstrate cord compression or lesions within the spinal canal, but a paraspinal mass will be visible in most cases if the appropriate exposure is used, although this finding may also be due to infection. When the vertebrae are involved, the principal radiographic findings are collapse or loss of height of the vertebral body, abnormally high or low density of the body, rarefaction or absence of a pedicle, or loss of definition of a spinous process (Fig. 1). Adjacent vertebrae may be affected and acute angulation of the spine may be seen at the site of vertebral body destruction. Plain radiography of the chest should also be undertaken, as bronchial carcinoma is one of the commonest primary tumours in patients with spinal metastasis. Presentation with spinal cord compression as the first sign of undiagnosed bronchial carcinoma carries a very poor prognosis.

In the non-urgent situation, isotope bone scan is a useful adjunct to the more specific investigation methods in suspected spinal tumour. It is more sensitive than plain radiographs in the demonstration of bone destruction and often areas thought to be normal on radiographs will be shown to harbour tumour deposits. It may be falsely negative, particularly in lymphoma and myeloma and because it is effectively demonstrating active new bone formation

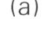
(a)

(b)

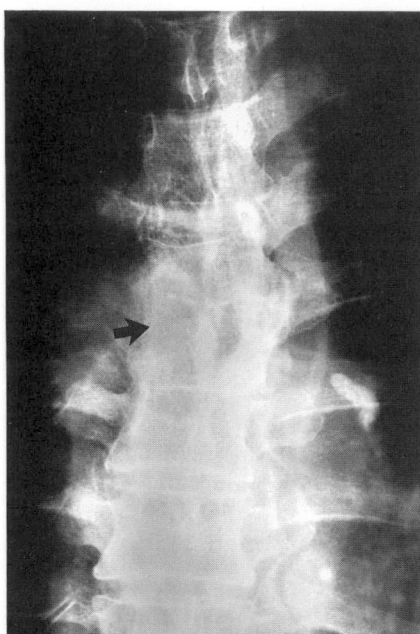

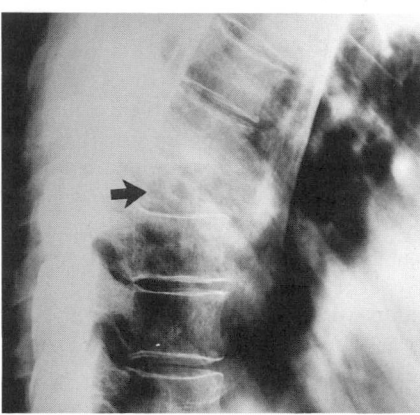

Fig. 1 (a) Anteroposterior and (b) lateral radiographs showing high density change in a single vertebra with loss of height and of pedicle definition.

it may be falsely positive in trauma, infection, Paget's disease, etc. Probably its real value lies in the diagnosis of extraspinal bone involvement and of the involvement of multiple areas in the spine.

Myelography is best performed in specialist centres, where the diagnostic requirements for appropriately targeted treatment are more often appreciated. The equipment is frequently more up to date and should include the facility of combined CT and myelography; magnetic resonance imaging is also more likely to be available. The potential complications of the technique can also be dealt with more speedily. Myelography was until recently the most rapid and sensitive mode of investigation in spinal compression but developments in magnetic resonance imaging have greatly reduced its use. One other investigation should be performed in all patients with back pain who have neurological signs or characteristic plain radiograph abnormalities.

Oil-soluble intrathecal contrast media are no longer used. With modern water-soluble media, the procedure is extremely safe, although seizures may occur rarely if the contrast material is allowed to escape into the intracranial cerebrospinal fluid compartment.

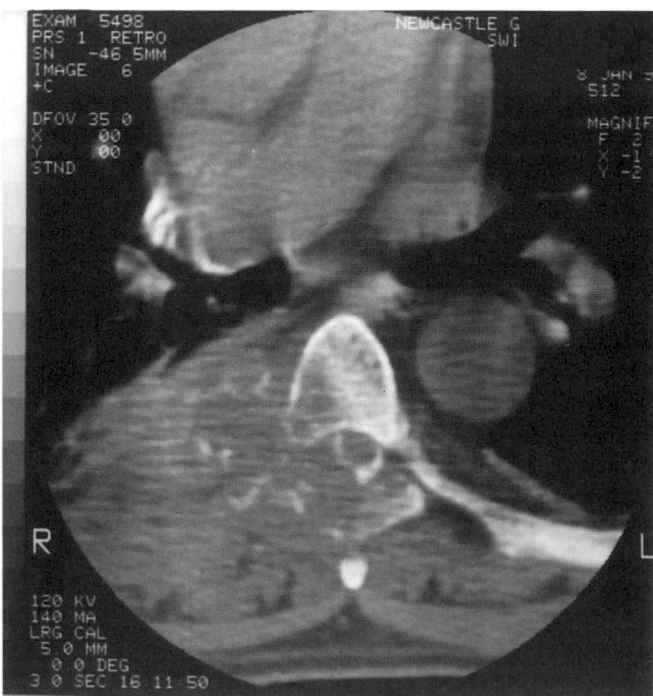

Fig. 2 Unenhanced axial CT scan showing destruction of a vertebral body by metastasis.

Fig. 3 Axial CT myelogram of a vertebra showing metastatic disease in the body with spread to the extradural space and distortion of the contrast-filled spinal theca.

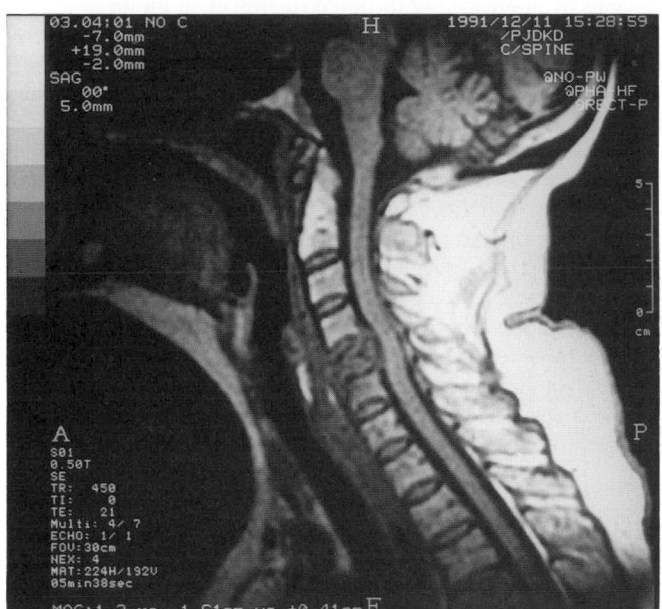

Fig. 4 Sagittal magnetic resonance image of the spine showing a single diseased vertebra with extradural compression.

Occasionally, a patient with spinal compression will deteriorate abruptly during or following myelography owing to impaction of the compromised cord onto surrounding structures. This necessitates immediate surgical decompression.

The procedure is initiated by lumbar puncture, unless a lumbar or cranial tumour is suspected, with withdrawal of cerebrospinal fluid and instillation of contrast medium. The withdrawn cerebrospinal fluid should be examined for malignant or inflammatory cells and for the high protein and xanthochromia which follow stagnation of cerebrospinal fluid loculated by tumour at a higher level or secretion of protein by the tumour itself. The contrast medium is then run throughout the spinal canal and films are taken at all levels. The presence of spinal compression will be demonstrated by a complete or partial hold-up (block) to the passage of contrast and the direction of impingement of an extra- or intradural mass upon the cord will be seen. If the block is complete, repositioning of the patient may allow some contrast to pass, but if this manoeuvre is unsuccessful it will be necessary to demonstrate the upper extent of the block (which may run for several segments) by injection of further contrast medium from above via cervical puncture. The relationship of the intraspinal mass to vertebral and/or extraspinal abnormalities can then be assessed. The myelogram should be scrutinized for the presence of other spinal deposits. Occasionally myelography will demonstrate a benign and treatable cause of neurological compromise in cancer patients.

CT scanning of the spine is more sensitive than either bone scanning or plain radiography in delineating spinal disease within bone (Weissman et al. 1985; Colman et al. 1988). Because of bone-hardening artefact, however, structures within the spinal canal are not well defined and for this reason intrathecal contrast medium must be used in most cases. In cases of vertebral collapse unenhanced CT can help to differentiate between osteoporosis, where the cortex of the vertebral body will appear intact on transverse images and tumour, where it is usually extensively disrupted (Fig. 2). An additional disadvantage of CT is that images are obtained in the axial plane only; reconstruction in other planes

is time-consuming, incomplete, and subject to artefact, while acquisition of data on the whole spine is laborious. Thus, CT scanning is not generally accepted as a first-line investigation or screening tool. However, it is extremely useful in patients in whom a lesion and its spinal level have already been shown. When performed within 12 h of myelography, contrast medium still present in the theca will help to delineate the cord and the extra- and intradural structures and compressive lesions will be seen in far greater detail than with myelography (Fig. 3). Thus, scanning is performed around the level shown to be abnormal on myelography; additional information gained would include the direction of cord compression, the presence of bony disease, and any paravertebral extension. Paraspinal lymph node enlargement can also be seen and with little extra time penalty the lungs and liver may be imaged. In patients with normal plain radiographs and myelography in whom spinal metastasis is suspected because of characteristic pain and a known primary, CT is a sensitive way of showing bone involvement; in addition, CT has demonstrated lesions not contiguous with a known spinal secondary in 38 per cent of patients (Colman et al. 1988).

Magnetic resonance imaging (MRI) of the spine is becoming established as routine practice in most specialist centres and in skilled hands this technique may soon replace all others (Godersky et al. 1987). Because it reflects changes in the amount and binding of tissue water, MRI is extremely sensitive to oedema caused by any pathological process and to the presence of pathological tissue (Fig. 4). Imaging may be performed in any plane and thus a small series of sagittal images covering the whole spine used to localize pathology may be followed by axial images at appropriate levels. Because of its complex curvature in the anteroposterior plane, coronal imaging is of limited use in the spine; similarly, imaging of the scoliotic patient can be difficult. Other disadvantages include the discomfort of lying still through the comparatively long image acquisition time for patients with severe back pain and the relative insensitivity of the method in the demonstration of intradural extramedullary lesions. In most cases, however, MRI will provide more information than myelography and has the advantages of being non-invasive and well tolerated and of demonstrating bony and paraspinous disease as well as extradural compression. The use of multiple imaging parameters and of paramagnetic contrast agents such as gadolinium-DTPA (Sze et al. 1988), increase its sensitivity but require experienced radiological direction as certain pulse sequences may fail to reveal secondary deposits with or without contrast. MRI should now be regarded as the definitive investigation in suspected metastatic spinal disease.

In order for appropriate treatment plans to be formulated, accurate tissue diagnosis must be available. In 40–50 per cent of these patients, far more if only presentation to neuroscience units is considered, spinal compression is the first sign of malignant disease; if an obvious primary lesion is not found by examination or simple tests such as chest radiography, then histology may be obtained from the spinal lesion. Further delay will inevitably result in neurological deterioration.

Tissue may be obtained at open operation for decompression. In the past few years, however, opinion has swung away from posterior decompressive surgery as it is no more effective than radiotherapy in improving neurology. In cases not undergoing surgery, biopsy confirmation of the diagnosis is mandatory. If CT or MRI show involvement of the paraspinal muscles, a trocar biopsy can be a simple and effective means of obtaining a diagnosis. When the vertebral body is affected, tissue can be obtained by percutaneous needle biopsy. This technique is safe and swift and tissue diagnosis can be obtained by smear examination with more than 95 per cent accuracy within minutes (Findlay *et al.* 1988). It is almost always possible to obtain sufficient soft tissue for the smear technique when bone pathology exists.

The technique was first described in Ottolenghi (1955) and is appropriate for vertebrae from T4 to the sacrum. It is feasible, but more difficult, to biopsy the bodies of C3 to C7 by this method, but the proximity of the great vessels renders the procedure too dangerous in the intervening segment. A core biopsy is preferable to fine-needle aspiration; Fyfe *et al.* (1983) showed fine-needle aspiration to have a lower diagnostic yield (50 per cent). Under local anaesthesia and with the patient in the lateral position, a localizing needle is advanced under radiographic control to the posterolateral surface of the body of the abnormal vertebra. An introducer is then advanced alongside this needle and a trocar run over it is impacted on the vertebra. The biopsy cannula (internal diameter 3 mm) is inserted through the trocar and rotated so that its toothed edge cuts a core of bone which is removed for analysis. Half the specimen can be kept for decalcification and conventional sectioning and staining, while the other half can be examined directly by smearing and staining. A portion may be sent for bacteriological analysis if infection is thought to be a possible diagnosis. It is now usual to perform such biopsies under CT control.

If the compressive lesion is purely extradural, the only recourse is to open biopsy and decompression as described in the next section.

Neoplastic meningitis

The definitive diagnosis of meningeal carcinomatosis is no more straightforward than the clinical assessment and similarly may be arrived at by piecing together fragments of information from various tests.

The finding of malignant cells in the cerebrospinal fluid is pathognomonic. These may be seen in isolation or in clumps. However, it is not uncommon for the cerebrospinal fluid to be normal, particularly in the early stages of the disease. Non-specific cerebrospinal fluid findings include raised protein content, reduced glucose, and lymphocytes or polymorphs. This may lead to a mistaken diagnosis of infective or inflammatory meningitis. Biochemical markers specific to the primary tumour, if known, may be sought.

Electroencephalography is abnormal in more than 50 per cent of patients with neoplastic meningitis, reflecting its widespread nature. Again, this is a non-specific finding.

Contrast myelography and spinal CT scanning are relatively insensitive except in advanced disease. Myelography may show nodular filling defects or prominence or crowding of the nerve roots of the cauda equina. Cranial CT with intravenous contrast medium may show enhancement around the tentorium, cerebral sulci, or basal cisterns, and hydrocephalus is not uncommon.

MRI is useful, demonstrating clumping of lumbar nerve roots and nodules in the cauda equina. Changes in protein content of the cerebrospinal fluid will be evident on appropriate pulse sequences. Meningeal enhancement with intravenous contrast agents such as gadolinium-DTPA may be seen (Sze *et al.* 1988).

MANAGEMENT

The diagnosis of spinal metastasis is a very serious factor of poor prognosis in a patient with cancer. Nevertheless, it is vital to appreciate that all efforts must be made to improve the quality of remaining life in these unfortunate patients and not to increase their problems by ill-advised or ill-timed treatment. With mass lesions, it is generally felt that surgery purely for neurological compromise is only justified if life expectancy is likely to be greater than 3 months; even with optimal neurological response in a motivated patient, at least 2 months of physiotherapy will generally be required to re-establish good walking ability. However, surgery for the relief of severe pain may be appropriate in all but the moribund and should always be considered even if the neurological outlook is hopeless. The presence of systemic disease which would render aggressive management hazardous should not necessarily be a contraindication, as most patients will accept fearsome odds for the ability to remain mobile or for the relief of pain. It is this consideration, together with the poor results of lesser procedures, which has led to a reappraisal of the rôle of major decompressive and/or reconstructive surgery in selected patients.

Mass lesions

All patients should be started on corticosteroids as soon as the clinical diagnosis is made. The mechanism of action of steroids is still uncertain. Experimentally, vasogenic oedema resulting from epidural venous obstruction is reduced (Ushio *et al.* 1977). Corticosteroids also inhibit prostaglandin synthesis and, thus, the formation of PGE_2, a mediator of inflammation and oedema (Siegal *et al.* 1988). However, it seems possible that steroids have in addition a specific antitumour effect, particularly in lyphoma (Posner *et al.* 1977).

A starting dose in adults of 12–20 mg dexamethasone intravenously followed by 4 mg four times daily is usually adequate. There is little evidence to support regimes of very high steroid dosage, although Marshall and Langfitt (1977) found clinical response to doses of 36–40 g/day in some patients who were resistant to conventional doses. They also suggested that there may be an association between the short-term response to steroid therapy and the probable benefit from or need for definitive decompressive treatment. However, they pointed out that failure to respond should not preclude surgery; three of their 29 patients deteriorated on steroid treatment but improved with laminectomy. Prompt steroid treatment will often also allow some time for fuller investigation. There is some evidence that prolonged steroid therapy can diminish the response to decompression and the side-effects of such therapy can be devastating. Steroids should be reduced from the above dose within 48–72 h after surgery, if performed and stopped over a period of up to 10 days. If the neurological state deteriorates during dose reduction, the dose should be raised again and the patient reinvestigated. If radiotherapy is proposed as a primary or secondary treatment, a small dose (1–2 mg twice daily) should be maintained until its completion to guard against radiation-induced oedema and swelling.

Until recent years, the diagnosis in a neurosurgical unit of a myelographic block due to malignancy was followed in most cases by decompressive laminectomy and subsequent radiotherapy. However, proper audit of results in terms of the number of patients regaining or retaining the ability to walk has led to a redefinition of the precise role of laminectomy (Findlay 1984, 1987; Siegal and Siegal 1986; Sundaresan *et al.* 1986). Several workers culminating in Gilbert *et al.* (1978), compared the results of laminectomy plus radiotherapy with those of urgent radiotherapy alone and found no effective difference except in the morbidity and mortality of surgery. Indeed, in patients with a more acute onset of weakness, Gilbert *et al.* found radiotherapy to be more effective in restoring power when used alone. Findlay (1984) reviewed all papers from 1960 onwards dealing with the treatment of spinal cord compression due to malignancy. No significant difference was found in the percentage of patients remaining ambulant or regaining ambulation, following laminectomy or radiotherapy and overall less than 40 per cent of patients were able to walk at the end of treatment. Even of those initially ambulant, 21 per cent were unable to walk after radiotherapy. In most series, the percentage of patients remaining ambulatory with either treatment is less than 50 per cent. Further difficulties regarding laminectomy arise if there is significant vertebral body disease or collapse and if cold compression is mostly anterior. Not only is laminectomy less likely to relieve the compression, it will often cause further instability with consequent pain and increased neurological deficit: over 20 per cent will be made unstable and symptoms will progress in 50 per cent (Findlay 1987). Similarly, radiotherapy should not be considered as a primary treatment if paraparesis is severe or if vertebral collapse or instability are demonstrated. Therefore it has become evident that the treatment plan and surgical approach should be carefully tailored to the site of the lesion, gaining maximum decompression with minimum cord displacement and including stabilization and subsequent radiotherapy where indicated.

The alternatives to laminectomy are approaches by the transpedicular route, costotransversectomy, and anterior resection (transthoracic, transabdominal, or retroperitoneal). Similarly, stabilization may be anterior, lateral, or posterior. The indications and method for each approach are outlined below.

Laminectomy

Laminectomy should be reserved for cases where the tumour is found to be posterior or posterolateral only. If laminectomy is indicated, it should include all involved levels and as much tumour tissue should be removed as is feasible without excessive traction on the cord or nerve roots. Soft tissue spread is more common than would be expected from radiography analysis, being better shown by MRI, and it is not unusual to cut through skin directly into tumour. Blood loss may be considerable in such circumstances and indeed even an isolated extradural tumour can bleed profusely. The facet joints should be spared wherever possible in order to increase stability. Where they have to be removed or where exploration reveals that they or the vertebral body are involved with tumour, posterior fixation should be employed. Laminectomy and posterior instrumentation may also be indicated where significant anterior disease is present as a palliative procedure in patients with advanced disease or a highly malignant and poorly responsive tumour. Early mobilization is possible and pain due to pressure and instability is well controlled, allowing such patients to go home early. The perioperative mortality of laminectomy is of the order of 3–5 per cent. Potential complications include venous thrombosis and pulmonary embolus, particularly in the immobile patient, extradural bleeding and compression, the production of spinal instability, and wound infection or delayed healing.

Instrumentation must be seen as a temporary measure and will always fail in time; it should be supplemented by bone grafting if longer-term survival is envisaged. Several techniques of posterior instrumentation are available. Hartshill or other shaped rectangular bars, such as Luque bars held in place by sublaminar wires, are routinely inserted in many centres. Harrington distraction rods, where hooks placed in the facet joint of the upper vertebra and on the lamina of the lower vertebra are distracted by a ratcheted steel bar, are now much less frequently used. Where laminar bone is of good quality, a rigid steel bar (for example, the Banks–Dervin rod (Miles *et al.* 1984)) may be used, fixed by translaminar screws and

acrylic. All these fixation methods should be anchored to at least two healthy vertebrae above and below the diseased area. Pedicle fixation with rods, screws, or plates may be used from the mid-thoracic area down and lateral mass fixation may be used in the neck. The advantage of this technique is that it results in fusion only at the affected segment.

Transpedicular and costotransversectomy approaches

Very good access to the lateral part of the spinal canal can be obtained by extending laminectomy to remove the pedicle(s) on the appropriate side; it must be noted that bilateral pedicle removal will render the spine unstable. Posterolateral approaches such as costotransversectomy in the thorax or transverse process osteotomy in the lumbar region allow reasonable access for palliative debulking of tumour. These techniques should generally be reserved for patients who are debilitated, who have a poor overall prognosis, or in whom vertebral body involvement is minimal.

Anterior approaches

For patients with anterior compression of the spinal cord from vertebral body tumour extension or collapse, an anterior surgical approach with vertebral body resection, tumour decompression, and stabilization must be considered. Although this type of approach was first reported in the 1950s (Hodgeson and Stock 1956) in the radical treatment of spinal tuberculosis, the extensive nature of the surgery and the poor prognosis of the patients did not encourage its use in malignant spinal disease. However, with the poor overall results of posterior and posterolateral approaches in terms of adequacy of decompression and stability, this attitude has undergone reappraisal during the last 10–15 years. Improved anaesthetic techniques together with growing surgical expertise, has meant that such operations are no longer so fearsome. Provided that lung function is good, the perioperative mortality of anterior surgery is similar to that of laminectomy at 4–8 per cent (Siegal and Siegal 1985*b*; Siegal *et al.* 1985; Sundaresan *et al.* 1985; Perrin and McBroom 1987) while the neurological complication rate is less.

In the upper cervical spine (C1–C2), anterior resection is technically difficult and dangerous. For short-term stability a halo brace and radiotherapy should suffice, while for more indolent lesions sublaminar wiring or Ransford loop fixation with bone graft or lateral mass fixation may be used. As mentioned above, lesions here are less likely to cause neurological problems. The bodies of C3–C7 and T1 are accessible through a standard anterior neck approach. The excised body may be replaced with bone graft or a methylmethacrylate prosthesis and may be strengthened by anterior plating. This method can be used if three or fewer vertebral levels are involved; posterior instrumentation is preferable if there is more extensive involvement.

The first, second, and third thoracic vertebrae are relatively inaccessible, with exposure often necessitating a sternal split and manipulation of the great vessels (Sundaresan *et al.* 1984). Excellent exposure of the remainder of the thoracic spine to T11 is available through a standard thoracotomy at the appropriate level, while T12 and L1 require a thoracoabdominal approach. The affected body or bodies are removed, together with extradural tumour, until the dura is seen to be well decompressed. The defect is replaced by bone graft or a methylmethacrylate or metallic 'spacer'. At the thoracolumbar junction, additional posterior stabilization is usually also necessary through a separate approach. Newer anterior fixation systems such as that described by Kaneda, which fix to the adjacent vertebral bodies, can be used to avoid an additional posterior instrumentation.

The bodies from L2 to the sacrum may be approached retroperitoneally or transabdominally and similar techniques used.

The drawbacks of anterior surgery in the thoracolumbar spine are principally those of major surgery in the less fit patient. However, perioperative mortality is little greater than that of laminectomy; the causes include pulmonary embolus, renal failure, pneumonia, and myocardial infarction. The incidence of non-fatal complications is similar to that after laminectomy, except that thromboembolism is more common because of the manipulation of the great veins and the period of post-operative immobilization. Pain can be severe, particularly following thoracotomy.

Radiotherapy

Radiotherapy remains necessary as a supplementary primary treatment in most operated cases. Where it is used in whole or in part as the definitive method of tumour decompression, it should be started as soon as possible and most units are prepared to give emergency radiotherapy within hours of diagnosis. Where surgery arrests or improves neurological compromise, it is preferable to wait for at least 10 days after operation to allow wounds to heal. The radiation portal should include the extent of the known tumour plus two vertebral levels above and below, together with any other deposits seen on radiographs or scans. In the cervical or lumbar spine, parallel-opposed anteroposterior fields are used as the spine is centrally situated in the body and cord overdosage is easier to avoid. In the thoracic spine a single posterior field is irradiated, prescribing to a depth of 6 cm. In medulloblastoma and neoplastic meningitis full craniospinal irradiation is necessary. This means that in the adult most of the functioning bone-marrow is irradiated, which can be particularly hazardous if adjunctive chemotherapy is being considered.

Neurological improvement with radiotherapy is a direct result of tumour shrinkage and may not be apparent for days or weeks. Where instability is not a major feature, however, pain is usually relieved extremely rapidly (less than 24 h) in many different tumour types by various applications such as local therapy, hemibody irradiation, or even pituitary irradiation. This suggests that tumour regression is not the only factor and that other mechanisms such as the inhibition of prostaglandin-secreting cells may play a part.

Protocols for radiotherapy in spinal metastasis vary between units and it is difficult to find hard data supporting different treatment methods. Conventional dosage regimes vary with the type of tumour and the expected survival of the patient. In a very ill patient with bronchial carcinoma, a single dose of 8–10 Gy may be used, while if the patient's condition is good but the expected survival fairly poor a total of 20 Gy may be given in five doses over 5–7 days. If survival is estimated as good, 30 Gy may be given over 10–14 days. In myeloma, 35 Gy over 14 days may be curative. Craniospinal irradiation in medulloblastoma or malignant meningitis from other tumours may be treated with 32 Gy in 16 fractions.

However, trials of single-dose therapy have shown pain relief to be rapidly achieved with a single dose of 8 Gy (Price et al. 1986) and maintained for as long as happens with multiple fractions to 30 Gy. Acute gastrointestinal symptoms were slightly more frequent in a group of patients receiving single doses of 8 Gy (Cole 1989) than in a group receiving six doses of 4 Gy, while mean survival was actually longer in the single-dose group. Neurological response is more difficult to assess but again seems to be little affected by dosage regimes. The use of single doses is easier for the patient and also permits reirradiation within the limits of cord tolerance if symptoms recur. Recent attempts to improve local control with high-dose fractionation or with radiation sensitizers such as metronidazole have met with some success. Chemotherapy is rarely used as a primary treatment in spinal compression, but tumour-specific treatment may be a useful adjunct in certain cases such as lymphoma and myeloma following definitive treatment.

Neoplastic meningitis

Treatment of patients with neoplastic meningitis is generally unsuccessful, principally because malignant disease is well advanced by the time that it is manifest. Treatment must be directed to the whole neuraxis.

CNS tumours with a propensity for leptomeningeal spread, such as medulloblastoma, are highly radiosensitive, as are tumours of the haemopoietic system. Therefore, craniospinal irradiation is effective in the short term in these tumours in the majority of patients and will halt the progression of symptoms or lead to clinical improvement. Radiotherapy should also be used in patients with other tumours or where the primary site is unknown.

Intrathecal chemotherapy has been studied extensively and is effective against many tumours; the blood–brain barrier prevents the accumulation in the cerebrospinal fluid of therapeutic concentrations of most drugs when administered by other routes. The folic acid antagonist methotrexate has been most commonly used and is the most effective drug to date (Sculier 1985). Combinations of drugs seem to offer no advantage.

RESULTS

Irrespective of the treatment used, up to 10 per cent of patients with symptomatic spinal metastasis will be dead within a month and by 3 months this figure rises to 30–45 per cent. Only 18–30 per cent of patients survive more than 1 year (Shaw et al. 1980; Constans et al. 1983). With the exception of surgical complications, or respiratory compromise in cervical lesions, survival is dependent on the aggressiveness of the primary disease. Most patients in whom neurological deterioration is arrested will die before local recurrence causes further deterioration. The mean survival in most series is approximately 7 months. If this is broken down into tumour type, lung cancer patients survive for a mean of 2.6 months, while those with prostatic, breast, or haematological malignancies can have more extended survival. The more aggressive therapies should thus be directed at lesions in patients known to harbour less aggressive tumours, particularly in view of data which show that neurological recovery is also related to tumour biology. In general, rapidly advancing tumours are less well controlled by radiotherapy and surgery is also less successful.

Increasing the quality of survival is thus the goal in most patients and two main factors must be considered in each case. Preservation or restoration of the ability to walk is the yardstick most commonly used in studies of comparative treatment outcomes. However, pain relief is increasingly a target of active treatment in its own right with the quality of survival being heavily dependent upon it. It must be remembered that bone or root pain are often difficult to control with analgesic medicines.

Overall, most studies suggest that the results of laminectomy plus radiotherapy are no better than those of radiotherapy alone, while the results of laminectomy alone are significantly less good (Gilbert et al. 1978; Shapiro and Posner 1983; Findlay 1984). This is the basis of the shift in recent years towards early radiotherapy as a primary treatment. However, if careful consideration is given to the nature of bone involvement and the direction of cord compression, as demonstrated by radiological studies, an appropriate surgical approach can be chosen with consequent improvement in outcome. This has been the main thrust of active treatment in the past few years.

The most important prognostic factors in the effect of any treatment on neurological recovery are the nature of the primary tumour and the extent of the deficit at the time treatment is started. Most series, but not all, suggest that the rate of deterioration also plays a part, with rapidly developing neurology being less recoverable. Interestingly, the more recent literature, such as a paper by Barcena et al. (1984), contradicts this long-held belief. Although exceptional cases regain useful function, it is generally accepted that the outlook regarding ambulation is hopeless if a patient has been completely paraplegic for longer than 24 h. In patients who can no longer walk, but who retain some leg power, walking will be restored in less than 50 per cent with either laminectomy plus radiotherapy or radiotherapy alone (Gilbert et al. 1978; Shapiro and Posner 1983; Findlay 1984) and even patients still walking when treatment starts have only a 60–80 per cent chance of remaining ambulant by the time of its completion (Shaw et al. 1980; Constans et al. 1983; Sundaresan et al. 1986). Patients with less aggressive tumours, such as myeloma, lymphoma, and prostatic carcinoma, have a better prognosis for functional recovery. The spinal level affected appears to have little effect on prognosis.

Several recent series show that an anterior surgical approach with vertebral body resection, dural decompression, and internal stabilization gives better results in terms of both mobility and pain relief than does laminectomy (Siegal and Siegal 1985a; Sundaresan et al. 1985, 1986; Turner et al. 1988). An 80–90 per cent rate of restoration or maintenance of ambulation has been reported and dramatic recovery of function has been achieved even in paraplegic patients. It seems likely that this should be the procedure of choice in selected cases.

Pain at the site of the metastasis is fairly responsive to all treatments. This implies that decompression itself is instrumental in relieving pain, as even unstabilized cases respond. Short-term pain reduction is reported in up to 75 per cent of patients undergoing laminectomy, radiotherapy, or both. Those whose pain fails to improve usually have a degree of instability which may be alleviated by instrumentation. Anterior surgery with posterior stabilization has the greatest likelihood of improving pain (up to 95 per cent). If the wrong surgical approach is chosen, pain may well be increased as the remaining stability is reduced.

CONCLUSION

With systematic critical appraisal of the results of traditional treatments, protocols for the management of malignant spinal disease have changed dramatically over the last 15 years. The aims of therapy as now stated are the restoration or maintenance of ambulation and the relief of pain. What is emerging is a treatment plan specifically designed for each type of patient, taking into account all variables known to have a significant effect on outcome: the age, fitness, and life expectancy of the patient, the primary tumour site, if known, the extent and progression of pain and neurological disturbance, the site and extent of the secondary tumour, using all imaging resources necessary, the presence of instability, etc.

For this to be successful requires a recognition of the syndrome, and in particular of its urgent nature, on the part of the clinicians who first encounter the patient. Immediate referral to a specialist centre is mandatory. Once there, a coordinated team will assess the patient clinically and radiologically, analysing the variables mentioned above, to emerge with a tailored treatment plan carrying the greatest chance of success. It cannot be stressed too strongly that the most important factors in this chain are early recognition of the problem and speed of referral and treatment. Only by attention to these can significant improvements be made in the quality of survival of these patients.

REFERENCES

Arseni CN, Simionescu MD, Horwath L (1959). Tumors of the spine: a follow-up study of 350 patients with neurological considerations. *Acta Psychiatrica Scandinavica*, **34**:398–410.

Barcena A, et al. (1984). Spinal metastatic disease: analysis of factors determining functional prognosis and the choice of treatment. *Neurosurgery*, **15**:820–7.

Barron KD, Hirano AS, Araki S, Terry RD (1959). Experiences with metastatic neoplasms affecting the spinal cord. *Neurology*, **9**:91–106.

Batson O (1940). The function of the vertebral veins and their role in the spread of metastases. *Annals of Surgery*, **112**:138–49.

Black P (1979). Spinal metastasis: Current status and recommended guidelines for management. *Neurosurgery*, **5**:726–46.

Bockman PS (1980). Hypercalcaemia in malignancy. *Clinics in Endocrinology and Metabolism*, **9**:317–33.

Brice J, McKissock W (1965). Surgical treatment of malignant extradural spinal tumours. *British Medical Journal*, **1**:1339–44.

Chason JL, Walker FB, Landers JW (1963). Metastatic carcinoma in the central nervous system and dorsal root ganglia. A prospective autopsy study. *Cancer*, **16**:781–7.

Cole DJ (1989). A randomized trial of a single treatment versus conventional fractionation in the palliative radiotherapy of painful bone metastases. *Clinical Oncology of the Royal College of Radiologists*, **1**(2):59–62.

Colman LK, Porter BA, Redmond J, et al. (1988). Early diagnosis of spinal metastases by CT and MR studies. *Journal of Computer Assisted Tomography*, **12**:423–6.

Constans JP, de Divitiis E, Donzelli R, et al. (1983). Spinal metastases with neurological manifestations. Review of 600 cases. *Journal of Neurosurgery*, **59**:111–18.

Costigan DL, Winkelman MD (1985). Intramedullary spinal cord metastasis. A clinicopathological study of 13 cases. *Journal of Neurosurgery*, **62**:227–33.

Evans AE, Gilbert ES, Zandstra R (1970). The increasing incidence of central nervous system leukaemia in children. *Cancer*, **26**:404–9.

Findlay GFG (1984). Adverse effects of the management of malignant spinal cord compression. *Journal of Neurology, Neurosurgery and Psychiatry*, **47**:761–8.

Findlay GFG (1987). The role of vertebral body collapse in the management of malignant spinal cord compression. *Journal of Neurology, Neurosurgery and Psychiatry*, **50**:151–4.

Findlay GFG, Sandeman DR, Buxton P (1988). The role of needle biopsy in the management of malignant spinal compression. *British Journal of Neurosurgery*, **2**:479–84.

Fyfe IS, Henry AP, Mulholland RC (1983). Closed vertebral biopsy. *Journal of Bone and Joint Surgery*, **65B**:140–3.

Gilbert RW, Kim JH, Posner JB (1978). Epidural spinal cord compression from metastatic tumour: diagnosis and treatment. *Annals of Neurology*, **3**:40–51.

Godersky JC, Smoker WRK, Knutzon R (1987). Use of magnetic resonance imaging in the evaluation of metastatic spinal disease. *Neurosurgery*, **21**:676–80.

Green DM, et al. (1980). Comparison of three methods of central-nervous-system prophylaxis in childhood acute lymphoblastic leukaemia. *Lancet*, i:1398–401.

Grem JL, Burgess J, Trump DL (1985). Clinical features and natural history of intramedullary spinal cord metastasis. *Cancer*, **56**:2305–14.

Hodgeson AR, Stock FE (1960). Anterior spine fusion for tuberculosis of the spine. *Journal of Bone and Joint Surgery*, **42A**:295–310.

Marshall LF, Langfitt TW (1977). Combined therapy for metastatic extradural tumors of the spine. *Cancer*, **40**:2067–70.

Miles J, Banks AJ, Dervin E, Noori Z (1984). Stabilisation of the spine affected by malignancy. *Journal of Neurology, Neurosurgery and Psychiatry*, **47**: 897–904.

Ottolenghi C (1955). Diagnosis of orthopaedic lesions by aspiration biopsy. Results of 1061 punctures. *Journal of Bone and Joint Surgery*, **37A**:443–64.

Perrin RG, McBroom RJ (1987). Anterior versus posterior decompression for symptomatic spinal metastasis. *Canadian Journal of Neurological Science*, **14**:75–80.

Posner JB, Howieson J, Cvitkovic E (1977. "Disappearing" spinal cell compression: oncolytic effect of glucocorticoids (and other chemotherapeutic agents) on epidural metastases. *Annals of Neurology*, **2**:409–13.

Price P, Hoskin PJ, Easton D, Austin D, Palmer SG, Yarnold JR (1986). Prospective randomized trial of single and multifraction radiotherapy schedules in the treatment of painful bone metastases. *Radiotherapy and Oncology*, **6(4)**:247–55.

Sculier JP (1985). Treatment of meningeal carcinomatous cancer. *Cancer Treatment Reviews*, **12(2)**:95–104.

Shapiro WR, Posner JB (1983). Medical versus surgical treatment of metastatic spinal cord tumors. In *Controversies in neurology* (eds RA Thompson and JR Green), pp. 57–65. Raven Press, New York.

Shaw MDM, Rose JE, Paterson A (1980). Metastatic extradural malignancy of the spine. *Acta Neurochirugica*, **52**:113–20.

Siegal T, Siegal T (1985a). Treatment of malignant epidural cord and cauda equina compression. *Progress in Experimental Tumor Research*, **29**:225–34.

Siegal T, Siegal T (1985b). Surgical decompression of anterior and posterior malignant epidural tumors compressing the spinal cord: a prospective study. *Neurosurgery*, **17**:424–32.

Siegal T, Tiqva P, Siegal T (1985). Vertebral body resection for epidural compression by malignant tumors. Results of forty-seven consecutive operative procedures. *Journal of Bone and Joint Surgery*, **67B**:375–82.

Siegal T, et al. (1988). Indomethacin and dexamethasone treatment in experimental neoplastic spinal cord compression. *Neurosurgery*, **22**:328–39.

Sundaresan N, Shah J, Foley K, Rosen G (1984). An anterior surgical approach to the upper thoracic vertebrae. *Journal of Neurosurgery*, **61**:686–90.

Sundaresan N, et al. (1985). Treatment of neoplastic epidural cord compression by vertebral body resection and stabilisation. *Journal of Neurosurgery*, **63**:676–84.

Sundaresan N, Digiacinto GV, Hughes JEO (1986). Surgical treatment of spinal metastases. *Clinical Neurosurgery*, **33**:503–22.

Sze G, Krol G, Zimmerman RD, Deck MDF (1988). Malignant extradural spinal tumors: MR imaging with Gd-DTPA. *Radiology*, **167**:217–23.

Torma T (1957). Malignant tumors of the spine and the spinal extradural space: a study based on 250 histologically verified cases. *Acta Chirurgica Scandinavica*, **225** (Suppl.):1–176.

Turner PL, Prince HG, Webb JK, Sokal MPJW (1988). Surgery for malignant extradural tumours of the spine. *Journal of Bone and Joint Surgery*, **70**:451–6.

Ushio Y, Posner R, Posner JB (1977). Experimental spinal cold compression by epidural neoplasms. *Neurology (Minneapolis)*, **27**:422–9.

Weissman DE, Gilbert M, Wang H, Grossman SA (1985). The use of computed tomography of the spine to identify patients at high risk for epidural metastases. *Journal of Clinical Oncology*, **3**:1541–4.

Winkelman MD, Adelstein DJ, Karlins NL (1987). Intramedullary spinal cord metastasis. Diagnostic and therapeutic considerations. *Archives of Neurology*, **44**:526–31.

Wright R (1963). Malignant tumors in the spinal extradural space: results of surgical treatment. *Annals of Surgery*, **57**:227–31.

19.7 Pathological fracture

CHARLES S. B. GALASKO

INTRODUCTION

Skeletal metastases may present with pain, hypercalcaemia, impending fracture, pathological fracture, spinal instability, and compression of the spinal cord or cauda equina. Impending and pathological fractures and spinal instability are discussed in this chapter.

IMPENDING FRACTURE

Impending fractures present with pain and usually a large lytic metastasis is seen on the radiograph. By the time a large lytic metastasis has developed, there is considerable bone destruction and the cortex has been involved. Skeletal metastases arise in the medulla and are not usually evident on plain radiographs until 50 per cent of the bone in the X-ray beam access has been destroyed (Edelstyn et al. 1967). The mechanism of pain in these lesions is not fully understood, but may be associated with infraction of the surrounding bone. The risk of fracture is high. Fidler (1981) found that the risk of fracture correlated with the degree of cortical destruction. If less than 25 per cent of the cortex was destroyed, the risk of fracture was virtually negligible. If more than 50 per cent of the cortex of a long bone was involved, there was a sudden rise in fracture incidence. Fidler reported a fracture incidence of 3.7 per cent when 25–50 per cent of the cortex was involved

and 61 per cent when the degree of involvement ranged between 50 and 75 per cent. CT scanning may be of help in assessing the degree of bone destruction.

Radiotherapy relieves pain but temporarily weakens the bone, probably owing to the associated transient osteoporosis and as a result may increase the risk of pathological fracture. However, Cheng et al. (1980) reported that fractures developed in only two out of 97 skeletal metastases during radiation therapy and in a further two after completion of treatment. Biopsy of a metastasis may also predispose to fracture.

Although most fractures are associated with large lytic metastases, they can also occur in other types. There are three types of bone destruction consequent upon skeletal metastases.

1. Geographic: these are large solitary well-defined lytic areas more than 1 cm in diameter and usually with a sharply demarcated edge.

2. Moth-eaten: there are multiple, smaller lytic areas (2–5 mm) which may coalesce to form larger confluent areas. Their margins are usually ill defined.

3. Permeative: there are multiple tiny lytic areas (usually 1 mm or less) seen principally in cortical bone. Figure 1 shows a pathological fracture in a bone riddled with permeative metastases.

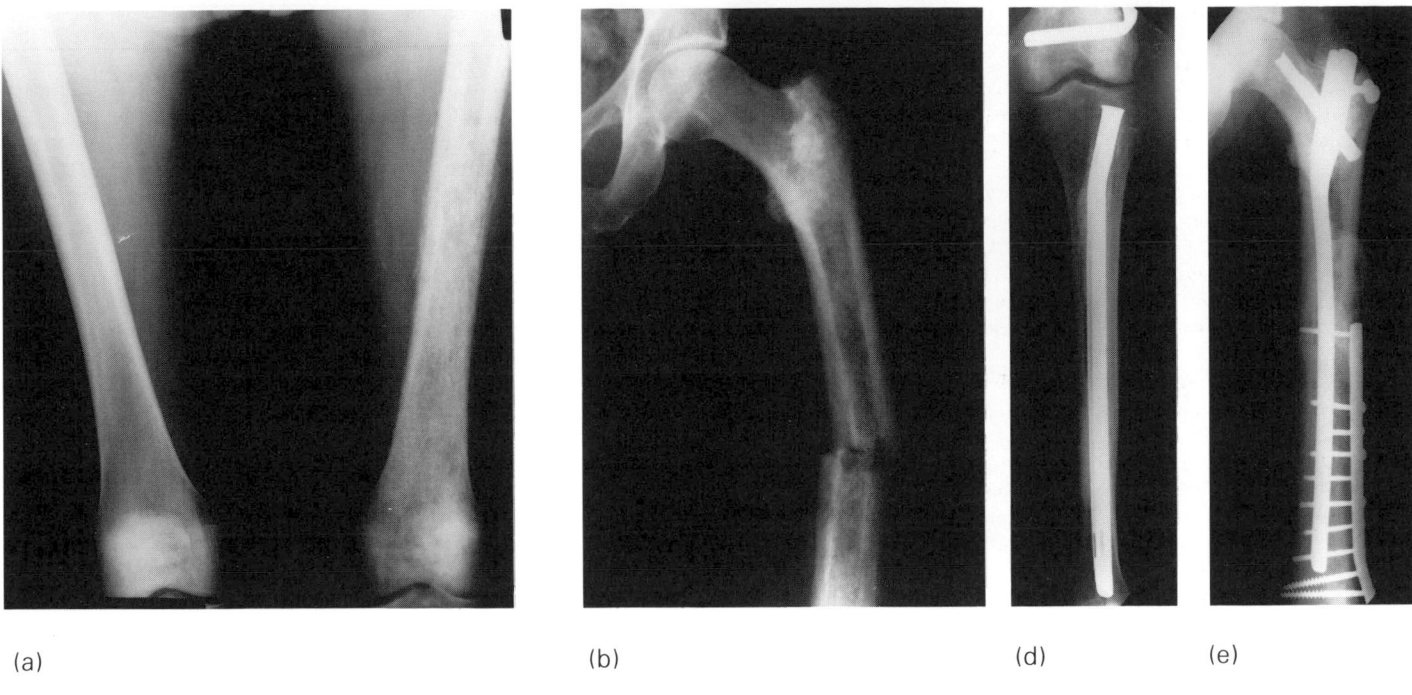

(a)　　　　　　　　　　　　　(b)　　　　　　　　　　(d)　　　　(e)

(c)

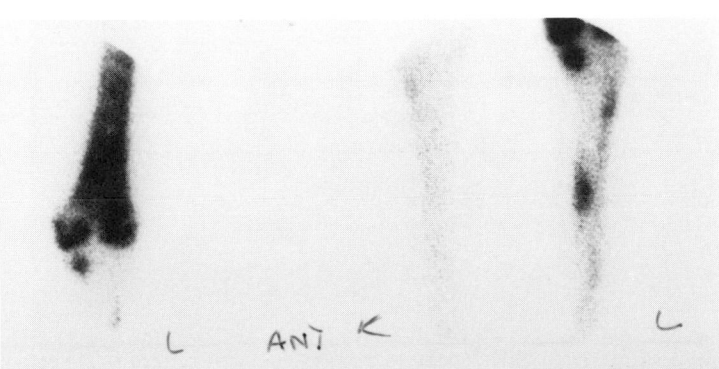

Fig. 1 Patient with carcinoma of the large bowel. The patient had been unsuccessfully treated for pain in his left thigh prior to referral to the orthopaedic clinic. (a) Multiple permeative metastases involving the left femur: the patient was advised to have the femur stabilized, but decided to go home for the weekend to think about surgery. (b) He was admitted as an emergency on Sunday evening with a pathological fracture through the left femur. (c) Skeletal scintigram shows involvement of the entire left femur and multiple lesions in the ipsilateral tibia. (d) and (e) He was treated by internal fixation of the pathological fracture, using a Zickel nail supplemented with methylmethacrylate, stabilization of the distal femur using a blade plate, and stabilization of the tibia using an intramedullary nail also supplemented with methylmethacrylate. All stabilizations were carried out under a single anaesthetic. It may not have been necessary to supplement one of the newer interlocking nails with a blade plate.

Geographic destruction is usually found in the slowest developing metasteses, whereas permeative destruction occurs in the most aggressive lesions. A patient with multiple metastases usually shows one of the three principal patterns.

Primary internal stabilization of the weakened bone has certain advantages (Fig. 2). It is easier to fix the bone whilst it is still intact and the rehabilitation and convalescence are much shorter and easier. The type of internal stabilization depends on the site of the lesion. It is the author's view that it should be the primary treatment in the vast majority of impending fractures, followed by irradiation. Where feasible, closed intramedullary nailing is preferred and, if indicated, a biopsy can be taken using bronchial biopsy forceps or through a separation incision. Care must be taken to avoid producing a fracture when positioning the patient or whilst stabilizing the lesion.

It is essential that the internal stabilization of the lesion provides sufficient strength to allow unsupported use of the limb, including weight bearing in the lower limb. If the implant alone is unlikely to provide this, the stabilization should be supplemented with

methylmethacrylate. The tumour is removed, the cavity is filled with methylmethacrylate whilst still soft, and the implant is fixed across the methylmethacrylate as well as the normal bone above and below the lesion. Filling a large defect with methylmethacrylate has been reported as significantly increasing both axial load and torque strength of the bone (Ryan and Begeman 1984).

Irradiation is an essential part of treatment to inhibit further tumour growth, since the latter will result in progressive bone destruction, resulting in loosening of the stabilization and an increased risk of fracture. Depending on the primary lesion, the patient may also require endocrine therapy or chemotherapy.

Internal fixation carries a theoretical risk of disseminating tumour cells both locally and into the circulation. However, this has never been proved, provided that the lesion is irradiated. Furthermore, there is no evidence that the combined effect of surgical intervention and general anaesthesia has affected the overall prognosis in these patients. On the contrary, there is some experimental evidence that pathological fracture is associated with an increase in the incidence of pulmonary metastases and that prophylactic stabilization of an

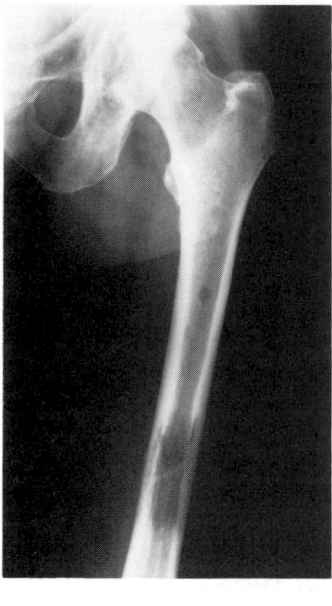
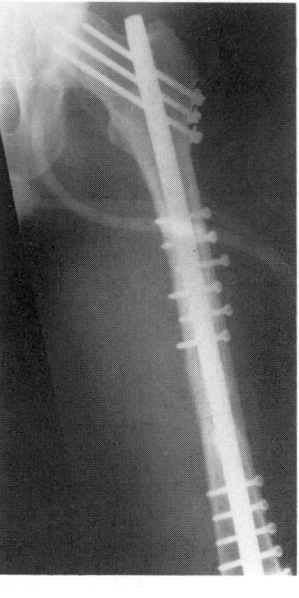

(a)   (b)

Fig. 2 Patient with myeloma who had multiple lytic deposits affecting his left femur. This was treated by internal stabilization using a locking nail and supporting the entire femur.

Table 1 Pathological fractures

Primary tumour	No. of patients	No. of fractures
Breast	101	116
Bronchus	21	22
Prostate	21	22
Kidney	7	7
Rectum	6	6
Bladder	3	3
Stomach	3	3
Melanoma	2	2
Uterus	2	2
Thyroid	1	1
Colon	1	1
Oesophagus	1	1
Bile duct	1	1
Cervix	1	1
Penis	1	1
Squamous cell	1	1
Lymphoma	4	5
Leukaemia	6	6
Myeloma	24	34
Not known	4	4
Total	211	239

Table 2 Pathological fractures

	Site	Number
Pelvis		2
Femur	Transcervical	57
	Intertrochanteric	25
	Subtrochanteric	26
	Shaft	40
	Distal	10
Humerus	Proximal	19
	Shaft	47
	Distal	3
Tibia	Proximal	2
	Shaft	1
Radius	Shaft	2
Ulna	Shaft	1
Clavicle		3
Mandible		1
Total		239

impending pathological fracture decreases the incidence of pulmonary metastases (Bouma *et al.* 1983).

It is important that radiographs and scintigrams of the entire length of the affected bone are obtained prior to treatment so that any other metastasis, which may subsequently develop into a pathological fracture, can be stabilized with the same implant and included in the radiotherapy field. A pathological fracture at the edge of an implant, particularly if the latter has also been fixed with methylmethacrylate, is more difficult to treat than if there were no implant in the bone. Furthermore, it is extremely difficult to irradiate a metastasis if part of the lesion has been included in a previous field.

PATHOLOGICAL FRACTURES

Although virtually every malignant tumour can metastasize to bone and may be associated with a pathological fracture, virtually half are secondary to mammary carcinoma (Table 1), probably because skeletal metastases occur more commonly from this cancer than in association with any other tumour. The commonest site of pathological fracture is in the femur (Table 2), but virtually any long bone is at risk.

The development of a pathological fracture is not necessarily a terminal event. There has been an improvement in survival over the years. In 1974 Galasko reported a mean survival of 10.1 months. Fifty-four per cent of patients survived for more than 3 months and 23 per cent for more than 1 year. The survival was related to the primary tumour, with none of the patients with bronchial carcinoma surviving for more than 6 months, but several of the patients with carcinoma of the breast lived for more than 1 year and some for 6 or 7 years. By 1981 the survival had apparently increased to 19 months (Harrington 1981*b*). Patients with metastatic

prostatic carcinoma survived the longest (29.3 months) compared with mammary carcinoma (22.6 months), renal carcinoma (11.8 months), and bronchial carcinoma (3.6 months). Gainor and Buchert (1983) also reported that none of their patients with fractures from metastatic bronchial carcinoma lived for more than 6 months.

There are three aspects to the treatment of pathological fractures:
(1) orthopaedic management;
(2) localized irradiation;
(3) treatment of the causative tumour.

Orthopaedic management will be discussed in this chapter. Irradiation, chemotherapy, and endocrine therapy are discussed in other chapters. However, it is worth emphasizing that post-operative irradiation is an essential part of management.

The evaluation of a patient with a pathological or impending fracture includes an assessment of the general fitness of the patient,

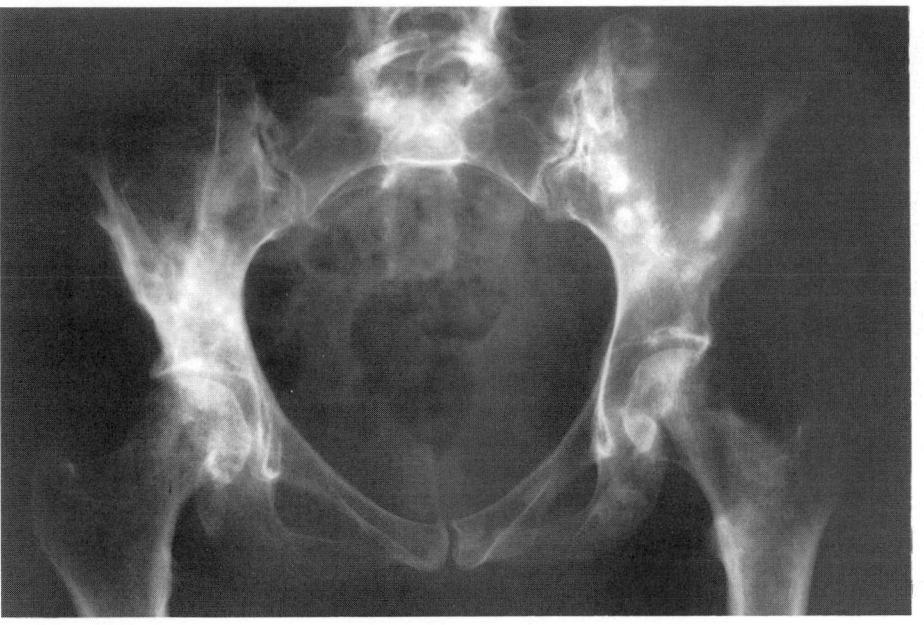

(a)

(b)

Fig. 3 Patient with mammary carcinoma: (a) undisplaced transcervical fracture of the right femur with metastatic involvement of the acetabulum; (b) treatment by total hip replacement arthroplasty using a long-stemmed femoral component.

the degree of dissemination of the tumour, the diagnosis of the primary tumour if not already known, and the presence of other complications. In addition to a careful clinical examination, the evaluation includes appropriate blood tests, radiographs, skeletal scintigrams, and other forms of radiographic imaging as required. If the primary lesion is not known or if there is any uncertainty about the origin of the pathological fracture, a biopsy of the lesion is essential. This can be carried out at the time of surgical stabilization. Biopsy is not an essential part of every internal stabilization, particularly if a closed method of intramedullary fixation is used.

Transcervical femoral fractures

Pathological transcervical femoral fractures do not unite, irrespective of the method of orthopaedic treatment (Galasko 1974), probably owing to the effect of irradiation on an area where fractures are associated with impaired vascularity. This failure of union occurs regardless of the degree of displacement. Replacement arthroplasty gives the best results; the type of arthroplasty depends on the degree of tumour involvement. If the acetabulum is intact, a hemiarthroplasty may be all that is required. It should be cemented into the femoral shaft with methylmethacrylate. If the acetabulum is involved, a total replacement arthroplasty is indicated; the tumour is curetted from the acetabulum and the defect is filled with methylmethacrylate. If there is more extensive involvement of the acetabulum, pelvic reconstruction may be required at the time of arthroplasty (Harrington 1981b). If more distal metastases are found in the femur on pre-operative radiographs or scintigrams, which should be obtained prior to stabilization, a long-stemmed femoral component is used (Fig. 3). It is reasonable to treat each fracture with a long-stemmed total replacement arthroplasty, in case there are acetabular or distal femoral metastases not revealed on the radiological

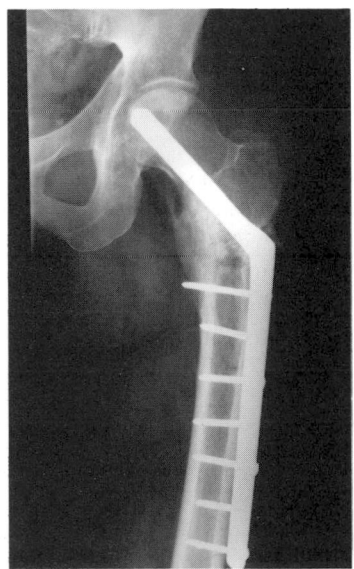

Fig. 4 Patient with mammary carcinoma. Pathological subtrochanteric fracture of the left femur was treated by internal stabilization and post-operative radiotherapy. The fracture was united by bone.

investigations. At the time of surgery the tumour is curetted from the neck of the femur and the defect filled with methylmethacrylate.

Other femoral and tibial fractures

Unlike transcervical femoral fractures, the majority of pathological fractures involving the rest of the femur or tibia are united by bone in patients who survive for more than 3 months, irrespective of the

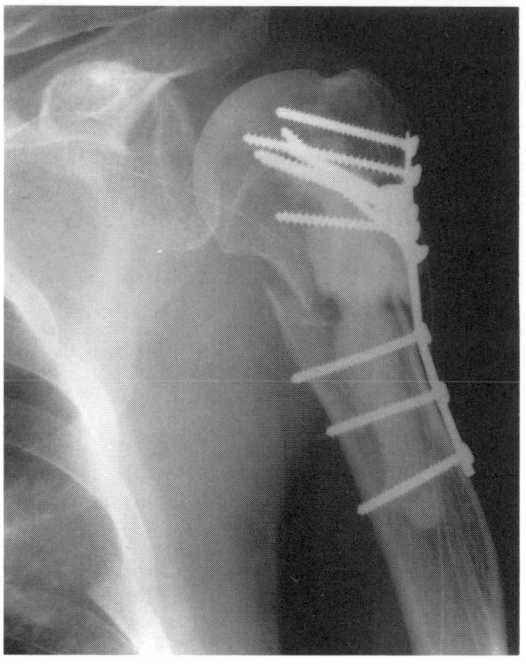

(a)

(b)

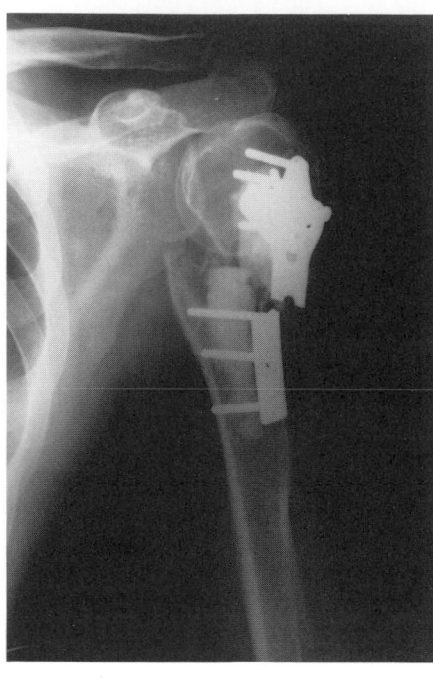

(c)

Fig. 5 (a) Patient with bronchial carcinoma who presented with a pathological fracture of the proximal humerus. (b) The fracture was stabilized with a plate, supplemented by methylmethacrylate. The stabilization is inadequate. (c) Because of the inadequate stabilization, it has given way. The fracture through the plate and the column of methylmethacrylate should be noted.

type of orthopaedic treatment (Galasko 1980) (Fig. 4). However, internal fixation provides definite advantages over external stabilization. It gives the patients greater and much more rapid relief of pain, it is associated with easier nursing, more comfortable turning of the patient, and prevention of pressure sores and it allows much earlier mobilization of the patient and discharge from hospital. As with impending fractures, it is essential to stabilize the bone adequately, sufficient for weight bearing, at the time of surgery. If necessary, the internal fixation must be supplemented by methylmethacrylate, even though this may interfere with callus formation. However, methylmethacrylate will not compensate for inadequate mechanical stability due to a poorly positioned or inadequate implant (Fig. 5). The type of implant depends on the site of the fracture and of other metastases in the same bone. In general terms, fractures of the shaft of the long bone should be fixed by an intramedullary nail, whereas fractures in the metaphysis may require fixation with a plate, blade plate, or locked nail. The method of fixation must also stabilize other metastases in the affected bone to avoid the risk of subsequent fracture adjacent to an implant. Closed intramedullary rodding can be supplemented by methylmethacrylate, but pressure injection of the latter carries the risk of fat embolism (Kunec and Lewis 1984). Gainor and Buchert (1983) reported that 67 per cent of pathological fractures from myeloma united, compared with 44 per cent secondary to metastatic renal cell carcinoma, 37 per cent in mammary carcinoma, and none in bronchial cancer. They also found that internal fixation improved the rate of fracture union by 23 per cent compared with cast immobilization.

Humeral fractures

Internal fixation is of benefit in that it provides the patients with much greater mobility and earlier use of the limb and more rapid and greater pain relief, but the advantages over conservative treatment are not as marked as with pathological fractures of the lower limb (Galasko 1980). McCormack *et al.* (1985) suggested that a functional cast brace was indicated if the patient had a limited life expectancy, but for those patients expected to survive for longer than 3 months internal fixation was the method of choice to ensure pain relief and restoration of function and to avoid later refracture.

Fractures of the proximal humerus may require replacement arthroplasty if they cannot be stabilized (Fig. 6). The indication for replacement arthroplasty is different from that in transcervical femoral fractures. In the humerus, replacement is indicated if it is not possible to stabilize the fracture because of its site or degree of bone destruction, whereas in the femur replacement is indicated because pathological fractures of the femoral neck do not unite irrespective of the method of treatment.

The vast majority of pathological fractures of the humerus, radius, or ulna can be treated by intramedullary nailing. Fractures around the metaphysis may require plate fixation. Where necessary, the implant must be supplemented with methylmethacrylate.

Multiple fractures

Some patients present with several pathological fractures and each must be treated on its merits (Fig. 6).

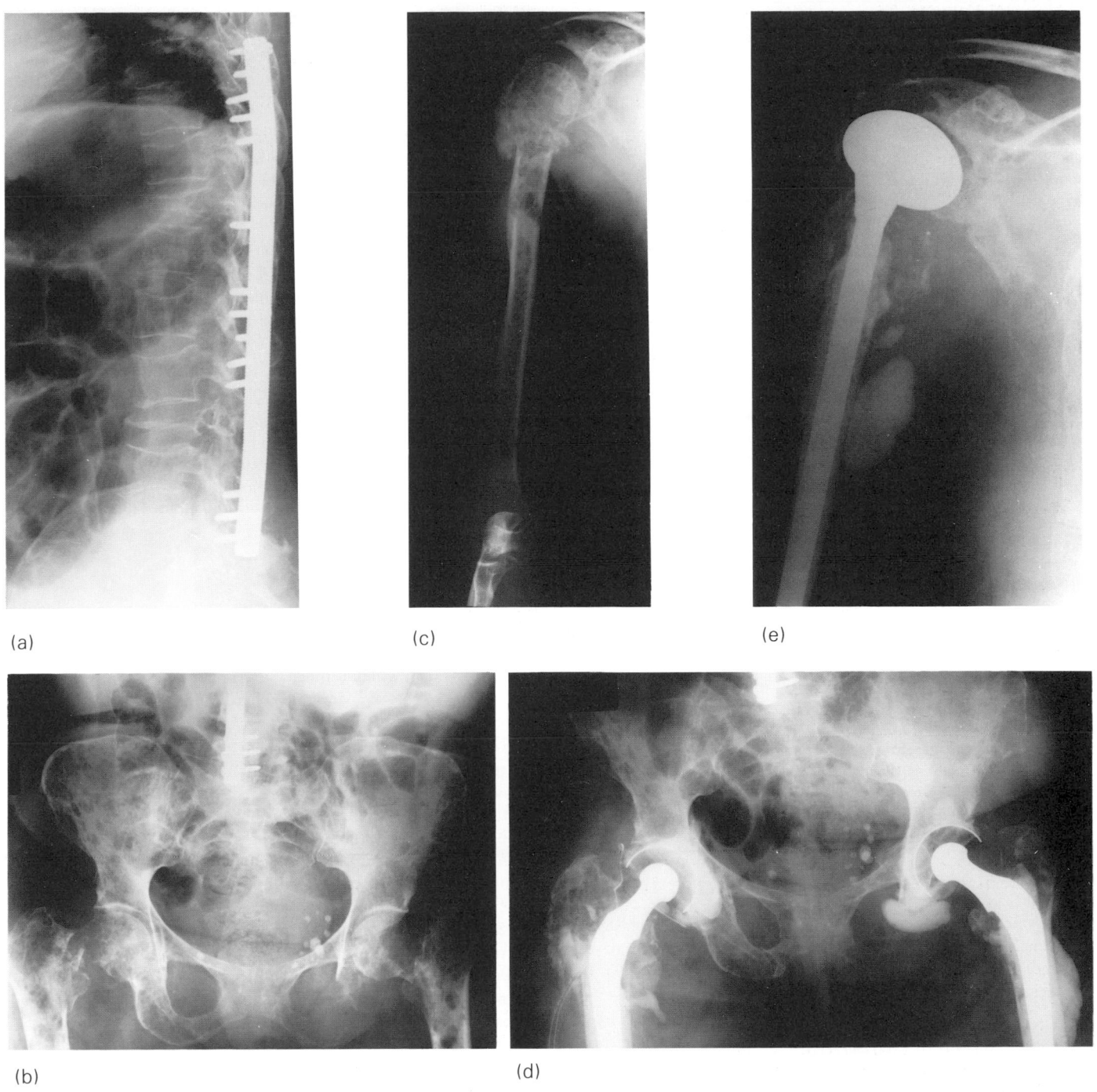

(a)

(c)

(e)

(b)

(d)

Fig. 6 Patient with multiple myeloma. (a) She initially presented with spinal instability which was treated by stabilization with a Banks rod. (b) and (c) Two years later she presented with bilateral pathological transcervical femoral fractures and a fracture of the neck of her right humerus.(d) and (e) She was treated with bilateral long-stemmed total hip replacement arthroplasties and a shoulder hemiarthroplasty.

Fractures through isolated metastasis

Occasionally patients present with an isolated skeletal metastasis. They usually present with pain, sometimes with an impending fracture and, occasionally, with a pathological fracture. The commonest primary is renal carcinoma and, provided that there is no other evidence of dissemination of the tumour, resection of the lesion should be considered, in the form of either localized resection and customized prosthetic replacement or amputation.

Highly vascular lesions

Occasional metastases, particularly those from renal carcinoma, may be highly vascular and surgery may be associated with massive blood

Table 3 Spinal instability

Primary tumour	No. of patients
Breast	30[a]+1[b]
Myeloma	8
Prostate	2
Melanoma	2
Bronchus	1
Kidney	1
Colon	1
Uterus	1
Cervix	1
Vagina	1
Stomach	1
Parotid	1
Lymphoma	1
Chondrosarcoma	1
Histiocytoma	1
Cordoma	1
Total	54+1[b]

[a] One patient's metastatic destruction was too extensive for surgical stabilization.
[b] Lumbar stabilization 22 months after successful dorsal stabilization.

Table 4 Spinal instability: results

Destruction too extensive for surgical reconstruction	1
Infection resulting in removal of implant	1
Loosening of implant	2
Pain relief	
Complete	49
Partial	2
Complications in the 51 patients with pain relief	
Infection (successfully treated)	1
Wound breakdown (successful secondary suture)	1
Fracture (L rod requiring additional anterior stabilization)	1
Fracture (Hartshill rectangle at 5 years)	1

loss. Pre-operative angiography is frequently indicated in metastases from renal carcinoma and pre-operative embolization may be indicated if the lesion is highly vascular (Roscoe *et al.* 1989). In such lesions amputation may be occasionally necessary.

Post-operative irradiation

Local irradiation is an essential part of treatment to control the tumour and to prevent progressive destruction of the bone and loosening and failure of the implant used to stabilize the fracture. Irradiation can be delayed until the wound has healed, but this is not essential. The implant does not appear to affect the irradiation, provided that megavoltage is used.

Radiotherapy does not interfere with fracture healing, provided that the fracture is adequately immobilized (Bonarigo and Rubin 1967; Gainor and Buchert 1983). Fracture of the humeral shaft treated by intramedullary nailing and post-operative radiotherapy healed more rapidly than non-pathological traumatic fractures at the same site and with greater amounts of bone (Galasko 1980).

The causative tumour must be treated on its merit by hormonal or endocrine therapy as indicated.

FRACTURE IN A PATIENT WITH MALIGNANT DISEASE BUT NO EVIDENCE OF DISSEMINATION

Patients with an underlying malignancy may develop a fracture like any other individual without a metastasis at the site of fracture. However, if the patient has a past history of malignancy and there is no evidence of dissemination, a biopsy should be taken from the fracture. In some instances this may be the first manifestation of dissemination of the disease, even though there has been a long disease-free interval.

Non-pathological fractures must be treated on their merits, as should other non-metastatic orthopaedic conditions (Galasko 1986).

The development of a non-pathological fracture in such a patient may subsequently be associated with dissemination of the cancer. The author has experience of two patients with mammary carcinoma, of whom one developed a transcervical femoral fracture 16 years after mastectomy and the other developed a fracture dislocation of a hip 22 years after mastectomy. In both patients there was no evidence of dissemination at the time of the fracture and histological examination of biopsies taken from the fractured bone end showed no tumour, yet both patients developed multiple metastases affecting lung and bone within 3 months of their fracture.

SPINAL INSTABILITY

Back pain is a frequent symptom in patients with disseminated carcinoma and in 10 per cent is due to spinal instability (Galasko and Sylvester 1978). Spinal instability can be associated with excruciating pain which is mechanical in nature. In the severe form the patient is only comfortable when lying absolutely still. Any movement, including log rolling by two or three trained nurses is associated with exquisite pain. The patient may not be able to sit, stand, or walk because of the pain, even with the use of a spinal orthosis.

In the milder form the patient may be relatively free from pain when wearing a rigid spinal orthosis, but any movement of the back (for example, turning in bed, sitting, or standing) may be impossible without the support. Radiographs show destruction of bone with some degree of vertebral collapse. No discrete fracture can be seen. Nevertheless, spinal instability should be considered the equivalent of a pathological fracture in a long bone because the pain is due to the instability and not the metastasis. Radiotherapy or chemotherapy will not alleviate the pain. As with pathological fracture of the long bones, immobilization is required for pain relief (Galasko 1991).

We have treated 54 patients with spinal instability secondary to spinal metastases. The primary tumours are shown in Table 3; the commonest is carcinoma of the breast. The survival is similar to that following pathological fractures of the long bones, with several of our patients being alive 4, 5, and 6 years after their stabilization. The results are shown in Table 4.

Several methods of spinal stabilization are available. The author prefers the use of a posterior implant that can be fixed to the spine at multiple levels with either screws or sublaminal wires (Figs 7–9). The implant must be fixed to at least two, but preferably three, vertebrae above the unstable segment and to two or three vertebrae below it. Pre-operative radiographs and skeletal scintigrams are important and if there are two areas of instability, the stabilization should support both areas. If posterior stabilization is not likely to provide sufficient support (for example, instability at the fifth lumbar level), it must be combined with an anterior stabilization. If the

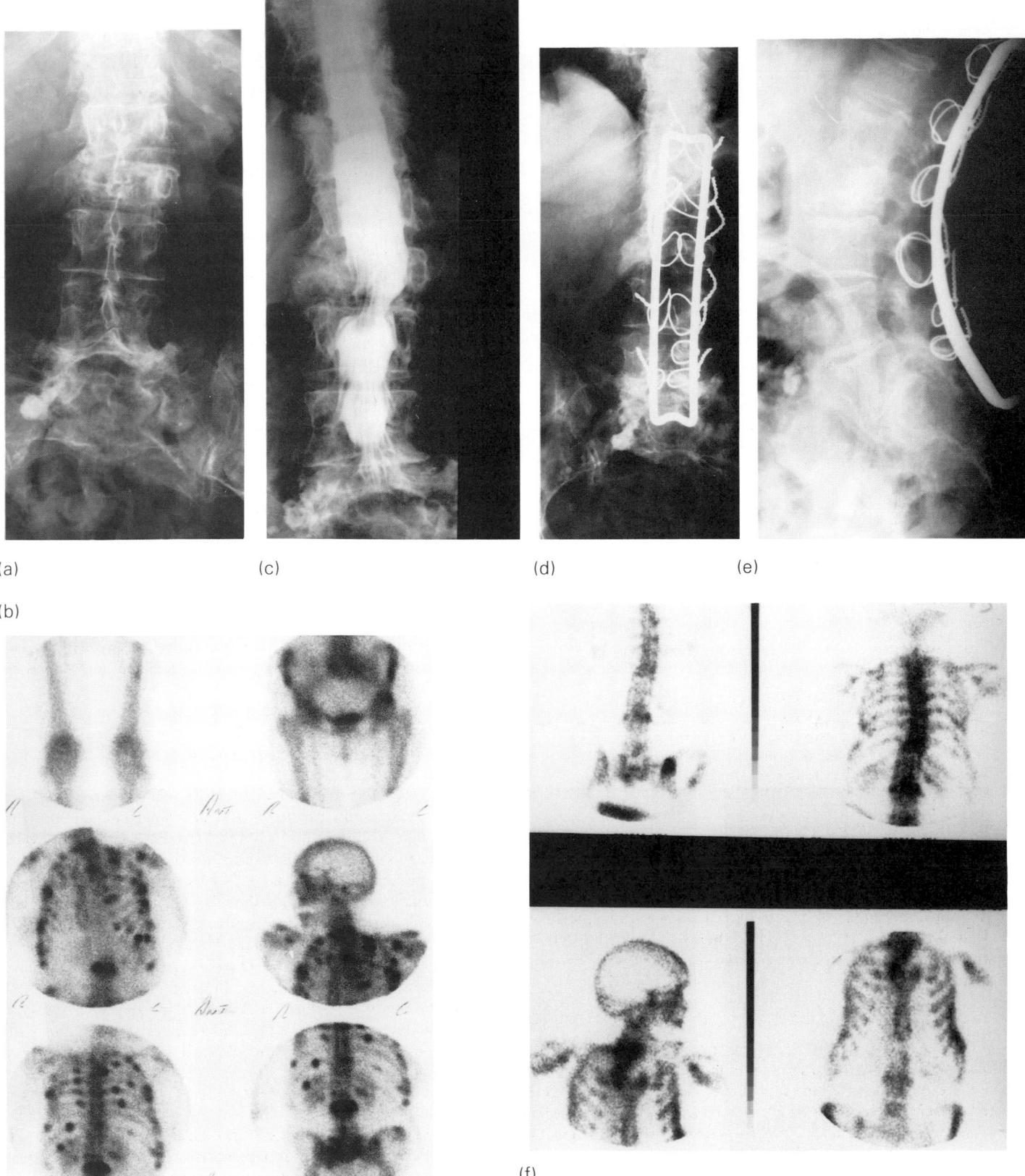

(a)

(b)

(c)

(d)

(e)

(f)

Fig. 7 Patient with mammary carcinoma who presented with severe low back pain and weakness affecting her left lower limb. (a) Anteroposterior radiograph of the lumbar spine indicating destruction of L3 with instability at that level. (b) ^{99m}Tc-MDP scintigram showing multiple skeletal metastases. (c) CT radiculogram showing compression of the cauda equina at the level of the lesion. (d) and (e) The patient was treated by decompression, stabilization using a Hartshill rectangle, localized irradiation, and endocrine therapy. Anteroposterior and lateral radiographs taken 3 years after surgery are shown. There has been reconstitution of the vertebral body. A lumbar lordosis has been moulded into the implant to maintain sitting balance post-surgery.(f) ^{99m}Tc-MDP scintigram taken 3 years after surgery. The metastases have responded to treatment. The patient is still alive 5 years after surgery.

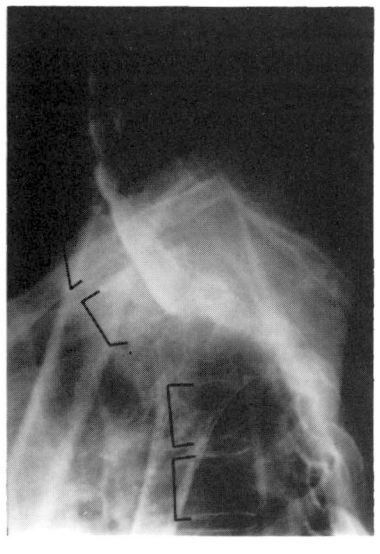

(a)   (b)

Fig. 8 Patient with carcinoma of the cervix who presented with back pain due to spinal instability and weakness of her lower limbs. (a) Lumbar myelogram. There is gross destruction of the L3 vertebra and complete obstruction to the column of dye seen on the lateral film. (b) She was treated by decompression, stabilization using a Banks rod, and post-operative radiotherapy. Following stabilization, she regained full power and her pain settled.

stabilization extends to the sacrum, a lumbar lordosis must be moulded into the implant to prevent a post-operative flat back which will interfere with sitting (Fig. 7).

Spinal instability can affect the cervical spine as well as the dorsal or lumbar spine. Anterior and/or posterior spinal stabilization may be required for the cervical spine (Fidler 1987). Minor degrees of cervical instability can usually be controlled by a surgical collar.

There was an associated neurological deficit in 28 of our patients with instability of their dorsal or lumbar spine. These patients did not present because of compression of the spinal cord or cauda equina but with pain due to spinal instability. However, evidence of cord or cauda equina compression was found on clinical examination. We routinely carry out a CT radiculogram or magnetic resonance imaging prior to spinal stabilization. Irrespective of any clinical evidence of cord or cauda equina compression, the cord or cauda equina is decompressed at the time of stabilization if there is any evidence of compression on the pre-operative CT radiculogram or magnetic resonance scan. Magnetic resonance imaging is preferable to CT radiculography. Both laminae and the spinous process are removed as the implant should provide sufficient stability. Twenty of the patients recovered significantly, although two developed recurrent signs of cord compression some months later. One other patient developed cord compression 9 months after stabilization. Eleven of the 17 patients reported by DeWald *et al.* (1985) had an associated neurological deficit. Five of these recovered significantly after spinal decompression and stabilization.

An alternative method of spinal decompression and stabilization is via an anterior approach with excision of the affected vertebral body, decompression of the dural sheath from the front, and subsequent stabilization of the spine using methylmethacrylate (Harrington 1981*a*).

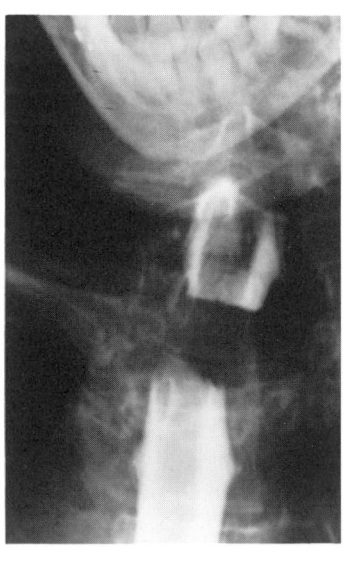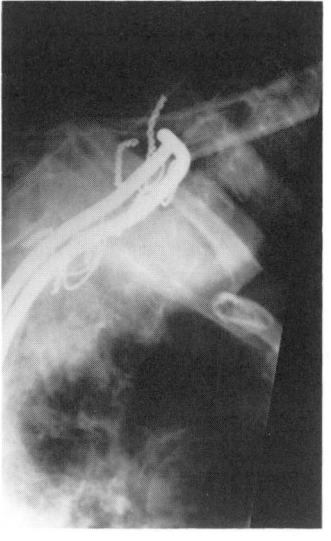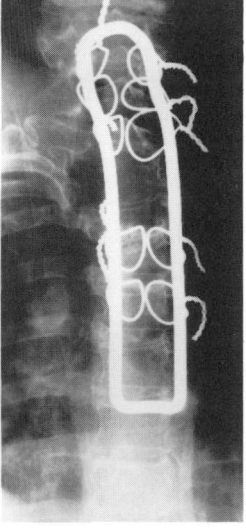

(a)   (b)   (c)   (d)

Fig. 9 Patient with mammary carcinoma who presented with severe upper thoracic pain due to spinal instability, paraplegia, and urine retention of 8 h duration. (a) Lateral radiograph showing destruction of D3 with subluxation of D2 upon D4. The anterior borders of the vertebral bodies are indicated. (b) Myelogram showing complete obstruction at the level of the lesion. The patient was treated by surgical stabilization using a Hartshill rectangle, posterior decompression, and post-operative irradiation. (c) and (d) Post-operative radiographs showing correction of the subluxation. Six weeks after surgery the patient walked out of hospital.

As with pathological fractures of the long bones, post-operative irradiation is an essential part of treatment. Pre-operative irradiation should be avoided, as it may be associated with delayed wound healing, wound breakdown, and infection. We have seen one patient who developed acute post-irradiation transverse myelitis with complete irreversible paraplegia before being referred for surgical stabilization of her metastasis. Spinal decompression revealed a swollen oedematous spinal cord with no intracanal spread from the vertebral metastasis.

Chemotherapy or endocrine therapy is also required where the metastases have occurred from primary tumours which are sensitive to these therapeutic modalities.

SUMMARY

The development of an impending fracture, pathological fracture, or spinal instability is not necessarily a terminal event. These lesions are associated with severe pain. The aims of treatment are to alleviate pain and restore mobility and the use of the affected limb or spine. With the exception of pathological transcervical femoral fractures, this is best achieved by internal stabilization. The former usually requires replacement arthroplasty. The type of stabilization depends on the site of the lesion and, if it is not adequate to provide unsupported use of the limb, it should be supplemented by methylmethacrylate.

Post-operative radiotherapy is an essential part of treatment, and the causative tumour should be treated by chemotherapy or endocrine therapy where indicated.

Before treating these lesions, the patient must be carefully evaluated to determine the degree of dissemination of his or her cancer, particularly any other areas of involvement in the affected bone, as this may influence the type of stabilization.

Optimum treatment of these lesions frequently requires major surgery, which probably should not be carried out if the patient is terminal. If the patient has only a few days to live, it is best to make them comfortable and immobilize the fracture or unstable spine with a suitable support. However, if the patient is likely to survive for at least some weeks, major surgery may be indicated to palliate the severe symptoms secondary to pathological fractures or spinal instability and to allow the patient to die with dignity. Finally, major surgery may also be required for non-neoplastic skeletal disorders to give the patient the optimum quality of life.

REFERENCES

Bonarigo BC, Rubin P (1967). Non-union of pathologic fracture after radiation therapy. *Radiology*, **88**:889–98.

Bouma WH, Mulder JH, Hop WCJ (1983). The influence of intramedullary nailing upon the development of metastases in the treatment of an impending pathological fracture: an experimental study. *Clinical and Experimental Metastasis*, **1**:205–12.

Cheng DS, Seitz CB, Eyre HJ (1980). Nonoperative management of femoral, humeral and acetabular metastases in patients with breast carcinoma. *Cancer*, **45**:1533–7.

De Wald RL, Bridwell KH, Prodromas C, Rodts MF (1985). Reconstructive spinal surgery as palliation for metastatic malignancies of the spine. *Spine*, **10**:21–6.

Edelstyn GA, Gillespie PJ, Grebbel FS (1967). The radiological demonstration of osseous metastases. Experimental observations. *Clinical Radiology*, **18**:158–62.

Fidler M (1981). Incidence of fracture through metastases in long bones. *Acta Orthopaedica Scandinavica*, **52**:623–7.

Fidler MW (1987). Pathological fractures of the spine including those causing anterior spinal cord compression. In *Recent developments in orthopaedic surgery* (ed. J Noble and CSB Galasko), pp. 94–103. Manchester University Press.

Gainor BJ, Buchert P (1983). Fracture healing in metastatic bone disease. *Clinical Orthopaedics and Related Research*, **178**:297–302.

Galasko CSB (1974). Pathological fractures secondary to metastatic cancer. *Journal of the Royal College of Surgeons, Edinburgh*, **19**:351–62.

Galasko CSB (1980). The management of skeletal meatastases. *Journal of the Royal College of Surgeons, Edinburgh*, **25**:143–61.

Galasko CSB (1986). *Skeletal metasteses*. Butterworths, London.

Galasko CSB (1991). Spinal instability secondary to metastatic cancer. *Journal of Bone and Joint Surgery*, **73B**:104–8.

Galasko CSB, Sylvester BS (1978). Back pain in patients treated for malignant tumours. *Clinical Oncology*, **4**:273–83.

Harrington KD (1981*a*). The use of methylmethacrylate for vertebral-body replacement and anterior stabilisation of pathological fracture-dislocations of the spine due to metastatic malignant disease. *Journal of Bone and Joint Surgery*, **63A**:36–46.

Harrington KD (1981*b*). The management of acetabular insufficiency secondary to metastatic malignant disease. *Journal of Bone and Joint Surgery*, **63A**:653–84.

Kunec JR, Lewis RJ (1984). Closed intramedullary rodding of pathologic fractures with supplemental cement. *Clinical Orthopaedics and Related Research*, **188**:183–6.

McCormack RR Jr, Glass DB, Lane JM (1985). Functional cast bracing of metastatic humeral shaft lesion. *Orthopaedic Transactions*, **9**:50–1.

Roscoe MW, McBroom RJ, St Louis E, Grossman H, Perrin R. (1989). Preoperative embolization in the treatment of osseous metastases from renal cell carcinoma. *Clinical Orthopaedics and Related Research*, **238**:302–7.

Ryan JR, Begeman PC (1984). The effects of filling experimental large cortical defects with methylmethacrylate. *Clinical Orthopaedics and Related Research*, **185**:306–10.

19.8   Complications related to radiotherapy

ALBERT J. VAN DER KOGEL AND K. KIAN ANG

GENERAL CONCEPT OF RADIATION-INDUCED COMPLICATIONS

Tolerance dose: definition and significance

It is stated repeatedly in standard textbooks that the aim of radiation treatment is to cure malignant tumours (that is, to eradicate malignant cells capable of indefinite proliferation) without producing unacceptable adverse effects to the surrounding normal tissues. When such a condition is satisfied, then it is said that the treatment has resulted in a favourable therapeutic ratio.

In reality, however, only a few tumours are so profoundly radiosensitive that they can be controlled locally by radiation doses carrying negligible or zero risk of normal tissue injury. Examples of these unusual tumours are seminoma and some lymphoma

This work was supported in part by the Dutch Cancer Society and by grant CA06294 awarded by the National Cancer Institute, United States Department of Health and Human Services.

subtypes. In the vast majority of cancers, a reasonable cure rate can only be obtained with radiation doses that are associated with a certain risk of normal tissue damage. In other words, radiation doses required to cure most cancers are close to the level that is 'tolerated' by the surrounding normal tissues. Under these circumstances no clear-cut or stringent rule can be applied to define the acceptability of adverse effects. In fact, whether a tissue injury is considered acceptable or excessive frequently depends on a large number of factors. The relative importance of these factors may differ in various clinical contexts. Therefore, the tissue 'tolerance dose' should be viewed as a guideline that has to be applied with clinical judgement in different sets of circumstances. Operationally, it could be defined as the radiation dose regimen that produces the largest therapeutic differential between the probability of cure and the incidence of complications in a given group of patients (Ang et al. 1985; Withers 1989).

The best known factor determining the tolerance of tissues to ionizing radiation is dose fractionation. This topic is dealt with in detail in the chapter on the biological basis of radiotherapy. The relevance of other factors will be discussed briefly in this chapter. For simplicity, they are divided into four categories, although it should be realized that these factors are frequently interrelated.

Functional reserve of tissues

Tissues differ markedly in their structural and functional organization. At one end of the spectrum are tissues such as the lung, liver, and bone-marrow that are composed of a very large number of identical functional units. In physiological conditions, such tissues have abundant functional reserve since the number of functional units they possess far exceeds what is needed for their proper functioning. Thus, loss of individual components is of no consequence in these tissues until their functional reserve is exhausted and the tolerance of such tissues to radiation depends very much on the volume irradiated. In the treatment of bronchial carcinoma, for instance, it is customary to deliver 60–66 Gy (in 2 Gy fractions) to a portion of the lung. This treatment results in total elimination of the function of the lung tissue within the radiation portal but it is tolerated, except in cases of severe emphysema, because respiration can be secured by the remaining lung tissue. In contrast, when both lungs are to be irradiated, such as in the elective treatment of patients with osteosarcoma of the limb (van der Schueren and Breur 1982), the dose has to be limited to 20 Gy in order to avoid fatal respiratory insufficiency. The same principle applies to the liver and bone-marrow. Thus, the tolerance of this class of tissues depends to a large extent on the volume irradiated.

The structural and functional organization of the kidney resembles that of the lung and bone-marrow. It has a large reserve with regard to its excretory function. Therefore, irradiation of a portion of a kidney to high doses will not compromise the exocrine function. However, the resultant small area of renal fibrosis could be detrimental through induction of malignant hypertension by endocrine (renin–angiotensin) perturbations (Kim et al. 1984). Hence, the relative tolerance dose for partial renal irradiation is not as high as that for the lung.

At the other end of the spectrum are tissues that are composed of specialized elements each carrying out very specific functions. A typical example is the nervous system. Radiation-induced damage even to a small area of the tissue invariably leads to a permanent deficit since the uninjured components are not able to take over the functions of the affected elements. As a consequence, the tolerance dose of such tissues is only slightly influenced by the volume of the tissue irradiated. The volume effect in this group of tissues relates more to the increased probability of inducing a lesion within the irradiated region as a larger volume is treated. In addition, irradiating a larger volume of tissues may result in a more severe functional failure because of elimination of a larger number of tissue elements.

Nature of radiation injury

The acceptability of a treatment-induced side-effect depends very much on its functional and cosmetic repercussions and on the possibility of remedying the tissue breakdown. Osteoradionecrosis of the mandible for example, is certainly annoying since it requires rigorous medical care, including therapy with hyperbaric oxygen. In refractory cases it may even be necessary to resort to a hemimandibulectomy. However, a good functional and cosmetic result can be obtained after partial mandible resection with modern reconstructive techniques. Thus, osteoradionecrosis of the mandible is generally considered more acceptable than, for instance, an optic chiasm injury leading to irreversible bilateral blindness or a cervical myelopathy resulting in permanent quadriplegia. Consequently, it is easier to accept a 5 per cent risk of developing mandibular necrosis as a trade-off for a chance of tumour control than a 5 per cent risk of bilateral blindness or quadriplegia.

Disease status

The disease status is a very important determinant in assessing the acceptability of adverse radiation effects. Elective treatment should carry a minimal risk of complications, particularly when the proportion of patients at risk for developing recurrence is not high (for example, elective nodal treatment in patients with T2 N0 carcinoma of the supraglottic larynx). In contrast, it is judicious to accept a higher risk of complications in the treatment of a disease for which failure to control or an alternative therapy modality, such as surgery, will produce major functional deficits (for example, intramedullary spinal tumour).

The general condition of patients also has to be taken into account in the assessment of the acceptability of side-effects. Severe transient radiation reactions are a minor price to pay in return for a good probability of cure. In fact, curative radiotherapy is frequently given at a pace that induces quite severe, but reversible, acute side-effects. Such acute toxicity is usually unacceptable for patients with a short life expectancy or in poor general condition.

Subjective factors

A given side-effect that is acceptable for one person may not be acceptable to another individual because of professional, social, or other factors. Similarly, it is also possible that one physician is prepared to take a higher risk than another. These factors frequently play a role in day-to-day therapeutic decision-making, but it is difficult to quantify their overall impact.

In summary, it is not realistic to define tissue tolerance doses without taking the whole clinical context into account. Therefore, the tolerance dose of a tissue in a given treatment situation is defined as a dose regimen that produces the maximum complication-free survival.

Time course and pathogenesis of radiation injury

Morbidities associated with irradiation of normal tissues are divided into acute reactions and late complications, depending on the time of manifestation of injury relative to radiation treatment. By definition, acute reactions occur during a course of fractionated irradiation. They are observed in rapidly proliferating tissues that are organized into stem cell (clonogen), maturation, and functional compartments such as epithelia and bone-marrow. In most cases radiation-induced injury in this class of tissues can be attributed to mitotic-linked reproductive killing of stem cells. The time of onset of acute radiation reactions correlates with the life-span of the differentiated functional cells and the intensity of reactions reflects the balance between the rate of stem cell killing and the rate of regeneration of surviving clonogens.

Late radiation sequelae appear months to years after therapy has been completed and occur in tissues characterized by slow cellular turnover, such as mature connective tissues and parenchyma of various organs. Since tissues that manifest late effects generally have less well-defined proliferative compartments, it is more difficult to ascribe injury to death of a single cell type. Therefore, it has not been established whether the final injury results predominantly from damage to the parenchymal elements or the stromal elements of slowly proliferating tissues (Hopewell 1980; Withers *et al.* 1980). It has been suggested that the late effects are more likely to be the consequence of damage to both elements (van der Kogel 1980).

The distinction between the radiation response characteristics of these two classes of tissues has important clinical implications. Since acute reactions are usually observed during the course of a conventionally fractionated radiotherapy schedule (1.8–2 Gy per fraction, five times a week), it is possible to adjust the dose regimen in the event that the reactions are too severe to allow a sufficient number of stem cells to survive. These surviving stem cells will repopulate and restore the structural and functional integrity of the rapidly proliferating tissues. However, if the overall treatment time is drastically reduced, the acute reactions may not reach the maximum intensity before completion of treatment. This precludes the possibility of adjusting the dose regimen to the grade of reactions. If intensive ultrashort fractionation schedules reduce the number of surviving stem cells to below what is needed for effective tissue restoration, acute reactions will persist for some time and may progress into chronic injury, which is referred to as consequential late complications (Peters *et al.* 1988). Examples of such complications are persistent mucosal ulceration and fistulae observed in patients with head and neck cancers treated with three fractions of 2 Gy per day, 4 h apart, to total doses of 48–56 Gy over 9–10 days (Peracchia and Salti 1981).

Obviously, since late effects never have their onset before completion of radiation treatment, therapeutic decisions can be made only on a probability basis based on empirical data. By careful clinical observation in patients treated with conventional fractionation schedules, a certain relationship has been established between the intensity of acute reactions and the severity of late complications. This relationship is sometimes applied for minor therapy adjustments because of concerns about late complications when an unexpected degree of acute reaction is observed. When unconventional regimens are used, this established relationship no longer applies because of the differential effects of changing the size of dose per fraction and overall time on the two classes of tissue (Peters *et al.* 1992). The unexpected occurrence of radiation myelopathy in patients who were treated with a concentrated hyperfractionated accelerated radiotherapy (CHART) schedule (Dische and Saunders 1989) emphasizes this.

Volume effects

Volume effect is an interesting but also a confusing issue in radiotherapy. The reason for the confusion is that the impact of radiation volume on the tolerance varies among tissues and organs because of differences in their structural and functional organization. As mentioned earlier, the tolerance dose for tissues with a large functional reserve (that is, those with functional units arranged in parallel), depends to a large extent on the volume irradiated. In contrast, the tolerance dose of tissues with limited functional reserve is only slightly affected by the radiation volume.

Other factors may also play a rôle in determining the volume effects. Notably, recovery through migration of stem cells from surrounding unirradiated areas has been demonstrated in the skin. It is obvious that this type of recovery is more efficient when only a small region of skin is irradiated. In addition, the subjective repercussions vary with the volume of tissue injury. For instance, the same degree of mucositis over a large area of oral cavity produces more symptoms than over a small area. In fact, the difference in the intensity of symptoms is frequently called upon by clinicians as evidence of a volume effect.

SITE-SPECIFIC COMPLICATIONS

In this section we address common and significant complications encountered in daily clinical practice rather than compiling an exhaustive list of all possible side-effects.

Skin and adnexae

From the earliest days of radiotherapy, skin has probably been investigated more than any other normal tissue. The orthovoltage X-rays used previously caused the highest dose to be deposited near the surface and, as a result, skin was often a dose-limiting structure. In the absence of radiobiological models to guide the radiotherapist, total doses were adjusted based on the appearance of a well-defined skin reaction; that is, the 'skin erythema dose'. This reflects the erythematous reaction starting in the second to third week of a fractionated course, which is believed to be a secondary inflammatory reaction to the depletion of the basal stem cell population. Depending on the level of depletion and interference with the continuous renewal of the differentiated epidermal cell layers, this reaction may progress to dry or moist desquamation of the epidermis after 4–6 weeks. When severe, moist desquamation may progress to a secondary ulceration.

However, with modern megavoltage radiotherapy, where the maximum dose deposition is 0.5–4 cm below the surface, epidermal reactions are usually limited to dry desquamation and increased pigmentation. This moderate skin response is seen after conventional irradiation with daily fractions of 2 Gy up to a total dose of approximately 60–65 Gy in the target volume, but only 40–50 Gy total in the basal layer of the epidermis. This dose is tolerated by the skin because a substantial part of the recovery takes place by stem cell proliferation during the 6–8 weeks of irradiation. The total tolerated dose for skin, as well as for several other acutely responding tissues such as the oral or gastrointestinal mucosa, depends to a much smaller extent on fraction size compared with most late-responding critical organs. In contrast, variations in overall time can have a large but less predictable influence on the tolerance of acutely responding tissues. As an approximation, skin tolerance doses decrease by approximately 3–4 Gy/week when treatment duration is shortened from the standard 6–8 weeks. An example of the most drastic reductions of treatment time to only 12 days is the CHART regimen for the management of carcinomas of the head and neck and bronchus (Saunders *et al.* 1991). With this strategy, a total dose of 54 Gy given in 36 fractions, three times a day, is well tolerated by the skin. However, acute mucosal reactions preclude dose escalation or further shortening of the duration of treatment (see below).

Epidermal recovery is usually complete within 2 weeks of completion of fractionated radiotherapy. Hair loss may occur after doses of 5–10 Gy. With doses of up to 50 Gy, in 2 Gy fractions, hair regrowth starts within a few months. Alopecia is likely to be permanent after higher doses. The sebaceous glands appear to be more sensitive and usually do not regain function after 40–50 Gy, resulting in a permanently dry skin (Trott and Kummermehr 1991).

With modern high-energy X-rays a higher dose is deposited below the surface and therefore late damage may occur in the dermis in the absence of acute reactions. These are characterized by atrophy leading to contraction of the irradiated area and a clinical appearance of induration. This so-called 'radiation fibrosis' is not really an accumulation of fibrous tissue but is mostly due to contraction (Hopewell 1990). In pig skin, which has been shown to be very similar to human skin in its radiation response, two separate phases of dermal thinning have been described (Hopewell 1990). The first phase, which takes place within a year, is believed to be the result of a loss of capillaries and a decline of dermal blood flow. The second phase, which is observed after approximately 1 year, may be due to the degeneration of the arteriolar smooth muscle cells, although the loss of fibroblasts could not be excluded as the underlying mechanism. The progressive occurrence of telangiectasia beyond 1 year points to the continuing involvement of the vasculature in the late phases of radiation injury to the dermis.

After initially having applied the Ellis formula to all types of skin effects, it was soon realized that different time–dose relationships applied to early and late effects in skin. The differential between early and late effects in a particular tissue was first demonstrated in extensive experimental studies in pig skin (Berry et al. 1974; Withers et al. 1978). This was subsequently confirmed in human skin, the most thoroughly studied human tissue (Turesson and Thames 1989). It was shown in patients with breast cancer receiving radiotherapy with 200 kV X-rays or 12–13 MeV electrons that spotty to confluent desquamation of the skin started to occur at epidermal doses of 35–40 Gy, with a 50 per cent incidence at approximately 50 Gy in 2 Gy fractions (Turesson and Thames 1989). The total dose for a ten fraction regimen was only approximately 5 per cent lower than that for a 25 fraction schedule delivered over the same overall time. In contrast, for late effects (that is, significant telangiectasia at 5 years in 50 per cent of the patients), the difference in the equivalent total doses between the two fractionation schemes was 24 per cent.

Although these findings are conceptually important, it should be realized that in modern radiotherapy the dose to the subcutis with resulting fibrosis or telangiectasia is in general more of a limiting factor rather than acute epidermal reactions. After irradiations of vocal cord cancer, subcutaneous fibrosis was observed to occur above a threshold dose of 68.5 Gy in 25–28 fractions, with a steep rise in incidence between 69 and 75.4 Gy (Parsons 1984). A threshold of 60–65 Gy in 2 Gy fractions was reported for fibrosis of the breast (van Limbergen et al. 1989); this may be due to a larger irradiated volume, but other factors such as differences in dosimetry may also contribute.

The influence of treatment volume on skin tolerance is a disputed issue. For acute skin reactions it seems logical to ascribe the volume effect to differences in regeneration rate and intensity of symptoms. Severe moist desquamation over 10 cm² of skin heals rapidly by migration of basal cells from the edges of the field and is tolerable to the patient. A similar effect over a larger area is less likely to heal by cell migration and is more bothersome to the patient. Correspondingly, a large area of skin fibrosis is more annoying

and also more prone to trauma with a secondary tissue breakdown.

No specific treatment is available for radiation-induced acute and late skin injuries. Dry desquamation is managed by moisturizing ointments commencing after completion of radiation. Supportive care, such as rinsing with diluted hydrogen peroxide to prevent infection and regular application of moisturizing ointments, may promote healing of moist skin desquamation. Care should be taken to prevent traumatic injury to atrophic skin.

Haemopoietic tissues

The effects of radiation on haemopoiesis depend on the radiation dose and, even more, on the volume of the marrow and lymphoid tissues irradiated. The age of the individual is important in view of the differences in the distribution of the active marrow throughout the skeleton (Custer and Ahfeldt 1932). As a consequence, when a given anatomical site is irradiated, the proportion of active marrow encompassed in the field varies with the age of the individual.

Localized irradiation, such as that used in the local-regional treatment of breast cancer, head and neck tumours, or pelvic malignancies, does not usually produce appreciable changes in the blood counts, except for lymphopenia. The magnitude and duration of lymphopenia and the alteration in the distribution of various lymphocyte subsets depends on the total radiation dose, the volume of tissue, and the area of the body treated (Blomgren et al. 1983). This effect on the lymphoid system has no clear clinical consequences.

Significant reduction in blood counts occurs when large radiation portals are used, such as mantle and inverted-Y fields for the management of lymphomas and craniospinal irradiation for medulloblastoma (Plowman 1983). These side-effects may necessitate an interruption of treatment. Lymphopenia usually manifests itself within 1–3 days of starting fractionated wide-field radiotherapy and reaches its nadir during the second week of treatment. The rapid fall in the lymphocyte count is the result of the unique intermitotic cell killing (Anderson and Warren 1976). After total nodal irradiation, the initial absolute lymphopenia persists for approximately 1 year. This is followed by T-lymphocytopenia and compensatory B-lymphocytosis for up to 10 years. In addition to the changes in the counts of lymphocyte subsets, there is a long-term impairment of T-cell-mediated immune functions (Fuks et al. 1976). Surprisingly, these alterations do not lead to major complications, except for an increased susceptibility to herpes zoster infection.

Neutrophil and platelet counts begin to decrease 1 week into treatment, reaching a nadir in the second or third week, and generally returning to near normal values 1–2 months after completion of therapy (Plowman 1983). There is usually little change in the haemoglobin level. Transient reduction in monocyte counts and relative eosinophilia are sometimes observed during wide-field irradiation. These haematological effects of radiation are largely the consequence of the elimination of uncommitted marrow stem cells within the portals.

Repopulation of marrow, mainly through migration of stem cells from an unirradiated area into the irradiated volume, occurs after doses of 35–40 Gy ($\sim$ 2 Gy fractions) or less (Maloney and Patt 1972; Hill et al. 1980). The magnitude of marrow regeneration is greater in young children than in adults.

Bone-marrow failure is one of the causes of death after acute whole-body exposure. A dose of 4 Gy to the whole body causes lethality, within 30 days of exposure, in 50 per cent of affected individuals (Vriesendorp and van Bekkum 1984).

The nervous system: central and peripheral

The nervous system is less sensitive to radiation injury than some other critical organs such as the lung or kidney. Damage to this organ results in dramatic consequences and therefore should be avoided whenever possible.

Brain

Radiation injury to the central nervous system has been the topic of several extensive reviews (Sheline *et al.* 1980; Leibel and Sheline 1991) and monographs (Gilbert and Kagan 1980; Gutin *et al.* 1991). Irradiation of the brain may lead to one or more syndromes traditionally distinguished on the basis of their time of appearance. This does not necessarily imply separate pathogenetic mechanisms.

The only acute form of injury is the occurrence of brain oedema within days to weeks of the start of therapy. The oedema is reversible and is usually ameliorated by steroids. Its occurrence is generally associated with irradiation of large volumes in large dose fractions over a short duration. Conventional treatments with 2 Gy or less per fraction to doses as high as 70–80 Gy are infrequently accompanied by acute oedema (Salazar *et al.* 1976; Linstadt *et al.* 1991).

The 'delayed syndromes' cover a time span of a few months to several years after therapy. Traditionally, they have been separated into 'early' or 'late' delayed injuries based on the time of onset. This separation appears to lose its basis as different types of lesions are being recognized with overlapping time distributions. For instance, early delayed reactions occurring within the first 6 months comprise transient demyelination (somnolence syndrome) or the much more severe leucoencephalopathy. Early leucoencephalopathy is generally associated with high-dose chemotherapy (intravenous and intrathecal) combined with whole-brain irradiation (Bleyer and Griffin 1980). The more classical radiation necrosis may also occur near the end of the first period of 6 months, particularly after irradiation with high doses per fraction (Safdari *et al.* 1985).

The use of CT and magnetic resonance imaging (**MRI**) diagnostic procedures allows earlier recognition and potential discrimination between the transient and the more severe progressive injuries and, hence, contributes to removing the boundaries between early and late delayed reactions. Within the 'early delayed' category, changes ranging from a mild form of transient cerebral oedema without CT contrast enhancement to pronounced oedema with contrast enhancement or even frank radiation necrosis have been described (Watne *et al.* 1990).

Histopathologically, changes in the early delayed syndrome are mostly restricted to the white matter. After 6–12 months the grey matter may also become involved, together with more pronounced vascular lesions (telangiectasia, focal haemorrhages). Thus, the late delayed radionecrosis of the brain with latent times clustering between 1 and 2 years usually shows a mixture of histological features.

The functional repercussions of brain injury depend on the location and size of the lesions. There is no specific treatment for these complications. However, when brain necrosis is accompanied by severe oedema and, hence, intracranial hypertension, surgical debridement can result in a rapid relief of symptoms.

The time–dose–fractionation relationships for radiation necrosis of the brain have been reviewed extensively, notably by Sheline *et al.* (1980). These studies show a negligible risk after a dose of 50 Gy in 2 Gy fractions and an approximately 5 per cent risk of complication after a dose of 60 Gy. The tolerance varies greatly as a function of fraction size, with a predicted equivalence to 60 Gy (2 Gy fractions) ranging from 35 to 80 Gy at fraction sizes decreasing from 5 to 1 Gy. The preliminary results of an ongoing trial suggest that hyperfractionated treatments of the brainstem to total doses of up to 72 Gy, given as two daily fractions of 1 Gy, were well tolerated (Shrieve *et al.* 1991). With doses above 72 Gy a loss of effectiveness was noted, possibly because of increasing normal brain injury. This is in keeping with the estimation using the linear quadratic model of dose response. However, caution should be exercised with such interpretations until firm data (longer follow-up and post-mortem studies) are available because it is difficult to distinguish radiation necrosis from tumour recurrence on clinical and radiological findings.

In addition to the classical early and late delayed brain injuries, a systematic use of CT scanning in the follow-up leads to the detection of more subtle, progressive, and diffuse changes in the white matter presenting as hypodense areas without contrast enhancement. These changes have been observed after relatively low doses, such as in patients treated for benign brain tumours and those receiving prophylactic cranial irradiations for small cell lung cancer (Lee *et al.* 1986). Histologically, the lesions range from clear diffuse glial atrophy to leucoencephalopathy, with minimal involvement of the vasculature. The clinical significance of these changes in the central nervous system is still unclear. Time–dose relationships are not well established, but from several reports it appears that these lesions occur at higher frequencies than previously thought.

Spinal cord

Adverse effects in the spinal cord are similar to those in the brain in terms of latent period, histology, and dose–incidence relationship. Among the early delayed syndromes, the Lhermitte sign is a frequently occurring but usually reversible type of injury, which becomes manifest between one and several months after completion of treatment and lasts for a few months to more than a year. The characteristics of this syndrome were well described by Jones (1964). It appears to occur more often and at dose levels well below the tolerance for permanent radiation myelopathy (35–40 Gy), when a long segment of cord is included in the radiation portal, such as for mantle field irradiations. Its occurrence does not herald impending permanent myelopathy. The pathogenesis of this side-effect is probably a transient demyelination (van der Kogel 1991).

As in the brain, the more permanent delayed types of myelopathy seem to show a bimodal distribution suggestive of two underlying mechanisms (Schultheiss *et al.* 1984). The early delayed type, occurring from approximately 6 to 8 months after treatment, is generally limited to demyelination and necrosis of the white matter, whereas the late variety, with a distribution of 1–4 years or even longer, shows predominantly vascular damage. These two types of injury have also been amply documented for the rat spinal cord (van der Kogel 1980).

The clinical manifestations of progressive radiation myelopathy are a subacute development of spinal cord signs, often as a Brown-Séquard syndrome with unilateral weakness and pyramidal signs and contralateral sensory signs from injury in the spinothalamic tracts. There are no specific signs of radiation myelopathy and diagnosis is usually by exclusion of other causes such as intraspinal metastases. Since the lesions are located in specific cord segments, the progression of symptoms into a transverse syndrome usually reflects the affected cord level. There is no specific treatment for radiation myelopathy, although corticosteroids have been used to reduce oedema.

Time–dose relationships for the spinal cord are mostly based on extensive animal experiments, which have shown that the tolerance dose depends to a large extent on the size of the dose per fraction, while variations in overall duration of the treatment have a negligible impact on tolerated dose in conventional irradiations with one fraction per day. It should be noted that in accelerated schedules with more than one fraction per day a loss of tolerance may occur when the time between fractions is less than 6–8 h and repair of so-called sublethal damage is incomplete. The relationship between fraction size and total dose can be expressed using various simple mathematical expressions, allowing calculations of the adjustment in total dose as a function of dose per fraction (for a more detailed description see van der Kogel (1991)). A widely used formulation in clinical radiotherapy is the 'neuret' (Sheline *et al.* 1980), in which the total tolerated dose is correlated with $N^{0.4-0.45}$, where N is the number of fractions, multiplied by a single-dose reference value. Such power law formalisms seem safe to apply at doses per fraction of 2 Gy and higher, but increasing the dose above 60–70 Gy for fraction doses of less than 2 Gy should be done with caution. The human data are largely derived from anecdotal cases supplemented by recent analyses of a few large groups of long-term survivors which show a minimal risk for myelopathy at a total dose of 50 Gy and a less than 5 per cent probability at 60 Gy (2 Gy per fraction). These tolerance dose estimates are supported by a study in rhesus monkeys (Schultheiss *et al.* 1990).

The peripheral nervous system

Perhaps because of its less dramatic nature, the incidence of complications in peripheral nerves, mainly plexuses and nerve roots, is less well documented than for the spinal cord. There seems to be no firm evidence for the dogma that cranial or peripheral nerves are more resistant to radiation than their central counterparts, although this issue is still open to debate. As mentioned earlier, new diagnostic techniques and more specific searches frequently detect discrete structural changes after doses which were previously regarded as safe, such as the 50 Gy limit usually adopted for optic nerves and retina (Minehan *et al.* 1991). The clinical relevance of these findings remains to be clarified.

The best documented series of radiation-induced peripheral neuropathy is the brachial plexopathy. The brachial plexus lies within the portals encompassing axillary and supraclavicular nodes in breast cancer patients. From the times that treatments with large fraction doses (more than 3 Gy) were still fashionable, high incidences of plexopathies were reported (Stoll and Andrews 1966; Westling *et al.* 1972). However, when radiation is given in 2 Gy fractions the incidence of plexopathy is negligible after a total dose of 50 Gy and is approximately 5 per cent after 60 Gy. A recent report indicates a similarity between the spinal cord and brachial plexus in terms of tolerance dose and fractionation sensitivity (Powell *et al.* 1990). The latter is supported by experimental studies on radiculopathy and myelopathy in the rat showing α/β values in the range of 2–4 Gy (van der Kogel 1991). The responses of the cauda equina and lumbosacral plexus are similar to that of the brachial plexus.

Clinically, plexopathy is characterized by mixed sensory and motor deficits, developing after a latent time ranging from 6 months to several years. The latent period varies with the radiation dose. Higher biological dose (high total doses or treatments with large dose fractions) are associated with latent periods of 6–24 months in contrast with latencies of 1–4 years after lower doses. The pathogenesis involves progressive vascular degeneration, fibrosis,

and demyelination with loss of nerve fibres. The presence of lymphoedema does not appear to increase the incidence of brachial plexopathy (Olsen *et al.* 1990).

It is interesting that, analogous to the Lhermitte sign after spinal cord irradiation, transient paraesthesias in the lower extremities have been noted 2–3 months after irradiation of the sacral plexus (Schiødt and Kristensen 1978). As in the cord, this phenomenon is probably due to reversible demyelination.

Head and neck structures

Radiation-induced changes in the cutis, subcutaneous tissues, and nervous systems (central and peripheral) have been discussed earlier. In this section we focus on the effects on the mucosa of the upper aerodigestive tracts, salivary glands, and facial bones.

Mucous membranes

The intensity of acute mucous membrane reactions is a major factor limiting the rate of dose accumulation, that is, the daily and weekly dose rate, in modern radiotherapy with skin-sparing megavoltage equipment. The features of mucositis were clearly documented by Fletcher and colleagues in the early 1960s. These investigators showed that when a total dose of 55 Gy was given in 6–6.5 weeks (~1.8 Gy/day, ~9 Gy/week) to the mucous membranes of the oropharynx, the resulting mucosal reactions ranged from marked erythema to patchy mucositis. When the same total dose was delivered in 5–5.5 weeks (~2.2 Gy/day, ~11 Gy/week), some patients developed confluent mucositis whereas the majority experienced spotted mucosal denudation lasting for approximately 4 weeks. Upon further reduction of overall duration of treatment to 4–4.5 weeks (~2.6 Gy/day, ~13 Gy/week) all patients developed confluent mucositis, starting in the third week of treatment, which lasted for 3–6 weeks before recovery set in. The difference in the intensity and duration of mucositis induced by the three regimens reflects the magnitude of imbalance between the rate of stem cell killing and the pace of regeneration of surviving clonogens.

One of the commonly used radiation schedules in the curative management of head and neck cancers is administered in five 2 Gy fractions per week to 70 Gy over 7 weeks. This regimen induced confluent mucositis in almost all patients for a mean duration of 5 weeks (Van den Bogaert *et al.* 1985). Rigorous nutritional support, such as feeding through a nasogastric tube or parenteral alimentation, is required in approximately 5 per cent of patients because of profound weight loss or a lengthy healing process. Therefore, such a degree of mucositis is generally considered as the upper limit tolerated by patients. Young patients and those in excellent general condition may tolerate higher doses, but these are rather exceptional.

Several other schedules have been used in the management of patients with head and neck cancers. The following regimens have a long tradition and have been found to be tolerated:

(1) 54–55 Gy delivered in 15–16 fractions over 3–3.5 weeks over a relatively small volume;
(2) 50 Gy in 20 fractions over 4 weeks;
(3) 55 Gy in 25 fractions over 5 weeks.

More recently, a variety of unconventional fractionation schedules have been tested in clinical trials in an attempt to improve the control rate of a number of head and neck primaries. The two basic strategies applied are hyperfractionation and accelerated fractionation. The rationales of these strategies are outlined elsewhere in this book. The experience to date with hyperfractionated schedules reveals that doses of 76–80.5 Gy delivered in 1.1–1.2 Gy fractions twice a day over 6.5 and 7 weeks are reasonably well tolerated. Approximately 15 per cent of patients so treated experienced mucositis lasting for 2 months or more and 5 per cent of patients needed hospital admission for nutritional support (Wendt et al. 1989). Three prototypes of accelerated fractionation have been tested (Ang et al. 1990). Type A is referred to as the condensed fractionation schedule or CHART and is characterized by a drastic reduction of overall time of treatment from 7 weeks to approximately 1.5 weeks. With this approach, a dose of 54 Gy delivered in 36 fractions over 12 consecutive days (three fractions per day more than 6 h apart) appears to reach the maximum mucosal tolerance. In contrast, a dose of 48–54 Gy delivered in three fractions of 2 Gy per day, separated by 4 h, over 9–11 days was found to result in mucosal necrosis and fistula in 13 out of 22 patients treated (Peracchia and Salti 1981). Type B is referred to as split-course accelerated fractionation and is marked by two courses of intensive treatment (two or three fractions a day) separated by a rest period to allow acute reactions induced by the first course to subside. A relative safe schedule using this principle is 67.2 Gy delivered in two fractions of 1.6 Gy per day over an overall time of 6 weeks (including a 2 week treatment break period after 38.4 Gy). A few patients treated in this way required hospital admission for rehydration. Type C, the concomitant boost technique, is characterized by delivering the boost (10–12 fractions) as second daily treatments during, rather than following, the basic wide-field irradiations. By limiting the number of twice daily treatments to 10–12 days and the volume of tissues exposed to accelerated irradiations, it is possible to administer 72 Gy in 42 fractions over 6 weeks. Only 4 per cent of patients receiving such treatment had to be admitted for rehydration.

It can be concluded from the available clinical data that, in addition to fraction size and overall treatment time, the distribution of individual fractions is an important factor in determining the tolerance of mucosa to radiation treatment.

Salivary gland

Major salivary glands are located in the vicinity of the majority of primary head and neck cancers or their lymphatic spread pathway. Therefore, it is frequently impossible to exclude these glands from the radiation portals without risking a geographical miss. Common and distressing side-effects of radiotherapy of head and neck tumours result from injury to the major salivary glands.

The most consistent and annoying side-effect of salivary gland irradiation is xerostomia. Dry mouth begins to develop within the first week of fractionated irradiations (Kashima et al. 1965; Parsons 1984) and is the result of the killing of serous acinic cells in the intermitotic phase (apoptosis) (Sholley et al. 1974; Sodicoff et al. 1974; Stephens et al. 1986). Xerostomia is characterized by a decreased saliva flow and a change in saliva composition secondary to a reduction in watery serous secretion. Thus, the saliva becomes viscous and acidic because of an increase in mucinous material (Shannon et al. 1978). In addition, there is a reduction in protein content, including secretory immunoglobulin SIgA produced by plasma cells in the stroma and regional lymphoid tissues (Marks et al. 1981).

The severity of xerostomia is determined by the volume of salivary gland irradiated and radiation dose. This is particularly true for parotid glands, since they are the main source of alkaline serous secretions and are most sensitive to radiation injury. Significant xerostomia occurs when over half of both parotid glands together with other major glands are irradiated (Parsons 1984). In contrast,

irradiation of submandibular and sublingual glands, while sparing most parotid tissue, rarely induces dry mouth (Mira et al. 1981). Radiation doses to major salivary glands reported to result in permanent xerostomia vary from 4.5 to over 60 Gy. This wide range of tolerance is attributable to the variation in individual pre-treatment salivary flow (Mira et al. 1981). In general, a total dose of 40–60 Gy, given in fractions of approximately 2 Gy, to a large volume of salivary tissue was found to induce permanent xerostomia in 80 per cent of cases. A dose of over 60 Gy causes dry mouth in all individuals (Marks et al. 1981). No specific management is available for dry mouth. Some patients are helped with artificial saliva.

The two major consequences of xerostomia are dental decay and taste dysfunction. Dental caries is the result of enamel and dentine breakdown caused by acids produced by metabolism of indigenous oral flora. Reduced salivary flow and secretion of viscous acidic material with a reduced amount of secretory immunoglobulin promote the growth and metabolism of cariogenic bacteria and yeast, leading to breakdown of teeth (Brown et al. 1975; Marks et al. 1981). Fortunately, dental decay can be prevented by careful dental prophylaxis before commencement of radiation treatment and by rigorous oral hygiene and topical fluoride application during and after treatment.

The pathogenesis of dysgeusia is more complex. It is believed to result from the combination of direct radiation injury to taste buds and xerostomia (Mossman 1983; Kuten et al. 1986). Recovery of taste acuity usually begins 60–120 days after completion of radiotherapy.

Facial bones

Teeth-bearing facial bones (the maxilla and particularly the mandible) are susceptible to complications. Although radiation is a causative factor of osteoaradionecrosis, several other factors promote or precipitate its development. These are dental decay secondary to xerostomia, traumatic injury (for example, post-irradiation extraction or sharp objects), and bone destruction by tumour invasion. This explains the diversity in the reported incidence of osteoradionecrosis. Because the mandible has a less abundant vascular supply and is more prone to trauma, it exhibits a far greater frequency of osteoradionecrosis than does the maxilla.

Even though reported rates vary, the 'threshold' dose for osteonecrosis appears to be between 60 and 65 Gy for conventionally fractionated high-energy photon irradiation. Bedwinek et al. (1976) observed no necrosis in 29 patients who received 50–60 Gy to their mandibles. The incidences of spontaneous osteonecrosis (unrelated to dental extraction) were 2/111 (2 per cent) and 10/111 (9 per cent) for those receiving 60–70 Gy and 70–80 Gy, respectively.

Dentulous patients are at higher risk of developing osteonecrosis than their edentulous counterparts because of the possibility of dental decay occurring after radiotherapy which may lead to infection or necessitate extraction. However, this risk can be minimized by stringent oral hygiene and prophylactic fluoride application. Therefore, routine extractions of healthy teeth prior to radiation is not recommended. Patients with a large oral cavity or oropharyngeal primaries (T3 and T4) are also more prone to developing radiation-induced osteonecrosis than are those with small tumours (Wong et al. 1989). It is not clear whether this increased incidence is a result of a greater extent of normal tissue destruction by large tumours or is due to larger treatment volumes.

The treatment of osteonecrosis depends on the extent of the lesion and the presence or absence of infection. Conservative management is indicated in cases of small uninfected osteonecrosis. This includes strict oral hygiene and removal of bony irritants while awaiting bone sequestration. Treatment with hyperbaric oxygen to enhance the revascularization may promote healing (Marx 1983). Advanced infected lesions require surgical debridement, which usually involves hemimandibulectomy, together with administration of antibiotics. A myocutaneous flap may be used to cover the surgical defect after removal of necrotic tissues in order to aid in the restoration of vascularity to the irradiated region.

Thoracic structures

Lung

The lung is an intermediate to late responding tissue in which at least two separate radiation-induced syndromes are recognized:

(1) acute pneumonitis which manifests itself 2–6 months after treatment;
(2) fibrosis which develops slowly over a period of several months to years.

The lung is among the most sensitive late responding organs, but because of the structural organization of the functional units it only becomes dose limiting when large volumes are irradiated; that is, when the remaining lung is not capable of providing a minimal supportive function. The volume threshold above which debilitating complications occur depends on the magnitude of the functional reserve. Except in patients with severe emphysema, lung tolerance is critically dose limiting only when both lungs are irradiated, such as in upper half-body irradiations (as palliative treatment) and whole-body irradiations (in preparation for bone-marrow transplantation).

Clinical signs or symptoms of acute radiation pneumonitis are a reduced pulmonary compliance, progressive dyspnoea, decreased gas exchange, and dry cough. When there is insufficient volume of unaffected lung, these symptoms and signs deteriorate steadily within a few weeks, leading to death due to cardiorespiratory failure. Radiation pneumonitis may be a major component of the so-called 'idiopathic pneumonia' after whole-body irradiation, which may be exacerbated by the presence of graft versus host disease. The course of late fibrosis is that of progressive respiratory insufficiency.

Extensive experimental studies of the pathogenesis and time–dose–fractionation relationships have been performed by various groups notably by Travis and colleagues in mouse lung (Travis et al. 1980; Terry et al. 1988). These investigators have clearly demonstrated the development of two or three separate waves of injury and have established the evidence that late fibrosis could be dissociated from earlier pneumonitis by altering the pace of dose delivery. The cellular basis of the early and late radiation changes is still being investigated. The type II pneumocyte and/or the endothelial cell are considered to be most directly involved in early pneumonitis. For instance, one of the earliest changes observed is the reduced production of surfactant by the type II pneumocytes. It has also become clear that the fibrosis is not merely the formation of scar tissue developing after acute injury, but is the result of an imbalance in collagen production and degradation by fibroblasts. Although fibroblasts may be the effector cells of late injury, the effect of radiation may be mediated through growth factors produced by type II cells or macrophages.

Tolerance doses for whole-lung irradiation delivered in single treatments have been accurately established (van Dyk et al. 1981). When irradiation is carried out at high dose rates (0.5–4 Gy/min), a dose of 8 Gy induces a 5 per cent incidence of acute pneumonitis and a dose of 9.3 Gy carries a 50 per cent probability of complication (ED_{50}). Thus, the dose–response curve is very steep. Reducing the dose rate of 0.05–0.1 Gy/min increases the ED_{50} to approximately 11.5 Gy. Estimation of the tolerance to fractionated irradiations using the linear quadratic model by applying a low α/β ratio of 2–3 Gy reveals that nine or ten fractions of 2 Gy are equivalent to a single dose of 8 Gy delivered at a high dose rate. This is in agreement with the available data on prophylactic whole-lung irradiations in patients with osteosarcoma of the limb (van der Schueren and Breur 1982). These clinical data are supported by a large number of experimental studies showing an α/β ratio of approximately 3 Gy. The extent of the time factor during 6–8 week treatment times is still under discussion. It is noteworthy that the lungs have a large capacity to recover from occult radiation injury.

For partial volume irradiations, attempts were made to quantitate the level of early and late lung injury based on changes in CT density such that equivalent doses could be derived for various fractionation schedules (Mah et al. 1987). For observable CT changes this study yielded an ED_{50} of 24.7 Gy in 15 fractions for irradiated lung volumes varying from 25 to 75 per cent of the total lung. These doses, as defined by CT changes, were thus at most 10 per cent higher than determined for the induction of clinical signs of pneumonitis after whole-lung irradiation (van Dyk et al. 1981).

Heart

Relative to the lung and kidney, the heart is resistant to irradiation. Radiation-induced heart disease occurs predominantly in patients who receive irradiation for breast cancer or Hodgkin's disease. An excellent overview of the clinical and experimental studies on the heart was provided by Stewart and Fajardo (1984) and more recently by Schultz-Hector (1991).

The most common type of heart injury is pericarditis, which presents as variable degrees of pericardial effusions. This complication has a relatively early onset (approximately 50 per cent of the cumulative incidence manifests itself within the first 6 months and the remainder within 2 years of treatment). It is asymptomatic and clears spontaneously in the majority of patients. Approximately 20 per cent of the cases evolve by developing into constrictive pericarditis which may require surgical intervention for relief of symptoms. The remaining patients show asymptomatic pericardial fibrosis, detectable by echocardiography. Based on a literature survey, Schultz-Hector (1991) demonstrated a clear dose–response relationship for this side-effect. The incidence is very low after doses of less than 35–40 Gy to the anterior pericardium, but is over 50 per cent after doses in the 50–60 Gy range. With the availability of precise treatment planning and field shaping, the incidence of pericarditis seems to have been drastically reduced.

Radiation-induced cardiomyopathy is another form of complication that presents as either reduced ventricular ejection or conduction blocks and develops slowly over a period of 10–20 years. A significantly reduced cardiac function was demonstrated in approximately 15–20 per cent of patients treated for Hodgkin's disease after receiving a dose of 30–36 Gy to most of the heart (Schultz-Hector 1991). Histopathologically, this is characterized predominantly by diffuse interstitial fibrosis (Stewart and Fajardo 1984).

A final consequence of heart irradiation is an increased susceptibility to coronary artery disease detectable 10 years or more after therapy. An increased incidence of severe coronary artery stenosis was noted in relatively young patients on the average 4–5 years after receiving radiotherapy for Hodgkin's disease (Brosius et al. 1981).

As demonstrated for most late effects, the tolerance dose for radiation-induced heart disease also depends strongly on the dose per fraction. After a dose of 44 Gy given in 2.5 Gy fractions to patients with Hodgkin's disease no case of pericarditis occurred, while the same dose delivered in 3 Gy fractions was associated with a 9 per cent incidence of pericarditis (Cosset *et al.* 1988). This observation suggests a low α/β ratio which is substantiated by the results of experimental studies on dogs (McChesney *et al.* 1988). An important variable which significantly affects the tolerance of the heart to induction of pericarditis is the volume. Generally volumes of 60 per cent or more are included in mantle field irradiations, in contrast with 40 per cent or less for breast cancer patients. Despite the usually higher doses given to breast cancer patients, reported incidences of pericarditis were not higher than approximately 5 per cent, in contrast with an incidence of up to 50 per cent when the whole heart was irradiated with a dose of 30–40 Gy (Schultz-Hector 1991). These differences in complication rates after partial or whole-heart irradiation have led to definitions of the pericardial tolerance dose as 40 Gy for large volumes and 60 Gy for small volumes in daily fractions of 2 Gy (Stewart and Fajardo 1984).

Abdominal and pelvic structures

Gastrointestinal tract

Substantial parts of the gastrointestinal tract are included in the irradiated fields in the treatment of abdominal tumours. As in the skin and oral mucosae, both acute and late complications are observed. Acute mucositis frequently occurs with clinical symptoms such as diarrhoea or gastritis depending on the regions primarily involved. When limiting the dose to approximately 50–54 Gy in 2 Gy fractions, acute reactions are usually not dose limiting and if they occur, interruption of the treatment for a few days is often sufficient to overcome acute problems. Acute toxicity can also be largely prevented by limiting the total irradiated intestinal volume, while the intestinal mobility effectively reduces the total volume of tissue receiving the full dose. In this respect previous laparotomies may enhance the risk of intestinal complications by reducing the mobility due to formation of adhesions.

More serious side-effects on the gastrointestinal tract are the various types of chronic injury, which may either be the result of persistent severe acute reactions such as ulcerations or develop independently of acute damage in the submucosal, muscular, and serosal layers. Histological features include mucosal atrophy, submucosal fibrosis, and cystica profunda, with progression to severe ulceration and necrosis. Macroscopically the severe lesions present as deep ulcers, fistulae, or stenosis, which usually develop within a time frame of 1–2 years. Experimental studies of the pathogenesis of late gastrointestinal toxicity strongly suggest that, in the clinical dose range, chronic injuries develop independently from acute mucosal change, with progressive microvascular alterations leading to mucosal atrophy and secondary ulcers (Trott and Hermann 1991).

Although acute and late responses of the various parts of the gastrointestinal tract are basically similar, clinical differences in radiation tolerance are generally observed. With respect to the induction of late complications, the stomach and small intestine are the most sensitive, with a complication probability of 5 per cent or less associated with doses of 45–50 Gy in 25 fractions. Tolerance doses for late complications in the colon, rectum, and anus are approximately 55–60 Gy, while the tolerance of the oesophagus seems to be approximately 5 Gy higher (Gunderson and Martenson 1989). Combining radiotherapy with chemotherapy may reduce the tolerance, ranging from a minimal effect with 5-fluorouracil to a marked effect with drugs such as bleomycin or cisplatin. A highly significant influence of fractionation was observed in connection with severe late gastrointestinal morbidity (Cosset *et al.* 1988). A dose of 40 Gy in less than 5 weeks gave a very low incidence of late gastrointestinal injuries when administered in daily 2 Gy fractions, while the same dose of 40 Gy in fractions of 3.3 Gy resulted in a 22 per cent complication rate. No such difference was noted for acute injuries, supporting the independent pathogenesis of the acute and late changes and indicating a low α/β ratio for late gastrointestinal morbidity.

Kidney

Like the lung, the kidney is one of the most sensitive late responding critical organs. Because of its large reserve capacity, the slowly developing injury may take years to be recognized or may not be detected at all with routine assays such as serum urea or creatinine clearance. Clinical data on tolerance limits and time–dose–fractionation relationships are scarce. The Manchester group was the first to define the tolerance dose for the kidneys at 23 Gy when administered in small dose fractions over 5 weeks (Kunkler *et al.* 1952). Subsequent clinical experience revealed that a dose of 20 Gy delivered in 2 Gy or less per fraction to both kidneys carried a very low risk of injury. As discussed earlier, owing to the abundant functional reserve, parts of one or both kidneys can receive much higher doses without repercussions on the excretory function. However, a recognized possible side-effect following partial kidney irradiation is the development of hypertension after latent periods of 10 years or more which may require medical management.

The clinical syndromes of radiation nephropathy were described by Luxton (1961). By definition, acute nephritis occurs within a year of irradiation and presents as proteinuria and hypertension. In contrast, chronic nephritis is seen after a latent period of more than a year and manifests itself as proteinuria and progressive impairment in urine concentration. Anaemia is usually present and has been attributed to both haemolysis and a decreased production of erythropoietin. Finally, a mild form of nephritis, presenting as a sustained proteinuria only, may be observed over a period of many years.

These different clinical syndromes do not necessarily reflect different pathogenetic processes. They may be consistent with the findings from animal experiments indicating that radiation-induced renal failure is a slowly progressing process, the rate of which is dose dependent. It was shown in animal studies, notably in pigs and rodents, that hyperaemia occurs within a few days of irradiation and is followed by a dose-dependent gradual decrease in renal function, as measured by glomerular filtration and renal plasma flow, during an observation period of 6–12 months (Robbins and Hopewell 1987; Stewart and Williams 1991). These functional changes have been observed after single doses as low as 8–9 Gy. The pathogenesis of radiation nephropathy is complex and still controversial. Many authors favour tubular injury as the culprit accompanied by secondary glomerulosclerosis, while others argue for a predominant glomerular injury or primary arteriosclerosis (Stewart and Williams 1991).

Extensive animal experiments yielded a number of clinically relevant observations. The fractionation sensitivity of the kidney was found to be similar to that of other late responding tissues, with the α/β value being between 2 and 3 Gy. Applying this parameter, fractionated doses of 20–24 Gy given in fractions of 1–2 Gy are predicted to be equivalent to a single dose of 8–9 Gy which was determined as the threshold in animals. This estimation agrees with the tolerance doses set by Kunkler *et al.* (1952).

Unlike many organs and tissues, the dose tolerated by the kidney does not increase with increasing overall duration of treatment which indicates the absence of slow repair processes and repopulation. In contrast, even after doses well below the threshold for induction of functional deficits the tolerance of reirradiation was even lower, as expected in the absence of any recovery (Stewart and Oussoren 1990). These experimental studies suggest that retreatment involving the kidney should be avoided, even in absence of any signs of renal damage from the first treatment.

Liver

The liver ranks immediately behind the kidney and the lung in radiosensitivity for whole-organ irradiation. Because all these organs have their functional units organized in parallel structures, the tolerance of partial organ irradiation is substantially higher than that to whole-organ treatment, except when the functional reserve is depleted by pre-existing ailments. Therefore, liver tolerance is generally dose limiting when the whole organ is to be irradiated. A typical example is whole-body irradiation in preparation for bone-marrow transplantation. In most of the earlier studies the lung has been singled out as the dose-limiting organ, but more recently liver and kidney injury have been reported, particularly after conditioning regimes employing single doses of 10 Gy or higher.

Two phases of radiation hepatopathy can be discriminated, with acute radiation hepatitis as the most dominent. The acute phase develops approximately 2–6 weeks after irradiation and is accompanied by signs of liver enlargement and ascites. Most routine laboratory liver function tests are abnormal, particularly alkaline phosphatase. The hallmark lesion of acute hepatitis is veno-occlusive disease, characterized by central vein haemostasis. Progressive occlusion of the centrilobular veins causes atrophy and loss of the surrounding hepatocytes. Inflammation and necrosis are not usually present. The late or chronic hepatopathy has a variable latency ranging from 6 months to more than 1 year post-irradiation and is characterized by progressive fibrotic changes in both centrilobular and periportal areas. These alterations are accompanied by blood flow redistribution through recanalization or newly formed veins and regenerative proliferation of hepatocytes and bile ducts. Clinical signs are variable and may even be absent if the irradiated volume was small (Lewin and Millis 1973).

The pathogenetic mechanisms underlying the two phases of liver injury are yet to be clarified. Unfortunately, there have been no suitable animal models for assessing the pathogenesis and time–dose relationships of radiation hepatopathy.

The tolerance for whole-liver irradiation was established by Ingold *et al.* (1965) to be 30–35 Gy given in fractions of 2 Gy or less over 3–4 weeks. With fraction sizes of more than 2 Gy, a 20 per cent incidence of hepatitis was noted over a dose range of 25–30 Gy. Because of the architecture of the functional units and the large regenerative capacity, partial liver irradiation can be carried out to much higher doses. For instance, in addition to irradiation of the whole liver with doses of 20–30 Gy in fractions of less than 2 Gy, individual lobes have been treated with an additional 20–30 Gy with only transient signs of liver malfunction but no development of generalized hepatitis. It should be noted that in more recent studies employing dose–volume histogram analysis, a more conservative estimate of liver tolerance was suggested as 18 Gy in 2 Gy fractions to the whole liver or 30–35 Gy to volumes limited to 30 per cent of the liver (Austin-Seymour *et al.* 1986).

Adverse effects of radiation may be enhanced by chemotherapy, in particular vincristine, adriamycin, CCNU, and perhaps mitomycin-C. Other drugs such as 5-fluorouracil, hydroxyurea, or cyclophosphamide do not seem to enhance the effect of radiation on the liver.

The combination of radiation with agents such as actinomycin-D, adriamycin, or vincristine seems to produce more untoward effects in children than in adults. Children irradiated to the whole liver with doses above 20 Gy in combination with these drugs were reported to develop signs of radiation hepatitis (Cassady *et al.* 1979).

Bladder

The bladder and ureter are usually within the target volume for the treatment of many tumours of the pelvis such as prostate, uterine cervix, and rectum. In contrast with most other epithelia, the mucosal lining of the bladder and ureters, the urothelium, has a very slow turnover. As a result, radiation-induced desquamation takes a long time to develop unless precipitated by other injury such as infection or drug-related toxicity (Stewart and Williams 1991). In clinical studies, three phases of damage have been described (Gowing 1960). An acute phase occurs 4–6 weeks after irradiation and is characterized by hyperaemia and mucosal oedema. Infection may complicate this early damage, which may then progress to desquamation and ulceration. A subacute or early delayed phase develops from approximately 6 months to 2 years and presents as vascular ischaemia accompanied by progressive mucosal breakdown, ranging from superficial denudation to ulceration and even formation of fistulae. In contrast, late delayed damage may occur up to 10 years after irradiation and manifest as a reduced bladder capacity due to fibrosis of the wall. Late phases of bladder injury are also associated with an enhanced risk of urinary infection.

The available clinical data suggest that 50–54 Gy in 20 fractions with a field size of 10 cm^2 or less is tolerated by the bladder with respect to the delayed types of injury (Quilty *et al.* 1985). Part of the bladder is usually included in treatment of carcinoma of the cervix with combined intracavitary and external-beam irradiations. Several authors have concluded that if the maximum dose in the bladder was limited to 65–70 Gy, complications were less than 5 per cent, even if most of this dose was given by external beam (Rotman *et al.* 1989). In a review of complications after treatment of prostatic tumours by external beam the incidence of chronic cystitis and bladder ulcers was shown to be less than 5 per cent if anterior bladder wall doses were limited to 65 Gy (Dewit *et al.* 1983).

These clinical data are insufficient to determine the fractionation sensitivity of the bladder. Studies in rodents revealed an α/β value of 5–10 Gy, which is unusually high for a late responding tissue (Stewart *et al.* 1981), indicating a smaller dependence of the tolerance dose on fraction size in comparison with late effects.

REFERENCES

Anderson RE, Warren NL (1976). Ionizing radiation and the immune response. *Advances in Immunology*, **24**:215–35.

Ang KK, Xu FX, Vanuystel L, van der Schueren E (1985). Repopulation kinetics in irradiated mouse lip mucosa: the relative importance of treatment protraction and time distribution of irradiation. *Radiation Research*, **101**:162–9.

Ang KK, *et al.* (1990). Concomitant boost radiotherapy schedules in the treatment of carcinoma of the oropharynx and nasopharynx. *International Journal of Radiation Oncology—Biology—Physics*, **19**:1339–45.

Austin-Seymour MM, *et al.* (1986). Dose volume histogram analysis of liver radiation tolerance. *International Journal of Radiation Oncology—Biology—Physics*, **12**:31–5.

Bedwinek JM, Leonard MD, Shukovsky LJ, *et al.* (1976). Osteonecrosis in patients treated with definitive radiotherapy for squamous cell carcinomas of the oral cavity and naso- and oropharynx. *Radiology*, **119**:665–7.

Berry RJB, Wiernik G, Patterson TJS, Hopewell JW (1974). Excess late subcutaneous fibrosis after irradiation of pig skin consequent upon the application of the NSD formula. *British Journal of Radiology*, **47**:277–81.

Bleyer WA, Griffin TW (1980). White matter necrosis, mineralizing microangiopathy, and intellectual abilities in survivors of childhood leukemia: associations with central nervous system irradiation and methotrexate therapy. In *Radiation-damage to the nervous system* (ed. HA Gilbert and AR Kagan), pp. 155–74. Raven Press, New York.

Blomgren H, Edsmyr F, Naslund I, *et al.* (1983). Distribution of lymphocyte subsets following radiation therapy directed to different body regions. *Clinical Oncology*, **9**:289–98.

Brosius, FC, Waller BF, Roberts WL (1981). Analysis of 16 young (aged 15–33 years) necropsy patients who received over 3500 rads to the heart. *American Journal of Medicine*, **70**:519–30.

Brown LR, Dreizen S, Handler S, Johnston DA (1975). Effect of radiation-induced xerostomia on human oral microflora. *Journal of Dental Research*, **54**:740–50.

Cassady JR, Carabell SC, Jaffe N (1979). Chemotherapy-irradiation related hepatic dysfunction in patients with Wilms' tumor. In *Combined effects of chemotherapy and radiotherapy on normal tissue tolerance: frontiers of radiation therapy and oncology* (ed. JM Vaeth and JL Meyer), Vol. 13, pp. 147–60. Basel, New York.

Cosset JM, Henry-Amar M, Girinski T, *et al.* (1988). Late toxicity of radiotherapy in Hodgkin's disease. *Acta Oncologica*, **27**:123–9.

Custer RP, Ahfeldt FE (1932). Studies on the structure and function of bone marrow — II. Variation in cellularity in various bones with advancing years of life and their relative response to stimuli. *Journal of Laboratory and Clinical Medicine*, **17**:960–2.

Dewit L, Ang, KK, van der Shueren E (1983). Acute side effects and late complications of the prostate. A critical literature review. *Cancer Treatment Review*, **10**, 79–89.

Dische S, Saunders MI (1989). Continuous, hyperfractionated, accelerated radiotherapy (CHART). An interim report upon late morbidity. *Radiotherapy and Oncology*, **16**:65–72.

Fuks Z, Strober S, Bobrove AM, *et al.* (1976). Long term effects of radiation on T and B lymphocytes in peripheral blood of patients with Hodgkin's disease. *Journal of Clinical Investigation*, **58**.803–14.

Gilbert HA, Kagan AR (1980). *Radiation damage to the nervous system*. Raven Press, New York.

Gowing NFC (1960). Pathological changes in the bladder following irradiation. *British Journal of Radiology*, **33**:484–7.

Gunderson LL, Martenson JA (1989). Gastrointestinal tract radiation tolerance. In *Radiation tolerance of normal tissues. Frontiers of radiation therapy and oncology* (ed. JM Vaeth and JL Meyer), Vol. 23, pp. 277–98. Basel, New York.

Gutin P, Leibel SA, Sheline GE (1991). *Radiation injury to the nervous system*. Raven Press: New York.

Hill DR, Benak SB, Phillips TL, Price DC (1980). Bone marrow regeneration following fractionated radiation therapy. *International Journal of Radiation Oncology — Biology — Physics*, **6**:1149–55.

Hopewell JW (1980). The importance of vascular damage in the development of late radiation effects in normal tissues. In *Radiation biology in cancer research* (ed. RE Meyn and HR Wathers), p. 44–59. Raven Press, New York.

Hopewell JW (1990). The skin — its structure and response to ionizing radiation. *International Journal of Radiation Biology*, **57**:751–73.

Ingold JA, Reed GB, Kaplan HS, Bagshaw MA (1965). Radiation hepatitis. *American Journal of Roentgenology Radium Therapy and Nuclear Medicine*, **93**:200–8.

Jones A (1964). Transient radiation myelopathy. *British Journal of Radiology*, **37**:727–44.

Kashima HK, Kirkham WB, Andrews JF (1965). Postirradiation sialadenitis: a study of the clinical features, histopathologic changes and serum enzyme variation following irradiation of human salivary glands. *American Journal of Roentgenology, Radiotherapy and Nuclear Medicine*, **94**:271–91.

Kim TH, Somerville PJ, Freeman CR (1984). Unilateral radiation nephropathy — the long-term significance. *International Journal of Radiation Oncology — Biology — Physics*, **110**:2053–9.

Kunkler PB, Farr RF, Luxton RW (1952). The limit of renal tolerance to X-rays. An investigation into renal damage occurring following the treatment of tumours of the testis by abdominal baths. *British Journal of Radiology*, **25**:190–205.

Kuten A, Ben-Aryeh H, Berdicevsky I, *et al.* (1986). Oral side effects of head and neck irradiation: correlation between clinical manifestations and laboratory data. *International Journal of Radiation Oncology — Biology — Physics*, **12**:401–5.

Lee YY, Nauert C, Glass JP (1986). Treatment-related white matter changes in cancer patients. *Cancer*, **57**:1473–82.

Leibel SA, Sheline GE (1991). Tolerance of the brain and spinal cord to conventional irradiation. In *Radiation injury to the nervous system* (ed. P. Gutin, SA Leibel, and GE Sheline), pp. 239–56. Raven Press, New York.

Lewin K, Millis RR (1973). Human radiation hepatitis. A morphologic study with emphasis on the late changes. *Archives of Pathology*, **96**:21–6.

Linstadt DE, Edwards MSB, Prados M, *et al.* (1991). Hyperfractionated irradiation for adults with brain stem gliomas. *International Journal of Radiation Oncology — Biology — Physics*, **20**:757–60.

Luxton RW (1961). Radiation nephritis: a long term study of 54 patients. *Lancet*, **ii**:1221.

McChesney SL, Gillette EL, Powers BE (1988). Radiation-induced cardiomyopathy in the dog. *Radiation Research*, **113**:120–32.

Mah K, Van Dyk J, Keane T, Poon PY (1987). Acute radiation-induced pulmonary damage: a clinical study on the response to fractionated radiation therapy. *International Journal of Radiation Oncology — Biology — Physics*, **13**:179–88.

Maloney MA, Patt HM (1972). Migration of cells from shielded to irradiation marrow. *Blood*, **39**:804–8.

Marks JE, Davis CC, Gottsman VL, *et al.* (1981). The effects of radiation on parotid salivary function. *International Journal of Radiation Oncology — Biology — Physics*, **7**:1013–19.

Marx RE (1983). Osteoradionecrosis: a new concept of its pathophysiology. *Oral Maxillofacial Surgery*, **47**:283–8.

Minehan KJ, Martenson JA, Garrity JA, *et al.* (1991). Local control and complications after radiation therapy for primary orbital lymphoma: a case for low-dose treatment. *International Journal of Radiation Oncology — Biology — Physics*, **20**:791–6.

Mira JG, Westcott WB, Starcke EN, Shannon JL (1981) Some factors influencing salivary function when treating with radiotherapy. *International Journal of Radiation Oncology — Biology — Physics*, **7**:535–41.

Mossman KL (1983). Quantitative radiation dose-response relationships for normal tissues in man. 11. Response of the salivary glands during radiotherapy. *Radiation Research*, **95**:392–8.

Olsen NK, Pfeiffer P, Mondrup K, Rose C (1990). Radiation-induced brachial plexus neuropathy in breast cancer patients. *Acta Oncologica*, **29**:885–90.

Parsons JT (1984) The effect of radiation on normal tissues of the head and neck. In *Management of head and neck cancer* (ed. RR Million and NJ Cussisi), pp. 173–207. JB Lippincott, Philadelphia.

Peracchia G, Salti C (1981). Radiotherapy with twice-a-day fractionation in a short overall time. *International Journal of Radiation Oncology — Biology — Physics*, **7**:99–104.

Peters LJ, Ang KK, Thames HD (1988). Accelerated fractionation in the treatment of head and neck cancer: a critical comparison of different strategies. *Acta Oncologica*, **27**:185–94.

Peters LJ, Ang KK, Thames HD (1992). Altered fractionation schedules. In *Principles and practice of radiation oncology* (2nd edn) (ed. CA Perez and LW Brady), pp. 97–113. JB Lippincott, Philadelphia.

Plowman PN (1983). The effects of conventionally fractionated, extended portal radiotherapy on the human peripheral blood count. *International Journal of Radiation Oncology — Biology — Physics*, **9**:829–39.

Powell S, Cooke J, Parsons C (1990). Radiation-induced brachial plexus injury: follow-up of two different fractionation schedules. *Radiotherapy and Oncology*, **18**:213–20.

Quilty PM, Duncan W, Kerr GR (1985). Results of a randomized study to evaluate influence of dose on morbidity in radiotherapy for bladder cancer. *Clinical Radiology*, **36**:615–18.

Robbins MEC, Hopewell JW (1987). Radiation-related renal damage. In *Nephrotoxicity in the experimental and clinical situation*, part 2 (ed. PH Bach and EA Lock), pp. 817–46. Nijhoff, Dordrecht.

Rotman M, Aziz H, Choi KN (1989). Radiation damage of normal tissues in the treatment of gynecological cancers. In *Radiation tolerance of normal tissues. Frontiers of radiation therapy and oncology* (ed. JM Vaeth and JL Meyer), Vol. 23, pp. 349–66. Basel, New York.

Sacks EL, Goris ML, Glatstein E, *et al.* (1978). Bone marrow regeneration following large field radiation: influence of volume, age, dose, and time. *Cancer,* **43**:1057–65.

Safdari H, Fuentes JM, Dubois JB, *et al.* (1985). Radiation necrosis of the brain: time of onset and incidence related to total dose and fractionation of radiation. *Neuroradiology,* **27**:44–7.

Salazar OM, Rubin P, McDonald JV, Feldstein ML (1976). High dose radiation therapy in the treatment of glioblastoma multiforme: a preliminary report. *International Journal of Radiation Oncology — Biology — Physics,* **1**:717–27.

Saunders MI, Dische S, Grosch EJ, *et al.* (1991). Experience with CHART. *International Journal of Radiation Oncology — Biology — Physics,* **21**:871–8.

Schiødt AV, Kristensen O (1978). Neurologic complications after irradiation of malignant tumors of the testis. *Acta Radiologica Oncologica,* **17**:369–78.

Schultheiss TE, Higgins EH, El-Mahdi AM (1984). The latent period in radiation myelopathy. *International Journal of Radiation Oncology — Biology — Physics,* **10**:1109–15.

Schultheiss TE, Stephens LC, Jiang GL, *et al.* (1990). Radiation myelopathy in primates treated with conventional fractionation. *International Journal of Radiation Oncology — Biology — Physics,* **19**:935–40.

Schultz-Hector S. (1991). Heart. In *Radiopathology of organs and tissues* (ed. E Scherer, C Streffer, and KR Trott), pp. 347–68. Springer-Verlag, Berlin.

Shannon IL, Trodahl JN, Starcke EN (1978). Radiosensitivity of the human parotid gland. *Proceedings of the Society for Experimental Biology and Medicine,* **157**:50–3.

Sheline GE, Wara WM, Smith V (1980). Therapeutic irradiation and brain injury. *International Journal of Radiation Oncology — Biology — Physics,* **6**:1215–28.

Sholley, MM, Sodicoff M, Pratt NE (1974). Early radiation injury in the rat parotid gland. *Laboratory Investigation,* **31**:340–54.

Shrieve DC, Wara WM, Larson DA, *et al.* (1991). Hyperfractionated radiotherapy for brainstem gliomas in children and in adults. In *Radiation research: a twentieth-century perspective* (ed. JD Chapman, WC Dewey, and GF Whitmore). Academic Press, San Diego.

Sodicoff M, Pratt NE, Sholley MM (1974). Ultrastructural radiation injury of rat parotid gland: a histopathologic dose–response study. *Radiation Research,* **58**:196–208.

Stephens LC, Ang KK, Schultheiss TE, *et al.* (1986) Target cell and mode of radiation injury in rhesus salivary glands. *Radiotherapy and Oncology,* **7**:165–74.

Stewart JR, Fajardo LF (1984). Radiation-induced heart disease: an update. *Progress in Cardiovascular Diseases,* **27**:173–94.

Stewart FA, Oussoren Y (1990). Re-irradiation of mouse kidneys — a comparison of re-treatment tolerance after single and fractionated partial tolerance doses. *International Journal of Radiation Biology,* **58**:531–44.

Stewart FA, Williams MV (1991). The urinary tract. In *Radiopathology of organs and tissues* (ed. E. Scherer, C. Streffer, and KR Trott), pp. 405–32. Springer-Verlag, Berlin.

Stewart FA, Randhawa VS, Denekamp J (1981). Repair during fractionated irradiation of the mouse bladder. *British Journal of Radiology,* **54**:799–804.

Stoll BA, Andrews JT (1966). Radiation-induced peripheral neuropathy. *British Medical Journal,* **1**:834–7.

Terry NHA, Tucker SL, Travis EL (1988). Residual radiation damage in murine lung assessed by pneumonitis. *International Journal of Radiation Oncology — Biology — Physics,* **14**:929–38.

Travis EL, Down JD, Holmes SJ, Hobson B (1980). Radiation pneumonitis and fibrosis in mouse lung assayed by respiratory frequency and histology. *Radiation Research,* **84**:133–43.

Trott KR, Hermann T (1991). Radiation effects on abdominal organs. In *Radiopathology of organs and tissues* (ed. E. Scherer, C. Streffer, and KR Trott), pp. 313–46. Springer-Verlag, Berlin.

Trott KR, Kummermehr J (1991). Radiation effects in skin. In *Radiopathology of organs and tissues* (ed. E. Scherer, C. Strafer, and KR Trott), pp. 33–66. Berlin: Springer-Verlag.

Turesson I, Thames HD (1989). Repair capacity and kinetics of human skin during fractionated radiotherapy: erythema, desquamation, and telangiectasia after 3 and 5 years' follow-up. *Radiotherapy and Oncology,* **15**:169–88.

Van den Bogaert W, van der Schueren E, Tongelen CV, *et al.* (1985) Late results of multiple fractions per day (MFD) with misonidazole in advanced cancer of the head and neck. A pilot study of the EORTC radiotherapy group. *Radiotherapy and Oncology,* **3**:139–44.

van der Kogel AJ (1980). Mechanisms of late radiation injury in the spinal cord. In *Radiation biology in cancer research* (ed. RE Meyn and HR Withers), pp. 461–70. Raven Press, New York.

van der Kogel AJ (1991). The nervous system: radiobiology and experimental pathology. In *Radiopathology of organs and tissues* (ed. E. Scherer, C. Streffer, and KR Trott), pp. 191–212. Springer-Verlag, Heidelberg.

van der Schueren E, Breur K (1982). Role of lung irradiation in the adjuvant treatment of osteosarcoma. *Recent Results in Cancer Research,* **80**:98–102.

van Dyk J, Keane TJ, Kan S, *et al.* (1981). Radiation pneumonitis following large single dose irradiation: a re-evaluation based on absolute dose to lung. *International Journal of Radiation Oncology — Biology — Physics,* **7**:461–7.

van Limbergen E, Rijnders A, van der Schueren E, *et al.* (1989). Cosmetic evaluation of breast conserving treatment for mammary cancer. 2. A quantitative analysis of the influence of radiation dose, fractionation schedules and surgical treatment techniques on cosmetic results. *Radiotherapy and Oncology,* **16**:253–67.

Vriesendorp HM, van Bekkum DW (1984). Susceptibility to total body irradiation. In *Response to total body irradiation in different species* (ed. JJ Broerse and T MacVittie), pp. 43–53. Nijhoff, Dordrecht.

Watne K, Hager B, Heier M, Hirschberg H (1990). Reversible oedema and necrosis after irradiation of the brain. *Acta Oncologica,* **29**:891–895.

Wendt CD, Peters LJ, Ang KK, *et al.* (1989). Hyperfractionated radiotherapy in the treatment of squamous cell carcinomas of the supraglottic larynx. *International Journal of Radiation Oncology — Biology — Physics,* **17**:1057–62.

Westling P, Svensson H, Hele P (1972). Cervical plexus lesions following postoperative radiation therapy of mammary carcinoma. *Acta Radiologica,* **11**:209–16.

Withers HR (1989). Contrarian concepts in the progress of radiotherapy. *Radiation Research,* **119**:395–412.

Withers HR, Thames HD, Flow BL, *et al.* (1978). The relationship of acute to late skin injury in 2 and 5 fraction/week X-ray therapy. *International Journal of Radiation Oncology — Biology — Physics,* **4**:595–601.

Withers HR, Peters LJ, Kogelnik HD (1980). The pathobiology of late effects of irradiation. In *Radiation biology in cancer research* (ed. RE Meyn and HR Withers), pp. 439–48. Raven Press, New York.

Wong CS, Ang KK, Fletcher GH, *et al.* (1989). Definitive radiotherapy for squamous cell carcinoma of the tonsillar fossa. *International Journal of Radiation Oncology — Biology — Physics,* **16**:657–62.

19.9   Complications of cytotoxic therapy

GILBERTO SCHWARTSMANN, ADRIAAN W. DEKKER, AND JAN VERHOEF

INTRODUCTION

Anticancer agents generally exhibit a narrow therapeutic index, leading to significant toxicity to the normal tissues even at the doses used in routine patient care. Since most agents discovered so far exert their cytotoxic effects through the inhibition of DNA synthesis and/or its replication, it is not surprising that their side-effects are mainly observed in tissues with a high self-renewal rate, such as the bone-marrow and the digestive tract (Schwartsmann *et al.* 1988). Several studies evaluating the impact of the intensity of treatment in the outcome of malignancies are in progress at present (Hryniuk 1988). A clear correlation between chemotherapeutic dose intensity and the number of complete remissions, relapse-free survival, and overall survival has been already demonstrated in various tumour types, such as lymphomas and breast and ovarian carcinomas (Peters *et al.* 1990; Rankin *et al.* 1990). Therefore, it is very important for the practising oncologist to be aware of the risks of complications due to anticancer therapy. This may allow a more careful utilization of the available agents, preventing and/or decreasing the frequency of serious complications. The most frequent toxic effects of anticancer agents are discussed in this chapter.

COMPLICATIONS IN THE BONE-MARROW AND LYMPHOID TISSUE

Cytotoxic agents can lead to major complications in the bone-marrow and lymphoid tissues. Reduction of the phagocytic capacity of granulocytes and monocytes, as well as damage to the immune system, can result in the occurrence of severe infectious complications. The decrease in peripheral blood thrombocytes and disturbances in the coagulation system can produce life-threatening haemorrhagic complications. Anaemia can result from damage to the erythroid precursors in the bone-marrow as well as from drug-related haemolysis. In addition, cytotoxic agents can induce the occurrence of secondary malignancies in the bone-marrow and other tissues.

The severity and duration of bone-marrow suppression generally depends on the type of agent and the dose administered to the patient. These toxic effects are summarized in Table 1. Prior exposure to cytotoxic drugs, extensive prior irradiation, widespread bone metastases, and a poor performance status are important risk factors that may indicate a diminished tolerance to chemotherapy. Several experimental regimens, in which high-dose chemotherapy is being administered to cancer patients in association with bone-marrow stimulatory factors and/or protective agents, are being studied at present. Agents which are usually non-myelotoxic at standard doses may exhibit significant bone-marrow effects at higher doses.

Alkylating agents can produce significant bone-marrow effects. Busulphan and melphalan lead to both severe leucopenia and thrombocytopenia at standard doses. Although cyclophosphamide may cause severe leucopenia, it has less toxic effects on the megakaryocytes and, thus, is a better choice for patients planned to receive alkylating therapy but presenting with thrombocytopenia prior to the start of therapy. Ifosfamide (given in combination with the uroprotector mesna) leads to moderate myelosuppression. Chlorambucil has only moderate bone-marrow toxicity when given by standard oral administration. The nitrosoureas CCNU, BCNU, and methyl-CCNU are highly myelotoxic and lead to delayed bone-marrow suppression, with recovery usually after 6–8 weeks.

Cisplatin causes only moderate myelosuppression at standard doses; its dose-limiting toxicities are kidney damage and peripheral neuropathy. However, severe leucopenia has been observed in patients receiving high-dose cisplatin in experimental regimens (Ozols *et al.* 1984). In contrast with cisplatin, carboplatin is not nephrotoxic but has its dose-limiting toxicity in the bone-marrow, usually manifesting as thrombocytopenia (Von Hoff 1987).

Antitumour antibiotics produce significant myelotoxicity at conventional doses. Doxorubicin and daunorubicin cause both leucopenia and thrombocytopenia, which are observed around days 10–14, with recovery by the end of the third week. Significantly less bone-marrow toxicity has been observed when doxorubicin is

Table 1 Factors contributing to infection in cancer patients

Disruption of natural physical barriers
  Skin and mucosal damage due to cytotoxic therapy
  Indwelling catheters, hyperalimentation lines, or haemodynamic monitoring devices
  Mechanical obstruction of natural drainage pathways and physiological disturbance due to the tumour
  Colonization by new pathogens due to antibiotics

Decrease of phagocytic capacity
  Qualitative and quantitative defects of granulocytes and monocytes due to cytotoxic therapy
  Qualitative defects in phagocytic function due to the disease

Disturbances in cellular immune function
  Defects related to specific neoplasms (for example, Hodgkin's disease) or advanced malignancy
  Prolonged corticosteroid therapy
  Prolonged cytotoxic therapy

Disturbances in humoral immune function
  Defects related to specific neoplasms (for example, multiple myeloma or chronic lymphocytic leukaemia)
  Prolonged cytotoxic therapy

Disturbances in the reticuloendothelial system
  Defects in macrophage function
  Splenectomy

Malnutrition
  Defects in phagocytic capacity, B- and T-cell function (for example, cachexia)
  Bone-marrow defects (for example, severe vitamin and iron deficiency)
  Poor integrity of integumental and mucosal barriers

given by weekly divided doses or by continuous infusion over 24 h. The latter strategy has also been shown to reduce the risk of cardiotoxicity. However, the usefulness of this approach has to be balanced against the need for a central catheter and the risk of local complications due to drug extravasation (Benjamin *et al.* 1988).

Mitomycin C is also highly myelotoxic and, as in the case of the nitrosoureas, causes more delayed bone-marrow depletion, with recovery only after 6–8 weeks. Mithramycin causes relatively more severe thrombocytopenia than leucopenia at the doses utilized as an anticancer agent. However, only mild toxicity is observed at lower doses in the management of malignant hypercalcaemia. In contrast, bleomycin is only rarely associated with the development of myelosuppression. For this reason, it has been utilized in several combination chemotherapy regimens for the treatment of aggressive non-Hodgkin's lymphomas in order to prevent tumour regrowth in the intervals between the administration of highly myelosuppressive agents.

Methotrexate causes mild to moderate bone-marrow toxicity at standard doses. However, severe toxicity can occur with high-dose regimens or with standard doses in the presence of renal impairment. This adverse effect is probably related to the prolonged exposure of sensitive tissues to the drug. The administration of adequate doses of leucovorin can prevent this complication. 5-Fluorouracil produces moderate myelosuppression by conventional weekly intravenous administration. Severe myelotoxicity has been observed after the utilization of 5-fluorouracil in combination with leucovorin. In contrast, a marked reduction in the incidence of this side-effect has been documented in patients receiving 5-fluorouracil by continuous intrahepatic infusion, probably because of the significant metabolism of this agent in its first pass through the liver (Pinedo and Peters 1988).

Ara-C is rapidly inactivated by cytidine deaminase and single-dose administration causes only modest biological effects. Thus, continuous infusion and/or repeated injections daily for several days is preferable. When the latter schedules are used Ara-C causes severe leucopenia and thrombocytopenia. Recently, high-dose Ara-C has been studied in patients with haematological malignancies, where it produces severe myelosuppression (Donehower *et al.* 1986). 5-Azacytidine and hydroxyurea are highly myelotoxic at conventional doses.

Vincristine has only mild effects in the bone-marrow at conventional doses. Notably, it may lead to an elevation of thrombocyte counts owing to its inhibitory effect on mitosis and the consequent induction of megakaryocyte endoreduplication. In contrast, vinblastine causes significant leucopenia and thrombocytopenia. Vindesine leads to moderate leucopenia, but has only mild effects on thrombocytes (Schwartsmann and Bender 1988). The epipodophylotoxins (etoposide and teniposide) are also more closely associated with the development of leucopenia, with thrombocytopenia occurring in only a minority of patients. Miscellaneous agents such as dacarbazine, procarbazine, hexamethylmelamine, amsacrine (M-AMSA), and mitoxantrone can cause mild to moderate myelotoxicity at conventional doses.

Infectious complications

Granulocytes and monocyte–macrophages are the major defences of the organism against bacteria and fungi. Granulocytes are present in the bone-marrow and are also distributed between two pools in the peripheral blood, namely those that are marginated and those that are circulating. The half-life of a circulating granulocyte is approximately 6 h. Thereafter, cells either marginate along the

vascular endothelium or migrate to the extravascular space. During an infectious episode, both the marginating and the bone-marrow pools are released into the circulation and signals are given from the periphery to enhance the production of new precursor cells by the bone-marrow (Schaffner *et al.* 1982).

Since normal bone-marrow is capable of supplying the peripheral blood with mature cells for 7–10 days after the precursor cells have been damaged by cytotoxic agents, drug effects tend to be documented in the peripheral blood counts a few days after drug administration. Changes in cell counts are evident between days 7 and 14, with recovery observed in most cases between days 21 and 28. With agents which cause severe damage to the stem cell population, such as the nitrosoureas and mitomycin C, more delayed myelosuppression is usually observed, with complete recovery of blood counts about days 28–42. The risk of infection tends to increase linearly with the degree and duration of granulocytopenia. Bacteraemia is particularly frequent if granulocyte counts are

Table 2 Myelosuppressive effects of anticancer agents

Type of agent	Leucocytes	Thrombocytes
Alkylating agents		
Busulfan	+++	+++
Melphalan	+++	+++
Cyclophosphamide	+++	+
Ifosfamide	++	++
Chlorambucil	++	++
Nitrosoureas	+++[a]	+++[a]
Cisplatin	++	++
Carboplatin	+++	+++
Antitumour antibiotics		
Doxorubicin	+++	+++
Daunorubicin	+++	+++
Actinomycin D	+++	+++
Mitomycin C	+++[a]	+++[a]
Mithramycin	+	+++
Bleomycin	—	—
Antimetabolites		
Methotrexate	++	++
5-Fluorouracil	++	++
Ara-C	+++	+++
6-Mercaptopurine	++	++
6-Thioguanine	++	++
5-Azacytidine	+++	+++
Hydroxyurea	+++	++
Deoxycoformycin	+	+
Vinca alkaloids		
Vincristine	+	+
Vinblastine	+++	+++
Vindesine	++	+
Epipodophylotoxins		
Etoposide	++	+
Teniposide	++	+
Miscellaneous		
Dacarbazine	+	+
Procarbazine	++	++
Hexamethylmelamine	+	+
m-AMSA	++	++
Mitoxantrone	++	++

Toxicity scored at conventional doses: — not reported or rare; +, mild; ++, moderate; +++, severe; recovery usually between weeks 2 and 4.
[a]Delayed recovery usually between weeks 6 and 8.

Table 3 Most common microorganisms in granulocytopenic patients

Gram-negative bacilli	Gram-positive bacteria	Fungi
E. coli	*Staphylococcus aureus*	*Candida* spp.
Klebsiella spp.	*Staphylococcus epidermidis*	*Aspergillus* spp.
Enterobacter spp.	*Streptococcus pneumoniae*	Mucorales
Proteus spp.	Viridans streptococci	
P. aeruginosa	Enterococci	
	Corynebacterium	

below 500/mm³. Therefore, empirical antibiotic treatment has been recommended in this situation (Bodey *et al.* 1986).

Qualitative abnormalities in granulocyte function, such as defects in chemotaxis, migratory capacity, phagocytosis, and bactericidal properties, have been reported in patients with malignancy, mainly in the case of acute leukaemias and lymphomas (Curnette and Boxer 1985). Cytotoxic agents in combinations (particularly those including corticosteroids) or as part of high-dose chemotherapy regimens can produce a significant decrease in the phagocytic and bactericidal activity of granulocytes.

The mature monocyte–macrophage is rather more resistant to the damaging effects of anticancer agents and contributes to the phagocytic capacity of white cells during severe granulocytopenia. Macrophages have a fundamental role in the initiation of the immune response; the identification, processing, and presentation of foreign antigens to T and B lymphocytes. The activated macrophage is critically important for the host defences against microbacteria, fungi, protozoans, and viruses (Nossal 1987).

Cytotoxic therapy can affect both B-cell and T-cell functions, causing a decrease in opsonizing activity, disturbances in agglutination and lysis of bacteria, and reduced neutralization of toxins. In fact, cancer patients can be extremely susceptible to infections, considering that chemotherapeutic agents can cause the violation of natural barriers such as the skin and mucosal surfaces, affect the phagocytic capacity of granulocytes and monocytes, disturb macrophage function and impair cellular and humoral immunity. These complications of chemotherapy are summarized in Table 2. Corticosteroids are often prescribed to cancer patients, and may contribute significantly to impairment of granulocyte and macrophage function, and also interfere with T-cell function. In addition, cancer patients can develop malnutrition due to the cancer itself or the toxicity of the treatment (Bodey 1986; Nossal 1987).

In general, bacterial infections are more commonly diagnosed during periods of severe granulocytopenia after chemotherapy. The risk of infection increases rapidly when the granulocyte count drops below 500/mm³. The majority of severe infections are observed when granulocyte counts are below 100/mm³. The most common pathogens are the Gram-negative bacteria (*Escherichia coli*, *Klebsiella* spp., *Enterobacter* spp., and *Pseudomonas aeruginosa*) and staphylococci. Fungal infections (*Candida* spp., *Aspergillus* spp., *Cryptococcus neoformans*, and Phycomycetes) are seen mainly in immunosuppressed patients who have experienced prolonged granulocytopenia and persistent fever despite initial empirical treatment with antibiotics (Sculier 1984). The most common microorganisms infecting granulocytopenic patients are summarized in Table 3.

Infections due to intracellular pathogens such as Mycobacteria and *Listeria monocytogenes*, viruses (herpes simplex, varicella zoster, cytomegalovirus, and adenoviruses), protozoa (*Pneumocystis carinii* and *Toxoplasma gondii*), and yeasts (such as *C. neoformans*), are more frequent in patients with severe T-cell dysfunction, such as occurs

after prolonged treatment with corticosteroids or multiple courses of cytotoxic drugs or in patients with diseases affecting predominantly T-cell function (AIDS or disseminated histoplasmosis).

Patients with an impaired opsonizing capacity of their serum due to hypogammaglobulinaemia or splenectomized patients are susceptible to infections caused by encapsulated bacteria such as pneumococcus, meningococcus or *Haemophilus influenzae*. Splenectomized patients present a selective deficiency in tufsin (phagocytosis-promoting peptide) and have decreased levels of immunoglobin M (IgM) and properdin. Fulminant septicaemia has been reported in patients with Hodgkin's disease after staging laparotomy and splenectomy. Patients with chronic lymphocytic leukaemia and multiple myeloma also have defective antibody production and are particularly susceptible to pyogenic infections, even in the absence of granulocytopenia as are patients previously treated with broad-spectrum antibiotics, particularly β-lactams, which permit colonization of the intestinal flora by new pathogens. *Staphylococcus aureus* and the coagulase-negative staphylococci, as well as *P. aeruginosa*, are particularly frequent causal agents in patients with intravenous catheters. Tumour-related obstruction leading to stasis and overgrowth of microorganisms may also be a cause of infection (Bodey 1986).

The management of infections in patients receiving cytotoxic therapy depends on the underlying malignancies and the degree of treatment-related host compromise, such as the violation of integumentary and mucosal barriers, damage to the phagocytic defences, impairment in cellular and/or humoral immunity, prior exposure to antibiotics, and the general condition of the patients.

Infecting micro-organisms

The most common micro-organisms which cause infection in granulocytopenic patients are aerobic Gram-negative bacilli, such as *E. coli*, *Klebsiella* spp., *Enterobacter* spp., *Serratia* spp., *Proteus* spp., and *P. aeruginosa*, and Gram-positive bacteria, particularly *S. aureus*, *S. epidermidis*, and viridans streptococci (Table 3). Infections caused by anaerobic bacteria are relatively rare in granulocytopenic patients without intra-abdominal disease. More than 80 per cent of infections are caused by microorganisms colonizing the patient at the site of infection (Schimpff 1972). These bacteria belong to the patient's own microflora or have been acquired during hospitalization and may colonize the mucosa of the alimentary tract, the respiratory tract, the urinary tract, and the skin. Therefore, the most common infections in these patients are oropharyngeal infections including periodontal infection, oesophagitis, perianal and perirectal lesions, pneumonia, cellulitis, and bacteraemias caused by microorganisms originating from the alimentary tract, which is the main reservoir (Schimpff 1980). The major fungal pathogens in cancer patients are *Candida* and *Aspergillus*. The value of surveillance cultures for predicting infections seems more useful in bacterial than in fungal infections. It is important to note that the spectrum of infection in granulocytopenic patients is continually changing. In the last two decades the incidence of infections caused by Gram-negative bacilli, particularly *P. aeruginosa* infections, has been decreasing, while infections caused by Gram-positive bacteria have increased (Rubin *et al.* 1988). The emergence of infections caused by *S. epidermidis* or JK Corynebacterium, which are part of the normal skin flora, may be due to the intrinsic antibiotic resistance of these microorganisms and the frequent use of central venous catheters. An increase in bacteraemias caused by viridans streptococci has also been reported, possibly as a consequence of the use of cytotoxic regimens with a high degree of mucosal toxicity.

Evaluation and treatment of fever in the cancer patient

Fever is a common occurrence in cancer patients. Although it is usually regarded as a sign of infection, it may also be caused by the underlying malignancy or cancer therapy. Advanced stages of cancer with tumour necrosis, inflammation, or the production of mediators such as interleukin 1, tumour necrosis factor, and other cytokines may be responsible for the aetiology of neoplastic fever (Dinarello et al. 1988; Chang 1989). However, the majority of fevers, particularly when the patient is granulocytopenic (that is, granulocytes below 500/mm^3), have an infectious cause. Fever is the most prominent sign of infection in the granulocytopenic patient, with many classic signs and symptoms of infection being absent because the inflammatory response is diminished or delayed (Sickles et al. 1975). Repeated physical examinations are mandatory. Special attention should be drawn to subtle signs of infection of the mouth, skin, and perianal region (Lazarus et al. 1989). Blood cultures should be collected prior to the administration of antibiotic therapy. In patients who have indwelling venous catheters, blood cultures should be taken simultaneously from the catheter as well as from a peripheral vein. It is important to obtain urine, stool, sputum, or other fluids for culturing. In the case of a respiratory tract infection, sputum production is frequently absent in granulocytopenic patients and this makes microbiological documentation difficult. Another problem is that positive cultures from respiratory tract samples may not always reflect the infecting pathogens but only those that colonize the oropharynx. The patient with pneumonia can have a normal chest radiography examination at the onset of infection; therefore repeated chest radiographs are needed in the granulocytopenic patient with fever. When an infection is not treated adequately at a very early stage, it can rapidly be fatal to those patients.

In patients developing fever and granulocytopenia during the post-chemotherapy period, a detailed evaluation including history, physical examination, urinalysis and culture, blood cultures, baseline chemistry, and chest radiography is mandatory. The empirical administration of antibiotics is recommended. In most centres, a combination of an aminoglycoside plus a β-lactam antibiotic is administered as soon as cultures are collected (Markman and Abeloff 1983).

If granulocytopenia resolves within a week, antibiotics can be discontinued when the granulocyte counts show definite signs of recovery. In patients exhibiting clinical improvement and the disappearance of fever within a week, but still remaining granulocytopenic, antibiotics should be maintained for longer periods. If fever does not reappear by day 14, antibiotics can be discontinued regardless of the granulocyte counts. Failure to control fever within 48 h in a severely granulocytopenic patient should be regarded as an indication to reconsider antibiotic policy. Culture data should be received and additional material obtained for reculturing. Antistaphylococcal agents (flucloxaciline or vancomycin) and antibiotics covering anaerobics (metronidazole) should be considered. If fever persists or signs of fungal infection become apparent, antifungal agents such as amphotericin B should be added to the scheme (Pizzo et al. 1982).

Persisting fever and empiric antifungal therapy

Invasive fungal infections are a major cause of morbidity and mortality in granulocytopenic patients with cancer. At autopsy,

disseminated fungal infections are much more common than clinically suspected. The major pathogens are Candida or Aspergillus spp.; other organisms such as cryptococcus, Torulopsis glabrata, and other fungi occasionally cause severe infections. Fungal infection should be considered particularly during persistent granulocytopenia or after the previous use of broad spectrum antibiotics or corticosteroids. The diagnosis of invasive fungal infections is very difficult. It usually requires a tissue biopsy which is hazardous to perform in patients with a low platelet count. Serological tests for the diagnosis of fungi are still unreliable (Rogers 1986). Bronchoalveolar lavage is a safe technique which can provide useful diagnostic information in the immunocompromised patient with suspected pulmonary infections (Martin et al. 1987). However, this approach is unsatisfactory for diagnosing fungal infections. The prognosis of an untreated invasive fungal infection in a granulocytopenic patient is very poor. Therefore, the early use of amphotericin B is recommended for the granulocytopenic patient who has persistent unexplained fever for more than 7 days or has non-responsive pulmonary infiltrates despite appropriate antibiotic therapy. The new oral antifungal drugs, such as itraconazole or fluconazole, may be alternatives for Candida infections. More recently, focal hepatosplenic candidiasis has been seen with increased frequency. Characteristics are persistent fever in a granulocytopenic patient, despite recovery of the granulocytes to normal and often abdominal pain with an elevated serum alkaline phosphatase level (Thaler et al. 1988). The lesions seen with ultrasound examination or CT are not detectable until granulocyte recovery has occurred. Diagnosis can be established only by histopathological demonstration of Candida. Early and prolonged antifungal therapy is needed. Cure is difficult to achieve.

Antiviral therapy and prophylaxis

Viral infections are common in cancer patients. Herpes viruses are the most frequent pathogens in those patients and include herpes simplex, varicella-zoster virus, Epstein–Barr virus, and cytomegalovirus. The last two viruses may result in a broad spectrum of diseases, mainly in transplanted patients. The primary cytomegalovirus infection can be prevented by use of leucocyte-poor blood components. Reactivation of cytomegalovirus in seropositive transplant patients is more common and pneumonitis is an important cause of mortality (Meyers et al. 1986; Davey 1990). The possibilities for prevention and treatment of cytomegalovirus pneumonitis has been improved since the introduction of ganciclovir and intravenous immune globulin (Ho 1991). Herpes simplex may cause recurrent vesicles and ulcerations, but rarely disseminated disease (Correy and Spear 1986). Extensive ulcerations of the skin and mucosa can predispose to bacterial and/or fungal infections. Therapy or, in the severely immunocompromised patient, prophylaxis with oral acyclovir is very effective against herpes simplex. The incidence of varicella-zoster infection in cancer patients is five times greater than in the general population (Rusthoven et al. 1988). Patients with haematological malignancies are particularly at risk and they also have an increased risk of disseminated disease. In those cases prompt treatment with high-dose acyclovir is indicated. However, in patients with solid tumours, reactivation of varicella-zoster leads to only localized infection (shingles). Although acyclovir is the most effective treatment of the acute phase, infection in these patients is generally self-limiting and it is uncertain whether acyclovir will prevent post-therapeutic neuralgia (Anonymous 1990).

Granulocyte transfusions

There is little evidence that granulocyte transfusions have substantial benefit in addition to optimal antimicrobial therapy in granulocytopenic patients with documented infections (Winston *et al.* 1982). However, they may be useful in Gram-negative bacteraemia which persists despite appropriate antibiotic therapy. The adverse effects of granulocyte transfusions, such as alloimmunization causing platelet refractoriness, transmission of cytomegalovirus, or the development of pulmonary infiltrates, are considerable.

Immunoglobulin therapy

Immunoglobulin substitution may be indicated in patients with major infections and severe hypogammaglobulinaemia. With the exception of patients with chronic lymphocytic leukaemia and multiple myeloma, cancer patients do not usually have significant hypogammaglobulinaemia. Although human immunoglobulins are now available for intravenous administration, their use in the prevention and treatment of infections in cancer patients are still limited (Co-operative Group 1988). However, in two very recent clinical trials the use of monoclonal antibodies against the lipid A region of the endotoxin molecule of Gram-negative microorganisms has been shown to decrease mortality in patients with Gram-negative bacterial infections. These studies did not include a significant number of granulocytopenic patients. Thus, additional studies are needed to confirm the value of the above approach.

Haematopoietic growth factors

Colony-stimulating factors are glycoprotein hormones which stimulate the proliferation of precursor cells and enhance the function of mature leucocytes. Recombinant granulocyte colony-stimulating factor and granulocyte–macrophage colony-stimulating factor are being investigated as an adjunct to chemotherapy. They accelerate granulocyte recovery and could potentially reduce the morbidity and mortality of myelosuppressive chemotherapy. However, it is yet to be determined whether a significant reduction of infections during cancer therapy can be achieved. The growth factors are promising factors for stimulating the bone-marrow. In the future it is likely that combinations of early-acting factors, such as interleukin-3 (multi-colony-stimulating factor) and later-acting factors, such as granulocyte colony-stimulating factor, will be used (Groopman *et al.* 1989).

Specific infections

Sinus infection

Sinusitis is primarily caused by bacteria in cancer patients with obstructive tumours and in this regard anaerobic infections deserve special consideration and appropriate therapy (for example, clindamycin). Granulocytopenic patients are also susceptible to fungal infections such as *Aspergillus* spp. Diagnosis can be made by a biopsy and amphotericin B is the most effective therapy.

Pulmonary infection

The lung is the most common site of severe infection in the immunocompromised host (Table 4). Unfortunately, specific clinical or radiological signs are often absent. Examination of sputum in granulocytopenic patients is only possible in relatively few cases. A pulmonary infection early in the course of a chemotherapy-induced granulocytopenia is usually of bacterial origin. However, when no response occurs to broad spectrum antibiotics, further investigation by the use of bronchoscopy and bronchoalveolar lavage is needed. After conventional and specific staining techniques including immunofluorescence, opportunistic infections such as *P. carinii*, Legionella, Nocardia, Mycobacteria, herpes virus, varicella zoster virus, cytomegalovirus, and occasionally fungi can be diagnosed. Patients with an impaired cellular immunity are particularly at risk for pulmonary infections caused by *P. carinii* or cytomegalovirus. These patients often present with fever, cough, tachypnoea, and hypoxaemia, with few auscultatory findings. The chest radiograph shows bilateral diffuse infiltration. Rapid treatment with high-dose trimethoprim-sulfamethoxazole or with pentamidine is mandatory when *P. carinii* is suspected. Candidiasis of the lung often develops after previous bacterial infections treated by antibiotics. *Aspergillus* pneumonia often presents an invasive necrotizing bronchopneumonia with signs of acute pulmonary embolism. *Aspergillus* spp. invade the blood vessels, with consequent thrombosis and infarction. Without prompt initiation of amphotericin B therapy, invasive aspergillosis is fatal. The prognosis remains poor when no bone-marrow recovery occurs.

The value of an open-lung biopsy for diagnosing unexplained pulmonary infiltrates in granulocytopenic and non-granulocytopenic cancer patients is not clear (Rogers 1986; Browne *et al.* 1990). In addition to infectious aetiologies, cytotoxic-induced injury, radiation

Table 4 Causes of pneumonia in the immunocompromised patient

Bacteria
    Gram-positive cocci
    Gram-negative bacilli
    Legionella
    Mycobacteria
    Nocardia

Mycoplasma
    M. pneumoniae

Protozoa
    P. carinii
    T. gondii

Viruses
    Cytomegalovirus
    Herpex simplex, varicella zoster
    Adenovirus, influenza, respiratory syncytial virus

Fungi
    Candida spp.
    Aspergillus spp.
    Cryptococcus
    Histoplasma

Others
    Radiation
    Cytoxicity
    Bleeding
    Malignancy

pneumonitis, pulmonary haemorrhage or oedema, and non-specific pneumonitis may cause diffuse interstitial infiltrates. However, in only a minority of cases will it establish a treatable diagnosis after previous bronchoalveolar lavage and transbronchial lung biopsies have been performed. The combination of signs of a pulmonary and central nervous system infection may indicate aspergillosis, cryptococcosis, toxoplasmosis, or nocardiosis.

Oropharyngeal infection

Oral mucosal damage frequently results from the use of cytotoxic drugs. Colonization by pathogenic bacteria and *Candida* may result in local infections or bacteraemias in granulocytopenic patients. Preventive measures such as treatment of periodontal disease (Peterson *et al.* 1987) and mouth washing are probably helpful. The most common oral infection is candidiasis (thrush). These local infections respond well to topical agents, such as amphotericin B or nystatin suspensions. Infection caused by herpes simplex virus can be an important pathogen in transplanted patients but occurs infrequently in granulocytopenic cancer patients. In that case oral or intravenous acyclovir is a very effective drug. *Candida albicans* and herpex simplex may cause infections of the oesophagus which may produce dysphagia and severe retrosternal pain. Topical or intravenous amphotericin B or azole derivates such as ketoconazole, itraconazole, and fluconazole are effective in candidiasis of the oesophagus.

Gastrointestinal infection

Some special problems involving the gastrointestinal tract sometimes occur in cancer patients and granulocytopenic patients. Enterocolitis secondary to the production of a toxin by *Clostridium difficile* may occur, presumably as a consequence of previous antibiotic therapy. The only treatment is oral vancomycin. Another very serious infection is typhlitis, which usually presents as an acute abdomen in granulocytopenic patients, particularly in children and adults with leukaemia (Katz *et al.* 1990). Necrotizing cellulitis of the caecum, possibly caused by Gram-negative bacilli, is responsible for this disease. It is not clear whether surgical excision is of extra benefit to intensive medical management. Perianal and perirectal infections are particularly common in patients with acute leukaemia. The majority are caused by aerobic Gram-negative bacilli; the morbidity of these infections is impressive and bacteraemias are frequent.

The therapy consists of continued use of antibiotic therapy during granulocytopenia, sit-baths, and stool softeners. Surgical drainage is difficult to achieve and possibly of no benefit to the patient during the granulocytopenic period.

Urinary tract

The incidence of urinary tract infections in granulocytopenic patients is low unless obstruction, atony, or a catheter is present. Bacterial infections are caused by enteric pathogens. Occasionally superficial candidiasis of the bladder occurs in catheterized patients.

Central nervous infection

Most infections occur as a result of bacteraemia or fungaemia. Nevertheless, meningitis is surprisingly infrequent in granulocytopenic patients. The most likely pathogens are Gram-negative bacilli, particularly *P. aeruginosa*. Pneumococcus, meningococcus,

and *H. influenzae* are the most common pathogens in asplenic patients. *Listeria monocytogenes* may cause meningitis in patients with an immune dysfunction. High-dose amoxycillin is the therapy of choice. Cryptococcal meningitis is the most common fungal meningitis in severely immunocompromised patients. It presents as an insidious disease with few symptoms. Diagnosis can be made after detection of cryptococcal antigen in the cerebrospinal fluid; cultures are often negative. Treatment consists of amphotericin B and flucytosine or fluconazole.

Skin infections

The skin has an important barrier function which is frequently damaged as a result of underlying disease or intravenous procedures. Local infections are caused by *S. aureus* and *S. epidermidis* or by Gram-negative bacilli which have colonized the alimentary tract. Skin hygiene by regular washing with soap or pvodine–iodine solutions will remove most of the transient pathogens and diminish the infection risk (Wade and Schimpff 1988). The skin can also become infected during bacteraemias. A characteristic lesion is ecthyma gangrenosum (with central necrosis) caused by invasion of capillary walls by microorganisms such as *P. aeruginosa*. Herpes zoster is not common in patients with solid tumours, but occurs in approximately 25 per cent of patients with Hodgkin's disease or non-Hodgkin's lymphoma. It is caused by reactivation of varicella-zoster virus. Radiation therapy contributes to the risk of reactivation; the involved dermatome is often the site of previous irradiation. Cutaneous and visceral dissemination may occur in immuno-suppressed patients. These patients should be treated with intravenous acyclovir. Unfortunately, this drug does not seem to prevent the troubling post-therapeutic neuralgia.

Central catheter-related infections

The use of Hickman catheters and other permanent indwelling venous catheters has been associated with an increase in the incidence of infections. In granulocytopenic infection at the exit site of the catheter, tunnel infections and particularly catheter-associated bacteraemias can be expected in 20 per cent of the patients. The most common microorganisms are coagulase negative staphylococci, but some are caused by *Corynebacterium*, *Bacillus* spp. or even Gram-negative bacilli. Appropriate antibiotic therapy for Gram-positive microorganisms, such as with vancomycin, may prevent removal of the catheter. However, when catheter-associated infections are caused by Gram-negative bacilli, *Bacillus* species, multiresistant JK Corynebacteria, or *Candida*, or in the case of a tunnel infection, initial catheter removal is recommended (Newman *et al.* 1989).

Prevention of infections

Various measures can be taken to prevent infection in granulocytopenic patients. Simple handwashing, the use of disinfectants, good housekeeping cleaning procedures, and the control of water and food are often underestimated (Dekker *et al.* 1989). In particular, handwashing before and after contact with the patient is frequently neglected. A rational approach to the prevention of infection is to suppress the potential pathogens already colonizing the patient and to reduce the acquisition of new microorganisms from the environment (Schimpff *et al.* 1972, van der Waaij and Berghuis-de Vries 1974; Dekker *et al.* 1989).

Reverse isolation

The effectiveness of simple protective isolation or complete reverse isolation with laminar air flow alone is not convincing. The main reservoir for infections is the patient's own alimentary tract flora. Use of isolation procedures requires expensive equipment, skilled nursing staff, and other services. In addition, strict isolation is a psychological burden to the patient.

Total decontamination

The basic method of total microbial suppression is the use of non-absorbable antibiotics, such as gentamicin, vancomycin, and nystatin, in conjunction with topical antiseptics. The results of this approach have not been particularly successful, probably because of poor compliance, overgrowth of pathogens, and acquisition of resistant strains from the hospital environment.

Selective decontamination

Another approach was developed by van der Waaij and Berghuis-de Vries (1974), namely selective decontamination of the alimentary tract. The aim is to suppress only the potentially pathogenic aerobic Gram-negative rods without affecting the anaerobic flora. With the anaerobic flora left intact, the resistance to colonization by aerobic Gram-negative bacilli is considered to be maintained and subsequent infection prevented. Agents such as trimethoprim–sulphamethoxazole, colistin, nalidixic acid, and the new fluorinated quinolones can be used for selective decontamination of the alimentary tract. These drugs are more palatable, leading to better compliance and are much cheaper than aminoglycosides and vancomycin. Another advantage of this approach is that there is no need to nurse the granulocytopenic patient in isolation rooms. One of the potential problems of using trimethoprim–sulphamethoxazole alone as a prophylactic agent is the emergence of resistant Gram-negative bacilli and the development of hypersensitivity reactions (Dekker et al. 1989; Verhoef et al. 1989). The addition of colistin can reduce the number of infections due to resistant Enterobacteriaceae (Winston et al. 1986), but a disadvantage of this combination is the large number of tablets that have to be taken. Results from recent randomized studies showed that the new fluorinated quinolines such as norfloxacin (Dekker et al. 1987; Karp et al. 1987), ciprofloxacin (Winston et al. 1990), and ofloxacin (Laing et al. 1990) are the most efficacious agents for the prevention of Gram-negative infections in granulocytopenic patients.

Antifungal prophylaxis

Invasive fungal infections are an increasing cause of mortality in granulocytopenic patients. Patients with refractory disease, prolonged granulocytopenia, or corticosteroid therapy are at particularly high risk for the development of these infections. However, there are no proven effective prophylactic measures which prevent cryptococcosis, mucormycosis, or aspergillosis. The use of prophylactic drugs such as polyenes (nystatin, amphotericin B) or imidazoles (miconazole, clotrimazole, ketoconazole) have diminished the incidence of localized candidiases, but their efficacy in reducing disseminated candidiasis in granulocytopenic patients remains controversial (Meunier 1987). A disadvantage of the orally administered polyenes is their unpleasant taste, leading to poor compliance. Two new triazole antifungal drugs (fluconazole and itraconazole) have recently been developed (Davey 1990). They have a wider range of antifungal activity and seem to be promising agents for prevention and treatment of *Candida* infections in the immunocompromised patient.

Haemorrhagic and thrombotic complications

The bleeding time increases as the thrombocyte count drops from approximately $100\,000/mm^3$ to $10\,000-20\,000/mm^3$, below which it is definitely prolonged. Thus, the risk of haemorrhage follows linearly the severity of thrombocytopenia. In studies performed in patients with acute leukaemia, there was a clear correlation between the degree of thrombocytopenia and the risk of intracranial bleeding. Therefore, platelets should be transfused prophylactically in patients with thrombocyte counts below $20\,000/mm^3$.

The benefit of preventing life-threatening haemorrhagic episodes by prophylactic platelet transfusions should be balanced against the chances of the development of alloantibodies against the transfused platelets, which may affect its efficacy in future haemorrhagic episodes. Therefore, it is routine practice in some centres to recommend prophylactic platelet transfusions in the induction of remission of acute leukaemias (to maintain thrombocyte counts above $20\,000/mm^3$), but to save it for the case of haemorrhagic episodes in patients with chronic thrombocytopenia, such as in post-chemotherapy myelodysplasia (Malpass and Harker 1980).

After platelet transfusion, approximately 30 per cent of the platelets will be retained in the spleen. Obviously, that percentage will be higher in patients with hypersplenism and minimal in asplenic individuals. Depending on the conditions of the transfused platelets, the rate of consumption, or degree of alloimmunization, their half-lives will vary from 2 to 7 days. Usually, one unit of transfused platelets produces an elevation of $6000-10\,000$ platelets/mm^3. In the routine, one unit per 10 kg of body weight is administered to the patient. For patients showing modest elevations of peripheral thrombocyte counts after transfusion (less than $4000/mm^3$ increase per unit), HLA-matched single-donor platelets should be considered. In patients showing an increased bleeding time in the presence of normal thrombocyte counts, the diagnosis of von Willebrand's disease or a qualitative platelet defect should be strongly considered (Day and Rao 1986).

In addition to the development of severe thrombocytopenia, anticancer agents may disturb the normal coagulation process, leading to an excessive risk of bleeding as well as increasing the risk of thromboembolic events. L-Asparaginase can cause inhibition of the synthesis of clotting factors, leading to thrombotic and haemorrhagic complications, depending on the depletion of vitamin-K-dependent factors, antithrombin III, and factors II, VII, IX, and X. Depletion of protein C, which occurs shortly after drug exposure might also lead to thrombotic complications (Homans et al. 1987).

Mithramycin is also associated with haemorrhagic complications, particularly in patients receiving daily treatments. It is characterized by a drop in thrombocyte counts, an increase in prothrombin time, and a decrease in clotting factors II, V, VII, and X. Deaths due to gastrointestinal bleeding have been reported.

Rarely, dacarbazine has been associated with hepatic veno-occlusive disease. The cause of this complication is still unknown, but it has been reported in several patients receiving the drug as adjuvant treatment for malignant melanoma. Acute hepatic failure has also been described (Feaux de Lacroix et al. 1983).

Suramin is a novel antineoplastic agent which has shown activity against hormonally refractory prostatic cancer and nodular lymphomas. Significant anticoagulation, as measured by elevations in the prothrombin and partial thromboplastin time, was observed in various patients receiving this agent during initial clinical trials (Myers *et al.* 1990).

Drug-induced haemolysis

Erythrocytes have a life-span of approximately 120 days in the peripheral blood and are usually unaffected by a single chemotherapy course. Anaemia due to a toxic effect on the erythroid precursors of the bone-marrow is more often observed after prolonged therapy. Indeed, the occurrence of anaemia in oncological patients results from a combination of several factors such as poor nutrition and blood loss as well as disease progression. Therefore, the oncologist should be aware that an acute drop in red cell counts shortly after cytotoxic therapy is usually due to other causes such as haemolysis and/or massive blood loss.

Haemolytic anaemia has been described in some patients in association with exposure to certain anticancer agents. Mitomycin C can cause a form of haemolytic–uraemic syndrome, characterized by a microangiopathic haemolytic anaemia and acute renal failure. Renal endothelial injury has been suggested as the cause of this complication. This form of haemolytic–uraemic syndrome is more common in patients who received total doses of the drug above $70 \, \text{mg/m}^2$ and it can be exacerbated in some cases by blood transfusion. It is rarely reversible and does not respond to corticosteroids and/or plasmapheresis (Cantrell *et al.* 1985).

Cisplatin can also cause a form of haemolytic anaemia, usually after extended periods of treatment. This toxic effect appears to be related to direct damage to the red cell membrane (Doll and Weiss 1985). Rare cases of haemolytic–uraemic syndrome have also been reported in patients who received cisplatin therapy.

2'-Deoxycoformycin is a purine nucleoside analogue which inhibits adenosine deaminase and has produced significant objective responses in hairy cell leukaemia. Occasional reports of probable drug-induced haemolysis correlated with dATP accumulation have been described (Johnston *et al.* 1986).

Elliptinium acetate is an experimental cytotoxic agent derived from the indole plant alkaloid ellipticine. It has shown objective antitumour activity (approximately 25 per cent objective responses) in patients with advanced breast cancer. Acute haemolytic anaemia has been documented in some patients who received this agent during phase II evaluation. Free-radical damage to the red cell membrane has been suggested as the cause of this complication (Mondesir *et al.* 1985).

COMPLICATIONS IN THE DIGESTIVE TRACT

Cytotoxic agents can affect the digestive tract by inducing emesis or by causing damage to the gastrointestinal mucosa after systemic or regional drug delivery. Since drug-induced emesis is discussed elsewhere, this discussion is restricted to the other types of complications.

Direct cytotoxic damage to the digestive tract

Cytotoxic agents tend to produce significant morbidity to the mucosa of the digestive tract. Epithelial cells are normally undergoing intense self-renewal and are particularly affected by agents that interfere with DNA replication. These cytotoxic effects are usually observed 7–14 days after drug administration and tend to recover completely by days 14–21. It is very important not to underestimate this form of complication, as it can lead to a significant reduction in the intake of nutrients and fluids, worsening the clinical condition of the patients. In severe cases it may also contribute to secondary infections and violation of natural barriers, increasing the risk of bowel perforation and septicaemia. More recently, changes in small bowel function associated with malabsorption have been described in children receiving chemotherapy for various types of malignancies (Brunneto 1990).

Mucositis is a common toxicity of methotrexate therapy, even at standard intravenous weekly administrations. It can be more severe and sustained in patients receiving high-dose regimens. It is important to remember that more severe and life-threatening toxicity can occur in patients with renal dysfunction. In this situation leucovorin rescue should be considered (Evans *et al.* 1986).

5-Fluorouracil can cause mucositis and diarrhoea. These toxic effects are more pronounced in patients receiving the drug as part of a regimen including repeated daily intravenous administrations or continuous infusion. In contrast, mucositis is quite tolerable in patients receiving weekly administrations or intrahepatic infusion for the treatment of hepatic metastasis. A higher incidence of severe mucositis and sepsis secondary to drug-related intestinal perforation has been described in patients receiving 5-fluorouracil plus leucovorin, particularly in the elderly population (Petrelli *et al.* 1987). Although the latter combination seems to increase response rates compared with 5-fluorouracil alone, it is also associated with a higher risk of toxicity to the normal tissues. Recently, major toxicity to the gastrointestinal tract was observed in a randomized trial of 5-fluorouracil plus leucovorin given at either high or low dose (Grem *et al.* 1987a). Severe diarrhoea was documented in 25 per cent versus 13 per cent of patients in the high-dose and low-dose leucovorin groups, respectively. Nine patients died as a result of severe gastrointestinal damage, including haemorrhagic enterocolitis.

Gastrointestinal damage is one of the main dose-limiting toxicities of Ara-C. Patients can develop ulcerations in the intestinal mucosa, which can progress to intramural haematomas and gastrointestinal perforation. Apart from mucositis, diarrhoea, nausea, and vomiting are significant toxic effects of Ara-C (Rustum *et al.* 1987). 6-Mercaptopurine and 6-thioguanine exert their cytotoxic effects mainly against rapidly growing precursor cells. Therefore, it is not surprising that mucositis and, less frequently, diarrhoea are observed after exposure to these agents.

Mucositis is one of the main dose-limiting toxicities of the anthracyclines doxorubicin and daunorubicin. It tends to appear around days 5–7 and shows complete recovery between days 14 and 21. When any of these agents are included in combination regimens, mucositis might be a frequent cause of treatment delay and/or discontinuation. The gastrointestinal toxicity of actinomycin D is infrequent but can be quite distressing, with ulceration of the mucosa throughout the digestive tract and abdominal pain and diarrhoea. It can produce severe toxic damage to the organs exposed previously and/or simultaneously to irradiation. Mithramycin can cause mucositis and diarrhoea. However, this agent is only used in specific situations such as malignant hypercalcaemia and refractory germ cell tumours.

Etoposide and teniposide lead to gastrointestinal complaints in only a minority of patients. However, the digestive toxicity of etoposide has been reported to be substantially increased when the oral route is utilized. The main dose-limiting toxicity of hexamethylmelamine is nausea and vomiting, which tends to worsen as the drug is continuously administered orally over a period of weeks. Gastrointestinal toxicity might be partially attenuated by giving the drug at higher doses for a shorter period.

Dacarbazine causes significant nausea and vomiting at standard doses. In patients suffering from severe toxicity, doses may be reduced initially and then gradually increased to the desirable dose. This might improve drug tolerance in some patients. Procarbazine is commonly used with nitrogen mustard, vincristine, and prednisolone in the MOPP combination in Hodgkin's disease as well as in the palliative treatment of brain tumours, mostly by daily oral administrations. When administered by this route, procarbazine is often associated with the development of anorexia and food intolerance.

Damage due to the regional delivery of cytotoxic drugs

Patients receiving regional chemotherapy for the treatment of liver metastasis may sometimes present catheter slippage into the gastroduodenal artery, leading to ischaemia and/or necrosis of the gastrointestinal epithelium. Abdominal pain, ileus, and gastrointestinal perforation with sepsis can occur in patients with this complication. Hepatic portal perfusion appears to be a less preferable form of regional therapy for liver metastasis since most tumour deposits in this organ receive their blood supply via the arterial circulation.

5-Fluorouracil is perhaps the most commonly used agent in this approach, since approximately half the total administered drug is clearly in its first pass through the liver and the occurrence of systemic toxicity is significantly reduced. The use of mitomycin C by hepatic arterial administration in association with 5-fluorodeoxyuridine has recently been reported in patients with previously resected liver metastases. Transient hepatitis and gastrointestinal ulcerations occurred in 50 per cent of patients (Patt et al. 1987).

COMPLICATIONS IN THE LIVER, PANCREAS, AND BILIARY TRACT

Methotrexate has been reported to cause both acute and chronic liver toxicity. After high-dose administration, elevations of liver enzymes and hyperbilirubinaemia have been described. This type of toxic effect is usually reversible and is probably related to the high drug concentrations in plasma. Lipid infiltration has been described in liver biopsy material obtained from affected patients. A chronic form of hepatic damage has been documented after prolonged daily oral administration in patients with psoriasis. Liver biopsy obtained in patients developing this complication has revealed hepatic fibrosis. Cirrhosis has been diagnosed in isolated cases. The risk appears to be lower in patients receiving the drug weekly or at longer intervals.

Hepatic damage has been described in patients receiving high-dose Ara-C. This syndrome is characterized by moderate enzyme elevations, which usually return to normal levels in most patients. Severe liver impairment leading to drug discontinuation has been documented in only a minority of patients who received Ara-C (Preisler et al. 1986). 6-Mercaptopurine and 6-thioguanine can cause acute cholestasis, with elevation of bilirubin, alkaline phosphatase, and transaminases. This syndrome is usually reversible on cessation of treatment.

Bleomycin has occasionally been associated with the development of hyperbilirubinaemia. Mithramycin has been associated with the development of severe liver damage. Although this seems to be a rare event, it has been recommended that liver enzyme levels should be closely monitored and treatment discontinued in the case of such enzyme elevations. Dacarbazine has been shown to cause acute liver necrosis in melanoma patients as a result of acute veno-occlusive disease. Fever and eosinophilia have also been described in association with this syndrome. In addition, fatal hepatic necrosis has been associated with the use of the doxorubicin, bleomycin, vinblastin, and dacarbazine (ABVD) regimen in Hodgkin's disease (Feaux de Lacroix et al. 1983). This complication appears to occur more often when dacarbazine is given daily for 5 days instead of every 14 days (Joensuu et al. 1986).

L-Asparaginase has been associated with the development of acute elevations of serum amylase in approximately 10 per cent of cases. Haemorrhagic pancreatitis has been documented in some of these patients. In addition, fatty changes in the liver have frequently been reported in patients treated with this agent (Clavell et al. 1986). Clinically, hyperbilirubinaemia and elevation of alkaline phosphatase and transaminases in the plasma were reported. Carboplatin was also shown to induce acute reversible liver damage in initial clinical studies in childhood malignancies (Allen et al. 1987). The experimental agent suramin was also shown to cause the elevation of bilirubin, transaminases, and alkaline phosphatase in initial clinical trials (Myers et al. 1990).

COMPLICATIONS IN THE KIDNEY AND URINARY TRACT

Oncological patients are particularly susceptible to developing kidney and urinary tract toxicity. Drug-induced nephropathy and haemorrhagic cystitis have been observed after cytotoxic therapy. In addition to renal damage due to cytotoxic agents, other factors may be of importance, such as the concomitant use of antibiotics with nephrotoxic potential, such as aminoglycosides or amphotericin B, the presence of radiation nephropathy, hypercalcaemia, hyperuricaemia, disseminated intravascular coagulation, and microangiopathic haemolytic anaemia. Furthermore, cancer patients are at risk of the development of other forms of kidney disease, such as immune-complex-mediated glomerulopathy, amyloidosis, or paraprotein-related nephropathy, and also of direct tumour infiltration of the kidney or obstructive nephropathy (Ries and Klastersky 1986). Examples of cytotoxic agents that can produce kidney damage are given in Table 5.

Table 5 Examples of anticancer agents causing kidney toxicity

Alkylating agents
  Cisplatin
  Methyl-CCNU

Antitumour antibiotics
  Mitomycin C
  Mithramycin

Antimetabolites
  Methotrexate
  5-Azacytidine

Miscellaneous
  Streptozotocin
  Gallium nitrate

Kidney toxicity

The nephrotoxic potential of cisplatin has been extensively documented in many studies. Animal studies performed in mice, rats, dogs, and monkeys have consistently shown a dose-dependent acute tubular damage, progressing from laboratory changes, such as urea and creatinine elevation, proteinuria, and urinary concentration defects, to proximal tubular necrosis, uraemia, and death. In rats, the S3 segment of the proximal tubules in the outer part of the medullary region of the kidney was more often affected, showing signs of cytoplasmic vacuolization, tubular dilatation, pyknotic nuclei, and hydropic degeneration. After repeated drug exposure, cyst formation, interstitial fibrosis, and thickening of the tubular basement membranes were documented.

Initial descriptions of platinum kidney toxicity in humans were comparable with those described in large animals, such as dogs and monkeys. A dose-related, cumulative, and partially reversible nephropathy with cessation of drug exposure was reported. The main pathological features consisted of acute tubular necrosis, tubular degeneration, and vacuolized mitochondria, with disruption of the brush border microvilli. Glomerular morphology was rarely affected (Safirstein et al. 1986).

Functional studies performed in patients receiving cisplatin have shown a decrease in renal blood flow and consequent drop in glomerular filtration rate within a few hours of drug administration. These effects may be due to an elevation of renal vascular resistance. However, when pre-hydration is given to the patients, the serum creatinine or creatinine clearance are not sensitive enough to detect subclinical cisplatin-related renal damage.

Several enzymatic changes can be used as indirect markers of drug toxicity. The alanine aminopeptidases may show elevation, reflecting damage to the brush-border membrane of proximal tubules. N-Acetyl-β-D-glucosaminidase (NAG) is a lysosomal enzyme with high activity in the proximal tubule, although it can also be elevated in cases of damage to the distal tubules. The above mentioned enzymes are usually detected in the urine 36–48 h after drug administration. Other enzymes that might also show elevation are β-glucuronidase, leucine aminopeptidase, and β_2-microglobulin. The last mentioned can be detected in the urine for up to 5 days after therapy (Litterst et al. 1986).

Hydration is the most important measure in preventing cisplatin-related nephrotoxicity. There is convincing experimental evidence that hydration should always be given using chloride-containing solution, such as normal saline or glucose 5 per cent in saline solution. Indeed, preclinical studies performed in rats have shown no protective effect of pre-hydration with tap-water as opposed to normal saline. Furthermore, animal studies have suggested that nephrotoxicity is significantly higher when cis-platinum is administered to chloride-deprived rats, while protection is achieved by pharmacologically induced chloriuresis (Earhart et al. 1983).

It appears that saline hydration alone is effective in preventing kidney damage for patients receiving cisplatin at doses of 20 mg/m²/days administered by infusion for 1–2 h/day for 5 days. Experience has also been gained with either higher doses of cisplatin as a single short-term infusion (100–120 mg/m²) or 40 mg/m²/day for 5 days, using pre-hydration with normal saline plus mannitol or frusemide. As a general rule, cisplatin should only be given to patients with an urinary output of at least 100 ml/h during and immediately after drug administration.

In very high-dose cisplatin regimens (180–220 mg/m²), intensive parenteral hydration with hypertonic saline, divided into five daily doses with close monitoring of urinary output (at least 200–250 ml/h), has proved to be devoid of significant nephrotoxicity. Notably, thrombocytopenia is the main dose-limiting toxicity reported with such a type of cisplatin regimen. More recently, studies evaluating the continuous intravenous administration of cisplatin with adequate hydration during the total duration of drug infusion have demonstrated a significant reduction in renal and gastrointestinal toxicity (Gandara et al. 1986).

Recently, studies performed on animal models as well as humans have suggested that administration of the thiol compound WR-2721 (S-2-(3-iminoprophylamino)-ethylphosphorothionic acid) has a protective effect on cisplatin toxicity without a significant reduction in antitumour activity. WR-2721 is now undergoing evaluation in patients with ovarian and lung cancer receiving cisplatin therapy (Glover et al. 1987).

Diethyldithiocarbamate is a strong SH group chelator which has also been shown to protect cisplatin nephrotoxicity in animal models. This effect probably depends on the competition with cisplatin for protein-bound SH groups in the renal tubules (Murthy et al. 1987).

Sodium thiosulphate can react covalently with cisplatin, reducing its cytotoxicity. However, it may also protect tumour cells from drug effects. Sodium thiosulphate is highly concentrated in the renal tubules and may be particularly useful if administered intravenously while cisplatin is given intraperitoneally, as for instance in the case of patients with ovarian cancer. Under the latter conditions, it might allow the administration of significantly higher doses of cisplatin (up to 270 mg/m²) without significant renal toxicity. Other thiol-related compounds such as thiourea, penicillamine, or L-methionine may also inhibit toxicity (Howell et al. 1982).

Probenecid appears to inhibit the active secretion of cisplatin by the para-aminohippurate system, decreasing cisplatin toxicity in animal models (Osman and Litterst 1983). Acetazolamide, which is a carbonic anydrase inhibitor in addition to its diuretic effect, may compete with cisplatin for tubular reabsorption, thus facilitating cisplatin excretion. In addition, it could enhance the detoxification of cisplatin through the chemical interaction of sulphur atoms with the drug. Superoxide radical formation could also be involved in cisplatin nephrotoxic effects, as the enzyme copper–zinc superoxide dismutase can decrease kidney damage in animals. Selenium might also decrease cisplatin toxicity either by increasing its detoxification and/or by preventing cisplatin tubular reabsorption. The angiotensin inhibitor captopril and the calcium-channel blocker verapamil have also been shown to reduce cisplatin toxicity. This effect may be related to an inhibitory effect on cisplatin-related reduction of renal plasma flow (Offerman et al. 1985).

Methotrexate is mainly excreted by the kidneys. Consequently, patients with decreased renal function can suffer from increased toxicity due to the higher tissue exposure to the drug, particularly the gut and bone-marrow. Methotrexate-related nephrotoxicity can be caused by drug precipitation in the renal tubules, direct cytotoxic effects in the kidney cells, and changes in the glomerular filtration rate. Tubular precipitation of the drug is particularly likely in the presence of concentrated and acid urine, leading to a form of obstructive nephropathy. This can cause acute renal failure and has been implicated in approximately 20 per cent of deaths during high-dose methotrexate therapy. However, the fact that most patients developing renal damage are not oluguric or anuric at diagnosis suggests that other nephrotoxicity mechanisms, such as direct cytotoxic effect in the renal tubules, might have an important role (Abelson and Garnick 1982).

In order to prevent methotrexate-induced kidney damage, hydration and urine alkalinization are recommended. This is particularly important in patients receiving high-dose methotrexate.

Therefore, it is critical to maintain an adequate urinary output during therapy, keeping the urinary pH above 7 by means of oral or parenteral bicarbonate administration. If elevations of serum creatinine are documented, more vigorous hydration and folinic acid rescue should be considered. In addition, drug plasma levels should be monitored and folinic acid given accordingly. In exceptional cases, methotrexate levels can be reduced by means of peritoneal dialysis or haemodialysis. However, the value of such an approach has not yet been proved (Weiss and Poster 1982).

Methyl-CCNU may cause progressive renal tubular atrophy, with glomerulosclerosis and interstitial fibrosis. It is particularly likely in patients who have received a total cumulative dose above 1400 mg/m^2 and is characterized by elevation of serum creatinine levels that might progress to irreversible renal failure. In practice, it only occurs in patients responding to the drug who are maintained on treatment for prolonged periods, usually more than a year. The management of this complication is essentially palliative (Schacht et al. 1981; Weiss et al. 1983).

Initial reports on the nephrotoxic properties of mitomycin C revealed microangiopathic changes in the renal vessels, haematuria, proteinuria, renal failure, and circulatory congestion, in association with red cell fragmentation and haemolytic anaemia in a so-called haemolytic–uraemic syndrome. These changes occurred after repeated doses of the drug, particularly in patients exposed to a total dose above 70 mg/m^2 and ranging from 40 to 115 mg/m^2 in one series (Verweij et al. 1987). Histopathological studies performed in necropsy material obtained from patients who received mitomycin C have shown microangiopathic lesions with fibrous thrombi in the glomeruli and small arteries, thickened basement membrane, glomerular nuclear degeneration, glomerular necrosis, hyperplasia of the intima in arterial vessels, and mesangial changes. Immune complexes have been detected in patients with mitomycin C-related haemolytic–uraemic syndrome (Pavy et al. 1982).

The management of this complication is still not satisfactory. Corticosteroids, anticoagulants, platelet inhibitors, immuno-suppressive agents, and plasmapheresis have all been tried in this disorder, showing no effect or only a temporary benefit. In patients developing severe renal impairment, haemodialysis may be necessary for symptomatic relief. Therefore, it is important to monitor renal and haematological function in patients receiving mitomycin C. If renal damage or haemolysis are detected, the drug has to be discontinued immediately. Transient worsening of this syndrome has been reported after blood transfusion in some series. Therefore, blood or blood products should be administered with caution.

Kidney damage is the main dose-limiting toxicity of streptozotocin. This complication appears to be dose related, occurring more often at doses above 1500 mg/m^2/week. It consists of proteinuria which progresses to a Fanconi-like syndrome characterized by renal tubular acidosis, hypocalaemia, renal glycosuria, hyphosphataemia, nephrogenic diabetes, and oliguria. Streptozotocin-related nephrotoxicity may be prevented by avoiding the administration of high cumulative doses of the drug and by repeated examinations for proteinuria. Treatment should be discontinued if proteinuria or renal impairment are documented. After resolving these abnormalities, streptozotocin may be administered again in patients showing therapeutic benefit from the treatment (Weiss 1982).

Nephrotoxicity has been reported in patients receiving mithramycin therapy. It is dependent on the total cumulative dose administered to the patients and is irreversible in some cases. The clinical picture consists of proteinuria and renal failure. Histopathological changes include renal tubular oedema, degeneration, necrosis, and atrophy, with minimal or no glomerular damage. 5-Azacytidine can cause azotemia and renal tubular damage. Proximal, distal, and collecting ducts may be affected, giving rise to polyuria, aminoaciduria, renal glycosuria, sodium wasting, and a defect in phosphate reabsorption (Peterson et al. 1981).

Gallium nitrate has shown objective antitumour activity against refractory lymphomas and small cell lung carcinoma during initial clinical trials. It has also shown activity against cancer-related hypercalcaemia. Kidney damage has been reported as one of the main dose-limiting toxicities of this compound, which seems to be at least partially circumvented by vigorous pre-hydration and osmotic diuresis. Continuous infusion regimens have also been reported to produce less nephrotoxicity (Foster et al. 1986; Keller et al. 1986).

Bladder toxicity

Haemorrhagic cystitis is a well-described complication after ifosfamide and, less often, cyclophosphamide therapy. After drug administration, these agents undergo metabolic transformation into active alkylating metabolites (phosphoramide mustard), which are responsible for its antitumour activity and acrolein, which causes local irritation in the bladder. Haemorrhagic cystitis is more frequent in high-dose cyclophosphamide protocols and after prolonged oral administration.

The most effective procedure for preventing the above complication is to provide adequate hydration to the patients during cyclophosphamide therapy and the administration of the protective agent sodium-2-mercapto-ethane sulphonate (mesna). This agent forms an inactive dimer in plasma, causing no interference with the effect of hydroxycyclophosphamide. However, it undergoes hydrolysis in the urinary tract and can neutralize cyclophosphamide metabolites, preventing the occurrence of haemorrhagic cystitis, without interfering with its antitumour properties. Mesna is not usually needed when the cyclophosphamide dose is below 1 g/m^2. For patients showing persistent and/or severe haematuria despite the above measures, local instillation of alum solution (1 per cent) into the bladder should be considered. Cystectomy should also be considered in patients with life-threatening haemorrhage that does not respond to non-surgical manouevres (Andriole et al. 1987).

COMPLICATIONS IN THE NERVOUS SYSTEM

Cytotoxic agents can cause several forms of complications in the central and peripheral nervous system. Acute central nervous toxicity is usually related to the presence of high concentrations of the drug or a toxic metabolite in the brain tissues. In contrast, peripheral neuropathy is mostly dependent on the total cumulative dose administered to the patients. The most common anticancer agents causing neurotoxicity are shown in Table 6.

The neurotoxicity of 5-fluorouracil appears to be due to the presence of the neurotoxic metabolite 5-fluorocitrate. It can cause somnolence, cerebellar ataxia, and upper motor neurone syndrome. These complications are particularly prevalent in patients receiving 5-fluorouracil by intracarotid infusion.

Intrathecal methotrexate has caused various forms of complications (Kaplan and Wiernik 1982). An acute arachonoiditis has been documented in some patients during the first days after intrathecal drug administration. This syndrome has to be

Table 6 Examples of anticancer agents causing neurotoxicity

Central nervous system syndromes
  5-Fluorouracil
  Methotrexate
  Ifosfamide
  High-dose Ara-C
  Hexamethylmelamine
  Procarbazine
  L-Asparaginase
  Fludarabine[a]
  Hexamethylene bisacetamide[a]
  Suramin[a]

Peripheral neuropathy
  Cisplatin
  Vincristine
  Vindesine
  Etoposide
  Ara-C
  Procarbazine
  Methotrexate
  Taxol[a]

[a]Experimental agents.

distinguished from the syndrome that occurs after repeated intrathecal drug administrations. It is characterized by motor dysfunction, cranial nerve palsy, convulsions, and, more rarely, coma. A syndrome of brain damage associated with prophylactic cranial irradiation plus methotrexate has been reported in children with acute lymphoblastic leukaemia. Ventricular dilatation, intracerebral calcification, and a reduced cortex to medulla ratio could be documented by CT of the brain (Morse et al. 1985b).

Patients receiving ifosfamide can develop a form of central nervous complication characterized by cerebellar dysfunction, mental disturbance, drowsiness, coma, and eventually seizures. This complication appears to be due to the presence of a neurotoxic metabolite chloroacetaldehyde and is more frequent in patients receiving high-dose ifosfamide and presenting liver function abnormalities (Meanwell et al. 1986) and also when the drug is administered orally.

Neurological complications, characterized mainly by ataxia and mental disorientation, have been described in patients who received high-dose Ara-C. The cerebellar dysfunction appears in approximately 20 per cent of patients more than 50 years old, while occurring in only 3 per cent of patients aged less than 50 years. In addition, it is more common in patients receiving a total dose above $48 \, \text{g/m}^2$ per course, with lethality in approximately 1 per cent of patients. Reducing the dose of Ara-C to $2 \, \text{g/m}^2$ 12 times per course in patients over 50 years has been recommended (Herzig et al. 1987).

Modifications of the commonly utilized high-dose regimen, giving Ara-C by continuous infusion at the rate of $250 \, \text{mg/m}^2$ for 18 h, have recently been studied; high sustained drug concentrations were obtained. However, the mean steady state concentration was several times lower than the peak levels achieved after a 2 h infusion of $3 \, \text{g/m}^2$. Only one episode of cerebellar toxicity was documented in this study. Efforts to reduce the risk of neurological toxicity of high-dose regimens by avoiding the presence of high levels of Ara-C in the brain are ongoing (Watson et al. 1985).

Ara-C also causes aseptic meningitis when given intrathecally. On rare occasions, aseptic meningitis has been associated with high-dose systemic therapy. This syndrome is characterized by fever, nucal rigidity, and leucocytosis in the cerebrospinal fluid. The

related experimental compound Ara-A can also cause neurotoxicity, which is clearly dose limiting. It is characterized by dementia, seizures, vision disturbances, and coma. These complications are the main reason why Ara-A has not gained a place in the routine management of haematological malignancies, such as chronic lymphocytic leukaemia, despite its significant antitumour activity (Thordarson and Talstad 1986).

Cisplatin can cause a very disabling form of distal sensory neuropathy, which usually occurs after repeated drug administrations. With the effective utilization of pre-hydration programmes for the prevention of nephrotoxicity, neuropathy became the main dose-limiting toxicity in patients exposed to cisplatin for prolonged periods. Ototoxicity has also been reported in patients receiving cisplatin therapy. It is usually characterized by a hearing impairment for high-frequency sounds (Roelofs et al. 1984). The concomitant utilization of protective agents such as WR-2721 has been suggested as a way of reducing the risk of neurotoxicity from cisplatin. In addition, in recent studies in which cisplatin was adminstered by prolonged infusion significantly less neurotoxicity than the conventional short-term intravenous infusions has been described (Glover et al. 1987; Kemp et al. 1990).

Vincristine can cause a progressive form of neurotoxicity after repeated drug injections. Animal experiments on the pathogenesis of vincristine-induced neuropathy have revealed alterations of microtubule morphology and membrane organelle system in rat sciatic nerve fibres exposed to the drug. Microtubule-length histograms from vincristine-treated animals showed that exposed axons had a shorter length compared with controls. Treated axons had a decrease in the number of microtubules per square micrometre of axonal area, loss of portions of microtubules, accumulation of free vesicles, and fragmentation of smooth endoplasmic reticulum (Sahenk and Mendell 1983). In clinical studies, a decrease in deep tendon reflexes associated with paraesthesias in the extremities was documented after repeated exposure to vincristine. In severe cases, cranial nerve palsy and severe weakness of the hands and feet have been described. Autonomic neuropathy has been also described, with cases of constipation and paralytic ileus. These complications are more frequent in older patients, with concomitant neurological disorders. Unfortunately, only a partial improvement can be obtained following cessation of drug administration. Most patients who develop these types of complications suffer from some form of permanent disability (Miller 1985).

No agents capable of providing significant protection against vinca alkaloid neurotoxicity are available at present. Preclinical studies suggesting a protective effect by the concomitant administration of leucovorin were not confirmed in the clinic (Thomas et al. 1986). In addition, the results obtained using pyridoxine during vincristine administration in humans were also disappointing (Jackson et al. 1986).

Both etoposide and teniposide can cause peripheral neuropathy, with reduction of deep tendon reflexes and paraesthesias. Although this complication is not usually as severe or as frequent as with the vinca alkaloids, it can be very disabling in patients previously exposed to repeated courses of the latter drugs. Hexamethylmelamine and pentamethylmelamine can cause severe types of neurological manifestation. Hexamethylmelamine may cause hallucinations, changes in behaviour, and peripheral neuropathy after successive drug administrations, with complete recovery on cessation of drug administration. Pentamethylmelamine was reported to induce coma after rapid intravenous administration during initial clinical studies.

Procarbazine can cause paraesthesias, confusion, and a depressive syndrome. Some of these effects may be due to the inhibition of monoamine oxidase. Therefore, inhibitors of this enzyme should be avoided in patients receiving procarbazine, such as the tricyclic antidepressive and sympathomimetic agents. The concomitant use of strong hypnotics should also be avoided owing to the possible additive hypnotic effect of procarbazine.

L-Asparaginase can produce a syndrome of cerebral disturbances, with mental confusion and coma, probably related to serum elevations of ammonia. Nitrogen mustard can produce a syndrome characterized by cholinergic effects such as lacrimation, sweating, and diarrhoea.

Fludarabine phosphate is a purine derivative of adenosine arabinoside and has shown interesting antitumour activity against haematological malignancies, particularly chronic lymphocytic leukaemia. Neurotoxicity was reported in several clinical studies with this compound. It seems to be more common at doses above 96 mg/m^2/day for 5–7 days. Most patients developed a form of delayed neurotoxicity, consisting of visual symptoms, blindness, changes in mental status, and coma, 1–3 months after drug cessation. At necropsy, diffuse or focal demyelination was observed in the brain and spinal cord, particularly in the occipital lobes and optic tracts.

Taxol is a plant product derived from the western yew *Taxus brevifolia*. It is a mitotic inhibitor that enhances microtubular assembly and prevents its depolymerization. Peripheral neuropathy, consisting of dysaesthesias, loss of deep-tendon reflexes, and distal sensory loss, as well as motor disturbances and paralytic ileus at higher dose levels, was one of its main dose-limiting toxicities during early clinial trials (Donehower *et al.* 1987).

Hexamethylene bisacetamide is an experimental polar-planar compound related to *N*-methylformamine with differentiation-inducing properties in experimental models. One of its dose-limiting toxicities in initial clinical studies was neurotoxicity, manifested as agitation, confusion, and coma (Egorin *et al.* 1987). Recently, neurotoxicity was also described in patients receiving suramin in initial clinical trials, particularly in those achieving high peak concentrations in the cerebrospinal fluid (Myers *et al.* 1990).

COMPLICATIONS IN THE CARDIOVASCULAR SYSTEM

The complications of cytotoxic therapy in the cardiovascular system can be divided into two distinct groups: damage to the heart muscle, pericardium, and/or conduction system and toxic effects in the blood vessels. Examples of agents that can cause cardiovascular complications are given in Table 7.

Damage to the heart muscle, the pericardium, and/or the conduction system

Doxorubicin and daunorubicin may lead to two distinct forms of cardiac toxicity. The so-called myocarditis–pericarditis syndrome can occur immediately after drug administration or up to 2–3 days thereafter and consists of rhythm disturbances or less often acute congestive heart failure. In some cases, pericarditis with pericardial effusion is observed. Electrocardiographic changes such as supraventricular and/or ventricular arrhythmias and heart block can be documented. In patients with more severe abnormalities, a drop in left-ventricular ejection fraction can be observed (Ahmed and Slayton 1980).

Table 7 Examples of anticancer agents causing cardiovascular toxicity

Myocarditis–pericarditis
  Doxorubicin
  Daunorubicin
  Mitomycin C
  Mitoxantrone
  M-AMSA
  Bleomycin
  Actinomycin D
  Ara-C
  Cyclophosphamide (high dose)

Vascular changes
  5-Fluorouracil
  Cisplatin
  Vinblastine
  Mitomycin C
  Bleomycin
  Dacarbazine
  Procarbazine
  Flavone acetic acid[a]

[a]Experimental agent.

The second type of cardiac complication of anthracycline therapy is the development of a cumulative dose-dependent cardiomyopathy. This form of toxicity is more frequent at total cumulative doses over 550 mg/m^2. Indeed, up to 10 per cent of patients receiving this total dose were shown to develop congestive heart failure in various series. Prior exposure to other cardiotoxic agents and/or irradiation in the mediastinum can cause the appearance of this complication at lower total cumulative doses. In order to diagnose it at an earlier stage, repeated measurements of left-ventricular ejection fraction and the use of endomyocardial biopsy have been advocated. For obvious reasons, the use of ECG-gated pool scan measurement of the ejection fraction can produce results comparable with those obtained by radionuclide angiocardiography (Kramer *et al.* 1990).

The mechanism of cardiac damage due to the anthracyclines is not yet fully understood. It seems that doxorubicin is able to stimulate oxygen-radical formation in the cardiac muscle and also to reduce the ability of this organ to detoxify these radicals. Notably, the heart has relatively lower levels of catalase compared with other tissues and doxorubicin has been shown to interfere with the activity of glutathione peroxidase. Perhaps the most important step in the chain of reactions leading to the formation of free radicals involves doxorubicin, iron, and peroxide. In animal studies, tocoferol has been effective in preventing doxorubicin free-radical damage. However, these results could not be reproduced in humans. Recently, experiments using isolated hepatocytes have demonstrated that tocoferol protects cells in proportion to its available concentrations in the cells (Pascoe and Reed 1987).

Interestingly, the iron chelator ICRF-187 has been shown to be an effective cardioprotector. Initial reports of randomized trials have demonstrated that this agent significantly reduces the cardiotoxicity of doxorubicin in humans. Laboratory and initial clinical experience with ICRF-187 supports the concept that anthracycline-related cardiotoxicity can be circumvented without significantly affecting its antitumour activity. Other possible ways of reducing the cardiotoxicity of anthracyclines are by the use of continuous infusion or repeated small doses. Clinical studies using this approach have shown significantly less cardiotoxicity while maintaining comparable antitumour effects. Furthermore, analogues such as 4'-epidoxorubicin have been developed which possess similar antitumour activity but less risk of cardiac damage (Legha et al. 1982; Benjamin et al. 1988; Myers 1988).

Although the data on the cardiotoxicity of mitomycin C alone are scanty, this agent has been reported to accelerate the appearance of doxorubicin-related cardiomyopathy. This additive effect is probably due to the capacity of both agents to induce free-radical formation. Mitoxanthrone is a hydroxyquinone that appears to possess less risk of myocardial damage. It interferes with topoisomerase II function. In preclinical studies it was shown not to induce free-radical formation, which might explain its lower cardiotoxicity. Further studies are needed to confirm this observation in the clinic (Shenkenberg et al. 1986). M-AMSA has been shown to induce both acute and chronic cardiotoxicity. After drug administration, patients can develop supraventricular and ventricular arrhythmias, with prolongation of the Q–T interval. Rarely, acute heart failure can occur minutes to hours from drug injection. Although it has been demonstrated that M-AMSA can have significant antitumour activity in anthracycline-resistant patients, it is not yet clear whether prior exposure to anthracyclines increases the risk of cardiac toxicity. In view of the frequency of ECG abnormalities (Q–T prolongation), special care should be taken in patients presenting with hypocalaemia (Cassileth and Gale 1986).

Myocardial ischaemia, arrhythmias, and congestive heart failure have been reported in isolated patients after 5-fluorouracil administration, particularly during intravenous infusion of the drug alone or in combination with cisplatin. The mechanism involved in this toxic effect is not yet known (Labianca et al. 1982). An increased incidence of cardiomyopathy has also been reported in children treated with doxorubicin plus dacarbazine. However, this observation needs confirmation by further studies.

Haemorrhagic myocarditis has been described in patients receiving high-dose chemotherapy with cyclophosphamide-containing regimens. It appears to be related to a direct toxic effect on endothelial cells by the drug. However, an acquired form of platelet secretion and aggregation which might contribute to the development of this complication has recently been described (Panella et al. 1990). Furthermore, an acute lethal form of pericarditis–myocarditis has been observed after high-dose cyclophosphamide regimens employed in bone-marrow transplantation programmes (Cazin et al. 1986).

Isolated cases of documented myocardial infarction a few hours after the administration of vinblastine plus cisplatin have been documented. Angina can again be observed after reinstitution of therapy, even at a reduced dose. This complication may be related to a direct effect of the drug on platelets, causing coronary artery thrombosis and/or coronary spasm. Dose reductions have been recommended during initial treatment of patients with previous diagnosis of coronary insufficiency (Subar and Muggia 1986). Pericarditis has also been described after exposure to Ara-C, bleomycin, and actinomycin D (Vainckus and Letendre 1984).

Toxic effects in the blood vessels

As previously discussed in this chapter, mitomycin C can induce endothelial damage to the kidney vessels, leading to the development of haemolytic–uraemic syndrome. Hypertension can be diagnosed as a complication of this syndrome. Raynaud's phenomenon has been described in patients receiving cisplatin-containing regimens,

particularly in the treatment of testicular cancer. Although this phenomenon has previously been reported with other cytotoxic agents, it is unclear if there is a significant increase with drug combinations. However, the incidence of vascular complications is less than 5 per cent in most series of patients receiving cisplatin-containing regimens for the treatment of germ cell tumours. Also, some patients did not show evidence of Raynaud's phenomenon after retreatment. Furthermore, the influence of other agents and of cisplatin-related electrolyte disturbances with potential influence on cardiac function and vascular tone (such as hypomagnesaemia) has not been properly assessed.

Bleomycin has been shown to cause changes in the endothelium of capillary vessels and arterioles. Raynaud's phenomenon has been reported in patients receiving bleomycin plus vincristine for the treatment of germ cell tumours in the 1970s. Acute hypertension has also been reported in patients receiving this drug at relatively high doses (above 25 mg/day). Hypotension has been described in patients receiving etoposide by bolus intravenous administration. This acute complication can be avoided in the vast majority of patients by giving the drug by a short-term infusion (30–60 min).

As previously described, dacarbazine can cause fulminant hepatic veno-occlusive disease which can result in acute hepatic necrosis and death. Procarbazine inhibits monoamine oxidase. Therefore, hypertensive crisis can develop after the ingestion of significant quantities of tyramine-containing food, such as wine and cheese. Also, this syndrome can be precipitated by the concomitant administration of other inhibitors of monoamine oxidase such as tricyclic antidepressants.

The experimental agent flavone acetic acid is one of a series of compounds developed on the basis of the flavone ring. Initial clinical studies in which the compound was administered by short-term intravenous infusion have shown that acute hypotension is the main dose-limiting toxicity. This complication was reversible on cessation of drug administration (Kerr et al. 1986). It is believed that the vascular problems induced by drugs such as bleomycin and flavone acetic acid are caused by the secondary in vivo release of cytokines such as interleukins 1 and 6 and tumour necrosis factor, all of which have potent effects on vascular endothelium.

COMPLICATIONS IN THE RESPIRATORY TRACT

Several anticancer agents can produce damage to the lungs, as illustrated in Table 8. Acute and chronic pneumonitis have been described in patients receiving bleomycin. This complication appears to be related to a reduced availability of the enzymes involved in the metabolism of the drug in certain tissues, such as skin and lung. Notably, interspecies differences in the susceptibility to lung damage due to bleomycin have been correlated with the concentration of the inactivating enzymes. Bleomycin toxicity has also been studied in cultured bovine pulmonary arterial endothelial cells, suggesting an important rôle for iron-catalysed superoxide formation in lung damage (Martin and Kachel 1987). In addition, the surfactant-induced ambroxol has been shown to reduce bleomycin-related pulmonary toxicity in a rat model. However, conflicting results were obtained with the use of N-acetylcysteine (Berend 1985; Pozzi et al. 1987).

Histopathological studies performed in lung tissue obtained from affected patients have revealed an acute inflammatory infiltrate, interstitial and intra-alveolar oedema, hyaline membrane formation, squamous metaplasia of the alveolar lining cells, and lung fibrosis.

Table 8 Examples of anticancer agents causing lung damage

Antitumour antibiotics
  Bleomycin
  Mitomycin C

Alkylating agents
  Busulfan
  BCNU
  Cyclophosphamide
  Chlorambucil
  Melphalan

Antimetabolites
  Methotrexate
  Ara-C

Miscellaneous
  Procarbazine
  4-Ipomeanol[a]

[a]Experimental agent.

Clinically, patients develop cough, dyspnoea, and sometimes fever. A bilateral pulmonary infiltrate, distributed at the basilar segments in particular, is diagnosed at chest radiography. These abnormalities can include linear and nodular densities, which may become confluent. These symptoms and the radiological findings are not easily distinguished from other common complications occurring in cancer patients, such as opportunistic infections or carcinomatous lymphangitis.

The clinical manifestations of bleomycin-induced lung toxicity may become evident before any radiological abnormality is observed. The CT scan may uncover pulmonary changes in up to a third of patients exhibiting a normal chest radiograph (Bellamy et al. 1985). The same seems to hold for gallium scans. Asymptomatic patients may show a decrease in carbon monoxide diffuse capacity as the total drug exposure increases. However, the latter test cannot be considered a reliable predictor of impending severe toxicity in the asymptomatic patient.

It has been suggested that chemoluminescence allows the detection of singlet oxygen production by bleomycin in a comparative way to haem-mediated catalysis and that this may be due to bleomycin-induced lung damage (Kanofsky 1986). The diagnosis of bleomycin lung toxicity should be based on the clinical, laboratory, and radiological picture, confirmed by the presence of a form of polymorphonuclear alveolitis on bronchoalveolar lavage and transbronchial or open lung biopsy (Ginsberg and Comis 1982).

In most documented cases of bleomycin toxicity to the lungs, a close correlation can be established between the total cumulative dose of the drug and the risk of toxicity. In general, this complication is observed at a dose of over 450 mg. However, severe toxicity can be demonstrated at lower doses, particularly in elderly patients, in patients with lung fibrosis or emphysema, in patients with impaired renal function, or in patients previously exposed to irradiation to the lungs. The definitive diagnosis of bleomycin-related pneumonitis involves the above clinical and radiological picture plus the histopathological confirmation by lung biopsy. With the discontinuation of therapy in asymptomatic patients, normalization of the chest radiograph and the carbon diffusion capacity test are frequent. However, only partial recovery can be expected in symptomatic patients (Sorensen et al. 1985).

Interstitial and alveolar infiltration by lymphocytes, eosinophils, and plasma cells, sometimes associated with granuloma formation,

can occur shortly after exposure to methotrexate. This form of acute pneumonitis is uncommon and has been associated with peripheral eosinophilia. In the rare reports of this complication, retreatment has not always been associated with reappearance of lung abnormalities. A form of drug-induced hypersensitivity reaction has been suggested. This syndrome can respond dramatically to corticosteroids (Eigen 1985).

Chronic lung fibrosis can develop after long-term busulphan therapy. This complication has been described mostly in patients with chronic myelogenous leukaemia. Initially, the chest radiograph may not reveal significant abnormalities or may develop a picture consisting of a bilateral basal reticular pattern. In rare cases, responses to high-dose corticosteroids were observed. BCNU has also been associated with a form of lung fibrosis similar to that observed after bleomycin therapy. The chest radiograph may show a bilateral basal recticular infiltrate. Corticosteroids are usually of no benefit in this complication (Selker et al. 1980).

Mitomycin C can produce a diffuse reticular infiltrate in the lungs, on some occasions associated with pleural effusion. Histopathologically, it resembles bleomycin toxicity. Patients may develop a dry cough and dyspnoea. The definitive diagnosis is usually based on clinicoradiological findings and confirmed by lung biopsy (Gunstream et al. 1983). Rarely, cyclophosphamide, melphalan, and chlorambucil can produce lung toxicity, which is usually characterized by a bilateral basal reticular infiltrate. Less often, diffuse alveolar infiltrate and pulmonary oedema have been observed (Morse et al. 1985a).

Isolated cases of lung toxicity have been reported after exposure to Ara-C. Histopathologically, a proteinaceous exudate with extravasation of blood cells and no inflammation has been described. Clinically, patients may develop acute dyspnoea and signs of pulmonary oedema. The chest radiograph reveals a diffuse interstitial and alveolar pattern. Rarely, procarbazine can produce acute pulmonary toxicity, characterized by a mononuclear cell infiltration. This syndrome resembles a hypersensitivity reaction and resolves rapidly following drug discontinuation.

Fatal episodes of acute respiratory distress syndrome have recently been reported after intensive combined modality chemotherapy with doxorubicin, cyclophosphamide, and etoposide plus radiation therapy in patients with small-cell lung cancer. The intensity of chemotherapy (number of courses) and the inclusion of doxorubicin in the combination were associated with a higher risk of pulmonary toxicity (Maurer et al. 1990).

4-Ipomeanol is an experimental naturally occurring lung toxin isolated from cultures of the common sweet potato infected with the fungus Fusarium solani which is presently undergoing initial clinical evaluation. It has remarkable lung-specific toxicity in several animal species. When activated by mixed-function oxidase enzymes present at the Clara cells of the lung, it causes interstitial inflammation and multifocal necrosis of the bronchiolar epithelium. At present the lung tissue specificity of 4-ipomeanol is being explored as a means of providing a novel approach to the treatment of lung cancer (Christian et al. 1989).

COMPLICATIONS IN THE HOMEOSTASIS OF FLUIDS AND ELECTROLYTES

Abnormalities in the homeostasis of fluids and electrolytes can be produced in cancer patients by a direct effect of chemotherapy in the tumour cells or as a consequence of the cytotoxic effects of therapy on the organs involved in the absorption and/or elimination of these body constituents.

Cisplatin can also cause electrolytic disturbances, the most frequent being hypomagnesaemia and a form of renal magnesium wasting syndrome. Hypomagnesaemia develops in approximately 50 per cent of patients receiving cisplatin. Patients with this complication can present with neuromuscular toxicity, central nervous system toxicity, and cardiac disturbances, particularly when the serum magnesium levels are below 1 mmol/l. In this situation, magnesium sulphate should be administered intravenously.

Hypomagnesaemia is often complicated by the development of hypocalcaemia. The latter is secondary to a decrease in parathyroid hormone release and/or due to end-organ resistance to parathyroid hormone-induced hypomagnesaemia. In this context, hypocalcaemia should be treated by magnesium sulphate replacement, in that it is not usually responsive to calcium replacement alone. More rarely, hypokalaemia is observed in patients with cisplatin-induced nephrotoxicity. The management of this complication consists of potassium and magnesium replacement (Blachley and Hill 1981).

Hyperuricaemia has been observed in patients with rapidly growing malignancies which are highly responsive to cytotoxic therapy, such as the acute leukaemias and lymphomas. In this situation, patients should receive pre-hydration, urine alkalinization with sodium bicarbonate, and/or prophylactic allopurinol before starting chemotherapy to avoid the deposition of uric acid in the kidneys and the occurrence of life-threatening acute renal failure. In more severe cases, a tumour lysis syndrome is characterized with acute hyperuricaemic nephropathy, hypercalcaemia, and hyperphosphataemia owing to the sudden destruction of large numbers of neoplastic cells.

Tumour lysis syndrome is generally observed after the successful therapy of bulky non-Hodgkin's lymphomas and acute leukaemias. The latter cells tend to have high phosphate concentrations and, thus, seem to be more prone to cause hyperphosphataemia compared with solid tumour cells (Stapleton et al. 1988). However, this syndrome has also been reported after the treatment of non-haematological malignancies such as germ cell tumours and breast cancer. As a rule, bulky tumours, with rapid growth and spontaneous evidence of tumour lysis, are predisposing factors. This syndrome is managed preferably by preventing its occurrence through the vigorous utilization of the measures mentioned above. Haemodialysis has been attempted in severe cases.

Cyclophosphamide, melphalan, and vincristine can cause a syndrome of inappropriate secretion of antidiuretic (SIADH), probably due to a direct stimulatory effect in the release of the hormone. This complication is particularly prevalent in patients who have fluid overload. It consists of dilutional hyponatraemia, mental confusion, seizures, and sometimes death. Clinically, drug-related SIADH is suspected in patients without signs of volume depletion and/or oedema, with normal or diminished serum creatinine, and with a urinary sodium concentration that usually exceeds 20 mmol/l unless fluid intake has been restricted. Asymptomatic hyponatraemia does not need specific treatment.

The management of the above complication in symptomatic patients involves cessation of drug administration, water restriction, and sometimes the administration of demeclocycline. If severe symptomatic hyponatraemia is documented, intravenous treatment is indicated. The amount of sodium to be administered should be calculated by multiplying the deficit in plasma sodium concentration in millimoles per litre by the total body water (approximately 50–60 per cent of body weight) and infused over several hours. Isolated cases of brain damage due to central pontine myelinolysis have been

associated with the rapid correction of hyponatraemia (Hainsworth et al. 1983). Mithramycin can effectively reduce serum calcium levels in patients with several forms of hypercalcaemia through the induction of a decrease in bone resorption. This apparent complication has proved to be of therapeutic use in cases of malignant hypercalcaemia. However, the toxic effects of this agent to the gastrointestinal system, the liver and kidney, and coagulation has precluded its widespread routine utilization.

ENDOCRINE AND METABOLIC COMPLICATIONS

Endocrine complications of chemotherapy can lead to significant morbidity to patients. As discussed above, an Addison-like syndrome has been described in patients receiving chronic busulphan therapy. However, this syndrome is not related to any significant adrenal disturbance. Owing to its toxic effects on pancreatic islet cells, streptozotocin can cause hyperglycaemia in a significant number of patients. L-Asparaginase may cause a decrease in serum insulin leading to hyperglycaemia. It may also cause a decrease in serum lipoproteins and thyroxine-binding globulin. These effects are due to its inhibitory effects on protein synthesis. In addition, the experimental differentiation-inducing agent hexamethylene bisacetamide has been shown to produce hyperchloraemic metabolic acidosis in initial clinical trials (Egorin et al. 1987).

CUTANEOUS COMPLICATIONS

The complications of cytotoxic agents in the skin can be caused by direct cytotoxic damage, local reactions, hypersensitivity and hypersensitivity-like reactions, alterations in pigmentation, or infectious complications related to immunosuppression by cytotoxic agents. Examples of cytotoxic agents which may lead to cutaneous complications are given in Table 9.

Toxic non-immunologically mediated dermatitis is an example of a direct cytotoxic effect of anticancer agents. It has been reported after the administration of various anticancer agents, such as the antimetabolites. Alopecia is another form of direct cytotoxic damage of chemotherapy. It is dependent on the type of agent, the dose, and the frequency of drug administration and is more common after anthracycline and cyclophosphamide therapy. Chemotherapy-induced alopecia is reversible, but the colour and texture of the hair may be changed after regrowth. Usually, hair starts to fall out approximately 1–2 weeks after drug administration and reaches a maximum loss during the first 6–8 weeks. It involves mainly the scalp, but loss of pubic, axillary, or facial hair can also occur after prolonged drug therapy (Hood 1986).

Methotrexate can cause acute dermatitis, with skin irritation and desquamation. Photosensitization has also been described with this agent. Isolated cases of severe skin reaction, leading to a form of Stevens–Johnson syndrome (lesions affecting the oral mucosa and skin of arms and feet, characterized by ruptured bullae surrounded by an inflammatory area and haemorrhagic crusts, as well as so-called 'target lesions'), have been reported (Bronner and Hood 1983).

5-Fluorouracil can produce acute skin reaction and hyperpigmentation at the site of drug injection and proximally, following the venous return. The latter complication tends to persist for months, slowly fading away after prolonged periods. In contrast, Ara-C does not produce local injury after drug extravasation and is often given to patients by the subcutaneous route (Donagin 1982).

Table 9 Examples of anticancer agents causing skin toxicity

Direct cytotoxic damage
  Acute dermatitis
    Methotrexate
    5-Fluorouracil
    Bleomycin
    Trimethexate[a]
    PALA[a]
    DUP-785[a]
  Alopecia
    Doxorubicin
    Daunorubicin
    Mitomycin C
    Melphalan
    Vinca alkaloids

Local reactions
  Cellulitis/necrosis
    Doxorubicin
    Daunorubicin
    Mitomycin C
    Nitrogen mustard
    Vinca alkaloids
  Phlebitis
    5-Fluorouracil
    Doxorubicin
    Daunorubicin
    Nitrogen mustard
    Mitomycin C

Hypersensitivity (-like)
  Bleomycin
  Doxorubicin
  Procarbazine
  L-Asparaginase
  DUP-785[a]

Alterations in pigmentation
  5-Fluorouracil
  Bleomycin
  Busulfan
  DUP-785[a]

Infectious/secondary tumours due to immunosuppression
  Cyclophosphamide

Miscellaneous reactions
  Recall phenomenon
    Doxorubicin
    Daunorubicin
    Actinomycin D
    Trimetrexate[a]
  Photosensitivity
    Methotrexate
    5-Fluorouracil
    DUP-785[a]

[a]Experimental agents.

Doxorubicin and daunorubicin are commonly associated with the development of alopecia. This complication occurs in virtually all patients treated at standard doses. In addition, anthracyclines can cause severe skin reactions at the site of drug administration. Drug extravasation often leads to local inflammation and tissue necrosis. More rarely, local allergic reaction can be observed at the site of doxorubicin administration. In patients who received prior irradiation a type of recall phenomenon, characterized by an erythematous reaction at the previous irradiation field, has been described with both doxorubicin and daunorubicin.

Mitomycin C is also frequently associated with the development of alopecia. It is also vesicant, causing severe tissue damage after drug extravasation. Isolated cases of late development of tissue necrosis months after drug extravasation have been reported. Actinomycin D also shows interaction with the radiation therapy, probably because of its inhibitory effect on DNA repair induced by radiation. The combined use of this agent with radiation may cause severe skin and gastrointestinal toxicity. Apart from that, actinomycin D causes recall phenomenon later at the irradiated fields, as described for doxorubicin (Bronner and Hood 1983).

Nitrogen mustard is highly reactive chemically and is a potent vesicant. Drug extravasation at the site of injection leads to severe local tissue damage and skin necrosis. The management of extravasation lesions consists basically of immediate cessation of drug administration, symptomatic treatment against pain and to avoid secondary infection, and early surgical debridgement of necrotic areas. Over the past years, several agents have been investigated in an attempt to protect against local injury due to the extravasation of cytotoxics, always with conflicting results. Rarely, both nitrogen mustard and cyclophosphamide have been associated with the development of hypermelanosis.

Melphalan is often associated with the development of alopecia after prolonged drug administration. Busulphan can produce an Addison-like state characterized by hyperpigmentation of the skin and muscle weakness. This syndrome does not seem to be related to any detectable changes in adrenal function and was initially observed in patients with chronic myeloid leukaemia after prolonged therapy (Hood 1986).

Bleomycin often causes skin reaction, characterized by erythema, induration, and desquamation of the skin. The lesions usually progress to hyperpigmentation and tend to occur in areas of previous scratching. Again, bleomycin-inactivating enzymes have been shown to be at low concentrations in the skin (Sehti and Lazo 1987).

Vincristine, vinblastine, and vindesine can cause moderate to severe alopecia. In addition, these agents are highly vesicant causing inflammation and skin necrosis after drug extravasation at the injection site. With a mouse model, the local vesicant effect of extravasated vinca alkaloids was diminished by the local administration of hyaluronidase, saline, and leucovorin and by the application of heat locally. In contrast, skin cooling and topical corticosteroids increased local toxicity. Dyphenidramine and sodium bicarbonate were considered ineffective (Buchanan et al. 1985).

Procarbazine can produce hypersensitivity reactions characterized by cutaneous maculopapular rash and pulmonary infiltrates. The skin reaction usually subsides with the administration of corticosteroids. L-Asparaginase can cause a syndrome of immunological sensitization characterized by urticariform lesions in the skin, particularly after repeated drug administrations.

PALA and DUP-785 are experimental agents which act through the inhibition of pyrimidine biosynthesis. Both agents have been shown to cause severe skin reactions. These reactions were characterized by a widespread maculopapular erythematous cutaneous rash, probably because of a direct toxic effect on the skin. These lesions usually appeared during the second week after drug administration, with resolution after 2–3 weeks. The histopathological picture of DUP-785-induced toxic dermatitis usually consists of parakerathosis, acanthosis with elongation of the epidermal papillae, migration of inflammatory cells through the epidermis, vacuolar degeneration of basal cells, and destruction of the basal membrane. Intercellular oedema with focal intraepidermal and subepidermal vesicles are common. Sometimes, the upper dermis shows oedematous changes and mononuclear infiltration (Hart *et al.* 1980; Schwartsmann *et al.* 1989).

Trimexate is a lipid-soluble folate antagonist that is a strong inhibitor of dihydrofolate reductase. It appears to enter cells independently of the methotrexate carrier system. Initial clinical trials have documented three forms of skin toxicity: radiation recall, cellulitis at the injection site, and widespread erythematous reaction (Weiss *et al.* 1986).

Cytotoxic therapy can also facilitate the occurrence of secondary infections in the skin as a consequence of the breakage of natural barriers and the immunosuppressive effects of prolonged treatment. Bacterial and fungal infections, such as cellulitis caused by *P. aeruginosa*, *E. coli*, *S. epidermidis*, *C. albicans*, or *S. aureus*, have been observed during chemotherapy. Varicella zoster can occur mainly in children receiving intensive cytotoxic therapy (Kingston and Mackey 1986).

COMPLICATIONS IN THE SENSORY ORGANS

Ocular toxicity has been reported in patients with ovarian carcinoma following the administration of high-dose cisplatin. Blurred vision and altered colour perception in association with cone dysfunction have been documented (Wilding *et al.* 1985). Retinopathy has also been observed after intracarotid cisplatin and BCNU therapy in malignant gliomas (Miller 1985).

Acute conjunctivitis can develop after 5-fluorouracil therapy. In some cases chronic changes such as tear duct stenosis can occur. These complications are usually reversible with cessation of therapy (Griffin and Garnick 1981). Acute conjunctivitis was also observed in patients with acute leukaemia receiving Ara-C in high doses. This complication was seen within days of drug administration and recovered spontaneously after the drug was discontinued.

Ototoxicity has frequently been described after cisplatin therapy. It is usually dose related and irreversible, and mainly occurs at higher frequencies (Melamed *et al.* 1985). Vestibular toxicity is less common after cisplatin therapy. Animal studies have suggested that fosfomycin can decrease ototoxicity when administered simultaneously with cisplatin in a guinea-pig model. The inhibition of the enzyme phosphoenopyruvate transferase by the antibiotic has been associated with this protective effect (Schweitzer *et al.* 1986).

Disturbances of smell and taste have also been reported in patients receiving cytotoxic therapy. The latter has been associated with an injury to receptor cells and gustatory loss caused by cytotoxic therapy (Snow 1983).

HYPERSENSITIVITY(-LIKE) REACTIONS

Hypersensitivity reactions have occasionally been reported in patients receiving cisplatin therapy. This complication is characterized by urticaria, bronchospasm, and hypotension immediately after drug administration. The prophylactic utilization of corticosteroids and/or antihistamines has been shown to prevent this reaction, allowing retreatment of patients.

Bleomycin-induced hypersensitivity reactions are sometimes observed within 48 h of drug administration. They usually consist of fever, urticaria, and bronchospasm. As discussed above,

pre-treatment with corticosteroids and/or antihistamines can protect the patients from the occurrence of this complication and are recommended in the case of patients considered for drug readministration (Donagin 1982).

Procarbazine can produce hypersensitivity reactions, which are characterized by the development of widespread maculopapular skin rash and lung infiltrates. This syndrome can be prevented by the concomitant administration of corticosteroids. Furthermore, procarbazine may also cause a disulfiram-like reaction after the ingestion of alcholic beverages. As observed with the administration of disulfiram, flushing, headache, sweating, nausea, and vomiting are sometimes seen (Hood 1986).

Immunological sensitization to L-asparaginase can cause hypersensitivity phenomenoma in approximately one-third of patients and is characterized by urticaria, bronchospasm, abdominal pain, and, more rarely, laryngeal oedema, hypotension, and anaphylaxis. In patients hypersensitive to L-asparaginase derived from *E. coli*, other preparations of the enzyme, such as the one derived from Erwinia, can be utilized. Dacarbazine can produce an influenza-like syndrome that may persist throughout treatment. The cause of this side-effect is not yet known.

Initial clinical trials with taxol showed anaphylactoid reactions, characterized by flushing, urticaria, bronchospasm, and hypotension in approximately 20 per cent of patients. These reactions were more frequent in short-term intravenous administrations and were probably related to the rapid infusion of the polyoxyethylated castor oil vehicle (cremophor EL) used in the drug formulation. Significant reduction in this complication was documented after a more prolonged intravenous infusion (6–24 h) was chosen, with prophylactic administration of corticosteroids and antihistamines (Grem *et al.* 1987*b*).

REFERENCES

Abelson HT, Garnick MB (1982). Renal failure induced by cancer chemotherapy. In *Cancer and the kidney* (ed. RE Riselbach and MB Garnick), pp. 769–813. Lea and Febiger, Philadelphia.

Ahmed M, Slayton RE (1980). Report on drug-induced pericarditis. *Cancer Treatment Reports*, 64:353–5.

Andriole GL, *et al.* (1987). The efficacy of Mesna (2-mercaptoethane sodium sulfonate) as a uroprotectant in patients with hemorrhagic cystitis receiving further oxazaphosphorine chemotherapy. *Journal of Clinical Oncology*, 5:799–803.

Anonymous (1990). Postherpetic neuralgia (editorial). *Lancet*, 336:537–8.

Bellamy EA, Husband JE, Blaquiere RM, Law MR (1985). Bleomycin-related lung damage: CT evidence. *Radiology*, 156:155–8.

Benjamin RS, *et al.* (1988). Adriamycin cardiac toxicity: an assessment of approaches to cardiac monitoring and cardioprotection. In *Organ directed toxicities of anticancer drugs* (ed. MP Hacker, JS Lazo, and TR Triton), pp. 41–55. Nijhoff, The Hague.

Berend N (1985). Inhibition of bleomycin lung toxicity by *N*-acetylcysteine in the rat. *Pathology*, 17:108–10.

Blachley JD, Hill JB (1981). Renal and electrolytic disturbances associated with cisplatin. *Annals of Internal Medicine*, 95:628–32.

Bodey GP (1986). Infection in cancer patients: a continuing association. *American Journal of Medicine* 81, 11–26.

Bronner AK, Hood AF (1983). Cutaneous complications of chemotherapy agent. *Journal of the American Academy of Dermatology*, 9:645–63.

Browne MJ, *et al.* (1990). A randomized trial of open lung biopsy versus empiric antimicrobial therapy in cancer patients with diffuse pulmonary infiltrates. *Journal of Clinical Oncology*, 8:222–9.

Brunneto AL (1990). Small-bowel mucosal function in children with malignancy. Thesis, University of Newcastle upon Tyne.

Buchanan GR, Buchsbaum HJ, O'Banion K, Goje B (1985). Extravasation of dactinomycin, vincristine and cisplatin: studies in an animal model. *Medical and Pediatric Oncology*, **13**:375–80.

Cantrell JE, Phillips TM, Schein PS (1985). Carcinoma-associated hemolytic uremic syndrome: a complication of mitomycin C chemotherapy. *Journal of Clinical Oncology*, **3**:723–34.

Cassileth PA, Gale RP (1986). Amsacrine: a review. *Leukemia Research*, **10**:1257–65.

Cazin B, *et al.* (1986). Cardiac complications after bone marrow transplantation: a report on a series of 63 consecutive transplantations. *Cancer*, **57**:2061–9.

Chang JC (1989). Neoplastic fever. A proposal for diagnosis. *Archives of International Medicine*, **149**:1728–30.

Christian MC, *et al.* (1989). 4-Ipomeanol: a novel investigational new drug for lung cancer. *Journal of the National Cancer Institute*, **81**:1133–43.

Clavell LA, *et al.* (1986). Four-agent induction and intensive asparaginase therapy for the treatment of childhood acute lymphoblastic leukaemia. *New England Journal of Medicine*, **315**:657–63.

Co-operative Group for the Study of Immunoglobulin in Chronic Lymphocytic Leukemia (1988). Intravenous immunoglobulin for the prevention of infection in chronic lymphocytic leukemia. *New England Journal of Medicine*, **319**:902–7.

Correy L, Spear PB (1986). Infections with herpes simplex viruses: parts I and II. *New England Journal of Medicine*, **314**:686–91, 749–57.

Curnette JT, Boxer LA (1985). Clinically significant phagocytic cell defects. In *Current clinical topics in infectious diseases* (ed. J Remington and M Swartz), Vol. 6, pp. 103–56. McGraw-Hill, New York.

Davey PG (1990). New antiviral and antifungal drugs. *British Medical Journal*, **300**:793–8.

Day HJ, Rao AK (1986). Platelets and megakaryocytes. *Seminars in Hematology*, **23**:89–101.

Dekker AW, Rosenberg-Arska M, Verhoef J (1987). Infection prophylaxis in acute leukemia: a comparison of ciprofloxacin with trimethoprim-sulfamethoxazole and colistin. *Annals of Internal Medicine*, **106**:7–12.

Dekker AW, Verhoef J, Rozenberg-Arska M (1989). Prevention of bacterial and fungal infections in granulocytopenic patients. *European Journal of Clinical Oncology*, **25**:1345–50.

Dinarello CA, Cannon JG, Wolff SM (1988). New concepts on the pathogenesis of fever. *Reviews of Infectious Diseases*, **10**:168–89.

Doll DC, Weiss RB (1985). Hemolytic anemia associated with antineoplastic agents. *Cancer Treatment Reports*, **69**:777–82.

Donagin WG (1982). Clinical toxicity of chemotherapeutic agents: dermatologic toxicity. *Seminars in Oncology*, **9**:14–22.

Donehower RC, Karp JE, Burke PJ (1986). Pharmacology and toxicity of high-dose cytarabine by 72-hour continuous infusion. *Cancer Treatment Reports*, **70**:1059–65.

Donehower RC, *et al.* (1987). Phase I trial of taxol in patients with advanced cancer. *Cancer Treatment Reports*, **71**:1171–7.

Earhart RM, *et al.* (1983). Improvement in the therapeutic index of cisplatin (NSC 119875) by pharmacologically induced chloriuresis in the rat. *Cancer Research*, **43**:1187–94.

Egorin MJ, *et al.* (1987). Phase I clinical and pharmacokinetic study of hexamethylene bisacetamide (NSC 95580) administered as a five-day continuous infusion. *Cancer Research*, **47**:617.

Eigen H (1985). Bleomycin lung injury in children: pathophysiology and guidelines for management. *American Journal of Pediatric Hematology and Oncology*, **7**:71–8.

Evans WE, *et al.* (1986). Clinical pharmacodynamics of high-dose methotrexate in acute lymphocytic leukemia: identification of a relation between concentration and effect. *New England Journal of Medicine*, **314**:471–7.

Feaux de Lacroix W, *et al.* (1983). Acute liver dystrophy with thrombosis of hepatic veins: a fatal complication of dacarbazine treatment. *Cancer Treatment Reports*, **67**:779–84.

Foster BJ, Clegett-Carr K, Hoth D, Leyland-Jones B (1986). Gallium nitrate: the second metal with clinical activity. *Cancer Treatment Reports*, **70**:1311–19.

Gandara DR, *et al.* (1986). High-dose cisplatin in hypertonic saline: reduced toxicity of a modified dose schedule and correlation with plasma pharmacokinetics. A Northern California Oncology Group pilot study in non-small cell lung cancer. *Journal of Clinical Oncology*, **4**:1787–93.

Ginsberg SJ, Comis RL (1982). The pulmonary toxicity of antineoplastic agents. *Seminars in Oncology*, **9**:34–51.

Glover D, *et al.* (1987). WR-2721 and high-dose cisplatin: an active combination in the treatment of metastatic melanoma. *Journal of Clinical Oncology*, **5**:574–8.

Grem JL, *et al.* (1987a). Overview of current status and future direction of clinical trials with 5-fluorouracil in combination with folinic acid. *Cancer Treatment Reports*, **71**:1249–64.

Grem JL, *et al.* (1987b). Phase I study of taxol administered as a short IV infusion daily for 5 days. *Cancer Treatment Reports*, **71**:1179–84.

Griffin JD, Garnick MD (1981). Eye toxicity of cancer chemotherapy. *Cancer*, **48**:1539–49.

Groopman JE, Molina JM, Scadden DT (1989). Hematopoietic growth factors. Biology and clinical applications. *New England Journal of Medicine*, **321**:1449–59.

Gunstream SR, *et al.* (1983). Mitomycin-associated lung disease. *Cancer Treatment Reports*, **67**:301.

Hainsworth JD, Workman R, Greco FA (1983). Management of the syndrome of inappropriate antidiuretic hormone secretion in small cell lung cancer. *Cancer*, **51**:161–5.

Hart DD, Ohnuma T, Holland JF (1980). Initial clinical study with *N*-(phosphonacethyl)-L-aspartic acid (PALA) in patients with advanced cancer. *Cancer Treatment Reports*, **64**:617–24.

Herzig RH, *et al.* (1987). Cerebellar toxicity with high-dose cytosine arabinoside. *Journal of Clinical Oncology*, **5**:927–32.

Ho M (ed) (1991). Cytomegalovirus infections in the immunocompromised transplant patient: diagnosis and treatment. *Transplantation Proceedings*, **23**(2) (Suppl. 1):35.

Homans AC, *et al.* (1987). Effect of L-asparaginase administration on coagulation and platelet function in children with leukemia. *Journal of Clinical Oncology*, **5**:811–7.

Hood AF (1986). Cutaneous side-effects of cancer chemotherapy. *Medical Clinics of North America*, **70**:187–209.

Howell SB, *et al.* (1982). Intraperitoneal cisplatin with systemic thiosulfate protection. *Annals of Internal Medicine*, **97**:845–51.

Hryniuk WM (1988). The importance of dose intensity in the outcome of chemotherapy. In *Important advances in oncology* (ed. VT DeVita, S Hellman, and SA Rosenberg), pp. 121–42. JB Lippincott, Philadelphia.

Jackson DV Jr, *et al.* (1986). Clinical trials of folinic acid to reduce vincristine neurotoxicity. *Cancer Chemotherapy and Pharmacology*, **17**(3):281–4.

Joënsuu H, Soderstrom KO, Nikkanen V (1986). Fatal necrosis of the liver during ABVD chemotherapy for Hodgkin's disease. A case report. *Cancer*, **58**:1437–40.

Johnston JB, *et al.* (1986). The treatment of hairy cell leukaemia with 2'-deoxycoformycin. *British Journal of Haematology*, **63**:525–34.

Kaplan RS, Wiernik P (1982). Neurotoxicity of antineoplastic agents. *Seminars in Oncology*, **9**:103–30.

Kanofsky JR (1986). Singlet oxygen production by bleomycin. A comparison with heme-containing compounds. *Journal of Biological Chemistry*, **261**:135–46.

Karp JE, *et al.* (1987). Oral norfloxacin for prevention of Gram-negative bacterial infections in patients with acute leukemia and granulocytopenia. *Annals of Internal Medicine*, **107**:1–7.

Katz JA, Wagner ML, Gresik MV, Mahoney DH Jr, Fernbach DJ (1990). Typhlitis. An 18 year experience and postmortem review. *Cancer*, **65**:1041–7.

Keller J, Bartolucci A, Carpenter JT, Feagler J (1986). Phase II evaluation of bolus gallium nitrate in lymphoproliferative disorders: a South-Eastern Cancer Study Group trial. *Cancer Treatment Reports*, **70**:1221–3.

Kemp GM, Glover DJ, Schein PS (1990). The role of WR-2721 in the reduction of combined cisplatin and cyclophosphamide toxicity. *Proceedings of the American Society of Clinical Oncology*, **9**:67.

Kerr DJ, *et al.* (1986). Phase I and pharmacokinetic study of LM985 (flavone acetic acid ester). *Cancer Research*, **46**:3142–6.

Kingston ME, Mackey D (1986). Skin clues in the diagnosis of life-threatening infections. *Reviews of Infection Diseases*, **8**:1–11.

Labianca R, *et al.* (1982). Cardiac toxicity of 5-fluorouracil: a study of 1083 patients. *Tumori*, **68**:505–10.

Lazarus HM, Creger RJ, Gerson SL (1989). Infectious emergencies in oncology patients. *Seminars in Oncology*, **16**:543–60.

Legha SS, *et al.* (1982). Reduction of doxorubicin cardiotoxicity by prolonged continuous infusion. *Annals of Internal Medicine*, **96**:133–9.

Liang RHS, Yung RWH, Chan T-K, Chau P-Y, Klam W, So S-Y, Todd D (1990). Ofloxacin versus co-trimoxazole for prevention of infection in neutropenic patients following cytotoxic chemotherapy. *Antimicrobial Agents and Chemotherapy*, **9**:408–16.

Litterst C, *et al.* (1986). Sensitivity of urinary enzymes as indicators of renal toxicity of the anticancer drug cisplatin. *Uremia Investigation*, **9**:111–17.

Malpass TV, Harker LA (1980). Acquired disorders of platelet function. *Seminars in Hematology*, **17**:242–58.

Markman M, Abeloff M (1983). Management of hematologic and infectious complications of intensive induction therapy for small cell carcinoma of the lung. *American Journal of Medicine*, **74**:741–6.

Martin WJ II, Kachel DL (1987). Bleomycin-induced pulmonary endothelial cell injury: evidence for the role of iron-catalyzed toxic oxygen-derived species. *Journal of Laboratory and Clinical Medicine*, **110**:153.

Martin WJ II, *et al.* (1987). Role of bronchoalveolar lavage in the assessment of opportunistic pulmonary infections: utility and complications. *Mayo Clinic Proceedings*, **62**:549–57.

Maurer H, *et al.* (1990). Adult respiratory distress syndrome (ARDS) after combined modality chemotherapy and radiation therapy in limited disease small cell lung cancer. *Proceedings of the American Society of Clinical Oncology*, **9**:229.

Meanwell CA, *et al.* (1986). Prediction of ifosfamide/Mesna-associated encephalopathy. *European Journal of Cancer and Clinical Oncology*, **22**:815–19.

Melamed LB, Selim MA, Schuchman D (1985). Cisplatin ototoxicity in gynecological cancer patients. *Cancer*, **55**:41–3.

Meunier F (1987). Prevention of mycoses in immunocompromised patients. *Reviews of Infectious Diseases*, **9**:408–16.

Meyers JD, Flournoy N, Thomas ED (1986). Risk factors for cytomegalovirus infection after human marrow transplantation. *Journal of Infectious Diseases*, **153**:478–88.

Miller BR (1985). Neurotoxocity and vincristine. *Journal of the American Medical Association*, **253**:2045.

Mondesir JM, *et al.* (1985). Drug-induced antibodies during 2-*N*-methyl-9-hydroxyellipticinium acetate (NSC-264137) treatment: schedule dependency and relationship to hemolysis. *Journal of Clinical Oncology*, **3**:735–40.

Morse CC, *et al.* (1985a). Pulmonary toxicity of cyclophosphamide: a 1 year study. *Experimental and Molecular Pathology*, **42**:251–60.

Morse M, *et al.* (1985b). Altered central nervous system pharmacology of methotrexate in childhood leukemia: another sign of meningeal relapse. *Journal of Clinical Oncology*, **3**:19–24.

Murthy MS, Rao LN, Khandakar JD, Scanlon EF (1987). Enhanced therapeutic efficacy of cisplatin by combination with dethyldithiocarbamate and hyperthermia in a mouse model. *Cancer Research*, **47**:774–9.

Myers C (1988). Anthracyclines. In *Cancer chemotherapy and biological response modifiers annual 10* (ed. HM Pinedo, DL Longo, and BA Chabner), pp. 33–9. Elsevier, Amsterdam.

Myers C, *et al.* (1990). Treatment of hormonally refractory prostate cancer with suramin. *Proceedings of the American Society of Clinical Oncology*, **9**:133.

Newman KA, Reed WP, Bustamante CI, Schimpff SC, Wade JC (1989). Venous access devices utilized in association with intensive cancer chemotherapy. *European Journal of Clinical Oncology*, **25**:1375–8.

Nossal GJV (1987). Current concepts: immunology: the basic components of the immune system. *New England Journal of Medicine*, **316**:1320–5.

Offerman JJG, *et al.* (1985). The influence of verapamil on renal function in patients treated with cisplatin. *Clinical Nephrology*, **24**:249–55.

Osman NM, Litterst CL (1983). Effect of probenecid and *N'*-methyl-nicotinamide on renal handling of *cis*-dichloro diammineplatinum-II in rats. *Cancer Letters*, **19**:107–11.

Ozols RF, *et al.* (1984). High-dose cisplatin in hypertonic saline. *Annals of Internal Medicine*, **100**:19–24.

Panella TJ, *et al.* (1990). Platelets acquire a secretion defect after high-dose chemotherapy. *Cancer*, **65**:1711–16.

Pascoe GA, Reed DJ (1987). Vitamin E protection against chemical-induced cell injury. *Archives of Biochemistry and Biophysics*, **256**:159–66.

Patt Y, *et al.* (1987). Adjuvant perioperative hepatic arterial mitomycin C and floxuridine combined with surgical resection of metastatic colorectal cancer in the liver. *Cancer*, **59**:867–73.

Pavy MD, Wiley EL, Abeloff MD (1982). Hemolytic–uremic syndrome associated with mitomycin therapy. *Cancer Treatment Reports*, **66**:457–61.

Peters WP, Shpall EJ, Jones RB, Ross M (1990). High-dose combination cyclophosphamide, cisplatin, carmustine with bone marrow support as initial treatment for metastatic breast cancer: three–six year follow-up. *Proceedings of the American Society of Clinical Oncology*, **9**:10.

Peterson BA, *et al.* (1981). 5-Azacytidine and renal tubular dysfunction. *Blood*, **57**:182–5.

Peterson DE, *et al.* (1987). Microbiology of acute periodontal infection in myelosuppressed cancer patients. *Journal of Clinical Oncology*, **5**:1461–8.

Petrelli N, *et al.* (1987). A prospective randomized trial of 5-fluorouracil versus 5-fluorouracil and methotrexate in previously untreated patients with advanced colorectal carcinoma. *Journal of Clinical Oncology*, **5**:1559–65.

Pinedo HM, Peters GF (1988). Fluorouracil: biochemistry and pharmacology. *Journal of Clinical Oncology*, **6**:1653–64.

Pizzo PA, *et al.* (1982). Fever in the pediatric and young adult patient with cancer. A prospective study of 1001 episodes. *Medicine (Baltimore)*, **61**:153–65.

Pozzi E, *et al.* (1987). Role of alveolar phospholipids in bleomycin-induced pulmonary fibrosis in the rat. *Respiration (Supplement)*, **51**:23–32.

Preisler HD, *et al.* (1986). High-dose cytosine arabinoside in the treatment of preleukemic disorder. *American Journal of Hematology*, **23**:131–4.

Rankin EM, *et al.* (1990). The degree of myelosuppression experienced with standard dose carboplatin mirrors progression-free survival in advanced ovarian cancer. *Proceedings of the American Society of Clinical Oncology*, **9**:156.

Ries F, Klastersky J (1986). Nephrotoxicity induced by cancer chemotherapy with special emphasis on cisplatin toxicity. *American Journal of Kidney Diseases*, **5**:368–79.

Roelofs RI, *et al.* (1984). Peripheral sensory neuropathy and cisplatin chemotherapy. *Neurology*, **34**:934–8.

Rogers TR (1986). Investigation of infection in immunocompromised patients. *British Journal of Haematology*, **61**:195–201.

Rozenberg-Arska M, Dekker AW, Verhoef J (1989). Prevention of infections in granulocytopenic patients by fluorinated quinolones. *Review of Infectious Diseases*, Suppl. 5:1231–6.

Rubin M, Hathorn JW, Marshall D, Gress JH, Steinberg SM, Pizzo PA (1988). Gram-positive infections and the use of vancomycin in 550 episodes of fever and neutropenia. *Annals of Internal Medicine*, **108**:30–5.

Rusthoven JJ, Ahlgren P, Elhakim T, Pinfold P, Refd J, Stewart L, Feld R (1988). Varicella-zoster infection in adult cancer patients. A population study. *Annals of Internal Medicine*, **148**:1561–6.

Rustum YM, Riva C, Preisler HD (1987). Pharmacokinetic parameters of 1-beta-D-arabinofuranosylcytosine and their relationship to intracellular metabolism of ara-C, toxicity, and response of patients with acute nonlymphocytic leukemia treated with conventional and high-dose ara-C. *Seminars in Oncology (Supplement)*, **14**:141–8.

Safirstein R, *et al.* (1986). Cisplatin nephrotoxicity. *American Journal of Kidney Diseases*, **8**:356–67.

Sahenk Z, Mendell JR (1983). Studies on the morphologic alterations of axonal membraneous organelles in neurofilamentous neuropathies. *Brain Research*, **268**:239–47.

Schacht RG, *et al.* (1981). Nephrotoxicity of nitrosoureas. *Cancer*, **48**:1328–34.

Schaffner A, Douglas H, Braude A (1982). Selective protection against *Candida* and against *Mycelia* by polymorphonuclear phagocytes in resistance to *Aspergillus*. *Journal of Clinical Investigation*, **69**:617–31.

Schimpff SC (1980). Infection prevention during profound granulocytopenia. New approaches to alimentary canal microbial suppression. *Annals of Internal Medicine*, **93**:358–61.

Schimpff SC, Young VM, Greene WH, Vermeulen GD, Moody MR, Wiernik PH (1972). Origin of infection in acute nonlymphocytic leukemia. Significance of hospital acquisition of potential pathogens. *Annals of Internal Medicine*, **77**:707–14.

Schwartsmann G, Winograd B, Pinedo HM (1988). The main steps in the development of new anticancer agents. *Radiotherapy and Oncology*, **12**:301–13.

Schwartsmann G, Bender RA (1988). Vinca alkaloids. In *Cancer chemotherapy and biological modifiers annual 10* (ed HM Pinedo, DL Longo, and BA Chabner), pp. 50–6. Elsevier, Amsterdam.

Schwartsmann G, *et al.* (1989). Mucocutaneous side-effects of Brequinar sodium. A new inhibitor of pyrimidine *de novo* biosynthesis. *Cancer*, 63: 243–8.

Schweitzer VG, *et al.* (1986). Amelioration of cisplatin-induced ototoxicity by fosfomycin. *Laryngoscope*, 96:948–58.

Sculier JP, Weerts D, Klastersky J (1984). Causes of death in febrile granulocytopenic cancer patients receiving empiric antibiotic therapy. *European Journal of Cancer and Clinical Oncology*, 20:55–60.

Sehti SM, Lazo JS (1987). Separation of the protective enzyme bleomycin hydrolase from rabbit pulmonary aminopeptidases. *Biochemistry*, 26: 432–7.

Selker RG, Jacobs SA, Moore PB (1980). BCNU (1,3-bis[2-chloroethyl]-1-nitrosourea) induced pulmonary fibrosis. *Neurosurgery*, 7:560–5.

Shenkenberg TD, *et al.* (1986). Mitoxantrone: a new anticancer drug with significant clinical activity. *Annals of Internal Medicine*, 105:67–70.

Sickles EA, Greene WH, Wiernik PH (1975). Clinical presentation of infection in granulocytopenic patients. *Archives of Internal Medicine*, 135:715–19.

Snow JB (1983). Clinical problems in chemosensory disturbances. *American Journal of Otolaryngology*, 4:224–7.

Stapleton FB, *et al.* (1988). Acute renal failure at onset of therapy for advanced stage Burkitt lymphoma and B cell acute lymphoblastic lymphoma. *Pediatrics*, 82:863–9.

Subar M, Muggia FM (1986). Apparent myocardial ischemia associated with vinblastine administration. *Cancer Treatment Reports*, 70:690–1.

Thaler M, Pastakia B, Shawker TH, O'Lear T, Pizzo PA (1988). Hepatic candidiasis in cancer patients: the evolving picture of the syndrome. *Annals of Internal Medicine*, 108:88–100.

Thordarson H, Talstad I (1986). Acute meningitis and cerebellar dysfunction complicating high-dose cystosine arabinoside therapy. *Acta Medica Scandinavica*, 220:493–5.

Tucker MA, *et al.* (1987). Leukemia after therapy with alkylating agents. *Journal of the National Cancer Institute*, 78:459–64.

Vainckus L, Letendre L (1984). Pericarditis induced by high-dose cytarabine therapy. *Archives of Internal Medicine*, 144:1868–9.

van der Waaij D, Berghuis-de Vries JM (1974). Selective elimination of Enterobacteriaceae species from the digestive tract in mice and monkeys. *Journal of Hygiene, Cambridge*, 72:205–11.

Verweij J, De Vries J, Pinedo HM (1987). Mitomycin C-induced renal toxicity, a dose-dependent side-effect? *European Journal of Cancer and Clinical Oncology*, 23:195–9.

Von Hoff DD (1987). Whither carboplatin? A replacement for or an alternative to cisplatin? *Journal of Clinical Oncology*, 5:169–71.

Wade JC, Schimpff SC (1988). Epidemiology and prevention of infection in the immunocompromised host. In *Clinical approach to infection in the compromised host* (2nd edn) (ed. RH Rubin and LS Young), pp. 5–40. Plenum, New York.

Watson PR, Brubaker LH, Yaghmai F (1985). Severe central nervous system toxicity from high-dose cytarabine: expressive aphasia occurring after the second day of treatment. *Cancer Treatment Reports*, 69:313–14.

Weiss RB (1982). Streptozotocin: a review of its pharmacology, efficacy and toxicity. *Cancer Treatment Reports*, 66:427–38.

Weiss RB, Poster DS (1982). The renal toxicity of cancer chemotherapeutic agents. *Cancer Treatment Reports*, 9:37–56.

Weiss RB, *et al.* (1983). Nephrotoxicity of semustine. *Cancer Treatment Reports*, 67:1105–12.

Weiss RB, *et al.* (1986). Skin reactions induced by trimetrexate, an analog of methotrexate. *Investigational New Drugs*, 4:159–63.

Wilding G, *et al.* (1985). Rectinal toxicity after high-dose cisplatin therapy. *Journal of Clinical Oncology*, 3:1683–9.

Winston DJ, Ho WG, Gale RP (1982). Therapeutic granulocyte transfusions for documented infections. A controlled trial in ninety-five infectious granulocytopenic episodes. *Annals of Internal Medicine*, 97:509–15.

Winston DJ, Ho WG, Nakao SL, Gale RP, Champlin RE (1986). Norfloxacin versus vancomycin/polymixin for prevention of infections in granulocytopenic patients. *American Journal of Medicine*, 80:884–90.

Winston DJ, Ho WG, Bruckner DA, Gale RP, Champlin RE (1990). Ofloxacin versus vancomycin/polymixin for prevention of infections in granulocytopenic patients. *American Journal of Medicine*, 88:36–42.

19.10 Effects of cancer chemotherapy on fertility

CLAIRE BARTON AND JONATHAN WAXMAN

INTRODUCTION

Radical improvements in the treatment of malignant disease have resulted in the long-term survival of people of reproductive age and with their survival the effects of therapy on reproductive function have become apparent.

The incidence and importance of gonadal toxicity is easily underestimated but is of immense significance to the patient. Infertility, hormonal imbalance, and sexual dysfunction are a high price to pay for the successful treatment of malignant disease. We need to recognize gonadal damage and treat it appropriately in order to improve the quality of our patients' lives.

GONADAL TOXICITY: HISTOLOGICAL AND ENDOCRINE EFFECTS

In the testis, cytotoxic drugs predominantly affect the germinal epithelium. Histologically there is variable loss of the developing spermatozoa with relative sparing of Sertoli and Leydig cells. These changes are demonstrated in Fig. 1. When damage is severe the seminiferous tubules may show Sertoli cells only. Clinically, there are corresponding abnormalities in sperm count, morphology, and motility, but testosterone levels and libido tend to be maintained. Baseline luteinizing hormone (LH) concentrations are generally unchanged, although dynamic testing with gonadotrophin-releasing hormone (GnRH) may demonstrate supraphysiological release (Waxman *et al.* 1982). Basal follicle-stimulating hormone (FSH) levels are usually elevated, reflecting decreased spermatogenesis. In women, gross destruction of normal ovarian follicular structures may result ultimately in a fibrotic 'streak ovary' as shown in Fig. 2. Normal ovulation may cease and the woman is rendered infertile and at risk of premature osteoporosis. Serum levels of 17-oestradiol and progesterone fall into the post-menopausal range, whilst LH and FSH levels rise.

The investigation of pre-treatment fertility has been largely limited to Hodgkin's disease and testicular cancer, as these are the

(a)

(b)

Fig. 1 (a) Normal testis before treatment. (b) Testis after chemotherapy for Hodgkin's disease, showing germ cell aplasia.

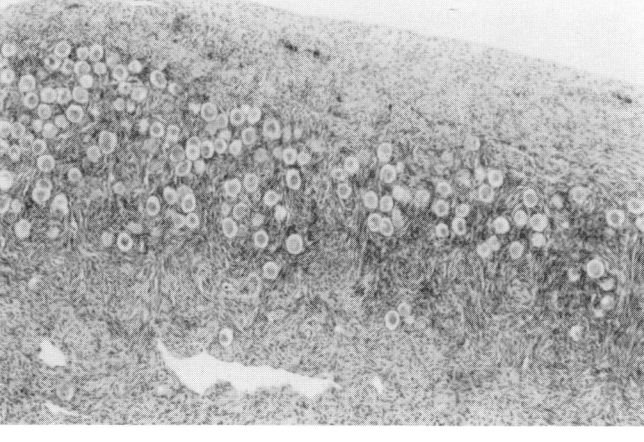

(a)

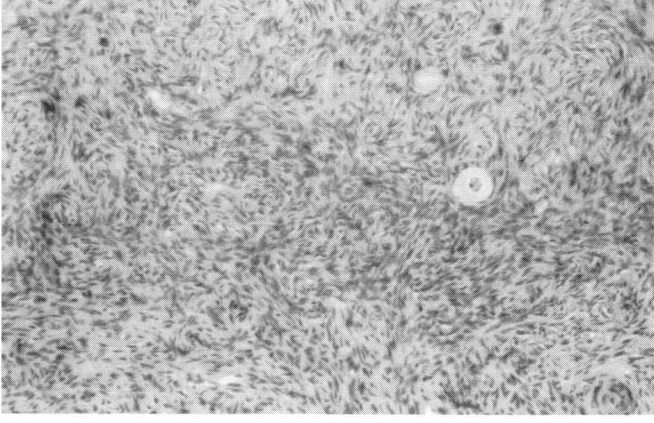

(b)

Fig. 2 (a) Normal ovary before treatment. (b) Ovary after chemotherapy for Hodgkin's disease, showing gross follicular destruction.

most important curable tumours which occur in young people of reproductive age.

PRE-TREATMENT FERTILITY IN MEN: SPERM BANKING

Artificial insemination is used frequently in the United States and in general pregnancy occurs in approximately 60 per cent of cases (Curie-Cohen *et al.* 1979). The success rate depends predominantly upon the number of inseminations, prior pregnancy, and physician experience. In a small study of 22 couples, Scammell *et al.* (1985) analysed fertilization using cryopreserved semen from cancer patients. A near normal conception rate was achieved, with sperm concentrations before cryopreservation of at least 20×10^6/ml, a sperm motility of 40 per cent or more and a post-thaw motility greater than 30 per cent. Unfortunately, a high proportion of patients with Hodgkin's disease or germ cell tumours do not have suitable semen for cryopreservation, particularly when post-thaw motility is considered (Sanger *et al.* 1980; Mahadevan *et al.* 1983). Selby *et al.* (1988) have published guidelines for cryopreserving semen. They suggest it should be offered if the patient wishes to

have children, when there is a greater than 30 per cent chance of survival at 2 years and a substantial risk of infertility beyond 2 years, when the patient is fit enough to provide at least three adequate samples, and when treatment can safely be delayed for a week. *In vitro* fertilization, sperm microinjection, and embryo transfer techniques now allow pregnancy to be achieved with cryopreserved semen of poorer quality and these criteria may be challenged (Rowland *et al.* 1985).

Hodgkin's disease

Pre-treatment fertility has been reviewed by Hendry *et al.* (1983) who found that only 27 per cent of 49 patients with Hodgkin's disease had initial sperm counts over 10×10^6/ml. Chapman *et al.* (1981) studied 47 men with Hodgkin's disease prospectively, none of whom had a history of infertility. Forty-three per cent (16/37) were subfertile due to impotence (four patients) and inadequate sperm counts (12 patients). FSH was elevated in 16 per cent and there was hormonal evidence of compensated Leydig cell failure in 40 per cent. Nine patients had a pre-treatment testicular biopsy and only one was normal. Redman *et al.* (1987) performed pre-treatment seminal analysis in 79 men with Hodgkin's disease. Sperm concentration, fresh motility, fresh progression, post-thaw motility, and post-thaw progression were all significantly decreased compared with normal controls, but these changes did not correlate with clinical status.

Germ cell tumours

Several studies have shown a reduced semen quality in patients with germ cell tumours of the testis. Hendry *et al.* (1983) analysed the pre-treatment sperm characteristics after orchidectomy of 208 patients with germ cell tumours of the testis. Only 22 per cent of 55 patients with seminomas and 29 per cent of 154 patients with teratomas or mixed tumours had sperm counts greater than 10×10^6/ml. Hansen *et al.* (1989) investigated 97 similar patients with testicular tumours. Fifty-eight per cent had a total sperm count of less than 8×10^6/ml, 81 per cent had reduced sperm motility, 35 per cent had more than 40 per cent abnormal head forms, and 33 per cent had elevated serum FSH levels. Androgen levels were below the normal range in only 5 per cent of patients, but LH values were elevated in 14 per cent, suggesting compensated mildly impaired Leydig cell function. A primary germ cell disorder (Carroll *et al.* 1987), elevated human chorionic gonadotrophin (hCG) levels (Cochran *et al.* 1975; Hurdadli *et al.* 1984), cryptorchidism (Hansen *et al.* 1989) carcinoma *in situ* (Berthelsen *et al.* 1979; von der Maase *et al.* 1986), raised scrotal temperature (Weissbach *et al.* 1980), and immunological mechanisms (Bartsch *et al.* 1980; Harrison *et al.* 1981) have all been implicated in the impaired spermatogenesis of patients with testicular cancer. Fever (Marmor *et al.* 1986) and immunological dysfunction (Redman *et al.* 1987) are likely to be important contributing factors in patients with Hodgkin's disease.

PRE-TREATMENT FERTILITY IN WOMEN: OOCYTE BANKING

Infertility appears to be less frequently associated with malignant disease in women than in men, but estimates may be inaccurate since some women may be subfertile despite persistent menses because of anovulatory cycling. This may be a 'non-specific' effect of illness or be related to the production of cachetin/tumour necrosis factor (TNF) or other unidentified factors by the tumour.

Whitehead *et al.* (1983) studied 44 adult females with Hodgkin's disease. Four were pregnant at presentation and a further six were amenorrhoeic for between 3 and 24 months before treatment. Each of these women had lost more than 10 per cent of her body weight and had symptoms of systemic disease. None had menopausal symptoms and all experienced a rapid return of menses within the first or second treatment cycle.

Two studies describe an association of infertility with female breast cancer. Eighty-seven pre-menopausal women with breast cancer underwent endometrial curettage during the luteal phase around the time of mastectomy (Grattarola 1964). Only 17 per cent were found to have a secretory endometrium compared with 68 per cent of matched controls with benign breast disease, suggesting that the cancer patients were having anovulatory cycles. A later study, involving 10 000 normal women in Guernsey, showed that pre-menopausal women at high risk of the development of breast cancer were more likely to have anovulatory cycling, as shown by low levels of luteal phase progesterone (Bulbrook *et al.* 1978).

Oocyte or embryo cryopreservation is theoretically possible for women about to be treated with cytotoxic chemotherapy, but oocyte harvest is considerably more invasive and technically demanding than harvesting sperm. Oocyte yield is poor unless the ovaries have been artificially stimulated and retrieval has to be timed, which may delay treatment. In addition, failure of ovulation is almost invariably associated with failure of ovarian hormone production. Recently, successful pregnancies have been brought to term in women with ovarian failure or absent ovaries using surrogate embryo transfer, synchronized endometrial stimulation, and exogenous hormone support (Navot *et al.* 1986; Sauer *et al.* 1987). It is to be hoped that such techniques will become more widely available.

SINGLE-AGENT CHEMOTHERAPY AND GONADAL FUNCTION

The gonadal toxicity of cytotoxic chemotherapy was first reported in 1948 (Spitz 1948). At post-mortem, 27 out of 30 men who had been treated with nitrogen mustard for lymphoma were noted to have absent spermatogenesis. Louis *et al.* (1956) reported amenorrhoea in four pre-menopausal women with chronic myeloid leukaemia who were treated with busulphan at a daily dosage of 10 mg for 3 months. In the early 1970s the gonadal toxicity of chlorambucil and cyclophosphamide was recognized. Cyclophosphamide has been widely used in non-malignant conditions, such as glomerulonephritis and rheumatoid arthritis and its gonadal effects are well described. Many of the features of cyclophosphamide-related gonadal toxicity have been found to apply to alkylating agents in general.

Alkylating agents

Cyclophosphamide and male infertility

Cyclophosphamide, like other alkylating agents, predominantly affects the germinal epithelium in men. In a study of 31 men treated for nephrotic syndrome with daily doses of cyclophosphamide ranging from 50 to 100 mg, a reduction in sperm count was noted in some patients as early as 3 weeks after initiating treatment (Fairley *et al.* 1972). None of the men developed azoospermia unless at least 4 months of treatment had been given. Testicular biopsies from these men showed survival of Sertoli cells only, suggesting that all generations of germ cells were destroyed. Serial semen analysis post-treatment revealed recovery of spermatogenesis in two and ten patients after 3 and 19 months, respectively. Sperm counts continued to fall in two patients for 2–3 months after stopping treatment and biopsies showed reduced spermatogenesis 1 year and 15 months after treatment. Many subsequent studies have produced similar results, demonstrating a general dose and duration dependence with individual variation in susceptibility (Kumar *et al.* 1972; Buchanan *et al.* 1975).

Early reports based on the histological findings from small numbers of patients suggested that cyclophosphamide did not affect the pre-pubertal testis (Arneil 1972; Berry *et al.* 1972; Rapola *et al.* 1973). Hormone data from later studies without seminal analysis supported this concept, revealing normal serum FSH, LH, and testosterone levels in pre-pubertal boys treated with cyclophosphamide some years earlier (De Groot *et al.* 1974; Pennisi *et al.* 1975; Kirkland *et al.* 1976; Parra *et al.* 1978). However, more recently it has become apparent that the pre-pubertal testis is vulnerable to chemotherapeutic agents. Lentz *et al.* (1977) evaluated 19 male patients who received cyclophosphamide for nephrotic syndrome before, during, and after puberty. They found that decreased spermatogenesis was related to total cyclophosphamide dose and was more frequent with doses greater than 365 mg/kg. Normal FSH levels did not exclude gonadal damage in pre- or post-pubertal boys. Etteldorf *et al.* (1976) studied gonadal function in adult or late adolescent men who had received cyclophosphamide for nephrotic syndrome before or during puberty. Doses of cyclophosphamide between 2 and 4.6 mg/kg/day for periods of 2 months or less were associated with normal fertility. However, doses of 3.5–3.7 mg/kg/day for 3 months or longer produced oligospermia and azoospermia. Testosterone levels were normal, but both LH and FSH levels were elevated in azoospermic men. Penso *et al.* (1974) studied seven patients treated with cyclophosphamide before puberty, 1–4 years post-treatment. Six had normal secondary sexual characteristics and one had testicular atrophy, but only two had normal semen. In these patients the FSH level appeared to correlate with the severity of testicular damage.

In a study of the long-term effects of cyclophosphamide on testicular function, 30 men treated in childhood with doses of 2–3 mg/kg/day for 6–12 months were assessed approximately 12 years after treatment (Watson *et al.* 1985). Four patients were azoospermic, nine were oligospermic, and 17 had normal sperm counts. All had normal secondary sexual characteristics, serum androgens, prolactins, and libido, but even those with normal sperm counts had significantly elevated basal and stimulated FSH levels consistent with impaired spermatogenesis. Dynamic LH responses to GnRH suggested compensated Leydig cell failure. There was a significant inverse correlation between sperm density and cyclophosphamide dosage and duration of treatment. After a further mean follow-up of 7.2 years, three previously oligospermic and one previously azoospermic patient had normal sperm counts, indicating that late recovery of spermatogenesis is possible. The return of spermatogenesis is unpredictable and may occasionally occur after long periods of treatment, even when biopsies show Sertoli cells only (Buchanan *et al.* 1975).

Confusion over the susceptibility of the immature testis to chemotherapy-induced damage may have arisen because of a reliance on 'normal' baseline hormonal tests in the pre-pubertal child to indicate normal gonadal function. Normal basal gonadotrophin levels may be found in this group because the control of gonadotrophin levels is different before puberty (Shalet *et al.* 1981). At this stage, inhibin may be less important than androgens in the feedback inhibition of FSH. Since Leydig cells are relatively spared cytotoxic damage, androgen levels and, hence, gonadotrophin levels remain normal.

Cyclophosphamide and female infertility

Uldall *et al.* (1972) reported amenorrhoea in 18 out of 24 women treated with 40–120 mg/day of cyclophosphamide for renal disease. Twelve patients developed amenorrhoea within 1 month and the majority within 7 months of starting treatment. Urinary oestrogens were low, with elevated serum FSH and LH levels. Nine patients discontinued treatment but in only one, aged 21 years, did menstruation return after 6 months off therapy. Warne *et al.* (1973) reviewed ovarian biopsy specimens in 22 patients who had received cyclophosphamide for glomerulonephritis or rheumatoid arthritis. Seventeen patients had developed premature ovarian failure, which recovered in one patient 10 months after treatment ceased. None of the ovarian biopsies was normal; primordial follicle development and maturation were absent and ova were seen in only two specimens. These histological appearances suggested that cyclophosphamide has an early effect on thecal cells, preventing follicle formation, whilst ova are directly affected after greater

doses. Alternatively, destruction of surrounding follicle cells might lead to premature resumption of meiosis and senescence and death of the denuded ova (Edwards 1966; Biggers *et al.* 1967; Donahue 1968). Patient age correlates with susceptibility to gonadal toxicity. In one series of patients treated for breast cancer, the total dose of cyclophosphamide received before the onset of amenorrhoea in women aged 40 years or older was 5.2 g, in patients aged 30–39 years it was 9.3 g, and in women aged 20–29 years it was 20.4 g (Koyama *et al.* 1977). Recovery of ovarian function after cessation of cyclophosphamide has been reported (Belohorsky *et al.* 1960; Uldall *et al.* 1972). Kumar *et al.* (1972) noted the return of menses in six out of eight patients rendered amenorrhoeic by treatment with daily doses of cyclophosphamide, starting at 3 mg/kg/day, including one woman who was still taking cyclophosphamide. None of the patients in this study received therapy for more than 9 months. There have been few studies of the effects of cyclophosphamide on gonadal function in the pre-pubertal and pubertal female. In six pre-pubertal and pubertal girls, cyclophosphamide in doses of 525 mg/kg or less did not prevent ovulation as detected by basal body temperature graphs (Lentz *et al.* 1977). Etteldorf *et al.* (1976) noted no histological changes in the ovaries of two pre-pubertal girls who died of the complications of nephrotic syndrome after two courses of cyclophosphamide, but Miller *et al.* (1971) reported ovarian follicular atresia at post-mortem in a 13 year old girl who had received cyclophosphamide for 29 months.

Chlorambucil

Richter *et al.* (1970) examined testicular morphology in eight men with lymphoma who were treated with single-agent chlorambucil and found a close relationship between the total dose and the severity of germinal epithelial damage. Increased dosages led to the disappearance of the germinal cell line, leaving only Sertoli cells with moderate peritubular fibrosis but without damage to vascular or interstitial cells. Spermatogenesis recovered if a total dose of less than 400 mg was given. Guesry *et al.* (1978) reported similar findings in 21 adolescent and adult men treated with chlorambucil for nephrotic syndrome before or during puberty. Patients received daily doses of 0.1–0.2 mg/kg with or without azathioprine for a mean period of 10 months and were assessed 2–9 years later. Fertility was preserved with total dosages under 7 mg/kg and azoospermia appeared to be irreversible with total dosages of 25 mg/kg or greater. Ten patients completed treatment before puberty, six of whom also received mustine. Nine were azoospermic and one had severe oligospermia, suggesting that the pre-pubertal testis is as vulnerable as the adult testis to damage by alklyating agents. In this study FSH levels were significantly elevated in 13 patients but did not correlate with sperm count. Testosterone levels were normal in 15 patients even after very high dosages and when testicular atrophy was present. Serial seminal analysis showed no sign of recovery, in contrast with the findings of other workers (Cheviakoff *et al.* 1973).

Less information is available for the gonadal effects of chlorambucil in women. Ezdinli and Stutzman (1965) noted amenorrhoea in two women who took 6–12 mg of chlorambucil daily for 4–8 weeks for lymphoma. Freckman *et al.* (1964) reported chemical castration in three pre-menopausal women aged 41–45 years receiving 14–20 mg of chlorambucil daily for breast cancer. At autopsy no follicles were detected in the ovaries of these patients.

Nowadays, chlorambucil tends to be given in interrupted cycles rather than continuously and the gonadal toxicity under these circumstances may be different.

Other alkylating agents

All alkylating agents appear to damage the gonad similarly and there appears to be a general relationship for each compound between dose, patient age, and gonadal toxicity, with individual variation in susceptiblity.

Pre-menopausal women participating in a trial of adjuvant melphalan for breast cancer developed menstrual disturbances (Fisher et al. 1979). Seventy-three per cent of those aged 40–49 years became amenorrhoeic, compared with 22 per cent of younger women and none resumed normal menstruation on cessation of therapy. In a small trial of adjuvant melphalan versus combination chemotherapy in breast cancer, three patients taking 0.15 mg/kg/day of melphalan for 5 days every 6 weeks for an unspecified period retained normal menses and five became amenorrhoeic (Rose and Davies 1977). Hormone profiles in the amenorrhoeic patients were consistent with primary ovarian failure.

Mustine may be one of the most gonadotoxic single agents. It kills mature sperm cells in addition to their precursors, rapidly causing infertility (Spitz 1948). All of ten young women treated with mustine for Hodgkin's disease developed amenorrhoea or profound oligomenorrhoea within 1 or 2 months of starting treatment (Sobrinho et al. 1971). However, ovarian function was maintained in two patients despite these menstrual abnormalities and one became pregnant during therapy.

Vinca alkaloids

Vincristine and vinblastine have been studied in male rats and compared with cyclophosphamide and nitrogen mustard (Cooke et al. 1978). All four drugs impaired fertility and produced similar histological changes in the testis. Vinca alkaloids would not be expected to affect the non-dividing ova, but experimental studies have not been published. In humans, fertility in both sexes has only rarely been reported to be affected by the vinca alkaloids (Sobrinho et al. 1971; Shamberger et al. 1981a).

Antimetabolites

Methotrexate

Since methotrexate affects the availability of DNA precursors and is cycle specific, it would not be expected to destroy either the slowly replicating spermatogonial cells or the non-dividing oocytes, but it might suppress replication of the more rapidly dividing differentiated spermatogonia. In humans methotrexate is rarely associated with disturbance of reproductive function (Weinblatt 1985). Even at high doses, methotrexate alone or with vincristine had no adverse effects on menstrual function or the hormone profiles of women receiving adjuvant therapy for osteosarcoma (Shamberger et al. 1981b). Four out of ten men receiving the same regimen developed severe oligospermia during and immediately after treatment and five had transient elevations of FSH with normal LH levels. Testicular function returned to normal in all men tested after treatment. In a small study of women treated with combination chemotherapy and radiotherapy for soft tissue sarcoma, menstruation returned to three patients while they were still receiving high-dose methotrexate (Shamberger et al. 1981b).

Doxorubicin

Doxorubicin does not appear to cause permanent infertility in humans although there are few data on its use as a single agent. Da Cunha et al. (1983) examined the testicular morphology and semen of 14 patients who had been treated with a variety of drug regimens, which all included doxorubicin. Total doses of 145–625 mg/m^2 were given and testicular function was assessed 7–79 months after treatment. Five patients had normal sperm counts and three were oligospermic with sperm motility of 20–80 per cent, showing that recovery of spermatogenesis is possible even after high doses of doxorubicin. Shamberger et al. (1981) were unable to demonstrate increased gonadal toxicity with maximal doses of doxorubicin in younger women treated with adjuvant doxorubicin, cyclophosphamide, and high-dose methotrexate for soft tissue sarcoma. Recovery of testicular function occurred in younger men treated with maximal doses, suggesting that, in humans, doxorubicin gonadal toxicity is relatively slight and reversible.

5-Fluorouracil

In mice 5-fluorouracil has an effect on post-spermatogonial cell types in addition to earlier forms (Meistrich et al. 1982). It has virtually no effect on reproductive function in humans (Koyama et al. 1977; Fisher et al. 1979).

Etoposide

Short intensive courses of etoposide are associated with ovarian failure. Twenty-two patients with refractory or recurrent gestational trophoblastic tumours were treated with repeated courses of etoposide at a dosage of 200 mg/m^2/day for 5 days fortnightly (Yew et al. 1985). After a mean total dosage of 5 g, five young patients developed transient ovarian failure, two older women became permanently menopausal, two patients developed anovulatory cycles, and two developed oligomenorrhoea.

Corticosteroids

Corticosteroids are a common constituent of chemotherapeutic regimens for lymphomas, are occasionally used for breast cancer, and are frequently used in high doses for short periods of time as anti-emetics. Their effects on female ovarian function are variable (Kay and Mattison 1985). In men steroids may have either inhibitory or stimulatory effects. Mancini et al. (1966) examined the effects of prednisolone in small groups of normal men and patients with oligospermia or azoospermia of unknown aetiology and with oligospermia secondary to hypogonadism as a consequence of hypophysectomy. There were no changes in patients taking 10 mg/day, but patients taking 30 mg/day had a decrease in sperm number and motility which was apparent at 15 days and maximal at 30 days. Recovery took 6 months after a 1 month course of prednisolone, suggesting a decrease in spermatogonial proliferation. Testicular histology showed arrested spermatogenesis but no change in the appearance of Sertoli or Leydig cells. No stimulation of spermatogenesis was observed in patients with azoospermia. The mechanism of these steroid effects is not known.

COMBINATION CHEMOTHERAPY AND GONADAL FUNCTION

A considerable body of data are now available describing the effects of combination chemotherapy programmes on gonadal function. In this section we review the effects of these programmes in specific malignant diseases.

Hodgkin's disease

Adults

Treatment of patients with Hodgkin's disease causes permanent infertility in the majority of patients and may be associated with significant hormonal and psychological changes. Chapman et al. (1979b) assessed testicular function and libido in 74 men who had completed 6–16 cycles of MVPP (mustine, vinblastine, procarbazine, prednisolone) chemotherapy for Hodgkin's disease. All were azoospermic after treatment, FSH levels were consistently raised, and testicular biopsies showed germinal aplasia. Only four patients regained spermatogenesis during a mean follow-up period of 27 months, but two men managed to father children despite oligospermia. Prolactin levels were raised in 42 per cent and in some this was associated with an elevated thyroid-stimulating hormone (TSH) level. In a later study, Chapman et al. (1981) prospectively examined the effects of MVPP in 47 men with Hodgkin's disease. A significant proportion were subfertile and had abnormal hormonal profiles before treatment. After only two cycles all the men tested had become persistently azoospermic with elevated FSH levels. There was hormonal evidence of Leydig cell failure in some patients. Serum prolactin levels fluctuated widely and two patients were diagnosed as having pituitary microadenomas after completing therapy.

Whitehead et al. (1982) reported similar results with MVPP in 93 men with Hodgkin's disease. The incidence of infertility post-treatment was high: 42 out of 49 patients were azoospermic and five were severely oligospermic after six cycles of MVPP. Eleven patients were studied 6–8 years after treatment and ten were still azoospermic, suggesting that the potential for recovery is very small. Median basal and luteinizing-hormone-releasing hormone (LHRH)-stimulated FSH and LH levels were significantly elevated and testosterone levels were depressed compared with controls. Testicular volumes were significantly decreased but no patients required androgen replacement. There was no evidence of hyperprolactinaemia in this study, but gynaecomastia occurred in seven patients. Decreased libido and sexual activity were common during treatment, but the majority noticed no overall change after treatment compared with before. Changes in sexual interest or activity did not correlate with Leydig cell dysfunction and libido seemed to decline only in the older men.

The long-term effects of 6–16 cycles of MVPP on gonadal function were assessed 2–12.5 years after chemotherapy in 41 male patients in prolonged remission from Hodgkin's disease (Waxman et al. 1982). Azoospermia or profound oligospermia was found in 36 men (88 per cent). The remaining five patients had counts between 20×10^6/ml and 88.4×10^6/ml. Three patients with azoospermia and one with a count of 10×10^6/ml following treatment had further recovery of spermatogenesis with counts ranging from 20×10^6/ml to 88.4×10^6/ml. All three patients were aged less than 30 years at the time of therapy. The vast majority of patients had basal or stimulated gonadotrophin profiles typical of primary testicular dysfunction, but all had testosterone levels within the normal range. Three men had normal basal FSH levels despite azoospermia and eight patients had abnormal serum prolactin concentrations. These results emphasize that 'normal' baseline hormone levels do not necessarily reflect normal spermatogenesis and suggest that recovery of spermatogenesis after MVPP may occur

in up to 20 per cent of patients after a delay of as much as 10 years. There are anecdotal reports of paternity after even longer periods of sterility (Stricker et al. 1981).

Combination chemotherapy for Hodgkin's disease is also associated with severe gonadal toxicity in females. The patient's age at treatment is an important determinant of ovarian damage. Chapman et al. (1979a) studied ovarian function in 41 women treated with MVPP, all of whom had normal pre-treatment fertility. After treatment patients could be grouped into three categories according to their ovarian function. Forty-nine per cent of women had complete ovarian failure with amenorrhoea, elevated gonadotrophins, menopausal serum oestradiol concentrations, and menopausal symptoms. Seventeen per cent had normal cyclical ovarian activity and 34 per cent fell into an intermediate group with irregular menstruation, some menopausal symptoms, and hormonal patterns suggestive of failing ovaries. Over the next 16 months, six women with failing ovaries progressed to complete ovarian failure. By the end of the study, only 11 per cent had normal ovarian function, 26 per cent had failing ovaries, and 62 per cent had complete ovarian failure. The pattern of ovarian response was clearly age related. Only 31 per cent of women less than 30 years old had ovarian failure, whereas 84 per cent of those aged 30–51 years developed complete ovarian failure and amenorrhoea occurred after fewer cycles of MVPP in the older women. Ovarian biopsies after treatment showed severe depletion of primordial follicles with two to three follicles per biopsy compared with 55 observed pre-treatment. Even the biopsies from two patients with apparently normal gonadal function had fewer follicles than expected. Subsequently, one of these patients developed signs of failing ovaries and one patient with failing ovaries progressed to total ovarian failure. In females proliferation of germ cells is completed during intrauterine life and, after approximately 20 weeks' gestation, numbers progressively fall, so that younger patients have a greater reserve of follicles. Since there is no way of replenishing the oocytes and follicles after destruction, one might expect all patients to progress to premature ovarian failure with time.

Chapman and co-workers (Chapman et al. 1979c; Chapman 1982) also assessed the effects of treatment for Hodgkin's disease on the sexual activity and interpersonal relationships of the same 41 women. Divorce or separation occurred in 30 per cent of 33 women at risk, which was four times the rate of a matched population of the same age. Irritability, family rows, and loss of friendships were reported and some patients failed at work or left their jobs through lack of confidence. Frequently the patients told no-one of these problems and were unaware that their symptoms might be related to their treatment. Hormone replacement therapy resulted in dramatic relief of symptoms in almost all cases.

Some of the observations in the study by Chapman and co-workers were supported by Whitehead et al. (1983) who found that all patients over the age of 36 years stopped menstruating during MVPP chemotherapy and became permanently amenorrhoeic 3–6 months after completion of treatment. The overall rate of amenorrhoea after treatment was 39 per cent and the very high rate of sexual dysfunction and divorce was not substantiated.

In a series reported by Horning et al. (1981) the outlook for female reproductive capacity after treatment for Hodgkin's disease appeared better. In particular, a significant proportion of patients regained fertility. Overall, 69 per cent of patients had regular or irregular menstruation after treatment and 31 per cent were amenorrhoeic. Menses were present in 18 out of 19 patients treated with total lymphoid irradiation alone, 29 out of 34 patients treated with chemotherapy without pelvic irradiation, and 24 out of 50 patients treated with total lymphoid irradiation and cytotoxic drugs. Only age was found to be predictive for the effects of treatment and the increased probability of regular menses in younger patients was particularly marked in patients under the age of 30 years. Eight (40 per cent) of the patients who became pregnant had experienced temporary amenorrhoea and menopausal symptoms for up to 3.5 years. Part of the explanation for the discrepancy between Chapman's results and those of Horning et al. (1981) lies in the younger age and the inclusion of patients who did not receive chemotherapy in the latter study.

COPP (cyclophosphamide, vincristine, procarbazine, prednisolone) chemotherapy is reported to have even more gonadal toxicity than MOPP (nitrogen mustard, vincristine, procarbazine, prednisolone) and MVPP (Kreuser et al. 1987). All 19 men studied up to 11 years after receiving COPP were found to be azoospermic with significantly elevated FSH levels, but none had abnormal testosterone or basal LH concentrations. The incidence and severity of ovarian failure was approximately the same as reported for MOPP and MVPP. Six out of seven (86 per cent) women over the age of 24 years at the time of treatment had permanent amenorrhoea compared with two out of seven (28 per cent) younger women. None of these patients showed any recovery of ovarian function in up to 17 years of follow-up.

Children

There have been two major studies on the effects of treatment for Hodgkin's disease in childhood. Whitehead et al. (1982) assessed 15 boys and two girls after receiving MOPP, five of whom also had abdominal radiotherapy. Almost all the boys in late puberty or early adulthood had abnormally small testes. Basal testosterone levels were normal in each case, but eight patients had raised basal LH or exaggerated LH responses to LHRH. Nine out of 12 tested had elevated basal or stimulated FSH concentrations. All four pre-pubertal boys had normal basal FSH and peak FSH responses to LHRH, but three had impaired testosterone responses to hCG. One patient had normal pre-pubertal levels of FSH but abnormally high levels in early puberty. Six patients provided semen samples up to 8 years after treatment and all were azoospermic. These observations suggest that pre-pubertal boys are susceptible to testicular damage by MOPP, but this may not be detectable until puberty or after. Both the girls treated during childhood subsequently developed regular menstrual cycles with evidence of ovulation. The onset and progression of puberty in both sexes did not appear to be affected by treatment. One boy in this study developed gynaecomastia.

In an earlier study, Sherins et al. (1978) noted an exceptionally high incidence of gynaecomastia associated with Leydig cell dysfunction which occurred in nine out of 13 Ugandan boys treated with MOPP for Hodgkin's disease. Elevated serum oestradiol and prolactin did not appear to be responsible.

Non-sterilizing regimens for Hodgkin's disease

In an attempt to reduce the gonadal toxicity of MVPP, MOPP, and COPP, mustine, cyclophosphamide, and procarbazine have been substituted with non-alkylating drugs of similar efficacy but less gonadal toxicity. One example is the ABVD combination (adriamycin, bleomycin, vinblastine, dacarbazine). Viviani et al. (1985) randomized 53 men with Hodgkin's disease to receive either three cycles of MOPP or three cycles of ABVD before and after nodal irradiation. MOPP produced azoospermia in 97 per cent of patients with significantly increased FSH levels and ABVD induced oligospermia in 54 per cent of patients with normal FSH concentrations in 77 per cent. Recovery of spermatogenesis was demonstrated in three out of 21 cases who received MOPP and in all 13 cases tested who were given ABVD and occurred sooner in the ABVD-treated patients. Sixty-one women less than 45 years old were randomized in the same trial. In women above 30 years amenorrhoea lasting more than 6 months occurred in six out of 14 MOPP-treated patients but in none of the eight patients treated with ABVD. A number of prospective randomized trials have shown that ABVD is as effective a treatment as MOPP and, since the incidence of second malignancies is also less with ABVD, this combination should perhaps be used more widely (Bonadonna 1982; Bonadonna and Santoro 1982; Kaldar et al. 1987).

Germ cell tumours in men

The advent of cisplatin-based combination chemotherapy in the late 1970s has resulted in the cure of over 70 per cent of patients with testicular cancer, with an additional 10–15 per cent achieving complete remission following surgical resection of residual disease. In these patients ejaculatory failure caused by retroperitoneal lymph node dissection is the major contributory factor to the infertility of survivors. Although the chemotherapy used does have deleterious effects on the gonads, fewer patients are affected and more recover fertility than is the case with patients treated for Hodgkin's disease. Roth et al. (1988) estimate that over one-third of patients are able to father healthy children after treatment.

PVB/BEP chemotherapy

Fossa et al. (1985b) reported that 50–60 per cent of their patients regained active spermatogenesis 1–3 years after treatment for testicular cancer. Semen analysis was performed on 35 patients, of whom 13 had node dissection only and 22 had cisplatin-based chemotherapy (PVB: cisplatin, vinblastine, bleomycin) with or without other treatment including abdominal radiotherapy and node dissection. Fourteen patients, nine of whom had had retroperitoneal lymph node dissection, successfully impregnated their wives. Four who were azoospermic and one who had highly impaired spermatogenesis before treatment recovered normal spermatogenesis after treatment and five patients who initially had highly impaired spermatogenesis subsequently fathered a child, indicating that even patients with very poor semen characteristics before treatment may achieve normal fertility. In this study abdominal irradiation and the addition of other cytotoxic agents decreased the chances of recovery. Serum testosterone and LH were virtually unaffected in these patients.

Kreuser et al. (1986) reported similar results in 45 patients with testicular cancer but recovery of spermatogenesis was delayed for longer and sperm motility was significantly impaired. Patients received PVB with or without doxorobucin and 33 had primary or delayed retroperitoneal lymph node dissection. Twenty per cent had elevated FSH levels and 60 per cent had oligospermia with reduced sperm motility before treatment. In the first year after treatment all patients were azoospermic and 95 per cent had significantly elevated FSH concentrations. By the third year eight out of 10 patients tested (80 per cent) had normal FSH levels and all seven tested had recovery of spermatogenesis. However, there was a high percentage of immotile sperm and only one patient fathered a child. Ejaculation was disturbed in 57 per cent of patients who had had node dissection and this was believed to be the major cause of infertility.

Drasga et al. (1983) reported low serum testosterone in 25 per cent of their patients treated with PVB. In this study 80 per cent of patients had some recovery of spermatogenesis 18 months after completing treatment.

POMB/ACE chemotherapy

Rustin et al. (1987) assessed gonadal function in 59 men who completed chemotherapy with the POMB/ACE regimen (cisplatin, vincristine, methotrexate, bleomycin, actinomycin D, cyclophosphamide, etoposide). Forty-nine per cent had sperm present but only 12 patients had counts greater than 20×10^6/ml. Spermatogenesis returned 11–68 months (median 17 months) after the completion of chemotherapy. Eleven men, including two who were oligospermic, fathered children after treatment. No patient who received abdominal radiotherapy recovered spermatogenesis and patients with bulky disease, liver, or brain metastases were less likely to recover, as were those who received chemotherapy for more than 6 months. Pre-treatment sperm count, age, and laparotomy were not found to be predictive factors.

VAB-6 chemotherapy

Bosl and Bajorunas (1987) reported significant deleterious effects of chemotherapy on Leydig cell function. Twenty-two patients had hormonal assessments 9–24 months after completing chemotherapy with the VAB-6 (cyclophosphamide, vinblastine, bleomyin, cisplatin, actinomycin D) or EP (etoposide, cisplatin) regimens. All but one had had a unilateral orchidectomy and more than two-thirds had had a retroperitoneal lymph node dissection which precluded seminal analysis. Six patients who had not received chemotherapy were studied for comparison. In 21 out of 22 treated and untreated patients baseline testosterone levels were normal, but basal LH levels were elevated in both groups. Peak dynamic LH levels were markedly higher in the treated patients and eight out of 13 treated patients also had a subnormal rise in serum testosterone in response to hCG stimulation. Those studied less than 18 months after treatment had higher LH levels than those assessed later. These data indicate that nearly all the patients treated with the VAB-6 and EP regimens had defective testicular hormone production which improved with time.

Surgery and infertility

Surgical disruption of the thoracolumbar sympathetic plexus causes sympathetic denervation of the bladder neck, seminal vesicles, prostate, and vasa deferentia. Ejaculatory failure may be caused by failure of emission, in which case no sperm or seminal vesicle secretions will be found in the urine or by failure of synchronous bladder neck contraction so that semen is ejaculated partially or totally retrogradely into the bladder. Differences in operative technique and individual anatomical variation in the function and position of the sympathetic ganglia probably account for the difference in the proportion of patients reported to have retrograde ejaculation and those with failure of seminal emission. Kedia et al. (1975) found that 35 out of 36 patients examined more than 1 year after retroperitoneal lymph node dissection had absent or 'dry' ejaculation only. None of these patients had sperm in the urine, suggesting that there was failure of emission due to loss of peristalsis of the ductus deferens and seminal vesicles. All these patients had

normal potency and orgasm. Ejaculation returned spontaneously to one patient after 7 years and he was able to father a child successfully. Kom et al. (1971) showed that, in their patients, ejaculatory loss after surgery was due to failure of seminal emission with spermatozoa progressing only as far as the prostate gland. Lack of fructose in the urine suggested that the seminal vesicles also failed to contract. Narayan et al. (1982) analysed 55 patients with ejaculatory failure after retroperitoneal lymph node dissection for testicular teratoma. Care was taken to preserve the presacral plexus at operation and subsequently retrograde ejaculation was more common than failure of emission. In this series of 25 men, an exceptionally high proportion spontaneously recovered antegrade ejaculation 3 months to 3 years after surgery, and seminal analysis in 20 of them ranged from 35×10^6/ml to 190×10^6/ml with normal sperm morphology and motility.

Attempts to avoid the complication of ejaculatory failure by careful preservation of at least part of the sympathetic plexus at the time of operation have reduced the incidence of this complication, but this operative manoeuvre may not always be feasible particularly in patients having debulking procedures post-chemotherapy. Fossa et al. (1985a) found that none of their patients who underwent a right-sided staging node dissection developed ejaculatory disturbance, compared with seven out of 21 patients who had a left-sided dissection and 51 out of 61 who had bilateral surgery. Dissection around the inferior mesenteric artery tends to be wider during operations on the left side, which may account for the better results after right-sided unilateral dissections. In this series, retrograde ejaculation was more frequent than failure of emission and spontaneous recovery was rare. Pizzocaro et al. (1985) reported similar results in 61 patients. The effectiveness of surveillance (Colls et al. 1992; Horwich et al. 1992) and the success of current chemotherapy regimens has reduced the need for staging retroperitoneal lymph node dissections, which are now rarely performed.

Personal perception and adjustment

Gritz et al. (1989) examined the effects of treatment for testicular tumours on body image, self-esteem, sexual function, and intramarital relationships of married long-term survivors. Fifty per cent of 34 couples did not wish for children in the future, mainly because they already had as many as they wanted. Forty-one per cent expected to have to adopt children in the future and only three patients and one spouse thought that inability to conceive children naturally would create problems in their marriage. Libido was decreased in approximately 50 per cent of patients after surgery, but generally this was a transient phenomenon lasting 2 or 3 months. Overall, this study suggests that patients adjust reasonably well after surviving testicular cancer and, in contrast to female patients with Hodgkin's disease, marital relationships may even be strengthened, despite slightly impaired sexual functioning in a significant proportion of patients.

Germ cell tumours in women

Malignant germ cell tumours are extremely rare in females and long-term survival was relatively uncommon until the advent of cisplatin-containing chemotherapy regimens. Few series have been published and the numbers of patients included are necessarily small. Generally, the outlook for the return of fertility after chemotherapy seems to be good, although some patients will become sterile as a result of surgery to remove residual tumour. There are several anecdotal reports of pregnancies occurring in young women after unilateral oophorectomy or adnexectomy together with chemotherapy regimens which include 5-fluorouracil, cyclophosphamide, actinomycin D, and melphalan (Forney 1978; Rosenshein et al. 1979; Schwartz and Vidone 1981; Ward et al. 1982). Gershenson et al. (1983) retrospectively reviewed 41 patients with ovarian germ cell tumours treated between 1944 and 1981. Twenty-two of these patients were treated with vincristine, actinomycin D, and cyclophosphamide, and 16 patients with a median age of 19 years had a prolonged survival. Three of these patients subsequently had successful pregnancies. More recently, Pektasides et al. (1987) noted the return of menstruation in 16 out of 17 women successfully treated with the POMB/ACE regimen. All patients were amenorrhoeic during treatment, but menses returned after a median of 4 months post-chemotherapy. Seven pregnancies occurred in five women after treatment. Recovery of fertility was not expected in 11 other patients owing to pelvic surgery, radiotherapy, or an abnormal karyotype and three patients were pre-pubertal. These observations suggest that there is a high probability of fertility returning to patients with ovarian germ cell tumours after treatment.

Gestational trophoblastic tumours

In the majority of cases treated for gestational trophoblastic tumours there is a high chance of retaining normal fertility. Van Thiel et al. (1970) reviewed 91 women with intact uteri and ovaries treated with chemotherapy between 1956 and 1969 for gestational trophoblastic tumours. Patients received single-agent therapy with methotrexate, actinomycin D, vinblastine, mustine, and 6-diazo-norleucine or multiagent combinations containing chlorambucil and actinomycin D or methotrexate, chlorambucil, and actinomycin D. Within this group there were 88 pregnancies in 50 women. Ten of the 41 who did not conceive were using some form of contraception and four had other gynaecological reasons for infertility. Details were not available for the remaining 27 patients. In this series there was no correlation between the amount of chemotherapy and the ability to conceive or with fetal abnormalities or fetal loss. The incidence and type of congenital abnormalities were no different to those of the normal population. In another series (Richter et al. 1987) nine women became pregnant after treatment with methotrexate or with methotrexate and actinomycin D. Normal children were born to eight and the ninth had an elective termination.

Leukaemia in males

The treatment of patients with leukaemia, of whatever type, involves the use of several drugs, frequently in complex regimens given for long periods and often in combination with radiotherapy. Comparison of the effects of different regimens on gonadal function is difficult because of the variety of protocols which exist. The picture which emerges is similar to that found in other diseases treated with multiagent chemotherapy. Infertility is by no means universal but occurs in a significant proportion of patients. In males tubular function is primarily affected but hormone production may be damaged to a lesser extent. The severity of gonadal injury correlates roughly with the amount of chemotherapy received but with great individual variation and recovery may occur unpredictably and after several years. Regimens without alkylating agents are significantly less harmful to the testes and ovaries and there is less potential for recovery of ovarian function than testicular function. In females, age is important in determining how gonadal toxicity is manifest. In older women it manifests as a premature menopause,

but in younger women and children it may only be apparent histologically with maintenance of menstruation. In both sexes the pre-pubertal gonad is not spared the injurious effects of treatment, but the initiation and progress of puberty appear to pass undisturbed.

Lendon et al. (1978) studied the testicular histology of 44 boys who were receiving or had finished treatment for acute lymphoblastic leukaemia with several regimens, all including vincristine, prednisolone, 6-mercaptopurine, and methotrexate. Some also received asparaginase, cyclophosphamide, cytosine arabinoside, and doxorubicin. Their testes were compared with those of 16 boys with acute leukaemia who died within 3 weeks of starting therapy and who had received little if any chemotherapy. In the testes of the extensively treated boys, a leukaemic infiltrate was identified in 11 per cent, interstitial fibrosis in 55 per cent, and basement membrane thickening in 14 per cent. The mean tubular fertility index was 50 per cent of that of controls. Previous treatment with cyclophosphamide or more than $1 \, g/m^2$ of cytosine arabinoside was associated with a reduced tubular fertility index. Age, pubertal status, and total dose of other cytotoxic agents did not appear to relate to the tubular fertility index, but it improved with time from chemotherapy. The tubular fertility index was also significantly depressed in those boys who died before receiving much treatment, suggesting that the disease itself or a generally debilitated state might account for some or all of the abnormal tubular morphology. Abnormally elevated FSH levels were found in a much higher proportion of pubertal than pre-pubertal patients despite similar degrees of histological damage, which supports the contention that elevated gonadotrophin levels are an unreliable way of detecting tubular dysfunction in pre-pubertal boys. Median basal gonadotrophin and testosterone levels and stimulated gonadotrophin and testosterone levels were similar to age-matched controls of the same pubertal status. Only two patients showed an absent or blunted response of testosterone to hCG (Shalet et al. 1981).

Kuhajda et al. (1982) studied autopsy gonadal tissue from 183 patients treated for leukaemia and compared them with matched controls. Cyclophosphamide, vincristine, methotrexate, and prednisolone were the drugs most commonly used for patients with acute lymphoblastic leukaemia, cyclophosphamide, cytosine arabinoside, and daunorubicin for patients with acute non-lymphoblastic leukaemia, chlorambucil, vincristine, and prednisolone for patients with chronic lymphoblastic leukaemia, and busulphan, chlorambucil, daunorubicin, and cytosine arabinoside for chronic myeloid leukaemia. Most of the patients were post-pubertal at the time of death. Significantly decreased spermatogenic activity and tubular fertility index and increased interstitial fibrosis were seen in 103 male leukaemic patients. There was no clear correlation between the severity of morphological changes and the sexual maturity of the patient, type of leukaemia, dose or type of chemotherapy, or time since the last dose of any antineoplastic agent. This wide difference in individual susceptibility suggests that other factors may affect spermatogenesis. The testes of pre-pubertal patients were damaged at least as much as their more mature counterparts. Testicular involvement with leukaemia was demonstrable in 25 per cent of patients, all of whom had disease in other organs. Nevertheless, there was histological evidence of residual reproductive potential in 65 per cent of patients.

Despite the severity of morphological damage demonstrated in histopathological studies, Blatt et al. (1981) observed normal pubertal progression in boys treated with similar antileukaemic regimens for acute lymphoblastic leukaemia and, like Shalet et al. (1981), found virtually no hormonal evidence of gonadal toxicity. Testosterone and gonadotrophins were normal in each case and only one out of six patients who provided semen for analysis had a low normal sperm count.

Even after prolonged periods of treatment for leukaemia patients may retain normal fertility, but this depends upon the agents used. Evenson et al. (1984) assessed six adult men who had received treatment with the L10 protocol for acute lymphoblastic leukaemia. This protocol includes cyclophosphamide, carmustine, vincristine, actinomycin D, methotrexate, cytosine arabinoside, thioguanine, and asparaginase. No cranial radiotherapy is given and there are relatively long intervals between alkylating agents. Semen analysis was performed 10–52 months after completion of at least 3.5 years of continuous therapy. Only one of the patients was found to have a sperm concentration below normal, but he had a near normal total sperm count and normal motility. The other patients had normal semen.

Nowadays, the treatment of leukaemia and other malignant diseases may involve the use of 'biological' agents. Little is known about the potential gonadal effects of these new treatments. Schilsky et al. (1987) evaluated 81 male patients with stable hairy cell leukaemia. Thirty-three were receiving no treatment at the time and 48 were receiving recombinant 2b-interferon. Minor abnormalities in testicular function were noted in a small proportion of patients in both treated and control groups. However, most patients appeared to have normal testicular and sexual function, with 2b-interferon exerting no obvious adverse effect.

The importance of alkylating agents given over prolonged periods as maintenance therapy to men with leukaemia has been shown by Waxman et al. (1983). Patients with acute lymphoblastic leukaemia had induction therapy with daunorubicin, vincristine, and L-asparaginase, with cyclophosphamide, 6-mercaptopurine, and methotrexate maintenance. Patients with acute non-lymphoblastic leukaemia received six courses of treatment with daunorubicin, cytosine arabinoside, and 6-thioguanine. Infertility occurred in men with acute lymphoblastic leukaemia who had maintenance chemotherapy for up to 3 years and normal fertility was seen in patients with acute non-lymphoblastic leukaemia who received short-term therapy.

Leukaemia in females

The gonadal problems associated with antileukaemic therapy have also been addressed in females and there are varying reports of ovarian dysfunction. In a post-mortem study Kuhajda et al. (1982) examined 80 females and found that there was no significant difference in the number of primary follicles in the ovaries of patients compared with age-matched controls. However, the number of secondary follicles was markedly decreased in both pre- and post-pubertal patients, suggesting impairment of follicle maturation without loss of germ cells. As in males, these changes were largely idiosyncratic and did not reflect the type or amount of chemotherapy or the time elapsed since the last treatment. Ovarian involvement with leukaemia occurred but, as with testicular infiltration, reflected more widespread disease; the gonads did not appear to be a sanctuary site in either sex. These histological findings do not concur with clinical studies which tend to show a closer relationship between the dose of cytotoxic drug, particularly alkylating agents, patient age, and ovarian failure. Moreover, one would expect maturation arrest to be a reversible condition and, with primary follicles still present, ovarian failure to be transient.

Siris et al. (1976) explored the effects of antileukaemic therapy on puberty and reproductive function in girls. Thirty-five girls were studied, seven of whom had evidence of disrupted puberty. Four

patients had reduced levels of circulating gonadotrophins owing to pituitary dysfunction which in three followed cranial irradiation. Three patients had features of primary ovarian dysfunction with abnormally elevated circulating gonadotrophins. One of these girls had received busulphan, but surprisingly an autopsy study of her ovaries did not show atrophy or oocyte depletion but maturation arrest. The other two patients developed secondary amenorrhoea with a perimenopausal gonadotrophin pattern which resolved spontaneously. The remaining 28 patients progressed normally through puberty. In this study pubertal progression was more likely to be affected if puberty had already started at the time of treatment and pre-pubertal patients were relatively spared. Pubertal status was a stronger predictor than amount or duration of treatment. The effects of meningeal involvement and cranial irradiation could not be discerned from this study because of the small numbers involved. Other studies (Shalet et al. 1977) have shown that hypothalamic/pituitary function may be affected by cranial irradiation given as part of treatment for leukaemia, but growth hormone, TSH, and ACTH secretion are usually affected before the gonadotrophins and infertility is generally associated with primary ovarian dysfunction due to cytotoxic drugs, particularly alkylating agents.

Sanders et al. (1988) assessed ovarian function in 187 females after bone-marrow transplant for aplastic anaemia or leukaemia. Age at transplant was the only significant factor in the recovery of ovarian function. After high-dose cyclophosphamide, recovery occurred in all women less than 26 years old and in five out of 16 older women. After cyclophosphamide and total-body irradiation only nine out of 76 younger patients but none out of 68 older patients recovered. With increasing age at transplantation, the probability of recovery after total-body irradiation was calculated to decrease by a factor of 0.8 per year of age. Sixty-four per cent of patients experienced menopausal symptoms which were helped by hormone replacement therapy. Beard and Clark (1984) reported similar results from a small series of patients treated with a variety of regimens for a selection of haematological and related malignancies. Ovarian failure occurred in over half the patients and was more frequently observed in those aged over 25 years and those on continuous low dosages of alklyating agents.

Intracranial tumours

There is some controversy about the relative contribution of radiotherapy and chemotherapy to the infertility observed in long-term survivors of childhood brain tumours. The situation is complicated by the fact that hypothalamic and pituitary damage may occur in addition to primary gonadal injury.

Ahmed et al. (1983) first ascribed primary gonadal damage in children treated for medulloblastoma to their adjuvant chemotherapy. They found that all children treated with adjuvant chemotherapy developed clinical and biochemical evidence of primary gonadal dysfunction compared with none of the patients who had not received chemotherapy. Carmustine or lomustine was given to all the children receiving adjuvant therapy and some received vincristine and/or procarbazine in addition. The evidence strongly suggests that the nitrosoureas were responsible. Clayton et al. (1988) confirmed these findings in a study of 50 boys treated for childhood brain tumours with adjuvant chemotherapy including nitrosoureas and in some cases vincristine and/or procarbazine, for 0.9–2.2 years. All boys entered and proceeded through puberty normally except for two who were gonadotrophin deficient as a result of cranial irradiation. However, only one out of 19 evaluable boys treated in the pre-pubertal years and only one out of eight boys treated between the ages of 12 and 16 years had no sign of testicular damage. In 18 out of 21 girls there was evidence of primary ovarian dysfunction at some stage after the same treatment. One developed secondary amenorrhoea due to gonadotrophin deficiency secondary to radiation-induced hypothalamic dysfunction (Clayton *et al.* 1989). As in boys, pubertal progression appeared to be unaffected by treatment but, unlike the boys, serum gonadotrophin levels eventually returned to normal in some patients. Scatter from spinal irradiation may have contributed to the ovarian toxicity, but chemotherapy was believed to have been the major factor since patients from the same centre, treated with craniospinal radiotherapy alone, were much less likely to develop ovarian dysfunction. Livesey and Brook (1988) investigated gonadal function in 93 children treated for intracranial tumours and also found that primary gonadal dysfunction was relatively common and secondary dysfunction was rare. Eighty-one patients were pre-pubertal at the time of treatment. All received cranial radiotherapy, 59 had spinal irradiation, and 28 had adjuvant chemotherapy with lomustine, vincristine, and methotrexate singly or in combination. Primary ovarian dysfunction occurred in 64 per cent and was significantly associated with spinal irradiation, particularly in younger patients. The incidence was not increased by the addition of chemotherapy, but in patients who did not receive spinal irradiation chemotherapy was associated with ovarian dysfunction in two out of three patients compared with none out of 14 who received cranial radiotherapy alone. Testicular dysfunction only occurred in boys who received chemotherapy, although there was no obvious relation to dose or duration of treatment. In addition, five boys had delayed or arrested puberty owing to gonadotrophin deficiency. Overall, it is apparent that adjuvant treatment with nitrosoureas in particular may have harmful effects on the gonads and where possible treatment should be kept to a minimum or confined to high risk groups.

Breast cancer: adjuvant therapy

There has been increasing evidence that adjuvant chemotherapy improves relapse-free and overall survival in pre-menopausal women with operable primary breast cancer (Early Breast Cancer Trialists' Collaborative Group 1988). Most adjuvant chemotherapy trials involve combinations of drugs, particularly CMF (cyclophosphamide, methotrexate, 5-fluorouracil) or similar regimens or single-agent alkylating agents such as cyclophosphamide, melphalan, and thiotepa. Approximately 60–80 per cent of patients develop age-related irreversible amenorrhoea and hormonal studies have confirmed that this is due to primary ovarian failure (Koyama *et al.* 1977; Rose and Davis 1980; Hortobagyi *et al.* 1986; Padmanabhan *et al.* 1987). It is debatable whether the beneficial effects of adjuvant chemotherapy are due to the induction of an early menopause alone or whether there is an additional cytotoxic effect (Ludwig Breast Cancer Study Group 1985*a,b*; Goldhirsch and Gelber 1986; Beex *et al.* 1988). In one study CMF improved relapse-free survival in subsets of patients without amenorrhoea, with oestrogen-receptor-negative tumours, and with tumours of low histological differentiation (Brincker *et al.* 1987). Similarly, the Milan group testing adjuvant CMF in pre-menopausal women with oestrogen-receptor-negative tumours found significantly improved relapse-free and overall survival compared with control patients (Bonadonna *et al.* 1983; Bonadonna and Valagussa 1987). Fisher *et al.* (1979) found a discrepancy between the effects of adjuvant melphalan on gonadal function and the beneficial effects in terms of relapse-free survival. Ovarian failure occurred in 73 per cent of pre-menopausal patients aged 40–49 years and in 22 per cent of younger

patients. Yet adjuvant chemotherapy reduced the incidence of treatment failure in both age groups and the effect was greater in the younger patients relative to their controls (69 per cent disease-free survival at 4 years versus 32 per cent in those aged less than 40 years and 61 per cent versus 48 per cent in the age group 41–49 years). Further evidence that adjuvant chemotherapy does not work by chemical castration alone comes from the failure of surgical oophorectomy to improve outcome in some clinical trials (Kennedy *et al.* 1964; Ravolin *et al.* 1970; Tengrup *et al.* 1986) and the less dramatic beneficial effects of adjuvant chemotherapy in post-menopausal patients.

The effects of chemotherapy on hormonal and reproductive function in patients with breast cancer cannot be regarded in the same light as in other patients with cancer. Ovarian ablation is likely to contribute a major part of the therapeutic effect in this hormone-responsive disease and consequently cannot strictly be regarded as a side-effect of treatment.

Prostate cancer

Prostate cancer usually occurs at an age when fertility is no longer desired but potency usually is. Bladder neck dysfunction results from transurethral resections of the prostate for benign or malignant disease and it is possible that it may respond to manoeuvres used for patients with retrograde ejaculation secondary to sympathetic plexus damage. Radical prostatectomy may result in impotence due to damage to the pelvic plexus, particularly the branches passing to the corpora cavernosa and spongiosa (Walsh and Donker 1980), with loss of erection and emission but preservation of penile sensation and orgasm. Fortunately, recently developed nerve-sparing operative techniques have reduced the likelihood of this complication from 100 per cent to approximately 25 per cent of patients after surgery.

Unfortunately, most treatments for advanced disease involve interruption or antagonism of the normal androgenic hormonal pathways. Therefore almost all hormone manipulations for prostatic carcinoma are associated with loss of libido and frequently, although not universally, with impotence, in addition to reduced spermatogenesis. Some newer anti-androgens are claimed not to impair potency. α-Blocker injection has a role in those patients who wish to maintain potency and this is discussed further in the next section.

MANAGEMENT OF TREATMENT-RELATED INFERTILITY

Sphincter dysfunction following retroperitoneal lymph node dissection

Mechanical strategies

A reduced or absent ejaculate with semen in the post-coital urine is suggestive of bladder neck dysfunction and the ability to void urine whilst having an erection is virtually pathognomonic of this disorder. Since potency and orgasm are unaffected, treatment is usually only required when there is a wish to conceive. Various strategies have been investigated in the management of this problem.

Attempts have been made to retrieve spermatozoa from the urine and use it for insemination. Unfortunately, few pregnancies have been reported, mainly because of the deleterious effects of urine on sperm. Spermatozoa may remain motile for 3 h or more in urine provided that it is not too dilute or acidic (pH < 6.2); therefore sodium bicarbonate (5 g by mouth) 1 or 2 h before intercourse may improve the chances of obtaining viable sperm (Brindley 1981). Early attempts to improve results included pre-ejaculation bladder wash outs followed by retrieval of sperm with a catheter (Hotchkiss *et al.* 1955; Rieser 1961). Later methods involved immediate dilution to wash away the urine, followed by centrifugation and resuspension in various media containing human serum albumin (Scammell *et al.* 1982) and carefully selected electrolytes (Cameron and Gillett 1985). With these methods it is usual to recommend completely emptying the bladder before ejaculation to reduce urine contamination to a minimum. However, by increasing the pressure within the bladder, ejaculation with a full bladder in the standing position may enable patients to produce sufficient antegrade ejaculate, relatively uncontaminated with urine, for artificial or natural insemination of their partners (Crich and Jequier 1978).

Pharmacological strategies

α-Adrenergic drugs have been applied to patients with retrograde ejaculation in order to increase bladder neck tone. Stockamp *et al.* (1974) treated six patients with intravenous synephrine, an α-adrenergic receptor agonist. One patient had full restoration of antegrade ejaculation, three were unchanged, and two became worse with treatment. Treatment failure was believed to have arisen from excessive adrenergic stimulation causing ductus deferens spasm. There have been anecdotal reports of restoration of antegrade ejaculation and fertility in patients after systemic self-administration of adrenaline (Lynch and Maxted 1983). This has obvious practical problems and α-adrenergic agents which are orally active have been investigated. Nijman *et al.* (1982) treated 12 patients with oral imipramine (25 mg twice daily). Five out of ten patients with retrograde ejaculation had antegrade ejaculation restored and achieved pregnancies. Narayan *et al.* (1982) reported a return of antegrade ejaculation in five out of ten patients during treatment with sympatho-mimetic drugs and an improvement in semen volume in a further two patients. Fossa *et al.* (1985b) observed a significant improvement in ejaculation in seven out of ten men with the use of imipramine. From these studies it seems that those patients who are likely to benefit from treatment with sympathomimetic drugs have FSH within the normal range and demonstrable sperm in the urine after masturbation or sexual intercourse. If treatment with imipramine (25 mg twice daily) fails, it may be worth increasing the dose to 50 mg twice daily, but further increases are likely to be counterproductive because of receptor blockade.

Impotence

Potency may be achieved in some patients with intrapenile injections of papaverine and phentolamine (Virag 1982; Brindley 1983; Davis *et al.* 1985; Morley 1986; Balducci *et al.* 1988). Alternatively, semi-rigid or inflatable penile prostheses may be surgically implanted (Kudish 1983; Beutler *et al.* 1984; Nelson 1988).

Prevention of cytotoxic damage: experimental approaches

Obvious strategies for reducing the gonadal toxicity of antineoplastic therapy include the substitution of alternative drugs for alkylating agents, limiting the total dose of alkylating agents and keeping the dose and duration of treatment to a minimum without compromisng the therapeutic outcome. However, these manoeuvres will still leave

a substantial proportion of patients at risk of infertility. The main thrust of attempts to reduce gonadal side-effects comes from the contentious observation that the pre-pubertal testis and ovary are relatively more resistant to damage than the mature gonad and that this may be due to their 'inactive' state. Unfortunately, many reports already outlined have shown that the difference in vulnerability to chemotherapy between the mature and immature gonad is not great. Moreover, we still do not know whether oocyte depletion in very young patients will lead to premature ovarian failure in time. It is likely that any protection conferred by returning a mature gonad to a pre-pubertal quiescent state will be relative and not absolute.

Steroid hormones

It has been suggested that the combined oestrogen–progestogen contraceptive pill is protective in patients having chemotherapy for Hodgkin's disease (Chapman *et al.* 1981). No protective effect was seen when these patients were reassessed (Waxman, unpublished data). Nine women treated with MVPP for Hodgkin's disease (Whitehead *et al.* 1983) took the oral contraceptive pill throughout treatment and there was no evidence of protection against subsequent ovarian failure.

Gonadotrophin-releasing hormone agonists

Glode *et al.* (1981) pre-treated male mice with a GnRH agonist analogue before administering a single dose of cyclophosphamide and found that the testicular germinal epithelium was histologically less severely damaged than in control animals given cyclophosphamide alone. However, spermatogenesis is different in mice and a single dosage of cyclophosphamide is not sterilizing (Waxman 1987). Pre-treatment with GnRH analogues before receiving regular doses of cyclophosphamide over a prolonged period has been investigated in male beagles and baboons and the results suggest that there is a protective effect (Goodpasture *et al.* 1984; Lewis *et al.* 1985). In these experiments, the animals were pre-treated for several weeks before receiving the cytotoxic drug.

Protection using gonadotrophin analogues has been attempted in man (Waxman *et al.* 1987a,b). Thirty men and 18 women with Hodgkin's disease were randomly allocated to receive buserelin before and during chemotherapy. Two different dose schedules were used. Unfortunately, there was no evidence of any benefit at follow-up assessment up to 3 years later. All the men, whether treated with buserelin or not, were profoundly oligospermic and four out of eight women were amenorrhoeic compared with six out of nine female controls. In all patients peak LH response to GnRH was suppressed throughout treatment, but the initial suppression of peak FSH response to GnRH was not maintained. As patients were only pre-treated for a short period before starting chemotherapy, it may be that the pre-treatment period was inadequate for protection.

Treatment of gonadal failure

In women, early gonadal failure causes premature osteoporosis, amenorrhoea, dyspareunia, infertility, flushing, and decreased libido. These symptoms may be helped by steroid hormone replacement therapy using sequential oestrogens and progestrogens. This may not adequately restore libido and androgen replacement is frequently required. In men, androgen replacement is generally unnecessary owing to the relative resistance of the Leydig cells to chemotherapeutic agents. Unfortunately, at present there is no way of restoring fertility to either sex.

CONCLUSION

The luxury of cure allows us to contemplate the disadvantages of treatment. Although infertility might be considered a minor issue in the context of the successful treatment of malignancy, its importance to the patient should not be underestimated. Recognition and treatment of this complication are essential if clinicians are to care adequately for their patients.

REFERENCES

Ahmed SR, Shalet SM, Campbell RHA, Deakin DP (1983). Primary gonadal damage following treatment of brain tumours in childhood. *Journal of Pediatrics*, 103(4):562–5.

Arneil GC (1972). Cyclophosphamide on a prepubertal testis. *Lancet*, ii:1259–60.

Balducci L, *et al.* (1988). Sexual complications of cancer treatment. *Association of Family Practitioners*, 37(3):159–72.

Bartsch G, Frank LT, Marberger H, Mikuz G (1980). Testicular torsion: late results with specific regard to fertility and endocrine function. *Journal of Urology*, 124:375–8.

Beard BEJ, Clark VA (1984). Ovarian failure following cytotoxic therapy. *New Zealand Medical Journal*, 97:759–62.

Beex LVAM, *et al.* (1988). Adjuvant chemotherapy in premenopausal patients with primary breast cancer; relation to drug induced amenorrhoea, age and the progesterone receptor status of the tumour. *European Journal of Cancer and Clinical Oncology*, 24:719–21.

Belohorsky B, Siracky J, Sandor L, Kaluber E (1960). Comments on the development of amenorrhoea caused by myleran in cases of chronic myelosis. *Neoplasma*, 4:397.

Berry CL, *et al.* (1972). Cyclophosphamide and the prepubertal testis. *Lancet*, ii:1033–4.

Berthelsen JG, Shakkebaek NE, Morgensen P, Sorensen BL (1979). Incidence of carcinomas *in situ* of germ cells in contralateral testis of men with testicular tumours. *British Medical Journal*, 2:363–4.

Beutler LE, *et al.* (1984). Women's satisfaction with partners' penile implant. Inflatable versus non-inflatable prosthesis. *Urology*, 24:552–8.

Biggers JD, Whittingham DG, Donahue RP (1967). The pattern of energy metabolism in mouse oocyte and zygote. *Proceedings of National Academy of Sciences USA*, 58:560–7.

Blatt J, Poplack DJ, Sherins RJ (1981). Testicular function in boys after chemotherapy for acute lymphoblastic leukemia. *New England Journal of Medicine*, 304:1121–4.

Bonadonna G (1982). Chemotherapy strategies to improve the control of Hodgkin's disease. The Richard and Hinda Rosenthal Foundation Award Lecture. *Cancer Research*, 42:4309–20.

Bonadonna G, Santoro A (1982). ABVD chemotherapy in the treatment of Hodgkin's disease. *Cancer Treatment Reviews*, 9:21–35.

Bonadonna G, Rossi A, Tancini G, Valagussa P (1983). Adjuvant chemotherapy in breast cancer. *Lancet*, i:1157.

Bonadonna G, Valagussa P (1987). Current status of adjuvant chemotherapy for breast cancer. *Seminars in Oncology*, 14:8–22.

Bosl GJ, Bajorumas D (1987). Pituitary and testicular hormonal function after treatment for germ cell tumours. *International Journal of Andrology*, 10:381–4.

Brincker H, *et al.* (1987). Evidence of a castration mediated effect of adjuvant cytotoxic chemotherapy in premenopausal breast cancer. *Journal of Clinical Oncology*, 5:1771–8.

Brindley GS (1981). Electroejaculation: its technique, neurological implications and uses. *Journal of Neurology, Neurosurgery and Psychiatry*, 44:9–18.

Brindley GS (1983). Cavernosal alpha blockade: a new technique for investigating and treating erectile impotence. *British Journal of Psychiatry*, 143:332–7.

Buchanan JD, Fairley KF, Barrie JU (1975). Return of spermatogenesis after stopping cyclophosphamide therapy. *Lancet*, ii:156–7.

Bulbrook RD, *et al.* (1978). Plasma oestradiol and progesterone levels in women with varying degrees of risk of breast cancer. *European Journal of Cancer*, 14:1369–75.

Cameron MC, Gillett WR (1985). The recovery of sperm, insemination and pregnancy in the treatment of infertility because of retrograde ejaculation. *Fertility and Sterility*, 44:844–5.

Carroll PR, *et al.* (1987). Fertility status of patients with clinical stage 1 testis tumour on a surveillance protocol. *Journal of Urology*, 138:70–2.

Chapman RM (1982). Effect of cytotoxic therapy on sexuality and gonadal function. *Seminars in Oncology*, 9(1):84–94.

Chapman RM, Sutcliffe SB, Malpas JS (1979a). Cytotoxic induced ovarian failure in women with Hodgkin's disease. I. Hormone function. *Journal of the American Medical Association*, 242:1877–81.

Chapman RM, Sutcliffe SB, Malpas JS (1979b). Cytotoxic induced ovarian failure in Hodgkin's disease. II. Effects on sexual function. *Journal of the American Medical Association*, 242:1882–4.

Chapman RM, *et al.* (1979c). Cyclical combination chemotherapy and gonadal function. *Lancet*, i:285–9.

Chapman RM, Sutcliffe SB, Malpas JS (1981). Male gonadal dysfunction in Hodgkin's disease. A prospective study. *Journal of the American Medical Association*, 245:1323–8.

Cheviakoff S, Calamera JC, Morgenfeld M, Manchini RE (1973). Recovery of spermatogenesis in patients with lymphoma after treatment with chlorambucil. *Journal of Reproduction and Fertility*, 33:155.

Clayton PE, Shalet SM, Price DA, Campbell RHA (1988). Testicular damage after chemotherapy for childhood brain tumours. *Journal of Pediatrics*, 112:922–6.

Clayton PE, Shalet SM, Price DA, Morris Jones PH (1989). Ovarian function following chemotherapy for childhood brain tumours. *Medical and Pediatric Oncology*, 17:92–6.

Cochran JS, *et al.* (1975). The endocrinology of human chorionic gonadotrophin-secreting testicular tumours: new methods in diagnosis. *Journal of Urology*, 114:549–55.

Colls BM, *et al.* (1992). Results of the surveillance policy of stage I non-seminomatous germ cell testicular tumours. *British Journal of Urology*, 70:423–8.

Cooke RA, Nikles A, Roeser HP (1978). A comparison of the anti-fertility effects of alkylating agents and vinca alkaloids in male rats. *British Journal of Pharmacology*, 63:677–81.

Crich JP, Jequier AM (1978). Infertility in men with retrograde ejaculation: the action of urine on sperm motility and a simple method for achieving antegrade ejaculation. *Fertility and Sterility*, 30:372–6.

Curie-Cohen M, Luttrell L, Shapiro S (1979). Current practice of artificial insemination by donor in the United States. *New England Journal of Medicine*, 300:585–90.

Da Cunha MF, *et al.* (1983). Active sperm production after cancer chemotherapy with doxorubicin. *Journal of Urology*, 130:927–30.

Davis SS, *et al.* (1985). Evaluation of impotence in older men. *Western Journal of Medicine*, 142:499–505.

De Groot GW, Fairman C, Winter JDS (1974). Cyclophosphamide and the prepubertal gonad: a negative report. *Journal of Pediatrics*, 84:123–5.

Donahue RP (1968). Maturation of mouse oocyte *in vitro*. I. Sequence and timing of nuclear progression. *Journal of Experimental Zoology*, 169:237–49.

Drasga RE, *et al.* (1983). Fertility after chemotherapy for testicular cancer. *Journal of Clinical Oncology*, 1:179–83.

Early Breast Cancer Trialists Collaborative Group (1988). Effects of adjuvant tamoxifen and of cytotoxic therapy on mortality in early breast cancer. *New England Journal of Medicine*, 319:1681–92.

Edwards RG (1966). Mammalian eggs in the laboratory. *Scientific American*, 215:72–81.

Etteldorf JM, West CD, Pittcock JA, Williams DL (1976). Gonadal function, testicular histology and meiosis following cyclophosphamide therapy in patients with nephrotic syndrome. *Journal of Pediatrics*, 88:206–12.

Evenson DP, *et al.* (1984). Male reproductive capacity may recover following drug treatment with the L-10 protocol for acute lymphocytic leukemia. *Cancer*, 53:30–6.

Ezdinli EZ, Stutzman L (1965). Chlorambucil therapy for lymphomas and chronic lymphocytic leukaemia. *Journal of the American Medical Association*, 191:444–50.

Fairley KF, Barrie JU, Johnson W (1972). Sterility and testicular atrophy related to cyclophosphamide therapy. *Lancet*, i:568–9.

Fisher B, Sherman B, Rockette H (1979). L-Phenylalanine mustard (L-PAM) in the management of premenopausal patients with primary breast cancer; lack of association of disease free survival with depression of ovarian function. *Cancer*, 44:847–57.

Forney JP (1978). Pregnancy following removal and chemotherapy of ovarian endodermal sinus tumour. *Obstetrics and Gyneology*, 52:360–2.

Fossa SD, Ous S, Abyholm T, Loeb M (1985*a*). Post treatment fertility in patients with testicular cancer. I. Influence of retroperitoneal lymph node dissection on ejaculatory potency. *British Journal of Urology*, 57:204–9.

Fossa SD, *et al.* (1985*b*). Post treatment fertility in patients with testicular cancer. II. Influence of cisplatin based combination chemotherapy and of retroperitoneal surgery on hormone and sperm cell production. *British Journal of Urology*, 57:210–14.

Freckman HA, Fry HL, Mendez FL, Maurer ER (1964). Chlorambucil–prednisolone therapy for disseminated breast carcinoma. *Journal of the American Medical Association*, 189:23–6.

Gershenson DM, Dei Junco G, Herson J, Rotledge FN (1983). Endodermal sinus tumour of the ovary: the MD Anderson Experience. *Obstetrics and Gynecology*, 61:194–202.

Glode LM, Robinson J, Gould SF (1981). Protection from cyclophosphamide induced testicular damage with an analogue of gonadotrophin releasing hormone. *Lancet*, i:1132–4.

Goldhirsch A, Gelber R (1986). Adjuvant treatment for early breast cancer: the Ludwig breast cancer studies. *National Cancer Institute Monographs*, 1:55–70.

Goodpasture JC, Bergstrom K, Waller DP, Vickery BM (1984). Interactions between an LHRH analogue and cancer chemotherapeutic agents at the testicular level. In *LHRH analogues 1984* (ed. F Labrie, A Belanger, and A Du Pont), pp. 156–72. Excerpta Medica, Amsterdam.

Grattarola R (1964). The premenstrual endometrial pattern of women with breast cancer: a study of progestational activity. *Cancer*, 17:1119–22.

Gritz ER, *et al.* (1989). Long term effects of testicular cancer on sexual functioning in married couples. *Cancer*, 64:1560–7.

Guesry P, Lenoir G, Broyer M (1978). Gonadal effects of chlorambucil given to prepubertal and pubertal boys for nephrotic syndrome. *Journal of Pediatrics*, 92:299–303.

Hansen PV, Trykker H, Andersen J, Helkjaer PE (1989). Germ cell function and hormonal status in patients with testicular cancer. *Cancer*, 64:956–61.

Harrison RG, de Marval MJM, Lewis-Jones DI, Connelley RC (1981). Mechanism of damaged contralateral testis in rats with an ischaemic testis. *Lancet*, ii:723–5.

Hendry WF, *et al.* (1983). Semen analysis in testicular cancer and Hodgkin's disease: pre and post treatment findings and implications for cryopreservation. *British Journal of Urology*, 55:769–73.

Horning SJ, Hoppe RT, Caplan HS, Rosenberg SA (1981). Female reproductive potential after treatment for Hodgkin's disease. *New England Journal of Medicine*, 304:1377–82.

Hortobagyi GN, Buzdar AU, Marcus CE, Smith TL (1986). Immediate and long term toxicity of adjuvant chemotherapy regimens containing doxorubicin in trials at MD Anderson Hospital and Tumor Institute. *National Cancer Institute Monographs*, 1:105–9.

Horwich A, *et al.* (1992). Surveillance following orchidectomy for stage I testicular seminoma. *British Journal of Cancer*, 65:775–8.

Hotchkiss RS, Pinto AB, Kleegman S (1955). Artificial insemination with semen recovered from the bladder. *Fertility and Sterility*, 6:37.

Hurdadli KS, Arbatt NJ, Mehta S, Sheth AR (1984). Serum inhibin levels after administration of human chorionic gonadotrophin. *Archives of Andrology*, 12:45–8.

Kaldar JM, *et al.* (1987). Second malignancies following testicular cancer, ovarian cancer and Hodgkin's disease: an international collaborative study among cancer registries. *International Journal of Cancer*, 39:571–85.

Kay H, Mattison D (1985). How radiation and chemotherapy affect gonadal function. *Contemporary Obstetrics and Gynaecology*, 109:106.

Kedia KR, Markland C, Fraley EE (1975). Sexual function following higher retroperitoneal lymphadenectomy. *Journal of Urology*, 114:237–9.

Kennedy BJ, Mielke PLW, Fortuny IE (1964). Therapeutic castration versus prophylactic castration in breast cancer. *Surgery, Gynecology and Obstetrics*, 118:524–40.

Kirkland RT, *et al.* (1976). Gonadotrophin responses to luteinising releasing factor in boys treated with cyclophosphamide for nephrotic syndrome. *Journal of Pediatrics*, 89:941–4.

Kom C, Mulholland SG, Edson M (1971). Etiology of infertility after retroperitoneal lymphadenectomy. *Journal of Urology*, 105:528–30.

Koyama H, *et al.* (1977). Cyclophosphamide-induced ovarian failure and its therapeutic significance in patients with breast cancer. *Cancer*, 39:1403–9.

Kreuser ED, Harsch U, Hetzel WD, Schreml W (1986). Chronic gonadal toxicity in patients with testicular cancer after chemotherapy. *Journal of Cancer and Clinical Oncology*, 22(3):289–94.

Kreuser ED, Xiros N, Hetzel WD, Heimpel H (1987). Reproductive and endocrine gonadal capacity in patients treated with COPP chemotherapy for Hodgkin's disease. *Journal of Cancer Research and Clinical Oncology*, 113:260–6.

Kudish HG (1983). Treatment of impotence. Proven and promising methods. *Postgraduate Medicine*, 74(4):233–40.

Kuhajda FP, Haupt HM, Moore GW, Hutchins GM (1982). Gonadal morphology in patients receiving chemotherapy for leukemia. Evidence for reproductive potential and against a testicular tumor sanctuary. *American Journal of Medicine*, 72:759–67.

Kumar R, Biggart JD, McEvoy J, McGeown MG (1972). Cyclophosphamide and reproductive function. *Lancet*, i:1212–14.

Lendon M, *et al.* (1978). Testicular histology after combination chemotherapy in childhood for acute lymphoblastic leukaemia. *Lancet*, ii:439–41.

Lentz RD, *et al.* (1977). Post pubertal evaluation of gonadal function following cyclophosphamide therapy before and during puberty. *Journal of Pediatrics*, 91:385–94.

Lewis RD, Dowling KJ, Schally AV (1985). D-Tryptophan-6 analog of luteinizing hormone releasing hormone as a protective agent against testicular damage caused by cyclophosphamide in baboons. *Proceedings of the National Academy of Sciences USA*, 82:2975–9.

Livesey EA, Brook CGD (1988). Gonadal dysfunction after treatment of intracranial tumours. *Archives of Disease in Childhood*, 63:495–500.

Louis J, Limirz LR, Best WR (1956). Treatment of chronic granulocytic leukemia with myeleran. *Archives of Internal Medicine*, 97:299–308.

Ludgwig Breast Cancer Study Group (1985*a*). Adjuvant chemotherapy (CMF) with or without low dose prednisolone (P) in premenopausal patients (PTS) with metastases in one to three axilliary lymph nodes. *Cancer Research*, 45:4454–9.

Ludwig Breast Cancer Study Group (1985*b*). Chemotherapy with or without oophorectomy in high risk premenopausal patients with operable breast cancer. *Journal of Clinical Oncology*, 3:1059–67.

Lynch JH, Maxted WC (1983). Use of ephedrine in post lymphadenectomy ejaculatory failure: a case report. *Journal of Urology*, 129:379.

Mahadevan MM, Trounson AO, Leeton JF (1983). Successful use of human semen cryobanking for *in vitro* fertilisation. *Fertility and Sterility*, 40:340–3.

Mancini RE, *et al.* (1966). Effect of prednisolone upon normal and pathologic human spermatogenesis. *Fertility and Sterility*, 17:500–13.

Marmor D, Elefant E, Dauchez C, Rouk C (1986). Semen analysis in Hodgkin's disease before the onset of treatment. *Cancer*, 57:1986–7.

Meistrich ML, *et al.* (1982). Damaging effects of 14 chemotherapeutic drugs on mouse testis cells. *Cancer Research*, 42:122–31.

Miller JJ, Williams GF, Leissring JC (1971). Multiple late complications of therapy with cyclophosphamide including ovarian destruction. *American Journal of Medicine*, 50:530–5.

Morley JE (1986). Impotence. *American Journal of Medicine*, 80:897–905.

Narayan P, Lange PH, Fraley EE (1982). Ejaculation and fertility after extended retroperitoneal lymph node dissection for testicular cancer. *Journal of Urology*, 127:685–8.

Navot D, *et al.* (1986). Artificially induced endometrial cycles and establishment of pregnancies in the absence of ovaries. *New England Journal of Medicine*, 314:806–11.

Nelson RP (1988). Non-operative management of impotence. *Journal of Urology*, 139:2–6.

Nijman JM, *et al.* (1982). The treatment of ejaculation disorders after retroperitoneal lymph node dissection. *Cancer*, 50:2967–71.

Padmanabhan N, Wang DY, Moore JW, Rubens RD (1987). Ovarian function and adjuvant chemotherapy for early breast cancer. *European Journal of Cancer and Clinical Oncology*, 23:745–8.

Parra A, *et al.* (1978). Plasma gonadotrophins and gonadal steroids in children treated with cyclophosphamide. *Journal of Pediatrics*, 92:117–24.

Pektasides D, *et al.* (1987). Fertility after chemotherapy for ovarian germ cell tumours. *British Journal of Obstetrics and Gynaecology*, 94:477–9.

Pennisi AJ, Grushkin CN, Lieberman E (1975). Gonadal function in children with nephrosis treated with cyclophosphamide. *American Journal of Diseases of Children*, **129**:315–18.

Penso J, Lippe B, Ehrlich R, Smith FG (1974). Testicular function in prepubertal and pubertal male patients treated with cyclophosphamide for nephrotic syndrome. *Journal of Pediatrics*, **84**:831–6.

Pizzocaro G, Salvinoi R, Zanoni F (1985). Unilateral lymphadenectomy in intra-operative stage I non-seminomatous germinal testis cancer. *Journal of Urology*, **134**:485–9.

Rapola J, *et al.* (1973). N. Cyclophosphamide and the prepubertal testis. *Lancet*, i:98–9.

Ravolin RG, *et al.* (1970). Results of a clinical trial concerning the work of prophylactic oophorectomy for breast carcinoma. *Surgery, Gynecology and Obstetrics*, **131**:1055–64.

Redman JR, *et al.* (1987). Semen cryopreservation and artificial insemination for Hodgkin's disease. *Journal of Clinical Oncology*, **5**(2):233–8.

Richter P, *et al.* (1970). Effects of chlorambucil on spermatogenesis in the human with malignant lymphomas. *Cancer*, **25**:1026–30.

Richter VP, Buchholz K, Lotze W (1987). Schwangerschaftsverlauf und Geburt nach zytostatischer Behandlung von Throphoblasttumoren. *Zentralblatt für Gynäkologie*, **109**:586–9 (English abstract).

Rieser C (1961). The etiology of retrograde ejaculation and a method for insemination. *Fertility and Sterility*, **12**:488–92.

Rose DP, Davies TE (1980). Effects of adjuvant chemohormonal therapy on the ovarian and adrenal function of breast cancer patients. *Cancer Research*, **40**:4043–7.

Rosenshein NB, Grumbine SC, Woodruff JD, Ettinger DS (1979). Pregnancy following chemotherapy for an ovarian immature embryo or teratoma. *Gynecologic Oncology*, **8**:234–9.

Roth BJ, Ironhorn LH, Greist A (1988). Long term complications of cisplatin based chemotherapy for testis cancer. *Seminars in Oncology*, **5**(4):345–50.

Rowland GF, Cohen J, Steptoe PL, Hewitt J (1985). Pregnancy following *in vitro* fertilisation using cryopreserved semen from a man with testicular teratoma. *Urology*, **26**:33–6.

Rustin GJF, *et al.* (1987). Fertility after chemotherapy for male and female germ cell tumours. *International Journal of Andrology*, **10**:389–92.

Sanders JE, *et al.* (1988). Ovarian function following marrow transplantation for aplastic anemia or leukemia. *Journal of Clinical Oncology*, **6**:813–18.

Sanger WG, Armitage JO, Schmidt MA (1980). Feasibility of semen cryopreservation in patients with malignant disease. *Journal of the American Medical Association*, **244**:789–90.

Sauer MV, *et al.* (1987). Pregnancy following non-surgical donor ovum transferred to a functionally agonadal woman. *Fertility and Sterility*, **48**:324–5.

Scammell GE, Stedronska J, Dempsey A (1982). Successful pregnancies using human serum albumin following retrograde ejaculation. A case report. *Fertility and Sterility*, **37**:277–9.

Scammell GE, *et al.* (1985). Cryopreservation of semen in men with testicular tumour or Hodgkin's disease: results of artificial insemination of their partners. *Lancet*, ii:31–2.

Schilsky RL, *et al.* (1987). Gonadal and sexual function in male patients with hairy cell leukemia: lack of adverse effects of recombinant alpha 2-interferon treatment. *Cancer Treatment Reports*, **71**:179–81.

Schwartz PE, Vidone RA (1981). Pregnancy following combination chemotherapy for a mixed germ cell tumour of the ovary. *Gynecologic Oncology*, **12**:373–8.

Selby P, *et al.* (1988). Semen cryopreservation for patients surviving malignant disease: implications of proposed legislation. *Lancet*, ii:1197.

Shalet SM, *et al.* (1977). Endocrine function following the treatment of acute leukemia in childhood. *Journal of Pediatrics*, **90**:920–3.

Shalet SM, *et al.* (1981). Testicular function after combination chemotherapy in childhood for acute lymphoblastic leukaemia. *Archives of Disease in Childhood*, **56**:275–8.

Shamberger RC, Rosenberg SA, Seipp CA, Sherins RJ (1981a). Effects of high dose methotrexate and vincristine on ovarian and testicular functions in patients undergoing post-operative adjuvant treatment of osteosarcoma. *Cancer Treatment Reports*, **65**(9–11):739–46.

Shamberger RC, *et al.* (1981b). Effects of post-operative adjuvant chemotherapy and radiotherapy on ovarian functioning in women undergoing treatment for soft tissue sarcoma. *Journal of the National Cancer Institute*, **67**(6):1213–18.

Sherins RJ, Olweny CLM, Ziegler JL (1978). Gynecomastia and gonadal dysfunction in adolescent boys treated with combination chemotherapy for Hodgkin's disease. *New England Journal of Medicine*, **299**:12–16.

Siris ES, Leventhal BG, Vaitukaitis JL (1976). Effects of childhood leukemia and chemotherapy on puberty and reproductive function in girls. *New England Journal of Medicine*, **294**:1143–6.

Sobrinho LG, Levine RA, De Conti RC (1971). Amenorrhea in patients with Hodgkin's disease treated with anti-neoplastic agents. *American Journal of Obstetrics and Gynecology*, **109**:135–9.

Spitz S (1948). The histological effects of nitrogen mustards on human tumors and tissues. *Cancer*, **1**:383–98.

Stockamp K, Schreifer F, Altwein J (1974). Alpha adrenergic drugs in retrograde ejaculation. *Fertility and Sterility*, **25**:817–20.

Stricker S, Crosby K, Carey RW (1981). Paternity after chemotherapy induced sterility in Hodgkin's disease. *New England Journal of Medicine*, **304**:1175.

Tengrup I, Nitby LT, Landberg T (1986). Prophylactic oophorectomy in the treatment of carcinoma of the breast. *Surgery, Gynecology and Obstetrics*, **162**:209–14.

Uldall PR, Kerr DNS, Tacchi D (1972). Amenorrhoea and sterility. *Lancet*, i:693–4.

Van Thiel DH, Ross GT, Lipsett MB (1970). Pregnancies after chemotherapy of trophoblastic neoplasms. *Science*, **169**:1326–7.

Virag R (1982). Intracavernous injection of papaverine for erectile failure. *Lancet*, ii:938.

Viviani S, *et al.* (1985). Gonadal toxicity after combination chemotherapy for Hodgkin's disease. Comparative results of MOPP versus ABVD. *British Journal of Cancer and Clinical Oncology*, **21**:601–3.

von der Maase H, *et al.* (1986). Carcinoma *in situ* of contralateral testis in patients with testicular germ cell cancer: study of 27 cases in 500 patients. *British Medical Journal*, **293**:1398–1401.

Walsh PC, Donker PJ (1980). Impotence following radical prostatectomy. Insight into etiology and prevention. *Journal of Urology*, **128**:492–7.

Ward BG, Harvey VJ, Shepherd JH (1982). Pregnancy after treatment of endodermal sinus tumour. Case report with 5 years survival. *British Journal of Obstetrics and Gynaecology*, **89**:769–70.

Warne GL, Fairley KF, Hobbs JB, Martin FIR (1973). Cyclophosphamide induced ovarian failure. *New England Journal of Medicine*, **289**:1159–62.

Watson AR, Rance CP, Bain J (1985). Long term effects of cyclophosphamide on testicular function. *British Medical Journal*, **291**:1457–60.

Waxman J (1987). Preserving fertility in Hodgkin's disease. *Baillière's Clinical Haematology*, **1**(1):185–90.

Waxman JHX, *et al.* (1982). Gonadal function in Hodgkin's disease: long term follow up of chemotherapy. *British Medical Journal*, **285**:1612–13.

Waxman JH, Terry YA, Rees LH, Lister TA (1983). Gonadal function in men treated for acute leukaemia. *British Medical Journal*, **287**:1093–4.

Waxman JH, *et al.* (1987a). Failure to preserve fertility in patients with Hodgkin's disease. *Cancer Chemotherapy and Pharmacology*, **19**:159–62.

Waxman J, *et al.* (1987b). The effects of a gonadotrophin-releasing hormone agonist on testicular histology. *Fertility and Sterility*, **48**(6):1067–9.

Weinblatt ME (1985). Toxicity of low dose methotrexate in rheumatoid arthritis. *Journal of Rheumatology*, **12** (Suppl. 12):35–9.

Weissbach L, Vahlensieck W, Fitte M, Grauthoff H (1980). Diagnostik bei Hodentumoren. *Urologe (Ausg. B)*, **20**:106.

Whitehead E, *et al.* (1982). Gonadal function after combination chemotherapy for Hodgkin's disease in childhood. *Archives of Disease in Childhood*, **47**:287–91.

Whitehead E, *et al.* (1983). The effect of combination chemotherapy on ovarian function in women treated for Hodgkin's disease. *Cancer*, **52**:998–93.

Yew CC, Chan SYW, Wong LC, Ho K (1985). Ovarian dysfunction in patients with gestational trophoblastic neoplasia treated with short intensive courses of etoposide. *Cancer*, **55**:2348–52.

19.11 The teratogenic effect of cancer treatment

YVONNE D. SENTURIA

INTRODUCTION

More effective chemotherapeutic regimens and improvements in supportive therapy for children with acute leukaemia and Wilms' tumour and for adolescents and young adults with choriocarcinoma, Hodgkin's disease, chronic myelogenous leukaemia, and testicular teratoma have led to increased survival rates. In many cases permanent sterility may be an outcome of treatment. However, in other cases reproductive capacity may be restored. It then becomes relevant, in a population of young people wishing to have their own families, to determine whether there is any long-term damage to gonadal tissue. It is of prime importance to this population that an accurate assessment be made of the impact of treatment with cytotoxic agents on subsequent offspring. While the production of fetal abnormalities through effects exerted after conception (terato-genesis) is the primary subject of this chapter, information concerning exposures prior to conception (mutagenesis) is increasingly becoming available.

While in some cases it may be possible to delay treatment of the pregnant cancer patient until completion of pregnancy, in other cases this is neither feasible or desirable. Advising patients whether to continue or terminate pregnancy during cancer chemotherapy must be based on all available information, as should the recommendations made to young men and women contemplating starting a family after surviving cancer treatment.

TERATOGENESIS

Dorland's Illustrated medical dictionary defines a teratogen as 'an agent or factor that causes the production of physical defects in the develop-ing embryo'. Cytotoxic agents are most likely to affect the developing fetus during the first trimester in the period of organ differentiation. However, within this framework there are differences in the timing and degree of susceptibility of various fetal organs to cytotoxic agents. The teratogenic potential of a particular drug is then related to how well it crosses the placenta, the dose and duration of treatment, the route of administration, and the stage of pregnancy during which treatment occurs. In most cases current treatment regimes involve administration of more than one agent, either sequentially or in combination. This decreases the likelihood of being able to implicate a single drug as the causative agent for any ensuing defects. Although the bulk of experience in this field has been with animal models, there are further problems with extrapolating from this experience. The human embryo appears to be less susceptible to damage and the timing of injury seems to differ when human experience is compared with animal models (Sokal and Lessmann 1960).

EFFECT OF EXPOSURE TO THERAPEUTIC AGENTS DURING PREGNANCY: ANIMAL MODELS AND CASE REPORTS IN HUMANS

Busulfan

Treatment of rat fetuses on days 12 and 13 of gestation led to numerous abnormalities: cleft palate, digital defects, ovarian dysgenesis, and destruction of seminiferous tubules.

Nine out of 13 cases involving treatment for chronic leukaemia included therapy in the first trimester (Sieber and Adamson 1975). One infant died at 1 month with pulmonary atelectasis and a second, whose mother was treated with 6-mercaptopurine at 1 month, busulfan at 2–8 months, 6-mercaptopurine at 9 months, and 2 Gy died at 10 weeks with multiple anomalies including microphthalmia, corneal opacities, and cleft palate.

Chlorambucil

Defects of the central nervous system, skeleton, and palate were noted after exposure of the rat fetus on days 11–12 of gestation.

There has been a report of unilateral absence of ureter and kidney in a fetus after chlorambucil treatment and radiation for Hodgkin's disease at 5–11 weeks (Shotton and Monie 1963) and two normal births after treatment at 4.5 and 7 months.

Cyclophosphamide

Cleft lip/cleft palate, reduction defects of the extremities and encephalocele/exencephaly have been noted in the rat, mouse, rabbit, and rhesus monkey. The organ system affected in the rhesus monkey differed based on the timing of the insult, whereas days 11–13 seemed the period of greatest toxicity for the rat, mouse, and rabbit models. Hydrocephalus and micrognathia were observed in the offspring of male rats treated at 7–9 weeks, along with a dose-dependent increase in fetal wastage (Trasler 1985).

Cyclophosphamide has been shown to have a higher fetal to maternal toxicity ratio than chlorambucil. A woman who conceived and delivered a normal female after radiation for Hodgkin's disease subsequently became pregnant while being treated with cyclo-phosphamide for a relapse. Treatment was received throughout gestation, with the highest dosage (27–28 mg/kg) during weeks 7–8. Since this is the period of differentiation of the limb buds, the presence of multiple anomalies, including absent toes, hypoplastic fifth finger, and flattening of the nasal bridge, was believed to be consistent with damage secondary to cyclophosphamide treatment (Greenberg and Tanaka 1964).

5-Fluorouracil

This pyrimidine analogue interferes with RNA and DNA synthesis. Exposure on days 11–12 results in defects of the palate, skeleton, and central nervous system in the rat and mouse.

Radial aplasia, imperforate anus, oesophageal aplasia, and hypoplasia of the duodenum, lung, and aorta were noted after a pregnant woman received 600 mg of 5-fluorouracil five times weekly at 11–12 weeks' gestation (Stephens *et al.* 1980).

6-Mercaptopurine

This purine analogue produced defects of the tail and extremities when rat fetuses were exposed on days 11–12.

Sixteen women treated during pregnancy produced offspring without evidence of congenital malformations, although one of four babies born after treatment in the first trimester died in the neonatal period of problems related to prematurity (Sieber and Adamson 1975).

Methotrexate

Normal offspring have been reported following exposure of rabbits and rats to low doses, while 25–50 mg/kg produced exencephaly, omphalocele, ectrodactyly, and cleft palate in the mouse.

This folic acid antagonist is a methyl derivative of aminopterin. Absence of the frontal bones, premature craniosynostosis, rib defects, and absence of digits were reported after a regime of 2.5 mg daily for 5 days at 8–10 weeks gestation (Milunsky et al. 1968). Two women treated for leukaemia with methotrexate and 6-mercaptopurine after the first trimester produced normal offspring (Sokal and Lessmann 1960).

Nitrogen mustard

Exposure of the rat on days 11–12 of gestation has been reported to result in exencephaly, encephalocele, skeletal defects, and cleft palate.

Two women treated for Hodgkin's disease with this alkylating agent in the first month and two treated at 4–5 months produced offspring without malformations (Sokal and Lessmann 1960).

Procarbazine

Treatment between days 8 and 12 in the rat produced eye defects, whereas treatment between days 12 and 14 produced limb defects.

A woman treated with this hydrazine for the first 38 days delivered a normal male infant (Wells et al. 1968), while another woman who received 100 mg daily on days 28–35 of gestation (and a single dose of nitrogen mustard and vincristine on day 28) had a fetus with small pelvic kidneys. A normal newborn was delivered after treatment in the first two trimesters (Shepard 1986).

Vincristine and vinblastine

Teratogenic effects, including microcephaly, neural tube closure defects, eye defects, and skeletal defects, have been demonstrated in the rat, rabbit, monkey, and hamster after treatment during pregnancy with these vinca alkaloids.

Four women produced normal infants after treatment during pregnancy for Hodgkin's disease, even though two began treatment in the first trimester (Sieber and Adamson 1975).

Radiation

X-irradiation during pregnancy has a documented ability to damage the fetal central nervous system, with microcephaly and mental retardation as outcomes (Brent 1980).

Russell (1950), using radiation doses of 1–4 Gy, found the timing of exposure of mice determined the target organ for the teratogenic effect. As would be expected, when the mouse was irradiated before implantation, the effect was extreme: either embryonic demise or no evident abnormality. A continuum, in relation to gestational age at time of treatment, resulted in microphthalmia and coloboma (days 7.5–9.5), renal abnormalities (day 9.5), or skeletal malformations (days 9.5–12.5).

The incidences of embryonic death (spontaneous abortion), microcephaly, and mental retardation following irradiation of the fetus seem to have a dose–response effect. The timing of exposure

is also important, with mental retardation most prevalent when exposure had occurred 8–15 weeks post-fertilization. Most investigators have failed to see an increase in congenital malformations in the offspring of male and female radiologists. However, there is controversy over whether irradiation during pregnancy results in an increased incidence of Down's syndrome, although the bulk of evidence suggests maternal exposure as a risk factor.

Summary

Few malformations have been reported after single-agent treatment in humans. Severe malformations after chemotherapy without radiotherapy have been associated with cyclophosphamide, 5-fluorouracil, and methotrexate, although normal offspring have been reported when methotrexate was given after the first trimester of pregnancy. It is difficult to implicate busulfan or chlorambucil definitively as causative agents as therapy in cited cases included irradiation in addition to chemotherapy. The abnormalities seen after procarbazine were mild.

Problems arise with attempts to draw any conclusions from the clinical case reports presented. Anecdotal findings may be the result of case selection or may actually represent genetic effects of cancer or cancer treatment. Case ascertainment is unlikely to be systematic; it would be difficult to ensure that children with malformations were not more likely to be reported in the literature than children with no abnormal findings on examination. With case reports there is also the problem of the absence of a denominator or base population to use as a reference for establishing the frequency with which certain abnormalities occur.

PREGNANCY OUTCOME AFTER CANCER TREATMENT

Hodgkin's disease

Women with Hodgkin's disease are likely to have received courses of chemotherapy lasting for a period longer than 6 months and concomitant radiation damage to the ovaries increases the likelihood of ovarian failure. Thus, impaired fertility is the major effect of treatment for Hodgkin's disease. However, there are some women who do conceive after treatment or whose treatment has occurred during an existing pregnancy.

Retrospective review: treatment 1944–1975 (Holmes and Holmes 1978)

The study population included 29 women who became pregnant after beginning treatment and 19 men who fathered children following treatment. They were located from record review and contact with patients or families of those 'who could have produced offspring after diagnosis of Hodgkin's disease'. Sixty-nine of the 77 siblings were located and served, with their offspring, as controls. Information was obtained from the study population or their families regarding pregnancies and their outcome.

There was no difference in the proportion of abnormalities noted when comparing children born to patients (8/84 abnormal) and children born to controls (26/209 abnormal). From the information available, the patients had fewer pregnancies (1.93 compared with 3.3 for controls) and fewer term/near-term deliveries (1.7 compared with 3 for controls). This decreased exposure would tend to make their pregnancy experience more favourable and perhaps mask any increased risk. Choosing the first child conceived after treatment, matched to the most age-appropriate control child, would be an alternative analytic approach to address this.

The study period involved various radiotherapeutic techniques and chemotherapy regimes. It was not feasible, with the size and heterogeneity of the study population, to subdivide the analysis by type of chemotherapy received.

All children were conceived at least 1 year post-treatment. The problems noted in the offspring of patients ranged from stillbirth (two), absent Fallopian tube, and rectal stenosis, to amblyopia, autism, learning difficulties, and scleroderma. Five of these children were born to women who had been treated with irradiation and chemotherapy.

It is difficult to generalize from the results of this study. Although for a subgroup of women treated with irradiation and chemotherapy there seemed to be a relationship between type of treatment and presence of malformations in offspring, this did not hold for the larger group nor for the wives of men treated with irradiation and chemotherapy.

Retrospective survey: treatment 1968–1979 (Horning et al. 1981)

In this survey 103 out of 129 women successfully treated for Hodgkin's disease responded to a postal questionnaire about their reproductive function pre- and post-treatment. The median age at time of treatment was 23 years, with a median of 64 months having elapsed from the end of treatment to completion of the questionnaire. Almost all the 84 patients treated with chemotherapy (75) received nitrogen mustard, vincristine, and prednisolone (MOP) or nitrogen mustard, vincristine, prednisolone, and procarbazine (MOPP) and the majority (50/84) received adjuvant irradiation. It is noteworthy that outcome of post-treatment pregnancies was verified by record review, personal interview, and/or contact with physicians, although it is not stated whether any children were specifically examined with a view to excluding the presence of congenital malformations.

Of the 34 women who resumed normal menses and did not use birth control, 20 conceived. There were nine births after irradiation, seven after chemotherapy, and eight after combined treatment. No congenital malformations have been seen in these children, whose median age is 2.3 years (range 1 month–7.5 years).

Retrospective survey (McKeen et al. 1979)

Thirty-seven women treated for Hodgkin's disease who had conceived or were pregnant at or after diagnosis were identified from a survey of oncologists and questioned about their reproductive history. Five of the 10 women treated with chemotherapy during the first trimester had pregnancy terminations, one had a spontaneous abortion, and two had normal term infants. There were two children with congenital malformations: cleft palate and hydrocephalus. The two women who received chemotherapy after the first trimester had normal offspring. A child born after first-trimester radiotherapy had hearing loss and the offspring of a patient given radiotherapy in the second trimester was educationally subnormal.

When conception occurred after treatment, 23 out of 34 live births were normal children born at term, six were premature, and three had significant malformations (hydrocephalus, tracheomalacia, and dark hairy naevus). There were no malformations noted in two stillbirths. The proportion of live births with major malformations was higher in women treated during pregnancy (2/9 compared with 3/34 of those who conceived after treatment). A large sample size and knowledge of maternal characteristics, such as age and parity, would be useful before attempting to generalize from these results.

Case reports of normal children following MOPP

A 27 year old woman became pregnant 1 month after completing chemotherapy for stage IIIB disease and received a booster dose of MOPP in the second month. Premature delivery (24 weeks) of a male with minor skeletal malformations (absence of two toes and some webbing) resulted. However, ten other women are reported to have conceived and delivered 'normal children' after MOPP therapy (Garrett 1973). Two other women, treated with radiotherapy and 6–15 courses of MOPP, conceived and delivered offspring without abnormalities more than 2 years after cessation of chemotherapy (Johnson et al. 1979).

Summary

Interpretation of the findings from the above studies is difficult. Some cases represented gonadal exposure to radiation therapy and/or cytotoxic chemotherapy, whereas others represented preconception exposure; some subjects were women and some were the wives of treated men. The diversity of the study groups was increased further by the heterogeneity of the treatment regimes and drug dosages employed. The number of subjects was small enough to decrease further the likelihood of being able to document a statistically significant positive association. Larger populations of patients who have received similar treatment with uniform surveillance over an extensive time period would probably be necessary to determine a specific effect.

Gestational trophoblastic tumours

Chemotherapeutic regimes have been increasingly successful in treatment of gestational trophoblastic tumours, with a proportion of these women going on to subsequent conceptions. Analysis of the results of these pregnancies is relevant to consideration of these chemotherapeutic agents as possible mutagens.

Retrospective review: treatment 1956–1973 (Van Thiel et al. 1970; Ross 1976)

Fifty-eight women reported 96 conceptions at least 1 year after treatment with various single and combination agent regimes. Of 78 live births, congenital malformations were noted in three: Pendred syndrome (goitre and congenital deafness), tetralogy of Fallot, and a child with haemangiomata, eczema, and strabismus. One of three stillbirths had multiple malformations, but the other two were reported to have no apparent abnormalities by the physician who managed the pregnancy.

Maternal age, maternal parity, and the chemotherapeutic agents and dosage received in individual cases resulting in offspring with congenital malformations are not delineated. It is therefore difficult to make any specific associations between the malformed offspring and particular treatments. There was no correlation between methotrexate dose and the proportion of conceptions resulting in spontaneous abortion or stillbirth. Ross (1976) found no increase in congenital malformations on comparing his sample with Swedish population data.

The agents most commonly used to treat gestational trophoblastic neoplasms (methotrexate and actinomycin D) are most likely to exert their effect on cells undergoing DNA synthesis. Therefore it is possible that by instituting a waiting period of 1 year following treatment before attempted conception, wastage of the more mature ova which might have been damaged by chemotherapy will have been accomplished and subsequent conceptions will involve genetic material unaffected by the previous cancer therapy.

Chromosomal analyses (Cohen et al. 1971)

Review of chromosomes of five mother–child pairs and one additional child revealed an increase in chromosomal breaks in the offspring compared with their mothers. All analyses were performed post-treatment. It is unclear how the subjects were recruited or what quantitative measures were used to compare the groups with reference to chromosomal breaks. With the small sample used, it would be difficult to demonstrate a statistically significant difference.

These results add to the feeling that even if defective ova are produced following chemotherapy, they are not often utilized in the production of viable offspring, which would explain the demonstrated teratogenic effect of various agents in animal models while treatment of human subjects can result in normal births.

Treatment with etoposide: 1977–1984 (Adewole et al. 1986)

This potent antineoplastic has been used with hydroxyurea, 6-mercaptopurine, actinomycin D, methotrexate, vincristine, and cyclophosphamide in medium- and high-risk regimes. Fifty-seven out of 66 treated women who wished to conceive post-treatment delivered 78 live-born infants and one stillbirth, with 11 spontaneous abortions and seven elective pregnancy terminations in the same reference population. The only congenital malformation noted was microcephaly in a child suspected of having congenital cytomegalovirus infection, although there is no information on whether laboratory confirmation of this presumptive diagnosis was achieved. This series militates against a significant mutagenic effect for etoposide, at least in the first generation.

Retrospective review: treatment 1958–1978 (Rustin et al. 1984)

One hundred and eighty-seven women delivered 275 liveborn infants and eight stillbirths. Two of the stillborn infants were anencephalic, five were premature (gestational ages less than 34 weeks), and one death was secondary to uterine rupture. Two of the liveborn infants died in the neonatal period, presumably from problems related to their prematurity (gestational age 32 weeks). Five other liveborn infants were noted to have congenital malformations: tetralogy of Fallot, spina bifida, talipes equinovarus, 'collapsed lung', and umbilical hernia. This did not represent a statistically significant increase over official estimates for population rates of congenital malformations in England and Wales. When three mothers of children who developed desquamative fibrosing alveolitis, mental retardation, and neonatal tachycardia were added to the mothers of the five liveborn and two stillborn children with congenital malformations, there were no statistically significant differences in age, time from completion of treatment to conception, drugs used, or dosage when compared with the other 177 mothers.

Thirty-two of the 187 women had conceived less than 1 year after completing treatment. These conceptions resulted in 31 live births, one of the two anencephalic stillbirths, and seven spontaneous abortions. In the overall sample of 217 women who wished to conceive, 23 had pregnancies which always ended either in stillbirth or spontaneous abortion. The proportion of non-viable pregnancies reported in the first year after treatment (8/39) was higher than in the overall sample over the total period of follow-up (23/217). This is consistent with an increase in prevalence of damaged ova in this early period after treatment.

Methotrexate was part of the therapeutic regime in all the women in this series and those who were prescribed a multidrug regime tended to receive the different drugs in sequence rather than as simultaneously administered combination chemotherapy. Rustin et al. (1984) believe that this timing may be relevant to the preservation of fertility.

Long-term follow-up: treatment 1959–1980 (Song et al. 1988)

In this study 303 out of 355 pregnancies to 205 women after treatment resulted in live births. Three of these 303 offspring had congenital malformations (anencaphaly, hydrocephalus, and congenital heart disease (type unspecified)) and 20 were premature. No malformations were noted in the two second-trimester intrauterine deaths nor in the three stillbirths (prolapsed umbilical cord, placenta previa, and post-term asphyxia). Comparisons were made with population data and no increase was found in the incidence of fetal wastage (23 spontaneous abortions, two ectopic pregnancies, two intra-uterine deaths, and three stillbirths), prematurity, or congenital malformation. Cytogenetic studies performed on the peripheral lymphocytes of 94 children showed 'no significant abnormalities'.

All the mothers had been followed for at least 5 years post-treatment, with 40 women having 20 years of observation after treatment. Children were seen regularly for follow-up, with 80 per cent of the 295 living children over 5 years of age when last examined. Therefore, this well-conducted follow-up study suggests that there is no evidence for a mutagenic effect in the first generation of offspring. However, further observation of subsequent generations would provide more definitive information on this subject.

Summary

With excellent survival rates with current treatment and reasonable resumption of fertility with many of the chemotherapeutic regimes, the outlook is good for child-bearing after successful treatment of gestational trophoblastic tumours. Theoretical considerations, together with the data of Rustin et al. (1984), support continuing to counsel avoidance of pregnancy for the first year after completion of treatment as the incidence of fetal wastage seems to be higher during this time and the risk of fertilization of a damaged ova may also be increased. A significant mutagenic effect in the population of women conceiving over a year after treatment for this tumour has not yet been proved. However, with changes in chemotherapeutic regimes over time and the utilization of more potent treatments, it is difficult to extrapolate from past studies and more data are definitely needed.

Childhood cancer patients: is there any mutagenic effect demonstrable in their offspring?

Retrospective review: 5 year survivors diagnosed under age 18 (Li et al. 1979)

The median age of the reference population was 30 years, with a median survival of 21 years. Each of the survivors was contacted by letter, telephone, or during a clinic visit to obtain information on any conceptions. Those who reported at least one pregnancy were asked for information as to parity, gravidity, and health of offspring. An attempt was made to confirm any reports of abnormalities by medical records, although it is unclear in what proportion this was successful. Medical records were not searched if no problems were reported, which could introduce bias in case ascertainment. The subjects also provided health information on their nieces and nephews for use as controls, leading to the possibility of differential ascertainment of abnormalities, thereby tending to exaggerate any difference between the two groups.

Eighty-four women and the wives of 62 men reported conceptions after treatment. Of 242 live births, the majority occurred after treatment for lymphoma (59 births to 34 patients), bone tumour (39 births to 20 patients), or brain tumour (30 births to 19 patients). Median survival after diagnosis was 21 years and 78 of the 242 offspring had reached the age of 10 years. The seven deaths to date included five children with congenital malformations: hereditary retinoblastoma, trisomy 18, and cardiac, brain, and multiple malformations. Four major malformations were noted among the 20 survivors with birth defects: Hirschsprung's disease, Marfan's syndrome, pyloric stenosis, and congenital deafness. The survival curve and the incidence of congenital malformations was compared with United States population data; no significant increase was seen. The method of data collection utilized for the controls could have tended to lead to under-reporting, thus exaggerating any real differences in the cases and controls. Therefore, the absence of a significant difference would tend to support there being no real difference, as suggested by comparison with population data.

Li et al. (1979) suggest that sterility may be the major genetic effect of cancer treatment in childhood and that damaged cancer cells are not viable and, thus, do not participate in subsequent successful fertilizations. Neither the number of malformed offspring born to women patients and to the wives of male patients, nor the gravidity, parity, or age of the women at time of conception are clear. It is also not clear whether any of the nine abnormal offspring were born to patients whose treatment included radiation.

Childhood leukemia treatment (Siris et al. 1976)

The hypothalamic–pituitary–ovarian axis was evaluated in a group of 35 girls, all of whom had been exposed to methotrexate, vincristine, mercaptopurine, and prednisolone in several protocols. One of the seven who was over 10 years of age but not yet pubertal at the time of leukaemia diagnosis and treatment became pregnant 7 years after completing treatment, with subsequent birth of a normal, term infant. One of the seven who was post-pubertal at the time of diagnosis became pregnant 3 years after completing treatment, with the subsequent birth of a normal term infant. Another in this post-pubertal group conceived twice while on maintenance chemotherapy and had voluntary terminations each time.

It is unclear how this group of 35 was assembled, so that the generalizability of this information is unknown, but it does represent anecdotal data on pregnancy outcome after childhood treatment with a common combination of agents.

Summary

It is difficult to generalize from the results of these two studies, particularly when the treatments for childhood cancers have changed since many of these individuals were treated.

Children fathered after treatment for testicular cancer

Testicular cancer is the most common malignancy in men aged 20–34 years in England and Wales. With modern chemotherapy, survival rates of over 90 per cent with metastatic non-seminomatous germ cell tumours and seminomas are to be expected. Both chemotherapy and radiotherapy give rise to azoospermia, indicating a profound effect on the germinal epithelium. At least two-thirds of men treated with platinum-based chemotherapy for testicular cancer recover spermatogenesis and can then go on to father children. Whether changes in the germinal epithelium result in viable but defective spermatozoa capable of fertilizing the ovum and producing abnormalities in the fetus is a question of concern.

Case-control study: treatment 1964–1986 (Senturia et al. 1985)

Children fathered by 27 testicular cancer patients treated with radiotherapy, 25 treated with chemotherapy, and 57 control men were examined for evidence of congenital malformations. These children represented the offspring of all men known to have fathered at least one live-born child after starting treatment for testicular tumour at one treatment centre. There were no statistically significant differences between the three groups in mother's age at birth of the index child, father's social class, or birth order of the first child born after treatment. When these index children were compared with the control children, there was no difference in the proportion with malformations.

In addition to the comparison of treated and control groups, the rates for specific malformations in the complete cohort of 40 children born after radiotherapy and 30 children born after chemotherapy were compared with known national rates. The observed rates were not statistically different from the national rates. There was also no difference in time from completion of treatment to birth of the index child between children with and without malformations.

When this study was expanded to include 131 children born to 107 men treated with chemotherapy in 25 centres in England and Wales (Senturia and Peckham 1990), again there was no evidence of an increased risk of malformations in the treatment group when compared with stage I patients treated with surveillance (controls) or with incidence rates for malformations in the general population. The following malformations were noted in the chemotherapy group: strabismus, cor biloculare, inguinal hernia (two), laryngomalacia, talipes and testicular maldescent, ventricular septal defect, total anomalous pulmonary venous drainage, sagittal synostosis, and kyphosis and marfanoid features. Cisplatin, vinblastine, and bleomycin were the most common agents involved in treatment, although different treatment regimes were utilized over the time period.

Although there was no evidence for an increase in malformations when the children fathered by radiotherapy patients or chemotherapy patients were compared with community or population controls, larger samples would be needed to eliminate a small increase in risk or to implicate particular chemotherapeutic agents or combinations.

Case reports: children fathered after treatment

Seventy-four men have been reported to have fathered 88 children after radiotherapy for testicular cancer. Their offspring are presumed to be normal, yet only Sandemann (1966) described the children as being free of malformations. Another centre recorded

11 established pregnancies after chemotherapy, six of whom were known to have resulted in the birth of a 'healthy child' (Drasga *et al.* 1983). Another centre reported three men to have 'fathered children' within 18 months of completion of chemotherapy but gave no details concerning the offspring (Lange 1983).

Summary

Based on available information, it does not appear that chemotherapy for testicular malignancy should be a reason for advising termination of pregnancy.

COUNSELLING: CANCER TREATMENT AND REPRODUCTIVE OUTCOME

Certain characteristics of person, place, and time are pertinent to the interpretation of possible risks after exposure to cancer treatment agents. Maternal age at conception and parity have a proven effect on pregnancy outcome. The disease for which the individual was treated, the treatment agents used, the dose and duration of treatment, and the stage of gestation during which treatment occurs or the time from completion of treatment to conception are important factors. Unfortunately, owing to considerations of sample size and heterogeneity of treatment regimes over time, quantitation of the influence of these factors is difficult.

In most cases single-agent treatments have been supplanted by multiple drug regimes, some in sequence and some simultaneously delivered. Whether radiation therapy is used alone or as an adjunct to chemotherapy and in what doses is known to affect outcome.

There is little doubt that radiation given in the first trimester is a potent teratogen, as are the alkylating agents. However, the major affect of cancer treatment is still probably a decrease in fertility, rather than an influence on the genetic material in those fertilized ova which are successfully carried to term. Pregnancies with exposure to cancer treatments present risks. However, in order to demonstrate the presence of new dominant mutations, it is necessary to be able to measure the teratogenesis/mutagenesis of particular agents. Since these are rare effects, it would be difficult to observe sufficient cases with specific malformations, particularly when those presumed most at risk (treatment during the first trimester) often undergo pregnancy termination. Voluntary terminations in each population studied and the difficulty of accurately counting spontaneous abortions also complicate the documentation of any significant increase in fetal wastage.

There are problems with illustrating an effect when dealing with a rare event. If a new teratogen or mutagen can affect only a proportion of the cases of a birth defect, the total incidence of the defect may not show any increase even though the incidence in the subgroup is greatly increased. Larger groups of subjects will need to be studied by pooling information from various treatment centres with careful classification of birth defects into aetiologically homogeneous subgroups.

It is possible that the paucity of demonstration of teratogenic effects arises from the fact that few pregnant women have received relatively large doses of chemotherapeutic agents during the first trimester. The teratogenic potential of alkylating agents and irradiation is clear. Reaching conclusions regarding mutagenesis is more difficult, as the absence of an effect in the first generation does not exclude some potential for harm. Valid denominators are needed, with sufficiently large groups to evaluate these probably rare effects. It is also difficult to make assessments of risk based on prior generations of treatment, when current treatments tend to be more intense with perhaps more toxicity to genetic material. There is always the possibility, raised by several investigators, that the ova and sperm which are able to participate in subsequent viable pregnancies have not been damaged. In the absence of more definitive information, precautions against administering any cytotoxic agent during the first trimester of pregnancy still seem prudent.

REFERENCES

Adewole LE, Rustin GJS, Newlands ES, Dent J, Bagashawe KD (1986). Fertility in patients with gestational trophoblastic tumors treated with etoposide. *European Journal of Cancer and Clinical Oncology*, 22:1479–82.

Brent RL (1980). Radiation teratogenesis. *Teratology*, 21:281–98.

Cohen MM, Gerbie AB, Nadler HL (1971). Chromosomal investigation in pregnancies following chemotherapy for choriocarcinoma. *Lancet*, i:219.

Drasga RE, Einhorn LH, Williams SD, Patel DN, Stevens EE (1983). Fertility after chemotherapy for testicular cancer. *Journal of Clinical Oncology*, 1(3):179–83.

Garrett MJ (1973). Teratogenic effects of combination chemotherapy. *Annals of Internal Medicine*, 80(5):667.

Greenberg LH, Tanaka KR (1964). Congenital anomalies probably induced by cyclophosphamide. *Journal of the American Medical Association*, 188(5):423–6.

Holmes GE, Holmes FF (1978). Pregnancy outcome of patients treated for Hodgkin's disease. *Cancer*, 41:1317–22.

Horning SJ, Hoppe RT, Kaplan HS, Rosenberg SA (1981). Female reproductive potential after treatment for Hodgkin's disease. *New England Journal of Medicine*, 304:1377–82.

Johnson SA, Goldman JM, Hawkins DF (1979). Pregnancy after chemotherapy for Hodgkin's disease. *Lancet*, ii:93.

Lange PH, Narayan P, Vogelzang NJ, Shafer RB, Kennedy BJ, Fraley EE (1983). Return of fertility after treatment for nonseminomatous testicular cancer: changing concepts. *Journal of Urology*, 129:1131–5.

Li FP, Fine W, Jaffe N, Holmes GE, Holmes FF (1979). Offspring of patients treated for cancer in childhood. *Journal of the National Cancer Institute*, 62(5):1193–7.

McKeen EA, Mulvihill JJ, Rosner F, Zarrabi MH (1979). Pregnancy outcome in Hodgkin's disease. *Lancet*, ii:590.

Milunsky A, Graef JW, Gaynor MF (1968). Methotrexate-induced congenital malformations with a review of the literature. *Journal of Pediatrics*, 72:790–5.

Ross GT (1976). Congenital anomalies among children born of mothers receiving chemotherapy for gestational trophoblastic neoplasms. *Cancer*, 37:1043–7.

Russell LB (1950). X-ray induced developmental abnormalities in the mouse and their use in the analysis of embryological patterns. *Journal of Experimental Zoology*, 114:545–602.

Rustin GJS, Booth M, Dent J, Salt S, Rustin F, Bagashawe KD (1984). Pregnancy after cytotoxic chemotherapy for gestational trophoblastic tumours. *British Medical Journal*, 288:103–6.

Sandeman TF (1966). The effects of X irradiation on male human fertility. *British Journal of Radiology*, 39:901–7.

Senturia YD, Peckham MJ (1990). Children fathered by men treated with chemotherapy for testicular cancer. *European Journal of Cancer*, 26(4):429–32.

Senturia YD, Peckham CS, Peckham MJ (1985). Children fathered by men treated for testicular cancer. *Lancet*, ii:766–9.

Shepard TH (ed.) (1986). *Catalog of teratogenic agents.* Johns Hopkins University Press, Baltimore.

Shotton D, Monie IW (1963). Possible teratogenic effect of chlorambucil on a human fetus. *Journal of the American Medical Association*, 186:74–5.

Sieber SM, Adamson RH (1975). Toxicity of antineoplastic agents in man: Chromosomal aberrations, antifertility effects, congenital malformations and carcinogenic potential. *Advances in Cancer Research*, 22:57–155.

Siris ES, Leventhal BG, Vaitukaitis JL (1976). Effects of childhood leukemia and chemotherapy on puberty and reproductive function in girls. *New England Journal of Medicine*, 294:1143–6.

Sokal JE, Lessmann EM (1960). Effects of cancer chemotherapeutic agents on the human fetus. *Journal of the American Medical Association*, 172:1765–71.

Song H, Wu P, Wang Y, Yang X, Dong S (1988). Pregnancy outcomes after successful chemotherapy for choriocarcinoma and invasive mole: long-term follow-up. *American Journal of Obstetrics and Gynecology*, **158**: 538–45.

Stephens TD, Golbus MS, Miller JR, Wilber RR, Epstein CJ (1980). Multiple congenital anomalies in a fetus exposed to 5-fluorouracil during the first trimester. *American Journal of Obstetrics and Gynecology*, **137**: 747–9.

Trasler JM, Hales BF, Robaiee P (1985). Paternal cyclophosphamide treatment of rats causes fetal loss and malformations without affecting male fertility. *Nature*, **316**:144–6.

Van Thiel DH, Ross GT, Lipsett MB (1970). Pregnancies after chemotherapy of trophoblastic neoplasms. *Science*, **169**:1326–7.

Wells JH, Marshall JR, Carbone PP (1968). Procarbazine therapy for Hodgkin's disease in early pregnancy. *Journal of the American Medical Association*, **205**:935–7.

19.12 Carcinogenic effects of cancer treatment

PINUCCI A. VALAGUSSA AND GIANNI BONADONNA

During the last quarter of a century, cancer treatment has undergone considerable development. Single-agent and multiple-drug chemotherapies, which were proved to be effective in the treatment of advanced tumours, have been adopted as an important part of the multidisciplinary approach to the management of a large number of malignancies. Modern cancer treatment has increased the duration of survival as well as the potential for cure of certain tumour types, but it has also increased the possibility of long-term complications including treatment-induced second malignancies.

Initial publications describing the carcinogenic effects of anticancer agents consisted of studies of laboratory animals or reports of single cases or small series of patients. Such observations emphasized the treatments administered and the risk of a second cancer with respect to a specific agent. Today, studies are available on large population bases from which a better assessment of the risk can be estimated using proper epidemiological and statistical methods. However, even when examining well-documented series of patients in which the agents utilized, doses, routes, time course of administration, and association with other treatment modalities are detailed, problems remain in positively relating the occurrence of second neoplasms to cancer treatment alone. The possibility of metabolic interactions when anticancer agents are delivered together with other drugs, previous or concomitant occupational or environmental exposure to other carcinogens, life-style, and other possible predisposing factors all remain confounding variables. Paradoxically, it is only when the primary treatment is successful that a discussion of late effects and second cancers is possible. Toxic treatments should be avoided, but not at the expense of decreasing the potential cure rate and without exploring all possible co-factors.

In this chapter we first summarize the data available on individual treatment modalities. However, it is important to emphasize that not all reports on the carcinogenic potential of either irradiation or chemotherapy clearly state whether only one modality was administered or whether a combination of both was delivered during the course of the disease. Studies of large population bases, (Hodgkin's disease, ovarian cancer, resectable breast cancer, and paediatric neoplasms) as well as host-related factors and methods for assessing the risk of second cancers are also discussed.

RADIATION CARCINOGENESIS

Ionizing radiation is perhaps the most extensively investigated carcinogen and epidemiological studies have been conducted on human populations exposed to many sources including natural background, nuclear weapons production and testing, uranium mining and milling, routine emissions from nuclear power plants, and medical practices (National Research Council 1980; Kohn and Fry 1984; Preston *et al.* 1987). Investigators have examined the types of tumours induced by radiation and the time for tumours to develop. In the case of medical irradiation, the effect of dosage and the modifying influence of dose rate, fractionation, and quality of radiation have also been evaluated. Experimental studies with animals and cell culture have led to inferences about carcinogenic mechanisms (Upton 1977) and models have been developed to suggest how the transfer of energy at the cellular level might induce malignant transformation (Kellerer and Rossi 1978). Despite this wealth of knowledge, there is considerable controversy concerning the magnitude of the biological effects of ionizing radiations, such as gamma rays, X-rays, or beta rays, which are of primary interest in medical practice.

The largest population studies on the carcinogenicity of ionizing radiation are of survivors of the atomic bomb explosions. Radiation exposure produced an increased absolute risk of death (excess death/10^6 person-year cGy) from leukaemia, multiple myeloma, and cancers of the lung, female breast, stomach, colon, oesophagus, and urinary tract. For the period 1950–1954, the absolute risk of leukaemia was 4.13, while the risk for all other cancers was 1.58 (Kato and Schull 1982). These data have recently been updated using newer statistical techniques (Preston *et al.* 1987). Significant dose responses were confirmed for the malignancies mentioned above. Owing to diagnostic difficulties, results for liver and ovarian cancers, while suggestive of significant dose responses, have not provided convincing evidence for radiogenic effects. No significant dose responses were seen for cancers of the gall bladder, prostate, rectum, pancreas, uterus, or for malignant lymphomas. Both excess and relative risks of leukaemia decreased between 1959 and 1982 (approximately 11 per cent/year) following the peak at

5–10 years; conversely, the excess relative risk for all other cancers increased at approximately 5 per cent/year during the same period (Preston *et al.* 1987). As will be discussed later, it is quite tempting to extrapolate from atomic bomb data to the clinical situation, but caution should be exercised, particularly for the different types of exposure and the different underlying conditions of the populations under study (Kohn and Fry 1984).

Data derived from populations exposed to medical irradiation at moderate to high levels for both malignant and non-malignant diseases have been reviewed in detail (Boice 1981). These data have contributed greatly to the estimation of radiation risks and to the development of models of radiation carcinogenesis. Some conclusions can be drawn from these studies. The dose–hazard relationship for radiation in humans cannot be stated with precision and dose–effect curves reflect complex radiation and biological interactions. In the lower dose range (hundreds of centigrays) the risk that a second cancer will develop seems to increase with dose, whereas this may not be true in the higher dose ranges used clinically (National Research Council 1980; Kohn and Fry 1984). There are two possible explanations for this phenomenon. First, the higher the dose, the more likely is oncogenesis, but this is counterbalanced by the greater probability of killing the involved cells. Second, the tissue damage which occurs after 'high' dosage often leads to fibrosis which may impede cellular development (Kohn and Fry 1984).

There is no unique radiogenic cancer and, unlike certain environmental neoplasms, radiation-induced tumours cannot be distinguished from naturally occurring cancer. The data suggest that the bone-marrow, thyroid, and breast appear particularly radio-sensitive, but also that cancer can be induced in other tissues under the appropriate conditions. The period of life in which radiogenic cancers appear tends to be similar to that during which naturally occurring cancers develop. Generally, the minimum latency period for solid tumours is approximately 10 years. However, it can vary for individuals in the population under investigation and generalizations concerning the different types of tumours cannot be made with certainty because of the incomplete lifetime follow-up of exposed populations. In contrast, excess incidence of leukaemia begins within 2–4 years, has a peak around 6–8 years, and decreases to normal levels approximately 25 years later (Boice 1981).

Age at exposure may influence the risk of radiogenic cancer. The developing evidence suggests that persons exposed at younger ages tend to be at greater risk than those exposed later, however, this may not be true for all types of cancers. As already mentioned, radiogenic cancers do not generally occur before the ages normally associated with the peak incidence of the equivalent naturally occurring cancer. Thus, the 'latent period' may simply reflect the age at exposure, with young people having longer latent periods than older persons before the excess cancers will be expressed.

CHEMOTHERAPY CARCINOGENESIS

The carcinogenic potential of antineoplastic drugs was first demonstrated experimentally in 1948 (Haddow *et al.* 1948). Since then, a considerable number of similar experimental investigations have been conducted and hundreds of chemical compounds have been evaluated (Weisburger *et al.* 1975; Sieber 1977; Schmähl and Habs 1978; Rieche 1984). Despite the fact that different experiments were carried out using different methods to answer different questions, some common features allow relatively convincing statements to be made. Of all antitumour drugs, a relatively strong carcinogenic action must be attributed to alkylating agents, nitrosourea derivatives, procarbazine, and dacarbazine. However, the carcinogenicity of the antimetabolites and antimitotic agents examined so far has produced contradictory results. Carcinogenic effects have been reported for antitumour antibiotics, androgen compounds, and oestrogen compounds. Obviously not all individual drugs bear the same carcinogenic potential, but comparative quantitative statements are difficult because of different daily doses, times of exposure, and animal species in which the substances were tested (Schmähl and Habs 1978).

So far, a positive correlation between administration of antineoplastic drugs and the subsequent occurrence of a second cancer in humans has been observed for only a few agents (Tomatis *et al.* 1978). However, as previously mentioned for ionizing radiations, long-term follow-up of patients successfully treated for their first cancer is mandatory to exclude entirely the potential carcinogenicity of anticancer drugs in humans.

The predominant malignancy reported to be associated with cancer chemotherapy has been acute non-lymphocytic leukaemia (Koeffler and Rowley 1985; Pedersen-Bjergaard 1985). As summarized in Table 1, chemotherapy with alkylating agents or nitrosoureas is the most frequent inducer of leukaemia. Whereas

Table 1 Actuarial risk of therapy-related acute non-lymphocytic leukaemia (data derived from representative studies reported in medical literature)

Primary disease	Actuarial risk		Agents considered responsible
	Per cent	Years	
Polycythemia vera	>20	8	Chlorambucil
Multiple myeloma	10–17	10	Melphalan, carmustine, cyclophosphamide
Hodgkin's disease	6–8	10	Nitrogen mustard, procarbazine±radiotherapy
Non-Hodgkin's lymphomas	5–10	10	Total body irradiation+alkylating agents
Ovarian cancer	7.6	5	Dihydroxybusulfan±radiotherapy
	9.6	7	Melphalan, chlorambucil, cyclophosphamide±radiotherapy
Breast cancer	1.3	10	Melphalan
Lung cancer	5.8	5	Busulphan
Gastrointestinal cancer	4	6	Nitrosourea derivatives

acute non-lymphocytic leukaemia may be part of the natural history of polycythemia vera, no other malignancy has so far been shown to predispose to this type of leukaemia. The median latency period for the development of this second malignancy has been estimated as approximately 3–4 years from the start of primary treatment, with possible minimal variations according to the type of first cancer and the cumulative risk has been reported to increase almost constantly up to at least 8–10 years. Secondary leukaemia, frequently called therapy-related leukaemia because the patients had previously received radiotherapy and/or chemotherapy for a primary disease, is considered the most serious long-term complication of current cancer therapy. Thus, extensive investigations have been undertaken and a few conclusions can be drawn from these data. Therapy-related leukaemia is a recognizable syndrome with the acute non-lymphocytic leukaemia having a pre-leukaemic phase beginning several years after the delivery of antineoplastic agents, a distinct chromosomal abnormality in the pre-leukaemic and leukaemic cells, and usually a very short survival after the development of leukaemia (Koeffler and Rowley 1985). The occurrence of unexplained pancytopenia and the loss of part or all of chromosomes 5 and/or 7 in the bone-marrow cells of previously treated patients is almost pathognomonic of pre-leukaemia which occurs in approximately 70 per cent of such cases. Progression to overt leukaemia may be universal if the patient survives the complication of haemorrhage or infection.

Various theories have been proposed to explain leukaemias developing in cancer patients. It has been claimed that certain diseases have an intrinsic predisposition to leukaemic transformation, but before the era of aggressive therapy patients did not live long enough to develop leukaemias. However, several reports from 1931 to 1970 suggest that no patients with Hodgkin's disease developed acute leukaemia if no radiotherapy or chemotherapy was given. Similarly, no increased incidence of leukaemia was reported in patients with all stages of ovarian cancer, the majority of whom never received chemotherapy (Koeffler and Rowley 1985). Untreated patients with polycythemia vera or lymphoproliferative diseases have a low background incidence of acute leukaemia transformation. In a review paper (Rosner and Grunwald 1980), 19 out of 145 cases of leukaemia were reported to have occurred almost simultaneously with the diagnosis of multiple myeloma. These data could be consistent with the notion that the same aetiological factor caused both malignancies. There is convincing evidence that leukaemic transformation does not occur in the cells of the patient's primary disease and the karyotype of the cells from the primary malignancy is different from the karyotype of the leukaemic cells. In addition, many patients are in complete remission when acute leukaemia develops and therapy-related leukaemia occurs in some patients who have never had a malignancy, such as those receiving immuno-suppressive therapy. The immune system is frequently impaired by neoplasia or by aggressive therapy with growth-inhibiting agents. Nevertheless, immune suppression *per se* probably does account for the subsequent development of acute leukaemia. Patients with congenital or acquired immunodeficiency states show a markedly increased incidence of malignancies, but most of these are lymphoid (Penn 1990) and almost no cases of acute non-lymphocytic leukaemia are associated with immunodeficiency conditions. Leukaemias that develop after the use of antineoplastic drugs, particularly the alkylating agents and radiation exposure are believed to be caused by a direct effect of these agents on susceptible cells. Most agents also have immunosuppressive side-effects. Thus, the question arises as to whether they are carcinogenic through their immunosuppressive properties or by a direct effect on cells or

through both mechanisms. Animal experiments have provided conflicting data. Clinical data on patients with Hodgkin's disease who have an abnormality of the immune system, particularly of the T lymphocytes, suggest that this probably does not account for their high risk of acute leukaemia. Prior to the availability of chemotherapy and radiotherapy, some of the patients survived for a long time and did not develop leukaemia. The majority of cases of acute leukaemia have occurred within the last two decades, together with the introduction of aggressive curative treatments. Therefore it can be concluded that immunosuppression may play a rôle in the leukaemogenic effect that is principally caused by antineoplastic agents. Although formal proof is lacking, the most plausible mechanism of therapy-related non-lymphocytic leukaemia is an alteration of cellular DNA in a myeloid haematopoietic progenitor cell. The alteration of DNA might represent a change in a structural gene or a change in its expression (Koeffler and Rowley 1985).

Le Beau *et al.* (1986) studied chromosome 5 deletions in 17 patients with therapy-related leukaemia and found that these deletions were on the internal (interstitial) segment of the long arm of chromosome 5. This smallest interstitial segment was consistently deleted in all 17 patients and was referred to as the 'critical region'. This region extends from band 5q23 distally to 5q32 and contains the genes that encode various haematopoietic growth factors (granulocyte–macrophage colony-stimulating factor, multiple colony-stimulating factor, eosinophil colony-stimulating factor, and platelet-derived growth factor) as well as the myelomonocytic differentiation antigen CD14 (Human Gene Mapping 1988). In addition, the gene for erythropoietin has been mapped to 7q22 and, although the critical region of chromosome 7 is not known, the erythropoietin gene may also be deleted in this syndrome. The exact relation between these deletions and the occurrence of acute non-lymphocytic leukaemia is yet to be elucidated. None the less, the deletions of these genes, which are critical to the proliferation and differentiation of haematopoietic tissue, should have a central role in the basic biology of therapy-related leukaemia.

The explanation for the long latency period in acute non-lymphocytic leukaemias is not clear. Ionizing radiations or drugs may cause random chromosomal breaks including chromosome 5 and/or 7. A break on these chromosomes of a pluripotent myeloid stem cell might stimulate expression of the transformed phenotype only after the cell is stimulated to divide, which may occur some time after the initial mutagenic event. Moreover, the initial deletion of chromosome 5 and/or 7 may not be enough to cause leukaemia, but a further mutation of the myeloid stem cell in the normal allele on chromosome 5 and/or 7 is also needed. The requirement for several non-random mutagenic insults to produce leukaemic transformation would explain the long latency period for leukaemo-genesis (Koeffler and Rowley 1985).

Another class of acute leukaemia has been more recently related to therapy with anticancer drugs targeting DNA topoisomerase II. These leukaemias differ from those that follow treatment with alkylating agents in that they occur sooner (approximately 15 months after treatment), there is no period of pancytopenia, they respond more favourably to chemotherapy, and show balanced chromosome aberrations, primarily translocations involving chromosome bands 11q23 and 21q22 (Pedersen-Bjergaard and Philip 1991).

Cytotoxic drugs may be responsible for inducing other types of tumours in addition to leukaemia. Reports of these long-term complications have been constantly increasing during the last few years, but data to assess the magnitude of the problem are still scanty and, as for radiation-induced cancers, long-term follow-up of the exposed populations is mandatory. From the available reports, the median latency period from starting anticancer therapy appears to be approximately 8–10 years and, apart from a few cases of bladder cancer following treatment with cyclophosphamide, the spectrum of second tumours reported is quite broad so far. In addition, many of the second tumours were observed in patients receiving both chemotherapy and radiotherapy. Owing to the paucity of available data, no generalizations can be attempted as yet on whether the period of life during which drug-induced second tumours occur tends to be similar to that of naturally occurring cancer and whether first cancer and age at exposure is an important host factor.

SECOND MALIGNANCIES AFTER THERAPY FOR HODGKIN'S DISEASE

The modern treatment strategy for patients with Hodgkin's disease is relatively standard in major centres and has produced an excellent cure rate in what is a relatively young population (Bonadonna 1982). Therefore, long-term follow-up of large case series is available and has provided important data on the risk of developing second cancers. Since the first report in 1972 by investigators of the National Cancer Institute of United States (Arseneau et al. 1972), many research groups have published their data. This discussion will essentially focus on the series from the Milan Cancer Institute (Valagussa et al. 1982, 1986), Stanford University (Coleman et al. 1982; Tucker et al. 1988), and the National Cancer Institute (Tester et al. 1984; Blayney et al. 1987) as these address the major clinical issues. References to other case series are available in these reports.

The series of 1329 patients from the Milan Cancer Institute (Valagussa et al. 1986) has recently been updated and the overall actuarial risk for all types of second tumours (basal cell carcinomas excluded) was 16±2.2 per cent at 15 years. Table 2 details the actuarial risk of secondary leukaemia, solid tumours, and non-Hodgkin's lymphomas according to the treatment modalities utilized during the course of Hodgkin's disease. Secondary leukaemia (27 cases) was largely associated with combined radiotherapy and chemotherapy. We have documented only one case of leukaemia following chemotherapy alone (Valagussa et al. 1980) and no leukaemias were observed after radiotherapy alone. It is worth mentioning that in the major case series of patients with Hodgkin's disease treated with irradiation alone, secondary leukaemia has been documented in only a few cases. Overall, our data on therapy-related acute leukaemia are consistent with the findings reported by other investigators (Tester et al. 1984; Tucker et al. 1988), particularly when the same drug combinations are taken into consideration. In patients treated with MOPP (nitrogen mustard, vincristine,

procarbazine, prednisolone) and radiotherapy, the risk of leukaemia was 6.2 per cent in the Stanford series treated with adjuvant chemotherapy (Tucker et al. 1988), 9.5 per cent in the Milan series given either adjuvant or salvage MOPP, and 17 per cent in the series from the National Cancer Institute who also included in the analysis the myelodysplastic syndromes (five out of 12 cases) (Blayney et al. 1987). It is important to emphasize a particular aspect of the case series from the Milan Cancer Institute. A drug combination entirely different from MOPP, that is, ABVD (doxorubicin, bleomycin, vinblastine, dacarbazine) which does not include alkylating agents, was first designed by our group in 1973 and subsequently introduced into clinical practice because it was found to be at least as effective as MOPP (Bonadonna 1982). Of 180 patients who received both irradiation and ABVD alone, we documented only one case of acute leukaemia for a risk of 0.7 per cent. The difference between the MOPP and ABVD groups was statistically significant at $p=0.04$ (Table 2). Similar findings, that is, a decreased incidence of secondary leukaemias, were also observed at Stanford after treatment with radiotherapy and PAVe (procarbazine, melphalan, vinblastine), despite the fact that this drug regimen contains an alkylating agent (Tucker et al. 1988). In contrast with the Stanford results, we observed an increased risk of secondary leukaemia in patients in whom salvage MOPP was given after radiotherapy failures compared with patients who received combined MOPP and radiotherapy as a first treatment (Table 3). Our findings are in line with the previous experience reported by the National Cancer Institute (Tester et al. 1984). In the series reported by Tucker et al. (1988), the risk of secondary leukaemia was 4.9 per cent after initial combined modality treatment and 1.8 per cent for salvage chemotherapy, respectively (Table 3). However, it is important to emphasize that in the Stanford series patients treated with external irradiation and intravenous radioactive colloidal gold, a treatment in use before 1975 (Tucker et al. 1988), were examined separately from the main treatment group. The authors reported that the risk for secondary leukaemia after salvage MOPP in patients failing on radiotherapy and radioactive gold was 12.3±6.8 per cent, whereas no cases of leukaemia were documented in the group treated with external radiotherapy and radioactive gold who had no subsequent MOPP. As also reported by other research groups (Coleman et al. 1982; Coltman and Dixon 1982; Glicksman et al. 1982; Pedersen-Bjergaard and Larsen 1982), in our series we documented an increased risk of leukaemia in patients aged more than 40 years at diagnosis of Hodgkin's disease (18.6±6.4 per cent following radiotherapy plus MOPP) compared with younger adults

Table 2 Actuarial risk of second malignancy in 1329 patients with Hodgkin's disease treated at the Milan Cancer Institute (data at 15 years)

	Secondary leukaemia±SE (%)	Solid tumours[a]±SE (%)	Non-Hodgkin's lymphoma±SE (%)
Total	4.1±0.9	11.3±2.1	1.2±0.5
RT	0	9.9±2.8	2.4±1.3
CT	1.4±1.6	1.8±1.8	0
RT+CT	5.9±1.4	12.8±2.9	0.8±0.4
RT+MOPP	9.5±3.8	4.9±1.6	0.8±0.6
RT+ABVD	0.7±0.7	3.8±2.1	0

SE, standard error; RT, radiotherapy; CT, chemotherapy.
[a] Basal cell cancers excluded.

Table 3 Cumulative risk of therapy-related leukaemia following MOPP and extensive irradiation (data at 15 years)

	Cumulative risk±SE (%)	
	Milan Cancer Institute	Stanford University
Total	9.5±3.8	
17–40 years	8.7±5.8	NR
>40 years	18.6±6.4	
Combined treatment modality	4.3±1.7	4.9±1.5
Salvage MOPP after radiation failure	17.7±7.8	1.8±1.3
Salvage MOPP after failure following radiation and radioactive gold	—	12.8±6.8

SE, standard error; NR, not reported, but increased risk for ages >50 years.

(8.7±5.8 per cent, $p < 0.001$). The possible association between leukaemia and splenectomy has been evaluated and it has been reported that splenectomy increases the risk of secondary leukaemia (van Leeuwen *et al.* 1989). This observation of the increased risk of leukaemia in patients with Hodgkin's disease subjected to splenectomy has been emphasized in a recent report from an international collaborative group of 12 population-based cancer registries and six large oncology hospitals (Kaldor *et al.* 1990*a*). A total of 163 cases of therapy-related leukaemia were documented in a total of 29 552 patients. To investigate the effect of different treatments, for each case patient with leukaemia three matched controls were chosen who had been treated for Hodgkin's disease but in whom leukaemia had not developed. However, caution should be exercised in extrapolating data into different subsets with particular features because the well-known bias related to the selection of matched controls can be overemphasized. We have observed similar findings (that is, higher risk of leukaemia after splenectomy) in patients treated with radiation plus MOPP, but it is worth noting that in our experience most patients who underwent splenectomy and eventually developed leukaemia were over 40 years of age and had received salvage MOPP following radiotherapy failures. It is also worth mentioning that in the majority of reported case series the length of follow-up is probably shorter in patients not undergoing staging laparotomy because many centres have only recently abandoned the routine use of staging laparotomy with splenectomy. Thus, additional data with an appropriate follow-up are needed prior to claiming as definitive the association between splenectomy and leukaemia in Hodgkin's disease. In fact, in two recently published reports (Andrieu *et al.* 1990; Cosset *et al.* 1991) splenectomy was not found to play any role in the risk of secondary leukaemia. Although the peak incidence of therapy-related leukaemia is estimated to be approximately 5–6 years after initial treatment, it has been reported that the risk decreases after 9–10 years (Blayney *et al.* 1987; Tucker *et al.* 1988). While this may be true, additional follow-up is required; cases of leukaemia have been documented more than 15 years after initial therapy (van Leeuwen *et al.* 1989) and in our series the risk is still appreciable after 10 years. In almost all reported case series, therapy-related acute leukaemias have a short fatal course.

In addition to secondary leukaemia, non-Hodgkin's lymphomas and a variety of solid tumours have also been documented in patients treated for Hodgkin's disease. In the initial report by Krikorian *et al.* (1979), the risk of developing secondary non-Hodgkin's lymphomas was 4.4 per cent. Subsequent studies have demonstrated that the risk is substantially lower, in the range of 1–2 per cent after 10 years; however, some cases may have a long latency period, suggesting that the true risk of this secondary malignancy awaits definition. It is still not clear whether the secondary lymphomas are related to treatment carcinogenicity or to disease-related or treatment-induced immunosuppression or whether this event is merely due to a chance association. However, it is worth mentioning that in a recent report on secondary cancers after bone-marrow transplantation for leukaemia or aplastic anaemia (Witherspoon *et al.* 1989), 16 cases of non-Hodgkin's lymphoma were observed among 35 patients with secondary tumours. Unlike the secondary leukaemias, non-Hodgkin's lymphomas are curable in approximately 50 per cent of patients (Coleman *et al.* 1982; Valagussa *et al.* 1986).

As the follow-up time over which survivors have been observed has lengthened, an excess risk of developing second solid tumours has become apparent and all investigators who previously reported on therapy-related leukaemias have acknowledged the occurrence of non-haematological malignancies (Coleman *et al.* 1982; Tester

et al. 1984; Valagussa *et al.* 1986). The risk appears independent of the type of chemotherapy, but almost all second solid tumours were observed in patients who received radiation therapy during the course of their treatment. In both the Milan and Stanford case series, approximately two-thirds of the tumours were documented within the radiation fields. However, it is still unclear whether all solid tumours are due directly to the radiation, to the altered immunity from treatment, to the disease process itself, or to other risk factors such as heavy smoking in patients developing lung cancer (Coleman *et al.* 1982; Valagussa *et al.* 1986) or the presence of dysplastic naevus syndrome in the development of secondary melanoma (Tucker *et al.* 1985). As recently reported, the risk of thyroid cancer following mantle or cervical irradiation varies greatly by age at radiation therapy; among children, the risk is increased 67-fold (Tucker *et al.* 1991) compared with a 16-fold increase among a predominantly adult group (Hancock *et al.* 1993). The Stanford group (Hancock *et al.* 1993) also documented a 4-fold increased risk of developing breast cancer following mantle irradiation. The risk varied dramatically by age and time interval since treatment, young women being at a markedly increased risk more than 15 years later (<20 years at the time of radiation, relative risk 38; 20–29 years at the time of radiation, relative risk 17). Other frequently documented second tumours are lung cancer, bone and soft tissue sarcomas, and melanoma (Valagussa *et al.* 1986; Tucker *et al.* 1988, van Leeuwen *et al.* 1989). In our series of patients we documented 50 cases of second solid tumours with an actuarial risk of 11.3±2.1 per cent within 15 years. Eighteen cases of lung cancer were observed (actuarial risk 4.1±0.5 per cent), with 13 being documented in patients aged over 40 years at the time of the diagnosis of Hodgkin's disease (actuarial risk 9.4±3.4 per cent). In contrast with what has been reported by List *et al.* (1985), we documented only one case of small-cell lung carcinoma. All but one patient had received radiotherapy to the mediastinal lung area and a history of smoking was recorded in the majority of patients. In the Stanford series (Tucker *et al.* 1988), 46 second solid tumours occurred more than 1 year after diagnosis of Hodgkin's disease and at 15 years the actuarial risk was 13.2 per cent. On the basis of tumour incidence rates specific for sex, age, and calendar year obtained from the Connecticut Tumor Registry, 14.5 cases of solid tumours were expected in the Stanford series for a relative risk of 3.2 (95 per cent confidence interval 2.3–4.2). Among these second solid tumours, 14 were lung cancer (relative risk 7.7) and four were melanoma (relative risk 8.9). The Netherlands Cancer Institute (van Leeuwen *et al.* 1989) has reported a similar analysis based on tumour incidence rates specific for sex and age obtained from the Cooperative Association of Hospitals in Oncology cancer registry. A total of 32 second solid tumours were documented and 12.76 were expected for a relative risk of 2.5 (95 per cent confidence interval 1.7–3.5); the relative risk for lung cancer was 4.9. The median latency period for solid tumours is longer than that reported for secondary leukaemias and it is estimated that the risk will increase with lengthening of follow-up. As mentioned in the two previous sections, both radiotherapy and chemotherapy have potential carcinogenic effects in humans, but whether the association of the two modalities can additionally increase the risk of solid tumours in the population exposed still awaits definition.

How should the occurrence of second malignancies change our approach to the treatment of Hodgkin's disease? Drug selection may be important, particularly as far as therapy-related leukaemias are concerned. Despite the wealth of data available, the relative role of different intensities of treatment, namely radiation doses and fields, doses and time schedule of chemotherapy, sequences of irradiation and chemotherapy, length of total therapy, and potential additive effects of salvage treatment, are still under investigation. As far as chemotherapy is concerned, less leukaemogenic but equally effective regimens, such as ABVD, are now available. None the less, the choice of treatment should not be based merely on the risk of developing a secondary malignancy. While cure remains of primary importance and the unnecessarily prolonged delivery of potentially toxic regimens must be avoided, it should be emphasized that suboptimal initial therapy may be detrimental in the long-term. Treatment failure following initial therapy with less intensive regimens may subsequently require the administration of the same or potentially more carcinogenic regimens which could increase the risk of second malignancy.

SECOND MALIGNANCIES AFTER THERAPY FOR OVARIAN CANCER

It has been demonstrated that patients who have received chemotherapy with alkylating agents for ovarian cancer have an increased risk of acute leukaemia, particularly the myeloid type. However, most of the initial studies have not been large enough to allow detailed analysis of the risk and the time of occurrence of leukaemia according to the amount and type of chemotherapy received.

Green et al. (1986) were the first to explore in detail the association between risk of leukaemia and specific alkylating agents as well as the relationship between cumulative drug dose and the eventual development of leukaemia. The study included a large cohort of 3363 women who had survived for 1 year after treatment for ovarian cancer in five randomized clinical trials and at two large medical centres in North America. The 10 year cumulative risk of secondary leukaemia was 8.5 ± 1.6 per cent after treatment with any alkylating agent, 11.2 ± 2.6 per cent after treatment with melphalan, and 5.4 ± 3.2 per cent after cyclophosphamide treatment. More recently, a similar analysis (Kaldor et al. 1990b) has been conducted by a collaborative group comprising 11 population-based cancer registries in Europe and Canada and two large oncology hospitals in Europe. Among 99 113 patients with ovarian cancer, 114 women developed leukaemia. For each case patient three matched controls were sought who had not developed this second malignancy. Despite differences in the methods of reporting on secondary leukaemia, Table 4 attempts a comparison of the findings from the two studies. In the report by Green et al. (1986) the

cumulative dose for each agent was calculated by multiplying dose by duration for each drug exposure and adding results, whereas in the study by Kaldor et al. (1990b) low and high doses were defined with respect to the median dose in the controls. As can be seen from Table 4, melphalan may be a more potent inducer of leukaemia than cyclophosphamide, but a dose–response relationship was apparent for both agents.

Other studies have confirmed the increased risk of leukaemia in patients with ovarian cancer treated with alkylating agents. In contrast, the risk of second solid tumours seems to be only marginally increased and apparently not associated with a particular type of treatment.

The actual trend in treatment for ovarian cancer is towards more use of chemotherapy and in particular increased reliance on drug combinations. However, there is limited evidence so far that the effectiveness of such chemotherapy improves with increasing the number of drugs. In the case of Hodgkin's disease, the risk of therapy-related leukaemia following combination chemotherapy is clearly counterbalanced by gains in survival. The extent to which the increased risk of leukaemia after ovarian cancer is offset remains unclear.

SECOND MALIGNANCIES AFTER ADJUVANT THERAPY FOR BREAST CANCER

The moderate but consistent benefit of systemic adjuvant therapy in high-risk resectable breast cancer has been clearly established (Early Breast Cancer Trialists' Collaborative Group 1992). Thus, it is increasingly important to measure the immediate and delayed toxicity costs of given drug treatments to determine the cost–benefit ratio. The data available on second malignancies for breast cancer are still scanty, since at present the follow-up is more limited than that for the Hodgkin's disease populations. None the less, since many patients will be treated with adjuvant chemotherapy and/or tamoxifen, some considerations of the potential risk of second cancers are warranted. Leukaemia subsequent to the diagnosis of breast cancer has been observed after treatment by surgery alone or followed by radiation therapy (Rosner et al. 1978), by prolonged adjuvant chlorambucil (Lerner 1978), by thiotepa (Chan et al. 1977), or by mitomycin C and cyclophosphamide given for a few years (Koyama et al. 1980). These were essentially case reports and, thus, lacked not only estimates of risk but even denominators of treated patients. More recently, some case-control studies based on tumour registries have reported an increased risk of leukaemia following adjuvant cyclophosphamide therapy (Haas et al. 1987) or an alkylating regimen with or without post-operative irradiation (Curtis et al. 1992). Although it was possible to analyse large patient numbers in such studies, there is still the possibility of bias being introduced by over- or undermatching and details of single or total doses delivered and duration of treatments were usually lacking.

Prospective controlled studies aimed at evaluating the efficacy of adjuvant therapy for breast cancer offer the almost unique possibility of comparing the risk of second malignancies in a population undergoing extensive long-term follow-up. A subgroup of this population has been randomly allocated to receive only surgery as initial treatment, whereas the other subgroup also received post-operative radiotherapy or anticancer drugs or both. Because of randomization, all other factors should ideally be

Table 4 Risk of leukaemia in patients with ovarian cancer

	Cumulative risk at 10 years$\pm$SE[a] (%)	Relative risk (95% confidence interval)[b]
No radiation or chemotherapy	0	1.0
Radiation only	0.1 ± 0.1	1.6 (0.5–4.8)
Chemotherapy only	8.6 ± 2.2	12.0 (4.4–32)
Radiation plus chemotherapy	8.3 ± 2.4	9.8 (3.4–28)
Cyclophosphamide	5.4 ± 3.2	NR
Low dose	0	2.2
Medium dose	0	
High dose	11.2 ± 6.2	4.1
Melphalan	11.2 ± 2.6	NR
Low dose	1.1 ± 1.1	12
Medium dose	5.0 ± 2.9	
High dose	19.5 ± 4.9	23

SE, standard error; NR, not reported.

[a] Green et al. (1986).

[b] Kaldor et al. (1990b).

Table 5 Actuarial risk of second malignancies after adjuvant therapy for operable breast cancer

Research group	Follow-up (years)	Second tumour investigated	Treatment after surgery	Actuarial risk (%)
NSABP	10	Acute leukaemia	No treatment	0.1
			Radiotherapy	1.4
			L-PAM regimens	1.3
Milan	15	Acute leukaemia	No treatment	0
			CMF regimens	0.23
		Solid tumours[a]	No treatment	8.4
			CMF regimens	6.5
Stockholm	4.5	Infiltrating endometrial cancer	No treatment	<0.5
			TAM×2 years	1.0
			TAM×5 years	5.5

L-PAM, melphalan; TAM, tamoxifen 40 mg daily.
[a] Basal cell carcinoma and contralateral breast cancer excluded.

comparable. Thus, it is possible to investigate whether the underlying first cancer may be an important host factor or whether potentially carcinogenic agents are responsible for the occurrence of second cancers. The data detailed so far in the medical literature and from which a few conclusions can be drawn are those of the National Surgical Adjuvant Breast Project (NSABP) (Fisher et al. 1985) and from the Milan and Stockholm trials (Valagussa et al. 1987; Fornander et al. 1989).

The NSABP investigators (Fisher et al. 1985) analysed data from a very large patient population presenting with positive axillary nodes to assess the risk of secondary leukaemia. Briefly, three cases of leukaemia were documented within 10 years among 2068 patients initially treated with surgery alone, six cases among 1116 who received post-operative irradiation, and 27 in 5299 patients given adjuvant melphalan with or without methotrexate, fluorouracil, and tamoxifen. The comparative actuarial risk is reported in Table 5. Although the 10 year risk is relatively small, the difference has been reported to be statistically significant between surgery alone and surgery plus chemotherapy and of borderline significance between surgery and surgery plus irradiation.

At the Milan Cancer Institute, we have recently updated our previous findings (Valagussa et al. 1987) on a larger series of 2465 cases, 91 per cent of whom received cyclophosphamide, methotrexate, fluorouracil, or CMF chemotherapy and 18 per cent were subjected to breast irradiation after conservative surgery (Valagussa et al. 1994). In the chemotherapy-treated group, three patients developed acute non-lymphocytic leukaemia (cumulative risk at 15 years, 0.23 per cent; relative risk, 2.3). The data reported so far for breast cancer (Fisher et al. 1985; Curtis et al. 1992; Valagussa et al. 1994) suggest that, as in ovarian cancer (Green et al. 1986), melphalan may be a more potent leukaemogenic drug than cyclophosphamide. However, additional studies are required to assess the relative rôle in breast cancer patients of different alkylating agents with or without local–regional irradiation in inducing secondary leukaemia.

As far as second solid tumours are concerned, our findings suggest that within 15 years there is not an increased risk of second malignancies in patients receiving surgery plus adjuvant CMF compared with women undergoing surgery alone (Table 5). It is probably still too early to assess definitely the actual risk of solid neoplasms, but the similarity of tumour types, time to development, and median survival from diagnosis of second malignancies in both treatment groups suggest that, in breast cancer, second tumours cannot be entirely ascribed to treatment with adjuvant CMF. The malignancies most frequently observed were gynaecological and gastrointestinal cancers and only five cases of bladder cancers have

been documented so far (actuarial risk, 0.31 per cent), despite the use of cyclophosphamide (Habs et al. 1981).

Adjuvant tamoxifen has been utilized by many investigators in the adjuvant treatment of breast cancer (Early Breast Cancer Trialists' Collaborative Group 1992). After a median follow-up of 4.5 years, investigators from Stockholm (Fornander et al. 1989) have reported an increased risk of infiltrating endometrial cancer in women receiving tamoxifen (40 mg daily) compared with women treated with only local–regional modality. The greatest cumulative frequency was seen among patients allocated to 5 years of tamoxifen (Table 5), but even in women who received tamoxifen for 2 years the risk of infiltrating endometrial cancer was doubled compared with patients in the control group. Other research groups have failed to confirm this important finding, but detailed data are still lacking and in many series the follow-up remains short. In addition, the majority of patients are receiving tamoxifen at a daily dose of 20 mg. However, it is important to mention that in athymic mice transplanted with a hormone-dependent breast tumour and endometrial tumour and treated with tamoxifen, the oestrogen-stimulated growth of the breast tumour is controlled but that of the endometrial tumour is not (Jordan 1988). Thus, occult endometrial carcinoma may not be controlled in women receiving tamoxifen therapy for breast cancer. The spectrum of other solid tumours reported by the Swedish group was not different from what has been observed in the Milan series (Fornander et al. 1989; Valagussa et al. 1994).

Although additional reports on second tumours developing in patients cured of their first breast cancer may be expected during the next few years, there is no reason at present to regard treatment-related carcinogenicity as a necessary complication of successful adjuvant therapies. None the less the indiscriminate prolonged use of potentially toxic therapy must be avoided and efforts should be made to identify subsets of breast cancer patients for whom cytotoxic treatments really resulted in a survival gain. Also, data on long-term complications from tamoxifen are mandatory before this treatment modality becomes commonplace in patients probably cured by optimal local–regional treatment alone (Bonadonna and Valagussa 1989).

SECOND MALIGNANCIES AFTER THERAPY FOR PAEDIATRIC NEOPLASMS

In this section data on second malignancies developed in children who survived for 2 years or more after a diagnosis of a cancer will rely heavily on reports from the Late Effects Study Group (LESG). Thirteen centres in the United States, Canada and Western Europe are participating in this group and the medical records of 9170 patients are available (Tucker *et al.* 1987), thus representing an almost unique case series. In 1985, the LESG reported on 292 patients who had developed at least one second malignancy (Meadows *et al.* 1985) and data were available regarding the types of first and second neoplasms, the therapy administered, and the predisposing factors. In 292 patients, the most common primary was retinoblastoma, followed by Hodgkin's disease, soft tissue sarcomas, and Wilms' tumour. Clearly, this distribution is not similar to the relative frequency of paediatric primary cancers and the association between the first and the second neoplasm seems not just a chance or merely a treatment-related effect (Meadows *et al.* 1985). Thus, some specific risk factors or predisposing conditions can be postulated, despite the fact that the majority of second malignancies (68 per cent) developed in tissue exposed to ionizing radiation. Fifty-two patients presented with primary retinoblastoma and bone or soft tissue sarcomas developed in 20 and 16 of them, respectively. In a more recent LESG study (Tucker *et al.* 1987), the actuarial risk that a patient with retinoblastoma would develop osteosarcoma was higher than the risk for patients with all other cancers. In addition, there is a well-known association between familial retinoblastoma and osteosarcoma (Abramson *et al.* 1984), with both tumours showing similar chromosomal abnormalities (Hansen *et al.* 1985). It is important to note that the series reported by Meadows *et al.* (1985) included 44 children who had been treated with neither radiation nor chemotherapy and 24 patients with known predisposing conditions. Of interest in the LESG group is the association between primary leukaemia and secondary brain tumours, a finding also reported by other investigators (Rimm *et al.* 1987). However, it remains to be elucidated whether this association is related to treatment or to some predisposing factors. In contrast, secondary leukaemias were most commonly documented in children with primary Hodgkin's disease treated with chemotherapy with or without irradiation and these findings are in agreement with data previously discussed for adult patients.

A more recent report from the LESG group estimated the risk of subsequent bone cancer among 9170 patients who had a diagnosis of cancer in childhood and were treated with radiotherapy and/or chemotherapy (Tucker *et al.* 1987). As expected, the overall risk was highest among children treated for retinoblastoma, followed by those with Ewing's sarcoma and rhabdomyosarcoma. The authors concluded that both radiotherapy and chemotherapy including alkylating agents for childhood cancer increase the subsequent risk of bone tumours. The risks increased with greater amounts of chemotherapy and were not confounded by the high rate of 'spontaneous' bone sarcomas associated with genetic retinoblastoma. This study also provided an opportunity to quantify the risk of bone sarcoma according to the estimated dose of radiation to the bone. No increased risk was associated with doses of less than 1000 cGy to the osseous site, but the risk increased to 38.3 following the delivery of 6000 cGy or more. Thus, radiogenic bone sarcoma appears to be a high-dose effect following external-beam exposure (Tucker *et al.* 1987).

The National Wilms' Tumor Study Group (Breslow *et al.* 1988) has recently reported that a substantial number of second malignancies occur as patients are followed more than 10 years from diagnosis. A total of 15 second cancers were observed among 2438 patients who contributed 14 381 person years of observation. According to the United States incidence rates for 1973–1977, only 1.77 cancers would have been expected for a relative risk of 8.5

(95 per cent confidence interval 4.7–14.0). The relative risk was 10.8 for those who received radiation as part of the initial course of treatment and 5.0 for those who did not, but the difference was not statistically significant.

HOST-RELATED FACTORS

Second malignancies may be due to factors other than the agents used to treat cancer patients who, similarly to the general population, are exposed to environmental and occupational carcinogens that can affect multiple organs. It is not unusual to document multiple tumours of the same organ system in patients with head and neck, lung, and bladder cancers. Multiple tumours in different organ systems have also been observed when the two cancers share common risk factors, such as breast and endometrial cancers or may be caused by common exposure, such as lung and bladder cancers. In addition, single-gene traits are associated with an increased risk of producing tumours at multiple sites. More than 200 single-gene disorders have been associated with the development of benign or malignant tumours in humans (Mulvihill 1977; Lynch and Frichot 1978) and a few of these genetic diseases, chiefly autosomal dominant diseases, predispose to more than one form of cancer. For example, von Recklinghausen's neurofibromatosis and tuberous sclerosis are associated with neural tumours, Gardner's syndrome is associated with colon cancers and sarcomas, in the multiple-endocrine neoplasia syndromes, the component neoplasms appear to share common progenitor cells in the embryonic neural crest, chromosome instability syndromes, such as Bloom's or Fanconi's syndromes have been associated with the development of leukaemia, and neurofibromatosis has also been described in association with childhood non-lymphocytic leukaemia, Wilms' tumour, and rhabdomyosarcoma (McKeen *et al.* 1979).

Some cancers tend to aggregate in families and genetic influences have been postulated for this occurrence; families have been reported with clusters of adenocarcinomas of the breast, ovary, colon, and endometrium in several generations (Fraumeni 1977). Apart from family cancer syndrome in childhood neoplasms (Fraumeni 1977), other constellations have also been reported in small series but chance aggregation may be the plausible explanation (Moertel 1977).

Undoubtedly there is an important interrelation between the immune system and susceptibility to the development of cancer. The association between cases of Hodgkin's disease in multiple-case families with HLA-linked or unlinked determinants of susceptibility has been investigated (Chakravarti *et al.* 1986). Findings suggested that a recessive susceptibility gene tightly linked to the HLA complex was responsible for 60 per cent of cases, with the remaining 40 per cent being due to environmental or other factors. An association with HLA-DR5 in white populations has been suggested for both endemic and epidemic Kaposi's sarcoma (Pollack *et al.* 1984) but not for endemic sarcoma in Africa (Melbye *et al.* 1987).

The association between immunodeficiency states and the development of cancer is relevant to the study of therapy-related malignancies since the primary disease and its treatment can lead to permanent defects in the immune system. Genetically determined immunodeficiency states have been associated with secondary neoplasms (Coleman 1982). More importantly, organ transplantation with iatrogenic immunodeficiency (Coleman 1982; Penn 1990) and acquired immunodeficiency syndrome (Fauci *et al.* 1984) is associated with increased risk of developing specific cancers. A common malignancy observed in these settings is intermediate or high grade non-Hodgkin's lymphoma, almost universally of the B-cell type and these lymphomas are similar to those seen after treatment for Hodgkin's disease (Coleman 1982).

Advances in molecular biology techniques demonstrated that certain malignancies are related to specific DNA damage (for example, alterations in the retinoblastoma locus, germ-line mutations in p53). A cancer can develop through the loss of expression of a gene by the deletion of both alleles and at least one of them is required to prevent the development of a cancer. These new discoveries are important in allowing improved understanding of the underlying mechanisms of carcinogenesis and to define better the role of treatment in inducing second malignancies. It is beyond the scope of this chapter to summarize techniques and findings from investigations of molecular biology. However, retinoblastoma, to which predisposition can be inherited as an autosomal dominant trait, may serve as an example. The occurrence of retinoblastoma as both heritable and sporadic forms has allowed detailed statistical analyses (Knudson 1983) which indicate a relationship between the two forms of the disease. A locus RB1, which plays a role in the development of this tumour, has been localized to the q14 band of human chromosome 13 through segregation analysis and by the identification of specific deletions of this chromosomal region in some retinoblastoma patients or their tumours. A model to unify these observations has been proposed (Nordenskjold and Cavenee 1988) based on the previous hypothesis that as few as two mutations are required for malignant transformation (Knudson 1983). In this model, bilateral retinoblastoma cases have inherited a germinal mutation of the RB1 locus which predisposes each cell to transformation by a further event. Heritable cases of retinoblastoma also seem to be at greatly increased risk for the development of second primary tumours, particularly osteogenic sarcoma. Molecular genetic evidence indicates that the development of these two disparate tumour types involves specific somatic loss of constitutional heterozygosity for the region of human chromosome 13 that includes the RB1 locus (Hansen *et al.* 1985). Furthermore, these same chromosomal mechanisms eliciting losses of constitutional heterozygosity have been observed in sporadic osteosarcoma, suggesting a genetic similarity in pathogenetic causality. The consolidation of formal genetic, epidemiological, and molecular genetic data has provided a complementary model that invokes the unmasking of recessive predisposing mutations by aberrant mitotic events. This model first proposes the fixation of monoallelic genetic damage and subsequently its elucidation through mitotic malsegregation or recombination. The net result of these two sequential events is a single somatic tumour progenitor that is homozygously defective at the relevant tumour locus. These events have been reasonably well delineated in the cases of retinoblastoma and Wilms' tumour and limited studies indicate the applicability of the model to other solid tumours (Nordenskjold and Cavenee 1988). At present, the involvement of various environmental or chemical agents in these processes is unknown. None the less, it is conceivable that the abnormalities in gene expression needed to produce a malignant tumour could be induced by therapy for a first malignancy. Using a technique for measuring somatic mutations in lymphocytes, it has been demonstrated that the mutation frequency in untreated patients with cancer did not differ from that of controls. In contrast, an elevated mutation frequency in lymphocytes was observed in patients treated previously with chemotherapy or chemotherapy plus radiotherapy (Dempsey *et al.* 1985). In a setting in which one DNA lesion is already present, it might be expected that the risk of developing a second tumour would be high as only one additional DNA lesion would be required. Further studies will be needed to confirm increased mutation frequency and to show whether the degree of increase is of any value in predicting which patients will develop second malignancies.

METHODS OF REPORTING SECOND MALIGNANCIES

Several methods have been used to report findings on second cancers. Individual cases or limited case series are important in establishing the occurrence of second malignancies but not in quantifying risks. The use of population-based tumour registries has some advantages, particularly because relatively large numbers of patients can allow the detection of even small risks. None the less, these registries do have some disadvantages, namely differential reporting of cancers, variable follow-up, limited data on treatment, and different diagnostic criteria for second cancers. As previously mentioned, clinical trials are an extremely valuable source of information on the risks of secondary tumours. Individuals within each arm have received comparable treatments, and the risk of second cancers can be directly compared between treatment arms. Complete treatment information, including therapies administered at disease progression, is generally available, so that the risk of misclassification at exposure is minimized. This controls for any intrinsic risk of a second malignancy associated with the first cancer and also allows the comparison of risks from specific drug therapies or radiation exposure. The major disadvantage of most of the clinical trials is the relatively small number of patients that can be studied in a given institution or research group.

Two types of analysis are usually adopted to evaluate the association between treatment of a primary cancer and subsequent development of a second malignancy. The first consists of the person-year method used by epidemiologists. For this type of analysis, the risk of developing a second malignancy is implicitly assumed to remain constant during each patient's follow-up period (Makuch and Simon 1979), but this assumption may be inappropriate. The advantage of this method is that tumour incidence rates from the general population specific for age, sex, race, and calendar year are available and the number of expected tumours to be compared with those of the cancer population under study can be derived. None the less, comparisons of rates of second malignancies in cancer patients with rates in the general population can be criticized because, as previously mentioned, some types of cancer may have an intrinsically increased risk of specific secondary cancers. Despite these limitations, we should recognize that these studies are informative even if they give minimal estimates of risk because of the relatively incomplete follow-up. However, some additional caution is required when the matched case-control approach is utilized. In this situation, individuals who develop second cancers (cases) are compared with those who do not (controls). The selection of the appropriate controls is critical in that they should be representative of the entire group; bias in the selection of the control group can lead to spurious associations or can obscure a true association.

Another type of analysis that is appropriate for these studies is the actuarial or life-table approach (Makuch and Simon 1979). This analysis provides the cumulative risk expressed as a percentage for a particular time period. The actuarial risk of a secondary cancer occurring can be compared between treatment arms using methods similar to those employed for the comparison of survival. It has been claimed that the major limitation of this method is that it does not account for the baseline tumour rates in the general population, however, when the oncogenic potential of different treatments are compared in patients with a first primary cancer who are taking part in clinical trials, then both the baseline tumour rates in the general population and those that can be intrinsically related to the first cancer itself are ideally alike 'on the average' among the various treatment groups.

CONCLUSION

It is our hope that examination of the multiple factors responsible for inducing secondary cancers and the use of appropriate methods of reporting these complications will result in more adequate evaluation concerning the risks of second malignancies. Curative modern cancer treatment has called our attention to the long-term complications of therapy and it is ironic that second malignancies are only seen because the primary treatment is so successful. Clearly, attempts should be made to reduce these complications, but not at the price of cure. Changes in therapy to minimize second cancers should be made in carefully designed studies through which current treatments can be made less toxic while maintaining or even improving their efficacy.

REFERENCES

Abramson DH, et al. (1984). Second nonocular tumors in retinoblastoma survivors: are they radiation-induced? Ophthalmology, 91:1351–5.

Andrieu JM, et al. (1990). Increased risk of acute nonlymphocytic leukemia after extended-field radiation therapy combined with MOPP chemotherapy for Hodgkin's disease. Journal of Clinical Oncology, 8:1148–54.

Arseneau JC, et al. (1972). Non-lymphomatous malignant tumors complicating Hodgkin's disease: possible association with intensive therapy. New England Journal of Medicine, 287:1119–22.

Blayney DW, et al. (1987). Decreasing risk of leukemia with prolonged follow-up after chemotherapy and radiotherapy for Hodgkin's disease. New England Journal of Medicine, 316:710–14.

Boice JD (1981). Cancer following medical irradiation. Cancer, 47:1081–90.

Bonadonna G (1982). Chemotherapy strategies to improve the control of Hodgkin's disease: the Richard and Hinda Rosenthal Foundation Award Lecture. Cancer Research, 42:4309–20.

Bonadonna G, Valagussa P (1989). Systemic therapy in resectable breast cancer. In Diagnosis and therapy of breast cancer, Hematology/Oncology Clinics of North America (ed. IC Henderson), pp. 727–42. WB Saunders, Philadelphia.

Breslow NE, et al. (1988). Second malignant neoplasms in survivors of Wilms' tumor: a report from the National Wilms' Tumor Study Group. Journal of the National Cancer Institute, 80:592–5.

Chakravarti A, et al. (1986). Etiological heterogeneity in Hodgkin's disease: HLA linked and unlinked determinants of suscepibility independent of histological concordance. Genetics and Epidemiology, 3:407–15.

Chan PYM, Sadoff L, Winkley HJ (1977). Second malignancies following first breast cancer in prolonged thiotepa adjuvant chemotherapy. In Adjuvant therapy of cancer (ed. SE Salmon and SE Jones), pp. 597–607. North-Holland, Amsterdam.

Coleman CN (1982). Secondary neoplasms in patients treated for cancer: etiology and perspective. Radiation Research, 92:188–200.

Coleman C, et al. (1982). Leukemias, non-Hodgkin's lymphomas and solid tumors in patients treated for Hodgkin's disease. Cancer Surveys, 1:733–44.

Coltman CA, Dixon DO (1982). Second malignancies complicating Hodgkin's disease: a Southwest Oncology Group 10-year follow-up. Cancer Treatment Reports, 66:1023–33.

Cosset JM, Henry-Amar M, Meerwaldt JH, for the EORTC Lymphoma Cooperative Group (1991). Long-term toxicity of early stages of Hodgkin's disease therapy: the EORTC experience. Annals of Oncology, 2 (Suppl. 2):77–82.

Curtis RE, et al. (1992). Risk of leukemia after chemotherapy and radiation treatment for breast cancer. New England Journal of Medicine, 326:1745–51.

Dempsey JL, Seshadri RS, Morley AA (1985). Increased mutation frequency following treatment with cancer chemotherapy. Cancer Research, 45:2873–7.

Early Breast Cancer Trialists' Collaborative Group (1992). Systemic treatment of early breast cancer by hormonal, cytotoxic or immune therapy: 133 randomised trials involving 31,000 recurrences and 24,000 deaths among 75,000 women. Lancet, 339:1–15, 71–85.

Fauci AS, et al. (1984). Acquired immunodeficiency syndrome: epidemiologic, clinical, immunologic, and therapeutic considerations. Annals of Internal Medicine, 100:92–106.

Fisher B, et al. (1985). Leukemia in breast cancer patients following adjuvant chemotherapy or postoperative radiation: the NSABP experience. Journal of Clinical Oncology, 3:1640–58.

Fornander T, et al. (1989). Adjuvant tamoxifen in early breast cancer: occurrence of new primary cancer. Lancet, i:117–19.

Fraumeni JF Jr (1977). Clinical patterns of familial cancer. In Genetics of human cancer (ed. JJ Mulvihill, RW Miller, and JF Fraumeni Jr), pp. 223–33. Raven Press, New York.

Glicksman AS, et al. (1982). Second malignant neoplasms in patients successfully treated for Hodgkin's disease: a Cancer and Leukemia Group B study. Cancer Treatment Reports, 66:1035–44.

Green MH, et al. (1986). Melphalan may be a more potent leukemogen than cyclophosphamide. Annals of Internal Medicine, 105:360–7.

Haas JF, et al. (1987). Risk of leukaemia in ovarian tumour and breast cancer patients following treatment by cyclophosphamide. British Journal of Cancer, 55:213–18.

Habs M, Schmähl D, Lin PZ (1981). Carcinogenic activity in rats of combined treatment with cyclophosphamide, methotrexate and 5-fluorouracil. International Journal of Cancer, 28:91–6.

Haddow A, et al. (1948). The growth-inhibitory and carcinogenic properties of 4-aminostilbene and derivatives. Philosophical Transactions of the Royal Society of London, Series A, 241:247.

Hancock SL, Cox RS, McDougall RI (1991). Thyroid diseases after treatment for Hodgkin's disease. New England Journal of Medicine, 325:599–605.

Hancock SL, Tucker MA, Hoppe RT (1993). Breast cancer after treatment for Hodgkin's disease. Journal of the National Cancer Institute, 85:25–31.

Hansen FM, et al. (1985). Osteosarcoma and retinoblastoma: a shared chromosomal mechanism revealing recessive predisposition. Proceedings of the National Academy of Sciences USA, 82:6216–20.

Human Gene Mapping 9.5: New Haven Conference (1988). Update of the Ninth International Workshop on Human Gene Mapping. Cytogenetics and Cell Genetics, 49:1–258.

Jordan VC (1988). Tamoxifen and endometrial cancer. Lancet, ii:1019.

Kaldor JM, et al. (1990a). Leukemia following Hodgkin's disease. New England Journal of Medicine, 322:7–13.

Kaldor JM, et al. (1990b). Leukemia following chemotherapy for ovarian cancer. New England Journal of Medicine, 322:1–6.

Kato H, Schull WJ (1982). Studies of the mortality of A-bomb survivors. Radiation Research, 90:395–432.

Kellerer AM, Rossi HH (1978). A generalized formulation of dual radiation action. Radiation Research, 75:471–88.

Koeffler HP, Rowley JD (1985). Therapy-related acute non lymphocytic leukemia. In Neoplastic diseases of the blood (ed. PH Wiernik, GP Canellos, and RA Kyle, et al.), pp. 357–81. Churchill Livingstone, New York.

Kohn HI, Fry RJM (1984). Radiation carcinogenesis. New England Journal of Medicine, 310:504–11.

Koyama H, et al. (1980). Surgical adjuvant chemotherapy with mitomycin C and cyclophosphamide in Japanese patients with breast cancer. Cancer, 46:2373–9.

Knudson AG Jr (1983). Hereditary cancers of man. Cancer Investigations, 1:187–93.

Krikorian JG, et al. (1979). Occurrence of non-Hodgkin's lymphoma after therapy for Hodgkin's disease. A study of 21 patients. New England Journal of Medicine, 300:452–8.

Le Beau MM, et al. (1986). Clinical and cytogenetic correlations in 63 patients with therapy-related myelodysplastic syndromes and acute nonlymphocytic leukemia: further evidence for characteristic abnormalities of chromosomes no. 5 and 7. Journal of Clinical Oncology, 4:325–45.

Lerner HJ (1978). Acute myelogenous leukemia in patients receiving chlorambucil as long-term adjuvant chemotherapy for stage II breast cancer. Cancer Treatment Reports, 62:1135–8.

List AL, Doll DC, Greco FA (1985). Lung cancer in Hodgkin's disease: association with previous radiotherapy. *Journal of Clinical Oncology*, 3: 215–21.

Lynch HT, Frichot BC III (1978). Skin, heredity, and cancer. *Seminars in Oncology*, 5:67–84.

McKeen EA, *et al.* (1979). Rhabdomyosarcoma complicating multiple neurofibromatosis. *Journal of Pediatrics*, 94:173–4.

Makuch R, Simon R (1979). Recommendations for the analysis of the effect of treatment on the development of second malignancies. *Cancer*, 44:250–3.

Meadows AT, *et al.* (1985). Second malignant neoplasms in children: an update from the Late Effects Study Group. *Journal of Clinical Oncology*, 3:532–8.

Melbye M, *et al.* (1987). HLA studies of endemic African Kaposi's sarcoma patients and matched controls: no association with HLA-DR5. *International Journal of Cancer*, 39:182–4.

Moertel CG (1977). Multiple primary malignant neoplasms. *Cancer*, 40:1786–92.

Mulvihill JJ (1977). Genetic repertory of human neoplasia. In *Genetics of human cancer* (ed. JJ Mulvihill, RW Miller, and JF Fraumeni Jr), pp. 137–43. Raven Press, New York.

National Research Council, Committee on the Biological Effects of Ionizing Radiations (1980). *The effects on populations of exposure to low levels of ionizing radiation*. National Academy of Science, Washington, DC.

Nordenskjold M, Cavenee WB (1988). Genetics and the etiology of solid tumors. In *Important advances in oncology 1988* (ed. VT De Vita Jr, S Hellman, and SA Rosenberg), pp. 83–101. JB Lippincott, Philadelphia.

Pedersen-Bjergaard J (1985). Incidence, previous treatment and chromosome characteristics of secondary acute non-lymphocytic leukemia. *Cancer Treatment Reviews*, 12:65–75.

Pedersen-Bjergaard J, Larsen SO (1982). Incidence of acute nonlymphocytic leukemia, preleukemia, and acute myeloproliferative syndrome up to 10 years after treatment of Hodgkin's disease. *New England Journal of Medicine*, 307:965–71.

Pedersen-Bjergaard J, Philip P (1991). Two different classes of therapy-related and *de-novo* acute myeloid leukemia? *Cancer Genetics and Cytogenetics*, 55:119–24.

Penn I (1990). Cancers complicating organ transplantation. *New England Journal of Medicine*, 323:1767–8.

Pollack MS, *et al.* (1984). Classical and AIDs Kaposi sarcoma. In *Histocompatibility testing 1984* (ed. ED Albert, MP Baur, and WR Mayr), pp. 403–6. Springer-Verlag, New York.

Preston DL, *et al.* (1987). Studies of the mortality of A-bomb survivors. *Radiation Research*, 111:151–78.

Rieche K (1984). Carcinogenicity of antineoplastic agents in man. *Cancer Treatment Reviews*, 11:39–67.

Rimm IJ, *et al.* (1987). Brain tumors after cranial irradiation for childhood acute lymphoblastic leukemia. *Cancer*, 59:1506–8.

Rosner F, Grunwald H (1980). Multiple myeloma and Waldenstrom's macroglobulinemia terminating in acute leukemia. *New York State Journal of Medicine*, 80:558.

Rosner F, Carey RW, Zarrabi MH (1978). Breast cancer and acute leukemia: report of 24 cases and review of the literature. *American Journal of Hematology*, 4:151–72.

Schmähl D, Habs M (1978). Experimental carcinogenesis of antitumour drugs. *Cancer Treatment Reviews*, 5:175–84.

Sieber SM (1977). The action of antitumor agents: a double-edged sword? *Medical and Pediatric Oncology*, 3:123–31.

Tester WJ, *et al.* (1984). Second malignant neoplasms complicating Hodgkin's disease: the National Cancer Institute experience. *Journal of Clinical Oncology*, 7:762–9.

Tomatis L, *et al.* (1978). Evaluation of carcinogenicity of chemicals: a review. *Cancer Research*, 38:877–85.

Tucker MA, *et al.* (1985). Cutaneous malignant melanoma after Hodgkin's disease. *Annals of Internal Medicine*, 102:37–41.

Tucker MA, *et al.* (1987). Bone sarcomas linked to radiotherapy and chemotherapy in children. *New England Journal of Medicine*, 317:588–93.

Tucker MA, *et al.* (1988). Risk of second cancers after treatment for Hodgkin's disease. *New England Journal of Medicine*, 318:76–81.

Tucker MA, *et al.* (1991). Therapeutic radiation at a young age is linked to secondary thyroid cancer. *Cancer Research*, 51:2885–8.

Upton AC (1977). Radiological effects of low doses: implications for radiological protection. *Radiation Research*, 71:51–74.

Valagussa P, *et al.* (1980). Second malignancies in Hodgkin's disease: a complication of certain forms of treatment. *British Medical Journal*, 280:216–19.

Valagussa P, *et al.* (1982). Absence of treatment-induced second neoplasms after ABVD in Hodgkin's disease. *Blood*, 59:488–94.

Valagussa P, *et al.* (1986). Second acute leukemia and other malignancies following treatment for Hodgkin's disease. *Journal of Clinical Oncology*, 4:830–7.

Valagussa P, Tancini G, Bonadonna G (1987). Second malignancies after CMF for resectable breast cancer. *Journal of Clinical Oncology*, 5:1138–42.

Valagussa P, *et al.* (1994). Second malignancies following CMF-based adjuvant chemotherapy in resectable breast cancer. (In press.)

van Leeuwen FE, *et al.* (1989). Increased risk of lung cancer, non-Hodgkin's lymphoma, and leukemia following Hodgkin's disease. *Journal of Clinical Oncology*, 7:1046–58.

Weisburger JH, *et al.* (1975). The carcinogenic properties of some of the principal drugs used in clinical cancer chemotherapy. *Recent Results in Cancer Research*, 52:1–17.

Witherspoon RP, *et al.* (1989). Secondary cancers after bone marrow transplantation for leukemia or aplastic anemia. *New England Journal of Medicine*, 321:784–9.

19.13 Supportive care, anti-emetics, and alimentation

MAURIZIO TONATO AND FAUSTO ROILA

Nausea and vomiting are the most distressing symptoms experienced by cancer patients submitted to chemotherapy (Coates *et al.* 1983). Possible consequences of vomiting are impairment of nutritional status, metabolic complications (metabolic alkalosis, dehydration, hyperazotemia), gastric/oesophageal bleeding, negative psychological and sociological implications, refusal of treatment, and choice of less emetogenic but also less effective chemotherapeutic agents.

During the last few years considerable progress has been made in the pharmacological treatment of nausea and vomiting induced by antineoplastic agents. Despite this, emesis remains a critical problem in cancer chemotherapy, particularly in some subgroups of patients and with certain drugs.

As illustrated in Table 1, antineoplastic agents vary considerably in their emetic potential. In addition, the emetic activity and pattern

Table 1 Emetogenic potential of cancer chemotherapeutic agents

High	Moderate	Low
Cisplatin	Cyclophosphamide	Methotrexate
Dacarbazine	Cytosine arabinoside	Mitomycin C
Mechlorethamine	Anthracyclines	Bleomycin
Dactinomycin	Carboplatin	Busulphan
	Nitrosoureas	Chlorambucil
	Procarbazine	Melphalan
		Hydroxyurea
		Etoposide
		Teniposide
		Fluorouracil
		Vinca alkaloids

of drugs vary according to their dose and administration schedule. For example, cisplatin induces nausea and/or vomiting in almost 100 per cent of patients. Vomiting usually begins 2–3 h after its administration, reaches its maximal intensity after 5–6 h, and thereafter appears only sporadically. Patients who do not vomit within the first 8 h rarely vomit during the following 16 h (approximately 1.2 per cent of treated patients) (Roila *et al.* 1989). However, delayed emesis, beginning 24 h after chemotherapy, is an adjunctive problem in 20–85 per cent of patients treated with the drug.

Low doses of cisplatin (for example, 20 mg/m^2) induce less vomiting than doses of 50 mg/m^2 or above and therefore emesis due to such doses can be more easily prevented. When doses greater than 50 mg/m^2 are used there is an increase in emetogenic potential as the dose increases (Roila *et al.* 1985, 1987*a*). The schedule of cisplatin administration is also important. Lengthening the duration of its infusion from 1 to 8 h results in a significant decrease in vomiting episodes (Jordan *et al.* 1985) and when the drug is administered in divided doses during consecutive days a tolerance to emetic effect is observed. In fact, nausea and vomiting may peak during the first 2 days of chemotherapy but then gradually decrease until they disappear on days 4 or 5.

Cyclophosphamide induces vomiting beginning 6–12 h after its administration (Fetting *et al.* 1982*a*). The latency of the emetic effect can be explained by the time required for the production in the liver of phosphoramide mustard and other metabolites which have strong emetic potential (Fetting *et al.* 1982*b*). Again, in this case the dose and administration schedule are important. Nausea and vomiting are more frequent after intravenous CMF (cyclophosphamide, methotrexate, 5-fluorouracil) than after 'standard' CMF where the cyclophosphamide is given orally for 2 weeks.

PATHOPHYSIOLOGY OF CHEMOTHERAPY-INDUCED EMESIS

The sites of emetic action of antineoplastic agents have not been well defined. The act of vomiting is controlled by the vomiting centre which is located in the lateral reticular formation in the floor of the fourth ventricle. Stimulated by afferent impulses, it coordinates the emetic response. Impulses arrive at the vomiting centre from the following regions:

(1) the chemoreceptor trigger zone located within the area postrema on the fourth ventricle, which can be stimulated by substances contained in either the blood or the cerebrospinal fluid;

(2) the gastrointestinal tract via sympathetic and vagal pathways;

(3) the higher cortical centres which transmit psychogenic stimuli;

(4) the vestibular apparatus of the middle ear (this does not seem to be important for chemotherapy-induced nausea and vomiting).

The precise neurotransmitters involved in nausea and vomiting due to antineoplastic agents have not yet been identified. However, various neuroreceptors have been pinpointed in or around the area postrema and in the gastrointestinal tract, including dopaminergic, cholinergic, and H_1 and H_2 histaminergic, opioid, and serotoninergic receptors. These 5-hydroxytryptamine (5-HT) receptors have recently been classified into three main types with evidence of subtypes in some of them (Bradley *et al.* 1986) (Table 2).

Among the 5-HT receptors, 5-HT$_3$ seems to play a determinant role in chemotherapy-induced nausea and vomiting (Tyers *et al.* 1989). In fact, in experimental studies in animals some anti-emetic drugs such as sulpiride or domperidone, which are potent antagonists of dopamine (D$_2$) receptors, have been shown to be ineffective in the prevention of cisplatin-induced nausea and vomiting, while the selective 5-HT$_3$ receptor antagonists induced a high rate of complete protection from vomiting.

The precise site of action of 5-HT$_3$ receptor antagonists has not yet been identified, but two hypotheses have been formulated. The

Table 2 Classification of 5-HT receptors

Receptor type	Selective agonist	Available antagonists	Comment
5-HT$_1$	5-Carboxamidotryptamine	Methiotepin	At least four subtypes identified
5-HT$_1$-like		Methysergide	
5-HT$_2$	Methyl-5-HT	Ketanserin	No definitive evidence of subtypes
		Methiotepin	
		Methysergide	
5-HT$_3$	2-Methyl-5-HT	Ondansetron	Species-specific subtypes identified
		Granisetron	
		Tropisetron	
		Batanopride	
		Dolasetron	

2359

first, based on the fact that damage of gastrointestinal mucosa and modifications of its 5-HT and 5-hydroxyindolacetic acid levels have been shown in the ferret after cisplatin administration, has suggested a peripheral action. Indeed, chemotherapeutic agents determine 5-HT release from the enterochromaffin cells in the upper gastrointestinal mucosa. 5-HT, stimulating $5-HT_3$ receptors on vagal afferent fibres, acts centrally on the chemoreceptor trigger zone and/or the vomiting centre and induces nausea and vomiting (Andrews *et al.* 1988).

The second hypothesis, which suggests a central mechanism of action of the $5-HT_3$ receptor antagonists, is based on the presence of several neurones containing 5-HT and a high concentration of $5-HT_3$ receptors in the area postrema. The depletion of 5-HT from the area postrema and injection of $5-HT_3$ receptor antagonists in the same area inhibits cisplatin-induced emesis (Higgins *et al.* 1989).

A possible role for the $5-HT_1$ receptors has recently been suggested (Lucot and Crampton 1989). The administration of $5-HT_1$ antagonists (buspirone, 8-OH-DPAT) in the cat suppresses the vomiting induced by different emetic stimuli (cisplatin, motion sickness, etc.). This suggests that $5-HT_1$ antagonists exert their action on a common convergent structure that could be the vomiting centre. No studies verifying this hypothesis in man have yet been published. Finally, it is also possible that the antineoplastic agents act on different sites and stimulate different receptors so that a combination of anti-emetic agents may produce better results than single drugs (Peroutka and Snyder 1982).

ANTI-EMETICS

A classification of the most common anti-emetic agents is shown in Table 3. Their efficacy has been demonstrated in many studies, although these vary significantly in their design, patient selection, and methods of evaluation. The following is a concise description of the drugs used in the most frequently encountered emetic problem, that is, emesis due to cisplatin chemotherapy. Anti-emetics used in patients treated with chemotherapy without cisplatin will then be considered.

Table 3 Anti-emetic agents

Antidopaminergics	$5-HT_3$ antagonists
Phenothiazines	Ondansetron
Prochlorperazine	Granisetron
Chlorpromazine	Zacopride
Thiethylperazine	Batanopride
Perphenazine	Tropisetron
	Dolasetron
Butyrophenones	**Antihistamines**
Haloperidol	Diphenhydramine
Droperidol	
	Corticosteroids
Metoclopramide	Methylprednisolone
Domperidone	Dexamethasone
New benzamide derivatives	**Benzodiazepines**
Alizapride	Lorazepam
Clebopride	Diazepam
Dazopride	
	Cannabinoids
	Tetrahydrocannabinol
	Nabilone
	Levonantradol

Anti-emetics in patients submitted to cisplatin chemotherapy

Metoclopramide

This procainamide derivative is minimally effective at standard doses (10–20 mg) for the prevention of nausea and vomiting induced by cisplatin chemotherapy.

On the basis of a dose–response correlation shown in animal experiments, metoclopramide has been tested in a pilot study at increasing doses (from 0.4 to 3 mg/kg). The drug was moderately toxic and an optimal anti-emetic activity was obtained with a single dose of at least 1.5 mg/kg (Gralla *et al.* 1981*a*). Subsequently, two placebo-controlled trials (Gralla *et al.* 1981*b*; Homesley *et al.* 1982) and several open trials confirmed that metoclopramide at doses of 1–3 mg/kg administered every 2 h three to six times per day was significantly superior to placebo and induced a complete protection from vomiting in approximately 30–40 per cent of cisplatin-treated patients.

The main side-effects of this treatment were sedation, which was generally mild and well accepted by the patient, diarrhoea (10–20 per cent of cases), which can also be caused by cisplatin, and particularly extrapyramidal reactions (akathisia, trismus, osculogyric crisis). The incidence of this last side-effect, which is rapidly reversible with diphenhydramine administration, is low (3–5 per cent) except in patients less than 30 years old in whom it can reach 25–30 per cent (Kris *et al.* 1983).

The optimal dose and schedule of metoclopramide have not yet been defined. Only a few clinical trials have compared different high doses and their design was frequently inadequate and the population studied too small to draw definitive conclusions. Furthermore, pharmacokinetic data show that metoclopramide at doses of 2 mg/kg repeated every 2 h accumulates in the body, while an intravenous bolus followed by continuous infusion produces constant plasma concentrations even though there are interpatient variations.

Three studies have compared intermittent administration versus continuous infusion of metoclopramide. The results, concerning efficacy, toxicity, and patient preference, are contradictory (Warrington *et al.* 1986; Dana *et al.* 1987; Navari 1989).

Steroids

The mechanism of action of steroids is unknown, although a possible antiprostaglandin effect has been suggested. In four double-blind trials steroids (dexamethasone and methylprednisolone) have not been demonstrated to have superior efficacy to placebo (Dana *et al.* 1985; D'Olimpo *et al.* 1985; Schallier *et al.* 1985; Metz *et al.* 1987), although two of these studies did report a minor difference in the duration of nausea (Dana *et al.* 1985; D'Olimpo *et al.* 1985). Other studies, all including only a few patients, compared steroids with high-dose intravenous metoclopramide. In two trials steroids had the same efficacy as metoclopramide, while in two others they were statistically less efficacious (Cognetti *et al.* 1984; Benrubi *et al.* 1985; Frustaci *et al.* 1986; Shinkai *et al.* 1986).

Steroid toxicity is mild, although the possibility of a potential negative interaction with the antitumour effect of chemotherapy and of a risk of infectious complications should be considered. At present, however, these possibilities have not been clearly demonstrated in man. Owing to their low toxicity and limited activity, steroids are probably most useful in combination with other anti-emetic drugs.

Combination of high-dose MTC plus steroids

Several trials (Allan *et al.* 1984; Kris *et al.* 1985*a*; Strum *et al.* 1985; Bécouarn *et al.* 1986; Roila *et al.* 1987*a*) have evaluated the activity of the association of metoclopramide with dexamethasone or methylprednisolone versus metoclopramide alone. The anti-emetic combination significantly increased complete protection from vomiting (from 30–40 per cent with metoclopramide alone to 45–55 per cent with metoclopramide plus steroids). Furthermore, a significant decrease in the incidence of diarrhoea was shown in some studies (Allan *et al.* 1984; Kris *et al.* 1985*a*).

Combination of three or more anti-emetic drugs

It has been postulated that more drugs with different mechanisms of action and toxicity might improve efficacy. This concept is based on the presence of different neuroreceptors in or around the chemoreceptor trigger zone and on the differences in the potency of the various drugs in blocking them (Peroutka and Snyder 1982). In an attempt to increase complete protection from emesis in cisplatin-treated patients, several studies using three or more anti-emetic combinations have been performed. Open studies in patients with vomiting who are refractory to high-dose metoclopramide have shown that some patients could be protected with a combination of three or more anti-emetic drugs (metoclopramide, dexamethasone, diphenhydramine, a phenotiazine, and sometimes benzodiazepine). When these combinations were evaluated in open studies using untreated patients, the rate of complete protection from vomiting was usually above 60 per cent.

Only a few double-blind trials comparing various anti-emetic combinations have been published. Three of these merit attention as they add important knowledge about the optimal prevention of cisplatin-induced emesis as well as the limitations of these anti-emetic regimens. In the first trial (Roila *et al.* 1989) involving 367 patients the metoclopramide (3 mg/kg×2 i.v.) plus dexamethasone (20 mg) plus diphenhydramine (50 mg) combination was significantly superior to metoclopramide (1 mg/kg×4 i.v.) plus methylprednisolone (250 mg×2 i.v.). Complete protection from vomiting was obtained in 72 per cent and 56 per cent of patients, respectively. Furthermore, the use of diphenhydramine, while increasing the rate of mild sedation, significantly decreases the incidence of extrapyramidal reactions, nervousness, and sweating. These results are probably due to the higher single dose of metoclopramide (resulting in an antiserotoninergic effect as shown in animal experiments), although a diphenhydramine anti-emetic action cannot be excluded. Unfortunately, with both anti-emetic regimens, complete protection from vomiting decreases significantly after the first subsequent cycle of chemotherapy (Roila *et al.* 1989) making the efficacy of the metoclopramide combination regimens even less satisfactory in non-chemotherapy-naïve patients.

In the second trial involving 120 patients, where the same three-drug combination was compared with metoclopramide plus dexamethasone at the same doses plus lorazepam (1.5 mg/m² i.v.), a similar complete protection from vomiting was shown (56 per cent and 63 per cent, respectively), with lorazepam decreasing the incidence of agitation and akathisia (Kris *et al.* 1987). The third trial was a double-blind cross-over study aimed at identifying the best metoclopramide dosage and schedule. It compared one single higher dose of intravenous metoclopramide (4 mg/kg 0.5 h before cisplatin) with two separate doses of metoclopramide (3 mg/kg), both combined with dexamethasone and diphenhydramine, in 56 cancer patients (Roila *et al.* 1991*a*). The efficacy and tolerability of the two regimens were found to be similar, making the single-dose metoclopramide, dexamethasone, and diphenhydramine regimen preferable because of patient convenience and the lower cost.

Cannabinoids

Anecdotal experiences of decreased emesis in younger patients who used marijuana while receiving chemotherapy have stimulated the clinical evaluation of cannabinoids. In a double-blind trial, delta-9-tetrahydrocannabinol showed less anti-emetic efficacy and more toxicity than high-dose intravenous metoclopramide in cisplatin-treated patients (Gralla *et al.* 1984). The other two cannabinoids, nabilone and levonantradol, have not been compared with high-dose intravenous metoclopramide.

Phenotiazines

Prochlorperazine, the most studied of this class of drugs, has been ineffective at standard oral or parenteral doses in preventing nausea and vomiting induced by cisplatin and is significantly inferior to high-dose intravenous metoclopramide (Gralla *et al.* 1981*b*). Moreover, the activity of prochlorperazine is dose dependent and a single dose of 30–40 mg, when combined with diphenhydramine, seems to increase its anti-emetic efficacy without increasing toxicity (Carr *et al.* 1987). A double-blind trial comparing high-dose prochlorperazine with high-dose intravenous metoclopramide, both combined with dexamethasone and lorazepam, has recently been reported. The two anti-emetic regimens were equally effective and safe (Carr *et al.* 1989).

Butyrophenones

Haloperidol and, more often, droperidol have been evaluated in patients treated with cisplatin. The results of double-blind trials comparing droperidol with high-dose metoclopramide are contradictory. Two studies (Lewis *et al.* 1984; Saller and Hellenbrecht 1986) have shown an inferior activity, and two others (Cronin *et al.* 1985; Govil *et al.* 1985), published as abstracts only, showed a similar activity. In all these trials droperidol was used at doses lower than those identified as being optimal in pilot studies (Kelley *et al.* 1986).

Domperidone

Data on the efficacy of domperidone have been conflicting. Because of serious side-effects associated with its parenteral administration (unexpected deaths, seizures, and cardiovascular arrests) further clinical evaluation has been suspended.

Benzodiazepines

Although lorazepam may have an intrinsic anti-emetic action, this still has not been definitely demonstrated in cisplatin-treated patients. However, it does increase the tolerability of nausea and vomiting by inducing an amnesic anxiolytic effect. Furthermore, because it reduces the risk of extrapyramidal reactions from high-dose intravenous metoclopramide, lorazepam can be useful in anti-emetic combination regimens. Its main side-effect is moderate sedation in all patients.

Table 4 Ondansetron versus metoclopramide in cisplatin-treated patients

No. of patients	Cisplatin doses (mg/m²)	Anti-emetics	Dose	CP (%)	Result	Reference
97	80–100	Ondansetron	8 mg bolus+1 mg/h CI for 24 h	46	OND>MTC	Marty et al. (1990)
		Metoclopramide	3 mg/kg bolus+0.5 mg/kg/h CI for 8 h	17	<Toxicity >preference	
121	50–100	Ondansetron	8 mg bolus+1 mg/h CI for 24 h	72*	OND>MTC	Van Liessum et al. (1989)[a]
		Metoclopramide	3 mg/kg bolus+0.5 mg/kg/h CI for 8 h	41*	<Toxicity >preference	
307	100	Ondansetron	0.15 mg/kg×3	40	OND>MTC	Pendergrass et al. (1990)[a]
		Metoclopramide	2 mg/kg×6	30	<Toxicity	

CP, complete protection; CI, continuous infusion.
[a] Complete plus major responses

New benzamide anti-emetics

In an attempt to separate the therapeutic activity of metoclopramide from its undesirable side-effects, new drugs have been synthesized by modifying its basic side chain (clebopride, dazopride, etc.) as well as by substituting its aromatic ring (alizapride, sulpiride, etc.). Except for alizapride, benzamides have not been extensively studied with respect to the prevention of cisplatin-induced nausea and vomiting.

In pilot studies alizapride showed a good anti-emetic activity with very low toxicity. When it was compared with high-dose intravenous metoclopramide in double-blind trials, alizapride was significantly less efficacious and induced more side-effects (hypotension, diarrhoea, sweating) (Saller and Hellenbrecht 1985; Joss et al. 1986; Basurto et al. 1988a).

5-HT₃ receptor antagonists

These new compounds have been obtained by modification of the 2-substituent on the benzene ring of metoclopramide. They are devoid of dopamine antagonist activity and their anti-emetic activity is mediated by a selective antagonism of $5-HT_3$ receptors. Ondansetron (GR38032F), granisetron (BRL43694), zacopride, tropisetron, batanopride and dolasetron are the most representative drugs of this new class. In animal experiments they have proved to be potent and effective antagonists of cisplatin-induced emesis.

Ondansetron

Ondansetron is the most widely studied compound and has been marketed in various countries in oral and intravenous formulations.

In several pilot studies of patients submitted to cisplatin chemotherapy at doses of 50 mg/m² or above, ondansetron gave 35–55 per cent complete protection from vomiting. Optimal doses of ondansetron for prevention of cisplatin-induced vomiting are believed to be 0.15 mg/kg (or 8 mg) in bolus followed by a continuous infusion of 1 mg/hour for 24 hours or by two further bolus doses every 2 or 4 h.

Three controlled studies (Van Liessum et al. 1989; Marty et al. 1990a; Pendergrass et al. 1990) comparing ondansetron with high-dose metoclopramide in cisplatin-treated patients have been published (Table 4). In all three, ondansetron showed more anti-emetic activity and fewer adverse effects than metoclopramide and in the two cross-over studies was preferred by the patients. Complete protection from vomiting was obtained in 40–45 per cent of patients.

An increase in the anti-emetic efficacy of ondansetron when combined with dexamethasone has recently been shown in both ferrets and man (Cunningham et al. 1989; Hawthorn and Cunningham 1990; Smith et al. 1990). Based on this information, a double-blind cross-over study comparing ondansetron alone with ondansetron plus dexamethasone (20 mg i.v.) was carried out in an Italian cooperative study (Roila et al. 1991b). The combination was significantly superior to the single drug (91 versus 64 per cent complete protection from vomiting) and was preferred by the patients. The next logical step in the search for the best treatment in the prevention of cisplatin-induced acute emesis was to compare ondansetron plus dexamethasone with a standard three-drug anti-emetic combination containing meto-clopramide.

The first of these studies has recently been reported (Roila et al. 1992a). It was a multicentre randomized double-blind study including 289 patients receiving cisplatin ≥50 mg/m². Ondansetron+dexamethasone was shown to be significantly more efficacious than metoclopramide+dexamethasone+diphenhydramine. Complete protection from vomiting was obtained in 78.7 and 59.5 per cent of patients, respectively, on day 1 after cisplatin adminstration. Furthermore, complete protection from vomiting was significantly better with ondansetron+dexamethasone versus the three-drug combination even on day 2 (83.9 versus 68.0 per cent) and day 3 (86.3 versus 7.12 per cent) after cisplatin administration, while all patients were receiving the same anti-emetics for prophylaxis of delayed emesis. Adverse events were also significantly less frequent with the ondansetron+dexamethasone regimen. In particular, slight sedation was reported by 2.1 per cent of patients treated with ondansetron versus 11.8 per cent of those receiving the high-dose metoclopramide regimen, while extrapyramidal reactions were observed only with metoclopramide (2.7 per cent).

In conclusion, ondansetron plus dexamethasone seems to be the most efficacious and least toxic anti-emetic therapy presently available for prevention of cisplatin-induced acute emesis. Furthermore, the anti-emetic efficacy of ondansetron, unlike metoclopramide, can be maintained in subsequent cycles of cisplatin chemotherapy (Italian Group for Antiemetic Research 1993).

Recently, three large studies have re-evaluated the problem of the optimal dose and schedule of ondansetron (Marty et al. 1990a; Beck et al. 1992; Seynaeve et al. 1992). In two double-blind studies (Marty et al. 1990a; Seynaeve et al. 1992) a single 32 mg intravenous dose of ondansetron administered before cisplatin showed a similar efficacy and toxicity compared with an 8 mg loading dose followed by a 24 h infusion of 1 mg/h.

One of these studies (Seynaeve *et al.* 1992) involving 535 patients included a third treatment arm in which patients received only a single 8 mg intravenous dose before cisplatin chemotherapy. Control of emesis was similar in all three groups, with complete protection from vomiting in approximately 55 per cent of patients.

However, these results were not confirmed in a double-blind study evaluating 699 patients (Beck *et al.* 1992). In fact, the efficacy of an 8 mg intravenous single dose and that of intravenous ondansetron 0.15 mg/kg every 4 h for three doses was shown to be inferior to a 32 mg intravenous single dose.

More studies are therefore needed to clarify the optimal dose and schedule of ondansetron.

When cisplatin is administered at low doses (20–40 mg/m^2) for several days (a condition in which repeated high doses of metoclopramide induce a high rate of extrapyramidal reactions) ondansetron could be particularly helpful. Initial experiences (Nagy *et al.* 1988; Hainsworth *et al.* 1989) using 0.15 mg/kg three times daily for 4–5 days showed a range of complete protection from vomiting in 42–83 per cent of patients.

Two double-blind comparative studies have been published in which ondansetron was compared with metoclopramide used alone (Sledge *et al.* 1992*b*) or both in combination with dexamethasone (Weissbach 1991). Ondansetron in both studies was more efficacious than metoclopramide when used alone and in combination with dexamethasone. Furthermore, while the incidence of extrapyramidal reactions in metoclopramide recipients was very high, resulting in one study (Weissbach 1991) in the interruption of anti-emetic treatment after the first 2 days of cisplatin in 23 per cent of patients, the tolerability of repeated doses of ondansetron was very good. Therefore, in this particular group of patients, the combination of ondansetron plus dexamethasone, offering good efficacy and low toxicity, should probably be considered the anti-emetic therapy of choice.

Adverse effects are generally mild and infrequent. Only three cases of extrapyramidal reactions have been reported (Dobrow *et al.* 1991; Halperin and Murphy 1992; Garcia-del-Muro *et al.* 1993). In the first, the patient had already received an antidopaminergic drug (droperidol) as an anti-emetic and therefore the relationship between ondansetron and the extrapyramidal reaction is questionable (Kanarek *et al.* 1992). In the third case the extrapyramidal reaction occurred immediately after the seventh dose of ondansetron (0.15 mg/kg three times daily). The episode lasted 1–2 min and resolved spontaneously. The reaction did not recur after subsequent doses of ondansetron administered as a 15 min intravenous infusion.

The most frequent adverse effects are headache (approximately 20 per cent of patients) and constipation (5–10 per cent). The transitory increase in transaminase levels shown in pilot studies was probably secondary to cisplatin itself. In fact, when ondansetron was compared with metoclopramide the incidence of this adverse effect was similar in the two groups of patients (Smith 1989). Furthermore, a retrospective study showed a dose-related effect and cumulative dose effect of cisplatin on hepatic transaminase values (Hesketh *et al.* 1990).

Recently, a possible relationship between ondansetron and angina has been reported in seven patients receiving various antineoplastic agents (Ballard *et al.* 1992). Thrombocytopenia, renal insufficiency and thrombotic episodes in eight patients receiving ondansetron and cisplatin chemotherapy have also been described (Coates *et al.* 1992). On the other hand, an analysis of all patients entering comparative clinical trials of ondansetron has shown that vascular occlusive events were uncommon and occurred with equal frequency in patients receiving ondansetron and those receiving comparator drugs (Castle *et al.* 1992; Gralla 1991).

Granisetron

This drug is marketed in several countries, but only as an intravenous formulation. There is, however, less published data concerning its pharmacological and clinical profile in patients undergoing chemotherapy than for ondansetron. Granisetron has a more prolonged half-life (approximately 9–11 h) than ondansetron (Addelman *et al.* 1990) but this is not important in terms of dose and schedules.

When used as a single-dose administration of 40 or 100 μg/kg, granisetron induced 16–50 per cent complete protection from vomiting in pilot studies in cisplatin-treated patients. In two large controlled studies (Chevallier 1990; Warr 1991) granisetron showed similar efficacy and less toxicity than a combination of metoclopramide+dexamethasone (±diphenhydramine) (Table 5); however, metoclopramide and dexamethasone doses were different from those still considered optimal. In another study of cisplatin-treated patients a single dose of 40 μg/kg gave results similar to those using a single dose of 160 μg/kg (Soukop 1990). Recently, the efficacy of granisetron was compared with that of alizapride plus dexamethasone in the control of emesis in 142 patients receiving 5 consecutive days of cisplatin therapy. Complete protection from vomiting was obtained in a greater percentage of patients treated with granisetron (49 per cent) than with the combination (35 per cent), although this difference was not statistically significant (Bremer 1992).

Studies where intravenous granisetron has been evaluated in combination with corticosteroids have not yet been published. An oral formulation of the drug is under investigation. Preliminary results have been published in abstract form (Dott 1993) showing that in cisplatin recipients the addition of dexamethasone to granisetron (1 mg twice daily) increased the occurrence of complete protection from acute emesis compared with granisetron alone.

The tolerability profile of granisetron appears to be similar to that of ondansetron.

Tropisetron

Experience accumulated to date with tropisetron is very limited. Most studies have been published in sponsored symposium proceedings (van Oosterom and Bianco 1992; Joss 1993) and their design and methodology are far from satisfactory.

This drug has a long half-life (8–15 h). In patients undergoing high-dose cisplatin treatment, tropisetron has been evaluated in some pilot studies in doses varying from 5 to 48 mg/m^2, with complete protection from vomiting in 30–66 per cent of patients. On the basis of phase I–II studies an intravenous dose of 5 mg immediately before cisplatin administration was chosen for phase III studies. Only one multicentre randomized study has been published regarding prevention of acute emesis caused by cisplatin (Sorbe *et al.* 1994). In 260 patients 5 mg intravenous tropisetron was compared with a combination of high-dose intravenous metoclopramide (3 mg/kg in two doses) plus 20 mg intravenous dexamethasone with or without two doses of 1 mg intravenous lorazepam. The same percentage of patients (63 per cent) obtained complete protection from vomiting with the two treatments. The results of this study, however, must be interpreted with extreme caution as the percentage of complete responses among the various participating centres was extremely variable (from

Table 5 Granisetron: randomized studies in cisplatin-treated patients

Type of study	No. of patients	Cisplatin doses (mg/m^2)	Anti-emetic	CP (%)	Result	Reference
Single-blind	234	50	Granisetron 40 mg/kg	70	Granisetron=metoclopramide+dexamethasone	Chevallier (1990)
			Metoclopramide 3 mg×4 i.v. bolus+ 0.5 mg/kg/h for 8 h+ dexamethasone 12 mg i.v.	68	>Headache with granisetron Extrapyramidal reactions only with metoclopramide+ dexamethasone	
Double-blind	149	50	Granisetron 80 mg/kg	46	Granisetron=metoclopramide+dexamethasone+ diphenhydramine	Warr (1991)
			Metoclopramide 2 mg/kg×5 i.v.+ dexamethasone 10 mg i.v.+ diphenhydramine 50 mg i.v.	44	>Somnolence with metoclopramide+dexamethasone+ diphenhydramine	

CP, complete protection

30 to 100 per cent). Further studies are needed to clarify the therapeutic rôle of this drug.

Prognostic factors of cisplatin-induced acute emesis

Gender is probably the most important prognostic factor in conditioning the response to anti-emetic treatment. Consistent data from three large double-blind randomized clinical trials support this hypothesis and show that, irrespective of anti-emetic treatment, females vomit and experience nausea more frequently than males (Roila et al. 1985, 1987a, 1989). The gender of the patient also appears to affect the incidence of nausea and vomiting, irrespective of both chemotherapy regimen and primary cancer site.

The age of patients is another important variable in predicting the risk of nausea and vomiting. In one very large study (Roila et al. 1989), complete protection from vomiting and nausea was significantly better in older patients ($\geqslant$65 years, 73.9–78.3 per cent) than in younger patients (<50 years, 43.4–54.7 per cent). At present, the reasons for the effects of age on the results of anti-emetic therapy are unknown.

It is common opinion and experience that poorly controlled emesis in previous courses of chemotherapy predisposes a patient to unsatisfactory anti-emetic results in subsequent treatments. In a large multicentre double-blind trial patients were randomized to receive the same anti-emetic treatment for three consecutive cycles. Complete protection from vomiting on the first cycle of chemotherapy was 35 per cent for metoclopramide plus methylprednisolone and 67.6 per cent for metoclopramide plus dexamethasone plus diphenhydramine in patients who had received chemotherapy previously, whilst in those who had no protection it was observed in 62.1 per cent and 73.9 per cent of patients respectively (Roila et al. 1989). Furthermore, during the second and third cycle, irrespective of anti-emetic treatment, the probability of vomiting or experiencing nausea was significantly greater for those patients who had experienced vomiting or nausea in previous cycles. The fact that protection obtained in previous cycles of chemotherapy is one of the most important prognostic factors of cisplatin-induced emesis had been recently confirmed in another large double-blind study from our group (Italian Group for Antiemetic Research 1993).

Administration of antineoplastic agents on an out-patient basis is considered to be very convenient for many reasons. However, some studies have shown that in-patients experience less nausea and vomiting. This may very well be due to environmental factors which make them feel more protected.

Alcohol intake is another factor that can influence chemotherapy-induced emesis. Two trials, one prospective and the other retrospective (Sullivan et al. 1983; D'Acquisto et al. 1986), have shown that patients with a history of chronic heavy alcohol intake experience less cisplatin-induced nausea and vomiting than those who are not heavy drinkers. Complete protection from vomiting decreased from 93 per cent to 52 per cent. It has been postulated that long-term alcohol exposure decreases the sensitivity of the chemoreceptor trigger zone. However, these data should be accepted with caution as a selection bias related to the gender of heavy drinkers cannot be excluded. In fact, men, particularly those with head and neck cancer, also have a more frequent history of chronic ingestion of alcohol. At present, it is not known whether gender and chronic ingestion of alcohol are independent prognostic variables.

Delayed emesis from cisplatin

The importance of delayed emesis is increasing as its mechanism and natural history are better understood. Between 20 and 85 per cent of patients submitted to cisplatin chemotherapy present this form of emesis (Kris et al. 1985b; Grunberg et al. 1986). This large range is probably related to prognostic factors conditioning the phenomenon. In particular, it seems that patients treated with higher doses of cisplatin and patients who vomit during the first 24 h after cisplatin are more predisposed to it.

Few studies have evaluated anti-emetic drugs in the prevention of delayed emesis. However, a combination of oral dexamethasone and metoclopramide may be useful in patients submitted to cisplatin at doses of 120 mg/m^2 (Kris et al. 1989). Oral ondansetron has been evaluated in some pilot studies and has shown good anti-emetic efficacy. In one double-blind study (Gandara et al. 1991) ondansetron was shown to be superior to placebo for prevention of delayed emesis when administered orally at doses of 16 mg three times daily. However, another double-blind study (Grunberg et al. 1990) did not show any difference in anti-emetic efficacy between 2 and 16 mg of ondansetron three times daily.

Larger double-blind trials evaluating the role of the new 5-HT$_3$ antagonists administered orally both alone or combined with steroids are warranted.

Anticipatory emesis

Anticipatory emesis begins before the administration of chemotherapy. It is generally observed in patients who have suffered from poor anti-emetic control in previous courses of chemotherapy and is believed to be triggered by the hospital environment or other treatment-related factors (odours, sights, etc.). The best way to avoid this phenomenon is to prevent post-chemotherapy nausea and vomiting by using the most effective anti-emetic regimens available from the very first cycle of chemotherapy. The behavioural therapy approach can be successful in the control of anticipatory emesis.

Anti-emetics in patients treated with chemotherapy without cisplatin

Relatively few anti-emetic therapy trials have been conducted in selected patients submitted to antineoplastic agents without cisplatin. Dacarbazine, alone or in combination with cyclophosphamide, vincristine, and doxorubicin (CYVADIC), is considered one of the most emetic anticancer agents, with virtually all patients receiving it experiencing nausea and vomiting.

In a pilot trial and then in a double-blind trial (Tyson et al. 1982; Basurto et al. 1989), high-dose intravenous metoclopramide (2 mg/kg) induced complete protection from vomiting in over 60 per cent of patients. When metoclopramide was combined with methylprednisolone (250 mg×2 i.v.) an increase in anti-emetic activity was demonstrated in patients submitted to consecutive days of dacarbazine chemotherapy (Basurto et al. 1989).

Doxorubicin, either alone or in combination with cyclophosphamide and vincristine or with 5-fluorouracil and cyclophosphamide, has been reported to produce vomiting in approximately 60 per cent of patients. Conflicting data have been published regarding the efficacy of metoclopramide in preventing emesis due to doxorubicin (Mellink et al. 1984; Edge et al. 1987; Basurto et al. 1988b). Two double-blind trials have shown a high rate of complete protection with dexamethasone (20 mg i.v. followed by 10 mg×4 os every 6 h) (Markman et al. 1984) or methylprednisolone (125 mg i.v.×3 every 6 h) (Basurto et al. 1988b). Moreover, when compared with metoclopramide, methylprednisolone seems to have lower toxicity (Basurto et al. 1988b). An important prognostic factor for vomiting induced by doxorubicin is gender, with males vomiting less frequently than females (Mellink et al. 1984).

The intravenous CMF combination is frequently used to treat breast cancer induces emesis in 70–90 per cent of patients. Metoclopramide at standard oral doses (Morran et al. 1979) or high intravenous doses (David et al. 1984), as administered to cisplatin-treated patients, is no more efficacious than placebo. Instead, the use of 20 mg intravenously every 3 h for five doses induces complete protection in approximately 65 per cent of patients (Roila et al. 1988). This is probably due to the prolonged duration of anti-emetic treatment which allows protection from late vomiting episodes induced by cyclophosphamide.

Intravenous or intramuscular methylprednisolone induces complete protection from vomiting in approximately 70–80 per cent of CMF-treated patients (Chiara et al. 1987; Roila et al. 1987b, 1988). An open randomized trial comparing two different doses of methylprednisolone (40 mg and 125 mg) showed similar efficacy and tolerability (Chiara et al. 1987). Age is an important variable with younger CMF-treated patients vomiting significantly more than older ones (Roila et al. 1988). In conclusion, except for the prevention of dacarbazine-induced emesis, a highly emetogenic drug requiring a combination of high-dose metoclopramide plus steroids, it appears clear that corticosteroids are the most efficacious and well-tolerated anti-emetic agents for the preventive treatment of emesis induced by some of the most widely utilized regimens such as those containing doxorubicin and/or cyclophosphamide.

The availability of the new antiserotoninergic compounds has prompted many researchers to employ them in the prevention of emesis induced by moderately emetogenic antineoplastic agents. In several pilot studies, ondansetron was shown to have good efficacy even in patients refractory to the usual anti-emetic drugs. Recently, two studies comparing different oral dosages of ondansetron have been published. One of these (Fraschini et al. 1991), with 60 patients treated with doxorubicin plus cyclophosphamide, compared oral doses of 1, 4, and 8 mg three times daily. Ondansetron was very efficacious and its efficacy appeared to be dose related over this dose range, with an 8 mg dose inducing complete protection from vomiting in 85 per cent of patients. The other (Dicato 1991), performed in 324 patients receiving cyclophosphamide, doxorubicin, or epirubicin plus other non-cisplatin cytostatics, compared 8 mg ondansetron intravenously prior to chemotherapy followed by 8 mg orally two or three times daily. Both the two and three times daily schedules provided similar good control of nausea and emesis and were well tolerated. Therefore, from these studies it can be concluded that an 8 mg twice daily oral regimen of ondansetron could be a good and convenient choice in the prevention of emesis in out-patient treatment with these chemotherapy regimens.

At present, three multicentre double-blind trials have been performed in breast cancer patients treated with the fluorouracil+cyclophosphamide and fluorouracil+epirubicin+cyclophosphamide combinations (Bonneterre et al. 1990; Kaasa et al. 1990; Marschner et al. 1991b). In these studies 8 mg oral ondansetron three times daily was compared with 20 mg oral metoclopramide three times daily (first dose 60 mg intravenously). Complete protection from vomiting was always greater with ondansetron, although it reached a statistically significant difference in only one study. Both drugs were well tolerated, but metoclopramide induced extrapyramidal adverse effects in 5 per cent of patients.

Only one comparative double-blind trial has so far been published comparing ondansetron with dexamethasone (Jones et al. 1991). In 112 patients receiving intravenous anthracycline and/or cyclophosphamide and/or etoposide, dexamethasone (8 mg intravenously before chemotherapy and 4 mg orally four times daily on days 1 and 2, reduced to 2 mg four times daily on days 3 and 4 and to 1 mg four times daily on day 5) was shown to have similar efficacy as ondansetron (4 mg intravenously and 4 mg orally every 6 h on days 1–5) in controlling acute and delayed emesis. Both anti-emetic regimens were well tolerated.

Less clinical experience has been accumulated with other 5-HT$_3$ antagonists. Granisetron has been evaluated in some pilot studies and in three large controlled studies (Marty 1990b; Smith 1990; Warr et al. 1991).

The first trial (Smith 1990) was a double-blind study comparing two different doses of the drug (40 and 160 μg/kg). The complete protection from vomiting achieved was similar with the two dosages (76 and 81 per cent, respectively). The other two comparative studies, one single-blind (Marty 1990b) and the other double-blind (Warr et al. 1991), showed that intravenous granisetron had greater anti-emetic activity (40 or 80 μg/kg) than the combination of chlorpromazine or prochlorperazine plus dexamethasone (administered in a single dose before chemotherapy). Complete protection from vomiting was achieved in 70, 49, and 34 per cent of patients, respectively, and tolerability was also better in granisetron-treated patients. At present, no studies have been published comparing granisetron with steroids used at repeated doses every 4–6 h, probably the optimal treatment for the prevention of vomiting caused by drugs other than cisplatin.

On the basis of these data and considering the cost of 5-HT$_3$ antagonists, dexamethasone or methylprednisolone may remain the anti-emetics of choice for prevention of emesis induced by moderately emetogenic antineoplastic drugs.

ALIMENTATION AND CHEMOTHERAPY-INDUCED EMESIS

The alimentation of the patient undergoing chemotherapy, particularly with very emetogenic drugs, is an extremely difficult task despite the active anti-emetic treatments available. A patient affected by cancer is usually already in a malnourished state. Many possible factors contribute to this problem. These include the presence of a tumour obstructing the gastrointestinal tract, an altered sense of taste, depression, stress and the anxieties that accompany cancer, and an altered host metabolism. The nausea and vomiting induced by chemotherapy and radiotherapy add significantly to this malnutrition.

Other possible causes of decreased oral intake of food in cancer patients receiving chemotherapy are the mucositis that often accompanies the use of certain drugs, the learned food aversion, the intense dislike that develops as a result of the association of various foods with unpleasant gastrointestinal symptoms, the hepatotoxicity secondary to methotrexate and asparaginase, and infections both in the sense of dysphagia due to candidiasis and the severe catabolic state that exists during periods of sepsis (Kokal 1986). All these factors may contribute significantly to nutritional deficiencies.

The rôle of nutritional support of the cancer patient, with all its problems and perspectives, will be addressed in another chapter in this book. Here we would like to discuss some general concepts regarding alimentation of patients receiving chemotherapy and presenting with nausea and vomiting and to give some practical advice.

It is common experience that patients who receive highly emetogenic chemotherapy find it difficult to ingest any substantial amount of food on the same day as chemotherapy and therefore it is advisable that such patients do not eat for at least 8 h after treatment. A clear liquid diet may be best after this period, particularly fruit juices, effervescent sweet drinks, gelatin desserts, tea, or iced tea. It may be helpful to take beverages chilled. Ice lollipops, salty snacks, light soups with soda crackers, toast, and puddings are often well tolerated. We have found the general recommendation of taking frequent small meals, as opposed to three large meals a day, to be a most important factor in helping the patient who has difficulty in tolerating food. Food and drink should be taken slowly and food should not be forced past the point of tolerance. Rest after eating, possibly without lying down, is recommended. Excessively sweet, greasy, hot, or spicy foods and foods with strong odours should be avoided. Cold meat, sandwiches, cottage cheese, and other cold foods may be more appealing because they have less odour (Kelly 1986). If nausea occurs in the morning, techniques used for morning sickness during pregnancy, such as eating melba toast, dry toast, or crackers first thing in the morning, may also be helpful. Furthermore, an attractive table setting, foods with eye appeal, garnishes, and a good smell can also make a difference.

Considering the impact on the nutritional status and the psychological mood of the patient, every effort should be made to attempt to reduce nausea and vomiting with anti-emetic therapy and dietary measures. In the case of persistent deficient food intake, nutritional support should be provided. The type and amount of nutritional support will be determined by the patient's degree of weight loss, the rapidity of disease progression, the ultimate prognosis, the type of antineoplastic therapy in use, and the facilities available for the delivery and supervision of nutritional therapy. We believe that if antineoplastic therapy is to have a favourable outcome, aggressive nutritional support, such as total parenteral nutrition for leukaemic patients undergoing bone-marrow transplantation, is entirely justified. However, patients with progressive metastatic disease, although malnourished, will probably be better served by maintaining and supplementing their oral intake rather than starting parenteral hyperalimentation (Fearon and Calman 1986). However, aggressive nutritional support in these conditions has not been able to improve the response rate to treatment and overall survival or to reduce the chemotherapy-related toxicity. With total parenteral nutrition, only weight loss can be controlled; nausea and vomiting have been shown to be reduced in only one small study (Evans et al. 1987; Valdivieso et al. 1987).

Conclusions

In the last decade important advances have been made in the prevention of chemotherapy-induced nausea and vomiting. This has been a gradual process and at this point, some guidelines on the choice of the best anti-emetic treatments for different clinical situations can be given.

Cisplatin-induced acute emesis

For the prevention of acute emesis induced by a high single dose of cisplatin (>50 mg/m^2) or by low doses ($20-40$ mg/m^2) repeated for 4–5 days, the combination of ondansetron plus dexamethasone is the most efficacious and least toxic anti-emetic therapy available today. It is likely that this could also be true for other $\geqslant$ 5-HT$_3$ antagonists, but comparative data are still lacking. However, the metoclopramide plus dexamethasone combination, although significantly inferior and more toxic than ondansetron plus dexamethasone, also protects many patients from nausea and vomiting. Furthermore, the incidence of extrapyramidal reactions is low and generally easily controlled by appropriate therapy. Therefore, considering the high acquisition cost of ondansetron or other 5-HT$_3$ antagonists, the definitive choice can be based only on an appropriate pharmacoeconomic analysis, which is still lacking.

The combination of a 5-HT$_3$ antagonist plus dexamethasone should, instead, be routinely used in all patients receiving cisplatin on consecutive days because of the high extrapyramidal toxicity caused by high-dose metoclopramide-containing regimens when given for several days.

Cisplatin-induced delayed emesis

Orally administered metoclopramide plus dexamethasone is the standard treatment for delayed emesis induced by cisplatin used at doses of 120 mg/m^2. Whether this combination also works well with lower doses of cisplatin should be evaluated by double-blind comparative studies with placebo.

Other emetogenic chemotherapy

For the prevention of emesis induced by moderately emetogenic drugs, orally administered 5-HT$_3$ antagonists, although as efficacious as dexamethasone, are indicated only in those patients refractory to corticosteroids or in those who cannot use them because of their higher acquisition cost.

It is desirable that the knowledge acquired during the last few years find the widest possible clinical application in order to provide the best available anti-emetic treatment for every patient undergoing chemotherapy. At the same time, it is necessary to pursue new avenues of research to resolve definitively the problems of emesis induced by chemotherapy.

REFERENCES

Addelman M, *et al.* (1990). Phase I/II trial of granisetron: a novel 5-hydroxytryptamine antagonist for the prevention of chemotherapy-induced nausea and vomiting. *Journal of Clinical Oncology*, 8:337–41.

Allan SG, *et al.* (1984). Dexamethasone and high-dose metoclopramide: efficacy in controlling cisplatin induced nausea and vomiting. *British Medical Journal*, 13:235–7.

Andrews PLR, Rapeport WG, Sanger GJ (1988). Neuropharmacology of emesis induced by anti-cancer therapy. *Trends in the Physical Sciences*, 9:334–41.

Ballard HS, Bottino G, Bottino J (1992). Ondansetron and chest pain. *Lancet*, 340:1107.

Basurto C, *et al.* (1988*a*). A prospective randomized double-blind crossover study comparing the antiemetic activity of alizapride and metoclopramide in patients receiving cisplatin chemotherapy. *Cancer Investigation*, 6:475–9.

Basurto C, *et al.* (1988*b*). A double-blind trial comparing antiemetic efficacy and toxicity of metoclopramide versus methylprednisolone versus domperidone in patients receiving doxorubicin chemotherapy alone or in combination with other antiblastic agents. *American Journal of Clinical Oncology*, 11:594–6.

Basurto C, *et al.* (1989). Antiemetic activity of high-dose metoclopramide combined with methylprednisolone versus metoclopramide alone in dacarbazine-treated cancer patients. *American Journal of Clinical Oncology*, 12:235–8.

Beck TM, *et al.* (1992). Stratified, randomized, double-blind comparison of intravenous ondansetron administered as a multiple-dose regimen versus two single-dose regimens in the prevention of cisplatin-induced nausea and vomiting. *Journal of Clinical Oncology*, 10:1969–75.

Bécouarn Y, *et al.* (1986) Improved control of cisplatin-induced emesis with a combination of high doses of methylprednisolone and metoclopramide: a single-blind randomized trial. *European Journal of Cancer and Clinical Oncology*, 22:1421–4.

Benrubi GI, Norvell M, Nuss RC, Robinson H (1985). The use of methylprednisolone and metoclopramide in control of emesis in patients receiving cisplatinum. *Gynecologic Oncology*, 21:306–13.

Bonneterre J, *et al.* (1990). A randomized double-blind comparison of ondansetron and metoclopramide in the prophylaxis of emesis induced by cyclophosphamide, fluorouracil, and doxorubicin or epirubicin chemotherapy. *Journal of Clinical Oncology*, 8:1063–9.

Bradley PB, *et al.* (1986). Proposals for the classification and nomenclature of functional receptors for 5-hydroxytryptamine. *Neuropharmacology*, 25:563–76.

Bremer K on behalf of the Granisetron Study Group (1992). A single-blind study of the efficacy and safety of intravenous granisetron compared with alizapride plus dexamethasone in the prophylaxis and control of emesis in patients receiving 5-day cytostatic therapy. *European Journal of Cancer*, 28A:1018–22.

Carr BI, *et al.* (1987). High doses of prochlorperazine for cisplatin-induced emesis. A prospective, random, dose-response study. *Cancer*, 60:2165–9

Carr BI, *et al.* (1989). Combination antiemetic therapy based on high doses of either prochlorperazine or metoclopramide give complete protection against platinum-induced emesis. *Proceedings of the American Society for Clinical Oncology*, 8:325.

Castle WM, Cunningham K, Kanarek BB (1992). Ondansetron is not associated with vascular adverse events, thrombocytopenia or renal failure. *Annals of Oncology*, 3:773–4.

Chevallier B, on behalf of the Granisetron Study Group (1990). Efficacy and safety of granisetron compared with high-dose metoclopramide plus dexamethasone in patients receiving high-dose cisplatin in a single-blind study. *European Journal of Cancer*, 26(Suppl.):33–6.

Chiara S, *et al.* (1987). Methylprednisolone for the control of CMF-induced emesis. *American Journal of Clinical Oncology*, 10:264–7.

Coates A, *et al.* (1983). On the receiving end—patient perception of the side-effects of cancer chemotherapy. *European Journal of Cancer and Clinical Oncology*, 19:203–8.

Coates AS, *et al.* (1992). Severe vascular adverse effects with thrombocytopenia and renal failure following emetogenic chemotherapy and ondansetron. *Annals of Oncology*, 3:719–22.

Cognetti F, *et al.* (1984). Randomized open cross-over trial between metoclopramide (MCP) and dexamethasone (DXM) for the prevention of cisplatin induced nausea and vomiting. *European Journal of Cancer and Clinical Oncology*, 20:183–7.

Cronin C, *et al.* (1985). A randomized, double-blind, crossover comparison of metoclopramide (MCP) and droperidol (DPD) in patients (PTS) receiving cisplatin chemotherapy (CT). *Proceedings of the American Society for Clinical Oncology* 4:270.

Cunningham D, Turner A, Hawthorn J, Rosin RD (1989). Ondansetron with and without dexamethasone to treat chemotherapy-induced emesis. *Lancet*, i:1323.

D'Acquisto RW, *et al.* (1986). The influence of a chronic high alcohol intake on chemotherapy-induced nausea and vomiting. *Proceedings of the American Society of Clinical Oncology*, 5:257.

Dana BW, Everts EC, Dickinson D (1985). Dexamethasone vs placebo for cisplatin induced emesis. A randomized cross-over trial. *American Journal of Clinical Oncology*, 8:426–8.

Dana BW, McDermott M, Everts E, Abdulhay G (1987). A randomized trial of high dose bolus metoclopramide versus low-dose continuous infusion metoclopramide in the prevention of cisplatin-induced emesis. *American Journal of Clinical Oncology*, 10:253–6.

David M, *et al.* (1984). Cyclophosphamide, methotrexate, and 5-FU (CMF)-induced nausea and vomiting: a controlled study with high-dose metoclopramide. *Cancer Treatment Reports*, 68:921–2.

Dicato M (1991). Oral treatment with ondansetron in an outpatient setting. *European Journal of Cancer*, 27(Suppl. 1):518–19.

Dobrow RB, Coppock MA, Hosenpud JR (1991). Extrapyramidal reaction caused by ondansetron. Correspondence. *Journal of Clinical Oncology*, 9:1921.

D'Olimpo JT, *et al.* (1985). Antiemetic efficacy of high-dose dexamethasone vs placebo in patients receiving cisplatin-based chemotherapy: a randomized double blind controlled clinical trial. *Journal of Clinical Oncology*, 3:1135–5.

Dott C (1993). Comparison of the effects of oral (po) granisetron, alone and with dexamethasone, and a conventional antiemetic treatment for the prevention of nausea and vomiting for 24 hours following cisplatin therapy. *Proceedings of the American Society of Clinical Oncology*, 12:460 (Abstract 1602).

Edge SB, *et al.* (1987). High-dose oral and intravenous metoclopramide in doxorubicin/cyclophosphamide-induced emesis. *American Journal of Clinical Oncology*, 10:257–63.

Evans WK, *et al.* (1987). A randomized study of oral nutritional support versus *ad lib* nutritional intake during chemotherapy for advanced colorectal and non-small-cell lung cancer. *Journal of Clinical Oncology*, 5:113–24.

Fearon KCH, Calman KC (1986). Methods of nutritional support for cancer patients. *Clinics in Oncology*, 5:317–35.

Fetting JH, *et al.* (1982*a*). The course of nausea and vomiting after high-dose cyclophosphamide. *Cancer Treatment Reports*, 66:1487–93.

Fetting JH, McCarthy LE, Borison HL, Colvin M (1982*b*). Vomiting induced by cyclophosphamide and phosphoramide mustard in cats. *Cancer Treatment Reports* 66:1625–9.

Fraschini G, *et al.* (1991). Evaluation of three oral dosages of ondansetron in the prevention of nausea and emesis associated with cyclophosphamied-doxorubicin chemotherapy. *Journal of Clinical Oncology*, 9:1268–74.

Frustaci S, *et al.* (1986). Randomized cross-over antiemetic study in cisplatin treated patients. Comparison between high-dose IV metoclopramide and high-dose IV dexamethasone. *Cancer Chemotherapy and Pharmacology*, 17:75–9.

Gandara DR, *et al.* (1991). Efficacy of ondansetron in the prevention of delayed emesis following high dose cisplatin. *Proceedings of the American Society for Clinical Oncology*, 9:328.

Garcia-del-Muro X, Cadenal F, Ferrer P (1993). Extrapyramidal reaction associated with ondansetron. *European Journal of Cancer*, 29A:288.

Govil M, *et al.* (1985). Antiemetic efficacy of high dose droperidol versus high dose metoclopramide in a double blind randomized trial of patients receiving cisplatinum containing chemotherapy. *Proceedings of the American Society for Clinical Oncology*, 4:261.

Gralla RJ, *et al.* (1981*a*). Metoclopramide: initial clinical studies of high dosage regimen in cisplatin-induced emesis. In *The treatment of nausea and vomiting induced by cancer therapy* (ed. D Poster), pp. 167–76. Masson, New York.

Gralla RJ, *et al.* (1981*b*). Antiemetic efficacy of high-dose metoclopramide: randomized trials with placebo and prochlorperazine in patients with chemotherapy-induced nausea and vomiting. *New England Journal of Medicine*, **305**:905–9.

Gralla RJ, *et al.* (1984). Antiemetic therapy: a review of recent studies and a report of a random assignment trial comparing metoclopramide with delta-9-tetrahydrocannabinol. *Cancer Treatment Reports*, 68:163–72.

Grunberg SM, *et al.* (1986). Comparison of metoclopramide and metoclopramide plus dexamethasone for complete protection from cisplatinum-induced emesis. *Cancer Investigation*, 4:379–85.

Grunberg SM, *et al.* (1990). Double blind randomized study of 2 doses of oral ondansetron (GR38032F) for the prevention of cisplatin-induced delayed nausea and vomiting. *Proceedings of the American Society for Clinical Oncology*, 9:327.

Hainsworth JD, *et al.* (1989). GR38032F: a new antiemetic effective in multiple day regimen of cisplatin. *Proceedings of the American Society for Clinical Oncology*, 8:328.

Halperin JR, Murphy B (1992). Extrapyramidal reaction to ondansetron. *Cancer*, 69:1275.

Hawthorn J, Cunningham D (1990). Dexamethasone can potentiate the anti-emetic action of a 5HT₃ receptor antagonist on cyclophosphamide induced vomiting in the ferret. *British Journal of Cancer*, 61:56–60.

Hesketh PJ, Twaddell T, Finn A (1990). A possible role for cisplatin in the transient hepatic enzyme elevations noted after ondansetron administration. *Proceedings of the American Society for Clinical Oncology*, 9:323.

Higgins GA, *et al.* (1989) 5-HT₃ receptor antagonists injected into the area postrema inhibit cisplatin-induced emesis in the ferret. *British Journal of Pharmacology*, 97:247–55.

Homesley HD, *et al.* (1982). Double-blind placebo-controlled study of metoclopramide in cisplatin-induced emesis. *New England Journal of Medicine*, 307:250–1.

Italian Group for Antiemetic Research (1993). Difference in persistence of efficacy of two antiemetic regimens on acute emesis during cisplatin chemotherapy: results of a prospective study. *Journal of Clinical Oncology*, 11:2396–404.

Jones AL, *et al.* (1991). Comparison of dexamethasone in the prophylaxis of emesis induced by moderately emetogenic chemotherapy. *Lancet*, 338:483–7.

Jordan NS, *et al.* (1985). The effect of administration rate in cisplatin induced emesis. *Journal of Clinical Oncology*, 3:559–61.

Joss RA (1993). Tropisetron and the 5-HT₃ antiemetics in perspective. Proceedings of an international symposium October 2, 1992 — Vienna, Austria. *Annals of Oncology*, 4(Suppl. 31):1–47.

Joss RA, *et al.* (1986). The antiemetic activity of high-dose alizapride and high-dose metoclopramide in patients receiving cancer chemotherapy: a prospective, randomized, double-blind trial. *Clinical Pharmacology and Therapy*, 39:619–24.

Kaasa S, *et al.* (1990). A comparison of ondansetron with metoclopramide in the prophylaxis of chemotherapy-induced nausea and vomiting: a randomized, double-blind study. *European Journal of Cancer*, 26:311–14.

Kanarek BB, *et al.* (1992). Ondansetron: confusing documentation surrounding an extrapyramidal reaction. *Journal of Clinical Oncology*, 10:506–7.

Kelley SL, *et al.* (1986). Trial of droperidol as an antiemetic in cisplatin chemotherapy. *Cancer Treatment Reports*, 70:469–72.

Kelly K (1986). An overview of how to nourish the cancer patient by mouth. *Cancer*, 58:1897–1901.

Kokal WA (1986). Effects of antineoplastic therapy on nutritional status: surgery, chemotherapy, and radiotherapy. *Clinics in Oncology*, 5:277–92.

Koretz RL (1984). Parenteral nutrition: is it oncologically logical? *Journal of Clinical Oncology*, 2:534–8.

Kris MG, *et al.* (1983). Extrapyramidal reactions with high-dose metoclopramide. *New England Journal of Medicine*, 309:433.

Kris MG, *et al.* (1985*a*). Improved control of cisplatin induced emesis with high dose metoclopramide and with combinations of metoclopramide, dexamethasone and diphenhydramine. Results of consecutive trials in 255 patients. *Cancer*, 55:527–34.

Kris MG, *et al.* (1985*b*) Incidence, course, and severity of delayed nausea and vomiting following the administration of high-dose cisplatin. *Journal of Clinical Oncology,* 3:1379–84.

Kris MG, *et al.* (1987). Antiemetic control and prevention of side effects of anticancer ·therapy with lorezapam or diphenhydramine when used in combination with metoclopramide plus dexamethasone. A double-blind, randomized trial. *Cancer*, 60:2816–22.

Kris MG, *et al.* (1989). Controlling delayed vomiting: double-blind, randomized trial comparing placebo, dexamethasone alone, and metoclopramide plus dexamethasone in patients receiving cisplatin. *Journal of Clinical Oncology*, 7:108–14.

Lewis GO, Bernath AM, Ellison NM, *et al.* (1984). Double-blind crossover trial of droperidol, metoclopramide, and prochlorperazine as antiemetics in cisplatin therapy. *Clinical Pharmacy*, 3:618–21.

Lucot JB, Crampton GH (1989). 8-OH-DPAT suppresses vomiting in the cat elicited by motion, cisplatin or xylazine. *Pharmacology Biochemistry and Behavior*, 33:627–31.

Markman M, *et al.* (1984). Antiemetic efficacy of dexamethasone. Randomized, double-blind, crossover study with prochlorperazine in patients receiving cancer chemotherapy. *New England Journal of Medicine*, 311:549–52.

Marschner N, Adler M, Nagel GA, Christmann D (1991*a*). Double-blind randomized trial of the anti-emetic efficacy and safety of ondansetron and metoclopramide in advanced breast cancer patients treated with epirubicin and cyclophosphamide. *Journal of Cancer Research and Clinical Oncology*, **116** (Suppl.):641.

Marschner NW, *et al.* (1991*b*). Double-blind randomised trial of the antiemetic efficacy and safety of ondansetron and metoclopramide in advanced breast cancer patients treated with epirubicin and cyclophosphamide. *European Journal of Cancer*, 27:1137–40.

Marty M on behalf of the Granisetron Study Group (1990*a*). A comparative study of the use of granisetron, a selective 5-HT₃ antagonist, versus a standard anti-emetic regimen of chlorpromazine plus dexamethasone in the treatment of cytostatic-induced emesis. *European Journal of Cancer and Clinical Oncology*, 26(Suppl.):28–32.

Marty M, d'Allens H et le Groupe Multicentrique Français (1990*b*). Etude randomisée en double-insu comparant l'efficacité de l'ondansetron selon deux modes d'administration: injection unique et perfusion continue. *Cahiers Cancer*, 2:541–6.

Marty M, *et al.* (1990*c*). Comparison of the 5-hydroxytryptamine 3 (serotonin) antagonist ondansetron (GR38032F) with high-dose metoclopramide in the control of cisplatin-induced emesis *New England Journal of Medicine*, 322:816–21.

Mellink WA, Blijham GH, Van Deyk WA (1984). Amitriptyline plus fluphenazine to prevent chemotherapy-induced emesis in cancer patients: a double-blind randomized cross-over study. *European Journal of Cancer and Clinical Oncology*, 20:1147–50.

Metz CA, Freedman RS, Magrina JF (1987). Methylprednisolone in cisplatinum induced nausea and emesis: a placebo-controlled trial. *Gynecologic Oncology*, 27:84–9.

Morran C, Smith DC, Anderson DA, McArdle CS (1979). Incidence of nausea and vomiting with cytotoxic chemotherapy. A prospective randomized trial of antiemetics. *British Medical Journal*, 1:1323–4.

Nagy C, Einhorn L, Werner K, Chubb J (1988). GR-C507/75: a new effective antiemetic for patients receiving cisplatin chemotherapy. *Proceedings of the American Society for Clinical Oncology*, 7:281.

Navari RM (1989). Comparison of intermittent versus continuous infusion metoclopramide in control of acute nausea induced by cisplatin chemotherapy. *Journal of Clinical Oncology*, 7:943–6.

Pendergrass K, *et al.* (1990). Ondansetron (OND): more effective than metoclopramide (MCP) in the prevention of cisplatin (DDP)-induced nausea (N) and vomiting (V). *Proceedings of the American Society for Clinical Oncology*, 9:319.

Peroutka SJ, Snyder SH (1982). Antiemetics: nuerotransmitter receptor binding predicts therapeutic actions. *Lancet*, i:658–9.

Roila F, *et al.* (1985). Antiemetic activity of two different high doses of metoclopramide in cisplatin-treated cancer patients: a randomized double-blind trial of the Italian Oncology Group for Clinical Research. *Cancer Treatment Reports*, **69**:1353–7.

Roila F, *et al.* (1987*a*). Antiemetic activity of high doses of metoclopramide combined with methylprednisolone versus metoclopramide alone in cisplatin-treated cancer patients: a randomized double-blind trial of the Italian Oncology Group for Clinical Research. *Journal of Clinical Oncology*, **5**:141–9.

Roila F, *et al.* (1987*b*). Double-blind controlled trial of the antiemetic efficacy and toxicity of methylprednisolone (MP), metoclopramide (MTC) and domperidone (DMP) in breast cancer patients treated with iv CMF. *European Journal of Cancer and Clinical Oncology*, **23**:615–17.

Roila F, *et al.* (1988). Methylprednisolone versus metoclopramide for prevention of nausea and vomiting in breast cancer patients treated with intravenous cyclophosphamide, methotrexate, 5-fluorouracil: a double-blind randomized study. *Oncology*, **45**:346–9.

Roila F, *et al.* (1989). Protection from nausea and vomiting in cisplatin-treated patients: high-dose metoclopramide combined with methylprednisolone versus metoclopramide combined with dexamethasone and diphenhydramine: a study of the Italian Oncology Group for Clinical Research. *Journal of Clinical Oncology*, **7**:1693–1700.

Roila F, *et al.* (1990). A double-blind multicenter randomized crossover study comparing the antiemetic efficacy and tolerability of ondansetron (OND) vs OND plus dexamethasone (DEX) in cisplatin (CDDP) treated cancer patients (PTS). *Proceedings of the American Society for Clinical Oncology*, **9**:339.

Roila F, *et al.* (1991). Double-blind cross-over trial of single vs divided dose of metoclopramide in a combined regimen for treatment of cisplatin-induced emesis. *European Journal of Cancer*, **27**:119–21.

Roila F, *et al.* (1992). Ondansetron+dexamethasone vs metoclopramide+dexamethasone+diphenhydramine in prevention of cisplatin-induced emesis. *Lancet*, **340**:96–9.

Saller R, Hellenbrecht D (1985). Comparison of the antiemetic efficacy of two high-dose benzamides, metoclopramide and alizapride, against cisplatin-induced emesis. *Cancer Treatment Reports*, **69**:1301–3.

Saller R, Hellenbrecht D (1986). High doses of metoclopramide or droperidol in the prevention of cisplatin-induced emesis. *European Journal of Cancer and Clinical Oncology*, **22**:1199–203.

Schallier D, Van Belle S, De Greve J, Willekens A (1985). Methylprednisolone as an antiemetic drug. A randomized double blind study. *Cancer Chemotherapy and Pharmacology*, **14**:235–7.

Seynaeve C, *et al.* (1992). Comparison of the anti-emetic efficacy of different doses of ondansetron, given as either a continuous infusion or a single intravenous dose, in acute cisplatin-induced emesis. A multicentre, double-blind, randomised, parallel group study. *British Journal of Cancer*, **66**:192–7.

Shinkai T, *et al.* (1986). Antiemetic efficacy of high-dose intravenous metoclopramide and dexamethasone in patients receiving cisplatin-based chemotherapy: a randomized controlled trial. *Japanese Journal of Clinical Oncology*, **16**:279–87.

Sledge GW, *et al.* (1992*a*). Randomized trial of ondansetron and metoclopramide as antiemetic therapy for cisplatin-based chemotherapy. *Proceedings of the American Society for Clinical Oncology*, **9**:323.

Sledge GW, Einhorn L, Nagy C, House K (1992*b*). Phase III double-blind comparison of intravenous ondansetron and metoclopramide as antiemetic

therapy for patients receiving multiple-day cisplatin-based chemotherapy. *Cancer*, **70**:2524–8.

Smith DB, *et al.* (1990). Ondansetron (GR38032F) plus dexamethasone: effective anti-emetic prophylaxis for patients receiving cytotoxic chemotherapy. *British Journal of Cancer*, **61**:323.

Smith IE on behalf of the Granisetron Study Group (1990). A comparison of two dose levels of granisetron in patients receiving moderately emetogenic cytostatic chemotherapy. *European Journal of Cancer and Clinical Oncology*, **26**(Suppl.):19–23.

Smith RN (1989). Safety of ondansetron. *European Journal of Cancer and Clinical Oncology*, **25**:47–50.

Sorbe B, *et al.* (1994). A randomized, multicenter study comparing the efficacy and tolerability of tropisetron, a new 5-HT₃ receptor antagonist, with a metoclopramide-containing antiemetic cocktail in the prevention of cisplatin-induced emesis. *Cancer*, **73**(2):445–54.

Soukop M on behalf of the Granisetron Study Group (1990). A comparison of two dose levels of granisetron in patients receiving high-dose cisplatin. *European Journal of Cancer*, **26**(Suppl.):S15–19.

Strum SB, McDermed JE, Liponi DF (1985). High-dose intravenous metoclopramide vs combination high-dose metoclopramide and intravenous dexamethasone in preventing cisplatin-induced nausea and emesis: a single-blind cross-over comparison of antiemetic efficacy. *Journal of Clinical Oncology*, **3**:245–51.

Sullivan JR, Leyden MJ, Bell R (1983). Decreased cisplatin-induced nausea and vomiting with chronic alcohol ingestion. *New England Journal of Medicine*, **309**:796.

Tyers MB, Bunce KT, Humphrey PPA (1989). Pharmacological and anti-emetic properties of ondansetron. *European Journal of Cancer and Clinical Oncology*, **25**(Suppl. 1):15–19.

Tyson LB, Clark RA, Gralla RJ (1982). High-dose metoclopramide: control of dacarbazine-induced emesis in a preliminary trial. *Cancer Treatment Reports*, **66**:2108.

Valdivieso M, *et al.* (1987). Long-term effects of intravenous hyperalimentation administered during intensive chemotherapy for small cell bronchogenic carcinoma. *Cancer*, **59**:362–9.

Van Liessum P, *et al.* (1989). A multicentre double-blind comparison of GR38032F and high dose metoclopramide in the prophylaxis of acute vomiting induced by cisplatin. *Proceedings of the American Society for Clinical Oncology*, **8**:328.

van Oosterom AT, Bianco AR (ed.) (1992). First international symposium on tropisetron. Proceedings of a satellite symposium to the 6th European Conference on Clinical Oncology held in Florence, Italy, 27 October, 1991. *Drugs*, **43**(Suppl. 3):1–44.

Warr D, *et al.* (1991). Superiority of granisetron to dexamethasone plus prochlorperazine in the prevention of chemotherapy-induced emesis. *Journal of the National Cancer Institute*, **83**:1169–73.

Warrington PS, *et al.* (1986). Optimising antiemesis in cancer chemotherapy: efficacy of continuous versus intermittent infusion of high dose metoclopramide in emesis induced by cisplatin. *British Medical Journal*, **293**:1334–7.

Weissbach L and Multi-day Cisplatin Emesis Study Group (1991). Ondansetron. *Lancet*, **338**:753.

19.14 Nutritional support of cancer patients

MATTI S. AAPRO

Anorexia and the ensuing malnutrition are two of the many factors complicating treatment of cancer patients. Cancer patients often present with poor nutritional status, which will decrease their resistance to surgery (Meguld *et al.* 1986), radiation therapy (Copeland *et al.* 1977), and chemotherapy (deWys *et al.* 1980). Malnutrition leads to increased complications of these treatments in patients whose underlying deficient immune status is further debilitated by malnourishment. This inadequate nutrient intake is

Table 1 Non-metabolic causes of reduced nutritional status in untreated cancer patients

Altered taste and smell
Odynophagia, dysphagia
Mechanical obstruction
 Oesophageal, gastric, intestinal
Hepatic insufficiency
Pancreatic tumours
Blind-loop syndromes
Psychological factors leading to
 Anorexia
 Diarrhoea
 Early satiety
 Malabsorption
 Nausea and vomiting

Table 2 Metabolic causes of weight loss in cancer patients

Elevated energy expenditure related to
 Abnormal glucose metabolism
 Insulin resistance
 Elevated protein turnover
 Increased fat oxidation

Inappropriate response to decreased nutrient intake

related to complex mechanisms whereby the tumour also modifies body metabolism, a modification which cannot be reversed without appropriate treatment of the underlying disease. This chapter will review some of these mechanisms and describe the means and the results of nutritional support.

ANOREXIA

Cancer patients often complain of meat aversion and generally decreased appetite as presenting symptoms of their disease. Decreased or modified taste and smell, in the absence of the confounding effects of therapy-induced mucositis or loss of saliva, have been associated with the reduced food intake of these patients. Changes in sensitivity to sucrose and urea have been described and the latter seems related to the meat aversion (deWys and Walters 1975).

Other factors related to anorexia can be mechanical, with early repletion of an operated stomach or of a stomach compressed by liver enlargement or ascites and other causes listed in Table 1.

Hepatic insufficiency, whether caused by cancer or viral hepatitis, is also associated with the impossibility of ingesting adequate nutrients. There does not seem to be a modification of the mechanisms of satiety, as hypothalamic surgery does not alter cachexia in tumour-bearing rats submitted to this treatment (Baillie *et al.* 1965). Psychological factors, from depression to learned food aversion (Bernstein and Berstein 1981), may also play a key rôle in this particular type of anorexia.

Therapy-related anorexia is discussed in the appropriate chapters. It is sufficient to state here that therapy-related nausea and vomiting is one of the main causes of anorexia and that stomatitis, loss of saliva, gastric surgery, and intestinal bypasses all contribute to decreased nutrient intake or absorption.

CACHEXIA

Although cachexia is a common observation among cancer patients and a possible direct cause of death in approximately 20 per cent (Warren 1932), it remains poorly understood. Anorexia, as discussed

Table 3 Cytokines and hormones in cancer cachexia

	Production by	Effect/observation	Treatment results
TNF	Macrophages Human tumour	Anorexia Weight loss	Anti-TNF antibodies reverse anorexia, decrease tumour growth
IL-1	Macrophages Mouse tumour	Anorexia Weight loss	Anti IL-1 receptor antibodies reverse anorexia, decrease tumour growth
IL-6	Macrophages	Anorexia Fever Acute phase hepatic response	Indomethacin reverses animal weight loss
γ-IFN	Macrophages	Anorexia Weight loss	Antibody to IFN reverses cachexia
Insulin	Pancreas	Glucose intolerance (a) Decreased tissue sensitivity (b) Decreased production	Insulin increases rat survival
Catecholamine	Adrenal	Increased sensitivity Overproduction	No study

TNF, tumour necrosis factor; γ-IFN, γ-interferon.

above, is one of the causes of this syndrome. However, anorexia does not explain the disproportionately profound state of nutritional impairment observed in some patients, which is often unrelated to food intake or tumour burden and is observed with almost any tumour type. Thus, it can be argued that anorexia is just one of the manifestations of the cachexia syndrome. There are many changes in the way that cancer patients handle their food intake and several mediators have been suggested.

Metabolic changes

There is considerable debate about the actual changes in energy metabolism that are observed in cancer patients (Heber *et al.* 1992). Measurements of energy expenditure by indirect calorimetry (Knox *et al.* 1983) in 200 malnourished cancer patients has provided contrasting results. Resting energy expenditure was increased in 26 per cent of the patients and decreased in 33 per cent, with no significant changes in the remaining 41 per cent. Another group has looked at lung cancer patients and has also failed to find increases in resting energy expenditure (Heber *et al.* 1982). However, this same group described elevated protein turnover in these patients and other metabolic changes, including abnormal carbohydrate metabolism (insulin resistance and glucose intolerance, increased Cori cycle activity, etc.) and increased fat oxidation, have been well documented (Table 2) (Holroyde and Reichard 1981; Holroyde *et al.* 1984; Hansell *et al.* 1986; Hyltander *et al.* 1991*a*).

The abnormal adaptation of the basic metabolic rate of cancer patients to the decreased nutrient intake resembles in many ways the responses observed during acute inflammatory and injury processes (Norton *et al.* 1980; Albert *et al.* 1986). Cancer patients have significant reductions in skeletal muscle mass compared with malnourished non-tumour-bearing patients, suggesting impaired fat mobilization and proteolysis (Cohn *et al.* 1981). These observations have led to some recommendations concerning the way that cancer patients and severely injured patients should receive their supplemental nutrition, and this is discussed later in this chapter.

Cytokines and hormones as mediators of cachexia (Table 3)

Anorexia and the metabolic disturbances described above may be mediated by toxic products from the injured tissues or cancer cells. This proposal has now been replaced by the suggestion that certain cytokines and hormones released by the tumour and host cells are probable mediators of the anorexia–cachexia syndrome.

On the basis of the observation that the metabolic disturbances of cancer patients resemble those of patients with severe injuries, present research suggests that the same mediators may be playing a rôle in both classes of patients. Cancer, infections, septic states, and inflammatory diseases all lead to cachexia and several mediators that induce cachexia in experimental animals are related to these disease processes. This tumour necrosis factor (cachectin), interleukin-1 (IL-1), interleukin-6 (IL-6), and γ-interferon have been considered (Langstein and Norton 1991; McNamara *et al.* 1992; Moldawer *et al.* 1992).

Tumour necrosis factor (cachectin) induces cachexia, anaemia and inflammation (Tracey *et al.* 1988). Although tumour necrosis factor is produced mainly by macrophages, tumour cell production of this factor has been documented by *in situ* hybridization techniques (Naylor *et al.* 1990). IL-1 is produced by macrophages in cancer patients (Moldawer *et al.* 1988) and has also been shown

to be produced by a mouse sarcoma (Lönnroth *et al.* 1990). Administration of antibodies to either tumour necrosis factor or IL-1 has been shown to result in increased food intake by tumour-bearing animals (Gelin *et al.* 1991). IL-6 produces anorexia and gives rise to acute phase hepatic response (Busbridge *et al.* 1989) and has been suggested to be a mediator of the distant effects of tumour necrosis factor and IL-1 which seem to act locally. Indeed, there are no detectable circulating levels of tumour necrosis factor and IL-1 in most cancer patients (Moldawer *et al.* 1988), whereas increased levels of IL-6 are observed in parallel with increasing tumour burden (Langstein and Norton 1991). The effects of these cytokines can be blocked both by antibodies directed against them or their receptors and by prostaglandin inhibitors like indomethacin (Gelin *et al.* 1991). Prostaglandins are recognized as the key effectors of cytokine activity. Animal studies have been conducted showing that antibodies to γ-interferon can reverse cancer cachexia (Langstein *et al.* 1989).

Decreased peripheral tissue sensitivity to insulin and decreased insulin response to glucose administration are one of the features of cancer cachexia (Waterhouse and Kemperman 1971) and may be related to mechanisms induced by tumour necrosis factor (Walton and Cronin 1989). Another group of hormones proposed as mediators of the increased energy expenditure of cancer patients are the catecholamines, for which both increased sensitivity and overproduction have been documented (Drott *et al.* 1989; Hyltander *et al.* 1991*a*).

Treatment as a cause of cachexia

In addition to the nausea and vomiting mentioned previously, which may be related to chemotherapy, pain therapy (morphine), abdominal surgery, or radiation therapy, as well as mechanical problems due to tumour invasion of the gastrointestinal tract, cancer therapies have hundreds of other ways of promoting anorexia or enhancing the underlying tumour-related cachexia. Xerostomia after radiation therapy, post-surgical blind-loop syndromes, dumping syndromes after gastric surgery, restricted gastric capacity, therapy-related diarrhoea (after radiation therapy and chemotherapy), intestinal strictures after radiation therapy, and adhesions and subocclusive status after abdominal surgery are only the most evident therapy-related factors which add to the complexity of the anorexia–cachexia syndrome.

Table 4   Presentation of the cachectic patient

Signs
    Weight loss
    Muscle atrophy and myopathy
    Loss of fat deposits
    Oedema

Symptoms
    Anorexia
    Fatigue
    Malaise

Laboratory
    Anaemia
    Decreased albumin
    Decreased transferrin
    Glucose intolerance
    Deficiencies in trace metals, vitamins

Table 5 Factors suggesting a need for nutritional support

Any two of the following three parameters
Recent weight loss more than 10 per cent of prior weight
Serum albumin level below 34 g/l
Serum transferrin level below 1.5 g/l

EVALUATION OF THE CACHECTIC PATIENT

Cachectic patients are by definition in bad general condition (*Kakos*: poor, bad; *hexis*: state). Table 4 gives the usual full-blown clinical picture, but most patients will present, initially at least, with only some of the features. The surgeon, medical oncologist, or radiation therapist will not conduct a detailed nutritional evaluation of their patient, but fortunately there is an excellent correlation between a good anamnesis and physical examination and the complex methods used by nutritionists (Baker *et al.* 1982). Patient weight *per se* is not a good parameter, but a loss of prior body weight of more than 10 per cent within the previous 3 months is a good indicator of the severity of the underlying cancer and is correlated with significant protein-calorie malnutrition. Patient examination should include a search for signs of albumin loss (oedema) and muscle wasting (often difficult and best elicited by questioning the patient for signs of decreased strength, for example when walking upstairs). Obviously, pelvic obstruction can lead to inferior limb oedema and an Eaton–Lambert syndrome will decrease muscle strength and these causes must be excluded. Although many objective tests have been described, their complexity or non-availability render their use impossible in daily practice. Others, such as the evaluation of delayed hypersensitivity with a demonstration of anergy in severely malnourished patients which will be restored to normal after parenteral nutrition, are of limited interest. Combinations of objective tests, including albumin level, delayed hypersensitivity skin test result, transferrin level, and measurement of the triceps skinfold, have been suggested for the determination of prognostic indices (Rugby *et al.* 1980). Some measurements in serum are of major interest and the measurement of albumin levels is well correlated with the nutritional status of the patient (Brinson *et al.* 1987; Tayek 1988). Pre-albumin, which has a much shorter half-life (0.5 days compared with 20 days) is an interesting factor for the evaluation of recent dietary deficiencies. Transferrin has also been well correlated with the nutritional status of patients. As shown in Table 5, nutritional support will be discussed clinically if two out of three of the above major signs or tests is abnormal.

NUTRITIONAL SUPPORT

Patients who have to undergo major elective surgery, debilitating intensive chemotherapy (for example, bone-marrow transplantation), or suffer from the side-effects of radiation therapy should receive nutritional support in order to tolerate the procedure. However, it should be emphasized that such support will not modify the ultimate outcome of the cancer.

Perioperative total parenteral nutrition is beneficial in terms of reduced complication rates, but does not appear to modify mortality, although this is debated (Klein *et al.* 1986). The same authors have also addressed the rôle of total parenteral nutrition in chemotherapy or radiation therapy and found no benefit. It should be noted that these patients were often normally nourished at the start of

Table 6 Data for cancer cachexia and nutritional support

Basal energy expenditure (Harris–Benedict formula)
Males: $66+13.7\times$weight(kg)$+5.0\times$height(cm)$-6.8\times$age(years) kcal
Females: $655+9.6\times$weight(kg)$+1.7\times$height(cm)$-4.7\times$age(years) kcal

Nutritional non-protein caloric needs
1.5–1.8×basal energy expenditure, and more if fever or other factors are present

Proteins
To represent 1.5–2.0 g/kg

Glucose
Up to 7 g/kg/day (consider insulin)

Lipids
To represent 30–50 per cent of calories and up to 2 g=9 kcal/kg/day

Essential amino acids, vitamins, and trace elements
To be supplemented (commercial preparations available)

Electrolytes
Sodium, 60–120 mEq; potassium, 60–100 mEq; chloride, 60–120 mEq; magnesium, 8–10 mEq; calcium, 5–10 mmol; phosphorus, 10–40 mmol

treatment and that many of the support regimens were inadequate (McGeer *et al.* 1990).

The daily caloric requirements of patients are usually evaluated as a multiple (1.5–1.8 times in the absence of fever and other complicating factors, which add 10–40 per cent to the requirement) of the basal metabolic expenditure of 30–40 non-protein kcal/kg calculated by the Harris–Benedict equation (Table 6) (Harris and Benedict 1919). It has been proposed that patients should receive double the value calculated according to this formula (Hyltander *et al.* 1991*b*). In addition to the caloric content, nutritional support has to restore protein deficits and 1.5–2.0 g of protein (0.2–0.33 g of nitrogen) per kilogram of current weight is recommended, at least for malnourished patients. Supplementation with essential amino acids is done using commercial preparations. Administration of insulin together with the glucose infusions will be necessary for patients with high caloric requirements. Lipid administration should represent, at least in intravenous support, 30–50 per cent of the total caloric intake. Patients can usually tolerate up to 7 g/kg/day of glucose intake and 2 g/kg/day of fat. Serum lactescence and triglyceride levels must be monitored regularly. Recommended daily allowances of electrolytes (National Academic Press 1989) are indicated in Table 6. Commercial preparations of vitamins and trace elements generally supply sufficient quantities of these factors when the manufacturers' recommendations are followed. Increased requirements for folic acid and vitamin K may be necessary in patients undergoing, respectively, chemotherapy and transfusion or hepatotoxic treatment. Zinc is a particularly important trace element as deficits affect taste and immune status (Prasad *et al.* 1988).

Route of nutritional support

Patients who have very severe nutritional impairment (albumin levels below 28 g/l) usually suffer from diarrhoea (Brinson *et al.* 1987), as do those with severe calcium deficiencies. These patients should first be treated parenterally. All other patients should be considered for continuous enteral feeding via a nasogastric tube. Placement of this tube, which should be small bore (CH8-10 or 8-10 Fr) and made of silicone or polyurethane, should be assessed radiologically, as it should lie 5–10 cm below the cardial margin. A high placement induces regurgitation and too low a tube induces diarrhoea. The osmolality of the enteric feeding may also determine diarrhoea, as may the rapidity and temperature of the flow. Formulae of various types are available in every country. Ideally, polymeric or semi-modular, isotonic, and fibre-enriched formulae should be used and they can be adapted to the patient's individual needs with a specialized nutritional consultation. It is recommended that nutrition is started with flows of 25 ml/h and increased by 25 ml/h every 24–48 h. Gastrostomy or jejunostomy should be used if nutritional support is to be of long duration. Patients who achieve the desired weight gain can be maintained on intermittent nightly enteral nutrition.

Total parenteral nutrition is reserved for patients with severely increased requirements or who are unable to tolerate enteral feeding. Extreme care to avoid any type of infection is mandatory and whenever possible the route of parenteral nutrition should be different from that used for chemotherapy or antibiotic administration. Hyperosmolar parenteral nutrition solutions are necessary for most patients and, thus, central lines have to be used. The desired caloric administration is achieved with a progressive introduction of the mixture, usually at 1000 ml on the first day and then by 500 ml increments. Discontinuation of total parenteral nutrition should also be gradual to avoid hypoglycaemia. Patients exhibiting changes in their status should be checked for abnormal glucose, ammonium, phosphorus, and magnesium levels.

Major disturbances can occur after starting enteral or intravenous nutrition and patients have to be monitored closely (Solomon and Kirby 1990).

Support in the advanced patient

Treatment of cachexia associated with advanced incurable cancer is of a palliative nature and should be directed towards the patient's complaints and not the anxiety of the family who insists that he or she should eat or the physician who cannot tolerate his or her progressive emaciation. Thus, the first step is to check the reality of the clinical problem. Is the patient really suffering from his or her advancing cachexia or is the suffering merely related to the whole process of dying? Once this first step is taken and if a dietary consultation with assessment of possible improvements in food intake, even using commercially available supplements (which provide around 100 kcal/100 ml and 4–10 g of protein per 100 ml), shows that simple measures do not permit an adequate caloric supplementation, some kind of pharmacological support can be considered.

Corticosteroids provide short-term relief and improve not only appetite but also general well-being (Bruera *et al.* 1985). When used at doses of approximately 0.5 mg/kg of prednisone or its equivalents, these agents are limited by their many side-effects and there is little impact on objective measurements. However, they remain a cheap and powerful tool in the management of the terminally ill patient. Hydrazine sulphate has been the subject of some controversy. It has been claimed to improve patient survival in cases of non-small cell carcinoma of the lung (Chlebowski *et al.* 1990), but other studies have been negative (Kosty *et al.* 1992). Cyproheptadine sulphate inhibits gluconeogenesis, which is one of the possible mechanisms of cachexia.

Of interest is the observation that progestational agents increase appetite, food intake, and weight, as first shown in breast cancer patients, independently of any tumour response (Tchekmedyian *et al.* 1987). Many other studies have subsequently confirmed this initial observation and weight gain seems to be related to increased body fat and body cell mass and not just fluid retention (Loprinzi *et al.* 1990). The effective dosage of this compound is probably approximately 480–800 mg/day, although it is already active in half of patients at daily doses of 160 mg (Loprinzi *et al.* 1993). The side-effects of progestational agents in male and female patients have to be weighed against the possible symptom relief and as there is no demonstration of a survival benefit, the choice remains a question of subjective feelings.

REFERENCES

Albert JD, *et al.* (1986). Peripheral tissue amino acid metabolism in humans with varied disease states and similar weight loss. *Journal of Surgical Research*, 40:374–81.

Baillie P, Millar FK, Pratt AW (1965). Food and water intakes and Walker tumor growth in rats with hypothalamic lesions. *American Journal of Physiology*, 209: 293–300.

Baker JP, Detsky AS, Wesson D (1982). Nutritional assessment. A comparison of clinical judgment and objective measurements. *New England Journal of Medicine*, 306:969–72.

Bernstein IL, Bernstein ID (1981). Learned food aversions and cancer anorexia. *Cancer Treatment Reports*, 65 (Suppl. 5):43–7.

Brinson RR, Byron E, Kolts E (1987). Hypoalbuminemia as an indicator of diarrheal incidence in critically ill patients. *Critical Care Medicine*, 15:506–9.

Bruera E, *et al.* (1985). Action of oral methylprednisolone in terminal cancer patients. A prospective randomized double-blind study. *Cancer Treatment Reports*, 65:751–4.

Busbridge J, *et al.* (1989). Acute central effects of interleukin-6 on body temperature, thermogenesis and food intake in the rat. *Proceedings of the Nutritional Society*, 38:48A.

Chlebowski RT, *et al.* (1990). Hydrazine sulfate influence on nutritional status and survival in non-small cell lung cancer. *Clinical Oncology*, 8:9–15.

Cohn SH, *et al.* (1981). Body composition and dietary intake in neoplastic disease. *American Journal of Clinical Nutrition*, 34:1997–2004.

Copeland EM, *et al.* (1977). Intravenous hyperalimentation as an adjunct to radiation therapy. *Cancer*, 36:609–16.

deWys WD, Walters K (1975). Abnormalities of taste sensation in cancer patients. *Cancer*, 36:1888–96.

deWys WD, *et al.* (1980). Prognosis of weight loss prior to chemotherapy in cancer patients. *American Journal of Medicine*, 69:491–7.

Drott C, Persson H, Lundholm K (1989). Cardiovascular and metabolic response to adrenalin infusion in undernourished patients with and without cancer. *Clinical Physiology*, 9:427–39.

Gelin J, Anderson C, Lundholm K (1991). Effects of indomethacin, cytokines and cyclosporin A on tumor growth and the subsequent development of cancer cachexia. *Cancer Research*, 51:415–21.

Hansell DT, *et al.* (1986). Body fuel oxidation in cancer patients and controls. *Clinical Nutrition*, 15(Suppl.):62.

Harris JA, Benedict FD (1919). *A biometric study of basal metabolism in man.* Carnegie Institute, Publication 279, Washington, DC.

Heber D, *et al.* (1982). Abnormalities in glucose and protein metabolism in non-cachectic lung cancer patients. *Cancer Research*, 42:4815–19.

Heber D, Byerley L, Tchekmedyian NS (1992). Hormonal and metabolic abnormalities in the malnourished cancer patient: effects on host–tumor interaction. *Journal of Parenteral and Enteral Nutrition*, 16:605–45.

Holroyde CP, Reichard A (1981). Carbohydrate metabolism in cancer cachexia. *Cancer Treatment Reports*, 65(Suppl.):55–9.

Holroyde CP, *et al.* (1984). Glucose metabolism in cachectic patients with colorectal cancer. *Cancer Research*, 44:5910–14.

Hyltander A, *et al.* (1991*a*). Elevated energy expenditure in cancer patients with solid tumours. *European Journal of Cancer*, 27:9–15.

Hyltander A, *et al.* (1991*b*). Effect on whole-body protein synthesis after institution of intravenous nutrition in cancer and non-cancer patients who lose weight. *European Journal of Cancer*, 27:16–21.

Klein S, Simes S, Blackburn GL (1986). Total parenteral nutrition and cancer clinical trials. *Cancer*, **58**:1378–86.

Knox LS, *et al.* (1983). Energy expenditure in malnourished cancer patients. *Annals of Surgery*, **197**:152–62.

Kosty M, *et al.* (1992). Cisplatin, vinblastine and hydrazine sulfate in advanced non-small cell lung cancer. A randomized, placebo controlled, double-blind phase III study. *Proceedings of the American Association of Clinical Oncology*, **11**:294.

Langstein H, Fraker D, Norton J (1989). Reversal of cancer cachexia by antibodies to interferon-gamma but not cachectin/tumor necrosis factor. *Surgical Forum*, **40**:408–10.

Langstein HN, Norton JA (1991). Mechanisms of cancer cachexia. *Hematology and Oncology Clinics of North America*, **5**:103–23.

Lönnroth C, *et al.* (1990). Tumor necrosis factor alpha and interleukin-1 alpha production in cachectic, tumor-bearing mice. *International Journal of Cancer*, **46**:889–96.

Loprinzi CL, *et al.* (1990). Controlled trial of megestrol acetate for the treatment of cancer anorexia and cachexia. *Journal of the National Cancer Institute*, **82**:1127–32.

Loprinzi CL, *et al.* (1993). Phase III evaluation of four doses of megestrol acetate as therapy for patients with cancer anorexia and/or cachexia. *Journal of Clinical Oncology*, **12**:762–7.

McGeer AJ, Detsky AS, O'Rourke K (1990). Parenteral nutrition in cancer patients undergoing chemotherapy. A meta-analysis. *Nutrition*, **6**:233–40.

McNamara M, Alexander R, Norton J (1992). Cytokines and their role in the pathophysiology of cancer cachexia. *Journal of Parenteral and Enteral Nutrition*, **16**:50S–5S.

Meguld M, *et al.* (1986). Influence of the nutritional status on the resumption of adequate food intake in patients recovering from colorectal cancer operations. *Surgical Clinics of North America*, **66**:1167–76.

Moldawer LL, Drott C, Lundholm K (1988). Monocytic production and plasma bioactivity of interleukin-1 and tumour necrosis factor in human cancer. *European Journal of Clinical Investigation*, **18**:486–92.

Moldawer L, Rogy M, Lowry S (1992). The role of cytokines in cancer cachexia. *Journal of Parenteral and Enteral Nutrition*, **16**:435–95.

Naylor MS, Stramp GWH, Balkwill FR (1990). Investigation of cytokine gene expression in human colorectal cancer. *Cancer Research*, **46**:889–96.

Norton JA, Stein TP, Brennan MF (1980). Whole body protein turnover studies in normal humans and malnourished patients with and without cancer. *Annals of Surgery*, **31**:94–6.

Prasad AS, Meftah S, Abdallah J (1988). Serum thymulin in human zinc deficiency. *Journal of Clinical Investigation*, **82**:1202–10.

Rugby GP, *et al.* (1980). Prognostic nutritional index in gastrointestinal surgery. *American Journal of Surgery*, **139**:160–7.

Solomon SM, Kirby DF (1990). The refeeding syndrome. A review. *Journal of Parenteral and Enteral Nutrition*, **14**:90–7.

Tayek JM (1988). Albumin synthesis and nutritional assessment. *Nutrition and Clinical Practice*, **3**:219–20.

Tchekmedyian NS, *et al.* (1987). High-dose megestrol acetate: a possible treatment for cachexia. *Journal of the American Medical Association*, **257**:1195–8.

Tracey KJ, *et al.* (1988). Cachectin/tumor necrosis factor induces cachexia, anemia and inflammation. *Journal of Experimental Medicine*, **167**:1211–27.

Walton PE, Cronin MJ (1989). Tumor-necrosis factor inhibits growth hormone secretion from cultured anterior pituitary cells. *Endocrinology*, **125**:925–9.

Warren S (1932). The immediate causes of death in cancer. *American Journal of Medical Science*, **184**:610–15.

Waterhouse C, Kemperman JH (1971). Carbohydrate metabolism in subjects with cancer. *Cancer Research*, **31**:1273–8.

Section 20
End-points, quality of life, and economic issues

20.1 Clinical trial methodology

MARC E. BUYSE

CLINICAL TRIALS IN PERSPECTIVE

The scientific evaluation of new cancer therapies

Over the last few years, clinical trials have become the method of choice for evaluating new therapies and randomization is now considered almost indispensable to establishing the superiority of new therapeutic approaches over standard ones. Such strong reliance on carefully designed and strictly controlled experiments is recent in the history of medicine (Bull 1959). In 1946, a sample of papers taken at random from general medical journals contained no reports of clinical trials; in 1976, 5 per cent of the papers described results of trials (Fletcher and Fletcher 1979). The proportion would assuredly be far larger today and this trend reflects the increasingly scientific nature of clinical practice (Begg *et al.* 1987).

The purpose of this chapter is to give a detailed exposition of the fundamentals of clinical trials, but alternative methods which have been suggested for the evaluation of cancer treatments must first be briefly mentioned.

Trends in cancer mortality

A controversial paper in a leading journal recently indicated that, despite spectacular advances in the treatment of uncommon tumours such as Hodgkin's lymphomas, germ cell tumours, choriocarcinomas, and various solid tumours of childhood, the overall cancer mortality had increased over the last 30 years. The authors concluded that research on cancer treatment had failed to achieve its promises (Bailar and Smith 1986). While it is obvious that the war against cancer is not won by a long way, such a simplified evaluation of current therapies presents definite dangers (Correspondence 1986). In fact, whether oncologists' views on the achievements of cancer therapy tend to be pessimistic (Kearsley 1986), optimistic (DeVita 1989), or simply ambivalent (Wittes 1988), they basically agree that properly conducted clinical trials are the surest way of testing new therapeutic regimens and identifying small, but worthwhile, treatment benefits.

Historical control series

Some authors have advocated comparison of a group of patients treated using a new therapy with a supposedly comparable group of 'historical control' patients treated using standard therapies (Gehan and Freireich 1974). The main difficulty with this approach is that there may be systematic differences between the historical and the treated series because of changes over time in patient characteristics, supportive care, diagnosis, and skill of the clinicians, as well as biases in patient selection. These problems can be partially alleviated when there has been a sequence of studies admitting similar kinds of patients, but even in such situations comparability cannot be guaranteed. Statistical modelling can account for the most obvious discrepancies between the historical and the treated series in terms of the known prognostic factors, but no similar adjustments can be made for the many unknown or unmeasured factors which may have a substantial bearing on patient outcome.

An excellent example of the dangers of using historical controls was given by Byar *et al.* (1976) who compared two large series of patients selected by the same criteria at the same institutions, both given placebo and yet differing substantially in survival. Pocock (1977) studied 19 pairs of consecutive randomized trials carried out under identical conditions at the same institutions. In each pair of trials, the same treatment was used as control. Little difference between the control groups of each pair of trials would be expected and yet there were major differences; in four cases, the comparison was even statistically significant ($p < 0.05$).

Historical controls are sufficient only in those instances in which the new treatment is so clearly beneficial that no formal comparison with a control group is needed. Such instances are exceptional and it is unreasonable to conduct clinical research under the assumption that they will occur. However, there is a role for historical controls in the interpretation of the results of clinical trials. For instance, if the patients in the control group of a randomized experiment fared much worse than expected on the basis of previous series, one could suspect that a small treatment advantage identified in this trial might be due to chance.

Uncontrolled studies

Comparison with a historical control group is only one of the many attempts that have been made to overcome the difficulty of randomization. It has been suggested that computerized databases containing prognostic, treatment, and outcome information on every patient seen in an institution can be used to draw conclusions about the value of alternative therapies. Here the opportunity for bias is even greater than in historical comparisons because the choice between therapeutic alternatives is made on the basis of patient prognosis and no adjustment can make patients in different prognostic groups directly comparable (Byar 1980).

Randomized experiments

Randomization in clinical trials consists of assigning treatments to patients using a chance procedure. This concept was first introduced by R. A. Fisher in his famous work on experimental design in the 1920s and implemented in medical trials by A. B. Hill in the 1940s. The fundamental feature of randomization is to provide comparability of the treatment groups with respect to all known and unknown factors, thus permitting an unbiased comparison between treatment groups (Armitage 1982). Many benefits follow directly from randomization: simple, unadjusted statistical tests provide valid treatment comparisons which are more likely to be convincing than adjusted comparisons based on elaborate models; changes over time in the patient population under study, in diagnostic procedures or even in the evaluation of therapeutic response will affect all randomized groups equally and will therefore not invalidate the treatment comparisons.

Some authors have argued that new treatments should be compared with the standard treatment through randomization from the very first patient (Chalmers 1975). Indeed, one may question the ethical validity of 'pilot' studies in which patients are submitted to potentially inferior or harmful experimental procedures without being given the chance, through randomization, of receiving the

Table 1 The successive phases in testing a new therapeutic regimen

	Type of trial		
	Phase I	Phase II	Phase III
Purpose	Determination of tolerated dose	Screen for clinical activity	Comparison with standard therapy
Main end-point	Toxicity	Response	Survival, time to disease progression
Typical number of patients	5–15+	15–50+	50–5000+
Typical duration	Weeks	Months	Years
Randomized?	Never	Sometimes	Always
Multicentre?	Never	Sometimes	Often
Site-specific?	Sometimes	Often	Always

standard procedure. As a clinical investigator put it eloquently: 'I need permission to give a new drug to half of my patients but not to give it to them all' (Chalmers 1990). Space is too limited to discuss ethics in detail here, but the prevailing pressure towards double standards, which purport to impose tyrannical rules on clinical trials and no rules at all on the remainder of clinical practice, is clearly misguided and unjustified (Baum 1986). Some clinicians have suggested that the decision not to enter an eligible patient in a clinical trial approved by an institution should be subject to the same ethical requirements as trial entry (Segelov *et al.* 1992). While this proposal is unlikely to be readily adopted at most institutions, it does stress the point that ethical dilemmas exist both within and outside of randomized clinical trials (Buyse 1991; Cavalli 1992; Williams 1992).

Types of trial

New cancer treatments are usually studied in a sequence of clinical trials. There are basically three phases in this sequence: phase I trials purport to determine the dose at which the treatment is to be administered, phase II trials are used as a screen to reject inactive treatments from further study, and, finally, phase III trials compare the new treatment to a standard, established treatment. Every phase of clinical testing has its own objectives and as a consequence each type of trial has distinct characteristics which are summarized in Table 1.

Phase I

The phase I trial is the earliest trial in humans with a new compound that has shown activity *in vitro* and in animal screening systems. It is essentially a dose-finding experiment in patients who are no longer expected to benefit from any known therapy. The purpose of the phase I trial is to determine the maximum tolerated dose, which is the maximum dose of the compound that can be administered according to a specific route and schedule with an acceptable toxicity.

While the purpose of phase I trials is not to evaluate clinical activity, there is a chance, albeit small, that some of the patients will respond to the new compound. A recent review of all phase I trials published between 1972 and 1987 showed an overall response rate of 4.5 per cent among over 6500 patients treated (Decoster *et al.* 1990).

Phase II

The phase II trial is essentially a screen to reject drugs which have insufficient activity to warrant further investigation in specific cancer types. The most serious error in such a trial is to reject an effective drug from further study since this could mean that a drug of potential interest is lost forever. The end-points of a phase II trial are response rate (that is, the proportion of patients with measurable lesions in whom tumour regression is observed) and toxicity.

While the purpose of phase II trials is not to compare the new treatment with an established treatment, they may be randomized to provide some control over the selection of patients included in the study (Simon *et al.* 1985). Indeed, a low response rate for a new drug may be due to either a true lack of activity of the drug or the selection of poor prognosis patients in the trial. In a randomized phase II trial where half the patients receive a standard drug and half receive the new drug, the response rate for the standard treatment is a rough but useful indicator of the patient population entered in the trial; if this response rate is close to what was expected from previous experience, it is likely that the new drug was given a fair chance of showing its activity. Randomization may also be used when several dose regimens or routes of administration are studied in a single phase II trial. The number of patients entered in a randomized phase II trial is usually insufficient to permit an informative statistical comparison between the treatment groups, but the trial may be continued as a proper phase III trial if such a comparison is warranted.

Phase III

The phase III trial is a comparative trial involving two or more treatments with the primary purpose of determining the relative merits of each. Some phase III trials attempt to show that a new treatment is more effective than a standard treatment; others attempt to show that a new treatment is as effective as a standard therapy but with less morbidity. The objectives and end-points of a phase III trial are different in studies of adjuvant (prophylactic) treatments in patients clinically free of disease after 'curative' removal of the tumour, and in studies of treatments for advanced (metastatic) disease.

Trials with biological response modifiers

One of the most active areas of research in recent years has been the identification of biological response modifiers such as interferons, interleukins, colony-stimulating factors, etc. These agents are designed to improve the therapeutic benefit by modifying the host response to the tumour and/or cytotoxic drugs. The phase I trials described above are often inappropriate to test biological response modifiers because the maximum tolerated dose may not be the optimum dose. Phase I trials with biological response modifiers should attempt to determine the dose which achieves optimum modification of the host biological response; that is, the maximum effective dose. The criteria needed to determine the maximum effective dose depend on the mechanism of action of the agent under study.

The end-point for a phase II trial of a cytotoxic drug is objective tumour regression; this end-point is inappropriate for a phase II trial of a biological response modifier which does not produce tumour regression. Sometimes the effect of the biological response modifier can be measured by the modulation of the host response through some laboratory or clinical examination, but often the effect of the biological response modifier can only be measured by a benefit on survival. In this case, a control group is required and a comparative trial must be contemplated. In fact, many immune modulating agents such as BCG, levamisole, or *C. parvum* have been used in phase III comparative trials without proper phase I/II

Table 2 The life-cycle of a phase III trial and the problems most frequently encountered

Frequent sources of bias	Frequent sources of problems
Design	
Post-randomization exclusions	Optimistic treatment benefit
	Optimistic patient accrual
	Stringent selection criteria
Conduct	
Losses to follow-up	Administrative burden
'Significant' interim results	Diminishing interest
Analysis	
Exclusion of patients	Inadequate statistical tests
Analysis by actual treatment	Multiple comparisons
Interpretation	
Data-derived results	$p > 0.05$ does not imply no benefit
Overemphasis of subgroups	$p < 0.05$ does not imply large benefit

Table 3 Protocol contents

1. Title page
2. Introduction and scientific background
3. Objectives
4. Patient selection criteria
5. Trial design and schema
6. Therapeutic regimens, dose modifications, and toxicity
7. Required clinical evaluations and laboratory tests
8. Criteria for evaluating the effect of treatment
9. Registration and randomization of patients
10. Case report forms and procedures for data collection
11. Statistical considerations
12. Ethical considerations and informed consent
13. Administrative responsibilities, addresses, and telephone numbers
14. References
15. Appendices

evaluation; this may partly explain why the potential role of these agents in cancer treatment is still so unclear. Biological response modifiers introduced more recently, such as interferons, have been evaluated more appropriately, but a uniform trial methodology for these agents is still badly needed.

The life-cycle of a trial

A clinical trial is typically a major undertaking which must satisfy a number of scientific and ethical requirements and which is only feasible if appropriate logistic and financial support is available (Pocock 1983). In the remainder of this chapter, the life-cycle of a trial is broken down into four chronological stages corresponding to the design of the experiment, the conduct of the trial, the analysis of the data, and the interpretation of the results (Buyse *et al.* 1985). The problems that frequently occur at each stage are summarized in Table 2 and will be discussed further in the remainder of this chapter.

DESIGN OF CLINICAL TRIALS

In this chapter we place a rather strong emphasis on the design of trials, as opposed to their conduct or analysis. Indeed, a poor design ruins an experiment irretrievably (and this is sometimes realized after years of painstaking data collection), while a poor analysis can always be repeated and improved upon if necessary. Moreover, too often the advice of an expert statistician is sought at the time of data analysis rather than before data collection. For these reasons it is important that clinicians be aware of the issues involved in designing a study, rather than of the technicalities of data analysis.

The trial protocol

The most important document in a clinical trial is the protocol, which is a self-contained written description of the rationale, objectives, and logistics of the study (Buyse *et al.* 1985). Particular care must be taken to define the objectives of the trial and the hypothesis to be tested as clearly as possible; the objectives must be such that the trial will yield useful information no matter what its results turn out to be. A typical table of contents for a protocol is given in Table 3.

Phase III clinical trial protocols should be precise and detailed, but they should not attempt to provide exhaustive guidelines for patient management since many of the routine examinations and procedures which would be performed outside the clinical trial contribute no useful information to the end-points. Rather, phase III clinical trial protocols should emphasize the few key aspects that make comparative trials trustworthy, such as the treatment allocation procedures and the need to provide minimal follow-up information on all randomized patients.

End-points

Response end-points

Response to treatment is a relevant end-point in assessing treatment effectiveness against measurable advanced disease. The achievement of a response is an important marker of biological therapeutic effect and is often associated with both objective and subjective improvements in patient condition. However, the achievement of a higher response rate is not sufficient *per se* to establish treatment superiority. The net therapeutic benefit to the patient must also take account of treatment toxicities and the duration of survival or other time-related end-points.

Response must be assessed at regular intervals, usually before the beginning of each treatment course, but in any case at least every 4 weeks (WHO 1979).

Complete response

Complete response is defined as the disappearance of all malignant disease for at least 4 weeks. Complete response is often established clinically, but it may also be demonstrated pathologically when rebiopsy of the malignant areas or second-look surgery is possible.

Partial response

Partial response is defined as a decrease in tumour size of at least 50 per cent over at least 4 weeks, without an increase of more than 25 per cent in the size of any area of known malignant disease or the appearance of new areas of malignant disease. The 50 per cent decrease is measured in terms of the tumour area of an organ site or as the sum of the products of perpendicular diameters of multiple lesions at the same organ site.

No change

No change, sometimes called 'stable disease', is defined as a decrease in tumour size of less than 50 per cent or an increase in tumour size of less than 25 per cent at all sites, without the appearance of new areas of malignant disease. In practice, no change tends to be a catch-all category between clear response and clear progression; for instance, if there are multiple measurable sites and if one of them shows a complete response but not the others, the overall assessment may end up as no change despite disappearance of the tumour at one site.

Progression

Progression or progressive disease is defined as an increase in tumour size of more than 25 per cent at any site or the appearance of new areas of malignant disease.

Non-evaluable response

The four categories of response defined above (complete response, partial response, no change, progression) cover all possible situations for patients in whom response can be evaluated, but there are frequently patients in whom response cannot be evaluated. The most common reasons are early patient death, loss to follow-up or unavailable data, and failure to complete therapy. In all these cases the patients must be considered as treatment failures irrespective of the reason for their being non-evaluable. It might be felt desirable to exclude at least some of these patients, for instance those who did not receive enough treatment to have a fair chance of responding to treatment, but the exclusion of the patients who did not fare well may bias the response rate and casts doubts on the objectivity of the trial results.

Time end-points

In many clinical trials, the end-point of interest is the period of time from some arbitrary origin to the occurrence of some well-defined event, usually indicating treatment failure, such as death or disease relapse. Patients who have not yet failed at the time of the analysis constitute so-called censored observations, because their time to failure will eventually be longer than that observed at the time of the analysis.

Overall survival

Overall survival is the time period between some well-defined origin (usually the time of entry to the trial) and patient death, whatever its cause.

Overall survival is often regarded as the most important end-point to establish treatment benefit, particularly in rapidly lethal tumours. It is an easily and objectively measurable end-point, but one which is extremely hard to affect. Comparative trials seldom show survival differences between the treatment groups, in part because the treatments under investigation are often too similar to differ in terms of survival and in part because small survival differences are swamped in random errors due to patient heterogeneity.

Cancer survival

Cancer survival is the time period between some well-defined origin and patient death from malignant disease. Patients who die from other causes, such as intercurrent diseases, are regarded as censored observations.

Cancer survival is a more sensitive indicator of treatment effect than overall survival, particularly if the competing risks of dying from other causes are high (for example, in old age groups or with highly curable diseases). Zelen and Gelman (1986) discuss this problem in trials of early breast cancer and show that any beneficial effect of adjuvant chemotherapy for breast cancer is 'diluted' by

the other causes of mortality and therefore may be missed unless some allowance is made for the dilution by increasing the number of patients required in the trial. The analysis of cancer survival may provide valuable insight into the effects of treatment, but any evidence thus obtained may be biased. Indeed, causes of death are notoriously difficult to ascertain, so that misclassification between cancer and non-cancer causes may occur. Moreover, if treatment affected the non-malignant causes of death (perhaps because of some toxicity), an analysis of cancer survival could be misleading; for instance, an aggressive treatment might cure more patients of their cancer but kill them because of toxicity, resulting in no net benefit. In such cases, the overall survival analysis would correctly conclude that there was no benefit, while the cancer survival analysis would show a treatment benefit. Both analyses would have to be considered simultaneously for a reliable and informative conclusion to be drawn.

Time to progression and disease-free interval

Time to progression is the time period between some well-defined origin and a clear-cut disease progression, either clinical or pathological. Patients who die without evidence of disease progression are regarded as censored observations. In situations of adjuvant treatment, patients who have undergone curative therapy are declared free of disease until recurrence of the malignant process and time to progression is then called the disease-free interval.

In most cases time to progression is a worthwhile end-point in addition to survival. As for cancer survival, it is a more sensitive biological marker of treatment effect but a less reliable indicator of net benefit to the patient. The type of progression can yield useful information on the disease process. Therefore time to progression is usually subdivided into time to local progression (with distant progressions regarded as censored observations) and time to distant progression (with local progressions regarded as censored observations). These times can be as relevant as survival if disease recurrence has a major impact on the patient's condition and if no treatment is available on recurrence; for instance, time to local recurrence is an important end-point after radical surgery of rectal cancer because recurrences in the pelvis can be very painful and difficult to remove surgically.

Disease-free survival

Disease-free survival is defined in adjuvant therapy trials as the time period between curative therapy and either recurrence of the malignant process or death, whichever comes first. Disease-free survival combines both survival and time to recurrence information into a single end-point.

Duration of response

Duration of response is defined in advanced disease as the time period between the appearance of a treatment response and a recurrence of the disease. Because it is often difficult to measure precisely when the response started, duration of response may alternatively be defined in responding patients as the time period between the beginning of treatment and a recurrence of the disease.

Other end-points

Other end-points include toxicity and side-effects of treatment. Toxicities should be measured as objectively as possible, preferably on widely used scales such as those recommended by the World Health Organization (WHO 1979).

Quality of life is an increasingly important end-point of cancer trials, although its definition and measurement are fraught with difficulties. The reader is referred to the book edited by Aaronson and Beckmann (1987) for state of the art reviews.

Target population and eligibility criteria

The target population for a clinical trial is defined by a list of eligibility criteria. These are usually checked at the time that a patient is entered by comparing his or her characteristics with a list of inclusion and exclusion criteria.

Narrow versus broad eligibility criteria

Two diverging attitudes can be adopted in defining eligibility criteria for a clinical trial: they can be very precisely and narrowly defined, so that only a small fraction of available patients are eligible or at the other extreme they can be left as broad as possible so that most available patients are eligible.

Advantages of narrow eligibility criteria

Narrow eligibility criteria make the patient sample as homogeneous as possible. Homogeneity of the patient sample may be a desirable aim in identifying treatment benefits unequivocally in a subgroup of patients with well-defined prognostic features. All future patients in the same prognostic group can then be offered the treatment, should it prove effective in the clinical trial. Narrow eligibility criteria are preferable to broad criteria when there are good *a priori* reasons for believing that the treatment will be beneficial only to a subgroup of patients; this is typically the case when the treatment is potentially active but too toxic to be administered to patients with good prognosis. For instance, patients with a Dukes A rectal cancer are usually not submitted to adjuvant radiotherapy since most of them are cured after tumour resection.

Advantages of broad eligibility criteria

Broad eligibility criteria generally result in a larger accrual in the trial, therefore reducing the total duration of the study (Buyse 1990b). They also result in a patient sample which is more closely representative of the total patient population, and therefore their results can be extrapolated more readily to all future patients outside the trial. Broad eligibility criteria are preferable to narrow criteria when at the time of designing the trial little is known about the possible benefit that may be expected from the treatment under investigation in different subgroups of patients. In this (common) situation, the most plausible hypothesis is that the treatment is beneficial in different subgroups of patients and the best strategy is to choose eligibility criteria which are as broad as possible.

Uncertainty as to the main eligibility criterion

There is often a lack of agreement as to which patients may or may not benefit from a given therapy. When designing a trial, the investigators may try to reach a consensus about the exact eligibility criteria that they all believe to be appropriate or they may leave all participating clinicians to decide for themselves which patients may ethically be randomized, thus leaving uncertainty on the clinician's part as the main eligibility criterion (Stenning 1992). The latter approach may result in a somewhat unpredictable patient mix, for different clinicians may have diverging views as to which patients should be included. However, this approach, which is perfectly consistent with ethics, may be needed to overcome endless disputes in situations of genuine uncertainty.

Study designs

Phase I designs

The design of phase I trials has received little attention so far (Geller 1984). The standard phase I design consists of entering consecutive groups of patients, usually three, at a series of prespecified dose levels (Carter 1977). The starting dose is chosen as some proportion of the toxic dose in animals. The successive dose levels are usually determined using a 'modified Fibonacci' series, whereby dose escalations are initially rapid with smaller increments as the toxic range is approached. If no unacceptable toxicity is seen at a given dose level, then the next group of patients is treated at the next-highest dose level. However, if unacceptable toxicity is seen in one or more patients, then an additional group of three patients is entered at the same dose level. The trial is stopped when at least two out of six patients experience unacceptable toxicity at a given dose level, which is then taken as the maximum tolerated dose. This design, although widely used, can be criticized on statistical grounds (Storer and DeMets 1987).

Phase II designs

Several approaches have been proposed for the design of phase II trials. A classical approach is based on the work of Gehan (1961). Gehan's design consists of two stages: if no response is observed in the first stage, the trial is stopped and the drug rejected from further study; however, if one or more responses are observed in the first stage, additional patients are entered in the second stage to obtain an estimate of the response rate to a given precision (standard error). The major criticism of this design is that its second stage is not consistent with the overall aim of a screening trial since estimation of the response rate will not provide any formal rule to decide whether or not the drug should be tested further.

Another approach was suggested by Fleming (1982) to take better account of the two types of errors (type I and type II errors) in the decision-making process. In this approach two response rates are chosen: a response rate p_0 which is definitely unworthy of further investigation and a response rate p_1 which is definitely worthy of further investigation. For example, if the standard treatment of a given tumour has a 10 per cent response rate, p_0 could be chosen as 5 per cent and p_1 as 20 per cent for an investigational drug. Limits are also set on the probability of accepting the drug if its true response rate is lower than p_0 (type I error) and the probability of rejecting the drug if its true response rate is higher than p_1 (type II error). This design can have one or several stages; at each stage, the trial is stopped if the number of responses is less than some minimum or more than some maximum and is continued otherwise. At the end of the trial, the number of responses allows one to decide where the response rate lies with respect to p_0 and p_1.

A very attractive design using a decision-theoretical approach was studied by Sylvester (1988). A detailed description of this and several other designs is beyond the scope of this general chapter (see Herson (1985) for a review).

As mentioned earlier, phase II trials can be randomized, for instance when two or more drugs become available simultaneously, when screening analogues or when a comparative phase III trial of the new agent versus the standard treatment is considered to be highly likely. It should be emphasized that randomized phase II trials are not comparative trials; for this reason Herson and Carter (1986) prefer to call them 'calibrated' phase II trials.

Phase III designs

Many designs can be adopted for phase III trials (Staquet and Dalesio 1985). A few important examples are discussed in this section. The scheme used for treatment allocation, which is a particularly critical feature of phase III designs is discussed below.

Factorial designs

A factorial design is useful when two or more questions are simultaneously of interest for the same patient population. For instance, if one were interested in testing the worth of pre-operative radiotherapy and of adjuvant post-operative chemotherapy in resectable rectal cancer, a factorial design would consist of randomizing each patient to either radiotherapy or control before surgical resection and then randomizing each patient again to either chemotherapy or control after surgery. Thus, half of the patients would receive radiotherapy and the other half would not; likewise half the patients would receive chemotherapy and the other half would not. In effect, these two randomizations would create four groups of patients: one group receiving no adjuvant treatment, one receiving only radiotherapy, one receiving only chemotherapy, and one receiving both adjuvant treatments. This design allows one to study both the radiotherapy and the chemotherapy questions with the same number of patients as would be needed to study either one of these questions alone. In other words, studying each question separately would require twice as many patients as studying them both in a single factorial design (Byar and Piantadosi 1985). That factorial designs should result in such huge savings in terms of patient numbers is somewhat counterintuitive, but it is merely due to the fact that every patient contributes to both questions independently.

The two or more randomizations of a factorial design do not have to be performed at different times, as in the previous example. For instance, in a study of two drugs suppressing androgens in prostatic cancer, say A and B, each patient would be randomized between no antiandrogen therapy, A, B, or A and B. Factorial designs can also be used to answer an ancillary question (for example, on supportive care) at the same time as a main therapeutic question is being studied.

Sequential and group sequential designs

Most cancer trials are designed to accrue a predetermined number of patients. In such 'fixed-sample' designs the statistical analysis of the trial data is performed at the end of the follow-up period. Even if interim analyses are performed, they are seldom formally incorporated in the trial design (although they should be). In a sequential clinical trial, the data are analysed continuously as they become available in an effort to reach an early conclusion (Armitage 1975; Whitehead 1992). The basic idea is to stop the trial as soon as the observed treatment effect is large enough to cross a pre-calculated boundary. This approach is conceptually appealing, but it has rarely been used in cancer trials for two main reasons: first, in many cases the event of interest occurs after a long time, so that a reasonable estimate of the treatment effect will only be available long after the accrual into the trial is over; second, sequential designs are most useful to safeguard against large treatment effects, since in such situations they are likely to call for earlier termination than fixed-sample designs. While these situations may occur (for example, in the treatment of AIDS patients with AZT), they tend to be rather exceptional in cancer treatment where small differences are more likely to be expected. Group sequential

designs, in which the data are not analysed continuously but at several predetermined stages of the trial, may offer a reasonable compromise between pure sequential designs and fixed-sample designs; their main advantage is to build interim analyses formally into the trial design (O'Brien and Fleming 1979; Lan and DeMets 1983).

Pre-randomization

Clinicians often find it difficult to seek consent from patients before randomizing them into a trial, because many patients resent the uncertainty (however genuine) about which treatment is best for them. Zelen (1979) proposed a class of designs to alleviate this problem. In one version the patients are randomized prior to giving their consent. Clinicians will then find it easier to explain to patients that they will receive the treatment assigned by randomization unless they have a definite preference for the alternative treatment. This approach avoids the most overt difficulties of choosing treatment 'by the flip of a coin'. Therefore, it may encourage clinicians to enter more patients in the trial; however, the possibility that some patients will refuse the treatment assigned and choose the alternative treatment must be taken into account. In the analysis of the trial, these patients must be analysed by 'intention to treat' rather than by actual treatment to avoid bias. These cross-overs dilute any true treatment effect and cause a loss of power in the statistical tests. Thus, the number of patients required in this design is greater than in a conventional design in which patients who have a clear preference for either treatment may refuse to enter the trial and are not randomized. Another possible concern with this design is that the patients may be less informed about the alternative treatment when the randomization has already occurred (Ellenberg 1984).

Sources of bias in phase III designs

Bias will generally be avoided in the comparison between several randomized treatments under the following conditions:

(1) investigators are unaware, before deciding to enter a patient in the trial, of the treatment which will be assigned next;

(2) no randomized patient is excluded from the trial or from the statistical analyses for any reason.

Randomized trials must be designed with these two objectives in mind. If condition (1) does not hold, the investigators who know (or can guess) which treatment their next patient will receive may create a bias by selecting the patient accordingly. This is called selection bias. Investigators who carefully select the patients for entry in the trial without foreknowledge of the next treatment assignment do not create any selection bias (even though the term seems to imply that they do). If condition (2) does not hold, the excluded patients may differ between the various treatment groups, which again may bias the treatment comparisons. This is called exclusion bias. The most obvious form of exclusion bias occurs when patients who cannot receive their full treatment dose, that is, those faring worse than the average, are excluded from the analysis or taken 'off-study' and no longer followed up. It may be argued that these patients should not have entered the trial, but if they have, they must be followed up just like all others.

Even when no selection bias nor exclusion bias has occurred, there may be a chance maldistribution of important prognostic factors between the treatment groups. Such maldistribution could confound the effect of treatment and, thus, create a bias. This is called accidental bias. The likelihood of an accidental bias decreases dramatically as the number of patients increases. It is often useful to safeguard against accidental bias by stratifying the treatment allocation.

Treatment allocation schemes

When a comparative study is contemplated, the way in which the various treatments will be assigned to the successive patients who enter the study must be carefully defined. Pure randomization, that is, simply choosing the treatment at random every time a new patient enters the study, is only one possible method among various others, which are collectively called treatment allocation schemes (Kalish and Begg 1985).

Aims of treatment allocation schemes

Many methods have been proposed for allocating treatments to patients in clinical trials. Some are as simple as flipping a coin to choose between two treatments; others are fairly complex and require knowledge of some patient characteristics before the treatment is assigned. The important aims to keep in mind when choosing a method are as follows.

1. Treatment assignments should be unpredictable (otherwise selection bias may take place; investigators who know the next treatment assignment may select the next patient they enter in the trial accordingly).

2. A good balance should exist between the number of patients assigned to each treatment, both overall and if possible in subsets of particular interest (otherwise statistical efficiency may be lost, accidental bias may take place, and the imbalance may raise suspicion about the validity of the allocation procedure).

3. The distribution of patients in the treatment groups should be such that the efficiency of the treatment comparisons is maximized (otherwise the number of patients needed will have to be increased to ensure the same statistical power).

4. The randomization procedure should be simple and rapid (otherwise investigators may be reluctant to enter patients in the trial).

5. The randomization procedure should be foolproof (otherwise distortions may ruin the very purpose of randomization, which is to ensure comparability between treatment groups).

These various goals are to some extent conflicting and no method of treatment allocation is uniformly better for all of them.

Unequal allocation

It is generally advisable, irrespective of the allocation technique adopted, that all treatments be chosen with equal probability, but in some cases it may be preferred to allocate more patients to one treatment than to the others (Peto et al. 1976). For instance, if a very promising experimental therapy is compared with a standard method, it may be preferred to allocate twice as many patients to the former than to the latter.

Simple randomization

Simple randomization consists of choosing the treatment at random irrespective of the patient characteristics. The advantage of simple randomization, in addition to simplicity, is that it completely eliminates selection bias since the next treatment assignment is never

predictable. The disadvantage is that chance imbalances between the different treatments may occur. With simple randomization the likelihood of an overall chance imbalance is negligible if the number of patients is large enough (several hundred patients), but it may not be negligible in all subgroups of patients of clinical interest (say, in elderly patients without prior therapy). If balance in such subgroups is desired, stratification of the treatment allocation should be considered.

Stratification

Treatment allocation is said to be stratified if it depends on certain patient characteristics known as stratifying factors (for example, age, sex, disease stage, prior therapies, etc.) The cross-classification of all stratifying factors defines distinct strata (for example, if sex and age are stratifying factors, one stratum could be females under 50 years of age). The purpose of stratified randomization is to reduce the likelihood of chance imbalances in the treatment assignments among strata. There are three principal advantages to stratified randomization:

(1) the potential for accidental bias resulting from imbalances between treatment groups is reduced;

(2) the results of the trial may be more convincing because treatment groups look alike in terms of the important prognostic factors;

(3) the precision of the estimates of treatment effect and the efficiency of the statistical tests for treatment effect are increased (although the gain is usually quite small).

If stratification is adopted, it is advisable to stratify only for factors of known prognostic value. For instance, if histology were of no prognostic impact on the patient outcome, it would be pointless to stratify for histology. It is also advisable to stratify only for factors that are known with certainty at the time of randomization. For instance, if histology were only confirmed several weeks after randomization, it would be hazardous to stratify for histology. The number of stratifying factors should not be so large as to discourage patient entry into the trial. In multicentre trials it is also advisable to include institution as a stratifying factor to limit treatment imbalance within each institution.

Permuted blocks

Permuted blocks are used to reduce the effect of chance by ensuring perfect balance between the treatment groups after a fixed number of patients have been entered. For instance, if one compares a treatment (T) with a control group (C), one may wish to have exactly two patients allocated to treatment and two allocated to control after four patients have been entered. In this case the block size is four. Within a block, the sequence of treatment assignments is chosen at random from all possible permutations. In the example these permutations are CCTT, CTCT, CTTC, TCCT, TCTC, and TTCC. The block size is usually chosen as a small multiple of the number of treatments. Permuted blocks extend easily to the situation where stratification is required; independent permuted blocks are then used within each stratum. The advantage of permuted blocks is that they force periodic balance in the number of patients assigned to each treatment group. This may be particularly desirable if patient characteristics change with time. The disadvantage is that the last treatment assignment(s) in a block are predictable. Thus, selection bias due to foreknowledge of the next treatment assignment can be substantial if the block size is small and known to the

Table 4 Treatment allocation using a minimization algorithm

Prognostic factor values	Number of patients	
	Control	Treatment
Age: between 55 and 65 years	23	22
Sex: male	58	54
Institution: ABC	16	20
	Imbalances If next patient is assigned to	
	Control	Treatment
Age: between 55 and 65 years	2	0
Sex: male	5	3
Institution: ABC	−3	−5
Total	4	−2

The treatment assigned to the next patient is chosen so as to minimize the total imbalance between the control group and the treatment group with respect to some important prognostic factors (here age, sex, and institution).

investigators. In our example, if two patients have been assigned to the control group in a block, then the next two patients who enter the trial will with certainty be assigned to the treatment group.

Minimization

Minimization is a method that attempts to achieve optimum treatment balance on several factors simultaneously, not within the separate strata. The method is best explained by means of an example. Suppose that in a certain trial comparing a new treatment with control, age, sex, and institution are stratifying factors. A 62 year old male patient presents for randomization in institution ABC when the numbers of patients already assigned to each treatment are as shown in Table 4.

Minimization consists of choosing the treatment that minimizes the total imbalance on some scale (Freedman and White 1976). In our example, assigning the next patient to the control group results in a larger total imbalance; therefore the patient will be assigned to the treatment group.

The major advantage of using minimization is that good treatment balance can be achieved across a (possibly large) number of stratifying factors. One disadvantage is that the balance is achieved in the levels of the stratifying factors and not in the strata. For instance, in our example balance will be achieved for male patients and for those aged 55–64 years, but perhaps not for male patients who are aged 55–64 years. Another problem is that the method is deterministic so that it is not guaranteed to provide the randomness assumed by the statistical tests used to analyse the trial results. It can be used safely only if the entry of patients in the trial can be assumed to be random. Some randomness can easily be introduced in the assignment process, for instance by choosing the treatment at random if the imbalance is lower than a specified limit.

Other schemes

Various other treatment allocation schemes have been proposed to achieve the aims listed above, among which are biased coin schemes (Efron 1971), urn models (Wei 1978), optimum sampling schemes (Begg and Iglewicz 1980), and many variations on related themes. In practice the major choice is between simple randomization and one of the methods that take prognostic features into account. Kalish and Begg (1985) have reviewed all methods and their statistical properties have been studied by Lachin *et al.* (1988).

Trial outcomes, error types, significance, and power

Some fundamental statistical concepts which will be needed for the calculation of the number of patients required in clinical trials, and for a proper interpretation of their results are now introduced. The interested reader should consult Armitage (1971) for further details or Folks (1981) for an introduction to statistical concepts.

Trial outcomes

In its simplest form, the outcome of a trial can be viewed as either positive or inconclusive. The outcome of a phase II trial is positive if the drug is declared effective; the outcome is inconclusive if the drug cannot be declared effective. The outcome of a phase II trial is never that a drug is ineffective, but merely that there is insufficient evidence to claim that it is effective. This distinction is important in the interpretation of negative results (Freiman *et al.* 1978). The outcome of a phase III trial is positive if one treatment arm is declared superior to the others; it is inconclusive if no treatment arm can be declared superior to the others. The outcome of a phase III trial is never that the treatment arms are equivalent, but merely that there is insufficient evidence to claim that there is a difference between them.

Error types

The purpose of a trial is to uncover the true state of nature (which is, of course, unknown). If the trial concludes that there is a significant treatment benefit when in truth there is none, the error made is called a type I error or false-positive. Conversely, if the trial concludes that there is no treatment benefit when in truth there is, the error made is called a type II error or false-negative. Obviously both types of error must be minimized for the trial to yield useful information. Equally obviously, a price must be paid for this minimization. One type of error can be minimized at the expense of the other: declaring no treatment benefit regardless of the actual data always minimizes the type I error but maximizes the type II error; conversely, declaring a treatment benefit regardless of the actual data always minimizes the type II error but maximizes the type I error. Neither of these extreme attitudes would be very sensible. A sensible approach would consist of controlling both types of errors simultaneously by acting on the number of patients entered in the trial; that is, the sample size.

When a clinical trial is being planned, a probability is specified somewhat arbitrarily for each error type. It is customary to set the probability α of a type I error at 0.05 (5 per cent) and the probability β of a type II error at 0.20 (20 per cent); α is called the significance level and $1-\beta$ the power. These values for α and β are only indicative and different values could make perfect sense. In fact, α and β should be set according to the problem at hand. If one compared a new promising treatment with an established treatment, one would not want to miss a real benefit of the new treatment

Table 5 Types of errors and their corresponding probabilities α and β[a]

Truth	Outcome of trial	
	Treatment benefit	No treatment benefit
Treatment benefit	Correct, $1-\beta$	Type II error (false-negative), β
No treatment benefit	Type I error (false-positive), α	Correct, $1-\alpha$

[a] The power; that is, the probability of detecting a true treatment benefit, is $1-\beta$.

and therefore one would choose low values for β (perhaps 0.10 or less). However, if one compared a very toxic new treatment with an established treatment, one would not want to subject future patients to the new treatment unless there were a high probability that it is really effective and therefore one would choose low values for α (perhaps 0.01 or less).

Significance

When data are available at the end of a comparative clinical trial, a statistical test is performed to compare the various treatments under investigation. The hypothesis which is being tested, called the null hypothesis, is that all treatments are equivalent. In general terms, the statistical test calculates the probability under the null hypothesis of observing data at least as extreme as those observed. This probability is called the statistical significance of the test or its p value. If the p value is less than the significance level α which was specified before the trial, the test is said to be statistically significant and the null hypothesis of treatment equivalence is rejected. Imagine, for instance, that one has observed long survival times more frequently in a treatment group than in a control group: how likely is this observed difference due to chance? The way to answer this question is to assume that both treatments are equivalent, to perform a statistical test appropriate for survival times (a log rank test) and to claim that the observed difference is unlikely to be due to chance and therefore is likely to be due to a real treatment benefit, if the p value of the log rank test is less than $\alpha=0.05$.

Power

If the null hypothesis of treatment equivalence is untrue, then an alternative hypothesis must be true. The alternative hypothesis specifies some difference between the treatments on an appropriate scale (for example, rate difference, rate ratio, etc.) For instance, if a treatment group is compared with a control group, an alternative hypothesis could specify that treatment is better than the control by 20 per cent (one-sided alternative) or that there is a 20 per cent difference in either direction between the treatment and the control (two-sided alternative). The statistical power of a comparative clinical trial is the probability of detecting a postulated treatment difference if in truth it exists. Using the notation of Table 5, the power is equal to $1-\beta$. The power is obviously a function of the magnitude of the postulated benefit: the same trial may have good power (that is, high probability) to detect a huge treatment difference, but poor power (that is, low probability) to detect a small treatment difference.

Number of patients needed

Phase II trials

If Gehan's classical two-stage plan is used, the number of patients required in the first stage depends on the minimum response rate one is interested in detecting. Suppose, for instance, that the minimum response rate of interest is 20 per cent. If the drug has a true response rate of 20 per cent, then the probability that the first patient will fail to have a response is 80 per cent, the probability of the first two patients failing is 64 per cent (80 per cent×80 per cent), the probability of the first three patients failing is 51 per cent (80 per cent×80 per cent×80 per cent), ..., and the probability of the first 14 patients failing is just under 5 per cent. Thus, if no response is observed in the first 14 patients, the drug can be rejected from further study. This ensures a 5 per cent probability for the type II error of falsely rejecting a drug which has a true response rate of at least 20 per cent. In general, if β is the probability of a type II error and r is the response rate of interest, the minimum number of patients in the first stage is given by $\log \beta / \log (1-r)$. The number of patients required in the second stage depends on how many responses were observed in the first stage and the degree of precision (standard error) desired for the estimate of the response rate (Gehan 1961).

Theoretical objections can be raised against this approach, which is inadequate for planning efficient phase III trials (Storer and DeMets 1987). In fact, a review of phase II trials performed between 1970 and 1985 showed that many of them had an insufficient sample size to allow an adequate evaluation of the new drugs being tested (Marsoni et al. 1987).

Phase III trials

The number of patients entered in a phase III trial, called its sample size, is usually calculated to ensure reasonable power (say 0.80, that is, 80 per cent probability) of detecting a postulated treatment effect at a pre-specified significance level α. Treatment effects can be measured in various ways depending on the end-point of interest, for example response to treatment or some time-related end-point. If, for instance, one were interested in the effect of some adjuvant therapy on colorectal cancer, an appropriate measure of treatment effect could be the survival benefit at 5 years. The 5 year survival without any adjuvant therapy is of the order of 50 per cent. The upper curve of Fig. 1 gives the sample size that would be needed to detect 5 year survival benefits with power equal to 0.80, assuming a significance level of $\alpha=0.05$ (Freedman 1982).

To have an 80 per cent chance of detecting a 5 year benefit of 45 per cent, only 40 patients need to be randomized. However, it is clearly unreasonable to plan a trial in the hope of improving the proportion of patients still alive at 5 years from 50 to 95

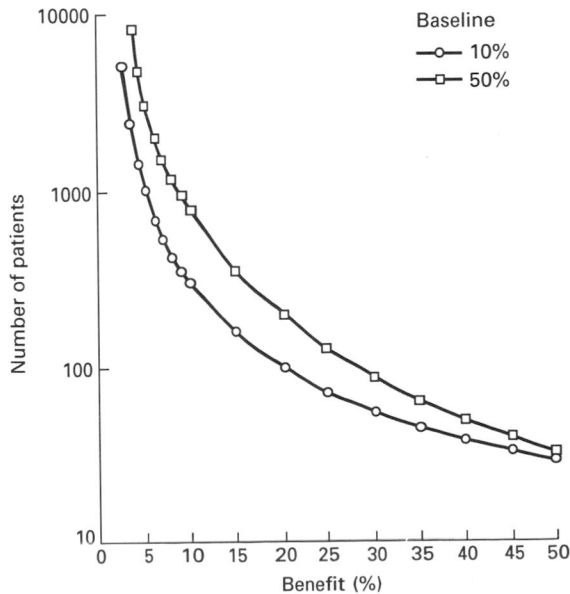

Fig. 1 Number of patients required (vertical axis) to detect a postulated survival benefit (horizontal axis) with a statistical power of 80 per cent using a two-sided log rank test at significance level 5 per cent. The vertical axis is drawn on a logarithmic scale. The two curves correspond to two different assumptions on the baseline survival in the control group: 10 per cent (lower curve) and 50 per cent (upper curve).

Table 6 Total number of patients required to compare the response rate in a treatment group with that in a control group ($\alpha=0.05$, $\beta=0.20$, two-sided test)

Response rate in treatment group	Response rate in control group							
	0.10	0.20	0.30	0.40	0.50	0.60	0.70	0.80
0.15	1450	—	—	—	—	—	—	—
0.20	440	—	—	—	—	—	—	—
0.25	230	2270	—	—	—	—	—	—
0.30	144	630	—	—	—	—	—	—
0.35	102	310	2830	—	—	—	—	—
0.40	76	182	750	—	—	—	—	—
0.45	60	124	350	3150	—	—	—	—
0.50	50	90	210	820	—	—	—	—
0.55	40	70	136	380	3210	—	—	—
0.60	34	56	98	220	820	—	—	—
0.65	30	44	74	140	370	3020	—	—
0.70	26	38	58	98	210	760	—	—
0.75	22	32	46	72	132	330	2580	—
0.80	20	26	38	56	90	182	630	—
0.85	18	22	30	44	66	114	270	1890
0.90	16	20	26	34	50	76	144	440
0.95	14	16	22	28	38	54	86	176

Table 7 Total number of patients required to compare the survival rate in a treatment group with that in a control group ($\alpha=0.05$, $\beta=0.20$, two-sided test)

Survival rate in treatment group	Survival rate in control group							
	0.10	0.20	0.30	0.40	0.50	0.60	0.70	0.80
0.15	970	—	—	—	—	—	—	—
0.20	300	—	—	—	—	—	—	—
0.25	156	1830	—	—	—	—	—	—
0.30	100	510	—	—	—	—	—	—
0.35	74	250	2490	—	—	—	—	—
0.40	58	150	660	—	—	—	—	—
0.45	46	104	310	2900	—	—	—	—
0.50	40	78	182	750	—	—	—	—
0.55	34	60	122	340	3030	—	—	—
0.60	30	50	88	196	760	—	—	—
0.65	28	42	68	128	340	2900	—	—
0.70	26	36	54	92	192	710	—	—
0.75	24	32	44	68	124	310	2490	—
0.80	22	28	38	54	86	172	600	—
0.85	20	26	32	44	64	108	250	1820
0.90	20	24	28	36	50	74	134	410
0.95	20	22	26	32	40	54	80	160

per cent and therefore small trials are doomed to failure in this disease. To detect a more realistic 5 year benefit of 5 per cent, over 3000 patients need to be randomized. Many past clinical trials in colorectal cancer accrued less than 500 patients; as can be seen from Fig. 1, these trials had adequate statistical power to detect a 5 year survival benefit of at least 12 per cent but insufficient power to detect any smaller benefit. The number of patients increases sharply as the treatment benefit of interest decreases. In this example, the baseline survival rate was taken as 50 per cent; Fig. 1 also shows the number of patients needed to detect postulated treatment benefits over a baseline rate of 10 per cent.

Comparison of proportions (for example, response rates)

The number of patients needed to detect a postulated difference in response rate between a treatment group and a control group (in either direction) is given in Table 6. Formulae and tables appropriate for more than two groups, and for different values of α and β, are given by George (1985) and by Machin and Campbell (1987).

Comparison of survival times

The number of patients needed to detect a postulated difference in survival rate between a treatment group and a control group (in either direction) is given in Table 7. Formulae and tables appropriate for more than two groups and for different values of α and β, are given by Freedman (1982), George (1985), and Machin and Campbell (1987).

Equivalence trials

The purpose of phase III trials is not always to show that treatment is superior to the control in terms of response rate or survival; sometimes they aim to demonstrate that an investigational treatment is equivalent to the control as far as the main end-points are concerned, while being less toxic, less mutilating, more widely available, less expensive, etc. In such cases the statistical considerations must be adapted accordingly (Blackwelder 1982).

The need for some large phase III trials

Phase III clinical trials should be planned for the reliable detection of small to moderate treatment effects and not for the identification of major breakthroughs. Large treatment benefits have seldom been reported and should not generally be expected in cancer clinical trials. As a consequence, small trials (a few dozen patients) should be the exception and large trials (several hundred or even thousand patients) the rule (Peto 1978). The minimum treatment benefit which is considered clinically worthwhile depends primarily on the severity of the disease and the undesirable side-effects of the therapy. While a large survival improvement may be demanded of aggressive therapy for a fatal condition (say polychemotherapy for primary liver cancer), it is self-defeating to hope for more than a small survival improvement with an adjuvant therapy in patients with good prognosis (say chemotherapy after curative resection of a colon tumour) (Freedman 1989). Some investigators claim that small treatment effects, such as a 5 per cent improvement in 5 year survival after adjuvant chemotherapy of colorectal cancer, are unimportant (Buyse et al. 1988). This claim is disputable, because it is blatantly incorrect to claim that a treatment which offers a small overall benefit is of no value to the individual patient (Letters 1988). Moreover, such small effects, if real, might be of great public health importance. The widespread application of marginally effective treatments for frequent diseases might indeed result in the saving of thousands of lives every year (Yusuf et al. 1984). Recent adjuvant trials in cancer have been planned to accrue many more patients than in the past; recent intergroup studies in the United States have accrued thousands of patients over a few months. It has been suggested that a meta-analysis of several small trials could replace one large trial; in fact, even if some trials with a few thousand patients were performed, a meta-analysis of all related trials would still be needed for a true assessment of the value of an adjuvant therapy (Levin and O'Connell 1988).

CONDUCT OF CLINICAL TRIALS
Patient entry

One of the essential elements of a properly controlled trial is a reliable mechanism for patient entry. In phase II trials patients must be registered into the trial before their treatment begins (otherwise investigators may be tempted not to report patients who do not fare well). In phase III trials, whichever treatment allocation scheme (see above) is used must be implemented in a foolproof manner. Methods such as providing each investigator with lists of random treatment assignments or sealed envelopes are not foolproof and should be avoided. Central patient registration is by far the best way of ensuring that treatments are allocated properly and of keeping tight control over the progress of the trial (Lange and MacIntyre 1984). Central registration is usually done by telephone, but more recently computer networks have also been used (EuroCODE Steering Committee 1990).

In multicentre trials it is often useful to build an institutional factor into the treatment allocation scheme. There are several reasons for doing this. First, patient recruitment patterns may differ substantially between institutions and it may be useful to account for these differences by treating the institution as a stratifying factor. Second, it is sometimes necessary to exclude all patients entered by an institution from a clinical trial, for example if no follow-up was received from this institution. Third, participating investigators usually like to view the clinical trial within their institution as if it were a single-centre trial.

Patient follow-up

Patient follow-up is usually a major difficulty in trials extending over long periods of time. It is usually sufficient to ensure regular follow-up of a few essential parameters, such as disease recurrence or death, using routine clinical examinations. It is counterproductive to impose highly sophisticated follow-up techniques, as this may lead to reluctance to enter patients in the trial and is not even warranted from a statistical viewpoint (Peto 1980).

However, it is essential to minimize the number of patients who are lost to follow-up during the course of the trial. Such losses may bias the trial results if they are related to the treatment itself. For instance, some patients on more aggressive treatment may be so sick that they never come back. National mortality records, where they exist in sufficient detail to trace individual patients, may provide an alternative way of collecting dates of deaths for patients lost to follow-up (Peto 1978).

In comparative trials some patients are not given the treatment allocated by the randomization for a variety of reasons (patient refusal, fear of toxicity, etc.). These patients must be followed up like the others and analysed by 'intention to treat' rather than by actual treatment. If such deviations occur frequently, they may cause a substantial loss in power of the statistical tests. The number of patients must then be multiplied by an 'inflation' factor to preserve the nominal power of the trial (Ellenberg 1984). Figure 2 shows the value of the inflation factor as a function of the proportion of patients who are crossed over to the other treatment in the case of a two-arm trial. If half the patients cross over, any treatment effect is entirely diluted and can no longer be detected regardless of the number of patients.

Trial monitoring

The success or failure of a clinical trial depends critically on the study coordinator who must first 'sell' the trial concept to potentially interested colleagues, then monitor the ongoing trial and check all incoming data and finally report the trial results (Dodion and Abele 1989). This is a heavy responsibility for a single individual, particularly when he or she is a busy clinician with competing

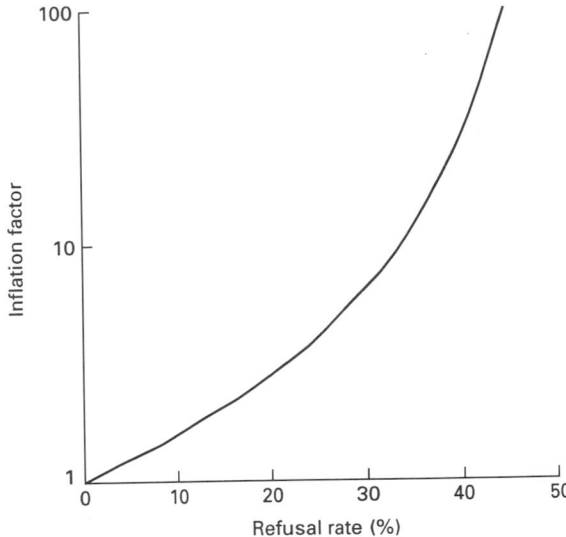

Fig. 2 Factor by which the number of patients must be increased to maintain the statistical power of a clinical trial if some proportion of the patients refuse the treatment assigned by randomization and choose the other treatment instead. The vertical axis is drawn on a logarithmic scale.

demands and priorities. As well as a dedicated coordinator, the successful conduct of a clinical trial typically requires substantial logistic support from a team specializing in data management, computer science, and biostatistics.

In phase II and limited phase III trials in advanced disease, it is often important to control the way in which the trial is conducted at the various participating institutions by performing extramural reviews of pathological material and on-site checks of treatment administration, end-point assessment, and other features which may have an impact on the trial results. In these trials one is interested in giving investigational therapies their best chance of showing an activity. In large phase III trials, however, such quality control checks are useless, given the pragmatic nature of the trials. In these trials, one is interested in accruing large numbers of patients treated as they would be outside of the trial (Buyse 1993a). Such trials are variously known as confirmatory, pragmatic, or public health trials, in contrast to early trials which are known as explanatory or regulatory trials (Schwartz and Lellouch 1967).

It is often desirable to monitor the results of a trial in order to stop it early should any of the following circumstances occur.

1. An unexpected and serious toxicity has been observed.

2. An unexpectedly large treatment difference has emerged, and continued accrual into the trial is felt to be unethical.

3. Absolutely no therapeutic advantage has been observed and continued accrual into the trial is felt to be unnecessary.

These circumstances may be noticed on the occasion of an interim analysis, but the play of chance must be borne in mind when interpreting interim results, even if these appear to be quite extreme. In trials of substantial size or importance, an independent Data Monitoring Committee is normally appointed to assess the interim results and to advise the study coordinator about the desirability to stop or to continue patient accrual (Buyse 1993b).

Sources of bias in the conduct of phase III trials

Follow-up should be available for all randomized patients and should be identical in thoroughness and frequency in the various treatment groups. For instance, seeing treated patients more frequently than control patients could bias the assessment of disease-free interval because recurrences would be detected earlier in the treated group. Softer end-points, such as disease recurrence, are more subject to bias than harder end-points, such as death. For instance, if an untreated control group is compared with a treatment group, there may be pressure to scrutinize the untreated patients much more thoroughly than the treated patients in order to identify and treat disease recurrences as early as possible (Buyse 1989). Some have advocated blind assessment of the end-points, that is, assessment by investigators not aware of the treatment actually received, but this practice has limited applicability in clinical trials of treatments with noticeable toxicities (Horwitz 1987).

Missing information can be a major cause of bias. Really important data items are more likely to be obtained if the amount of information requested is minimized. The follow-up form of a phase III clinical trial can generally be kept very simple, with information on the major end-points only (Buyse 1989). When treatments reach the phase III trial, they are usually well known in terms of their feasibility, toxicities, side-effects, etc. Collecting information on these aspects is at best a waste of time and confuses the real issue of the trial (unless, of course, the purpose of the trial is to compare toxicities). In contrast, clinical trials offer a unique opportunity to evaluate prospectively the frequency and severity of rare or unexpected toxicities. Late effects of therapy, such as MeCCNU-induced leukaemias, are best documented in the context of clinical trials.

ANALYSIS OF CLINICAL TRIALS

A reasonable coverage of the statistical techniques appropriate for clinical research would fill an entire volume (see, for instance, Armitage (1975)). In this section we provide a superficial introduction to the techniques that are most commonly used for the analysis of clinical trials (Table 8).

Techniques appropriate for response data

Estimation of response rates

Assume that some treatment was given to N_T patients, of whom R_T experienced a 'response' (Table 9). An estimate of the response rate is given simply by R_T/N_T. Suppose that $R_T=33$ and $N_T=59$,

Table 8 Statistical procedures most commonly used in the analysis of cancer clinical trials

Type of analysis	Type of end-point Response	Time-related
Estimation	Response rate (and 95% confidence limits)	'Survival' curve: Kaplan–Meier estimate (and 95% confidence limits)
Hypothesis testing	Chi-square test Fisher's exact test	Log rank test
Stratified analysis	Mantel–Haenszel test	Stratified log rank test
Multivariate analysis	Logistic regression	Cox's proportional hazards regression

Table 9 The 2×2 table used to compare the response rates in a control group and a treatment group

	Control	Treatment	
Response	R_C	R_T	$R_C+R_T=R$
No response	P_C	P_T	$P_C+P_T=P$
	$R_C+P_C=N_C$	$R_T+P_T=N_T$	$N_C+N_T=R+P=N$

then the response rate is $33/59=0.56$. It is informative to report not only the response rate, but also its confidence limits. The 95 per cent confidence limits are defined as those two response rates which, in the long run, would include the true (unknown) response rate 95 per cent of the time. The interval between the lower and the upper confidence limit is called the 95 per cent confidence interval. The width of the confidence interval is a function of the number of patients N_T: the larger is N_T, the smaller is the confidence interval. The 95 per cent confidence limits of the response rate are given approximately by $R_T/N_T \pm 1.96$ $(R_T P_T/N_T^3)^{1/2}$. In the example, it is easily verified that the 95 per cent confidence interval for the response rate is $(0.43, 0.69)$. If ten times more patients had been observed (590 patients) with the same proportion of responses (0.56), the confidence interval would have been considerably smaller $(0.52, 0.60)$, thus providing a much better idea of where the true response rate is likely to be. The confidence interval is easily computed, but the above formula is an approximation which is valid only if the numbers of patients with and without response (R_T and P_T) are both larger than ten (otherwise the binomial distribution should be used). Further details are given by Armitage (1971).

Comparison of response rates

The response rates in several groups and their corresponding confidence intervals, can be estimated as described above. However, the question of interest when there are several groups is whether their response rates are 'significantly different' from each other.

In the example in Table 10 CHOP has a higher response rate than BCOP (0.56 versus 0.36), but is the observed difference statistically significant (Bartolucci 1985)? The statistical test usually employed to answer this question is called the chi-square test and can be computed as follows. The number of responses observed in the treatment group is defined as the 'observed' number O. In the notation of Table 9, $O=R_T$. If there were no difference between treatment and control, the same response rate would be expected in both groups. The overall response rate for all patients is R/N and since there are N_T patients in the treatment group, the expected number of responses in this group would be $N_T R/N$. This 'expected' number of responses is denoted E. The variance of the number of responses can be computed by the approximate formula

$$V=N_C N_T RP/[N^2(N-1)]$$

Table 10 The 2×2 table used to compare the response rates in two groups of patients with non-Hodgkin's lymphoma receiving CHOP or BCOP

	BCOP	CHOP	
Response	19 (36%)	33 (56%)	52
No response	34	26	60
	53	59	112

CHOP, cytoxan, adriamycin, vincristine, and prednisone;. BCOP, BCNU, cytoxan, vincristine, and prednisone.

The chi-square statistic is then given simply by $(O-E)^2/V$, which can be compared with a table of the chi-square distribution with one degree of freedom. In our example, the values are

$$O=33, \quad E=52\times59/112=27.39, \quad V=53\times59\times52\times60/(112)^3=6.94$$

giving a chi-square statistic of

$$(33-27.39)^2/6.94=4.53$$

A table of the chi-square distribution with one degree of freedom indicates that a value at least as large as the statistic is observed with probability $p=0.03$. Because this p value is less than 0.05, we can conclude that the difference between 0.56 and 0.36 is unlikely to be due to chance and therefore is statistically significant. The chi-square statistic is easily computed, but the chi-square test is only valid if the number of patients in each cell of the table (R_C, R_T, P_C, P_T) is greater than five (otherwise Fisher's exact test should be used). Further details are given by Armitage (1971).

It is important to emphasize that the p value indicates the probability that a finding is due to chance; it tells us nothing about the magnitude of the observed benefit. This caveat has led some authors to distinguish between statistical significance, quantified by the p value and clinical significance, quantified by the observed benefit. In our example, the difference between 0.56 and 0.36 is statistically significant (there is a 3 in 100 chance that the difference is due to chance); whether a 0.20 benefit in response rate is also clinically worthwhile depends on other considerations such as the toxicity, inconvenience, long-term risks, etc.

Stratified comparison of response rates

In practice, some patient characteristics are strong predictors of response to treatment; for instance, heavily pre-treated patients are less likely to respond than previously untreated patients. In this case it may be desirable to construct a separate subtable similar to Table 9 for each prognostic category or stratum. Even if subtables are examined, the greatest interest is still in testing the overall effect of treatment. Mantel and Haenszel (1959) proposed a method for estimating and testing the effect of treatment within each subtable as well as overall through a 'stratified' (or 'adjusted') analysis. In our example, one subtable would compare treatment effectiveness in pre-treated patients and the other in previously untreated patients. The estimates of treatment effect from each subtable could then be combined to provide an overall 'stratified' estimate (and test of significance). The Mantel–Haenszel approach has the intuitive advantage of comparing 'like with like' within each subtable. It also has the interesting statistical property, in some circumstances, of improving the estimate of treatment effect and of increasing the power of the statistical tests for treatment effect.

Multivariate models for response rates

It is often required to assess the predictive power of several variables simultaneously on treatment response. A commonly used approach to this problem is to model the probability of a response given the patient characteristics. Specifically, a linear regression can be performed with the prognostic factors as independent variables and some suitable transformation of the probability of response as the dependent variable. A popular model in this class is the logistic regression model (Armitage 1975).

Techniques appropriate for survival data

Survival data usually present two features which make their analysis somewhat complicated: first they tend to be highly 'skewed' (that is, they do not comply with the assumption of normality that is required by many conventional statistical techniques) and, second, they may be censored (that is, they may be incomplete for some individuals in the data set).

Censoring of time-related data may be due to two distinct mechanisms: first some patients may not yet have suffered the event of interest at the time of the analysis (for instance, if the event of interest is death, some patients may still be alive at the time of the analysis) and, second, some patients may have suffered another event which will forever prevent them from having the event of interest (for instance, if the event of interest is disease recurrence, some patients may have died without evidence of the disease).

Estimation of survival curves

Suppose that we have observed a group of ten patients over a period of time: four patients have died after 3, 7, 11, and 14 months, while the six patients who are still alive have been followed for 9+, 10+, 12+, 13+, 15+, and 18+ months (the plus sign indicates that these are censored observations). How can we use these data? Simply computing their mean and variance would be erroneous because of the six censored observations; indeed, we know that the survival times for these six observations will eventually be longer than at the time of the analysis. The standard method of handling the problem is to estimate a survival cure, which gives the probability of survival as a function of time (Kaplan and Meier 1958).

The method used to compute the survival curve is as follows (Table 11):

(1) sort the observed survival times in increasing order (column a);

(2) the number of patients 'at risk', that is, still known to be alive, decreases at each censored time and at each death time by the number of patients lost to follow-up or dead at that time (columns b and c);

(3) the probability of surviving past a death time is estimated by the number of patients at risk just after that time divided by the number of patients at risk just before that time; the probability of surviving past a censored time is unity (column d);

(4) the survival curve gives the probability of survival past the nth death time and, thus, is equal to the product of the probabilities of surviving the first, the second, the third, etc., until the nth death time (column e).

Table 11 Estimation of the survival curve for a group of patients with survival times of 3, 7, 9+, 10+, 11, 12+, 13+, 14, 15+, and 18+ months

a Times (months)	b Patients at risk		d Probability of surviving past this time	e Proportion surviving
	Before	After		
<3	10	10	1.000	1.000
3	10	9	0.900	0.900
7	9	8	0.888	0.800
9+	8	7	1.000	0.800
10+	7	6	1.000	0.800
11	6	5	0.833	0.667
12+	5	4	1.000	0.667
13+	4	3	1.000	0.667
14	3	2	0.667	0.444
15+	2	1	1.000	0.444
18+	1	0	1.000	0.444

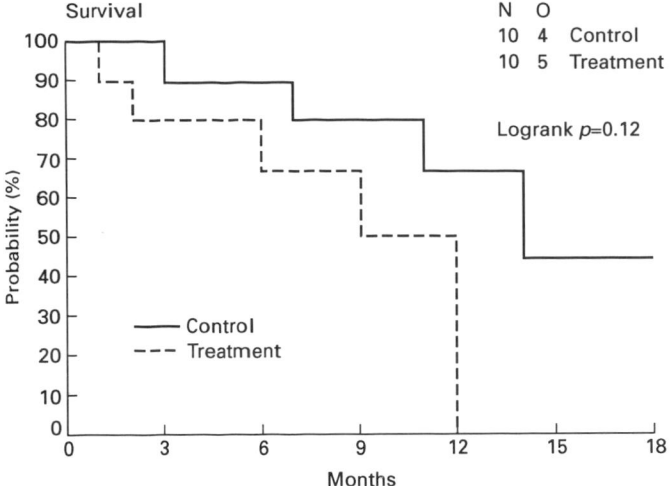

Fig. 3 Survival curves estimated in a 'control' group and a 'treatment' group and the *p* value of the log rank test comparing these two curves (see calculations in Tables 11 and 12)

These computations for our example are summarized in Table 11 and the resulting survival curve is shown as 'Control' in Fig. 3. As for the estimation of response rates, it may be useful to compute a confidence interval for the survival curve at each point in time. The standard error of the survival curve can be computed using Greenwood's formula (Cox and Oakes 1984). The survival curve drops only at death times; censored times are indicated by a tick on the curve.

Care should be taken in interpreting the shape of the survival curve, notably 'plateaux' which can occur in the tail of the survival curve (see the 'Control' group on Fig. 3). Because very few patients are usually at risk in the tail of the curve, its variability is too great to conclude that a given proportion of patients is cured and will enjoy very long survivals. Similarly, a sharp drop at the end of the curve (see the 'Treatment' group on Fig. 3) is no cause for worry if few patients are at risk of dying at that time.

Comparison of survival curves

Now suppose that we have observed two groups of patients, say a control group and a treatment group and that we have estimated their survival curves as above (Fig. 3). How can we compare these two curves and claim that they are or are not 'significantly different'? The standard way of making such a comparison is to use a non-parametric statistical test; that is, a test which makes no assumption about the distribution of survival and yet uses all available survival times as efficiently as possible. A test which is commonly used because it has been shown to be statistically optimum in many situations is the log rank test, also called the Mantel–Haenszel test (Mantel and Haenszel 1959). Other rank tests frequently used in situations where it is important to detect early differences between survival curves are the generalized Wilcoxon tests (Cox and Oakes 1984).

The method of computing the log rank test is as follows (Table 12).

1. Sort all observed survival times in increasing order (column a).

2. Let N be the number of patients at risk at each death time (N_C on control, N_T on treatment) and D be the number of deaths at each death time (D_C on control, D_T on treatment) (columns b–d).

3. Compute the number of deaths (column e) that would be expected in the treatment group at each death time under the null hypothesis of no difference between control and treatment using the formula

$$E_T = DN_T/N$$

and its variance (column g) by the formula

$$V_T = DN_C N_T (N-D) / [N^2(N-1)]$$

4. Compute the difference between the observed and the expected number of deaths in the treatment group at each death time (column f) and sum these differences over all death times: $GD = \text{sum } (D_T - E_T)$.

Table 12 Computation of the log rank test to compare the survival times in a control group and a treatment group

a Times (months)	b Control N_C	D_C	c Treatment N_T	D_T	d Total N	D	e E_T	f $D_T - E_T$	g V_T
1	10		10	1	20	1	0.500	0.500	0.250
2	10		9	1	19	1	0.474	0.526	0.249
3	10	1	8		18	1	0.444	−0.444	0.247
4+	9		8		17				
5+	9		7		16				
6	9		6	1	15	1	0.400	0.600	0.240
7	9	1	5		14	1	0.357	−0.357	0.230
8+	8		5		13				
9	8		4	1	12	1	0.333	0.667	0.222
10+	7		3		10				
11	6	1	2		8	1	0.250	−0.250	0.188
12	5		1	1	6	1	0.167	0.833	0.139
13+	4		0		4				
14	3	1	0		3	1	0.000	0.000	0.000
15+	2		0		2				
18+	1		0		1				
Total				5			2.925	2.075	1.765

Control survival times: 3, 7, 9+, 10+, 11, 12+, 13+, 14, 15+, and 18+ months. Treatment survival times: 1, 2, 4+, 5+, 6, 8+, 9, 10+, 11+, and 12 months.

5. Sum the variances V_T over all death times: $GV=\text{sum}(V_T)$.

6. The log rank statistic is given by $X=GD^2/GV$.

Under the null hypothesis of no difference between control and treatment, this statistic has a chi-square distribution with one degree of freedom and, thus, the p value can be read from a table of chi-square values.

Table 12 shows the computations for the two curves of Fig. 3. Thus in our example the log rank statistic is given by $X=(2.075)^2/(1.765)=2.44$ and a table of the chi-square distribution shows that the corresponding p value is 0.12. For a standard type I error rate α of 0.05, the difference between the two groups in Fig. 3 would not be declared significant since 0.12 is larger than 0.05.

These computations generalize to the comparison of more than two groups, in which case either an overall test or a test for linear trend can be performed. The former would be appropriate for comparing three different treatments, while the latter would be appropriate for testing the effect of increasing doses of the same treatment.

Stratified comparison of survival curves

As for response rates, survival analysis can be 'stratified' (or 'adjusted') to account for important prognostic factors. The approach used to stratify the log rank test is an extension of the Mantel–Haenszel approach (Peto *et al.* 1977).

Multivariate models for survival data

It is often required to assess the predictive power of several variables simultaneously on survival. If the data were not censored, a classical way of approaching this problem would be to perform a linear regression with the prognostic factors as independent variables and the survival time as the dependent variable. Because of the censoring of the survival time, the linear regression cannot be performed without modifications which introduce major difficulties in the analysis.

A convenient way of avoiding these difficulties is to model not survival times but hazard functions. The hazard function, which is also called the time-specific mortality rate, is the mortality rate at any given time among the individuals who have survived until that time (this definition can naturally be extended to events other than death). It can be estimated over a period of time by dividing the number of deaths occurring during that period by the total follow-up time in that period. An analysis of hazard functions usefully complements the analysis of the corresponding survival curves by revealing patterns in mortality over time (Simes and Zelen 1985).

A simple yet powerful way of modelling hazard functions to account for several variables consists of assuming that the effect of each variable is to multiply some 'baseline' hazard by a constant factor; this is called a proportional hazards regression model or simply Cox's regression model (Cox 1972). This regression model has become the preferred way of modelling survival data in the presence of several variables because of its generality; indeed, no assumption need be made about the baseline hazard which can be left completely unspecified. Another reason for the popularity of the proportional hazards model is that when there is only one variable (say treatment), testing the significance of that variable in a proportional hazards model is equivalent to a log rank test.

Sources of bias in clinical data analysis

Analysis by treatment received

The results of a trial should always be analysed by comparing patients according to the treatment that they were assigned to by randomization irrespective of the treatment that they actually received. What this analysis actually compares is two different policies or 'intentions to treat' (Peto *et al.* 1977). The analysis by treatment actually received is inherently biased. The analysis by intention to treat is not, but it may lack power to detect a true treatment benefit if many patients did not in fact receive the treatment.

Length-biased analyses

Survival comparisons involving an event which is itself dependent on the length of survival are 'length biased'. For instance, it is inappropriate to compare the survival curves of responders and non-responders to chemotherapy because the length of survival itself influences the likelihood of a patient being a responder or a non-responder (Anderson *et al.* 1983; Oye and Shapiro 1984). Likewise, it is incorrect to compare the survival of patients receiving their full dose of chemotherapy with those receiving less than full dose in order to claim that treatment is effective only if full dose is given. Patients who fare well tend to tolerate full doses and it is no surprise that their survival is better than the survival of those who do not fare well.

Multiple analyses

A clinical trial is a major undertaking extending over long periods of time. Therefore it is reasonable to perform multiple analyses on the data collected. There will usually be multiple end-points to examine, multiple prognostic factors to adjust for, multiple subgroups of clinical relevance, and multiple times at which all these analyses seem reasonable. The problem with multiple analyses is that the probability of any one of them being significant just by chance is much higher than 5 per cent even when all analyses are performed at the 5 per cent significance level. Thus, the probability of a type I error (false-positive result) is substantially increased. This problem has been extensively studied in the context of 'interim analyses', and several rules have been suggested for incorporating interim analyses in the trial design (Rubinstein and Gail 1982; Geller and Pocock 1987). These planned interim analyses allow accrual to be stopped as soon as a major difference emerges in favour of one of the treatment groups while preserving the overall probability of a type I error. In the absence of a formal allowance for multiple analyses, it is safe to believe the results of some interim look at the data only if the difference is highly significant (say $p<0.001$) as opposed to just significant (say $p<0.05$).

INTERPRETATION OF CLINICAL TRIALS

The presentation and interpretation of clinical trial results is far from trivial (Glatstein and Makuch 1984). Several authors have issued useful guidelines on how results should be reported (Tannock and Murphy 1983; Zelen 1983; Simon and Wittes 1985). Even if such guidelines are followed, there is ample room for distortion and misinterpretation. Baar and Tannock (1989) illustrated the difficulty of reporting results impartially by writing two papers describing the results of the same (hypothetical) trial. The two papers differ drastically in their conclusions and could conceivably have opposite consequences on clinical practice.

Generalizability of trial results

External validity

The results of a clinical trial are only useful if its results can be generalized to some population of future patients. Some authors suggest distinguishing between the 'internal' validity of the trial, which concerns the unbiasedness and precision of its results and its 'external' validity, which concerns the extent to which its results can be extrapolated to future patients (Nicolucci *et al.* 1989). The latter is a matter of judgment, not of statistics and depends primarily on the patient sample entered in the clinical trial: the more representative the sample, the safer is the extrapolation. Begg and Engstrom (1987) reviewed several trials run by major cooperative groups and noticed that only a small fraction of all available patients were eligible for these trials. Limiting the accrual into clinical trials not only curtails the power of the statistical tests for comparing treatments, but also casts serious doubt on the generalizability of the trial results. Broadening the eligibility criteria as much as is medically justified is an option that should in general be given more serious consideration.

Subgroup analyses

If a clinical trial succeeds in showing an overall treatment benefit, it does not follow that this treatment will be beneficial or even harmless in all future patients. Conversely, if a clinical trial does not succeed in showing treatment benefit overall, it does not follow that this treatment would be useless in all future patients. Which patients benefit from the treatment and which do not? In general, a single trial cannot answer this question reliably (unless it is really enormous or the true treatment effects are qualitatively different among clearly distinct subgroups of patients). Subgroup analyses, which attempt to estimate the effect of treatment in different subgroups of patients, are in general very misleading because of the surprisingly high probability that any observed difference between subgroups is due solely to chance (Byar 1985). Moreover, if many subgroups are examined, it is almost certain that the observed treatment effect will be exceedingly large, unusually small, or perhaps even in the wrong direction in at least one of these subgroups (Peto 1982). Yet the identification of true differences in treatment effectiveness among subgroups of patients is a question of paramount clinical importance (Buyse 1990*a*). New approaches to subgroup analyses are needed and it is probable that meta-analyses will play an increasing role in this respect.

Sources of bias in interpreting trial results

Clinical trial results may be misinterpreted in two basic ways. First, the results of a single trial are often taken as reflecting some absolute truth, yet even when these results are free from bias, they are inevitably subject to random error. All other things being equal, smaller trials have a larger random error than larger trials. The best way of reducing the random error to a minimum is to consider the results of all related trials, as opposed to one, a few carefully selected trials, or those which happen to be in the news at major conferences. The problem of reviewing all evidence unbiasedly is made worse by publication bias, through which studies showing a significant benefit from experimental therapies, including those where such a benefit occurred just by chance, tend to be published sooner than those failing to show an effect (Begg and Berlin 1988). Simes (1986) demonstrated publication bias in the reported results of randomized trials comparing combination chemotherapy with a single agent in the treatment of advanced ovarian cancer and of multiple myeloma.

In both cases, a review of the published trials showed a larger effect in favour of combination therapy than was shown in a review of trials prospectively registered in a database of protocol summaries.

Second, many 'negative' trials are too small to detect realistic treatment benefits and their results do not in any way imply that there is no treatment benefit, nor even that the benefit is too small to be of clinical value; in fact 'negative' results should more appropriately be called 'inconclusive' results. A review of 71 'negative' trials indicated that half of them had no more than one chance in four of detecting a true 25 per cent treatment effect, which would represent a major step forward in cancer therapy and an even lower chance of detecting smaller treatment benefits (Freiman *et al.* 1978).

Meta-analyses

'Meta-analysis' and 'overview' are synonymous terms to denote the combination of results from several related studies (Boissel *et al.* 1989; Stewart 1992). When addressing an important clinical question, such as the value of some new therapy, clinicians informally combine items of knowledge from various sources. In a sense, a meta-analysis is just a rigorous quantitative approach to this combination process. An increasing number of meta-analyses of clinical trials have appeared recently. Sacks *et al.* (1987) reviewed all meta-analyses of randomized clinical trials in the medical literature: they found four prior to 1970, 13 in the 1970s, and 69 between 1980 and 1985.

Rationale

The great majority of randomized clinical trials reported so far in cancer are too small to supply definitive answers to the questions of clinical interest. The results of individual trials are often at best inconclusive or at worst mutually conflicting. A meta-analysis of all available trials may then be the only way to reach large enough numbers of patients to ensure that the power of the statistical tests ceases to be a limiting factor (Collins *et al.* 1987). A meta-analysis is also a way of removing, at least in part, some of the biases that affect the results of individual trials, because it is unlikely that all the trials being combined are equally affected by the same sources of bias (Wachter 1988). Meaningful subgroup analyses are rarely possible in single randomized control trials but can be undertaken prospectively using meta-analysis. Meta-analysis is not a way of identifying treatment effects at all costs. In fact, it can lead to one of the following conclusions: the treatment effect is worthwhile and established beyond reasonable doubt (for example, adjuvant therapies of early breast cancer (Early Breast Cancer Trialists Collaborative Group 1988)), the treatment effect is so small as to be clinically negligible (for example, adjuvant chemotherapies of head and neck tumours (Stell 1989)), and the treatment effect remains unclear even when all available evidence is combined (for example adjuvant chemotherapies of colorectal cancer (Buyse *et al.* 1988)).

Statistical methods

The validity of a meta-analysis of clinical trials rests on the assumption that the true treatment effect, if any, differs in magnitude but not in direction among different subgroups of patients. A situation in which the treatment is actually beneficial for some patients but harmful for the others is called a qualitative interaction. Although this situation can occur, it does so only in exceptional circumstances. A far more frequent situation is that of quantitative interaction, in which the treatment effect is in the same direction in all patient subgroups although its exact magnitude can be expected to depend on the patient characteristics. If the situation under study is one of quantitative interaction, it is legitimate to combine the results obtained with similar treatments in somewhat different patient populations. However, simply pooling the data from all studies is likely to give a misleading result. What is needed instead is a stratified analysis in which a treatment effect is estimated within each study and then individual effects are combined to estimate an overall effect and test for its statistical significance. In this way the treated patients of a study are compared only with the control patients of the same study. Thus, the methods outlined above for the stratified analysis of a single trial (Mantel–Haenszel test and stratified log rank test) are appropriate for meta-analysis.

Some authors argue that, even after studies have been selected as suitable for meta-analysis because of their similarity, their possible heterogeneity must be taken into account explicitly through the use of 'random effects' models (DerSimonian and Laird 1986). In these models it is assumed that the variability observed in the treatment effects among the various studies is not due just to random fluctuations, but to underlying differences between the true treatment effects in these studies. The general issue of whether and when random effects models are preferable to fixed effects models akin to those described above is still unresolved. In practice, the two approaches would yield materially different answers only in the presence of substantial variability in treatment effects among the various trials (in which case random effects models are more conservative than their fixed effects counterparts). However, substantial variability in treatment effects may reflect genuine heterogeneity in the design of the various trials that are combined with regard to treatment schedules, supportive care, etc. Such heterogeneity makes the whole exercise of combining information from different sources questionable, regardless of the model that is being used to carry out the combination.

Finally, because meta-analyses usually combine evidence from very different sources, not all of which are equally trustworthy, it may be informative to take the quality of the individual studies into account (Chalmers *et al.* 1981). It is technically straightforward to weigh each study in proportion to its quality, but since there is no universal yardstick to assess the quality of individual studies such weighted analyses may be viewed with some scepticism.

Potential for meta-analyses

There is little doubt that meta-analysis of controlled trials is still in its infancy and will play an increasingly important role in the clinical evaluation of new cancer treatments. Louis *et al.* (1985) and L'Abbé *et al.* (1987) have discussed the potential impact of meta-analyses on public health and clinical research, respectively. However meta-analyses are the last step in a long process. They can contribute to a better knowledge of cancer therapy only if properly designed and conducted clinical trials, which address questions of significant clinical interest, have been performed.

REFERENCES

Aaronson NK, Beckmann JH, ed. (1987). *The quality of life of cancer patients.* Raven Press, New York.

Anderson JR, Cain KC, Gelber RD (1983). Analysis of survival by tumor response. *Journal of Clinical Oncology*, 1:710–19.

Armitage P (1971). *Statistical methods in medical research.* Blackwell, Oxford.

Armitage P (1975). *Sequential medical trials* (2nd edn). Wiley, New York.

Armitage P (1982). The role of randomization in clinical trials. *Controlled Clinical Trials*, 1:345–52.

Baar J, Tannock I (1989). Analyzing the same data in two ways: a demonstration model to illustrate the reporting and misreporting of clinical trials. *Journal of Clinical Oncology*, 7:969–78.

Bailar JC III, Smith EM (1986). Progress against cancer? *New England Journal of Medicine*, 314:1226–32.

Bartolucci A (1985). Estimation and comparison of proportions. In *Cancer clinical trials. Methods and practice* (ed. ME Buyse, MJ Staquet, and RJ Sylvester), pp. 337–60. Oxford University Press.

Baum M (1986). Do we need informed consent? *Lancet*, ii:911–12.

Begg CB, Berlin JA (1988). Publication bias: a problem in interpreting medical data (with discussion). *Journal of the Royal Statistical Society A*, 151:419–63.

Begg CB, Engstrom PF (1987). Eligibility and extrapolation in cancer clinical trials. *Journal of Clinical Oncology*, 5:962–8.

Begg CB, Iglewicz B (1980). A treatment allocation procedure for sequential clinical trials. *Biometrics*, 36:81–90.

Begg CB, Pocock SJ, Freedman L, Zelen M (1987). State of the art in comparative cancer clinical trials. *Cancer*, 60:2811–15.

Blackwelder WC (1982). "Proving the null hypothesis" in clinical trials. *Controlled Clinical Trials*, 3:345–53.

Boissel JP, Peyrieux JC, Sacks, H (1989). Considerations for the meta-analysis of randomized clinical trials. Summary of a panel discussion. *Controlled Clinical Trials*, 10:254–81.

Bull JP (1959). The historical development of clinical therapeutic trials. *Journal of Chronic Diseases*, 10:218–48.

Buyse M (1989). Potential and pitfalls of randomized clinical trials in cancer research. *Cancer Surveys*, 8:91–105.

Buyse M (1990*a*). Some comments on subgroup analyses. *Controlled Clinical Trials*, 10:187S–94S.

Buyse M (1990*b*). The case for loose inclusion criteria in clinical trials. *Acta Chirurgica Belgica*, 90:129–31.

Buyse M (1991). Randomized clinical trials in surgical oncology. *European Journal of Surgical Oncology*, 17:421–8

Buyse M (1993*a*) Regulatory versus public health requirements in clinical trials. *Drug Information Journal*, 27:977–84.

Buyse M (1993*b*). Interim analyses, stopping rules and data monitoring in clinical trials in Europe. *Statistics in Medicine*, 12:509–20.

Buyse ME, Staquet MJ, Sylvester RD, ed. (1985). *Cancer clinical trials. Methods and practice.* Oxford University Press.

Buyse M, Zeleniuch-Jacquotte A, Chalmers TC (1988). Adjuvant therapy of colorectal cancer: why we still don't know. *Journal of the American Medical Association*, 259:3571–8.

Byar DP (1980). Why databases should not replace randomized clinical trials. *Biometrics*, 36:337–42.

Byar DP (1985). Assessing apparent treatment-covariate interactions in randomized clinical trials. *Statistics in Medicine*, 4:255–63.

Byar DP, Piantadosi S (1985). Factorial designs for randomized clinical trials. *Cancer Treatment Reports*, 69:1055–63.

Byar DP, *et al.* (1976). Randomized clinical trials: perspectives on some recent ideas. *New England Journal of Medicine*, 295:74–80.

Carter SK (1977). Clinical trials in cancer chemotherapy. *Cancer*, 40:544–57.

Cavalli F (1992). Randomized trials: what's the problem? *Annals of Oncology*, 3:96.

Chalmers (1990). Report of Meeting of Open Section. *Journal of the Royal Society of Medicine*, 83:337–9.

Chalmers TC (1975). Symposium on diseases of the liver: randomization of the first patient. *Medical Clinics of North America*, 59:1035–7.

Chalmers TC, *et al.* (1981). A method for assessing the quality of a randomized control trial. *Controlled Clinical Trials*, 2:31–49.

Collins R, Gray R, Godwin J, Peto R (1987). Avoidance of large biases and large random errors in the assessment of moderate treatment effects: the need for systematic overviews. *Statistics in Medicine*, 6:245–50.

Correspondence. Progress against cancer? *New England Journal of Medicine*, 315:963–8.

Cox DR (1972). Regression models and life-tables (with discussion). *Journal of the Royal Statistical Society B*, 34:187–220.

Cox DR, Oakes D (1984). *Analysis of survival data.* Chapman and Hall, London.

Decoster G, Stein G, Holdener EE (1990). Responses and toxic deaths in phase I clinical trials. *Annals of Oncology*, 1:175–81.

DerSimonian R, Laird N (1986). Meta-analysis in clinical trials. *Controlled Clinical Trials*, **7**:177–88.

DeVita VT Jr (1989). Breast cancer therapy: exercising all our options. *New England Journal of Medicine*, **320**:527–9.

Dodion P, Abele R (1989). The role of the study coordinator in cancer clinical trials. In *Data management and clinical trials* (ed. N Rotmensz), pp. 163–73. Elsevier, Amsterdam.

Early Breast Cancer Trialists Collaborative Group (1988). The effects of tamoxifen and of cytotoxic therapy on mortality in early breast cancer: an overview of 61 randomized trials among 28,896 women. *New England Journal of Medicine*, **190**:1681–92.

Efron B (1971). Forcing a sequential experiment to be balanced. *Biometrika*, **58**:403–17.

Ellenberg S (1984). Randomization designs in comparative clinical trials. *New England Journal of Medicine*, **310**:1404.

EuroCODE Steering Committee. EuroCODE: a new approach to collaborative research in clinical oncology. *European Journal of Cancer and Clinical Oncology*, **25**:1905–6.

Fleming TR (1982). One-sample multiple testing procedures for phase II clinical trials. *Biometrics*, **38**:143–51.

Fletcher R, Fletcher S (1979). Clinical research in general medical journals—a 30-year perspective. *New England Journal of Medicine*, **301**:180–3.

Folks JL (1981). *Ideas of statistics*. Wiley, New York.

Freedman LS (1982). Tables of the number of patients required in clinical trials using the logrank test. *Statistics in Medicine*, **1**:121–9.

Freedman LS (1989). The size of clinical trials in cancer research—what are the current needs? *British Journal of Cancer*, **59**:396–400.

Freedman LS, White SJ (1976). On the use of Pocock and Simon's method for balancing treatment numbers over prognostic factors in the controlled clinical trial. *Biometrics*, **32**:691–4.

Freiman JA, Chalmers TC, Smith H Jr, Kuelbler RR (1971). The importance of beta, the type II error and sample size in the design and interpretation of the randomized control trial. Survey of 71 'negative' trials. *New England Journal of Medicine*, **299**:690–4.

Gehan EA (1961). The determination of the number of patients required in a preliminary and follow-up trial of a new chemotherapeutic agent. *Journal of Chronic Diseases*, **13**:346–53.

Gehan EA, Freireich EJ (1974). Non-randomized controls in cancer trials. *New England Journal of Medicine*, **290**:198–203.

Geller N (1984). Design of phase I and phase II clinical trials in cancer. *Cancer Investigations*, **2**:483–91.

Geller NL, Pocock SJ (1987). Interim analyses in randomized clinical trials: ramifications and guidelines for practitioners. *Biometrics*, **43**:213–23.

George S (1985). The required size and length of a phase III clinical trial. In *Cancer clinical trials. Methods and practice* (ed. ME Buyse, MJ Staquet, and RJ Sylvester), pp. 287–310. Oxford University Press.

Glatstein E, Makuch RW (1984). Illusion and reality: practical pitfalls in interpreting clinical trials. *Journal of Clinical Oncology*, **2**:488–97.

Herson J (1985). Statistical aspects in design and analysis of phase II clinical trials. In *Cancer clinical trials. Methods and practice* (ed. ME Buyse, MJ Staquet, and RJ Sylvester), pp. 239–57. Oxford University Press.

Herson J, Carter SK (1986). Calibrated phase II clinical trials in oncology. *Statistics in Medicine*, **5**:441–7.

Horwitz RI (1987). Complexity and contradiction in clinical trial research. *American Journal of Medicine*, **82**:498–510.

Kalish LA, Begg CB (1985). Treatment allocation methods in clinical trials: a review. *Statistics in Medicine*, **4**:129–44.

Kaplan EL, Meier P (1958). Nonparametric estimation from incomplete observations. *Journal of the American Statistical Association*, **53**:457–81.

Kearsley JH (1986). Cytotoxic chemotherapy for common adult malignancies: 'the emperor's new clothes' revisited? *British Medical Journal*, **293**:871–6.

L'Abbé KA, Detsky AS, O'Rourke K (1987). Meta-analysis in clinical research. *Annals of Internal Medicine*, **107**:224–33.

Lachin JM, Matts JP, Wei LJ (1988). Randomization in clinical trials: conclusions and recommendations. *Controlled Clinical Trials*, **9**:365–74.

Lan KKG, DeMets DL (1983). Discrete sequential boundaries for clinical trials. *Biometrika*, **70**:659–63.

Lange N, MacIntyre J (1984). A computerized patient registration and treatment randomization system for multi-institutional clinical trials. *Controlled Clinical Trials*, **6**:38–49.

Letters to the Editor. *Journal of the American Medical Association*, **261**:987–9.

Levin B, O'Connell MJ (1988). Colorectal cancer chemotherapy: meta-analysis or large-scale trials? *Journal of the American Medical Association*, **259**:3611.

Louis TA, Fineberg HV, Mosteller F (1985). Findings for public health from meta-analyses. *Annual Reviews of Public Health*, **6**:1–20.

Machin D, Campbell MJ (1987). *Statistical tables for the design of clinical trials*. Blackwell, Oxford.

Mantel N, Haenszel W (1959). Statistical aspects of the analysis of data from retrospective studies of disease. *Journal of the National Cancer Institute*, **22**:719–48.

Marsoni S, Hoth D, Simon R, Leyland Jones B, De Rosa M, Wittes RE (1987). Clinical drug development: an analysis of phase II trials, 1970–1985. *Cancer Treatment Reports*, **71**:71–80.

Nicolucci A, Grilli R, Alexanian AA, Apolone G, Torri W, Liberati A (1989). Quality, evolution, and clinical implications of randomized, controlled trials on the treatment of lung cancer. A lost opportunity for meta-analysis. *Journal of the American Medical Association*, **262**:2101–7.

O'Brien PC, Fleming TR (1979). A multiple testing procedure for clinical trials. *Biometrics*, **35**:549–56.

Oye RK, Shapiro MF (1984). Does response make a difference in patient survival? *Journal of the American Medical Association*, **252**:2722–5.

Peto R (1978). Clinical trial methodology. *Biomedicine Special Issue*, **28**:24–36.

Peto R (1980). Monitoring of cancer patients in clinical trials need not be precise. In *Cancer: assessment and monitoring* (ed. T Symington, AE Williams, and JG McVie). Churchill Livingstone, Edinburgh.

Peto R (1982). Statistical aspects of cancer trials. In *Treatment of cancer* (ed. KE Halnan), pp. 867–71. Chapman and Hall, London.

Peto R, *et al.* (1976). Design and analysis of randomized clinical trials requiring prolonged observation of each patient. I. Introduction and design. *British Journal of Cancer*, **34**:585–612.

Peto R, *et al.* (1977). Design and analysis of randomized clinical trials requiring prolonged observation of each patient. II. Analysis and examples. *British Journal of Cancer*, **35**:1–39.

Pocock SJ (1977). Randomized clinical trials. *British Medical Journal*, **6077**:1661.

Pocock SJ (1983). *The controlled clinical trial*. Wiley, New York.

Rubinstein LV, Gail MH (1982). Monitoring rules for stopping accrual in comparative survival studies. *Controlled Clinical Trials*, **3**:325–33.

Sacks HS, Berrier J, Reitman D, Ancona-Berk VA, Chalmers TC (1987). Meta-analysis of randomized controlled trials. *New England Journal of Medicine*, **316**:450–5.

Schwartz D, Lellouch J (1967). Explanatory and pragmatic attitudes in therapeutic trials. *Journal of Chronic Diseases*, **20**:637–48.

Segelov E, Tattersall MHN, Coates AS (1992). Redressing the balance—the ethics of *not* entering an eligible patient on a randomized clinical trial. *Annals of Oncology*, **3**:103–5.

Simes RJ (1986). Publication bias: the case for an international registry of clinical trials. *Journal of Clinical Oncology*, **4**:1529–41.

Simes RJ, Zelen M (1985). Exploratory data analysis and the use of the hazard function for interpreting survival data: an investigator's primer. *Journal of Clinical Oncology*, **3**:1418–31.

Simon R, Wittes RE (1985). Methodologic guidelines for reports of clinical trials. *Cancer Treatment Reports*, **69**:1–3.

Simon R, Wittes RE, Ellenberg SS (1985). Randomized phase II clinical trials. *Cancer Treatment Reports*, **69**:1375–81.

Staquet M, Dalesio O (1985). Designs for phase III trials. In *Cancer clinical trials. Methods and practice* (ed. ME Buyse, MJ Staquet, and RJ Sylvester), pp. 261–75. Oxford University Press.

Stell PM, Rawson NSB (1990). Adjuvant chemotherapy in head and neck cancer. *British Journal of Cancer*, **61**:779–87.

Stenning S (1992). "The uncertainty principle": selection of patients for cancer clinical trials. In *Introducing new treatments for cancer* (ed. CJ Williams), pp. 161–72. John Wiley and Sons.

Stewart L (1992). The role of overviews. In *Introducing new treatments for cancer* (ed. CJ Williams), pp. 383–401. John Wiley and Sons.

Storer B, DeMets D (1987). Current phase I/II designs: are they adequate? *Journal of Clinical Research and Drug Develolpment*, 1:121–30.

Sylvester RJ (1988). A Bayesian approach to the design of phase II clinical trials. *Biometrics*, 44:823–36.

Tannock I, Murphy K (1983). Reflections on medical oncology: an appeal for better clinical trials and improved reporting of their results. *Journal of Clinical Oncology*, 1:66–9.

Wachter KW (1988). Disturbed by meta-analysis? *Science*, 241:1407–8.

Wei LJ (1978). An application of an urn model to the design of sequential controlled clinical trials. *Journal of the American Statistical Association*, 73:559–63.

Whitehead J (1992). *The design and analysis of sequential clinical trials*. Ellis Horwood, Chichester.

WHO (1979). *WHO Handbook for reporting results of cancer treatment*. WHO Offset Publication No. 48, Geneva.

Williams CJ (ed.) (1992). *Introducing new treatments for cancer*. Wiley, New York.

Wittes RE. Progress in a desert: oasis or mirage? *Journal of the National Cancer Institute*, 80:5–7.

Yusuf S, Collins R, Peto R (1984). Why do we need some large, simple randomized trials? *Statistics in Medicine*, 3:409–20.

Zelen M (1979). A new design for randomized clinical trials. *New England Journal of Medicine*, 300:1242–5.

Zelen M (1983). Guidelines for publishing papers on cancer clinical trials: responsibilities of editors and authors. *Journal of Clinical Oncology*, 1:164–9.

Zelen M, Gelman R (1986). Assessment of adjuvant trials in breast cancer. *NCI Monographs*, 1:11–17.

20.2   Data management

NICOLE ROTMENSZ

INTRODUCTION

In oncology, clinical trials are a key practice in achieving new advances. They are based on a great deal of cooperation involving many researchers from different backgrounds. Clinicians, statisticians, computer analysts, and data managers have to collaborate closely to produce the most reliable results.

'Data management' is perhaps an obscure function, which is frequently neither well understood nor well identified. In practice, it covers several different kinds of activities:

(1) data collection, that is, collection of data in the hospital and transfer from the local chart to standard case report forms;

(2) data control, that is, computerization and analysis, in a coordinating data centre.

The first activity is related to what is arbitrarily defined in this chapter as 'local data management', in contrast with 'central data management' which applies to the tasks performed in a (coordinating) data centre for multicentre or single-centre trials.

Most of the examples given in this chapter are based on the latter type of activity and on experience acquired at the European Organization for Research and Treatment of Cancer (EORTC) Coordinating and Data Centre and at the Istituto Nazionale Tumori, Milan.

BACKGROUND

Profile

As 'data management' is still a vaguely defined procedure, the people performing this role come from a variety of backgrounds. In order to investigate this a survey was performed in 1986, involving a group of data managers working in centres collaborating with the EORTC (therefore it is related to what has been defined as local data management). Eighty-five questionnaires were sent out and 60 were completed and returned. The results showed that 27 per cent (16 out of 60 respondents) had a university degree of some type (excluding MD), 23 per cent had a nursing diploma (this category

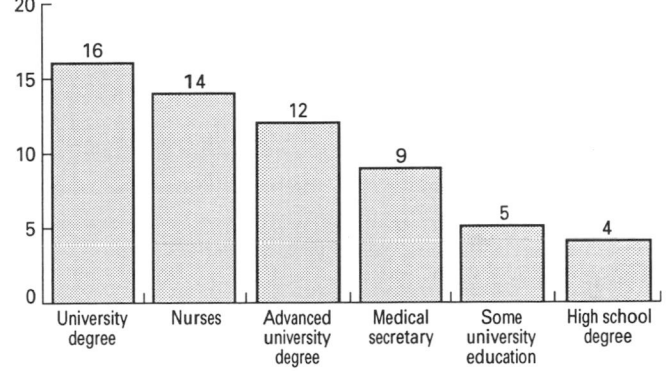

Fig. 1   Background of data managers.

also included physiotherapists), and 20 per cent had an 'advanced university degree' (a PhD in various fields or physicians). Fifteen per cent were medical secretaries, 8 per cent had 'some university education', that is, they had not completed their degree course, and 7 per cent had high school leaving qualifications (Fig. 1).

To establish a definition of the profession, we examined the exact nature of the activities of data managers and Table 1 shows the responses (obviously, the respondents could tick as many activities as applicable). The main task of data managers working in local centres is the collection of data and the transcription of information on forms. Sixty per cent perform administrative duties, consisting mainly of department organization and more than half are involved in the design of forms, preparation of reports, and publication of results. As a general comment, the majority of respondents expressed the need for recognition of their role and the difficulties often encountered in cooperating with physicians.

Education

The training of a data manager should primarily concentrate on the fundamental principles of oncology (that is, mechanisms of the disease, various treatment modalities, etc.) and the interpretation

Table 1 Nature of data management activities

Activity	Percentage of respondents
Collection of medical information	82
Data transcription	77
Administration	60
Designing forms	58
Preparation of reports	55
Publication of results	55
Collection of forms	47
Data entry on computer	45
Statistical analysis	43
Design of the protocol	35
Collection of quality of life data	28
Computer programming	23

of clinical data. Data managers should understand aetiology, diagnosis, staging and treatment of solid tumours, and haematological malignancies. Some medical background is essential before this training is given. When working in a hospital environment, it is important to collaborate closely with the medical staff. Thus, data managers should attend ward meetings where the evaluation of the patient's disease status is discussed, so that they have the opportunity to acquire a better understanding of the disease under study. In addition, although no courses in oncology are specifically designed for data managers, it is possible for them to attend courses intended for oncology nurses or tumour registrars. Furthermore, national and international workshops have been launched over the last years, offering an excellent opportunity to learn and exchange new concepts (Van der Putten and Boon 1989). Clinical trial methodology and simple statistics should also be part of a data manager's basic education. Again, training is rather empirical, based on attendance to courses and symposia or 'self-education' by reading books (Bland 1987) and scientific journals.

RUNNING A TRIAL

The results of a trial strongly depend on the quality of the data collected. The data manager's function is to standardize and optimize all steps of this activity.

The first task is to design case report forms which will record the patient's data. The next requirement is to ensure efficient collection, checking, and processing of all patients' forms so that the statistical analysis will be based on accurate data (Pocock 1983). Quality control includes methods aimed at maintaining or enhancing data reliability and validity. Preparation of interim reports to be presented to trialists provides up-to-date information on all relevant aspects of the trial. Publication of the results is the last step involving the trial office.

Form design

Well-designed forms make an important contribution to the success of a trial, whether multicentre or single-centre. Missing information as well as collection of too much data are pitfalls which may jeopardize the whole analysis. Therefore, forms should be developed by people experienced in form design who are also familiar with methods of data collection and data processing in prospective studies (Meinert 1986).

Data managers are responsible for form design but they should work in close cooperation with the physician coordinating the study and the statistician in charge of the analysis.

EORTC BREAST CANCER COOPERATIVE GROUP TRIAL 10881 ON STUDY FORM   JUNE 1988
INSTRUCTIONS: to be completed and return within one week of randomisation to:
EORTC DATA CENTER, 83 Av. Mounier, 1200 Brussels, Belgium

Patient's name: _____ Hospital chart No: _____

Institution: _____ Responsible physician: _____

1 ☐☐☐☐☐☐ Birthdate *(day/month/year)*

2 ☐ Menstrual status: *1=Normal, 2=Menses<than once every 3 months*

3 ☐☐☐☐☐☐ Date 1 of last menstruations *(day/month/year)*

4 ☐☐☐☐☐☐ Date of first histological diagnosis of primary breast cancer
(day/month/year)

PRIOR TREATMENT

5 ☐ Surgery: *1=No, 2=Yes*

6 ☐ Chemotherapy: *1=No, 2=Yes, adjuvant, 3=Yes, for advanced disease*

7 ☐☐☐☐☐☐ Date last treatment stopped *(day/month/year)*

8 ☐ Hormonotherapy: *1=No, 2=Yes, adjuvant, 3=Yes, for advanced disease*

9 ☐☐☐☐☐☐ Date last treatment stopped *(day/month/year)*

RECEPTOR STATUS

10 ☐☐☐☐ fmol/mg protein for Estrogen Receptors

11 ☐☐☐☐ fmol/mg protein for Progesterone Receptors

DISEASE STATUS

12 ☐ *1=Locally advanced, 2=Metastatic disease*

13 ☐ *Disease free interval: 1=None, 2=<2 years, 3=>2 years*

TREATMENT FOR THE PRESENT PROTOCOL

14 ☐ *1=LHRH-agonist, 2=LHRH-agonist & Tamoxifen, 3=Tamoxifen*

COMMENTS: ....
....
....
....

DATE: .... SIGNATURE: ....

Fig. 2 On-study form for a breast cancer trial of the EORTC.

General principles

Case report forms must have four main qualities: they must be clear, be easy to complete, contain all relevant information, and not contain unnecessary information (Rotmensz 1989).

Clarity

It should be possible to identify the following easily (Fig. 2).

1. The kind of information requested: is the form related to anamnesis and to prognostic factors, or to treatment and side-effects, or to laboratory data, etc.?

2. The schedules for completing this form: once at entry, on a sequential basis, at the end of treatment?

3. In the case of a multicentre trial, the person (or organization) to whom the form has to be returned and the complete address for return.

In addition, the display should be attractive and well laid out. The form should not be overloaded with questions, there should not be excessive explanatory text, and the method of answering questions should be immediately understandable, otherwise respondents will be discouraged.

Simplicity

When designed for a single-centre trial, the forms can be organized according to the logic of the local medical files. However, it is impossible to follow this principle in forms prepared for multicentre trials because each centre has a different organization. Therefore the minimum requirements are as follows.

1. The questions should be clearly formulated so as to avoid misinterpretation. For example, when enquiring about menopausal status, the definition of the term should be summarized on the form, assuming that a complete definition has been detailed in the protocol.

2. The dates requested should be well defined. For example, does 'date of tumour diagnosis' refer to the clinical or the pathological date?

3. The form should not take too long to complete in order to prompt the local data manager (or physician) to return it rapidly.

Inclusion of relevant information

All the end-points of the study should be properly requested in the set of forms. When asked to prepare forms for a new study, data managers should read the protocol carefully and indicate all relevant items to be included. A draft is then prepared in collaboration with the study coordinator and the statistician. That draft is circulated amongst the people most involved in the protocol under study. It can be subjected to a pilot study to check its adequacy and completeness. It is always advisable to leave a blank space for 'Comments' on the forms to allow the local investigator or data manager to report on unexpected events.

Exclusion of unnecessary information

This is usually a very difficult task that requires a great deal of tact when designing the forms. Physicians coordinating studies frequently request 'just-in-case' data, which are of limited interest or irrelevant to the study objectives, thus overloading the computer. In addition, the costs of data management (error checking, correction, and analysis) increase with the number of variables and there is the risk of losing touch with the primary objective of the trial (Greenberg 1984).

Types of form

Depending on whether the trial is phase II or phase III, forms should contain different types of information. As a general principle, at least five types of forms are required to follow a patient enrolled in a clinical trial.

1. A registration form completed at the time of registration or randomization in a trial, aimed at identifying the patient, giving the stratifications (if any), confirming the most important eligibility criteria, and defining the treatment received by random assignment (if applicable). It will also serve as a basis for all future reference to this patient.

2. A baseline form collecting information on the patient's characteristics at entry in a clinical trial. This is the only way to give an adequate description of the population under study when publishing the results. The minimum data requirements may vary according to the type of trial, but it should always be possible to verify whether the patient satisfies the selection criteria stipulated by the protocol. It is also important at this stage to double check the information supplied at the time of randomization such as

stratification (if any) and the treatment assigned (De Pauw and Buyse 1988).

3. A treatment form which will vary according to the type of therapy. It will be completed once for a surgical trial or periodically for chemotherapy or radiotherapy protocols. This form will also include information regarding the side-effects due to the treatment and the response, if applicable.

4. A follow-up form is necessary to record information on the progress of the patient during the trial. It includes data on physical examination, biochemistry, haematology, radiography, scans, and any other information pertaining to recurrence, progression, or survival. This form is usually completed both during and after treatment as long as the patient remains on study.

5. An off-study form is completed when the investigator, for whatever reason, is unable to further treat the patient or to follow him or her according to the protocol requirements. It includes the date and reason for going off study, the response to treatment, the date and site of progression, if applicable, the patient's survival status with the date of death or the date last known to be alive (whichever is applicable), and eventually the cause of death.

Additional information on pathology, compliance, unexpected toxicities, or other side studies can be recorded on separate sheets, depending on the aims of the protocol.

In phase II trials more attention has to be paid to side-effects and laboratory values, as checks should often be performed on a weekly basis to detect changes. Phase III forms should be simple, particularly when the study is large and does not require intense monitoring.

Standardization

Standardization of the coding system is of great importance. First widely accepted international coding systems, such as coding of the performance status according to the Karnofsky scale (Karnofsky *et al.* 1948), the World Health Organization (WHO) reporting system for toxic effects of chemotherapy or response to treatment (WHO 1979), or the International Classification of Diseases in Oncology (ICD-O) (WHO 1976), should be used whenever possible for recording the topography and morphology of tumours. Second the codes adopted should be consistent throughout one specific form, throughout all forms of a specific trial, and preferably throughout all forms used in a cooperative group.

For instance, once the code '1=No, 2=Yes', has been used, all no and yes answers should be recorded as 1 and 2, respectively. Moreover, it seems logical to extend this consistency to forms designed for all clinical trials monitored in the same coordinating centre. Other key questions, such as response to treatment, survival status, cause of death, etc., can easily be standardized throughout all trial forms (De Pauw and Buyse 1988). There are several methods for recording the date and explicit guidance must be given as to the order of days and months. In the United States 11/12/79 means 12 November 1979, while in Europe it would have been understood as 11 December 1979 (Wright and Haybittle 1979).

Data collection

Local setting

In each centre the data manager transfers data reported on the patient's hospital chart to standard case report forms. This requires good training and understanding of the disease and should always be done under the supervision of a physician. However, the local data manager must also remind the clinician about the kind of data to be collected and at what interval. Again, only good and close cooperation within the team can produce reliable information.

(Coordinating) data centre

Whereas data in single-centre trials should be immediately available, data collected in multicentre trials are sent by the participating institutions to the coordinating data centre for computerization and processing. The data manager will be in charge of the data collection and experience has shown that the following problems may occur.

1. Data may be missing because of inadequate physical examination, laboratory failure, or carelessness in completion of forms (Friedman *et al.* 1981). Therefore, when designing the forms, the temptation to ask for information which is likely to be frequently overlooked by the investigators should be resisted. Only data that are strictly necessary for the study should be requested, so that important information is not lost in a vast array of less relevant items (Peto *et al.* 1977; Buyse 1988).

2. Erroneous data may not be detected. Computer checks are reliable provided that all situations where wrong information could occur have been examined. Software equipment offers data managers a wide variety of systems for organizing range checks (data must fall in a predefined range of values or are rejected), consistency checks (cross-check of two or more types of data, for example stage of the disease and nodal involvement or age and menopausal status), and sequence checks (the date of death should be posterior to the date of progression). However, reality is more complex and manual controls by experienced data managers are always necessary. Sometimes erroneous data cannot be detected because they fall within the limits of the accepted values; only in-depth data quality control can solve this problem (see next section).

3. Variability of the observations due to physician bias can occur when the data to be collected are not strictly objective. For instance, information on side-effects due to treatment depends not only on the complaints reported by the patients but also on the questions asked by the clinician and the way that these are reported in the clinical files. Buyse (1988) reported a study run on 111 patients enrolled in a phase II trial involving 15 European institutions. He showed that the differences in reports of toxicity were not attributable to apparent variations in the patient population (age, extent of disease, etc.) or in treatment administration, but to the differing attitudes of the investigators. To minimize this risk, recommendations (WHO 1979) have been made in an attempt to improve the reporting of toxicities.

Quality control

Continuous efforts have to be made to maintain a high quality of the data and the role of the data manager is 2-fold: to use all means available to the coordinating data centre to ensure correctness and completeness of the data and to audit the participating centres in order to evaluate the quality of the data collected.

Computer checks

We have seen in the previous section how to monitor data collection and the possible problems that may result. Many of the computerized checks can be organized interactively during data entry and sometimes inconsistency can be corrected immediately, provided that confirmation by the responsible physician is requested. Other more sophisticated data verification should then be performed

and will often highlight the necessity for requesting feedback to the local institutions or directly to the laboratories or treating physicians in the context of single-centre trials. However, it is necessary to establish which data should be checked.

1. Dates are often wrongly reported, particularly in January when people automatically report the previous year. Consistency checks of dates should also be performed when an evident chronology of events has apparently not been respected.

2. Ideally, the questions on the forms should be clear to avoid any misunderstanding. Sometimes this is difficult as an item is still subject to controversy. For example, menopausal status may be an important prognostic factor in some trials, but when no agreement can be reached on its definition it may be necessary to cross-check this item with age and prior surgeries to establish the true status.

3. International coding systems, such as the TNM, are periodically updated and therefore disease stage may vary according to a new classification. Hence, it is important to maintain a coherent system throughout the trial.

4. In general, the main eligibility criteria have to be checked periodically during the course of a trial. For instance, age is frequently a limiting factor, but if this criterion is frequently 'violated' the next version of the protocol may be modified.

5. Toxicities must always be checked. This is easy in the case of extreme laboratory values, as a simple 'slip of the pen' or utilization of a different unit may be revealed. Other unexpected side-effects are often the subject of additional comments in the space provided on the forms and if these are missing an additional investigation has to be conducted.

6. Relapse and disease progression must be confirmed by radiological or pathological methods. No mistakes can be accepted at this stage as it is often one of the main end-points of a study.

This list is not exhaustive but attempts to give some indication as to what can be done using the computerized data.

In phase II trials it is recommended that all eligibility and baseline data are checked, as well as all data from treatment administration, toxicity, and main end-points. In phase III trials, even though fewer data are required, the most important check is to secure a regular follow-up and to keep patient loss to a minimum. This is done by making regular requests for missing forms.

Site visits

In multicentre trials, visits to the participating centres are very useful. Such visits may have a number of objectives such as controlling the radiotherapy material, the administration of chemotherapy, compliance with the protocol, response assessment, etc. However, when data managers are involved, the audit will consist of checking data collection and transfer to the case report forms.

A quality control protocol was implemented by the EORTC Study Group on Data Management. It consisted of organizing visits of a team composed of two experienced data managers and the physician in charge of the coordination of the protocol under review to the main participating centres in ongoing trials. Their task was to check item by item the correctness of all the data collected for a random number of patients. Results have shown that whatever the internal structure of the local institutions, the quality of data transfer was satisfactory (91.4 per cent correct data). However, one conclusion was that local data management support was not a

Table 2 Data to be reported during group meetings

1. Patient accrual: number of patients entered in the study, sorted by participating centres; entry by month, year, treatment, etc.
2. Ineligible patients and protocol violations: description of the causes of non-adherence to study criteria
3. Patients' characteristics: distribution of patients according to main prognostic factors (age, sex, stage, prior treatment, etc.)
4. Toxicities and side-effects: description of all side-effects due to treatment
5. Report on treatment interruptions: summary of treatment failures or other reasons for suspending treatment
6. Miscellaneous: problems of missing forms, missing data, etc.

guarantee of correctness. Rather, the main requirements were a good understanding of the disease and the trial procedures and good communications, both internally and with the coordinating data centre (Vantongelen *et al.* 1989). Another important result of this review was that local investigators considered the site visits as a kind of supervision of their work and took advantage of it by discussing and resolving some local problems.

Data reporting

In order to maintain the investigator's interest in and commitment to the trials, periodic meetings with the whole team of trialists are essential. They should be held before the beginning of the trial to outline protocol requirements and data collection procedures and t a later stage to follow the progress of the trial. At that time, it is good practice to report summaries of the trial advances. These are prepared and presented by the data manager and possible problems occurring in the study process should then be discussed. Some of the data to be reported are listed in Table 2. Preferably, the information to be presented should be discussed prior to the meeting with the physicians in charge of the coordination of each study. They will then decide on whether (or not) to present data which could influence (damage) the accrual rate.

Patient accrual is an indicator of the interest raised by a study. The number of cases entered by each participating centre is also key information as it has been shown that the quality of participation of an institution is correlated with the quantity of patients enrolled in terms of both compliance and the accuracy of the forms sent to the coordinating data centre (Sylvester *et al.* 1981). An overall drop in the accrual rate is a warning as to the feasibility of a study and, if confirmed, can lead to early termination of a protocol.

A detailed description of ineligible cases or protocol violations is useful for determining the accessibility of a trial. An abnormally large number of wrong inclusions or deviations may reflect overly strict eligibility criteria and perhaps the unfeasibility of a study.

A summary of the patients' characteristics will provide insight into the population under study, allow a check on any bias in selecting the patients, and ascertain that there is no imbalance in the main prognostic factors.

Toxicities and side-effects of the treatment under investigation should be reported. Care should be taken to avoid any confusion with the symptoms related to the disease itself.

All treatment or follow-up interruptions should be discussed. Again, if there are relatively high numbers of disease recurrences, refusal of patients to continue in the protocol, or loss of patients to follow-up, the causes should be evaluated and solutions to the problems proposed.

Finally, miscellaneous topics, such as the number of forms returned, the number of forms missing, improper data reporting,

etc., should be presented in order to consider the eventual need of an audit of the coordinating data centre.

These group meetings have a positive impact, as the diffusion of this kind of information may encourage centres with poor performances to improve their activity.

Publication of results

At the end of the follow-up or when it is considered that the main end-points have been reached, it is time for publication. Although this is a starting point of new therapeutic attitudes for many clinicians, it constitutes the final step of involvement for a coordinating data centre.

The data on the subjects under study and their outcome are the most important information communicated in a clinical trial publication. Readers may scan the paper looking for this information before reading the text and they will appreciate data that are organized and presented clearly (Greenberg *et al.* 1983). Therefore, data managers and biostatisticians play a key role. The most widely accepted method of reporting results in publications is as follows (Kisner and Sylvester 1980): (1) Introduction; (2) Materials and methods; (3) Results; (4) Toxicity of treatment; (5) Discussion.

The role of the data centre team starts with the section on 'Materials and methods', including the rationale for choosing a specific trial design and description of the randomization technique. The method used to calculate the required sample size should also be reported here. For the other sections, the data manager should provide a careful description of the population studied, including all the patients' characteristics, distribution of main prognostic factors by treatment, side-effects, response, criteria for withdrawal and the outcome for the withdrawn subjects, etc. Later, he or she should check that the data submitted have not been misinterpreted. In recognition of this role, he or she should be included as a co-author of the publication.

LOCAL ORGANIZATION

As specified in the Introduction, most of the methodology described above applies to the management of multicentre or single-centre trials, reflecting the standpoint of the (coordinating) data centre. However, the 'data manager' is also the person acting as 'trial referring point' in the hospital and this is briefly described here. One of the main tasks is the collection of data and their transfer to the appropriate case report forms as discussed previously. However, from the start of a new study, the local data manager should also create a practical administrative structure in which the trial can be organized within the hospital. This structure should include the following.

1. The distribution of guidelines to the medical staff, summarizing the main issues of the protocol under study and the preparation of check lists aimed at preventing the randomization of ineligible patients.

2. The randomization of the patients in the studies, ensuring that no bias is created by selecting patients for the trials. Priority should be given to centralizing this task so that the data manager will be permanently aware of the patients entered in the studies.

3. The organization of medical files, specifically designed for trial purposes, in order to guarantee adequate compliance with the protocol (Vantongelen 1989).

4. Providing a periodic report to the clinical team in order to clarify and explain possible problems in patient recruitment and follow-up.

In addition, all the other tasks previously described, such as form design, data computerization and control, etc., for local trials can be included.

CONCLUDING REMARKS

A number of topics have been discussed in this chapter, but only in a general manner. The dynamic aspect of this profession, the continuous update of international rules, the new computer systems and procedures allowing sophisticated construction of databases and data analysis, and the various managerial approaches due to cultural differences ensure that there is no definite description or assertion of a single right way of conducting data management.

The complexity of cancer clinical studies demands close interaction between the trialists. In this respect data managers provide essential administrative, technical, and scientific support throughout the whole process of a trial. Locally, they are necessary members of the medical team, as they can stimulate physicians to undertake clinical studies. Centrally, they organize and coordinate the trials in the (coordinating) data centre, thereby ensuring good support and reliable results.

REFERENCES

Bland M (1987). *An introduction to medical statistics*. Oxford University Press.
Buyse M (1988). Quality control in multi-centre cancer clinical trials. In *Cancer clinical trials. Methods and practice* (ed. ME Buyse, M Stanquet, and RJ Sylvester), pp. 120–3. Oxford University Press.
De Pauw M, Buyse M (1988). Design of forms for cancer clinical trials. In *Cancer clinical trials. Methods and practice* (ed. ME Buyse, M Stanquet, and RJ Sylvester), pp. 64–82. Oxford University Press.
Friedman LM, Furberg CD, De Mets DL (1981). *Data collection and quality control*, pp. 112–21. John Wright, Boston, MA.
Greenberg G (1984). Logistics and management. In *Current problems in clinical trials* (ed. DM Chaput de Saintonge and DW Vere), pp. 29–34. Blackwell, Oxford.
Greenberg EG, Baron JA, Colton T (1983). Reporting the results of a clinical trial. In *Clinical trials. Issues and approaches* (ed. SH Shapiro and TA Louis). Dekker, New York.
Karnofsky DA, Abelman WH, Craver LF, Burchenal JH (1948). The use of nitrogen mustards in the palliative treatment of carcinoma. *Cancer*, 1:634–56.
Kisner DL, Sylvester RJ (1980). Guidelines for reporting cancer clinical trials. In *Colloque INSERM/Direction de la Pharmacie. INSERM 96*, pp. 477–88.
Meinert CL (1986). *Clinical trials. Design, conduct, and analysis*. Oxford University Press.
Peto R, *et al.* (1977). Design and analysis of randomised clinical trials requiring prolonged observation of each patient. II. Analysis and examples. *British Journal of Cancer*, 35:1–39.
Pocock SJ (1983). *Clinical trials. A practical approach*. Wiley, New York.
Rotmensz N (1989). Behind the clinical trial. The data manager's supportive role. In *Data management and clinical trials* (ed. N Rotmensz, K Vantongelen, and J Renard), pp. 219–32. Elsevier, Amsterdam.
Sylvester RJ, *et al.* (1981). Quality of institutional participation in multicentre clinical trial. *New England Journal of Medicine*, 305:852–5.
Van der Putten E, Boon MC (1989). Data managers, skill and training. In *Data management and clinical trials* (ed. N Rotmensz, K Vantongelen, and J Renard), pp. 51–5. Elsevier, Amsterdam.
Vantongelen K (1989). Organisation of a local clinical trial office. In *Data management and clinical trials* (ed. N Rotmensz, K Vantongelan, and J Renard), pp. 57–71. Elsevier, Amsterdam.
Vantongelen K, Rotmensz N, van der Schueren E (1989). Quality control of validity of data collected in clinical trials. *European Journal of Cancer and Clinical Oncology*, 25(8):1241–7.
WHO (1976). *International classification of disease for oncology (ICD-O)*, 1st edn. WHO, Geneva.
WHO (1979). *WHO handbook for reporting results of cancer treatment*. WHO Offset Publication No. 48. Geneva
Wright P, Haybittle J (1979). Design of forms for clinical trials II. *British Medical Journal*, 2:590–2.

20.3   Quality of life

J. C. J. M. DE HAES AND ROBERT A. ZITTOUN

INTRODUCTION

The concept of quality of life became popular in the 1950s and 1960s in a political rather than a scientific context (Szalaï 1980). It was used to emphasize the necessity of promoting well-being as well as prosperity in society. Later, studies were designed to investigate how this aim could be achieved and which objective or subjective indicators would enhance the quality of life of the population at large.

In medicine 'the conscious and unconscious estimation of a patient's quality of life has always played a role' (Troidl *et al.* 1987). However, the concept has only received explicit attention in recent decades. The concept was introduced in the *Index medicus* under the heading of philosophy in 1975 and became a separate keyword in 1977. After 1977 the number of papers on quality of life increased rapidly. This increase was predicted by Elkington in 1966. He

suggested that it was a result of 'the power of the new weapons against disease', the question being whether all available new technologies should be used in clinical practice (Elkington 1966). What are the benefits for patients with respect to cure, survival, or quality of life? What are the concomitant drawbacks? Are these in balance with the costs involved? When making decisions about treatment policies, these consequences have to be weighed. Therefore, as in the general population, it became necessary to collect data to support decisions about medical care. Thus, the intuitive tradition began moving towards a more scientific approach to quality of life and decision-making.

Two main problems have been debated. First, how is the concept of 'quality of life' defined (Calman 1987)? It is generally accepted that this concept involves several dimensions such as physical well-being, psychological or emotional aspects, and social interactions including family, professional life, and economic aspects. All these dimensions interact and sometimes one of them can be predominant, overwhelming, and/or strongly modifying the others. In addition, it has been emphasized that the concept should take into account the values of the individual and the level of satisfaction or happiness when comparing the existing situation with personal aims. Second, the assessment of quality of life raises a fundamental epistemological issue: not only is it frequently emphasized that nobody can assess the quality of life of another person, but also the ability to measure, that is, to quantify, qualitative dimensions is questioned. A pragmatic approach to these arguments has been adopted, leading to a semi-quantitative evaluation of consensual dimensions by the patients themselves.

Quality of life has been the subject of much attention in oncology. Approximately half the quality of life studies published between 1980 and 1985 were related to different modes of cancer treatment (Hollandsworth 1988). This is in line with the question raised by Elkington (1966). First, the effect of cancer treatment on survival is often uncertain. Age-adjusted survival in the common types of cancer has not improved significantly in recent decades (Bailar and Smith 1986) and many patients still die as a result of the disease. Second, cancer treatment is often burdensome. Paradoxically, to have an effect on survival, toxicity may have to be maximized in chemotherapy and radiotherapy regimens. For these reasons, when nitrogen mustard was found to have an effect on tumour growth, Karnofsky and Burchenal (1949) suggested that the well-being of cancer patients should be studied along with their survival. Recently, many authors have proposed the integration of quality of life studies in clinical cancer research (Greer 1984; Brinkley 1985; Clark and Fallowfield 1986).

Quality of life can be studied in two ways: a descriptive method in which the consequences of disease or treatment interventions are mapped and an integrating approach where quality of life is taken as an end-point in medical decision-making and weighting processes are studied. These approaches are described in the following sections.

MAPPING THE CONSEQUENCES OF DISEASE AND TREATMENT

The consequences of cancer and cancer treatment are investigated for several reasons. First, data can be used to inform the patient about the probable experience of the disease. On the basis of this information patients can prepare themselves emotionally and socially and, thus, be capable of adjusting to the situation. Second, these data can be used to improve the rehabilitative care of patients. Third, data on specific consequences of different treatment options may help in making decisions on the policy to be chosen. For example, studies of the impact of mastectomy and lumpectomy on the quality of life in early breast cancer patients have supported the decision to introduce breast-conserving therapy as standard treatment in a number of institutions (Kiebert et al. 1991).

Which dimensions should be measured?

Quality of life is a general concept and must be specified when it is to be included in a description of the consequences of disease and treatment. Different frameworks have been proposed in the literature on quality of life research, some wide-ranging and some limited. The model suggested by Hörnquist (1982) is the most comprehensive. It includes physical, psychological, social, activity, financial, and structural dimensions. Spitzer (1987) considered five dimensions as a minimum requirement for quality of life research:

physical function, social function, emotional state, experience of symptoms, and sense of well-being. Aaronson et al. (1988) proposed four dimensions: physical function, physical symptoms, psychological function, and social function. Selby and Robertson (1987) used the World Health Organization (WHO) definition of health as a starting point and proposed including the physical, psychological, and social dimensions, while Donovan et al. (1989) suggested that assessment of the spiritual domain should also be incorporated. Finally, Moinpour et al. (1989) proposed, from a pragmatic point of view, that a physical and a psychological dimension are the minimum that should be investigated.

Which model is chosen depends on the specific clinical situation involved. For example, in a clinical trial comparing the side-effects of two chemotherapy regimens, the use of long questionnaires might lead to significant loss of data as a result of patient fatigue and difficulties in the organization of the trial. However, in a study of the late effects of bone-marrow transplantation, aspects such as employment status and cognitive function may be relevant and should be investigated more thoroughly. Thus, the choice depends on the comprehensiveness of the research and the practical possibilities. Following Moinpour et al. (1989), studying the physical and psychological consequences of disease or treatment is a minimum standard. However, it should be noted that the impact of treatment often reaches further. For example, Houts et al. (1984) have provided evidence of the major financial consequences of chemotherapy for patients in the United States. Therefore a broader approach, if possible, may yield more complete and more interesting results.

Once the dimensions to be measured are established, the specific variables and methods that should be used must be selected. In the physical domain, the functional status or activity level and the physical symptoms are generally relevant. In the psychological domain, symptoms giving an indication of the psychological distress or anxiety and depression level are often studied. A positive sense of well-being may also be included. From the social point of view, the structural aspect, the social network and any changes therein, or the functional aspect of the social experiences of patients can be evaluated. Negative and positive social experiences are generally independent and measuring the negative ones only will give a limited impression of the patient's situation (Tempelaar et al. 1989).

Self-reporting versus external evaluation

Some phenomena, such as alopecia, are easily observable: therefore when studying their occurrence agreement between external observers and the patients themselves will be high. However, caution should be applied as the subjective tolerance of the same grade of alopecia may differ markedly from one individual to another. Even on the Karnofsky performance index patients give ratings different from those provided by their carers (Mercier et al. 1987).

Other phenomena are more directly related to the personal experience of patients; their occurrence and, thus, the judgement of observers should be deduced from behaviour or verbal reports. Depressive feelings, for example, are less visible. In these areas the effects of treatment are less evident and discrepancies between observer and patient are more likely. Traditionally, the quality of life of cancer patients, their performance status, and the toxicity of treatments have been established by physicians. Bardelli and Saracci (1978) reviewed clinical cancer studies to determine whether quality of life had been considered. They found that, if it had, the Karnofsky and Zubrod indexes were used most frequently. These indexes (Karnofsky et al. 1948; Zubrod et al. 1960), like the usual

WHO toxicity grading system, are scored by physicians, although ratings provided by nurses could be more reliable (Yates *et al.* 1980). However, they concentrate on the physical dimensions. Recently, Sprangers *et al.* (1993) found proxies, external judges, to be generally more negative than patients in their quality of life evaluations.

More recently, an attempt has been made to provide health care providers with quality of life scales covering physical, psychological, and social domains (Spitzer *et al.* 1981). This approach has been criticized. It has been argued that the patient is the only person able to weigh the importance of benefits and adverse effects of treatment (Van Dam *et al.* 1983). However, this point of view leads to another dilemma. As shown by Michalos (1985), adaptation processes influence the subjective perception of a situation. The experience of having cancer and being treated is related to the coping style of the patient and his or her ability to adjust to adverse events. If adaptation is good, any situation may lead to satisfaction in patients and as a consequence it would not be possible to differentiate between more or less difficult situations. Therefore, a subjective evaluation may veil the intrusive character of treatment. However, studying an objective evaluation only does not take into account the patient's right to value his or her own life. Therefore, as has been proposed (Hollandsworth 1988), the ideal solution seems to be to measure the patient's experience together with the situation as observed by others, such as the physician or other carers.

It should be noted that in some instances, such as confused or terminal patients, it may be impossible to study the patient's own point of view. If this is the case, proxy measures, such as interviewing significant others or carers may be necessary (Morris *et al.* 1986). Information provided by family members, such as the parents of a sick child or the partner, can be important in quality of life studies in other situations. However, they give rise to supplementary methodological and ethical problems and in most cases proxy measures should not replace self-reporting by patients.

Self-administered questionnaires

The most frequent method of assessing quality of life in cancer patients is the self-administered questionnaire.

Response alternatives

The response alternatives can be limited to a simple choice between 'Yes' and 'No'. However, offering a range of alternatives will make the scale more responsive to changes in quality of life (Donovan *et al.* 1989). Two types of methods for quoting and quantifying more elaborate responses are utilized: the visual analogue scales use continuous 10 cm lines between two extreme answers, whereas the Likert scales offer a range of answers (three to seven) from 'never' or 'not at all' to 'always' or 'very much'. An example of such scales is given in Fig. 1. From a statistical point of view, visual analogue scales are preferable to Likert-type questions, since they represent the interval level of measurement more correctly and may be more suitable for some multivariate analyses. However, difficulties in the application of visual analogue scales have been reported (Ganz *et al.* 1988). Questions of the Likert type are more easily posed in a clinical situation. For example, they are used in the European Organization for the Research and Treatment of Cancer (EORTC) quality of life questionnaire (Aaronson *et al.* 1993) and in the Rotterdam Symptom Checklist (De Haes *et al.* 1990).

Number of items

The number of items varies markedly between methods. The more items that a scale has within each of the dimensions explored, the

Visual analogue scale

Did you feel tired over the last week

Not at all _____ Extremely
tired   tired

Likert-type scale

Did you feel tired over the last week

Not at all/A little/Quite a bit/Very much

Fig. 1 Comparison of two types of scale (visual analogue and Likert) for the same item.

more responsive to change it will be; five items per domain is generally regarded as satisfactory for detecting changes (Donovan *et al.* 1989). However, too many items results in an excessively long time for completion, which could limit feasibility in clinical studies. Most of the scales reviewed by Donovan *et al.* (1989) can be completed in 15 min or less, except for the Cancer Inventory of Problem Situations which consists of a total of 131 items and is reported to take 20 min to complete (Heinrich *et al.* 1984).

Time frame of the questions

Assessment of the short-term consequences of cancer disease and treatment implies the use of questions related to the last (few) day(s). The use of a short time frame (for example, 1 week) has been recommended even for long-term effects in order to minimize problems associated with memory loss and to avoid confusion of specific symptom experience with personality traits (Huisman *et al.* 1987).

Specificity of the instrument

Questionnaires developed for a particular study should be adapted to the problems raised (Schain *et al.* 1983). However, the use of more general questionnaires, which have already been assessed for their psychometric properties and allow comparison with other groups of patients or the normal population, is generally recommended. However, the use of generic methods has other drawbacks. They have been developed for a wide range of populations (normal, psychiatric, or chronically disabled) and may have little relevance to the cancer population under study; in addition they are sometimes lengthy, time-consuming, and, if so, unsatisfactory for repeated applications over time.

An interesting approach has been proposed by the EORTC Quality of Life Study Group (Aaronson *et al.* 1988). A core questionnaire is developed for the cancer patients, covering the functional status, the disease- and treatment-related symptoms, and the psychological and social function. This questionnaire is complemented by additional modules depending on the type of disease or treatment to be studied.

Examples of modular questions are those concerning fluid retention in patients receiving hormonal therapy, breathlessness and haemoptysis in lung cancer, cognitive functions following brain irradiation, and sexuality and fertility following treatment of gynaecological or testicular cancer. Some pilot work among physicians, nurses, and patients is necessary to establish which relevant questions should be raised.

The psychometric properties

It is generally preferable to use methods with established reliability and validity. Reliability refers to the amount of measurement error, that is, the extent to which a test will yield the same results when measuring an unchanged characteristic. Validity refers to the extent to which a method measures what it is intended to measure.

The reliability and validity of many generic methods used for health status and quality of life measurement have been investigated. For example, the Sickness Impact Profile (Bergner *et al.* 1981), the Nottingham Health Profile (Hunt *et al.* 1981), and the SF.36 were developed to investigate the health or illness situation of different patient populations. The Sickness Impact Profile has been successfully used with cancer patients (Ware and Sherbourne 1992). These methods enable comparisons to be made across disease groups. However, they do not take into consideration the specific symptoms that are relevant in cancer treatment and important to the cancer patient's experience. Therefore, either a specific method may have to be chosen or a combination may have to be used.

Specific methods for cancer patients have been devised over the past 15 years (for reviews see Van Knippenberg and De Haes 1988; Donovan *et al.* 1989; Maguire and Selby 1989; Moinpour *et al.* 1989; Cella and Tulsky 1990). These methods represent different approaches. A common factor in most of them is assessment of the situation as perceived by the patient. Different areas are covered and different measurement techniques are used.

Donovan *et al.* (1989) reviewed 17 scales and found only five with demonstrable reliability (Priestman and Baum 1976; Spitzer *et al.* 1981; Gough *et al.* 1983; Padilla *et al.* 1983; Selby *et al.* 1984) and five with at least two types of validity (content, construct, or concurrent) (Spitzer *et al.* 1981; Padilla *et al.* 1983; Schipper *et al.* 1984; Selby *et al.* 1984). None of these scales clearly demonstrated predictive validity through an external indicator such as frequency of request for medical help, use of psychotropic drugs, or use of psychiatric services (Donovan *et al.* 1989). Only two methods, the FLIC (Schipper *et al.* 1984) and the CARES (Heinrich *et al.* 1984), used the patients as a main source of generating problems, rather than the literature or the perception of professionals. More recently the psychometric of other instruments was described such as the EORTC-QLO (Aaronson *et al.* 1993), the FACT (Cella *et al.* 1993), and the RSCL (De Haes *et al.* 1990).

It is also possible for clinical trials to combine established instruments with known psychometric properties (for example, Hospital Anxiety and Depression Scales, Profile of Mood States, Social Adjustment Scale, etc.) with one of the existing scales for assessment of quality of life in cancer patients. This approach has been adopted by the EORTC (Aaronson *et al.* 1988) and by the Eastern Cooperative Oncology Group (Skeel 1989).

Interviews

The use of semi-structured or unstructured open interviews may be useful. In the open interview, starting from a general framework the patient is invited to describe his or her situation in a broad sense. In this way, each patient's experience is investigated most completely. Mechanisms underlying adaptation may be better understood if an open interview technique can be used in at least a few patients. They lead to problems of generalizability. Also, these methods are unsuitable for group comparisons and for use in cross-cultural studies. In such cases, stricter and more rigid methods are necessary although their content is less rich. In semi-structured standardized interviews, questions are established at the start of the study and are expressed in the same words for all subjects approached. Interviews can be applied to a broad range of patients

and quantification of answers is simplified. They may help to understand the specific aspects of the clinical situation under study.

Patient diaries

Patient diaries are particularly useful if a frequent (for example, daily) assessment of change in symptoms such as pain, nausea and vomiting, activity level, mood, and overall well-being is required (Fayers and Jones 1983). However, there is a strict limitation on the number of questions asked and serious problems of compliance occur, with a risk of retrospective completion after an initial period of enthusiasm.

Data collection

Oral interviews can be held either in the clinical setting or at the patient's home, directly or by telephone. The patient often uses the attention given by the interviewer as an opportunity to express the many aspects of his or her experience of the disease. The proportion of patients refusing to participate in these studies is less than when written questionnaires are used. Open interviews are generally tape-recorded and transcribed. Therefore, the method is time-consuming. Written questionnaires, which patients fill in without the help of an interviewer, can be given to the patient in the hospital or the out-patient clinic or be mailed to his or her home. They have the advantage of being less costly and therefore more feasible, particularly in large multicentre clinical trials. Two drawbacks of mailed questionnaires are that the exact date of completion is less easily controlled and that members of the patient's social network may assist in completion, which could bias the results of the study. However, in this less personal situation, the answers are also less likely to be socially desirable.

Design of the study

Cross-sectional studies limited to a unique assessment point are only relevant for the evaluation of long-term quality of life in patients cured of cancers. Even then it is impossible to compare the present status with that which prevailed before the onset of the disease. This could only be evaluated retrospectively by the patient. Therefore, a parallel study of a control group of normal subjects using the same methods is warranted.

In all other cases, a longitudinal study with repeated assessment is necessary. The relevant phases occurring as a consequence of the disease or treatment should be covered in the measurement procedure. The physical symptoms and the prevalence of depression and anxiety differ in the diagnostic phase, in the first months after surgery or radiotherapy and after the first year(s) of treatment. They also differ over the chemotherapy cycle and the number of cycles received (De Haes *et al.* 1987*b*). This implies that both the time schedule and the expected toxicity should be taken into account if full insight into the concomitant effects of disease and treatment is to be gained. An example of such design is given in Fig. 2.

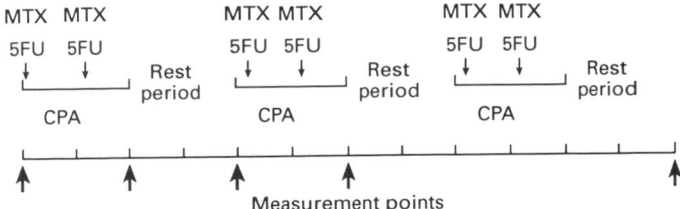

Fig. 2 An example of points at which quality of life could be measured during adjuvant CMF chemotherapy in early breast cancer.

Some comments are necessary. First, for treatment evaluation it is important to assess, whenever possible, the patient's quality of life at baseline. Thus, the patients' starting points and the original variance within the patient group can be established. This is not possible with respect to the experience of illness as the diagnostic phase will have already had an impact on the patient's life. Therefore, the use of a control group may be necessary. Second, it is important that the methods used are sensitive to the changes occurring over time. Sensitivity has not always been established for the methods discussed in this chapter and further work is necessary in this area. Third, there are some problems associated with data collection and analysis when using multiple measurement points. Short intervals between measurements may lead to scores being influenced by the memory of earlier answers. Also, multiple measurement points will result in a burden on the data collection organization and on the patients, with an increased risk of missing data. An optimum level should be established between the coverage of all relevant points in time and practicability.

ASSIGNING A SINGLE VALUE FOR QUALITY OF LIFE: WEIGHTING AND DECISION MAKING

Assigning a single value to quality of life for weighting processes

Assigning a single value to quality of life may be useful in clarifying weighting procedures. It allows a determination to be made, based on specific indicators and personal characteristics or coping behaviour, of how patients reach an overall evaluation of their life. Thus, the weight of concomitant effects of disease and treatment and the burden placed on patients by different symptoms, can be established (Troidl et al. 1987). In addition, the background of variance in reactions between patients can be studied.

A possible solution adopted in some of the approaches utilized in oncology has been to include specific scale(s) of the overall quality of life (Izsak and Medalie 1971; Irwin et al. 1982; Coates et al. 1987; Aaronson et al. 1988). Patients may be asked to rate their quality of life on scales based on affective representation (very good–very bad, very happy–very unhappy) and/or cognitive representation (very satisfied–very dissatisfied). There is evidence that the affective component of quality of life is more responsive to external changes inflicted upon the patient (De Haes et al. 1987a, 1992) and therefore is more sensitive to change.

Another method used to establish the weights of different symptoms or side-effects of the disease and treatment has been to ask patients to rate their importance directly, according to intensity and duration. It is thus possible to establish sum scores of the burden experienced by patients. This procedure could clearly be applied in deciding whether to use three or nine cycles of CMF (cyclophosphamide, methotrexate, 5-fluorouracil) treatment in stage II breast cancer (Levine et al. 1988). Corder and Ellwein (1984) have proposed using such weighting procedures in order to explain quality of life information to patients with the aim of providing an improved basis for informed consent and eliciting individual preferences.

Weighting factors could also be derived from regression analysis investigating the relation between side-effects and the overall evaluation. This procedure should be investigated for cancer patients. However, it could yield different results from those obtained by weighting the symptoms directly (Campbell et al. 1976). Again, a decision should be made as to who is to value the situation,

as differences in values assigned by different populations to the same disease states have been reported (Sackett and Torrance 1978). Therefore, the valuation should be made by individual patients. Groups of patients may also be asked to give their valuations of their situation; these values can be used for similar groups to be treated in the future. Ideally, these studies should be replicated to determine whether values change over time.

The only cases in which patients should not perform the evaluations themselves are those in which they are unable to make their valuations explicit, for example young children, terminal care, and severe neurological impairment. Proxy measures can be used successfully in such cases (Morris et al. 1986).

Integration of quality of life in decision making

When choosing between different treatment options, for individual patients as well as groups of patients, the different outcomes of such options (survival or quality of life or both) must be weighted and integrated so that a final decision can be made.

In some cases the difference in survival between treatment options is such that the quality of life is a less prominent factor in the decision to be taken. For example, treatment of testicular cancer with chemotherapy is very toxic. However, it has a major positive effect on survival and therefore the temporary impairment for some patients in quality of life is not a major issue in the choice of policy (Peckham 1988).

In contrast, in other cases treatment policies do not differ in their effect on survival but have very different effects on quality of life: for example, when comparing breast-saving procedures and mastectomy in early breast cancer, the quality of life is the most important consideration.

Finally, in oncology, trade-offs between duration and quality of life are made continuously, particularly in advanced disease. This is because the treatment options are generally intrusive but withholding treatment will usually lead to progression of the disease. Therefore, it may be necessary to define the quality of life after different treatments for the same disease using a value which can be related to the resulting duration of survival. An example of such an integration is outlined in Fig. 3: the quality of life is better after one treatment alternative, whereas the patient will survive for longer after the other. An example of this situation is treatment of lung cancer patients using chemotherapy. In this case quality of life and duration of survival must be weighed against each other.

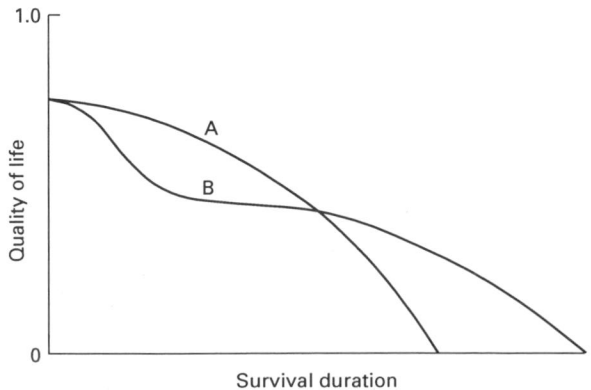

Fig. 3 Relative values of two types of treatment following integration of duration of survival and quality of life: treatment B prolongs the survival despite an initial impairment of quality of life.

Another situation is when a toxic treatment regimen prolongs the progression-free survival but not the overall survival. An example is the treatment of advanced breast cancer patients using chemotherapy (De Haes *et al.* 1993). In this case quality of life under chemotherapy should be weighed against quality of life during progression-free survival.

Quality of life as the main end-point in decision making

Many prospective randomized trials in oncology fail to demonstrate the superiority of one treatment option over the other(s) in terms of disease-free and/or overall survival. Quality of life should be considered as an important, and sometimes the main, end-point in these trials.

The results are frequently those which are intuitively expected, for example better quality outcome of conservative breast treatment compared with mastectomy. However, counter-intuitive findings are sometimes obtained, for example failure to demonstrate an increased fear of recurrence in breast cancer patients following conservative surgery (De Haes and Welvaart 1985) or better quality of life with intermittent rather than continuous chemotherapy in advanced breast cancer (Coates *et al.* 1987) or amputation not considered to be inferior to limb-sparing procedure in soft tissue sarcoma (Sugarbaker *et al.* 1982).

Some phase II trials would be equally appropriate for quality of life assessment (Skeel 1989); gathering information about a phase II programme which is expected to result in major effects and dysfunction can provide critical data. These could be helpful in changing the design of a subsequent phase III trial or building in checkpoints for early intervention to minimize symptoms and dysfunction during the phase III study. The knowledge gained from these evaluations could result in an increase in the number of patients who complete and benefit from the prescribed regimen, as well as easier completion of studies.

When quality of life is the main end-point, three possible solutions can be given. First, treatment options differ in only one respect. If so, the most favourable outcome is to be chosen. Second, more dimensions of quality of life are involved. If so, these different outcomes may be weighed as described above. Third, an overall value for the treatment options may be asked from patients and used to support decision making.

Integration of quality of life and survival

Decisions are made either for individual patients, or for groups of patients in the frame of a clinical trial.

Individual patients can weigh outcomes regarding quality of life and survival on the basis of good information. On a group level, different methods like decision trees and models have been developed. In a decision tree the value of each treatment option can be derived from the value or utility of the various outcomes multiplied by the probability of their occurrences. Utility is expressed in a score from zero for the worst state or death to unity for the best state imaginable. When designing a decision tree, the main difficulty is in the assignment of the utilities of the outcomes. Again, these can be determined by the patients or others on the basis of both the transient deterioration of their quality of life and the permanent somatic, psychological, and social impairment in the case of cure. When facing a decision-making problem, the degree of risk acceptance, which may vary according to age (McNeil *et al.* 1978) and other patient variables (Ciampi *et al.* 1982), must be taken into account. An example of a decision tree is given in

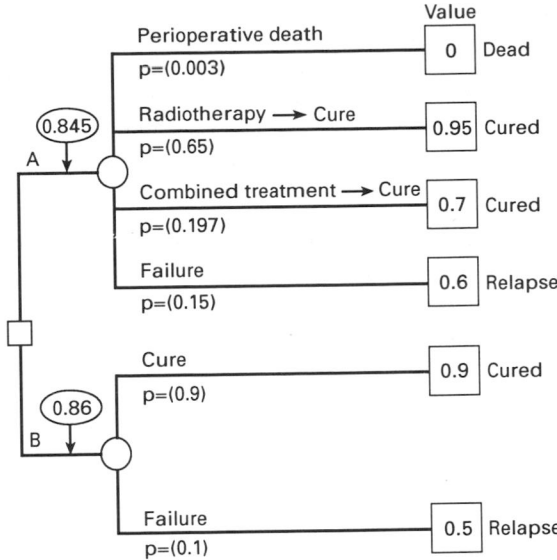

Fig. 4 Decision tree comparing two types of treatment in early stages of Hodgkin's disease. □ choice node; ○ chance node; ☐ outcome. The probabilities of the possible events at the chance nodes are shown in parentheses. The utilities of the various outcomes are shown in the boxes to the right of the decision tree. The expected utilities of the chance nodes are encircled with arrows pointing to the chance nodes. Treatment A is based on staging laparotomy, with radiotherapy or combined modality according to the findings at laparotomy. Treatment B is based on combined chemoradiotherapy without staging laparotomy.

Fig. 4, where two different treatments for the early stage of Hodgkin's disease are compared. The utilities must be derived from the data available in the literature or on a data basis; the relative value of each treatment option will vary according to its duration and side-effects (Corder and Ellwein 1984). The cost–benefit ratio could also include the total period of hospital which is an indicator of both quality of life and economic burden. A decision tree does, contrary to a Mairkov model (Hillner *et al.* 1991), not include time in different states.

Other methods have been developed to integrate values with respect to quality and duration of life. A simple model, the Q-TWIST (time without symptoms of disease and subjective toxicity), has been proposed by Goldhirsch *et al.* (1984) for the evaluation of adjuvant chemotherapy in early breast cancer. Another model, based on quality of life measurement, has been proposed by Asselain *et al.* (1986). They computed 'time quality of life' or 'quality adjusted life' after palliative treatment. This can be done by assigning values to the quality of life during successive time periods. The 'area under the curve' can be computed by multiplying the length of the time periods under consideration by their quality of life factor, thus establishing the number of quality-adjusted life years (QALYs). In fact the QALY model was not originated in oncology but described first by Miyamoto and Eraker (1985).

The independence of quality of life and survival duration, a requirement for their multiplication, is not always confirmed in the literature. Empirical evidence of dependence has been reported: a relation between the valuation of a health state and the duration of that state has been observed (Sackett and Torrance 1978; Sutherland *et al.* 1982); in a study of advanced breast cancer, the change in quality of life scores during chemotherapy was a significant independent predictor of subsequent survival (Coates *et al.* 1987).

In fact, also for a QALY model the use of 'utilities' is more appropriate than quality of life measures. Various methods have been proposed for utility measurement (Weinstein and Fineberg 1980). In the *standard gambling method* the utility of a disability is assessed by adjusting the odds for the gamble between immediate death and the gain of a perfect health until the decision-maker is indifferent between the gamble and the disability. Another possibility is the *time trade off method*. The respondent is asked to make a trade-off between an imperfect health state for a certain period followed by death and a perfect health for a varying shorter period of time. In *direct scaling methods* the respondent is asked, through a series of questions, to value different health states.

Comprehension is one of the difficulties in utility measurement, whether using the standard gambling method (Torrance 1987) or other techniques (Rosser and Kind 1978). In addition, systematic differences were found when using different methods, with the standard gambling technique yielding higher values than the time trade-off method and even higher values than the direct scaling methods (Read *et al.* 1984; Torrance 1987; Stiggelbout *et al.* 1994). Finally, the concurrence of the results of these valuation methods, which are restricted to a limited number of dimensions, and the values of patients in real life is uncertain. External judges and patients assign different values to health states (Sackett and Torrance 1978) and the way in which patients cope and adopt to the actual situation can modify the value primarily assigned (Calman 1984; De Haes and Van Knippenberg 1985).

There have been few studies of the utility of different health states after disease or treatment options in oncology. McNeil *et al.* (1978, 1981) reported the values for different treatment options and survival in lung cancer and laryngeal cancer using the gambling technique. The samples used consisted not of cancer patient populations. More recently cancer patients have been asked for utilities but not yet about their actual health (Llewellyn-Thomas *et al.* 1982, 1984; Sutherland *et al.* 1982, 1983; O'Connor *et al.* 1987; Boyd *et al.* 1990; Stiggelbout *et al.* 1994).

Despite objections, decision trees and QALY or Markov models based on current medical knowledge including survival and quality of life for each treatment option will help in making treatment choices or ascertaining the value of the treatment alternatives before enrolling a patient in a clinical trial. Thus, medical decision-making based on quality of life adjusted survival and risk acceptance may provide a scientific basis and facilitate the informed consent procedure. However, further ethical problems could arise: using utilities for group or policy decisions has been said to result in discrimination against individuals with a lower quality of life or a shorter life expectancy and they may receive less care as the expected gain could be lower (Ciampi *et al.* 1982; Harris 1987).

CONCLUSION

Quality of life is one of the important end-points of cancer treatment. It is particularly important in phase III trials, whereas the measurement of physical toxicity using the WHO score could be sufficient in phases I and II. In view of the number of phase III trials failing to show differences between the treatment arms for tumour response and survival, quality of life could be a major or even the first end-point in many of them.

Before embarking on a study implying measurement of quality of life, one should carefully identify the research question(s) based on the present knowledge and hypotheses. It is then necessary to analyse existing methods from both a psychometric and a clinical point of view in order to select those which are most relevant to the study. The design of the study should also take into account the appropriate time(s) for the measurement and identify the persons and techniques necessary for data collection as well as competent statisticians who can produce the scores and analyse the results.

The potential benefits of such measurements are numerous. There is already one positive impact which is seldom emphasized: the individual patient's awareness that staff and researchers are paying attention to his or her main concerns on the basis of his or her subjective perception and assessment. Any written questionnaire should be supplemented by the possibility of free comments and the most relevant answers should be transmitted to the carers in order to identify individual requirements for help and to improve support from staff and psychotherapeutic intervention. In addition, as has been shown in this chapter, in the near future the conclusions of studies on quality of life could be integrated in the measurement of survival in groups of patients and therefore help in medical decision-making and treatment strategy. An individual weighting of toxicities and the psychosocial burden of treatment is also possible, and this could help carers and patients to select the best treatment alternative.

REFERENCES

Aaronson NK, Bullinger M, Ahmedzai S (1988). A modular approach to quality of life assessment in cancer clinical trials. *Recent Results in Cancer Research*, 111:231–49.

Aaronson NK, *et al.* (1993). A quality-of-life instrument for use in international clinical trials in oncology. *Journal of the National Cancer Institute*, 85:365–76.

Asselain B, Gremy F, Nguyen L (1986). Peut-on intégrer qualité et durée de vie? Proposition d'un nouveau critère de décision. *Bulletin du Cancer*, 73:709–12.

Bailar JC III, Smith EM (1986). Progress against cancer? *New England Journal of Medicine*, 314:1226–32.

Bardelli D, Saracci R (1978). Measuring the quality of life in cancer clinical trials: a sample survey of published trials. In *Methods and impact of controlled therapeutic trials in cancer*. UICC Technical Report Series 36:75–97.

Bergner M, Bobbitt RA, Carter WB, Gilson BS (1981). Impact profile: development and final revision of a health status measure. *Medical Care*, 19:787–805.

Boyd NF, Sutherland HJ, Heasman KZ, Trichler DL, Cummings BJ (1990). Whose utilities for decision analysis? *Medical Decision Making*, 10:58–67.

Brinkley D (1985). Quality of life in cancer trials. *British Medical Journal*, 291:685–6.

Calman KC (1984). Quality of life in cancer patients—an hypothesis. *Journal of Medical Ethics*, 10:124–7.

Calman KC (1987). Definitions and dimensions of quality of life. In *The quality of life of cancer patients* (ed. NK Aaronson, J Beckman, JL Bernheim, and R Zittoun), pp. 1–9. Raven Press, New York.

Campbell A, Converse PE, Rodgers WL (1976). *The quality of American life*. Sage, New York.

Cella DF, Tulsky DS (1990). Measuring quality of life today: methodological aspects. *Oncology*, 4:29–33.

Cella DF, *et al.* (1993) The functional assessment of cancer therapy scale: development and validation of the general measure. *Journal of Clinical Oncology*, 11:570–9.

Ciampi A, Silberfeld M, Till JE (1982). Measurement of individual preferences. The importance of 'situation-specific' variables. *Medical Decision Making*, 2:483–95.

Clark A, Fallowfield LJ (1986). Quality of life measurements in patients with malignant disease: a review. *Journal of the Royal Society of Medicine*, 79:165–9.

Coates A, *et al.* (1987). Improving the quality of life during chemotherapy for advanced breast cancer. *New England Journal of Medicine*, 317:1490–5.

Corder MP, Ellwein LB (1984). A decision-analysis methodology for consideration of morbidity factors in clinical decision-making. *American Journal of Clinical Oncology*, 6:19–32.

De Haes JCJM, Van Knippenberg FCE (1985). The quality of life of cancer patients: a review of the literature. *Social Science and Medicine*, 20:809–17.

De Haes JCJM, Welvaart K (1985). Quality of life after breast cancer surgery. *Journal of Surgical Oncology*, **28**:123–5.

De Haes JCJM, Pennink BJU, Welvaart K (1987a). The distinction between affect and cognition. *Social Indicators Research*, **19**:367–78.

De Haes JCJM, *et al.* (1987b). Evaluation of the quality of life of patients with advanced ovarian cancer treated with combination chemotherapy. In *The quality of life of cancer patients* (ed. NK Aaronson and J Beckmann), pp. 215–26. Raven Press, New York.

De Haes JCJM, van Knippenberg FCE, Neijt JP (1990). Measuring psychological and physical distress in cancer patients: structure and application of the Rotterdam Symptom Checklist. *British Journal of Cancer*, **62**:1034–8.

De Haes JCJM, de Ruiter JH, Tempelaar R, Pennink BJW (1992). The distinction between affect and cognition in the quality of life of cancer patients—sensitivity and stability. *Quality of Life Research*, **1**:315–22.

De Haes JCJM, Nooy MA, Beex LVAM (1993). Quality of life and decision making, the treatment policy in advanced breast cancer. *European Journal of Cancer*, **29A**:S17.

Donovan K, Sanson-Fisher RW, Redman S (1989). Measuring quality of life in cancer patients. *Journal of Clinical Oncology*, **7**:959–68.

Elkington JR (1966). Medicine and the quality of life. *Annals of Internal Medicine*, **64**:711–14.

Fayers PM, Jones DR (1983). Measuring and analysing quality of life in cancer clinical trials: a review. *Statistics in Medicine*, **2**:429–46.

Ganz PA, *et al.* (1988). Estimating the quality of life in a clinical trial of patients with metastatic lung cancer using the Karnofsky Performance Status and the Functional Living Index—Cancer. *Cancer*, **61**:849–59.

Goldhirsch A, Gelber RD, Simes RJ, Glasziou P (1989). Costs and benefits of adjuvant therapy in breast cancer: a quality-adjusted survival analysis. *Journal of Clinical Oncology*, **7**:36–44.

Gough IR, Furnival CM, Schilder L, Grove W (1983). Assessment of the quality of life of patients with advanced cancer. *European Journal of Cancer and Clinical Oncology*, **19**:1161–5.

Greer S (1984). The psychological dimension in cancer treatment. *Social Science and Medicine*, **18**:345–9.

Heinrich RL, Schag CC, Ganz PA (1984). Living with cancer: the cancer inventory of problem situations. *Journal of Clinical Psychology*, **40**:972–80.

Hillner BE, Smith TJ (1991). Efficacy and cost-effectiveness of adjuvant chemotherapy in women with node-negative breast cancer. A decision-analysis model. *New England Journal of Medicine*, **324**:160–8.

Hollandsworth JG Jr (1988). Evaluating the impact of medical treatment on the quality of life: a 5-year update. *Social Sciences and Medicine*, **26**:425–34.

Hörnquist JO (1982). The concept of quality of life. *Scandinavian Journal of Social Medicine*, **10**:57–61.

Houts PS, *et al.* (1984). Non-medical costs to patients and their families associated with outpatient chemotherapy. *Cancer*, **53**:2388–92.

Huisman SJ, Van Dam FSAM, Aaronson NK, Hanewald G (1987). On measuring complaints of cancer patients: some remarks on the time span of the question. In *The quality of life of cancer patients* (ed. NK Aaronson, J Beckmann, J Bernheim, and R Zittoun), pp. 101–9. Raven Press, New York.

Hunt SM, *et al.* (1981). The Nottingham Health Profile: subjective health status and medical consultations. *Social Sciences Medicine*, **15a**:221–9.

Irwin PH, Gottlieb A, Kramer S, Danoff B (1982). Quality of life after radiation therapy: a study of 309 cancer survivors. *Social Indicators Research*, **10**:187–210.

Iszak FC, Medalie JH (1971). Comprehensive follow-up of carcinoma patients. *Journal of Chronic Diseases*, **24**:179.

Karnofsky DA, Burchenal JH (1949). The clinical evaluation of chemotherapeutic agents in cancer. In *Evaluation of chemotherapeutic agents* (ed. CM Macleod), pp. 192–205. Columbia University Press, New York.

Karnofsky DA, *et al.* (1948). The use of nitrogen mustards in the palliative treatment of carcinoma. *Cancer*, **1**:634–56.

Kiebert GM, de Haes JCJM, van de Velde CJH (1991). Quality of life after mastectomy and breast conserving surgery: a review. *Journal of Clinical Oncology*, **9**:1059–70.

Levine M, *et al.* (1988). Quality of life in stage II breast cancer, an instrument for clinical trials. *Journal of Clinical Oncology*, **6**:1798–1810.

Llewellyn-Thomas H, *et al.* (1982). The measurement of patient's values in medicine. *Medical Decision Making*, **2**:449–62.

Llewellyn-Thomas H, *et al.* (1984). The assessment of values in laryngeal cancer: reliability of measurement methods. *Journal of Chronic Diseases*, **37**:283–91.

McNeil BJ, Weichselbaum R, Pauker SG (1978). Fallacy of the five year survival in lung cancer. *New England Journal of Medicine*, **299**:1397–1401.

McNeil BJ, Weichselbaum R, Pauker SG (1981). Speech and survival, trade-offs between quality and quantity of life in laryngeal cancer. *New England Journal of Medicine*, **305**:982–7.

Maguire P, Selby P (1989). Assessing quality of life in cancer patients. *British Journal of Cancer*, **60**:437–40.

Mercier M, Schraub S, Bourgeois P (1987). Quality of life. *Lancet*, 161–2.

Michalos AC (1985). Multiple discrepancies theory (MDT). *Social Indicators Research*, **16**:347–413.

Miyamoto JM, Eraker SA (1985). Parameter estimates for a QALY utility model. *Medical Decision Making*, **5**:191–213.

Moinpour CM, *et al.* (1989). Quality of life endpoints in cancer clinical trials: review and recommendations. *Journal of National Cancer Institute*, **81**:485–95.

Morris JN, *et al.* (1986). Last days: a study on the quality of life of terminally ill cancer patients. *Journal of Chronic Diseases*, **39**:47–62.

O'Connor AMC, Boyd NF, Stolbach WL, Till JE (1987). Eliciting preferences for alternative drug therapies in oncology: influence of treatment outcome description, elicitation technique and treatment experiences. *Journal of Chronic Diseases*, **40**:811–18.

Padilla GV, *et al.* (1983). Quality of life index for patients with cancer. *Research in Nursing and Health*, **6**:117–26.

Peckham M (1988). Testicular cancer. *Acta Oncologica*, **27**:439–52.

Priestman TJ, Baum M (1976). Evaluation of quality of life in patients receiving treatment for advanced cancer. *Lancet*, i:899–901.

Read JL, *et al.* (1984). Preferences for health outcomes, comparison of assessment methods. *Medical Decision Making*, **4**:315–29.

Rosser R, Kind P (1978). A scale of valuations of states of illness: is there a social consensus? *International Journal of Epidemiology*, **7**:347–58.

Sackett DL, Torrance GW (1978). The utility of different health states as perceived by the general public. *Journal of Chronic Diseases*, **31**:697–704.

Schain W, *et al.* (1983). Psychosocial and physical outcomes of primary breast cancer therapy: mastectomy vs excisional biopsy and irradiation. *Breast Cancer Research Treatment*, **3**:377–82.

Schipper H, Clinch J, McMurray A, Levitt M (1984). Measuring the quality of life of cancer patients. The Functional Living Index—Cancer: the development and validation. *Journal of Clinical Oncology*, **2**:472–83.

Selby P, Robertson B (1987). Measurement of quality of life in patients with cancer. *Cancer Surveys*, **6**:521–43.

Selby PJ, *et al.* (1984). The development of a method for assessing the quality of life of cancer patients. *British Journal of Cancer*, **50**:13–22.

Skeel RT (1989). Quality of life assessment in cancer clinical trials. It's time to catch up. *Journal of National Cancer Institute*, **81**:472–3.

Spitzer WO (1987). State of science 1986: quality of life and functional status as target variables for research. *Journal of Chronic Diseases*, **40**:465–71.

Spitzer WO, *et al.* (1981). Measuring the quality of life of cancer patients. A concise QL-index for use by physicians. *Journal of Chronic Diseases*, **34**:585–97.

Sprangers MAG, Aaronson NK (1992). The role of health care providers and significant others in evaluating the quality of life of patients with chronic disease: a review. *Journal of Clinical Epidemiology*, **45**:743–60.

Stiggelbout AM, Kiebert GM, Kievit J, Leer JWH, Stoter G, de Haes JCJM (1994). Utility assessment in cancer patients: adjustment of time tradeoff scores for the utility of life years and comparison with standard gamble scores. *Medical Decision Making*, **14**:82–90.

Sugarbaker PH, Baroksky I, Rosenberg SA, Gianoma FJ (1982). Quality of life assessment of patients in extremity sarcoma clinical trials. *Surgery*, **91**:17–23.

Sutherland HJ, Llewellyn-Thomas H, Boyd NF, Till JE (1982). Attitudes toward quality of survival, the concept of 'maximal endurable time'. *Medical Decision Making*, **2**:299–309.

Sutherland HJ, Dunn V, Boyd NF (1983). Measurement of values for states of health with linear analog scales. *Medical Decision Making*, **3**:477–87.

Szalaï A (1980). The meaning of comparative research on the quality of life. In *The quality of life: comparative studies* (ed. A Szalaï and FM Andrews), pp. 7–21. Sage, London.

Tempelaar R, de Haes JCJM, de Ruiter JH, Bakker D, van den Heuvel WJA, van Nieuwen-huijzen MG (1989). The social experiences of cancer patients under treatment. *Social Science and Medicine*, 29/5:635–42.

Torrance GW (1987). Utility approach to measuring health related quality of life. *Journal of Chronic Diseases*, 40:593–600.

Troidl H, *et al.* (1987). Quality of life: an important endpoint both in surgical practice and research. *Journal of Chronic Diseases*, 40:523–8.

Van Dam FSAM, Van Linssen ACG, Couzijn AL (1983). Evaluating 'quality of life' in cancer clinical trials. In *Cancer clinical trials, methods, and practice* (ed. M Buyse, M Staquet, and R Sylvester), pp. 26–43. Oxford University Press.

Van Knippenberg FCE, De Haes JCJM (1988). Measuring the quality of life of cancer patients, psychometric properties of instruments. *Journal of Clinical Epidemiology*, 11:1043–53.

Ware J, Sherbourne C (1992). The MOS 36-Item Short-Form Health Survey. Conceptual framework and item, selection. *Medical Care*, 30:473–83.

Weinstein MC, Fineberg HV (1980). *Clinical decision analysis*. WB Saunders, Philadelphia.

Yates JW, Chalmer B, McKegney FP (1980). Evaluation of patients with advanced cancer using the Karnofsky performance status. *Cancer*, 45:2220–4.

Zubrod CG, *et al.* (1960). Appraisal of methods for the study of chemotherapy of cancer in man: comparative therapeutic trial of nitrogen mustard and triethylene thiophosphoramide. *Journal of Chronic Diseases*, 11:7–33.

20.4 Psychological sequelae of cancer and its treatment

PETER MAGUIRE

INTRODUCTION

Studies using standardized assessment methods have confirmed that the diagnosis and treatment of cancer is associated with a substantial psychiatric morbidity (Greer 1985). Anxiety and depression are found in up to a third of patients (Derogatis *et al.* 1983). This represents an increase in relative risk of three to four times compared with the prevalence of affective disorders in the general population. Body image problems and sexual difficulties are also more common (Anderson 1985). Even when cancer patients are disease free and no longer under treatment, they may fail to return to their former level of social and occupational adjustment. Therefore, the factors contributing to this increased morbidity need to be considered.

AETIOLOGY
Impact of diagnosis
Uncertainty

In some patients psychiatric morbidity develops because they fail to come to terms with the diagnosis of cancer. They continue to fear that the cancer will return, and will cause physical and mental suffering and premature death. They are unable to control these fears or distract themselves. Any reminder that they have cancer, like a magazine article or television programme, further intensifies their fears. Their worries are particularly intense if they have had an adverse experience of cancer in a close friend or relative, particularly if the friend or relative was reassured that all would be well but died later. Regular follow-up visits also reactivate worries that evidence of recurrence or progression will be found.

Search for meaning

People faced with serious illness try to find an explanation for it. Psychological adaptation is more likely if an adequate explanation can be found. This is relatively easy with coronary heart disease. Clear risk factors have been identified, such as a strong family

history, faulty diet, lack of exercise, or heavy smoking. No such explanations are available for most cancers. Therefore, this leaves a vacuum into which patients and relatives project non-scientific theories. Popular lay theories about why cancer develops include the ideas that it is due to some basic personality flaw, inability to cope with stress, or difficulty in expressing emotions like anger. Patients accepting these theories blame themselves for their predicament. This leads to lowered self-esteem and demoralization. This demoralization persists if they see no way of changing their personality, situation, or life-style.

Claims that cancer is caused by stress lead some patients to blame key relatives or employers because they judge them to be the source of their stress. Their bitterness hinders their ability to adapt and causes a serious breakdown in personal relationships.

Stigma

Some patients feel stimatized by their disease and use words like 'unclean', 'contagious', or 'leprosy' to convey this. Feelings of stigma are likely when the cancer has been linked with undesirable behaviour, as in women with cervical cancer where it has been claimed that it is due to sexual promiscuity. Stigma is also evident when the cancer has been linked with viruses as in leukaemia. Hence, mothers of children with leukaemia may fear that the child will be viewed as infectious and this fear is reinforced when they notice that other parents keep their children away from the affected child. Such feelings of stigma are associated with subsequent psychiatric morbidity.

Being secretive

When patients worry about the acceptability of their diagnosis to close friends, relatives, or employers they may decide to keep their diagnosis secret. They may also keep it secret to protect a loved one from anguish. Such secretiveness is associated with a poor psychological adaptation because it precludes their receiving emotional support. In contrast, promoting openness within families facilitates a good psychological outcome.

Loss of control

Patients cope better with life-threatening illnesses if they believe that they can contribute something towards the outcome. In coronary heart disease there are obvious risk factors that patients can modify such as their weight, diet, and level of exercise. However, patients with cancer have no strong risk factors apart from smoking. What can they contribute towards their own survival? They may feel helpless and this is associated with later depressive illness. Helplessness is probable if patients believe that they have already done their best to preserve their health. Thus, a woman who presents as soon as she finds a breast lump and is initially told that it is benign but is later found to have cancer will feel particularly let down and helpless.

Other patients decide to fight their disease. They change one or more aspect of their life-style (such as diet), utilize psychological techniques (such as relaxation, visualization, yoga, or meditation), and/or become involved in volunteer organizations and self-help groups. They usually cope well, unless their method of fighting cancer becomes an overriding obsession.

Treatment

Loss of a body part

Treatment may involve the surgical removal of a body part such as a breast or a limb. The patient then has to come to terms with the change in body image. This will be difficult if the body part is important to their sense of psychological well-being. For example, up to 25 per cent of women fail to adapt to the loss of a breast despite being given an adequate external breast prosthesis (Maguire et al. 1983). Three types of problem may develop singly or in combination. The patient cannot accept that she is no longer physically whole. This loss of physical integrity causes her to feel psychologically vulnerable. She then finds it harder to adapt to other stressful life events. Another patient may feel a heightened self-consciousness and worry that people only have to look at her to realize that she has lost a breast even when she conceals her shape by wearing baggy clothes. Finally, some women feel less attractive and feminine and are not reassured by their partner's claims that they love them as much as before surgery.

Continued inability to adapt to the loss of a body part or mutilation whether it be due, for example to breast loss, head and neck surgery, or amputation of a limb is highly correlated with subsequent psychiatric morbidity. Body image problems are also linked with later sexual difficulties. The sexual difficulties are due to a fear of rejection and to mood disturbance which lowers libido.

Loss of body function

This is associated with later psychiatric morbidity. Up to 32 per cent of patients who have a stoma formed after a cancer of the large bowel is removed become morbidly anxious and/or depressed (Williams and Johnson 1983; Thomas et al. 1987a). They cannot accept the stoma because it represents an 'obscene part of themselves' or their problems centre on the bag. They fear that it will cause a bulge, leak, smell, burst, or make a noise. They worry that it could have serious effects on personal relationships and employment. Those who have yet to form a close relationship and/or are homosexual face a difficult dilemma. Should they mention their stoma to a potential partner and at what point? While fears associated with the bag and fears of rejection contribute to their sexual difficulties, surgical destruction of the nerve supply to

the genital organs results in impotence, difficulties in ejaculation, frigidity, or inability to have an orgasm.

Loss of other bodily function such as the loss of voice after laryngectomy causes similar problems in adaptation.

Radiotherapy

Radiotherapy is explained to patients on the basis that it will destroy any residual cancer cells. This can have a paradoxical effect when patients were led to believe that they had a good prognosis. ('They said that all they needed to do was to remove the lump. I thought I was clear. Then they said I needed radiotherapy as an insurance. How do I square the two? I am getting more and more worried that the cancer is still there.')

Radiotherapy also increases the risk of depression via a fatigue syndrome. Patients complain of feeling exhausted towards the end of a course of radiotherapy. This fails to lift and biological symptoms of depression (see later) then develop. These indirect and direct effects of radiotherapy may explain why women undergoing breast conservation followed by radiotherapy experience as much psychiatric morbidity as those undergoing mastectomy (Fallowfield et al. 1986; Mansell et al. 1989). Radiotherapy also causes morbidity through direct physical damage. Thus, in women with cancer of the cervix, delivering radiotherapy through internal sources causes anatomical damage to the vagina including stenosis, fibrosis, and fistulae. This results in sexual problems, anxiety, and depression (Bos Branolte 1988). There is a strong relationship between adverse effects caused by radiotherapy and subsequent psychiatric morbidity (Devlen et al. 1986).

Chemotherapy

Chemotherapy also increases psychological morbidity and sexual problems, particularly when combinations are used. Psychiatric morbidity is linked to adverse side-effects, particularly gastro-intestinal effects like nausea, vomiting, and diarrhoea (Devlen et al. 1986) and the length of treatment (Hughson et al. 1986). Conditioned nausea and vomiting occurs in up to 25 per cent of patients (Morrow 1982) and this also contributes to the development of anxiety and depression. Characteristically, a patient experiences nausea and vomiting during the first two courses of treatment. Then they find that any sound, sight, or smell which reminds them of treatment provokes the same adverse effects reflexively. This can lead to phobic avoidance of treatment.

In other patients the mood disturbance is better explained in terms of a direct and rapid effect on the brain. Some patients become acutely anxious and depressed within a few hours of an infusion and may develop a depressive stupor. Other patients develop subtle but important impairment of short-term memory (Devlen et al. 1986). When mood disturbance develops it can set up a vicious circle. It lowers the threshold at which patients experience adverse effects and these then intensify the mood disturbance.

Body image problems like hair loss are usually temporary and have little effect on psychological morbidity. However, chemotherapy can depress oestrogen levels and elevate follicle-stimulating and luteinizing hormones. This causes infertility and a premature menopause in pre-menopausal women. Such effects are most likely when chemotherapy is used as an adjuvant. There is uncertainty about the extent to which these changes are reversible after chemotherapy. In women treated with chemotherapy for Hodgkin's disease and non-Hodgkin's lymphoma persistent sexual problems were found in over one-third of these patients who had had a satisfactory sexual relationship beforehand (Devlen et al. 1986).

The main effect of chemotherapy in men is on the germinal epithelium of the testis and leads to a reduced ability to produce sperm and to infertility. Chemotherapy may also reduce Leydig cell function. The extent to which these functions recover over time after chemotherapy have still to be determined by longer term follow-up studies. While persistent sexual problems were found in one-quarter of men treated with combination chemotherapy for Hodgkin's disease and non-Hodgkin's lymphoma (Devlen et al. 1986) sexual problems were more temporary in men treated for testicular cancer (Moynihan 1988). Alkylating agents are most likely to cause sexual problems (Whitehead et al. 1982).

Other treatments

Steroids can cause depression, mania, confusional states, a paranoid reaction, or a combination of these. Early studies of the effects of bone-marrow transplantation have suggested that fears about treatment-related mortality, concerns about the donor, and the experience of prolonged isolation increase psychiatric morbidity in the short- and longer term. Larger scale and longer term studies are needed to clarify the nature of these problems and their aetiology.

Disease status

Hughes (1985) found that 16 per cent of patients being treated for lung cancer had severe depression. This compares with a rate of 7 per cent found in women treated for early breast cancer (Maguire et al. 1978). This suggests that the incidence of psychiatric morbidity is greater in patients with advanced disease. This is confirmed by a study of patients with advanced cancer which found a prevalence of 33 per cent (Plumb and Holland 1981).

Disorders of cognition characterized by difficulty in sustaining attention, disorientation in time, place, and date, impairment of short-term memory and registration, perceptual distortions ranging from misperceptions to hallucinations, an increase or decrease in psychomotor activity, and insomnia or daytime drowsiness are more likely as the cancer progresses. A confusional state may herald a recurrence of cancer or metastatic spread, particularly to the brain. It may also be due to metabolic changes such as hypercalcaemia, liver failure, hyponatraemia, and hypomagnesaemia caused by the tumour or secretion of atopic hormones and other substances.

IMPROVING RECOGNITION

Psychological problems are recognized by those involved in cancer care in 20–40 per cent of cancer patients. Patients and health professionals both contribute to this problem.

Patient-led barriers

Patients believe that psychological and social problems are an inevitable consequence of having cancer and being treated for it. Therefore nothing can be done to relieve these problems and there is no point in mentioning them. They worry that if they disclose psychological concerns this will detract from their physical care. They could also be viewed as ungrateful, inadequate, or uncooperative. They notice that doctors and nurses are busy and have many patients to look after. Hence, they do not want to burden them further. They worry that it is not legitimate to mention psychological concerns since they perceive that few doctors and nurses ask directly about these. They also claim that when they attempt to disclose key problems like a change in mood ('Since my operation I have felt increasingly low'), body image problems ('I can't stand my stoma'),

or sexual difficulties ('Things are no longer the same between us'), these are ignored or dealt with superficially.

Professional-led barriers

In-depth interviews with doctor and nurses and direct observation of their consultations with cancer patients and relatives through audio and video recording, have confirmed that patients' perceptions are correct (Maguire 1985). Questions which focus directly on psychological aspects like 'How have you been feeling about your illness?', 'How have you felt about losing a breast?', or 'Has your operation had any effect on your relationship with your partner?' are rarely asked.

Consequently, patients and relatives try to signal that they are struggling to adapt by giving verbal and/or non-verbal cues such as 'I'm worried about the future' or 'I don't think I'll ever get used to this stoma'. Doctors and nurses then tend to deflect the dialogue into neutral areas by using distancing tactics. Thus, they may try to explain away a patient's distress as normal: 'I can see you are upset. You are bound to be. Everybody is when they come into hospital for this kind of surgery.'

It is also tempting to offer reassurance by saying, 'Don't worry, I'm sure we can sort it all out. You will soon feel better.' This is premature because the reasons for the patient's distress have not been established.

When faced with a distressed patient the doctor or nurse may respond by moving into 'information and advice mode'.

Doctor	I have explained to you that you have a form of cancer of the lymph glands, that is a lymphoma. I am confident that it will respond to treatment with strong drugs, that is chemotherapy.
Patient	Yes, but . . .
Doctor	I think we should get on with chemotherapy straight away so that we can get the best response. Is that all right?
Patient	I am not . . .
Doctor	Let me tell you exactly what this chemotherapy will involve.

This patient did not heed what was being said because he had important concerns that would have emerged had the doctor acknowledged and explored the basis of his distress.

Doctor	I have explained to you that you have a form of cancer of the lymph glands, that is a lymphoma. I am confident that it will respond to treatment with strong drugs, that is chemotherapy.
Patient	Yes but . . .
Doctor	But?
Patient	I am terrified of chemotherapy.
Doctor	Why?
Patient	I have heard it can make you sterile. We are so desperate to have a child. It can also make you very sick.

The doctor can now discuss what he can do to minimize the risk of sickness and sterility in the longer term.

When a patient signals that he wishes to discuss a major problem the doctor or nurse may switch the topic.

Doctor	How have you been getting on since your mastectomy?
Patient	Getting on, I haven't. It's been awful. I just can't bear to look at myself.
Doctor	How has the pain in your arm been?

When doctors and nurses realize that patients are worried about their prognosis they may offer false reassurance in a genuine bid to ease suffering.

Patient I am not going to get better am I?
Doctor Of course you are. You must stop being so pessimistic.

These data about distancing tactics came to light because doctors and nurses involved in cancer care were willing to have their practice observed directly and to discuss their experiences (Maguire 1985). Therefore, distancing cannot be attributed to a lack of concern or ignorance of psychological problems. It is often used instinctively. In-depth interviews revealed several major reasons for this.

The doctors and nurses considered that their professional training had not equipped them to deal with psychological aspects. They feared that asking questions like 'How do you see things working out?' would raise patients' anxieties about their futures. They were reluctant to ask questions like 'How have you felt about having a stoma?' or 'How is chemotherapy going?' because they worried that these might unleash strong emotions. They did not know how to alleviate this and feared that they would cause more harm than good. Therefore it was best to try and 'keep the lid on'. They believed that patients were psychologically fragile and that saying 'the wrong thing' would disorganize the patient.

Encouraging patients to discuss their concerns might lead them to ask difficult questions like 'I am not going to get better, am I?' or 'Why didn't my own doctor diagnose the cancer sooner?'. They did not know how to respond safely.

If doctors and nurses encourage patients to disclose how their lives were being affected by cancer and its treatment, they would have to face reality too frequently. How often could they confront this before they were affected adversely? Deaths of younger patients or of those who reminded them of persons to whom they were close were particularly difficult. It could lead them to question the value of medicine in general and their own rôle in particular. For all these reasons distancing tactics were preferable. Therefore, it is important to consider how doctors and nurses involved in cancer care can promote greater disclosure of patients' problems within their daily practice and survive themselves.

IMPROVING RECOGNITION

Taking the initial history

Persuading patients of a genuine interest in what they are thinking and feeling about their illness will usually lead them to disclose key concerns.

Surgeon Your doctor tells me that you found a lump in your left breast. Is that right?
Patient Yes.
Surgeon How did you come to notice it?
Patient I was having a bath and, as usual, I examined my breasts to check that I was OK.
Surgeon And?
Patient I felt this lump. It was hard. Like a brazil nut.
Surgeon What did you think it was?
Patient What does any sensible woman think these days? I thought it was cancer. That's why I went to my doctor. He agreed that it might be a cancer and sent me here.
Surgeon How did you feel when you thought you had cancer?
Patient Very worried, but hopeful that something could still be done.

When patients give cues that they have been distressed it is important that the nature and intensity of any distress and the reasons for it are explored.

Surgeon You say that you have been very worried. Just how worried have you been?
Patient I can't stop thinking that it could be cancer.
Surgeon What state of mind do you get into when you think that?
Patient I get extremely tense and anxious. I am having difficulty getting off to sleep and I am not functioning as well as I should.
Surgeon Why are you so anxious?
Patient My mother had this cancer. She wasted away, had horrendous pain, and died a horrible death.
Surgeon Any other reasons for your anxiety?
Patient She became confused toward the end.
Surgeon Any other reasons?
Patient No.

It is also worth enquiring how the illness has affected the patient's daily functioning.

Surgeon Has your illness been affecting your ability to function day to day?
Patient Oh, I still keep going but it has been an increasing strain.
Surgeon In what way?
Patient I find it harder to get up in the morning and face work. I have lost interest in doing my chores. My concentration isn't as good as it should be. I am constantly thinking that I could die from cancer.
Surgeon Any other effects?
Patient Yes, I have been much more irritable. I have gone on at my husband for no reason. I blow up at the children.
Surgeon Any other changes?
Patient No, I don't think so.

By establishing a patient's perceptions, feelings, and the impact of illness the patient realizes that the doctor is interested in her as a whole person. She is then more likely to disclose any subsequent psychological and social concerns.

Key skills

When taking an initial history certain key skills enhance disclosure. Most patients give verbal or non-verbal cues about their problems. It is important to be alert to these and to clarify them.

Medical oncologist You say you are worried about chemotherapy. (Acknowledgement)
Patient Yes, I am terrified.
Medical oncologist Why are you so terrified? (Clarification)
Patient I have heard that it causes severe vomiting. I don't think I could stand that, I have always been so squeamish.
Medical oncologist Are there any other reasons why you dread chemotherapy? (Screening question)
Patient No, it's just the sickness.
Medical oncologist Well, we ought to be able to control any sickness, but I can't pretend it might not happen. Would you like me to discuss it further?

The oncologist has acknowledged and explored the patient's concern about chemotherapy. He then reassures them that they should be able to do something about it but cannot guarantee success. In this way confidence is established.

Patients often sense that it will be painful to discuss their concerns. Therefore, if they are allowed to be vague in their history, they will avoid connecting with and revealing their true feelings. Encouraging patients to be precise about when key illness events occurred and what they experienced can overcome their reluctance.

Medical oncologist	You said that your sister died of melanoma. Could you bear to tell me about it. (Negotiation)
Patient	Not really.
Medical oncologist	Could you try? It would help me to know when she died.
Patient	She died last summer.
Medical oncologist	When exactly? (Precision)
Patient	In August.
Medical oncologist	When in August?
Patient	The first week.
Medical oncologist	Could you bear to tell me what happened? (Negotiation)
Patient	It had gone to her brain. For a few days she was very confused. Then she went into a coma. I couldn't bear to see her like that. It still distresses me to think about it.
Medical oncologist	I guess you have been worrying you could go the same way? (Educated guess)
Patient	Yes.

Thus, the oncologist has allowed their patient to share a terrible experience as well as their fears about their own future.

The use of precision helps the patient to get in touch with and express painful feelings. It is then necessary to decide if it is safe to continue. Here, the patient will be the guide.

Radiotherapist	I know that you have been told that you were referred here because you have cancer of the cervix. I noticed in talking with you that the moment we started discussing your cancer you became very distressed. I would like to talk to you about this further but can you bear to do so? (Negotiation)
Patient	I'm not sure. It is so painful
Radiotherapist	Why?
Patient	Life was going so well. I had just got married and we had a child. I can't believe that I have cancer.
Radiotherapist	I can understand that this is very upsetting. Can you bear to talk about it further? (Negotiation)
Patient	I am terrified that you will not be able to treat it.
Radiotherapist	That's what I am here for. I want to discuss with you what we might be able to do for you.

Doctors often have strong intuitions about what the patient or relative is feeling during the consultation. However, they tend to keep their intuitions private. They fear that if they voice them and are wrong, their relationship with a patient or relative will be damaged. Paradoxically, patients and relatives perceive such efforts as furthering understanding of their predicament as empathic, even if the intuition is wrong.

Medical oncologist	I get the feeling that you are not keen on more drug treatment?
Patient	You are right, I am terrified, I don't think I could cope with it. (Confirmation)
Medical oncologist	Why not?

Patient	I dread being so sick again. I used to get terrible panics and I had to be dragged into the car before coming to the hospital.

Many doctors and nurses claim that they avoid focusing on psychological aspects because they have insufficient time. However, observation of consultations has indicated that much time is wasted. For example, when patients are asked to give a history of their presenting problems they may wander off the point and talk about experiences unrelated to the present illness or discuss why they have become ill.

When patients are asked to describe the onset and development of their symptoms they often shift the time focus or topic. It is important that they are brought back to the point.

Medical oncologist	When did you first notice there was anything wrong with you?
Patient	I started having these sweats last October. My pyjamas were saturated. It reminded me of the time I had glandular fever. I thought it was that again. I was studying architecture. It came on just before finals. The doctor said it was due to worry about my exams.
Medical oncologist	What you say about glandular fever is helpful. But can I focus on this latest episode of sweating. What exactly are your sweats like?

Subsequent assessment

There is a danger that the initial assessment will result in bias. Thus, one might start by saying, 'Last time we met you were experiencing pain and swelling in your left arm. How has that been since?' This risks limiting the dialogue to physical concerns. It is more effective to start by asking, 'Since I last saw you have you had any problems?' If pain in the arm has continued to be the main problem, the patient will volunteer this first. If there have been other problems, these will also be disclosed. It is then important to establish how the patient has responded to any treatment that has been given by asking directive questions. ('How have you felt about losing a breast?', 'How has radiotherapy been going?', 'Have there been any problems with chemotherapy?') If the patient discloses only physical problems, it is worth shifting the focus once these have been explored. ('So, you are still troubled by pain in your ribs and your breathing has not been so good. Have you had any other problems?') Concern can be made explicit by saying, 'So far I have only touched on physical aspects. Have there been any other problems?'.

DIAGNOSIS AND MANAGEMENT
Anxiety

Anxious mood should be diagnosed when a patient complains of a persistent inability to relax or stop worrying; this represents a significant change both qualitatively and quantitively and the patient cannot distract himself or herself or be distracted by others. An anxiety state should be diagnosed if there are four or more other symptoms including initial insomnia, irritability, sweating, tremor or nausea, impaired concentration, indecisiveness, and spontaneous panic attacks. Patients with such generalized anxiety may also have irrational fears of specific situations like meeting people (social phobia) or leaving the house alone lest they collapse (agoraphobia).

If the patient is unable to cope from day to day or comply with treatment an anxiolytic drug (such as lorazepam) is necessary. To forestall dependence it should be given for only 3–4 weeks and taken only when necessary; thus, to cover each infusion of chemotherapy, a patient may be advised to take it 2 days beforehand. If this is not sufficient a major tranquillizer (such as chlorpromazine) or a tricyclic antidepressant (such as amitriptyline) is indicated. Beta blockers such as propanalol have a place when somatic symptoms of anxiety predominate.

Once anxiety is controlled the patient should be taught anxiety management techniques (Jannoun *et al.* 1982). These involve training in progressive muscular relaxation and positive imaging. These techniques can be taught immediately when the anxiety is not disorganizing. If the anxiety is provoked by irrational fears of recurrence or concerns about body image, cognitive therapy may be used in which antecedents of any irrational beliefs and their consequences are analysed critically and challenged (Goddard 1982).

When anxiety is maintained by realistic uncertainty about prognosis, this should be acknowledged and patients asked whether they wish to be given markers of what signs and symptoms might herald deterioration. They should also be asked how often they would like to be monitored physically. Few patients abuse this offer. Those who elect to be given indications of their progress must be given the results of tests and will adapt psychologically even if the news is bad. Those who decline the offer of indicators of progress should not have them imposed.

Depression

Depressed mood should be diagnosed when a patient complains of persistent low mood for 2–4 weeks, which is significantly greater quantitively and qualitatively compared with periods when the patient has been unhappy. Depressive illness should be diagnosed when this is accompanied by four or more other symptoms including sleep disturbance (repeated or early morning waking, excessive sleep), irritability, impairment of attention and concentration, restlessness or retardation, loss of energy, social withdrawal, negative ideation (ideas of hopelessness, self-blame, guilt, worthlessness, feeling a burden, seeing no future, pointlessness of life), suicidal ideation, diurnal variation of mood, loss of appetite or weight, and constipation.

Allowance should be made for the possibility that physical symptoms, such as loss of energy, appetite, and weight, could be due to the progression or recurrence of cancer. However, these symptoms, which are attributed to cancer, often disappear when depression is treated. The understandability of depression in the context of cancer and its treatment should not be used to argue against the need for treatment.

Depressive illness should be treated promptly with antidepressants which are effective but cause least side-effects, like dothiepin (prothiaden) or fluoxetine (Prozac). Otherwise, experiencing side-effects may hinder compliance or cause the patient to attribute them wrongly to cancer. In prescribing antidepressant medication it is important to emphasize several points to the patient.

Antidepressants do not cause physical or psychological dependence. They are necessary because the depression is due to changes in the body chemistry caused by the cancer or its treatment. They encourage the body to start producing the necessary chemicals again and need to be continued for 4–6 months to forestall relapse. Prescribing them is only the first step in helping the patient and any residual difficulties like body image problems will be dealt with once the patient's mood has begun to lift. The antidepressant must be taken as prescribed and not just when the patient feels low. No improvement is likely to occur for 2–4 weeks.

An alerting antidepressant like imipramine (Tofranil) is useful when a patient complains of being slowed down or has depression and phobic anxiety. Those who are agitated benefit from a more sedating agent (for example, amitriptyline or clomipramine). Such tricyclic antidepressants are associated with side-effects like sedation, postural hypotension, and atropine effects (dry mouth, blurred vision, difficulty with micturition, and constipation). Therefore, patients should be warned about these effects and the risks of driving and taking alcohol.

Most patients respond well to antidepressant medication but if they fail to do so psychiatric referral is indicated. Maintaining factors like inappropriately negative views of prognosis or body image can then be dealt with by cognitive therapy. Few patients will need admission to a psychiatric unit as suicidal risk is usually low, but if there is any possibility of suicide an urgent psychiatric opinion should be sought.

Body image problems

Behavioural treatments are often effective. They involve teaching patients anxiety management techniques and then using graded exposure. Patients are asked to spend increasing amounts of time looking at the affected body part after relaxing. When patients have irrational views of their image and its impact on people close to them cognitive therapy should be tried.

When surgical reconstruction is possible it is effective provided that the patient understands the possible complications and wants the surgery for himself or herself and there is evidence of visual avoidance of the affected body part.

Sexual problems

Patients with cancers which are not hormone dependent can be helped by hormone replacement when this is indicated. In those with hormone-dependent tumours or sexual problems due to anatomical damage through surgery or radiotherapy practical aids like the use of dilators, lubricating creams, prostheses, or discussion of alternative modes of pleasuring (as advised in the early stages of Masters and Johnson therapy) should be considered.

In the therapy described by Masters and Johnson (1970) the underlying premise is that sexual intercourse has come to be associated with anxiety. Therefore, the therapist begins by advising a couple to ban sexual intercourse and, instead, to educate each other about the kind of caressing, other than that of genital areas, which gives them most pleasure. Once this is achieved, the couple are advised to proceed to caressing genital areas before proceeding to full intercourse.

Illness behaviour

A substantial proportion of disease-free patients fail to return to their former level of adjustment and employment (Devlen *et al.* 1986). In some patients this is due to their reluctance to accept that they are cured of cancer. They need an explanation of their predicament and behavioural programmes to re-establish their functioning through referral to a clinical psychologist or psychiatrist.

REDUCING MORBIDITY
Giving information

The key is to determine how much information each patient wants about their illness and treatment. If the initial history has elicited their perceptions about their illness it will have revealed whether they are aware of their diagnosis. When they are aware, the task of the doctor is to confirm that they are right.

When the patient does not realize that they have cancer the doctor faces the problem of how to break the bad news without disorganizing them psychologically or provoking strong denial. First, a warning shot should be fired ('You will remember that I said the pain in your abdomen was due to an infection. Now I think it is more serious'). Then pause to allow them time to take this in and respond. Their response will indicate whether they wish to know more ('What do you mean you think it is more serious?') or prefers denial ('That's up to you, you are the expert'). When patients indicate that they wish to go on another clue should be provided ('You know we X-rayed your bowel. Some areas looked abnormal'). The patient can still pull out ('That's all right, that's up to you') or pursue it ('What do you mean abnormal?'). Thus, what is said can be tailored to what patients indicate that they wish to know and so facilitate psychological adjustment.

Identifying key concerns

Any resultant distress should be acknowledged ('I can see this has upset you') and negotiation should be attempted ('Would you mind telling me just what is upsetting you?'). This enables the patient to change their perception from feeling overwhelmed to identifying key concerns which can be resolved in part or whole.

Doctor	You seem very upset? (Acknowledgement)
Patient	I am.
Doctor	Can you bear to say what is distressing you? (Negotiation)
Patient	I am shattered. I have heard that melanomas can spread and cause havoc.
Doctor	How did you hear this. (Exploration)
Patient	I had a neighbour who had it and died. It went to her brain and she ended up in a coma.
Doctor	No wonder you are so upset. Are there any other concerns. (Screening question)
Patient	No, it's just the thought that it will get me quickly and horribly.

The doctor can now reassure the patient that their melanoma is likely to be more controllable and will make every effort to prevent such complications.

Each concern should be elicited before giving information or advice. Otherwise, important concerns will remain hidden and hamper the patient's ability to take in what is said. When tackling these concerns it is important to pitch comments appropriately. Thus, for a patient concerned about dying in pain, it is best to say 'I am hopeful that we can help you with your pain' rather than 'I can guarantee that you will have no pain'.

Whenever possible, let the patient indicate what they want to know rather than rely on a relative's opinion. Witholding information from patients who want it is as damaging psychologically as giving it to patients who wish to remain in ignorance. Having a relative or close friend accompany the patient appears to facilitate adaptation when bad news is broken (Fallowfield *et al.* 1986). They can both discuss what was communicated about the nature of the illness and treatment and can correct any misperceptions. Giving patients audiotapes of this 'announcement' also facilitates adaptation and is acceptable to most patients (Fallowfield *et al.* 1989).

Further information

It is important to check next if the patient wishes to have any information about any further investigations and treatments. This can be done by asking, for example, 'Would you like me to explain the tests that we need to do?'.

Be honest about possible adverse effects of treatment instead of minimizing them. If adverse effects develop, patients may feel let down and distrust subsequent advice and treatment. If they have serious worries about treatment the reasons should be explored. They are often rooted in adverse experiences of cancer in others.

Treatment choice

Some patients can be offered options. Therefore, it is important to establish whether a patient wishes to choose or leave it to the doctor. For example, some patients with early breast cancer wish to leave it to the doctor to decide whether to perform breast conservation or mastectomy. Other patients have a clear treatment preference and want this heeded. The offering of choice reduces psychiatric morbidity (Ashcroft *et al.* 1985; Morris and Royle 1988) in the short-term. However, these early advantages might be offset by problems which arise when women who opted for a specific procedure develop recurrence.

Other information

It has been suggested that all patients should be given a 'package' of information about their illness, investigation procedures, and treatment in the form of a booklet, audiotape, or videotape. This ignores variations between patients in their needs for information and how they like it presented. Therefore, it is important to negotiate with each patient: 'Would you like me to give you a booklet or videotape which will tell you more about the tests we need to do and the treatment'.

Training

A key uestion is how best to help those already involved in cancer care and improve their interviewing, assessment, and counselling skills. Short intensive residential and multidisciplinary workshops which utilize videotape demonstrations, practise key tasks under controlled conditions and include feedback and discussion of performance appears to increase these skills in the short-term (Maguire and Faulkner 1988). Workshops can also improve attitudes to psychological aspects of care (Razavi *et al.* 1988). However, longer courses are needed to ensure that this learning is maintained and applied.

Use of volunteers

Other patients are an important source of information, advice, and practical and emotional support. If they are to facilitate rather than hinder psychological adaptation, they need to belong to a credible volunteer organization. Credibility should be judged on the group's willingness to select and train volunteers, audit their work over time, and cooperate with professionals in cancer care. Training should focus on basic listening and responding skills, but avoid the trap of changing volunteers into 'professionals'. Fortunately, some major volunteer organizations now meet these criteria.

Although there are many anecdotal reports of the values of face-to-face contact between volunteers, there has been little study of their effectiveness.

Support groups

Only 10–20 per cent of patients with cancer utilize self-help groups. Groups have an important role in facilitating sharing of experiences and concerns, giving support, and reducing isolation. When they are led by or in cooperation with people who have a professional knowledge of group dynamics, they appear effective in alleviating distress. Such leaders are able to facilitate discussion even when it is between people with varying prognoses. They are also able to maintain discussion at a safe but constructive level (Yalom and Grieves 1977; Spiegel et al. 1981; van den Borne et al. 1986). Groups that meet, say, once a month and include patients, relatives, and staff also appear to be effective (Plant et al. 1987).

Specialist workers

Many cancer centres have appointed specialist nurses or social workers to provide information, advice, and practical and emotional support to individual patients or groups. The hope has been that this would reduce psychological and social morbidity. It has still yet to be proved that they have a preventative effect (Watson 1983). However, specialist workers can achieve a marked reduction in morbidity through the early recognition and psychiatric referral of those whom they detect as having problems. This can only be achieved if they are trained in the relevant interviewing, assessment, and counselling skills (Maguire et al. 1980).

Ongoing support from a nurse manager and the provision of regular supervision and clinical back-up by a psychologist or psychiatrist are necessary for such schemes to be fully effective. Unfortunately, specialist workers are often put into post without the relevant training, support, or supervision. They then distance themselves from psychological aspects of care and focus on physical issues like the provision of a breast prosthesis or stoma bag. Alternatively, they may become emotionally overinvolved, carry too large a case load, and become psychological casualties. Some workers become too autonomous and give little feedback to the treating clinician about psychological aspects. They may resist the involvement of others. There is also a danger that clinicians will leave psychological care to the specialist worker.

In a healthy system the specialist worker gives regular feedback to the clinical team about problems that patients are experiencing and discuss the action to be taken. A clinical psychologist, psychiatrist, and/or general practitioner is involved when appropriate.

Such specialist workers can make effective links with and encourage the development of volunteer organizations and self-help groups. They can also play a vital role in helping upgrade the psychological assessment and counselling skills of non-specialist nurses involved in cancer care. This can free them to concentrate on those who have more complex difficulties.

Limited contact

It is only necessary to assess cancer patients once after discharge to determine whether they have developed social or psychological problems. After a systematic psychosocial assessment has been carried out, patients realize that there is a member of the treating team who is prepared to deal with these problems. Up to 90 per cent of patients who develop problems after this first assessment can be relied on to contact a specialist worker. Therefore, there is no need to monitor every patient regularly (Wilkinson et al. 1988). Specialist workers could use their time even more efficiently if they could identify those at risk of psychosocial morbidity.

Groups at risk

Worden (1983) pioneered this approach. Questionnaires were used to identify those patients who were likely to show high levels of emotional distress subsequently. 'At-risk' patients were characterized by suppression of feelings, passivity, stoic acceptance, reducing tension through cigarette smoking or alcohol consumption, social withdrawal, blaming themselves or others for their predicament, and being unduly irritable. When they tested this predictive model prospectively 80 per cent of the 'at-risk' group were identified correctly, but only a minority accepted and completed the interventions offered. This highlights a major problem in such 'at-risk' approaches. Few of those 'at risk' accept they need help.

Alternatively, those people who are not coping could be identified before they become anxious or depressed. Promising markers include a past history of psychiatric illness, perceiving that friends and relatives are not supportive, finding it difficult to adapt to the loss of a body part or function, adverse effects of treatment, and feelings of helplessness (Thomas et al. 1987b; Maguire 1982; Dean 1987). Preventative schemes aimed at patients who show one or more of these markers have still to be evaluated.

Screening questionnaires

Self-rating questionnaires could be used to identify patients with anxiety or depression. Those scoring above a recommended threshold could then be interviewed by a specialist worker to determine if they required intervention. The Hospital Anxiety and Depression Questionnaire (Zigmond and Snaith 1985; Razavi et al. 1990) and the Rotterdam Symptom Check List (de Haes et al. 1983) seem promising in this regard. Their efficacy will depend on how well they identify those who need help without producing too many false-positives. Otherwise, the specialist worker would have to interview too many distressed but psychiatrically well patients to detect those with an affective disorder.

PSYCHOLOGICAL FACTORS AND SURVIVAL

Greer et al. (1979) found that patients who responded to their diagnosis by 'denial' or with 'fighting spirit' survived longer than those who reacted with 'stoic acceptance' or 'helplessness'. This may reflect patients' awareness of the biological aggressiveness of their disease. However, if these reactions influence survival, the best test would be to change 'helplessness' and 'stoicism' into 'denial' or 'fighting spirit' and determine if survival improved.

Recently, Ramirez et al. (1989) found a link between the experiencing of major stressful life events and subsequent recurrence of breast cancer. If this link was replicated in a larger study, an intervention study which aimed to target and help cancer patients who experienced life events would be justified.

In patients with advanced disease the provision of support through regular group meetings appears to lengthen survival (Spiegel et al. 1989). More intensive individual psychotherapy has been claimed to have a greater effect (Gossarth-Maticek et al. 1982). Concerns have been expressed about both studies because there was insufficient matching of key biological and treatment variables between the index and control groups. A long-term multicentre trial of psychological intervention is required in order to allow adequately for all the key variables that could influence survival. A similar rigorous scrutiny is required of the 'counselling' offered by cancer help centres. The case for improving psychological care would be even stronger if it improved the length as well as the quality of survival.

SUPPORT

If doctors, nurses, and social workers improve their psychological skills, they will elicit more problems and become even closer to the suffering of patients and their families. Therefore, they will need opportunities to discuss the problems they encounter and their feelings about these. They will also need advice and support so that they can further improve their knowledge and skills. It is not yet clear what methods of support are best. Is it better offered informally or through support groups?

Support groups can be helpful provided that certain conditions are met (Moynihan and Outlaw 1984). The leader should have a good knowledge of group dynamics and give guidance about the nature and function of the group, the importance of regular attendance (when possible), and confidentiality. The leader should be able to facilitate discussion, maintain the focus on work-related problems, and prevent disclosure of personal problems, for staff are not patients and support groups should not be turned into therapy groups.

There has been little evaluation of such groups. They can have a negative effect for staff become more aware of suffering of patients and families (Silberfarb *et al.* 1980).

REFERENCES

Anderson BL (1985). Sexual functioning morbidity among cancer survivors. *Cancer*, 55:1835–42.

Ashcroft JJ, Leinster SJ, Slade PD (1985). Breast cancer—patient choice of treatment: preliminary communication. *Journal of the Royal Society of Medicine*, 78:43–6.

Bos Branolte G, Rijshouwer YM, Zielstra EM, Duivenvoorden, HJ (1988). Psychologial morbidity in survivors of gynaecological cancers. *International Journal of Gynaecological Oncology*, 9:61–76.

Dean C (1987). Psychiatric morbidity following mastectomy: preoperative predictors and type of illness. *Journal of Psychosomatic Research*, 31:385–92.

de Haes JCJM, Pruyn TFA, Van Knippenberg FCE (1983). Klachten-lijst voor kanker patienten: erste ervaringen. *Nederlands Tijdschrift voor de Psychologie*, 38:403–22.

Derogatis LR, *et al.* (1983). The prevalence of psychiatric disorders among cancer patients. *Journal of the American Medical Association*, 249:751–7.

Devlen J, Maguire P, Phillips P, Crowther D, Chambers H (1986). Psychological problems associated with diagnosis and treatment of lymphomas. II: prospective study. *British Medical Journal*, 295:955–7.

Fallowfield LJ, Hogbin B (1989). Getting it taped—'Bad News'. Consultation with cancer patients. *British Journal of Hospital Medicine*, 41:330–4.

Fallowfield LJ, Baum M, Maguire GP (1986). Effects of breast conservation on psychological morbidity associated with diagnosis and treatment of early breast cancer. *British Medical Journal*, 293:1331–4.

Goddard A (1982). Cognitive behaviour therapy and depression. *British Journal of Hospital Medicine*, 27:248–50.

Greer S (1985). Cancer: psychiatric aspects. In *Recent advances in clinical psychiatry* (ed. K Granville-Grossman), pp. 87–104. Churchill Livingstone, London.

Greer S, Morris T, Pettingale KW (1979). Psychological response to breast cancer: effect on outcome. *Lancet*, ii:785–7.

Grossarth-Maticek R, Kanazin DI, Schmidt P, Vetter H (1982). Psychosomatic factors in the process of cancerogenesis. *Psychotherapy and Psychosomatics*, 38:284–302.

Hughes JE (1985). Depressive illness in lung cancer. I. Depression before diagnosis. II. Follow up of inoperable patients. *European Journal of Oncology*, 11:15–20.

Hughson AVM, Cooper AF, McArdle CS, Smith DS (1986). Psychological impact of adjuvant chemotherapy in the first two years after mastectomy. *British Medical Journal*, 293:1268–71.

Jannoun L, Oppenheimer C, Gelder M (1982). A self help treatment programme for anxiety state patients. *Behavioural Therapy*, 13:103–11.

Maguire P (1982). Psychiatric morbidity associated with mastectomy. In *Clinical trials in early breast cancer* (ed. M Baum, R Kay, and H Scheurlen), pp. 373–80. Birkhauser Verlag, Basel.

Maguire P (1985). Barriers to psychological care of the dying. *British Medical Journal*, 291:1711–13.

Maguire P, Faulkner F (1988). How to do it: improve the counselling skills of doctors and nurses in cancer care. *British Medical Journal*, 297:847–9.

Maguire GP, Lee EG, Bevington DJ, Kuchemann CS, Crabtree RJ, Cornell CR (1978). Psychiatric problems in the first year after mastectomy. *British Medical Journal*, 29:963–5.

Maguire P, Tait A, Brooke M, Thomas C, Sellwood RA (1980). The effect of counselling on the psychiatric morbidity associated with mastectomy. *British Medical Journal*, 281:1454–6.

Maguire P, Brooke M, Tait A, Thomas C, Sellwood RA (1983). The effect of counselling on physical disability and social recovery after mastectomy. *Clinical Oncology*, 9:319–24.

Mansell E, Brisson J, Deschenes L (1989). Psychological distress after initial treatment for breast cancer: A comparison of partial and total mastectomy. *Journal of Clinical Epidemiology*, 42:765–71.

Masters WH, Johnson VE (1970). *Human sexual inadequacy*. Churchill, London.

Morris J, Royle GT (1988). Offering patients a choice of surgery for early breast cancer: a reduction in anxiety and depression in patients and their husbands. *Social Science and Medicine*, 26:583–5.

Morrow GR (1982). Prevalence and correlates of anticipatory nausea and vomiting in chemotherapy patients. *Journal of the National Cancer Institute*, 68:585–8.

Moynihan C (1988). The psychosocial effects of the diagnosis and treatment of testicular cancer: a retrospective study. *Cancer Topics*, 198:18–20.

Moynihan RT, Outlaw E (1984). Nursing support groups in a cancer centre. *Journal of Psychosocial Oncology*, 2:33–47.

Plant H, Richardson J, Stubbs L, Lynch D, Ellwood J, Slevin M, de Haes H (1987). Evaluation of a support group for cancer patients and their families and friends. *British Journal of Hospital Medicine*, 10:317–20.

Plumb M, Holland J (1981). Comparative studies of psychological function in patients with advanced cancer II. Interviewer rated current and past psychological symptoms. *Psychosomatic Medicine*, 43:243–54.

Ramirez A, Craig TK, Watson, JP, Fentimon, IS, North WRS (1989). Stress and relapse of breast cancer. *British Medical Journal*, 298:291–3.

Razavi D, Delvaux N, Farvacques C, Robaye E (1988). Immediate effectiveness of brief psychological training for health professionals dealing with terminally ill cancer patients: a controlled study. *Social Science and Medicine*, 27:386–95.

Razavi D, Delvaux N, Farvacques C, Robaye E (1990). Screening for adjustment disorders and major depressive disorders in cancer patients . *British Journal of Psychiatry*, 156:79–83.

Silberfarb PM, Levine P (1980). Psychosocial aspects of neoplastic disease III. Group support for the oncology nurse. *General Psychiatry*, 3:192–7.

Spiegel D, Bloom JR, Yalom I (1981). Group support for patients with metastatic cancer. *Archives of General Psychiatry*, 38:527–33.

Spiegel D, Bloom JR, Kraemer HC, Gottheil E (1989). Effect of psychological treatment on survival of patients with metastatic breast cancer. *Lancet*, ii:888–91.

Thomas C, Madden F, John D (1987a). Psychological effects of stomas—I. Psychosocial morbidity one year after surgery. *Journal of Psychosomatic Research*, 31:311–16.

Thomas C, Madden F, John D (1987b). Psychological effects of stomas—II. Factors influencing outcome. *Journal of Psychosomatic Research*, 31:317–24.

van den Borne HW, Pruyn JFA, van dam de Mey K (1986). Self-help in cancer patients: a review of studies on the effects of contacts between fellow patients. *Patient Education and Counselling*, 8:367–85.

Watson M (1983). Psychosocial intervention with cancer patients: a review. *Psychological Medicine*, 13:839–46.

Whitehead E, Shalet SM, Blackledge G, Todd I, Crowther D, Beardwell C (1982). The effects of Hodgkin's disease and combination of chemotherapy on gonadal function in the adult male. *Cancer*, 49:418–22.

Wilkinson S, Maguire P, Tait A (1988). Life after breast cancer. *Nursing Times*, 84:34–7.

Williams NS, Johnston D (1983). The quality of life after rectal excision for low rectal cancer. *British Journal of Surgery*, **70**:460–2.

Worden JW (1983). Psychosocial sreening of cancer patients. *Journal of Psychosocial Oncology*, **1**:1–10.

Yalom ED, Grieves C (1977). Group therapy with the terminally ill. *American Journal of Psychiatry*, **134**:396–400.

Zigmond AS, Snaith RP (1983). The Hospital Anxiety and Depression Scale. *Acta Psychiatrica Scandinavica*, **67**:361–70.

20.5 Pain and symptom control in advanced cancer

G. W. HANKS AND P. J. HOSKIN

INTRODUCTION

In recent years much attention has been focused on the 'quality of life' of cancer patients. This reflects both a greater awareness of the need to balance the morbidity of intensive treatment against the potential gains and a recognition that much can be done even for patients with incurable disease. Particular improvements have been achieved in the alleviation of pain and other symptoms in patients with advanced cancer.

This area of cancer care has now acquired the status of a subspeciality of 'palliative medicine', a development which recognizes that there is a definable body of knowledge and expertise related to the management of incurable and end-stage disease. The components of palliative medicine in the context of advanced malignant disease are symptom management, rehabilitation, continuity of care, and terminal care and this chapter and the two which follow it are concerned with these topics.

There is a danger inherent in any move towards specialization that the knowledge and expertise contained therein may be made available or may be seen to be applicable only to a particular category of patients, in this case those with advanced or terminal malignancies. However, palliative medicine in its broadest sense has always been an important and integral part of the care of cancer patients and it is no less necessary now that recent knowledge and improvements in care are widely disseminated and applied. The principles of effective palliation of pain and other symptoms are applicable to cancer patients at every stage of their disease and should be familiar to all those involved in their care.

SYMPTOM MANAGEMENT

General principles

Although the aim of treatment may have moved from cure to palliation, the essentials of medical management remain the same. Appropriate and individualized treatment based on an accurate diagnosis is the cornerstone.

Few patients with advanced disease will present with a single symptom and careful assessment and analysis of individual problems is required, with due consideration given to both the physical and emotional components. A careful clinical history, a thorough physical examination, and selective investigations to elucidate the cause of each symptom are the basis of successful management.

Extensive investigations will be inappropriate in many cases, but simple blood tests and radiography examinations will often contribute useful information. In selected cases access to more sophisticated investigations is necessary.

The patient with advanced cancer is in a dynamic state in which his or her symptoms and their response to treatment are continually changing. Therefore, once a particular line of treatment has been instituted, careful surveillance and regular reassessment of the patient is vital in order to achieve and maintain control of both current symptoms and new problems that may arise. Many patients may suffer treatment-related morbidity, such as nausea and constipation when strong analgesics are used; early recognition and remedial action may avoid discarding a potentially useful therapy because of unwanted side-effects.

Although cure or local control of a tumour may no longer be possible, it is important that specific anticancer therapy is still considered as a treatment option in symptom management. A balance should be found between overtreatment with toxic agents at one extreme and, at the other, denying the use of a simple palliative therapy such as local irradiation for bone pain. Up to 30 per cent of patients may benefit from specific tumouricidal therapy (Hoskin and Hanks 1988).

SPECIFIC SYMPTOMS

Pain

'For many patients the fear of cancer is the fear of pain' (Morris *et al.* 1986). Many people believe that cancer is always associated with pain, but not all patients with cancer will suffer pain. The overall incidence of pain in patients with advanced disease is 60–70 per cent (Twycross and Lack 1983).

Considerable progress has been made in the management of pain in cancer patients, particularly over the last two decades. We now have the means and the knowledge to relieve pain effectively in the majority of patients with cancer. Problems remain in disseminating the knowledge and putting the means into practice, so that many patients will have pain that goes unrelieved. However, the situation continues to improve and there have been significant changes in the attitudes and knowledge of doctors, particularly regarding the use of strong opioid analgesics (White *et al.* 1990).

Assessment and diagnosis

Pain is not a simple sensation: it has both a cognitive and an affective component. The perception of painful stimuli is always modified by an emotional response to that perception. Changes in mood may considerably alter the experience of pain. Therefore the successful treatment of cancer pain cannot ever rely merely on analgesics or nerve blocks. Explanation and reassurance lead to understanding and hope and have an important 'analgesic' effect. Uncertainty, despair, fear, tiredness, and sleepless nights may be amenable to simple remedy, but will have a profound negative effect on morale and pain experience if ignored.

Patients with advanced cancer rarely have only one pain. Often three or four separate pains can be identified and each may have a

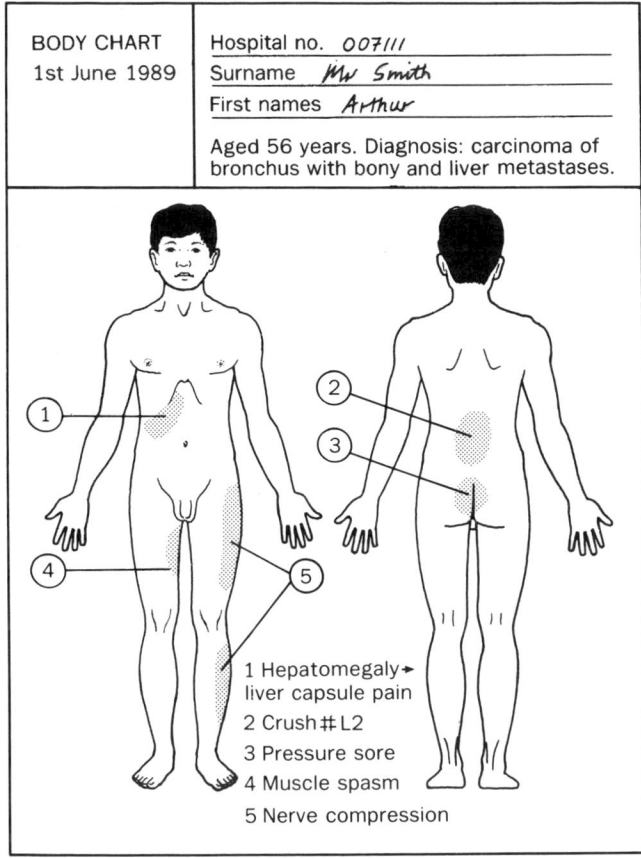

Fig. 1 A body chart may be useful in separating individual pains and aiding the diagnosis of each pain. (Reproduced with permission from Mansi and Hanks (1989).)

different cause. In up to one-third of patients pain may not be due to the cancer itself. Anticancer treatment may be the cause (for example, chemotherapy-induced neuropathy, post-radiation fibrosis, post-operative neuralgia) or the pain may be unrelated to the cancer or its treatment (for example, arthritis) (Twycross and Fairfield 1982).

The first step in the management of the patient in pain is a careful assessment and evaluation of the underlying cause or mechanism of the pain. In complicated cases this initial assessment may be greatly aided by a pain chart, so that individual pains can be identified and their subsequent progress monitored (Fig. 1). An attempt should always be made to make a diagnosis for each pain so that the most appropriate treatment strategy can be selected. This may require investigations such as radiography, bone scan, or occasionally CT or magnetic resonance imaging.

Bone pain is the most common type of pain in cancer (Foley 1985); nerve compression, soft tissue, visceral, and muscle spasm pain are also frequently encountered. The approach to the management of these different types of pain will follow a similar basic pattern but will differ in detail.

Objectives

Realistic objectives should be set using three stages of pain control: to be pain free at night, pain free at rest, and pain free on movement. It is almost always possible to achieve the first two, but for the patient with widespread metastatic bone disease it may not be possible to achieve complete control of pain on movement (so-called 'incident' pain). The other major problem area is pain associated with nerve damage. Neuropathic pain is the most difficult type of pain to treat in cancer patients because it does not respond in a straightforward way to conventional analgesics. Alternative drugs and treatment strategies are usually required in conjunction.

Analgesics

The choice of analgesic is primarily determined by the severity of the pain. This stepwise approach to the use of analgesics in cancer pain has been adopted by the World Health Organization (WHO) in its Cancer Pain Relief Programme (WHO 1986) and is illustrated in Table 1. The administration of whichever analgesic is chosen is governed by the principle that continuous pain requires continuous prophylactic treatment. The pain is brought under control and is not allowed to return. This means giving an adequate dose to relieve

Table 1 The analgesic ladder

Pain severity	Class of analgesic	Preferred drug	Dose
Mild pain	Simple ('mild') analgesic	Paracetamol (acetaminophen) (preferable to aspirin because of lack of gastrointestinal side-effects and lack of effect on platelet function)	1 g (two tablets) up to every 4 h
Moderate pain	Weak opioid analgesic (alone or in combination with simple analgesic)[a]	Dextropropoxyphene 32.5 mg+paracetamol 325 mg (coproxamol) or codeine 30 mg+paracetamol 500 mg	Two tablets up to every 4 h[b]
Severe pain	Strong opioid analgesic	Morphine	See text

Dihydrocodeine is a semi-synthetic analogue of codeine which is said to be 30 per cent more potent. Theoretically, equianalgesic doses are likely to be more constipating than the combination preparations shown in the table. A long-acting formulation (dihydrocodeine 60 mg) is available and may be advantageous for some patients.

The agonist—antagonist buprenorphine (a potent partial agonist at mu opioid receptors) can be used as a substitute for coproxamol or low-dose morphine. In some patients its sublingual administration and long duration of action (6–8 h) may be an advantage. Progression to morphine will be required in the majority of patients because of its limited therapeutic range. For more detailed consideration of these drugs see Hanks and Hoskin (1987).

[a]There is good evidence that the combination of analgesics with differing modes of action permits enhanced analgesia without the dose-related side-effects which might occur if the individual drugs were used in higher doses (Beaver 1981).

[b]This may exceed the manufacturer's recommendations.

the pain (which may vary considerably for individual patients) and giving the next dose before the first has worn off so that the pain is prevented from returning.

Strong opioid analgesics

Strong opioid analgesics are the final step on the 'analgesic ladder'. Morphine remains the strong opioid analgesic of choice for the management of severe chronic cancer pain. It is available for oral, rectal, and parenteral use. For many years the standard preparation has been the oral aqueous elixir and in some countries an immediate release tablet formulation is also available.

Peak plasma concentrations are achieved within the first hour after administration of morphine elixir and the duration of analgesia is approximately 4 h. Most patients require a 4 hourly regimen and doses must be tailored to individual needs according to response. A low dose is used initially and titrated against the pain until control is achieved. The dose range employed is very wide: from 2.5 to 1000 mg every 4 h or higher in a few patients, but 60–70 per cent of patients will not require more than 200 mg/day. It is important to remember that there is no arbitrary ceiling dose and that the need for a dose in the middle of the night can usually be avoided by giving a double dose at bedtime. Should pain return before the next scheduled dose of morphine, then a predetermined 'breakthrough dose' (usually the same as the 4 hourly dose) can be given.

If a patient has been receiving a regular weak opioid combination, such as coproxamol in a dose of two tablets every 4 h, the starting dose of morphine elixir should be 10 mg every 4 h. A higher starting dose will be required if patients are being converted from an alternative strong opioid analgesic. Equivalent doses are shown in Table 2. Once a stable dose of aqueous morphine has been reached for an individual patient, this can be substituted by controlled-release tablets. These are as effective as the elixir but need to be taken only twice daily (although a few patients may need to take them every 8 h).

Controlled-release morphine is designed for maintenance therapy and is not suitable during the dose titration phase or for the management of acute pain or breakthrough pain. Peak plasma concentrations are achieved 2–4 h after administration. The

bioavailability is the same as aqueous morphine elixir so that an identical daily dose of controlled-release morphine should be substituted. The first dose of controlled-release morphine can be started 4 h after the previous dose of aqueous morphine; a loading dose of aqueous morphine is not required (Hoskin *et al.* 1989). If patients experience breakthrough pain on controlled-release morphine, then morphine elixir or immediate release tablets can be used to cope with this using the equivalent of the 4 hourly dose repeated as often as is necessary.

Diamorphine (diacetylmorphine) was the traditional strong opioid analgesic for cancer pain in the United Kingdom. However, recent pharmacokinetic data indicate that diamorphine by mouth acts merely as a prodrug for morphine and may be an inefficient way of getting morphine into the systemic circulation (Inturrisi *et al.* 1984). It is rapidly deacetylated in the gut and liver to monoacetylmorphine and morphine. There is no evidence of any advantages over morphine when given by mouth for cancer pain.

The great majority of patients will be well controlled on oral medication until the final hours or days of their illness. Rectal administration is a good alternative route if a patient is unable to take oral drugs. Morphine suppositories are available in various strengths and may be directly substituted for oral morphine (same dose and time interval). Oxycodone suppositories have a longer duration of action (6–8 h) and may be preferable for some patients, but are not as readily available. Oxycodone and morphine are approximately dose equivalent (Table 2).

When parenteral medication is required, diamorphine has an advantage over morphine in that it is much more soluble so that a smaller-volume injection can be used for equivalent doses. In countries where diamorphine is not available, hydromorphone also has advantages over morphine in being both more potent and more soluble and therefore preferable for parenteral administration.

Opioid analgesics are subject to extensive first-pass metabolism when taken by mouth. This means that they are relatively more potent when given parenterally (Hanks *et al.* 1987). The dose of oral morphine should be divided by three to obtain the corresponding dose of subcutaneous diamorphine and halved if converting to parenteral morphine.

In some situations, for example the patient with terminal intestinal obstruction, prolonged parenteral administration of analgesics may be required. A battery-operated syringe driver or other slow infusion device with a subcutaneous butterfly needle is useful in these circumstances and can be managed easily in domiciliary practice (Oliver 1985). There has been a tendency for these syringe drivers to be overused. Opioid analgesics given in this way are not inherently more effective than when administered by the oral route and the indications for subcutaneous infusions are limited, the main one being when patients are unable to take oral or rectal medication.

Epidural and intrathecal opioids

Since the discovery of opioid receptors in the spinal cord it has been shown that both epidural and intrathecal administration of opioids in very small doses will produce effective and long-lasting analgesia. The putative advantage of this route of administration is that equivalent or better analgesia may be achieved with a reduction in side-effects by avoiding systemic administration. The evidence that opioids given in this way are any more effective than when given by the oral or parenteral routes is unconvincing (Morgan 1989). However, some patients who experience excessive side-effects with systemic opioids are able to obtain equivalent analgesia with fewer side-effects when the drugs are given epidurally or intrathecally.

Table 2 Equivalent oral doses of morphine relative to other opioid analgesics

Drug and dose (4 hourly unless stated)		Equivalent 4 hourly dose of morphine
Weak opioids		
Coproxamol (dextropropoxyphene 32.5 mg+paracetamol 325 mg)	Two tablets	< 10 mg
Dihydrocodeine	60 mg	< 10 mg
Strong opioids		
Pethidine	50 mg	6 mg
Methadone	5 mg 8 hourly	5 mg[a]
Dipipanone (with cyclizine 30 mg in Diconal)	10 mg	5 mg
Dextromoramide	5 mg	10 mg
Papaveretum	10 mg	7 mg
Nepenthe 1:10 (1 ml undiluted)	10 ml	12 mg
Phenazocine	5 mg	25 mg
Oxycodone suppository	30 mg 6 hourly	20 mg
Buprenorphine	0.4 mg 8 hourly	20 mg

[a]Probably considerably more in chronic dosage owing to accumulation of methadone.
Reproduced with permission from Hanks and Hoskin (1987).

This technique is potentially hazardous and can only be undertaken by skilled personnel in units experienced in its use, but when used selectively it can fulfil a useful function. In general, epidural administration will be preferable to intrathecal, particularly if long-term administration is contemplated and in this latter situation the catheter can be tunnelled under the skin to an implanted subcutaneous reservoir.

Side-effects of morphine

The most common side-effects of morphine are drowsiness, constipation, nausea and vomiting, and dry mouth. Drowsiness is usually only a problem when first starting morphine or when the dose is increased. Patients can generally be reassured that it will improve within a few days, although it may persist in some. Drowsiness is not an indication to reduce or stop therapy and should be dealt with by careful explanation and reassurance to both the patient and relatives. In occasional patients drowsiness can be a major problem which may necessitate using an alternative drug or route of administration. Stimulant drugs may be helpful in selected patients (Bruera *et al.* 1987), but they have the potential to cause hallucinations and occasionally bizarre psychological reactions. They cannot be generally recommended at present.

Constipation is almost universal and should be anticipated by giving laxatives. Codanthramer suspension contains a peristaltic stimulant (danthron) and a faecal softener (poloxamer). This preparation has a wide effective dose range (from 5–10 ml at night to 20 ml twice daily of strong codanthramer suspension; this represents a 24-fold increase in danthron and a 40-fold increase in poloxamer) and can be titrated against response.

A third to a half of patients receiving morphine do not require an anti-emetic and in those patients in whom nausea and vomiting does occur the symptoms may be only transient. Haloperidol given once or twice daily (1.5 mg nightly or twice daily) is usually an effective anti-emetic with fewer side-effects (sedation, anticholinergic, and cardiovascular) than the phenothiazines.

Unfounded fears about opioids

Failure to use strong opioid analgesics when they are properly indicated or to use an adequate dose is usually due to fears of respiratory depression or addiction. Respiratory depression is not a problem in cancer patients receiving oral opioid analgesics. Pain acts as a physiological antagonist of the depressant effect of morphine on the central nervous system, so that as long as a patient has pain the dose of morphine can be safely titrated upwards without fear of respiratory depression (Hanks *et al.* 1981). There is always a separation between the dose that will relieve the patient's pain and the dose that will cause significant depression of respiratory function.

Addiction does not occur in patients receiving strong opioid analgesics because they do not become psychologically dependent or develop 'drug craving'. Both tolerance and physical dependence can occur, but these are not problems in clinical practice. Tolerance is relatively uncommon, but if it does develop it can easily be coped with by appropriate dose adjustment or the careful use of adjuvant analgesic drugs. Physical dependence probably develops in the majority of patients receiving regular opioid analgesics for more than a week or two. However, this does not prevent reduction in dose in patients whose pain ameliorates, for whatever reason or discontinuation in those patients whose pain completely resolves. The patient is weaned off the opioid over 2–3 weeks or more quickly if treatment with the opioid has been relatively short. No special measures are required.

Adjuvant drugs

Adjuvant drugs or 'co-analgesics' are drugs which may not have intrinsic analgesic activity but which, when used with a conventional analgesic, may contribute significantly to pain relief.

Non-steroidal anti-inflammatory drugs

Non-steroidal anti-inflammatory drugs (NSAIDs) are primarily utilized for their anti-inflammatory activity. They block the action of cycloxygenase and thereby inhibit the production of prostaglandins from arachidonic acid. This action is believed to be the basis of their anti-inflammatory and antipyretic effect and may also be at least part of the explanation for their analgesic effect.

NSAIDs were found empirically to relieve bone pain in metastatic breast cancer and haematological malignancies and this was subsequently attributed to their antiprostaglandin action. However, the rôle of prostaglandins in the pathogenesis of bone pain is complex and the effectiveness of these drugs (when they work) may not be directly related to the inhibition of prostaglandin synthesis (Bennett 1988).

As in the treatment of rheumatic disorders the effect of NSAIDs in bone pain is not predictable or consistent. At present there is insufficient data to indicate why some patients respond to particular drugs and others do not and why responders to one drug may be non-responders to another. A trial of an NSAID is indicated in any patient with bone pain, but the use of these drugs must be regularly reassessed. If the first agent used does not produce any apparent benefit, it is worth changing to an alternative. In the absence of clear benefit despite an adequate trial the drug should be discontinued.

The most frequent side-effects associated with NSAIDs are symptoms of upper gastrointestinal irritation and fluid retention. In patients who derive benefit from an NSAID but who develop troublesome dyspeptic symptoms, an H_2 blocker or misoprostol may allow continued use of the drug (Simon *et al.* 1988).

Corticosteroids

Corticosteroids have an important rôle in the management of patients with advanced cancer and a frequent indication is as an adjuvant analgesic. They may be helpful wherever local pressure associated with a tumour mass is causing pain, for example nerve compression, raised intracranial pressure, hepatomegaly, pelvic or intra-abdominal masses, and head and neck tumours. The mode of action of corticosteroids is presumed to be related to their anti-inflammatory effect. Corticosteroids inhibit the production of prostaglandins and leucotrienes, in the latter case by blocking the action of lipo-oxygenase. The reduction of inflammatory oedema and hyperaemia surrounding a tumour mass or involved bone may reduce the pressure and relieve the pain.

Dexamethasone is generally preferable to prednisolone; it is equal in efficacy but more potent (4 mg is approximately equal to 30 mg prednisolone) so that few tablets are necessary and it has fewer mineralocorticoid effects resulting in less oedema and weight gain.

Psychotropic drugs

Anxiety, depression, fear, restlessness, and sleeplessness may all significantly lower a patient's pain threshold and exacerbate pain complaints. All of these symptoms may respond to psychotropic medication with a consequent reduction in pain or a greater ability to tolerate or cope with it.

Benzodiazepines are the most useful group of drugs for the management of these symptoms in cancer patients because of their wide therapeutic index and small potential for interacting with other agents. Diazepam is still preferable to other members of the group. It need be administered only once a day because of its long duration of action, although more frequent dosing will be required in some circumstances.

Phenothiazines have traditionally been used as adjuncts to opioids in cancer patients because of their anti-emetic and sedative effects and because it has been widely believed that they have a specific analgesic-potentiating action. The evidence for any analgesic or analgesic-potentiating effect of these drugs has been exaggerated and is generally unconvincing (Hanks 1984). Phenothiazines can cause excessive sedation, are associated with anticholinergic and cardiovascular side-effects, and lower seizure threshold. Benzodiazepines do not produce these side-effects and thus have significant advantages in cancer patients where an anxiolytic or sedative effect is desired.

Antidepressants are widely used in the management of chronic pain both in patients who have chronic pain and are depressed and in the absence of depression. The data relating to cancer pain are equivocal, but it is possible that antidepressants may have an opioid-sparing effect in this situation.

Calcitonin

Calcitonin is a single-chain polypeptide secreted by the parafollicular or C cells of the thyroid gland which lowers blood calcium and inhibits osteoclastic bone resorption. It has been used widely for the treatment of Paget's disease and in the management of hypercalcaemia.

Calcitonin has been promoted for the relief of metastatic bone pain. A critical review of the evidence suggests that a minority of patients with bone pain may respond, sometimes very well, to treatment with calcitonin (Hanks 1988). However, there are a number of disadvantages: calcitonin must be administered parenterally, there is no agreement on dosage or regimen, it is very expensive, and there is no way of identifying the small percentage of patients likely to respond. Side-effects of nausea and vomiting, flushing, and feelings of faintness are common following each injection. Calcitonin does not have a place in the routine management of bone pain.

Bisphosphonates

Bisphosphonates are analogues of pyrophosphate and are potent inhibitors of osteoclastic bone resorption. Bisphosphonates have an established place in the treatment of Paget's disease and they have now become the first-line treatment for cancer-associated hypercalcaemia (Ralston 1992). There is some evidence that these drugs can relieve pain from bone metastases associated with breast cancer (Elomaa et al. 1983) and myeloma and may significantly reduce skeletal morbidity in breast cancer patients (Paterson et al. 1993). There is substantial anecdotal experience to suggest that regular infusions of pamidronate (60 mg at 2 weekly intervals) may improve bone pain specifically but data from randomized controlled trials are not yet available to support this.

Anticonvulsants and other membrane stabilizers

Anticonvulsants may be helpful in the management of lancinating or stabbing dysaesthetic pains associated with nerve infiltration or compression, post-surgical neuralgias, post-herpetic neuralgia, or other forms of neuropathic pain. Drugs and doses are shown in Table 3. Burning dysaesthesiae may also respond.

Other 'membrane-stabilizing' drugs, notably anti-arrhythmic agents, have been used in the management of neuropathic pain.

Table 3 Anticonvulsants for neuropathic pain

Drug	Starting dose	Maintenance dose (mg/day)	Side-effects
Carbamazepine	100 mg twice daily	300–800	Drowsiness, confusion, ataxia, nystagmus, nausea
Sodium valproate	200 mg twice daily	600–1200	Increased appetite, weight gain, nausea, epigastric pain, ankle swelling, tremor, hair loss
Clonazepam	0.5 mg twice daily (or nightly)	1–4	Drowsiness, ataxia

NB: most patients need only a twice daily regimen. Side-effects are generally dose related; therefore increase the frequency of dosing if side-effects are a problem.

The most dramatic results have recently been reported with flecainide, an orally active congener of lignocaine. Experience with only a small number of patients was described and there has been recent concern about the safety of flecainide in post-myocardial infarction patients. Therefore caution should be exercised but drugs such as mexiletine or flecainide may be worthy of a trial in patients unresponsive to other drug treatments.

Muscle relaxants

Painful muscle spasm frequently occurs, particularly in association with metastatic bone disease in the axial skeleton. Baclofen and diazepam are equally effective, but diazepam is more sedative, whilst baclofen causes gastrointestinal disturbance more frequently (Young and Delwaide 1981). Muscle spasm may also respond to acupuncture, massage, or heat.

Non-drug measures

A variety of physical and other non-drug measures may have a part to play in the management of cancer pain. There has been a general move away from destructive nerve-blocking procedures and a greater emphasis on pharmacological or other non-invasive treatment. However, carefully selected patients may benefit from procedures such as coeliac plexus block for severe abdominal pain, particularly that associated with carcinoma of the pancreas (Hanna et al. 1989), percutaneous cordotomy for any unilateral pain below the C5 dermatome, or a neurolytic nerve block for patients with pain confined to one or two dermatomes (Wells 1989) and these options need to be kept in mind.

Chronic lymphoedema of both upper and lower limbs may be due to surgery, radiotherapy, or recurrent disease. It is a difficult problem to treat and often produces considerable pain and discomfort. In the first instance an elastic stocking or sleeve should be used in conjunction with other measures including massage, limb exercises, compression bandaging, and the use of intermittent compression sleeve devices (Mortimer et al. 1993).

Transcutaneous nerve stimulation and occasionally acupuncture may be helpful in some patients with difficult neuralgic or neuro-pathic pain. Simpler measures such as heat pads, massage, and relaxation therapy may also play an important role (Filshie 1998).

Gastrointestinal symptoms

Gastrointestinal symptoms are common in patients with advanced cancer. Constipation is almost universal and anorexia, nausea, and

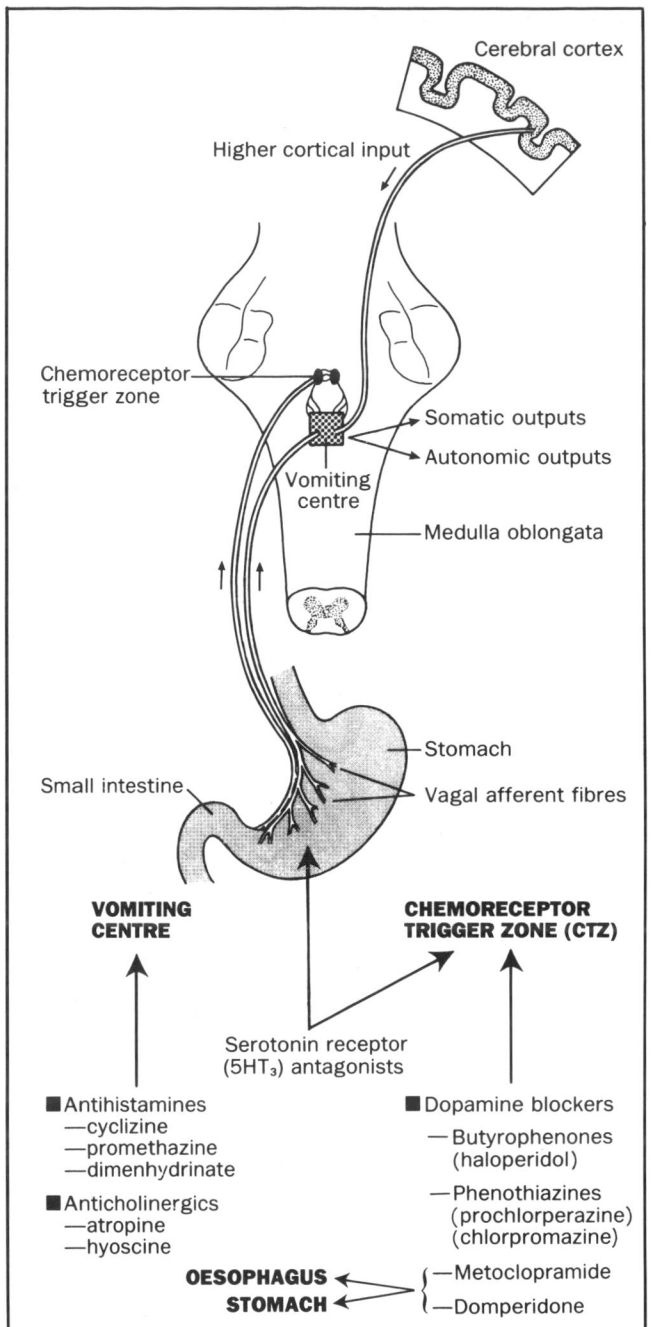

Fig. 2   The putative sites of action of anti-emetic drugs. Anti-emetics can be classified by their main site of action into those acting on the chemoreceptor trigger zone and those acting on the vomiting centre. However there is a considerable overlap. (Reproduced with permission from Mansi and Hanks (1989).)

vomiting will be a problem at some time in the majority of patients. Management is based on detecting the cause for each symptom so that a rational therapeutic regimen can be worked out.

Nausea and vomiting

There are many possible causes of nausea and vomiting in patients with advanced cancer and frequently several may be implicated in an individual patient. If the underlying mechanism can be determined it is possible to choose an appropriate anti-emetic on the basis of the predominant site of action of the drugs.

The physiology of vomiting involves the coordination of a number of stimulatory pathways in an area of the brainstem commonly referred to as the vomiting or emetic centre, which is in the region of the nucleus tractus solitarius, the dorsal motor nucleus of the vagus, and the nucleus ambiguus. When stimulated, vomiting occurs via efferent pathways to the abdominal muscles, diaphragm, stomach, vasomotor centres, salivary centre, respiratory centre, and cranial nerves. Anti-emetic drugs can be divided by their main site of action into those that act on the vomiting centre and those whose main effect is on the chemoreceptor trigger zone which is situated in the area postrema of the medulla in the floor of the fourth ventricle (Fig. 2). Some drugs also have peripheral sites of action and enhance gastric emptying and increase tone in the gastroesophageal sphincter (metoclopramide and domperidone).

In the majority of patients a careful history with particular attention to current medication, together with a few simple blood tests, will establish the underlying diagnosis. Table 4 demonstrates how a rational initial choice of anti-emetic can then be made. Alongside the use of anti-emetic drugs, simple modifications to life-style should also be considered. Avoidance of food preparation and cooking smells and changes in drug regimens so that specific emetogenic drugs and unpleasant formulations are replaced by alternatives, may be all that is required.

In situations where vomiting may be anticipated, such as during abdominal irradiation or in the management of chronic raised intracranial pressure or subacute intestinal obstruction, prophylactic anti-emetics may be most effective. Once nausea and vomiting has become established, drug administration can become a problem.

Table 4   Choice of initial anti-emetic drug related to cause of symptoms in advanced cancer

Cause	Drugs(s) of choice
Mediated via	
Chemoreceptor trigger zone	
Drugs (e.g. morphine, chemotherapy)	Haloperidol
Metabolic causes (e.g. uraemia, liver	Phenothiazines
failure, hypercalcaemia)	Metoclopramide or domperidone
	5-HT$_3$ antagonists
Mid-brain receptors for intracranial pressure	
Raised intracranial pressure	Dexamethasone
Vestibular nuclei	
Movement-related nausea and vomiting	Cyclizine
	Hyoscine
	Dimenhydrate
Peripheral sites (*via vagus*)	
i.e. gut, pharynx, heart	
Gut stasis	Metoclopramide or domperidone
Other causes (e.g. radiation, drugs with	Drugs acting on vomiting
gastrointestinal toxicity, mechanical irritation)	centre
Vomiting centre	
Emotion (e.g. fear, anxiety)	Benzodiazepine (e.g. lorazepam)
All other causes detailed above are mediated	Antihistamine
via the vomiting centre	(e.g. cyclizine)
	Anticholinergic
	(e.g. hyoscine)

The rectal route is much neglected but is useful for many patients and most of the common anti-emetics (except metoclopramide) are available in suppository form. If the rectal route is not available or not acceptable to the patient, regular parenteral administration for a short period may be required and continuous subcutaneous infusion of drugs such as metoclopramide or haloperidol may be preferable to repeated injections.

A small proportion of patients will require more than one anti-emetic. Routine use of two- or three-drug cocktails is not recommended and will only result in excessive side-effects in the majority of patients. There is little value in giving more than one drug with the same mode of action, such as a phenothiazine with haloperidol or metoclopramide with domperidone. When more than one anti-emetic is required, drugs acting on both the chemoreceptor trigger zone and vomiting centre should be combined, with the subsequent addition of steroids if necessary.

A new family of anti-emetic drugs with antagonist activity at 5-hydroxytryptamine (5-HT$_3$) receptors has recently been introduced for the treatment of chemotherapy-associated nausea and vomiting. Extensive experience has confirmed that these are highly effective agents for the treatment of chemotherapy and radiation-induced emesis, but they have yet to be investigated in the treatment of other causes of emesis encountered in a palliative care setting. Some patients have intractable nausea and vomiting. It is important to keep in mind that psychogenic factors may be involved and may require appropriate psychotropic medication. Acupuncture, hypnotherapy, and relaxation may also be useful adjunctive measures.

Constipation

Constipation, as defined by the passage of small hard faeces infrequently and with difficulty (Twycross and Lack 1987), will occur in most patients with advanced cancer and may be associated with anorexia, abdominal and rectal pain, and nausea and vomiting. Common causes of constipation in cancer patients are shown in Table 5 together with an outline of initial management. For many patients there will be more than one cause and for most some form of laxative will be required. As with other symptoms, where there is a continuing cause of constipation such as morphine, prophylactic use of a laxative is far more satisfactory than allowing a difficult problem to develop before initiating treatment.

Laxatives may be considered broadly in four main groups: bulking agents such as bran and methylcellulose, osmotic agents such as lactulose and magnesium salts, lubricants such as liquid paraffin, and stimulant or contact laxatives acting primarily by increasing intraluminal fluid and the activity of bowel smooth muscle (senna, cascara, danthron, and bisacodyl). The last group also includes drugs such as castor oil and docusate which not only have a contact laxative action but also are stool-softening agents. The choice of laxative for an individual patient can be guided by the considerations outlined in Table 5. For many of these patients the introduction of large quantities of bulking agents is both unwelcome and unsuccessful, compounding other problems of anorexia, nausea, and dry mouth. For most a combination of a faecal softening agent with a contact smooth muscle stimulant will be effective and codanthramer suspension contains both (see above). The dose can be titrated over a wide range and the addition of an osmotic agent such as magnesium sulphate is recommended in resistant cases.

In general, oral preparations are to be preferred, but drugs given by suppository may be required. Local irritation can become a problem with regular use of such preparations as bisacodyl suppositories and may even occur with simple glycerol suppositories.

Enemas will be required for stubborn constipation and faecal impaction. For patients who have stomas local suppositories or enemas may be used through the stoma, but retention may be poor and rectal or colonic washouts may be more useful.

Diarrhoea

Diarrhoea can be defined as an increased frequency and/or fluidity of bowel motions. A common cause in patients with advanced cancer is faecal impaction with overflow. Therefore a careful history, rectal examination, and review of the laxative regimen, together with local measures to relieve the faecal impaction, will resolve the problem for many patients.

Excessive use of laxatives is not uncommon in this group of patients and drugs other than laxatives may also cause diarrhoea. Antacids containing magnesium salts, antibiotics, and NSAIDs, including indomethacin and flurbiprofen, are commonly implicated. Certain chemotherapeutic agents, including 5-fluorouracil, mitomycin-C, methotrexate, and cisplatinum, may cause diarrhoea. Diarrhoea is also a recognized complication of radiotherapy where the bowel is included in the radiation field, such as occurs during treatment of the pelvis or lumbar spine. Other causes are intestinal obstruction and fistula formulation between the bowel, rectum, bladder, or vagina.

For the majority of patients antidiarrhoeal drugs, together with dietary advice (to avoid high fruit and vegetable intake), will be appropriate. Opioid derivatives, such as codeine, diphenoxylate, or loperamide, may also be required. The role of these drugs in patients already receiving morphine is unclear; theoretically, there is little value in adding a second weaker opioid agonist. Loperamide may be an exception to this rule because of its specific peripheral opioid agonist action. This drug also has the advantage of a flexible dose schedule, allowing dose titration according to the severity of the diarrhoea.

Where bowel malabsorption is thought to be an important component of the diarrhoea, as may occur after small bowel surgery or in chronic radiation enteritis, bile-salt-chelating drugs such as cholestyramine may help. If pancreatic disease or obstruction is present, pancreatic supplements (Pancrex) may help prevent diarrhoea due to fat malabsorption.

Diarrhoea resulting from fistulae which does not respond to simple constipating measures may be an indication for a proximal defunctioning colostomy.

Table 5 Management of constipation

Pathophysiology	Cause	Remedy
Low bulk	Anorexia	Dietary fibre
	Poor diet	supplements
Hard stool	Dehydration	Fluids
	Drugs (e.g. diuretics, anticholinergics)	Modify drug regimen
		Lubricant laxative
Reduced colonic motility	Drugs (e.g. morphine, anticholinergics, vincristine)	Modify drug regimen
	Hypercalcaemia	Correct electrolyte or calcium imbalance
	Hypokalaemia	Stimulant laxative
Local anal dysfunction	Anal fissure	Local measures
	Haemorrhoids	Lubricant laxative
Social inhibition	Lack of privacy	Provision of appropriate facilities and support
	Immobility and debility	
	Depression	
	Confusion	

Intestinal obstruction

Intestinal obstruction is a common complication of advanced intra-abdominal pelvic malignancy, being reported in 10 per cent of patients with colorectal carcinomas and in 25 per cent of ovarian carcinomas. Other common primary tumours are carcinomas of the uterus and stomach, although in one reported series of patients with malignant intestinal obstruction a third of the patients had extra-abdominal primaries including melanoma, breast, bronchus, and lymphomas. Intestinal obstruction in patients with cancer may also be unrelated to the cancer. In up to 25 per cent of patients with a known cancer developing intestinal obstruction, an unrelated pathology has been demonstrated and in over one-third of these a new primary carcinoma was diagnosed (Ketcham *et al.* 1970).

An autopsy study of patients dying from advanced cancer (mainly colorectal or ovarian) with intestinal obstruction showed that the small bowel is most commonly involved with multiple sites of obstruction in approximately 80 per cent of patients. The cause of obstruction in the majority is extrinsic compression and adhesions due to extensive serosal and mesenteric disease. In only two out of 18 patients was the large bowel the sole site of obstruction (Baines 1993).

Occasionally, functional obstruction, sometimes termed 'pseudo-obstruction', may be encountered, presenting with signs and symptoms of intestinal obstruction in the absence of mechanical occlusion. Possible causes in cancer patients include silent perforation or peritonitis, painful lumbar conditions including retroperitoneal tumour infiltration or haemorrhage, pneumonia, drugs (for example, vinca alkaloids or anticholinergic drugs), and hypokalaemia.

Conventional management of intestinal obstruction involves resuscitation with intravenous fluids and nasogastric suction, followed by laparotomy and appropriate surgical correction. In the patient with advanced cancer, a more selective surgical policy is indicated, balancing the morbidity and mortality of such procedures against the likelihood of a surgically correctable cause and subsequent survival from the underlying cancer. Surgical mortality in patients with advanced cancer is reported to be between 20 and 35 per cent, with faecal fistulae developing in up to 10 per cent, whilst the mean survival from onset of obstruction in one series was only 2.5 months (Piver *et al.* 1982). Therefore for many patients, particularly those with documented metastatic intra-abdominal disease and widespread metastases, a conservative approach to management will be more appropriate.

A regimen based on that developed at St Christopher's Hospice will enable the majority of patients to remain comfortable and in some cases to survive for many months (Table 6). The most recent development has been the use of octreotide, a synthetic analogue of somatostatin, to control troublesome vomiting in obstructed patients. The drug is administered by continuous subcutaneous infusion, is well tolerated, and may dramatically reduce the frequency and volume of vomiting (Riley and Fallon 1994).

Anorexia

Anorexia is a common symptom of cancer and may be particularly troublesome in patients with advanced disease. It may be primary or secondary (Table 7). The problem of anorexia is often compounded by anxious relatives pressing the anorexic patient to eat in the misplaced belief that this will in some way build up the patient and arrest the cancer. Careful explanation and reassurance is required that the patient with advanced cancer is likely to require less food

Table 6 The medical management of intestinal obstruction

Symptoms	Treatment
Pain/colic	Opioid analgesics (weak/strong) +antispasmodic (loperamide or hyoscine)
Anti-emetic	Cyclizine and/or haloperidol (or a phenothiazine) **Avoid** metoclopramide and domperidone[a] (may exacerbate vomiting or pain because of increase in gastrointestinal motility)
Constipation	Faecal softener (docusate sodium) Rectal measures **Avoid** stimulant laxatives (may exacerbate pain)

In early/subacute obstruction consider dexamethasone 4 mg four times daily (intravenously for 4–5 days) which may resolve the obstruction.
Chemotherapy may be an option for ovarian or colorectal cancers.
Avoid intravenous infusions if possible.
Nasogastric tubes are only indicated if there is significant gastric stasis, distension, and copious vomiting.
[a]Except in the presence of subacute obstruction when a subcutaneous infusion of metoclopramide may in some cases hasten resolution of the obstruction.

Table 7 Aetiology of anorexia in advanced cancer

Primary
　Cancer cachexia

Secondary

(a) Social causes		Presentation and type of food
		Environment
(b) Physical causes		
	Local	**General**
	Dry mouth	Metabolic
	Sore mouth	Hypercalcaemia
	Dysphagia	Hypokalaemia
	Nausea	Hyponatraemia
	Vomiting	Uraemia
	Abdominal mass	Hepatic failure
	Ascites	Ratiotherapy
	Malodorous tumour	Chemotherapy
		Pain
		Depression

and that no harm will result from irregular small meals taken when the patient feels comfortably able to do so. Diets should be individualized for each patient and made as palatable as possible with adequate food intake to prevent dehydration. There is no objective evidence that specific dietary supplements or exclusions are of value, but they need not be discouraged if found helpful by some individuals.

More specific management of anorexia lies in exploring possible aetiological factors as outlined in Table 7 with appropriate correction where possible. If required, appetite can be actively stimulated using simple measures such as an alcoholic drink before meals. Corticosteroids improve well-being and stimulate appetite in a proportion of patients though this effect is usually short-lived. Several other drugs have been demonstrated to improve appetite, including progestogens, anabolic steroids, phenothiazines, cyproheptadine, prolintane, and tetrahydrocannabinoids. Of these, the progestogens and particularly megesterol may significantly improve appetite and lead to weight gain and these drugs generally lack the side-effects associated with corticosteroids. Where early satiation and distension or other evidence of gastric stasis is prominent, metoclopramide or domperidone, which enhance gastric emptying, together with frequent small meals may help.

Table 8 Causes and management of dysphagia

Pathology	Management
Neurological	
Bulbar palsy	Steroids±local irradiation if due to
Pseudobulbar palsy	metastases
	Eating aids and dietary management
Mouth	
Major surgery	Mouthcare
Radical radiotherapy	Eating aids and dietary modification
	Artificial saliva
Mucositis	Topical steroids
Aphthous ulceration	Anti-inflammatory mouthwash (e.g.
	benzydamine)
	Topical anaesthetic
Loose dentures	Dental advice
Candidiasis	Oral antifungal (e.g. nystatin)
Oesophagus and cardia	
Tumour	Systemic steroids
	Irradiation
	Surgery
	Intubation
Stricture following surgery or	Surgical dilatation/intubation
radiotherapy	
Candidiasis	Oral antifungal (e.g. nystatin)

Aggressive nutritional support using nasogastric tube feeding or intravenous nutrients is rarely, if ever, indicated in patients with advanced cancer. Nutritional intake should be largely guided by the patient's desire for food and worries about a reduced food intake allayed by explanation and reassurance. Local symptoms of dehydration in the final days of life are more appropriately dealt with by attentive mouth care, sips of iced water, ice cubes, or fruit rather than by intravenous drips or parenteral feeding.

Dysphagia

Difficulty in swallowing has been described in 12 per cent of patients admitted to one hospice unit and almost half of these patients died within a week of presentation (Sykes et al. 1988). Common causes for dysphagia, together with appropriate management, are shown in Table 8.

Again, careful diagnosis is important. Up to two-thirds of patients will have oral candidiasis, treatment of which is simple and highly effective. In those patients with a life expectancy of several weeks and no obvious cause for their dysphagia on examination of the mouth or oropharynx, a barium swallow is indicated to enable accurate localization of the site and nature of the obstruction. In one series limited autopsy showed that the cause of dysphagia is related to local tumour obstruction in 81 per cent of patients, with multiple sites of obstruction in almost a quarter of these (Sykes et al. 1988). In this situation, both external-beam irradiation and surgical intubation will relieve dysphagia in approximately half of the patients. However, surgery is associated with greater mortality and morbidity in this group of patients, with an operative mortality of over 20 per cent being reported in one series (Pfleiderer 1982). Problems with 'tube malfunction', requiring readmission for a further procedure, occurred in over one-third of patients. Against this must be balanced reports of post-irradiation strictures requiring dilatation in up to 50 per cent of patients receiving external-beam radiation treatment of the oesophagus, and the risk of fistula formation into the trachea or bronchus where there is extensive tumour infiltration of these structures. Surgery provides more rapid symptom relief, but radiotherapy may be better tolerated.

Nasogastric intubation should only be considered as a temporary measure whilst definitive treatment is given and only rarely is it necessary perioperatively or during radiotherapy in this group of patients. Similarly, for the patient with advanced cancer in the last few weeks of life, gastrostomy is neither kind nor useful, even in the face of complete dysphagia when appropriate symptomatic measures are far more effective in keeping the patient comfortable with no detriment to his or her ultimate survival.

Newer techniques, such as the use of endoscopic laser therapy or intracavity irradiation to the oesophagus, may be applicable in selected patients.

Respiratory symptoms

Dyspnoea

Some reports have indicated that approximately half of all patients admitted to hospices complain of shortness of breath (Heyes Moore 1984).

Dyspnoea is the unpleasant awareness of difficulty in breathing and is a subjective sensation. The pathophysiological mechanisms involved are complex and have not been fully worked out. In patients with advanced cancer, dyspnoea has many causes and may be multifactorial. As with pain, dyspnoea may be related to the cancer itself, may result from the treatment of the cancer, or may arise from concurrent conditions.

Treatment should be directed towards altering the underlying pathological process if possible and this should be accompanied by symptomatic measures (Cowcher and Hanks 1990).

Pleural effusion

Pleural effusions are most common with tumours of the lung and breast and may be asymptomatic. If the effusion is causing dyspnoea, the treatment of choice is to drain the pleura dry and if it recurs to inject sclerosant. Comparative studies have not demonstrated any outstanding advantage with any one agent and tetracycline is the cheapest.

Lymphangitis carcinomatosa

Diffuse tumour invasion of the small lymphatics of the lungs can occur in a retrograde fashion from tumour in the hilar lymph nodes. Changes in chest radiography usually develop late and the patient may present with breathlessness disproportionate to the clinical or radiograph findings. A small proportion of patients may respond to treatment with corticosteroids, but for the majority only symptomatic measures will be available.

Pneumonia

The management of pneumonia should not present a dilemma even in patients with advanced disease. Life-threatening chest infections should be treated aggressively with parenteral antibiotics and physiotherapy if the patient has been active with a good quality of life prior to the infective episode. In patients who are less well but who have troublesome symptoms associated with the infection, oral antibiotics will often produce considerable symptomatic relief. If the patient is dying, then antibiotics are not helpful and the symptoms are best controlled by other means.

Pulmonary embolus

The management of recurrent small pulmonary emboli causing dyspnoea in advanced cancer patients may present a difficult choice. In the majority of patients the risks and burden of anticoagulation are likely to outweigh the benefits. Patients are usually taking several different drugs, many of which will have the potential to interact with anticoagulants and some of which, such as NSAIDs and corticosteroids, may be potential causes of haemorrhage from the gastrointestinal tract. Anticoagulation will also increase the likelihood of bleeding from a tumour and patients may be thrombocytopenic because of either the disease or its treatment. For all these reasons long-term treatment with anticoagulants will rarely be indicated. In patients for whom anticoagulants are being considered, confirmation of the diagnosis should be sought with a ventilation perfusion scan.

Ascites

Malignant ascites may be severe enough to cause diaphragmatic splinting and result in dyspnoea. Paracentesis may produce dramatic improvement in the breathlessness.

Symptomatic treatment of dyspnoea

Opioid drugs

Opioid analgesics have been shown to relieve dyspnoea in both cancer patients and non-cancer patients with chronic obstructive airways disease (Woodcock *et al.* 1981). The precise mechanism is not known, although morphine and related drugs have demonstrable effects on respiratory function; in normal subjects they reduce respiratory rate, alveolar ventilation, and the response to hypercapnia and hypoxia. In patients with chronic obstructive airways disease opioids decrease oxygen consumption and increase exercise tolerance. Both central and peripheral mechanisms are probably involved. There is evidence that part of the effect of morphine on respiration is mediated via opioid systems in the lung. This is in addition to a depressant effect on the respiratory centres in the medulla and possibly also an anxiolytic effect mediated via opioid receptors in the thalamus, amygdala, and frontal cortex.

In cancer patients the usual starting dose of morphine when used to treat dyspnoea is 5 mg every 4 h. In the elderly, cachectic, or debilitated patient a smaller starting dose of 2.5 mg may be advisable. The dose can be titrated upwards if necessary, although in general doses in excess of 15 mg every 4 h in the absence of pain will cause unwanted effects with little further symptomatic improvement. A laxative is necessary to counteract opioid-induced constipation and an anti-emetic may also be required.

Bronchodilators

Bronchodilators are useful where dyspnoea is exacerbated by reversible airways obstruction. Before commencing treatment the degree of reversibility should be assessed by measuring peak flow before and 30 min after a standard dose of a bronchodilator such as salbutamol. An improvement of greater than 15 per cent indicates that the patient is likely to derive significant clinical benefit.

Salbutamol, delivered by aerosol or via a nebulizer, is commonly used and generally acceptable. Tremor and tachycardia are the most common side-effects. Slow-release preparations of xanthine derivatives such as aminophylline or theophylline are useful alternatives.

Nebulized local anaesthetics

Nebulized local anaesthetics were first employed in the hope that anaesthesia of the pulmonary receptors mediating the sensation of dyspnoea would produce some relief. Studies with isotope-labelled local anaesthetics have shown that a particle size of less than 0.2 nm is necessary to reach the alveoli and the so-called 'J receptors'. An ultrasonic nebulizer is necessary to produce such a fine particle size. If the particles are larger (as produced by standard nebulizers), they are deposited in the larger airways and will be ineffective.

The published data on the use of nebulized local anaesthetics in dyspnoea in cancer patients are conflicting, but there is anecdotal evidence which suggests that the technique is useful for some patients. Both lignocaine and bupivacaine have been used, but the latter is more likely to cause bronchoconstriction. The dose of lignocaine is 5 ml of 2 per cent solution which can be repeated at intervals of 4 h. Patients may complain about the unpleasant taste of the local anaesthetic, and some anaesthesia of the mucous membranes of the mouth is likely. Patients should be warned not to eat or drink for 1 h following each administration, because the gag reflex is anaesthetized.

Anxiolytic agents

Cancer patients with dyspnoea are frequently anxious and a benzodiazepine or phenothiazine may produce some improvement. Neither of these groups of drugs appear to have a specific effect on dyspnoea distinct from their anxiolytic action.

Oxygen

The use of oxygen to relieve dyspnoea is controversial. Large changes in Pa_{O_2} are necessary in order to stimulate a ventilatory response to hypoxia. Because of this, hypoxia has generally been disregarded as a significant cause of dyspnoea and increased ventilation rate in breathless patients. However, recent work has shown that severe hypoxia does result in dyspnoea and an increased ventilatory response (Chronos *et al.* 1988).

Oxygen should not be offered to every dyspnoeic cancer patient as a panacea. It is often only of placebo benefit and encourages higher dependence, but there is no doubt that some patients find it helpful.

Non-drug measures

Dyspnoea related to advanced cancer is particularly anxiety provoking and frightening and this tends to exacerbate the symptom. Careful explanation and discussion of the patient's fears and clarification of the measures that are to be instituted to deal with the symptom, will help to alleviate anxiety. Relaxation exercises and particularly techniques involving breathing control can be helpful for some patients. Many patients find that facial cooling with cold air produces some symptomatic relief and this has also been demonstrated in normal subjects with exercise-induced dyspnoea. Patients should be offered a well-ventilated room and a fan may also be helpful.

Cough

Cough is the forcible expulsion of air and other substances from the lungs. Cough is both reflexly stimulated and under some degree of voluntary control. Irritant receptors in the upper airways can be stimulated by mechanical or chemical stimuli and initiate a coughing response.

Symptomatic treatment of cough

Simple measures such as humidification with steam or nebulized saline may relieve cough and many patients also find a simple linctus helpful. Expectorants have been widely used to treat viscid sputum, but their efficacy is not supported by controlled clinical studies, nor is there any evidence that proprietary cough syrups are any more effective than simple linctus.

Opioid drugs such as morphine, codeine, methadone, and pholcodine suppress the cough reflex centrally. They can be conveniently given in linctus form.

Nebulized local anaesthetics may diminish cough by producing anaesthesia of laryngeal and tracheobronchial irritant receptors and can be used in the same way as in the treatment of dyspnoea.

Paralysis of one of the vocal cords resulting from infiltration or compression of the recurrent laryngeal nerve produces a characteristic bovine cough associated with hoarseness and occasionally dyspnoea. The cough becomes ineffective because of incomplete closure of the cords. If the symptoms are troublesome and the patient has a reasonable prognosis, injection of Teflon into the affected cord may produce considerable improvement and is a simple procedure for a specialist surgeon.

Haemoptysis

Haemoptysis is the expectoration of blood of bronchopulmonary origin. It is common in bronchogenic lung cancer with an incidence of 50 per cent. Haemoptysis can also accompany pulmonary embolus or severe cardiac failure.

Minor degrees of haemoptysis are common where there is lung tumour and need no treatment other than reassurance. Troublesome haemoptysis that is attributable to an identifiable lesion can be alleviated by palliative radiotherapy in the majority of patients (Arnott 1987).

Stridor

Stridor is a high-pitched harsh inspiratory sound caused by partial obstruction of the main air passages. It may be one of the components of the syndrome of mediastinal obstruction, result from bilateral vocal cord paralysis, or occur with any cause of extrinsic compression of the larynx, trachea, or bronchi. Extrinsic compression by tumour may respond to high-dose corticosteroids (dexamethasone 4 mg four times daily). If the stridor is not amenable or does not respond to this treatment, a mixture of oxygen and helium may produce symptomatic relief for some patients (but will also result in a peculiar metallic voice).

Stridor can be a distressing and anxiety-provoking symptom and anxiolytic drugs are also an important part of its management.

Urinary symptoms

Bladder tenesmus

Severe spasms of pain arising from the bladder and sometimes radiating down the urethra usually arise from the detrusor muscle. They may be caused by tumour or infection, blood clots, or an indwelling catheter. These spasmodic pains are often difficult to treat pharmacologically and the first and most effective step is to see whether the precipitating cause can be dealt with. Radiotherapy should be considered if tumour bulk or bleeding is responsible and a catheter may relieve the symptoms if related to tumour infiltration or the passage of blood clot. Catheters themselves may result in painful spasm and a change in size (of catheter or balloon) should be considered if this is the case. Infection should be treated appropriately and bladder washouts given if pain is related to the passage of debris. A good state of hydration and urinary flow should be maintained.

Conventional analgesics should be used according to the usual principles but often will not be very effective. Occasionally a NSAID

may be helpful, as may corticosteroids if symptoms are related to bulky tumour where no further radiotherapy can be given. Experience with more specific drugs such as flavoxate, an anti-spasmodic agent and phenazopyridine, a so-called urinary analgesic, has generally not been very encouraging. Diazepam may prove to be more helpful, but there is no evidence that more sedative anxiolytic drugs such as chlorpromazine are any better. Lumbar sympathetic block has been reported to be effective in some patients, but other nerve blocks are not likely to be helpful.

Generally this is a difficult symptom to treat, but it will usually respond, at least partially, to some combination of the above measures.

Haematuria

Some drugs can discolour the urine so that it appears to contain blood and danthron is a frequent offender in this patient population. Thus, the first step in the management of apparent haematuria is to review drug therapy.

Frank haematuria may be an indication for radiotherapy if it is heavy, persistent, or causes the formation of clots. Less severe bleeding can usually be dealt with by explanation and reassurance.

Occasionally an antifibrinolytic agent such as tranexamic acid (1 g twice or four times daily) can be used to reduce heavy haematuria if radiotherapy cannot be given. However, this may cause excessive clotting which may result in increased discomfort or even ureteric obstruction. Side-effects of nausea, vomiting, and diarrhoea are also common, but tend to be dose related.

Urinary incontinence

Urinary incontinence may have a simple cause which is easily dealt with. This includes faecal impaction or constipation, urinary infection, excessive sedation, or weakness and inability to reach the toilet.

If simple measures are ineffective, drugs with anticholinergic activity may be indicated. A tricyclic antidepressant such as amitriptyline (25–75 mg at night) or imipramine (10–25 mg thrice daily) should be tried first. Propantheline (15–30 mg twice or thrice daily) may also be used but is more likely to cause excessive side-effects, particularly dry mouth, constipation, and blurring of vision. Some patients will require catheterization which may need to be permanent. Others may not be able to tolerate a catheter and will be managed with absorbant pads and other incontinence aids.

Incontinence of urine via the vagina or rectum may occur as a result of fistula formation. This may be extremely distressing for patients, and urinary diversion may be appropriate in patients who still have a reasonable life expectancy.

Urinary retention

Urinary retention may be an early sign of spinal cord compression and should immediately alert to this possibility. Careful neurological examination and appropriate investigations should be instigated.

Anticholinergic drugs (including phenothiazines and tricyclic antidepressants) and morphine can cause hesitancy or frank retention of urine and constipation is another common cause in cancer patients. Severe outflow obstruction may require urethral or suprapubic catheterization, but less severe symptoms may respond to phenoxybenzamine (10 mg at night), an α-adrenergic blocker which relaxes the internal sphincter. It may occasionally cause troublesome hypotension and tiredness. An alternative for patients with retention caused by a neuropathic bladder is distigmine (5 mg daily or on alternate days). Again, catheterization may be required if drugs fail to improve the symptoms.

Neurological symptoms

Headache

Headache in patients with advanced cancer may have many causes and not infrequently is unrelated to the cancer. One study of 100 consecutive hospice admissions found that migraine was as common as raised intracranial pressure (Twycross and Fairfield 1982). A careful clinical history will often enable the distinction between a typical tension headache or migraine and headaches suggestive of raised intracranial pressure when the pain is dull, continuous, wakes the patient at night, and is worse on coughing, sneezing, or straining. Where these features are present or where vomiting or focal neurological signs accompany the headache, cerebral metastasis or progression of a known primary brain tumour are likely and may be confirmed on brain scan.

Initial treatment is with simple analgesics, anti-emetics, and steroids, using dexamethasone in doses of up to 16 mg/day orally. In a patient with intracranial tumour and a prognosis of several weeks or months, cranial irradiation should be considered as the optimum means of controlling headache and also to prevent progressive neurological symptoms. Over 80 per cent of patients will benefit from a palliative course of cranial irradiation given over 1–2 weeks.

Where symptoms of raised intracranial pressure recur or fail to respond to the above treatment, the outlook is poor. Transient improvements may be gained using very high doses of steroids (up to 96 mg dexamethasone daily) or osmotic agents such as mannitol or glycerol, but such responses are short-lived and rarely worthwhile. Where there is no response to steroids these should be reduced over a relatively short period and pain controlled with appropriate and adequate analgesia.

Confusion

Confusion is a complex symptom in which the patient loses touch with his or her environment, causing a spectrum of disorder from mild disorientation to frank psychosis. Unlike dementia, which may also occur in up to 8 per cent of cancer patients (Derogatis *et al.* 1983), confusion is both avoidable and reversible in many cases and therefore should be carefully evaluated and investigated before resorting to treatment with sedatives or major tranquillizers.

A useful model of confusion proposes that the basis of the symptoms is a loss of ability to regulate and filter incoming stimuli into the conscious awareness (Stedeford 1985). This arises against a background of clouding of consciousness as a result of which simple environmental stimuli, both visual and auditory, become amplified and misinterpreted. The patient then becomes distressed and often terrified, with consequent behaviour disturbance. The principle of management using this model is to identify probable causes for the initial clouding of consciousness and to intervene at an early stage in the process of misinterpretation with reassurance, explanation, and drug therapy as appropriate.

Common causes of confusion in cancer patients are drugs, in particular opioids, steroids, and sedatives, drug withdrawal (for example, alcohol, diazepam, and benzodiazepine hypnotics), metabolic causes such as hypercalcaemia, hyponatraemia, uraemia, and liver failure, infections, particularly urinary and chest, hypoglycaemia, hypoxia, and cerebral metastases. A careful drug history and routine biochemical screen are important before instituting treatment in

a confused patient and a mid-stream urine specimen and chest radiography may be indicated.

During the period of investigation, where no particular cause is found or where confusion persists despite attention to underlying causes, psychotropic drugs may be required as the patient becomes increasingly disturbed and agitated. Haloperidol in oral doses of 1.5 mg to 3 or 5 mg twice daily is usually effective, but intramuscular administration may be necessary if the patient is acutely disturbed or distressed. If anxiety or agitation is prominent without hallucinations or disturbed behaviour, diazepam may be adequate.

In some patients a more sedative drug is required, in which case thioridazine or chlorpromazine may be given orally, rectally, or intramuscularly.

Terminal restlessness

Some patients who are near to death are restless despite what appears to be adequate pain control. Patients in this situation are often managed with subcutaneous infusions of an opioid analgesic. Methotrimeprazine added to the infusion may be helpful if restlessness is a problem. Midazolam (a water soluble benzodiazepine) may also be used in this way and is generally less sedative than methotrimeprazine.

Insomnia

In the light of the many symptoms which the patient with advanced cancer may suffer, it is hardly surprising that difficulty in sleeping also occurs. Common underlying causes include persisting pain, nausea, vomiting, anxiety, depression, cough, dyspnoea, urinary frequency, or pruritis. Identification and modification of such problems is the mainstay of treatment, but for many a regular hypnotic drug will be required. When choosing night sedation it is important to select a drug which has a short half-life, producing sleep for the required 8 h or so without a hangover effect throughout the next day. The most appropriate drugs in this setting are temazepam, triazolam, and chlormethiazole. If the sleep disturbance is related to depression, a sedative antidepressant such as dothiepin or mianserin may be preferable to a simple hypnotic.

Weakness

General debility and increasing withdrawal from active tasks is a recognized feature of progressive cancer. This must be distinguished from the physical weakness due to specific pathological processes such as cerebral metastasis, spinal cord or cauda equina compression, peripheral neuropathy, myopathy, myositis, or the Eaton–Lambert syndrome. Despite the presence of advanced disease a careful history and examination to identify those patients with a specific reversible cause of weakness is important, since early diagnosis and appropriate treatment may prevent progressive neurological deterioration.

Where there is progressive generalized weakness with advanced disease, other underlying causes should also be considered and, if appropriate, corrected. These include anaemia, dehydration, hypokalaemia, hypomagnesaemia, hyponatraemia, acute or chronic infection, and depression. The cycle of increasing weakness, resulting in prolonged immobilization, muscle wasting, and further weakness, may be prevented by appropriate physiotherapy and occupational therapy. Specific measures may include the use of steroids to elevate mood and stimulate appetite, although even relatively short-term use may lead to proximal myopathy, reducing mobility further.

Alongside the physical aspects of weakness, the psychological impact of increasing debility, helplessness, dependence, and loss of self-respect and identity will require careful and sympathetic support. With patients who have come to terms with their impending death, many of the above measures will be both inappropriate and unwelcome as they undergo a peaceful decline in physical capacity. For others there will be a continued need to strive against their decline as they seek to continue the fight against their cancer. Therefore, as for all symptoms, careful analysis and diagnosis is required before deciding on treatment for an individual patient. A balance should be sought between preventing unnecessary and reversible disability and enabling a peaceful decline in physical activity.

Fits

Fits are relatively rare compared with many of the symptoms discussed above, but are the cause of considerable distress and anxiety to the sufferer and his or her relatives and to fellow patients. Causes include intracranial tumour, either primary or metastatic, metabolic disturbances such as hypoglycaemia, hyponatraemia, hypercalcaemia, hypomagnesaemia, and hypoxia, or drugs including opioids, phenothiazines, and antidepressants.

Management is aimed at prevention by correction of metabolic disturbances or modification of the drug regimen, together with the use of anticonvulsants.

CONCLUSIONS

Much can be done to alleviate the symptoms of patients with advanced and terminal cancer. The principles of symptom management are to make a diagnosis of the cause or mechanism underlying each problem, to tailor the treatment to the individual patient, and to use the simplest effective measures.

Symptom control is the cornerstone of palliative medicine, but it should not be seen as an end in itself. The purpose is to return the patient to as normal a life as possible. This will involve not only restoration of function and relief of symptoms, but also physical, emotional, and practical support. The essence of palliation in cancer when cure is not possible is to enable patients to live whatever life remains to them as fully as possible. In order to achieve this, a logical and integrated approach is required with coordination and cooperation from the various disciplines which may be involved.

Palliative care does not imply that no further active treatment is available. Rather it should be part of a spectrum of treatment whose focus has changed from attempting to cure the disease to enabling patients to live well despite it. Patients with incurable cancer may feel that medicine has failed them. Even if their distressing symptoms are relieved, they may be worried about what is to come and can often feel isolated and hopeless. Great comfort can be given merely by showing a commitment to share the burden with them and by reassurance that they will not be abandoned. Continuity of care, support, and follow-up are just as important as any pharmacological or physical treatment. These sentiments are reflected in the way in which palliative care services are developing, with an emphasis on rehabilitation and home care wherever possible. These subjects are discussed in the following chapters.

REFERENCES

Arnott S (1987). Role of radiotherapy in the treatment of metastatic cancer. In *Management of metastases* (ed. M Slevin), pp. 537–50. Baillière Tindall, London.
Baines M (1993). The pathophysiology and management of malignant intentional obstruction. In *Textbook of palliative medicine* (ed. D Doyle, GWC Hanks, and N MacDonald). Oxford University Press, Oxford.
Beaver WT (1981). Aspirin and acetaminophen as constituents of analgesic combinations. *Archives of Internal Medicine*, **141**:293–300.

Bennett A (1988). The role of biochemical mediators in peripheral nociception and bone pain. *Cancer Surveys*, **7**:55–67.
Bruera E, Chadwick S, Brenneis S, Hanson J, MacDonald RN (1987). Methylphenidate associated with narcotics for the treatment of cancer pain. *Cancer Treatment Reports*, **71**:67–70.
Chronos N, Adams L, Guz A (1988). Effect of hyperoxia and hypoxia on exercise induced breathlessness in normal subjects. *Clinical Science*, **74**:531–7.
Cowcher K, Hanks GW (1990). Long term management of respiratory symptoms in advanced cancer. *Journal of Pain and Symptom Management*, **5**:320–30.
Derogatis LR, *et al.* (1983). The prevalence of psychiatric disorders among cancer patients. *Journal of the American Medical Association*, **249**:751–7.
Elomaa I, *et al.* (1983). Long-term controlled trial with diphosphonate in patients with osteolytic bone metastases. *Lancet*, i:146–9.
Filshie J (1988). The non-drug treatment of neuralgic and neuropathic pain of malignancy. *Cancer Surveys*, **7**:161–93.
Foley K (1985). The treatment of cancer pain. *New England Journal of Medicine*, **313**:84–93.
Hanks GW (1984). Psychotropic drugs. *Clinics in Oncology*, **3**:135–51.
Hanks GW (1988). The pharmacological treatment of bone pain. *Cancer Surveys*, **7**:87–101.
Hanks GW, Hoskin PJ (1987). Opioid analgesics in the management of pain in patients with cancer. A review. *Palliative Medicine*, **1**:1–25.
Hanks GW, Twycross RG, Lloyd JW (1981). Unexpected complication of successful nerve block: morphine induced respiratory depression following removal of severe pain. *Anaesthesia*, **36**:37–9.
Hanks GW, Hoskin PJ, Aherne GW, Turner P, Poulain, P (1987). Explanation for potency of repeated oral doses of morphine? *Lancet*, ii.723–5.
Hanna M, Peat SJ, Woodham MJ, Latham J, Gouliaris A, Di Vadi P (1989). The use of coeliac plexus blockade in patients with chronic pain. *Palliative Medicine*, **4**:11–16.
Heyes Moore L (1984). Respiratory symptoms. In *Management of terminal malignant disease* (2nd edn) (ed. C Saunders), pp. 113–18. Arnold, London.
Hoskin PJ, Hanks GW (1988). The management of symptoms in advanced cancer: experience in a hospital-based continuing care unit. *Journal of the Royal Society of Medicine*, **81**:341–4.
Hoskin PJ, Poulain P, Hanks GW (1989). Controlled-release morphine in cancer pain: is a loading dose required when the formulation is changed? *Anaesthesia*, **44**:897–901.
Inturrisi CE, Max MB, Foley KM, Schultz M, Shin SU, Houde RW (1984). The pharmacokinetics of heroin in patients with chronic pain. *New England Journal of Medicine*, **310**:1213–17.
Ketcham AS, Hoye RC, Pilch YH, Morton DL (1970). Delayed intestinal obstruction following treatment of cancer. *Cancer*, **25**:406–10.
Mansi J, Hanks GW (1989). Management of symptoms in advanced cancer. *Update*, **39**:82–94.
Morgan M (1989). The rational use of intrathecal and extradural opioids. *British Journal of Anaesthesia*, **63**:165–88.
Morris JN, Mor V, Goldberg RJ, Sherwood S, Greer DS, Hiris J (1986). The effect of treatment setting and patient characteristics on pain in terminal cancer patients: a report from the national hospice study. *Journal of Chronic Disease*, **39**:27–35.
Mortimer PS, Badger C, Hall JG (1993). Lymphoedema. In *Oxford textbook of palliative medicine* (ed. D Doyle, GWC Haule, and N MacDonald). Oxford University Press, Oxford.
Oliver DJ (1985). The use of the syringe driver in terminal care. *British Journal of Clinical Pharmacology*, **20**:515–16.
Paterson AHG, Powles TJ, Kamis JA, McCloskey E, Hanson J, Ashley S (1993). Double-blind controlled trial of oral clodronate in patients with bone metastases from breast cancer. *Journal of Clinical Oncology*, **11**:59–65.
Pfleiderer AG, Goodall P, Holmes, GKT (1982). The consequences and effectiveness of intubation in the palliation of dysphagia due to benign and malignant strictures affecting the oesophagus. *British Journal of Surgery*, **69**:356–8.
Piver MS, Barlow JJ, Lele SB, Frank A (1982). Survival after ovarian cancer-induced intestinal obstruction. *Gynecologic Oncology*, **13**:44–9.
Ralston SH (1992). Medical management of hypercalcaemia. *British Journal of Clinical Pharmacology*, **34**:11–20.

Riley J, Fallon MT (1994). Octreotide in terminal malignant obstruction of the gastrointestinal tract. *European Journal of Palliative Care*, 1:23–5.

Simon B, Damman HG, Lenght U, Muller P. Ranitidine in the therapy of NSAID-induced gastroduodenal lesions. *Scandinavian Journal of Gastroenterology*, 23 (Suppl. 154):18–21.

Stedeford A (1985). *Facing death*. Heinemann, London.

Sykes NP, Baines M, Carter RL (1988). Clinical and pathological study of dysphagia conservatively managed in patients with advanced malignant disease. *Lancet*, ii:726–8.

Twycross RG, Fairfield S (1982). Pain in far-advanced cancer. *Pain*, 14:303–10.

Twycross RG, Lack SA (1983). *Symptom control in far advanced cancer: pain relief*. Pitman, London.

Twycross RG, Lack SA (1987). *Symptom control in far advanced cancer: alimentary symptoms*. Pitman, London.

Wells JCD (1989). The use of nerve destruction for relief of pain in cancer: a review. *Palliative Medicine*, 3:239–47.

White ID, Hoskin PJ, Hanks GW, Bliss JM (1991). Analgesics in cancer pain: current practice and beliefs. *British Journal of Cancer*, 63:271–4.

Woodcock AA, Gross ER, Gellert A, Shah S, Johnson M, Geddes DM (1981). Effects of dihydrocodeine, alcohol and caffeine on breathlessness and exercise tolerance in patients with chronic obstructive airways disease and normal blood gases. *New England Journal of Medicine*, 305:1611–16.

WHO (1986). *Cancer pain relief*, pp. 5–70. WHO, Geneva.

Young RR, Delwaide PJ (1981). Spasticity. *New England Journal of Medicine*, 304:96–9.

20.6   Rehabilitation of the cancer patient

R. TIFFANY, CLAIRE MOYNIHAN, AND MICHAEL BRADA

INTRODUCTION

> Rehabilitation broadly conceived, is the restoration of a patient with residual defects as a result of his disease, or its treatment, to as normal a functional state as possible. (Gunn 1984).

Improvements in early diagnosis and greater effectiveness of modalities of treatment ensure that many of those diagnosed with malignant disease will be long-term survivors. The life which has been preserved through treatment must have quality and meaning.

The rehabilitation needs of people with cancer were considered of secondary importance to curative treatments or were not recognized until they had become chronic and more difficult to treat. If the developments in treating malignant disease are to be truly effective we must ensure that rehabilitation is assigned greater importance in the individual's plan of treatment. There are three major groups in cancer care where rehabilitation has a vital rôle.

The first group includes patients with good life expectancy whose treatment has left no residual disfigurement or disability. They may require some physical services and psychological support to enable them to resocialize and break away from their rôle of cancer sufferer.

The second group also have a good life expectancy, but have become physically or psychologically disabled and may require intensive multidisciplinary rehabilitation to redress physical and psychological deficits.

The third group are those who have failed to respond to treatment and for whom life expectancy is limited. They will require access to a full range of rehabilitation services to restore optimum function and allow them to return home and, if possible, to return to work and enjoy an enhanced quality of life for the remainder of their lives.

Successful rehabilitation for all groups must be seen to be proactive. In all stages, types, and treatments of malignant disease we should be aware of the sequelae of the disease and treatment; rehabilitation should be instituted at the onset of treatment and form part of the initial and ongoing treatment plan.

The development of multidisciplinary oncology teams has ensured greater collaboration between the various medical and surgical specialties in cancer care and this has encouraged the use of a variety of treatment modalities to control the disease. Similar progress is necessary in rehabilitation, with the formation of multiprofessional teams who can devise and implement relevant strategies for each patient. The creation of a rehabilitation department within cancer centres would ensure geographical proximity and facilitate multiprofessional rehabilitation planning and practice. It would also encourage research into the outcomes of rehabilitation and the introduction of innovative strategies to improve patient care.

The rehabilitation problems vary between individuals and the types of cancer and rehabilitation must be able to offer a flexible multidisciplinary service with interdisciplinary referrals, use of joint care plans, and regular multidisciplinary meetings. Ideally, a rehabilitation oncology team should include physiotherapy, dietetics, occupational therapy, speech therapy, patient education and health promotion, chaplaincy (all faiths), appliance fitting, chiropody, dental hygiene, therapeutic arts, diversional therapy, nursing, including specialists in breast care, community liaison, lymphoedema, psychological support, stoma care and massage, and all disciplines of medicine. Patients referred to the rehabilitation team should remain the responsibility of their primary medical practitioner who will monitor their progress and meet regularly with rehabilitation practitioners.

Regarding patients with cancer in the same way as any individuals with other chronic disease helps to recognize what recovery or cure will mean if they are destined to spend the remainder of their life secluded from society or totally dependent upon others. Therefore, rehabilitation cannot be viewed as a functional phenomena; rather it is a care philosophy which must be understood by and relevant to all health care providers.

PSYCHOLOGICAL THERAPY

The traumatic effects of cancer treatment on a patient's emotional well-being has been well documented. Although most people cope remarkably well, it is clear that cancer exacts a severe toll in some patients and their families. Cancer-related psychological and social morbidity may persist for many years, even in the absence of any signs of disease (Fobair *et al.* 1986; Moynihan 1987). A vivid description of such patients has been given by Naysmith *et al.* (1983).

> ... One sees a patient whose confidence in life has been completely destroyed by the experience of cancer. From seeing himself as a fit person, he has suddenly been faced with a terrifying and life-threatening illness, often when he is still at a relatively young age. His image of himself becomes that of an invalid, liable at any time to be overwhelmed by a further episode of illness or by death. He is often very slow to regain a belief in a worthwhile future. Such patients typically do not go back to work, even when physically well, and are inappropriately distressed by a host of very minor physical symptoms. They are frequently anxious, guilty and depressed.

The need for psychological therapy

What can be done to prevent or ameliorate such evident morbidity? Often it is assumed that, since emotional distress is an inevitable and understandable consequence of cancer, psychological treatment is neither feasible nor indicated. This assumption is now thought to be incorrect and is reflected in the increasing attention given to the construction of appropriate instruments and evaluation of the physical and emotional well-being of cancer patients, both in the short- and long-term. However, while the quality of a patient's life is generally considered to be an essential end-point to treatment and/or survival, those involved in cancer clinical trials have, hitherto given this aspect of care only 'lip service'. This, and the fact that the psychological aspects of medical care have been given low priority has made it difficult to (1) systematically establish the prevalence of morbidity and (2) to evaluate psychological interventions in an effort to alleviate such morbidity. In the last few years, however, there has been an attempt to conduct methodologically sound trials in order to demonstrate the efficacy of psychological therapy.

Methodological issues

Any evaluation of a psychological intervention is beset with daunting methodological problems. Difficulties centre around a lack of any clear counselling model being employed; an inadequately trained counsellor providing intervention and the use of outcome measures of efficacy that are too gross to pick up subtle but meaningful and important change (Fallowfield *et al.* 1992). Other important information such as how frequency of contact is determined or how patients are recruited or referred for counselling is omitted in the reporting (Fallowfield 1993). In addition, much of the research available that purports to show benefit often does not use a control group; intervention and assessment is administered by the same researcher; inappropriate statistics are used and the sample is too small for formal statistical analysis. Refusal to participate in studies can be high, due to a belief that to talk is to exacerbate the problem. People are known to feel stigmatized as a result of psychological 'labelling' and other barriers such as geographical location of the patient, financial and transport difficulties makes it difficult to recruit adequate numbers for results to be valid. Interestingly randomization is seldom given as the reason for refusal (Greer *et al.* 1992). Difficulties in recruiting sufficient patients for psychological intervention trials can be overcome to some extent by screening large numbers for psychological morbidity and carefully explaining

the rationale of randomized trials. One of the most important factors, however, is the support of clinicians; their active encouragement to patients to take part in trials of this kind may possibly increase patient compliance.

Current status of psychological therapy

Several randomized controlled trials of psychological therapy with cancer patients have been reported (Farash 1979; Maguire *et al.* 1980; Spiegel *et al.* 1981; Linn *et al.* 1982; Cain *et al.* 1986; Telch and Telch 1986; Watson *et al.* 1988; Greer *et al.* 1992, 1994) but it is difficult to make categorical statements regarding the efficacy of psychological therapy in alleviating psychosocial morbidity in cancer patients for the reasons discussed above. In general, results of studies carried out in oncology settings are equivocal (Massie *et al.* 1989). A few methodologically sound studies report benefit (Spiegel *et al.* 1989; Greer *et al.* 1992, 1994), rendering it possible to make some provisional conclusions.

1. While a few randomized controlled trials demonstrate that psychological therapy is associated with improvement in psychological and/or social adjustment, other studies have also failed to show any improvement.
2. Patients with advanced metastatic disease, as well as those with local or locoregional disease, have been shown to benefit from psychological therapy.
3. Psychological therapy is (i) acceptable to the majority of cancer patients who show evidence of significant psychological distress and (ii) feasible in oncology units.
4. There is insufficient evidence upon which to judge the relative merits of individual versus group therapy.
5. Further research is required to determine which specific psychotherapeutic procedures produce the greatest benefit.
6. Therapies which are based on cognitive theory and include the teaching of active coping strategies appear more effective in patients who have high levels of psychological morbidity than simple counselling intervention.

Specific treatments have been developed to enable patients to cope with a variety of cancer-related symptoms (Watson 1991). Adjuvant psychological therapy (APT) has been devised for cancer patients and has been subjected to randomized controlled trials (Greer *et al.* 1992, 1994).

Adjuvant psychological therapy

Adjuvant psychological therapy (APT) is not related to so-called 'alternative treatments' but is used only in conjunction with orthodox medical treatment for patients with cancer. It is also not counselling, although this may be included when necessary as a part of the therapy. ATP is based on cognitive therapy and on empirical data obtained from systematic clinical studies of cancer patients (for a detailed description see Moorey and Greer 1989).

Aims

1. To reduce anxiety, depression and other psychiatric symptoms.
2. To improve mental adjustment to cancer by inducing a positive 'fighting spirit' attitude.
3. To promote in patients a sense of personal control over their lives and active participation in the treatment of their cancer.
4. To assist patients to develop effective coping strategies for dealing with cancer-related problems and with other stressful situations.

5. To improve communication between the patient and the spouse or partner.

6. To encourage open expression of feelings, particularly anger and other negative feelings.

Theoretical basis

Cognitive therapy, as developed by Beck (1976) and others, aims to improve emotional disorders by identifying and altering maladaptive thinking. This tenet may be applied to cancer-related psychological morbidity. According to cognitive theory, such morbidity depends not only on the medical consequences of cancer (and its treatments) but also on two crucial factors.

1. The personal meaning of the disease; that is, how the individual perceives cancer and its implications.

2. The individual's coping ability; that is, the cognitive and behavioural attempts to reduce the threat posed by cancer.

For example, a diagnosis of breast cancer will be perceived as a challenge by patient A who will then cope by adopting a fighting spirit ('How can I beat this disease?'). For patient B, however, the same diagnosis denotes a death sentence; she will be unable to cope and her quality of life will be greatly reduced by feelings of helplessness and hopelessness.

The personal perceptions of cancer and coping ability are crucial determinants of psychological adjustment of the disease. It is these aspects on which adjuvant psychological therapy is focused. Since the patient's perceptions of cancer and ability to cope are influenced by the emotional support of those closest to him or her (Lichtman and Taylor 1986), the spouse or partner is included in therapy where possible.

As a general rule, cancer patients do not show evidence of psychopathology; their psychological disorders are regarded as those of essentially normal persons under severe stress. It follows that adjuvant psychological therapy should be directed primarily at current problems and that it should highlight and foster the patient's personal strengths.

Description

APT is conducted with individual patients and, where possible, with the spouse or partner. Approximately six sessions, each lasting 1 h, are held; occasionally more sessions are required. The therapeutic relationship is a collaborative one in which the therapist and patient set an agreed agenda, defining the specific problems to be addressed. Depression, anxious preoccupation with cancer, feelings of helplessness and uncertainty about the future, difficulties in communicating with one's spouse and family, loss of self-esteem, and sexual dysfunction associated with mutilating surgery and chemotherapy are among the major problems encountered. Before such problems can be addressed in therapy, a clinical psychiatric examination is carried out to determine the degree of depression and consequent need for antidepressant medication. Having defined the major problems, these are tackled using a variety of cognitive and behavioural techniques (see below). However, as with other psychotherapies, the adjuvant psychological therapist requires the qualities of empathy, warmth, and genuineness, as well as the ability to listen closely and to reflect accurately what the patient feels and thinks. These qualities are essential for a collaborative therapeutic relationship upon which the success of cognitive and behavioural techniques depends.

During adjuvant psychological therapy sessions patients are taught new coping strategies; this process is reinforced by homework assignments. The main procedures used are as follows.

1. Cognitive techniques. Patients are taught to identify and keep a record of illogical negative thoughts. They are then shown how to challenge them using reality testing: 'What is the evidence?'. In this way the negative thoughts can be replaced by more realistic adaptive coping responses (Moorey and Greer 1989). Among other techniques used is cognitive rehearsal. Impending stressful events and ways of coping with them are rehearsed, in imagination and rôle play.

2. Behavioural techniques. Relaxation training is a useful coping strategy for anxious patients. Patients who feel helpless are given behavioural assignments to enable them to develop a sense of self-esteem. They are encouraged to carry out various activities which give (i) a sense of mastery or control over some aspects of their lives and (ii) a sense of pleasure. The patient's personal strengths are identified and fostered as a means of overcoming feelings of helplessness and replacing these with a positive attitude.

3. Ventilation of feelings. Throughout adjuvant psychological therapy, the importance of open emotional expression is emphasized. This applies particularly to anger, since many cancer patients feel that they should not burden their families and friends with negative feelings about the illness. Where the partner can be included in therapy, frank mutual communication of feelings is encouraged during joint sessions.

PHYSIOTHERAPY IN CANCER REHABILITATION

At some stage during their disease many cancer patients will experience either a decline in their physical ability or an increase in symptoms. Physiotherapy is frequently necessary to overcome such problems and all oncology units should have access to a physiotherapy service. The rôle of physiotherapy in oncology can be divided into restoration of function, symptom control, and respiratory care.

Restoration of function

Physiotherapy aims to maintain and improve functional ability and, hence, independence. Causes of loss of function include hemiplegia arising from disease in the brain, shoulder stiffness following surgery or radiotherapy to the axilla, peripheral neuropathy with muscle atrophy as a side-effect of chemotherapy, or amputation of a limb. Physiotherapy will play a major part in restoring patients to their usual life-style or enabling them to manage any residual disability. The following two examples show how this can be achieved.

Physiotherapy in management of soft tissue sarcomas of the extremities

Combined modality treatment with radiotherapy and surgery has become standard in the management of patients with soft tissue sarcomas of the extremities. This may lead to lymphoedema, pain, decreased joint mobility and muscle power, causing mobility problems particularly with lesions of the lower limb (Marsha et al. 1984). Physiotherapy can reduce or eliminate many such problems. Passive stretching and active and resisted exercise prevent joint contractures, increase joint range of movement, and rebuild muscle power. Gait re-education can often restore a normal walking pattern and orthoses (for example, foot-drop appliances and knee braces) can help compensate for any permanent dysfunction that may occur as a result of surgical excision of a major nerve or muscle group. Early advice on the long-term management of swelling can prevent lymphoedema formation.

Physiotherapy management of primary spinal cord tumour

The level of the spinal cord tumour will be an important determinant of potential functional ability (Blocker 1972). Cervical lesion causing quadriplegia will dictate that the patient will require very substantial assistance. Patients with lower cervical lesions (C5–C7) may eventually be able to feed or partly groom themselves with the assistance of adapted hand devices. Lesions in the upper thoracic region and below cause paraplegia, but such patients may achieve complete wheelchair independence. In all instances a programme of passive movement and chest physiotherapy should be instigated as early as possible to prevent joint contracture and pulmonary infection. The main thrust of treatment is directed towards building up existing muscle groups and teaching activities such as wheelchair transfers in order to maximize independence. If any improvement of the paralysis takes place, physiotherapy techniques first to initiate muscle contraction (for example, proprioceptive neuromuscular facilitation) and then to strengthen muscles are used and the patient is taught how to use mobility aids (for example, walking frames and crutches) safely.

Symptom control

The palliative rôle of physiotherapy is important and is demonstrated in two examples.

Pain

Cancer pain may have many different components and the assessor should always consider physical methods of relief as they are often both effective and inexpensive. These include electrotherapy (for example, interferential and ultrasonic therapy), hot and cold therapies (for example, infrared and ice), massage, exercise, and transcutaneous electrical nerve stimulation.

Physiotherapy may effectively alleviate pain of spasm of the paraspinal muscles secondary to metastatic vertebral collapse, where relief is gained with the use of gentle massage or heat. Metastatic bone pain in the lower limb can be considerably relieved by supplying walking aids (for example, crutches). Providing a suitable sling to a patient with a upper limb lymphoedema can reduce pain caused by traction on the brachial plexus. Transcutaneous electrical nerve stimulation has been demonstrated to control incisional pain (Vander Ark and McGrath 1975) and interferential therapy is effective in the management of neurogenic pain such as post-herpetic neuralgia and phantom limb pain (Wells et al. 1988).

Pain prevention is also an important area for the physiotherapist; a painful 'dropped shoulder' syndrome can arise following radical neck dissection with removal of the spinal accessory nerve and consequent paralysis of the trapezius muscle (Short et al. 1984). Advice, together with exercise regimes designed to prevent contractures of the pectoralis major and strengthen the levator scapulae, rhomboid, and serratus anterior muscles, can reduce the incidence.

Respiratory care

Physiotherapy can be used to prevent and treat atelectasis and sputum retention. Patients undergoing major oncological surgery, particularly to the thorax or upper abdomen, will require respiratory physiotherapy from the first post-operative day as pulmonary function will be impaired as a result of long anaesthesia, surgical interruption of respiratory musculature, and pain. Chest physiotherapy may also be useful in the management of bacterial chest infection (for example, in the immunosuppressed patient) and when ventilatory dysfunction occurs as a result of neurological deficit. Techniques include breathing exercises, chest manipulation (for example, percussion, vibrations, rib springing), postural drainage, forced expiratory techniques, incentive spirometry, intermittent positive pressure breathing, and continuous positive airways pressure.

OCCUPATIONAL THERAPY IN CANCER REHABILITATION

From a rehabilitation point of view, cancer presents in much the same way as other conditions (for example, cerebral vascular accidents, fractures, and paraplegia) and the occupational therapist could use techniques and skills appropriate to treat them. However, the approach to cancer rehabilitation is different. The patient may be severely ill, suffering from the side-effects of chemotherapy and radiotherapy, often has an uncertain prognosis, and has to cope with the psychological implications of the disease.

Using techniques of observation, interviewing, and physical examination the occupational therapist should assess:

(1) physical abilities;

(2) functional abilities (for example, self-care activities, work);

(3) psychological state;

(4) social environment.

It is important to consider the patient's perception of his or her abilities and problems. A treatment programme should take into account previous life-style, his or her own aims, the desires of the family, and the problem areas identified by the occupational therapist.

Cancer is an illness which can lead to feelings of having lost control over oneself and one's environment. It is important to include the patient to provide a sense of control and thereby increase motivation. Assessment of the cancer patient needs to continue as treatment begins before the medical condition is stabilized.

Occupational therapists specialize in activity analysis. For example, a basic activity of daily living such as dressing can be analysed in terms of:

(1) motivation;

(2) concentration;

(3) coordination;

(4) balance;

(5) gross and fine range of movement in the upper and lower limbs;

(6) unimpaired body image;

(7) spatial awareness;

(8) figure–ground discrimination;

(9) sequencing.

Treatment of the specific dysfunction may involve the following.

1. Correcting the underlying problems, for example using a specific activity with the intention of encouraging a specific movement.

2. Teaching alternative methods, for example energy conservation.

3. Provision of adaptive equipment to enable function.

Part of discharge planning may include an assessment of the environment in which the patient has to function. This may be school, work, or home.

Cancer is an illness which has a large psychological component. Decreasing ability and loss of former rôle in life can lead to feelings of anger, frustration, hopelessness, and inadequacy. The occupational therapist can use techniques such as projective art and rôle play to help the patient acknowledge and express these feelings. The aim of occupational therapy intervention is to enable a person to lead as purposeful and satisfying a life as possible within the constraints of the disability, regardless of life expectancy.

NUTRITIONAL REHABILITATION OF THE PATIENT WITH CANCER

Cancer is often associated with the development of weight loss or malnutrition. In its extreme manifestation it is referred to as cancer cachexia. Weight loss is an easily measurable entity. Cancer-induced malnutrition can be described as an imbalance of energy intake and energy expenditure resulting in changes in body composition (von Meyenfeldt et al. 1988). This definition covers not only weight loss but loss of body fat or protein stores combined with unaltered weight.

Between 3 and 38 per cent of cancer patients show signs of severe malnutrition and up to 80 per cent showing signs of mild malnutrition (von Meyenfeldt et al. 1980). The mean incidence of severe malnutrition is approximately 10 per cent (Muller et al. 1986; Busby et al. 1988).

The presence of poor nutritional status has been associated with increased complication rates, decreased performance status, and decreased survival. There is a good correlation between weight loss and performance status: the more severe the weight loss, the worse the performance status (De Wys et al. 1980). Weight losses associated with decreased responses to chemotherapy (Carbonne et al. 1971; Bonadonna et al. 1986). In surgical cases, Muller et al. (1986) reported complication rates of up to 70 per cent in malnourished patients, with mortality reaching 90 per cent in severely malnourished patients.

Malnutrition in patients with cancer is caused by changes in metabolism and food intake (Wesdorp et al. 1983; von Meyenfeldt et al. 1988). These alterations result in increased energy expenditure through changes in intermediate metabolism and a failure to adapt to starvation.

A reduction in food intake may be caused by anorexia, dysgeusia, ageusia, nausea, vomiting, dysphagia, or malabsorption. These may be due to the disease itself, the side-effects of treatment, or a combination of both.

Anorexia is the most frequent eating difficulty found in cancer patients (De Wys 1979; Calman 1982). In a study of 110 patients admitted for primary treatment, 50 per cent of those with gastric cancer and 40 per cent of those with colorectal cancer were eating less than 80 per cent of their total energy intake before illness (von Meyenfeldt et al. 1988). Several explanations have been proposed for the aetiology of anorexia in cancer patients. De Wys (1979) suggested that the normal appetite control mechanism may be negatively affected by taste changes, decreased gastric secretions, and increased satiety, leading to a diminished appetite. Psychological factors such as anxiety or depression may also influence appetite (Holland 1977). Common side-effects of disease or treatment, such

Table 1 Nutritional problems associated with cancer and its treatment

Problem	Cause	Suggested dietary advice
Loss of appetite	Disease state	Small nourishing meals
	Chemotherapy	Between-meal snacks and/or nourishing drinks
	Radiotherapy	Energy/protein supplements, appetite stimulants (e.g. alcohol, steroids)
		Supplementary nasogastric feeding may be necessary
Nausea	Disease state	Small frequent meals
	Chemotherapy	Avoidance of cooking smells
	Radiotherapy to upper gastrointestinal tract	Short walk before meals, if possible
		Dry meals
		Drinks separate from meals
		Plain biscuits, dry toast
		Cold foods
		Reduce very sweet or very fatty foods
		Fizzy drinks may help
Dysphagia	Carcinoma of oesophagus	Small frequent meals of soft liquid diet
	Oral surgery	Nourishing drinks
	Oesophageal tubes	Fizzy drinks may clear oesophageal tubes
	Radiotherapy to mouth	Tube feeding may be necessary
Ageusia/dysgeusia	Some chemotherapy regimes	Avoidance of foods which accentuate unpleasant taste
Diarrhoea	Radiotherapy to lower abdomen	Low-fibre diet with high fluid intake
	Some chemotherapy regimes	Suggest use of antidiarrhoea agents
Constipation	Some chemotherapy regimes	High-fibre diet
	Use of narcotic drugs in pain relief	Plenty of fluids
		Suggest possible use of laxatives
Malabsorption	Radiotherapy or surgery to lower gastrointestinal tract	Low-fat diet
	Fistula	Low-fibre diet
		Lactose-free diet
		Chemical defined fluid diet (e.g. Vivonex, Flexical, Nutranel, etc.)
		Total parenteral nutrition
		All above as appropriate for type of malabsorption problem

as bowel obstruction, constipation, diarrhoea, and nausea, all tend to lead to poor appetite.

Correcting poor nutritional states is an important part of rehabilitation. This reduces complications and may improve well-being and quality of life. Even in the palliation of advanced disease, nutritional support may help to correct problems arising from anorexia and weight loss and relieve some of the symptoms associated with the cachectic state.

Nutritional support can range from simple encouragement and general dietary advice to complex enteral and parenteral feeding regimes. Some of the commonest nutritional problems and appropriate nutritional solutions are given in Table 1.

REHABILITATION FOR WOMEN UNDERGOING BREAST CANCER SURGERY

The aim of rehabilitation for women undergoing surgery for primary breast cancer is to facilitate the restoration of previous levels of physical and psychosocial health where possible. This will begin prior to surgery and continue for a variable period beyond it, with the involvement of many members of the multidisciplinary team within both the hospital and community settings.

Physical rehabilitation

Physical rehabilitation will depend on the type of operation and the type of adjuvant therapy. Both chemotherapy and radiotherapy can be expected to cause fatigue and lengthen the period of physical rehabilitation.

The two most common physical problems experienced following breast surgery are impaired shoulder movement and arm oedema (see below) following axillary dissection or radiotherapy to the axilla. The incidence is reduced with post-operative physiotherapy and instruction on exercises (Pollard et al. 1976; Wingate 1985). The combination of radiotherapy and surgery to the axilla is associated with worse problems (Atkins et al. 1972; Pollard et al. 1976; Swedborg and Wallgren 1981; Rytlor et al. 1983).

Although general agreement exists regarding the value of post-operative physiotherapy there is controversy on the most appropriate timing. Loitz et al. found that women who had performed extensive abduction and flexion exercises from the first post-operative day had more wound drainage, delayed wound healing, and a longer hospital stay than women starting exercises 7 days later. There was no difference in shoulder movement or oedema at 1, 3, or 6 months. However, Wingate (1985) reported that early physiotherapy did not increase wound complications and improved the rate at which shoulder function returned to normal.

Early but limited shoulder movement is encouraged, with the amount of abduction, adduction, flexion, and external rotation exercises gradually increased once wound drainage has significantly reduced. Restrictions may be imposed if the scar is very tight or after breast reconstruction.

Where possible, a physiotherapist should see a woman pre-operatively to assess shoulder movement and discuss post-operative exercises. Information sheets with diagrams are helpful reinforcers of what exercises to do, when, and for how long. Initially exercises may include full hand, wrist, and elbow movements, shoulder shrugging, and moving hands from shoulders to head, gradually moving on to brushing hair, doing up back fastenings on brassieres and clothes, and walking fingers up the wall. Exercises are recommended at least four times a day for 2 months and then once

or twice a day for a year to ensure that full movement is maintained whilst scar contraction is occurring. If previous normal movement is not attained after approximately 6 weeks, the woman should know how to contact the physiotherapist or doctor for further assessment. Many women may need reassurance that exercises will not cause the wound to burst although they may cause discomfort and regular mild analgesia may be necessary for 2 weeks or more. However, pain is a limiting factor and no shoulder exercise should be forced.

Prior to discharge every woman should receive information about hand and arm care to reduce the likelihood of lymphoedema and cellulitis and information concerning parasthaesia if axillary surgery has been performed. Many women are concerned about how long it will take to attain their 'normal' energy level, when they will be able to undertake work and household duties again, and when they can drive a car. Information in these areas is likely to reduce the anxiety experienced and increase the feelings of control the woman has over the recovery of her arm.

Everyone recovers from surgery at a different rate, but many women find that it takes many months or even a year before they feel that they are physically completely back to normal. A lack of energy seems to be the most frustrating factor and reassurance that nothing else is wrong may be needed.

Breast prosthetics and clothing advice

Fitting a woman with a breast prosthesis to wear in her brassiere is an essential part of rehabilitation after surgery where all or a substantial part of her breast has been removed. The prosthesis should ensure that she looks completely normal in clothing and feels confident about her appearance.

A soft temporary prosthesis should be fitted before leaving hospital and worn for 5 weeks until the wound is healed or until 2 weeks after radiotherapy has finished. A silicone prosthesis can then be fitted to achieve a virtually identical appearance to the other breast. Silicone prostheses usually last for 2–3 years. Silicone nipples are also available and may be particularly desired for use with swimsuits, T-shirts, or evening wear or following breast reconstruction where no nipple has been created.

The standard of prosthetic service varies widely. Thirty per cent of women in 34 areas did not receive temporary prostheses and 46 per cent were not happy with the permanent prosthesis they received. Most (67 per cent) had only been shown one prosthesis and had been fitted in less than 15 min. Fitting areas were often offices with no blinds, lacked privacy, and had no mirrors, which are the basic requirements for such an intimate procedure. Dissatisfaction is lower in women seen by a specialist nurse (Maguire et al. 1983). At present, surgical appliance officers, visiting company fitters, and specialist nurses may all fit prostheses.

There are several advantages of the fitting being carried out by a specialist nurse. The woman already knows the nurse and, hence, there is continuity and less likelihood of embarrassment at the scar being seen, the nurse is a contact for any future problems that occur, and the fitting provides an opportunity for the specialist nurse to assess how well the woman is coping following surgery. For these reasons it is felt that fitting by a specialist nurse is likely to provide a more acceptable and comprehensive service.

Psychological rehabilitation

For many women a diagnosis of breast cancer brings fear of death and of mutilating surgery to a part of their body intimately linked to perceptions of their femininity, sexuality, and motherhood.

Feelings similar to those of bereavement may be experienced, for example shock, denial, anger, and depression and frequently a state of inner turmoil is described, which affects both the woman and her family.

The prime concern at the time of diagnosis and initial treatment appears to be the cancer. However, most are concerned to some degree about a change in body image and this is the major concern for a minority (Maguire et al. 1978; Denton and Baum 1983).

The incidence of anxiety, depression, and sexual problems following mastectomy is high. Maguire et al. (1978) found that 25 per cent of women had symptoms of clinical anxiety or depression and 33 per cent had sexual problems in the first year after mastectomy. Other studies have shown similar results (Morris et al. 1977; Jamieson et al. 1978). With the advent of conservative surgery it was hoped that psychological morbidity would be reduced. Although body image disturbance is less, anxiety levels remain high, with particular concern about possible recurrence of cancer in the same breast and about adjuvant radiotherapy (Schain et al. 1983; Fallowfield et al. 1986).

The process of psychosocial rehabilitation may be painful and distressing and may take longer than physical rehabilitation. Some women require psychiatric help or sexual counselling, but all need time to adjust and opportunities to express their feelings and gather the information that they need to understand and cope with their situation. It is important that those close to the woman also have their needs met to be able to support the person they love and the family unit can continue to function. Husbands have very similar fears, concerns, and information needs to their wives, but do not feel as supported (Northouse 1988). Support for the husband may act as a buffer to stress, enabling women to cope better with their diagnosis and treatment. Specialist nurses in breast cancer care may help to support women through this distressing time and identify and refer those who have problems (Maguire et al. 1983).

Many women find it very helpful to talk to another woman who has had a similar operation and the Breast Care and Mastectomy Association have a register of volunteers. Others find great support from self-help groups or from complementary therapies such as meditation and relaxation. Others may find breast reconstruction is necessary for them to come to terms with and manage their feelings surrounding breast loss. This can frequently be offered at the time of mastectomy and there is evidence that it may help some women to take up their normal social activities again more quickly (Dean et al. 1983; Meyer and Ringberg 1986).

Most women return to their normal social activities in the first 3–4 months after surgery and reach a state of emotional equilibrium within 12 months (Maguire et al. 1978). However, a minority will not do so and will require help. Sensitivity, honesty, the provision of appropriate information, and opportunities to express feelings and make decisions will help to smooth the passage of women through this traumatic experience and facilitate rehabilitation.

THE MANAGEMENT OF LYMPHOEDEMA

Twenty-five per cent of breast cancer patients will develop lymphoedema of the arm following treatment (Kissin et al. 1986) and lymphoedema of the leg is common in patients with sarcoma, melanoma, and pelvic tumours.

Chronic oedema leads to reduced mobility, pain and discomfort (Badger et al. 1987), and increased susceptibility to acute inflammatory attacks.

Although lymphoedema is not curable, it can be controlled. Treatment is aimed at directing fluid away from swollen and congested areas of the body towards unaffected parts where it can be drained by normal functioning lymphatics.

Treatment is in two phases (Badger and Twycross 1988; Mortimer 1990). The first phase aims to reduce limb volume and to restore normal shape to the limb; the aim of the second phase is to maintain the smaller size and preserve normal shape.

In the first phase the treatment consists of multilayer compression bandaging, manual lymph drainage, exercises, and strict skin hygiene. Bandages are applied to give an evenly distributed high pressure which gradually diminishes towards the root of the limb. Manual lymph drainage is employed to stimulate the movement of fluid through all possible drainage pathways (tissue planes, veins, and functioning lymphatic routes) towards unaffected areas of the body. Exercise and normal use of the limb are encouraged. Physiotherapy may be required to improve joint mobility and strict skin hygiene is essential. This last phase lasts for 2–3 weeks, depending on the severity of oedema and the response to treatment.

In the second or maintenance phase (Regnard et al. 1988), patients are fitted with strong compression hosiery and are taught a simplified form of trunk massage. Normal use of the limb is encouraged with gentle exercise. Patients who have suffered more than one infection in the limb in the previous 12 months are given prophylactic antibiotics. The hosiery should be periodically checked and adjusted. Patients with mild oedema and normal-shaped limbs may be effectively treated with hosiery alone.

In patients with advanced cancer the same treatment techniques can be adapted to palliative symptoms associated with chronic oedema (Badger 1987; Badger and Regnard 1989). The application of external pressure usually results in a decrease in discomfort from tense distended tissues. The application of high pressure is not indicated and the overriding requirement is improved comfort. Gentle massage can help in reducing tissue tension but the effect is temporary, so that to be of benefit sessions need to be repeated frequently throughout the day.

SPEECH REHABILITATION

Speech requires good hearing, cognitive skills, the ability to decode the message, and the ability to formulate and generate ideas and to encode these into language. It is affected by respiration, the vocal cords, the soft palate, the facial muscles, the tongue, and the lips. In addition, the ability to learn and access a vocabulary is essential. Speech disorders in cancer arise most commonly where there is disease in the larynx, requiring its removal with subsequent loss of voice or anywhere else in the vocal tract (for example, the tongue, the floor of the mouth, the jaw, or the soft palate) affecting the intelligibility of speech, eating, and swallowing. The presence of a brain tumour may affect the language centres in the brain and the nervous pathways carrying complex messages to speech muscles, resulting in both language disturbance (dysphasia) and slurred incomprehensible speech (dysarthria). In children, the problems are present and are complicated by the developmental needs of the child and the effect on emotional and intellectual development of prolonged and repeated periods in hospital.

Rehabilitation in laryngectomy should begin at diagnosis, so that the patient is immediately aware that there is a supportive team looking to the future and to restoration of function. Patients vary in the amount of information that they desire pre-operatively, but all benefit from at least meeting the therapist and establishing a rapport. Such explanation as they want may be reinforced in writing (for example, a booklet) for reference and discussion with spouse, family, and friends.

Speech restoration in the laryngectomized patient may take place by the traditional method of air regurgitation, using the muscles of the pharynx as the new sound source (or pseudolarynx) or by tracheo-oesophageal puncture which involves the creation of a fistula through the back wall of the trachea into the top of the oesophagus. This enables pulmonary air to be shunted through the fistula into the pharynx, again using the pharyngeal muscles as the source of sound vibration. Patency of the fistula is maintained by the insertion of a small silicone valve. This method produces a vastly superior voice to the traditional method much more rapidly (for example, 10 days after the operation).

A few patients opt for an external communication aid, usually an artificial larynx. However, these aids have a rather harsh mechanical tone with little pitch variation or volume modulation and deny the patient the emotional release through their own voice. The speech therapist works closely with the patient and team throughout these procedures and takes primary responsibility for ensuring that each laryngectomee has some method of effective communication. There is no reason for any patient to remain silent, except from choice. Where no complications arise, patients may be discharged home 2 weeks after surgery with a good new voice. Nevertheless, there will be regular contact with the speech therapist, ideally in combination with routine out-patient checks, to deal with any technical problems and monitor progress.

Other speech problems arising from head and neck cancer such as glossectomy demand an individual approach and a tailored programme as well as a team approach including close liaison with the dietitian. Regaining socially acceptable patterns of deglutition together with adequate nutritional levels restores independence and control to the patient.

Technological advances and computerization have contributed enormously to objective measurement and evaluation of new procedures. For instance, using laryngography and videofluoroscopy it is possible to see the reconstructed vocal tract in action, to diagnose problems, and to note developments in form and structure.

Language disorders arising from cerebral disease require a quite different approach. Patients will often be confused and easily fatigued because of interference by the disease and treatment with the linguistic and intellectual processes, or because of oedematous pressure following surgery or radiotherapy.

The speech therapist needs to assess and monitor speech output at each stage of treatment, provide therapy and communication aids and ensure that others are aware of the true nature of the speech problem and communicate with the patient in an appropriate and dignified way. Loss of expressive speech does not mean that the patient cannot comprehend, but he or she may become mentally fatigued more quickly and easily distracted by extraneous noise.

Realistic aims can make everyone's task less stressful and bring comfort and reassurance to the patient and family.

REHABILITATION OF PATIENTS REQUIRING STOMAS

Cancer in any organ occupying the abdomen or pelvis could lead to stoma formation.

There are three main types of abdominal stoma (artificial opening).

1. Colostomy: an opening into the large colon.

2. Ileostomy: an opening into the ileum.

3. Urostomy, where a conduit is made from the ileum to which the ureters are attached. This small length of ileum is isolated from the rest of the small intestine (but keeps its own blood supply) and urine is conveyed to the surface of the abdomen via the stoma.

As there are no sphincters present the patient has no control over the effluent and therefore it is necessary to wear an appliance. Continent reservoirs (internal pouches) are made where possible to eradicate the need for an external appliance.

A stoma is a 'hidden' disability and therefore patients may go to great lengths to conceal their changed body image.

The aim in stoma care is self-care and even if the stoma has been provided for palliative reasons and patients will be unable to care for it themselves in the long-term, a certain amount of initial independence should be encouraged. Therefore, it is essential that patients receive help as soon as it is known that they will need a stoma. Often someone of the same age and sex who has experienced similar surgery and who has recovered well can be incorporated into the rehabilitation process.

Pre-operative preparation should include information about the stoma itself, about the life-style following stoma surgery, and counselling.

Pre- and post-operative counselling includes adaption to a change in body image and any sexual or psychological implications that this may have.

Pre-operative siting should be marked on a flat surface of the abdomen and the patient asked to sit, lie, and stand to enable the best site to be assessed. The patient should be told what the stoma will look like and warned that it could bleed a little on friction and should be taught a simple technique for cleaning and caring for the skin around the stoma.

Whilst it is hoped that a patient has been prepared emotionally as well as physically for stoma surgery, it is of benefit to assess continually how they and their family feel about life with a stoma. Non-invasive questions can often open the floodgates to problems that may have arisen.

A brave young woman speaking at an ostomy conference said, 'I am alive today, spending this time with my husband and children because this "hole" in my side makes it possible. Even if it is only for a short while, I am living a happy and fulfilling life'. This patient was truly rehabilitated, because it can be suggested that a patient's acceptance of their changed body image is not complete until they can look in the mirror and accept the person they see there.

REFERENCES

Anderson J (1989). The nurse's role in cancer rehabilitation. *Cancer Nursing*, **12**(2):85–94.
Atkins H, Hayward JL, Klugman DJ, Wayte AB (1972). Treatment of early breast cancer: a report after ten years of a clinical trial. *British Medical Journal*, **2**:423–9.
Badger C (1987). Lymphoedema: management of patients with advanced cancer. *Professional Nurse*, January, 100–2.
Badger C, Regnard C (1989). Oedema in advanced disease: a flow diagram. *Palliative Medicine*, **3**:213–15.
Badger C, Twycross RG (1988). *The management of lymphoedema*. Sobell Study Centre, New York.
Badger C, Twycross RG, Mortimer PS (1987). Pain in chronic obstructive lymphoedema of the upper limb. *Proceedings of the International Congress of Lymphology*.
Barkley V (1981). Cancer in an ageing society. *Cancer nursing update—Proceedings of 2nd International Conference on Cancer Nursing*. Baillière Tindall, London.
Beck AT (1976). *Cognitive therapy and the emotional disorders*. International Universities Press, New York.

Blocker WP Jr (1972). Rehabilitation of the paralysed patient with a spinal cord tumour. *Cancer Bulletin*, 24:76–9.

Bonadonna G, Valagussa P, Santora A (1986). Alternating non-cross-resistent combination chemotherapy or MOPP in stage IV Hodgkin's disease. A report of 8 year results. *Annals of Internal Medicine*, 104:739–46.

Bransfield DD, Horiot J-D, Nabid A (1984). Development of a scale for assessing sexual function after treatment for gynecologic cancer. *Journal of Psychosocial Oncology*, 2:3–19.

Buzby GP, *et al.* (1980). Prognostic nutritional index in gastro-intestinal surgery. *American Journal of Surgery*, 10:53–63.

Cain EN, *et al.* (1986). Psychosocial benefits of a cancer support group. *Cancer*, 57:183–9.

Calman KC (1982). Malignancy: cancer cachexia. *British Journal of Hospital Medicine*, January:28–31.

Carbonne PP, *et al.* (1971). Report of the Committee on Hodgkin's Disease Staging Classification. *Cancer Research*, 31:1860–1.

Collyer H (1984). *Facial disfigurement*. Macmillan, London.

Dean A, Chetty N, Forrest APM (1983). Effects of immediate breast reconstruction on psycho-social morbidity after mastectomy. *Lancet*.

Denton S, Baum M (1983). Psycho-social aspects of breast cancer. In *Breast cancer* (ed. R Marolese). Churchill Livingstone, Edinburgh.

De Wys W (1979). Anorexia as a general effect of cancer. *Cancer*, 43:2013–19.

De Wys WD, *et al.* (1980). Prognostic effect of weight loss prior to chemotherapy in cancer patients. *American Journal of Medicine*, 69:491–7.

Dietz J (1980). Adaptive rehabilitation in cancer: a program to improve quality of survival. *Postgraduate Medicine*, 68:145–7.

Dietz J (1981). *Rehabilitation oncology*. Wiley, New York.

Donvan MI, *et al.* (1987). Incidence and characteristics of pain in a sample of hospitalised cancer patients. *Cancer Nursing*, 10(2):85–92.

Dudley H, cited by Swaffield L (1979). Living with a stoma—finding the problems. *Nursing Times (Community Outlook)* 8 March.

Edels Y, ed. *Laryngectomy—diagnosis to rehabilitation*. Croom Helm, London.

Ell K, *et al.* (1989). A longitudinal analysis of psychological adaptation among survivors of cancer. *Cancer*, 63:406–13.

Fallowfield L. (1993). Evaluation of counselling in the NHS. *Journal of the Royal Society of Medicine*, 86:429–30.

Fallowfield LJ, Roberts RK (1992). Cancer counselling in the UK. *Psychological Health*, 6:107–17.

Fallowfield L, Baum M, Maguire GP (1986). Effects of conservation on psycho-social morbidity associated with the diagnosis and treatment of early breast cancer. *British Medical Journal*, 293:1331–4.

Farash JL (1979). Effect of counselling on resolution of loss and body image following a mastectomy. *Dissertation Abstracts International*, 39:4027B.

Fobair P, *et al.* (1986). Psychosocial problems among survivors of Hodgkin's disease. *Journal of Clinical Oncology*, 4:805–14.

Goffman E (1963). *Notes on the management of spoiled identity*. Prentice Hall, Englewood Cliffs, NJ.

Greer S, Burgess C (1987). A self-esteem measure for patients with cancer. *Psychology and Health*, 1:327–40.

Greer S, *et al.* (1992). Adjuvant psychological therapy for patients with cancer: a prospective randomised trial. *British Medical Journal*, 304:675–80.

Greer S, *et al.* (1994). Adjuvant psychological therapy for patients with cancer: outcome at one year. *Psycho-oncology*, 3:39–46.

Groher ME. *Dysphagia—diagnosis and management*. Butterworths, London.

Gunn A (1984). *Cancer rehabilitation*. Raven Press, New York.

Heyward J (1975). *Information—a prescription against pain*. RCN Series 2, No. 5. Royal College of Nursing, London.

Holland JCB (1977). Anorexia and cancer: psychological aspects. *Cancer*, 27:363–7.

Jamieson KR, Wellisch DK, Pasnara RO (1978). Psycho-social aspects of mastectomy: the woman's perspective. *American Journal of Psychiatry*, 135:434–6.

King's Fund Forum (1986). Consensus development conference: treatment of primary breast disease. *British Medical Journal*, 293:946–7.

Kissin MW, Quercis Della Rovere G, Easton D, Westbury G (1986). Risk of lymphoedema following the treatment of breast cancer. *British Journal of Surgery*, 73:580–4.

Langley J. *Working with swallowing disorders*. Winslow Press.

Levine MN, Guyatt GH, Gent M (1988). Quality of life in stage II breast cancer: an instrument for clinical trials. *Journal of Clinical Oncology*, 6(12):1798–1810.

Lichtman RR, Taylor SE (1986). Close relationships and the female cancer patient. In *Women with cancer* pp. 233–56. Springer, New York.

Lichtman RR, Taylor SE, Wood JV (1987). Social support and marital adjustment after breast cancer. *Journal of Psychosocial Oncology*, 5:47–74.

Linn MW, Linn BS, Harris R (1982). Effects of counselling for late stage cancer patients. *Cancer*, 49:1048–55.

Logeman J (1983). Evaluation and treatment of swallowing disorders. College-Hill Press, San Diego.

Maguire GP, *et al.* (1978). Psychiatric problems in the first year after mastectomy. *British Medical Journal*, 963–5.

Maguire GP, *et al.* (1980). Effect of counselling on the psychiatric morbidity associated with mastectomy. *British Medical Journal*, 281:1454–6.

Maguire GP, *et al.* (1983). The effect of counselling on physical disability and social recovery after mastectomy. *Clinical Oncology*, 9:319–24.

Mair A (1972). *Medical rehabilitation: the pattern for the future. Report of Sub-committee of Standing Medical Advisory Committee, Scottish Health Services Council*. Her Majesty's Stationery Office, Edinburgh.

Marsha H, *et al.* (1984). Soft tissue sarcoma: functional outcome after wide local excision and radiation therapy. *Archives of Physical Medicine and Rehabilitation*, 65:477.

Massie MJ, Holland J, Straker N (1989). Psychotherapeutic interventions. In *Handbook of psycho oncology* (ed. J Holland and JH Rowlands). Oxford University Press, New York.

Meyer L, Ringberg A (1986). A prospective study of psychiatric and psycho-social sequelae of bilateral subcutaneous mastectomy. *Scandinavian Journal of Plastic and Reconstructive Surgery*, 20:101–7.

Moorey S, Greer S (1989). *Psychological therapy for patients with cancer: a new approach*. Heinemann, Oxford.

Morris T, Greer SH, White P (1977). Psychological and social adjustment to mastectomy: a two year follow up study. *Cancer*, 40:2881.

Mortimer PS (1990). The management of lymphoedema. *Vascular Medicine Review*, in press.

Moynihan C (1987). Testicular cancer: the psychosocial problems of patients and their relatives. *Cancer Surveys*, 6:477–510.

Muller JM, *et al.* (1986). Indications and effects of pre-operative parenteral nutrition. *World Journal of Surgery*, 10:53–63.

Naysmith A, *et al.* (1983). Surviving malignant disease: psychological and family aspects. *British Journal of Hospital Medicine*, 30:22–7.

Northouse (1988).

Oncology Nursing Society Congress (1979). *Instructional session: patient education tapes*. Oncology Nursing Society, New Orleans.

Pollard R, Callum KG, Bates T (1976). Shoulder movement following mastectomy. *Clinical Oncology*, 2:343–9.

Pruyn JFA, van den Borne HW, Stringer P (1984). Theories, methods and some results on coping with cancer and contact with fellow sufferers. *Proceedings British Psychosocial Oncology Group 1st Annual Conference, November 1984*.

Regnard C, Badger C, Mortimer PS (1988). *Lymphoedema—advice on treatment*. Beaconsfield Publishers.

Rytlor N, Blichert-Toft M, Madsen EL, Weber J (1983). Influence of adjuvant irradiation on shoulder joint function after mastectomy for breast carcinoma. *Acta Radiologica Oncology*, 22:29–33.

Salter M (1984). Helping stoma patients at home. *Primary Health Care*, June.

Salter M, (ed.) (1988). *Altered body image*. Wiley, Chichester.

Schain W, *et al.* (1983). Psycho-social and physical outcomes of stage I breast cancer therapy: mastectomy V excision biopsy and irradiation. *Breast Cancer Research and Treatment*, 3:377–82.

Selby P, Robertson B (1987). Measurement of quality of life in patients with cancer. *Cancer Surveys*, 6:521–43.

Short SO, *et al.* (1984). Shoulder pain and function after neck dissection with or without preservation of the spinal accessory nerve. *American Journal of Surgery*, 148:478–82.

Simpson G (1985). Are you being served? *Senior Nurse*, 2(6):14–16.

Skelly M. *Glossectomee speech rehabilitation*. Thomas, Springfield, IL.

Spiegel D, Bloom JR, Yalom I (1981). Group support for patients with metastatic cancer. *Archives of General Psychiatry*, 38:527–33.

Spiegel D, Bloom J, Kraemer H, Gottheil E (1989). Effect of psychosocial treatment on survival of patients with metastatic breast cancer. *Lancet*, ii:888–91.

Sutherland AM (1967). Psychological observations in cancer patients. *International Psychiatric Clinics*, 4:75–92.

Swedborg I, Wallgren A (1981). The effects of pre and post mastectomy radiotherapy on the degree of oedema, shoulder joint morbidity and gripping force. *Cancer*, 47:877–81.

Taylor SE, *et al.* (1985). Illness-related and treatment-related factors in psychological adjustment to breast cancer. *Cancer*, 55:2506–13.

Telch CF, Telch MJ (1986). Group coping skills. Instruction and supportive group therapy for cancer patients: a comparison of strategies. *Journal of Consulting and Clinical Psychology*, 54:802–8.

Vander Ark GD, McGrath KA (1975). Transcutaneous electrical stimulation in the treatment of post-operative pain. *American Journal of Surgery*, 130:338–40.

von Eschenbach A, Schover L (1984). The role of sexual rehabilitation in the treatment of patients with cancer. *Cancer*, 54(Suppl.):2662–7.

von Meyenfeldt MF, Frederix EWHW, Haagh WAJJM (1988). The aetiology and management of weight loss and malnutrition in cancer patients. *Baillière's Clinical Gastroenterology*, 2(4):869–85.

Watson M (ed.) (1991). *Cancer patient care: psychosocial treatment methods*. The British Psychological Society.

Watson M, *et al.* (1988a). Development of a questionnaire measure of adjustment to cancer: the MAC scale. *Psychological Medicine*, 18:203–9.

Watson M, *et al.* (1988b). Counselling breast cancer patients: a specialist nurse service. *Counselling Psychology Quarterly*, 1:25–34.

Welch-McCaffrey D (1989). Geriatric oncology: nursing concerns in cancer nursing. A revolution in care. *Proceedings of 5th International Conference on Cancer Nursing*. Macmillan, London.

Wellisch DK, Jamieson KR, Pasnan RO (1978). Psycho-social aspects of mastectomy II: the man's perspective. *American Journal of Psychiatry*, 135:543.

Wells PE, Frampton NV, Bowshee D (1988). *Pain: the management and control in physiotherapy*, p. 164. Heinemann, London.

Wesdorp RIC, Krause R, von Meyenfeldt MF (1983). Cancer cachexia and its nutritional implications. *British Journal of Surgery*, 70:352–5.

Wingate L (1985). Efficacy of physical therapy for patients who have undergone mastectomies. *Physical Therapy*, 65(6):896–900.

20.7   Care of the dying patient

TOM WEST

INTRODUCTION

Why is skilled terminal care needed?

A majority of patients suffering from cancer will die of the disease. In the United Kingdom from the time of diagnosis 55 per cent of all cancer patients enter the palliative stream and only 45 per cent head towards cure (Bates 1985). During treatment in either mode there is a 15 per cent chance of crossover in one direction or the other, but the final figures speak for themselves: there is a hope for cure in 30 per cent of cases and a need for terminal care in 70 per cent (Fig. 1). It must be added that of this second larger group, perhaps only one-third endure what is dreaded by all; prolonged painful dying and inevitable death (Twycross and Lack 1983). In most cases this suffering is unnecessary.

When does terminal care begin?

Each potential advance in the cure or control of cancer complicates still further the decision-making that is needed before a change of direction can be taken from attempted cure to concentration on care. Decisions should be influenced by what treatment is still appropriate

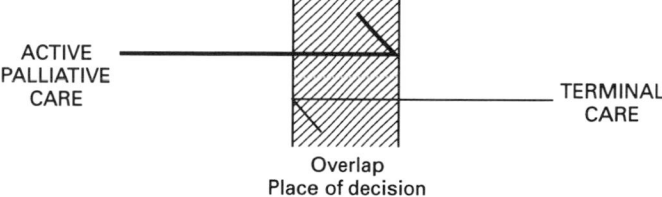

Fig. 2   Decision-taking in cancer care (reproduced from Saunders (1978), with permission).

and what is now becoming inappropriate; too often no real decisions are taken (Fig. 2). Those involved in cure as well as those concerned with care need to note that frequently there are no clear cut-off points and that the skilled control of problems in advanced and terminal disease does not necessarily have to wait until all hope for cure has been abandoned. Equally, the possibility that patients could still benefit from re-entering a more aggressive mode of treatment must never be forgotten (Fig. 3).

When clinicians are involved with chemotherapy and at the same time with the control of pain and nausea, it will be easier for them to recognize diminishing returns from the former and therefore

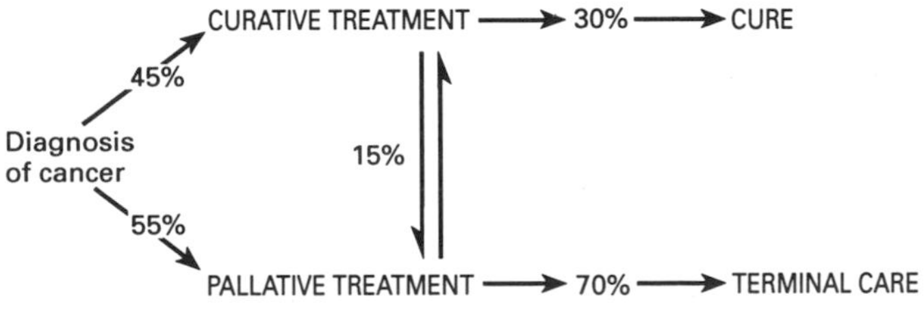

Fig. 1   Diagram demonstrating passage through treatment of all cancer patients (adapted from Bates (1985), with permission).

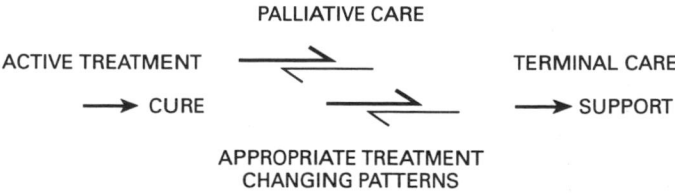

Fig. 3   Changing patterns of appropriate treatment (reproduced from Saunders (1984), with permission).

discontinue it, if they are still successfully addressing the problem of the pain and the nausea. Accepting a situation when treatment is directed to the relief of symptoms and the alleviation of general distress will then no longer mean an implicit 'there is nothing more that I can do' but an explicit 'everything possible is being done' (Saunders 1987).

Where should terminal care take place?

The appropriate place for terminally ill cancer patients to die should be a matter of concern. An increasing awareness of the need to give patients and their families information (and therefore choice) has to be offset against the hard facts of available medical services and of modern society. For patients with far advanced cancer the place of death will be hospital, home, hospice, or nursing home.

A majority of cancer patients will die in acute care hospitals (Cartwright *et al.* 1973). When the primary medical team know the patient well and have established good communication while the patient is still receiving active treatment, for example in patients with head and neck cancer or when the patient deteriorates rapidly, this may well be the place of choice. However, it necessitates an awareness by the busy ward staff of the needs of the dying and of the support that junior doctors and nurses should be given. The presence of a well-trained support team in the hospital can transform the situation (Dunlop *et al.* 1989).

A majority of people will state that they wish to die at home. However, this must depend on the home care services available, including the skill and willingness of the general practitioner to be fully involved, the family strengths, and the duration of the terminal phase of the illness. To provide sufficient security for the patient's family and care-givers well-staffed back-up beds must be immediately available.

The increase in the numbers of hospices often make them or a continuing care unit a realistic alternative. Patients and families may well be anxious about the thought, but by discussing the proposal weeks rather than days before the transfer and perhaps by arranging a visit to the hospice, fears can almost always be allayed. At the same time hospice staff can be a useful source of support and advice to those working in hospitals or the community.

With an ageing population the use of nursing homes needs to be carefully monitored. The dying patient not only needs considerate nursing care but also skilled, regular, and available medical input.

The place of death for a patient with terminal cancer should be included in the overall plan of care and wherever possible patient and family need to be involved in making the decision.

What is involved in terminal care?

The care of a patient with terminal cancer involves a continuing awareness of the primary site of the disease. For example, the metastatic spread from bronchus to brain, with the possibility of fits or from breast to bone, with the possibility of severe pain or a pathological fracture, needs to be kept in mind. In addition, it is important to remember that even patients with a terminal disease may suffer from conditions unrelated to the cancer. Haemorrhoids or heart failure can often be easily alleviated.

However, there is more to consider. The disease is contained in a person capable of a wider range of suffering than just that of physical pain. Mental anguish, family distress, and spiritual pain can all be present and in addressing the care of the dying person the concept of total pain remains an essential starting point. For effective management of this total pain the need for appropriate

Table 1 Total pain

Physical
Mental
Social
Spiritual
Staff

staff involvement and, therefore, of staff support, also has to be recognized (Table 1).

HOSPICE OR PALLIATIVE MEDICINE

In order to achieve sufficiently good care for those dying of terminal cancer the modern hospice movement was founded by Dame Cicely Saunders with the establishment of St Christopher's Hospice, London, in 1967. In less than one generation it is remarkable how her ideas have circled the world and given rise to the concept of hospice or palliative medicine.

Skills in addressing the problems of total pain are now available and are slowly being absorbed into mainstream medicine. It is being increasingly understood that terminal care for the patient dying from cancer will need as much careful planning and coordination as did the earlier attempts to cure and that it should be based on the tripod of good symptom control, improved communication, and relevant family support. Because no one person can be an expert in all three components, the other essential element must be an interdisciplinary team approach. These four components of good terminal care will now be addressed.

Symptom control

Although, with good reason, pain remains the symptom most dreaded by the cancer patient, their family, and the professional care-giver, dyspnoea can be more frightening and nausea and vomiting more distressing. A list of symptoms reported in patients on admission to St Christopher's Hospice in 1985 illustrates the wide range of the physical causes of suffering in a patient dying from cancer (Table 2). Skilfully addressing such symptoms provides enough scope to help prevent that sad report so often heard: 'The doctor said nothing more could be done'.

Three major problems in the symptom control of far-advanced cancer pain, dyspnoea, and nausea and vomiting, have already been considered in detail. They remain sufficiently important in the management of the terminal stages to warrant a further reference

Table 2 Symptoms on admission to St Christopher's Hospice of 722 cancer patients in 1985

Symptom	Total (%)	Men (%)	Women (%)
Weakness	91	93	90
Anorexia	76	78	74
Pain	62	61	64
Dyspnoea	51	58	47
Constipation	51	56	47
Cough	45	60	33
Nausea and vomiting	44	42	47
Dysphagea	25	28	22
Insomnia	24	25	24

Source: Baines (1988).

in the context of those at the very end of life. Bowel obstruction, confusion, and terminal restlessness will also be considered.

Pain

Pain and the fear of pain remains a major problem in the management of the dying patient. The element of fear, particularly when it has been reinforced in the past by poorly controlled chronic pain, enhances many other symptoms. This fact underlines the importance of taking a cancer patient's complaints of pain seriously and responding with early and effective intervention even if good results from chemotherapy are being confidently awaited.

The successful use of analgesics in controlling the chronic pain even of terminal disease continues to depend on a correct diagnosis of the cause of the pain (or pains) being made and then prescribing an appropriate drug in the correct dose at regular intervals. Perhaps this is the single most important message that those working in hospices have given the medical world. It has been well set out in the WHO publication *Cancer pain relief* (WHO 1986).

Fears that morphine will depress the respiration or result in addiction are still widespread. It has usefully been said that 'pain itself is the best antagonist to the side-effects of morphine' and it can be added that, when properly prescribed, respiration is not affected (Walsh 1984) and addiction (which in any case is irrelevant) does not occur (Saunders 1987).

Even in the terminal stages the underlying mechanism of the pain must be determined if possible, as the correct choice of analgesic drug, adjuvant medication, or non-medical treatment is often dependent on the cause. For doctors trained in acute medicine it is important to understand the different ways in which analgesic drugs are used in the management of chronic pain and pain in acute situations (Table 3).

Other methods of pain control

While analgesic drugs, properly administered, remain the fundamental weapon in controlling the physical components of a dying patient's pain, they are not the only means available. Adjuvant analgesic drugs, palliative radiotherapy, anaesthetic and neurological approaches, and the psychological support of patient and family may still be appropriate and have an important part to play (Baines 1989) (Fig. 4).

Table 3 Analgesic theory of acute versus chronic pain

	Acute	Chronic
Pain character	Meaningful, linear, reversible	Meaningless, cyclical, irreversible
Therapeutic goal	Pain relief	Pain prevention
Sedation	Often desirable	Usually undesirable
Rapid onset of effect	Important	Unnecessary
Desired duration of effect	2–4 h	As long as possible
Timing	As needed (on demand)	Regularly (in anticipation)
Dose	Usually standard	Individually titrated
Route	Parenteral	Oral
Adjuvant medication	Uncommon	Common

Source: Levy (1985).

The use of the adjuvant analgesic drugs may mean that analgesics are not required or can be given at a lower dose. Palliative radiotherapy is commonly used to control pain from bony metastases and it is now recognized that a single treatment can be as effective as multiple fractions (Price *et al.* 1986). Even at the end of life a few patients may benefit from a carefully considered and skilful nerve block (Lipton 1989).

As well as the physical component, psychosocial and spiritual elements of pain may need to be considered. Teasing out such components of a patient's 'total pain' and then attempting to prescribe appropriately for these different factors, while never losing sight of the fact they are contained in a human being, sums up the art and the science of good palliative medicine.

While no drugs can take the place of staff and family support, people who need comparatively large doses of drugs for their pain and physical distress may also need regular medication for their very understandable mental anxiety and anguish. When morphine is first commenced, a weak phenothiazine such as prochlorperazine should always be prescribed to prevent nausea and vomiting. Although this can often be stopped after a few days, if the patient is under increasing mental stress it can be replaced by a stronger drug, for example haloperidol. This may well be more appropriate than simply increasing the dose of morphine. The use of opioids (or other analgesics) for the physical components of pain and

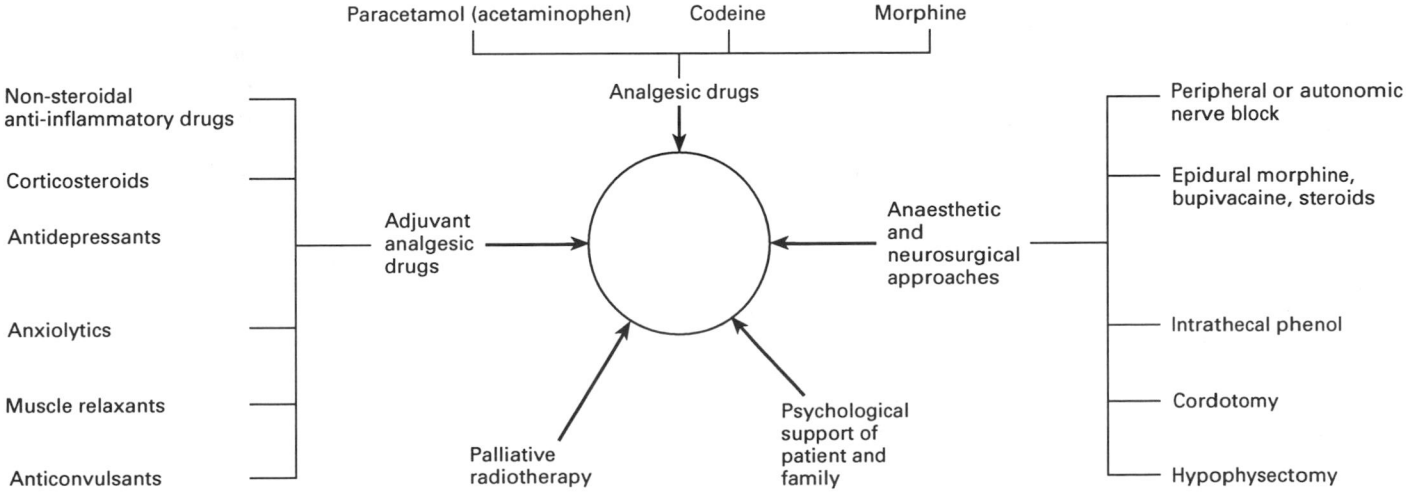

Fig. 4 Five-prong approach to cancer pain (reproduced from Baines (1989), with permission).

phenothiazines (or other psychotrophics) for the mental components is a balancing act and they may need to be kept in some sort of proportion to each other.

Dyspnoea

Dyspnoea (distressing difficulty in breathing) occurs in many patients suffering from advanced cancer other than those involving lung or pleura (Hoy 1987). The fear of suffocating or choking to death is common in patients at the end of life and can be a major component of their suffering.

A thorough physical examination will probably reveal the cause or causes. It will certainly reassure the patient. If the patient's general condition warrants it, reversible conditions should of course be treated: heart failure with diuretics, bronchospasm with bronchodilators, and pneumonia with antibiotics and physiotherapy. However, before prescribing drugs the whole patient rather than just the symptom must be considered. Transfusions for anaemia are seldom useful in far-advanced cancer, simply overloading an already failing heart, lung, and kidneys, while tapping a pleural effusion is seldom worthwhile as the rigid-walled space quickly refills.

The choice of appropriate treatment for dyspnoea in the terminally ill is usually limited to opiates, tranquillizers, hyoscine, and (less usefully) oxygen.

Morphine

Just as morphine takes away the feeling of pain, it also takes away the feeling of breathlessness and the anxiety that accompanies it. The common fear that the opiates, if given to a dyspnoeic patient, inevitably cause severe respiratory depression is not true if the dose is titrated carefully. Studies have shown that the great majority of cancer patients, even on high-dose morphine for pain control, continue to have a normal P_{CO_2} even if they have pre-existing respiratory disease (Baines 1987a). In treating dyspnoea, the starting dose of morphine should be low (for example, 2.5–5 mg every 4 h). This can be increased slowly if necessary.

Diazepam

The anxyiolitic and muscle-relaxant effects of diazepam are useful in reducing dyspnoea. Treatment starts with 5–10 mg at night; a smaller dose may also be needed during the day.

Hyoscine (scopolamine)

By drying up secretions and relaxing smooth muscle, hyoscine is most useful in abolishing the so-called 'death rattle'. It also relieves bronchospasm. It is markedly sedative and, to prevent the rare occurrence of agitation following its use, an opiate is commonly prescribed with it. The dose of hyoscine is 0.4–0.6 mg intramuscularly every 4–8 h.

Oxygen

Although used routinely for acute episodes of dyspnoea, oxygen is not often helpful in controlling the chronic dyspnoea of the terminally ill and the mask is a barrier between patient and family. By using the treatments described above with confidence, the majority of patients can be weaned off oxygen.

In helping a patient with dyspnoea, the importance of reassurance and diversion cannot be overemphasized. Both need the unhurried presence of competent carers or family.

Nausea and vomiting

Feeling sick and being sick are two of the most common and distressing symptoms of the terminally ill patient, occurring in almost 50 per cent of those with advanced cancer. Successful treatment depends on an understanding of the mechanisms involved in vomiting. Only then can specific treatment and/or the correct anti-emetic be prescribed (Baines 1988).

The causes of nausea or vomiting can be iatrogenic, metabolic, organic, or psychological. Amongst reversible causes, two of the commonest and simplest to treat are constipation and oral *Candida* infection. They are often missed.

Until the symptoms are brought under control it may be necessary to give the anti-emetic by injection or, better, by suppository. The pharmacist can supply a list of drugs available in this form or may even be able to make them up him/herself.

If the nausea or vomiting is not brought under control, then the dose of anti-emetic may need to be increased or a second anti-emetic with a different site of action may be added or the anti-emetic may be changed. Sometimes resistant nausea and vomiting will respond to steroids (dexamethasone 6–8 mg once daily) and, if successful, this can be reduced to a maintenance dose.

If the vomiting is intractable, continuous subcutaneous administration of an anti-emetic using a syringe driver may be necessary.

In helping a patient with nausea and vomiting, the importance of an explanation of the problem, reassurance, and the provision of small attractive meals cannot be overemphasized.

Obstruction

Twenty-five per cent of patients with ovarian carcinoma will obstruct and a proportion of patients with other gynaecological or large bowel malignancies may also do so. The obstruction may be due to a single site, but frequently multiple sites in the ileum and colon are involved. The following guidelines will be of help in deciding what is the appropriate treatment for a patient who is obstructing.

1. Every cancer patient who develops intestinal obstruction should be considered for palliative surgery. However, results are poor, mortality is high, and complications are frequent.

2. It should be noted that while intravenous fluids and nasogastric suction are of value prior to surgery they become inappropriate as long-term measures.

3. Almost always the symptoms in an obstructed patient at the end of life can be controlled medically as follows. The colicky pains respond to an antispasmodic drug such as hyoscine. The visceral pain responds to morphine. The nausea can usually be controlled and vomiting reduced to once or twice daily by an appropriate anti-emetic (for example, haloperidol or methotrimeprazine). The most effective route is often with a syringe driver giving a subcutaneous infusion over the 24 h period (Baines 1987b).

The syringe driver and controlled-release morphine sulphate tablets

Good symptom control for the terminally ill has been greatly facilitated by the introduction of the subcutaneous syringe driver and by controlled-release morphine sulphate tablets. Both methods of delivering drugs need to be correctly used.

Apart from the medical management of malignant bowel obstruction, the principal indications for the use of a continuous subcutaneous infusion include conditions such as nausea and vomiting, dysphagia, severe weakness, and coma, when oral medication can no longer be taken. Sometimes it is useful in the control of pain when other methods have failed (Oliver 1988).

Controlled-release morphine tablets are now available in a range of strengths. These represent a considerable practical advance (Dixon *et al.* 1989). Once a patient has been stabilized with doses of liquid morphine every 4 h, the total 24 h dosage is halved and the tablets substituted on a milligram for milligram basis; that is, 20 mg every 4 h×six doses=120 mg per 24 h=60 mg of controlled-release tablets every 12 h. They are not satisfactory for titrating morphine dosage (except perhaps in the home and when very small doses are required) and should be avoided in patients who have severe gastrointestinal abnormalities or swallowing difficulties (Walsh and West 1988).

Although back-up medication should always be available for patients with terminal disease, a consistent requirement for it when either of these two routes is being used is an indication that they are either inappropriate or being administered incorrectly.

Confusion and terminal restlessness

The differential diagnosis and management of confusion in a terminally ill patient are two of the most difficult problems that a doctor concerned with care of the dying has to face. Confusion is particularly common in elderly patients when their environment is changed and is a source of particular distress not only to the patient himself but also to his family.

As with all other symptoms, an accurate diagnosis of the underlying cause of the confusion must be attempted. Common causes include drugs, pain, discomfort (for example, full bladder or impacted faeces), infection, biochemical imbalance, brain damage, and psychogenic causes. Sometimes specific treatment can then be successfully prescribed, but even if the underlying cause cannot be treated a careful explanation to the family (and sometimes to the patient) will help to reassure them that it is 'the disease' and not that the patient is going mad (Baines 1984). The disorientation and flooding of consciousness by normally unconscious material experienced by a confused patient can create the living nightmare of not knowing what is real and what is unreal and of feeling completely 'out of control'. The resulting agitated or aggressive behaviour and confusion needs to be contained by re-establishing clear boundaries between the individual's conscious and unconscious world and between them and their external environment. Their fear and agitation may then be reduced (M. Kearney, personal communication).

The management of confusion is achieved by the correct use of sedative medication and by simple practical measures. Many confused patients require no medication, for example in the 'quietly muddled' patient sedative drugs may actually worsen the confusion by depressing the function of the already depleted brain cells (Stedeford 1984). Nevertheless, psychotrophic drugs can help to make a restless and aggressive patient easier to manage.

Practical measures include caring for the confused patient whenever possible in familiar surroundings, including the patient's family and staff that they know in their care and providing a quiet well-lit room.

Communicating with confused patients involves neither confrontation nor collusion but should respond to the emotional theme of what the patient is saying: for example, 'The hospital is on fire—I must get out of here'—'That sounds very frightening, as though you were trapped'—'That's how I feel' (M. Kearney, personal communication).

Terminal restlessness in the last hours of life may well need active treatment because of the distress it causes to family and staff. Adequate medication must be given for pain. Midazolam is probably the sedating drug of choice. The dose range is 5–10 mg immediately and, usually, 30–60 mg/24 h. Diazepam 5–10 mg by injection or suppository is used to control muscle twitching. Hyoscine 0.4–0.6 mg by injection will dry up excessive secretions as well as being a most effective sedative in an emergency (Baines 1984).

The last hours of life

Unless a catastrophic incident intervenes, the time will come when the patient can be said to be dying. Recognizing this time is a matter of experience as well as observation. Often the nursing staff are far more realistic than their medical colleagues and it is they who will collect and prepare the family as well as know what comfort and even suggest what medication the patient most needs.

At this stage most patients need their medication by injection. It can be important to explain to relatives (and sometimes staff) that the medicine now being given by injection is an equivalent dose to that given by mouth and that the deterioration in the patient's condition is due to the disease process and not to the drugs. This is also the time to review all the patient's medication. Steroids, diuretics, and antibiotics are examples of drugs that will probably no longer be appropriate, as the deteriorations they were prescribed to prevent are now inevitably occurring.

The main symptoms to distress patients dying from cancer are as follows:

(1) pain;

(2) breathlessness;

(3) restlessness;

(4) accumulation of secretions.

Although there is never any point in withholding necessary opioids, pain does not usually increase markedly over the last 24 h. If the patient's symptoms had already been reasonably well controlled, a simple increase of the analgesic and continuing it regularly will not only bring the pain under control again but will also help to cope with any increase in breathlessness or restlessness.

Increasing the dose of medazolam or changing to methotrimiprazine will help combat mental distress. In some cases, particularly in younger patients, the combination of both drugs may be necessary. Diazepam can be useful if physical restlessness is disturbing the patient and those sitting with him. Accumulation of secretions and the 'death rattle' can often be controlled by an injection of hyoscine 0.4–0.6 mg. Hyoscine, when combined with an opioid and a phenothiazine, is also a most effective sedative and tranquillizer.

If a haemorrhage is feared, diamorphine and a sedating drug in a slightly higher dose than that being regularly given, together with hyoscine, should be prescribed in anticipation and be immediately available.

Terminal pneumonia is usually a peaceful and indeed almost a natural way to die. Distressing symptoms such as copious phlegm can be treated with hyoscine.

Isolation can be the most distressing complication of all. If the family are unable, for whatever reason, to be with the patient during their final hours, every effort should be made for one of the team to sit with the patient, holding their hand and demonstrating that just because they are now dying they have not been abandoned (West 1987).

Guidelines for further active treatment

It is a function of those specializing in palliative medicine both to give appropriate advice to patients and families and to cooperate with and learn from colleagues who are specialists in other fields. Members of a hospital support team, hospice staff, and family doctors may well find themselves acting as the patient's advocate in discussing with the primary medical team either the continuation of therapy or the introduction of new ways to control the disease. A baseline for such discussion can be useful (Table 4).

Ethical considerations

Feeding

It becomes increasingly important to recognize the ethical dilemmas that accompany caring for patients who are dying (Wulf *et al.* 1986). The problem of nutrition can be summed up by the question 'Must patients always be given food and water?' The distinction was usefully drawn by a British Medical Association (BMA) Working Party (BMA 1988) between, on the one hand, '. . . simple care offering comfort, dignity and company and providing such sustenance as the patient can easily take' and, on the other hand, '. . . the imposition of medical interventions such as a naso-gastric tube or a gastrostomy'. They believed that the latter are 'medical treatments and are warranted only when they make possible a decent life in which the patient can reasonably be thought to have a continued interest'.

There are perhaps three situations when food and water need not be pressed: first, when the procedures that would be required are so unlikely to achieve nutritional and fluid levels that they could correctly be considered futile; second, when the improvement in nutritional and fluid balance cannot benefit the patient; third, when, for the patient, the burdens of receiving the treatment may outweigh the benefit (Lynn and Childless 1986). There is no evidence that alimentation prolongs life in patients with advanced cancer, while the common association of hyperalbuminaemia and advanced cancer means that replacement of fluid with crystalloids will precipitate serious problems with fluid overload.

The pressure to feed a dying person usually comes from the care-givers and family rather than from the patient, who no longer feels hunger or even thirst once their whole body is failing. If this can be recognized and discussed with all those involved, including whenever appropriate the patient him/herself, keeping the patient comfortable can take precedence over artificial feeding. Distressing dryness of the mouth may remain, but has been found to be better relieved by good mouth care and sips of fluid given naturally than

Table 4 Further active therapy: suggested guidelines for discussion

Nerve blocks	Relief can be immediate; patients with only a few days of life left may have their pain satisfactorily relieved
Radiotherapy	The patient may have to survive for 2 weeks before the benefits of symptom control are seen
Cytotoxic chemotherapy	Response may be rapid, as in the lymphomas or may take 4–8 weeks to become apparent in solid tumours
Surgery	A balance has to be sought between realistic benefit for the patient and resources available (for example, pinning of a pathological fracture may be the only way to control pain)
Hormones	Generally slower than cytotoxic chemotherapy

by the added burden of an intravenous line or even nasogastric tube. It is also relieved by opioids.

Euthanasia

The problem of euthanasia is compounded by confused thinking. Withholding active but inappropriate treatment is not euthanasia. Administering drugs needed for the control and alleviation of painful symptoms in a dying person is not euthanasia. However, deliberately killing a person must remain a matter of serious concern that no legal act could safely cover (BMA Working Party on Euthanasia 1988).

When patients say that they want to die they must be listened to with total attention and the real meaning behind their words carefully explored. Often all they are asking is that they should now be allowed to die and that inappropriate treatment be discontinued.

However, if they are in fact stating 'I want to die', they are expressing an anguish needing the interdisciplinary team approach to a situation of total pain. Physical symptoms may need further control and occasionally a treatable depression will be uncovered. Sadness (and anger) at all that is being lost can be acknowledged and then, with the support of family members and the team, some continuing sense of purpose may be looked for. Family distress can be shared and hidden strengths revealed. Rage against God can be absorbed and sometimes transformed.

The specific request 'Kill me' or 'My mother should not wake up again' is uncommon in practice. Again, it must be listened to with care, the situation and the fears must be explored, and a clear statement made that the doctor (or nurse) may not embark on any conduct with the primary intention of causing the patient's death (Kennedy 1984).

By responding with both concern and honesty continued skilful care for the patient and his family is made possible. The mutual support that members of the team are able to give each other in such situations is essential.

Communication

Only if distressing physical symptoms have been brought under reasonable control is it possible to communicate with patients suffering from terminal disease. When it is accepted that a patient has only a limited time left to live, those now responsible for providing terminal care must reassess the patient's current knowledge of the likely course of the disease and insight into the probable prognosis. Although there is evidence to suggest that most people would like to know if they have a terminal illness, there is also evidence that there are still many doctors who believe that it is not always wise to tell patients that they are dying (Gilhooly *et al.* 1988).

While it may well have been correct to present the best possible outcome earlier in the disease, at the same time it should be accepted that it is hardly ever right or necessary to lie. Once a lie has been discovered it is hard for those now responsible for the care of the patient to re-establish a proper degree of trust. This fact may need to be explained to relatives who themselves may well be fixed at the moment of diagnosis and denial: 'Don't tell him doctor; he'd give up if he knew'. Meanwhile, it often has not been recognized that the patient has pursued a lonely path towards knowledge: 'You don't go to radiotherapy ten times without knowing what is going on!'

Although the wishes and needs of the dying patient should take precedence over those of the family (and also of the staff) in these difficult situations, by acknowledging the problem and then discussing with those concerned their own anxieties a more realistic resolution can almost always be reached.

Although continuity of care is looked upon as the ideal, an advantage for a team taking over the care of a patient (whether it be in a hospital, hospice, or general practice) is the opportunity to ask questions such as 'What did they tell you at the other place' and for the patient to take this as an indication that they and the new doctor can start afresh and need no longer continue to engage in 'mutual pretence' (Glasser and Strauss 1965). 'They didn't tell me what it was' may not be strictly true. However, if it is followed by the question 'But do you know?', the beginning of a useful dialogue may have been established.

When a difficult question is asked, for example 'Is it cancer doctor?', it is often wise to check what sort of response is really wanted. Asking in return 'I wonder what made you ask me that question?' enables the patient either to back away from information that they are not yet ready to receive or to confirm that a clear statement is expected: 'Because you might give me an honest answer' (Buckman 1988).

It is important to listen attentively to the detail in each question, to answer this in as appropriate language as possible, to check comprehension, and then to stop. It is the patient (or family) who have the right to ask the next question or to call a halt. The truth does not always have to be the whole truth—even if one adds 'So help me God'!

The question 'How long?' should never be answered with a specific length of time. Days rather than weeks, or months rather than years, is usually about as far as it is wise to forecast. Often the real question is not 'How long?', but just 'How?'. 'Am I going to choke or suffocate to death?' 'Will you run out of painkillers?' 'When the end comes will I be isolated or abandoned?' Uncovering and taking such questions seriously and then responding with some confidence that this is not how it will be, can enable a patient and family to use the time left for living rather than merely in anticipating death (Lichter 1987).

Questions may well be asked of those aware of a spiritual dimension to life that will have little to do with religious practice or specific belief. At such moments it is not profound answers that are useful but rather an acknowledgement that all of us are travellers 'living and partly living', searching for a meaning to life and to death and perhaps learning how to trust in a God who loves and cares and forgives (Taylor 1986).

Family support

Every effort must be made by those caring for patients with advanced and terminal disease to ensure that family members are appropriately involved. Insufficient or confused information is often the major problem facing relatives in the acute hospital setting and, whenever possible, dying should be a family affair and not an isolated event.

But just as it is difficult to talk with a patient who is still in severe pain or who is continuously nauseated, so it is also hard to involve a family before distressing symptoms have come under some control.

Admission

The welcome given to the patient and his family by the team who will be responsible for the final phase sets the tone for all that will follow. There is now more than ever a need to create a safe and friendly space where people can reflect on their pain and suffering without fear and find the confidence to look for new ways in the centre of their confusion (Nouwen 1988).

In a hospital or hospice setting the reception staff and the nursing staff have an important rôle to play in ensuring that the patient and their family are expected and are made comfortable as quickly as possible. When the doctor arrives to admit the patient the ward staff may well be able to give them important information including advice on whether to take the history from the patient alone or whether it would be appropriate (and make a clear statement of family involvement) if the closest relative or friend is included in this initial dialogue.

It is still necessary to give the family their own time so that fears can be expressed, questions asked, and, most importantly, they can be reassured and congratulated: 'I just don't know how you managed so well and for so long. Your husband now needs full-time professional care. It would have been irresponsible to have kept him at home any longer.'

Families need to know that they are not being a nuisance when they telephone the ward and that they will receive a considered response and not a meaningless 'As well as can be expected'. Few people these days have seen anyone die. Reassurance is needed that symptoms can and will be controlled and that dying is usually a lessening of consciousness and increase in sleepiness and a running down of all the vital functions.

Family meetings

Increasingly, perhaps as the physical components of pain are better understood and controlled, the psychosocial aspects surrounding dying and death are being recognized. Drawing a family tree or genogram with the family is a good way of involving them and, at the same time, highlighting their strengths and their weaknesses. A number of deaths in the family, perhaps also from cancer, underline both what the family have had to cope with in the past and also what they have survived. Key members in this family's dynamics will emerge and so will family members at particular risk.

When a family is disintegrating rather than integrated, to call a family meeting may feel intrusive but can be most constructive. When a family can be assembled to meet the medical, nursing, and social work team they will feel that they are being supported rather than threatened as it becomes obvious that the two sides have a common objective and are working out how to form themselves into one united team. Such an exercise also avoids the problems that arise when family members are given information separately.

Among matters that may need to be brought out into the open and discussed are guilt from the past and fears for the future, the difficulties that a change in body image can produce in the patient and effect on the family around them and anger that this outrage should have been allowed 'by God'. At this point it may be helpful to ask the family if they would like to discuss matters with the chaplain.

The need to feed and the need to let go and, if it has not already been decided, where the patient should die may also need to be talked through.

At such a meeting with the family, children should not be excluded. Children are realists and in practice it is often the child who asks the question that adults do not dare to voice. At the end of the meeting, if the patient was not present, in order to avoid family secrets from further isolating them, it is important to discuss with the family how much they are going to share.

Dying, death, and bereavement

When a patient is dying they must be kept comfortable and any signs of distress noted and dealt with promptly and effectively as the emergency which they now are. Family members should be encouraged to be present, although if the family is large it can be helpful to suggest some sort of rota. People sitting round the bed should be helped to talk quietly but normally, to hold the patient's hand, and to report any anxieties that they may have to the staff.

When death occurs the family should be clearly informed and if it is wished prayers can be said. After the family have had time to sit with the body then the last offices should be carried out. Members of different faiths should have their beliefs respected and their rituals observed (Neuberger 1987). It is often helpful to encourage the family to view the body. Children as well as adults may need to know that the person really has died before they are able to say a sad but appropriate 'farewell'.

The staff caring for the patient and their family should already have a good idea of any family members under particular strain. The day after the death of a patient, when the family return to collect the death certificate and the possessions and to view the body, is a further important occasion to assess their needs. If at all possible a member of the team should be available to spend time with them, living through the past days (or sometimes years) and making some estimate of the family's ability to cope with all that lies ahead.

An in-patient's general practitioner should always be telephoned by the ward doctor and informed of the patient's death. If it is considered that the family are at risk, then they can be alerted at the same time.

A major bereavement is a bewildering and sometimes a very frightening experience (Stedeford 1987). Although a majority of families will cope well enough, it has been estimated that perhaps one-third of those losing a loved one may need bereavement counselling. If trained people are available, appropriate follow-up should be organized as a continuation of the original caring team (Yorkstone 1981).

The interdisciplinary team

Helping people with far-advanced cancer calls for more skills than any one individual can command. The interdisciplinary team approach has been developed in disciplines such as paediatrics where the whole family needs to be involved. Nowhere is it more essential than in response to the expressed and perceived needs of patients and their families in the terminal stages of cancer.

In interdisciplinary work responsibility is shared. Each member of the team brings to the day's work his or her professional skills with all the confidence that this produces. However, professional traditions will also be present and may well need adjusting. The doctor who is able to step aside for the social worker and the nurse who knows when they do not need to call the chaplain represent effective functioning by all four of these different disciplines.

In practice, no team can afford to be leaderless, but there is an important if less clear distinction between the leader and the manager of an interdisciplinary team. On a hospital or hospice ward although the doctor leads clinical decision-making it is the ward sister who is the obvious manager, while in a family meeting it may be the social worker who is the orchestrator, allowing different people to take the lead at appropriate points in the discussion. Good communication together with good recording is as essential to the smooth functioning of the team as it is to competent patient and family care.

Regular interdisciplinary meetings, when an honest audit of both successes and failures can take place and where vital information (frequently coming from unexpected members of the team) is collected, provide much of the team's necessary support and helps to maintain morale and a proper degree of job satisfaction.

Physiotherapists and occupational therapists amongst others can help to banish boredom and demonstrate how ever-diminishing aims can still be meaningful. Volunteers and the administrative staff have vital rôles to play. Too often lip service is paid to their membership of the team, when in practice not enough care has been taken in first carefully defining their special functions and then including them appropriately in the team (Zimmerman and Roche 1986).

Crisis points

During the course of a cancer patient's disease, starting from the time of the appearance of the first symptom (be it a lump in the breast or the coughing up of blood) and ending with the resolution of the situation (be it cure or terminal care), there are certain times of crisis which are predictable and therefore might have been anticipated.

A crisis situation is accompanied by a sense of increasing anxiety and a feeling of inability to cope with a changing and threatening situation. If this can begin to be acknowledged, the person is then able to search for solutions or a meaning to these overwhelming problems and use all the help that is available, including the mobilization of internal resources. At this point there is now a maximum potential for change and the introduction of a small amount of professional help can act as a catalyst to produce a positive and sometimes dramatic change in the person's attitude to the situation (Kaye 1989).

At each of the crisis points in a cancer patient's progress increased support is needed (Table 5). Too often it is not provided, either because the crisis has not been recognized or anticipated or perhaps because individual care-givers simply do not know how to give appropriate help. Two further examples of crisis are important enough to be mentioned. The early signs of spinal cord compression and the request for a solicitor to help remake a will are both emergencies that will not hold until after the weekend.

By mobilizing the interdisciplinary team (including the patient's family) competent symptom control, good lines of communication, and relevant family involvement can be provided at those times when they are most useful.

Table 5 Potential crisis points for cancer patients

First symptom	'Should I worry my husband?'	Panic
Medical appointment	'I don't think the doctor knows either.'	Uncertainty
Hospital investigations	'No one looked at me.'	Loneliness
Diagnosis	'Don't tell him doctor, he'd give up if he knew.'	Isolation
Side effects	'Why should this happen to me?'	Anger
Remission	'They say its all right.'	Anxiety/depression
Appearance of secondary	'Who has failed: treatment, doctor, or me?'	Failure
Stopping treatment	'The doctors said nothing more could be done.'	Abandonment
Hospice	'Dead End or Place of Hope?'	Fear

SUMMARY

Hospice and palliative medicine is concerned with improving the quality of life remaining for the patient and their family. The interdisciplinary team approach ensures that appropriate skills are available to control the different components of total pain. The team should be easily available to support and to advise on what it is possible to do and what ought to be done, not only at the end of life but also at any of the crisis points that mark a cancer patient's progress.

Competent teamwork will provide enough job satisfaction to change a time that is too often seen as one of failure into one that brings its own worthwhile rewards. Patient, family, and staff, by paying total attention to each other and to what is going on, can then find some meaning in an otherwise impossible situation.

REFERENCES

Baines M (1984). Control of other symptoms. In *The management of terminal malignant disease* (2nd edn) (ed. C Saunders), pp. 123–31. Arnold, London.

Baines M (1987a). Terminal illness. In *Textbook of medical treatment* (15th edn) (ed. RH Girdwood and JC Petrie), p. 11. Churchill Livingstone, London.

Baines M (1987b). Medical management of intestinal obstruction. In *Contemporary palliation of difficult symptoms* (ed. TD Bates), pp. 357–71. Baillière Tindall, London.

Baines M (1988). Nausea and vomiting in the patient with advanced cancer. *Journal of Pain and Symptom Management*, 3(2):81–5.

Baines M (1989). Pain relief in active patients with cancer: analgesic drugs are the foundation of management. *British Medical Journal*, 298:36–8.

Bates TD (1985). A clinician's view on palliative care, terminal care and quality of life. *Effective Health Care*, 2(5):211–15.

BMA (British Medical Association) (1988). *BMA Working Party on Euthanasia*, pp. 43–4. BMA, London.

Buckman R (1988). *'I don't know what to say': how to help and support someone who is dying*, pp. 68–9. Key Porter, Toronto.

Cartwright A, et al. (1973). *Life before death*, pp. 63–81. Routledge & Kegan Paul, London.

Dixon PJV, et al. (1989). Use of controlled release morphine sulphate tables by a terminal care support team: a retrospective cohort study. *Proceedings of the Symposium on Pain Control and Medical Education*, Edinburgh, October 1988, pp. 32–3. International Congress and Symposium Series No. 149, RSM Services.

Dunlop J, Davies RJ, Hockley JM (1989). Preferred v. actual place of death: a hospital palliative care support team experience. *Palliative Medicine*, 3(3):197–201.

Gilhooly MLM, et al. (1988). Truth telling with dying cancer patients. *Palliative Medicine*, 2(1):64–5.

Glasser BG, Strauss AL (1965). *Awareness of dying*, pp. 64–78. Aldine, Hawthorne, NY.

Hoy AM (1987). Dyspnoea. In *Contemporary palliation of difficult symptoms* (ed. TD Bates), p. 277. Baillière Tindall, London.

Kaye P (1989). *Notes on symptom control in hospice and palliative care*, p. 95. Hospice Education Institute, Essex, USA.

Kennedy I McC (1984). The law relating to the treatment of the terminally ill. In *The management of terminal malignant disease* (2nd edn) (ed. C Saunders), p. 230. Arnold, London.

Levy MH (1985). Pain management in advanced cancer. *Seminars in Oncology*, 12(4):396.

Lichter I (1987). *Communication in cancer care*, pp. 92–4. Churchill Livingstone, London.

Lipton S (1989). Pain relief in active patients with cancer: the early use of nerve blocks improves the quality of life. *British Medical Journal*, 298:37–8.

Lynn J, Childless JF (1986). Must patients always be given food and water? In *By no extraordinary means: the choice to forgo life-sustaining food and water* (ed. J Lynn), p. 47. Indiana University Press, Bloomington, IN.

Neuberger J (1987). *Caring for dying people of different faiths*, pp. 4–6. Austen Cornish with Lisa Sainsbury Foundation Series, London.

Nouwen HJM (1988). *Reaching out*, p. 90. Collins, London.

Oliver DJ (1988). Syringe drivers in palliative care: a review. *Palliative Medicine*, 2(1):21–6.

Price P, et al. (1986). Prospective randomised trial of single and multifunction radiotherapy schedules in the treatment of painful bony metastases. *Radiotherapy and Oncology*, 6:247–55.

Saunders CM (ed.) (1978). *The management of terminal disease*, p. 2. Arnold, London.

Saunders CM (ed.) (1984). *The management of terminal malignant disease* (2nd edn), p. 1. Arnold, London.

Saunders CM (1987). Terminal care. In *Oxford textbook of medicine*, Vol. 2 (2nd edn) (ed. DJ Weatherall, JGG Ledingham and DA Warrell), pp. 28.1, 28.9. Oxford University Press.

Stedeford A (1984). *Facing death: patients, families and professionals*, pp. 134–6. Heinemann, London.

Stedeford A (1987). Bereavement. *Medicine International*, July, 1779–85.

Taylor JV (1986). *A matter of life and death*, pp. 15–31. SCM Press, London.

Twycross RG, Lack SA (1983). *Symptom control in far advanced cancer: pain relief*, pp. 7–12. Pitman, London.

Walsh TD (1984). Opiates and respiratory function in advanced cancer. In *Pain in the cancer patient* (ed. M Zimmerman, P Drings, and G Wagner), p. 116. Springer, Berlin.

Walsh TD, West TS (1988). Controlling symptoms in advanced cancer. *British Medical Journal*, 296:478–9.

West TS (1987). In *Scott-Brown's otolaryngology* (5th edn) (ed. AG Kerr), p. 441. Butterworths, London.

WHO (World Health Organization) (1986). *Cancer pain relief*, pp. 18–21. WHO, Geneva.

Wulf HR, Pedersen SA, Rosenberg R (1986). *Philosophy of medicine: an introduction*, p. 172. Blackwell, Oxford.

Yorkstone P (1981). Bereavement. *British Medical Journal*, 282:1224–5.

Zimmerman JM, Roche KA (1986). The hospice care team. In *Hospice: complete care for the terminally ill* (2nd edn), pp. 99–117. Urban and Schwarzenberg, Baltimore, MD.

20.8 The organization of cancer services

JERZY EINHORN

The first part of this chapter describes the development of cancer services over the past 25 years, the demands which have prompted this development, and the present-day situation. Rapid scientific progress in recent years has made new demands on the organization of cancer services. The effects on the future structure of services are hard to predict. However, they will be discussed in the second part of the chapter.

DEMANDS ON CANCER SERVICES

Many national and international surveys in the past 25 years have led to decisions concerning the reorganization of cancer services. These surveys were prompted mainly by three facts:

(1) the growing number of cancer patients;

(2) the demands generated by medical progress;

(3) a newly aroused interest in the psychological and psychosocial aspects of cancer care.

Number of cancer patients

The first population-based cancer registers, offering a dependable basis on which to assess the incidence of cancer diseases, were started approximately 40 years ago in the Nordic countries, parts of the United Kingdom, Poland, and individual states of the United States and Canada. The Nordic registers in particular cover all cancer cases in an entire population with relatively low mobility and are of high proven dependability (Mattsson 1984). This documentation, together with more sporadic information from other countries, is sufficient to provide a convincing demonstration of the scope of the problem. The number of cancer patients is increasing rapidly. This also applies, to a lesser extent, to the age-adjusted incidence. If nothing happens to change the current trends, between one in four and one in three of the present inhabitants of the Nordic countries will develop a cancer disease at some time during their lives.

For example, approximately 19 300 new cancer cases were registered in Sweden in 1958, while the figure for 1985 was 38 000; that is, the incidence doubled in 27 years (Swedish Cancer Registry 1958, 1985). The figure for 1990 is < 10 300 (Swedish Cancer Registry 1990). Approximately half this increase is due to the fact that we are living longer. When this is adjusted for, the residual unexplained rate of increase comes to approximately 40 per cent in 27 years. It is not known to what extent this represents a real increase or is partially due to improved diagnostics. However, whatever the reasons for the increase, the medical care organization is faced with an increasing number of patients with diagnosed cancer.

Progress in treatment

In the 1950s there were essentially two methods available for the treatment of cancer: surgery and radiotherapy. The interest was focused on primary curative treatment. In this situation it was acceptable for many countries to have almost no structured organization for cancer care. With the exception of a few cancer hospitals and well-equipped radiotherapy centres, most cancer patients were diagnosed and cared for within the ordinary medical system. Specialized cancer services, if available, were usually responsible for primary treatment with a curative aim only. When cure was impossible or proved unsuccessful, patients in large parts of the world were seldom admitted to specialized units. Even then structured interdisciplinary consultations were common when important decisions had to be made on the choice of treatment method. However, this was usually restricted to the choice of the primary treatment with an attempt to cure.

Since then surgery and radiotherapy have undergone development. Advances in surgery have resulted in increased conservation and improved reconstruction. Radiotherapy has developed from a rough method with uneven dose distribution to a method with a degree of precision which no pharmacological method can rival. In addition,

methods for endocrine manipulation of the most common types of tumours and more than 30 clinically useful cytotoxic drugs have been developed. Old approaches have been refined and given new names such as adjuvant and neoadjuvant therapy.

These developments have contributed to making cancer care more complicated. It has become obvious that no individual specialist can master all aspects of modern cancer care and therefore it is essential that important decisions on treatment of cancer be arrived at by an interdisciplinary team of specialists. Not infrequently the patient can be offered several alternative modes of treatment, which has augmented the demands on diagnosis and on the documentation underlying clinical decisions. In addition, the volume of cancer care has expanded in response to demands for improvements in the care given to patients who cannot be offered curative treatment.

This enormous development of treatment possibilities within two decades was the main factor triggering demands for a better organization of cancer services.

Psychosocial aspects

During the 1970s more interest began to be taken in psychological and, in certain countries, psychosocial care of severely ill patients and their relatives. Here again, cancer care has often had a spearhead rôle.

It became obvious that having time and being sympathetic alone was not sufficient. The reactions of patients, relatives, the physician, and other personnel to a potentially fatal disease is a field of research and development like any other and physicians and nurses are better equipped to help if they understand these reactions. They need not only instruction but also support in order to satisfy new demands. This has highlighted the demands on having cancer services in a dedicated environment where such needs can be catered for and where knowledge can be developed.

CANCER CENTRES

The enormous development of cancer care and its complexity has led to new demands for resources in the form of trained staff and apparatus. Facilities for modern radiotherapy are often cited as examples of expensive instrumental requirements. Demands have come to be made for an environment in which new knowledge can be developed and personnel can receive continuous training and necessary support.

The requisite resources of specialized personnel teams and apparatus cannot be provided in a multiplicity of hospitals. As early as 1966, the World Health Organization (WHO) asserted that 'to deal with the cancer problem, the aim should be to establish a network of specialized cancer treatment centres'. The same conclusion has been reached in all major national and international surveys during the past two decades.

There is a surprising degree of congruence in the basic demands which cancer centres are requested to meet. These centres should be responsible for treatment, education, training, research, and development. Some reports recommend that the centres be assigned additional responsibilities. However, there is less unanimity regarding the organization of cancer centres and, accordingly, cancer care in general.

Organization of cancer centres

In recommendations and decisions published in various countries, the following principles for possible organizational models can be identified:

(1) cancer hospitals;

(2) comprehensive cancer centres;

(3) coordinating cancer centres.

A cancer hospital is a separate entity in which all the clinical disciplines, laboratories, and other facilities are specialized for and concerned only with the diagnosis and treatment of cancer patients.

A comprehensive cancer centre is, in most of the descriptions, a geographic entity offering comprehensive cancer care. This centre may be a cancer hospital or an autonomous unit within a large hospital or medical school.

A coordinating cancer centre is a functional and not a geographic entity. It should offer comprehensive cancer care by coordinating existing resources. However, it must have a sufficiently large nucleus specialized in cancer management in addition to resources for coordination.

The essential models appear to be comprehensive cancer hospitals and coordinating cancer centres.

The present situation

It is not easy to gauge reliably the present developmental state of cancer centres or the organization of cancer services in different countries (Einhorn 1987a,b). This is only natural, since organizations are passing through a dynamic development process as a result of recently identified needs and recent decisions. Results do not always turn out according to plan. This can be due to unexpected experiences of the organization or lack of resources, but sometimes also to political or regional conflicts. The structure, organization, and resources of the large established cancer hospitals are relatively well known, but they are not necessarily representative of the whole fabric of cancer care in an individual country.

Many countries have published guidelines laid down by governments and/or parliaments for cancer care and the organization of cancer centres. However, the network is, at best, in the process of being built up. Situation reports, experience feedback, and published corrections made on this basis are available from only a few countries. It is hard to arrive at a firm view of, for example, the degree of centralization of cancer care, the scope of specialist resources, etc.

The former Soviet Union, Hungary, Bulgaria, Poland, and other East European countries reported a consistently organized hierarchical system ranging from well-equipped internationally known national cancer centres and hospitals to dispensaries staffed by specially trained personnel, often from a regional cancer centre. France reports a more or less complete network of some 20 comprehensive cancer hospitals. The best known of these, both nationally and internationally, are the Institut Curie in Paris and the Institut Gustave-Roussy in Villejuif. Decisions are reported for the development of some 20 cancer centres in Germany. The best known of these are the centre in Essen and, as an establishment mainly dedicated to research, the Deutsches Krebsforschungzentrum in Heidelberg. It is reported that six or seven cancer centres are planned in The Netherlands and four cancer hospitals in Portugal. Italy has a number of internationally known cancer hospitals, the most eminent being the Istituto Nazionale per lo Studio e la Cura dei Tumori in Milan and more are under construction. The United Kingdom has two of the world's oldest and best-known cancer hospitals, the Royal Marsden Hospital in London and in Sutton, Surrey and the Holt Radium Institute in Manchester. However, ongoing expansion in the United Kingdom is confined to coordinating cancer centres. The United States has a number of the world's largest, best-equipped, and best-known cancer hospitals: the Memorial Sloan-Kettering Cancer Center in New York, the Roswell Park Memorial Institute in Buffalo, NY, and, of more recent origin, the MD Anderson Hospital and Tumor Institute in Houston, Texas. The continuing expansion of cancer services in the United States is based on the 1971 National Cancer Act (Public Law 92-218). Under this Act and with assistance from the National Cancer Institute Cancer Program, a network of, at present, 20 comprehensive cancer centres has been built up (Steckel 1985), most of which are integrated with general care hospitals, unlike the three original 'categorical' centres mentioned above. The Nordic countries have one cancer hospital, Det Norske Radiumhospital, in Montebello near Oslo. Otherwise cancer services are based on coordinating cancer centres.

The organization of coordinating centres is more complicated and so 'coordinating centre' is a rather abstract concept in many cases. Since all the Nordic countries have decided to base their cancer services on this model and have been developing it fairly consistently for 15 years, the organization in one of those countries, Sweden, will be described here by way of example.

It should be noted that, in practice, there is not all that much difference between cancer hospitals and coordinating cancer centres. Few of the existing cancer hospitals are truly comprehensive. Cancer hospitals are also building up a coordinating network within their regions. Demands in this direction are growing rapidly.

Organization of cancer services in the Nordic countries

Regionalization of the Swedish health services was accomplished in the 1950s. Sweden's population is approximately 8 million and six regional hospitals are responsible for the most resource-demanding services. The guidelines for the organization of cancer care in Sweden were formulated in 1974 by the Swedish National Board of Health and Welfare (National Board of Health and Welfare 1974). Similar guidelines have been developed in other Nordic countries. A coordinating cancer centre has been established in each regional hospital in Sweden and these centres are currently at various stages of development. Their task is to provide modern comprehensive cancer care by coordination and specialization of existing resources. Therefore, the centres are functional units rather than geographical entities.

Each oncology centre has a nucleus specializing in cancer care, including a department of (non-surgical) oncology, a regional cancer registry, and facilities for external consultations (oncologists and some cancer nurses), for development of cancer programmes, and for teaching and training of medical and paramedical personnel within the region and an oncological library. Some centres also include special units for psychosocial cancer care, tumour pathology, cancer prevention, coordination of screening programmes, telephone counselling services, etc. Many have facilities for laboratory research.

Formation of subunits specializing in cancer care is encouraged within other departments of the regional hospital, where many cancer patients are treated and also in other major hospitals. The national recommendations include staffing of such subunits by personnel with special experience of cancer care and provision by the cancer centre of appropriate training. These subunits are associated with the cancer centre but remain an integrated part of their parent departments (Fig. 1).

The activities performed by these centres in Sweden are manifold and increasing (Table 1). The overall purpose of cancer centres is to coordinate and improve cancer care in the health service region.

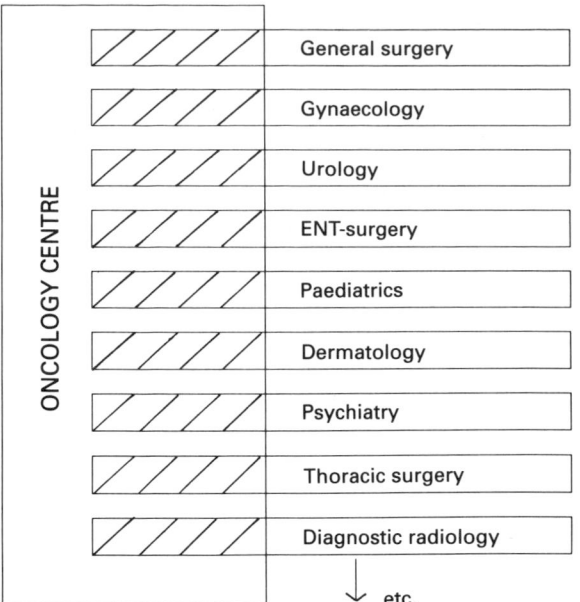

Fig. 1 Schematic organization of a coordinating cancer centre in Sweden.

Table 1 Responsibilities of cancer centres in Sweden

To organize registration and follow-up of cancer patients within the health service region

To coordinate the region's resources for cancer care by designing programmes for management and follow-up (core programmes)

To establish specialized interdisciplinary groups for cancer care

To meet requirements for training of all staff categories involved in cancer care

To be attentive to socio-medical aspects of cancer care

To promote integration of basic and clinical research on cancer

To advise on prevention of cancer and on screening for early detection

Source: Swedish National Board of Health and Social Welfare (1974).

The aim is to ensure a minimum standard of care in every case of cancer and optimum use of available resources.

Important aids to coordination include care (or management) programmes, regular interdisciplinary conferences concerning individual patients, a regional cancer register, consultation and information activities, telephone counselling services, and a special unit for psychological and socio-medical aspects of cancer care. All centres have access to biostatistical and epidemiological expertise associated with their regional cancer registers.

Care programmes

Coordination of cancer care within a region is aided by specially designed care or management programmes. A care programme is a statement of agreed policy, usually relating to a specific type of cancer. It covers referral routes and principles concerning examination, treatment, and follow-up, a system for evaluation of the results, and a mechanism for revision of the programme. Since care programmes must take into consideration the geography and resources of the region and since the clinicians responsible for cancer care within the same region must approve the principles outlined, there will inevitably be regional variations. Even so, there are an increasing number of national and also some pan-Nordic care programmes. A controlled clinical trial within the framework of the programme has proved to be a strong incentive for agreeing on and adhering to a care programme.

Oncological consultation service

In addition to the consultation service to hospitals, consultation services covering primary, home, and long-term care are also provided at some cancer centres.

These services include regular conferences at primary care centres. Patients attending these centres because of suspicion of neoplastic disease can be discussed, as can patients with known cancer who have been referred from hospitals to primary care physicians for treatment or follow-up. Measures for early diagnosis and cancer prevention can be discussed. This collaboration increases the scope for participation by primary care services in overall cancer management.

Cancer patients in long-term care clinics often have advanced disease. Regular consultancy visits of physicians and oncology nurses reduce the need for these patients to travel to specialist centres. The aim is to improve the quality of care by closer and more directed contact with the physicians and nurses attending the patients in these departments. The consulting physicians and nurses have similar functions for cancer patients in their homes.

Consultants should only give advice and not take over the responsibility for patients from attending physicians and nurses participating in regular home-care service, long-term care clinics, or primary care.

Management and evaluation of cancer centres

To gain acceptance for the coordinating functions of centres, it has proved appropriate for a policy-making steering group to be dominated by representatives of fields of activity outside the oncological centre whose activities the centre is to coordinate.

Since the network of cancer centres began to be built up in 1974, two nationwide evaluations of their development and performance have been made. The first, requested by the Swedish Government, was presented to the Riksdag (Parliament) in 1984 and the second, initiated by the National Board of Health and Welfare, Sweden, was conducted in 1993.

Current state of planning of cancer services

A large number of national and international reports, recommendations, and policy decisions exist concerning the future organization of cancer services. Perhaps the best-known is *Guidelines for developing a comprehensive cancer centre* (UICC 1978). The most realistic of the international reports, although not comprehensive, is the European Communities' Action Programme Against Cancer (CEC 1985, 1989). This programme also conveys the strongest impression of political determination to reduce the anticipated impact of cancer diseases on a wide front and on a basis of concerted international cooperation.

Few of these action programmes dare to define the amount of resources needed for specialized cancer care or to address the question of the optimal degree of centralization and decentralization. This is natural in view of the problems encountered when applying any form of generalized guidelines. Each country and region is likely to have variable levels of need, expertise, resources, and philosophy for the delivery of medical care. Moreover, the problems differ fairly widely according to the size and wealth of the countries and the type of existing health services (socialized, regionalized, etc.).

The WHO has attempted to estimate the resources needed on the basis of inquiries by groups of experts recruited from various countries. For example, bed requirements for cancer care in the mid-1960s were estimated in a WHO report to be 650 per million population (WHO 1985). Since then the numbers of cancer patients and the resource requirements per patient have increased. Current bed occupancy for cancer in various European countries seems to range from 600 to 900 per million population. In most countries with a system of cancer centres or cancer hospitals, the number of beds at these centres is much lower than the total occupied by cancer patients within the region. In the Stockholm-Gotland region (population 1.6 million) the mean bed occupancy for cancer is 1400–1500 (900 per million). Less than 200 of these beds are in units specializing exclusively in cancer care. The situation in most other countries appears to be much the same.

Therefore, in the great majority of countries only a fraction of cancer patients have the benefit of treatment at a cancer centre. At the same time there appears to be a widespread political determination to build up a viable network of cancer centres. Patients with curable cancer disease generally have only one chance of definitive cure and that is related to primary treatment. Therefore, this chance has to be put to the best possible use.

Author's conclusions

The author of this chapter has had the opportunity, as an expert engaged by the WHO, the UICC, and individual European, African, Asian, and North American states, to study what are considered to be the most important, relevant, and difficult problems connected with an ongoing organization of cancer services. These are as follows.

1. What is a realistic short-term objective in the absence of a network of cancer centres?

2. What is the minimum size for a functioning centre?

3. What are the mechanisms by which a coordinating centre can influence the community?

Although there are no generally accepted answers to these questions, there is growing agreement with regard to the size of a cancer centre. The aim should be to establish a network of regional cancer centres which can admit at least two-thirds of all cancer patients in the region at least once during their disease. However, even this aim may be difficult to attain. What, then, should be the realistic short-term objective with highest priority? The consensus appears to be that in most cases of cancer the important decisions on therapy should not be made by a single clinician but by an interdisciplinary team, preferably a team of physicians specializing in cancer care.

Progress towards a blanket organization for regional comprehensive cancer care can be made by concentrating management within specialist centres (a cancer hospital or a comprehensive cancer centre) or by coordinating existing resources. Both methods are valid. The balance between these two is difficult to strike, depending as it does on the geography of the region, the importance of proximity to the social network offered by the residential locality, the existing organization for medical care, the resources available, and the prestige and excellence of the cancer centre.

Concentration currently provides a highly sophisticated service, but in most countries only for a minority of patients. Agreements reached by coordination involve difficulties of a magnitude that can be appreciated only by those who have tried to surmount them. The boundaries between these extreme models are not rigid and in fact it seems as though they will be obliterated with the passage of time.

FUTURE DEMANDS ON CANCER SERVICES

The rapid development of our understanding of the causes, diagnosis, treatment, rehabilitation, and psychosocial needs of cancer patients and the requirements for 'total care' of the patient and the family will, before long, result in new demands on cancer services. It will not be easy to gain acceptance for these demands. An organization recently decided on for catering for present-day needs is in the process of being built up. Special problems arise when new demands, which can necessitate a revision, are presented during this build-up phase.

Cancer services have the aim of counteracting the effects of cancer. Theoretically, this can be achieved as follows:

(1) prevention;

(2) early diagnosis;

(3) treatment and rehabilitation;

(4) research which increases our knowledge in these fields.

Epidemiology and prevention

The first major discovery in cancer epidemiology was made in the United Kingdom in 1775, when Sir Percival Pott pointed out that boy chimney sweeps had a high incidence of what was otherwise a very uncommon type of tumour: skin cancer of the scrotum. This gave the signal for clinical and, later, experimental research based on this observation and, finally, effective prevention. Almost all subsequent major discoveries in cancer epidemiology concerned the causes of such signal tumours, that is, tumours of an uncommon type that suddenly increase in a small limited population, often as a result of an occupation exposure. The only exception concerning rarity was the discovery, also in the United Kingdom, of the relationship between smoking and lung cancer.

The advent of modern computer technology in recent decades has made possible developments in cancer epidemiology by allowing large quantities of information on large populations to be handled in a way that was previously quite inconceivable. As a result it has been observed that there are major differences in the incidence of different types of tumours between different countries and geographical regions. There are also large differences between regions with regard to the availability of medical care, diagnostic criteria, and the reliability of cancer registration. However, these cannot explain the magnitude of the differences that have been observed. These differences are also corroborated by the results of studies of emigrants who frequently approach the incidence rate of their new country for different forms of tumour, not infrequently within one or a few generations, despite consistent intermarriage between immigrants from the same region. The possibility cannot be excluded that the explanation as to why cancer of the prostate is 40 times more common in the United States than in Japan, primary cancer of the liver is 100 times more common in Mozambique than in the United Kingdom, or cancer of the nasopharynx is 40 times more common in Singapore than in the United Kingdom could provide us with a basis for rational and, it is hoped, realistic preventive measures.

Even more important is the fact that in countries with a reliable cancer registration kept over several decades, it has been found that the incidence of some types of tumours may increase or decrease dramatically over a relatively short period of time (Fig. 2).

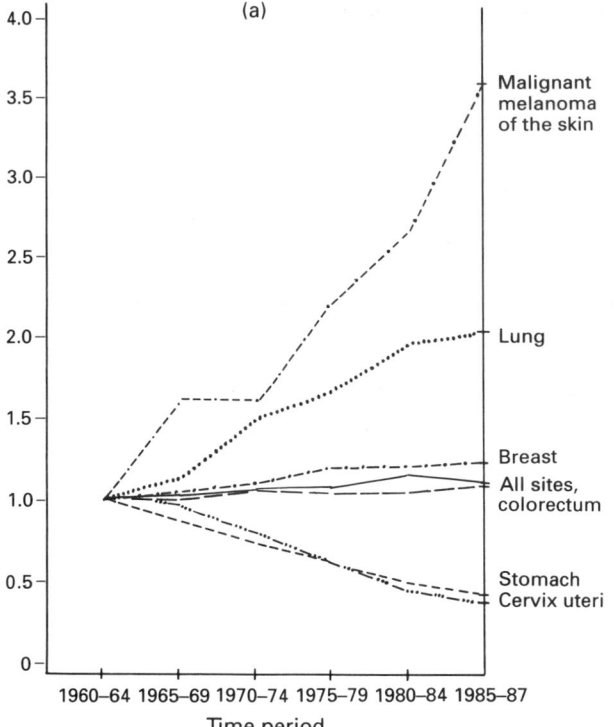

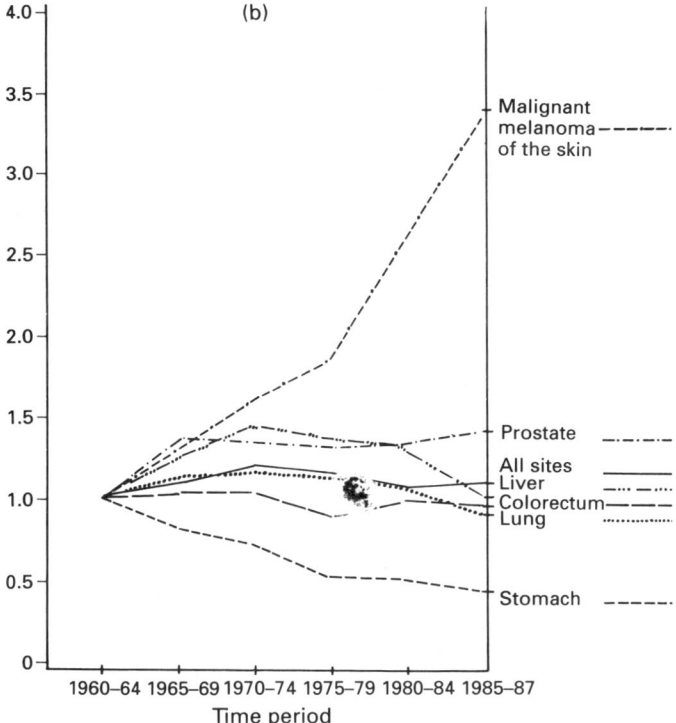

Fig. 2 Relative changes in the age-adjusted incidence of some tumours in (a) females and (b) males in Stockholm between 1960 and 1987. (Based on figures from the Regional Cancer Registry for the Stockholm-Gotland Region 1989.)

Table 2 Best estimates of the relative importance of different factors for the incidence of cancer in Sweden

Factor	Percentage of all cancer incidence
Diet	30
Tobacco	15
Sex and reproduction	10
Sun and UV light	5
Ionizing radiation (including radon)	3
Infections	2
Occupation	2
Air pollution	1

Source: Swedish Cancer Committee (1984).

cancer of the stomach has decreased by 50 per cent over the same period of time in both women and men (Fig. 2), this might provide us with a useful basis for realistic preventive measures.

Several researchers and research groups have tried to establish the relative importance of different factors governing the incidence of cancer. One of the best known is the estimate by Doll and Peto (1981) of factors governing cancer mortality in the United States. A corresponding estimate concerning cancer incidence in Sweden has been prepared by the Cancer Committee appointed by the Swedish Government (Swedish Cancer Committee 1984) (Table 2). Both must be regarded as the best possible guess based on incomplete information. However, there is a good degree of fit between these and other similar assessments. Almost all reports are in full agreement as to the importance of our living habits.

Cancer epidemiology has provided a rapidly increasing number of observations related to the common types of tumours: in developed countries these are cancer of the breast, prostate, lung, colorectum, nasopharynx, cervix, and endometrium (Doll and Peto 1981; Swedish Cancer Committee 1984). These reports, based on descriptive studies, correlation studies, and studies of the cohort or case-control type, are often insufficient to demonstrate causal relationships. However, when they are supported by the results of independent studies, for example using exposure of animals under controlled conditions, it must be accepted that there are strong indications for the existence of a causal relationship. This will create a new and often difficult situation for society to deal with. When the data linking cancer and living habits become more certain, the problem will be how to use the information. This background and the ethics and realism of the resultant conditions governing cancer prevention are described at greater length elsewhere in this book. However, it should be made clear that there is a generally accepted and well-substantiated view that the knowledge which we now possess and which is growing rapidly will soon have to be used (Committee on Diet, Nutrition, and Cancer 1982; Swedish Cancer Committee 1984; CEC 1985; NCI 1986).

Society must be very careful when using the ever-greater flow of scientifically more or less proven information on prevention of cancer as a basis for efforts to change attitudes, standards, and habits of the population. The most important method available at present for reducing the total cancer incidence is information on health. One of the questions which then arises is who should have the delicate responsibility for formulating and spreading this public health information. There is a growing awareness that the practising oncologists and nurses, who have daily contact with human cancer, have acquired knowledge and insights which ought to be utilized by society when formulating and disseminating this information.

These observations indicate that factors other than genetic are responsible for the observed rapid changes in incidence during a short period. For example, if it was known why the age-adjusted incidence of malignant melanoma in Stockholm has increased by approximately 350 per cent over 23 years and the incidence of

In addition, participation by cancer centres and by staff actively involved in cancer care has been found to enhance the credibility of preventive campaigns. To this end, however, oncologists and cancer nurses will have to familiarize themselves with the scientific, ethical, and human aspects of the problems involved in disseminating this new knowledge to the public and the responsibilities of cancer centres will have to be expanded.

Mass screening for early detection of cancer

Encouraged by the improvement in results due to earlier clinical diagnosis, we are trying to make diagnoses earlier still, preferably before the tumour gives rise to any symptoms. It is reasonable to suppose that, if we could detect tumours at this preclinical stage, even more cancer patients would be cured. However, the prerequisites are many: for example, access to a reliable diagnostic method which can be used to identify preclinical disease stages of a common type of tumour, reasonably effective methods of treating preclinical disease, and readiness to apply mass screening of healthy populations. In Europe at present the necessary criteria are believed to be satisfied in two or three types of common tumours. Mass screening projects are in progress for early detection of carcinoma of the uterine cervix and the breast and of colorectal cancer. Large-scale screening is in progress in China for early diagnosis of cancer of the liver (Shanghai) and oesophagus (Peking region) and in Japan for early diagnosis of cancer of the stomach and oesophagus.

The results of major prospective randomized trials in the United States (Shapiro et al. 1982) and Sweden (Tabar et al. 1985) have been published, as well as other interesting trials (Verbeek et al. 1984) using mass screening by mammography. All show a significant reduction of approximately 30 per cent of the breast cancer death rate for the study groups compared with a control group not offered screening. The gain appears to be greater after a longer observation period.

We have had even longer experience, more than 30 years, of mass screening for early diagnosis of cancer of the uterine cervix and its precursor lesions. Unfortunately, there is no controlled study of the usefulness of this procedure. Retrospective analyses cannot replace the information that is provided by prospectively randomized studies. However, the results of retrospective statistical analyses strongly indicate that cervical cancer mortality can be reduced as a result of mass screening (Pettersson et al. 1985, 1986). However, the 'price' paid by the screened population is high. Eight hundred and eighty new cases of invasive carcinoma of the uterine cervix were registered in Sweden in 1959. By 1985 the figure had dropped to 520. There was a reduction of more than 350 cases per year and also a reduction in the overall mortality in cervical cancer. We cannot be sure that this reduction is wholly due to mass screening. At the same time, screening has required more than a million smears and generated more than 7000 surgical operations every year.

Mass screening with mammography (Shapiro et al. 1982; Tabar et al. 1985; Verbeek et al. 1986) and vaginal cytology (Pettersson et al. 1985, 1986) can probably considerably reduce the mortality in breast and cervical cancer. Although this seems reassuring, many important questions remain unanswered.

We have no experience of the natural history of preclinical lesions. Some of them will proliferate rapidly, whereas others will not develop into clinical tumours during the patient's lifetime. Until we have methods for differentiating between these lesions, all patients with preclinical lesions must be offered treatment. Therefore, mass screening inevitably results not only in many people being worried but also in many being treated unnecessarily. Society and above all the screened population is subjected to unpleasantness and often is also burdened with considerable expense. Mass screening is based on a different ethical principle from routine medical care. By encouraging healthy persons with neither symptoms nor discomfort to attend mass screening, society takes upon itself a special responsibility.

When a new method which can alleviate the effects of a potentially fatal disease is discovered, it is natural that strong demands should be raised for its introduction. Given the periodicity characterizing standpoints on medical advances, enthusiasm followed by scepticism, one must expect the value of mass screening for early diagnosis of cancer to become a topic of debate after a few years, with special reference to the disadvantages to the individual and to the community. In addition, to the questions asked at present:

(1) how is morbidity and mortality of the disease reduced?

(2) how often has treatment been made less of an ordeal by early discovery?

(3) which are the optimum age groups and appropriate intervals between examinations?

The following questions will also be asked:

(1) how many people are frightened or treated unnecessarily?

(2) what medical care is generated by mass screening?

(3) what are the psychosocial effects of screening?

All these questions are aimed at assessing whether the drawbacks are reasonable in proportion to the benefits to the individual and whether the cost to society is reasonable in proportion to the benefits to the population. It is essential that answers be found to these justifiable questions concerning the advantages and disadvantages of mass screening. Answers must also be found to the questions that are asked by the patients selected for recall and treatment.

There are many actors involved, but it is cancer centres above all which ought to feel responsible for making reasonable documentation available for answering these questions. This calls for prompt appropriate prospective action to ensure that documentation is available for a future assessment based on dependable statistical and epidemiological data.

It is not certain that when all the facts are known they will favour the continuation of mass screening. However, in the short-term (that is, for the next decade or two), medical services and society in many countries will be involved in large-scale mass screening for early detection of various forms of cancer. Demands will then be made for cancer centres to take part in compiling the documentation on which to base the inauguration and evaluation of these measures. In several regions these centres are already being entrusted with the organization and coordination of mass screening and the administration of summons routines, follow-up, and evaluation.

FUTURE DEMANDS ON TRAINING

Growing demands from society for total care of cancer patients, including adequate psychological care and support for relatives, are making new and increasing demands on cancer services. In those countries where demands for optimum assessment at critical stages of a cancer disease will be fulfilled, the majority of cancer patients will pass through a cancer centre. Even then, however, the greater part of cancer care will be provided away from centres. Centres should be required to take part in the coordination of such care. Moreover, in the near future centres will be required to take part not only in care and rehabilitation but also in screening and preventive measures, including information to the public. This will mean demands for interaction with the community and new demands on the knowledge possessed by physicians and other personnel, particularly nurses working in cancer centres and subcentres.

Training of oncologists

Discoveries in fundamental science during the past decade have produced a breakthrough in several fields of cancer research. This has been brought about by the invention of recombinant DNA technology followed by the discovery of oncogenes and the development of technology for the production of monoclonal antibodies. We are beginning to understand one basic change in the cell that leads to malignancy. Tools are available for analysing malignant cells by isolating individual genes and identifying the proteins that they encode. We have the potential for biosynthesis of substances occurring in normal and in tumour cells, including products of oncogenes, anti-oncogenes, and regulatory proteins. Individual growth factors, antigrowth factors, and factors influencing cell function can be produced in large quantities. The possibilities for recognition, separation, purification, and production of cellular components and biologically active substances of the cells are apparently endless. With new biological techniques, analysis of the pattern of gene expression and of growth-control proteins, for example, may help us to predict the biological behaviour of the tumour. Information concerning the response of the tumour to treatment may in future be obtainable within a few days. These possibilities have profoundly influenced medical science and particularly those aspects relating to cancer.

Although few patients have experienced any benefit from these, achievements and limitations for future application in clinical practice are becoming obvious and it is necessary for tomorrow's oncologists to be acquainted with this new and expanding knowledge concerning the nature of cancer, the potential for developments in diagnosis, the advantages and limitations of the new 'biological' methods of treatment, and the scope for future development in these fields. This calls for a major expansion of the content of the education received by future oncologists. This is happening at a time when demands are being made for the participation of cancer services in prevention and mass screening for early diagnosis.

The responsibilities of future oncologists will extend far beyond the treatment of cancer patients. They will be required to have adequate knowledge of basic research as applied to clinical practice in oncology. Future oncologists (and cancer nurses) will have to be prepared to assume responsibility for 'total cancer care'. In addition, they will need to take part in cancer prevention and will require a sound knowledge of the advantages and disadvantages of mass screening for early diagnosis of cancer and provision of information to the public on all these problems. The education will have to be adapted to these requirements in a realistic way. It is essential to plan the training adapted for these future needs today.

Education and training of cancer nurses

There is a growing awareness of the need to acknowledge a changed rôle and identity for the nurse. The way ahead is obstructed by a myth: the doctor knows everything and the nurse knows a part of what the doctor knows. Of course, this is not true. Physicians

and nurses have different fields of knowledge. These fields overlap, but only partially. Nurses have their own field of knowledge and the best possibilities for developing it. It is essential for this and its consequences to be generally accepted, otherwise the development of an important field of clinical knowledge will be hampered. This development is another process which has been spearheaded by cancer care.

The growth of interest in caring issues is increasing the importance of the knowledge and rôle of the nurse. Nurses often have the best understanding of the physical and emotional needs of the patients and their relatives. Nurses have developed information and training programmes for patients and relatives. Nurses in specialized units are being allotted increasing responsibilities as teachers in primary, long-term, and home care. In several hospitals, nurses have their own consulting hours for dealing with practical aspects of care. Nurses are often best qualified to staff a telephone counselling service for the general public and to develop and evaluate supportive programmes for relatives. Nurses have played an important part in the development of measures to reduce the adverse effects of heavy treatment programmes, not least for cancer patients. They ought to play a rôle in the transmission of technology and methods from research to clinical practice and in the comprehensive evaluation of new clinical methods. Nurses in an increasing number of cancer centres are being allowed to contribute actively towards the planning and evaluation of the results of controlled clinical trials. This entails some new requirements and, accordingly, will demand additional knowledge. Therefore, nurses should be given increasing opportunities to develop their expanding field of knowledge and to undertake formalized research training.

The European Community has recently accepted an ambitious programme for training in cancer nursing which comprises a basic course and the opportunity of further training for oncology nurses (CEC 1986, 1988; Tiffany *et al.* 1987; European Oncology Nursing Society 1989). However, the most important factor in the long term will be the Common Core defined for structured higher education in cancer nursing. Among other things, the participants will undergo targeted research training. The European School of Oncology organizes national and international cancer nursing courses. Plans exist for a European School of Cancer Nursing. A separate Cancer Nursing section was recently set up within the National Institutes of Health (National Cancer Institute in the United States) and generous funds were set aside for research and development projects in cancer nursing, scholarships for nurses, funds for travel, etc. A growing number of national and international scientific congresses on cancer nursing are being organized.

When these questions are being debated, one feels bound to draw attention to other categories of medical care workers, for example medical secretaries and documentalists. Post-basic training of qualified medical secretaries adapted to the increasingly diversified needs of cancer centres would streamline the activities of those centres and relieve the load on other categories of personnel.

CONCLUSIONS

The history of clinical oncology and of cancer research is a history of unrealistic hopes followed by periods of unjustified pessimism. We are currently passing through a period of high optimism. Not all our hopes will come true, but some will.

Cancer has hitherto been given a low priority in our health care system. Therefore, the organization of cancer care and cancer services is often fragmented and the same is true for teaching the subject at most medical and nursing schools (Robèrt *et al.* 1988;

CEC and EORTC 1988). To the general public, cancer is often a mysterious disease, more feared than any other. The general attitude is that cure can only be offered to a few patients and that the remainder must die painfully. The facts are different and attitudes are changing.

During the past two decades, oncology has been one of the most rapidly developing fields of medicine. Progress has been made towards a better understanding of the nature of the disease, the possibilities of its prevention, and better and earlier diagnosis and treatment. We have a growing store of experience, practical knowledge, and motivation for taking care of the 50 per cent of cancer patients whom we cannot cure. This rapid progress is expected to continue, which is bound to affect requirements for cancer services.

The political powers appear to be well aware of the outlook for the future and the potential for development in cancer services. Cancer control programmes have been worked out in many countries and regions. Important components are the political determination to make the necessary policy decisions and to promote developments which will limit the effects of cancer diseases.

The concept of specialized cancer centres is gaining ground. It is acknowledged that cancer centres offer a base for the comprehensive expertise representing clinical and laboratory disciplines specializing in cancer care and necessary for the optimization of evaluation and treatment. They offer sufficient patient material to advance knowledge, for the education of specialists and students, and to provide a stable base for visiting consultants. There is also a growing awareness that cancer centres are needed in order to provide a credible base for cancer prevention campaigns. There appears to be cause for a certain amount of optimism concerning the future development of cancer services.

REFERENCES

CEC (Commission of the European Communities) (1985). *European action programme against cancer*. Document UKCCCR 86/8 COM (85), final, annex 1, 5 and 6; Document 495312/85 EN. CEC, Brussels.

CEC (Commission of the European Communities) (1986). *Europe against cancer. Programme: proposal for a plan of action 1987–1989*. Document COM 86/717 final. CEC, Brussels.

CEC (Commission of the European Communities) (1988). *Advisory Committee on Training in Nursing. Report on training in cancer nursing*. Document III/D/248/3/88. CEC, Brussels.

CEC (Commission of the European Communities) (1989). *Europe against cancer programme: outline for an action plan 1990–1994*. Document SEC (89) 648. CEC, Brussels.

CEC (Commission of the European Communities) and EORTC (1988). *A curriculum in oncology for medical students in Europe*. A report to the Commission of European Communities from the Consensus Workshop jointly organized by the EEC and EORTC, Bonn. CEC, Brussels.

Committee on Diet, Nutrition, and Cancer (1982). *Diet, nutrition, and cancer*. National Academy Press, Washington, DC.

Doll R, Peto R (1981). The causes of cancer: quantitative estimates of avoidable risks of cancer in the United States today. *Journal of the National Cancer Institute*, **66**:1191.

Einhorn J (1987*a*). Recent advances in radiotherapy and oncology and expectations for the future. In *Investigational techniques in oncology* (ed. NM Bleehen). Springer Verlag, Berlin.

Einhorn J (1987*b*). Recent developments in oncology and prospects for the future. *Lectures and Symposia, 14th International Cancer Congress, Budapest*, Vol. 1, p. 125. Karger, Basel.

Einhorn J, Holm LE (1987). Europe against cancer. *Lancet*, i:1208.

Eklund G, Carstensen J (1987). The Unit for Cancer Epidemiology of the Karolinska Institute, Stockholm. Communication based on *Cancer incidence in Sweden 1982, Swedish Department of Health and Welfare, and Swedish Mortality Statistics, Life Tables, 1976–1980*. Statistiska Centralbyrån.

European Oncology Nursing Society (1989). *A core curriculum for a post-basic course in cancer nursing*. Haigh and Hochland, Manchester.

Mattsson B (1984). Cancer registration in Sweden. Studies on completeness and validity of incidence and mortality registers. Dissertation, Stockholm.

National Board of Health and Welfare, Sweden (1974). Planering av onkologisk sjukvård. *Råd och anvisningar från Socialstyrelsen*, no. 32.

National Board of Health and Welfare (1993). Alliuèune rad supreude cancerroteleus orpevisetion.

NCI (National Cancer Institute), Division of Cancer Prevention and Control (1986). Cancer control objectives for the nation: 1985–2000. Executive Summary. *NCI Monograph*, **2**.

Pettersson F, Björkholme E, Näslund I (1985). Evaluation of screening for cervical cancer in Sweden: trends in incidence and mortality 1958–1980. *International Journal of Epidemiology*, **14**(4):521.

Pettersson F, Näslund I, Malker B (1986). Evaluation of the effect of Papanicolaou screening in Sweden: record linkage between a central screening registry and the National Cancer Registry. *IARC Scientific Publications*, **76**:91.

Regional Cancer Registry (1989). Stockholm-Gotlands Onkologiska Centrum, Radiumhemmet, Karolinska Hospital, Stockholm, Sweden.

Robèrt KH, Einhorn J, Kornhuber B, Peckham M, Zittoun R (1988). European undergraduate education in oncology. A report of the EORTC Education Branch. *Review in Oncology*, 1:423.

Shapiro S, Vennet W, Strax L, Roeser R (1982). Ten–fourteen-year effect of screening on breast cancer mortality. *Journal of the National Cancer Institute*, **69**:349–55.

Steckel JS (1985). The NCI's cancer centers program: past, present, and future. *Medical and Pediatric Oncology*, **13**:59–64.

Swedish Cancer Committee (1984). *Cancer, causes, prevention etc.* SOU 1984:67. Cancer Committee, Swedish Department of Health and Welfare, Stockholm.

Swedish Cancer Registry (1958). *Cancer incidence in Sweden*. National Board of Health and Welfare, Stockholm.

Swedish Cancer Registry (1985). *Cancer incidence in Sweden*. National Board of Health and Welfare, Stockholm.

Swedish Cancer Registry (1990). *Cancer incidence in Sweden*. National Board of Health and Welfare, Stockholm.

Tabar L, *et al.* (1985). Reduction in mortality from breast cancer after mass screening with mammography. Randomized trial from the breast cancer screening working group of the Swedish National Board of Health and Welfare. *Lancet*, i:829–32.

Tiffany R, Webb P, Copp K, Pritchard AP (1987). *Report of the ad-hoc Working Group on Training in Cancer to the Advisory Committee on Training in Nursing*. CEC, Brussels.

UICC (International Union Against Cancer) (1978). *Guidelines for developing a comprehensive cancer centre*. Committee on International Collaborative Activities (CICA), Geneva.

Verbeek AL, Hendriks JH, Holland R, Mrvunac M, Sturmans F, Day NE (1984). Reduction of breast cancer mortality through mass screening with modern mammography: first results of the Nijmegen project 1975–1981. *Lancet*, ii:1222–4.

WHO (World Health Organization) (1985). *Targets for health for all*. WHO Regional Office for Europe, Copenhagen.

20.9 Economic considerations in cancer care
JANE HALL AND MARTIN TATTERSALL

INTRODUCTION

Economics will feature increasingly in cancer research and in the allocation of resources for cancer prevention, diagnosis, and treatment. Clinicians are now expected not just to provide patient care but also to manage budgets. Consequently, clinicians concerned with giving the best possible care to their patients will need to understand something of what health care costs are and how they can be estimated. This is not as bad as some may fear, for health economics is as much concerned with health benefits as with costs. Health economists strongly advocate measurement of outcomes along with costs in considering how best to allocate scarce resources. Ineffective treatment cannot be cost-effective, however little it costs.

The treatment of cancer patients is being affected by economic considerations (Stoll 1988; Timothy *et al.* 1988). Costs are being considered in choosing treatment for patients with localized cancers. Until recently, in the development of new cancer treatments, assessment has included only an evaluation of treatment efficacy. As resources are limited it is increasingly clear that clinicians should now be concerned about costs in clinical practice and in the evaluation of new treatments (Wiltes 1987; McVie 1988; Timothy *et al.* 1988).

Examples of attempts to introduce cost factors into treatment considerations include the estimation of possible savings resulting from bone-marrow growth factor support, even though the charges for these new products are high. The costs of bone-marrow transplantation for patients with acute leukaemia in remission have been assessed and it was stated that 'at 6000 pounds each it [bone-marrow transplantation] must be a bargain' (Kay *et al.* 1980). The costs of anticancer drugs are easily itemized and, thus, many medical oncologists are aware of some of the costs of cancer treatment (Friedlander and Tattersall 1982; Rees 1985; Goodwin *et al.* 1988). Less easily identified are the costs of the attendant in-patient stay, antimicrobial therapy, and blood product support. High charges and fewer in-patient services have led to the replacement of in-patient care with ambulatory services. However, the costs of the elements of out-patient management are even less clear (Calman *et al.* 1978).

As well as treatment, costs of investigations are being scrutinized in, for instance, the identification of the primary tumour site in patients with metastases from an unknown primary (Levine *et al.* 1985; Shaha *et al.* 1988). Screening for cancer (for example, mammography) is being evaluated not only for its effectiveness but also for its financial and community costs.

In this chapter we outline what doctors should know about costs and introduce methods of economic evaluation. It is our hope that clinicians who are more economically aware will learn to communicate easily with health economists (and vice versa) and that this will lead to better health economics for the promotion of better health and better health services.

We start by working through an example that will illustrate the principles involved in economic evaluation in a context that may be familiar to clinicians.

REDUCING THE BURDEN OF BREAST CANCER: AN EXAMPLE

Let us assume that as part of a national programme for better health, the government has promised funds to reduce breast cancer mortality. Funds are available for this objective but the sum of money is fixed and limited. How should this money be spent? Enthusiastic radiologists point to the studies which show reduced mortality from mammographic screening (Shapiro *et al.* 1982; Taber *et al.* 1985). Should a national screening programme be established? The purpose of this section of the chapter is not to answer that question but rather to show how it can and indeed, in our opinion, should be answered. To do this we shall need to consider the costs, benefits, and risks of screening and alternative uses for the money to achieve the aim of reduced breast cancer mortality.

Costs

What are the costs of mammography screening? Most obviously, there are the costs of recruiting women for screening, taking the mammograms, and then reading them. However, these are not the total costs.

Screening mammograms will separate those women with radiologically suspicious features of breast cancer from those without these signs. Those who are suspected of having breast cancer will be investigated further until a diagnosis is reached. For every woman eventually diagnosed with breast cancer, ten others without breast cancer will require investigation. Of the women who proceed to surgical biopsy, one to two will not have cancer for every one who does (Forrest 1986; Mitchell 1987). These investigations would not have been undertaken without the screening programme. Therefore, the costs of the further investigations must also be counted in the costs of screening.

Following a positive diagnosis, women will require treatment for breast cancer and that also incurs costs. Breast cancer would be detected and treated (generally at a more advanced stage) in the absence of a screening programme, so some costs of breast cancer management would be incurred anyway, although later. In counting the treatment costs of screening, it is important to offset the savings from cancer treatment that would have been given ultimately in the absence of screening.

Most screening tests will detect various conditions other than the disease or condition in question. Often these other conditions would not have become evident and so would not have been treated without the screening. Mammography is no exception to this; non-malignant tumours and cysts in the breast, which would not have been discovered in the absence of screening, may be revealed. If these are deemed to require surgery or other interventions, these treatment costs will also add to the costs of the screening programme.

The costs of screening are more than the costs of taking and reading mammograms. The costs of subsequent investigations and treatment should also be counted. This is illustrated in Fig. 1.

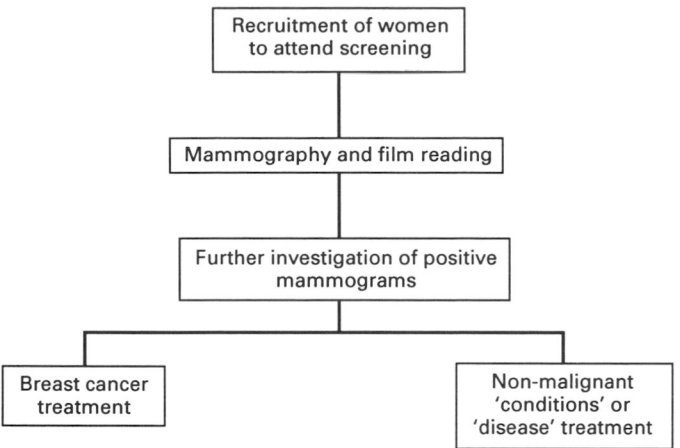

Fig. 1 Costs of mammographic screening.

There are several decisions to be made about how to operate a screening programme: to what age groups should screening be offered, how frequently should women be screened, should one-view or two-view mammograms be taken, and so on. Let us consider the choice of screening interval, for example. Women could be screened annually, once every 2 years, or once every 3 years. A more frequent screening interval will detect more cancers and reduce the number of cancers becoming symptomatic between screening rounds, but it will also be more expensive. The choice of screening interval is not just a clinical decision, but is also an economic one particularly if the funds available will not allow all women to be screened as frequently as desired by clinicians. Which is the best buy? The objective for which the funds were provided is the reduction of breast cancer mortality; therefore it follows that the best buy is the option which gives the greatest decrease in breast cancer deaths for the funds available.

Benefits (and risks)

Assessment of the total costs of screening shows how much screening can be funded from the hypothetical fixed budget, but it does not show whether screening represents value for that money. That requires an assessment of the benefits and risks involved.

The benefits of early treatment of screening-detected cancers, it is suggested, are not just better chances of survival but also improved quality of life. Conservative surgery might result in improved physical functioning and less psychological distress. Therefore, in choosing the best buy for interventions which reduce the burden of breast cancer, ideally both quantity and quality of life should be considered.

Very few medical interventions come with no risks or side-effects attached. There is substantial evidence that some new medical technologies have been adopted widely before adequate evaluation (Cochrane 1972; Frazier and Hiatt 1978) and that some new treatments have, on balance, done more harm than good (Barnes 1977; McPherson and Fox 1977; Banta and Thacker 1979). In the case of mammography, the hazards of radiation exposure are so low as to be considered negligible (Forrest 1986) but there are other costs and risks for the women being screened.

The examination itself requires women to give up their time, it is embarrassing and uncomfortable for most, and distinctly painful for some. Some women will suffer not only the time loss and discomfort associated with further investigations, but also the anxiety of a possible diagnosis of breast cancer. Yet, as discussed earlier,

most of these women will not have cancer. Breast disease, whether malignant or not, is associated with lower self-esteem, poorer body image, and impaired sexual relationships (Morris and Sherwood 1977) and surgery is associated with fear of disfigurement (Knobf 1986).

In assessing health outcomes, both gains and losses (both benefits and risks) should be made explicit as far as possible and taken into account. Furthermore, an analysis of risks should be broad, and include psychosocial, logistic, and other considerations which will impact on the population.

The 'best buy' in terms of screening strategies will be the one that provides the greatest increase in net health benefits in terms of quality and quantity for its additional net costs; in other words the most extra health for the available funds.

Alternatives

So far, we have considered a choice only between different screening strategies. Still working with our hypothetical example, let us say that whilst some breast clinicians advocate screening, others suggest that more effective treatment of micrometastatic disease at the time of clinical presentation, that is, adjuvant therapy after local control, will lead to a greater reduction in mortality.

Therefore, would more adjuvant chemotherapy be a better buy than establishing screening programmes? Chemotherapy following local treatment by surgery or radiotherapy is more expensive than local treatment alone. If this treatment delays the development of metastatic disease and/or reduces its incidence, then there will be some treatment cost savings in the future which will partially or possibly completely offset the higher initial treatment costs. Increasing the use of adjuvant therapy will have health gains in terms of both survival and quality of life.

Of course, in real life the decision would be how much more adjuvant chemotherapy should be provided against how much to extend a screening programme. The funds available are rarely sufficient to do everything. However, to keep matters simple in this hypothetical example let us restrict it to an either/or decision: either breast cancer screening or increased adjuvant therapy. In real life, as in our hypothetical example, a choice has to be made and the principles which can help in analysing the consequences of that choice are the same.

The best buy is the one that delivers the most health gains for the funds available. Therefore, we want to compare the cost per 'unit' of health gained from investing in screening with the cost per 'unit' of health gained from investing in more adjuvant therapy.

SOME ECONOMIC PRINCIPLES

Everyone who works in health care knows that more could be done if more money were available. However, there are never enough health care resources available for everyone who could benefit from health care interventions. Scarcity of resources (and money is just a convenient measure of resources) relative to the opportunities for their use is the principal tenet of economics (Table 1).

There are many other examples that could be drawn from modern cancer care to illustrate the choices that have to be made. However, as long as there are not enough resources to do everything, choice is inevitable. Although choices are often framed in terms of spending money, they are in essence about competing 'goods'. In the example discussed above, the competing alternatives were breast cancer screening or adjuvant therapy in breast cancer management. Both alternatives are 'good' in that they offer the potential to reduce breast cancer mortality and improve quality of life. The cost of choosing

Table 1 Some economics

Resources are scarce
Choice is inevitable
Opportunity costs are benefits forgone
Costs include the initial intervention and its consequences
Incremental costs, that is, the costs of moving from one programme to another, are usually the relevant costs
Efficiency maximizing health gains for funds available

a screening programme is forgoing the benefits of more adjuvant therapy or of some other health programme, for example palliative care, cardiac rehabilitation, neonatal intensive care, community services for the elderly, and so on. This notion of cost as benefits forgone is the concept of opportunity cost. The opportunity cost of a health care programme is the health gains missed by not using the available funds (that is, resources) in the next-best health care programme.

Another important aspect of costs was illustrated by the screening example. Costs include not just the resources used in doing something, but also the costs of the consequences of doing that thing. The costs of screening include recruitment, mammography, follow-up investigations, and treatment for breast cancer and for other conditions discovered by screening.

Of course some costs, such as treatment costs of breast cancer in the screening example, would eventually be incurred. Thus, the estimate of the costs of the screening programme should take into account any savings due to treatment that would have been given anyway. This illustrates another important concept, that of the margin. What extra resources will be used in moving to a world with a screening programme from a world without one? The difference is the marginal or incremental cost. It is the relevant cost because these are the resources that could have been used for some other good purpose.

Given that choice is inevitable and that it means giving up some health benefits for other health benefits, how should the choice be made? In the example above, where funds were made available to reduce breast cancer mortality, it was suggested that the best buy with those funds would be the programme that resulted in the lowest cost per 'unit' of health gained. (We shall come back to what those units might be.) This is the economic concept of efficiency. It has nothing to do with saving money or making health care cheaper. It is about health outcomes achieved for money spent.

ECONOMICS IN HEALTH CARE EVALUATION

A programme may cost more, less, or the same as the alternative use of funds and it may provide greater, fewer, or the same health benefits. Clearly, if a new programme can reduce costs but yield the same health outcomes it is more efficient. It is not difficult to decide that the new programme is preferable to the old way of doing things and is therefore better. It is not necessary to be trained as a health economist to see that a programme that fits into cell a in Fig. 2 is better than its alternative.

Figure 2 shows that the programmes that give unequivocally more health gains per pound are preferable to their alternatives (cells a, b, and d). Programmes that give clearly less health gains per dollar than their alternatives are not to be preferred (cells f, h, and i). Difficulties arise when a new treatment or programme, such as mammographic screening, offers improved health outcomes but at a higher cost. Is this programme delivering more or less health gains

It can ⟶ provide health benefits that are:

Cost	GREATER	SAME	LESS
LESS	a	b	c
SAME	d	e	f
MORE	g	h	i

Better: a, b, d; worse: f, h, i.

Thus 'a' indicates programmes that cost less but provide greater health benefits, 'b' programmes that cost less and provide the same health benefits, and so on to 'i', programmes which cost more but provide fewer health benefits. Programmes which cost less for more or the same health benefits are clearly better, as programmes which cost more for the same or fewer health benefits are clearly worse.

Fig. 2 Consequences of a new health programme.

per dollar? It is more difficult to judge the efficiency of these programmes (cell g).

It is in decisions such as these that the techniques of economic appraisal or economic evaluation or the cost–benefit approach are useful. The essence of economic evaluation is the comparison of costs and benefits so that the most efficient alternative (that is, the one providing greater gain in benefits for the funds invested), can be identified.

Types of economic appraisal

Economic evaluation is generally regarded as comprising three techniques: cost–benefit analysis, cost-effectiveness analysis, and cost–utility analysis (Table 2). They differ in their approach to measuring benefits. Studies that consider costs only are a partial economic evaluation.

Cost–benefit analysis

In cost–benefit analysis, all benefits are measured and valued in money. This technique has been widely applied in such areas as agriculture where benefits may accrue to a wide range of parties but are not difficult to value. The approach has proved less useful in health economics because of the problems inherent in valuing health outcomes. What value can be placed on the relief of pain, improved mobility, or even of extending life itself?

In practice, this has often been done by estimating the value of an individual's contribution to national productivity, as measured by his or her lifetime earnings. This is called the human capital approach to valuing human life. It does not account for differences in the quality of life beyond an individual capacity to work. It values those with a working life-span ahead of them more highly than the old and men as more valuable than women. Not surprisingly, most health care workers find it difficult to accept economic productivity as the goal of medical care and so do most health economists!

The other main approach to valuing benefits in money uses contingent valuation methods. Individuals are surveyed to elicit the values placed on benefits which may not be directly measurable, thus the resultant values are based on those individuals' willingness to pay. The use of this approach in valuing health care benefits has been increasing, particularly as a means of encompassing benefits

Table 2 Types of economic appraisal

Type	Benefits	Analysis	Advantages	Disadvantages
Cost benefit	All benefits measured in money	Is this programme worthwhile?	Programmes with different aims can be compared One programme can be considered versus do nothing	Difficult to measure health in money Intangible benefits often omitted
Cost effectiveness	Benefits measured in clinical units, for example life years saved, deaths averted, cases detected	Comparison of programmes with same health aims	Life and health do not have to be valued Wide range of alternative health programmes can be considered	Ignores quality of life Cannot compare health programmes with other programmes
Cost utility	Benefits measured in QALYs	Comparison of health programmes	Incorporates quality and quantity of life All health programmes can be compared	Cannot compare health programmes with other programmes Problems in measuring quality of life

of health care which may not be captured in health status measures, such as information (Morrison and Gyldmark 1992).

Cost-effectiveness analysis

The problems with valuing human life and health are avoided by cost-effectiveness analysis. With this technique, benefits are measured in their naturally occurring clinical units, most usually life years saved, although it could be heart attacks prevented, cases of cancer diagnosed, and so on. Cost-effectiveness analysis was developed primarily by the United States military which also met the problem of valuing human life, although with a rather different objective than the health services! The phrase 'more bang for the buck' is a reminder of the military contribution.

Cost-effectiveness analysis has been much more widely accepted in health care evaluation than cost–benefit analysis. However, it runs into problems when comparing interventions with quite different objectives: how do you choose between £5000 for a heart attack prevented and £150 for a cancer detected? This can be overcome if the outcomes can be transformed into the same measure of health benefit, such as life years saved. It allows a wide range of interventions to be compared on the basis of cost per life years saved. But how should a life year spent in a wheelchair after a motor vehicle accident be compared with a life year of chemotherapy for breast cancer? There is still a problem if quality of life as well as or instead of quantity of life is important.

Measuring quality of life

Improving quality of life is the primary aim of many cancer treatments. Research has shown that there are health states, such as being unconscious or confined to bed on life support systems in severe pain, which are widely regarded as worse than death (Torrance 1987). Concern with quality has prompted the development of another technique of economic evaluation: cost–utility analysis (Drummond *et al.* 1987). In this form of analysis, life years saved are counted but they are adjusted for quality less than full health. The resultant outcome measure is known generally as quality-adjusted life years (QALYs) and the results of the analysis are presented as cost per QALY.

There are two ways of approaching the estimation of QALYs. One can start with a generalized health status measure that is applied to the specific health outcomes being considered. Alternatively, one can develop the description of the health state and the QALY weight attached to it for the specific condition being considered.

Neither approach relies on health economists to value quality of life. The values for different health states are determined by the community: potential patients and/or patients.

Generalized measures are those that can apply to a wide range of age groups and disease conditions; they should incorporate at least the physical and mental aspects of health-related quality of life (Hall and Masters 1986). The scale that is used to measure QALYs must have interval properties, that is, a movement from 3 to 5 on the scale must be equivalent to a move from 8 to 10. As QALYs measure both survival and quality of life, the scale must be anchored to the reference states of death and good health. Generalized measures often have existing weighting scales derived from some form of community survey. One which is gaining widespread acceptance is the SF36 (Ware and Sherbourne 1992). However, the weighting scales do not always have interval properties, nor are they always anchored to the reference states. The Index of Well-Being (Kaplan and Bush 1982), the Rosser scale (Rosser and Kind 1978), and the Euroqol (Euroqol Group 1990) meet these criteria; all have been used to estimate QALYs.

These measures may not be sufficiently sensitive to all aspects of health-related quality of life that are significant in cancer treatment and prevention. For example, cancer patients often report that their friends feel uncomfortable talking about their illness and prognosis (Morris *et al.* 1977; De Haes and Welvaart 1985). The diagnosis of breast cancer has implications for a woman's self-esteem, femininity, and sexuality. In this situation, descriptions of health-related quality of life outcomes should be developed and weights derived for them from some means of community survey. These techniques are fully described by Drummond *et al.* (1987).

Cost–utility analysis is not without its difficulties and many criticisms have been levelled at QALYs. To some extent, these are based on poor assessment of quality of life or lack of rigour in the application of the methods rather than the methodology itself (Gerard and Mooney 1993). The next best alternative is to rely on cost-effectiveness analysis using life years saved alone as the measure of health outcomes. Yet it is clear that some health states are better than others and so when quality of life is an important aim of treatment or when one treatment offers better quality of life but lower survival, this approach is not satisfactory.

It is our view that QALYs are the preferred approach to measuring health gains, but only when health-related quality of life is adequately defined and described.

Both cost-effectiveness analysis and cost–utility analysis investigate efficiency (that is, health outcomes related to costs) and can answer the question as to which of the alternatives is the best buy. Therefore it follows that no programme considered alone can be 'cost effective'; it can only be more or less cost effective than an alternative. Cost–benefit analysis, by valuing benefits in units of money, shows whether the benefits are worth more than the costs and, hence, can answer the question: 'Is this programme worthwhile?'

Measuring costs

In all types of economic appraisal, costs are measured in money. Money is a convenient means of counting costs, particularly as costs often match expenditure. Note that we said 'often' and remember the concept of opportunity cost; actual expenditure does not always match the resources used.

The prices charged for health care services, such as the charge per day in hospital or the charge for a chest radiograph, rarely reflect the opportunity cost of resource use which are the theoretically correct costs to use. Charges are set with more consideration of health insurance arrangements than resource use.

To avoid this problem in costing hospital services, the mean per diem rate is frequently but again, inappropriately used. The problem with the per diem rate is that it is generally calculated by including all the hospital expenditure and dividing by all hospital days. This would be satisfactory if all hospital days were equally expensive. However, as per diem rates cannot distinguish obstetric patients from cardiac surgical patients or days in the intensive care ward from days in the medical ward, they rarely measure opportunity costs for any particular ward, patient group, or type of treatment.

The key issue in measuring costs of a hospital stay, a diagnostic method, or any other health care service is to compare the costs in a world with that service with those in a world without it. The difference, the incremental cost, is the relevant cost (Hall and Mooney 1990a,b). In calculating this, it is more important to have an imprecise estimate of the 'right' cost than a precise, but quite wrong, figure.

Estimating costs

Clinicians and health administrators often want to know the cost of health care services. So how can clinicians estimate costs? The steps to follow are summarized in Table 3 and described below.

Step 1. Specify the question

The first answer to the question 'How do I calculate the cost of my new improved course of chemotherapy?' is another question: 'Why do I want to know?' Is it to compare the cost of one chemotherapeutic regimen with that of another? Or to compare chemotherapy with radiotherapy? Or will the new regimen provide treatment for patients who were not previously treated with curative intent? The key issue, as stated, is defining the difference in resource use/benefits forgone in a world with this activity and a world without it. Therefore the alternatives must be specified.

Step 2. Identify the point of view

Whose costs are to be considered? The costs of health care fall on four main groups: patients, insurers, providers, and governments. From the providers' viewpoint the cost of a hospital stay is a measure of the resources that could otherwise be available to other patients. From the patients' viewpoint the cost of a hospital stay is the charge raised for that stay and the patient is interested in how much of that will be paid by the insurance fund and how much remains to be met by the patient himself or herself.

Step 3. Identify the relevant inputs

What resources are used in the services being considered and how will they change? For example, from the providers' viewpoint the surgical treatment of oesophageal cancer involves operating theatre time, nursing and medical time, days occupying a hospital bed, and antibiotic and chemotherapeutic agents (see Walker et al. (1989) for an example of estimating costs following these steps). It includes the treatment of complications in a proportion of patients. If oesophageal cancer patients were not treated at all, these resources would be available for other patients.

Some resources 'used' by these patients may not be released for other applications, at least not immediately. These are fixed costs; that is, costs which do not vary with changes in workload. If the workload in a hospital ward drops suddenly because of a surgeons' strike, there will be few cost savings. Nursing and other staff will still be in the wards; cleaning, lighting, and power will still be provided. However, the longer the surgeons are on strike, the fewer the costs that are fixed. In a week, almost all costs are fixed; over 20 years almost everything, even hospital buildings, can be varied.

Step 4. Count the quantities of the inputs

The amount of each input used should be measured in its naturally occurring unit. For example, hours of operating theatre time, hours of doctor time, number of doses of drugs, and number of fields of radiation therapy should be counted. Wherever possible, these quantities should be derived from actual amounts used rather than from subject estimates, which are usually unreliable. The information can be collected from patient record review or direct observation, or from both.

Step 5. Estimate opportunity cost for each input

A unit value for each input must be determined. This can usually be based on the prices of inputs, such as hourly wage rate of nurses, cost of drugs, or cost of meals, where the inputs can be identified with the particular group of patients being considered. Prices are appropriate when they reflect the opportunity cost of the resources being used. However, there are some inputs whose use is shared commonly by several groups of patients. These are known as joint costs. In a hospital, for example, the services of the personnel department, the power and lighting, and the information and reception desks are used by all and cannot be identified with particular patient groups. They are, by definition, shared. They can be apportioned to different patient groups and there are several accepted conventions for doing this (Drummond et al. 1987). In estimating incremental costs, shared costs are often fixed and therefore not relevant (to economists anyway; on this point economists and accountants will almost always differ).

Table 3 Estimating health service costs

Step 1	Specify the question
Step 2	Identify the point of view
Step 3	Identify the relevant inputs
Step 4	Count the quantities of each input
Step 5	Estimate an opportunity cost for each input
Step 6	Calculate cost estimates: total costs=(opportunity cost×quantity)

A piece of equipment, such as a linear accelerator, will be used over a long period of time and for many patients. Its acquisition price is paid only once. Opportunity cost is important in determining how much is used in any given time-span. Could the building or piece of equipment have been used for anything else? If not, the opportunity cost is zero. If it could, the opportunity cost is its value in that alternative use. When the opportunity cost is zero, the amount already paid for it is irrelevant, it is a sunk cost. If there is an opportunity cost, that is, if there are benefits forgone because more patients wait to use the machine beyond the group now using it, how should the value of the use of the linear accelerator be calculated? Although the payment is once only, the value of the capital is regarded as decreasing over time and with use. The opportunity cost of capital needs to be expressed in terms of the building or equipment use. For example, the capital depreciation of a linear accelerator may be converted to the cost per treatment fields given. (A detailed discussion of estimating depreciation is given by Drummond *et al.* (1987).)

Step 6. Calculate cost estimates

Calculation of the cost estimates is now a matter of simple arithmetic (opportunity cost multiplied by quantity).

OTHER ASPECTS OF THE CONSEQUENCES OF ILLNESS

This discussion of health care costs has looked at costs from the point of view of the health sector. These are the major costs of detecting and treating cancer and caring for those who have it. However, the costs of treating cancer can also comprise non-health service costs, such as the cost for the patient travelling to the treatment centre, or time spent by the patient in treatment, or time spent by family members looking after the patient.

It is particularly important to consider costs outside the health sector when the extent of these varies significantly from one programme to another. A good example of this is that community care for the elderly is often proposed as a cheaper alternative to institutional care. However, these analyses rarely take into account the costs borne by those providing the care at home, often the wives and daughters. It is not that community care is necessarily more costly from a social viewpoint; rather it transfers costs from the health sector to the non-health sector.

If one of two alternative treatments returns patients to work sooner, should the earnings generated by the earlier return to work be counted as cost savings? There are two issues involved here. The first is the distinction between costs and benefits; the second, the inclusion of productivity gains.

It is erroneous but not uncommon to categorize all the positive effects as benefits and all the negative ones as costs. The results of economic evaluation are often presented as ratios, a cost per unit of benefit and changing whether a particular item is classified as a 'cost' or a 'benefit' can alter the results. Consequently, classifying costs and benefits correctly is crucial. The aim here is to maximize something (perhaps health status) out of some limit. Costs are what is limited or constrained; that is, resources. Benefits are what is being maximized. So both costs and benefits can be positive and negative.

What is health care seeking to maximize? This brings us to the second issue which is whether the productivity gains from people participating in the workforce for longer should be included in estimating the benefits of health care. This is a thorny issue with some complex arguments for and against. It depends on clarifying what health is for, then determining the most appropriate means of measuring that, at the same time avoiding any double counting. However, it should be noted that these productivity gains, sometimes called indirect benefits, are frequently as large or larger than the value of resource use, so that their inclusion will significantly affect the results. Their inclusion also raises the issue of equity as they are greatest for those with greatest earning potential.

Return to work is sometimes suggested as a measure of recovery, an indicator of return to normal activities. Whilst this may be so, actual return to work will depend on social and economic circumstances such as the availability of jobs and the provision of pensions, as well as physical and mental function. In our view, the capacity to resume normal activities is better measured through estimating health gains and treated as a benefit in QALY terms.

It is sometimes suggested that the costs of providing pensions or social security benefits should also be counted as cost savings. Although these payments are costs to the government, it is generally agreed that they are not opportunity costs. From the viewpoint of society as a whole they represent not a loss of production but a transfer of purchasing power from one group to another. These are known as transfer payments.

The term 'economic costs of illness' is sometimes used to refer to the sum of the direct costs and the earning losses due to premature mortality and morbidity. Illness *per se* does not cost society anything; it is what society chooses to do about it that uses resources. Therefore, the term 'cost of illness' is misleading. In addition, this notional sum is not relevant to the approach of evaluating health interventions described here, that is, making explicit the additional health gains and costs of new or alternative health care programmes.

The results of economic evaluation will only be as good as the methods of analysis and the data on which they are based. While health economists understand the analytical principles, they are rarely familiar with the clinical realities of the programme being evaluated; while clinicians understand the medical problem and its treatment, they have rarely been trained in economics. Good economic evaluation requires clinicians and economists to work together.

IS EFFICIENCY ETHICAL?

The rationale for economic evaluation is that the health care budget is limited. Perhaps it should not be limited. After all, how can one value human life and well-being? Or, at least, perhaps it should not be so limited. In our example, more money should be spent on breast cancer control so that both screening and adjuvant therapy could be expanded.

The opportunity costs of expanding the share of national resources devoted to health care are other programmes that contribute to human well-being; better housing, education, opera companies. This is not a question of the most health gains for the funds available but, rather, whether the gains in health are worth the additional cost. As long as the resources available to society are limited, then these choices between health and other aspects of well-being have to be confronted at a societal level. They are confronted at a personal level, too, every time a decision is made to do something enjoyable even though it is not good for one's health.

What about the clinical level? Should doctors take costs and benefits into account in their clinical practice? Is it ethical to consider costs in caring for one's patients? Or is it the clinician's responsibility to prescribe the best care irrespective of cost?

Several recent articles have directed attention to the need for cancer clinicians to be aware of the costs of cancer care and control (Friedlander and Tattersall 1982; McVie 1988; Markman 1988; Stoll 1988; Timothy *et al.* 1988). Leading medical journals have begun to point out that consideration of costs must be integrated into clinical decision-making (Anonymous 1986, 1987). Others have suggested that the conflict between economics and clinical practice is misconstrued. After all, what makes good economic sense also coincides with what is best, in balancing probable benefits and risks, for the individual patient (Jennett and Buxton 1990).

The opposite point of view, that economics and cost-effectiveness should be kept completely out of clinical decision making, is still held strongly by several clinicians. As one physician wrote to the *New England Journal of Medicine*:

A physician who changes his or her way of practising medicine because of cost rather than purely medical considerations has indeed embarked on the 'slippery slope' of compromised ethics and waffled priorities. (Loewy 1980)

Yet, as Williams (1988) has pointed out, doctors already take economic considerations into account in making clinical decisions. Clinicians who consider the time and income that patients will lose from work or the time, travel costs, and family disruption suffered by patients from remote rural areas while undergoing a course of radiotherapy or balance the time spent with one patient against the needs of others in the waiting room are all having regard to economics.

So the issue is not whether or not it is ethical to count costs but rather where the line should be drawn between costs that may be counted and costs that may not. (Williams 1988)

'Clinical economics' can only develop if clinicians are aware of the costs and are able to count the benefits of specific interventions (Eisenberg *et al.* 1989). Two British articles have called for the development of specific guidelines defining appropriate and inappropriate care for tumours of different sites and stages (Timothy *et al.* 1988; Whitehouse 1989).

Timothy *et al.* (1988) reported the views of a group of oncologists, epidemiologists, and economists who considered priorities in resource allocation for cancer treatment. Two principles were believed to be central. Most felt that consensus was possible in determining what is 'appropriate or inappropriate treatment'. They also felt that 'unfettered clinical freedom' was not appropriate in cancer management. Indeed 'clinical freedom' has been labelled as 'at best . . . a cloak for ignorance and at worst an excuse for quackery' (Hampton 1986).

Whitehouse (1988) has also proposed the establishment of 'best documented practice' which could be displaced only if randomized trials showed that a different treatment was better. Others have adopted the consensus conference format to promote uniform standards in cancer control and management. Jennett and Buxton (1990) have argued that clinicians are driven to overuse cancer treatments in the hope of unrealistic outcomes. As every cancer treatment involves individual burdens and social costs, management requires the balancing of probable benefits and probable costs. According to Jennett and Buxton, the problem of the costs of cancer management lies not in the use of currently effective treatments but in the use of expensive therapies without demonstrated benefit.

Although these approaches to developing standard treatment have rarely discussed issues of cost, the costs of recommended standard treatments can be readily assessed and any new interventions or competing claims for allocation of health resources can be gauged against these standards.

Simply exhorting doctors to be aware of costs or providing them with cost data has been shown to have little or no effect on changing their patterns of practice (Eisenberg 1977; Wickings *et al.* 1983). This should not be surprising. Unless there is a real and immediate opportunity cost, that is, unless the resources saved (or expended) can be used (or not available) for other identified patients, why should clinicians bother?

Using financial incentives to change patterns of health care has been successful: capitation payments in health maintenance organizations have reduced hospital admission rates (Luft 1978); case mix payment and Diagnosis Related Group (DRG)-based reimbursement have reduced hospital stays (Davis *et al.* 1985). However, there is a danger that these mechanisms will be used to make arbitrary reductions, such as a 10 per cent reduction in length of stay across all cases. Without information about costs and outcomes, the efficient will be cut as much as the inefficient. This may result in cheaper but not more cost-effective health care.

The key to encouraging greater use of economic evaluation and, hence, to more efficient health care, lies on the one hand with more economically aware clinicians and on the other with incentives, within health care systems. It is not enough to count costs and outcomes; costs and outcomes must count.

REFERENCES

Anonymous (1986). Improving use of clinical resources. *Lancet*, ii:319–20.

Anonymous (1987). Why doctors must grapple with health economics. *British Medical Journal*, **294**:326.

Banta HD, Thacker SB (1979). *Costs and benefits of electronic fetal monitoring: a review of the literature.* (PHS) 79-3245, National Center for Health Services Research, Washington, DC.

Barnes BA (1977). Discarded operations: surgical innovation by trial and error. In *Costs, risks, and benefits of surgery* (ed. JP Bunker, BA Barnes, and F Mosteller). Oxford University Press.

Calman KC, McVie JG, Soukop M, Richardson M, Donald J (1978). Costs of out-patient chemotherapy. *British Medical Journal*, i:493–4.

Cochrane AL (1972). *Effectiveness and efficiency: random reflections on health services.* Nuffield Provincial Hospitals Trust, London.

Davis K, *et al.* (1985). Is cost containment working? *Health Affairs*, 4(3):81–94.

De Haes JC, Welvaart K (1985). Quality of life after breast cancer surgery. *Journal of Surgical Oncology*, 29(2):123–5.

Drummond MF, Stoddart GL, Torrance GW (1987). *Methods for the economic evaluation of health care programmes.* Oxford University Press.

Eisenberg JM (1977). An educational program to modify laboratory use by house staff. *Journal of Medical Education*, 52:578–81.

Eisenberg JM, *et al.* (1989). Clinical economics education in the International Clinical Epidemiology Network. *Journal of Clinical Epidemiology*, 42(7):689–95.

Euroqol Group (1990). EuroQol—a new facility for the measurement of health-related quality of life. *Health Policy*, 16(3):199–208.

Friedlander ML, Tattersall MHN (1982). Counting the costs of cancer therapy. *European Journal of Cancer and Clinical Oncology*, 18:1237–41.

Forrest P (1986). *Breast cancer screening: report to the health ministers of England, Wales, Scotland and Northern Ireland.* Department of Health and Social Security, London.

Frazier HS, Hiatt HH (1978). Education of medical practices. *Science*, 200:875–8.

Gerard K, Mooney G (1993). QALY league tables: handle with care. *Health Economics*, 2(1):59–64.

Goodwin PJ, Feld R, Evans WK, Pater J (1988). Cost effectiveness of cancer chemotherapy; an economic evaluation of a randomised trial in small-cell lung cancer. *Journal of Clinical Oncology*, 6:1537–47.

Hall J, Masters G (1986). Measuring outcomes of health services: a review of some available measures. *Community Health Studies*, 10:147–55.

Hall J, Mooney G (1990a). What every doctor should know about economics: the benefits of costing. *Medical Journal of Australia*, 152:29–31.

Hall J, Mooney G (1990b). What every doctor should know about economics: the benefits of economic appraisal. *Medical Journal of Australia*, **152**:80–2.

Hampton JR (1986). The end of clinical freedom. *British Medical Journal*, **287**:1237–8.

Jennett B, Buxton M (1990). When is treatment for cancer economically justified? Discussion paper. *Journal of the Royal Society of Medicine*, **83**:25–8.

Kaplan RM, Bush JW (1982). Health related quality of life measurement for evaluation research and policy analysis. *Health Psychology*, **1**:61–8.

Kay HEM, Powles RC, Lawler SD, Clink HG (1980). Cost of bone-marrow transplant in acute myeloid leukaemia. *Lancet*, **i**:1067–9.

Knobf MT (1986). Physical and psychologic distress associated with adjuvant chemotherapy in women with breast cancer. *Journal of Clinical Oncology*, **4**(5):678–84.

Levine MN, Drummond MP, Labelle RJ (1985). Cost-effectiveness in the diagnosis and treatment of carcinoma of unknown primary origin. *Canadian Medical Association Journal*, **33**:977–87.

Loewy EH (1980). Cost should not be a factor in medical care. *New England Journal of Medicine*, **302**:697.

Luft HS (1978). How do Health Maintenance Organisations achieve their 'savings'? *New England Journal of Medicine*, **298**:1336–43.

McPherson K, Fox MS (1977). Treatment of breast cancer. In *Costs, risks, and benefits of surgery* (ed. JP Bunker, BA Barnes, and F Mosteller). Oxford University Press.

McVie JC (1988). Counting costs of care. *Journal of Clinical Oncology*, **6**:1529–31.

Markman M (1988). An argument in support of cost-effective analysis in oncology. *Journal of Clinical Oncology*, **6**:937–9.

Mitchell H (1987). Organised mammographic screening programs: a benign or malignant neglect. *Medical Journal of Australia*, **146**:87–9.

Morris JN, Sherwood S (1977). Quality of life of cancer patients at different stages in the disease trajectory. *Journal of Chronic Diseases*, **40**(6):545–53.

Morris T, Steven-Greer H, White P (1977). Psychological adjustment after mastectomy (a 2 year follow up study). *Cancer*, **40**:2381–7.

Morrison GC, Gyldmark M (1992). Appraising the use of contingent valuation. *Health Economics*, **1**(4):233–44.

Parkerson GR, *et al.* (1981). The Duke–UNC Health Profile: an adult health status instrument for primary care. *Medical Care*, **19**:806–28.

Rees GJG (1985). Cost-effectiveness in oncology. *Lancet*, **ii**:1405–8.

Rosser RM, Kind P (1978). A scale of valuations of states of illness: is there a social consensus? *International Journal of Epidemiology*, **7**(4):347–55.

Shaha A, Hoover E, Marti J, Krespi Y (1988). Is routine triple endoscopy cost-effective in head and neck cancer? *American Journal of Surgery*, **155**:750–3.

Shapiro S, Venet W, Strax P, Venet L, Rosser R (1982). Ten to fourteen year effect of screening on breast cancer mortality. *Journal of the National Cancer Institute*, **2**:349–55.

Shibley L, Brown M, Schuttinga L, Rothenberg M, Whalan J (1990). Cioplatin-based combination chemotherapy in the treatment of advanced stage testicular cancer: cost benefit analysis. *Journal of the National Cancer Institute*, **82**(3):186–92.

Stoll BA (1988). Balancing cost and benefit in treatment of late cancer. *Lancet*, **i**:578–80.

Taber GA, *et al.* (1985). Reduction in mortality from breast cancer after mass screening with mammography. Randomised trial from the breast cancer screening working group of the Swedish National Board of Health and Welfare. *Lancet*, **i**:829–39.

Timothy AR, *et al.* (1988). Cost versus benefit in non-surgical management of patients with cancer. *British Medical Journal*, **297**:471–2.

Walker QJ, Salkeld G, Hall J, O'Rourke I, Bull CA, Tiver KW, Langlands AO (1989). The management of oesophageal carcinoma: radiotherapy or surgery? Cost considerations. *European Journal of Cancer and Clinical Oncology*, **25**(11):1657–62.

Ware JE, Sherbourne CD (1992). The MOS 36 item short form health survey (SF-36). Conceptual framework and item selection. *Medical Care*, **30**(6):473–83.

Whitehouse JNA (1989). Best documented practice. Time to set down a few benchmarks. *British Medical Journal*, **298**:1536–7.

Wickings I, *et al.* (1983). Review of clinical budgeting and costing experiments. *British Medical Journal*, **287**:576–7.

Williams A (1988). Health economics: the end of clinical freedom? *British Medical Journal*, **297**:1183–6.

Wiltes RE (1987). Paying for patient care in treatment research—who is responsible? *Cancer Treatment Reports*, **71**:107–13.

20.10   Cancer and society: health education

CAROLYN M. FAULDER

'KICKING CANCER OUT OF THE CLOSET'

Cancer has ceased to be the taboo word that no one dares utter, the disease that people talk about behind closed doors and in hushed tones. No longer does it automatically carry the cruel connotations of dirt, contagion, and creeping corruption. Nor, any longer, is it inevitably viewed as a killer.

In little more than a decade we have seen a remarkable change in public perceptions and attitudes. Greater openness, much more readiness to enquire, a stronger demand for information, and an increased expectation that the truth will be available for those who want it are all manifestations of this transformation. The emergence of AIDS as the final scourge for this tortured century has also

had an influence. The nature of this terrible new disease has forced us all into unremittingly frank discussions about private sexual behaviour; one toppling taboo tends to knock down others.

It is sometimes easier to chart the course of change than explain the causes. Thus, the methods and effects of the many agents of change can readily be observed, although the order which follows here is not to be taken as of any particular significance: the hospice movement, the cancer charities, particularly the newer ones with their emphasis on support and information, the health professionals, health educationalists and promoters, lay as well as medical, the women's movement, the media, health consumerism, support groups and patient associations, commercial interests in medical technology and pharmacology, some politicians, and, finally, a few outstanding individuals, usually cancer patients, whose experience has fired them with the determination to improve the lot of their fellow sufferers by fundraising or starting an organization or just by talking or writing about what happened to them.

All these groups have had a major influence on our thinking about cancer but they have been as much led by the prevailing *Zeitgeist* as they have led towards it. Their messages and their examples have fallen on fertile thirsty ground. The public psyche, even if not always fully aware of the depth of its need, has been longing for cancer to come out of the shadows. While it is true, of course, that many people would still prefer to know as little as possible about cancer, even when it affects them or others close to them, there are undoubtedly at least as many and probably more who now realize that they do want to be informed if only to retain some measure of control over their lives. The myths, mysteries, and horror stories surrounding this disease have caused untold anguish in the past and, sadly, continue to do so where ignorance is allowed to flourish. However, there is a new reality which is becoming more widely recognized. It is embodied in the medical advances which, in the first place, have given us cures for certain cancers while at the same time enabling us to believe, on good grounds, that more are on the way; second, they have substantially improved the quality of treatment for all patients at whatever stage of the disease and, concomitantly, their quality of life. Hope has finally entered the arena of cancer. With hope comes the realization that there is a chance to do better than just survive; it is possible to live positively with cancer.

'Kicking cancer out of the closet', was a favourite saying of the late Dr Vicky Clement-Jones. She was, of course, referring specifically to BACUP, the cancer information service which she founded in 1985 following her experience of cancer. The response to this service graphically indicates the expanding measure of need that it was set up to meet (Slevin *et al.* 1988). Other organizations which have been formed to meet similar or related needs but have not used such a systematic method of recording and evaluating the use made of them by their clients would certainly testify to the continual stream of enquiries and requests for help that they receive.

The demand increases quite significantly every time there is a newspaper article or television programme on some aspect of cancer. In the main the media look to the scientific and medical professions for factual information and to patients and other concerned parties for the essential 'human interest' angle. Obviously this selection of different sources coming from quite different directions and often with quite different ends in mind can appear arbitrary and insufficiently discriminating, particularly to any party which may feel that its viewpoint has been either unfairly or inaccurately represented. The frequently testy relationship between the media and the health industry will be examined at greater length later in this chapter when we are looking at the role of the various health educators. The point worth making here is that the media, whatever its perceived faults and shortcomings, plays an essential part in the two-way dissemination of information. Both sides, the professionals and the lay public, would be considerably deprived without its mediation. That the popular press and the mass media in general still have much room for improvement in their style of communication is indisputable, but this applies equally to the professionals.

Cancer has gone public in a big way. We have cancer weeks, cancer years, cancer phone-ins, and cancer events. People write books about their personal experience of 'conquering cancer' and books and articles proliferate about 'alternative cures' and treatments, but there are also an increasing number of carefully written explanatory books and pamphlets for those who want to be informed about orthodox treatments. In short, for those who seek it there is no dearth of information about cancer in all its aspects, although what is on offer may not always meet individual needs or be appropriately presented. There is a further caveat. Those living in certain areas, not necessarily remote, where the prevailing health ethos is that the less patients know the better or those who belong to particular socio-economic groups may find it almost impossible to obtain the kind of information that is suited to their needs.

KNOWLEDGE, BELIEF, AND BEHAVIOUR

Given that, for the most part, useful information about cancer is now widely available, how far has this knowledge affected either attitudes or behaviour in relation to the disease? Put another way, how far has this information, regardless of the way it is presented, increased understanding? Knowing something in your head is not the same as believing something in your heart, but even when belief is supported by knowledge this is no predictor of behaviour, nor does it guarantee protection against the fear and dread of cancer. Our emotions rise like water from a deep source beyond our control; it is only once they have made themselves manifest, whether internally or visibly, that we can attempt to suppress or divert them.

A rare quantitative study of public perceptions about serious illnesses and cancer in particular illustrates this point very clearly (Cancer Relief Macmillan Fund 1988). A carefully matched representative sample of the present United Kingdom population involving nearly 1000 respondents in 40 min interviews in their own homes showed that the level of 'overall knowledge [of cancer] is high and reasonably accurate' particularly in the higher social groups and among younger people. Seventy-two per cent of the population think that cancer is at least sometimes curable and 58 per cent know that heart disease is the major killer in the United Kingdom today, yet it is cancer which is the most personally feared disease (52 per cent). When asked to describe what cancer meant to them, more than one-third mentioned death and 41 per cent expressed the opinion that the fear of cancer is worse than the fear of death. Almost two-thirds (63 per cent) said that they would prefer to know whether or not they have cancer.

The smoking conundrum

Smoking is a classic illustration of the paradoxical and complex relationship between knowledge and behaviour. Most people in the Macmillan survey (86 per cent) recognized smoking as the most common cause of cancer; a similar proportion saw giving up smoking as the best way of reducing the risk of contracting cancer. However, more than half those respondents would have been smokers themselves, since 36 per cent of the total sample admitted to being regular smokers at the time of the interview and a further 20 per cent (the converted?) had smoked regularly, defined as one or more cigarettes a day, at some time in their lives.

Smoking as 'a bad thing' for health in general and the cause of many other diseases apart from cancer is now accepted by the majority of people. Interestingly, those who own to this or indeed any other 'unhealthy' habit such as overindulgence in alcohol or food, are also likely to be more rather than less aware of the specific risks that they run than the non-indulgers. Thus, the Health and Lifestyle Survey, a considerably larger population study than the Macmillan survey which was carried out in England, Wales, and Scotland during 1984 and 1985, revealed that many more smokers than non-smokers knew, for instance, about the relationships between smoking and heart disease (31 per cent compared with 20 per cent) and between smoking and bronchitis (62 per cent compared with 46 per cent) (Blaxter 1990).

Then there are the particular paradoxes relating to patterns of smoking in women. Overall the figures for both sexes are declining, from 65 per cent in 1948 to 35 per cent in 1985 for men and from 41 per cent to 34 per cent for women during the same period with a steep fall starting in 1974, but this reduction is due more to smokers giving up than to young adults never starting. Today there are indications that smoking consumption among women is once more on the increase, particularly among teenage girls of whom one in four (27 per cent) aged 15–16 years can be classified as a regular smoker compared with one in five boys (18 per cent) of the same age (Cancer Research Campaign 1989). Buried within these figures is this further highly significant fact: smoking in both sexes is closely associated with education and social class and this is a modern phenomenon. Whereas 30 years ago smokers were evenly distributed among all classes, today smoking has become predominantly a working-class habit and it is particularly prevalent in low-income socially disadvantaged households (ASH Women and Smoking Group 1990). The proportion of smoking women in households classified by manual occupations is nearly double that of women in the higher socio-economic groups: 35 per cent compared with 19 per cent (OPCS 1989). Research has shown that women of all classes are now well aware of the major ill effects of smoking, for themselves and their children, which leads us to ask: what is it that makes the very people who are least able to afford the habit, but are sufficiently informed of the risks, most likely to persist in it? One then has to follow this up with the supplementary question: how is it that among the better educated and more advantaged social groups there are now any smokers at all, given the overwhelming case against tobacco?

Complex factors affecting behaviour

A study of the vagaries of smoking behaviour provides a particularly unambiguous example of the difficulties facing the health educators. However, this is just one exclusive example of life-style behaviour: drinking, diet, and exercise are some of the other key behavioural factors affecting our health. We need to know much more about why some people behave in the way that they do while others in similar circumstances will react in a completely different fashion. We also need to understand in greater depth the effect that changing one particular behaviour may have on an individual's total behavioural pattern before we can begin to make statements about the benefits of health education or even plan a health promotion programme.

Cultural, social, and environmental influences are of similar importance and are much more difficult to measure, but their interaction with each other and their combined effect on behaviour have to be taken into consideration. Finally, there are the material circumstances of people's lives, often beyond their control, which no one involved in health education can afford to ignore. We know that people living in certain areas and certain groups of the population within and without these areas are at greater risk of suffering serious illness of all kinds; they also appear to be more prone to developing certain forms of cancer. Housing, employment, and schooling are among the most important social conditions affecting people's lives and therefore their health. It is not only the physical influence of these conditions that we have to consider but also the mental stress that they may induce.

What should we expect from health education?

This assortment of considerations at many levels makes it obvious that there are no simple answers. Had there been, by now we would

have solved the problem of delivering a successful health education message. How do we measure success in this context? In the final analysis it can only be decided by the degree of active take-up the particular message stimulates. If a sizeable proportion of the targeted audience is not responding 'appropriately' to the information, then everything has to be reviewed: concept, content, style, location, delivery, feedback, the target itself, all must be re-assessed. Force-feeding an undifferentiated mass population with health facts 'for their own good' is a guaranteed turn off and quite as expensive a waste of time as shrouding the message in images either so mysterious or so menacing, such as the coffins and icebergs of the notorious 1987 AIDS television campaign sponsored by the British Government, that everyone is left bewildered and probably even more fearful.

Before deciding on the ways and means of delivering any particular health message, the health educationalists must be clear in their own minds about three things: their aims, their target outcome and the best means to achieve it, and, finally, their order of priorities. Thus, their declared aims must include providing accurate and useful information followed through by realistic recommendations and backed up by adequately funded resources. This essential exercise of clarification and justification must be done at the planning stage of any health campaign because this is the moment for the health educationalists to be aware of the limits as well as the scope of their determined task. They may, so to speak, have 'seen the light' and wish to convince as many people as possible of the rightness of following a recommended 'healthy' course of action, but evangelistic fervour based on shaky foundations can prove to be an expensive and even dangerous folly, when it is not an actual deterrent.

Of course, all this must be done in the context of the particular category of health education which is at issue. Cancer education, for example, will have quite different goals from birth control education; it will be aimed at a population which may overlap to some extent, but will require quite different motivation triggers and the information should be tailored and presented accordingly.

These points may seem too obvious to state, but the resounding failure of too many health promotion campaigns suggests that they may have been insufficiently heeded in the enthusiasm 'to get the show on the road'. A prominent example is the long-running inability to achieve a comprehensive efficient national cervical screening programme in the United Kingdom.

DECIDING THE AIMS

In cancer education, like any other health education programme, the aims can only be formulated when those in charge of presenting the initiative know what they want to say and believe it to be valuable information which should be as widely disseminated as possible. Again this might appear to be an obvious truism, but think about it. The whole topic of cancer is mined with disagreements. The experts argue at length and loudly about facts, statistics, relative merits of treatments, and the virtues or otherwise of screening, to take a few broad examples. The effect of so much uncertainty is to leave the general public feeling confused and unhappy. Undoubtedly, it does not inspire them with confidence to heed the advice being offered.

Information: the enabling factor

It is not necessary to adopt a naïvely simplistic approach to appreciate how important it is that the content of the message, once decided upon, should have maximum support from the health professionals who will be charged with seeing it through. Furthermore, the information must be properly exploited to achieve its full effect. An intrinsic element of any cancer education campaign must be that it enables people to act upon what they have been taught is a health benefit for them.

The health educator is a reformer and not a revolutionary, possibly a campaigner, and unlikely to be a legislator. His or her rôle is to state the facts and present the case in such clear compelling terms that others in positions to effect change will feel obliged, if not inspired, to take the appropriate action. An illustration of how this can work in real life is the progress achieved by the antismoking lobby. Only a few years ago the small number of brave objectors to smoking in public places such as trains and restaurants were dismissed as cranky spoilsports. Today they have neatly turned the tables on the smoker who is now the one to be branded as antisocial and, increasingly, is being debarred from lighting up in public areas. Furthermore, this swing in public opinion has been achieved with figurative peanuts compared with the hundreds of millions of pounds poured into advertising and other promotions by the tobacco industry.

Before we smug lung savers all pat ourselves on our collective back, it is worth recording that there is a downside to this moral tale. The 'failures' in this instance tend to be the very people who, as we saw earlier in this chapter, find it hardest to give up what has become, for many of them, a necessity as well as their only luxury. They are poor and they are trapped. They live in substandard housing 'on their nerves' and probably on supplementary benefits. They certainly cannot afford to eat out and they only travel when they have to. Of course they do not represent the entire smoking population, but there are enough of them to make us realize that social disapproval is not an appropriate method of persuasion for this group. It could even drive them into heavier guilt-induced smoking.

Specific goals

Prevention

Prevention logically takes precedence over other cancer goals and would seem to be the most obviously desirable, but it can only operate within a limited range. The environment, diet, tobacco, and alcohol are all accorded varying degrees of responsibility for cancer. Of course, these are not the only causes, but they are the ones over which an individual can have some control. Unfortunately, apart from tobacco, they are difficult to quantify. The environment, for instance, can be almost anything one wants to make of it. It can include working conditions (asbestos, nuclear installations), pesticides and other chemicals leaching into water and the food chain, and a whole host of other carcinogenic substances occurring both naturally and artificially which we may unwittingly inhale, ingest, or touch. The world is a dangerous place and most of the time we have no idea how dangerous it is. The nature of epidemiological research is such that it can only tell us what to beware of after it has occurred sufficiently often to be able to link cause and effect.

Therefore, the emphasis in preventive education has to be almost entirely on life-style. Advice on avoiding obvious excesses is the most familiar model, along the lines of too much drinking, eating, smoking, sex, or sunbathing could run you into trouble, but care has to be taken that these warnings do not become merely bland and boring from endless repetition. People want to be reassured that they will experience some positive immediate benefits if they are to be persuaded to give up longstanding pleasures. Attempts

to shame them into denial by making them feel guilty or embarrassed tend to work in the short-term only. A lurid catalogue of facts and effects may be temporarily alarming but actually drive the individual back to his or her favourite indulgence for comfort. No matter how accurate, information that is delivered with too heavy a hand can be paralysing rather than enabling in its effects.

The best preventive measure is plainly never to start. Hence, it is important to educate children and young people to enable them to make informed choices about their life-style at an age before they have formed habits. Breaking a bad habit is much harder than deciding against starting. Peer pressures at this age cannot be underestimated and will often outweigh home and school combined; therefore they must be enlisted rather than antagonized by the educators.

Screening and early detection

Screening and early detection, that is, diagnosis, go together in the medical mind but not so readily in the lay one. There still exists a widespread presumption that if you submit yourself to a health check your reward will be a clean bill of health. This is a serious misunderstanding of the purpose of screening which, if not exactly encouraged, has certainly not been cleared up by some enthusiastic promoters of private services, nor has it been helped by ill-informed media reports of well woman screens, executive check-ups, and the like. One of the greatest challenges in cancer education lies in convincing a targeted population of the benefits of screening, when the end result for an individual may be that he or she will enter 'well' and exit 'ill', then enduring a profoundly stressful period of anxiety while waiting for the results of a biopsy.

Clearly, the value of an early diagnosis leading to a higher probability of cure has to be stressed and it has been proved for several of the more common cancers; cervix, breast, endometrial, testicular, and bowel to name a few. However, there is also the difficult subtext to explain: it does not always follow that an 'early' diagnosis means 'early' detection or, even if it is genuinely early, that it will prove to be a curable cancer. This requires sensitive and careful explanation and may have to be repeated at different times and in different ways.

Before the advent of machines self-screening through self-examination was regarded as the best way of discovering an early cancer. Women's organizations, encouraged by the medical profession, put out leaflets and ran campaigns teaching women how to examine their own breasts. Now, just as young men are learning how to examine their testicles and both sexes are being urged to keep an eye on their moles and their bowel habits and report any changes immediately, a vocal group among breast specialists is declaring that women should be discouraged from breast self-examination. They take the view that the practice is of doubtful value now that it has been superseded by mammography which can detect changes in the breast at a much earlier stage. They also believe that it encourages women to be overanxious. Is this a sensible thing to be saying to women who, although below the age band for National Health Service screening, know that none the less they could develop breast cancer, whether or not they are at special risk?

Until many of the current uncertainties about breast screening such as the optimum screening interval and the best age to start have been resolved, breast self-examination will continue to have a place in health care for those women who want to practise it. Not all do, but what we can be sure about is that women who have been discouraged from taking what appear to be sensible precautions at an earlier period of their lives will be even less likely to respond to an invitation for screening at the age of 50.

Screening continues to be a controversial subject. While it is right that the medical profession should constantly question its own procedures, the current debate about breast screening is causing a major headache for those who are trying to inform the clients and the family doctors (Roberts *et al.* 1989). If it goes on for too long it could erode public confidence and consequently the compliance that is essential to make the programme a success. It should be axiomatic that by the time a programme is *in situ* and receiving public funding, the basic philosophical and scientific questions about its merits are, if not totally resolved, at least accepted in broad outline so that future discussion can be focused on fine tuning. There is also a different 'Catch 22' situation that may develop. Any mass screening programme must attract sufficient numbers of the target population to justify its cost, but if the take-up is greater than anticipated, the follow-up service may not be able to meet the demand. The resulting backlog of delayed appointments and treatments will cause frustration and dangerous disillusion. These are clearly not problems which lie solely within the remit of the health educationalists to solve but they do have to be considered when planning the order of priorities.

Information: the empowering factor

Some information enables people to choose between courses of action that are within their control: they can choose whether or not to adopt a recommended 'healthy' life-style; they can accept or refuse an invitation to be screened. Other information empowers people to make decisions about things they either do or do not wish to have done to them. In the context of health care this means the health professionals sharing information with the patients and, on the basis of that information, inviting them to participate in making decisions about their treatment.

Informed decisions about treatment

Informed decisions about treatment can only be made by patients who have a reasonably complete understanding of their illness and the implications of its treatment. Clearly, much depends on the type of illness and the nature of the proposed interventions: whether it is short-term, curable, chronic, or life-threatening, what treatments are possible, and whether their side-effects are more or less acceptable. Much also depends on the individual patient: their age, sex, personality, social class, and educational background all play a part. Some patients are better able to ask for information and make their wishes known. Others may be intimidated by the hospital environment, be relatively inarticulate, or feel inhibited for a whole host of other reasons which make it difficult for them to seek information, particularly if they are not given any encouragement to do so. Some patients will make it quite clear they do not want to be informed or want only minimal information and that they expect their doctors to take all the decisions on their behalf. The nature of the relationship between doctor and patient is such that these 'permissions' are often granted implicitly, but the doctor always has to be sure that he or she is not taking them for granted.

In the case of a life-threatening condition like cancer, where the outcomes are more uncertain and the treatment intentions more difficult to explain, it would seem all the more important that patients be offered the opportunity to participate in the decision-making process. Research has shown that patients requiring surgery for less serious conditions who are informed about hospital procedures and have a good idea about what to expect pre- and post-operatively show reduced levels of anxiety and depression. They also often recover faster with less medication and pain (Morris

et al. 1989). The whole area of educating patients about their illness needs more refined investigation and Morris *et al.* (1989) offer some useful suggestions for future research. However, even at their present stage these are interesting results. It appears that while information increases consumer (patient) satisfaction, it also enhances the medical skills of the professionals. There is an additional bonus: because it hastens recovery and therefore speeds up the bed occupancy turnover, it can also be cost-effective.

Informed consent in clinical trials

This is another example in health care where information offered carefully and with respect for the patient's autonomy can turn out to be a surprisingly positive experience for those providing the information. At a very simple level, most patients will appreciate the consideration that is being shown for them by the doctor who seeks their permission. Later, when they have grasped the implications for themselves that a consent would involve, their decision to participate in a trial may well be tipped in its favour if the quality of the information has enabled them to place the request in its wider context of medical research directed at benefiting future patients. Probably more people than some doctors realize would like to contribute to research, as a way of showing their gratitude for the care they are receiving, always providing of course that it does not involve them in too great a personal sacrifice. However, patients also fear displeasing their carers. Information may be empowering, but in the patient–doctor relationship the doctor always retains the ultimate position of vantage: it is the doctor who offers the treatment and can withhold it. This makes it particularly important that doctors do not yield to the temptation to manipulate their patients' vulnerability to achieve ends of their own, however laudable they may appear to be.

Information: the ethical dimension

This element is implicit in any analysis of the purpose of health education, whether in a health care or health promotion context. The very process of providing adequate good quality information is a way of acknowledging the individual's autonomy and according respect for each individual's personal dignity and right to make decisions about his or her body. This is the primary ethical component of health education in any form.

A secondary ethically inspired motivation for a health education programme is that it should be planned in such a way as to help people feel more able to take responsibility for their own health. However, this assumes that people value health and regard it as important in their lives; a substantial number of people do not. Even where people are apparently receptive to health education, a careful balance of encouragement and support has to be maintained if they are not to feel victimized because they 'fail' to follow the advice that they have been given or decide to refuse it outright. This can be difficult to achieve, particularly if they suffer disadvantage and deprivation in their personal circumstances which reinforces their feelings of helplessness and hopelessness. People who believe that they are not in control of their lives will feel even less capable of taking positive measures about their health.

In the summarizing final chapter of her detailed analysis of the Health and Lifestyle Survey mentioned earlier, Blaxter (1990) makes two interesting points: first that 'few people's lifestyles are totally healthy or unhealthy: most are mixed' and second that 'Unhealthy behaviour does not reinforce disadvantage to the same extent as healthy behaviour increases advantage. This seems to suggest that *the prior effect on health is the general life-style associated with economic or occupational position*' (my emphasis). She accepts that this latter, for her, inescapable conclusion, given the evidence, is contrary to received wisdom. Later in the same chapter she points out that most people seem to have learnt the lessons of health education very well and 'believe strongly that voluntary behaviours are the most important determinants of health.' However, if Blaxter is correct in her deductions that social class and environment outweigh the individual's own regulation of their life-style, where does this leave health education? What kind of a rôle does it have? Should we not, at the very least, be considering alternative strategies?

THE EVER-MOVING TARGET
Fixing the target

The target is the population, but this is a shifting changing entity, segmented as we know into a variety of groupings based on various demographic, social, and educational factors, to give it its broadest definition. The needs and expectations of these groups also vary considerably, but unless they are understood and the messages are appropriately framed and delivered to meet those demands, the health educators are to all intents and purposes wasting their time.

There will always be an important place for health education at the personal level. The general practitioner who gives 5 extra minutes during a patient's surgery visit to explain why it would be sensible to accept the breast screening invitation or stop smoking will probably have more effect than any number of campaigns, articles, or posters that may have swum through the consciousness of the smoker. Any one-to-one encounter which demonstrates personal concern is powerful medicine, but there is a drawback. Unless this is group practice policy and supported by a good back-up system, it tends to be random and may be missing some of the more needy targets. It may also be unsuitable for some people who could feel that the doctor is taking liberties: 'I didn't come here for a lecture, just give me the tablets'. Others may feel picked upon and keep away from the surgery thenceforward.

Health education and health promotion are frequently used as interchangeable terms, but this blurs an important semantic distinction. Health education has the connotation of teaching and informing a specific group, whereas health promotion is much closer to persuading and 'selling' something to as many people as possible. In the lay mind you 'promote' a product to potential buyers but you 'educate' a person about subjects selected from a particular pool of knowledge. There is every good reason for health educationalists to be equally aware of this distinction when they are planning their campaigns. The skills required to conceive a health promotion campaign, for example 'a healthy diet week' or a 'no-smoking day' and design it to have maximum impact are very similar to those enlisted for an advertising campaign and with good reason. The aim is much the same: to persuade as many punters out there that the product on offer is their 'best buy'.

There is an obvious danger in packaging and promoting health like just another cereal or packet of soap powder: only too easily the public will begin to develop a cynical resistance to all such broad-brush campaigns. Good health itself, whatever that may mean, begins to come into disrepute if it is oversold, particularly if the experts appear seriously at odds with each other as we have seen in recent years, for example between the competing food factions. Health education must be regarded as being above these divisions, certainly not to be mixed up with any commercial interests, but to be offering impartial information about something that is recognized to be intrinsically good, may be worth even something of a struggle to achieve. At the same time it must be seen to be attainable, and this is where devising flexible alternative strategies to suit the different target groups becomes so important.

Strategies

The prevailing model of health education has been individualistic and the message has been unequivocal: it is your responsibility to look after your own health. While this may be true for those in a position to care for themselves, it is unrealistic for many, particularly the large numbers caught in the poverty trap and in some instances it is so unimaginative as to verge on the cruel, as for instance when it is addressed to the long-term unemployed, mothers struggling in bad housing, or elderly pensioners eking out meagre means.

There is obviously a strong case for encouraging self-responsibility but not to the point that behaviour deemed to be 'irresponsible' becomes an excuse for blaming the victim. However tempting it may be to say to the heavy smoker, for instance, 'it's your own fault if . . .', a judgemental attitude is likely to be counterproductive as far as changing behaviour is concerned. Where the individualistic style of health education proves to be inappropriate it will obviously also be ineffective and this means that alternative strategies must be devised.

The community approach embraces a variety of different initiatives, many of which have been identified by the Community Health Initiatives Resource Unit (CHIRU 1985). They are invariably based on the particular needs of a defined local community, usually inner city and often an ethnic minority and because they spring from the community itself they are precisely tailored and cheap to run. The health professionals can make a very positive contribution by using their influence to provide educational input, facilities, and ideally acquire some funding, but essentially the organization and development of the initiative remains with the community. It is essential for the success of these initiatives that the health professionals are enlisted as partners, not as teachers.

In cancer education this concept of like-minded people with particular needs combining for support and information has been crystallized in the cancer self-help groups, which now have an annual conference and an organization (CancerLink) which acts as a liaison body and provides training for group leaders when it is requested. The genesis of these groups ranges from a highly motivated individual starting a group for patients and relatives to a health professional, often a nurse, who has seen an unfulfilled need among hospital patients going back into the community. Some of these groups flourish and grow into national organizations; others last as long as the members themselves want them.

A remarkable example of the former is Breast Cancer Care, formerly the Breast Care and Mastectomy Association which was founded in 1973 by a breast cancer patient who realized after her own alienating experience that what women crave above all is an opportunity to talk through their practical and emotional problems with someone who has had similar problems and can share her solutions. Today Breast Cancer Care is a professional organization with volunteers throughout the United Kingdom who are available on the telephone to help any woman who rings in and asks for help with a wide range of problems. Care is taken to match volunteer and client for age, social class, and type of treatment. Helping people to live with their cancer is a valuable part of cancer education and it can be done very well by people who are willing to contribute their personal experience.

The rôle of the media

There is a curious love–hate relationship between health professionals and those working in the media. Health educators attribute a degree of power and influence to television in particular, 'going into all those millions of homes', which the programme makers are pleased to accept, although privately they may have some reservations. A closer look at the outcome of many of the health campaigns run in the media suggests that although people are quite good at absorbing a message, for example smoking causes cancer, what they do with that information is another matter. Indeed, being told what is good for you can heighten feelings of guilt and inadequacy even if it does not cause resentment, whereas a programme which combines useful information with an invitation to find out more, perhaps by ringing a help-line or writing in for leaflets, may be a positive encouragement to do something for yourself (Karpf 1988).

When the popular press carries banner headlines proclaiming an imminent cure for cancer which then fails to materialize, the doctors blame the journalists for irresponsible reporting. The hype surrounding these stories and the false hopes they raise certainly damage everyone: the general public, cancer patients and their families, and everyone working in the cancer field (researchers, carers, and fundraisers). However, the question must also be asked: who has given the story to the journalists? Often it emanates from someone working on the 'cure' who sees it as a way of pre-empting rival researchers; an alternative source is quite likely to be a keen researcher microscanning the scientific journals.

The problem for all health journalists, print or broadcast, is that they must rely on official medical and scientific sources for their information and on official goodwill to gain access to them. In an ideal world they would be sifting through everything that they read and checking everything that they were told; they would be comparing and questioning endlessly before they presented their report or programme. Indeed, the best science and health reporters do this most of the time, but they also have to meet deadlines and answer to editors. Of course, there are also the ranks of the less committed and the less scrupulous who will always be more concerned with a story than the truth. Time for the serious journalist is a major problem, just as it is for doctors who cannot possibly read all the papers relating to their particular interests. Therefore, to play safe, the harried journalist tends to reproduce the report or the carefully rehearsed medical briefing, often staged by a public relations company in the august setting of a Royal College or to rewrite the press release which has been interlarded with quotes from respected medical experts.

The medical profession, far from losing respect because of the media, has become its authority figure wheeled on to furnish magisterial statements on a wide range of topics, many of which would not previously have been regarded as within its ambit, such as ageing or bereavement (Karpf 1988). Nor should it be overlooked that doctors are seldom averse to some judicious media manipulation when it suits them. If, for instance, they can demonstrate that children or cancer 'victims' are being denied life-saving facilities for lack of funds, then their unrestrained 'shroud waving' in the tabloids is guaranteed to evoke a generous response from the public.

Media bashing is a popular sport and one that anyone can play, but on the occasions when a journalist or broadcaster presents a serious criticism of some aspect of medicine or medical practice the profession tends to take offence as part of its defence. For example, an exposure by a senior correspondent of *The Observer* that some cancer patients were being entered into clinical trials without seeking their informed consent, a fact well known to the medical profession but confined largely to private debate, aroused this kind of outraged reaction (Raphael 1988). The story ran for three consecutive Sundays and included a half-page rebuttal from one of the doctors involved, a lengthy 'right to reply' not usually granted to aggrieved parties. Journalists who spotlight a medical disagreement as, for instance, in the controversial 1980 BBC Television *Panorama* programme about brain death, are likely to bring the whole wrathful medical establishment tumbling about their ears. As Anne Karpf, the shrewd critic already cited in this section, points out: 'At the heart of many crises in medico-journalist relations are medical disagreements, with the messenger [i.e. journalist] as scapegoat.'

Educating the educators

These debates about the rôle of the media remind us that in health education as in other areas of health there are no single 'correct' answers. Health campaigners who find it difficult to explain the complexities surrounding killers like heart disease or cancer can fall into 'a form of worthy dishonesty' which the general public quickly sees through, thus creating a climate of cynicism rather than acceptance (Davidson 1990). Nor should we think that there is only one best way of delivering the message. A continuing programme of successful health education requires cooperation between the orthodox health educators whose professional status is represented by the Health Education Authority and all the other sectors of the community who could play a part. General practitioners, hospital doctors, nurses, other health professionals, school teachers, publicists, market researchers, journalists, editors, women's organizations, community leaders, employers, and trades unions are all channels through which useful information can be relayed. All are potential educators, but in order to educate effectively, they must first be educated themselves about cancer.

Cancer education covers all aspects: causes, prevention, and types of treatment including, very necessarily, palliative care, support networks, counselling, and financial and social advice. The information can be given orally, visually, or in written form or be a combination using teacher packs, booklets, interactive videos, and tapes. There is a growing amount of such resource material, particularly for the primary health care team, much of it financed by cancer charities such as Cancer Research Campaign, Marie Curie Cancer Care, and the Cancer Relief Macmillan Fund. Research into using teachers as cancer educators has shown that, if they are committed to good health and can see ways of integrating it into their pastoral rôle, they can be very effective. A few well-researched smoking-prevention programmes for school children of different ages are already in use (Charlton 1988, 1989). Several of the cancer charities are now producing their own leaflets, videos, and tapes and they offer a particularly good information resource for the media.

COUNTING THE COST

The initiatives are springing up all about us and there is no shortage of creative thinking about cancer education but, to be wholly successful, the strategies for its implementation must be shown to be cost effective as well as beneficial in their outcome. This means costing out the burden of illness, defining the end purpose of any given health promotion activity (as a simple example, is it purely informational or is it intended to change behaviour?), and evaluating both strategies and outcomes. Finally, it is necessary to set the priorities for an effective programme of cancer education, while remembering that it in turn has to be ranked for importance along with all the other health promotion activities which are competing for funding.

That there is a need for much more education about cancer in all its aspects is indisputable. It has been estimated that approximately 85 per cent of cancer could be avoided, and that smoking and diet are major risk factors (Doll and Peto 1981). Half the life years lost prematurely (before 65 years) for women are due to cancer, of which the predominant forms are breast and lung, whereas cancer accounts for less than one-third of male life years lost up to the same age. This is a significant sex difference which also has to be taken into consideration when deciding on priorities and strategies.

As outlined above, this is a major task and one which requires continuing cooperation between the health economists, health educationalists, and health carers. A comprehensive databank is essential so that all the relevant information can be evaluated and assessed according to agreed criteria. Only then will it be possible to make 'best buy' decisions about health education which are based on rational assessment of need and outcome, as opposed to what happens so often at the moment: an *ad hoc* response to an emotive appeal.

For an illuminating and in-depth analysis of these and other economic considerations for appraising health promotion policies the interested reader is referred to a discussion paper which has been produced jointly by the Health Education Authority and the Centre for Health Economics at York University (Godfrey *et al.* 1989).

An undivided house

Cancer may have been kicked out of the closet but its visible acknowledged presence has not yet markedly reduced the fear with which it is regarded. It remains the most dreaded disease and it continues to arouse negative attitudes in most people, including many of the health professionals most closely concerned with it. Information plain and simple will not be enough to counteract these emotional reactions; people need to be convinced that the information they are receiving has a positive content and that acting on it will bring them worthwhile benefits.

This conviction will not be achieved unless it is matched by an equal conviction and commitment from those in charge of planning and executing a continuing programme of cancer education. Any suggestion of half-hearted approaches or divided opinions among the professionals will immediately percolate through to the general public. The economic approach may be hard-headed but it need not be hard-hearted; a judgement based on a sound economic appraisal of what works in health education must include a humane appreciation of real needs and how best to meet them.

REFERENCES

ASH Women and Smoking Group (1990). *Women, smoking and poverty: an expert report*. ASH, London.

Blaxter M (1990). *Health and lifestyles*. Tavistock/Routledge, London.

Cancer Relief Macmillan Fund (1988). *Public attitudes to and knowledge of cancer in the UK—a quantitive study conducted by Thornton Drummond and Brett Limited*. Cancer Relief Macmillan Fund, London.

Cancer Research Campaign (1989). *Facts on cancer*. Factsheet 11.3, Cancer Research Campaign, London.

Charlton A (1988). *Cells, cancers and communities. Teacher's book and pupil's resource pack*. Thornes, Cheltenham.

Charlton A (1989). *The problems of C932: a smoking prevention programme for 9+10 year olds*. Nottingham Education Supplies Ltd.

CHIRU (Community Health Initiatives Resource Unit) (1985). NHS support for CHIs. *Community Health Initiatives Resource Unit Newsletter*, No. 3:1–2. Available from CHIRU, 26 Bedford Square, London WC1B 3HU.

Doll R, Peto R (1981). *The causes of cancer*. Oxford University Press.

Godfrey C, et al. (1989). *Priorities for health promotion—an economic approach*. Discussion Paper 59, Centre for Health Economics, University of York.

Karpf A (1988). *Doctoring the media: the reporting of health and medicine*. Routledge, London.

Morris J, et al. (1989). *The benefits of providing information to patients*. Discussion Paper 58, Centre for Health Economics, University of York.

Raphael A (1988). Wanted: human guinea pigs. *The Observer*, 2–16 October.

Roberts M (1989). Breast screening: time for a rethink?, *British Medical Journal*, 299:1153–5, and subsequent correspondence in later issues.

Slevin ML, *et al.* (1988). BACUP—the first two years: evaluation of a national cancer information service. *British Medical Journal*, 297:669–72.

20.11 Support systems for cancer patients

MARY M. H. CODY AND MAURICE L. SLEVIN

INTRODUCTION

For most patients and their families, the experience of cancer is intensely stressful. Maguire (1981) summarizes it well when he comments that cancer patients 'face the threats that they may lose their health, rôle, and life. They also have to live with the uncertainty as to whether and when those losses will occur.' Clinical research supports the idea that the diagnosis and treatment of cancer carries with it considerable psychological morbidity. Studies consistently report that 25–30 per cent of patients have significant emotional problems (Morris *et al.* 1977; Maguire *et al.* 1978) and that many of these could be alleviated through some form of intervention (Maguire *et al.* 1980). Psychosocial studies, which

highlight patient's perceptions of their illness, have helped to shape the development of support services for cancer patients. In practice, support systems are limited by the human and financial resources available.

Our aim in this chapter is to describe the many diverse systems that promote psychological adaptation to cancer which are increasingly available to patients within the framework of conventional medicine. Other resources, including family, friends, family doctor, work, church, and community, constitute valuable systems of support, but it is not intended to describe them any further here. Finally, a section of the chapter is devoted to consideration of the rôle of alternative/complementary treatments.

WHAT CONSTITUTES SUPPORT AND WHAT DO PATIENTS WANT?

The problems of attempting to define support have been well described. Most authors agree that it is a multidimensional construct and most acknowledge the importance of information, emotional support, material aid and services, and the maintenance of social identity and affiliation (Bloom 1982; Wortman 1984). Analyses of calls to cancer telephone helplines tend to support this all-embracing definition. During 1985 and 1986, BACUP, the national cancer information service, received 30 000 calls (Slevin *et al.* 1988). Fifty per cent of the callers requested specific medical information, while 40 per cent wanted supportive information about coping, support groups, communication problems, and emotional support. In a similar survey in the United States, 50 per cent of the telephone calls concerned psychosocial issues, with requests for referral to support groups, anxiety/depression about the diagnosis, family problems, doctor–patient communication problems, and the financial demands of the illness being the most frequent topics of conversation (Rainey 1985). These data suggest that a range of services and expertise is necessary if the needs of cancer patients and their families are to be met adequately.

THE ROLE OF THE CANCER DOCTOR

Increasingly, patients are looking not just for technical and medical expertise from their doctors, but for someone with whom they can discuss all aspects of their illness and the treatment options available (Morton 1987). Reports of dissatisfaction with doctor–patient communication suggest that there is some discrepancy between what patients want and what they actually receive (Gould and Toghill 1981). Brewin (1977) suggests that it is not what patients are told but the manner in which they are told. The majority of patients want information (Cassileth *et al.* 1980), but they do not want it delivered in a way that is incomprehensible or in an amount that is more than they can assimilate. They do not want to hear 'You have cancer and I'm afraid there is nothing more we can do for you'. Few appear to want specific information about the prognosis (Slevin *et al.* 1988). How the initial interview is handled is crucial and may well determine the patient's future adjustment to his or her illness. This is the ideal opportunity for the cancer doctor to commence a supportive relationship built on trust and openness. Information-giving that is accurately timed and aimed at the appropriate pitch can be extremely supportive because people experience less anxiety when they know what to expect and have mentally prepared themselves. Information should be tailored to the needs of the individual patient and sensitively imparted at a rate that the patient can manage (Slevin 1987). It needs to be consistent and repeated frequently. (For useful articles on doctor–patient communications, see Brewin (1977), Buckman (1984), Slevin (1987), and Maguire (1988).)

On hearing their diagnosis, some patients ask for a second opinion. Rather than viewing such individuals as difficult or demanding, it must be remembered that patients feel extremely threatened by the diagnosis of cancer and the first reaction may be to doubt the diagnosis or the recommended treatment. In fact, referral to other consultant colleagues is a very useful method of allaying anxiety and promoting a trusting doctor–patient relationship.

Enquiries about the emotional, social, and financial impact of the disease reassure the patient that the doctor is interested in them as an individual and not just another cancer case. Informational support which is not reinforced by emotional support is considered 'unhelpful' by patients (Dunkel-Schetter 1984). Plans of action need to be discussed with the patient and every effort should be made to involve the patient in all aspects of care (Cassileth *et al.* 1980). However, it is important to take into account individual preferences for the degree of involvement. Giving an anxious patient responsibility for decisions regarding choices of treatment may only heighten their anxiety.

Relapses are particularly difficult for patients and they often fear that they will be abandoned by their doctors. However, as Brewin (1977) points out, even in advanced cases 'it is seldom true to say that nothing can be done'. Focusing on plans for symptom relief and continuing care, even if it is of a palliative nature, can be very reassuring.

THE ROLE OF COUNSELLING

With the increasing recognition of the emotional burden of cancer patients, it is becoming customary for cancer treatment centres to provide counselling services. Designated nurse specialist/nurse counsellors have extensive knowledge of cancer and its treatment and are thus well equipped to deal with the practical worries and concerns of cancer patients. They are usually trained in communication skills and in eliciting symptoms of psychological distress. Nurse counsellors are not intended to absolve physicians of their responsibility to communicate with their patients. However, within the constraints of a busy practice, it may be impossible to spend as much time as is optimally desirable with the patient and his or her relatives. Furthermore, patients are frequently in such turmoil on hearing their diagnosis that they retain little of the initial information imparted to them. Nurse counsellors reinforce diagnostic and prognostic information from the physician and, in the case of breast cancer, help women to make an optimal decision regarding treatment. Misconceptions about cancer and its treatment are readily identified by nurse counsellors and methods of solving both practical and emotional problems are explored with the patient.

A broader counselling approach may also be undertaken by social workers, hospital chaplains, or indeed lay people with a training in counselling. Since these people have less specific knowledge of cancer and its treatment, this approach is more suitable for patients with interpersonal or emotional problems which may have predated the diagnosis. The British Association for Counselling has a large membership nationwide and can provide the names of counsellors working locally.

It has been suggested that the counselling approach is more suited to alleviating acute transient mood states than more severe protracted disturbance. For example, counselling failed to prevent psychiatric morbidity in mastectomy patients but led to increased recognition and early psychiatric referral, thus reducing the overall level of morbidity 12–18 months later (Maguire *et al.* 1980). Linn *et al.* (1982) evaluated the effects of counselling on 62 late-stage cancer patients and found that the quality of life was enhanced after 3 months of psychosocial counselling but not after 1 month. They stressed the importance of continuing counselling for more than 1 month.

Many patients have sufficient personal or social resources to buffer the stressful effects of cancer and therefore have no need for professional counselling. Furthermore, not all of those who are distressed will elect to discuss their problems with a counsellor. In one study of newly diagnosed patients, the uptake for counselling services among those deemed to be at risk of psychological problems was only 60 per cent (Worden *et al.* 1980). On the evidence of present data, there appears to be little to support the provision of counselling services for all. More research is needed to identify who should receive counselling, who should provide it, when it should occur, and the most effective form of intervention.

PSYCHOTHERAPY

Psychotherapy may be indicated when the emotional reaction to cancer is intense and protracted. Psychotherapy aims to bring about enduring changes in the patient's way of dealing with stressful situations. Many cancer patients are unable to benefit from in-depth psychoanalytic therapies because they are lengthy and emotionally demanding. However, brief forms of psychotherapy focusing on immediate problems and aimed at improving the patient's quality of life can be very helpful. Spouses and partners are frequently included in these sessions because of the far-reaching effects that the disease and its treatment have on people around the patient. In some cases, the added emotional burden of the illness may highlight and exacerbate pre-existing deficiencies in relationships. Psychiatrists and psychologists with a special interest in the emotional aspects of cancer are increasingly available in general hospitals to provide psychotherapeutic services (Ramirez 1989).

Adjuvant psychological therapy is a form of cognitive psychotherapy specifically adapted for cancer patients by psychiatrists at the Royal Marsden Hospital, London. In psychiatry, cognitive therapy has been shown to be effective in reducing depression (Blackburn *et al.* 1981). In adjuvant psychological therapy, the same principles have been applied to patients with cancer to enable them to overcome negative attitudes and to adopt more positive coping strategies. Patients become familiar with techniques such as calming self-instruction, positive self-statements, methods of distraction, reality testing, and cognitive rehearsal. Behavioural techniques such as relaxation and activity scheduling are also employed. The therapy is carried out over six to 12 sessions and the aim is to maximize the patient's involvement in the rewarding aspects of life (Moorey and Greer 1989). It has the advantage that, with some training, it can be practised by health professionals with diverse backgrounds and not just by psychiatrists and psychologists.

BEHAVIOURAL INTERVENTIONS

Stress management techniques from behavioural psychotherapy have been successfully applied to cancer medicine to reduce anxiety associated with the illness and also to reduce the side-effects associated with treatment. The aim of most of these approaches is to bring about a state of relaxation on the basis that relaxation and fear/tension are incompatible. Many different approaches have been used to elicit the relaxation response including progressive muscle relaxation, visual/guided imagery, hypnosis, biofeedback, meditation, yoga, autogenic training, and massage. (A summary of these techniques is given by Sims (1987).) Relaxation tapes and booklets on stress management are usually available from nurse counsellors and through many commercial outlets.

Recently, a number of studies have been carried out to evaluate the efficacy of some of these approaches. In a randomized controlled study of patients with early breast cancer, progressive muscle relaxation combined with mental imagery had a positive effect on mood state (Bridge *et al.* 1988). Imagery involved recalling a pleasant calming scene, rather than the more cancer-specific type described by Simonton. Relaxation was also thought to be helpful to patients with advanced cancer, although no objective outcome measures were possible in this study (Fleming 1985). In her review of studies on relaxation, Sims (1987) highlights the methodological shortcomings

and the anecdotal nature of much of the research and emphasizes the need for well-conducted controlled studies.

Relaxation has also been suggested as an adjuvant method of pain control because it reduces muscle tension and alleviates co-existing anxiety. Again, progressive muscle relaxation, breathing exercises, imagery, meditation, yoga, and biofeedback are used to bring about relaxation. Studies have not revealed any advantage of one specific method of relaxation over another, although patients may have individual preferences (Graffam and Johnson 1987). Hypnosis has also been shown to be effective in helping patients to experience pain relief and improved quality of life (Spiegel and Bloom 1983). Effective hypnotic strategies include blocking awareness through suggestion of anaesthesia, substituting another feeling, moving the pain perception to a similar but less vulnerable area, altering the meaning of the pain, and dissociating perception of the affected bodily part (Barber and Gitelson 1980).

Behavioural strategies have been used to reduce nausea and vomiting associated with chemotherapy. Redd *et al.* (1982) demonstrated that hypnosis combined with guided imagery significantly reduced anticipatory nausea and vomiting. In a controlled-outcome study, Morrow and Morrell (1982) showed that systematic desensitization, another behavioural technique, produced significant reduction in anticipatory nausea and vomiting compared with counselling or no treatment other than the standard anti-emetic regimen. Burish *et al.* (1988), in a follow-up study, showed that patients who had learnt progressive muscle relaxation to reduce the side-effects of chemotherapy continued to use this technique for a variety of stress-related problems 2 years after chemotherapy had ended.

Behavioural methods have beneficial effects when anxiety is of mild or moderate severity, but are less likely to be effective for severe anxiety when there may be no alternative to the use of an anxiolytic drug. Nor can they be used in the acute situation since it takes some time for the patient to acquire the techniques. Finally, a degree of motivation and perseverance is necessary on the part of the patient and some individuals either cannot or will not make this commitment.

Traditionally, behavioural approaches have been confined to the specialities of psychiatry and psychology, but there is no reason why they should not be incorporated into routine medical care as adjuvant complementary modes of practice. Many of the techniques are easily learnt and can readily be taught to patients by ward staff (Copley Cobb 1984).

PSYCHOPHARMACOLOGY

Psychotropic medication has an important role to play in the emotional support of the cancer patient. Many emotional problems associated with cancer can be resolved by counselling or psychotherapy, but occasionally patients are so distressed that they are not accessible to these forms of psychological intervention. Depressive and anxiety disorders constitute the most common psychiatric problems found in cancer patients (Derogatis *et al.* 1983). Major depressive illness should be suspected if there is severe and persistent lowering of mood. In making the diagnosis, it is important to enquire about the following: loss of interest and enjoyment, social withdrawal, anxiety, irritability, agitation, self-blame, hopelessness, and suicidal ideation. The physical symptoms of depression such as anergia, anorexia, weight loss, sleep disturbance, and somatic preoccupation are not very useful diagnostically unless they are disproportionate to the medical illness or are temporally related to the psychic symptoms (Cavanaugh 1984). As in all medically ill patients, organic mental states that mimic depression must be identified and treated appropriately before a primary psychiatric diagnosis is made. Tricyclic antidepressants are the mainstay of treatment for major depressive disorders and should be coupled with supportive psychotherapy. Amitriptyline is strongly sedative and is particularly suitable where agitation, insomnia, and anxiety are problems. Imipramine, in contrast, is less sedative and is more appropriate for the withdrawn retarded patient. In general, the therapeutic dose range varies from 75 to 150 mg/day, but it is wise to start with a low dose (for example, 30 mg/day) in the debilitated or elderly patient. All antidepressants have unwanted side-effects but some of the newer ones (for example, lofepramine) are reported to be less troublesome.

A recent development has been the introduction of a new class of antidepressant, the selective serotonin reuptake inhibitors. These drugs act specifically on the serotonin system and therefore avoid many of the unpleasant anticholinergic and cardiovascular side-effects of the tricyclic drugs. They are well tolerated by patients although nausea, vomiting, sweating, and tremor are seen in some patients. These drugs are given as a once daily dose, for example fluoxetine 20 mg mane or paroxetine 20 mg mane or sertraline 50 mg mane. They are as efficacious as the older tricyclic drugs but are more expensive. It is likely that these drugs will be widely used in the treatment of depression in medically ill patients in the future because of the low incidence of side-effects.

Tricyclic antidepressants with sedative properties such as dothiepin and amitriptyline are also useful for treating anxiety disorders. The anxiolytic dose is usually approximately half that of the antidepressant dose. Benzodiazepines have been criticized in recent times because of the potential for addiction and serious withdrawal effects (Ashton 1984). Nevertheless, they remain effective anxiolytic agents and are helpful when the patient is experiencing such overwhelming fear that a behavioural or counselling approach is impossible. Short-acting compounds such as lorazepam or oxazepam are appropriate when a brief duration of action is required. Long-acting compounds, which include diazepam and chlordiazepoxide, are appropriate for frequent episodes of anxiety when a sustained action is needed. Benzodiazepines should be used for the shortest time possible and in the lowest effective dosage. They are well tolerated by patients, but can lead to oversedation, ataxia, and confusion in the elderly.

SUPPORT GROUPS

Support groups in oncology are a relatively new phenomenon in the United Kingdom but are rapidly gaining in popularity. At the time of writing there were at least 250 cancer support or self-help groups throughout the United Kingdom (Alderson et al. 1989). Support groups help to reduce the sense of alienation and isolation often engendered by the diagnosis of cancer and its treatment. They differ in the range and type of service offered, depending on the needs and resources of the local community. Some support groups are hospital based, led by doctors and nurses. These are educational as well as supportive (Plant et al. 1987). Others are true self-help groups set up in the community, often by people who have experience of cancer personally or in family members or friends. Self-help groups tend to emphasize self-reliance and self-care. Finally, there are the rarer psychotherapeutic groups run by a mental health professional with a training in group dynamics. These explore the wider psychodynamic implications of the illness (Yalom and Greaves 1977). It is not a question of which system, self-help or professional, is better. Both have a role to play in helping patients

with the psychosocial problems related to cancer. Choice will largely depend on the preference of the individual and the hospital and community resources. Some groups are limited to those with a specific type of experience (for example, laryngectomy, colostomy, or mastectomy groups), while others welcome patients with a variety of cancer types.

The potential benefits of a support group include opportunities for sharing experiences, the ventilation of feelings in a supportive atmosphere, and the exchange of information about the physical, psychological, and social consequences of cancer and its treatment. Few patients report feeling more depressed as a result of attending a group, even when a group member dies. This may be because those who attend them are a self-selected highly motivated minority of cancer patients generally (Plant et al. 1987). An up-to-date directory listing the various support groups is available through CancerLink. The Groups Support Service set up by CancerLink provides training, finances, and support to those who are in the process of setting up new groups.

CANCER INFORMATION SERVICES

One of the most frequent sources of dissatisfaction for medical patients is the lack of information provided about their illness (Fletcher 1980). Cancer information services were developed specifically to redress this situation. They act as an adjunctive support system but they do not replace a doctor's professional advice to the individual patient.

The British Association for Cancer United Patients (BACUP) was founded in 1984 by Vicky Clement-Jones, a medical practitioner who developed cancer and subsequently recognized that there was little in the way of support and information for cancer patients (Clement-Jones 1985). BACUP is a national cancer information service which provides up-to-date information on all types of cancer by telephone or letter from a team of specially trained oncology nurses. The staff are supported by a medical and specialist advisory board which they can consult for specialized information. Confidential information is given on every aspect of cancer including treatment and care, support groups, and other services. The telephone service is free to patients inside and outside London on weekdays only. BACUP also produces leaflets and booklets on different types of cancer and cancer treatments and how to cope with them. A newsletter which is published three times a year focuses on new developments in cancer care. It acts as an important communication link for cancer patients and their families. Doctors and other health care professionals are invited to use the information and resources which are maintained on a computerized database. BACUP also has a cancer counselling service which is staffed by a number of volunteers who have been trained in counselling skills and the problems of living with cancer. This service is available to people living in the London area.

CancerLink was founded by a group of people with personal and professional experience of cancer. Trained staff provide telephone and written information about cancer, including practical and emotional help. A variety of booklets and leaflets has been prepared by CancerLink and they are freely available to cancer patients. A Directory of Useful Organizations includes addresses of the head offices of national organizations for information about specific types of cancer, counselling, hospice care, and bereavement services.

Other information services deal with specific types of cancer. The Breast Care and Mastectomy Association (BCMA) offers women specific information about prostheses, breast reconstruction, concealing blemishes after radiotherapy, etc. The association has a useful list of the many shops around the country which stock prostheses and related items as well as several mail order firms. The BCMA operates a telephone helpline 5 days a week. It also produces its own selection of books and leaflets on topics such as breast surgery, lymphoedema, and breast self-examination which are freely available to individuals.

The Leukaemia Research Fund is the national charity for the support of research into leukaemia and allied blood diseases. It runs an up-to-date practical information service on all aspects of these diseases for patients and their families.

The Hodgkin's Disease Association provides information and support to sufferers of Hodgkin's or non-Hodgkin's lymphoma and their relatives. Relevant literature and a video are available.

The Colostomy Welfare Group (CWG) provides a telephone and postal advice service and also welcomes personal callers. The CWG publishes a series of leaflets on living with a colostomy, how to cope with constipation and diarrhoea, travelling, etc. Advice is given on the suitability and availability of various appliances.

A comprehensive list of all the information services is available through BACUP and CancerLink.

BEFRIENDING

Many of the charitable organizations operate a system of visiting patients in hospital or in their own homes. Visitors are usually volunteers who have had personal experience of cancer themselves. Patients often find it difficult to confide in relatives who may be overly involved or very distressed (Dunkel-Schetter 1984) and they find it easier to talk to someone who shares a common experience and who can provide support in a caring but more objective manner. The BCMA has a list of volunteer helpers who can be called upon to visit women undergoing breast surgery or later at home. The British Colostomy Association (BCA) also operates a personal visiting system. The volunteers are often selected by stoma care nurses located in general hospitals and are then registered with the BCA after a period of training. Members of the National Laryngectomy Association Clubs, which promote the rehabilitation of laryngectomy patients, are frequently invited by surgeons and nursing staff to lecture and demonstrate speech aids and to talk to patients before and after their operation to show what can be achieved. The Leukaemia Care Society is an organization set up by parents and children who have had leukaemia. It provides a range of services such as visiting at home and in hospital, financial assistance, holidays, and support in times of stress.

FINANCIAL SUPPORT

Many patients with cancer, particularly those who are the main providers in a family, experience considerable financial difficulty as a result of loss of income and the many unplanned expenses that a chronic illness can incur. Sometimes it is the additional stresses such as inadequate housing or financial worry that lead to emotional decompensation. Many units have social workers who are able to advise sick patients about the benefits to which they may be entitled. Employers will usually be required to pay employees during the first 28 weeks of sick leave. Thereafter, invalidity benefit is payable from the Department of Social Security as long as National Insurance has been paid for the previous year. Income support may be obtainable from the Department of Social Security for unemployed patients. In addition, patients may be eligible for the Attendance Allowance which is a weekly tax-free benefit for people who require looking after at home. This is paid regardless

of income, savings and National Insurance contributions. The Mobility Allowance is another tax-free benefit which is not means tested and can be claimed by people under the age of 65 years who are unable or almost unable to get about.

Grants are also available to needy patients from various charitable organizations. The Cancer Relief Macmillan Fund gives money towards the cost of many different items including home helps, day and night nursing at home, fares for out-patient visits, nursing home fees, domestic appliances, meals on wheels, heating, telephone installations, and even holidays in some instances. Marie Curie Cancer Care also has a welfare grant scheme through which a limited amount of money is available for necessities. It is assumed that statutory resources have been explored first. The Malcolm Sargent Cancer Fund for Children provides cash grants to parents of children under the age of 21 years who have cancer. Patients can apply for grants through the medical social worker or through the social services.

Another useful agency is the Society for the Prevention of Asbestos and Industrial Diseases (SPAID), which offers advice on Department of Social Security Industrial Benefits, inquest procedures, and claims for compensation from employers.

Some of the cancer information services provide valuable information about mortgages, personal insurance, and holiday insurance. The Association of British Insurers can also provide cancer patients with advice and guidance on insurance matters.

SPECIALIZED ONCOLOGY UNITS

The organization and provision of psychosocial support services has been greatly facilitated by the recent development of specialized oncology units which concentrate medical and paramedical expertise. Many of these units have their own counsellors, social workers, and psychiatrists or psychologists who are skilled in the use of the psychotherapeutic and behavioural interventions outlined earlier in this chapter.

Specialized oncology units constitute minisupport systems in their own right because patients quickly build up relationships with the other patients as well as with members of staff. Thus, they help to alleviate the alienation experienced by so many cancer patients on general wards. They also function as the nucleus for supportive activities often run by the patients themselves (for example, support groups, relaxation groups, fund-raising concerns, etc.).

Specialized oncology units generally have strong links with local community services such as Macmillan nurses, community support teams, and local hospices, thus ensuring continuity of care from shortly after diagnosis through to the final stages of the illness.

THE ROLE OF ALTERNATIVE/ COMPLEMENTARY THERAPY
General comments

Alternative/complementary therapy is the name given to a system of health care which lies for the most part, outside the mainstream of conventional medicine. It is used to denote those therapies which are considered unorthodox by the medical establishment because they are unproven and have no scientific basis. The terminology is confusing in this area because the words alternative and complementary are frequently used interchangeably. In addition, counselling and relaxation techniques are often grouped together with complementary therapies. For the purposes of this chapter, complementary treatments are those unorthodox treatments which do not preclude the use of conventional treatments and which are claimed to have a specific anticancer effect by proponents. Alternative therapies, by definition, are those unorthodox treatments which specifically exclude conventional treatments. Psychological approaches such as psychotherapy, counselling, and the various relaxation techniques are regarded as part of conventional treatment and are not included in this definition.

Alternative/complementary therapy is currently enjoying a surge in popularity of unprecedented proportions. It has been described as one of the growth industries of the decade (Smith 1983). In 1985, it was estimated that there were approximately 12 practitioners per 100 000 population in the United Kingdom with annual consultation rates of 19.5–25.7 per 100 population (Fulder and Monro 1985).

A British Medical Association (BMA) Working Party, which was set up to investigate the reasons for this phenomenon, identified the dissatisfaction of the general public with the increasingly mechanistic technical approach to medicine, the fragmentation of care due to specialization, and the loss of bedside skills such as time spent with the patient, touch, and compassion (British Medical Association 1986). It is worth noting that the mean length of the consultation with a complementary practitioner is 36 minutes, six times longer than that with the average general practitioner (Fulder and Monro 1985). The BMA Working Party report also noted the heightened expectations of the general public, fostered by the unbalanced reporting of medical cases in the media. Patients and their families who have become accustomed to miracle cures and life-saving techniques find it difficult to accept that there is no effective treatment. Probably the single most important reason for the success of alternative medicine is the failure of science and medicine to produce curative treatment for the commonly occurring types of cancer or indeed the other incurable diseases of mankind, such as AIDS and multiple sclerosis (Lerner 1984). People turn to unscientific and untested approaches because alternative practitioners offer hope and involve patients as active participants in their own management. Furthermore, cancer patients are easily influenced by the claims made for the efficacy of alternative medicine and are often unaware of the difference between the anecdotal evidence produced by alternative practitioners and the scientific data obtained from carefully conducted controlled clinical trials. It is very difficult to accept the results produced by alternative practitioners without properly designed randomized clinical trials because, as Mapother commented, 'among those "cured" by any novel remedy, are those who never had the disease, those who still have it, those who never had the treatment, and those who would have recovered equally well without it' (quoted by Goldberg 1982).

Extent of the use of alternative/ complementary therapy

The prevalence of the use of alternative/complementary therapies varies widely from study to study. It is impossible to provide accurate figures because some patients opt solely for alternative treatment and never enter the hospital system or abandon it shortly after initial contact. Other patients may be reluctant to disclose their involvement for fear of incurring their physician's wrath. A survey of paediatric oncology out-patients in the United States showed that 8.7 per cent had tried at least one remedy, 5.8 per cent had additionally considered trying some remedy, and 24.6 per cent had received recommendations to do so from family and friends. Laetrile, faith-healing, and diets were the most commonly mentioned therapies (Faw et al. 1977). A multicentre trial in New Zealand revealed that 32 per cent of 463 patients had received advice

about alternatives to ordinary medical treatment. Sixty-five per cent of these had followed or intended to follow this advice (Clinical Oncology Group 1987). A recent study of 304 cancer patients attending a cancer centre and 356 attending alternative practitioners in the United States revealed that 54 per cent of all patients received both conventional therapy and unorthodox treatments. Thirteen per cent of patients attending the conventional cancer centre had used or were using unorthodox treatments. Patients who used both treatments or unorthodox treatments exclusively were predominantly White and better educated than those who used conventional treatments alone (Cassileth et al. 1984).

Types most commonly used

The popularity of different unorthodox treatments down through the ages seems to reflect underlying social trends and values (for a historical perspective see Cassileth (1986, 1989)). Treatments which are fashionable today emphasize a holistic self-care 'gentle' approach to cancer. They are the antithesis of the 'high-tech' conventional therapies with all their attendant toxicities. In descending order of frequency, treatments most commonly used in a recent study of 1000 patients in the United States were metabolic therapy, diet treatments including megavitamins, mental imagery used for antitumour effect, spiritual healing or faith-healing, and immune therapy (Cassileth et al. 1984). The most popular diets in the New Zealand study mentioned earlier were the Bristol, macrobiotic, and grape diets and the most popular vitamin supplements were C, E, A, and B complex.

Laetrile or amygdalin

Laetrile was used as a treatment for cancer in Germany in the late 1800s, but was abandoned because of its toxicity and lack of efficacy. It was rediscovered by Ernest T. Krebs, a physician in California and a 'new non-toxic' form termed laetrile was synthesized by his son, Ernest Krebs Jr, in the late 1940s. He later called it vitamin B 17 to manoeuvre it past the Food and Drug Administration, which had rejected laetrile as a safe and effective drug for cancer. However, vitamin B 17 (marketed as Bee 17 or Aprikern) has no food value and meets none of the criteria for a vitamin. Krebs asserted that all cancers stemmed from vitamin B 17 deficiency and could be cured by laetrile administration. Laetrile quickly gained in popularity and was widely used during the 1970s for the prevention, palliation, and cure of cancer. It is estimated that more than 70 000 people in the United States used laetrile as an anticancer remedy during the 1960s and 1970s (Ellison et al. 1978). More correctly known as amygdalin, laetrile is a cyanogenetic glycoside found in the seeds of apricots, peaches, and plums. Two different modes of action have been proposed for the substance, but neither are very convincing (Dorr and Paxinos 1978).

In 1973, the National Cancer Institute carried out two studies of laetrile in animals. Unfortunately, an interim report showing superiority of laetrile was leaked to the press and the journal Science and this led to an upsurge of interest among the public. Further well-controlled animal studies revealed no evidence of an anticancer effect. Nevertheless, a retrospective analysis of laetrile treatment was undertaken by the National Cancer Institute in 1978 in response to public demand. A panel of cancer specialists who were blind to the treatment received by a conventionally treated group of patients with cancer and a group who had received laetrile, judged that out of 68 courses of laetrile, six might have produced a response. The methodological difficulties of the retrospective design were highlighted in this study (Ellison et al. 1978). Finally, in order to establish the truth about laetrile, a multicentre prospective clinical trial was undertaken in the United States (Moertel *et al.* 1982). One hundred and seventy-eight patients who were considered to have a good performance status participated in the study. Only one patient met the criteria for a partial response and some patients developed symptoms of cyanide intoxication. The authors concluded that laetrile was of no clinical value in the treatment of cancer. Laetrile, once the most commonly used alternative anticancer remedy, subsequently diminished in popularity during the 1980s.

Homoeopathy

Although the practice of homoeopathy dates back to Hippocrates and Paracelsus, homoeopathy as it is known today was developed in the eighteenth century by the German doctor Samuel Hahnemann. Based on experiments carried out on himself and friends, Hahnemann developed a number of theories about disease and its treatment. One of these, the similarity theory, forms the basis of homeopathy (Greek *homoios*, similar; *pathos*, disease). The principle involves matching the symptoms of the patient to the symptoms produced in healthy individuals by a 'proven' drug which is then used to treat the patient. In other words, patients are treated with substances which produce much the same symptoms as the ones that they originally suffered, for example purgatives to cure diarrhoea. Hahnemann built up a homoeopathic pharmacopoeia of alkali and metallic salts after he had tested and noted the symptoms that each one produced in healthy volunteers. He believed that the minimum dose should be used and carried out serial dilutions of the drug which were often so great that it is unlikely that any of it remained. He also believed that by shaking the remedies vigorously he could enhance their potency; the succussion theory. After serial dilutions and succussions, Hahnemann believed that the remedy contained the 'dynamic energy of the vital force' which activates the body and promotes healing (Brunton 1989). Disease is viewed as a disturbance of the vital force rather than as an entity in itself. Homoeopaths are thus not just interested in symptoms but in aspects of the patient's life-style and personality. General advice is usually given about diet and other aspects of healthy living. Thus, treatment is aimed at the person rather than the disease.

Homoeopathy has a strong following in the United Kingdom and is available on the National Health Service in a limited number of homoeopathic treatment centres. Although it has been suggested that homoeopathy is best suited to conditions that are considered reversible, such as constipation, arthritis, cystitis, and stress (Braunton 1989), cancer and its manifestations are treated by some homoeopaths. Given the dosages used in homoeopathic remedies and the fact that they are diluted thousands of times, it is unlikely that this approach would have any ill-effects provided that conventional treatment is not abandoned. Claims have been made for the efficacy of homoeopathy as a primary treatment modality for cancer, but no scientific data exist to support this claim. The BMA Working Party on Alternative Medicine concluded that the value of homoeopathy lay in its placebo effect.

Herbalism

Although many homoeopathic remedies are herbal in origin, fundamental differences exist between herbalism and homoeopathy. Herbalists believe that only plant materials should be used in the treatment of disease, whereas many homoeopathic remedies are derived from mineral or even animal sources. Herbalists do not espouse the similarity theory of homoeopathy and they use substantially larger doses than are used by homoeopaths (Brunton

1989). The effectiveness of the herbal remedy depends crucially on the site and time of collection and the part of the plant used in the remedy. Medicines are specially prepared for the individual patient, based on an in-depth analysis of a full life history including the patient's customary diet. Herbal remedies are presumed to work by enhancing natural healing, normalizing body chemistry, and eliminating toxic substances. They appeal to patients because of their healthy natural image, but the BMA Working Party produced evidence of occasional adverse reactions and interference with conventional medicines.

Mistletoe (*Viscum album*), also known as iscador, was originally proposed as a treatment for cancer by Rudolph Steiner, founder of anthroposophy in the 1920s and is still widely used as an anticancer agent throughout the world. Diagnosis is made on the analysis of crystallized blood which, apparently, also gives the location of the tumour (Schraub and Bernheim 1987). The host tree on which the mistletoe grows is considered important in the treatment of specific types of cancer. Different forms of mistletoe are mixed with metals and are then prescribed for the individual patient. There is no reputable evidence to support the use of iscador as a cancer treatment.

Psychological approaches

The Simonton method

A form of psychological therapy for patients with cancer was devised by Carl Simonton and his wife Stephanie in 1971. Simonton, a radiotherapist in the United States, believed that a person's psychic energy could be harnessed to enhance the body's natural defence system, which would then bring about healing and, it was hoped, lead to prolongation of survival. This view was based on Simonton's clinical observations of patients who appeared to have beaten the odds and who had lived longer than expected. He noted that these patients had a strongly positive attitude to life and a determination to fight their illness (Simonton *et al.* 1978). Simonton later reported longer median survival times in patients who had received a standard individual and group counselling programme in addition to the appropriate medical treatment (Simonton and Mathews-Simonton 1981). However, this paper is based on a comparison with historical controls with all the inherent pitfalls of this approach.

Simonton's therapy emphasizes the importance of body, mind, and emotions working in harmony together. The treatment package consists of counselling, relaxation exercises, and visualization. It is adjunctive in that it takes place alongside conventional medicine and it is not intended to replace conventional methods. The visualization procedure requires the patient to picture their cancer in a symbolic way and then to imagine the defence systems of the body mobilizing against the tumour, eventually conquering it. The patient is instructed to carry out visualization for approximately 15 min three times daily. Important components of the programme are information and advice about diet, physical exercise, stress management, and reorganization of personal goals.

No convincing evidence has been produced that the Simonton method prolongs the lives of cancer patients. In addition, some believe that the suggestion of personal responsibility, for both the causation and the course of the illness, inherent in this type of approach may be psychologically harmful to some patients (Holland 1981). Simonton himself appears to have altered his views considerably (Scarf 1980), but his therapy remains popular with many patients. Its merits lie in the potential for improving quality of life by enhancing personal effectiveness and self-confidence, promoting relaxation, and instilling hope.

Healing

Healing is an ancient art which dates back to at least 500 BC, the time of Hippocrates who was renowned for his healing gift. With the advent of Jesus Christ, who was perhaps the most famous healer of all time, healing largely became the domain of churches and clergymen. Lay healers were liable to be executed as witches and heretics (Harvey 1983). To this day an uneasy relationship exists between those in the healing ministry of the Christian church and the growing body of unaffilliated lay healers, although increasingly the church recognizes a form of healing based on a strong life energy which is apparently possessed by some individuals (MacNutt 1974). Healing which occurs under the auspices of Christianity is based on the strong religious faith of the sick person or the healer. Four basic kinds of healing are recognized and prayers are offered accordingly for repentance, inner healing, physical healing, and deliverance. Perhaps the many-faceted nature of the process accounts for the relief that many patients experience with this form of healing even if their disease is not directly affected.

Spiritualism, although usually considered to be a result of divine intervention, is not unique to any religion, nor is it used to promote any religion. The healing powers of God or some other force are said to work through the healer who is merely instrumental or intermediary in the process. The recipient of the healing process often describes a feeling of tingling or warmth flooding through their body. Distance creates no problems. Absent or distant healing is believed to be equally effective (Edwards 1975).

Healing is one of the most popular complementary therapies used in the United Kingdom today, with an estimated 20 000 healers practising the art (Fulder and Monro 1985). Registered groups of healers such as the National Federation of Spiritual Healers try to maintain standards and a code of ethics, recognizing the potential for abuse in the wrong hands. Registered healers recommend that the patient seeks a doctor's advice beforehand and are anxious to cooperate with the medical profession, believing that each operates in different ways to achieve the same purpose (Edwards 1975). While there are no scientific studies to demonstrate the efficacy of healing, the experience often gives patients an emotional boost and there is no evidence that it is ever harmful.

Meditation

Meditation involves the induction of a state in which all or nearly all conscious mental activity ceases. Claims have been made for the success of intensive meditation as a means of controlling cancer. In one study of 73 patients with advanced cancer, approximately 10 per cent of patients were said to show a remarkable regression in the growth of the tumour after meditation, although most patients finally succumbed. It is difficult to comment on the validity of this study since no information was provided on the type of treatment that the patients had received or how the disease was assessed. The majority of patients reported greatly improved quality of life through reduction of anxiety and depression and they experienced less pain and discomfort. Meditation was said to act via the immune system, although the author had no data on which to base this hypothesis (Meares 1980). In a later paper, the same author states that chemotherapy and radiotherapy hinder the therapeutic effect of meditation by weakening the immune system (Meares 1983).

By utilizing meditation techniques, cancer patients may experience all the benefits that are associated with an intensive form of relaxation (for example, less anxiety) and possibly less discomfort and pain and better tolerance of the side-effects of treatment. Meditation is unlikely to have any ill effects, but it is important that it is seen as an adjunctive approach rather than a primary mode of treatment.

Dietary methods

'Let food be your medicine' (Hippocrates)

Dietary treatments are commonly used by cancer patients, either in conjunction with conventional treatments or exclusively for the treatment of cancer. Proponents believe that cancer results from some form of dietary deficiency or imbalance and can be cured or halted by the addition of the missing nutrient or by alteration of the diet in some way. Claims of dramatic cures, together with mass media publicity and successful marketing techniques, make them very attractive to cancer patients.

Unproven methods of dietary treatment often consist of high-fibre low-calorie vegetarian diets in combination with other substances (for example, megavitamins) or attended by certain rituals designed to boost natural healing such as detoxification. Each has its own underlying philosophy of cancer causation which is often presented in a quasi-scientific way. It is the simplistic explanation of cancer and its treatment, so easily understood by patients in this nutrition-conscious age, that makes the dietary option seem the 'logical' natural remedy for cancer. In contrast, conventional explanations, where they exist, often seem remote and inaccessible. The most popular regimes in the United Kingdom are the Bristol diet and the macrobiotic diet.

The Bristol approach

The Bristol Cancer Help Centre was opened in 1980 as a new approach to the treatment of cancer. Central to the Bristol philosophy is the belief that the body's natural defences, in particular the immune system, can be mobilized against cancer through a combination of diet, healing, and psychological therapy. It is assumed that chemicals, additives, and fats in our contemporary diet have contributed to the causation of cancer by weakening the immune system. The Bristol diet is designed to maximize the patient's self-healing ability and in its original form, consisted of an initial detoxification phase during which all meat, fish, and dairy produce were prohibited. Thereafter, fish and poultry could be eaten in moderation but clients were encouraged to adhere to vegetarianism if possible. The emphasis has changed more recently from the concept of detoxification to that of healthy eating based on a wholefood, largely vegetarian diet supervised by a dietary therapist.

Medical counselling from doctors who support the holistic approach to patient care is available at the Bristol Centre. The importance of the role of stress in weakening the body's defences is emphasized and more effective ways of coping with it are explored. Psychological techniques such as guided meditation and mental imagery are said to stimulate natural healing. Biofeedback, art, and music are used to promote calm and inner peace. Spiritual healing is also offered as well as advice on appropriate life-style changes and exercise. The emphasis throughout is on self-help and self-healing. Orthodox medical treatments can be used in conjunction with the Bristol approach, and indeed are said to be enhanced by it.

Currently no data are available to support the anticancer effects which are claimed for this therapy. A case-controlled study (Bagenal 1990) suggested that patients fared worse than controls but the study has subsequently been criticized for its methodology. Patients often claim to have received emotional support from the Bristol treatment approach but some feel unwell on the diet.

The macrobiotic diet

Zen macrobiotics, taken in its broadest context, is a philosophy of life which has its origins in a number of oriental religions and theories. Zen promises longevity and self-discovery based on a life-style that includes meditation and adherence to strict diet. Central to the philosophy is the idea of two opposing but complementary energy forces in nature, yin and yang, which seek to achieve balance. When balance is attained, a state of harmony, order, and health is said to result.

The macrobiotic diet (or Zen macrobiotic diet) consists largely of cereal products such as brown rice, wheat, and millet. Liquids are used sparingly and sugar, red meat, and animal products are forbidden, as are stimulant beverages such as tea and coffee. The diet is supposed to counteract the imbalance between the yin and yang elements of an unhealthy diet, thought to be responsible for carcinogenesis. Yin cancers (for example, breast), result from excessive intake of yin foods (alcohol, citrus fruits, tea, and coffee) while yang cancers (for example, colon), result from excessive intake of yang foods (red meat, smoked fish, and eggs). A range of macrobiotic diets varying in the balance of yin–yang foodstuffs, was originally devised by George Ohsawa (1893–1966), a Japanese writer and philosopher, who was the founder of macrobiotics. The most restrictive forms of these diets provide well below the recommended daily nutritional intake and clinical cases of nutritional deficiency have been documented (Bowman et al. 1984). The macrobiotic diet gained prominence as an anticancer therapy with the publication of a book about Dr Anthony Sattilaro MD who placed himself on the diet while undergoing treatment for prostatic cancer. The National Cancer Institute clinicans who reviewed his case believed that Dr Sattilaro's longevity could be attributed to the surgery and hormone therapy he received rather than the diet (National Cancer Institute Statement 1983).

There is no evidence at present to support the use of macrobiotics as a primary treatment for cancer. Fit cancer patients can tolerate the macrobiotic diet, but it is likely to be hazardous for malnourished patients (Bowman et al. 1984).

The Gerson diet

The Gerson diet was devised by Dr Max Gerson, a German physician who emigrated to the United States in the 1930s. The therapy was an adaptation of a treatment he had originally devised for tuberculosis and which had seemingly brought about the miraculous recovery of a patient with advanced cancer (Gerson 1978). This was followed by further highly publicized successes. Gerson viewed cancer as a degenerative disease, as indeed he had viewed tuberculosis and believed that the many diverse symptoms of cancer were simply manifestations of dysfunction or poisoning of the digestive and hepatic systems. Detoxification, he noted, had originally been recommended by Hippocrates and this became a most important component of the Gerson approach. Patients are prescribed a wide variety of substances, including thyroid extracts and Lugols solution and are recommended to adhere to a high-potassium, low-salt diet. Only fresh fruit and vegetables can be eaten for the first 6 weeks of treatment and these have to be specially prepared and cooked. No liquidizers, pressure-cookers, or aluminium utensils are allowed and no steam should escape during the cooking process. The idea of such an elaborate regime is to purify the internal milieu, alter the conditions in which the cancer cells are thought to thrive, and at the same time restore the function of the liver by means of liver extracts and carrot juice. Frequent caffeine enemas are used to stimulate the flow of bile and to facilitate the excretion of toxic cancer degradation products. Orthodox treatments are considered harmful and patients are not even allowed to use painkillers.

The Gerson diet demands considerable effort on the part of the patient and, if followed in full, is likely to preoccupy much of his life. The National Cancer Institute in the United States, after reviewing a number of cases submitted by Dr Gerson, found no evidence of a therapeutic effect (American Cancer Society 1973). Max Gerson died in 1955 but his therapy centre in Tijuana, Mexico, supervised by his daughter, Charlotte Gerson, continues to attract patients from all over the world.

The grape diet

Grapes have been used as anticancer agents since at least the 1500s. Interest in the grape diet as a cure for cancer was renewed by a book called The grape cure by Johanna Brandt published in 1928 (Brandt 1928). By 1968 the 24th edition had been printed. A leaflet advertising the book states that 'the secret of the cure lies in the fact that the Grape is not mixed with any other food'. Proponents believe that poisonous substances are formed in the stomach if non-grape foodstuffs are also ingested. The diet consists solely of good quality grapes, in quantities varying from 2 to 8 ounces, to be consumed every 2 h. Unsweetened grape juice can be substituted for very weak patients. Water is the only beverage allowed. After 2 weeks on this regime other raw vegetables, nuts, honey, and milk products are introduced. Grape poultices, compresses, enemas, and douches are also recommended, depending on the site of the cancer. The American Cancer Society reviewed the available information about the grape diet and concluded that there was no evidence of a therapeutic effect in humans (American Cancer Society 1974). The grape diet is less popular as an anticancer diet today, but it is still occasionally promoted by the non-medical Press.

Orthomolecular or megavitamin therapy

Nearly all the vitamins have been promoted as individual anticancer agents at some time or another (Young and Newberne 1981). Of all those considered, vitamin C has received the most attention, largely as a result of the combined work of Ewan Cameron, a Scottish surgeon and Linus Pauling, the Nobel prize winner. Vitamin C plays a key role in many of the processes involved in cellular repair, as well as in the maintenance of the intercellular matrix and it also influences immune function (Young and Newberne 1981). Therefore, it was not unreasonable to consider it as a possible enhancer of the body's natural healing potential. In several articles published individually and collectively, Cameron and Pauling, using historical controls, cited evidence of the value of megadose vitamin C in the treatment of advanced cancer (Cameron et al. 1975; Cameron and Pauling 1976, 1978). However, a study at the Mayo Clinic supported by the National Cancer Institute failed to show a therapeutic benefit for high-dose vitamin C in a double-blind placebo-controlled study to evaluate the effects on symptoms and survival (Creagan et al. 1979). Although this study has been criticized by the proponents of vitamin C therapy, evidence for its role in cancer treatment remains lacking.

Vitimin A has also been promoted as an anticancer therapy. This compound has long been the subject of scientific investigation, based on the fact that a large number of cancers are epithelial in origin and vitamin A is necessary for epithelial cell growth and differentiation. Epidemiological studies suggest a relationship between vitamin A intake and cancer risk. In addition, possible antineoplastic mechanisms for vitamin A have been described (Mills

1983). However, in clinical studies of cancer patients, the potential of vitamin A has been limited by unacceptable toxicity and minimal efficacy (Lippman and Meyskens 1989). In terms of an anticancer effect, it therefore seems unlikely that patients would benefit significantly from vitamin A dietary supplements.

Conclusions about dietary treatments

Although dietary therapies are promoted as safe innocuous alternatives to conventional cancer treatment they are not without harmful effects. Many are seriously deficient in basic nutrients and do not meet the calorific requirements of cancer patients. Strict adherence to them can lead to profound weight loss and weakness. Patients frequently report that the diets are tedious and unpalatable, but some feel obliged to persevere in the belief that they would be responsible for any relapse that might occur when they discontinue. Other patients undoubtedly benefit from these regimes, but the benefit is largely psychological, gained from renewed hope and the feeling of having some personal control over treatment of the cancer itself. While there is some evidence that diet plays a part in the causation of some cancers (Doll and Peto 1981), there is no evidence that a change in dietary habits will actually alter the course of the disease.

Thus, on the basis of current evidence, there is no reason to recommend substantial changes in diet in the hope that such changes will have curative potential. However, it is reasonable to provide sensible dietary advice in order to maximize general health and well-being. Referral to the hospital dietitian may help to reassure those patients who are worried about their diet. This approach has the advantage of involving patients in their own care and promoting a sense of personal control over management. It is possible that measures might also dissuade patients from the more restrictive alternative/complementary diets.

Guidelines for the physician

Some practitioners of unorthodox medicine see it as complementing rather than competing with conventional medicine and argue for its inclusion in the National Health Service system (Cosh and Sikora 1989). Many doctors have grave reservations about the ethics and potential health hazards associated with the more extreme unorthodox therapies. The most worrisome aspect is the possibility that patients will have their diagnosis delayed whilst pursuing alternative remedies or that they will opt out of conventional treatments when they could still be effective either curatively or palliatively. These concerns are borne out by a study in the United States which reports that 8 per cent of 600 patients never received any conventional treatment but proceeded directly to unorthodox methods (Cassileth et al. 1984). A substantial percentage also discontinued conventional treatment entirely in favour of alternative regimens after a mean of 8 months on standard therapy.

Another concern expressed by doctors is the needless expense to the patient and their family incurred by these treatments. It is not uncommon to hear of patients travelling great distances around the world in search of the latest miracle cure which, in itself, may be prohibitively expensive. Although some of the alternative/complementary specialities have professional bodies to govern standards of training and codes of practice, including the regulation of fees, there is no legislation to prevent any unqualified person from setting up in practice and charging whatever they wish. A multidisciplinary organization called the Campaign Against Health Fraud has been set up in the United Kingdom to protect the public from fraudulent or dangerous treatments by promoting scientific evaluation of all alternative/complementary treatments and better regulation of practitioners.

The tendency to seek alternative treatments could be lessened if, at the outset, physicians took time to explain the nature of the illness and aspects of its management. It is vitally important to establish rapport and to create an atmosphere in which patients believe that they can ask for and receive information about all aspects of their illness. A good doctor–patient relationship is well known to enhance compliance with treatment. Patients are often disproportionately alarmed at the thought of radiotherapy and chemotherapy and the 'safe natural' methods of alternative practitioners may seem more appealing in comparison. Thus, it is important to attempt to elicit and dispel any misconceptions that patients may have about their treatment. Confusing or puzzling aspects of management should be explained. Patients need to know that there are many different types of cancer and many different approaches to treatment. With some patients it may not be appropriate to commence therapy immediately. Nevertheless, they need to be assured of the doctors' continued interest and support and not to feel abandoned by them. In the meantime, advice on diet, exercise, and life-style allows patients to participate in their own management and to feel that something is being done between treatments. Patients are most vulnerable when they have failed to respond to standard treatment. Anything that offers the remotest chance of cure is likely to be accepted gratefully. It may be appropriate at this stage to offer patients the opportunity to participate in an ethically approved clinical trial of a new promising treatment which allows them to maintain hope in the outcome and to contribute to the understanding of cancer and its treatment.

When patients mention alternative/complementary treatments, it is best to demonstrate a willingness to discuss the subject and to present the relevant information as objectively as possible. Cancer physicians need to be conversant with the popular forms of unorthodox treatments and to be ready to make inquiries if necessary on behalf of their patients in order to present the facts clearly. Dismissing these treatments out of hand may alienate the patient and may make them turn away from conventional medicine. As long as the treatment is not pursued to the exclusion of conventional regimes, there is no reason to object to it, provided that it is not harmful, particularly if it gives the patient hope and improves the quality of their life. The patient should be the best judge of these possible benefits. If, after discussion of the advantages and disadvantages of each treatment modality, the patient elects solely for an alternative therapy, an angry judgemental response will only strengthen the patient's resolve and make him or her feel unable to return for conventional therapy in the future if he or she wishes to do so. Instead, recognition and acknowledgement of the patient's need to explore all avenues of treatment is more helpful for all concerned, although occasionally the issue may be resolved by referring the patient for a second opinion.

CONCLUSION

Malignant disease is the second commonest cause of death in adults in the United Kingdom today. Modern technology has produced significant advances in the treatment of some types of cancer, but has done little so far to alter the prognosis of the commonly occurring ones. It is vitally important that cancer research continues. Society demands a cure for cancer and it is hoped that current advances in our understanding of this disease will result in a steady improvement in outcome. It is equally important that we deal with the needs of those patients today who may not be fortunate enough to benefit from science. It is essential that the resources are made available to provide adequately for them. Supplying accurate information and emotional support in the form of counselling, relaxation training, and support groups has beneficial psychological effects and helps patients and their families to cope with what is undoubtedly a most traumatic experience.

USEFUL ADDRESSES

Association of British Insurers, 51 Gresham Street, London EC2 V7HQ
  Telephone 071 600 3333
BACUP, 3 Bath Place, Rivington Street, London EC2A 3JR
  Telephone 071 696 9003
Breast Care and Mastectomy Association, 15–19 Britten Street, London SW3 3TZ
  Telephone 071 867 1103
Bristol Cancer Help Centre, Grove House, Cornwallis Grove, Clifton, Bristol, Avon BS8 4PG
  Telephone 0272 743216
British Association for Counselling, 1 Regent Place, Rugby, Warwickshire CV21 2PJ
  Telephone 0788 550899
British Colostomy Association, 15 Station Road, Reading, Berkshire RG1 1LG
  Telephone 0734 391537
CancerLink, 17 Britannia Street, London WC1X 9JN
  Telephone 071 833 2818
Cancer Relief Macmillan Fund, Anchor House, 15–19 Britten Street, London SW3 3TZ
  Telephone 071 351 7811
Hodgkin's Disease Association, PO Box 275, Haddenham, Aylesbury, Bucks
  Telephone 0844 291500
Leukaemia Research Fund, 43 Great Ormond Street, London WC1N 3JJ
  Telephone 071 405 0101
Malcolm Sargent Cancer Fund for Children, 14 Abingdon Road, London W8 6AF
  Telephone 071 937 4548
Marie Curie Cancer Care, 28 Belgrave Square, London SW1X 8QG
  Telephone 071 235 3325 ext 253
National Association of Laryngectomy Clubs, Ground Floor, 6 Rickett Street, Fulham, London SW6 1RU
  Telephone 071 381 9993
Society for the Prevention of Asbestosis and Industrial Diseases (SPAID), 38 Drapers Road, Enfield, Middlesex EN2 8LU
  Telephone 0707 873025

REFERENCES

Alderson P, Ritchie S, Kingsmill S (1989). Cancer support groups: a friend at hand. *Nursing Standard*, 3:30–2.
American Cancer Society (1973). Unproven methods of cancer management: Gerson method of treatment for cancer. *CA: A Cancer Journal for Clinicians*, 23:314–17.
American Cancer Society (1974). Unproven methods of cancer management: the grape diet. *CA: A Cancer Journal for Clinicians*, 24:144–6.
Ashton H (1984). Benzodiazepine withdrawal: an unfinished story. *British Medical Journal*, 288:1135–40.
Bagenal FS, Easton DF, Harris E, Chilvers CE, McElwain TJ (1990). *Lancet*, 336 (8715):606–10.
Barber J, Gitelson J (1980). Cancer pain: psychological management using hypnosis. *CA: A Cancer Journal for Clinicians*, 30:130–6.
Blackburn IM, *et al.* (1981). The efficacy of cognitive therapy in depression: a treatment trial using cognitive therapy and pharmacotherapy, each alone and in combination. *British Journal of Psychiatry*, 139:181–9.
Bloom JR (1982). Social support systems and cancer: a conceptual view. In *Psychosocial aspects of cancer*. Raven Press, New York.
Bowman BB, *et al.* (1984). Macrobiotic diets for cancer treatment and prevention. *Journal of Clinical Oncology*, 2(6):702–11.
Brandt J (1928). *The grape cure*. Harmony Centre, New York.
Brewin TB (1977). The cancer patient: communication and morale. *British Medical Journal*, ii:1623–7.
Bridge LR, *et al.* (1988). Relaxation and imagery in the treatment of breast cancer. *British Medical Journal*, 297:1169–72.
British Medical Association-Report of the Board of Science and Education (1986). *Alternative therapy*. Chameleon Press, London.
Brunton N (1989). *Homeopathy*. Macdonald Optima, London.
Buckman R (1984). Breaking bad news: why is it still so difficult? *British Medical Journal*, 288:1597–9.
Burish TG, *et al.* (1988). Posttreatment use of relaxation training by cancer patients. *Hospice Journal*, 4(2):1–8.
Cameron E, Pauling L (1976). Supplemental ascorbate in the supportive treatment of cancer: prolongation of survival times in terminal human cancer. *Proceedings of the National Academy of Sciences USA*, 73(10):3685–9.
Cameron E, Pauling L (1978). Supplemental ascorbate in the supportive treatment of cancer: re-evaluation of prolongation of survival times in terminal human cancer. *Proceedings of the National Academy of America*, 75(9):4538–42.
Cameron E, Campbell A, Jack T (1975). The orthomolecular treatment of cancer. III. Reticulum cell sarcoma: double complete regression induced by high-dose ascorbic acid therapy. *Chemico-Biological Interactions*, 11:387–93.
Cassileth BR (1982). After laetrile, what? *New England Journal of Medicine*, 306(24):1483–5.
Cassileth BR (1986). Unorthodox cancer medicine. *Cancer Investigation*, 4(6):591–8.
Cassileth BR (1989). The social implications of questionable cancer therapies. *Cancer*, 63:1247–50.
Cassileth BR, *et al.* (1980). Information and participation preferences among cancer patients. *Annals of Internal Medicine*, 92:832–6.
Cassileth BR, *et al.* (1984). Contemporary unorthodox treatments in cancer medicine: a study of patients, treatments and practitioners. *Annals of Internal Medicine*, 101:105–12.
Cavanaugh S (1984). Diagnosing depression in the hospitalised patient with chronic medical illness. *Journal of Clinical Psychiatry*, 45(3(s 2)):13–16.
Clement-Jones V (1985). Cancer and beyond: the formation of BACUP. *British Medical Journal*, 291:1021–3.
Clinical Oncology Group (1987). New Zealand cancer patients and alternative medicine. *New Zealand Medical Journal*, 110–13.
Copley Cobb S (1984). Teaching relaxation techniques to cancer patients. *Cancer Nursing*, April, 157–61.
Cosh J, Sikora K (1989). Conventional and complementary treatment for cancer: time to join forces. *British Medical Journal*, 298:1200–1.
Creagan ET, *et al.* (1979). Failure of high dose vitamin C (ascorbic acid) therapy to benefit patients with advanced cancer. *New England Journal of Medicine*, 301(13):687–90.
Derogatis LR, *et al.* (1983). The prevalence of psychiatric disorders among cancer patients. *Journal of the American Medical Association*, 249(6):751–7.
Doll R, Peto R (1981). *The causes of cancer*. Oxford University Press.
Dorr RT, Paxinos J (1978). The current status of laetrile. *Annals of Internal Medicine*, 89(3):389–97.
Dunkel-Schetter C (1984). Social support and cancer: findings based on patient interviews and their implications. *Journal of Social Issues*, 40:77–98.
Edwards H (1975). The science of spiritual healing. *Nursing Times*, 171:2008–10.
Ellison NM, Byar DP, Newell GR (1978). Special report on laetrile: results of the National Cancer Institute's retrospective laetrile analysis. *New England Journal of Medicine*, 299(10):549–52.
Faw C, Ballentine R, Ballentine L (1977). Unproved cancer remedies. A survey of use in pediatric outpatients. *Journal of the American Medical Association*, 238:1536–8.
Fleming U (1985). Relaxation therapy for far-advanced cancer. *Practitioner*, 229:471–5.
Fletcher C (1980). Listening and talking to patients. *British Medical Journal*, 281:994–6.
Fulder SJ, Monro RE (1985). Complementary medicine in the United Kingdom: patients, practitioners and consultations. *Lancet*, ii:542–5.
Gerson M (1978). The cure of advanced cancer by diet therapy: a summary of 30 years of clinical experimentation. *Physiological Chemistry and Physics*, 10, 449–64 (posthumous publication).
Goldberg D (1982). Cognitive therapy for depression. *British Medical Journal*, 284:143–4.

Gould H, Toghill PJ (1981). How should we talk about acute leukaemia to adult patients and their families? *British Medical Journal*, 282:210–12.

Graffam S, Johnson A (1987). A comparison of two relaxation strategies for the relief of pain and its distress. *Journal of Pain and Symptom Management*, 2(4):229–31.

Harvey D (1983). *The power to heal: an investigation of healing and the healing experience*. Aquarian Press, London.

Holland JC (1981). Patients who seek unproven cancer remedies: a psychological prospective. *Clinical Bulletin*, 11(3):102–5.

Jukes TH (1976). Laetrile for cancer. *Journal of the American Medical Association*, 236(11):1284–6.

Lerner IJ (1984). The whys of cancer quackery. *Cancer*, 1 (Suppl.), 815–19.

Linn MW, Linn BS, Harris R (1982). Effects of counseling for late stage cancer patients. *Cancer*, 49:1048–55.

Lippman SM, Meyskens FL (1989). Results of the use of vitamin A and retinoids in cutaneous malignancies. *Pharmacology and Therapeutics*, 40(1):107–22.

MacNutt F (1974). *Healing*. Ave Maria Press, Notre Dame, IN.

Maguire P (1981). Psychological and social consequences of cancer. *Recent Advances in Clinical Oncology*, 376.

Maguire P, Faulkner A (1988). How to do it: communicate with cancer patients: 1. Handling bad news and difficult questions. *British Medical Journal*, 297:907–9.

Maguire P, Faulkner A (1988). How to do it: communicate with cancer patients: 2. Handling uncertainty, collusion and denial. *British Medical Journal*, 297:972–4.

Maguire GP, et al. (1978). Psychiatric problems in the first year after mastectomy. *British Medical Journal*, i:963–5.

Maguire P, et al. (1980). Effect of counselling on the psychiatric morbidity associated with mastectomy. *British Medical Journal*, 281:1454–6.

Meares A (1980). What can the cancer patient expect from intensive meditation? *Australian Family Physician*, 9:322–5.

Meares A (1983). Psychological mechanisms in the regression of cancer. *Medical Journal of Australia*, 11 June, 583–4.

Mills EED (1983). The role of vitamin A in cancer. *South African Medical Journal*, 63:74–7.

Moertel CG, et al. (1982). A clinical trial of amygdalin (laetrile) in the treatment of human cancer. *New England Journal of Medicine*, 306(4):201–6.

Moorey S and Greer S (1989). *Psychological therapy for patients with cancer: a new approach*. Heinemann, London.

Morris T, Greer HS, White P (1977). Psychological and social adjustment to mastectomy: a two year follow-up study. *Cancer*, 40:3281–7.

Morrow GR, Morrell C (1982). Behavioural treatment for the anticipatory nausea and vomiting induced by cancer chemotherapy. *New England Journal of Medicine*, 307(24):1476–80.

Morton J (1987). Personal view. *British Medical Journal*, 295:1482.

National Cancer Institute Statement (1983). *Macrobiotic diet*. Cancer Information Service, Memorial Sloan-Kettering Cancer Center.

Plant H, et al. (1987). Evaluation of a support group for cancer patients and their families and friends. *British Journal of Hospital Medicine*, October, 317–22.

Rainey LC (1985). Cancer counseling by telephone help-line: the UCLA psychosocial cancer counselling line. *Public Health Reports*, 100(3):308–15.

Ramirez AJ (1989). Liaison psychiatry in a breast cancer unit. *Journal of the Royal Society of Medicine*, 82:15–17.

Redd WH, Andresen GV, Minagawa RY (1982). Hypnotic control of anticipatory emesis in patients receiving cancer chemotherapy. *Journal of Consulting and Clinical Psychology*, 50(1):14–19.

Scarf M (1980). Images that heal: a doubtful idea whose time has come. *Psychology Today*, September, 32–46.

Schraub S, Bernheim J (1987). Quackery in the quest of quality. In *The quality of life of cancer patients*. Raven Press, New York.

Simonton OC, Matthews-Simonton S (1981). Cancer and stress: counselling the cancer patient. *Medical Journal of Australia*, 679–83.

Simonton OC, Simonton S, Creighton J (1978). *Getting well again*. Tarcher, Los Angeles, CA.

Sims SE (1987). Relaxation training as a technique for helping patients cope with the experience of cancer: a selective review of the literature. *Journal of Advanced Nursing*, 12:583–91.

Slevin ML (1987). Talking about cancer: how much is too much? *British Journal of Hospital Medicine*, July, 56–9.

Slevin ML, et al. (1988). BACUP—the first two years: evaluation of a national cancer information service. *British Medical Journal*, 297:669–72.

Smith T (1983). Alternative medicine. *British Medical Journal*, 287:307–8.

Spiegel D, Bloom JR (1983). Group therapy and hypnosis reduce metastatic breast carcinoma pain. *Psychosomatic Medicine*, 45(4):333–9.

Worden JW, Weisman AD (1980). Do cancer patients really want counselling? *General Hospital Psychiatry*, 2:100–3.

Wortman CB (1984). Social support and the cancer patient. *Cancer*, 53(Suppl.) 2339–60.

Yalom ID, Greaves C (1977). Group therapy with the terminally ill. *American Journal of Psychiatry*, 134(4):396–400.

Young VR, Newberne PM (1981). Vitamins and cancer prevention: issues and dilemmas. *Cancer*, 47:1226–40.

Subject index

Page numbers in bold refer to major discussions in the text and include major sections, subsections and principal headings. Page numbers in *italics* refer to pages on which tables are to be found. 'vs' denotes differential diagnosis.

Indexing style/conventions used
Alphabetical order. This index is in letter-by-letter order, whereby hyphens and spaces within index headings are ignored in the alphabetization. Terms in brackets are excluded from initial alphabetization eg.
  cell(s)
  cell adhesion molecule
  cell-cell
  cell culture

Cross-references. Cross-reference terms in *italics* are either general cross-references, or refer to subentry terms within the same main entry (the main entry term is not repeated, in order to save space) i.e. they are not main entry terms.

Index entries. Entries follow a hierarchical system, where possible, from a general tumour type to a specific tumour eg.
  1. *General*—Leukaemia; *Specific*—Leukaemia, chronic myeloid:
  2. *General*—Lymphoma; *Specific*—non-Hodgkin's lymphoma; *More specific*—B-cell lymphoma
If the required reference is not found under the specific tumour, please consult the more generalized tumour type or relevant organ. Cross-references are inserted, in places, as a reminder.

Index entries have been restricted to two subentry levels. Entries have therefore been reorganized/reworded or relocated where further levels have been required.
  eg. Lung cancer, small-cell *reworded/relocated to* Small-cell lung cancer
Cross-references are inserted to indicate correct keyword term or location of entry.

Some index subentries, particularly those referring to individual pages within a page grouping, have been included more to indicate the extent of the discussion in the text rather than the actual location of the reference.

Histology. Entries under common types of tumours eg adenocarcinoma, carcinoma have been restricted to generalized references and readers are advised to seek the specific tumour entry. Under less common histological types of tumours, an organ-by-organ listing is included.

Finally, entries under 'cancer', 'malignancy', 'tumour(s)' have been kept to a minimum and readers should consult more specific topics.

Abbreviations used in subentries (without explanation):

ADCC	Antibody-dependent cell-mediated cytotoxicity
CIN	Cervical intraepithelial neoplasia
CMV	Cytomegalovirus
CT	Computed tomography
EBV	Epstein-Barr virus
EGF	Epidermal growth factor
FSH	Follicle-stimulating hormone
G-CSF	Granulocyte colony-stimulating factor
GFR	Glomerular filtration rate
GhRH	Gonadotrophin releasing hormone
GM-CSF	Granulocyte-macrophage colony-stimulating factor
hCG	Human chorionic gonadotrophin
HIV	Human immunodeficiency virus
HPV	Human papilloma virus
HTLV	Human T-cell leukaemia virus
IFN	Interferon
IL	Interleukin
LAK	Lymphokine-activated killer cell
LH	Luteinizing hormone
LHRH	Luteinizing hormone-releasing hormone
MAbs	Monoclonal antibodies
MEN	Multiple endocrine neoplasia
MRI	Magnetic resonance imaging
MRS	Magnetic resonance spectroscopy
NSAIDs	Non-steroidal anti-inflammatory drugs
PCR	Polymerase chain reaction
PDGF	Platelet-derived growth factor
PET	Positron emission tomography
POMC	Pro-opiomelanocortin
SIADH	Syndrome of inappropriate antidiuretic hormone secretion
TGF	Transforming growth factor
TNF	Tumour necrosis factor